Contents in Brief

Bringing this manuscript to fruition has brought me a great deal of satisfaction and pride. With each topic I have read and each page written I am in awe of nursing and all it encompasses. None of this would have been possible without the unwavering support of my family, friends, and colleagues.

To my husband Anthony and my daughter Jaelyn Elizabeth, whose love and cheers have encouraged me in this process, I appreciate your support and understanding of the long hours and hard work needed to bring this book to publication. I love you both. To the boys, Andy Claude and Festus, your unwavering loyalty has been invaluable.

To my writing partner, Kelly Gosnell, words cannot express my respect for your hard work and dedication to our dream to produce a work we are infinitely proud of. You have been a source of strength and friendship in this endeavor. I look forward to many future chapters of writing adventures.

Kim Cooper

To my husband Ed and my daughters Katelyn and Kinsey, I thank you for your love, patience, and understanding during the time it took to complete this endeavor. Your acceptance of the demands on my time made it all possible. To the two newest members of my family, Jared and Miles Robert, this latest edition was your first exposure to the life of a nursing textbook author. I appreciated all you have done to support and brighten the road along the way.

To all my wonderful family, friends, and colleagues, your constant support and belief in me while completing this project mean more to me than I can express.

To my writing partner, Kim Cooper, without you getting me into the crazy world of ancillary writing years ago, I would not have had the opportunity to tackle this fantastic opportunity of nursing textbook authorship with you. It has been, and hopefully will continue to be, an awesome ride.

Kelly Gosnell

EDITION

8

Foundations and Adult Health Nursing

Kim Cooper, RN, MSN
Associate Professor and Dean
School of Nursing
Ivy Tech Community College
Terre Haute, Indiana
President, Indiana State Board of Nursing

Kelly Gosnell, RN, MSN
Associate Professor and Department Chair
School of Nursing
Ivy Tech Community College
Terre Haute, Indiana

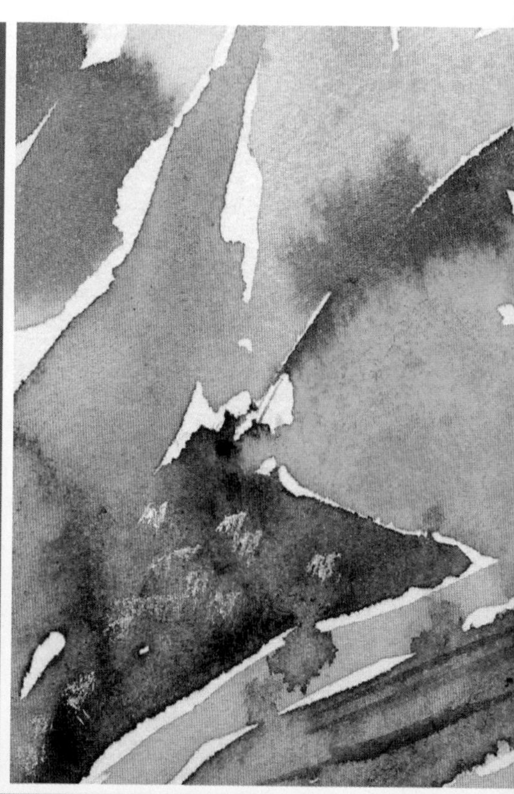

ELSEVIER

ELSEVIER

3251 Riverport Lane
St. Louis, Missouri 63043

FOUNDATIONS AND ADULT HEALTH NURSING, EIGHTH EDITION ISBN: 978-0-323-48437-4

Previous editions copyrighted 2015, 2011, 2006, 2003, 1999, 1995, and 1991.

Library of Congress Control Number: 2018961545

Senior Content Strategist: Nancy O'Brien
Senior Content Development Manager: Luke Held
Senior Content Development Specialist: Diane Chatman
Publishing Services Manager: Julie Eddy
Book Production Specialist: Carol O'Connell
Design Direction: Renee Duenow

Printed in the United States of America

Last digit is the print number: 9 8 7 6 5 4

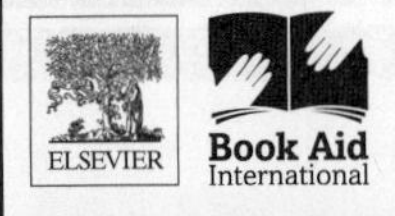

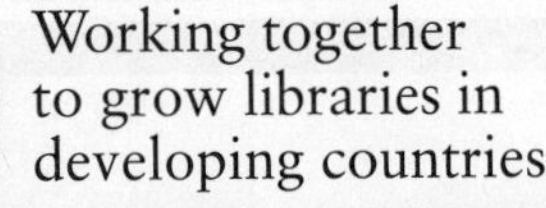

Acknowledgments

The eighth edition of this textbook has seen a great deal of change with updated material, new alignment of chapters, and the addition of an increased number of alternate format NCLEX questions at the end of each chapter. Material has been extracted from one chapter resulting in the addition of two new chapters. Oxygenation is now Chapter 14, and Elimination is now Chapter 15. With consideration for the increasing impact of social media on both society as a whole and the influences it has on the healthcare environment recommendations for safe, responsible, legal practice has been added to Chapter 2. Recognition of the need to approach heath care with an emphasis on all elements of the patient updates have been made to share holistic and complementary care initiatives in Chapter 20.

The nurturing of the youth is a focus for nursing. Chapter 30 with its focus on Health Promotion for children outlines potential barriers to health care for children. In addition, areas of growing concern to today's youth including obesity, media exposure, and the use of alternative smoking devices is investigated. At the same time, this edition has maintained the strong foundation that it has had since Barbara Christensen and Elaine Kockrow authored the first edition. We are grateful for the expertise that they have shared through the first six editions. Special thanks to our photographer Katelyn Gosnell Richey for her hard work in adding over 300 new photographs between *Foundations* and *Adult Health Nursing*, to our many family, friends, and colleagues for volunteering to be our models. and to Ivy Tech Community College, Terre Haute, Indiana, for their willingness to share their facility setting for many of the updated photographs.

We are thankful for Tiffany Trautwein, Developmental Editor, and Teri Hines Burnham, Director of Content Development, for reaching out to us and believing in our abilities to assume authorship of this outstanding textbook in the seventh edition. The tireless work behind the scenes has been immeasurable in the quest to bring this edition to fruition. Nancy O'Brien shared her keen oversight and guidance for the revision. Diane Chatman joined the team and provided positivity and support. Mary Stueck assisted us in the kick off to the copy editing process and later stepped aside to begin her much deserved retirement. She left capable hands behind as Carol O'Connell came aboard to provide tireless efforts to keep the needed pace in the final stages of the text development and production.

The role of the practical nurse is a key member of the health care team. The education of these dedicated men and women is needed to prepare them for entry to practice. Those contributors, reviewers, and dedicated colleagues have shared invaluable expertise in this journey in bringing this work to life and we are forever indebted.

Contributors and Reviewers

CONTRIBUTORS

Margaret Barnes, DNP, MSN, RN
Associate Professor
Division of Post-Licensure Nursing
Indiana Wesleyan University
Marion, Indiana

Terra Ripple Baughman
Assistant Professor
Nursing
Ivy Tech Community College of Indiana
Wabash Valley Region, Indiana

Tracy Blanc, RN, MSN
Associate Professor
Nursing
Ivy Tech Community College of Indiana
Terre Haute, Indiana

Emily J. Cannon, DNP, RN
Assistant Professor
School of Nursing
Indiana State University
Terre Haute, Indiana

Charlotte Connerton, EdD, RN, CNE-BC
Assistant Professor
Nursing
University of Southern Indiana
Evansville, Indiana

Jeffrey A. Coto, DNP, MS-CNS, RN, CCRN
Assistant Professor and Special Assistant to the Provost
Valparaiso University
College of Nursing and Health Professions
Valparaiso, Indiana

Sarah Fagg, BSN, MSN
Faculty
Nursing
Ivy Tech Community College
Terre Haute, Indiana

Pat Floro, RN, BSN
PN Instructor
Apollo Career Center
Lima, Ohio

Emma Hopson, ADN, BSN, MSN Ed
Nursing Instructor
Nursing
Tennessee College of Applied Technology at Elizabethton
Unicoi, Tennessee

Jamie Houchins, PhD, MSN, RN
School of Nursing
Ivy Tech Community College
Sellersburg, Indiana

Mary Joan Lavelle, MSN, RN
Nursing Instructor
Career Technology Center School of Practical Nursing
Scranton, Pennsylvania

Elizabeth L. Law, MSN, RN
Nursing Education Specialist
Community Health Network
Indianapolis, Indiana

Traci McNeil, RN, MSN
Associate Professor
School of Nursing
Ivy Tech Community College
Terre Haute, Indiana

Tammy Ortiz, MSN/Ed, PHN
Clinical Supervisor
Maxim Healthcare and Staffing
San Jose, California

REVIEWERS

Darlene Baker, RN, MSN
Program Director
Practical Nursing Department
Green Country Technology Center
Okmulgee, Oklahoma

Sandy Barker
Master Instructor, Nursing
Tennessee College of Applied Technology
Elizabethton, Tennessee

Melody Corso, MSN, RN, CNE
Executive Director, Nursing & Health Sciences
Florida Gateway College
Lake City, Florida

Fleurdeliza Cuyco, BS
Instructor
Preferred College of Nursing
Los Angeles, California

C. Michelle Doleyres, MSN/ed, RN
Department Chair
Health Science Department
Miami Lakes Educational Center & Technical College
Miami Lakes, Florida

Susan England, MS, RN
PN Coordinator
Practical Nursing
Tulsa Tech
Tulsa, Oklahoma

Sally Fitzgerald, MSN, RN
Professor of Nursing
Community College of Nursing
Monaca, Pennsylvania

Sally Flesch, RN, BSN, MA, EdS, PhD
Professor Emerita
Practical Nursing Program
Black Hawk College
Moline, Illinois

Paula Franden, RN, Bachelors in Vocational Education
Director, Nursing Programs
CTE
El Monte Rosemead Adult School
El Monte, California

Donald Laurino, MSN, CCRN, CMSRN, PHN, RN-BC
Faculty Development Coordinator
American Career College
Lynwood, California

T. Camille Lindsey Killough, RN, BSN
Instructor Nursing Department
Pearl River Community College
Hattiesburg, Mississippi

Carolyn McCune, RN, MSN, CRNP, CEN
LPN Director at Columbiana County Career and Technical Center
Adult Education
Columbiana County Career and Technical Center
Lisbon, Ohio

Pauline C. Morris, MA
Nursing Educator
Health Science Department
Miami Lakes Educational Center & Technical College
Miami Lakes, Florida

L. Jubeth Pascua, ESQ, RN, BSN, MSN, PHN, CCRN, DSD
Independent Nurse Educator
Los Angeles, California

Patricia L. Pence, EdD, MSN, RN
Assistant Professor
Illinois State University
Normal, Illinois

Trena Rich, RN, MSN, APRN, CIC
Director Quality Assurance, Patient Care Center
Western University of Health Sciences
Pomona, California

Laurie Sanders, BSN, MA, LCCE
Nursing Instructor
Loudoun County School of Practical Nursing
Leesburg, Virginia

Elaine K. Strouss, MSN, RN
Professor of Nursing
Coordinator: PN program, First Year of ADN program
Community College of Beaver County
Monaca, Pennsylvania

Audrey Tolouian, MSN, BSW, EdD
Clinical Instructor, School of Nursing
University of Texas
El Paso, Texas

Sister Ann Wiesen, RN, BSN, MRA
Director of Practical Nursing
Erwin Technical College
Tampa, Florida

Mary Albaugh Williams, DC, ADN/RN, BS
Doctor of Chiropractic, Psychiatric Technician Instructor
Health Occupations Department
Napa Valley College
Napa, California

LPN/LVN Advisory Board

Nancy Bohnarczyk, MA
Adjunct Instructor
College of Mount St. Vincent
New York, New York

Sharyn P. Boyle, MSN, RN-BC
Instructor, Associate Degree Nursing
Passaic County Technical Institute
Wayne, New Jersey

Nicola Contreras, BN, RN
Faculty
Galen College
San Antonio, Texas

Dolores Cotton, MSN, RN
Practical Nursing Coordinator
Meridian Technology Center
Stillwater, Oklahoma

Patricia Donovan, MSN, RN
Director of Practical Nursing and Curriculum Chair
Porter and Chester Institute
Rocky Hill, Connecticut

Nancy Haughton, MSN, RN
Practical Nursing Program Faculty
Chester County Intermediate Unit
Downingtown, Pennsylvania

Dawn Johnson, DNP, RN, Ed
Practical Nurse Program Director
Great Lakes Institute of Technology
Erie, Pennsylvania

Mary E. Johnson, RN, MSN
Director of Nursing
Dorsey Schools
Roseville, Michigan

Bonnie Kehm, PhD, RN
Faculty Program Director
Excelsior College
Albany, New York

Tawnya S. Lawson, MS, RN
Dean, Practical Nursing Program
Hondros College
Westerville, Ohio

Kristin Madigan, MS, RN
Nursing Faculty
Pine Technical and Community College
Pine City, Minnesota

Hana Malik, DNP, FNP-BC
Academic Director
Illinois College of Nursing
Lombard, Illinois

Mary Lee Pollard, PhD, RN, CNE
Dean, School of Nursing
Excelsior College
Albany, New York

Barbara Ratliff, MSN, RN
Program Director, Practical Nursing
Cincinnati State
Cincinnati, Ohio

Mary Ruiz-Nuve, RN, MSN
Director of Practical Nursing Program
St. Louis College of Health Careers
St. Louis, Missouri

Renee Sheehan, RN, MSN/Ed
Director of Nursing, Vocational Nursing
Nursing Assistant Programs
Summit College
Colton, California

Faye Silverman, RN, MSN/ED, WOCN, PHN
Nursing Education Consultant
Online Nursing Instructor
Lancaster, California

Fleur de Liza S. Tobias-Cuyco, BSc, CPhT
Dean, Director of Student Affairs, and Instructor
Preferred College of Nursing
Los Angeles, California

To the Instructor

The eighth edition of *Foundations and Adult Health Nursing* was developed to educate the practical/vocational nursing student in the fundamentals of nursing required to care competently and safely for a wide variety of patients in various settings. As the level of knowledge and responsibility increases for LPN/LVNs in all health care settings from acute to community-based care, it is essential that a text such as *Foundations and Adult Health Nursing* be available to educate the student for the growing demands of this profession.

This full-color text provides all of the fundamentals and skills, maternal and neonatal, pediatric, geriatric, mental health, community, and anatomy and physiology content needed in the LPN/LVN curriculum. This new edition was revised to incorporate the most current and clinically relevant information available on the following topics:

- Historical, legal, and ethical aspects of nursing
- Communication
- Physical assessment
- Nursing process and critical thinking
- Documentation
- Cultural and ethical considerations in nursing interventions
- Growth and development across the life span
- Death and dying
- Safety
- Medical-surgical asepsis
- Pain management, comfort, rest, and sleep
- Complementary and alternative therapies
- Basic nutrition and nutritional therapy
- Fluids and electrolytes
- Mathematics review and medication administration
- Emergency first aid nursing, including terrorism and bioterrorism interventions
- Maternal, neonatal, and pediatric care
- Gerontologic nursing and care of the older adult
- Mental health and community health
- Role of the LPN/LVN and leadership

Finally, it is our belief that nursing will always be both an art and a science. This philosophy is reflected throughout the text.

ORGANIZATION AND STANDARD FEATURES

The organization of the eighth edition continues to follow the strengths of the previous edition, based on positive comments from educators and students. The basic nursing skills are provided in Units II, III, and IV. Two new chapters have been added to provide the student with greater focus on individual concepts. Oxygenation concepts are now found in Chapter 14, and elimination concepts are housed in Chapter 15. Some additional changes include moving eye, ear, and vaginal irrigations to the medication chapter, nasogastric feedings to the nutrition chapter, and heat and cold therapy has moved the newly named Hygiene and Care of the Patient's Environment chapter. Medical-surgical nursing—with an overview of anatomy and physiology and a separate chapter on care of the surgical patient—are available in Unit VII.

TABLE OF CONTENTS

The text is divided into 8 units with 58 chapters. Chapters have been reorganized for easy, logical association of content. Updates have been made to ensure that students have access to the most current information. To match a growing emphasis on holistic care there are significant updates to alternative and complementary therapy information presented. The legal, ethical and professional aspects of nursing practice have been updated. Revision to health care and nursing practice have been made to provide students with an updated viewpoint.

CHAPTER ORGANIZATION

Disorders chapters in Unit VII typically are organized in the following format for more effective learning:

- Etiology and Pathophysiology
- Clinical Manifestations
- Assessment (with subjective and objective data)
- Diagnostic Tests
- Medical Management
- Nursing Interventions (including relevant medications)
- Nursing Diagnoses
- Patient Teaching
- Prognosis

NURSING PROCESS

The nursing process as applied to specific disorders is integrated throughout. A special nursing process summary section appears at the end of appropriate chapters, enabling the reader to see more clearly its application to the chapter content as a whole. For this text the authors have replaced nursing diagnoses with a patient problem list to better describe health problems the patient experiences. These statements provide a problem centered approach to nursing care. We have emphasized the role of the LPN/LVN in the nursing process as follows:

- The LPN/LVN will participate in planning care for the patient based on the patient's needs.
- The LPN/LVN will review the patient's plan of care and recommend revisions as needed.
- The LPN/LVN will follow defined prioritization for patient care.
- The LPN/LVN will use clinical pathways, care maps, or care plans to guide and review patient care.

REFERENCES

References are grouped by chapter and listed at the end of the book for easy access. *Additional Resources* such as websites and agencies are included where applicable.

In the appendixes, *Common Abbreviations* are listed along with The Joint Commission's *Lists of Dangerous Abbreviations, Acronyms, and Symbols* to promote safety in clinical practice in such areas as avoiding dosage errors, and *Laboratory Reference Values* provide quick access to important information. *Answers to the Review Questions* for the NCLEX® Examination are provided in Appendix C.

LPN THREADS

The eighth edition of *Foundations and Adult Health Nursing* shares some features and design elements with other Elsevier LPN/LVN textbooks. The purpose of these *LPN Threads* is to make it easier for students and instructors to use the variety of books required by the relatively brief and demanding LPN/LVN curriculum. *LPN Threads* include the following:

- Efforts are continually made to keep the *reading level* of our LPN texts around 10th grade to increase the consistency among chapters and ensure the text is easy to understand.
- *Full-color design, cover, photos,* and *illustrations* are visually appealing and pedagogically useful.
- *Objectives* (numbered) begin each chapter. Chapter objectives provide a framework for content and are especially important in providing the structure for the TEACH Lesson Plans for the textbook.
- *Key Terms* with phonetic pronunciations and page number references are listed at the beginning of each chapter. Key terms appear in color in the chapter and are defined briefly, with full definitions in the *Glossary.* Simple phonetic pronunciations accompany difficult medical, nursing, or scientific terms or other words that may be difficult for students to pronounce.
- A wide variety of *special features* related to critical thinking, clinical practice, care of the older adult, health promotion, safety, patient teaching, complementary and alternative therapies, communication, home health care, delegation and assignment, and more. Refer to the To the Student section of this introduction on page xii for descriptions of each of these features.
- *Critical Thinking Questions* with each Nursing Care Plan give students opportunities to practice critical thinking and clinical decision-making skills with realistic patient scenarios. Answers are provided in the Instructor Resources section on the Evolve website.
- *Key Points,* located at the end of chapters, follow the chapter objectives and serve as a useful chapter review.
- A full suite of *Instructor Resources* including TEACH Lesson Plans and Lecture Outlines, PowerPoint Lecture Slides, Test Bank, and an Image Collection. Each of these teaching resources is described in detail below.
- In addition to consistent content, design, and support resources, these textbooks benefit from the advice and input of the *Elsevier LPN/LVN Advisory Board.*

TEACHING AND LEARNING PACKAGE

FOR STUDENTS

- An *Evolve website* provides free student resources, including additional review questions for the NCLEX Examination for every chapter, calculators, and animations and video clips.
- The *Study Guide for Foundations and Adult Health Nursing* is designed to promote learning, understanding, and application of the content in the textbook. Each chapter ties specific activities to specific objectives rather than simply listing objectives and activities separately. Activities include hundreds of labeling, matching, and fill-in-the-blank questions, each with textbook page references; critical thinking questions with clinical scenarios; and multiple-choice and alternate-format questions for NCLEX review. The complete answer key is provided to instructors in the Instructor Resources section of the Evolve website. *Sold separately.*
- *Virtual Clinical Excursions* is an interactive workbook/online package that guides the student through a multifloor virtual hospital in a hands-on clinical learning experience. Students can assess and analyze information, diagnose, set priorities, and implement and evaluate care. NCLEX-style review questions provide immediate testing of clinical knowledge. *Sold separately.*

FOR INSTRUCTORS

The comprehensive *Evolve Resources With TEACH Instructor Resource* provides a rich array of teaching tools and includes the following:

- *TEACH Lesson Plans With Lecture Outlines,* based on the textbook learning objectives, provide ready-to-use lesson plans that tie together all of the text and ancillary components provided for *Foundations of Nursing.*

- A collection of more than 200 *PowerPoint Lecture Slides* are specific to the text.
- A *Test Bank,* delivered in ExamView, provides approximately 1500 multiple-choice and alternate-format NCLEX-style questions. Each question includes the correct answer, rationale, topic, objective, cognitive level, step of the nursing process, and NCLEX category of patient needs, as well as corresponding textbook page references.
- An *Image Collection* contains nearly 500 images from the textbook. Images are suitable for incorporation into classroom lectures, PowerPoint presentations, or distance-learning applications.
- *Answer Keys* are provided for the Critical Thinking Questions in Nursing Care Plans and for the activities in the Study Guide.

To the Student

Designed with you in mind, *Foundations and Adult Health Nursing* presents fundamental nursing concepts in a visually-appealing and easy-to-use format. Here are some of the numerous special features that will help you understand and apply the material.

READING AND REVIEW TOOLS

Objectives introduce the chapter topics, and *Key Terms* are listed with page number references, and difficult medical, nursing, or scientific terms are accompanied by simple phonetic pronunciations. Key terms are in color where they are briefly defined in the text, and complete definitions are provided in the Glossary.

Each chapter ends with a *Get Ready for the NCLEX® Examination!* section. *Key Points* follow the chapter objectives and serve as a chapter review. An extensive set of *Review Questions for the NCLEX® Examination* provides immediate opportunity for testing your understanding of the chapter content. *Answers* are located in Appendix C in the back of the book.

ADDITIONAL LEARNING RESOURCES

The online *Evolve Resources* at *http://evolve.elsevier.com/Cooper/foundations* give you access to even more Review Questions for the NCLEX Examination, animations, and much more.

CHAPTER FEATURES

Skills are presented in a logical step-by-step format with accompanying full-color illustrations. Clearly defined *nursing actions* followed by *rationales* in italicized type show you how and why skills are performed. Each skill includes icons that serve as a reminder to perform the basic steps applicable to *all* nursing interventions:

Check orders.

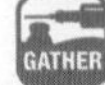

Gather necessary equipment and supplies.

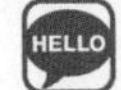

Introduce yourself.

Check patient's identification.

Provide privacy.

Explain the procedure/intervention.

Perform hand hygiene.

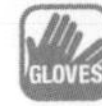

Don gloves (if applicable).

Nursing Care Plans, developed around specific case studies, include patient problem statements in place of nursing diagnoses. These patient problem statements better describe health problems the patient experiences. These statements provide a problem centered approach to nursing care. An emphasis is placed on patient goals and outcomes and questions to promote *critical thinking.* These sample care plans are valuable tools that can be used as a guideline in the clinical setting. The critical thinking aspect empowers you to develop sound clinical decision-making skills.

Patient problem statements and interventions are screened and set apart in the text in a clear, easy-to-understand format to help you learn to participate in the development of a nursing care plan.

Evidence-Based Practice boxes summarize the latest research findings and highlight how they apply to LPN/LVN practice.

Medication tables developed for specific disorders provide quick access to action, dosage, side effects, and nursing considerations for commonly used medications.

Safety Alert! boxes emphasize the importance of maintaining safety in patient and resident care to protect patients, residents, family, health care providers, and the public from accidents and the spread of disease.

Health Promotion boxes emphasize a healthy lifestyle, preventive behaviors, and screening tests to assist in the prevention of accidents and disease.

Patient Teaching boxes appear frequently in the text to help develop awareness of the vital role of patient/family teaching in health care today.

Coordinated Care boxes throughout the text promote comprehensive patient care with other members of the health care team, focusing on prioritization, assignment, supervision, collaboration, and leadership topics.

Complementary and Alternative Therapies boxes in nearly every chapter give a breakdown of specific nontraditional therapies, along with precautions and possible side effects.

Cultural Considerations boxes explore broad cultural beliefs and how to address the needs of a culturally diverse patient and resident population when planning nursing care.

Communication boxes focus on communication strategies with real-life examples of nurse-patient dialogue.

Life Span Considerations for the Older Adult boxes bring a gerontologic perspective to nursing care, focusing on the nursing interventions unique to the older adult patient or resident.

Home Care Considerations boxes discuss the issues facing patients and caregivers in the home setting.

Contents

APPENDIXES

The Evolution of Nursing

1

http://evolve.elsevier.com/Cooper/foundationsadult/

Objectives

1. Describe the evolution of nursing and nursing education from early civilization to the 20th century.
2. Identify the major leaders of nursing history in America.
3. Discuss the significant changes in nursing in the 21st century.
4. Discuss societal influences on nursing.
5. Identify the major organizations in nursing.
6. Define the three purposes of the National Association for Practical Nurse Education and Service (NAPNES) and the National Federation of Licensed Practical Nurses (NFLPN).
7. Identify the components of the health care system.
8. Describe the complex factors involved in the delivery of patient care.
9. Identify the participants in the health care system.
10. Define practical and vocational nursing.
11. Describe the purpose, role, and responsibilities of the practical and the vocational nurse.

Key Terms

accreditation (ŭ-CRĔD-ĭ-TĀ-shŭn, p. 10)
approved program (p. 10)
articulation (ăr-tĭc-ū-LĀ-shŭn, p. 10)
certification (sĕr-tĭ-fĭ-KĀ-shŭn, p. 13)
health (p. 17)
health care system (p. 12)
holistic (hō-LĬS-tĭk, p. 14)
holistic health care (p. 12)
illness (p. 1)
licensure (LĪ-sĭn-shŭr, p. 4)
patient (p. 17)
pesthouses (p. 2)
portfolio (p. 11)
wellness (p. 12)

Nursing is one of today's most exciting and challenging careers. Each nurse receives a formal education in an institution with a set curriculum that has been approved by each state's board of nursing. Degrees and certificates are awarded by the school. Licensure is conferred by the individual state. On completion of the nursing program, individuals are eligible to request permission to sit for the National Council Licensing Examination (NCLEX®). The nursing profession has not always had such an organized body of knowledge or a regulated process for licensure. To best understand the position of today's nursing profession and nursing education, a look back at the history of nursing is warranted.

HISTORY OF NURSING AND NURSING EDUCATION

The word *nursing* can be traced back to the Latin word *nutrire,* "to nourish." Throughout the ages, the perception of nursing has evolved as the profession has grown and changed. Many influences have led to changes in nursing and nursing education: the methods our society uses to care for the sick, the way people live, the relationship of people to their environment, the search for knowledge and truth through education, and technological advances. Nursing evolves as society and health care needs and policies change. The field responds and adapts to these changes, meeting new challenges as they arise.

CARE OF THE SICK DURING EARLY CIVILIZATION

The concepts of health, wellness, and illness and their relationships with one another and with nursing have evolved throughout history. **Illness** (an abnormal process in which aspects of the social, emotional, or intellectual condition and function of a person are diminished or impaired) was considered to be an indicator of how one stood with God; it was understood as a direct outcome of divine disfavor. Primitive people believed that a person became sick when an evil spirit entered the body and that the presence of a good spirit kept disease away.

Medicine men performed witchcraft and rituals to induce the bad spirits to leave the body of the ailing person. Some of their methods involved the use of frightening masks, noises, incantations, vile odors, charms, spells, and even sacrifices. They used purgatives (laxatives) and emetics, application of hot and cold substances, cautery, cupping (the use of suction on the skin to promote blood flow), and massage directly on the body or the affected part. Although others assisted the medicine men in treating illnesses, few were women. The role of women in health care was focused on helping other women during childbirth.

NURSING EDUCATION IN THE 19TH CENTURY

The hospitals of the early 19th century were very different from those of today. Hospitals, or **pesthouses** as they were called, were dirty, overcrowded facilities filled with patients. The scope of care delivered was limited. The providers of care typically were untrained. Hygienic practices were poor. These factors resulted in high infection and mortality rates. Hospitals of this era were places to contract diseases rather than be cured of them. Societal interest in care of the sick and disabled was limited. Training programs for health care providers were scarce, which led to recruitment of care providers with questionable qualifications. Women of "proper upbringing" did not work outside of the home. The ranks of workers loosely referred to as nurses were filled with women who drank heavily, engaged in prostitution, or were inmates in jails and prisons. Although religious orders did train and educate a small number of nurses, they were unable to meet the health care needs of communities.

Under the guidance of Theodor Fliedner, a German pastor in Kaiserswerth, Germany, the Lutheran Order of Deaconesses established the first school of nursing in the mid-1800s. The reputation of the school soon spread throughout Europe. It reached a young woman in England, Florence Nightingale, whose interest in nursing spurred her to overcome the opposition of her family, her friends, and the social class to which she belonged.

Florence Nightingale (1820 to 1910)

Florence Nightingale (Fig. 1.1), a strong-minded, intelligent, and determined young woman, joined the Kaiserswerth program in 1851 at age 31 years and became the superintendent of a charity hospital for ill governesses in 1853. The quality of patient care improved, but the governing board of the hospital was not always pleased with the changes and innovations she made and the guidance she gave her uneducated nurses.

In the following year, concerned by the news of the number of casualties and deaths among soldiers in the Crimean War and the atrocious conditions suffered by the wounded, Nightingale sent the secretary of war, a long-time friend, a letter offering her services. Ironically, it crossed with his request for her to lead a group of nurses to Scutari, Turkey, to care for the wounded. Within a week of receiving the secretary's letter, she and 38 other nurses were on their way.

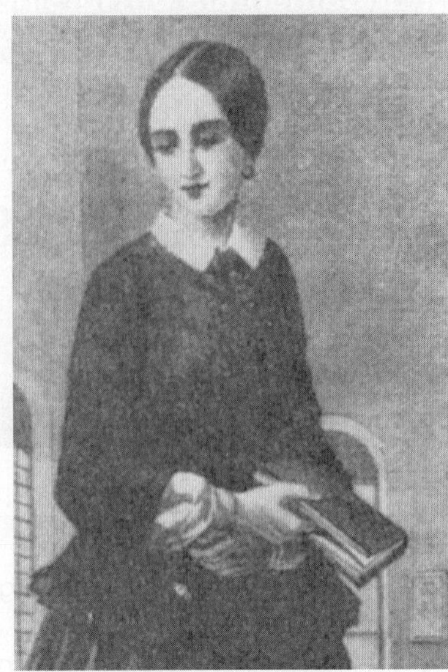

Fig. 1.1 Florence Nightingale, the first nursing theorist. (From the Dolan Collection, *Nursing Times* photograph.)

With use of the principles she learned at Kaiserswerth, Nightingale began to provide care to the wounded soldiers. Her nursing skills, dedication, and leadership turned the tide at the Barrack Hospital. Sanitary conditions, nonexistent before her arrival, were established. The hospital units were cleaned, and clothes were washed regularly. The mortality rate dropped significantly. The changes did not end with the physical environment of the hospital. Through Nightingale's patience, dedication, and empathic treatment of the soldiers, a psychological change took place as well. The soldiers grew to respect her and looked forward to her presence on the wards. They looked for her smile and took strength from her personality. When she made her rounds late at night through the rows of the injured and sick, she carried a lamp to light her way. Soon she was known as the "Lady with the Lamp." The small lamp became her trademark and continues to be the symbol of the nursing profession around the world (Fig. 1.2).

The standards of nursing care Nightingale established gained the respect of the medical community and led to improved care for the sick and a much-improved image of nursing in general. She is credited as the first nursing theorist. The need for educated and trained nurses had become painfully evident, and the time was right for a shift in the approach to nursing education (Ellis, 2008).

Nursing From Occupation to Profession

In 1860 Florence Nightingale began the reformation of nursing from occupation to profession by establishing the nursing school at Saint Thomas Hospital in London. With a reputation as a progressive medical facility, it was the ideal place to promote the new standards of nursing in which she so strongly believed.

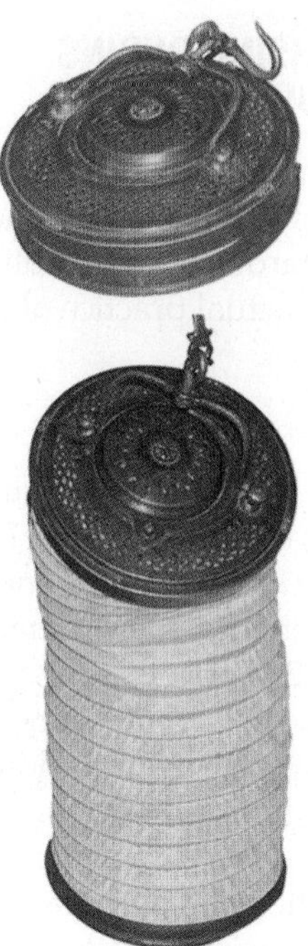

Fig. 1.2 The Nightingale lamp. (Courtesy the College and Association of Registered Nurses of Alberta Museum and Archives P-650.)

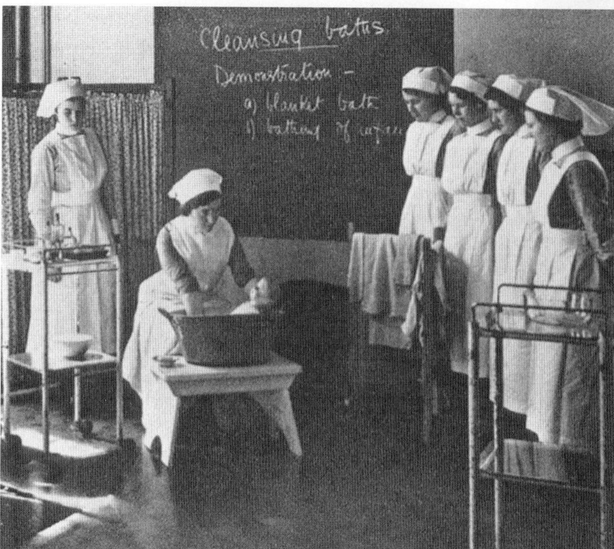

Fig. 1.3 Nursing students in an early training program. (Courtesy the National Library of Medicine.)

The nursing program operated separately from the hospital. It was financially independent to ensure that the major emphasis of its activity was placed squarely on the education of nursing students (Fig. 1.3). Students had to pass strict procedures for admission, and a residence was provided for them. The nurses' training lasted 1 year and included formal instruction and practical experience. Complete records were kept on each student's progress. This practice was known as the "Nightingale Plan," which became the model for nursing education in the 20th century. After the students graduated, records were also kept on their places of employment. The "register" that resulted was the beginning of a movement to exercise control over the nursing graduate and to establish a standard for the practicing nurse.

Students admitted into the nursing program at Saint Thomas had to provide excellent character references, show a strong commitment to a career in nursing, and demonstrate that they were intellectually capable of passing the course of study before them. The new "Nightingale nurses" improved patient care by such measures as good hygiene and sanitation, patient observation, accurate record keeping, nutritional improvements, and the introduction and use of new medical equipment. The demand for their services was overwhelming.

DEVELOPMENT OF NURSING EDUCATION IN THE UNITED STATES

At the same time Florence Nightingale was active in Europe, circumstances in the United States were creating similar patient care problems. The American Revolution and the Civil War involved severe casualties, disease, infected wounds, and archaic medical care. As in the Crimean War, nurses were scarce, and those who were available were poorly trained to handle the horrors of war.

In 1849 Pastor Theodore Fliedner of Germany, who had established Nightingale's alma mater, traveled to the United States with four of his highly trained nurse deaconesses. He was instrumental in the establishment of the first Protestant hospital on American shores. Located in Pittsburgh, it was called the Pittsburgh Infirmary and is still in existence under the name Passavant Hospital. While Fliedner was busy with the hospital, his deaconesses began the first formal education of nurses in the United States.

As hospitals in the large cities grew to meet the demands for health care, a shortage of nurses developed. Most early nursing programs were supported by these large hospitals. In 1869 the American Medical Association recommended that every large hospital should establish and support its own school of nursing to meet the need for patient care. Schools of nursing would be established by the turn of the century, all modeled after the Nightingale Plan.

In May 1873 the Bellevue Hospital School of Nursing in New York was established as the foremost proponent of the Nightingale Plan in the United States. In October of that same year, the Connecticut Training School opened in New Haven. In November, the Boston Training School began operating at the Massachusetts General Hospital.

Isabel Hampton Robb (Fig. 1.4) and Lavinia Dock organized the American Society of Superintendents of Training Schools of Nursing in 1893. The primary goal of these dedicated women was to set educational standards for nurses. The organization became the first of its kind for nursing. The structure of the organization was modeled after that of the American Medical Association. See Table 1.1 for a list of American nursing leaders.

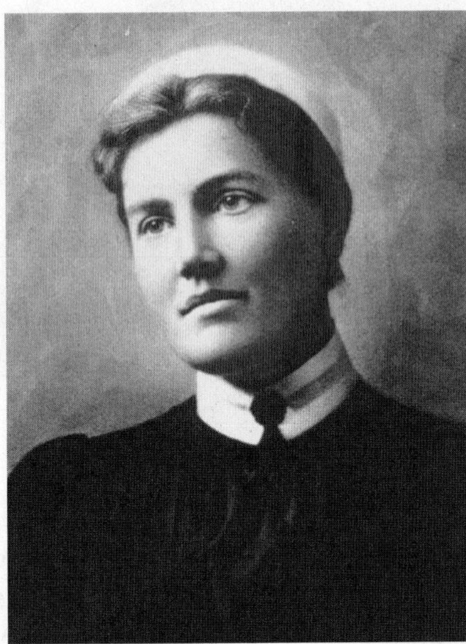

Fig. 1.4 Isabel Hampton Robb. (Courtesy the National Library of Medicine.)

CHANGES IN NURSING DURING THE 20TH CENTURY

Like the superintendents who operated at the national level, the graduates of the training schools also attempted to establish standards. They established the alumnae association for the actual practice of nursing at the local level.

LICENSING

At the beginning of the 20th century, more than 400 schools of nursing were in existence in the United States, with variations in the curricula and program lengths and differences between the competencies of program graduates. In 1903 North Carolina, New Jersey, New York, and Virginia became the first states to mandate **licensure** (the granting of permission by the overseeing authority to engage in practice or activity that would otherwise be illegal) as a criterion for entry to professional practice. The nursing organizations recognized the need to amend their purpose and redirect their focus. As part of the reorganization that followed, in 1911 the American Society of Superintendents of Training Schools became the National League for Nursing Education (NLNE, n.d.). In the years that followed the organization developed and released their first nursing curriculum plan.

Table 1.1 Leaders in the Development of Nursing in America

NURSE	CONTRIBUTION TO NURSING
Dorothea Dix (1802–1887)	Pioneer crusader for elevation of standards of care for the mentally ill. Superintendent of Female Nurses of the Union Army.
Clara Barton (1821–1912)	Developed the American Red Cross in 1881.
Mary Ann Ball (1817–1901)	One of the greatest nurse heroines of the Civil War. Championed the rights and comforts of the soldiers; organized diet kitchens, laundries, ambulance service; and supervised the nursing staff.
Linda Richards (1841–1930)	First trained nurse in America. Responsible for the development of the first nursing and hospital records. Credited with the development of our present-day documentation system.
Isabel Hampton Robb (1859–1910)	Organized the first graded system of theory and practice in the schools of nursing. One of the founders of the *American Journal of Nursing*.
Lavinia Dock (1858–1956)	Responsible, with Robb, for the organization of the American Society of Superintendents of Training Schools, which evolved into the National League for Nursing Education.
Mary Eliza Mahoney (1845–1926)	Graduated from the New England Hospital for Women and Children in 1879, becoming the first African-American professional nurse. Worked for acceptance of African Americans in the nursing profession.
Lillian D. Wald (1867–1940)	Responsible for the development of public health nursing in the United States through the founding of the Henry Street Settlement in New York City.
Mary Adelaide Nutting (1858–1948)	A leader in nursing education. Developed curriculum concepts and guidelines for student nurses. Assisted in the development of the International Council of Nurses.
Mary Breckenridge (1881–1965)	Pioneer in nurse-midwifery. Established the Frontier Nursing Service to deliver obstetric care to mothers in the hills of Kentucky; these nurses traveled on horseback to reach the mothers.

WORLD WAR I

In 1917 the United States' entry into World War I brought an increased demand for nurses. The newly formed Army and Navy Nurse Corps sought nurses who certifiably demonstrated "good moral character and professional qualifications." The available supply of nurses could not meet the demand, so once again, untrained women volunteered their services. Nursing leaders, concerned that these untrained personnel would be caring without adequate training for wounded and ailing soldiers, moved quickly to establish the Army School of Nursing. At the height of their service, more than 20,000 women are estimated to have served in the Nurse Corps (Army Heritage Center Foundation, n.d.).

After the war, most of the women who had served as military nurses returned to their homes and their previous jobs and careers. The image of professional nurses still posed a problem for most women, and few had the desire to remain in nursing as civilians. Furthermore, they were disenchanted because nurses' training still focused heavily on "service to the patient" rather than on a comprehensive professional education, which was far removed from what the Nightingale Plan had proposed for aspiring nurses.

WORLD WAR II

Twenty-five years later, World War II escalated the demand for trained nurses once again. The number of patient casualties and level of acuity skyrocketed. Early in the war, the Cadet Nurse Corps was established to provide an abbreviated training program designed to meet the needs of the war effort. In addition, federally subsidized programs in nursing were developed and implemented to offer women and, for the first time, men an education and a career in nursing while serving their country in the war.

After the war, many of the nurses trained by these programs remained in military service. Prestige, pay, and the opportunity for advancement were much greater in military service than for civilian nurses. In the major hospitals, particularly in urban areas, civilian nurses received low pay and worked long shifts in atrocious conditions. These conditions were hardly likely to attract those who became nurses as a result of the war and who, ironically, enjoyed a certain lifestyle that war provided. The aftereffects of World War I, the Great Depression, and World War II led to an increased nursing shortage.

Further, state boards of nursing, which had licensure responsibility, came under increasing pressure to mandate requirements for nurses. State-administered licensing examinations no longer seemed adequate for the country's needs. The parochial state examinations were in no way standardized and allowed people with a wide spectrum of competence to enter nursing. National norms of competence were sorely needed.

Contemporary Nursing

The focus of health care from care of the sick to an ever-expanding profit-driven industry resulted in a change in its culture and characteristics. Growth and diversity of services became the major emphases as the industry became increasingly lucrative. Contemporary nursing was born as the demand for nurses increased at a rate greater than could be met. This demand was accompanied by a growth in specialized inpatient services and an intensive growth in community-based services such as occupational and home health nursing. The number of advanced practice nursing roles, including nurse anesthetists, nurse practitioners, and midwives, has surged in recent decades.

The future of nursing as a profession has remained a source of deliberation. In 1903 Isabel Hampton Robb and Adelaide Nutting published a position paper recommending the baccalaureate degree level as the minimum acceptable preparation for entry into the profession. The associate degree was recommended as the minimum for technical nursing practice. Decades later, in 1965 the American Nurses Association (ANA) took a position recommending that nursing education take place in institutions of learning within the general system of education, much as Robb and Nutting had proposed.

Since that time there has been a change in the settings for nursing education. Although many early nursing programs were managed by hospitals, in the mid-1960s, hospitals began moving away from operating schools of nursing. Today registered nursing and licensed practical nursing programs are conducted primarily in technical schools, colleges, and universities. Licensed practical nurse (LPN) and licensed vocational nurse (LVN) programs may also be administered by high schools in some parts of the country. The shift toward colleges and universities provides the student nurse a broader educational base with an emphasis on not only skill development but also the integration of nursing theory and related general education courses (Box 1.1). More recently, the Institute of Medicine (IOM) has generated conversation with their publication *The Future of Nursing: Focus on Nursing Education*. The document presents the coming challenges to the health care and the nursing professions. The IOM has taken the position of promoting the need for changes in the nursing workforce, with a goal for 80% of working nurses to be prepared with a baccalaureate degree. The emphasis is on smoother transitions to higher degrees by nurses.

The National League for Nurses (NLN) released a position paper in 2014 recognizing the LPN/LVN as a valued member of the professional nursing team. The NLN voiced the need for LPN/LVNs to have continued support for their entry into practice. The education of the LPN/LVN should contain experiences of acute and long-term settings. Colleges and universities have been challenged further to develop programming geared to promote smooth transitions into increasingly advanced

Box 1.1 The Patient Care Partnership: Understanding Expectations, Rights, and Responsibilities

When you need hospital care, your doctor and the nurses and other professionals at our hospital are committed to working with you and your family to meet your health care needs. Our dedicated doctors and staff serve the community in all its ethnic, religious, and economic diversity. Our goal is for you and your family to have the same care and attention we would want for our families and ourselves.

The sections below explain some of the basics of how you can expect to be treated during your hospital stay. They also cover what we will need from you to care for you better. If you have questions at any time, please ask them. Unasked or unanswered questions can add to the stress of being in the hospital. Your comfort and confidence in your care are very important to us.

WHAT TO EXPECT DURING YOUR HOSPITAL STAY

- **High-quality hospital care.** Our first priority is to provide you the care you need, when you need it, with skill, compassion, and respect. Tell your caregivers if you have concerns about your care or if you have pain. You have the right to know the identity of doctors, nurses, and others involved in your care, and when they are students, residents, or other trainees.
- **A clean and safe environment.** Our hospital works hard to keep you safe. We use special policies and procedures to avoid mistakes in your care and keep you free from abuse or neglect. If anything unexpected or significant occurs during your hospital stay, you will be told what happened, and any resulting changes in your care will be discussed with you.
- **Involvement in your care.** You and your doctor often make decisions about your care before you go to the hospital. Other times, especially in emergencies, those decisions are made during your hospital stay. When decision making takes place, it should include the following:
  1. Discussing your medical condition and information about medically appropriate treatment choices. To make informed decisions with your doctor, you need to understand the following:
     - The benefits and risks of each treatment.
     - Whether your treatment is experimental or part of a research study.
     - What you can reasonably expect from your treatment and any long-term effects it might have on your quality of life.
     - What you and your family will need to do after you leave the hospital.
     - The financial consequences of using uncovered services or out-of-network providers.

     Please tell your caregivers if you need more information about treatment choices.
  2. *Discussing your treatment plan.* When you enter the hospital, you sign a general consent to treatment. In some cases, such as surgery or experimental treatment, you may be asked to confirm in writing that you understand what is planned and agree to it. This process protects your right to consent to or refuse a treatment. Your doctor will explain the medical consequences of refusing recommended treatment. It also protects your right to decide if you want to participate in a research study.
  3. *Getting information from you.* Your caregivers need complete and correct information about your health and coverage so that they can make good decisions about your care. That includes the following:
     - Past illnesses, surgeries, or hospital stays.
     - Past allergic reactions.
     - Any medications or dietary supplements (such as vitamins and herbs) that you are taking.
     - Any network or admission requirements under your health plan.
  4. *Understanding your health care goals and values.* You may have health care goals and values or spiritual beliefs that are important to your well-being. They will be taken into account as much as possible throughout your hospital stay. Make sure your doctor, your family, and your care team know your wishes.
  5. *Understanding who should make decisions when you cannot.* If you have signed a health care power of attorney that states who should speak for you if you become unable to make health care decisions for yourself, or a "living will" or "advance directive" that states your wishes about end-of-life care, give copies to your doctor, your family, and your care team. If you or your family need help making difficult decisions, counselors, chaplains, and others are available to help.
  6. *Protection of your privacy.* We respect the confidentiality of your relationship with your doctor and other caregivers, and the sensitive information about your health and health care that are part of that relationship. State and federal laws and hospital operating policies protect the privacy of your medical information. You will receive a Notice of Privacy Practices that describes the ways that we use, disclose, and safeguard patient information and that explains how you can obtain a copy of information from our records about your care.
  7. *Preparing you and your family for when you leave the hospital.* Your doctor works with hospital staff and professionals in your community. You and your family also play an important role in your care. The success of your treatment often depends on your efforts to follow medication, diet, and therapy plans. Your family may need to help care for you at home. You can expect us to help you identify sources of follow-up care and to let you know if our hospital has a financial interest in any referrals. As long as you agree that we can share information about your care with them, we will coordinate our activities with your caregivers outside the hospital. You can also expect to receive information and, where possible, training about the self-care you will need when you go home.
  8. *Help with your bill and filing insurance claims.* Our staff will file claims for you with health care insurers or other programs such as Medicare and Medicaid. They will also help your doctor with needed

Box 1.1 The Patient Care Partnership: Understanding Expectations, Rights, and Responsibilities—cont'd

documentation. Hospital bills and insurance coverage are often confusing. If you have questions about your bill, contact our business office. If you need help understanding your insurance coverage or health plan, start with your insurance company or health benefits manager. If you do not have health coverage, we will try to help you and your family find financial help or make other arrangements. We need your help with collecting needed information and other requirements to obtain coverage or assistance.

While you are here, you will receive more detailed notices about some of the rights you have as a hospital patient and how to exercise them. We are always interested in improving. If you have questions, comments, or concerns, please contact: ____________.

From American Hospital Association: *The patient care partnership: Understanding expectations, rights, and responsibilities,* Chicago, 2003, AHA. Reprinted with permission from the American Hospital Association.

levels of education upon the LPN/LVN's return to school. Growing the practical and vocational nursing curricula to incorporate roles and content characteristic of associate of science and baccalaureate level education was discouraged (NLN Board of Governers, 2014).

Challenges in Nursing Education

Nursing education has come an incredible distance since the days of Florence Nightingale. Expectations of the profession have expanded beyond the management of the activities of daily living and medication administration. Nurses are responsible for providing care to increasingly complex health conditions and managing complicated treatment modalities. Educating nurses who are able to meet the challenges of the health care environment can be difficult for nursing schools. Identified concerns include issues related to health care reform, defining the scope of practice, high stakes testing, diversity, academic progression, and faculty shortages.

Nursing Caps, Uniforms, and Pins

Originally, nurses wore the practical white, pleated cap and the apron of the maidservant, which signified respectability, cleanliness, and servitude. As the nursing profession gained recognition, nurses' caps became less utilitarian and more symbolic, a badge of office and achievement.

Since World War II, the nurse's cap has lost much of its significance. The "capping ceremony," a ritual in which junior nurses receive their first cap, has disappeared. The movement of nurses away from wearing the traditional nursing cap can be attributed to several reasons. The cap began its gradual decline in popularity around the same time as a movement toward a more informal uniform made the cap a dated piece of apparel. Nurses often reported that the cap interfered with the care being provided because it caught on equipment in the patient care area. Some nurses even reported hair loss from the constant friction of the hat. The movement of men into the profession, for whom there was no cap, was accompanied by discontent. Washing and starching the hat was a chore, and there were growing concerns about the caps harboring bacteria (Medscape Today News, n.d.) (Fig. 1.5).

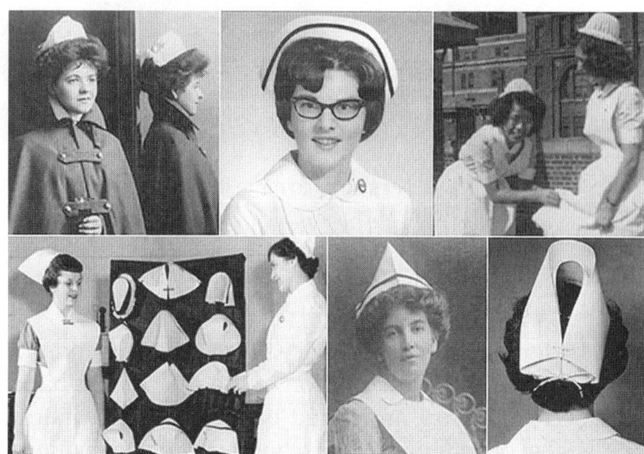

Fig. 1.5 Nursing caps in history. (Courtesy Ona Wilcox College of Nursing Records, Archives & Special Collections at the Thomas J. Dodd Research Center, University of Connecticut Libraries.)

The nursing uniform is another area that has seen and will continue to see change. Today controversy exists within the medical profession about the need for nursing uniforms. Many nurses do not approve of mandatory dress codes. They argue that other health care professionals do not depend on uniforms for their authority (Fig. 1.6).

A professional appearance is nonetheless important. Patients feel more comfortable and confident when they can easily find and distinguish nurses from other staff members. Agencies typically have dress codes in place. Some mandate the style of uniform; others assign certain colors to different health care groups. Facilities require staff members to wear nametags and identification badges and dress to promote professionalism. As a result of technological advances and the need for security, some facilities use fingerprint scans for access into the record-keeping and medication administration systems.

Pinning ceremonies began as a means to demonstrate successful program completion by nursing students. The practice of awarding a pin at the time of graduation dates back to the later 1800s in England (Early, 2015). In the United States the first nursing pins were awarded in New York's Bellevue Hospital in 1880. This first pin had a symbolic design. The center displayed a crane,

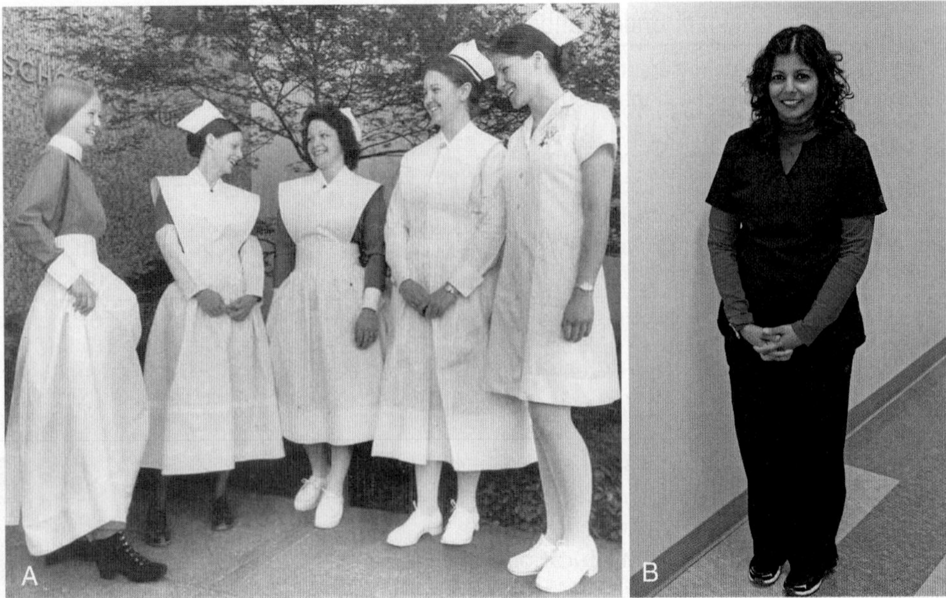

Fig. 1.6 A, Nursing uniforms in the early years. B, Nursing uniforms today. (A, Copyright the Royal Columbian Hospital, New Westminster, B.C.)

which demonstrated vigilance. There were bands of color around the outer portion of the pin. A blue band signaled constancy and a red band illustrated mercy and a relief of suffering. Most schools of nursing continue to award a nursing pin to the graduate nurse. Pinning does not bestow credentials such as degree completion or state licensure but is considered a rite of passage by many in the profession. Today, many of these pins bear the Nightingale lamp as a common component, along with an emblem of the school of nursing.

SIGNIFICANT CHANGES IN NURSING FOR THE 21ST CENTURY

Nursing practice is affected by various societal factors, along with developments that are more internal to the field. Demographics of the population, women's health care issues, men in nursing, rising numbers of people with fewer socioeconomic advantages seeking health care, and bioterrorism threats are a few of the societal factors that influence nursing today.

DEMOGRAPHIC CHANGES

Because the demographics of the population are changing, nursing education and practice must also change and adapt. Life expectancy of the population is increasing, and growing numbers of older adults are seeking health care for chronic illnesses.

WOMEN'S HEALTH CARE ISSUES

The unique health care needs of women are recognized. The number of research studies specific to these needs has increased, in part as a result of federal mandates that require inclusion of women in studies. Areas of interest for women's health include reproductive health, heart disease, and cancer (Agency for Healthcare Research and Quality, 2011).

Nursing is responding in two ways to women's health care issues and the women's movement. Nurses, most of whom are women, are increasingly asserting their equal rights as humans, employees, and health care professionals. Encouraged by the women's movement, they have sought greater autonomy and responsibility in providing care. In addition, the women's movement has helped women to become more aware of their own unique needs. Nurses have learned to encourage female patients to seek more responsibility for and control over their bodies, health, and lives in general.

MEN IN NURSING

Men have had a role in nursing throughout its history. However, in more modern times the number of men in nursing has decreased. The influences of war promoted the profession for women rather than men. Some critics also associate Florence Nightingale with the decreasing number of men in nursing. She recommended that "gentlewomen" replace workers who were unskilled. This verbiage promoted the idea that nursing was more "woman's work." Fortunately, the past few decades have shown increases in the number of men in nursing. Fewer than 10% of nursing program graduates are male (Payne, 2013). Smaller still is the percentage of men who are actively licensed and working. The majority of men in nursing are registered nurses.

To combat the shortage of men in nursing, education and professional settings have programs to attract and recruit men to the profession. Studies are showing that drawing men to the profession is not where the challenge ends. The attrition rate for men in nursing education is higher than that of women. Men are also more likely than their female counterparts to leave the profession once licensed. Reports indicate that challenges related to feelings of social isolation, stereotypes about men who choose nursing, nursing instructors' inability to incorporate masculine styles of caring into the curriculum, and a lack of male role models in the profession may be to blame.

HUMAN RIGHTS

Nursing advocates for the rights of all individuals. Beyond this basic requirement, the profession has promoted the rights of specific segments of the population through the creation of bills of rights. Such bills address the rights of hospitalized patients, those who are dying, older adults, and pregnant women. These bills of rights address the need to respect all patients as individuals and ensure quality care for all.

MEDICALLY UNDERSERVED

Soaring rates of unemployment, homelessness, undocumented workers, and poverty, combined with the enormous rise in health care costs, have led to an increased number of individuals in the United States who are unable to afford health care. These groups, when combined, represent a sizable population of those who are potentially unable to obtain health insurance or pay outright for health care.

Presently, health care costs account for nearly 17.1% of the nation's gross domestic product (GDP) (The Commonwealth Fund, 2015). The average spending on health care in the United States was just more than $9000 per person. Health care spending in the United States is significantly greater than in other industrialized nations. France is next in line for health care spending at 11.6% of their GDP. In 2015 the rate of uninsured in the United States was 9%. There are regional differences noted with the percentages of uninsured. Several southern states show higher rates than others. Overall the Northeast has lower rates of uninsured. Limited access to health care is another concern that hinders individuals with mental health disorders and those who live in rural areas. Initiatives to provide increased services in rural and community-based clinics offer assistance to these populations. Nursing engagement in health promotion activities to prevent and manage illness and chronic conditions is one such solution.

Frequently, nurses who work in these settings have a higher degree of training and function as advanced practice nurses, so they have the capability to provide direct health care. This area of nursing is expanding rapidly as more nurses seek to work with this underserved population.

NURSING SHORTAGE

The United States continues to face a nursing shortage. The nation is expected to need an increase of 16% LPN/LVNs (Bureau of Labor Statistics, 2018). This increase will require more than 117,000 more LPN/LVNs. Despite strategies to reduce the shortfall of nurses, the supply is not expected to meet the growing demand. The nursing workforce is aging; the average age of nurses is 42.6 years. In the coming decade, many nurses who currently are working are expected to retire.

Nursing, once considered a prime career choice for women, now faces competition as women look at other promising career options (American Association of Colleges of Nursing, 2012). Schools of nursing also are facing a shortage of qualified educators, which further hinders growth of the profession.

DEVELOPMENT OF PRACTICAL AND VOCATIONAL NURSING

ATTENDANT NURSES

The first school for training practical nurses opened in Brooklyn, New York, in 1892 under the auspices of the Young Women's Christian Association (YWCA). The Ballard School, as it was known, gave a course that lasted approximately 3 months and trained its students to care for invalids, children, the chronically ill, and the elderly. The main emphasis was on home care and included cooking, nutrition, basic science, and basic nursing procedures. Graduates of this program were referred to as attendant nurses.

Two other programs were patterned after the Ballard School. In 1907 the Thompson Practical Nursing School opened in Brattleboro, Vermont (still in operation and accredited by the National League for Nursing [NLN]), and in 1918 the Household Nursing Association School of Attendant Nursing (later changed to the Shepard-Gill School of Practical Nursing) opened in Boston. Hospital experience was not a part of the training in the early programs. The focus was on home nursing care and light housekeeping duties.

PRACTICAL NURSING PROGRAMS

Practical nursing programs developed slowly during the first half of the 20th century, with only 36 schools opening. The practical nursing schools before 1940 had few controls, little educational planning, and minimal supervision. Between 1948 and 1954, a sharp increase in the formation of practical and vocational nursing programs was attributed to the increased demand for nursing services in World War II and the postwar years and the excellent bedside nursing care demonstrated by the practical nurse. These programs varied in administrative design. Some were affiliated with hospitals or chronic care institutions, whereas others aligned themselves with private agencies or private schools. Students in these programs provided nursing services while they were obtaining their education and training. Technical and vocational education emphasized apprentice training. Federal funds allocated for training practical and vocational nurses helped recruit men and women.

FUTURE OF THE LICENSED PRACTICAL NURSE AND LICENSED VOCATIONAL NURSE

There are an estimated 825,000 LPN/LVNs in the United States (The Henry J. Kaiser Family Foundation, 2017). Their practice settings are vast. Although they once were a visible member of the health care team in acute care facilities, today only an estimated 25% are working in hospital settings. The position of the LPN/LVN has been in many areas of the country removed or sharply limited in acute care settings. With a looming nursing shortage there is a need for the LPN/LVN to be a key member of the team addressing this nationwide concern.

ORGANIZATIONAL INFLUENCE

As practical nursing programs continued to grow in number, the need to establish standards of curricula became increasingly evident. The Association of Practical Nurse Schools was founded in 1941 and was dedicated exclusively to practical nursing. Its membership was multidisciplinary and included licensed practical nurses, registered nurses, physicians, hospital and nursing home administrators, students, and public figures. Together they planned the first standard curriculum for practical nursing. By 1942 they saw the need to change the name to the National Association of Practical Nurse Education (NAPNE). They broadened their focus to include education and practice and established an accrediting service for schools of practical and vocational nursing in 1945. The association changed its name once more in 1959 to the National Association for Practical Nurse Education and Service (NAPNES). Today, NAPNES remains a guiding force in the development of practical nursing education.

In 1949 the National Federation of Licensed Practical Nurses (NFLPN) was founded by Lillian Kuster. Limited to LPNs and LVNs, this association is the official membership organization for the LPN/LVN. Working together, NAPNES and NFLPN set standards for practical and vocational nursing practice, promote and protect the interests of LPN/LVNs, and educate and inform the general public about practical and vocational nursing.

In 1961 the NLN broadened its scope of service because of the growth of practical and vocational nursing programs. The NLN established the Department of Practical Nursing Programs and developed an accreditation service for these programs, which is now called the Council of Practical Nursing Programs.

For 20 years, the NLN and the NAPNES provided accreditation services. Nursing programs had the option of seeking accreditation from either organization. In recent years, however, NAPNES has discontinued this service.

PROGRAM CREDENTIALING

Accreditation of a program differs from program approval. Approval is required for a program to open and operate. An **approved program** is one that satisfies the minimum standards set by the state agency responsible for overseeing educational programs: for example, it meets the needs of the student, has adequate course content and qualified faculty, is of sufficient length, has adequate facilities, and provides clinical experience. To protect the welfare of the public, the state requires programs to demonstrate all these elements for graduates to be eligible for licensure. **Accreditation** is a higher standard that signifies that the accrediting organization has judged that a program has met its preestablished criteria. The administrators of the program seeking accreditation submit voluntarily to the accreditation process; they do so because of the recognition of quality it confers. Often the standards established by professional organizations that give accreditation are far higher than those established by the state. Although graduates of nonaccredited programs can take the licensure examination required in most states, accreditation is extremely important when programs seek federal funding. Graduates from nonaccredited programs may face challenges when attempting to transfer completed course work to another institution for further education.

CONTEMPORARY PRACTICAL AND VOCATIONAL NURSING EDUCATION

Practical nursing programs are offered by various organizations, including high schools, trade or technical schools, hospitals, junior and community colleges, colleges and universities, and private education agencies. Programs are required to meet the minimum state standards. The length of the programs is usually 12 to 18 months, with a focus on nursing skills and theory that is correlated with clinical practice.

Educational programs in nursing today offer various creative approaches to the education of student LPN/LVNs. The combination of practical and vocational nurse education with associate degree programs in 2-year colleges is available. At the successful completion of the first academic year and of the requirements for the practical nursing portion of the program, the student can either exit and take the licensure examination for practical or vocational nursing or continue for another year and earn an associate degree in nursing, becoming eligible to take the licensure examination for registered nursing. Many other programs offer other combinations of education and degrees throughout the United States. Most states have some type of articulation plan.

Articulation allows nursing programs to plan their curricula collaboratively; the purpose is to lessen duplication of learning experiences and support a process of progressive buildup. Thus one program becomes the foundation for another program. An LPN/LVN may receive as much as 50% credit toward the associate degree; the associate degree–prepared registered nurse (RN) may receive as much as 50% credit toward the bachelor of science in nursing (BSN) degree. This process is sometimes referred to as a 1-plus-1 program or a 2-plus-2 program, respectively. Articulation acknowledges the student's existing knowledge base and permits the student to continue her or his advancement in education without repeating previous course work.

CAREER ADVANCEMENT

The career ladder is a model that some institutions use to allow for professional advancement. A career ladder recognizes the clinical expertise of the nurse and provides a mechanism for financial compensation. Each institution clearly lists and defines its criteria for advancement on the ladder. Items generally include adherence to facility policies, completion of mandatory education programs, and demonstration of leadership and clinical skills. Nurses make application for consideration of the career ladder by submitting a portfolio illustrating their accomplishments. A **portfolio** is an organized account of an individual's education and professional accomplishments.

FACTORS THAT INFLUENCED PRACTICAL AND VOCATIONAL NURSING

Before 1860 nursing care in the United States was provided generally by people who were self-taught and who gained what knowledge they could through experience. Registration, licensing, and title differentiation were unclear or nonexistent. Duties and responsibilities were not defined clearly. The term *nurse* was used only in the broadest sense as "a person who takes care of the sick."

NEED FOR TRAINED CAREGIVERS

Practical nursing in the United States evolved from the need for caregivers who could be trained and ready for service in a short time. The cost of the services provided by these caregivers was expected to be reasonable and easily affordable by the patient. There was also the need to provide a vocation for the many unskilled women who were migrating to the larger cities to seek better opportunities. Women generally were not skilled or trained for jobs other than manual labor.

WORLD WAR I

World War I increased the need for trained nurses abroad, and in the United States, the Spanish influenza epidemic strained the resources of the nursing community. The Smith-Hughes Act was passed in 1917 to provide vocational and public education. Federal funding then provided the means for vocational-based practical and vocational nursing programs throughout the country. Even with these resources, the demand for nurses caused by the war and the epidemic could not be met.

SELF-TAUGHT PRACTICAL NURSE

By 1940 thousands of self-taught "practical nurses" were working to meet the needs of the country. They lacked the education and experience obtainable only under supervision in an established program. Few states had minimum standards for the practice of practical and vocational nurses. There was no agreement on the duties, the role, and the responsibilities of practical and vocational nurses, and they were known by many job descriptions and titles. The absence of standards and licensing created difficulties and safety concerns.

The state of New York was the first to have mandatory licensure laws. A state pool of test questions was adopted in 1945 by the State Boards of Nursing Examiners in 25 states (Smith, 2009). By 1950 all states had joined the momentum and required testing and licensure for entry into practice.

DUTIES OF LICENSED PRACTICAL NURSES AND LICENSED VOCATIONAL NURSES

In 1944 the US Department of Vocational Education commissioned an intensive study of practical and vocational nursing tasks. The outcome of this study differentiated the tasks performed by the LPN/LVN in relation to those tasks performed by the registered nurse. As a result of this study, individual state boards of nursing began to specify the duties and responsibilities that could be accomplished by each group of nurses.

POSITION PAPER OF THE AMERICAN NURSES ASSOCIATION

In 1965 the *American Nurses Association's First Position on Education for Nursing* was released. The document outlined recommendations for the educational levels for the nurse to enter practice. It recommended a 2-year technical education be provided in vocational and community college settings. Graduates of these programs would earn an associate of science degree. The professional nurse would earn a baccalaureate degree. The paper did not specifically discuss the LPN/LVN. Practical and vocational nurses nonetheless have proved their worth. Under the supervision of a registered nurse or physician, they provide excellent bedside nursing skills in many areas of service. The 1965 position paper of the ANA was another influence that brought about a change in attitude toward practical and vocational nursing.

LICENSURE FOR PRACTICAL AND VOCATIONAL NURSING

Licensing laws have been passed to protect the public from unqualified practitioners in most fields and professions. In the mid-1950s, states moved toward mandatory licensure for nurses. The laws passed were managed by state agencies such as the state boards of nursing. The state's nurse practice acts provide specific information about the scope of practice for the differing nursing levels. On completion of a nursing program, the graduate is eligible to take the National Council Licensing Examination for Practical Nursing (NCLEX-PN®). Once the examination is completed successfully, licensure is awarded by the state of application.

LAWS THAT MONITOR THE LICENSED PRACTICAL NURSE AND THE LICENSED VOCATIONAL NURSE

Licensing for practical and vocational nurses in the United States began in 1914, when the state legislature in Mississippi passed the first laws pertaining to that group. This licensing followed the passage of laws on licensing for RNs. The passage of such laws governing practical and vocational nursing in other states did not rapidly follow. After the outbreak of World War II and the opening of a large number of practical and vocational nurses training programs, all the states were forced to pass legislation concerning their licensure. By 1955 all states had passed laws in this area in consonance (agreement) with the standards set by NAPNE. The State Board Test Pool of the NLN Education Committee established a testing mechanism for all states and administered the examination several times a year throughout the country. Graduates of a state-approved practical or vocational nursing education program were eligible to sit for the examination; if they passed, they became LPNs, or LVNs as they are called in Texas and California. Each state set its own required passing score on the examination.

Today graduates of an approved LPN/LVN education program are eligible to apply to take the licensure examination. This application must be approved by the individual's state board of nursing. On completion of the computerized examination with a "pass" score (numerical scores are no longer given), the graduate is issued a license to practice as an LPN or an LVN.

HEALTH CARE DELIVERY SYSTEMS

LPN/LVNs practice within the health care delivery system as a whole. To achieve their greatest potential, nurses must be aware of the complexity of this system and the vital role that nursing plays in its functioning.

HEALTH CARE SYSTEM DEFINED

The **health care system** consists of a network of agencies, facilities, and providers involved with health care in a specified geographic area. Many categories of health care professionals operate within this system, including the LPN/LVN. This health care environment includes the patient, the patient's family, the community in which the system operates, technology, governmental and regulatory agencies, the medical profession, third-party participants (e.g., insurance companies), and many other forces that affect the patient's care. The major goal of the system is to achieve optimal levels of health care for a defined population. The means of achieving this goal is provision of adequate and appropriate health care services. The LPN/LVN is an integral member of the team of health care professionals who provide these services within the scope of practice as defined by the state's nurse practice act.

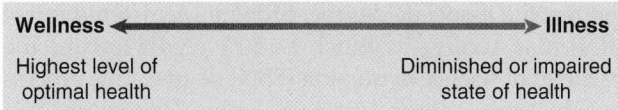

Fig. 1.7 Health care continuum.

WELLNESS-ILLNESS CONTINUUM

The range of a person's total health is described along the *wellness-illness continuum.* One's position on this continuum is ever changing and is influenced by the individual's physical condition, mental condition, and social well-being. At one end of the spectrum is **wellness** (a dynamic state of health in which an individual progresses toward a higher level of functioning, achieving an optimal balance between internal and external environment). Wellness represents the highest level of optimal health. Illness, at the opposite end of the spectrum, represents a diminished or impaired state of health (Fig. 1.7).

A balance of all aspects of life is the key to maintaining one's health. Factors that affect the level of wellness include age, gender, family relationships, emotional stressors, ethnic and cultural influences, and economic status. Consideration of the interrelationships among these variables is paramount when the nurse is planning and providing care. An all-inclusive approach to health care is known as **holistic health care** (a system of comprehensive or total patient care that considers the physical, emotional, social, economic, and spiritual needs of a person).

MASLOW'S MODEL OF HEALTH AND ILLNESS

Several models of the wellness-illness continuum have been developed. These models enable the nurse to understand the patient's individual level of wellness and position on the continuum. The most common model was developed in the 1940s by Abraham Maslow. He believed that an individual's behavior is formed by the individual's attempts to meet essential human needs, which he identified as physiologic, safety and security, love and belongingness, and esteem and self-actualization. Maslow placed these needs into a conceptual hierarchy, or pyramid, that ranks them according to how basic each one is. A person has to meet needs at the base of the pyramid before advancing

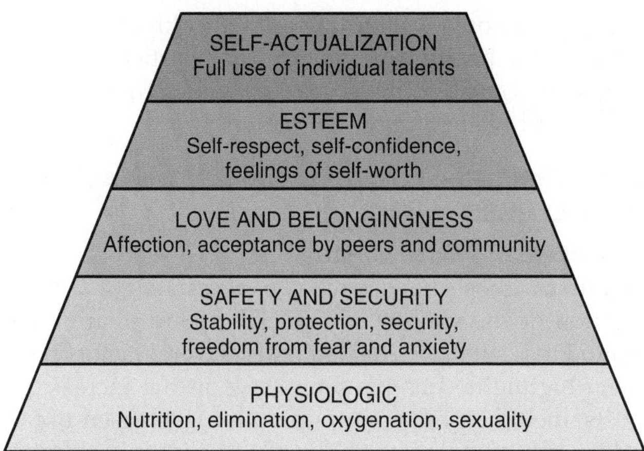

Fig. 1.8 Maslow's hierarchy. (Data from Maslow A: *Motivation and personality*, ed 2, New York, 1970, Harper & Row.)

to the needs higher on the pyramid. Those needs placed higher on the pyramid are not requirements for life but rather enhance it. Remember that each patient may view or prioritize individual needs according to his or her own value system (Fig. 1.8).

HEALTH PROMOTION AND ILLNESS PREVENTION

From the earliest recorded civilizations to the 20th century, the primary focus of health care was on the care of the sick. Today's focus has broadened to include an emphasis on an awareness of the causes of disease and the prevention of its spread through the use of health-promotion activities.

In contrast to their origins as dirty, unsanitary, and ill-kept institutions where unsuspecting patients acquired diseases, hospitals have become clean, increasingly safe locations where patients and their families are cared for with limited fear that they will be exposed to additional illness and medical problems. The US Department of Public Health works to help in the identification of disease types and related risk factors. These statistics identify problem areas for researchers and health care providers, who then direct their efforts at developing treatment for the illness, isolating its cause, and establishing methods to decrease its spread. The determination of cause-and-effect relationships provides a starting point for the development and implementation of health promotion initiatives.

Today three levels of health promotion are recognized. Their purpose is to promote health through maintaining wellness, preventing disease-related complications, and reducing the infirmity associated with disease states. *Primary prevention* seeks to avoid disease states through wellness activities and preemptive screening programs such as mammograms, colonoscopies, and glucose screening. *Secondary prevention* recognizes the presence of disease but seeks to reduce the impact of the condition by encouraging behaviors to promote health. An example of this type of prevention is dietary teaching to a patient with diabetes with the intention to reduce episodes of hyperglycemia. The management of care activities for those with serious health problems who seek to improve the quality of life and reduce further loss of function are captured by *tertiary prevention*.

CONTINUITY OF CARE

The patient is the focus of the health care system. However, many factors in our holistic health care system determine what actually happens in the care of each patient. The number of health care providers and health care agencies involved in the care and treatment of a single patient is extensive. Increased specialization by health care providers and health care institutions, reimbursement procedures by third-party payers (e.g., insurance companies), cumbersome federal regulatory organizations, and state health care regulatory agencies affect the consumer (the patient) and the type and quality of care provided.

One of the greatest challenges for the consumer of medical care is artful navigation of the health care delivery system. The consumer faces challenges to maintain autonomy and obtain continuity of care. Patients who already are weakened by the stressors of actual or potential medical conditions can become frightened as they attempt to understand the medical care and related choices available to them.

DELIVERY OF PATIENT CARE

The care of patients is a humanistic enterprise. It involves not only treating disease and injury but also preventing disease, restoring optimal wellness through rehabilitation, caring for the chronically ill, and educating patients and families. To identify the individual needs of the patient and to plan a systematic approach to meet those needs, nurses participate in developing an individualized care plan with use of the nursing process (see Chapter 5). The purpose of the care plan is to meet the expressed needs of the patient. Its development involves the patient and all health care providers who, through a coordinated and cooperative effort, work toward meeting the patient's total needs in a holistic, caring manner.

PARTICIPANTS IN THE HEALTH CARE SYSTEM

Professional Health Care Specialists

The patient is the central focus of activities performed by more than 200 types of health care providers identified in the health care system in the United States. Many professions require **certification** or licensure of their members. Within many disciplines are subspecialties of individuals who have advanced training and licensure.

Registered Nurses

The RN is a direct health care provider who is licensed after completion of one of three types of nursing education programs: a 4-year baccalaureate degree program, a 2-year associate degree program, or a 3-year diploma program. RNs practice in a variety of settings inside and outside of the care facility. The RN's duties and tasks vary according to educational background and the state's nurse practice act. Educational and career opportunities exist for the registered nurse beyond initial licensure. Nurses with master's degrees or doctorates represent a small but growing segment of the profession. These individuals often are termed advanced practice nurses. Their roles are expanded and may involve educator, administrator, and prescriptive authority.

Licensed Practical and Licensed Vocational Nurses

The LPN/LVN practices under the supervision of the RN or the physician. Working together, the LPN/LVN and the RN are the direct patient caregivers in most institutions. The role of the LPN/LVN is based on the scope of practice outlined in each state's nurse practice act (see Chapter 40 for more information on nurse practice acts).

Other Caregivers

Other caregivers also are required to be registered or licensed and to have the specialized education and training dictated by their professional organizations. **Holistic** care requires that professionals from differing areas come together to provide comprehensive care. When a patient's condition dictates, referral to other care providers may be indicated. For example, social workers are trained to counsel patients who have social, emotional, or environmental problems. Physical therapists use precise methods of massage, exercise, and hydrotherapy to help restore physical function of the body. Dietitians are trained to determine the foods that meet the nutritional requirements of the patient. Respiratory therapists assist the patient by administering oxygen, monitoring and maintaining ventilators, drawing blood for blood gas analysis, and performing other pulmonary function tests.

Technologists, Medical Technicians, and Paraprofessionals

Diagnostic personnel work in the laboratory and radiology departments. Their roles involve assisting the medical professional staff in testing for disease states and injury. The term *technologist* refers to those who have a baccalaureate degree, whereas the term *technician* refers to those who have had training and have earned an associate degree or certificate. Paraprofessionals are educated to assist the professional in providing care for patients. Unlicensed assistive personnel (UAP) are educated in basic nursing techniques and perform under the supervision of the RN. The unit secretary prepares and maintains patient records, orders supplies, schedules tests, and performs receptionist duties on the care unit.

These are only a sampling of the health care participants in the health care system. Each participant has a valuable contribution to make toward ensuring the safety and well-being of the patient.

ECONOMIC FACTORS THAT AFFECT HEALTH AND ILLNESS

Rising Health Care Costs

Health care costs have reached a critical height. A large portion of the country's financial resources are committed to health care–related costs. Several factors have been highlighted as playing a role in the increase in costs, including an aging population, increased use of advanced technologies, rising cost of private health care insurance, the rising cost of medical malpractice insurance, and a struggling economy.

Increasing number of aging Americans. As the baby boomer generation nears the age of retirement, their health problems increase; this onset of chronic diseases in a large segment of the population strains the health care system. Diseases associated with aging include heart disease, diabetes, and osteoporosis. As the US population ages, an increasing number of older adults need nursing home care, which is costly and has limited coverage under traditional insurance plans.

Advances in technology. Advances in technology have led to better diagnosis and treatment of illness, but such progress carries a large price. Research and the development of technology cost millions of dollars, a price that is passed on to the patient in the cost of the individual tests or treatments. Technological advances have resulted in concerns for patient privacy as electronic piracy has become an increasing threat. Safeguards for the electronic health records add to the costs for health care.

Health care insurance. Private health care insurance initially was developed to defray some or all of the cost of health care. It made health care more affordable, but it also raised the demand for it. As more individuals sought care, the price of health care services and insurance costs spiraled. This trend continues at an alarming and seemingly uncontrollable speed. The underinsured and uninsured populations face hardship when health care is needed. Determination of who receives care and who does not is becoming an ethical issue at all levels of the health care delivery system. To further compound the current economic problems, nearly 16% of Americans or 48.6 million people are without health care coverage (United States Census Bureau, 2011). Although this number has declined for the first time in several years, it is still a cause for concern because these individuals too often avoid preventive and routine care and are seen only in crisis situations.

Malpractice insurance. Nurses and doctors carry medical malpractice insurance to protect themselves in the event a malpractice claim is filed against them. As malpractice claims have increased in frequency and amount, the premiums for this insurance have also risen. In response, physicians sometimes resort to practicing "defensive medicine." That is, they become overly cautious out of fear of a claim, ordering costly tests and procedures not because they are medically necessary but to protect themselves. These behaviors have resulted in higher medical costs for the patient.

These issues are alarming for health care providers. Nurses can help keep costs to a minimum by using materials and time economically and providing knowledgeable efficient care.

CHANGES IN DELIVERY SYSTEM

Hospitals throughout the United States are changing delivery systems to make care more cost effective. Case management and cross-training are two commonly encountered methods for modifying the systems used to deliver care.

Case management nursing revolves around the use of clinical pathways, which map out expectations of the hospitalization according to a designated time frame. The RN functions as a case manager, coordinating and planning the care of a group of patients, or caseload. An LPN/LVN works with the RN to assist the patient in attaining desired outcomes of care. Case management nursing has been proven to reduce the length of stay for the patient, which in turn reduces the overall cost of the patient's health care.

Cross-training allows employers to maximize the use of available staff. Workers are trained to perform duties that cross traditional role boundaries. Cross-training may involve combining the roles of differing categories of workers or expanding the responsibilities of staff members to cover multiple care units. Two groups of workers that frequently cross-trained to expand their roles are clerical support staff and UAP. This training enables a single worker to perform UAP-related tasks (e.g., ambulating patients and taking vital signs) as well as clerical support duties (e.g., transcribing orders and ordering unit supplies). Another type of cross-training involves linking patient care units, frequently identified as sister units. Common sister units are maternal child care and women's health, and the nursing staff are trained to work in both areas. Individuals receive training to perform duties that vary according to the needs at a given time. This training can be as narrowly defined as medical training to care for surgical patients or as broadly defined as housekeeping personnel training to give basic morning care to patients. The scope of cross-training usually is defined by the individual institution, and the purpose is to reduce the number or cost of employees without compromising the quality of patient care.

Other trends that affect the economics of health care include the development of multisystem health care chains or networks that may include several hospitals, clinics, nursing homes, and pharmacies. These systems share expenses and generally achieve an overall reduction in operating expenses. Health maintenance organizations (HMOs) or group health care practices provide health care to members for a fixed prepaid rate. This service includes medical care, nursing care, diagnostic tests, hospitalization, and various inpatient and outpatient treatments. This service has shown a high quality of low-cost health care.

SOCIAL AND ENVIRONMENTAL FACTORS THAT AFFECT HEALTH AND ILLNESS

Social and environmental factors do not necessarily cause illness, but they do influence the development or progression of an illness. Financial hardship, lifestyle choices, and social pressures all influence an individual's willingness or ability to actively maintain health or prevent illness. In addition, personal behavior choices such as smoking, drug abuse, alcoholism, and obesity affect an individual's health and wellness. The individual's mental state has an influence on patient outcomes. Emotions associated with fear, loss of identity, and loss of control commonly are experienced during illness. An imbalance in body functions can affect one's physical condition and ultimately the position along the wellness-illness continuum. Although there is often a tendency to separate social factors from physical factors, remember that the two areas affect each other reciprocally.

Each patient possesses a unique personality, background, lifestyle, and level of education. Early recognition of the effect of environmental factors on a patient and prompt intervention by family, health care providers, or the patients can decrease or minimize any negative impact.

HEALTH PROMOTION

Most people in the United States believe that everyone has a right to health care, regardless of race, color, creed, or economic status. This health care includes the treatment of disease and health promotion and preventive medicine. In many cases, treatment of illness is less of a concern than its prevention. The acute awareness of preventive medicine has resulted in today's emphasis on education about issues such as smoking, heart disease, drug and alcohol abuse, weight control, and mental health and wellness promotion activities.

During illness or after a change in health status, people often feel they are not in control of their health, but they typically do trust in the health care system. The presumption is that care will be highly satisfactory and lead to a cure. Health care providers are expected to provide service in a knowledgeable, safe, and expeditious manner and to work in a cooperative manner for their benefit. Patients also expect the cost of care to be reasonable and, most importantly, paid by somebody else (an insurance company or the government).

Patients' Rights

In 1972 the American Hospital Association (AHA) issued the *Patient's Bill of Rights* in an effort to ensure the patient's fundamental rights for treatment with dignity and compassion were protected. The trailblazing document was revised again in the 1990s and finally was replaced in 2003 when the AHA adopted the *Patient Care Partnership* (Box 1.2). According to the terms of this document, patients are assured that they can expect high-quality hospital care, a clean and safe environment, involvement in their care and the decision-making process, protection of privacy, help when leaving the hospital, and help with billing concerns (American Hospital Association, 2003). Nursing home patients' rights also are protected. The *Resident's Bill of Rights* is a document developed to provide clarity to the needs and rights of the individual who resides in a long-term care environment. It is the responsibility of the facility staff to provide copies of these rights and to explain them to the residents (Centers for Medicare and Medicaid Services, n.d.).

Box 1.2 Nursing Conditions in the Past

The following job description was given to floor nurses by a hospital in 1887.

In addition to caring for your 50 patients, each nurse will follow these regulations:

- Daily sweep and mop the floors of your ward, dust the patient's furniture and windowsills. Maintain an even temperature in your ward by bringing in a scuttle of coal for the day's business.
- Light is important to observe the patient's condition. Therefore, each day fill kerosene lamps, clean chimneys, and trim wicks. Wash the windows once a week.
- The nurse's notes are important in aiding the physician's work. Make your pens carefully; you may whittle nibs to your individual taste.
- Each nurse on day duty will report every day at 7 a.m. and leave at 8 p.m., except on the Sabbath, on which day you will be off from 12 noon to 2 p.m..
- Graduate nurses in good standing with the director of nurses will be given an evening off each week for courting purposes or two evenings a week if you go regularly to church.
- Each nurse should lay aside from each payday a goodly sum of her earnings for her benefits during her declining years so that she will not become a burden. For example, if you earn $30 a month, you should set aside $15.
- Any nurse who smokes, uses liquor in any form, gets her hair done at a beauty shop, or frequents dance halls will give the director of nurses good reason to suspect her worth, intentions, and integrity.
- The nurse who performs her labors and serves her patients and doctors without fault for 5 years will be given an increase of 5 cents a day, providing there are no hospital debts outstanding.

It is interesting to compare current practical and vocational nursing tasks with those that were expected in 1887. Practical and vocational nursing has indeed come a long way.

From Hill SS, Howlett HA: *Success in practical/vocational nursing: From student to leader,* ed 7, St. Louis, 2013, Saunders.

Health Care Providers' Rights

The delivery of health care must be a process of mutual exchange between patients and health care providers. Patients expect their rights to be respected, but health care workers have expectations as well. Health care professionals expect that patients will do the following to actively participate in their care as much as possible: take an active role in the planning process, understand the care and the treatment given, ask questions, follow the treatment plan prescribed, act responsibly with respect to their own conditions, and give health care workers the same respect to which patients are entitled.

INTERDISCIPLINARY APPROACH TO HEALTH CARE

The primary goal of the health care team is the optimal physical, mental, and social well-being of the patient. This goal is achieved by promoting and restoring health within the wellness-illness continuum. Health care personnel, when working to meet the needs of the patient, must work together as a health care team. Following this interdisciplinary approach to treatment prevents the fragmentation of patient care. Just as the plan of care for patients is developed in a holistic manner, so is the actual delivery of health care. All health care providers must remember that the central focus of all their activity is the patient.

Each member of the team is responsible for coordinating activity with every other member of the team by developing a comprehensive care plan, effectively communicating, and keeping accurate records (Fig. 1.9).

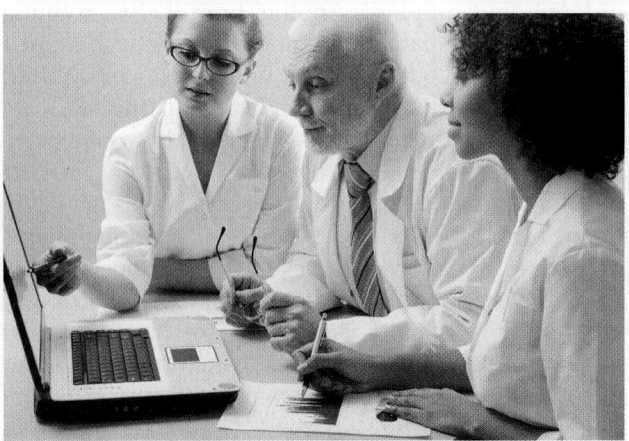

Fig. 1.9 Nurse collaborating with other members of the interdisciplinary team. (Copyright 1999–2012 Thinkstock. All rights reserved.)

Care Plan

The care plan is a document that outlines the individual needs of the patient and the approach of the health care team to meet these needs. It is developed in cooperation with the patient and, in some cases, the patient's family. It further identifies who will assist in treating the patient. The plan of care is a "living document" that is updated as the patient's condition warrants. The goal of the document is to guide and direct the activities surrounding the patient's care, ensure continuity and consistency of care, and eliminate duplication of services. (See Chapter 5 for further discussion of use of the nursing care plan in the nursing process.)

Communication

Good communication is essential for the exchange of information among the members of the health care team. Communication is the prerequisite for meeting the needs of the patient or, if necessary, making appropriate changes to do so. (See Chapter 4 for further discussion of communication.)

Documentation

Documentation in any form is the permanent record of the patient's progress and treatment. It constitutes the formal and legal record of care received by the patient and the patient's response to that care (Fig. 1.10). The information recorded during the entire course of treatment serves many purposes. It provides a progress record of treatment so that all the involved health care members are aware of what treatment the patient is receiving. It also provides a chronicle of events, which becomes a valued piece of the patient's health history that may be referenced for future health care needs. (See Chapter 3 for further discussion of documentation.)

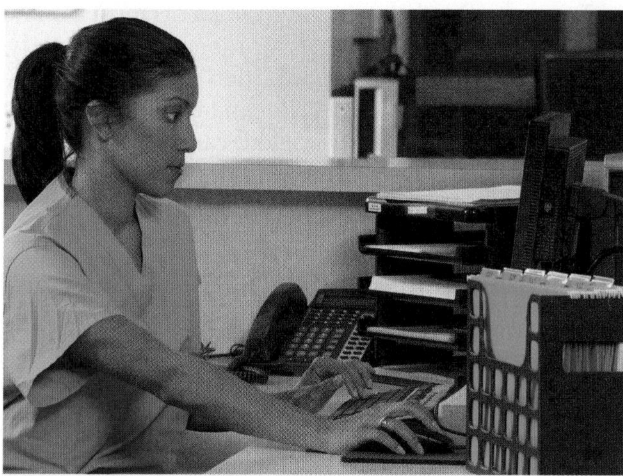

Fig. 1.10 Nurse documenting patient care at a computer. (Copyright 1999–2012 Thinkstock. All rights reserved.)

NURSING CARE MODELS

Since the time of Florence Nightingale, nursing and health care technology have continued to change to meet the needs of the patient. Initially, nursing education was like an apprenticeship. Experienced nurses demonstrated skills, and the student nurse practiced these skills until technical competence was achieved. Little emphasis was placed on development of a knowledge base to enable the nurse to solve future problems or to adapt the skills learned to various complex situations. Through research, nursing theorists have developed several models to assist with problem solving and organization of care. Many schools of nursing loosely base their curriculum or philosophy on a specific nursing model to help their students learn about and understand the nursing process (see Chapter 5).

As early as the 1970s, nursing leaders identified the following four major concepts that were the basis for all nursing models of care:

- *Nursing:* Encompasses the roles and actions of the nurse
- **Patient:** The individual who receives the care
- **Health:** The area along the wellness-illness continuum that the patient occupies
- *Environment:* The setting for the nurse-patient interaction

Several leading nurse theorists have developed nursing models of care, and their work is ongoing. Table 1.2 shows six leading nursing theories that incorporate those basic concepts.

CONTEMPORARY PRACTICAL AND VOCATIONAL NURSING CARE

As stated earlier, the existence of the LPN/LVN in the health care delivery system is not new. What is new is the expansion of the LPN/LVN's role and responsibilities from bathing patients and doing light housekeeping to performing skilled tasks needed to provide health care to people along the wellness-illness continuum.

The ongoing evolution of the role is influenced by various state nurse practice acts, individual changes within the health care agencies, the availability of health care workers, and the needs of patients. LPN/LVNs are finding careers in hospitals, clinics, outpatient agencies, home health agencies, long-term care facilities, insurance companies, physician offices, and the military services.

PRACTICAL AND VOCATIONAL NURSING DEFINED

Practical and vocational nursing is defined as the activity of providing specific services to patients under the direct supervision of a registered nurse or licensed physician.

Table 1.2 Leading Theories

THEORIST	NURSING OBJECTIVE	SETTING
Nightingale (1860)	To facilitate "the body's reparative processes" by arranging the patient's environment.	Patient's environment is arranged; includes appropriate noise control, nutrition, hygiene, lighting, comfort, socialization, and hope.
Orem (1971)	To care for and help patient attain total self-care.	This is self-care deficit theory. Nursing care becomes necessary when patient is unable to fulfill biologic, psychological, developmental, or social needs.
Leininger (1978)	To provide care consistent with nursing's emerging science and knowledge, with caring as the central focus.	In this transcultural care theory, caring is the central and unifying domain for nursing knowledge and practice.
Roy (1979)	To identify types of demands placed on patient, assess adaptation to demands, and help patients adapt.	This adaptation model is based on the physiologic, psychological, sociologic, and dependence-independence adaptive modes.
Parse (1981)	To focus on humans as unitary living beings and humanity's qualitative participation with the health experience (nursing as science and art).	Humans continually interact with environment and participate in maintenance of health. Health is a continual open process rather than a state of well-being or absence of disease.
Benner and Wrubel (1989)	To focus on patient's needs for caring as a means of coping with stressors of illness.	Caring is central to the essence of nursing. Caring creates the possibilities for coping and enables possibilities for connecting with and concern for others.

The services are provided in a structured setting surrounding the caring for the sick, the rehabilitation of the sick and injured, and the prevention of sickness and injury.

The nurse has a unique function: to assist individuals, sick or well, in the performance of those activities that contribute to health, to their recovery, or to a peaceful death—activities that patients would perform unaided if they had the necessary strength, will, or knowledge—and, if feasible, to do this in such a way as to help patients gain independence as rapidly as possible. The practical or vocational nurse is educated to be a responsible member of a health care team, performing basic therapeutic, rehabilitative, and preventive care to assigned patients. Currently, there are slightly fewer than 700,000 LPN/LVNs working in the United States (Bureau of Labor Statistics, 2016).

The practice of discharging patients from acute care facilities for continued recuperation in extended care units and nursing homes, places of employment for LPN/LVNs, is evident in the increasing number of patients who need more complex care. Every 3 years, the National Council of State Boards of Nursing performs a job analysis. This analysis helps to determine the content areas for the NCLEX-PN. The findings of the latest job analysis indicate that newly licensed LPN/LVNs are continuing to provide care in all types of settings, with the majority continuing to be employed in long-term care settings. No statistically significant changes have occurred in work settings since the last job analysis.

OBJECTIVES AND CHARACTERISTICS OF PRACTICAL AND VOCATIONAL NURSING EDUCATION

The objectives for practical and vocational nursing education are the following:

- To acquire the specialized knowledge and skills needed to meet the health care needs of patients in a variety of settings
- To be a graduate of a state-approved practical or vocational nursing program
- To take and pass the NCLEX-PN examination
- To acquire a state license to practice

To accomplish these objectives, students must assume responsibility for their own education, intensive study, and dedication to duty. Organization of time effectively helps accomplish these objectives and ultimately ensures the patient of safe and competent care.

Distinguishing characteristics, roles, and responsibilities for the LPN/LVN are shown in Box 1.3.

ROLES AND RESPONSIBILITIES

NAPNES (2007) issued the following statement of responsibilities required for practice as an LPN/LVN:

- Demonstrate professional behaviors of accountability and professionalism according to the legal and ethical standards for a competent licensed practical/vocational nurse.
- Effectively communicate with patients, significant support person(s), and members of the interdisciplinary

Box 1.3 Characteristics, Roles, and Responsibilities of the Practical or Vocational Nurse

- Is a responsible and accountable member of the health care team
- Maintains a current license
- Practices within the scope of the state's nurse practice act
- Practices under the supervision of the registered nurse, or physician
- Supervises other practical and vocational nurses and unlicensed assistive personnel
- Participates in continuing education activities
- Uses the nursing process to meet patients' needs
- Promotes and maintains health, prevents disease, and encourages and assists in rehabilitation
- Maintains a professional appearance
- Subscribes to recognized ethical practices
- Participates in activities of professional organizations
- Assists in developing the role of the licensed practical nurse and licensed vocational nurse of tomorrow

health care team incorporating interpersonal and therapeutic communication skills.

- Collect holistic assessment data from multiple sources, communicate the data to appropriate health care providers, and evaluate patient responses to interventions.
- Collaborate with the registered nurse or other members of the health care team to organize and incorporate assessment data to plan/revise patient care and actions based on established nursing diagnoses, nursing protocols, and assessment and evaluation data.
- Demonstrate a caring and empathic approach to the safe, therapeutic, and individualized care of each patient.
- Implement patient care, at the direction of a registered nurse, licensed physician or dentist through performance of nursing interventions or directing aspects of care, as appropriate, to UAP.

LPN/LVNs are required to be aware of the content of the nurse practice act of the state in which they are employed. The role of the LPN/LVN is found in this law, and the law differs from state to state.

A major criterion in differentiating between the roles of the RN and the LPN/LVN is the level of independence for the practice activities. The LPN/LVN never functions independently. LPN/LVNs provide care in basic and complex situations under the general supervision of an RN or physician. They are responsible for functioning safely and are accountable for their actions.

LPN/LVNs function interdependently when they offer input to the RN about the effectiveness of care or offer suggestions to improve the patient's care. Because LPN/LVNs provide actual care at the bedside in acute care situations, the data collected during the giving of care are valuable in determining whether progress is being made toward meeting patient goals.

Practical and vocational nursing is an exciting, challenging career that provides an opportunity to care for others while receiving personal satisfaction. The focus is on bedside and personal care of patients in a variety of settings. Performance in a responsible and accountable manner calls for knowledge, skill, and expertise.

Get Ready for the NCLEX® Examination!

Key Points

- The evolution of nursing was influenced greatly by the way care was given to the sick and injured.
- The influence of Florence Nightingale on nursing practice and nursing education was highly significant in the 19th century.
- Nursing practice and education in the United States were influenced significantly by the activities of Florence Nightingale.
- The Association of Practical Nurse Schools was organized in Chicago in 1941 to address the needs of practical nursing education. Its name was changed in 1942 to the National Association of Practical Nurse Education (NAPNE).
- NAPNE changed its name again in 1959 to the National Association for Practical Nurse Education and Service (NAPNES).
- In 1949 the National Federation of Licensed Practical Nurses (NFLPN) was founded by Lillian Kuster.
- Mandatory licensure laws were established for practical and vocational nursing education and practice.
- The wellness-illness continuum is a range that comprises the entirety of a person's health.
- Prevention of illness and injury and continuity of patient care are integral components of holistic health care.
- The practical or vocational nurse is one of many of the large groups of health care workers who provide health care services.
- The practical and vocational nursing community functions in accordance with several states' nurse practice acts.
- Roles and responsibilities of the nurse are varied and complex and evolve with new technologies and research advances.
- Ongoing education is valued, expected, and required for continued licensure.

Additional Learning Resources

SG Go to your Study Guide for additional learning activities to help you master this chapter content.

evolve Be sure to visit the Evolve site at *http://evolve.elsevier.com/Cooper/foundationsadult/* for additional online resources.

Review Questions for the NCLEX® Examination

1. A prospective nursing student questions what program accreditation means. What should be included in the information provided?
   1. Accreditation is a voluntary review by a given organization to determine whether the program meets that organization's preestablished criteria.
   2. An accredited program is one that meets the minimal standards set by the respective state agencies responsible for overseeing educational programs.
   3. Program accreditation is necessary before the graduate is eligible to take the National Council Licensing Examination for Practical Nursing (NCLEX-PN).
   4. Nursing program accreditation is a federally funded health care program that educates practical nurse students.
2. The nursing student is discussing the impact of preventative medicine. Which change has resulted from this focus?
   1. Anxiety over diagnostic workups such as colonoscopies or gynecologic examinations
   2. The number of admissions for inpatient services
   3. The length of a hospitalization stay
   4. Knowledge and services to promote health and prevent illness (wellness-illness continuum)
3. Growth and advancement of the nursing profession in the 21st century can be attributed to:
   1. growth of cities.
   2. better education of nurses.
   3. teachings of Christianity.
   4. improved conditions for women.
4. Nursing education programs may seek voluntary accreditation by which agency?
   1. American Nurses Association
   2. International Council of Nurses
   3. Congress for Nursing Practice
   4. National League for Nursing
5. When developing a definition of "health," a person should consider that health is:
   1. a condition of physical, mental, and social well-being and absence of disease.
   2. the ability to pursue activities of daily living.
   3. a function of the physiologic state.
   4. a static condition; the absence of pathology.
6. Which philosophy is described as comprehensive or total patient care that considers the physical, emotional, social, economic, and spiritual needs of the person; the person's response to the illness; and the impact of the illness on the person's ability to meet self-care needs?
   1. The wellness-illness continuum
   2. The Patient Care Partnership
   3. Holistic nursing
   4. The health care delivery system
7. The student nurse reviewing the history of nursing knows that the "Lady with the Lamp" is:
   1. Clara Barton.
   2. Florence Nightingale.
   3. Phoebe.
   4. Lavinia Dock.
8. The American Society of Superintendents of Training Schools of Nursing was established in 1894. What was the major goal of the organization?
   1. To promote development of new schools of nursing
   2. To train nursing leaders
   3. To set educational standards for nurses
   4. To develop standards for licensure
9. Nurses correctly recognize what as the key determinant of their scope of practice?
   1. The nursing process
   2. The agency's policies
   3. The Hippocratic Oath
   4. The nurse practice act
10. Nursing theorists are helpful in enabling the nursing profession to problem solve and establish standards. Who is largely recognized as the first nursing theorist?
    1. Phoebe
    2. Clara Barton
    3. Florence Nightingale
    4. Sister Calista Roy
11. The most commonly used model that assists in the understanding of the patient's place on the wellness-illness continuum is that of:
    1. Abraham Maslow.
    2. Dorothea Dix.
    3. Clara Barton.
    4. Theodore Fliedner.
12. Which person was the first nurse to train in America?
    1. Lavinia Dock
    2. Linda Richards
    3. Clara Barton
    4. Mary Breckenridge
13. Which was the first school dedicated to the training of the practical nurse in the United States?
    1. The Ballard School
    2. The Young Women's Christian Association (YWCA)
    3. The Thompson Practical Nursing School
    4. The Shepard-Gill School
14. What is health?
    1. The absence of illness
    2. A state of complete physical, mental, and social well-being
    3. A condition between disease and good health
    4. The opposite of disease
15. Which statement about men in nursing is the most correct description?
    1. Men were not permitted to serve in the military.
    2. The prominence of men in nursing increased during the Civil War.
    3. The number of men in the profession is decreasing.
    4. Men are regaining their historical position in the profession as nurses.

16. The nurse is reviewing the planned health promotion activities for a local community center. Which primary prevention activities may be included? *(Select all that apply.)*
1. Screening for complications of diabetes
2. Dietary teaching focused on prevention of obesity
3. Support group development for the victims of partner violence
4. Weight loss programs for patients with diabetes
5. Exercise programs for teens

17. Which factors affect male students' success in nursing programs? *(Select all that apply.)*
1. Men have more difficulty studying for examinations.
2. Men may feel isolated in the nursing program.
3. Many men have difficulty showing their feelings of care and empathy.
4. There are limited role models for men in nursing.
5. Instructor attitudes may not embrace male students.

2 Legal and Ethical Aspects of Nursing

http://evolve.elsevier.com/Cooper/foundationsadult/

Objectives

1. Summarize the structure and function of the legal system.
2. Compare and contrast nursing negligence and malpractice.
3. Discuss the legal relationship that exists between the nurse and the patient.
4. Explain the importance of maintaining standards of care.
5. Give examples of ways the nursing profession is regulated.
6. Give examples of legal issues in health care.
7. Discuss federal regulations of the Health Insurance Portability and Accountability Act of 1996 (HIPAA) privacy rule and its impact on the health care system.
8. Give examples of ways the licensed practical/vocational nurse can avoid being involved in a lawsuit.
9. Differentiate between a legal duty and an ethical duty.
10. Explain advance directives.
11. Summarize how culture affects an individual's beliefs, morals, and values.
12. Identify how values affect decision making.
13. Distinguish between ethical and unethical behavior.
14. Explain the meaning of a code of ethics.
15. Explain the nurse's role in reporting unethical behavior.
16. Give examples of ethical issues common in health care.

Key Terms

accountability (ăk-kŏwnt-ă-BĬL-ĕ-tē, p. 25)
advocate (ĂD-vō-kăt, p. 25)
deposition (dĕ-pō-SĬ-shŭn, p. 24)
doctrine of informed consent (p. 27)
ethical dilemmas (ĔTH-ĭ-kăl, p. 35)
ethics (ĔTH-ĭks, p. 33)
euthanasia (ūth-ĕn-Ā-zhă, p. 31)
laws (p. 23)
liability (lī-ă-BĬL-ĕ-tē, p. 25)
liable (LĪ-ă-bl, p. 24)
malpractice (p. 24)
nonmaleficence (nŏn-mă-LĔF-ĭ-sĕns, p. 36)
standards of care (p. 26)
value clarification (p. 35)
values (p. 34)
verdict (p. 24)

Today's health care system is dynamic and complex. It has undergone significant changes over the decades. Health care providers are guided by established laws, rules, regulations, and ethical principles. The rising cost of health care and growing consumer awareness have had an impact on the practice of nursing and the distribution and use of available health care resources. Additional challenges are presented by the rapid advances in technology and communication. Practice opportunities and settings for the licensed practical/vocational nurse (LPN/LVN) are changing with the focus on managed care, community health, and home health care.

Nursing practice of the LPN/LVN is guided by a combination of legal principles, established laws, moral standards, and ethical principles. Nurses must understand the legal standards and ethical principles that affect practice. Each state has laws that govern the scope and practice of nursing that are referred to as nurse practice acts. The law sets an obligatory minimum standard in any given situation. Ethical principles, which evolve out of society and culture, frequently impose an even higher duty. These legal standards and ethical principles serve as a support for all members of the health care system and help protect the rights of all members of society.

LEGAL ASPECTS OF NURSING

The legal relationship that exists between the nurse, patient, and family is influenced by the existing laws, rules, and regulations that govern nursing practice. Acting outside the established scope of practice or failing to meet the established standard of care has the potential to result in injury to the patient and give rise to legal liability and the potential loss or sanction of the nursing license. Nurses must be aware of their scope of nursing practice and the standards of care that constitute professional duties.

Many legal issues are related to health care, and health care–related litigation that involves nurses is common. Today's patients are more educated, are more aware of their rights, and have higher expectations regarding the care they receive than patients from previous generations. To practice safely, the nurse must have a familiarity with common legal issues in nursing. Reviews of nursing errors often find a series of preventable failures in performance.

OVERVIEW OF THE LEGAL SYSTEM

The legal system is a complex set of rules and regulations that has developed in response to the needs of society. **Laws** prescribe proper behavior in society; they sanction acceptable behavior and prohibit unacceptable behavior. Nurses must have a basic understanding of the legal system, which mandates and protects. The law assigns fundamental legal duties and provides protection for all members of the health care system.

The two primary categories of law are criminal and civil (Box 2.1). Matters related to criminal law are those that involve the needs of the public. Cases that concern matters of criminal law are charged by agents that represent either the federal or the state government. Civil cases are between individuals. The charges involved in a civil matter are brought by an individual or agency. Some degree of overlap may exist with the cases. For example, a criminal matter may result in individuals filing a civil lawsuit. The penalties that result from the cases also differ. Criminal cases are resolved with a finding of guilt or innocence. The penalty may involve fines, incarceration, or a combination of the two. Civil matters conclude with a determination of accountability or innocence. Monetary settlements are assigned based on the type of liability assessed. Civil law and criminal law are established in one of two ways: (1) federal, state, and local governments develop *statutory law;* and (2) *common law,* or case law, evolves in response to specific legal questions that come before the court and usually follows *precedent* (previous rulings on an issue).

Box 2.1 Characteristics of Criminal and Civil Law

CRIMINAL

- Conduct at issue is offensive to society *in general.*
- Conduct at issue is detrimental to society *as a whole.*
- The law involves *public* offenses (such as robbery, murder, assault).
- The law's purpose is to *punish* for the crime and deter and *prevent* further crimes.

CIVIL

- Conduct at issue violates a *person's* rights.
- Conduct at issue is detrimental to that *individual.*
- The law involves an offense that is against an *individual.*
- The law's purpose is to *make the aggrieved person whole again,* to restore the person to where he or she was.

Negligence

The terms negligence and malpractice often are used interchangeably. However, this is incorrect. There are distinct differences between them. *Negligence* refers to the absence of due care. It is more of a general action that often can be attributed to being careless. Nurses and unlicensed assistive personnel may be charged with negligence. Professional-level accountability and judgment are not required elements to establish negligence. Negligence refers to the failure to act in a manner demonstrating the care and knowledge any prudent individual would. Examples of negligence may include medication errors, patient falls, use of restraints, and equipment injuries (Motacki and Burke, 2011). An example of negligence can be found in Box 2.2.

Box 2.2 *Busta v Columbus Hospital Corporation* (1996)

While he was a postoperative patient at Columbus Hospital in Great Falls, Mr. Busta died from injuries sustained in a fall from his third-floor window; apparently, he had tried to climb down on an improvised rope. At trial, the nurse assigned to care for Mr. Busta testified that during her last evening visit with him, he had experienced an episode of tachycardia and hypertension. He had also behaved atypically, desiring isolation and refusing all nursing care and his prescribed medication, known to have adverse effects, including confusion, anxiety, and psychosis. The nurse did not report the symptoms and the change in behavior to the physician. She also testified that when she observed the patient at midnight, he appeared to be sleeping; she did not reassess his vital signs.

Mr. Busta's surgeon testified that, because of the mind-altering adverse effects of the patient's medication, he would have reassessed his patient if he had been notified of the changing signs and symptoms. Expert testimony opined that the nurse was negligent in failing to adequately monitor Mr. Busta on the evening and night before he died and in failing to report the constellation of signs and symptoms to the surgeon and that the hospital was negligent in failing to maintain a safe environment (evidence presented at trial showed that the hospital had not acted on a directive from The Joint Commission [TJC] to restrict the opening of windows in patients' rooms).

The jury found that the negligence of Columbus Hospital combined with the patient's contributory negligence caused the patient's injuries and death; the jury apportioned 70% of the liability to the hospital and 30% to Mr. Busta. The jury found that Mr. Busta and his estate were damaged in the amount of $5000 and his heirs $800,000. On the basis of the jury's apportioned liability, the district court entered a judgment in favor of Mr. Busta's estate in the amount of $3500 and in favor of his heirs $560,000.

From Croke E: Nurses, negligence and malpractice. *Am J Nurs* 103(9):59–60, 2003.

Malpractice

Malpractice refers to professional negligence. Nursing responsibilities include actions taken and those omitted. The concept of malpractice must contain four key elements. Each of the elements must be present for liability to be established.

1. *Duty* refers the established relationship between the patient and the nurse.
2. *Breach* of duty is failure to perform the duty in a reasonable, prudent manner.
3. *Harm* has occurred; this does not have to be physical injury.
4. The breach of duty was the *proximate cause* of the harm; the occurrence of harm depended directly on the occurrence of the breach.

If the court finds that malpractice has occurred, the nurse is subject to legal punishment or restitution as the court determines. The best way to avoid being charged with malpractice is to practice within the rules and regulations, the standards of care, and the employing agency's policies and procedures. The nurse-patient relationship is also very important; strive to maintain a positive relationship. A poor nurse-patient relationship has been identified as a leading factor in whether a patient seeks legal action.

There are four options for establishing the levels of responsibility. The individual may be personally responsible for the act of negligence or malpractice committed. A manager or supervisor may be implicated if there was inappropriate supervision or delegation by another member of the health care team. The employer may be found responsible for the employee's actions if there are deficits in education or inappropriate credentials for the role. The employer is also responsible for ensuring the staff members have the needed supplies and equipment (Missouri Department of Health & Human Services, n.d.).

OVERVIEW OF THE LEGAL PROCESS

Civil litigation involves the legal exchange between individuals as opposed to legal concerns that involve a criminal matter, which would involve the state or federal government bringing charges. Most legal suits in health care involve civil litigation. The process for filing a claim begins when an individual believes that a breach of duty has taken place and resulted in pain, suffering, or injury. At that time, the plaintiff (the complaining party) typically seeks legal representation. In some states, a prelitigation panel may meet to ascertain the validity of the suit being proposed. If this process results in a finding that litigation in this case has a legal basis, the plaintiff writes a statement called a *complaint* and files it in the appropriate court. The complaint names the *defendant* (the person alleged to be **liable** [legally responsible]), states the facts involved in the case, defines the legal issues the case raises, and outlines the *damages* (compensation that the plaintiff is seeking). The defendant (the person accused of the crime) is served a *summons* (a court order that notifies the defendant of the legal action), which constitutes the necessary legal notice, and the defendant usually hires an attorney to represent him or her in the lawsuit. The defendant is asked to provide a response to the charges. This response is either an admission of guilt or a denial of allegations listed in the complaint.

Discovery is the next step in the process. Discovery allows both sides of the case to review documents and interview witnesses. The witnesses may be the defendant being named in the suit or individuals who have facts about the case. Witnesses are required to undergo questioning by the attorneys. This process is referred to as the **deposition**. Witnesses are under oath. The statements made are recorded. This transcript becomes a part of the evidence.

Other tools also serve the process of discovery. The *interrogatory* is a written question that one party sends to the other party, to which an answer is legally required. A *Request for Production of Documents and Things* is a formal request by the agents filing the charges for all items that are deemed to be related to the case at hand. In a health care–related case, these items may include policies and procedures, standards of care, medical records, assignment sheets, personnel files, equipment maintenance records, birth certificates, marriage certificates, medical bills, and other documents pertinent to the issues at hand. A fourth discovery technique is the admission of facts. This tool requests the party to admit or deny certain statements to streamline the factual presentation of the case.

Once the evidence has been presented, the court renders a **verdict** (decision) based on the facts of the case, the evidence and testimony presented, the credibility of the witnesses, and the laws that pertain to the issue. Either party has the right, in case of disagreement with the outcome of the lawsuit, to file an *appeal* (request a review of the decision) asking that a higher court review the decision. The outcome of litigation is never certain.

In a criminal trial, the question is whether the defendant is answerable for a crime against the people (because criminal law concerns crimes against society rather than individuals). At trial, the people's attorney and the defendant's attorney present their cases. The judge or the jury (if a jury trial) then *deliberate* (consider and decide) the guilt or innocence of the defendant. If the judge or jury reaches a verdict of *not guilty*, the defendant is cleared of the charges. If the verdict is *guilty*, the judge passes a *sentence* (penalty) based on the severity of the crime, the defendant's past criminal record, and applicable laws. The defendant who receives a guilty verdict may appeal if there has been an error either: (1) in the process in which the conviction was obtained or (2) by the court during the proceedings. Box 2.3 presents some common legal terminology.

Box 2.3 Common Legal Terminology

Term	Definition
Abandonment of care	Wrongful termination of providing patient care
Assault	An intentional threat to cause bodily harm to another; does not have to include actual bodily contact
Battery	Unlawful touching of another person without informed consent
Competency	A legal presumption that a person who has reached the age of majority can make decisions for herself or himself unless proved otherwise (if she or he has been legally declared incompetent)
Defamation	Spoken or written statements made maliciously and intentionally that may injure the subject's reputation
Harm	Injury to a person or the person's property that gives rise to a basis for a legal action against the person who caused the damage
Libel	A malicious or untrue writing about another person that is brought to the attention of others
Malpractice	Failure to meet a legal duty, thus causing harm to another
Negligence	The commission (doing) of an act or the omission (not doing) of an act that a reasonably prudent person would have performed in a similar situation, thus causing harm to another person
Slander	Malicious or untrue spoken words about another person that are brought to the attention of others
Tort	A type of civil law that involves wrongs against a person or property; torts include negligence, assault, battery, defamation, fraud, false imprisonment, and invasion of privacy

LEGAL RELATIONSHIPS

Legal liability for alleged harm may be held solely or shared between multiple parties. The patient or family may choose to pursue charges against the facility, nursing personnel, medical staff, or ancillary departments. Each may be charged separately or in a group. In the past, nurses did not hold legal liability for alleged harm suffered by a patient while receiving medical care, but the physician and/or the hospital did. As nurses gained recognition for their expertise and gained more autonomy, dissatisfied patients (and their attorneys) began to look at nurses as potential defendants and to seek to hold nurses accountable under the law. **Accountability** (being responsible for one's own actions) is a concept that gives rise to a legal duty, and thus **liability** (legal responsibility), in nursing.

Indeed, the nurse is not immune from liability in the practice of nursing. An analysis of statistics shows sharp increases in the amount of litigation against nurses by patients. A variety of reasons explain the increases (Boxes 2.4 and 2.5). Nurses are facing increased responsibilities in the health care arena. Technological advances require more knowledge and competence. Staffing shortages and budgetary constraints also may play a role. High levels of patient acuity and an emphasis on early discharge may result in the need for more comprehensive referrals and improved discharge teaching. Flaws in either may result in litigation. Finally, insurance experts believe that some responsibility may rest with the large payout to litigants. Legal findings against nurses can be categorized. The most common areas of litigation against nurses involve performance failures in the following areas: standards of care, use of equipment, documentation, and patient advocacy (Reising and Allen, 2007).

When a nurse accepts a patient care assignment, the nurse-patient relationship is initiated. This relationship, beyond its more personal human component, has a legal basis: the duty to provide professional care. A failure to provide care to the expected level of expertise gives rise to legal liability (see the discussion on standards of care in the next section). In the nurse-patient relationship, the nurse accepts the role of advocate for the patient. An **advocate** is one who defends or pleads a cause or issue on behalf of another. A nurse advocate has a legal and ethical obligation to safeguard the patient's interests.

Box 2.4 Preventable Omissions in Nursing

Nursing errors can be tied to seven largely preventable omissions. These involve failures to:

1. Collaborate with other health care team members
2. Clarify interdisciplinary orders
3. Ask for and offer assistance
4. Utilize evidence-based performance
5. Communicate information to patients and families
6. Limit overtime
7. Adequately staff patient care units with appropriately credentialed staff

Source: Nursing Made Incredibly Easy. How to avoid the top seven nursing errors. Deamont, Ann MSN, RN, VHA-CM. March/April 2013 Volume 11, Issue 2, pages 8–10. Retrieved from *http://journals.lww.com/nursingmadeincrediblyeasy/Fulltext/2013/03000/How_to_avoid_the_top_seven_nursing_errors.4.aspxhttp://journals.lww.com/nursingmadeincrediblyeasy/Fulltext/2013/03000/How_to_avoid_the_top_seven_nursing_errors.4.aspx.*

A landmark case that addressed nursing liability was *Darling v Charleston Community Memorial Hospital.* In this case, an 18-year-old man fractured his leg and had a cast applied in the hospital. He was admitted to a room, and the nurses caring for the patient noticed that the toes on his casted leg were edematous and discolored. The patient reported decreased feeling in his toes to the nursing staff. Over the next few days, gangrene developed, and the man's leg had to be amputated. The Illinois Supreme Court heard the case and held that the nurses were liable, along with the physician, because the nursing staff had failed to adhere to the

Box 2.5 Common Breaches of the Standard of Care

PRACTICE

Failure to:

- Use proper judgment
- Properly assess
- Properly administer medication
- Protect patients from burns
- Properly maintain the airway
- Restock crash cart
- Honor advance directives
- Take an accurate and thorough history
- Provide a safe environment
- Properly administer injections
- Go through hierarchy to get the care needed
- Detect that the patient has an allergy
- Protect the patient from abuse
- Prevent abuse, neglect, or injury by other patients
- Obtain physician orders—practicing outside the scope of nursing practice by writing orders
- Practice safely (by using drugs or alcohol while working)
- Protect and prevent falls

MONITORING

- Properly monitor
- Recognize and report signs and symptoms of patient's deteriorating condition
- Properly use monitoring equipment
- Protect against injuries from monitoring equipment
- Detect or prevent decubitus ulcers
- Monitor and detect polypharmacy effects on patient
- Detect signs and symptoms of a medical condition in a timely and proper fashion
- Detect signs and symptoms of drug toxicity
- Properly use restraints

COMMUNICATION

- Document in a timely and proper fashion
- Notify physician of laboratory values in a timely and proper fashion
- Report child or elder abuse
- Notify physician of a change in status
- Communicate with other health care personnel about advance directives
- Properly give discharge instructions
- Document patient's status or condition in a timely and proper fashion
- Document communications between health care providers in a timely and proper fashion
- Document the need for restraints in a timely and proper fashion
- Properly to properly document (precharting)

standards of care. This case established a precedent that almost every state has adopted.

REGULATION OF PRACTICE

Standards of care define acts whose performance is required, permitted, or prohibited. These standards of care derive from federal and state laws, rules, and regulations and codes that govern other professional agencies and organizations such as the American Nurses Association (ANA) and the Canadian Nurses Association (CNA). These organizations regularly evaluate existing standards and revise them as needed. Standards of care coupled with the *scope of nursing practice* give direction to the practicing nurse. They define the obligations of the nurse, including those activities that are obligatory and those that are prohibited. Failure to adhere to these standards gives rise to legal liability. Ignorance of the requirements and limitations does not absolve liability.

Nursing liability falls into several areas: practice, monitoring, and communication. Box 2.5 shows common breaches of the standards of care. The legal test is the comparison with the hypothetical actions under similar circumstances of a reasonably *prudent* (careful, wise) nurse of similar education and experience. The standards of care follow those laws of the individual state. In reality, application of the standards is not always easy. Nursing shortages in some states have led to a need for individual nurses to take on increased responsibilities and work more hours. Personnel cutbacks often leave units short staffed, and nurses feel pressure to take on expanded duties; this increases their risk for liability considerably. In addition, special challenges face entry-level licensed nurses when they enter the workforce. Orientation programs often fail to adequately cover all the skills needed to be a competent practitioner. It is the nurse's responsibility to seek additional instruction and supervision when faced with an unfamiliar practice or procedure. Remember that it is not possible for the nurse to meet every patient's needs.

The laws that formally define and limit the scope of nursing practice are called *nurse practice acts.* All state, provincial, and territorial legislatures in the United States and Canada have adopted nurse practice acts, although the specifics they contain often vary. It is the nurse's responsibility to know the nurse practice act that is in effect for the geographic region. A free copy of the state's nurse practice act can be obtained by writing to the board of nursing in a given state or accessing its website.

In addition to the boundaries made by the state's nurse practice act, the employing institution often places limitations on practice. The institution has the right to establish policies and procedures for nursing activities within the confines of the state's nurse practice act. When a question comes before the court regarding whether the standard of care was met in a particular situation, the court uses a variety of resources to answer the question (Box 2.6).

LEGAL ISSUES

Many legal issues affect the LPN/LVN and influence the level of care delivered to the patient. Statutory and common law play important roles in defining the rights and responsibilities of the patient and the nursing professionals. The patient has a right to expect the nurse to act in the patient's best interest by providing care

Box 2.6 Evidence of Nursing Standards

- Accreditation criteria of The Joint Commission (formerly the Joint Commission on Accreditation of Healthcare Organizations [JCAHO])
- Agency policy and procedure manuals
- American Nurses Association Code for Nurses (2001)
- American Nurses Association Standards of Practice (1995)
- Customs and usual community practices
- Education, continuing education, staff development, and orientation
- Experience
- Expert nurse witness, other experts, and peers
- Nursing literature, textbooks, and journals
- Nursing specialty standards of care and certification
- Other accreditation standards depending on the practice setting (e.g., National League for Nursing, National Association of Home Care)
- Practice protocols, contracts, practice agreements, employment agreements, and personnel or employee manuals
- State and federal licensing laws and regulations that govern health care agencies: state, professional, and occupational legislation and regulations
- State nurse practice acts and regulations

that meets and is consistent with the established legal standards and principles.

Patients' Rights

Patients have expectations regarding the health care services they receive. In 1972 the American Hospital Association (AHA) developed the Patient's Bill of Rights. Since its inception, the Patient's Bill of Rights has undergone revisions; the modified version of 2003 is called The Patient Care Partnership: Understanding Expectations, Rights, and Responsibilities (see Box 1.1). The AHA encourages health care institutions to adapt the template bill of rights to their particular environments. This involves considering the cultural, religious, linguistic, and educational backgrounds of the population the institution serves. In 1980 the Mental Health Patient's Bill of Rights and the Pregnant Patient's Bill of Rights were adopted into law. The goal of the AHA is to promote the public's understanding of their rights and responsibilities as consumers of health care. Failure of the nurse to embrace the outlined rights of the patient can promote breaches in the relationship between the nurse and the patient.

The Joint Commission is an independent accrediting agency responsible for accrediting and certifying more than 19,000 facilities in the United States. The Joint Commission has developed a brochure titled *Know Your Rights,* which is a statement on the rights and responsibilities of patients. The Patient Self-Determination Act (included in the Omnibus Budget Reconciliation Act of 1990, U.S. Code vol. 42, sec. 1395 cc[a][1]) regulates any institution that receives federal funding. The Patient Self-Determination Act requires that institutions maintain written policies and procedures regarding advance directives (including the use of life support if the patient is incapacitated), the right to accept or refuse treatment, and the right to participate fully in health care–related decisions.

The Health Insurance Portability and Accountability Act (HIPPA) was passed into legislation in 1996. In the years that followed there were modifications. Then, agencies and facilities had until 2003 to become compliant with the mandates. Health care providers who maintain and transmit health care information must provide reasonable and appropriate administrative, technical, and physical safeguards on a patient's health information. The law sets rules and limits on who has permission to look at and receive health information and assigns penalties for wrongful disclosure of individually identifiable health information. All health care providers must be knowledgeable about the HIPAA standards and protect the privacy rights of patients and residents *(www.hhs.gov/ocr/hipaa).*

Health care institutions are obligated to uphold the patient's rights to (1) access to health care without any prejudice, (2) treatment with respect and dignity at all times, (3) privacy and confidentiality, (4) personal safety, and (5) complete information about one's own condition and treatment.

Patients' responsibilities to the health care institution include (1) providing accurate information about themselves, (2) giving information regarding their known conditions, and (3) participating in decision making regarding treatment and care.

Informed Consent

The Patient Care Partnership establishes the patient's right to make decisions regarding his or her health care. The **doctrine of informed consent** refers to full disclosure of the facts the patient needs to make an intelligent (informed) decision before any invasive treatment or procedure is performed (Fig. 2.1). The patient has the right to accept or reject the proposed care but only after understanding fully what is being proposed—that is, the benefits of the treatment, the risks involved, any alternative treatments, and the consequences of refusing the treatment or procedure. The explanation of the procedure must be in nontechnical terms and in a language the patient can understand. Failure to secure informed consent may result in civil liability for battery. *Civil battery* (also called technical battery) is the unlawful touching of a person; an intent to harm is not necessary. Consent must be given freely. Coercion negates the spirit of informed consent. Patients who seek treatment sign forms to indicate acceptance of care interventions. Additional consent for treatment may be needed for further invasive actions. Patients may withdraw or limit consent at any time. Consent may be communicated in a variety of ways. Patients may imply consent by their actions. Patients may verbalize their acceptance of

AUTHORIZATION FOR AND CONSENT TO OPERATION. ADMINISTRATION OF ANESTHETICS, SPECIAL DIAGNOSTIC OR THERAPEUTIC PROCEDURES AND THE RENDERING OF OTHER MEDICAL SERVICES

Patient Jaelyn Cooper Date January 9, 2018 Time 0800

1. **Operation or Procedure and Alternatives**
   a. I hereby authorize Dr. Kelly Gosnell and whomever she may designate as her assistants to perform the following procedure and/or alternative procedure necessary to treat my condition: (state nature of procedure(s) to be performed).

   Right total hip replacement
   OK for blood transfusion
   (LIST PROCEDURE(S))

   b. I understand the reason for the procedure is: to replace my right hip joint and the head of my right hip bone. OK to receive blood transfusion

   c. For the purpose of advancing medical education and care, I consent to the admittance of observers to the operating room.
   d. It has been explained to me that conditions may arise during this procedure whereby a different procedure or an additional procedure may need to be performed and I authorize my physician and her assistants to do what they feel is needed and necessary.
   e. I understand that no guarantee or assurance has been made as to the results of the procedure and that it may not cure the condition.
   f. I consent to the examination and disposal by hospital authorities of any tissues or body parts that may be removed.
2. **Risks:** This authorization is given with the understanding that any operation or procedure involves some risks and hazards. The more common risks include: infection, bleeding, nerve injury, blood clots, heart attack, allergic reactions, and pneumonia. These risks can be serious and possibly fatal. Specific risks for this procedure and alternative methods of care have been explained to me by my physician.
3. **Anesthesia:** The administration of anesthesia also involves risks, most importantly a rare risk of reaction to medications causing severe injury or death. I consent to the use of such anesthetics as may be considered necessary by the person responsible for these services.
4. **Photography:** I consent to the photographing of operations to be performed, including appropriate portions of my body for medical, scientific, or educational purposes, providing my identity is not revealed by the pictures or by the descriptive texts accompanying them.
5. **Patient's Consent:** I have read and fully understand this consent form, and I understand I should not sign this form if all items, including all my questions, have not been explained or answered to my satisfaction or if I do not understand any of the terms or words contained in this consent form.

   IF YOU HAVE ANY QUESTIONS AS TO THE RISKS OR HAZARDS OF THE PROPOSED SURGERY OR TREATMENT, OR ANY QUESTIONS CONCERNING THE PROPOSED SURGERY OR TREATMENT ASK YOUR SURGEON NOW! **BEFORE SIGNING THIS CONSENT FORM.**

   DO NOT SIGN UNLESS YOU HAVE READ AND THOROUGHLY UNDERSTAND THIS FORM!
6. I certify that I have read and fully understand the above consent after adequate explanations were made to me, and after all blanks were filled in or crossed out before I signed.

Kim Richey
(Witness to Signature only)

Signed Jaelyn Cooper
(Patient, Parent, or Legal Guardian's Signature)

Betty Berg RN
(Second Witness Signature if needed)
(i.e., Telephone Consent)

(Doctor Signature)

AUTHORIZATION AND CONSENT

Kell-Russell Memorial Hospital
12 West Industrial Blvd.
Terre Haute, IN 47805
(800) 555-0000

NS-81 (Rev. 2/01)

LABEL

4532

Fig. 2.1 Sample consent form for a special procedure.

treatment interventions. Invasive procedures may require a written consent document to be completed.

Consent must be provided by the appropriate person. To provide consent, the patient must be at least 18 years of age. Minors under the age of 18 years may consent for treatment if they meet certain criteria, including the following:

- Marriage
- Court-approved emancipation
- Living apart from parents or guardians for at least 60 days and independent of parental support
- Service in the armed forces

In some situations, a minor may consent for care, including treatment for sexually transmitted infections, drug and alcohol abuse, sexual assault, and family planning.

There also must be competence to consent for care. Competence requires that the patient be of sound mind to accept the treatment. In addition, consent cannot be obtained from one who is impaired or under the influence of alcohol or drugs. If the patient is deemed incompetent to provide consent, a legal process exists for the determination of the individual legally eligible to provide the consent. In many cases, consent is provided by the spouse. In the absence of the spouse, this role may be passed to another legally identified individual.

It is the duty of the physician or nurse practitioner who is performing the procedure or treatment to provide the needed information to the patient. The nurse often has the responsibility to witness the patient signing the consent. In this case, the nurse's responsibility is limited to the actual witnessing of the signature, not provision of information. The nurse does not discuss with the patient the elements of disclosure that the physician or the nurse practitioner are required to make. Involvement in providing this type of information to the patient potentially places the nurse in a position of liability. Answers to any unanswered questions that the patient has about the procedure are the responsibility of the health care provider who will perform the procedure.

Certain situations may require consent for treatment to be obtained over the telephone. Health care facilities have policies that govern telephonic consent. This type of consent traditionally is needed in management of emergency procedures.

Confidentiality

Nurses have a duty to protect information about a patient regardless of how the information is kept. Information should be accessed only on a need-to-know basis. For example, on a patient care unit only those health care personnel directly involved in an individual's care should be able to access that patient's information. Failure to maintain patient confidentiality risks legal liability, and civil and criminal filings may result. Employers consider violations of confidentiality an offense that justifies termination. The responsibility of maintaining confidentiality is not limited to the work shift. All matters committed to the nurse's keeping are to be held in confidence. Securing the materials that contain confidential information is a responsibility of the nurse. These materials include not only the physical chart forms but also the technological resources as well. When accessing computerized patient files, the nurse must ensure the appropriate log-out information is entered to prevent others from viewing the records. Written notes and chart forms must be stored in restricted areas. Information that can be used to identify a patient is considered protected health information (PHI) (Box 2.7). These identifiers extend well beyond the patient's name and include admission and discharge dates; social security number; photographs; addresses and phone numbers; and date of birth. The age of patients who are 89 years of age or older also is considered an identifier and PHI. Conversations discussing patients and their personal information should be held in private conference rooms. Discussions away from the patient care areas, such as the elevator or cafeteria, are problematic and should be avoided.

Box 2.7 HIPAA Patient Identifiers

1. Names
2. Geographic locations smaller than a state—includes zip code, city, county, precinct
3. Dates—includes admission date, discharge date, date of death, and all ages over 89
4. Phone numbers
5. Fax numbers
6. Electronic mail addresses
7. Social security numbers
8. Medical record number
9. Health plan beneficiary
10. Account numbers
11. Certificate/license numbers
12. Vehicle identifiers
13. Device identifiers and serial numbers
14. URLs
15. Internet protocol (IP) addresses
16. Biometric identifiers, including fingerprints and voice prints
17. Full face photographic images
18. Any other unique identifying number, characteristic, or code

HIPAA, Health Insurance Portability and Accountability Act of 1996.
Modified from HIPAA PHI: List of 18 Identifiers and Definitions. UC Berkeley Human Research Protection Program.

Social Media

"Social media describes the online and mobile tools that people use to share opinions, information, experiences, images and video or audio clips and includes websites and applications used for social networking" (InfoNurses, 2015). The advances of social media have an impact on health care. Smartphones and handheld devices are common. Nurses have ready access to a variety of social media sites. Social media access is not

Box 2.8 Common Myths About the Use of Social Media for the Health Care Professional

1. Posted communication is private between the individual posting it and the initial intended recipient.
2. Content is deleted easily from a social media site.
3. If transmitted information is shared with a few people and the patient does not find out, it is acceptable.
4. If names are not used in posted communication, the patient's privacy is protected and violations are avoided.

without merit. The use of the Internet allows for nurses to have access to educational materials and stay abreast of advances within the profession. There is an ability to connect with other nurses and establish mentoring relationships. Social media and Internet access negate the barriers of time and location. Nurses can connect at any time with either a minimal or no cost (Stokowski, 2011).

The ready access to these sites and personal electronic devices has resulted in a serious situation. Most health care facilities have policies about the use and accessibility of smartphones and handheld devices in the care environment. Violations relating to the use of social media most often result when nurses violate or blur the boundaries between themselves and their patient (Box 2.8). Simply taking a picture or uploading information about patients, families, or the facility can be tempting. Nurses who violate social media policies established by their employers can be disciplined up to and including termination. The nursing board may choose to take sanctions against the license. Discipline can range from fines and changes in the status of the license to other sanctions.

In a case that caught national attention an established emergency department nurse photographed the scenes from the emergency trauma room while empty that was in disarray from the recent treatment of a victim who had been hit by a New York subway train. She titled the photo #Man vs 6 Train. After 7 years on the job, she was terminated. Some violations may not involve what many would consider a violation by divulging personal information but instead likely may be considered poor judgment. A nurse was terminated from her place of employment after posting on Facebook while at the same time providing patient care (Stokowski, 2011).

Social media violations are not limited to patient care delivery nor to privacy issues. Discussing the care facility in a disparaging manner can be viewed negatively by employers. Making comments about sensitive subjects such as staffing or airing concerns or opinions about management may result in a sanction by the agency.

In response to growing concerns the American Nurses Association (ANA) and National Council State Boards of Nursing (NCSBN) worked together in 2011 to release a position paper discussing social media (ANA and NCSBN, 2011). They outlined the benefits of social media and warned nurses of pitfalls that can result from inappropriate use of the forum. In addition they have posters, pamphlets, and videos available to nurses and students at *http://www.ncsbn.org/NCSBN_SocialMedia.pdf.*

Medical Records

Laws govern the collection, maintenance, and disclosure of information in medical records. Each health care institution also has policies and procedures regarding patient medical records. Medical records are not public documents, and the information they contain must be kept secure. Any breach in the confidentiality of information kept in a patient's medical record risks legal liability.

In a lawsuit, both parties are permitted to use the patient's medical record to argue facts of the case. Entries made in the chart often show whether the standards of care were met in each situation. It is essential that the employing institution's policies and procedures regarding the patient's medical record be followed. All entries in the medical record must be permanent, accurate, complete, and legible. Two current trends potentially affect patient confidentiality. Many smaller health care organizations are merging to form large corporations to save resources while continuing to provide services. Also, computer-based health care records are becoming common. Together, these two trends have the potential to increase drastically the number of people with access to confidential patient information. Those implementing these trends are required to take federal HIPAA privacy standards into consideration and prevent unauthorized disclosure of medical records and patient information.

Invasion of Privacy

The legal concept of invasion of privacy involves a person's right to be left alone and remain anonymous if he or she chooses. Consent for treatment does not waive the right to privacy. Privacy-related concerns may include the physical exposure or disclosure of patient information to others. When providing care, protect the patient from unnecessary exposure with the use of drapes and remember to close the door or use available signage to restrict admission to rooms during procedures as needed. Handle calls and inquiries concerning the patient with care. Providing information to callers can result in a breach in confidentiality. Refer calls to the charge nurse or available family members. Nurses frequently take notes during change of shift report. Monitor these notes closely during the shift. Destroy report sheets and communication tools at the end of the shift before leaving the worksite. Use of any patient information (name, photograph, specific facts regarding an illness, and so on) without authorization is a violation of the patient's legal rights. Safeguard the patient's right to privacy at all times.

Reporting Abuse

There are exceptions to the right to privacy. The law stipulates that the health care professional is required to report certain information to the appropriate authorities. The report should be given to a supervisor or directly to the police, according to agency policy. When acting in good faith to report mandated information (e.g., certain communicable diseases or gunshot wounds), the health care professional is protected from liability.

To respond to the growing problem of child abuse, the federal Child Abuse Prevention Treatment Act of 1973 made the reporting of child abuse *mandatory.* Health care professionals are mandated reporters. Failure to report suspected cases to the appropriate authorities may result in fines or imprisonment. Facilities have procedures in place to assist the nurse when making reports. Withholding medical treatment to an infant born with serious life-threatening handicaps is a form of child abuse. Congress enacted the Child Abuse Amendments in 1984 to protect the rights of these handicapped newborns to proper treatment and care. These regulations make any institution that receives federal funds legally responsible to investigate the withholding of medical treatment to an infant. In general, withholding of lifesaving treatment and care is a form of passive **euthanasia** (letting a person die) and medical neglect. This act carries the risk of professional neglect (medical malpractice) charges.

Spousal and elder abuse also may be a hidden problem within a family. Populations at increased risk include women and older adults (see the Lifespan Considerations box). Most states have responded to the issue of spousal and elder abuse by enacting laws to protect victims. Fines, restraining orders that prohibit contact by the abusing person, and even imprisonment are some of the ways often attempted to protect the victims of abuse. Abuse is an underreported crime. Only a portion of abuse cases are ever reported. It is the responsibility of the nurse to know the signs of abuse and the procedures for reporting suspected cases.

Workplace violence is another form of abuse that occurs at times in the health care setting. This form of violence includes verbal abuse, emotional abuse, sexual harassment, physical assault, and threatening behavior. Health care institutions are implementing policies and procedures to promote a safe work environment, and education is an important component of the awareness and prevention measures. Strategies to provide adequate supervision, employ security personnel, monitor work areas, and facilitate reporting of incidents represent efforts to decrease the incidence of workplace violence.

HOW TO AVOID A LAWSUIT

The best defense against a lawsuit is to provide compassionate, competent nursing care. The nurse-patient relationship should be based on trust and respect. Open and honest communication is the key to building a therapeutic relationship and often helps resolve patient dissatisfaction before the patient resorts to legal action (Fig. 2.2). Following the standards of care and the policies and procedures of the facility and adhering to the scope of practice for the LPN/LVN reduce the likelihood of lawsuit. Remaining current on practice developments and taking advantage of continuing education opportunities help to ensure competence.

Nurses may be in settings outside of the worksite in which an individual is injured and needs assistance. Concerns may result about the responsibility of the nurse and the decision to offer assistance to a victim. Nurses are not required to offer assistance when they are acting as a "private citizen." If the nurse chooses to offer help, liability may be limited under Good Samaritan laws. These statutes have been developed to provide immunity from liability in certain circumstances. The goal of this protection (except in cases of gross negligence) is to encourage assistance in emergencies that occur outside of a medical facility. State and provincial laws vary, so it is important to know the Good Samaritan laws that apply.

Proper documentation in the medical record is another important factor in assessment of liability. The medical

Lifespan Considerations

Older Adults

Elder Adults

Factors that put older adults at risk for physical, emotional, or financial abuse include the following:

- Declining physical health
- Declining mental ability
- Decreased strength and mobility
- Loss of independence
- Isolation
- Loss of loved ones, friends, and relatives

These factors often make the older adult feel helpless and frightened. Impaired communication, decreased hearing acuity, and anxiety make assessment of an older adult more difficult. Nonetheless be sure to watch for the signs of abuse.

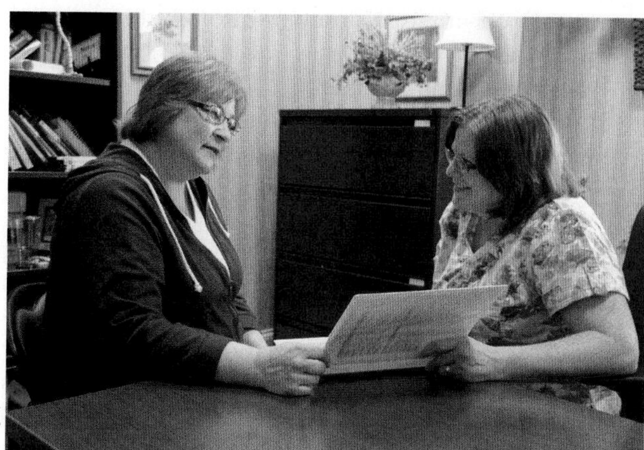

Fig. 2.2 A patient-nurse relationship built on trust and open communication is the best way to prevent a lawsuit.

record is examined thoroughly in the event of a lawsuit, and its use is permitted to demonstrate in court the level of care that was provided to the patient. An important legal presumption to remember is, "Care was not given if it was not charted." Simply stating care was provided does not provide legal protection. Omissions in charting provide a great boost to the team bringing the lawsuit.

INSURANCE

Obtaining insurance is an important part of being a professional and protecting personal assets or garnishment of wages. The determination about carrying insurance is personal, but nurses must evaluate their personal level of vulnerability when making a decision.

Professional Liability Insurance

Employers carry insurance for their facilities. This coverage provides insurance to the employees. Still, many nurses choose to purchase individual coverage. Many experts support the decision to have professional liability insurance. A careful review of policy options before purchase is important to ensure that the terms of the policy meet the needs of the individual nurse. The two types of policies are as follows:

- *Claims-made policy:* This type of policy provides protection when the claim for nursing or negligence is made while the policy is in force (during the policy period or during extended coverage).
- *Occurrence-basis policy:* This type of policy protects against claims made about events that occurred during the policy period or extended coverage period.

A *"tail" agreement* offers extended coverage for periods when a nurse is exposed to professional liabilities but no longer has a claims-made policy.

Disciplinary Defense Insurance

Disciplinary defense insurance or license protection insurance provides the following if a nurse is brought before the LPN/LVN board of nursing for disciplinary actions and problems with the license:

- A qualified nurse attorney or attorney to represent the nurse
- Wage loss reimbursement
- Travel, food, lodging reimbursement
- Legal fees paid or reimbursement for payment

DISCIPLINARY PROCESS

If a nurse receives a letter from the board of nursing alleging breaches of the standards of care or infractions of patient safety practices, it is best to seek legal representation. Every state has a variation of the disciplinary process. The process plays on various levels, such as investigation of the allegations, meeting with investigators, hearings with the board, and appeals through the court system. Licensure issues fall under administrative law (Box 2.9).

Box 2.9 Common Grounds for Licensure Proceedings

- Aiding and abetting a criminal
- Aiding and abetting someone in violating the nurse practice act
- Attempting to sell or selling, or falsely obtaining or providing, a nursing diploma or license to practice as a registered nurse
- Being convicted of a crime or offense that shows the inability of a nurse to practice without due regard for the safety and health of patients or clients
- Being found to be legally insane or mentally incompetent by the courts
- Being guilty of moral turpitude
- Committing Medicare/Medicaid fraud
- Diverting or stealing narcotics
- Documentation errors
- Entering a plea of guilty or *nolo contendere* to a criminal charge regardless of the disposition of the proceeding (e.g., expungement)
- Failure to exercise technical competence
- Failure to maintain confidentiality of patient information
- Failure to practice nursing according to the legal standards of nursing practice
- Failure to properly cooperate with the state board of nursing
- Failure to properly delegate or assign nursing care, treatment, or duties
- Failure to properly notify appropriate person when leaving or refusing an assignment
- Failure to report health care providers who are practicing in an illegal, unethical, or incompetent manner
- Failure to report previous criminal actions
- Failure to report to the state board of nursing status as a carrier of HIV or hepatitis B when participating in or performing exposure-prone procedures
- Failure to use good nursing judgment
- Falsifying information on a renewal or application
- Falsifying records
- Having a license in nursing or in another health care profession that has been revoked, suspended, probated, denied, or restricted
- Having a mental or physical impairment that interferes with nursing skills, abilities, judgment, or a combination of these
- Misappropriating patient, facility, or individual items
- Patient abuse
- Performing duties when competency has not been attained, maintained, or achieved
- Practicing outside the scope of the nurse practice act
- Practicing without a valid license
- Sexual misconduct
- Using, when on duty, alcohol, illegal drugs, or drugs that impair nursing judgment
- Violating rules or orders adopted by the state board of nursing
- Violating state or federal law relating to nursing practice
- Violating state or federal narcotics or controlled substance laws

Potential Sanctions Against a Nursing License

Any of the following may result from investigation of a claim by the state board of nursing regarding licensure issues or disciplinary actions:

- Dismissed charge
- Investigations agreement
- Letter of reprimand, formal or informal
- Probation with stipulations (e.g., education, fines, monitoring fees, worksite monitors, and evaluation by psychiatrist, psychologist, or drug addiction specialists)
- Mandated diversion program for drug-related or alcohol-related charges or mental condition
- Suspension with stipulations
- Revocation of license

ETHICAL ASPECTS OF NURSING

The science of ethics studies the relationships between moral actions and values and how these affect society. The word **ethics** refers to values that influence a person's behavior and the individual's feelings and beliefs about what is right or wrong. Nursing ethics involve moral values and principles that affect personal and professional conduct. As previously mentioned, the LPN/LVN has the responsibility to practice within the legal and ethical boundaries of nursing practice. Nursing ethics propose the duties and obligations of nurses to their patients, other health care professionals, the profession, and society.

ADVANCE DIRECTIVES

Advance directives are signed and witnessed documents that provide specific instructions for health care treatment if a person is unable to make these decisions personally at the time they are needed.

The two basic types of advance directives are living wills and durable powers of attorney for health care. Many patients have instituted one or both.

The Patient Self-Determination Act (PSDA; 1991) requires health care institutions to provide written information to patients concerning the patient's rights under state law to make decisions, including the right to refuse treatment and formulate advance directives (Levin, 1990). It is especially important to understand patients' cultural beliefs and values when explaining advance directives. Regulatory mandates to benefit the public are based on the dominant value in American society of self-determination, which may conflict with a patient's cultural heritage.

Under the act, whether the patient has signed an advance directive must be documented in the patient's record. The hospital also is required to ensure that state law is followed. The institution must provide education for the staff and the public concerning living wills and durable powers of attorney. For either type of advance directive to be enforceable, the patient must be legally incompetent or lack capacity to make decisions regarding health care treatment. The termination of legal competency is made by a judge, and the determination of decisional capacity usually is made by the physician and the family. Therefore the advance directive is implemented within the context of the health care team and the health care institution. Be familiar with the institution's policies involving the act.

A *living will* is a written document that directs treatment in accordance with a patient's wishes in the event of a terminal illness or condition (Fig. 2.3). Living wills are often difficult to interpret and are not clinically specific in unforeseen circumstances. Each state has its own requirements for executing living wills. Generally, the presence of two witnesses is required when the patient signs the document; neither may be a relative or physician. If health care workers follow the directions of the living will, they are immune from liability.

A *durable power of attorney* for health care designates an agent, surrogate, or proxy to make health care decisions on the patient's behalf based on the patient's wishes.

In addition to federal statutes, the ethical doctrine of autonomy ensures the patient the right to refuse medical treatment. This right was upheld in the *Bouvia v Superior Court* case in 1986. That case allowed the discontinuation of the patient's tube feedings per the patient's prior request. The courts also have upheld the right of a legally competent patient to refuse medical treatment based on religious beliefs. Jehovah's Witnesses, for example, accept medical treatment but refuse blood transfusions. In the absence of a truly compelling reason otherwise, the right to make such choices is protected. The US Supreme Court stated in the *Cruzan v Director, Missouri Department of Health* case in 1990, "We assume that the United States Constitution would grant a competent person a constitutionally protected right to refuse lifesaving hydration and nutrition" (Cornell University Law School, 1990). In cases that involve the patient's right to refuse or withdraw medical treatment, the courts balance the patient's interest with the state's interest in protecting life, preserving medical ethics, preventing suicide, and protecting innocent third parties. Children generally are considered innocent third parties. Although the courts do not force adults to undergo treatment that is refused for religious reasons, they do grant an order that allows hospitals and physicians to treat children of Christian Scientists or Jehovah's Witnesses who have denied consent for treatment of their minor children.

When patients are legally incompetent and are unable to make health care decisions, the court intervenes. Balancing the state's interest with that of the patient, the court attempts to deliver a judgment that represents what the patient would have chosen if competent. The Supreme Court held in the Cruzan case that states had the right to require "clear and convincing evidence" of a legally incompetent patient's prior wishes when

LIVING WILL DECLARATION OF

If I should lapse into a persistent vegetative state or have an incurable and irreversible condition that, without the administration of life-sustaining treatment, will, in the opinion of my attending physician, cause my death within a relatively short time and I am no longer able to make decisions regarding my medical treatment, I direct my attending physician, pursuant to the Rights of the Terminally Ill Act, to withhold or withdraw life-sustaining treatment that is not necessary for my comfort or to alleviate pain.

Declarant Signature

Signed this________ day of __________, 20____

Social Security Number: __________ Date of Birth: ________

Address: __________ Signature: ________

City/State: __________

The declarant voluntarily signed this writing in my presence.

Signature of witness: __________ Printed name/Date: ________

Signature of witness: __________ Printed name/Date: ________

-OR-
NOTARY

The declarant voluntarily signed this document in my presence.

STATE OF NEBRASKA)
) SS.
COUNTY OF________) Notary Public

Fig. 2.3 Example of a living will.

making determinations to discontinue life-sustaining treatment. In that case, nutrition and hydration were recognized as life-sustaining medical treatment that could be withdrawn.

Every state now requires "clear and convincing" evidence of the patient's choice, but individual states differ as to what standard satisfies the requirement. In the absence of evidence indicating the patient's prior choice, most states allow treatment to be stopped based on other factors, including the best interest of the patient balanced with the state's interest (Box 2.10).

DEVELOPMENT OF ETHICAL PRINCIPLES

Values are personal beliefs about the worth of an object, an idea, a custom, or an attitude. Values vary among people and cultures; they develop over time and undergo change in response to changing circumstances and necessity. Each individual adopts a value system that governs what is deemed right or wrong (or good and bad) and influences behaviors in a given situation.

Values influence everyday decisions. Each person has many values and at times has to choose between competing or conflicting values. Some values are more important than others, and the choices made are based on the priority placed on each value. A person's values are learned through experience, observation, and reasoning. Some values are consciously chosen; others are adopted unconsciously. Society has a strong influence on children's behaviors and values retained and learned. Acceptable behavior is rewarded, and unacceptable behavior is punished. The development of an individual value system occurs with maturity and largely reflects culture (see the Cultural Considerations box).

Cultural Considerations

Culture and Ethics

People of different cultural backgrounds often define health and illness in different ways. Culture is learned as the individual grows up and is influenced (usually subconsciously) by the surrounding environment. The nurse must be aware of cultural differences and should avoid: (1) transferring personal expectations to patients; (2) making generalizations based on personal views; (3) assuming patients can understand what is being said just because they speak English; and (4) treating each patient the same. To meet patients' needs, respect for their cultural heritage is vital.

Box 2.10 The Living Will and Durable Power of Attorney

- People who receive extraordinary measures to prolong life are often unconscious or mentally incompetent by the time these measures are put into effect. Therefore only by deciding ahead of time what kind of care you want and communicating these decisions to others can you ensure that you receive the extent of care that you want. This can be done through such documents as a living will and a medical durable power of attorney. If your state has adopted legislation for either or both documents, you should use the legally approved wording.
- Address the living will and send copies of it to your family physician, your attorney, and close family members. It specifies that if the time comes when you can no longer take part in decisions for your own future, this statement will stand as an expression of your wishes and directions while you are still of sound mind.
- You may, for example, direct that if a situation should arise in which there is no reasonable expectation of recovery from extreme physical or mental disability, you be allowed to die and not be kept alive by medications, artificial means, or "heroic measures." You may also, of course, use a living will to request such measures to keep you alive as long as possible. You may request pain-relieving medication, even though it may shorten your life. You may spell out specific provisions regarding, for example, cardiac resuscitation, mechanical respiration, antibiotics, tube feeding, and permission to offer your organs as transplants to other people.
- Some "living will" legislation applies only to terminally ill patients, not to patients who are incapacitated by illness or injury but may live many years in severe pain, who are in a coma, or who are in some other greatly disabled state. Thus it is advisable to draw up a durable power of attorney, an instrument that appoints another person (a health care surrogate) to make decisions in the event of your incompetence. Some states have enacted statutes expressly for decisions about health care, known as a "medical durable power of attorney." In these states, filling out a form is all that is required; you do not have to consult an attorney.
- Depending on the statute, the agent you appoint (someone you trust and have confidence in) may give, withdraw, or withhold consent to specific medical or surgical measures; hire and fire medical personnel; gain access to your medical records; go to court to carry out your wishes; spend or withhold funds for treatment; and interpret your living will.

REMEMBER

- Both documents must be signed and dated before two witnesses who are not blood relatives and to whom you are not leaving property.
- For the durable power of attorney, you must have your signature notarized. If you choose more than one proxy for decision making on your behalf (a good idea in case your first choice is not available), give an order of priority (1, 2, 3).
- Give a copy to your physician to keep in your medical file, and be sure that the physician agrees with your wishes.
- Give copies to close relatives, friends, or both.
- Tell these people about your intentions now.
- Look over your living will once a year. Redate it and initial the new date to make it clear that your wishes are unchanged.

Nurses must reflect on and assess their own values. **Value clarification** is the process of self-evaluation that helps gain insight into personal values. To clarify values, do the following: (1) select the belief or behavior and consciously examine it; (2) decide its value; and (3) incorporate the value into everyday responses and behaviors. These steps exercise freedom of choice and determine which values are most important. Nurses are in a unique position of having the ability to assist in value clarification as well, by encouraging the patient to express feelings and thoughts related to a situation, without contributing personal opinions. Patients need to act on their own values, not those of the nurse. Sometimes the patient may be referred to a clergy member or other professional who can help deal with ethical issues. Most health care institutions have an ethics committee to help resolve ethical questions that arise and to act as an advising body for issues encountered.

Ethical dilemmas are situations that do not have a clear right or wrong answer (Box 2.11). They are complex, confusing, and often frustrating situations that call for

Box 2.11 Ethical Dilemmas

WHAT WOULD YOU DO?

The following are scenarios with an ethical dilemma. What would you do or say in each one?

1. You see a nursing assistant stealing the patient's ring. She says she needs money to pay her house note or the bank will foreclose. What should you do?
2. The patient has a do-not-resuscitate order and a living will. He has not designated a health care proxy or representative. The patient goes into arrest, and the daughter who has not seen her dad in 10 years yells, "Do something, or I will sue you if he dies!" Whose wishes should you follow?
3. You know your friend at work is diverting drugs. You have confronted her, but she says it is not for her but for a friend. What should you do?
4. You suspect elder abuse by a family member of one of your relatives. What should you do?
5. You made a mistake, and your charge nurse tells you to just rewrite the nurse's notes to protect the unit and the hospital. What should you do?

careful rational analysis. First, the problem must be identified as an ethical one. This means that the question presented cannot be answered by applying external laws, rules, policies, and procedures. Many situations present a combination of legal and ethical questions. It is important to sort out the questions and seek guidance as needed. The next step is complete assessment of the situation, with as much information as possible gathered to aid in the decision-making process. Before a decision is finalized, any ethical principles that may apply to the situation should be considered. Ethical principles are general, but they provide a framework for decision making.

ETHICAL PRINCIPLES IN NURSING PRACTICE

Several common ethical principles are important for consideration when health care professionals are confronted with an ethical question. The first, most fundamental principle is *respect for people.* This principle leads us to view all human life as sacred, with each individual having inherent worth as a person. To the nurse, this principle means that no one person is more important than another; each patient has the same worth and always is entitled to respect. *Autonomy* is another ethical principle; it refers to freedom of personal choice, a right to be independent and make decisions freely. Frequently the patient may ask the nurse for opinions or assistance in making decisions. The nurse does not have the authority to make decisions for the patient. *Beneficence* means doing good or acting for someone's good; this principle is one of primary importance to nurses. The nurse has an ethical duty to protect life and promote the well-being of all patients. Another ethical principle is **nonmaleficence,** which means to do no harm. It is paramount to nursing practice to act in the patient's best interest and an ethical and legal duty to do nothing that has a harmful effect on the patient. Finally, there is the principle of *justice,* or the concept of what is fair. In the context of nursing, justice means that all patients have the same right to nursing interventions.

It is a great challenge to the nurse to balance these ethical principles when they seem in conflict. Rarely are options clear or black and white. Decisions often come down to choosing what seems more right and less wrong, more good and less bad.

CODES OF ETHICS

As a member of society and the health care community, nurses use personal and professional ethical principles to govern professional practice. Professional organizations have developed codes of ethics for the nursing profession that serve as a way to regulate the nurses' actions and give guidelines for ethical behavior. By helping health care practitioners become more competent, trustworthy, and accountable, such codes of ethics help safeguard society. The National Federation of Licensed Practical Nurses (NFLPN) has developed a code for LPN/LVNs. This code specifies what is expected: (1) to know and function within the scope of practice for a licensed LPN/LVN; (2) to maintain patient confidences; (3) to provide health care without discrimination; (4) to maintain a high degree of professional and personal behavior; and (5) to take an active role in the development of the LPN/LVN profession. The ANA and the CNA also have developed codes of ethics that specify the ethical duties required of the nursing professional.

REPORTING UNETHICAL BEHAVIOR

Nurses have a duty to report behavior witnessed that does not meet the established standards. Unethical behavior involves failing to perform the duties of a competent, caring nurse. Making a decision to report unethical behaviors can be stressful. When making a decision about reporting unethical behaviors, the nurse must consider key issues, including asking if the behavior or practice (NCSBN, n.d.):

- Puts the patient or facility at risk
- Demonstrates incompetence
- Involves the use of alcohol or drugs
- Is related to a physical or mental condition
- Violates a nursing statute

When reporting unethical behavior, always follow the proper chain of command and explain the facts as clearly as possible. Any documentation of the incident must be objective and accurately state what occurred, when and where it occurred, and any other pertinent facts. The state's board of nursing can provide direction to the complainant. Reporting a coworker is never an easy task. However, always remember that a nurse's first duty is to the patient's health, safety, and well-being.

ETHICAL ISSUES

Ethical issues are difficult for the nurse, as for everyone, because there is no absolutely right nor absolutely wrong answer to the question the issue presents. Like many other issues in health care, ethical issues change as society changes. Some of the current ethical issues in nursing include practitioner-assisted suicide (PAS), the right to refuse treatment, the nurse's right to refuse to provide care, and genetic research.

Practitioner-Assisted Suicide

Health care professionals and patient advocacy groups on both sides of the issue are debating the ethics of PAS. Also called physician-assisted suicide, this is a form of active euthanasia in which a health care provider takes an active role in ending a patient's life. Two cases, *Vacco v Quill* and *Washington v Glucksberg,* were brought before the US Supreme Court regarding the legality of state bans on assisted suicide. The Supreme Court ruled in 1997 that there is no constitutional right to assisted suicide. This ruling allows each state to decide whether to legalize or ban assisted suicides. The ANA has taken a firm stand on the issue of PAS: PAS is not consistent with the philosophy of nursing. ANA's specific objections to PAS are based on the principle of nonmaleficence, to do no harm, and beneficence, the duty to protect life.

In 1944 the ANA adopted a position statement concerning PAS. The ANA wrote that such an act is in violation of the *Code of Ethics for Nurses* and the ethical tradition of the profession. Nurses have an obligation to provide compassionate end-of-life care that includes providing comfort and pain relief. However, proponents of PAS cite the ethical principles of the right to autonomy and the right to self-determination in support of their position.

Right to Refuse Treatment

In the context of health care, competent adults have the right to refuse treatment. This right derives from their right to determine what is done, or not done, to them. Medicine's technical capacity to sustain life and postpone death further complicates this complex issue. It is the right of the patient to accept or refuse a treatment, even if the refusal has the potential to or is certain to result in death. To exercise the right to refuse treatment, many patients prepare advance directives. Living wills, one kind of advance directive, become effective when patients are incapacitated and are not able to make their own wishes known; these documents specify which lifesaving treatments are acceptable and which are not. Some patients choose to designate a *health care proxy* (assign durable power of attorney) to make decisions regarding medical treatment if the patient becomes unable to make them. The proxy is another person who will speak for the patient and make decisions regarding the patient's care. The proxy is obligated to act on the patient's behalf according to the patient's expressed wishes. State laws vary on the legalities of the various forms of advance directives, and nurses need to know the applicable laws in their state.

Do-Not-Resuscitate Orders

The patient usually is not involved directly at the time a *do-not-resuscitate (DNR) order* is written. Although many people make their wishes regarding DNR status known in an advance directive, at this stage the patient usually is incapacitated with little hope for recovery. The physician, after consultation with the patient's family, writes the DNR order in the medical record. The physician is responsible for following the applicable policies and procedures for writing DNR orders. When a DNR order is written in the chart, the nurse has the duty to follow the order.

Refusal to Treat

Refusal to treat is an issue that arises when a patient's care requires a nurse to do something that conflicts with his or her personal moral beliefs. A typical example of this dilemma involves assisting in or caring for a woman having an abortion. There is a legal right to abortion, but this does not establish whether abortion is morally right or wrong. If the nurse has a strong moral or religious belief regarding abortion, these concerns must be communicated with the appropriate supervisor. Do not abandon the patient; instead, ask for another assignment. Remember that the right to disqualify oneself from assisting with an abortion does not extend to the complete ability to avoid caring for the patient after the abortion. Disagreement with care decisions made by patients does not allow the nurse to refuse to care for them.

Patient diagnoses and lifestyles do not allow the nurse the legal right to refuse to care for a person. Examples include an infectious disease, such as HIV, or sexual orientation. The rationale is that the need for standard precautions (infection control measures) applies to every patient, and therefore the nurse is at no greater risk for infection from one patient than from another. The ethical principle of respect for all people without discrimination underlies this issue. The patient has the right to receive care, and the nurse has the responsibility to provide nursing interventions.

CONCLUSION

There are no easy, quick answers to legal or ethical issues. The nurse has the charge of working to manage difficult situations effectively. Today's health care system is facing many challenges, as is the profession of nursing. The health care system will continue to undergo changes in response to the enormous problem of containing health care costs while improving quality of care. The nursing profession will be called on to adjust and adapt to these changes. The legal system also is undergoing changes. Members of the legal community and the health care system have to work together to ensure that the legal and ethical rights of all individuals are considered and protected.

Get Ready for the NCLEX® Examination!

Key Points

- Laws regulate the practice of the licensed practical/vocational nurse (LPN/LVN).
- The Patient Care Partnership and other legislative directives outline what the patient can expect from the health care system.
- LPN/LVNs are legally and ethically obligated to know the scope of practice and the standards of care that apply in the state or province where they are licensed.
- Every patient has the right to receive care that meets the established standards of care.
- Malpractice (professional negligence) is when the health care professional fails to meet the standard of care.

- Prevention is the best defense to a lawsuit. A competent, caring nurse who follows the standards of care is less likely to be sued.
- Values systems have developed over the history of civilization.
- Ethical decisions regarding health care are influenced by a person's culture, beliefs, attitudes, and values.
- A code of ethics and ethical principles helps guide the practice of nursing.
- On April 14, 2003, the Health Insurance Portability and Accountability Act of 1996 (HIPAA) for regulating patient privacy standards took effect; these federal regulations have had an impact on the field of health care.

Additional Learning Resources

SG Go to your Study Guide for additional learning activities to help you master this chapter content.

evolve Be sure to visit the Evolve site at *http://evolve.elsevier.com/Cooper/foundationsadult/* for additional online resources.

Review Questions for the NCLEX® Examination

1. The newly licensed practical/vocational nurse (LPN/LVN) has reviewed the nurse practice act (NPA) of the state of licensure. What is the purpose of this documentation?
   1. Determine the quality of nursing care
   2. Enforce the standards of nursing practice
   3. Define the scope of nursing practice
   4. Set the nurse's educational requirements
2. The nurse working in a nursing home correctly recognizes that duties include patient advocacy. Which role is considered a primary duty of patient advocacy?
   1. To complete all nursing responsibilities on time
   2. To maintain the patient's right to privacy
   3. To safeguard the well-being of every patient
   4. To act as the patient's legal representative
3. The health care provider's order read "assist the patient with walking." The nurse allowed the patient to walk alone. The patient fell, fracturing the humerus. Which verdict is the most likely occurrence?
   1. The nurse will be found guilty of malpractice.
   2. The nurse will be guilty of negligence.
   3. The nurse will be charged with technical battery.
   4. The nurse will not be found liable for any harm.
4. The patient refused to take the medication his doctor ordered for relief of pain. The LPN/LVN knows this is a patient right established by:
   1. the principle of beneficence.
   2. the doctrine of negligence.
   3. specific nurse practice acts.
   4. the Patient Self-Determination Act.
5. The LPN/LVN knows that one of the best defenses against a lawsuit is for a nurse to:
   1. work only in a large hospital or nursing home.
   2. provide for every patient's needs as quickly as possible.
   3. promote a positive nurse-patient relationship.
   4. carry individual professional liability insurance.
6. The nurse believes that all patients should be treated as individuals. The ethical principle that this belief reflects is:
   1. autonomy.
   2. beneficence.
   3. nonmaleficence.
   4. respect for people.
7. LPN/LVNs have a code of professional and personal ethics to follow. The purpose of a code of ethics is to:
   1. establish penalties for any unethical behavior.
   2. promote trustworthy, accountable LPN/LVNs.
   3. make certain that all nurses are competent and always honest.
   4. give the nurse guidelines for ethical decision making.
8. The patient admitted for surgery has a lump in her breast. The patient's daughter asks the LPN/LVN if her mother should have the surgery. Which issue must be considered before responding?
   1. Confidentiality and invasion of privacy
   2. Informed consent, beneficence, and respect
   3. Respect for people and personal autonomy
   4. Nonmaleficence, justice, and liability
9. The nurse's first job as an LPN/LVN is on a unit that cares for terminally ill children. What action should be taken by the nurse before helping families cope with their children's illnesses?
   1. Study the nurse practice act to find rules relating to the medical care of terminally ill children
   2. Spend time performing value clarification to aid in identifying her feelings about this new role
   3. Evaluate her own personal mores and customs that may affect the practice of nursing in general
   4. Review the state and federal laws that prescribe how a child may be treated when near death
10. The LPN/LVN is reviewing the patient's medical record. The nurse notes the presence of an advance directive. The nurse recognizes that the purpose of this documentation is to:
    1. help every person exercise the right to die with dignity.
    2. encourage a person to determine how he or she will die.
    3. allow a patient to exercise the right of autonomy.
    4. provide a means to prevent medical maltreatment.
11. The nurse knows that all patients have the right to nursing interventions regardless of their race, religion, or gender. The ethical principle that best describes this concept is:
    1. nonmaleficence.
    2. justice.
    3. autonomy.
    4. beneficence.

12. An alert adult patient has refused an intramuscular injection. The nurse waits until the patient is asleep and gives the injection anyway. The nurse could be charged with:
1. civil battery.
2. malicious homicide.
3. criminal assault.
4. invasion of privacy.

13. The nurse loves photography and brings his camera to work at the nursing home. He takes a picture of one of his coworkers walking a patient. What best describes the actions taken by the nurse?
1. He violated the patient's right to privacy.
2. He failed to get proper medical clearance.
3. He performed an act of nursing malpractice.
4. He legally obtained a realistic picture.

14. The nurse gets a report, puts his patient assignment notebook in his pocket, and goes on break. His notebook has very specific information about his patients and is missing from his pocket when he returns to the unit. The book is found later on the floor in the cafeteria by a visitor and is returned to the information desk. The nurse:
1. may have breached the Patient Self-Determination Act.
2. is guilty of criminal misconduct.
3. could be fired for malpractice.
4. has violated the Health Insurance Portability and Accountability Act of 1996 (HIPAA).

15. The newly licensed nurse is assigned a patient who needs catheterization. The nurse has not performed the procedure before. What would be the best action for the nurse?
1. Contact the nursing supervisor and explain that the procedure will need to be done by another nurse.
2. Review the agency procedure for catheterization in the unit's resource area and see the assistance of another experienced nurse for help during the procedure.
3. Immediately advise the charge nurse that someone else will need to assume care of this patient.
4. Promptly notify the staff development office that an instructor needs to do this procedure.

16. A nurse who has recently been promoted to unit manager questions her immediate supervisor if there is any potential liability for her as a result of the actions of her nursing staff member. What information included in the supervisor's response would be appropriate? *(Select all that apply.)*
1. "An individual nurse is solely responsible for their actions."
2. "As long as you are working in good faith you cannot be found liable."
3. "As a supervisor there is some liability if measures are not followed to ensure staff understand how to utilize the care equipment."
4. "A supervisor is required to assess the performance of their staff to ensure competency."
5. "Employer liability is limited to cases in which a death occurs."

17. Social media use can have positive benefits including which outcomes? *(Select all that apply.)*
1. Networking between professionals
2. Reduction in the amount of lateral violence between staff members
3. Provides readily available education opportunities
4. Access to mentoring answer
5. Use of social media is an inexpensive answer

18. A nurse reported that she did post on a social media site about her clinical experiences. The nurse reports she did not use the patient's name. Which information should be given to the nurse? *(Select all that apply.)*
1. "Names are the only identifiers that are of concern when considering patient privacy."
2. "Any patient information that can aid in the identification of the patient's identity can be problematic and a violation."
3. "As long as the information is erased there is not a problem."
4. "Any distribution of information regarding the patient or clinical assignment is a violation of confidentiality."
5. "Personal emails are lesser violations than posting on large websites."

3 Documentation

http://evolve.elsevier.com/Cooper/foundationsadult/

Objectives

1. List the five purposes for patient records.
2. Describe the electronic health record (EHR) and the personal health record (PHR).
3. Determine when the use of Situation, Background, Assessment, and Recommendation is beneficial.
4. State important legal aspects of chart ownership, access, confidentiality, and patient care documentation.
5. Describe differences between traditional and problem-oriented medical records.
6. Describe the basic guidelines for and the mechanics of charting.
7. Describe the differences in documenting care with activities of daily living and physical assessment forms, narrative, SOAPE, and focus formats.
8. Discuss documentation and clinical (critical) pathways.
9. Discuss home health care documentation.
10. Discuss long-term health care documentation.
11. Discuss issues related to computerization in documentation.

Key Terms

auditors (p. 41)
chart (health care record) (p. 40)
charting (p. 40)
charting by exception (p. 48)
computer on wheels (p. 42)
database (DĀ-tă-bās, p. 46)
diagnosis-related groups (p. 41)
documenting (p. 40)
electronic health record (p. 40)
electronic medical record (p. 40)
informatics (p. 43)
Kardex (or Rand) (p. 49)
narrative charting (p. 45)
nomenclature (NŌ-mĕn-klā-chŭr, p. 43)
nursing care plan (p. 49)
nursing notes (p. 42)
peer review (p. 41)
personal health record (p. 43)
point-of-care (p. 42)
problem list (p. 46)
problem-oriented medical record (p. 46)
quality assurance, assessment, and improvement (p. 41)
recording (p. 40)
SBAR (p. 43)
SOAPE (SŌP, p. 46)
SOAPIER (SŌP-ē-ŭr, p. 46)
traditional (block) chart (p. 44)

The **chart (health care record)** has never been more important in the health care system than it is today; it is a legal record that is used to meet the many demands of the health, accreditation, medical insurance, and legal systems.

The process of adding information to the chart is called **charting, recording**, or **documenting**. Documenting involves recording the interventions carried out to meet the patient's needs. In the charting of interventions, documenting the type of intervention, the time care was rendered, and the signature and title of the person providing care is essential. Anything written or printed that is a record or proof of activities will play a role in this process. Although many details are necessary to remember when documenting in the chart, the process is not difficult but is often time consuming. Good documentation reflects the nursing process. Documentation is an integral part of the implementation phase of the nursing process (see Chapter 5) and is necessary for the evaluation of patient care and for reimbursement for the cost of care provided. In the past, all documenting in the patient's health records involved written documentation. Today a majority of facilities use some form of **electronic health record** (EHR), also sometimes referred to as **electronic medical record** (EMR). EHRs are used in various settings, including hospitals, long-term care settings, health care provider's offices, clinics, and home care agencies.

The licensed practical/vocational nurse (LPN/LVN) must understand how to use medical records effectively

Table 3.1 **Essential Elements of Documentation**

NURSING PROCESS	OBSERVATION SOURCES	WHERE TO DOCUMENT
Assessment		
Physiologic status Functional status Knowledge Psychosocial well-being Family Safety	Patient and family interview History and physical examination Laboratory and radiology results Medication records Environment	Discharge and transfer forms Progress notes Flow sheets
Diagnosis	Nursing judgment	Patient care plan Critical pathways Protocols Progress notes Patient problem lists Admission sheets
Outcomes Identification/Planning		
Outcome definition Defining care priorities Defining intervention strategy Activation of care plan	Patient care plan Critical pathways Projected length of stay Standards of care Admission assessment data Staff reports	Patient care plan Critical pathways Protocols Progress notes Patient problem lists
Implementation	Progress notes Patient rounds Direct patient care	Progress notes Critical pathways Protocols
Evaluation	Patient and family interview Physical assessment Staff reports Progress notes Diagnostic test results Flow sheets	Patient care plan Critical pathways Progress notes Protocols Patient problem lists

and efficiently. This chapter addresses the purposes for health records, the common types of records, the basic guidelines and rules for documentation, and legal concerns. Knowledge of these guidelines and the ability to chart completely, accurately, and legibly (when using written records) are requirements for licensure and employment as a nurse. See Table 3.1 and Chapter 5 for information on the nursing process and documentation.

PURPOSES OF PATIENT RECORDS

The five basic purposes for accurate and complete patient records are (1) documented communication; (2) permanent record for accountability; (3) legal record of care; (4) teaching; and (5) research and data collection.

The patient's chart provides a concise, accurate, and permanent record of past and current medical and nursing problems, plans for care, care given, and the patient's responses to various treatments. The record facilitates accurate communication and continuity of care among all members of the health care team. Recorded information is not as easily lost or altered as the spoken word. Proper charting covers all areas of patient needs and concerns: physical, emotional, psychological, social, and spiritual.

This permanent record sometimes is used by various government and other agencies to evaluate the institution's patient care, to justify cost reimbursement for care provided, and to establish or review accreditation. Current regulations require chart audits (review of specific chart components for completion and appropriateness) by officially appointed **auditors** (people appointed to examine patient charts and health records to assess quality of care). Auditors check to see whether all ordered care was charted as given and whether responses to specific care plan items and treatments are noted. Institutions have medical and **peer review** systems (an appraisal by professional coworkers of equal status). Peer review appraises the manner in which an individual nurse conducts practice, education, or research. Institutions also have specific procedures to provide for **quality assurance, assessment, and improvement**, which is an audit in health care that evaluates services provided and the results achieved compared with accepted standards. Accurate and legible records are the only means institutions have to prove that they are providing care to meet patient needs and established standards.

Cost reimbursement rates by the government plans (Medicare, Medicaid) are based on the prospective payment system of **diagnosis-related groups** (DRGs; a system that classifies patients by age, diagnosis, surgical procedure, and other information with hundreds of different categories to predict the use of hospital resources, including length of stay, resulting in a fixed payment amount) (CMS, 2016). Many private insurance companies now use similar illness categories when setting hospital payment rates. Institutions are reimbursed by insurance companies or government programs only for documented patient care. The payers carefully review various items in patient medical records, including the **nursing notes** (the form on the patient's chart on which nurses record their observations, the care given, and the patient's responses), when deciding whether the necessary and ordered care is being given or was given.

The patient chart or health record is a legal document; when necessary and appropriate, it is used in court proceedings. Although the physician or institution owns the original record, lawyers and courts are able to gain access to it. Therefore it is important to chart in a very detailed manner to protect those involved in patient care.

Patient health records also are used for teaching. Students in the health care professions learn more quickly and easily if examples of good charting are shared. Individuals also learn from their mistakes and the mistakes of others. It is important for students to remember that the patient's information is to be held confidential.

Patient records that involve research and data collection have many uses in the health field. For example, the government periodically publishes data on certain diseases and the effectiveness of new treatments. In addition, the pressure to contain or limit health care costs has made data regarding the usual length of hospitalization and the cost of treatment for specific illnesses or surgeries important for governmental and other health insurance providers.

ELECTRONIC HEALTH RECORD

In many health care settings, the EHR facilitates delivery of patient care and supports the data analysis necessary for coordinating patient care. EHRs contain information that is identical to that found in traditional records but eliminate repetitive entries and allow more freedom of access to the database (Fig. 3.1). In general, EHRs increase efficiency, consistency, and accuracy and decrease costs. Legibility is a further benefit of these systems.

The scope of the use of EHR for documentation in health care agencies varies depending on the agency. In addition to documentation of nursing care and interventions, most health care agencies have incorporated information systems for management of admissions, billing, and the communication of orders for diet, pharmacy, and diagnostic tests. A benefit of the EHR is the ability for all health care providers to view a patient's records, encouraging increased continuity of care. In addition, agency-wide computer information systems are more efficient because information entered in the system can be transferred automatically to other areas. In regard to nursing documentation, systems often include options for generating individualized care plans, automated Kardex forms, acuity levels, and medication administration records (MARs). Although the terms EMR and EHR often are used interchangeably, a key difference between the EHR and the EMR is that the EHR allows the exchange of patient data not only within a facility but also from one facility to another. The EMR typically is set up to exchange patient data within a facility (Office of the National Coordinator for Health Information Technology, 2011).

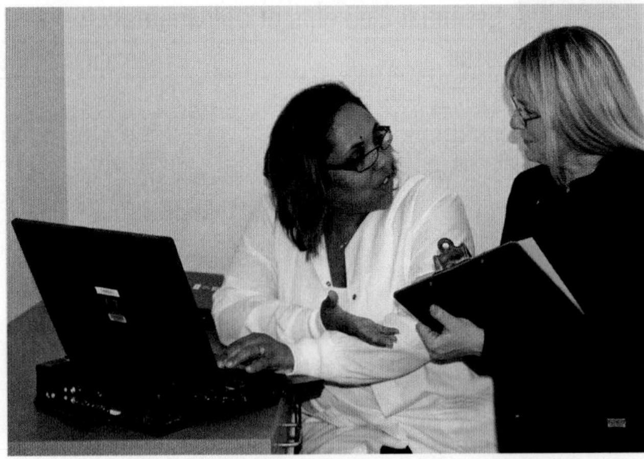
Fig. 3.1 Nurses use computers for documentation.

EHR systems vary in the way they are accessed, depending on the facility. Some systems permit computer input only at the nurses' station; some facilities have bedside systems, also referred to as **point-of-care** (POC) systems; and others use handheld systems. POC systems are sometimes housed on wheeled carts referred to as **computers on wheels**, or COWs. Charting at the bedside saves time and allows current information to be immediately available to all who need it. Some systems automatically retrieve and record information from electronic devices (e.g., vital signs) and simultaneously enter the data in all relevant locations in the record, which cuts down on duplication of effort. In addition, some systems prompt for certain data to be entered, which results in more accurate and complete record keeping.

Electronic charting procedures vary by agency. Data often are recorded in flow-sheet format for easy storage and retrieval. Some agencies incorporate the use of free-text narratives in addition to standardized phrases to allow specific and individualized documentation. The standard phrases indicate information such as patient health problems, interventions, and outcomes classification systems. Assessment data, for instance, are entered by selecting from a list of preformulated choices, which means that the accuracy and pertinence of the data entered depend on the nurse's familiarity with the language the system uses to name the patient problems, the lists of data for assessment, and anything else that is entered by picking from a list.

Naming conventions, or **nomenclature** (a classified system of technical or scientific names and terminology), must be considered when choosing computer-based documentation. The field of medical or nursing **informatics** (the study of information processing) is evolving constantly, which requires that software programs be updated on a regular basis to stay current with changes in terminology. In addition, considerable time must be invested in training personnel in charting procedures and the terminology the system uses and in conducting ongoing refresher training. Newly hired personnel need to learn a new system even if they already have had considerable experience in the field.

In addition to the EHR, the **personal health record** (PHR) is an extension of the EHR that allows patients to input their information into an electronic database. Although the PHR allows for a more comprehensive profile of the patient, points of contention for the PHR are how the information is going to be stored, who is going to store the information, and what economic costs are involved (NLM, 2017). Not only may the PHR contain information submitted by the patient but also some systems may allow input of information from other health care personnel such as pharmacists, laboratories, and the patient's primary health care provider. PHR applications may be managed by various institutions such as private vendors, hospitals, primary care health care providers, and insurance companies. These vendors may choose whether to charge a fee for storage of this information (AHIMA, 2017).

SBAR

SBAR (situation, background, assessment, and recommendation) is a method of communication among health care workers and a part of documentation (Kaiser Permanente, 2007). SBAR is considered a safety measure in preventing errors from poor communication during interactions between health care personnel, the communication between nurses that occurs from one shift to the next, or when a nurse phones a health care provider with information about a patient. SBAR is recognized by The Joint Commission as one method of meeting National Patient Safety Goals (TJC, 2018). When SBAR occurs between a nurse and a health care provider over the telephone and an order is received from the health care provider, a facility often mandates using an additional "R" in the communication exchange. The additional "R" (SBARR) represents "read back." This occurs when the nurse reads back the order to the health care provider to ensure what the nurse heard was accurate. See Box 3.1 for an example of the use of SBARR.

Box 3.1 SBARR

S *Situation:* "Hello, Dr. Reads. This is Nurse Schwenk. I am calling you about Mr. Walter's predischarge laboratory results."

B *Background:* "All his laboratory results are within normal range, except for his serum potassium level. It is 3.1."

A *Assessment:* "When I was speaking with him about his home medications, he said he has not been taking his potassium supplement for about 2 weeks. He says he forgot to refill the potassium but has continued taking his Lasix."

R *Recommendation:* "Could we give him a new prescription for potassium and include this information on his discharge instructions?"

R *Read back:* "Let me read that order back to you to make sure I understood you correctly. 'Prescription for K-tab, 10 mEq, p.o. B.I.D. and include on discharge instructions.' "

BASIC GUIDELINES FOR DOCUMENTATION

The quality and accuracy of the nursing notes are extremely important. They have a decisive impact on the success or failure of communication. Sometimes the nursing notes clearly and concisely convey the intended message; sometimes, in contrast, they cause confusion and errors in communication and patient care. Correct choice of words and spelling; grammar and punctuation; and good penmanship and other writing skills (with non–computer-based systems) are critical. The LPN/LVN must ensure the information recorded in the chart is clear, concise, complete, and accurate.

The registered nurse (RN) has primary responsibility for each patient's initial admission nursing history, physical assessment, and development of the care plan based on the patient health care problem identified. Contributions by all team members during this initial process as well as during later updating sessions are important.

The forms used to provide documentation of patient care vary based on each health care institution's policy. Each facility uses a combination of graphics, care flow sheets, and narrative or SOAPE notes (see description in later material) to document observations, care, and responses. The LPN/LVN should be sure that nursing notes correlate with the medical orders, Kardex information, and nursing care plan.

CHARTING RULES

See Box 3.2 for generally accepted documentation rules that provide consistency in documentation between health care providers and facilities. These rules also meet the standards expected by the individuals and the agencies that use the charts. Some of the rules apply to handwritten documentation. With a computerized documentation system, as is used with an EHR or EMR,

Box 3.2 Basic Rules for Documentation

- All documents should have the correct patient name, identification number, date of birth, date, and time if appropriate.
- Avoid use of generalized empty phrases such as "status unchanged" or "had good day."
- Be objective in charting: only what you hear, see, feel, smell.
- Be timely, specific, accurate, and complete.
- Chart after care is provided, not before.
- Chart all ordered care as given or explain the deviation (e.g., nothing by mouth [NPO] for laboratory, off unit, refused).
- Chart as soon and as often as necessary.
- Chart facts; avoid judgmental terms and placing blame.
- Chart only your own care, observations, and teaching; never chart for anyone else.
- Describe each item as you see it: for example, "white metal ring with clear stone" (rather than "diamond ring"). Do not speculate, guess, or assume.
- Document only what you observe, not opinions. Never use charting to accuse someone else.
- Fill all spaces; leave no empty lines. Chart consecutively. Go line by line. Do not indent left margin.
- Follow each institution's policies and procedures for charting.
- Follow rules of grammar and punctuation.
- If a charting error is made, identify the error according to facility policy and make the correct entry.
- If you question an order, record that clarification was sought. For example, do not record "physician made error," but chart "Dr. Bradley was called to clarify order for ______."
- Note patient response to treatments and response to analgesics or other special medications.
- Sign each block of charting or entry as directed by the agency policy.
- Use direct quotes when appropriate.
- Use only approved abbreviations and medical terms.
- Use only hard-pointed, permanent black ink pens; no erasures or correcting fluids are allowed on charts for written patient records.
- When a patient leaves a unit (e.g., to go to x-ray, laboratory, or office), chart the time and the method of transportation on departure and return.
- When making a late entry, note it as a late entry and then proceed with your notation: for example, "Late entry ____________," or as dictated by the facility policy.
- Write legibly (for written documentation).

the LPN/LVN should follow the guidelines for that particular system.

LEGAL BASIS OF DOCUMENTATION

Accurate documentation is one of the best defenses in the event of legal claims associated with nursing care (see Chapter 2). To limit nursing liability, the nursing documentation must indicate clearly that individualized, goal-directed nursing care was provided to a patient based on the nursing assessment. The record has to describe exactly what happened to a patient. This is best achieved when the chart is updated immediately after providing care. Although nursing care may have been excellent, if the care was not documented, a court of law will consider that care was not provided. It is the nurse's responsibility to indicate all assessments, interventions, patient responses, instructions, and referrals in the medical record.

Inappropriate documentation may lead to nursing malpractice. Some examples of inappropriate documentation include not charting the correct time that events occurred or that an event occurred at all, failing to record verbal orders, charting nursing care in advance, and documenting incorrect data. Table 3.2 lists some legal guidelines for documentation to be kept in mind. Again, some of the rules apply to handwritten documentation. With a computerized documentation system, follow the guidelines for that particular system.

COMMON MEDICAL ABBREVIATIONS AND TERMINOLOGY

Use standard medical abbreviations and terminology for effective documentation. Avoid using abbreviations or terms that are not standard or in question. Use of the complete word is always better if unsure of the proper abbreviation. Many abbreviations that once were accepted are now found on "abbreviations to avoid" lists because of the probability of error if these terms are used. Most facilities have a published list of generally accepted medical abbreviations and the terms approved for use in charting. The use of abbreviations when charting can be confusing if a facility's approved abbreviations are not followed. For example, is "BS" breath sounds, bowel sounds, or blood sugar? In addition, abbreviations used for communication outside of the health care facility, such as cell and smartphone texting abbreviations, must never be used in patient records. (See Appendix A for a list of commonly used abbreviations and The Joint Commission's list of abbreviations to avoid.)

METHODS OF RECORDING

The documentation system selected by a health care facility optimally reflects the philosophy of the facility and the way nursing care is implemented. Professionally executed charting is legal proof of care given and communicates the patient's status and progress. The nursing process shapes the approach to providing care, and in turn, effective documentation of the care the nurse provides reflects the nursing process.

TRADITIONAL CHART

The **traditional (block) chart** is divided into sections or blocks. Emphasis is placed on specific sections (or sheets

Table 3.2 Legal Guidelines for Documentation

GUIDELINES	RATIONALE	CORRECTIVE ACTION
Do not erase, apply correction fluid, or scratch out errors made while recording when using handwritten records.	Charting becomes illegible. It may appear as though there was an attempt to hide information or deface the record.	Draw a single line through error, and follow agency policy for identifying errors. Then record note correctly.
Do not document retaliatory or critical comments about patient or care by other health care professionals.	Statements can be used as evidence for unprofessional behavior or poor quality of care.	Enter only objective descriptions of patient's behavior; record patient comments as quotations.
Correct all errors promptly.	Errors in recording often lead to errors in treatment.	Avoid rushing to complete charting; be sure information is accurate.
Record all facts.	Record is required to be accurate and reliable.	Be certain entry is factual; do not speculate or guess.
Do not leave blank spaces in nursing notes when using handwritten records.	It is possible for another person to insert additional or incorrect information in the space.	Chart consecutively, line by line; if space is left, draw line horizontally through it and sign at the end.
Record all entries legibly and in black ink when using handwritten records.	Illegible entries are open to misinterpretation, which causes errors and lawsuits. Ink is not subject to erasure; black ink is more legible when records are photocopied.	Never erase entries or use correction fluid, and never use pencil.
If an order was questioned, record that clarification was sought.	Seeking clarification is the correct action to take because the nurse is just as liable for prosecution as the health care provider is if an order was carried out that is known to be improper. It is not professional to criticize another professional in the notes (see previous entry).	Do not record "physician made error." Instead, chart that "Dr. Smith was called to clarify order for analgesic."
Chart only for yourself.	You are accountable for information you enter into chart.	Never chart for someone else. (EXCEPTION: If caregiver has left unit for day and calls you with information that has to be documented, include the name of the source of information in the entry and include that information was provided via telephone.)
Avoid using generalized, empty phrases, such as "status unchanged" or "had good day."	Specific information about patient's condition or case is sometimes accidentally deleted or overlooked if information is too generalized.	Use complete, concise descriptions of care.
Begin each entry with time of entry, and end with your signature and title as specified by facility policy.	This guideline ensures that correct sequence of events is recorded; signature documents who is accountable for care delivered.	Do not wait until end of shift to record important changes that occurred several hours earlier; be sure to sign each entry.
Keep computer passwords for documentation confidential.	Maintains security and confidentiality.	Once logged into the computer, do not leave the terminal unattended.

for noncomputerized charts) of information. Typical sections are the following: admission information, physician's orders, progress notes, history and physical examination data, nurse's admission information, care plan and nursing notes, graphics, and laboratory and x-ray examination reports. The order, the content, and the number of the sections vary among institutions. Nurses use flow sheets, graphics, and **narrative charting** (recording of patient care in descriptive form) (Fig. 3.2) to chart observations, care, and responses. Narrative charting is used for computerized and noncomputerized nurse's notes. Narrative charting includes the data (subjective, objective, or both) about the basic patient need or problem, whether anyone has been contacted or consulted, care and treatments provided (implementation), and the patient's response to treatment (evaluation). Information obtained from the nurse's assessment of the patient is clustered (see Chapter 5) and organized in a head-to-toe manner. This type of charting is documented in an abbreviated story form instead of in the outline style of the problem-oriented medical record format described in the following section.

PROBLEM-ORIENTED MEDICAL RECORD

The **problem-oriented medical record** (POMR) is organized according to the scientific problem-solving system or method. The principal sections are database, problem list, care plan, and progress notes. The accumulated data, or **database**, from the history, the physical examination, and the diagnostic tests are used to identify and prioritize the health problems on the master medical and other problem lists.

This **problem list** (Fig. 3.3) of active, inactive, potential, and resolved problems serves as the index for chart documentation. Together, representatives of all the disciplines involved with the patient's care develop a care plan with identified patient problems (Fig. 3.4). All health care providers—physicians, nurses, social workers, and therapists—chart on the same progress notes with forms such as narrative notes, flow sheets, and discharge summaries to document patient progress. This is done to facilitate and enhance communication between care providers.

SOAPIER (SOAPE documentation) (Box 3.3) is an acronym for seven different aspects of charting. For notes on specific patient problems, only the necessary parts needed for completeness are used.

S *Subjective* information is what the patient states or feels; only the patient can provide this information.

O *Objective* information is what the nurse can measure or factually describe.

A *Assessment* refers to an analysis or potential diagnosis of the cause of the patient's problem or need.

P *Plan* is the general statement of the plan of care to be given or action to be taken.

I *Intervention* or implementation is the specific care given or action taken.

E *Evaluation* is an appraisal of the response and effectiveness of the plan.

R *Revision* includes the changes that may be made to the original plan of care.

SOAPE is the briefer adaptation of the charting format for the POMR. In this more compact form, the care given or action taken (intervention [I]) is included in the notations under planning. The needed plan revisions (R) are noted in the evaluation section after the evaluation of the response to treatment is recorded. Fig. 3.5 shows the SOAPE charting forms in the progress notes that commonly are used in the patient's medical record.

Nurse's Notes: *0800 Alert and oriented x 3, pt. is conversing with nurse. B/P 132/84, P 88 and regular, R 20 and unlabored, T 98.7. Reports 2/10 pain is tolerable to right anterior chest wall incision, states "PCA is controlling my pain well." Hand grip and arm strength strong to right, weak on the left. Push pull strength to lower extremities strong to right and weak to left. PERRL. Oral mucosa pink, moist, and intact. Apical pulse auscultated for 1 min at 88bpm, strong and regular rhythm, lungs clear anterior and posterior in all fields. O_2 sat. 95% with O_2 @2L via N/C. Using incentive spirometer every hour with 10 breaths reaching a maximum of 1300 mL. Abdomen soft and non-distended with bowel sounds x 4 quads. No edema to extremities, skin turgor immediate return, capillary refill less than 3 seconds. Dressing to chest wall incision dry and intact, due to be changed today. Jackson-Pratt has 75 mL of serosanguinous fluid. IV D5 ½ NS infusing into right forearm with no signs of infiltration, PCA infusing Morphine as ordered. Family members at bedside. Pt. voicing no c/o @ this time. Call light within reach. L. Coffey, RN*

0900 Assisted x 1 to BR. Gait was steady. Voided 225 mL of clear yellow urine with no odor present. Returned to chair with call light in reach. L. Coffey, RN

N-135 11/10 Nurse's Record

Fig. 3.2 Example of narrative charting.

MASTER PROBLEM LIST

Date	Problem	Resolved	Reviewed	Reactivate
7/4/18	#1 Insufficient knowledge R/T preoperative and postoperative procedures.	7/6/18		
7/5/18	#2 Recent onset of pain R/T incision.	7/6/18		
7/5/18	#3 Inability to regulate body temperature 2° due to bladder infection.			

Addressograph
000-123, DOB 11/1/1954
Serbane, Donna M. - Room 348A
Female - 63
Dr. Janeston

Fig. 3.3 Master problem list.

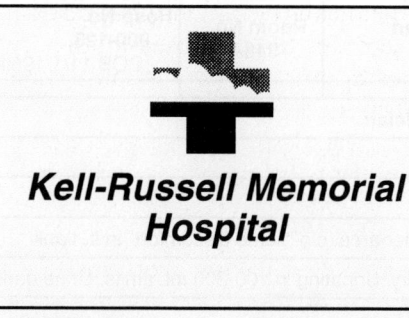

000-123, DOB 11/1/1954
Serbane, Donna M. - Room 348A
Female - 63
Dr. Janeston

PATIENT CARE PLAN

Admitting Diagnosis: Cholelithiasis — Operation: Cholecystectomy — Surgery Date: 7/4/18

Additional Diagnosis: UTI — Surgeon: Dr. Janeston — Adm. Date: 7/3/18 Dism. Date:

Patient Problem Statement with Goal	Start Date	Nursing Interventions	Date D/Cd	Init	Reassessment	Date D/Cd	Init
#3 Inability to regulate body temperature r/t	7/4/18	Vital signs q̄ 4 and PRN		MH			
infection		Encourage fluids as tolerated					
in bladder AEB (as		I & O, provide high calorie in					
evidenced by)		between meal snacks. Assess comfort					
T 101.2, urine		Medicate for temperature > 102° (0)					
becoming cloudy,		q̄ 4 PRN					
report of burning on							
urination. Goal: #1							
Temp will remain							
within normal limits							
within 48 hours of							
starting ordered							
antibiotic; #2 Urine							
will begin turning							
clear with no burning							
within 48 hours of							
starting ordered							
antibiotic							

INITIALS AND SIGNATURE M.H., Michaela Heldeman, RN

Fig. 3.4 Patient care plan.

Box 3.3 SOAPE and SOAPIER Documentation Formats

SOAPE	SOAPIER
Subjective	**S**ubjective
Objective	**O**bjective
Assessment	**A**ssessment
Plan	**P**lan
Evaluation	**I**ntervention
	Evaluation
	Revision

FOCUS CHARTING FORMAT

In the *focus charting format* (Box 3.4), which was developed by nurses, a modified list of patient problems statements is used as an index for nursing documentation. Note the similarity of this list to the problem list used for the POMR. Focus charting can be used with traditional and POMR charting.

Focus charting uses the nursing process and the more positive concept of the patient's needs rather than medical diagnoses and problems. The focus is sometimes a current patient concern or behavior and sometimes a significant change in patient status or behavior or a significant event in the patient's therapy. A focus is not a medical diagnosis.

DARE is the acronym for four different aspects of charting using the focus format (see Box 3.4). Data *(D)* are subjective and objective and are equivalent to the assessment step of the nursing process. Action *(A)* is a combination of planning and implementation. Response *(R)* of the patient is the same as evaluation of effectiveness. Some facilities include education or patient teaching *(E)*. The nurse does not need to use all the DARE steps each time notes are documented on a particular focus (Fig. 3.6).

CHARTING BY EXCEPTION

Some facilities require the narrative notes for each shift to include a minimum of three entries and a flow sheet on which the nurse charts care given. Behind this policy is the legally derived charting concept that if the care was not documented it is considered that care was not provided. All care must be charted, but this is a time-consuming, detailed, and defensive method.

Last name: Serbane	First name: Donna M.	Attending Physician Dr. Janeston	Room No. 348A	Hosp No. 000-123, DOB 11/1/1954

Date	Notes Should Be Signed by Physician
7-5-18	0930 Problem #1 Inability to regulate body temperature
	(Patient problem: elevated body temperature)
	S Feels hot & flushed. Has burning on urination and heavy feeling over bladder area. c/o "some discomfort" in lt. flank
	O Temperature 101^2 (0) elevated from 99^8 @ 0730 AM. Skin warm, flushed, dry. Urinating in 100-200 mL am'ts. Urine dark,
	amber and cloudy. Foley Cath. dc'd 7/4 @ 2200. Lungs clear.
	A Possible bladder infection secondary to Foley catheter.
	P Notify Dr. Janeston of temperature elevation, dysuria and back discomfort. Assess for other signs of infection. To x-ray
	for chest evaluation. Begin oral antibiotics after catheterization and urine specimen to laboratory for C & S per Dr. Janeston
	orders. Encourage increased oral fluids.
	E Urine to laboratory, x-ray of chest ordered, chest and breath sounds clear. Nonproductive cough. Drank 500 mL of water this
	shift. 2230 urine less concentrated.

Fig. 3.5 SOAPE charting progress notes.

EXAMPLE OF FOCUS CHARTING

Date	Time	Focus		Data, Actions, Patient Response, and Education
7/5/18	0820	Hypotension	D	BP in left arm 90/60, patient's skin diaphoretic, patient responds to name
			A	Placed patient in Trendelenburg position, increased IV fluid rate to 100 mL/hr per protocol, called Dr. Janeston.
			R	Patient remains responsive, BP in left arm 94/68 3 min after increasing fluid S Wilson, RN
7/5/18	1620	Pain	D	Twisting in bed, grimacing with movement, states "has sharp lower back pain"
			A	Administered morphine sulfate 10 mg IV in RVL
			R	Verbalized relief within 15 min, lying quietly.
			E	Instructed patient to move slowly when getting out of bed and to call for assistance T. Newson, RN

Fig. 3.6 Focus charting nurse's notes.

Box 3.4 Focus Charting Format

Data
Action
Response and evaluation
Education and patient teaching

To alleviate this problem, many facilities now have a policy called **charting by exception** (CBE). The nurse charts complete physical assessments, observations, vital signs, intravenous (IV) site and rate, and other pertinent data at the beginning of each shift. During the shift, the only notes the nurse makes are for additional treatments done or planned treatments withheld, changes in patient condition, and new concerns. Notations are made reflecting progress or revisions for all active patient problems on the nursing care plan.

With the CBE method of documentation, the nurse uses more detailed flow sheets, which enhances the focus on existing concerns. One format that may be used is the problem, intervention, and evaluation (PIE) format. It is a problem-solving approach, so PIE is similar to the SOAPE format; the main difference is that SOAPE charting originated from the medical model, whereas PIE charting arose from the nursing process. The SOAPE method of documentation also is oriented to the problems, interventions, and evaluations involved in nursing care. It was designed to provide an ongoing plan of nursing care with daily documentation. The care and assessment flow sheets consist of standardized assessment criteria and interventions. With this method, the nurse assesses all areas and compares the results with normal standards. The PIE format may be written in several ways, so the nurse should use the format dictated by the agency's policy. At each shift, the nurse evaluates each patient problem at least once, and if the problem remains unresolved, the nurse ensures it is addressed continually until resolution is reached. After the patient problem is resolved, it no longer is covered by the daily documentation.

Sometimes the nurse uses a variation of the PIE format that includes assessment *(A)* data before the PIE (APIE). These assessment data include subjective *(S)* and

Date	Time	Progress notes
7/6/18	0900	A - Assessment: (s) states -"sharp shooting pain in epigastric region" Patient reports 7/10 on pain scale (o) guarding abdomen and refuses lunch tray. States "I am nauseated."
	0915	P - Problem: Pain related to unknown cause
	0920	I - Intervention: Demerol 100 mg given IM in R ventral gluteal region
	1000	E - Evaluation: States "the pain is gone." C. Sommers, LPN

Fig. 3.7 APIE (assessment, problem, intervention, and evaluation) documentation.

objective *(O)* data. This assists the nurse to follow the steps of the nursing process (Fig. 3.7).

RECORD-KEEPING FORMS AND EXAMPLES

Different facilities use a variety of forms to make medical record documentation easy and quick, yet comprehensive. Many forms help eliminate the need to duplicate data repeatedly in the nursing notes. The forms present several types of information in a format more accessible than compilation of all progress notes. Most of the forms are self-explanatory regarding the type of information required from the nurse (Fig. 3.8). It is unnecessary to chart a narrative note each time a medication is given (see Chapter 17) or a bath (see Chapter 9) or measurement of vital signs (see Chapter 12).

The nursing **Kardex (or Rand)** system is used by some facilities to consolidate patient orders and care needs in a centralized, concise way. The cumulative care file or Rand is kept at the nursing station for quick reference or is part of the EHR or EMR. Forms vary among institutions based on information required for care (Fig. 3.9).

The **nursing care plan** (which outlines the proposed nursing care based on the nursing assessment and the identified patient problems to provide continuity of care) is developed to meet the nursing care needs of a patient. Many facilities use standardized care plans for certain conditions or surgeries; however, individualization of the plan of care based on each patient's own needs or circumstances is also important. This kind of plan, developed by nurses for nurses, is based on nursing assessment and identified patient problems. Standardized nursing care plans include the pertinent patient problems, goals, and plans for care and specific actions for care implementation and evaluation.

Incident Reports

An *incident report* (form used to document any event not consistent with the routine operation of a health care unit or the routine care of a patient, Fig. 3.10) is sometimes necessary in response to an unplanned occurrence within a health care facility. For example, if a nurse neglects to give a medication or treatment or gives an incorrect dose of a drug, an incident report must be filed. Either of these events has the potential to cause injury. Incident reports also are filled out for any unusual event in a hospital (e.g., injuries to a patient, visitor, hospital personnel). Many staff members are reluctant to fill out these forms, but this information helps the facility risk manager and unit managers to track occurrences of incidents. One of the benefits of tracking particular incidents is to prevent future problems through education and other corrective measures.

When filling out an incident report, give only objective, observed information. Do not admit liability or give unnecessary details. Include in the incident report care given to the patient in response to the incident and the name of the health care provider notified. When charting the incident in the patient's nursing notes, do not mention the incident report, because doing so makes it easier for an attorney to request that document for a court case (Table 3.3).

Twenty-Four–Hour Patient Care Records and Acuity Charting Forms

The nursing records may be consolidated into a system that accommodates a 24-hour period. A 24-hour record-keeping system helps eliminate unnecessary record-keeping forms. It is easier to obtain accurate assessment information and documentation of activities of daily living with 24-hour notations. In addition, 24-hour patient care records often use flow sheets and checklists to enhance efficiency further.

Twenty-four–hour patient care records provide the foundation for an acuity charting system. *Acuity charting* uses a score that rates each patient by severity of illness. With documentation and analysis of nursing interventions, an overall level of acuity for each patient is determined. For example, perhaps an acuity system rates patients from 1 to 5 (1 is high, 5 is low). A patient returning from surgery with multisystem problems is an acuity level 1. On the same continuum, another patient awaiting discharge after a successful recovery from surgery is an acuity level 5. One benefit is the ability to determine efficient staffing patterns according to the acuity levels of the patients on a particular nursing unit. The patient-to-staff ratios depend on a composite gathering of data in regard to the 24-hour interventions necessary for implementing care.

Discharge Summary Forms

Much emphasis is placed on preparing a patient for a timely discharge from a health care institution. Ideally, discharge planning begins at admission, and in some cases, even before admission, as is necessary with same-day surgery admissions and childbirth. Nurses continue discharge planning as the patient's condition changes. Patients and family should be involved in the discharge planning process.

Text continued on p. 54

PHYSICAL ASSESSMENT (HEAD TO TOE) TIME OF ASSESSMENT: ______	NOTES:
1. NEUROLOGIC: Level of consciousness	
Confused	
Oriented x 1. person 2. place 3. time 4. purpose	
PERRLA—Babinski: Positive or Negative	
Hand strength: Strong or Weak	
Leg movement: Strong or Weak	
2. INTEGUMENTARY	
Condition: Moist or Dry	
Temperature:	
Turgor	
Tenting	
Incision	
Location:	
Without erythema	
Exudate:	
Sutures/staples intact	
Sutures/staples not intact	
Open wound	
Hemovac: Color Amt	
Davol: Color Amt	
Jackson-Pratt: Color Amt	
Penrose: Color Amt	
Wound vac: Color Amt	
Dressing	
Clean & dry	
Needs changed	
3. CARDIOVASCULAR	
Apical pulse rate:	
Capillary refill <3 sec: Yes or No	
Pedal pulses (1-4+): L & R	
Pedal edema (1-4+): L & R	
Nonpitting edema	
IV	
Solution	
Peripheral	
Central line	
Rate:	
Site & condition:	
4. RESPIRATORY	
Anteriorly	
Posteriorly	
O_2 Saturation level: %	
Crackle	
Wheezes: Sonorous or Sibilant	
Pleural friction rub	

Fig. 3.8 Nursing care record.

Dyspnea Tachypnea Orthopnea	
O_2 Therapy: type:	
Rate: Liters per:	
Incentive spirometer	
Inspiratory capacity: mL	
Chest tube to H_2O seal ____ cm	
Chest tube to H_2O seal and wall suction ____ mm Hg	
Color and amount ____ mm Hg	
5. GASTROINTESTINAL	
Appetite ____ Type of diet ____	
Dentures: Yes or No	
Oral fluid intake:	
Bowel sounds *4:	
Active Hyper Hypo Absent	
Distention Tympanic Tenderness	
Flatulence	
BM #: Color: Consistency:	
Stoma pink & viable: Yes or No	
N/G	
Amt: mL	
Color of drainage	
Peg tube ____	
Site condition ____ Flush ____ Feeding ____	
Gastrostomy tube ____	
Site condition ____ Flush ____ Feeding ____	
Jejunostomy ____	
Site condition ____ Flush ____ Feeding ____	
6. URINARY	
Output amount: ____ hours of output ____	
Color:	
Odor:	
Catheter	
Type: Foley Ureterostomy	
Suprapubic Nephrostomy	
Urostomy	
CBI credit:	
True urine:	
7. MOBILITY	
Activity level:	
Bed rest. chair. up with assistance. walker.	
crutches. cane	
Up ad lib: Yes or No	
Gait: Unsteady or Steady	
Level of tolerance:	
Traction: Kind: Weight:	

Fig. 3.8, cont'd Nursing care record.

Continued

8. REPRODUCTIVE	
Prostate problems: Yes or No	
Hysterectomy: Yes or No	
Breast—monthly breast self-exam: Yes or No	
Mastectomy:	
____ Rt ____ Left ____ Appearance	
Vaginal drainage: Yes or No	
9. SENSORY	
Hard of hearing: Yes or No	
Hearing aid: Yes or No	
Glasses	
Contacts	

VITALS	VITALS	ADLs
TIME TAKEN: hr	TIME TAKEN: hr	BED BATH-TIME:
Temp:	Temp:	Supplies needed: 1 linen bag
Pulse:	Pulse:	2-3 towels
Respirations:	Respirations:	2-3 washcloths
Blood pressure:	Blood pressure:	4-5 disposable washcloths
How taken:	How taken:	Soap, shampoo, deodorant, comb
Level of pain:	Level of pain:	1disposable garbage bag
NOTES:	NOTES:	Cotton swabs
		Orange stick/nail file
		Lip conditioner
		Toothbrush, toothettes, toothpaste
		Denture supplies
CHECK:	CHECK:	Other supplies need by pt:
Water filled & cool	Water filled & cool	
Bed straightened	Bed straightened	
Patient comfortable?	Patient comfortable?	LINEN CHANGE OF BED:
Patient requests:	Patient requests:	1 linen bag (if not doing @ bedtime)
		1 contour sheet
		1 flat sheet
		1 pull sheet
		Pillow case(s) - How many pillows?
		1 blanket
		1 bedspread
		Add'l supplies needed for pt:
___ **ALL INFO CHARTED**	___ **ALL INFO CHARTED**	___ **ALL INFO CHARTED**

Fig. 3.8, cont'd Nursing care record.

Date Activities	Date Elimination	Date Supportive	Date Wounds	Date Hygiene	Date	Diet
7/5 Bed rest 7/6 BRP ___ Dangle ___ Chair ___ w/Chair ___ Crutched ___ Walker ___ Ad. Lib. ___ Turn 7/7 Up with Assistance	7/5 Catheter dc'd 7/6 ___ Commode ___ Adult Diaper ___ Colostomy Old/New ___ Ileostomy Old/New ___ Hematest ___ Save Stools ___ Strain all Urine ___ Urostomy 7/5 Intake/Output ___ Ileo Conduit ___ Enema/Flush PRN ___ CBI	___ Cradle/Footboard ___ Overhead Frame ___ TED Hose ___ Telemetry #___ ___ NG Tube ___ Tracheotomy ___ Traction ___ Oxygen ___ Siderails ___ Restraints ___ Egg Crate 7/5 IV's/Int. lock ___ Isolation ___ PCA Pump ___ Oral Suction ___ K-Pad	___ Packing ___ Hemo drain ___ Drain 7/5 Incision ___ Suction ___ Solcotrans 7/5 T-Tube ___ Chest Tube	7/6 Bed Bath 7/7 Assist ___ Self Bath ___ Shower/Tub ___ Sitz ___ Towel Bath ___ Oral ___ Hair ___ Skin/Decubitus	7/6 Snacks Food Allergies: milk	Clear liquids Beverages B Hot tea D Hot tea S Hot tea

LABORATORY and RADIOLOGY

7/5 Chest x-ray ECG CBC	7/7 Chest x-ray UA/C&S			

DATE	TREATMENTS	DISC.
	DAILY WEIGHT SCALE	
7/5	Incentive spirometer every hour while awake.	
7/5	Vital signs q 4 hr.	
7/5	Turn, cough, and deep breath q 2 hr.	
7/5	Reinforce dressings PRN.	
7/6	Chg. abdominal dressings PRN.	
7/6	Record T-tube drainage.	

CONTACT (next of kin)	BLUE DOT:	RECENT/PRESENT SURGERY:	ADDITIONAL DIAGNOSIS:
W.L. Spaur - husband 534-3974 Chaplain/Minister G Timmons		Open Cholecystectomy 7/5/18	UTI 7/7

Room:	Date of Birth (DOB):	Name:	Sex:	S(M)W.D.	Religion	Diagnosis:	Attending Physician:	Consulting Physician:
348A	11/1/1954	Serbane, Donna M.	Fe		Prot	Cholelithiasis & Cholecystitis	D. Janeston, MD	J.W. Richtey, MD

Fig. 3.9 Nursing Kardex (or Rand) card.

Table 3.3 Examples of Incident Report Entries

PROPER ENTRY	INCORRECT ENTRY
1900 Resident found on floor in a sitting position beside table in activity room. Complete assessment performed. Vital signs stable; 1-cm abrasion on anterior left forearm noted. No complaints by resident. Abrasion recorded on skin assessment record. Notified Dr. Reads per phone. Orders received to perform neurologic assessment every 2 hours for 24 hours and place on fall risk protocol.	1900 Resident found on floor in activity room. Apparently missed chair when trying to move chair and sit down. Minor abrasion on left arm. Dr. Reads notified and orders received.
0800 Administered hydrochlorothiazide 25 mg p.o. Hydrochlorothiazide 12.5 mg ordered. Vital signs measured and remain stable. Dr. Reads notified. Order received to continue monitoring vital signs every hour × 4 hours. If stable, monitor every 4 hours for 24 hours.	0800 Administered 25 mg hydrochlorothiazide by mistake. Patient had no complaints and states he "feels fine." Notified Dr. Reads and orders received.
1700 Felt sharp pain in lower back, 8/10, after assisting patient from bed to chair. Gait belt used to assist in patient transfer. Notified employee health department.	1700 Injured back while helping patient transfer from bed to chair. Notified employee health department.

KELL-RUSSELL MEMORIAL HOSPITAL

Report of Medication, Patient (Visitor) Safety Variance

To be completed by the person most closely involved or the person discovering the incident/occurrence.

PATIENT NAME: Longe, John AGE: 70 SEX: male

ADDRESS: 59 W Bass Ave

TYPE OF PATIENT: ____ Inpatient ____ Outpatient ____ Emergency
(check one) X Visitor ____ Employee

Date and time of variance: 07/07/2018

Exact location of variance: Room 3001

Description of variance: Visitor found lying on floor at foot of patient's bed. "I got light headed when I saw all of the tubes and machines on my dad."

What was the nature of the injury to the patient (visitor), etc.: no injuries noted

Equipment or supplies involved: none

ID # & Present Location: 3001

Why did variance occur? Visitor states "I got light headed when I saw all of the tubes and machines on my dad. I didn't get hurt because my brother caught me and eased me down to the floor." Visitor refuses to see a physician.

Physician notified? ____ yes ____ no X when? ____

Signature Sandra Suey, RN Physician: Dr. Janeston

Witness Mary Pinkton, RN

If the incident is related to patient care, this sheet must remain on inpatient medical record for 24 hours, after which it shall be taken to the Risk Management Department.

CONFIDENTIAL - NOT PART OF THE MEDICAL RECORD

Fig. 3.10 Incident report.

A discharge summary form provides important information that pertains to the patient's continued health care after discharge. A discharge summary always should be provided to the patient or the family (or both) so that there is written documentation of instructions given to the patient and so that the patient can refer to those instructions after being discharged. Discharge summary forms (see Fig. 11.5) make the summary concise and instructive. Often the form includes a copy that is given to the patient, a family member, or a home health care nurse and a copy that is kept with the patient records. Home health care agencies or extended nursing care facilities also benefit from receiving information on these summary forms and use it to provide better continuity of care.

DOCUMENTATION AND CLINICAL (CRITICAL) PATHWAYS

Documentation tools that integrate the standards of care of multiple disciplines have been developed to meet the needs of managed care. Managed care is a systematic approach to care that provides a framework for the coordination of medical and nursing interventions.

These documentation tools are called *clinical (critical) pathways*. Clinical (critical) pathways allow staff from all disciplines to develop standardized, integrated care plans for a projected length of stay for patients of a specific case type. The case types that have clinical (critical) pathways are usually those that occur in high volume and are predictable. A clinical (critical) pathway

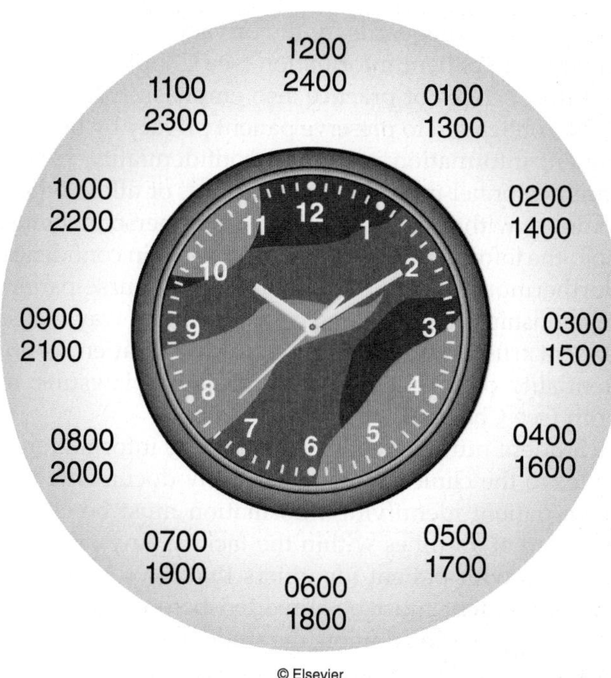

Fig. 3.11 Military time clock.

for a total hip repair may recommend on a day-to-day basis the level of activity, pain control therapy, advancement in diet, and educational topics necessary for a patient's recovery.

The exact contents and format of these clinical (critical) pathways vary among institutions. The contents include a care plan, interventions specific for each day of hospitalization, and a documentation tool. The clinical (critical) pathway replaces other nursing forms such as the nursing care plan.

The LPN/LVN and other team members use the pathways to monitor a patient's progress and as a documentation tool. CBE is frequently the method used with pathways. Staff members document only when anticipated interventions are not provided as projected.

Many agencies use military time, a 24-hour system that uses digit numbers to indicate morning, afternoon, and evening times regardless of which method of documentation is used (Fig. 3.11).

HOME HEALTH CARE DOCUMENTATION

The home health care industry continues to grow in our society for a number of reasons. Limitations in coverage within the acute care setting are a major cause for the growth, as is the desire patients have to be cared for in their home rather than in a health care facility.

Documentation in the home health care system has different implications than in other areas of nursing. The primary difference is the nature of the home setting, which dictates that a narrower scope of people (e.g., patient, family, direct health care provider) witness the majority of care. Home health care requires that the entire health care team work closely together. The documentation of care must be accurate and complete so that all members of the team are able to ascertain what care is rendered in the home. In addition, the documentation provides the quality control and the justification for reimbursement from Medicare, Medicaid, or private insurance companies. Nurses have to document all their services for payment (e.g., direct skilled care, patient instructions, skilled observations, evaluation visits). The nurse is the pivotal person in the documentation of the delivery of home health care.

Home health care documentation has several components that the nurse must consider. Medicare, Medicaid, and private insurance typically have similar requirements in regard to documentation. The patient's eligibility for home care must be assessed thoroughly and documented. The nurse must document in detail any procedures, treatments, or medications administered and response to these interventions. Another important aspect of health care documentation is noting any patient education and demonstration of learning. Home health documentation also must reflect coordination of services by all members of the health care team and evidence of compliance with regulations (Medicare and Medicaid Services, n.d.). Home health care is discussed in more detail in Chapter 37.

LONG-TERM HEALTH CARE DOCUMENTATION

An ever-increasing number of older adults need care in long-term health care facilities. Because many individuals live in this setting for the rest of their lives, they are referred to as residents rather than as patients. The acuity of residents' conditions, and the number of their disabilities, continues to escalate commensurate with their age. Nursing personnel often face challenges much different from those in the acute care setting. These differences establish a significantly different basis for nursing documentation.

Outside agencies are instrumental in determining the standards and policies for documentation in long-term health care. For example, the Omnibus Budget Reconciliation Act (OBRA) of 1987 instituted significant Medicare and Medicaid requirements for long-term care provision and documentation. Among the requirements of OBRA are minimum data sets (MDS) and regulated standards for resident assessments, individualized care plans, and qualifications for health care providers (RNs and LPN/LVNs). In addition, the department of health in each state governs the frequency of the required nursing entries in the records of residents in long-term care facilities. Long-term care documentation supports a multidisciplinary approach in the assessment (referred to as the MDS) and the planning process (referred to as resident assessment protocols) of the residents. Often long-term care agencies also have skilled care units where patients or residents stay when, in response to mandates for shorter hospital stays, they need increased levels of care and are not able to return directly to their usual residence after a hospital admission. Multidisciplinary communication among such health care providers as nurses, unlicensed assistive personnel (UAP), social workers, physical therapists, and dietitians is essential in the regulated documentation process. The fiscal management of long-term care hinges on the justification of nursing care as demonstrated in sound documentation of the services rendered. Additional documentation information in long-term care is discussed in Chapter 38.

SPECIAL ISSUES IN DOCUMENTATION

RECORD OWNERSHIP AND ACCESS

The original health care record or chart is the property of the institution or the health care provider. On admission to the health care facility, the patient usually is asked to sign a form granting permission for appropriate people, such as insurance carriers, to have access to the record as necessary. Patients may not have immediate access to their full records, depending on the agency policy. Lawyers, with the patient's written permission, are given access to the patient's medical records. Courts have the legal right to obtain records for review and use in the case of a lawsuit.

Patients have gained access rights to their records in most states, but only if they follow the established policy of each facility. A written request for chart access may be required, and institutions can specify a period that allows the physician and the facility to review the record and give a response. Sometimes the institution requires that a staff member or physician be present while the individual looks through the chart to answer questions and to protect the integrity of the record. Patients also may ask for a copy of their medical records. The Office of the National Coordinator for Health Information Technology (ONC), which is part of the Department of Health and Human Services, is working continually on making access to medical records easier and less time consuming for patients, including electronic access. The department currently is focusing on the issue of personal health records (PHR) (NLM, 2017).

CONFIDENTIALITY

Health care personnel are required to respect the confidentiality of the patient's record. The Patient Care Partnership (patients, when admitted to a facility, receive this information regarding their rights and responsibilities) and the law guarantee that medical information is kept private, unless the information is needed in providing care or the patient gives permission for others to see it (American Hospital Association, n.d.). The Health Insurance Portability and Accountability Act (HIPAA), an act of Congress passed in 1996, affords certain protections to persons covered by health care plans, including continuity of coverage when changing jobs, standards for electronic health care transactions, and primary safeguards for the privacy of individually identifiable patient information (see Chapter 2).

Ethical codes of practice also emphasize the LPN/LVN's obligation to preserve patient privacy by holding patient information in highest confidentiality. Health care personnel may not read a record, or allow others to do so, without a clinical reason, and personnel must hold the information regarding the patient in confidence. Furthermore, trust is necessary for good nurse-patient relationships, and breaking confidences is a way to lose patient trust. Breaking laws concerning patient confidentiality often leads to job termination, lawsuits, or both (see Chapter 2).

Student nurses are reminded that no information is to leave the clinical site and that any documents that have patient identifying information must be closely guarded at all times within the facility. Any printouts or notes with patient identifiers that have been used by the student must be shredded before leaving the clinical agency. In addition, the student must be vigilant in keeping documents in a safe place when in the clinical agency; documents with patient identifiers never should be left anywhere unattended, such as on bedside tables in the patient's room, at the nurses' station, or on conference room tables. Any information that the student does need for course assignment purposes regarding assigned patients should have no identification information on the documents. Identification information is not limited to the patient's name, age, or identification number. Any unique information about the patient, such as medical diagnosis or past medical history, is considered a patient identifier.

ELECTRONIC DOCUMENTATION SAFEGUARDS

Charting with an electronic system is an efficient method of documentation, but the security of the system must be considered when considering legal and ethical issues. Confidentiality, access to information, and inappropriate alterations in patient records are areas of concern. Networks typically are protected by a firewall from illegitimate outside access. Some computer systems permit online access from remote sites, but this further complicates the task of keeping the system secure. To protect the patient's rights and keep the patient's record confidential, anyone who enters data into or consults a computerized record has to log on to the system with a secure password. The institution may require the user to change passwords at certain time frames, such as every 90 days, to maintain security. Because the password is assigned only to individual health care personnel, any data entered are credited automatically to whoever signed in; thus personnel must never share the password with anyone. Be sure to log off the system before leaving the terminal to ensure that information about a patient does not remain on the monitor display for others to view.

It is also necessary to protect computer-generated printouts and prevent the indiscriminate duplication or

Box 3.5 Guidelines for Safe Computer Documentation

- Do not share with another caregiver the password that you use to enter and sign off computer files. (NOTE: A good system requires frequent changes in personal passwords to prevent unauthorized people from accessing and tampering with records. Some facilities use fingerprint scanners instead of passwords.)
- After logging on, never leave the computer terminal unattended without first logging off.
- Follow the correct protocol for correcting errors. To correct an error after storage, follow the facility policy for identifying documentation errors, then add the correct information and date and initial the entry. If you record information in the wrong chart, follow facility policy for identifying this error.
- Make sure that stored records have backup files, an important safety check. If you inadvertently delete part of the permanent records, type an explanation into the computer file with the date, the time, and your initials and submit an explanation in writing to your manager.
- Do not leave information about a patient displayed on a monitor where others have the opportunity to see it.
- Follow the agency's confidentiality procedures for documentation.
- Printouts of computerized records also have to be protected. Shredding of printouts and keeping a log that accounts for every copy (whether electronic or printed) of a computerized file that you have generated from the system are ways to keep waste and creation of duplicate records to a minimum and protect the confidentiality of patients.

distribution of information about patients. Most facilities that use computer charting incorporate a system for logging and tracking computer printouts (Box 3.5) and have protocols for shredding the copies that are made.

USE OF FAX MACHINES

Fax machines send written documents over telephone lines to transmit data quickly between health care facilities, such as health care provider's offices, hospitals, long-term care facilities, and laboratories. HIPAA rules allow for a patient's medical records and information to be faxed. Information can be transmitted from health care providers to health care facilities and vice versa. For example, laboratory results can be sent via fax, email, or phone to a health care provider, or a health care provider may fax medical information to another professional for consultation. Various safeguards must be in place to maintain patient confidentiality and privacy. Some facilities require that the sender verify the fax number with the recipient. Similarly, a facility may preprogram frequently faxed numbers into the system to prevent incorrect dialing of the intended number. Although fax machines are still used, they are being used less by facilities that have an EHR system in place.

Get Ready for the NCLEX® Examination!

Key Points

- Documentation is part of the implementation phase of the nursing process and is used in evaluation.
- Only approved abbreviations and medical terms should be used when charting in a patient's record. Knowledge of the common abbreviations and terms is required.
- The five purposes for patient records are (1) a means of communication to facilitate continuity of care; (2) a permanent record for accountability purposes (audits, accreditation, and cost reimbursement); (3) a legal record; (4) usage in teaching; and (5) usage for research and data collection.
- Many facilities have an electronic health record (EHR) or electronic medical record (EMR) system in place to facilitate documentation and coordination of patient care.
- SBAR (*s*ituation, *b*ackground, *a*ssessment, and *r*ecommendation) aids in communication during "hand-off" or "handover" interactions with other health care personnel.
- Two common types of medical records or charts are the traditional (block) chart and the problem-oriented medical record (POMR).
- The POMR uses a master patient problem list as an index to the chart. These listed problems are usually medical diagnoses.
- SOAPIER is one format for charting in the POMR. The letters stand for subjective *(S)*, objective *(O)*, assessment *(A)*, plan *(P)*, implementation *(I)*, evaluation *(E)*, and revision *(R)*.
- Two other common formats for charting nursing notes are narrative and focus. Focus charting includes data *(D)*, action *(A)*, response and evaluation *(R)*, and education and patient teaching *(E)*.
- Charting must be legible (with handwritten documentation), clear, concise, accurate, and complete. These guidelines serve as a national standard for licensed nurses.
- The specific institution or unit often has specific forms and charting formats; in addition, the general guidelines and rules for charting should be followed.

- Medical records are legal documents. The health care provider or institution owns the original record.
- Lawyers, courts, and patients are able to gain access to the record by following specified access procedures.
- The contents of a health record are confidential information protected by the law and the Patient Care Partnership.
- The nursing Kardex or Rand is a card-filing system used in some facilities by nurses to condense all the orders and other care information needed quickly for each patient. It is updated frequently.
- Computerized information systems provide information about a patient in an organized and easily accessible fashion.
- Clinical pathways allow staff from all disciplines to develop integrated care plans for a projected length of stay for patients of a specific case type.
- Many agencies use military time. This system uses four-digit numbers to indicate morning, afternoon, and evening times.
- A 24-hour record-keeping system helps eliminate unnecessary record-keeping forms.
- The acuity level determined by analyzing what nursing care is necessary allows patients to be rated in comparison with one another. Staffing patterns then can be determined by examining the acuity levels for the patients on a particular nursing unit.
- Fax machines are used to send written documents over telephone lines to transmit data quickly between hospitals and other facilities, such as health care provider offices.

Additional Learning Resources

SG Go to your Study Guide for additional learning activities to help you master this chapter content.

evolve Be sure to visit the Evolve site at *http://evolve.elsevier.com/Cooper/foundationsadult/* for additional online resources.

Review Questions for the NCLEX® Examination

1. The nursing preceptor is preparing to speak with the new licensed practical/vocational nurse (LPN/LVN) regarding documentation. Which statement by the preceptor is correct?
   1. "It is important to use only approved medical terms and abbreviations when documenting in the electronic health record (EHR)."
   2. "Our facility discourages nurses from using complete words when documenting because it takes up too much space in the chart."
   3. "To prevent errors, our facility does not allow the use of abbreviations for documentation."
   4. "The physician uses more abbreviations when writing orders than the nurse uses when documenting."
2. The patient asks the LPN/LVN if he can take his chart with him on discharge from the hospital. Which response by the nurse is most accurate?
   1. "The chart has confidential information in it and cannot be taken out of the facility."
   2. "The chart belongs to you, so I will check to see whether this is permissible."
   3. "We need to complete the proper forms for you to take your chart with you."
   4. "The chart is the property of the hospital, but if you need copies of your records, we can arrange that for you."
3. When reviewing information regarding the problem-oriented medical record (POMR), the LPN/LVN correctly identifies which guideline?
   1. The problem list has only active and resolved problems.
   2. Only the physician charts on the progress notes.
   3. The charting format is SOAPE or SOAPIER.
   4. Focus charting format is used with this type of record.
4. The LPN/LVN is using the SOAPE method to chart. When documenting the *S* portion, which entry demonstrates correct documentation? *(Select all that apply.)*
   1. Patient's vital signs are stable.
   2. Patient reports left hip pain 8/10.
   3. Patient's wife was present during patient teaching.
   4. Patient ambulated 20 ft unassisted with steady gait.
   5. Patient reports a feeling of nausea after eating.
5. The student nurse is correct when identifying which concept regarding documentation as being correct?
   1. Chart as soon and as often as necessary.
   2. Remember to chart only basic care information.
   3. Leave blank lines for others if asked.
   4. Chart facts with use of judgmental terms if needed.
6. Understanding that health care personnel must respect the confidentiality of patient records, which action by the nurse is appropriate?
   1. Looking at a friend's chart to see the diagnosis
   2. Stating that only the Patient Care Partnership advocates confidentiality
   3. Reading charts only for a professional reason
   4. Sharing information from a chart to protect a friend
7. Following orientation to the facility's computer system, which statement by the new nurse is most accurate?
   1. "I can save on charting time once I am comfortable using this system."
   2. "The computer system is not that efficient."
   3. "Documentation can be done only on a shared terminal at the desk."
   4. "Most computerized systems lack security measures to protect confidentiality."
8. The nurse demonstrates knowledge of correctly completing an incident report with which action?
   1. Documenting in the chart that the incident report has been filed
   2. Having all parties involved sign the report
   3. Asking the supervising nurse to complete the incident report
   4. Documenting facts regarding the incident

9. Which statement is correct about formats for documentation? *(Select all that apply.)*
   1. Focus charting is a goal-oriented system.
   2. Clinical pathways are the most commonly used format now.
   3. Charting by exception documents those conditions, interventions, or outcomes outside the norm.
   4. Standardized care plans are not cost effective.
   5. EHR systems allow for patient data to be shared for collaboration of care.
10. Which statement is a recommended guideline for charting?
    1. Documentation should be lengthy and detailed.
    2. Content that suggests a risk situation should be included.
    3. One should skip lines between charting entries.
    4. The patient's name and identification number should be on all documents.
11. Which statement is a safe principle of computerized charting?
    1. It is acceptable to chart in advance of care being given.
    2. Each unit or department has its own password.
    3. There is no room for mistakes in computerized charting.
    4. Do not leave patient information displayed on the monitor.
12. Which accreditation agency specifies guidelines for documentation?
    1. The Joint Commission (TJC)
    2. American Nurses Association
    3. National League of Nursing
    4. American Academy of Colleges of Nursing
13. What is the primary purpose of Title II of the Health Insurance Portability and Accountability Act (HIPAA)?
    1. Ensure proper documentation in patient's medical records
    2. Maintain privacy and confidentiality of patient's health information
    3. Regulate the availability and range of group insurance plans
    4. Limit restrictions on insurance coverage based on preexisting conditions
14. Which statement is correct about abbreviations? *(Select all that apply.)*
    1. The nurse should be aware of any abbreviations on the "do not use" list.
    2. Creating abbreviations saves time for the reader.
    3. Abbreviating drug names and dosages helps reduce medication errors.
    4. When in doubt, the nurse should use the complete word and not the abbreviation.
    5. The nurse should include medical abbreviations on discharge instructions.
15. The nurse documents in the patient record, "0830 patient appears to be in severe pain and refuses to ambulate. Blood pressure and pulse are elevated, physician notified, and analgesic administered as ordered with adequate relief. J. Doe RN." Which statement about the documentation is most accurate?
    1. The documentation is inadequate because the pain is not described on a scale of 1 to 10.
    2. The documentation is good because it shows immediate responsiveness to the problem.
    3. The documentation is acceptable because it includes assessment, intervention, and evaluation.
    4. The documentation is unacceptable because it is vague, nondescriptive data without supportive data.
16. The nurse works in a facility that uses narrative charting for nurse's notes. Identify which documentation is an example of narrative charting. *(Select all that apply.)*
    1. "Patient alert and oriented ×3, PERRLA, hand grips strong and equal."
    2. "S—The patient complains of pain in the lower back, 6 out of 10."
    3. "Patient ambulated 60 ft in the hall, unassisted with steady gait. Currently resting in chair with no complaints."
    4. "Problem #1—Elevated blood glucose. Plan—Measure patient's blood glucose with finger stick method before meals and at bed time."
    5. "Patient asking for pain medication for incisional pain 7/10. Hydrocodone 10–325, 2 tablets administered by mouth while patient was eating lunch. Patient resting in bed with side rails up × 2, and call light in reach."
17. In most states, patients can gain access to their medical records by which means?
    1. Asking the nursing staff to allow them to view each entry in the record
    2. Submitting a written request to the facility to view the record
    3. Requesting the state board of health to allow access to the record
    4. Asking the staff for copies of their records
18. The charge nurse in a long-term care facility has been asked by the facility administrator to be sure that the staff documents in a way that will help ensure appropriate reimbursement for services provided. The charge nurse should instruct the staff to chart using what system as a guide?
    1. Minimum data sets (MDS)
    2. Charting by exception (CBE)
    3. DARE (*d*ata, *a*ction, *r*esponse, *e*ducation)
    4. Problem-oriented medical record (POMR)
19. An elderly patient with pneumonia is in an acute care hospital. Medicare will pay for 4 days of care in the facility. What prospective payment system is responsible for determining this reimbursement?
    1. Evaluation of nursing documentation
    2. Submission of appropriate physician progress notes
    3. Clinical (critical) pathways
    4. Diagnosis-related groups (DRGs)

4 Communication

http://evolve.elsevier.com/Cooper/foundationsadult/

Objectives

1. Recognize that communication is inherent in every nurse-patient interaction.
2. Discuss the concepts of verbal and nonverbal communication.
3. Discuss the impact of nonverbal communication.
4. Recognize assertive communication as the most appropriate communication style.
5. Use various therapeutic communication techniques.
6. Identify various factors that have the potential to affect communication.
7. Discuss potential barriers to communication.
8. Recognize trust as the foundation for all effective interaction.
9. Apply the nursing process to patients experiencing difficulty with verbally communicating.
10. Apply therapeutic communication techniques to patients with special communication needs.

Key Terms

active listening (p. 65)
aggressive communication (p. 63)
altered cognition (p. 73)
assertive communication (p. 63)
assertiveness (p. 63)
clarifying (p. 69)
closed posture (p. 62)
closed question (p. 67)
communication (kŏ-MYŪ-nĭ-KĀ-shŭn, p. 60)
connotative meaning (kŏn-nō-TĀ-tĭv, p. 61)
denotative meaning (dĭ-nō-TĀ-tĭv, p. 61)
expressive aphasia (ă-FĀ-zhă, p. 76)
focusing (p. 69)
gestures (p. 62)
jargon (JĂR-gŏn, p. 61)
minimal encouragement (p. 66)
nontherapeutic communication (nŏn-thĕr-ă-PYŪ-tĭk, p. 64)
nonverbal communication (p. 61)
one-way communication (p. 61)
open posture (p. 62)
open-ended question (p. 68)
paraphrasing (p. 69)
passive listening (p. 65)
posture (p. 62)
receive, receiver (p. 60)
receptive aphasia (p. 76)
reflecting (p. 69)
restating (p. 69)
send, sender (p. 60)
therapeutic communication (p. 64)
two-way communication (p. 61)
unassertive communication (p. 64)
verbal communication (p. 61)

Communication is one of the most important aspects of care in nursing. Some form of communication occurs each time an interaction takes place. Interactions occur between two parties, such as the nurse and the patient or the nurse and a family member, a physician, or a coworker, or other combinations. Remember that the message intended is not always the message received. The licensed practical/licensed vocational nurse (LPN/LVN) should aways strive to communicate effectively and minimize miscommunication. This chapter explores various aspects of communication.

Communication can be described simply as the exchange of information. The way in which information is exchanged may vary greatly. Communication takes verbal and nonverbal forms and conveys a variety of messages (e.g., information, emotions, humor, acceptance, rejection). Many variables influence the effect of the message.

OVERVIEW OF COMMUNICATION

For communication to occur, a sender and a receiver of a message are necessary. The **sender** is the one who conveys the message, whereas the **receiver** is the person or people to whom the message is conveyed. The individual who receives the message is sometimes the intended receiver and sometimes an unintended receiver. Consider the following scenario:

> The night nurse, reporting to the day nurse outside Ms. B.'s room: "Ms. B. was on her call light all night. She's a real complainer!"
>
> Ms. B overhears the exchange.

The day nurse is the intended receiver, or the one with whom the night nurse means to communicate regarding Ms. B.'s behavior. Because Ms. B. also hears the statement, she becomes an unintended receiver. Consider the possible effect of this message on the relationship between Ms. B. and the night nurse. Negative consequences for the relationship between Ms. B. and the day nurse are another possible outcome, if Ms. B. believes that the day nurse shares the night nurse's view of her.

Communication can be one-way or two-way; which type of communication actually occurs depends partly on the roles of the people in the interaction. One-way communication is highly structured; the sender is in control and expects and gets little response from the receiver. A lecture to a large audience is an example of one-way communication. **One-way communication** is of limited use in the nurse-patient relationship. **Two-way communication** requires that the sender and the receiver participate in the interaction. It allows for exchange between the nurse and the patient, and its purpose is to meet the needs of the nurse and the patient and to establish a trusting relationship. It is important to always strive to seek and accept the patient's input and feedback rather than simply talk to the patient.

VERBAL COMMUNICATION

Verbal communication involves the use of spoken or written words or symbols. It may seem that there is little room for misunderstanding or misinterpretation of the intended message as long as the receiver understands the words and symbols being used. Frequently this is not the case. Sometimes words have very different meanings, or connotations, for different people. The **connotative meaning** of a word is subjective and reflects the individual's perception or interpretation. There is a potential for miscommunication that lies in such subjective variation. Take, for example, the word *stable*. If the family members are informed that their loved one's condition is stable, they perhaps may understand that for the moment, the patient's condition is not deteriorating. On the other hand, they may hear a different message, not the one that was intended: the patient is doing well and is out of danger.

Denotative meaning refers to the commonly accepted definition of a particular word. For example, the word *telephone* means the same thing to anyone who is familiar with the English language. The key word here is *familiar*. No guarantee exists that both parties know the word or assign the same definition to it. Consider the situation in which the nurse asks the patient when he last voided or had a stool. Although these terms and phrasing are familiar to health care professionals, the patient may have no idea that the nurse is asking when he last urinated or had a bowel movement. This is an example of the nurse using hospital jargon. **Jargon** is commonplace "language" or terminology unique to people in a particular work setting, such as a hospital, or to a specific type of work, such as nursing. It is as though the nurse and the patient have different dictionaries for what is thought to be a shared language. The nurse must be cautious of the terminology used when communicating with patients.

NONVERBAL COMMUNICATION

Messages transmitted without the use of words (either oral or written) constitute **nonverbal communication.** Nonverbal cues include tone and rate of voice, volume of speech, eye contact, physical appearance, and use of touch (Table 4.1). Some degree of nonverbal communication usually accompanies verbal communication.

Voice

Aspects of the voice affect nonverbal messages, including tone, volume, and the rate of speech. Characteristics of people's voices vary depending on their emotions, familiarity with a situation, confidence, and geographic and cultural influences. Meaning cannot be interpreted accurately on the basis of tone, rate, and volume alone. For example, a high-pitched, loud voice and rapid speech may indicate that an individual is frightened, but people also speak that way out of excitement or enthusiasm. In fact, some people always tend to use this speech pattern, and thus no conclusions are appropriate at all. The nurse should consider the voice characteristics in the context of the situation as a whole so that interpretation of the message is accurate.

Eye Contact

Eye contact is responsible for much communication and miscommunication. Generally, eye contact communicates an intention to interact. However, the nature of the interaction and the results of eye contact are not necessarily always positive. Extended eye contact sometimes implies aggression and arouses anxiety. On the other hand, the person who maintains eye contact for 2 to 6 seconds during an interaction helps involve the other person in what is said without being threatening or intimidating. An absence of eye contact communicates many things: shyness, lack of confidence, disinterest, embarrassment, or hurt, or in contrast, deference and respect. Sensitivity to eye contact of each communication partner helps with perceiving what actually is occurring in an interaction. Culture significantly affects how people interpret eye contact. Most Americans view eye contact in a positive manner, whereas some cultures may view eye contact differently. Some people of Middle Eastern, Latin American, Asian, and Native North American

Table 4.1 Nonverbal Cues

ATTRIBUTE OR BEHAVIOR EXHIBITED BY SENDER (CUE)	COMPONENTS	POSSIBLE INTERPRETATION OR PERCEPTION BY RECEIVER
Voice	Tone, volume, pitch, rate of speech	Fear, excitement, enthusiasm, stress, anger, comfort, concern, confidence, calm
Eye contact	Extended (longer than 6 s)	Aggression, intimidation, disrespect
	Brief but direct (2–6 s)	Interest, respect, caring
	Absent or fleeting	Shyness, lack of confidence, low self-esteem, disinterest, anxiety, fear, uneasiness, hurriedness, or deference or respect (culture-specific)
Physical appearance	Size, color of skin, dress, grooming, body carriage, age, gender	Professional or nonprofessional, trust or distrust, respect or disrespect, comfort or intimidation, interest or disinterest, competence or incompetence
Gestures	Distinct movements of hands, head, body	Emphasis, clarification, pleasure, helpfulness, anger, threat, disrespect
Posture	*Open:* Relaxed stance, facing receiver, uncrossed arms and legs, slight shift toward receiver, direct eye contact, smile	Warmth, acceptance, caring
	Closed: Formal, distant stance; arms and possibly legs tightly crossed	Disinterest, coldness, nonacceptance, authority, control, intimidation, condescension

descent may view eye contact as impolite, aggressive, or improper (Maier-Lorentz, 2008; Scudder, 2014).

Physical Appearance

The physical appearance of the participants in an interaction has the potential to greatly influence the perceptions they form of each other. Physical appearance includes attributes of size, color of skin, dress, grooming, posture, and facial expression. Although often these attributes have absolutely nothing to do with any messages the sender intends to convey, they can have a major impact on the receiver's interpretation. Consider, for example, the patient with a personal bias against individuals with numerous tattoos or body piercings. Although the tattoos and piercings have no impact on the competency of the nurse, the patient with a bias against these may have difficulty establishing a trusting and therapeutic relationship with a nurse who has tattoos or piercings.

A professional appearance conveys self-respect and competence. How the nurse chooses to dress while on duty sends a strong message to the patient. The LPN/LVN who chooses to wear wrinkled uniforms or soiled shoes may risk sending the message that the patient is not worth the time it would take for the nurse to look professional. This may lead the patient to view the nurse as uncaring or incompetent.

Many health care facilities have adopted specific dress codes to convey professionalism in the workplace. Scrubs of one design or color often are worn by specific personnel as a means of communicating to the patient the role of that professional. In some facilities, the nurse may wear one color of scrubs, and the unlicensed assistive personnel (UAP) may wear another. Jewelry, piercings, tattoos, and hair also may be addressed in dress codes within health care facilities.

Gestures. **Gestures** are movements people use to emphasize the idea they are attempting to communicate. Gestures also play a useful role in clarifying. A patient is often better able to express where pain is on the body by pointing to a particular area than trying to describe it in words. However, many gestures affect communication negatively. For example, a nurse who frequently looks at a watch while interviewing a patient conveys disinterest in what the patient is saying or that the nurse has a limited amount of time to spend with the patient. Also, gestures often have different meanings from individual to individual and from culture to culture. It is essential to be constantly aware of gestures the participants use during interactions and to consider the implication of gestures used.

Posture. The way that an individual sits, stands, and moves is called **posture.** Posture has the potential to convey warmth and acceptance or distance and disinterest. A person is considered to display an **open posture** when taking a relaxed stance with uncrossed arms and legs while facing the other individual. A slight shift in body position toward an individual, a smile, and direct eye contact are consistent with open posturing and convey warmth and caring (Balzer Riley, 2017). **Closed posture** is a more formal, distant stance, generally with the arms, and possibly the legs, tightly crossed. A person often interprets closed posture as disinterest, coldness, and even nonacceptance. Standing at the bedside looking

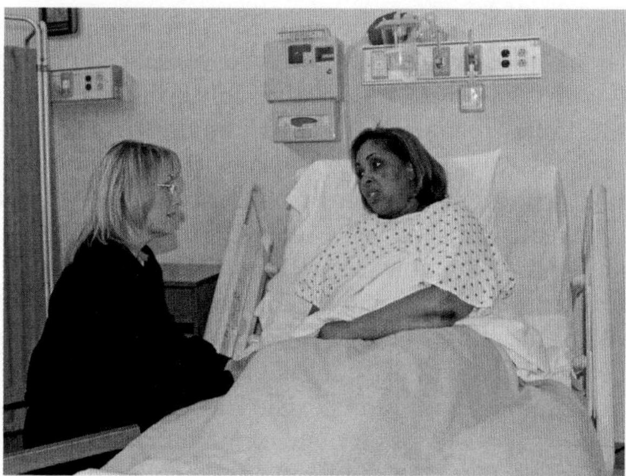

Fig. 4.1 Whenever possible, place yourself level with the patient.

down at the patient in the bed places the nurse in a position of authority and control. The patient is likely to experience this as intimidating and condescending. Whenever possible, the nurse should be at the same level as the patient during conversations; this is especially important with pediatric patients. Sitting at the bedside in a relaxed and open posture is one example (Fig. 4.1).

Consistency of Verbal and Nonverbal Communication

No definitive studies prove what percentage of communication is verbal or nonverbal; however, most people and communication experts believe that nonverbal communication is often more accurate and makes up the largest percentage of our communication. Nonverbal communication is very powerful. If nonverbal cues are inconsistent or incongruent with the verbal message, the nonverbal message is most likely the one received. At the very least, this incongruence frequently is the cause of misinterpretation and misunderstanding. The following scenario is an example of incongruence between what the nurse is stating and what she is demonstrating.

> Nurse M. has been having a very busy morning. While trying to get Ms. D. ready to go to surgery, Nurse M. has been interrupted several times by staff members asking for help or advice. Now Mr. R., a patient also assigned to Nurse M., has put on his call light. As she enters Mr. R.'s room in an obvious hurry, Mr. R. states, "I'm very sorry to bother you, but could you refill my water pitcher?" Nurse M. grabs the pitcher from the bedside stand and takes it to the sink, while muttering through tight lips, "It's no bother, Mr. R. I'm happy to do it!"

The words Nurse M. used are appropriate. However, Nurse M.'s nonverbal cues are "speaking" much louder than her words, and Mr. R. is sure to pick up on her anger and frustration from her posture, tone of voice, and facial expression. How is it possible for him to really believe that he has not been a bother and that Nurse M. is "happy" to help him?

Box 4.1 Assertive Communication for Nurses

Communicating assertively means:
- Being able to express your needs while being aware of others' needs
- Being confident in communicating directly and honestly
- Feeling comfortable and in control of anxiety, tenseness, shyness, or fear
- Honoring the fact that you and the other person have rights

An assertive nurse:
- Appears self-confident and composed
- Ensures that verbal and nonverbal communication is congruent
- Is unapologetic
- Maintains eye contact
- Speaks firmly and with a positive attitude
- Speaks genuinely, without sarcasm
- Takes initiative to guide situations
- Uses clear, concise speech

Modified from Balzer Riley J: *Communication in nursing*, ed 8, St. Louis, 2017, Mosby.

STYLES OF COMMUNICATION

The manner, or style, in which a message is communicated greatly affects the mood and the overall outcome of an interaction. Every time an interaction occurs between a nurse and a patient the tone is set for the nurse-patient relationship. The style of communication the nurse demonstrates is often what makes the difference between a positive or negative interaction.

ASSERTIVE COMMUNICATION

Assertiveness is one's ability to confidently and comfortably express thoughts and feelings while still respecting the legitimate rights of the patient. An **assertive communication** style is interaction that considers the feelings and needs of the patient yet honors the nurse's rights as an individual (Box 4.1). It makes interactions more even and has positive benefits for all involved (Balzer Riley, 2017).

AGGRESSIVE COMMUNICATION

Aggressive communication occurs when an individual interacts with another in an overpowering and forceful manner to meet one's own personal needs at the expense of the other. Aggressive communication is destructive and nontherapeutic. In the situation just described, Nurse M. responds to Mr. R. in an aggressive manner. Neither party benefits from such an interaction. After the fact, Nurse M. most likely feels guilty and disrespectful for having responded to Mr. R. in this harsh manner, and Mr. R. undoubtedly feels humiliated and unworthy.

UNASSERTIVE COMMUNICATION

Another choice for Nurse M., although not a favorable one, would have been to respond unambiguously to Mr. R. but in an **unassertive communication** style. In this style, the nurse agrees to do what the patient requests, even though doing so creates additional problems for the nurse. Use of this style sacrifices one's legitimate personal rights to the needs of the patient, and there is a price to pay: resentment.

Imagine that Nurse M. had responded like this to Mr. R.'s request to have his water pitcher refilled:

> "Well, I'm really busy right now, but … well, I guess I can do it if I hurry. I just don't know how I'm ever going to get my other patient ready for surgery in time. Here, give me your pitcher."

This interaction is much like the previous one, although more open. The problem with this interaction is that no one really benefits from the interaction. Mr. R. now has fresh water but probably feels like he has imposed on the nurse unduly. Perhaps he even feels angry, thinking that his needs are not as important as those of another patient. Nurse M. now is even further behind than before and is likely to feel resentment toward Mr. R. and as guilty or ashamed as before for giving Mr. R. the impression he is a "bother."

The most effective way for Nurse M. to address the situation is with an assertive communication style. Perhaps the interaction sounds like this:

> "Well, Mr. R., if you don't mind waiting about 10 minutes, I will be glad to fill your water pitcher with fresh ice and water. If you need it filled before that, I can ask one of the nursing assistants to fill it for you now."

With assertive communication, the needs of Nurse M. and Mr. R. can be met, with neither of them feeling unworthy, belittled, resentful, or guilty.

ESTABLISHING A THERAPEUTIC RELATIONSHIP

A therapeutic nurse-patient interaction is one in which the nurse demonstrates caring, sincerity, empathy, and trustworthiness. If the patient senses that the nurse is not being genuine in conveying these feelings, a therapeutic, trusting relationship does not develop. If the nurse appears hurried or detached from the interaction, a message is sent that the patient is not as important as the other things on the nurse's mind, which very likely leaves the patient feeling frustrated and diminished in self-worth.

Ensure that the *patient* is the focus of each interaction, not the equipment or the task. On entering a patient's room, look at and address the patient before assessing or adjusting any equipment. In addition, be diligent in following through with commitments. If you have promised to assist the patient with a bath in 15 minutes, then this commitment should be fulfilled. If this is not going to be possible, explain this to the patient and establish another mutually agreeable plan for completing the bath. Failure to follow through on commitments undermines the relationship and erodes trust.

Trust is essential to effective nurse-patient interaction. Much of the information that the patient shares with the nurse is personal and often highly sensitive. The patient must be able to trust the nurse to treat the information confidentially and share it only with those individuals who need it to provide safe and competent care for the patient. Although confidentiality is critical to maintain, certain limits exist. The nurse is obligated to report a patient's statement of intent to do self-harm or to harm others. This obligation should be made clear to all patients.

Be careful to maintain professional boundaries in nurse-patient relationships. Sharing of personal information, such as address and phone number, is not advisable. Doing so often leads to situations that the nurse is not prepared to handle.

COMMUNICATION TECHNIQUES

Communication in nursing has the potential to be therapeutic or nontherapeutic. **Therapeutic communication** is the ideal. It consists of an exchange of information that facilitates the formation of a positive nurse-patient relationship and actively involves the patient in all areas of care. In contrast, **nontherapeutic communication** usually blocks the development of a trusting and therapeutic relationship.

Specific communication techniques are used to facilitate the development of therapeutic interaction. Some techniques are verbal, and others are nonverbal. Individual nurses are more or less comfortable with the various techniques, and the LPN/LVN should choose a communication technique that fits the nurse's style and the patient's, and a given situation. The use of therapeutic communication techniques does not guarantee that therapeutic communication will occur. Therapeutic communication requires the nurse to have an awareness of the patient's feelings and the ability to respond to the patient's needs through the use of verbal and nonverbal communication skills (see the Coordinated Care box).

NONVERBAL THERAPEUTIC COMMUNICATION TECHNIQUES

Listening

Listening is an acquired skill that is vital to the nurse-patient relationship. Nurses who have mastered this skill are quiet while the patient is speaking, pay attention to not only the verbal but also the nonverbal communication of the patient, and truly focus on what the patient is saying. One of the most effective methods of therapeutic communication, listening also can be one of the most difficult to master (Table 4.2). It often feels awkward and uncomfortable at first. This nonverbal

Table 4.2 **Therapeutic Communication Techniques: Nonverbal**

NONVERBAL TECHNIQUES	BENEFITS
Active listening	Conveys interest and caring; gives patient full attention; allows feedback to verify understanding of the message
Maintaining silence (often used in conjunction with touch)	Allows time to organize thoughts and formulate an appropriate response; often conveys respect, understanding, caring, and support; allows observation of patient's nonverbal responses
Minimal encouragement by nodding occasionally and maintaining eye contact (usually also involves brief verbal comments; e.g., "Yes, go on" or "Then what happened?")	Communicates to the patient that the nurse is interested and wants to hear more
Touch	Often conveys warmth, caring, comfort, support, and understanding
Conveying acceptance (usually also involves a verbal component)	Demonstrates acceptance of patient's rights to current beliefs and practices without condoning them; nonjudgmental, therefore encourages honesty and openness on the part of the patient; provides an opportunity to bring about change in health behaviors while still maintaining the patient's personal integrity

Coordinated Care

Supervision

Communication Skills

- Nurses who have many years of education and experience continue to develop and improve effective communication skills, particularly cross-cultural communication.
- New and inexperienced unlicensed assistive personnel (UAP) often need guidance to make their communication skills more effective.
- It is a responsibility of the nurse to monitor how effective the UAP are when communicating with patients and ancillary personnel from other departments such as x-ray, laboratory, and dietary departments.
- Two methods to help UAP become better communicators are role modeling effective communication techniques and in-service education programs.

communication technique is a behavior that conveys interest and caring toward the patient. It is not always the result that counts the most: it is possible to *hear* without *listening*.

Listening is sometimes active and sometimes passive. **Active listening** requires full attention to what the patient is saying. The nurse hears the message, interprets its meaning, and gives the patient feedback, indicating understanding of the message. The patient has an opportunity to validate that the message was received or not received as intended.

In **passive listening,** listening to the speaker is indicated either nonverbally through eye contact and nodding, or verbally through encouraging phrases such as "Uh-huh" and "I see" (Balzer Riley, 2017). Although it is not possible for the patient to be sure that the nurse has received or understood the message accurately, passive listening lets the patient know that the nurse is interested and being attentive to what is being said by the patient. The nurse's level of confidence affects the ability to listen attentively. Novice nurses often are "thinking ahead" to the most appropriate response to the patient and, by so doing, miss what the patient really is trying to communicate. As experience and confidence are attained, the LPN/LVN gains the capacity to give full attention to the patient's message, thus allowing for more appropriate intervention.

Silence

Maintaining silence is an extremely effective, yet sometimes difficult, therapeutic communication technique. In American society, silence often feels awkward, which leads to the desire to interrupt silence by making conversation. This impulse does not always allow the people involved in an interaction time to organize their thoughts sufficiently to communicate their needs or response. A person commonly needs several seconds after hearing a verbal message to interpret what has been stated and to formulate the most appropriate response. Unfortunately, the receiver often does not get this amount of time before a response is necessary. In many cases, the sender becomes uncomfortable with the silence and begins speaking again before the receiver has had an opportunity to formulate a response.

The ability to use silence effectively requires skill and timing. Prolonged silence is often difficult to maintain but is vital to an interaction. Silence conveys support, compassion, and caring. Holding the patient's hand or placing one's hand on the shoulder of a patient or loved one when combined with silence conveys caring and concern. An example of effective use of silence is when a patient dies. The nurse can communicate support and compassion by remaining with the family after relaying the news to them. Allowing family members time to express their feelings while remaining silent and using therapeutic touch communicates that the nurse cares about the family without trying to talk away the situation.

In some cases, it is helpful for nurses to let patients know that they do not have to speak and to convey that they are willing to just sit and wait until patients feel ready to respond. However, the nurse's nonverbal cues must be congruent with this willingness to wait. Actions such as fidgeting, writing, and looking at one's watch communicate the opposite message. Therapeutic silence requires practice to master the skill in a way that it becomes easy and natural.

Touch

Touch is another form of nonverbal communication that is inherent in the practice of nursing. Nearly every nursing intervention for the purpose of providing physical care calls for touch. When a nurse provides nursing care, touch is often highly personal or intimate (e.g., giving a bed bath, assisting a patient on or off a bedpan, inserting a urinary catheter). Because of the intimate nature of touch in the nursing context, it must be used with great discretion to fit into sociocultural norms and guidelines. Some nurses are uncomfortable with touch because of a fear of its seeming inappropriate or being misinterpreted. When the nurse is comfortable with physical contact with a patient, touch has the potential for conveying warmth, caring, support, and understanding (Fig. 4.2). For the nurse to convey warmth, the nature of touch must be sincere and genuine. However, if the nurse is not comfortable with touch, or the nurse touches the patient in a manner that communicates hesitancy or reluctance, a very strong negative message, such as rejection, is sent to the patient.

Interpretation of touch depends on several factors, such as the duration and intensity of the contact; the body part touched; the culture, gender, and age of the patient and the nurse; the environment; and the stage of development of the relationship. Depending on the patient's culture, holding the hand of a patient who does not speak English during a difficult procedure may be more effective and comforting than efforts to communicate verbally. A small child who is frightened by the hospital environment often responds better to being cuddled than to a verbal explanation of what is taking place. Older adult patients frequently reach out to touch the person caring for them. Many patients who are sad find a warm embrace to be very comforting. A back rub for the patient who is in pain often promotes relaxation and eases the pain. However, because of sociocultural differences, the nurse must always be alert to and aware of the possible variations in interpretation of touch. When used appropriately, touch has powerful potential as a communication technique.

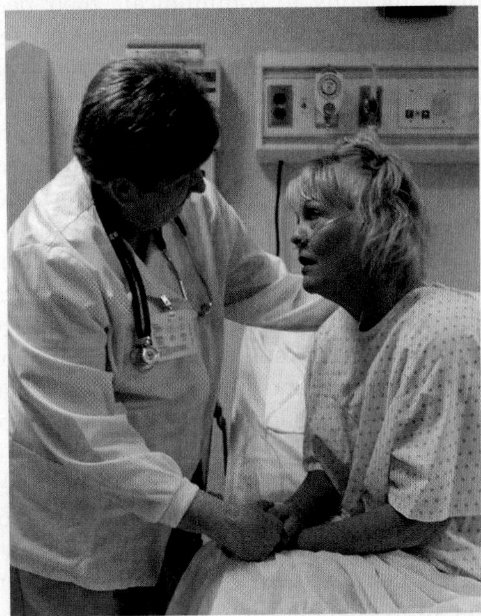

Fig. 4.2 Touch has the potential to communicate caring and comfort.

VERBAL THERAPEUTIC COMMUNICATION TECHNIQUES

Conveying Acceptance

Many issues in the nurse-patient relationship are highly personal. Some patients are hesitant to give the nurse complete information, particularly as it relates to values, beliefs, lifestyles, and practices. Often this reluctance has to do with a fear of disapproval from the nurse in regard to the patient's values, beliefs, or practices, or even rejection of the individual as a person.

The nurse's acceptance and willingness to listen and respond to what a patient is saying without passing judgment on the patient is key to the development of a therapeutic nurse-patient relationship. It is likely that, given variances in sociocultural influences (e.g., economic status, religion, upbringing, cultural background, and age), a patient's values, beliefs, and practices will differ from that of the nurse. The nurse must be cognizant of conveying disapproval or communicating disapproval nonverbally through gestures or facial expressions.

Minimal encouragement is a subtle therapeutic technique that communicates to the patient that the nurse is interested and wants to hear more. It indicates acceptance of the patient as a person. It usually involves nonverbal cues, such as maintaining appropriate eye contact, nodding occasionally, and verbal comments such as "Yes, go on" to encourage the patient to continue.

The nurse may be confronted with a patient whose practices are harmful to a healthy lifestyle. Acceptance of the patient and the lifestyle is not synonymous with approving of the lifestyle choices. The challenge for the nurse is to facilitate changes in the patient's health behaviors while helping the patient to maintain personal integrity. Keep in mind that the nurse and the patient have the right to their own beliefs. The nurse can demonstrate acceptance of the patient's right to his or her present beliefs and practices without condoning them. The next step is to communicate a healthier alternative to the present behavior and assist patients in initiating the new behavior if they choose to make these practices a part of their life.

Questioning: Closed

Much of the information gathered by the nurse about a patient comes from questioning the patient directly. The type of information sought determines what type of questioning is most appropriate (Table 4.3). A **closed question** is focused and seeks a particular answer. For example, when interviewing a newly admitted patient with diabetes, the nurse asks, "What is your insulin dosage in the morning?" A specific question with a specific answer, it is typical of closed questions, which generally require only one or two words in response. This direct type of questioning is useful if this is the

Table 4.3 Therapeutic Communication Techniques: Verbal

VERBAL TECHNIQUES	BENEFITS	EXAMPLES
Closed Questioning		
Focused and seeks a particular answer; usually requires and elicits only a "yes" or "no" or one-word to two-word answer	Provides a very specific answer to a very specific question	"How old are you?" "How many children do you have?" "Have you had a tetanus shot in the past 5 years?"
Open-Ended Questioning		
Does not require a specific answer and cannot be answered by "yes," "no," or a one-word response; usually begins with words such as "how," "what," "can you tell me about," "in what way"	Allows the patient to elaborate freely; useful in assessing feelings; elicits the patient's thoughts without influencing the response	"How do you feel about having surgery tomorrow?" "What concerns do you have about going home?" "How are these symptoms different from the last time you were ill?"
Restating		
Repeating to the patient what the nurse believes to be the main point that the patient is trying to communicate; tone of voice rises slightly at the end of the phrase as if asking a question	Lets the patient know whether the nurse heard what was said; encourages the patient to offer additional information	*Patient:* "I'm not sure how I will manage the housework when I get home. My husband will expect me to do the cooking and cleaning just like always, and I don't think I'll be able to do it so soon after my surgery." *Nurse:* "Your husband will expect you to do the cooking and cleaning when you get home?" *Patient:* "Yes. I don't think he understands how difficult this surgery has been for me, and how weak and tired I feel."
Paraphrasing		
Restatement of the patient's message in the nurse's own words	Verifies that the nurse's interpretation of the message is correct	*Patient:* "I wish I was having a general anesthetic instead of a spinal. My neighbor had a relative who had a spinal anesthetic and never walked again." *Nurse:* "You are concerned that you might have complications from the spinal anesthetic?" *Patient:* "I sure am." *Nurse:* "I can have the anesthesiologist come talk to you some more about the risks and benefits of a spinal anesthetic. Would that be helpful?" *Patient:* "Oh, yes. Would you do that, please?"
Clarifying		
Seeks to understand the patient's message by asking for more information or for elaboration on a point; expressed as a question or statement followed by a restatement or paraphrasing of part of the patient's message	Allows the patient to verify that the message received is accurate; particularly useful when the message is ambiguous or not easily understood	*Nurse:* "How are you getting along with the new blood pressure medication?" *Patient:* "Well, the doctor told me to take one every day, but they are so darned expensive, I've only been taking them every other day. It seems to be working out okay." *Nurse:* "Let me make sure I understand this correctly. The cost of the medication is keeping you from being able to take it each day?" *Patient:* "Yes, I just can't afford it on my fixed income."

Continued

Table 4.3 Therapeutic Communication Techniques: Verbal—cont'd

VERBAL TECHNIQUES	BENEFITS	EXAMPLES
Focusing		
The nurse encourages the patient to select one topic over another as the primary focus of discussion	Allows the nurse to gather more specific information when the patient's message is too vague; focuses on specific data	*Patient:* "Don't let them give me any morphine. The last time they gave me that I almost died!" *Nurse:* "Will you please tell me, as accurately as you can, what you experienced the last time you were given morphine?"
Reflecting		
Assists the patient to reflect on feelings and thoughts rather than seeking answers and advice from another	Promotes independent decision making; allows the patient to see that her or his ideas and thoughts are important	*Patient:* "Sometimes I think my family is falling apart. All we ever do is fight and argue. My kids don't take responsibility for themselves, much less help out around the house. This makes my husband furious, and we all end up in a shouting match with everyone feeling miserable. What should I do? Sometimes I just feel like walking out." *Nurse:* "What do you think you should do?" *Patient:* "I don't know. I would like for us to go to counseling, but I'm afraid my husband won't hear of it." *Nurse:* "Have you discussed this with him?" *Patient:* "No. I suppose that is where I need to start."
Stating Observations		
The nurse makes observations of the patient during an interaction and communicates these observations back to the patient	Allows for clarification of the intended message when verbal cues do not match nonverbal cues; allows for more accurate interpretation of patient concerns	(Ms. C. denies having any concerns about her upcoming hysterectomy. However, the nurse notes that Ms. C.'s posture and facial expression are tense, her eye contact is brief and darting, and she is fidgeting about in bed. The nurse shares these observations with Ms. C.) *Nurse:* "Ms. C., you seem to understand the information about your surgery that we have discussed, but you still seem to be quite tense and anxious. Can you tell me what is bothering you?" *Patient:* "Well, it's just that my husband and I always wanted to have one more child and now that will never happen. It all seems so final."
Offering Information		
The nurse provides the patient with relevant data and asks for feedback to determine the patient's level of understanding	Useful for patient teaching; promotes informed decision making	Preoperative teaching Diabetes education Discharge instruction
Summarizing		
Concise review of main ideas from a discussion	Focuses on key issues and allows for additional information that was perhaps omitted; particularly useful when interaction has been lengthy or has covered several topics	"We've covered a lot of information in the past few minutes. The main things to keep in mind are ____________________." (Review the primary topics covered in the interaction.)

type of information desired. However, if the LPN/LVN wants the patient to give more details on a subject, an open-ended question is a more effective communication technique.

Questioning: Open-Ended

Open-ended questions do not require a specific response and allow the patient to elaborate freely on a subject when replying. This type of question is useful in assessing the patient's feelings. Consider the different responses possible for a patient who is asked the following questions:

Closed: "Mr. A., are you worried about your scheduled surgery?"

Open-ended: "How you are feeling about having surgery tomorrow, Mr. A.?"

The closed question requires only a yes or no answer and probably elicits a very short response. The open-ended question invites Mr. A. to elaborate in whatever direction he chooses with regard to his feelings about having surgery. Given the opportunity to explore his feelings, Mr. A. may reveal information about other aspects of his life or questions and concerns he may have regarding his upcoming surgery. Open-ended questions also convey the message that the nurse is interested in the patient as an individual, not just in obtaining information.

Restating

When using the technique of **restating,** the nurse repeats to the patient what is believed to be the main point that the patient is trying to convey. It is another way of letting the patient know that the nurse is listening. Simply by repeating the central theme of the patient's comments, the nurse encourages the patient to provide more information. If the nurse also slightly raises the tone of his or her voice at the end of the restatement, the patient probably will take this as a signal that the nurse is interested in hearing more information.

Restating often feels awkward to the nurse who is not experienced in using this technique. Avoid overuse of this technique, because this sounds as though you are "parroting" what the patient is saying. Parroting can sound like a planned response and often is annoying to the patient. When used selectively, restating is a valuable technique to encourage the patient to offer helpful information.

Paraphrasing

Although **paraphrasing** bears some similarity to restating, it differs in intent. Paraphrasing is the restatement of the patient's message in the nurse's own words in an attempt to verify that the nurse has interpreted the patient's message correctly.

Clarifying

Clarifying takes restating and paraphrasing a step further and is useful when the patient's message is incomplete or confusing or does not go deeply enough into the area being explored. When clarifying, the LPN/LVN suggests to the patient some of his or her own ideas about what the patient is trying to communicate in a manner that asks the patient to verify that the nurse's understanding of the message is accurate. Clarifying prevents misinterpretation of the patient's comments.

Focusing

The technique of **focusing** also is used when more specific information is needed to understand the patient's message accurately. The patient may be providing the nurse with important information, but if the message is too vague or strays from the topic being discussed, it is difficult for the nurse to identify the actual message.

Reflecting

Reflecting is like restating, but it involves feelings and thoughts more than facts. This therapeutic technique is used to assist patients to explore their own feelings, often about a choice that lies before them, rather than seeking answers or advice from someone else, such as the nurse. The nurse allows for the expression of the patient's feelings but, rather than offering advice, reflects the thoughts back to the patient. This empowers the patient to verbalize a possible solution and at the same time places the patient in a position of control and promotes self-esteem and autonomy.

Reflecting allows patients to see that their ideas and thoughts are important and have worth. Patients gain confidence in their own decision making instead of feeling the need to rely on others for decision making.

Stating Observations

While interacting with a patient, the nurse also is observing the patient. Communicating the nurse's observations to the patient is called *stating observations* and is often useful in validating the accuracy of observations. This technique can be especially helpful when the patient's verbal message does not seem to match the nonverbal behaviors witnessed by the nurse. With description of the patient's observed behavior, feedback is provided, and the patient is invited to verify that the message received was the one the patient intended to send. Clarification of the confusion between verbal and nonverbal cues allows the nurse to address the patient's concerns more effectively.

Offering Information

Much of the communicating that the nurse does takes the form of *offering information.* Preparing a patient for what to expect before, during, and after an invasive diagnostic procedure is one example of how the nurse uses this communication technique. Discharge teaching to prepare the patient for self-care at home is another example. The nurse should use the patient's feedback to determine whether the information given has been understood. Offering information is not the same as giving advice. Giving advice takes decision making away from the patient and puts the nurse-patient relationship at risk.

Summarizing

Summarizing means providing a review of the main points covered in an interaction. This technique is used most often after a lengthy interaction or one that has covered several issues (e.g., at the end of a patient teaching session). It helps the patient to separate the essential information from the "nice to know" information and gives a sense of closure to the session.

Use of Humor

The power of humor during interactions with patients should not be underestimated as an effective

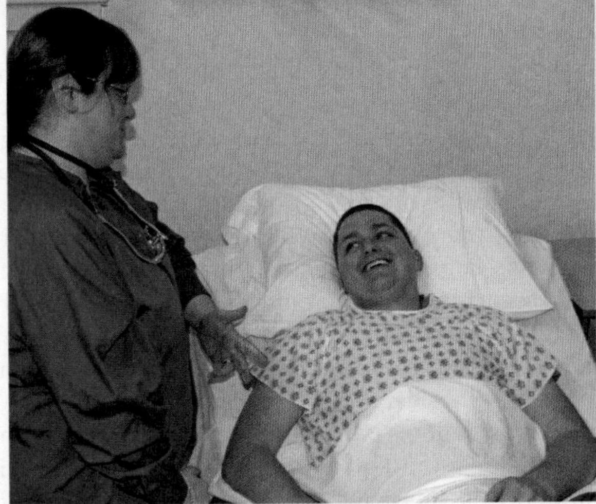

Fig. 4.3 Help reduce stress and support a therapeutic relationship by sharing a joke or laughing with patients.

communication tool. Old (2012) notes that laughter provides a positive psychological and physiologic effect on the body by increasing catecholamine levels, relaxing smooth muscles, and stimulating the release of endorphins and serotonin. These responses lead to enhanced feelings of well-being and can help reduce anxiety, pain, and the level of stress hormones (Fig. 4.3).

Humor can help put the nurse and the patient at ease. However, it is important for the nurse to know when humor is appropriate and when it is inappropriate. It is never appropriate to laugh *at* a patient; it is only appropriate to laugh *with* a patient. The timing and context of humor are also important. In some serious situations, humor is not appropriate, such as when a patient has just received a serious diagnosis or when a patient is trying to convey thoughts or feelings. In general, get to know the patient before using humor. Correct perception of the patient and situation allows you to take cues from the patient or the patient's significant others to predict how the patient may respond to humor. In some situations, remember to be especially cautious with the use of humor (e.g., when the patient is from a different culture or background or is confused or cognitively impaired). Another pitfall to watch out for is use of humor to avoid confronting or dealing with issues. Rather than allowing yourself or the patient to resort to humor to mask fears and other difficult emotions, try to find a more appropriate technique that helps the patient communicate effectively. Humor is certainly effective and therapeutic in some situations, but it becomes a hindrance, and potentially destructive, if it is the only tool used by the nurse.

FACTORS THAT AFFECT COMMUNICATION

POSTURING AND POSITIONING

Where and how the nurse sits or stands conveys a message to the patient. Standing at the bedside while the patient lies in the bed sends the message that the LPN/LVN has power and the patient does not. The crossing of arms over the chest may convey a lack of openness to the patient. Assuming a position of total relaxation, such as leaning back into the chair, possibly even slouching, sends a message of disinterest.

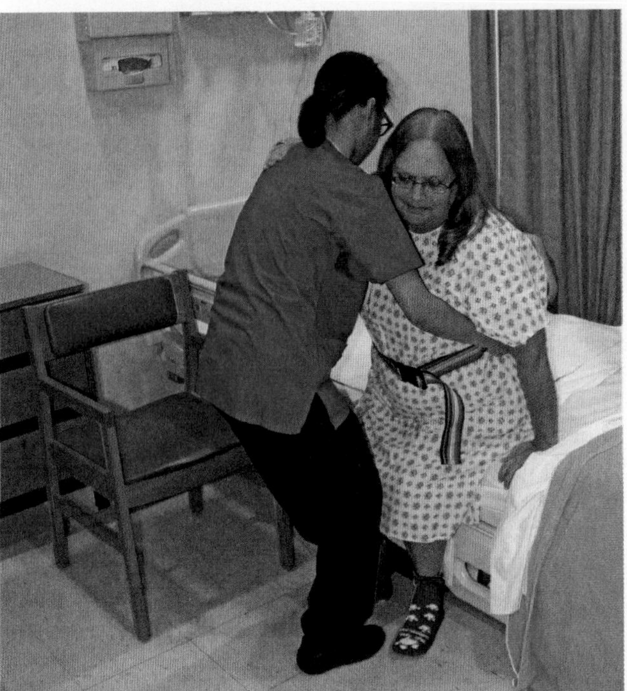

Fig. 4.4 Much of the nursing care provided to a patient occurs in the intimate space.

The most therapeutic posture and positioning is the same position and level as the patient, or as close to it as feasible. For example, if the patient is lying in bed, the nurse should sit on a chair at the bedside facing the patient during a conversation. In addition, the head of the bed should be elevated, unless contraindicated, so that the patient is at same level as the nurse. Sitting in a comfortable position and leaning slightly forward toward the patient convey a message of interest and openness.

SPACE AND TERRITORIALITY

Generally, Western cultures recognize four zones of personal space. From the face to about 18 inches away is the *intimate space*. Because of the nature of many nursing interventions, the LPN/LVN must enter the patient's personal space. Bathing, inserting urethral catheters, and changing dressings are just a few examples. Entering this space can cause uneasiness for the nurse and the patient. Approaching these interventions in a professional manner can help alleviate much of the uneasiness felt by the nurse and patient (Fig. 4.4). The *personal space* comprises the area from 18 inches to 4 feet away from a person. Sitting and talking with a patient is an example of an interaction in the personal space. This area tends to be a comfortable space for most people during an interaction such as that between a nurse and patient. The *social space* is 4 to 12 ft from a person. An example of a social space is a nurse conducting a diabetes class for a group of patients. Beyond 12 ft from a person is considered *public space* (Krauss Whitbourne, 2012). Factors such as the patient's culture, individual preferences, and the situation determine the level of comfort with the various types of space. The nurse should be especially aware of the patient's nonverbal communication when interacting with the patient in these zones of personal space.

ENVIRONMENT

The general environment surrounding an interaction often has a significant impact on the interaction's effectiveness. A therapeutic interaction between the nurse and the patient is extremely difficult if a lot of commotion is occurring in the room. Key elements for a successful interaction are a calm, relaxed atmosphere and privacy. Ideally, the initial interaction should take place in a private room with the door closed. However, this degree of privacy is not always possible. If the patient has a roommate, taking the patient to a private conference room is sometimes a good option, depending on the status of the patient and the nature of the interaction. At the very least, the privacy curtain should be pulled between the two patients during interaction with a patient.

LEVEL OF TRUST

A trusting relationship is essential to an effective nurse-patient interaction. Without trust, interaction does not progress past superficial social interaction. The nurse first must gain the patient's trust before expecting to have a meaningful or therapeutic interaction. One way for the LPN/LVN to build trust is by demonstrating confidence and competence. A trusting relationship is often difficult to establish with a patient who has had negative encounters with other health care providers. The LPN/LVN should be sensitive to the patient's previous experiences and demonstrate a sincere effort to make the current situation a positive experience for the patient.

LANGUAGE BARRIERS

In today's culturally diverse society, care of a patient who speaks a different language is not unusual. Language barriers can pose a major threat to effective communication and development of a therapeutic nurse-patient relationship. Some larger hospitals or hospitals where the community has a very diverse population often have a translator on staff or one who is easily accessible. If the LPN/LVN is employed in a health care facility that does not have a translator available, the nurse should use all available means (e.g., social services) to find one. If an interpreter cannot be located, the nurse may rely on the patient's family members or friends to assist with communication if they speak the same language as the nurse. The nurse should be very cautious that misinterpretation does not occur with use of family members as interpreters and should avoid use of younger children as the interpreter. Keeping messages simple and avoiding the use of medical terminology can help in preventing misinterpretations. Use of gestures and pictures also may be helpful in communicating with the patient. The LPN/LVN also must comply with Health Insurance Portability and Accountability Act of 1996 (HIPAA) regulations and guidelines when using a family member or friend as an interpreter.

Some health care institutions may have resources such as translation dictionaries in the languages most common to its geographic location available, or the nurse may use an online resource (Boxes 4.2 and 4.3). Use these resources with caution. There is a high risk of mispronouncing words or using incorrect words, and doing so can convey unintended or inaccurate messages. Consider information concerning barriers in language and communication that may exist between subcultures of a group, including the use of slang terms.

Box 4.2 Guidelines for Communicating With Patients Who Are Partially Fluent in English

- Ask for feedback. Provide the patient with paper and pencil.
- Assess the patient's nonverbal and verbal communication.
- Avoid using medical terms.
- Remain at eye level with the patient. Assess whether the patient is comfortable with eye contact.
- Remember that patients usually understand more than they can express. They need time to process the discussion and to determine what they want to respond.
- Remember that stress interferes with the patient's ability to think and speak in English.
- Speak slowly and never loudly (unless the patient has a hearing impairment).
- Use pictures when possible.

Modified from Balzer Riley J: *Communication in nursing*, ed 8, St. Louis, 2017, Mosby.

CULTURE

Nursing is concerned with holistic care of the patient. Culture is a significant component of a patient's psychosocial well-being. The nurse must attempt to seek specific information regarding cultural practices and beliefs of the patients being cared for, especially when the patient is from a culture different from that of the nurse. The effect of culture on communication is immense, and a complete discussion is beyond the scope of this chapter. Julia Balzer Riley (2017) offers useful guidelines when relating to patients of different cultures (see the Cultural Considerations box). For more complete information, refer to Chapter 6.

Box 4.3 Guidelines for Communicating With Non–English-Speaking Patients

If an interpreter is available:

- Address questions to the patient, not the interpreter.
- Avoid using children and relatives as interpreters.
- Be aware that more time will be needed for interactions to allow for translation and interpretation.
- Give the patient and interpreter time alone together.
- Select same-age and same-gender interpreters if possible.
- Use dialect-specific interpreters, not translators.

If an interpreter is *not* available:

- Be aware of the patient's nonverbal communication. This helps in determining if the translation is accurate of the patient's feelings.
- Determine whether there is a third language that you and the patient speak. In many cultures, it is common for patients to speak several languages.
- Pantomime simple words and actions to help the patient understand the desired message.
- Talk with your facility's administration about the importance of using trained medical interpreters when caring for the non–English-speaking patient.
- Until medical interpreters are available, use formal and informal networking to locate a suitable interpreter.
- Use a translator.
- Use picture boards.

Modified from Balzer Riley J: *Communication in nursing*, ed 8, St. Louis, 2017, Mosby.

AGE AND GENDER

The effects of *age* and *gender* on communication are influenced strongly by cultural or societal beliefs and attitudes. A significant age difference between the nurse and the patient does, in some cases, raise a barrier to communication. Nurses who have had limited interaction with children may find it difficult to communicate effectively with children in the health care setting. Teenagers also may present a unique challenge when communicating with nurses. Their vocabulary and expressions are often unique to their age group and include the use of slang terms. At the other end of the spectrum, the nurse may encounter an older adult who does not have confidence in a very young nurse or has some physiologic or cognitive impairment that hampers effective communication. Communication is most effective if the nurse tries to understand as much about patients across the lifespan as possible and selects the most appropriate communication techniques for a variety of circumstances.

When communicating with older adults who may have communication barriers because of hearing loss or cognitive barriers, consider ways to improve communication. Speaking directly to patients by getting their attention and facing them enhances the interaction. If the patient wears a hearing aid, be sure it is in place and in working order. Eliminate background noise when speaking with the patient and do not shout at the patient. Also give the patient time to process what has been said and allow ample time for the patient to respond. Last, do not talk to the patient as a child, or in a simplified and slow manner, with terms of endearment such as "honey" or "sweetie," commonly referred to as "elder speak."

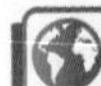 **Cultural Considerations**

Communicating With Patients of Different Cultures From Your Own

DOMINANT LANGUAGE AND DIALECTS

- Identify the dominant language of the group.
- Identify dialects that have the potential to interfere with communication.
- Explore contextual speech patterns of the group. What is the usual volume and tone of speech?

CULTURAL COMMUNICATION PATTERNS

- Explore the willingness of individuals to share thoughts, feelings, and ideas.
- Explore the practice and meaning of touch in the given society: within the family, among friends, with strangers, with members of the same gender, with members of the opposite gender, and with health care providers.
- Identify typical personal spatial and distancing characteristics during one-to-one communication. Explore how distancing changes with friends compared with strangers.
- Explore the use of eye contact within the group. Does avoidance of eye contact have special meaning? How does eye contact vary among family, friends, and strangers? Do eye contact practices change when communication occurs between members of different socioeconomic groups?
- Explore the meaning of various facial expressions. Do specific facial expressions have special meanings? Do people tend to smile a lot? How are emotions displayed or not displayed in facial expressions?
- Are there acceptable ways of standing and greeting outsiders?

ATTITUDES TOWARD TIME

- Explore attitudes in the group toward time. Are individuals oriented primarily to the past, present, or future? How do individuals see the context of past, present, and future?
- Identify differences in the interpretation of social time versus clock time.
- Explore how time factors are interpreted by the group. Are individuals expected to be punctual in arrival to jobs, appointments, and social engagements?

FORMAT FOR NAMES

- Explore the format for personal names.
- How does the individual expect to be greeted by strangers and health care practitioners?

From Balzer Riley J: *Communication in nursing*, ed 8, St. Louis, 2017, Mosby.

Male and female patterns of communication often are related closely to cultural, familial, and lifestyle patterns developed over a lifetime. The beliefs, values, and attitudes that an individual or a society in general holds regarding male or female status and expectations are likely to affect how messages are sent and received (Balzer Riley, 2017).

PHYSIOLOGIC FACTORS

Many physiologic factors may interfere with the patient being able to communicate effectively. *Pain* is a common example. While a patient is experiencing pain, all available energy is focused on coping with the pain; it is difficult, if not impossible, for the patient to communicate about anything except the pain. The LPN/LVN first should address the patient's pain before trying to communicate with the patient, especially before performing any patient teaching.

Altered cognition is another physiologic factor that frequently hinders effective communication. If the patient lacks the cognitive ability to receive, process, and send information, communication is disrupted. Several factors have the potential to affect a patient's cognitive ability. A cerebrovascular accident (stroke), sedative effects of medication, dementia, and developmental delays are examples of such factors.

Careful assessment of a patient's level of cognitive function is important when beginning any interaction. The nurse should assist with keeping the patient's sensory abilities operating at their maximum potential. For example, if the patient wears glasses or a hearing aid, the nurse should ensure these assistive devices are in place to help the patient process information accurately. If there is decreased ability to comprehend, the environment should be kept quiet during communicating. Box 4.4 lists strategies for communicating with patients who are cognitively impaired.

Impaired hearing is another common physiologic factor that impedes communication. Hearing impairment may lead to misinterpretation of messages and frustration for the sender and the receiver. The LPN/LVN should be sure that all efforts are made to ensure that effective communication is not sacrificed because of a patient's impaired hearing. See Box 4.5 for strategies for communicating with the patient with a hearing impairment.

Box 4.4 Communicating With Patients Who Are Cognitively Impaired

- Allow time for patient to respond.
- Ask one question at a time.
- Be attentive when listening to the patient speak.
- Get the patient's attention before speaking.
- Include family and friends in conversations.
- Reduce environmental distractions while talking with the patient.
- Use simple sentences and avoid long explanations.

Modified from Potter PA, Perry AG: *Fundamentals of nursing*, ed 9, St. Louis, 2016, Mosby.

PSYCHOSOCIAL FACTORS

A multitude of factors place patients under stress. The patient may be frightened, in pain, deprived of sleep, nauseated, or experiencing a host of other unpleasant circumstances. Stress can lead to problems with communication between the patient and the nurse. While experiencing increased stress, the patient may respond with anger, impatience, or even withdrawal. Realize that these behaviors are not directed at you personally but are coping mechanisms used by the patient.

When the patient is experiencing stress, especially extreme stress, you may need to modify communication methods. Keep information simple, basic, and concrete and offer only essential information. Let the patient direct the conversation. Being supportive of the patient aids in keeping the lines of communication open and effective.

An illness often is accompanied by some degree of *grieving* as a result of actual or perceived loss. This loss can take many possible forms, including role or lifestyle change, physical change, altered function, terminal prognosis, and anticipated or actual loss of a loved one.

Nurses often feel uncomfortable interacting with a grieving patient for fear of not knowing what to say or saying the wrong thing. Because of this uneasiness, nurses may sometimes say nothing or avoid the subject entirely. The challenge for the LPN/LVN in dealing with patients and their loved ones who are grieving is to attempt communication with them despite any feelings of personal inadequacy. A silent presence is often all that is necessary. The grieving process may be facilitated by using therapeutic touch, displaying warm

Box 4.5 Communicating With Patients Who Have Hearing Impairment

- Be sure to get the patient's attention when entering the room before you begin speaking.
- Ensure the patient is wearing hearing aids and/or glasses if he or she has them.
- Ensure the patient can see your lips because many lip-read.
- Face the patient.
- If the patient hears better from one ear, stand nearer to that ear when speaking.
- Reduce environmental noise, such as the television or radio.
- Rephrase comments rather than repeating if the patient continues to have difficulty understanding.
- Speak at a normal volume rather than shouting.
- Try to lower the tone of your voice. Hard-of-hearing individuals usually have difficulty with high-pitched sounds and voices.
- Use sign language or provide a sign language interpreter if needed.

and caring behaviors, listening, and using open-ended statements to assist those who are grieving to understand their own feelings and behaviors.

BLOCKS TO COMMUNICATION

Just as therapeutic techniques enhance the quality of an interaction, barriers to communication block its effectiveness. The list of possible responses that block communication is extensive. The most common are presented in Table 4.4.

❖ NURSING PROCESS

When a patient experiences difficulty with verbally communicating, the care plan is geared toward assisting the patient with communicating by other means. With input from the patient, significant others, and members of the intraprofessional health care team, the nurse determines which methods of communication will best work for each individual patient.

◆ ASSESSMENT

Any of the factors that affect communication discussed previously in this chapter potentially are related to difficulty with verbally communicating. Factors that indicate difficulty with verbally communicating include the patient's inability to produce words (either by complete aphasia or expressive aphasia), lack of nonverbal communication, struggle with speech pattern, and being disoriented to person, place, or time.

PATIENT PROBLEM

If one or more of certain patient factors are present, the patient problem of *Compromised Verbal Communication* may be indicated. For example, a patient with an endotracheal tube in place to relieve respiratory distress that occurred after a traumatic chest injury will have this patient problem. The presence of the endotracheal tube renders him unable to speak. The loss of speech hampers his abilities to express his needs and supports the identification of the patient problem of difficulty with verbally communicating.

◆ SETTING PATIENT GOALS AND PLANNING

The goal for any patient experiencing difficulty with verbally communicating is that the patient will be able to communicate effectively with others in the environment by sending and receiving clear, concise, and understandable messages. The patient goals must be specific and realistic for the patient and address the patient's needs and concerns. In general, the desired patient goals include:

- The patient will use effective communication techniques.
- The patient will use alternative methods to communicate.
- The patient's verbal communication will match nonverbal communication.

◆ IMPLEMENTATION

Nursing interventions appropriate to the patient difficulty with verbally communicating depend on the type of communication problem that exists and the factors contributing to the problem. Thus nursing interventions may vary greatly from one patient to another. See Box 4.6 for examples of helpful nursing interventions related to specific types of difficulty with communication.

◆ EVALUATION

The nurse evaluates the effectiveness of communication based on the patient's ability to meet the established goals. A good way to accomplish this is by observing the patient's response to an interaction and considering what kind of message is received from the patient's verbal and nonverbal communication. Does the patient appear to have received the message, and is the patient satisfied with it? If the patient goals have been achieved but the impairment is ongoing, continue with the current plan of care. If the impairment no longer exists, on the other hand, consider the patient problem to be resolved. If the goals have not been met, reexamine the phases of the nursing process to determine what revisions are necessary.

COMMUNICATION IN SPECIAL SITUATIONS

The communication techniques discussed thus far are generally applicable to any type of nurse-patient interaction. Some patients have unique communication needs. Three examples of such situations follow.

PATIENTS WITH VENTILATOR DEPENDENCE

Patients who receive mechanical ventilation via endotracheal tube or tracheostomy experience an inability to speak because the trachea is obstructed by the tube. Patients often find this inability to speak devastating, and it often disrupts their sense of well-being and control. When the patient is unable to produce sound, it is essential to identify and implement *alternative methods of communication.*

To determine which communication method is most appropriate, the nurse should assess carefully the patient's ability (e.g., cognitive level, literacy, visual acuity, consciousness level, primary language, gross motor skills, and fine motor skills) to use a particular alternative. One valuable tool is a *communication board.* Depending on the patient's literacy, a communication board includes the alphabet, commonly used phrases, pictures, or a combination of all three. If able to point, the patient points to pictures or phrases on the board to communicate a need or thought. If the desired picture or phrase is not on the board, the patient points to the letters that spell out the message. This method is not feasible for the patient who does not read or cannot see well enough to select from the board.

Table 4.4 Responses That Block Communication

CATEGORY OF RESPONSE	EXPLANATION OF CATEGORIES	EXAMPLES	OUTCOME
False reassurance	Using falsely comforting phrases in an attempt to offer reassurance	"It will be okay." "Don't worry. Everything will be just fine." "You'll be fine."	You promise something that will not occur or is unrealistic
Giving advice or personal opinions	Making a decision for a patient; offering personal opinions; telling a patient what to do with phrases such as "should do," "ought to"	"If I were you I would …" "I think you should …" "Why don't you …"	Takes decision making away from the patient; impairs decision making; creates doubt; encourages blaming the nurse if decision has unwanted outcome
False assumptions	Making an assumption without validation; jumping to conclusions	"It seems like you don't care to learn about your diagnosis." "Your husband isn't very supportive." "You aren't really trying."	Easily leads to a wrong conclusion; often viewed as accusatory or argumentative
Approval or disapproval	Trying to impose the nurse's own attitudes, values, beliefs, and moral standards on a patient about what is right and wrong	"I don't agree with your decision to not try this treatment option!" "Having cosmetic surgery seems like a waste of money." "You shouldn't even think that." "He really is a good doctor."	Easily leads the patient to doubt personal values; creates feelings of guilt and resentment; causes friction between you and the patient
Automatic responses	Stereotyped or superficial comments that do not focus on what the patient is feeling or trying to say	"You can't win them all." "Isn't that nice?" "I don't make the rules; I just follow them." "The doctor knows best."	Tends to belittle the individual's feelings and minimize the importance of the message; communicates the message that you are not taking the patient's concerns seriously
Defensiveness	Responding negatively to criticism; often in response to feelings of anger or hurt on your part; usually involves making excuses	"I'm doing the best I can." "We are never short staffed." "You must have misunderstood what I said."	Implies that the patient has no right to an opinion; results in ignoring or minimizing the patient's concerns; displays defensive behavior
Arguing	Challenging or arguing against the patient's statements or perceptions	"How can you say you didn't sleep all night? You were sleeping every time I came into your room." "How could your pain level be so high? You were just talking and laughing with your visitor."	Denies that the patient's perceptions are real and valid; implies that the patient is not being truthful, is misinformed, or uneducated
Asking for explanations	Asks the patient to explain her or his actions, beliefs, or feelings with "why" questions	"Why aren't you following the directions your primary care provider gave you?" "Why do you feel that way?" "Why didn't you go to the doctor sooner?"	Frequently viewed by the patient as accusatory; puts patient on the defensive; risks causing resentment, insecurity, and mistrust of the nurse
Changing the subject	Inappropriately focusing the discussion on something other than the patient's concern	"We'll worry about that later. It's time for you to go to physical therapy." "Let's talk about something happier. Talking about your cancer diagnosis is making you too sad."	Rude and shows lack of empathy; blocks further communication, and sometimes makes patient feel uncomfortable about expressing feelings; interrupts thoughts, and often inhibits the sharing of important information

Modified from Potter PA, Perry AG: *Fundamentals of nursing,* ed 9, St. Louis, 2016, Mosby; Arnold E, Boggs KU: *Interpersonal relationships: Professional communication skills for nurses,* ed 7, Philadelphia, 2016, Saunders.

Box 4.6 Nursing Interventions for Patients Experiencing Difficulty Verbally Communicating

1. Determine language spoken; obtain language dictionary or interpreter if possible and accepted by the patient.
2. Listen carefully. Validate verbal and nonverbal expression, particularly when dealing with pain.
3. Anticipate patient's needs until effective communication is possible.
4. Use simple communication; speak in a well-modulated voice, smile, and show concern for the patient.
5. Maintain eye contact at patient's level if culturally appropriate.
6. Use touch as appropriate and if culturally appropriate. Holding a patient's hand or stroking the arm is a simple, unobtrusive way of showing empathy and concern.
7. Spend time with the patient, allow time for responses, and make the call light readily available.
8. Explain all health care procedures.
9. Determine the patient's literacy status.
10. Obtain communication equipment such as electronic devices, paper and pen, letter boards, picture boards, and magic slates as indicated.
11. With an individualized approach, establish an alternative method of communication, such as writing or pointing to letters, words, phrases, picture cards, or simple drawings of basic needs.
12. If there is a comprehension deficit, keep environment quiet when communicating and get the patient's attention before attempting to communicate (e.g., touch patient's shoulder, call patient's name).
13. Give praise for progress noted. Ignore mistakes and watch for frustration or fatigue.
14. Never raise your voice or shout at a patient.
15. Be persistent in deciphering what the patient is saying, and do not pretend to understand when the message is unclear.

Modified from Ackley BJ, Ladwig GB: *Nursing diagnosis handbook: An evidence-based guide to planning care*, ed 11, St. Louis, 2016, Mosby.

If the patient is unable to move well enough to point, alternative selection methods are necessary. Possibilities include setting up a "signal" system, such as one eye blink for "yes" and two blinks for "no." The receiver (e.g., the nurse or a family member) systematically points to items or letters on the board, and the patient "signals" when the correct item is selected. This is a slow and rather cumbersome process for communicating and requires patience of the patient and the receiver of the message. In many cases, it is also very tiring for the patient. Nevertheless, it has the potential to be a helpful tool when no other means of communicating is available or feasible. Box 4.7 lists additional alternative methods of communication to use with the patient who is unable to speak.

Box 4.7 Alternative Methods of Communicating With Patients Who Are Unable to Speak

- *Clock face communicator:* Messages placed at intervals around the clock face; clock hand scans the messages, and the patient presses a button to stop the hand on the desired message.
- *Computer-assisted communication:* Patient uses keyboard to type messages.
- *Eye blinks:* Predetermined system in which the number of times a patient blinks in response to a question indicates yes or no answer.
- *Lip-reading:* Patient mouths words to be interpreted by the receiver.
- *Magnetic boards with plastic letters:* Patient moves letters around on board to spell words or phrases.
- *Paper and pencil or magic slate:* Patient writes messages to communicate needs.
- *Picture board:* Patient points to pictures on a board or poster of typical patient needs.
- *Sign language:* Hand and finger signals used to indicate letters; used throughout the world for hearing-impaired patients.
- *Word or picture cards:* 3 × 5 cards with words or pictures on them; patient picks appropriate card or sorts cards into short phrases or sentences.

PATIENTS WITH APHASIA

Aphasia is a deficient or absent language function that results from ischemic insult to the brain, such as stroke (cerebrovascular accident), brain trauma, or anoxia. Some patients experience **expressive aphasia,** in which they are unable to *send* the desired verbal message; and some suffer **receptive aphasia,** or an inability to recognize or interpret the verbal message being *received.* Communication methods recommended for the patient with aphasia are summarized in Box 4.8.

UNRESPONSIVE PATIENTS

It is not certain whether, or how much, the unresponsive patient is able to hear or interpret verbal stimuli. Some patients, after regaining consciousness, have reported hearing actual statements that were made in the room while the patient was still in an unconscious state. Because of this, anyone interacting with the unresponsive patient must assume that all sound and verbal stimuli may be heard by the patient. Caution people nearby about making negative or anxiety-producing statements. Encourage health care providers and family and friends to speak to the unresponsive individual as if he or she were awake. This sometimes feels awkward, and family members and friends often need support and encouragement to talk with the patient as they would have before the illness or accident. Talking about daily activities and reading books, cards, and newspapers is beneficial. Also, always explain to the patient any procedure or activity that involves the patient. Remember not to have conversations with other health care providers about

Box 4.8 Communicating With Patients With Aphasia

- Avoid patronizing and childish phrases.
- Collaborate with a speech pathologist.
- Do not shout or speak loudly (hearing loss is not the problem).
- Encourage patients to speak as much as possible when they are able and ready, not to provide just yes or no answers.
- Give the patient time to understand; be calm and patient; do not pressure or tire the patient.
- If the patient has expressive aphasia, ask questions that require simple yes or no answers or blinking of the eyes. Offer pictures or a communication board to which the patient can point.
- If the patient has problems with comprehension, use simple, short questions and facial gestures to give additional clues.
- Listen to the patient, and wait for the patient to communicate.
- Speak of things familiar and of interest to the patient.
- Use communication aids (see Box 4.7).

Modified from Potter PA, Perry AG: *Fundamentals of nursing,* ed 9, St. Louis, 2016, Mosby.

topics that do not place the patient at the center of the discussion or that may cause stress or anxiety if the patient were to hear it.

CONCLUSION

No interaction takes place that does not involve communication. Every time the LPN/LVN interacts with a patient, there is opportunity for a positive or negative outcome. By becoming familiar with therapeutic communication techniques and practicing them to become proficient in their use, the nurse can promote a helping relationship with the patient. By also being aware of factors that affect communication and of blocks to communication, the LPN/LVN succeeds in preventing interactions that may negatively affect the patient's self-esteem and sense of worth.

Get Ready for the NCLEX® Examination!

Key Points

- All interactions result in the occurrence of some form of communication.
- Communication is verbal and nonverbal.
- Nonverbal communication is very powerful.
- The manner, or style, in which a message is communicated greatly influences the mood and the overall outcome of an interaction.
- Communication in nursing should be therapeutic.
- Trust is essential to effective nurse-patient interaction.
- Active listening is one of the most effective methods of therapeutic communication.
- Touch is a form of nonverbal communication that is inherent to the practice of nursing.
- Humor is potentially a powerful tool in promoting the well-being of an individual.
- Numerous factors affect communication.
- Impaired verbal communication requires alternative methods for communicating effectively.

Additional Learning Resources

SG Go to your Study Guide for additional learning activities to help you master this chapter content.

evolve Be sure to visit the Evolve site at *http://evolve.elsevier.com/Cooper/foundationsadult/* for additional online resources.

Review Questions for the NCLEX® Examination

1. The patient is fearful concerning his upcoming surgery. Which statement by the nurse is most therapeutic?
   1. "Sometimes anxiety is not easy to deal with. Can you tell me what is bothering you the most about your upcoming surgery?"
   2. "Don't worry. Everyone has some anxiety about having surgery."
   3. "Just try to think about the positive results from the surgery. You'll recover quickly."
   4. "I had surgery once, and it still scares me to think about it, so I know how you feel."
2. During an admission interview, the patient refers several times to "all the problems I had last time." What is the most appropriate communication technique for the nurse to use in this situation?
   1. Reflection
   2. Paraphrasing
   3. Minimal encouragement
   4. Focusing
3. The patient states, "I'm so nervous about being hospitalized." Which statement is the nurse's best response to get the patient to elaborate?
   1. "It's normal to be nervous, but we'll take good care of you."
   2. "You're feeling especially nervous?"
   3. "How many times have you been hospitalized?"
   4. "Nurses will be here all the time to check on you."

4. The nurse is talking with the patient about her husband's death 2 years ago. Tears form in the patient's eyes, and she stops talking. What is the most appropriate therapeutic response by the nurse?
   1. Change the subject to something less difficult for the patient.
   2. Remain silent and hold the patient's hand.
   3. Leave the room to provide privacy.
   4. Pretend not to notice the tears and continue the conversation.
5. Which question is an example of clarification? (*Select all that apply.*)
   1. "You will take your medicine now, won't you?"
   2. "Does this headache have anything in common with your previous headaches?"
   3. "In other words, you feel that your stomach aches are associated with stress at work?"
   4. "What do you mean by that?"
   5. "Do I understand you correctly that you are saying that you don't understand why the doctor prescribed this medication for you?"
6. The newly admitted Vietnamese patient speaks almost no English. The nurse needs to obtain from the patient a urine specimen for culture and sensitivity. An interpreter is not readily available. What is the best nursing action to assist in obtaining the specimen?
   1. Speak very slowly and distinctly.
   2. Show the patient the equipment and illustrations of the process.
   3. Obtain a physician's order to catheterize the patient to collect the specimen.
   4. Delay the collection of the specimen until an interpreter can be found.
7. Abdominal surgery has revealed that the patient, a young mother, has advanced metastatic colon cancer. While the nurse is changing her dressing, the patient begins to cry and states, "If I had just gone to the doctor sooner, my kids wouldn't have to grow up without a mother." Which response by the nurse is most therapeutic?
   1. "It's natural to blame yourself in situations like this."
   2. "Is their father available to care for the children?"
   3. "Don't give up. The chemotherapy and radiation might be very effective."
   4. "You feel that if you had been diagnosed earlier, the situation might be different?"
8. During his admission interview, an older patient states, "I can't hear you very well." After determining that the patient does not have a hearing aid, which action assists with communicating with this patient? (*Select all that apply.*)
   1. Speak in a higher pitched voice.
   2. Speak loudly into his "good" ear.
   3. Exaggerate lip movement while speaking.
   4. Face the patient and speak slowly and distinctly.
   5. Be sure to get the patient's attention before speaking.
9. Which statement by the student nurse is an example of assertive communication? (*Select all that apply.*)
   1. "It's time for your morning care. Do you prefer to use the shower chair, or do you think you are strong enough to stand during your shower today?"
   2. "I'd like you to take your shower now, but if you'd rather do it later, I guess that would be okay."
   3. "It would be best if we completed your morning care now, but since you want to wait until tonight, I'll ask my instructor if that would be okay."
   4. "I'm sure you'll feel better after you have your morning care. Will you please take your shower now?"
   5. "Since you will be going to physical therapy soon, it's important we get your morning care completed. Do you want to take a sponge bath or a shower?"
10. The patient has a long history of smoking and has just been diagnosed with lung cancer. He states to the nurse, "There's no point in trying to stop smoking now. I might as well enjoy the time I have left." Which is the best response by the nurse?
    1. "You're probably right. It won't do much good to stop smoking now."
    2. "You feel that there is no reason to stop smoking now?"
    3. "It's never too late to stop smoking."
    4. "I know it's hard, but if you stop smoking now, your condition might improve."
11. The patient tells the nurse that he is frightened about having cancer. Which response by the nurse is most effective in getting the patient to vent his concerns?
    1. "Fear is a common reaction to having cancer."
    2. "Tell me more about being frightened by having cancer."
    3. "Have you told your wife you are afraid?"
    4. "Would you like me to call the chaplain to visit with you?"
12. The nurse is admitting a patient with long-standing type 1 diabetes. Which communication technique is most efficient in ascertaining the number of units of insulin the patient usually takes?
    1. Closed question
    2. Reflection
    3. Minimal encouragement
    4. Paraphrasing
13. The patient is being seen in the clinic for a follow-up visit after fracturing her ankle. The nurse notes that she is not using her crutches correctly. Which statement by the nurse is most appropriate?
    1. "You are not using your crutches correctly."
    2. "Let me show you some ways to make crutch walking easier for you."
    3. "Who taught you to use your crutches like that?"
    4. "Do your crutches seem to fit you properly?"
14. Which method is most appropriate for communicating with an alert patient on a ventilator with an endotracheal tube in place?
    1. Open-ended questions
    2. Communication board
    3. Reflection
    4. Restatement

15. The patient is in a coma after a motor vehicle accident. Which statement regarding communication with the patient is most appropriate? *(Select all that apply.)*
    1. Speak to the patient as if he can hear what is being said.
    2. Avoid verbal stimulation because of its potential to trigger excitability.
    3. Encourage family members to limit visitation to no more than 5 minutes per hour.
    4. Leave the television on continuously to stimulate the patient.
    5. Encourage family members to read a book or newspaper to the patient.
16. Which statement about communication is most accurate?
    1. Use of therapeutic communication techniques guarantees that a therapeutic interaction takes place.
    2. Some form of communication takes place each time there is an interaction between individuals.
    3. The intended receiver is always the person receiving the communication.
    4. Verbal communication is more effective than nonverbal communication.
17. Which communication technique is considered appropriate in all interactions?
    1. Listening
    2. Clarifying
    3. Touch
    4. Eye contact
18. The nurse is providing discharge instructions to a patient. Which action provides the most accurate assessment of understanding by the patient?
    1. Asking the patient whether he understands the instructions
    2. Repeating the instructions a second time
    3. Providing the patient with written instructions
    4. Asking the patient to repeat the instructions
19. Which nurse-patient interaction usually occurs in the "personal zone" of space surrounding the patient? *(Select all that apply.)*
    1. Urethral catheterization
    2. Complete bed bath
    3. Discharge instructions
    4. Injection administration
    5. Admission interview
20. Which approach is most appropriate for effective communication with a patient with cognitive impairment?
    1. Repeating a phrase until the patient indicates understanding
    2. Asking friends and family to step out of the room to decrease distraction
    3. Using simple sentences and avoiding detailed explanations
    4. Directing communication to significant others rather than the patient

5 Nursing Process and Critical Thinking

http://evolve.elsevier.com/Cooper/foundationsadult/

Objectives

1. Explain the use of each of the six phases of the nursing process.
2. List the elements of each of the six phases of the nursing process.
3. Describe the establishment of the database.
4. Discuss the components of a patient problem statement.
5. Differentiate between types of health problems.
6. Describe the development of patient-centered goals.
7. Discuss the creation of nursing orders.
8. Explain the evaluation of a nursing care plan.
9. Demonstrate the nursing process by preparing a nursing care plan.
10. Explain North American Nursing Diagnosis Association International (NANDA-I), *Nursing Interventions Classification (NIC)*, and *Nursing Outcomes Classification (NOC)*.
11. Describe the use of clinical pathways in managed care.
12. Discuss critical thinking in nursing.
13. Define evidence-based practice.

Key Terms

assessment (p. 80)
biographic data (bī-ō-GRĂF-ĭk DĀ-tă, p. 82)
case management (kās MĂN-ĭj-mĕnt, p. 91)
clinical pathway (CLĬN-ĭ-căl PĂTH-wā, p. 91)
collaborative problems (kŏ-LĂB-ŭr-ă-tĭv PRŎB-lĕmz, p. 85)
cue (kyū, p. 82)
database (p. 82)
defining characteristics (dē-FĪN-ĭng kăr-ăk-tŭr-ĬS-tĭks, p. 84)
diagnose (dī-ăg-NŌS, p. 82)
evaluation (ē-văl-yū-Ā-shŭn, p. 89)
goal (p. 85)
implementation (ĭm-plĕ-mĕn-TĀ-shŭn, p. 89)
managed care (p. 91)
medical diagnosis (MĔD-ĭ-kăl dī-ăg-NŌ-sĭs, p. 85)
NANDA-I (p. 83)
nursing diagnosis/patient problem statement (p. 83)
nursing interventions (p. 86)
nursing process (p. 80)
nursing-sensitive patient outcomes (p. 90)
objective data (ŏb-JĔK-tĭv DĀ-tă, p. 82)
outcome (goal) (p. 81)
planning (p. 86)
potential patient problem statement (p. 81)
standardized language (p. 90)
subjective data (sŭb-JĔK-tĭv DĀ-tă, p. 82)
variance (VĂR-ē-ăns, p. 91)

According to the American Nurses Association (ANA), the current definition of nursing states, "Nursing is the protection, promotion, and optimization of health and abilities, prevention of illness and injury, facilitation of healing, alleviation of suffering through the diagnosis and treatment of human response, and advocacy in the care of individuals, families, groups, communities, and populations" (ANA, n.d.a). This broad definition seeks to illustrate nursing's growth as a profession. The nursing process serves as the organizational framework for the practice of nursing.

The **nursing process** is a systematic method by which nurses plan and provide care for patients. This involves a problem-solving approach that enables the nurse to identify patient problems and potential problems. Once these problems are identified, the nurse is then able to plan, deliver, and evaluate nursing care in an orderly, scientific manner. The nursing process consists of the following six dynamic and interrelated phases: assessment, diagnosis, outcomes identification, planning, implementation, and evaluation (Fig. 5.1). Box 5.1 describes how the nursing process is carried out by the registered nurse (RN) and licensed practical/vocational nurse (LPN/LVN). The LPN/LVN has a significant role in the nursing process, which is discussed subsequently in the chapter.

ASSESSMENT DATA

The ANA defines **assessment** as "a systematic, dynamic way to collect and analyze data about a client, the first step in delivering nursing care. Assessment includes not only physiological data, but also psychological, sociocultural, spiritual, economic, and life-style factors as well" (ANA, n.d.b). Information is gathered by the nurse to identify the condition of the patient's health. The nurse

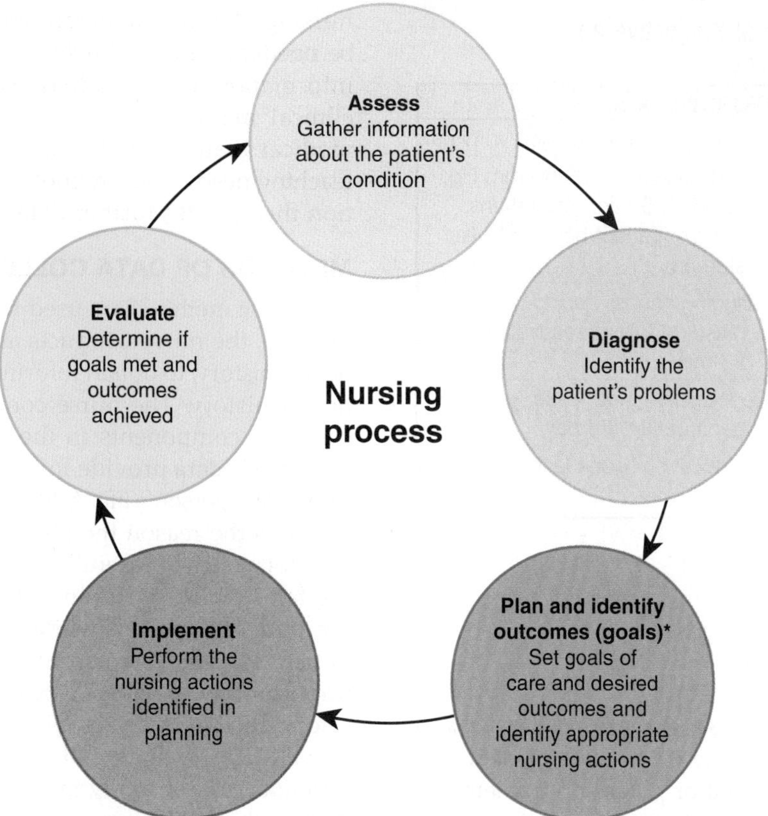

Fig. 5.1 Relationships among the steps of the nursing process. *Note: Combined American Nurses Association (ANA) standards 3 and 4.

> **Box 5.1 Implementation of the Nursing Process by the Registered Nurse (RN) and Licensed Practical/Vocational Nurse (LPN/LVN)**
>
> *Assessment:* The RN is responsible for the initial assessment of the patient; the LPN/LVN assists the RN with ongoing assessments.
>
> *Diagnosis:* The RN is responsible for identifying the appropriate nursing diagnosis (patient problem) for the patient with the assistance of the LPN/LVN.
>
> *Outcomes Identification:* The RN develops individualized goals or expected outcomes directly associated with the nursing diagnoses. The LPN/LVN also can assist the RN with identifying these outcomes.
>
> *Planning:* The RN, with assistance from the LPN/LVN, plans interventions that will help meet the patient's desired goals/expected outcomes.
>
> *Implementation:* The RN and LPN/LVN implement the proposed plan.
>
> *Evaluation:* The RN and LPN/LVN perform ongoing assessments, allowing the RN to determine whether proposed goals/outcomes have been met.

performs a patient assessment on initial contact with the patient, with the remaining phases of the nursing process dependent on the accuracy and completeness of this initial data collection. Either a complete assessment or a focused assessment is performed, depending on the patient's status and the type of facility. The LPN/LVN assists the RN by performing ongoing complete and focused assessments of patients, depending on the facility and scope of practice within a state.

A complete assessment involves a review and physical examination of all body systems (e.g., musculoskeletal, respiratory, gastrointestinal) (see Chapter 13). This type of assessment also includes cognitive, psychosocial, emotional, cultural, and spiritual components and is appropriate for a patient with a stable condition who is not in acute distress. Information about functional abilities, lifestyle, and developmental concerns is also important.

A focused assessment is advisable when the patient is critically ill, disoriented, or unable to respond. A focused assessment is used to gather information about a specific health problem. For example, if the patient reports abdominal distention, lack of appetite, and straining to have a bowel movement, one possible patient problem statement might be *Infrequent or difficult bowel elimination*. To further investigate the situation, the nurse may ask additional questions about intake of foods high in fiber, fluid intake, and amount of exercise.

Focused assessments also are performed continually throughout nurse-patient contact. The nurse who monitors intake and output, skin turgor, and oral mucous membranes is performing a focused assessment for inadequate fluid volume. Assessments made to determine progress toward the achievement of desired **outcomes**

Table 5.1 Comparison of Subjective and Objective Data

SUBJECTIVE DATA	OBJECTIVE DATA
"I feel nauseated."	50 mL dark green–tinged vomitus
"My chest hurts."	Blood pressure, 100/60 mm Hg; pulse, 100/min; respirations, 32/min; patient holds fist over sternum
"I'm nervous."	Wringing hands, pacing in hall; pulse, 112/min; respirations, 28/min
"I'm tired."	Dark circles under eyes, yawning, naps during the day
"My foot hurts."	1-cm × 2-cm open lesion on left heel

(outcomes, or goals, are something that a person strives to achieve) are also focused assessments.

TYPES OF DATA

In an assessment, the nurse gathers subjective and objective data. A **cue** is a piece or pieces of data that often indicate that an actual or potential problem has occurred or will occur. **Subjective data** are information that is provided by the patient. Statements about nausea and descriptions of pain, fatigue, and anxiety are examples of subjective data. Other terms for subjective data are *symptoms* and *subjective cues*. Subjective data are hidden until shared by the patient.

Objective data are observable and measurable signs. For example, the LPN/LVN is able to observe capillary refill, measure a patient's blood pressure, and observe and measure edema. Other terms for objective data are *signs* and *objective cues*. Table 5.1 shows a comparison of subjective and objective data.

SOURCES OF DATA

Data are obtained from primary or secondary sources. The primary source of data is the patient. In most instances, the patient is considered the most accurate reporter. The alert and oriented patient is able to provide information about past illnesses and surgeries as well as present symptoms and lifestyle.

When the patient is unable to supply adequate information because of deterioration of mental status, age, or seriousness of illness, the nurse turns to secondary sources. Secondary sources include family members, significant others, medical records, diagnostic procedures, and previous nursing progress notes. Members of the patient's support system often are able to furnish information about the patient's past health status, current illness, allergies, and current medications.

Health team professionals are also helpful secondary sources. Health care providers, nurses, dietitians, respiratory and physical therapists, and others frequently provide data about the patient. The nurse should review nursing literature to determine what information may be needed. Nursing textbooks are a good resource for information about etiology (cause), pathophysiology, clinical manifestations, assessment, diagnostic tests, medical management, nursing interventions, patient teaching needs, and prognosis. This important information then guides further data collection.

METHODS OF DATA COLLECTION

Two basic methods are used to collect data. In the first method, the nurse conducts an interview, the nursing health history, to obtain information about the patient's health history. The nurse commonly assesses several common components in the course of the interview. **Biographic data** provide information about the facts or events in a person's life. Additional information collected includes the reason the patient is seeking health care, a history of the present illness, the health history, and the family history. Because the environment in which the patient lives and works often plays a part in the patient's health status, an environmental history is important to obtain. A psychosocial history yields information about a combination of psychological and social factors. When gathering information about the function of each body system, the nurse follows the nursing health history with a review of systems.

The second method of data collection is the physical examination. The physical examination often is guided by subjective data provided by the patient. For example, the nurse should follow up with a thorough assessment of any body part or system for which the patient has reported symptoms or concerns. A head-to-toe format provides a systematic approach that helps avoid omission of important data (see Chapter 13).

A completed nursing health history and a physical examination allow the nurse to establish a **database** (a large store or bank of information) for the patient. Analysis of the database leads to the identification of nursing diagnoses. In addition, the database makes information available for the health care provider who assists in the medical management of the patient and all health care personnel who are involved in the patient's care.

DATA CLUSTERING

Data obtained from the health history, physical examination, and related diagnostic procedures are analyzed in development of a plan of care. Data clustering is one method of data organization. The clustering of related data helps to identify patterns that assist with the identification of patient's health problems. Some schools of nursing or health care facilities use the term *defining characteristics* as a synonym for data clustering.

DIAGNOSIS

To **diagnose** is to identify the type and cause of a health condition. Only the physician or other medically qualified

Table 5.2 **Determination of Significant Cues**

PATIENT VALUES	NORM[a]	CONCLUSION
42-year-old man with blood pressure 165/92 mm Hg	<120/80 mm Hg	High blood pressure
18-year-old patient with respirations of 32/min	16/min to 22/min	Tachypnea
Small-frame woman with weight of 178 lb, height 5′1″	105 to 118 lb	Weight above accepted normal standard
22-month-old child not walking	12 months	Walking delayed
Male adult patient with hemoglobin of 8 g/dL	14 to 18 g/dL	Below normal limits
Female adult patient with hemoglobin of 12 g/dL	12 to 16 g/dL	Within normal limits
25-year-old patient with pulse of 120 beats/min	60 to 100 beats/min	Tachycardia
Newborn patient with pulse of 132 beats/min	130 to 150 beats/min	Within normal limits
Adult patient with thrombocyte count of 20,000/mm^2	150,000/mm^2 to 400,000/mm^2	Thrombocytopenia

[a]Conclusion is based on the appropriate norm for the age and gender of the patient.

health care provider such as a nurse practitioner can provide a medical diagnosis. The LPN/LVN and the RN observe and collect data. Once the initial assessment has been completed, the data require analysis. In most situations, the RN is responsible for analyzing and interpreting data to identify health problems that the nurse can treat, referred to as the nursing diagnosis or patient problem statement (Table 5.2). The RN often collaborates with the LPN/LVN when determining the nursing diagnosis.

NURSING DIAGNOSIS/PATIENT PROBLEM STATEMENT

A **nursing diagnosis/patient problem statement** is a type of health problem that can be identified by the nurse. In 1990 the North American Nursing Diagnosis Association (NANDA) was created; in 2002 NANDA became NANDA International **(NANDA-I)** to reflect nursing diagnosis terminology used around the world. NANDA-I approves the official definition for a nursing diagnosis. In 2013 NANDA-I updated the definition of a nursing diagnosis as "a clinical judgment concerning a human response to health conditions/life processes, or a vulnerability for that response, by an individual, family, group or community. A nursing diagnosis provides the basis for selection of nursing interventions to achieve outcomes for which the nurse has accountability" (NANDA-I, 2018). The assessment and development of nursing diagnoses or patient problem statement are the responsibility of the RN. These are the foundational elements for the patient care plan. The RN is permitted legally to identify and prescribe the primary interventions to treat or prevent problems that are identified as nursing diagnoses or patient problems. Nurses must be aware of this important point. If the nurse is not able to prescribe the primary treatment, the problem is *not* a nursing diagnosis or a patient problem statement. As a member of the health care team, the LPN/LVN actively participates in patient care planning. This role includes collaboration with the RN to update the care plan and to implement prescribed nursing interventions.

Components of a Patient Problem Statement

The nursing community views the NANDA-I nursing diagnosis designations as being RN focused. In this text, *patient problem statements* are used to guide the development of a nursing care plan. This terminology allows for active participation in the care planning process by the LPN/LVN and other members of the intra-professional health care team. When identifying patient problems, consider the following factors: the patient's presenting signs and symptoms; contributing, etiologic (causative), and related factors; and defining characteristics.

Patient problem statement. Patient problems may be actual or potential. The nursing assessment determines how to classify the problem. If the patient's condition is expected to change, add the phrase "potential for" before the patient problem statement. For example, it is reasonable to expect that a patient being prepared for surgery will experience pain, alteration in mobility, or the need for education. Therefore, a patient problem statement would be *Potential for Discomfort.* This problem is identified based on a pattern of related cues or data that support the patient problem statement. A list of the most commonly seen patient problem statements to be used throughout *Foundations of Nursing and Adult Health Nursing* may be found on the back inside cover.

Adjectives add meaning to the patient problem statement by describing or modifying the statement. Examples of adjectives include *inability, insufficient, impaired,* and *willingness.* The patient problem statement given in the nursing care plans and nursing process sections of this text include the appropriate adjectives. Similarly, if assessment findings of the identified patient problem characterize it to be a potential problem, *Potential for* is placed in front of the patient problem statement. Examples include *Inability to Clear Airway* or *Potential for Inability to Clear Airway.*

Definition. Chronic conditions are something that are always present or consistently recur. These conditions commonly last 3 months or longer. Acute problems are typically rapid in onset and are limited in the duration of time. Acute problems can become chronic if the condition is not resolved. For this text, the patient problems that are acute will be labeled as either *acute* or *recent*. Chronic patient problems will be labeled as either *chronic* or *prolonged*. The definition presents a clear, precise description of the patient problem statement. This description helps identify the difference between similar patient problems. An example of an acute patient problem related to a recent injury is *Recent Onset of Pain*. A patient with a debilitating illness whose pain is present on some level for more than 3 months would have the patient problem *Prolonged Pain*.

Contributing, etiologic, and related factors and risk factors. Contributing, etiologic, and related factors are conditions that often are involved in the development of a problem. The factors may become the focus for nursing interventions. These authors will refer to a contributing factor as a "related to." Contributing, etiologic, and related factors are written as the "related to" in actual patient problem statements. A patient who has limited mobility and refuses to get out of bed would have the patient problem statement *Potential for Pressure Injury, related to lack of mobility and refusal to get out of bed.*

Defining characteristics. **Defining characteristics** are the clinical cues, signs, and symptoms that furnish evidence that the problem exists. The cues, signs, and symptoms identified in the patient's assessment are prefaced with "as evidenced by" in the patient problem statement. Examples are presented in the following discussion of the writing of patient problem statements. If utilizing NANDA-I nursing diagnoses, the defining characteristics for each nursing diagnosis title or label is listed in nursing diagnosis handbooks.

Data Clustering

Data obtained from the health history, physical examination, psychosocial history, and related diagnostic procedures are analyzed in the development of a plan of care. Data clustering is one method of data organization. The clustering of related data helps to identify patterns that assist with the identification of the patient problem statement. Some schools of nursing or health care facilities use the term *defining characteristics* as a synonym for data clustering. Examples of data clustering and the related patient problem include the following:

- Urine loss associated with physical exertion, such as lifting a heavy object, and urine loss associated with increased abdominal pressure, such as with pregnancy, are cues for the patient problem *Inability to Control Urination Due to Physical Stress*.
- Abnormal blood pressure, increased heart rate response to activity, exertional dyspnea, and verbal report of fatigue or weakness are cues for the patient problem *Inability to Tolerate Activity*.

Actual patient problem statement. An actual patient problem statement identifies health-related problems that exist and are discovered during the nursing assessment. These health problems can be treated by the nurse, which is how they differ from a medical diagnosis. In an educational setting, the actual patient problem statement usually is represented by a three-part statement. In a clinical setting, only the first two parts of the statement typically are used. The three parts are written in the following order: (1) the patient problem statement; (2) the contributing, etiologic, or related factor(s); and (3) the specific cues, signs, and symptoms from the patient's assessment that support the patient problem stateent. Connecting phrases are used to join the three parts of the statement. "Related to" (r/t) links the first and second parts of the statement. "As evidenced by" (AEB) joins the second and third parts of the patient problem statement. Note the bold italicized connecting words of an actual patient problem statement in the following example.

- *Infrequent or Difficult Bowel Elimination,* ***related to*** *insufficient fluid intake* ***as evidenced by*** *increased abdominal pressure, no bowel movement for 5 days, and straining with defecation*

Potential patient problems. Potential patient problem statements are health-related problems that the nurse deems as having a strong possibility of occurring. The nursing assessment indicates that risk factors are present that are known to contribute to the development of the problem. **Potential patient problems** are written as two-part statements: (1) the patient problem statement with the adjective "potential" in front of it, and (2) the risk factor(s). As in an actual patient problem statement, the two parts are connected by the words "related to." An example of a potential patient problem statement is as follows:

- *Potential for Compromised Skin Integrity,* ***related to*** *physical immobilization*

Note that no third part (as evidenced by) is seen in this statement. If signs or symptoms were found, an actual problem would exist.

Health promotion patient problem statements. A health promotion patient problem statement refers to the willingness of the patient, caregiver, or significant others to participate in activities that will aid in keeping the patient well. Health promotion problem statements are identified with the adjective *"willingness."* An example of a health promotion patient problem statement is *Willingness to Learn Breastfeeding, related to delivery of infant AEB mother's interest in meeting with the lactation consultant.*

OTHER TYPES OF HEALTH PROBLEMS

Collaborative problems and medical diagnoses must be distinguished from patient problem statements. These two types of problems are defined and discussed separately.

Collaborative Problems

Collaborative problems are health-related problems that the nurse anticipates based on the condition or diagnosis of a patient. Both health care provider–prescribed and nursing-prescribed interventions (discussed subsequently in this chapter) are used in the management of collaborative problems (Carpenito, 2016). An example of a collaborative problem is the care of a patient with hypertension who is taking a new medication for the condition. The potential for hypotension is considered a collaborative problem because prevention uses physician-prescribed interventions (e.g., adjustment of the hypertensive medications as needed) and nursing-prescribed interventions (e.g., monitoring of the patient's blood pressure, assistance when the patient goes from a sitting to standing position). If the prevention or treatment of the problem is primarily the nurse's responsibility, the problem is identified as a patient problem statement. *Potential for Infection* for the new postoperative surgical case is a potential complication that is a nursing responsibility.

Medical Diagnosis

A **medical diagnosis** is the identification of a disease or condition with evaluation of physical signs, symptoms, patient interview, laboratory tests, diagnostic procedures, review of medical records, and patient history. The health care provider is licensed to make and treat medical diagnoses. Examples of medical diagnoses are congestive heart failure, pneumonia, diabetes mellitus, and hepatitis B.

Differentiation of Medical and Patient Problems

Students often have difficulty with the distinction between a medical and a patient problem statement. Health care providers, including physicians and advanced practice nurses, diagnose diseases or disorders such as those listed previously. These diseases or disorders are the result of changes in the structure or the function of an organ or body system. Diagnostic studies such as x-ray examinations and laboratory studies help with identification of medical diagnoses. Although the patient is often able to recover from a medically diagnosed condition, the diagnosis does not change. The patient who recovers from a heart attack (myocardial infarction) has a history of a myocardial infarction. The patient who was diagnosed with diabetes is likely to still have diabetes.

In the case of a patient problem statement, the situation is different. Patient problem statements address *human responses* to health problems and life processes. The nurse addresses the patient's concerns about the medical problem. If a patient is diagnosed with cancer, the nurse has the opportunity to address the patient's responses to the diagnosis; responses to the disease may include anxiousness, fear of the disease or treatment, grief, inability to tolerate activity, and nausea associated with treatment. These problems often change as the LPN/LVN carries out interventions. The nurse may assist the patient who is concerned about dying with grief resolution or perhaps teach the patient coping strategies. A patient problem statement may change or resolve as care is provided or the condition changes. The medical diagnosis of cancer may not go away; however, the goal for the patient may be the ability to resolve feelings of fear regarding the diagnosis, prognosis, and treatment through nursing interventions addressed in the care plan.

GOAL IDENTIFICATION

The nurse, in collaboration with the patient, develops expected outcomes for the established patient problem. The goal statement indicates the degree of wellness desired, expected, or possible for the patient to achieve and contains a patient goal statement. The ANA uses the term *outcome identification,* but alternative terms for this statement are a patient goal, a patient-centered goal, an objective, a behavioral objective, or a patient outcome. The authors of this text have chosen to use the term patient goal statement. A patient goal statement provides a description of the specific, measurable behavior (outcome criteria) that the patient will be able to exhibit in a given time frame after the interventions. The nurse must avoid writing a goal statement that is centered on nursing interventions because this indicates what the nurse is meant to do rather than what the patient is to do.

Desired patient goal statements serve two functions. First, they guide the selection of nursing interventions. Nursing interventions are selected to promote the achievement of the desired outcome. Second, the goal statement establishes the measuring standard that is used to evaluate the effectiveness of the nursing interventions. Therefore the goal statement has to provide the specific details that can be used as the benchmark to judge progress or the solution of the problem.

A well-written patient-centered **goal** statement does the following:

- Uses the word *patient* or a part of the patient as the subject of the statement
- Uses a measurable verb
- Is specific for the patient and the patient's problem
- Does not interfere with the medical plan of care
- Is realistic for the patient and the patient's problem
- Includes a time frame for patient reevaluation

Because the subject of the patient goal statement is meant to be the patient or a part of the patient, the goal statement should begin with the words, "The patient will" or "The patient's ... will."

Measurable verbs indicate the precise behavior that the nurse anticipates hearing or seeing. *Define, describe, list, walk, demonstrate,* and *verbalize* are examples of measurable verbs.

The properly written patient goal statement is specific to the patient and the patient's health problem. A patient who is in traction because of a bone fracture has mobility restrictions. A goal statement indicating that all joints will be moved through full range of motion is not safe for this patient's problem.

The patient goal statement also must be realistic for the patient and the patient's health problem. Although some 88-year-old patients are joggers, the expectation that an 88-year-old patient will learn to jog is probably not reasonable.

A time frame is written into the patient goal statement to provide a deadline for evaluation of the patient's progress. Nursing experience assists the nurse in accurate prediction of realistic time frames.

Patient goal statements indicate a reversal of the patient problem statement, as shown in the following example:

PATIENT PROBLEM STATEMENT	GOAL STATEMENT
Compromised Skin Integrity, related to prolonged immobility as evidenced by (AEB) 2-cm–diameter excoriated area on coccyx	Patient will have intact skin within 3 wk. (NOTE: Intact skin is a reversal of the impaired skin.)

Patient goal statements can be written in two ways. The previous example illustrates the simple reversal of the problem statement in a concise fashion. A second approach is to list the desired behavior in broader terms and then list exact criteria or standards; this also may be referred to as a long-term and short-term goal. In the following list, the first example is the long-term goal, and the second and third examples are short-term goals:

- The patient will use her walker to ambulate at all times rather than using her wheelchair within the next 2 months. (Long-term goal)
- The patient will participate in range-of-motion exercises on her lower extremities bilaterally two times a day. (Short-term goal)
- The patient will ambulate 20 feet every day with assistance of her walker, increasing distance ambulated by 5 feet daily. (Short-term goal)

PLANNING

During the **planning** phase of the nursing process, priorities of care are established and nursing interventions are chosen to best address the patient problem statement. This information typically is communicated through the care plan so that all health care personnel directly involved in care of the patient can follow the same plan, resulting in continuity of care. The nurse must work with the patient and significant others in choosing appropriate interventions and in considering evidence-based practice guidelines. The plan of care should comprise standardized languages or recognized terminology to document and effectively communicate the plan.

PRIORITY SETTING

The nurse in today's busy health care facility is caring for many patients with complex problems and is challenged daily to use time and effort wisely. Priorities must be established to provide care for each patient.

Once patient problem statements have been identified, the RN must prioritize the patient problem statements according to the patient's current health status. The framework most often used to guide the prioritization is Maslow's hierarchy of needs. This structure is based on the principle that lower-level needs must be met before higher-level needs can be satisfied. The physiologic needs are more vital than the safety and security needs, and the safety and security needs are more critical than the love and belonging needs. Review Maslow's hierarchy in Fig. 1.8. Life-threatening and health-threatening problems are ranked before other types of problems. Actual problems often are ranked before potential problems, unless the potential problems, if they were to develop, are life threatening. For example, *Potential for Inability to Clear Airway* may be prioritized higher than an actual problem of *Inability to Control Urination* due to urgency. With use of Maslow's hierarchy, the nurse can determine whether the actual or *potential* patient problem statement has the highest priority. The nurse also must take into consideration the patient's thoughts and feelings regarding prioritization of problems. If patients are not active participants in the plan of care, they are not likely to be driven to work toward meeting the agreed-upon goals.

Time factors and severity of illness are important considerations in the determination of which problems to address initially. The patient who is admitted to the emergency department with a possible heart attack (myocardial infarction) is not ready at that time to contemplate dietary instructions to reach a goal of reducing cholesterol.

Priorities change as the patient progresses through time in a health care facility. As some problems are resolved, the approach to other problems comes into focus. Consider the following scenario and how the concerns of nursing change during one patient's hospital stay.

A 28-year-old woman admitted for an abdominal hysterectomy may have the preoperative patient problem of *Fearfulness*. *Recent Onset of Pain* is an important patient problem in the first few days after surgery. As the pain is controlled, *Deficient Nutrition* and *Potential for Infrequent or Difficult Bowel Elimination* are managed. When the patient approaches discharge, teaching about wound care and activity restrictions becomes the focus for patient problems. Because of the loss of reproductive ability, self-esteem problems have to be confirmed or ruled out as possible patient problems for this patient. Note how the patient problems changed, but the medical procedure did not.

SELECTING NURSING INTERVENTIONS

Nursing interventions are those activities that promote the achievement of the desired patient goal. Interventions include activities that the nurse selects, in partnership with the patient, to resolve a patient problem, monitor for the development of a potential problem, or carry out physician orders. Nursing interventions are classified as physician prescribed or nurse prescribed.

Physician-prescribed interventions are those actions ordered by a physician for a nurse or other health care professional to perform. Remember that physician orders are not orders for nurses but are prescriptive instructions for patients (Carpenito, 2016). Although the physician has given the order, nursing judgment must still be used. The LPN/LVN must follow orders when administering medications, performing wound care, and ordering diagnostic tests. Assessing, teaching, and validating the safety of physician orders are important nursing responsibilities. In this text, the term "health care provider" has been used to encompass those health care professionals who have prescriptive authority, such as physicians, advanced practice nurses, and physician assistants. The term "physician-prescribed interventions" applies to these individuals.

Nurse-prescribed interventions are any actions that a nurse is legally able to order or begin independently. Nurses write interventions for themselves or other nursing staff (Carpenito, 2016). Examples of independent nursing interventions are providing a back massage, turning a patient every 2 hours, and monitoring for complications. When determining appropriate nursing interventions, the nurse should consider the contributing, etiologic, and related factors; risk factors; the patient-centered goal; and the patient problem itself. Nursing interventions are focused on any or all of these areas.

Nursing interventions often are aimed at reducing or eliminating the causative factor. For example, for the patient problem statement *Anxiousness, related to lack of knowledge about hospital procedures,* an appropriate nursing intervention is to teach the patient about typical routines and procedures. Providing information addresses any knowledge deficit, which helps to reduce the fear of the unknown, thereby reducing anxiety.

The patient goal also is considered when selecting nursing interventions. For example, when the patient goal statement says, "The patient will plan a week's menu for an 1800-calorie diabetic diet within 1 week," the interventions are selected to increase the patient's knowledge about planning for a diabetic diet.

The patient problem statement also may direct the interventions. If the patient problem is *Recent Onset of Pain,* interventions to relieve acute pain are selected.

A variety of sources list nursing interventions. Nursing textbooks, periodicals, and care planning books are helpful sources of information. The *Nursing Interventions Classification (NIC)* may be another helpful source for nursing interventions and activities. (The *NIC* is discussed subsequently in this chapter.) Nursing colleagues and previous experience in nursing care are also good sources of ideas for interventions, as are patient suggestions regarding care. In addition, nursing conferences held to plan patient care often provide an environment for the development of creative approaches to patient care.

WRITING NURSING INTERVENTIONS

Because nursing interventions offered in textbooks and care planning resources are often broad, general statements that indicate an activity to be performed, these nursing interventions must be converted to more specific instructional statements when writing a care plan for an actual patient. Suggested interventions for constipation may include increase dietary bulk, increase activity, and encourage fluids.

This information is helpful because it prescribes a direction for care, but the information provided is lacking in specific details. The nurse must determine specific information regarding interventions so that any person following the direction of the care plan can carry out interventions without question. For care planning purposes, the nurse must be able to change the guiding general statement about the nursing intervention to a more specific statement. Nursing interventions have to be written to reduce the likelihood of misinterpretation. Details are provided to convey the intended meaning. Written nursing interventions should include the subject (the nurse is assumed unless stated otherwise), action verb, and qualifying details. Consider the following interventions:

- Ambulate the patient three times a day at 0900, 1400, and 1900.
- Ambulate the patient 30 feet three times a day at 0900, 1400, and 1900.

The correctly written nursing intervention is the second one because it contains the subject (the nurse is assumed), the action verb (ambulate), and the qualifying details (30 feet three times a day). This intervention is specific and easily interpreted by any health care professional following the care plan.

A properly written nursing intervention is specific for the problem, realistic for the patient, compatible with the medical plan of care, and based on scientific, evidenced-based principles. The following examples illustrate appropriate conversion of general nursing interventions into specific nursing interventions:

- Add four servings of fruits and vegetables of patient's choice to daily menu, one extra serving per meal and one snack.
- Turn the patient every 2 hours with the assistance of two personnel and the lift sheet.
- Offer water and juices up to 2000 mL per day according to the following schedule: 7 to 3 shift, 1200 mL; 3 to 11 shift, 600 mL; 11 to 7 shift, 200 mL.

COMMUNICATING THE NURSING CARE PLAN

After completing the initial assessment, analyzing the data, writing the patient problem statement, selecting goals, and selecting appropriate nursing interventions (which are then made more specific with written nursing

Table 5.3 Nursing Care Plan Form

PATIENT PROBLEM STATEMENT	NURSING ORDER	SCIENTIFIC PRINCIPLE	EVALUATION
Patient 1 *Recent Onset of Pain, r/t tissue trauma from broken fibula and tibia, AEB grimaces, reports right leg pain at 8/10, and has elevated blood pressure 140/100 mm Hg.* DESIRED PATIENT GOAL: Patient will demonstrate improved comfort level as evidenced by relaxed facial expression, statements of pain relief, and return of vital signs to patient's normal range within 30 min of nursing interventions.	1. Assess verbal and nonverbal indications of pain. 2. Monitor blood pressure and pulse for increase over baseline value q 4 hr. 3. Elevate right leg on two pillows at all times except meals. 4. Offer back rub and position change when statements of pain are made.	1. Fractures cause swelling and pressure on nerves. Patient pain report establishes need for intervention. 2. Pain increases heart rate and blood pressure. 3. Gravity helps reduce edema, which reduces pain. 4. Sensory nerve impulses from the skin "close the gate" and prevent pain transmission.	Goal achieved. D = States pain in lower right leg 8/10. Blood pressure 140/100 mm Hg. A = Right leg elevated on two pillows. Back rub given for 10 min. R = States pain improved to 2/10. Blood pressure 132/88 mm Hg; no facial grimacing.
Patient 2 *Potential for Compromised Skin Integrity, r/t pressure on bony prominences, impaired circulation, and physical immobilization.* DESIRED PATIENT GOAL: Short-term goal: Patient will remain free of any skin impairments, such as reddened areas, by 10/28/2018. Long-term goal: Patient will have no skin breakdown with q 2 hr turning during duration of stay in facility.	1. Monitor skin condition for skin color and texture changes q 2 hr with turning. 2. Identify areas that are more at risk for skin impairment, such as bony prominences (e.g., elbows, heels, and sacral area). 3. Use lotions or moisturizers to prevent dry skin with a.m. care and PRN. 4. Change patient's position at least q 2 hr	1. Early identification of any skin impairment can prevent breakdown. 2. Identifying problem areas makes knowing where to look and how often to look for skin impairment a more effective process. 3. Dry skin can lead to cracks in the skin and infection. 4. Changing position in immobile residents prevents pressure ulcers from forming.	Goal achieved. D = Patient has no areas of skin impairment. A = Patient's position changed q 2 hr and lotion applied in a.m. and PRN. R = Voices no reports of discomfort regarding skin condition.

Critical Thinking Questions

1. The patient experiencing pain (patient 1) asks why he has an elevated blood pressure. How should the nurse respond?
2. What interventions can the nurse initiate to prevent this patient's pain from reaching an 8/10 level in the future?
3. What nutritional measures can the nurse include in the plan of care for the patient who is at risk for impaired skin integrity (patient 2)?

A, Action; *AEB*, as evidenced by; *D*, data; *PRN*, as needed; *q 2 hr*, every 2 hours; *R*, response/evaluation; *r/t*, related to.

interventions), the nurse has the responsibility to communicate the detailed plan of care for the patient. The written nursing care plan is the tangible product of the nursing process (Table 5.3). (Refer to Chapter 3 for additional information on charting and documentation.)

Because the nursing staff constantly changes (nurses work different shifts and have days off), written guidelines are important for continuity of patient care. Continuity increases patient trust in the nursing staff and promotes outcome achievement.

Nursing care plans may be written specifically for a patient, or the nurse may use a standardized care plan for a patient. The nurse must individualize each care plan to the patient, even with use of standardized care plans. Individually prepared care plans are the most time consuming but often provide care that is best matched to the specific patient's needs and situation. An individualized plan of care takes into consideration pertinent patient characteristics such as age, culture, and medical diagnosis.

Standardized nursing care plans are appropriate for patient populations with routine, expected care requirements. Women who have had a vaginal delivery or a cesarean delivery are ideal patient populations for standardized care plans. Many standardized care plans include blank spaces that the nurse fills in to individualize to some degree.

Linear Care Plans Versus Concept Maps

Among nursing faculty, a range of different expectations often exists for the care planning process. Formats for the written nursing care plan vary from school to school. Components that are common in an educational setting are NANDA-I diagnostic labels, patient-centered goals and desired patient outcomes, and nursing interventions and orders.

Nursing faculty may require students to submit the care plan in a four-column or five-column format that is referred to as a *linear style*. With this system, rationale is often necessary to explain why the intervention is needed or how the intervention will work. This encourages the student to use critical thinking skills and evidence-based practice for supporting the nursing interventions chosen.

Other nursing faculty may prefer the care plan to be represented as a concept map. Concept maps typically use different shapes, and sometimes colors, that are connected with lines when there is a relationship between one or more items. A concept map is especially beneficial for visual learners. With concept mapping, the student may put the patient problem statement into a rectangular shape in the middle of the page; interventions are in circles that branch off from the nursing diagnosis, and outcomes are placed into a triangle. The student should follow the specific guidelines of the nursing program for topics to be included on a concept map and its organization.

IMPLEMENTATION

During the **implementation** phase of the nursing process, the nurse and other members of the team put the established plan into action to promote goal achievement. This is the fifth phase of the nursing process. With evidence-based interventions, the nurse should ensure that the plan is implemented in a timely and safe manner.

In emergency situations, the nursing process as a means of problem solving is accelerated. The nurse proceeds directly from assessment of the problem to intervention. If a patient has gone into cardiac or respiratory arrest, the nurse initiates cardiopulmonary resuscitation immediately.

Nursing interventions include nurse-prescribed and physician-prescribed activities. (See the discussion of selecting nursing interventions in the previous "Planning" section in this chapter.) According to the ANA Scope and Standards of Practice (2010), implementation for nursing intervention includes activities such as teaching, monitoring, providing, counseling, delegating, and coordinating.

EVIDENCE-BASED PRACTICE

Nursing research is the basis for evidence-based practice. Nursing research was cultivated in the 1950s, leading to the development of nursing theories in the 1960s and 1970s. In the 1990s nursing theories were researched and further tested to expand the field of nursing and evidence-based practice. Nursing research today continues to solidify theories and practice and introduce new theories. Other disciplines such as sociology, psychology, biology, and physics are incorporated into nursing theory.

The ANA Scope and Standards of Practice (2010) defines evidence-based practice as: "a scholarly and systematic problem-solving paradigm that results in the delivery of high-quality health care. In order to make the best clinical decisions using EBP, external evidence from research is blended with internal evidence (i.e., practice-generated data), clinical expertise, and healthcare consumer values and preferences to achieve the best outcomes for individuals, groups, populations, and healthcare systems."

EVALUATION

Evaluation is a determination made about the extent to which the established goals have been achieved. The nurse takes several steps to complete the evaluation phase. (1) Review the patient-centered goals or desired patient outcomes that were established previously. These goal statements present standards and criteria that are observable and measurable. (2) Reassess the patient to gather data that indicate the patient's actual response to the nursing interventions. (3) Compare the actual outcome with the desired outcome and make a critical judgment about whether the patient-centered goal or desired patient outcome was achieved.

This critical judgment leads the nurse to make one of three conclusions or decisions: the goal was achieved, the goal was not achieved, or the goal was partially achieved. Evaluation of the desired patient goal is illustrated in the following statement:

PATIENT GOAL STATEMENT	EVALUATION AND DOCUMENTATION
1. The patient will demonstrate self-administration of insulin with sterile technique and selection of correct site by 10/21/2018.	1. 10/21/2018: Patient goal achieved. Patient correctly administered regular insulin into upper thigh with sterile technique.
2. Patient's left hip ulcer will measure 1 cm (W) × 2.5 cm (L) in 3 wk (10/28/2018).	2. 10/28/2018: Patient goal partially achieved. Patient's left hip ulcer measures 0.3 cm (W) × 0.5 cm (L).

The plan of care generally undergoes changes during this phase of the nursing process. The nurse makes modifications according to whether the goal has been achieved, partially achieved, or not achieved. When a problem has been resolved, it is removed from the nursing care plan.

When the goal has been achieved partially or not achieved, further analysis is needed. At this point, the nurse should review all phases of the nursing process. The following are examples of questions the nurse should consider to ensure the accuracy of the nursing process:

- Was the assessment complete and accurate?
- Was the problem identified correctly?
- Was the desired patient goal realistic and specific?
- Were the interventions realistic, and did all personnel implement them consistently?

- Did new problems develop?
- Was adequate time allowed?

Once the nurse has determined the answers to these questions, the nursing care plan can be modified accordingly.

STANDARDIZED LANGUAGES: NANDA-I, *NIC*, AND *NOC*

Effective communication in the health care setting is vital to provide consistent quality care for patients. Nurses work in a variety of settings, and patients may be cared for in a variety of settings, sometimes with transfer from one facility to another. The use of a **standardized language** (terms that have the same definition and meaning regardless of who uses them) fosters communication regarding aspects of patient care.

NANDA-I, *Nursing Interventions Classification (NIC)*, and *Nursing Outcomes Classification (NOC)* provide standardized nursing diagnoses (patient problem statements), nursing interventions, and nursing-sensitive patient outcomes (goals). These classification systems further provide research-based information regarding nursing treatments and judgments. NANDA-I, *NIC*, and terminology are used internationally in all patient settings, including acute care hospitals, long-term care facilities, outpatient and ambulatory settings, rehabilitation facilities, and home care. These systems aid in supporting clinical decisions, provide evidence-based practice used in plans of care, and support of effective staffing, student learning, and staff education. NANDA-I, *NOC*, and *NIC* (NNN) comprise the components of a care plan by identification of the nursing diagnosis, nursing outcome(s), and nursing interventions. In this text the authors illustrate this process as follows:

PATIENT PROBLEM	GOAL STATEMENT	NURSING INTERVENTION
Inefficient Oxygenation	Arterial blood gases within normal limits	Ensure use of incentive spirometer 10 breaths every hour

NURSING INTERVENTIONS CLASSIFICATION

This standardized language, developed at the University of Iowa, encourages enhanced communication between nurses regarding nursing interventions. The current edition of *Nursing Interventions Classification (NIC)* lists more than 500 interventions and 13,000 activities. Each *NIC* intervention has a label, a definition for that label, a list of activities that can be used for that intervention, and background information. The label and definition should not be altered when they are used, but the activities must be individualized to the patient's needs. The title given to nursing interventions is concise. Examples of nursing interventions are *Airway management; Analgesic administration; Teaching: prescribed diet;* and *Therapeutic play.* Some *NIC* interventions are called *indirect interventions* because they occur away from the bedside but on behalf of the patient. Examples of indirect care interventions are *emergency cart checking, shift report, staff development,* and *supply management* (Butcher et al, 2019).

The list of activities is a helpful guide for beginning nurses. The following example shows a *NIC* intervention and lists 3 of the 36 possible activities for the intervention (Butcher et al, 2019). NOTE: The definition given and the indicated number that can be retrieved with computer systems. These numbers "run in the background" and are not for memorization.

NIC intervention: 6540

Infection control: Minimizing the acquisition and transmission of infectious agents

Activities:

- Isolate individuals exposed to communicable disease.
- Wash hands before and after each patient-care activity.
- Ensure appropriate wound care technique.

NURSING OUTCOMES CLASSIFICATION

Nursing Outcomes Classification (NOC), which measures the effects of nursing care, is the effort of a group of researchers working at the University of Iowa. These researchers have developed a standardized system with an organized structure to name and measure **nursing-sensitive patient outcomes.** Identification of outcomes that are responsive to nursing care is important work for nursing, especially in connection with efforts to contain costs and establish best practices (Moorhead et al, 2018). There are currently 385 outcomes with accompanying definitions, measurement standards, indicators, and references (Moorhead et al, 2018).

The *NOC* outcomes use brief phrases to describe the result of nursing care. Indicators are given as subheadings for each outcome. These indicators use a measurement scale to evaluate the degree of outcome attainment. The outcome statement and indicator can be described with selected key words from a patient goal statement ("The patient will demonstrate beginning *grief resolution* as evidenced by the ability to *verbalize reality of loss* after nursing interventions"). NOTE: The coded nature of the outcome and indicators that are used to enhance entry and retrieval of information from a computer database.

Grief resolution (outcome 1304). Verbalizes reality of loss (indicator 130403). The scale used for this indicator measures from "never demonstrated" to "consistently demonstrated" (1 to 5 scale) (Moorhead et al, 2018).

These measurement scales can be used to establish a baseline assessment and then the scale can be applied again during the evaluation phase. Some facilities use these indicators to plan for patient discharge. For example, if the patient does not achieve a 4 or 5 on a scale, then a referral is sometimes necessary.

Box 5.2 Role of the Licensed Practical/Vocational Nurse in the Nursing Process

ASSESSMENT

- Observe and report significant cues to the nurse in charge or to the health care provider.

DIAGNOSIS

- Assist with the determination of accurate patient problem statements.
- Gather further data to confirm or eliminate problems.

GOAL IDENTIFICATION AND PLANNING

- Assist with setting priorities.
- Suggest interventions.
- Assist with the development of realistic patient-centered goals and desired patient outcomes.

IMPLEMENTATION

- Assist with the establishment of priorities.
- Carry out health care provider and planned nursing interventions.
- Evaluate the effectiveness of nursing activities.

EVALUATION

- Assist with reevaluation of the patient's health state after nursing interventions.
- Suggest alternative nursing interventions when necessary.

ROLE OF THE LICENSED PRACTICAL/VOCATIONAL NURSE

The LPN/LVN plays a vital role in the collaborative care of the patient. The role of the LPN/LVN in the nursing process may vary from state to state and with different institutions. All practical and vocational student nurses should be knowledgeable regarding their own state's practice. In many states, the RN is responsible for the coordination of care, initiation of the nursing care plan, and evaluation of patient outcomes with the assistance of the LPN/LVN. The LPN/LVN is frequently responsible for providing direct bedside nursing care. This direct care position allows the LPN/LVN to closely observe, prioritize, intervene, and evaluate the care provided to and for the patient. See Box 5.2 for a summary of the role of the LPN/LVN in the nursing process.

MANAGED CARE AND CLINICAL PATHWAYS

To practice in the changing world of health care today, nurses are called on to go beyond performing technical skills and providing direct patient care. Responsibilities include working with outcomes, cost, resources, and other members of the health care team. One way of addressing cost containment issues is through managed care. **Managed care** refers to health care systems that have control over primary health care services and attempt to trim down health care costs by reducing unnecessary or overlapping services; an emphasis is placed on health promotion, education, and preventive medicine. Case management is one way managed care is achieved in a health care setting. **Case management** encompasses planning, coordination of care, and patient advocacy in providing quality, cost-effective outcomes for the patient. The case management system of care allows for continuity in care because one person coordinates the plan of care for an individual patient within the health care setting, including discharge planning.

Case management usually depends on the use of clinical pathways. A **clinical pathway** is a multidisciplinary plan that incorporates evidence-based practice guidelines for high-risk, high-volume, high-cost types of cases while providing for optimal patient outcomes and maximized clinical efficiency. Synonyms for clinical pathways are critical pathways, multidisciplinary action plans, action plans, and care maps. The clinical pathway guides care with coordination of actions from all disciplines in a health care facility, such as nursing, respiratory therapy, medicine, pharmacy, social services, dietary therapy, occupational therapy, speech therapy, and physical therapy, to develop the plan of care. Clinical pathways, like any method of planning care for a patient, are aimed at providing continuity of care, efficiency in care provided, and reducing facility costs. Clinical pathways are generally standardized documents, so it is important for the nurse to be sure to individualize them to the patient's needs. If a patient does not achieve the projected outcome, it is considered a **variance**. A variance must be evaluated to determine why the patient did not meet the outcome. Possible reasons an outcome was not achieved include the patient's condition changed, interventions were not performed or were not effective, or a new problem developed. Variance analysis then is used to promote continuous quality improvement. Repetition of variances often leads the health care team to revise a clinical pathway.

Whether the health care facility uses the traditional care plan, clinical pathways, or another system for organizing care, the goal remains the same: efficient care with positive patient outcomes. In addition, the nurse and all health care professionals must be cognizant of cost containment when providing care.

CRITICAL THINKING

"Thinking with a purpose" describes the term *critical thinking*. Critical thinkers question information, conclusions, and points of view and look beneath the surface. They are logical and fair in their thinking. The skills related to critical thinking are applied to reading, listening, and writing across all subjects. Critical thinking is a complex process, and no single simple definition explains all aspects of critical thinking. Each author who writes about critical thinking has his or her own definition. The National League for Nursing (2000) defines critical thinking for nursing as "a discipline-specific, reflective reasoning process that guides a nurse in generating, implementing, and evaluating approaches for dealing with client care and professional concerns."

Critical thinking is essential to providing quality nursing care for patients in various situations. One of the first skills a nursing student learns is to take a temperature. The student nurse must choose among obtaining tympanic (ear), oral, rectal, skin, temporal, or axillary measurements. Critical thinking enables the nurse to use the nursing process in choosing the appropriate method. One consideration is the need for accuracy in the results. Also, certain medical or surgical problems may interfere with the accuracy of the reading. If a patient has an ear infection, the results of a tympanic reading may not be accurate. The nurse avoids a rectal thermometer when the patient is recovering from hemorrhoid surgery. If the patient is likely to have a seizure, an oral thermometer is contraindicated because the patient may bite down on the device. The condition of the site to be used also should be taken into consideration. Heavy perspiration often interferes with axillary temperature readings; oral temperature is affected by ingestion of hot or cold beverages. All of these variables are taken into consideration by the student nurse who uses critical thinking skills in the decision-making process.

It is crucial for nurses to not only be able to *perform skills* (the "doing" of nursing) but also *think about* what they are doing. Nurses use a knowledge base to make decisions, generate new ideas, and solve problems. Nursing students add to their knowledge base by studying facts, principles, evidence-based practice guidelines, and theories. Knowledge of psychology, anatomy, physiology, pharmacology, and other related course work helps the student to gain the scientific knowledge base to think critically.

Nurses also must reflect on situations or care given to determine what was effective and what was not effective. Critical thinkers are able to analyze this information and adjust care accordingly, if necessary. Critical thinkers are also able to explore the relationships between concepts and ideas and apply these concepts to unique patient care situations.

To help determine the difference between thinking and critical thinking, consider the following nonclinical situations:

- *Situation 1:* On the day before classes begin, the student is anxious about getting started and is unsure of her chances of success. She is thinking, "I hope I don't get lost. I hope the teachers are nice. I wonder if I will be able to pass the tests. Will I succeed?" On the day classes begin, she drives to school, finds a parking space, and enters the building to locate her classroom.
- *Situation 2:* On the day before classes begin, the student is anxious about getting started and is unsure of her chances of success. She is thinking, "I will drive to the school so that I can judge how much time to allow for travel. I want to go early and locate my classroom today so that I will have an easier time tomorrow. Maybe I can get some course materials early so that I can organize my notebook."

Both of these situations involve individuals who are thinking. The student in situation 1 is experiencing a mental activity, but it is aimless and without purpose. The student in situation 2 has recognized the need to gain control and get organized. This student is beginning to think critically and with a purpose, which is to decrease the anxiety associated with her first day of class.

The following clinical situations provide examples of some aspects of critical thinking at the bedside.

- *Situation 1:* The nurse was caring for a patient with chronic obstructive pulmonary disease and peripheral vascular disease. During the assessment, the nurse used a pulse oximeter on the patient's finger to measure the patient's oxygen saturation level. The measurement yielded an oxygen saturation of 87%. The assessment revealed clear lung sounds, no difficulty with respirations or reports of shortness of breath, capillary refill less than 2 seconds, and extremities cool to the touch. The nurse demonstrates critical thinking skills by realizing that the assessment does not match the oxygen saturation measurement and decides to recheck the oxygen saturation level with the earlobe probe because the patient's hands were cool to the touch. The oxygen saturation level with the earlobe probe was 93%, which matched the assessment findings. With use of critical thinking skills, the nurse was able to make comparisons between the assessment findings and the oxygen saturation level and problem solve by determining how to address the situation.
- *Situation 2:* A patient with diabetes was admitted to the hospital for a bladder infection. At the change of shift, the oncoming nurse entered the room to perform an assessment. The nurse noted that the patient was unresponsive. The nurse demonstrates critical thinking skills by realizing the patient is most likely experiencing one of two problems: hypoglycemia or hyperglycemia. The nurse first performed a quick "ABC" assessment and determined that the patient's airway was open, the patient was breathing, and the patient's heart was circulating blood. Then, because the patient was admitted with an infection, the nurse suspected that the patient was experiencing a rise in blood glucose levels, or hyperglycemia. He obtained a finger-stick blood glucose reading of 346. The nurse also noted that the patient's skin was warm, dry, and flushed. The patient's respirations were deep, and her breath smelled "fruity." The nurse quickly called the physician to report these findings and anticipated receiving orders to give the patient more insulin. Critical thinking skills enabled the nurse to deal with this patient situation appropriately.

Anticipating questions, asking an expert, and asking *why* are examples of other strategies to improve critical thinking. The more experience the student nurse or nurse gains, the better their critical thinking skills become. Hearing others think aloud also may help the student learn how other people reason. The student should take advantage of every learning opportunity and realize that every experience, mistake, and encounter is a potential learning opportunity.

Get Ready for the NCLEX® Examination!

Key Points

- The nursing process consists of six interconnected phases: assessment, diagnosis, outcome identification, planning, implementation, and evaluation. In this text, diagnosis is frequently referred to as *patient problem statement*, and outcome identification is frequently referred to as *patient goal.*
- A complete and valid assessment influences the remaining phases of the nursing process.
- The patient is the primary source of data; all others are secondary sources.
- The nurse prescribes the primary interventions to treat a nursing diagnosis or patient problem statement.
- The nurse uses assessment data to develop the nursing diagnosis (patient problem statement).
- The nurse projects end results that are measurable, desirable, and observable during outcome identification or patient goal.
- The nurse develops an individualized plan of care that considers pertinent patient characteristics such as age, culture, medical diagnosis, and mutual interest.
- Nursing interventions are planned activities to promote outcome (patient goal) achievement.
- Evaluation is an ongoing component of each phase of the nursing process.
- During evaluation, the actual patient outcome (goal) is compared with the desired patient outcome (goal), and a judgment is made about outcome (goal) achievement.
- The plan of care is changed according to evaluation and the resulting identification of needs.
- NANDA-I, *NIC,* and *NOC* continue to develop standardized nursing languages to aid communication and research.
- The LPN/LVN has a significant role in the nursing process.
- Managed care and case management systems have emerged in response to rising health care costs.
- A clinical pathway is a multidisciplinary plan that schedules clinical interventions over an anticipated time frame for specific types of patient health problems.
- Critical thinking involves thinking with a purpose and using reasoning with decision making.
- Evidence-based practice provides the latest guidelines for patient care based on best practices provided by research.

Additional Learning Resources

SG Go to your Study Guide for additional learning activities to help you master this chapter content.

evolve Be sure to visit the Evolve site at *http://evolve.elsevier.com/Cooper/foundationsadult/* for additional online resources.

Review Questions for the NCLEX® Examination

1. The student nurse correctly identifies which as a medical diagnosis? *(Select all that apply.)*
   1. Acute pain
   2. Pneumonia
   3. Inability to tolerate activity
   4. Inability to clear airway
   5. Neuropathy, secondary to type 2 diabetes mellitus
2. A patient is admitted to a hospital for coronary artery bypass graft surgery. His wound continues to drain, and when he is discharged, home health nurses will visit to continue to care for him. Who is most likely responsible for coordinating the patient's discharge plans?
   1. RN team leader
   2. Social worker
   3. Case manager
   4. Physician
3. Which patient problem statement includes all appropriate components of an actual patient problem statement? *(Select all that apply.)*
   1. *Inefficient Oxygenation*
   2. *Potential Complication: Gastric Bleeding, related to gastric ulcer*
   3. *Fearfulness, related to separation from support system as evidenced by statements of being scared, pallor, and increased respirations*
   4. *Potential for Falling, related to confusion as evidenced by calling nurse by name of aunt*
   5. *Anxiousness, related to upcoming surgery as evidenced by the patient stating, "I am very worried that something is going to go wrong."*
4. *Prolonged Infrequent or Difficulty With Bowel Elimination, related to the effects of analgesic medications on the bowel as evidenced by statements of straining to have a bowel movement and no bowel movement in 5 days* is an example of which type of patient problem statement?
   1. An actual patient problem statement
   2. A potential patient problem statement
   3. A wellness patient problem statement
   4. A patient problem statement
5. Based on Maslow's hierarchy of needs, which patient problem statement label has the highest priority?
   1. *Potential for Aspiration Into Airway*
   2. *Insufficient Knowledge*
   3. *Recent Onset of Pain*
   4. *Inability to Control Urination Due to Physical Stress*
6. Which patient goal statement is best stated and contains necessary criteria? *(Select all that apply.)*
   1. The patient will identify the types of foods to include in a high-fiber diet.
   2. The nurse will teach the patient about constipation prevention.
   3. The nurse will increase total fluids during hospitalization.
   4. The patient will have a soft, formed bowel movement on the third day after surgery.
   5. The patient will ambulate 50 feet three times per day, with the assistance of 1, starting on postoperative day 1.

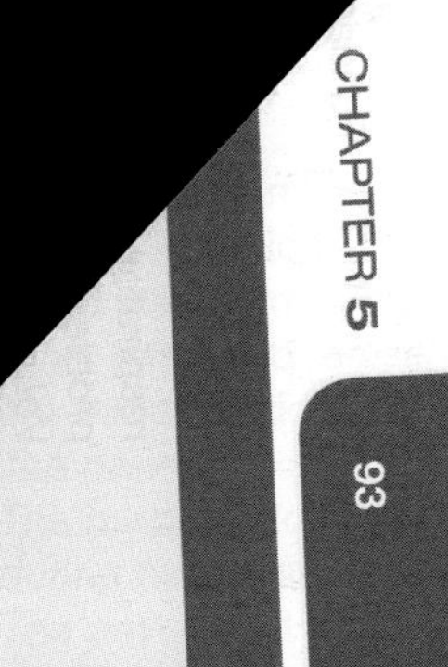

he hospital with an upper
rse writes the following
l for Inadequate Fluid
drink fluids, secondary to
est patient goal statement

mL of fluids per day

e a less sore throat in 8

3. The nurse will maintain an intravenous infusion of fluids for the ordered length of time.
4. The patient will maintain adequate hydration as evidenced by moist mucous membranes, elastic skin turgor, and voiding of clear dilute urine.

8. A woman who has had four children comes to the clinic. She tells the nurse that when she laughs or coughs she loses control of some urine. Which nursing intervention is properly written in the care plan?
1. The nurse will teach the patient Kegel exercises.
2. The patient will perform Kegel exercises 10 times a day with four to six repetitions each time.
3. The nurse will teach the patient how to perform Kegel exercises 10 times a day with four to six repetitions each time.
4. The patient will not experience stress incontinence after 2 months of performing Kegel exercises 10 times per day.

9. A 14-year-old patient is admitted to the emergency department with a possible medical diagnosis of acute appendicitis. Who should the nurse interview first when performing the assessment?
1. The patient's parents
2. The patient
3. The physician
4. The admissions nurse

10. Which statement by the student nurse best demonstrates knowledge of the nursing process when describing defining characteristics?
1. "Defining characteristics are a description of the patient problem."
2. "Defining characteristics tell how the nursing diagnosis was determined."
3. "Defining characteristics are a cluster of clinical cues."
4. "Defining characteristics are factors such as signs and symptoms that support the nursing diagnosis."

11. Which phrases are most appropriate to use to connect the parts of a patient problem statement?
1. "Related to" and "due to"
2. "Due to" and "as evidenced by"
3. "Related to" and "as evidenced by"
4. "Due to" and "as evidenced by"

12. What occurs during the last phase of the nursing process?
1. The nurse gathers data to use in planning care.
2. The nurse selects nursing interventions to achieve the desired outcomes.
3. The nurse compares the desired outcome with the actual outcome.
4. The nurse prioritizes nursing interventions.

13. Which statement best describes a patient problem statement?
1. Statement of the patient's needs according to Maslow's hierarchy
2. Description of the patient's disease process
3. Listing of the required nursing interventions
4. A patient's health-related problem that can be treated by the nurse.

14. The patient is experiencing severe respiratory distress that is related to his chronic obstructive pulmonary disease. The patient is alert and oriented and is capable of answering questions. Which source of information is most accurate when performing a nursing history during the admission assessment?
1. The patient
2. The patient's wife
3. The physician
4. The medical record

15. The student nurse is correct in identifying which statement as objective data? *(Select all that apply.)*
1. "When I walk to the mailbox, I get very short of breath."
2. "My legs ache when I climb stairs."
3. 4-cm Transverse abdominal incision
4. Report of pain 6 on a scale of 0 to 10
5. B/P 178/90

16. A newborn has the nursing diagnosis of *Potential for Inability to Regulate Body Temperature.* What is the most accurate patient goal for this patient problem statement?
1. Parents state that they will keep the infant's room warm.
2. Parents state that they will wrap their infant in two blankets.
3. Parents state that they will keep their infant's temperature between 97.5°F and 98.6°F.
4. Parents state that they will be sure that their infant wears something on her head at home.

17. While giving a bath, the nurse notes skin breakdown on a patient's coccyx. What part of the patient problem statement is this observation?
1. The patient problem statement
2. The etiologic or related factor
3. The patient goal
4. The defining characteristic

18. Which example includes all appropriate components of a *potential* patient problem statement? *(Select all that apply.)*
1. *Potential for Inability to Tolerate Activity*
2. *Potential for Aspiration Into Airway, related to difficulty swallowing*
3. *Potential Complication: Hemorrhage*
4. *Potential for Inability to Clear Airway, related to accumulation of mucus in trachea*
5. *Potential for Compromised Skin Integrity, related to immobility as evidenced by 2-cm abrasion*

Cultural and Ethnic Considerations

6

http://evolve.elsevier.com/Cooper/foundationsadult/

Objectives

1. Identify the importance of transcultural nursing.
2. Describe ways that culture affects the individual.
3. Explain how personal cultural beliefs and practices affect nurse-patient and nurse-nurse relationships.
4. Identify and discuss cultural variables that potentially influence health behaviors.
5. Explain how cultural data can be used to help develop therapeutic relationships with the patient.
6. Discuss cultural and religious influences as they relate to the older adult.
7. Discuss the use of the nursing process in the care of culturally diverse patients.

Key Terms

biomedical health belief system (Table 6.2, p. 108)
cultural competence (KŬL-chŭr-ăl KŎM-pĕ-tĕns, p. 96)
culture (p. 95)
ethnic stereotype (p. 96)
ethnicity (ĕth-NĬS-ĭ-tē, p. 97)
ethnocentrism (ĕth-nō-SĔN-trĭz-ŭm, p. 96)
folk health belief system (Table 6.2, p. 108)
holistic health belief system (Table 6.2, p. 108)
race (p. 96)
society (p. 95)
stereotype (STĔR-ē-ō-tīp, p. 96)
subculture (p. 95)
transcultural nursing (p. 96)

The United States has been described as a "melting pot" of people from many different countries. This description implies that people are blended so completely together that everyone shares the same values, beliefs, health practices, communication styles, and religion. A better description is to say the country is like a pot of vegetable soup—many different, but distinct, pieces are combined to form a rich assortment. This assortment makes up our **society** (a nation, community, or broad group of people who establish particular aims, beliefs, or standards of living and conduct). In addition, the "soup recipe" is no longer what it had been; as a result, our societal "flavor" is changing.

US Census projections anticipate a decrease in the percentage of the population identifying as the majority, designated as "white only," over the next 40 years. Before the 2000 US Census, respondents had no way to select more than one race. Because of this, the comparison to previous years is not completely accurate. However, the prediction of a decreasing "white only" population is supported by recent data that showed increases in the percentage of minority children under the age of 5. In fact, more than half the population under the age of 1 are a racial minority. The racial composition of the United States will continue to be influenced by immigration as well as family size and multiple race identification. More people are identifying as biracial, Hispanic, and black (US Census Bureau, 2012).

CULTURE DEFINED

Culture is a set of learned values, beliefs, customs, and practices that are shared by a group and are passed from one generation to another. Because of the influx of diverse cultures, the United States rapidly is becoming multicultural and multilingual. Many immigrants have come from areas of the world devastated by wars, natural disasters, famine, and poverty. They have had little preparation or time to learn English or American culture before arriving. Many of these immigrant populations have formed subcultures in US society.

Often separate subcultures exist within a given group. A **subculture** shares many characteristics with the primary culture but has characteristic patterns of behavior and ideals that distinguish it from the rest of a cultural group. Even among Americans who have lived here for several generations, these subcultures exist. For example, a person who grew up in the mountains of Appalachia has very different cultural practices than a person from New York City. Understanding of these variables and acceptance of each person as an individual are the first steps in giving holistic care to patients.

Although cultures often differ considerably from one another, they share certain basic characteristics. Box 6.1 identifies four common characteristics of all cultures.

All members of a culture do not exhibit the same behaviors. These variations within a cultural group

Box 6.1 Common Characteristics of Cultures

- Culture is learned, beginning at birth, through language and socialization. Behaviors, values, attitudes, and beliefs are learned within the cultural family system.
- Culture tends to be dynamic and ever changing. Language, traditions, and norms of customs may act as stabilizers for a culture.
- Members of the same cultural group may share patterns that are present in every culture. These include communication, means of economic and physical survival, transportation systems, family systems, social customs and mores, and religious systems. (Morals are accepted traditional customs, moral attitudes, or manners of a particular social group.)
- Culture is an adaptation to specific factors or conditions in a specific location, such as the availability of natural resources. When people are removed from that location, their customs continue even though they are no longer called for in the new setting.

occur because of individual differences. Examples of these differences are as follows:

- Age
- Amount and type of interaction between younger and older generations
- Degree to which values in current country are adopted
- Dialect or language spoken
- Gender identity and roles
- Geographic location of country of origin or current residence
- Religion
- Socioeconomic background

Cultural influences vary with each individual. It is best to deliver culturally competent care and avoid stereotyping behaviors. Culture influences each person in various ways. The nurse is advised to avoid stereotyping members of any cultural group. A **stereotype** is a generalized expectation about forms of behavior, an individual, or a group. An **ethnic stereotype** is a fixed concept of how all members of an ethnic group act or think. Stereotypes sometimes do and sometimes do not have any relationship to reality.

CULTURAL COMPETENCE AND TRANSCULTURAL NURSING

Most people look at the world from their own cultural viewpoint. They often believe that the beliefs and practices of their particular culture are best. This belief is called **ethnocentrism.** The nurse must learn to value the beliefs of others and realize that practices of other cultures can be valuable in health care.

In the care of patients from many different cultures, the licensed practical/vocational nurse (LPN/LVN) must develop **cultural competence:** the awareness of one's own cultural beliefs and practices and their relation to those of others, which may be different. One way to identify these beliefs and practices is through a self-assessment. This self-assessment is important. Personal beliefs and practices influence, and sometimes put some limitations on, the ability to care for those from other cultures. Understanding personal beliefs enables one to respond to those from different cultures with openness, understanding, and acceptance of cultural differences.

The nurse needs to accept that it is not possible to act the same with all patients and still give effective, individualized, holistic care. Rather than ignore the differences, the nurse should include questions about cultural practices during the nursing process. This information is critical and is important in developing a plan of care to meet patient needs. Box 6.2 gives some guidelines for cultural information that can be gathered in the patient assessment.

Because of the many variations in cultural and subcultural practices, culturally appropriate nursing care is a challenge in the 21st century. Understanding these variables and integrating an understanding into all aspects of nursing care is referred to as **transcultural nursing.** The LPN/LVN should strive to achieve a high level of transcultural nursing in day-to-day practices.

It is important to understand that people from different cultures have a variety of practices related to health care, treatment methods, and responses to illness and death (see the Evidence-Based Practice box). In many cases, these differences extend to practices related to childbirth and the ways people of different age groups are cared for (see the Lifespan Considerations for Older Adults box). In addition, cultural beliefs frequently affect diet and nutrition. Remember to assess areas that potentially are influenced by cultural factors.

In addition to caring for people from various cultures, nurses find that many other health care providers come from different ethnic, cultural, and religious backgrounds than their patients. Some of these nurses have received their education in foreign countries and have moved to the United States for better opportunities. Others were born in this country but are part of a different cultural or racial group.

Learning about cultural differences that exist improves working relationships between members of the health care team. In much the same way that this kind of openness helps in caring for patients, it helps in understanding and accepting differences among nurses and their colleagues.

RACE AND ETHNICITY

There are various reasons why a given individual demonstrates a given cultural practice. Perhaps the person is from a foreign country or a region of the United States where that practice is common. Perhaps the person's practice is related to **race** (a group of people who share biologic physical characteristics) and

Box 6.2 Cultural Assessment for Health Care

NURSING DATA COLLECTION (OBTAINED THROUGH INTERVIEW OR OBSERVATION)

- What language is used? If the patient does not commonly use English, how well does the patient understand English? Whom does the patient depend on to translate information?
- What cultural practices have the potential to interfere with receiving health care?
- Differences in health care beliefs
- Difficulty with care being performed by members of the opposite sex
- Modesty and privacy concerns
- Personal space practices
- Use of folk medicines or treatments
- What dietary practices have the potential to interfere with treatment for this illness?

INTERVIEW QUESTIONS

- Who will make decisions about your treatment?
- Who is the person in your family who must be involved with health care decisions?
- Will members of your community be asked to help with making decisions about your care?
- Can you describe what is wrong?
- What do you think has caused your problem (illness, condition)?
- Why do you think this has happened at this time?
- Why did it happen to you?
- Why did it affect your (body part)?
- How long have you had this problem?
- Why did you come for help now?
- What do you think will help to clear up your problem?
- Who else do you think can help you?
- Have you gone to this person for help?
- What did the person do?
- Did this treatment help?
- What results do you hope to get from your care?
- How will your illness affect your family?

Modified from Potter PA, Perry AG, Stockert P, et al: *Fundamentals of nursing,* ed 9, St. Louis, 2017, Mosby.

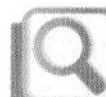 **Evidence-Based Practice**

Cultural Beliefs and Rituals Regarding Death

EVIDENCE SUMMARY

Although culture and religion are important to people who are dying, and to their families, practices regarding the death of a loved one vary among cultures and religions. Focus groups were used in this research study to find similarities and differences among cultural and religious beliefs, ceremonies, and rituals about death. Many cultures and religions use beliefs for praying, talking, and remembering loved ones. Rituals often accompany ceremonies and are used to delay death, ward off evil, ensure that the dying person is remembered, and help the family cope with the death. All participants in the study indicated that respect and protection of the dying person's soul were important. Many practices that surround death are influenced by religion and culture. Hispanic and Latino rituals often are influenced heavily by Catholicism. African-American and Caribbean participants identified the importance of faith, hope, and prayer and similarities were found between Hindu and Buddhist beliefs about funeral arrangements, afterlife, family customs, and Karma.

APPLICATION TO NURSING PRACTICE

- Be aware of religious and cultural preferences when helping patients and families prepare for death.
- Ask families about the rituals and ceremonies they use to help them cope with the death of a loved one.
- Allow patients and families the ability to participate in planning which rituals will be done at the patient's bedside.
- Be sensitive to cultural perceptions regarding organ donation, viewing the body, and preparing for burial.

REFERENCE

Lobar SL, Youngblut JM, Brooten D: Cross-cultural beliefs, ceremonies, and rituals surrounding death of a loved one. *Pediatr Nurs* 32(1):44–50, 2006.

From Potter PA, Perry AG, Stockert P, et al: *Fundamentals of nursing: Concepts, process, and practice,* ed 9, St. Louis, 2017, Mosby.

hereditary factors. **Ethnicity** refers to a group of people who share a common social and cultural heritage based on shared traditions, national origin, and physical and biologic characteristics. They often share social practices such as language, religion, dress, music, and food. Factors related to culture, race, and ethnicity often overlap, and many people combine a variety of practices related to several of these factors. It is important to understand that not everyone in a cultural, racial, or ethnic group has identical practices and that each person should be treated in an individual, holistic manner.

ETHNIC AND RACIAL GROUPS IN THE UNITED STATES

The United States is home to people from many cultures. Do not make assumptions about a patient's beliefs or practices based on the person's name, skin color, or language.

Assumptions commonly are made about the predominant cultures and subcultures in our country based on one's own family or community. A larger view of our society is necessary for a better understanding of our country.

Changes in the nation's demographic are illustrated in Table 6.1. Significant decreases are noted in the white population accompanied by increases in most other racial groups. The largest increase has occurred in the Hispanic population, which rose from 12.5% to 16.3% of the population between 2000 and 2010. Predictions for the future indicate that this trend will continue and that the minority cultures will, in combination, make up a majority of the US population by the middle of this century (US Census Bureau, Census 2010).

One significant aspect of this diversity is the language used to communicate. Many new immigrants from these diverse cultures may not speak English or may have a limited grasp of the language. Often the younger members of the family are the ones who help the adults communicate with others outside of the cultural community. Adults frequently bring a young child along as a translator when shopping or seeking health care. A professional translator is preferable as opposed to a friend or family member to prevent bias, inaccuracy, or compromises in confidentiality. Adults who are asked about personal health issues may be reluctant to answer these questions if answers are translated through their children or grandchildren.

Lifespan Considerations

Older Adults

Cultural Background

- Cultural background has an impact on family dynamics and plays an important role in determining the role and the status of the older person.
- Older adults form a unique cultural group based on shared historical experiences. Often fewer differences are found between two older individuals of diverse cultural backgrounds than between two people of the same culture but from different age groups because of shifts in value systems that occurred over time.
- Some older adults are less tolerant of other cultures as a result of influences or experiences early in their lives, which raises the possibility of misunderstandings and distrust when the caregiver is of a cultural group different from the older person.
- Older people experiencing disturbed cognitive function from Alzheimer's disease or other conditions sometimes speak without regard for the cultural sensitivity of others and thus make hurtful comments to caregivers and other people.
- Older adults may value home remedies and cultural practices regarding health care and sometimes resist the attempts of caregivers to change even their harmful practices. Practices that are not harmful are left alone out of respect for their wishes.

CULTURALLY RELATED ASSESSMENTS

To care for a patient from a different culture, the nurse should assess the patient's beliefs. Patients cannot be expected to accept care and health teaching if they do not believe that the practices will help them to recover.

Brief examples of specific beliefs and practices of some cultures are presented later in this chapter. Stereotyping an individual according to common cultural practices should be avoided. The individual may or may not accept all of the practices within a culture or subculture.

When the nurse assesses a patient, several areas should be explored: communication, space, time, social organization, religious beliefs, health practices, and biologic variations.

COMMUNICATION

The most apparent communication variation is the language spoken. Whether the nurse and the patient can understand each other must be determined. When patients do not understand what is being said, they sometimes say yes or nod the head nonetheless, giving the mistaken impression of agreeing with the nurse. Many people do this to avoid embarrassment or to be polite. The nurse must not assume that the patient or the family understands.

Sometimes the patient understands some English, or the nurse speaks some of the patient's language. If patients have a poor grasp of English, they may tire quickly when trying to understand what is being said. In addition, medical terminology potentiates an even greater risk without a medical interpreter in the native language of the client. Questions and directions should be kept brief and simple. It is better to provide more information later than to give long explanations. Sometimes, the patient's ability to read written English is

Table 6.1 Changes in Racially Designated and Hispanic Populations, 2000–2010

	2000		2010		
RACE	NUMBER	PERCENTAGE OF TOTAL POPULATION	NUMBER	PERCENTAGE OF TOTAL POPULATION	PERCENT CHANGE
Total population	281,421,906	100.0%	308,745,538	100.0%	+9.7%
White	211,460,626	75.1%	223,553,265	72.4%	–5.7%
Black or African American	34,658,190	12.3%	38,929,319	12.6%	+12.3%
American Indian or Alaska Native	2,475,956	0.9%	2,932,248	0.9%	+18.4%
Asian	10,242,998	3.6%	14,674,252	4.8%	+43.3%
Native Hawaiian and other Pacific Islander	398,835	0.1%	540,013	0.2%	+35.4%
Some other race	15,359,073	5.5%	19,107,368	6.2%	+24.4%
Two or more races	6,826,228	2.4%	9,009,073	2.9%	+32%
Hispanic or Latino (of any race)	35,305,818	12.5%	50,477,594	16.3%	+3.8%

From US Bureau of the Census: Table DP-1: General population and housing characteristics, 2010; US Bureau of the Census: Profile of general population and housing characteristics, 2010. Retrieved from *http://factfinder2.census.gov*.

better than his or her speaking ability. In such cases, the patient benefits from written explanations accompanied by pictures when possible.

The preferred approach is the use of a professional interpreter. Many health care facilities have employees on call to translate when a language barrier exists. Availability of a translator may require that the nurse work with a family member who is able to translate. Note that this intervention affects confidentiality surrounding the patient's care. The patient must understand essential information such as why care is being given and why medications are ordered. The nurse's responsibility is to make every effort to provide this information to the patient. Use of effective communication techniques is beneficial as the nurse cares for patients from different cultures (Box 6.3).

Even among English-speaking people, different cultural groups assign different meanings to the same words. For example, a person from the United Kingdom may say he is going to take the "lift." An American may not understand that this refers to an elevator. Within the United States, the variety of regional accents further complicates communication. People from different areas of the country (e.g., people from the north and the south) often struggle to understand each other because of the different accents or regional expressions they use. Some cultural or regional groups speak very rapidly, which adds to the difficulty of understanding. In addition, people from Spain use many words with different meaning than that of Spanish people from Central America.

Other cultural patterns also play a role in communication. In some cultural groups, many family members commonly accompany a person to the health care setting. Large groups of family members tend to make communication difficult. They sometimes all try to assist by answering at once. Or perhaps, when in the presence of strangers, a person from another group only answers direct questions and thus appears rude or uncommunicative. Unfortunately, the appearance of rudeness is a common by-product of a cross-cultural mismatch in communication. Sometimes a person speaks more loudly to emphasize a point out of the mistaken belief that this helps the hearer understand better. In fact, it often has the opposite effect of the one desired. Members of some cultures interpret the raised voice as rudeness or aggression and shut out the sound altogether.

Consider, in contrast, the use of silence. Silence indicates many things to many cultures: a lack of understanding, stubbornness, apprehension, discomfort, agreement, disagreement, respect, or disdain. In some cultures, the presence of silence may result in feelings of discomfort and anxiety. It is not uncommon for people to make attempts to fill periods of silence with conversation. Among American Indian, Chinese, and Japanese cultures, silence sometimes is used to allow the listener to consider what the speaker has said before continuing. Members of other cultures, such as Russians, the French, and the Spanish, tend to become silent to indicate consensus between parties. In Asian cultures, people often use silence as a sign of respect, especially to elders (see the Cultural Considerations box). In contrast, people from other cultures, such as those of Mexican descent, may use silence when they disagree with a person of authority.

Box 6.3 Strategies for Communication With Patients From Different Cultures

- Take a little extra time to establish a level of comfort between you and the patient.
- Ask questions in an unhurried and calm manner. Rephrase a question and ask it again if the answer seems inconsistent with other information the patient has provided.
- Observe the cultural differences in communication, and honor those differences. Use eye contact, touch, and seating arrangements that are comfortable for the patient.
- Ask patients about the meaning of health and illness and their understanding of treatments and planned care. Investigate how the illness is likely to affect their life, relationships, and self-concept. Find out what patients consider to be the cause of their illness. Ask how patients prefer to manage their illness.
- To establish a therapeutic relationship, listen to the patients' perceptions of their needs, and respect the patients' perspectives.
- Listen actively and attentively; try not to anticipate the patient's response.
- Talk to patients in an unhurried manner that considers social and cultural amenities.
- Give patients time to answer.
- Use validation techniques to verify that the patient understands. Remember that smiles and head nodding may indicate that the patient is trying to please the nurse, not necessarily that the nurse is understood.
- Sexual concerns may be difficult for patients to discuss. Having a nurse of the same gender may facilitate communication.
- Use alternative methods of communication, such as a foreign language phrase book, an interpreter, gestures, or pictures, for patients who do not speak English.
- Learn key phrases in languages that are commonly spoken in your community.

From Harkreader H, Hogan MA, Thobaben M: *Fundamentals of nursing: Caring and clinical judgment,* ed 4, Philadelphia, 2007, Saunders.

NONVERBAL COMMUNICATION

Nonverbal communication usually is expressed through body language. Some groups are more comfortable than others with touching or maintaining eye contact. Touch is particularly culturally or regionally related. In parts of the United States, many people consider even casual touching inappropriate. In other regions, casual touch and embracing between acquaintances is the norm. Recent immigrants from England and Germany may be less likely to touch each other in public or allow casual touching by strangers. Spanish, French, Italian,

> **Cultural Considerations**
>
> **Culturally Sensitive Communication**
>
> - It should be noted that any reference to cultural practices among a specific culture are commonalities. Individuals within a culture may or may not possess the same practices, beliefs, or values.
> - Ask all patients how they like to be addressed. If in doubt, address them formally.
> - Determine the patient's preferences for touch. For example, Americans often greet each other with a firm handshake. Many Native Americans, however, see this as a sign of aggression. Touch outside of marriage sometimes is forbidden in older adults from the Middle East.
> - Investigate the patient's preferences for silence. Generally, Eastern cultures value silence, whereas Western cultures are uncomfortable with silence.
> - Be aware of the patient's beliefs about eye contact during conversation. Direct eye contact in European American cultures is a sign of honesty and truthfulness. Older Native Americans may avoid eye contact. Asian adults sometimes avoid eye contact with authority figures because this is considered disrespectful, and direct eye contact between the sexes in Middle Eastern cultures sometimes is forbidden except between spouses.
>
> From Potter PA, Perry AG, Stockert P, et al: *Fundamentals of nursing*, ed 9, St. Louis, 2017, Mosby; Meiner SE: *Gerontologic nursing*, ed 4, St. Louis, 2010, Mosby.

Jewish, and South American individuals are likely to be much more comfortable about touching each other and being touched.

Eye contact also has significant cultural interpretations. Many people in the United States regard maintaining eye contact as an indication of openness, interest in others, attentiveness, and honesty. Lack of eye contact thus is interpreted as a sign of shyness, humility, guilt, embarrassment, rudeness, thoughtlessness, or dishonesty. Other cultures have various other reasons for not maintaining eye contact. Some Asian cultures and American Indians relate eye contact to impoliteness or an invasion of privacy. Certain East Indian cultures avoid eye contact with people of lower or higher socioeconomic classes. Among some Appalachian people, maintaining eye contact indicates hostility or aggressiveness.

Body language and gestures often are related culturally. In the United States, certain gestures generally are understood by most people who have lived in the United States for an extended period of time. However, some commonly used gestures have the potential to offend someone from another culture. For example, a "thumbs up" hand gesture conveys acceptance or a "good job" in the United States. To someone from another culture this may mean something else that may not have a positive connotation. Traditionally, Italian people use a great deal of hand gestures when communicating.

Assessing the communication variables of a patient from another culture is important. First, an assessment of cultural factors is performed; then the nurse has to respond appropriately. Every effort should be made to communicate with others at their personal level of comfort to establish good rapport. If the patient is from a culture that avoids eye contact, try to look away when talking with the patient. If touch is unacceptable among casual acquaintances, avoid patting the shoulder or touching a hand when talking with the patient. The nurse should be sensitive to any difficulty a patient is having with the more intimate touching that inevitably accompanies many nursing interventions.

Violations of cultural beliefs and practices by the nurse are likely to interfere with establishing a therapeutic relationship with the patient and the patient's family. Do not expect to completely adjust individual personal cultural practices, but try to understand and accept the differences among practices in various cultures. Do not judge the patient's behavior according to personal practices.

SPACE

Cultural interpretation of space varies and is an important element of assessment. Cultures assign different comfort areas and meanings to personal space. In the United States, people are often more comfortable when given a larger amount of personal space than what is common in many other countries. Closer contact is reserved for more intimate relationships. Members of some cultures are accustomed to more close contact, which may be interpreted as an invasion of one's space in other cultures. A nurse who is receptive to the patient's interpretation of a comfortable space may find it easier to establish a therapeutic relationship. Occasionally, the need for personal space also is manifest in a desire to use a certain space. For example, perhaps a resident in a nursing home always wishes to sit in a particular chair or in a specific part of the room. Another resident chooses to sit at the same table for each meal. A change in any of these arrangements may cause either of these residents to become upset.

TIME

The measurement of time and the rhythms of people's activities and interactions often have different meanings in various cultures. These different meanings have the potential to create some problems in the care of patients from other cultures. Traditional nursing practice emphasizes that medications and treatments are provided on a rigid schedule. The United States and many Northern European cultures generally give a high priority to being on time for appointments, and people typically expect everyone to follow this pattern. Japanese American culture also places emphasis on promptness and the adherence to fixed schedules, especially when meeting with a person who is regarded highly. People in many cultures believe that other concerns regarding time are more important. In Eastern cultures, including Chinese, East Indian Hindu, Filipino, and Korean, schedules and time are much more flexible concepts. Some Asians spend a lot of time getting to know someone and view abrupt endings to a conversation as rude. Mexican Americans may be late for an appointment because they focus more on a current activity and are less concerned about a previously planned meeting. According to Giger (2017), this concept, known as "elasticity," implies that future activities are possible to recover but not present ones. If these cultural differences are not understood, the nurse may feel angry when a patient is late for an appointment, fails to come at all, or does not follow therapeutic schedules. Similarly, health care providers should strive to plan for and communicate realistic wait times for procedures and appointments. In lower-income areas, patients may rely more heavily on public transportation or family and friends to get to appointments. In communities where patients have less control over transportation, patients may have a more relaxed outlook about schedules. In areas with fewer transportation barriers, appointments may be seen as more rigid. Long wait times may be seen as a lack of respect for the patient's time.

Perception of time or time orientation also varies among cultures. Many people in the United States tend to be future oriented. Present actions are taken based on a future outcome. An example is a person who takes medication to treat hypertension to prevent illness. Among members of other cultures, notably African American or black, Hispanic, and American Indian, individuals tend to be more present oriented. Sometimes, like people described previously who prolong a current encounter rather than rushing off to be on time for another one, a present-oriented person chooses to satisfy a current, more urgent need rather than prepare for a less immediate one that is in the future. A pregnant woman, for instance, may miss her own health care provider's appointments to take care of her family; if her older child needs a ride to school, the mother skips the appointment and drives the child. A patient with this belief system is often difficult to encourage to follow through on treatment for a chronic illness. Such a patient perhaps views the cost of a medication for hypertension to prevent future problems as an optional expense. Paying the rent or buying food for the family is a current need that takes precedence.

SOCIAL ORGANIZATION

Cultural behavior is socially acquired, not genetically inherited. How nurses react to members of other cultures reflects an internalized response that is part of their own culture. Often we are not aware of the strong impact these patterns of cultural behavior have each day in our lives. We may behave in a hostile manner toward a person of a particular ethnic group or a person with a different skin color merely because of a culture-related belief. It is important to recognize these biases and to deal with them rationally. Understanding other cultures and that one culture is not superior over another helps to overcome prejudices that have nothing to do with an individual.

Self-concept also is influenced by culture and cultural identity. Individuals view themselves as part of a particular social group. They describe themselves in terms such as "African American" or "black," "Hispanic," "German American," "Irish Catholic," or "Texan." Clearly, these descriptions vary greatly. What is important is to understand how the person sees herself or himself. A good cultural assessment takes this self-description into account.

The varying social structures within a culture also have an impact on how individuals and families function. Some cultures are patriarchal, and the men (often the oldest) make most of the decisions. In a culture that is matriarchal, the women usually make the decisions about health care, provide the care, and discipline the children. The structure of the family is important to determine in a health care setting. For example, a family in a patriarchal society sometimes delays any decision making regarding health care for one of the family members until the oldest man in the family is consulted. Another family, in a matriarchal society, expects the women to give care to a family member in the hospital.

The description of family may differ among cultures. Some family structures are based on biologic relationships. Others are based on meeting basic needs for family by forming a group among unrelated individuals. Knowledge of the family structure assists the nurse to better understand the patient. A common mistake is to assume that every family is a traditional nuclear family. In fact, this family structure is becoming increasingly rare. Knowing who the patient depends on for comfort and decision making and how the patient describes the family or support system is more important.

RELIGIOUS BELIEFS AND HEALTH CARE

Religious beliefs frequently are entwined with cultural beliefs. Some cultures expect all members to adhere to a particular religion. In these societies, religious and cultural beliefs are difficult to separate. In the United States, wide variations are found in religious practices (Box 6.4). In addition, as people from varying cultures intermarry, religious practices also become more varied.

Data for religious affiliations are not collected by the US Bureau of the Census, making an accurate way to determine the numbers of followers of the various religions in the United States difficult. Despite the inability to quantify the religious preferences in the country, nursing care clearly is affected by patients' religious beliefs and practices. The nurse must be aware of and open to the wide range of such beliefs to ensure that care provided is sensitive to the needs of individual patients.

Text continued on p. 106

Box 6.4 Religious Beliefs and Practices That Affect Health Care in the United States

It should be noted that any reference to cultural practices among a specific culture are commonalities. Individuals within a culture may or may not possess the same practices, beliefs, or values.

AMERICAN MUSLIM MISSION

Baptism: No baptism is practiced.

Death: The family is contacted before any care of the deceased is performed. Special procedures are observed for washing and shrouding the body.

Dietary habits: In addition to refusing pork, many do not eat foods traditional in black culture such as cornbread and collard greens.

Other practices: Quiet time is necessary to permit prayer.

ASSEMBLIES OF GOD (PENTECOSTAL)

Anointing the sick: Members believe in divine healing through prayer and the laying on of hands. Clergy is notified if the patient or family desires this.

Baptism: Water baptism with complete immersion is practiced when an individual has received Jesus Christ as Savior and Lord based on Acts 2:38.

Death: No special practices are observed.

Dietary habits: Abstinence from alcohol, tobacco, and all illegal drugs is encouraged strongly.

Holy Communion: Notify clergy if the patient desires to receive this sacrament.

Other practices: Faith in God and in the health care providers is encouraged. Members pray for divine intervention in health matters. Encourage and allow patients time for prayer. Members sometimes "speak in tongues" during prayer.

BAPTIST (MORE THAN 27 DIFFERENT GROUPS IN THE UNITED STATES)

Baptism: Baptists do not practice infant baptism.

Death: No general service is provided, but the clergy does minister through counseling, prayer, and Scripture as requested by the patient or family, and the patient is encouraged to believe in Jesus Christ as Savior and Lord.

Dietary habits: Total abstinence from alcohol is expected.

Holy Communion: Notify clergy if the patient desires to receive this sacrament.

Other practices: The Bible is held to be the word of God, so either allow quiet time for Scripture reading or offer to read to the patient.

CHRISTIAN CHURCH (DISCIPLES OF CHRIST)

Baptism: These members do not practice infant baptism but do have dedication service. Believers are baptized with immersion.

Death: No special practices are observed.

Holy Communion: Open communion is celebrated each Sunday and is a central part of worship services. Notify the clergy if the patient desires it; sometimes the clergy member suggests it.

Other practices: Church elders and clergy are appropriate to notify to assist with meeting the patient's spiritual needs.

CHRISTIAN SCIENCE

Birth: Physician or nurse-midwife is present during childbirth. No baptism ceremony is practiced.

Death: Autopsy usually is declined unless required by law. Organ donation is unlikely but is an individual decision.

Dietary habits: Because alcohol and tobacco are considered drugs, they are not used. Coffee and tea often are declined.

Other practices: Members normally do not seek medical care because they approach health care in a different, primarily spiritual, framework. They commonly use the services of a surgeon to set a bone but decline drugs and, in general, other medical or surgical procedures. Hypnotism and psychotherapy also are declined. Family planning is left to the family. They seek exemption from vaccinations but obey legal requirements. They report infectious diseases and obey public health quarantines. Nonmedical care facilities are maintained for those needing nursing assistance in the course of a healing. The *Christian Science Journal* lists available Christian Science nurses. When caring for a Christian Science believer, allow and encourage time for prayer and study. Patients often request that a Christian Science practitioner be notified to come.

CHURCH OF THE BRETHREN

Anointing the sick: This is practiced for physical healing and spiritual uplift and held in high regard by the church. The clergy is notified if the patient or the family desires.

Baptism: These members do not practice infant baptism but have dedication service.

Death: The clergy is notified for counsel and prayer.

Holy Communion: This usually is received within church, but clergy give it in the hospital when requested.

CHURCH OF JESUS CHRIST OF LATTER-DAY SAINTS (MORMONS)

Anointing the sick: Mormons frequently are anointed and given a blessing before going to the hospital and after admission by laying on of hands.

Baptism: If a child over age 8 years is very ill, whether baptized or unbaptized, call a member of the church's priesthood.

Birth control and abortion: Abortion is opposed except when the life of the mother is in danger. Only natural means of birth control are recommended. Artificial means are permitted when the health of the woman is at stake (including emotional health).

Death: Mormons prefer burial of the body. Notify a church elder to assist the family. If need be, the elder assists the funeral director in dressing the body in special clothes and gives other help as needed.

Dietary habits: Mormons practice abstinence from the use of tobacco; beverages with caffeine such as cola, coffee, and tea; and alcohol and other substances considered injurious. Mormons eat meat but encourage the intake of fruits, grains, and herbs.

Holy Communion: Hospitalized patients often desire to have a member of the church priesthood administer this sacrament.

Personal care: Cleanliness is very important to Mormons. A sacred undergarment may be worn at all times by Mormons and is removed only in emergency situations.

Other practices: Allowing quiet time for prayer and the reading of the sacred writings. The church maintains a welfare system to assist those in need. Families are of great importance, so visiting is important to encourage.

Box 6.4 Religious Beliefs and Practices That Affect Health Care in the United States—cont'd

CHURCH OF THE NAZARENE

Baptism: Parents have the choice of baptism or dedication for their infant. Emphasis is on the believer's baptism, which is regarded as a symbol of the New Covenant in Jesus Christ.

Death: Cremation is permitted, and stillborn term infants are buried.

Dietary habits: The use of alcohol and tobacco is forbidden.

Holy Communion: Pastor administers if the patient wishes.

Other practices: The members believe in divine healing but not to the exclusion of medical treatment. Patients sometimes desire quiet time for prayer.

EASTERN ORTHODOX

Anointing the sick: The priest conducts this in the hospital room.

Birth: The infant must be baptized within 40 days after birth. If sprinkling or immersion into water is not possible, baptism is performed by moving the baby in the air in the sign of the cross. Only an ordained priest or a deacon may perform the ritual in this manner.

Birth control and abortion: Birth control and abortion are not permitted.

Dietary habits: Fasting from meat and dairy products is required on Wednesdays and Fridays during Lent and on other holy days. Hospital patients are exempt if fasting is detrimental to health.

Death: Last rites are obligatory and handled by an ordained priest who is notified while the patient is conscious. The Russian Orthodox Church does not encourage autopsy or organ donation. Euthanasia, even for the terminally ill, is discouraged, as is cremation.

Holy Eucharist: The priest is notified if the patient desires this sacrament.

Special days: Christmas is celebrated on January 7, and New Year's on January 14. This is important to the care of a patient who is hospitalized on these days.

EPISCOPAL (ANGLICAN)

Anointing the sick: A priest often administers this rite when death is imminent, but it is not considered mandatory.

Baptism: Infant baptism is practiced and is considered urgent if the infant is critically ill. The priest is notified to administer the sacrament. Laypersons are permitted to baptize in an emergency.

Death: No special practices are observed.

Dietary habits: Some patients abstain from meat on Fridays. Others fast before receiving the Eucharist, but fasting is not mandatory.

Holy Communion: Notify the priest if the patient wishes to receive this sacrament.

Other practices: Confession of sins to a priest is optional; if the patient desires this, the clergy should be notified.

ISLAM

Birth: A baby is bathed immediately after birth, before being given to the mother. The father (or mother if the father is not available) then whispers the call to prayer in the child's ears so that the first sounds heard are about the Muslim faith. Circumcision is recommended culturally before puberty. A baby born prematurely but at least at 130 days of gestation is given the same treatment as any other infant.

Birth control and abortion: Abortion is forbidden, and many conservative Muslims do not encourage the use of contraceptives because they believe that it interferes with God's purpose. Others believe that it is best for a woman to have only as many children as her husband can afford. Contraception is permitted by Islamic law.

Care of women: Because women are not allowed to sign consent forms or make a decision regarding family planning, it is mandatory for the husband to be present. Women are very modest and frequently wear clothes that cover all of the body. During a medical examination, the woman's modesty must be respected as much as possible. Muslim women prefer female doctors. For 40 days after giving birth and also during menstruation, a woman is exempt from prayer because this is a time of cleansing for her.

Death: Before death, family members ask to be present so that they can read the Koran and pray with the patient. An Imam comes if requested by the patient or family but is not required. Patients face Mecca and confess their sins and beg for forgiveness in the presence of their family. If the family is unavailable, any practicing Muslim is permitted to provide support to the patient. After death, Muslims prefer that the family wash, prepare, and place the body in a position facing Mecca. If necessary, health care providers are allowed to perform these procedures as long as they wear gloves. Burial is performed as soon as possible. Cremation is forbidden. Autopsy is also prohibited except for legal reasons, and then no body part is to be removed. Donation of body parts or organs is not allowed because, according to culturally developed law, people do not own their bodies.

Dietary habits: No pork nor alcoholic beverages are allowed. All halal (permissible) meat must be blessed and killed in a special way. This is called zabihah (correctly slaughtered). Daytime fasting is practiced during Ramadan.

Personal devotions: At prayer time, washing is required, even by those who are sick. A patient on bed rest sometimes requires assistance with this task before prayer. Provision of privacy is important during prayer.

Religious objects: The Koran is not to be touched by anyone ritually unclean, and nothing is to be placed on top of it. Some Muslims wear taviz, a black string on which words of the Koran are attached. These should not be removed and must remain dry. Certain items of jewelry such as bangles may have religious significance; do not allow them to be removed unnecessarily.

JEHOVAH'S WITNESS

Baptism: No infant baptism is practiced. Baptism with complete immersion of adults is done as a symbol of dedication to Jehovah because Jesus was baptized.

Birth control and abortion: Use of birth control is a personal decision. Abortion is opposed based on Exodus 21:22–23.

Blood transfusions: Blood transfusions violate God's laws and therefore are not allowed. Patients do respect

Continued

Box 6.4 Religious Beliefs and Practices That Affect Health Care in the United States—cont'd

physicians and accept alternatives to blood transfusions. These include the possible use of nonblood plasma expanders, careful surgical techniques to decrease blood loss, use of autologous transfusions, and autotransfusion through use of a heart-lung machine. Be sure to check unconscious patients for medical-alert cards or bracelets that state that the person does not want a transfusion. Because Jehovah's Witnesses are prepared to die rather than break God's law, you need to be sensitive to the spiritual as well as the physical needs of the patient.

Death: Autopsy is a private matter to be decided by the persons involved. Burial and cremation are acceptable.

Dietary habits: Use of alcohol and tobacco is discouraged because these harm the physical body.

Organ transplants: Use of organ transplant is a private decision; if used, it is required that the organ be cleansed with a nonblood solution.

JUDAISM, OBSERVANT (ORTHODOX JUDAISM AND SOME CONSERVATIVE GROUPS)

Birth: For observant Jews, babies are named by the father. Male children are named 8 days after birth, when ritual circumcision is done. A mohel performs the circumcision. Circumcision is often postponed if the infant is in poor health. Female babies usually are named during the reading of the holy Torah. Nurses need to be sensitive to the wishes of the parents when caring for babies who have not yet been named.

Birth control and abortion: Artificial methods of birth control are not encouraged. Vasectomy is not allowed. Abortion is permitted only to save the mother's life.

Care of women: A woman is considered to be in a ritual state of impurity whenever blood is coming from her uterus, such as during menstrual periods and after the birth of a child. During this time, her husband does not have physical contact with her. When this time is completed, she bathes herself in a pool called a mikvah. Nurses need to be aware of this practice and be sensitive to the husband and wife because the husband does not touch his wife. He cannot assist her in moving in the bed, so the nurse has to do this. An Orthodox Jewish man does not touch any woman other than his wife, daughters, and mother. Home health care workers need to be aware of these practices.

Death: Judaism defines death as occurring when respiration and circulation are irreversibly stopped and no movement is apparent. (1) Euthanasia is strictly forbidden by Orthodox Jews, who advocate the strict use of life-support measures. (2) Before death, Jewish faith indicates that visiting of the person by family and friends is a religious duty. The Torah and Psalms are often read, and prayers are recited. A witness must be present when a person prays for health so that if death occurs God protects the family and the spirit is committed to God. Extraneous talking and conversation about death are not encouraged unless initiated by the patient or visitors. In Judaism, the belief is that people should have someone with them when the soul leaves the body, so allow family and friends to stay with dying patients. After death, the body is not to be left alone until burial, usually within 24 hours. (3) When death occurs, the body is to remain untouched for 8 to 30 minutes. Medical personnel are not to touch or wash the body; only an Orthodox person or the Jewish Burial Society is permitted to care for the body. Handling of a corpse on the Sabbath is forbidden to Jewish persons. If need be, the nursing staff is permitted to provide routine care of the body while wearing gloves. Water receptacles in the room must be emptied, and the family often requests that mirrors be covered to symbolize that a death has occurred. (4) Orthodox Jews and some conservative Jews do not approve of autopsies. If an autopsy is necessary, all body parts are required to remain with the body. (5) For Orthodox Jews, the body is required to be buried within 24 hours. No flowers are permitted. A fetus is required to be buried. (6) A 7-day mourning period is required by the immediate family. They stay at home except for Sabbath worship. (7) Ensure that organs or other body parts such as amputated limbs are made available for burial for Orthodox Jews because they believe that all of the body must be returned to the earth.

Dietary rules: (1) Kosher dietary laws include the following: no mixing of milk and meat at a meal; no consumption of food or any derivative thereof from animals not slaughtered in accordance with Jewish law; use of separate cooking utensils for meat and milk products; and if for medical reasons a patient requires milk and meat products for a meal, the dairy foods should be served first, followed later by the meat. (2) During Yom Kippur (Day of Atonement), a 24-hour fast is required, but exceptions are made for those who cannot fast because of medical reasons or age. (3) During Passover, no leavened products are eaten. (4) Observant Jewish patients often wish to say prayers over the bread and wine before meals. Time and a quiet environment should be provided for this.

Head covering: Orthodox men wear skullcaps at all times, and women cover their hair after marriage. Some Orthodox women wear wigs as a mark of piety. Conservative Jews cover their heads only during acts of worship and prayer.

Organ transplants: Donor organ transplants generally are not permitted by Orthodox Jews but with rabbinical consent are sometimes allowed.

Prayer: Praying directly to God, including a prayer of confession, is required for Orthodox Jews. Provide quiet time for prayer.

Sabbath: Observed from sunset Friday until sunset Saturday. Orthodox law prohibits riding in a car, smoking, turning lights on and off, handling money, and using television and telephone. Nurses need to be aware of this when caring for observant Jews at home and in the hospital. Medical or surgical treatments should be postponed if possible.

Shaving: The beard is regarded as a mark of piety among observant Jews. For very Orthodox Jews, shaving is never done with a razor, but with scissors or an electric razor, because no blade is to contact the skin.

LUTHERAN (10 DIFFERENT BRANCHES [SYNODS])

Anointing the sick: Patients sometimes request an anointing and blessing from the minister when the prognosis is poor.

Box 6.4 Religious Beliefs and Practices That Affect Health Care in the United States—cont'd

Baptism: Lutherans baptize only living infants any time but usually 6 to 8 weeks after birth. Adults are also baptized, and modes of baptism, as appropriate, include sprinkling, pouring, and immersion.
Death: A service of Commendation of the Dying is performed at the patient's or family's request.
Holy Communion: Notify the clergy if the patient desires this sacrament. Clergy sometimes also inquire about the patient's wishes.

MENNONITE (12 DIFFERENT GROUPS)
Baptism: No infant baptism is observed, but the child is sometimes dedicated if requested by the parents.
Death: Prayer is important at time of crisis, so contacting a minister is important.
Dietary habits: Abstinence from alcohol is urged for all.
Holy Communion: Communion is served twice a year, with foot washing as part of the ceremony.
Other practices: Women sometimes wear head coverings during hospitalization. Anointing with oil is administered in harmony with James 5:14 when requested.

METHODIST (MORE THAN 20 DIFFERENT GROUPS)
Anointing of sick: If requested, the clergy comes to pray and sprinkle the patient with olive oil.
Baptism: Notify the clergy if the parent desires baptism for a sick infant.
Death: Scripture reading and prayer are important at this time. Donation of one's body or part of the body at death is encouraged.
Holy Communion: Notify the clergy if a patient requests communion before surgery or another health crisis.

PRESBYTERIAN (10 DIFFERENT GROUPS)
Baptism: Infant baptism is practiced with pouring or sprinkling. Immersion is also practiced at times for adults.
Death: Notify a local pastor or elder for prayer and Scripture reading if desired by the family or patient.
Holy Communion: Communion is given when appropriate and convenient, at the hospitalized patient's request.

QUAKER (FRIENDS)
Baptism and Holy Communion: Friends have no creed; therefore a diversity of personal beliefs exists, one of which is that outward sacraments are usually not necessary because there is the ministry of the Spirit inwardly in such areas as baptism and communion. A few Friends baptize with water.
Death: Friends believe that the present life is part of God's kingdom and generally have no rite of passage from this life to the next. Ascertain the patient's personal beliefs and wishes, and then act on the patient's wishes.
Other practices: The name of the Quaker infant is recorded in official record books at the local meeting.

ROMAN CATHOLIC
Anointing the sick: The priest anoints the forehead, hands, and, if desired, the affected area. The rite is performed on any who are ill and desire it. People receiving the sacrament seek complete healing and strength to endure suffering. Before 1963 this sacrament was given only to people at time of imminent death, so the nurse must be sensitive to the meaning this has for the patient. The priest should be called before the patient becomes unconscious but also may be called in the case of sudden death; the sacrament also may be given shortly after death. The nurse should document that this sacrament has been administered.
Birth: Because Roman Catholics believe that unbaptized children are cut off from heaven, infant baptism is mandatory. For newborns with a grave prognosis, stillborns, and all aborted fetuses (unless evidence of tissue necrosis and prolonged death are present), emergency baptism is required. The nurse calls a priest to perform the baptism unless the possibility exists that death will occur before the priest arrives. In that case, anyone is permitted to baptize by pouring warm water on the infant's head and saying, "I baptize you in the name of the Father, of the Son, and of the Holy Spirit." All information about the baptism is recorded on the chart, and the priest and family are notified.
Birth control: Contraception is prohibited except for abstinence or natural family planning methods. Referral to a priest for questions about this is often of great help. Nurses teach the techniques of natural family planning if they are familiar with them; otherwise, the nurse should make referral to the physician or to a support group of the Church that instructs couples in this method of birth control. Sterilization is prohibited unless an overriding medical reason exists.
Death: Each Roman Catholic is to participate in the anointing of the sick and the Eucharist and penance before death. The body is not to be shrouded until after these sacraments are performed. All body parts that retain human quality are required to be appropriately buried or cremated.
Dietary habits: Obligatory fasting is excused during hospitalization. However, if no health restrictions exist, some Catholics still observe the following guidelines: (1) Anyone 14 years of age or older has to abstain from eating meat on Ash Wednesday and all Fridays during Lent. Some older Catholics still abstain from meat on all Fridays of the year. (2) In addition to abstinence from meat, people 21 to 59 years of age are required to limit themselves to one full meal and two light meals on Ash Wednesday and Good Friday. (3) Eastern Rite Catholics are stricter about fasting and fast more frequently than Western Rite Catholics, so the nurse should know whether a patient is Eastern or Western.
Holy Eucharist: For patients and health care providers who are to receive communion, abstinence from solid food and alcohol is required for 15 minutes (if possible) before reception of the consecrated wafer. Medicine, water, and nonalcoholic drinks are permitted at any time. If a patient is in danger of death, the fasting requirement is waived because the reception of the Eucharist at this time is very important.
Organ donation: Donation and transplantation of organs are acceptable as long as the donor is not harmed and is not deprived of life.
Religious objects: Rosary prayers are said using rosary beads. Medals bearing the images of saints, relics, statues, and scapulars are important objects that are often pinned to a hospital gown or pillow or kept at the

Continued

Box 6.4 Religious Beliefs and Practices That Affect Health Care in the United States—cont'd

bedside. Ensure that extreme care is taken not to lose these objects because they have special meaning to the patient.

SEVENTH-DAY ADVENTIST

Anointing the sick: The clergy are contacted for prayer and anointing with oil.
Baptism: No infant baptism is practiced, but dedication services are.
Death: No special procedures are required.
Dietary habits: Because the body is viewed as the temple of the Holy Spirit, healthy living is essential. Therefore the use of alcohol, tobacco, coffee, and tea and the promiscuous (careless) use of drugs are prohibited. Some are vegetarians, and most avoid pork.
Holy Communion: Although this is not required of hospitalized patients, the clergy is notified if the patient desires.
Special days: The Sabbath is observed on Saturday.
Other practices: Use of hypnotism is opposed by some. People of homosexual or lesbian orientation are ministered to in the hope of "correction" of these practices, which are believed to be wrong. Ensure that a Bible is always available for Scripture reading.

UNIFICATION CHURCH

Baptism: No baptism is practiced.
Death: Members believe that after death one's place of destiny depends on his or her spirit's quality of life and goodness while on Earth. In the afterlife, one will have the same aspirations and feelings as before death. Hell is not a concern because it will not be a place as heaven grows in size. People who leave the Unification Church are warned of the possibility that Satan will try to possess them.
Special days: Sunday mornings are used to honor Reverend and Mrs. Moon as the true parents, and members get up at 5 a.m., bow before a picture of the Moons three times, and vow to do what is needed to help the Reverend accomplish his mission on Earth.
Other practices: All marriages are required to be solemnized by Reverend Moon to be part of the perfect family and have salvation. The church supplies its faithful members with life's necessities. Members sometimes use occult practices to have spiritual and psychic experiences.

UNITARIAN UNIVERSALIST ASSOCIATION

Baptism: No baptism is practiced.
Death: Cremation is often preferred rather than burial.
Other practices: Use of birth control is advocated as part of responsible parenting. Strong support for a woman's right to choice regarding abortion is maintained. Unitarian Universalists advocate donation of body parts for research and transplants.

UNITY CHURCH

Baptism: Baptism is symbolically practiced. Heaven and hell are states of consciousness. People are spiritual beings that are in God's image. God is inherently good; therefore spiritual beings created by God are also inherently good. The church does not believe there are sins to wash away. Christening of newborns are common as a celebration of the newborn's Christ-like nature.
Death: At death, the physical body is left behind and the soul continues on a spiritual journey. Memorial services are "Celebrations of Life." Reincarnation is not taught but is a common belief.
Prayer: Prayer requests may be made 24 hours a day/7 days a week by calling 1-800-NOW–PRAY, by using the uPray mobile prayer app, or by submitting an online prayer request form at https://www.unity.org/prayer
Other practices: Unity is nondiscriminatory and actively supports diversity and acceptance. The focus in on supporting a positive and active spiritual life. Unity does not reject any medical practice. Affirmative prayer, meditation, and metaphysical practices may be used to enhance physical and spiritual health.

UNITED CHURCH OF CHRIST

Baptism: Members practice infant and adult baptism. Three modes are used as appropriate: pouring, sprinkling, and immersion.
Death: If the patient desires counsel or prayer, notify the clergy.
Holy Communion: Clergy is notified if the patient desires to receive this sacrament.

Modified from Carson VB, Koenig HG: *Spiritual dimensions of nursing practice,* revised ed, Philadelphia, 2008, Templeton.

Assessment of family and social organization becomes increasingly more complicated as our society brings together more and more diverse cultures. It is not unusual for a family to be bicultural or biracial or to follow two different faith practices. Be constantly on guard against making assumptions about patients based on appearance, language, ethnic origin, names, or religious practices. Assessment of the individual and family on their own terms helps the nurse to understand each person.

HEALTH PRACTICES

For many years, the belief popular in the United States was that modern biomedical health care was the best and only way to treat diseases. Today many health care providers still find it difficult to believe that any alternative therapies are as effective as the biomedical methods that they have seen used for many years. In recent years, a variety of alternative health services such as folk remedies, holistic therapies, and spiritual interventions have aroused attention in the traditional medical community. Scientific research is being done in these areas to determine the effectiveness of these methods. Some are now accepted more readily and sometimes are used concurrently with biomedical methods (see Chapter 20).

Several factors are driving this change in thinking about health care. Some of the long-established methods have become less effective, notably antibiotics used to treat infections. A number of complementary therapies and folk remedies have been proven effective in treatment of certain diseases. More health care providers with varied backgrounds and beliefs about health and illness now practice in the United States. Increasing mobility and use of electronic media have resulted in more sharing of information, which has promoted diversity. Movement of cultural groups to new areas provides exposure of new information and methods of managing health issues (Fig. 6.1). Some health care practices among cultures are benign and ineffective, and others are therapeutic and useful. The concern lies with those that can pose danger to health and wellness. It is important to allow patients to follow practices that are in accordance with their cultural identity and personal beliefs when they are receiving health care in the traditional health care system, without allowing the effectiveness of either approach to be compromised. The characteristics of four basic concepts of health beliefs are described in Table 6.2. For many years, Western cultures have used almost universally the biomedical method of treating illness and maintaining health. Folk medicine encompasses many different traditions in cultures around the world. It often includes native healers who use a variety of methods in treating disorders (Fig. 6.2). At times, this belief system also incorporates religious practices and magic. Within this system, methods are used to manipulate the environment to improve health.

Do not assume that patients born in the United States accept the biomedical view of health care. Individuals in many subcultures of the United States practice folk medicine. These people sometimes avoid seeking care from health care providers or practice folk medicine while also receiving traditional care.

As our medical system becomes more open to considering a variety of alternative health care systems, the nurse is expected to understand the relationships between different views. Assessing the health practices of patients is an important part of achieving this

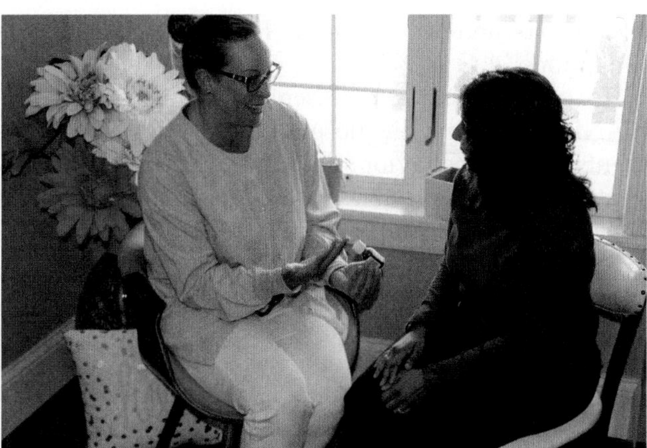

Fig. 6.1 While providing information in a home care setting, a nurse compares traditional and Western remedies. Culture influences how people perceive health, illness, and pain. The nurse must take cultural variations into account to effectively communicate with patients and their families.

understanding. If individual beliefs are discussed openly, the patient probably will be more willing to tell the nurse about using other health care methods in addition to those directed by the health care provider. Be aware that this information must be shared with the doctor to prevent conflicts among treatments.

BIOLOGIC VARIATIONS

Cultural groups are identified in a variety of ways. In some instances, the members share strong biologic characteristics. This is especially true if the cultural group is made up primarily of individuals from a particular race or geographic region. When assessing these individuals, include these characteristics. Some of the obvious ones are body structure, skin color, and hair color and texture. For example, the nurse probably expects a cultural group from the Scandinavian region to have many people with blond hair and blue eyes. Asians are likely to have straight, coarse, dark hair. More important to health care practice is a family history of diseases that are common within the ethnic group. Some diseases, such as sickle cell anemia, are found more frequently among those of African ancestry. Other diseases, such as diabetes, asthma, or heart disease, tend to be more prevalent among certain cultural groups. Even with consideration of diet, diabetes occurs more frequently among American Indians.

Another important health consideration is the effect of culturally determined dietary practices. Many traditional foods are high in saturated fats, sodium, and sugar. If these foods are eaten frequently, they have the potential to affect patients' health and the health of their family members. In some cases, members of some cultural groups have dietary deficiencies caused by low intake of protein, complex carbohydrates, and fresh fruits and vegetables. When assessing the patient, include questions to determine whether the patient follows cultural dietary practices or eats a more general diet. Several diverse cultural groups (Chinese, Korean, Mexican, Puerto Rican, and Vietnamese) have beliefs that diseases and foods are classified as either "hot" or "cold." The diet is adjusted according to the perceived balance, and thus diseases are treated with the proper foods. This practice sometimes leads to a failure to meet basic nutritional needs and to dietary problems (see Chapter 19).

NURSING PROCESS AND CULTURAL FACTORS

When caring for patients, the nurse typically uses the nursing process to develop a plan of care. With use of the information gathered in an assessment, cultural behaviors can be determined and included in a plan of care accordingly.

North American Nursing Diagnosis Association–International (NANDA-I) nursing diagnoses and similar patient problem statements may be difficult to appropriately apply to culturally diverse patients. People from other cultures often do not share the

Table 6.2 Health Belief Systems

BELIEF SYSTEM	CHARACTERISTICS
Biomedical health belief system	Life is regulated by biomedical and physical processes. Life processes can be manipulated by humans with mechanical interventions. Health is the absence of disease or signs and symptoms of disease. Disease is an alteration of the structure and function of the body. Disease has a specific cause, onset, course, and treatment. It is caused by trauma, pathogens, chemical imbalances, or failure of body parts. Treatment focuses on the use of physical and chemical interventions.
Folk health belief system	This commonly is referred to as "third-world" beliefs and practices. It often is called strange or weird by nurses and other health professionals who are unfamiliar with folk medicine beliefs. In most instances, these practices do not seem "strange or weird" once health care providers become acquainted with them. This system classifies illnesses or diseases as natural or unnatural. According to this belief system, natural events have to do with the world as God made it and as God intended it to be. Thus there is a certain amount of predictability for daily life. Unnatural events imply the exact opposite because they upset the harmony of nature. Thus unnatural events are those events that interrupt the plan intended by God and at their very worst represent the forces of evil and the machinations of the devil. They have no predictability and are beyond the control of ordinary mortals. Treatment is done by carrying out rituals or repentance or giving in to the supernatural force's wishes.
Holistic health belief system	Religious experiences are based on cultural beliefs and may include such things as blessings from spiritual leaders, apparitions of dead relatives, and even miracle cures. Healing powers also may be ascribed to animate or inanimate objects. Religion dictates social, moral, and dietary practices designed to assist an individual in maintaining a healthy balance and in playing a vital role in illness prevention (e.g., burning of candles, rituals of redemption, and prayer). Baptism may be seen as a ritual of cleansing and dedication and prevention of evil. Anointing the sick may be seen as preparation for death and also may be performed as the hope of a miracle. Circumcision also is viewed as a religious practice. Treatment is designed to restore balance with physical, social, and metaphysical worlds. It may extend beyond treating the person to treating the environment to decrease pollution or prevent hunger, homelessness, etc.
Alternative or complementary belief system	Today many Americans use one or more nonmedical forms of therapy to treat an illness. Acupuncture, aromatic therapy, meditation, therapeutic touch, and a variety of other techniques provide feasible alternative therapies (see Chapter 20). Most of the individuals who use an alternative therapy do so without informing their health care provider. Alternative therapies address the whole patient by viewing symptoms as the tip of the iceberg and as the body's means for communicating to the mind that something must be changed, removed, or added to one's life. The mind and body are seen as a whole unit.

Data from Giger JM: *Transcultural nursing: Assessment and intervention*, ed 7, St. Louis, 2017, Elsevier.

biomedical health belief system on which these diagnoses or problems are based. Classifying patient problems and needs according to a rigid standard is unrealistic. Unfortunately, a patient's behavior may be labeled as abnormal when it is actually normal in the person's own cultural context. The difficulties go even further, however. The goal of the nursing diagnosis or patient problem system is to help change patient behavior; however, doing so by imposing biomedically based health care beliefs and practices without regard to cultural identity violates the basic tenets of nursing's patient-centered approach.

Certain nursing diagnoses or problem statements are particularly difficult to tailor to particular patients. It is necessary to be cautious with using nursing diagnoses or patient problem statements such as *Insufficient Knowledge, Compromised Verbal Communication, Impaired Health Maintenance,* and *Noncooperation.* Table 6.3 discusses these limitations.

To provide care and lessen the limitations of the NANDA-I nursing diagnoses or patient problem statements, patient behavior should be evaluated from the perspective of the individual's culture. The nurse, the health care system, or both may be required to change to accommodate, maintain, or reinforce the patient's health beliefs and practices. Perhaps the nurse will do this by reprioritizing nursing goals and changing procedures. A compromise is important between individual health beliefs and practices and those of the patient. The patient and family or support system are unlikely to accept any of the health teaching or treatments the nurse attempts to provide if their own beliefs are not recognized. A mutually acceptable alliance with the patient is imperative. Equally important is a mutual respect between the patient and nurse. If the patient defers health care decisions to clergy, a family member, or a significant other, it is also important for the nurse to recognize and communicate respectfully with that person if possible under the guidelines of the Health Insurance Portability and Accountability Act (HIPAA). If the nurse or health care team does not recognize this relationship and respect the dynamics, then compliance is in jeopardy in the event of a conflict. Remember that the ultimate goal is to assist the patient to achieve optimal health. One possible implication of this is that the nurse needs to adjust many of the accepted nursing interventions to accommodate patients and their cultures.

Because of a patient's cultural background, the nurse sometimes must modify how an assessment is performed or care is provided or must adapt the usual routines of the institution to the patient's needs. For instance, consideration should be given when accommodating cultural practices among Muslim patients. The nurse should allow Muslim women to keep the head, arms, and legs covered as much as possible. In addition, every attempt should be made to assign female staff members to care for Muslim women. Because Muslims pray several times each day, care should be scheduled around these times to allow the patient privacy and the necessary leisure to pray. The nurse should be ready to consider similar accommodations to meet the needs of patients in other culturally dependent, special circumstances.

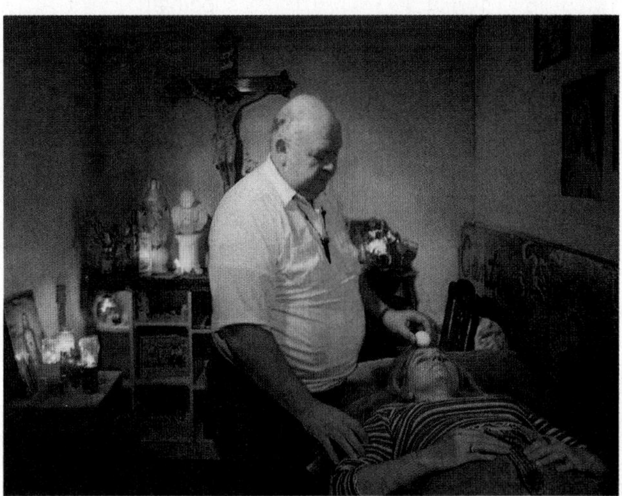

Fig. 6.2 Within the Mexican American folk medicine system, the *curandero* is the folk healer. (From Harkreader H, Hogan MA: *Fundamentals of nursing: Caring and clinical judgment*, ed 3, Philadelphia, 2007, Saunders.)

CULTURAL PRACTICES OF SPECIFIC GROUPS

Hispanics make up a large percentage of the population in the United States and account for as much as 50% of the population in some counties (Fig. 6.3). Subcultures also exist within the Hispanic culture, and Hispanics' origins vary as well. According to the 2010 US Census Bureau report, the largest Mexican populations are found in areas of California, Texas, Illinois, and Arizona. Puerto Ricans are concentrated in New York, Florida, Illinois, and Pennsylvania. About two thirds of all Cubans in the United States live in Florida (US Census Bureau, Census 2010). Although these groups share some common beliefs, they each have distinct practices. The place of origin is important to determine when caring for a Hispanic patient.

Numerous tribes of American Indians live throughout various regions of the United States (US Census Bureau, Census 2010). Nursing care of this population is complicated by the fact that each nation or tribe of American Indians has its own language, religion, and belief system. Practices differ significantly among groups and among members of the same tribe. When the term "American Indian" is used, it is intended to refer to tribes residing within the continental United States.

A complete picture of all cultural practices and beliefs for groups living in the United States is impossible in the context of this chapter. Table 6.4 gives examples

Text continued on p. 114

Table 6.3 Patient Problem Statements and Cultural Limitations

PATIENT PROBLEMS	LIMITATIONS
Insufficient Knowledge	Patient decision-making and health-seeking behavior is directed by a different health belief system. Nurse also has knowledge deficit if care plan and nursing interventions are based solely on nurse's own health belief system.
Compromised Verbal Communication	Ability to understand each other is the problem; communication is not impaired. Patients sometimes seem unable to speak normally when they attempt to respond to someone speaking another language. Nonverbal communication between patient and nurse is likely to become more significant.
Impaired Health Maintenance	Patient is very possibly following acceptable guidelines for health maintenance in his or her culture. Nurse expects person to change behavior to meet nurse's cultural view.
Noncooperation	Patient makes decisions based on a health belief system that is different from the nurse's. Concept of time possibly delays implementation. Religious beliefs sometimes affect adherence to biomedical treatment regimens. Perhaps others in the patient's cultural context counsel the patient to follow alternative health practices.

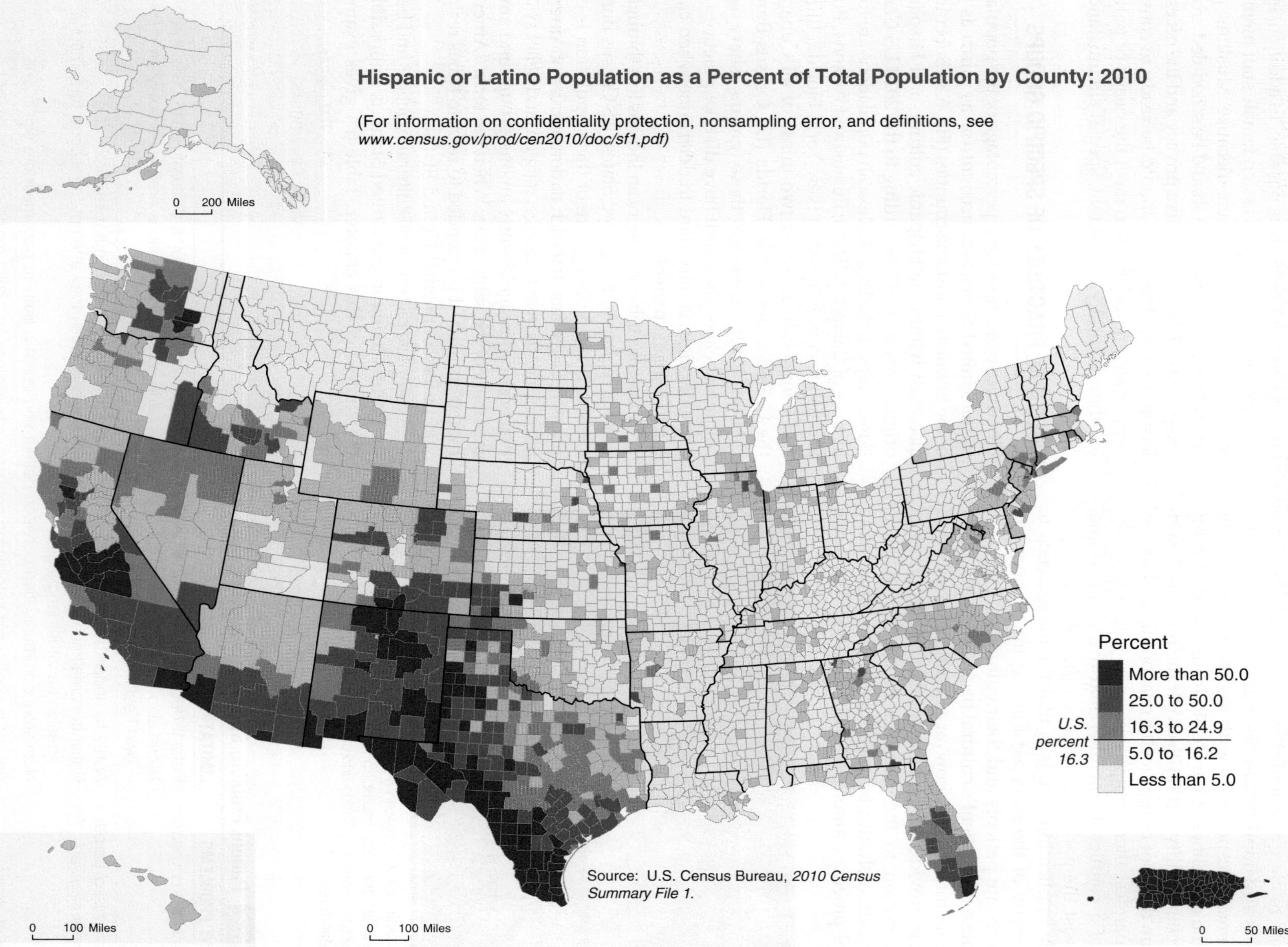

Fig. 6.3 Hispanic percentage of the US population according to Census 2010. (From the US Census Bureau.)

Table 6.4 Cultural Beliefs and Practices

MEXICAN AMERICANS	BLACKS (AFRICAN AMERICANS)	CHINESE AMERICANS	MUSLIM AMERICANS	AMERICAN INDIANS
Predominant Health Belief System				
Sometimes accept biomedical, but belief system is often heavily mixed with folk practices.	Highly diverse. Many adhere to biomedical system. Others, particularly from rural areas, more closely follow folk health beliefs. Often the two belief systems are practiced concurrently. Prayer is important.	Holistic belief system is primary influence. Accept biomedical interventions for serious illness, but possibly continue to practice traditional methods to reestablish natural balance.	Holistic. Essential to preserve modesty and privacy. Obligatory to keep body parts covered as much as possible. Use same-sex health care providers if at all possible. Always examine a female patient in presence of another female. Patient may wish to have doctor consult with Imam (religious leader) when planning care.	Historically, American Indians have been guided by sacred myths and legends that describe the tribes' evolution from inception to the present time. Supernatural beings portrayed in these stories symbolize the culture, in which religion and healing practices are blended. Values and beliefs intrinsic to culture and religion form the day-to-day living experiences. Traditional American Indian concepts focus on the need for the individual to be in harmony with the surrounding environment and with the family. Health and religion cannot be separated within the American Indian culture.
Language				
Spanish, often mixed with English. Children often are better able to speak English and sometimes translate for adults. Many adults never learn English.	English is understood and used when speaking with those outside of cultural group. Black English dialect sometimes is used when speaking with family and friends. Words commonly used in this dialect sometimes are intermixed with standard English when speaking with those in outside community.	Sometimes continue to speak native language even after many years in United States. It is possible to view this as honoring ancestors and native country. Learning to speak English is often difficult because there is little common basis for pronunciation, written characters, or word order.	Varies with country of origin. New immigrants often need family member or community leader to help with translations.	American Indian language has been shown to be derived from the languages used by the people in northwestern Canada. It is also similar to the language spoken by some people living in Alaska, some on the northern coast of the Pacific Ocean, and some in northern California. The language involves tonal speech in which the pitch is of great importance. Every vowel and consonant are fully sounded, regardless of how many times they are doubled or tripled within a word. Vowels are often interchanged, creating several variations and meanings of a word. Even today, many American Indians still speak the native language and are fluent in English, but some do not speak English and need the assistance of an interpreter.

Continued

Table 6.4 Cultural Beliefs and Practices—cont'd

MEXICAN AMERICANS	BLACKS (AFRICAN AMERICANS)	CHINESE AMERICANS	MUSLIM AMERICANS	AMERICAN INDIANS
Communication				
Sustained direct eye contact is considered rude, immodest, or dangerous. Women and children are susceptible to *mal ojo* (evil eye) and so avoid eye contact. Touch is used often. Touch has potential to neutralize mal ojo. Closeness and physical contact are valued in familiar situations. Modesty is highly valued, so it is possible that men and women will be embarrassed when exposure of body is necessary.	Personal space comfort area tends to be close. Eye contact is sometimes uncomfortable, especially among older generation.	Maintaining eye contact often is considered ill mannered and disrespectful. Uncomfortable when face to face. Prefer to sit side-to-side or at right angles to carry on conversation. Touching is not usual during conversation; it is regarded as disrespectful or impolite. Touch possibly acceptable among same-sex acquaintances, but touching in public between opposite sexes is not acceptable.	Women do not usually shake hands with men. Women prefer to keep head, arms, and legs covered. Allow Imam to visit. Allow privacy to pray. Identify Muslim patients on chart and bracelet. Post signs to alert male staff members to avoid room with female Muslim patient.	Until recently, the Navajo language was unwritten. In World War II, a special branch of the US Marine Corps was developed for Navajos who served as Navajo code talkers. It has been estimated that this highly esteemed group saved millions of lives because the enemy was unable to understand the Navajo language or infiltrate the code. Instead of shaking hands, people of this culture extend a hand and lightly touch the hand of the person they are greeting. Initially these people are silent and reserved, but once they become familiar, warm behavior usually is demonstrated. When introducing themselves by name, they give honor to ancestors by stating the clan and the location of their home area. They avoid eye contact, which is considered a sign of disrespect.
Family Roles				
Families sometimes expect to help care for patient. Male family members usually are consulted before health care decisions are made. Only a wife is permitted to give care to husband at home if genitalia are touched.	Women are primary decision makers in family and are frequently head of the household. Extended family plays important role. Even when not related by blood, close ties exist. May refer to these people as "Aunt," "Uncle," "Grandmother," and include them in family decisions.	Loyalty and devotion to family is more important than individual feelings. Taking care of family members brings honor to family. Older children have authority over younger children in family. Decision making is organized in this way, and younger siblings must show respect and deference or it shames the family.	Decision-making unit is the family, not the individual. Husband is consulted in any decisions about family. Imam often included in health-related decisions.	This culture is extremely family oriented, but "family" has a much broader meaning than just father, mother, and children. The biologic family is the center of social organizations and includes all members of the extended family. They are traditionally a matriarchal society. Thus, when a couple marries, the husband makes his home with his wife's relatives and his family becomes one of several units that live in a group of adjacent hogans or other type of dwelling.

Table 6.4 Cultural Beliefs and Practices—cont'd

MEXICAN AMERICANS	BLACKS (AFRICAN AMERICANS)	CHINESE AMERICANS	MUSLIM AMERICANS	AMERICAN INDIANS
				Usually, a male family member who is looked on as having the greatest amount of prestige rises as leader for the extended family and provides necessary direction. However, in settling issues, all sides are listened to and the entire group determines the outcome. To be without relatives is to be really poor.
Birth Rites				
Inappropriate for husband to be present during birth. Father not expected to see wife or baby until both are cleaned and dressed. Female family members sometimes request to be present during labor and delivery.	Many folk customs potentially influence birth. Mother often supported through birth process by female family members. Breast-feeding is not readily accepted by new mothers or encouraged by older generations.	Fathers generally are not present in labor and delivery areas. Some mothers prefer acupuncture for birth rather than Western pain-control methods. Traditionally, mother does not see child for 12 to 24 hours.	Men are not present during labor and delivery. Some husbands wish to be present during the birth process. Women seek a female physician. Pregnant women are exempt from fasting during Ramadan, the sacred ninth month during which Muslims fast from food and drink from dawn to dusk.	The tradition of massaging the newborn baby as a bonding experience between the mother and baby is still practiced. Assistance with ceremonies, particularly those associated with birth, is shared and has great importance. After delivery, the umbilical cord is taken from the newborn, dried, and buried near an object or place that symbolizes what the parents want for the child's future. The infant death rate remains disproportionately high for American Indians.
Death Rites				
Small children are shielded from the dying and death scene. Families take turns staying around the clock with the dying person. Grief sometimes is expressed with hyperkinetic or seizure type of behavior that serves to release emotions.	Extended family is very supportive during final illness. Family members generally take turns staying with dying person. Some fear touching the body or being present when a person has died.	Often have aversion to death and anything concerning death. Donation of body parts is encouraged. Eldest son is responsible for all arrangements for the deceased. White, yellow, or black clothing is worn as sign of mourning.	Life is unique and precious; any intervention to hasten death is forbidden. Autopsy is acceptable with medical and legal need. It is important to allow family and Imam to follow Islamic practices to prepare body for funeral. Organ donations are permitted.	Assistance with ceremonies, particularly those associated with death, is a shared responsibility and has great importance. People of this culture have a taboo against touching a dead person or any article associated with the deceased individual. Taboos associated with death in a hogan include the need to seal the entry and warn others to stay away; frequently the need to abandon or burn the hogan is observed.

Continued

Table 6.4 Cultural Beliefs and Practices—cont'd

MEXICAN AMERICANS	BLACKS (AFRICAN AMERICANS)	CHINESE AMERICANS	MUSLIM AMERICANS	AMERICAN INDIANS
Dietary Practices				
Lactose intolerance is sometimes present. Rice, corn, and beans are good sources of protein. Meats include beef, pork, poultry, and goat. Diet is high in fat because frying is common method of cooking. Fruits and vegetables that are native are included in diet. Sometimes there is an inadequacy in calcium, iron, vitamin A, folic acid, and vitamin C.	High incidence of lactose intolerance, so intake of milk and milk products is low. Many celebrations and rites revolve around food and feasting on traditional dishes (soul food). Traditional dishes such as collard greens, other leafy and yellow vegetables, legumes, beans, rice, and potatoes are high in nutritive value. Overall, the diet tends to be low in fiber, calcium, and potassium and high in fat. Dietary restrictions sometimes related to religious practices.	Diet is low in fat and sugar. Fat intake is limited because of cooking methods. Fish, pork, and poultry, and nuts, dried beans, and tofu, are protein sources. Milk products are avoided because of lactose intolerance. Salt intake sometimes high as a result of eating preserved foods and seasoning with soy sauce. Rice is eaten with almost every meal.	Fasting during daylight hours during Ramadan. Medical condition often exempts person from fasting. Allow family to provide meals if allowed with treatment. Alcohol and drugs are forbidden. Ensure that no pork products are included in foods.	Lack of food and food storage sometimes contributes to nutritional deficiencies. Lactose intolerance is extremely prevalent, affecting 79% of the American Indian population. One hypothesis suggests that some have a predisposition for diabetes that is seemingly triggered by changes in dietary practices and increasing obesity. Contemporary American Indian diet combines food indigenous to the areas with modern processed foods. Food practices are also influenced by tribal beliefs, practices, geographic area, and local availability of selected food. Foods preferred by many include meat and blue cornmeal. Milk is not a preferred food. The fat intake is primarily of saturated fats, and fiber intake is low. Commodity foods are supplied by the US Department of Agriculture's food distribution program.

It should be noted that any reference to cultural practices among a specific culture are commonalities. Individuals within a culture may or may not possess the same practices, beliefs, or values.

of common cultural practices of prevalent minority groups. Always keep in mind the strong influence culture has on patients, colleagues, and the nurse. An awareness of the community in which the nurse practices is especially important. If the LPN/LVN resides in an area that is populated heavily by a culture that is unlike his or her own, it is the nurse's responsibility to learn as much as possible about the people and the culture.

Get Ready for the NCLEX® Examination!

Key Points

- Transcultural nursing is practiced when the nurse consistently attempts to apply knowledge about culture to all aspects of care.
- To achieve cultural competence, the nurse needs an understanding of individual cultural beliefs and practices and an ability to perceive the health care setting from the patient's point of view. This understanding helps the nurse to be more open and sensitive to the patient's cultural values.
- The impact of culture on behaviors, attitudes, and values depends on individual factors and varies among members of a specific cultural group.
- Beliefs and practices vary among and within cultures.
- Ethnocentrism can interfere with development of cultural competence. It is essential to be open to other cultures and value their beliefs and to recognize that your own cultural beliefs are not necessarily superior to those of others.
- A preconceived idea that all members of a particular group possess the same attributes is known as stereotyping.
- Ethnic and racial stereotyping can lead to assumptions about an individual that are often inaccurate.
- Recognition of different health belief systems assists the nurse to develop a plan of care that incorporates varying beliefs.
- Nursing diagnoses and patient problems are based on the biomedical health belief system and may have limitations when used to develop a plan of care for culturally diverse patients with different health beliefs.
- Increased knowledge about cultural groups is imperative as transcultural nursing continues to be important in health care.

Additional Learning Resources

SG Go to your Study Guide for additional learning activities to help you master this chapter content.

evolve Be sure to visit the Evolve site at *http://evolve.elsevier.com/Cooper/foundationsadult/* for additional online resources.

Review Questions for the NCLEX® Examination

1. The nurse works in a community with many Mexican American families. What is the best method for the nurse to learn about the Mexican American culture?
   1. Eat at Mexican American restaurants in the area.
   2. Schedule a home visit with a Mexican American family.
   3. Conduct a library study or Internet search of information on the culture.
   4. Observe cultural behaviors in a movie theater in the area.
2. The patient is admitted to the hospital with reports of diffuse symptoms such as nausea, vomiting, weight loss, headaches, insomnia, and chest pain, which she describes by saying, "My heart aches." Which intervention is appropriate for this patient, whose cultural beliefs may differ from the nurse's beliefs about physical illness?
   1. Adhere to the philosophy, "I treat all my patients the same."
   2. Encourage the patient to describe her symptoms using only English.
   3. Contact an adviser who is familiar with the cultural beliefs of the patient.
   4. Allow the patient to continue taking herbal preparations while she is hospitalized.
3. A Muslim patient visiting the health care provider's office was told she had to remove her clothes and put on an examination gown. The patient said she preferred to remain in her own clothes. Why should the nurse allow the patient to remain in her clothes?
   1. The patient is embarrassed.
   2. Her beliefs may require her to keep as much of her body covered as possible during the examination.
   3. The patient is being uncooperative.
   4. The patient cannot disrobe in front of another female.
4. The patient explains to the nurse that he became ill because the natural balance in his body was upset when he moved into a new apartment. He has been taking herbs and rearranging objects to change the environment. The patient is most demonstrating what health belief system?
   1. Biomedical
   2. Folk
   3. Holistic
   4. A combination of all three
5. A patient, who speaks a language different from the nurse's, asks that her daughter remain with her while the nurse performs a history and physical examination. What action by the nurse is most appropriate?
   1. Ask the daughter to leave to maintain privacy for the patient.
   2. Explain to the patient that family members are not allowed to stay in the examining room because of infection control.
   3. Consider that the daughter may be there to serve as an interpreter for her mother.
   4. Ignore the daughter while performing the history and physical examination.
6. The student nurse tells her instructor that she does not understand why a Chinese American family is not grieving for their dying father. What behaviors are being demonstrated by the student nurse?
   1. Subculture orientation
   2. Stereotyping
   3. Ethnocentric
   4. Culturally racist

7. A male nurse is assigned to care for a female patient. The patient's husband tells the nurse that he cannot care for his wife due to religious reasons. Which statement best describes the patient's spouse's position?
   1. The couple are prejudiced against the nurse's race.
   2. The patient's religion requires that women should be assigned to care for her.
   3. The nurse is not the same religion as the patient and therefore cannot care for the patient.
   4. The couple does not speak English.
8. The nurse is planning to do a cultural assessment of an elderly Chinese American patient. What position of the nurse is most therapeutic?
   1. The nurse sits facing the patient.
   2. The nurse touches the patient frequently to convey concern.
   3. The nurse positions the chair so that the nurse sits at a right angle to the patient.
   4. The nurse maintains good eye contact while asking questions.
9. A female nurse who is black is assigned to care for a new 86-year-old resident in a long-term care facility. When she enters his room, he makes several racially offensive remarks. What is an appropriate response?
   1. The nurse should refuse to give care to the patient.
   2. The nurse should understand that he is possibly less tolerant of other races because of his own cultural experiences or he perhaps has disturbed cognitive functions.
   3. The nurse should become angry and retaliate by making racial statements directed at the patient.
   4. The nurse should tell her supervisor that she will not take care of any other white patients.
10. Upon entering a patient's room the nurse realizes that the patient is praying. What action by the nurse is most appropriate?
    1. The nurse should stay in the room and wait until the patient is finished with his prayers.
    2. The nurse should quietly leave the room and give the patient privacy to pray.
    3. The nurse should interrupt the patient and tell him it is time for his care to be given.
    4. The nurse should tell the patient that he cannot pray while he is in the hospital.
11. A Mexican American is pregnant with her second child. When the nurse is reviewing her diet, the patient states that she never drinks milk. What culturally related factor may explain this?
    1. The patient does not like the taste of milk.
    2. Milk is forbidden in her cultural diet.
    3. Lactose intolerance occurs often among Mexican Americans.
    4. The patient cannot afford to buy milk.
12. An elderly patient has been diagnosed with type 2 diabetes and hypertension. The student nurse tells the patient that her vegetables should be steamed and served plain. The patient responds, "I always cook my green beans with ham and salt and pepper. How can I eat them plain?" Which response by the nurse is most culturally sensitive?
    1. "I'm sorry, but you will just have to change your method of cooking."
    2. "I guess you will just have to give up eating green beans."
    3. "You must follow the health care provider's order if you want to get better."
    4. "Could you try cooking the beans with half as much ham and not add salt?"
13. When caring for a patient who speaks a foreign language, the patient problem statement *Compromised Verbal Communication* would be inappropriate for what reason?
    1. An inability to understand each other is the problem, not impaired verbal communication.
    2. The patient is using a different health belief system that interferes with communication.
    3. The patient is perhaps following acceptable communication guidelines within his or her culture.
    4. The patient has deficient knowledge, not impaired verbal communication.
14. What term describes a nurse who is aware of her or his own cultural beliefs and the beliefs and practices of other cultures and who has the ability to interact effectively with people from other cultures?
    1. Stereotyping
    2. Ethnocentric
    3. Culturally aware
    4. Culturally competent
15. Before implementation of any newly prescribed procedure, the nurse notices that the family of an older adult patient always consults the eldest son. What is the social organization of this family? *(Select all that apply.)*
    1. Hispanic in origin
    2. Patriarchal
    3. Male dominated
    4. Traditional nuclear
    5. Matriarchal
16. The nurse caring for a Chinese American woman after an appendectomy can anticipate which intervention?
    1. Maintaining eye contact with education
    2. Sitting side-by-side to communicate
    3. Touching the patient frequently to comfort
    4. Providing a same-gender caregiver
    5. Allowing the patient to keep head, arms, and legs covered
17. ____________________ means the nurse is aware of his or her own cultural beliefs and practices and how they relate to those of others.

Asepsis and Infection Control

7

http://evolve.elsevier.com/Cooper/foundationsadult/

Objectives

1. Explain the difference between medical and surgical asepsis.
2. Explain how each element of the chain of infection contributes to infection.
3. List five major classifications of pathogens.
4. Identify the body's normal defenses against infections.
5. Discuss nursing interventions used to interrupt the chain of infection.
6. Describe the signs and symptoms of a localized infection and those of a systemic infection.
7. Discuss the events in the inflammatory response.
8. Discuss standard precautions.
9. Demonstrate the proper procedure for hand hygiene.
10. Demonstrate technique for gowning and gloving.
11. Identify principles of surgical asepsis.
12. Describe the accepted techniques of preparation for disinfection and sterilization.
13. Discuss patient teaching for infection prevention and control as an element of health promotion.
14. Discuss infection prevention and control measures in the home.

Key Terms

antiseptic (ăn-tĭ-SĔP-tĭk, p. 118)
asepsis (ā-SĔP-sĭs, p. 118)
carrier (KĀR-ē-ŭr, p. 122)
Centers for Disease Control and Prevention (CDC) (SĔN-tĕrz fŏr dĭ-ZEZ kŏn-trol ănd prē-VĔN-shŭn, p. 127)
contamination (kŏn-tăm-ĭ-NĀ-shŭn, p. 122)
disinfection (dĭs-ĭn-FĔK-shŭn, p. 118)
endogenous (ĕn-DŎJ-ĕn-ŭs, p. 126)
exogenous (ĕks-ŎJ-ĕn-ŭs, p. 126)
fomite (FŌ-mīt, p. 123)
health care-associated infection (hĕlth kār ā-SŌ-sē-ā-tĭd ĭn-FĔK-shŭn, p. 125)
host (HŌST, p. 123)
infection prevention and control (ĭn-FĔK-shŭn prē-VĔN-shŭn, p. 118)
medical asepsis (MĔD-ĭ-kăl ā-SĔP-sĭs, p. 118)
microorganisms (mī-krō-ŎR-găn-ĭz-ĕmz, p. 117)
reservoir (RĔZ-ŭr-vwăhr, p. 122)
spore (spōr, p. 119)
standard precautions (STĂN-dŭrd prē-KĂW-shŭnz, p. 127)
sterilization (stĕr-ĭ-lĭ-ZĀ-shŭn, p. 152)
surgical asepsis (SŬR-jĭ-kăl ā-SĔP-sĭs, p. 118)
vector (VĔK-tŭr, p. 122)
vehicle (VĒ-ĭ-kĕl, p. 122)
virulent (VĬR-ū-lĕnt, p. 125)

With the discovery that microorganisms cause infection came the realization that illness or disease caused by infection is prevented by inhibiting or stopping growth and reproduction of microorganisms. Aseptic technique is a method developed by Joseph Lister (1827–1912) to reduce morbidity and mortality from infection. Lister is known as the father of aseptic technique, although many researchers contributed to its development.

In today's health care environment, nurses and other health care workers must practice effective infection prevention and control measures to protect patients. In addition to protecting patients, nurses and health care workers must be aware of the risk involved with drug-resistant microorganisms and occupational exposure to infectious material. Diligent attention to infection prevention reduces the incidence of patient deaths, disabilities, and extended health care days of admission. Health care delivery costs are reduced when infection prevention is implemented at all facilities.

ASEPSIS

The increase of transmissible infections, not only in health care facilities but also in the home, is an issue of great societal concern. **Microorganisms** (tiny, usually microscopic, entities capable of carrying on living processes) are naturally present on and in the human body and in the environment. Many of these microorganisms are harmless (nonpathogenic) and in most individuals do not produce disease. Some are even helpful. If an individual is highly susceptible to infection, the nonpathogenic microorganisms can be dangerous.

Any patient who enters a health care facility has a greater risk of an infection because of reduced immunologic function. Increased stressors to the patient's immune system are the presenting illness, exposure to disease-causing microorganisms, and portals created by invasive procedures. In addition, health care facilities are conducive to the spread of these microorganisms because of the many ill carriers within their walls. The nurse's knowledge about infection and the application of infection prevention and control principles help protect patients from infection. With each patient care activity, the nurse should ensure that infection prevention and control are routine.

Infection prevention and control involve the implementation of policies and procedures in hospitals and other health care facilities to minimize the spread of health care–associated or community-acquired infections to patients and other staff members. During patient care, the nurse may be exposed to pathogenic microorganisms. The nurse is a chief player in the prevention of the spread of infection, which is accomplished with learning and continued observation of routine and specialized practices of cleanliness and disinfection. These techniques aid in accomplishing **asepsis** (the absence of pathogenic microorganisms). Asepsis is divided into the following two categories:

1. **Medical asepsis** consists of techniques that inhibit the growth and transmission of pathogenic microorganisms. Medical asepsis is also known as *clean technique* and is used in many daily activities, such as hand hygiene and changing of patient bed linens.
2. **Surgical asepsis** consists of techniques designed to destroy all microorganisms and their spores (the reproductive cell of some microorganisms, such as fungi or protozoa). Surgical asepsis is known as sterile technique and is used in specialized areas, such as the operating room, or during invasive procedures, such as urinary catheter insertion.

INFECTION

For an infection to develop, a specific cycle or chain of events must occur. The following six elements are necessary for infection and are referred to as the chain of infection (Fig. 7.1):

1. *Infectious agent:* A pathogen
2. *Reservoir:* Where the pathogen can grow
3. *Portal of exit (exit route):* Exit route from the reservoir
4. *Mode (method) of transmission:* Method or vehicle of transportation, such as exudate, feces, air droplets, hands, and needles
5. *Portal of entry (entrance):* Entrance through skin, mucous lining, or mouth

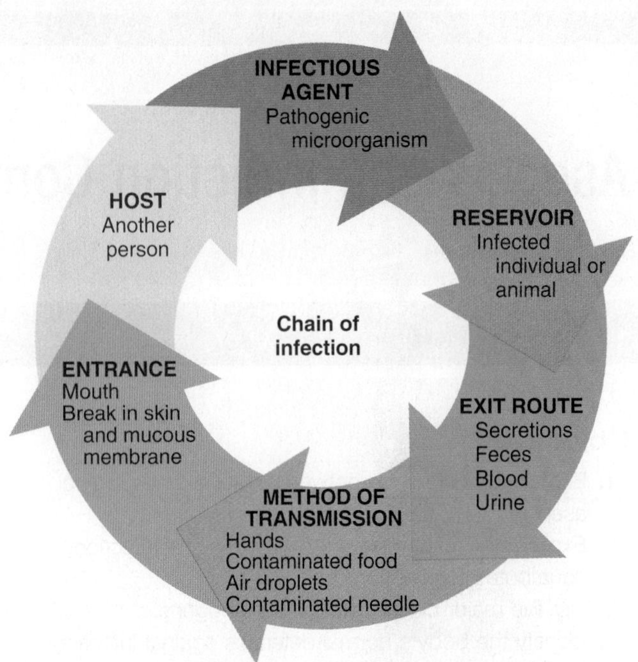

Fig. 7.1 The chain of infection.

6. *Host:* Another person or animal that is susceptible to the pathogen

For prevention of the transmission of an infection, the cycle must be interrupted. Medical asepsis is an effective way to disrupt the chain of infection. This practice helps to inhibit (to stop or slow a process) the growth and reduce the number of microorganisms.

INFECTIOUS AGENT

Pathogenic microorganisms are infectious agents. Pathogens can be bacteria, viruses, yeasts, fungi, and protozoa. All these microorganisms need food for growth and a suitable environment in which to live. Unwashed hands, wound drainage, soiled linen, and decaying teeth provide ideal areas for pathogenic growth. The microorganism strength, the number of microorganisms present, the effectiveness of a person's immune system, and the length of exposure to the microorganisms determine the ability to produce disease. The role of the nurse is to provide a safe environment by working to prevent the transmission of infection.

Health care workers have several ways to help their patients remain free of infection. Proper **disinfection** (the use of a chemical that can be applied to objects to destroy microorganisms), appropriate use of an **antiseptic** (a substance that tends to inhibit the growth and reproduction of microorganisms and may be used on humans), and use of surgical asepsis when indicated are important ways to help reduce the presence of microorganisms.

Bacteria

Bacteria have many different characteristics. In addition to their three basic shapes (round, oblong, and spiral),

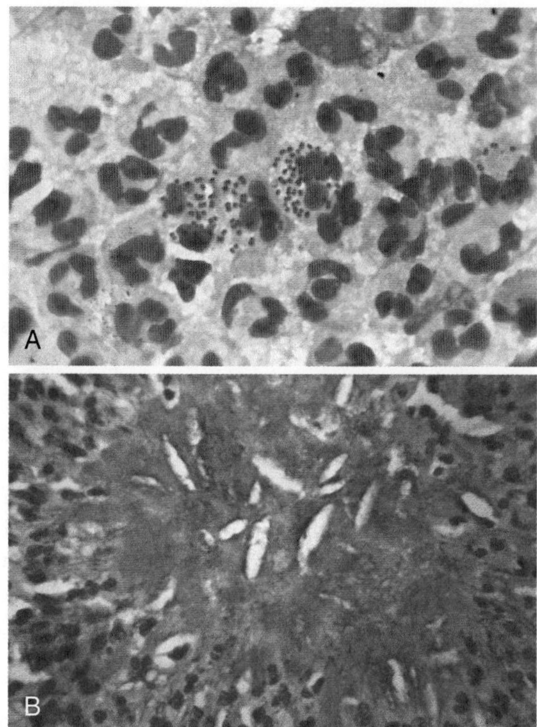

Fig. 7.2 A, Aerobic bacteria. B, Anaerobic bacteria. (Courtesy the Centers for Disease Control and Prevention. A, Bill Schwartz; B, Dr. Richard L. Levin, Greater Southeast Community Hospital, Washington, DC.)

there are many variations. Some are elongated or have pointed ends, and some are flattened on one side. Some are shaped like commas, and others appear square. Spirilla are often tightly coiled, like a corkscrew. During cell division, some bacteria remain together to form pairs, whereas others form long chains. Diagnostic testing focuses on the unique characteristics for identification of specific types of bacteria.

Bacteria also can be differentiated by their chemical compositions, the nutrients that they need to grow, and the waste products the bacteria form. *Aerobic* bacteria grow only in the presence of oxygen, whereas *anaerobic* bacteria grow only in the absence of oxygen (Figs. 7.2A and B). Some bacteria are capable of movement. Motility is possible because of fine, hairlike projections—flagella—that extend from the bacterial cell. These projections move in a wavelike fashion to propel the cell. Some bacteria have only one flagellum attached to one end of the cell, and others have many flagella surrounding the cell. Locomotion of the spirochete is achieved with a wiggling motion that involves the entire cell body.

Some bacteria form a specialized structure called a **spore.** The spore is a round body that is formed by the bacterium when conditions are unfavorable for growth of the bacterium. The spore enlarges until it is as large as the bacterial cell and is surrounded by a capsule. Eventually, the portion of the cell that surrounds the spore disintegrates. The spore remains dormant until environmental conditions become favorable for growth. Then the spore germinates and begins reproducing. Characteristically, spores have a high degree of resistance to heat and disinfectants. Some bacteria have the ability to form capsules around the cell wall. These mucilaginous (of a thick, sticky, slimy substance) envelopes form when the bacterial environment is hostile. The formation of the capsule is a defense mechanism to help protect the bacteria. As with spores, staining in the laboratory usually requires special procedures. Capsule formation also contributes to the development of multidrug resistance. When capsules are present, antibiotic therapy is sometimes ineffective because the capsule prevents the drug from reaching the bacteria within the capsule and destroying it.

Identification of the specific organism is vital to the development of the appropriate plan of treatment. Antimicrobial therapies provide a system of attack that is individualized to specific microorganisms. Specially trained laboratory personnel perform this identification. In some instances, they examine a specimen before staining it, but this method is usually less satisfactory. Most bacteria are not visible without a special staining process, in which a dye is applied to a specially prepared glass slide that contains a small amount of the material to be examined. Identification of most bacteria is possible with this simple process; however, other bacteria necessitate additional staining.

Depending on whether a color can be removed with a solvent or the color is retained after the use of the solvent, the organism is identified as gram positive or gram negative. Special staining techniques are required for bacteria that have flagella, spores, or capsules.

The nurse collects specimens of body fluids and secretions suspected of containing pathogenic organisms in sterile containers and sends them to the laboratory for culture and sensitivity testing. Laboratory personnel transfer the specimen to a special culture medium that promotes growth. They then study the culture and identify the pathogens. The results of the sensitivity tests assist the practitioner in determining which antimicrobial (antibiotic) medication will inhibit the pathogens' growth effectively. The practitioner then orders appropriate antimicrobial agents on the basis of these tests, which typically take 48 to 72 hours to complete. Different organisms require different antibiotics to be destroyed effectively.

Bacterial infections are transmitted from person to person by direct contact, by inhalation, and by indirect contact with articles contaminated with the pathogen. Some also are transmitted through the ingestion of contaminated food and drink (Fig. 7.3).

The *Streptococcus* bacterium is responsible for more diseases than any other organism, but methicillin-resistant *Staphylococcus aureus* (MRSA) has been proven responsible for a number of serious and sometimes fatal infections. Patients with immunocompromised conditions who are admitted to health care facilities have an increased risk of exposure to strains of MRSA that are multidrug resistant and therefore more difficult to treat.

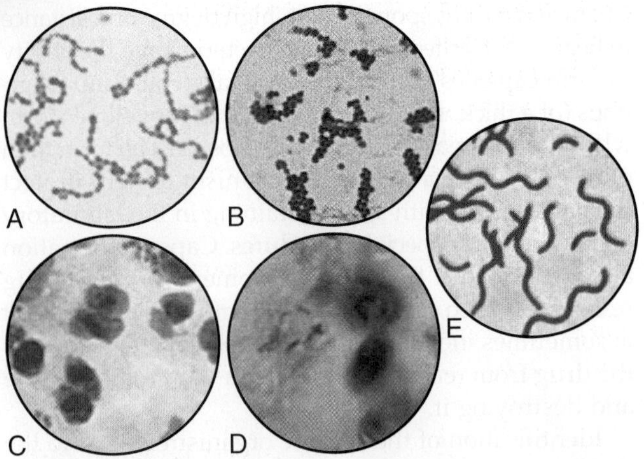

Fig. 7.3 Some common disease-producing bacteria. A, Streptococci. B, Staphylococci. C, Diplococci. D, Bacilli. E, Spirilla. (Courtesy the Centers for Disease Control and Prevention. A, Dr. Gilda Jones; B, Dr. Richard Facklam; C, Dr. Norman Jacobs; D, Dr. Roger Feldman.)

Rocky Mountain spotted fever has been found in almost every area of the United States, and its prevalence continues to increase. It is transmitted to humans through the bite of an infected tick. Several varieties of ticks carry the disease. The ticks live on many different kinds of animals found in rural and wooded areas. They are also able to live on common house pets, such as cats and dogs. People who work in areas where ticks are known to be abundant are more likely to become infected. The tick attaches itself to the skin, and the longer it remains attached, the more likely the person is to become infected. Great care must be taken not to crush or squeeze the tick on removal from the skin.

The spore-forming bacterium *Bacillus anthracis* causes the acute infectious disease of anthrax. Anthrax infection occurs in three forms:

- Cutaneous (skin) (Fig. 7.4)
- Gastrointestinal
- Inhalation

Anthrax occurs more commonly in animals, but it also can infect humans. It is seen more often in agricultural regions of South and Central America, southern and eastern Europe, Asia, Africa, the Caribbean, and the Middle East, where it is found in animals. It rarely infects domesticated animals in the United States.

B. anthracis spores can live in the soil for many years. Casual contact from person to person does not spread anthrax. In cases of intentional exposure (e.g., during a biologic terrorism event), the most likely routes of infection are inhalation of the spores and spore contact with skin. *B. anthracis* is considered by the Centers for Disease Control and Prevention (CDC, 2016) to be one of the most likely agents that may be used during a biologic terrorism event (see Chapter 10).

Anthrax infection is diagnosed when *B. anthracis* is detected in blood, skin lesions, or respiratory secretions by means of a laboratory culture or measurement of specific antibodies in the blood of infected people.

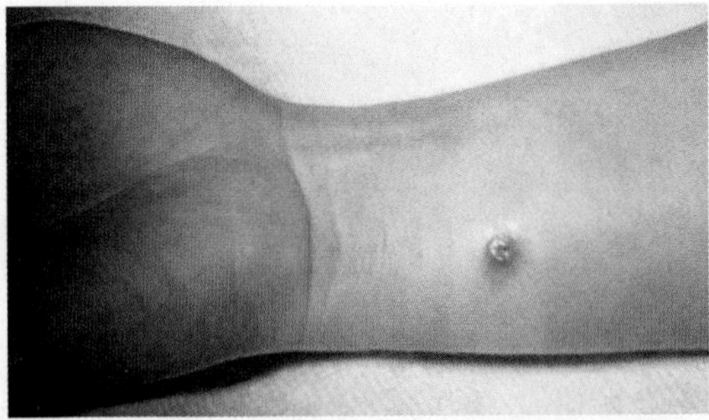

Fig. 7.4 Cutaneous anthrax infection. (Courtesy the Centers for Disease Control and Prevention.)

Treatment consists of antibiotics such as ciprofloxacin (Cipro) or doxycycline (Vibramycin) (US FDA, 2016; 2017). A vaccine is available for prevention of anthrax infection. Vaccination is recommended for those at high risk of exposure, such as laboratory personnel who handle the bacterium or members of the armed forces. If left untreated, anthrax can be fatal (Mayo Clinic, 2017).

Viruses

Viruses are the smallest known agents to cause disease. They are not complete cells but are composed of either RNA or DNA. They consist of a protein coat around a nucleic acid core and depend on the metabolic processes of the cell they enter. Before 1900 scientists discovered that certain agents, unlike bacteria, can pass through a laboratory filter. In addition, they were unable to observe these tiny bodies with the ordinary microscope. In 1898 Martinus W. Beijerinck called these small bodies *viruses*, and they became known as filterable viruses.

For years, scientists knew little about viruses, even though they were able to observe their effect on humans and animals. In 1941 the electron microscope became available. With this advancement, the science of virology was born, and a whole new era in the study of human disease was opened. In addition, the development of other tools and techniques has resulted in rapid advances in the study of viruses: the use of certain dyes that become luminous when exposed to ultraviolet light (fluorescent microscopy), tissue culture methods, ultracentrifuge, cytochemistry, and the development of other technical laboratory aids.

Viruses gain entrance to the body through various portals such as the respiratory tract, the gastrointestinal tract, and broken skin. Sometimes a virus can infect a susceptible host through a mosquito bite or during an accidental needlestick with a contaminated needle. Viruses are selective in the type of body cells they attack, but once they have found cells for which they have an affinity, they enter the cell and reproduce rapidly. As they multiply, they interrupt the cell activities and use the cell material to produce new virus material.

Viral infections are usually self-limiting. They run a given course, and recovery usually occurs. One exception is acquired immunodeficiency syndrome (AIDS). Without adequate treatment with specific types of medication, the human immunodeficiency virus (HIV) reproduces, and the immune system continues to be stressed to the point at which it can no longer fight off even the most common infection; the patient then receives the diagnosis of AIDS.

Other viral diseases have the capacity to cause death if complications occur or if they attack individuals with extremely weak or debilitated conditions. People who are at either end of the age spectrum are also at increased risk for complications. The common cold is caused by a virus. Symptoms of the common cold usually are relieved by bedrest and taking over-the-counter remedies. No medicine cures the cold; medicine only relieves the discomfort. Antibiotics do not alter the course of the majority of viral diseases.

Viruses are classified in various ways, either according to the diseases they cause or by the characteristics of a specific group. In the latter classification system, each subgroup often has many types or strains (Table 7.1).

Fungi

Fungal (mycotic) infections are among the most common diseases found in humans. Fungi are among the most plentiful forms of life. They belong to the plant kingdom, and although many of them are harmless, some are

Table 7.1 Common Pathogens, Reservoirs, and Infections or Diseases

ORGANISM	PRIMARY RESERVOIR	INFECTION OR DISEASE
Bacteria		
Staphylococcus aureus	Skin, hair, anterior nares	Wound infection, pneumonia, food poisoning
β-Hemolytic group A streptococci	Oropharynx, skin, perineal care	Strep throat, rheumatic fever, scarlet fever, impetigo
β-Hemolytic group B streptococci	Adult genitals	Urinary tract infection, wound infection, neonatal sepsis
Escherichia coli	Colon	Enteritis
E. coli serotype O157:H7	Colon—food and water	Hemolytic-uremic syndrome (HUS)
Neisseria gonorrhoeae	Genitourinary tract, rectum, mouth, eye	Gonorrhea, pelvic inflammatory disease, conjunctivitis
Staphylococcus epidermidis	Skin	IV line infection, bacteremia, endocarditis
Tubercle bacillus *(Mycobacterium tuberculosis)*	Lungs	Tuberculosis infection Tuberculosis disease
Bacillus anthracis	Infected animals or their products; bioterrorist release	Cutaneous anthrax Inhalation anthrax Gastrointestinal anthrax
Rickettsia rickettsii	Wood tick	Rocky Mountain spotted fever
Viruses		
Herpes simplex virus I and II	Lesions of the mouth, skin, adult genitals	Cold sores, sexually transmitted infections
Hepatitis A and E	Food or water, feces	Hepatitis A and E
Hepatitis B, C, D, and G	Blood, body fluids, and excretions	Hepatitis B
Human immunodeficiency virus (HIV)	Blood, semen, vaginal secretions, breast milk	HIV-positive status, HIV infection
Varicella zoster virus	Vesicle fluid, respiratory tract infections	HIV disease Varicella (chickenpox) primary infection, herpes zoster (shingles) reactivation
Fungi		
Pneumocystis jiroveci (carinii)	Intestinal tract, genitourinary tract, respiratory tract, and circulatory system of humans and animals	Pneumonia referred to as an opportunistic infection in acquired immunodeficiency syndrome (AIDS)
Candida albicans	Mouth, skin, colon, genital tract	Thrush, dermatitis, sexually transmitted diseases
Cryptococcus species	Bird feces	Pneumonia-like illness, meningoencephalitis
Protozoa		
Plasmodium falciparum	Mosquito	Malaria
Entamoeba histolytica	Intestinal tract (specifically the large intestine)	Diarrhea, colitis

IV, Intravenous.

responsible for infections. Fungus types that many people are familiar with include the fuzzy black, green, or white growth on stale bread. Mycotic infections are diseases caused by yeasts and molds. Some are superficial and involve the skin and the mucous membranes. Most frequently, the infections involve the external layers of the skin, the hair, and the nails.

Fungi also may invade the deeper tissues of the body. These types of infections may produce no signs or symptoms; however, some become serious and potentially fatal, especially in a patient with severe immunocompromise. Coccidioidomycosis (valley fever) and histoplasmosis (a systemic fungal respiratory disease) are examples of systemic fungal infections.

Protozoa

Protozoa are single-celled animals; in some form, they exist everywhere in nature. Some of the parasitic forms of protozoa are found in the intestinal tract, the genitourinary tract, the respiratory tract, and the circulatory system of humans and other animals. Protozoa are responsible for malaria, amebic dysentery, and African sleeping sickness (see Table 7.1).

RESERVOIR

To thrive, organisms need a proper atmosphere. Characteristics of an environment that supports organism growth include an available food source, oxygen, water, light, and desirable temperatures and levels of acidity or alkalinity. Any natural habitat of a microorganism that promotes growth and reproduction is a **reservoir.** Many areas of the body typically host a variety of microorganisms, but the presence of these microorganisms does not always cause illness. Reservoirs include humans, animals, and environmental sources. Within the health care environment, infection may breed and thrive in soiled dressings and medical equipment, including stethoscopes, bedside tables, and overbed tables.

A **carrier,** or **vector,** is a person or animal that does not become ill but harbors and spreads an organism, causing disease in others.

The nurse must be aware of the potential risk presented within the health care environment. Ensuring cleaning between patient use, prompt changing of soiled materials, and proper disposal of contaminated materials are critical (Box 7.1).

Box 7.1 Measures to Reduce Reservoirs of Infection

BATHING

- Use soap and water to remove drainage, dried secretions, excess perspiration, or sediment from disinfectants.

DRESSING CHANGES

- Change wet or soiled dressings.

CONTAMINATED ARTICLES

- Place used tissues, soiled dressings, and soiled linen in moisture-resistant bags for proper disposal. Place dressings that can be poured, dripped, or squeezed in biohazard bags.

CONTAMINATED NEEDLES AND SHARPS

- Place syringes, uncapped hypodermic needles, and sharps such as scalpels in moisture-resistant, puncture-proof containers (often called "sharps containers"). Keep these in patients' rooms or treatment areas so that carrying exposed, contaminated equipment any distance is not necessary.
- Do not recap needles or attempt to break them.

BEDSIDE UNIT

- Keep table surfaces clean and dry.

BOTTLED SOLUTIONS

- Do not leave bottled solutions open for prolonged periods.
- Keep solutions tightly capped.
- Date bottles when opened.
- Use only as directed by the manufacturer.

SURGICAL WOUNDS

- Maintain the patency of drainage tubes and collection bags to prevent accumulation of serous fluid under the skin surface.

DRAINAGE BOTTLES AND BAGS

- Empty and dispose of drainage suction canisters according to agency policy.
- Empty all drainage systems on each shift unless otherwise ordered by a physician.[a]
- Never raise a drainage system (e.g., urinary drainage bag) above the level of the site being drained unless it is clamped off.

[a]Closed, water-sealed chest drainage system receptacles are never emptied, only replaced if necessary, per hospital protocol.

PORTAL OF EXIT

A microorganism does not have the capacity to cause disease in another host without finding a point of escape from the reservoir. Examples of exit routes in humans are any body fluids produced from the patient, such as those from the gastrointestinal, respiratory, and genitourinary systems or from an open area on the patient's body.

With hand hygiene, the nurse can help prevent the spread of microorganisms. Also, the nurse should teach the patient to cover the nose and mouth when coughing or sneezing.

MODE OF TRANSMISSION

A contaminated **vehicle** is the means by which microorganisms are carried about and transported to the next host, once they have left the reservoir. **Contamination** means a condition of being soiled, stained, touched by, or otherwise exposed to harmful agents (i.e., the entry of infectious materials into a previously clean or sterile environment), which makes an object potentially unsafe for use. If the vehicle is a living carrier, it is called a vector. If the vehicle is an inanimate (nonliving) object, it is called a **fomite.** Some examples of fomites found in health care facilities are computers (many people touch the computer throughout the day), medical records and charts, stethoscopes, thermometers, bandage scissors, used tissues, drinking glasses, needles, and soiled dressings.

Transmission via this kind of common contact with a fomite or vector is known as the indirect method of transmission. Transmission through direct contact is also possible, such as when the nurse uses poor hand hygiene technique and then touches a patient while providing care such as assessing, bathing, or repositioning the client or during medication administration.

Air currents can carry microorganisms. To help reduce the number of microorganisms in the air, do not shake the linens when making a bed. Use of a dampened or treated cloth when dusting can help prevent circulation of dust particles.

The floor is one of the dirtiest areas in any building. Do not use anything that has been dropped on the floor. Linens that have been dropped on the floor should be treated as soiled and placed in the appropriate container to be sent for laundering. Supplies (such as dressings) should be discarded. During care, it may be necessary to squat to provide care such as emptying an indwelling urinary catheter or to assist in bathing the patient's legs and feet. During such situations, squat in a way to avoid the knees touching the floor. Feet and furniture are the only items that belong on the floor.

Because so many factors can promote the spread of infection to a patient, all health care workers who provide direct care (physical therapists, physicians, nurses) and those who perform diagnostic and support services (laboratory technicians, respiratory therapists, dietary workers) must follow infection prevention and control practices to prevent or minimize the spread of infection.

PORTAL OF ENTRY

Once the microorganism has exited the reservoir and has been transmitted to a susceptible host, it has to find a way to enter the host. When the host's defense mechanisms are reduced (see the section "Host"), the microorganism has a greater chance to gain entry to the host and produce infection. If the patient's skin is punctured with a contaminated needle, microorganisms are able to enter into the bloodstream. If the nurse is not careful when changing a wound dressing, contamination of the new dressing or the wound could occur and could introduce possibly pathogenic microorganisms into the open wound and cause an infection.

Many of the entrance and exit routes microorganisms take are the same, and methods used to prevent or control both processes are also similar. The skin is the first line of defense. It should be kept intact, lubricated, and clean. Observe the patient's skin closely for any open areas and treat them accordingly (see Chapter 9).

Accidental needlesticks are a potential hazard for all personnel who work in a health care facility. Any injury caused by a sharp piece of possibly dirty equipment (such as a used needle or scalpel) should be reported immediately so that procedures can be initiated to help prevent development of specific types of infections (such as hepatitis B and HIV). Available and appropriate waste containers are essential for safe disposal of sharp instruments, often referred to as "sharps containers." Needles should never be recapped.

An indwelling urinary catheter or another type of drainage equipment often provides an entrance for microorganisms. Ensure that tubes remain connected and intact. Take care when turning, positioning, or transferring a patient to prevent any tubes from becoming tangled or pulling apart.

In the care of open areas of the skin or mucous membranes, specific techniques can be used to prevent the entrance of microorganisms. Wear gloves when handling soiled dressings, and place the dressings in the appropriate type of waste container for disposal per facility policy.

HOST

A **host** is an organism in which another organism is nourished and harbored.

Susceptibility to an infection is defined by the amount of resistance that the host can exhibit against the pathogen. Microorganisms are constantly in contact with people, but an infection does not develop unless a person is susceptible to the microorganism's strength and numbers. As the pathogen's strength and numbers increase, the person becomes more susceptible. Factors that affect a person's immunologic defense mechanisms are described in Box 7.2.

Immunizations have proven effective in reducing susceptibility to some types of infectious diseases. These are given before a person has been exposed to a disease (to provide protection before contact) or after exposure

Box 7.2 Factors That Affect Immunologic Defense Mechanisms

- Chemotherapy
- Diagnostic procedures
- Disease processes
- Environmental factors
- Fatigue
- Hereditary factors
- Increasing age and extreme youth
- Lifestyle
- Medical therapy
- Nutritional status
- Occupation
- Radiation
- Stress
- Trauma
- Travel history

Table 7.2 Normal Defense Mechanisms Against Infection

DEFENSE MECHANISMS	ACTION	FACTORS THAT MAY ALTER DISEASE
Skin		
Intact multilayered surface (body's first line of defense against infection)	Provides barrier to microorganisms	Cuts, abrasions, puncture wounds, areas of maceration
Shedding of outer layer of skin cells	Removes organisms that adhere to skin's outer layers	Failure to bathe regularly
Sebum	Contains fatty acid that kills some bacteria	Excessive bathing
Mouth		
Intact multilayered mucosa	Provides mechanical barrier to microorganisms	Lacerations, trauma, extracted teeth
Saliva	Washes away particles that contain microorganisms Contains microbial inhibitors (e.g., lysozyme)	Poor oral hygiene, dehydration
Eye tearing and blinking	Provides mechanisms to reduce entry (blinking) or to assist in washing away (tearing) particles that contain pathogens, thus reducing number (dose) of organisms	Injury, exposure—splash or splatter of blood or other potentially infectious material into the eye
Respiratory Tract		
Cilia lining upper airway coated by mucus	Trap inhaled microbes and sweep them outward in mucus to be expectorated or swallowed Engulf and destroy microorganisms that reach lungs' alveoli	Smoking, high concentration of oxygen and carbon dioxide, decreased humidity, cold air
Urinary Tract		
Flushing action of urine flow	Washes away microorganisms on lining of bladder and urethra	Obstruction to normal flow by urinary catheter placement, obstruction from growth or tumor, delayed micturition Introduction of urinary catheter, continual movement of catheter in urethra
Gastrointestinal Tract		
Acidity of gastric secretions	Chemically destroys microorganisms incapable of surviving low pH	Use of antacids
Rapid peristalsis in small intestine	Prevents retention of bacterial contents	Delayed motility resulting from impaction of fecal contents in large bowel or mechanical obstruction by masses
Vagina		
At puberty, normal flora cause vaginal secretions to achieve low pH	Inhibit growth of many microorganisms	Antibiotics, excessive douching, and oral contraceptives disrupting normal flora

(if the person's history indicates possible contact with an infectious microorganism). Table 7.2 lists the normal defense mechanisms against infection.

Health care facility policies may mandate that workers be current with immunizations. Many facilities also recommend preventive medications and vaccines. As role models, nurses should provide teaching and encouragement to their patients concerning the benefits of these practices.

INFECTIOUS PROCESS

When the nurse understands the chain of infection, the nurse gains the ability to intervene to prevent infections from developing. When the patient acquires an infection, the nurse can observe certain signs and symptoms and take appropriate actions to prevent its spread. Infections follow a progressive course (Box 7.3). The severity of the patient's illness depends on the extent of the infection, the virulence (disease-causing power) of the microorganisms, and the susceptibility of the host.

If infection is *localized* (e.g., a superficial wound infection), proper care helps control its spread and minimizes the illness (Fig. 7.5). The patient usually experiences localized symptoms such as pain and tenderness at the wound site. An infection that affects the entire body instead of just a single organ or part is *systemic* and has the potential to be fatal.

The course of an infection influences the level of nursing care that must be provided. The nurse is responsible for the administration of prescribed antimicrobial

Box 7.3 Stages of an Infectious Process (Localized or Systemic)

INCUBATION PERIOD
Interval between entrance of pathogen into body and appearance of first symptoms (e.g., chickenpox, 1 to 3 weeks; common cold, 1 to 2 days; influenza, 1 to 3 days; mumps, 12 to 26 days). The host may be infectious during this period.

PRODROMAL STAGE
Interval from onset of nonspecific signs and symptoms (malaise, low-grade fever, fatigue) to more specific symptoms; during this time, microorganisms grow and multiply, and patient is more capable of spreading disease to others. For example, herpes simplex begins with itching and tingling at the site during the prodromal stage, before the lesion appears.

ACUTE STAGE
Interval when patient manifests signs and symptoms specific to type of infection (e.g., common cold manifested by sore throat, sinus congestion, rhinitis; mumps manifested by earache, high fever, parotid and salivary gland swelling). This is often the period in which the individual is most contagious.

CONVALESCENCE
Interval when acute symptoms of infection disappear; length of recovery depends on severity of infection and patient's general state of health, and recovery takes from several days to months.

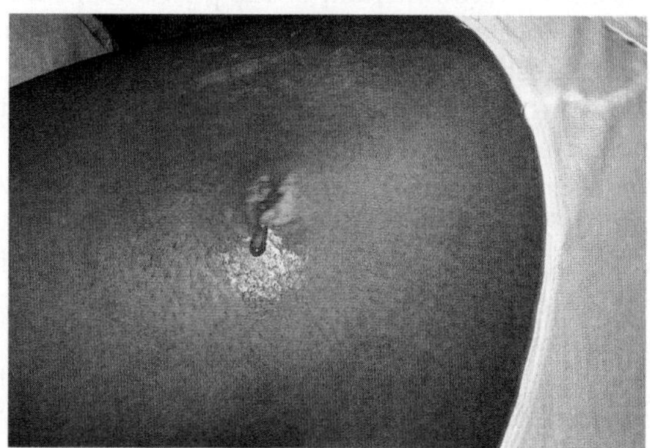

Fig. 7.5 Localized skin infection. (Courtesy the Centers for Disease Control and Prevention/Bruno Coignard, MD; Jeff Hageman, MHS.)

agents (antibiotics, antivirals, or antifungals). Monitoring patients to assess their response to the therapies includes the objective nursing assessment and vital signs, laboratory studies (e.g., white blood cell levels and albumin values), and subjective reports from the patient. Supportive therapy includes providing adequate nutrition and rest to bolster the body's defense against the infectious process. The complexity of care further depends on body systems affected by the infection.

Regardless of whether infection is localized or systemic, the nurse plays a critical role in minimizing its spread. For example, the organism that causes a simple wound infection often spreads to involve an incisional wound site if the nurse uses improper technique during the dressing change. If nurses have a break in their own skin, they may acquire infections from patients if the technique for controlling infection transmission is inadequate.

INFLAMMATORY RESPONSE

Inflammation is the body's response to injury or infection at the cellular level. Inflammation is a protective vascular reaction that delivers fluid, blood products, and nutrients to interstitial tissues in the area of an injury. The process neutralizes and eliminates pathogens or necrotic (dead) tissues and establishes a means of repairing body cells and tissues. Signs of inflammation frequently include edema (swelling), rubor (redness), heat, pain or tenderness, and loss of function in the affected body part. When inflammation becomes systemic, other signs and symptoms develop, including fever, leukocytosis (increased white blood cell count), malaise (generalized discomfort), anorexia, nausea, vomiting, and lymph node enlargement.

The inflammatory response is triggered by physical agents, chemical agents, or microorganisms. Mechanical trauma, temperature extremes, and radiation are examples of physical agents. Chemical agents include external and internal irritants, such as harsh poisons or gastric acid. Microorganisms trigger this response as well, as previously discussed. The inflammatory response sometimes occurs in the absence of an infectious process.

HEALTH CARE–ASSOCIATED INFECTIONS

Approximately 1 in every 25 patients admitted to the hospital has development of a **health care–associated infection** (HAI) (CDC, 2018a). These infections previously were referred to as nosocomial infections and include infections patients get when undergoing medical treatment in a health care facility. Much attention has been given to the prevention of HAIs, including monitoring and surveillance by the CDC (2018b) and The Joint Commission's National Patient Safety Goal standards (TJC, 2017). Nurses will be involved in monitoring and preventing HAIs, such as central line–associated bloodstream infections (CLABSIs), catheter-associated urinary tract infections (CAUTIs), surgical site infections (SSIs), and ventilator-associated pneumonia (VAP) (CDC, 2018b). These infections pose a far-reaching and serious problem. Hospitals harbor microorganisms that are often highly **virulent** (exceedingly pathogenic), which makes them more likely places for infection. The hospitalized patient's immune system is probably already weakened from disease or invasive procedures, which makes the patient more susceptible to pathogens. HAIs not only necessitate longer hospital (or any health care facility) stays for the patient and increase costs for the patient and the hospital but also can result in disability and death.

An **exogenous** (growing outside the body) infection is caused by microorganisms from another person (e.g., an infection transmitted to the patient by a health care worker). An **endogenous** (growing within the body) infection is caused by the patient's own normal microorganisms, which become altered and overgrow or are transferred from one body site to another (e.g., microorganisms in fecal material are transferred to skin by hands and infect a wound).

HAIs are most commonly transmitted via direct contact between health care workers and patients or from patient to patient. For this reason, a strong emphasis must be placed on the prevention of transmission with measures such as hand hygiene and environmental cleaning.

The nurse is responsible for providing the patient with a clean and safe environment. The nurse must be conscientious and thorough while performing clean and aseptic procedures to reduce the transmission of infection. To decrease the occurrence or duration of HAIs, many facilities have an infection prevention and control department, which investigates and establishes policies to ensure that all personnel maintain aseptic techniques while performing a procedure on a patient. These procedures include clean technique, which is used in all areas, and sterile technique, which is used in invasive procedures.

HAIs significantly increase health care costs. Extended lengths of stay in health care facilities increase disability, and prolonged recovery times add to the expenses the patient has to bear, and to those of the health care facility and any funding bodies (e.g., health insurance companies, Medicare, and Medicaid). The Centers for Medicare and Medicaid Services (CMMS) require hospitals to collect and report data regarding the incidence of HAIs to receive funding. This position encourages facilities to focus on activities that prevent HAIs to avoid financial penalties.

INFECTION PREVENTION AND CONTROL TEAM

Infection prevention and control is a valuable discipline in the health care arena. The Occupational Safety and Health Administration (OSHA), hospital accrediting agencies, and hospital administration place a strong emphasis on infection prevention and control. Administratively, infection control nurses and other members of the infection prevention and control team function within the hospital via the infection prevention and control committee.

INFECTION CONTROL NURSE

Many facilities employ nurses or other professionals who are specially trained in infection prevention and control. They are responsible for advising hospital personnel on the development and implementation of safe patient care delivery practices and for monitoring infection within the health care agency. Duties of an infection control nurse are as follows:

- Assessing microorganism sensitivity to antibiotics presently in use and communicating with medical staff regarding current sensitivity and resistance patterns.
- Compiling data and analyzing the results regarding the epidemiology of health care–associated (or health care–acquired) infections.
- Conferring with various hospital departments and other resources to investigate unusual events or clusters of infection.
- Consulting with occupational health departments concerning recommendations to prevent and control the spread of infection among health care personnel, such as testing for tuberculosis.
- Educating patients and families in the prevention and control of infection.
- Identifying infection control problems associated with medical or patient equipment.
- Notifying the local public health department of incidences of specific reportable communicable diseases.
- Providing staff education on infection prevention and control.
- Reviewing and revising infection prevention and control policies and procedures to ensure they are in compliance with local, state, and federal regulations and with hospital accrediting agencies.
- Reviewing patient medical records and laboratory reports and recommending appropriate transmission-based isolation procedures.
- Screening patient records for community-acquired infections (those that are acquired outside of the health care setting). These infections often are distinguished from HAIs by the type of organisms that affect patients who are recovering from a disease or injury.

An infection control nurse is a valuable resource in the prevention and control of HAIs.

OCCUPATIONAL HEALTH SERVICE

The occupational health service plays an important role in the prevention or the control of an infection in a health care setting by taking measures to protect the health care worker and patients from certain infections. Federal law requires that health care employers make available the hepatitis B vaccine and vaccination series to all employees who have the risk for occupational exposure.

When any needlestick occurs, the health care worker must report it immediately. Hepatitis B, or serum hepatitis, is the most commonly transmitted infection from contaminated needles. Health care agencies require workers who have had a needlestick to complete an injury report and seek appropriate treatment (Box 7.4).

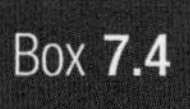

Box 7.4 Vaccination and Follow-Up Care for Health Care Workers

HEPATITIS B

1. Federal law requires that health care employers make available at no cost the hepatitis B vaccine and vaccination series to all employees who have occupational exposure. If an employee declines the vaccine, the employee is required to sign a declination form. Evaluation and follow-up care are available to all employees who have been exposed.
2. A blood test (titer) is offered in some facilities 1 to 2 months after completion of the three-dose vaccine series (check the health care facility or agency policy).
3. After exposure, no treatment is needed if a positive blood titer is on file. If no positive titer is on file, it is mandatory to follow the CDC guidelines.

HEPATITIS C

1. The employee is offered a baseline blood test to test for the presence of the disease within 48 hours.
2. Additional testing is conducted to monitor for the disease approximately 3 weeks after exposure (check the health care facility or agency policy). If the source patient is identified and tests positive for hepatitis C (HCV), the employee may receive a baseline test (CDC, 2017).
3. If results are positive, the employee is started on treatment. (No prophylactic treatment exists for HCV after exposure.)
4. Early treatment for infection has the potential to prevent chronic infections.

HUMAN IMMUNODEFICIENCY VIRUS

1. If the patient tests positive for HIV infection, a viral load study is performed to determine the amount of virus present in the blood.
2. If the exposure meets the CDC criteria for HIV prophylactic treatment, or postexposure prophylaxis (PEP), it optimally is started as soon as possible to establish a baseline, preferably within hours rather than days after exposure. Follow-up postexposure testing should occur at 6 weeks, 12 weeks, and 6 months. All medical evaluations and procedures, including the vaccine and vaccination series and evaluation after exposure (prophylaxis), are made available at no cost to at-risk employees. A confidential written medical evaluation is available to employees who have experienced exposure incidents.

From Centers for Disease Control and Prevention (CDC): Updated US Public Health Service Guidelines for the management of occupation exposures to HIV and recommendations for postexposure prophylaxis, 2005. Retrieved from *www.cdc.gov/mmwr/preview/mmwrhtml/rr5409a1.htm;* Occupational Safety and Health Administration, Occupational Safety and Health Act of 2001. Retrieved from *https://www.osha.gov/OshDoc/data_BloodborneFacts/bbfact04.pdf.*

Many facilities mandate that all workers and students obtain titers as proof of immunity against varicella, measles, mumps, and rubella. Titers are laboratory tests that measure the amount of an antibody in the bloodstream. If the amount of the antibody is not high enough, the health care agency often requires personnel to receive a vaccination or be revaccinated to prevent the disease.

STANDARD PRECAUTIONS

With the understanding that exposure to bloodborne pathogens (e.g., hepatitis B virus, HIV) can produce illness and infection came the realization that specific precautions can be used to help prevent infections.

The **Centers for Disease Control and Prevention (CDC)**, part of the US Department of Health and Human Services, provides facilities and services for investigation, prevention, and control of disease. The CDC has conducted studies on health care workers with documented skin or mucous membrane exposure to blood or body fluids of infected patients (Siegel et al, 2007). The studies show that infection is much more likely to occur when health care workers do not use appropriate protective measures.

Accurate identification of all patients infected with bloodborne pathogens is difficult. In the past, the CDC recommended that health care workers use "universal blood and body fluid precautions," or "universal precautions," and body substance isolation when caring for all patients. These two sets of precautions have now been incorporated into one standard set of guidelines, called **standard precautions** (Box 7.5).

The increased incidence of tuberculosis (TB) has led to a heightened stress, along with these precautions, on wearing the particulate respirator mask (Fig. 7.6) to protect against airborne pathogens.

The CDC guidelines for transmission-based precautions in hospitals, revised in 2007, have been adopted by many health care facilities (Siegel et al, 2007). The goal of these guidelines is to interrupt the chain of infection and reduce transmission of bloodborne pathogens and other potentially infectious materials. The guidelines apply to (1) blood; (2) all body fluids, secretions, and excretions except sweat, regardless of whether they contain visible blood; (3) nonintact skin; and (4) mucous membranes. Standard precautions are designed to reduce the risk of transmission of microorganisms from recognized and unrecognized sources of infections.

These precautions promote hand hygiene and use of gloves, masks, eye protection, and gowns when appropriate for patient contact.

HAND HYGIENE

Hand hygiene is the single most important and basic preventive technique that health care workers can use to interrupt the infectious process. Box 7.6 indicates when initiation of hand hygiene is essential.

Performing hand hygiene (Skill 7.1) provides the necessary protection before the nurse cares for a patient. For effective cleansing of hands soiled with dirt or organic matter, or if the nurse has handled a contaminated item, soap or detergents that contain antiseptic and water are required. The standard is to wash for at least 20 seconds with facility-approved soap, running hands under water (CDC, 2015a; Mayo Clinic, 2018).

Box 7.5 Standard Precautions

HAND HYGIENE

- Hand hygiene is considered of utmost importance when practicing standard precautions. Hands are to be washed before patient care and after touching blood, body fluids, secretions, excretions, and contaminated items, regardless of whether gloves are worn. Perform hand hygiene immediately after gloves are removed, between patient contacts, and when otherwise indicated to prevent transfer of microorganisms to other patients or environments. Washing hands may be necessary between tasks and procedures on the same patient to prevent cross-contamination of different body sites.
- Use approved soaps and alcohol-based hand sanitizers and lotions.

GLOVES

- Wear clean gloves when the potential for touching blood, body fluids, secretions, excretions, and contaminated items exists. Put on clean gloves just before touching mucous membranes and nonintact skin. Change gloves between tasks and procedures on the same patient after contact with material that possibly contains a high concentration of microorganisms. Remove gloves promptly after use, before touching noncontaminated items and environmental surfaces. Perform hand hygiene immediately after removing gloves to prevent transfer of microorganisms to other patients or environment.

MASK, EYE PROTECTION, FACE SHIELD

- Wear a mask and eye protection or a face shield to protect mucous membranes of the eyes, the nose, and the mouth during procedures and patient care activities that are likely to generate splashes or sprays of blood, body fluids, secretions, and excretions.

GOWN

- Wear a fluid-resistant gown (a clean, unsterile gown is adequate) to protect skin and prevent soiling of clothing during procedures and patient care activities that are likely to generate splashes or sprays of blood, body fluids, secretions, or excretions or cause soiling of clothing. Select a gown that is appropriate for the activity and amount of fluid likely to be encountered. Remove the soiled gown as promptly as possible and perform hand hygiene to prevent transfer of microorganisms to other patients or environments.

MISCELLANEOUS GUIDELINES

- Place used sharps, such as needles or scalpels, in a designated sharps disposal container.
- Do not purposefully bend, break, or recap needles.
- Place disposable wastes and articles contaminated with blood or large amounts of body fluids in a biowaste container for a trash pickup.
- Clean up spills of blood or body fluids per facility protocol (i.e., blood spill kit).
- Place all soiled linen in a laundry bag. Do not overfill the bag, to prevent contamination of the environment.
- For patients with diarrhea, strongly recommend soap and water for hand hygiene in place of alcohol-based hand cleansers because the spores of *Clostridium difficile* are not killed by alcohol (CDC, 2007).
- For patients who are coughing, wear a face mask if within 3 feet of patient and teach patient about respiratory hygiene.
- Use mouthpieces, resuscitator bags, or other ventilation devices if resuscitation is needed.
- Health care workers: If you have exudative (draining) lesions, refrain from all direct patient care and from handling patient care equipment until wound is healed.
- Handle laboratory specimens from all patients as if they are infectious (refer to agency manual).
- Use private rooms for patients with communicable diseases subject to airborne transmission or patients who soil their environment uncontrollably with body substances. For certain diseases (e.g., meningococcal meningitis), personnel and family entering the patient's room are to wear masks. This is true for the first 24 hours until antibiotics have been started, then is no longer required per the CDC. Roommates who are immune to the patient's disease or who currently are infected with the same disease are permitted to share rooms (institutional policy may vary on this specific procedure).

From Siegel JD, Rhinehart E, Jackson M, et al: Guideline for isolation precautions: Preventing transmission of infectious agents in healthcare settings, 2007. Retrieved from *www.cdc.gov/ncidod/dhqp/pdf/isolation2007.pdf;* Centers for Disease Control and Prevention: Healthcare-associated infections: Frequently asked questions about *Clostridium difficile* for healthcare providers, 2012. Retrieved from *http://www.cdc.gov/HAI/organisms/cdiff/Cdiff_faqs_HCP.html.*

Box 7.7 contains an overview of the CDC hand hygiene guidelines, and Box 7.8 addresses the use of alcohol-based waterless antiseptics for hand hygiene. All forms of HAIs can result from improper hand hygiene and use of contaminated equipment.

Increased use of artificial fingernails and nail polish has prompted several research studies. A variety of regulatory agencies, including the CDC, The Joint Commission, and the Association of Perioperative Registered Nurses (AORN), have adopted position statements concerning their use. Only natural nails should be worn in the health care setting; these should be no longer than ¼ inch. The use of artificial and acrylic nails should be avoided because of their potential status as carriers of harmful microorganisms.

In addition to hand hygiene, other actions can be taken to reduce the chance of transmitting microorganisms. Teach patients and visitors about appropriate times for hand hygiene (see the Patient Teaching box on infection prevention and control). Provide patients with their own set of personal care articles, such as a bedpan, urinal, bath basin, water pitcher, and drinking glass, to prevent cross-contamination. Because microorganisms are also transmitted by indirect contact with contaminated equipment and soiled linen, place these articles in special waste containers or laundry bags. Keep

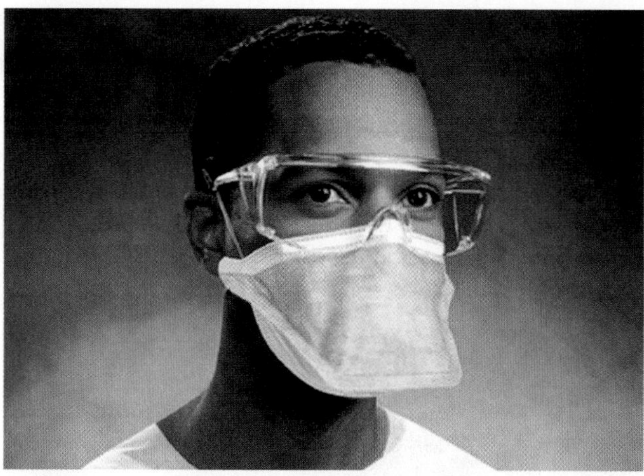

Fig. 7.6 Nurse wearing particulate respirator mask. (From Ignatavicius DD, Workman ML: *Medical-surgical nursing across the health care continuum*, ed 8, Philadelphia, 2013, Saunders.)

Box 7.6 Essential Hand Hygiene

Hand hygiene is essential:

- After contact with organic material, such as feces, wound drainage, and mucus.
- After removing disposable gloves or handling contaminated equipment.
- At the beginning and end of the shift.
- Before and after caring for a patient.
- Before and after eating.
- Before and after using the toilet.
- Before changing a dressing or having contact with open wounds.
- Before preparing and administering medications.
- In preparation for an invasive procedure, such as suctioning, catheterization, or injections.
- When hands are visibly soiled.

Skill 7.1 Performing Hand Hygiene With Soap and Water

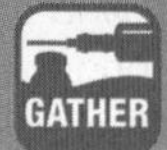

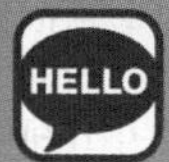

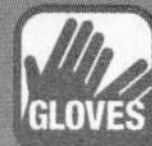

NURSING ACTION *(RATIONALE)*

1. Inspect hands, observing for visible soiling, breaks, or cuts in the skin and cuticles. *(Poor personal hygiene and an open area of the skin provide areas in which microorganisms are able to grow.)*
2. Determine amount of contaminant on hands. *(Determines the type of hand hygiene needed.)*
3. Assess areas around the skin that are contaminated. *(Prevents contamination of hands during and after hand hygiene procedure.)*
4. Adjust the water to appropriate temperature and force. *(Water that is too hot can chap skin, and too much force causes splashing and may spread microorganisms to other areas, especially your clothing.)*
5. Wet hands and wrists under the running water, always keeping hands lower than elbows. *(Hands are the most contaminated part of the upper extremities; water should flow from the wrists [least contaminated area] over the hands, and then down the drain.)*
6. Lather hands with liquid soap (about 1 teaspoon). *(Soap lather emulsifies fat and aids in cleansing.)*
7. Wash hands thoroughly with a firm, circular motion and friction on back of hands, palms, and wrists. Wash each finger individually, paying special attention to areas between fingers and knuckles by interlacing fingers and thumbs and moving hands back and forth, causing friction. *(Helps to loosen soil and microorganisms, both resident [normally present] and transient [acquired from contamination].)*

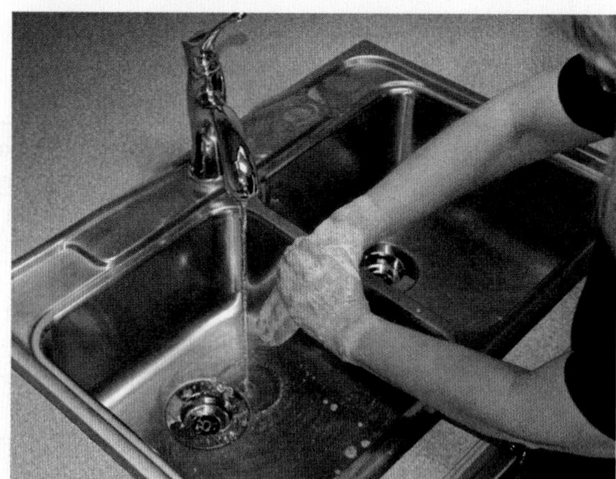

8. Wash for at least 20 seconds (CDC, 2015a). *(The greater the contamination, the more need for longer washing.)*
9. Rinse wrists and hands completely, again keeping hands lower than elbows. *(Water should run from cleaner area [the wrists] over the hands, and then down the drain, rinsing the dirt and microorganisms away.)*

Continued

Skill 7.1 Performing Hand Hygiene With Soap and Water—cont'd

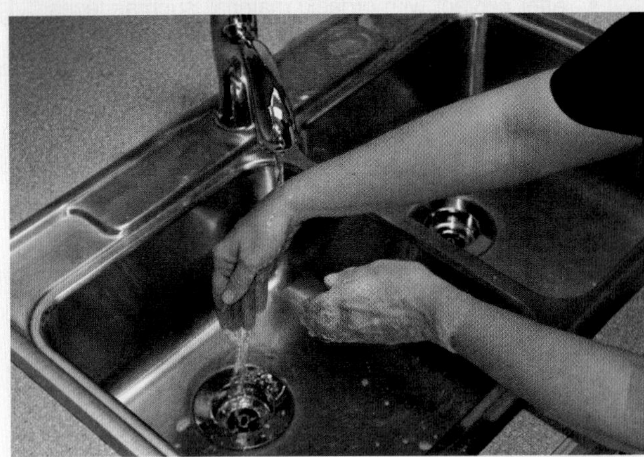

10. Dry hands thoroughly with paper towels. Start by patting at fingertips, then hands, and then wrists and forearms. *(Prevents chapping. Drying should progress from clean to less clean, and the cleanest areas are now your fingers and hands.)*
11. If it is necessary to turn off faucets manually, use a dry paper towel. *(Keeps clean hands from touching contaminated handles.)*
12. Use hospital-approved hand lotion if desired. *(Keeps skin soft and lubricated so it does not crack easily.)*
13. Inspect hands and nails for cleanliness. *(Ensures cleanliness of hands and nails.)*
14. If hands are not visibly soiled, use an alcohol-based waterless antiseptic for routine decontamination of hands in all clinical situations, unless you are caring for a patient with *Clostridium difficile* or *Candida* infection. These spores are unaffected by alcohol, so soap and water must be used in these instances (see Box 7.8).

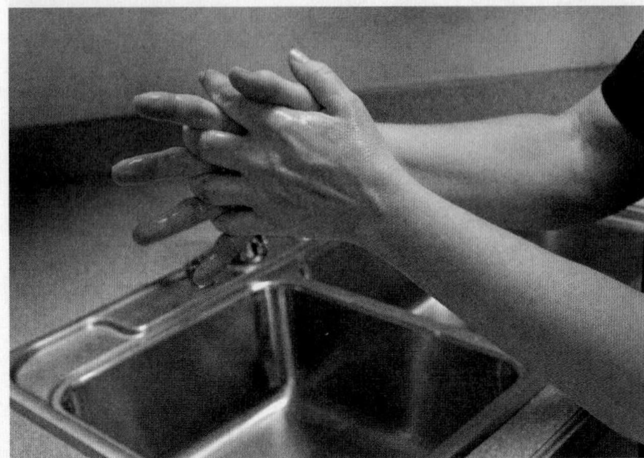

15. Provide patient teaching (see the Patient Teaching box on infection prevention and control).
16. Explain to the patient the importance of hand hygiene. *(Helps the patient understand that hand hygiene slows down the spread of infection.)*
17. If contamination occurs, it is necessary to reassess technique.

From Centers for Disease Control and Prevention (CDC): Handwashing: clean hands save lives: Show me the science–how to wash your hands, 2015. Retrieved from *https://www.cdc.gov/handwashing/show-me-the-science-handwashing.html.*

Box 7.7 Overview of CDC Hand Hygiene Guidelines

The Centers for Disease Control and Prevention (CDC) makes recommendations for hand hygiene in health care settings. Hand hygiene is a term that applies to hand washing, use of an antiseptic hand sanitizer, and surgical hand antisepsis. Evidence suggests that hand antisepsis, the cleansing of hands with an antiseptic hand sanitizer, is more effective in reducing HAIs than is plain hand washing.

FOLLOW THESE GUIDELINES IN THE CARE OF ALL PATIENTS

- Continue practice of washing hands with either facility-approved soap or antimicrobial soap and water whenever hands are visibly soiled.
- Use an alcohol-based hand sanitizer to routinely decontaminate the hands in the following clinical situations: (NOTE: If alcohol-based hand sanitizers are not available, the only alternative is hand washing; see Skill 7.1, step 14.)
  - Before and after patient contact.
  - Before donning sterile gloves when inserting central intravascular catheters.
  - Before performing nonsurgical invasive procedures (e.g., urinary catheter insertion, nasotracheal suctioning).
  - After contact with body fluids or excretions, mucous membranes, nonintact skin, and wound dressings.
  - If moving from a contaminated body site (rectal area or mouth) to a clean body site (surgical wound, urinary meatus) during patient care.
  - After contact with inanimate objects (including medical equipment) in the immediate vicinity of the patient.
  - After removing gloves.
  - Before eating and after using a restroom, wash hands with facility-approved soap and water.
- Antimicrobial-impregnated wipes (i.e., towelettes) are not a substitute for using an alcohol-based hand sanitizer or antimicrobial soap.
- If exposure to *Bacillus anthracis* is suspected or proven, wash hands with facility-approved soap and water. The physical action of washing and rinsing hands is

Box 7.7 Overview of CDC Hand Hygiene Guidelines—cont'd

recommended because alcohols, chlorhexidine, iodophors, and other antiseptic agents have poor activity against spores.

FOLLOW THESE GUIDELINES FOR SURGICAL HAND ANTISEPSIS
(See Skill 7.6)

- Surgical hand antisepsis reduces the resident microbial count on the hands to a minimum.
- The CDC recommends using an antimicrobial soap to scrub hands and forearms for the length of time recommended by the manufacturer. Refer to agency policy for time required.
- When using an alcohol-based surgical hand-scrub product with persistent activity, follow the manufacturer's instructions. Before applying the alcohol solution, prewash hands and forearms with a non-antimicrobial soap and dry hands and forearms completely. After application of the alcohol-based product as recommended, allow hands and forearms to dry thoroughly before donning sterile gloves.

GENERAL RECOMMENDATIONS FOR HAND HYGIENE

- Use facility-approved hand lotions or creams to minimize the occurrence of irritant contact dermatitis associated with hand antisepsis or hand washing.
- Do not wear artificial fingernails or nail polish when having direct contact with patients at high risk (e.g., those in intensive care units or operating rooms).
- Keep natural nail tips less than ¼ inch long.
- Wear gloves when contact with blood or other potentially infectious materials, mucous membranes, and nonintact skin could occur.
- Remove gloves after caring for a patient. Do not wear the same pair of gloves for the care of more than one patient, and do not wash gloves between uses with different patients.
- Change gloves during patient care if moving from a contaminated body site to a clean body site.

HAIs, Health care–associated infections.
Modified from Boyce JM, Pittet D; Healthcare Infection Control Practices Advisory Committee; Society for Healthcare Epidemiology of America; Association for Professionals in Infection Control Infectious Diseases Society of America Hand Hygiene Task Force: Guideline for hand hygiene in health-care settings: Recommendations of the Healthcare Infection Control Practices Advisory Committee and the HICPAC/SHEA/APIC/IDSA Hand Hygiene Task Force. *Infection Control and Hospital Epidemiology,* 23(12 Suppl):S3–S40, 2002.

Box 7.8 Using an Alcohol-Based Waterless Antiseptic for Routine Hand Hygiene

The Centers for Disease Control and Prevention (CDC) recommends the use of alcohol-based waterless antiseptics to improve hand hygiene practices, protect health care workers' hands, and reduce transmission of pathogens to patients and personnel in health care settings. Alcohols have excellent germicidal activity and are more effective than either plain soap or antimicrobial soap and water. Emollients are added to alcohol-based antiseptics to prevent drying of the skin.

If hands are not visibly soiled, use an alcohol-based waterless antiseptic for routine decontamination of hands in most clinical situations.

1. Apply an ample amount of product to palm of one hand. *(Enough product is needed to thoroughly cover the hands.)*
2. Rub hands together, covering all surfaces of hands and fingers with antiseptic.
3. Rub hands together for several seconds until alcohol is dry. Allow hands to dry before applying gloves. If an adequate volume is used, 15 to 25 seconds are needed for hands to dry. *(Drying ensures full antiseptic effect.)*
4. If hands are dry or chapped, a small amount of facility-approved lotion or barrier cream can be applied. *(Use the hospital-provided container of lotion because other lotions possibly interfere with antimicrobial action or disintegrate gloves.)*

NOTE: Alcohol-based waterless antiseptics are not recommended if caring for a patient with *Clostridium difficile* (C. diff) diarrhea or *Candida* species infections. The spores are unaffected by the alcohol in the hand sanitizer.

NOTE: Because of the risk of alcohol poising with ingestion of large amounts, alcohol-based waterless antiseptics should be kept out of reach of children who may swallow them.

Data from Boyce JM, Pittet D; Healthcare Infection Control Practices Advisory Committee; Society for Healthcare Epidemiology of America; Association for Professionals in Infection Control Infectious Diseases Society of America Hand Hygiene Task Force: Guideline for hand hygiene in health-care settings: Recommendations of the Healthcare Infection Control Practices Advisory Committee and the HICPAC/SHEA/APIC/IDSA Hand Hygiene Task Force. *Infection Control and Hospital Epidemiology,* 23(12 Suppl):S3–S40, 2002.

these items should be kept away from your uniform. The risk of transmitting HAIs or infectious diseases among patients is high when standard precautions are not followed. Health care workers need to stay informed about patients who have a known source of infection and communicate the information with other health care workers as appropriate. By following recommendations for infection prevention and control practices, health care workers experience more protection from exposure and reduce the patient's risk for acquiring an HAI.

GLOVING

Nurses and other health care personnel should don gloves if any possibility exists of contact with infectious material with their hands. The CDC (Boyce, Pittet et al, 2002) gives the following advice regarding gloves:

- Wear gloves only once, and then place them into the appropriate waste containers for safe disposal.
- If you have not completed the patient's care but have come into contact with infectious material, change the gloves before continuing the patient's care.

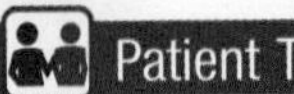

Patient Teaching

Infection Prevention and Control

- Teach the patient about the infection process, especially how an infection is transmitted, and stress the importance of interrupting the process. Use a simple diagram to illustrate this (see Fig. 7.1). Teaching caregivers is extremely important as well.
- Use an example for each step that is familiar to the patient.
- Provide a simple explanation of clean and contaminated items.
- Although hand hygiene is a basic hygiene technique, emphasize when and how the procedure should be performed to be effective in preventing infection. Demonstrate hand hygiene within sight of the patient whenever possible.
- Instruct the patient about the signs and symptoms of infection.
- Teach the applications of aseptic principles to self-care activities, such as wound care and medication administration.
- When isolation apparel (such as mask, gown, or gloves) is to be used, demonstrate the procedures for the patient and visitors.
- Instruct the patient to place contaminated dressings and other disposable items that contain infectious body fluids in a leak-resistant bag. At home, needles should be placed in bleach bottles with the cap taped or glued on or placed in a sharps container and taken to a local hospital for disposal.

Always allow a question-and-answer session for the patient (some patients need special assistance in understanding the precautions).

- Because of the risk of perforating the gloves during use, perform hand hygiene after removing the gloves (Skill 7.2).

Family members need to understand the importance of the use of gloves. Explain that gloves become contaminated if they touch infected material or a contaminated object (see the Patient Teaching box on gloving technique).

Patient Teaching

Gloving Technique

- Ensure that the patient understands the rationale for the use of gloves.
- Some patients need special assistance in understanding the precautions.
- Demonstrate to the patient how to don gloves.

Latex Allergy

Latex allergy causes an individual to have a reaction to certain proteins found in natural rubber latex, a product manufactured from a milky fluid derived from the rubber tree found in Africa and Southeast Asia. The latex proteins can enter the body through the skin and mucous membranes, intravascularly, and by inhalation. Suspect the presence of a latex allergy and obtain an evaluation by a physician when anyone has development of red, watery, itchy eyes; sinus or nasal congestion; tachycardia; or hypotension after exposure to latex. Anaphylaxis is a potentially life-threatening condition that can develop when someone is exposed to latex and has a severe latex allergy.

Skill 7.2 Gloving

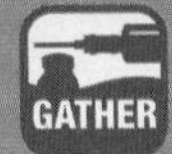

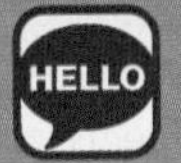

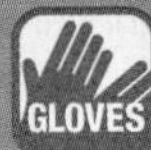

NURSING ACTION *(RATIONALE)*

Donning Gloves

1. Remove gloves from dispenser. *(Keeps gloves handy and ready for use.)*
2. Inspect gloves for perforations. *(Prevents pathogenic microorganisms from entering through perforation in gloves.)*
3. Don gloves when ready to begin patient care. Wearing gloves with a gown does not necessitate any special technique for putting them on; wear them pulled over cuffs of gown. *(Ensures full coverage of your wrists.)*
4. Change gloves after direct handling of infectious material such as wound drainage. *(Prevents cross-contamination.)*
5. Do not touch side rails, tables, or bed stands with contaminated gloves. *(Prevents spread of microorganisms throughout environment.)*

Removing Gloves

6. Remove first glove by grasping outer surface at palm with other gloved hand and pulling glove inside out and off. Place this glove in the hand that is still gloved. *(Prevents you from touching your own skin with contaminated glove.)*

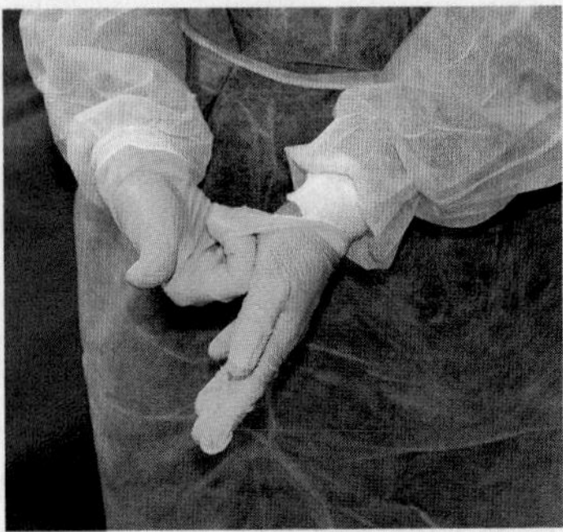

Skill 7.2 Gloving—cont'd

7. Remove second glove by placing finger under cuff and turning glove inside out and over other glove. Drop gloves into waste container. *(Prevents you from touching contaminated glove; wraps contamination inside gloves to help protect others.)*

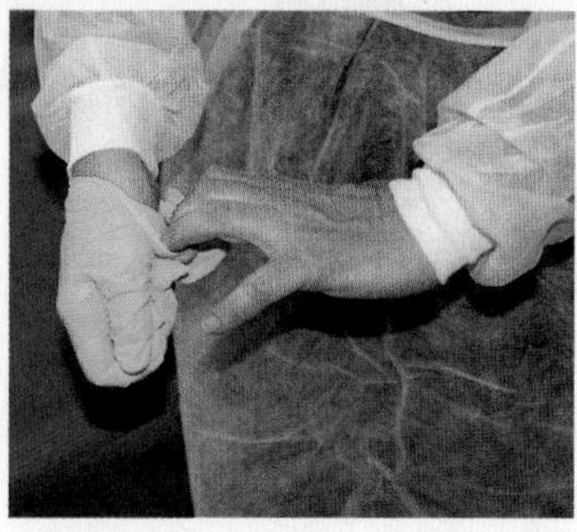

8. Perform hand hygiene. *(Helps prevent cross-contamination.)*
9. Provide patient teaching (see the Patient Teaching box on gloving technique).
10. If contamination occurs, it is necessary to reassess technique.

Box 7.9 Preventing Latex Allergy

The American Nurses Association (ANA) provides the following suggestions for nurses to avoid becoming allergic to latex:

1. Whenever possible, wear powder-free gloves (they are lower in protein allergens).
2. Wear gloves that are appropriate for the task (e.g., avoid use for cleaning).
3. Wash with a pH-balanced soap immediately after removing gloves.
4. Apply only non–oil-based hand care products (oil-based products break down latex).
5. If a reaction or dermatitis occurs, report to employee health or seek medical treatment immediately.

Some medical products contain latex. Synthetic versions of many products are available. Even though an individual product is "latex free," an environment is "latex safe" only when all items of latex that have the potential to come in contact with the allergic individual are removed (Box 7.9).

GOWNING

The nurse should don a gown when preparing to provide care for a patient in isolation to help protect the nurse's clothing from becoming soiled. The gown also provides protection against unknown infectious microorganisms. Recommendations are that the nurse discard the gown when leaving the patient's room rather than reuse it. This aids in preventing the spread of pathogens to other patients or personnel. This procedure also applies to visitors.

Another rationale for use of a gown is protection of a patient whose immune system is inadequate. In this situation, health care workers and visitors wear a gown to prevent the transfer of microorganisms from themselves to the patient.

There are several types of isolation. Some necessitate the wearing of a gown, whereas others do not. Donning of an isolation gown is indicated in the care of patients with diseases characterized by heavy drainage or exudate, infectious and acute diarrhea, other gastrointestinal disorders, respiratory disorders, skin wounds or burns, and urinary disorders.

Isolation gowns open at the back and have ties at the neck and the waist to keep the gown securely closed, protecting the back and the front of the nurse's uniform. The gown must be long enough to cover the uniform and, for added protection, have long sleeves with cuffs.

To don gowns correctly, follow the procedure listed in Skill 7.3.

MASK AND PROTECTIVE EYEWEAR

When a mask is applied correctly, it fits snugly below the health care worker's chin and securely over the nose and mouth; the top edge fits below eyeglasses, if worn (this prevents fogging of glasses). Masks are available with eye shields to cover the wearer's eyes (or glasses). Goggles are another way to protect eyes (see Fig. 7.6). Nurses should change their masks at least every 20 to 30 minutes and/or when they become moist. Nurses should not reuse their masks or allow them to dangle around their necks and then reuse them (Skill 7.4). Masks and protective eyewear guard members of the health care team in the following ways:

- They protect the wearer from inhaling microorganisms that travel on airborne droplets for short distances or that remain suspended in the air for longer periods and from splashing if it should occur. Masks also prevent the mucous membranes of the nose and mouth from coming into contact with contaminants.

Skill 7.3 Gowning for Isolation

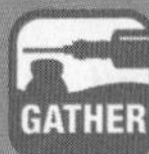

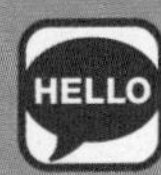

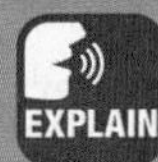

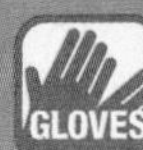

NURSING ACTION *(RATIONALE)*

1. Push up long sleeves, if you have them. *(Ensures that uniform sleeve is under gown sleeve for protection.)*
2. Perform hand hygiene. *(Reduces spread of microorganisms.)*
3. Don gown and tie it securely at neck and waist. *(Provides protective covering of the entire uniform.)*

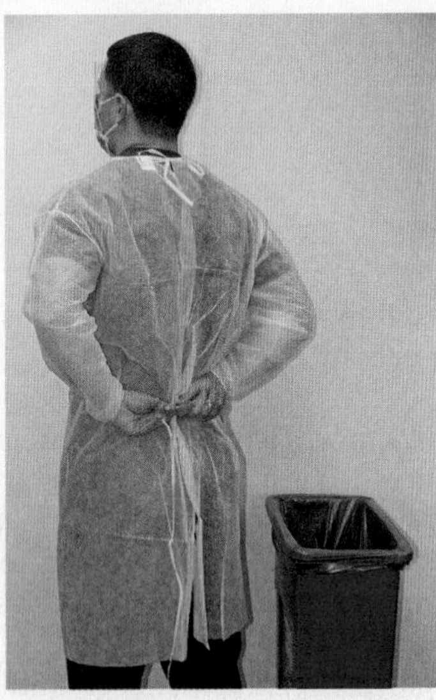

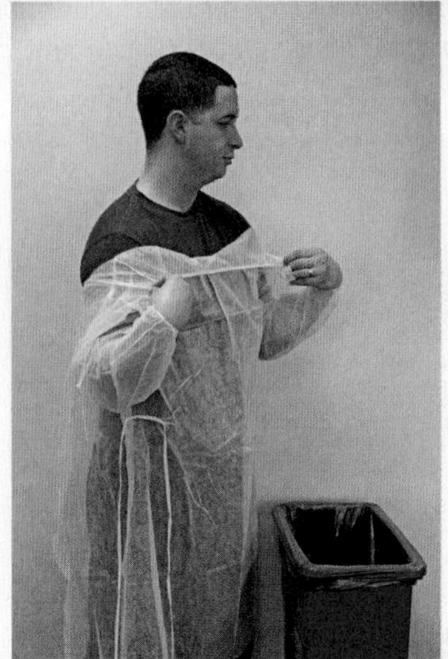

4. Remove gown after providing necessary patient care. *(Has protected the nurse.)*

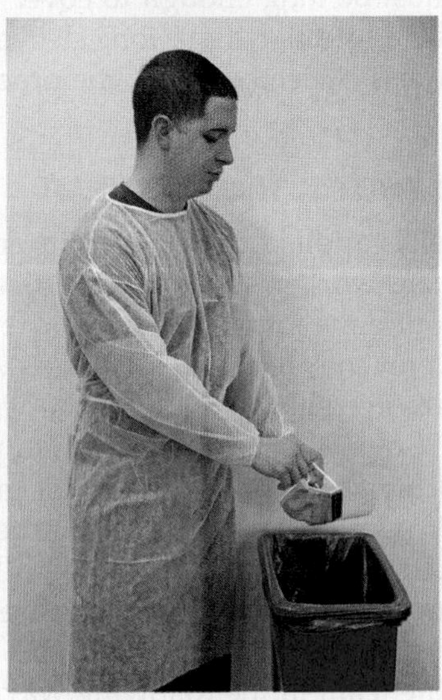

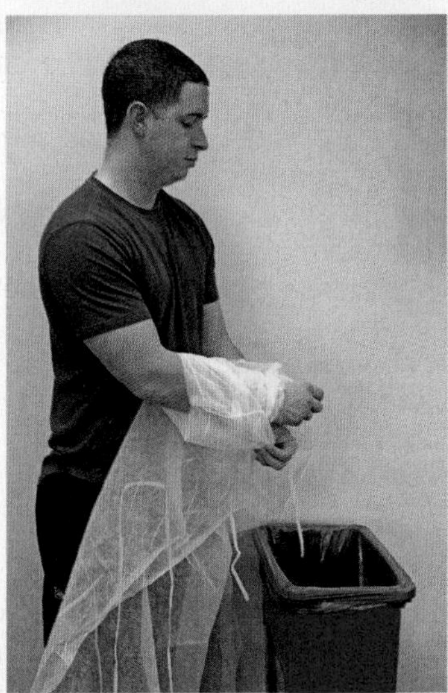

5. Discard soiled gown appropriately. *(Prevents contamination.)*

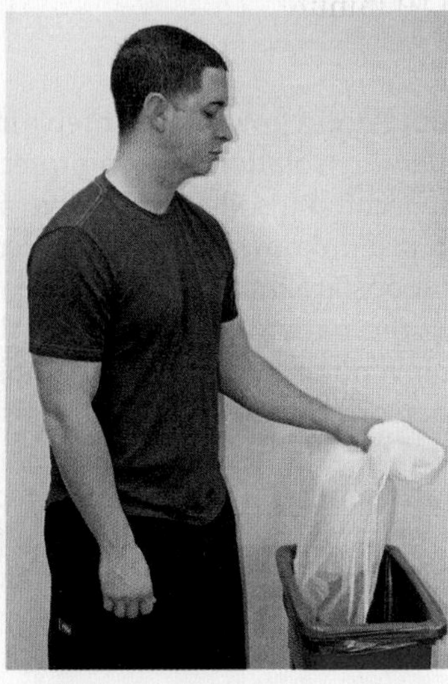

Skill 7.3 Gowning for Isolation—cont'd

6. Perform hand hygiene. *(Prevents spread of microorganisms.)*
7. Record use of gown in isolation procedure if required by the health care agency. *(Provides proof that appropriate procedure was followed.)* Some agencies charge a daily rate for isolation precautions. This is noted on a daily basis in the patient's record. Therefore repeated notations throughout the 24 hours are not necessary.
8. Provide patient teaching (see the Patient Teaching box on infection prevention and control).
9. If contamination occurs, it is necessary to reassess technique.

Skill 7.4 Donning a Mask

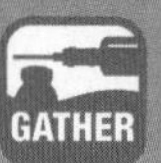

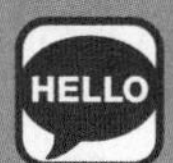

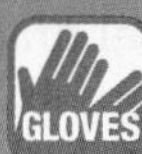

NURSING ACTION *(RATIONALE)*

The nurse should perform the following steps when donning a mask:

1. Remove mask from container. *(Mask is readily available for use.)*
2. Don mask when ready to begin patient care by covering your nose, mouth, and eyes (or glasses) with the device. Wear a mask with a protective eye shield when there is risk of splashing. Secure mask in place with elastic band or by tying the strings behind your head. *(Provides protection from microorganisms.)*

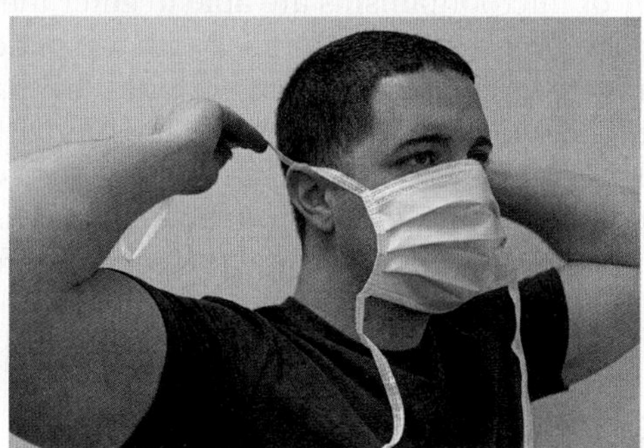

3. Wear mask until it becomes moist, but no longer than 20 to 30 minutes. *(Moisture renders a mask ineffective.)*
4. Remove mask by untying the strings or moving the elastic. Be certain not to touch contaminated area *(Prevents your contact with contaminated mask)*.

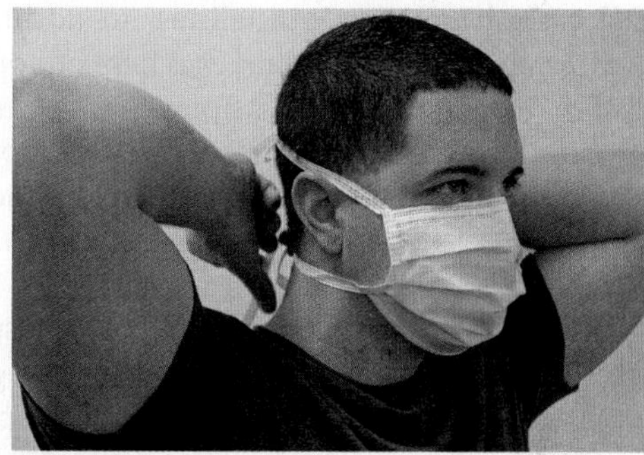

5. Dispose of soiled mask in appropriate container. *(Protects other health care workers.)*
6. Wash hands thoroughly. *(Removes microorganisms.)*
7. Record use of mask during patient care (some agencies require documentation of specific barriers used). *(Provides proof of wearing mask for protection of patient and nurse.)*
8. Provide patient teaching (see the Patient Teaching box on infection prevention and control).
9. If contamination occurs, it is necessary to reassess technique.

- They prevent the patient from inhaling pathogens if resistance is reduced or if a patient with an airborne respiratory infection is being transported to another care area.
- Eyewear shields protect the membranes and conjunctiva of the eye.

DISPOSING OF CONTAMINATED EQUIPMENT

Health care facilities generate immense quantities of contaminated materials, some of which are disposable and some of which are reusable. It is essential to design and implement an effective mechanism to handle this material within the facility. The process for the disposal of contaminated materials is reviewed by the infection control nurse and the infection prevention and control committee. Some facilities manage the waste onsite, and other facilities rely on waste haulers to remove the waste. A major risk to health care workers and facility personnel is in the improper disposal of sharps (needles, scalpels), which often are contaminated by blood or bodily fluid. When left in linens, these sharp items have the potential to injure workers cleaning patient care areas. For prevention of this problem, all patient care areas in which sharps are ever used must be provided with puncture-proof containers into which health care workers place used disposable sharp items.

HANDLING LINEN

The CDC recommends the following guidelines for handling linen:

- Place soiled linen in a laundry bag in the patient's room.
- Treat all linen as though it were infectious.

Note that double bagging (placing a plastic bag that contains contaminated linen into another clean plastic bag) is no longer recommended as a universal practice, unless a cloth bag is being placed in a plastic bag. In most cases, a single bag is adequate if it is possible to place the contaminated articles in the bag without contamination of the outside of the bag.

ISOLATION TECHNIQUE

The CDC issued isolation guidelines, in addition to standard precautions, that contain two tiers of approach (CDC, 2015b). The first tier contains precautions designed for health care workers to use when caring for all patients in health care facilities regardless of their diagnosis or presumed infectiousness. This first tier is called *standard precautions.*

The second tier condenses the disease-specific approach to isolation into transmission categories: airborne, droplet, and contact precautions. These precautions are designed to be used in the care of patients with a specific type of confirmed or suspected infection (Box 7.10 and Figs. 7.7 to 7.9).

The type of isolation techniques followed for a given patient depends on how transmissible the pathogen in question is. The nurse should follow some basic principles regardless of which technique is used:

- Perform thorough hand hygiene before and after caring for a patient.
- Have an adequate understanding of the disease process and the method of transmission of the infectious microorganism to help determine which protective barriers to use.
- Dispose of contaminated equipment and articles in a safe and effective manner to prevent transmission of pathogens to other individuals.
- If the patient is to be transported to other areas in the agency (away from the isolation room), take necessary measures to protect those who potentially will be exposed. The patient should be transported in accordance with hospital protocol.

Environmental barriers keep pathogens in a confined area. Examples of such barriers are placing a patient in a private or isolation room, closing the patient's door, and wearing personal protective equipment (e.g., gown, mask, goggles, gloves).

The patient with an infectious disease should be placed in a private or isolation room equipped with the appropriate hand hygiene and toilet facilities. Private rooms used for airborne illness isolation have negative-pressure airflow that prevents infectious particulates from flowing out of the closed environment. Special rooms with positive-pressure airflow also are used for patients with immunocompromised conditions, such as transplant recipients or patients who are receiving certain kinds of chemotherapy. In this case, a reduced number of microorganisms are able to enter the room. All articles that come into contact with the patient are contaminated, and these items should be handled appropriately to help reduce the transmission of microorganisms. Dedicated equipment for assessment of vital signs remains in the room if possible. Otherwise it is mandatory for the health care worker to disinfect the

Box 7.10 Types of Precautions and Patients Who Require Those Precautions

STANDARD PRECAUTIONS (TIER 1)

Use standard precautions for the care of all patients. This general mandate is necessary because whether the patient is colonized or infected with certain pathogenic microorganisms is sometimes not known. Barrier precautions reduce the need to handle sharps.

TRANSMISSION PRECAUTIONS (TIER 2)

Airborne Precautions (See Fig. 7.7)

In addition to standard precautions, use airborne precautions for patients known or suspected to have serious illnesses transmitted by airborne droplet nuclei. Examples of such illnesses include the following:

- Measles
- Varicella zoster virus (including disseminated zoster), responsible for chickenpox and shingles
- Tuberculosis
    - Airborne precautions should be practiced for all patients with known or suspected TB. (Suspected TB is defined by agency policy and generally means any patient with a positive acid-fast bacillus [AFB] smear, a cavitated lesion seen on a chest x-ray, or identification as high risk with a screening tool.)
    - Isolation is mandatory in a single-patient room designated as negative-pressure airflow and having at least 6 to 12 air exchanges per hour. It is necessary to vent room air to the outside and to ensure that the door is closed (before and after entering the room) to maintain negative pressure.
    - It is mandatory that health care workers wear an N-95 or higher particulate respirator mask or a

Box 7.10 Types of Precautions and Patients Who Require Those Precautions—cont'd

powered air purifying respirator (PAPR) when entering an AFB isolation room (check agency's policy for type of mask).
- It is mandatory for health care workers to undergo a fit-test before using a respirator for the first time. This ensures that the type and the size of the respirator are appropriate for the individual.
- It is mandatory for health care workers to fit-check the respirator's fit before each use.
- Respirators are permitted to be reused and stored according to manufacturer recommendations and agency policy.

- Fit-test: Procedure to determine adequate fit of respirator, usually with qualitative measure (wearers are exposed to a concentrated saccharin solution and asked if they can detect taste while wearing respirator).

DROPLET PRECAUTIONS (See Fig. 7.8)

In addition to standard precautions, use droplet precautions for patients known or suspected to have serious illness transmitted by large particle droplets. Examples of such illnesses include the following:

- Invasive *Haemophilus influenzae,* including meningitis, pneumonia, epiglottitis, and sepsis
- Invasive *Neisseria meningitidis* disease, including meningitis, pneumonia, and sepsis

Examples of other serious bacterial respiratory infections spread by droplet transmission include the following:

- Diphtheria (pharyngeal)
- Mycoplasma pneumonia
- Pertussis
- Pneumonic plague
- Streptococcal pharyngitis, pneumonia, and scarlet fever in infants and young children

Examples of serious viral infections spread by droplet transmission include the following:

- Adenovirus
- Influenza
- Mumps
- Parvovirus B19
- Rubella

CONTACT PRECAUTIONS (See Fig. 7.9)

In addition to standard precautions, use contact precautions for patients known or suspected to have serious illnesses easily transmitted by direct patient contact or by contact with items in the patient's environment. Examples of such illnesses include the following:

- Gastrointestinal, respiratory, skin, or wound infections or colonization with multidrug-resistant bacteria judged by the infection prevention and control committee, and current state, regional, and national recommendations, to be of special clinical and epidemiologic significance
- Enteric infections with a low infectious dose or prolonged environmental survival, including the following:
  a. *Clostridium difficile*
  b. Diapered or incontinent patients with the following:
     1. *Escherichia coli* O157:H7
     2. Shigella
     3. Hepatitis A
     4. Rotavirus
- Respiratory syncytial virus, parainfluenza virus, and enteroviral infections in infants and young children
- Skin infections that are highly contagious or that tend to occur on dry skin, including the following:
  a. Diphtheria (cutaneous)
  b. Herpes simplex virus (neonatal or mucocutaneous)
  c. Impetigo
  d. Major (noncontaminated) abscesses, cellulitis, or decubitus ulcers
  e. Pediculosis
  f. Scabies
  g. Staphylococcal furunculosis in infants and young children
  h. Methicillin-resistant *Staphylococcus aureus* (MRSA)
  i. Vancomycin-resistant enterococci (VRE)
  j. Extended-spectrum beta-lactamase (ESBL); this enzyme attaches to the cell wall of *E. coli* and some *Klebsiella* organisms, which in turn makes the organisms multidrug resistant
  k. Varicella zoster virus (disseminated or in the immunocompromised host)
  l. Viral or hemorrhagic conjunctivitis
  m. Viral hemorrhagic infections (Ebola, Lassa, Marburg)

PATIENTS WITH IMMUNOCOMPROMISED CONDITIONS

Patients with immunocompromised conditions vary in their susceptibility to health care–associated infections depending on the severity and the duration of immunosuppression. They are generally at increased risk for bacterial, fungal, parasitic, and viral infections from endogenous and exogenous sources. In general, the use of standard precautions for all patients and transmission-based isolation precautions for specified patients reduces the acquisition by these patients of institutionally acquired organisms from other patients and environments. Patients with leukopenia sometimes require protective measures in addition to standard precautions. In such instances, the physician or infection control nurse instructs nursing staff about the necessary protective measures (e.g., masks, private room). They place an isolation sign on the door, which lists the additional protective measures that staff and visitors are required to follow for the safety of the patient.

MONITORING OF ISOLATION

Transmission-based isolation practices are monitored on an ongoing basis by the infection control nurse.

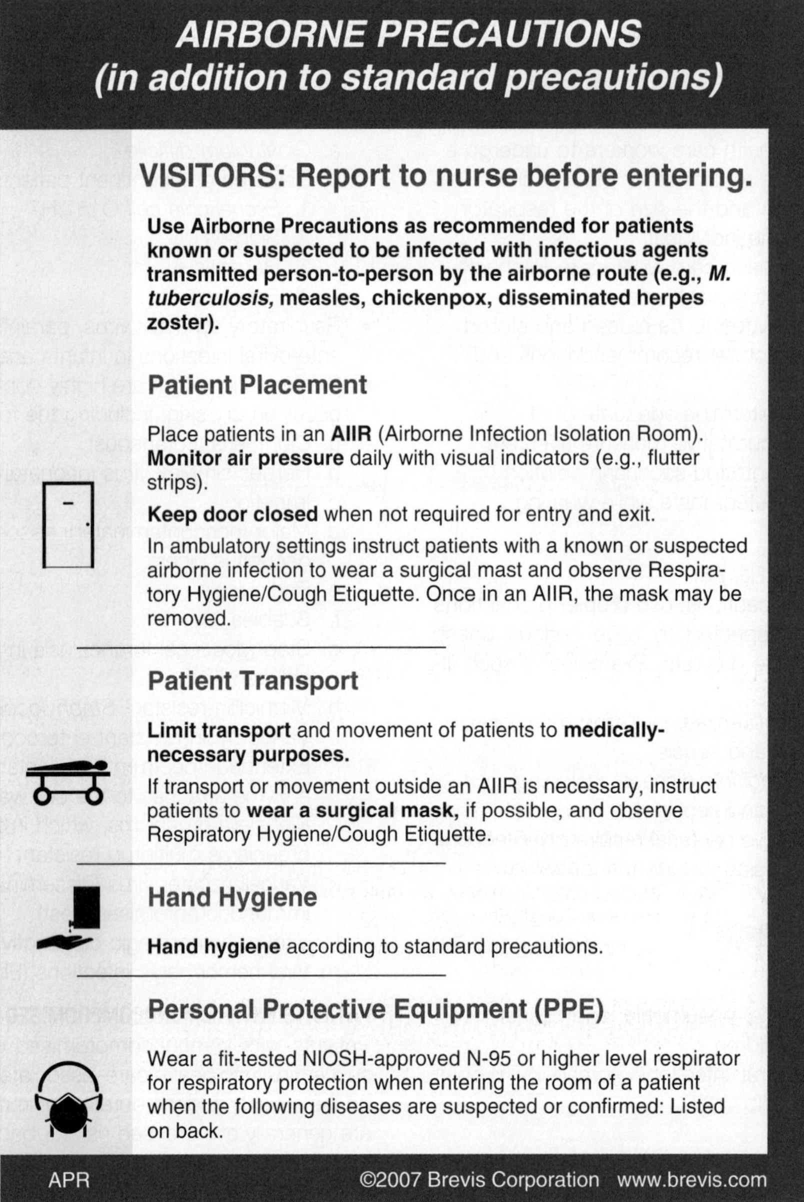

AIRBORNE PRECAUTIONS
(in addition to standard precautions)
VISITORS: Report to nurse before entering.
Use Airborne Precautions as recommended for patients known or suspected to be infected with infectious agents transmitted person-to-person by the airborne route (e.g., M. tuberculosis, measles, chickenpox, disseminated herpes zoster).
Patient Placement
Place patients in an AIIR (Airborne Infection Isolation Room). Monitor air pressure daily with visual indicators (e.g., flutter strips).
Keep door closed when not required for entry and exit.
In ambulatory settings instruct patients with a known or suspected airborne infection to wear a surgical mast and observe Respiratory Hygiene/Cough Etiquette. Once in an AIIR, the mask may be removed.
Patient Transport
Limit transport and movement of patients to medically-necessary purposes.
If transport or movement outside an AIIR is necessary, instruct patients to wear a surgical mask, if possible, and observe Respiratory Hygiene/Cough Etiquette.
Hand Hygiene
Hand hygiene according to standard precautions.
Personal Protective Equipment (PPE)
Wear a fit-tested NIOSH-approved N-95 or higher level respirator for respiratory protection when entering the room of a patient when the following diseases are suspected or confirmed: Listed on back.
APR
©2007 Brevis Corporation www.brevis.com

Fig. 7.7 Airborne precautions. (Copyright 1997–2007 Brevis Corporation. Courtesy Brevis Corporation, Salt Lake City, Utah.)

equipment when it must be removed from the room to use on another patient.

The psychological or emotional deprivation that may result with use of these transmission-based isolation precautions must be considered in the care of the patient. The patient is forced into solitude and deprived of normal social contacts. If possible, spend extra time with the patient to reduce feelings of isolation. Keep the room clean and pleasant. Provide instruction about the rationale for the precautions to the patient and family members. Teach the family and visitors how to apply and dispose of any personal protective equipment that they may need to wear and ensure that the procedure is followed (Skill 7.5).

PULMONARY TUBERCULOSIS PRECAUTIONS

Pulmonary tuberculosis (TB) infections continue to concern health care workers. Some strains of these bacteria are multidrug resistant, which makes treatment of the infection very difficult. The best way to prevent the transmission of pulmonary TB is to quickly identify, isolate, and treat patients with TB. The nurse should suspect a patient has pulmonary TB if the patient has respiratory symptoms that last longer than 2 weeks. Other suspicious symptoms include fatigue, unexplained weight loss, dyspnea, fever, night sweats, and hemoptysis (a cough that can be productive of blood). Good assessment skills hasten the possibility of a diagnosis,

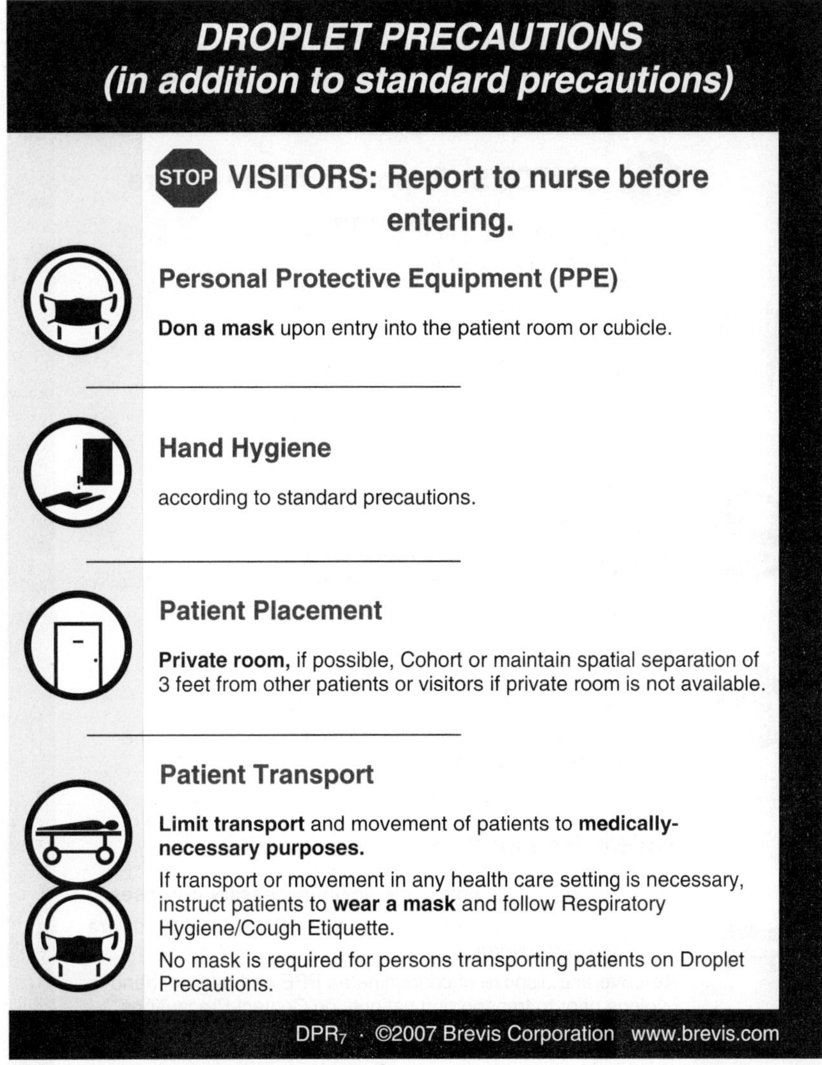

Fig. 7.8 Droplet precautions. (Copyright 1997–2007 Brevis Corporation. Courtesy Brevis Corporation, Salt Lake City, Utah.)

which is essential because the risk of exposure is greatest before a diagnosis is made and isolation precautions are implemented. Isolation for patients with known or suspected TB includes a negative-pressure isolation room (see Box 7.10). Such rooms have negative pressure in relation to surrounding areas in the facility so that room air is vented directly to the outside or through special high-efficiency particulate air (HEPA) filters, if recirculation is unavoidable. High-risk procedures on patients with suspected or confirmed infectious TB must be performed in negative-pressure rooms.

OSHA and CDC guidelines require health care workers who care for patients with known or suspected TB to wear an N-95 (or higher) respirator or mask (CDC, 2007). The respirators have the capacity to filter particles smaller than 5 μm with a filter efficiency of 95% or higher. The masks of health care employees who work with TB cases must undergo a fit-test to obtain a face-seal leakage of 10% or less. To ensure correct fit and efficiency, workers who experience a significant weight loss or weight gain should repeat the fitting process. Under National Institute for Occupational Safety and Health (NIOSH) criteria, the minimally acceptable level of respiratory protection for TB is the N-95 respirator (see Skill 7.5). Training in the wearing and storage of the respirator is required for hospital staff. OSHA also requires employers to provide training concerning transmission of TB, especially in areas where risk of exposure is high, such as areas where bronchoscopies are performed. Other requirements include annual TB skin testing for health care workers and appropriate follow-up when a previously negative skin test becomes positive.

Another option for health care workers who work around patients with known or suspected airborne infections such as TB is called a powered air purifying respirator (PAPR). A PAPR may be selected instead of an N-95 respirator if an N-95 respirator does not fit

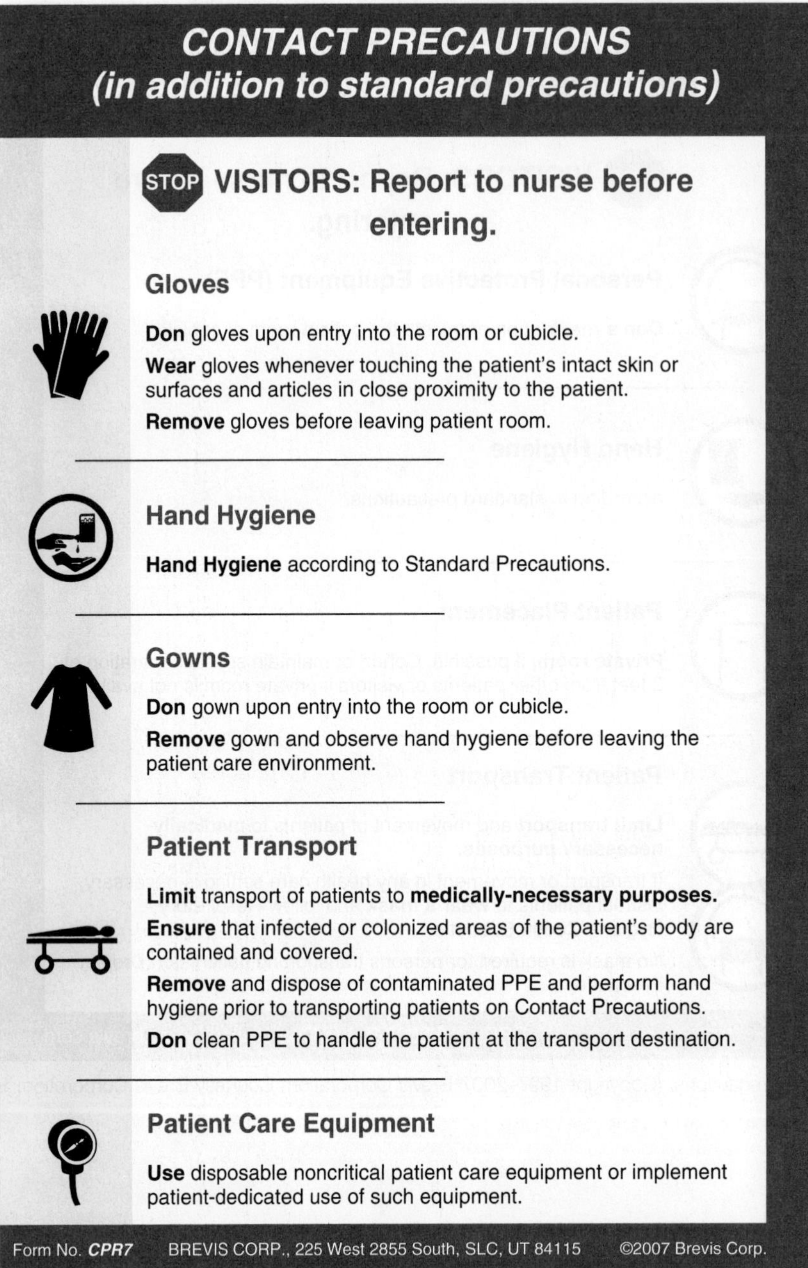

CONTACT PRECAUTIONS
(in addition to standard precautions)
STOP
VISITORS: Report to nurse before entering.
Gloves
Don gloves upon entry into the room or cubicle.
Wear gloves whenever touching the patient's intact skin or surfaces and articles in close proximity to the patient.
Remove gloves before leaving patient room.
Hand Hygiene
Hand Hygiene according to Standard Precautions.
Gowns
Don gown upon entry into the room or cubicle.
Remove gown and observe hand hygiene before leaving the patient care environment.
Patient Transport
Limit transport of patients to medically-necessary purposes.
Ensure that infected or colonized areas of the patient's body are contained and covered.
Remove and dispose of contaminated PPE and perform hand hygiene prior to transporting patients on Contact Precautions.
Don clean PPE to handle the patient at the transport destination.
Patient Care Equipment
Use disposable noncritical patient care equipment or implement patient-dedicated use of such equipment.
Form No. CPR7
BREVIS CORP., 225 West 2855 South, SLC, UT 84115
©2007 Brevis Corp.

Fig. 7.9 Contact precautions. (Copyright 1997–2007 Brevis Corporation. Courtesy Brevis Corporation, Salt Lake City, Utah.)

adequately. Facial hair and facial deformities may interfere with the face seal of an N-95. A PAPR also may be worn if an N-95 respirator is unavailable.

SURGICAL ASEPSIS

Surgical asepsis, or sterile technique, requires that the nurse use different precautions from those of medical asepsis. *Surgical asepsis* is the complete removal of all microorganisms, including spores, from an object. The slightest break in technique, when working with a sterile field or with sterile equipment, results in contamination. The nurse must practice surgical asepsis during the period of care to keep microorganisms away from the area.

Although surgical asepsis is practiced in the operating room, the labor and delivery area, and major diagnostic or procedure areas, the nurse also sometimes uses surgical aseptic techniques at the patient's bedside. This includes, for example, when the nurse inserts intravenous (IV) lines or urinary catheters, suctions the patient's lower airway, and applies sterile dressings. In an operating room, the nurse follows a series of steps to maintain sterile techniques, including donning a mask, protective eyewear, and a cap; performing surgical hand hygiene; and donning a sterile gown and gloves. In contrast,

Skill 7.5 Isolation Precautions

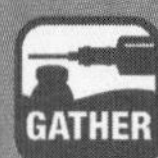

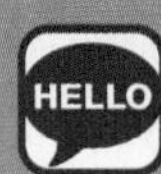

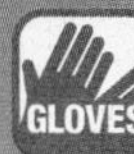

NURSING ACTION *(RATIONALE)*

1. Determine causative microorganism and patient's immune system status. *(Determines virulence of causative pathogen and how well the patient's immune system is working.)*
2. Recognize mode of transmission and how the microorganism may exit the body. *(Determines the category or type of isolation to use.)*
3. Follow agency policy for specific type of transmission-based precautions used. *(Increases awareness of isolation categories available in the agency.)*
4. Ensure that the environment has the equipment and supplies for the type of isolation:
   a. Private or isolation room with anteroom. *(Reduces spread of pathogens.)*
   b. Adequate hand hygiene facilities. *(All workers and visitors are to perform hand hygiene before entering and leaving the area.)*
   c. Containers for trash, soiled linen, and sharp instruments (such as needles). *(Ensures safe disposal of contaminated articles.)*
5. Provide explanation of isolation precautions to patient, family, and visitors. *(Relieves apprehension and promotes cooperation of those involved.)*
6. Post sign on door of patient's room or wall outside room stating the type of protective measures in use for patient care. *(Informs personnel, patient, family, and visitors entering room of precautions to be followed and encourages cooperation.)*
7. Be certain to supply the room with lined containers designated for soiled linens and for trash. *(Prevents transmission of pathogens from seepage through container.)*
8. Assess vital signs with designated equipment if possible, administer medications, administer hygiene, and collect specimens (Table 7.3). *(Administers patient care.)*
9. Report any changes in patient's health status to primary health care provider or supervisor. *(Ensures continuity of care and helps determine patient progress.)*
10. Record assessments and performance of transmission-based precautions. *(Provides proof of appropriate patient care.)* Document per agency policy.
11. Determine patient's understanding of activities in room. *(Increases patient's comfort and feeling of well-being.)*
12. Provide patient teaching (see the Patient Teaching box on infection prevention and control).
13. Additional techniques for acid-fast bacillus (AFB) isolation (airborne precautions):
    a. Before entering room, don N-95 respirator mask that for which you have undergone a fit-test. *(Reduces transmission of airborne droplet nuclei.)*
    b. Educate patient, family, and other visitors about how AFB is transmitted. *(Improves ability of patient to participate in care. TB cannot be transmitted through contact with clothing, bedding, food, or eating utensils.)*
    c. Explain to patient that TB is transmitted by inhalation of droplets that remain suspended in the air when patient coughs, sneezes, or speaks (CDC, 2006). Offer opportunity for questions. *(Improves ability of patient to participate in care.)*
    d. Instruct patient to cover mouth with tissue when coughing, educate patient about when to perform hand hygiene, and educate about the importance of wearing a regular disposable surgical mask while out of the room. *(Reduces spread of droplet nuclei.)*
    e. Record assessments and performance of patient care. *(Promotes continuity of care.)*

when changing a dressing at a patient's bedside, the nurse often only performs hand hygiene, dons sterile gloves, and maintains a sterile area during the procedure.

Because surgical asepsis requires exact techniques, the nurse needs the patient's cooperation. For this reason, the nurse should prepare the patient before any procedure. Some patients may fear moving or touching objects during a sterile procedure, whereas other patients may try to assist. The nurse should explain how a procedure is to be performed and instruct the patient how to avoid contaminating sterile items, including the following measures:

- The patient should try not to make sudden movements of body parts covered by sterile drapes.
- The patient should refrain from touching sterile supplies, drapes, and the nurse's gloves and gown.
- The patient should avoid coughing, sneezing, or talking over a sterile area.

Table 7.3 **Specimen Collection Techniques for the Patient in Isolation**

AMOUNT NEEDED[a]	COLLECTION DEVICE[a]	SPECIMEN COLLECTION AND TRANSFER
Wound (Culture) Specimen		
As much as possible (after cleaning surface of skin or wound bed to remove flora or debris)	Sterile cotton-tipped swab or syringe	Clean site with sterile water or saline solution before wound specimen collection. Don gloves and place clean test tube or culturette tube on clean paper towel. After swabbing center of wound site, grasp collection tube by holding it with paper towel. Carefully insert swab without touching outside of tube. After removing gloves, washing hands, and securing tube's top, transfer labeled tube into bag for transport to laboratory. Document that procedure was performed.
Blood (Culture) Specimen		
This specimen usually is obtained by the laboratory technician 10 mL per culture bottle, from two different venipuncture sites (volume may differ based on collection containers and age of patient)	Syringes, needles, and culture media bottles	Don gloves and perform venipuncture per hospital protocol at two different sites to decrease likelihood of both specimens being contaminated by skin flora. Inject 10 mL of blood into each bottle. Remove gloves and wash hands. Secure tops of bottles, label specimens, complete requisition, and send to laboratory. Document that procedure was performed.
Stool (Culture) Specimen		
Small amount, approximately size of a walnut	Clean specimen cup with seal top (not necessary to be sterile) and sterile tongue blade	Don gloves and place cup on clean paper towel in patient's bathroom. With tongue blade, collect needed amount of feces from bedpan, not the toilet. Transfer feces to specimen cup without touching cup's outside surface; cover with lid provided. Remove gloves, wash hands, and place seal on cup. Repeat hand washing. Transfer specimen cup into clean bag for transport to laboratory after ensuring cup is correctly labeled. Document procedure was performed.
Urine (Culture) Specimen		
5–15 mL for adults	Syringe and sterile cup	Don gloves and place cup or tube on clean towel in patient's bathroom. Use alcohol swab pad, syringe, and needle to collect specimen if patient has an indwelling urinary catheter. (All indwelling urinary catheters are equipped with needleless ports, which must be cleaned per manufacturer guidelines; alcohol swabs are not sufficient.) Otherwise, have patient follow procedure to obtain clean-voided specimen (see Chapter 23). Transfer urine into sterile container by injecting urine from syringe or pouring it from container. Secure top of labeled container, remove gloves, and wash hands. Transfer labeled specimen into clean bag for transport to laboratory, after ensuring container is labeled correctly. Document procedure was completed.

[a]Agency policies may differ on type of container. Ensure that all specimen containers used have the biohazard symbol on the outside and amount of specimen required and are bagged for transport to a laboratory.
From Pagana KD, Pagana TJ: *Mosby's diagnostic and laboratory test reference,* ed 7, St. Louis, 2005, Mosby.

PRINCIPLES OF STERILE TECHNIQUE

When beginning a surgically aseptic procedure, follow the principles listed in Box 7.11 to ensure maintenance of surgical asepsis. Failure to follow each principle conscientiously endangers patients by placing them at risk for infection.

Assemble all the equipment necessary for a sterile procedure before the procedure begins. By doing so, avoid the need to leave a sterile area unattended to locate missing equipment or supplies. Have a few extra supplies available in case something accidentally becomes contaminated. If an object becomes contaminated during the procedure, it should be discarded immediately per facility policy.

SURGICAL HAND SCRUB

In the operating room setting, effective hand washing or use of appropriate surgical hand rub to achieve surgical hand hygiene is imperative. To reduce patients' risk of postoperative infection, the nurses and other surgical personnel use an antimicrobial solution for hand hygiene as an integral part of the presurgical scrubbing procedure. Although sterilizing the skin is not possible,

Box 7.11 Principles of Sterile Technique

1. *A sterile object remains sterile only when touched exclusively by other sterile objects.* (This principle guides your placement of sterile objects and how you handle them.)
   a. Sterile touching sterile remains sterile; for example, wear sterile gloves and use sterile forceps to handle objects on a sterile field.
   b. Sterile touching clean becomes contaminated; for example, if the tip of a syringe or other sterile object touches the surface of a clean disposable glove, the object is contaminated.
   c. Sterile touching contaminated becomes contaminated; for example, when you touch a sterile object with an ungloved hand, the object is contaminated.
   d. Sterile touching questionable is contaminated; for example, when you find a tear or break in the covering of a sterile object, discard the object regardless of whether it appears untouched or not.
2. *Place only sterile objects on a sterile field.* Properly sterilize all items before use. It is essential to keep the package or container holding a sterile object intact and dry. A package that is torn, punctured, wet, or open is unsterile.
3. *A sterile field out of the range of vision or an object held below a person's waist is contaminated.* Never turn your back on a sterile field or leave it unattended. Contamination can occur accidentally from a dangling piece of clothing, falling hair, or an unknowing patient touching a sterile object. Consider any object below waist level contaminated because you are not able to keep it in constant view. Keep sterile objects in front of you with your hands as close together as possible.
4. *A sterile object or field becomes contaminated by prolonged exposure to air.* Avoid activities that potentially create air currents, such as excessive movements or rearranging linen after a sterile object or field becomes exposed. When opening sterile packages, keep to a minimum the number of people walking into the area. Microorganisms also travel by droplets through the air. Be sure no one talks, laughs, sneezes, or coughs over a sterile field or when gathering and using sterile equipment. Never perform sterile procedures if you have a cold or other respiratory ailment unless you are wearing a specialized mask. Microorganisms have the potential to travel through the air and fall on sterile items or fields if you reach over the work area. When opening sterile packages, hold the item or piece of equipment as close as possible to the sterile field without touching the sterile surface. Do not continue to rearrange the sterile items on the sterile field to help reduce the contamination that can occur by microorganisms traveling through the air.
5. *When a sterile surface comes in contact with a wet, contaminated surface, the sterile object or field becomes contaminated.* Moisture seeping through a sterile package's protective covering permits microorganisms to travel to the sterile object. When stored sterile packages become wet, discard the objects immediately or send the equipment for resterilization. When working with a sterile field or tray, you sometimes have to pour sterile solutions. Any spill is a possible source of contamination unless the object or field rests on a sterile surface impervious to moisture. For example, urinary catheterization trays contain sterile supplies that rest in a sterile, plastic container. Any sterile solution spilled within the container does not contaminate the catheter or other objects. In contrast, if you place a piece of sterile gauze in its wrapper on a patient's bedside table and the table surface is wet, consider the gauze to be contaminated.
6. *Fluid flows in the direction of gravity.* A sterile object becomes contaminated if gravity causes a contaminated liquid to flow over the object's surface. To prevent contamination during a surgical hand scrub, raise and hold your hands above your elbows. This allows water to flow downward without contaminating your hands and fingers. The principle of water flow by gravity is also the reason for drying in a sequence from fingers to elbows, with hands held up, after the scrub (see Skill 7.6).
7. *Consider the edges of a sterile field or container to be contaminated.* Frequently, you place sterile objects on a sterile towel or drape. Because the edge of the drape touches an unsterile surface, such as a table or bed linen, a 1-in (2.5-cm) border around the drape must be considered contaminated. The edges of sterile containers become exposed to air after they are open and thus are contaminated. After you remove a sterile needle from its protective cap or after removing a forceps from a container, do not allow the objects to touch the container's edge. The lip of an opened bottle of solution also becomes contaminated after it is exposed to air. When pouring a sterile liquid, first pour a small amount of solution and discard it. The solution thus washes away microorganisms on the bottle lip. Then pour a second time on the same side to fill a container with the desired amount of solution.

the number of microorganisms can be reduced greatly by chemical, physical, and mechanical means.

The surgical hand scrub (Skill 7.6) is the traditional method for surgical asepsis. With the use of an antimicrobial agent and sterile brushes, the surgical hand scrub removes debris and transient microorganisms from the nails, the hands, and the forearms. This technique also reduces the resident microbial count to a minimum and inhibits rapid or rebound growth of microorganisms. Use of an alcohol-based surgical hand rub is also acceptable as long it has met US Food and Drug Administration requirements to be used for this purpose. Both hand antiseptic methods currently are used in operating room settings. Skill 7.6 addresses both techniques. Surgical personnel wear surgical attire (i.e., scrubs) in the operating room to reduce the chance for contamination from themselves to patients and vice versa. Fingernails should be short, clean, and natural. Do not wear artificial nails.

Skill 7.6 Surgical Hand Hygiene

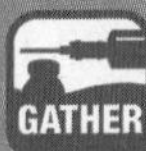

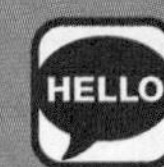

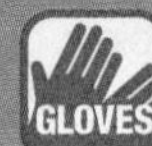

NURSING ACTION *(RATIONALE)*

1. Inspect hands for presence of abrasions, cuts, or open lesions. *(These conditions increase likelihood of more microorganisms residing on skin surfaces.)*
2. Apply surgical shoe covers, cap or hood, face mask, and protective eyewear. *(Mask prevents escape into air of microorganisms that can contaminate hands. Other protective wear prevents exposure to blood and body fluid splashes during the procedure.)*
3. Perform surgical hand hygiene (traditional method):
   a. Turn on water using knee or foot controls and adjust to comfortable temperature.
   b. Wet hands and arms under running lukewarm water and lather with detergent to 5 cm (2 inches) above elbows. (Keep hands above elbows at all times.) *(Hands become cleanest part of upper extremity. Keeping hands elevated allows water to flow from least to most contaminated areas because water runs by gravity from fingertips to elbows. Washing a wide area reduces risk of contaminating gown that you will don later.)*
   c. Rinse hands and arms thoroughly under running water. **Remember to keep hands above elbows.** *(Rinsing removes transient microorganisms from fingers, hands, and forearms.)*
   d. Under running water, clean under nails of both hands with nail pick. Discard after use. *(Removes dirt and organic material that harbor large numbers of microorganisms.)*

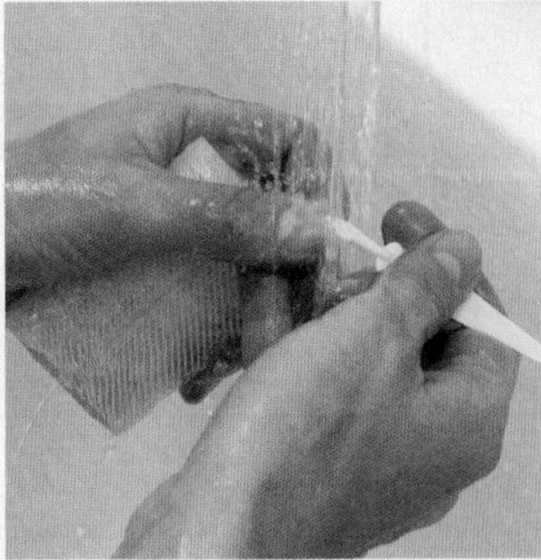

   (1) Wet clean sponge and apply antimicrobial detergent. Scrub nails of one hand with 15 strokes. Holding sponge perpendicular to hand, scrub palm, each side of thumb and fingers, and posterior side of hand with 10 strokes each.

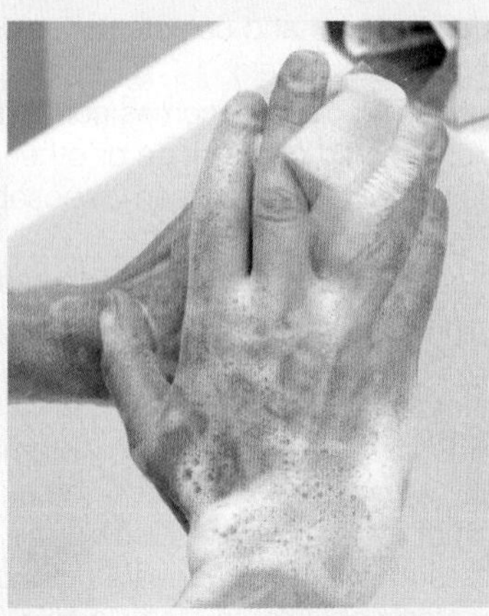

   (2) Mentally divide your arm into thirds, and scrub each third 10 times. Entire scrub should last 5 to 10 minutes. Rinse sponge and repeat sequence for other arm. It is permitted to substitute with a two-sponge method. Check agency policy. *(Friction loosens resident bacteria that adhere to skin surfaces. Ensures coverage of all surfaces. Scrubbing is performed from cleanest area [hands] to marginal area [upper arms.])*

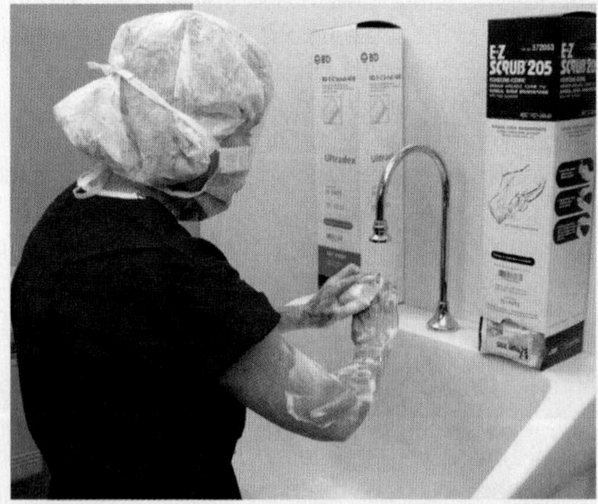

   e. Discard sponge and rinse hands and arms thoroughly. Turn off water with foot or knee control and back into room entrance with hands elevated in front of and away from the body. *(After it has touched skin, consider the sponge contaminated. Rinsing removes resident bacteria. Prevents accidental contamination.)*

Skill 7.6 Surgical Hand Hygiene—cont'd

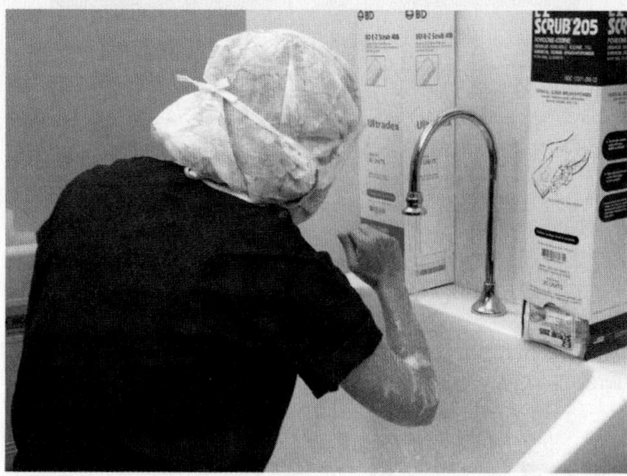

(1) Walk up to sterile tray and lean forward slightly to pick up a sterile towel.

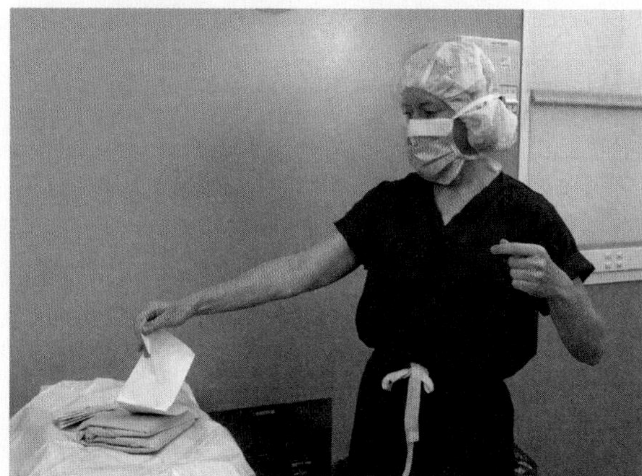

(2) Dry one hand thoroughly, moving in sequence from fingers to elbow. Dry in a rotating motion. Dry from cleanest to least clean area. *(Drying prevents chapping and facilitates donning of gloves. Leaning forward prevents accidental contact of arms with scrub attire.)*

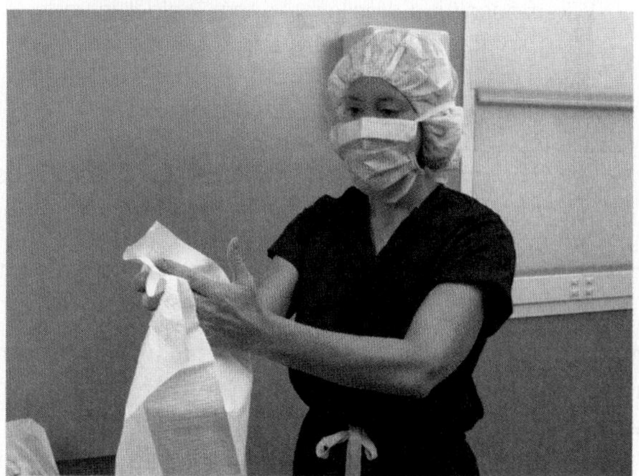

f. Repeat drying method for other hand by carefully reversing towel or using a new sterile towel. *(Prevents accidental contamination.)*

g. Discard towel. *(Prevents accidental contamination.)*

h. Proceed with sterile gowning.

4. Alternate method of surgical hand hygiene using alcohol-based antiseptic:

a. Wash hands with soap and water for 15 to 30 seconds to remove soil. *(Removes dirt and organic material that harbor large numbers of microorganisms.)*

b. Under running water, clean under nails of both hands with nail pick. Discard after use and dry hands with a paper towel. *(Removes dirt and organic material that harbor large numbers of microorganisms.)*

c. Apply enough alcohol-based waterless antiseptic to one palm to cover both hands thoroughly. Spread the antiseptic over all surfaces of the hands and the fingernails. Follow product instructions for length of time to rub over hand surfaces. Allow to air dry. *(Ensures coverage of all surfaces. Air drying ensures complete antisepsis.)*

d. Repeat the process and allow hands to air dry before applying sterile gloves.

Figures from Potter PA, Perry AG: *Fundamentals of nursing: Concepts, process, and practice,* ed 9, St. Louis, 2016, Elsevier.

Artificial nails harbor microorganisms and fungus. Remove all rings, watches, and bracelets before the surgical scrub and while assisting with procedures that require surgical asepsis.

The Association of Perioperative Registered Nurses (AORN, 2013) has a revised set of policies and procedures; in addition, refer to agency policy on surgical hand hygiene (refer to *Adult Health Nursing*, Chapter 2).

MANAGING STERILE PACKAGES

Sterile items such as syringes, gauze dressings, and catheters are packaged in paper or plastic containers that are impervious to (unable to be penetrated by) microorganisms as long as the items remain dry and intact. Paper packages are permeable to steam and thus allow for steam autoclaving. A disadvantage of paper wrappers is that they tear or puncture relatively easily. Sterile items should be placed in clean enclosed storage cabinets and never kept in the same room as dirty equipment.

Sterile supplies have dated labels or chemical tapes that indicate the date when the sterilization expires. The tapes change color during the sterilization process. Failure of the tapes to change color means the item is not sterile. Never use or allow use of a sterile item or piece of equipment after the expiration date. Some agencies use the "event-related" contamination rule. If the integrity of the sterile package is questionable (i.e., wet, torn, discolored), the item is discarded or resterilized per policy. If the nurse finds moisture present after a sterile tray is opened, the item is either discarded or returned to the institution's supply area for resterilization.

Before opening a sterile item, perform thorough hand hygiene. Assemble the supplies at the work area, such as the bedside table or in the treatment room, before packages are opened. A bedside table or countertop provides a large, clean working area for opening of items. Ensure that the work area is above your waist level. Sterile supplies should not be opened in a space where a dirty object may fall on or come into contact with them.

Sterile packaged items can be opened without contamination of the contents even when you are not wearing sterile gloves. Commercially packaged items usually are designed so that you only have to tear away or separate the paper or plastic cover from the rest of the tray or kit. Hold the item in one hand while pulling the wrapper with the other (Fig. 7.10). Be careful after opening to keep the inner contents sterile before use. When opening items packed in linen and some commercially prepackaged items, use the steps described in Box 7.12 and illustrated in Figs. 7.10 and 7.11.

PREPARING A STERILE FIELD

Performing sterile procedures requires a sterile work area that provides room for handling and placing sterile items. A sterile field is an area that is free of microorganisms and has been prepared to receive sterile items.

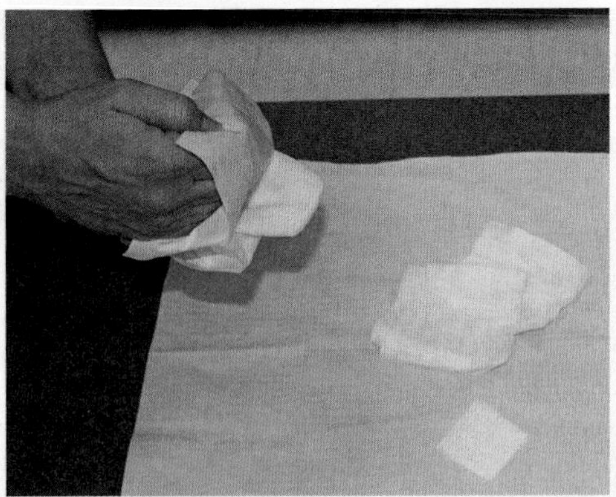

Fig. 7.10 When opening a commercially packaged sterile item, tear the wrapper away from your body.

Box 7.12 Opening Sterile Packages

1. Perform hand hygiene.
2. Place the item flat in the center of the work surface.
3. Remove the tape or seal that indicates the sterilization date.
4. Grasp the outer surface of the tip of the outermost flap.
5. Open the outer flap away from your body, keeping your arm outstretched and away from the sterile field.
6. Grasp the outside surface of the first side flap.
7. Open the side flap, allowing it to lie flat on the table surface. Keep your arm to the side and not over the sterile surface. Do not allow flaps to spring back over the sterile contents.
8. Grasp the outside surface of the second side flap and allow it to lie flat on the table surface.
9. Grasp the outer surface of the last and innermost flap.
10. Stand away from the sterile package and pull the flap back, allowing it to fall flat on the surface.
11. Use the inner surface of the package cover (except for the 1-in border around the edges) as a sterile field to handle this or additional sterile items (see Fig. 7.10). Grasp the 1-in border to maneuver the entire field on the table surface.
12. When opening a small sterile item, hold it in your hand so that you can pass it to a person wearing sterile gloves or transfer it to a sterile field. Hold the package in your nondominant hand while you open the top flap and pull it away from you. With your dominant hand, carefully open the side and top flaps away from the enclosed sterile item in the same order in the previous steps (see Fig. 7.9).

The nurse should prepare the field by using the inner surface of a sterile wrapper as the work surface or by using a sterile drape (Skill 7.7).

Sometimes nurses choose to wear sterile gloves while preparing items on the field. The nurse is then able to touch the entire drape, but an assistant has to open and pass sterile items to the nurse unless the nurse applies new sterile gloves to prevent contamination of the sterile

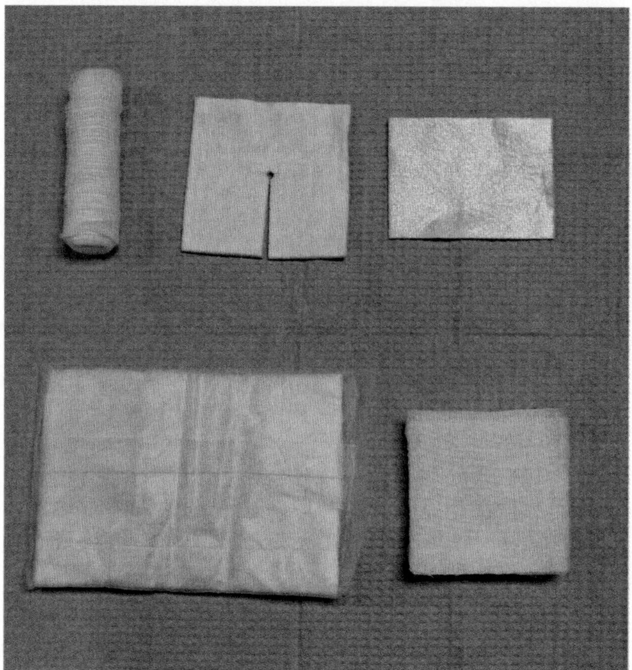

Fig. 7.11 Placement of items on a sterile field.

items. The nurse should not allow the gloves to touch the outside wrapping of the package that contains the sterile items.

POURING STERILE SOLUTIONS

The nurse may be required to pour sterile solutions into sterile containers. A bottle that contains a sterile solution is sterile on the inside and contaminated on the outside. The bottle's neck is also contaminated, but the inside of the bottle cap is sterile. After opening a cap or lid, hold it in the hand or place it, sterile side (inside) up, on a clean surface. Thus you can see the inside of the lid as it rests on the table surface. Never allow a bottle's cap or lid to rest sterile side down on a sterile surface because the cap's outer edge is unsterile and will contaminate the surface. Likewise, placement of a sterile cap down on an unsterile surface increases the chances of the inside of the cap becoming contaminated.

Hold the bottle with its label in the palm of the hand to prevent the solution from wetting the label. If the solution is allowed to wet the label, it may cause it to fade and reduce its legibility. Keep the edge of the bottle from touching the edge or the inside of the receiving

Skill 7.7 Preparing a Sterile Field

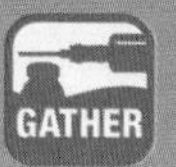

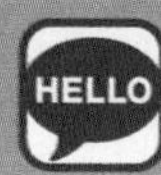

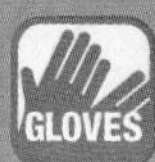

NURSING ACTION *(RATIONALE)*

1. Prepare sterile field just before planned procedure. *(Prevents exposure of sterile field and supplies to air contamination.)* Be sure to use supplies immediately.
2. Select clean work surface that is above waist level. *(Consider sterile objects held below waist contaminated.)*
3. Assemble necessary equipment. *(Preparing equipment in advance prevents breaks in technique.)*
   - Sterile drape
   - Assorted sterile supplies
4. Check dates, labels, and condition of package for sterility of equipment. *(Consider equipment stored beyond expiration date, or a package that is damaged, unsterile.)*
5. Wash hands thoroughly. *(Prevents spread of microorganisms.)*
6. Place package containing sterile drape on work surface and open. *(Ensures sterility of packaged drape.)*
7. With fingertips of one hand, pick up folded top edge of sterile drape. *(Up to the 1-inch border around drape is unsterile and permitted to be touched.)*
8. Gently lift drape up from its outer cover and let it unfold by itself without touching any object. Discard outer cover with your other hand. *(If sterile object touches any unsterile object, it becomes contaminated.)*
9. With other hand, grasp adjacent corner of drape and hold the entire edge straight up and away from your body. Now, properly place drape while using two hands and be sure to keep the drape away from unsterile surfaces. *(Prevents contamination.)*
   a. Holding drape, first position the bottom half over intended work surface. *(Prevents from reaching over sterile field.)*
   b. Allow top half of drape to be placed over work surface last. *(Creates a flat, sterile work surface.)*
10. Perform procedure using sterile technique. *(Prevents contamination.)*

container, which is unsterile. Pour the solution slowly to avoid splashing the underlying drape or field. Never hold the bottle so high above the recipient container that even slow pouring causes splashing. Hold the bottle over the outside of the edge of the sterile field (Fig. 7.12).

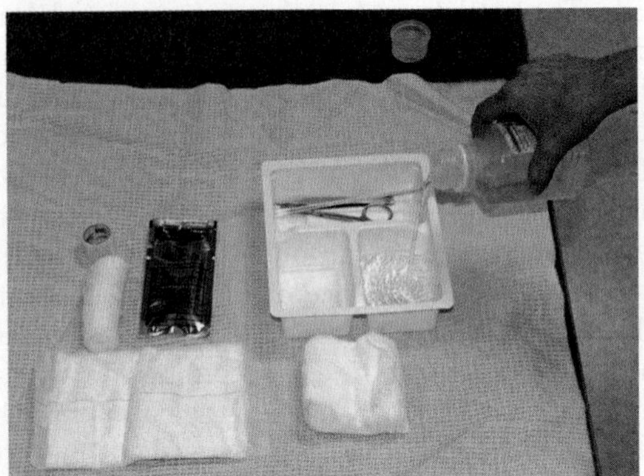

Fig. 7.12 Place receptacle into which you pour fluids near edge of sterile table to prevent the need for reaching over the sterile field to pour.

DONNING A STERILE GOWN

A nurse must don a sterile gown (Skill 7.8) before working in the operating room and before assisting with certain sterile procedures or working in special treatment areas. The sterile gown decreases the risk of contaminating sterile objects when the nurse handles them. In addition, the sterile gown prevents contamination of sterile objects or sterile fields by microorganisms shed from the nurse's skin (Potter, et al., 2019).

DONNING STERILE GLOVES

Sterile gloves are an additional barrier used to prevent the transmission of microorganisms. The two methods of donning gloves are open (Skill 7.9) and closed (Fig. 7.13). Nurses who work on general nursing divisions use open gloving before procedures such as dressing changes or urinary catheter insertions. Nurses should use the closed gloving method when donning a sterile gown before procedures in the operating room and special treatment areas.

When donning sterile gloves, select the proper glove size. The glove must be snug enough for you to pick

Skill 7.8 Donning a Sterile Gown

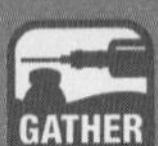

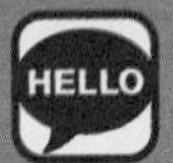

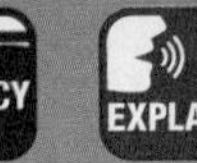

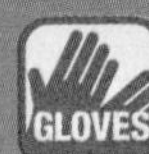

NURSING ACTION *(RATIONALE)*

The nurse should perform the following steps when applying a sterile gown:

1. Don surgical cap, shoe covers, protective eyewear, and mask, and then perform surgical hand hygiene. *(Prevents contamination of the surgical field and protects the nurse from blood and body fluid exposure.)*

2. Ask the circulating nurse to open the sterile gown package and the sterile glove package. *(Prevents contamination of the hands after the surgical hand wash because the outer wraps are not sterile.)*

3. Don the gown.

a. If available, the scrub nurse assists by pulling the gown over your extended hands and arms. If no assistance from a scrub nurse is available:

(1) Pick up the gown touching only the inner surface below the neck. *(Touching the outer, sterile surface causes the gown to become contaminated because the hands are not yet gloved and thus unsterile.)*

(2) Maintain constant control of the folded layers of the gown. *(Prevents the gown from brushing against unsterile surfaces.)*

(3) While holding the gown at arm's length, allow the gown to unfold from top to bottom. Be sure that the gown does not touch the floor. *(Prevents contamination.)*

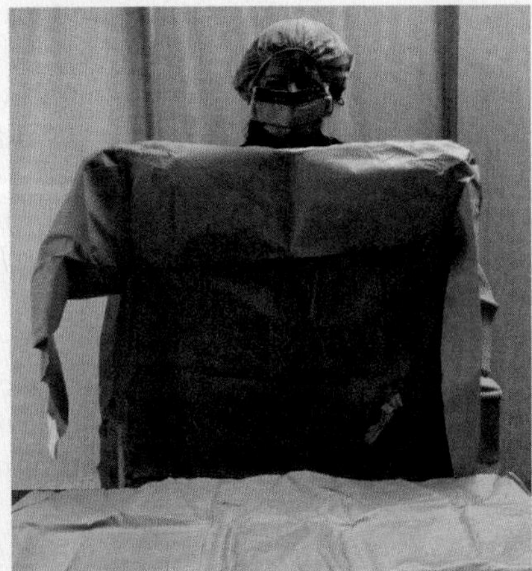

(4) While holding the inside of the gown near the shoulders and below the neckband, slide hands and arms into the sleeves with your fingers stopping at the end of the cuffs. *(The fingers remain inside the sleeves to don the sterile gloves by means of closed gloving.)*

Skill 7.8 Donning a Sterile Gown—cont'd

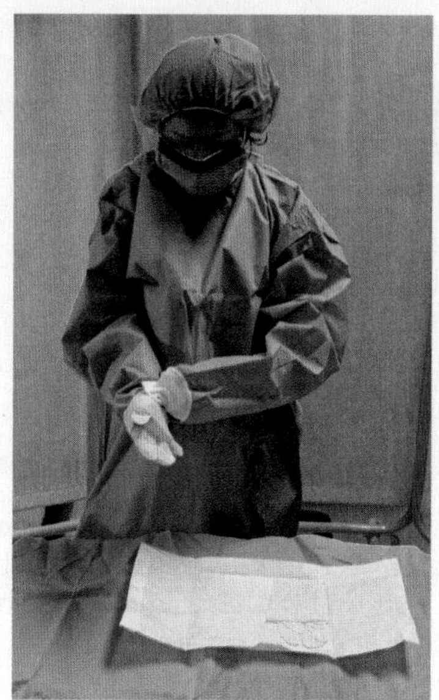

(5) Ask another staff member to grasp the cord that is attached to the ties of the gown to draw the ties around to the back with the gown overlapping itself. The staff member should now tie the gown, avoiding touching any part of the gown except the ties. *(Do not allow the front or the sides of the gown to be touched by the staff member because these areas are sterile.)*

Skill 7.9 Performing Open Sterile Gloving

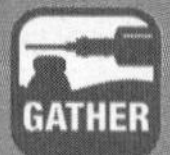

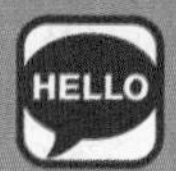

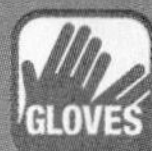

NURSING ACTION *(RATIONALE)*

1. Have package of properly sized sterile gloves at treatment area. *(Facilitates procedure.)*
2. Perform thorough hand hygiene. *(Removes bacteria from skin surfaces.)*
3. Remove outer glove package wrapper by carefully separating and peeling apart sides. *(Prevents inner glove package from accidentally opening and touching contaminated objects.)*

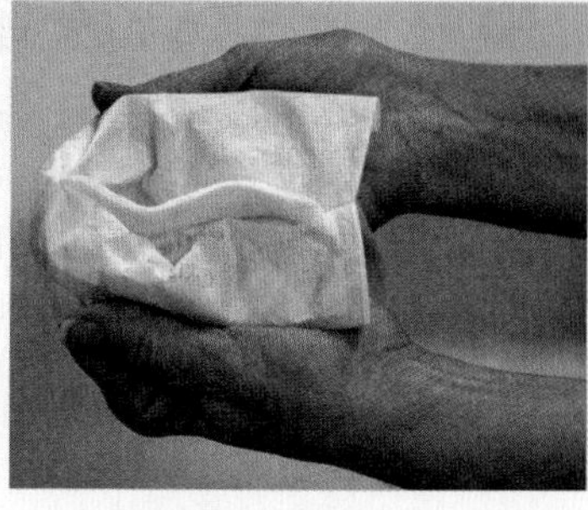

4. Grasping inner side of package, lay package on clean flat surface just above waist level. Open package, keeping gloves on wrapper's inside surface. *(Inner surface of glove package is sterile. Sterile objects held below the waist are considered contaminated.)*

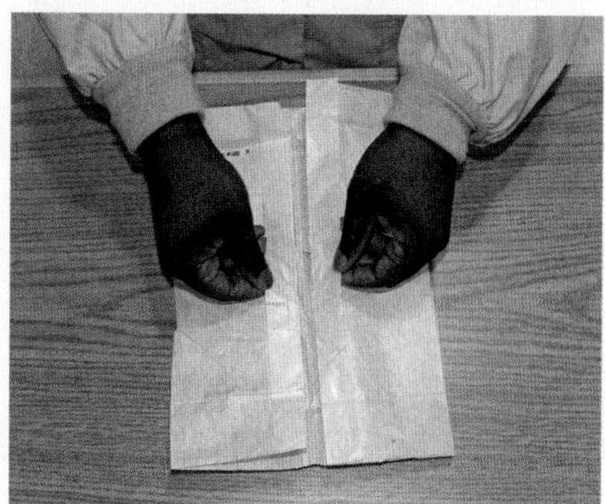

Continued

Skill 7.9 Performing Open Sterile Gloving—cont'd

5. Identify right and left gloves. Each glove has a cuff approximately 2-in (5-cm) deep. *(Proper identification of gloves prevents contamination by improper fit.)*

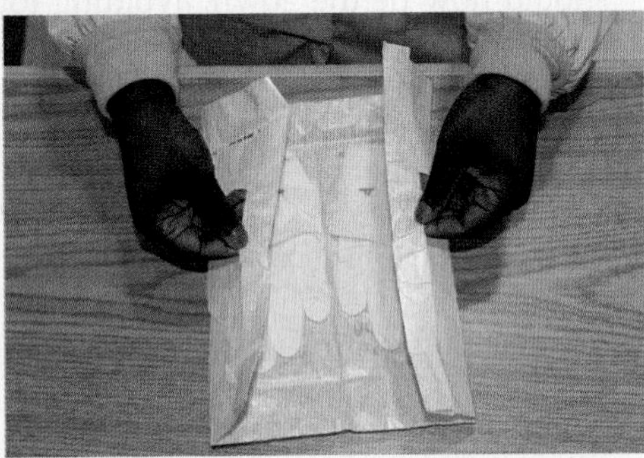

6. Glove dominant hand first. With thumb and first two fingers of nondominant hand, grasp edge of cuff of glove for dominant hand. Touch only glove's inside surface. *(Gloving of dominant hand first improves dexterity. Touching inside surface is permitted because inner edge of cuff will lie against skin. If glove's outer surface touches hand or wrist, it is contaminated.)*

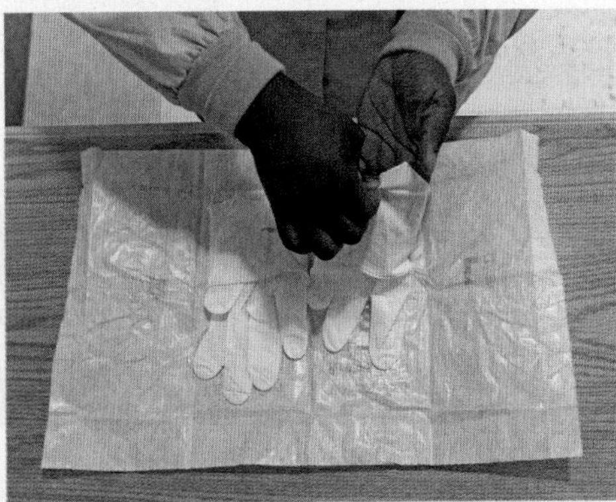

7. Carefully pull glove over dominant hand, leaving cuff; be sure cuff does not roll up wrist. Be sure thumb and fingers are in proper spaces. *(If glove's outer surface touches hand or wrist, it is contaminated.)*

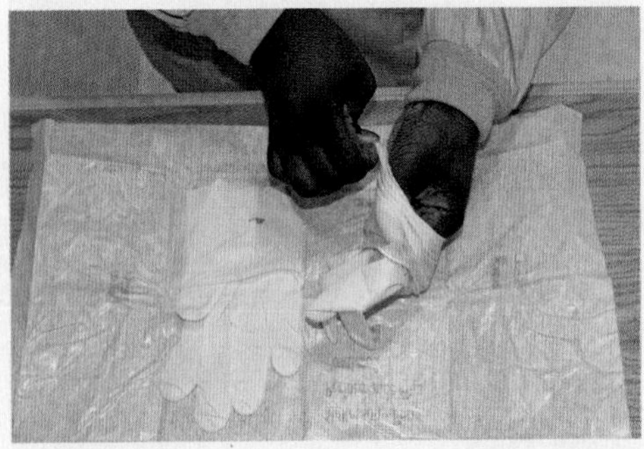

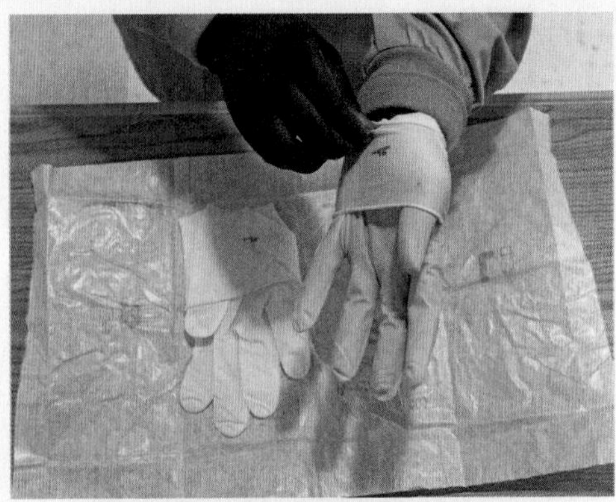

8. With gloved dominant hand, slip fingers underneath second glove's cuff in such fashion that the cuff will protect the gloved fingers. *(Sterile touching sterile prevents glove contamination.)*

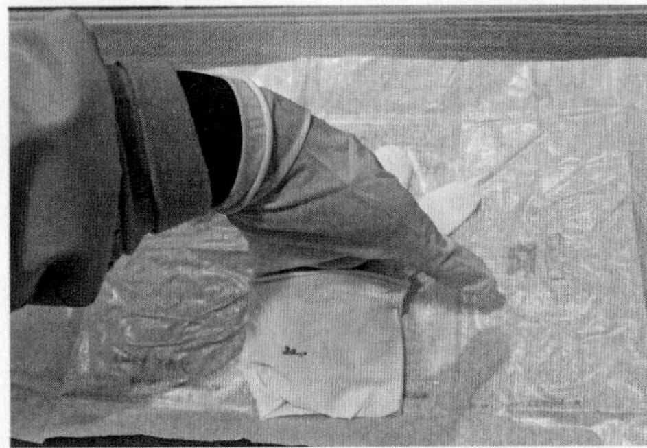

9. Carefully pull second glove over nondominant hand. Do not allow fingers and thumb of gloved dominant hand to touch any part of exposed nondominant hand. Keep thumb of dominant hand abducted back. *(Contact of gloved hand with exposed hand results in contamination.)*

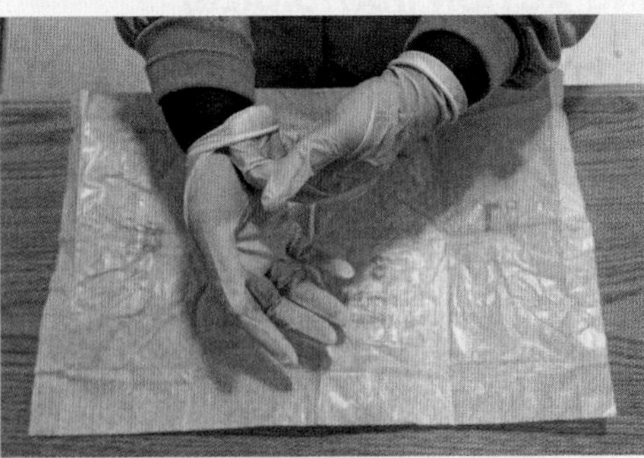

10. After second glove is on, interlock hands. *Be sure to touch only sterile sides.* The cuffs usually fall down after application. *(Ensures smooth fit over fingers.)*

Skill 7.9 Performing Open Sterile Gloving—cont'd

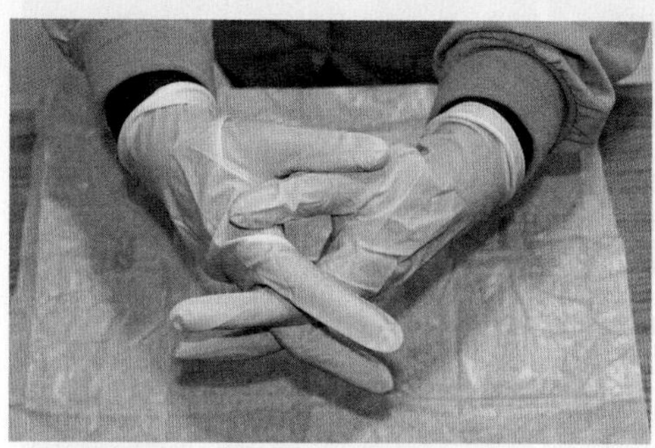

GLOVE REMOVAL AND DISPOSAL

11. Grasp outside of one cuff with other gloved hand; avoid touching wrist. *(Minimizes contamination of underlying skin.)*

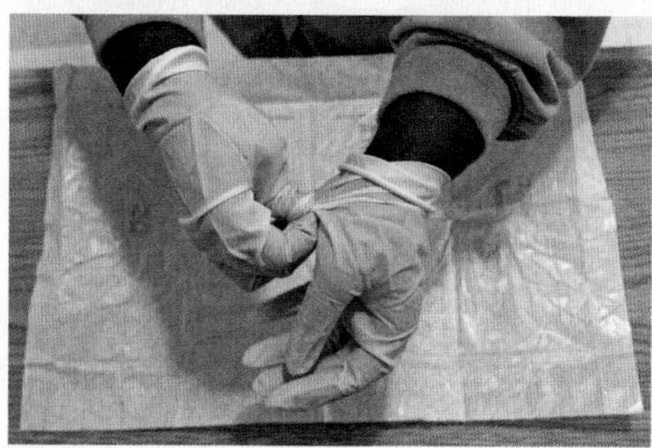

12. Pull glove off, turning it inside out. Discard in receptacle. *(The outside of glove does not touch skin surface.)*

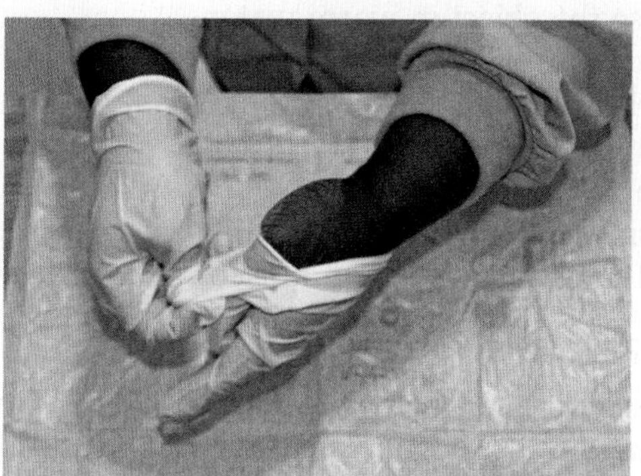

13. Take fingers of bare hand and tuck inside remaining glove cuff. Peel glove off, inside out. Discard in receptacle. *(Reduces spread of microorganisms.)*

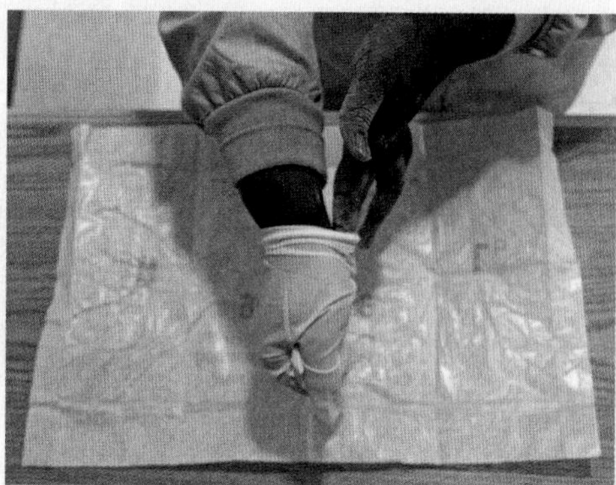

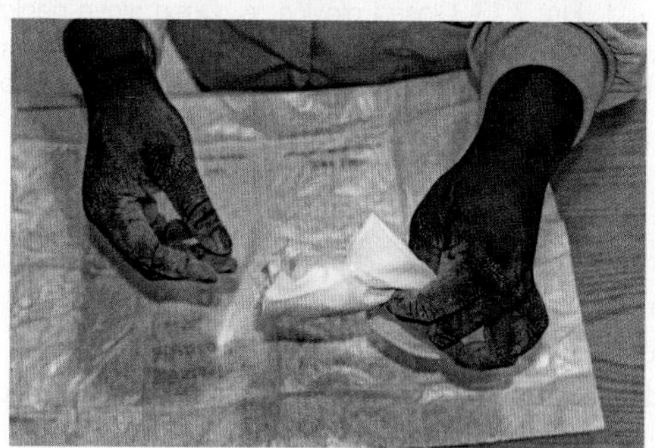

up things easily and yet not so tightly stretched that it tears easily.

Closed Gloving

Closed gloving is practiced when the nurse also needs to wear a sterile gown. With closed gloving, contamination of the sterile gown is prevented. The wearer of a sterile gown and sterile gloves can safely handle sterile materials and instruments during surgery or other types of sterile procedures.

CLEANING, DISINFECTION, AND STERILIZATION

Microorganisms are present on items in the home and public areas, including health care agencies. By following basic clean or aseptic technique, the nurse can help interrupt the spread of infection. Antiseptics are a means to inhibit the growth of microorganisms, although killing them this way is not possible. Antiseptics also are referred to as *bacteriostatic* solutions. *Bacterio-* means "microorganism," and *static* means "referring to that

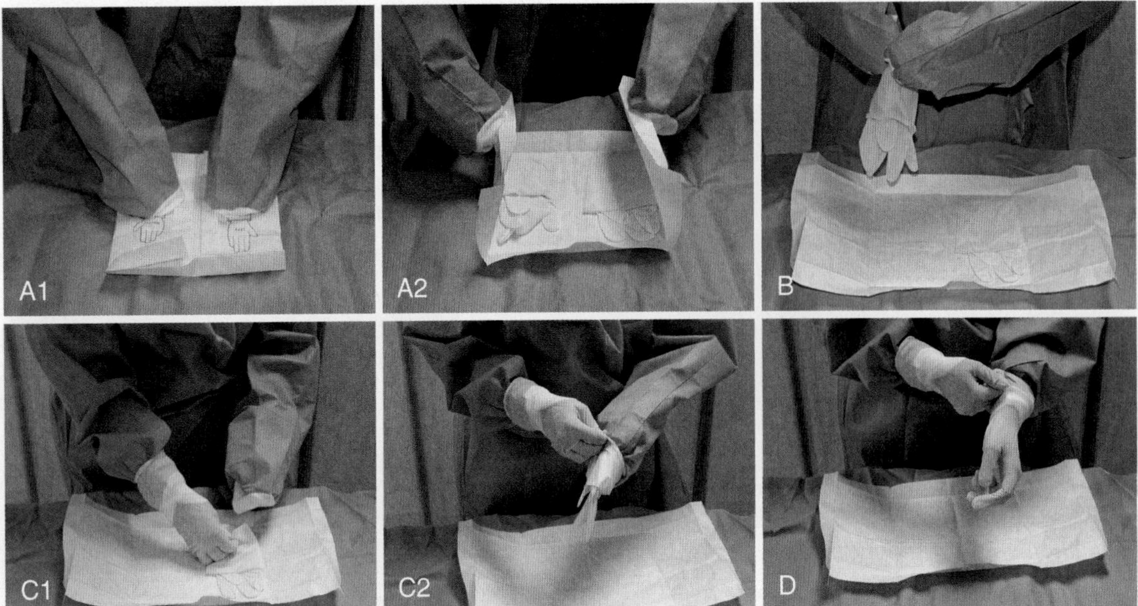

Fig. 7.13 Closed gloving. A, Open glove package. B, Grasp back of dominant hand's glove cuff with nondominant hand and stretch over end of dominant hand's sleeve. C, Glove nondominant hand in same manner. D, Use gloved dominant hand to pull on glove, keeping nondominant hand inside sleeve until it emerges into glove.

which cannot move or grow." Use of antiseptics (e.g., alcohol or chlorhexidine gluconate) on human tissue is acceptable and often is performed before sterile procedures such as surgery and during wound care. Antiseptics can be used for mouth care and when performing hand hygiene.

CLEANING

Cleaning is the removal of foreign materials, such as soil and organic material, from objects. Generally, cleaning involves use of water and mechanical action with or without detergents.

When an object comes in contact with potentially infectious material, the object is contaminated. If the object is disposable, it is discarded per facility policy. Reusable objects must be cleaned thoroughly and then either disinfected or sterilized before reuse, per facility policy.

When cleaning equipment that is soiled by organic material such as blood, fecal matter, mucus, or pus, put on a mask and protective eyewear or goggles (or a face shield), a fluid-resistant gown, and waterproof gloves. These barriers provide protection from infectious organisms (as discussed previously). A stiff-bristled brush and detergent or soap are necessary for cleaning.

Perform the following steps when cleaning equipment:

1. Rinse a contaminated object or article with cold running water to remove organic material. Hot water causes the protein in organic material to coagulate and stick to objects, making removal difficult.
2. After rinsing, wash the object with soap and warm water. Soap or detergent reduces the surface tension of water and emulsifies dirt and remaining material. Rinse the object thoroughly to remove the emulsified dirt.
3. Use a brush to remove dirt or material present in the equipment's grooves or seams. Friction dislodges contaminated material for easy removal. Open any hinged items for cleaning.
4. Rinse the object in warm water.
5. Dry the object and prepare it for disinfection or sterilization if indicated by the intended use of the item.
6. The brush, the gloves, and the sink in which the equipment is cleaned are considered contaminated and must be cleaned and dried per facility policy.

DISINFECTION

Disinfection is used to destroy microorganisms. However, it does not destroy spores. The solutions used during disinfection are called *disinfectants,* or possibly *bactericidal solutions* (the suffix *-cidal* is derived from a Latin word meaning "to kill"). These solutions are too strong to use on human skin and are appropriate to use on inanimate objects. If a disinfectant solution comes in contact with human tissue, the tissue may feel "slippery." This is the first step of tissue breakdown. When using a disinfectant, use clean gloves to protect the skin (Skill 7.10).

STERILIZATION

Sterilization refers to methods used to kill all microorganisms, including spores. The two types of sterilization methods are physical and chemical (Box 7.13).

Most health agencies have a central supply department that disinfects and sterilizes reusable equipment

Skill 7.10 Preparing for Disinfection and Sterilization

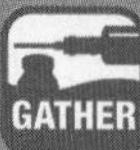

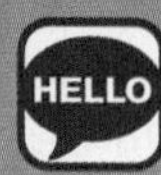

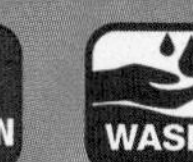

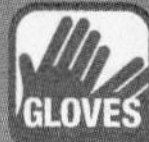

NURSING ACTION *(RATIONALE)*

1. Prepare equipment and supplies. *(Ensures organization of procedure.)*
    - Disinfectant to use for cleansing. *(Aids in appropriate care of equipment and reusable supplies.)*
    - Method of sterilization. *(Ensures that appropriate method is used.)*
    - Gloves. *(Protects you from contamination.)*
    - Running water. *(Aids in cleansing and rinsing of articles.)*
    - Scrub brush. *(Aids in cleaning grooves.)*
    - Cloth wrapper. *(Provides the means for wrapping articles that require sterilization.)*
2. Don gloves. *(Protects you from contamination.)*
3. Rinse article under cool running water. *(Emulsifies or softens soil for removal.)*
4. Wash article with detergent. *(Emulsifies or softens dirt for easy removal.)*
5. Use scrub brush to remove material in grooves. *(Friction loosens material in corners and grooves.)*
6. Dry article thoroughly. *(Prevents the growth of microorganisms.)*
7. Prepare article for sterilization by wrapping it in cloth wrapper. *(Promotes appropriate sterilization of the article.)*
8. Clean work area and put in order. *(Prevents the spread of microorganisms.)*
9. Perform patient teaching (see the Patient Teaching box on disinfection and sterilization in the home).

Box 7.13 Methods of Disinfection and Sterilization

PHYSICAL METHOD

1. Steam under pressure, or moist heat, is the most practical and dependable method for destruction of all microorganisms. This process is called sterilization. Examples of sterilization equipment are the autoclave, which is used in hospitals and other agencies, and the pressure cooker, which is used in a home environment.
2. Boiling water is the best method for home use and is the least expensive. However, this technique does not destroy bacterial spores and some viruses. The article must be boiled for a minimum of 15 to 20 minutes for disinfection.
3. Radiation is used to sterilize pharmaceutical goods, foods, and heat-sensitive items. It is extremely effective on articles that are difficult to sterilize with other methods.
4. Dry heat is a method used for disinfecting articles that are destroyed by moisture. Health agencies seldom use this method, but in the home, an article can be disinfected by being placed in the oven for 2 hours at 320°F (160°C) or for 45 minutes at 350°F (176.7°C).

CHEMICAL PROCESS

1. Gas (ethylene oxide) is used for sterilization. It destroys spores formed by bacteria.
2. Chemical solutions often are used to disinfect instruments because they are effective in destroying microorganisms. One way to store clinical thermometers is in a chemical solution, and some articles are soaked in a solution to prepare them for another, more definitive method of disinfection or sterilization.

and supplies. Although most supplies used today for patient care are disposable, some supplies and equipment still require the use of disinfection and sterilization. The patient and family members should be taught the principles of cleansing and disinfecting in the home environment (see the Patient Teaching box on disinfection and sterilization).

There are two accepted methods of disinfection and sterilization (see Box 7.13). One is a physical process that uses heat or radiation; the second process uses chemicals. Both methods destroy microorganisms. The method used depends on the following factors: (1) the type of microorganisms present (spore-forming bacteria are resistant to destruction); (2) how many microorganisms may be present (it takes longer to kill a large number); and (3) the type of item that must be disinfected and sterilized (some materials are so sensitive that heat or certain chemicals destroy them). Other determinants of the sterilization method used are (1) the intended use for the article (e.g., surgery requires that all organisms be destroyed, whereas medical asepsis consists of techniques that inhibit the growth and transmission of pathogenic microorganisms) and (2) the methods of sterilization available.

Liquid and gaseous chemicals are used to sterilize and disinfect equipment. Examples may include iodine, alcohol, dialdehyde, and chlorine bleach compounds. Chlorine bleach is useful for household disinfection and disinfection of water, but it must never be mixed with ammonia because of the resulting emission of toxic fumes. Chlorine bleach has a tendency to corrode some metals. Iodine is a good bactericidal agent (i.e., it kills bacteria but not spores). Iodine leaves behind stains and is not used as widely as it was previously.

PATIENT TEACHING FOR INFECTION PREVENTION AND CONTROL

Patients and families often have to learn to use infection prevention and control practices at home. Aseptic technique becomes almost second nature to the nurse, who practices it daily. However, the patient is less aware of the factors that promote the spread of infection and of the ways to prevent its transmission. The nurse should educate patients about the nature of infection and the techniques to use in planning or controlling its spread (see the Lifespan Considerations for Older Adults and Cultural Considerations boxes regarding infection control).

Lifespan Considerations

Older Adults

Infection Prevention and Control

- The older adult experiences an alteration in integrity of the oral mucosa. Promote careful oral hygiene and emphasize the importance of routine dental care.
- The older adult experiences a decrease in the production of digestive acid. Teach the older patient to wash hands carefully before food preparation, to cook foods adequately, and to refrigerate unused portions promptly.
- The dermal and epidermal skin layers of the older adult become thinner, and elasticity is decreased. Turn the bedridden patient frequently, and carefully observe the skin for impairment.
- The older adult may experience urethral stricture, neurogenic bladder, and prostatic enlargement (in males). In the older patient with an indwelling urinary catheter, assess for adequate drainage and maintain cleanliness of the urethra and the perineal area.
- Older adults experience a decrease in rib cage movement during inspiration. When caring for older adults after surgery, elevate the head of the bed (if indicated) and encourage the patient to cough and breathe deeply and to get out of bed as soon as possible to prevent postoperative complications such as pneumonia.

INFECTION PREVENTION AND CONTROL FOR HOME AND HOSPICE SETTINGS

Patients commonly are discharged from acute care to their homes more quickly than in the past. Thus they often require care from home health personnel. An infection that develops within 30 days after discharge, such as a wound infection at an operative site, may be an outcome of hospitalization, and the acute care facility's infection control department must receive a report. As more patients elect to die at home, care for the dying will make similar care and reporting measures necessary more often. The epidemiologic (pertaining to the study of the occurrence, distribution, and causes of disease in humankind) basis of infections that develop in homes sometimes is related to the diseases that affect a community. The patient develop of influenza, an enteric infection, or a streptococcal pharyngitis as it passes through the community.

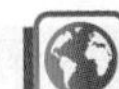

Cultural Considerations

Infection Prevention and Control

- Cultural heritage affects all dimensions of health. The patient's cultural background must be considered when educating a patient about infection prevention and control measures.
- The way that culture influences behaviors, attitudes, and values depends on many factors and is often not the same for every member of a cultural group.
- Clean water may be a difficult commodity for many Alaskan Eskimos to obtain reliably. In some villages near the ocean, drinking water is brought in as ice from several miles upriver. In this process, the chunks of ice destined for human consumption often are handled by many people and must be melted, boiled, and cooled.
- Some Japanese Americans have a traditional belief that disease is caused by contact with contaminated agents such as blood, corpses, and skin diseases.
- The germ theory can be confusing to individuals with animistic beliefs (a belief in the existence of spirits and demons). They may believe that the supernatural or spirit world causes disease.
- Observant Jews have customs that promote good hygiene or have been proven medically sound practices, such as washing the hands on awakening from sleep, after elimination of body wastes, after hair cutting, after touching vermin (insects and small animals), after being close to a dead body, and before eating or drinking.
- In Cajun culture, people may trust faith healers and be less likely to take preventive health measures.

As home care and hospice programs continue to expand, questions emerge about infection prevention and control in these settings. The reliability of hospital infection rates depends directly on accurate identification of the source of infection. Such accuracy tends to be problematic when rapid hospital discharges leave the source of an infection unclear. Hospitalized patients need to receive education and instruction at discharge about reporting the occurrence of any signs and symptoms of infection such as pain, erythema (redness), edema (swelling), drainage or exudate, and fever to the appropriate acute care personnel after discharge (see the Health Promotion box).

❖ NURSING PROCESS

The role of the LPN/LVN in the nursing process as stated is that the nurse:

- Participates in planning care for patients based on patient needs.

 Health Promotion

Prevention of Infection in the Home Setting

The basic principles of hygiene are bathing; not sharing personal articles such as combs, toothbrushes, razors, and washcloths; and covering the mouth when coughing and sneezing. These practices are important to help prevent the spread of infection in the home setting. Patient education about the risk of spreading microorganisms responsible for hospital-acquired infections to family or friends is important, especially when family members are assisting at home in changing dressings or managing hygiene for patients with incontinence.

The licensed practical/vocational nurse (LPN/LVN) helps educate patients and family members about the following activities:

- *Hand hygiene.* Wash hands after using the bathroom, after contact with any secretions, before eating, and before and after patient care. Use water, soap, and friction for at least 20 seconds, and dry hands thoroughly (CDC, 2015a; Mayo Clinic, 2018).
- *Food preparation.* Ensure the patient has the resources needed to maintain basic food safety such as indoor plumbing with hot and cold water and power for a refrigerator (electricity or gas). Do not allow any person with an infectious gastrointestinal disease to prepare food until symptoms resolve. Do not thaw and then refreeze foods. Be sure cooked foods are stored immediately in clean containers in the refrigerator. Wash hands before food preparation. Do not allow raw meat items to come in contact with other food items because of a risk of spreading disease. Using a dishwasher or washing dishes in hot soapy water decreases the risk of contamination (CDC, 2017).
- *Tube feedings.* Prepare enough formula for only 8 hours (commercially prepared) or 4 hours (home prepared). Contaminated enteral feeding may cause infections in patients (e.g., *Salmonella* or staphylococcal infections). The feeding bag and tubing should be cleansed or replaced per manufacturer recommendations.
- *Linens.* Wash linens that are contaminated with blood or body fluids separately in hot, soapy water with 1 cup of bleach per load, and dry them in a dryer on the hot cycle.
- *Waste containers.* Keep waste containers available in the patient contact area for the disposal of dressings, diapers, tissues, and other disposable items. Place a sturdy bag inside the waste container to prevent spilling and leakage. Flush body fluids such as urine, vomitus, feces, and blood down the toilet.
- *Body fluid spills.* Clean up any accidental body fluid spill as soon as possible, while wearing gloves. To disinfect, spray a solution of 1 cup of bleach diluted with 10 cups of water over the spill, and clean up with paper towels. Then place the paper towels in the plastic-lined waste container.

- Reviews patient's plan of care and recommends revisions as needed.
- Reviews and follows defined prioritization for patient care.
- Uses clinical pathways, care maps, or care plans to guide and review patient care.

◆ ASSESSMENT

By evaluating signs and symptoms revealed during assessment, the nurse can determine whether a patient's clinical condition indicates a risk for infection. Early recognition of infection helps the nurse identify a patient problem and thus establish an appropriate treatment plan. In addition, the nurse should consider how well the patient is dealing with the disease and whether any resources could benefit the patient. It is important to include the patients: how does the infection affect them?

Prompt assessment of laboratory data will provide information about potential infections. Laboratory values such as increased white blood cell count or a positive blood culture often indicate infection. In assessment of laboratory data, the nurse should consider the age of the patient. For example, in the older adult, smaller amounts of bacteria such as *Salmonella* have the potential to cause gastrointestinal infections because of the decrease in bactericidal gastric acids and deterioration of the mucosal layer of the stomach.

Sometimes positive laboratory results indicate the need to use transmission-based isolation precautions. In this case, the nurse should consult the infection control nurse or refer to the facility's infection prevention and control policy manual.

◆ PATIENT PROBLEMS

The selection of patient problems is based on data collected during the assessment. Possible patient problems for patients susceptible to or affected by an infection include the following:

- *Compromised Tissue Integrity*
- *Potential for Infection* (Nursing Care Plan 7.1)
- *Social Seclusion*

◆ EXPECTED OUTCOMES AND PLANNING

The plan of care focuses on achieving specific goals and outcomes related to the patient problems chosen. Interventions are determined with the aid of the patient, the family, the physician, and other members of the health care team. These goals and outcomes possibly include the following:

Goal 1: Transmission of infectious organism is prevented.
Outcome: Patient does not experience onset of health care–associated infection (HAI).

Goal 2: Progress of infection is controlled or decreased.
Outcome: Inflammation or signs and symptoms over an involved site decrease in 5 days.

Nursing Care Plan 7.1 The Patient With an Infection

This care plan has been created for the patient who is at risk for infection. Mr. R. is a 68-year-old man in the nursing unit for 8-hour postoperative care after a bowel resection. He has intravenous fluids infusing and a urethral catheter in place.

PATIENT PROBLEM

Potential for Infection, related to presence of abdominal incision, intravenous devices, age, presence of indwelling catheter

Patient Goals and Expected Outcomes	Nursing Interventions	Evaluation
Patient remains free of the signs and symptoms of infection as evidenced by normal vital signs and absence of purulent drainage from abdominal incision, tubes, and catheter	Assess for presence or existence of risk factors, such as abdominal incision, indwelling catheter, and venous or arterial devices. Monitor white blood count (WBC). Monitor the following for signs and symptoms of infection: • Erythema (redness) • Edema (swelling) • Increased pain • Purulent exudates (drainage) at incision, exit sites of IV, indwelling urinary catheter • Elevated temperature • Color of respiratory secretions • Appearance of urine Assess nutritional status. Perform asepsis for wound care, catheter care, and IV access management. Maintain hand hygiene before patient contact and between procedures with patient. Encourage diet and fluid intake (contact dietitian as necessary). Encourage coughing and deep breathing; consider use of incentive spirometer. Teach patient and family how to perform hand hygiene correctly.	Patient demonstrates understanding of necessary precautions to prevent infection. Patient remains free of infection.

CRITICAL THINKING QUESTIONS

1. Mr. R. has a peripheral IV infusing and reports discomfort at the site of insertion. What should the nurse do?
2. Mr. R. has a urinary catheter connected to continuous drainage. He reports burning at the site of insertion, and the nurse notes dark, concentrated urine in the tubing. What should the nurse do next?
3. The nurse notes on the sheet of laboratory results for the patient that his WBC count is 2800/mm^3. Why is this a concern, and what is recommended as a precautionary measure?

◆ IMPLEMENTATION

The nurse's role is to prevent the onset and spread of infection and promote healing. By recognizing and assessing a patient's risk factors and implementing appropriate measures, the nurse has the capacity to help reduce the risk of transmitting infections. Use good hand hygiene techniques, properly use sterile supplies, and wear appropriate personal protective equipment, as indicated.

◆ EVALUATION

The success of the nurse who practices infection prevention and control techniques is measured according to the extent to which the goals are achieved for reducing or preventing infection. Evaluation is by nature ongoing because a patient's condition can change at any time. The nurse is then in a position to decide to continue nursing interventions, revise them as necessary, or determine that the problem has been resolved. This is accomplished by referring to the goals and outcomes identified when planning care.

Goal 1: Transmission of infectious organisms is controlled.
Evaluative measures: Assess patient's temperature; observe wound sites for erythema, edema, tenderness, or exudate.

Goal 2: Progression of infection is controlled or decreased.
Evaluative measures: Inspect size of inflamed area over consecutive intervals; gently palpate involved site to note reduction in tenderness.

See the Coordinated Care box for infection prevention and control procedures.

 Coordinated Care

Delegation

Infection Prevention and Control

Hand hygiene or antisepsis involves a set of basic procedures that all caregivers are obliged to perform correctly. If you observe other caregivers or family caregivers cleanse their hands incorrectly, reinforce the importance of the correct technique and procedural steps.

OBSERVE THE CONSISTENCY AND THOROUGHNESS OF STAFF IN WASHING OR DISINFECTING HANDS

Application of disposable gloves is a basic procedure that should be performed correctly by unlicensed assistive personnel (UAP). If you observe UAP failing to use gloves when necessary, reinforce the importance of the procedure.

CLARIFY FOR THE UNLICENSED ASSISTIVE PERSONNEL THE TYPE OF ISOLATION PRECAUTIONS TO USE (see Figs. 7.7 to 7.9)

Basic care procedures (e.g., bathing and feeding) that are performed for patients in transmission-based isolation can be delegated to UAP. The nurse is responsible for assessing whether it is more effective to provide direct care or delegate care activities, depending on the patient's clinical status. Procedures such as medication administration and care of IV lines require the application of critical thinking knowledge unique to the nurse.

CLARIFY FOR UNLICENSED ASSISTIVE PERSONNEL SPECIAL PRECAUTIONS IN USE OF A FITTED RESPIRATOR MASK

Basic care procedures (e.g., bathing, feeding) that are performed under airborne infection isolation (see Skill 7.5) can be delegated to UAP. The nurse is responsible for assessing whether it is more effective to provide direct care or delegate care activities, depending on the patient's clinical status. Procedures such as medication administration and care of IV lines require the critical thinking and knowledge application unique to the nurse.

Get Ready for the NCLEX® Examination!

Key Points

- The mucous membranes of the respiratory, gastrointestinal, and genitourinary tracts provide primary defense against pathogenic microorganisms, as does intact skin.
- An infection has the potential to develop as long as the six elements that compose the infectious chain are uninterrupted.
- A microorganism's virulence depends on its ability to resist attack by the body's normal defenses.
- Age, poor nutrition, stress, inherited conditions, chronic disease, and treatments or conditions that compromise the immune system increase susceptibility to infection.
- The signs of local inflammation and infection are similar, but the inflammatory response can occur in the absence of an infectious process.
- Surgical asepsis requires more stringent techniques than medical asepsis and is directed toward eliminating all microorganisms and their spores.
- Contamination of a sterile object or field occurs when it comes into contact with a wet surface that contains microorganisms or when it is exposed to airborne microorganisms.
- The CDC recommends that health care workers consider all patients as infectious and that health care workers use standard precautions to reduce the risk of exposure to blood and body fluids.
- Following aseptic principles is the key to a nurse's success in preventing patients from acquiring infection.
- Some types of equipment (e.g., sphygmomanometer or blood pressure cuff) are designated best for use in a patient who has been placed in transmission-based precautions. The item should be disinfected per hospital policy before use on other patients or discarded if it is disposable.
- Lack of proper hand hygiene is the main cause of the spread of infections.
- An infection control nurse monitors the incidence of infections within an institution and provides educational and consultative services to maintain aseptic practices to staff, patients, and their caregivers.
- Isolation transmission–based precautions are used to prevent personnel and patients from acquiring infections and prevent transmission of microorganisms to other people.
- Wearing gloves, gowns, and masks in combination with eye protection devices such as goggles or glasses with solid side shields is mandatory when contact with blood or potentially infectious material is possible or whenever splashing or spraying of blood or potentially infectious material is possible.
- The restricted environment subjects a patient in transmission-based isolation to psychological and emotional deprivation.
- Standard precautions are used to prevent the spread of organisms present in blood, all other body fluids, nonintact skin, and mucous membranes.
- Standard precautions are used with all patients because it is often unknown which patients have an infection. This includes the use of barrier protection when appropriate.
- If the skin is broken or if the nurse performs an invasive procedure into a body cavity normally free of microorganisms, surgical aseptic practices are followed.
- The major sites for health care–associated infections include the urinary and respiratory tracts, the bloodstream, and surgical or traumatic wounds.
- Nurses must be role models and keep up to date with their own immunizations and teach patients to do so.

- Proper cleansing requires mechanical removal of all foreign materials from an object or area.
- Cultural influences play a major role in patient education and follow-up care.

Additional Learning Resources

SG Go to your Study Guide for additional learning activities to help you master this chapter content.

evolve Be sure to visit the Evolve site at *http://evolve.elsevier.com/Cooper/foundationsadult/* for additional online resources.

Review Questions for the NCLEX® Examination

1. A young adult patient is admitted to a medical unit with the diagnosis of hepatitis A and placed in contact precautions. What is the primary goal of this action?
   1. To prevent transmission of infectious microorganisms
   2. To control the environment of the patient during hospitalization
   3. To protect the patient from infectious microorganisms
   4. To protect only the family from the transmission of the disease

2. The nurse is working in a clinical medical area with a census of 15. Each patient has a different illness. When planning care, the nurse recognizes which as the most important action to provide protection to each patient from health care–associated infections?
   1. Wearing a gown
   2. Placing each patient in isolation
   3. Hand hygiene
   4. Wearing gloves

3. The nurse is caring for the patient in isolation and plans to wear latex gloves. Which is an important consideration?
   1. Assess the patient and the patient's record for potential latex allergy.
   2. Vinyl gloves actually provide higher barrier protection than latex.
   3. The cost of latex gloves is significantly higher than that of synthetic gloves.
   4. Latex gloves are so reliable as barriers that hand hygiene is not required.

4. The nurse is speaking with a patient about the need to prevent infection. The nurse recognizes the patient understands proper hand hygiene when the patient makes what statement?
   1. "The water I wash my hands with should be as hot as I can tolerate to kill all of the germs on my skin."
   2. "If there isn't time to completely wash my hands, it will be all right to rinse them quickly in warm water."
   3. "After washing my hands with soap for at least 20 seconds, I will rinse them thoroughly under running water."
   4. "I will put soap into a basin of warm water, lather my hands for 15 seconds, and then rinse them in the basin."

5. The nursing instructor is discussing the chain of infection to a group of student nurses. What is the most important information about identifying the chain of infection for the health care provider?
   1. Understanding of the chain of infection allows for tests to be performed to assess resistance to communicable diseases.
   2. Recognition of the chain of infection provides information about which patients will most benefit from isolation precautions.
   3. The need for antibiotic therapy can be determined by assessing the chain of infection.
   4. Points at which the infection can be stopped or prevented can be located by identifying the chain of infection.

6. A patient in isolation is experiencing signs of social deprivation. Which intervention by the nurse is appropriate?
   1. Allow visitors to remove masks while in the patient's room.
   2. Leave the door of the negative-pressure room open slightly.
   3. Remind the patient that the isolation is for his or her own benefit.
   4. Set specific times when the nurse will return to the patient's room.

7. A middle-aged client is admitted to the hospital with cellulitis of the right foot. Three days later, the patient develops bacterial pneumonia. How would the patient's bacterial pneumonia be classified?
   1. Acute primary
   2. Health care–associated
   3. Interstitial
   4. Mycoplasmic

8. The student is reviewing sterile technique. When using the technique, the student nurse remembers to hold sterile objects in which location?
   1. Close to shoulder level
   2. Just below waist level
   3. Over the patient's bed
   4. Above waist level

9. The nurse is planning care for several patients undergoing procedures. For which procedure will the nurse gather supplies to implement surgical asepsis? *(Select all that apply.)*
   1. Inserting an IV line
   2. Performing perineal care
   3. Performing oral care
   4. Obtaining a sputum specimen
   5. Inserting an indwelling catheter

10. The nurse is performing a surgical hand scrub. During a surgical hand scrub, how are the hands to be held?
   1. Above the elbows
   2. With the fingers pointing downward
   3. Whichever way is convenient
   4. Just below the waist

11. To practice strict surgical asepsis, the nurse:
    1. adheres to principles of sterile technique.
    2. performs routine environmental cleaning.
    3. disinfects surfaces that come into contact with body fluids.
    4. maintains proper hand hygiene before and after patient care.
12. The student nurse is preparing to don sterile gloves. What action by the student indicates understanding of the needed procedure?
    1. Touch only the inside surface of the first glove while pulling it onto the hand.
    2. Place the fingers of the dominant hand into the outside cuff of the first glove.
    3. Let the cuff of the glove roll up over the hand as it is being pulled onto the hand.
    4. Begin the procedure by pulling the first glove upward and over the nondominant hand.
13. The nurse has completed a sterile procedure and is preparing to remove the soiled gloves. Place the steps in the correct order:
    1. Grasp the outer surface of the glove.
    2. Place the glove in the hand that is still gloved.
    3. Peel the second glove off, turn inside out, and discard.
    4. Take fingers of bare hand and tuck inside remaining glove cuff.
14. To remove the gloves, what action is required of the nurse?
    1. Pull each finger from each of the gloves first, then roll the glove back over the hand.
    2. Remove the glove from the nondominant hand by reaching inside the glove and pulling it off.
    3. Remove one glove, then use the bare fingers to push the remaining glove off from inside the cuff.
    4. Hold both gloved hands under running water and roll the gloves down to keep microorganisms contained.
15. Which is a principle of surgical asepsis?
    1. Any sterilized item is considered unsterile once it is allowed to fall below knee height.
    2. Sterile fields and sterilized items are no longer sterile if they contact a clean surface.
    3. A person not wearing sterile garments can come no closer to a sterile field than 3 ft.
    4. The front and back of a sterile gown being worn are considered sterile from shoulders to knees.
16. A patient isolated for pulmonary tuberculosis is expressing anger at the nurse. What action by the nurse is most appropriate? *(Select all that apply.)*
    1. Provide a dark, quiet room to calm the patient.
    2. Explain isolation procedures and provide meaningful stimulation.
    3. Reduce the level of precautions to keep the patient from becoming angry.
    4. Limit family and other caregiver visits to reduce the risk of spreading the infection.
    5. Talk with the patient about how they are feeling.
17. The nurse is assisting the physician with an irrigation of a draining abdominal wound by preparing the sterile tray. To maintain sterility of the tray, which action by the nurse is correct?
    1. Use sterile forceps while reaching across it to move the contents around.
    2. Wear clean gloves to open and touch the contents of the tray.
    3. Allow the open tray to stand unattended for 20 minutes, then cover it with a towel.
    4. Put on sterile gloves before handling the contents of the tray.
18. The nurse is presenting an educational program on the CDC's hand hygiene recommendations for implementation in a hospital. Which statement by the nurse demonstrates an understanding of the CDC's recommendation? *(Select all that apply.)*
    1. Health care providers will wear gloves at all times when providing patient care.
    2. Disinfecting hands after glove removal is not necessary according to the guidelines.
    3. Alcohol-based hand cleaner is effective on hands that are not visibly soiled with blood and body fluids.
    4. It is necessary to remove waterless alcohol-based hand cleaner with paper towels to remove pathogens from hands.
    5. The nurse should use water and soap to wash hands after caring for a patient diagnosed with *Clostridium difficile*.
19. The nurse is preparing to open the outer sterile wrap of a indwelling catheter tray. Which flap of the wrap (in which direction) should be opened first?
    1. The flap that opens away from the nurse
    2. The flap that opens to the left
    3. The flap that opens to the right
    4. The flap that opens toward the nurse
20. The patient asks the nurse how his skin will be sterilized before his surgery. What is the best response by the nurse?
    1. "We will use alcohol to sterilize your skin."
    2. "It is not possible to sterilize skin, but we will use an antimicrobial solution to eliminate most microorganisms."
    3. "There are a series of steps used in sterilizing your skin to prevent you from getting an infection."
    4. "We will use Betadine solution to sterilize your skin."

8 Body Mechanics and Patient Mobility

http://evolve.elsevier.com/Cooper/foundationsadult/

Objectives

1. State the principles of body mechanics.
2. Explain the rationale for use of appropriate body mechanics.
3. Discuss considerations related to mobility for older adults.
4. Discuss the complications of immobility.
5. Demonstrate the use of assistive devices for proper positioning.
6. State the nursing interventions used to prevent complications of immobility.
7. Demonstrate placement of patient in various positions, such as Fowler's, supine (dorsal), Sims, side-lying, prone, dorsal recumbent, and lithotomy positions.
8. State the assessment for the patient's neurovascular status, including the phenomenon of compartment syndrome.
9. Describe and demonstrate range-of-motion exercises and explain their purpose.
10. Identify complications caused by inactivity.
11. Relate appropriate body mechanics to the techniques for turning, moving, and lifting the patient.
12. Discuss use of the continuous passive motion machines.
13. Discuss the nursing process and how it relates to patient mobility.

Key Terms

abduction (ăb-DŬK-shŭn, Table 8.4, p. 171)
adduction (ă-DŬK-shŭn, Table 8.4, p. 171)
alignment (ă-LĪN-měnt, p. 161)
base of support (p. 161)
body mechanics (p. 161)
compartment syndrome (p. 169)
contracture (kŏn-TRĂK-chŭr, p. 174)
disuse syndrome (p. 174)
dorsal (supine) (DŎR-săl, sū-PĪN, p. 164)
dorsal recumbent (DŎR-săl rē-KŬM-běnt, p. 164)
dorsiflexion (dŏr-sĭ-FLĔK-shŭn, Table 8.4, p. 173)
ergonomics (p. 160)
extension (Table 8.4, p. 171)
flexion (Table 8.4, p. 171)
Fowler's (p. 164)
genupectoral (jĕ-nyū-PĔK-tŏr-ăl, p. 166)
hyperextension (hī-pŭr-ĕk-STĔN-shŭn, Table 8.4, p. 171)
immobility (p. 167)
joint (p. 171)
lithotomy (lĭ-THŎT-ō-mē, p. 166)
mobility (p. 167)
musculoskeletal disorders (MSDs) (p. 160)
orthopneic (ŏr-thōp-NĒ-ĭk, p. 165)
pronation (prō-NĀ-shŭn, Table 8.4, p. 172)
prone (p. 165)
range-of-motion (ROM) (p. 171)
semi-Fowler's (p. 165)
Sims (p. 165)
supination (sū-pĭ-NĀ-shŭn, Table 8.4, p. 172)
Trendelenburg's (Trĕn-DĔL-ĕn-bŭrgz, p. 166)

The two concepts of body mechanics and patient mobility are directly related to one another. Nursing personnel must learn and practice proper principles of body mechanics to prevent injury to themselves and injury to their patients. When assisting patients in mobility, nurses must be constantly aware of their own body mechanics. According to the Bureau of Labor Statistics (*www.bls.gov*), nursing personnel (which includes unlicensed assistive personnel [UAP], such as certified nurse assistants [CNAs], orderlies) rank second in the number of occupational injuries requiring days away from work. Nurses fall just below the top five occupations that require days away from work resulting from injuries. The majority of these injuries are classified as **musculoskeletal disorders (MSDs),** with back injuries prominent among health care personnel.

Most injuries occur when nursing personnel perform tasks that require repetitive movement, uncomfortable posture, and exertion to assist patients in activities such as feeding, dressing, bathing, toileting, repositioning, and ambulation. Awareness of proper ergonomic principles (**ergonomics** is the science of matching workplace conditions and job demands to the capabilities of workers, especially in regard to MSDs and their prevention) and good body mechanics help prevent injury.

Mechanical lifting devices (sling and standing lifts) and assistive patient-handling equipment, such as roller boards, sliders, friction-reduction pads, transfer chairs, and gait belts, work by taking on the energy and force that otherwise are imposed on the nurse during the lifting, transferring, or repositioning of a patient. Regular use of lifts and other assistive devices reduces the risk of injury (see the Evidence-Based Practice box). When a mechanical lift with a sling is used, the patient's head must be supported during transfer. To ensure safety, most facilities require two staff members be present during patient transfer with a mechanical lift. The patient should be informed of what is happening continually during the process because mechanical lifts can be frightening to the patient.

Safe patient transfer requires adequate staffing, the right mix of personnel, and appropriate, readily available, well-maintained patient-lifting equipment. The licensed practical/vocational nurse (LPN/LVN) is responsible for being competent in the appropriate and safe use of equipment and for ensuring that UAP are knowledgeable regarding proper use of assistive devices.

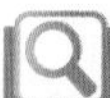 Evidence-Based Practice

Evaluation of Safe-Lift Programs

EVIDENCE SUMMARY

This study surveyed 200 long-term care facilities that used mechanical lifting devices for a 3-year period. Ninety-five percent of the facilities had mechanical lifts available for use, with an 80% compliancy of the staff using the devices. All of the facilities reported a decrease in the number of work-related injuries and worker's compensation claims after implementing a safe-lift program. Safe-lift programs incorporated the director of nursing (DON) and nursing staff to ensure that mechanical lifts were used consistently and that all nurses and UAP were trained properly in the use of the devices.

APPLICATION TO NURSING PRACTICE

- All nursing personnel must be trained in proper use of mechanical lifting devices.
- Nursing personnel should strive to use mechanical lifting devices 100% of the time that the patient's condition warrants a mechanical lift.
- DONs must convey the importance of safe-lift programs and ensure that all nursing personnel use mechanical lifts when necessary.

REFERENCE

Sheehan P: Safe-lift programs require commitment, *Long-Term Living* 60(6):46, 2011.

Equally important is the use of appropriate body mechanics or movements that protect large muscle groups from injury and provide safety for patients during ambulation assistance. Special care should be taken in the care of older adults (see the Lifespan Considerations for Older Adults box regarding mobility). Assistive devices such as splints, crutches, braces, canes, gait belts, and walkers are available to aid in promotion of patient activity. Also important is the need to teach the patient appropriate positioning for home care and to help a family member to learn how to assist the patient at home.

USE OF APPROPRIATE BODY MECHANICS

Understanding of **body mechanics** (the area of physiology for the study of muscle action and how muscles function in maintaining the posture of the body and prevention of injury during activity) includes knowledge of how certain muscle groups are used. The nurse uses body mechanics daily in making beds, assisting the patient to walk, carrying supplies and equipment, lifting, providing patient care, and carrying out other procedures.

For prevention of injury to the nurse and the patient, principles of body mechanics for health care workers (Table 8.1) should be followed by all health care professionals and personnel. Patients also should be taught principles of good body mechanics to protect themselves. The appropriate use of body mechanics should be practiced consistently in the workplace and outside the workplace so that MSDs do not occur. Maintenance of appropriate body alignment is the key factor in proper body mechanics. The term **alignment** refers to the relationship of various body parts to one another. Alignment helps balance and helps coordinate movements smoothly and effectively.

Maintenance of a wide **base of support** (a stance with feet shoulder width apart) when standing is one of the basic concepts of good body mechanics and alignment that should be followed because it helps in providing better stability (Fig. 8.1). Better stability prevents the nurse from losing proper balance while carrying out patient care, which could result in strain or injury to muscles.

The skeletal muscles and the nervous system maintain equilibrium, or balance, which facilitates appropriate body alignment when lifting, bending, moving, and performing other activities. Bending the knees and hips before attempting these activities protects the back from the stress and potential injury inherent to the physical work of nursing. When stooping, flex the hips and/or bend the knees and maintain appropriate body alignment (i.e., the back kept straight). Bending from the waist should be avoided because this will, in time, strain the lower back (Fig. 8.2). Work at a height or level that is comfortable to help prevent undue stress and strain on the back muscles. Adjust the height of the bed to a level appropriate for your height.

Use of large muscle groups (such as arm and shoulder muscles, hips, and thigh muscles) helps to perform a bigger workload more safely. The more muscle groups that are used, the more evenly the workload is distributed. If the base of support is widened in the direction of movement, less effort is needed to carry out an activity. To avoid twisting the spine, nurses should stand directly

Lifespan Considerations

Older Adults

Mobility

- The skin of older adults is more fragile and susceptible to injury. When moving or transferring older adults, avoid pulling them across bed linens because this has the potential to cause shearing or tearing of the skin.
- Always support older adults under the joints when moving them in bed. Lifting in any other manner increases the stress on the joint and causes increased pain, particularly if some degenerative joint disease exists. Explain each step in simple language, and avoid jerky, sudden movements.
- Aging tends to result in loss of flexibility and joint mobility, which often interferes with normal transfer techniques and necessitates modifications to protect patient and nurse.
- Weakness and hypotension are common signs and symptoms noted in an older adult on bed rest. Proceed slowly and cautiously when helping a patient ambulate for the first time after prolonged immobility. While facilitating independence and proper utilization of patient's body mechanics, use assistive devices such as canes, walkers, and trapeze bars. Provide adequate help to ensure patient safety when moving a patient from a lying to a sitting position and from a sitting to a standing position.
- Older adults who have many diseases or have undergone prolonged bed rest have greater risk for hypotension with postural change (orthostatic hypotension).
- Patients who use medications to reduce blood pressure are at greater risk for orthostatic hypotension.
- Older adults, particularly those with altered sensory perception, sometimes become fearful when hydraulic lifts are used for transfers. Provide eyeglasses and basic instructions.
- Limited positioning alternatives are available for the older adult who has arthritis, neuropathies, or other restrictive conditions.
- Discourage older adult patients from sitting for prolonged periods of time without stretching and moving. Lack of movement presents a risk for contractures of joints.
- Ensuring good body alignment when the patient is sitting is a way to prevent joint and muscle stress.
- Provide patient teaching that includes use of strong joints and large muscle groups for activities that require extra strength to prevent strain and pain in joints.
- For older adult patients with osteoporosis, encourage appropriate exercise programs that prevent fractures and reduce bone loss.
- Encourage exercise programs for those older adults who do not participate in regular exercise. Ensure that patients consult with their health care provider before beginning any exercise program.
- Special adjustments to an exercise program are often necessary to prevent any problems for those older adults in advanced age.
- Older adults who are not able to participate in a structured exercise program are frequently able to achieve improved circulation and joint mobility by stretching and by exaggerating normal movements.

Data from Potter PA, Perry AG, Stocket PA, et al: *Fundamentals of nursing: Concepts, process, and practice*, ed 9, St. Louis, 2017, Mosby.

Table 8.1 Body Mechanics for Health Care Workers

ACTION	RATIONALE
When planning to move a patient, arrange for adequate help. Use mechanical aids if help is unavailable.	Two workers lifting together divide the workload by 50%.
Encourage patient to assist as much as possible.	This promotes patient's abilities and strength while keeping workload to a minimum.
Keep back, neck, pelvis, and feet aligned. Avoid twisting.	Twisting increases risk of injury.
Flex knees; keep feet shoulder length apart.	A broad base of support increases stability.
Position yourself close to patient (or object being lifted).	This minimizes strain and undue stress on the lifter. Holding an object or patient away from the body increases the workload.
Use arms and legs (not back).	The leg muscles are stronger larger muscles capable of greater work without injury.
Slide patient toward yourself using a pull sheet.	Sliding requires less effort than lifting. Pull sheet keeps to a minimum any shearing forces, which can damage patient's skin.
Set (tighten) abdominal and gluteal muscles in preparation for move.	Preparing muscles for the load limits strain to the least possible level.[a]
Person with the heaviest load coordinates efforts of team involved by counting to 3.	Simultaneous lifting keeps the load for any one lifter to a minimum.

[a]Back injuries are still the most common occupational injury among nurses.

in front of the person or object with which they are working.

Nurses have numerous other ways to protect themselves and the patient from injury. Carrying objects close to the midline of the body (see Fig. 8.2), avoiding reaching too far, avoiding lifting when other means of movement are available (such as sliding, rolling, pushing, or pulling), using devices instead of or in combination with lifting, and using alternating periods of rest and activity are just a few of the ways to prevent injury. Knowing the maximum weight that is safe to carry is also important. Many facilities suggest a 50-lb weight limit on lifting for their staff.

Nurses should assess their own abilities and limitations and those of the person helping, if working in pairs. Correct use of body mechanics is essential to provide efficient care while preventing injury (Box 8.1).

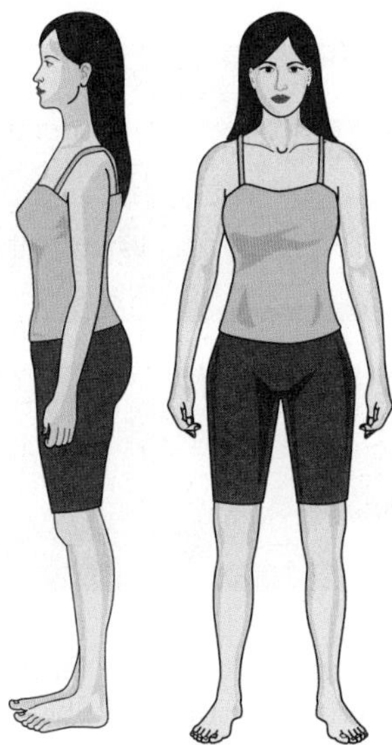

Fig. 8.1 Good position for body mechanics: chin is high and parallel to the floor, abdomen is tightened (internal girdle) in and up with the gluteal muscles tucked in, and feet are spread apart for a broad base of support.

POSITIONING OF PATIENTS

Positioning of patients is a common intervention performed by nursing personnel. Many positions can be used to prevent patients from development of complications (Skill 8.1 and the Patient Teaching box on mobility). Inappropriate positioning poses the risk of causing permanent disability.

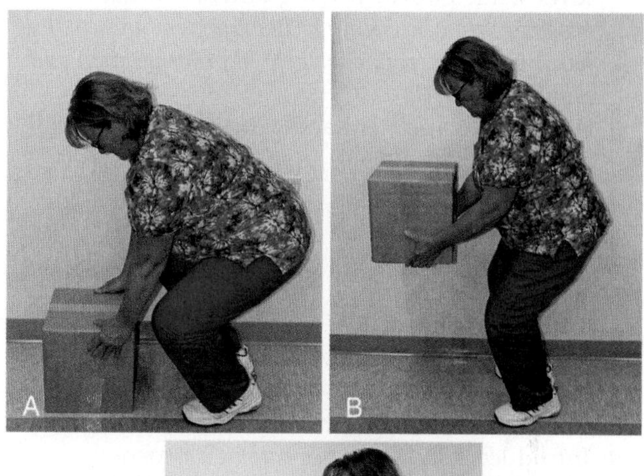

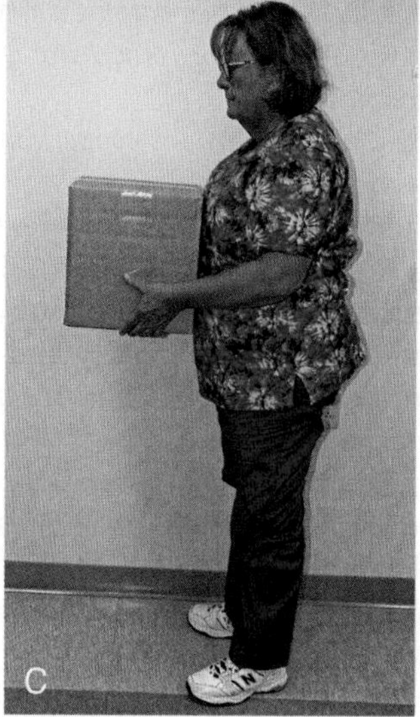

Fig. 8.2 Picking up a box with use of good body mechanics. Box is carried close to the nurse's body and base of support.

Box 8.1 Correct Use of Body Mechanics

Actions to promote proper body mechanics *(Rationale)*:

- Position feet shoulder width apart. *(Provides adequate base of support.)*
- Align and balance weight on both feet. *(Distributes weight evenly.)*
- Flex knees slightly. *(Prevents hyperextension [extreme or abnormal stretching].)*
- Tilt pelvis forward by pulling buttocks inward so that gluteal muscles are contracted in and down. *(Helps straighten the lumbar curve of the spine, increasing power and reducing strain.)*
- Contract abdominal muscles in and up. *(Provides support and reduces muscle strain.)*
- Hold chest up. *(Allows adequate lung expansion.)*
- Keep head erect. *(Helps maintain appropriate alignment of the spine.)*
- Use appropriate body mechanics in all activities: standing, sitting, bending, and lifting. *(Produces most efficient body movement.)*
- Face your work area. *(Prevents unnecessary twisting.)*
- Push, slide, or pull heavy objects. *(Places less strain on body than lifting does.)*
- Lift twice—first mentally, and then physically. *(Helps determine whether assistance is needed.)*
- Do not lift objects higher than chest level. Do not reach above your shoulders. *(Use of a step stool to reach an object higher than chest level is much safer.)*

Skill 8.1 Positioning Patients

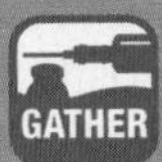

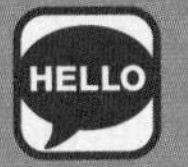

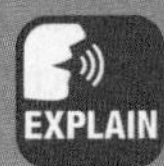

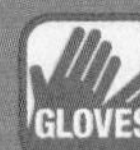

NURSING ACTION *(RATIONALE)*

1. Assess patient's body alignment and comfort level while patient is lying down. *(Provides baseline data concerning body alignment and comfort level. Helps determine ways to improve position and alignment.)*
2. Assemble equipment and supplies. *(Organizes procedure.)*
    - Pillows
    - Footboard
    - Trochanter roll
    - Splinting devices
    - Hand rolls
    - Safety reminder devices
    - Side rails
3. Request assistance as needed. *(Provides for safety.)*
4. Introduce self. *(Decreases patient's anxiety.)*
5. Identify patient. *(Ensures procedure is performed with correct patient.)*
6. Explain procedure. *(Enlists cooperation from patient and decreases patient anxiety.)*
7. Perform hand hygiene. Wear gloves as necessary according to agency policy and guidelines from the Centers for Disease Control and Prevention (CDC) and Occupational Safety and Health Administration (OSHA). *(Reduces spread of microorganisms.)*
8. Prepare patient. *(Prepares for procedure.)*
    a. Close door or pull curtain. *(Provides privacy.)*
    b. Raise level of bed to comfortable working height. *(Promotes good body mechanics in the nurse and safety for the patient.)*
    c. Remove pillows and devices used in previous position. *(Makes access to patient easier.)*
    d. Put bed in flat position, or as low as patient can tolerate, and lower side rail closest to you. *(Facilitates procedure.)*
9. Position patient.
    a. **Dorsal (supine)** position (lying flat on the back) (see illustration).
        (1) Place patient on back with head of bed flat. *(Necessary for placing patient in supine position.)*
        (2) Place small rolled towel under lumbar area of back. *(Provides support for lumbar spine.)*
        (3) Place pillow under upper shoulder, neck, and head. *(Maintains correct alignment and prevents flexion contractures of cervical lumbar spine.)*
        (4) Place trochanter rolls parallel to lateral surface of thighs. *(Reduces external rotation of hip.)*
        (5) Place small pillow or roll under ankle to elevate heels. *(Reduces pressure on heels, helping to prevent skin impairment.)*
        (6) Support feet in dorsiflexion with firm pillow, footboard, or high-top sneakers. *(Prevents foot drop.)*
        (7) Place pillows under pronated forearms, keeping upper arms parallel to patient's body (see illustration). *(Reduces internal rotation of shoulder and prevents extension of elbows. Maintains correct body alignment.)*
        (8) Place hand rolls in patient's hands. *(Reduces extension of fingers and abduction of thumb.)*

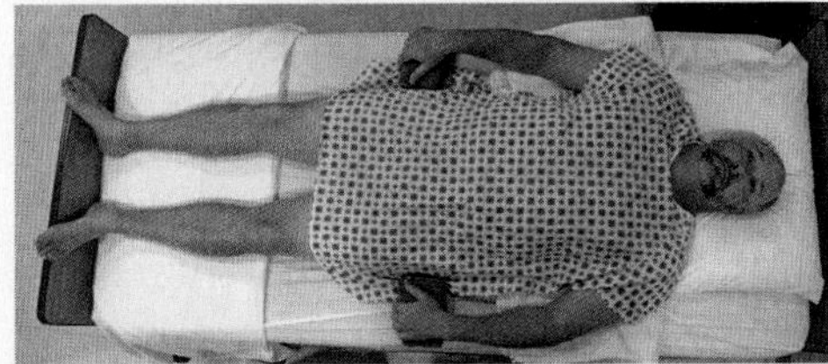

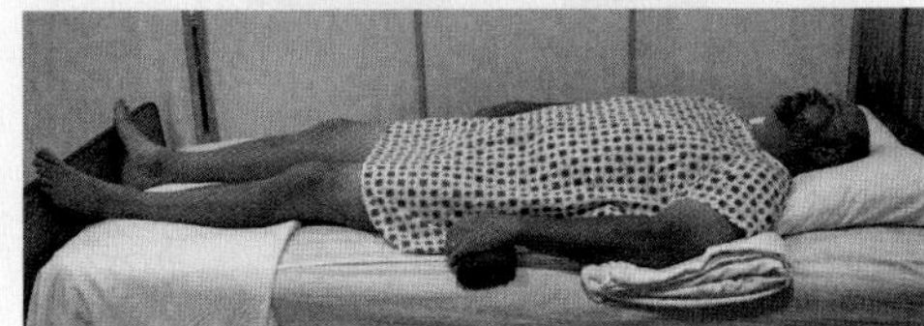

    b. **Dorsal recumbent** position (supine position with patient lying on back, head, and shoulder with extremities moderately flexed; legs are sometimes extended).
        (1) Move patient and mattress to head of bed. *(Ensures appropriate body alignment.)*
        (2) Turn patient onto back. *(Appropriately positions patient.)*
        (3) Assist patient to raise legs, bend knees, and allow legs to relax. *(Puts patient in dorsal recumbent position.)*
        (4) Replace pillow. Patient sometimes needs a small lumbar pillow. *(Provides comfort.)*
    c. **Fowler's** position (posture assumed by patient when head of bed is raised 45 to 60 degrees) (see illustration).
        (1) Move patient and mattress to head of bed. *(Ensures appropriate body alignment.)*
        (2) Raise head of bed to 45 to 60 degrees. *(Positions patient appropriately.)*
        (3) Replace pillow. *(Provides comfort, maintains proper body alignment, and ensures skin integrity.)*

Skill 8.1 Positioning Patients—cont'd

(4) Use footboard or firm pillow. *(Prevents patient from slipping down in bed.)*
(5) Use pillows to support arms and hands. *(Provides comfort and maintains correct alignment.)*
(6) Place small pillow or roll under ankles. *(Reduces risk of skin impairment over heels.)*

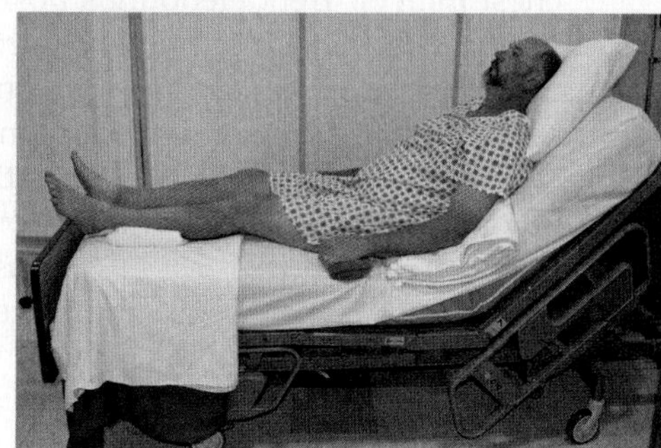

d. Semi-Fowler's position (posture assumed by patient when head of bed is raised approximately 30 degrees).
(1) Move patient and mattress to head of bed. *(Ensures appropriate body alignment.)*
(2) Raise head of bed to about 30 degrees. *(Positions patient appropriately.)*
(3) Replace pillow. *(Provides patient comfort.)* See Step 9c for positioning of pillows.

e. Orthopneic position (posture assumed by the patient sitting up in bed at 90-degree angle, or sometimes resting in forward tilt while supported by pillow on overbed table) (see illustration). Often used for the patient with a cardiac or respiratory condition.
(1) Elevate head of bed to 90 degrees. *(Facilitates positioning.)* Patient sometimes sits on side of bed with legs dangling or propped on a chair.
(2) Place pillow between patient's back and mattress. *(Provides back support.)*
(3) Place pillow on overbed table and assist patient to lean over, placing head on pillow. *(Facilitates ease of breathing. Women are more comfortable with arms on pillow and head on arms.)*

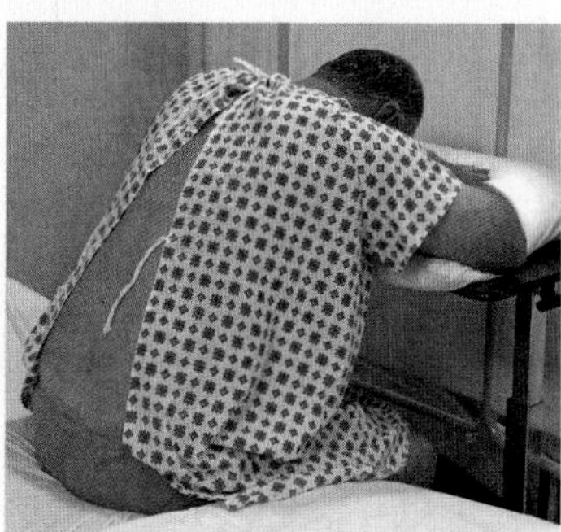

f. Sims position (position in which patient lies on side with knee and thigh drawn upward toward chest) (see illustration). The left Sims position is appropriate for the enema procedure and administration of a rectal suppository.
(1) Place patient in supine position. *(Prepares patient for position.)*
(2) Position patient in lateral position, lying partially on the abdomen. *(Patient is rolled only partially on abdomen.)*
(3) Draw knee and thigh up near abdomen and support with pillows. *(Positions patient appropriately.)*
(4) Place patient's lower arm along the back. *(Provides appropriate body alignment.)*
(5) Bring upper arm up, flex elbow, and support with pillow. *(Provides comfort and decreases strain on joints.)*
(6) Allow patient to lean forward to rest on chest. *(Provides maximum comfort.)*

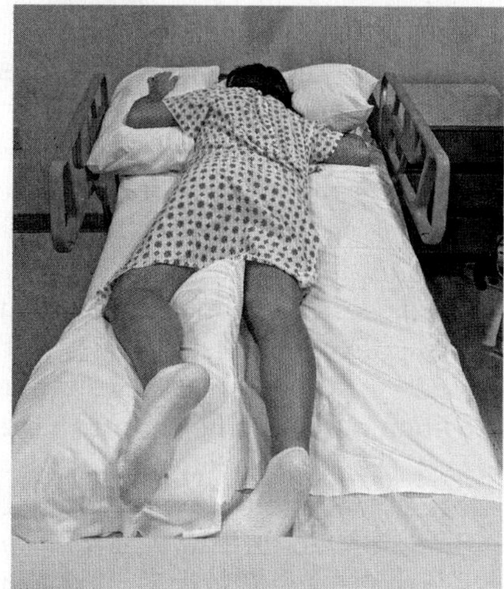

g. Prone position (lying face down in horizontal position) (see illustration).
(1) Assist patient onto abdomen with face to one side. *(Facilitates positioning.)*
(2) Flex arms toward the head. *(Provides appropriate body alignment.)*
(3) Position pillows for comfort. Place a pillow under lower leg to release any "pull" on the lower back, or place a pillow under the head as shown (or both). *(Increases comfort and maintains proper body alignment.)*

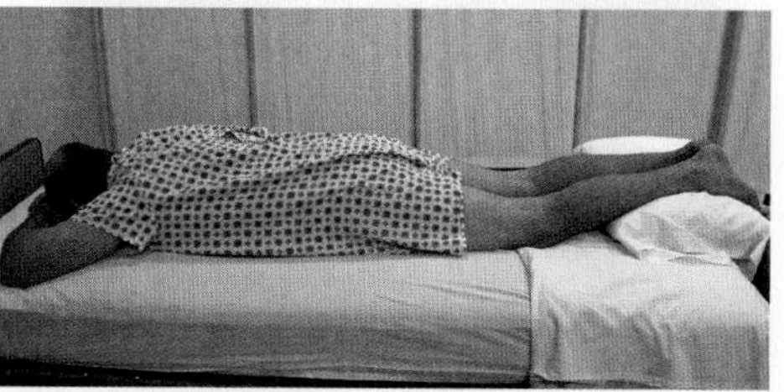

Continued

Skill 8.1 Positioning Patients—cont'd

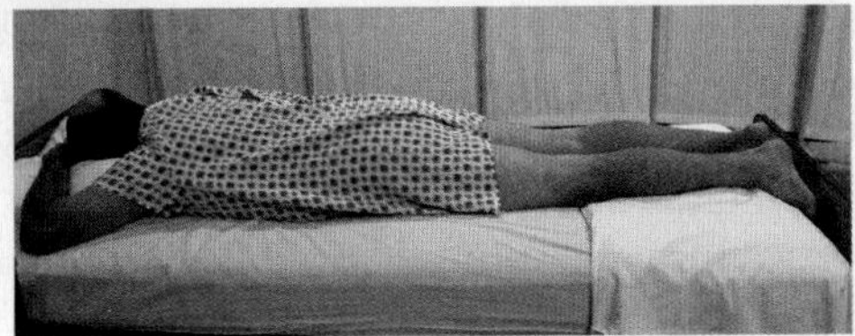

h. Knee-chest (**genupectoral**) position (patient kneels so that weight of body is supported by knees and chest, with abdomen raised, head turned to one side, and arms flexed) (see illustration).

(1) Turn patient onto abdomen. *(Facilitates positioning.)*

(2) Assist patient into kneeling position; arms and head rest on pillow while upper chest rests on bed. *(Allows for as much comfort as possible in this position.)*

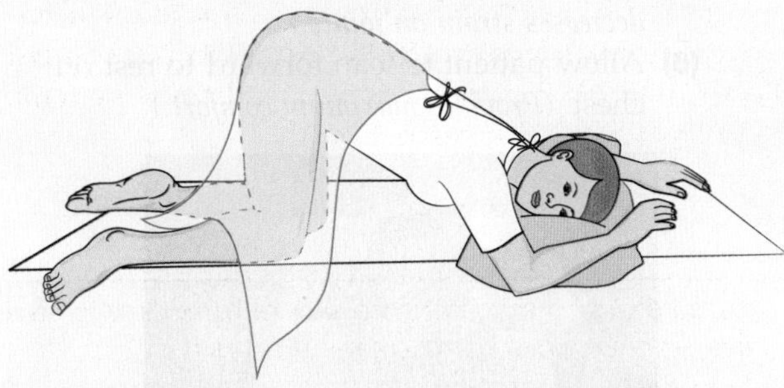

i. Lithotomy position (patient lies supine with hips and knees flexed and thighs abducted and rotated externally [sometimes feet are positioned in stirrups]) (see illustration).

(1) Position patient to lie supine (lying on the back). *(Facilitates positioning.)*

(2) Request patient to slide buttocks to edge of examining table. *(Facilitates positioning.)*

(3) Lift both legs; have patient bend knees and place feet in stirrups. *(Positions patient appropriately.)*

(4) Drape patient. *(Provides privacy.)*

(5) Provide small lumbar pillow if desired. *(Provides comfort. Pillow under head also provides comfort.)*

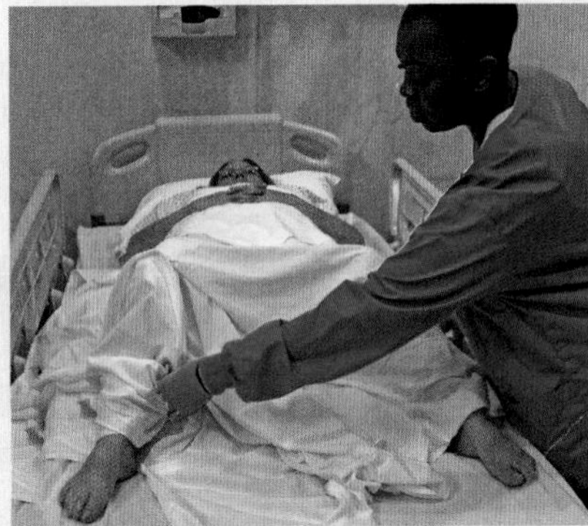

j. Trendelenburg's position (patient's head is low and the body and legs are on inclined plane) (see illustration).

(1) Place patient's head lower than body, with body and legs elevated and on an incline. Foot of bed is sometimes elevated on blocks (not used if patient has a head or chest injury). Trendelenburg's position was used to treat shock but now is used less often because it causes pressure on the diaphragm by organs in the abdomen and shunts more blood to the brain rather than all of the vital organs. This position is sometimes used to assist in venous distention during central line placement.

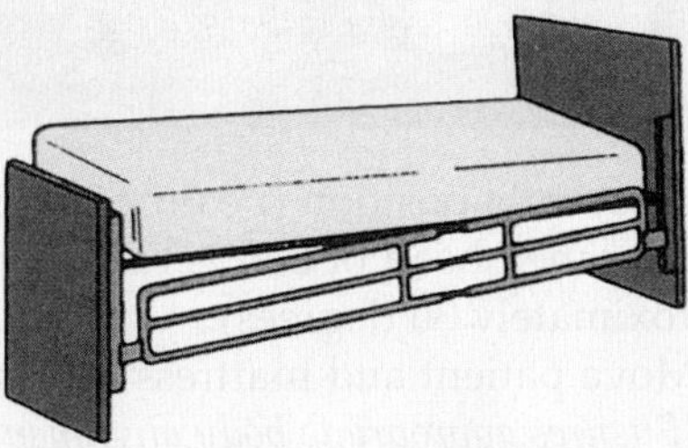

k. Lateral position (see Chapter 9).

10. Assess patient for the following: *(Provides follow-up with appropriate nursing interventions.)*
- *Proper body alignment.* Small children often need to be propped with pillows to help them maintain a position.
- *Comfort.* Performing a back massage after turning from one position to another helps prevent impaired skin integrity.
- *Skin integrity.* Skin of older adults is often thin, lacks elasticity, and needs special care to prevent tearing and further impaired skin integrity.
- *Breathing.* Additional support is necessary in some positions if patient finds ease of respiratory effort difficult to maintain.
- *Tolerance of position.* Ongoing observations regarding patient's activity tolerance is provided, and complications of immobility are indicated.
- *Repositioning.* Reposition debilitated, unconscious, or paralyzed patients at least every 2 hours.

11. Perform hand hygiene. *(Reduces spread of microorganisms.)*

12. Document. *(Records procedure, patient's response, and effectiveness of nursing interventions.)*
- Procedure
- Observations (e.g., skin condition, joint movement, patient's ability to assist with positioning)
- Patient teaching (see the Patient Teaching and Home Care Considerations boxes).

Patient Teaching

Mobility

- Instruct the patient and the family on proper mobility techniques.
- Teach the patient ways to assist with positioning.
- Provide the opportunity for return demonstration.
- Teach the patient and the family signs and symptoms of skin impairment and contractures.
- Teach the patient to avoid prolonged sitting. Frequent stretching decreases joint and muscle contractures.
- Teach the importance of maintaining skin integrity.
- Explain the importance of proper body alignment.
- Explain the importance of rising slowly from lying to sitting, from sitting to standing, and after stooping (prevents orthostatic hypotension).
- Provide time for questions and answers.
- Emphasize the importance of the patient performing active range-of-motion (ROM) exercises when possible.
- If the patient's height prevents the feet from touching the floor when sitting, teach the patient to rest feet on a footstool.
- For prevention of thrombophlebitis, teach patients not to cross their legs when sitting and to avoid prolonged immobility. Teach those at increased risk the signs and symptoms of thrombophlebitis.

MOBILITY VERSUS IMMOBILITY

Mobility is a person's ability to move around freely in his or her environment. Moving about serves many purposes, including exercising, expressing emotion, attaining basic needs, performing recreational activities, and completing activities of daily living (ADLs; those activities of physical self-care such as bathing, dressing, and eating). In addition, mobility is fundamental to maintaining the body's normal physiologic activities. For normal physical mobility, the body's nervous, muscular, and skeletal systems must be intact, functioning, and used regularly. Although a person may welcome a rare day to lie in bed and rest, the person who is *immobile* (experiencing **immobility,** the inability to move around freely) is predisposed to a wide variety of complications (Box 8.2).

Many types of health problems potentially lead to a decline in a patient's mobility. Patients with certain illnesses, injuries, or surgeries sometimes experience a period of immobilization as a result of changes in medical and physical status. In some cases, immobilization also is used therapeutically to limit the movement of the whole body or a body part, and some patients are under ambulation restrictions.

Box 8.2 Complications of Immobility and Preventive Measures

COMPLICATIONS

- *Anorexia* (decreased appetite): Lack of mobility slows the digestive process and slows the metabolic rate, causing decreased appetite.
- *Constipation:* Immobility slows peristalsis, resulting in stool remaining in the colon longer and muscle atrophy in the abdominal muscles that aid in expulsion of stool.
- *Contractures:* When muscles, ligaments, and tendons are not shortened and lengthened with movement, a permanent shortening of these structures may occur.
- *Disorientation:* Lack of stimulation, decreased endorphin production, decreased need for thought processes, and decreased socialization may lead to disorientation.
- *Disuse osteoporosis:* Lack of weight bearing on bones causes bone demineralization, allowing fractures to occur more easily.
- *Hypostatic pneumonia:* Decreased aeration and accumulation of secretions lead to inflammation and infection in the lungs.
- *Insomnia:* Decreased stimuli, depression, and frequent napping during the day as a result of immobility may cause difficulty sleeping at night.
- *Muscle atrophy and asthenia* (muscle weakness): Muscles decrease in size and strength when not continually used.
- *Orthostatic hypotension* (drop in systolic blood pressure of 20 mm Hg or a decrease of 10 mm Hg in diastolic blood pressure within 3 minutes of standing when moving from lying or sitting to standing position): Immobility can lead to a decrease in venous return or decreased cardiac output in response to postural change.
- *Pressure ulcer:* Tissue ischemia (lack of blood flow to an area) from unrelieved pressure results in skin breakdown.
- *Pulmonary embolism* (blood clot that has traveled to the lungs): Deep vein thrombosis (DVT) that has broken loose from vessel and has traveled to the lungs, causing a blockage in a pulmonary vessel.
- *Renal calculi* (kidney stones): Urinary stasis from immobility leads to slowed calcium metabolism, thus leading to stone formation.
- *Thrombophlebitis and DVT* (blood clot with accompanying inflammation of the involved vein, usually of the lower extremity): Decrease in venous circulation allows blood to pool in lower extremities, leading to inflammation of vessels and clot formation.
- *Urinary tract infection:* Urinary stasis causes changes in pH and allows bacterial growth.

INTERVENTIONS

- Reposition at least every 2 hours
- Ensure adequate intake; encourage fluids
- Encourage a well-balanced diet
- Prevent deformities (e.g., footboard or other measures to prevent foot drop)
- Handle and transfer patients carefully; maintain proper body alignment
- Position lower extremities properly (a pillow or wedge between the legs, never under knees)
- Early ambulation
- Antiembolism measures (thromboembolic deterrent [TED] hose or decompression boots)
- Progressive ambulation

Continued

Box 8.2 Complications of Immobility and Preventive Measures—cont'd

- Roll up head of bed
- Dangle over side of bed
- Stand
- Take a few steps
- Sit in the chair
- Up to bathroom
- Up and about the room
- Up and out in the hallway
- Up as desired

DURING AMBULATION

1. Observe the patient closely.
2. Encourage the patient to do the following:
   - Take slow, deep breaths
   - Keep eyes open and look straight ahead
   - Keep head up

   (These measures aid in preventing vertigo, syncope, weakness, and nausea and vomiting.)
3. If the patient starts to fall, do not attempt to prevent the fall. Ease the patient to the floor. This allows you to break the fall, control its direction, and protect the patient's head. Follow these steps when assisting a patient's fall:
   - Stand with your feet apart. Keep your back straight.
   - Bring the patient close to your body as quickly as possible. Use the gait belt if one is worn. If not, wrap your arms around the patient's waist. Move your leg so that the patient's buttocks rest on it. Move the leg near the patient (see illustration).
   - Lower the patient to the floor by letting the patient slide down your leg. Bend at your hips and knees as you lower the patient (see illustration). *(The gravitational pull allows the patient to be lowered to the floor with a minimal amount of strain to your musculoskeletal system.)*
   - Call for assistance.
   - Assist patient to return to bed.
   - Report and document the following:
     - How the fall occurred
     - How far the patient walked
     - How activity was tolerated before the fall
     - Any report of symptoms before the fall
     - The amount of assistance needed by the patient while walking
     - Complete an incident report, if required. *(Know agency policy.)*
4. On a daily basis encourage the following:
   - Deep breathing and coughing exercises (spirometry)
   - Careful use of medications
5. Be certain to provide the following:
   - Suitable diversion
   - Meticulous skin care
   - Range-of-motion exercises
   - Reality therapy

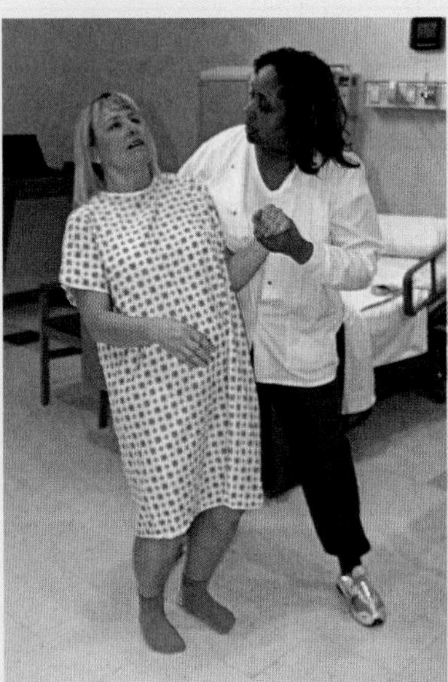

May support the falling patient under the arms as shown.

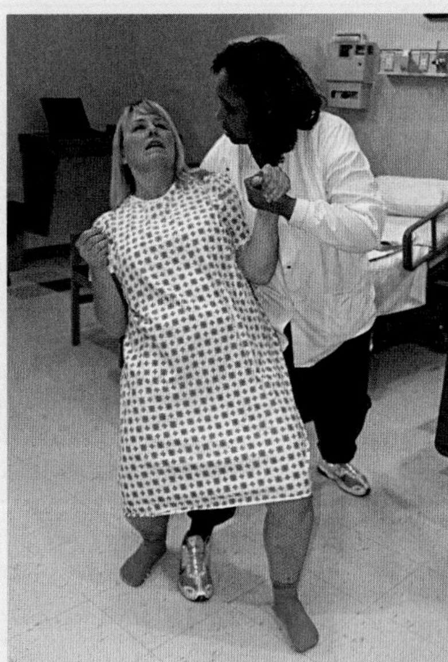

The patient's buttocks rest on your leg.

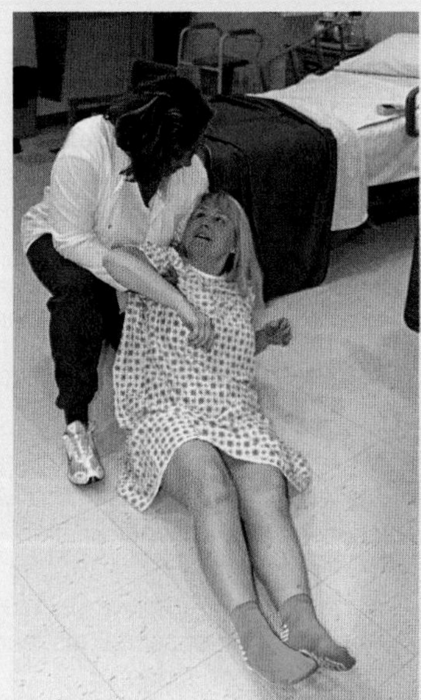

Slide the patient down your leg to the floor.

Interventions to prevent complications of immobility are varied, and many do not require a physician's order (see Box 8.2).

Various assistive devices help maintain correct body positioning and prevent complications that commonly arise when a patient needs prolonged bed rest (Table 8.2). Several of the devices are especially useful in the care of patients who have a loss of sensation, mobility, or consciousness (Figs. 8.3 to 8.5).

NEUROVASCULAR FUNCTION

One of the responsibilities of the nurse is frequent monitoring of the patient's neurovascular function, or

Table 8.2 Common Assistive Devices Used for Proper Patient Positioning

ASSISTIVE DEVICE	COMMON USES
Pillow	Provides support of body or extremity (e.g., placing behind the patient's back when in lateral position); elevation of body parts (e.g., the arm or leg; splinting of the incision in the postoperative patient during activity or coughing and deep breathing)
Foot drop boots or foot boards	Maintains the foot in dorsiflexion position, which prevents foot drop (plantar flexion)
Trochanter roll (see Fig. 8.3)	Prevents external rotation of legs when patient is in supine position
Hand roll (see Fig. 8.4)	Maintains hand in a normal position; prevents skin-to-skin contact of palm of hand; maintains fingers in slightly flexed position
Hand-wrist splint	Maintains proper alignment of the lower arm and hand; maintains wrist in slight dorsiflexion
Trapeze bar (see Fig. 8.5)	Allows the patient to raise the trunk from bed to assist in movement; allows patient to perform exercises that strengthen upper arms
Side rail	Helps the patient to roll from side to side or to sit up in bed; gives a sense of security in a hospital bed
Bed board	Provides additional firmness to mattress
Abductor splint	Used to maintain the legs in abduction after total hip replacement surgery (see Fig. 8.6)

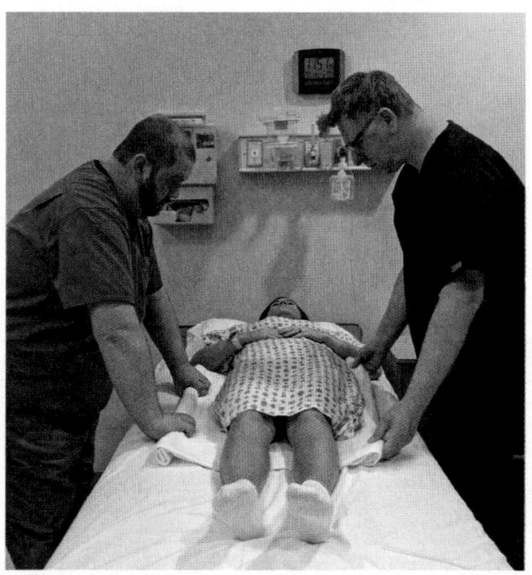

Fig. 8.3 Trochanter roll.

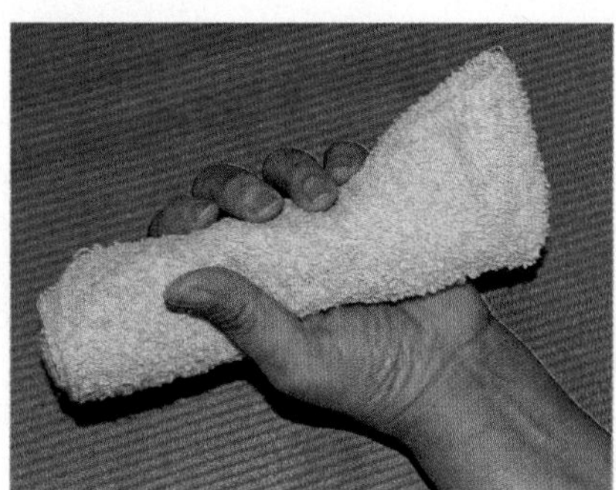

Fig. 8.4 Hand roll.

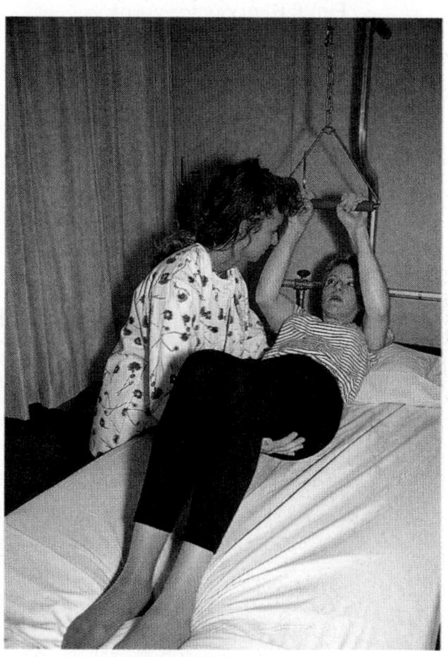

Fig. 8.5 Patient using a trapeze bar. (From Potter PA, Perry AG: *Essentials for nursing practice,* ed 8, St. Louis, 2015, Mosby.)

circulation, movement, and sensation (CMS) assessment. The LPN/LVN checks for skin color, temperature, movement, sensation, pulses, capillary refill, and pain. The affected limb should be compared with the unaffected one (Table 8.3).

This assessment is especially important when compression from external devices, such as casts and bulky dressings, creates the risk of acute **compartment syndrome,** which has the potential to cause extensive tissue damage. Acute compartment syndrome occurs in the extremities, especially the legs, where a sheath of inelastic fascia partitions blood vessel, nerve, and muscle tissue. Normally, the pressure in this compartment is less than capillary pressure. However, compression created by external pressure or the accumulation of excessive tissue fluid from severe burns, fractures, crushing injuries, or severely bruised muscles increases compartmental pressure and in some cases leads to compartment syndrome. Permanent nerve damage with irreversible muscle function can occur within 12

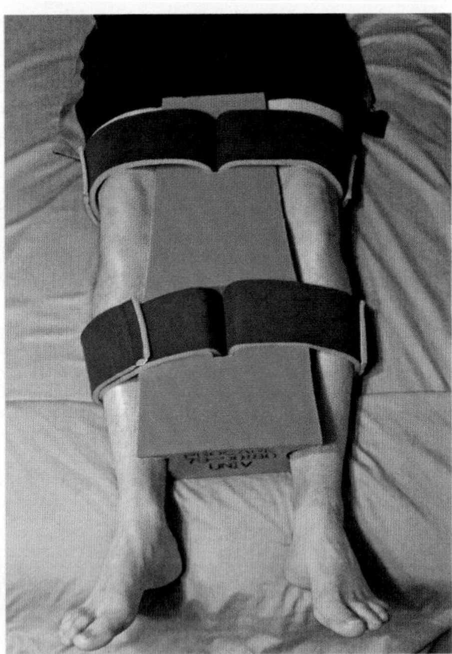

Fig. 8.6 Abductor splint.

to 24 hours if the compression of these structures is not reversed (NLM, 2014).

Symptoms of acute compartment syndrome include pain within the muscle, especially when stretched, which is more intense than expected from the injury or causative factor; tingling and burning or a feeling of pins and needles in the affected area (paresthesias); and a full or tight feeling in the muscle. Numbness and paralysis are late signs of compartment syndrome and may be indicative of permanent damage.

Acute compartment syndrome is an emergency situation. The earlier compartment syndrome is treated, the better the prognosis. If acute compartment syndrome is caused by an external device, such as a cast or tight bandage, the pressure should be removed immediately by cutting away these devices. If the syndrome is caused by other factors, surgical intervention may be required. A fasciotomy may be necessary, in which the surgeon makes an incision into the skin and fascia to release the pressure. This incision is sometimes left open until swelling subsides.

Table 8.3 Assessment of Neurovascular Status

CHARACTERISTIC	ASSESSMENT TECHNIQUE	NORMAL FINDINGS
Skin color	Inspect the color of the skin distal to the injury.	The skin color should match that of the unaffected body part.
Skin temperature	Palpate the area distal to the injury to determine whether any change in skin temperature has occurred compared with other body parts.	The skin is warm to the touch.
Movement	Ask the patient to move the affected area or the area distal to the injury, unless contraindicated.	The patient is able to move with minimal difficulty and with minimal, if any, discomfort.
	Move the area distal to the injury if the patient is unable to move the body part on his or her own.	No difference in comfort is found compared with the patient actively moving the body part.
Sensation	Ask the patient if numbness or tingling is present (paresthesia), and assess with proper devices as necessary, such as a cotton-tipped applicator or tongue blade.	No numbness or tingling occurs; no difference in sensation is seen in the affected and unaffected body parts.
	Assess sensation with a cotton-tipped applicator, tongue blade, or other device as indicated.	Loss of sensation may indicate nerve or circulatory impairment.
Pulses	Palpate the pulses distal to the site of injury.	Pulses are strong and easily palpated; no difference is found in the affected and unaffected extremities.
Capillary refill	Press the nail beds distal to the injury until blanching occurs (or until the skin near the nail blanches, if nails are thick and brittle); pressure should be applied for approximately 3 to 5 sec.	Blood returns (return to usual color) within 3 sec (5 sec for older adult patients).
Pain	Ask the patient about the location, the nature, and the frequency of pain and to rate the pain with a pain scale.	The patient should have no or minimal reports of pain.

Chronic compartment syndrome is not an emergency situation and usually is caused by exercise that involves repetitive movement, such as bicycling or running. The symptoms include pain and cramping during exercise, visible muscle bulging, and numbness. These symptoms usually are alleviated by discontinuing the activity and by rest.

PERFORMANCE OF RANGE-OF-MOTION EXERCISES

Regardless of whether the causes of immobility are permanent or temporary, the immobilized patient needs some type of exercise to prevent excessive muscle atrophy and joint contracture. The nurse and other health care personnel, including members of the physical therapy department, help the patient with decreased mobility to perform **range-of-motion (ROM)**; movement of the body that involves the muscles and joints in natural directional movements) exercises. *Passive* ROM exercise is performed by caregivers, and *active* ROM by patients. The designated **joint** (any one of the connections between bones) is moved actively or passively to the point of resistance or pain, with avoidance of injury. ROM exercises are increased with subsequent exercises as tolerated (Table 8.4 and Skill 8.2).

Table 8.4 Joint Range-of-Motion Exercises

BODY PART	TYPE OF JOINT	TYPE OF MOVEMENT
Neck and cervical spine	Pivotal	*Flexion*[a]*:* Bring chin to rest on chest. *Extension*[b]*:* Return head to erect position. *Hyperextension*[c]*:* Bend head back as far as possible. Use caution with older adults. *Lateral flexion:* Tilt head as far as possible toward each shoulder. *Rotation:* Turn head as far as possible to right and left.
Shoulder	Ball and socket	*Flexion:* Raise arm from side position forward to position above head. *Extension:* Return arm to position at side of body. *Hyperextension:* Move arm behind body, keeping elbow straight.
Shoulder—cont'd		*Abduction*[d]*:* Raise arm to side to position above head with palm away from head. *Adduction*[e]*:* Lower arm sideways and across body as far as possible. *Internal rotation:* With elbow flexed, rotate shoulder by moving arm until thumb is turned inward and toward back. *External rotation:* With elbow flexed, move arm until thumb is upward and lateral to head. *Circumduction*[f]*:* Move arm in full circle. (Circumduction is combination of all movements of ball-and-socket joint.)

[a]Flexion: Movement of certain joints that decreases angle between two adjoining bones.
[b]Extension: Movement of certain joints that increases angle between two adjoining bones.
[c]Hyperextension: Extreme or abnormal extension beyond normal joint ability.
[d]Abduction: Movement of the arm or leg away from body.
[e]Adduction: Movement of the arm or leg toward axis of body.
[f]Circumduction: Movement of a body part in a 360-degree circular motion, usually involves the arm or leg.

Continued

Table 8.4 Joint Range-of-Motion Exercises—cont'd

BODY PART	TYPE OF JOINT	TYPE OF MOVEMENT
Elbow	Hinge 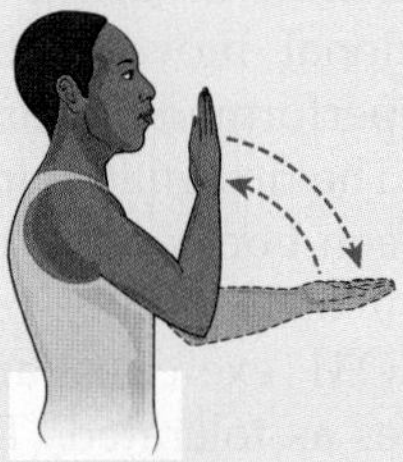	*Flexion:* Bend elbow so that lower arm moves toward its shoulder joint and hand is level with shoulder. *Extension:* Straighten elbow by lowering hand. *Hyperextension:* Bend lower arm back as far as possible.
Forearm	Pivotal 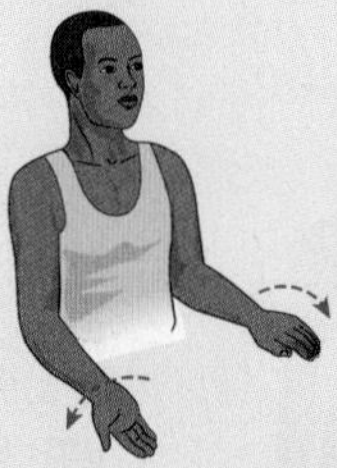	*Supination*[g]: Turn lower arm and hand so that palm is up. *Pronation*[h]: Turn lower arm so that palm is down.
Wrist	Condyloid 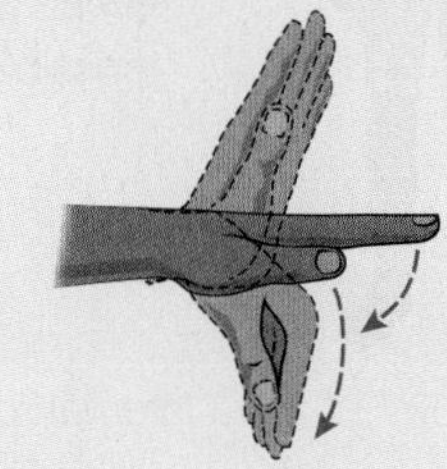 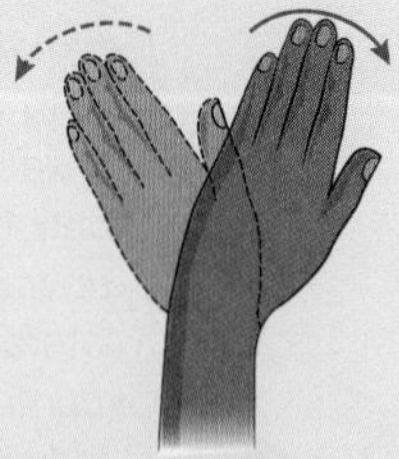	*Flexion:* Move palm toward inner aspect of forearm. *Extension:* Move fingers so that fingers, hands, and forearm are in same plane, in a straight line. *Hyperextension:* Bring dorsal surface of hand back as far as possible. *Radial flexion:* Bend wrist medially toward thumb. *Ulnar flexion:* Bend wrist laterally toward fifth finger.
Fingers	Condyloid hinge 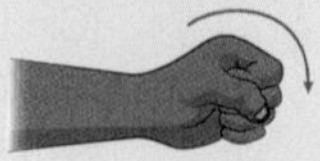 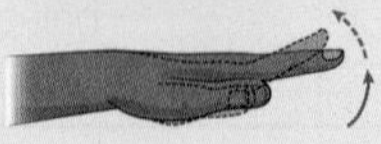	*Flexion:* Make fist. *Extension:* Straighten fingers. *Hyperextension:* Bend fingers back as far as possible.
Fingers—cont'd	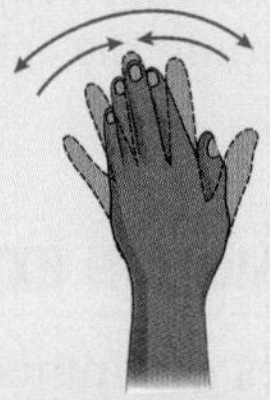	*Abduction:* Spread fingers apart. *Adduction:* Bring fingers together.
Thumb	Saddle 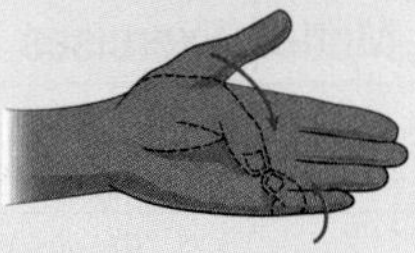 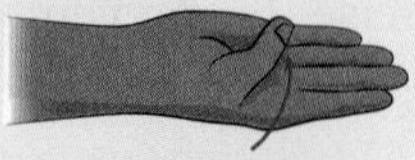	*Flexion:* Move thumb across palmar surface of hand. *Extension:* Move thumb straight away from hand. *Abduction:* Extend thumb laterally (usually done when placing fingers in abduction and adduction). *Adduction:* Move thumb back toward hand. *Opposition:* Touch thumb to each finger of same hand.
Hip	Ball and socket 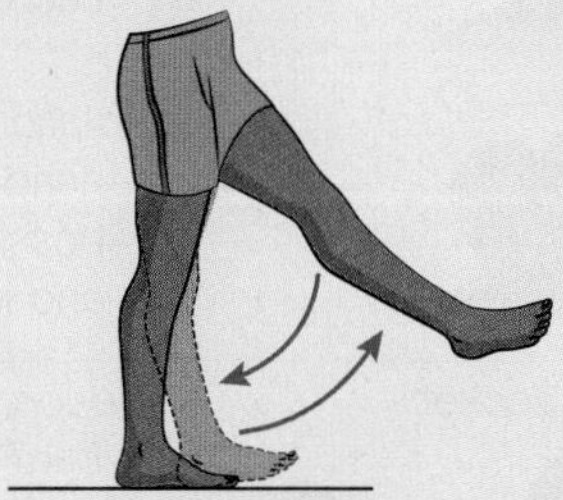 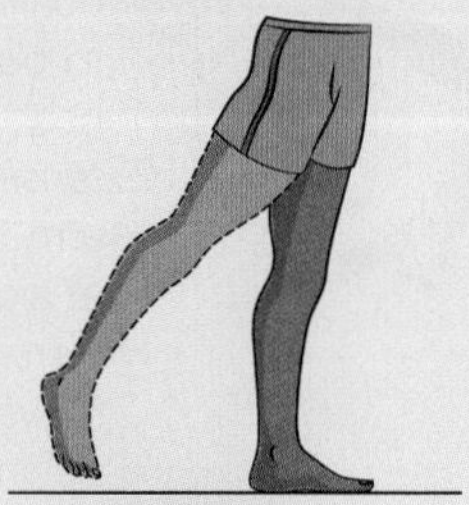 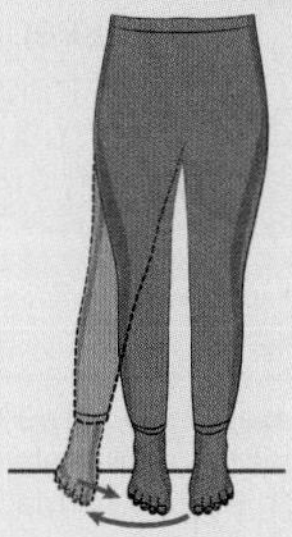	*Flexion:* Move leg forward and up with knee in extension. *Extension:* Move leg back beside other leg while knee joint remains in extension. *Hyperextension:* Move leg behind body. *Abduction:* Move leg laterally away from body. *Adduction:* Move leg back toward medial position and beyond if possible.

[g]Supination: Movement of the palm of the hand from facing downward to facing upward.
[h]Pronation: Movement of the palm of the hand from facing upward to facing downward.

Table 8.4 Joint Range-of-Motion Exercises—cont'd

BODY PART	TYPE OF JOINT	TYPE OF MOVEMENT	BODY PART	TYPE OF JOINT	TYPE OF MOVEMENT
Hip—cont'd		*Internal rotation:* Turn foot and leg toward other leg. *External rotation:* Turn foot and leg away from other leg. *Circumduction:* Move leg in circle.	Ankle	Hinge	*Dorsiflexion*[i]: Move foot so that toes are pointed upward. *Plantar flexion:* Move foot so that toes are pointed downward.
			Foot	Gliding	*Inversion:* Turn sole of foot medially. *Eversion:* Turn sole of foot laterally.
Knee	Hinge	*Flexion:* Bring heel back toward back of thigh. *Extension:* Return heel to floor.	Toes	Condyloid hinge	*Flexion:* Curl toes downward. *Extension:* Straighten toes. *Abduction:* Spread toes apart. *Adduction:* Bring toes together.

[i]Dorsiflexion: Backward flexion of the hand of foot.

Skill 8.2 Performing Range-of-Motion Exercises

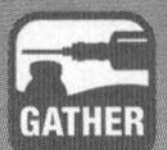

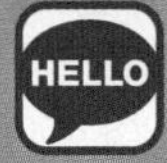

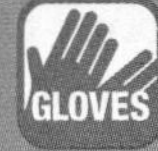

NURSING ACTION *(RATIONALE)*

1. Refer to medical record or care plan for special interventions. *(Provides basis for care.)*
2. Assemble equipment. *(Organizes procedure.)*
   - Clean gloves, if necessary (see Step 6).
3. Introduce self. *(Decreases patient's anxiety.)*
4. Identify patient. *(Ensures procedure is performed with correct patient.)*
5. Explain procedure. *(Enlists cooperation and decreases patient's anxiety.)*
6. Perform hand hygiene and don clean gloves according to agency policy and guidelines from CDC and OSHA. *(Reduces spread of microorganisms.)*
7. Prepare patient for intervention:
   a. Close door to room or pull curtain. *(Provides privacy.)*
   b. Drape for procedure if appropriate. *(Prevents unnecessary exposure of patient.)*
   c. Raise bed to comfortable working level. *(Promotes good body mechanics in the nurse and safety for the patient.)*
   d. Assist patient to a comfortable position, either sitting or lying down. *(Ensures patient's comfort.)*
   e. Medicate patient as needed for pain. *(Promotes patient comfort.)*

Continued

Skill 8.2 Performing Range-of-Motion Exercises—cont'd

8. Support the body part above (proximal to) and below (distal to) the joint by cradling the extremity or by using cupped hand to support the joint being exercised. *(Protects the weaker joints and muscles.)*

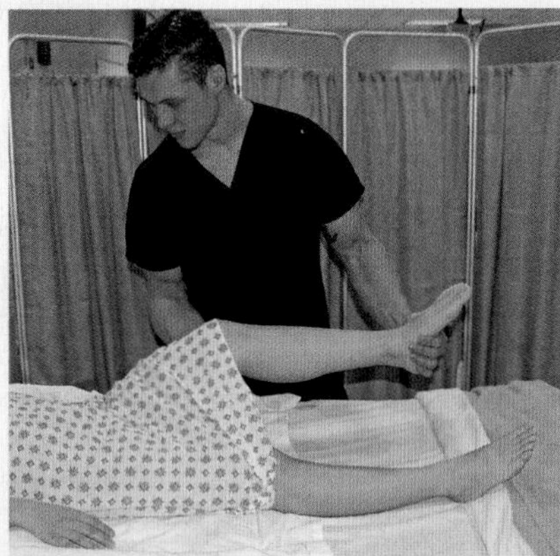

9. Begin by doing exercises in normal sequence (see Table 8.4). Repeat each full sequence five times during the exercise period. *(Exercises are easiest to perform in head-to-toe manner.)* Discontinue exercise if patient reports pain or if resistance or muscle spasm occurs.
10. Assist patient by putting each joint through full range of motion (see Table 8.4). *(Provides baseline for joint movement.)*
11. Position patient for comfort. To prevent **contracture** (an abnormal shortening of a muscle), do not allow patients with joint pain to remain continuously in position of comfort; joints must be exercised routinely. *(Immobility contributes to contractures.)* Periodically provide back massage. *(Provides comfort.)*
12. Adjust bed linen. *(Provides comfort and privacy.)*
13. Remove and dispose of gloves and wash hands. *(Reduces spread of microorganisms.)*
14. Document the following: *(Records procedure and patient's response.)*
    - Joints exercised
    - Presence of edema or pressure areas
    - Any discomfort resulting from the exercises
    - Any limitations of ROM
    - Patient's tolerance of the exercises
    - Patient teaching (see Patient Teaching and Home Care Considerations boxes)

Some patients who are weak or partially paralyzed are able to move a limb partially through ROM, and the nurse then may assist the patient to finish the full ROM. This is referred to as *passive assisted* ROM. *Active assisted* ROM occurs when the patient uses the strong arm to exercise the weaker or paralyzed arm. The LPN/LVN best meets the needs of the patient by encouraging the patient to be as independent as possible.

Assessment by the nurse and the physical therapy department determines the patient's current mobility status. The patient who is able to move about freely independently performs ADLs and active ROM exercises. Patients who are partially immobile or unable to move about freely (from paraplegia, quadriplegia, weakness, or fatigue) need the nurse and other health care personnel to assist with passive ROM exercises.

Encourage and assess active ROM every day (see the Lifespan Considerations for Older Adults box). The total amount of activity required to prevent **disuse syndrome** (a state in which an individual is at risk for deterioration of body systems as a result of prescribed or unavoidable inactivity) is only about 2 hours for every 24-hour period. Schedule this activity throughout the day to prevent the patient from remaining inactive for long periods (Ackley and Ladwig, 2017).

Lifespan Considerations

Older Adults

Range-of-Motion Exercises

- Some older adults who have chronic illnesses need to separate range-of-motion (ROM) exercises into two or more sessions to control fatigue.
- Inadequate intake of calcium or exposure to sunlight increases older adults' risk of bone loss and increases the need for ROM and weight-bearing exercise.
- Older people who fear falling often display reluctance to move about freely. Encouragement, reassurance, and assistance from family members and caregivers decrease anxiety.
- Older adult patients who are depressed often prefer to stay in bed, especially when they were accustomed to being very independent and active and now need assistance.
- Many older adults with arthritis require additional time in the morning before resuming activities.
- Even without arthritis, older adults often need more time in the morning to resume activity.

CONTINUOUS PASSIVE MOTION MACHINES

Continuous passive motion (CPM) machines flex and extend joints for passive mobilization without the strain of active exercises (Fig. 8.7). This therapy sometimes is used immediately after total knee replacement surgery (knee arthroplasty), but CPM also can be used in outpatient or home physical therapy programs. The CPM machine's settings must be adjusted according to the

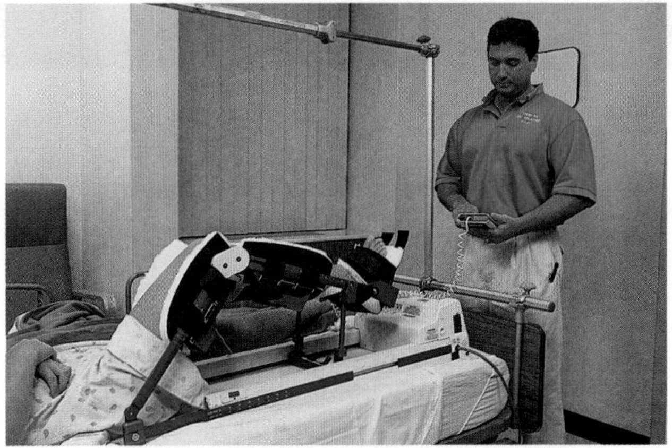

Fig. 8.7 Continuous passive motion (CPM) machine. (From Perry AG, Potter PA, Elkin MK: *Nursing interventions and clinical skills*, ed 5, St. Louis, 2012, Mosby.)

health care provider's orders for the degree and the speed of flexion and extension for each individual patient to prevent damage to the joint or surgical site. Some recent studies question the necessity of CPM machines and encourage the use of immediate physical therapy instead. Many orthopedic surgeons have adopted the practice of immediate physical therapy over CPM therapy.

CPM machines can be used on joints other than the knee, including the hip, the shoulder, and the ankle. Mobilization of the joint prevents complications, such as joint contracture, atrophy of surrounding muscles, and thromboembolism. Physical therapy typically accompanies CPM therapy. Ongoing CPM therapy can be accomplished in a rehabilitative facility or at home with the oversight of a home care agency.

MOVING THE PATIENT

A common nursing action is assisting patients in movement. Patients may need assistance in various ways, such as moving the patient up in bed, out of bed, or from a chair or wheelchair; turning the patient; and assisting the patient in and out of the bed for ambulation (Skill 8.3). For some situations, the nurse uses mechanical

Text continued on p. 180

Skill 8.3 Moving the Patient

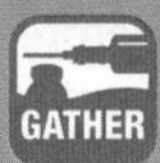

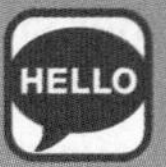

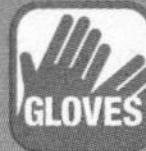

NURSING ACTION *(RATIONALE)*

1. Refer to the medical record or care plan for special interventions. *(Provides basis for care.)*
2. Assemble equipment. *(Organizes procedure.)*
   - Hospital bed
   - Chair
   - Side rails
   - Patient's slippers
   - Cotton blanket
   - Pillows
   - Extra personnel
   - Lifting devices (see Skill 8.4)
3. Introduce self. *(Decreases patient's anxiety.)*
4. Identify patient. *(Ensures procedure is performed with correct patient.)*
5. Explain procedure. *(Enlists cooperation and assistance from patient and decreases patient's anxiety.)*
6. Perform hand hygiene. *(Reduces spread of microorganisms.)*
7. Prepare patient for interventions.
   a. Close door or pull curtain. *(Provides privacy.)*
   b. Adjust bed level for safe working height. *(Promotes good body mechanics in the nurse and safety for the patient.)*
   c. Medicate patient as needed. *(Promotes patient comfort.)*
8. Arrange for assistance as necessary. *(Provides for safety.)*
9. Lift and move patient up in bed (sometimes requires one nurse and sometimes more):
   a. Place patient supine with head flat. *(Creates less resistance on flat surface.)*
   b. Face the patient and establish base of support. *(Protects your back.)*
   c. Use a lift (draw) sheet to assist patient up in bed. *(Supports patient, assists staff, and prevents shearing of patient's skin.)*
      (1) Roll patient first to one side and then the other, placing lift sheet underneath patient from shoulders to thighs. *(Facilitates the position change.)*
      (2) Flex knees and face body in the direction of the move. The foot farthest away from the bed faces forward for broader base of support.
      (3) With one nurse on each side of patient, grasp lift sheet firmly with hands near patient's upper arms and hips, rolling the sheet material until hands are close to the patient. *(The closer the nurse is to the patient, the less the nurse needs to raise the patient up to clear the bed during the move.)*

Skill 8.3 Moving the Patient—cont'd

(4) Instruct patient to rest arms over body and to lift head on the count of 3; at the same time, pull the sheet to move the patient up to head of bed.

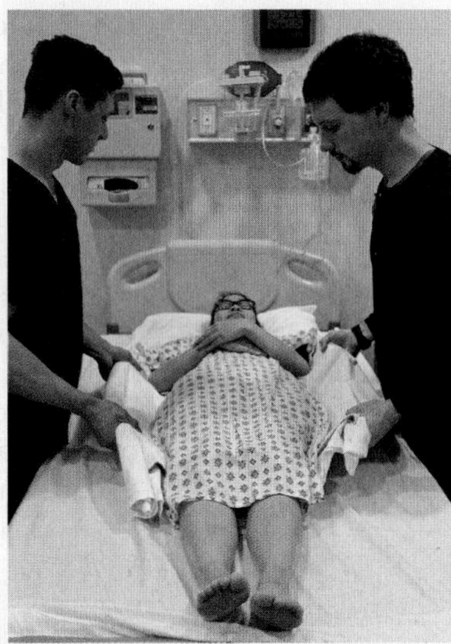

10. Turning the patient:
  a. Stand with feet slightly apart and flex knees. *(Provides base of support.)*
  b. If the patient is unable to assist in turning, two people should use the lift sheet to turn the patient. *(Provides patient safety and support and protects the back of the persons assisting with the turn.)*
  c. Move patient's body to one side of the bed. *(Allows room for the patient to turn in the bed.)*
  d. If patient is assisting in turning, turn the patient on side facing raised side rail, toward the nurse. *(Prevents patient from falling out of bed.)* If patient is not assisting, then use the lift sheet to turn the patient.
  e. Flex one of patient's legs over the other. Place pad or pillow between legs. *(Reduces pressure on lower leg and prevents skin breakdown by avoiding skin on skin.)*
  f. Align patient's shoulders; place pillow under head. *(Ensures proper body alignment.)*
  g. Support patient's back with pillows as necessary. A "tuck back" pillow is made by folding pillow lengthwise. Tuck smooth area slightly under patient's back. *(Helps keep patient in position.)*

11. Dangling patient:
  a. Assess pulse and respirations. *(Provides baseline for assessing patient's response to dangling.)*
  b. Move patient to side of bed toward the nurse. *(Makes it easier for patient to sit up. Request patient do by self if possible.)*
  c. Lower bed to lowest position. *(Provides patient safety when getting up.)*
  d. Raise head of bed. *(Patient can swing around more easily to sitting position.)*
  e. Support patient's shoulders and help to swing legs around and off bed; do this all in one motion by simply pivoting patient. Ensure patient's feet touch floor. *(Prevents strain on patient, especially if patient has an incision.)*

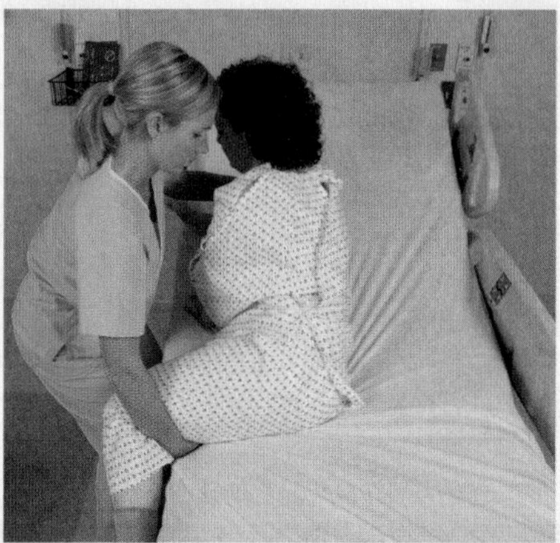

  f. Another way to accomplish this is by rolling the patient onto his or her side before sitting the patient up. *(Decreases the amount the nurse needs to lift because the patient's body weight actually helps the patient to sit upright.)* The nurse then stoops and, when standing, brings the patient along with the nurse. *(This causes less back strain for the nurse and the patient does not feel pulled.)*
  g. Help patient place slippers on; cover legs. *(Prevents patient from becoming chilled.)* For safety, have patient place slippers on while in bed.
  h. Assess patient's pulse and respirations. *(Determines patient's response to procedure.)*

12. Log-rolling the patient (back, neck, or head conditions sometimes necessitate logrolling after injury or surgery):
  a. Enlist the help of at least one additional person. *(Ensures patient safety.)*
  b. Lower the head of the bed as much as the patient can tolerate. *(Maintains alignment of the spinal column.)*
  c. Place a pillow between the patient's legs. Use of a pull sheet placed between shoulders and knees facilitates turning (see Step 9c[4]). *(Maintains position of the lower extremities.)*
  d. Extend the patient's arm over the patient's head unless shoulder movement is restricted. *(Prevents rolling over it during the turn.)* If shoulder movement is restricted, keep the arm in extension next to the body.

Skill 8.3 Moving the Patient—cont'd

e. With both nurses on the same side of the bed, one of the nurses places one hand on the patient's shoulder and the other on the hip, while the other nurse places one hand to support the patient's back and the other behind the knee. If a lift sheet is used, space hands in such a way to provide even support for the length of the rolled sheet and to distribute weight evenly.

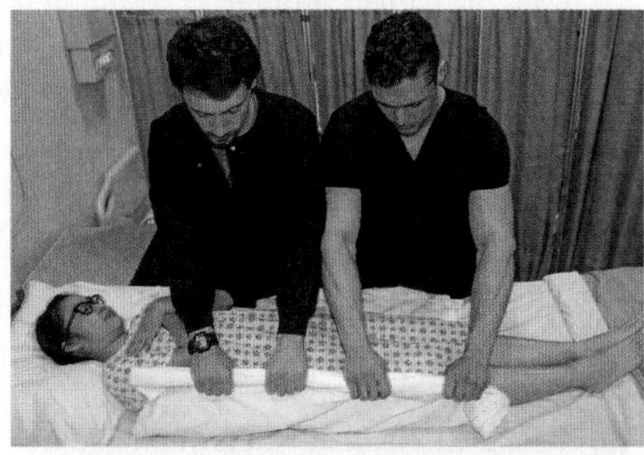

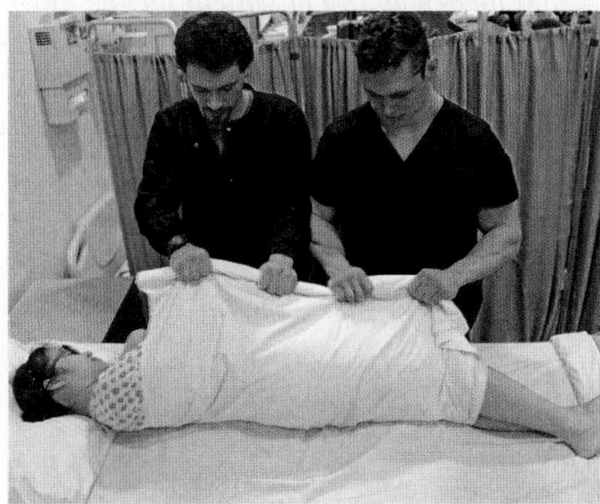

f. On a count of 3, turn the patient with a continuous, smooth, and coordinated effort. *(Maintains body alignment, preventing stress on any part of the body.)*

g. Support the patient with pillows as previously discussed (see Step 10g). *(Promotes patient comfort.)*

13. Transferring the patient from bed to straight chair or wheelchair:

a. Lower bed to lowest position. *(Provides patient safety when getting up.)*

b. Raise head of bed. *(Patient can more easily swing around to sitting position.)*

c. Support patient's shoulders and help swing legs around and off bed; perform all in one motion (see Step 11e). *(Prevents strain on patient, especially if patient has incision.)*

d. Help patient don robe and slippers (or do this before beginning procedure). *(Prevents chilling.)*

e. Have chair positioned beside bed with seat facing foot of bed. *(Provides easy access to chair.)*

(1) Place wheelchair at right angle to bed and lock wheels after bed is lowered. *(Provides safety.)*

(2) Place straight chair against wall or have another nurse hold the chair. *(Provides safety.)*

f. Stand in front of patient and place hands at patient's waist level or below; allow patient to use his or her arms and shoulder muscles to push down on the mattress to facilitate the move. *(Prepares the patient for movement to chair.)*

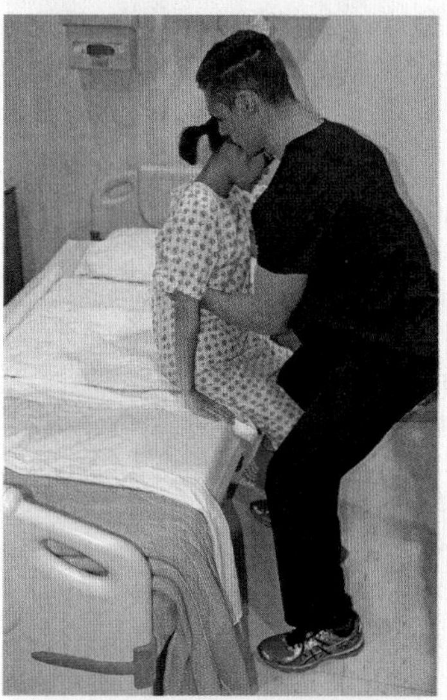

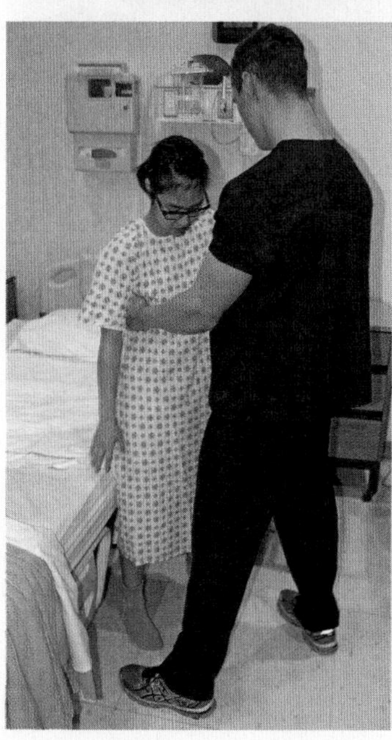

Continued

Skill 8.3 Moving the Patient—cont'd

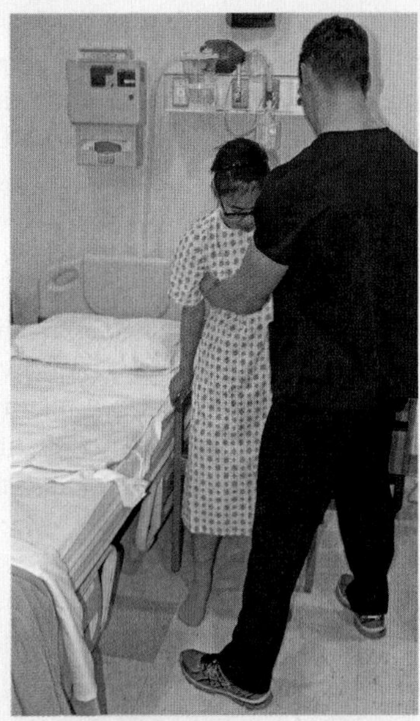

g. Assist patient to stand and swing around with back toward seat of chair. Keep the strong side toward the chair. *(Provides safety.)*

h. Help patient to sit down as the nurse bends his or her knees to assist process. *(Prevents patient from slipping and falling. If patient begins to fall, prevent patient injury by holding patient and allowing patient to sit down gently on floor;* see Box 8.2, Step 3.)

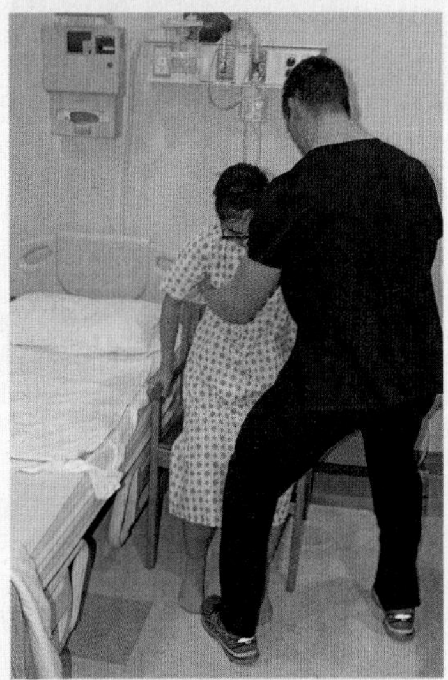

i. Apply blanket to legs. *(Provides extra warmth.)*

j. If transfer belt is used, apply after patient is sitting on side of bed and follow these guidelines:

(1) Stand in front of the patient. *(Permits excellent view of patient.)*

(2) Have the patient hold on to the mattress, or ask the patient to place his or her fists on the bed by the thighs. *(Any assistance from the patient minimizes strain on you.)*

(3) Be sure the patient's feet are flat on the floor. *(Provides balance and stability for patient.)*

(4) Have the patient lean forward.

(5) Instruct the patient to place his or her hands on the nurse's shoulders, not around the nurse's neck or at the side as shown. *(Arms around the neck could result in neck injury to nurse.)*

(6) Grasp the transfer belt at each side. *(Offers stability of patient for the nurse.)*

(7) Brace knees against the patient's knees. Block the patient's feet with the nurse's feet. *(Provides safety and prevents patient's foot from slipping.)*

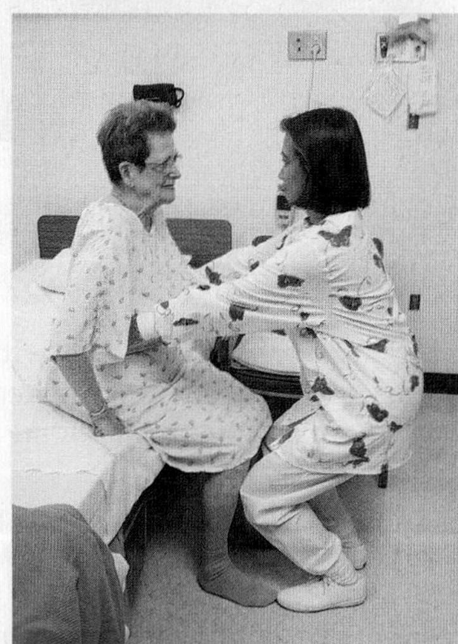

Skill 8.3 Moving the Patient—cont'd

(8) Ask the patient to push down on the mattress and to stand on the count of 3. Pull the patient into a standing position as you straighten your knees. *(Provides for less strain on your back.)*

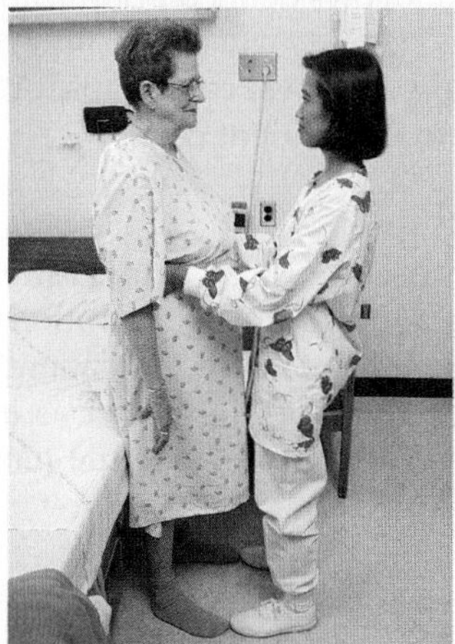

(9) Pivot the patient so that he or she is able to grasp the far arm of the chair. Back of the legs will be touching the chair. *(Enables patient to assist in the transfer.)*

(10) Continue to turn the patient until the other arm rest is grasped.

(11) Gradually lower the patient into the chair as you bend your hips and knees. The patient assists if able by leaning forward and bending his or her elbows and knees. *(Encourages patient to assist in transfer and increases muscle strength and a sense of control.)*

(12) Ensure buttocks are to the back of the chair. *(Ensures patient safety.)*

(13) Cover patient's lap and legs. *(Promotes patient's comfort and privacy.)*

14. Transferring from bed to stretcher or gurney back to bed:

a. Position bed flat and raise to the same height as stretcher or gurney. Lower side rails. *(Facilitates procedure.)*

b. Cover patient with top sheet or blanket and remove linens without exposing patient. *(Provides privacy.)*

c. Assess for IV line, Foley catheter, tubes, or surgical drains, and position them to avoid tension during the transfer. *(Prevents accidental tension and possible removal of tubes.)*

d. Position the gurney as close to the bed as possible, and lock the wheels of the bed and gurney (with side rails lowered). *(Ensures patient's safety.)*

e. When patient is able to assist, stand near side of gurney and instruct patient to move feet, then buttocks, and finally upper body to the gurney, bringing blanket along. Be certain patient's body is centered on the gurney. *(Promotes safety and security.)*

f. When patient is unable to assist, place a folded sheet or bath blanket under the patient so that it supports patient's head and extends to mid-thighs. Roll the sheet or bath blanket close to the patient's body. Assist patient to cross arms over chest. Two nurses reach over the bed to patient, and two more nurses stand as close to the gurney as possible. A fifth nurse stands at the foot to transfer the feet. Using a coordinating count of 3, all five nurses lift the patient to the edge of the bed. With another effort, lift the patient from edge of bed to gurney. Roller devices are available in some facilities to facilitate this transfer.

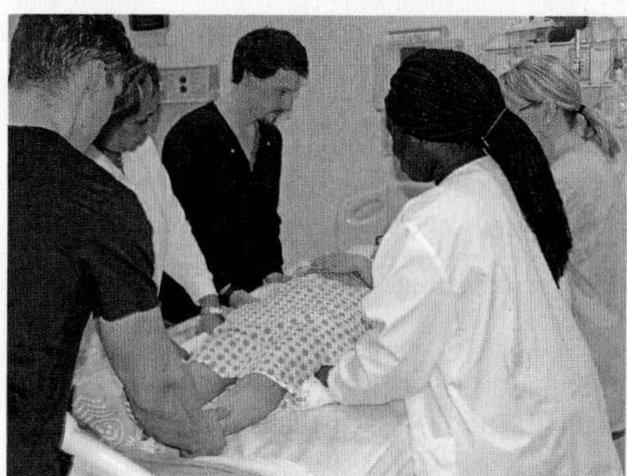

15. Perform hand hygiene. *(Reduces spread of microorganisms.)*

16. Assess patient for appropriate body alignment after move. When repositioning, always assess previously dependent skin surfaces (pressure areas). Position pillows for comfort. Do not overtire patient during ambulation. As in all transfers, be certain call device is in easy reach. *(Evaluates, determines, and promotes patient safety and comfort.)*

17. Document procedure. *(Notes procedure and patient's response.)*

- Patient's response
- Expected and unexpected outcomes
- Patient teaching (see the Patient Teaching and Home Care Considerations boxes)

Step 11e figure from Perry AG, Potter PA, Ostendorf WR, et al: *Clinical nursing skills and techniques,* ed 9, St. Louis, 2018, Elsevier.

equipment for lifting patients, such as the hydraulic lift, roller board, and gurney lift. The nurse first should think through the lift to be prepared for lifting the patient and then physically perform the lift. The nurse must ensure that patients do not become too dependent on assistance with mobility. Frequent assessment of the patient's ability to assist with mobility is necessary to prevent overdependence. The LPN/LVN should also assess the patient for pain and administer pain medications before activities that cause further pain (Box 8.3 and the Coordinated Care box).

Coordinated Care

Delegation

Mobility

The following information is needed when delegating the skill of position changes to UAP:

- Have the patient wear shoes with a nonslip surface during transfer or ambulation.
- Make slow, gradual position changes.
- Help the patient sit in a chair or return to bed if the patient has symptoms of orthostatic hypotension.
- When assisting with ambulation:
  - Do not try to hold patients if they become dizzy or faint. Ease them into a sitting position in a chair or onto the floor.
  - Use assistive devices such as walkers, crutches, gait belt, or cane when appropriate.
  - Be sure the area is free of clutter, wet areas, and rugs that may slide.

UAP, Unlicensed assistive personnel.

USE OF THE LIFT FOR MOVING PATIENTS

Mechanical devices, such as the patient lift with a sling (Fig. 8.8), are useful for moving patients safely and protecting the nurse's back and for full-weight lifting of patients who cannot assist. Follow agency policy for use of the lift (Skill 8.4).

❖ NURSING PROCESS FOR PATIENT MOBILITY

The role of the LPN/LVN in the nursing process as stated is that the LPN/LVN:

- Participates in planning care for patients based on patient needs.
- Reviews the patient's plan of care and recommends revisions as needed.
- Reviews and follows defined prioritization for patient care.
- Uses clinical pathways, care maps, or care plans to guide and review patient care.

◆ ASSESSMENT

Assessment focuses on ROM, muscle strength, activity tolerance, gait, and posture. Observation during ADLs enables the nurse to estimate the patient's fatigability, muscle strength, and ROM. Further assessment helps determine the type of assistance the patient needs to

Box 8.3 Long-Term Care Considerations for Mobility

- Patients who have maintained bed rest for a long time sometimes revert to a favorite position. Frequently assess these patients, and turn them more often as needed.
- Use a lift (draw) sheet as often as possible to prevent shearing force on fragile skin.
- Allow the patient to assist with moving and positioning whenever possible to promote independence.
- Perform safety and maintenance checks of ambulation devices on a routine basis.
- Perform periodic assessments to ensure that the patient is using ambulation device properly.
- Consult the physical therapist for additional assistance or exercises and to ascertain the patient's response to the exercise program.
- Group activities (e.g., simple games, walking, tossing a ball in a large circle) are useful in maintaining ROM.

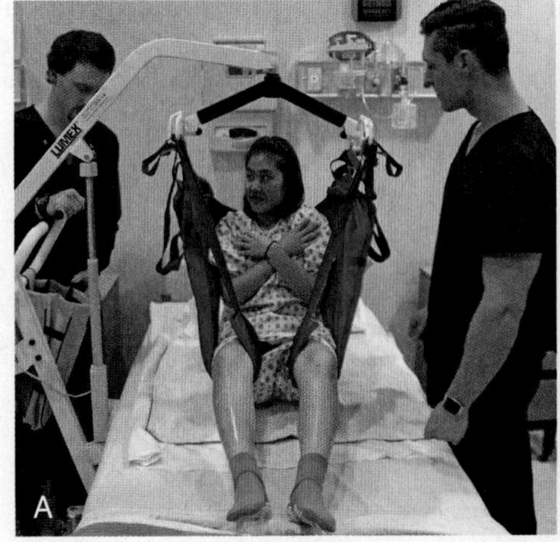

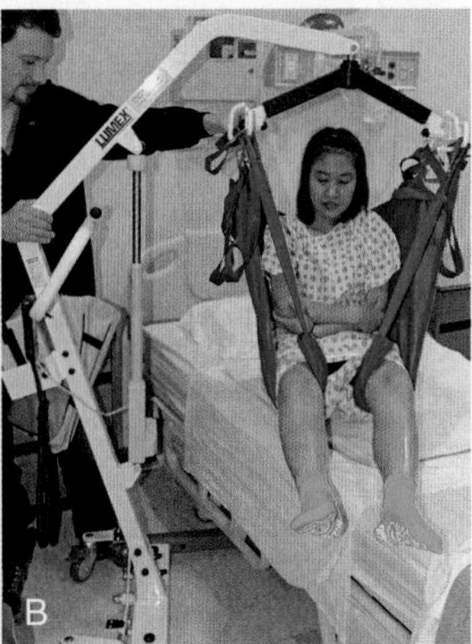

Fig. 8.8 A, Motorized lift. B, Use of a mechanical lift to lower patient into chair.

Skill 8.4 Using Lifts for Moving Patients

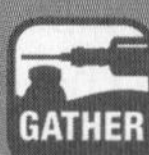

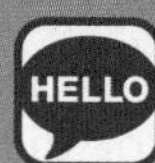

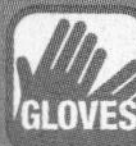

NURSING ACTION *(RATIONALE)*

1. Refer to medical record or care plan for special interventions. *(Provides basis for care.)* Read manual for direction.
2. Assemble equipment:
   - Mechanical lift frame (see Fig. 8.8)
   - Seat sling attachment (may be one piece or two) or a standing frame
   - Two cotton bath blankets
3. Introduce self. *(Decreases patient's anxiety.)*
4. Identify patient. *(Ensures procedure is performed with correct patient.)*
5. Explain procedure. *(Enlists cooperation and assistance from patient and decreases patient's anxiety.)*
6. Perform hand hygiene. *(Reduces spread of microorganisms.)*
7. Prepare patient for interventions.
   a. Close door or pull curtains. *(Provides privacy.)*
   b. Adjust bed level to working height (even with level of arm of chair [of lift] if chair is not removable or level with seat if chair is removable). *(Promotes safety.)*
   c. Medicate patient as needed. *(Promotes patient comfort.)*
   d. Place cotton bath blanket over chair for patient's comfort.
   e. Cover patient with remaining bath blanket.
8. Secure adequate number of personnel. *(Provides necessary assistance and patient safety.)*
9. Place chair near bed. *(Prepares seat for patient.)*
10. Appropriately place canvas seat under patient; support head and neck. *(Helps in lifting safely.)*
11. Slide horseshoe-shaped bar under bed on one side. *(Places lift close to bed.)*
12. Lower horizontal bar to level of sling. *(Places lift close to patient.)*
13. Fasten hooks on chain to openings in sling. *(Attaches lift to sling seat.)*
14. Raise head of bed. *(Places patient in sitting position.)*
15. Fold patient's arms over chest. *(Prevents patient injury.)*
16. Pump lift handle until patient is raised off bed. *(Ensures patient safety during lifting.)*
17. With steering handle, pull lift off bed and down to chair. *(Places patient safely in chair provided.)*
18. Release valve slowly to lift and lower patient toward chair. *(Appropriately places patient in chair.)*
19. Close off valve and release straps. *(Prevents patient injury from boom.)*
20. Remove straps and lift. *(Provides safety and comfort.)*
21. Perform hand hygiene. *(Reduces spread of microorganisms.)*
22. Document procedure. *(Note procedure and patient's response.)*
    - Evaluate body alignment to help prevent skin impairment.
    - Evaluate patient's response to movement to help determine patient's mobility potential.
23. Perform patient teaching (see the Patient Teaching and Home Care Considerations boxes).

change position or transfer from bed to chair or wheelchair. These assessments give the LPN/LVN an understanding of the patient's overall level of mobility and coordination (see the Cultural Considerations box).

It is acceptable to delegate the skills of safe and effective transfer from bed to chair to UAP who have demonstrated successfully good body mechanics and safe transfer techniques for patients involved.

Teaching patients how to use assistive devices requires critical thinking and knowledge application unique to a nurse. However, UAP are able to assist ambulatory patients with assistive devices.

- Have the patient wear shoes with a nonskid surface during ambulation.

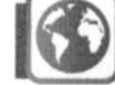

Cultural Considerations

Promotion of Patient Mobility

- Assess and listen carefully to patient's expressions of health and illness beliefs and practices.
- Be aware of the patient's personal space; seek permission before intruding in the patient's territory.
- The nursing process enables the nurse to provide individualized care; adapt care to be culturally sensitive.
- When speaking with a patient (or family member) who does not understand English, many people try to compensate for the lack of understanding by speaking more loudly. Speaking slowly, distinctly, and at a normal volume is more effective (see Chapter 4).

- Be sure the area is free of clutter, wet areas, and rugs that may slide or buckle.
- Ensure UAP knows how to use an intravenous (IV) pole to assist in ambulation for a patient with continuous IV therapy.
- Be sure the patient uses the correct gait and weight bearing during ambulation.
- Ease the patient to a sitting position in a chair or on the floor if he or she becomes dizzy or faint.
- Have UAP alert the LPN/LVN if the patient becomes dizzy or lightheaded or suffers a fall.

The skill of performing ROM exercises can be delegated to UAP. Patients with spinal cord injury or orthopedic trauma or surgery usually require exercise to be performed by nurses or physical therapists. When delegating this skill, instruct UAP to perform exercises slowly and provide adequate support to the joint being exercised. In addition, remind UAP not to exercise joints beyond the point of resistance or to the point of fatigue or pain. In addition, if muscle spasms occur, exercise should stop until the spasms have subsided.

The LPN/LVN may delegate the skill of safe and effective transfer with a mechanical lift to UAP who have demonstrated the ability to use good body mechanics and safe transfer techniques and equipment (mechanical lift).

◆ PATIENT PROBLEMS

Assessment enables the nurse to cluster relevant data and develop actual or potential (risk) problem statements related to the patient's needs. The patient problems are listed along with the probable causes "related to (r/t)." Identification of the cause of the problem further individualizes the care plan and leads to selection of appropriate care.

Example: *Compromised Physical Mobility, r/t left shoulder pain, as evidenced by patient pain 8/10 and patient unable to assist in dressing self.*

◆ EXPECTED OUTCOMES AND PLANNING

The nurse should set goals and expected outcomes with the patient to direct interventions. Care planning is individualized to the patient, with the patient's most immediate needs taken into consideration. These goals are based on the patient problem statement formulated.

Goal: Patient will demonstrate ability to assist in dressing self within 3 days.

Expected outcomes: Patient reports pain level decreased to 4/10 for 3 consecutive days and assists with dressing self each of these 3 days.

◆ IMPLEMENTATION

Nursing interventions should be individualized according to the level of risk to the patient. The nurse, the patient, and other members of the health care team work together to determine the most effective interventions (Nursing Care Plan 8.1). While implementing the established goals, the nurse also should assess the patient's readiness to learn and teach appropriate body mechanics (see the Home Care Considerations box on mobility).

The nurse is aware of the patient's motor deficits, ability to aid in transfer, and body weight. As suggested by the National Institute for Occupational Safety and Health's (NIOSH) Division of Safety Research, health care personnel should never attempt to lift more than 35 pounds of a patient's body weight, or should use the Revised NIOSH Lifting Equation (CDC/NIOSH, 2017). For the safety of the staff and the patient, additional assistance always should be secured when the transferability of a patient is in doubt.

Many special problems are to be considered in transfer. Patients who have been immobile for several days or longer may be weak or have vertigo (dizziness) and sometimes have orthostatic hypotension (a drop in blood pressure) when transferred. A patient with neurologic deficits perhaps has paresis (muscle weakness) or paralysis unilaterally or bilaterally, which complicates safe transfer. A flaccid arm easily can sustain injury during transfer if unsupported. The nurse must be creative when necessary in the transfer of trauma patients. As a general rule, a gait (transfer) belt should be used and assistance obtained for mobilization of such patients.

◆ EVALUATION

The success of interventions is evaluated with a comparison of the patient's response with the outcome established for each nursing goal, such as the following:

1. Ask the patient to rate pain on a scale of 1 to 10 (determines need for additional pain control).
2. Note the patient's behavioral response to transfer (reveals level of pain, motivation, and self-care potential).

For evaluation of the patient's perception of the interventions, knowledge of the patient's expectations concerning joint mobility, posture, or body alignment is necessary first. What is acceptable or anticipated on the nurse's part is sometimes very different from what the patient and family members anticipate or are able to accept.

Nursing Care Plan 8.1 The Patient With Activity Intolerance

Mr. D., a 56-year-old patient hospitalized with multiple orthopedic traumas, reports pain in his left shoulder during movement. He also reports difficulty extending his shoulder joint in carrying out activities of daily living. The nurse observes that he limits motion in his left arm. Range of motion (ROM) is reduced 30 degrees during abduction of arm.

PATIENT PROBLEM

Compromised Physical Mobility, related to (r/t) left shoulder pain as evidenced by (AEB) limited mobility of left arm, c/o (complaints of) pain and favoring left arm

Patient Goals and Expected Outcomes	Nursing Interventions	Evaluation
Patient will gain optimal ROM of left shoulder within 4 months. Patient will perform self-care activities using left arm within 2 days. Patient will report decreased pain by at least 2 on a scale of 0 to 10 within 2 days. Patient will increase ROM in upper extremity joints by 20 degrees. Patient will follow a regular exercise program by discharge.	Offer analgesic 30 min before ROM exercises (peak action of analgesic will occur as patient begins exercises). Schedule active ROM exercises between meals and hygiene activities (promotes frequent exercise to affected joints and reduces risk of contracture development). Teach patient specific ROM exercises for left shoulder and arm. (Teaching provides the patient with opportunity and knowledge to maintain and increase ROM.) (See Patient Teaching and Home Care Considerations boxes on mobility.)	Ask patient to report changes in perception of left shoulder pain, using a scale of 1 to 10. Observe patient while doing ROM exercises in upper extremities and while doing self-care to determine increase of 20 degrees of upper extremities by time of discharge.

CRITICAL THINKING QUESTIONS

1. The nurse is in the process of transferring Mr. D. from his bed to a chair with use of a mechanical lift. The nurse has prepared the chair and placed it near the bed. The nurse turns Mr. D. to his side, places the sling under Mr. D. to ensure adequate support of his head, returns Mr. D. to his back, and slowly begins to lift him from his bed. What has the nurse forgotten to do, and why is it important?
2. The patient has a trapeze bar across the bed, trochanter rolls, and a footboard. Explain the rationale for use of each of these devices to maintain proper body alignment.

Home Care Considerations

Mobility

- Instruct family or caregiver about the rationale for slow, gradual position changes.
- Instruct family or caregiver about the use of a gait belt and correct body mechanics for transfer of patient.
- Instruct family or caregiver to not attempt ambulation if patient reports dizziness or lightheadedness.
- Transfer ability at home is greatly enhanced by prior teaching of family, assessment of home for safety risks and functionality, and provision of applicable aids.
- Have family practice transfer in hospital and achieve success before taking patient home.
- Alternatively, have the patient who lives alone practice activities he or she will use at home to manage toileting and showering. Teach patients to transfer to armchairs for ease of rising and sitting.
- Be sure the home is free of risks (e.g., throw rugs, electric cords, slippery floors). If a wheelchair is used, see that access is possible through all doors and that space for transfer is available in bedroom and bathroom.
- Ensure arrangements are made for a home health nurse or support person to continue to assist the family at home.
- Instruct patient about how to use the ambulation aids on various terrains (e.g., carpet, stairs, rough ground, inclines).
- Instruct patient in how to maneuver around obstacles, such as doors, and how to use the aid when transferring, such as to and from a chair, toilet, tub, and car.
- Attach a carrying bag to patient's walker to carry objects; caution patient not to overfill the bag to prevent forward tipping of walker.
- Assess family member or primary caregiver's ability, availability, and motivation to assist patient with exercises that patient is unable to perform independently.
- Assist family or primary caregiver to arrange home environment to promote exercise program (e.g., space allocation, lighting, temperature, safety precautions).
- Teach family members about body mechanics.
- In the absence of a hospital bed and equipment, creative adaptation is necessary.
- Consider the need for a bed that places the bedridden patient at caregiver's waist level.
- Teach caregivers to change patient's position every 1 to 2 hours, if possible, to maintain musculoskeletal alignment and to reduce pressure on bony prominences. Develop and post a realistic turning schedule.

Get Ready for the NCLEX® Examination!

Key Points

- Protection of the musculoskeletal system is essential to prevent injury to patient and nurse.
- Less effort is needed to carry out an activity if the base of support is widened in the direction of movement.
- Appropriate body mechanics should be practiced consistently.
- Maintenance of correct body alignment is the key to proper body mechanics.
- Correct body alignment promotes balance and helps coordinate movements.
- Permanent disability can occur from inappropriate positioning.
- Proper positioning permits activity, enhances comfort, and prepares patients for procedures.
- Immobility sometimes results from illness or trauma, and sometimes it is prescribed for therapeutic reasons. Whatever the reason, immobility poses the risk of serious complications. Interventions to avoid these complications are possible.
- The nurse performs range-of-motion exercises to promote circulation, prevent contractures, and provide joint mobility.
- When turning, moving, lifting, or carrying a patient, the nurse should secure adequate assistance to reduce strain and prevent injury to the nurse and the patient. The nurse should perform procedures safely and properly, facilitating the patient's independence, and should teach the patient and others safety in moving.
- Mechanical devices such as a mechanical lift, roller board, and gurney lift are used for moving patients safely.
- Use the nursing process to provide care for patients who are at risk for or are experiencing activity intolerance and impaired mobility.

Additional Learning Resources

SG Go to your Study Guide for additional learning activities to help you master this chapter content.

evolve Be sure to visit the Evolve site at *http://evolve.elsevier.com/Cooper/foundationsadult/* for additional online resources.

Review Questions for the NCLEX® Examination

1. The nurse is assigned to care for an 82-year-old patient who weighs 252 pounds (lb) (114.54 kilograms [kg]) and has undergone a bilateral below-the-knee amputation. Which transfer method is the safest for the patient and the nurse?
   1. Logrolling
   2. A gurney lift
   3. A mechanical lift with a sling
   4. Two nurses to lift the patient without assistive equipment
2. The nurse helps ambulate an 84-year-old female patient who has peripheral vascular disease that caused a severe stasis ulcer. The patient becomes very weak, reports feeling faint, and begins to fall. What is the most appropriate action to prevent injury to the patient?
   1. Support her while she is falling and allow her to sit on the floor.
   2. Carefully attempt to return her to her room.
   3. Tell her to hold on to the wall and that you will get more assistance.
   4. Ask her to take deep breaths and look straight ahead.
3. A 56-year-old patient had an open cholecystectomy. The nurse is going to assist the patient with dangling on the side of the bed before ambulation. After sitting the patient on the edge of the bed, which nursing intervention should the nurse perform before proceeding with the ambulation?
   1. Measurement of the patient's temperature
   2. Assessment of the patient's pulse and respirations
   3. Auscultating the patient's lung sounds
   4. Removal of the patient's anti-embolism stockings
4. The patient accidentally knocks the emesis basin to the floor. When picking up the emesis basin, which movement demonstrates proper body mechanics by the nurse?
   1. The nurse lowers the body by flexing the knees and bending the hips.
   2. The nurse bends from the waist and hips.
   3. The nurse flexes the knees and bends at the waist.
   4. The nurse keeps the legs straight and flexes the waist.
5. A patient who was admitted with the diagnosis of a stroke has slid to the foot of the bed. With use of appropriate body mechanics, the nurse maintains a wide base of support and faces the patient in the direction of movement. What do these actions allow the nurse to do?
   1. Use the back muscles
   2. Use the gluteal muscles
   3. Exert less physical effort
   4. Use the large muscles across the scapula
6. An 82-year-old patient has had a cerebrovascular accident that affects her right side. The nurse repositions the patient to her left side, placing a pillow between her legs and another behind her back. What is the primary purpose of this intervention?
   1. Maintaining the patient's comfort
   2. Ensuring the patient's proper body alignment
   3. Keeping the patient in the desired position for at least 2 hours
   4. Preventing the patient from development of contractures

7. It is the patient's first night after an abdominal hysterectomy. She has not voided for 9 hours, and the nurse is to insert a 16 French Foley catheter into her bladder. What patient position best allows insertion of the catheter?
   1. Dorsal recumbent
   2. Lithotomy
   3. Sims
   4. Prone
8. The nurse is assigned to care for a patient who was admitted for exacerbation of chronic obstructive pulmonary disease and pneumonia. The patient is experiencing dyspnea and is unable to rest in a supine position. The nurse elevates the head of the bed to 90 degrees, places a pillow on the overbed table, and assists the patient to lean forward, placing the patient's head on the pillow. What position should the nurse document the patient as being in?
   1. Semi-Fowler's
   2. Dorsal
   3. Sims
   4. Orthopneic
9. The nurse explains to the patient that the log-rolling technique will be used to help the patient change position. The patient asks why this is necessary. Which response is accurate?
   1. "Logrolling will help you keep your hips slightly flexed toward your chest."
   2. "By having you dangle your legs at the bedside, you will be more comfortable."
   3. "Because of your injury, it is extremely important that the head of your bed remain up at all times."
   4. "It is important to keep your neck and spine in straight alignment while we help you move onto your side."
10. The nurse and a UAP are to move a dependent patient from the supine to the lateral position. Which action should be performed first?
    1. Move the patient to the side of the bed.
    2. Turn the patient with use of a lift sheet.
    3. Ensure that the upper arm and leg are supported with pillows.
    4. Explain to the patient what actions the nurse and UAP are going to perform.
11. An older adult patient has been lying in the supine position for 3 hours and tells the nurse that she is too uncomfortable to move right now. What is the best response by the nurse?
    1. The nurse should express concern that she is uncomfortable and promise to come back later.
    2. The nurse should assess the patient's need for pain medication before helping her change position.
    3. The nurse should explain to the patient that if she does not move now, she will develop pneumonia.
    4. The nurse should find another nurse to help move the patient to the lateral position immediately.
12. The student nurse demonstrated principles of good body mechanics with which activity? *(Select all that apply.)*
    1. Keeping the knees in a locked position
    2. Maintaining a wide base of support and bending at the knees
    3. Bending at the waist to maintain one's balance
    4. Holding objects away from the body for improved leverage
    5. Asking for help when deemed necessary when assisting a patient with transfers
13. A patient becomes faint and diaphoretic while sitting on the side of the bed in preparation to ambulate. To prevent injury to the patient and nurse, which action should the nurse take? *(Select all that apply.)*
    1. The nurse should call for assistance.
    2. The nurse should not allow the patient to get out of bed at this time.
    3. The nurse should allow the patient to lower the head to rest on the nurse's abdomen.
    4. The nurse should find an emesis basin because the patient will probably vomit.
    5. The nurse should continue to assist the patient to a standing position, looking forward and taking deep breaths.
14. A patient has been immobilized for 5 days because of extensive abdominal surgery. When this patient is helped out of bed for the first time, which patient problem related to safety applies to this patient? *(Select all that apply.)*
    1. *Recent Onset of Pain*
    2. *Compromised Skin Integrity*
    3. *Compromised Blood Flow to Tissue*
    4. *Potential for Inability to Tolerate Activity*
    5. *Potential for Falling*
15. Which assistive device allows patients to pull with the upper extremities to raise their trunk off the bed, to assist in transfer from bed to wheelchair, and to perform upper arm exercises?
    1. Trapeze bar
    2. Trochanter roll
    3. Hand rolls
    4. Footboard
16. In which position is the patient lying face down or chest down?
    1. Supine
    2. Lateral
    3. Prone
    4. Fowler's
17. What is a necessary safety precaution when helping a patient who has an unsteady gait to ambulate? *(Select all that apply.)*
    1. Have family members present.
    2. Have patient wear well-fitting nonskid shoes or slippers.
    3. Have at least two people present to assist the patient.
    4. Be sure no pain medication was given for at least 3 hours before ambulation.
    5. Use a gait belt when assisting the patient to stand and to ambulate.

18. What is a major benefit of active ROM exercises? *(Select all that apply.)*
1. Preventing contractures
2. Preventing the patient from getting arthritis
3. Maintaining joint movement and mobility
4. Preventing atrophy of muscle near the joints
5. Increasing the patient's self-esteem and motivation

19. The nurse is receiving a report on a patient. The nurse giving the report states that the patient has foot drop. The nurse receiving the report knows that which is the correct terminology for foot drop?
1. Plantar flexion of the foot
2. Dorsiflexion of the foot
3. Ankle extension
4. Ankle hyperextension

20. When using a lift sheet to assist in moving a patient up in bed, what should the nurse ask the patient to do? *(Select all that apply.)*
1. Bend the knees to assist in moving
2. Keep the hands at sides of the body
3. Raise the arms above the head
4. Maintain good body alignment
5. Place the arms across the chest

Hygiene and Care of the Patient's Environment

9

http://evolve.elsevier.com/Cooper/foundationsadult/

Objectives

1. Discuss the therapeutic hospital room environment.
2. Describe personal hygienic practices.
3. Discuss variations of the bath procedure determined by a patient's condition and physician's orders.
4. Describe the procedure for a bed bath.
5. Identify nursing interventions for the prevention and treatment of a pressure ulcer/injury.
6. Discuss heat and cold therapy and related procedures.
7. Describe the procedures for oral hygiene, shaving, hair care, nail care, and eye, ear, and nose care.
8. Outline the procedure for a back rub.
9. Summarize the procedure for perineal care for a male patient and a female patient.
10. Discuss the procedures for skin care.
11. Describe the procedure for making an unoccupied bed.
12. Describe the procedure for making an occupied bed.
13. Discuss assisting a patient in the use of the bedpan, the urinal, and the bedside commode.

Key Terms

axilla (ăk-SĬL-ă, p. 195)
bedpan (BĔD-păn, p. 225)
canthus (KĂN-thŭs, p. 195)
cerumen (sĕ-RŪ-mĕn, p. 220)
circumorbital (sŭr-kŭm-ŎR-bĭ-tăl, p. 219)
dentures (DĔN-chŭrs, p. 211)
febrile (p. 201)
hygiene (HĪ-gēn, p. 187)
labia majora (LĀ-bē-ă mă-JŎR-ă, p. 218)
labia minora (LĀ-bē-ă mĭ-NŎR-ă, p. 218)
medical asepsis (ā-SĔP-sĭs, p. 188)
oral hygiene (ŎR-ăl HĪ-gēn, p. 211)
pathogenic (păth-ō-GĔN-ĭk, p. 188)
perineal care (pĕr-ĭ-NĒ-ăl, p. 214)
personal hygiene (PŬR-sŭn-ăl HĪ-gēn, p. 187)
pressure injury (PRĔ-shŭr ĬN-jŭ-rē, p. 201)
pressure ulcer (PRĔ-shŭr ŬL-sĕr, p. 201)
prone (prōn, p. 196)
range of motion (ROM) (rānj ŏv MŌ-shŭn, p. 192)
Sims position (SĬMZ pŏ-zĭ-shŭn, p. 196)
supine (SŪ-pīn [noun], sū-PĪN [adjective], p. 196)
syncope (SĬN-kō-pē, p. 192)
umbilicus (ŭm-BĬL-ĭ-kŭs, p. 195)
urinal (Ū-rĭn-ăl, p. 225)
vasoconstriction (vā-zō-kŏn-STRĬK-shŭn, p. 206)
vasodilation (vā-zō-dī-LĀ-shŭn, p. 206)
vertigo (VŬR-tĭ-gō, p. 192)

Hygiene (the principles of health) includes care of not only the skin but also the hair, the hands, the feet, the eyes, the ears, the nose, the mouth, the back, and the perineum. This chapter discusses the bath, components of the bath, bed making, and assisting the patient in the use of the bedpan, the urinal, and the bedside commode. Many factors influence the practice of an individual's personal hygiene (Box 9.1 and the Cultural Considerations box about personal hygiene).

When assisting with the patient's hygiene needs, the licensed practical/vocational nurse (LPN/LVN) has an opportunity to observe the patient's ability to perform self-care. Assisting a patient with hygiene care gives the nurse an opportune time to perform a complete and thorough physical assessment. During the bath, the nurse is able to assess the patient's physical and emotional state and assess all body systems. Assisting a patient with bathing involves close contact with the patient and offers an opportunity to communicate with the patient to enhance a therapeutic relationship and learn about the emotional needs of the patient.

Patients often are in a dependent role and need assistance from the nurse in carrying out **personal hygiene** (the self-care measures people use to maintain health and prevent disease). The nurse's responsibility is to preserve the patient's well-being, encourage as much of the patient's independence as possible, and respect the patient's privacy when assisting with hygiene measures.

Sometimes the nurse needs to teach health promotion practices, and the performance of hygienic care provides an excellent opportunity for this. An attitude of acceptance during care for a patient with poor hygiene allows for development of the nurse-patient relationship.

Box 9.1 Factors That Influence a Patient's Personal Hygiene

- *Body image.* Body image is a person's subjective concept of physical appearance. This body image affects the manner in which hygiene is maintained. The nurse must provide education to the unclean patient about the importance of hygiene. Nurses must be careful not to convey feelings of disapproval when caring for the patient whose hygiene practices differ from others.
- *Cultural variables.* Patients from diverse cultural backgrounds follow different self-care practices. In North America, people typically take daily baths (tub or shower), but in many European countries, it is not unusual to bathe completely only once a week. Avoid being judgmental when caring for patients with different hygienic practices (see the Cultural Considerations box).
- *Knowledge.* Knowledge alone is not enough. The patient also must be encouraged to maintain self-care. Often, learning about an illness or condition encourages patients to improve hygienic practices. For example, teaching the patient with diabetes the importance of foot care helps prevent infections. It is important to maintain a nonjudgmental attitude while providing hygiene for the patient.
- *Personal preference.* Individual patients have individual desires and choices as to when to bathe, shave, and shampoo. Patients choose different shampoos, deodorants, and toothpastes according to personal needs or selections. Do not try to change the patient's preferences unless the patient's health is affected.
- *Physical condition.* Patients in the late stages of terminal illness or those who have undergone surgery often lack the physical energy or dexterity to perform personal hygiene. Some disease conditions exhaust or incapacitate patients, thereby requiring you to perform all aspects of hygiene. Other disease conditions, such as serious cardiac or pulmonary problems, cause severe activity intolerance.
- *Social practices.* Social groups, family customs, age, friends, and work groups influence practices of personal hygiene.
- *Socioeconomic status.* The patient's economic resources often influence the type or extent of hygienic practices used.

Different types of hygienic care usually are performed at certain times throughout the day. These times depend on various factors, including patient schedules and staff responsibilities (Box 9.2). Sometimes scheduling of hygiene measures at the same time as other care measures is most convenient.

The nurse's own conscientious practice of personal hygiene is essential (Box 9.3). Nurses are role models and teach by example. Hygienic practices promote **medical asepsis,** also known as clean technique. This technique inhibits the growth and spread of **pathogenic** (disease-producing) microorganisms (see Chapter 7).

 **Cultural Considerations**

Personal Hygiene

- Cultural practices vary within a culture. The authors of this text are describing common cultural practices. Please note that these practices are not demonstrated by all members of a particular culture.
- Touch or lack of touch has cultural significance and symbolism and is a learned behavior. Cultural uses of touch vary. Although the rules of touch are typically unspoken and unwritten, they are usually visible to the observer. Stay within the rules of touch that are culturally prescribed.
- Chinese Americans sometimes view tasks associated with closeness and touch as offensive. Vietnamese Americans are likely to feel very uneasy during a back rub. Ask patients what makes them most comfortable during a bath.
- Use touch with discernment and avoid forcing touch on anyone. A momentary and seemingly incidental touch has the capacity to establish a positive, temporary bond between strangers, making them more compliant, helpful, positive, and giving.
- Be mindful of the patient's reaction to touch and avoid being perceived as intrusive.
- Consider the individual patient's beliefs, values, and habits.
- Individual preferences usually do not affect health in any significant manner and usually fit without problem into the plan of care.
- East Indian Hindus consider personal hygiene to be extremely important. A daily bath is part of their religious duty. Some Hindus believe bathing after a meal to be injurious. Likewise, a bath that is too hot has the potential to injure the eyes. Hot water may be added to cold water, but cold water is not to be added to hot water when preparing a bath. Once a bath is completed, the individual carefully dries the body thoroughly with a towel.

PATIENT'S ROOM ENVIRONMENT

Many patients with limitations such as traction, casts, or monitoring equipment may not leave their rooms as frequently as other patients. Patients who are critically ill may be confined to their rooms for an extended period of time. These rooms must be kept comfortable and safe (Fig. 9.1). By controlling factors such as room temperature, ventilation, noise, and odors, the LPN/LVN creates a more therapeutic environment. Keeping the room clean, neat, and orderly contributes to a sense of well-being.

MAINTAINING COMFORT

Consider the patient's age, severity of illness, and activity tolerance to maintain optimal patient comfort. The recommended room temperature is 68° to 74°F (20° to 23°C). Infants, older adults (see the Lifespan Considerations for Older Adults box), and the acutely ill are likely to need warmer temperatures. Physically active

Box 9.2 Hygiene Care Schedule

- *Early morning care.* Nursing personnel provide basic hygiene to patients getting ready for breakfast, scheduled tests, or early morning surgery. "a.m. care" includes offering a bedpan or urinal if the patient is not ambulatory, washing the patient's hands and face, and assisting with oral care.
- *Morning care, or after-breakfast care.* This care is performed after breakfast. Offer a bedpan or urinal to patients confined to bed; provide a bath or shower; provide oral, foot, nail, and hair care; give a back rub; change the patient's gown or pajamas; change the bed linens; and straighten the patient's bedside unit and room. This often is referred to as complete a.m. care.
- *Afternoon care.* Because hospitalized patients often undergo many exhausting diagnostic tests or procedures in the morning, they tend to greatly appreciate afternoon care. This is also true for the long-term care resident. Many of these residents have participated in exercise, physical therapy, or activities throughout the day. Afternoon hygienic care includes washing the hands and face, assisting with oral care, offering a bedpan or urinal, and straightening bed linen.
- *Evening care, or hour-before-sleep (HS) care.* Before bedtime, offer personal hygienic care that helps a patient relax to promote sleep. "p.m. care," sometimes referred to as HS care, typically includes changing soiled bed linens, gowns, or pajamas; assisting the patient in washing the face, hands, and back; providing oral hygiene; giving a back massage; and offering the bedpan or urinal to nonambulatory patients.

patients and patients with chronic pulmonary problems tend to be more comfortable in a cooler environment.

Good ventilation is necessary to keep stale air and odors from lingering in the room. Take care to protect the patient from drafts. Ensure that odors are kept to a minimum. Promptly emptying and cleaning bedpans, urinals, and commodes helps to eliminate odors.

Noises are unpleasant intrusions. Ill patients are more sensitive to the noises commonly heard within the hospital environment. Work with other hospital personnel to monitor the noise level that results from the moving of metal equipment on and off the elevator and from televisions and radios, telephones ringing, loud talking, and laughter at the nurses' station. Manage equipment properly, answer phones immediately, and control voice volume. Ask patients to keep televisions and radios turned down.

Proper lighting is necessary for the safety of the nurse and the patient. Reduce lighting levels to encourage sleep, and brighten the room for stimulation. Adjust the lighting by closing or opening the drapes, adjusting overbed and floor lights, and opening or closing room doors.

The nurse must help the patient conserve energy for the recovery process. Controlling stimuli within the patient's personal environment is one way to help

Box 9.3 Personal Hygiene for Nurses

- Take a daily bath or shower.
- Use a strong, odorless, and effective deodorant every day.
- Wear clean undergarments every day.
- Wear a clean uniform every day.
- Shampoo hair as often as necessary to maintain cleanliness.
- Keep hair off the collar or at least pulled back away from the face and in a contained hairstyle. Wear barrettes and bows that blend in with your hair.
- Wear clean, comfortable shoes that follow facility policy.
- Keep fingernails short, clean, and well manicured. Nail polish and artificial nails are not allowed in many facilities. Pathogens get trapped underneath polish or artificial nails and have the potential to cause serious infections, especially in newborns.
- Wear makeup only in moderation.
- Wear only an engagement ring or wedding ring (or both) without stones (stones harbor microorganisms). In departments such as the operating and delivery rooms, rings are not worn at all.
- Wear only small unobtrusive earrings; wear only one pair. Large or dangling earrings are not recommended. These are considered hazardous because they can be pulled out easily and damage the ear.
- Avoid perfumes or colognes (many patients are allergic to these).
- Wear the standard departmental uniform.
- Keep beards and mustaches clean, short, and well trimmed.
- Use breath mints; the smell of coffee, foods, or nicotine is often offensive to patients.

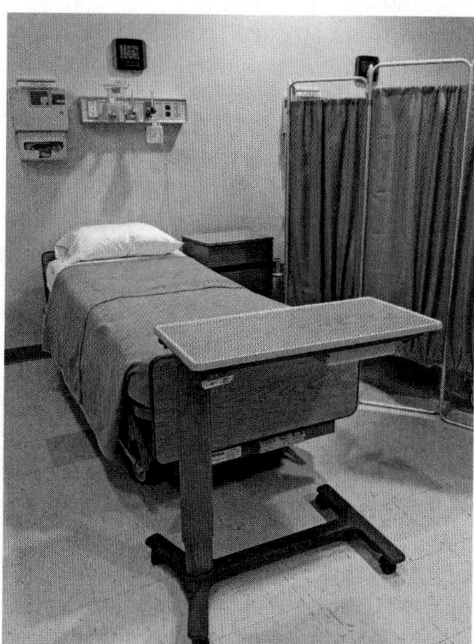

Fig. 9.1 A typical hospital room.

Lifespan Considerations

Older Adults

Hygiene Practices

- Older individuals are more likely to become chilled during bathing or when left uncovered. Maintain a warmer room temperature than for younger people, and keep drafts to a minimum.
- Drape older adults properly during care to prevent chilling and provide for modesty.
- Older adults with limited mobility may need assistance in perineal care. Use of a side-lying position increases the patient's comfort and provides the nurse with opportunity to provide perineal care and inspect surrounding skin. Perineal care should be performed daily and after each episode of incontinence.
- Impaired circulation or neurologic changes sometimes decrease the older person's ability to sense temperature changes in water, so use caution to prevent burns during tub or shower bathing.
- Too-frequent bathing and use of detergent soaps have harmful effects on the skin of most older adults. Determine the type and frequency of baths and the choice of soap based on individual needs.
- Rehydrate patient's skin with lotions and fluids.
- Immobility, incontinence, and poor nutrition increase the risk of skin impairment in older adults. Adequate diet, frequent change of position, use of pressure-reducing devices, regular toileting, and prompt cleansing of the skin after incontinence reduce the risks.
- Older adults with urinary incontinence need meticulous skin care to reduce skin irritation from urine and feces.
- The aging process contributes to changes in voiding and defecating. Often the aging patient needs immediate response to a request for the bedpan or urinal or assistance to the toilet.
- Incontinence of urine or stool is *not* an expected result of the aging process.
- Decreased production of saliva in aging necessitates more frequent oral hygiene. Good cleaning of the oral cavity and teeth or dentures helps reduce the alteration in taste common with aging.
- Good oral hygiene practices help older adults preserve their ability to eat. Patients with diabetes need to visit the dentist a minimum of every 6 months. Older adults, especially those at risk for oral problems, should avoid spicy, coarse, acidic, and sugary foods, which tend to cause dental caries.
- Treat older adults with respect. Keep grooming, including hair care and use of cosmetics, age appropriate.
- Because of normal changes in the nails and an increased incidence of circulatory problems or diabetes mellitus, older individuals are more likely to require special foot care.
- Changes in aging skin include thinning of epidermis and subcutaneous fat and dryness because of decreased activity of oil and sweat glands. These changes become visible in the feet. In addition, nails become opaque, tough, scaly, brittle, and hypertrophied.
- Individuals who have not participated in regular exercise often experience a laxity of foot ligaments and musculature, which leads to instability and impaired mobility.
- Common foot problems of older adults include heel pain caused by tearing of plantar fascia and foot musculature, metatarsalgia (pain beneath metatarsal head), hammertoes and claw toes, corns and calluses, pathologic nail conditions (e.g., ingrown toenails, fungal infections), arthritis, and neuropathies that cause diminished sensation in the foot.
- Older persons are also more vulnerable to bunions because feet tend to spread with aging.
- Usually the facial hair of the older adult does not grow quickly; thus a shave is not necessarily required every day.
- Older adults have fragile skin and require more protection. Be sure bed linens are clean, dry, and free of wrinkles.
- Encourage older adults to spend as much time out of bed as possible.
- Use draw sheets and waterproof pads with caution. Accumulation of moisture creates a risk for skin maceration and impairment, so these items must be changed as needed.

conserve energy. This promotes a sense of security and enhances the patient's ability to gain needed rest and sleep (see Chapter 21).

ROOM EQUIPMENT

The usual hospital room contains certain basic furniture: bedside stand, bed, overbed table, chairs, and lights (see Fig. 9.1). In addition, the standard hospital room has either a closet or drawer space. Room equipment and furniture for the long-term care facility differs somewhat, often incorporating more personal furniture and decor (see Chapter 38).

The bedside stand stores the patient's personal articles and hygienic equipment, such as towels, the emesis and bath basins, toothpaste and toothbrush, and comb and brush. The telephone, the drinking glass, and the water pitcher ordinarily are kept on the patient's bedside stand.

The overbed table is on wheels and is adjustable to various heights over the bed or a chair. Usually a storage area is located under the tabletop. This tabletop is ideal to use as a working space when performing procedures. It also serves as a surface for meal trays, toileting items needed during hygienic care, and other objects frequently used by the patient. The tabletop should be cleaned before and after procedures and before meals.

Chairs are a necessity in the hospital room. Straight chairs and lounge chairs are typical. The patient and visitors make use of the lounge chair. Straight chairs are more maneuverable than lounge chairs. They are also more convenient when temporarily transferring the patient from the bed, such as during bed making. Relatives who sit with the patient are apt to use recliner chairs.

Lights in each patient's room provide comfort, safety, and ease. A call light is available at each bedside. The call signal indicates that a patient needs assistance. Many facilities are designed so that the call light from a patient's bathroom flashes off and on quickly, denoting a call of a more serious nature. In contrast, the bedside call light typically does not flash. Respond as soon as possible when a patient indicates a need for assistance.

Critically ill patients often remain in bed for longer periods of time. Hospital beds are designed for comfort and safety and their capacity to accommodate position changes (Table 9.1). The standard hospital bed has a firm water-repellent mattress on a metal frame that is raised and lowered horizontally as needed. An even surface provides for the greatest comfort. Bariatric beds are available in most facilities to accommodate obese patients. Handles on the sides of the mattress are helpful with removing or turning the mattress.

Different bed positions are used to promote lung expansion, postural drainage, and other interventions. Most beds are powered by electricity, but some are operated manually. These beds are convenient to raise while working at the bedside and then lower when the patient is being transferred or when leaving the patient's room. Furthermore, the nurse or patient can raise and lower the head or the foot of the bed independently. In most cases, the controls are situated conveniently on the side of the bed or in the side rail. Teach the patient the proper use of the controls, and caution the patient to leave the bed at its lowest level to prevent injuries from falls.

Hospital beds have a number of safety features. Locks on the wheels prevent unwanted movement. Side rails (adjustable metal frames that are raised and lowered by pushing or pulling a knob) are located on both sides of the bed. These side rails protect patients from falling, aid patients in positioning themselves, and provide upper extremity support as the patient gets out of bed. Never leave the bedside of a patient in bed if the side rail is lowered. Full side rails are considered a form of restraint in a long-term care setting (see Chapter 38). Another safety feature is the special removable headboard on some beds, which is important when the medical team needs easy access to the patient's head during cardiopulmonary resuscitation.

Table 9.1 Bed Positions

POSITION	DESCRIPTION	USES
Fowler's to high Fowler's	Head of bed raised to angle of 45 degrees or more (up to 90 degrees); semi-sitting to full upright sitting position	Appropriate position for eating or drinking to prevent aspiration; beneficial during breathing exercises to promote full lung expansion
Semi-Fowler's (also referred to as low Fowler's)	Head of bed raised approximately 30 degrees	Often used for patients who cannot tolerate Fowler's or high Fowler's; position sometimes ordered after lumbar puncture has been performed
Trendelenburg's	Entire bed tilted downward toward head of bed with no break in the middle of the bed	Facilitates removal of secretions with postural drainage; facilitates venous return in patients with poor peripheral circulation; sometimes used to aid in dilation of large vessels for central line placement
Reverse Trendelenburg's	Entire bed frame tilted downward toward foot of bed with no break in the middle of the bed	Not commonly used position; promotes gastric emptying and prevents esophageal reflux; facilitates arterial circulation to lower extremities
Flat	Entire bed frame parallel with floor	For patients with vertebral injuries, immediately after lumbar puncture, and in cervical traction; generally preferred by patients for sleeping

Modified from Potter PA, Perry AG: *Essentials for nursing practice*, ed 8, St. Louis, 2015, Mosby.

BATHING

The extent of the patient's bath and methods used for bathing depend on the patient's capabilities, the degree of hygiene required, and the physician's order, as in the case of therapeutic baths. The types of therapeutic baths are outlined in the following sections. Some hygiene skills are acceptable to delegate to unlicensed assistive personnel (UAP; see the Coordinated Care box on bathing and other hygienic care measures), unless UAP are not available or are not part of the staff of a particular unit or facility.

Maintain a water temperature of 110°F (about 43°C) if the purpose is to apply heat to the affected area. If the purpose is to promote healing or to produce relaxation, use a water temperature of about 98° to 102°F (34° to 39°C). Remember to prevent chilling by covering the patient's legs with a bath blanket and the shoulders with a towel. Place a towel behind the patient's back for comfort.

Optimally, the sitz bath lasts from 20 to 30 minutes; it usually is ordered three times daily. The time seems to pass more quickly when the patient has reading material.

Observe the patient for signs and symptoms of weakness, such as a rapid or weak pulse, tachypnea, or **vertigo** (dizziness) or **syncope** (fainting). Never leave the patient alone unless you are sure the patient is safe;

Coordinated Care

Delegation

Hygiene Care Measures

BATHING

The skilled task of bathing often is delegated to UAP; however, skin and **range of motion (ROM)** (normal movement that any given joint is capable of making) assessment require the critical thinking and knowledge application unique to the nurse.

- Instruct the UAP in what type of bath (e.g., complete, partial assist, tub, shower) is appropriate to the patient's diagnosis and needs.
- Remind the UAP to notify you of any skin integrity problems so that you can inspect areas of impairment or potential impairment.
- Remind the UAP to use an organized approach and reassuring tone of voice so that the patient feels safe and comfortable during bathing.
- Instruct the UAP to encourage the patient to report any concerns or discomfort during the bath.
- Instruct the UAP to encourage as much independence in the patient's self-care skills as appropriate and to provide positive feedback.

ORAL CARE

Skills of oral care, toothbrushing, and denture care are appropriate to delegate to UAP, but the patient's gag reflex should be assessed first.

- Instruct the UAP in the proper way to position the patient if the patient is unconscious or debilitated.
- Remind the UAP to report any changes in oral mucosa.
- Review with the UAP the use of oral suction for cleansing oral secretions (if allowed by facility policy), if the patient is likely to need it.

HAIR CARE AND SHOWERING

The skills of shampooing and shaving are appropriate to delegate to UAP, unless the patient has a trauma or injury of the cervical spine.

- Instruct the UAP how to properly position individual patients and use any special products indicated.
- Be sure the UAP knows how to correctly use medicated shampoos for lice or other conditions and the appropriate steps to prevent transmission to other patients.
- Remind the UAP to report how the patient tolerated the procedure and any changes that indicate possible inflammation or injury.

HAND, FOOT, AND NAIL CARE

The skill of care of the fingernails and foot care for patients without diabetes or any circulatory compromise, anticoagulant therapy, or bleeding disorder is appropriate to delegate to UAP.

- Instruct UAP in the proper way to use nail files and clippers (check agency policy on whether UAP are permitted to use nail clippers on patients).
- Caution UAP to use warm water.
- Remind UAP to report any changes that indicate possible inflammation or injury.

BED MAKING

Bed making usually is delegated to UAP.

- Instruct UAP on whether an unoccupied or occupied bed is to be made.
- Review with UAP the safety precautions or activity restrictions for the patient; stress the use of side rails in the acute care setting and the call system in the event that staff assistance is needed.
- Instruct UAP to notify the nurse immediately if wound drainage, dressing material, drainage tubes, or intravenous (IV) tubing is found in the linen or becomes dislodged.
- Instruct UAP to allow the patient rest periods and notify the nurse if the patient becomes fatigued.

CARE OF THE PATIENT WITH INCONTINENCE

The skill of providing care for patients with incontinence is appropriate to delegate to UAP. The following measures are all particularly important when assisting the patient with incontinence:

- Caution UAP to be aware of the patient's dignity and self-esteem needs and to take measures to prevent violating these needs.
- Ensure that UAP know standard precautions guidelines related to handling of body fluids.
- Be sure UAP report information such as abdominal pain, increased episodes of incontinence, changes in appearance of urine or stool, and evidence of skin breakdown.
- The nurse is responsible for ensuring that all patients are given adequate privacy for elimination and that cultural modesty standards are observed.

a call signal should be placed within easy reach. Instruct the patient to stay out of drafts and to rest after a sitz bath.

COOL WATER TUB BATH

The cool water tub bath is an option to relieve tension or lower body temperature. Take precautions to prevent the patient from chilling. The water temperature is tepid, 98.6°F (37°C). Cold water should not be used because it causes chilling and shivering.

WARM WATER TUB BATH

A warm water tub bath is given primarily to reduce muscle tension. The recommended water temperature is approximately 110°F (43°C).

HOT WATER TUB BATH

The hot water tub bath helps relieve muscle soreness and muscle spasms. This procedure is not recommended for children. The proper water temperature for adults is 113° to 115°F (45° to 46°C). Keep in mind the danger of burns, and take precautions to prevent them. This bath is not used for patients with neurologic disorders or circulatory impairment because of the risk of causing burns.

SITZ BATH

A sitz bath cleanses and aids in reducing inflammation of the perineal and anal areas of the patient who has undergone rectal or vaginal surgery or childbirth. Discomfort from hemorrhoids or a fissure also is relieved with a sitz bath.

The appliance for the sitz bath is shown in Fig. 9.2. Depending on the patient's diagnosis and the health care provider's order, the desired results are possible to obtain from a tub bath. The water in the tub should be kept to a minimum so that the warm water will be concentrated in the perineal area. The tub is the least desirable method because heat also is applied to the legs, thus reducing the effects on the pelvic region.

OTHER BATHS

A complete bed bath is for patients who are totally dependent and require total assistance (Skill 9.1). As the patient's condition improves, only partial assistance becomes necessary. Assist with bathing those body parts that are inaccessible to the patient.

Text continued on p. 201

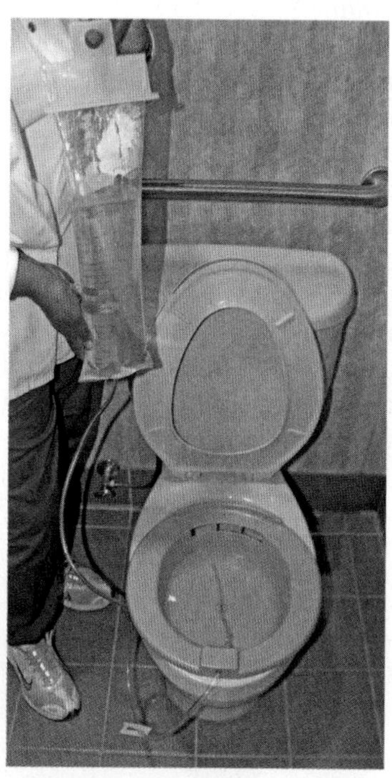

Fig. 9.2 The portable sitz bath.

Skill 9.1 Bathing the Patient and Administering a Back Rub

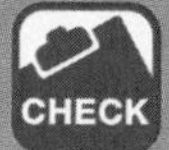

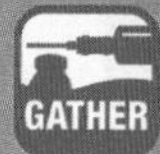

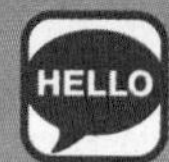

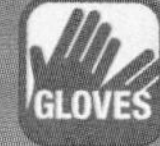

NURSING ACTION *(RATIONALE)*

1. Refer to medical record, care plan, or Kardex for special interventions. *(Provides basis for care.)*
2. Assemble the necessary supplies. *(Organizes procedure.)*
   - Bath blanket
   - Bath towels (2)
   - Disposable gloves
   - Drapes
   - Gown or patient's own pajamas or nightgown
   - Hygiene articles, such as lotion, powder, and deodorant
   - Laundry bag or hamper
   - Soap and soap dish
   - Washbasin
   - Washcloths (2)
3. Introduce self. *(Decreases patient's anxiety.)*
4. Identify patient. *(Ensures procedure is performed with correct patient.)*
5. Explain procedure to patient. *(Enlists cooperation and decreases anxiety.)*
6. Perform hand hygiene and, as appropriate, don clean gloves. Know agency policy and guidelines from the Centers for Disease Control and Prevention (CDC) and Occupational Safety and Health Administration (OSHA). *(Reduces spread of microorganisms.)*

Continued

Skill 9.1 Bathing the Patient and Administering a Back Rub—cont'd

7. Prepare patient for intervention.
   a. Close door or pull curtain. *(Provides privacy.)*
   b. Drape for procedure as appropriate. *(Prevents unnecessary exposure.)*
   c. Suggest use of bedpan, urinal, or bathroom. *(Prevents interruptions during procedure and provides for patient's comfort.)*
   d. Arrange supplies. *(Provides convenient access to equipment.)*
   e. Adjust room temperature. *(Prevents patient from chilling.)*
   f. Raise bed to comfortable working position. *(Promotes proper body mechanics.)*
8. Bed bath.
   a. Lower side rail; position patient on side of bed closest to you. *(Ensures proper body mechanics.)*
   b. Loosen top linens from the foot of the bed; place bath blanket over the top linens. Ask patient to hold bath blanket while you remove top linens. If patient is unable, hold bath blanket in place while removing linens. *(Provides warmth and privacy.)*
   c. Place soiled laundry in laundry bag; do not touch uniform with soiled laundry. *(Reduces spread of microorganisms.)*
   d. Assist patient with oral hygiene. *(Prevents mouth diseases, improves self-image, and improves appetite.)* If patient is unable, the nurse performs the procedure (see Skill 9.3).
   e. Remove patient's gown, all undergarments, and jewelry. *(Facilitates a more effective bed bath.)* If an extremity is injured or has reduced mobility, begin removal of the gown from the unaffected side. If the patient has an IV tube, remove gown from the arm without IV first, then lower IV container or remove tubing from pump and slide gown covering down over the affected arm and over tubing and container. Rehang IV container and check flow rate or reset pump. Do not disconnect tubing. *(Undressing the unaffected side first makes manipulating gown over body part easier with reduced range of motion [ROM] [normal movement that any given joint is capable of making].)*

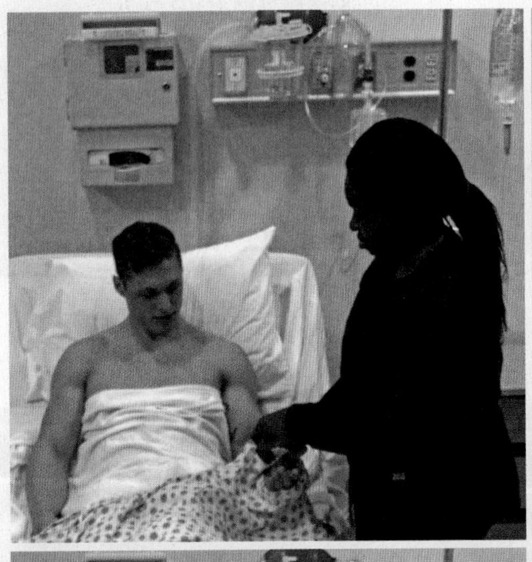
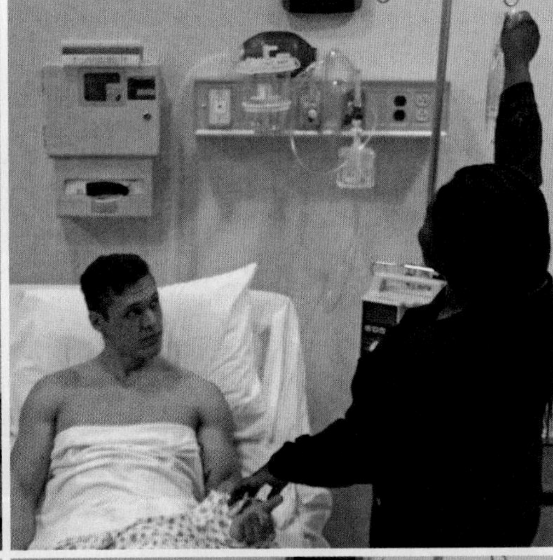
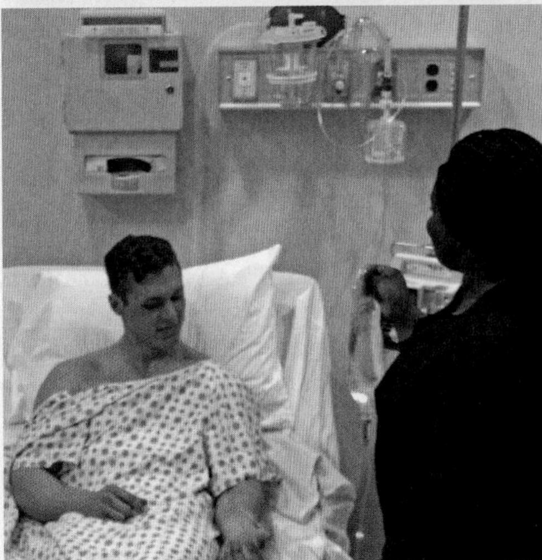
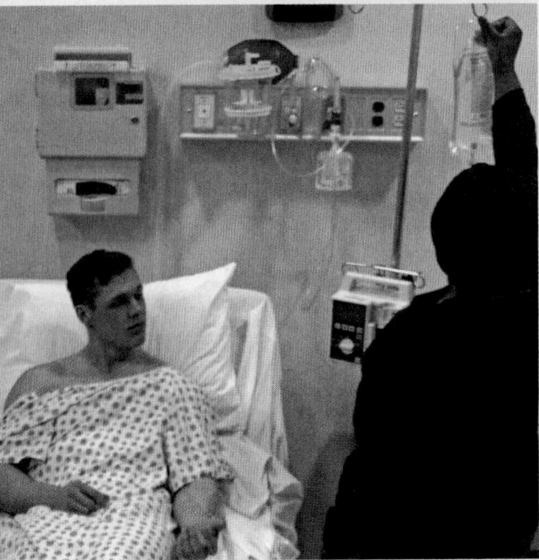

Skill 9.1 Bathing the Patient and Administering a Back Rub—cont'd

f. Raise side rail and fill washbasin two-thirds full with water at 110° to 115°F (43° to 46°C). To prevent spillage, do not overfill basin. *(Maintains patient's safety.)*

g. Remove pillow and raise head of bed to semi-Fowler's position if patient is able to tolerate it. *(The patient's face, ears, and neck are more accessible for cleansing. Patients with breathing difficulties need a pillow or elevation of head of bed during bath.)*

h. Form mitt with bath cloth around your hand (see illustration); dip mitt and hand into bath water. Squeeze out excess water. *(Facilitates handling of bath cloth and prevents corners from brushing against patient. Do not place soap in bath water—too many suds prevent adequate rinsing.)*

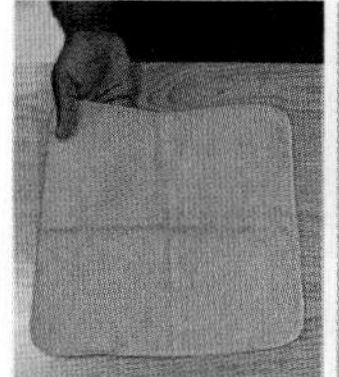
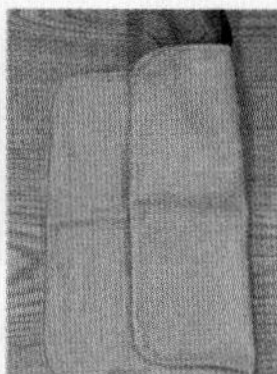
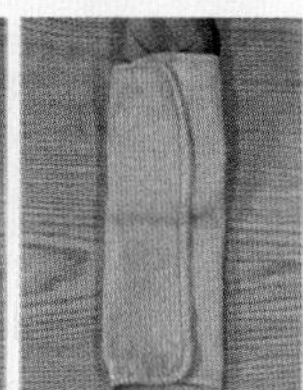
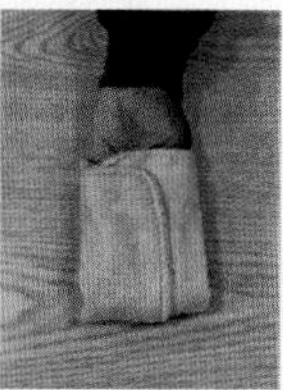

i. Wash around patient's eyes, using a different portion of washcloth for each eye. Cleanse from inner to outer **canthus** (corner of eye; see illustration). Dry gently. *(Prevents irritation, spread of infection, and injury.)*

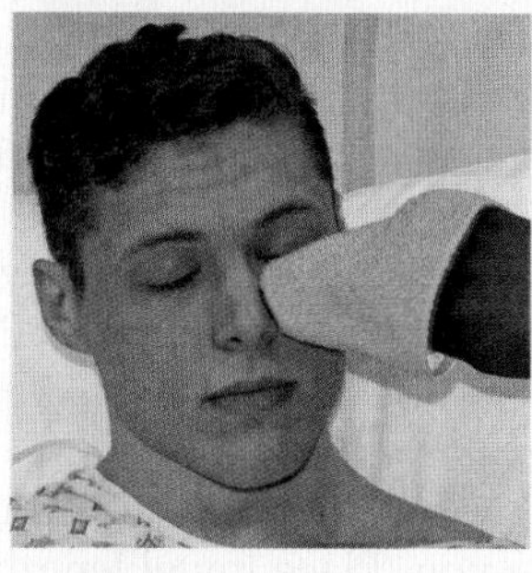

j. Rinse bath cloth (then continue to use as mitt) and finish washing face. (Ask patient about use of soap on face because some patients, especially female patients, do not use soap on face.) Wash ears and neck. Cleanse pinna (the projecting part of the external ear) with cotton-tipped applicators. *(Rinsing cloth well helps reduce any skin irritation from the soap. Do not place soap in washbasin to keep rinse water from getting soapy.)*

k. Expose arm farthest from you. Place towel lengthwise under patient's arm. To cleanse the hands, the nurse can place washbasin on towel and place patient's hand in basin of water, or the hands can be cleansed with the washcloth (be sure to clean between the fingers). Bathe arms with long, firm strokes; a firm stroke rather than a light stroke prevents tickling the patient. Supporting arm, raise it above patient's head to bathe the **axilla** (the underarm area or armpit). Rinse and dry well. In most cases, provide nail care at this time (see next step), although if desired, it is possible to do separately (see Skill 9.4). Apply deodorant if desired. *(Beginning on far side prevents reaching over clean area; long, firm strokes stimulate circulation. Raising arm promotes ROM and exposes axilla. Deodorant controls body odor. Axilla is bathed last because it is considered less clean than arm.)*

l. When doing nail care, allow patient's hand to soak for 3 to 5 minutes; push back cuticles gently with washcloth. Clean under nails and file smoothly as needed. Dry thoroughly. *(Enhances feeling of self-worth and decreases spread of infection. Soaking softens cuticles and loosens debris under nails.)*

m. Bathe arm closest to you. Follow Steps k and l.

n. Cover patient's chest with bath towel; fold bath blanket down to waist and wash chest with circular motion. Be certain to cleanse and dry well in skin folds and under breasts. *(Use of circular motion while bathing chest prevents injury to delicate breast tissue. Covering chest with towel prevents unnecessary exposure. Cleansing well in skin folds and under breasts maintains skin integrity.)* Continue to observe the condition of the patient's skin, degree of mobility, and behavior and encourage the patient to verbalize concerns.

o. Fold bath blanket down to pubic area, keeping chest covered with dry towel. Wash abdomen, including **umbilicus** (the depressed point in the middle of the abdomen; wash umbilicus with cotton-tipped applicators), and skin folds. Dry thoroughly. *(Maintains privacy. Prevents unnecessary exposure and prevents skin impairment.)*

p. Raise side rail; empty basin into hopper or stool. *(Flushes microorganisms down the stool and does not contaminate sink.)*

q. Rinse basin and washcloth. Refill basin two-thirds full with water at 110° to 115°F (43° to 46°C). *(Promotes patient's safety and comfort.)*

Continued

Skill 9.1 Bathing the Patient and Administering a Back Rub—cont'd

r. Expose leg farthest away from you, keeping *perineum* (the genital area) covered. Place bath towel lengthwise on bed under patient's leg. Place washbasin on towel and place patient's foot in basin. Patients with diabetes mellitus need special foot care. Be certain to support patient's leg properly; flex knee and grasp heel. If patient is unable to place foot in washbasin, wash leg and foot with mitted washcloth. *(Beginning on the far side prevents reaching over clean area; bath towel prevents wetting bottom linens; supporting patient's leg properly prevents injury.)*

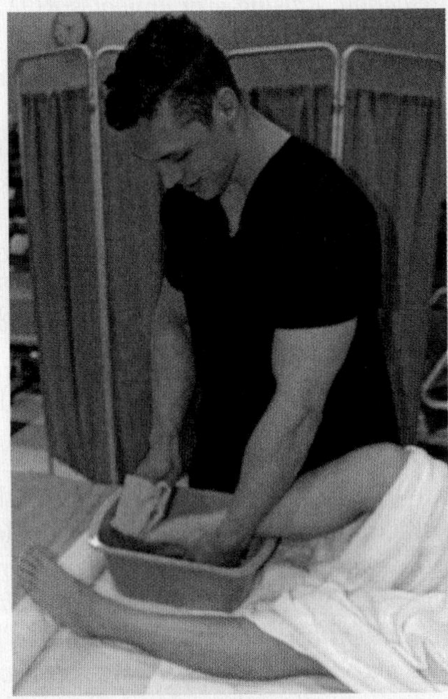

s. With long firm strokes, bathe the leg. *(Promotes circulation.)* However, note that bathing the lower extremities of patients with history of deep vein thrombosis (DVT) or hypercoagulation disorders with long firm strokes is contraindicated; use circular, gentle strokes for these patients so that the clot is not dislodged. After soaking, perform nail care (may be done at a separate time; see Skill 9.4). If skin is dry, apply lotion if desired. Do not massage legs. **Never massage lower extremities.** *(Prevents possible embolus [a moving blood clot].)*

t. Bathe leg and foot closest to you as in Steps r and s.

u. Raise side rail. Be sure patient is covered with bath blanket. Be certain to expose only those body parts being bathed. Change water (see Steps p and q). *(Provides clean water and promotes good hygiene.)* Lower side rail. If patient tolerates, position **prone** (lying face-down) or in **Sims position** (side-lying position). Place towel lengthwise on bed along back. Wash and dry back from neckline down to buttocks. If patient tolerates a massage action, do so while washing back. *(Promotes circulation, thus preventing skin impairment, and promotes relaxation.)*

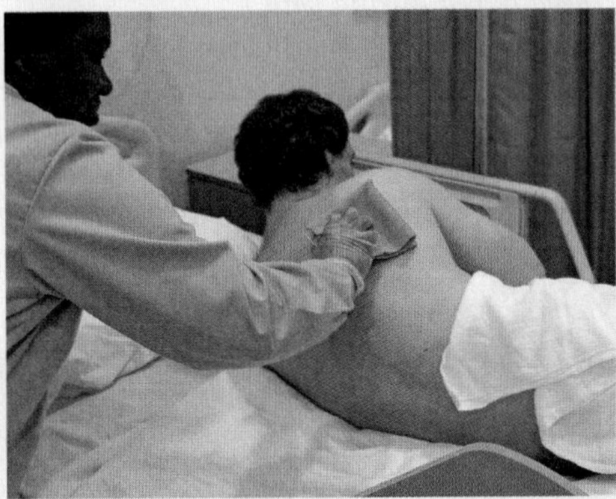

v. Reposition patient **supine** (lying face up). Provide basin of water, soap, washcloth, and towel, and instruct patient to cleanse perineal area. (Give patient privacy to do this.) If patient is unable to finish bath, don new gloves and complete this aspect of patient care (see Skill 9.5). *(Completes the bath procedure, decreases infection, and prevents skin impairment.)*

w. Be certain patient is covered with blankets. *(Prevents chilling.)* Raise side rail. *(Promotes safety.)* Empty, wash, and rinse basin. Replace basin in bedside stand. Place washcloth in laundry bag for soiled linen. *(Practice of medical asepsis reduces spread of microorganisms.)*

x. Position patient in Sims or prone position close to you. Place towel lengthwise along patient's back. Give back rub (see Step 14). *(Facilitates back care; provides comfort and promotes skin integrity.)* Never massage reddened areas. *(Potentially causes further skin breakdown.)*

y. Assist patient into clean gown. If ordered, assist patient to ambulate to chair; place towel over shoulders, and comb hair. *(Promotes positive self-image.)* Women sometimes wish to apply makeup at this time. While patient is in chair, make unoccupied bed (see Skill 9.6). If patient is not ambulatory, make the occupied bed (see Skill 9.6). *(Maintains clean environment.)*

Skill 9.1 Bathing the Patient and Administering a Back Rub—cont'd

z. Place all soiled linen into laundry bag. Be certain all bath equipment is clean and put it away as necessary. *(Reduces spread of microorganisms.)*

aa. Place call light, overbed table, nightstand, and telephone within easy reach. *(Promotes safety.)*

bb. Position patient for comfort, and provide warmth. *(Promotes patient's well-being.)*

cc. Remove gloves, if wearing any; discard them in proper receptacle, and perform hand hygiene. *(Reduces spread of microorganisms.)* Maintain a neat, clean work area.

9. The partial bed bath differs from the bed bath only in that the patient does not need assistance bathing many anatomic regions. Help by bathing those areas that the patient cannot reach (e.g., feet, back, perineal area). All steps of the bath are followed, with the same considerations. Place supplies within easy reach. Change water as noted in the bed bath procedure, and give back care, skin care, nail care, and hair care. A partial bath, in which face, neck, hands, axilla, and perineum are washed, is practiced in some agencies. The feet may be included in a partial bed bath if necessary.

10. Towel bath.[a]
  a. Follow Steps 1 and 3 to 7.
  b. Assemble supplies. *(Organizes procedure.)*
    - Articles for personal hygiene: comb, toothbrush, lotion, toothpaste, and mouthwash
    - Bath blankets (3)
    - Bath towel
    - Clean gown
    - Concentrate or no-rinse solution
    - Disposable gloves
    - Large plastic bag
    - Linens for bed making
    - Measuring device, such as plastic medication cup or liter-calibrated container
    - Towel–bath towel (3 × 7.5 ft)
    - Washcloths (2)
  c. Prepare patient. *(Ensures that bath towel will be warm enough for patient's comfort and for effective towel bath. It is necessary to ready the patient before the bath towel is prepared; the temperature cools down quickly.)*
    (1) Remove patient's clothing and excess bedding (top linens, bedspread). Place patient on bath blanket, and cover patient with bath blanket. *(Provides privacy and prevents unnecessary exposure of patient; provides for patient warmth.)*
    (2) Cover with plastic any surgical dressings, casts, or areas that are not to be gotten wet. *(Maintains integrity of dressing or cast.)*
    (3) Fanfold a clean bath blanket at foot of the bed. *(Provides easy access to clean blankets.)*
    (4) Position patient supine with legs partially separated and arms loosely at sides. *(Facilitates the towel bath.)*
  d. Prepare towel. *(Prevents unnecessary cleanups and promotes effective procedure.)*
    (1) Fold towel in half, top to bottom; fold in half again, top to bottom; fold in half again, side to side. Then roll towel–bath towel with bath towel and washcloths inside, beginning with folded edge.

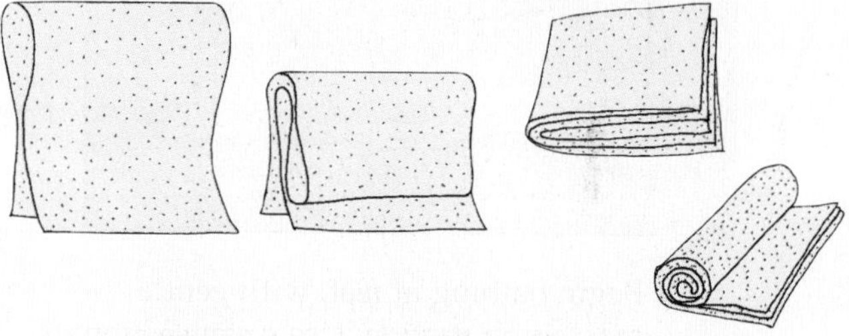

    (2) Place rolled-up towel–bath towel (with bath towel and washcloths inside) in plastic bag with selvage edges toward open end of bag.
    (3) Draw 2000 mL of water at 115° to 120°F (46° to 49°C) into plastic pitcher. If the towel is not warm, the sauna-like effect is not produced and the patient is chilled. Measure 30 mL of concentrate with a pump (a single stroke measures 30 mL). Mix 2000 mL of water and no-rinse solution.
    (4) Pour mixture over towel in plastic bag.

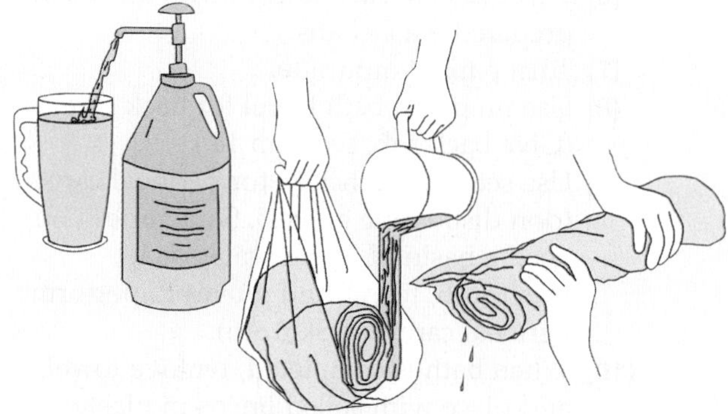

    (5) Knead the solution quickly into towel; position plastic bag with open end in sink and squeeze out excess water.

Continued

[a]An alternative to the towel bath is "bath-in-a-bag." This is similar to the towel bath except the washcloth is presoaked with no-rinse soap. The bag is placed in a warmer, and the patient is bathed. Some facilities use disposable cloths for bath-in-a-bag.

Skill 9.1 Bathing the Patient and Administering a Back Rub—cont'd

e. Bathe patient with the following procedure. *(Promotes effective towel bath, provides warmth, and keeps bed dry, avoiding chilling the patient.)*

(1) Fold bath blanket down to waist. Remove warm moist towel from plastic bag and place on patient's right or left chest with open edges up and outward. Unroll towel across chest.

(2) Open towel to cover entire body while removing top bath blanket. Tuck towel–bath towel in and around body (leave bath towel and washcloths in plastic bag to keep warm).

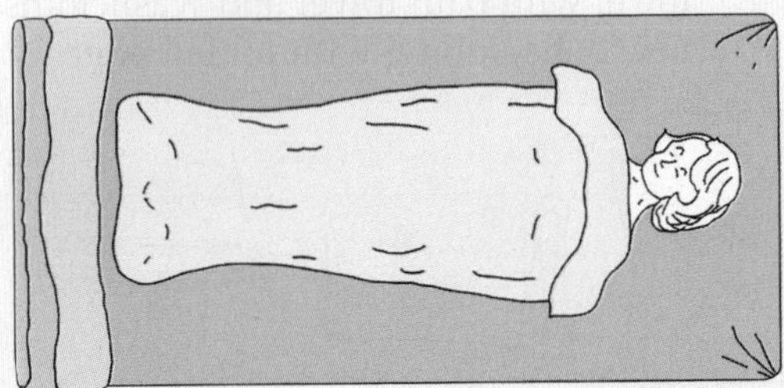

(3) Begin bathing at feet, with gentle massaging motion. Use clean section of towel for each part of body as you move toward patient's head.

(4) Fold lower part of towel upward away from feet as bathing continues. Help from an assistant makes the bath process more effective.

(5) Continue to draw clean bath blanket upward and place over patient as you move upward. Leave 3 inches of exposed skin between towel and bath blanket. Skin dries in 2 or 3 seconds. If towel bath is given properly, the patient is refreshed and relaxed.

(6) Wash face, neck, and ears with one of the prepared washcloths.

(7) Turn patient onto side.

(8) Use prepared bath towel for back care. (Give back rub; see Step 14.)

(9) Use second washcloth for perineal care (don disposable gloves). Sometimes you need a basin of warm water, soap, washcloth, towel, and gloves to perform perineal care (see Skill 9.5).

(10) When bath is completed, remove towel and place with soiled linens in plastic laundry bag. *(Promotes medical asepsis.)*

(11) If top bath blanket is not soiled, fold for reuse later.

f. Make occupied bed (see Skill 9.6). *(Provides comfort and promotes practices of medical asepsis.)*

11. Tub bath or shower.

a. Follow Steps 1 and 3 to 7.

b. Determine whether activity is allowed by consulting patient's activity order.

c. Be certain tub or shower appliance is clean. See agency policy. Place nonskid mat on tub or shower floor if necessary and disposable mat outside of tub or shower. *(Promotes patient's safety. Conditions that place patients at risk for falls in the bathtub include neurologic impairment, arthritis, and poor balance.)*

d. Assemble all items necessary for bathing. *(Prevents unnecessary interruptions.)*

- Clean gown or patient's own pajamas or nightgown
- Deodorant
- Lotion
- Soap
- Towel
- Washcloth

e. Assist patient to tub or shower. Shower chairs are available in most facilities to transport patients from the bedside to the shower, bathe and dry patients, and return them to bed. Be certain patient wears robe and slippers. *(Promotes patient's safety and prevents patient from chilling.)*

f. Instruct patient on how to use call signal. Place "in use" sign on tub or shower door if not using private bath. *(Provides for patient's safety and privacy.)*

g. If tub is used, fill with warm water, 109.4°F (43°C). Have patient test water, if able, then adjust temperature. Instruct patient on use of faucets—which is hot and which is cold. If shower is used, turn water on and adjust temperature. *(Prevents accidental burns and promotes safety.)*

h. Caution patient to use safety bars. Discourage use of bath oil in water. Safety must be maintained at all times. Check on patient every 5 minutes (q 5 min). Do not allow to remain in tub more than 20 minutes. *(Maintains patient's safety and prevents vertigo and syncope.)*

i. Return when patient signals. Make an unoccupied bed while the patient bathes unless patient condition is such that you are required to remain with the patient. Return to the tub or shower room and offer to wash the patient's back. Knock before entering. *(Provides privacy and promotes comfort.)*

Skill 9.1 Bathing the Patient and Administering a Back Rub—cont'd

- **j.** Assist patient out of tub and with drying. Observe the patient for signs and symptoms of weakness, such as rapid pulse, paleness, diaphoresis, unsteady gait, tachypnea, vertigo, and syncope. If patient reports weakness, vertigo, or syncope, drain tub before patient gets out and place towel over patient's shoulders. *(Prevents falls and promotes comfort.)*
- **k.** Assist patient into clean gown, robe, and slippers. Accompany to room, position for comfort, and give back rub (see Step 14). *(Maintains warmth and safety.)*
- **l.** Make unoccupied bed if patient can tolerate sitting in chair. Perform back, hair, nail, and skin care. *(Maintains clean environment to promote positive self-image and medical asepsis and promotes patient's well-being.)*
- **m.** Return to shower or tub. Clean according to agency policy. Place all soiled linens in laundry bag and return all articles to patient's bedside. *(Promotes orderly environment and reduces spread of microorganisms.)*
- **n.** Perform hand hygiene. *(Reduces spread of microorganisms.)*

12. Give tepid sponge bath for temperature reduction.

- **a.** Follow Steps 1 and 3 to 7.
- **b.** Assess patient for elevated temperature. *(Provides basis for care.)*
- **c.** Explain to patient; outline steps of the procedure. *(Reduces patient's anxiety.)*
- **d.** Assemble equipment. *(Promotes organization.)*
  - Bath basin
  - Bath blanket
  - Patient thermometer
  - Tepid water (98.6°F [37°C])
  - Washcloths (4)
- **e.** Cover patient with bath blanket, remove gown, and close windows and doors. *(Prevents chilling and provides privacy.)*
- **f.** Test water temperature. Place washcloths in water, then apply wet cloths to each axilla and groin (the depressed area between the thigh and trunk). If patient is in tub, allow to stay in water for 20 to 30 minutes. *(Promotes cooler temperature and allows for more effective heat loss because blood vessels are close to the surface of the body in the axilla and the groin.)*
- **g.** Gently sponge an extremity for about 5 minutes. If patient is in tub, gently sponge water over upper torso, chest, and back. *(Prevents sudden drop in body temperature.)*
- **h.** Continue sponge bath to other extremities and back, for 3 to 5 minutes each. Assess temperature and pulse q 15 min. *(Minimizes risk of patient chilling.)*
- **i.** Change water and reapply freshly moistened washcloths to axilla and groin as necessary. *(Maintains tepid water temperature and continues to promote cooling.)*
- **j.** Continue with sponge bath until body temperature falls to slightly above normal. Keep body parts that are not being sponged covered. *(This prevents shivering, which causes temperature to rise.)* Discontinue procedure according to agency policy. *(Prevents body temperature from falling below normal; body temperature will continue to drop.)*
- **k.** Dry patient thoroughly and cover with light blanket or sheet. *(Prevents chilling.)* Avoid rubbing the skin too vigorously because that may cause an increase in heat production. Leave patient in comfortable position.
- **l.** Clean and return equipment to storage, clean area, and change bed linens as necessary. Perform hand hygiene. *(Reduces spread of microorganisms.)*

13. Give medicated bath.

- **a.** Follow Steps 1 and 3 to 7.
- **b.** Prepare tub bath (see Steps 11c, f, g). *(Promotes orderly procedure.)*
- **c.** Add agent as ordered by physician. *(Follows physician's orders.)*
- **d.** Don gloves as necessary.
- **e.** Assist patient to tub. *(Maintains patient's safety.)*
- **f.** Allow patient to remain in tub for required time. *(Promotes effective procedure.)*
- **g.** Assist patient out of tub. *(Maintains patient's safety.)*
- **h.** Gently pat dry. *(Allows medication to remain on patient's skin.)* Teach patient not to scratch lesions. *(Avoids further irritation and prevents infection.)*
- **i.** Assist patient into gown, pajamas, or clothes. *(Prevents patient from chilling.)*
- **j.** Assist patient to return to bed, and position for comfort. *(Allows patient to rest and relax. Promotes well-being.)*
- **k.** Remove and dispose of gloves and perform hand hygiene. *(Reduces the spread of microorganisms.)*

14. Give back rub.

- **a.** Prepare supplies. *(Organizes procedure.)*
  - Bath blanket (optional)
  - Bath towel

Continued

Skill 9.1 Bathing the Patient and Administering a Back Rub—cont'd

- Skin lotion, powder. If powder is used, apply sparingly. *(Lotion lubricates skin, whereas powder absorbs body moisture and clumps, which could result in skin irritation.)*

b. Follow Steps 1 and 3 to 7 and provide quiet environment.

c. Lower side rail. Position patient with back toward you. Cover patient so that only parts to massage are exposed. *(Prevents unnecessary exposure.)*

d. Warm hands if necessary. Warm lotion by holding some in hands. Explain that lotion often feels cool. *(Enhances relaxation.)*

e. Begin massage by starting in sacral area using circular motions. Stroke upward to shoulders. Massaging over bony prominences is no longer recommended because this may cause skin breakdown.

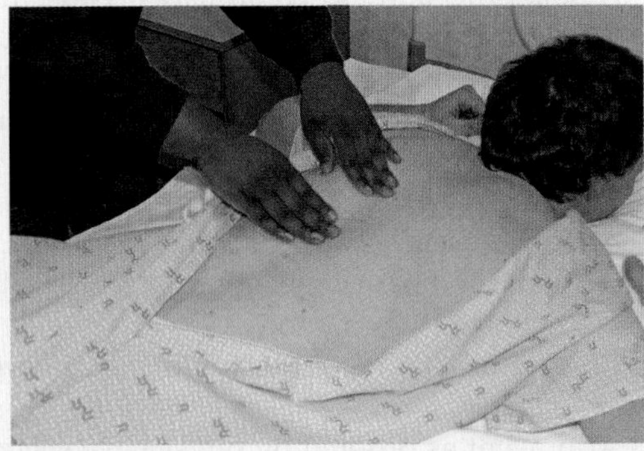

f. Use firm, smooth strokes to massage over scapulae. Continue to upper arms with one smooth stroke and down along side of back to iliac crest. Do not break contact with patient's skin. Complete massage in 3 to 5 minutes. *(A firm, gentle pressure promotes relaxation. Use of firm pressure prevents tickling the patient. Continuous contact with skin surface is soothing and stimulates circulation.)*

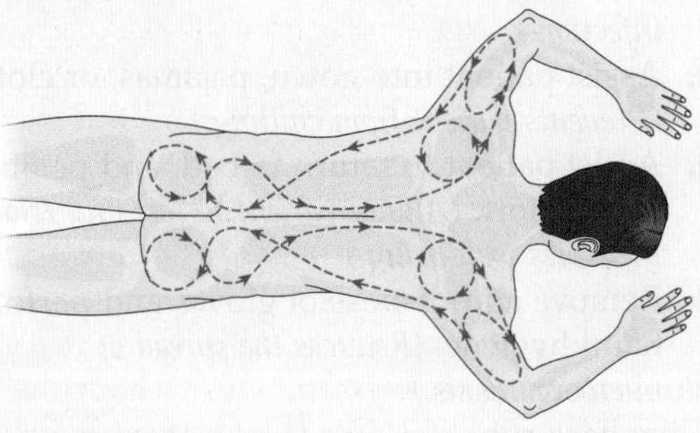

g. Gently but firmly knead skin by grasping area between thumb and fingers. Work across each shoulder and around nape of neck. Continue downward along each side to sacrum. *(Kneading increases circulation; motion is soothing and relieving.)*

h. With long smooth strokes, end massage, remove excess lubricant from patient's back with towel, and re-tie gown. *(These strokes are relaxing and the most soothing of all massage movements.)* Position for comfort. Lower bed and raise side rail as needed and place call button within easy reach. *(Promotes patient's safety. Excess lotion often irritates skin. Comfortable position enhances the back rub's effect.)*

i. Place soiled laundry in proper receptacle, and perform hand hygiene. *(Reduces spread of microorganisms.)*

15. Assess patient. *(Determines patient's ability to perform self-care and level of assistance required from staff.)*

- Knowledge of importance of skin hygiene
- Level of cognitive ability
- Level of discomfort
- Musculoskeletal function; extent of joint ROM
- Risk for compromised skin integrity (e.g., presence of paralysis or large casts or traction, or those patients who are weakened and disabled)
- Tolerance of activity
- Vital signs *(Helps detect an unexpected outcome of an elevation in heart rate and systolic blood pressure.)*

16. Document. *(Timely documentation maintains accuracy of patient's record; condition of skin documents response to therapy [e.g., turning and positioning].)*

- Type of bath (e.g., sitz bath, medicated bath, or tepid sponge bath), water temperature, and solution used, when appropriate
- Duration of treatment
- Level of assistance required
- Condition of skin; any significant findings (e.g., erythematous [pertaining to erythema or redness] skin areas, bruises, nevi [moles], joint or muscle pain, or exudate [drainage])
- Vital signs if applicable (e.g., sponge bath for temperature reduction)
- Patient's response
- Patient teaching (see the Patient Teaching box)

17. Report alterations in skin integrity to nurse in charge or physician. *(Special medical treatment is sometimes necessary.)*

Box 9.4 Bathing Patients Who Have Dementia

- When caregivers maintain a more relaxed demeanor and smile frequently while bathing patients with dementia, the patients demonstrate greater degrees of calmness and cooperation. Use language appropriate to the patient's level of comprehension, and try to determine which words and phrases the patients uses in reference to bathing—some say "washing up" rather than "having a bath," for example. Explain what you intend to do. If the patient reports pain or discomfort, apologize and try to determine and address the cause: for example, "I'm sorry that I hurt you. I won't scrub as hard. Is that better?" Offer reassurance frequently, such as, "You are doing really well; we'll be finished soon," or "As soon as we're finished, I'm going to wrap you in a warm towel and put some of the lotion that you like on your skin."
- Use distraction and negotiation instead of demands.
- Minimize noise in the bathing area.
- Be sure bathing environment is warm.
- Set priorities as to which body parts need bathing and which can be "skipped."
- Use as few staff members as possible.

If the patient's condition warrants it and ambulation has been ordered, the patient may be allowed to take a tub bath; however, in most facilities, a patient showers.

A tepid sponge bath is administered to reduce the elevated temperature of patients who are **febrile** (condition characterized by an elevated body temperature).

A medicated bath sometimes is ordered. This bath is likely to include agents such as oatmeal, cornstarch, Burow's solution, and sodium bicarbonate (alkaline bath). The medicated bath helps reduce tension, relax the patient, and relieve the pruritus caused by certain skin disorders.

When bathing patients who have dementia, the nurse may find it necessary to adjust the style of interaction (Box 9.4).

BACK CARE AND BACK RUB

The nurse or UAP typically administers the back rub after the patient's bath. Offer this opportunity to the patient because it promotes relaxation, relieves muscular tension, and stimulates circulation. To give an effective back rub, massage for 3 to 5 minutes (see Skill 9.1). During the back rub, observe the skin for abnormalities. Monitor pulse and blood pressure of those patients with a history of hypertension or dysrhythmias. The back rub is contraindicated if the patient has conditions such as fractures of the ribs or vertebral column, burns, pulmonary embolism, or open wounds.

COMPONENTS OF THE PATIENT'S HYGIENE

CARE OF THE SKIN

When a person's physical condition changes, the skin often reflects this by alterations in color, thickness, texture, turgor, temperature, and hydration. As long as the skin remains intact and healthy, its physiologic function remains optimal. Intact skin is the first line of defense against infection by invasion of pathogenic organisms.

Data Collection

Determine the condition of the patient's skin by observing its color, texture, thickness, turgor, temperature, and hydration. Be certain to use ample lighting. Natural or halogen lighting is suggested. Normal skin has the following characteristics:

- Good turgor (elastic and firm); generally smooth and soft
- Intact without abrasions
- Localized changes in texture across surface
- Skin color variations from body part to body part
- Warm and moist

Pressure Ulcers and Pressure Injuries

The National Pressure Ulcer Advisory Panel (NPUAP) has announced that the term **pressure injury** will be used to replace the former term, **pressure ulcer,** in the staging system. The NPUAP has determined that the term pressure injury more accurately describes injuries to intact and ulcerated skin, especially because stage 1 previously was referred to as a pressure injury and the remaining stages were referred to as ulcers. The numbering system also was changed to Arabic numbers (NPUAP, 2016).

The patient problem of *Compromised Skin Integrity,* either *actual* or *risk for,* is a common diagnosis for any patient in a health care facility. Prevention and treatment of skin impairment is one of the nurse's highest priorities of care. Prevention is the ultimate goal, but when this is not possible, good nursing interventions can result in (1) optimal healing of the impaired skin without complications; (2) a decrease in the patient's discomfort; (3) a decrease in length of stay in the facility if a discharge is planned; and (4) a decrease in the cost of ongoing care.

Approximately 2.5 million hospitalized patients develop pressure injuries each year despite national guidelines regarding their prevention and treatment (AHRQ, 2014). The incidence of pressure injuries in acute care facilities is detrimental to the health of patients. The development of pressure injuries leads to longer hospital stays, resulting in increased chance of not only infection to the pressure injury but also other infections related to the extended stay in the facility.

To encourage acute care facilities to become more aggressive in the prevention of pressure injury development, as of October 2008, the Centers for Medicare and Medicaid stopped covering the costs of treatment of pressure injuries that develop during the patient's hospitalization. The goal is to prevent patients from experiencing the pain, loss of function, complications such as infection, prolonged hospital stays, and the

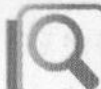 Evidence-Based Practice

Evaluation of Hospital Acquired Pressure Ulcers

(NOTE: This study was conducted before the introduction of the new "pressure injury" terminology.)

EVIDENCE SUMMARY

Lyder et al conducted a retrospective study of 51,842 randomly selected Medicare patients in hospital settings. The study found that 5.8% of these patients were admitted with pressure ulcers, and 4.5% developed at least one new pressure ulcer during their hospitalization. These patients were hospitalized longer (4.8 versus 11.2 days) and were 11.2% more likely to die during this stay (increase from 3.3% during normal stay). The study also found that these patients were more likely to die within 30 days of discharge (4.4% versus 15.3%) and were more likely to be readmitted within 30 days of discharge (17.6% versus 22.6%), and the facilities incurred significantly more costs resulting from the extended care and stay in the facility.

REFERENCE

Lyder CH et al: Hospital-acquired pressure ulcers: Results from the National Medicare Patient Safety Monitoring System (MPSMS) study, *J Am Geriatr Soc* 60:1603–1608, 2012.

increased costs associated with the development of pressure injuries (Medscape, 2008). The same is true for long-term care facilities.

Pressure injuries occur when sufficient pressure on the skin causes the blood vessels in an area to collapse. The flow of blood and fluid to the cells is impaired, resulting in ischemia, or lack of oxygen and nutrients, to the cells. When the external pressure against the skin is greater than the pressure in the capillary bed (network of capillaries), blood flow decreases to the adjacent tissue. If the pressure continues without relief for more than 2 hours, cells in the involved layers of skin tend to undergo necrosis (death of tissue). Pressure is usually most severe over bony prominences (e.g., sacrum, scapulae, ears, elbows, heels, inner and outer malleoli, inner and outer knees, back of head, ischial tuberosities, trochanteric areas of the hips, and heels).

In addition to unrelieved pressure, two mechanical factors play a common role in the development of pressure injuries. The first is *shearing force.* This occurs when the tissue layers of skin slide on each other, causing subcutaneous blood vessels to kink or stretch and resulting in an interruption of blood flow to the skin (Fig. 9.3).

The second mechanical factor is *friction.* The rubbing of skin against another surface produces friction, which may remove layers of tissue. This may occur when moving patients in bed by sliding them across the bed linen, when improperly lifting patients, and when improperly placing bedpans.

The appearance of pressure injuries is a major manifestation of impaired skin integrity. A patient who stays in one position without relief of pressure, especially over bony prominences, is at risk for development of a pressure injury. Patients especially at risk are chronically ill, debilitated, older, disabled, or incontinent and those with spinal cord injuries, limited mobility, circulatory impairment, or poor overall nutrition.

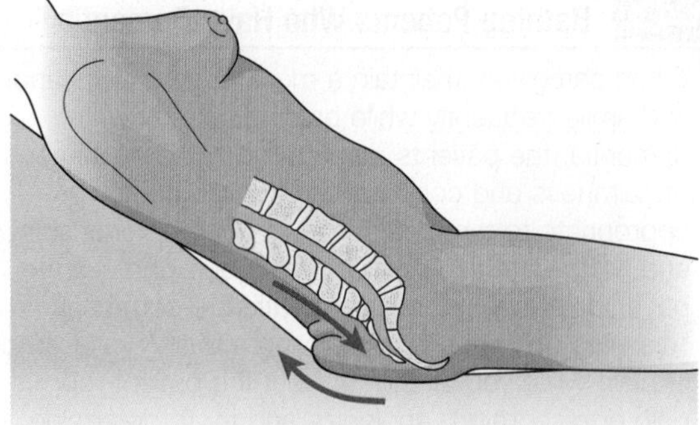

Fig. 9.3 Diagram of shearing force exerted against sacral area.

Those who are incontinent are at risk because continual contact of the skin with urine and feces often causes chemical irritation, which frequently leads to impaired skin integrity. Nutritional factors play a role for those who are overweight and those who are underweight. Obesity increases the risk because fat tissue has less vascularity and resilience, and the added bulk and weight increase the pressure on bony prominences. Obesity also causes increased skin-on-skin contact, especially in skin folds. Being underweight increases the risk because of a lack of cushion over the bones and muscles and lack of nutrition to the skin cells. In addition, any condition that results in a decreased supply of oxygen and nutrients to the cells, such as anemia, atherosclerosis, or edema (swelling), increases the risk of skin impairment because the cells are not adequately nourished.

Patients who are at increased risk for any reason need careful ongoing assessment and a plan of care aimed at preventing skin impairment (see the Coordinated Care box on skin care).

Definition and staging. The definition of a pressure injury was revised by the NPUAP in 2016. The NPUAP also added definitions to the six category staging system for pressure injuries. These definitions are for deep tissue injury, medical device pressure-related injury, and mucosal membrane pressure injury. The NPUAP defines a pressure injury as:

> localized damage to the skin and/or underlying soft tissue usually over a bony prominence or related to a medical or other device. The injury can present as intact skin or an open ulcer and may be painful. The injury occurs as a result of intense and/or prolonged pressure or pressure in combination with shear. The tolerance of soft tissue for pressure and shear may also be affected by microclimate, nutrition, perfusion, co-morbidities and condition of the soft tissue.

 Coordinated Care

Collaboration

Skin Care

Although assessment for the presence of skin impairment is a nursing responsibility and is not to be delegated, UAP provide hygienic care in many settings. Therefore UAP should be instructed in the following areas:

- Report any changes in the patient's skin condition, such as redness, irritation, dryness, maceration, or discomfort.
- Provide care to prevent the patient from exposure to body fluids such as urine, feces, wound drainage, and gastric secretions.
- Observe bony prominences (e.g., sacrum, scapulae, ears, elbows, heels, inner and outer malleoli, inner and outer knees, back of head, ischial tuberosities, trochanteric areas of the hips, and heels) for any signs of redness, irritation, or skin breakdown.
- Observe and prevent any areas of pressure from external devices such as oxygen tubing, nasogastric tubing, casts, braces, urinary catheter tubing, or drainage tubing.
- Provide perineal care as needed and observe the area for any signs of skin breakdown. Apply protective barrier creams as allowed by facility policy.

Assess any reports from the UAP regarding potential or actual skin integrity issues. If reddened areas are found, assess the area by noting any blanching of the area (by gently pressing on the reddened area with a gloved finger; if the area does not blanch when pressure is applied, injury to the tissue is likely). Document and report such findings to the health care provider. If actual skin impairment has occurred already, measure and document the area according to facility protocol and report the findings to the health care provider.

The following sections summarize the revised stages of pressure injury development according to the NPUAP 2016. Additional information regarding pressure injuries can be found at *www.npuap.org*.

Stage 1. A stage 1 pressure injury is a localized area of skin, typically over a bony prominence, that is intact with nonblanchable redness. Skin with darker tones may not have visible blanching, but its color is likely to differ from the surrounding area. The wound characteristics vary: areas may be painful, firm, soft, warm, or cool compared with adjacent tissue. This stage is typically difficult to detect in patients with dark skin tones.

Stage 2. A stage 2 pressure injury involves partial-thickness loss of dermis. It appears as a shallow open injury, usually shiny or dry, with a red-pink wound bed without slough or bruising. (Bruising raises the suspicion of deep tissue injury.) Some stage 2 injuries manifest as intact or open (ruptured) serum-filled blisters. Do not use the term stage 2 to describe skin tears, tape burns, perineal dermatitis, maceration, or excoriation.

Stage 3. A stage 3 pressure injury involves full-thickness tissue loss, in which subcutaneous fat is sometimes visible, but bone, tendon, and muscle are not exposed. If slough is present, it does not obscure the depth of tissue loss. Possible features are undermining and tunneling. The depth of a stage 3 pressure injury varies depending on its anatomic location. On the bridge of the nose, the ear, the occiput, and the malleolus, which lack subcutaneous tissue, these injuries are shallow. Extremely deep stage 3 pressure injuries develop in areas with significant layers of deep adipose tissue.

Stage 4. A stage 4 pressure injury involves full-thickness tissue loss with exposed bone, tendon, cartilage, or muscle. Sometimes slough or eschar is present on some parts of the wound bed. The injury often includes undermining or tunneling. As with stage 3 pressure injuries, stage 4 pressure injuries vary in depth depending on their location. Because these injuries extend into muscle and supporting structures, the patient is at risk for osteomyelitis.

Unstageable/unclassified. An unstageable pressure injury involves full-thickness tissue loss, a wound base covered by slough (yellow, tan, gray, green, or brown), and eschar in the wound bed that usually is tan, brown, or black. The true depth and stage of the injury cannot be determined until the base of the wound has been exposed. Stable eschar on the heels provides a natural biologic cover: do not remove it.

Suspected deep tissue pressure injury. During this stage, the wound appears as a localized purple or maroon area of discolored intact skin or a blood-filled blister. This is caused by underlying soft tissue damage from pressure or shear. Characteristics of the area range from painful, firm, mushy, boggy, or warm to cool compared with adjacent tissue. In patients with dark skin tones, deep tissue injury is sometimes difficult to detect but often starts with a thin blister over a dark wound bed. The wound sometimes becomes covered with thin eschar. Even with prompt treatment, some wounds evolve rapidly, exposing additional layers of tissue.

Interventions. Nursing interventions for patients with pressure injuries include ongoing assessment and evaluation of improvement. Assessment data include the size and the depth of the injury (Fig. 9.4), the presence of any undermining, the amount and the color of any exudate, the presence of pain or odor, and the appearance of the exposed tissue. Healing is a long-term process; therefore be sure the plan of care is consistent over time and evaluate it for effectiveness. Interventions are determined according to the stage of the injury (Boxes 9.5 and 9.6 and Figs. 9.5 through 9.7).

HEAT AND COLD THERAPY

Patients who have experienced injury to some part of the body often benefit from the application of heat or cold therapy, or both. The heat or cold can be either dry or moist, depending on the injury, or need, and on

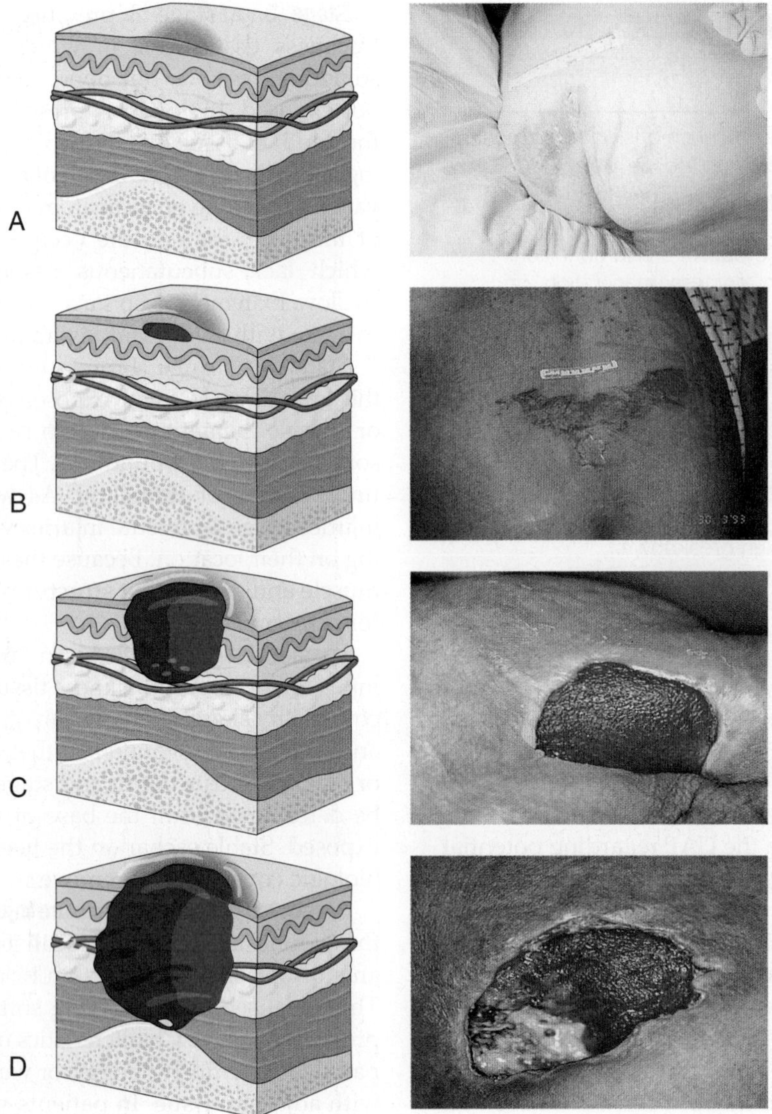

Fig. 9.4 Pressure injuries. A, Stage 1 pressure injury. B, Stage 2 pressure injury. C, Stage 3 pressure injury. D, Stage 4 pressure injury. (Photos courtesy Laurel Wiersma, RN, MSN, Clinical Nurse Specialist, Barnes-Jewish Hospital, St. Louis. From Potter PA, Perry AG: *Fundamentals of nursing,* ed 7, St. Louis, 2009, Mosby.)

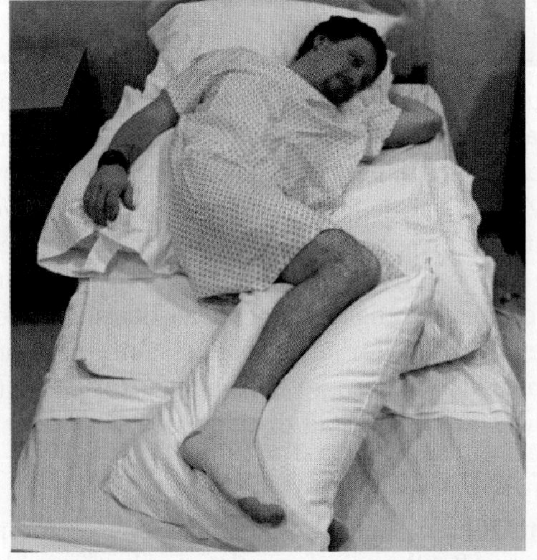

Fig. 9.5 Thirty-degree lateral position to avoid pressure points.

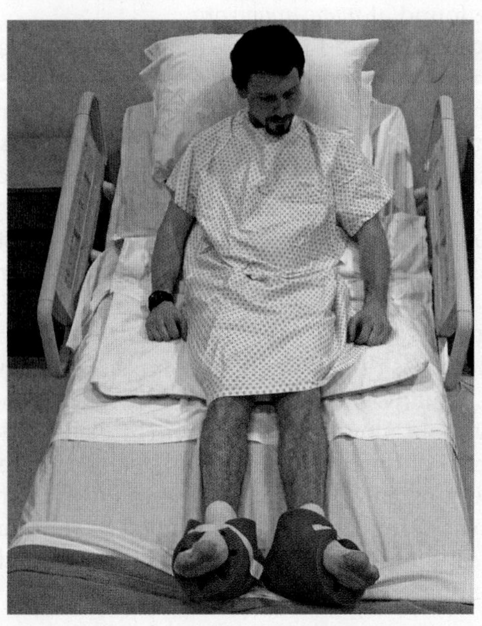

Fig. 9.6 Use of pressure-reducing boots to prevent pressure on heels.

Box 9.5 General Guidelines for Care of Pressure Injuries

- Never massage reddened areas (risk of further skin breakdown). Massage over bony prominences is no longer recommended. *(Massage results in decreased blood flow and tissue damage in some patients.)*
- Nutritional support, which promotes healthy tissue repair, is likely to be as important as local wound care for the patient.
- Observe the patient's hydration. If it is inadequate or if signs of dehydration (decreased skin turgor and recessed eyes) are present, carefully observe the patient's intake and output (I&O) and monitor fluid replacement therapy as ordered.
- Turn patients who are on complete bed rest or unable to reposition themselves every 2 hours. It is important to avoid the full lateral position, which results in direct pressure on the trochanteric region. The 30-degree lateral-incline position is preferable (see Box 9.6).
- Reposition chair-bound patients every hour. If chair-bound patients are able to shift their weight, teach them to do so every 15 minutes.
- Place patients who are at risk for skin impairment on a pressure-relieving mattress or chair cushion. Doughnut types of cushions are not advisable because they sometimes cause a congestion of blood to the area, resulting in edema and decreased blood flow to the area. Placement of a rolled bath blanket under the distal extremity helps prevent pressure injuries on the heel by "floating" the heel (raises the heel off the bed) (see Figs. 9.6 and 9.7).
- Other pressure-relieving devices to try are therapeutic beds and mattresses. Examples of pressure-relieving beds are low-air-loss beds and oscillating support surface beds. In addition, there are the alternating air mattress and the water mattress.
- Many kinds of topical agents to facilitate healing are available to apply to the wound and edges of the wound. Take care to evaluate the effectiveness of any product used on the injury. Use with caution any products that have the capacity to damage fragile skin and prevent epithelialization (formation of new cells), such as hydrogen peroxide or alcohol.

Box 9.6 Moving Dependent Patient to 30-Degree Lateral (Side-Lying) Position

This move removes pressure from bony prominences of the entire back but especially the greater trochanters. (If patient is able to move freely, a side-lying position with upper and lower shoulders aligned is acceptable.)

PROCEDURE *(RATIONALE)*

1. Lower the head of the bed as much as patient can tolerate, keeping head of bed below 30-degree angle. Lower side rail. *(Reduces shear. Prevents working against gravity.)*
2. Using a pull sheet, move patient to the side of the bed opposite the one toward which the patient will be turned. Raise side rail. Go to opposite side of the bed and lower side rail. *(Ensures that patient is in center of the bed when turned.)*
3. Assist patient to raise arm nearest you above head, adjusting pillow if needed.
4. Grasp patient's shoulder and hip, and assist patient to roll toward you onto side. *(Turning patient toward you promotes patient's sense of security.)*
5. Flex both of the patient's knees after the turn, and support upper leg from knee to foot with a pillow or folded blanket. *(Keeps spine in good alignment.)*
6. Ease lower shoulder forward, and bring upper shoulder back slightly. Assess patient's comfort. *(Prevents excessive pressure directly on shoulder.)*
7. Support upper arm with pillows so that arm is level with shoulder. *(Improves respiratory effort by reducing pressure on chest to a minimum.)*
8. Optional: Place pillow behind and under patient's back so that it is tucked smoothly against back (see Fig. 9.5). *(Provides support and prevents patient from rolling onto back.)*
9. Make certain patient's back is straight without evidence of twisting. Adjust as needed for comfort.
10. Pressure points to assess include the ear, the shoulder, the anterior iliac spine, the trochanter, the lateral side of the knee, the malleolus, and the foot. *(Prevents further skin impairment.)*

the health care provider's order. Because the application of heat or cold affects the blood circulating throughout the body, it is the nurse's responsibility to ensure patient safety during this therapy. Systemic reaction to heat therapy can include a rapid pulse, faintness, or difficulty breathing, and the systemic reaction to cold therapy includes shivering. Therefore it is important to monitor the patient closely during the administration of heat or cold therapy. The nurse must be able to evaluate the skin integrity of the body part being treated and determine the patient's ability to perceive temperature variations to the body part affected.

The body's thermoreceptors generally can adapt well to temperatures between 59°F (15°C) and 113°F (45°C). Typically patients exposed to temperatures below 59°F

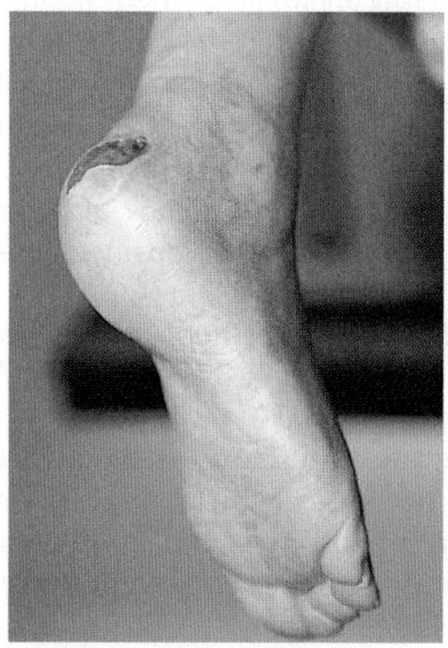

Fig. 9.7 Pressure injury on heel. (From Potter PA, Perry AG: *Basic nursing,* ed 7, St. Louis, 2011, Mosby.)

(15°C) experience numbness followed by pain, and when exposed to temperatures above 113°F (45°C), patients experience pain and burning. Initially, healthy patients are able to sense these temperature changes, but within a short time, the patient's skin adapts to the temperature, and the patient no longer feels sensations of warmth or coolness. This wide range of adaptability, along with decreased sensitivity to temperature extremes, creates the risk of injury. Therefore it becomes imperative to identify patients at greatest risk for developing injuries related to heat and cold applications (see the Lifespan Considerations box on cold applications).

Lifespan Considerations

Older Adults/Young Children

Cold Applications

- Older adults and young children are more sensitive to cold because skin layers are thin and delicate.
- Remain with the patient for the first 5 minutes of treatment to evaluate subjective response.
- If the patient response to the therapy is poor, shorten the duration of the therapy and notify the health care provider.
- Evaluate skin every 2 to 3 minutes after first 10 minutes of therapy.
- Older adults and young children frequently require more covering for warmth.

Other factors that influence the likelihood of damage to the skin include any diseases or disorders that would impede feeling temperature extremes or changes (e.g., neuropathy, peripheral vascular disease, and spinal cord injury). Damage from heat and cold therapy is also more likely to occur with unconscious or confused patients because they may not be able to report or sense feelings of discomfort. Open wounds should be avoided because heat may cause bleeding and cold may impair circulation because of lack of skin as a barrier.

Local Effects of Heat and Cold

Heat applications generally are used to provide comfort and to speed healing. Patients with musculoskeletal discomfort, such as joint or back pain, may benefit from application of heat to the area. Cold normally is used to decrease swelling and to reduce pain. Cold often is used for sprains, fractures, and nosebleeds or after some surgical procedures, such as tonsillectomies.

Systemic effects of heat application. Heat produces **vasodilation** (dilation of the blood vessels). Vasodilation causes increased blood flow to the area of the body being treated; as a consequence, blood flow to the rest of the body decreases, which potentially can result in increased pulse, dizziness, and shortness of breath. In addition, more nutrients are brought to the area, which produces an increase in metabolism and tissue growth. In situations in which infection is involved, the application of heat brings more antibodies and leukocytes to the area to fight infection and speed healing. If heat applications are left in place for more than 1 hour, a heat-conserving mechanism sets in, and vessels begin to constrict, which decreases blood flow to that area. Extended heat application also may cause damage to epithelial cells and produce erythema, tenderness, and blistering. The health care provider's order should include frequency and duration of heat therapy, and it even may specify a temperature (Table 9.2). If it does not, the facility's policy should be followed to prevent systemic complications.

Table 9.2 Temperature Ranges for Hot and Cold Applications

TEMPERATURE	FAHRENHEIT RANGE	CENTIGRADE RANGE
Very hot	105° to 115°F	41° to 46°C
Hot	98° to 105°F	37° to 41°C
Warm	93° to 98°F	34° to 37°C
Tepid	80° to 93°F	26° to 34°C
Cool	65° to 80°F	18° to 26°C
Cold	50° to 65°F	10° to 18°C

Systemic effects of cold application. Exposure of the skin to cold results in **vasoconstriction** (narrowing of blood vessels). Vasoconstriction decreases blood flow to the area; as a consequence, blood flow to the other organs and tissues increases, which causes the body to shiver in an attempt to produce heat. If the cold application is left in place for too long, or if the temperature is too low, the cold interferes with adequate circulation to the area, and the tissue involved is damaged. Such damage to the skin often is accompanied by a burning type of pain. If exposure to extreme cold continues for an extensive period, the skin could freeze and necrose, as in frostbite. Again, the health care provider's order or facility policy should be followed to prevent complications.

Patient Safety

To prevent injuries related to heat or cold application, it is important for the nurse to determine the patient's ability to distinguish heat and cold temperature variations before application. It is also important for the nurse to check for any contraindications to therapy or intolerance to heat or cold before applying either therapy.

Contraindications to heat therapy include any bleeding because vasodilation increases bleeding; inflammation, which sometimes worsens as a result of the vasodilation; and cardiovascular problems because heat applied to large areas of the body has the potential to interrupt blood flow to vital organs.

Cold therapy should not be used if edema has occurred already. The cold decreases circulation to the area, prevents absorption of the interstitial fluid that has accumulated, and prolongs resolution of the edema. Anyone with impaired circulation or an acute injury

Box 9.7 Factors Influencing Heat and Cold Tolerance

The body's response to heat and cold applications depends on the following factors:

- *Age and physical condition:* Tolerance to temperature variations changes with age. Patients who are very young and older adults are most sensitive to the heat and cold. If a patient's physical condition reduces the perception of sensory stimuli, tolerance to temperature extremes is high, but the risk of injury is also high.
- *Body part:* Certain areas of the skin are more sensitive to temperature variations. These areas include the neck, the inner aspect of the wrist and forearm, and the perineal region. The foot and the palm of the hand are less sensitive.
- *Body surface area:* People have less tolerance to temperature changes when a large area of the body is exposed to heat or cold.
- *Damage to body surface:* Exposed skin layers are more sensitive to temperature variations.
- *Duration of treatment:* Short exposure to temperature extremes is better tolerated than is lengthy exposure.
- *Prior skin temperature:* The body responds best to minor temperature adjustments. If a body part is cool and a hot stimulus touches the skin, the response is greater than if the stimulus is warm. (A gradual change in temperature is preferred.)

From Potter PA, Perry AG: *Basic nursing: Essentials for practice*, ed 7, St. Louis, 2011, Mosby.

in which nerve damage is suspected should not receive cold therapy because cold decreases blood supply further and increases complications. Furthermore, cold tends to increase shivering, which results in a significant increase in body temperature; therefore patients with an already increased temperature may suffer complications from cold therapy.

Patients who have an altered level of consciousness or are disoriented should be observed frequently during heat or cold application because they are at increased risk of injury from either type of application. In addition, the nurse must ensure that the equipment being used for heat and cold applications is in proper working order. Equipment must be checked for leaks, and electrical equipment must be inspected for damaged cords or wires before use. It is also necessary to check for even distribution of temperature of the equipment because uneven temperature distribution may suggest that the equipment is not functioning properly. By making sure the patient and the equipment are prepared appropriately before application of heat or cold therapy, the nurse can determine the effectiveness of therapy and identify any complications after the application of heat or cold (Box 9.7 and see the Coordinated Care box on heat and cold therapy).

The task of applying cold therapy to intact skin also may be delegated to UAP. Again, the nurse must evaluate the condition of the patient's skin and protect the patient from harm.

 **Coordinated Care**

Delegation

Heat and Cold Therapy

In some states, the task of applying moist heat, or warm, moist compresses may be delegated to UAP under the supervision of the nurse. When you delegate this task, keep in mind that the nurse is responsible for evaluating the condition of the patient's skin and preventing injury to the patient. The nurse should remind the UAP to observe the following guidelines:

- Maintain proper temperature of heat or cold applications.
- Maintain application only for the prescribed length of time.
- Check patient's skin for excessive redness and pain during application and to report any such adverse reactions to the nurse.
- Report to the nurse when the treatment is complete so that the nurse may evaluate the patient's response.

Hot, Moist Compresses

When hot, moist compresses are ordered, the solution is heated to the appropriate temperature, gauze or cloth is dipped in the solution, and the damp gauze or cloth then is applied to the designated area. If a wound is open, sterile technique and sterile gauze must be used. Hot, moist compresses increase circulation to the affected area, decrease edema, and consolidate any purulent exudate that may be present.

To maintain the temperature of a compress, it may be necessary to change the compress frequently or wrap the compress in an aquathermia pad (K-pad), a waterproof heating pad, a piece of plastic, or a dry towel. Moist heat is a better conductor of heat than is dry heat; therefore it may be necessary to lower the temperature settings for moist heat. Because moist heat causes evaporation of heat from the skin, it is important to cover the patient with a blanket and minimize drafts in the room to keep the patient warm, especially for elderly patients (Skill 9.2 and see the Home Care Considerations box on heat and cold applications).

Warm Soaks

Warm soaks are accomplished by immersing a body part in a warm solution or wrapping a body part in dressings that have been saturated with a warm solution. A whirlpool treatment also may be used to apply a warm soak (Fig. 9.8). Warm soaks increase circulation to the affected area, reduce edema, aid in the débridement of wounds, relax muscles, and can be used to apply a medicated solution to large areas.

To administer a warm soak, heat the solution to 105° to 110°F (40.5° to 43°C) and then immerse the patient's affected body part in the solution. Place waterproof pads under the container and cover the container with towels or waterproof pads to minimize heat loss. The solution usually retains the desired temperature for

Skill 9.2 Applying a Hot, Moist Compress to an Open Wound

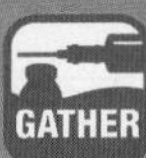

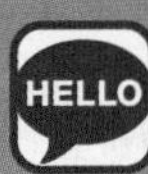

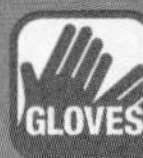

NURSING ACTION *(RATIONALE)*

1. Refer to standard steps 1 to 9.
2. Assemble equipment:
   - Aquathermia or heating pad (optional)
   - Bath blanket
   - Bath thermometer
   - Commercially prepared compresses (optional)
   - Disposable gloves
   - Dry bath towel
   - Petroleum jelly (optional)
   - Prescribed solution warmed to appropriate temperature, approximately 110° to 115°F (43° to 46°C)
   - Sterile container for solution
   - Sterile cotton swabs
   - Sterile gauze dressings
   - Sterile gloves
   - Tape or ties
   - Waterproof pad
3. Explain purpose of therapy to patient, and describe sensations to be felt (e.g., feeling of warmth and wetness). Explain precautions to prevent burning, and instruct patient to report changes in sensation immediately. *(Promotes patient cooperation, decreases patient's anxiety, and prevents injury to patient.)*
4. Evaluate condition of exposed skin and wound on which compress is to be applied. *(Provides baseline for determination of changes in skin during heat application. Very thin or impaired skin is more susceptible to injury from heat.)*

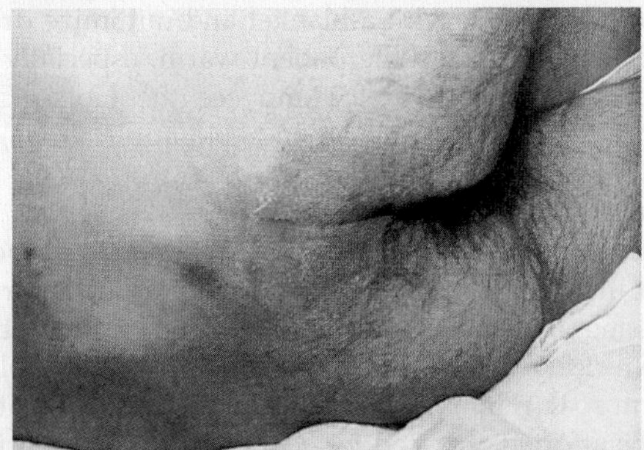

5. Place waterproof pad under area to be treated. *(Protects bed linens.)*
6. Assemble equipment. Pour warmed solution into sterile container. (If a portable heating source is to be used, keep solution warm. It is acceptable to leave commercially prepared compresses under infrared lamp until just before use.) Open sterile packages, and drop gauze into sterile container to immerse in solution. Set aquathermia pad (if used) to correct temperature and assess fluid level of unit. *(It is necessary for compresses to retain warmth for therapeutic benefit. Refer to health care provider's order or facility policy for appropriate temperature of solution.)*
7. Don disposable gloves. Remove any existing dressings covering wound. Dispose of gloves and dressings in proper receptacle. *(Reduces spread of microorganisms.)*
8. Apply sterile gloves. *(Allows the nurse to manipulate sterile dressing and touch open wound.)*
9. Apply sterile petroleum jelly, if it is ordered, with cotton swab to skin around wound. Do not apply jelly on impaired skin. *(Protects undamaged skin from possible burns and maceration.)*
10. Pick up one layer of immersed gauze and squeeze out excess water. *(Excess moisture macerates skin and increases risk of burns and infections.)*
11. Apply gauze lightly to open wound. Observe patient's response, and instruct patient to report any discomfort. After a few seconds, lift edge of gauze to check site for erythema. *(Enables the nurse to determine appropriate temperature and tolerance of treatment. It also prevents burns.)*
12. If patient tolerates temperature of the compress, pack gauze snugly against wound. Be certain all wound surfaces are covered by hot compress. *(Prevents rapid cooling from underlying air currents and allows all areas to be treated uniformly.)*
13. Wrap or cover moist compress with dry bath towel. If necessary, pin or tie in place. *(Insulates compress to prevent heat loss.)*
14. Change hot compress frequently according to order or facility policy. *(Prevents cooling and maintains therapeutic benefit of compress.)*
15. Apply aquathermia or waterproof heating pad over compress, if applicable, and keep it in place for desired duration of application (20 to 30 minutes). *(Promotes consistent temperature of compress. Local application of heat for more than 60 minutes often results in vasoconstriction. Removing hot compress after 30 minutes and reapplying in 15 minutes, if desired, maintains vasodilation and positive therapeutic effects.)*

Skill 9.2 Applying a Hot, Moist Compress to an Open Wound—cont'd

16. Provide the patient with a timer, clock, or watch. *(Allows patient to assist with timing the treatment; increases independence and compliance.)* Make sure call light is within patient's reach. *(Allows patient to call for assistance if needed and decreases potential for injury.)*

17. Instruct patient not to move compress, adjust temperature settings, or touch the wound site. *(Prevents patient injury and infection.)*

18. Check patient periodically for discomfort or burning sensation. Never leave the patient unattended if temperature sensations are impaired. Observe area of skin not covered by compress. *(Helps prevent injury. Continued exposure to heat poses risk of burns to skin.)*

19. Remove pad, towel, and compress in 30 minutes. Again, evaluate wound and condition of skin. *(Continued exposure to moisture will macerate skin. Action prevents injury.)*

20. Ask patient whether an unusual burning sensation is noticed that was not felt before. *(It is often difficult to determine the presence of a burn merely by color changes or the presence of inflammation or exudate.)*

21. Apply dry, sterile dressing as ordered. *(Prevents entrance of microorganisms into wound site.)*

22. Refer to standard steps 10 to 17.

23. Document the following: *(Verifies performance of procedure and ensures continuity of care.)*
- Date and time
- Type of application
- Temperature of application
- Location and duration of application
- Condition of wound and skin before and after application
- Patient's response to therapy.

See Chapter 12 for additional wound care techniques.

Illustration for Step 4 from Ignatavicius DD, Workman ML: *Medical-surgical nursing across the health care continuum,* ed 6, Philadelphia, 2009, Saunders.

Home Care Considerations

HEAT APPLICATIONS
- Do not apply heat immediately after an injury; heat will increase bleeding and edema.
- A washcloth or towel soaked in hot or warm water can be used as a moist compress in emergency situations.
- Never put washcloths or linen in the microwave because this may cause a fire.
- Check electrical cords on lamps and heating pads if they are to be used for heat therapy.
- Instruct patient not to lie on heating pads; the heat cannot disperse appropriately and may cause burns.
- Never use the high setting on heating pads.
- Instruct patients not to sleep with a heating pad on; this may increase the risk for burns.
- Use a cloth or towel between the heating device and the skin to prevent burns and skin damage.

COLD APPLICATIONS
- Keeping gel packs in the freezer at home makes at-home cold treatments easy.
- Instruct patients never to use cold packs designed for use in freezer chests for food or beverages on the skin.
- Suggest using a bucket filled with ice and water to immerse foot, hand, or elbow. Use a bath thermometer to test temperature.
- Freeze water in a plastic foam cup, and use it to treat a sprain or strain. Peel off the rim of the cup to or below the level of the ice, and apply ice in a circular motion.
- A bag of frozen vegetables conforms readily to a body part needing cold therapy for a brief time.
- Put ice and water in a zipper-locked bag to quickly make an ice bag for home use.
- Use a cloth or towel between the cooling device and skin to prevent skin damage.

approximately 10 minutes; it is necessary afterward to add more of the heated solution to maintain a constant temperature. To prevent injury to the body part, remove it from the water while the heated solution is added. Upon completion of the soak, dry the body part completely.

Another form of warm soak is a paraffin bath. A paraffin bath consists of a warmed mixture of heated paraffin wax and mineral oil. Patients with painful arthritis or other joint discomforts of the hands and feet may benefit from these baths. In many institutions, physical therapists administer the paraffin bath, but there are now appliances available for home use. It is important to instruct patients not to allow the bath temperature to exceed 128° to 130°F (53.3° to 54.5°C), to prevent burns and skin damage.

Aquathermia (Water-Flow) Pads (K-Pads)

In health care institutions, the aquathermia pad, also known as a *water-flow pad* or *K-pad* (Fig. 9.9), is used as

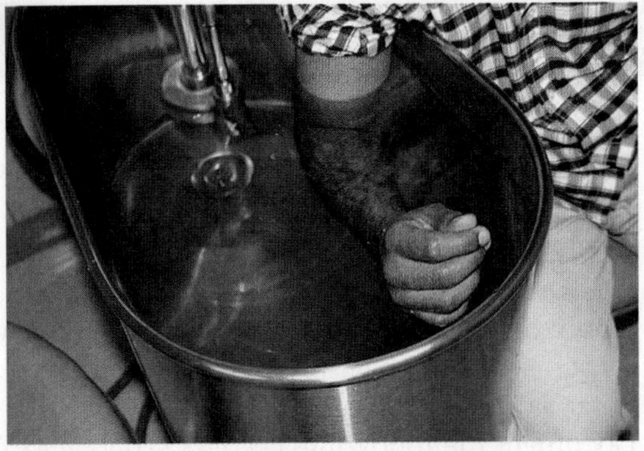

Fig. 9.8 Whirlpool moist heat therapy. (From Szekeres M, Chinchalkar S, King G: Optimizing elbow rehabilitation after instability. *Hand Clinics*, Feb 2008, Elsevier.)

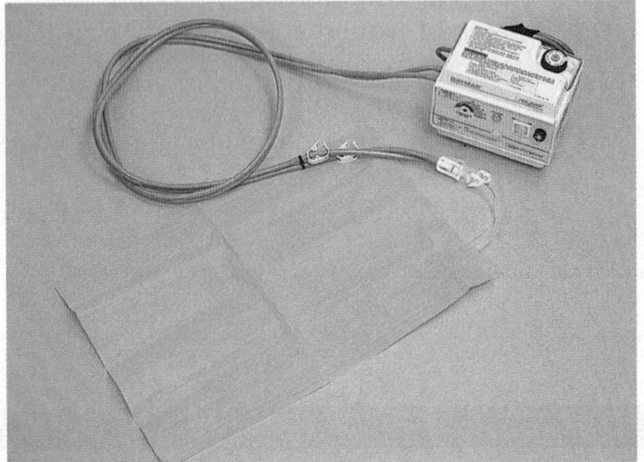

Fig. 9.9 Aquathermia pad. (From Sorrentino SA & Remmert LN: *Mosby's textbook for nursing assistants*, ed 9, St. Louis, 2017.)

a source of moist or dry heat application in lieu of conventional heating pads. Aquathermia pads, which are waterproof, tend to be safer than heating pads because a precise temperature is set by inserting a plastic key into the temperature regulator, or the temperature is preset before use. In aquathermia pads, distilled water is circulated through internal channels in the pad via hoses connected to an electrical unit that houses a heating element and motor.

The recommended temperature setting for the aquathermia pad is between 105° and 110°F (40.5° and 43°C). To ensure proper functioning and safety of the unit and even distribution of water circulation, make sure the tubing is kept even with the unit and is secured in place. When the water reservoir runs low, the unit should be filled with distilled water rather than tap water to prevent mineral deposits from forming in the unit.

As with all heat or cold applications, a thin towel or pillowcase is placed next to the patient's skin so that the pad is not in direct contact with the patient. The pad may be secured with tape, ties, or gauze rolls. An aquathermia pad must never be secured with safety pins because those may cause the pad to leak. In addition, patients should not be allowed to lie on the pad because this prevents even heat distribution, and burns may occur. Applications typically last for 20 to 30 minutes. Some health care providers may order the application to be applied for longer periods of time, depending on the reason and the patient's condition. No matter how long the application is on, it is always important to check the patient's skin periodically during the application for any signs of burning.

Dry Heat Application

Warm, dry heat can be applied with commercially available disposable hot packs, electric heating pads, or hot water bottles. With the commercially prepared hot packs, the heat is released when the chemicals contained in the pack are mixed by squeezing, kneading, or breaking the internal container according to package directions.

Hot water bottles are not recommended in acute care facilities, but they may be used in the home setting. If they are used in the home, it is essential to instruct the patient to practice extreme caution to prevent burns.

Heating pads also are used frequently in the home setting but are not recommended for use in acute care or long-term care facilities. Heating pads contain an electrical coil surrounded by a waterproof pad covered by cotton or flannel fabric. The temperature regulation for these units is limited to the choice of low, medium, and high settings instead of exact temperatures. Safety precautions include teaching the patient to avoid lying on the pad, to avoid using the high setting, and to avoid securing the pad with a safety pin, which may cause an electrical shock.

Cold, Moist, and Dry Compresses

Cold compresses typically are used to treat inflammation and prevent edema. They can be either clean or sterile and usually are applied for 20 minutes at 59°F (15°C). The procedure for application of cold compresses is similar to that used for warm compresses (see Skill 9.2). A thin towel or cloth should be applied between the skin and the compress, and the health care provider orders frequency and duration of treatment.

Commercially prepared disposable cold packs work like disposable hot packs. They are packaged in various sizes and shapes and permit dry cold application. The nurse is responsible for evaluating the patient for signs of complications from cold therapy, including erythema, burning sensation, numbness, mottling, extreme paleness, and cyanosis. The nurse also must teach the patient the normal progression of sensations experienced during cold therapy; first cold, then pain relief followed by burning skin pain, and finally numbness. Make sure to apply towels (sterile towels over an injured area) between the cold application and the skin (Fig. 9.10). To prevent frostnip or frostbite, remove the cold pack or compress after 20 minutes, and inspect the skin for signs of complications.

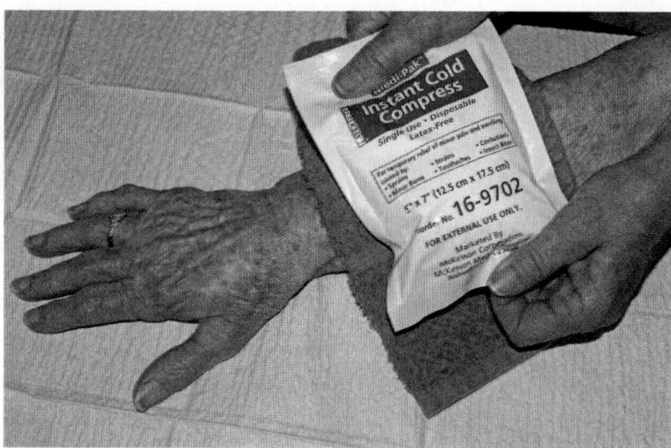

Fig. 9.10 Commercial cold pack used for therapy.

Ice Bags or Collars

Ice bags or ice collars can be used to reduce edema formation and bleeding and provide an anesthetic effect to areas of hemorrhage and hematoma formation, as well as for patients who have undergone dental surgery or those with muscle strain. When these devices are used, the nurse must make sure there are no leaks by filling the device with water before use. The device is filled two-thirds full of crushed ice. This allows the device to mold well to the body part, and it does not apply too much pressure on the area being treated. Excess air must be expelled from the device before the cap is secured because conduction of cold is interrupted by excess air in the device. Excess moisture should be dried from the device, and the device is covered with flannel material, a towel, or a pillowcase. The ice pack or collar is applied according to the health care provider's order or facility policy.

ORAL HYGIENE

Oral hygiene (care of the oral cavity) helps maintain a healthy state of the mouth, the teeth, the gums, and the lips. Brushing the teeth removes food particles, plaque, and bacteria; massages the gums; and relieves discomfort that results from unpleasant odors and tastes. Complete oral hygiene gives a sense of well-being and thus can stimulate appetite. Proper care prevents oral disease such as gingivitis or periodontitis and tooth destruction. Certain patients are at risk for oral disorders (Box 9.8).

Patients should brush their own teeth when possible. When the patient is unable to do so, the nurse must perform this procedure (Skill 9.3).

Dentures (a set of artificial teeth not permanently fixed or implanted) are the patient's personal property. Dentures must be handled with care because they easily can be broken and they can be very expensive. Use an enclosed, labeled cup to soak dentures or to store them when they are not being worn (e.g., during surgery or a diagnostic procedure, or at night). Patients who return from surgery or a diagnostic test and patients who have just woken up in the morning usually prefer to have their dentures reinserted as quickly as possible. Many people find the change in appearance that results when dentures are removed to be embarrassing.

Box 9.8 Conditions That Place Patients at Risk for Oral Disorders

- Alteration in the integrity of teeth and mucosa resulting from disease or treatments
- Inability to perform oral care
- Lack of knowledge about oral hygiene
- Patients in hospitals or long-term care facilities often do not receive appropriate oral care. Patients who are particularly at risk are those experiencing the following:
  - Chemotherapy drugs
  - Diabetes
  - Disorientation
  - Nothing-by-mouth (NPO) status
  - Paralysis
  - Radiation therapy
  - Serious illness
  - State of unconsciousness
  - Upper-extremity activity limitations

Most patients prefer to clean their dentures themselves; encourage them to do so as often as for natural teeth to prevent infection and irritation. However, when the nurse must assist with denture care, always consider the patient's preference of cleanser and soaking (see Skill 9.3).

Provide oral care on a regular basis; frequency of hygiene measures depends on the condition of the patient's mouth. The beneficial outcomes of oral hygiene are probably not seen for several days. Repeated cleansing often is needed to remove tenacious, dried exudate of the tongue and to restore the mucosa's hydration to normal. For patients whose condition warrants turning and repositioning by the staff on a scheduled basis (e.g., every 2 hours), oral care may be provided at these times.

HAIR CARE

Proper hair care is important to the patient's self-image. Combing, brushing, and shampooing are basic hygiene measures needed by all patients. Illness or disability often prevents patients from performing their own daily hair care. A bedfast patient's hair soon becomes tangled. Remember that most patients always are aware of their appearance. Good hair care should be performed routinely, at least daily, to meet the hygiene needs of the patient. If the patient is not able to carry out this part of self-care, the nurse must assist. If the patient is able to take a shower or tub bath, the hair can be shampooed easily at this time. One option is to use a portable chair in the shower, and another is to place a chair in front of a sink.

For the helpless bedfast patient, the shampoo must be performed with the patient in bed. Check whether a health care provider's order is necessary. Most facilities

Skill 9.3 Administering Oral Hygiene Care

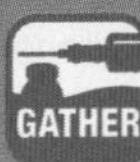

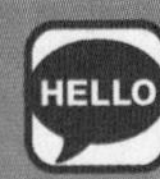

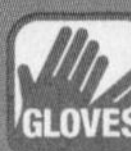

NURSING ACTION *(RATIONALE)*

1. Refer to medical record, care plan, or Kardex for special interventions. *(Provides for basis of care.)*
2. Assemble supplies. *(Organizes procedure.)*
   a. For oral care
      - Cleansing solution, such as diluted hydrogen peroxide, toothpaste, normal saline solution, baking soda solution, or mouthwash
      - Dental floss (optional)
      - Disposable gloves
      - Emesis basin
      - Flashlight
      - Toothette, soft-bristled toothbrush, or tongue blade wrapped with gauze
      - Towel

   b. For denture care
      - 4 × 4 gauze
      - Cleansing agent
      - Denture brush
      - Denture cup
      - Disposable gloves
      - Emesis basin or sink
      - Soft-bristled toothbrush
      - Washcloth
      - Water glass
3. Introduce self. *(Decreases patient's anxiety.)*
4. Identify patient. *(Ensures procedure is performed with correct patient.)*
5. Explain procedure to patient. *(Enlists cooperation and decreases patient's anxiety.)*
6. Assess patient for the following: *(Determines special needs and level of assistance required from nurse; wear gloves when in contact with the patient's mucosa or body fluids.)*
   - Ability to perform own oral care (independence is to be encouraged)
   - Aging
   - Chemotherapeutic drugs or radiation therapy to head and neck
   - Diabetes mellitus
   - Integrity of lips, teeth, buccal mucosa, gums, palate, and tongue
   - Oral surgery; trauma to mouth
   - Presence of artificial airway
   - Presence of nasogastric or oxygen (O_2) tubes
   - Risk of dehydration (NPO status)
7. Perform hand hygiene and don clean gloves according to agency policy and guidelines from the CDC and OSHA. *(Reduces spread of microorganisms.)*
8. Prepare patient for intervention.
   a. Close door or pull privacy curtain. *(Provides privacy.)*
   b. Raise bed to comfortable working position. *(Promotes proper body mechanics.)*
   c. Arrange supplies. *(Provides convenient access to equipment.)*
   d. If patient tolerates the activity, provide supplies in the bathroom and allow patient privacy.
   e. If patient is on bed rest but tolerates the activity while remaining in bed, arrange overbed table in front of patient; provide supplies, and allow patient privacy. *(Patient involvement with procedure keeps anxiety to a minimum.)*
   f. If you are performing the procedure with an unconscious patient, position patient's head to the side toward you (dependent side if possible) and close to you (see Step 9a). *(Proper positioning of head prevents aspiration.)*
9. Oral care.
   a. Place towel under patient's face and emesis basin under patient's chin. *(Facilitates procedure and prevents soiling of bed.)*

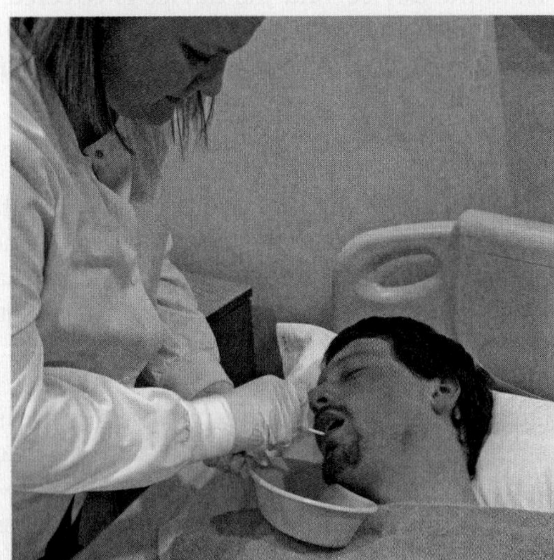

   b. Carefully separate patient's jaws. *(Protects your fingers.)*
   c. Cleanse mouth using brush, tongue blade, or toothette moistened with cleansing agent. Clean inner and outer tooth surfaces. Swab roof of mouth and inside cheeks. Use flashlight for better visualization of oral cavity. Gently swab tongue. Rinse and repeat. Rinse several times. *(Removes food particles, secretions, and dried exudate. Moistens mucosa; leaves mouth fresh.)*

Skill 9.3 Administering Oral Hygiene Care—cont'd

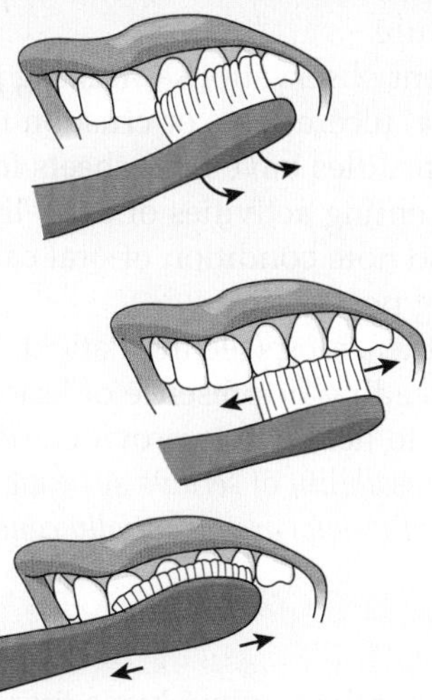

d. Apply lubricant to lips. *(Provides moisture to prevent drying and cracking [cheilosis].)*

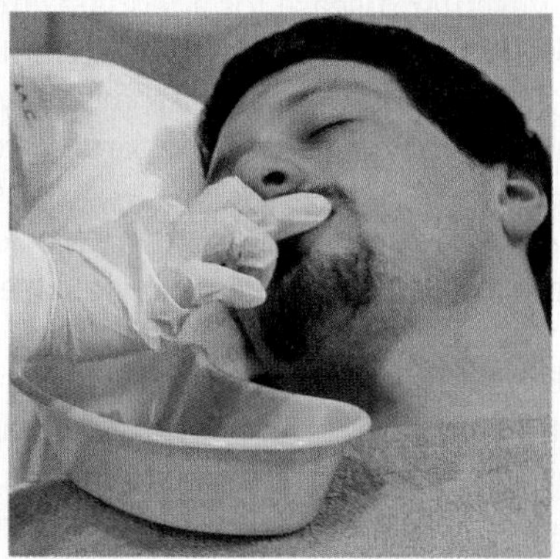

10. Cleaning dentures.

a. Fill emesis basin half full of tepid water or place a washcloth in the bottom of the sink. *(Acts as a cushion for the dentures if accidentally dropped, preventing damage to dentures. Temperature extremes harm dentures.)*

b. Ask patient to remove dentures and place in emesis basin. If patient is unable to remove own dentures, break suction that holds upper denture in place by using thumb and finger. With gauze, apply gentle downward tug and carefully remove from patient's mouth. *(Gauze prevents slipping while handling dentures.)* Next, remove lower denture by carefully lifting up and turning sideways. Remove and place in emesis basin.

c. Cleanse biting surfaces. Cleanse outer and inner tooth surfaces. Be certain to cleanse lower surface of dentures. *(Prevents bacteria, odor, and stain formation from lodged food particles.)*

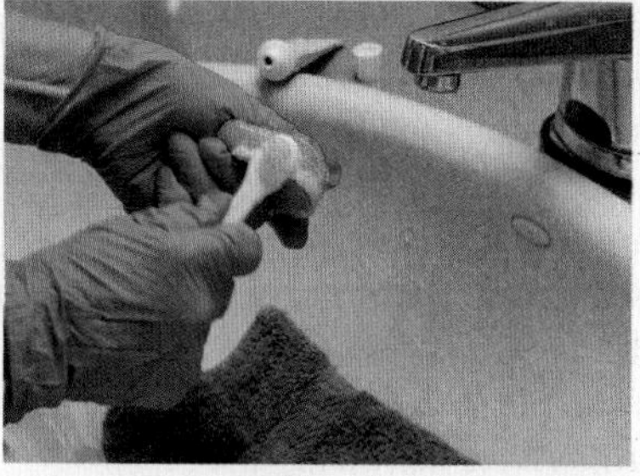

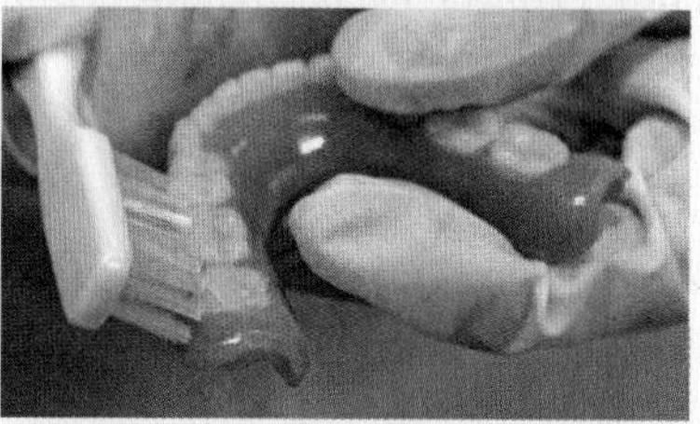

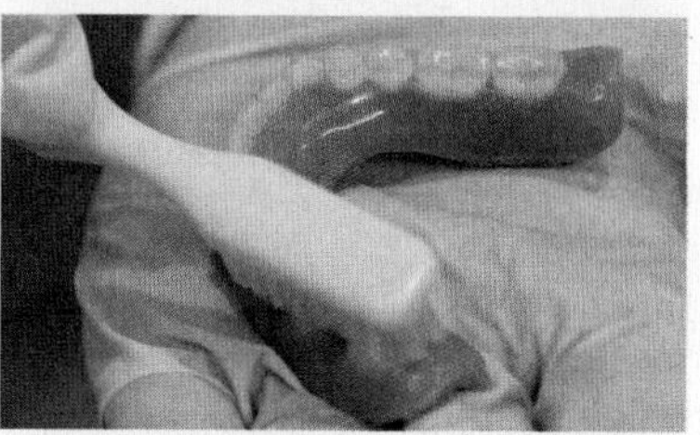

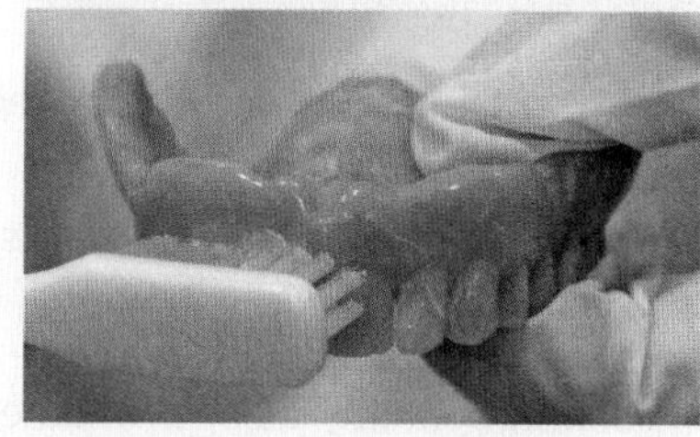

d. Rinse dentures thoroughly with tepid water. *(Warm water is more effective than cold water.)*

e. Before replacing dentures in patient's mouth or after storing dentures properly, gently brush patient's gums, tongue, and inside of cheeks and rinse thoroughly. *(Cleansing of the oral cavity is also necessary to promote healthy gums and mucosa.)*

f. Replace dentures either in patient's mouth or in container of solution placed in safe place. *(Dentures may become brittle and warped if not kept moist. Dentures are costly and must be handled with care.)*

g. When reinserting the dentures, replace the upper denture first if patient has both dentures. Apply gentle pressure to reestablish the suction. Moisten dentures for easier insertion. Be certain dentures are comfortably

Continued

Skill 9.3 Administering Oral Hygiene Care—cont'd

situated in patient's mouth before leaving the bedside. *(Promotes comfort.)*

11. Dispose of gloves in proper receptacle. Clean and store supplies. Perform hand hygiene. *(Reduces spread of microorganisms.)*
12. Position patient for comfort, raise side rail, and lower bed. *(Promotes comfort and safety.)*
13. Assess for patient comfort. *(Helps determine whether dentures are fitting properly.)*
14. Document. *(Timely documentation maintains accuracy of patient's record and communicates interventions given.)*
    - Procedure
    - Pertinent observations (bleeding gums, dry mucosa, ulcerations, or crust on tongue)
    - Most facilities have flow sheets for documenting activities of daily living (ADLs) but also note condition of oral cavity in nursing notes
    - Patient teaching (see the Patient Teaching box)
15. Report bleeding or presence of lesions to nurse in charge or to health care provider. *(Bleeding indicates possibility of serious systemic problems. Certain oral lesions are potentially cancerous.)*

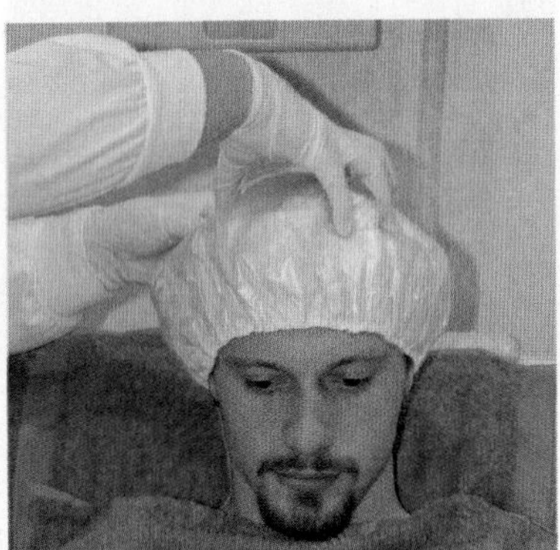

Fig. 9.11 Bed shampoo using a shampoo cap.

have portable blow dryers and curling irons available and shampoo boards (Skill 9.4). Shampoo caps (Fig. 9.11) are often available (cap with no-rinse shampoo inside). Dry shampoos are also available in most facilities.

SHAVING THE PATIENT

Many patients prefer to shave at the time of bathing. Remember that an electric razor should be used for those patients who have a bleeding disorder or who are undergoing *anticoagulant therapy* (medications that increase the tendency to bleed). Do not allow a disoriented or depressed patient to use a razor with a blade, to prevent accidental or self-inflicted injury. A male patient's beard, mustache, or sideburns are never removed without consent of the patient, except for emergency purposes.

The patient needs to be shaved if unable to perform this himself (e.g., the patient is too ill or has an arm immobilized in traction or a cast) (see Skill 9.4).

HAND, FOOT, AND NAIL CARE

Hands and feet often need special attention to prevent infection, odors, and injury. Problems arise from abuse or poor care of the hands and feet (e.g., biting the nails or wearing ill-fitting shoes).

Assessment of the feet involves a thorough examination of all skin surfaces. Carefully assess the area between the toes. Observe patients with diabetes mellitus or peripheral vascular disease for adequate circulation to the feet. The elderly are also at risk for foot disorders because of poor vision or decreased mobility. Consider whether a podiatry consult is in order; consult the physician.

Administer care of the hands and feet during the morning bath, or at another time if desired (see Skill 9.4).

PERINEAL CARE

Perineal care (pericare, or care of the genitalia) is part of the complete bed bath. Those patients most in need of meticulous pericare are those at risk for acquiring an infection: for example, patients with indwelling catheters, patients recovering from rectal or genital surgery, and postpartum patients. If patients can perform their own pericare, allow them to do so. A professional, dignified attitude helps diminish embarrassment and puts patients at ease when providing this care for patients who are unable to do so themselves. Catheter care is provided at least two times daily for all patients with indwelling catheters, unless otherwise ordered by the health care provider.

Be alert for signs of vaginal or urethral exudate (discharge), skin impairment, unpleasant odors, reports of burning during urination, or localized tenderness or pain of the perineum. Also observe for skin impairment in the perineal area, especially in those patients with urinary or fecal incontinence, rectal and perineal surgical dressings, and indwelling urinary catheters (Skill 9.5).

Perineal Care for the Patient With an Indwelling Catheter

As stated earlier, catheter care is provided twice daily for all patients with indwelling catheters, unless otherwise ordered by the health care provider. Daily catheter care includes cleansing of the meatal-catheter junction

Text continued on p. 219

Skill 9.4 Care of the Hair, Nails, and Feet

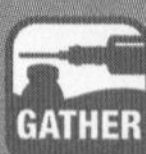

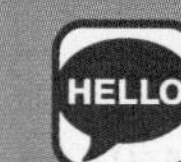

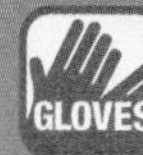

NURSING ACTION *(RATIONALE)*

1. Refer to medical record, care plan, or Kardex for special interventions. *(Provides basis for care.)*
2. Assemble supplies. *(Organizes procedure.)*
   a. Bed shampoo
      - Bath blanket
      - Bath towels (2)
      - Comb and brush
      - Hair dryer and curling iron (optional)
      - Shampoo
      - Shampoo board or shampoo cap
      - Wash basin
      - Washcloth or hand towel
      - Water pitcher

   b. Shaving
      - Aftershave lotion or powder, if desired
      - Basin with hot water, 115°F (46°C), or as patient prefers
      - Bath blanket
      - Bath towel
      - Face towel
      - Mirror
      - Safety razor with sharp blade or electric razor
      - Shaving cream or soap and brush for safety razor
      - Washcloth

   c. Nail and foot care
      - Disposable bath mat
      - Disposable gloves (optional)
      - Emesis basin
      - Hand towel
      - Lotion
      - Nail clippers, emery board, and orangewood stick
      - Wash basin
      - Washcloth
3. Introduce self. *(Decreases patient's anxiety.)*
4. Identify patient. *(Ensures procedure is performed with correct patient.)*
5. Explain procedure. *(Enlists cooperation and reduces patient's anxiety.)*
6. Assess patient for the following: *(Determines special interventions necessary.)*
   - Ability to care for own hair, nails, and feet. *(Encourages independence.)*
   - Condition of scalp, hair, nails, and feet; color and temperature of toes, feet, and fingers.
   - Contraindications to shampooing, shaving, or nail care. (In some facilities, only RNs are permitted to trim the toenails of a patient with diabetes. Follow agency policy.)
   - Knowledge of foot and nail care practices.
   - Restrictions to positioning.
7. Perform hand hygiene and don clean gloves according to agency policy and guidelines from the CDC and OSHA. *(Reduces spread of microorganisms.)*
8. Prepare patient for intervention. *(Readies patient for procedure.)*
   a. Close door or pull privacy curtain. *(Provides privacy.)*
   b. Raise bed to a comfortable working height. *(Promotes proper body mechanics.)*
   c. Arrange supplies at bedside or, if patient is able to perform procedure, have supplies available in the bathroom and offer assistance as needed. *(Patient's involvement with procedure reduces anxiety to a minimum.)*
9. Bed shampoo.[a]
   a. Position patient close to one side of bed. Place shampoo board under patient's head and washbasin at end of spout. Ensure spout extends over edge of mattress. *(Prevents wetting of bed linens.)*
   b. Position rolled-up bath towel under patient's neck. *(Reduces discomfort.)* Certain conditions such as cervical neck injuries, open incisions, or tracheostomy place the patient at risk for injury, in which case a modified position is used.
   c. Brush and comb patient's hair. If hair is matted with blood, hydrogen peroxide is effective as a cleansing agent. *(Removes tangles and loosens dried secretions.)*
   d. Obtain water in pitcher at about 110°F (43°C). *(Prevents burns.)*
   e. If patient is able, instruct patient to hold washcloth over eyes. Completely wet hair and apply small amount of shampoo. *(Prevents water and shampoo from getting into eyes.)*
   f. Massage scalp with pads of fingertips, not nails. Shampoo hairline, back of neck (lift head slightly), and sides of hair. *(Ensures thorough cleansing and increases scalp circulation. Use of pads of fingertips prevents injury to scalp.)*

Continued

[a]Some facilities use shampoo caps. These caps contain a no-rinse shampoo; they are placed on the patient's head, and the shampoo is massaged into the patient's hair and scalp.

Skill 9.4 Care of the Hair, Nails, and Feet—cont'd

g. Rinse thoroughly and apply more shampoo, repeating Steps e and f. Rinse, and repeat rinsing until hair is free of shampoo. *(Prevents scalp irritation.)*

h. Wrap dry towel around patient's head. Dry patient's face, neck, and shoulders. Dry hair and scalp with second towel. *(Prevents patient from chilling.)*

i. Comb hair and dry with hair dryer as quickly as possible. *(Prevents patient from chilling.)*

j. Complete styling hair and position patient for comfort. *(Promotes sense of well-being.)*

10. Shaving the patient.

a. Assist patient to sitting position if patient is able. *(Simulates the natural position.)*

b. Observe face and neck for lesions, moles, or birthmarks. *(Cutting poses risk to cause infection, bleeding, or irritation.)*

c. Use shaving cream or soap. *(Lathering softens beard and facilitates shave.)*

d. Shave in direction hair grows. Use short strokes. Start with upper face and lips, and then extend to neck. If patient is able, hyperextending (tilting backward) his head is helpful to shave curved areas. *(Provides for closer shave without irritation.)*

e. Pull skin taut with nondominant hand above or below the area being shaved. *(Promotes uniform shaving.)*

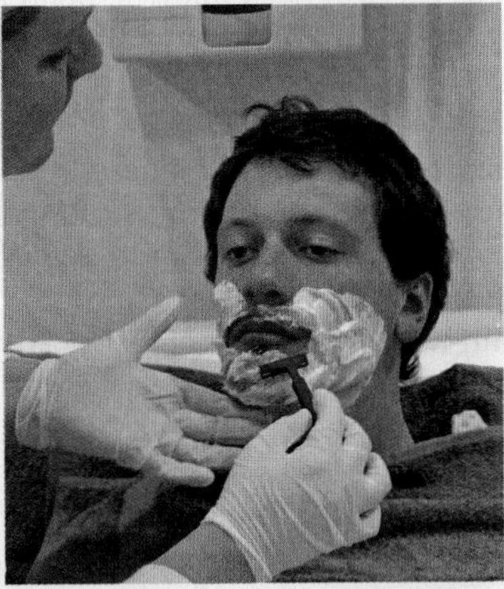

f. Rinse razor after each stroke. *(Keeps cutting edge clean.)*

g. Rinse and dry face. *(Removes remnants of lather and shaved hair.)*

h. If patient desires, apply lotion or cologne. *(Causes cooling sensation that feels refreshing.)*

i. Dispose of blades in sharps container. *(Protects others from accidental injury.)*

11. Hand and foot care.

a. Position patient in chair. If possible, place disposable mat under patient's feet. *(Protects bare feet from floor.)*

b. Fill basin with warm water and test temperature. Place basin on disposable mat and assist patient to place feet into basin. **(Do not soak hands and feet of a patient with diabetes for extended periods of time; soaking increases risk of infection by skin breaking down from maceration.)** Allow to soak 10 to 20 minutes. Rewarm water as necessary. *(Soaking in warm water softens nails and ensures easy manipulation of cuticles. Keeping water warm prevents chilling the patient.)*

c. Place overbed table in low position in front of patient. Fill emesis basin with warm water and test water temperature. Place basin on table, and place patient's fingers in basin. Allow fingernails to soak 10 to 20 minutes. Rewarm water as necessary. *(Soaking loosens foreign particles under nails and ensures easy manipulation of cuticles. Keeping water warm prevents chilling the patient.)*

d. Using orangewood stick, gently clean under fingernails. *(Orangewood stick removes debris that harbors microorganisms from under nails.)* With clippers, trim nails straight across and even with tip of fingers. With emery board, shape fingernails. Push cuticles back gently with washcloth or orangewood stick. *(Prevents injury to delicate nail beds.)*

e. Don gloves, and with washcloth scrub areas of feet that are calloused. *(Reduces spread of microorganisms. Scrubbing after soaking helps remove dead skin layers.)*

f. Trim and clean toenails following Step d instructions.

g. Apply lotion or cream to hands and feet. Return patient to bed and position for comfort. Dry fingers and toes thoroughly to impede fungal growth and prevent maceration (a softening and breaking down of tissue resulting from prolonged exposure to moisture). *(Creams and lotions lubricate dry skin.)* Do not apply lotion between toes of patients with diabetes. *(Organisms may be harbored and increase the chance of infection.)*

h. On completion of procedure, observe the nails and the surrounding tissue for condition of skin and any remaining rough edges.

i. If the patient's nails are extremely hard or if the patient is unable to perform personal nail care, have a podiatrist (a person trained in the

Skill 9.4 Care of the Hair, Nails, and Feet—cont'd

treatment of nail and foot problems) provide nail care.

j. Teach the patient with diabetes about appropriate foot care. The teaching plan includes inspecting the feet daily for breaks, wearing shoes at all times, wearing socks, drying feet completely, and noting any areas of numbness, tingling, or pain.

12. Dispose of gloves in proper receptacle. Clean and store supplies. Place soiled laundry in hamper. Perform hand hygiene. *(Reduces spread of microorganisms.)*
13. Assess for patient's comfort, lower bed level, raise side rails, and place call button within easy reach. *(Promotes safety.)*
14. Document. *(Timely recording maintains accuracy of patient's record and communicates interventions given.)*
    - Procedure
    - Pertinent observations (e.g., breaks in the skin, inflammation, or ulcerations)
    - Most facilities have flow sheets for ADLs; shaving, and nail and foot care are usually not recorded in nursing notes; know agency policy
    - Patient teaching (see the Patient Teaching and Home Care Considerations boxes)
15. Report abnormal findings (breaks in the skin or ulcerations) to nurse in charge or physician. *(Additional interventions are sometimes required.)*

Skill 9.5 Perineal Care: Male and Female and the Catheterized Patient

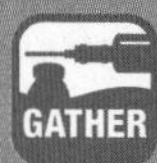

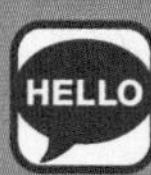

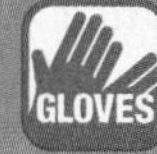

NURSING ACTION *(RATIONALE)*

1. Refer to medical record, care plan, or Kardex for special interventions. *(Provides basis for care.)*
2. Assemble supplies. *(Organizes procedure.)*
    a. Perineal care
        - Bath blanket
        - Bath towel
        - Bedpan
        - Disposable gloves
        - Mild soap
        - Solution bottle
        - Toilet tissue
        - Washbasin and warm water
        - Washcloths (2)
        - Waterproof pad
    b. Additional supplies that may be needed for the catheterized patient:
        - Antimicrobial ointment (only if ordered by the health care provider)
        - Sterile package of cotton-tipped applicators
3. Introduce self. *(Reduces patient's anxiety.)*
4. Identify patient. *(Ensures procedure is performed with correct patient.)*
5. Explain procedure. *(Enlists cooperation and reduces patient's anxiety.)*
6. Assess patient for the following, wearing gloves when in contact with mucous membranes or secretions: *(Determines whether additional interventions are necessary.)*
    - Ability to perform self-care
    - Accumulated secretions
    - Extent of care required by patient
    - Knowledge of importance of perineal care
    - Lesions
    - Surgical incision
7. Remove and dispose of soiled gloves and perform hand hygiene and don clean gloves according to agency policy and guidelines from the CDC and OSHA. *(Reduces spread of microorganisms.)*
8. Prepare patient for interventions. *(Readies patient for procedure.)* Allow postpartum patients to perform this procedure by themselves while sitting on the stool, using a pericare squeeze bottle. Patients allowed tub or shower baths do this by themselves. Be certain supplies are close by. *(Patient's involvement with procedure reduces anxiety.)*
    a. Close door or pull privacy curtain. *(Provides privacy.)*

Continued

Skill 9.5 Perineal Care: Male and Female and the Catheterized Patient—cont'd

b. Raise bed to comfortable working height and lower side rail. *(Promotes proper body mechanics.)*

c. Arrange supplies at bedside. *(Facilitates procedure.)*

d. Assist patient to desired position in bed: dorsal recumbent for female or supine for male. *(Facilitates procedure.)*

e. Drape for procedure. *(Reduces patient's embarrassment.)*

9. Female perineal care

a. Raise side rail and fill basin two-thirds full of water at 105° to 109°F (41° to 43°C). *(Promotes patient safety. Filling basin only two-thirds full prevents unnecessary splashing.)*

b. Position waterproof pad or towel under patient's buttocks with patient lying in the dorsal recumbent position in bed. Drape patient with bath blanket placed in the shape of a diamond. One corner is under the patient's chin; one corner is on each side of the patient, with the bath blanket wrapped around each foot and leg; and the last corner is between the patient's legs. This corner can be lifted to expose the patient's perineum. *(Draping in this manner keeps exposure to a minimum, decreasing the patient's anxiety.)*

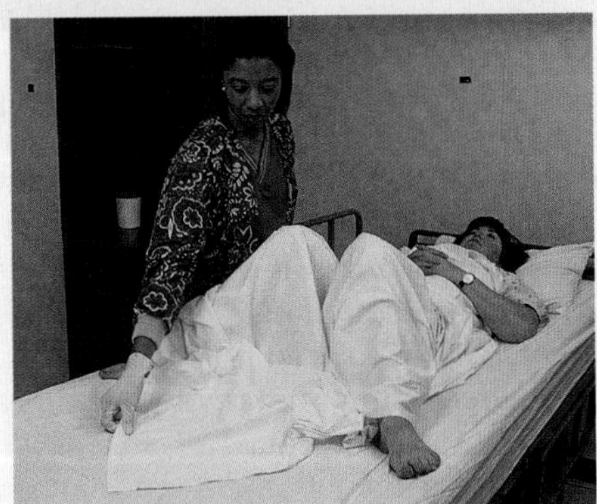

c. With a washcloth or disposable washcloth wrapped around one hand, wash and dry patient's upper thighs. *(Surrounding skin surfaces need cleansing also.)*

d. Wash **labia majora** (larger fold or lip) and **labia minora** (smaller fold or lip). Wash carefully in skin folds. Cleanse in direction anterior to posterior. Use separate corner of washcloth for each skin fold. *(Prevents microorganisms around the anus from entering the meatus or vagina.)*

e. Separate labia to expose the urinary meatus (opening) and the vaginal orifice. Wash downward toward rectum with smooth strokes. Use separate corner of washcloth for each smooth stroke. *(Reduces spread of microorganisms.)*

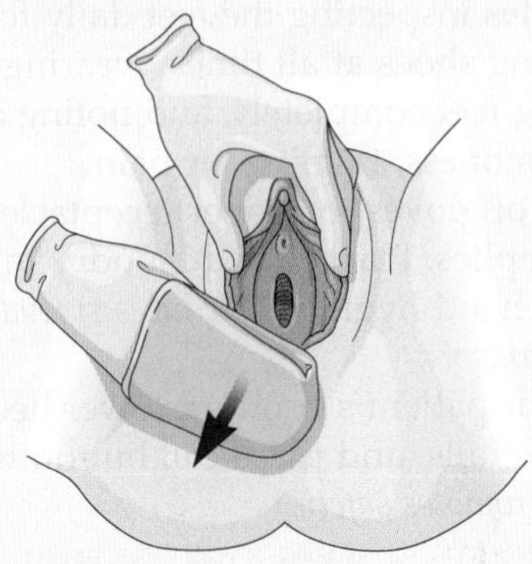

f. Cleanse, rinse, and dry thoroughly. *(Retained moisture harbors microorganisms.)*

g. Assist patient to side-lying position and cleanse rectal area with toilet tissue, if necessary. Wash area by cleansing from perineal area toward anus. You often may need several washcloths. Many facilities have disposable wipes. If so, use them. Wash, rinse, and dry thoroughly. *(Reduces spread of microorganisms and risk of skin impairment.)*

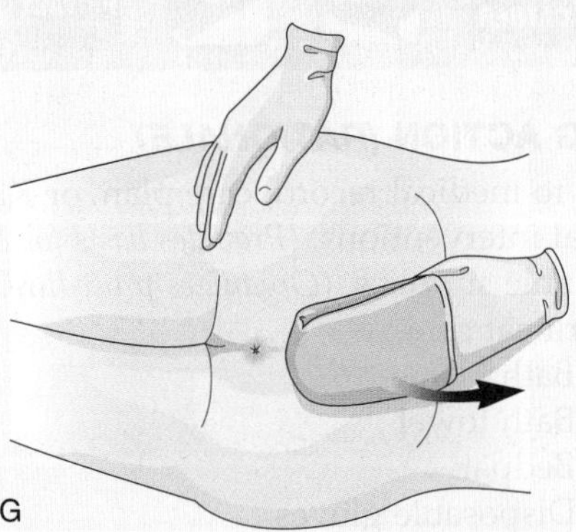

10. Male perineal care

a. Raise side rail and fill basin two-thirds full of water at about 105° to 109°F (41° to 43°C). *(Promotes patient safety and prevents unnecessary spillage.)*

b. Gently grasp shaft of penis. Retract foreskin of uncircumcised patient. *(Secretions collect under foreskin.)*

c. Wash tip of penis with circular motion.

d. Cleanse from meatus outward. *(Prevents microorganisms from entering urethra.)* Two washcloths are often necessary. Wash, rinse, and dry gently.

Skill 9.5 Perineal Care: Male and Female and the Catheterized Patient—cont'd

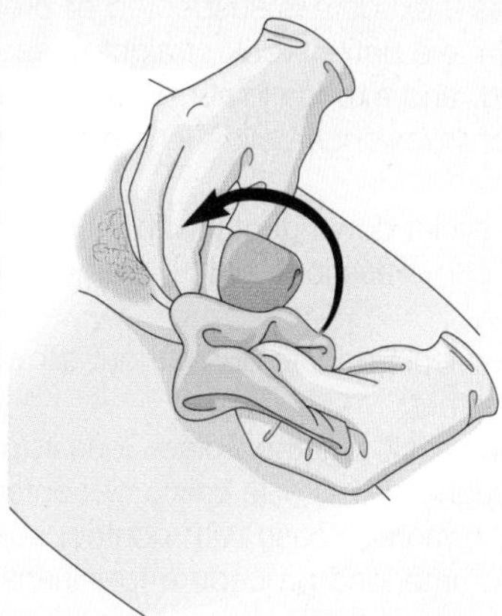

e. Replace foreskin, and wash shaft of penis with a firm but gentle downward stroke. Replace the foreskin of the uncircumcised male patient after thorough cleansing. *(Prevents edema and discomfort.)*
f. Rinse and dry thoroughly. *(Retained moisture harbors microorganisms.)*
g. Cleanse scrotum gently. Cleanse carefully in underlying skin folds. Rinse and dry gently. *(Pressure on scrotal tissue is often very painful.)*
h. Assist patient to a side-lying position. *(Facilitates procedure.)* Cleanse anal area. Follow Step 9f of female perineal care.

11. Catheter care
    a. Raise side rail and fill basin two-thirds full of water at about 105° to 109°F (41° to 43°C). *(Promotes patient safety and prevents unnecessary spillage.)*
    b. Position and drape the patient. (Supine position with gown to pubic area and bath blanket up over legs, exposing only the perineum.)
    c. Cleanse around urethral meatus and adjacent catheter. Cleanse entire catheter with soap and water. *(Reduces risk of urinary tract infections.)*
    d. Repeat cleansing to remove all exudate from meatus and catheter. *(Exudates are often irritating and are medium for infectious organisms.)*
    e. If ointment is ordered, open package of sterile cotton-tipped applicators. Do not touch cotton tip. Apply ointment to applicator. Do not touch wrapper to cotton tip. *(Maintains sterility.)*
    f. Apply ointment to junction of catheter and urethral meatus. *(Reduces irritation and reduces spread of microorganisms.)*
12. Remove gloves. Clean and store equipment. Dispose of contaminated supplies in proper receptacle. Perform hand hygiene. *(Reduces spread of microorganisms.)*
13. Position patient for comfort. *(Promotes relaxation.)*
14. Document. *(Timely recording maintains accuracy of patient's record and communicates interventions given.)*
    - Procedure
    - Pertinent observations such as the following:
        - Character and amount of discharge and odor if present
        - Condition of genitalia (erythema, edema, or discomfort)
    - Patient's ability to perform own care
    - Patient teaching (see the Patient Teaching and Home Care Considerations boxes)
15. Report abnormal findings to nurse in charge or health care provider. *(Additional interventions are sometimes necessary.)*

Figure for Step 9b from Potter PA, Perry AG: *Essentials for nursing practice*, ed 8, St. Louis, 2015, Mosby.

with a mild soap and water and sometimes application of a water-soluble microbicidal ointment (only if ordered by the health care provider; this is not routinely performed) (see Skill 9.5).

EYE, EAR, AND NOSE CARE

Special attention is given to cleansing the eyes, the ears, and the nose during the patient's bath. The nurse often has the responsibility of assisting patients in the care of eyeglasses, contact lenses, or artificial eyes. For patients who wear eyeglasses, contact lenses, artificial eyes, or hearing aids, assess the patient's knowledge and methods used to care for the aids, and any problems caused by the aids. Patients who cannot grasp small objects, have limited mobility in the upper extremities, have reduced vision, or are seriously fatigued need the nurse's assistance.

The eyes, ears, and nose are sensitive; therefore take extra care to prevent injury to these tissues.

Care of the Eyes

The **circumorbital** (circular area around the eye) area of the eyes usually is cleansed during the bath, typically by washing with a clean washcloth moistened with clear water. Do not use soap because it often causes burning and irritation. Cleanse the eye from the inner to the outer canthus. Use a separate section of the washcloth each time to prevent spread of infection. If the patient has dried exudate that is not removed easily with gentle cleansing, first try placing a damp cotton ball or gauze on the lid margins to loosen secretions. Never apply direct pressure over the eyeball; doing so has the potential to cause injury. Remove any exudate from the eyes carefully and as often as necessary to keep the eye clean.

The eyes are well protected with eyelashes, tearing, and a split-second blink reflex and usually do not need special care. However, the unconscious patient is likely to need frequent special eye care. Secretions often collect along the margins of the lid and the inner canthus when the blink reflex is absent or when the eyes do not completely close.

Many patients wear eyeglasses. They represent a large financial investment; therefore use care when cleaning glasses and protect them from breakage or other damage when not worn.

Store eyeglasses in the case and place them in the drawer of the bedside stand when not in use to prevent accidental damage. Eyeglasses may require special cleansing solutions and drying tissues. Do not use washcloths, towels, tissue paper, or paper towels when cleaning eyeglasses.

Most patients prefer caring for their own contact lenses. A contact lens is a small, round, sometimes colored disk that fits on the cornea of the eye over the pupil. If the patient's condition does not permit self-removal of the lenses, seek assistance if necessary from someone who is familiar with the procedure (Box 9.9). The lenses need not be reinserted until the patient is more capable of caring for the lenses. Protect those patients who are unable to care for their lenses properly, because prolonged wearing of contact lenses is likely to cause damage to the cornea. A large variety of products are available for lens care.

Box 9.9 Contact Lens Removal and Care

SOFT LENSES

- Wear gloves if exudate is suspected or present.
- If possible, have patient look straight ahead. Retract lower eyelid, and expose lower edge of lens.
- With pad of index finger, slide lens off cornea to white of eye.
- Pull upper eyelid down gently with thumb of other hand, and compress lens slightly between thumb and index finger.
- Gently pinch lens, and lift out without allowing edges to stick together.
- If lens edges stick together, place lens in palm and soak thoroughly with sterile saline or contact solution.
- Place lens in storage case with contact solution.
- Follow recommended procedure for cleansing and disinfecting.

RIGID LENSES

- Wear gloves if exudate is suspected or present.
- Be sure lens is positioned directly over cornea. If it is not, have patient close eyelids. Place index and middle fingers of one hand beside the lens, and gently but firmly massage lens back over cornea.
- Place index finger on outer corner of patient's eye, and draw skin gently back toward ear.
- Ask patient to blink. Do not release pressure on lids until blink is completed.
- If lens fails to pop out, gently retract eyelid beyond edges of lens. Press lower eyelid gently against lower edge of lens.
- If patient is unable to assist, use a specially designed suction cup. Place cup on center of lens, and while applying suction, gently remove lens off patient's cornea.
- Place lens in storage case.
- Follow manufacturer's recommended procedure for cleansing and disinfecting.

Care of the Ears

The ears are cleaned during the bed bath. A clean corner of a moistened washcloth rotated gently into the ear canal works best. Also, a cotton-tipped applicator is useful for cleansing the pinna. Teach patients never to use bobby pins, toothpicks, cotton-tipped applicators, or any device to clean the internal auditory canal. These objects easily damage the tympanic membrane (eardrum) or cause **cerumen** (wax) to become impacted in the canal.

Hearing aids. Hearing loss is a common health problem. The ability to hear enables patients to communicate and react appropriately to stimuli in their environment. The care of the hearing aid involves routine cleanings, battery care, and proper insertion technique. Assess the patient's knowledge of and routines for cleaning and caring for the hearing aid. Determine whether the patient hears clearly with the use of the aid by talking slowly and clearly in a normal voice tone. Advise restricting initial use of a hearing aid to quiet situations in the home. Patients need to adjust gradually to voices and household sounds. Have the patient suggest any additional tips for care of the hearing aid. When not in use, see that the hearing aid is stored where it will not become damaged. Take care to turn off the hearing aid or remove the battery when not in use to prolong the life of the battery, depending on the type of hearing aid and battery. Some hearing aid batteries will begin draining power upon exposure to air; turning off the hearing aid for this type of battery will not prolong the battery life. Clean the outside of the hearing aid with a dry, soft cloth (Fig. 9.12 and see the Coordinated Care box on care of the hearing aid).

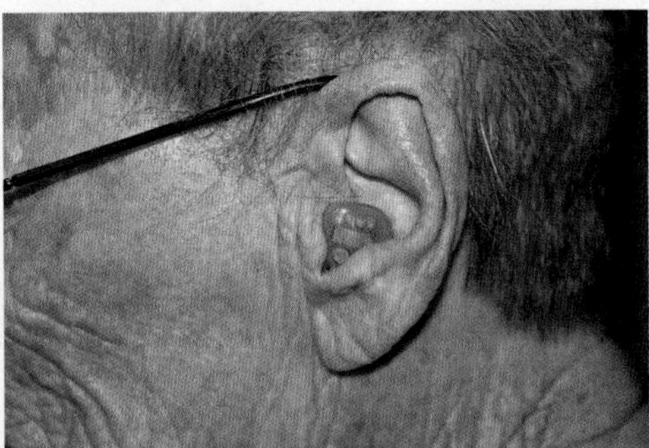

Fig. 9.12 Hearing aid. (From Elkin MK, Perry AG, Potter PA: *Nursing interventions and clinical skills*, ed 4, St. Louis, 2008, Mosby.)

 Coordinated Care

Delegation

Care of the Hearing Aid

The skill of caring for a hearing aid is appropriate to delegate to assistive personnel.

- Confirm that patient knows proper way to care for prosthetic device.
- Clarify communication tips to use for individual patient while aid is being cleaned.
- Have care provider report presence of any drainage to registered nurse (RN).
- The small size of hearing aids (see Fig. 9.11) frequently makes handling and manipulating the devices difficult for older adults. Have patients with this difficulty contact their hearing aid specialist for assistance. Family members often can assist with care of device.
- High-pitched signals associated with consonants *f, p, t, k, ch, sh,* and *st* are more difficult to hear clearly as people age.
- Inappropriate responses to questions or situations, inattentiveness, difficulty following instructions, and monopolization of conversation often are red flags for hearing loss that may require evaluation. Be sure that you and family members remain alert to this possibility, instead of incorrectly assuming that the patient is confused.
- Be alert for patient assessment findings that indicate some possible depression. Hearing loss in association with depression is common, and correction of hearing loss actually resolves depression in some patients.
- Age-related hearing loss, presbycusis, is common. Patients and their families often compensate adequately for this auditory change by speaking slowly and clearly. Not all patients with this type of hearing loss need a hearing aid.
- Avoid exposure of hearing aid to extreme heat or cold. Do not leave it in its case near stove, heater, or sunny window. Do not use with hair dryer on hot settings or with sunlamp.
- Remove hearing aid for bathing and when at hair stylist. Hair spray tends to clog hearing aid.
- Because of the typically high number of hearing aids in long-term care facilities, patients and their families need to clearly mark the hearing aid.
- Always store the hearing aid according to facility policy.
- Instruct family to buy an extra battery to keep in patient's bedside table, whenever possible.
- Instruct patients not to remove their hearing aids in common rooms of the facility (e.g., sunroom, recreation areas).

Care of the Nose

The patient is usually able to remove secretions from the nose by gently blowing into a soft tissue. This is often the only daily hygiene necessary. Teach the patient that harsh blowing causes pressure capable of injuring the tympanic membrane (eardrum), the nasal mucosa, and even sensitive eye structures. If the patient is not able to clean the nose, give assistance, using a saline solution–moistened washcloth or cotton-tipped applicator. Never insert the applicator beyond the cotton tip. If nasal secretions are excessive, suctioning sometimes is necessary. When the patient receives oxygen per nasal cannula or has a nasogastric tube, cleanse the nares every 8 hours with a cotton-tipped applicator moistened with saline solution. Because secretions are more likely to collect and dry around the tube, the tube should be cleansed with water and a mild soap.

BED MAKING

The patient's bed usually is made in the morning after the bath. When possible, make the bed while it is not occupied, when the patient is in the tub, showering, or out of the room for a diagnostic examination or procedure. When the patient is unable to be out of bed, you make an occupied bed (Skill 9.6).

Patient safety is a top priority. Comfort and privacy are also important. Remember to use side rails, to keep the call light within easy reach, and to maintain the bed in the proper position: high position while working at the bedside, and low position when work is completed, to protect the patient from accidental falls.

The nurse's responsibility is to keep the bed as clean and comfortable as possible. This is likely to require frequent inspections to ensure bedding is clean, dry, and wrinkle free. Check the linens for food particles after meals and for urine incontinence or involuntary stool. If linens are soiled with urine, feces, blood, or emesis, change them. Use waterproof pads with caution. Accumulation of moisture creates a risk for skin maceration and impairment.

Follow basic principles of medical asepsis (Box 9.10).

Use proper body mechanics while making the bed: for example, raise the bed to a working level to avoid bending down or stretching. Also, apply the principles of body mechanics while turning and repositioning the patient.

The two ways to make an unoccupied bed are open and closed. In the open bed, the top linens are fanfolded toward the foot of the bed to allow the patient to return to bed more easily. A closed bed is prepared after a patient's dismissal or transfer, or when the patient dies, before another patient is admitted. Closed beds frequently are made in long-term care settings because many patients do not return to bed until night time. Housekeeping personnel clean the mattress and bed and apply fresh linens (see Skill 9.6).

The postoperative bed is a form of the open bed. The top sheet and the spread are not mitered or tucked in at the corners. The top linens usually are fanfolded lengthwise or crosswise at the foot of the patient's bed. Arrange the top bed linens in such a way that they allow easy transfer of the surgical patient from the gurney to the bed. A complete linen change is done if the patient is returning from surgery (Fig. 9.13).

Skill 9.6 Bed Making

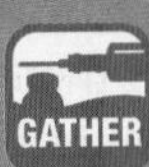

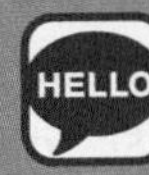

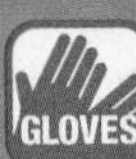

NURSING ACTION *(RATIONALE)*

1. Refer to medical record, care plan, or Kardex to determine potential for orders or specific precautions for mobility and positioning. *(Provides basis for care.)*
2. Assemble supplies. *(Organizes procedure.)*
   - Bedside chair or table
   - Blanket
   - Bottom sheet—many facilities use the contour or fitted sheet
   - Disposable gloves (optional)
   - Laundry bag
   - Linen draw sheet
   - Mattress pad (optional)
   - Pillowcase(s)
   - Protective draw sheet (optional)
   - Spread
   - Top sheet, flat
   - Waterproof cloth or disposable underpad, or bath blanket, or both (2)
3. Introduce self. *(Reduces patient's anxiety.)*
4. Identify patient. *(Ensures procedure is performed with correct patient.)*
5. Explain procedure. *(Enlists cooperation and reduces patient's anxiety.)*
6. Perform hand hygiene and don gloves according to agency policy and guidelines from the CDC and OSHA. *(Reduces spread of microorganisms.)*
7. Prepare patient. *(Readies patient for procedure.)*
   a. Close door or pull privacy curtain. *(Provides privacy.)*
   b. Raise bed to appropriate height and lower side rail on the side closest to you. *(Promotes proper body mechanics.)*
   c. Lower head of bed (HOB) if patient tolerates it. *(Patient with a respiratory disorder frequently is not be able to tolerate lying flat. The use of contour sheets makes it easier to make hospital beds with the HOB elevated.)*
   d. Assess patient's tolerance of procedure. Be alert for signs of discomfort and fatigue. *(Use judgment in providing the opportunity for rest and comfort measures.)*
8. Occupied bed.
   a. Remove spread and blanket separately and, if soiled, place in laundry bag. If linens will be reused, fold neatly and place over back of chair. (Keep linens away from uniform.) Do not fan or shake linens. *(Reduces spread of microorganisms.)*
   b. Place bath blanket over patient on top of sheet.
   c. Request patient to hold on to bath blanket while you remove top sheet by drawing sheet out from under bath blanket at foot of bed. If patient is unable to assist, hold bath blanket in place while removing sheet. *(Prevents unnecessary exposure of patient.)*
   d. Place soiled sheet in laundry bag. *(Reduces spread of microorganisms.)*
   e. With assistance from coworker, slide mattress to top of bed. *(If mattress has shifted to foot of bed, it is difficult to tuck in linens.)*
   f. Position patient to far side of bed with the back toward you. Assure patient that he or she will not fall out of bed. Adjust pillow for comfort. Be sure side rail is up. *(Provides for patient's safety.)*
   g. Beginning at head and moving toward foot, loosen bottom linens. Fanfold linen draw sheet, protective draw sheet, and bottom sheet, tucking edges of linens under patient. *(Provides maximal work space.)*
   h. Apply clean linens to bed by first placing mattress pad (if used). Fold lengthwise, ensuring crease is in center of bed. Likewise, unfold bottom sheet and place over mattress pad. Place hem of bottom sheet (if flat sheet is used) with rough edge down and just even with bottom edge of mattress (see illustration of Step 9g). *(Keeps energy and time you need for bed making to a minimum. Rough edge of hem away from patient prevents skin impairment to patient's heels.)*
   i. Miter corners (if flat sheet) at head of bed. Continue to tuck in sheet along side toward front, keeping linens smooth. *(Prevents linens from becoming easily loosened.)*

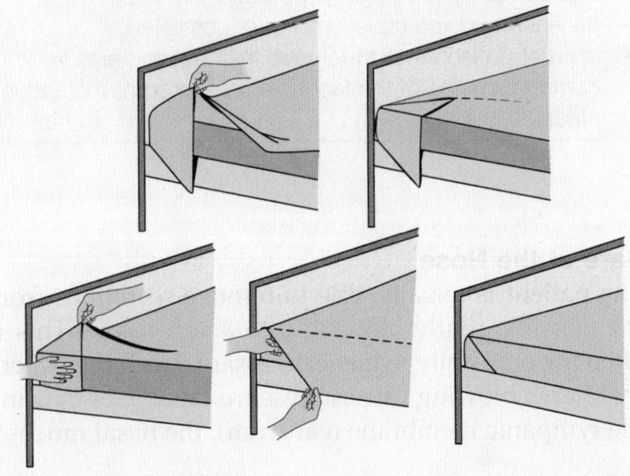

Skill 9.6 Bed Making—cont'd

j. Reach under patient to pull out protective draw sheet (if used), and smooth out over clean bottom sheet. Tuck in. Unfold linen draw sheet and place center fold along middle of bed, smooth out over protective draw sheet, and tuck in. Tuck in folded linens in center of bed so they are under patient's buttocks and torso.

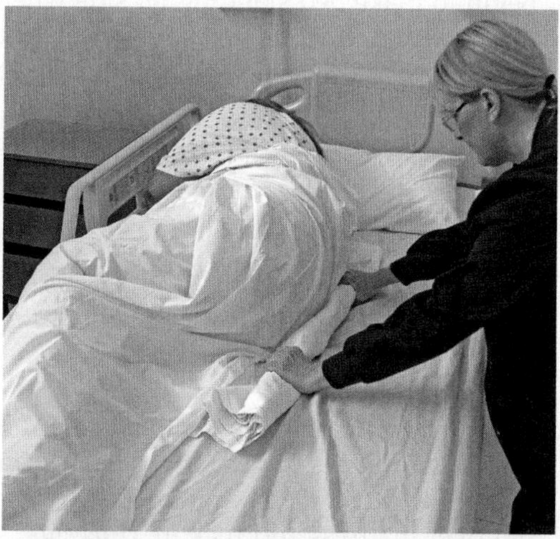

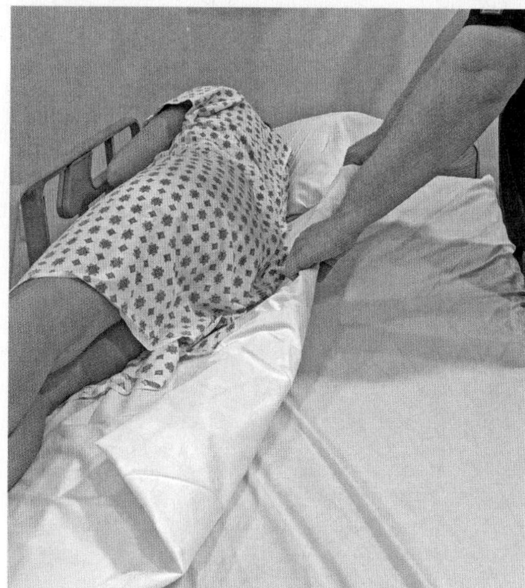

k. Keep palms down as linens are tucked under mattress. *(Provides for patient's comfort.)*

l. Raise side rail and assist patient to roll slowly toward you over folds of linen. Go to opposite side of bed and lower side rail. *(Maintains patient's safety.)*

m. Loosen edges of all soiled linens. Remove by folding into a bundle, and place in laundry bag. *(Reduces spread of microorganisms.)*

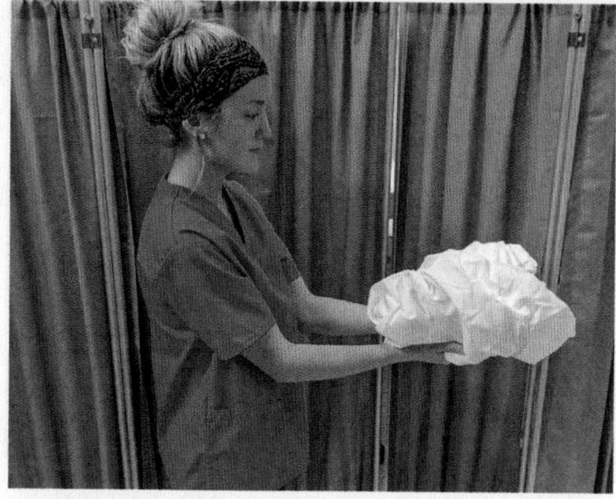

n. Spread clean linens, including protective draw sheet, out over mattress and smooth out wrinkles. Assist patient to supine position and position pillow for comfort. *(Maintains patient's comfort.)*

o. Miter top corner of bottom sheet, pulling sheet taut. Tuck bottom sheet under mattress all the way to foot of bed. *(Maintains smooth linens. Avoid lifting mattress too far. Ensures tight fit.)*

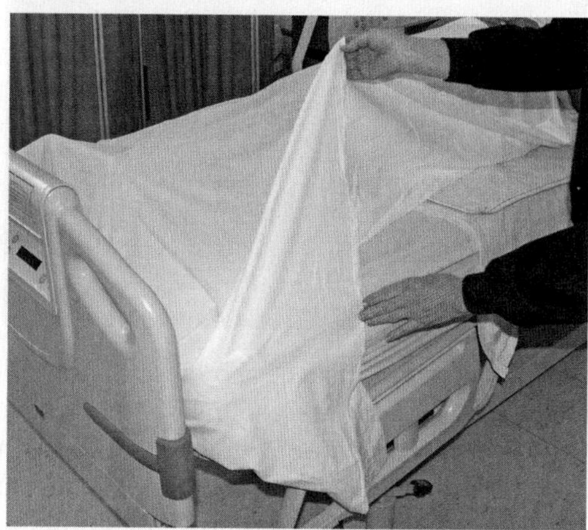

p. Smooth out draw sheets. Pulling sheet taut, tuck in protective draw sheet and then tuck in linen draw sheet, first in center, then top, and bottom last. *(Ensures tight fit.)*

q. Place top sheet over bath blanket that is over patient. Request patient to hold top sheet while you remove bath blanket. Place blanket in laundry bag. (Be sure center fold of sheet is in center of bed.) If blanket is used, place over sheet and place spread over blanket. Form cuff with top linens under patient's chin. *(Provides for patient's comfort and warmth.)*

Continued

Skill 9.6 Bed Making—cont'd

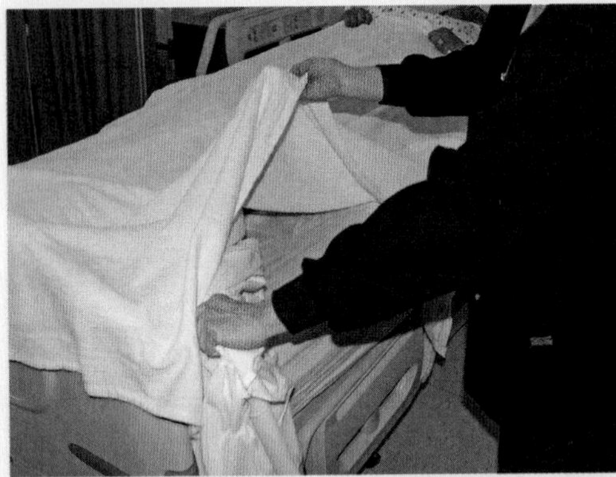

r. Tuck in all linens at foot of bed, making modified miter corner (see illustration). Raise side rail and make opposite side of bed. Remember to allow for toe pleat. Make toe pleat by placing fold either lengthwise down center of bed or across foot of bed. *(Prevents unnecessary pressure on patient's feet, possibly causing foot drop.)*

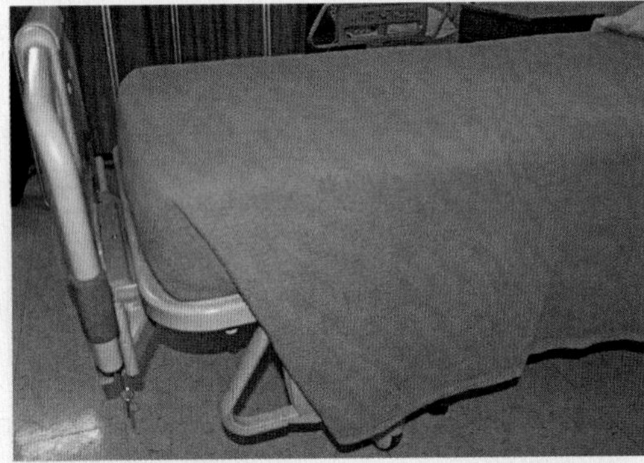

s. Change pillowcase. Grasp closed end of pillowcase, turning case inside out over hand. Now grasp one end of pillow with your hand in the case and smooth out wrinkles, ensuring pillow corners fit into pillowcase corners. *(Never place pillow on top of patient while changing its cover.)* As pillow is removed from under patient, support neck muscles. *(Prevents injury.)* Never hold pillow under your chin. *(Reduces spread of microorganisms.)*

9. Unoccupied bed

a. Starting at head of bed, loosen linens all the way to foot. Go to opposite side of bed, loosen linens, roll all linens up in ball (see illustration of Step 8m), and place in soiled laundry bag. Do not permit linens to come in contact with uniform. Do not shake or fan linens. Wash hands after handling soiled linens. Perform hand hygiene. *(Reduces spread of microorganisms.)*

b. If blanket and spread are to be reused, fold neatly and place over back of chair. Remove soiled pillowcase.

c. Slide mattress to head of bed. *(It is easier to tuck in linens.)*

d. If necessary, clean mattress with cloth moistened with antiseptic solution, and dry thoroughly. *(Reduces spread of microorganisms.)*

e. Begin to make bed standing on side where lines are placed. Unfold bottom sheet, placing fold lengthwise down center of bed. Be certain rough edge of hem lies down away from patient's heels and even with edge of mattress. Smooth out sheet over top edge of mattress and miter corners (see Step 8i). Tuck remaining sheet under mattress all the way to foot. Keep linens smooth. *(Time is saved if one side of bed is made at a time. Fanfolding all linen lengthwise down bed promotes neatness and prevents wrinkling.)*

f. Place draw sheet on bed so that center fold lies down middle of bed. If protective draw sheet is to be used, place it on first. Smooth out over mattress and tuck in. *(Prevents loosening and wrinkling.)* Keep palms down. *(Prevents stones in wedding rings from catching in bed springs.)*

g. Place top sheet over bed and smooth out. Place blanket over top sheet. Smooth out. Place spread over blanket and smooth out. Make cuff with top linens. *(Provides for patient's comfort.)*

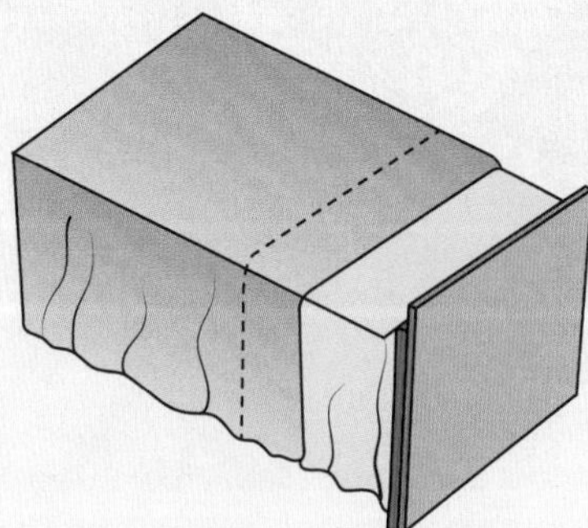

h. Allow for toe pleat. Make modified mitered corner by not tucking tip of sheet under mattress. *(Provides for patient comfort.)*

i. Move to opposite side of bed and complete making bed as described in Steps 9e to 9h. *(Saves your time and energy.)* Pull linens tight and keep taut as linens are tucked in.

j. Put on clean pillowcase (see Step 8s). Place pillow at head of bed and position for comfort. Place call light within easy reach and lower bed level. *(Promotes patient's safety.)*

Skill 9.6 Bed Making—cont'd

k. If patient is to return to bed, fanfold top linens down to foot of bed. Be sure cuff at top of linens is easily accessible to patient. *(It is easier for patient to return to bed.)*

10. Arrange personal items on bed table or bedside stand and place within patient's easy reach. *(Promotes patient's safety.)*
11. Leave area neat and clean. *(Promotes patient's sense of well-being.)*
12. Place all soiled linens in proper receptacle. Perform hand hygiene. *(Reduces spread of microorganisms.)*
13. Assist patient to bed, and position for comfort. *(Promotes patient's safety and comfort.)*
14. Documentation.
    - Bed making does not have to be recorded in most facilities.
    - Record patient's vital signs, signs, and symptoms only if changes occur.
15. Report any abnormal findings to nurse in charge or physician.

Box 9.10 Principles of Medical Asepsis for Bed Making

- Keep soiled linens away from uniform.
- Place soiled linens in hamper or plastic bag.
- Never fan linens in the air. *(This causes air currents, which spread microorganisms.)*
- Never place soiled linens on the floor. If clean linens touch the floor, place in laundry hamper immediately.
- Remove all unnecessary equipment and maintain a neat work area.

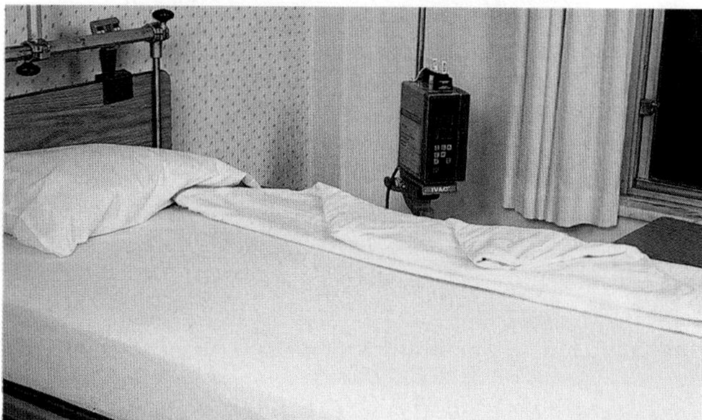

Fig. 9.13 The postoperative bed. (From Potter PA, Perry AG, Stockert WR, et al: *Fundamentals of nursing: Concepts, process, and practice*, ed 9, St. Louis, 2016, Elsevier.)

ASSISTING THE PATIENT WITH ELIMINATION

A patient who is unable to get up to the bathroom or bedside commode for the purpose of *urination* (the act of emptying the urinary bladder) or of *defecation* (the act of eliminating feces) uses a **bedpan** (device for receiving feces or urine from either male or female patients confined to bed) or **urinal** (a device for collecting urine from male patients; urinals for female patients are also available). Use of a bedpan or urinal is a private and personal procedure. Be sure to afford patients as much privacy as their condition allows.

Offer the bedpan or urinal frequently because patients risk accidentally soiling bedclothes if their elimination needs are not met. Patients often procrastinate using a bedpan because it is uncomfortable and embarrassing. Patients sometimes try to get to the bathroom unassisted even if their condition prohibits ambulation. Remind patients of the possibility of accidents or falls (Box 9.11).

Report and record in the nursing notes any abnormalities in urine or stool (Box 9.12). Flow sheets usually are provided for documentation of normal voiding and stools.

Bedpans are made of plastic. Of the two types of bedpans, one type has a high back, and the second type is flat and smaller and is called a fracture pan (Fig. 9.14A).

A urinal is made of plastic; there are two types of urinals. One type serves the male patient for voiding (see Fig. 9.14B). The other type is called a *female urinal,* which has an adapter that accommodates the female anatomy. If the male patient is unable to place the urinal for himself, assist him.

1. Request that the patient abduct his legs a slight distance.
2. Holding the urinal by the handle and directing the urinal at an angle, place the urinal between the patient's legs, making certain the long flat side, which is opposite the handle of the urinal, is resting on the bed.
3. Gently raising the penis, place it fully within the urinal.

Empty the bedpan and the urinal immediately after use, and cleanse and store it properly. If the patient's intake and output are being monitored, measure urine and record result. Estimate liquid stool on the appropriate form according to the agency's policy. See Skill 9.7 for positioning the bedpan.

Box 9.11 Assisting the Patient With Elimination

- Allow the patient enough time for elimination. Ignoring the urge to defecate or urinate or not taking time to eliminate completely is a common cause of constipation or urine retention.
- Be prompt when called to assist the patient to the bathroom or onto the bedpan or bedside commode.
- When the patient shares a room with another patient, be certain to curtain off the patient's area. This enables the patient to relax, knowing that interruptions will not occur.
- Close the bathroom door. If it is necessary to remain nearby, stand outside door or curtain.
- For those patients unable to assume the normal squatting position, stool risers can be used, which call for less effort to sit or stand.

Box 9.12 Characteristics of Normal Urine and Normal Stool

NORMAL URINE
- Has a characteristic odor: faintly aromatic
- Is transparent at the time of voiding
- Ranges from a pale to straw color
- Yields negative results when tested for protein, glucose, ketone bodies, red blood cells, white blood cells, and bacteria

NORMAL STOOL
- Brown
- Contains undigested food, dead bacteria, fat, bile pigment, living cells, intestinal mucosa, and water
- Frequency ranges from once a day to two or three times a week
- Has soft, formed consistency
- Odor is affected by food types
- Resembles the shape of the rectum

Another option for elimination, instead of the bedpan or the urinal, is the bedside commode (Fig. 9.15). It is useful at night and for the patient who is not able to ambulate as far as the bathroom easily.

Care of the Incontinent Patient

Incontinence is a very common problem, especially among older adults and adults who are debilitated. Regardless of the cause, incontinence is psychologically distressing and socially disruptive.

Urinary incontinence occurs because pressure in the bladder is too great, because the sphincters are weak, or because neurologic function has been compromised

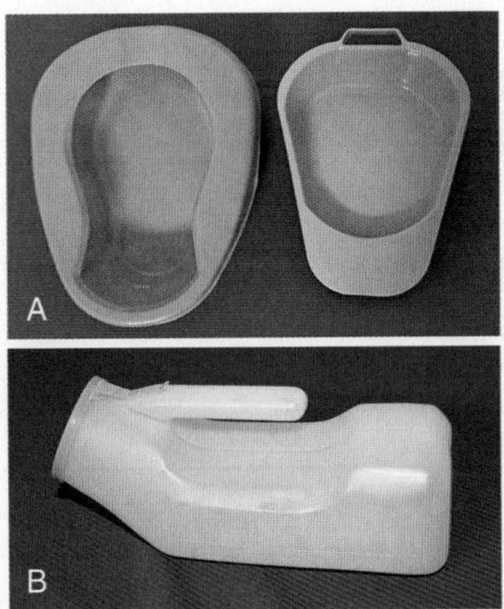

Fig. 9.14 Selected equipment and supplies for elimination. A, Regular bedpan *(left)* and fracture pan *(right)*. B, Male urinal.

Skill 9.7 Positioning the Bedpan

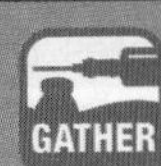

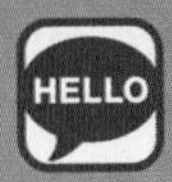

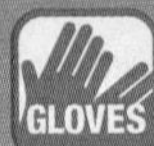

NURSING ACTION *(RATIONALE)*

1. Refer to medical record, care plan, or Kardex. *(Provides basis for care.)*
2. Assess patient's needs. *(Allows nurse to note any potential problems with patient's environment.)*
3. Assemble supplies according to patient's needs (see Fig. 9.10). *(Organizes procedure.)*
4. Introduce self. *(Reduces patient's anxiety.)*
5. Identify patient. *(Ensures procedure is performed with correct patient.)*
6. Explain procedure. *(Enlists cooperation and reduces patient's anxiety.)*
7. Prepare patient. *(Facilitates procedure.)*
    a. Close door or pull privacy curtain. *(Elimination is a personal function and is greatly facilitated by providing privacy.)*
    b. Arrange supplies close to the bedside. *(Provides easy access to supplies.)*
    c. Place protective pad under patient's buttocks, if necessary. *(Protects linens from soiling.)*
8. Perform hand hygiene and don clean gloves according to agency policy and guidelines from the CDC and OSHA. *(Reduces spread of microorganisms.)*
9. When patient is able to assist self onto bedpan, nurse positions patient in supine position with knees flexed and bottom of feet flat on bed

Skill 9.7 Positioning the Bedpan—cont'd

surface. As patient raises hips, nurse supports patient's lower back with arm and positions bedpan under patient. When patient has finished with elimination, nurse removes bedpan in same manner. *(Allows for some measure of independence.)*

10. For patient unable to assist self on bedpan.

a. Turn patient away from nurse toward opposite side rail, moving linens out of way. *(Provides for patient safety and maintains clean linens.)*

b. Fit bedpan to patient's buttocks. *(Prevents injury to patient's skin.)*

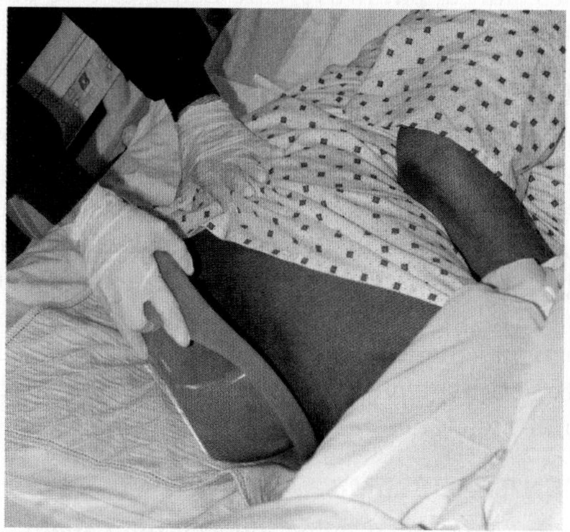

c. Assist patient to turn over onto bedpan while nurse secures bedpan. *(Allows nurse to use appropriate body mechanics.)*

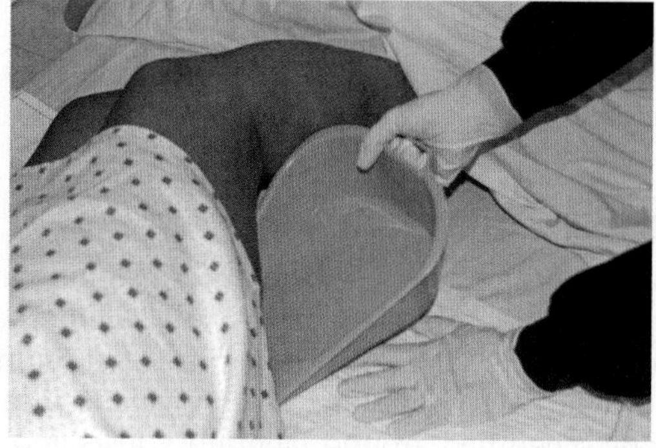

d. Raise head of bed 30 degrees. *(Promotes patient's comfort.)*

e. Place toilet tissue and call light within easy reach. *(Provides for patient's convenience and promotes certain measure of independence.)*

11. For those patients who can be out of bed but are unable to ambulate far, the bedside commode can be used (see Fig. 9.14). Some are equipped with wheels, which allow the patient to be moved to the bathroom. *(Provides privacy.)*

12. When transferring a patient to the commode, assist the patient in the same manner as if assisting to a chair. *(Maintains proper body mechanics.)*

13. Provide a means for the patient to wash hands; either assisting to the sink or providing hand washing while patient is in the bed.

14. Document according to agency policy: *(Verifies patient's care.)*

- Amount
- Color
- Consistency
- Abnormal findings such as blood, unusual odor, or color

15. Report unusual findings. *(Further interventions may be necessary.)*

as a result of illness or injury. Collaborate with other members of the health care team to assess the cause and the extent of incontinence and to assist in managing the problem. The physical therapist, for example, is prepared to assess the extent of musculoskeletal involvement and determine methods of treatment.

Incontinence sometimes involves a small leakage of urine that occurs when a person laughs, coughs, or lifts something heavy. This type of incontinence is referred to as stress incontinence. Teach the patient exercises to strengthen muscles around the external sphincters to help manage this type of incontinence. Pelvic floor

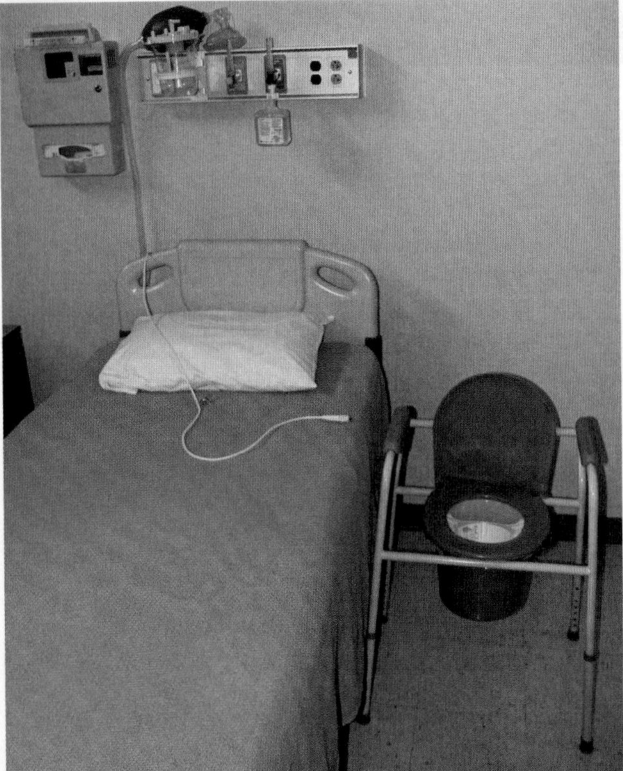

Fig. 9.15 The bedside commode has a toilet seat with a container underneath. The container slides out from under the toilet seat for emptying and cleaning.

exercises (Kegel exercises) involve tightening the ring of muscle around the vagina and anus and holding the muscle contraction for several seconds. Have the patient do this a minimum of 10 times, 3 times a day.

Alert patients need an incontinence product that is discreet and promotes self-care. Some incontinence products are designed for small amounts of leakage. Persistent urge, stress, or overflow incontinence most likely necessitates referral for urologic evaluation (refer to Chapter 15 for types of incontinence).

Incontinence characterized by urine or fecal flow at unpredictable times necessitates the use of disposable adult undergarments or underpads as the primary means of management. Urine and feces are very irritating to the skin. Skin that is continually exposed quickly becomes inflamed and irritated. Cleanse the skin thoroughly after each episode of incontinence with warm, soapy water and dry it thoroughly to help prevent skin impairment. Many facilities use a protective barrier cream for patients with incontinence to prevent skin breakdown.

When urinary incontinence results from decreased perception of bladder fullness or impaired voluntary motor control, bladder training may be helpful. Bladder training consists of assisting the patient to the bathroom or commode at certain time intervals in an attempt to strengthen the urinary sphincter muscles, typically every 2 hours initially for the first several times, then at increased time intervals as the patient tolerates until the point of bladder control is reached.

❖ NURSING PROCESS FOR HYGIENE

The role of the LPN/LVN in the nursing process as stated is that the LPN/LVN:

- Participates in planning care for patients based on patient needs
- Reviews patient's plan of care and recommends revisions as needed
- Reviews and follows defined prioritization for patient care
- Uses clinical pathways, care maps, or care plans to guide and review patient care

◆ ASSESSMENT

Nursing assessment is an ongoing process. It is important to determine whether the patient can perform hygienic care independently or whether assistance is required. Also, observe the patient's physical condition and the integrity of the patient's skin, oral cavity, and sensory organs. Explore any developmental factors that influence the patient's hygiene needs. Note the patient's self-care ability and hygiene practices. Determine the patient's cultural preferences as well.

◆ PATIENT PROBLEMS

Nursing assessment helps identify the patient's need for and ability to maintain personal hygiene. Interventions are based on the identified patient problem. Patient problem statements possibly include the following:

- *Compromised Oral Mucous Membranes*
- *Compromised Physical Mobility*
- *Compromised Skin Integrity* (Nursing Care Plan 9.1)
- *Inability to Bathe Self*
- *Inability to Dress Self*

◆ EXPECTED OUTCOMES AND PLANNING

Considering the patient's preferences before planning is important. The hygiene measures that the patient desires or requires determine the supplies and equipment that are necessary. In some cases, hygiene measures must be scheduled around laboratory tests and diagnostic procedures and involve the family in planning and adapting approaches for home care, and in hygiene instruction. Be aware of community resources that will be of assistance to meet the patient's needs.

Nursing interventions are focused on specific goals and outcomes that pertain to the identified patient problems, such as the following:

Goal: Patient's skin integrity remains intact during stay in facility.

Outcome: Patient's skin remains pink and warm and with good turgor and no open areas noted.

Goal: Patient assists with hygienic measures by washing face, neck, and hands.

Nursing Care Plan 9.1 Skin Care

Mr. P. is a 48-year-old patient immobilized because of trauma to the spinal cord. He has periods of diaphoresis. He has had liquid diarrhea for the past 48 hours. The skin on Mr. P.'s back, sacral regions, and buttocks is dry and intact, with a 2-cm area of erythema around the sacrum.

PATIENT PROBLEM

Compromised Skin Integrity, related to immobilization and secretions

Patient Goals and Expected Outcomes	Nursing Interventions	Evaluation
Skin will remain intact during hospitalization Skin will remain free of pressure Skin will have reduced or absent secretions Skin will be dry, warm, and smooth	Provide perineal care after each diarrheal episode. Change linen after diaphoresis or diarrheal episode. Apply lotion to areas that easily become dried and chapped. Monitor length of time any areas of erythema persist. Determine turning interval (e.g., 2 h). Place oscillating air mattress on patient's bed. Do not massage erythemic (reddened) area or bony prominences. Reassess skin area daily. Assess for history of preexisting chronic diseases (diabetes, malignancy, acquired immunodeficiency syndrome [AIDS], peripheral or cardiovascular conditions). Assess surface that patient spends majority of time on (mattress for bedridden patient, cushion for wheelchairs). Specifically assess skin over bony prominences (sacrum, scapulae, ears, elbows, heels, inner and outer malleoli, inner and outer knees, back of head, ischial tuberosities, trochanteric areas of the hips, and heels).	Observe and time the duration of erythemic area after each position change; palpate underlying and adjacent tissues after each position change.

CRITICAL THINKING QUESTIONS

1. Mr. P. has a poor appetite, and his chemistry profile reveals low protein, low albumin, and low anion gap (A/G) ratio. Explain why poor nutrition predisposes to impairment of skin integrity and poor tissue healing.
2. With Mr. P.'s history of diarrhea, explain the possible complication that could evolve if the dry intact skin develops an open lesion.

Outcome: Patient was able to wash face, neck, and hands without difficulty.

◆ IMPLEMENTATION

Nursing interventions that promote the patient's personal hygiene include bed making, bathing, and care of hair, eyes, ears, nose, nails, and skin.

Hygiene is a basic part of a patient's care. Learn and use care practices that help alleviate the patient's anxiety and promote comfort and relaxation while performing each hygiene measure. For example, while giving a patient a bath and changing a gown, use a gentle approach in turning and repositioning. Use of a soft, gentle voice while conversing with the patient helps relieve any fears or concerns. Inform the patient of all care being performed. For patients experiencing symptoms such as pain or nausea, administering symptom relief before hygiene procedures better prepares the patient.

The nurse is in a unique position to assess the patient's readiness to learn and to teach health promotion practices whenever possible (see the Patient Teaching and Home Care Considerations boxes). This includes educating patients on proper hygiene techniques and connecting patients with the community resources necessary to enable them to perform hygienic care in the home setting when assistance is required. The nurse should always encourage the patient's independence and privacy and foster the patient's physical well-being.

◆ EVALUATION

Assess the success of the nursing interventions on completion of the hygienic measures. Reassess the condition of the patient's skin, nails, oral cavity, and sensory organs. Determine whether the patient's comfort level has improved. Ask the patient to demonstrate hygiene self-care skills, and ask the patient whether expectations are being met.

Always be prepared to revise the care plan based on the evaluation. Systematic evaluation requires you to determine whether expected outcomes have been met. Refer to the identified goals and outcomes when planning interventions.

Goal: Patient's skin integrity remains intact during stay in facility.

Evaluative measure: Assess for pink skin that is warm, moist, without abrasions, and with immediate color return on blanching.

Goal: Patient assists with hygienic measures by washing face, neck, and hands.

Evaluative measure: Evaluate patient's ability to assist with hygienic measures.

Patient Teaching

Hygiene

GENERAL PRINCIPLES

- Initiate patient teaching at the beginning of the hygienic procedure and continue throughout the intervention.
- Teach and encourage independence no matter how minimal it seems to be (e.g., washing the face and perineal area, brushing teeth, combing hair).
- Explain steps of procedure in which patient will be participating.

TEACHING POINTS

Teaching points include the following:

- How to assess temperature of the bath water, especially for elderly and other patients with reduced sensation (e.g., bath thermometer).
- How to inspect surfaces between skin folds for signs of irritation or impairment (breakdown; e.g., erythema, scalding).
- Proper cleansing of the perineum (e.g., female patients: cleansing from front to back; uncircumcised males: retracting foreskin to adequately cleanse underneath, then replacing foreskin).
- How to use a trapeze bar on beds to assist in bed mobility.
- Importance of washing hands before and after performing catheter care or after urinating and defecating.
- If patient achieves relaxation from back rub, teaching family members how to perform procedure.
- Stressing importance of consistent use of sunscreen with a protective factor of at least 15 and avoidance of unnecessary sun exposure.
- Methods to prevent tooth decay (e.g., reduce intake of carbohydrates between meals [sweet snacks], brush within 30 minutes of eating sweets, rinse mouth thoroughly with water or eat acid-containing fruit such as an apple, use fluoridated water).
- How to prevent or heal dry lips by applying lip ointment or lubricant and avoiding licking the lips.
- Proper storage methods for dentures, stressing techniques of cleaning that avoid damage to dentures (e.g., use brush with soft bristles; carry dentures in a container; hold dentures with cloth to avoid dropping).
- How to remove dentures at bedtime to give gums a rest and to store dentures in water or cleansing solution to prevent drying and warping.
- Signs and symptoms of oral infection or irritation (e.g., erythematous or whitened areas, bleeding, lesions).
- Advise patient to brush teeth at least two times daily and to rinse well after brushing.
- Advise patients with diabetes to visit their dentist every 3 to 4 months and to handle tissues gently. *(Diabetes depresses the immune system and decreases circulation to the mucosa.)*
- Proper hair care: regular shampooing, avoidance of chemicals and hot combs for straightening hair. *(May result in scalp burns, hair loss, or allergic reaction.)*
- Primary caregiver safety precautions for shaving, especially if patient is receiving anticoagulant therapy, and the technique to follow in the event a patient is nicked accidentally.
- Proper foot care:
  - Wash and soak feet daily with lukewarm water; thoroughly pat feet dry and dry well between toes. Soaking the feet of a patient with diabetes or a patient with peripheral vascular disease is not recommended. This potentially leads to maceration (excessive softening of the skin), skin breakdown, and infection.
  - File nails; never clip them if patient is diabetic or has circulatory issues.
  - Caution against self-treating corns or calluses. Consult a physician or podiatrist.
  - If needed, apply a mild foot powder.
  - Inspect feet daily.
  - Wear clean socks or stockings daily (change twice a day if feet perspire).
  - Do not walk barefoot.
  - Wear properly fitting shoes.
  - Wash and dry minor cuts immediately. Use only mild antiseptic (e.g., triple antibiotic ointment).
- Cleansing the eye by going from the inner corner or canthus to the outer corner or canthus.
- Never inserting hairpins, toothpicks, cotton-tipped applicators, or any device into the ear canal. If necessary, consult a physician.
- Skin care:
  - Process of wound healing and expected wound appearance.
  - Signs and symptoms of pressure ulcers to report to health care team.
  - Prevention guidelines to halt further breakdown.
  - Importance of good nutrition and adequate fluid intake.

Home Care Considerations

Hygienic Care

BATHING

- Include family members in discussion about patient's hygienic care, before discharge if possible.
- Set up equipment according to established routine.
- Advise installing grab bars around tub, carpeting bathroom floor, and using a portable shower seat for safety.
- The three types of baths for the home-bound patient are the complete bed bath; the abbreviated bed bath, during which only the parts of the patient's body are washed whose neglect will potentially cause illness, odor, or discomfort; and the partial bath, which takes place at the sink, in the tub, or in the shower with a shower chair.

 Home Care Considerations—cont'd

Hygienic Care

- The kind of bath chosen depends on assessment of the home, availability of running water, and condition of the bathing facilities.
- If beds do not have side rails, positioning is possible with pillows or by placing bed against the wall.
- Never leave bathing patient unattended. Adhesive strips on bottom of tub or shower, handrails, chairs, or stools in tub or shower further protect patient.
- Follow patient's usual bathing and skin care routines.
- Assess patient to see whether a home health aide or other assistance is needed after discharge.

SKIN CARE

- Assess perineum at every visit because of risk for infection and skin breakdown.
- Protect patient from falling off bed during back rub.
- The 30-degree lateral position or the prone position is sometimes useful at night to prolong the time needed between position changes, resulting in less sleep disruption for the patient and the caregiver.
- Identify community resources such as neighbors and relatives for assistance should patient need help with position changes.
- Customize pressure-relief maneuvers for the independent patient. Some individuals find it useful to use a watch with timer, mark even or odd hours, and use television commercials as guidelines to remember when to complete pressure-relief techniques.
- Identify clean storage area for dressing supplies.
- Determine availability of required supplies.
- Discuss need for home pressure-relief surface or bed.
- Identify adaptive equipment needed to care for patient at home, such as stool risers.

ORAL CARE

- Assess state of dental health of patient and family members and attitudes toward oral hygiene.
- Family members need instruction in oral care so that family understands how to protect the patient from aspirating while ensuring thorough cleansing of the oral cavity.
- Irrigate oral cavity with a bulb syringe; if unavailable, a clean gravy baster is acceptable to use as a substitute. A large syringe is another possibility.
- Cleanse mouth at least twice a day. If patient breathes through mouth, use a sponge-tipped applicator or wrap gauze or soft linen around a tongue blade, moisten, and use every 1 to 2 hours to keep mouth moist and fresh.
- On regular visits, assess for signs and symptoms of infection or irritation, including erythematous, bleeding lesions of the gums.
- Provide special care to patients undergoing head and neck radiation because the gums are usually dry and edematous and are likely to interfere with proper denture fit.

HAIR CARE

- Assess temperature of the room, availability of water, and the most satisfactory position of the patient for the procedure.
- Provide extra protection from wetness for patients with casts.
- Obtain dry shampoo preparations or a shampoo cap when a wet shampoo is contraindicated.
- Construct a trough by arranging a plastic shower curtain or tablecloth under the patient's head and then tapering the cloth to form a narrow end that can drain into a container or basin next to the patient's bed.
- In the home setting, you need to find ways the patient can shampoo the hair without causing injury. Some patients with a long leg cast need to wash the hair at a sink until it is safe to shower or until the cast is removed and resumption of tub baths is permitted.
- Caution patients about use of chemicals and hot combs for straightening hair. Such practices often cause considerable damage to the hair. Misuse results in possible scalp burns, hair loss, and allergic reactions that cause severe skin rashes, urticaria, and conjunctivitis.

SHAVING AND FACIAL HAIR REMOVAL

- Provide enough towels around the patient's neck to help prevent spilling shaving cream or water on chest or bed.
- Provide adequate lighting for the procedure.
- Perform the procedure in a comfortable setting, such as the bathroom or bedroom.
- Usually the facial hair of the older patient does not grow quickly, so a shave may not be necessary every day.
- If patient is on anticoagulant therapy, use an electric razor.
- Facial hair for females should be addressed according to the patient's preference. Methods of facial hair removal include clipping, tweezing, shaving, hair removal lotions, and use of a depilatory.

NAILS AND FEET

- Alternative therapies: moleskin applied to areas on feet that are under friction is less likely to cause local pressure than corn pads; spot adhesive bandages guard corns against friction but do not have padding to protect against pressure; wrapping small pieces of lamb's wool around toes reduces irritation of soft corns between toes.
- Assess use of patient's bathroom sink for soaking patient's hands and tub for soaking patient's feet.
- Financial constraints are often why patients wear poorly fitted shoes, which can cause foot problems.

BED MAKING

- Assess primary caregiver's ability and willingness to maintain a clean environment for the patient.
- Assess home laundry facilities to plan with the primary caregiver the most reasonable frequency with which linens will be laundered.
- Assess amount of linens in the home to establish with the primary caregiver the number of changes of sheets that it is possible to reserve for the patient's use.

Get Ready for the NCLEX® Examination!

Key Points

- Hygiene is a personal matter; all factors that influence the personal hygiene routine must be considered.
- Be sure the patient's room is comfortable, safe, and large enough to allow the patient and visitors to move around freely.
- Assume the responsibility for providing the daily hygienic needs of patients if they are unable to care for themselves adequately.
- Providing hygienic care gives you the opportunity to assess all external body surfaces and the patient's emotional state.
- Assisting or providing the patient with daily hygienic needs allows you to use teaching and communication skills to develop a meaningful relationship with the patient.
- Consider the patient's personal preferences as you plan the daily hygienic care.
- Be sure to maintain the patient's privacy and comfort when providing daily care.
- Various sociocultural, economic, and developmental factors influence patients' hygiene practices.
- During assessment of the skin, observe the characteristics most influenced by hygienic measures.
- Patients who are immobilized, who are poorly nourished, and who have reduced sensation are at risk for impaired skin integrity.
- External pressure, shearing force, moisture, impaired peripheral circulation, edema, and obesity contribute to the development of pressure injuries.
- When the external pressure against the skin is greater than the pressure in the capillary bed, blood flow decreases to the adjacent tissues.
- Pressure injuries tend to occur initially in the superficial layers of the skin.
- Meticulous assessment of the skin and underlying tissue and identification of risk factors are important in preventing the circumstances favorable to development of pressure injuries.
- Preventive skin care is aimed at controlling external pressure on bony prominences and keeping the skin clean, well lubricated, hydrated, and free of excess moisture.
- Proper positioning reduces the effects of pressure and guards against shearing force.
- Cleansing and topical agents used to treat pressure injuries vary according to the stage of the ulcer.
- When applying heat or cold therapy, properly assess the patient's ability to sense variation in temperatures, know factors that place the patient at risk for complications, and understand the physiologic effects of the applications to use the therapies safely.
- Patient teaching is important in assisting the patient to take responsibility for his or her own care.
- Wear gloves during hygienic care when there is risk of contacting body fluids.
- Techniques used during tepid sponging are designed to minimize the risk of a patient becoming chilled.
- Patients with diabetes mellitus need special consideration when you provide nail and foot care.
- When administering oral care to unconscious patients, take measures to prevent aspiration.
- The evaluation of hygienic care is based on the patient's expression of a sense of relaxation and well-being and an understanding of personal hygienic techniques.

Additional Learning Resources

SG Go to your Study Guide for additional learning activities to help you master this chapter content.

evolve Be sure to visit the Evolve site at *http://evolve.elsevier.com/Cooper/foundationsadult/* for additional online resources.

Review Questions for the NCLEX® Examination

1. The nurse is supervising a new UAP providing hygiene care to a patient. Which action by the UAP requires the nurse to provide additional instruction regarding hygiene care? *(Select all that apply.)*
   1. The UAP performs hand hygiene before providing care.
   2. The UAP holds the clean linens against the uniform.
   3. The UAP places soiled linens on the floor.
   4. The UAP places clean linens on the patient's clean overbed table.
   5. The UAP places soiled linens in a linen bag for transport.
2. During the bed bath, the nurse covers the patient with a bath blanket. The patient asks what the bath blanket is for. What is the nurse's best response?
   1. "The bath blanket helps to prevent skin irritation."
   2. "The bath blanket is part of our bathing procedure."
   3. "The bath blanket helps to prevent chilling during the bath."
   4. "The bath blanket is used to prevent the spread of microorganisms."
3. A patient with severe crippling rheumatoid arthritis is confined to bed for extended periods. An erythematous area over the coccyx that has the potential to become an open lesion is noted. The nurse is correct in reporting this area to the health care provider as having the potential to become what?
   1. An inflammatory injury
   2. A pressure injury
   3. A stasis injury
   4. An arterial injury
4. A patient is too weak to perform her own perineal care. The student nurse includes bathing which areas as part of perineal care?
   1. Back and buttocks
   2. Lower back, upper thighs
   3. Upper torso and thighs
   4. Upper thighs, genitalia, and anal area
5. Which patient is at greatest risk for skin impairment?
   1. A 12-year-old on bed rest
   2. A 7-month-old with cool skin temperature
   3. A 26-year-old with diarrhea
   4. A 60-year-old in a body cast

6. A patient is in her second postoperative day after an abdominal hysterectomy. The nurse plans to give the patient a bed bath. Which action is appropriate when caring for the patient's face? *(Select all that apply.)*
   1. Use only water on the patient's face.
   2. Ask the patient if she prefers soap or plain water.
   3. Use soap in all areas of the face except the eyes.
   4. Use a cleansing cream to cleanse her face and neck.
   5. Use a different area of the wash cloth for each eye
7. The nurse is teaching the patient proper hygiene measures. What should the nurse include when teaching the patient about eye care?
   1. Wash from the inner canthus to the outer canthus.
   2. Cleanse dried exudate with hot water.
   3. Avoid drying the circumorbital area after washing.
   4. Use a cotton-tipped applicator for each eyelid.
8. An 11-month-old infant is admitted with a tympanic temperature of 105°F (40.6°C). The physician orders a tepid sponge bath. The infant's mother asks, "What is the purpose of this bath?" Which is the best response by the nurse?
   1. "The bath helps reduce your baby's body temperature."
   2. "The bath is used to help prevent febrile seizures."
   3. "The bath stimulates circulation to the skin."
   4. "The bath helps calm and relax your baby."
9. An uncircumcised man is in the first postoperative day after a transurethral prostatectomy. When administering perineal care, which action by the nurse is correct?
   1. Retract the foreskin, cleanse the penis, and allow the foreskin to return to its former position.
   2. Retract the foreskin, cleanse the penis, and sprinkle powder under the foreskin to facilitate retraction.
   3. Retract the foreskin, cleanse the penis, and leave the foreskin slightly damp to allow retraction to its former state.
   4. Retract the foreskin, cleanse the penis, and return the foreskin with a gentle forward motion.
10. A patient was discharged home with a Foley catheter. The student nurse instructs the patient in the proper procedure for cleansing the female perineal area. What teaching point should the nurse include in discharge instructions?
    1. Cleanse the area in circular motions around the rectum.
    2. Cleanse from the rectum toward the pubis.
    3. Cleanse from the pubis toward the anal area.
    4. Cleanse in circular motions around the vaginal area.
11. The nurse is reviewing the teaching plans of several patients on a medical unit. Which patient does the nurse correctly identify as most at risk for development of complications of the feet?
    1. A 55-year-old disoriented patient
    2. A 30-year-old patient whose career requires extensive standing
    3. A 60-year-old patient with a 30-year history of diabetes mellitus
    4. A 62-year-old patient who had a total hip replacement 2 years ago
12. The nurse is providing oral care to a patient who is unconscious. The optimal position for providing oral hygiene to this patient is _________ to prevent choking.
    1. High Fowler's position
    2. High Fowler's position with head hyperextended
    3. Supine with the head lowered
    4. Side-lying with head facing to the side
13. A patient has diffuse pancreatitis causing severe weakness. The CNA is bathing the patient. While the CNA cleanses the patient's ears, which action by the CNA will prompt the nurse to intervene? *(Select all that apply.)*
    1. Cleansing the outer ear with the washcloth during the bath
    2. Retracting the outer ear downward to loosen visible cerumen
    3. Irrigating the ear with cool water to remove tenacious cerumen
    4. Using cotton-tipped applicators to cleanse the pinna of each ear
    5. Placing an otoscope in the ear canal to visualize any areas that need cleaning
14. The student nurse has completed her educational instructions on the correct procedures for bed making. Which intervention is correct for bed making? *(Select all that apply.)*
    1. Preparing a closed bed for receiving postoperative patients
    2. Shaking soiled linen before placement in the hamper
    3. Mitering the corners of the bottom fitted sheet
    4. Washing hands thoroughly after making a patient's bed
    5. Folding and reusing the patient's bedspread if it is not soiled
15. A patient is in his first postoperative day. As part of his morning care, the nurse removes and cleanses his dentures. Which action demonstrates proper denture care?
    1. Brushing the dentures over an open sink with the water running
    2. Rinsing dentures thoroughly with hot water before brushing
    3. Brushing dentures with a soft toothbrush or denture brush
    4. After cleaning, storing dentures in a dry denture cup
16. The nurse is providing instruction to the UAP who is assisting with caring for an immobile patient who requires turning every 2 hours. The UAP asks the nurse why it is best to place the patient in the 30-degree lateral position. Which response by the nurse is correct?
    1. "This position helps prevent pressure injuries on spinous processes."
    2. "This position helps prevent pressure injuries on the ischial tuberosities."
    3. "This position helps prevent pressure injuries on the greater trochanters."
    4. "This position helps prevent pressure injuries on the occipital prominence."

17. The nurse is reviewing documentation from the previous shift. The nurse is correct when determining the patient has a stage 3 pressure injury based on which note?
    1. Nonblanchable reddened areas where the skin is intact
    2. Full-thickness tissue loss extending through subcutaneous tissue and muscle
    3. Extensive destruction of skin and adipose tissue with possible tunneling
    4. Areas of full-thickness skin loss with extension to the bone
18. The patient has been changing a dressing on a pressure injury for several days and is now being seen in the physician's office. The patient states, "There is a lot of pink tissue at the base of the wound." The nurse explains to the patient that this is the result of what process?
    1. Improper dressing technique and probable infection
    2. Presence of a layer of eschar that has to be removed
    3. Development of a fungal overgrowth interfering with healing
    4. The normal process of healing with healthy granulation tissue
19. The nurse is most concerned when applying heat therapy to which patient?
    1. A patient who has been diagnosed with high blood pressure
    2. A patient who is unconscious as the result of an automobile accident
    3. A patient who has just returned from physical therapy for back pain
    4. A patient who was recently diagnosed with type 2 diabetes mellitus
20. The nurse is providing discharge instructions for a patient who will be using cold therapy after knee replacement surgery. What statement by the patient indicates the need for further instruction? *(Select all that apply.)*
    1. "I don't have a cold pack at home like the one I had in the hospital. I will use the cold pack I use in my cooler to ice my knee."
    2. "I will use a cloth or towel to wrap my cold pack in when I get home so that I don't damage my skin when I'm applying it to my knee."
    3. "My friend says that using a bag of frozen vegetables works well as an ice pack as long as you wrap it in a cloth."
    4. "I will leave the cold pack on my knee for 1 hour, leave it off for 30 minutes, and then apply it again for 1 hour all day long so that my knee won't swell."
    5. "The cold pack really helps the pain in my knee. I will use it at home so that I hopefully won't have to take a lot of pain medication."

Safety

10

http://evolve.elsevier.com/Cooper/foundationsadult/

Objectives

1. Summarize safety precautions to help prevent falls.
2. Relate specific safety considerations to the developmental age and needs of individuals across the lifespan.
3. Identify nursing interventions that are appropriate for individuals across the lifespan to ensure a safe environment.
4. Describe safe and appropriate methods for the application of safety reminder devices and nursing interventions when caring for patients.
5. Discuss nursing interventions that promote a restraint-free environment.
6. Discuss safety concerns in the health care environment.
7. Cite the steps to be taken during a fire.
8. Describe nursing interventions to treat accidental poisoning.
9. Discuss the role of the nurse in disaster planning and active shooter situations.
10. Discuss terrorism.
11. Discuss high-risk syndromes of bioterrorism and the role of the nurse.

Key Terms

bioterrorism (p. 253)
Centers for Disease Control and Prevention (CDC) (SĔN-tĕrz fŏr dĭ-ZĒZ kŏn-TRŌL ănd prē-VĔN-shŭn, p. 247)
codes (p. 252)
disaster manual (p. 252)
disaster situation (p. 251)
elopement (ē-LŌP-mĕnt, p. 242)
endemic (ĕn-DĔM-ĭk, p. 255)
epidemic (ĕp-ĭ-DĔM-ĭk, p. 255)
Hazard Communication Act (p. 247)
Occupational Safety and Health Administration (OSHA) (p. 247)
PASS (p. 250)
poison (p. 250)
RACE (p. 250)
safety reminder device (SRD) (p. 241)
sentinel event (SĔN-tĭ-nĕl, p. 236)
terrorism (p. 252)

Safety of the patient is a primary concern of the nurse. Ensuring a safe physical environment, administering medications safely, and helping patients feel safe in their environment are goals for nurses within a health care facility. The nurse also is concerned with safety of patients within the community setting. Numerous factors can endanger the patient's safety physically and psychologically. This chapter explores potential threats to a patient's safety in various environments and how the nurse can meet the safety needs of the patient.

SAFETY IN THE HOSPITAL OR HEALTH CARE ENVIRONMENT

Traditionally, the patient's overall safety in the hospital or other health care environment has been a primary concern of nursing. Today the focus on a safe environment has expanded as we have come to recognize and identify potential hazards and threats faced by hospital and long-term care facility personnel, patients, and visitors (Box 10.1).

A safe environment implies freedom from injury and prevention of falls, electrical injuries, fires, burns, and poisoning. The nurse must be alert to potential safety problems, including workplace violence, and must know how to report and respond when safety is threatened.

Providing and maintaining a safe environment involves the patient, visitors, and members of the health care team. Protection and education are primary nursing responsibilities, and the nurse is involved directly and actively in ensuring a safe health care environment. Checking to see that the call light or signal system is working and accessible is an example of how the nurse helps maintain a safe environment.

Each year, The Joint Commission releases national patient safety goals for health care facilities. These goals are based on evidenced-based practices developed from a review of national databases and assist facilities in

Box 10.1 Precautions to Promote Safety

- Assist patients when they get out of bed if they have had surgery, have received narcotics for analgesia, have an unsteady gait, or have been in bed for an extended period.
- Demonstrate the proper use of emergency call buttons or cords.
- Encourage patients to wear nonslip slippers or shoes when ambulating.
- Encourage the use of hand rails in the bathrooms and halls.
- Follow facility policies regarding the use of side rails.
- If bed is equipped with an alarm, turn on for the restless, disoriented patient.
- Instruct patient to use the call bell for assistance.
- Keep adjustable beds in the low position except when giving care.
- Keep environment free of clutter because such items as books, magazines, and shoes sometimes cause the patient to trip and fall.
- Lock wheels on beds, wheelchairs, and gurneys.
- Orient patient to the environment to provide familiarity.
- Place bedside table and overbed table within reach. Ensure that frequently used items, such as the telephone, eyeglasses, or other personal belongings, are easily accessible.
- Provide adequate lighting.
- Some institutions have adopted "fall precaution" policies in which every patient is evaluated on admission to determine the degree of likelihood for a potential fall (see Box 10.2).
- Wipe or mop up spilled liquids promptly. Personnel and patients must be alert to signs warning of wet or slippery floors.

Box 10.2 Sample Questions Found on a Fall Assessment Tool

	YES	NO
1. Is there a history of a fall(s) in the past year?		
2. Does the patient have an unsteady gait or difficulty ambulating?		
3. Is the patient on any high-risk medications?		
4. Does the patient require equipment to assist in ambulating?		
5. Does the patient have an altered mental status?		
6. Is the patient experiencing blood pressure problems, dizziness, or vertigo?		
7. Is the patient age 70 years or older?		
8. Does the patient experience bowel or bladder incontinence?		
9. Does the patient have an intravenous (IV), chest tube, or oxygen line or attachment to any other tubing?		
10. Does the patient have any vision or other sensory problems?		

maintaining patient safety. A component of these goals includes the identification of sentinel events. The Joint Commission defines a **sentinel event** as "any unexpected occurrence involving death or serious physical or psychological injury, or the risk thereof" (TJC, n.d.). The reporting of certain sentinel events to The Joint Commission is required, including a thorough review of the event and the plan for improvements that will prevent the event from occurring again. Examples of sentinel events include medication errors and errors in procedures and treatments that led to the death of an individual and inappropriate application of safety reminder devices (SRDs; formerly referred to as *restraints*).

FALLS

Falls are a common problem in health care facilities, requiring the nurse to be alert to patients who are at an increased risk for falls. A fall risk assessment is important to perform on admission to the unit and whenever a significant change in the patient's condition has occurred. Patient falls are a major safety consideration for *all* institutions (see the Coordinated Care box). The very young and older adults are not the only individuals at risk in the health care environment. Individuals who become ill or who are injured are also at risk. An unfamiliar environment and the various symptoms and signs associated with the patient's diagnosis often place an individual at risk. The use of anesthesia, sedatives, or narcotics increases the risk of falling, as does an unstable gait or a problem with balance. A fall risk assessment is necessary on admission to a facility or if a significant change in the patient's condition has occurred. Box 10.2 is a sample list of questions found on a fall risk assessment tool. Facilities require fall precautions if the answer is "yes" to a specified number of questions on a fall risk assessment tool.

Gait belts are an effective way to help patients ambulate safely. A gait belt is a canvas (or other very strong material) belt that encircles the patient's waist (some belts have handles attached for the staff to grasp) while the patient ambulates. Correct technique in the use of the gait belt is as follows:

1. Apply gait belt securely around the patient's waist. The health care worker should be able to fit two fingers between the gait belt and the patient's waist.
2. Walk to the side of patient, grasping the gait belt toward the patient's back. The other hand may either support the patient's arm or grasp the gait belt toward the patient's side. Unless the patient has a tendency to lean toward one particular side, walk on the

Coordinated Care

Delegation

Patient Safety and Fall Prevention

Although preventing falls is the responsibility of all caregivers, including unlicensed assistive personnel (UAP), assessment for risk of fall or injury requires the critical thinking and knowledge application unique to the nurse and is not delegated. When delegating safety measures, stress the importance of the following:

- The patient's mobility limitations and any specific measures to minimize risks
- Environmental safety precautions (e.g., bed locked and in low position, call bell and personal items within reach, clear pathway, nonskid footwear)
- What to do when a patient starts to fall while being assisted with ambulation (i.e., ease patient into a sitting position in a chair or on the floor and alert the nurse)

Monitoring patient behavior for risk of injury and promoting a safe environment are acceptable to delegate as a responsibility of UAP and of nursing staff. Assessment of a patient's behaviors and decisions about less restrictive interventions require the critical thinking and knowledge application unique to the nurse.

Although the application of SRDs is acceptable to delegate to UAP, assessment of when SRDs are needed and the appropriate type to use requires the critical thinking and knowledge application unique to the nurse and is not delegated. The importance of the following factors should be emphasized:

- Correct placement of the SRD
- Observation for constriction of circulation, skin integrity, and adequate breathing
- When and how to change position and provide range-of-motion exercises, skin care, toileting, and opportunities for socialization

Care of the patient receiving internal radiation therapy is acceptable to delegate to UAP. Care measures that should be highlighted include the following:

- Patient's activity limitations
- Safety regulations (e.g., use of dosimeter, time and distance limits)
- Use of protective equipment (shields, gloves)
- Visitor restrictions (no one younger than 18 years of age or who is or may be pregnant)
- Care and handling of patient care–related items and substances (e.g., linen, trash, dietary tray, specimens, urine, feces)

The setting up of seizure precautions and protection for patients at risk for seizures is acceptable to delegate to UAP if they have been trained appropriately. Stress the importance of protection from falls, avoiding attempts to restrain, and not placing anything in the patient's mouth. Interventions for a patient experiencing a seizure are not to be delegated. Assessment of the patient's airway patency, breathing, and circulatory status requires the critical thinking and knowledge application unique to the nurse and cannot be delegated. Refer to *Adult Health Nursing,* Chapter 14, for further care of the patient with seizures.

patient's weaker side so that you are able to give assistance if the patient starts to fall. See the illustration for Skill 10.1, Step 6d(1).

3. Have patient support self by leaning on or holding your arm.
4. Walk slightly behind the patient for better support.
5. Walk with your knees and hips flexed.
6. After ambulation, loosen or remove the gait belt.
7. Document procedure.

INFANTS AND CHILDREN

Ensuring the safety of the environment of infants and children requires protecting the child and educating the parents to do so. The nurse is responsible for anticipating potential injuries and individualizing patient care and teaching. Accidents involving children are largely preventable, but parents and caregivers need to be aware of specific dangers at each stage of growth and development. Growth and the acquisition of new motor skills place the child at great risk for injury. See Chapters 24, 30, and 31 for a more detailed discussion.

Many dangers exist in a child's environment. All household cleaning items are potentially poisonous when ingested and must be kept out of children's reach. Remind parents that most younger children are not able to read or understand labels on cleaning materials or medication containers. Educate parents that infants in the oral stage of development put almost anything into their mouths and that as infants learn to crawl, electrical sockets and cords also become a danger. Toddlers and young children can be protected from burns by turning pot handles on a stove away from the child's reach. Bath water can be another potential hazard for children because of the temperature of the water or from leaving children unattended for any length of time. Pool safety also should be emphasized to parents and caregivers. Protecting infants and toddlers from falling out of bed while in the health care facility is a concern. Keeping side rails up or using a pediatric crib are safety measures to prevent falls. When giving care, place your hand on the infant or toddler when you turn to obtain supplies; this prevents the infant or child from falling off a bed or examination table. See Chapters 24, 30, and 31 for a more detailed discussion.

OLDER ADULTS

Changes associated with aging significantly affect the ability of older adults to protect themselves from injury (see the Lifespan Considerations for Older Adults box). Unsteady gait, age-related vision changes, and medication side effects (such as vertigo) pose a threat to the older adult's safety. Ensuring that older adults wear their eyeglasses and hearing aids and use assistive devices for ambulating when necessary are important nursing interventions to promote patient safety.

Assisting weak or disoriented older patients when drinking hot liquids such as soups, coffee, or tea can prevent burns. People in this age group are more

Skill 10.1 Applying Safety Reminder Devices

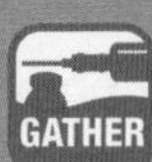

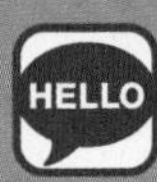

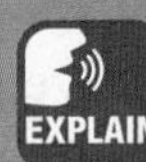

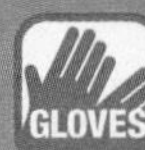

NURSING ACTION *(RATIONALE)*

1. Refer to medical record, care plan, and Kardex. Review agency policy. *(Provides basis of care; a physician's order is required before SRDs are applied.)*
2. Perform hand hygiene. *(Reduces spread of microorganisms.)*
3. Introduce self. *(Decreases patient's anxiety.)*
4. Identify patient. *(Identifies correct patient for procedure.)*
5. Procedure:
   a. Explain procedure. *(Enlists cooperation or assistance from patient and family and decreases anxiety.)*
   b. Prepare for procedure by providing privacy and assembling necessary supplies. *(Organizes procedure and decreases patient's anxiety.)*
   c. Assess patient for need for SRD (a comprehensive nursing assessment of the patient's potential for injury and treatment in relation to the need for an SRD is crucial before applying SRD). *(Restraining a patient without a physician's order or without reasonable cause incurs risk of charges of false imprisonment. Some facilities have specific requirements for SRD use in certain situations [e.g., the presence of an endotracheal tube].)*
6. Apply appropriate type of SRD:
   a. Wrist or ankle (extremity) SRD designed to immobilize one or more extremities
      (1) If using Kerlix gauze, make a clove hitch by forming a figure of 8 and picking up the loops. *(The clove hitch does not tighten when pulled.)*
      (2) Place gauze or padding around the extremity. *(Decreases risk of injury to underlying skin.)*
      (3) Slip the wrist(s) or ankle(s) through loops directly over the padding; if using a commercially made SRD, wrap the padded portion of the device around affected extremity, thread tie through slit in device, and fasten to second tie with a secure knot. *(Decreases risk of injury to underlying skin.)*

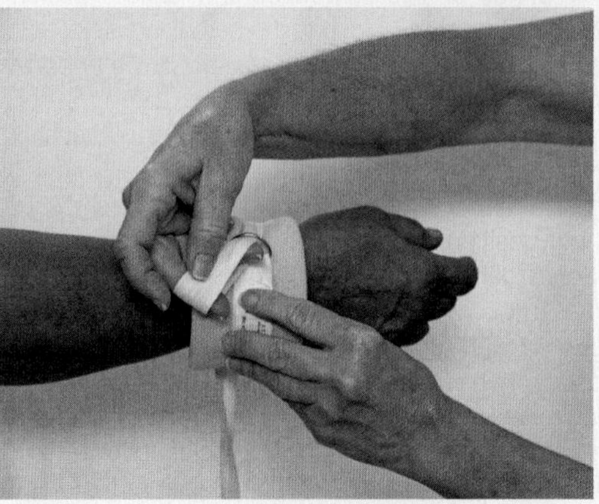

      (4) Secure ends of ties to the movable portion of the bed frame that moves with the patient when the bed is adjusted, **not to side rails**. *(If side rails are lowered with the SRD attached, injury is a possible result.)*

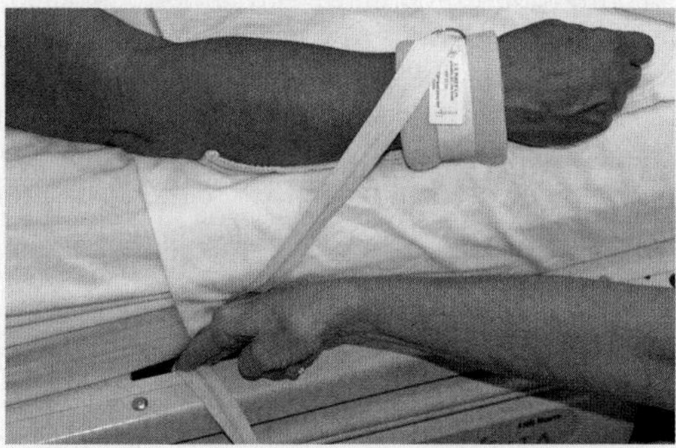

      (5) Leave as much slack as possible (1 to 2 inches). *(Provides for movement.)*
      (6) Palpate pulses below the SRD. *(Ensures that the device is not so tight as to occlude circulation.)*
   b. Elbow SRD
      (1) Place SRD (a piece of fabric with slots for the insertion of tongue blades to keep the elbow straight) over the elbow or elbows. *(Elbow SRDs often are used with children to prevent elbow flexion so that they cannot disturb tubes, catheters, and dressings.)*

Skill 10.1 Applying Safety Reminder Devices—cont'd

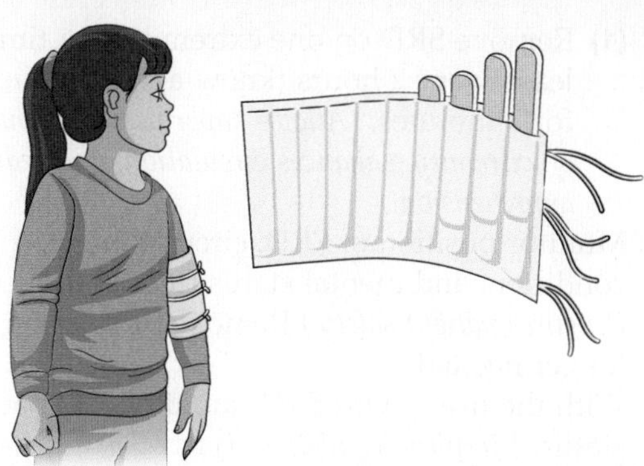

(2) Wrap SRD(s) snugly, tying them at the top. For small infants, tie or pin SRDs to their shirts. *(Tying or pinning the restraint to the infant's shirt ensures a secure fit.)*

c. Vest (sometimes referred to as a wrap jacket or chest SRD)

(1) Apply device over the patient's gown. *(Protects the skin.)*

(2) Put vest on patient with V-shaped opening in the front. *(If vest is on backward and patient becomes restless, choking is possible result.)*

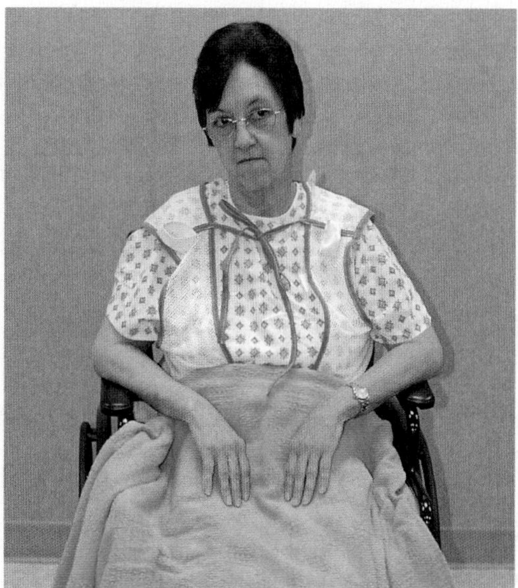

(3) Pull tie at end of vest flap across the chest and slip tie through slit on opposite side of vest.

(4) Wrap the other end of the flap across patient and tie the straps to frame of bed or behind wheelchair. *(Helps secure vest SRD to the patient.)* Use the quick-release knot. *(A tight restraint potentially causes constriction and impedes circulation. Assessment for constriction prevents neurovascular injury.)*

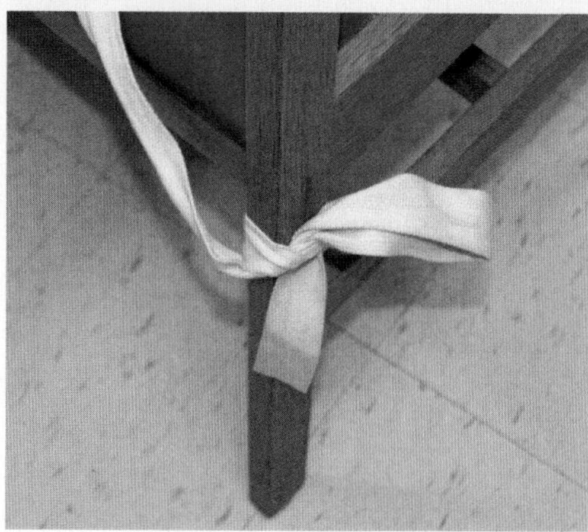

(5) With a proper fit, there is room for a fist in the space between the vest and the patient. *(This determines that the vest is not too tight.)*

d. Gait or safety reminder belts

(1) Apply belt over the patient's gown. *(Protects the skin.)*

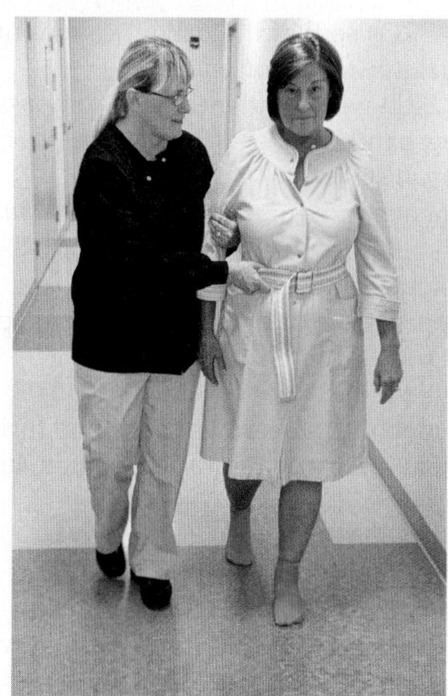

(2) If patient is ambulating, place belt around the patient's waist. The belt usually has a buckle to secure the belt in place. *(Provides a snug fit and prevents slipping.)*

(3) If the belt does not have a buckle, use a slip knot. *(Allows for quick removal in case of emergency.)*

7. Use a quick-release knot rather than a regular knot to secure the safety reminder device to bed frame. *(A quick-release knot is quick to undo in an emergency.)*

Continued

Skill 10.1 Applying Safety Reminder Devices—cont'd

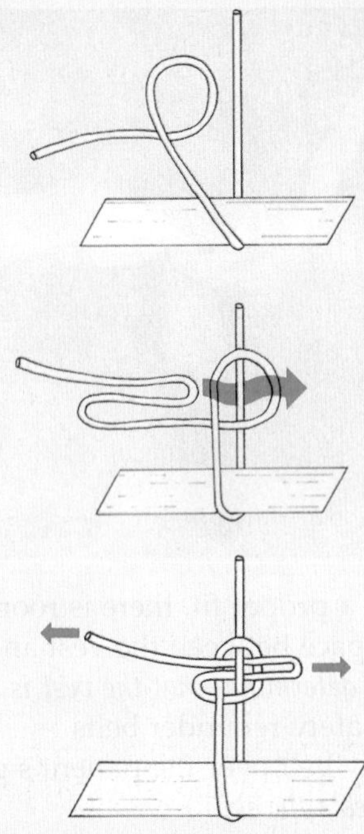

8. Secure SRDs so that the patient cannot untie them. *(Prevents patient injury.)*
9. Apply SRD with gentleness and compassion.
10. Perform hand hygiene. *(Reduces spread of microorganisms.)*
11. Document procedure. *(Notes procedure and patient's response.)*
    - Reason(s) SRD needed
    - If appropriate, the notification of the physician and time order obtained
    - The time and type of SRD applied
    - The ongoing assessment and monitoring of the patient's skin, extremity circulation, and mental status
    - The response(s) of the patient
    - The periodic removal of the SRD and any skin care performed
    - If SRD removed, note time and follow-up assessments
    - If reapplication is needed, note reasons, time, and patient assessment
    - A flow sheet is an excellent tool for this documentation (see Fig. 3.8 for an example of a flow sheet)
12. Follow-up
    a. Monitor for skin impairment. *(Excessive pressure potentially leads to loss of skin integrity.)*
    b. With the use of extremity SRD, assess extremity distal to SRD every 30 minutes or more often according to agency policy. *(Identifies any problems or need to remove or adjust SRD.)*
        (1) Remove SRD on one extremity at a time at least every 2 hours (know agency policy) for 5 minutes. *(Allows supervised movement of extremity, enhances circulation, and reduces apprehension.)*
    c. Monitor position of SRD, circulation, skin condition, and mental status frequently. *(Ensures patient safety.)* Remove SRD when no longer needed.
    d. With the use of vest SRD, monitor respiratory status. *(Respiratory distress is possible if there is restriction from the vest.)*
    e. Do NOT leave the patient unattended during temporary removal of SRD. *(An unattended patient is at risk for injury.)* Do take advantage of removal to change patient's position and inspect skin.
    f. Gently massage the skin beneath SRD; apply lotion or powder if desired. *(A gentle massage of the skin increases circulation to area.)*
    g. Change SRD when soiled or wet. *(Reduces risk of skin impairment and infection.)*
    h. Assess frequently for tangled ties or pressure points from knots; adjust SRD device(s) as needed. *(Excess pressure leads to loss of skin integrity and impaired circulation.)*
13. Evaluation
    a. The SRD is adequate and appropriate for the individual patient's condition. *(Prevents interruption of treatment or therapy; prevents patient from falling from bed, chair, or wheelchair, and possibly from harming others.)*
    b. SRDs are applied correctly. *(Correct application prevents injury to the patient or to others.)*
    c. Quick-release knots are released easily. *(Ensures quick access to the patient in case of an emergency.)*
    d. Related problems (e.g., of the skin or of the musculoskeletal system) are identified. *(Complications are prevented by performing timely interventions.)*
14. Provide patient teaching (see the Patient Teaching box on safety promotion).
15. Pediatric considerations
    a. When a child must be restrained for a procedure, it is best that the person applying the restraint not be the child's parent or guardian.
    b. A mummy restraint is a safe, efficient, short-term method to restrain a small child or infant for examination or treatment.
        (1) Open a blanket, and fold one corner toward the center. Place the infant on the blanket with shoulders at the fold and feet toward the opposite corner.

Skill 10.1 Applying Safety Reminder Devices—cont'd

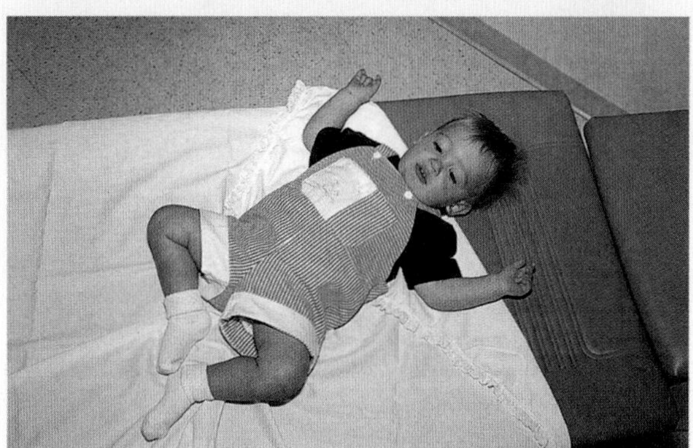

(2) With infant's right arm straight down against body, pull the right side of the blanket firmly across the right shoulder and chest, and secure beneath the left side of body.

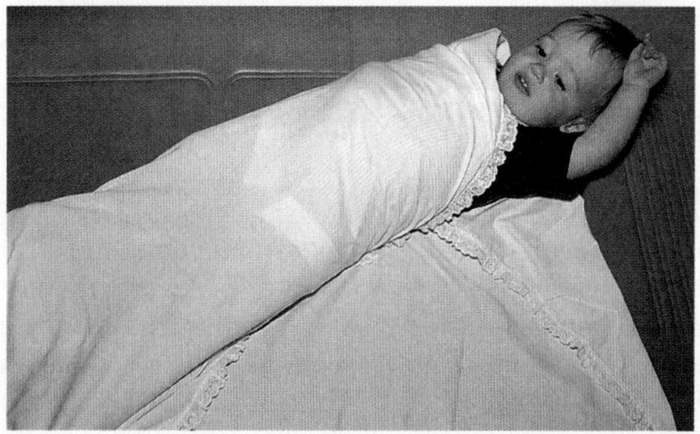

(3) Place the left arm straight against the body, bring the left side of the blanket across the shoulder and chest, and lock beneath the infant's body on the right side.

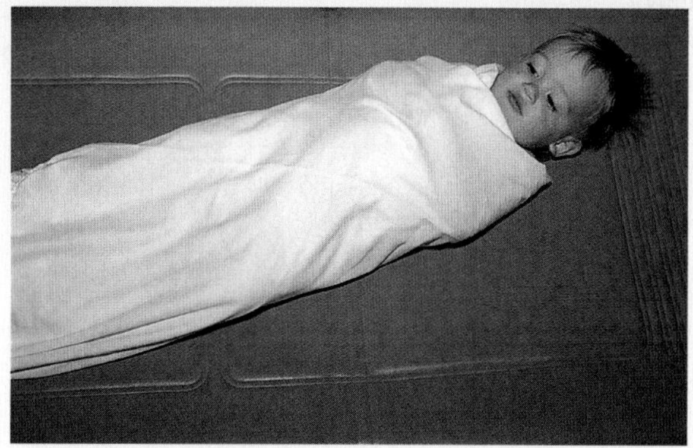

(4) Align the infant's legs, pull the corner of the blanket near the feet up toward the body, and tuck snugly in place or fasten securely with safety pins.

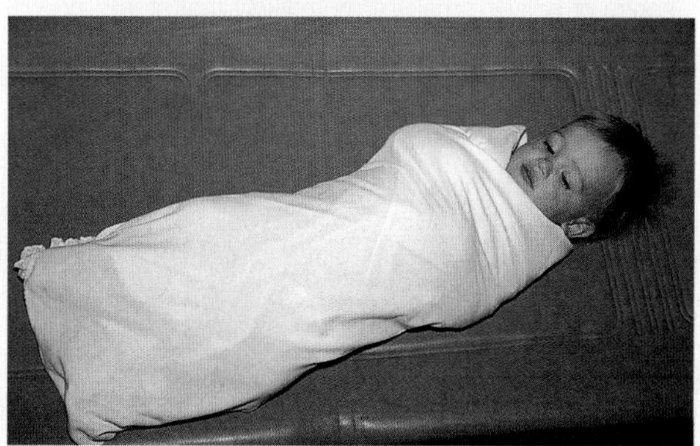

(5) Remain with the infant during restraint, and remove the restraint immediately after treatment is complete. If restraint is required for an extended period, remove it at least every 2 hours and perform range-of-motion exercises on all extremities.

Steps 15a(2) through 15a(5) from Elkin MK, Perry AG, Potter PA: *Nursing interventions and clinical skills*, ed 4, St. Louis, 2008, Mosby.

vulnerable to burns from spilled hot liquids and from heating pads and electric blankets.

SAFETY REMINDER DEVICES

A **safety reminder device (SRD)** is defined as any of the numerous devices used to immobilize a patient or part of the patient's body, such as arms or hands. Many facilities have adopted a restraint-free environment, thus eliminating the use of any type of SRD. This is especially true in long-term care facilities. The long-term care setting is the permanent home for many residents, so maintaining a safe environment while protecting the individual's dignity is a priority.

The use of SRDs also tends to result in increased restlessness, disorientation, agitation, anxiety, and a feeling of powerlessness. It contributes to patient immobility and associated problems with immobility such as dehydration, health care–associated infection, and incontinence. The resulting disuse of body parts has the potential to increase disability and lead to further patient weakness and unsteadiness. Patients often pull against the SRDs, causing skin and circulation problems.

SRDs may be used for various reasons but are primarily for considerations of patient safety. SRDs that restrain the use of a limb (e.g., a wrist restraint) are used primarily in the mental health setting to protect the patient and the staff from harm, pediatric setting to prevent such incidents such as displacement of intravenous lines by the patient, and the intensive care setting to prevent the patient from pulling out medical devices such as an endotracheal tube. Certain patient populations, such as the disoriented patient, are more likely to need SRDs

Lifespan Considerations

Older Adults

Safety

Physiologic changes in aging increase the need for safety precautions:

- Changes in vision, including altered depth perception, increased sensitivity to glare, and decreased visual acuity in dim light, increase the risk of falls because of misperception of visual cues.
- Changes in hearing, including varying degrees of deafness and tinnitus (ringing in the ears), increase the risk of injury from hazards in the environment because certain warnings that commonly are detected with auditory cues, such as motor vehicle horns, alarms, or even spoken warnings, are not heard.
- Prevent sensory overload in older adults because reflexes and the ability to respond to multiple stimuli slow with aging.
- Changes in muscle strength and joint function that result in slowed reaction time, altered gait, and altered sense of balance make it more likely that stumbling will result in a fall.
- Changes in the cardiovascular system, such as anemia, orthostatic hypotension, and heart block, increase the risk of syncope, which increases the risk of falls.
- Changes in the peripheral vascular system sometimes result in loss of sensitivity to heat, cold, or foreign objects, which increases the risk of tissue damage from burns, frostbite, and pressure.
- Older adults take many medications that increase the need for safety precautions. Sedatives, hypnotics, and tranquilizers affect reaction time and increase the risk of injury. Antihypertensives, diuretics, and antihistamines increase the risk of orthostatic hypotension (a drop of 25 mm Hg in systolic pressure and 10 mm Hg in diastolic pressure), which increases the risk of falls.
- Keep to a minimum the use of SRDs with older adults and, when necessary, the amount of any restraint used. SRDs reduce mobility and result in a loss of strength that can increase the risk of falls or injury.
- Accidental poisoning is a significant problem in older adults. Visual changes raise the potential for misreading of labels on medication or other package labels and lead to overdose or other errors in administration. Medication organizers or dispensers help reduce the risk of medication errors in the home. In addition, many older adults do not consider over-the-counter medications to be "real" medicine, so they take them freely and fail to mention them when questioned regarding drug use. Many over-the-counter medications increase the risk of injury to the older adult by potentiating or interfering with the effects of prescription drugs.

in the forms of bed or chair alarms. A bed or chair alarm alerts the staff if a patient attempts to get out of a bed or chair without assistance. This helps reduce the risk of the patient falling from a bed, chair, or wheelchair (Fig. 10.1). For patients or residents in a long-term care setting who are at risk for **elopement** (leaving the health care facility without permission or necessary supervision), a device referred to as a wander guard may be needed. This device is worn on the wrist or ankle and sets off an alarm when the person leaves the facility. These devices are especially beneficial for the confused or disoriented patient or resident who would be at risk for attempting to leave the facility.

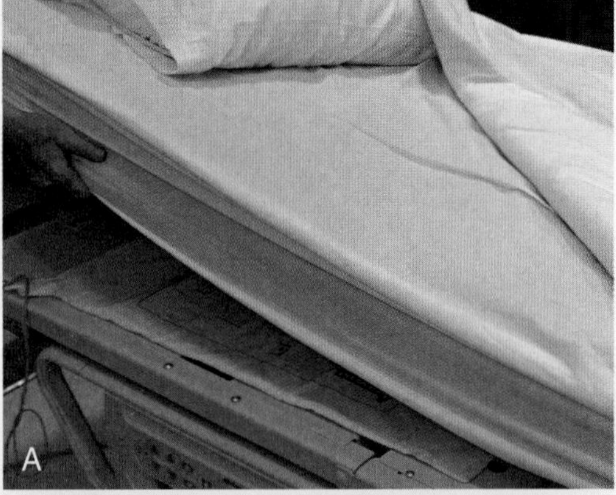

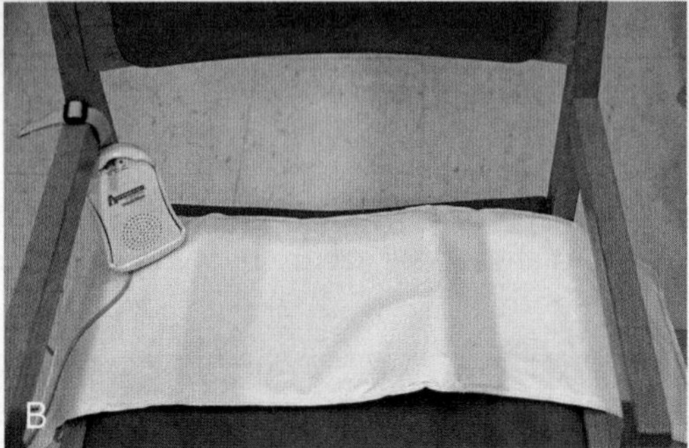

Fig. 10.1 A, Weight-sensitive alarm. B, Chair alarm.

The focus of patient care is on attempting alternative strategies before turning to the use of SRDs (Box 10.3). By assessing individual patient needs, characteristics of the environment, and organizational change, the licensed practical/vocational nurse (LPN/LVN) often is able to plan interventions that reduce or eliminate the need for SRDs. Patient safety and the safety of others are the only reasons an SRD is used. Most health care facilities have specific policies and procedures related to the use of SRDs (Box 10.4 and see Skill 10.1), and most require a specific order from a health care provider. Some facilities require that a health care provider order for SRDs be renewed every 24 hours. Explain to the patient the need for the devices even if the patient does not seem to understand the explanation. Also, inform family members about the need for SRDs (see the Cultural Considerations box and the Patient Teaching box). Include information about the specific device used and the approximate period for use.

Documentation about the need for the SRDs, the type of device used, and the patient's response is crucial (see Box 10.4). Perform a comprehensive assessment that focuses on the patient's behavior, activity, and skin

Box 10.3 Designing a Restraint-Free Environment

Care of the patient who may be prone to threats to safety and security requires a creative, systematic, and attentive approach. A wide variety of electronic devices have been developed to alert staff to a patient's need for assistance. A weight-sensitive alarm can be placed under a patient in bed or in a chair. When the patient tries to get up, an alarm sounds (see Fig. 10.1A). A chair alarm may be used to remind the patient or alert the staff when a patient who requires assistance when standing or ambulating tries to get up without assistance (Fig. 10.1B).

To design a restraint-free environment:

- Orient patient and family to surroundings; explain all procedures and treatments.
- Encourage family and friends to stay, or use sitters for patients who need supervision.
- Assign confused or disoriented patients to rooms near the nurses' station. Observe these patients frequently.
- Provide appropriate visual and auditory stimuli (e.g., family pictures, clocks, radio).
- Eliminate bothersome treatments as soon as possible. For example, discontinue tube feedings and begin oral feedings as quickly as the patient's condition allows.
- Use relaxation techniques (e.g., massage).
- Institute exercise and ambulation schedules as the patient's condition allows.
- Encourage participation in diversional activities (e.g., long-term care facilities typically have daily activities planned for the residents, such as games, movies, entertainment).
- Maintain toileting routines.
- Consult with physical and occupational therapists to enhance patient's abilities to carry out activities of daily living.
- Evaluate all medications patient is receiving to determine whether the medication is having the desired therapeutic effect.
- Conduct ongoing assessment and evaluation of patient's care and patient's ongoing response to care.

Box 10.4 Long-Term Care Variations for Safety Reminder Devices

Legislation has affected greatly the use of safety reminder devices (SRDs) in the long-term care facility. Under the Omnibus Budget Reconciliation Act (OBRA) of 1987, residents' rights are addressed specifically in terms of SRDs. This act, effective October 1, 1990, mandates specific guidelines and prohibits routine use of SRDs in long-term care facilities. The act regulates the use of extremity SRDs, hand mitts, safety vests, and wheelchair safety bars. SRDs may be used only to ensure the physical safety of the resident or other residents. A written order by the physician must detail the duration and circumstances under which the SRDs are to be used.

OBRA states the following as acceptable reasons for the use of physical restraints:

- All other interventions have been attempted before the use of restraints.
- Other disciplines have been consulted for their assistance.
- Supporting documentation has been completed.

ESSENTIALS OF SRD DOCUMENTATION

- Reason for the physical restraint
- Explanation given to patient and family
- Date and time of the patient's response to treatment
- Duration
- Frequency of observation and patient's response
- Safety
- Release the physical restraint at least every 2 hours
- Routine exercise of extremities, including range-of-motion exercises
- Assessment for circulation and skin integrity
- Assessment for continued need for the physical restraint
- Patient outcome

condition. Note all nursing interventions, including patient and family teaching about the SRDs.

LATEX SENSITIVITY

Question all patients regarding allergies, and ask specifically about latex allergies. A latex allergy can precipitate a respiratory arrest, which is a life-threatening event (Box 10.5). This potential reaction must be kept in mind at all times. Do not wear, or permit others to wear, latex gloves when caring for patients with latex allergies. For individuals at high risk of or with suspected sensitivity to latex, use exclusively latex-free products, including gloves, and inspect the contents of all patient care supply kits for items that contain latex (e.g., catheters, tubing). Institutions have latex-free procedure kits available for use.

ELECTRICAL HAZARDS

Much of the equipment used in health care settings is electrical and requires maintenance. Use of properly grounded and functional electrical equipment decreases the risk of electrical injury and fire. Teaching patients and family how to reduce their risk of electrical injury in the home (e.g., prevention of electrical shock, avoidance of use of electrical appliances near water source, methods of grounding appliances, avoidance of operating unfamiliar equipment) is a responsibility of the home health nurse.

RADIATION

Radiation presents a health hazard, if used incorrectly, in health care settings and the community. Radiation

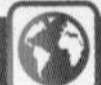

Cultural Considerations

Safety in Health Care Settings

- Cultural heritage affects all dimensions of health; the nurse must consider cultural background when planning for patient safety.
- The way that culture influences behaviors, attitudes, and values depends on many factors and thus may not be the same for individual members of a cultural group.
- Before assessing the cultural background of a patient, assess the influence of the nurse's own culture.
- Adapt the planning and implementation of nursing interventions for safety as much as possible to a patient's cultural background.
- Evaluate attitudes and emotions toward providing nursing interventions for safety to patients from diverse sociocultural backgrounds.
- Patients from some cultures may seem unfriendly and distant in terms of space. It is often very difficult for them to have an outsider in their home who is suggesting changes with regard to their personal belongings, even though the purpose is to reduce physical hazards.
- Determination of a patient's attitude toward the home is particularly difficult when another language is spoken. Use an interpreter or engage the patient's family to interpret if available. Attentiveness to the patient's nonverbal communication becomes extremely important as you assess the home.
- Another culturally sensitive issue is the patient's sense of environmental control. Be aware of health beliefs and practices that affect the outcome of interventions. For example, reliance on family and religious organizations, as opposed to community resources, is likely to affect compliance with nursing interventions and referrals.

Patient Teaching

Safety Promotion

- Teach the primary caregiver the dangers associated with restraining a patient with a history of seizures and how to modify the environment for the patient's protection.
- Instruct the primary caregiver how to position correctly a patient who is nauseated and vomiting if a restraint is in use.
- Instruct the primary caregiver how to routinely change the patient's position and use passive range of motion.
- Explain to the patient and members of the family why SRDs are necessary.
- Provide information about the type of SRD to be used and the approximate time frame for use.
- Inform patient and family that the patient will still receive comfort measures such as repositioning and limb exercises.
- Inform patients and parents about potential sources of poisoning found in the home and appropriate safety precautions (see Box 10.11).
- Inform patients and parents about poison control centers. Provide number of closest center or instruct to call 911.
- Teach basic interventions to follow in the case of a poisoning.
- See that safety items, such as stickers with poison center information, are available.
- Teach parents and caregivers not to try home remedies. When ingestion of a dangerous substance is suspected, appropriate medical intervention must be sought immediately (see the Cultural Considerations box).
- Removal of poisonous and toxic substances does not take the place of education as a means to prevent accidental poisoning.
- Instruct family to place bedside tables and overbed tables close to the patient.
- Encourage the patient to rise from the bed or chair slowly to prevent vertigo (dizziness) that results from postural hypotension.
- Advise the family to remove clutter from bedside tables, hallways, bathrooms, and grooming areas.
- Encourage family to mount grab bars around toilets and showers; instruct the patient how to use them.
- Recommend that rugs and carpets be attached securely to floors and stairs.
- Recommend that bath mats and nonskid strips be attached to bathtubs and the floors of shower stalls.
- Recommend that electrical cords be secured against baseboards so that the patient will not trip over them easily.
- Ensure that the call bell is within easy reach of the hospitalized patient, and show patient the location of emergency call bells in bathrooms. (The nurse must respond to call lights quickly, especially for patients who need assistance to the bathroom.)
- See that wheelchairs remain locked when transporting a patient from bed to wheelchair or back to bed.
- Instruct caregivers to check that side rails are up and safety straps secured around the patient who is on a gurney (stretcher; see the Coordinated Care box).
- Use the fire drill procedure as an opportunity to talk about fire safety.

and radioactive materials are used in the diagnosis and treatment of patients. Hospitals have strict guidelines on the care of patients who are receiving radiation and on the handling of radioactive materials. To reduce the amount of exposure to radiation, the nurse must limit time spent near the source, keep as great a distance from the source as possible, and use shielding devices such as lead aprons. Staff members who work near radiation on a routine basis are required to wear devices that track their cumulative exposure to radiation. After

Box 10.5 Levels of Latex Sensitivity

- *Contact dermatitis:* A nonallergic response characterized by skin redness and itching.
- *Type IV hypersensitivity:* Cell-mediated allergic reaction to chemicals used in latex processing. Delayed reaction, including redness, itching, and hives, up to 48 hours is possible. Localized swelling, red and itchy or runny eyes and nose, and coughing often develop.
- *Type I hypersensitivity:* A true latex allergy that is possibly life threatening. Reactions are likely based on type of latex protein and degree of individual sensitivity, including local and systemic. Symptoms include hives, generalized edema, itching, rash, wheezing, bronchospasm, difficulty breathing, laryngeal edema, diarrhea, nausea, hypotension, tachycardia, and respiratory or cardiac arrest.

From Asthma and Allergy Foundation of America: Types of latex reactions. Retrieved from *www.aafa.org/display.cfm?id=9&sub=21&cont=428*.

collection and processing of these devices, those staff members whose radiation exposure readings fall above a set limit frequently are assigned to an alternative work area away from radiation exposure. Follow-up medical attention often is mandated for them as well.

The community is put at risk for radiation exposure if radioactive waste products are disposed of or transported incorrectly. Community health agencies, the Environmental Protection Agency (EPA), the Nuclear Regulatory Commission (NRC), the Department of Energy (DOE), and the Department of Transportation (DOT) have established specific, strict guidelines for the disposal of radioactive waste (EPA, 2015). If a radioactive leak occurs, these agencies institute measures to prevent exposure of surrounding neighborhoods, to clean up radioactive leaks as quickly as possible, and to ensure that anyone injured receives prompt medical care.

MERCURY SPILL

The nurse must know whom to contact when exposure to a hazardous chemical such as mercury occurs in the health care setting. Exposures in a health care facility include broken thermometers or sphygmomanometers, although these devices are seldom used or allowed in most health care facilities. Mercury enters the body through inhalation and absorption through the skin. Exposures that occur in a health care facility setting are usually brief but still have the potential to affect the brain or kidney. Full recovery is likely once the body cleans itself of the contamination. Box 10.6 summarizes steps to take in the event of a mercury spill. Although a mercury spill is not likely to occur in the health care setting, it is important to be aware of the facility's policy for proper cleanup of a mercury spill. Mercury-containing equipment may be used in factory settings, so the occupational health nurse should be aware of mercury spill safety in case an employee comes into contact with mercury while on the job.

Box 10.6 Mercury Spill Cleanup Procedure

In the event of a mercury spill, follow these steps while waiting for trained personnel to arrive:

1. Evacuate the room except for a housekeeping crew (if available).
2. Ventilate the area. Close interior doors and open any outside windows.
3. DO NOT VACUUM THE SPILL.

After the mercury has been recovered:

4. Mop the floor with a mercury-specific cleanser (see agency policy).
5. Dispose of collected mercury according to local environmental safety regulations.

WORKPLACE SAFETY

The health care environment is a source of potential safety hazards to health care workers. Of significant impact is the threat of workplace violence (Box 10.7). Active shooters are also a concern in the health care setting. An active shooter is defined by the US Department of Homeland Security (2008) as "an individual actively engaged in killing or attempting to kill people in a confined and populated area; in most cases, active shooters use firearms(s) and there is no pattern or method to their selection of victims." In July 2016 The Joint Commission issued Planning and Response Guidelines in Health Care Settings from the FBI. It was recognized that active shooter guidelines were geared toward schools, government, and business settings but not toward the health care setting. The environment within the health care setting has several potentially dangerous areas in the presence of an active shooter. The patient population is a vulnerable and potentially large target for an active shooter. Another area of concern is departments that house hazardous materials. Suggested response guidelines to an active shooter can be found at *https://www.jointcommission.org/emergency_management_resources_violence_security_active_shooter/*.

Workplace safety also addresses other various biologic, chemical, radiologic, and physical hazards. The increased use of lasers in the health care setting requires specific safety precautions because a laser has the potential to cause skin and eye injury and start a fire, if used improperly. Therefore eye protection is necessary for the patient and the staff working with the laser. Personnel involved with laser-based procedures wear specially designed eyewear. Because a laser beam generates an enormous amount of energy, dry combustibles in the surgical field can accidentally ignite, posing a threat to the patient and staff. Ensure that water and a halon fire extinguisher are readily available. For prevention of injury to patients, staff, and equipment, sufficient and appropriate fire extinguishers must be located in magnetic resonance imaging (MRI) areas.

Hospital workers frequently are exposed to blood and body fluids, contaminated needles, radiation, and

Box 10.7 Workplace Violence

Violence does not always involve physical injury, especially in relation to workplace violence. The term workplace violence refers to any intense extreme behavior used to frighten, intimidate, threaten, or injure a person or damage or destroy property. The behavior is sometimes physical, sometimes verbal, and sometimes even nonverbal, such as a gesture. Legally, if by either threat or gesture, someone causes a person to fear being struck, an assault has occurred. Any unwelcomed physical contact from another person is battery. In other words, one does not have to be physically "hurt" to get protection under the law.

According to the most recent statistics from the US Safety and Health Topics in 2010 more than 11,300 assaults occurred against health care and social assistance workers, with nearly 19% occurring in nursing and residential care facilities. Most workplace violence, including in the health care setting, results in nonfatal injuries (*https://www.osha.gov/SLTC/healthcarefacilities/violence.html*).

Unfortunately, these statistics do not provide the full picture because many workplace violence incidents are not reported. Sometimes nurses do not report a violent incident because they are unsure what constitutes violence, do not know of the requirement to report the incident, or do not know whom to inform; sometimes they do not file a report because the injuries do not require emergency treatment or time off from work.

Risk factors for work-related assaults in health care agencies include the following:

- On-site presence of patients, families, friends, and coworkers in the possession of handguns
- Patients who are hospitalized and under police custody at the same time (people arrested or convicted of crimes)
- On-site presence of acutely disturbed and violent people seeking health care
- On-site presence of mentally ill people who do not take medicine, do not receive follow-up care, and are not hospitalized unless they are an immediate threat to themselves or others
- On-site presence of upset, agitated, and disturbed family members and visitors
- Long emergency department waits that increase a person's agitation and frustration
- On-site agency pharmacies that are a source of drugs and therefore a target for robberies
- Gang members and substance abusers having access to agencies as patients or visitors
- Staff being alone with patients during care or transport to other agency areas during examination or treatment
- Low staffing levels during meals, during emergencies, and at night
- Poorly lighted parking areas or distant parking areas
- Lack of staff training in recognizing and managing potentially violent situations

OSHA provides guidelines for violence identification and prevention programs with a goal of eliminating or reducing employee exposure to situations that have potential to cause death or injury. These guidelines can be found at the OSHA Workplace Violence Safety and Health Topics page. The worksite is analyzed for hazards. Prevention strategies are developed and implemented. Furthermore, employees are required to receive safety and health training per facility protocol. The nurse's responsibility in violence prevention programs include the following:

- Understand and follow the workplace violence prevention program.
- Understand and follow safety and security measures.
- Voice safety and security concerns.
- Report violent incidents promptly and accurately.
- Serve on health and safety committees that review incidents of workplace violence.
- Take part in training programs that focus on recognizing and managing agitation, assaultive behavior, and criminal intent.
- Practice the following safety measures when dealing with agitated or aggressive people:
  - Stand away from the person. Judge the length of the person's arms and legs. Stand far enough away that the person will not be able to hit or kick you.
  - Position yourself close to the door. Do not allow yourself to become trapped in the room.
  - Note the location of panic buttons, call bells, alarms, closed-circuit monitors, and other security devices.
  - If you wear your identification badge around your neck, be sure it will break away if pulled.
  - Keep your hands free.
  - Stay calm. Talk to the person in a calm manner. Do not raise your voice or argue, scold, or interrupt the person.
  - Do not touch the person.
  - Tell the person that you will get the supervisor to speak to the person.
  - Leave the room as soon as you are able. Be sure the person is safe.
  - Notify the supervisor or security officer of the situation.
  - Complete an incident report according to agency policy.

From the US Department of Labor Occupational Safety and Health Administration (OSHA): Workplace violence. Retrieved from *https://www.osha.gov/SLTC/healthcarefacilities/violence.html*.

vaccine-preventable diseases. Immunization programs help protect hospital personnel and, in turn, patients at risk of being infected by hospital personnel. The Centers for Disease Control and Prevention (CDC; 2017) have published health care personnel vaccination recommendations (Box 10.8). These recommendations also apply to student nurses because they are fulfilling clinical requirements in health care facilities.

Needlesticks are another source of potential injury to health care personnel. Intravenous tubing and accessories that do not require needles are available, thus reducing the risk of needlesticks. Needlesticks can be

Box 10.8 Centers for Disease Control and Prevention Health Care Personnel Vaccination Recommendations

VACCINES	RECOMMENDATIONS IN BRIEF
Hepatitis B	If you do not have documented evidence of a complete hepatitis B (HB) vaccine series, or if you do not have an up-to-date blood test that shows you are immune to hepatitis B (i.e., no serologic evidence of immunity or prior vaccination) then you should • Get the 3-dose series (dose #1 now, #2 in 1 month, #3 approximately 5 months after #2). • Get anti-HBs serologic tested 1–2 months after dose #3.
Flu (influenza)	Get 1 dose of influenza vaccine annually.
MMR (measles, mumps, and rubella)	If you were born in 1957 or later and have not had the MMR vaccine, or if you do not have an up-to-date blood test that shows you are immune to measles or mumps (i.e., no serologic evidence of immunity or prior vaccination), get 2 doses of MMR (1 dose now and the 2nd dose at least 28 days later). If you were born in 1957 or later and have not had the MMR vaccine, or if you do not have an up-to-date blood test that shows you are immune to rubella, only 1 dose of MMR is recommended. However, you may end up receiving 2 doses, because the rubella component is in the combination vaccine with measles and mumps. For health care workers (HCWs) born before 1957, see the MMR Advisory Committee on Immunization Practices (ACIP) vaccine recommendations.
Varicella (chickenpox)	If you have not had chickenpox (varicella), if you have not had varicella vaccine, or if you do not have an up-to-date blood test that shows you are immune to varicella (i.e., no serologic evidence of immunity or prior vaccination) get 2 doses of varicella vaccine, 4 weeks apart.
Tdap (tetanus, diphtheria, pertussis)	Get a one-time dose of Tdap as soon as possible if you have not received Tdap previously (regardless of when previous dose of Td was received). Get Td boosters every 10 years thereafter. Pregnant HCWs need to get a dose of Tdap during each pregnancy.
Meningococcal	Those who routinely are exposed to isolates of *Neisseria meningitidis* should get one dose.

Modified from Centers for Disease Control and Prevention (CDC): Vaccine information for adults: Recommended vaccines for healthcare workers, 2017. Retrieved from *https://www.cdc.gov/vaccines/adults/rec-vac/hcw.html.*

reduced further by never recapping needles and following proper disposal of needles into sharps containers after use. A stray needle lying in bed linens or carelessly thrown into a wastebasket is a prime source of exposure to bloodborne pathogens. Overfilling a sharps container is another source of needlestick injuries. A staff member may try to deposit a needle into the overfilled container, thus causing a stick to occur. Many facilities use safety devices that prevent the need to recap needles (see Fig. 21.10). Bloodborne diseases that can be transmitted through accidental needlesticks include hepatitis B and C and HIV. Current guidelines and recommendations by the CDC and Occupational Safety and Health Administration (OSHA) and safety needle devices have reduced dramatically the number of health care worker (usually nurses and laboratory technicians) needlestick injuries. Studies by the CDC indicate a 95% reduction in health care workers (HCWs) infected with hepatitis B (HBV) from needlesticks from 1983 to 2001; 400 HCWs were infected in 2001 compared with 17,000 in 1983 (CDC, 2011). This time period and statistics are significant because precautions related to bloodborne pathogens were initiated in the early 1980s. Current statistics indicate that the rate of HIV transmission to a health care worker from a needlestick is approximately 0.3% and 0.1% if contaminated blood is exposed to mucous membranes (i.e., the nose, eye, or mouth) of the health care worker. For hepatitis B, if the health care worker is not immunized the statistics indicate that the rate of transmission from a needlestick injury is 6% to 24% and 1% to 8% for hepatitis C (Stobart-Gallagher, 2017).

The National Institute for Occupational Safety and Health (NIOSH) focuses on safety and issues related to health. Identifying risks associated with the preparation of certain drugs and looking at ways to control exposure during preparation and administration is just one example of how this group works to ensure a safe health care environment for health care workers. The **Hazard Communication Act** of the **Occupational Safety and Health Administration (OSHA)** (a federal organization that provides guidelines to help reduce safety hazards in the workplace) requires health care facilities to inform employees about the presence of or potential for harmful exposures and how to reduce the risk of exposure. The **Centers for Disease Control and Prevention (CDC)** (a federal agency that provides facilities and services for the investigation, identification, prevention, and control of disease) also provides guidelines for working with infectious patients (e.g., standard precautions; see Chapter 7). Referring to this information and following recommended guidelines for reducing exposure to the variety of hazards present in the health care environment are the responsibility of the nurse.

FIRE SAFETY

In 2016 the National Fire Protection Association reported that from 2009 to 2013 fire departments in the United

States responded to 5650 health care facility structural fires; 65% of those were caused by cooking. Only 4% of health care facility fires spread beyond the room in which the fire originated. The reports indicate that 4 deaths and 160 injuries resulted from these fires (Campbell, 2017).

An established fire safety program is mandatory for all health care facilities (Box 10.9). Most facilities have a safety committee that is actively involved in establishing and monitoring prevention and fire education programs. Fire prevention includes good housekeeping, maintenance, and employee discipline (Box 10.10).

Box 10.9 Fire Safety Interventions and Safe Evacuation of Patients

ACTION *(RATIONALE)*

1. Follow facility fire plan in the event of a fire. *(Fire plan outlines procedures to follow.)*
   a. Ascertain patient's age, sensory impairments, level of mobility, ability to comprehend instructions, and overall need for protection. *(Protects and assists patient in interpreting environmental stimuli relevant to safety.)*
   b. If indicated, assess patients for type of evacuation assistance needed. *(Move individuals at risk for injury to a safer area.)*
   c. Provide clear explanations to patients and visitors in a calm manner. *(Anxiety hinders understanding of situation and ability to follow instructions.)*
   d. Assist with evacuations if needed:
      (1) Usually patients are moved horizontally (e.g., out of rooms, across halls, and through the next set of fire doors). *(The fire and its potential for spreading often necessitate movement to a safer area. Some agencies have fire doors that are normally held open by magnets and close automatically when a fire alarm sounds. It is important to keep equipment away from these doors.)*
      (2) If smoke or fire prevents you from moving patients across the hall, proceed vertically down to a lower level. **Never use elevators as an exit route. A fire spreads very quickly up through the elevator shaft.**
      (3) If a patient cannot walk or be moved by bed, stretcher, or wheelchair from the fire area, the patient often must be carried. (Use the carrying method that is safe for you and the patient; fire department personnel will help with the evacuation.)
      (4) Infant and child removal.
         (a) Place a blanket or sheet on floor.
         (b) Place two infants in each bassinet, using diapers or small blankets for padding.
         (c) Place the bassinet in the middle of the blanket.
         (d) Use the baby vest if available or fold the blanket over one end, fold the corners in, then roll the sides in to form a pocket.
         (e) Grasp the folded corners of the blanket and pull the infants to safety. Two people (or, if necessary, one person) are able to drag eight babies to the prescribed area.
         (f) Alternatively, place as many children as possible in one crib and pull the crib to the prescribed area.
      (5) Universal carry: The universal carry is a method of removing a patient from a bed to the floor. It is a quick and effective method for removing a patient who is in immediate danger. This carry can be used by anyone, regardless of patient size.
         (a) Spread a blanket, sheet, or bedspread on the floor alongside the bed, placing one-third of it under the bed and leaving about 8 inches to extend beyond the patient's head.
         (b) Grasp the patient's ankles, and move the patient's legs until they fall at the knee over the edge of the bed.
         (c) Grasp each shoulder, slowing pulling the patient to a sitting position.
         (d) From the back, encircle the patient with your arms, place your arms under the patient's armpits, and lock your hands over the patient's chest.
         (e) Slide the patient slowly to the edge of the bed, and lower the patient to the blanket. If the bed is high, instruct the patient to slide down one of your legs.
         (f) Taking care to protect the patient's head, gently lower the head and upper torso to the blanket and wrap the blanket around the patient.
         (g) At the patient's head, grip the blanket with both hands, one above each shoulder, holding the patient's head firmly in the 8 inches of blanket. Do not let the patient's head snap back.
         (h) Lift the patient to a half-sitting position, and pull the blanketed patient to safety.
      (6) Blanket drag: If vertical or downward evacuation by an interior stairway is necessary, in many cases one person can handle a helpless patient by using the blanket drag.
         (a) Double a blanket lengthwise, and place it on the floor parallel and next to the bed, leaving 8 inches to extend above the patient's head.
         (b) Using cradle drop, kneel drop, universal carry, or other suitable means, remove the patient from the bed to the folded blanket on the floor alongside the bed.
         (c) Grasp the blanket above the patient's head and pull to the stairway; start down the stairs with patient coming headfirst onto the stairway.
         (d) Position yourself one, two, or three steps lower than the patient, depending on your height and the patient's height. The patient's lower body inclines upward.

Box 10.9 Fire Safety Interventions and Safe Evacuation of Patients—cont'd

(e) Place your arms under the patient's arms, and clasp your hands over the patient's chest.
(f) Back slowly down the stairs, constantly maintaining close contact with the patient, keeping one leg against the patient's back.

(7) When considering the two-person swing, and all evacuation methods, take into consideration the patient's size and weight.
(a) Two staff members grasp each other's forearms to form a seat for the patient to sit in (Fig. 10.2A).
(b) Other personnel lift the patient into the seat formed and patient is removed from area (see Fig. 10.2B).

2. Follow-up
   a. Listen to the "All clear" announcement after a drill or follow specific instructions from the fire department or supervisor regarding the return of patients. ("This area is safe for patients and staff.")
   b. Reduce the potential for fire-related injuries by doing the following:
      (1) Follow and enforce the smoking policy. Most facilities have adopted a *No Smoking* policy to promote a smoke-free environment for patients and employees.
      (2) Know the location of fire alarm boxes and type of fire extinguishers available.
      (3) Know the location of the fire exits.
      (4) Be familiar with the hospital fire safety program and protocols for evacuation.
      (5) Keep hallways free of unnecessary supplies, furniture, and other obstacles.
      (6) Check to see that electrical equipment is operating safely. *(Planning saves valuable time and improves overall performance.)*
   c. Participate, when possible, in fire drills. Fire safety education programs are necessary to meet the requirements of accrediting agencies, such as The Joint Commission. *(Learning experiences are provided through participation in fire drills and formal critiques of the activity.)*
3. Evaluation
   a. The immediate environment of the patient is safe from potential fire hazards. *(Fire safety practices help prevent fires.)*
   b. In the event of a fire, established protocols are followed. *(The emergency will be handled rapidly and appropriately.)*

Box 10.10 Fire Prevention Guidelines for Nurses

- Keep the phone number for reporting fires visible on the telephone at all times.
- Know the agency's fire drill and evacuation plan.
- Know the location of all fire alarms, exits, and fire extinguishers.
- Use the mnemonic *RACE* to set priorities in case of fire:
  R Rescue and remove all patients in immediate danger.
  A Activate the alarm. Always do this before attempting to extinguish even a minor fire.
  C Confine the fire by closing doors and windows and turning off all oxygen and electrical equipment.
  E Extinguish the fire using an extinguisher.
- Memorize the mnemonic *PASS* to operate the fire extinguisher:
  P Pull the pin to unlock the handle.
  A Aim low at the base of the fire.
  S Squeeze the handle.
  S Sweep the unit from side to side.

Housekeeping responsibilities include eliminating all unnecessary combustible material; and maintenance responsibilities include ensuring the proper functioning of fire protection devices, such as alarms, extinguishers, and sprinklers. It is mandatory to identify, light, and unlock exits. Cooking and laundry equipment, filters, and air ducts are to be kept free of lint and grease. It is obligatory to inspect and maintain all mechanical and electrical equipment regularly to keep fire hazards to a minimum.

All employees need to know the telephone number or procedure for reporting a fire and the location of the nearest alarms and firefighting equipment. In addition, health care workers must know their roles in the overall hospital evacuation plan. Checking for fire hazards on an ongoing basis is a must.

An important element in any fire safety program is an understanding of what type of fire extinguisher to use on different types of fires. Use the appropriate fire extinguisher for each type of fire:

- Paper, wood, and cloth fires require a type A fire extinguisher.
- Flammable liquid fires, such as those caused by grease and anesthetics, require a type B fire extinguisher.
- Electrical fires require a type C fire extinguisher.
- Fire extinguishers marked ABC are acceptable for use on any type of fire.

Knowledge of which type of extinguisher is on the unit before a fire occurs is vital. Most fire safety programs afford health care workers the opportunity to handle the different types of fire extinguishers.

Certain areas of the health care facility require additional fire safety programs and precautions. Fire and smoke inhalation are potential problems associated with the use of lasers in surgery and with oxygen therapy. Other common ignition sources in the operating area are electric cautery equipment and high-intensity light cords. In the event of a fire, patients on life-support

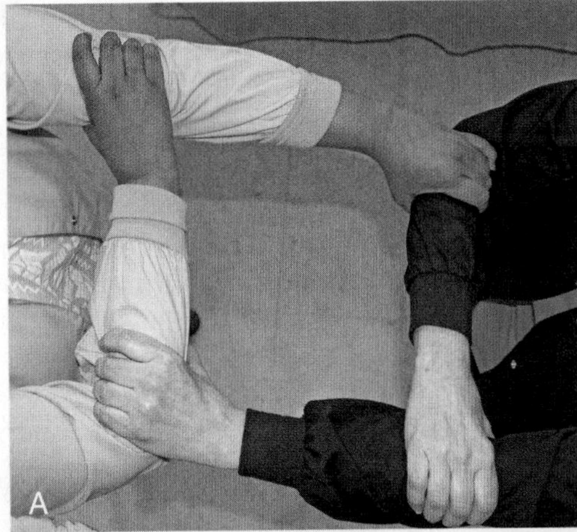

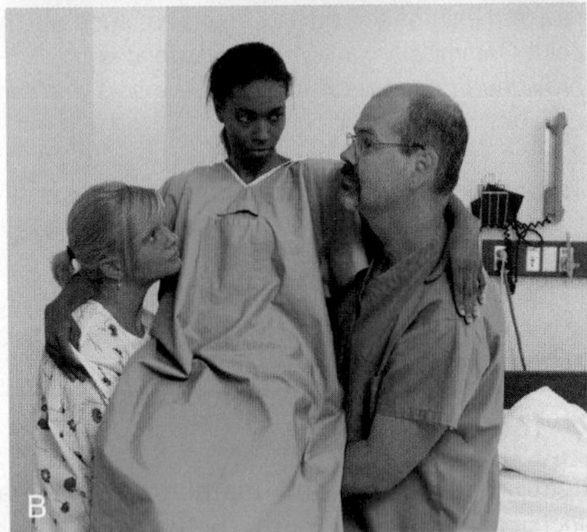

Fig. 10.2 The two-person evacuation carry. A, Hands positioned to form two-person evacuation swing. B, Patient is seated firmly on swing and holds nurses by shoulders for emergency evacuation.

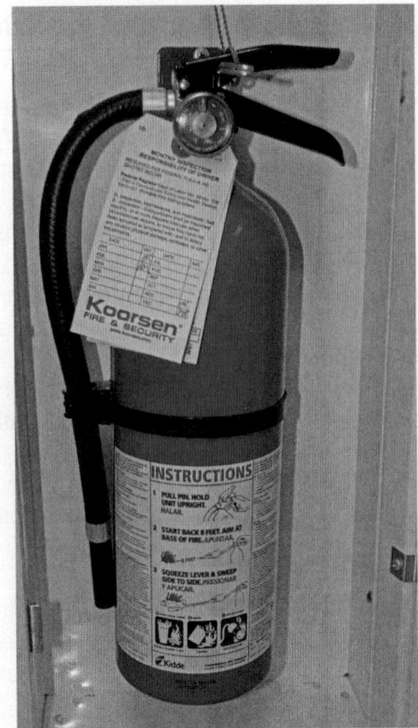

Fig. 10.3 Fire extinguisher.

systems may need manual respiratory support with an Ambu bag.

By remembering the mnemonic **RACE** (**R**escue patients, sound the **A**larm, **C**onfine the fire, and **E**xtinguish or **E**vacuate), the LPN/LVN is prepared when safety is threatened by fire. In the event of fire, rescue patients in *immediate* danger, and then follow the facility's procedure for activating the fire alarm and reporting the location and extent of the fire. Then take measures to contain or extinguish the fire if no immediate threat to safety exists. These measures include closing doors and windows, turning off oxygen and electrical equipment, and using the appropriate fire extinguisher (Fig. 10.3). The mnemonic **PASS** (**P**ull the pin, **A**im low, **S**queeze handle, **S**weep the unit) will help the nurse remember how to operate the fire extinguisher (see Box 10.10).

Enforcement of the facility's smoking policy and monitoring for potential electrical hazards help prevent fires. Frayed or broken electrical cords or a faulty piece of equipment should never be used. Notify the maintenance department of any defects in the equipment, and report any shocks felt while using equipment. The nurse must enforce no smoking policies. The safety of patients and caregivers depends on the staff's knowledge of fire prevention guidelines and fire procedures (see the Home Care Considerations box).

ACCIDENTAL POISONING

The CDC defines a **poison** as "any substance that is harmful to your body when ingested (eaten), inhaled, injected, or absorbed through the skin. Any substance can be poisonous if too much is taken." Poisoning (refers to the condition or physical state produced by the ingestion, injection, inhalation, or exposure of a poisonous [toxic] substance) continues to be an issue in the United States. According to the National Capital Poison Center the 2016 poison statistics show that 2.159 million Americans contacted poison control centers by phone. Of those calls 6.6 poison exposures/1000 population occurred with 41.3 poison exposures in children younger than 6 years/1000 children (Poison Control, 2016). Although legislation passed in the early 1970s required the use of child safety packaging for certain substances, a significant number of accidental poisonings continue to occur. Emergency department visits for medication poisoning are twice as common as household substance poisonings among children. Statistics for children under the age of 6 years for emergency department visits for accidental poisoning is 41.9 per 1000 children (Poison Control, 2016). Specific antidotes and treatments are now available for all types of poisons. Note that syrup of ipecac is no longer recommended for use (see the Patient Teaching box on nonuse of ipecac). The 2016 statistics from the CDC (2016) indicate that the 25-year to 64-year age group saw the highest death rate caused

 Home Care Considerations

Fire Safety

- Today, as more patients are discharged with follow-up care to be provided in the home, the nurse has an excellent opportunity to evaluate fire safety practices in the home environment. Patients who are elderly or who have mobility limitations often need your assistance to achieve an environment free of potential fire hazards.
- Give instructions about the proper use of monitoring or therapy equipment used.
- See that several electrical circuits are used to prevent overloading of any single one.
- Do not use electrical appliances and equipment near sinks, bathtubs, or showers.
- Review smoking practices, and give instructions to not smoke in bed or when sleepy.
- Do not permit smoking by the patient, family, or visitors in areas where oxygen is used.
- Advise against the use of electrical appliances (e.g., electric razors) around oxygen.
- Encourage the installation of fire alarms, smoke detectors, and carbon monoxide detectors and the purchase of a portable fire extinguisher.
- Have the family plan fire escape routes from each room and practice exit drills. Establish a place to meet outside to verify that everyone is safe.
- Teach *stop, drop,* and *roll* to extinguish fire on clothing.
- Do not place electrical cords under carpeting.
- Allow only certified electricians to work on wiring.
- Avoid using candles for light or heat, and never leave a burning candle unattended.

by unintentional poisonings. Ninety-one percent of all unintentional poisonings are related to drugs (over-the-counter and prescription).

 Patient Teaching

Nonuse of Ipecac at Home

According to the National Capital Poison Center:

- The American Academy of Pediatrics and the American Association of Poison Control Centers recommend that ipecac syrup not be kept in homes for available use.
- The US Food and Drug Administration (FDA) is considering making ipecac syrup available to the public by prescription only.
- Most pharmacies no longer carry ipecac syrup.
- The first action recommended in the event of ingestion of a poison is to call the poison control center at 1-800-222-1222.

From National Poison Control Center: *Ipecac syrup.* Retrieved from *www.poison.org/prepared/ipecac.asp*.

The older adult is also at risk. Changes associated with aging interfere with the individual's ability to absorb and excrete drugs. Some older adults share medications with friends or limit their medications because of the expense. Changes in eyesight sometimes lead to an accidental ingestion. If elderly patients have any memory impairment, they are likely to forget when they last took either prescribed or over-the-counter medication.

Hospitalized patients and those in other types of health care facilities are at risk for accidental poisoning because of poisonous substances in the environment. Cleaning solutions and disinfectants must be labeled and stored properly. To prevent poisoning, toxic agents are removed from areas where accidental poisoning is possible. Do not remove toxic or poisonous substances from their original containers because incorrect labeling is one of the likely results, and never use substances from unmarked containers.

Drugs are potentially hazardous if prepared or administered inappropriately. Human carelessness causes errors of both types. Always follow medication administration procedures (see Chapter 17). Be sure to attend staff in-service programs that present new drugs or provide updated information on frequently used drugs.

Poison control centers are valuable sources of information when poisoning occurs or is suspected. Nurses must ensure that the closest poison control center phone number is posted clearly in the patient's home and in the health care facility. Information received from the center helps in treatment and in referral. Most health care facilities also have posted instructions about how to handle poisoning cases (Box 10.11). Additional information on poisoning can be found in Chapter 16.

DISASTER PLANNING

Disaster planning, or emergency preparedness, enables rescuers to respond effectively and efficiently when confronted with a disaster situation. A **disaster situation** is an uncontrollable, unexpected, psychologically shocking event that is unique and likely to have a significant impact on a variety of health care facilities. Examples of natural threats to safety are earthquakes, hurricanes, floods, and tornados. Bombings, arson, riots, shootings, and hostage taking represent acts of violence carried out by people and do not always affect a facility's day-to-day operations.

Factors that affect disaster response include the time of the day; the scope and duration of the triggering event; readiness of the health care facility, personnel, and equipment; preparations for appropriate procedures; and the extent to which the various community agencies and institutions collaborate with one another. Health care facilities are expected to receive victims and survivors and to assist rescuers.

Disasters are referred to as external or internal. The external disaster originates outside the health care facility and results in an influx of casualties brought to the facility (e.g., an explosion in a chemical plant, a tornado, a train accident). The emergency department is the main

Box 10.11 Accidental Poisoning Interventions

ACTION *(RATIONALE)*

1. When a poisoning occurs:
   a. Obtain an accurate history. *(Identifies possible antidote[s] and method of treatment needed.)*
      (1) Identify the route (e.g., injected, ingested, inhaled), type, and amount of poisonous substance(s) received.
      (2) Determine how long ago the poisoning happened.
      (3) Obtain a history of allergies, prescribed medications, medical problems, and general state of physical and mental health.
   b. Assess for changes in mental status and the presence of motor and sensory deficits. *(Incomplete data possibly result in incorrect identification of patient's health needs.)*
   c. Notify the poison control center and follow facility protocols (see the Patient Teaching box on nonuse of ipecac). *(Treatment guidelines will be furnished.)*
   d. Do not induce vomiting if poisoning is related to the following substances: household cleaners, lye, furniture polish, grease, or petroleum products. *(Vomiting increases risk of internal burns.)*
   e. Do not induce vomiting in an unconscious individual. *(Vomiting increases danger of aspiration.)*
2. Perform hand hygiene. *(Reduces spread of microorganisms.)*
3. Document procedure. *(Note procedure and patient's response.)*
4. Follow-up
   a. Continue to monitor vital signs and response to treatment. *(Ongoing assessment is a part of the treatment.)*
   b. Reduce the potential for accidental poisoning by doing the following:
      (1) Be aware of potentially poisonous substances (e.g., drugs, plants, and cleaning solutions).
      (2) Inform patients and families about how to handle a poisoning emergency.
      (3) Ensure that poisonous substances are labeled, locked, and out of the reach of children. *(It is possible to greatly reduce the risk of accidental poisoning. Quick and appropriate action often decreases the effects of the poisoning.)*
   c. Know where emergency instructions are located. *(Procedures and guidelines for handling the emergency are outlined.)*
   d. Know the number of the poison control center (National Poison Control Center: 1-800-222-1222; *www.poison.org*) or call 911 and be prepared to provide information about the poison. *(The poison control center provides information needed to treat the patient, and all dispatchers offer referral assistance.)*
   e. The immediate environment is safe from potential poisoning hazards when poisonous substances are labeled, locked, and properly stored. *(Safety practices reduce the risk of accidental poisoning.)*

SPECIAL CONCERNS

- Always follow drug administration policies and procedures. Have your dosage calculations checked, especially if a mixed or prepared drug is to be infused.
- Keep informed of new medications and recommended dosages.
- Properly label and store cleaning solutions and disinfectants.
- Never use substances from unmarked containers.

focus of activity. Typically, no immediate safety threat to staff, patients, or hospital property exists.

The internal disaster represents an extraordinary situation that is brought about by events within the health care facility, such as a fire. In many cases, the organization's ability to function normally is threatened. An internal disaster has the ability to threaten the safety of patients, visitors, staff, and facility property.

Disaster planning consists of putting appropriate measures into place to ensure that health care facilities and personnel have the capacity to manage a disaster effectively (Boxes 10.12 and 10.13). Most state and federal regulators require health care personnel to conduct disaster drills on a routine basis to prepare to meet their responsibilities effectively. Personnel must be familiar with the location and the contents of the facility's **disaster manual** (sometimes called the Emergency Response Plan or Emergency Management Plan). This manual specifies chain of command, callback procedures, assignment procedure, departmental responsibilities, patient evacuation procedure and routes, procedures for the receipt and management of casualties, and policies related to the overall management of supplies and equipment.

Various **codes** (a system of notification to be transmitted rapidly) are used by health care facilities to alert personnel to the various emergencies affecting the facility. All personnel in a health care facility must be knowledgeable of the code system and how to act in response to codes.

TERRORISM

Terrorism or the possibility of a terrorist attack is viewed as an environmental health threat. **Terrorism** is a violent or dangerous act used to intimidate or coerce a person or government to further a political or social agenda. Before 1990 and the Gulf War, the possibility of the United States coming under attack from terrorist groups using biologic, chemical, or nuclear weapons seemed remote. After the terrorist attacks on the World Trade Center in New York City and the Pentagon on September 11, 2001, the government implemented the Homeland

Box 10.12 Disaster Planning Interventions

ACTION *(RATIONALE)*

1. **Planning**
   a. Review facility disaster plan frequently to update knowledge. The development of the disaster preparedness plan is an evolving and ongoing process. The purpose of disaster preparedness planning is to prepare the facility and health care workers for external and internal disasters. *(Information helps health care workers anticipate their roles in the event of a disaster.)*
   b. Know your own particular responsibilities in a disaster emergency. *(Valuable time is saved and overall performance improved.)*
   c. Participate, when possible, in disaster drills. Learning experiences are provided through disaster drills and formal critiques of the responses. *(Drills are helpful in evaluating the overall safety program and are required by accrediting agencies.)* Disaster drills may be initiated on a particular nursing unit, facility wide, community wide, or even statewide.
   d. Participation in a crisis support group is desirable if directly involved in a disaster or a disaster response. Individuals often experience some level of emotional or critical incident stress. *(Crisis support teams or groups encourage staff to share thoughts and feelings related to the experience [debriefing].)*
2. **Follow facility disaster plan in the event of a disaster.** *(Disaster plan outlines procedures to follow and is most effective when personnel respond appropriately.)*
   a. Identify the type of disaster emergency by recognizing the code that is used to announce it. *(Unfamiliarity with the codes tends to result in loss of valuable time and injury to patients or personnel.)*
   b. Identify each patient's age, sensory impairments, level of mobility, ability to comprehend instructions, and overall need for protection. *(Helps you to protect and assist patients in interpreting environmental stimuli relevant to safety.)*
   c. If indicated, assess patients for possible discharge or transfer. Protection of inpatients, and casualties from a disaster, is a top priority. *(Space may be needed for disaster victims.)*
   d. Provide clear explanations to patients and visitors in a calm manner. *(The amount of information patients and families have about the situation [drill, disaster event] affects their ability to cooperate and participate in any planned or unplanned activity.)*
   e. If a disaster occurs when you are off duty, follow your facility protocols for reporting in (i.e., some facilities require you to report for duty at your regularly scheduled times, whereas others require you to contact your manager for instruction). Community agencies and resources are incorporated into the overall plan. *(Additional personnel [e.g., student nurses and clinical faculty] in some cases assist with inpatient care to free staff for more critical disaster victims.)*
   f. If an internal disaster occurs, assist with planned evacuations as needed. *(Some disasters necessitate moving patients to a safer area.)*
   g. Listen for the "All clear" announcement after a disaster drill. *(This indicates that the drill is over.)*
3. **Evaluation.** Compare actual outcomes and performances with disaster preparedness plan (usually a critique session is held). *(Evaluation allows facility to examine whether plan accomplished goals and objectives; permits necessary changes to be made.)*

Box 10.13 Variations for Disaster Planning: Nursing Home

Nursing home residents also sometimes need evacuation and relocation in the case of an internal disaster. The successful nursing home disaster preparedness plan, like those for hospitals, outlines the sequence of events to be followed:

- Residents need some type of identification (picture identification or identification bracelet, such as those used in the memory support unit for patients diagnosed with Alzheimer's disease).
- At the designated triage site, nurses decide where residents will go.
- Residents sometimes need admission to a hospital or other building, such as a school or church, for temporary shelter and care.
- The disaster plan must include instructions and guidelines for what is to be done after the relocation is completed.
- Notification of families and physicians is critical.
- A log is kept to document events. List the name of the patient, who and how transported, and where patient was sent so family and physicians are aware of the patient's location and transfers as they occur.

Security Act of 2002. Its purpose was to have a single agency to oversee the development of a comprehensive approach to a large domestic incident. The Department of Homeland Security is concerned primarily with preventing and managing potential attacks by an individual or small group on one of our cities, a large sporting event, a school, or a unit of our military forces.

BIOTERRORISM

Bioterrorism is the use of biologic agents to create fear and to threaten. Health care facilities must be prepared to treat mass casualties from such an attack. A facility's emergency management plan provides details on how to respond to a terrorist attack: for example, determining the agent used, determining the time and location of the attack and the affected population, obtaining and delivering supplies, and providing treatment. Education and training is required to prepare nurses to respond to an attack by taking the necessary steps to initiate an agency's emergency management plan.

Bioterrorist Attacks

The nurse must be prepared to make accurate and timely assessments in any type of setting in the event of a bioterrorist attack. OSHA has health safety and topics information concerning the biologic agents plague, ricin, anthrax, tularemia, smallpox, and viral hemorrhagic fever (VHF). A bioterrorist attack may resemble a natural outbreak initially, but sometimes the microorganism used is modified to obtain increased virulence or have resistance to antibiotics or vaccines. Biologic attacks sometimes are *overt* (announced) and sometimes *covert* (unannounced). In the case of an overt attack, rapid assessment of its real scope is necessary, followed by an appropriate response. Covert attacks become obvious only after victims seek medical care, that is, after the incubation period has passed and clinical signs begin to appear. In both cases, the nurse must recognize and understand how to manage high-risk syndromes (groups of signs and symptoms that result from a common cause or appear together to present a clinical picture of a disease) (Box 10.14). Acutely ill patients representing

Box 10.14 High-Risk Syndromes for Bioterrorism

1. **Anthrax** (acute infectious disease caused by *Bacillus anthracis,* a spore-forming, gram-positive bacillus). Humans become infected through skin contact, ingestion, or inhalation. Person-to-person transmission of inhalational disease does not occur. Direct exposure to vesicle secretions of skin anthrax potentially results in secondary cutaneous infection.
   Clinical Features. Inhalation: Incubation period is usually less than a week but can be up to 2 months. Symptoms include flulike symptoms (e.g., low-grade fever, nonproductive cough, fatigue, diaphoresis) with possible brief interim improvement; within 2 to 4 days, abrupt onset of respiratory failure and hemodynamic collapse occur. Gram-positive bacilli are found on blood culture tests. *Cutaneous:* Local skin involvement is common on head, forearms, and hands; localized itching is followed by a papular lesion that becomes vesicular and within 2 to 6 days becomes a depressed black eschar. *Gastrointestinal:* Incubation period is usually 1 to 7 days and causes abdominal pain, nausea, vomiting, anorexia, and fever after eating contaminated food (usually meat); bloody diarrhea, hematemesis; gram-positive bacilli are found on blood culture. Abdominal pain becomes severe as symptoms progress.
2. **Botulism** (caused by *Clostridium botulinum,* an encapsulated anaerobic gram-positive, spore-forming bacterium that produces a potent neuroparalytic). Food-borne botulism is the most common form. Airborne and wound are other forms of botulism that may occur.
   Clinical Features. Food-borne botulism symptoms can occur within 6 hours to 10 days after exposure and cause abdominal cramping, diarrhea, and other gastrointestinal symptoms. Food-borne and inhalation botulism cause the following: drooping eyelids, weakened jaw clench, difficulty swallowing or speaking; blurred vision and double vision; symmetric paralysis of arms first, followed by respiratory muscles, then legs; respiratory dysfunction from respiratory muscle paralysis; *no sensory deficits or change in alertness or body temperature.* Neurologic symptoms often begin 12 to 36 hours after ingestion of food-borne botulism and 24 to 72 hours after inhalation of the airborne form. The disease is not transmitted from person to person.
3. **Plague** (an acute bacterial disease caused by the gram-negative bacillus *Yersinia pestis).* Bubonic plague occurs from a flea bite or through a break in the skin. A bioterrorism-related outbreak is likely to be airborne (pneumonic plague) and can spread among people via large aerosol droplets.
   Clinical Features. Features include fever, cough, headache, chest pain, weakness, hemoptysis, and mucopurulent or watery sputum with gram-negative rods in a Gram stain test. Pneumonia develops rapidly after exposure to the bacteria and may cause respiratory failure and death if early treatment is not initiated.
4. **Smallpox** (an acute viral illness caused by the variola virus). Disease has the potential to cause severe morbidity in a nonimmune population. Transmission via the airborne route is most common, but transmission can occur through direct contact. A single case of smallpox is a public health emergency.
   Clinical Features. Incubation period is 7 to 17 days, in which time the infected person is not contagious. Initial symptoms last 2 to 4 days and include fever, malaise, and myalgia (muscle aches). The symptoms then progress to a rash that starts on the tongue and in the mouth and throat. The rash progresses into pustules and spreads to the face and extremities (including palms and soles). During this time, the infected person is most contagious. The rash typically scabs over in 1 to 2 weeks. Smallpox is transmitted by large and small respiratory droplets. Patient-to-patient transmission is likely from airborne and droplet exposure and by contact with skin lesions or secretions.

Data from Centers for Disease Control and Prevention (CDC): *Bioterrorism agents/diseases.* Retrieved from *http://emergency.cdc.gov/agent/agentlist.asp#.*

the earliest cases after a covert attack usually seek care in emergency departments. Less ill patients or those at the onset stage of an illness sometimes seek care in primary care settings or try to manage the signs and symptoms on their own.

Basic epidemiologic (the distribution and determinants of health-related states and events in populations) principles are used to assess whether a patient's presentation of symptoms is typical of an **endemic** (the expected or normal incidence native to or occurring naturally to a specific area or environment) disease or is an unusual event that calls for investigation. The possibility of a bioterrorism-related outbreak should be considered if trends or events such as the following are observed:

- A rapidly increasing incidence of a disease (e.g., within hours or days) in a normally healthy population
- An unusual increase in the number of people seeking care, especially with fever or respiratory or gastrointestinal symptoms
- An **epidemic** disease, or a disease that emerges rapidly at an uncharacteristic time or in an unusual pattern
- Lower incidence among patients who had been indoors, in areas with filtered or closed ventilation, compared with people who had been outdoors
- Clusters of patients arriving from a single locale
- Large numbers of rapidly fatal cases
- Any patient with development of a disease that is relatively uncommon and has bioterrorism potential

The nurse must have the ability to recognize a casualty of a biologic attack and to carry out roles and responsibilities quickly and efficiently. Timely communication is critical for alerting the medical and the general community to a bioterrorist attack. Health care agencies' emergency plans outline the departments to contact in the event of an attack and who is responsible for reporting the suspected occurrence to the local public health authorities.

Infection prevention and control practices are critical in the event of a biologic attack. Manage all patients with suspected or confirmed bioterrorism-related illnesses with standard precautions (see Chapter 7). For certain diseases, such as smallpox or pneumonic plague, airborne and contact isolation precautions are needed. Although a number of infections associated with biologic agents are not transmissible from patient to patient, in general, be sure to limit the transport and movement of patients to what is essential for treatment and care. Also ensure that staff uses all safety precautions necessary to protect themselves and those in the immediate surroundings.

TERRORISM BY NUCLEAR EXPOSURE

One example of how the threat of nuclear terrorism possibly would manifest is an attack on a domestic nuclear weapon facility. Another is the use of a so-called "dirty bomb," which is a radiation-dispersal device that couples nuclear waste with a conventional bomb.

A patient is contaminated by radiation from a source on the body or the clothing, from ingesting it, or by absorbing it through a skin opening. The effects on the patient are determined by the amount of radiation absorbed (absorbed radiation is measured by the gray [Gy], equal to 100 rads). When less than 0.75 Gy is absorbed, patients usually do not have any symptoms. Patients who absorb 8 Gy usually die, and an absorption of 30 Gy is always fatal.

The patient who absorbs more than 0.75 Gy is at risk for development of acute radiation syndrome; the severity and nature of symptoms vary, depending on the amount of radiation absorbed:

- *Cerebrovascular and central nervous systems:* Cerebral edema, hyperpyrexia, hypotension, confusion, and disorientation.
- *Gastrointestinal:* Loss of mucosal barrier and cells that line the intestine, which results in fluid and electrolyte loss, vomiting, hematemesis, diarrhea, melena, loss of normal flora, and sepsis.
- *Hematopoietic:* Deficiency of white blood cells and platelets, which leads to bleeding, anemia, infections, impaired wound healing, and immunodeficiency.
- *Skin:* Loss of epidermis and possibly the dermis.

During the prodromal phase immediately after exposure, signs and symptoms in more than one of these areas typically appear. The latent phase, when all symptoms generally disappear for a few days to a few weeks, follows in 1 or 2 days. Then, in the illness phase, the signs and symptoms reappear and intensify. After this peak, the patient either begins to recover or dies. Death typically occurs from infection or other complications related to the exposure. OSHA requires that hospitals have an emergency plan for treating patients contaminated with radioactive substances. A decontamination unit is set up near the emergency department.

CHEMICAL TERRORISM

Chemical terrorism or exposure occurs by several different methods. Health care facilities have specific guidelines that must be followed in the event of patient exposure to chemical agents. Gross decontamination and formal and fine decontamination are methods that the nurse may be involved in implementing in the event of chemical exposure. *Gross decontamination* refers to a continuous shower of low-volume and high-volume water and removal of the patient's clothing. *Formal decontamination* and *fine decontamination* follow gross decontamination. Formal decontamination may incorporate several steps in the cleaning process, including water spray, cleaning solution, and scrubbing the patient with brushes. Fine decontamination is performed in specific isolated areas of the facility and includes cleaning of the eyes, ears, and fingernails and inspecting body orifices and swabbing mucous membranes of the nose and mouth (OSHA, n.d.).

The following are several types of agents that may possibly be used in chemical terrorism:

- *Pulmonary agents:* Include the gases chlorine (Cl), phosgene, ammonia, and hydrochloric acid. These agents cause shortness of breath, chest tightness, and wheezing and, in some cases, pulmonary edema. Symptoms sometimes take up to 2 to 24 hours to appear. Fluid in the lungs leads to hypovolemia and hypotension. Patients often need mechanical ventilation and supportive care.
- *Incapacitating agents:* Include 3-quinuclidinyl benzilate, a glycolate anticholinergic compound typically known by its NATO code *BZ* and *agent 15* (an Iraqi version of BZ). These agents impair rather than kill or seriously injure victims. The effects include decreased organ function, hyperthermia, hallucinations, altered perceptions, and erratic behavior.
- *Cyanide agents:* Hydrogen cyanide is one example; these agents form cyanide when metabolized and are either ingested or inhaled. A patient in severe respiratory distress without cyanosis has probably been exposed to cyanide. Cyanide has a pungent odor similar to bitter almonds or peaches. When an individual is exposed to a high concentration, death occurs within 5 to 10 minutes.
- *Nerve agents:* Taubin, sarin, soman, and V-agents are some of the most toxic nerve agents, and they cause death in a matter of minutes. Symptoms include increased saliva production, chest pressure, rhinorrhea, vomiting, muscle weakness, incontinence, and convulsions. Symptoms usually appear up to 10 hours after exposure to a low concentration.
- *Vesicant agents:* Sulfur mustard (H), distilled mustard (HD), nitrogen mustard (HN 1, 3), mustargen (HN 2), lewisite (L), and phosgene oxime (OX) are in this group. Vesicants are more lethal than pulmonary agents and cyanide agents because they sometimes remain in the environment for weeks, which results in a continuing source of exposure. Sulfur mustard smells like mustard or garlic, whereas another agent smells like geraniums, and yet another has a peppery smell. Vesicants affect the skin, the eyes, and the airway, and large doses damage the bone marrow. These agents have the capacity to cause the formation of vesicles that progress to severe tissue necrosis and sloughing. Symptoms of sulfur mustard exposure appear in 4 to 8 hours, but cellular damage occurs in 2 minutes with agents such as lewisite and phosgene.

❖ NURSING PROCESS FOR PATIENT SAFETY

The role of the LPN/LVN in the nursing process as stated is that the LPN/LVN will:

- Participate in planning care for patients based on patient needs.
- Review patient's plan of care and recommend revisions as needed.
- Review and follow defined prioritization for patient care.
- Use clinical pathways, care maps, or care plans to guide and review patient care.

◆ ASSESSMENT

Using the nursing process, the LPN/LVN can reduce the risk of injury to patients and staff. Seek to determine which patients are at risk for injury as soon as possible. Identify actual and potential threats to the patient's safety, the effect of the underlying illness on the patient's safety, and the risks for the patient's developmental stage. Specific interventions help ensure a safe environment. If safety is threatened, follow established guidelines to resolve the situation (Nursing Care Plan 10.1).

◆ PATIENT PROBLEMS

Identification of defining characteristics from the data directs the LPN/LVN's efforts to identify appropriate patient problems. Include specific causes of a patient's safety risk among the patient problems to individualize nursing care. For example, a patient with an unsteady gait is at risk for falling or injury. Patient problems related to patient safety could include the following:

- *Compromised Physical Mobility*
- *Potential for Falling*
- *Potential for Harm or Damaage to the Body*

◆ EXPECTED OUTCOMES AND PLANNING

In the plan of care, identify nursing interventions that prevent threats to safety and meet safety needs. Perform planning and goal setting with the patient, the family, and other members of the health care team. Goals and priorities are based on the risk to patient safety and health promotion. The overall goal for a patient with a threat to safety is remaining free from injury (see (Nursing Care Plan 10.1).

◆ IMPLEMENTATION

Nursing interventions are designed to promote the safety of the patient in the home and the health care setting. These interventions include health promotions, developmental considerations, environmental protection, and education of family members or patient caregivers (see (Nursing Care Plan 10.1).

◆ EVALUATION

Evaluate nursing interventions for reducing threats to safety by comparing the patient's response to the expected outcomes for each goal of care. Assess patient for signs and symptoms of injury and assess the environment for physical hazards continually throughout hospitalization. Remove the hazards and modify the environment as necessary.

Observe for correct application of SRDs. Observe skin, monitor pulses, assess the restrained body part every 30 minutes, and release the restrained body part every 2 hours. Continuously monitor for complications of immobility.

 Nursing Care Plan 10.1 **Patient Safety**

This care plan has been adapted for the patient who is at risk for injury.

PATIENT PROBLEM

Potential for Harm or Damage to the Body, related to disease process, weakness, lack of mental acuity, medications, or age

Patient Goals and Expected Outcomes	Nursing Interventions	Evaluation
Patient or caregiver will demonstrate knowledge and understanding of potential hazards and will practice preventive measures or will be protected from injury as necessary during hospitalization	Assess the following: 1. Patient's mental, visual, and auditory acuity (fall assessment, see Box 10.2). 2. Patient's level of consciousness. 3. Patient's ability to perform activities of daily living (ADLs), exercise, and ambulation. Prevent clutter; wipe up spills; provide adequate lighting. Orient patient to surroundings and assess effectiveness of reality orientation. Maintain side rails (depending on facility policy) and bed alarm. Maintain bed in low position when care is not being given. Place patient in room close to nurses' station. Assist patient with ADLs as needed. Determine the need for assistive devices such as a walker, cane, or wheelchair. Obtain medication history and administer medications according to agency policy. Document nursing interventions for medications and monitor side effects. Offer fluids q 2 hr while awake unless contraindicated. Offer use of commode, bedpan, or urinal q 2 hr while awake.	Patient demonstrates understanding of potential health hazards. Patient practices injury prevention for self. Patient remains injury free.

CRITICAL THINKING QUESTIONS

1. The nurse walking down the hall hears a patient calling out for help. The nurse assesses the situation and realizes that the patient does not remember how to use the call light. What factors possibly contribute to the patient's inability to remember, and how should the nurse teach the patient to use the call light?
2. The nurse enters the patient's room to answer the call bell and sees the patient frantically pointing to the trash can next to the bed. The nurse smells smoke and sees small flames. What should be done to help prevent fires, and what should the nurse do in this situation?

Get Ready for the NCLEX® Examination!

Key Points

- Discuss safety measures for coping with violence in the workplace.
- Prevention of falls, electrical injuries, fires, burns, and accidental poisoning is key to maintaining a safe environment.
- Infants, young children, older adults, and the ill or injured patient are at risk for falling.
- Proper patient orientation includes information about the use of the call light and bed controls. Place frequently used items within reach of patients.
- Question all patients regarding allergies. Ask specifically about food and latex allergies.
- Keep adjustable beds in the low position except when care is given.
- Gait belts are an added safety feature to use when assisting patients to ambulate.
- Consider designing a restraint-free environment before applying an SRD.
- Ensure your priority is patient safety or the safety of others when applying an SRD.
- SRD use has the potential to result in increased restlessness, disorientation, agitation, anxiety, and feelings of powerlessness.
- Once SRDs are applied to a patient, document the position of the device, circulation, physical and mental status, and ongoing need for the device.
- When extremity SRDs are applied, place gauze or padding around the extremity and secure the ends of the ties to the bed frame, not to the side rails.
- Remove SRDs at least every 2 hours and assess the skin. Do not leave the patient unattended during this time.
- Know agency policy and procedures regarding SRD use and documentation.
- Electrical accidents often are prevented by reporting frayed or broken electrical cords or any shocks felt when using equipment.
- Fire-related injuries can be reduced by knowing the location of exits, fire alarm boxes, and fire extinguishers.
- By remembering the mnemonic RACE (**R**escue patients, sound the **A**larm, **C**onfine the fire, and

Extinguish or **E**vacuate), you will be prepared when safety is threatened by a fire.

- Participation in fire and disaster drills helps staff become familiar with established protocols.
- Poison control centers are valuable sources of information when poisoning is suspected or has occurred.
- A terrorist attack is a potential environmental health threat.
- Bioterrorism, or the use of biologic agents to create fear and threat, is the most likely form a terrorist attack will take.
- Several national organizations, including OSHA, NIOSH, and the CDC, provide guidelines that help reduce safety hazards in the workplace.

Additional Learning Resources

SG Go to your Study Guide for additional learning activities to help you master this chapter content.

evolve Be sure to visit the Evolve site at *http://evolve.elsevier.com/Cooper/foundationsadult/* for additional online resources.

Review Questions for the NCLEX® Examination

1. The nurse is caring for a patient on a ventilator and reads the order "restrain prn." The nurse considers which factor when caring for this patient? *(Select all that apply.)*
   1. SRDs often decrease anxiety because the patient feels safer.
   2. All older adult patients need some type of SRD at night.
   3. Allow as much freedom of movement as possible when applying SRDs.
   4. When using soft SRDs to prevent pulling of the ventilator tubing, tie them to the side rail.
   5. Ensure that the nurse's two fingers can be inserted between the SRD and the patient's skin.
2. The LPN/LVN is reviewing the care plan of the patient who has an SRD applied for personal safety. Which is the highest priority goal for this patient?
   1. Patient will remain free of injury.
   2. Patient will allow SRDs to be used.
   3. Nurse will check SRD every 30 minutes.
   4. Use least restrictive form of SRD possible.
3. The nurse is documenting on a patient with an SRD. What information must the nurse include in this documentation?
   1. The nurse's feelings about having used the SRD.
   2. The specific type of SRD used and assessment of the patient.
   3. Confirmation of a prn order for use of the SRD.
   4. Evidence that the patient was assessed every 8 hours.
4. When caring for the patient who requires the use of an SRD, what should be included in the patient's plan of care? *(Select all that apply.)*
   1. Monitor the skin for signs of impairment.
   2. Remove the SRD once every 2 hours.
   3. Secure the ends of the ties to the side rails.
   4. Ensure that the SRD is in place at all times.
   5. Reevaluate the need for the SRD frequently.
5. The nurse discovers smoke in a soiled utility room across the hall from a patient's room. What should the nurse's initial action be?
   1. Sound the fire alarm.
   2. Disconnect the oxygen supply.
   3. Use any extinguisher on the fire.
   4. Remove the patient from the area.
6. The nurse is observing the UAP who is assisting a resident in a long-term care facility ambulate with a gait belt. Which action by the UAP indicates to the nurse that further instruction is necessary? *(Select all that apply.)*
   1. The UAP loosely fastens the gait belt around the patient's waist.
   2. The UAP places the gait belt on the resident before assisting the resident to a standing position.
   3. The UAP grasps the gait belt while assisting the resident out of bed.
   4. The UAP fastens the belt around the arm of the chair to prevent the resident from slipping out of the chair.
   5. The UAP explains to the resident that the gait belt is used to prevent injury to the resident and the UAP when assisting with ambulation.
7. A type C fire extinguisher is required for which type of fire?
   1. Paper
   2. Cloth
   3. Grease
   4. Electrical
8. When the staff's knowledge of the fire safety precautions is assessed, which action indicates the need for further fire safety instruction? *(Select all that apply.)*
   1. Fire exits and corridors are kept clear.
   2. A *No Smoking* sign is posted when oxygen is in use.
   3. A heating pad cord is taped when a frayed area is noted.
   4. Facility smoking policies are a part of the admission procedure for patients.
   5. An UAP evacuated critically ill patients on the elevator during a fire drill.
9. The home health nurse is assessing a child for the risk of injury. Which factor places a child at greatest risk for specific types of injuries?
   1. Gender of the child
   2. Overall health
   3. Educational level
   4. Developmental level

10. During the 7 a.m. to 3 p.m. shift on the adult surgical unit, the code is announced for an external disaster emergency. Which event best represents this type of situation?
1. A school bus accident
2. A bomb threat in the mail room
3. A hostage-taking event in the emergency department
4. An electrical fire in the maintenance department

11. The nurse is providing home poison control instruction to the parent of a 2-year-old boy. Which statement by the parent indicates the need for further teaching?
1. "I will call the national poison control center if my child ingests a poisonous substance."
2. "I will call 911 immediately if my child ingests medication that is not intended for him."
3. "Child safety caps on household cleaner can still be opened by some children."
4. "I will give my child syrup of ipecac if he ingests a poisonous substance that is not caustic."

12. An adult patient is brought to the emergency department for treatment of an unintentional poisoning. What is the nurse's first action in caring for this patient?
1. Induce vomiting.
2. Assess the patient.
3. Place the patient in an upright position.
4. Notify the poison control center.

13. The home health nurse is visiting an older adult patient and her husband. What safety concern is of the highest priority when the nurse is assessing this patient's home environment?
1. Accidental poisoning
2. Electrical shock
3. Accidental falls
4. Thermal burns

14. The LPN/LVN is reviewing the admission information of a patient. Which information is of most concern to the nurse that this patient is at high risk for falling?
1. The patient has diabetes.
2. The patient had a stroke 3 years ago with no complications.
3. The patient becomes disoriented in the evening hours.
4. The patient wears eyeglasses and a hearing aid.

15. The occupational health nurse learns of a mercury spill that occurred in the factory in which she is employed. Which action by the nurse is correct?
1. The nurse cleans the mercury spill with alcohol and ordinary cleaning cloths.
2. The nurse closes all windows and doors to prevent the mercury spill from spreading out of the area.
3. The nurse instructs the housekeeping staff to vacuum up the spill.
4. The nurse evacuates the area and contacts trained personnel to clean up the spill.

11 Admission, Transfer, and Discharge

http://evolve.elsevier.com/Cooper/foundationsadult/

Objectives

1. Identify guidelines for admission, transfer, and discharge of a patient.
2. Discuss the concepts of the Health Insurance Portability and Accountability Act (HIPAA).
3. Describe common patient reactions to hospitalization.
4. Identify nursing interventions for common patient reactions to hospitalization.
5. Discuss the nursing process and how it pertains to admitting, discharging, and transferring the patient.
6. Discuss the nurse's responsibilities in performing an admission.
7. Describe how the nurse prepares a patient for transfer to another unit or facility.
8. Discuss discharge planning.
9. Explain how the nurse prepares a patient for discharge.
10. Identify the nurse's role when a patient chooses to leave the hospital against medical advice.

Key Terms

admission (p. 260)
against medical advice (AMA) (p. 275)
continuity of care (p. 269)
discharge (p. 269)
discharge planning (p. 269)
disorientation (dĭs-ŏr-rē-ĕn-TĀ-shŭn, p. 260)
empathy (ĔM-pă-thē, p. 261)
health care facility (p. 260)
home health agency (p. 273)
separation anxiety (p. 260)
third-party payers (p. 269)
transfer (p. 268)

COMMON PATIENT REACTIONS TO ADMISSION TO A HEALTH CARE FACILITY

Admission (entry of a patient into the health care facility) to a hospital or other **health care facility** (any agency that provides health care) is an anxious time for patients and their families. The patient usually is concerned about health problems or possible health problems and the potential outcome of treatment. Often the patient is having pain or other discomfort. The first contact with nurses and health care workers is important. It provides an opportunity to lessen anxiety and fears and initiate a positive attitude regarding the care to be received.

A way to significantly ease the patient's anxiety and promote cooperation and positive response to treatment is to convey concern for the patient while implementing efficient admission routines. Admission routines that the patient perceives as careless or excessively impersonal tend to heighten anxiety, reduce cooperation, impair response to treatment, and possibly aggravate symptoms.

The nurse's responsibility is to assist the patient in maintaining dignity and a sense of control and in becoming comfortable in the new environment of the health care facility. This environment differs from a patient's home and has new sights, sounds, and smells that may interfere with the patient's comfort.

Each person's reaction to admission to a health care facility is unique. Some common reactions include fear of the unknown, loss of identity, **disorientation** (mental confusion characterized by inadequate or incorrect perception of place, time, and identity), **separation anxiety** (fears and apprehension caused by separation from familiar surroundings and significant people), and loneliness. These reactions are related to some of the needs described by Maslow (1970) (see Fig. 1.8).

Fear of the unknown, which causes insecurity, is often the most common reaction. This relates to the need Maslow calls safety. Explanations about facility policies, information about medical orders and procedures, and simple direct answers to common questions from the patient or family help the person feel more comfortable and in control of the situation. Questions the patient may have include: "How do I work the bed?"; "How do I call the nurse?"; "How or when do I get some food?"; "When can my family visit?"; and "What are they going to do to me next?" Orienting the patient to the new environment and answering these simple questions can alleviate much of the fear and anxiety felt by the patient on admission to the facility.

During the admission process to a health care facility, many patients feel a loss of identity that reflects a need for esteem, love, and belonging. Recognition, as described by Maslow, is part of this need. Sometimes putting the identification (ID) band on the patient's wrist reduces the patient to feeling like the number and name on the ID rather than a person. Explain that the ID is a necessary procedure to provide a positive means of identification and maintain the safety of the patient.

Learn new patient names quickly. Address patients with Mr., Mrs., Ms., or Miss with the last name, and only use a first name at the patient's request. Use of terms such as "honey," "dear," "Gramps," and "Grandma" is never appropriate.

 Lifespan Considerations

Older Adults

Admission, Transfer, and Discharge

- The older adult admitted to the health care facility today is likely to be seriously ill.
- In a normally alert and oriented older adult, medical conditions that necessitate admission to a health care facility often result in some level of disorientation.
- Older adults, who often have some limitation of vision or hearing, are more likely to become agitated or fearful on admission to a health care facility. Many experience relocation stress.
- Transfers, even within the facility, tend to be confusing and upsetting to older adults.
- Hospitalized older adults frequently are concerned that they will be unable to return to their homes and will need institutional placement.
- Appropriate referrals for home nursing, therapy, homemaking, home nutrition programs, or other services are essential for older adults.
- Older adult patients need health care professionals to converse with them slowly and clearly because hearing may be less acute and information may take longer to process. Do not rush older patients; wait for patients to answer questions rather than letting family members answer.
- The change in environment and daily routine sometimes causes disorientation, loss of appetite, or reversal of sleeping-waking patterns.
- The stress of being in a health care facility sometimes is serious for the older patient because of a reduction in adaptive capacity. Helplessness, lack of control, and dependency often emerge, although a large degree of personal control possibly can be restored.
- When an older adult patient is transferred to a new facility, the relocation is also stressful. Ensure that significant support people are still accessible, the patient is oriented thoroughly to new surroundings, the patient is allowed to take along important memorabilia, and the patient has an opportunity to make decisions about care.

Separation anxiety and loneliness are reactions that reflect the needs Maslow identified as belongingness and love. Separation anxiety is very common in young children, but adults and older adults often have this reaction as well. In children, it generally is expressed by crying; with adults, behaviors may include the patient being withdrawn or being very talkative; the older adult sometimes exhibits disorientation or depression.

The company of friends and loved ones is the best antidote to separation anxiety. Liberal visiting hours in health care facilities encourage family and friends to visit. Many facilities allow small children to visit relatives (facility policy and the patient's condition must be considered). Parents should be encouraged to stay with their hospitalized child to prevent the anxiety separation causes and to give the child a feeling of security. In some facilities, pets are allowed to visit. Many long-term facilities have pet therapy visits from organizations or actually have pets that live in the facility.

The licensed practical/vocational nurse (LPN/LVN) has the ability to help reduce the severity of these common reactions to hospitalization with a warm, caring attitude and with courtesy and **empathy** (ability to recognize and to some extent share the emotions and state of mind of another and to understand the meaning and significance of that person's behavior). To help patients adapt, treat them with respect; maintain their dignity; involve them in the plan of care; and whenever possible, adjust facility routines to meet their desires. Special considerations for the older adult are listed in the Lifespan Considerations for older adults box.

CULTURAL CONSIDERATIONS FOR THE HOSPITALIZED PATIENT OR LONG-TERM CARE RESIDENT

If the patient does not speak English and is not accompanied by a bilingual family member on admission, contact the appropriate resource (usually the social services department) to secure an interpreter. Culture plays a vital role in the patient's ability to cope with stress and illness. Assist the patient with maintaining cultural practices as much as possible (see Chapter 6 for an in-depth discussion of cultural issues in health care).

ADMITTING A PATIENT

The admission procedure generally begins in the admitting department. The admission department representative is responsible for obtaining vital information from the patient, such as demographic information, insurance information, identifying information (social security number), and emergency contacts. Privacy and confidentiality must be maintained while this information is obtained. An interpreter should be used if the patient does not speak English. Depending on the facility and the time of admission, the collection of this information may become the responsibility of the nurse.

Once the necessary identifying information has been collected, an ID band is placed on the patient's wrist. The ID band usually contains the patient's full name

Cultural Considerations

Admission, Transfer, and Discharge

- It should be noted that any reference to cultural practices among a specific culture are commonalities. Individuals within a culture may or may not possess the same practices, beliefs, or values.
- Consider the decision-making process of the family. Some patients may need extra time for decisions regarding care and procedures if the family unit is important in this process. Other patients may refer to whomever is the authority figure for decision making.
- Appalachians (found chiefly in the Eastern and some Southern states) often intertwine religion and culture; therefore, in the interests of cultural sensitivity, include the assessment of the patient's religious beliefs on admission to the health care system. Because some Appalachians tend to be fundamental and fatalistic in their religious beliefs, this belief must be considered an influencing variable.
- Chinese Americans often value personal relationships over rules and procedures. Be sure to consider the importance of the patient's loved ones when planning care.
- Many Haitians believe that leaves have a special significance in healing. The nurse may sometimes find leaves in the clothes and on various parts of the body. Leaves are thought to have mystical power related to regaining or keeping health.
- Some Haitian American patients are more likely to feel they are receiving effective treatment when a nurse is seen. In some Haitian cultures, a nurse is given more authority and status than a physician, and the patient may be more cooperative with directions given by a nurse. When nursing measures are implemented (e.g., taking the patient's blood pressure), tell the patient what you are doing and that it is for the patient's benefit. Nursing actions are seen as caring and helpful.
- Some Haitian Americans associate wheelchairs with sickness. Therefore the patient who is allowed to walk out of the hospital at discharge is more likely to feel that care has been effective.
- A traditional Japanese belief is that contact with blood, skin disease, and corpses causes illness. Some Japanese also believe improper care of the body, including poor diet and lack of sleep, causes illness.
- Orthodox Jewish patients observe sundown Friday to sundown Saturday as the Sabbath, which is a time of rest. These patients may avoid the use of any electronic equipment during that time, so the nurse should find alternatives to the use of this equipment if possible.

and date of birth. Some facilities may assign a facility number that also is included on the ID band. Patient allergies typically are identified on a separate red wrist band. This information should be checked and verified by looking at the ID band and asking the patient to state this information (if capable) before procedures and medication administration. Identification of the patient who is unconscious on admission to the facility is delayed until a family member or legal guardian is present.

On admission to a health care facility, the patient signs a consent form that gives permission for general treatment. The Joint Commission and Medicare and Medicaid Services require that all hospitals and other health care facilities present a Patient's Bill of Rights to the patient or the patient's legal guardian at the time of admission. Facilities also may have other written forms that are presented, which contain policies and procedures that further inform patients of their rights and of the nurse's responsibilities in ensuring these rights are honored.

The Patient Self-Determination Act of 1991 and the Health Insurance Portability and Accountability Act (HIPAA) also are presented on admission to a health care facility. Facilities that accept Medicare and Medicaid reimbursement are required to present information on The Patient Self-Determination Act. It addresses the patient's right to refuse or accept medical treatment and information regarding advance directives. The facility must refer the patient who requests information about advance directives to the appropriate resources. All patients, regardless of the type of health care facility, must be given and sign a document that verifies receipt of information regarding HIPAA (see Chapter 2 for an explanation of HIPAA).

Some hospitals or surgery centers have telephone admitting. The day before a planned admission, a representative from the admitting office calls the patient at home and gathers all the information needed to begin the records. Instructions are given regarding time to arrive at the facility, items to bring to the facility, and items that are better to leave at home (e.g., jewelry and large sums of money). When the patient arrives the next day, the records and ID band must be verified with the patient for accuracy.

People brought to the emergency department of a hospital sometimes are admitted directly to a patient care room or a special care unit (SCU), intensive care unit (ICU), coronary care unit (CCU), or burn unit. In these situations, a family member, usually the next of kin or the patient's health care representative, provides the admitting office with the necessary information.

When the unit staff are notified that a new patient is en route, they prepare the room for admission of the patient. A room that is neat and clean, of appropriate temperature, with lighting and personal care items in place, makes the patient feel expected and welcome. This makes a good first impression and facilitates the development of a therapeutic nurse-patient relationship.

If special equipment is needed by the new patient, such as oxygen, have it in place and ready when the patient arrives. A patient who arrives on a stretcher needs the bed in the high position; the low bed position is best for a patient who arrives by wheelchair or walking.

Greeting the patient by name and making the patient feel welcome is one of the most important aspects of

Box 11.1 Patient Room Orientation

Orientation should include the following:
- Explanation of policies applicable to the patient
- How to adjust the bed and the lights
- How to call the nurse from the bed and the bathroom
- How to operate the telephone and the radio
- How to operate the television
- How to use the intercom system if one is present
- The location of lounge areas
- The location of shower and bathroom facilities
- The relationship of the room to the nurses' station

the admission procedure. Call patients by their surname unless otherwise directed by the patient. To introduce yourself, give your first name and title. A person who is warmly welcomed is more at ease in this new environment.

Remember that patients do not get ill and need hospitalization at the nurse's convenience. The patient's admission to the unit may occur at any time. Regardless of the time or the activity occurring on the nursing unit, the staff must be courteous to, interested in, and receptive of the new patient. The new patient needs an orientation to the unit and the room (Box 11.1).

The routine of the facility must be explained to the patient and family. Knowledge of when meals are served (or in some facilities the time frame for the patient to call the dietary department to order food to be delivered), when family and friends are allowed to visit, when laboratory tests or diagnostic imaging evaluations are scheduled, when the health care provider usually makes rounds, and the policy on side rails gives the patient a sense of security and lessens anxiety. Many facilities have booklets for patients that explain these routine activities so that patients have a reference for this information. Some booklets include information about the availability of various social services, religious services, and facilities such as cafeteria, library, and gift shop. Some degree of patient teaching also may occur during the admission process (see the Patient Teaching box).

The electronic health record (EHR) may expedite the admission process in the admitting department and on the nursing unit. Information in the EHR is transferred into the admission form used by the admitting department and the nursing admission form. The admission department and the admitting nurse must verify information found in the EHR with the patient to verify that the data are current and accurate. This time-efficient practice benefits staff and the patient.

The admitting procedure on the patient care unit is much more extensive than that in the admitting department (Skill 11.1). Check the ID band and verify the information with the patient. Assess immediate needs such as pain, shortness of breath, or severe anxiety, and report the results. If another patient is in the room, introduce the two patients.

Patient Teaching

Patient Admission to the Health Care Facility

- Some teaching occurs during the admission process. The nurse provides information regarding physical assessment findings, planned diagnostic procedures, and facility routines. A formal teaching plan does not begin until assessment is completed and a care plan is developed.
- In an emergency situation, instruct family members on the rationale for any procedures and routines to expect in the patient's care.
- Teaching begins early in a patient's admission to a facility. Introduce instruction when the patient is able to be attentive and learn from the information. This is sometimes difficult in an acute care setting. Keep information specific, and focus on topics such as nature of the patient's illness, medications needed for treatment, and use of equipment in self-care (e.g., dressing, ambulatory devices).
- Explain shift times and shift changes to the patient.
- Consider how hospitalization influences an adult patient's occupational status. Will the illness seriously delay work that the patient is assigned to complete? Will there be a considerable delay before the patient can return to work?
- Confirm the patient's understanding of transfer and procedures through discussion and questions. Explain the reason for the transfer, the time it is to occur, and what procedures are planned.
- Be prepared to repeat information and instructions to the patient and significant others during the transfer of a patient because transfers often elicit feelings of anxiety.
- Before the patient leaves the facility, provide for return demonstration of any skills taught.
- Patients who have short stays in health care facilities often do not receive teaching until the day of discharge.
- Anticipation of some prescriptions is not always possible. The day of discharge is sometimes the only opportunity to teach patient about medications. Some facilities have standardized information material that provides specific information about individual medications (see Fig. 11.4).
- Obtain the help of social services or discharge planners to ensure the transfer of a patient to a long-term care facility or home care agency is appropriate in meeting the patient's physical and mental needs.

Encourage the patient to give jewelry, money, and medications to the family to take home as long as the patient feels comfortable with doing so. If no family member is present, valuables are placed in the facility safe. Carefully follow the facility policy for patient valuables. Loss of a patient's valuables incurs serious legal implications for the nurse and the facility. Documentation of disposition of valuables must be in the medical record. In an Alzheimer's unit of a long-term care facility or in a mental health unit, the facility does assume some responsibility for patient belongings because the patient

Skill 11.1 Admitting a Patient

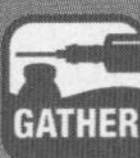

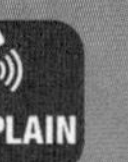

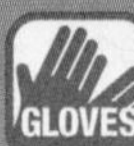

NURSING ACTION *(RATIONALE)*

1. Perform hand hygiene. *(Reduces spread of microorganisms.)*
2. Prepare the room before the patient arrives: care items in place; bed at proper height and open; light on. *(This makes patient feel expected and welcome.)*
3. Courteously greet the patient and family. Introduce yourself. Project interest and concern. Introduce roommate. *(The patient and family are more at ease when they know the people around them.)*
4. Check the ID band and verify its accuracy. *(Ensures identification before tests or surgery are performed or medication is given. In long-term care facilities, the residents may not wear ID bands. A picture of the resident is used for identification purposes.)*
5. Assess immediate needs. *(Establishes trust when needs are recognized and met.)*
6. Orient the patient to the unit, the lounge, and the nurses' station. *(Promotes safety.)*
7. Orient the patient to the room. Explain the use of equipment, call system, bed, telephone, and television. *(Allows the patient some control over the environment and promotes safety.)*
8. Explain facility routines, such as visiting hours and meal times. *(Decreases fear of unknown and gives a feeling of security.)*
9. Provide privacy if the patient desires or if abuse is suspected. Family members are sometimes asked to leave the room. *(This allows the patient to answer questions openly and honestly without fear of the family member hearing the answers.)* Admission of an infant or small child requires emotional support for child and parents. Parents generally are encouraged to stay with their child to prevent separation anxiety. The most reliable source of admission information is the parent. Assist the patient to undress if necessary. *(Helps maintain dignity and shows respect for the patient. Helping the patient undress prevents fatigue and falls. Provides opportunity to assess range of motion and the skin.)*
10. Follow facility policy for care of valuables, clothing, and medications. *(Helps prevent loss of valuables, clothing, or medications, which is disturbing to the patient and family and potentially results in legal problems.)*
11. Obtain the patient's health history and perform the initial nursing assessment. *(Provides a basis for individualized care.)* When a patient is admitted in critical condition, only the most pertinent information must be collected immediately. The remaining information can be obtained later. Young children are very curious about what is happening to them and the environment around them. Encourage the child to use equipment on dolls to help reduce anxieties. Encourage children to express how they feel. Invasive procedures (e.g., obtaining blood specimens, starting intravenous lines) generally are performed best in a treatment room. *(Enables children to perceive their room as a safe area.)*
12. Provide for safety: bed in low position, side rails up (unless admission is to a long-term care facility), call light within easy reach. *(Promotes patient safety.)*
13. Begin care as ordered by the health care provider. *(The patient and family develop a positive attitude about the institution when care is started immediately.)*
14. Invite family back into the room if they left earlier. *(Decreases family anxiety when they observe the patient is settled.)*
15. Perform hand hygiene. *(Reduces spread of microorganisms.)*
16. Record the information on the patient's health care record according to agency policy. *(Provides information that also can be used by other health professionals. It is the beginning of the permanent record.)*
17. Allow patient and family time alone together, if desired. *(Admission procedure is often stressful and fatiguing. Allows time for decision making.)*
18. Perform patient teaching (see the Patient Teaching box).

is not competent to do so. In this case, the careful listing and description of the patient's property become even more important. In some cases, hospitals are required to reimburse the patient for lost items. In these units, patients generally are not allowed to keep any jewelry (other than a wedding ring) or any money at the bedside. Medications brought in by the patient should be sent home if possible. If this is not possible, these medications typically are locked in a designated area following the same process as valuables.

Coordinated Care

Delegation

Assessment and Data Collection

The Joint Commission (TJC) requires each hospitalized patient to have an admission assessment prepared by a registered nurse (RN) within 24 hours of admission (TJC, n.d.). The RN then is allowed to delegate aspects of data collection, for example, to the LPN/LVN. Preadmission assessment and screening for a patient who is hospitalized with a planned admission to a long-term care (LTC) setting usually is performed by the LTC's admissions coordinator, who is typically a registered nurse. Admission requirements for long-term care facilities are directed by each state's governing agency.

The patient usually is asked to put on a hospital gown for the admission process so that a physical assessment can be completed. If the patient does not need help with dressing, the nurse provides privacy for the patient to change. An inventory is made of clothing along with other personal items the patient uses, such as glasses, contacts, dentures, prostheses, canes, or hearing aids. If the patient is keeping any jewelry or money in the room, these items also must be recorded. Fig. 11.1 shows sample clothing and valuables on an inventory checklist.

Once the patient is established in the room, the nurse obtains the health history and the initial nursing assessment (see the Coordinated Care box). The health history generally includes the reason for admission; signs and symptoms the patient is experiencing; past illnesses, surgical procedures, and hospitalizations; medications (prescription and nonprescription); allergies (food, medications, other); eating habits; urinary and bowel patterns; sleep routine; and activity and exercise habits and routine. Other information to be included in a history is the language spoken (and languages understood), family members or significant others, home situation, interests, abilities, activities of daily living, and occupation.

The initial assessment includes level of consciousness, vital signs, height, weight, and a review of body systems (see Chapter 13). Fig. 11.2 is an example of a record used to collect this information. Fig. 11.3 shows a typical medication record to keep track of the medications a patient is taking on admission.

Box 11.2 Managing Emergency Admissions

- For the patient admitted through the emergency department (ED), immediate treatment takes priority over routine admission procedures. After ED treatment, the patient arrives on the nursing unit with a temporary ID bracelet, a physician's order sheet, and a record of treatment. Read this record and confer with the nurse who cared for the patient in the ED to gain insight and to ensure continuity of care.
- Document any ongoing treatment, such as an intravenous infusion, in the nursing notes. Obtain and record the patient's vital signs, and follow the health care provider's orders for treatment. If the patient is conscious and not in great distress, explain any treatment orders. If family members accompany the patient, ask them to wait in the lounge while assessing the patient and beginning treatment. Permit them to visit the patient after the patient is settled in the room. When the patient's condition allows, proceed with routine admission procedures.

The health care provider is notified when the patient has been admitted. If no orders have been received yet, the health care provider gives orders at this time. In some acute care settings, a hospitalist is assigned to the patient's care if the primary health care provider chooses not to follow patient care in the hospital setting.

Skill 11.1 identifies the general steps to follow in admitting a patient. Specific facility policies and the patient's condition may necessitate some alterations to these steps. See Box 11.2 for managing emergency admissions.

NURSING PROCESS FOR PATIENT ADMISSION

The role of the LPN/LVN in the nursing process as stated is that the LPN/LVN will:

- Participate in planning care for patients based on patient needs
- Review patient's plan of care and recommend revisions as necessary
- Review and follow defined prioritization for patient care
- Use clinical pathways, care maps, or care plans to guide and review patient care

ASSESSMENT

Assessment of the patient begins at admission. Subjective and objective data are collected during the assessment. Most facilities have a patient database form to assist in organizing these data (see Figs. 11.2 and 11.3). Facility policy mandates the time frame in which the admission assessment must be completed and what the RN and LPN/LVN responsibilities are concerning the admission process.

CLOTHING LIST		
[] Clothing [] Belt [] Blouse [] Boots [] Bra [] Coat/jacket [] Dress/skirt [] Hat/cap gloves	[] Hose/socks [] Jeans/slacks [] Luggage [] Nightgown/pajamas [] Robe [] Shirt [] Shoes [] Shorts [] Slip	[] Slippers [] Sweatpants [] Sweatshirt [] Sweater [] Tie [] Underwear [] Other clothing [] Clothing sent with family [] No clothing items
[] Personal items [] Bible/book [] Crutches [] Curling iron [] Dentures, upper [] Dentures, lower [] Dentures, partial [] Hair dryer [] Right hearing aid [] Left hearing aid	[] Prosthesis [] Radio/tape player [] Razor [] Toothbrush [] Walker [] Other personal items	[] Personal items sent with family [] All personal items sent with family [] No personal items
[] Valuables [] Bracelet [] Contacts [] Earrings [] Glasses/case [] Medals/rosary [] Money	[] Necklace [] Purse [] Rings [] Wallet [] Wrist watch [] Other valuables	[] Valuables sent with family [] All valuables sent with family [] Valuables sent to safe (receipt on chart) [] Valuables in Same Day Surgery locker number

I take full responsibility for retaining in my possession the items/clothing listed above and any others brought to me while I am a patient at Regional Medical Center.

Admission signatures completed at time admission		**Discharge signatures completed at time of discharge**	
Patient/Family:	Date/Time:	Patient/Family:	Date/Time:
Staff 1: Staff 2:	Date/Time:	Nurse:	Date/Time:

Fig. 11.1 Example of a clothing and personal belongings list.

◆ PATIENT PROBLEM

The patient being admitted to most health care facilities is required to have a nursing care plan initiated by the RN within the first 24 hours of admission. Although care plans must be individualized, common patient problems for a newly admitted patient include *Anxiousness and Potential for Injury, Insufficient Knowledge Regarding Admission Process/Illness,* and *Fearfulness, related to admission to health care facility.*

◆ EXPECTED OUTCOMES AND PLANNING

Planning involves the development of patient-centered goals based on the patient problem statements formed. Expected outcomes and planning are discussed further in Chapter 5.

Goal 1: Patient will voice understanding of care planned while in facility.

Goal 2: Patient will not suffer accidental injury while in facility.

◆ IMPLEMENTATION

Nursing interventions related to admission include the following:

- Orient or acquaint the patient to the facility to ease the patient's anxiety.
- Establish nurse-patient rapport directed at fostering a therapeutic nurse-patient relationship.

NURSING ADMISSION STATEMENT

Admitted: Ambulatory, Cart, Wheelchair, Arms, Ambulance

From: Office, ER, Surgery, Radiology, Recovery Room Transferred From: ______

Oriented to Room: Call Light, Side Rails, TV, Phone, Safety/Smoking Policy: Yes____ No____

Vital Signs: T____ P____ R____ BP____ HT____ WT____ Dentures____

Diet at Home ______

Allergies: Drug ______ Reaction ______

Other ______ Organ Donor: Yes____ No____

Reason for Admission ______ Signature ______

Date: ______ Time: ______

EYES: Impaired vision, blind, cataract, glaucoma, contacts, glasses, prosthesis R.L.
Comments: ______

EARS, NOSE, THROAT: Hard of hearing, deaf, lesions, hearing aid R.L., tracheotomy
Comments: ______

RESPIRATORY: Pain, dyspnea, wheeze, asthma, sinusitis, COPD, cough,
Productive____ Nonproductive____
Oxygen needed, smoker
Comments: ______

CIRCULATION: Apical, radial, strong, weak, thready, bounding, regular, palpitations, chest pain, numbness, bruising, edema, hypertension, Hx MI, CHF, pacer, bypass surgery
Comments: ______

ENDOCRINE: Thyroid, diabetes
Comments: ______

GI TRACT: Heartburn, ulcers, pain, hernia, dysphagia, nausea, vomiting, loss of appetite, distention, diverticulitis
Comments: ______

ELIMINATION: Last BM____ Normal, constipated, diarrhea, tarry, bright red, clay colored, hemorrhoids, involuntary, use of laxatives: Yes/No, enema: Yes/No, ileostomy, colostomy
Comments: ______

URINARY: Incontinence, nocturia, hematuria, dysuria, burning, frequency, urgency, dribbling, infections, cath: Yes/No
Comments: ______

NEUROLOGIC: Convulsions, paralysis, syncope, paresthesia, dizziness, coordination, weakness, headaches
Comments: ______

SKIN: Color____ Turgor____ Temp____
Describe any rashes, lesions, ecchymosis, petechiae, scars, diabetic sores
Comments: ______

MUSCULOSKELETAL: Pain, stiffness, contractures, deformities, tremors, backaches, weight bearing, amputation
Comments: ______

FEMALE REPRODUCTION: L MP____ EDC____
Menopause, breast pain, breast tenderness, vaginal discharge
Comments: ______

PREVIOUS SURGERIES: ______

MEDS TAKEN AT HOME:

Med: Dose: Last taken:

DISPOSAL OF MEDS:

Did not bring ______

Pt. has____ Family took home ______

Retained/taken to pharmacy ______

Other: ______

Signature: ______

Time: ______

Fig. 11.2 Nursing admission assessment form.

MEDICAL INFORMATION	MEDICATION RECORD
Medical Conditions: HF and Hypertension	Name: Mable Lauritsen
My Doctor(s): Dr. J. Bernard	Address (street): 28 West Park
Allergies: Darvocet-N 100	City: Spencer, State: Iowa, Zip: 59101
Pharmacy or Pharmacist: James Manning	My Birth Date: 8-28-1933
	My Weight: 262 lb; My Height: 5′-4″

MEDICATION (Prescription and Over-the-Counter)	FOR WHAT CONDITION	DOSAGE	WHEN and HOW TO TAKE
1. Lasix	HF	40 mg	by mouth every AM
2. Lanoxin	HF	0.125 mg	by mouth every AM
3. Micro-K	HF	8 mEq	by mouth twice a day
4. Metamucil	constipation	$\bar{\text{II}}$ Tbs.	at bed time
5. Mycolog	leg ulcers	topical	apply to lesions daily
6.			
7.			
8.			
9.			
10.			
11.			
12.			

Fig. 11.3 Example of a patient's medication record.

- Identify risk behaviors or limitations to assist the staff in making the environment safe (see Skill 11.1).
- Confirm through discussion and questions that the patient understands the diagnostic tests and procedures.
- Monitor the patient's ability to ambulate alone.
- Monitor the patient's ability to operate the hospital bed, the call light, and the emergency button.

◆ EVALUATION

Determine whether the patient has met the previously established goals.

Goal 1: Patient demonstrates understanding of procedure (specify).

Goal 2: Patient has remained injury free.

TRANSFERRING A PATIENT

The changing condition of a patient, whether improving or becoming more critical, frequently necessitates **transfer** (moving a patient from one unit to another [intra-agency transfer] or moving a patient from one health care facility to another [interagency transfer]). Transfers are sometimes to another unit in the hospital and sometimes to another health care institution, such as a long-term care facility or rehabilitation hospital (Box 11.3 and Fig. 11.4).

Often a patient whose condition becomes critical while in the hospital is moved to special care areas, such as the ICU or the CCU. A patient whose condition improves is likely to be moved from a special care area to a general care area or a step-down unit. Other patients are transferred to a long-term care facility if they need continued care. Transfers also may be done at the patient's request; for example, some patients wish to have a private room or a quieter room.

The patient transfer requires thorough preparation and careful documentation. Preparation includes an explanation of the transfer to the patient and family, discussion of the patient's condition and plan of care with the staff of the receiving unit or facility, and

Box 11.3 Long-Term Care Considerations

Admission to a long-term care facility sometimes occurs as a transfer from the hospital (see Skill 11.2) and sometimes as a direct admission. Perform a health history and initial nursing assessment to determine the patient's condition. Encourage the patient to bring clothing and other personal items, such as pictures; even personal furniture may be brought to place in the room to give a feeling of familiarity (see Chapters 33, 38, and 39). Agency policies and requirements of **third-party payers** (entities [people or elements] other than the giver or receiver of service responsible for payment; e.g., Medicare or insurance company) must be followed so that benefits are not lost. Discharge from a nursing home is essentially the same as discharge from a hospital. There are more personal belongings to gather and pack.

arrangements for transportation, if necessary. Documentation of the patient's condition before and during transfer and adequate communication among nursing staff ensures **continuity of care** (continuing of established patient care from one setting to another) and provides legal protection for the transferring facility and its staff.

Transfer combines admission and discharge. The patient is discharged from one unit and received on the new unit, much like an admission. An order from the health care provider is necessary to begin the transfer process. An interagency transfer requires documentation from the accepting facility and health care provider and a signed consent from the patient indicating an understanding of the risks and benefits associated with the transfer. Failure to follow these procedures instituted by COBRA and EMTALA (discussed in Chapter 2) may result in monetary fines to both facilities. Skill 11.2 gives general steps to follow when transferring a patient. Box 11.4 lists special considerations for transferring patients.

NURSING PROCESS FOR PATIENT TRANSFER

ASSESSMENT

The nurse determines the patient's understanding of the reason for the transfer and gives explanations as necessary. The patient's condition must be assessed before transfer to determine the necessary method of transfer. The nurse receiving the patient after a transfer also assesses the patient because the patient is now his or her responsibility.

PATIENT PROBLEM

Patient problems that the patient had before the transfer may still be current after the transfer. The nurse's assessment helps in determining whether revisions to the care plan are necessary. If the patient has been transferred from one facility to another, new patient problem statements are likely to be necessary. As with admission, the patient commonly has the nursing problem of *Anxiousness* and *Potential for Injury* because of the new environment.

Box 11.4 Special Considerations for Transferring Patients

- Arrange transportation via ambulance with social services department, if the patient requires it, for transfer to another facility. Ensure that the necessary equipment is assembled to provide care during transport.
- Be especially careful that all documentation is complete when the patient is being transferred to another facility. (A communication breakdown carries high potential to interfere with continuity of the patient's care.)
- If the patient is being transferred to a different facility, be sure that all of the appropriate patient care measures have been performed (e.g., suctioning of airway, administration of prescribed medication, changing of soiled dressings, bathing of an incontinent patient, and emptying of collection devices).

EXPECTED OUTCOMES AND PLANNING

Transfer planning involves the development of patient-centered goals based on the nursing diagnosis formed.

Goal 1: Patient will voice an understanding of the reason for and the process involved with the transfer.

Goal 2: Patient will incur no injury during or after transfer.

IMPLEMENTATION

Nursing interventions include the following:

- Explain to patient and family the reason for the transfer, when it is to occur, and what procedures are planned.
- Encourage questions (see Skill 11.2).
- Confirm the patient understands the transfer and procedures through discussion and questions.
- Inspect the patient's positioning in or on transport vehicle.
- During final assessment, compare present data with previous findings.

EVALUATION

Goal 1: Patient states the reasons for the transfer.

Goal 2: Patient is secured into wheelchair or gurney and remains injury free.

DISCHARGING A PATIENT

DISCHARGE PLANNING

Planning for a patient's discharge is just one aspect that aids in providing continuity of care for a patient in a health care facility. **Discharge planning** is defined as the systematic process of planning for patient care after discharge from a hospital or health care facility.

Although **discharge** from a facility usually is considered routine, effective discharge requires careful planning and continued assessment of the patient's

Patient Transfer Form

Patient Transfer Form	Date: 1-31-19	Medical record no.: 432-612-1111
Patient's name: Sandra Knox — Phone # 555-1263	Diet on transfer: Low sodium	Date of transfer: 1-31-19
Address: 28 West Park, Spenser, Iowa	Attending physician at time of transfer: Dr. J.W. Short	

Diagnosis:
Primary: myocardial infarction
Secondary: heart failure
All other conditions: ______ Allergies: penicillin

Current medications: (date and time last dose)
Bumex 1 mg po daily
Lanoxin 0.25 mg po daily
Colace tabs po H.S.
Slow-K 10 mEq po B.I.D.
Procardia XL 30 mg po B.I.D.
Nitrostat 6.5 mg po daily

Nursing evaluation

a. Speech	☒ Normal	☐ Impaired	☐ Unable to speak	
b. Hearing	☐ Normal	☒ Impaired	☐ Deaf	
c. Sight	☐ Normal	☒ Impaired	☐ Blind	
d. Mental status	☒ Always alert	☐ Occasionally confused	☐ Always confused	
e. Feeding	☒ Independent	☐ Help with feeding	☐ Cannot feed self	
f. Dressing	☒ Independent	☐ Help with dressing	☐ Cannot dress self	
g. Elimination	☐ Independent	☒ Help to bathroom	☐ Bedpan or urinal required	☐ Incontinent
h. Bathing	☒ Independent	☒ Help with bathing	☐ Bed bath with help	☐ Bed bath
i. Ambulatory status	☐ Independent	☒ Walks with assistance	☐ Help from bed to chair	☐ Bed bound

Appliances or support: walker, up c̄ assistance

Physical activity: ______

Nursing assessment and other pertinent information: grieving the loss of husband 2 months ago, alert and oriented × 3, crackles in right apex, last BM this AM - brown semiformed stool, last set of vitals = 97°-80-22 100/60. Abdomen soft and nondistended, pedal pulse + 2 bilaterally

Nurse's signature: Kelly J. Russell Title: RN, MSN Date: 1-31-19

Fig. 11.4 Example of a patient transfer form.

needs during the stay in the facility. Ideally, discharge planning begins shortly after admission. Discharge planning has several purposes, including teaching the patient and the family about the patient's illness and its effect on lifestyle; providing instructions for home care; communicating dietary or activity instructions; and explaining the purpose, adverse effects, and scheduling of medication treatment. It also can include arranging for transportation, follow-up care when necessary, and coordination of outpatient or home health care services.

Good discharge planning involves the patient from the beginning, uses the strengths of the patient and caregivers in planning, provides resources to meet the patient's limitations, and is focused on improving the patient's long-term outcomes.

The Joint Commission (Kind and Smith, n.d.) suggests the following instructions be given to patients upon discharge from a health care facility:

- Reason for the admission
- Safe and effective use of medications and medical equipment
- Instruction on nutrition and modified diets
- Rehabilitation techniques to support adaptation to or functional independence in the environment
- Access to available community resources as needed
- When and how to obtain further treatment

Skill 11.2 Transferring a Patient

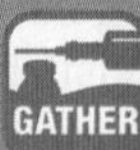

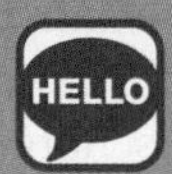

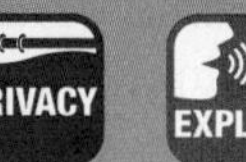

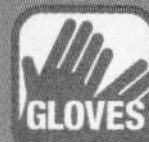

NURSING ACTION *(RATIONALE)*

1. Perform hand hygiene. *(Reduces spread of microorganisms.)*
2. Check health care provider's order for transfer. *(Verifies if and when a patient is to be transferred.)*
3. Inform patient and family of the transfer. *(Reduces the fear of the unknown and strengthens the nurse-patient relationship.)*
4. Notify the receiving unit of the transfer and when to expect the patient. *(Allows preparation time to best welcome the new patient and begin care in a courteous, thoughtful, and unhurried manner.)*
5. Gather all the patient's belongings and necessary care items to accompany the patient. *(Builds trust and prevents loss of items.)*
6. Assist in transferring the patient, usually via stretcher or wheelchair. *(Ensures patient safety. The patient's condition determines mode of transportation.)*
7. Introduce patient and family to nurses on new unit and to roommate. *(Establishes the beginning of new therapeutic nurse-patient relationship and gives a sense of belonging.)*
8. Provide a brief summary of medical diagnosis, treatment care plan, and medications. Review medical orders with nurse assuming care. Situation, background, assessment, and recommendation (SBAR) is the common format used for reporting this information (see Chapter 3 for information regarding SBAR). If transfer is to another facility, complete an interagency transfer form. *(Gives personnel on the receiving unit pertinent information for continuing care. Reviewing records together prevents errors.)*
9. Explain equipment, policies, and procedures that are different on the new unit. *(Gives the patient some control and reduces anxiety.)*
10. Perform hand hygiene. *(Reduces spread of microorganisms.)*
11. Record condition of patient and means of transfer. The nurse on the new unit also records an assessment of the patient's condition on arrival. *(Properly executed, the patient's medical record reflects all care given and the patient's response to that care while in the facility.)*
12. For an intra-agency transfer, other departments, such as diagnostic imaging, laboratory, admission department, physical therapy, dietary, and business offices, must be notified of the transfer. *(Keeps records current and prevents errors.)*
13. An interagency transfer usually is made via air or ground ambulance or via private car. Be sure the patient is dressed or covered appropriately for environmental comfort. If oxygen is necessary, a small transport tank usually is used. A nurse generally accompanies a critically ill patient who is being transferred. *(Promotes continuity of care.)*
14. Infants generally are transported in an isolette that is later returned to the sending health care facility. Parents usually accompany their child during transfer unless the transfer is via air ambulance. In this case, the parents generally follow in family transportation. *(Promotes continuity of care.)*
15. Perform patient teaching (see the Patient Teaching box). See Box 11.4 for special considerations for patient transfer.

- The patient's and family's responsibilities in the patient's ongoing health care needs and the knowledge and skills needed to carry out those responsibilities
- Maintenance of good standards for personal hygiene and grooming
- It is also necessary to identify risk factors for discharge planning, such as the following:
  - Older adult age group
  - Multisystem disease process
  - Major surgical procedure
  - Chronic or terminal illness

Discharge planning is a multidisciplinary process that involves participation by all members of the health care team, the patient, and the patient's family or significant others. Many larger hospitals have discharge planners or coordinators. The social worker is often in charge of discharge planning for the long-term care resident. Considered part of the health care team, these people orchestrate the discharge planning. This is especially important when the patient is considered at risk. Depending on the facility or acuity level of the patient, the staff or the charge nurse may be responsible for discharge planning. With the assistance of social workers or community-based nurses, the staff identifies and anticipates patient needs after discharge from the hospital and formulates a plan for meeting those needs (Box 11.5, Fig. 11.5, and the Home Care Considerations box).

Another approach to discharge planning is to perform transitional care with transition specialists. This role

Box 11.5 Discharge Teaching Goals

The goals of discharge teaching help to ensure that patients do the following:

- Carefully follow their diet
- Comply with their medication therapy
- Know about possible complications
- Know when to seek follow-up care
- Manage their activity level
- Recognize their need for rest
- Understand their illness
- Understand their treatments

Be certain that the discharge teaching includes the patient's family or other caregivers to ensure that the patient receives proper care at home.

was developed to facilitate the transition from hospital (where discharge planning is initiated) to recovery (in the home). The transition specialist begins discharge planning and usually makes a home visit before the patient is discharged. After discharge to the home, this specialist is available to the patient and family. This type of transitional care and coordination is cost effective and has improved the quality of care.

Communication among the patient, the family or caregivers, and health care agencies is essential for effective discharge planning. The nurse establishes a dialogue between these various people and coordinates the discharge plan before the patient leaves the facility. Any necessary referrals to other agencies are initiated

DISMISSAL INSTRUCTION SHEET

Name *Marjorie Oden* Allergies *NKA*

1. Diet: Regular ____ Soft *X* Liquid ____ Special instructions: ____
2. Activity: Walking *X* Rest *X* Lifting *10 lb.* Driving *no*
   Work ____ Other ____
3. Bowels: *Laxative of choice*
4. Bathing: Shower *X* Tub *no* Sponge *—*
5. Wound care: Incision care ____
   Dressing change ____
   Special instructions ____
6. Tubes, drains, saline lock, appliances: Special instructions *Leave Steri-Strips in place on abdomen until physician's visit*
   Saline lock patient instruction sheet given: yes ____ NA *X* Prescriptions sent: yes *X* NA ____
   Physician's instruction sheet given: yes *X* NA ____ Home med sent: yes *X* NA ____
7. Medications:

Drug	Dose	Frequency	Route	Special Instructions
Koflex	*250 mg*	*three times daily*	*by mouth*	*Take with food or milk*
Tylenol ES	*tabs 2*	*every 4 hr*	*by mouth*	*As needed for pain control*
Colace	*caps 2*	*daily*	*by mouth*	*At hours of sleep*
Halcion	*0.125 mg*	*daily*	*by mouth*	*As needed for sleep*

8. Other instructions: *Call physician if any redness, pain, or swelling of incision or temperature greater than 100° F*
9. Office visit: Call for an appointment on *5-9-14 at 2 PM* (date)
   Doctor *Edward Roberts* Address *1402 Indiana Street* Phone number *308-2890*

Please bring this instruction sheet to your first appointment with your doctor.

Instructions received and understood,

Patient or responsible party *Kinsey Nicoley* Signature *Daughter* Date *5-2-19*

Nurse signature *Kimberly Horrall, RN, MSN*

Label

Fig. 11.5 Example of a dismissal instruction sheet.

Home Care Considerations

The Discharged Patient

- A patient who needs care at home after discharge from a health care facility often is referred to a **home health agency** (an organization that provides health care in the home; see Chapter 37). Typical services include skilled nursing care or simply assistance with activities of daily living. A health care provider's order is necessary for these services to be reimbursable from insurance or Medicare and Medicaid. A health history and initial assessment are performed, just as in the hospital.
- Discharge from a home health agency involves the same kind of teaching as discharge from the hospital. The nurse is responsible to ascertain whether the patient or family is able to provide any care still needed.
- Assess availability and skill of the primary caregiver; assess time availability, ability, willingness, emotional and physical stamina, and knowledge.
- Perform the following assessments of immediate family members: attitude; ability to adjust to demands of patient care; impact of care demands on their lives; and impact of potential ongoing nature of the patient's needs. Family members who are not properly prepared for their role as caregivers are more likely to be overwhelmed by the patient's needs, resulting in caregiver role strain or readmission to a health care facility.
- Assess additional resources that may be available to help, such as close friends.
- Evaluate emergency preparations: for example, signaling device or phone is set up within patient's reach, and appropriate protocol is written out.

before the patient is discharged. The nurse, if no discharge planner is available, is responsible for coordinating such referrals, including signed health care provider's orders for specific care, treatments, or medications, to enable the patient to obtain reimbursement from third-party payers.

A discharge summary is part of the discharge plan. This summary includes the patient's learning needs, how well they have been met, the patient teaching completed, short-term and long-term goals of care, referrals made, and coordinated care plan to be implemented after discharge.

REFERRALS FOR HEALTH CARE SERVICES

Often a patient who is discharged needs the further services of various disciplines (departments) within a facility, such as dietary, social work, or physical therapy. The nurse is often the first to recognize the patient's needs, so it is important to recognize the specialized skills and knowledge of other health professionals. They are often in a position to give a patient services that the nurse is unable to offer. Referrals should be made as soon as possible after the patient's need is identified. In many facilities, a health care provider's order is needed for a referral, especially when specific therapies are planned (e.g., physical therapy) (see the Health Promotion box).

Health Promotion

Referrals and Discharge Planning

Continuity of care for the patient can be enhanced by approaching discharge planning with an interdisciplinary approach. The following list summarizes the role that various health disciplines play in referrals during discharge planning.

DIETITIAN

- Provides proper nutrient and food source requirements in patients' diets
- Instructs patients on meal planning and diet restrictions

SOCIAL WORKER

- Provides counseling for major life crises, such as terminal illness and family problems
- Assists in finding community resources, such as equipment for home health care or an agency that accepts patients after discharge from a facility
- Assists in finding financial resources to cover medical costs

PHYSICAL THERAPIST

- Assists in the examination and treatment of physically disabled people
- Assists in rehabilitating patients and restoring musculoskeletal function to a patient's greatest potential

OCCUPATIONAL THERAPIST

- Teaches patients to adapt to physical or cognitive challenges by learning new vocational skills or activities of daily living

SPEECH THERAPIST

- Assists patients with disorders that affect normal oral communication
- Assists patients with techniques that address swallowing disorders

CLINICAL NURSE SPECIALIST

- Consults with nursing staff on appropriate nursing interventions for complex nursing diagnoses
- Provides instruction to patients and family members who will assume patient care

HOME HEALTH CARE NURSE

- Provides follow-up discharge visits to a patient's home for the delivery of nursing services

DISCHARGE PROCESS

Many facilities have a form with written instructions and teaching documentation for the patient to sign acknowledging understanding of the instructions. These instructions serve as a guide for the patient to use at home (see Fig. 11.5). Skill 11.3 outlines the steps for discharging a patient. Box 11.6 discusses what to do if a patient decides to leave hospital facility against medical advice (Fig. 11.6).

Skill 11.3 Discharging a Patient

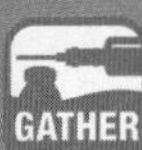

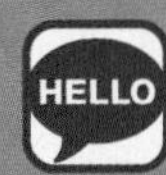

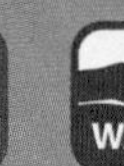

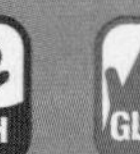

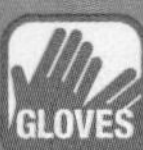

NURSING ACTION *(RATIONALE)*

1. Perform hand hygiene. *(Reduces spread of microorganisms.)*
2. Be certain there is a discharge order. *(Verifies health care provider's decision regarding time for the patient to be discharged.)*
3. If no discharge order has been written and the patient insists on leaving the facility, have the patient sign against medical advice (AMA) form (see Fig. 11.6). *(Generally patients cannot be held against their wishes.)* The patient's signature acknowledges full responsibility for what happens after the patient leaves. Be sure the health care provider is notified. Every effort should be made to encourage the patient to stay until speaking with the health care provider.
4. Notify the family or the person who will be transporting the patient home. *(Prevents delay in discharge.)*
5. Verify that the patient and the family or caregiver understand the instructions for care (e.g., medications, special diet, exercise, follow-up care). *(Ensures appropriate home care.)*
6. Gather equipment, supplies, and prescriptions that the patient is to take home. *(Provides service patient and family are unable to perform for themselves.)*
7. Assist the patient in dressing and packing items to go home. *(Conserves patient's strength.)*
8. Check clothing and valuables list made on admission according to policy. *(Prevents patient from leaving personal items at facility.)*
9. Transfer the patient and belongings to the vehicle outside.
   a. Many facilities escort the patient via wheelchair.

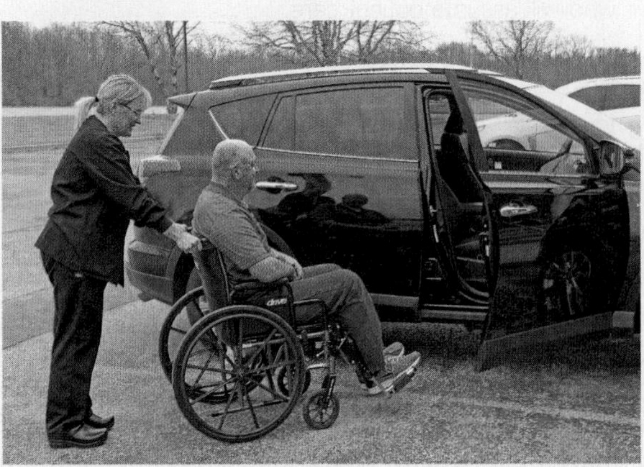

   b. Many patients are discharged via gurney.

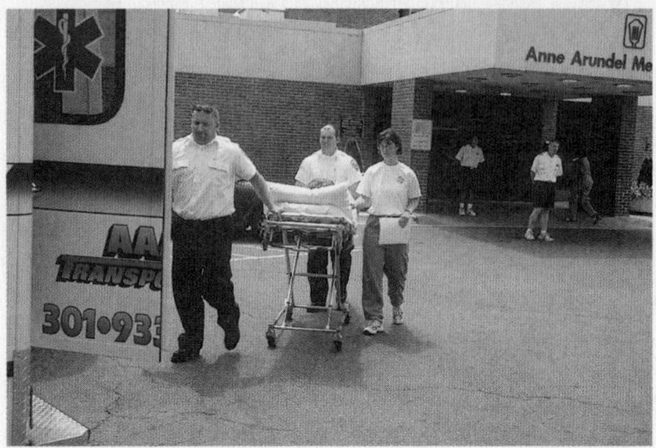

   c. Assist the patient into the vehicle. Help the family place personal belongings into car. As with all procedures, use good communication skills and wish patients well as they leave the facility. *(Provides patient safety and complies with policy of most health care facilities. Agency's liability ends once patient is safely in vehicle.)*
10. Perform hand hygiene. *(Reduces spread of microorganisms.)*
11. Document entire discharge procedure. *(Completes the record. Legally this is necessary to verify what occurred during the discharge process.)* Document the following:
    - Teaching
    - Patient's condition
    - Method of discharge
12. When the patient is a child, the parents must be included in all aspects of teaching and in the entire discharge procedure. Some facilities have a special form to be signed by the person legally responsible for taking the child away from the facility.

STATEMENT OF PATIENT LEAVING HOSPITAL AGAINST ADVICE

This is to certify that I am leaving ______________________________ Hospital at my own insistence and against the advice of the hospital authorities and my attending physician. I have been informed by them of the dangers of my leaving the hospital at this time. I release the hospital, its employees and officers, and my attending physician from all liability for any adverse results caused by my leaving the hospital prematurely.

Signed ______________________________

I agree to hold harmless the ______________________________ Hospital, its employees and officers, and the attending physician from all liability, with reference to the discharge of the patient named above.

____
(Husband, wife, parent, etc.)

Date ______________________________

Witness ______________________________

Fig. 11.6 Example of form used when a patient leaves the hospital against medical advice.

Box 11.6 Discharge Against Medical Advice

Occasionally, the patient or the patient's family may demand discharge **against medical advice (AMA;** when a patient leaves a health care facility without a health care provider's order for discharge). If this occurs, notify the health care provider immediately. If the health care provider fails to convince the patient to remain in the facility, the provider asks the patient to sign an AMA form (see Fig. 11.6) releasing the facility from legal responsibility for any medical problems the patient experiences after discharge.

If the health care provider is not available, discuss the discharge form with the patient and obtain the patient's signature. If the patient refuses to sign the AMA form, do not detain the patient. Doing so is a violation of the patient's legal rights.[a] After the patient leaves, document the incident thoroughly in your notes and notify the health care provider.

[a]Forcible detainment of a rational adult patient who will not sign the form is not permitted. Only if a court order was issued for the admission, as in some cases of mental illness, is it possible to forcibly detain a patient. A lawsuit for false imprisonment can be filed against the hospital or personnel for keeping patients against their wishes. The refusal to sign the form and the information given about the risks of leaving must be documented in the patient's health care record.

NURSING PROCESS FOR PATIENT DISCHARGE

ASSESSMENT

Every patient requires discharge planning, which is initiated on admission. Some conditions place a patient at greater risk for being unable to meet continuing health care needs after discharge. These conditions include multiple disease processes, major surgical procedures, chronic or terminal illness, emotional or psychologic instability, and advanced age.

Assess the patient's and family's needs for health teaching and collaborate with health care providers and staff in other disciplines to assess any needs for referral. This assessment is important in providing continuity of care to the patient.

PATIENT PROBLEM

When patients are discharged, they may still have nursing diagnoses that must be addressed. Common nursing diagnoses for the patient being discharged include *Compromised Maintenance of Health* and *Inability to Bathe Self*.

EXPECTED OUTCOMES AND PLANNING

Planning involves the development of patient-centered goals based on nursing diagnoses.

Goal 1: Patient or family member will be able to care for individual needs.

Goal 2: Health care resources regarding bathing and hygiene will be available at home.

IMPLEMENTATION

On the day of discharge, nursing interventions include the following:

- All equipment, supplies, and prescriptions that the patient is to take home are gathered.
- The nurse verifies that the patient and the caregiver understand the instructions for care.
- Have patient or family member perform any treatments to be continued in the home (return demonstration).
- Home health nurse inspects home environment to assess for obstacles or risks.

EVALUATION

Goal 1: Home health agency has been notified of patient's needs on arrival at home.

Goal 2: Home health agency's initial visit is completed before discharge or soon thereafter.

Get Ready for the NCLEX® Examination!

Key Points

- Admission into a health care facility begins with ensuring that patients are knowledgeable about routine procedures and activities that will occur during their stay.
- The Patient Self-Determination Act requires all Medicare-recipient and Medicaid-recipient hospitals to provide patients with information about their right to accept or reject medical treatment.
- The patient has the right to be treated with dignity, courtesy, and respect.
- The nurse's attitude often influences the patient's feelings about the care received.
- Common reactions to admission to a health care facility are fear of the unknown, loss of identity, disorientation, separation anxiety, and loneliness.
- An adult patient always should be addressed as Miss, Ms., Mrs., or Mr. (last name), unless the patient grants permission to do otherwise.
- Transfers may be intra-agency (patient is discharged from one unit and received on the new unit, much like an admission).
- Transfers also may be interagency (patient leaving one health care facility to enter another health care facility).
- Coordination is the key to the efficient and safe transfer of a patient.
- Discharge planning begins when a patient is admitted to a health care facility.
- Multiple medical conditions sometimes place a patient at risk for needing more thorough discharge planning.
- Nurses may find involvement of other health care professionals in discharge planning necessary when the expertise of those professionals is needed to help plan or provide ongoing care.
- Although discharge from a health care facility usually is considered routine, effective discharge requires careful planning and continuing assessment of patients' needs during their stay in the facility.
- Every patient in a health care facility requires discharge planning.
- Successful discharge planning is a centralized, coordinated, multidisciplinary process that ensures the patient has a plan for continuing care after leaving the health care facility.
- The ultimate goal of discharge planning is to give patients and families the knowledge, skills, and resources needed to assume self-care or patient care after discharge.
- When the patient is leaving without a health care provider's discharge order, the appropriate forms (AMA) must be signed and the health care provider notified.
- Generally, a person cannot be kept in a health care facility against his or her will.

Additional Learning Resources

SG Go to your Study Guide for additional learning activities to help you master this chapter content.

evolve Be sure to visit the Evolve site at *http://evolve.elsevier.com/Cooper/foundationsadult/* for additional online resources.

Review Questions for the NCLEX® Examination

1. When the patient is received from the admitting department, what does the nurse expect has been completed? *(Select all that apply.)*
   1. The patient has been informed of the Patient's Bill of Rights.
   2. A list of patient allergies has been recorded in the patient's record.
   3. The patient has been informed of current health care provider's orders.
   4. The patient has an allergy band in place.
   5. The patient has an ID band in place with proper identification information.
2. A patient is admitted for observation and various diagnostic tests. What is the initial nursing action in the admission process?
   1. The nurse introduces self and roommates.
   2. The nurse measures vital signs.
   3. The nurse helps the patient get undressed and into bed.
   4. The nurse notifies the physician.
3. A 90-year-old patient has been hospitalized with pneumonia and needs reorientation to his surroundings periodically. The nurse assisting him with his morning care hears the unlicensed assistive personnel (UAP) refer to the patient as "Gramps." What action should the nurse take?
   1. Tell the UAP it is okay to call him "Gramps" if he has grandchildren.
   2. Inform the UAP that it is acceptable if the UAP cannot remember his name.
   3. Explain that it is acceptable if the UAP feels comfortable calling him "Gramps."
   4. Educate the UAP that it is not acceptable to call the patient "Gramps" unless the patient has requested to be called this.
4. A patient has been transferred out of the ICU to a medical unit. A nurse has been assigned to complete the transfer. Which type of transfer is this?
   1. Patient-initiated transfer
   2. Interagency transfer
   3. Business office transfer
   4. Intra-agency transfer

5. A patient is being transferred to the surgical unit from the recovery room after extensive surgery as the result of trauma from an automobile accident. What concept should the nurse remember when transferring this patient?
   1. The patient is a human who deserves dignity, courtesy, and respect.
   2. The patient is ill and unable to make decisions or give accurate information.
   3. The nurse knows best and should tell the patient what to do.
   4. Families get in the way and should be encouraged not to get involved in the patient's care.
6. A patient has been recently diagnosed and hospitalized for type 1 diabetes. The multidisciplinary health care team has been preparing her for discharge. What is the primary purpose of discharge planning?
   1. Verifying prescribed medications
   2. Providing accurate medical treatment
   3. Supplying ongoing patient education
   4. Ensuring continuity of care
7. A patient has been hospitalized for 6 days with a diagnosis of a stroke. When should the nurse begin the patient's discharge planning?
   1. When his condition has stabilized
   2. On his admission to the hospital
   3. When he begins to ask questions
   4. When his family asks for information
8. A patient is determined to leave the hospital. His health care provider is not aware of his intent, nor is it in his best interest to be discharged at this time. When a patient chooses to leave a health care facility without a health care provider's order, what should the nurse do? *(Select all that apply.)*
   1. Call the family so that they can expect the patient at home.
   2. Allow the patient to leave because no one can be held against his or her will.
   3. Call security because a physician's order is necessary before a patient may leave.
   4. Notify the physician as soon as possible regarding the patient's intent.
   5. Explain the risks of leaving and request that the patient sign a paper accepting responsibility for problems that may occur.
9. The nurse is admitting a patient to the long-term care facility. What nursing diagnosis is most appropriate at this time?
   1. Self-care deficit, activities of daily living related to necessary admission to a long-term care facility
   2. Anxiety related to new living environment
   3. Ineffective coping related to admission to a long-term care facility
   4. Loneliness related to separation from family and friends
10. The patient is being discharged from the hospital to home and will be assisted with abdominal bandage changes by his wife. Which nursing action is most important?
    1. Ask the patient if he has any questions.
    2. Have the patient and wife read all discharge instructions.
    3. Demonstrate how to change the bandage every time the wife visits.
    4. After teaching, ask the patient and his wife to perform the bandage change and observe their technique.
11. A patient is being admitted to the hospital for stabilization of a heart condition. Before the patient arrives on the nursing unit, what tasks will the admissions department complete? *(Select all that apply.)*
    1. The patient will have signed consent for treatment.
    2. The admissions staff will itemize the patient's belongings.
    3. The patient's vital signs will be measured.
    4. The physician's orders will be reviewed.
    5. The admissions staff will place the hospital ID band on the patient's wrist.
12. During the admission of a patient to a long-term care facility, for what is the LPN/LVN most likely responsible?
    1. Admission charting
    2. Admission interview
    3. Formulating nursing diagnoses
    4. Obtaining vital signs and assisting with assessment
13. The nurse is discharging a patient for the first time. What documentation demonstrates that the nurse understands the discharge process? *(Select all that apply.)*
    1. A summary of the patient's stay
    2. An account of all financial obligations
    3. The method of discharge
    4. A summary of personnel who cared for the patient
    5. Where the patient is being discharged to
14. The services of a transition specialist for patient discharge are most important for which reason?
    1. Increasing insurance reimbursement rates for facilities
    2. Improving continuity of care from facility to home
    3. Ensuring completion of facility documentation requirements
    4. Preventing readmitting of patients to hospitals
15. What is the correct order of the steps for discharging a patient from a long-term care facility?
    1. Asking the patient what the home situation is in regard to people who can assist in care, levels of floors, and number of steps
    2. Giving the patient written discharge instructions
    3. Obtaining the order for the resident to be discharged
    4. Meeting with members of the health care team, such as the physical therapist or dietitian, to discuss the patient's discharge

12 Vital Signs

http://evolve.elsevier.com/Cooper/foundationsadult/

Objectives

1. Discuss the importance of accurate assessment of vital signs.
2. Identify the guidelines for vital signs measurement.
3. Accurately assess oral, rectal, axillary, and tympanic temperatures.
4. List the various sites for pulse measurement.
5. Accurately assess an apical pulse, a radial pulse, and a pulse deficit.
6. Describe the procedure for determining the respiratory rate.
7. Accurately assess the blood pressure.
8. State the normal limits of each vital sign.
9. List the factors that affect vital signs readings.
10. Accurately assess the height and weight measurements.
11. Discuss optimal frequency of vital signs measurement.
12. Discuss methods by which the nurse can ensure accurate measurement of vital signs.
13. Identify the rationale for each step of the vital signs procedures.
14. Describe the benefits of and the precautions to follow for self-measurement of blood pressure.
15. Accurately record and report vital signs measurements.

Key Terms

apical pulse (ĀP-ĭ-căl PŬLS, p. 293)
auscultate (ĂW-skŭl-tāt, p. 289)
blood pressure (p. 296)
bradycardia (brād-ĭ-KĂR-dē-ă, p. 290)
bradypnea (brād-ĭp-NĒ-ă, p. 295)
Cheyne-Stokes respirations (CHĀN STŌKS, p. 295)
diastolic (dī-ă-STŎL-ĭk, p. 296)
dyspnea (DĬSP-nē-ă, p. 295)
dysrhythmia (dĭs-RĬTH-mē-ă, p. 290)
febrile (FĔB-rĭl, p. 282)
hypertension (hī-pŭr-TĔN-shŭn, p. 297)
hyperthermia (hī-pŭr-THŬR-mē-ă, p. 282)
hypotension (hī-pō-TĔN-shŭn, p. 298)
hypothermia (hī-pō-THŬR-mē-ă, p. 283)
Korotkoff sounds (kŏ-RŎT-kŏf, p. 299)
orthostatic hypotension (ŏr-thō-STĂT-ĭk hī-pō-TĔN-shŭn, p. 298)
pulse (p. 290)
pulse deficit (p. 293)
pulse pressure (p. 297)
respiration (p. 294)
sphygmomanometer (sfĭg-mō-mă-NŎM-ĕ-tŭr, p. 298)
stethoscope (STĔTH-ō-skōp, p. 288)
systolic (sĭs-TŎL-ĭk, p. 296)
tachycardia (tăk-ĭ-KĂR-dē-ă, p. 290)
tachypnea (tăk-ĭp-NĒ-ă, p. 295)
temperature (p. 281)
tympanic (tĭm-PĂN-ĭk, p. 284)
vital signs (p. 278)

Vital signs include temperature, pulse, respirations, and blood pressure. The ability to obtain accurate measurements of vital signs is critical. Because vital signs are an indication of basic body functioning, it is appropriate to begin the physical assessment by obtaining these data. These data are called **vital signs** because of their importance.

The skills required to measure vital signs are simple, but the simplicity should never reduce the critical value of the task. Vital signs and other physiologic measurements often provide the basis for problem solving. Careful technique ensures accurate findings.

Many facilities have begun using a fifth vital sign: pain level or comfort level (see Chapter 21; Fig. 21.3 provides an example of a pain assessment guide). Nurses use a more descriptive format for documentation in their notes.

Assessment of vital signs enables the identification of nursing diagnoses, implementation of planned interventions, and evaluation of success when vital signs have returned to acceptable values (see the Health Promotion box).

A cultural assessment should be included in the overall assessment for all patients. This provides a better

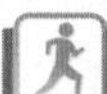

Health Promotion

Vital Signs

- Demonstrate measurement of vital signs on self or a family member. (Demonstrating on the patient prevents the patient from being able to observe entire procedure.)
- Explain rationale for each step during demonstration.
- Instruct patient and family in proper cleaning and storage of the thermometer in the home.
- Patients should be instructed to wait at least 20 minutes after smoking or eating to measure their vital signs.
- Instruct patient or primary caregiver to use fingertips, never thumbs, for counting the pulse. (The thumb has its own pulse.)
- Instruct in use of gentle pressure; reinforce not to press hard over the pulses because this obliterates the pulse.
- Instruct in use of a watch with a second hand to assess pulses.
- Patients who demonstrate decreased ventilation often benefit from being taught deep-breathing and coughing exercises.
- Advise family member to count patient's respiratory rate when patient is unaware of being observed. (If patient is aware of the assessment, respiratory rate sometimes is altered.)
- Instruct family member to notify health care provider if unusual fluctuations in respiratory rate occur.
- Educate patient about risks for hypertension. People with family history of hypertension are at significant risk. Obesity, cigarette smoking, heavy alcohol consumption, high blood cholesterol levels, and continued exposure to stress are factors linked to hypertension.
- Patients with hypertension should learn about blood pressure values, long-term follow-up care and therapy, the usual lack of symptoms that is responsible for hypertension's nickname, *the silent killer* (it cannot be felt), therapy's ability to control but not cure it, and the benefits of a consistently followed treatment plan.
- Patients often learn to take their own blood pressure.
- Instruct patient or primary caregiver to take blood pressure at the same time each day and after patient has had a brief rest. The blood pressure should be taken with the patient sitting or lying down; use same position and arm each time pressure is taken. (Advise patient not to cross legs.)
- Positioning and selection of arm site are potential causes of inaccurate readings.
- Place arm on a table or desk that is raised to the level of the heart.
- Instruct caregiver that if the pressure is difficult to hear, the cuff may be too loose, not big enough, or too narrow; the stethoscope may be misplaced; the cuff may have been deflated too quickly or too slowly; or the cuff may not have been pumped high enough for systolic readings. Wait 1 minute and try again.
- Teach patient risk factors for hypothermia and frostbite: fatigue; malnutrition; hypoxemia; cold, wet clothing; and alcohol intoxication.
- Teach patient risk factors for heat stroke: strenuous exercise in hot, humid weather; tight-fitting clothing in hot environments; exercising in poorly ventilated areas; sudden exposure to hot climates; and poor fluid intake before, during, and after exercise.
- Patients undergoing cardiac rehabilitation should learn to assess their own pulse rates to determine their response to exercise. Pulses should be taken before, during, and after exercise.
- Instruct patients on the importance of appropriate size and placement of blood pressure cuff for home use.
- Teach patient signs and symptoms of hypoxemia: headache, somnolence, confusion, dusky color, shortness of breath, and dyspnea.
- Teach patient effect of high-risk behaviors such as cigarette smoking on oxygen saturation.

understanding of each patient as an individual and thus assists with administering appropriate nursing care to the patient. See Chapters 6 and 13 for a more thorough discussion (see the Cultural Considerations box).

GUIDELINES FOR OBTAINING VITAL SIGNS

Vital signs are a part of the database obtained during assessment. The procedure for assessing vital signs is not routine. Part of the nurse's task is to individualize the procedure to each patient's needs and condition. Nurses must ensure their skills include all of the following:

- Measuring vital signs correctly
- Understanding and interpreting the values
- Communicating findings appropriately
- Beginning interventions as needed

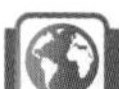

Cultural Considerations

Vital Signs

- Many cultures believe that certain natural or herbal products protect one's health or treat certain health conditions.
- Provide privacy when measuring vital signs.
- Procedures that may be considered routine in some cultures can produce anxiety because of cultural variables regarding touch, privacy, and gender of the health care worker.
- If the patient speaks a different language than the nurse, take extra steps to ensure that the patient understands the vital sign measurement procedure and findings.
    - Use an interpreter if needed and demonstrate the procedure to promote patient understanding.

Box 12.1 Guidelines for Measurement of Vital Signs

- The nurse who cares for the patient is ideally the one to assess vital signs, interpret their significance, and participate in decisions about care.
- Be sure equipment used to measure vital signs (e.g., thermometer, stethoscope, sphygmomanometer) is in proper working condition to ensure accuracy of findings.
- Use standard precautions and ensure equipment is clean. Be aware of the normal range for all vital signs. This knowledge helps detect abnormalities.
- Be aware of the patient's normal range of vital signs. The normal range of some patients differs from the standard range. These values serve as a baseline for comparison with findings obtained later.
- It is wise to know the patient's medical history, therapies, and medications prescribed. Some illnesses or treatments cause predictable changes in vital signs.
- Keep environmental factors that have potential to affect vital signs to a minimum. If you are not able to control these factors, values that are not true indicators of the patient's condition are likely to result (e.g., if assessing the patient's pulse after ambulation or an emotional trauma or obtaining a temperature reading in a warm, humid room).
- Approach the patient in a calm and caring manner while demonstrating proficiency in handling supplies needed for vital sign measurements.
- Use an organized, systematic approach when obtaining vital signs.
- The nurse and the health care provider decide the frequency of vital signs measurement on the basis of the patient's condition. Most acute care facilities have a policy of assessing a patient's vital signs at least once every shift. However, certain conditions dictate more frequent measurement of vital signs. For instance, after a patient has had surgery or a major diagnostic procedure, take frequent measurements until vital signs stabilize to the patient's baseline before the procedure. If a patient's physical condition begins to worsen, take vital signs more frequently, perhaps every 5 to 10 minutes.
- Evaluate the results of vital sign measurement. Vital signs are only one measurement of the patient's condition. It is also necessary to assess other signs and symptoms and be aware of the patient's ongoing health status. Vital signs are only a part of the assessment of the patient's physical and psychologic condition.
- Verify and communicate significant changes in vital signs. The baseline measurement allows the nurse to identify changes in vital signs. Report significant changes in vital signs to the health care provider. Also record and report any changes to the nurses working the oncoming shift.
- Before examination of a patient by the primary provider in an outpatient setting, the nurse or appropriate health care personnel measure the vital signs.
- Report abnormalities in vital signs to the health care provider.

Whether and how frequently vital signs are measured (Box 12.1) depend on the nurse's judgment of the need, the patient's condition, and the orders of the health care provider.

If a possibility of contact with body secretions exists, gloves should be worn while obtaining vital signs.

WHEN TO ASSESS VITAL SIGNS

Although this chapter presents assessing temperature, pulse, respiration, and blood pressure as separate procedures, they usually are assessed at the same time and at set intervals. A set of vital signs is taken when a patient is admitted to a facility and then as prescribed by the health care provider or as policy dictates (e.g., every 4 hours, once a shift, or even weekly in some extended-care facilities) (Box 12.2).

The more ill the patient, the more frequently the nurse takes vital signs. The nurse must use judgment in cases in which the patient's condition worsens, at which time it is necessary to obtain vital signs more frequently. Vital sign readings are interrelated. A rise in temperature of 1°F has potential to cause an increase in pulse rate of 4 beats per minute. Respiratory rate and blood pressure readings likewise increase with a rise in temperature; however, when blood pressure falls because of hemorrhage, the pulse and respirations

Box 12.2 When to Assess Vital Signs

- During admission and discharge to a health care facility
- On a routine schedule as determined by health care provider's order or agency policy
- Before and after surgical procedures
- Before and after invasive diagnostic procedures
- Before and after administering certain medications, especially those that affect cardiovascular, respiratory, and temperature control function
- When the patient's general condition changes (loss of consciousness, hemorrhage, cardiac dysrhythmias, or the onset of intense pain)
- Before and after certain nursing interventions (when a patient ambulates for the first time or after tracheal suctioning)
- When the patient reports nonspecific symptoms of physical distress (reports of "feeling funny" or "different")
- Routinely as part of a procedure (e.g., blood transfusion, liver biopsy, paracentesis, thoracentesis)
- When assessing patient during home health visit
- Pain is considered the fifth vital sign. Pain must be evaluated and documented each time other vital signs are taken. Refer to Chapter 21 for a more in-depth discussion of pain and the interventions available for pain control.

Table 12.1 Age-Related Variations in Vital Signs

AGE GROUP	HEART RATE (PER MINUTE)	RESPIRATORY RATE (PER MINUTE)	BLOOD PRESSURE (MM HG)[a]
Neonate	120–160	36–60	Systolic 20–60
Infant	125–135	40–46	Systolic 70–80
Toddler	90–120	20–30	Systolic 80–100
School-age (6–10 yr)	65–105	22–24	Systolic 90–100 Diastolic 60–64
Adolescent (10–18 yr)	65–100	16–22	Systolic 100–120 Diastolic 70–80
Adult	60–100	12–20	Systolic 100–120 Diastolic 70–80
Older adult	60–100	12–18	Systolic 130–140 Diastolic 90–95

[a]A blood pressure reading of 120/80 mm Hg is now considered prehypertension.

rates increase and the temperature usually decreases. Age-related differences in vital signs are also important to recognize (Table 12.1 and the Home Care Considerations and Lifespan Considerations for Older Adults boxes).

Home Care Considerations

Vital Signs

- Assess temperature and ventilation of environment to determine existence of any conditions that have the potential to influence patient's temperature.
- Assess home noise level to determine the room that provides the quietest environment for assessing pulse and blood pressure (BP).
- Assess family's financial ability to afford a sphygmomanometer for performing BP evaluation on a regular basis.
- Consider an electronic BP cuff with large digital display for home if patient or caregiver has hearing or vision difficulties.
- It is wise for patients taking certain prescribed cardiotonic or antidysrhythmic medications to learn to assess their own pulse rates to detect side effects of medications.
- Assess for environmental factors in the home that have the potential to influence patient's respiratory rate, such as secondhand smoke, inadequate ventilation, or gas fumes.
- Instruct patients who are using mercury-in-glass thermometers at home on their proper use, safety factors, and hazards (see Box 12.8).
- Monitor the effectiveness of home oxygen therapy with the noninvasive method of pulse oximetry.

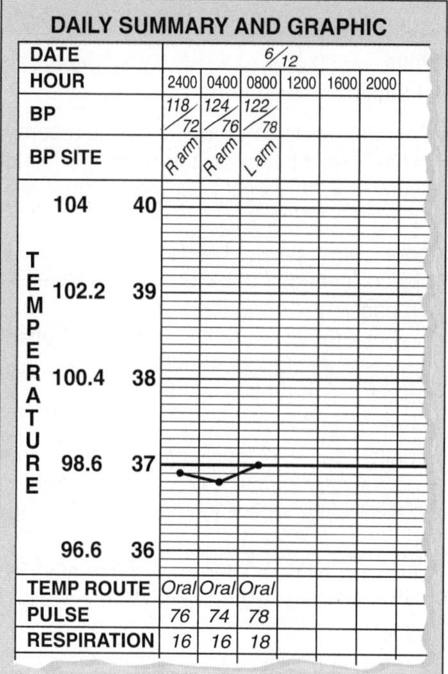

Fig. 12.1 Vital signs documented on flow sheet.

RECORDING VITAL SIGNS

Accuracy in documentation is important. Most facilities have graphic flow sheets for charting vital signs; Fig. 12.1 shows an example. In some facilities, a rectal temperature is indicated with a small circled *R*, and axillary temperature with a small circled *Ax* (see Fig. 12.1) next to the reading. The blood pressure is always written with the systolic first and the diastolic beneath: 120/80 mm Hg. A final /0 may be added (120/80/0) if the beat is clearly heard until the end. All abnormal findings must be reported immediately to the nurse manager or health care provider. In addition to actual vital signs values, any accompanying or precipitating signs and symptoms such as chest pain, vertigo, shortness of breath, flushing, and diaphoresis should be noted in the nurse's notes. Any interventions initiated as a result of vital signs measurement, such as tepid sponging (for temperature elevation), also should be documented.

TEMPERATURE

BODY'S REGULATION OF TEMPERATURE

The body strives to maintain a **temperature** (a relative measure of sensible heat or cold) of 98.6°F (37°C) (Box 12.3), which is considered normal. Variations from 97° to 99.6°F (36.1° to 37.5°C) are considered to be within normal range. Many factors have the potential to cause body temperature variances, including the environment, the time of day, the patient's state of health and activity levels, and the stage of the patient's monthly menstrual cycle (Box 12.4).

Lifespan Considerations

Older Adults

Taking Vital Signs

- An active older adult generally maintains a core body temperature within the accepted norms for younger adults. After age 75 years, core temperature averages 97.2°F (36°C).
- Older adults often have a baseline temperature that is not typical of the adult patient, so knowledge of each patient's baseline is important.
- Environmental temperature has more of an effect on body temperature in older than in younger adults and is more likely to contribute to hypothermia and hyperthermia.
- Older adults often have occlusive amounts of earwax in one or both ear canals. Consider this when assessing an older adult's tympanic temperature reading.
- The older adult with an infection is often afebrile. Be aware of other signs and symptoms of infection in the older adult.
- Manifestations of delayed or diminished febrile response to infection are subtle and variable and very difficult to assess. Be especially attentive to subtle temperature changes and other manifestations of fever in this population, such as tachypnea, anorexia, falls, delirium, and overall functional decline.
- The older adult has a decreased heart rate at rest.
- Once elevated, the pulse rate of an older adult takes longer to return to normal resting rate.
- Pulses can be occluded easily in older adults; therefore apply only gentle pressure.
- Pulse irregularities are seen more commonly in older adults. Apical pulses should be auscultated as part of a thorough assessment.
- When assessing older women with sagging breasts, gently lift the breast tissue and place the stethoscope at the fifth intercostal space (ICS) or the lower edge of the breast.
- Heart sounds are often muffled or difficult to hear in older adults because of an increase in air space in the lungs.
- With aging, depth of respirations typically decreases. Respiratory rate often increases to compensate.
- Decreased efficiency of respiratory muscles results in breathlessness at low exercise levels.
- Responses to hypoxia are reduced in older adults as compared with the young, which limits the ability of older adults to respond to hypoxia with respiratory changes.
- Often a standard adult cuff is too large for an older individual who has lost upper arm mass. Incorrect cuff sizing potentially results in significant errors.
- The skin of many older adults is more fragile and susceptible to cuff pressure when blood pressure measurements are frequent, as during the use of repeated electronic measurement. Perform more frequent assessment of the skin area under the cuff or increase rotation of blood pressure sites.
- Accurate measurement of blood pressure is essential for older adults receiving antihypertensive medication.
- Orthostatic hypotension (a sudden drop in blood pressure with positional change) commonly is observed in inactive older adults, particularly when rising after a period of bed rest.
- Closely monitor older adults receiving antihypertensives and vasodilators for orthostatic hypotension.
- An older adult's blood pressure often elevates with age. Do not consider such elevations a normal aspect of aging, but monitor minor elevations.
- Older adults have an increase in systolic pressure related to decreased vessel elasticity. The diastolic pressure remains the same, resulting in a wider pulse pressure.
- Older adults are instructed to change position slowly and wait after each change to avoid postural hypotension and prevent injuries.
- Identification of an acceptable pulse oximeter probe site on older adults is often difficult because of the possible presence of peripheral vascular disease, decreased cardiac output, cold-induced vasoconstriction, and anemia. Alternate pulse oximetry sites include the earlobe and toes.

Box 12.3 Normal Body Temperatures According to Measurement Sites

	Oral	Rectal	Axillary	Tympanic/ Temporal
Fahrenheit (F)	98.6°F	99.6°F	97.6°F	98.6°F
Celsius (C)	37.0°C	37.5°C	36.4°C	37.0°C

When it is necessary to convert temperature readings, formulas are available to use. To convert Fahrenheit to centigrade, subtract 32° from the Fahrenheit reading and multiply the results by 5/9: (98.6–32) × 5/9 = 37. To convert centigrade to Fahrenheit, multiply the Celsius reading by 9/5 and add 32° to the reading: 37 × 9/5 + 32 = 98.6.

Regulation of body temperature is the job of the hypothalamus, which is located in the brain and forms the floor and part of the lateral wall of the third ventricle. The hypothalamus helps maintain a balance between heat lost and heat produced by the body. A rise in metabolism, as occurs with exercise and digestion, is the primary mechanism the body uses to generate heat. Constriction of peripheral vessels prevents loss of heat through the skin surface and thus helps conserve heat.

Body temperature falls into two categories: *core temperature,* which is the temperature of the deep tissues of the body, and *surface temperature,* which is the temperature of the skin. Apart from pathologic disturbances, core temperature remains relatively constant unless a person is exposed to severe extremes in environmental temperature. Surface temperature, on the other hand, often varies a great deal in response to the environment.

Temperature elevations are frequently the first sign of illness (Box 12.5). The terms *pyrexia,* **febrile**, and **hyperthermia** are used to describe the condition of having above-normal body temperature. Fever is actually a body defense. Elevated body temperature helps destroy

Box 12.4 Factors That Affect Body Temperature

AGE
The neonate's temperature normally ranges from 96° to 99.5°F (35.5° to 37.5°C). Temperature regulation is labile (unstable) during infancy because of immature physiologic mechanisms. This often continues to be the case until puberty. In older adults, the normal range commonly lowers, and a body temperature of 95°F (35°C) is not unusual for some older patients in cold weather. With aging, sensitivity to temperature extremes develops because of deteriorating control mechanisms.

EXERCISE
Any form of exercise can increase body temperature. Prolonged strenuous exercise has the potential to temporarily raise body temperatures to as high as the 103.2° to 105.8°F (40° to 41°C) range.

HORMONAL INFLUENCES
Women generally have greater variations in body temperature than men. Hormonal changes during ovulation and menopause cause body temperature fluctuations.

DIURNAL (DAILY) VARIATIONS
Body temperatures normally change throughout the day, with the lowest reading occurring between 1 a.m. and 4 a.m. (97.7°F [36.5°C] on average). The temperature usually peaks around 4 p.m. to 6 p.m. The temperature patterns in people who work at night and sleep during the day do not reverse automatically. It generally takes 1 to 3 weeks for the cycle to reverse.

STRESS
Physical or emotional stress, such as anxiety, often raises body temperature.

ENVIRONMENT
Environmental temperature extremes have the potential to raise or lower the body temperature. The changes depend on the extent of exposure, air humidity, and the presence of convection currents.

INGESTION OF FOOD AND HOT AND COLD LIQUIDS
Drinking hot or cold liquids or ingestion of food can cause variations in oral temperature readings (e.g., by 20.2° to 21.6°F after drinking iced water).

SMOKING
Smoking cigarettes or cigars sometimes alters body temperature measurement (±0.2°F).

Box 12.5 Signs and Symptoms of Elevated Body Temperature

- Anorexia
- Disorientation, progressing to convulsions in infants and children
- Elevated pulse and respiratory rates
- Flushed, warm skin
- Glassy eyes or photophobia (sensitivity to light), or both
- Headache
- Increased perspiration
- Irritability
- Restlessness or excessive sleepiness
- Thirst

Box 12.6 Nursing Interventions for the Patient With an Abnormal Body Temperature

- If temperature reading is abnormal, repeat measurement. If indicated, select another site.
- Remove or reduce the patient's external coverings.
- Keep patient's clothing and bed linens dry.
- Monitor patient's temperature at least every 4 hours or prn.
- Administer medication (usually acetaminophen) as ordered by the health care provider.
- Limit patient's physical activity. Increase frequency of rest periods.
- Increase or encourage oral fluid intake if not contraindicated (i.e., heart failure [HF]). If temperature is elevated, assess for additional related data that suggest systemic infection such as anorexia, headache, thirst, and chills.
- If temperature is above normal, further assess for possible site of localized infection such as pain or tenderness, purulent exudates, erythema, edema, and area of unusual warmth.
- If temperature continues to be elevated, encourage oral hygiene because oral mucous membranes dry easily from dehydration.
- If patient's temperature is subnormal, cover patient with more blankets; close room doors or windows to eliminate drafts; encourage warm liquids; and remove wet clothes and replace with dry ones.

invading bacteria. Temperatures exceeding 105°F (40.5°C) also have the potential to damage normal body cells, and therefore intervention is often necessary (Box 12.6).

Fevers are classified as constant, intermittent, or remittent. Constant fevers remain elevated consistently and fluctuate very little. Intermittent fevers rise and fall; for example, temperature is normal or subnormal in the morning and "spikes" (is elevated) in the afternoon. Remittent fevers are similar to intermittent fevers except the temperature does not return to normal at all until the patient becomes well (Fig. 12.2).

When the body temperature is abnormally low, the condition is called **hypothermia.** Death is a risk when the body temperature falls below 93.2°F (34°C). Cases of people surviving with much lower temperatures have been documented. Patients may be placed intentionally in hypothermia for a surgical procedure. Certain conditions, such as hypothyroidism, produce a subnormal temperature.

OBTAINING TEMPERATURE MEASUREMENTS

Temperature measurements are obtained by several methods (Skill 12.1). When a patient has a normal body

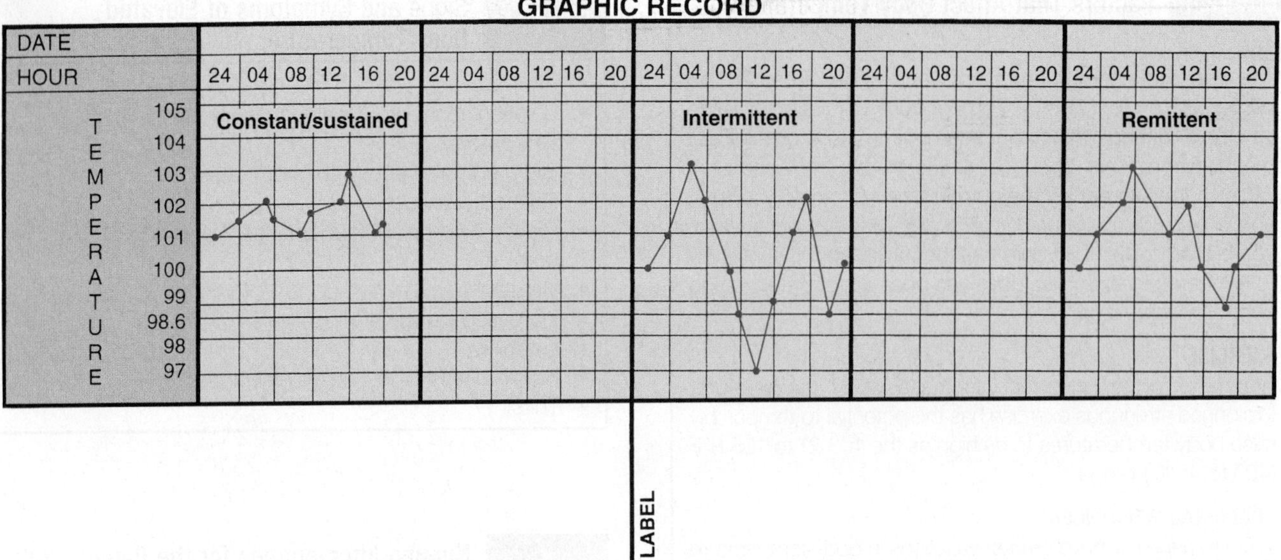

Fig. 12.2 Temperature measurements recorded on a flow sheet showing types of fevers.

temperature, a peripheral temperature gives a good estimate of core temperature. Touch the patient's skin and observe its moisture and warmth. For an actual reading of surface temperature, the use of heat-sensitive patches is one method (Fig. 12.3A). Place the patch on an area of skin, such as the forehead; the color change on the patch indicates the temperature.

If the patient's temperature is rising or falling rapidly, the body's thermoregulatory system affects peripheral sites, and temperatures can lag significantly behind true core temperature. Remember this when using one of the various types of thermometers to assess a patient's core temperature (Box 12.7). Experts no longer recommend the use of mercury-containing thermometers (Box 12.8). Electronic thermometers (Fig. 12.3B) consist of a rechargeable battery-powered display unit, a thin wire cord, and a temperature-processing probe that should be used only with a disposable cover. Separate probes are available for oral temperature measurement (blue tip) and rectal temperature measurement (red tip). Specially designated electronic thermometers are used to obtain the **tympanic** temperature by scanning the tympanic (eardrum) membrane (Fig. 12.3C).

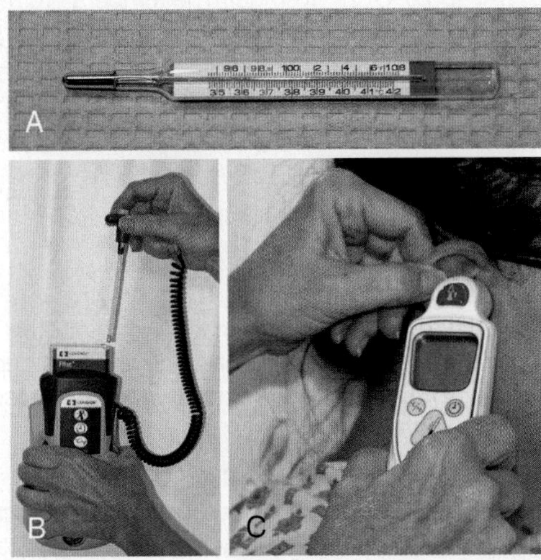

Fig. 12.3 A, Disposable, single-use thermometer. B, Electronic thermometer. C, Tympanic thermometer.

Tympanic thermometers have been available for many years and are now widely accepted. They are very likely more accurate than traditional thermometers, when placed correctly, because measurement is from an enclosed cavity unaffected by the environmental temperatures. The tympanic membrane shares its blood supply with the hypothalamus, the body's temperature control center, and thus is a good source for obtaining core-temperature readings. To obtain the reading, place the sensor probe on the tympanic thermometer in the external ear; the sensor measures infrared heat. These thermometers boast many advantages: they are easy to use and produce readings in a few seconds; they are suitable for patients of all ages, except infants less than 6 months old; they virtually eliminate the risk of cross-contamination; and they are cost effective (see Skill 12.1). In contrast to rectal and oral measurement, they necessitate neither the exposure of the patient nor the patient's active participation. An additional means of measuring core temperature is the temporal artery method, which provides a reliable noninvasive measurement. It uses an infrared sensor that is brushed over the temporal artery to measure the core temperature that is present in the blood passing through the temporal artery (see Skill 12.1).

Skill 12.1 Measuring Body Temperature

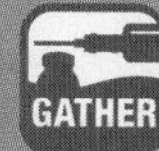

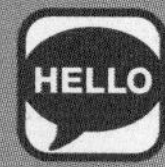

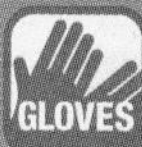

NURSING ACTION *(RATIONALE)*

1. Perform hand hygiene. *(Reduces spread of microorganisms.)*
2. Assess for signs and symptoms of temperature alterations and for factors that influence body temperature. *(Enables the nurse to more accurately assess nature of variations.)*
3. Introduce self to patient. *(Decreases patient's anxiety.)*
4. Identify patient by identification band. *(Ensures correct patient for procedure.)*
5. Explain the procedure to patient: site of temperature reading and importance of maintaining proper position until reading is complete. *(Gains patient's cooperation.)*
6. Prepare for procedure.
   a. Assemble the thermometer, soft disposable tissues, lubricant (for rectal temperature only), pen and note pad, disposable gloves, plastic sleeve, or disposable probe cover. *(Promotes an efficiently completed procedure.)*
   b. Provide for patient privacy. *(Decreases anxiety level.)*
   c. Determine whether patient has consumed hot or cold beverages or food or has been smoking; if so, wait 20 to 30 minutes before measuring oral temperature. *(Ensures accuracy.)*
7. Obtaining an oral temperature reading with an electronic thermometer.
   a. Follow Steps 1 through 6.
   b. Perform hand hygiene and don disposable gloves (optional). *(Reduces spread of microorganisms.)*
   c. Remove thermometer pack from charging unit. *(Adds maneuverability; battery power is available.)* Remove probe from storage well of recording unit. Grasp top of stem, being careful not to apply pressure to eject button. *(Ensures proper working order.)*
   d. Insert probe snugly into probe cover: red probe for rectal readings, blue probe for oral and axillary readings (see Fig. 12.3). *(Using probe cover helps reduce spread of microorganisms.)*
   e. Inspect digital display. *(Ensures that unit is ready for use.)*
   f. Request patient to open the mouth; gently insert probe into the posterior sublingual pocket. Request patient to hold thermometer in place with lips closed. *(Ensures an accurate reading.)*

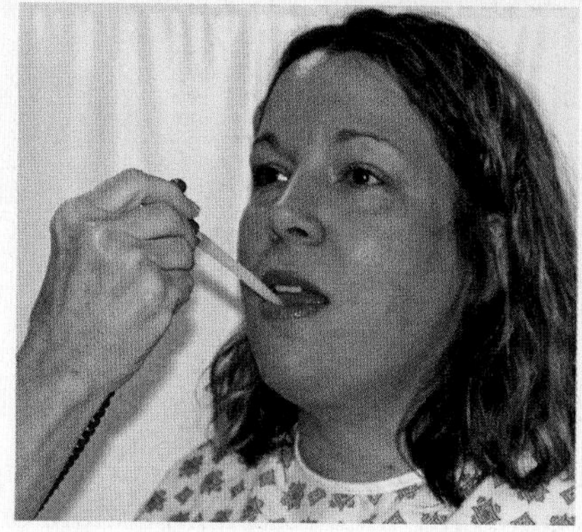

   g. Wait for audible signal. *(Indicates temperature reading is complete.)*
   h. Remove probe from patient's mouth and remove probe cover by pressing the eject button, directing probe cover into trash receptacle. *(Reduces spread of microorganisms.)*
   i. Provide for patient comfort.
   j. Read and write down reading from digital display before reinserting probe into holder. *(Ensures accurate recording.)*
   k. Perform hand hygiene. *(Reduces spread of microorganisms.)* Return electronic unit to charger. *(Maintains battery charge.)*
   l. Complete procedure by following Step 12, a through d.
8. Measuring rectal temperature with an electronic thermometer. CAUTION: If unable to insert thermometer adequately into the rectum, remove thermometer and consider alternative method for obtaining temperature. Never force thermometer.
   a. Follow Steps 1 through 6b.
   b. Don gloves. *(Maintains standard precautions.)*
   c. Assist patient to the Sims position with upper leg flexed. Move aside the bed linens to expose only the rectal area. *(Ensures correct thermometer placement and prevents unnecessary exposure of patient.)*
   d. Remove thermometer pack from charging unit. Be certain rectal (red) probe is attached to the unit and slide disposable plastic cover over thermometer probe until it locks into place. *(Reduces spread of microorganisms.)*
   e. With thermometer in probe cover, lubricate 1 inch of tip. *(Eases insertion.)*
   f. For an adult, with patient in the Sims position, gently spread buttocks and insert thermometer probe 1.5 inches into rectum. Hold on to thermometer throughout procedure. *(Ensures safety.)*

Continued

Skill 12.1 Measuring Body Temperature—cont'd

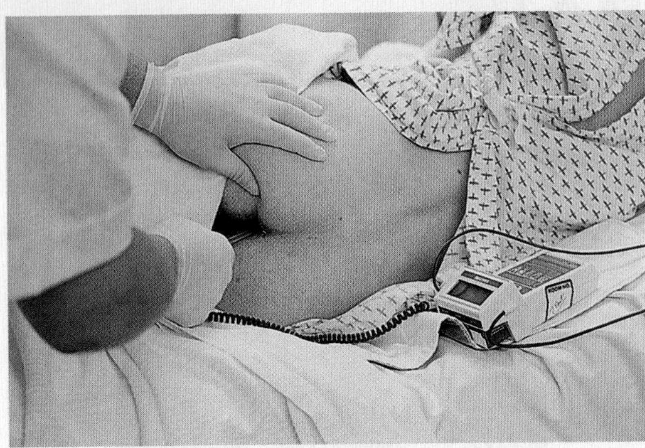

g. Hold electronic probe until audible signal occurs; only then read temperature on digital display (keep probe in place until signal occurs). *(Ensures accurate reading.)*

h. Carefully remove probe from rectum; push eject button to remove probe cover and dispose into appropriate receptacle. *(Reduces spread of microorganisms.)*

i. Return probe to storage unit, and later return the unit to its charging device. *(Prevents damage to the unit and ensures accurate working for the next assessment.)*

j. Clean anal area of lubricant and possible feces. Remove and dispose of gloves and perform hand hygiene. *(Provides comfort and hygiene and reduces the spread of microorganisms.)*

k. Assist patient to position of comfort. *(Restores self-esteem.)*

l. Write down reading for later documentation. *(Ensures accurate recording.)*

m. Complete procedure by following Step 12, a through d.

9. Measuring axillary temperature with an electronic thermometer.

a. Follow Steps 1 through 6b.

b. Don gloves. *(Maintains standard precautions.)*

c. Assist patient to supine or sitting position. *(Provides easy access to axilla.)*

d. Expose axilla; be certain the area is clean and dry. *(Ensures accurate reading.)*

e. Prepare electronic thermometer following Step 7, c through e.

f. Insert probe into center of axilla; lower arm over thermometer, placing arm across patient's chest. In an infant or young child, it is sometimes necessary to hold the arm against the child's side when using the axillary method. If infant is in a side-lying position, the lower axilla records the higher temperature. *(Maintains proper positioning of temperature probe.)*

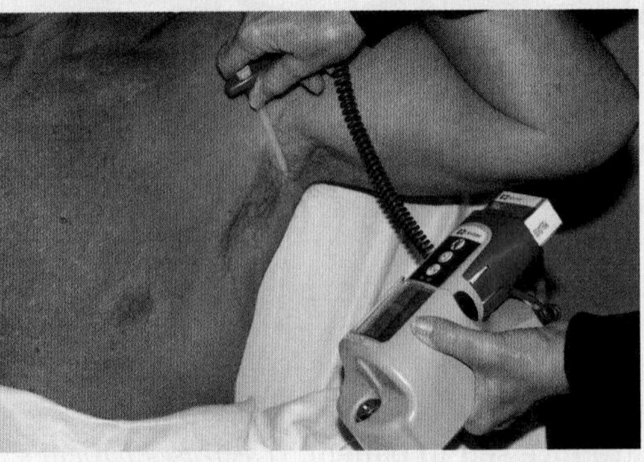

g. Hold electronic probe until audible signal occurs. Reading appears on digital display. *(Probe must stay in place for accurate reading to occur.)*

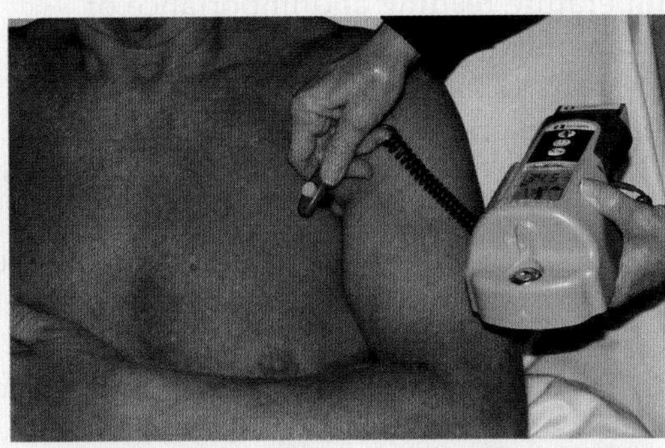

h. Remove probe from patient's axilla. Push eject button to remove probe cover and dispose into trash container. *(Reduces spread of microorganisms.)*

i. Return electric probe to storage well of recording unit. *(Prevents damage to unit.)*

j. Assist patient to regown and position for comfort. *(Restores a sense of well-being.)*

k. Remove and dispose of gloves in proper receptacle, and perform hand hygiene. *(Reduces spread of microorganisms.)*

l. Return thermometer to charger base. *(Maintains battery charge.)*

m. Write down reading for later documentation. *(Ensures accurate recording.)*

n. Complete procedure by following Step 12, a through d.

10. Measuring tympanic temperature with an electronic thermometer.

a. Follow Steps 1 through 6a.

b. Assist patient to a comfortable position with head turned toward the side, away from you. *(Ensures comfort and exposes auditory canal for accurate temperature reading.)*

c. Remove thermometer handheld unit from charging base. *(Provides easy access to thermometer.)*

Skill 12.1 Measuring Body Temperature—cont'd

- **d.** Slide disposable plastic speculum cover over otoscope-like tip until it locks into place. *(Prepares the unit to measure temperature; the plastic speculum reduces spread of microorganisms.)*
- **e.** Follow manufacturer's instructions for tympanic probe positioning.
  - **(1)** Gently tug ear pinna upward and back for an adult, down and back for a child. *(Difference is because of age-related anatomic differences).*
  - **(2)** Gently insert thermometer into ear. *(Ensures correct placement.)*
  - **(3)** Fit ear probe snugly into canal. Do not allow further movement. *(Ensures correct reading.)*
  - **(4)** Point digital readout toward you, following manufacturer's positioning recommendations. *(Steps [1] through [4] ensure correct positioning of the probe with respect to ear canal; the ear tug straightens the external auditory canal, allowing maximum exposure of the tympanic membrane.)*
- **f.** Depress scan button on handheld unit and read assessment. Temperature reading appears on digital display.
- **g.** Carefully remove sensor from ear and push release button to eject plastic speculum cover; discard into proper receptacle. *(Reduces spread of microorganisms.)*
- **h.** Return handheld unit to charging base. *(Maintains battery charge.)*
- **i.** Assist patient to a comfortable position. *(Restores sense of well-being.)*
- **j.** Perform hand hygiene. Dispose of gloves, if worn, into proper receptacle. *(Reduces spread of microorganisms.)*
- **k.** Write down reading (for documentation later).
- **l.** Complete procedure by following Step 12, a through d.

11. Measuring temporal artery temperature. (This skill can be delegated to unlicensed assistive personnel who are knowledgeable in the procedure, but it is the nurse's responsibility to assess the significance of the findings.)

- **a.** Follow Steps 1 through 6a.
- **b.** Ensure that forehead is dry. *(Decreases chance of moisture interfering with temperature measurement.)*
- **c.** Place probe flush on patient's forehead. *(Prevents measuring ambient temperature by mistake.)*
- **d.** Press the scan button. *(Continuous scanning for the highest temperature occurs until you release the scan button.)*
- **e.** Keeping the probe flush on the skin, slowly brush the thermometer straight across forehead. *(Promotes accuracy in measurement.)*
- **f.** Keeping the scan button pressed, sweep the probe across the forehead and continue to just behind the earlobe.
- **g.** The thermometer makes a clicking sound when highest temperature is reached. Read and document temperature.
- **h.** Wipe probe with alcohol, or remove and dispose of probe cover.
- **i.** Complete procedure by following Step 12, a through d.

12. Complete the procedure for body temperature measurement.

- **a.** Compare temperature findings with baseline and normal temperature range for patient's age group. *(Comparison reveals presence of abnormalities.)*
- **b.** If temperature is abnormal, repeat procedure. If indicated, choose an alternate site or instrument. *(Second reading confirms initial findings of abnormal body temperature.)*
- **c.** Record temperature on vital sign flow sheet, graphic flow sheet, or nurse's notes and report abnormal findings to nurse in charge or health care provider (see Fig. 12.1 and Box 12.5). *(Recording promptly prevents omissions from the record. Abnormalities often necessitate immediate therapy.)* When recording an axillary temperature, write *Ax* above your documentation. When recording a rectal temperature, write *R* above the reading.
- **d.** Do patient teaching (see patient teaching in the Health Promotion box on vital signs).

Figure for Step 8f from Potter PA, Perry AG, Stockert PA, et al: *Fundamentals of nursing,* ed 8, St. Louis, 2013, Mosby.

An assessment of the patient guides the choice of method to measure the temperature (Table 12.2). The method chosen to check the temperature must be documented along with the reading. Obtaining an oral temperature should not be attempted in the comatose or the disoriented patient, or in small infants, because this method requires the patient's cooperation. Rectal measurements are contraindicated for patients with recent rectal surgery or certain conditions of the perineum. Axillary measurement is considered the least accurate method and is used less frequently since the advent of the tympanic thermometer (see Skill 12.1). Rectal readings are normally 1°F higher, and axillary readings 1°F lower, than oral readings. When obtaining an oral or a tympanic reading, the nurse typically does not need to provide privacy for the. Use of the temporal artery scanner is appropriate in almost all situations. If the patient has diaphoresis, to increase the accuracy of the measurement, brush the scanner all the way across the forehead through to behind the ear.

Box 12.7 Assessing Tympanic Temperature Accurately

- Be certain the patient has been indoors for at least 10 minutes. Also be certain the patient has not been lying on the ear, which could warm it artificially.
- The base of the thermometer provides battery power.
- If the reading seems too low, replace the probe cover and repeat the procedure. Be certain that the lens and the probe cover are clean and intact. Reassess the temperature, paying close attention to technique. Follow manufacturer's recommendations.
- The eject button releases the plastic probe cover from the tip of the thermometer.
- Be alert to temperature variations from ear to ear, especially if the temperature does not fit the patient's clinical picture. Sometimes different readings are obtained in the patient's left and right ears. Document which ear was used for the temperature assessment.
- Fluctuations in normal body temperature are minimal; therefore, if a significant variation from normal is seen, a second measurement is necessary for comparison. Ensure that the probe is not placed improperly or moved during temperature measurement.

AUSCULTATING WITH THE STETHOSCOPE

A **stethoscope** (an instrument that is placed against the patient's chest or back to hear heart and lung sounds) (Fig. 12.4) is used to measure the apical rate of the heart (see definitions of *apical* and *radial* in the following section on the pulse). The major parts of the stethoscope are the earpieces, the binaurals, the tubing, and the chest piece.

The plastic or rubber earpieces should fit snugly and comfortably in the ears. If the fit is proper, the binaurals are angled and strong enough that the earpieces stay

Box 12.8 Elimination of Mercury-Containing Devices

- In 1714 Fahrenheit invented the constant reference point thermometer using mercury in glass.
- In 1868 Wunderlich established the normal range of body temperatures in humans as 97.25° to 99.5°F, using Fahrenheit's constant reference point thermometer. This remains the standard today.
- The mercury-in-glass thermometer was the only instrument available for use for more than 200 years. It was portable, accurate, and easy to use. However, we now know these thermometers are potentially dangerous if they break, posing a serious threat to not only the patient but also the environment. One gram of mercury, the amount contained in a mercury-in-glass thermometer, is enough to contaminate a lake with the surface area of 20 acres.
- A technical report from the American Academy of Pediatrics (Goldman, 2001) addresses the hazards of mercury and discusses possible measures for pediatricians to reduce children's exposure. One of the chief findings was the recommendation for pediatricians to stop using all mercury-containing devices, including thermometers, and encourage parents to do the same. If the thermometer breaks, the mercury vaporizes and can be inhaled, causing toxicity. The statement calls for an end to the use of all mercury-containing thermometers. **Most health care facilities, clinics, and health care providers' offices have discontinued the use of glass mercury thermometers, and mercury-calibrated sphygmomanometers. Most pharmacies no longer sell these products.** However, glass thermometers are still used in homes.

In the event of a mercury spill:

- Do NOT touch spilled mercury droplets. If skin contact has occurred, immediately flush area with water for 15 minutes.
- If possible, remove patient from immediate environment of contamination.
- Change any clothing or linen that has been contaminated with mercury. Perform hand hygiene thoroughly after changing. Wash clothing before reuse.
- Notify the environmental services department or obtain a mercury spill kit, if available.
- Follow procedures for mercury removal as directed by the Material Safety Data Sheet (MSDS). Spills are removed with special absorbent materials, filtered vacuum equipment, and protective clothing.
- Promote exhaust ventilation to reduce concentration of mercury vapors.
- Follow agency guidelines for laundering clothing.
- Complete occurrence or incident report as directed by institution procedure.

The Emergency Response Safety and Health Database, 2013. Retrieved from *www.cdc.gov/niosh/ershdb/EmergencyResponseCard_29750021.html.*

Table 12.2 Selection of Sites for Temperature Measurement

ADVANTAGES	DISADVANTAGES AND LIMITATIONS
Oral	
Most accessible site; comfortable for patient; necessitates no position change	Do not use for patients who could be injured by thermometer, who are unable to hold thermometer properly, or who may bite down on thermometer (glass thermometer); infants or small children; disoriented or unconscious patients; patients who have had oral surgery; patients with trauma to face or mouth; patients experiencing oral pain; patients who breathe only with mouth open; patients with history of convulsions; or patients experiencing a shaking chill.
Rectal	
Argued to be more reliable when oral temperature cannot be obtained	Use sensitivity because use is embarrassing. Do not use for patients after rectal surgery; patients who have a rectal disorder, such as tumor or hemorrhoids; or patients who cannot be positioned for proper thermometer placement, such as those in traction. There is a risk of body fluid exposure, and lubrication is required.
Axilla	
Safe method because noninvasive	This is the least accurate method.
Tympanic	
Noninvasive, accurate, safe; provides core reading	Excessive cerumen (earwax) has the possibility to interfere with accurate reading; continuous measurement of temperature is not possible; new disposable probe cover is necessary for each patient, which raises the cost; patients must remove hearing aid in the ear that temperature is being measured.
Temporal Artery	
Provides core temperature; rapid, noninvasive method; tolerated well by children; lessens need to handle newborns, which aids in preventing heat loss	Diaphoresis and airflow across the face may affect the accuracy; possible for any bandages or dressings on the face or head to prevent measurement with the device.

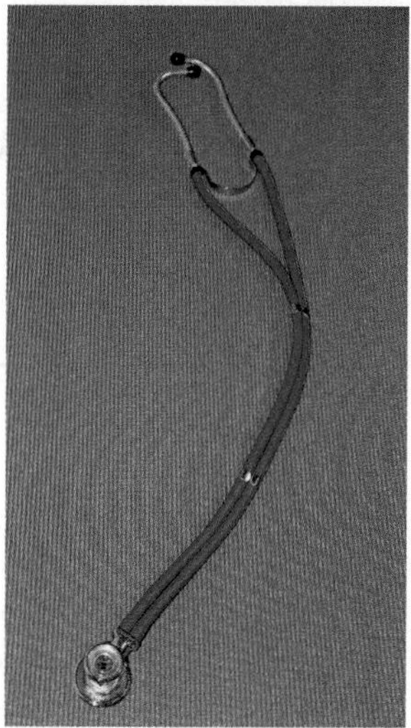

Fig. 12.4 Parts of a stethoscope. Chest piece must be placed firmly against the chest wall.

firmly in the ears without causing discomfort. For the best reception of sound, the earpieces follow the contour of the ear canal, pointing toward the user's face when the stethoscope is in place.

The proper polyvinyl tubing is flexible and 12 to 18 inches (30 to 40 cm) long. Longer tubing decreases the transmission of sound waves. The tubing is thick walled and moderately rigid to eliminate transmission of environmental noise and prevent the tubing from kinking, which distorts sound wave transmission. Some stethoscopes have single tubes, and some have dual tubes.

The chest piece consists of a bell and a diaphragm. According to which is chosen for use, the bell or the diaphragm is rotated into proper position on the chest piece so that the sounds are heard through the stethoscope. To test, lightly tap to determine which side is functioning.

The diaphragm is the circular, flat-surfaced portion of the chest piece covered with a thin plastic disk (see Fig. 12.4). It transmits the high-pitched sounds created by the high-velocity movement of air and blood. **Auscultate** (listen for sounds within the body to evaluate the condition of heart, lungs, pleura, intestines, or other organs or to detect fetal heart tones) bowel, lung, and heart sounds with the diaphragm. Position the diaphragm to make a tight seal against the patient's skin. Exert enough pressure to leave a temporary red ring on the patient's skin when the diaphragm is removed.

The bell is the bowl-shaped chest piece, usually surrounded by a rubber ring (see Fig. 21.4). The ring prevents the cold metal from chilling the patient's skin. The bell transmits low-pitched sounds created by the low-velocity movement of blood. Auscultate heart and vascular sounds using the bell. Apply the bell lightly, resting the chest piece on the skin. Compressing the bell against the skin reduces low-pitched sound amplification and creates a "diaphragm of skin."

When listening through the stethoscope, maintain a position that allows the tubing to extend straight and hang free. Movement creates the potential for tubing to rub or bump objects, creating extraneous sounds. Kinked tubing muffles sounds. When the nurse is using the stethoscope, the nurse and the patient should remain quiet.

The stethoscope is a delicate instrument and requires proper care for optimal function. Remove the earpieces regularly and clean them of cerumen (earwax). Clean the bell and diaphragm of dust, lint, and body oils after each patient contact for infection control purposes. Keep the tubing away from your body oils. Do not drape the stethoscope around your neck next to the skin. Cleaning the tubing or head with alcohol can dry and crack the material and is not recommended. Mild soap and water are preferred.

PULSE

BODY'S REGULATION OF PULSE

A **pulse** is a rhythmic beating or vibrating movement. In the body, it signifies the regular, recurrent expansion and contraction of an artery produced by the waves of pressure that are caused by the ejection of blood from the left ventricle of the heart as it contracts. Each pulse beat corresponds to a contraction of the heart. The adult pulse rate is normally between 60 and 100 beats per minute, with the approximate average being 80.

The condition of the heart and the patient's age, gender, emotional state, size, temperature, and amount of physical activity can influence the pulse rate. If the pulse is faster than 100 beats per minute, the adult patient has **tachycardia**; if it is slower than 60 beats per minute, the patient has **bradycardia**. Tachycardia has many potential causes: shock, hemorrhage leading to hypovolemia (an abnormally low circulating blood volume), exercise, fever, medication or substance abuse, and acute pain. Some drugs, such as epinephrine, also increase the pulse rate. One cause of bradycardia is unrelieved severe pain. Pain stimulates the parasympathetic nervous system, which slows the heart rate. Cardiac issues such as heart blocks also may cause bradycardia (see *Adult Health Nursing*, Chapter 8). Some drugs, such as beta blockers, lower the heart rate. Resting in a supine position also has the potential to decrease the heart rate, as does the cardiac condition called *heart block* (Box 12.9).

If the amount of time between beats varies, there is an irregular pulse or **dysrhythmia** (any disturbance or abnormality in a normal rhythmic pattern, specifically, irregularity in the normal rhythm of the heart). In the normal pulse, the amount of time between beats is even.

Box 12.9 Factors That Influence Pulse Rates

ACUTE PAIN, ANXIETY
These increase the pulse rate because of sympathetic stimulation.

AGE
The pulse rate decreases as the aging process progresses from infancy through adulthood. Pulse rate in the older adult is sometimes greater than 80 beats per minute because of weakened heart muscle or because of medication.

EXERCISE
Short-term exercise increases pulse rate. Long-term exercise strengthens heart muscle, resulting in a lower-than-normal rate at rest and a quicker return to resting rate after exercise.

FEVER, HEAT
Both increase the pulse rate because of increased metabolic rate. Hypothermia decreases pulse rate.

HEMORRHAGE
Loss of blood increases the pulse rate because of the sympathetic stimulation.

MEDICATIONS
Various medications alter pulse rate. For example, digitalis decreases the pulse rate; atropine and epinephrine increase the pulse rate.

METABOLISM
Certain diseases such as hyperthyroidism sometimes cause a chronic elevated pulse rate. Hypothyroidism sometimes causes a slowing of the pulse.

POSTURAL CHANGES
Lying down initially decreases the pulse rate. Standing or sitting increases the pulse rate.

PULMONARY CONDITIONS
Pulmonary conditions increase pulse rate because these diseases cause poor oxygenation.

UNRELIEVED SEVERE PAIN, CHRONIC PAIN
These decrease the pulse rate because of parasympathetic stimulation.

The volume of the pulse refers to the amount of blood pushing against the artery wall with each beat. A weak pulse is difficult to palpate; a bounding pulse is easily felt with light palpation. A pulse that you are unable to feel at all is imperceptible. Another means to communicate the volume of the pulse is by the use of numbers (Table 12.3). Follow agency policy when describing the pulse because some agencies may use a slightly different scale.

OBTAINING PULSE MEASUREMENTS

When taking the pulse, note the rate, the rhythm, and the volume, or strength, of the pulse. Palpate pulses using the pads of the index and middle fingers (Skill 12.2). Apply only slight pressure over the artery to avoid

Table 12.3 Pulse Volume Variations

NUMBER	TYPE	DESCRIPTION
0	Absent pulse	None felt
1+	Thready pulse	Difficult to feel; not palpable when only slight pressure applied
2+	Weak pulse	Somewhat stronger than a thready pulse but not palpable when light pressure applied
3+	Normal pulse	Easily felt but not palpable when moderate pressure applied
4+	Bounding pulse	Feels full and springlike even under moderate pressure

obliterating the pulse (by occluding blood flow). Assess pulses on both sides of the peripheral vascular system. Assess both radial pulses, for example, to compare the characteristics of each and compare the left with the right pulse. In many disease states (e.g., thrombus [clot] formation, aberrant [abnormal] blood vessels, cervical rib syndrome, or aortic dissection), a pulse in one extremity is unequal in strength or absent. Assessment of all symmetric pulses simultaneously is acceptable, except for the carotid pulse. Never measure both carotid pulses simultaneously because excessive pressure has the potential to occlude blood supply to the brain. Do not reach across the patient's neck to count the carotid pulse (the patient's airway can be occluded with the

Skill 12.2 Obtaining a Pulse Rate

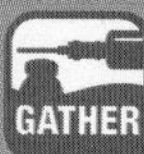

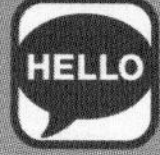

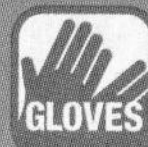

NURSING ACTION *(RATIONALE)*

1. Perform hand hygiene. *(Decreases spread of microorganisms.)*
2. Introduce self to patient. *(Decreases patient's anxiety.)*
3. Identify patient by identification band. *(Verifies correct patient for procedure.)*
4. Explain procedure. *(Seeks cooperation and assistance from the patient and decreases patient's anxiety.)*
5. Prepare for procedure by doing the following:
   a. Assemble all necessary supplies, including a wristwatch with second hand. *(Organizes procedure.)*
   b. Provide privacy for the patient if necessary. *(Decreases patient's anxiety.)*
6. Implement procedure: Count pulse for 60 seconds.
   a. Palpate pulse:
      (1) For *radial pulse,* lightly place tips of first and second fingers in groove formed along radial side of forearm, lateral to flexor tendon of wrist. *(Pulse is relatively superficial and should not require deep palpation.)*

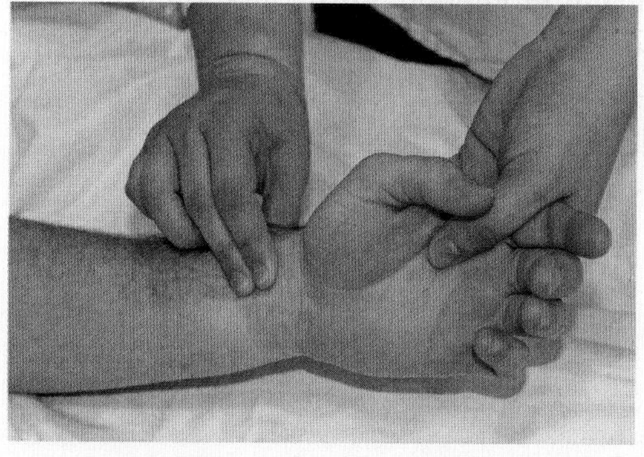

      (2) For ulnar pulse, place fingertips along ulnar side of forearm. *(Palpated when arterial insufficiency to hand is expected or when nurse assesses effects radial occlusion might have on circulation to hand.)*

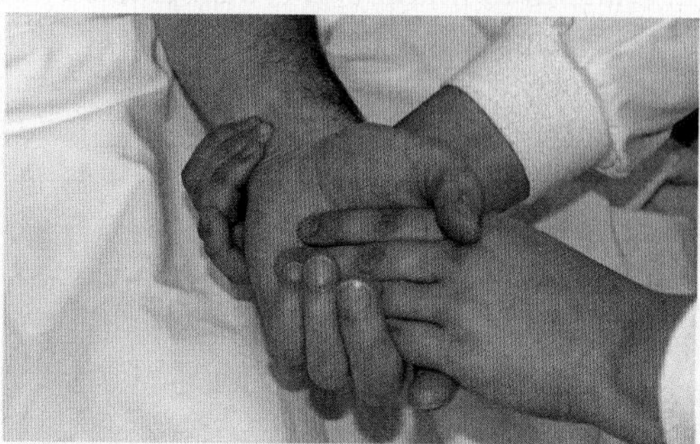

      (3) For *brachial pulse,* locate groove between biceps and triceps muscles above elbow at antecubital fossa. Place tips of first three fingers in muscle groove. *(Artery runs along medial side of extended arm, requiring moderate palpation.)*

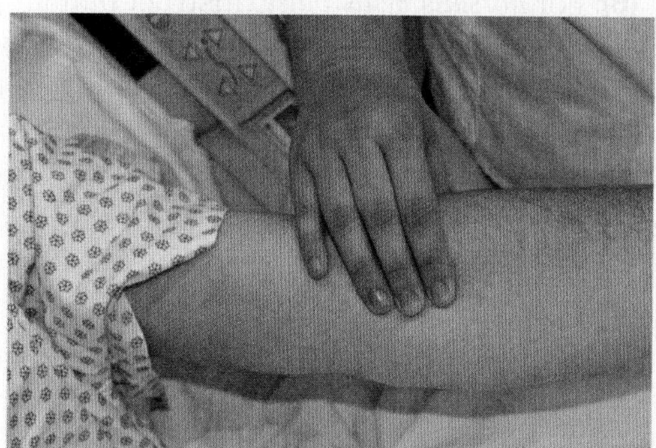

Continued

Skill 12.2 Obtaining a Pulse Rate—cont'd

(4) For *femoral pulse,* with patient supine, place first three fingers over inguinal area below inguinal ligament, midway between pubic symphysis and anterosuperior iliac spine. *(Supine position prevents flexion in groin area, which interferes with artery access.)*

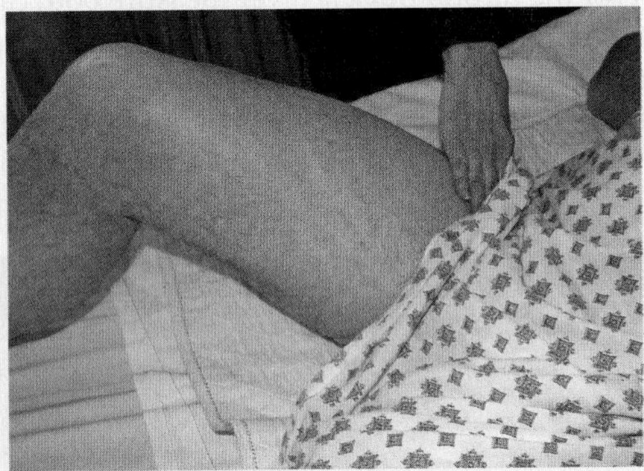

(5) For *popliteal pulse,* instruct patient to slightly flex knee with foot resting on table or bed. Instruct patient to keep leg muscles relaxed. Palpate deeply into popliteal fossa with fingers of both hands placed just lateral to midline. It is also possible for patient to lie prone to achieve exposure of artery. *(Flexion of knee and muscle relaxation improve accessibility of artery. Popliteal pulse is one of the more difficult pulses to palpate.)*

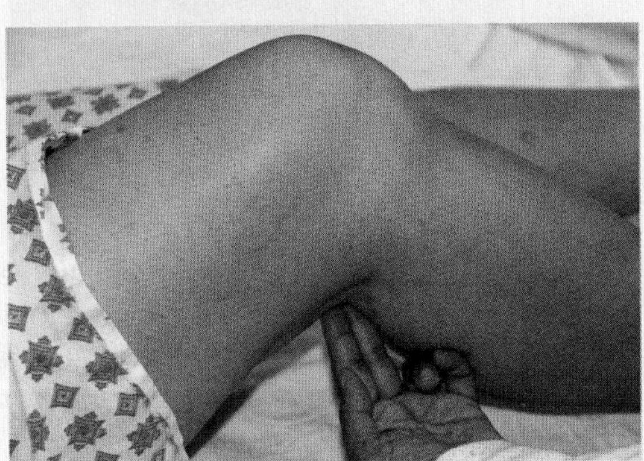

(6) For *dorsalis pedis pulse,* instruct patient to lie supine with feet relaxed. Gently place fingertips between great and first toes and slowly move them along groove between extensor tendons of great and first toes, until pulse is palpable. *(Artery lies superficially and does not require deep palpation. Pulse is sometimes congenitally absent in healthy adults.)*

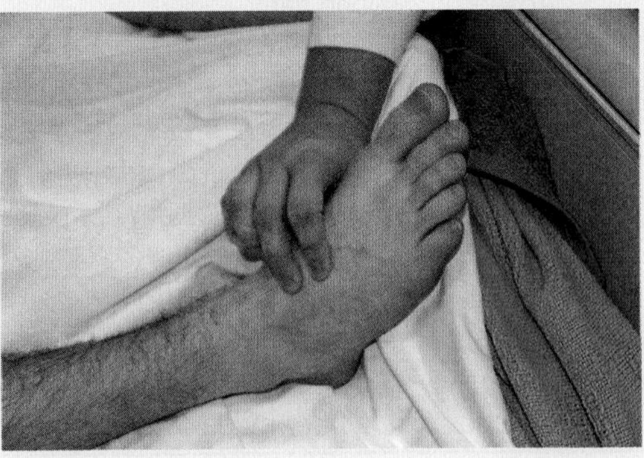

(7) For *posterior tibial pulse,* instruct patient to relax and slightly extend feet. Place fingertips behind and below medial malleolus (ankle bone). *(Artery is easily palpable with foot relaxed.)*

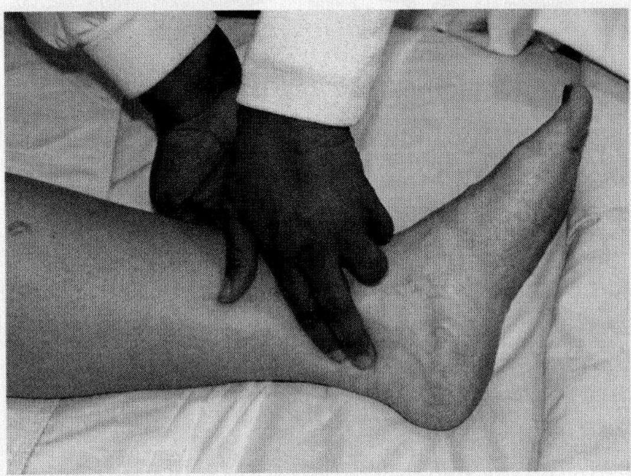

b. Determine strength of the pulse. Note thrust of vessel against fingertips. Strength equals volume of blood ejected against arterial wall with each heart contraction.

7. Write down radial pulse rate (for documentation later).

8. Perform hand hygiene. *(Reduces spread of microorganisms.)*

9. Document rate on graphic flow sheet (see Fig. 12.1). *(Records procedure.)*

10. Follow up by reporting any abnormal pulse rates. *(Rate sometimes has to be reassessed.)*

11. Do patient teaching (see patient teaching in Health Promotion box on vital signs and Skill 12.1).

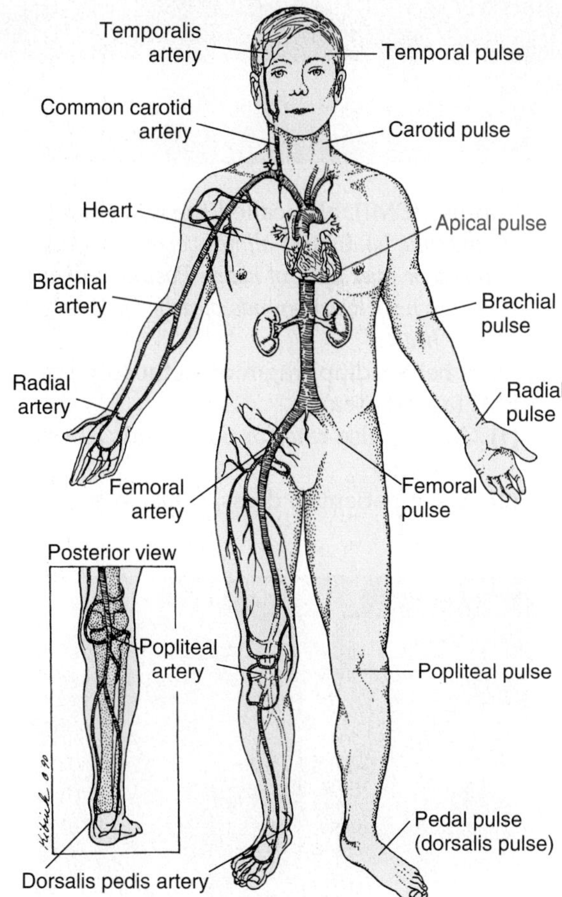

Fig. 12.5 Pulse sites.

pressure of your arm). Measure the carotid pulse in the patient's neck on the side facing you.

Any artery can be assessed for pulse rate, but the radial and carotid arteries are the most easily palpated peripheral pulse sites (Fig. 12.5). People learning to monitor their own heart rates, such as athletes, often use these sites. When a patient's condition suddenly deteriorates (Box 12.10), the carotid site is the best for finding a pulse quickly. The heart continues delivering blood through the carotid artery to the brain as long as possible. When cardiac output declines significantly, peripheral pulses weaken and are difficult to palpate. (See Chapter 13 for further identification of the pulse sites.)

The radial pulse rate is obtained at the radial artery, which is located on the thumb side of the inner wrist. On initial assessment, palpate all major pulses and auscultate the apical rate. Major pulses include temporal, facial, carotid, brachial, radial, femoral, popliteal, posterior tibial, and dorsalis pedis (see Fig. 12.5); the pulses provide general and specific information. A pulse palpated at the dorsalis pedis, for example, indicates blood flow to the foot.

Auscultation of the apical rate is essential on all cardiac patients, and when the radial pulse is irregular or is difficult to palpate or when certain medications such as digoxin (Lanoxin) make this necessary (Skill 12.3). *Apical* refers to apex (the tip, the end, or the top of a structure) of the heart. The **apical pulse** represents the actual beating of the heart. The apical pulse site is the best site to use when taking the pulse rate of an infant. In auscultation of the apical rate, the "lub-dub" that is heard represents one cardiac cycle, or heartbeat (Figs. 12.6 and 12.7).

At times, a difference is found between the radial and the apical rates. This is called a **pulse deficit.** A *pulse deficit* is confirmed by one nurse listening to the apical rate, and a second nurse palpating the radial pulse at the same time, using the same watch for 1 full minute. A deficit exists when the radial rate is less than the apical rate. For example, an apical rate of 92 beats per minute and a radial rate of 88 beats per minute means there is a pulse deficit of 4. A pulse deficit signifies that the pumping action of the heart is faulty or there is a peripheral vascular issue. This often is seen in atrial fibrillation because the heart is not pumping effectively

Box 12.10 Nursing Interventions for the Patient With an Abnormal Pulse

- If patient's pulse is weak or difficult to palpate, perform complete assessment of all peripheral pulses.
- Observe for symptoms associated with altered tissue perfusion, such as pallor or cyanosis of tissue distal to weak pulse, and for coldness of extremity and any change in level of consciousness (LOC).
- Observe for factors associated with a decrease in cardiac output, such as hemorrhage, hypothermia, or heart muscle damage, that result in diminished peripheral pulses.
- If pulse is above normal, assess for related data such as pain, fear, anxiety, recent exercise, low blood pressure, elevated temperature, or inadequate oxygenation.
- Observe for symptoms such as dyspnea, fatigue, chest pain, orthopnea, syncope, cyanosis, or pallor of skin.
- If pulse is below normal, assess apical pulse and ascertain the presence of such factors as digoxin and antidysrhythmic medications. It is sometimes necessary to withhold medication pending the health care provider's evaluation of the situation.
- If the pulse is weak or irregular, assess apical pulse for a pulse deficit. Sometimes the health care provider orders an electrocardiogram or 24-hour heart monitor.
- When assessing for a pulse deficit, which sometimes indicates alteration in cardiac output, count the apical pulse while your colleague counts the radial pulse. Begin the assessment, counting out loud so that you assess pulses simultaneously. The nurse with the watch should indicate when to begin counting, either by counting out loud or by another predetermined signal. This same nurse indicates when to stop counting. If pulse count differs by more than two, a pulse deficit exists.

Skill 12.3 Obtaining an Apical Pulse Rate

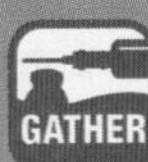

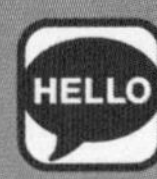

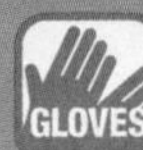

NURSING ACTION *(RATIONALE)*

1. Perform hand hygiene. *(Reduces spread of microorganisms.)*
2. Introduce self to patient. *(Decreases patient's anxiety.)*
3. Identify patient by identification band. *(Ensures correct patient for procedure.)*
4. Explain procedure. *(Seeks cooperation and assistance from patient and decreases patient's anxiety.)*
5. Prepare for procedure by doing the following:
   a. Assembling all necessary supplies: stethoscope and watch with second hand. *(Organizes procedure.)*
   b. Providing privacy for patient if necessary. *(Decreases patient's anxiety.)*
6. Implement procedure:
   a. Clean earpiece and diaphragm of stethoscope with alcohol swab as necessary. *(Ensures instrument is clean and promotes auscultation.)*
   b. With patient in supine or sitting position, expose sternum and left side of chest. *(Exposes portion of chest wall for selection of auscultation site.)*
   c. Palpate angle of Louis, located just below suprasternal notch at point where horizontal ridge is felt along body of sternum. Place index finger just to right (patient's left) of sternum and palpate second intercostal space. Place next finger in intercostal space below, and proceed downward until fifth intercostal space is located. Move index finger horizontally along fifth intercostal space to left midclavicular line. Palpate point of maximal impulse (PMI), also called the apical area. *(Use of anatomic landmarks allows correct placement of stethoscope over apex of heart. Position enhances ability to hear heart sounds clearly. PMI is over apex of heart.)*
   d. Place bell or diaphragm of stethoscope over PMI (apical area).
      (1) Count pulse rate for 60 seconds. *(Ensures accuracy.)*
      (2) Assist patient to dress. *(Provides for patient's comfort.)*

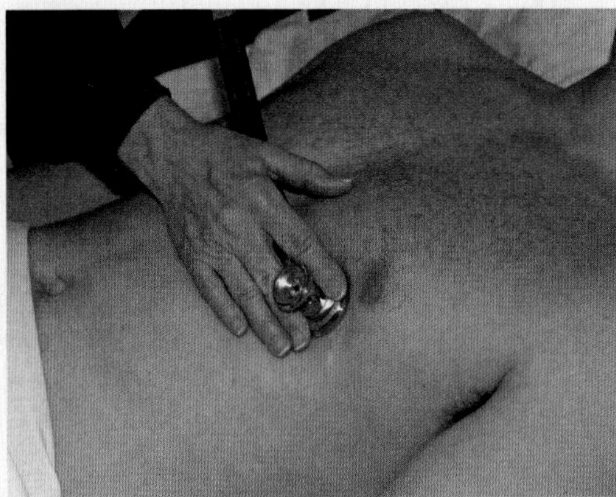

7. Write down pulse rate (for later documentation).
8. Perform hand hygiene. *(Reduces spread of microorganisms.)*
9. Document pulse rate on graphic flow sheet (see Fig. 12.1).
10. Follow up by reporting an abnormal pulse rate (see Box 12.9).
11. Do patient teaching (see patient teaching in the Health Promotion box on vital signs).

to distribute blood throughout the body (see *Adult Health Nursing*, Chapter 8).

RESPIRATION

RESPIRATORY FUNCTION

Respiration (the taking in of oxygen, its utilization in the tissues, and the giving off of carbon dioxide; the act of breathing [i.e., inhaling and exhaling]) is internal and external. Internal respiration refers to the exchange of gas at the tissue level caused by the process of cellular oxidation (any process in which the oxygen content of a compound is increased) and the gas exchange that occurs in the alveoli of the lungs. The breathing movements of the patient that are observed are called *external respirations*. The cycle of external respirations has two parts: inspiration and expiration. *Inspiration* is inhaling air with oxygen into the lungs, and *expiration* is exhaling air with carbon dioxide out of the lungs. The rate of respiration is controlled by the medulla oblongata in the brain.

Any activity that increases metabolism (the aggregate of all chemical processes that take place in living organisms resulting in growth, generation of energy, elimination of wastes, and other bodily functions as they relate to the distribution of nutrients in the body after digestion) increases the need for oxygen by the body and increases respiratory rate.

The normal respiratory rate for an adult is between 12 and 20 respirations per minute (Boxes 12.11 and 12.12). A rapid respiratory rate is called **tachypnea.** Exercise and fever increase respiratory rate. A slow respiratory rate, below 10 per minute, is called **bradypnea.** The depth of respiration is determined by the amount of air taken in with inhalation. Normally, 500 mL of air is inspired with each breath. The diaphragm (a dome-shaped fibrous muscle partition that separates the thoracic and abdominal cavities) aids respirations by moving down during inspiration and moving up during expiration. The proper rhythm of respiration is regular and uninterrupted. Occasional sighing is normal and allows all alveoli (plural for alveolus, an air cell of the lungs where gases are exchanged in respirations) to be aerated. Normal respirations are not audible except with the aid of a stethoscope.

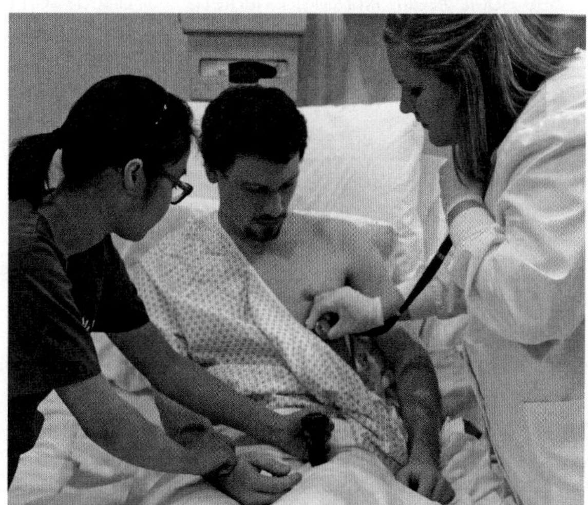

Fig. 12.6 Taking an apical or radial pulse. One worker takes the apical pulse, and the other takes the radial pulse. NOTE: Two nurses are using the same watch.

ASSESSMENT OF RESPIRATION

When assessing respirations, note the rate, the depth, the quality, and the rhythm (Skill 12.4). Assessment of the depth of respirations requires observing the movement by the diaphragm and the intercostal muscles. Shallow respirations make ventilation difficult to observe, and only a small amount of air is exchanged in the lungs. **Dyspnea** is breathing with difficulty. The patient may be laboring to get enough oxygen, with pursed lips, flared nostrils, and clavicular and costal retractions (the visible sinking in of the soft tissues of the chest between and around the firmer tissues of the cartilaginous and body ribs, as occurs with increased inspiratory effort).

Assessing patterns of breathing is another part of checking the respiratory status (Fig. 12.8). Apnea is a lack of spontaneous respirations. **Cheyne-Stokes respirations** are an abnormal pattern of respiration characterized by alternating periods of apnea and deep rapid breathing. The periods of apnea increase as time goes on. Cheyne-Stokes respirations are noted in the critically or terminally ill patient. Hyperventilation is when the rate of ventilation exceeds normal metabolic requirements for exchange of respiratory gases, such as during emotional trauma. Volume and depth of respirations increase. Hypoventilation occurs when the rate of ventilation entering the lungs is insufficient for metabolic needs. Respiratory rate is below normal, and depth of ventilation is depressed. A patient may experience hypoventilation after certain surgical procedures such as a cholecystectomy. In these cases, deep breathing results in discomfort.

The best time to assess respirations is immediately after counting a radial or an apical pulse. The patient

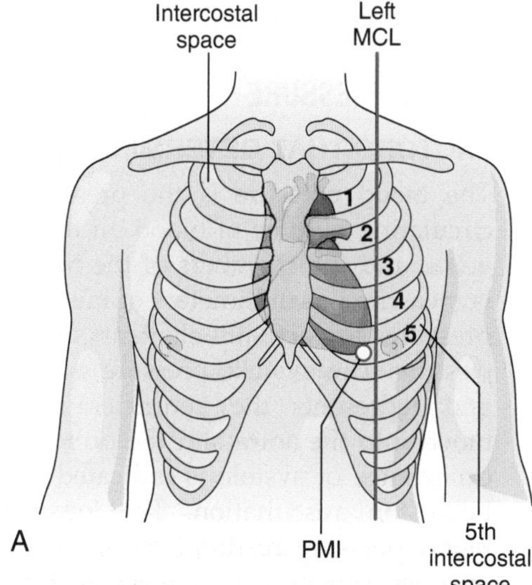

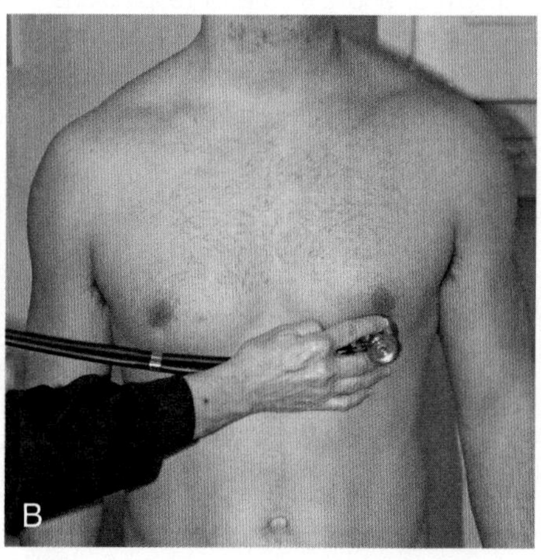

Fig. 12.7 A, Point of maximal impulse is at fifth intercostal space. *MCL*, midclavicular line; *PMI*, point of maximal impulse. B, Assessing apical pulse.

Box 12.11 Factors That Influence Respiration

ACUTE PAIN
Pain increases the rate and the depth of respirations as a result of sympathetic stimulation; breathing becomes shallow.

AGE
With growth from infancy to adulthood, the lungs' capacity increases and respiratory rate gradually declines. In older adults, lung capacity and depth of respirations decrease, and respiratory rate increases.

BODY POSITION
In slumped or stooped positions, ventilation often is impaired, with a reduced depth of respirations. A straight, erect posture promotes full chest expansion. Lying flat should be avoided because full chest expansion is limited in this position.

BRAINSTEM INJURY
Injury to the brainstem impairs the respiratory center and inhibits respiratory rate and rhythm.

DISEASE OR ILLNESS
Chronic lung disease (e.g., emphysema or bronchitis) alters the normal stimulus for ventilation. Lung tissue disease, reduced red blood cell levels, chest pain, kidney diseases, febrile disease, and diseases of the heart are a few of the conditions that alter the rate and the depth of respirations.

EXERCISE
Exercise increases the rate and the depth of respirations.

FEVER
Hyperpyrexia (greatly elevated temperature) results in an abnormally rapid rate of breathing.

GENDER
Men have a greater lung capacity than women.

HEMOGLOBIN FUNCTION
Respiratory rate and depth are increased by conditions caused by decreased hemoglobin function. Examples include anemia, in which the blood's oxygen-carrying capacity is limited, and increased altitude, in which the amount of saturated hemoglobin is reduced.

MEDICATIONS
Narcotic analgesics depress the patient's ability to increase the volume of air inspired, and the rate of respirations is decreased. Other medications have the potential to increase or decrease the rate and depth of respirations and affect the rhythm. The rate and depth of respirations is increased with the use of amphetamines and cocaine. Conversely, bronchodilators cause dilation of the airways, causing the respiratory rate to decrease.

SMOKING
Long-term smoking changes the lungs' airways, resulting in an increased respiratory rate.

STRESS
An anxious or fearful patient likely has increases in the rate and depth of respirations; as a result, hyperventilation can occur.

Box 12.12 Nursing Interventions for the Patient With Abnormal Respirations

- Occasional periods of apnea are a symptom of underlying disease in the adult and must be reported to the health care provider or nurse in charge. Irregular respirations and short apneic spells of less than 20 seconds are normal in a newborn.
- Positions of discomfort may cause patient to breathe more rapidly. Assess patients with difficulty breathing (dyspnea), such as those with heart failure or abdominal ascites or who are in late stages of pregnancy, in the position of greatest comfort.
- Repositioning may increase the work of breathing, which increases respiratory rate; allow for a period of rest.
- Respiratory rates of less than 10 or more than 20 breaths per minute or shallow and slow respirations (hypoventilation) are likely to necessitate immediate intervention.
- See *Adult Health Nursing,* Chapter 2, for discussion of inspirometry.
- See *Adult Health Nursing,* Chapter 9, for discussion of pulse oximetry and assessment of adequate oxygenation.
- Observe for related factors such as obstructed airway or stertorous (snoring) respirations.
- Observe for related signs and symptoms such as cyanotic nail beds, lips, or mucous membranes; restlessness; irritability; confusion; dyspnea; shortness of breath; productive cough; and abnormal breath sounds.
- Consider possible effects of anesthesia or medications such as opioids.
- Assist patient to a supported sitting position (semi-Fowler's or full Fowler's, unless contraindicated).
- Provide oxygen as ordered by health care provider (see Chapter 14) if patient shows signs of respiratory distress.

is unaware you are doing so and is less likely to consciously alter respirations.

BLOOD PRESSURE

FACTORS THAT DETERMINE BLOOD PRESSURE

The **blood pressure** is the pressure exerted by the circulating volume of blood on the arterial walls, the veins, and the chambers of the heart. Blood pressure is measured in millimeters of mercury (mm Hg). Two pressures are actually elements of what we call *blood pressure.* The **systolic** pressure is the higher number and represents the ventricles contracting, forcing blood into the aorta and the pulmonary arteries. The occurrence of systole is indicated by the first sound heard on auscultation. The lower number of the blood pressure reading, the second pressure, is the **diastolic** pressure. It represents the pressure within the artery between beats, that is, between contractions of the atria or the ventricles, when blood enters the

Skill 12.4 Obtaining a Respiratory Rate

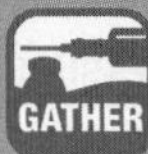

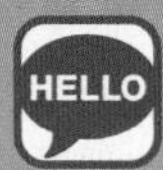

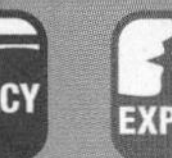

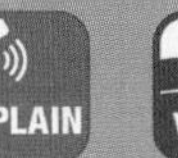

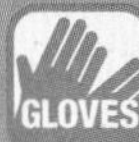

NURSING ACTION *(RATIONALE)*

1. Perform hand hygiene. *(Reduces spread of microorganisms.)*
2. Introduce self to patient. *(Decreases patient's anxiety.)*
3. Identify patient by identification band. *(Verifies correct patient for procedure.)*
4. Explain procedure. *(Seeks cooperation and assistance from patient and decreases patient's anxiety.)*
5. Prepare for procedure:
   a. Assemble all necessary supplies, including a wristwatch with a second hand. *(Organizes procedure efficiently.)*
   b. Provide privacy for patient if necessary. *(Decreases patient's anxiety.)*
   c. If patient has been active, wait 5 to 10 minutes. *(Exercise increases respiratory rate and depth.)*
   d. Be certain patient is in a position of comfort, preferably sitting or lying supine with the head of the bed elevated 45 to 60 degrees, if patient can tolerate it. *(Discomfort causes the patient to breathe more rapidly. The erect, sitting position promotes full ventilation.)*
6. Implement procedure:
   a. Place fingertip as if to obtain a radial pulse (see illustration). Because patients sometimes unconsciously alter the respiratory rate when being observed, it is best to obtain the respiratory rate at the same time as the radial pulse reading.

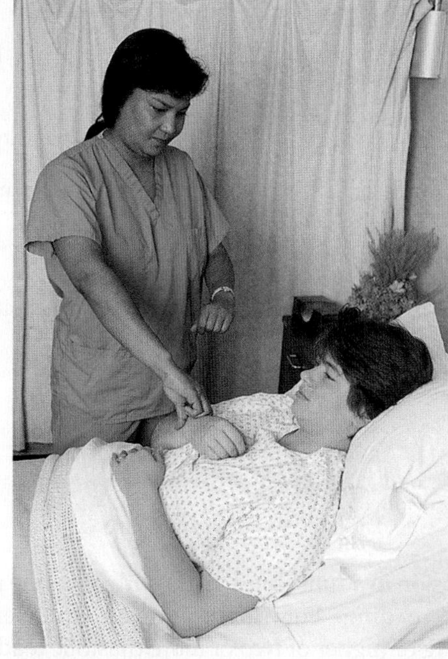

   b. Observe respiratory rate for 60 seconds. *(Ensures accuracy.)* Count each rise of the chest wall. One inhalation and exhalation = one respiration.
   c. Provide for patient comfort. *(Promotes patient's self-esteem.)*
7. Write down rate (for documentation later).
8. Perform hand hygiene. *(Reduces spread of microorganisms.)*
9. Document the rate on the graphic flow sheet (see Fig. 12.1).
10. Follow up by reporting any abnormal respiratory rates (see Box 12.11). *(Rate sometimes has to be reassessed.)*
11. Do patient teaching (see patient teaching in Health Promotion box on vital signs).

relaxed chambers from the systemic circulation and the lungs. The difference between the two readings is called the **pulse pressure.** A reading of 120/80 mm Hg reveals a pulse pressure of 40, which is a normal pulse pressure. Pulse pressure is an indication of cardiac function.

Blood pressure reflects *cardiac output* (the amount of blood discharged from the heart per minute), the quality of the arteries, the blood volume, and blood viscosity. When blood is pumped by the heart into the arteries, the pressure within the arteries rises. The greater the amount of blood pumped by the heart, the greater the pressure.

Likewise, if the blood volume is increased, the pressure within the artery increases. When the arteries' lumens (channels within the arteries) narrow and become less flexible, blood pressure rises because there is less space for the blood to enter. Increased viscosity (thickness) of the blood causes a slower flow of blood in the capillaries, which causes backup pressure in the larger vessels. See Box 12.13 for factors that influence blood pressure.

The optimal blood pressure reading for a healthy middle-aged adult is less than 120/80 mm Hg. Values of 120–139/80–89 mm Hg are considered *prehypertensive.* **Hypertension** occurs when the elevated pressure is sustained above 140/90 mm Hg. The diagnosis of

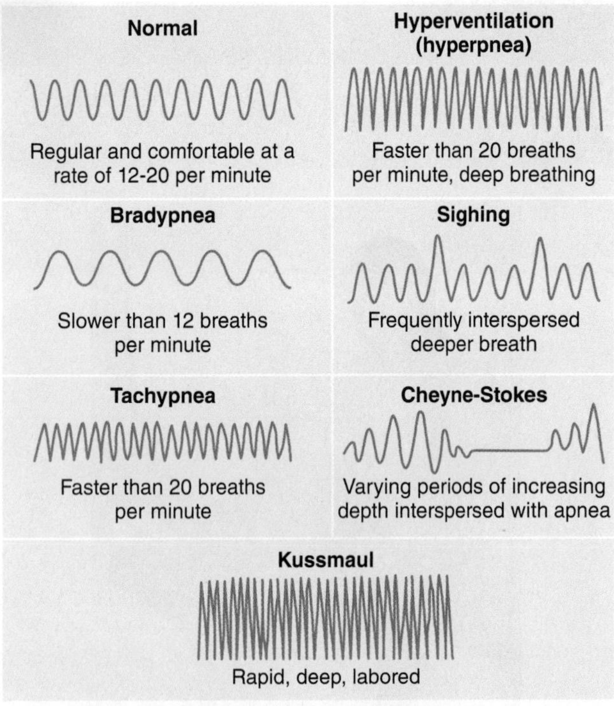

Fig. 12.8 Patterns of respirations.

hypertension in adults is not made with only one random elevated reading. For this diagnosis, an average of 90 mm Hg or higher of two or more diastolic readings on at least two subsequent visits is necessary, or an average higher than 140 mm Hg of two or more systolic readings on at least two visits. Primary, or essential, hypertension is the most common form. The cause for this type of hypertension is unknown. Risk factors also contribute; consider their significance when doing patient teaching. These risk factors include family history of hypertension, obesity, smoking, heavy alcohol consumption, elevated blood cholesterol level, and continued exposure to stress. Table 12.4 lists normal and hypertensive values. If an individual's blood pressure is normal, the blood pressure should be monitored once every 2 years starting at the age of 20. For prehypertension and hypertension, individuals should follow the recommendations of their health care provider for how often they should be monitored (American Heart Association, 2017).

A blood pressure below normal is **hypotension**. A low blood pressure is considered healthy, provided there are no ill effects, such as vertigo (dizziness) or syncope (fainting). **Orthostatic hypotension** (a drop of 25 mm Hg in systolic pressure and a drop of 10 mm Hg in diastolic pressure when a person moves from a lying to a sitting or from a sitting to a standing position) occurs when a person rises too quickly, usually from a supine position. The patient frequently feels lightheaded and unstable. Advise the patient to rise slowly from lying to sitting to standing, thus preventing blood volume from shifting suddenly (Box 12.14). Hypotension resulting from shock or massive hemorrhage is very serious and necessitates immediate medical intervention. See Table 12.5 for conditions that cause alterations in blood pressure.

Box 12.13 Factors That Influence Blood Pressure

Normal blood pressure levels vary throughout life.

AGE	BLOOD PRESSURE (mm Hg)
Newborn (3000 g [6.6 lb])	Mean 36–40
1 mo	85/54
1 y	95/65
6 yr	105/65
10–13 yr	110/65
14–17 yr	<120/75
18 yr and up	<120/80

In children and adolescents, hypertension is defined as blood pressure that is, on repeated measurement, at the 95th percentile or greater, adjusted for age, height, and gender.

Alcohol and tobacco use. Excessive use of alcohol and the use of tobacco raise the blood pressure.

Anxiety, fear, pain, and emotional stress. May increase blood pressure because of increased heart rate and increased peripheral vascular resistance. Stress also can lead to other activities that increase blood pressure, such as using tobacco or alcohol.

Diet. Eating a healthy diet can help maintain the blood pressure at normal levels; switching from an unhealthy to a healthy diet can sometimes lower the blood pressure. Diets high in sodium, fats, and sugars tend to raise the blood pressure.

Diurnal (happening daily). The blood pressure tends to vary through the day, starting low in the morning, rising during the day, then lowering at night.

Gender. Men are more likely to be hypertensive until the age of 45. From the age of 45 to 64 there is no difference in the rate of hypertension. After the age of 65 women have a higher rate of hypertension.

Hormones. Variations in blood pressure may be manifested as a person ages because of hormonal alterations. Pregnancy may cause mild to severe elevations in blood pressure.

Medications. Can either lower or increase blood pressure depending on their pharmacologic action. Common medications that raise blood pressure are over-the-counter cold medications. Diuretics are an example of medications that lower blood pressure.

Obesity and being overweight. Excess weight places extra workload on the heart, resulting in hypertension.

Race. The occurrence of hypertension is higher in African Americans than any other populations, and hypertension starts at an earlier age than other populations. The incidence of hypertension-related deaths is high in African Americans.

Data from the American Heart Association: Know your risk factors for high blood pressure, 2017. Retrieved from *http://www.heart.org/HEARTORG/Conditions/HighBloodPressure/UnderstandYourRiskforHighBloodPressure/Understand-Your-Risk-for-High-Blood-Pressure_UCM_002052_Article.jsp#.WI0aWflsOSo.*

OBTAINING BLOOD PRESSURE MEASUREMENTS

Blood pressure readings are taken with a **sphygmomanometer** and a stethoscope. A sphygmomanometer (a

Table 12.4 Values for Normal Blood Pressure and Hypertension Categories

BLOOD PRESSURE CATEGORY	SYSTOLIC MM HG (UPPER NUMBER)		DIASTOLIC MM HG (LOWER NUMBER)
Normal	Less than 120	and	Less than 80
Prehypertension	120–139	or	80–89
High blood pressure (Hypertension) stage 1	140–159	or	90–99
High blood pressure (Hypertension) stage 2	160 or higher	or	100 or higher
Hypertensive crisis (Emergency care needed)	Higher than 180	or	Higher than 110

Source: American Heart Association, Inc.

Box 12.14 Measurement of Orthostatic Blood Pressure

Some patients, especially those who are older or taking certain medications, experience a drop in blood pressure or an increase in pulse when changing from a lying to a sitting or from a sitting to a standing position.

Certain medications, including many antiseizure medications, antipsychotics, and antihypertensives, commonly cause orthostatic hypotension. Patients taking these medications often have a routine order to have orthostatic blood pressure readings taken.

1. Obtaining orthostatic blood pressure measurements requires critical thinking and ongoing nursing judgment; do not delegate this task.
2. Obtain supine patient's blood pressure in each arm. Select arm with highest systolic reading for subsequent measurements.
3. Leaving blood pressure cuff in place, assist patient to sitting position. After 1 to 3 minutes with patient in sitting position, obtain blood pressure. If orthostatic symptoms occur, such as dizziness, weakness, lightheadedness, feeling faint, or sudden pallor, terminate blood pressure measurement and assist patient to a supine position.
4. Leaving blood pressure cuff in place, assist patient to standing position and obtain blood pressure. If orthostatic symptoms occur (see previous), terminate blood pressure measurement and assist patient to a supine position. In most cases, orthostatic hypotension is detectable within 1 minute of standing.
5. Record patient's blood pressure in each position: for example, "140/80 supine, 132/72 sitting, 108/60 standing." Note any additional symptoms or reports.
6. Report findings of orthostatic hypotension or orthostatic symptoms to health care provider or nurse in charge. Instruct patient to obtain assistance when getting out of bed if orthostatic hypotension is present or orthostatic symptoms occur.

Evidence-Based Practice

Forearm Versus Upper Arm Blood Pressure Measurements

EVIDENCE SUMMARY

Blood pressure measurement is an important factor in determination of the diagnosis of hypertension and evaluation of therapies. Because hypertension leads to serious complications, eliminating errors in measuring blood pressure is important. When the upper arm is not accessible or when the blood pressure (BP) cuff does not fit the patient's upper arm, the forearm has been used for BP measurement. In this research study, BP measurements taken on the forearm and the upper arm were compared when patients were supine and when the head of the bed was elevated at 45 degrees. The researchers wanted to know whether placement of the BP cuff affected systolic and diastolic BP. The BP of 221 medical surgical inpatients was measured at both arm locations in the supine and head-elevated positions. Researchers selected cuff size based on forearm and upper arm circumference. Results indicated a significant difference between upper arm and forearm blood pressures in both positions. Systolic and diastolic blood pressure differed as much as 33 mm Hg.

APPLICATION TO NURSING PRACTICE

- A consistent approach to the placement of upper extremity blood pressure cuff allows accurate assessment of a change in condition.
- Appropriate cuff size is essential for accurate measurement.
- Forearm BP measurements cannot be substituted for upper arm blood pressure measurements and be considered accurate.

Schrauf CM: Monitoring blood pressure: Do method and body location matter? *Nephrol Nurs J* 39(6):502–512, 2012.

device for measuring the arterial blood pressure) consists of an inflatable cuff and a gauge. The gauge is aneroid (Figs. 12.9 and 12.10; see Box 12.8). Inflate the cuff around the patient's arm to compress the artery, which occludes blood flow; then, slowly deflate it, which allows blood flow to resume (see the Evidence-Based Practice box).

While doing this, listen at the brachial artery with the stethoscope to hear pulsating sounds. These are called **Korotkoff sounds.** The sounds go through five phases (Fig. 12.11). At the first audible sound, make a mental note of the point on the sphygmomanometer gauge at which it occurs, and note again the point at which the sound disappears. That first point is the systolic pressure, and the second is the diastolic pressure.

As the pressure is lowered, the Korotkoff sounds sometimes seem to disappear temporarily. In this case, listen for a subtle difference in the quality of what you

Table 12.5 Conditions That Cause Alterations in Blood Pressure

CONDITION	EFFECT	CAUSE
Hemorrhage	Lowers pressure	Decreased blood volume
Increased intracranial pressure	Raises pressure	Disturbance of cardiovascular control mechanisms in brainstem resulting from pressure exerted on the medulla oblongata
Acute pain	Raises pressure	Increased vasomotor tone and peripheral vascular resistance as a result of sympathetic stimulation
End-stage renal disease	Raises pressure	Increased blood volume resulting from increased retention of sodium and water; release of renin, a vasopressor that increases peripheral vascular resistance
Primary essential hypertension	Raises pressure	Increased peripheral vascular resistance resulting from progressive thickening of arterial walls
General anesthesia	Lowers pressure	Decreased vasomotor tone resulting from depression of vasomotor center in brainstem
Exercise	Raises pressure	Increased cardiac output
Postural change	Lowers pressure	Decreased blood volume as person moves from lying to sitting or standing position; normally, variations are minimal
Smoking	Raises pressure	Increased vasoconstriction

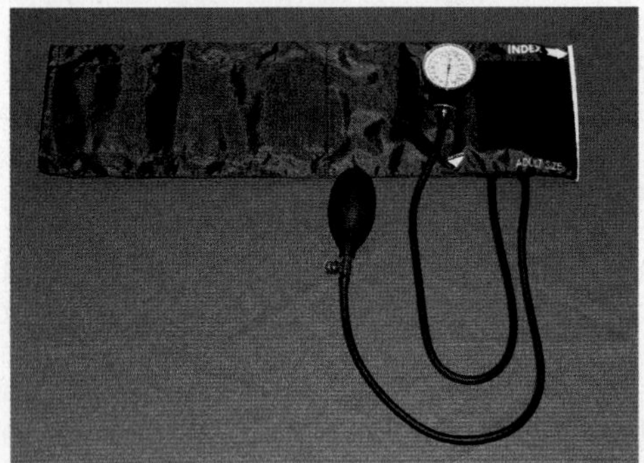

Fig. 12.9 Aneroid manometer and cuff.

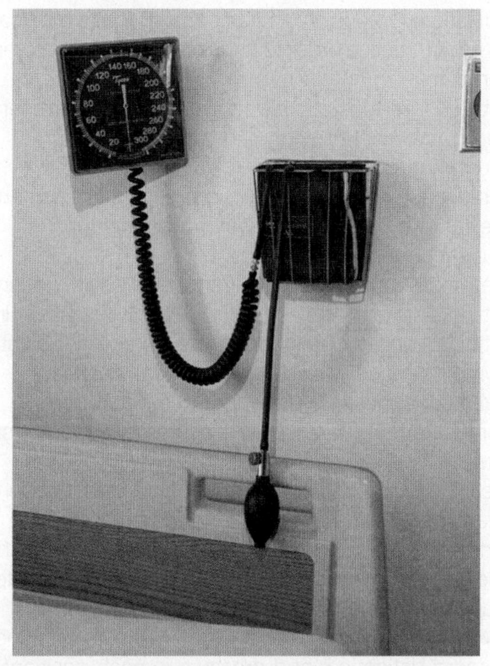

Fig. 12.10 Wall-mounted aneroid sphygmomanometer. (From Potter PA, Perry AG: *Fundamentals of nursing: Concepts, process, and practice*, ed 8, St. Louis, 2013, Mosby.)

hear as the manometer approaches the diastolic reading. In patients with hypertension, the sounds usually heard over the brachial artery disappear as pressure is reduced and then reappear at a lower level. This temporary disappearance of sound is the auscultatory gap. It typically occurs between the first and the second Korotkoff sounds. The gap in sound sometimes covers a range of 40 mm Hg and thus has the potential to cause an underestimation of systolic pressure or overestimation of diastolic pressure. Be certain to inflate the cuff enough to hear the true systolic pressure before the auscultatory gap. Palpation of the radial artery helps determine how high to inflate the cuff. Inflate the cuff 30 mm Hg above the pressure at which the radial pulse was palpated and disappeared. The range of pressures in which the auscultatory gap occurs is recorded (e.g., "blood pressure 190/94, with an auscultatory gap from 190 to 160").

If sounds are heard immediately after inflation of the cuff and the beginning of listening, the pressure should be released immediately and completely. After 60 seconds, the cuff then may be reinflated to a point 30 mm Hg above where the sounds were heard the first time. Reinflation of a partially deflated cuff is uncomfortable for the patient and often yields an inaccurate reading.

If sounds cannot be auscultated because of a weakened arterial pulse, use of a Doppler ultrasonic stethoscope may be possible. This stethoscope allows low-frequency sounds to be heard and is used commonly with adults who have very weak blood pressure and with infants and children (Fig. 12.12).

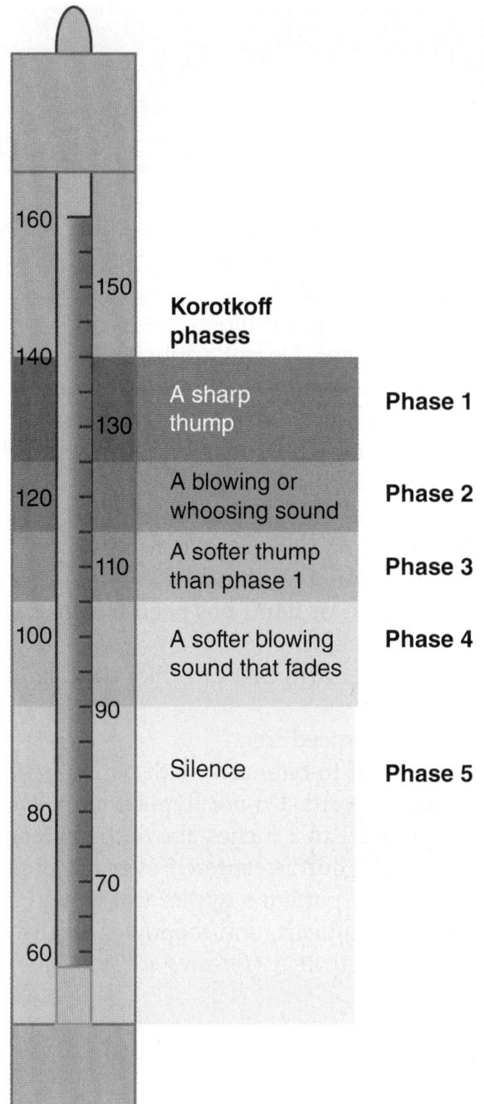

Fig. 12.11 The sounds auscultated during blood pressure measurement can be differentiated into five Korotkoff phases. In this example, blood pressure is 140/90 mm Hg.

For the blood pressure reading to be accurate, the environment must be quiet, the equipment should be in good working order, and the cuff must fit correctly on the arm and be at the level of the heart. The gauge must be in plain view, not off to the side of the arm. The patient should be lying down or sitting up with both feet flat on the floor (legs not crossed) (Skill 12.5). See Box 12.15 for nursing interventions for the patient with abnormal blood pressure reading. See Box 12.16 for assessment of blood pressure in both arms.

Assessment of Blood Pressure in the Lower Extremities

Occasionally dressings, casts, intravenous catheters, or other devices make the upper extremities inaccessible, so you have to measure blood pressure in the lower extremities. Also, in patients with certain circulatory abnormalities, a comparison of blood pressure in the upper extremities with that in the legs is helpful. The popliteal artery, located behind the knee in the popliteal space, is the site for auscultation. With a cuff that is wide and long enough to allow for the larger girth of the thigh, position the cuff with the bladder over the posterior aspect of the mid-thigh. Placing the patient in a prone position is best. If such a position is impossible, ask the patient to flex the knee slightly for easier access to the artery. The procedure is the same as that for brachial artery auscultation. Systolic pressure in the lower extremities is usually higher by 10 to 40 mm Hg than in the brachial artery, but the diastolic pressure is essentially the same (Figs. 12.13A and B).

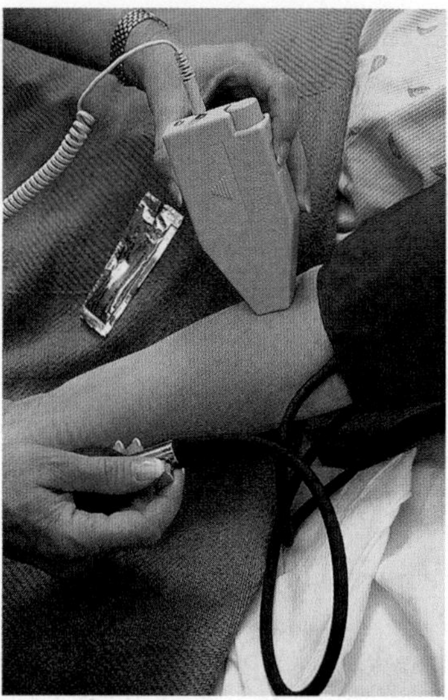

Fig. 12.12 Doppler stethoscope over brachial artery to measure blood pressure. (From Perry AG, Potter PA, Ostendorf WR, et al., *Clinical nursing skills and techniques*, ed 9, St. Louis, 2018, Elsevier.)

Electronic Measurement Devices

Many electronic devices determine blood pressure automatically (Figs. 12.14 and 12.15). The devices may be programmed to check blood pressure continuously or at set intervals. On medical-surgical floors and in operating rooms, postanesthesia care units, intensive care units, and postpartum units (see the Coordinated Care box), their use is now frequent.

Once the cuff is applied, the device can be programmed to obtain and record blood pressure readings at preset intervals. Alarm limits also can be programmed to alert the nurse if the blood pressure measurement is outside desired parameters. The system includes either a microphone or a pressure sensor built into the inflatable cuff. The microphone or acoustic system picks up Korotkoff sounds and registers systolic and diastolic readings. The pressure sensor or the ultrasonic system responds to the pressure waves generated by the movement of blood through the artery.

The advantages of automatic devices are the ease of use and efficiency when repeated or frequent measurements are needed. The automatic blood

Skill 12.5 Obtaining a Blood Pressure Reading

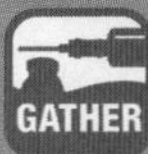

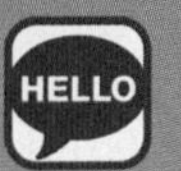

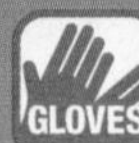

NURSING ACTION *(RATIONALE)*

1. Perform hand hygiene. *(Reduces spread of microorganisms.)*
2. Introduce self. *(Decreases patient's anxiety.)*
3. Identify patient by identification band. *(Verifies correct patient for procedure.)*
4. Explain procedure. *(Seeks cooperation and assistance from patient and decreases patient's anxiety.)*
5. Determine whether patient has ingested caffeine or has been smoking. (If so, wait 30 minutes before assessment, because caffeine and smoking can cause false elevations.)
6. Prepare for procedure:
   a. Assemble all necessary supplies, sphygmomanometer, and stethoscope. *(Organizes procedure efficiently.)* Determine the correct cuff size. *(An improper size gives an inaccurate reading.)* The cuff should be approximately 40% of the circumference of the extremity on which the cuff is to be used. *(A higher, inaccurate reading is obtained if too small a cuff is used; a lower, inaccurate reading is obtained if too large a cuff is used.)*
   b. Provide privacy. *(Decreases patient's anxiety.)*
   c. Request that patient assumes sitting or lying position. Be certain room is quiet and warm. *(Maintains comfort.)*
   d. Determine site for blood pressure measurement. Do not apply cuff to arm when in the following situations: *(Applying the cuff complicates these preexisting conditions.)*
      (1) Catheter is in antecubital fossa and fluids are infusing.
      (2) Arteriovenous shunt is in place.
      (3) Breast or axillary surgery has been performed on that side.
      (4) An arm or hand has been traumatized or is diseased.
      (5) A lower arm cast or bulky bandage is in place.
7. Implement procedure:
   a. Apply cuff to bare arm with patient's palm facing upward. Do not hyperextend. The cuff is applied 1 to 2 inches above the antecubital space. The cuff is centered over the brachial artery. The patient's upper arm is held at the level of the heart, and the lower arm is rested on a firm surface. *(Ensures accuracy of procedure.)*

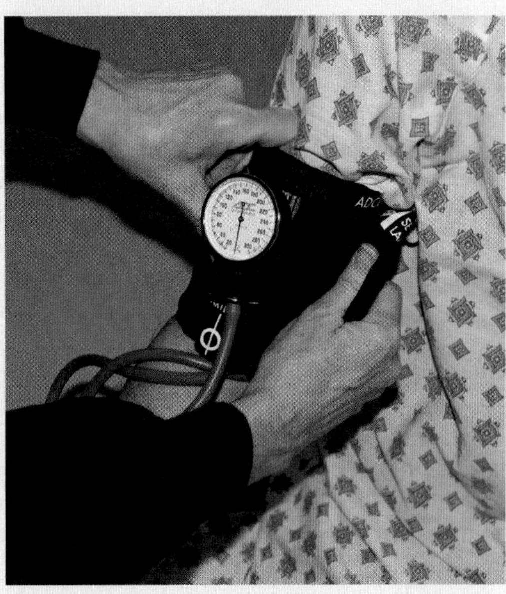

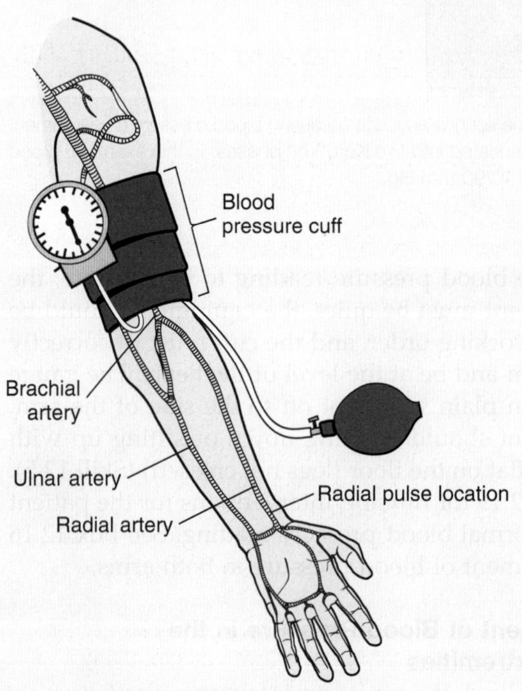

Skill 12.5 Obtaining a Blood Pressure Reading—cont'd

b. Palpate radial artery (see illustration in Skill 12.2).
c. Inflate cuff. Note the point on the manometer gauge when the radial pulse is obliterated. *(This is the approximate systolic pressure.)*
d. Deflate the cuff. *(Deflating the cuff allows congestion to leave the arm, preventing a false-high reading.)* Rest arm for 1 minute.
e. Palpate the brachial artery and place the bell or the diaphragm of the stethoscope over it.

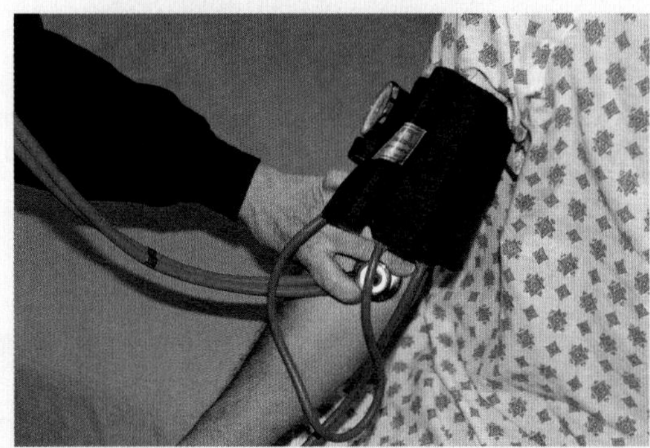

f. Reinflate cuff to 30 mm Hg above point at which radial artery was obliterated. *(Avoids the auscultatory gap.)* Estimating prevents false low readings that possibly result from the presence of this auscultatory gap (inaudible sounds below the systolic pressure). This phenomenon occurs in about 5% of adults and is prevalent in individuals with hypertension.
g. Slowly deflate cuff. Cuff is deflated at a rate of 2 mm Hg per second. Note the point at which the pulse is heard. *(This is the systolic pressure.)* Note the point at which no pulse is heard. *(This is the diastolic pressure.)*
h. When the Korotkoff sounds are no longer audible, continue to listen for another 10 to 20 mm Hg. *(Confirms blood pressure reading. Too-rapid deflation often causes a measurement error.)*
i. Completely deflate and remove the cuff.
j. Assist the patient to dress. *(Provides patient comfort.)*

8. Write down reading (for documentation later).
9. Perform hand hygiene. *(Reduces spread of microorganisms.)*
10. Document reading on graphic flow sheet (e.g., blood pressure 120/80 mm Hg; see Fig. 12.1).
11. Follow up by reporting abnormal readings immediately (see Box 12.16 for assessment of blood pressure in both arms and Box 12.14 for assessment of orthostatic blood pressure). *(Reading sometimes has to be reassessed.)*
12. Do patient teaching (see patient teaching in the Health Promotion box on vital signs).

Box 12.15 Nursing Interventions for the Patient With Abnormal Blood Pressure Reading

- Repeat assessment, but first eliminate extraneous noise, such as television and conversation. Noise interferes with accuracy. Falsely elevated readings are obtained if patient moves, talks, or coughs during blood pressure measurement.
- If you hear sounds, immediately release the pressure, wait 60 seconds, and estimate systolic pressure at higher reading. Reinflate cuff 30 mm Hg above the sound first heard. Reinflation of a partially deflated cuff is uncomfortable for the patient and often yields an inaccurate reading.
- Patient should be seated or lying in a quiet environment, free from temperature extremes, for at least 5 minutes before blood pressure is obtained. This is a good time to discuss with patient the benefits of exercise and weight control in reducing the risks for hypertension and coronary artery disease or lowering an existing blood pressure elevation.
- Electronic blood pressure cuff and machine must be matched by the manufacturer. Do not interchange blood pressure cuffs from machines of different manufacturers.
- Because blood pressure measurement can frighten children, this is a good time to prepare the child for the squeezing feeling of the inflated blood pressure cuff by saying, "This will feel like a tight hug for a minute," or "This will feel like a rubber band on your finger."
- If using an electronic blood pressure machine, tell the patient and family that these machines have audible alarm systems. Explain and allow the patient to hear the sound. Inform patient that "the alarms do not always mean you have a problem, but also show that the machine needs attention."
- If an abnormal blood pressure reading is obtained, measure blood pressure on the other arm or on a lower extremity or use an ultrasonic Doppler instrument (see Fig. 12.12). Ask another nurse to reassess abnormal readings.
- If blood pressure is above normal, observe for related symptoms such as headache (usually occipital), flushed face, and epistaxis (nosebleed). Older patients may notice fatigue.
- Be certain size of cuff is appropriate.
- Administer medications as ordered.
- Compare your current reading with the patient's baseline.
- If blood pressure is below normal, observe for symptoms such as weak, thready pulse; weakness; vertigo; confusion; pale, dusky, or cyanotic skin; or cool, mottled skin.
  - Position patient in supine position and limit activity.
  - Increase rate of intravenous fluid if infusing.

Box 12.16 Assessing Blood Pressure in Both Arms

- For the initial assessment, measure blood pressure in both arms, especially if the patient has heart disease or if the reading in the first arm is abnormal.
- Normally, a difference of 5 to 10 mm Hg exists between the arms. In subsequent assessments, the blood pressure should be measured in the arm with the higher pressure.
- Pressure differences higher than 10 mm Hg indicate conditions such as aortic stenosis or an arterial occlusion in the arm with the lower pressure.

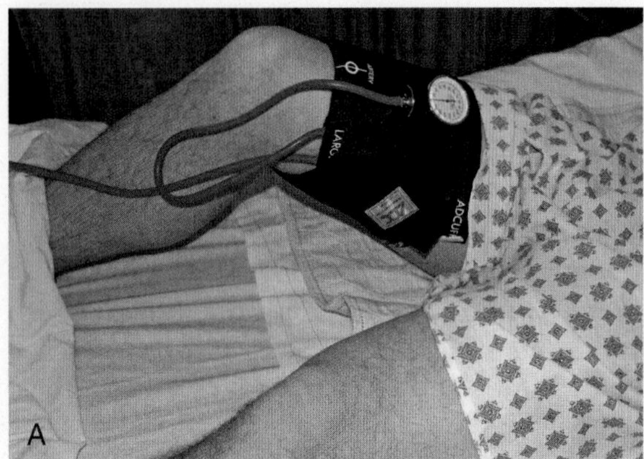

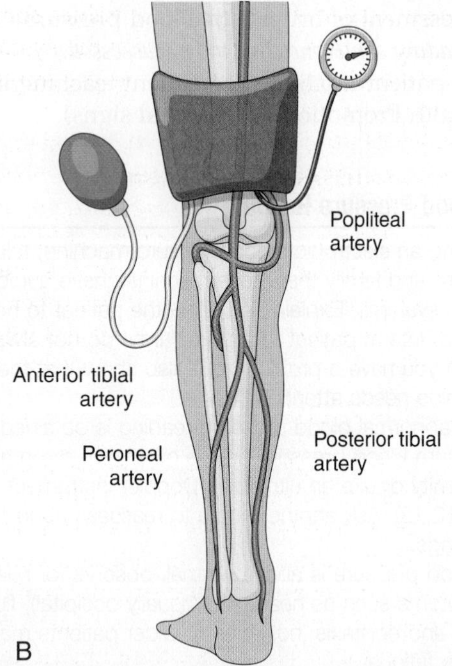

Fig. 12.13 A, Lower-extremity blood pressure cuff positioned above popliteal artery at mid-thigh. B, Location of the popliteal artery and placement of the cuff.

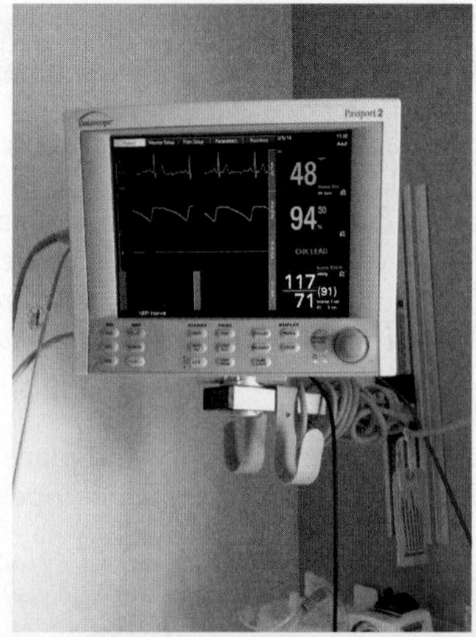

Fig. 12.14 Monitor displays blood pressure reading. (From Sorrentino SA, Remmert LN: *Mosby's textbook for nursing assistants*, ed 9, St. Louis, 2017, Elsevier.)

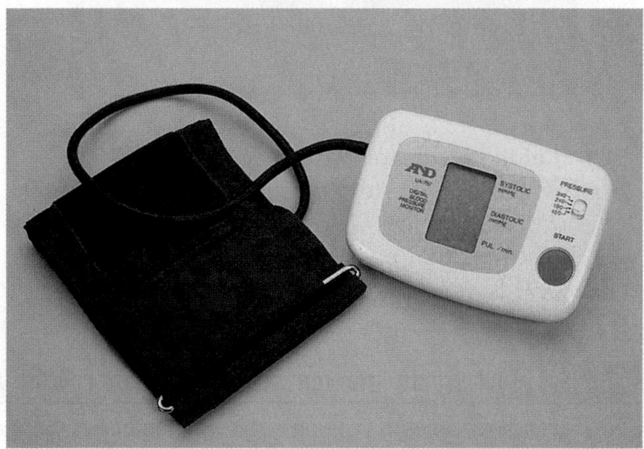

Fig. 12.15 Electronic sphygmomanometer.

pressure cuff is also useful for home use if the patient or caregiver has hearing difficulties. The ability to use a stethoscope is not required. Automatic devices are sensitive to outside interference and are susceptible to error. For proper function, the microphone or the pressure sensor must be positioned directly over the artery. Patient movements, vibration, or outside noise may interfere with the microphone or the sensor signal. Most automatic blood pressure devices are unable to process sounds or vibrations of low blood pressure (Box 12.17). In addition, the range of device quality sometimes makes comparing blood pressure measurements difficult.

The use of automatic blood pressure devices permits assessment of blood pressure during interpersonal interactions. Nonetheless, avoid speaking to the patient for at least a minute before initiating a blood pressure recording. Talking to a patient when the blood pressure is being assessed has the potential to increase readings.

Self-Measurement

More people today measure their own blood pressure, thanks to improved technology in home monitoring

Coordinated Care

Supervision

Vital Signs

The skill of vital signs measurement can be delegated to unlicensed assistive personnel (UAP). The nurse is responsible for assessing the effect of changes in the body's vital signs.

- Inform UAP of the following:
  - Appropriate route and device to measure temperature
  - Specific factors related to patient that can falsely raise or lower temperature
  - The frequency of temperature measurement for specific patient
  - Any factors that will affect the positioning of a patient when measuring a rectal temperature
  - Patient's history or risk of irregular pulse
  - Frequency of pulse measurement for specific patient
  - The proper positioning of the patient when measuring the apical pulse
  - Patient history or risk for increased or decreased respiratory rate or irregular respirations
  - Frequency of respiration measurement for specific patient
  - If patient has alterations that affect the appropriate limb for blood pressure measurement
  - Appropriate-size blood pressure cuff for designated extremity
  - Frequency of blood pressure measurement for specific patient
  - Before blood pressure measurement if the patient is at risk for experiencing orthostatic hypotension
- Determine that UAP is aware of the usual values of each vital sign for patient.
- Inform UAP of abnormalities of each vital sign that should be reported and reconfirmed by the nurse.
- The UAP is not responsible for using the Doppler. This is a skill for the registered nurse (RN) or licensed practical/vocational nurse (LPN/LVN) to perform.
- Explain which weight device to use for a specific patient.

devices and a greater interest in health promotion. Two of the more common types of devices the general public uses are portable home devices and stationary automated machines.

The portable home devices include the aneroid sphygmomanometer (see Fig. 12.9) and electronic digital readout devices that do not require use of a stethoscope. The electronic devices inflate and deflate cuffs with the push of a button (see Fig. 12.15). Although the electronic devices are often easier to manipulate, there are some disadvantages. They easily become inaccurate and require recalibration more than once a year. Because of their sensitivity, improper cuff placement or movement of the arm frequently causes electronic devices to give incorrect readings. A useful blood pressure device that overcomes these difficulties fits around the wrist, does not require a stethoscope, is easy to use, and is well adapted for home use. This device also inflates and deflates at the push of a button.

Box 12.17 Patient Conditions That Make Use of Electronic Blood Pressure Measurements Inappropriate

- Arrhythmias
- Excessive tremors
- Inability to cooperate to minimize arm motions
- Irregular heart rate
- Obese extremity
- Older adults
- Peripheral vascular obstruction (e.g., clots, narrowed vessels)
- Seizures
- Shivering

Stationary automated machines often are located in public places such as grocery stores, pharmacies, fitness clubs, banks, airports, and work sites. Users simply rest the arm within the machine's inflatable cuff, which contains a pressure sensor. The cuff fits over the clothing. A visual display tells users their blood pressure within 60 to 90 seconds. The reliability of the stationary machines is limited. Blood pressure values sometimes vary by 5 to 10 mm Hg or more (for the systolic and diastolic values) compared with the pressures taken with a manual sphygmomanometer.

If they have the information that they need to perform the procedure correctly, and if they know when to seek medical attention, consumers can learn to use self-measurement devices to their benefit. Patients should be advised of possible inaccuracies in the machines, how to understand the meaning and implications of readings, and the proper measurement techniques.

HEIGHT AND WEIGHT

With the initial measurement of vital signs, the patient's height (the vertical measurement of a structure, organ, or other object from bottom to top, when it is placed or projected in an upright position) and weight (the force exerted on a body by the gravity of the earth; normal weight depends on the frame of the individual) should be measured. Height and weight determination is important because it helps assess normal growth and development, aids in proper drug dosage calculation, and often is used to assess the effectiveness of drug therapy, such as diuretics. Only in cases of extreme illness is it acceptable to delay obtaining these valuable assessments. A stated height and weight should not be relied on because of the importance placed on these in the treatment process. Malnourished patients, patients who are undergoing diuretic therapy, and patients who have diseases that increase fluid retention, such as heart, liver, and kidney disease, may need to be weighed frequently (such as weekly or daily).

OBTAINING WEIGHT MEASUREMENTS

Patients are weighed to give the health care provider information for prescribing medication dosages and to determine nutritional status and water balance. Because 1 L of fluid equals 1 kg (2.2 lb), a weight change of 1 kg (2.2 lb) often reflects a loss or gain of 1 L of body fluids. A significant loss of weight frequently points to an underlying disease.

Patients should be weighed at the same time of day, on the same scale, and in the same type or amount of clothing to allow an objective comparison of subsequent weighings. An ideal time to weigh patients is in the morning after voiding and before breakfast.

Various types of weighing scales are available to meet the patients' needs. Patients capable of bearing their own weight use a standing scale (Skill 12.6). The patient must stand on the scale platform and remain still. Manual scales are calibrated by setting the weight at zero and noting whether the balance beam registers in the middle of the mark. To obtain the patient's weight, slowly adjust the scale weight on the balance beam until the tip of the beam registers in the middle of the mark. Scales with a digital display must read zero before each use. Digital scale readouts display weight in a matter of seconds.

Chair and sling scales are available for patients unable to bear weight (Fig. 12.16). The sling is placed under the patient and connected to the arms of the scale, the patient is lifted above the bed by a hydraulic device, and the weight is measured on a balance beam or digital display. Caution must be used to promote patient safety when transferring patients to and from the scales.

Bed scales may be available in some facilities for those patients who are unable to get out of bed. The nurse should ensure that the patient is not placed in the bed before the scale is zeroed. The patient always should be weighed in the same clothing and, if possible, during the same time of the day.

OBTAINING HEIGHT MEASUREMENTS

Height measurement is recorded in inches or centimeters, depending on agency policy. The calculation to use if transferring height from inches into centimeters is 1 inch is equal to 2.54 centimeters (cm). For example, a person who is 68 inches is 172.72 cm.

When measuring the height of a patient on a standing scale, ensure that the patient is standing upright with shoes removed. Most standing scales have a metal bar that is placed over the top of the patient's head. For the patient who is unsteady, there is often a hand rail attached to the wall for safety. Assist patients on and off the scale. Disinfect the scale after patient use.

Skill 12.6 Measuring Height and Weight

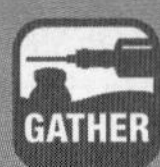

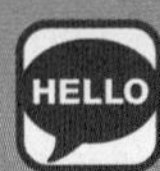

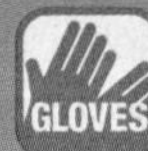

NURSING ACTION *(RATIONALE)*

1. Perform hand hygiene. *(Reduces spread of microorganisms.)*
2. Introduce self. *(Decreases patient's anxiety.)*
3. Identify patient by identification band. *(Verifies correct patient for procedure.)*
4. Explain procedure to patient. *(Gains cooperation and assistance and decreases patient's anxiety.)*
5. Prepare for procedure:
   a. Assemble supplies, including scale: standing, chair, or bed type. *(Organizes procedure efficiently.)*
   b. Provide privacy. *(Decreases patient's anxiety.)*
6. Implement procedure:
   a. Balance scale at zero. *(Ensures accurate reading.)*
   b. Place paper towel over base of scale where patient will stand, if patient is barefoot. *(Promotes medical asepsis.)*
   c. Have patient step onto scale. Patient should be weighed in same amount of clothing each time—preferably gown; slippers are optional. *(Promotes an accurate comparison.)*
   d. Measure height with patient standing upright, if patient can tolerate this. *(Promotes accurate measurement.)*
   e. Measure weight. *(Provides accurate measurement.)*
   f. Assist patient off scale by having patient step to side. *(Safer than stepping backward.)*
   g. Assist to bed or chair to provide for patient's comfort. *(Promotes patient's self-esteem.)*
7. Write down measurement (for documentation later).
8. Perform hand hygiene. *(Reduces spread of microorganisms.)*
9. Document measurements (e.g., height: 64 inches [162.56 cm], weight: 136 lb) (see Fig. 12.1).
10. Follow up by reporting measurement. *(Reading often varies and must be reassessed.)*

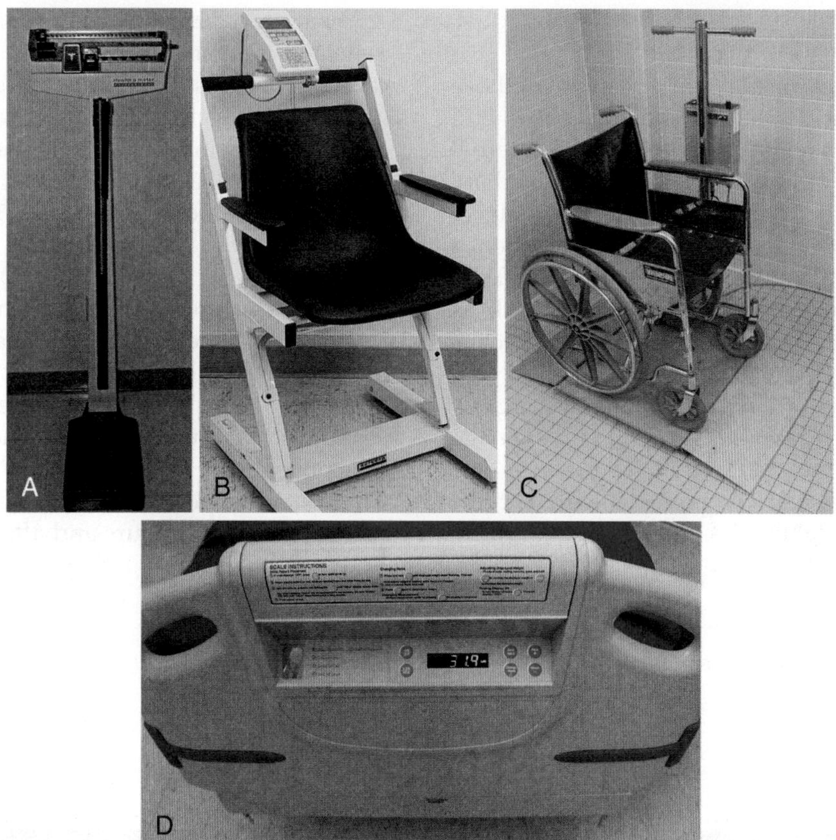

Fig. 12.16 Types of scales. A, Standing scale. B, Chair scale. C, Lift scale. D, Bed scale. (B and C from Sorrentino SA, Remmert LN: *Mosby's textbook for nursing assistants*, ed 9, St. Louis, 2017, Elsevier.)

❖ NURSING PROCESS

The role of the LPN/LVN in the nursing process as stated is that the LPN/LVN will:

- Participate in planning care for patients based on patient needs
- Review patient's plan of care and recommend revisions as needed
- Review and follow defined prioritization for patient care
- Use clinical pathways, care maps, or care plans to guide and review patient care

◆ ASSESSMENT

At initial contact with a patient, a baseline measurement of vital signs routinely is obtained to provide a means for comparison with subsequent vital signs values. These findings aid in determining whether more thorough assessment of specific body systems is necessary. For example, after assessment of an abnormal respiratory rate, the lung sounds also should be auscultated. In certain situations, the assessment of vital signs may be limited to measurement of a single vital sign for the purpose of reviewing a specific aspect of a patient's condition. For example, after the administration of an antihypertensive medication, measurement of the patient's blood pressure to evaluate the medication's effects is essential. Part of a nurse's clinical judgment involves deciding which vital signs to assess and measure and when and how frequently.

This assessment includes the following:

- Normal daily fluctuations
- Factors likely to interfere with accuracy of vital signs reading
- Medications that have potential to influence vital signs
- Factors that influence vital signs
- Conditions that precipitate fever, such as infections
- Previous baseline vital signs from patient's record; baseline information provides basis for comparison and assists in assessment of current status

◆ PATIENT PROBLEM

A review of all data gathered during assessment is required to determine the patient problem. Defining characteristics, when clustered, reveal this problem. The following are possible patient problems related to vital signs:

- *Inadequate Fluid Volume*
- *Elevated Body Temperature*
- *Below Normal Body Temperature*
- *Potential for Inability to Regulate Body Temperature*
- *Inefficient Oxygenation*

◆ EXPECTED OUTCOMES AND PLANNING

The appropriate focus for the plan of care is on those nursing interventions that identify abnormalities and restore homeostasis (a relative constancy in the internal environment of the body; naturally maintained by adaptive responses that promote healthy survival).

A possible patient-centered goal is often "patient's vital signs will be within normal range" or, for patients with chronic diseases that alter vital signs, such as chronic obstructive pulmonary disease (COPD), "baseline will be established."

Expected outcomes often include the following:

- Patient's vital signs are within normal range for age group.
- Baseline is established for patients with chronic diseases such as COPD.

◆ IMPLEMENTATION

The severity of an alteration in a vital sign influences the priorities in the care of the patient.

What procedures the health care team uses to intervene and treat an abnormal vital sign depends on the cause, any adverse effects, and the strength and intensity of the abnormal vital signs and how long the abnormality persists. Direct interventions toward providing comfort to the patient and to keeping complications to a minimum (see Boxes 12.6, 12.10, 12.12, and 12.15).

◆ EVALUATION

Evaluate all nursing interventions by comparing the patient's actual responses with the outcome of the care plan. An example follows:

Outcome: Patient's blood pressure, pulse, respirations, and temperature are within normal range for age group.

Evaluative measures: Assess vital signs on a regular basis, such as every 4 hours and after activity.

Get Ready for the NCLEX® Examination!

Key Points

- Vital signs include the physiologic parameters of temperature, pulse, respiration, and blood pressure.
- Vital signs often are measured as part of a complete physical examination or, more commonly, in a review of the patient's condition.
- Obtain vital signs whenever the patient's condition changes adversely.
- Knowledge of the factors that influence vital signs assists in interpreting abnormal values.
- Vital signs' measurements provide a basis for evaluating the patient's response to medical and nursing interventions.
- Approach the patient in a calm and caring manner while demonstrating proficiency in handling supplies needed for vital sign measurement.
- Vital signs are best measured when the patient is inactive (at rest) and the environment is controlled for comfort.
- A fever is one of the body's normal defense mechanisms.
- Temperatures are obtained via oral, rectal, axillary, and tympanic routes.
- The use of in-glass mercury thermometers and all mercury-containing devices for patient care is no longer advisable because of the danger of mercury toxicity.
- Do not perform rectal temperature measurements on newborns, infants, or adults with rectal alterations.
- The tympanic route is the most accessible and acceptable site for measuring core body temperature.
- Assess the presence and character of peripheral pulses to determine the adequacy of peripheral blood flow.
- For blood pressure assessment, having the proper equipment is as important as using the correct technique.
- Self-measurement of blood pressure is useful when it leads to detection of an elevated blood pressure in people previously unaware of a problem and in monitoring blood pressure in people already diagnosed with hypertension.
- No clinically significant difference in blood pressure levels are found between boys and girls. After puberty, males tend to have higher blood pressure readings. After menopause, women tend to have higher levels of blood pressure than men of similar age.
- The automatic blood pressure cuff is useful for home use if the patient or caregiver has hearing difficulties.
- Most facilities have developed a fifth vital sign: pain control or comfort level. Pain has an observable effect on vital signs.
- Temperature, pulse, respiration, and blood pressure are interrelated; a change in one has the potential to alter the others.

Additional Learning Resources

SG Go to your Study Guide for additional learning activities to help you master this chapter content.

evolve Be sure to visit the Evolve site at *http://evolve.elsevier.com/Cooper/foundationsadult/* for additional online resources.

Review Questions for the NCLEX® Examination

1. A patient is undergoing antibiotic therapy for pneumonia. His rectal temperature reading is 101.6°F. What is the expected oral temperature reading?
1. 101.6°F (38.7°C)
2. 100.6°F (38.1°C)
3. 99.6°F (37.5°C)
4. 97.6°F (36.4°C)

2. A patient has a postpartum temperature that is elevated in the evening but returns to a normal reading in the morning. This has occurred for several days. What is this type of fever classification?
1. Constant
2. Intermittent
3. Remittent
4. Crisis

3. A patient has a 10-year history of coronary artery disease. The patient is recovering from a myocardial infarction. What is the most accurate way for the nurse to assess the pulse rate?
1. Carotid pulse
2. Radial pulse
3. Apical pulse
4. Brachial pulse

4. An adult patient is admitted to the emergency department with an exacerbation of asthma. Respirations are 40 breaths per minute. After treatment, the rate returns to normal limits. What respiratory range is considered to be normal?
1. 30 to 60
2. 12 to 20
3. 16 to 22
4. 24 to 30

5. During a routine physical examination, a patient's blood pressure is noted at 180/90 mm Hg. The patient states, "Oh no, I didn't know I had high blood pressure." The nurse is aware that the patient's blood pressure must measure above what level at two separate office visits for the patient to be diagnosed with hypertension?
1. 160/100 mm Hg
2. 140/90 mm Hg
3. 130/70 mm Hg
4. 120/80 mm Hg

6. A 65-year-old man has a history of emphysema resulting from 30 years of cigarette smoking. He frequently reports dyspnea. What is dyspnea?
1. Pallor
2. Absence of retractions
3. Cyanosis
4. Difficulty breathing

7. A patient reports palpitations that result from anxiety over an impending surgery. The pulse rate is found to be 110 beats per minute. How will the nurse describe this heart rate?
1. Bradycardia
2. Tachycardia
3. Tachypnea
4. Hypertension

8. The nurse obtains a supine blood pressure reading of 130/64 mm Hg. One hour later, the nurse obtains a supine blood pressure reading of 134/62 mm Hg and a sitting blood pressure reading of 95/62 mm Hg. What should be the immediate action of the nurse?
1. Assist the patient to return to a supine position.
2. Obtain a blood pressure reading in the other arm.
3. Report the findings to the nurse in charge.
4. Question the patient about any symptoms.

9. The nurse is assessing a patient's blood pressure for the first time as part of the patient's postoperative assessment. After reaching the point at which the radial pulse is obliterated, what is the next action of the nurse?
1. Deflate the cuff slowly and wait 15 to 20 seconds before reinflating.
2. Deflate the cuff rapidly and wait 15 to 30 seconds before reinflating.
3. Deflate the cuff slowly and wait 1 minute before reinflating.
4. Deflate the cuff rapidly and wait 1 minute before reinflating.

10. The nurse has been assigned several patients. Which patient is most likely to have a higher-than-normal temperature? *(Select all that apply.)*
1. A depressed, apathetic patient
2. A patient assessed with hemorrhage
3. A patient who is recovering from surgery
4. A patient who just finished eating
5. A patient who has a temperature of 101.4°F

11. A patient is admitted after a motorcycle accident. The nurse is assessing the pulse pressure. The blood pressure reading is 140/102 mm Hg. What is the correct pulse pressure? ______________

12. The nurse is preparing to assess a 2-day-old infant's pulse rate. Which site should be used?
1. Scalp artery
2. Femoral artery
3. Apical site
4. Radial site

13. The nurse is assessing a postoperative patient's apical and radial pulses. Which statement is correct concerning this assessment of the patient's apical and radial pulse measurements?
1. The apical pulse and radial pulse should be taken for 1 full minute each.
2. The apical and radial pulse rates are lower when the temperature is elevated.
3. The apical and radial pulses are taken at the same time for 30 seconds.
4. The apical and radial pulses are taken at the same time for 60 seconds.

14. The health care provider has ordered an orthostatic blood pressure measurement. Place the following statements in correct order concerning the orthostatic method of assessing blood pressure.
1. The measurement is taken when the patient is standing.
2. The measurement is taken with the patient lying down.

3. The nurse assesses the blood pressure in the sitting position.
4. The nurse documents the blood pressure readings.

15. The patient's oral temperature is 37°C. What is the appropriated reporting of this temperature?
 1. Febrile
 2. Afebrile
 3. Hypotensive
 4. Hypertensive

16. Which is an important factor in the measurement of vital signs? *(Select all that apply.)*
 1. Ranges of normal for vital signs are very narrow and apply to all patients.
 2. The most significant aspect of measuring vital signs is their documentation.
 3. Environmental factors have an insignificant effect on the patient's vital signs.
 4. All measuring equipment is chosen on the basis of the patient's conditions and characteristics.
 5. Smoking can alter the temperature, pulse, respirations, and blood pressure by increasing each vital sign.

17. The patient has been hospitalized after a severe head injury. What is most likely the reason for the patient having difficulty in maintaining a normal body temperature when there is no infection present?
 1. Choosing the wrong time of day to obtain vital signs
 2. Errors by the nurse in measuring temperature
 3. Increased vasodilation of the superficial vessels contributing to excess heat loss
 4. The patient's head injury causing interference with the function of the hypothalamus

18. A pulse deficit provides information about the heart's ability to adequately perfuse the body. What is the definition of a pulse deficit?
 1. The difference between the radial and the apical pulse rates
 2. The digital pressure felt when taking radial and ulnar pulses
 3. The amount of pressure felt when taking radial and ulnar pulses
 4. The difference between the systolic and the diastolic blood pressure readings

19. The nurse finds that the patient's oral temperature is 98.8°F (37.1°C). What is the next nursing action?
 1. Administer an antiemetic drug.
 2. Offer the patient an additional blanket.
 3. Report that the patient's temperature is normal.
 4. Compare this with the patient's baseline.

20. The unlicensed assistive personnel reports that the patient is feeling "funny." What is the nurse's first action?
 1. Notify the health care provider.
 2. Obtain the patient's vital signs yourself.
 3. Delegate the assistant to retake the vital signs.
 4. Tell the assistant to keep assessing the patient and report any further symptoms.

21. The nurse is taking vital signs measurements and notes that the patient has a strong radial pulse that diminishes in intensity and that there are interruptions in rhythm about every four to six beats. What is the next action of the nurse?
 1. Report the findings to a health care provider.
 2. Measure a 60-second apical pulse.
 3. Connect the patient to a cardiac monitor.
 4. Obtain a 60-second apical-radial pulse.

22. When documenting a patient's blood pressure, at what point is the systolic pressure recorded?
 1. At the first Korotkoff sound
 2. At the second Korotkoff sound
 3. At the fourth Korotkoff sound
 4. At the fifth Korotkoff sound

23. Which method of measuring temperature reveals core temperature? *(Select all that apply.)*
 1. Skin
 2. Temporal
 3. Oral
 4. Axillary
 5. Tympanic

24. The nurse is providing discharge teaching to a patient who recently has been diagnosed with a cardiac condition. In teaching this patient how to assess the pulse, which is the best for the nurse to teach?
 1. Radial artery
 2. Pedal artery
 3. Brachial artery
 4. Femoral artery

25. When teaching the patient about monitoring his own pulse, the nurse informs the patient that the pulse may be elevated by which of the following? *(Select all that apply.)*
 1. Taking beta blockers
 2. Fever
 3. Sleeping
 4. Standing up too quickly
 5. Acute pain

26. The nurse begins to measure the blood pressure of an adult. The patient says that his doctor has instructed him to always use a large cuff. What is a reason for using a large cuff?
 1. A blood pressure cuff that is too small gives inaccurately high readings.
 2. A blood pressure cuff that is too small likely injures the brachial artery.
 3. Large cuffs are typically more accurate on adults than normal-size cuffs.
 4. Normal-size cuffs should be used for pediatric patients.

27. The nurse is developing a care plan for a patient taking a diuretic to treat fluid retention. The nurse knows that weighing the patient on a daily basis will assist in monitoring the effectiveness of the medication because a weight loss of 1 kg indicates a fluid loss of how much? ______________

Physical Assessment

13

http://evolve.elsevier.com/Cooper/foundationsadult/

Objectives

1. Discuss the difference between a sign and a symptom.
2. Compare and contrast the origins of disease.
3. List the four major risk categories for development of disease.
4. Discuss frequently noted signs and symptoms of disease conditions.
5. List the cardinal signs of inflammation and infection.
6. Describe the nursing responsibilities when assisting a physician with the physical examination.
7. List equipment and supplies necessary for the physical examination/assessment.
8. Explain the necessary skills for the physical examination/nursing assessment.
9. Discuss the nurse-patient interview.
10. List the basic essentials for a patient's health history.
11. Discuss the sequence of steps when performing a nursing assessment.
12. Discuss normal and abnormal assessment findings in the head-to-toe assessment.
13. Describe documentation of the physical examination/nursing assessment.
14. Explain ways to develop cultural sensitivity.

Key Terms

acute (p. 313)
anorexia (p. 332)
assessment (p. 314)
auscultation (ăw-skŭl-TĀ-shŭn, p. 318)
borborygmi (bŏr-bō-RĬG-mē, p. 333)
bruits (BRŪ-ē, p. 327)
chronic (p. 313)
crackles (p. 328)
disease (p. 312)
drainage (p. 312)
dullness (p. 318)
edema (p. 314)
erythema (ĕr-ĕ-THĒ-mă, p. 314)
etiology (ē-tē-ŎL-ĕ-jē, p. 312)
exudate (ĔKS-ū-dāt, p. 312)
flatness (p. 318)
focused assessment (p. 324)
functional disease (p. 313)
infection (p. 313)
inflammation (p. 313)
inspection (p. 318)
level of consciousness (LOC) (p. 323)
neoplastic (nē-ō-PLĂS-tĭk, p. 312)
nursing health history (p. 319)
nursing physical assessment (p. 323)
objective data (p. 311)
organic disease (p. 313)
palpation (p. 318)
percussion (pŭr-KŬ-shŭn, p. 318)
pruritus (prū-RĪ-tŭs, p. 312)
purulent (PYŪ-rū-lĕnt, p. 314)
remission (p. 313)
signs (p. 311)
subjective data (p. 312)
symptoms (p. 312)
thrill (p. 327)
turgor (TŬR-gŏr, p. 327)
tympany (TĬM-pă-nē, p. 318)
wheezes (p. 329)

Assessment of the patient is a key element of nursing care. The patient's well-being is a great responsibility that relies heavily on an accurate nursing assessment. The patient's baseline condition and changes in condition are monitored by the nurse; therefore strong assessment skills are imperative.

SIGNS AND SYMPTOMS

In a nursing assessment, **signs** are **objective data** as perceived by the examiner. What the nurse sees, hears, measures, and feels are considered objective data. More than one person can verify objective data with observation and measurement. Examples of signs are rashes, altered vital signs, abnormal lung or heart sounds, and visible drainage or exudate. **Drainage** refers to the passive or active removal of fluids from a body cavity, wound, or other source of discharge by one or more methods. Examples are the closed urinary drainage system or an open drainage system, such as a Jackson-Pratt drain. **Exudate** refers to fluid, cells, or other substances that are slowly exuded, or discharged, from cells or blood vessels through small pores or breaks in the cell membrane, usually as a result of inflammation or injury. Perspiration, pus, and serum sometimes are identified as exudates.

The senses of sight, hearing, touch, and smell are used to gather these objective data or signs. Objective data also include laboratory findings and diagnostic imaging and other diagnostic studies.

Symptoms are subjective indications of illness that the patient perceives. Examples of symptoms are pain, nausea, vertigo, pruritus, diplopia, numbness, and anxiety. These subjective data are what the patient describes related to pain, nausea, and others. An example is, "I feel like a knife is stabbing me in my stomach" as the patient points to the upper abdominal area.

In **subjective data** collection, the interviewer encourages a full description by the patient of the onset, the course, and the character of the problem and any factors that aggravate or alleviate it. Many signs accompany symptoms; for example, the nurse often sees erythema and a rash when a patient reports **pruritus** (itching). Objective confirmation of some symptoms is possible; for example, absence of response to a pinprick confirms patient reports of numbness of a body part.

DISEASE AND DIAGNOSIS

Disease, a pathologic condition of the body, is any disturbance of a structure or function of the body. A recognized set of signs and symptoms characterizes a given disease. How these signs and symptoms are clustered or grouped allows the health care provider to make a medical diagnosis. The nurse relies on assessment of signs and symptoms in this case to formulate a patient problem statement. Unlike the medical diagnosis, which deals with pathophysiologic factors and the cure of disease, the patient problem statement recognizes holistic needs of the patient that will be treated with nursing interventions. Some nursing interventions are made independently. To accomplish others, the nurse depends on or collaborates with other members of the health care team.

ORIGINS OF DISEASE

Disease or illness originates from many causes; these are sometimes hereditary and sometimes congenital, inflammatory, degenerative, infectious, deficiency, metabolic, neoplastic, traumatic, environmental, or some combination of these. For other diseases, no apparent cause is known. These illnesses, such as autoimmune diseases, are said to have an unknown **etiology,** or cause.

Hereditary diseases are transmitted genetically from parents to children. Some examples are cystic fibrosis, sickle cell anemia, color blindness, and hemophilia.

Congenital diseases appear at birth or shortly thereafter but are not caused by genetic abnormalities. These diseases result from some failure in development during the embryonic stage, or the first 2 months, of pregnancy. Contributing factors include inadequate oxygen, maternal infection, drugs, alcohol, malnutrition, and radiation. Structural and functional defects occur. Examples include absence of limbs (structural) and blindness (functional).

Inflammatory diseases are those in which the body reacts with an inflammatory response to some causative agent. Microorganisms are the cause in many instances, such as with pharyngitis or bronchitis. Other inflammatory diseases, such as hay fever, are manifestations of an allergic reaction. Still others have an unknown cause.

Degenerative disease implies degeneration, often progressive, of some part of the body. The aging process may play a role in these types of diseases. Osteoarthritis is a common example.

Infectious diseases result from the invasion of microorganisms into the body. Examples of infectious diseases include acquired immunodeficiency syndrome (AIDS), tuberculosis, measles, and pneumonia.

Deficiency diseases result from the lack of a specific nutrient. Nutrients are minerals, vitamins, proteins, fats, and carbohydrates. Iron deficiency anemia sometimes results from a severe deficiency of iron in the diet.

Metabolic disease is caused by a dysfunction that results in a loss of metabolic control of homeostasis in the body. The dysfunction usually involves endocrine glands, which secrete hormones to regulate body processes. Diabetes mellitus results from the dysfunction of the pancreatic islets. Other examples of metabolic disease are hypothyroidism and acromegaly, which involve the thyroid and pituitary glands.

Neoplastic disease is described as an abnormal growth of new tissues. The new growth is sometimes benign and sometimes malignant (cancerous). Malignant neoplasms are a serious threat to health because of the rapid growth of the cells and their ability to invade and metastasize.

Traumatic conditions result from physical and emotional trauma. Physical trauma, such as a motor vehicle accident, has the potential to result in traumatic brain injury (TBI). TBI frequently leaves the individual mentally and physically impaired. Individuals who suffer emotional trauma, such as the loss of a loved one, sometimes become unable to manage the activities of daily living (ADLs) they participated in before the trauma.

Environmental diseases are a group of conditions that develop from exposure to a harmful substance in the environment. Carbon monoxide (CO), an odorless, colorless gas that can cause sudden illness and death, is produced any time a fossil fuel is burned and is produced by cars and trucks, generators, stoves, lanterns, burning charcoal and wood, gas ranges, and heating systems (CDC, 2017a). Asbestos is another substance in the environment that potentially leads to lung problems and various cancers.

Although many disease conditions have an unknown cause, many now consider a number of conditions to result from *autoimmune responses.* In an autoimmune response, the body develops immunoglobulins (antibodies) against its own tissues or body substances. Autoimmune diseases include rheumatoid arthritis and ulcerative colitis.

RISK FACTORS FOR DEVELOPMENT OF DISEASE

A risk factor is any situation, habit, environmental condition, genetic predisposition, physiologic condition, or other variable that increases the vulnerability of an individual or group to illness or accident. Risk factors for the development of coronary artery disease, for example, include heredity, cigarette smoking, high blood levels of cholesterol, and stress. The presence of risk factors does not necessarily mean that a person will have a disease condition develop, only that the chance is higher. The nurse assesses the patient's risk factors and uses them to help formulate nursing diagnoses, because nursing diagnoses are made for the patient's potential, and actual, problems.

Risk factors fall into four major categories: genetic and physiologic, age, environment, and lifestyle (Box 13.1). Some, such as many environmental and lifestyle risk factors, are modifiable; others, such as age and family history, are not.

TERMS USED TO DESCRIBE DISEASE

Diseases are described in terms of duration. **Chronic** disease develops slowly and persists over a long period, often for a person's lifetime. Diabetes mellitus (inability of the body to use glucose) is an example of a chronic disease. Chronic disease frequently is described further as early, late, or terminal; another possibility is that it is in remission. **Remission** means a partial or complete disappearance of clinical and subjective characteristics of the disease has occurred. Remission is sometimes spontaneous and sometimes a result of therapy.

In comparison, a disease described as **acute** begins abruptly with marked intensity of severe signs and symptoms and then often subsides after a period of treatment. An episode of appendicitis is considered acute.

Disease is also often described as organic or functional. An **organic disease** results in a structural change in an organ that interferes with its functioning. Stroke is an organic disease of the brain. Manifestations of **functional disease** often appear to be those of organic disease, but careful examination fails to reveal evidence of structural or physiologic abnormalities. Many nervous and mental diseases are classified as functional.

Box 13.1 Risk Factors for Disease

GENETIC AND PHYSIOLOGIC

- A family history of cancer increases the risk that an individual will have cancer develop (genetic).
- Malnourishment predisposes an individual to illness (physiologic).

AGE

- Osteoporosis makes the older adult more prone to fractures, especially of the hip.
- Thinning skin in older adults makes this group more susceptible to skin trauma.

ENVIRONMENT

- Air, water, and noise pollution increase the risk of illness.
- Asbestos in building structures increases the risk of cancer of the pleura (in lung).
- Carbon monoxide (CO) with the burning of fossil fuels in generators, gas stoves, and heaters may lead to sudden illness and death.
- Extremes of heat and cold have potential to damage or destroy body cells.
- High crime rates and overcrowding also lead to stress, which makes individuals more susceptible to disease.
- Within the family, conflicts or other problems have the potential to create stressors that put individual members or the family as a whole at increased risk of illness.

LIFESTYLE

- Other habits that place a person at risk for illness include alcohol and substance abuse.
- Overeating or poor nutrition, insufficient rest and sleep, and poor personal hygiene also add to increased risk for illness for the individual.
- Prolonged emotional stress, especially with ineffective coping mechanisms, increases the risk of development of illness and disease.
- Smoking increases the risk of many diseases, including oral (mouth) cancer, pharyngeal cancer, laryngeal cancer, lung cancer, renal cancer, esophageal cancer, pancreatic cancer, bladder cancer, uterine and cervical cancer, cardiovascular disease, and osteoporosis. Smoking is the most preventable cause of death in our society.
- Sunbathing increases the risk of skin cancer.

FREQUENTLY NOTED SIGNS AND SYMPTOMS OF DISEASE

Although signs and symptoms of inflammation and infection are similar, it is important not to confuse the two. **Infection** is caused by an invasion of microorganisms, such as bacteria, viruses, fungi, or parasites, that produce tissue damage. **Inflammation** is a protective response of body tissues to irritation, injury, or invasion by disease-producing organisms. The cardinal signs of infection and inflammation include **erythema** (redness), **edema** (swelling), heat, pain, **purulent** drainage (pus), and loss of function (Table 13.1).

The inflammatory response is actually the body's defense against some causative agent. Erythema and heat are the result of increased blood flow to the area. The damaged tissue releases chemical substances that cause the capillary walls to become more permeable. This enables white blood cells and plasma to move from the blood to the affected area. The white blood cells (neutrophils) digest microorganisms and cellular debris, and the excess of fluid in the tissues, or edema, increases pressure on sensitive nerve endings, causing pain. Loss of function imposes a period of rest for the injured area. Purulent exudate is the accumulation of neutrophils, dead cells, bacteria, and other debris from the infectious process.

ASSESSMENT

A complete health **assessment** is an evaluation or appraisal of the patient's condition. The process involves the orderly collection of information concerning the patient's health status. It is performed by the health care provider and nursing personnel and usually involves taking a medical history and performing a physical examination. The data collected establish a baseline. This baseline allows the health care provider or the nurse to identify problems and plan care; in addition, ongoing assessments produce contrasting data that permit the evaluation of the effectiveness of care.

MEDICAL ASSESSMENT

When the health care provider conducts a physical examination, the licensed practical nurse (LPN) often

Table 13.1 Frequently Noted Signs and Symptoms of Disease Conditions

TERM	DEFINITION
Anorexia	Lack of appetite that results in the inability to eat. This symptom can occur in many disease conditions.
Asthenia	A condition of debility, loss of strength and energy, and depleted vitality.
Bradycardia	A circulatory condition in which the myocardium contracts steadily but at a rate of less than 60 contractions per minute.
Constipation	Difficulty in passing stools or an incomplete or infrequent passage of hard stools. There are many organic and functional causes.
Coughing	A sudden audible expulsion of air from the lungs. Coughing is an essential protective response that clears the lungs, the bronchi, and the trachea of irritants and secretions and prevents aspiration of foreign material into the lungs. It is a common sign of diseases of the larynx, the bronchi, and the lungs.
Cyanosis	Bluish discoloration of the skin and mucous membranes caused by an increase of deoxygenated hemoglobin in the blood.
Diaphoresis	The secretion of sweat, especially the profuse secretion associated with an elevated body temperature, physical exertion, exposure to heat, and mental or emotional stress.
Diarrhea	Frequent passage of loose, liquid stools; generally results from increased motility in the colon. This is usually a sign of an underlying disorder. The characteristics of the diarrhea give evidence as to the source. Dark black, tarry stools sometimes mean there is bleeding in the intestines. Bright red blood in the feces indicates active bleeding from the lower portion of the intestinal tract.
Dyspnea	A shortness of breath or difficulty in breathing that is sometimes caused by certain heart and lung conditions, strenuous exercise, or anxiety.
Ecchymosis	Discoloration of an area of the skin or mucous membrane caused by the extravasation of blood into the subcutaneous tissues as a result of trauma to the underlying blood vessels or by fragility of the vessel walls (also called a *bruise*).
Edema	An abnormal accumulation of fluid in interstitial spaces. Some causes include overhydration, excess sodium intake, capillary hyperpermeability, and loss of serum albumin (a protein), which causes fluid to leave the vessels and collect in the interstitial space. Skin that is edematous is taut and shiny. Pitting sometimes occurs when the skin is pressed; a small indentation remains after the finger is removed.
Erythema	Redness or inflammation of the skin or mucous membranes that is the result of dilation and congestion of superficial capillaries; erythema is seen in a mild sunburn.
Fetid	Pertaining to something that has a foul, putrid, or offensive odor. Also called *malodorous*.
Fever	An abnormal elevation of the temperature of the body above 98.6°F (37°C) because of disease; also called *pyrexia*. It results from an imbalance between the elimination and production of heat. Infection and many different diseases often lead to febrile condition, or elevated temperature.
Inflammation	The protective response of the tissues of the body to irritation or injury.
Jaundice	Yellow tinge to the skin; often indicates obstruction in the flow of bile from the liver.

Table 13.1 Frequently Noted Signs and Symptoms of Disease Conditions—cont'd

TERM	DEFINITION
Lethargy	The state or quality of being indifferent, apathetic, or sluggish.
Nausea	A sensation that often leads to the urge to vomit. Common causes include intense pain, gallbladder disease, inflammation of the stomach, paralytic ileus, and food poisoning.
Orthopnea	An abnormal condition in which a person has to sit or stand to breathe deeply or comfortably. Occurs in many disorders of the respiratory and cardiac systems.
Pain	An unpleasant sensation caused by noxious (extremely destructive or harmful) stimulation of the sensory nerve endings. It is a cardinal symptom of inflammation and is valuable in the diagnosis of many disorders and conditions. Pain has varied manifestations: mild or severe, chronic, acute, burning, dull or sharp, precisely or poorly localized, or referred.
Pallor	An unnatural paleness or absence of color in the skin; often results from a decrease in hemoglobin and erythrocytes (red blood cells).
Pruritus	A symptom of itching and an uncomfortable sensation that leads to an urge to scratch. Some causes are allergy, infection, jaundice, elevated serum urea, and skin irritation.
Purulent drainage (pus)	A creamy, viscous, pale yellow or yellow-green fluid exudate that is the result of fluid remains of liquefied necrosis of tissues. Bacterial infection is the most common cause. The character of the pus, including its color, consistency, quantity, or odor, often has diagnostic significance.
Sallow	Pertaining to an unhealthy, yellow color; usually said of a complexion or skin.
Scleral icterus	The color of the sclera is yellow. This jaundice is the result of coloring of the sclera with bilirubin that infiltrates all tissues of the body.
Tachycardia	An abnormal condition in which the heart contracts regularly but at a rate greater than 100 beats per minute. The heart rate accelerates in response to fever, exercise, or nervous excitement.
Tachypnea	An abnormally rapid rate of breathing seen in many disease conditions.
Vomit	To expel the contents of the stomach through the esophagus and out of the mouth. The quality of the vomitus often gives a clue to the underlying cause. "Coffee-ground" vomitus indicates bleeding in the stomach. The blood takes on a coffee-ground appearance because of the effect of the digestive juices. Vomiting of bright red blood is potentially a sign of gastric hemorrhage.

is expected to carry out certain assistive functions. Preparing the examining room, assisting with equipment, preparing the patient, and collecting specimens are a few examples of the nurse's responsibilities to facilitate the physical examination. The nurse has both preexamination and postexamination responsibilities.

When preparing the patient for the physical examination, verify that certain data have been obtained and specific requirements have been addressed. The following list addresses these requirements and data:

- Ensure that an informed consent has been obtained by the health care provider for necessary procedures and that the consent form contains appropriate signatures.
- Verify that all prerequisite tests have been completed and results are available.
- Confirm that all necessary supplies and equipment have been obtained for the health care provider to perform the examination (Fig. 13.1 and Box 13.2).
- A full set of vital signs should be measured and the results made available to the health care provider before the examination is performed.
- Explain what will occur during the examination to the patient. Determine whether the patient has any unanswered questions (Box 13.3).
- Determine whether the physical examination will be performed in the patient's room (when in the hospital or long-term care setting) or if an examination room must be reserved. If the examination is occurring in a health care provider's office, ensure that the room is appropriate for the examination (e.g., if a gynecologic examination is planned, an examination table with stirrups is necessary).
- Consider the patient's ability to assume the necessary positions (Table 13.2) for the examination and determine what assistance will be needed.
- Determine whether the nurse's assistance will be required during the examination. The nurse should not leave the patient alone. Most examiners appreciate a nurse in attendance. Many facilities require a female nurse to be present when a male health care provider is performing a gynecologic examination.
- If specimens are being obtained, determine what supplies will be necessary and where the specimens are being sent for testing (see Chapter 15).
- Document information regarding the procedure, including vital signs, pertinent signs and symptoms, reports of pain, anxiety level, and specimens; obtain the necessary specimens and send them to the laboratory.

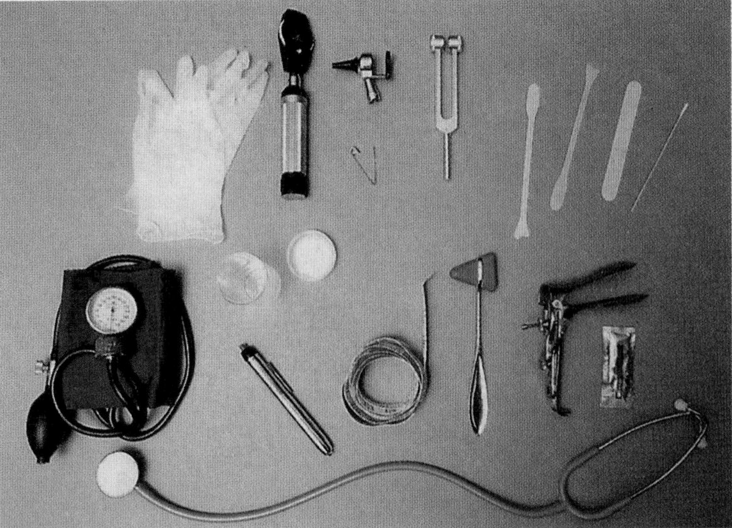

Fig. 13.1 Equipment used during a physical examination *(clockwise from upper left):* disposable gloves, ophthalmoscope, otoscope attachment, sterile safety pin, tuning fork, cervical spatulas, tongue depressor, cotton-tipped swab, lubricant, vaginal speculum, reflex hammer, tape measure, penlight, specimen cup, sphygmomanometer, and stethoscope *(bottom).* (From Elkin MK, Perry AG, Potter PA: *Nursing interventions and clinical skills,* ed 4, St. Louis, 2008, Mosby.)

Box 13.2 Equipment and Supplies for Physical Examination and Assessment

- Cotton applicators
- Cytobrush
- Disposable pad
- Drapes
- Eye chart (e.g., Snellen chart)
- Flashlight and spotlight
- Forms (e.g., physical examination results, laboratory requisitions)
- Gloves (sterile and clean)
- Gown for patient
- Lubricant
- Ophthalmoscope
- Otoscope
- Papanicolaou (Pap) smear slides
- Paper towels
- Percussion hammer
- Safety pins
- Scale with height measurement rod
- Spatula
- Specimen containers and microscope slides
- Sphygmomanometer and cuff
- Stethoscope
- Swabs or sponge forceps
- Tape measure
- Thermometer
- Tissues
- Tongue depressor
- Tuning fork
- Vaginal speculum
- Wristwatch with second hand

Perform an assessment to determine the actual or potential (risk for) patient problems that will require nursing interventions for the safety and well-being of the patient. For example, if during the examination you observe that the patient has a need for oxygen (a basic human need), take steps to ensure placement of oxygen, positioning, deep breathing, and coughing to meet this need.

Box 13.3 Psychological Preparation for a Physical Examination

Psychological preparation often is the nurse's highest priority before the examination. Patients become embarrassed when required to answer sensitive questions about body functions or when certain body parts are exposed and examined. The possibility of the examiner finding something abnormal also creates anxiety. Give the patient information about the examination in general terms. As each body system is examined, provide a more detailed explanation. Simple terms are used when describing the steps of the examination because complicated terminology confuses some patients and easily adds to their fears.

As the caregiver, the nurse is in constant contact with the patient and must perform accurate assessments to discover developing complications and to evaluate medical treatments.

NURSING ASSESSMENT

Nursing assessment comprises the gathering, verifying, and communicating of data about the patient. The purpose of the assessment is to establish a baseline database about the patient's level of wellness, health practices, past illnesses, related experiences, and health care goals. The information contained in the database is the basis for an individualized plan of nursing care developed throughout the nursing process.

Data collected during this process include the nursing health history, physical examination findings, results of laboratory and diagnostic tests, and information from health care team members and the patient's family or

Table 13.2 Positions for Examination

POSITION	AREAS ASSESSED	RATIONALE	LIMITATIONS
Sitting	Head and neck, back, posterior thorax and lungs, anterior thorax and lungs, breasts, axillae, heart, vital signs, and upper extremities	Sitting upright provides full expansion of lungs and provides better visualization of symmetry of upper body parts.	Some physically weakened patients are unable to sit. Use supine position with head of bed elevated instead.
Supine	Head and neck, anterior thorax and lungs, breasts, axillae, heart, abdomen, extremities, pulses	This is the most normally relaxed position. It provides easy access to pulse sites.	If patient becomes short of breath easily, consider raising head of bed.
Dorsal recumbent	Head and neck, anterior thorax and lungs, breasts, axillae, heart, abdomen	Position is used for abdominal assessment because it promotes relaxation of abdominal muscles.	Patients with painful disorders are more comfortable with knees flexed.
Lithotomy[a]	Female genitalia and genital tract	This position provides maximal exposure of genitalia and facilitates insertion of vaginal speculum.	Lithotomy position is embarrassing and uncomfortable, so minimize time that patient spends in it. Keep patient well draped.
Sims	Rectum and vagina	Flexion of hip and knee improves exposure of rectal area.	Joint deformities may hinder patient's ability to bend hip and knee.
Prone	Musculoskeletal system	This position is used only to assess extension of hip joint.	Patients with respiratory difficulties tolerate this position poorly.
Lateral recumbent	Heart	This position aids in detecting murmurs.	Patients with respiratory difficulties tolerate this position poorly.
Knee-chest[a]	Rectum	This position provides maximum exposure of rectal area.	This position is embarrassing and uncomfortable.

[a]A patient with severe arthritis or other joint deformity may be unable to assume this position.

significant others. Obtain the health history while initiating the nurse-patient relationship by interviewing the patient. Various techniques are used to progress through the interview (see Chapter 4). When assessing the patient, always pay special attention to areas about which the patient has expressed concern.

Once the interview is completed, proceed to the physical assessment. Use inspection, palpation, auscultation, and percussion to collect physical examination data (Box 13.4). Laboratory and diagnostic tests validate findings from the history and physical examination and often lead to identification of problems not previously noted (Box 13.5).

Initiating the Nurse-Patient Relationship

Perhaps the most challenging patient interview the nurse ever has to conduct is the first one with every patient. For some patients, being interviewed by a nurse is a

Box 13.4 Physical Assessment Techniques

INSPECTION

Visually inspect the patient's body and observe moods, including all responses and nonverbal behaviors. This **inspection,** or purposeful observation, is the technique the nurse uses most frequently. It begins with the nurse's first contact with the patient and continues throughout the gathering of the nursing history. Use inspection to collect data systematically about significant behaviors or physical features. It is important to be accurate and thorough, using a systematic approach such as a head-to-toe assessment.

PALPATION

With **palpation,** the nurse uses the hands and sense of touch to gather data. Hands are highly sensitive to texture, temperature, and moisture and thus help determine the quality of an area. Use palpation to detect tenderness, temperature, texture, vibration, pulsations, masses, and other changes in structural integrity. Palpate each body part, usually according to a systematic assessment pattern. Palpation rules out or confirms suspicions raised during interview and inspection. Because touching has the potential to elicit fear, embarrassment, pain, or other strong emotions, explain the nurse's actions and the reasons for them. In addition, instruct the patient to let the nurse know whether palpation produces sensations of tenderness, pressure, or pain. The three palpation techniques are light, moderate, and deep. Light and moderate palpations are illustrated in Figs. 13.10A and B.

When using palpation, be sure the fingernails are short, and warm the hands before touching the patient. Social conversation during palpation is appropriate at times to distract patients and help them relax. Use the pads of the fingers; place them flat against the patient's skin with slight pressure and gentle rotation of the area under examination. The thumb and forefinger can be used to palpate muscle mass on arms and legs. Palpate pulses with the pads of the fingers. Someone who is not appropriately trained to perform palpation can cause internal injuries. During palpation, also observe the patient's facial expressions; if you see a grimace indicating pain, for instance, ask the patient to describe it.

AUSCULTATION

Auscultation is the process of listening to sounds produced by the body. Three systems produce sounds the nurse will auscultate: the cardiovascular system, the respiratory system, and the gastrointestinal system. For auscultation of these systems, the nurse uses a stethoscope, an instrument that amplifies sounds produced by internal organs. The nurse also uses the technique of auscultation to detect the fetal heart sound.

To master the auscultation technique and gain experience at interpreting the sounds the nurse hears, the nurse needs repeated practice on healthy and ill patients. Accurate assessment requires a quiet environment. Television, sounds from nasogastric suction, movement of bed linen, and conversation can interfere with accurate auscultation. Try closing the eyes while listening to reduce visual distractions. Never rush auscultation. Take time to assess each area properly.

Place the diaphragm of the stethoscope gently over the patient's skin. If the area is hairy, dampening it sometimes decreases the sound of the hair rubbing against the diaphragm.

PERCUSSION

Percussion is use of the fingertips to tap the body's surface to produce vibration and sound. The sounds indicate the density of the underlying tissue and thus help the nurse detect the location of body organs and structures. For example, percussion over a hollow organ such as the stomach produces a high-pitched, drumlike sound called **tympany.** Percussion over a dense organ such as the liver produces a low-pitched, thudlike sound called **dullness.** Percussion over a muscle produces a soft, high-pitched, flat sound called **flatness.** To perform percussion, place the palmar surface of one hand against the patient's body while tapping with the fingers of the other hand. Tap each area two or three times. Properly performed, percussion is not painful for the patient, but if it does cause discomfort, discontinue it and document the results. This assessment technique is the one the nurse uses least frequently.

new experience. The nurse's first task is to establish an effective nurse-patient relationship before proceeding to the nursing health history.

 Communication

Before Assessment

Nurse: Good morning, Mr. C. I'm Ms. A., a student nurse. I'll be caring for you today. A portion of my nursing care is to conduct an assessment. My assessment will help me plan your nursing care. I will be including temperature, pulse, respirations, blood pressure, heart rate, orientation, pain scale, lung sounds, O_2 saturations, abdominal sounds, arterial pulses, and skin color in my assessment. It will take me about 30 minutes. Do you have any questions? (pause) May I begin now? (pause) I will start with your vital signs.

The first step in initiating the nurse-patient relationship is to introduce oneself, including name, position, and the purposes of the interview. In the Communication box, the nurse introduces herself, gives an estimate of the time needed for the assessment, and tells the patient the reason for the assessment. Indicating the length of time is important because it helps ensure cooperation. Do not consider the patient, even one in a hospital, a captive audience. Take steps to ensure that the patient's time is not used inappropriately. In the example, the nurse also gives the patient an opportunity to ask questions. Whether the patient has any pressing questions is important to determine before beginning the more targeted part of the interview. By answering these questions, the nurse meets some of the patient's immediate needs, and the patient may feel more comfortable answering the nurse's questions. For example, sometimes

Box 13.5 Common Laboratory and Diagnostic Tests

BLOOD ANALYSIS
- Arterial blood gas (ABG) analysis
- Blood chemistry profile
- Complete blood count (CBC), includes red blood cell (RBC), hemoglobin (Hgb), hematocrit (Hct), erythrocyte indices, platelets, white blood cell (WBC) with differential, and examination of peripheral blood cells
- Electrolyte tests: sequential multiple analysis–6 (SMA-6), SMA-12
- Fasting blood sugar (FBS) test
- International normalized ratio (INR)
- Megaloblastic anemia profile
- Partial thromboplastin time (PTT)
- Prothrombin time (PT)

URINE ANALYSIS
- 24-hour urine collection for creatinine clearance, protein content
- Urinalysis (UA)
- Urine culture and sensitivity test

DIAGNOSTIC IMAGING EXAMINATIONS
- Barium enema (BE) examination
- Chest roentgenogram (chest x-ray [CXR])
- Computed tomography (CT): scans of the body, the head, the chest, the abdomen, the pelvis, and the bones
- Intravenous pyelogram (IVP)
- Magnetic resonance imaging (MRI)
- Upper gastrointestinal (UGI) examination

STOOL ANALYSIS
- *Clostridium difficile*
- Culture and sensitivity
- *Escherichia coli* strain O157:H7
- Guaiac tests (Hematest stools)
- Ova and parasite tests

SPUTUM ANALYSIS
- Acid-fast bacilli (AFB) test
- Culture and sensitivity test
- Cytology tests

OTHER
- Colonoscopy examinations
- Endoscopy examinations
- Electrocardiogram (ECG), echocardiogram, transesophageal echocardiogram
- Stress test
- Tuberculosis (TB) skin test

a patient who is unsure of how the hospital bed operates is distracted and thinks more about the bed than about the questions being presented; this patient is less likely to provide complete information for the database. Finally, the nurse asks whether it is acceptable to conduct the interview at that time, thereby giving the patient a choice.

The next step in initiating the nurse-patient relationship is to communicate the nurse's trustworthiness and discretion to patients. Illnesses that cause people to seek help often are accompanied by anxiety, powerlessness, altered family processes, economic concerns, and changes in self-image. Patients frequently are asked to provide highly personal information about themselves and their families. Generally, people share such information only with family members or close friends. To be able to do so with the nurse, the patient must be comfortable that the information will be shared only with caregivers who need it to provide proper care. Assure patients that information concerning past or present levels of wellness or family relationships is strictly confidential.

The nurse-patient relationship is enhanced by the professionalism and competence conveyed. The nurse's professional manner, attitude, and appearance encourage a supportive therapeutic relationship with the patient that enables the nurse and the patient to communicate freely, thereby allowing identification of health care needs and goals.

Interview

Conduct the interview in a relaxed, unhurried manner in a quiet, private, well-lighted setting. Convey feelings of compassion and concern and, at the same time, remain objective. The patient must feel that the information being sought is truly important and that the nurse demonstrates an interest in the patient's state of wellness.

Determine by what name the patient wishes to be addressed, and then use that name during the interview. An accepting posture, sitting in a relaxed manner at eye level with the patient, is likely to enhance the interview. A pleasant facial expression promotes communication, and eye contact helps confirm to patients that they have the nurse's full attention.

One way to enhance communication is by using nonjudgmental language. Statements such as, "Yes, I see," or "What happened next?" encourage the patient to clarify without feeling threatened. Reflecting what the patient has stated clarifies statements, as does summarizing and restating what the patient has said. Approving nods and gestures facilitate the exchange of information. Be responsive to the patient's condition at all times. Pause the interview if necessary, stabilize the patient's condition, and ensure comfort and safety before proceeding. (Read more about interviewing in Chapter 4.)

NURSING HEALTH HISTORY

The **nursing health history** is the initial step in the assessment process. Data collected provide the nurse with information about the patient's level of wellness, changes in life patterns, sociocultural role, and mental and emotional reactions to illness. The objective is to identify patterns of health and illness, risk factors for physical and behavioral health problems, deviations from normal, and available resources for adaptation to life's changes.

Biographic Data

In most facilities, the admitting department obtains the biographic data; begin the interview by referring to this information. It generally includes data such as date of birth, gender, address, family members' names and addresses, marital status, religious preference and practices, occupation, source of health care, and insurance, Medicare, and Medicaid benefits. Verify this information with the patient to ensure that it is correct.

Reasons for Seeking Health Care

Ask why the patient has sought health care because the information contained on the admission form sometimes differs considerably from the patient's subjective reason for seeking health care. This often is referred to as the *chief complaint*. Perhaps ask simply, "What is the reason for the admission?" This allows the patient not only to describe the reason for admission but also to make expectations known to the nurse. To get the most information from the patient about health concerns, use the OPQRSTUV method (Box 13.6). Be sure to document this information in the patient's own words, using quotation marks. This helps remove the possibility of bias from later interpretation of the data.

Eliciting the patient's expectations of the health care providers is also appropriate. Determine whether patients expect to be "cured" or become "free of pain" or "able to care for self." This information assists in establishing the goals of nursing interventions and in determining whether patients' expectations of themselves and the health care providers are realistic. In addition, such expectations provide the nurse with information on patient perceptions about patterns of illness or changes in lifestyle.

Present Illness or Health Concerns

The data collected relate to the progression of the present illness from the onset to the current signs and symptoms. The data must be detailed and comprehensive to allow the nurse to plan appropriate interventions. To ensure that data collection is complete, examine the guidelines in Box 13.7.

Health History

Information from the health history provides data on the patient's health care experiences. Determine whether the patient has ever been hospitalized or has undergone surgery. Also essential in planning nursing interventions are descriptions of allergies, including allergic reactions to food, drugs, or pollutants. If an allergy is present, note the specific reaction and treatment on the assessment form.

Also use the health history to identify habits and lifestyle patterns. Use of alcohol, tobacco, illegal drugs, caffeine, herbal products, or over-the-counter drugs or prescription medications has potential to place the patient at risk for diseases involving the liver, the lungs, the heart, the nervous system, and thought processes. Note the type of habit, and the frequency and duration of use, to provide essential data. This is

Box 13.6 History of Present Illness

When discussing the history of the present illness with the patient, be sure the patient describes the problems fully. To do this, ask the patient the following questions about each symptom:

Time of onset. When was the first date (the problem) happened? What time did it begin?

Type of onset. How did (the problem) start: Suddenly? Gradually?

Original source. What were you doing when you first experienced or noticed (the problem)? What seems to trigger it: Stress? Position? Certain activities? Arguments?

Characteristics. What is (the problem) like? If describing a discharge: Thick? Runny? Clear? Colored? If describing a psychological problem: Do the voices drown out other sounds? Whose voice does it sound like?

Severity. How bad is (the problem) when it is at its worst? Does it interfere with your normal activities? Does it force you to lie down, sit down, slow down?

Radiation. In the case of pain, does it travel down your back or arms, up your neck, or down your legs? What is the pain intensity on a scale of 0 to 10?

Time relationship. How often do you experience (the problem): Hourly? Daily? Weekly? Monthly? When do you usually experience it: Daytime? At night? In the early morning? Are you ever awakened by it? Does it ever occur before, during, or after meals? Does it occur seasonally?

Duration. How long does an episode last?

Course. Does (the problem) seem to be getting better or getting worse, or does it remain the same?

Associations. Does (the problem) lead to anything else? Is it accompanied by other signs and symptoms?

Source of relief. What relieves it: Changing diet? Changing position? Taking medications? Being active?

Source of aggravation. What makes it worse?

The nurse can remember all these questions using the letters OPQRSTUV:

O Onset-Timing
Onset, duration

P Precipitating-Provocative-Palliative
What causes it? What makes it worse? What makes it better?

Q Quality-Quantity: describe it: sharp, dull …
How does it feel, look, or sound, and how much of it is there? How often, when, how long?

R Region-Radiation
Where is it? Does it spread?

S Severity scale
Does it interfere with activities? How does it rate on a severity scale of 0 to 10?

T Treatments
What helps? For how long?

U Understanding
What do you think is causing it? How does it affect you?

V Values
Goals of care; expectations

Box 13.7 Review of Systems

The nurse probably will not include questions pertaining to all the aspects of each system every time a nursing health history is taken. Nevertheless, include some questions regarding each system in every history. These essential areas are listed in italic type in the outline that follows. Whenever the patient gives positive responses to the first questions for that system, include questions about the more comprehensive and detailed areas relating to each system listed afterward. Keep in mind that these lists do not represent an exhaustive enumeration of questions; even more details are required frequently within an organ system, depending on the patient's problem.

A. *General constitutional symptoms:* Fever, chills, malaise, fatigability, night sweats; weight (average, preferred, present, change, appetite)
B. *Skin:* Rash or eruption, pruritus, pigmentation or texture change; diaphoresis (excessive sweating); abnormal nail or hair growth or loss; new growths or changes in moles
C. *Skeletal:* Joint stiffness, pain, restriction of motion, edema, erythema, heat, bone deformity
D. *Head*
    1. *General:* Frequent or unusual headaches, vertigo (sensation of the room spinning), dizziness (sensation of themselves spinning,) syncope (fainting), severe head injuries
    2. *Eyes:* Visual acuity, blurring, diplopia (double vision), photophobia (abnormal sensitivity to light), scotomas (spots before the eyes), nystagmus (involuntary rhythmic movements of the eye), pain, recent change in appearance or vision, glaucoma, use of eye drops or other eye medications, history of trauma or familial eye disease
    3. *Ears:* Hearing loss, pain, discharge, tinnitus (ringing in ears), vertigo
    4. *Nose:* Sense of smell, frequency of colds, obstruction, epistaxis (nosebleed), postnasal discharge, sinus pain
    5. *Mouth:* Bleeding or edema of gums; recent tooth abscesses or extractions; soreness of tongue or buccal mucosa, ulcers; disturbance of taste; throat: hoarseness or change in voice; dysphagia (difficulty swallowing); frequent sore throats
E. *Endocrine:* Thyroid enlargement or tenderness, heat or cold intolerance, unexplained weight change, diabetes mellitus (changes in thirst, urination and hunger), nervousness or depression, and fatigue
F. *Reproduction*
    1. *Males:* Onset of puberty, erections, emissions, testicular pain, libido, infertility
    2. *Females*
        a. *Menses:* Onset, regularity, duration of flow, dysmenorrhea (pain associated with menstruation), last period, intermenstrual discharge or bleeding, pruritus, date of last Papanicolaou (Pap) smear, age at menopause, libido, frequency of intercourse, sexual difficulties
        b. *Pregnancies:* Number, miscarriages, abortions, duration of pregnancy in each and any complication during any pregnancy or postpartum period; use of oral or other contraceptives
        c. *Breasts:* Pain, tenderness, discharge, lumps, mammograms; family history of breast cancer
G. *Respiratory:* Pain relating to respiration, dyspnea, cyanosis, crackles, wheezing, cough, sputum (character and quantity), hemoptysis (expectorating blood from respiratory tract), night sweats; date and result of last chest x-ray examination; dependence on supplemental oxygen, smoker (include how much and how long)
H. *Cardiac:* Chest pain or distress, precipitating causes, timing and duration, relieving factors, palpitations, dyspnea, orthopnea (number of pillows needed), edema, claudication (weakness of legs accompanied by cramplike pain), hypertension, previous myocardial infarction, heart failure, estimate of exercise tolerance, past electrocardiogram (ECG) or other cardiac tests; history of coronary artery bypass surgery, percutaneous transluminal coronary angioplasty, or percutaneous balloon valvuloplasty
I. *Hematologic:* Anemia, tendency to bruise or bleed easily, thromboses, thrombophlebitis, any known abnormality of blood cells, transfusions
J. *Lymph nodes:* Enlargement, tenderness, suppuration (to produce purulent material [pus])
K. *Gastrointestinal:* Appetite, digestion, intolerance for any type of foods, dysphagia (difficulty swallowing), heartburn, nausea, vomiting, hematemesis, regularity of bowels, constipation, diarrhea, change in stool color or contents (clay colored, tarry, fresh blood, mucus, undigested food), flatulence, hemorrhoids, hepatitis, jaundice, dark urine; history of ulcer, gallstones, polyps, tumor; previous x-ray examinations (where, when, findings)
L. *Genitourinary:* Dysuria, flank or suprapubic pain, urgency, frequency, nocturia, hematuria, polyuria, hesitancy, dribbling, loss in force of stream, passage of stone, edema of face, stress incontinence, hernias, sexually transmitted infection (inquire what kind and signs and symptoms, and list results of serologic test for syphilis [STS], if known)
M. *Neurologic:* Syncope (brief lapse in consciousness caused by transient cerebral hypoxia); history of stroke, seizures, weakness or paralysis, abnormalities of sensation or coordination, tremors, loss of memory; unusual frequency, distribution, or severity of headaches; serious head injury in past
N. *Psychiatric:* Depression, mood changes, difficulty concentrating, nervousness, tension, suicidal thoughts, irritability, sleep disturbances

sometimes an uncomfortable area for the patient and the nurse. To have a better chance of obtaining an accurate response, ask the patient, "How much alcohol do you drink?" rather than asking whether the patient drinks alcohol.

Assess the patient's ability to perform ADLs. Patterns of sleep, exercise, and nutrition are important to assess when planning nursing interventions. Correlate the patient's lifestyle patterns to how the nursing care plan will dictate these activities within a health care setting. If possible, see that variations in sleep, activity, and nutritional patterns are accommodated.

Family History

The purpose of the family history is to obtain health data about the patient's immediate family members and blood relatives. These data include health issues or cause of death and history of illnesses (e.g., diabetes mellitus, hypertension, heart disease, cancer). The objectives are to determine whether the patient is at risk for illnesses of a genetic or familial nature and to identify areas of health promotion and illness prevention. The family history also provides information about family structure, interaction, and function that are often useful in planning care. For example, a cohesive, supportive family is a possible resource in assisting a patient to adjust to an illness or disability; it is important in this case to incorporate the family into the plan of care. Conversely, if the patient's family is not supportive, it is often more therapeutic to refrain from involving them in care, particularly if the family history reveals that the patient is experiencing stress related to familial relationships.

Environmental History

The environmental history provides data about the patient's home and work environments. The environmental history identifies areas of concern such as exposure to pollutants that can affect health, high crime rates that prevent patients from walking around their neighborhoods, and resources available to assist patients in returning to the community.

Psychosocial and Cultural History

The psychosocial and cultural history includes data about the patient's primary language, cultural group, educational background, attention span, and developmental stage. It also provides information about the patient's and family's coping skills and support systems. It can help in identification of potential or actual problems in dealing with the present illness and in planning of appropriate interventions. Be certain to identify major values, beliefs, and behaviors related to particular health concerns. Individualize assessments and interventions to the patient and family. Avoid making assumptions about cultural beliefs and behaviors without receiving validation from the patient (see the Cultural Considerations box).

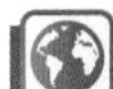

Cultural Considerations

Developing Cultural Sensitivity

Cultures are complex, integrated systems that include knowledge, skills, art, morals, law, customs, and any other acquired habits and capabilities of a group of people. Cultural beliefs and personal characteristics determine health behavior in individuals and families. More than half of all health problems are the result of behavior and lifestyle. If nursing's goal is to promote health while respecting individual value systems and lifestyles, culture-based behavior must be understood (see Chapter 6).

The following are ways to develop cultural and ethnic sensitivity:

- Recognize that cultural and ethnic diversity exists.
- Identify and examine the nurse's own cultural and ethnic beliefs.
- Demonstrate respect for people as unique individuals.
- Respect the unfamiliar.
- Recognize that some cultural and ethnic groups have definitions of health and illness, and practices aimed at promoting health and curing illness, that differ from the nurse's own.
- Interpret patients' signs and symptoms, and respond to them, in accordance with their cultural norms.
- Be willing to modify health care delivery in keeping with the patient's cultural background.
- Do not expect all members of one cultural group to behave in the same manner.
- Appreciate that each person's cultural values are ingrained and therefore very difficult to change.

Review of Systems

The review of systems (ROS) is a systematic method for collecting data on all body systems (see Box 13.7). During the ROS, the nurse asks the patient about normal functioning of each system and any changes the patient has noted. Such changes are usually subjective data because they are described in terms of how the patient perceives them.

As you proceed through the nursing health history, record the data obtained in a clear, concise manner with use of appropriate terminology. A clear, concise record is necessary because other health care professionals are likely to use the nursing health history when delivering health care. Fig. 13.2 illustrates the correct way to record such information.

When determining the status of each body system, ask the patient specific questions relating to the functioning of the system. For example, you may begin assessment of the respiratory system with the question, "Are you having any difficulty with breathing?" Remember to be alert to the patient's comfort and well-being in the moment; if the answer is "yes," the focus of the assessment may shift to the current situation before continuing with questions. Once the patient's respiratory status is stable, continue the questioning with, "Please explain," or more specific questions, such as, "Do you

NURSING ADMISSION ASSESSMENT

Admitted: Ambulatory, Cart, Wheelchair, Arms, Ambulance

From: Office, ER, Surgery, Radiology, Recovery Room Transferred From: physician's office

Oriented to Room: Call Light, Side rails, TV, Phone, Safety/Smoking Policy: Yes ✓ No ____

Vital Signs: T 101^2 P 92 P 24 BP 160/92 HT 5'4" WT 190 Dentures upper/lower

Diet at home: 2 g sodium

Allergies: Drug penicillin Reaction hives

Other: none Organ Donor: Yes ____ No X

Reason for Admission Elevated temperature & fluid retention Signature J.Doe, LPN Date: 1/9/18 Time: 2010

EYES: Impaired vision, Blind, Cataract, Glaucoma, Contacts, Glasses, Prosthesis R. L.
Comments: cataract surgery (rt eye) 2012 OD

EARS, NOSE, THROAT: Hard of hearing, Deaf, Lesions, Hearing Aid, R, L., Tracheotomy
Comments:

RESPIRATORY: Pain, Dyspnea, Wheeze, Asthma, Sinusitis, COPD, Cough, Productive ____ Nonproductive X Oxygen needed, Smoker
Comments: c/o shortness of breath upon exertion crackles right base

CIRCULATION: Apical, Radial, Strong, Weak, Thready, Bounding, Regular, Palpitations, Chest pain, Numbness, Bruising, Edema, Hypertension, Hx MI, CHF, Pacer, Bypass Surgery
Comments: st" 4 pound weight gain in the last 3 days 3+ pitting edema bilaterally

ENDOCRINE: Thyroid, Diabetes
Comments: no problems

GI TRACT: Heartburn, Ulcers, Pain, Hernia, Dysphagia, Nausea, Vomiting, Loss of Appetite, Distention, Diverticulitis
Comments:

ELIMINATION: Last BM 2 days ago, Normal, Constipated, Diarrhea, Tarry, Bright red, Clay colored, Hemorrhoids, Involuntary, Use of laxatives, Yes/No enema, Yes/No Ileostomy, Colostomy
Comments:

URINARY: Incontinence, Nocturia, Hematuria, Dysuria, Burning, Frequency, Urgency, Dribbling, infections, Cath: Yes/No
Comments:

NEUROLOGICAL: Convulsions, Paralysis, Syncope, Paresthesia, Dizziness, Coordination, Weakness, Headaches
Comments:

SKIN: Color pale Turgor poor Temp warm
Describe any Rashes, Lesions, Ecchymosis, Petechiae, Scars, Diabetic sores,
Comments: central abdominal scar

MUSCULOSKELETAL: Pain, Stiffness, Contractures, Deformities, Tremors, Backaches, Weight bearing, Amputation
Comments:

FEMALE REPRODUCTION: LMP EDC
Menopause, Breast pain, Breast tenderness, Vaginal discharge
Comments: post

PREVIOUS SURGERIES: herniorrhaphy ventral 2009
Rt eye Cataract surgery 2008

MEDS TAKEN AT HOME:

Med:	Dose:	Last Taken:
Cozaar	50 mg hour of sleep	Last PM
Coreg	12.5 mg BID	AM
Lasix	40 mgm qAM	AM
K-Lor	10 mEq BID	AM
Restoril	15 mg hour of sleep	Last PM

DISPOSAL OF MEDS:
Did not bring ✓
Pt. has ____ Family took home ____
Retained/taken to Pharmacy ____
Other: ____

Signature: S.Smith RN
Time:

Fig. 13.2 Nursing admission assessment.

have shortness of breath?" An ROS guide can be used to guarantee a complete interview.

The Communication box on admission assessment shows an example of an interview using the OPQRSTUV technique. However, the ROS carried out during the patient interview at the beginning of the physical assessment may give much more information about the patient than the content of the words spoken. The nurse observes patient mobility and gains insight about the patient's intellect, level of orientation, and emotional and psychological state.

Assess the appropriateness of the patient's answers. By asking questions such as "Can you tell me your name?" "Why are you here?" "What is the date?" and "Can you tell me where we are right now?" determine the patient's **level of consciousness (LOC)** and level of orientation. Is the patient oriented to person, place, time, and purpose?

Communication

Admission Assessment

Mr. J. is admitted to the hospital with a diagnosis of possible peptic ulcer.

Nurse: Mr. J., can you tell me about your pain? What brings on your pain?

Patient: I get the pain several times a day after I eat. *(Provocative) (Timing)*[a]

Nurse: What does it feel like?

Patient: It feels like burning. *(Quality)*

Nurse: Where does the pain occur?

Patient: In my stomach. *(Region)*

Nurse: How does the pain rate, on a scale of 0 to 10?

Patient: About an 8. *(Severity)*

Nurse: How long have you had this pain?

Patient: It began about 6 months ago. *(Timing)*

[a]See the description in Box 13.6 of the OPQRSTUV method of interviewing.

NURSING PHYSICAL ASSESSMENT

The physical examination performed sometimes also is referred to as the **nursing physical assessment** or the nursing assessment. Nurses are usually the first to detect changes in the patient's condition. The skills of physical assessment provide the nurse with powerful tools to detect subtle and obvious changes in a patient's health. The data collected comprise the first step of the nursing process. Remember that the purpose of the nursing assessment is to determine the patient's state of health or illness. It is the initial step used to form the nursing care plan, just as the physician performs a physical examination to determine the medical diagnosis and a proposed course of treatment. Many of the questions raised by the nurse in preparation to assist the physician are also a necessary part of the nursing physical assessment. Special considerations for assessing older adults are listed in the Lifespan Considerations box.

Lifespan Considerations

Older Adults

Assessment

- All systems manifest changes to a greater or lesser extent with aging. An awareness of how aging affects an older adult helps sort out expected changes from pathologic processes. Adapt assessments to uncover problems and intervene effectively. All older adults do not show the physical signs of aging at the same rate.
- Adequate time must be allowed for a thorough assessment. Several shorter sessions are likely to be better tolerated than one long session.
- During the assessment, monitor for signs of fatigue, such as slumping, sighing, or irritability.
- For comfort during the assessment, do the following:
  - Ensure privacy. If the older person has cognitive difficulty or wishes a family member's assistance, allow it. Be careful that the family member does not dominate the conversation.
  - Encourage the older person to void before the assessment.
  - Conduct the assessment in a room where bathroom facilities are readily available.
  - Verify that the temperature of the room is warm enough for the older person and free from drafts.
- Explain what is going to occur in terms the older person can understand and avoid the use of medical jargon. Speak slowly and clearly so that the older person is able to hear what is being said and has the opportunity to process the information.
- Be patient and listen. Older people often take longer to reply, but they should be allowed to complete ideas in their own words without interruption.
- Obtain objective and subjective data during the assessment.

When to Perform a Nursing Physical Assessment

The best time to assess the patient is as soon after admission as possible. In some facilities, policy dictates that the assessment be completed within 24 hours of admission. A registered nurse (RN) performs the initial baseline nursing assessment. The ongoing assessment is the responsibility of the registered nurse and the licensed practical/vocational nurse (LPN/LVN).

The formal head-to-toe assessment is completed initially when the patient is admitted. Portions of the assessment can be performed when observation of changes in the patient's condition are noted. This also is referred to as a **focused assessment:** attention is concentrated or focused on a particular part of the body, where signs and symptoms are localized or most active, to determine their significance. A nursing assessment is part of daily nursing care. By performing an assessment at the beginning of each shift, the nurse can identify changes in the patient's condition, anticipate potential problems, communicate those changes to other medical personnel, and alter the nursing plan of care accordingly.

Where to Perform a Nursing Physical Assessment

Regardless of the setting—hospital, clinic, extended care facility, or the patient's home—the location for performing the nursing assessment must be comfortable and safe for the patient. Ensure that an adjustable table or bed is available, and consider the patient's privacy. Be careful that the location is free of distracting sights, sounds, and odors. Keep the ambient temperature comfortable because the patient's body is exposed during the assessment. In most cases, the patient's own room works very well and is convenient for the nurse and the patient.

Methods of Performing a Nursing Physical Assessment

The assessment can be organized in head-to-toe order or system by system. In either case, proceed systematically. By performing the assessment in the same manner each time, the nurse can avoid inadvertently omitting a portion of the assessment. Box 13.8 is an example of a pocket guide to follow during the physical assessment, which can be useful when charting the assessment in the nursing notes.

If the patient expresses special concerns, or observation of changes in a patient's status is noted, it is necessary to analyze the system presented by performing a focused assessment. If a complete physical assessment is necessary, any painful areas are best assessed last. This ensures better cooperation from the patient.

Performing the Nursing Physical Assessment

Items essential to the nurse's assessment are a penlight or flashlight, a stethoscope, a blood pressure cuff, a thermometer, gloves, watch with second hand, scissors, black pen, and a tongue blade (see Fig. 13.1 and Box 13.2). The nurse also uses the senses of touch, smell, sight, and hearing. Thorough washing of the hands should be completed before beginning the physical assessment. Follow the Centers for Disease Control and Prevention (CDC) guidelines on standard precautions and hand hygiene guidelines (Centers for Disease Control, 2017b). Provide the patient the opportunity to empty the bladder before the examination. This makes the patient more comfortable and allows easier assessment of the bladder.

Obtain the patient's vital signs, including temperature, pulse, respirations, and blood pressure. Perform pain assessment to obtain the fifth vital sign (Box 13.9). The vital signs data gathered at the beginning of the

Box 13.8 Physical Assessment Guide

1. *Neurologic:* Level of consciousness: alert, drowsy, lethargic, oriented to: 1 (person); 2 (person, place); 3 (person, place, and time); 4 (person, place, time, and purpose)
2. *Integumentary:* Skin condition, color, temperature, turgor, skin impairments, moist, dry
3. *Cardiovascular:* Apical pulse (strength and regularity), capillary refill (less than 3 seconds) in upper and lower extremities, pedal pulses (1+ to 4+), pitting edema (1+ to 4+; see Box 13.10), nonpitting edema, type of intravenous fluid with rate, site condition (without edema or erythema)
4. *Respiratory:* Posteriorly (lower lobes), anteriorly (upper lobes), right axilla (right middle lobe); auscultate for crackles, wheezes (sibilant and sonorous), pleural friction rub, respiration characteristics (tachypnea, orthopnea, dyspnea [resting or exertional]); assess arterial oxygen saturation (SaO_2) via pulse oximeter; oxygen therapy with route (cannula, mask), and liters per minute of oxygen flow (e.g., O_2 2 L/min per nasal cannula)
5. *Gastrointestinal:* Diet, appetite, fluid intake; observe for distention; auscultate for presence of bowel sounds × 4 quadrants (active, hypoactive, hyperactive, absent by quadrants); palpate masses, tenderness, bowel movement with description, including colostomy or ileostomy stoma assessment, amount and consistency; nasogastric suction (color and amount)
6. *Urinary:* Urine amount, color, odor; presence of catheters (Foley, nephrostomy, suprapubic, ureteral); voiding; include ureterostomy stoma assessment
7. *Mobility:* Activity level: bed rest, chair, up ad lib; gait and level of tolerance; ambulation aids needed, such as walker, cane, or crutches

Box 13.9 Pain Assessment Scale

Use a pain rating scale to assess pain intensity systematically and manage pain. The most commonly used numeric scale is 0 to 10. Ask the patient to rate pain from 0 (no pain) to 10 (worst pain). Ratings of 3 to 5 are considered mild pain, ratings of 5 to 7 are considered moderate pain, and ratings greater than 7 are considered severe pain. Some agencies use a scale of 0 to 5. For children, use happy and sad faces to rate the pain. For clinical assessment, any of these scales is adequate and appropriate. However, always use the same scale with the same patient. See Fig. 21.8 for sample pain intensity scales.

assessment often provide clues to areas that warrant more critical evaluation. The beginning of the examination is also a good time to measure the patient's height and weight. For accuracy, measure height and weight on admission and then compare the results with the patient's stated height and weight. If a significant difference is found between these measurements, possible causes must be explored.

Head-to-toe assessment. When performing a head-to-toe assessment, begin with a neurologic assessment, followed by an assessment of the skin, the hair, the head, and the neck. The assessment of the head includes the eyes, ears, nose, and mouth. Examine the chest, the back, the arms, the abdomen, the perineal area, the legs, and the feet (in that order).

Note that the assessment does not stop after the completion of the head-to-toe assessment. It is a continuous process.

Neurologic. The neurologic assessment can be integrated into the rest of the assessment. For instance, after taking the radial pulse, have the patient grasp your hands to test for equal grip. Always begin the neurologic assessment with the patient's level of consciousness and level of orientation.

Consciousness is awareness of one's thoughts and feelings and of the environment. The levels of consciousness (responsiveness) generally are described according to the behavior exhibited by the individual (Table 13.3).

Careful assessment is critical of the neurologic status of patients who have a head injury or signs or symptoms of a neurologic deficit from a neurologic disease (Jarvis, 2016). Neurologic assessment includes the following:

1. *Level of consciousness.* The earliest and most important factor in neurologic assessment is a change in the level of consciousness. Determine whether the patient is oriented to: 1 (person); 2 (person and place); 3 (person, place, and time); or 4 (person, place, time, and purpose). Patients are alert if they can open their eyes spontaneously; if they are oriented to person, place, time and purpose; and if they are able to comply correctly to verbal clues (Jarvis, 2016).
2. *Motor function.* Ask the patient to move each extremity. Have the patient smile, frown, and lift the eyebrows.
3. *Pupillary response.* Check the pupils for size, equality, and shape. Use a penlight to shine into each pupil. Each pupil should constrict quickly. Pupils should be equal in size (3 to 7 mm in diameter). When the pupils are assessed and the reaction is normal in all examinations, record the letters PERRLA (pupils equal, round, reactive to light, and accommodation).

The third cranial nerve (cranial nerve III, or oculomotor nerve) runs parallel to the brainstem. The function of the oculomotor nerve is essential for eye movements (supplying extrinsic and intrinsic eye muscles). The intrinsic muscle affects the size and the equality of the pupils. A TBI often results in increased intracranial pressure and edema of the brainstem with pressure on cranial nerve III, causing the ominous sign of a unilateral, dilated, and nonreactive pupil (Jarvis, 2016).

Other major areas of neurologic examination include the following:

1. Proprioception (pertaining to the sensations of body movements and awareness of posture) and cerebellar function
2. Deep tendon reflexes
3. Cranial nerve assessment (performed by the RN)

Table 13.3 Level of Consciousness

LEVEL	BEHAVIORS
Consciousness	Level of awareness of oneself and the environment. Appropriate response to external stimuli; oriented to time, place, person, and purpose.
Confusion	Inappropriate response to stimuli and decreased attention span and memory; inappropriate reactions to simple commands.
Lethargy (hypersomnia)	Drowsiness or increased sleep time; is able to be aroused; responds appropriately; possibly falls asleep again immediately.
Delirium	Confusion, disordered perception, and decreased attention span; motor and sensory excitement; inappropriate reactions to stimuli; marked anxiety.
Coma	Loss or lowering of consciousness.
Stage I (stupor)	Arousable with vigorous repeated stimuli. See slowed verbal responses but deep tendon and superficial reflexes are intact.
Stage II (light coma)	Simple motor and verbal (moaning) response to painful stimuli; mass motor movement or flexion (avoidance) response.
Stage III (deep coma)	Decerebrate posturing to painful stimuli (extension of body and limbs and pronation of arms).
Stage IV	Flaccid muscles; papillary reflex absent, apneic; on ventilator; superficial and some deep tendon reflexes present.
Brain death	No responses noted, and reflexes are abnormal or absent.
Syncope	Temporary loss of consciousness (partial or complete) associated with increased rate of respiration, tachycardia, pallor, perspiration, and coolness of skin.
Fugue state	Dysfunction of consciousness (hours or days) in which the individual carries on purposeful activity that he or she does not remember afterward.
Amnesia	Memory loss over time or for specific subjects; individual affected responds appropriately to external stimuli.

From Estes MEZ: *Health assessment and physical examination*, ed 4, Clifton Park, NY, 2010, Delmar.

Table 13.4 Glasgow Coma Scale: Demonstrating Measurement of Level of Consciousness[a]

STIMULUS	RESPONSE	SCORE
Eye opening	Spontaneous—open with blinking at baseline	4
	To verbal stimuli, command, speech	3
	To pain only (not applied to face)	2
	None	1
Verbal response	Oriented	5
	Confused conversation, but able to answer questions	4
	Inappropriate words	3
	Incomprehensible speech	2
	No response	1
Motor response	Obeys commands for movement	6
	Purposeful movement to painful stimulus	5
	Withdraws in response to pain	4
	Flexion in response to pain (decorticate posturing)	3
	Extension response in response to pain (decerebrate posturing)	2
	No response	1

[a]The Glasgow Coma Scale provides a score in the range 3 to 15; patients with scores of 3 to 8 are usually said to be in a coma. The total score is the sum of the scores in three categories.
From the Centers of Disease Control and Prevention (2003). *http://www.bt.cdc.gov/masscasualties/gscale.asp.*

Vital signs. Vital signs are important in assessment of the patient as an indicator of overall status of the patient. The nurse may note an increase in systolic blood pressure with widening pulse pressure, bradycardia, and an irregular breathing pattern (Cushing's triad) late in the course of the development of increased intracranial pressure (Jarvis, 2016).

Glasgow Coma Scale. The Glasgow Coma Scale (GCS) is a standardized, objective measurement of the level of consciousness (Table 13.4). The scale has a numeric value. The scale is divided into three areas: eye opening, verbal response, and motor response. Assess each of the three areas separately, and give a number for the patient's correct response. Total the three numbers. A normal GCS demonstrating no brain trauma is 15. A score of 8 or less indicates severe brain injury (Jarvis, 2016).

Clues to areas of neurologic abnormality are sometimes evident during the patient's history, such as orientation, speech, and ability to interact with the examiner. Continue to evaluate the patient throughout the assessment process for a more accurate neurologic assessment. (Refer to *Adult Health Nursing,* Chapter 14 for a more detailed description of the neurologic system.)

Skin and hair. Observe the skin for color, temperature, moisture, texture, turgor, and evidence of injury or skin lesions. Normal skin tones vary with race, heredity, and sun exposure. Note the overall appearance and the color in the sclera, the mucous membranes, the tongue, the lips, the nail beds, and the palms and soles. A general uniformity of color from dark brown to light tan with pink or yellow overtones (depending on the patient's race) is normal. Changes in skin color that sometimes provide evidence of systemic disease include pallor, cyanosis, jaundice, erythema, and ecchymosis. The appearance of cyanotic (dusky blue) fingers, lips, or mucous membranes is abnormal in light-skinned and dark-skinned individuals. Jaundice in dark-skinned individuals sometimes appears as yellow staining in the sclera, the hard palate, and the palmar or plantar surfaces.

Normally, the skin is warm, dry, and smooth, with good turgor. **Turgor** refers to the elasticity of the skin caused by the outward pressure of the cells and interstitial fluid (Fig. 13.3). Dehydration results in *decreased* skin turgor and is manifested by lax skin that, when grasped and raised between two fingers, slowly returns to its previous position (skin "tenting"). Marked edema results in *increased* turgor, manifested by smooth, taut, shiny skin that cannot be grasped and raised.

Note any skin lesions or evidence of other skin impairments. Document their size, shape, color, pattern, and location and any presence of exudate.

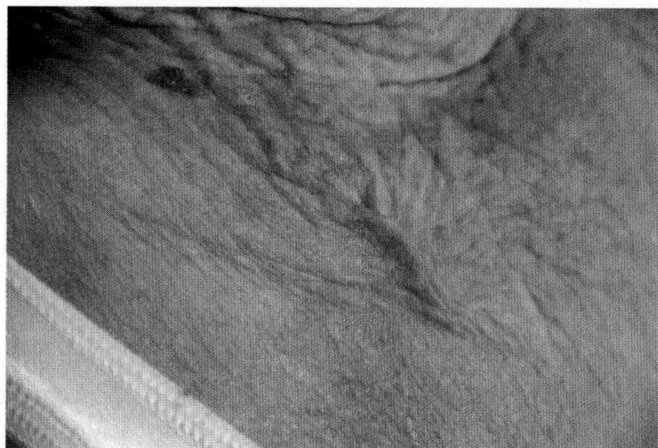

Fig. 13.3 Assess skin turgor by first grasping fold of skin on back of the patient's hand, sternum, forearm, or abdomen. Note ease and speed with which skin returns to place.

Examine the hair over the entire body to determine the distribution, the quantity, and the quality. Hairless lower extremities sometimes signify an arterial disorder with reduced arterial blood flow. The hair is normally of a smooth texture and not oily or dry. A healthy scalp is free of dandruff, lesions, and parasites. Wear gloves if you wish to inspect the hair and scalp. Abnormalities are sometimes related to external factors, such as the use of beauty products, and sometimes to internal factors, such as systemic or localized illnesses.

Head and neck. Assessment of the head includes the eyes, the ears, the nose, and the mouth. The neck assessment involves the arteries, the veins, and the lymph nodes. Facial expression and appearance are likely to be the first observations the nurse makes and often give clues to the emotional state of the patient. Note the symmetry of the face; normal facial movements are also symmetric and appropriate. The head is normally upright and still.

A gross assessment of range of motion (ROM) can be made by having the patient move the head from side to side and in a nodding motion. The patient should be able to move the head comfortably through these motions. With the pads of the fingers, palpate beneath the jaw and down each side of the neck to feel for enlarged lymph nodes. Although having an enlarged node may not be abnormal, tenderness is not normal. Palpate the carotid arteries gently and one at a time (Fig. 13.4). The normal carotid pulse is regular and palpable without a **thrill** (a vibrating sensation the nurse perceives during palpation along the artery).

Inspect for jugular venous distention. The jugular veins give information about activity on the right side of the heart. Specifically, they reflect filling pressure and volume changes. Distention results when ineffective pumping action of the right ventricle causes increased volume and pressure within the veins (Jarvis, 2016). Normally the veins are not observable with the patient in a sitting position. Jugular venous distention is seen in venous hypertension or right-sided heart failure. Auscultation of the carotid artery can be performed by listening with the bell of the stethoscope. Normally, no bruits are audible. **Bruits** are abnormal "swishing"

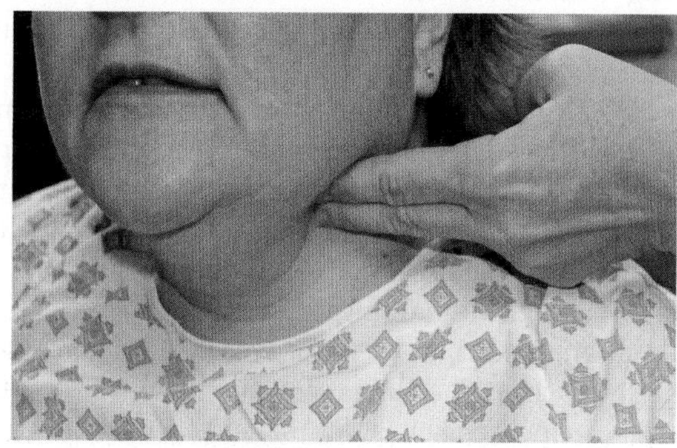

Fig. 13.4 Palpation of carotid artery.

sounds heard over organs, glands, and arteries. A bruit results from an abnormality in an artery that results from a narrow or partially occluded artery, such as occurs in atherosclerosis (Jarvis, 2016).

Mouth and throat. Inspect the lips and the mucous membranes of the mouth with a tongue blade and penlight, assessing all surfaces of the oral cavity. Normal mucous membranes are moist, pink, and free of lesions. With dehydration, mucous membranes look dry. The lips should be smooth, moist, and free of cracking. The condition of the teeth and gums gives the nurse insight into the health habits of the patient. Breath odors often indicate disease; foul, fruity, or musty breath is not normal.

Eyes. Note whether the eyes are symmetric. No exudate from the eyes is normally seen, and the lids should be open. The normal sclera of the eye is white, and the conjunctiva pink. The conjunctiva is observed by gently depressing the lower lid. Periorbital edema (edema around the eye) is abnormal.

Assess both eyes individually. Also observe the eyes for pupillary reflex. Do this by darkening the room and using the penlight to shine light into the pupil. Have the light come from the side of the eye; shine the light across the eye, with the patient looking straight ahead at a focal point. The normal eye shows the pupil constricting when the light is applied. The pupil toward which the light is directed normally constricts; this reaction is the direct papillary response to light. If normal, the other pupil also constricts; this reaction is the consensual response to light. When assessing accommodation, ask the patient to follow his or her finger when it is brought in toward the patient's eyes, directly between the eyes. A normal accommodation response is that both pupils constrict equally. The rate and degree of constriction should be equal. A tip to recall these findings is to use the acronym PERRLA, which stands for *pupils equal, round, reactive to light, and accommodation.*

Ears. First note whether the ears are symmetric. Pull back and up gently on the external ear to straighten and examine the ear canal with help from the penlight. With a child younger than 3 years of age, pull the pinna back and down. Normally no pain is associated with this movement. The ear canal is normally free of excess cerumen (earwax), blood, and any other discharge. During this assessment, note whether the patient is following commands appropriately, indicating an ability to hear.

Nose. The nose is usually symmetric, although variation in size is considered normal. To test for patency, press against one nostril and ask the patient to breathe. Air should flow through the nose. Assess both nostrils, observing for bleeding or drainage. Also note the appearance of a deviated septum.

Chest, lungs, heart, and vascular system. Perform assessment of the chest and lungs with the patient in a sitting position. Inspect the chest for bilateral chest expansion, which is normally symmetric. Note the rate and depth of respirations. The normal rate for an adult is 12 to 20 breaths per minute. Normal breathing is quiet.

Tachypnea is a rapid rate of breathing at a rate greater than 24 breaths per minute. Tachypnea occurs in fever, fear, exercise, pneumonia, alkalosis, and respiratory insufficiency. Bradypnea refers to slow breathing of fewer than 10 breaths per minute. Bradypnea occurs in increased intracranial pressure, or depression of the respiratory center in the medulla oblongata from the action of opioids. Cheyne-Stokes respiration is an abnormal cycle of respirations that begins with slow, shallow respirations that become rapid. Respirations become slower and are followed by periods of apnea (20 seconds) before the cycle repeats. The most common causes of Cheyne-Stokes respiration are heart failure, opioid overdose, renal failure, meningitis, and severe head injury (Jarvis, 2016).

Note any sounds that are audible without the stethoscope; later, auscultate them and determine their origin. Posture is often indicative of acute or chronic respiratory disease. The patient who is unable to lie supine or who must lean forward to breathe is showing signs of this distress. A large, rounded "barrel chest" is diagnostic for adults with pulmonary disease such as emphysema. Assess arterial oxygen saturation (SaO_2, the amount of oxygen bound to hemoglobin) via pulse oximetry, a noninvasive method of monitoring in which a sensor is attached to the person's finger or earlobe. An SaO_2 of 90% to 100% is needed to replenish O_2 in plasma.

Breasts. The breasts can be examined during a lung assessment. Many patients also do an examination on a monthly basis. Teach breast self-examination to male and female patients. Recommendations regarding breast self-examination are available at the National Breast Cancer Foundation *(www.nationalbreastcancer.org/breast-self-exam).* Note any changes in how the breast feels, the appearance of the nipples, or discharge from the nipples.

Lung sounds. Auscultation provides information about the functioning of the respiratory system and about the presence of any obstruction in the air passages. Most commonly, the nurse uses the diaphragm of the stethoscope, which is designed to transmit the usually higher pitch of abnormal breath sounds.

Auscultation of lungs is preferable with the patient in a sitting position. Place the patient in a sitting position, leaning forward with arms across the lap. Instruct the patient to breathe through the mouth quietly and more deeply and slowly than in a usual respiration. Place the stethoscope firmly but not tightly on the skin, and listen for one full inspiratory–expiratory cycle at each point. Never listen with a stethoscope over clothing. Systematically auscultate the apices and the posterior, lateral, and anterior chest. Use a zigzag approach, comparing the findings at each point with the corresponding point on the opposite side (Figs. 13.5 and 13.6).

Adventitious breath sounds are classified as either crackles or wheezes (Fig. 13.7). **Crackles,** produced by

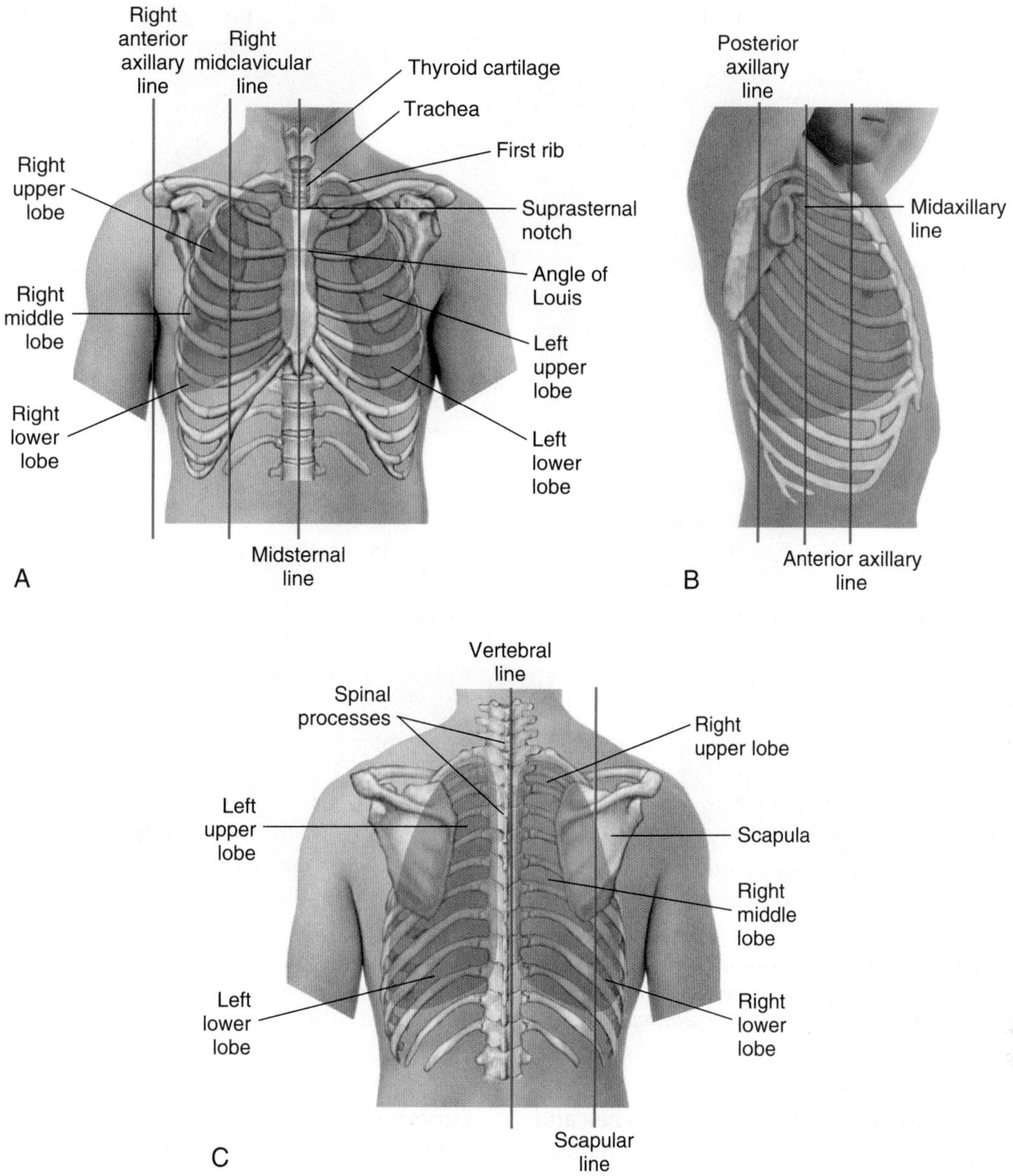

Fig. 13.5 Thoracic landmarks. A, Anterior thorax. B, Right lateral thorax. C, Posterior thorax. (From Ball JW, Dains JE, Flynn JA, et al: *Seidel's guide to physical examination,* ed 9, St. Louis, 2019, Elsevier.)

fluid in the bronchioles and the alveoli, are short, discrete, interrupted, crackling, or bubbling sounds that are heard most commonly during inspiration. The sound of crackles is similar to that produced by hairs being rolled between the fingers while close to the ear. Crackles are described further as fine, medium, or coarse. **Wheezes** are sounds produced by the movement of air through narrowed passages in the tracheobronchial tree. They predominate in expiration because bronchi are shortened and narrowed during this respiratory phase. However, they sometimes occur in the inspiratory and the expiratory phases of respiration, suggesting that lumina have been narrowed during both respiratory phases. Wheezes are classified as sibilant or sonorous (see the Coordinated Care box).

Sibilant wheezes have a high-pitched squeaking and musical quality and are produced by airflow through narrowed airways. *Sonorous* wheezes have a lower-pitched, coarser, gurgling, snoring quality and usually indicate the presence of mucus in the trachea and the large airways. *Stridor* is a high-pitched, inspiratory, crowing sound, louder in the neck than over the chest

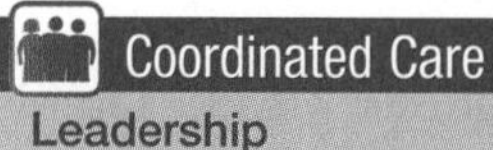

Leadership

Assessing Lung Sounds

Assessment of the lung and thorax requires application of skills and knowledge unique to a nurse. For these skills, delegation is inappropriate. If a patient has abnormal lung sounds, instruct certified assistive personnel (CAP) to observe a patient's respirations and report any changes in rate and depth to the nurse immediately and to keep the head of the bed elevated to assist the patient to breathe easier.

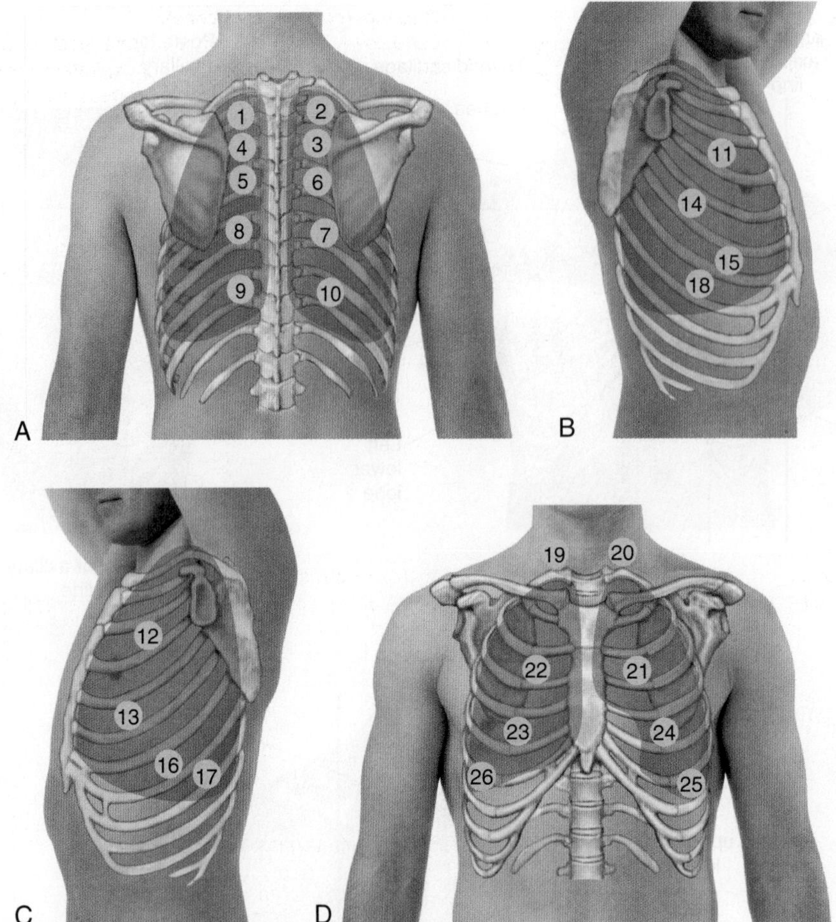

Fig. 13.6 Suggested sequence for systematic percussion and auscultation of the thorax. A, Posterior thorax. B, Right lateral thorax. C, Left lateral thorax. D, Anterior thorax. The pleximeter finger or the stethoscope is moved in the numeric sequence suggested; however, other sequences are possible. It is beneficial to be systematic. (From Ball JW, Dains JE, Flynn JA, et al: *Seidel's guide to physical examination*, ed 9, St. Louis, 2019, Elsevier.)

wall. Stridor originates in the larynx or the trachea and indicates upper airway obstruction from edematous, inflamed tissues or a foreign body. *Pleural friction rubs* are produced by inflammation of the pleural sac; the nurse hears a rubbing, grating, or squeaky sound on auscultation. The grating sounds as if two pieces of leather are being rubbed together.

Whenever you hear adventitious breath sounds during auscultation, instruct the patient to cough, and then listen again. Sonorous wheezes are the most likely to clear, at least somewhat, with cough. However, crackles, especially when patients are on bed rest, sometimes also clear somewhat with cough. Document this finding with the breath sounds.

Spine. With the patient in a sitting position, note the curvature of the spine. Also assess the patient's posture when standing. Run the fingers down the patient's spine, which should be straight, assessing for the normal lumbosacral curve. Common postural abnormalities include lordosis, kyphosis, and scoliosis. Kyphosis, or humpback, is an exaggeration of the posterior curvature of the thoracic spine. Lordosis, or swayback, is an increased lumbar curvature. Scoliosis is a lateral spinal curvature. Check that the skin of the back has normal color, temperature, and moisture.

Heart sounds. Heart sounds are auscultated with the stethoscope using both the bell and the diaphragm. The normal "lub-dub" sound of the heart is caused by the closure of the atrioventricular and the semilunar valves, respectively. The first normal heart sound, S_1, occurs with closure of the atrioventricular valves (AV) and thus signals the beginning of systole. S_1 usually is auscultated most clearly at the apex. The second normal heart sound, S_2, occurs with closure of the semilunar valves and signals the end of systole. S_2 is auscultated most clearly at the base (Jarvis, 2016). Extra heart sounds are S_3 and S_4. S_3, which sounds after S_2, is heard best at the apex. S_3 is sometimes normal in children but is usually abnormal in adults. S_3 has a dull, soft sound and is sometimes an early sign of heart failure. S_4 is heard late in diastole when the atria contract. It is auscultated most clearly at the apex and is heard immediately before S_1. The sound is soft with a low pitch. S_4 is sometimes normal and sometimes pathologic; it is heard in patients with coronary artery disease after myocardial infarction (MI) or cardiomyopathy (Jarvis,

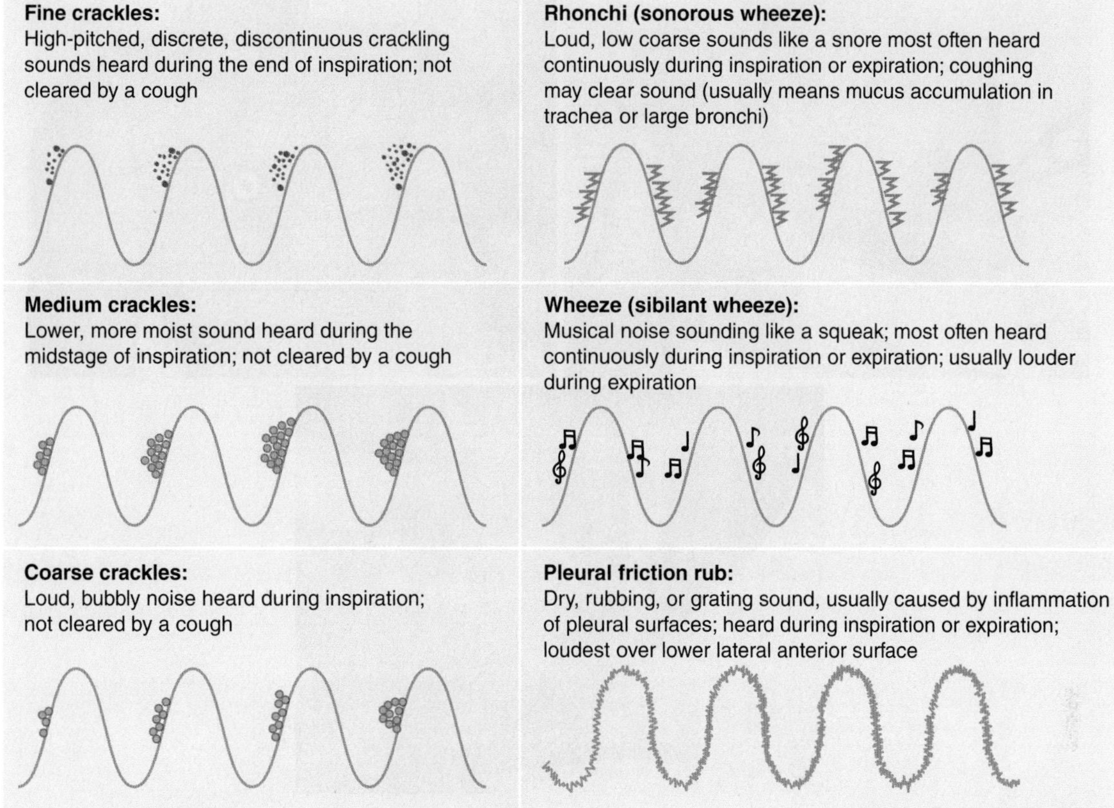
Fine crackles:
High-pitched, discrete, discontinuous crackling sounds heard during the end of inspiration; not cleared by a cough
Rhonchi (sonorous wheeze):
Loud, low coarse sounds like a snore most often heard continuously during inspiration or expiration; coughing may clear sound (usually means mucus accumulation in trachea or large bronchi)
Medium crackles:
Lower, more moist sound heard during the midstage of inspiration; not cleared by a cough
Wheeze (sibilant wheeze):
Musical noise sounding like a squeak; most often heard continuously during inspiration or expiration; usually louder during expiration
Coarse crackles:
Loud, bubbly noise heard during inspiration; not cleared by a cough
Pleural friction rub:
Dry, rubbing, or grating sound, usually caused by inflammation of pleural surfaces; heard during inspiration or expiration; loudest over lower lateral anterior surface

Fig. 13.7 Adventitious breath sounds.

2016). With the patient in various positions (Fig. 13.8), listen to the heart sounds for several cardiac cycles in each of the four points on the patient's chest (see Fig. 13.6). Listen for the intensity of the sound, ranging from faint to strong. Also determine the regularity of the rhythm: regular, regularly irregular, or irregularly irregular. For patients with faint heart sounds, very irregular rhythms, very rapid heart rates, or noisy respirations, palpation of the carotid or the radial pulses simultaneously with the auscultation of the heart sounds is helpful.

Peripheral vascular system. Arteries provide oxygen and nutrients to the tissues. The nurse assesses the peripheral arteries by palpating peripheral arterial pulses. An arterial pulse is a pressure wave transmitted through the arterial system with each contraction of the heart. Peripheral pulses that the nurse is able to assess are radial, brachial, ulnar, femoral, popliteal, dorsalis pedis, and posterior tibial (see Skill 11.2).

Using the pads of the fingertips, apply enough pressure at the pulse to gather information on the pulse rate, rhythm, and strength. Do not press so hard that the artery is occluded. If difficulty in locating the pulse is encountered, carefully move the fingers to slightly different positions in the area and vary the pressure exerted. Assess the pulse rate by counting the pulsation for 60 seconds. Check the rhythm for regularity. Measure the strength of the pulse by using the following scale: 0, absent; 1+, thready; 2+, weak; 3+, normal; and 4+, bounding. Follow agency policy when describing the pulse.

Begin with the most distal pulses to assess the arterial circulation at the farthest palpable point. Palpate the brachial pulse over the antecubital fossa (anterior surface of the elbow joint). Palpate the radial pulse by placing the pads of the first and second fingers on the palmar surface of the patient's relaxed and slightly flexed wrist medial to the radius bone. Palpate the femoral pulse midway between the anterosuperior iliac crest and the symphysis pubis, below and medial to the inguinal ligament. Palpate the popliteal pulse by pressing deeply into the dorsal aspect of the knee while the knee is slightly bent. Palpate the dorsalis pedis pulse by applying light touch between the first and second toes and slowly moving up the dorsum of the foot. The dorsalis pedis artery runs along the top of the foot in line with the groove between the extensor tendons of the great toe and the first toe. Palpate the posterior tibial pulse slightly below and posterior to the medial malleolus of the ankle. (*Ischemia* results if there is a decreased supply of oxygenated blood to the tissues; often this is caused by a narrowing of an artery.) An embolism sometimes results in complete occlusion of an artery and death of tissue distal to the occlusion. Atherosclerosis has the potential to cause a partial occlusion of an artery and thus an insufficient delivery of oxygenated blood

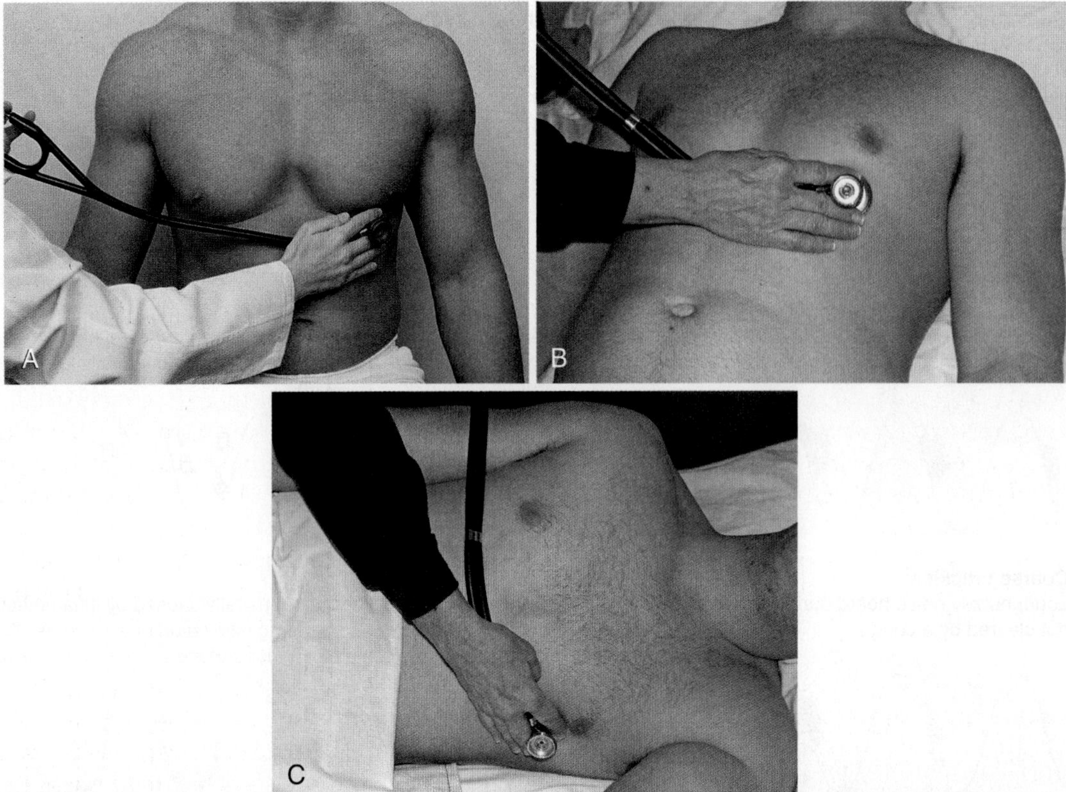

Fig. 13.8 Sequence of patient positions for auscultation of heart sounds. A, Sitting up, leaning slightly forward. B, Supine. C, Left lateral recumbent. (A from Seidel HM, Ball JW, Dains JE, et al: *Mosby's guide to physical examination*, ed 6, St. Louis, 2006, Mosby.)

to the tissues. This sometimes results in a condition called claudication, which results in cramplike pains in the lower extremities, usually occurring after walking. The pain is caused by insufficient oxygen to the leg muscles (Jarvis, 2016).

Inspect the extremities for symmetry, color, and varicosities. They are normally symmetric and without edema or discoloration. Palpate the hands and feet for temperature; normally, they are warm. Peripheral veins are normally fairly flat and barely visible.

Perform the capillary refill, or blanch, test by pressing firmly for 5 seconds on the fingernail or toenail and estimating the speed at which the blood returns (the tips of the fingers and toes can be used if the person has thick, unblanchable nail beds). In a person with good cardiac function and distal perfusion, capillary refill usually takes less than 3 seconds. A capillary refill of more than 3 seconds is considered a sign of sluggish digital circulation, and a time of 5 seconds is considered abnormal. Poor cardiac function, dehydration, and peripheral vascular diseases are examples of disease processes that often cause delays in capillary refill.

Gastrointestinal system. During the remaining portion of the examination, the patient may remain in the supine position with knees elevated. During this portion of the assessment, be sure the patient is properly draped to decrease exposure of the pubic area and the breasts. Interview the patient regarding expelling of flatus, the latest bowel movement, and any reports of nausea, vomiting, or altered or decreased appetite **(anorexia).** After the interview, examine the abdomen. First inspect the abdomen for shape, contour, lesions, scars, lumps, or rashes. Normally, the abdomen's contour is even, and skin color is the same as that of the thorax. Then auscultate for bowel sounds (NOTE: *before* palpating; palpating first can alter the bowel sounds) by placing the diaphragm of the stethoscope over the divisions of the abdomen (Fig. 13.9) and listening for the sounds of peristalsis (wavelike movements of the intestine). It is helpful, before beginning, to make sure the room is quiet. If the patient is on a nasogastric suction machine, or if a radio or television is on, turn them off. Light pressure on the stethoscope is sufficient to detect bowel sounds. Because peristalsis is continuous, sounds normally are heard in all quadrants. Bowel sounds occur every 15 to 60 seconds and are classified as active, hyperactive, hypoactive, or absent. The normal rate of bowel sounds is 4 to 32 per minute.

Listen to bowel sounds for 1 minute in all quadrants to ensure you do not miss any sounds and to localize specific sounds. It is especially important to be thorough and take time when evaluating for a silent abdomen (i.e., the absence of bowel sounds), which indicates the arrest of intestinal motility. Because peristaltic sounds are sometimes highly irregular, listen for at least 4 minutes before concluding that no bowel sounds are present.

The two significant alterations in bowel sounds are: (1) the absence of any sound or extremely soft and widely separated sounds and (2) increased sounds with a characteristically high-pitched, loud, rushing sound **(borborygmi)**:

- *Decreased bowel sounds.* Diminished or absent bowel sounds accompany inhibition of bowel motility. Decreased motility occurs with inflammation, gangrene, or paralytic ileus. Decreased peristalsis frequently accompanies peritonitis, electrolyte disturbances, the aftermath of surgical manipulation of the bowel, and late bowel obstruction. In addition, diminished bowel sounds often are correlated with lower lobe pneumonia.

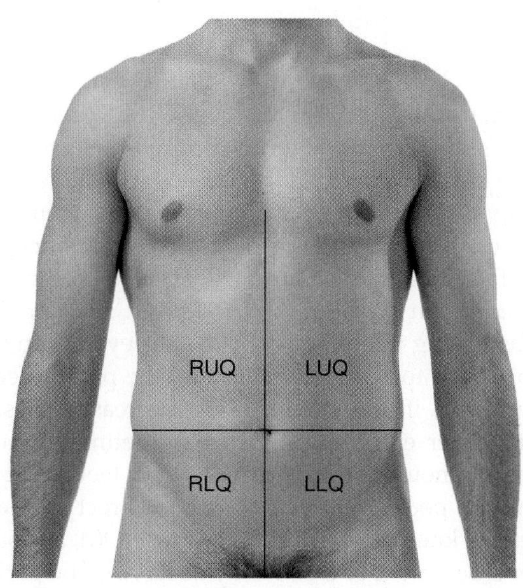

Fig. 13.9 Anatomic divisions of the abdomen (quadrants). (From Wilson SF, Giddens J: *Health assessment for nursing practice*, ed 5, St. Louis, 2013, Elsevier.)

- *Increased bowel sounds.* Loud, gurgling borborygmi often accompanies increased motility of the bowel, such as with diarrhea. Sounds of loud volume also are heard over areas of stenotic bowel. Sounds from an early bowel obstruction are high pitched. Frequently these are splashing sounds, similar to the emptying of a bottle into a hollow vessel. Fine, metallic, tinkling sounds are emitted as tiny gas bubbles break through the surface of intestinal juices. Common pathologic conditions associated with increased bowel sounds are gastroenteritis and subsiding ileus. Increased motility is sometimes caused by the use of a laxative and sometimes by gastroenteritis.

Assessment of the abdomen for distention, firmness, and tenderness is also very important. After auscultating for bowel sounds, palpate the underlying structures. Palpation comes after auscultation because the manipulation has potential to stimulate intestinal activity and thus alter bowel sounds. Use light and deep palpations, beginning with light palpation; note texture, temperature, and moisture of the skin in all regions (Fig. 13.10A). Normal skin of the abdomen is smooth, dry, and warm. Light palpation enables the nurse to detect superficial lesions just below the skin. Advanced practice nurses use deep palpation to detect tenderness or masses of the abdomen. In the upper right quadrant just below the rib cage, palpation of the liver is sometimes possible (Fig. 13.10B). If the liver is felt, it may be enlarged. The normal liver is smooth and nontender. The abdomen normally is free of masses, and palpation is not uncomfortable for the patient.

To ensure that the patient is relaxed during the palpation, be sure your hands are warm, and use conversation to distract the patient. Note the patient's face when palpating and check for grimacing. Sometimes patients also guard a tender area, which means they tighten up abdominal muscles when the area is touched. If a pulsating mass is detected in the abdomen, stop palpation immediately and notify the charge nurse or health care provider. This may indicate the presence of an aneurysm.

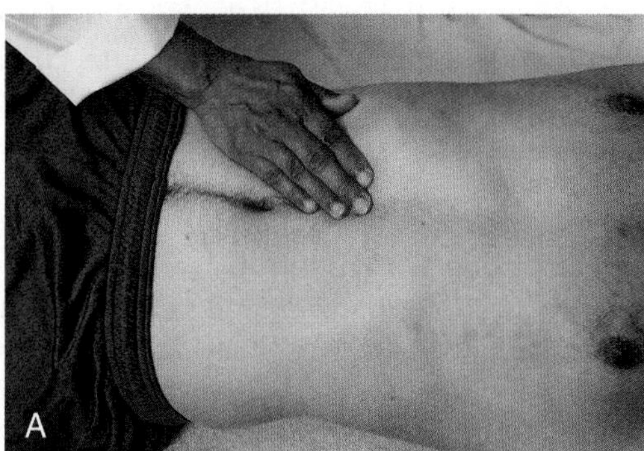

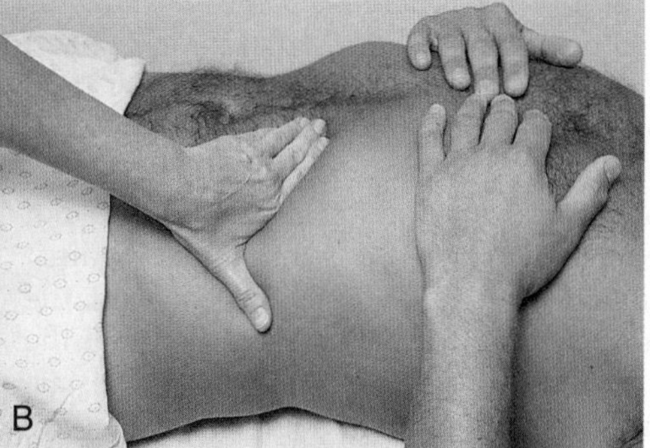

Fig. 13.10 A, Light palpation of the abdomen to assess for distention, masses, or tenderness. B, Palpation of the liver using moderate palpation. (From Seidel HM, Ball JW, Dains JE, et al: *Mosby's guide to physical examination*, ed 6, St. Louis, 2006, Mosby.)

Percussion on the abdomen is used to note the density of underlying tissue and to locate the margins of internal organs. The normal abdomen has a tympanic (drumlike) sound, with dullness noted over the liver. A hollow sound heard over the stomach or intestines indicates flatus. Percussion generally is performed by the physician or an advanced practice nurse.

Genitourinary system. Nurses do not perform the vaginal examination with a speculum unless they have had advanced training. Assessment of the urinary system is performed using observation and palpation. It is most convenient for the nurse to perform this inspection during the perineal care of the patient. Wear gloves when inspecting the labia for lesions. Inspect the pubic hair for lice, and note any vaginal discharge. Normal labia are pink, moist, and free of lesions. A normal white vaginal discharge known as leukorrhea is sometimes present.

Inspect the male genitalia for lesions and lice; look for discharge from the penis. Palpate the scrotum for lumps or hernias. If the male is uncircumcised, gently retract the foreskin to inspect for lesions on the glans penis.

While inspecting the genitalia on male and female patients, palpate the femoral artery in that area (see Skill 12.2). Use palpation of the suprapubic area to determine distention.

Rectum. The rectal area is best examined with the patient in a Sims position. Spread the buttocks to look for hemorrhoids or lesions. Normal skin around the anus is darker than the surrounding skin. To further assess the intestinal system, the health care provider may order a hemoccult test of occult blood (see Chapter 15). The results of the test usually indicate whether gastrointestinal bleeding is present.

Legs and feet. The legs and feet are the final area of assessment. Palpate femoral, popliteal, dorsalis pedis, and posterior tibial as described earlier (see Skill 12.2). Assess the extremities for temperature. Cold extremities signal possible peripheral vascular disease with inadequate arterial perfusion. Observe the legs and feet, and palpate them for edema. *Edema* is an excessive accumulation of fluid in the interstitial spaces caused by leakage of fluid from veins and capillary beds. This occurs as a result of many disease processes, such as heart failure, pathologic conditions of the kidneys, burns, lymphatic stasis, and trauma. Observe for edema in dependent parts of the body such as the feet, the legs, the scrotum, and the sacral area.

Pitting sometimes does and sometimes does not occur with edema. To check for pitting, press against a bony prominence for 5 seconds, and then lift the finger. Observe the skin for rebounding, and feel the area for the presence of an indentation. If the tissue rebounds immediately, the patient does not have pitting edema. An indentation indicates pitting edema, which usually graded is on a scale of 1 to 4 as shown in Box 13.10.

Box 13.10 Pitting Edema Scale

1+ *Trace:* A barely perceptible pit (2 mm)
2+ *Mild:* A deeper pit (4 mm), with fairly normal contours, that rebounds in 10 to 15 seconds
3+ *Moderate:* A deep pit (6 mm); lasts for 30 seconds to more than 1 minute
4+ *Severe:* An even deeper pit (8 mm), with severe edema that possibly lasts as long as 2 to 5 minutes before rebounding

If edema is not pitting, it cannot be given a grade on this scale. Edema without pitting often arises from arterial disease and arterial occlusion. Unilateral edema is likely the result of occlusion of a major vein.

Check the color, motion, sensation, and temperature (CMST) of both feet. Normal skin color on the legs is similar to that of the rest of the body. Test for sensation by asking the patient to close the eyes; then touch the patient's toes and ask whether the patient feels it. Ask patients if they have pain or decreased sensation in the lower extremities, which sometimes indicates peripheral neuropathy. Normally, both feet are equally warm and pedal pulses are present. Direct the patient to flex the knees and ankles to test for ROM, although a better assessment of ROM is by observing the patient's gait. Varicosities (enlarged veins) are not normally present.

Documenting the Interview and the Assessment

Most institutions have a standardized form to follow when completing the patient history and the physical assessment. It serves as the baseline for evaluation of subsequent changes in the patient's condition and for decisions related to therapy (see Fig. 13.2). Therefore the information must be objective, clear, complete, and concise.

Telephone Consultation

With the rapid changes taking place in health care, nurses work in a variety of new settings. One example is telephone consultation, especially in the health care provider's office or clinic. When patients call with a health problem, the nurse is usually the person to whom they talk. If the nurse takes a call like this, sometimes the nurse dispenses advice or instructions immediately, and sometimes the nurse directs the patient to come in for a visit, see another health care provider, or seek care in the emergency department. Any interventions the nurse makes are based on the nurse's assessment of the patient, despite the fact that all the assessment data the nurse uses come directly from the patient. Will the nurse always know the appropriate questions to ask? Several publications are currently available to use as a guideline to assist the nurse. Box 13.11 is an example of a tool to use when communicating between patient and health care provider and health care facility to health care facility. Health Insurance Portability and Accountability Act (HIPAA) guidelines must be followed to protect the privacy of patient information.

Box 13.11 Telephone Communication: SBAR

SBAR stands for **S**ituation, **B**ackground, **A**ssessment, and **R**ecommendation. SBAR was developed first by the US Military and the Federal Aviation Administration and later incorporated for use in health care; it provides a structured communication tool and has seen improved patient safety during routine care and transfer and in complex cases. A copy of this tool may be found at the website for the Institute for Healthcare Improvement *(www.ihi.org/resources/Pages/Tools/SBARToolkit.aspx)*.

This tool meets The Joint Commission safety goals and allows for the "standardized approach to hand off communications, including an opportunity to ask and respond to questions" (see Box 3.1 for an example of SBAR communication).

From The Joint Commission: Patient safety. Retrieved from *www.jointcommission.org/Patient-Safety*.

Get Ready for the NCLEX® Examination!

Key Points

- The health care provider perceives signs by using the senses of sight, touch, smell, and hearing.
- The patient feels symptoms, which are sensations such as pruritus (itching), pain, and dizziness.
- Diseases originate from several different causes and are hereditary, congenital, traumatic, neoplastic, infectious, inflammatory, degenerative, deficiency, or environmental.
- Risk factors for acquiring a disease include age, genetics, environment, and lifestyle variables.
- The universal signs of infection are erythema, edema, pain, heat, loss of function, and purulent, malodorous drainage.
- Some frequently noted signs and symptoms of disease are cyanosis, pallor, erythema, edema, pain, nausea, vomiting, diarrhea, dyspnea, tachycardia, and fever.
- When a physician conducts a physical examination, the nurse often is requested to assist the examiner. The nurse has certain responsibilities, such as preparing the examining room, assisting with equipment, and preparing the patient.
- Results of laboratory evaluation of specimens such as urine and stool often add to the information about the patient.
- Optimally a complete nursing physical assessment is performed as soon after admission as possible.
- Interviewing the patient initially helps to identify signs, symptoms, and areas of patient concern that the examination seeks to clarify.
- Properly performed, the physical assessment proceeds in an orderly fashion: head to toe or system by system.
- Perform assessment using specific skills of observation, palpation, percussion, and auscultation.
- The nurse's role requires the nurse to be familiar with normal assessments and thus able to identify abnormalities.
- Perform a physical assessment of each patient at the beginning of each nursing shift to determine actual or potential patient problems that will require medical or nursing interventions to promote the safety and well-being of the patient.

Additional Learning Resources

SG Go to the Study Guide for additional learning activities to help you master this chapter content.

evolve Be sure to visit the Evolve site at *http://evolve.elsevier.com/Cooper/foundationsadult/* for additional online resources.

Review Questions for the NCLEX® Examination

1. When preparing to perform an assessment, which elements need to be included to ensure the integrity of the nurse-patient relationship?
   1. Introduction of the nurse to the patient, which includes title (LPN/LVN) and purpose of visit
   2. Explanation of what the nurse will need to accomplish (i.e., vital signs, body system review) during the time with the patient
   3. An estimated time frame to complete the assessment
   4. Standing at the foot of the bed to get the best look at the patient and his and her responses
   5. Preparation of the room for the least amount of distractions so that the patient can remain focused to questions offered by the nurse

2. A patient has been admitted with acute bronchitis. When performing a lung assessment, the nurse is best able to auscultate the lower lobes by listening to what location on the body?
   1. Posterior
   2. Anterior
   3. Lateral
   4. Superior
3. A 90-year-old patient is having difficulty answering the nurse's questions while completing the patient history. What should the nurse keep in mind about caring for older adults?
   1. All older adults age at the same rate.
   2. The nurse should write down all of the questions and have the patient's family complete the information.
   3. The nurse should sit down at eye level with the patient and allow a longer period to answer each question.
   4. The nurse should talk more loudly and raise the pitch of the voice.
4. The nurse documents which finding while assessing a patient with heart failure where it is noted that the lower extremities have deep indentations that remain for 30 seconds when pressed?
   1. Nonpitting edema
   2. 2+ pitting edema
   3. 3+ pitting edema
   4. 4+ pitting edema
5. The patient reports severe abdominal pain. What type of assessment should the nurse perform?
   1. Head-to-toe assessment
   2. Focused assessment
   3. System-by-system assessment
   4. Complete assessment
6. An elderly male patient is admitted for chest pain. How does the nurse best document the information the patient gives about his symptoms?
   1. Use the patient's own words in quotation marks.
   2. Briefly summarize what the patient says.
   3. Interpret the patient's comments using medical terminology.
   4. Use the information for the chief complaint from the admission sheet.
7. The nurse asks the patient about which signs and symptoms experienced when reviewing the elderly patient's gastrointestinal system? *(Select all that apply.)*
   1. Changes in bowel habits
   2. Pyrosis (heartburn)
   3. Firmness of the abdomen
   4. Dyspnea
   5. Anorexia
8. What is the first area to be assessed after taking vital signs when performing a nursing assessment?
   1. Assess for level of consciousness and orientation.
   2. Assess the skin.
   3. Listen to lung sounds.
   4. Check for pitting edema.
9. A patient has been admitted for dehydration after a prolonged period of diarrhea. Which finding does the nurse expect to observe in this patient?
   1. Skin warm, moist, pink with good skin turgor
   2. Skin warm, dry, pale with decreased skin turgor
   3. Skin cool, dry, pink with increased skin turgor
   4. Skin cool, moist, pale with decreased skin turgor
10. The nurse assesses a vibration felt along the patient's carotid artery with palpation. How should the nurse describe this assessment finding?
    1. Palpation
    2. Thrill
    3. Bruit
    4. Aneurysm
11. The nurse is preparing a female patient for a gynecologic examination. Which patient position best assists the health care provider in this examination?
    1. High Fowler's
    2. Dorsal recumbent
    3. Lithotomy
    4. Sims
12. Which risk factor for cardiovascular disease can be modified? *(Select all that apply.)*
    1. Age
    2. Race
    3. Diet
    4. Family history
    5. Smoking
13. What is the term used to describe a patient's respiratory rate that exceeds 36 breaths per minute?
    1. Sonorous
    2. Bradypnea
    3. Tachypnea
    4. Apnea
14. The nurse is auscultating breath sounds on a patient and detects adventitious breath sounds. The nurse describes them as a loud, bubbly noise heard during inspiration. The nurse is correct when using which term for documenting this finding?
    1. Coarse crackles
    2. Sonorous wheezes
    3. Pleural friction rub
    4. Sibilant wheezes
15. The nurse is documenting a patient assessment. The nurse correctly identifies which information as being objective data? *(Select all that apply.)*
    1. "I have a headache and feel like the room is spinning."
    2. "When I eat I have horrible pain in my stomach."
    3. "It burns when I use the bathroom; what do you think is wrong with me?"
    4. "It is noted that the blood pressure (B/P) is high at 156/96."
    5. "Abdomen is distended and hypoactive bowel sounds are noted."

16. The nurse is performing a cardiovascular system assessment on a patient. Which is included in an assessment of the peripheral vascular system? *(Select all that apply.)*
1. Assessment of the apical pulse rate by counting the pulsations for 60 seconds
2. Assessment of the brachial, radial, ulnar, femoral, popliteal, dorsalis pedis, and posterior tibial pulses
3. Assessment of capillary refill in the nail beds of the fingers and toes
4. Determination of the rate, rhythm, and strength of the dorsalis pedis pulse
5. Assessment of the patient's skin turgor by counting the amount of time the skin remains tented

17. The patient has been admitted to the medical unit with a wound to the left lower extremity from a mowing accident 2 days ago. The inflammatory response present at this stage includes which signs and symptoms? *(Select all that apply.)*
1. Swelling
2. Pain
3. Coolness
4. Purulent drainage
5. Pale skin at injury site

18. The patient asks the nurse why all of the nurses always listen to his abdomen with the stethoscope before pressing on it. Which response is correct?
1. This prevents distortion of vascular sounds.
2. This prevents distortion of bowel sounds.
3. This determines any areas of tenderness or pain.
4. This allows the patient to relax and be comfortable.

14 Oxygenation

http://evolve.elsevier.com/Cooper/foundationsadult/

Objectives

1. Discuss nursing interventions and related procedures for the patient receiving oxygen therapy.
2. Identify safety precautions necessary when oxygen therapy is in use.
3. Differentiate the various types of oxygen therapy delivery devices.
4. Discuss transtracheal oxygen delivery.
5. Develop patient problem statements for the patient receiving oxygen therapy to direct nursing care.
6. Describe the process of suctioning a patient with a tracheostomy.
7. Describe the process of providing tracheostomy care.
8. Differentiate and describe oropharyngeal, nasopharyngeal, and nasotracheal suctioning.

Key Terms

apnea (ĂP-nē-ă, p. 346)
arterial partial pressure oxygen (PaO_2) level (p. 344)
endotracheal tube (ĕn-dō-TRĀ-kē-ăl tūb, p. 346)
flowmeter (p. 339)
fraction of inspired oxygen (FiO_2) (p. 339)
hypoxia (hī-pŎK-Sē-ăh, p. 338)
nasal cannula (NĀ-zŭl KĂN-yū-lă, p. 340)
nonrebreather mask (Table 14.1, p. 340)
partial rebreather mask (Table 14.1, p. 340)
patency (PĀ-tĕn-cē, p. 352)
simple face mask (Skill 14.1, p. 343)
tracheostomy (trā-kē-ŎS-tō-mē, p. 346)
Venturi mask (vĕn-TŪ-rē măsk, Skill 14.1, p. 343)

Oxygen is needed by all cells of the body to metabolize nutrients and produce energy needed to function. When **hypoxia** (reduced oxygen content in tissue and cells) occurs, cell metabolism slows down, and cells begin to die. Oxygen therapy is one method of preventing or relieving tissue hypoxia. Oxygen therapy must be ordered by a health care provider and closely monitored by the nurse to ensure proper administration (see the Coordinated Care box on oxygen administration). Oxygen is treated as a drug; therefore it is important to follow the six rights of drug administration when administering oxygen (see Chapter 17).

An accurate and thorough assessment of the respiratory system (see Chapter 13) is necessary when administering oxygen therapy to determine the need and the effectiveness of the treatment ordered. Knowledge of the respiratory system and related disorders (see *Adult Health Nursing,* Chapter 9) also will help the nurse care for the patient requiring oxygen therapy. Some oxygen delivery devices, such as the continuous positive airway pressure (CPAP) device, are discussed in *Adult Health Nursing,* Chapter 9.

STANDARD STEPS IN SELECTED SKILLS

To ensure patient safety, as well as nurse safety, during nursing procedures, it is important to understand the steps involved in specific skills. The skill boxes in this chapter list those steps for a variety of nursing procedures related to oxygen therapy. Certain steps performed before and after every procedure are listed as follows. The skill boxes that follow refer to them as *Standard Steps.* These steps must be followed before and after every procedure to provide the patient with safe, effective nursing care.

BEFORE THE PROCEDURE

The rationales for these steps are listed in italics in parentheses.

1. Check the health care provider's order. *(Provides basis for care. Many nursing interventions require a health care provider's order. Verification is essential before any procedure is started.)*
2. Introduce yourself to the patient; include your name and title or role. *(Decreases patient anxiety and aids in establishing rapport with the patient.)*
3. Identify the patient by checking his or her identification bracelet and requesting that the patient state his or her full name or birth date, or both (facility policy will determine the methods for patient identification). *(Ensures that procedure is performed on correct patient.)*
4. Explain the procedure and the reason it is to be done in terms that the patient is able to understand.

Advise the patient of any unpleasantness that may be involved with the procedure. Give the patient time to ask questions. *(Promotes cooperation, decreases patient's anxiety, and prepares patient.)*

5. Determine need for and provide patient education before, during, and after the procedure. *(Promotes patient's independence and compliance.)*
6. Evaluate the patient. Each skill box contains an assessment section that includes specific data to evaluate. *(Provides baseline information for later comparisons.)*
7. Perform hand hygiene. Don clean or sterile gloves and personal protective equipment as needed according to the procedure, agency policy, and guidelines from the Centers for Disease Control and Prevention (CDC) and the Occupational Safety and Health Administration (OSHA) (see Chapter 7). *(Reduces the spread of microorganisms and protects the patient and the nurse.)*
8. Assemble equipment, and complete necessary charges. Each skill box lists the specific equipment required. *(Organizes procedure so that it will go more smoothly. Some equipment is reusable and is kept at the patient's bedside. Some of the equipment is disposable and charged to the patient when used. Know agency policy.)*
9. Prepare the patient for the procedure:
   a. Close the door or pull the privacy curtain around the patient's bed. *(Provides privacy and promotes patient comfort.)*
   b. Raise the bed to a comfortable working height, and lower the side rail on the side nearest the nurse. *(Promotes proper body mechanics by minimizing nurse's muscle strain and preventing injury and fatigue.)*
   c. Position and drape the patient as necessary. Descriptions of specific positions are included in each skill. *(Shows respect for patient's privacy and dignity.)*

DURING THE PROCEDURE

10. Promote patient involvement as much as possible. *(Participation encourages the patient's cooperation and increases patient's knowledge of condition and care. It also may increase the patient's sense of independence and importance and increase the patient's compliance with treatment.)*
11. Determine the patient's tolerance of the procedure, being alert for signs and symptoms of discomfort and fatigue. If the patient cannot tolerate a procedure, describe this inability in the nursing notes. *(Patients' ability to tolerate interventions varies, depending on severity of illness and disability. It is necessary to determine when to provide the patient with an opportunity to rest and when to provide comfort measures.)*

AFTER THE PROCEDURE

12. Assist the patient to a position of comfort, and place needed items within easy reach. Ensure that the patient has a means to call for help and knows how to use it. *(Promotes comfort and safety. Patients often try to reach items and risk falling or injury.)*
13. Raise the side rails, and lower the bed to the lowest position. *(This minimizes the patient's risk in getting out of bed unattended. Use nursing judgment and facility policy to safely allow alert, cooperative patients to have their side rails down.)*
14. Remove gloves and all protective barriers such as gown, face shield, and masks. Store appropriately or discard. Remove and dispose of soiled supplies and equipment according to agency policy and guidelines from the CDC and OSHA. *(Reduces spread of microorganisms, maintains cleanliness of environment, and enhances patient comfort and safety.)*
15. Perform hand hygiene after removing gloves. *(Wearing gloves does not eliminate the need to perform hand hygiene. Hand hygiene is the most important technique for preventing and controlling the spread of microorganisms.)*
16. Document the patient's response to the procedure, expected or unexpected outcomes, and all patient teaching. Specific areas of documentation are indicated in each skill box. *(Timely and accurate documentation is legally required, records patient's progress, and promotes continuity of care.)*
17. Report any unexpected outcomes. Specific notes for reporting unexpected outcomes are included in each skill. *(Additional procedures or treatments may be necessary.)*

SKILLS FOR RESPIRATORY DISORDERS

OXYGEN THERAPY

Oxygen therapy consists of various devices, depending on the respiratory needs of the patient. The skill of the nurse with these therapies directly affects the patient's outcome of the prescribed therapy, as well as the confidence the patient has in the nurse's ability to perform a procedure. Being familiar with the various devices used in oxygen therapy is critical for the nursing student before providing care to the patient. The flow rate of oxygen is ordered in liters per minute (L/min). This determines how much oxygen the patient will receive; however, these numbers do not correlate directly with the percentage of oxygen delivered. The percentage or concentration of oxygen delivered is called the **fraction of inspired oxygen (FiO_2)**. The amount of oxygen delivered will depend on the type of device used (Table 14.1). An oxygen **flowmeter** (Fig. 14.1) is the device used to set the prescribed rate of oxygen.

There are many safety issues involved in the administration of oxygen. It is a colorless, odorless, and tasteless gas that does not burn or explode, but it does support combustion; that is, if it is combined with other factors, such as an electrical spark or fire, oxygen enables combustion, and nearby objects ignite. Therefore smoking, wool blankets, and friction toys should be

Table 14.1 Oxygen Delivery Devices With Percentage of Oxygen Delivered

DELIVERY DEVICE	AMOUNT OF DELIVERED FIO_2
Nasal cannula	1–6 L/min = 24%–44% O_2
Simple face mask	5–8 L/min = 35%–55% O_2
Venturi mask	4–10 L/min = 24%–55% O_2
Partial rebreather mask	6–12 L/min = 60%–90% O_2
Nonrebreather mask	6–15 L/min = 70%–100% O_2

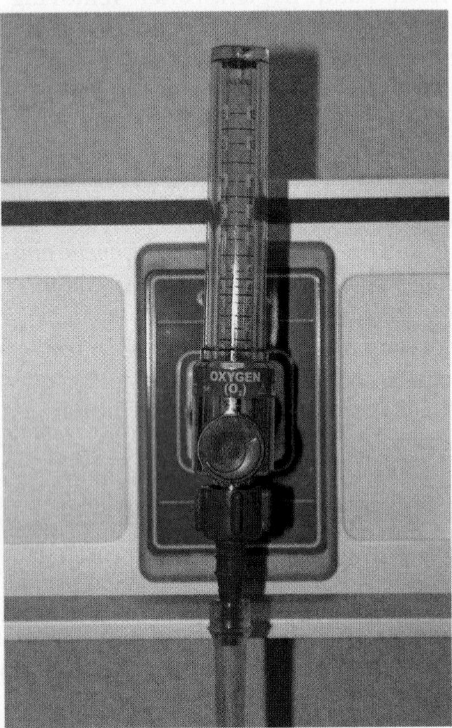

Fig. 14.1 Oxygen flowmeter.

Coordinated Care

Collaboration

Oxygen Administration

- Oxygen administration requires the critical thinking skills of a nurse. The nurse is responsible for ensuring that the oxygen is administered in the correct manner, adjusting oxygen flow rate and evaluating the patient's response to oxygen therapy.
- Correct placement and adjustment of oxygen devices may be delegated to unlicensed assistive personnel (UAP) after the care provider is instructed about the possible complications and outcomes associated with oxygen delivery and the need to report these to the nurse immediately if they occur. Adjustment of the oxygen flow rate is not delegated to UAP.

Box 14.1 Safety Precautions During Oxygen Use

- Place "No Smoking" or "Oxygen in Use" signs, or both, in the patient's room and where easily seen.
- Instruct the patient, the family, and visitors that smoking is not permitted because oxygen supports combustion (burning).
- Avoid the use of electrical appliances, such as razors, blankets, and heating pads while oxygen is administered.
- Avoid use of petrolatum products such as petroleum jelly when oxygen is administered because of the combustibility of oxygen.
- Secure portable oxygen delivery systems, such as cylinders or portable tanks, into proper portable oxygen carrying equipment to prevent falling or tipping because these delivery devices can become projectiles.
- Avoid placing oxygen cylinders near sources of heat, such as lamps or radiators.
- Avoid clothing that is not fire resistant.
- Ensure that all electrical equipment is functioning appropriately and is well grounded (three-prong plug). Avoid frayed, tangled, or cluttered cords, and do not overload circuits.
- Know the facility's fire procedure and the locations of fire extinguishers.
- Administer oxygen by the method and rate ordered by the health care provider.
- Ensure that the patient is aware if extension tubing is in use to prevent falls from tripping over the tubing.

avoided when oxygen is administered. The nurse must observe all safety precautions (Box 14.1). It also can be very drying to mucous membranes, which increases the risk of tissue cracking and opening, leaving the patient at risk for infection; humidification may be necessary. In addition, oxygen toxicity can cause scarring of the respiratory tract tissue and blindness.

Oxygen therapy may be initiated by a respiratory therapist, a nurse, an emergency medical technician (EMT), or any other licensed health care provider with an appropriate order for the oxygen. In some facilities, there is a respiratory care department, staffed by respiratory therapists who assume the responsibility of administering oxygen and delivering treatments that will improve a patient's ventilation and oxygenation.

Patients in need of oxygen may exhibit various symptoms in accordance with the degree of oxygen deprivation they are experiencing (Boxes 14.2 and 14.3). In caring for a patient having difficulty breathing or exhibiting any symptoms of hypoxia, the nurse must recognize the symptoms quickly and administer the oxygen via the appropriate mechanism as soon as possible. There are several ways to deliver oxygen. Delivering through a **nasal cannula** (device consisting of small tubes inserted into the nares) is the most common way to administer oxygen, but it also can be delivered by a Venturi mask (Fig. 14.2), by an oxygen hood or halo, or by an oxygen tent (Skill 14.1). Many

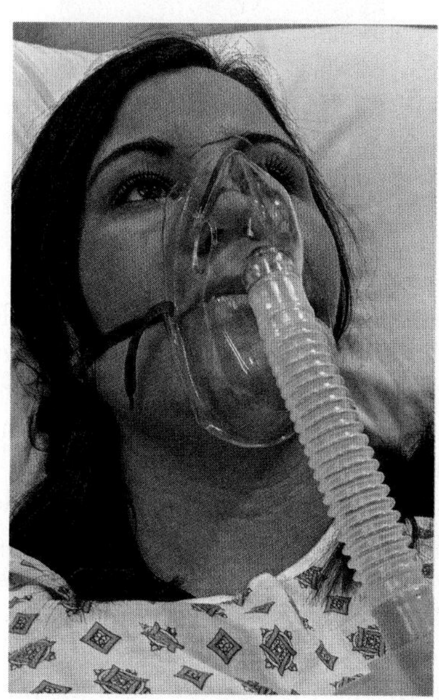

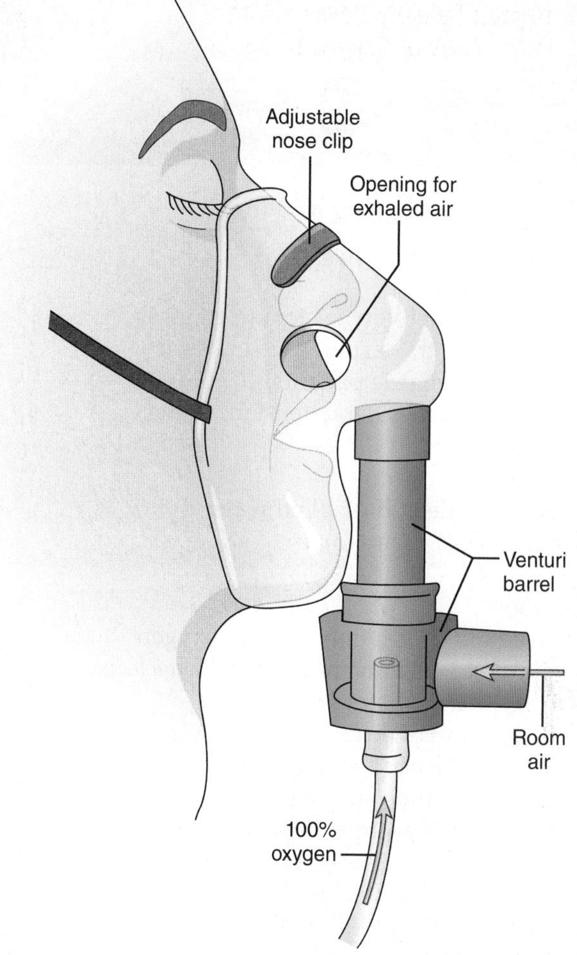

Fig. 14.2 Venturi mask.

Box 14.2 Signs and Symptoms of Hypoxia

- Apprehension, anxiety, restlessness
- Behavioral changes
- Cardiac dysrhythmias
- Cyanosis
- Decreased ability to concentrate
- Decreased level of consciousness
- Digital clubbing (with chronic hypoxia)
- Dyspnea
- Elevated blood pressure
- Increased fatigue
- Increased pulse rate: As hypoxia advances, bradycardia results, which in turn results in decreased oxygen saturation
- Increased rate and depth of respiration: As hypoxia progresses, respirations become shallow and slower, and apnea develops
- Pallor
- Vertigo

Box 14.3 Identifying Patient Problem Statements to Promote Oxygenation

Inability to Clear Airway
- Related to ineffective cough
- Related to excessive secretions

Inability to Maintain Adequate Breathing Pattern
- Related to respiratory muscle weakness
- Related to fatigue
- Related to abnormal breathing patterns

Inability to Tolerate Activity
- Related to imbalance between oxygen supply and demand

Anxiousness, Fearfulness, or Despair
- Related to dyspnea and feelings of suffocation
- Related to fear of dying

Compromised Verbal Communication
- Related to presence of tracheostomy
- Related to intubation

elderly patients and patients with chronic lung disease require oxygen in the home setting. See the Lifespan Considerations for Older Adults, Patient Teaching, and Home Care Considerations boxes for special considerations and instructions for these patients.

TRANSTRACHEAL OXYGEN DELIVERY

A method of oxygen delivery for the patient with a tracheostomy is the transtracheal catheter, which is inserted directly into the trachea between the second and third tracheal cartilages.

Skill 14.1 Oxygen Administration

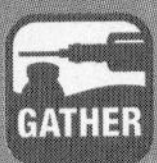

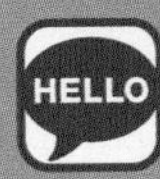

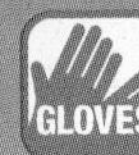

NURSING ACTION *(RATIONALE)*

1. Refer to Standard Steps 1 to 9.
2. Assemble equipment:
   - Specific oxygen delivery system (e.g., mask, cannula, or tent, the last of which is used primarily for pediatric patients)
   - Oxygen tubing (consider extension tubing)
   - Source of oxygen
   - Flowmeter
   - Humidifier bottle and distilled water
   - "Oxygen in Use" sign
   - Clean gloves
   - Stethoscope
3. Explain necessary precautions during oxygen therapy (see Box 14.1). *(Increases patient knowledge and compliance and promotes safety.)*
4. Position patient in Fowler's or semi-Fowler's position. *(Allows for maximum lung expansion.)*
5. Auscultate lung sounds and observe for signs and symptoms of hypoxia or respiratory distress (see Box 14.2). Review arterial blood gas results. *(Enables the nurse to confirm patency of airway and to determine need for oxygen.)* Suction any secretions obstructing the airway, and listen to lung sounds after suctioning (see Skill 14.2 and 14.5). *(Assists in clearing airway and increasing oxygenation.)*
6. Use a prefilled humidification container or fill the humidifier container with distilled water to designated level, if necessary. Humidify oxygen if flow rate is greater than 4 L/min. Use only distilled water in humidifier. *(Provides moisture to prevent drying of the nasal and oropharyngeal mucosa. Distilled water provides bacteria- and mineral-free water.)*
7. Attach flowmeter to humidifier and insert in proper oxygen source: central oxygen outlet, portable oxygen cylinder, or oxygen concentrator. The oxygen then is turned on to the prescribed liter flow. If the flowmeter has a metal ball, the oxygen is turned on until the middle of the metal ball is positioned on the line on the flowmeter for the prescribed oxygen flow. *(It is necessary to secure flowmeter properly to oxygen source for adequate delivery of oxygen.)* Verify that water is bubbling. *(Presence of bubbling indicates that oxygen is humidified before delivery to patient.)*
8. Administer oxygen therapy:
   a. A *nasal cannula* allows patient to eat and talk normally, and its use is appropriate for all age groups.

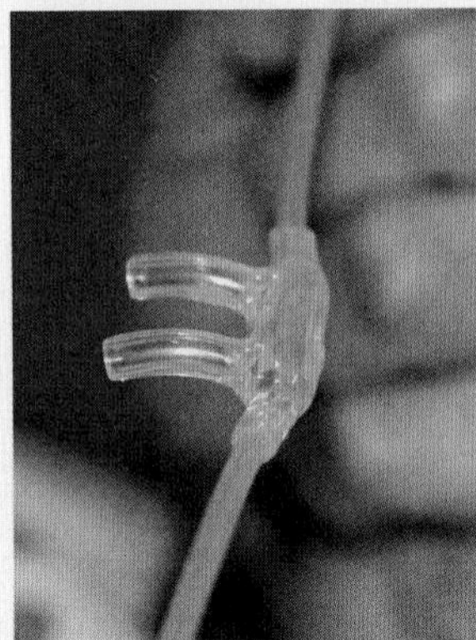

(1) Attach nasal cannula tubing to flowmeter. *(Oxygen delivery system must be continuous to ensure adequate supply of oxygen.)*

(2) Adjust flowmeter to 6 to 10 L/min to flush tubing and prongs with oxygen. Feel the oxygen on your skin to ensure flow. *(Enables the nurse to determine patency and removes any microscopic particles possibly in tubing.)*

(3) Adjust flow rate to prescribed amount; 1 to 6 L/min may be ordered. *(Ensures delivery of oxygen flow rate as directed by the health care provider.)*

(4) Place a nasal prong into each nostril of the patient in the direction that the prongs are curved (see illustration). *(Directs flow of oxygen into patient's upper respiratory tract.)*

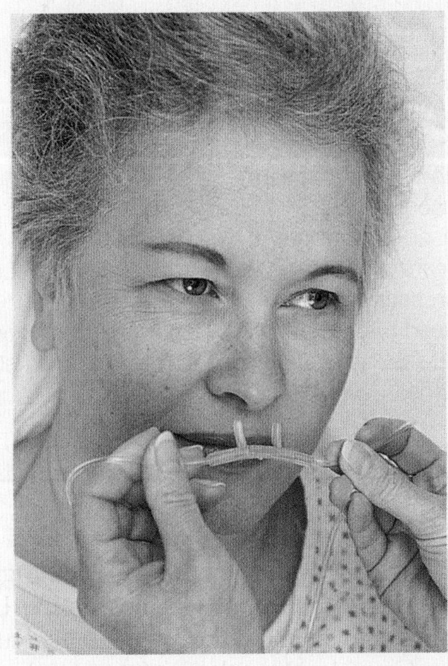

Skill 14.1 Oxygen Administration—cont'd

(5) Place cannula tubing over the patient's ears, and tighten under the chin (see illustration). *(Proper fit is snug and comfortable to prevent displacement of prongs.)*

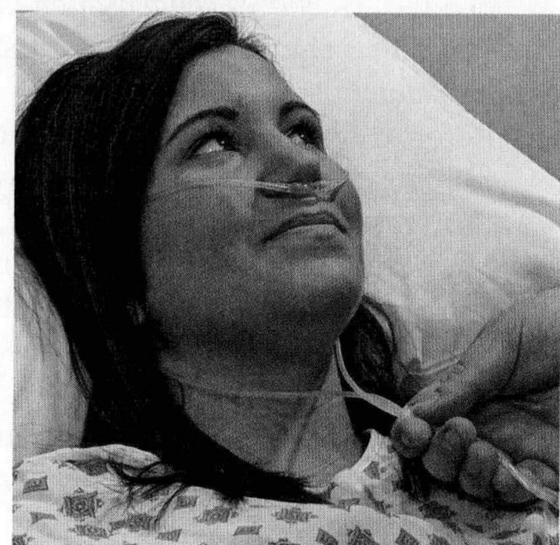

(6) Place padding between strap and ears if needed. Use lamb's wool, gauze, or cotton balls. Some nasal cannula tubing already has protective devices in place. *(Prevents skin irritation and breakdown.)*

(7) Ensure that the cannula tubing is long enough to allow for patient movement. *(Reduces risk that one or both prongs will cause pressure on the nares, as well as risk of displacement, as patient moves or is repositioned.)*

(8) Regularly evaluate equipment and patient's respiratory status. *(Ensures delivery of prescribed oxygen flow rate. Determines whether patient needs further respiratory interventions.)*

(a) Evaluate cannula frequently for possible obstruction.

(b) Observe external nasal area, nares, and superior surface of both ears for skin impairment every 6 to 8 hours.

(c) Observe nares and cannula prongs at least once a shift for irritation or breakage. Cleanse skin with cotton-tipped applicator as needed. *(Prevents skin irritation or trauma to the nares from damaged cannula prongs.)*

(d) Apply water-soluble lubricant to nares if needed. *(Prevents drying and irritation of nares. Water-soluble lubricant will not occlude the nasal cannula.)*

(e) Refer to health care provider's orders for any prescribed changes in flow rate.

(f) Maintain solution in humidifier container, if used, at appropriate level at all times. *(Prevents inhalation of dehumidified oxygen.)*

(g) Auscultate lung sounds. *(Verifies adequate oxygenation and patency of airway.)*

(h) Consult with health care provider regarding need for pulse oximetry if patient's oxygen level is unstable. *(Assists in determining oxygenation needs and helps prevent oxygen toxicity.)*

b. *Face mask:* Depending on patient's respiratory condition, the health care provider may prescribe delivery of oxygen by a mask. The mask is designed to fit snugly over the patient's nose and mouth. Different types of masks are used according to patient's needs, such as the **Venturi mask** (see Fig. 14.2), the partial rebreather mask (Step 8b[5a]), the nonrebreathing mask (Step 8b[5b]), and the **simple face mask**.

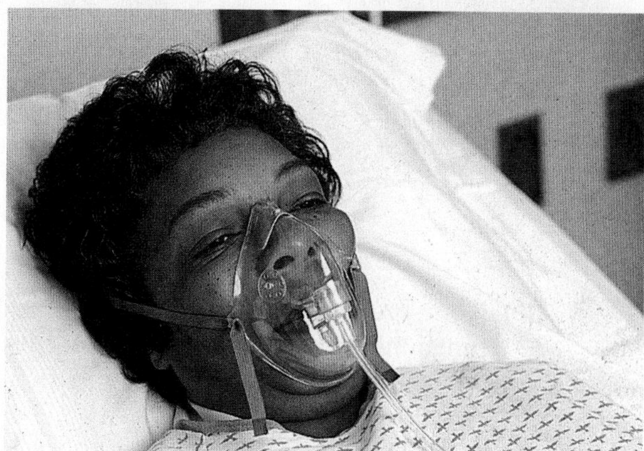

(1) Explain to the patient the need for oxygen mask. *(Decreases patient's fear and increases compliance.)*

(2) Adjust flow rate of oxygen per health care provider's order. Usually 6 to 10 L/min, which is measured in percentages (35% to 95%), is prescribed. In some facilities, the respiratory therapist assumes responsibility for maintaining proper flow. Observe for fine mist or bubbling in humidifier.

(3) Allow patient to hold the oxygen mask over the bridge of the nose and mouth, if he or she is able. Assist as necessary. *(Placing mask over patient's face sometimes causes feeling of suffocation and apprehension. Allowing patient to place the mask helps patient become accustomed to mask and to have some control over placing it on face.)*

(4) Adjust straps around patient's head and over ears. Place cotton ball or gauze over ears under elastic straps. *(Provides comfort and prevents skin impairment.)*

Continued

Skill 14.1 Oxygen Administration—cont'd

(5) Cover the reservoir hole in the mask and allow the reservoir bag to completely fill BEFORE placing on the patient. Observe reservoir bag for appropriate movement if one is attached to mask. *(Mask's expanding and collapsing with patient's breathing confirm appropriate fit and that oxygen delivery is maintained.)*

(a) Partial-rebreathing mask: When functioning properly, the reservoir fills on exhalation and almost collapses on inhalation.

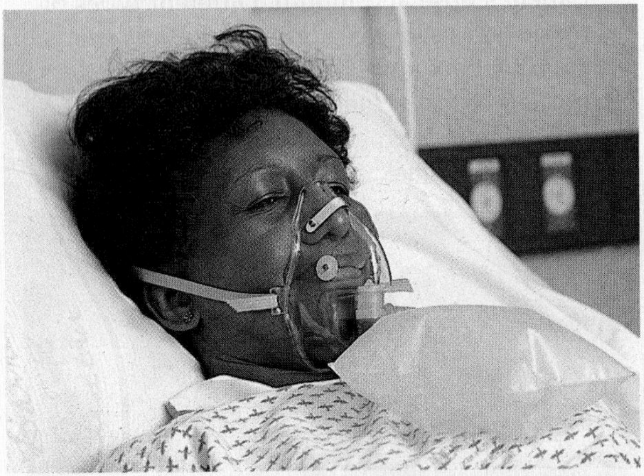

(b) Nonrebreathing mask: When functioning properly, the reservoir fills on exhalation but never totally collapses on inhalation.

(6) Evaluate equipment function regularly. *(Ensures that mask is working properly and that the patient is receiving appropriate amount of oxygen.)*

(a) Remove mask and evaluate skin every 2 to 4 hours. Clean and dry skin as needed. *(Removes condensation and other debris that may form and prevents skin breakdown.)*

(b) Refer to health care provider's orders for prescribed flow rate and any changes.

(c) Maintain solution in humidifier container, if used, at appropriate level at all times. Always use distilled, never tap, water. *(Prevents inhalation of dehumidified oxygen. Distilled water decreases the growth of microorganisms.)*

9. Refer to Standard Steps 10 to 17.

10. Document the following. *(Verifies performance of procedure and ensures continuity of care.)*

- Date
- Time
- Flow rate
- Method of oxygen delivery
- Evaluation of respiratory status
- Patient's response to oxygen therapy
- Changes in health care provider's orders
- Adverse reactions or side effects of oxygen therapy
- Assess condition of skin around oxygen device
- Patient teaching (see the Patient Teaching and Home Care Considerations boxes on oxygen therapy)

Figure for Step 8a(4) from Potter PA, Perry AG, Stockert P, et al: *Fundamentals of nursing: concepts, process, and practice*, ed 9, St. Louis, 2016, Elsevier. Figures for Step 8b and 8b(5)(a) from Perry AG, Potter PA, Ostendorf WR, et al: *Clinical nursing skills and techniques*, ed 9, St. Louis, 2018, Elsevier.

 Lifespan Considerations

Older Adults

Oxygen Therapy

- Normal arterial oxygen levels sometimes decrease with age but not usually low enough to fall outside the normal range. It may be possible for a 70-year-old person to have an **arterial partial pressure oxygen (PaO2) level** (the amount of oxygen found in the arterial circulation) between 80 and 85 mm Hg (normal range is 80 to 100 mm Hg) without experiencing significant alterations in health.
- The respiratory drive normally is initiated by arterial carbon dioxide ($PaCO_2$) levels rising, but in patients with chronic obstructive pulmonary disease (COPD), hypoxia tends to be the driving force behind respiratory effort (hypoxic drive). If the hypoxia is corrected in a patient with COPD, then the respiratory drive is reduced, and respiratory difficulty will occur. For this reason, oxygen flow rates greater than 2 L/min are to be given with great caution in these individuals. Flow rates higher than 2 L/min could eliminate the respiratory drive, and breathing may stop.
- The older adult is often at increased risk for skin impairment. Therefore frequent monitoring for erythema and skin breakdown over the ears is necessary when a nasal cannula is being used for oxygen delivery. Early interventions such as loosening the straps, repositioning the tubing, or adding padding over the ears often prevent impairment.

Patient Teaching

Oxygen Therapy

- Teach patient how to apply the oxygen equipment, such as the nasal cannula or oxygen mask, appropriately.
- Discuss safety precautions for oxygen use (see Box 14.1).
- Stress the dangers of adjusting the oxygen flow rate without notifying the health care provider. Emphasize that it is possible for the patient to be short of breath because of reasons other than hypoxia and to contact the health care provider if shortness of breath increases.
- Instruct patient to ambulate or change positions frequently to mobilize secretions.
- Teach the patient to cough and practice deep breathing, and encourage practicing these techniques frequently, as directed by the patient condition or provider's orders, to facilitate air exchange.
- Teach the patient to maintain adequate fluid intake to help liquefy secretions. Recommend fluids that are free of caffeine and sugar because drinks high in caffeine and sugar sometimes cause dehydration. Teach the patient to avoid dairy products, which tend to thicken secretions.
- Teach the rationale for prescribed medications, as well as side effects. This helps increase compliance.
- Teach that performing oral hygiene at regular intervals helps rid the mouth of any bad taste from secretions coughed up or expectorated.

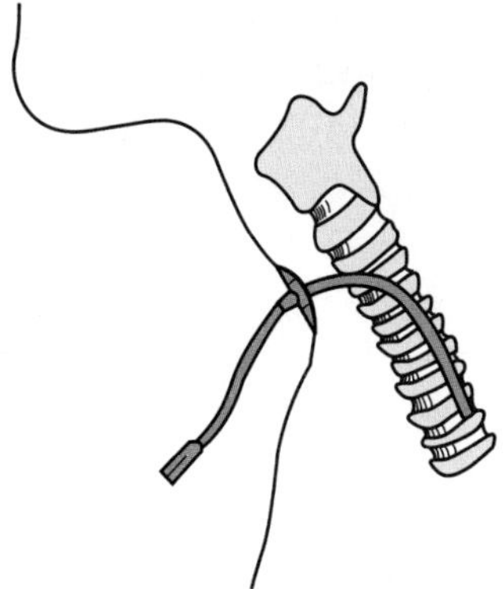

Fig. 14.3 A transtracheal catheter is inserted into the trachea between the second and third tracheal cartilages.

Unlike a tracheostomy tube, a transtracheal catheter (Fig. 14.3) does not interfere with drinking, eating, or talking. With a nasal cannula, oxygen is delivered only during inhalation. With the transtracheal oxygen delivery system, oxygen is delivered throughout the entire respiratory cycle. No oxygen is lost to the atmosphere; therefore oxygen delivery is less expensive. Additional humidification is unnecessary because the nasopharynx, the area most in need of supplemental humidity, is bypassed. This delivery system also allows the flow rate to be decreased for some patients. Patients who require 2 L/min with a cannula may need only 1 L/min with a transtracheal catheter. The low flow rates also enable patients to use portable oxygen delivery systems longer between refills.

Home Care Considerations

Oxygen Therapy

- If oxygen is used at home, instruct the patient's family to post a "No Smoking" sign on all entry doors of the house.
- When oxygen cylinders are used, it is necessary to secure them so that they will not fall over. Oxygen cylinders are stored upright, chained on appropriate holders.
- In home settings, oxygen tubing is sometimes as long as 50 feet (15.2 m), which presents a tripping hazard. Instruct patient on risks for falling that are associated with this length of tubing.
- Instruct patient's family on safety measures of oxygen therapy (see Box 14.1).
- Teach patient and family members how to use home equipment.
- Instruct patient and family members to observe level of oxygen in canister tanks and to use portable tanks when patient is not at home.
- Instruct patient and family members to fill plastic humidifier bottle with distilled water every 24 hours. Instruct patient and family members to use only distilled water, not tap water.
- Provide two complete sets of tubing so that one set of equipment is available for use while the other is being cleaned or repaired.
- Evaluate home for availability of a three-pronged outlet for the compressor, to prevent electric shock.
- Teach patient to maintain constant flow rate and to change flow rate only with the health care provider's knowledge and advice.
- Evaluate home for appropriate storage of equipment.
- Evaluate family's willingness to assist patient with home delivery system.
- Teach patient and family deep breathing and coughing exercises.
- Teach patient and family adequate nutritional and hydration needs based on the patient's diagnosis and current condition.

For transtracheal oxygen delivery, a small oxygen tube (8-French [Fr] or 9-Fr) is inserted through the transtracheal tract opening through which oxygen is administered. After the insertion tract has matured (healed), it is possible for the patient or a family member to remove the tube for cleaning. A single transtracheal catheter may last up to 3 months. After that period, the catheter is likely to become brittle and must be replaced. This method of oxygen delivery is suited especially for home use. It allows the individual to be more active and can be concealed under a shirt. Some transtracheal oxygen delivery systems even have a beaded chain necklace attached to help disguise the catheter. The patient should be instructed to inspect the transtracheal tract opening regularly for erythema, edema, or excessive exudate. (Small amounts of clear exudate are expected.) The area is cleaned twice daily with a cotton-tipped applicator. Hydrogen peroxide may be used to wash the neck and remove dried exudate. The transtracheal tract (like a tracheostomy) never truly heals as long as it is kept open with an oxygen delivery catheter. If the catheter is removed and not replaced within a timely manner, the opening may close over. If this occurs, the surgical procedure must be repeated.

ENDOTRACHEAL TUBES

An **endotracheal** (ET) **tube** (Fig. 14.4) is a tube inserted through the patient's mouth and into the upper airway to provide a patent airway. Oxygen is administered through an ET tube via an oxygen setup or through a ventilator. Suctioning of secretions also can be performed through an ET tube. An ET tube typically is used in an emergency situation to establish a patent airway or to provide an airway and oxygenation of a patient undergoing general anesthesia. ET tubes are used for short-term management of the airway. Typically an ET tube is replaced by a tracheostomy if an artificial airway is needed for longer than 2 weeks.

Care of the Tracheostomy

A **tracheostomy** is an artificial opening made by a surgical incision into the trachea. A tracheostomy may be created for patients who are experiencing **apnea** (cessation of breathing) or some form of respiratory obstruction. It also may be used to prevent aspiration of secretions and blood or to provide easier access to the lower airways. Many types of tracheostomy tubes are available; the one chosen depends on why it is being used and the condition of the patient. During a sterile surgical procedure, the health care provider makes an incision into the patient's trachea and inserts a tracheostomy tube into the opening. The tube then is secured in place by cotton tape or a specifically designed tie/strap wrapped around the patient's neck. This provides the patient with a patent airway. Sterile 4 × 4 precut drain gauze is placed around the opening in the neck, under the flange of the outer tube. This protects the skin during the healing process and decreases the risk for infection. An endotracheal or a tracheostomy tube provides a direct route for introduction of pathogens into the lower airway, which increases the risk of infection.

The primary nursing responsibilities for maintaining a tracheostomy tube are to keep the airway clear, keep the inner cannula clean, prevent impairment of surrounding tissue, and provide the patient with a means of communication (Skill 14.2 and see Fig. 14.4). The nursing interventions that follow enable the nurse to meet those responsibilities and adequately care for a patient with a tracheostomy tube.

- Minimize infection risk:
  - Evaluate the patient for excess secretions and suction as often as necessary.
  - Provide constant airway humidification.
  - Change or clean all respiratory therapy equipment every 8 hours.
  - Remove water that condenses in equipment tubing.
  - Provide frequent mouth care (apply moisturizing agents to dry, cracked lips).

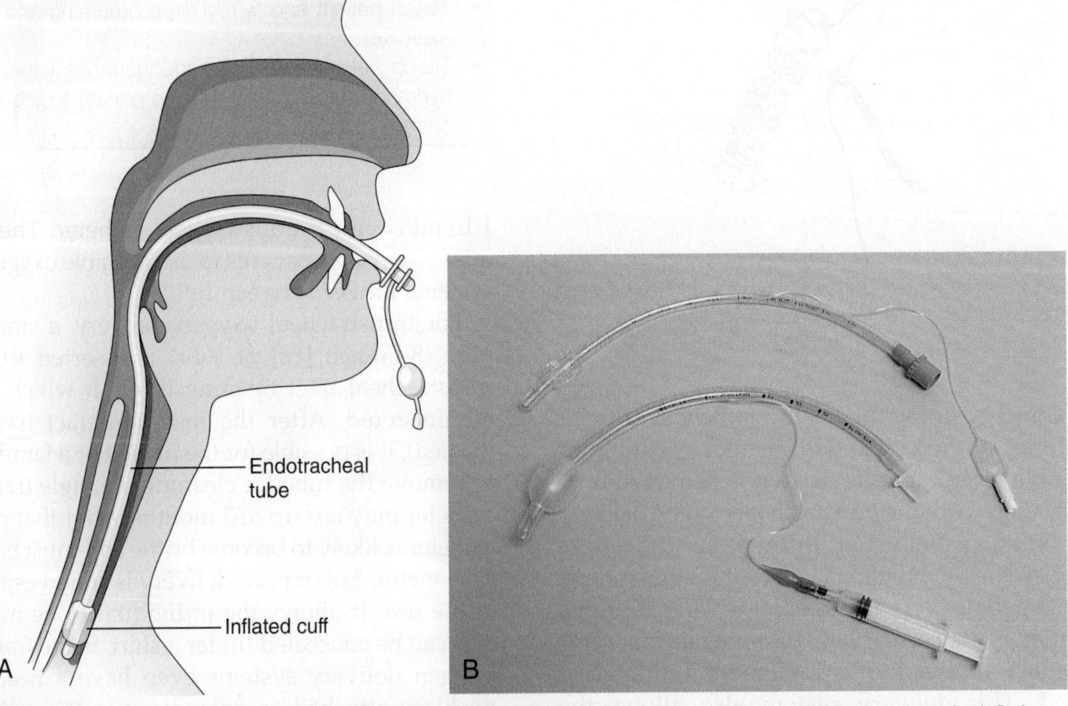

Fig. 14.4 A, Endotracheal tube with inflated cuff. B, Endotracheal tubes with uninflated cuffs and syringe for inflation. Patient is unable to speak while tube is in place because air cannot flow through the vocal cords. (B from Perry AG, Potter PA, Elkin MK: *Nursing interventions and clinical skills*, ed 5, St. Louis, 2012, Mosby.)

Skill 14.2 Tracheostomy Suctioning and Care

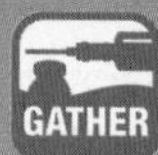

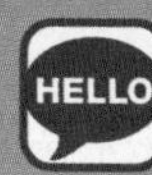

PRIVACY
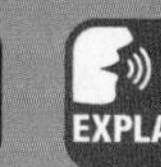

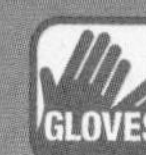

NURSING ACTION *(RATIONALE)*

Tracheostomy Suctioning

1. Refer to Standard Steps 1 to 9.
2. Assemble equipment:
   - Sterile suction catheter kit
   - Sterile water or normal saline if not contained in kit
   - Sterile gloves
   - Clean gloves
   - Clean, water-repellent gown, and mask with face shield (if indicated)
   - Stethoscope
3. Check patient's tracheostomy for exudate, edema, and respiratory obstruction; check that tracheostomy phalange is secure with the ties/strap. *(Allows the nurse to identify potential need for further nursing interventions.)*
4. Position patient in semi-Fowler's position. *(Allows for optimal lung expansion; during suctioning the patient may cough forcefully and dislodge the tracheostomy if it is not secure.)*
5. Provide paper and pencil or a communication board for patient. *(Because patient cannot speak, this offers a means of communication.)*
6. Position self at head of bed facing patient. Always face patient while cleaning or suctioning a tracheostomy. *(Enables close observation for respiratory difficulty and coughing, which could expel the tracheostomy cannula.)*
7. Auscultate lung sounds. *(Provides baseline information regarding airway for comparison after suctioning.)*
8. Place towel or prepackaged drape under tracheostomy and across chest. *(Protects patient's gown and the bed linens and provides a sterile field on the chest.)*
9. Perform hand hygiene. Prepare equipment and supplies on overbed table. *(Organizes procedure.)*

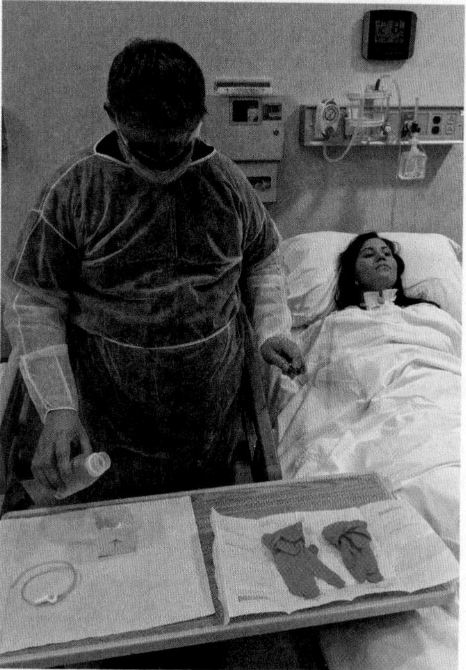

a. Open suction catheter kit but maintain sterility of contents, leaving the catheter in its wrapper. *(Maintains sterility.)* The order of steps depends on how the equipment is placed in the kit and if there is a prefilled container of sterile saline or water. Don sterile gloves if there is a prefilled container of saline or water. Open the container. If there is only an empty basin for saline to be added, open the basin and remove the lid from the bottle of sterile saline or water outside of the kit, then don sterile gloves. Fanfold or wrap suction catheter around dominant hand. *(Helps protect the sterility of the catheter tip.)* Pick up tubing from the machine with the nondominant hand and attach the end of the suction catheter to the suction machine tubing. *(This hand will no longer be sterile for the remainder of the procedure.)*

Continued

Skill 14.2 Tracheostomy Suctioning and Care—cont'd

b. If sterile saline or water is to be added to an empty basin inside the suction kit, use the nondominant hand to pour the sterile saline or water into the basin. *(Sterile saline or water is used to rinse suction catheter. The nondominant hand is no longer sterile and can be used to pour solution.)*

c. Turn on suction machine with nondominant hand and check that suction is working by suctioning a small amount of the sterile saline or water. This is accomplished by covering the port on the suction tubing with the thumb of the nondominant hand.

10. Preoxygenate patient by having patient take several deep breaths, by setting ventilator to deliver 100% oxygen with sigh breaths, or by having an assistant use a resuscitator bag. If patient is receiving oxygen, wait to remove oxygen delivery system until just before suctioning. *(Prevents oxygen depletion during procedure.)*

11. Suction tracheal cannula. *(Aids in maintaining patent airway.)*

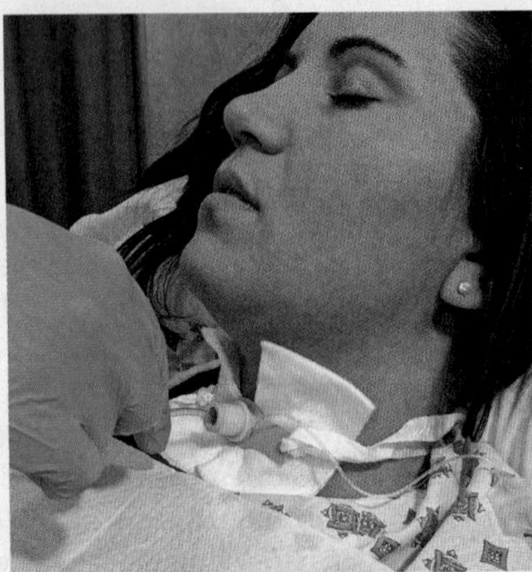

a. Place thumb over suction control vent; place tip of suction catheter in container of sterile rinse solution. Withdraw sterile rinsing solution through catheter by placing thumb over suction control. *(Moistens catheter and clears any mucus from the catheter tip.)*

b. Remove thumb from suction control; advance catheter gently through the tracheostomy while maintaining sterility until resistance is met, and then withdraw catheter approximately 1 cm. (Depth of catheter approximately equals the length of outer cannula, the distal end of which protrudes from the opening approximately 1 to 2 inches.) *(Keeping thumb off of suction vent prevents suctioning while inserting catheter, which has the potential to damage the mucosa. Resistance is met when the catheter reaches the junction of the main bronchi.)*

c. Apply intermittent suction by placing thumb on and off suction control, and gently rotate catheter as it is withdrawn. *(Secretions are suctioned around the circumference of the trachea.)*

d. Suction for a maximum of 10 seconds at a time, never longer. *(Prolonged suctioning depletes oxygen supply.)*

e. Rinse catheter with sterile solution by suctioning sterile solution through it. Repeat Steps 11b through 11e if needed. Most facilities' policies indicate no more than three suction attempts during the suctioning procedure.

f. Allow patient to rest between each suctioning effort. If patient was receiving oxygen previously, reapply it at the prescribed rate between each suctioning episode. *(Suctioning is often exhausting and frightening for patient. Resting helps patient regain depleted oxygen and decreases fear.)*

g. Turn off suction, and dispose of catheter appropriately by rolling catheter up into one gloved hand and pulling glove off over catheter; then placing glove with catheter into other hand and pulling glove off over the glove with the catheter.

h. Perform hand hygiene.

i. Auscultate lung sounds. *(Evaluate effectiveness of suctioning.)*

12. Refer to Standard Steps 10 to 17.

13. Document the following. *(Verifies performance of procedure and ensures continuity of care.)*
   - Date
   - Time
   - Respiratory evaluation before suctioning
   - Tracheostomy suctioned
   - Characteristics of material that was suctioned
   - Amount (it will not be possible to determine the exact amount suctioned because the sterile saline for rinsing the catheter is in the suction canister along with the respiratory secretions. This is a subjective measure noting the amount as small/moderate/large or copious.)
   - Color
   - Consistency
   - Respiratory evaluation after suctioning
   - Adverse reactions
   - Patient's response
   - If oxygen is administered, note flow rate and method used
   - Patient teaching

Tracheostomy Care

1. Refer to Standard Steps 1 to 9.
2. Check patient's tracheostomy for exudate, edema, and respiratory obstruction. *(Allows the*

Skill 14.2 Tracheostomy Suctioning and Care—cont'd

nurse to identify potential need for further nursing interventions.)

3. Perform suctioning if it is needed before performing tracheostomy care. *(Removes excess secretions and prevents soiling new dressing.)*
4. Position patient in semi-Fowler's position. *(Provides for optimal lung expansion.)*
5. Perform hand hygiene; then position self at head of bed, facing patient. Always face patient while cleaning or suctioning a tracheostomy. *(Hand hygiene prevents spread of microorganisms. Facing patient enables close observation for respiratory difficulty and coughing.)*
6. Don clean gloves. Remove old dressing from around tracheostomy stoma, and discard it in appropriate receptacle. *(Removes any exudate or drainage from stoma site.)*
7. Prepare equipment and supplies on overbed table (see Step 9 illustration under "Tracheostomy Suctioning"). *(Organizes procedure.)*
   a. Open tracheostomy cleaning kit with aseptic technique. *(Prevents contamination of supplies.)*
   b. If basins are packed with sterile gloves, apply one sterile glove to dominant hand. Separate basins with dominant hand. Use nondominant hand to pour cleansing solution (hydrogen peroxide) in one basin and rinsing solution (sterile saline) in another basin. *(Cleanses mucus and secretions from inner cannula and to rinse cannula.)* In some facilities, a third solution of half hydrogen peroxide and half normal saline is used to clean around the tracheostomy stoma. Check facility policy.
8. With nondominant hand, unlock and remove inner cannula; place in hydrogen peroxide cleansing solution. *(The nondominant hand has a clean glove on it and can remove contaminated inner cannula without breaking sterile technique.)* Never remove outer cannula. If it is expelled by patient, use hemostat to hold tracheostomy open, and call for assistance. Always have a sterile packaged hemostat, as well as an extra sterile tracheostomy set, available at bedside. *(Prevents closure of stoma until new outer cannula can be inserted.)*
9. Apply second sterile glove or apply new pair of sterile gloves if contamination has occurred. *(Reduces spread of microorganisms.)*
10. Clean inner cannula. *(Removes secretions and hydrogen peroxide from inner cannula.)*
    a. Use brush to clean inside and outside of inner cannula.
    b. Place inner cannula in sterile normal saline solution. *(Rinses away the hydrogen peroxide.)*
    c. At some facilities, pipe cleaners are used to dry inside of inner cannula. Check facility policy.
    d. Inspect inner and outer areas of inner cannula. Remove excess liquid (see Step 13a).
    e. Insert inner cannula in the direction of the tracheostomy and lock in place. *(Secures inner cannula and reestablishes oxygen supply.)*

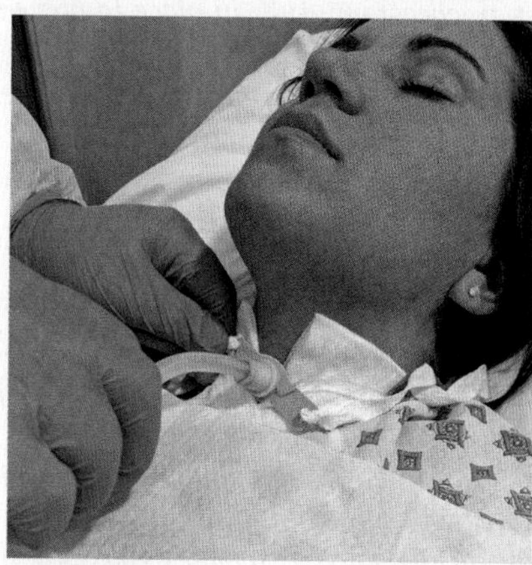

11. Clean skin around tracheostomy and tabs of outer cannula with hydrogen peroxide (or half-and-half mixture) and cotton-tipped swabs; clean away from the opening. Use wipes that are free of lint around the tracheostomy opening. *(Removes any remaining exudate or drainage. Inhaled lint [e.g., from cotton balls] irritates the respiratory passages and tends to cause undue coughing. Special tracheostomy dressings are available.)*
12. It may be necessary to rinse cleansing solution from skin. If so, use sterile 4 × 4 gauze. *(Aseptically removes secretions from stoma site.)* Place dry, sterile 4 × 4 drainage sponge around the tracheostomy opening. *(Prevents skin impairment caused by rubbing of flange of tracheostomy tube against the skin.)*

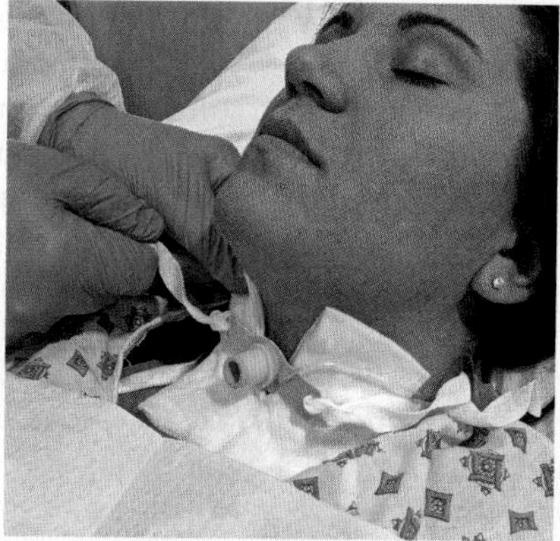

13. Change ties/straps holding tracheostomy in place if necessary. *(Always do this after cleaning inner and outer cannula to prevent cannula from being expelled.)*
    a. If assistance is not available, thread clean tie through opening in flange of outer cannula along old tie. If assistance is available, untie

Continued

Skill 14.2 Tracheostomy Suctioning and Care—cont'd

one side of cotton tape from outer cannula and replace with clean one while the assistant stabilizes the tracheostomy tube. *(Prevents accidental expulsion of outer cannula.)*

b. Bring clean tape under back of neck. *(Securely holds tracheostomy tube in place to prevent movement of cannula.)*

c. If assistance is not available, thread tie through opening in opposite flange of outer cannula along old tie. If assistance is available, remove other side from outer cannula and replace with clean tape.

d. Tie ends of clean cotton tapes together in a knot at side of neck. *(Secures ties and cannula in place. Putting knot at side of neck avoids pressure and skin irritation at back of neck.)*

14. Auscultate lung sounds. *(Enables the nurse to determine any change from baseline.)*

15. Provide mouth care. *(Promotes good oral hygiene. Patients with tracheostomies often have halitosis.)*

16. Refer to Standard Steps 10 to 17.

17. Place call light, paper, and pencil within easy reach of the patient. *(Enables patient to communicate needs.)*

18. Reassess patient's tracheostomy for signs of bleeding, edema, and respiratory obstruction. *(Patients with tracheostomy frequently have bloody secretions for 2 to 3 days after procedure or for 24 hours after each tracheostomy tube change.)*

19. Document the following: *(Verifies performance of procedure and ensures continuity of care.)*
- Date/time of tracheostomy care
- Type of tracheostomy care performed and solution used to clean around the stoma
- Patient's response
- Evaluation of respiratory status
- Adverse reactions
- Condition of tracheal stoma and peristomal skin
- If oxygen is administered, note flow rate and method used
- Patient teaching (see the Home Care Considerations box on tracheostomy care)

- Maintain nutritional levels:
  - Patients with ET tubes are allowed nothing by mouth (NPO). It is necessary to provide parenteral or enteral nourishment.
  - Patients with a tracheostomy may not be limited in regard to drinking fluids and eating once the initial healing phase of the new tracheostomy has passed. If a patient is able to eat, a cuffless tracheostomy tube is best. Not all patients have cuffless tracheostomy tubes. The patient may have a tracheostomy tube with a cuff to provide maximum sealing of the airway. Cuffed tracheostomy tubes generally are used for patients who are at risk for aspiration because of swallowing difficulties or who are receiving mechanical ventilation. The cuff must be deflated at prescribed intervals to prevent tissue necrosis of the trachea. Noncuffed tracheostomy tubes often are used to maintain the patient's airway when a ventilator is not needed or when the patient is being prepared to have the tracheostomy discontinued. The physician, often with consultation with the respiratory therapist, chooses the tube based on the patient's condition, neck shape, and size and purpose of the tracheostomy.
- Ensure adequate ventilation and oxygenation:
  - Listen to lung sounds regularly.
  - Elevate the head of the bed to assist with ventilation.
  - Turn and reposition the patient every 2 hours for maximal ventilation and lung expansion.
  - Evaluate the effects of respiratory therapy regularly.
- Provide safety and comfort:
  - Check tube placement at regular intervals; tracheostomy tubes are secured around the neck with tapes or specially designed ties/strap. Make sure they are snug and the tube is securely in the neck stoma.
  - Change the tapes or ties/strap whenever they are soiled to lessen the chances of skin impairment.
  - Always keep a spare tracheostomy tube at the bedside.
- Enhance communication:
  - Organize questions so that the patient can give simple "yes" or "no" responses by nodding the head or using hand signals.
  - Assess whether the patient can use an erasable board or notepad to communicate.
  - Talk to the patient and explain all procedures.
  - Reorient the patient frequently if necessary.
  - Encourage family and friends to talk to the patient.
  - Keep a call light (or tap bell) within patient's reach.

Currently many types of tracheostomy tubes are available; tube types can be specific to the patient who needs them. Tubes are available in cuffed and cuffless styles; some have only a single cannula, and others have an outer cannula and an inner cannula that can

Skill 14.3 Care of a Cuffed Tracheostomy Tube

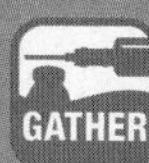

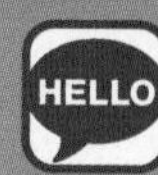

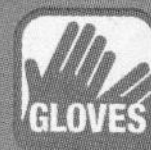

NURSING ACTION *(RATIONALE)*

1. Refer to Standard Steps 1 to 9.
2. Perform suction for patient as in Skill 14.2, Steps 1 to 11.
3. Connect syringe to pilot balloon valve. *(Provides inflation and deflation of tube balloon.)*
4. Clean the diaphragm of the stethoscope and position the stethoscope in sternal notch or above tracheostomy tube and listen for minimal amount of air leak at end of inspiration. *(Allows the nurse to confirm proper cuff inflation.)*

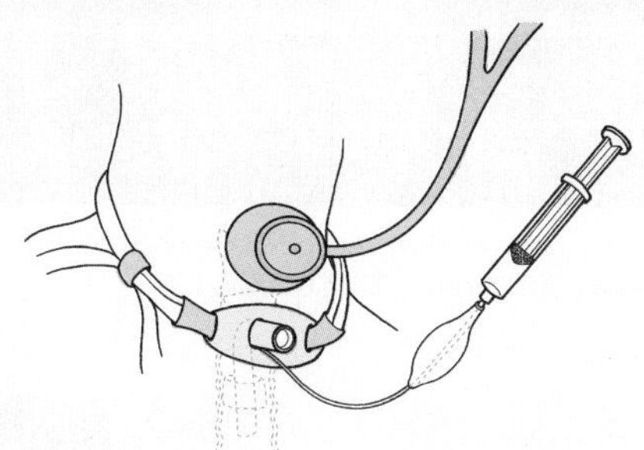

5. Remove all air from cuff if no air leak is auscultated. *(Releases excessive air pressure.)*
6. While you listen with stethoscope, slowly inflate cuff with 0.5 to 1 mL of air at a time. When no air leak is heard, stop injecting air and slowly withdraw up to 0.5 mL of air until air leak is auscultated with stethoscope.
7. If excessive air leak is heard, slowly add air as in Step 6. *(Air leak will sometimes prevent lung expansion and increases risk of aspiration.)*
8. Remove stethoscope and cleanse diaphragm with alcohol swab. *(Reduces spread of microorganisms.)*
9. Remove syringe from pilot balloon valve and discard in appropriate receptacle. Do not leave syringe attached to pilot balloon valve. *(Leaving the syringe attached may cause valve to break or stick open.)*
10. Follow Steps 17 to 19 in Skill 14.2.

be removed easily for cleaning. Being able to remove and clean the inner cannula reduces the risk of occlusion from a buildup of secretions (see Fig. 14.4).

Cuffed tracheostomy tubes are used routinely in patients who require mechanical ventilation. Step 14.3 describes how to care for a cuffed tracheostomy tube. A cuffless tube may be used for patients who require a long-term tracheostomy and for those in the process of being weaned from a tracheostomy tube. A single-cannula tracheostomy tube has one tube or cannula for airflow and suctioning of secretions. Uncuffed, single-cannula tubes are usually for neonates, infants, and young children. A double-cannula tube has a hollow outer cannula and a removable inner cannula. A fenestrated tube has holes (fenestrations) for air to flow upward through the vocal cords and mouth. This type of tracheostomy tube lets the patient talk and breathe naturally.

Although nursing interventions for patients with endotracheal and tracheostomy tubes are similar, patients with tracheostomies have additional nursing care needs and considerations related to respiratory status and suctioning (see Skill 14.2 and Skill 14.3 the Home Care Considerations and Coordinated Care boxes on suctioning for tracheostomy care). Some of these considerations are as follows:

- To prevent depression of the respiratory center, it is advisable to give analgesics and sedatives with caution.
- Suction is performed as often as necessary, possibly every 5 minutes during the first few postoperative hours. (Whenever respirations are noisy and the pulse and respiratory rates are increased, the patient needs suctioning.)
- Patients who are conscious are usually able to indicate when they need suctioning.
- A patient who is able to expectorate secretions requires less suctioning.
- The amount of mucus decreases gradually, and the nurse performs suctioning less frequently. A patient who remains apprehensive may require constant attendance and reassurance.

 **Home Care Considerations**

Tracheostomy Care

- Some patients with an artificial airway who are at home have a permanent tracheostomy, as well as a T piece or T tube or tracheostomy collar (Figs. 14.6 and 14.7).
- Determine patient's ability to perform tracheostomy care and suctioning techniques.
- Evaluate patient's home environment for presence of respiratory irritants, cleanliness, and location in which to clean suctioning equipment and hang it up to drain.
- Ensure that a humidifier is present: added moisture is important.

Care of the Patient With a Tracheostomy Collar and T Piece or T Tube

In a healthy person, the upper airway normally filters and humidifies air upon inspiration. The air taken in by a patient with a tracheostomy bypasses the upper

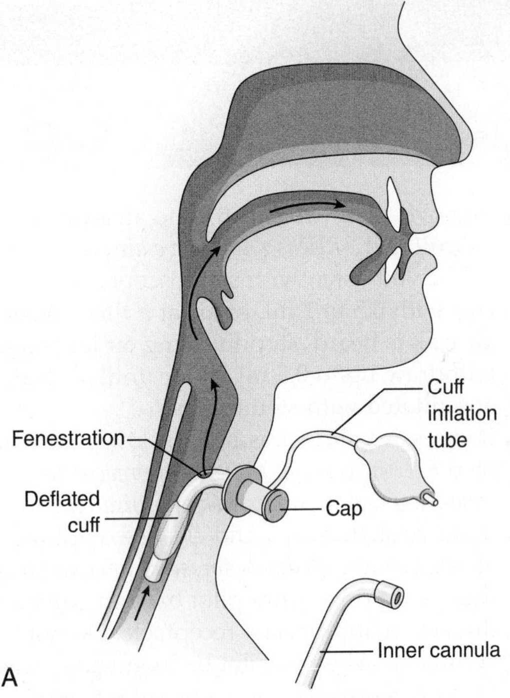

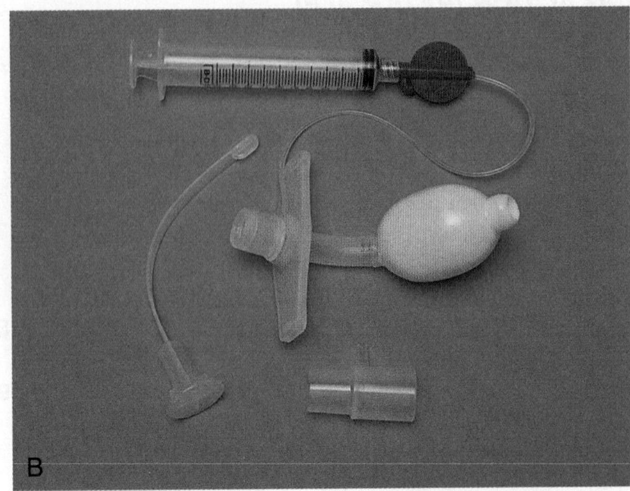

Fig. 14.5 A, Tracheostomy tube (fenestrated) with inner cannula removed and cap in place to allow speech. B, Tracheostomy tube with obturator for insertion and syringe for inflation of cuff. (B from Perry AG, Potter PA, Ostendorf WR, et al: *Clinical nursing skills and techniques*, ed 9, St. Louis, 2018, Elsevier.)

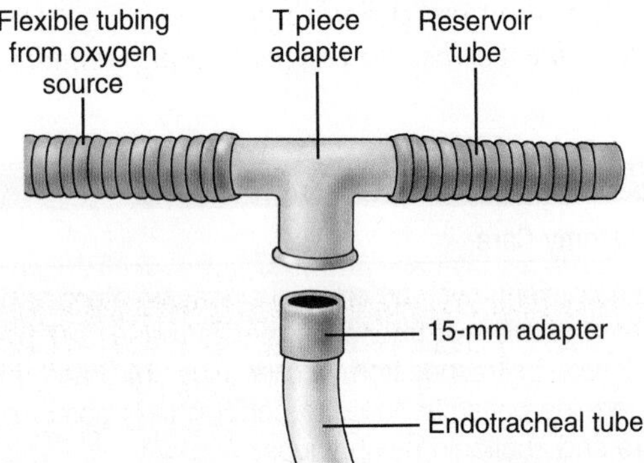

Fig. 14.6 T piece or T tube. (From Ignatavicius DD, Workman ML, Blair M, et al: *Medical-surgical nursing; patient-centered collaborative care*, ed 8, St. Louis, 2016, Elsevier.)

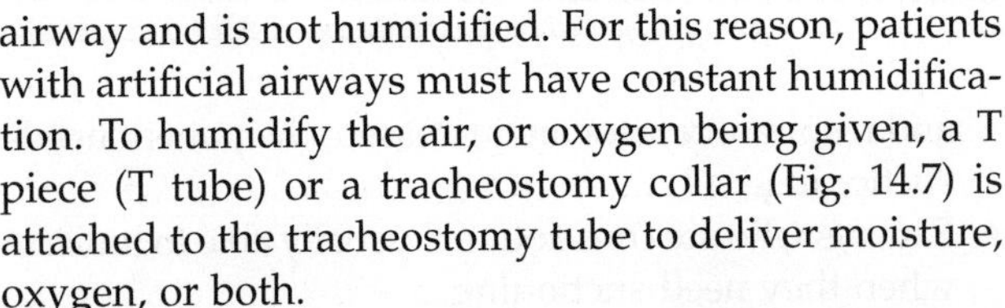

airway and is not humidified. For this reason, patients with artificial airways must have constant humidification. To humidify the air, or oxygen being given, a T piece (T tube) or a tracheostomy collar (Fig. 14.7) is attached to the tracheostomy tube to deliver moisture, oxygen, or both.

The T piece or T tube is a T-shaped device that is connected to large-bore tubing and then can deliver humidification, oxygen, or both (see Fig. 14.6). A tracheostomy collar also is designed to supply humidification and humidified oxygen to the lower respiratory tract. The collar covers the open end of the tracheostomy tube and has an adjustable strap that extends around the patient's neck (see Fig. 14.7). Refer to Skill 14.4 for procedures used to ensure adequate oxygenation and humidification via a T tube or tracheostomy collar. Refer to Skill 14.5 for the steps involved in clearing a patient's airway.

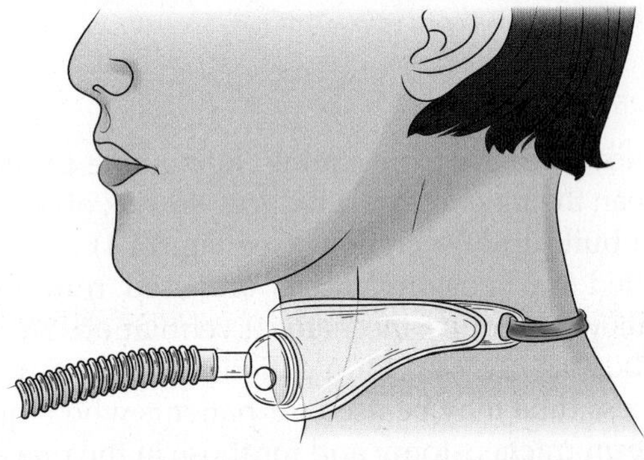

Fig. 14.7 Tracheostomy collar.

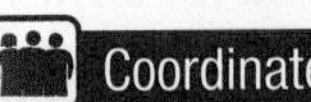

Coordinated Care

Collaboration

Suctioning a Tracheostomy

- The skill of suctioning, other than oropharyngeal suctioning, requires the critical thinking and knowledge of a nurse or other licensed health care professional.
- The task of oropharyngeal suctioning can be delegated to unlicensed assistive personnel (UAP), including the patient and family when appropriate. Check facility policy.
- In special situations, the task of performing a permanent tracheostomy tube suctioning can be delegated to UAP. These situations include those in which stable patients have a well-established permanent tracheostomy tube and patients are receiving mechanical ventilation at home.
- The nurse is responsible for evaluating the patient's airway **patency** (openness) and response to airway suctioning.

Skill 14.4 Care of the Patient With a T Tube or Tracheostomy Collar

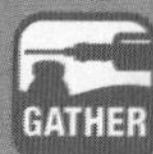

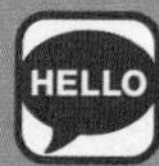

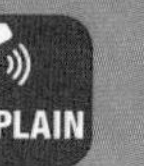

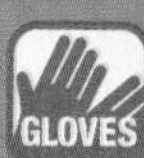

NURSING ACTION *(RATIONALE)*

1. Refer to Standard Steps 1 to 9.
2. Perform hand hygiene. *(Reduces transmission of microorganisms.)*
3. Position the patient for comfort, usually in a semi-Fowler's position. *(Helps patient relax and allows adequate access to tracheostomy and to T tube or tracheostomy collar.)*
4. Inspect the rate of flow and the solution level for humidification at regular intervals during the course of the patient's oxygen therapy. *(Ensures adequate oxygenation and humidification.)*
5. Provide nose and mouth care regularly during the course of the patient's therapy. *(Keeps the mucosa lubricated, moist, clean, and fresh.)*
6. Secure the collar or T piece at the neck over the tracheostomy. Make certain all tubing connections are secure. *(Prevents the T piece or collar from dislodging and depriving the patient of oxygen, humidification, or both.)*
7. Adjust the oxygen flow rate according to the health care provider's order. *(Provides adequate oxygenation for the patient.)*
8. Adjust the temperature of the humidified oxygen. *(Higher temperatures create more moisture and condensation.)*
9. Use large-lumen tubing from the oxygen source to the patient. *(Allows for adequate oxygenation and fewer complications from condensation.)*
10. Condensation occurs within the tracheostomy collar or T piece, so observe frequently. *(Too much condensation can create problems with oxygen delivery and cause respiratory distress in the patient.)*
11. The collar or T piece and tubing should be removed frequently to be drained and cleaned. *(Decreases risk of aspiration of the moisture and infection.)*
12. As moisture collects, suction the tracheostomy, and provide tracheostomy care as often as necessary. *(Helps to prevent excess moisture buildup and aspiration.)*
13. Make sure the nurse is always able to see the mist of the humidified oxygen. *(A visual way to determine whether the oxygen is being humidified.)*

Skill 14.5 Clearing the Airway

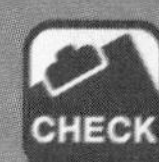

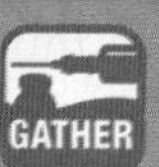

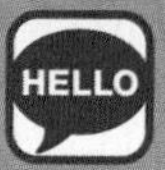

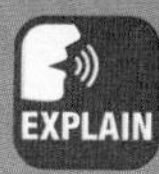

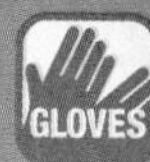

NURSING ACTION *(RATIONALE)*

1. Refer to Standard Steps 1 to 9.
2. Assemble equipment:
   - Appropriate suction catheter
   - Sterile gloves if not in kit
   - Clean gloves as indicated
   - Sterile equipment (suction kit)
   - Unsterile equipment (unsterile basin or cup)
   - Sterile water, or normal saline
   - Towel
   - Portable or wall suction apparatus
   - Connecting tubing
   - Face shield, if splashing is anticipated
3. Evaluate need for suctioning. *(Physical signs will indicate need for this procedure.)*
   - Gurgling respirations
   - Restlessness
   - Vomitus in mouth
   - Drooling
4. Explain procedure to the patient and that coughing, sneezing, or gagging is expected. *(Encourages patient's cooperation and reduces patient's anxiety.)*
5. Position patient.
   a. If patient is alert and conscious, place in semi-Fowler's position with head to one side. *(Promotes drainage of secretions.)*
   b. If patient is unconscious, place in side-lying position facing nurse. *(Promotes drainage of secretions.)*
      (1) Place towel lengthwise under patient's chin and over pillow. *(Protects bed linens from contamination.)*
6. Pour sterile normal saline solution into sterile container. *(For moistening and cleansing catheter.)*
7. Perform hand hygiene and don clean gloves. Turn on suction machine, and select appropriate

Continued

Skill 14.5 Clearing the Airway—cont'd

suction pressure. (Check facility policy.) Never suction with any more vacuum pressure than needed to remove the secretions, and use the smallest catheter that will remove the secretions well. *(Elevated pressure setting or using a too-large catheter increases risk of trauma to oral and nasal mucosa.)* Connect suction catheter to tubing.

a. Common vacuum settings for wall suction units:
  (1) Infants: 60 to 80 mm Hg
  (2) Children: 100 to 120 mm Hg
  (3) Adults: 120 to 150 mm Hg

b. Common catheter sizes:
  (1) Infant: 6-Fr to 8-Fr
  (2) Children: 10-Fr to 12-Fr
  (3) Adults: 12-Fr to 14-Fr

8. Suction solution through catheter by placing thumb over open end of connector or over vent. *(Enables the nurse to check patency of suction catheter and suction pressure and moistens catheter for ease of insertion.)*

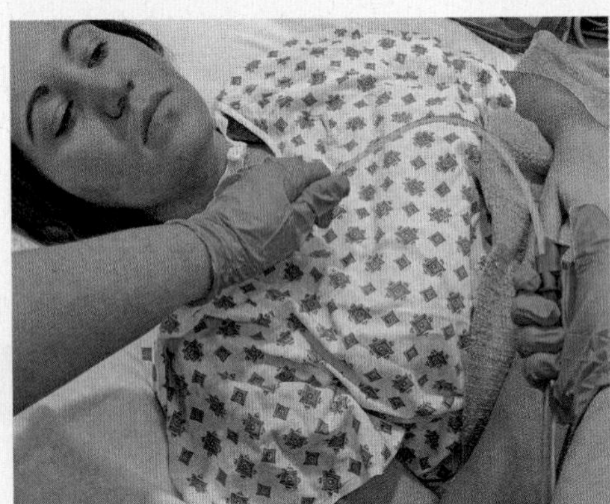

9. Remove thumb from open end of connector or vent, or pinch catheter with thumb and index finger if a continuous suction catheter is used. *(Stops suctioning and prevents injury to mucous membrane while catheter is being inserted.)*

10. Proceed with suctioning. (See specific suction guidelines.)

a. Oropharyngeal suctioning:
  (1) Don clean gloves if those are not already on. *(Prevents spread of microorganisms.)*
  (2) Gently insert Yankauer or tonsillar tip suction catheter into one side of mouth and glide it toward oropharynx without suction. *(Prevents tissue trauma.)*

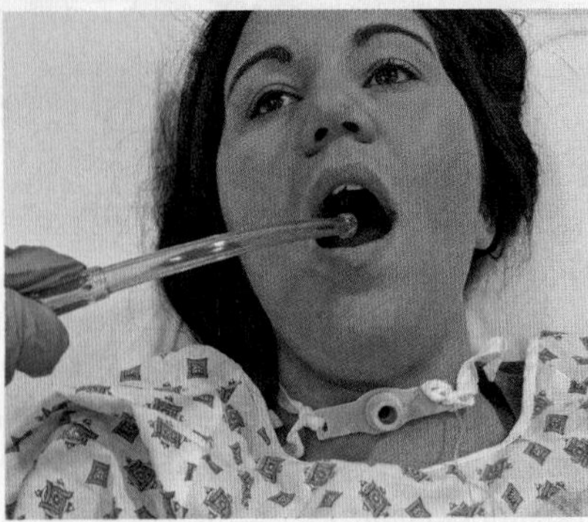

  (3) Move Yankauer or tonsillar tip catheter around mouth until secretions are cleared. *(Removes secretions without damaging tissue.)*
  (4) Encourage patient to cough. *(Moves secretions from lower airway into mouth and upper airway so that they can be suctioned.)*
  (5) Rinse Yankauer or tonsillar tip catheter with water in cup or basin until connecting tubing is cleared of secretions. Turn off suction. *(Rinses catheter and reduces probability of transmission of microorganisms.)*
  (6) Repeat procedure as necessary.

b. Nasopharyngeal suctioning:
  (1) Ask patient if either side of nose is obstructed; use unobstructed side. If patient is unable to answer this question cover one nostril and feel for air from the other nostril.
  (2) Open suction catheter kit and don sterile gloves. *(Prevents spread of microorganisms.)* Holding suction catheter with thumb and index finger, place nasal catheter near region between patient's earlobe and tip of nose. Do not touch side of face, nose, or earlobe. *(Marks correct length of catheter for insertion. Distance from earlobe to tip of nose approximates depth of insertion.)*
  Approximate length of insertion:
    (a) Adults: 16 cm
    (b) Older children: 8 to 12 cm
    (c) Infants and young children: 4 to 8 cm
  (3) Lubricate catheter with water-soluble jelly or dip the tip of the catheter into the sterile saline or water, depending on facility policy. *(Water-soluble lubricant dissolves, thus preventing possible buildup that could hinder airway. Lubricating catheter allows for easier insertion.)*

Skill 14.5 Clearing the Airway—cont'd

(4) Hold catheter angled up then downward with the anatomy of the nasopharyngeal area. Gently insert catheter into one side of nasal passage. *(Using the natural curvature of the catheter and gentleness facilitates easier and less traumatic insertion.)*

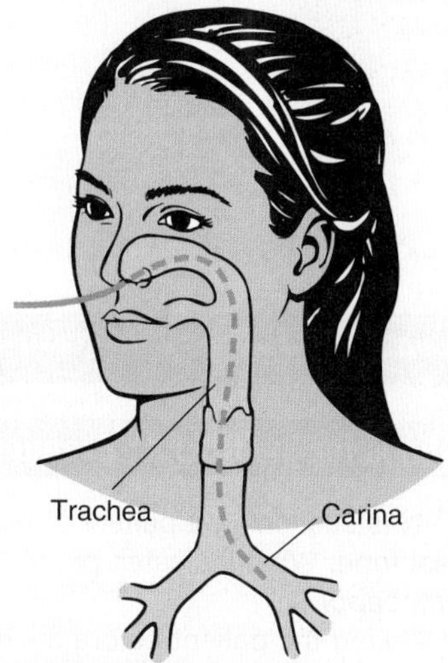

c. Nasotracheal suctioning:

(1) Ask patient if either side of nose is obstructed; use unobstructed side. If patient is unable to answer this question, cover one nostril and feel for air from the other nostril.

(2) Open suction catheter kit and don sterile gloves. Holding suction catheter with thumb and index finger, place nasotracheal catheter near region between earlobe to tip of nose and extend to trachea. Do not touch patient's side of face, nose, or earlobe. *(Maintains sterility. Marks correct length of catheter for insertion.)* Length of insertion:

(a) Adults: 20 to 24 cm
(b) Older children: 14 to 20 cm
(c) Young children and infants: 8 to 14 cm

(3) Lubricate catheter with a water-soluble jelly or dip the tip of the catheter into the sterile saline or water, depending on facility policy. *(Water-soluble lubricant dissolves, thus preventing possible buildup that could hinder airway. Lubricating catheter allows for easier insertion.)*

(4) Hold catheter angled up then downward with the anatomy of the nasopharyngeal area. Gently insert catheter into one side of nasal passage. *(Using the natural curvature of catheter and gentleness facilitates easier and less traumatic insertion.)*

(5) Stimulate coughing reflex, or ask patient to cough, to guide catheter into trachea. If no cough reflex is present or if patient is not able to assist, insert catheter when patient inhales (see illustration of Step 10b[4]). *(Helps prevent displacement of catheter into esophagus.)*

11. Apply intermittent suction by placing thumb over suction opening; withdraw catheter while rotating it gently. *(Intermittent suction and gentle rotation of the catheter prevents injury to mucosa.)*

12. Observe patient closely, and limit suction to 10 to 15 seconds. *(Suctioning longer than 10 to 15 seconds risks causing cardiopulmonary compromise.)*

13. Repeat suctioning if it is needed.

14. Allow 1 to 2 minutes of rest between suctioning if it is necessary to repeat procedure. If oxygen is administered by nasal cannula, mask, or other means, reapply oxygen during rest period. *(Provides rest and comfort and allows patient to regain oxygen supply. Time needed for patient to rest between suctioning varies, depending on patient's ability to tolerate procedure.)*

15. If patient is alert and is able to cooperate, instruct patient to breathe deeply and cough between suctioning attempts. *(Coughing moves secretions from lower airway into mouth and upper airway and allows them to be removed more easily.)*

16. When suctioning of catheter is complete, suction between cheeks and gum line and under tongue; suction mouth last to prevent contaminating catheter. *(Ensures that all secretions have been removed.)*

17. Place catheter in solution and apply suction. *(Flushes secretions from catheter and tubing to maintain patency in the event it is necessary to repeat procedure.)*

18. Discard catheter and used suction catheters: wrap catheter around gloved hand; pull glove off hand and over catheter. Remove face shield, if worn. Perform hand hygiene. *(Reduces the transmission of microorganisms and prevents direct contact with equipment and secretions.)*

19. Place sterile, unopened catheter at patient's bedside. *(Provides quick access to suction equipment if patient needs suctioning immediately.)*

20. Provide mouth care. *(Promotes patient comfort.)*

21. Evaluate patient's breathing patterns, fatigue, vital signs, level of consciousness, and color. Determine whether patient has a decrease in anxiety. *(Identifies successful suctioning attempt and patient's response to suction procedure.)*

Continued

Skill 14.5 Clearing the Airway—cont'd

22. Refer to Standard Steps 10 to 17.
23. Document the following. *(Verifies performance of procedure and ensures continuity of care.)*
- Date
- Time
- Method of suctioning
- Amount, consistency, color, and odor of secretions
- Respiratory assessment before and after procedure
- Patient's response
- Patient teaching

Get Ready for the NCLEX® Examination!

Key Points

- Oxygen therapy improves tissue oxygenation. Delivery devices include, but are not limited to, nasal cannulas, nasal catheter, and various types of oxygen masks.
- Teaching the patient effective coughing techniques and the implementation of suctioning will help keep the patient's airway patent.
- The Venturi mask offers a precise concentration of oxygen and is used for patients requiring a more controlled concentration of oxygen.
- Safety precautions must be followed in the clinical setting and in the home setting.
- Hypoxia signs and symptoms include neurologic changes, changes in vital signs, cardiac dysrhythmias, and changes in the color of the mucous membranes. Early and later signs of hypoxia differ.
- COPD patients require a lower concentration of oxygen therapy to not suppress their respiratory center.
- Endotracheal tubes are used for short-term airway maintenance.
- Tracheostomy is used for long-term airway maintenance.
- Tracheostomy tubes may be cuffed or noncuffed, depending on the patient's need.
- Tracheostomy care and suctioning can be performed by the nurse, or by the patient or caregivers.
- Tracheostomy care and suctioning requires sterile technique.
- The tracheostomy collar is used to supply oxygen to a patient with a tracheostomy.
- The Yankaur suction catheter is used to perform oropharyngeal suctioning.

Additional Learning Resources

SG Go to your Study Guide for additional learning activities to help you master this chapter content.

evolve Be sure to visit the Evolve site at *http://evolve.elsevier.com/Cooper/foundationsadult/* for additional online resources.

Review Questions for the NCLEX® Examination

1. The LPN/LVN is suctioning a patient through an endotracheal tube. What indicates proper technique? *(Select all that apply.)*
   1. Preoxygenating the patient before suctioning
   2. Dipping the suction catheter into sterile saline before suctioning
   3. Using a clean catheter with each suctioning attempt
   4. Withdrawing the catheter with the thumb continually covering the suction control vent
   5. Suctioning the tube for at least 30 seconds with each suctioning attempt

2. A patient's physician told the patient that she was suffering from hypoxia. The patient asks the nurse what that means. Which statement by the nurse is most accurate?
   1. "Hypoxia means that there is a deficient amount of oxygen in your blood."
   2. "It would be best if you asked your physician to explain hypoxia."
   3. "There is too much carbon dioxide in your blood."
   4. "Hypoxia means that the cells in your body's tissues are not receiving enough oxygen."

3. What is the maximum time suction should be applied during nasotracheal suctioning?
   1. 15 seconds
   2. 20 seconds
   3. 30 seconds
   4. 45 seconds

4. If a patient's condition requires a very precise delivery of oxygen concentration, the nurse anticipates that the health care provider will order oxygen to be delivered via which device?
   1. Venturi mask
   2. Simple face mask
   3. Nasal cannula
   4. Transtracheal cannula

5. A patient is being discharged to home with an order for oxygen. The order reads, "Continuous O_2 at 2 L per N/C." What is the best explanation of this order for the nurse to give the patient?
   1. "You will have oxygen on 24 hours a day at home by use of a nasal cannula, with the flow meter set at 2 liters."
   2. "You will need to wear your oxygen during the hours you are awake since your body uses more oxygen during the day. Your order is for 2 liters by nasal cannula."
   3. "Your doctor has ordered oxygen for you to use at home to keep your blood oxygen levels at a good level."
   4. "You will need to wear oxygen at home whenever you are feeling short of breath. Be sure to set your flowmeter at 2 liters and use your nasal cannula."
6. The home health nurse is visiting a patient who is on home oxygen therapy. What action by the patient and family members alerts the nurse that further teaching about home oxygen therapy is necessary? *(Select all that apply.)*
   1. The nurse notes a fire extinguisher in the kitchen.
   2. The patient's brother-in-law is in a separate room smoking a cigarette.
   3. The patient states that when shaving an electrical razor is used.
   4. The patient is using a water-soluble gel to help with lubricating dry mucous membranes.
   5. The oxygen tubing is coiled and secured with a rubber band to prevent the patient from tripping over the tubing.
7. The nurse encourages the patient to drink an adequate amount of fluids to help with dry mucous membranes and to liquefy secretions. What fluids should the nurse include in this teaching? *(Select all that apply.)*
   1. Coffee
   2. Milk
   3. Water
   4. Juice
   5. Tea
8. The nurse is reviewing the arterial partial pressure of oxygen (PaO_2) level on the patient's arterial blood gas report. Which level is most concerning to the nurse?
   1. PaO_2 75 mm Hg
   2. PaO_2 80 mm Hg
   3. PaO_2 85 mm Hg
   4. PaO_2 90 mm Hg
9. The home health care nurse is observing the patient while he is filling the humidifier bottle attached to the oxygen tank. Which action by the patient demonstrates knowledge of this procedure?
   1. The patient fills the bottle with distilled water.
   2. The patient fills the bottle with tap water.
   3. The patient fills the bottle sterile normal saline.
   4. The patient fills the bottle with spring water.
10. The nurse observes the student nurse suction the patient with a tracheostomy. Which action by the student nurse requires the nurse to intervene? *(Select all that apply.)*
    1. The student preoxygenates the patient before beginning suctioning.
    2. The student suctions the patient for 30 seconds during each suctioning attempt.
    3. The student uses tap water to clear the catheter tubing between suction attempts.
    4. The student applies intermittent suction when withdrawing the suction catheter from the airway.
    5. The student places the thumb over the suction control vent when advancing the catheter into the patient's airway.
11. The health care provider has ordered oxygen at 100% via a nonrebreathing mask. The nurse evaluates that the mask is working properly when making which observation?
    1. The reservoir bag collapses 50% when the patient inhales.
    2. The reservoir bag collapses completely when the patient inhales.
    3. The reservoir bag remains nearly full when the patient inhales.
    4. The reservoir bag inflates when the patient inhales.
12. The nurse is preparing to perform tracheostomy care and suctioning. What is the best order of actions when performing these two procedures? Place the steps in the correct order.
    1. The nurse performs tracheostomy suctioning.
    2. The nurse changes the tracheostomy ties/strap.
    3. The nurse changes the dressing around the tracheostomy.
    4. The nurse cleans around the tracheostomy with prescribed solution.
13. The nurse has just performed oropharyngeal suctioning. Which documentation is the most complete after this procedure?
    1. "Suctioned patient using a Yankaur suction catheter. Large amount of mucus suctioned. Patient tolerated procedure well and is breathing better."
    2. "Performed oropharyngeal suctioning using Yankaur suction catheter. Moderate amount of thick green, odorless, mucus suctioned. Tolerated procedure well and respirations are nonlabored."
    3. "Oropharyngeal suctioning performed due to patient being unable to expectorate secretions. Used Yankaur suction catheter to perform procedure. Patient breathing better following suctioning."
    4. "Patient requiring suctioning. Oropharyngeal suctioning performed. Patient unable to cough up thick mucus. Breathing improved after suctioning. Used a Yankaur suction catheter for procedure."

14. The health care provider has ordered a patient diagnosed with pneumonia to have oxygen via a simple face mask. The nurse is aware that the patient will be receiving a FiO_2 of what percentage depending on the flowmeter setting?
    1. 24%–44%
    2. 35%–55%
    3. 24%–55%
    4. 60%–90%

15. The nurse is assessing a patient who is displaying early signs of hypoxia. What signs and symptoms will the nurse observe? *(Select all that apply.)*
    1. Restlessness
    2. Increased pulse rate
    3. Decreased blood pressure
    4. Irregular apical pulse
    5. Dyspnea

Elimination and Gastric Intubation

15

http://evolve.elsevier.com/Cooper/foundationsadult/

Objectives

1. Discuss management of the patient with an indwelling catheter or urinary diversion:
   - Male catheterization
   - Female catheterization
   - Discontinuing an indwelling catheter
   - Catheter irrigation
2. Explain the procedure for external and internal vaginal irrigation (douche).
3. Explain nursing interventions for the patient with nasogastric intubation.
4. Discuss gastric and intestinal suctioning care.
5. Describe the procedure for nasogastric tube removal.
6. Identify the procedures for promoting bowel elimination:
   - Administering an enema
   - Inserting a rectal tube
   - Removing a fecal impaction
7. Describe nursing care necessary to maintain structure and function of a bowel diversion.
8. Discuss the need for and nursing care necessary to maintain an ostomy.

Key Terms

bladder training (BLĂD-ŭr TRĀ-nĭng, p. 372)
catheterization (kă-thĕ-tŭr-ĭ-ZĀ-shŭn, p. 361)
colostomy (kŏl-ŎS-tō-mē, p. 383)
defecation (dĕf-ĕ-KĀ-shŭn, p. 379)
dumping syndrome (DŬMP-ĭng SĬN-drōm, p. 375)
enema (ĔN-ŭ-mŭ, p. 382)
fecal impaction (FĒ-căl ĭm-PĂK-shŭn, p. 382)
flatulence (FLĂCH-yū-lĕns, p. 382)
ileostomy (ĭl-ē-ŎS-tō-mē, p. 383)
incontinence (ĭn-KŎN-tĭ-nĕns, p. 370)
irrigation (ĭr-ĭ-GĀ-shŭn, p. 361)
nasogastric (NG) tube (nā-zō-GĂS-trĭk TŪB, p. 373)
ostomy (ŎS-tō-mē, p. 383)
urinary catheter (YŪ-rĭn-ăr-ē KĂ-thĕ-tŭr, p. 361)
urostomy (yŭr-ŎS-tō-mē, p. 383)

Elimination includes the urinary system and the gastrointestinal system. Elimination is essential for the body to function properly. Both systems help the body detoxify and eliminate waste products. Disease, tumors, surgery, medications, or trauma may interfere with normal elimination. When elimination is interrupted, certain procedures may be ordered by the health care provider.

An accurate and thorough assessment of the urinary and gastrointestinal systems (see Chapter 13) is necessary when implementing ordered procedures to determine the effectiveness of the treatment ordered. Knowledge of these systems and related disorders (see *Adult Health Nursing,* Chapters 5 and 10) also help the nurse to care for the patient.

Nasogastric intubation procedures also are discussed in this chapter because they involve the gastrointestinal system. Insertion of a nasogastric tube, procedures involving a nasogastric tube, and care of a nasogastric tube are discussed. Mastering these skills is necessary for the nurse to provide competent care for the patient.

STANDARD STEPS IN SELECTED SKILLS

To ensure patient safety, as well as nurse safety, during nursing procedures involving elimination and gastric intubation, it is important to understand the steps involved in specific skills. The skill boxes in this chapter list those steps for a variety of nursing procedures. Certain steps performed before and after every procedure are listed in the next section. The skill boxes that follow refer to them as *Standard Steps.* These steps must be followed before and after every procedure to provide the patient with safe, effective nursing care.

BEFORE THE PROCEDURE

The rationales for these steps are listed in italics in parentheses.

1. Check the health care provider's order and review facility policy. *(Provides basis for care. Many nursing interventions require a health care provider's order. Verification is essential before any procedure is begun.)*
2. Introduce yourself to the patient; include your name and title or role. *(Decreases patient anxiety and aids in establishing rapport with the patient.)*
3. Identify the patient by checking his or her identification bracelet and requesting that the patient state his or her name or birth date, or both. *(Ensures that procedure is performed on correct patient.)*
4. Explain the procedure and the reason it is to be done in terms that the patient is able to understand. Advise the patient of any unpleasantness that may be involved with the procedure. Give the patient time to ask questions. *(Promotes cooperation, decreases patient's anxiety, and prepares patient. Also helps determine whether procedure is still appropriate.)*
5. Determine need for and provide patient education before and during procedure. *(Promotes patient's independence and compliance.)*
6. Evaluate the patient. Each skill box contains an assessment section that includes specific data to evaluate. *(Provides baseline information for later comparisons.)*
7. Perform hand hygiene and don clean gloves according to agency policy and guidelines from the Centers for Disease Control and Prevention (CDC) and the Occupational Safety and Health Administration (OSHA) (see Chapter 7). *(Reduces the spread of microorganisms and protects the patient and the nurse.)*
8. Assemble equipment, and complete necessary charges. Each skill box lists the specific equipment required. *(Organizes procedure so that it will go more smoothly. Some equipment is reusable and is kept at the patient's bedside. Some of the equipment is disposable and charged to the patient when used. Know agency policy.)*
9. Prepare the patient for the procedure:
   a. Close the door or pull the privacy curtain around the patient's bed. *(Provides privacy and promotes patient comfort.)*
   b. Raise the bed to a comfortable working height, and lower the side rail on the side nearest the nurse. *(Promotes proper body mechanics by minimizing nurse's muscle strain and preventing injury and fatigue.)*
   c. Position and drape the patient as necessary. Descriptions of specific positions are included in each skill. *(Shows respect for patient's privacy and dignity.)*

DURING THE PROCEDURE

10. Promote patient involvement as much as possible. *(Participation encourages the patient's cooperation and increases patient's knowledge of condition and care. It also may increase patient's sense of independence and importance and increase patient's compliance with treatment.)*
11. Determine the patient's tolerance of the procedure, being alert for signs and symptoms of discomfort and fatigue. If the patient cannot tolerate a procedure, describe this inability in the nursing notes. *(Patient's ability to tolerate interventions varies, depending on severity of illness and disability. It is necessary to determine when to provide the patient with an opportunity to rest and when to provide comfort measures.)*

AFTER THE PROCEDURE

12. Assist the patient to a position of comfort, and place needed items within easy reach. Ensure that the patient has a means to call for help and knows how to use it. *(Promotes comfort and safety. Patients often try to reach items and risk falling or injury.)*
13. Raise the side rails, and lower the bed to the lowest position. *(This minimizes the patient's risk in getting out of bed unattended. Use nursing judgment and facility policy to safely allow alert, cooperative patients have their side rails down.)*
14. Remove gloves and all protective barriers such as gown, goggles, and masks. Store appropriately or discard. Remove and dispose of soiled supplies and equipment according to agency policy and guidelines from the CDC and OSHA. *(Reduces spread of microorganisms, maintains cleanliness of environment, and enhances patient comfort and safety.)*
15. Perform hand hygiene after removing gloves. *(Wearing gloves does not eliminate the need to perform hand hygiene. Hand hygiene is the most important technique for preventing and controlling the spread of microorganisms.)*
16. Document the patient's response to the procedure, expected or unexpected outcomes, and all patient teaching. Specific areas of documentation are indicated in each skill box. *(Timely and accurate documentation is legally required, records patient's progress, and promotes continuity of care.)*
17. Report any unexpected outcomes. Specific notes for reporting unexpected outcomes are included in each skill. *(Additional procedures or treatments may be necessary.)*

SKILLS FOR URINARY TRACT PROCEDURES

URINARY ELIMINATION

Urinary elimination is a natural process that clears the body of waste material and helps maintain electrolyte balance. Therefore conditions that interfere with urinary function have the potential to create a health crisis. The urinary tract can be affected by a problem with the kidneys, the ureters, the bladder, the urethra, or surrounding organs. It is also very susceptible to infection.

Neurologic deficits also may lead to problems with the urinary system.

Patients at risk for problems with urine elimination include those who have undergone surgical procedures of the bladder, the prostate, or the vagina; patients with primary urologic problems, such as urethral stricture or tumor; neurologic trauma; and those who are critically ill with multisystem problems. When there is a problem with the urinary system, the health care provider often orders a urinary catheter to be inserted to monitor urinary output and the urinary system. Most often the nurse caring for the patient is responsible for inserting and monitoring the catheter and output (see the Coordinated Care box).

Coordinated Care

Delegation

Urinary Catheterization

- Urinary catheterization is a task that can be delegated to unlicensed assistive personnel (UAP) in some settings (check facility policy). In some facilities, first-time catheterization, catheterization of patients in an acute care setting, or catheterization of patients with urethral trauma requires the critical thinking and knowledge of a nurse, and delegation of this task to UAP is inappropriate.
- The task of removing a urinary catheter can be delegated to UAP in some facilities; however, patient evaluation and teaching must be performed by the nurse. After removal of the catheter, instruct UAP to measure amount of urine in patient's first voiding and to report time and amount to the nurse.
- It is acceptable to delegate the task of obtaining urine specimens from a catheter to UAP in some settings (check facility policy). Initial patient evaluation and coordination of repeated specimens require the knowledge of a nurse, and delegation of this task to UAP is inappropriate.
- The skill of catheter irrigation requires knowledge of a nurse. Delegation of this task to UAP is inappropriate.
- The skill of caring for a newly established suprapubic catheter requires the knowledge of a nurse. Delegation of this task to UAP is inappropriate.

Urinary Catheters

Most urinary catheters are made of soft plastic or rubber and can be used for treatment and diagnosis. Urinary catheters are used to maintain urine flow, to divert urine flow to facilitate healing postoperatively, to introduce medications by **irrigation,** and to dilate or prevent narrowing of some portions of the urinary tract. Catheters are used for intermittent and continuous urinary drainage. Urinary catheters can be placed in the bladder, the ureter, or the kidney. **Catheterization** of the bladder, which is usually the responsibility of the nurse, involves introducing a rubber or plastic tube (a **urinary catheter**) through the urinary meatus and the urethra into the urinary bladder. Catheterizing the ureters or kidneys

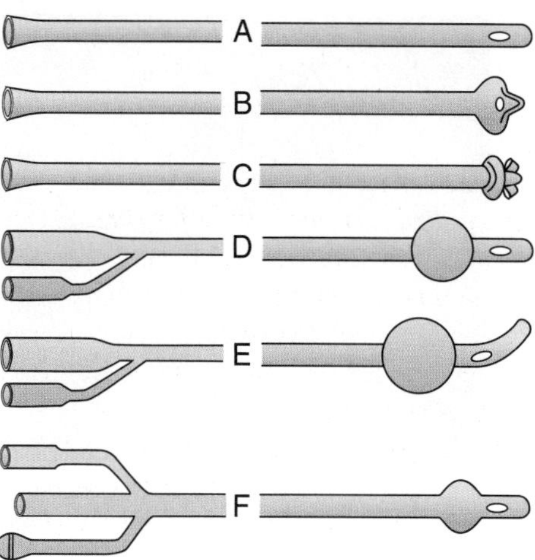

Fig. 15.1 Different types of commonly used urinary catheters. A, Simple urethral catheter. B, Mushroom, or de Pezzer, catheter (can be used for suprapubic catheterization). C, Winged-tip, or Malecot, catheter. D, Indwelling catheter with inflated balloon. E, Indwelling catheter with coudé tip, or Tiemann catheter. F, Three-way indwelling catheter (the third lumen is used for irrigation of the bladder).

is the responsibility of the health care provider. Catheters are measured by the French (Fr) system and range in size from 14-Fr to 24-Fr for adult patients.

Types of Catheters

Several types of catheters are used for different purposes (Fig. 15.1). The type and size of urinary catheter used are determined by the location being catheterized and the cause of the urinary tract problem. The coudé catheter has a tapered tip and is used when enlargement of the prostate gland is suspected. The curved stylet of the coudé catheter is used to assist the health care provider in the insertion of a urethral catheter in a male patient with prostate enlargement. The Foley catheter has a balloon near its tip that is inflated after insertion to hold the catheter in the urinary bladder for continuous drainage. Malecot and de Pezzer (mushroom) catheters are used to drain urine from the renal pelvis of the kidney, and the Robinson catheter has multiple openings in its tip to facilitate intermittent drainage. Catheters designed to be inserted into the ureters are long and slender to pass into the ureters more easily. In patients with blood in their urine, a whistle-tip catheter may be used because it has a slanted, larger orifice at its tip. The cystostomy, the vesicostomy, or the suprapubic catheter is inserted through the abdominal wall above the symphysis pubis to create a urinary diversion in cases of obstruction, strictures, or injury to the bony pelvis, the urinary tract, or surrounding organs. The catheter is inserted surgically, is connected to a sterile closed drainage system, and is secured to avoid accidental removal; the wound is covered with a sterile dressing. When the lower urinary tract has healed, the patient's ability to void is tested, and when the patient's residual urine is low enough, according to the health care provider, the catheter can be removed. Sometimes,

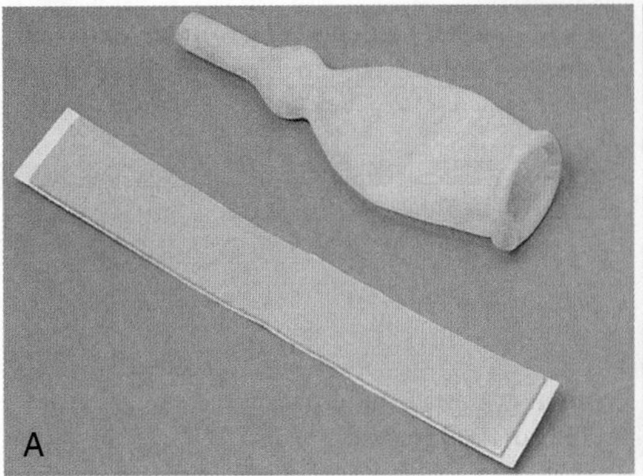

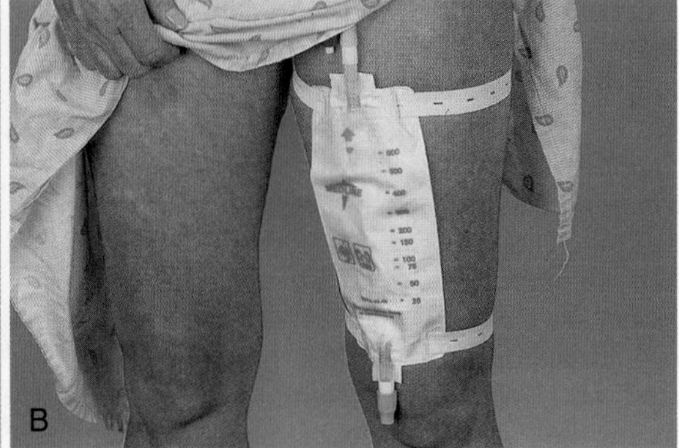

Fig. 15.2 A, Condom catheter. B, Condom catheter attached to leg bag. (From Elkin MK, Perry AG, Potter PA: *Nursing interventions and clinical skills*, ed 4, St. Louis, 2008, Mosby.)

the problem causing the need for a suprapubic catheter is permanent, and the catheter is left in place.

Another form of urinary drainage system that many refer to as a catheter is the condom, or Texas, catheter. This device is not a catheter but rather a drainage system connected to the external male genitalia (Fig. 15.2). This noninvasive appliance is used for incontinent men to minimize skin irritation from urine. One drawback to using this device is that it can become too constrictive. It is therefore important to remove the appliance daily for cleansing and inspection of the skin. Use of the external condom catheter allows for a more normal lifestyle for the patient and limits the risk for infection that an indwelling catheter may cause.

Nursing Interventions

Nursing interventions for the patient with a urinary drainage system are aimed at early detection and prevention of infection and trauma (Fig. 15.3 and see Skills 15.1, 15.2, and 15.3). When caring for urinary drainage systems, take the following actions:

1. Follow aseptic technique when inserting the catheter, and keep the collecting bag off the floor. This prevents the introduction of microorganisms into the body from the environment (Fig. 15.4).
2. Record fluid intake and urinary output (I&O), and check the drainage system for proper placement and function regularly (Fig. 15.5). For precision monitoring, such as hourly urine output, add a urometer to the drainage system.
3. Encourage the patient to drink plenty of fluids to flush the urinary tract.
4. Do not open the drainage system after it is in place except to irrigate the catheter, and then only with a specific order from the health care provider. It is important to maintain a closed system to prevent urinary infections (Fig. 15.6).
5. Perform catheter care twice daily and as needed, according to standard precautions (see Skill 15.2). Inspect insertion site for blood or exudate that could indicate infection or trauma.

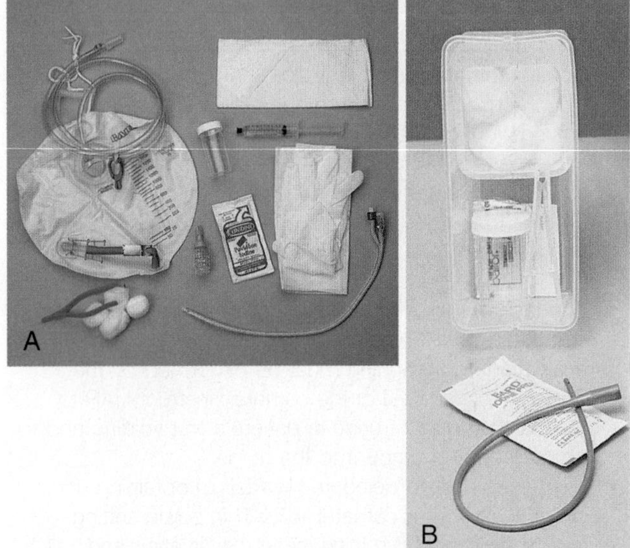

Fig. 15.3 A, Urinary drainage device, sterile specimen cup, sterile drape, sterile gloves, indwelling catheter, sterile cleanser, sterile saline, and sterile cotton balls with forceps. B, Catheter kit with straight catheter and iodine cleanser used for an indwelling catheter placement. (From Elkin MK, Perry AG, Potter PA: *Nursing interventions and clinical skills*, ed 4, St. Louis, 2008, Mosby.)

6. Check the drainage system daily for leaks. Know facility policy on replacing the system. Observe characteristics of the urine, noting blood or sediment. Note odor when draining collection bag.
7. Avoid placing the urinary drainage bag above the level of the catheter insertion. This will cause urine to reenter the drainage system and contaminate the urinary tract (see Fig. 15.4).
8. Secure the catheter to the patient to prevent tension on the system or backflow of urine.
9. Have the patient ambulate, if possible, to facilitate urine flow. If it is necessary to restrict the patient's activity, turn and reposition patient every 2 hours.
10. Avoid kinks or compression of the drainage tube to prevent pooling of urine within the system. Gently

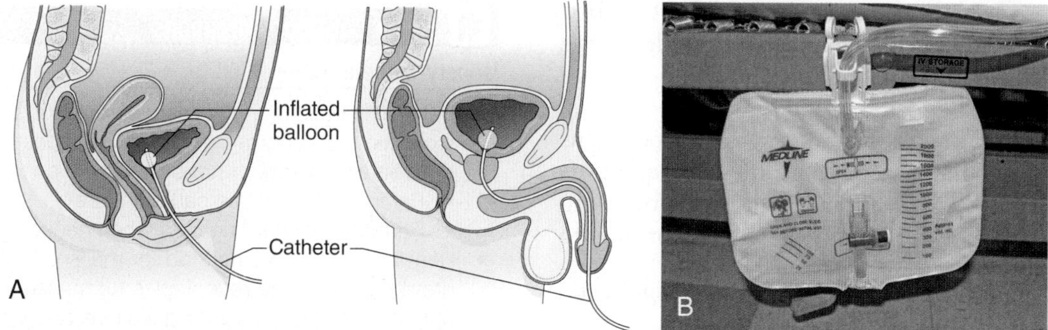

Fig. 15.4 Urinary drainage system. A, Balloon inflation in male and female patients. B, It is essential to keep drainage system below the level of the bladder. Do not place bag on side rails or allow it to rest on the floor. Attach drainage bag to bed or, while patient is ambulating, to intravenous pole.

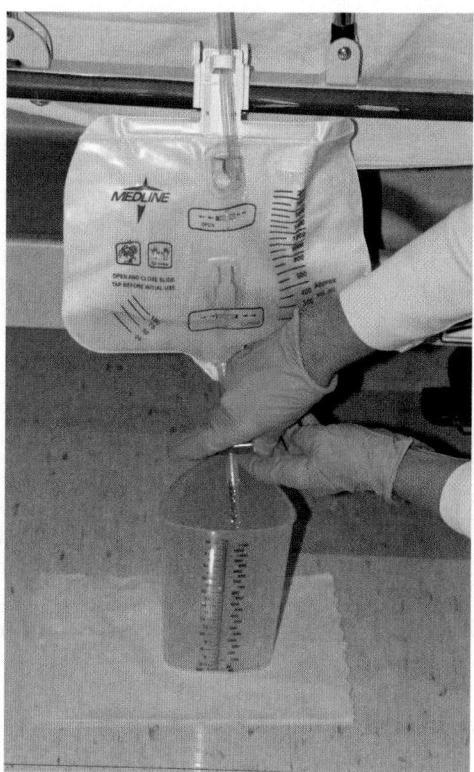

Fig. 15.5 Empty and record urine output from Foley catheter into clean graduated container. Clean the drainage port before draining and before recapping.

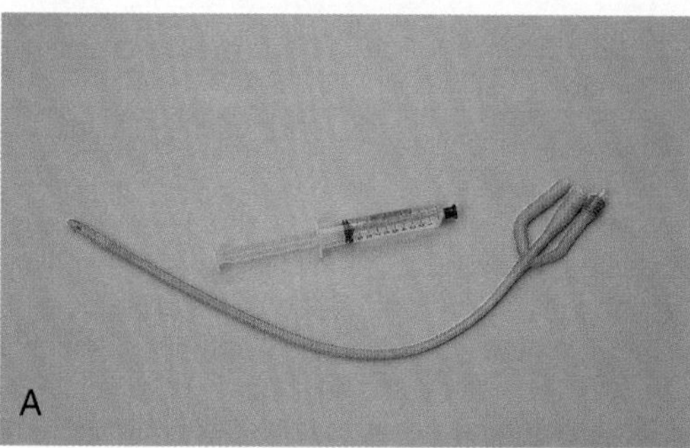

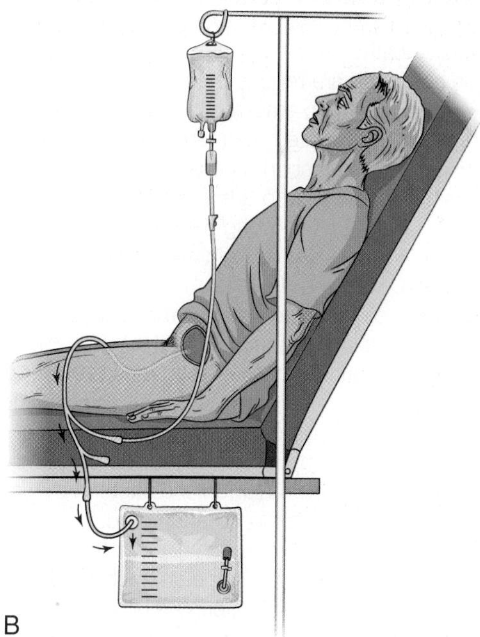

Fig. 15.6 Bladder irrigation. A, Triple-lumen catheter with sterile syringe to inflate catheter balloon. Note the port for inflating the balloon. B, Continuous sterile bladder irrigation setup. (A from Elkin MK, Perry AG, Potter PA: *Nursing interventions and clinical skills,* ed 4, St. Louis, 2008, Mosby.)

coil excess tubing and secure to the bottom bed linens with a clamp or pin to avoid dislodging the catheter. Remember to release the tubing before transferring or repositioning the patient.

11. When urine specimens are ordered, collect specimens from the catheter by cleansing the drainage port with alcohol, then withdrawing the urine by using a sterile needle and 10-mL syringe according to standard precautions.
12. Be sensitive to the patient's feelings regarding the catheter and the constant drainage from the system, and answer patient's questions and concerns when presented (see the Lifespan Considerations for older adults box on catheterization and the Home Care Considerations box on urinary catheter care).

Lifespan Considerations

Older Adults

Catheterization

- A patient with a catheter is especially vulnerable to urinary tract infections. Older adult patients who are physically compromised run the additional risk of developing septicemia, a potentially life-threatening infection that has spread to the blood. Therefore do not routinely catheterize an older patient who is incontinent.
- Encourage adequate oral fluid intake of at least 2000 mL/day, and assist the older adult to the bathroom on a regular, timed basis. This will help with bladder retraining and may prevent the need for excessive catheterization.
- When catheters are required, an older adult may be more cautious when ambulating. Encourage as much ambulation as tolerated, and remove the urinary drainage device as soon as possible.
- Suggest to patients who are at home or in long-term care that they use a leg bag during the day and switch to a large-volume bag at night so that sleep is not interrupted.
- Intermittent self-catheterization may be an option for some patients at home or in long-term care facilities. Discuss this option with the health care provider. Self-catheterization can be successful in maintaining continence and may enable more independence.
- External catheters may work well for patients with prostatic obstruction. An internal catheter may cause prostate trauma if insertion is attempted.
- Carefully evaluate patients with neuropathy before application of an external catheter; such patients may require more frequent monitoring related to the tissue damage that could occur.
- If a condom catheter is used on an older person, close monitoring is necessary. The skin of an older patient is frail and delicate, and the adhesive used on the condom catheter could damage the skin.

After the urinary catheter is removed, some patients may have difficulty voiding as a result of poor bladder tone and decreased sensation. If the patient complains of urinary retention, try stimulating urination by running water, placing the patient's hands in warm water, or pouring warm water over the perineum. Female patients should be encouraged to sit on a bathroom stool or commode and male patients to stand to void. Some patients may experience some dribbling of urine after voiding as a result of dilation of the sphincter from the catheter. Such patients should be reassured that this is normal and should improve as sphincter tone improves. Record the time of urination, the amount of urine output, and the color of the urine.

Home Care Considerations

Urinary Catheter Care

- Determine patient and primary caregiver's ability and motivation to perform the following actions:
  - Maintain accurate records of intake and output (I&O)
  - Participate in routine catheter care
  - Perform catheter irrigation when necessary
- Demonstrate proper method for measuring I&O, and provide appropriate receptacles for measuring urinary output if needed. Allow for questions and return demonstrations.
- Instruct on appropriate catheter care (see Skill 15.2).
- Teach signs and symptoms of urinary tract infection:
  - Urgency
  - Frequency
  - Hesitancy
  - Burning sensation
  - Bladder spasms
- Disposable supplies are best. If it is necessary to reuse catheters, teach patient and primary caregiver to boil rubber catheters 20 minutes and wrap in clean cloth.
- Teach catheterization techniques if necessary (see Skill 15.1).
- Evaluate patient's environment for appropriate space to store required materials and to perform procedure.
- Consult with health care provider for a home care agency referral for follow-up and to reinforce teaching concepts.

Self-Catheterization

Self-catheterization is a potential option for the patient who has had a spinal cord injury or other neurologic disorders that interfere with urinary elimination. Intermittent self-catheterization promotes independence for the patient and eliminates the need for an indwelling urinary drainage system. In the home, there are fewer foreign microorganisms and therefore less risk of cross-contamination. For this reason, it is possible to perform the catheterization procedure with clean technique rather than sterile technique. It is necessary to instruct the patient to be alert for signs of infection, and the patient should be encouraged to have periodic evaluations by the health care provider.

Routine Catheter Care

Routine catheter care is an important aspect of an indwelling urinary drainage system. Patients should receive routine catheter care and perineal hygiene at

Skill 15.1 Catheterization: Male and Female Patients

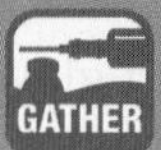

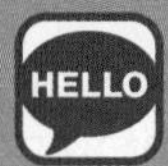

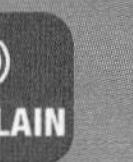

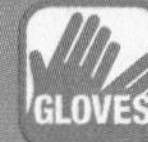

NURSING ACTION *(RATIONALE)*

1. Refer to Standard Steps 1 to 9.
2. Assemble equipment:
   - Sterile Foley catheterization or straight catheterization tray:
     - Antiseptic cleansing unit
     - Bed protector
     - Catheter of correct size and type for procedure
     - Cotton balls and pickup forceps
     - Drape
     - Lubricant
     - Prefilled syringe of sterile water
     - Receptacle or basin (usually bottom of catheterization tray)
     - Safety pins
     - Specimen container (optional)
     - Sterile drainage tubing and collection bag
     - Sterile gloves (may not be included in tray)
     - Tape
   - Light (flashlight or penlight)
   - Bath blanket
   - Disposable gloves, basin of warm water, soap, towel, and disposable washcloth
3. Determine the following. *(Enables the nurse to determine need for procedure and special interventions.)*
   a. When patient last voided
   b. Patient's level of awareness
   c. Mobility and physical limitation of patient
   d. Patient's sex and age
   e. Whether patient's bladder is distended
   f. Presence of any pathologic conditions that are likely to impair passage of catheter (especially enlarged prostate gland in men)
   g. Allergies (to antiseptic [iodine], tape, rubber, and lubricant)
   h. Patient's knowledge of the purpose of catheterization
4. Arrange for extra nursing personnel to assist if needed. *(Patients are not always able to assume positioning for procedure.)*
5. Position patient.
   a. Male patient: Supine position with thighs slightly abducted. *(Allows relaxation of muscles and easy access to urinary meatus.)*
   b. Female patient: Supine position with knees flexed and about 2 feet apart (see illustration). *(Allows relaxation of muscles and easy access to urinary meatus.)*

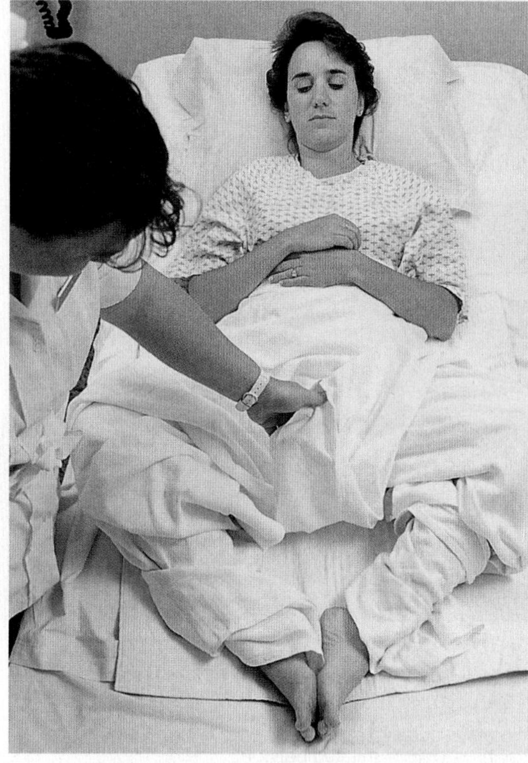

6. Drape patient with bath blanket, covering upper body and shaping over both knees and legs but leaving genital area exposed. *(Prepares patient for procedure and provides for patient's privacy.)*
7. Place waterproof absorbent pad under patient's buttocks. *(Protects bed linens.)*
8. Arrange supplies and equipment on bedside table. Provide a good light. *(Easy access prevents possible contamination.)*
9. Don clean gloves, and wash perineal area with mild soap and warm water. *(Decreases microorganisms at the site.)*
10. Remove disposable gloves, and place them in proper receptacle. *(Reduces the spread of microorganisms.)*
11. Facing patient, stand on left side of bed if right-handed (on right side if left-handed). *(Successful catheter insertion requires the nurse to assume comfortable position with all equipment close by.)*
12. Open packaging with the use of sterile technique. Don sterile gloves. *(Allows the nurse to handle sterile supplies without contamination and decreases spread of microorganisms.)*

Continued

Skill 15.1 Catheterization: Male and Female Patients—cont'd

13. If indwelling catheter is used, test balloon by injecting normal saline or sterile water into balloon lumen until balloon is inflated; then aspirate saline or sterile water out of balloon. *(Determines integrity of balloon. If balloon fails to inflate, obtain another sterile catheter. This step is omitted if the manufacturer indicates that balloon testing has already occurred before shipment of the equipment.)*

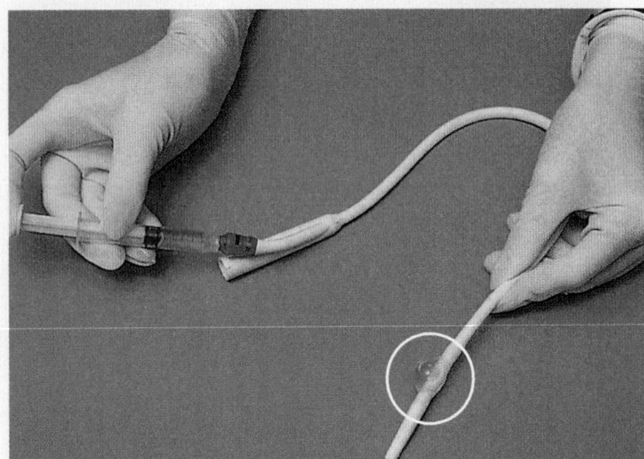

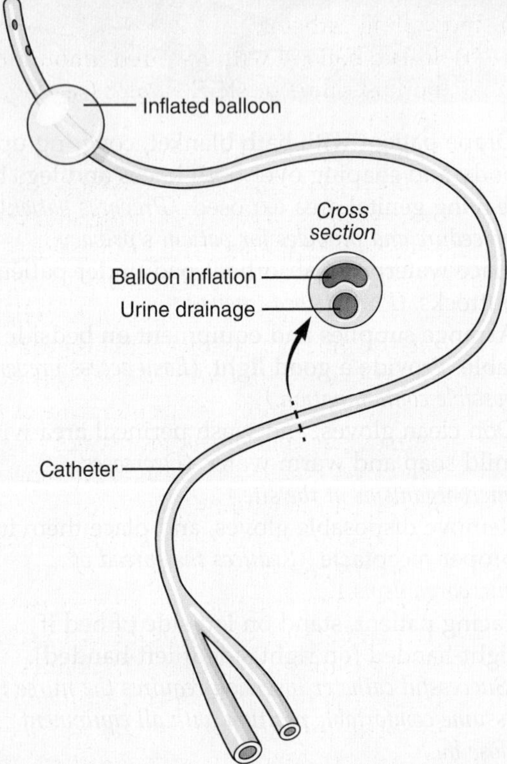

14. Add antiseptic to cotton balls; open lubricant container. Lubricate catheter approximately 1.5 to 2 inches (3.5 to 5 cm) for female patient and approximately 6 to 7 inches (15 to 18 cm) for male patient. *(Maintains sterility of supplies. Lubricating catheter reduces the chance that friction will cause trauma to the delicate mucous membranes of the urethra.)*

15. Wrap edges of sterile drape around gloved hands, and request patient to raise hips; then slide drape under patient's buttocks. *(Protects hands from contamination while towel is placed under edge of patient's buttocks.)*

16. Cleanse perineal area with forceps to hold cotton balls soaked in antiseptic solution. *(Cleansing reduces number of microorganisms at urethral meatus and decreases risk of urinary tract infection.)*

a. Male: If male patient is not circumcised, retract foreskin with nondominant hand. Be certain to replace foreskin when procedure has been completed. If erection occurs, discontinue procedure momentarily. This is normal but often embarrassing to patient. React in a professional manner. *(Release of foreskin or letting go of the penis during cleansing requires process to be repeated because area has been contaminated.)*

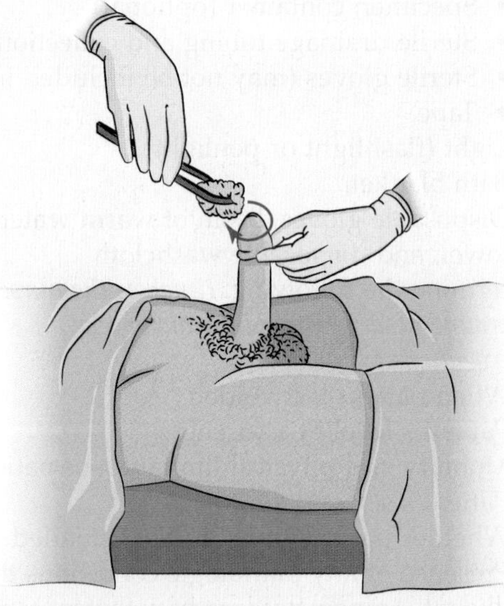

(1) Grasp penis at shaft below glans with nondominant hand; continue to hold throughout insertion of catheter. The nondominant hand is no longer sterile and must not come in contact with sterile supplies.

(2) With other hand, use forceps to pick up cotton balls soaked in antiseptic solution.

(3) Cleanse meatus by beginning at top of penis and moving in a circular motion down and around meatus one time. Discard cotton ball in appropriate receptacle. *(Decreases introduction of organisms into bladder.)*

(4) Repeat cleansing two more times with sterile cotton balls each time. *(Cleansing in this manner ensures optimal reduction of microorganisms from the area.)*

Skill 15.1 Catheterization: Male and Female Patients—cont'd

b. Female:

(1) Spread labia minora with thumb and index finger of nondominant hand to expose meatus; continue to hold throughout insertion of catheter. The nondominant hand is no longer sterile and must not come in contact with sterile supplies.

(2) With other hand, use forceps to pick up cotton balls soaked in antiseptic solution.

(3) Cleanse area from clitoris toward anus. Use a different sterile cotton ball each time: first to the right of the meatus, then to the left of the meatus, then down the center over meatus. *(Full separation of labia prevents contamination of meatus during cleansing. If the labia close, it is necessary to repeat the procedure.)*

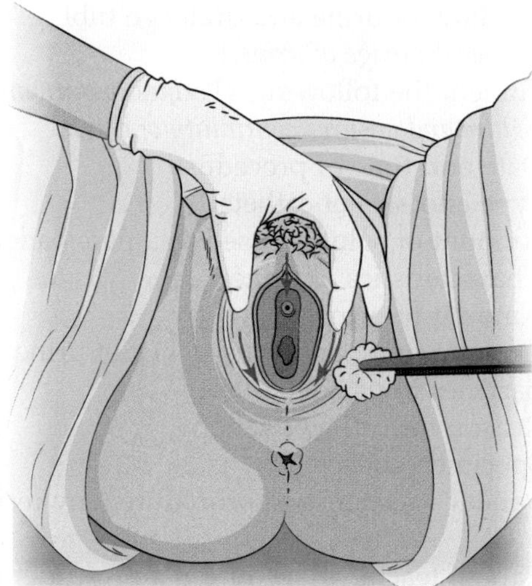

17. Pick up catheter with dominant sterile-gloved hand near the tip; hold remaining part of catheter coiled in hands; place distal end in basin. *(Placing distal end of catheter in basin allows for urine collection. Coiling catheter in hand and holding near the tip allows easier manipulation during insertion.)*

18. Insert catheter gently, about 6 to 7 inches (15 to 18 cm) for male patient or 2 to 4 inches (5 to 10 cm) for female patient. *(Asking patient to bear down gently as if to void causes relaxation of external sphincter, which aids in insertion of catheter.)* Once urine flow is established, insert catheter 1½ inches (3.5 cm) farther. *(Advancement of catheter ensures correct bladder placement.)* Inflate balloon with 10 mL of sterile water. Gently pull back on catheter until resistance is felt as balloon rests at orifice of urethra (see illustration and Fig. 15.5A). In a female patient, if no urine returns in a few minutes, observe whether catheter has been inserted by mistake into vagina. If so, leave catheter in place as landmark indicating where not to insert, and insert another sterile catheter. *(Use of the same catheter will introduce microorganisms into the bladder.)*

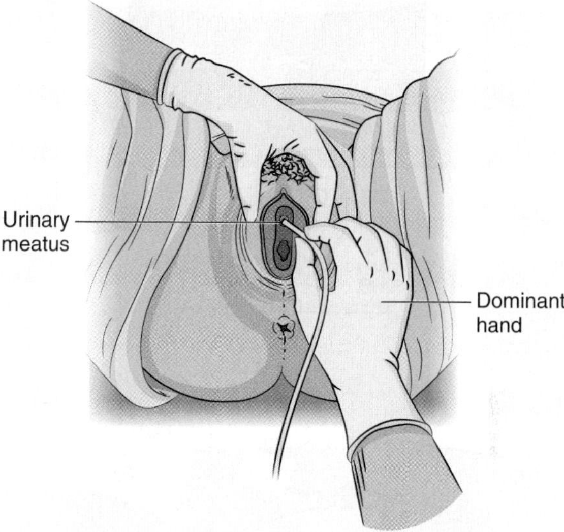

a. Indwelling catheter:

(1) Inflate balloon with required amount of normal saline or sterile water (see Fig. 15.4A).

(2) Pull gently to feel resistance.

(3) Collect urine specimen, if needed, by placing open lumen end of catheter into specimen container. *(Allows for sterile specimen to be obtained for testing.)*

(4) Attach open lumen of catheter to collecting tube of drainage system, holding drainage bag below bladder level. (Some catheters are presealed to the collecting tube of the drainage system. If catheter is not presealed, clean both the catheter and tubing end with antiseptic before reconnecting them, to maintain sterility of catheter and tube.)

(5) Attach collection bag to a nonmoveable part on the side of bed (see Fig. 15.4B).

(6) Secure catheter to patient. *(Minimizes tension and trauma to urethral opening.)*

(a) Male patient: Tape catheter to inner aspect of thigh or up over pubis, or apply leg strap (depends on health care provider's order); allow slack for body movement.

(b) Female patient: Tape catheter to inner thigh or apply leg strap; allow slack for body movement.

Continued

Skill 15.1 Catheterization: Male and Female Patients—cont'd

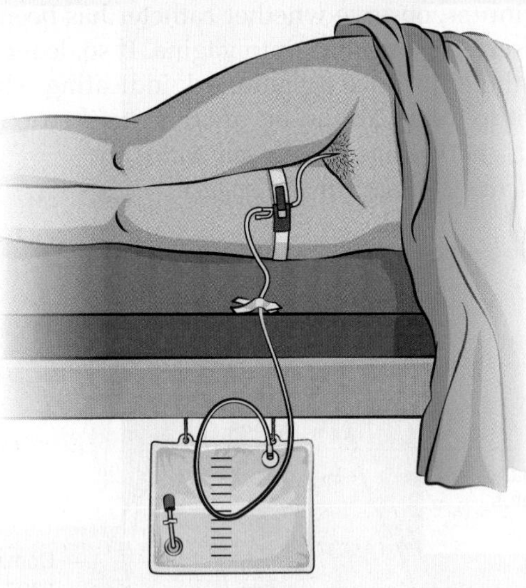

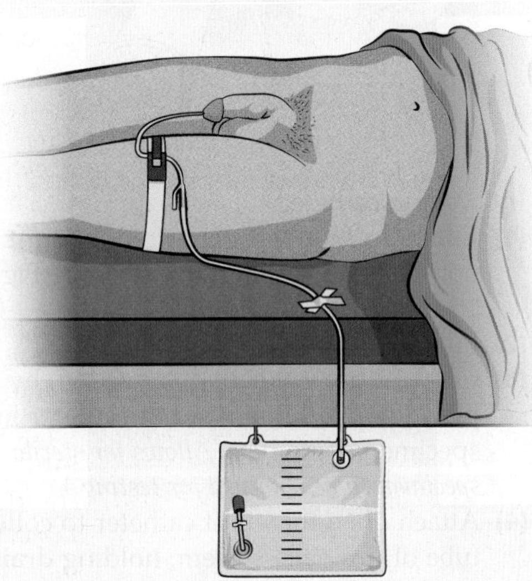

(7) Clip drainage tubing to bed linen; allow slack for body movement.

b. Straight catheter:

(1) Once urine flow is established, hold open lumen of catheter over basin.

(2) Empty bladder (approximately 700 to 1000 mL). Refer to facility policy to determine whether urine should be allowed to continue draining. *(If a distended bladder is drained too rapidly, the bladder may collapse into spasms, which are painful.)*

(3) Collect urine specimen, if needed, by placing open lumen end of catheter into specimen container. *(Allows for sterile specimen to be obtained for testing.)*

(4) Withdraw catheter slowly. *(Minimizes patient discomfort.)*

19. Wash and dry perineal area. *(Maintains patient comfort.)*

20. Refer to Standard Steps 10 to 17.

21. Label urine specimen with patient's name, date, health care provider's name, and other information as required by facility. *(Verifies correct specimen for laboratory.)* Ensure urine is transported to laboratory.

22. Check flow of urine and drainage tubing. *(Checks for proper drainage of urine.)*

23. Document the following. *(Verifies performance of procedure and ensures continuity of care.)*
- Date and time of procedure
- Type and size of catheter
- Amount of solution used to inflate balloon
- Characteristics of urine
- Amount of urine
- Color of urine and consistency of urine (note particles in urine)
- Reason for catheterization
- Specimen collected
- Patient's response to procedure (any resistance met)
- Patient teaching (see Lifespan Considerations for older adults box on catheterization)

24. Report any unusual findings immediately:
- No urine output
- Bladder discomfort despite catheter patency
- Leakage of urine from catheter
- Inability to insert catheter *(If it is not possible to advance catheter, report immediately. Discomfort indicates possible infection or trauma. Leakage around catheter indicates possibility of improper catheter placement or inflation of balloon.)*

Figure for Step 5b from Perry AG, Potter PA, Ostendorf WR, et al: *Clinical nursing skills and techniques*, ed 9, St. Louis, 2018, Elsevier. Figure for Step 13 from Potter PA, Perry AG, Stockert P, et al: *Fundamentals of nursing: concepts, process, and practice*, ed 9, St. Louis, 2016, Elsevier.

least every 8 hours to prevent urinary tract infections (Skill 15.2). During catheter care, cleanse the first 2 inches of the catheter to remove any secretions or encrustations from the catheter. Look for inflammation at and around the urethral meatus and check for swelling or discharge from the urethra. Some facilities discourage the use of powders and lotions in the perineal area of patients with catheters because these can lead to the growth of microorganisms that could enter the urinary tract and cause urinary tract infections. Perform perineal and catheter care after bowel movements, especially if the patient is incontinent of stool.

Skill 15.2 Performing Routine Catheter Care

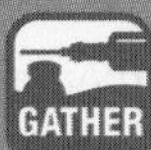

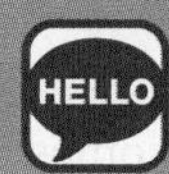

PRIVACY

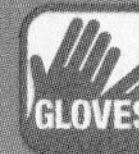

NURSING ACTION *(RATIONALE)*

1. Refer to Standard Steps 1 to 9.
2. Assemble equipment:
   - Bath blanket
   - Bed protector
   - Catheter care kit (if not using a kit, the following supplies are necessary):
     - Basin of warm water and mild soap
     - Towel and washcloth (disposable washcloths are acceptable)
     - Small plastic bag for trash
   - Disposable gloves
3. Evaluate patient for the following. *(Enables the nurse to determine patient's condition.)*
   a. Length of time catheter has been in place (follow facility policy)
   b. Encrustations or discharge around urethral meatus
   c. Complaints of pain and for allergies to antiseptic ointment
   d. Patient's temperature (check temperature every 4 hours for 24 hours if odor or exudate is present)
   e. Patient's intake (maintain adequate fluid intake to ensure free-flowing urine)
4. Position patient.
   a. Male: supine position in bed with thighs slightly abducted
   b. Female: supine position in bed with knees flexed and about 2 feet apart
5. Place waterproof disposable pad under patient's buttocks. *(Keeps bed linens dry.)*
6. Drape patient with bath blanket, exposing only perineal area. *(Keeps patient warm and protects privacy.)*
7. If sterile catheter care kit is to be used:
   a. Open supplies with sterile technique, and arrange them on bedside table. *(Organizes procedure.)*
   b. Don sterile gloves. *(Prevents transmission of microorganisms.)*
   c. Place cotton balls in sterile basin near the nurse, and saturate with antiseptic solution. *(Having supplies nearby prevents accidental contamination. Maintaining sterility of supplies reduces the possibility of introducing pathogens into the urinary tract.)*
   d. With one hand, expose urethral meatus:
      (1) Male: Retract foreskin if it is present, then hold penis erect; hold position.
      (2) Female: Gently retract labia minora away from urinary meatus and hold in position.
   e. Wash the area at the meatus and around catheter with cotton balls soaked in antiseptic solution.
      (1) Male:
         (a) With one cotton ball, cleanse around meatus and catheter in a circular motion, starting at top of penis.
         (b) Repeat twice more, using different cotton balls each time.
      (2) Female:
         (a) With one cotton ball, swab to one side of labia minora from anterior to posterior. *(Prevents microorganisms from rectum entering the urinary system.)*
         (b) Repeat with second cotton ball on opposite side.
         (c) Repeat with third cotton ball down middle over meatus and around catheter; do not bring cotton ball back up once descent has begun.
   a. Discard soiled cotton balls in other basin in kit.
   b. With forceps, pick up cotton ball soaked in antiseptic solution, or use mild soap and water, and cleanse around catheter from urethral opening to approximately 4 inches (10 cm) of the catheter from the urethral opening. *(Cleans catheter of exudate. The urethral opening is considered less contaminated than the catheter tube.)*
8. If a collection of sterile supplies is to be used:
   a. Open separate sterile packages, observing sterile technique.
   b. Don clean gloves. *(Prevents accidental contamination. Maintaining sterility of supplies reduces the possibility of introducing pathogens into the urinary tract.)*
   c. Arrange small plastic bag for used, contaminated supplies.
   d. Cleanse the perineal area with mild soap and warm water. Pat dry.
      (1) Male: Retract foreskin if it is present; then hold the penis erect.
      (2) Female: Gently retract labia away from urinary meatus.
   e. Release labia of female patient; replace foreskin of male patient after cleaning.

Continued

Skill 15.2 Performing Routine Catheter Care—cont'd

9. Observe meatus, catheter, and surrounding tissue to determine normal or abnormal condition. Note presence or absence of inflammation, edema, malodorous exudate, color of tissue, or burning sensation. *(Determines need for more aggressive therapy.)*
10. Dispose of equipment and linens, according to standard precautions and facility policy; remove gloves and dispose of them in proper receptacle. Perform hand hygiene. *(Reduces spread of microorganisms.)*
11. Retape catheter to thigh or use a catheter strap. *(Prevents trauma and pain from tension and pulling.)*
12. Refer to Standard Steps 10 to 17.
13. Observe flow of urine through drainage tubing; note the accumulation of urine in the collecting receptacle. *(Promotes accurate evaluation of urine.)* If the drainage tubing becomes cloudy or stained, change the tubing to aid accurate observations of urine. Empty drainage receptacle at least every 8 hours or as necessary to prevent backup of urine into the tubing or bladder (see Fig. 15.6).
14. Document the following. *(Verifies performance of procedure and ensures continuity of care.)*
    - Date and time
    - Procedure
    - Assessment of urinary meatus
    - Character of urine
    - Patient's response
    - Patient teaching
15. Report any unusual findings immediately. *(Further therapy may be required.)*

If a catheter strap or adhesive tape is used to secure the tubing to the abdomen or leg, it should be replaced after catheter care is given. If the tubing and collection device must be changed because of leakage, odor, or collection of sediment in the tubing or collection device, follow sterile technique (see the Patient Teaching and Home Care Considerations boxes). If patency of the catheter itself becomes interrupted by mucus, blood clots, or sediment, catheter irrigation may be necessary. This procedure requires a physician's order in most facilities (Skill 15.3).

 **Patient Teaching**

Indwelling Urinary Drainage System Care

- Explain the procedure and expected sensations associated with the procedure to the patient before you insert the catheter.
- Answer the patient's questions about the procedures.
- Explain the need for the patient to drink fluids to flush the urinary system.
- Instruct the patient about proper transfer from a bed, chair, or stretcher.
- Teach the principles of, and need for, catheter and perineal care.
- Instruct the patient how to perform Kegel exercises.
- Teach the patient the side effects that are possible with an indwelling catheter and symptoms of an infection. Encourage the patient to report symptoms immediately.
- Caution the patient not to lie on tubing and to keep the drainage bag below the level of the bladder.
- Discourage the use of lotions or powder during perineal care.
- Encourage using a leg bag during the day and a bedside drainage bag at night.
- Instruct patient to wear loose-fitting clothing to promote adequate drainage.

Incontinence and Its Management

Incontinence—the inability to control urine or bowel elimination—can be a psychologically distressing and socially disruptive problem, especially among older adults.

Urinary incontinence can occur because pressure in the bladder is too great or because the sphincters are too weak. It can involve a small leakage of urine when the person laughs, coughs, or lifts something heavy (stress incontinence), or it can be a constant leakage whenever the bladder contains urine (urge incontinence). Collaborating with other members of the health care team is important to identify the cause and the extent of incontinence and to assist in managing the problem.

Patients with urinary incontinence may be referred to a urologist for evaluation, and treatment may involve teaching the patient exercises to strengthen muscles around the external sphincters or employing bladder training. If a paralyzed patient has overflow incontinence or incontinence related to an overfull bladder, the Credé maneuver is helpful. This involves applying manual pressure over the lower abdomen to express urine from the bladder at regular intervals. When this technique is used, care must be taken to prevent injury to the bladder from excess pressure.

Fecal incontinence may result from diarrhea or constipation, muscle damage or weakness, nerve damage, a rectocele, or even inactivity. Patients with urinary or fecal incontinence may require disposable adult undergarments or underpads to help prevent soiling of clothing and embarrassment. Use of discreet incontinence products helps promote self-care and self-esteem.

Urine and feces are also very irritating to the skin. Skin that is exposed continuously becomes inflamed and irritated quickly. To help prevent skin impairment,

Skill 15.3 Catheter Irrigation

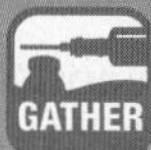
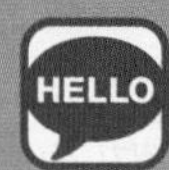
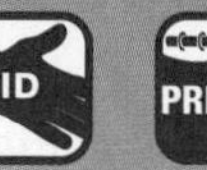

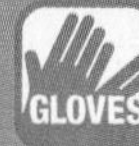

NURSING ACTION *(RATIONALE)*

1. Refer to Standard Steps 1 to 9.
2. Assemble equipment (exact equipment depends on method used):
   - Antiseptic cleanser
   - Clean gloves
   - Irrigation setup
   - Medication for instillation
   - Sterile basin
   - Sterile calibrated container
   - Sterile gloves
   - Sterile plug
   - Sterile solution
   - Sterile syringe
   - Waterproof pad
3. Observe the following. *(Enables the nurse to determine patient's condition.)*
   a. Color of urine and presence of mucus or sediment
   b. Patency of drainage tubing
   c. Patient's intake and output record
   d. Patient for presence of bladder spasms and discomfort
   e. Patient's knowledge regarding purpose of the catheter irrigation
4. Position patient:
   a. Male: supine position in bed
   b. Female: supine position in bed
5. Drape patient with bath blanket, exposing only perineal area; remove and dispose of gloves. *(Exposes catheter.)*
6. Place waterproof absorbent pad under patient's buttocks and perform catheter care (see Skill 15.2). *(Protects bed linens from soiling and cleans area before procedure.)*
7. Arrange supplies and equipment at bedside on overbed table. *(Easy access prevents possible contamination.)*
8. Perform irrigation:
   a. Open method:
      (1) Pour sterile irrigating solution (sterile normal saline unless otherwise specified) into sterile graduated container, and recap solution bottle. Have irrigating solution at room temperature.
      (2) Don sterile gloves. *(Maintains the sterile field.)*
      (3) Place sterile basin between patient's legs, close to perineal area.
      (4) Kink catheter and disconnect catheter from drainage system. Plug drainage tubing with sterile plug. *(Prevents urine from draining from catheter before procedure. Sterile plug maintains sterility of drainage tube during procedure.)*
      (5) Draw 30 mL of sterile solution into syringe.
      (6) Cleanse catheter end with antiseptic swab. *(Maintains sterility of equipment.)*
      (7) Place tip of syringe into end of catheter, and gently insert solution. *(A gentle approach reduces incidence of bladder spasms and clears catheter of obstruction.)*
      (8) Withdraw syringe, and allow solution to drain into basin by gravity.
      (9) If solution does not return, turn patient on side, facing the nurse. If solution still does not return, refer to facility policy for further action. *(Change in position sometimes moves tip of catheter in bladder, increasing the likelihood that instilled fluid will flow out.)*
      (10) Repeat injection of solution until amount ordered is instilled and returned; maintain sterility of equipment.
      (11) Clean end of catheter with antiseptic solution. Remove plug from drainage tubing, and connect tubing to catheter. Do not touch ends of catheter and tubing. *(Prevents contamination of the system.)*
      (12) Measure solution. *(Determines amount returned and amount of urine expelled.)*
   b. Closed intermittent method (repeat Steps 1 through 7 as described). *(Maintaining a closed system ensures against contamination that could result in a urinary tract infection.)*
      (1) Pour sterile irrigating solution into graduated container. *(Sterile normal saline is used unless otherwise specified.)*
      (2) Draw up sterile solution into syringe.
      (3) Clamp catheter below injection port.
      (4) Cleanse port with antiseptic. *(Decreases spread of microorganisms.)*
      (5) Insert needle of syringe into port. *(Needleless ports may also be present.)*
      (6) Inject solution into catheter slowly. *(Helps prevent bladder spasm while dislodging clots, sediment, or other material.)*

Continued

Skill 15.3 Catheter Irrigation—cont'd

c. Closed continuous method (continuous bladder irrigation). The health care provider must order the solution, the strength, and the flow rate of a continuous bladder irrigation. If the health care provider specifies only solution, check with facility policy for protocol for strength and rate. The irrigation solution infuses continuously through one port of a triple-lumen catheter, and the second port drains urine and irrigation solution.

(1) Set up irrigating solution by attaching tubing to bag.

(2) Clamp off tubing so that no solution flows through.

(3) Suspend bag on intravenous pole.

(4) Open clamp and allow solution to flow through tubing. *(Primes tubing to prevent air from entering the bladder and causing patient pain or discomfort.)*

(5) Cleanse irrigating lumen on end of triple-lumen catheter (see Fig. 15.6A). *(Necessary for system to remain sterile.)*

(6) Connect irrigating solution tubing to catheter lumen; maintain sterility of equipment.

(7) Open clamp on irrigation tubing, and calculate drip rate. *(Ensures continuous, even irrigation of catheter system. Prevents accumulation of solution in bladder, which can cause bladder distention and injury.)*

(8) When drainage bag is emptied, the amount of irrigation solution infused should be subtracted from total amount returned. *(Allows the nurse to compute accurate urine output.)*

d. Bladder instillation:

(1) Disconnect catheter from tubing; stabilize tubing to prevent touching the floor. NOTE: Using triple-lumen catheter makes it unnecessary to disconnect catheter from drainage tubing (see Fig. 15.6B).

(2) Cleanse end of catheter with antiseptic swab. *(Maintains sterility of equipment and decreases spread of microorganisms.)*

(3) Draw medication or solution into syringe. *(Prepares for instillation.)*

(4) Place tip of syringe into end of catheter, and slowly inject medication or solution. *(Proceeding slowly prevents trauma to bladder mucosa.)*

(5) Clamp off end of catheter for necessary period. *(Allows medication or solution to be absorbed by bladder.)* Clean catheter and tubing ends with antiseptic solution; then reconnect catheter and tubing, making certain the system is tightly connected. *(Decreases risk of infection.)*

(6) Measure solution returned. *(Enables the nurse to determine amount returned and amount of urine for accurate recording of input and output [I&O].)*

9. Observe flow of urine through drainage tubing (see Fig. 15.6B). *(Determines urine flow and effectiveness of therapy.)*

10. Refer to Standard Steps 10 to 17.

11. Record urine output on I&O sheet, and document the following:

- Date and time
- Solution used as irrigant
- Amount of solution used
- Amount returned as drainage
- Character of drainage
- Patient teaching (see the Patient Teaching boxes on catheter care and removing a urinary catheter)

12. Report any unusual findings immediately. *(More aggressive therapy may be necessary.)*

- If irrigant does not return
- Increased pain
- Occlusion
- Signs or symptoms of infection
- Sudden bleeding
- Unrelieved bladder spasms

make sure to change the undergarments or underpads frequently; cleanse the skin thoroughly after each episode of incontinence with warm, soapy water; and dry it completely (Box 15.1). Cleanse the perineum in a professional, caring, and matter-of-fact manner. The patient must not be reprimanded, scolded, or humiliated for having an "accident."

Bladder training. **Bladder training** is the achievement of voluntary control over voiding; it often involves developing the use of muscles in the perineum. When urinary incontinence results from decreased perception of bladder fullness or impaired voluntary motor control, bladder training is often helpful.

Before the removal of a urethral catheter, bladder training may be ordered by the health care provider and involves a clamp-unclamp routine to improve bladder tone. Kegel exercises also may be used to improve perineal muscle tone and sphincter control as part of a bladder training regimen. The patient is

Box 15.1 Patient Problem Statements for the Patient With a Urinary Tract Disorder

Functional Inability to Control Urination:
- Related to cognitive deficits
- Related to mobility deficits
- Related to sensory deficits

Potential for Compromised Skin Integrity:
- Related to presence of urine on skin

Impaired Self-Esteem due to Current Situation:
- Related to inability to control passage of urine

Inability to Control Urination due to Physical Stress:
- Related to changes in muscles and structure of urinary system associated with increased age

Inability to Control Urination due to Urgency:
- Related to decreased bladder capacity

Potential for Infection:
- Related to inadequate personal hygiene
- Related to lack of knowledge of care of a urinary stoma

instructed to perform Kegel exercises by trying to stop the flow of urine during voiding. Once the patient has identified the correct muscles and the feeling of their contraction, the patient can perform these exercises when not voiding by tightening the muscles of the perineum, holding the tension for 10 seconds, and then relaxing for 10 seconds. This should be done multiple times, several times a day. Because muscle control develops gradually, it sometimes takes 4 to 6 weeks to slow or stop urinary leakage.

Habit training is also a part of bladder training and involves establishing a voiding schedule. This provides cooperative patients with the opportunity to achieve continence by voiding at regular intervals (every 1.5 to 2 hours). Monitor the patient's voiding for a few days to identify patterns, or schedule voiding times to correlate with the patient's activities. Typical voiding times are upon rising, before each meal, and at bedtime. Assist the patient to void as scheduled, check the patient for wetness periodically, and remind or assist the patient to the toilet as scheduled. After a few days, evaluate the scheduled voiding pattern by identifying its effectiveness in keeping the patient continent. Then the schedule is modified until continence is established. Fluid intake and medications typically influence voiding patterns. Limiting fluids after the evening meal reduces the need for nighttime voiding and helps keep the patient dry.

REMOVAL OF AN INDWELLING CATHETER

It is always best to remove an indwelling catheter as soon as possible because its presence increases the risk for urinary tract infection (Skill 15.4). After surgery, the health care provider usually orders the catheter removed after 8 to 24 hours, depending on the type of surgery. In some situations, the catheter remains in place for days or even weeks. The longer a catheter has been in place, the greater is the risk that an infection will develop. Urinary tract infections are one of the most common types of *iatrogenic* (caused by treatments or diagnostic procedures) infections in health care. Symptoms of a urinary tract infection may not appear for 2 or more days after the catheter is removed. That means the patient may already be home before he or she begins displaying symptoms. For that reason, it is necessary to inform the patient of the risk for infection, how to prevent it, signs and symptoms to watch for, and when to call the health care provider.

Sometimes patients have difficulty voiding after the removal of a urinary catheter because the sphincter muscles are weakened. Patients with an overdistended bladder or who have altered sensory perception because of regional anesthesia, such as a spinal or epidural block, are likely to have difficulty voiding after catheter removal. Most patients should void adequately within 8 hours after catheter removal. If they do not, the health care provider must be notified and further orders received (see the Patient Teaching box on removing a urinary catheter).

 **Patient Teaching**

Removing Urinary Catheter

- Instruct the patient that it will take time for the urinary bladder to reestablish voluntary control of urine.
- Explain the need for collecting and measuring urine output, and teach the patient how to do so.
- Explain the need to drink at least 2 L (eight 8-oz glasses/cups) of fluid per day (to reduce risk of infection) unless this is contraindicated by the patient's condition.
- Explain that it is common to feel some burning sensation or discomfort when first voiding.
- Identify the side effects that are possible, and explain the need to report them immediately.
- Instruct patients that the use of over-the-counter medications, such as nasal decongestants and anticholinergic medications (e.g., diphenhydramine, acetaminophen PM), have the potential to cause urinary retention and that their use should be limited.

SKILLS FOR GASTROINTESTINAL PROCEDURES

INSERTING AND MAINTAINING NASOGASTRIC TUBES

A **nasogastric (NG) tube** is a flexible, hollow tube that is passed into the stomach via the nasopharynx. It can be used to remove gas, fluids, or toxic substances from the stomach; to diagnose gastrointestinal problems; to obtain secretions; or to administer fluids and nutrients into the stomach. It also can help prevent vomiting and abdominal distention and allow the digestive tract to rest and heal. There are various types of NG tubes, including percutaneous endoscopic gastrostomy (PEG), Button, and jejunal tubes. The physician determines which tube is best suited for the patient.

Skill 15.4 Removing an Indwelling Catheter

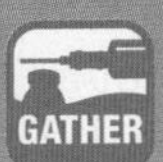

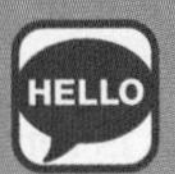

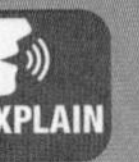

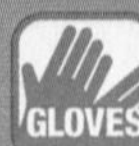

NURSING ACTION *(RATIONALE)*

1. Refer to Standard Steps 1 to 9.
2. Assemble equipment:
   - 10-mL syringe or larger (depending on volume of fluid used to inflate balloon) without a needle.

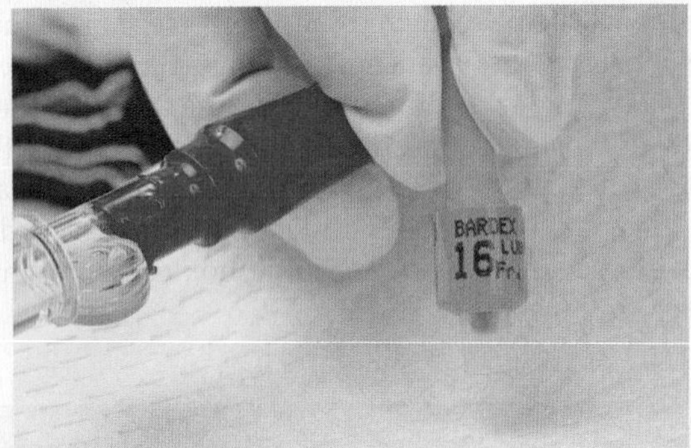

3. Determine the following:
   a. Length of time catheter has been in place. *(The longer the catheter has been in place, the greater the risk for decreased bladder muscle tone and inflammation of the urethra.)*
   b. Patient's knowledge of procedure and what to expect. *(Many patients anticipate discomfort or have fears about ability to void successfully after removal of the catheter.)* Educate patient if necessary.
4. Provide privacy. Position the patient supine, and place a waterproof pad under the patient's buttocks. *(Protects the bed linens.)* Female patients need to abduct their legs with the drape between their thighs (see Step 5b of Skill 15.1). For male patients, it is acceptable for drape to lie on the thighs.
5. Insert hub of syringe into inflation valve (balloon port), and aspirate until tubing collapses or resistance is felt. *(Indicates that entire contents of balloon have been removed.)*
6. Remove catheter steadily and smoothly (in female patients, the catheter is in about 2 to 3 inches [5 to 7.5 cm] and in male patients, about 6 to 7 inches [15 to 18 cm]). *(Decreases discomfort.)* Catheter usually slides out very easily. Do not use force. If any resistance is noted, repeat Step 5 to remove remaining water. *(Prevents trauma to the urethra.)*
7. Wrap catheter in waterproof pad. Unhook collection bag and drainage tubing from the bed. *(Prevents any leakage from the catheter onto the patient, the nurse, or bed linens.)*
8. Measure urine, and empty drainage bag. *(Promotes accurate reporting and recording.)*
9. Record output. *(Communicates patient care.)*
10. Cleanse the perineum with soap and warm water, and dry area thoroughly. *(Promotes comfort and a feeling of cleanliness.)*
11. Explain the following to patient:
    a. It is important to have a fluid intake of 1.5 to 2 L/day unless contraindicated.
    b. The patient must void within 8 hours, and each voiding should be measured. Some facilities and health care providers determine how much the patient should void to verify adequate emptying of the urinary bladder. *(Confirms the ability of the patient to empty the bladder adequately.)*
    c. Mild burning sensation or discomfort with first voiding is anticipated. Instruct patient to notify the nurse if it does not subside with subsequent voidings. *(Infection may be present, and treatment may have to be initiated.)*
    d. Signs of urinary tract infection are urinary urgency, burning sensation, urinary frequency, excretion of only small amount, and continued pain or discomfort. These symptoms may develop 2 to 3 days after removal of catheter.
12. Place the urine measuring device on the toilet seat. *(Facilitates accurate assessment of patient's output.)*
13. Refer to Standard Steps 12 to 17.
14. Document and report the following. *(Promotes continuity of patient care.)*
    - Date and time of catheter removal
    - Patient teaching related to increasing fluid intake and signs and symptoms of urinary tract infection
    - Time, amount, and characteristics of first voiding after catheter removal
    - Complete input and output record

Figure from Elkin MK, Perry AG, Potter PA: *Nursing interventions and clinical skills,* ed 4, St. Louis, 2008, Mosby.

Gastric Gavage

When used to deliver fluids or nutrients (gastric gavage), the NG tube can be attached to a feeding pump, or the feeding can be allowed to flow in by gravity via a bag or a syringe. If a patient is receiving feedings by way of an NG tube, it is essential to keep the head of the bed elevated at least 30 degrees to help prevent aspiration or gastric reflux.

Tube feedings usually are started slowly and gradually increased, or they may be diluted and gradually strengthened, to prevent **dumping syndrome.** Dumping syndrome is caused by too rapid an infusion of highly concentrated feedings. The symptoms are similar to those of shock and can be very disturbing to the patient. During tube feedings, the health care provider also may order additional water to be given through the tube. This helps meet the fluid needs of the patient, keeps the tube patent, and helps dilute the tube feeding.

Before introducing anything into an NG tube, verify placement of the tube to prevent contents from entering the lungs. Many facilities require injecting air into the tube while listening to the abdomen over the stomach with a stethoscope. If the tube is in the correct place, a swishing or gurgling noise will be heard. Aspirating gastric contents is also an appropriate way to check NG tube placement. While the nurse monitors patients receiving nutrients through an NG tube, it is also necessary to check occasionally for residual feeding left in the stomach. Excess residual formula could indicate a problem with peristalsis, and the health care provider must be notified. It also could cause gastric reflux, aspiration, or both. Each facility and health care provider has a policy for how often to check residual formula and how much is considered excessive.

Gastric Lavage

Gastric lavage often is used in cases of poisoning or to stop gastrointestinal bleeding. It involves instilling room-temperature medications or solutions into the stomach and then suctioning it back out. Iced or cooled solutions should not be used, especially when copious amounts are needed, as with gastrointestinal bleeding, because they may cause hypothermia, impair platelet production, and cause increase in bleeding.

When performing gastric lavage, the health care provider orders the type of solution, as well as the amount, to be instilled. Usually 500 mL of the solution is administered at a time and then siphoned back out of the stomach. This process is repeated until the ordered amount of solution has been used or the anticipated results have been achieved. Every time the solution is removed from the stomach, it must be measured and evaluated and the results documented. Sometimes the health care provider orders a specimen of the removed solution to be sent to the laboratory for analysis. Remember that this procedure is emotional and physically challenging for the patient. Provide appropriate support and reassurance.

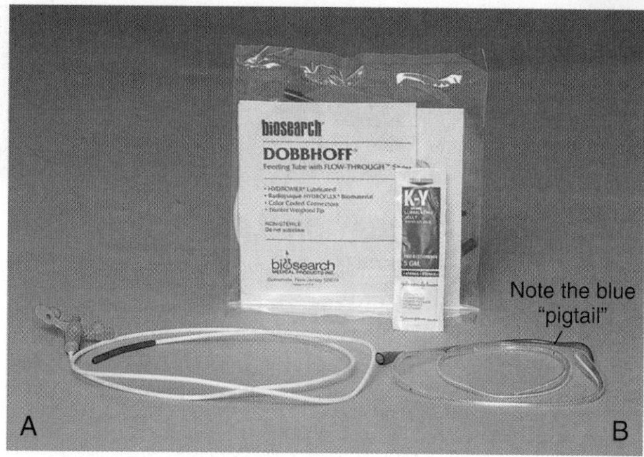

Fig. 15.7 Types of nasogastric tubes. A, Small-bore feeding tube. B, Salem sump tube. Note the blue "pigtail." This pigtail is an air vent that helps to prevent the tube from adhering to the gastric mucosa. (From Potter PA, Perry AG, Stocket PA, et al: *Fundamentals of nursing: Concepts, process, and practice*, ed 8, St. Louis, 2013, Mosby.)

Gastric Decompression

The purpose of gastric decompression is to remove the air and fluids that build up when gastrointestinal motility is slowed. It is used frequently after surgery to help with the distention that may occur and to prevent nausea and vomiting. When used for decompression, the NG tube usually is connected to an intermittent gastric suction device, and the nurse must routinely measure and evaluate the contents of the suction canister. The tubes most commonly used for decompression are the Levin and Salem sump tubes. The Levin tube has one lumen and several openings near the tip. The Salem sump tube is a double-lumen tube: one lumen provides an air vent, and the other is for removal of gastric contents (Fig. 15.7).

The patient with an NG tube presents several nursing challenges. Maintaining patient comfort is sometimes the biggest challenge. NG tubes continually irritate the nasal mucosa and can cause trauma to the tissue. To lessen this discomfort and potential trauma, the tube should be secured to the patient's nose with tape or a nose guard and then secured to the patient's gown with a pin to prevent unnecessary movement (Skill 15.5 and the Patient Teaching box on nasogastric tubes). Other comfort measures include removing excess secretions from around the nares and then lubricating the nostrils and the tube with a water-soluble lubricant to prevent crusting of secretions. Box 15.2 lists selected patient problem statements for the patient with a gastric tube.

After an NG tube is inserted, patients tend to breathe through their mouths because of the nasal occlusion by the tube, and the lips and tongue often become dry and cracked. Provide mouth care at least every 2 hours to increase comfort. Rinsing the mouth with cool water or oral swabs provides some comfort. Ensure that the patient does not swallow any water. Check the health care provider's orders to see whether the patient is

Skill 15.5 Inserting a Nasogastric Tube

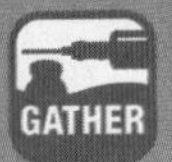

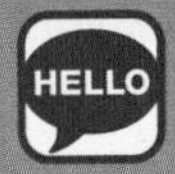

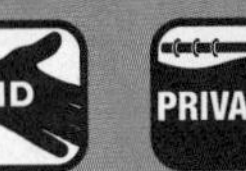

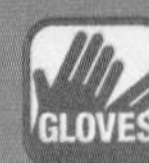

NURSING ACTION *(RATIONALE)*

1. Refer to Standard Steps 1 to 9.
2. Assemble equipment:
   - 14-Fr or 16-Fr nasogastric (NG) tube (smaller bore for child) or feeding type of tube (see Fig. 15.7)
   - Bath towel
   - Clamp
   - Clean gloves
   - Facial tissues
   - Felt tip marker
   - Flashlight
   - Glass of water with straw
   - Normal saline
   - Safety pin and rubber band
   - Stethoscope
   - Suction container
   - Suction machine
   - Syringe
   - Tape, nose guard, or both
   - Tincture of benzoin (optional)
   - Tongue blade
   - Water-soluble lubricating jelly
3. Evaluate condition of patient's oral cavity. *(Enables the nurse to determine need for special nursing measures and for oral hygiene after tube placement.)* Palpate patient's abdomen. *(Provides baseline data for later comparison after tube is inserted.)*
4. Position patient in high Fowler's position with pillow behind head and shoulders. *(Promotes patient's ability to swallow during procedure.)*
5. Stand at right side of bed if you are right-handed and left side if you are left-handed. *(Allows for easy manipulation of tubing.)*
6. Place bath towel over patient's chest; give tissues to patient. *(This prevents soiling of gown. Tube insertion through nasal passages sometimes causes eyes to tear up.)*
7. Instruct patient to relax and breathe normally while one nostril is occluded. Repeat this action for other nostril. Select nostril with greater airflow. *(The tube passes more easily through nostril that is more patent.)* Some institutions suggest nasogastric tubes be cooled in ice or saline, which stiffens them to facilitate passage. Know facility policy.
8. Measure distance to insert tube. Measure total distance from tip of nose to earlobe and from there to xiphoid process of sternum. Tube should extend from nostril to stomach; distance varies with each patient. *(Allows tube to be inserted completely into stomach and not end in esophagus.)*

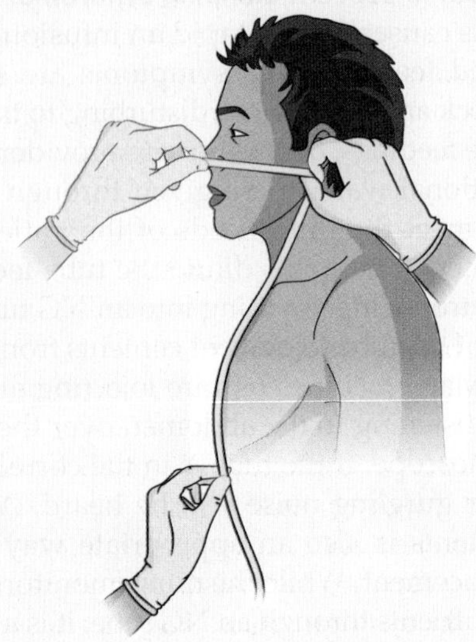

9. Mark off length of tube to be inserted with piece of tape or felt tip marker, or note distance from next tube marking. *(Helps ensure correct length of tubing will be inserted.)*
10. Curve 14 to 16 inches (10 to 15 cm) of tube tightly around fingers; release. *(Curving tube tip aids insertion.)*
11. Lubricate 3 to 4 inches (7.5 to 10 cm) of end of tube with water-soluble lubricating jelly. *(Minimizes friction against nasal mucosa.)*
12. Instruct patient to extend head against pillow; insert tube slowly through nostril with curved end pointing downward (see illustration). *(Facilitates initial passage of tube through nostril and maintains clear airway for open nostril.)*

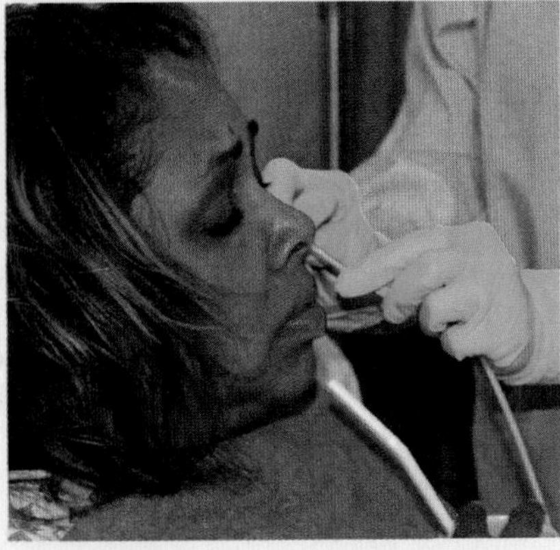

Skill 15.5 Inserting a Nasogastric Tube—cont'd

13. Continue to pass tube along floor of nasal passage, aiming down toward ear. When resistance is felt, apply gentle downward pressure to advance tube (do not force past resistance). *(Reduces discomfort of tube rubbing against upper nasal turbinates. Resistance is caused by posterior nasopharynx. Downward pressure helps tube curl around corner of nasopharynx.)*
14. If resistance continues, withdraw tube, allow patient to rest, relubricate tube, and insert into other nostril. *(Forcing against resistance has potential to cause trauma to mucosa. Pause also helps relieve anxiety.)*
15. Continue insertion of tube until just past nasopharynx by gently rotating tube toward opposite nostril.
    a. Stop tube advancement, allow patient to relax, and provide tissues. *(Relieves anxiety; tearing is natural response to mucosal irritation.)*
    b. Explain that the next step requires swallowing. *(Tube is about to enter esophagus.)*
16. With tube just above oropharynx, instruct patient to flex head forward and dry swallow or suck in air through straw. Advance tube 1 to 2 inches (2.5 to 5 cm) with each swallow. While advancing the tube in an unconscious patient (or in a patient who cannot swallow), stroke the patient's neck. *(Encourages the swallowing reflex and facilitates passage down the esophagus.)* If patient has trouble swallowing and is allowed fluids, offer glass of water. Advance tube with each swallow of water. *(The flexed position closes off upper airway to trachea and opens esophagus. Swallowing closes epiglottis over trachea and helps move tube into esophagus. Swallowing water reduces gagging or choking.)*
17. If patient begins to cough, gag, or choke, stop tube advancement. Instruct patient to breathe easily and take sips of water. *(Tubing sometimes accidentally enters larynx and initiates cough reflex. Gagging is eased by swallowing water.)*
18. If patient continues to cough, pull tube back slightly. *(It is possible for tube to enter the larynx and obstruct airway.)*
19. If patient continues to gag after tube is pulled back, check back of pharynx with flashlight and tongue blade. *(It is possible for tubing to accidentally enter larynx and initiate cough reflex.)*
20. After patient relaxes, continue advancing tube to desired distance. *(Tip of tube must be in the stomach to provide proper decompression.)*
21. Ask patient to talk. *(Patient is unable to talk if tube is passed through vocal cords.)*
22. Observe posterior pharynx for coiling of tube. *(The tube is pliable, and there is potential for it to coil up in back of pharynx instead of advancing into esophagus.)*
23. Attach syringe to end of tube. Aspirate gently back on syringe to obtain gastric contents. *(Begins determination of whether tube is correctly in place in the stomach.)*
24. Measure pH of aspirate with color-coded pH paper. Gastric aspirates have acidic pH values of 4 or less. *(Determines whether tube is correctly placed in the stomach.)* While returning gastric aspirates to stomach, place stethoscope over stomach area on abdomen and listen for swishing or gurgling sounds. *(Another check to determine correct placement of tube.)*
25. If tube is not in the stomach, advance another 1 to 2 inches (2.5 to 5 cm) and repeat Steps 23 and 24. *(Assesses for tube placement.)*
26. After tube is properly inserted, clamp end or connect it to suction. *(Refer to health care provider's order determining suction or clamp.)*
27. Secure tube to nose with tape or nose guard. Avoid putting pressure on nares. *(Anchors the tube securely.)* Clean the skin over the nose with alcohol to remove any skin oils or soil and coat with skin protectant solution before applying the tape or nose guard.

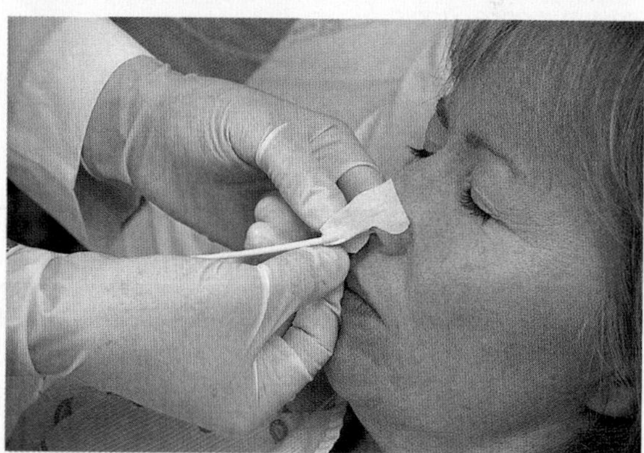

28. Fasten end of tube to gown by looping rubber band around tube in slip knot. Pin rubber band to gown. Provide slack in tubing to allow for movement. *(Reduces chance of putting pressure on nares by tube moving. Pinning provides slack for movement.)*

Continued

Skill 15.5 Inserting a Nasogastric Tube—cont'd

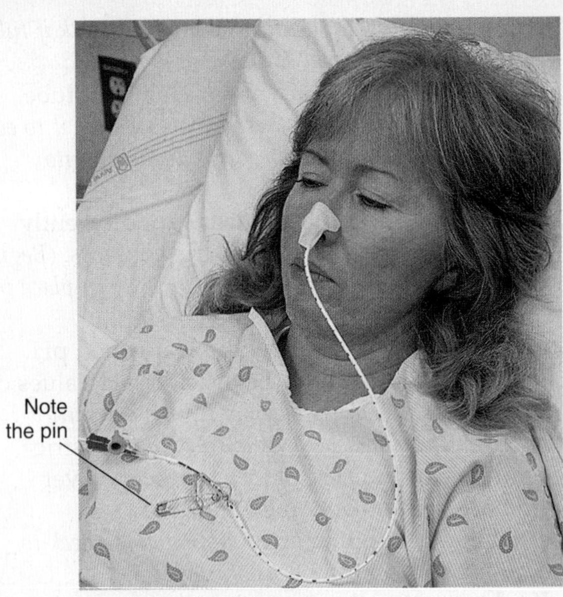

29. Unless health care provider orders otherwise, elevate head of bed 30 degrees. *(Helps prevent esophageal reflux and minimizes irritation caused by tube against posterior pharynx.)*
30. Refer to Standard Steps 10 to 17.
31. Document the following. *(Verifies performance of procedure and ensures continuity of care.)*
    - Date, time, and type of tube inserted
    - Patient's tolerance of procedure
    - Confirmation of placement
    - Character and amount of gastric contents
    - Whether tube is clamped or connected to suction
    - Patient teaching (see the Patient Teaching box on nasogastric tubes)
32. Report abnormalities:
    - Inability to advance tube *(Additional interventions or therapies may be necessary.)*

Step 27 and 28 figures from Elkin MK, Perry AG, Potter PA: *Nursing interventions and clinical skills,* ed 4, St. Louis, 2008, Mosby.

Box 15.2 Patient Problem Statements for the Patient With a Gastric Tube

Deficient Nutrition:
- Related to insufficient intake

Compromised Swallowing Ability:
- Related to neuromuscular impairment

Potential for Aspiration Into Airway:
- Related to inability to swallow effectively

Frequent, Loose Stools:
- Related to altered intake associated with tube feedings

Infrequent or Difficult Bowel Elimination:
- Related to altered intake associated with tube feedings

permitted to chew gum to increase salivation or to suck on small ice chips to help relieve throat dryness.

Another nursing concern is maintaining patency of the tube. Sometimes the tube becomes occluded with secretions, or the internal tip of the tube becomes occluded if the end of the tube is pressing against the gastric mucosa. Irrigate the nasogastric tube regularly with normal saline and a syringe (Skill 15.6). Turning the patient helps drain the stomach and may help reposition the tube so that it is not against the wall of the stomach. If necessary, try advancing the tube further or withdrawing it a little to reposition it. Keep in mind, however, that only a health care provider is permitted to reposition the tube when the patient has had gastric or esophageal surgery.

Patient Teaching

Nasogastric Tube

- Explain the need for a nasogastric tube.
- Explain how the tube will prevent nausea, vomiting, and abdominal distention.
- Teach patient and family how to care for the nasogastric tube at home, if this is appropriate.
- Explain the need to maintain moistness of mucous membranes with special mouth care.
- Explain to patient how to relax and communicate during tube insertion.
- Before insertion, explain the technique and sensations that the patient may feel.
- Allow time for, and address, patient's questions and concerns.
- Ensure adequate lubrication of the tube to decrease discomfort, especially with older adults.

Coordinated Care

Collaboration

Nasogastric Tube

- The skill of inserting a nasogastric tube requires the critical thinking and knowledge of a nurse. Unlicensed assistive personnel (UAP) are permitted to measure and record the drainage from the NG tube and provide oral and nasal hygiene. Teach UAP how to properly secure the NG tube.
- The skill of irrigating an NG tube requires the critical thinking and knowledge of a nurse; this task should not be delegated to UAP.
- The skill of removing an NG tube requires the critical thinking and knowledge of a nurse; this task should not be delegated to UAP.

Skill 15.6 Nasogastric Tube Irrigation

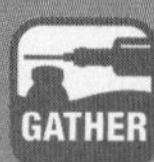

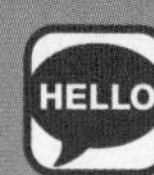

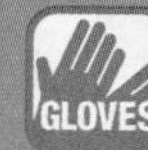

NURSING ACTION *(RATIONALE)*

1. Refer to Standard Steps 1 to 9.
2. Assemble equipment:
   - Clamp
   - Clean gloves
   - Container for irrigant
   - Irrigation set with syringe
   - Irrigation solution (usually normal saline)
   - Stethoscope
   - Syringe
   - Towel or waterproof pad
3. Place patient in semi-Fowler's position. *(Facilitates procedure.)*
4. Verify that tube is in right place:
   a. Attach syringe to end of tube and aspirate for stomach contents. Listen with stethoscope over stomach area on abdomen while returning aspirate for gurgling or swishing sounds. *(Confirms that tip of tube is in the stomach.)*
5. Evaluate abdomen. *(Provides baseline data for later comparison.)*
6. Pour normal saline into container; draw 30 mL (or amount ordered) into syringe. *(Use of saline minimizes loss of electrolytes from stomach fluid.)*
7. Clamp connection tubing distal to connection site. Disconnect tubing, and lay end on a towel. *(Reduces backflow of secretions and minimizes soiling of patient's gown and bed linens.)*
8. Insert tip of irrigating syringe into end of nasogastric (NG) tube. Hold syringe with tip pointed toward the floor, and instill 30 mL or ordered amount of saline slowly and evenly. Do not force solution; allow it to flow in by gravity. Never use air vent or pigtail on tubing of Salem sump for irrigation. *(Position of syringe prevents introduction of air into vent tubing, which has potential to cause gastric distention. Introducing solution under pressure may cause gastric trauma.)*
9. If resistance is met, check tubing for kinks, change patient's position, and repeat attempt; if resistance continues, confer with registered nurse (RN) or health care provider. *(Ensures that tip of tubing is not lying against wall of stomach. Buildup of secretions will cause distention.)*
10. Withdraw fluid into syringe and measure; continue irrigating with ordered amount of saline until purpose of irrigation has been accomplished. *(Clears the tubing.)*
11. Reconnect NG tube to suction or drainage tubing. To prevent leakage of fluid from airway vent of Salem sump tubes, introduce 30 mL of air into airway lumen to clear air vent tubing. Secure airway lumen above level of stomach to prevent siphoning effect. *(Reestablishes drainage collection.)*
12. Note amount of saline instilled and withdrawn. Subtract amount instilled from amount withdrawn and record difference as output. *(Fluid remaining in stomach is measured as intake.)*
13. Refer to Standard Steps 10 to 17.
14. Document the following. *(Description of gastric contents provides baseline to determine any change.)*
    - Date and time
    - Type and amount of solution
    - Character and volume of aspirate
    - Patient teaching (see the Patient Teaching box on nasogastric tubes)
    - Record balance of fluid instilled and aspirated on intake and output (I&O) sheet *(Balance reflects fluid gain or loss.)*
15. Report abnormalities. *(Abnormal findings indicate need to reposition tube or administer additional therapies.)*
    - Failure of tube to drain
    - Abdominal distention
    - Unusual characteristic of drainage (blood)

States and facilities vary on policy for who is authorized to insert NG tubes (see the Coordinated Care box on nasogastric tubes). Some states and facilities allow a licensed practical nurse or licensed vocational nurse (LPN/LVN) to insert NG tubes (see Skill 15.5). Most facilities allow the LPN/LVN to irrigate the NG tube (see Skill 15.5), administer feedings (see Chapter 19, Skill 19.1), care for the NG tube (Skill 15.7), and remove the NG tube (Skill 15.8). Check your state's scope of practice for the LPN/LVN and facility policy.

BOWEL ELIMINATION

Elimination of bowel wastes **(defecation)** is a basic human need and is essential for normal body function. Normal bowel elimination depends on several factors: a balanced diet, including high-fiber foods; a daily fluid intake of 2000 to 3000 mL; and activity to promote muscle tone and peristalsis. Each patient has an individual pattern of defecation, but every patient should have a bowel movement at least every 1 to 3 days. This pattern

Skill 15.7 Care of Gastric and Intestinal Suctioning

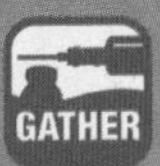

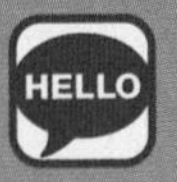

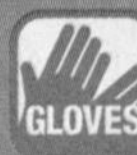

NURSING ACTION *(RATIONALE)*

1. Refer to Standard Steps 1 to 9.
2. Assemble equipment:
   - Clean gloves
   - Emesis basin
   - Stethoscope
   - Suction apparatus (if used)
   - Syringe
   - Towel
3. Determine that suction apparatus is working correctly.
   a. For suction machine (Gomco), check the following:
      (1) Machine is plugged in securely.
      (2) Light is blinking on and off.
      (3) Tubing connections are secured.
      (4) Setting is correct.
   b. For wall suction, check the following:
      (1) Pressure gauge connections are tight.
      (2) Pressure indicated on gauge is as ordered or according to facility policy. *(High pressure could lead to gastric bleeding.)*
      (3) Suction is set on intermittent or continuous as ordered.
4. Evaluate the following. *(Enables the nurse to determine need for any special care before or after procedure.)*
   a. Patient's oral and nasal cavities
   b. Patient's abdomen for bowel sounds and extent of distention. *(Provides baseline data for further assessments and may indicate tube malfunction.)*
   c. Patient's oral intake; nothing-by-mouth (NPO) status should be ordered
   d. Patient's lips and oral mucosa for dryness and cracking
5. Ensure that tubing is not kinked and that patient is not lying on tubing. *(Verifies that the patient or tube is not causing obstruction.)*
6. Pin nasogastric (NG) tube to patient's gown with enough slack to allow movement (see illustration for Step 28 of Skill 15.5). *(Prevents dislodging tube and patient discomfort.)*
7. Verify that drainage is moving through tubing to drainage collection bottle. *(Indicates that stomach or intestinal contents are being removed.)*
8. For Salem sump tube, ensure that vent is pointing upward. *(There is potential that vent pointing downward will promote drainage through vent via gravity.)* Listen at opening of blue air vent. *(Hissing sound indicates air vent is patent.)* If no hissing sounds are heard, instruct patient to cough, or reposition patient in the right or left Sims position or the supine position. *(Helps move distal opening of tube in the stomach away from the mucosa wall and enables the suction to resume.)* It may be necessary to momentarily disconnect the NG tube from the suction tubing; be certain to reconnect immediately.
9. Measure amount of drainage in bottle, noting color; empty when it becomes full and at end of each shift. *(Provides baseline data for further assessments, prevents overflow, and ensures accurate measurement.)*
10. Refer to Standard Steps 10 to 17.
11. Document the following. *(Description of gastric contents provides baseline data to determine any change.)*
    - Date and time
    - Procedure
    - Observations
    - Amount, color, and consistency of drainage
    - Abnormalities
    - Patient teaching (see the Patient Teaching box on nasogastric tubes)
12. Report any abnormalities to health care provider. *(Abnormal findings indicate need to reposition tube or administer additional therapies.)*
    - Failure of tube to drain
    - Abdominal distention
    - Unusual characteristics of drainage (blood)

should be determined on hospital admission, and an abdominal evaluation should be completed. Ask about any alterations in bowel elimination to determine patient problems related to elimination (Box 15.3).

To promote a normal pattern of elimination, establish a routine time for defecation, encourage the patient to heed the urge to defecate, and allow the patient to sit on a commode or, if he or she is in bed, in a Fowler's position because this is the customary position for defecation. Bowel elimination is a private activity. Afford the patient as much privacy as possible, and avoid continually "checking on" the patient, because this may make the patient uncomfortable and not provide an environment conducive for defecation. Some patients

Skill 15.8 Nasogastric Tube Removal

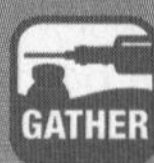

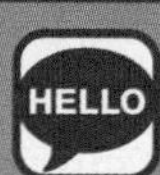

PRIVACY

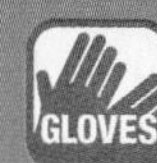

NURSING ACTION *(RATIONALE)*

1. Refer to Standard Steps 1 to 9.
2. Assemble equipment:
   - Clamp (optional)
   - Clean gloves
   - Facial tissues
   - Mask and goggles if splashing is expected (optional)
   - Plastic bag
   - Towel or waterproof pad
3. Reassure patient that nasogastric (NG) tube removal is less distressing than tube insertion. *(Reduces patient's anxiety and promotes cooperation.)*
4. Evaluate the following:
   a. Patient's abdomen for bowel sounds. *(Provides baseline abdominal data for future comparison.)*
   b. Patient's nasal and oral cavities. *(Enables the nurse to determine need for special interventions before or after procedure.)*
5. If tube is attached to suction, turn off suction and disconnect tubing, remove tape or nose guard from nose, and unfasten pin from patient's gown. *(Prevents pulling on tape or nose guard and damaging tissue on nose.)*
6. Place towel or waterproof pad across patient's chest, and give patient tissues. *(Protects bed linens and patient's gown. Patients often wish to wipe eyes and blow nose after tube removal.)*
7. Instruct patient to take deep breath and hold it; pinch tube with fingers or clamp. *(Prevents aspiration from any leakage and prevents tube from leaking during procedure.)* Quickly and smoothly remove tube while patient is holding breath. *(If patient begins to gag, continue to remove tubing. It is the tubing that is causing the patient to gag.)*
8. Place tubing in plastic bag or towel. *(Plastic bag or towel covers and conceals tube, which is not usually a pleasant sight.)*
9. Provide oral and nasal care; position patient for comfort. *(Promotes comfort.)*
10. Dispose of tube and equipment; measure drainage and note characteristics of drainage. *(Reduces transfer of microorganisms. Ensures accurate measure of fluid output.)*
11. Inspect condition of nares and oral cavity. Report abnormalities. *(Abnormal findings indicate need for additional therapies.)*
    - Absence of bowel sounds
    - Complaints of severe sore throat
    - Erythema
    - Excoriation
    - Irritation during swallowing
    - Nasal fullness
    - Tenderness
12. Palpate abdomen periodically, noting any distention, pain, or rigidity; auscultate abdomen for bowel sounds. *(Determines success of abdominal decompression and the return of peristalsis.)*
13. Refer to Standard Steps 10 to 17.
14. Document the following. *(Verifies performance of procedure and ensures continuity of care.)*
    - Date and time
    - Removal of NG tube and condition of tube
    - Characteristics of drainage
    - Condition of nasal cavity
    - Presence of bowel sounds
    - Abdominal distention
    - Patient's tolerance of procedure

Box 15.3 Patient Problem Statements for the Patient With Altered Bowel Elimination

Anxiousness:
- Related to bowel function
- Related to rejection by friends

Distorted Body Image:
- Related to presence of ostomy

Impaired Coping:
- Related to daily ostomy care requirements

Infrequent or Difficult Bowel Elimination:
- Related to decreased activity
- Related to decreased peristalsis
- Related to dehydration
- Related to inadequate dietary fiber

Insufficient Knowledge Regarding Condition, Treatment Program, and Self-Care:
- Related to lack of exposure and information
- Related to misinterpretation of information
- Related to unfamiliarity with information

Potential for Compromised Skin Integrity:
- Related to irritation of skin around stoma

Recent Onset of Pain:
- Related to bowel distention

may resist using a bedpan because of discomfort and lack of privacy. Reassure the patient as much as possible and make sure the bed is in Fowler's position.

Many people have their own established ritual to promote elimination, such as drinking warm water with lemon juice or drinking black coffee with breakfast. Be alert to patient habits that are detrimental to normal bowel function, such as long-term, routine use of laxatives and cathartics. Eventually these may cause the intestines to lose the ability to respond to the presence of stool in the rectum, which often results in chronic constipation. Overcoming dependency on these medications is often difficult to accomplish and requires cooperation and compliance from the patient (see the Lifespan Considerations box on altered bowel elimination in older adults).

 Lifespan Considerations

Older Adults

Altered Bowel Elimination

- Many older adult patients are especially prone to dysrhythmias and other problems related to vagal stimulation associated with defecation. Therefore it is important to monitor heart rate and rhythm closely.
- In many older adults, constipation results from insufficient dietary bulk, inadequate fluid intake, laxative abuse, diminished muscle tone and motor function, decreased defecation reflex, mental or physical illness, and the presence of tumors or strictures.
- For an older adult, a diet containing at least 6 to 10 g of dietary fiber per day adds bulk, weight, and form to stool and improves defecation.
- Older adults should develop a regular toileting routine in response to the urge to defecate.
- The older adult patient or a family member should keep a week's diary of meals and fluid intake. The nurse should determine whether dietary pattern contributes to constipation. The nurse should recommend an increase in fiber if it is needed.
- The nurse should encourage as much activity as tolerated to maintain peristalsis and decrease the risk for constipation.

CARE OF THE PATIENT WITH HEMORRHOIDS

Hemorrhoids are swollen and inflamed veins in the anus and lower rectum. They may result from straining during bowel movements or from increased pressure during pregnancy or with heavy lifting. Hemorrhoids can be internal (inside the rectum), or external (around the anus). They are frequently a source of discomfort and have the capacity to cause an alteration in elimination. The goal for patients with hemorrhoids is to decrease pain, prevent elimination problems, and prevent damage to the already swollen tissue. To facilitate these goals, it is necessary for the patient to maintain a proper diet high in fiber, ensure adequate fluid intake, and participate in regular exercise. If the hemorrhoids are particularly troublesome, localized heat in the form of a sitz bath, or witch hazel pads often provide some relief. Use extreme caution when inserting rectal suppositories for patients with hemorrhoids. Use a liberal amount of lubricant during insertion to prevent pain or trauma to the rectal tissue. In such patients, rectal thermometers and rectal tubes should not be used.

FLATULENCE

Flatulence, or the presence of air or gas (flatus) in the intestinal tract, typically occurs when a person consumes gas-producing liquids and foods such as carbonated beverages, cabbage, or beans; swallows excessive amounts of air; or is constipated. It also can be caused by decreased peristalsis, abdominal surgery, some narcotic medications, and decreased physical activity. Flatulence may cause distention of the stomach and abdomen and, in some cases, mild to moderate abdominal cramping, which can be painful. To promote peristalsis and passage of flatus, encourage the patient to ambulate. If ambulating does not help relieve the flatulence and the possible cause is not found, use of a rectal tube may be necessary. The presence of the tube in the rectum stimulates peristalsis and the movement of flatus, thus eliminating the discomfort (Skill 15.9).

ADMINISTERING AN ENEMA

An **enema** is the instillation of a solution into the colon via the anus. The primary reason for an enema is promotion of defecation in a patient with constipation. Enemas can be given for a number of reasons, such as cleansing the colon before a diagnostic procedure or abdominal surgery, management of constipation or fecal impaction, and administration of medication. The volume and type of enema administered depends on the reason for it and the health care provider's order.

A cleansing enema stimulates peristalsis by introducing large volumes of fluid to distend the bowel. This type of enema helps empty the colon completely and is used frequently before surgery or a GI diagnostic procedure.

An oil retention enema is used to soften the stool and lubricate the bowel to make defecation easier. It is used when a fecal impaction is suspected. A **fecal impaction** is a collection of feces in the rectum in the form of a mass that becomes so large or hard that the patient is unable to pass it voluntarily. Medicated enemas can be used for a variety of reasons but are used most frequently to bring down an extremely high potassium level (polystyrene sulfonate [Kayexalate] enema).

No matter what type of enema is used, caution patients to limit the number of enemas they use. The defecation reflex may become dependent on enemas with repeated use, which can cause constipation. It is better to determine the cause of bowel irregularity or constipation and treat the cause rather than relying on enemas (Skill 15.10).

Skill 15.9 Inserting a Rectal Tube

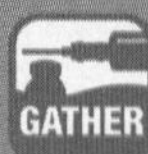

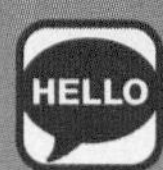

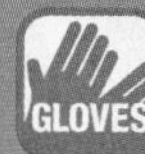

NURSING ACTION *(RATIONALE)*

1. Refer to Standard Steps 1 to 11.
2. Assemble equipment:
   - Clean gloves
   - Commercial kit with water-soluble lubricant, gloves, rectal tube, sponges, basin, and waterproof pad (if available)
   - Protector pad (Chux)
   - Stethoscope
   - Water-soluble lubricant
3. Auscultate bowel sounds. *(Provides basis for determining effectiveness of therapy.)*
4. Assist the patient to the left Sims position. Arrange gown and top linens to prevent soiling while still covering patient. *(Facilitates procedure and provides for patient privacy.)*
5. Place waterproof pad under buttocks. *(Protects bottom linen.)*
6. Don clean gloves. Lubricate tube well with water-soluble lubricant. *(Reduces spread of microorganisms and facilitates the insertion of tube.)*
7. Expose patient's anus. Insert tube 4 to 6 inches (10 to 15 cm) in the same manner as for an enema (see Skill 15.10).
8. Insert drainage end into receptacle or use commercially prepared set. *(The receptacle will contain any expelled stool.)*
9. Instruct the patient to lie quietly to prevent dislodging tube; leave tube in place no more than 30 minutes. If flatulence persists, notify the health care provider.
10. Remove tube and assist patient to bedpan, bedside commode, or toilet as necessary; stimulation of peristalsis often results in bowel movement.
11. Provide for patient hygiene; auscultate bowel sounds, and assist patient to bed or chair.
12. Refer to Standard Steps 12 to 17.
13. Document the following. *(Verifies performance of procedure and ensures continuity of care.)*
    - Date and time of tube insertion
    - Results
    - Patient's response to procedure
14. If flatulence, abdominal discomfort, or distention continues, reinsert tube as required or as ordered by health care provider. *(Continued use of rectal tubes has potential to cause irritation and eventual skin impairment of the anus and the rectal mucosa.)*

OSTOMIES

An **ostomy**, by definition, is an artificial opening. The site of the opening is called a *stoma.* Ostomies can be created because of trauma to the intestine, severe inflammation, or diseases such as cancer that involve part of the intestine. They can be temporary or permanent, depending on the reason they are present, and the characteristics of the fecal material vary according to where the ostomy is located along the intestine. Fecal material in the ileum is liquid, and fecal matter in the rectum is solid. Therefore the closer the ostomy is to either end determines what type of stool will be in the ostomy. Material coming out of the stomach contains many enzymes that increase the acidity of the material. Therefore stool in the ileum, cecum, and ascending colon tends to be more acidic and irritating to the skin surrounding the ostomy. As the material moves through the large intestine, water is removed, and the material becomes more solid and less acidic, causing less irritation to the skin surrounding the stoma.

An **ileostomy** is an opening in the ileum (the distal part of the small intestine). An ileostomy is needed when the entire colon must be removed or bypassed, as in cases of congenital defects, cancer, inflammatory bowel disease, or bowel trauma.

A **colostomy** is the surgical creation of a stoma on the abdominal wall to where the colon is normally attached. The colostomy then diverts stool through the stoma. Again, the stool may be liquid, semiformed, or formed, depending on the area of the colon incised. The procedure is performed for patients with cancer of the colon, intestinal obstructions, intestinal trauma, or inflammatory diseases of the colon. Some colostomies are permanent, and some are temporary measures used until intestinal healing occurs.

A **urostomy** is the diversion of urine away from a diseased or defective bladder through a surgically created opening or stoma in the skin. This may be necessary in the presence of a congenital anomaly or when the bladder must be removed because of disease, trauma, or obstruction.

Colostomy Care

To be able to provide the patient with optimal colostomy care, it is important for the nurse to know the correct use of various products used for colostomy care and to educate the patient about appropriate care and use

Skill 15.10 Administering an Enema

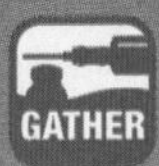

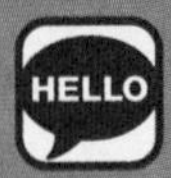

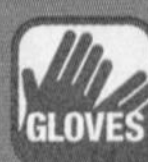

NURSING ACTION *(RATIONALE)*

1. Refer to Standard Steps 1 to 9.
2. Assemble equipment:
   - Bath blanket
   - Bedpan, bedside commode, or access to toilet
   - Clean gloves
   - Intravenous (IV) pole
   - Prepared kit or enema set
   - Solution
   - Toilet tissue
   - Wash basin, washcloth, towel, soap
   - Water-soluble lubricant

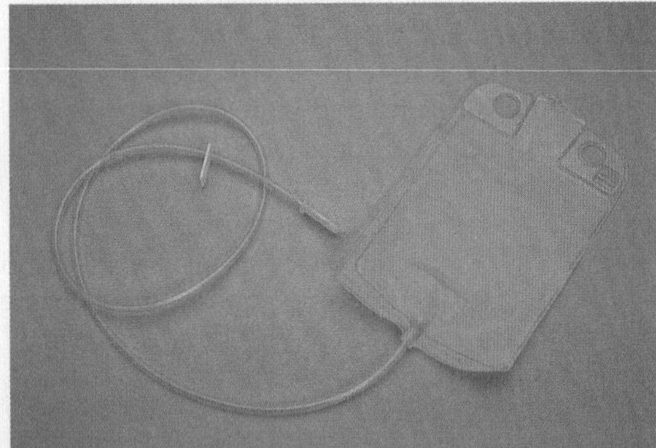

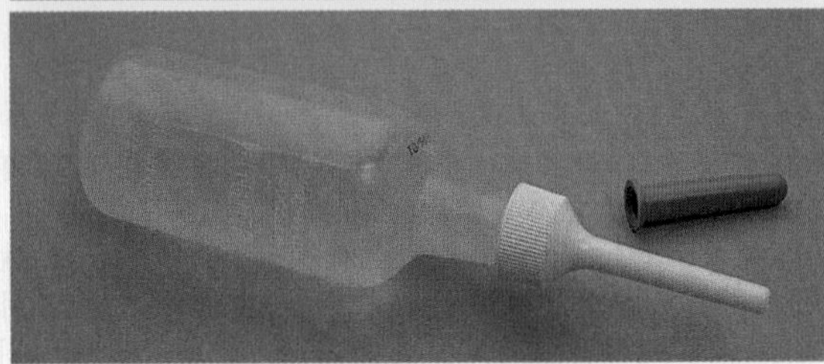

3. Determine the following. *(Determines need for enema.)*
   a. Most recent bowel movement
   b. Presence or absence of bowel sounds
   c. Ability to control rectal sphincter *(It is necessary to place patients with no sphincter control on a bedpan before the procedure because such patients cannot retain enema solution.)*
   d. Presence or absence of hemorrhoids *(Hemorrhoids may obscure the rectal opening and cause discomfort or bleeding.)*
   e. Presence of abdominal pain *(May preclude the use of enema. Never give an enema to patients with possible appendicitis because the appendix can rupture.)*
   f. Patient's level of understanding and previous experience with enemas *(Enables the nurse to provide for appropriate teaching and reassurance.)*
4. Prepare solution. There are several types of enema solutions. Cleansing enemas include tap water, normal saline, low-volume hypertonic solutions, and soapsuds solution. *(Prepares equipment for procedure.)*
5. Arrange equipment at patient's bedside. *(Organizes procedure.)*
6. Assist patient to the Sims position. *(Allows enema solution to flow downward by gravity along natural curve of sigmoid colon and rectum, thus improving retention of enema.)* When an enema is given to a patient who is unable to contract the external sphincter, position the patient on the bedpan. Avoid giving the enema with the patient sitting on the toilet; it is possible for the inserted rectal tubing to abrade the rectal wall, and the enema solution is forced uphill, which makes the enema less effective.
7. Place waterproof pad under patient. *(Protects bed linens.)*
8. Place bath blanket over patient and fanfold linen to foot of bed; adjust patient's gown to keep it from being soiled while it still provides privacy. *(Protects bed linens and patient's gown from soiling and provides warmth and privacy.)*
9. Clamp tubing; fill container with correctly warmed solution (usually 750 to 1000 mL at 105°F [41°C]) and any additives ordered. Administer a child's enema using appropriate equipment at 100°F to avoid burning rectal tissue (see illustration for Step 2, *top*); read disposable package for instructions. *(Hot water has capacity to burn intestinal mucosa. Cold water has capacity to cause abdominal cramping and is difficult to retain.)* Release clamp, allowing solution to flow through tubing to remove any air from the tubing; reclamp. Suggested maximal volumes are as follows:
   - Infant: 150 to 250 mL
   - Toddler: 250 to 500 mL
   - School-age child: 500 mL
   - Adolescent: 500 to 700 mL
   - Adult: 750 to 1000 mL

   a. For commercially prepared enema (see illustration for Step 2, *bottom*)
      (1) Remove cover from tip of enema (tip is prelubricated, but add additional lubricant if needed); insert entire tip into anus.
      (2) Squeeze container until it is empty. Usually a small amount of solution will remain in container. Most containers hold about

Skill 15.10 Administering an Enema—cont'd

250 mL. Continue to squeeze the container to prevent siphoning solution back into the container.

(3) Encourage patient to retain solution at least 5 minutes. *(Retention of solution promotes peristalsis and enhances defecation.)*

b. For standard enema:

(1) Lubricate 4 inches (10 cm) at end of tubing; spread patient's buttocks to expose anus; while rotating tube, gently insert it 3 to 4 inches (7 to 10 cm). Instruct patient to breathe out slowly through mouth. *(Breathing out promotes relaxation of external rectal sphincter.)*

(2) Elevate container 12 to 18 inches (30 to 45 cm) above level of anus (see illustration). *(Allows solution to flow at appropriate rate. Raising container too high causes rapid infusion and possible painful distention of colon. Holding container too low leads to inadequate instillation of enema solution.)*

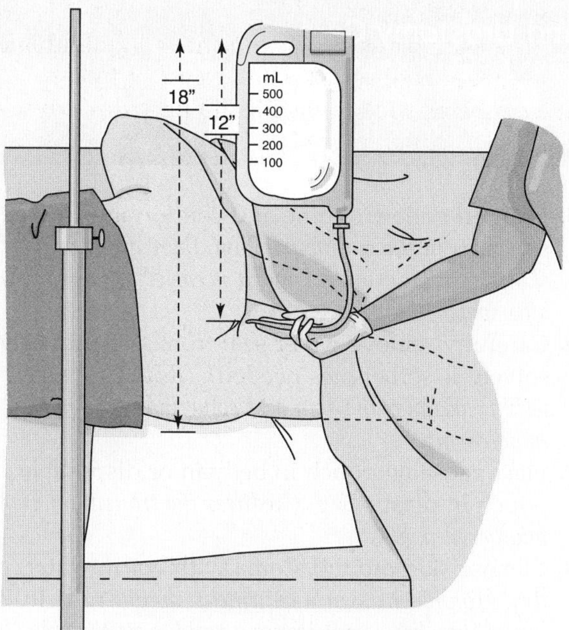

(3) Release clamp, and allow solution to flow slowly. Usually solution will flow for 5 to 10 minutes. *(Allowing solution to instill slowly enables patient to retain all of solution and minimizes discomfort.)*

(4) Lower container or clamp tubing if patient complains of cramping; encourage slow, deep breathing. Do not remove tubing tip. *(Temporary cessation of infusion reduces cramping and promotes ability to retain all of the solution.)* If severe cramping, bleeding, or sudden severe abdominal pain occurs and is unrelieved by temporarily stopping or slowing flow of solution, stop enema and notify health care provider.

(5) Clamp and remove tube when all the solution has been administered. Encourage patient to retain solution at least 5 minutes. *(Retention of solution promotes peristalsis and enhances defecation.)*

15. When patient is no longer able to retain solution, assist patient to bedpan, bedside commode, or bathroom. *(Normal squatting position promotes defecation; longer retention promotes more effective stimulation of peristalsis and defecation.)*

16. Instruct patient to call the nurse to inspect results before stool is flushed. Observe characteristics of feces or solution. *(Allows nurse to evaluate effectiveness of procedure.)* When enemas are ordered "until clear" in preparation for surgery, enemas are repeated until patient passes fluid that is clear and contains no fecal matter. Usually three consecutive enemas are adequate. If after three enemas the water is highly colored or contains solid fecal material, notify health care provider before continuing. *(Excessive loss of electrolytes is a dangerous possibility.)*

17. Refer to Standard Steps 10 to 17.

18. Provide for patient hygiene; assist patient to bed or chair. *(Patients sometimes need assistance to clean anal area. Fecal contents tend to irritate skin. Hygiene promotes patient comfort and decreases the risk of skin impairment.)*

19. Document the following. *(Verifies performance of procedure and ensures continuity of care.)*

- Date and time
- Type and volume of enema
- Temperature of solution
- Characteristics of results
- How patient tolerates procedure

Figure for Step 2 from Perry AG, Potter PA, Elkin MK: *Nursing interventions and clinical skills*, ed 5, St. Louis, 2012, Mosby. Figure for Step 9b(3) from Sorrentino SA & Remmert LN: *Mosby's textbook for nursing assistants*, ed 9, St. Louis, 2017, Elsevier.

of these products. There are various types of pouching systems and skin barriers available to patients. One-pouch systems have a skin barrier (wafer) that is preattached to the pouch; two-piece systems have a pouch that is separate from the wafer. Some skin barriers are precut, whereas others must be cut to fit the stoma. When skin barriers are cut to fit the stoma, ensure the ostomy appliance opening is small enough to form a proper seal, 1⁄16 inch larger than the stoma. Also, the appliance must not cause pressure on the stoma, because there is a blood and nerve supply in the stoma but no sensation. An ill-fitting appliance can cause a pressure sore and lead to gangrene (Fig. 15.8 and Skills 15.11 and 15.12; see also the Patient Teaching boxes on ostomy care and on urostomy care, and the Home Care Considerations, Lifespan Considerations, and Coordinated Care boxes on ostomy care).

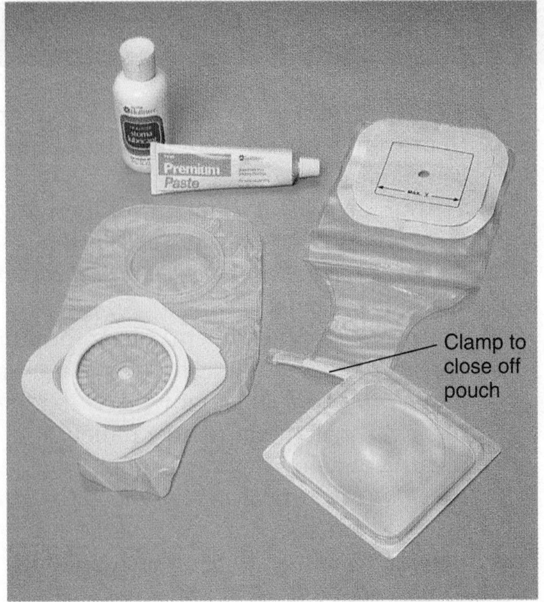

Fig. 15.8 Ostomy pouches and skin barriers. (From Elkin MK, Perry AG, Potter PA: *Nursing interventions and clinical skills*, ed 4, St. Louis, 2008, Mosby.)

Colostomy Irrigation

Colostomy irrigation sometimes is used to maintain a regular elimination pattern. It is used less frequently now than in the past: many patients have regular bowel

Skill 15.11 Performing Colostomy, Ileostomy, and Urostomy Care

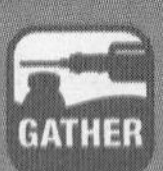

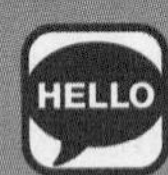

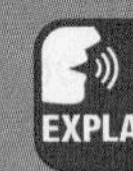

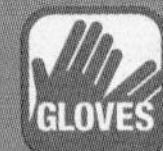

NURSING ACTION *(RATIONALE)*

Ostomy Care

1. Refer to Standard Steps 1 to 9.
2. Assemble equipment (see Fig. 15.8):
   - 1-inch–wide paper tape (optional)
   - Barrier paste
   - Basin with warm water
   - Bedpan or trash bag
   - Clean gloves
   - Measuring guide (if used)
   - Pouch clamp
   - Pouch with attached wafer seal
   - Scissors
   - Skin sealant wipes
   - Washcloth (disposable washcloth is acceptable)
3. Observe for the following. *(Enables the nurse to determine need for pouch change.)*
   a. Pouch leakage and length of time in place *(Pouches must be changed every 3 to 7 days to prevent skin impairment.)*
   b. Stoma for healing and color *(Proper stoma appearance is moist and reddish pink.)*
   c. Abdominal incision
4. Arrange supplies and equipment at patient's bedside or in bathroom (see Fig. 15.8). *(Promotes smooth flow of procedure.)*
5. Position patient supine and comfortable. *(When patient is in the supine position, there are fewer skinfolds and wrinkles, and it is easier to position and affix wafer.)*
6. Carefully remove wafer seal from skin (adhesive solvent is sometimes needed). *(Reduces trauma; jerking irritates the skin and sometimes causes skin impairment.)*
7. Place reusable pouch in bedpan or disposable pouch in plastic bag. *(Reduces the transmission of microorganisms.)*
8. Cleanse skin around stoma with warm water; pat dry. *(To prevent skin impairment, do not rub. Avoid use of soap because it leaves a residue on the skin that interferes with pouch adhesion to skin.)*
9. Measure stoma opening. *(Ensures proper fit.)*
10. Place toilet tissue over stoma; use gauze for ileostomy. *(Prevents expelled stool from leaking during procedure.)* Note color and viability of stoma. If skin sealant is to be used, apply to skin and allow to dry.
11. Apply protective skin barrier about 1⁄16 inch from stoma. *(Creates wrinkle-free, secure seal; decreases chance of skin irritation from adhesive on skin.)*

Skill 15.11 Performing Colostomy, Ileostomy, and Urostomy Care—cont'd

12. Cut an opening in the center of wafer to $\frac{1}{16}$ inch larger than stoma, and apply protective wafer with flange. *(Ensures proper fit.)*
13. Gently attach pouch to flange by compressing the two together. *(Ensures appropriate collection of feces and application of pouch reservoir.)*
14. Remove tissue or gauze from stoma and backing from protectant wafer; center opening over stoma, and press against skin for 1 to 2 minutes. *(Establishes contact between barrier adhesive and skin and ensures pouch adherence.)*
15. Fold over bottom edges of pouch once to fit clamp. Secure clamp. If bottom edge of pouch is folded over more than once, the plastic will be too thick for the clamp, thus springing the clamp and causing spillage of fecal matter. *(Creates secure seal to prevent leaking.)*
16. If patient uses belt, attach at this time. *(Supports pouch and enhances feelings of security.)*
17. Assist patient to comfortable position in bed or chair; remove equipment from bedside. *(Promotes comfort.)*
18. Empty, wash, and dry reusable pouch. *(Reduces odor and extends usefulness.)*
19. Refer to Standard Steps 10 to 17.
20. Document the following. *(Verifies performance of procedure and ensures continuity of care.)*
    - Date and time
    - Procedure
    - Type of pouch
    - Type of skin barrier
    - Amount and appearance of feces
    - Condition of stoma and peristomal skin
    - Patient's level of participation
    - Patient teaching (see the Patient Teaching boxes on urostomy and ostomy care and Home Care Considerations box on ostomy care)

Urostomy Care

Follow Steps 1 to 5 of ostomy care procedure. Then perform the following actions:

1. Empty urine into graduated pitcher; note amount and characteristics of urine. *(Provides nurse with data to determine further needs.)*
2. Carefully remove wafer seal from skin (use adhesive solvent if necessary), and place pouch in plastic bag. *(Reduces trauma; jerking movements irritate the skin and tend to cause skin impairment.)*
3. Cleanse skin with warm water and pat dry. *(To prevent skin impairment, do not rub. Avoid using soap because it may irritate the skin.)*
4. Measure stoma. Note color and viability of stoma. *(Ensures accurate fit. Careful observation provides data for later comparison.)*
5. Place gauze over stoma. *(Prevents urine from contacting skin.)*
6. If skin sealant is to be used, apply to skin and allow to dry; apply protective stoma paste about $\frac{1}{16}$ inch from the stoma. *(Ensures a snug fit.)*
7. Cut an opening in the center of wafer $\frac{1}{16}$ inch larger than stoma. Apply protective wafer with flange. *(Creates wrinkle-free seal; decreases chance that skin impairment will occur.)*
8. Refer to Steps 13 through 20 of ostomy care procedure to complete urostomy care.

Skill 15.12 Performing Colostomy Irrigation

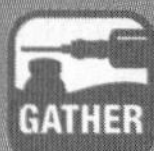

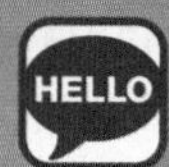

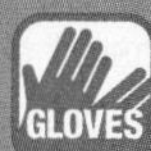

NURSING ACTION *(RATIONALE)*

Note that colostomy irrigation is no longer performed on a routine basis, but it may help patients achieve some regularity of elimination.

1. Refer to Standard Steps 1 to 9.
2. Assemble equipment and supplies:
    - Bed protector
    - Bedpan or toilet
    - Catheter with cone
    - Clamp
    - Clean gloves
    - Container
    - Irrigation set
    - Irrigation sleeve with or without belt
    - New pouch and wafer seal with flange
    - Tubing with clamp
    - Warm water and basin
    - Washcloth and towel (disposable washcloth is acceptable)
    - Water-soluble lubricant

Continued

Skill 15.12 Performing Colostomy Irrigation—cont'd

3. Determine the following. *(Enables the nurse to determine need for procedure.)*
   a. Level of comfort (on a scale of 0 to 10) and need for pain management
   b. Appropriateness of patient's condition for irrigation *(Only patients with a descending or sigmoid colostomy are appropriate candidates because stool is more formed and less liquid.)*
   c. Patient's ability to manipulate irrigation equipment and to understand concepts of bowel management
   d. Patient's readiness to learn self-irrigation of colostomy
4. Position patient.
   - Bathroom: Instruct patient to sit on toilet or on a chair in front of the toilet.
   - Bed: Have patient lie comfortably with head of bed slightly elevated. *(Do not overexpose patient.)*
   - NOTE: Allow the patient to perform as many of these steps as possible independently; provide teaching and assistance as needed. Be alert to patient's readiness to learn and perform self-care.
5. Remove pouch, cleanse skin, and place irrigation sleeve over stoma; attach belt if patient uses one; place end of sleeve in toilet. *(Provides for patient cleanliness and decreases risk for skin breakdown. Make sure irrigation sleeve is correctly attached. End of sleeve must be in toilet or bedpan to prevent spillage of feces.)*
6. Close clamp on irrigation tubing; fill irrigation container with 1000 mL of tepid water (or as otherwise ordered). It is acceptable to hang container on a hook at patient's shoulder level. *(This position prevents too high a pressure and reduces possibility of bowel damage.)* Allow a small amount of water to flow through tubing. *(Allow some solution to fill tubing to express air, which is otherwise forced into the bowel and causes cramps.)*
7. Attach cone to tubing; lubricate cone; insert cone into stoma through top of sleeve. Do not force cone into stoma. Use gentle pressure to hold tip in place in stoma. *(To prevent trauma to bowel, do not insert entire length of cone into stoma. Too little pressure causes the irrigation solution to flow out alongside of cone and not into patient. Too much pressure has capacity to block flow of irrigation solution into patient.)*

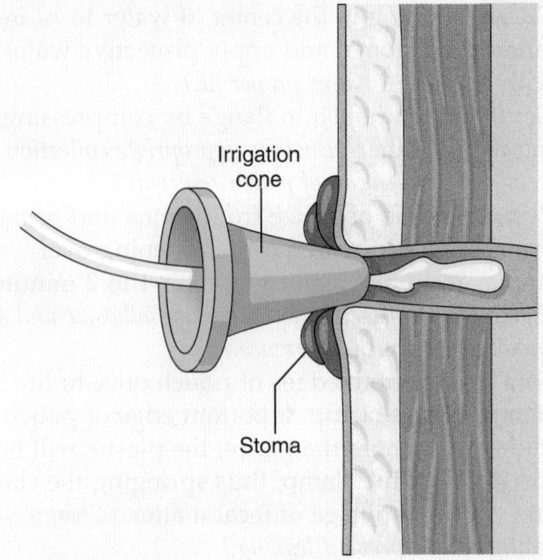

8. While you hold cone in place, allow solution to flow slowly into colon (500 to 1000 mL over 15 minutes). If patient complains of cramping, stop flow without removing cone until cramps subside. *(Stopping or slowing infusion allows patient to adjust to irrigation and tolerate the procedure better.)*
9. After all solution is instilled, remove cone and close top of sleeve. *(Prevents spillage of feces.)*
10. Instruct patient to sit about 15 to 20 minutes while the returning solution flows into toilet. *(If patient cannot sit this long, it is acceptable to close the end of the irrigation sleeve with a clamp and allow the patient to be up and walk around the room. Exercise stimulates the bowel.)*
11. Drain sleeve; rinse and remove it. *(Some irrigation sleeves are reusable and should be cleaned as directed by manufacturer.)*
12. Observe patient and results of irrigation; flush toilet. *(Provides data for comparison.)*
13. Perform colostomy care (see Skill 15.11). *(Provides for patient comfort.)*
14. Refer to Standard Steps 10 to 17.
15. Document the following. *(Verifies performance of procedure and ensures continuity of care.)*
    - Date and time
    - Solution used
    - Amount of solution
    - Results
    - Observations
    - Patient's tolerance of procedure

movements without irrigation. If the patient desires irrigation, the patient must be prepared to devote 60 to 90 minutes per day in the bathroom for the procedure.

Colostomy irrigation requires special equipment and is not without complications. The patient needs a cone-tipped irrigation device (see Step 7 of Skill 15.12), an irrigation sleeve, and irrigation solution or access to tap water. The patient places the cone-tipped irrigation device in the stoma through the sleeve. The sleeve is used to contain the drainage from the stoma as it passes into the commode. Approximately 500 to 1000 mL is instilled slowly into the stoma, and the patient must sit on the commode while it drains out (approximately 30 minutes). Complications associated with colostomy irrigation include damage or perforation of the bowel, which can lead to peritonitis. Other complications range from tissue damage as a result of the temperature of the irrigating solution to fluid and electrolyte imbalances if too much tap water is used.

Lifespan Considerations

Older Adults

Ostomy Considerations

- Evaluate the older adult's cognitive status and capacity to understand ostomy self-care instructions.
- Evaluate the older adult's motor and visual ability to prepare ostomy equipment.
- For patients who are unable to custom-cut the size of their skin barriers, consider having barriers precut by the ostomy equipment supplier or using a precut two-piece system.
- Avoid hot water and harsh soaps when washing the skin around the ostomy.
- Teach patients about the change in the number of bowel movements that may occur on a daily basis. With some irrigation routines, irrigation is not performed daily; therefore the patient may not have a daily bowel movement.
- The cost of ostomy supplies and reimbursement are often an important concern for older patients on limited incomes; referral to community resources may be necessary.

Patient Teaching

Ostomy Care

- Include family members or significant others in teaching; this tends to facilitate the patient's readiness to learn.
- Use every pouch change as an opportunity to teach even if the patient does not appear interested. Do not force the patient to look at the stoma; allow for a period of adjustment.
- Reinforce positive performance. Some patients are not willing to learn ostomy care for a period of time after receiving one. The patient may refuse to look at or touch the stoma and may not participate in ostomy care until he or she has accepted the ostomy.
- Many nurses are able to judge a patient's readiness to learn by the patient's willingness to look at the stoma and by the patient's asking questions. If the patient is apprehensive about touching or looking at stoma, have the patient hold a gauze pad over the stoma and clean around the stoma.
- Some patients acknowledge a stoma with minimal emotional difficulty; some never completely adjust to it. Individualize care according to the patient's situation and circumstances.
- Teach the patient to avoid constipation by eating a balanced diet or using a daily stool softener.
- If the patient has limitations affecting dexterity, select a pouching system that can be most easily managed.
- A teaching manual with clearly stated steps or audiotaped instructions may be helpful for the patient. Patients with a learning disability may benefit from a picture book of the steps involved in ostomy care.
- Give the patient a list of equipment and the name, address, and phone number of a supplier in the patient's community.
- In most cases, patients are able to wear their normal clothes; snug clothing does not interfere with ostomy function.
- Instruct patients not to leave pouches in extremely hot or cold locations because temperature has the potential to affect the barrier and adhesive materials.

Patient Teaching

Urostomy Care

- Teach the patient and caregivers to avoid touching the stoma with adhesive solvents to prevent irritating the stoma.
- Teach the patient and caregivers to wick the urine with an absorbent, lint-free material to prevent a constant flow of urine while they change the appliance.
- Teach the patient and caregivers to remove hair from the stoma area with scissors or an electric razor to prevent hair follicles from becoming irritated when the pouch is removed.
- Teach the patient and caregivers that the appliance should be able to remain in place 3 to 5 days.
- Teach the patient and caregivers to empty appliance through the drain valve when it is one third to one half full to prevent the weight of the urine from loosening the seal around the stoma.
- Teach the patient and caregivers to connect the appliance to a urine-collection container at night to prevent urine from stagnating in the appliance.
- Teach sanitary and dietary measures that will protect the skin around the ostomy and control odor.
- Offer positive reinforcement and written instructions or videos.

See the Patient Teaching box on ostomy care for further instructions.

Coordinated Care

Collaboration

Ostomy Care

- The skill of applying a pouch to a fresh stoma requires the critical thinking and knowledge of a nurse. Some facilities permit delegation of the task of pouching of an established ostomy. Instruct the care provider about the expected amount, color, and consistency of drainage from the ostomy. In addition, teach the care provider to report changes in the stoma and surrounding skin integrity.
- The skill of applying a pouch to an incontinent urinary diversion requires the critical thinking and knowledge of a nurse. In some facilities, a stoma nurse specialist is available to provide this care. Unlicensed assistive personnel (UAP) who provide personal care are instructed to report any leakage of urine and breakdown of skin to the nurse.
- The skill of irrigating a newly established colostomy requires the critical thinking and knowledge of a nurse. In some settings, UAP are trained to perform irrigations on established ostomies. Review facility policy.

Home Care Considerations

Ostomy Care

- Consult with the health care provider to obtain a referral to a home health agency or a visiting nurse before patient's hospital discharge.
- Pouches that wear well in the hospital will not necessarily wear well when the patient resumes a normal routine.
- If an irrigation routine is required, assist the patient to adapt the procedure to the home setting. Suggest hanging the irrigation solution container from a hook on the wall or from a shower curtain rod instead of an intravenous (IV) pole.
- Urostomy, colostomy, and ileostomy products are usually available for purchase at local pharmacies.
- Encourage the patient to become involved with local ostomy organizations.
- Teach the patient and caregivers to routinely inspect the stoma and the surrounding skin. The proper appearance of the stoma is moist, shiny, and dark pink to red, with minimal if any bleeding around it. Teach the patient and caregivers to report excessive bleeding, abnormal color, or swelling to the nurse or the health care provider.
- Teach the patient and caregivers to avoid using alcohol around the stoma, because alcohol dilates capillaries, causing bleeding, and may dry the skin excessively.
- Teach the patient and caregivers not to use lotions or creams around the stoma, because they may prevent pouches from adhering.
- Teach the patient and caregivers not to use peroxide on or around the stoma, because it may irritate the tissue.
- Instruct the patient and caregivers to wash the skin around the stoma with mild soap and water and rinse thoroughly. Soap is often irritating to the skin. Pat or blot the skin dry.
- Evaluate the patient's home toileting facilities for the following:
  - The presence of adequate functioning and accessible toileting facilities
  - Number and location of toileting facilities
  - Number of other people living in the home who have to share the toileting facilities
  - The pattern of use of the toileting facilities by the other people living in the home (time of day and amount of time spent in bathroom)
- Evaluate the patient's ostomy routine in relation to his or her usual lifestyle after discharge.
- Caution the patient not to flush ostomy pouches and barriers down the toilet; they clog the pipes. Dispose of used ostomy pouches according to local sanitation regulations.
- Make sure the patient understands that it is not necessary to use sterile gauze to cleanse the stoma. Using a washcloth made of any soft material is fine.
- Review the patient's dietary pattern. Help patient and family members learn the types of foods to avoid to prevent problems with stoma drainage or odor.
- Teach patients that if water is not drinkable, they should not use it for irrigations (e.g., as in another country).

Get Ready for the NCLEX® Examination!

Key Points

- Closed bladder drainage systems necessitate the use of aseptic technique during care.
- Intermittent urinary catheterization has a lower risk of infection than indwelling urinary catheterization because of the relatively shorter time the intermittent catheter remains in the bladder.
- Strict asepsis is necessary in caring for a closed urinary drainage system.
- It is possible to use closed urinary drainage systems for instillation of sterile solutions or medications into the bladder.
- When a nasogastric tube is to be inserted, it is necessary to lubricate the tube well with a water-soluble lubricant to prevent trauma to the mucous membranes.
- It is imperative for the nurse to check for proper nasogastric tube placement before an irrigation or a tube feeding.

- Proper administration of an enema consists of the slow instillation of the correct volume of a warm solution.
- Emotional support of the patient with an ostomy is important to foster eventual acceptance of the change in body image.
- Consistency of the feces is affected directly by which portion of the colon is brought out to the stoma.
- Even when an ostomy pouch is adhering well, it is best to change it at least every 3 to 5 days or according to pouch recommendations to allow for observation of the stoma and the skin around the stoma.
- Patients with urostomies are at high risk for skin impairment at the site because of the nearly continuous urine drainage.
- Irrigation of an ostomy follows the same principles as an enema administration, except that a special irrigating tube is needed and the patient is not able to control the passage of feces.
- Skin impairment is possible after repeated exposure to liquid stool. This is especially true in patients who have a stoma.

Additional Learning Resources

SG Go to your Study Guide for additional learning activities to help you master this chapter content.

evolve Be sure to visit the Evolve site at *http://evolve.elsevier.com/Cooper/foundationsadult/* for additional online resources.

Review Questions for the NCLEX® Examination

1. What would the nurse do to determine the correct distance to insert a nasogastric tube?
   1. Measure from center of forehead to top of nose to end of sternum.
   2. Measure from tip of nose to tip of earlobe to the xiphoid process.
   3. Measure from lips to tip of ear to just below the umbilicus.
   4. Measure from tip of ear to midway between end of sternum and umbilicus.
2. After inserting a nasogastric tube, the nurse would check for proper placement by which methods? *(Select all that apply.)*
   1. The fact that the patient no longer complains of pain or nausea
   2. The ability to inject 30 mL of normal saline with ease
   3. Gurgling or a swishing sound heard with a stethoscope over the stomach when air is injected into the tube
   4. The ability to aspirate gastric contents with a syringe
   5. Placement of the end of the tube in a glass of water and watching for bubbling
3. If the patient is suspected of having a fecal impaction, which type of enema would the nurse anticipate the health care provider to order?
   1. Soapsuds enema
   2. Polystyrene sulfonate (Kayexalate) enema
   3. Oil retention enema
   4. Tap water enema
4. Bladder training instructions are being given to a patient who has a history of urinary incontinence. The nurse should give the patient which instruction?
   1. "Wait until you feel the urge to void."
   2. "Don't void any more often than every 4 to 6 hours."
   3. "Void every 1.5 to 2 hours while you are awake."
   4. "Void any time you feel the urge."
5. A nurse is preparing to insert a nasogastric tube. The nurse should place the patient in which position?
   1. On the right side.
   2. Low Fowler's position.
   3. High Fowler's position.
   4. Supine with head of bed flat.
6. A male patient with urinary incontinence has been using an external (condom) catheter. The nurse is evaluating the patient's technique of applying the device. Which finding would indicate that the nurse should give the patient further instructions? *(Select all that apply.)*
   1. Washing the penis with warm, soapy water and drying the area well before applying the device
   2. Spiraling the tape around the penis to secure the device
   3. Using elastic tape and wrapping in a spiral pattern to secure the device
   4. Checking the penis carefully for any signs of irritation before applying the device
   5. Changing the catheter after each time of urination
7. What is considered a noninvasive method of collecting urine for the incontinent patient?
   1. Suprapubic catheterization
   2. Reinsertion of a Foley catheter
   3. Catheter irrigation
   4. Condom catheterization
8. A patient with a colostomy continues to worry about odor. Which statement would be appropriate for the nurse to tell the patient about colostomy odor?
   1. "It occurs only when the colostomy appliance is changed."
   2. "It is caused by certain foods that can be omitted from the diet."
   3. "It is mainly caused by poor hygiene and can be remedied."
   4. "It is far more noticeable to the patient than to others."

9. The nurse is instructing the patient in performing Kegel exercises. The patient should be instructed to contract the muscles he or she would use to stop the flow of urine. What is the proper technique for performing Kegel exercises?
1. Contract for 3 to 4 seconds and relax for 3 to 4 seconds.
2. Contract for 3 to 4 seconds and relax for 10 seconds.
3. Contract for 10 seconds and relax for 3 to 4 seconds.
4. Contract for 10 seconds and relax for 10 seconds.

10. A bladder retraining program for a patient in an extended-care facility should include which intervention? *(Select all that apply.)*
1. Providing negative reinforcement when the patient is incontinent.
2. Having the patient wear clothing protectors to help decrease embarrassment.
3. Putting the patient on q 2 hr toilet schedule during the day.
4. Promoting the intake of caffeine to stimulate voiding.
5. Encouraging the use of the bedpan.

11. The nurse is caring for a patient with a new ostomy. What is the best nursing strategy for encouraging patient self-care of an ostomy?
1. Plan to change the pouch when family members will be present, have the patient watch, and have the patient and family listen to the procedure.
2. Frequently tell the patient that if he or she does not learn stoma self-care, no one is going to do it for him or her.
3. Encourage the patient to watch the stoma care procedure, gradually encouraging participation.
4. Shield the patient from sight of the stoma until the patient actually asks to see it.

12. A patient has a nasogastric tube inserted. What type of patient teaching should the nurse give the patient about the NG tube? *(Select all that apply.)*
1. "Be careful to not pull on the tube."
2. "Call the nurse if you feel as if you are going to vomit."
3. "Turn the suction off if you feel as if you are going to vomit."
4. "Refrain from coughing while the tube is in place."
5. "Let the staff know if the tape holding the tube is irritating your skin."

13. To maintain proper drainage of an indwelling catheter, it is important to perform which action?
1. Irrigate the catheter every 2 to 4 hours.
2. Ensure that the collection device is below bladder level.
3. Place the tubing under the patient's leg to prevent pulling on the bladder neck.
4. Demonstrate to the patient how to disconnect the device while ambulating.

14. The nurse instructs the patient to be diligent in cleaning fecal matter from around the stoma because the fecal matter can cause which complication? *(Select all that apply.)*
1. Fungal infection
2. Bacterial infection
3. Yeast infection
4. Irritation of the stoma
5. Skin breakdown around the stoma

15. The nurse is administering a cleansing enema. Before administering the enema, the nurse assists the patient into which position?
1. Supine
2. On right side
3. Left Sims position
4. Left side with head of bed elevated 45 degrees

16. The nurse caring for a patient with a Foley catheter should perform which actions to lower the risk for infection? *(Select all that apply.)*
1. Keep bag below the level of the bed.
2. Provide perineal care twice a day.
3. Coil tubing on the bed.
4. Keep the drainage system closed.
5. Limit fluid intake to 300 mL per shift.

17. The nurse is administering a routine enema to an adult patient. The patient complains of cramping and the urge to defecate. Which nursing intervention is the best to carry out?
1. Quickly finish instilling the rest of the solution.
2. Briefly stop the instillation.
3. Instruct the patient to hold his or her breath and bear down.
4. Immediately discontinue the instillation and withdraw the enema tubing from the rectum.

18. When providing routine indwelling catheter care, the nurse should be most diligent in cleaning which areas?
1. The perineal area
2. The area surrounding the urinary meatus
3. The labia majora and the labia minora
4. The perineal area and 2 inches of the catheter

Care of Patients Experiencing Urgent Alterations in Health

16

http://evolve.elsevier.com/Cooper/foundationsadult/

Objectives

1. List the priorities of assessment to be performed in a situation in which first aid is necessary.
2. Discuss moral, legal, and physical interventions/implications involved in performing first aid.
3. List the reasons for performing cardiopulmonary resuscitation (CPR).
4. List the steps in performing one-rescuer and two-rescuer CPR on an adult, child, and infant victim.
5. Identify the steps in performing the abdominal thrusts on conscious and unconscious victims and pregnant victims.
6. Discuss management of airway obstruction in a child and an infant.
7. Discuss the signs and symptoms of shock and interventions to treat shock.
8. Discuss three methods of controlling bleeding.
9. Discuss the five general types of open wounds: abrasions, incisions, lacerations, punctures, and avulsions.
10. Discuss treatment of wounds.
11. Discuss methods of treating four common types of poisonings.
12. Describe the nursing interventions used when treating heat and cold emergencies.
13. List characteristics and first aid treatment of bone, joint, and muscle injuries.
14. Discuss emergency care for spinal cord injuries.
15. Define the classifications of burns and list nursing interventions used in the first aid treatment of burns.

Key Terms

air embolism (ār ĔM-bŏ-lĭzm, p. 403)
biologic death (p. 395)
brain death (p. 395)
CAB (circulation, airway, breathing) (p. 396)
cardiac arrest (p. 396)
cardiopulmonary resuscitation (CPR) (kăr-dē-ō-PŬL-mō-nā-rē rē-sŭs-ĭ-TĀ-shŭn, p. 394)
clinical death (p. 395)
contusions (kŏn-TŪ-zhŭnz, p. 406)
crepitus (KRĔP-ĭ-tŭs, p. 415)
cyanosis (sī-ă-NŌ-sĭs, p. 402)
ecchymoses (ĕk-ĭ-MŌ-sēz, p. 406)
emergency medical services (EMS) (p. 393)
epistaxis (ĕp-ĭ-STĂK-sĭs, p. 404)
epistaxis digitorum (ĕp-ĭ-STĂK-sĭs dĭj-ĭ-TŌR-ŭm, p. 405)
flail chest (p. 408)
Good Samaritan laws (p. 394)
hematemesis (hē-mă-TĔM-ĕ-sĭs, p. 406)
hematuria (hē-mă-TŪ-rē-ă, p. 406)
hemoptysis (hē-MŎP-tĭ-sĭs, p. 406)
hemothorax (hē-mō-THŌ-răks, p. 407)
melena (MĔL-ĕ-nă, p. 406)
oliguria (ŏl-ĭ-GŪ-rē-ă, p. 402)
pleural space (PLŪR-ăl spās, p. 407)
pneumothorax (nū-mō-THŌ-răks, p. 407)
shock (shŏk, p. 402)
stridor (STRĪ-dŏr, p. 401)
tachycardia (tăk-ĕ-KĂR-dē-ă, p. 402)
tetanus toxoid (TĔT-ă-nŭs TŎKS-ŏyd, p. 406)
triage (TRĒ-ăhzh, p. 393)

First aid is the immediate initial assistance given to a person who is injured or has become ill. First aid includes assessing the victim for life-threatening conditions, performing appropriate interventions to sustain life, and keeping the person in the best possible physical and mental condition until the assistance of **emergency medical services (EMS)** is obtained. EMS is a national network of services that provides coordinated aid and medical assistance from primary response to definitive care. First aid does not replace medical care but is used to preserve life until medical help is obtained. Because permanent disability and injury can occur within minutes, the nurse should be prepared to handle emergency conditions and administer first aid. In the case of multiple injuries, patients are surveyed quickly for severity of injuries so that health care providers can treat life-threatening problems first. This process of classifying a group of patients according to the severity of injury and need of care is called **triage.** The triage process is based on the premise that patients who have a threat to life, vision, or limb should be treated before other patients. In a disaster, triage is a process in which numerous patients are "sorted" so that it is possible to concentrate care and resources on those who are more likely to survive. In this chapter, the rescuer often is referred to as the nurse or you, the reader. However, any person certified to perform cardiopulmonary resuscitation (CPR) and first aid may assist with these activities.

OBTAINING MEDICAL EMERGENCY AID

The nurse's ability to recognize the need for medical assistance and understanding of how to obtain medical emergency aid can sometimes mean the difference between life and death to an injured or ill person. It is important for the nurse to know the right phone number to call in the community and in the institutional setting. In most communities, the emergency medical number is 911. However, in some areas and in some situations, it may be best to call the number for the fire department, police department, or local hospital. Box 16.1 provides information to convey when calling in a medical emergency from the community.

Health care providers must be prepared to provide **cardiopulmonary resuscitation (CPR)** (basic emergency procedure for life support) if needed until emergency medical assistance arrives. All health care providers should maintain CPR certification. Most health care institutions provide training. CPR certification is also available from local fire departments and local chapters of the American Red Cross and the American Heart Association.

The guidelines for administering CPR undergo periodic review and are subject to change. This chapter discusses CPR in accordance with the most current guidelines provided by the American Heart Association at the time of this text's publication. Further information on CPR can be found at *www.heart.org*.

Box 16.1 Information to Convey in a Medical Emergency

1. Name of the person making the call
2. Location of the emergency
3. What has happened (either by direct observation or by gathering data from other people)
4. Whether an immediate threat, such as fire or flood, or physical threat by someone, such as use of a gun or knife, still exists
5. Number of people who need assistance
6. Every victim's name and age
7. Obvious injuries and every victim's apparent condition
8. First aid measures that have already been administered
9. Presence of medical-alert bracelet or any known history
10. The physical characteristics of the scene of the rescue (stairs, elevators)

NOTE: Only hang up when instructed to do so by the emergency services operator.

MORAL AND LEGAL RESPONSIBILITIES OF THE NURSE

Good Samaritan laws (legal protection for those who give first aid in an emergency situation) have been enacted in most states to protect health professionals from legal liability when they provide emergency first aid. If a nurse follows a reasonable and prudent course of action, the chances of resulting legal problems are very small. Nurses are obliged to obtain permission to treat any conscious patient, even in an emergency situation. Before first aid is administered, verbal permission should be obtained from the victim, because the victim has the right to refuse first aid. The law assumes consent from an unconscious person. After the nurse has initiated first aid, there is a moral and legal obligation to continue the aid until someone with comparable or better training is able to care for the victim; for example, an emergency medical technician (EMT), or paramedic, or a health care provider may arrive at the scene and assume first aid care of the victim.

ASSESSMENT OF THE EMERGENCY SITUATION

Assessment of life-threatening problems is the priority in an emergency situation. Assess the scene for potential safety hazards. Sometimes you will need the aid of another person, whether to help care for victims with some injuries or illnesses or to call EMS. If necessary, shout to get someone's attention or request that someone call 911 or another emergency number. While seeking help, continue the primary survey by assessing the patient's circulation, airway, and breathing (CAB). An immediate life-threatening situation of highest priority is abnormal circulation; an absent or abnormal pulse is a life-threatening situation. Assess the rate, rhythm, and strength of the carotid pulse for no longer than 10 seconds. Monitor the victim for signs of external bleeding and internal bleeding, which may lead to shock. Additional assessment includes the person's skin color, temperature, pupil reaction, pulse, and respiration. Poisonings also may be life threatening. Observe for burns or stains in and around the person's mouth or hands. Depressed respirations and circulatory collapse are other possible results of poisoning.

Ensure that the victim's airway is open. The airway is opened with a head-tilt/chin-lift maneuver unless a neck injury is suspected. If a cervical spine injury is suspected, use a jaw-thrust maneuver without tilting the head to open the airway. Use caution not to move the neck out of proper alignment. Because of the potential for causing or exacerbating a cervical spine injury, do not hyperextend the patient's neck to establish an airway.

Assess the victim's ability to breathe by determining whether the chest is rising, listen for breath sounds, and place your cheek near the victim's mouth to feel the passage of air from the victim's breathing. Assess rhythm, depth, and rate of respirations. The following clinical manifestations indicate that the victim is having trouble breathing: cyanosis, gasping, wheezing, stridor, and snoring.

After the initial assessment for life-threatening problems, assess the victim for indications of skull injury and brain or spinal cord damage, which necessitate immediate interventions. A decreasing level of consciousness, abnormal pupil reaction, and lack of movement in the arms or the legs are indicative of a possible injury to the head or spinal cord. Focus on the victim's fractures, dislocations, and superficial ecchymoses or wounds only after treating the more serious conditions.

CARDIOPULMONARY RESUSCITATION (CPR)

ETHICAL IMPLICATIONS

Reasons that individuals choose not to become involved in performing CPR include feeling panicked, fear of incorrectly administering CPR, and fear of hurting the patient. However, once the nurse or anyone starts CPR, it should not be discontinued *except* for the following reasons:

- The victim recovers.
- An automated external defibrillator (AED) is available and CPR is discontinued before the equipment is applied.
- The scene becomes unsafe and evacuation of the victim is necessary.
- The rescuer is exhausted and is not able to continue CPR.
- Trained medical personnel arrive on the scene and take over CPR.
- A licensed health care provider arrives on the scene, has the authority to pronounce the victim dead, and orders CPR to be discontinued.

When a licensed practical nurse/licensed vocational nurse (LPN/LVN) is providing emergency care to a patient, this nurse should stay with the patient until care is taken over by a registered nurse (RN), a health care provider, or emergency medical personnel.

EVENTS NECESSITATING CARDIOPULMONARY RESUSCITATION

Many situations necessitate resuscitation efforts (Box 16.2). CPR is indicated when the patient is not responsive and not breathing. There are two purposes of CPR:

1. To keep the blood circulating and carrying oxygen to the brain, the heart, and other parts of the body
2. To keep the airway open and the lungs supplied with oxygen when breathing has stopped

Clinical death means that heartbeat and respiration have stopped. **Biologic death** results from permanent cellular damage caused by lack of oxygen. The brain is the first organ damaged by this lack of oxygen. If CPR is started within 4 minutes of cardiopulmonary arrest, it may help reverse clinical death. After 10 minutes without CPR, brain death most likely occurs. Therefore it is extremely important to begin CPR as quickly as possible. **Brain death** is an irreversible form

Box 16.2 Events Necessitating Cardiopulmonary Resuscitation

- *Anaphylactic reaction:* Exposure to a known allergen (e.g., food, poisons, and drugs) or an insect bite has the capacity to produce the severe allergic reaction known as *anaphylaxis.* This reaction often causes spasms or edema of the upper airway and, in some cases, progresses to cardiovascular collapse. It is necessary to initiate cardiopulmonary resuscitation (CPR) immediately, as with any other emergency situation.
- *Asphyxiation:* Asphyxiation or suffocation caused by inhaling a gas other than oxygen is possible as a result of fires, chemical spills, or gas leaks. In addition, children and adults sometimes suffer respiratory arrest and ultimately cardiac arrest from choking on food or small objects that are placed in the mouth. Abdominal thrusts and CPR are performed in this instance.
- *Cardiac arrest:* The most common cause of cardiac arrest is myocardial infarction (MI). In addition, shock from hemorrhage, trauma to the heart, respiratory arrest, and drugs have the potential to precipitate a cardiac arrest.
- *Drowning:* Children are common victims of drowning and boating accidents. People using alcohol or other drugs near bodies of water are often victims of drowning. It is important to note that near-drowning victims sometimes recover completely after long periods of submersion. The low water temperature that produces hypothermia reduces the metabolic rate and decreases oxygen demands. Because of this, it is necessary to initiate CPR even when 4 to 6 minutes of cardiac or respiratory arrest is known to have elapsed.
- *Drug overdose:* Intentional or accidental abuse of alcohol and drugs poses a risk for respiratory and cardiac arrest. Besides treating this as a poisoning emergency, perform CPR as necessary.
- *Electrical shock:* People who come near sources of high-voltage electricity run the risk of accidental electrocution. Electrical shock sometimes paralyzes the breathing muscles and causes cardiac arrest by interfering with the normal rhythm of the heart. It is essential for the rescuer who is initiating CPR to be careful not to inadvertently come into contact with the electric current. The rescuer must ensure that the current is de-energized before beginning CPR.
- *Sudden infant death syndrome (SIDS):* SIDS is the unexpected and sudden death of an apparently normal and healthy infant that occurs during sleep and with no evidence of disease on physical examination or autopsy. Aspects of prevention include readiness to perform early CPR and home monitoring systems.

of unconsciousness characterized by a complete loss of brain function while the heart continues to beat. The legal definition of this condition varies from state to state. Brain death statutes in the United States differ by state and institution. Some US state or hospital guidelines require the examiner to have certain expertise. Guidelines can be found at the University of Miami Health System website (*http://surgery.med.miami.edu/laora/clinical-operations/brain-death-diagnosis*). The usual clinical criteria for brain death include the absence of reflex activity, movements, and respiration. The pupils are dilated and fixed. Because hypothermia, anesthesia, poisoning, and drug intoxication have the capacity to cause a deep physiologic depression that resembles brain death, a diagnosis of brain death requires that the electrical activity be evaluated and shown to be absent on two electroencephalograms obtained 12 to 24 hours apart. Cerebral blood flow studies are permitted in some states to evaluate whether brain death has occurred. Brain death also is referred to as *irreversible coma.* Statutes in states and even health care facility procedures may vary concerning brain death determination. Refer to your state law and to facility policy and procedure manuals.

INITIAL ASSESSMENT AND RESPONSE

The initial assessment task in determining the need for CPR is to determine responsiveness. The trained rescuer—the nurse—should do this by gently shaking the victim and loudly asking, "Are you OK?" This precaution will prevent the nurse from injuring a person who is sleeping.

The nurse, or layperson, should call for help immediately when beginning a rescue. It is imperative to access the EMS as quickly as possible. Shout for help, make a phone call for help, or direct another person to make a phone call if another person is available. The American Heart Association (AHA) (2017) guidelines indicate that it may be reasonable for communities to incorporate social media technologies that summon rescuers who are in proximity to a victim of suspected out of hospital cardiac arrest (OHCA) and are willing and able to perform CPR. It is vital to obtain an AED if one is available. Use the AED to treat defibrillation if necessary.

For the most successful treatment of cardiac arrest, CPR and the use of an AED should be initiated within the first 3 to 5 minutes. AEDs are available in numerous nonhospital settings such as airports, schools, and business locations for use by laypersons who determine that someone has suffered cardiac arrest (Fig. 16.1). Basic life support education for health care providers, as well as for non–health care providers, includes instruction in CPR and in how to use an AED.

CABS OF CARDIOPULMONARY RESUSCITATION

To remember the steps of one-rescuer or two-rescuer CPR, remember to spell **CAB,** a mnemonic for assessing the status of patients in an emergency:

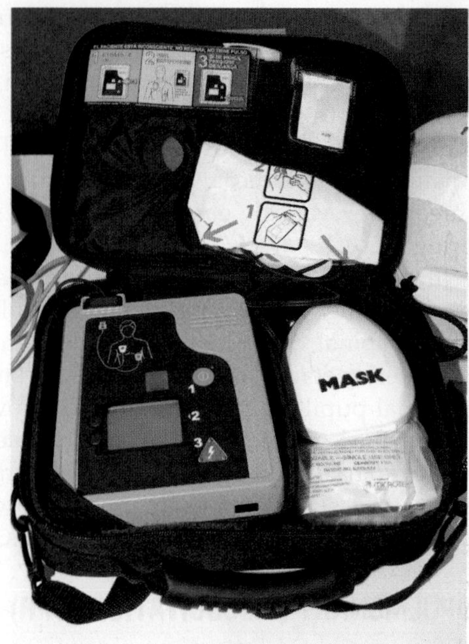

Fig. 16.1 A portable automatic external defibrillator (AED). (Copyright Thinkstock Photos.)

Circulation
*A*irway
*B*reathing

CPR performed by the health care provider differs slightly from that performed by the layperson. The health care provider and layperson verify unresponsiveness, activate the EMS, and retrieve an AED. Both determine whether there is no breathing or abnormal breathing. Only the health care provider assesses for a carotid pulse, taking no more than 10 seconds to palpate for the pulse. The layperson does not assess for a carotid pulse.

Circulation

Respiratory arrest is possible without cardiac arrest. Once the nurse has determined that the victim is not breathing, the nurse should assess the person's pulse. Pulselessness (cardiac arrest) indicates the need for external cardiac compressions. Performing external cardiac compressions on a victim with a pulse, however, has the potential to result in injury to the victim.

To determine pulselessness, the carotid pulse is the most reliable and accessible to the nurse. Maintain the head tilt with one hand resting on the victim's forehead while assessing for the presence of a pulse. With two or three fingers of the other hand, locate the victim's thyroid cartilage. Then gently slide the fingers into the groove between the trachea and the muscles on the side of the neck until the carotid pulse is felt. Palpate the pulse gently only on one side so as not to obliterate arterial blood flow to the brain (Fig. 16.2). The absence of a pulse confirms the diagnosis of **cardiac arrest** (sudden cessation of functional circulation).

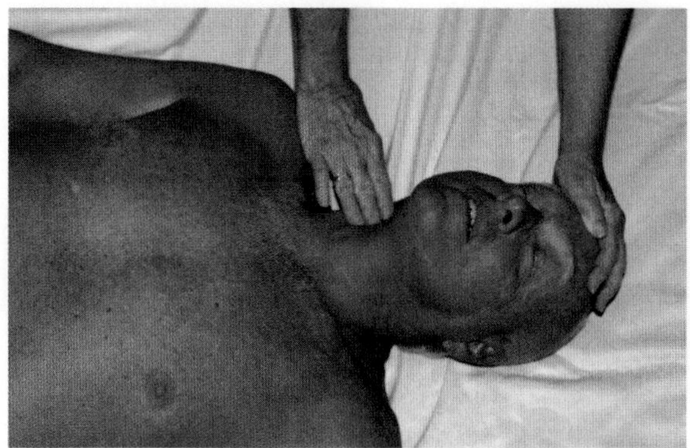

Fig. 16.2 Carotid pulse assessment.

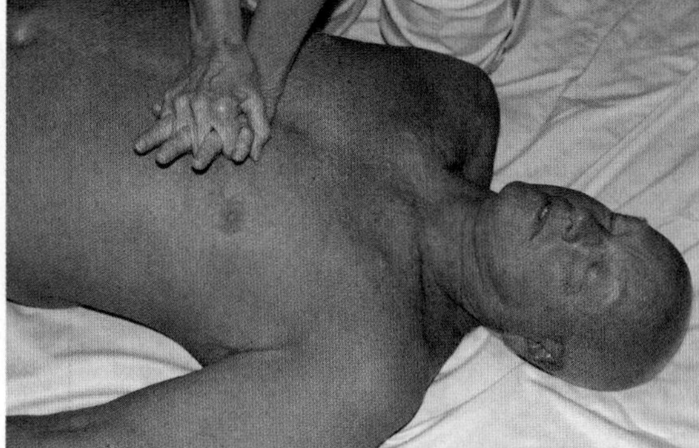

Fig. 16.3 Proper hand placement for chest compressions.

Performing external cardiac compressions helps blood circulate to the heart, the lungs, the brain, and the rest of the body. If external cardiac compressions are performed properly, it is possible to maintain 20% to 50% of the normal output of the heart. This provides enough oxygen to the body to sustain life. Proper hand position enables as much blood to be circulated as possible. Position your hands as follows (Fig. 16.3):

1. Compress the lower half of the victim's sternum in the center (middle) of the chest, between the nipples.
2. Place the heel of one hand on the victim's sternum in the center (middle) of the chest between the nipples, and then place the heel of the second hand on top of the first so that the hands overlap and are parallel.
3. It is acceptable to extend or interlace fingers, but keep them off the chest.

Proper compression technique is important for delivering the appropriate amount of force to simulate the pumping action of the heart. Compression techniques are as follows:

1. Lock elbows in place, with arms straight and shoulders positioned over hands so that the thrusts of external cardiac compressions are in a downward motion. Some of the force of the compressions will be lost if there is a rolling or rocking motion.
2. Lean forward and push, creating pressure to depress the sternum at least 2 inches (5 cm) in an adult (see the section "Pediatric Cardiopulmonary Resuscitation: Child or Infant" for the correlated information for children). This is difficult to estimate, but some give will be felt in the sternum. The motion is smooth, never rolling or jerking. Excessive depth of chest compressions (greater than 2.4 inches, or 6 cm) should be avoided in the adult to prevent damage to surrounding tissues.
3. 2015 AHA guidelines state that it is reasonable for rescuers to avoid leaning on the chest between compressions, to allow full chest wall recoil for adults in cardiac arrest. This allows blood to flow into the heart. Practice is necessary to learn how to deliver good chest compressions. (During a two-person rescue, trade off with another rescuer every few minutes to minimize fatigue, which contributes to inadequate chest compression depth and rate.) Keep the time allowed for compression to approximately equal to the time for chest recoil or relaxation. Do not pause between compressions. The proper compression rate is 100 to 120 compressions per minute.
4. Maintain hand position at all times; do not lift your hands or move them in any way. Keep hands in contact with the chest.

Complications of external chest compressions include lacerated liver, fractured ribs, and fractured sternum, as well as bruising or bleeding of the liver, the lungs, and the spleen. Do not let any concern for possible injuries from CPR interfere with its prompt and efficient application.

The sequencing of breathing to external compressions in one-rescuer and two-rescuer CPR is discussed next.

Airway

Assess the victim's airway to confirm the absence of breathing and to establish a patent airway. If there is no evidence of head or neck trauma, use the head-tilt/chin-lift maneuver to open the airway (Fig. 16.4A). Place one hand on the victim's forehead and apply firm backward pressure to tilt the head back. Place the fingers of the other hand under the jaw (avoiding the soft tissue under the chin) to lift the chin forward.

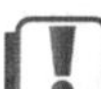

Safety Alert

If a neck injury is suspected, establish the airway by using the jaw-thrust (or chin-lift) maneuver without tilting the head. To perform the jaw-thrust maneuver, grasp the angle of the victim's lower jaw with your hands on both sides of the jaw and bring the mandible forward, while keeping the neck in straight alignment and not tilting the head back (see Fig. 16.4B). Attempt again to establish whether spontaneous breathing is present once the airway is open.

Breathing

Mouth-to-mouth ventilation is the quickest method of supplying oxygen to the victim's lungs. The rescuer's exhaled air has enough oxygen to supply the victim's needs until life-support systems take over. Maintain the head-tilt/chin-lift position and an airtight seal

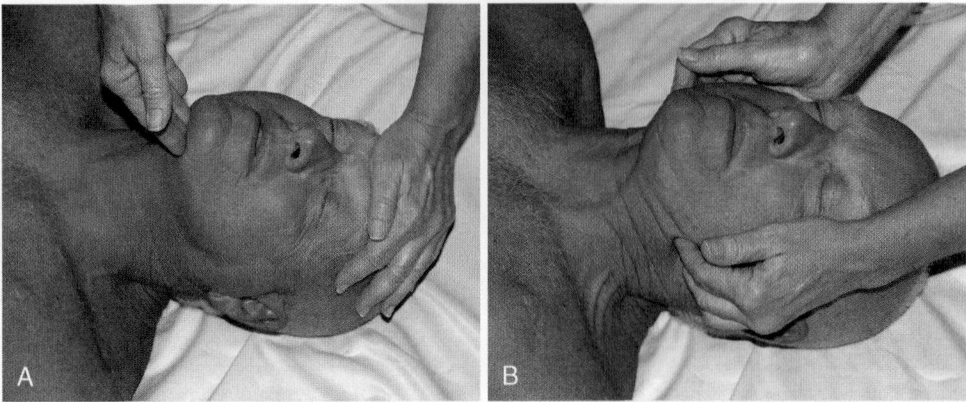

Fig. 16.4 A, Head-tilt/chin-lift maneuver. B, Jaw-thrust maneuver.

throughout rescue breathing. If the victim has a pulse, initiate rescue breathing at a rate of one breath every 6 to 8 seconds, or 8 to 10 times per minute, in an adult (see the section "Pediatric Cardiopulmonary Resuscitation: Child or Infant"). Cardiac arrest follows if respiratory arrest continues.

To preserve the open airway, kneel by the victim's shoulders. To gently pinch the nostrils closed, use the thumb and the index finger of the same hand that he or she is using to maintain the head tilt. Take a deep breath, seal the lips around the outside of the victim's mouth (creating an airtight seal), and give two full breaths lasting 1 second each. This method is used to keep gastric distention to a minimum and decrease the potential for the victim to vomit, which sometimes results from receiving rapid breaths and excessive air volume. Allow the victim to exhale passively. When a mask is available mouth-to-mask ventilation is performed (Fig. 16.5). Mouth-to-mask ventilation with a one-way valve prevents the transfer of microorganisms from the victim to the rescuer.

If your initial attempt to ventilate the victim is unsuccessful, reposition the head and again attempt to ventilate. Improper chin and head position is the most common reason for difficulty with ventilation. If the second attempt at ventilation is also unsuccessful, commence procedures to manage airway obstruction by a foreign body (see later discussion).

STEPS FOR ADULT ONE-RESCUER CARDIOPULMONARY RESUSCITATION

1. Determine unresponsiveness.
2. Determine breathlessness.
3. Call for help. Activate the EMS system.

Circulation

1. Determine pulselessness.
2. If pulse is present, continue rescue breathing about 8 to 10 times per minute, or one breath every 6 to 8 seconds. Activate the EMS system.
3. If pulse is not present, perform 30 chest compressions at a rate of at least 100 per minute. Count "one, two, three, four, five" until you have done 30 compressions, and follow them with two slow breaths. The rescuer must be sure to provide chest compressions of the proper depth and rate to provide 100 to 120 beats per minute. In order to maintain this rate of compressions the lay person may use songs such as "Stayin' Alive" by the Bee Gees, "Crazy in Love" by Beyoncé featuring Jay-Z, "Hips Don't Lie" by Shakira, or "Walk the Line" by Johnny Cash to maintain the rate.
4. Continue with 30 compressions and two slow breaths until an AED becomes available or help arrives.

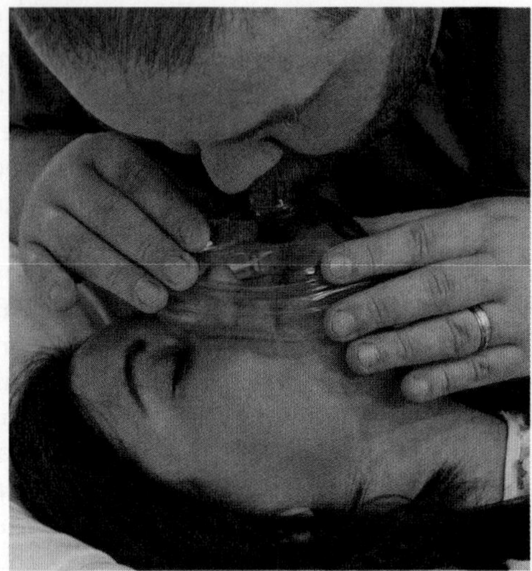

Fig. 16.5 Mouth-to-mask ventilation.

Airway

Open the victim's airway using the head-tilt/chin-lift maneuver. Gently lift the chin forward to help open the victim's airway. If the victim has a suspected neck injury, use the jaw-thrust (or chin-lift) maneuver without tilting the head.

Breathing

1. If the victim is not breathing, give two slow breaths (1 second each). Allow for exhalation between breaths.
2. If unable to give two breaths, reposition the victim's head and reattempt to ventilate.
3. If still unable to give two breaths, proceed with procedures to manage airway obstruction by a foreign body.

ADULT TWO-RESCUER CARDIOPULMONARY RESUSCITATION

Because CPR expends a great deal of energy, it is less fatiguing if two rescuers perform CPR. If the EMS system has not been activated already, direct the second rescuer to initiate CPR before starting to assist with CPR.

The rescuer at the victim's head is referred to as the "ventilator," and the rescuer at the victim's chest is referred to as the "compressor." The ventilator should determine responsiveness. If there is no response, the ventilator assesses for breathlessness for 5 to 10 seconds. The compressor or a bystander should activate the EMS and call for an AED. The ventilator should assess for pulselessness for 5 to 10 seconds. If the victim has a pulse, the ventilator should initiate rescue breathing at a rate of one breath every 6 to 8 seconds, or 8 to 10 times per minute, for an adult victim. If the victim does not have a pulse, then the compressor starts compressions. The compression:ventilation ratio for two-person CPR is 30 chest compressions for every 2 breaths. Exhalation occurs during chest compressions. The compression rate for two-person CPR is at least 100 per minute. The rescuer performing chest compressions is more likely to become fatigued. The rescuers should switch positions every five cycles of 2 minutes to continue effective CPR.

The switch is initiated by the rescuer performing chest compressions at the end of a 30:2 sequence. After giving a breath, the ventilator moves to the chest and gets into position to give compressions. The compressor moves to the victim's head and checks the pulse for 5 to 10 seconds. If no pulse is felt, he or she gives the command, "Resume CPR," and compressions are restarted, followed by breaths.

PEDIATRIC CARDIOPULMONARY RESUSCITATION: CHILD OR INFANT

The basic steps of CPR and procedures to manage airway obstruction by a foreign body are the same whether the victim is an infant, a child, or an adult. For the purpose of basic life support, an *infant* is defined as anyone younger than 1 year of age, and a *child* is defined as anyone between age 1 year and puberty. First determine unresponsiveness. A child may be gently shaken, but with an infant, try gently tapping the infant's heels.

Position the victim on a firm, flat surface for the best CPR effectiveness. It is sometimes advantageous to carry a small child or infant while performing CPR, although this technique is not as effective.

Use the head-tilt/chin-lift or jaw-thrust technique to open the airway of a child, while taking care not to hyperextend an infant's neck because this sometimes allows the infant's shorter trachea to become occluded. In the case of a head injury, do not tilt the head but use the jaw-thrust technique instead. Caution is necessary with suspected neck injuries in infants and children, as it is in adult cases.

After establishing that the airway is open, look for movement of the chest, listen for breath sounds, and feel for exhaled airflow. If the infant or child is not breathing, the nurse should begin the CAB sequence.

Circulation

Check for circulation by assessing the pulse on the carotid artery in a child and the brachial artery in an infant. If there is a pulse, continue rescue breathing at a rate of one breath every 6 to 8 seconds. If there is no pulse or if the pulse is less than 60 beats per minute, begin to perform external cardiac compressions.

Airway

Use the head-tilt/chin-lift or jaw-thrust technique to open the airway of a child or infant.

Breathing

When providing breathing, give two breaths (1 second per breath). The volume of air in an infant's lungs is smaller than that in an adult's, so adjust your breaths to allow for appropriate rise and fall of the chest. A good rule of thumb is usually to use the amount of air for the infant that an adult is able to hold in the cheeks. Gastric distention is common in infants and children during CPR as a result of overinflation of the lungs.

When performing external cardiac compressions in the infant, do the following (this technique is preferred for infants when two health care providers are present):

1. Visualize an imaginary line between the nipples.
2. Use two fingers to perform chest compressions.
   a. Place two fingers about one fingerbreadth below the nipple line. Fig. 16.6A, demonstrates position of fingers for proper compression technique for one-rescuer infant CPR; Fig. 16.6B demonstrates position of fingers for proper compression technique for two-rescuer infant CPR.
3. The breastbone is compressed to a depth of at least one third the diameter of the chest, or 1.5 inches (4 cm), at a rate of at least 100 times per minute. Count aloud very quickly: "one, two, three, four, five." Perform the compression-and-release action smoothly. It has been recommended to "think" the count rather than counting aloud; it is easy to lose count because the rate is so fast.
4. At the end of each compression, release pressure and allow the sternum to return to normal position without removing hands from their placement. Keep movements smooth, not jerky.
5. The sequence of compressions to ventilation is 30:2 (30 compressions to 2 breaths). If there are two health care provider rescuers, the sequence is 15:2 (15 compressions to 2 breaths).

When performing cardiac compressions in a child, do the following:

1. Compress the chest with the heel of one hand at the nipple line at a depth of at least one-third the diameter

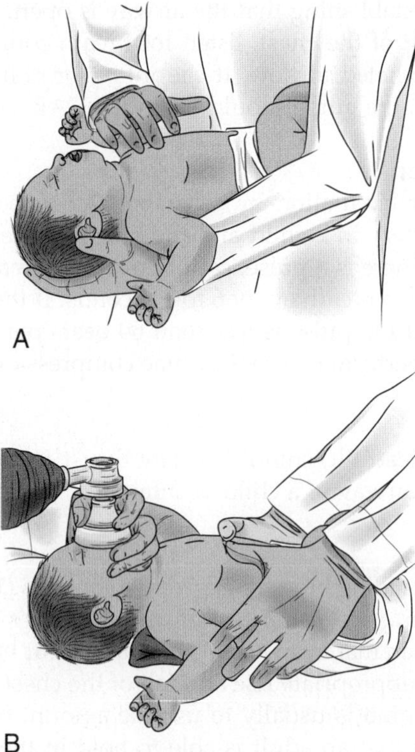

Fig. 16.6 A, Position of fingers for proper compression technique for one-rescuer cardiopulmonary resuscitation (CPR) in an infant. B, Position of fingers for proper compression technique for two-rescuer CPR in an infant.

of the chest, or 2 inches (5 cm), at least 100 times per minute. Make sure that the fingers do not touch the ribs.
2. Keep the compressions smooth, allowing the chest to return to the natural position after each compression.
3. The sequence is 30 compressions to 2 breaths. If two health care providers are performing the rescue, the sequence is 15:2 (15 compressions to 2 ventilations).

HANDS-ONLY CARDIOPULMONARY RESUSCITATION

In their 2017 update, the AHA recommends that bystanders who are not trained in conventional CPR use only their hands, without the rescue breathing, in the crucial moments after they witness an out-of-hospital sudden cardiac arrest. The AHA recommends that if a person witnesses a sudden collapse of an adult and the victim is unresponsive, it is best to call 911 and start chest compressions "hard and fast" in the middle of the chest. Many times people nearby do not help because they are not confident in what they are doing and fear that they will hurt the victim. If the bystander is not trained in CPR or is not confident in being able to perform rescue breathing, performing hands-only CPR is the best response. Optimally, this continues until EMS arrives or an AED is made available.

Several studies have found that among people with OHCA, survival numbers were comparable between those who received chest compressions only and those who received conventional CPR (AHA, 2017a). People probably are more likely to assist with CPR if hands-only is used because they are much less likely to come into contact with microorganisms from the victim.

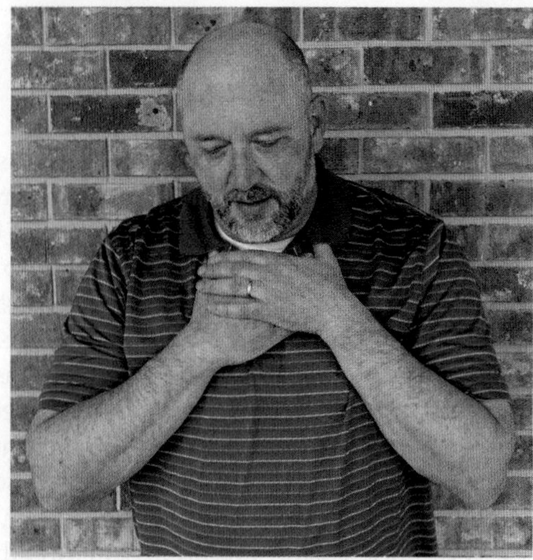

Fig. 16.7 Victims typically clutch the neck when experiencing airway obstruction.

PROCEDURES TO MANAGE AIRWAY OBSTRUCTION BY A FOREIGN BODY

Food, particularly meat, is the most common cause of choking or airway obstruction in adults. Factors that contribute to this include large or poorly chewed pieces of food, talking while eating, the ingestion of alcohol, the use of sedatives, loose-fitting dentures, and neurologic deficits. In addition to food, foreign objects (e.g., marbles, balloons, beads, buttons) are the most common cause of airway obstruction in children.

If the victim can cough forcibly, the air exchange is good, although there may be wheezing between coughs. The rescuer should *not interfere* with the victim at this point. Monitor the victim closely because it is possible that air exchange may regress to a poor state.

The victim experiencing poor air exchange is likely to have a weak, ineffective cough; make a high-pitched, "crowing" noise while inhaling; exhibit increased respiratory difficulty; and develop cyanosis. With complete airway obstruction, the victim is not able to speak, breathe, or cough and sometimes clutches the neck (Fig. 16.7). This sign is a universal distress signal. To assess the inability to speak, ask the victim, "Are you choking?" Complete airway obstruction will prevent oxygen from entering the lungs and being circulated to the brain and vital organs. Unless prompt action is initiated, the victim will become unconscious and death will result.

The following maneuver is the most effective method of removing foreign bodies that obstruct the airway.

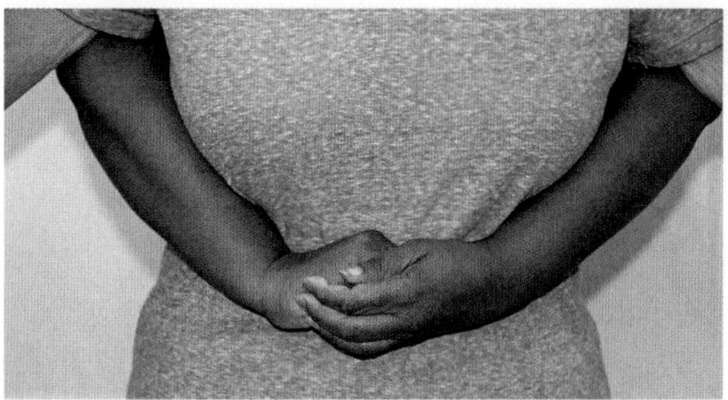

Fig. 16.8 Abdominal thrusts.

CONSCIOUS VICTIM

Abdominal thrusts given just above the victim's navel—an emergency procedure for dislodging a bolus of food or other obstruction from the trachea to prevent asphyxiation—are recommended for relieving airway obstruction by a foreign body. These thrusts put pressure on the diaphragm, forcing air from the lungs to move and expel the foreign object. If the victim is in a sitting position, stand behind the victim and wrap your arm around the victim's waist. Then make a fist with one hand and place the thumb of the fist against the middle of the victim's abdomen, slightly above the navel and well below the tip of the xiphoid process. Wrap the other hand over the fist to provide added force. Then press the fist into the victim's abdomen with a quick upward thrust (Fig. 16.8). Repeat each thrust until the foreign body is expelled or the victim becomes unconscious. If the victim is pregnant or obese, chest thrusts are acceptable instead of abdominal thrusts. To provide chest thrusts, place your hands in the same position that is used for chest compressions during CPR.

UNCONSCIOUS VICTIM

If a victim becomes unconscious, lay him or her down in a face-up (supine) position. Blind finger sweeps are no longer recommended. Attempt to remove an object from the victim's mouth only if the object is visible. Check for the object each time you prepare to provide breaths.

Open the airway and attempt to ventilate (if the foreign body has been successfully dislodged, the victim may require artificial respirations and possibly external cardiac compressions). If ventilation is unsuccessful, perform five abdominal thrusts. To perform abdominal thrusts on an unconscious victim, kneel astride the victim's thighs and place the heel of one hand against the victim's abdomen, in the midline slightly above the navel but well below the tip of the xiphoid process. Keep the second hand on top of the first hand for additional force. Press into the abdomen with a quick, upward thrust. Open the victim's mouth again and look for the foreign object. The steps should be repeated until the foreign body is dislodged and spontaneous breathing is restored. If spontaneous breathing is not restored, initiate CPR.

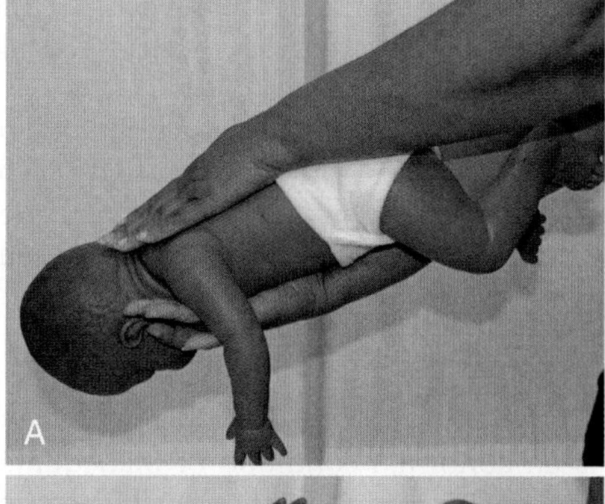

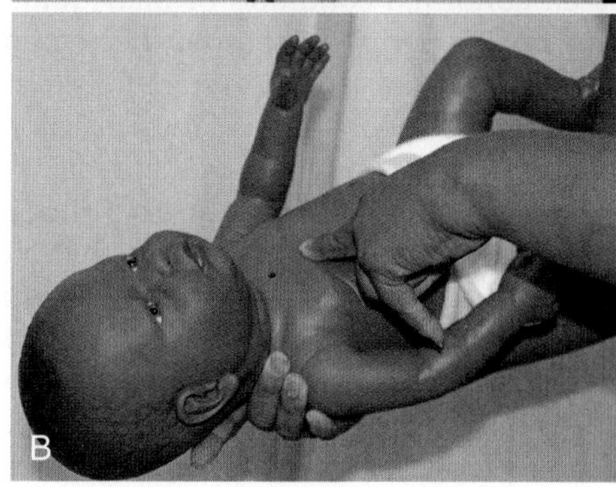

Fig. 16.9 Clearing airway obstruction in an infant. A, The infant is held face down and supported. Five quick, forceful blows are given with the heel of the hand. B, In the back-lying position, two fingers are placed in the center of the infant's breastbone and five quick downward thrusts are given.

INFANT

Of all deaths from foreign body aspiration, many occur in infants. Aspirated materials include food, such as candies and nuts, and small objects. Infants and children experience acute respiratory distress with coughing, gagging, and **stridor** (harsh sound during respirations, high-pitched and resembling the blowing of wind, caused by obstruction of the air passage). The victim often becomes unconscious.

If assisting a child who has aspirated a foreign body, treat the child in a manner similar to that for an adult with performance of abdominal thrusts. However, there is a potential for injury with use of this maneuver in an infant. Use a combination of back blows and chest thrusts with an infant, as follows:

1. Straddle the infant over your arm with the head lower than the trunk and the face down, and support the infant firmly at the jaw.
2. Rest the arm holding the infant on your thigh, and deliver five back blows between the infant's shoulders with the heel of the hand of the other arm (Fig. 16.9A).
3. Place the free hand on the infant's back so that the victim is sandwiched between the two hands, one supporting the neck, jaw, and chest while the other supports the back.
4. While continuing to support the head and neck, turn the infant and place the infant on the thighs, with the head lower than the trunk (see Fig. 16.9B).

5. Perform five chest thrusts with the hands in the same position as when performing external cardiac compressions (see Fig. 16.6).
6. Never use the blind finger-sweep technique because it is possible to cause the foreign body to become lodged within the airway. If you can see the object when the infant's mouth is open, attempt to remove it.

SHOCK

Shock is an abnormal condition of inadequate blood flow to the body's peripheral tissues (decreased tissue perfusion). The cardiovascular system fails to provide sufficient blood circulation (oxygen, nutrients, hormones, and electrolytes) to the body's tissues and major organs, and metabolic waste removal is decreased. Shock results in life-threatening cellular dysfunction, hypotension, and **oliguria** (diminished amount of urine formation, less than 500 mL of urine produced within 24 hours). To maintain circulatory homeostasis, there are several mechanisms that are necessary for the body to perform. The heart must function efficiently enough to circulate blood and a sufficient volume of blood must be available. The vascular system must be capable of maintaining adequate circulation. The heart pumps oxygen-rich blood to the capillaries and cells. Glucose, oxygen, and essential nutrients are provided to the cells, and carbon dioxide is returned to the right side of the heart. Inability of the body to compensate for failure of one or more of these mechanisms results in shock.

CLASSIFICATION OF SHOCK

Shock is classified according to its cause. The most common causes of shock are severe loss of blood, intense pain, extensive trauma, burns, poisons, emotional stress or intense emotions, extremes of heat and cold, electrical injury, allergic reactions, and a sudden or severe illness. Box 16.3 provides several examples of types of shock.

Box 16.3 Types of Shock

- *Anaphylactic shock:* Anaphylaxis (an exaggerated hypersensitivity reaction to a previously encountered antigen) results from a sudden, severe, allergic reaction to a foreign substance. Shock occurs because of the sudden decrease in the amount of circulating blood caused by the sudden release of histamine, which creates capillary hyperpermeability, which in turn causes the release of plasma through the capillary walls.
- *Cardiogenic shock:* This type results from poor heart function that results from various cardiovascular abnormalities. The heart is unable to maintain sufficient blood pressure to all body parts.
- *Hypovolemic shock* (also known as *hemorrhagic shock*): This type is caused by a decrease in fluid volume from bleeding, prolonged vomiting, or diarrhea, or by loss of fluid as a result of surgery, trauma, or burns.
- *Neurogenic shock:* This type is caused by the nervous system's failure to maintain normal contraction of the blood vessels. Common causes are spinal anesthesia, quadriplegia, or medications that cause vasodilation, which create a condition in which the blood pressure is lower because there is not enough blood to fill the dilated blood vessels.
- *Psychogenic shock syncope:* This type is caused by the nervous system's reaction to an emotional stimulus. The blood vessels dilate temporarily, decreasing blood flow to the brain, which results in unconsciousness, or syncope.
- *Septic shock:* This type results from severe infection. Toxins from the microorganisms cause loss of fluid through the blood vessel walls. This often is seen in people who have other infections such as a urinary tract infection or wound infection; in patients who recently have had surgery; in people receiving chemotherapy; or in other conditions that result in immunocompromised functioning, such as acquired immunodeficiency syndrome (AIDS).

ASSESSMENT

The signs and symptoms of shock are sometimes disguised by other signs of injury, and some often appear only in the late stages of shock. When assessing the patient for shock, monitor for the development of clinical manifestations in the following areas:

- *Level of consciousness:* The victim tends to experience changes in behavior, restlessness, anxiety, disorientation, syncope, and agitation. As the condition worsens, the victim becomes more lethargic. Coma and death are possible.
- *Skin:* The skin becomes cool and clammy. The skin and mucous membranes become pale and ashen. As shock progresses, **cyanosis** (slightly bluish, grayish, slatelike, or dark purple discoloration of the skin, especially of the lips and nail beds, caused by an excess of deoxygenated hemoglobin in the blood) develops, and the victim appears dehydrated.
- *Blood pressure:* Initially the blood pressure is often normal, but as shock progresses, there is a steady decrease in blood pressure, and capillary refill time is delayed. In hypovolemic shock, hypotension is a late manifestation.
- *Pulse:* The pulse rate usually increases (**tachycardia,** abnormal rapidity of heart action, usually defined as a heart rate of more than 100 beats per minute in an adult) in all types of shock. The pulse also becomes weak and thready.
- *Respirations:* The respiratory rate increases. Respirations are also frequently shallow, rapid, labored, or irregular as a result of vasoconstriction in the lungs, which causes fluid to accumulate.
- *Urinary output:* With decreased circulation of fluid volume, the patient may develop oliguria.

- *Neuromuscular system:* Decreased oxygen to the tissues results in weakness or tremors of the arms and legs. Eyelids close, and the pupils dilate.
- *Gastrointestinal system:* Because of loss of fluids and fluid shifts, the victim complains of thirst. Nausea, vomiting, and dryness of mucous membranes are also possible.

NURSING INTERVENTIONS

It is essential to treat shock immediately. Priority interventions are to establish an airway, control bleeding if present, and provide fluid replacement. Place the patient in a supine position with the legs slightly higher than the head (Fig. 16.10A). This position helps improve venous flow to the right side of the heart and to the vital organs and helps increase cardiac output.

When a patient is in shock, hypotension is possible. Trendelenburg's position is not recommended. If you suspect that the patient may have head, neck, or spinal injuries, keep the victim flat and do not move him or her unless absolutely necessary to prevent further injury (see Fig. 16.10B). If the victim is unconscious or is vomiting or bleeding around the nose and mouth, position him or her on the side to allow the airway to clear and to encourage drainage. Elevate the head and shoulders if the victim is having problems breathing (see Fig. 16.10C).

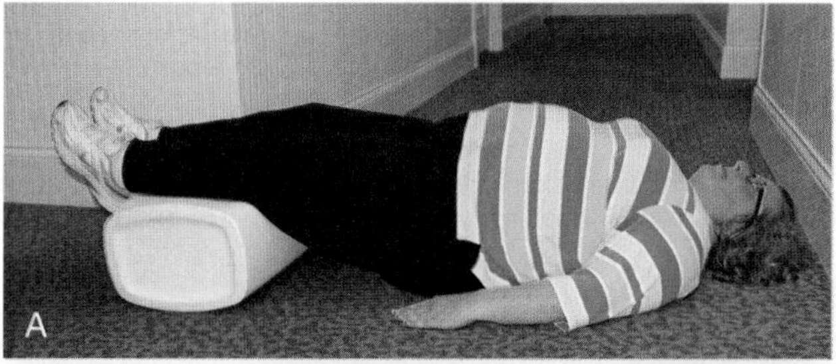

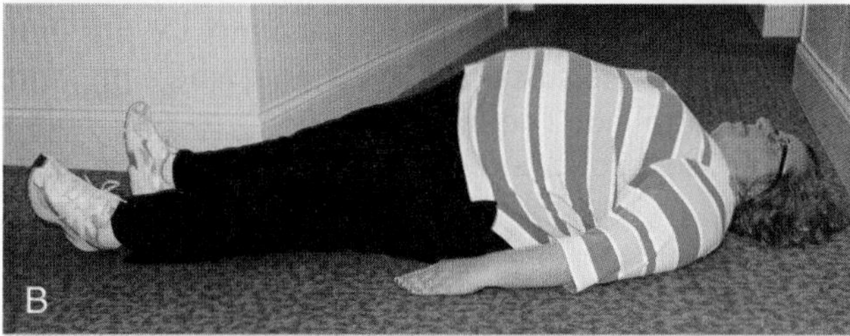

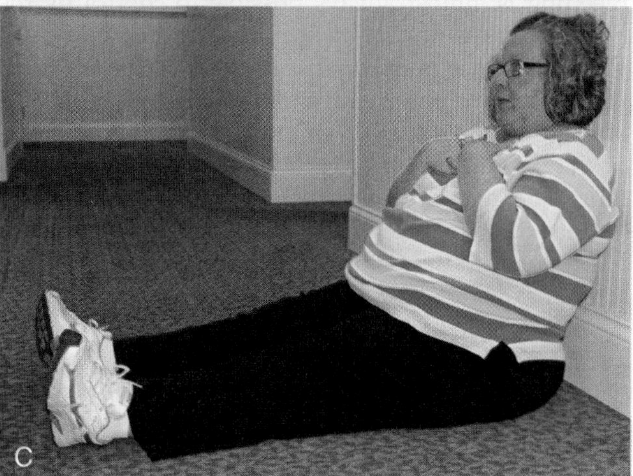

Fig. 16.10 Body positions for shock. A, Supine position with patient's legs elevated 6 to 8 inches (15 to 20 cm). B, Position for patients with suspected head, neck, or spinal injuries. C, Position for patients with breathing problems.

It is important to maintain the shock victim's body temperature. Wrapping the patient in blankets or other available material helps prevent heat loss. Foods and fluids are withheld in case internal injuries are present, which necessitate immediate surgical intervention. Provide the victim with a moistened cloth to help relieve dryness of the mouth or mucous membranes. In a clinical setting, venous access is established, usually with two large-bore intravenous catheters (ideally 14- to 16-gauge) to facilitate rapid administration of fluids and blood products, if needed.

If an injury is present, pain control should be addressed. Nursing interventions include positioning, adjusting tight or uncomfortable clothing or bandages, and avoiding rough handling. Do not give analgesics or drugs unless directed by a health care provider. Victims experiencing shock are likely to be very frightened, so it is essential for the nurse to give emotional support and reassurance.

BLEEDING AND HEMORRHAGE

An average adult has approximately 5 to 6 L (8 to 12 pints) of blood circulating in the bloodstream. Blood is necessary to transport oxygen and nutrients to all parts of the body. The body may compensate for some degree of blood loss without any changes noted, but at some point, the effects of blood loss become evident. The body attempts to cause clotting of the blood to halt bleeding. Clotting usually requires 6 to 7 minutes. Bleeding, if uncontrolled, can result in shock and death.

TYPES OF BLEEDING

Bleeding from a wound may occur through one or more of the following three sources: capillaries, veins, and arteries. Capillary bleeding results from damaged or broken capillaries and is characteristic from wounds such as the oozing that occurs with minor cuts, scratches, and abrasions. This is the most common type of external hemorrhage.

Venous bleeding occurs when a vein is severed or punctured. The result is a slow, even flow of dark red blood. Besides shock from blood volume loss, a danger of venous bleeding is the entrance of air into the severed vein, which creates the risk of an **air embolism** (an abnormal circulatory condition in which air travels through the bloodstream and becomes lodged in a blood vessel) that travels to the vital organs, including the heart, lungs, and brain.

Arterial bleeding is the least common type of injury because arteries are located deep in the body and usually are protected by bones, fat, and other structures. When

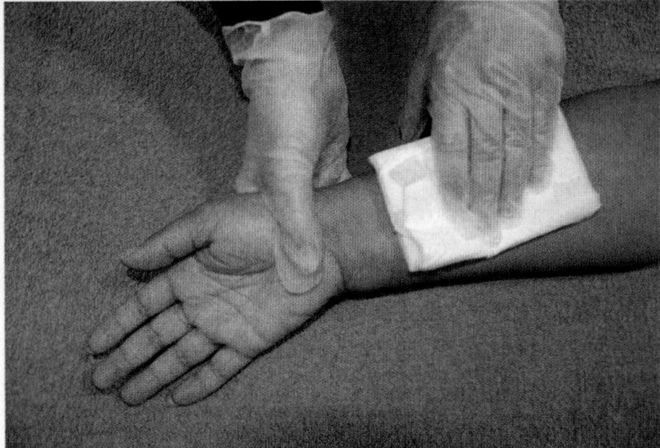

Fig. 16.11 Applying pressure to a wound site.

an artery is severed or punctured, the bleeding is characterized by the heavy spurting of bright red blood in the rhythm of the heartbeat. The following arteries are the most common sites of arterial bleeding:

- Brachial (in the medial aspect of the upper arm)
- Carotid (on either side of the neck)
- Femoral (in the upper thigh and groin)
- Radial (in the medial aspect of the lower arm)

NURSING INTERVENTIONS

Direct Pressure

The most effective general treatment of bleeding is to apply direct pressure over the bleeding site. Place a dressing or the cleanest material possible over the wound and apply firm pressure with a gloved hand (Fig. 16.11). Then apply a bandage and secure it snugly over the wound to exert direct pressure. This can be accomplished by tying a knot in the bandage over the wound or by using an elasticized securing bandage. If bleeding continues after the bandage is applied, resume pressure with a gloved hand over the bandage. Bleeding usually is controlled in 10 to 30 minutes. Do not allow anyone but a health care provider to remove the bandage while exerting direct pressure, even if it becomes saturated with blood. Instead, place an additional layer of dressing on top of the saturated bandage and continue firm pressure.

Raise the bleeding part of the body above the level of the heart to decrease blood flow and increase the victim's ability to clot at the injured site. This technique should be used only if there are no suspected or known fractures or conditions that are possible to exacerbate by use of this maneuver. It is acceptable to elevate a splinted fracture if no other contraindications are present.

Indirect Pressure

If direct pressure and elevation do not control bleeding, apply indirect pressure to any of the pressure points situated along the main arteries (Fig. 16.12). To apply indirect pressure, use the fingers or the heel of the hand to compress the artery against the underlying bone located between the heart and the wound. Do this only if no fractures are suspected in the area where pressure could be applied. The most common pressure points are over the carotid, subclavian, brachial, and femoral arteries.

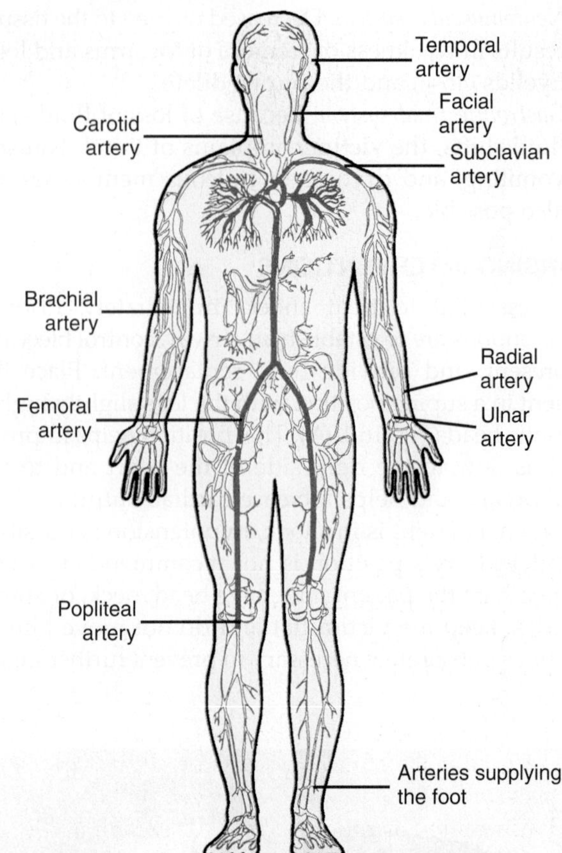

Fig. 16.12 Pressure points for bleeding control. (From Kidd PS, Stuart PA: *Mosby's emergency nursing reference*, St. Louis, 1996, Mosby.)

Application of a Tourniquet

Bleeding is almost always possible to control by the three-step measure of *direct pressure, elevation,* and *indirect pressure.* Use a tourniquet *only* when these methods have failed and the victim's life is in danger. Extensive damage to the affected extremity is possible because of the cessation of arterial blood flow to the area. A tourniquet also has the capacity to damage nerves and vessels directly below or under the tourniquet. An improperly, loosely applied tourniquet does not stop arterial flow but does hinder venous flow. Tourniquet use often is considered beyond the scope of first aid and of persons acting in good faith, such as a Good Samaritan, and usually is restricted to professionals such as health care providers and paramedics. Skill 16.1 provides steps to follow in applying a tourniquet.

EPISTAXIS

Epistaxis (nosebleed) is common but is seldom a serious emergency. However, profuse bleeding from

Skill 16.1 Applying a Tourniquet[a]

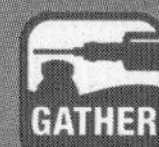

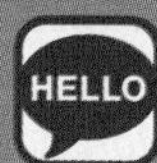

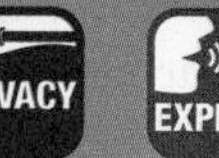

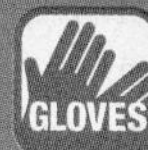

NURSING ACTION *(RATIONALE)*

1. Use a strong, wide, flat piece of material, if possible (e.g., towel, necktie, wide belt). *(Never use rope or wire, which has the potential to cut the skin.)*
2. Place pressure on the nearest pressure point. *(Controls bleeding while you are applying the tourniquet.)*
3. Apply a pad (piece of cloth, handkerchief, dressing) over the artery to be compressed. *(Prevents damage to the skin.)*
4. Place the tourniquet between the wound and the heart; allow some uninjured skin between the wound and the tourniquet. *(Prevents undue pressure on the injured site.)* Wrap the material around the limb twice, and tie a half-knot on the upper surface of the limb. *(Secures tourniquet in place.)*
5. Place a stick or rod (approximately 6 inches long) over the knot, and secure it in place. *(Enhances effect of tourniquet.)*
6. Twist the stick enough times to stop the bleeding. *(A tighter twist poses a risk for additional injury.)*
7. Secure the stick firmly with the free ends of the tourniquet. Do not cover the tourniquet. *(Tourniquet must be clearly visible to medical personnel.)*

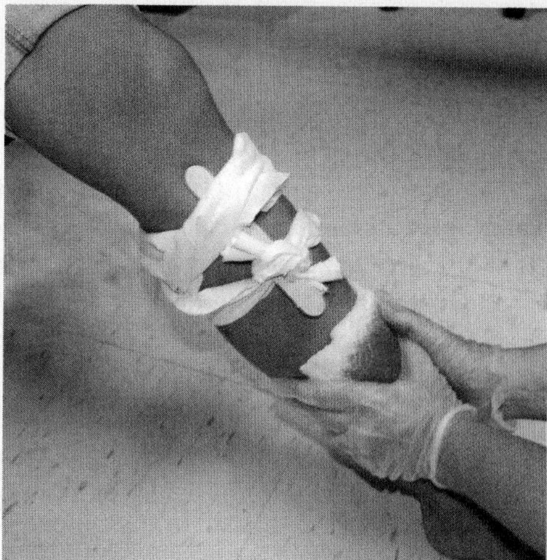

8. Write "T" (meaning tourniquet) and the time it was applied, on the victim's forehead. Attach a note to the victim's clothing describing the time and location of the tourniquet application. *(Ensures further interventions. A tourniquet allowed to remain in place too long poses the risk of further injury.)*
9. Treat the victim for shock, and transport him or her to the nearest medical facility. *(Ensures timely interventions.)*
10. Always seek medical attention once a tourniquet has been applied. *(Consistent treatment is necessary.)*

Note: Tourniquet use is often considered beyond the scope of first aid and of people acting in good faith, such as a Good Samaritan; placement is usually restricted to professionals such as health care providers and paramedics.

the nose does have the potential to lead to shock. Epistaxis has several causes: trauma (especially a direct blow to the nose); **epistaxis digitorum** (self-inflicted local digital trauma from nasal picking); infections, including the common cold; snorting cocaine; overuse of nasal sprays; high blood pressure; strenuous activity; hemophilia; and low humidity in winter months. Epistaxis in an older adult may be caused by underlying conditions, such as hypertension. Always assess an adult's blood pressure if epistaxis is present.

Nursing Interventions

The victim experiencing epistaxis is kept in a quiet sitting position, leaning forward. If the victim is unable to sit up, it is best that he or she remain supine with the head and shoulders raised (if this position is not contraindicated by other injuries).

Other interventions include the following:

- Keep the victim's head tilted slightly forward so that blood will not run down the back of the throat and cause choking or vomiting.
- With the thumb and forefinger, apply steady pressure to the bridge of the nose for 10 to 15 minutes before releasing.
- Remind the victim to breathe through the mouth and to expectorate any accumulated blood.
- Apply ice compresses over the nose, which may help control bleeding.
- Look in the victim's mouth at the back of the throat to assess for bleeding from a posterior site.

If bleeding continues despite interventions, seek medical assistance because it is possible that the victim is bleeding from a posterior site, which could necessitate fluid replacement and an emergency procedure to control bleeding.

INTERNAL BLEEDING

Internal bleeding is a potentially life-threatening situation. It is difficult to diagnose and often progresses rapidly. Common causes include fractures, knife or bullet wounds, crush injuries, organ injuries, and medical conditions such as aneurysm rupture.

Assessment

All the signs and symptoms of shock are often present. Initially, some victims experience only vertigo (dizziness). Some victims expectorate blood **(hemoptysis)** or vomit blood **(hematemesis).** Dark, tarry stool **(melena)** or blood in the urine **(hematuria)** may occur. Pain, tenderness, or a dislocation at the site of a suspected injury indicates possible internal bleeding, as does bleeding from the mouth, rectum, or any other body opening.

Nursing Interventions

Internal bleeding is a priority medical emergency. Make every effort to obtain medical care immediately. Victims receiving anticoagulant therapy are likely to develop significant blood loss from minor injury. Significant blood loss also occurs in some victims with a history of alcohol abuse, as well as victims with blood dyscrasias.

The victim is placed on a flat surface with legs slightly elevated if this is not contraindicated by other injuries. Initiate treatment for shock. Place a cold compress or ice on the area of the suspected injury. Do not apply the ice directly to the skin because it can damage the tissue; place a towel or clean cloth between the ice and the skin. The victim's body temperature should be maintained with blankets, and the victim's vital signs should be assessed every 5 minutes. Withhold foods and fluids in case surgical intervention is necessary. Administer oxygen as ordered by the health care provider. Provide the victim with emotional support and reassurance to help decrease his or her anxiety.

WOUNDS AND TRAUMA

A *wound* is an injury to the internal or external soft tissues of the body. The basic rules for first aid treatment of wounds are as follows:

1. Stop the bleeding.
2. Treat shock.
3. Prevent infection.

CLOSED WOUNDS

Closed wounds involve the underlying tissues of the body; the top layer of skin is not broken. Examples of closed wounds are **ecchymoses** (discolorations of an area of the skin or mucous membrane caused by the extravasation of blood into the subcutaneous tissues; also called *bruises*), **contusions** (injuries that do not break the skin, caused by a blow and characterized by edema [swelling], discoloration, and pain), strains, and sprains. They most commonly occur as a result of falls, automobile accidents, or contact sports.

The following signs and symptoms are most likely to occur with a closed wound: (1) *edema* usually appears within 24 to 48 hours; (2) *discoloration* is likely to result from the formation of a hematoma (swelling containing blood): initially the discoloration is blackish blue and then turns to green or yellow within a few days; (3) *deformity* of the limbs is caused by fractures and dislocations; (4) *shock* often follows from the force of the trauma; (5) *pain* and *tenderness* at the site are possible; and (6) signs of *internal bleeding* are sometimes present.

Nursing Interventions

If the wound is small, it may be best to apply an ice pack, along with padding, an elastic bandage, or a 4- × 4-inch abdominal dressing used for pressure. If the wound is large, monitor the patient for shock; apply cold compresses and a pressure bandage. Obtain medical assistance immediately.

OPEN WOUNDS

Open wounds are openings or breaks in the mucous membrane or skin. Regardless of the type, there is always danger of bleeding or infection. Infection is more common in wounds that do not bleed freely because active bleeding tends to flush microorganisms from the wound. There are five general types of open wounds: abrasions, punctures, incisions, lacerations, and avulsions. The following is a discussion of each of these open wound types and the appropriate nursing interventions that should be used (Fig. 16.13).

An injection of **tetanus toxoid** (an active immunizing agent prepared from detoxified tetanus toxin that produces an antigenic response in the body, conferring active immunity to tetanus infection) may be necessary as a general treatment for an open wound. The patient should receive the tetanus vaccine every 10 years to maintain immunity. The attending health care provider

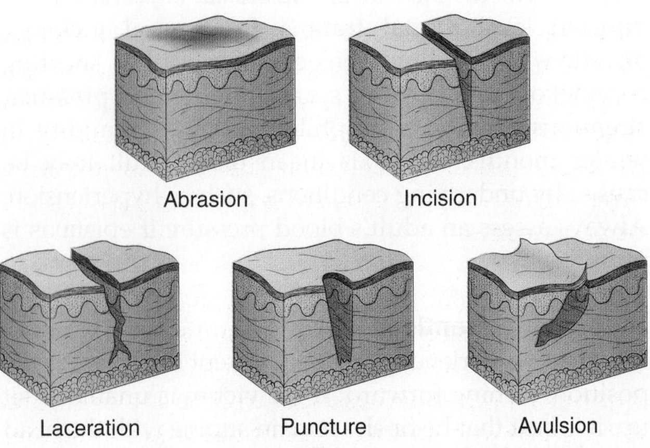

Fig. 16.13 Five types of open wounds.

ultimately decides on administration in a given case, especially for wounds that have occurred as a result of a soiled object or are dirty.

Abrasions

Abrasions are caused by a rubbing or scraping of the outer layers of the skin. Bleeding typically is limited to oozing of blood; there is danger of infection from contamination with dirt and microorganisms. Examples of abrasions include rope and road burns, scratches, and scrapes of knees and elbows.

Nursing interventions. Remove all dirt, if possible. Strong antiseptics should not be used because they easily can irritate the skin. Normal saline is safe and effective, and copious irrigation with saline helps remove debris. Clean the wound from the inside out. Povidone-iodine, unless properly diluted, actually causes tissue necrosis because it is too harsh. Cover the abrasion with a sterile dressing.

Advise the victim about the signs and symptoms of infection, such as edema, erythema, pain, and purulent exudate. Instruct the victim to seek medical attention if these signs and symptoms occur.

Puncture Wounds

Puncture wounds are piercing wounds of the skin. They typically are made by knives, nails, wood, glass, or other objects that penetrate the skin. Punctures often force dirt and microorganisms deep into the tissues. If the object remains firmly in the skin, do not attempt to remove it. Leave it in place for the health care provider to remove. Removal has the potential to cause significant bleeding or other types of complications that may necessitate emergency surgical intervention.

Nursing interventions. Thoroughly irrigate all puncture wounds to remove as much debris and as many microorganisms as possible. Patients often require a tetanus booster vaccination. As with abrasions, advise the victim about signs and symptoms of infection.

Incisions

Incisions are smoothly divided wounds made by sharp instruments. Infection is not as likely to occur because blood flows freely from the wound. However, bleeding is sometimes extensive, and muscle, tendon, and nerve damage is possible. Common examples of incisional wounds include cuts from knives, broken glass, razors, or paper edges.

Nursing interventions. Carefully clean the incision and cover it with a sterile dressing. An antiseptic should be used only with a health care provider's recommendation. Typically, a butterfly bandage, Steri-Strips, or sutures are applied to hold the edges of the wound together. Help control any bleeding by applying pressure. If the incision is deep, bleeding is profuse, and function is limited, seek medical care for the patient.

Lacerations

Lacerations are wounds that are torn with jagged, irregular edges. Bleeding is often profuse, and tissue destruction and infection are possible. Auto accidents, blunt objects, and heavy machinery accidents are common causes of lacerations.

Nursing interventions. Lacerations are cleaned in a manner similar to that for abrasions and puncture wounds. Bleeding should be controlled by applying pressure (see Fig. 16.11). Use adhesive strips, Steri-Strips, or butterfly bandages to close the edges of the laceration if possible. Cover the wound with a sterile dressing, and the victim should be seen by a health care provider.

Avulsions

An avulsion is a torn piece of tissue that results in a section being completely removed or left hanging by a flap. Avulsions are sometimes minor, with only a small amount of displaced skin, but sometimes they include large areas of tissue, with exposure of underlying bones, tendons, or muscles. Avulsions are often more difficult to heal than other types of wounds because wound edges are more difficult to approximate.

Nursing interventions. Bleeding should be controlled by direct pressure. Thoroughly cleanse the wound. Suturing is often necessary to repair an avulsion wound. Closely monitor the wound site for healing without complications.

CHEST WOUNDS

Chest wounds are extremely dangerous and necessitate immediate medical attention. In many chest wounds, air or blood escapes into the **pleural space** (the potential space between the visceral and parietal layers of the pleurae). Normally this space is a vacuum created by negative pressure; therefore air **(pneumothorax)** or blood **(hemothorax)** entering this space has the potential to cause an increase in pressure, which often results in collapse of lung tissue.

Assessment. Assess the patient for the following:

- Sharp pain at the site of the injury
- Pain associated with breathing
- Difficult and labored breathing
- Failure of one or both sides of the chest to expand normally with inspiration
- Expectoration of bright red or frothy blood (hemoptysis)
- Signs and symptoms of shock: rapid, weak, thready pulse; vertigo; and hypotension
- Cyanosis of the skin and mucous membranes

- A sucking or hissing sound as air flows in and out of the chest
- Distention of the neck and arm veins
- Anxiety
- Tracheal deviation

Nursing interventions. For the first aid treatment of penetrating chest wounds, if the chest wall has been penetrated by a sharp object, do *not* remove the object; this sometimes results in further bleeding and the entrance of air into the chest wound. Instead immobilize the object with dressings and tape. It is sometimes necessary to elevate the victim's head slightly to help facilitate breathing.

If there is a sucking chest wound (without the penetrating object in place), apply an airtight dressing. Any available material is acceptable to use: gauze, plastic wrap, clothing, or even a hand, if that is the only thing available. It is necessary for this dressing to be large enough that it is not sucked into the hole in the victim's chest and as airtight as possible. Monitor the victim for any signs and symptoms of a developing pneumothorax. Any signs of increased respiratory distress indicate the possible development of a tension pneumothorax. In that case, leave one side of the dressing untaped. Liquids should be withheld because aspiration is possible.

For the first aid treatment of crushing chest wounds, understand that the most common injury to the chest is fractured ribs. Severe blunt trauma sometimes results in **flail chest** (two or more ribs fractured in two or more places, resulting in instability in part of the chest wall) with associated hemothorax, pneumothorax, and pulmonary contusion (Fig. 16.14). Paradoxic motion develops as a result of the instability this brings about in part of the chest wall, with the lung underlying the injured area contracting on inspiration and bulging on expiration. If the condition is uncorrected, respiratory distress and hypoxia result. Elevate the victim's head and shoulders to facilitate breathing if a spinal injury is not suspected. Carefully apply dressings to any open wounds to avoid any pressure to the chest that has potential to impair breathing.

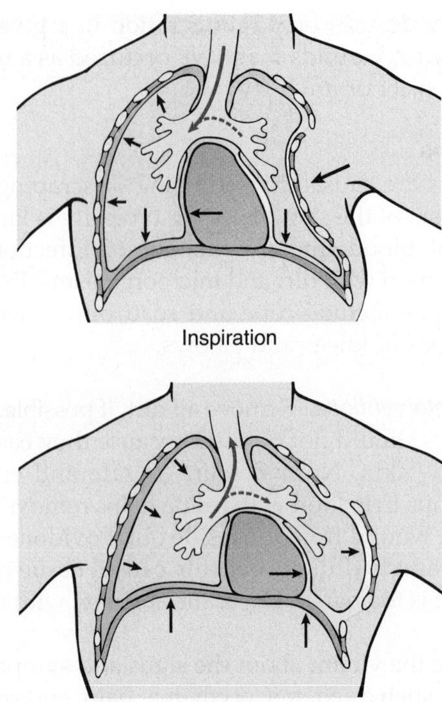

Fig. 16.14 Flail chest. (From Lewis SL, Butcher L, Heitkemper MM, et al: *Medical-surgical nursing: Assessment and management of clinical problems*, ed 10, St. Louis, 2017, Elsevier.)

DRESSINGS AND BANDAGES

General Principles of Bandaging

First control bleeding before applying a sterile bandage. If sterile equipment is not available, use the cleanest material possible. The dressing should cover the entire wound and be tight enough to control bleeding but not as tight as a tourniquet. Tourniquets have the potential to cause tissue and nerve damage.

Always bandage the part in the desired alignment; do not bend a joint after it is bandaged. Tips of the fingers and the toes should be left exposed, if possible, so that the victim's circulation can be assessed. It is critical to assess for edema and adequate circulation frequently. If loose material is used for the bandage, tie it with a knot over the top of open wounds to help apply pressure and control bleeding, unless this is contraindicated.

Application of Common Types of Bandages

Bandage compress. The bandage compress is the most common type of dressing. It consists of several thicknesses of gauze covered with tape, roller gauze, or other materials. These bandages are used to control bleeding.

Triangular bandage. The triangular bandage is made of a piece of cloth that is folded diagonally and cut along the fold. Nurses use this most commonly as a sling to support injured bones. Skill 16.2 describes the application of an arm sling with a triangular bandage.

Gauze bandage. Rolls of gauze bandage are used to support an injured part, apply pressure to a dressing for control of bleeding, or secure a splint to immobilize a part (Fig. 16.15). The roll of gauze bandages is applied uniformly to ensure even pressure. The skin should be covered completely. It is best to use a greater number of evenly spaced overlapping turns rather than fewer, tighter turns of the bandage. Begin application of the gauze bandage at the point of the dressing or at the part of the limb with the smallest circumference (e.g., the wrist or the ankle). Gauze bandages are secured with either tape or a square knot. A circular or spiral

Skill 16.2 Applying an Arm Sling With a Triangular (Sling and Swathe) Bandage

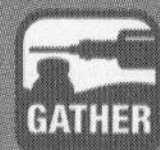

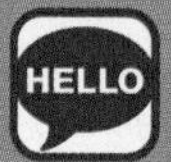

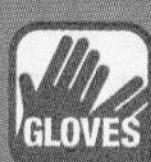

NURSING ACTION *(RATIONALE)*

1. Place one end of the base of the open triangle over the uninjured shoulder. *(Prevents undue pressure on injured side.)*
2. Place the apex of the triangle behind the elbow of the injured arm. *(Facilitates usefulness of sling.)*
3. Bend the arm at the elbow with the hand elevated slightly (4–5 in [10–13 cm]). *(Enables venous return from hand and forearm and facilitates drainage from edema.)*
4. Bring the forearm across the chest and over the bandage. *(Establishes position of arm in sling.)*

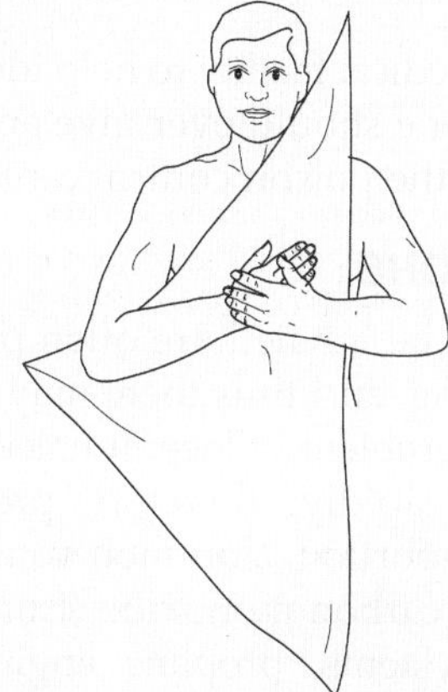

5. Take the lower end of the triangle and bring it over the shoulder of the injured side. Tie the bandage on the neck at the uninjured side so that the knot is on the side of the neck. *(Prevents pressure on cervical spine.)*

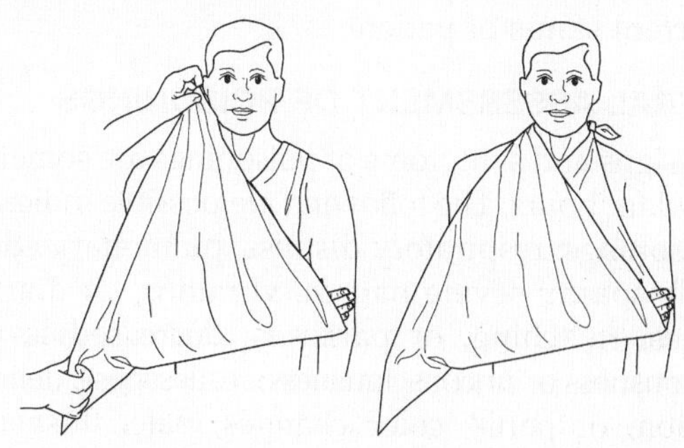

6. Twist the remaining end of the bandage and tuck it in at the elbow. *(Secures sling.)*

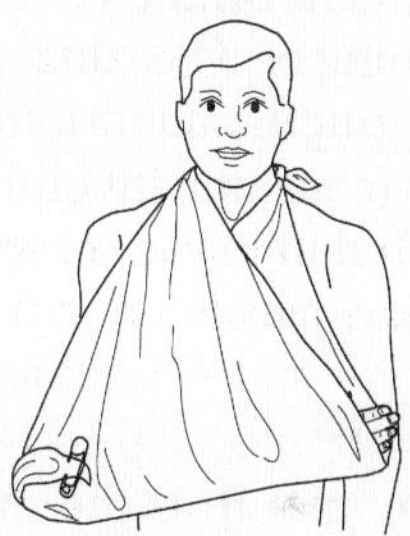

7. Remember to keep fingertips exposed. *(Secures sling and allows for easy assessment of circulation.)*

Figures from Proehl JA: *Emergency nursing procedures*, ed 4, St. Louis, 2009, Saunders.

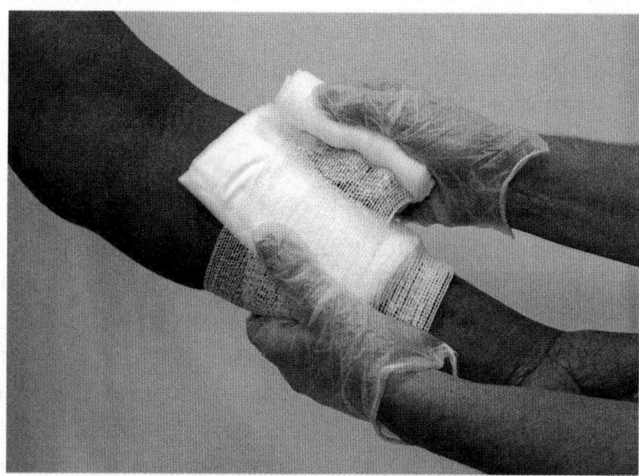

Fig. 16.15 Use of a roll of gauze bandage.

roll of gauze bandages is used to cover a cylindric part. A figure-8 bandage is another option, especially if splints are necessary or when a dressing is applied to an ankle (see Chapter 22).

POISONS

Each year thousands of people die from self-inflicted or accidental poisonings. The majority of these people are children. A *poison* is any substance (solid, liquid, or gas) that even in small amounts causes damage to the body or interferes with the function of its systems. Poison control centers throughout the United States are equipped to give information about poisons and methods of treatment on a 24-hour-a-day, 7-day-a-week basis. Most poisons act rapidly and thus necessitate immediate first aid.

Poison control centers need the following information:

- Patient's weight
- Patient's age
- Substance ingested, inhaled, or injected
- Amount of substance taken
- Time when substance was taken
- Any medications patient has taken
- Current status of patient

GENERAL ASSESSMENT OF POISONINGS

Acute signs and symptoms of poisonings are sometimes delayed for hours. The following are possible indications of poisonings: respiratory distress; pulmonary edema; bronchospasm; severe nausea, vomiting, or diarrhea; seizures, twitching, or paralysis; decreased level of consciousness or unconsciousness; restlessness, delirium, agitation, or panic; color changes; pale, flushed, or cyanotic skin; signs of burns or edema around the mouth or other areas of the body; pain, tenderness, or cramps on swallowing; characteristic odor on the breath; unusual urine color (red, green, bright yellow, black, bronze); slow, labored breathing or wheezing; abnormal constriction or dilation of pupils; abnormal eye movements, such as nystagmus (constant, involuntary, cyclic movement of the eyeball); skin irritation, erythema, or edema; and shock or cardiac arrest.

INGESTED POISONS

Poison ingestion by mouth is the most common type of poisoning, especially in children. Common substances include household cleaning products such as drain cleaners, oven cleaners, laundry detergents, floor or furniture polish, rat poison, cockroach sprays and baits, diaper pail deodorants, garden and garage supplies (e.g., insecticides, gasoline), drugs, medications, food, and plants, such as poinsettias. Older adults sometimes require special precautions (see the Lifespan Considerations for older adults box).

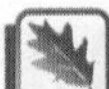

Lifespan Considerations

Older Adults

Accidental Overdose

Older adult patients are sometimes the victims of accidental overdose for the following reasons:

- Poor eyesight potentially leads to ingesting the wrong medication. Anyone assisting with the care of an older adult should ensure that all medications and other substances are marked clearly in large lettering.
- Confusion potentially leads to repeating a medication dosage accidentally. Use of medication boxes in which medications are organized for a week at a time helps eliminate duplicate dosing.
- Older patients often are prescribed several medications. Health care providers should be sure to document a good health history, including all medications, when providing emergency treatment.

Immediate Response

The person who determines that another person has been poisoned should call the poison control center immediately (1-800-222-1222) to describe the poison ingested and to receive instructions. The poison control center will give instructions for any treatment to start in the home or recommend immediately bringing the patient to an emergency center for treatment. The poison control center number should be kept by the telephone in the home and programmed into a person's cell phone for easy access. Keeping syrup of ipecac in the home to induce vomiting is no longer recommended (see Chapter 10).

Treat the patient for clinical manifestations associated with shock and, if necessary, administer CPR. Ensure that the substance's container and any vomitus are brought to the medical facility to help identify and treat the poison. No one should ever give an antidote until consulting with the poison control center.

INHALED POISONS

Poisons that can be inhaled are often present without anyone's knowing, and thus there may be no advance warning of a problem. Once inhaled, poisons are absorbed very rapidly; therefore prompt first aid measures are important. Common sources of inhaled poisons include carbon monoxide (from automobiles, fires, heating systems, propane engines, and paint remover), carbon dioxide (from sewers or industry), and refrigeration gases. Chlorine (used in cleaning and industry) and other spray and liquid chemicals also have the potential to give off poisonous fumes, typically when cleaning chemicals are mixed together.

Nursing Interventions

Before assisting any victim of an inhaled poison, first assess the danger. The victim should be removed from the area of exposure as soon as possible, but only if there is no danger to the nurse or any other rescuers. Loosen clothing from the victim's throat and chest, and assess the victim to determine whether CPR is necessary. The victim should be kept quiet and inactive while being transported immediately to the nearest medical facility.

ABSORBED POISONS

Poisons, caustic chemicals, and substances from poisonous plants that come in contact with the skin often are absorbed rapidly, causing burning, skin irritation, allergic responses, or severe systemic reactions. Most signs and symptoms occur within 1 to 2 hours after absorption. Signs and symptoms include nausea, vomiting, diarrhea, flushed skin, dilated pupils, cardiovascular abnormalities, and central nervous system and respiratory reactions.

Poison ivy, poison oak, and poison sumac are the plants that most commonly elicit a poison response.

Nursing Interventions

First, quickly remove the source of the irritation and then wash the contacted area with soap and water. Skin preparations that are effective in the treatment of contact poisonings include baking soda, Burow's solution, and oatmeal. Calamine lotion and hydrocortisone cream (5%) are effective in relieving pruritus.

INJECTED POISONS

A person can develop an allergic reaction if the person is injected with a drug to which the person is allergic or if the person receives a venomous sting or bite from an insect, reptile, or animal. In addition, immediate follow-up treatment is recommended because bites from animals, reptiles, or rodents may lead to infection. Many health care practitioners prescribe prophylactic antibiotic treatment to prevent infection. If an animal is thought to be rabid, the person should wash the bite immediately with soap and water for at least 5 minutes and then seek emergency care for treatment of rabies (Immunization Action Coalition, n.d.). Wound cleansing is especially important in rabies prevention because, in animal studies, thorough wound cleansing alone without other postexposure prophylaxis has been shown to reduce markedly the likelihood of rabies (CDC, 2016). Emergency care for bites from a reptile such as a snake include the following:

- Restrict the movement of the affected extremity and keep it below heart level to reduce the amount of toxin flowing toward the heart and recirculating. Remove rings and any restrictive clothing in case swelling occurs.
- Monitor the person for signs of shock and seek medical attention immediately.
- If the area around the bite begins to swell or change color, it is likely that the snake was poisonous.
- If the snake is dead, it should be brought to the hospital for testing only if it is safe to do so. Snakes can bite after being dead because of their reflexes (National Library of Medicine, 2017).

Minor Reactions to Insect Bites

If a person has been stung by a bee or wasp, remove the stinger with gauze or some other clean material in a scraping motion. An attempt to grasp the barbed stinger with tweezers sometimes forces venom further into the skin. Nursing interventions include washing the area with soap and water and applying cold packs to relieve pain and slow the absorption of the poison. A paste of baking soda and water sometimes relieves pruritus at the site.

Severe Reactions to Insect Bites

Within as little as 60 minutes or up to several hours afterward, a victim of a bite or sting sometimes experiences a severe allergic reaction. Urticaria, wheezing, edema of the lips and tongue, generalized pruritus, and respiratory arrest are the most common signs and symptoms of anaphylactic shock (severe allergic reaction).

Nursing interventions. People who know that they have an allergy sometimes wear medical alert tags and carry an epinephrine pen, an anaphylaxis kit, or antihistamines such as diphenhydramine (Benadryl) to take after a bite. The patient may self-administer these types of medications. A health care provider may direct the nurse to administer such medications in this type of emergency situation.

DRUG AND ALCOHOL EMERGENCIES

Drugs (including alcohol) are chemical substances that have the potential to affect body functioning and are subject to abuse and overdose.

ALCOHOL

Alcohol is the most commonly abused drug in the world. It is a central nervous system depressant that has the capacity to cause many signs and symptoms, even death (Table 16.1).

Assessment

Signs and symptoms of *mild* intoxication include nausea, vomiting, diarrhea, lack of coordination, and poor muscle control. Flushing, erythema of the face and eyes, visual disturbances, and rapid mood swings are often present. Slurred or inappropriate speech, inappropriate behavior, and lethargy (sleepiness) are also typical.

Serious alcohol intoxication usually is caused by consuming a large quantity of alcohol over a short period of time. Signs and symptoms include drowsiness that progresses to coma; rapid, weak pulse; and depressed, labored breathing or respiratory arrest. Loss of control of urinary and bowel functions, and disorientation, restlessness, and hallucinations are possible, as are tremors that have the potential to progress to grand mal seizures, nausea, vomiting, expectoration of blood from the respiratory tract, and diarrhea. Some affected people also experience loss of memory, visual disturbances, lack of muscle coordination, and depressed reflexes.

DRUGS

Abuse of drugs is a major problem worldwide. Not only illegal drugs but also prescription and over-the-counter medications are abused. When assessing the drug abuser, observe for signs and symptoms of disorientation, hallucinations, and changes in the victim's level of consciousness; coma and death are possible results. Slurred speech, extremes in mood swings, inappropriate behavior, and anxiety are also present in some cases. Sometimes the victim has a fever and flushed skin and experiences diaphoresis (sweating). Because

Table 16.1 Blood Alcohol Concentration (BAC) and Related Effects

BAC[a] mg/dL (mg%)	PSYCHOPHYSIOLOGIC EFFECT
20 (0.02)	Light and moderate drinkers begin to feel some effects. Approximate BAC is reached after one drink.
40 (0.04)	Most people begin to feel relaxed.
60 (0.06)	Judgment is mildly impaired. People are less able to make rational decisions about their capabilities (e.g., driving skills).
80 (0.08)	Definite impairment of muscle coordination and driving skills occurs. Person is considered legally intoxicated in some states.
100 (0.10)	Clear deterioration of reaction time and control is observed. Person is considered legally intoxicated in most states.
120 (0.12)	Vomiting occurs unless this level is reached slowly.
150 (0.15)	Balance and movement are impaired. The equivalent of one half pint of whiskey is circulating in the bloodstream.
300 (0.30)	Many people lose consciousness.
400 (0.40)	Most people lose consciousness, and some die.
450 (0.45)	Breathing stops; person eventually dies.

[a]BAC generally is recorded in milligrams of alcohol per deciliter (mg/dL) of blood or in milligrams percentage (mg%). Percentage is used for legal definitions of intoxication. BAC is dependent on how much alcohol is consumed, how fast it is consumed, and the person's weight and sex. Alcohol affects women differently than men. Women usually have substantially more alcohol-caused impairment than men at equivalent levels of consumption.
From Lewis SL, Heitkemper MM, Dirksen SR, et al: *Medical-surgical nursing: Assessment and management of clinical problems*, ed 7, St. Louis, 2007, Mosby.

of lack of coordination and impaired judgment, safety is typically an issue. Depending on the drug, the pulse and blood pressure often increase or decrease, the pupils constrict or dilate, and the appetite increases or decreases. Hypodermic needle marks ("track marks") on arms, legs, hands, feet, and neck are often obvious. Many victims complain of diarrhea or pain in the abdomen, legs, or joints and experience tremors or seizures.

Nursing Interventions

Because an accurate nursing history is important, obtain as much information as possible about the substance ingested and identify any containers that contained the substance if possible. Life-threatening situations should be handled first. Establish and maintain the airway. If the victim is unconscious, the victim is turned onto his or her side. Loosen the victim's clothing to assist with ventilation. If the victim is having muscle twitching and is drowsy, do not arouse the victim because this may precipitate a seizure. If a fever is present, attempt to reduce the victim's temperature by applying cool, wet compresses. Victims must be protected from self-injury during a seizure or hallucination by removing potentially harmful objects from the patient's vicinity. Do not attempt to restrain a victim during seizure activity or place anything within the victim's mouth.

A calm, supportive, nonjudgmental approach is best when a victim is very agitated or excited. An intoxicated person should not be left alone. Frequently perform a careful assessment of the victim's mental status and vital signs. It is possible for a victim of substance abuse to go into respiratory arrest quickly. Ensure the victim is transported promptly to a medical facility.

THERMAL AND COLD EMERGENCIES

HEAT INJURIES

Heat exhaustion or heatstroke results when the body is unable to cool itself when exposed to excessive environmental heat. Normally the body reacts to heat with excessive perspiration and slowing of muscle activity. If excessive perspiration occurs without rehydration of the body, heat exhaustion results. On the other hand, if the body is unable to cool itself, the internal body temperature rises, resulting in heatstroke. Heat exhaustion and heatstroke have different characteristics and treatment protocol.

Heat Exhaustion

Heat exhaustion is the most common type of heat injury and is the result of prolonged perspiration and the loss of large quantities of salt and water. It occurs most often in hot, humid weather when people do not adequately replace fluids (common in older adults, in whom the thirst mechanism is diminished even when they are dehydrated).

The nursing assessment of a victim of heat exhaustion includes assessing for signs and symptoms such as headache, vertigo, nausea, weakness, and diaphoresis.

Mental disorientation and brief loss of consciousness may occur. The victim has a normal body temperature with pale, cold, clammy skin. Some victims complain of abdominal cramps and loss of appetite. Breathing is typically rapid and shallow, and the pulse is weak and rapid. Blood pressure sometimes drops but usually returns to normal when the person assumes a recumbent position.

Nursing interventions. Move the victim to a cool area and cool off the victim as quickly as possible, without inducing chilling and shivering. Chilling and shivering would cause the body temperature to rise. Remove as much of the victim's clothing as possible and loosen constrictive clothing to allow the circulation of air to cool the body. Cold, wet compresses are used to cool the victim, as well as a fan or air conditioner if available.

If the victim is completely conscious and alert, give the victim fluids. Water and sports drinks are recommended. If the victim is drowsy or vomiting, do not give any fluids by mouth. In the clinical setting, intravenous fluids are given. The victim should be transported to a medical facility as soon as possible.

Heatstroke

Heatstroke is a more serious heat injury; death is possible if heatstroke goes untreated. The most common cause of heatstroke is vigorous physical activity in a hot, humid environment. The body becomes overheated, but the cooling mechanism of perspiration is not helpful because of the hot, humid conditions. The body stores excessive heat because it is unable to cool itself properly. Body temperature sometimes rises to 106°F (41°C) or greater. Damage to the victim's brain and central nervous system may result.

Assessment. The signs and symptoms of heatstroke include rapidly rising body temperature; hot, dry, erythemic skin; and no visible perspiration. The pulse is rapid initially and then slows and weakens as the blood pressure falls. Breathing becomes deep and rapid. The victim complains of headache, dry mouth, and nausea and may vomit; some victims experience vertigo and decreased level of consciousness and may collapse. Muscle twitching and convulsions may occur.

Nursing interventions. It is important for the nurse to cool the victim as quickly as possible and to move him or her to a cooler area. If the victim is alert, he or she should receive 0.5 cup (120 mL) of fluid every 15 minutes. Water and sports drinks are acceptable. Assist the victim to lie down with the feet 8 to 12 in (20.5 to 30.5 cm) higher than the head to avoid shock. Loosen the victim's clothing and remove excess clothing. Cool the victim's bare skin as quickly as possible with cool, wet cloths or with cool water directly on the victim's skin. Place cold packs around the neck, under the axillae, on the inguinal area, and around the ankles to cool the blood in the main arteries. Use a fan or air conditioner if available. Continue treatment until the victim's temperature falls below 100°F (37.7°C). Monitor the victim for chilling (control shivering because this will only increase the victim's body temperature) as the victim's temperature falls, and check the victim's temperature every 10 to 15 minutes to ensure that it does not rise again. Continue cooling efforts until the victim is able to obtain medical assistance.

EXPOSURE TO EXCESSIVE COLD

When the body is exposed to severe cold, body heat is lost, blood vessels constrict, and destruction of tissue sometimes results. Cold, moist air, fatigue, smoking, drugs, alcohol, dehydration, age, constricting clothing and footwear, and some diseases (such as diabetes mellitus or heart disease) accelerate the potential for injury.

Hypothermia

Hypothermia results when a person's body temperature drops lower than 95°F (35°C). The drop in body temperature affects all vital organs and body tissue because of lack of oxygenated blood perfusing tissues. Hypothermia occurs most frequently when the air is windy, cold, and moist or when precipitation is present. Submersion in cold water is a common cause as well. Common risk factors for hypothermia include exhaustion, mental illness, medical conditions such as hypothyroidism, and medications such as narcotics and sedatives. Age is also a common risk factor. The very young and elderly are susceptible to hypothermia because of the body's decreased ability to regulate body temperature (Mayo Clinic, 2018).

Assessment. Initially, the victim is likely to shiver uncontrollably; shivering ceases when the body temperature is less than 90°F (32.2°C). Additional symptoms include lethargy and drowsiness, weakness and clumsiness, and confusion. Victims often become irritable and combative and may experience hallucinations or delirium. Symptoms may progress to seizures, stupor, and coma. Respirations and heart rate slow, and the victim may go into respiratory or cardiac arrest or both. Finally, there is a loss of all reflexes, and the victim appears to be dead. Severe problems with electrolyte disturbances create the risk of serious dysrhythmias and cardiac arrest.

Nursing interventions. Although some people who are profoundly hypothermic may appear to be dead because of the effects of the lowered metabolic rate, it is possible to revive many of these victims. Attempt to treat hypothermia by instituting first aid. Initiate CPR and continue it until the body is warmed. Place the victim in a supine position with the head lower than the feet to treat possible shock. Warm the victim *slowly* because rapid exposure to warmth tends to precipitate shock. The victim should be moved to a warm area, and all the victim's wet clothes should be removed and replaced with dry ones. Cover the victim with warm blankets. For a patient experiencing profound hypothermia (core temperature below 30°C), active internal rewarming in addition to passive external rewarming effectively will raise the core body temperature. Administration of warm, humidified oxygen per mask or per ventilator; warmed blankets; heat lamps; and heated intravenous fluids such as 5% dextrose in normal saline (D_5NS) ranging in temperatures from 104° to 113° to 149°F (40° to 45° to 65°C). The temperature of the solution should be raised gradually, dependent on the patient's condition. Patients in the final stages of hypothermia sometimes develop atrial fibrillation and therefore need continuous electrocardiographic monitoring during treatment and immediately afterward. Cardiac arrest may occur if rewarming efforts are not successful (Li, 2017; Mareedo et al, 2008).

If the victim is completely conscious, provide the victim with warm fluids to drink. Rescuers should *never* give alcohol to the victim because of its vasodilatory effect on the peripheral vessels, which causes the central core temperature to drop further. Obtain medical help as soon as possible.

Frostbite

Frostbite is the most common and dangerous local cold injury involving freezing and damaging of body cells. Ice crystals form in the body's interstitial and cellular fluid spaces as a result of the cold temperature leading to decreased blood flow, inhibiting sufficient heat to the body's tissues, and causing destruction of tissue integrity. Common areas affected by frostbite are the ears, nose, fingers, toes, and lips. Deep tissue frostbite can result in tissue death. Hypothermia sometimes accompanies frostbite (Zonnoor B, 2018).

Assessment. Initially the frostbitten skin takes on a red flush, and the victim typically complains of numbness, tingling, or pain. The affected area becomes progressively hard and loses all sensation. The color of the affected area changes to grayish white as circulation diminishes further. If thawing occurs, the color often changes to bluish purple or black, indicating severe damage to or death of tissues. Edema often develops, followed by blisters. If frostbite damage is severe, complete loss of function of the part is possible.

Nursing interventions. If there is a possibility that the part will become refrozen after it has been thawed, it is better to leave it frozen until the victim arrives at a medical facility. Severe tissue damage is possible as a result of thawing and refreezing a frozen part. The victim may need to be treated for shock and hypothermia. It may be necessary to establish and maintain an airway. Remove any constricting clothing to encourage circulation.

If there is no risk that the part will become refrozen, warm it in the following manner: immerse the frozen part in warm water (preferably a bathtub) at 101° to 104°F (38.3° to 40°C) for approximately 30 minutes. Check the water temperature frequently and do not allow it to cool. If a tub is not available, use a very warm, moist towel. Be very careful *not* to rub the part because the friction may bruise and damage the underlying tissue. If water is not available, warm the part by placing it against a warm part of another person's body: the axilla, the abdomen, or between the legs. The frozen area should not be placed near an open flame or oven. Gentle warming is necessary to prevent burns and damage.

Once the part is warmed, the victim should be encouraged to gently move the part. If the legs or feet are involved, however, the victim should not be allowed to walk. The thawed part should be wrapped in clean towels or bulky dressings, and elevated. Try to keep the entire body warm and offer warm fluids to drink. Again, alcohol should not be provided to the victim. The victim also should not be allowed to smoke because this will cause further vasoconstriction and more damage. Never place ice, snow, or cold sources on a frostbitten area. A health care provider should evaluate all frostbite injuries, no matter how minor (University of Maryland Medical Center, 2010).

BONE, JOINT, AND MUSCLE INJURIES

The four major types of injuries that occur to bones, tendons, ligaments, and muscles are fractures, dislocations, sprains, and strains. Emergency care is initiated, and prompt medical care is obtained when these injuries occur.

FRACTURES

A *fracture* is a break in the continuity of a bone. Fractured bones are seldom an immediate threat to life, although they do have the potential to cause serious complications. When administering first aid to an injured victim, nurses may have to initiate CPR and treat hemorrhage. Fractures sometimes cause considerable blood loss (750 to more than 4000 mL from a fractured pelvis [Wheeless III, 2016] and up to more than 1000 mL from a fractured femur [Keany, 2015]).

There are several types of common fractures (refer to *Adult Health Nursing,* Chapter 4, Fig. 4.19 for diagrams of types of fractures):

- *Closed fracture:* The skin overlying the injury is intact.
- *Open or compound fractures:* An open wound exists over the fracture site. Often the affected bone is visible as it protrudes through the skin.
- *Comminuted fracture:* The bone is shattered into two or more fragments or pieces.
- *Spiral fracture:* Results from a twisting force.
- *Impacted fracture:* Results from trauma that causes the bone ends to jam together.
- *Greenstick fracture:* An incomplete break, occurring most commonly in children because their bones are more pliable.
- *Compressed fracture:* To the vertebrae as the result of pressure.
- *Depression fracture:* Results from blunt trauma to a flat bone, causing an indentation in the bone.
- *Displaced fracture:* Fracture in which the ends of the bones are not in alignment with each other.

- *Oblique fracture:* Break runs diagonally across the bone, at approximately a 45-degree angle to the shaft of the bone.

Assessment

The health care provider, using x-ray diagnostic procedures, will determine whether a bone is fractured. Fracture is suspected if there is pain and tenderness in the area of the fracture, if pain increases during movement, and if the victim complains of an inability to adequately move the affected part. A deformity of the limb may be obvious, with edema and discoloration (cyanosis, erythema) of the area. Fragments of bone sometimes protrude through the skin. If the affected part is moved, a grating sound may be heard. This is called **crepitus** and is caused by the broken bones scraping against each other. Sometimes victims report having heard or felt the bone snap.

Nursing Interventions

Do not move the victim unless he or she is in danger. Provide first aid and attempt to control bleeding in open fractures by cutting away the clothing around the wound and covering the wound with a large, sterile pressure dressing. No attempt should be made to reduce the fracture, because this may cause further damage to the bone and tissue. The victim may need to be treated for shock.

Immobilization of the fracture is necessary, but no attempt should be made to realign the bone. Splint the body part as it was found. It is possible to change a fracture from a simple break to a comminuted or splintered one by moving it improperly. Use a lightweight but rigid splint that is long enough to extend past the joints above and beyond the fracture and is wider than the thickest part of the injury. The splint should be padded on the inner surface to prevent contact with the skin. Support the fractures while sliding the splint under the limb. Roller gauze or similar material is used to secure the limb in place (Fig. 16.16). Monitor circulation in the affected limb by assessing color, temperature, movement, and pulses below the injury; complaints of numbness and tingling; and evidence of edema. Use ice or cold packs to reduce edema.

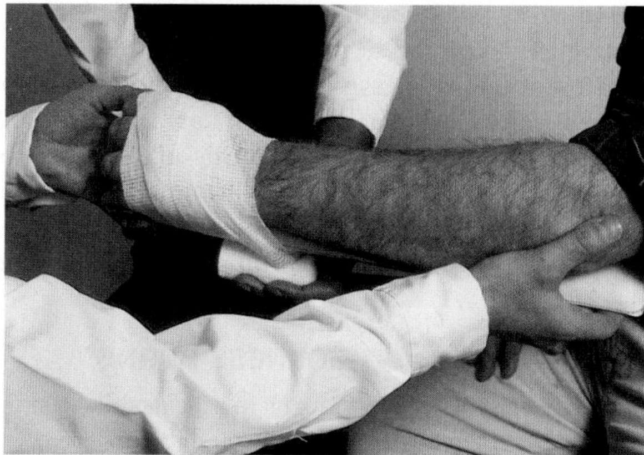

Fig. 16.16 Immobilization of a fractured arm. (From Henry MC, Stapleton ER: *EMT prehospital care*, ed 2, Philadelphia, 1997, Saunders.)

DISLOCATIONS

Dislocations occur in joints. They usually result from a blow or fall. Common sites of dislocations are the jaw, the shoulder, the elbow, the wrist, the finger, the hip, and the ankle.

Assessment

Victims usually complain of pain and edema in the area of the dislocation. Sometimes the nurse is able to observe a deformity of the part. Sometimes the part is rigid, and the victim is unable to move it.

Nursing Interventions

Never reduce dislocations, and never push dislocated joints back into place; this may further damage delicate ligaments, tendons, nerves (especially in the olecranon [elbow]), and the bone. Splint the joint in the same manner as a fracture. The splint should be large enough to support the limb in the line of the deformity. The limb should be bound to the body or supported in a sling. This is useful in dislocations of the shoulder and elbow. Apply ice or cold packs to reduce edema in surrounding tissues.

STRAINS AND SPRAINS

Strains are injuries to muscle tissue that result from stretching and tearing from overexertion. Sprains are injuries to joints resulting from stretched or torn ligaments, typically caused by twisting the joint beyond the normal range of motion. The joints most commonly affected are the knee and the ankle. Permanent damage to the tissue and joint are possible if sprains are left untreated.

Assessment

Injuries to muscle or ligaments result in the following signs and symptoms:

- *Strains:* Spasms or muscle "knots," acute pain, stiffness, and weakness on movement; back pain radiating down the leg; discoloration
- *Sprains:* Pain or tenderness around a joint; immobility of the joint; rapid and marked edema; discoloration around the joint

Nursing Interventions

Musculoskeletal injuries such as sprains and strains typically are treated initially according to the mnemonic RICE:

R *Rest* the affected extremity.

I *Ice* is applied to the part but not directly to the skin as soon as possible after the injury and for the next 48 hours, for 15 to 20 minutes, four to eight times a day. Ice should be followed with warm compresses to encourage healing by increasing the blood flow.

Skill 16.3 Moving the Victim With a Suspected Spinal Cord Injury

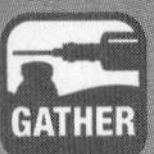

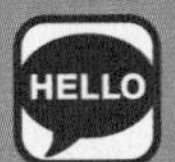

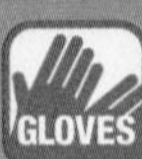

NURSING ACTION *(RATIONALE)*

1. Carefully roll the victim, with the assistance of at least three other trained people, supporting the entire length of the body, just enough to slip a solid board underneath the victim. It is necessary for the board to extend beyond the victim's head and feet. *(Supports the entire spine.)*
2. While another person steadies the victim's head, place a towel or padding in the space underneath the victim's neck (never put the head on a pillow). *(Immobilizes the head and neck.)*
3. Place additional padding (rolled-up blankets, towels, sandbags) around the head and neck, keeping the neck in line with the body. Using a cervical collar is acceptable. *(Holds the head in place.)*
4. Secure the victim to the backboard with something such as bandages. Tape the head in place. *(Immobilizes the entire body.)*
5. In an emergency situation in which the victim is wearing a helmet, immobilize the victim with the helmet left in place. *(Prevents further injury.)*

Assess the victim's skin frequently for any evidence of burns.

C *Compression:* An elastic bandage or compression bandage is used to support the injured part.

E *Elevation:* The injured part should be elevated above the level of the heart to promote venous flow and reduce edema.

Some recent studies have raised the question as to whether RICE is the ideal way to treat these types of injuries. Another strategy, with the mnemonic POLICE, is being suggested by some orthopedic specialists:

P *Protection:* Protecting the injured body part. This step consists of a shorter period of rest than with RICE. Movement of the injured extremity while maintaining protection with assistive devices such as crutches is suggested with POLICE. Rest should be limited to the first few days after injury with this principle.

O, L *Optimal Loading:* Weight-bearing to be determined by the primary care provider or orthopedic specialist (this may be an orthopedic physician, nurse practitioner, or physical therapist), either with or without a boot.

The remainder is unchanged: **I** (ice), **C** (compression), **E** (elevation) (Harrison, 2014).

SPINAL CORD INJURIES

Assessment

To assess for paralysis, ask the victim whether he or she is able to move the hands and feet and whether any pain or sensation is felt. Assess for sensation by touching or gently pinching the victim's skin. Any abrasions and ecchymosis, especially on the head, shoulders, back, and abdomen, indicate possible injury to the victim's spinal cord.

Nursing Interventions

Spinal cord precautions should be taken in all cases of head trauma and multiple traumas. In patients with facial lacerations, there is a high correlation between neck injuries and spinal cord injuries. Maintain the victim's airway and ensure that the victim's head remains in a neutral position (the neck should never be hyperextended). If the victim vomits, direct several people, acting together as one unit, to help logroll the victim onto his or her side to allow drainage (see Chapter 8, Skill 8.3). When the victim is transported to a health care facility, the victim's head and neck must be kept in line with the body. Even a slight movement of the individual's head out of line with the body can potentially cause spinal damage. Do not attempt to move the victim without at least three assistants (Skill 16.3).

BURN INJURIES

Burns are a leading cause of accidental injuries; 486,000 burns per year necessitate medical treatment in the United States (American Burn Association, 2016). Burns are caused by heat from fire, hot liquids or steam, electricity from faulty wiring, chemicals such as lye, strong cleaning products, acids, solar radiation, and radioactive materials. The initial management of the patient with burns begins at the time of injury. The priority is to stop the burning process.

Burns often are classified according to their depth or the extent of the body surface area burned. The principal complications of all burns are shock, from loss of fluids and electrolytes, and trauma and infection as results of the loss of the skin as a barrier. The extent of burns can be calculated according to the rule of nines (Fig. 16.17).

SHALLOW PARTIAL-THICKNESS BURNS

Shallow partial-thickness burns (also classified as first-degree burns) are the least serious of all burns, involving only the outer layer of the skin. The most common first-degree burns are simple sunburns or burns from contact with hot objects. Healing usually is spontaneous

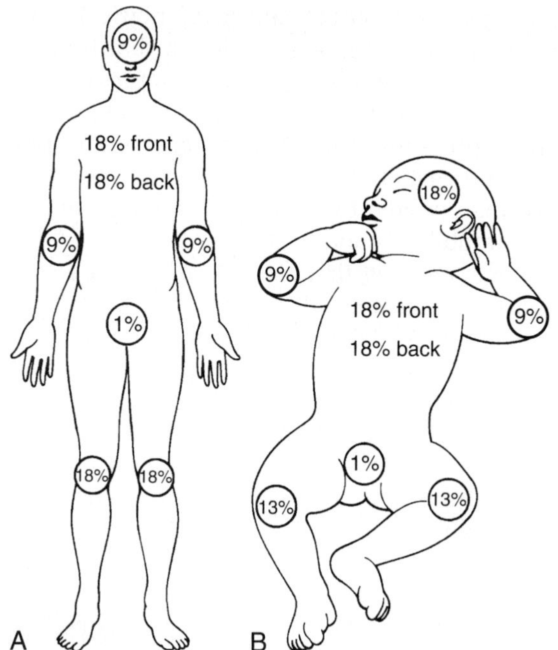

Fig. 16.17 Rule of nines. A, Adult. B, Child. (Modified from Sheehy SB, Lombardi J: *Manual of emergency care,* ed 4, St. Louis, 1995, Mosby.)

or occurs within 2 to 5 days and is uncomplicated. Signs and symptoms include erythema and pain.

Nursing Interventions

Cool the burn immediately by soaking the affected area in cold (not icy) water, or apply cold compresses to the area for as long as it takes to decrease pain (up to 30 minutes). Grease, butter, or salt water should not be applied to the burn. Place a sterile dressing over the burn site to help prevent infection.

DEEP PARTIAL-THICKNESS BURNS

Deep partial-thickness burns (also classified as second-degree burns) fully involve the first layer of skin (epidermis), as well as some of the underlying tissue (dermis); scarring from vesicles and infection is possible. Common causes of second-degree burns are severe sunburn, scalding liquids, direct flame, and chemical substances. Healing may take 5 to 21 days.

Assessment

Signs and symptoms include deep erythema or mottled skin with blister formation. Considerable edema often results, lasting several days. Fluid typically weeps through the skin surface (loss of plasma), and the patient complains of intense pain.

FULL-THICKNESS BURNS

Full-thickness burns (also classified as third-degree burns) involve destruction of the skin and underlying tissue, including fat, muscle, and bone. The area usually is charred, and healing is difficult. The skin is usually thick and leathery, with the presence of black or dark brown, cherry red, or dry and milky white colors. Many victims do not complain of pain because nerve endings are damaged so severely by the burn. Capillaries become hyperpermeable, so plasma seeps into the interstitial spaces, resulting in edema and vesiculation (blistering). The larger the burned area involved, the greater the shift of fluid from the intravascular area into the interstitial area. Fluid loss causes a fluid and electrolyte imbalance. Hypovolemic shock and infection are common complications. Medical attention is urgent. Common causes of full-thickness burns are direct flame (such as ignited clothing), explosions, and gasoline and oil fires.

Nursing Interventions for Moderate to Severe Burns (Deep Partial-Thickness and Full-Thickness Burns)

It is crucial to establish an airway before edema occurs. Assess respiratory and cardiac function. CAB are the priority concerns. Remove all of the victim's clothing, as well as shoes and jewelry, which may be constricting and even smoldering. It is possible to increase the severity of the burns by leaving clothing on the victim. The victim should be kept warm, with the burned area elevated. Inspect for burns or the presence of soot around the mouth and nose, which may indicate that the patient's respiratory status has been affected. Immediately flush chemical burns with copious amounts of water.

If medical help will arrive within 15 to 30 minutes, withhold oral fluids. If medical help is delayed, it may be advisable to give oral rehydration therapy with formulations suggested by the World Health Organization (WHO) or with sports drinks to replace electrolytes (Vyas and Wong, 2013). If vomiting occurs, do not provide the victim with fluids to drink. Attempt to cool a partial-thickness burn immediately, using cool compresses. It is not appropriate to do this for other types of burns. Cool compresses sometimes cause hypothermia in victims with more extensive burns. Vesicles (blisters) should not be broken intentionally; avoid touching the burn with anything except sterile dressings. It is not appropriate to apply antiseptics, ointments, sprays, or creams to the burn because they potentially may interfere with medical treatment and cause further complications. Apply loose, sterile dressings to the burned area. Monitor the victim frequently to be sure that edema has not caused further constriction of the area near the burn.

❖ NURSING PROCESS

The role of the licensed practical nurse/licensed vocational nurse (LPN/LVN) in the nursing process is that the LPN/LVN will:

- Participate in planning care for patients on the basis of patient needs
- Review patient's plan of care and recommend revisions as needed
- Review and follow defined prioritization for patient care
- Use clinical pathways, care maps, or care plans to guide and review patient care

◆ ASSESSMENT

Patients requiring first aid may be suffering from a variety of injuries, not just the immediately visible problem. It is necessary to perform a complete head-to-toe assessment on all patients to determine the extent of injury. Give primary consideration to CAB. Quick and accurate assessment of the situation is vital.

In all patients who have sustained head trauma, suspect spinal injuries. Automobile accidents and falls are injuries that often result in spinal injuries. Even though no visible injury is noted, severe damage is possible in the absence of proper immobilization.

Also assess the emotional status of patients needing first aid. Even minor accidents often cause emotional distress. This is true not only for the patient but also for the patient's family and friends.

◆ PATIENT PROBLEM

Identifying patient problems provides the basis for developing a plan of care for the patient. Patients receiving emergency care often have a variety of problems that are necessary to address. The nurse is then able to plan care of the patient. Possible patient problems for first aid may include the following:

- *Anxiousness*
- *Below Normal Body Temperature*
- *Compromised Blood Flow to Tissue (cerebral, cardiopulmonary, renal, gastrointestinal, peripheral)*
- *Compromised Skin Integrity*
- *Elevated Body Temperature*
- *Inability to Clear Airway*
- *Insufficient Cardiac Output*
- *Potential for Infection*
- *Problematic Spontaneous Breathing*
- *Recent Onset of Confusion*
- *Recent Onset of Pain or Prolonged Pain*

◆ EXPECTED OUTCOMES AND PLANNING

For patients who need first aid, focus the plan on life-threatening emergencies as a priority. Specific, measurable goals and outcomes are important for preventing further injury to the patient. Be prepared to provide care quickly and efficiently and be aware of complications as they become apparent.

The plan of care relates to the specific patient problem. Examples include the following:

Goal 1: The patient will develop no infection in the open wound during stay in facility.

Outcome: No signs or symptoms of infection are noted.

Goal 2: Patient remains free of complications such as dehydration after a burn injury.

Outcome: Patient's intake and output are balanced.

◆ IMPLEMENTATION

Depending on the patient's injuries, a variety of measures are possible to implement to meet the patient's needs (Nursing Care Plan 16.1). Priorities are always to ensure that the patient has adequate circulation, has an open airway, and is breathing. Ensuring cardiac functioning sometimes involves giving cardiac compression. Severe bleeding, such as arterial spurting, is possible to control by direct pressure, indirect pressure, or a tourniquet as a last resort. Stabilization of the spine in suspected spinal injuries is possible to accomplish through the use of neck immobilizers and backboards.

Patients needing first aid care also need emotional support. Family and friends are also likely to need the nurse's understanding and comforting. Keeping the patient and family informed of procedures and the arrival of emergency aid will help them keep their anxiety levels under control. See the Cultural Considerations and Home Care Considerations boxes for additional information regarding emergency nursing interventions.

Cultural Considerations

Effect of Culture During Emergencies

- At a time of emergency, patients often fall back on their language of origin. An interpreter is able help with language barriers.
- Emergency equipment is frightening to many people. Ensure that the patient understands the rationale for any nursing interventions that are being performed and the purpose of any equipment.
- People from some cultures believe in the use of a local medicine person and are distrustful of Western health care providers. Try to work within a patient's beliefs rather than contradicting them outright. In an emergency, patients will refer to what they know best.

Home Care Considerations

Emergencies in the Home

- If ice is not available in the home, look for a bag of frozen vegetables. Peas work especially well.
- Have patients keep a list of medications, allergies, and special needs with their list of emergency numbers. This often saves time and provides valuable information for emergency medical personnel.
- Advise all patients to equip their homes with an emergency first aid kit, kept in an easily accessible place. Properly supplied kits include adhesive bandages, antiseptic, gauze dressings, tape, tweezers, scissors, and antibiotic ointment. It is also a good idea to include directions for what to do in an emergency.
- Prevention is the key to eliminating emergencies in the home. Advise patients to "accident-proof" their homes. Advise patients to keep cleaning products and poisons, as well as medications, out of the reach of children. Handrails, nonskid surfaces, and adequate lighting help prevent falls. Advise older adults to avoid decorating with throw rugs and other objects that can cause them to trip. Keep electrical cords in good repair with no fraying.

Nursing Care Plan 16.1 The Patient With a Laceration

Ms. T., 75 years of age, is living in a long-term care facility. She accidentally cut herself with a knife during dinner. On examination, the nurse finds a 2-cm laceration in the patient's left hand that is actively bleeding.

PATIENT PROBLEM

Compromised Skin Integrity, related to trauma

Patient Goals and Expected Outcomes	Nursing Interventions	Evaluation
Bleeding wound will be controlled within 15 min Patient's wound will heal without complication within 7–10 days	Assess extent of wound, amount and type of bleeding, presence of dirt or contaminating substances. Cleanse wound, using normal saline. Apply direct pressure to control bleeding. Dress wound with sterile dressings.	Superficial 2-cm laceration to the palm of the left hand; moderate amount of bleeding noted. No visible dirt or food particles in wound. Wound irrigated with normal saline; bleeding controlled after 5 min of direct pressure. Wound dressed with a sterile 4- × 4-inch gauze secured with tape.

PATIENT PROBLEM

Potential for Infection, related to laceration

Patient Goals and Expected Outcomes	Nursing Interventions	Evaluation
Wound will heal within 7–10 days without signs of infection	Cleanse wound every shift with normal saline and apply treatment as specified by health care provider. Keep covered with sterile dressings until wound heals. Monitor the wound and resident daily for signs and symptoms of infection.	Wound edges well approximated; no bleeding, redness, swelling, or drainage from site.

CRITICAL THINKING QUESTIONS

1. Ms. T.'s wound was superficial. In contrast, what would be the nurse's actions if the wound appeared to be deep or was spurting blood?
2. What safety measures are indicated to ensure Ms. T. is not injured again?

◆ EVALUATION

Evaluation is an ongoing process. Injuries are not always visible on initial assessment. It is essential to constantly reevaluate the situation until the patient's condition is stable. The nurse will update the plan of care, depending on the evaluation. Refer to the goals and outcomes when planning care and perform procedures designed to meet those goals. Examples of goals and evaluative measures are as follows:

Goal 1: Patient will not have excessive bleeding from open wound.
Evaluative measure: No visible bleeding is noted after application of direct pressure.
Goal 2: Patient has no apparent spinal cord injury.
Evaluative measure: Patient is neurologically intact after immobilization of spine.

Get Ready for the NCLEX® Examination!

Key Points

- The goal of first aid is to preserve life until medical help arrives, not to replace medical care.
- Circulatory problems, airway problems, breathing problems, profuse bleeding, and poisonings are life-threatening situations that necessitate priority emergency care.
- Suspect shock in all situations involving traumatic injuries, diseases, and physical and emotional stress.
- Reactions to a poisonous bite often take a few minutes to several hours to appear. Take first aid measures immediately.
- Always splint a fractured part in the position it is in, and never attempt to realign it.
- Take spinal cord precautions in all cases of head trauma and multiple traumas. Even a slight movement of the individual's head creates the potential for causing spinal damage.
- The dangers from burn injuries are shock, loss of fluids, and infection.

- In heat emergencies, it is important to cool the victim as soon as possible.
- Personnel trained in CPR and a rapid-response EMS system are often able to resuscitate victims of cardiac arrest or apparent sudden death.
- All health care providers need to maintain current CPR certification.
- It is necessary for rescuers to perform CPR according to the standards designated by the American Heart Association or the American Red Cross.
- There is a moral obligation to continue CPR once it has been initiated unless the rescuer is exhausted and is not able to continue, trained medical personnel take over CPR, or a licensed health care provider pronounces the victim dead.
- Circulation, airway, and breathing (CAB) are the three steps to remember in one-rescuer and two-rescuer CPR.
- If external cardiac compressions are performed accurately, it is possible to supply enough oxygen to the heart, the lungs, the brain, and the rest of the body to sustain life.
- Two fingers are used during chest compressions in an infant.
- If a victim is choking but has good air exchange (is coughing forcibly), do not interfere.
- Performing abdominal thrusts is the most effective method of removing a foreign body obstructing the airway.
- Do not use the finger-sweep technique when managing airway obstruction by a foreign body in the infant.

Additional Learning Resources

SG Go to your Study Guide for additional learning activities to help you master this chapter content.

evolve Be sure to visit the Evolve site at *http://evolve.elsevier.com/Cooper/foundationsadult/* for additional online resources.

Review Questions for the NCLEX® Examination

1. A patient is developing shock. Which action should the nurse take?
   1. Elevate the victim's head.
   2. Elevate the victim's legs and feet.
   3. Elevate the victim's upper body.
   4. Leave the victim in a flat position.
2. The nurse finds a client in a burning car. The client is breathing with fractured arm and lacerations that are bleeding profusely. What action should the nurse take first?
   1. Splint the fractured arm.
   2. Get the client out of the car.
   3. Give mouth-to-mouth resuscitation.
   4. Stop the bleeding.
3. A neighbor tells the nurse that her 12-year-old child has been burned with scalding water. The arm is red and starting to blister. In addition to advising her to see a health care provider, what will the nurse tell the neighbor to apply to the burn?
   1. Hydrogen peroxide
   2. Petroleum jelly
   3. Cool compresses
   4. Salt water compresses
4. The nurse comes across a one-car automobile accident. The driver of the car is walking around with a dazed look on his face. He states that he was wearing his seatbelt but is unsure of what happened exactly. He has no visible injury. In checking his vital signs, the nurse finds his blood pressure is 84/56 mm Hg, his pulse is 110 beats per minute, and his respirations are 32 per minute. Another bystander says that an ambulance is on the way. What is the nurse's initial action?
   1. Complete a neurologic assessment.
   2. Instruct him to get back in the car and rest.
   3. Position him on his back on the ground with legs and feet elevated.
   4. Assess for any wounds that may be contributing to his memory loss.
5. The nurse is told in report that one of the patients has been very depressed lately. On checking the unit, the nurse finds the patient in the bathroom with one wrist bleeding profusely. The patient states that he broke a glass and used it to cut his wrist in a suicide attempt. What should the nurse do after sending someone to call for help?
   1. Attempt to find out what has been causing her depression.
   2. Apply a tourniquet above the injury.
   3. Use 4- × 4-inch gauze pads to apply direct pressure.
   4. Thoroughly wash the wound.
6. A neighbor tells the nurse that her 5-year-old son has ingested one of her liquid cleaning supplies. The child is in no distress at this time. The mother shows the nurse the bottle; the nurse is unfamiliar with the ingredients. Which action by the nurse is appropriate?
   1. Give syrup of ipecac to induce vomiting.
   2. Give milk to neutralize any acids.
   3. Give water to dilute the poison.
   4. Call the poison control center.
7. The nurse comes upon a victim who is unconscious. Place in order the interventions that the nurse should take.
   1. Administer 30 chest compressions.
   2. Give 2 mouth-to-mouth breaths.
   3. Check the carotid pulse.
   4. Activate the EMS.
   5. Open the airway.

8. The nurse is in the park and witnesses a child getting stung by a wasp. What action should the nurse implement first?
 1. Cleanse the site with soap and water.
 2. Remove the stinger with a scraping motion.
 3. Apply ice to the stung area.
 4. Determine whether the child has an allergy to wasps.

9. The nurse is assessing an adult patient who has been brought to the hospital with third-degree burns covering his head, right arm, and right leg. The nurse demonstrates accurate assessment skills by determining what to be the extent of the patient's burns?
 1. 27%
 2. 36%
 3. 45%
 4. 54%

10. A man suffers heat exhaustion while mowing the grass. The man's wife demonstrates knowledge of proper care of her husband with which action? *(Select all that apply.)*
 1. The wife calls 911 immediately.
 2. The wife encourages her husband to sit in a tub of cold water.
 3. The wife gives her husband cold water and a sports drink.
 4. The wife carefully monitors her husband while he finishes mowing.
 5. The wife loosens her husband's clothing.

11. The nurse is educating a group of hikers about how to treat frostbite. Which statement by one of the hikers indicates the need for further teaching?
 1. "I should place the frozen body part in hot water, around 110° to 114°F (43.3° to 45.6°C)."
 2. "I can wrap a frozen body part in a warm moist towel."
 3. "I should avoid vigorously rubbing the frozen body part."
 4. "After the frozen part is warmed, I should wrap it in clean material and elevate it."

12. A patient comes to a sports medicine clinic after twisting his ankle while playing soccer. The health care provider determines he has a sprain. What discharge instructions will the nurse include in discharge summary for the patient? *(Select all that apply.)*
 1. "Apply ice to the sprained area for 1 hour, then off for 1 hour."
 2. "Wrap your ankle with an ACE bandage each morning."
 3. "Elevate your leg as much as possible to prevent further swelling."
 4. "Exercise your ankle as soon as you get home to prevent stiffness."
 5. "You will use warm compresses to increase blood flow to the area after removing the ice."

13. The patient suffered a fracture of the tibia after crashing his motorcycle. He tells the nurse that his health care provider told him he shattered his tibia in three places and will need surgery. The nurse is aware that the patient has which type of fracture?
 1. Greenstick fracture
 2. Spiral fracture
 3. Comminuted fracture
 4. Compound fracture

14. Several high school teachers completed a CPR class. Which comment by one of the teachers demonstrates knowledge of proper CPR? *(Select all that apply.)*
 1. "The chest compression rate should be at least 100 per minute."
 2. "A jaw-thrust maneuver should be used on all patients when I open the airway."
 3. "The proper sequence for CPR is circulation, airway, and breathing."
 4. "I should look, listen, and feel for breathing for no more than 10 seconds."
 5. "The adult chest should be compressed at least 2 inches during compressions."

15. When the nurse is caring for a person who has developed a nosebleed, which nursing action is appropriate?
 1. Apply steady pressure to the bridge of the nose for 5 minutes.
 2. Remind the victim to try to breathe through the nose.
 3. Avoid using ice over the nose.
 4. Keep the victim's head tilted slightly forward.

17 Dosage Calculation and Medication Administration

http://evolve.elsevier.com/Cooper/foundationsadult/

Objectives

1. Demonstrate use of the most common equivalents of metric and apothecary measurement systems.
2. Correctly convert units of measurement within and between the metric, apothecary, and household measurement systems.
3. Apply mathematics skills to solve dosage calculation problems accurately.
4. Demonstrate the methods of calculating pediatric dosages.
5. Describe each phase of drug action.
6. Explain how decreased hepatic and renal functioning affect medication absorption and excretion.
7. Discuss the principles of drug action and interactions.
8. Discuss factors that affect a patient's response to medications.
9. Identify the nurse's responsibilities regarding medication administration.
10. List the six "rights" of medication administration.
11. Describe factors to consider in choosing routes of medication administration.
12. Discuss the use of the Joint Commission's abbreviations to prevent medication errors.
13. Explain the importance of accurately transcribing medication orders.
14. Define *controlled substance.*
15. Discuss the three preferred sites for intramuscular injections in adults.
16. Describe the correct techniques for locating intramuscular injection sites.
17. Describe the procedures for irrigating the eye, the ear, and the nose.
18. Describe the correct techniques for administration of vaginal and rectal medications.

Key Terms

adverse drug reaction (ĂD-vŭrs DRŬG rē-ĂK-shŭn, p. 434)
agonist (ĂG-ŏ-nĭst, p. 433)
anaphylactic shock (ăn-ă-fĭ-LĂK-tĭk, p. 478)
antagonist (ăn-TĂG-ŏ-nĭst, p. 433)
body surface area (BŎD-ē SŬR-fĭs ĂR-ē-ŭ, p. 431)
buccal (BŬK-ŭl, p. 449)
compatibility (kŭm-păt-ŭ-BĬL-ĭ-tē, p. 433)
cumulative (kyūm-yū-lŭ-tĭv, p. 432)
denominator (dē-NŎM-ĭn-ā-tŭr, p. 424)
dimensional analysis (dĭ-MĔN-shŭn-ŭl ŭ-NĂL-ĭ-sĭs, p. 430)
drip factor (DRĬP FĂK-tŭr, p. 477)
drug interaction (DRŬG ĭn-tŭr-ĂK-shŭn, p. 433)
enteral (ĔN-tŭr-ŭl, p. 442)
enteric-coated (ĕn-TĔR-ĭk KŌT-ĭd, p. 442)
extremes (ĕk-STRĒMZ, p. 429)
gauge (GĀJ, p. 467)
graduated (GRĂD-yū-ā-tĭd, p. 445)
idiosyncratic (ĭd-ē-ō-sĭn-KRĂT-ĭk, p. 433)
intermittent venous access device (ĭn-tŭr-MĬT-ĕnt VĒ-nŭs ĂK-sĕs dĭ-VĪS, p. 473)
irrigations (ĭr-rĭ-GĀ-shŭnz, p. 449)
lumen (LŪ-mĕn, p. 467)
means (MĒNZ, p. 429)
meniscus (mĕ-NĬS-kŭs, p. 445)
metabolite (mĕ-TĂB-ŏ-līt, p. 432)
milliequivalent (mĭll-ē-ĕ-KWĬV-ă-lĕnt, p. 423)
numerator (NŪ-mŭr-ā-tŭr, p. 424)
parenteral (păr-ĔN-tŭr-ŭl, p. 462)
patient-controlled analgesia (PCA) (PĀ-shŭnt kŭn-TRŌLD ăn-ŭl-JĒ-zē-ŭ, p. 474)
percent (pŭr-SĔNT, p. 429)
percutaneous (pŭr-kyū-TĀ-nē-ŭs, p. 449)
pharmacology (făr-mŭ-KŎL-ŭ-jē, p. 432)
potentiation (pō-tĕn-shē-Ā-shŭn, p. 433)
proportion (prŭ-PŌR-shŭn, p. 429)
pulverized (PŬL-vŭr-īzd, p. 444)
ratio (RĀ-shē-ō, p. 429)
souffle cup (sū-FLĀ CŬP, p. 447)
sublingual (sŭb-LĬNG-gwūl, p. 449)
therapeutic (thĕr-ŭ-PYŪ-tĭk, p. 433)
tolerance (TŎL-ŭr-ĭns, p. 434)
topical applications (TŎP-ĭ-kŭl ăp-lĭ-KĀ-shŭnz, p. 449)
toxicity (tŏk-SĬS-ĭ-tē, p. 433)

One of the nurse's roles is to calculate drug dosages accurately to administer medications safely to each patient. This chapter provides the student nurse with three measurement systems, several types of dosage calculations that the nurse should be able to perform, and methods used to determine the appropriateness of drug orders for patients.

MATHEMATICS AND DOSAGE CALCULATION REVIEW

METRIC SYSTEM

The metric system is the preferred system of weights and measures. It is more accurate than the imperial system in calculating dosage problems.

Like the US monetary system, which is based on the dollar, the metric system also is based on the decimal system. In the decimal system, the divisions and multiples of a unit are always in ratios of tens. For example:

1 dollar	= 10 dimes
10 dimes	= 20 nickels
20 nickels	= 100 pennies

All these units are multiples or divisions of ten.

In the metric system, the following basic units are used for volume, weight, and length:

liter (L)	volume (amount) of fluids
gram (g)	weight of solids
meter (m)	measure of length

Fractions of these units are designated by the following prefixes:

deci-	0.1 (one tenth) of the unit
centi-	0.01 (one hundredth) of the unit
milli-	0.001 (one thousandth) of the unit

Multiples of these units are designated with the following prefixes:

deca-	10 times the unit
hecto-	100 times the unit
kilo-	1000 times the unit

Units of Volume

1 liter (L)	= 1000 milliliters (mL)
0.001 liter (L)	= 1 milliliter (mL)
1 milliliter (mL)	= 1 cubic centimeter (cc)

Units of Weight

1 gram (g)	= 1000 milligrams (mg)
0.001 gram (g)	= 1 milligram (mg)
1 kilogram (kg)	= 1000 grams (g)
0.001 kilogram (kg)	= 1 gram (g)

In addition to the preceding units of measurement, nurses often encounter the term *milliequivalent,* abbreviated mEq. **Milliequivalent** refers to the concentration of electrolytes in a certain volume of solution, expressed as milliequivalents per liter (mEq/L). Potassium chloride (KCl) is an electrolyte that sometimes is ordered as an intravenous (IV) additive to a liter (1000 mL) of fluid.

EXAMPLE: The health care provider orders the following:

Add 40 mEq KCl to 1 L NS [normal saline] to infuse at 125 mL/h.

APPROXIMATE EQUIVALENTS OF THE METRIC SYSTEM

The basic unit of length in the metric system is the meter. The meter is equal to 39.37 inches, about 3½ inches longer than 1 yard (36 inches). A unit of measurement that nurses frequently use is the centimeter (cm). One inch is equivalent to 2.5 centimeters (cm). Some measurements that nurses obtain using the metric system are the following:

- Abdominal girth (obstetrics and patients with ascites and heart failure)
- Area size for topical applications
- Height, length, and head circumference (common tasks in obstetrics and pediatrics)
- Pressure ulcers
- Results of intradermal skin tests (size of drug or allergen reaction on the skin)
- Wound size

0.001 meter	= 1 millimeter (mm)
0.01 meter	= 1 centimeter (cm)
0.1 meter	= 1 decimeter (dm)
10 meters	= 1 decameter (dam)
100 meters	= 1 hectometer (hm)
1000 meters	= 1 kilometer (km)

The most frequently used equivalents are the following:

1 meter (m)	= 1000 millimeters (mm)
0.001 meter (m)	= 1 millimeter (mm)
1 meter (m)	= 100 centimeters (cm)
1 centimeter (cm)	= 10 millimeters (mm)
1 millimeter (mm)	= 0.1 centimeter (cm)

APOTHECARY SYSTEM

The apothecary system is a system of measurement still used by some health care providers and hospitals. It is being replaced by the metric system. Because its use does continue today, nurses occasionally need to use the following equivalents to convert dosages from one system to another. The conversions are only approximations, but they are acceptable equivalents with which to work. Nurses need to convert from one system to another to calculate dosage problems in the same measurement units.

VOLUME

METRIC	APOTHECARY
30 milliliters (mL)	= 1 fluid ounce (fl oz)
500 milliliters (mL)	= 1 pint (pt)
1000 milliliters (1 L)	= 1 quart (qt)

Weight

METRIC	APOTHECARY
60 milligrams (mg)	= 1 grain (gr)
1000 milligrams (mg)	= 15 grains (gr XV)
30 grams (g)	≈ 1 ounce (oz)
0.45 kilogram (kg)	≈ 1 pound (lb)
1 kilogram (kg)	≈ 2.2 pounds (lb)

HOUSEHOLD UNITS OF MEASURE

In the clinical setting, the use of metric dosages is most common. Most medication, however, is administered in home settings. In the home, patients may be confused by metric and apothecary units of measure. It is important for the nurse to review dosages and understand the correlation between household units of measure and metric units. Common conversions include the following:

1 teaspoon (tsp)	= 5 mL
1 tablespoon (tbsp)	= 15 mL
1 ounce	= 30 mL
1 cup	= 240 mL

BIG-TO-SMALL RULE

Whatever method is used to solve dosage problems, always convert the units of measurement in the problem to the same unit of measurement.

Some students find it difficult to convert dosages that contain decimal fractions. This section discusses a quick, easy method called the *big-to-small rule.* It is useful in converting dosages *within the same system* (the metric system).

Because there are 1000 mL in 1 L (and 1000 mg in 1 g), this method works for converting milliliters to liters (and milligrams to grams). Likewise, liters can be converted to milliliters (and grams to milligrams) by this method.

CONVERTING LARGER UNITS OF MEASUREMENT TO SMALLER UNITS OF MEASUREMENT (GRAMS TO MILLIGRAMS; LITERS TO MILLILITERS)

RULE 1: Write down "BIG → SMALL."

RULE 2: Place the large unit under the word "BIG" and the small unit under the word "SMALL."

EXAMPLE: BIG → SMALL
1.7 g = _______ mg

RULE 3: Move the decimal point three places in the direction of the arrow; add zeros.

EXAMPLE: BIG → SMALL
1.700 g = 1700. mg

CONVERTING SMALLER UNITS OF MEASUREMENT TO LARGER UNITS OF MEASUREMENT (MILLIGRAMS TO GRAMS; MILLILITERS TO LITERS)

RULE 1: Write down the big-to-small rule formula.

EXAMPLE: BIG → SMALL

RULE 2: Reverse the direction of the arrow.

EXAMPLE: BIG ← SMALL

RULE 3: Place the large unit under the word "BIG" and the small unit under the word "SMALL."

EXAMPLE: BIG ← SMALL
xg = 1700 mg

RULE 4: Move the decimal point three places in the direction that the arrow points.

EXAMPLE: BIG ← SMALL
1.7 g = 1700. mg

ROUNDING A NUMBER

RULE 1: Round up a number that follows the decimal point if it is 5 or larger, to increase the number before it by one whole number.

EXAMPLE 1: 7.55 is rounded up to 7.6 (rounded to the tenths place) or 8 (rounded to a whole number).

EXAMPLE 2: 7.42 is rounded down to 7.4 (rounded to the tenths place) or 7 (rounded to a whole number).

HINT: There are times when it is practical to round a volume of medication.

PROBLEM: How is it possible to give 1.85 tablets?

ANSWER: Round 1.85 to 2; give 2 tablets.

MATHEMATICS REVIEW AND PRINCIPLES

FRACTIONS

Fractions may be a challenging mathematical dilemma for some students. It helps to understand what fractions are. A fraction is a "part" of a whole number. Fractions consist of two parts: the numerator and the denominator.

Numerator: The "top" number of a fraction

Denominator: The "bottom" number of a fraction

TYPES OF FRACTIONS

Proper fractions: The numerator is less than the denominator.

EXAMPLE: $\frac{1}{2}$ 1 Numerator, 2 Denominator

Improper fractions: The numerator is larger than the denominator.

EXAMPLE: $\frac{2}{1}$ 2 Numerator, 1 Denominator

Mixed fractions: These consist of a whole number plus a fraction.

EXAMPLE: $1\frac{1}{2}$; 1 is the whole number, $\frac{1}{2}$ is the fraction.

CHANGING AN IMPROPER FRACTION TO A WHOLE OR MIXED NUMBER

RULE 1: Divide the denominator (bottom number) into the numerator (top number).

EXAMPLE 1: Change $\frac{10}{5}$ to a *whole* number.

$10 \div 5 = 2$ (a WHOLE number)

EXAMPLE 2: Change $\frac{40}{5}$ to a *whole* number.

$40 \div 5 = 8$ (a WHOLE number)

EXAMPLE 3: Change $\frac{20}{7}$ (an improper fraction) to a *mixed* number.

$$20 \div 7 = 7\overline{)20} = 2\frac{6}{7}\text{(a MIXED number)} \quad \begin{array}{r} 2 \\ 7\overline{)20} \\ \underline{14} \\ \underline{6} \\ 7 \end{array}$$

EXAMPLE 4: Change $\frac{54}{5}$ to a *mixed* number.

$$54 \div 5 = 5\overline{)54} \quad \begin{array}{r} 10 \\ 5\overline{)54} \\ \underline{50} \\ \frac{4}{5} \end{array} = 10\frac{4}{5}\text{(a MIXED number)}$$

CHANGING A MIXED NUMBER TO AN IMPROPER FRACTION

RULE 1: Multiply the denominator (bottom number) by the whole number.

RULE 2: Add the numerator to the product; this sum is now the new numerator.

EXAMPLE 1: Change $2\frac{6}{7}$ (a mixed number) to an improper fraction.

Multiply the denominator 7 by the whole number 2.

$7 \times 2 = 14$ (The answer from numbers multiplied is called the *product*.)

EXAMPLE 2: Add the original numerator to the product.

$6 + 14 = 20$ (The answer from numbers added is called the *sum*.)

EXAMPLE 3: Place the sum, 20, over the original denominator, 7, to obtain an improper fraction: $\frac{20}{7}$.

The mixed number is now the improper fraction.

REDUCING FRACTIONS TO THE LOWEST TERM

Fractions commonly are reduced to the lowest term in which they can be expressed, because it is easier to work with smaller numbers.

RULE 1: Find a number that will evenly divide into the numerator *and* the denominator.

EXAMPLE: $\frac{2}{10}$

What number will divide into the numerator, which is 2?

2 will divide evenly into the numerator 2 one time.

2 will divide into the denominator (which is 10) five times.

$\frac{2}{10} = \frac{1}{5}$ (reduce all fractions to their lowest terms)

DETERMINING WHICH FRACTION IS LARGER

RULE 1: If the denominators are the *same*, the fraction with the *larger numerator* is the larger fraction.

PROBLEM: Which is larger, $\frac{4}{6}$ or $\frac{2}{6}$?

ANSWER: $\frac{4}{6}$ is larger

RULE 2: If the denominators are *different*, as in $\frac{2}{5}$ and $\frac{1}{3}$, first find a "common denominator." (Finding a common denominator means to find a number into which both denominators can be divided.) Common, or equivalent, numerators will also be found.

PROBLEM: Which is larger, $\frac{2}{5}$ or $\frac{1}{3}$?

$$\frac{2}{5} = \frac{?}{15} \quad \frac{1}{3} = \frac{?}{15}$$

RULE 3: Find a common denominator. HINT: Try multiplying the denominators to get a common denominator.

$$\frac{2}{5} = \frac{?}{15} \quad \frac{1}{3} = \frac{?}{15}$$

Multiply the numerator and denominator by 3

$$\frac{2}{5} = \frac{6}{15} \quad \frac{1}{3} = \frac{5}{15}$$

-OR-

Find an equivalent numerator by dividing the first denominator into the equivalent denominator; multiply the answer by the first numerator.

$$\frac{2}{5} = \frac{6}{15}(15 \div 5 = 3; 3 \times 2 = 6)$$

$$\frac{1}{3} = \frac{5}{15}(15 \div 3 = 5; 5 \times 1 = 5)$$

RULE 4: Compare the two fractions; the one with the larger numerator is the larger fraction.

PROBLEM: Which is larger, $\frac{6}{15}$ or $\frac{5}{15}$?

ANSWER: $\frac{6}{15}$ is larger.

PROBLEM: Which is larger, $\frac{2}{3}$ or $\frac{6}{8}$?

$$\frac{2}{3}=\frac{16}{24}\quad\frac{6}{8}=\frac{18}{24}$$

ANSWER: $\frac{6}{8}$ is larger.

ADDING FRACTIONS WITH THE SAME DENOMINATOR

RULE 1: Add the numerators; place this sum of the numerators over the denominator, and reduce the new fraction if possible.

EXAMPLE: $\frac{1}{6} + \frac{1}{6} = \frac{2}{6}=\frac{1}{3}$

ADDING FRACTIONS WITH DIFFERENT DENOMINATORS

RULE 1: Find common denominators for all fractions in the problem.

EXAMPLE: $\frac{2}{4}=\frac{6}{12}$ (3 and 4 will divide into 12; 12 is the common denominator.)

ANSWER: $\frac{2}{4}=\frac{6}{12}$

RULE 2: Add the numerators.

EXAMPLE 1: $\frac{10}{12}=\frac{5}{6}$

EXAMPLE 2: $\frac{4}{18}+\frac{10}{18}=\frac{14}{18}=\frac{7}{9}$

ADDING MIXED NUMBERS

RULE 1: Add the fractions of the mixed number. Then add the sum of the fractions to the whole numbers.

EXAMPLE 1: $1\frac{2}{3} + 2\frac{1}{3} = 3\frac{3}{3}=4$

EXAMPLE 2: $1\frac{3}{5}=1\frac{6}{10}$

$+4\frac{5}{10}=4\frac{5}{10}$

$5\frac{11}{10}=5+1\text{ whole}+\frac{1}{10},$

which $=6\frac{1}{10}$

SUBTRACTING FRACTIONS WITH THE SAME DENOMINATOR

RULE 1: Subtract the numerators, and place the answer over the denominator in the answer.

EXAMPLE 1: $\frac{3}{5} - \frac{1}{5} = \frac{2}{5}$ EXAMPLE 2: $\frac{4}{7} - \frac{2}{7} = \frac{2}{7}$

SUBTRACTING FRACTIONS WITH DIFFERENT DENOMINATORS

RULE 1: First find a common denominator, and then subtract.

EXAMPLE 1: $\frac{3}{4}=\frac{9}{12}$, $-\frac{1}{3}=\frac{4}{12}$, $\frac{5}{12}$

EXAMPLE 2: $\frac{2}{3}=\frac{4}{6}$, $-\frac{1}{2}=\frac{3}{6}$, $\frac{1}{6}$

SUBTRACTING MIXED NUMBERS

RULE 1: When the numerator of the top fraction is smaller than that of the bottom fraction, borrow one whole number from the whole number of the mixed fraction, and express it as a fraction.

PROBLEM: $3\frac{9}{15} - 2\frac{10}{15}$ ANSWER: $3=2\frac{15}{15}$

RULE 2: Add the fraction of the original mixed number to the new fraction.

EXAMPLE: $3\frac{9}{15}=2\frac{15}{15}+\frac{9}{15}=2\frac{24}{15}$ ANSWER: 14/15

RULE 3: Subtract fractions and whole numbers, if any.

EXAMPLE: $5\frac{6}{10}=4\frac{10}{10}+\frac{6}{10}=4\frac{16}{10}$

MULTIPLYING FRACTIONS

RULE 1: Multiply the numerators by each other; multiply the denominators by each other.

EXAMPLE 1: $\frac{1}{2}\times\frac{3}{4}=\frac{1\times3}{2\times4}=\frac{3}{8}$

EXAMPLE 2: $\frac{4}{8}\times\frac{1}{3}=\frac{4\times1}{8\times3}=\frac{4}{24}=\frac{1}{6}$

MULTIPLYING FRACTIONS AND MIXED NUMBERS

RULE 1: Change the mixed number to an improper fraction. (See the section on changing mixed numbers to improper fractions.)

PROBLEM: Multiply $3\frac{1}{2}$ by $1\frac{2}{3}$.

EXAMPLES 1 AND 2: Change $3\frac{1}{2}$ and $1\frac{2}{3}$ to improper fractions.

$$3\frac{1}{2}=\frac{7}{2}=1\frac{2}{3}=\frac{5}{3}$$

MULTIPLY

ANSWER: $\frac{7}{2}\times\frac{5}{3}=\frac{35}{6}=5.8333$

PROBLEM: Multiply $1\frac{2}{3}$ by $2\frac{3}{4}$.

ANSWER: $\frac{5}{3}\times\frac{11}{4}=\frac{55}{12}=4\frac{7}{12}$

DIVIDING FRACTIONS

RULE 1: Write the problem down *correctly*.
RULE 2: Invert the second fraction, and multiply the two fractions; then reduce the answer to lowest terms.

PROBLEM: Divide $\frac{1}{2}$ by $\frac{3}{4}$

EXAMPLE: 1. Write the problem down *correctly*.

$$\frac{1}{2}\div\frac{3}{4}$$

2. Invert the second fraction; change the division sign to a multiplication sign; multiply the two fractions.

$$\frac{1}{2}\times\frac{4}{3}=\frac{4}{6}$$

3. Reduce the answer to the lowest terms.

$$\frac{4}{6}=\frac{2}{3}$$

DIVIDING FRACTIONS AND WHOLE NUMBERS

RULE 1: Change the whole number to a fraction.
RULE 2: Divide, and then reduce to lowest terms.

PROBLEM: Divide 4 by $\frac{3}{5}$

EXAMPLE: 1. Change 4 to a fraction. Make 4 the numerator, and use 1 as the denominator.

$$\frac{4}{1}$$

2. Invert second fraction; multiply.

$$\frac{4\times5}{1\times3}=\frac{20}{3}$$

3. Reduce the answer to lowest terms.

DECIMAL FRACTIONS

The decimal fraction is a type of fraction whose denominator is always some multiple (or division) of 10. The placement or position of the decimal point determines whether the denominator is 10, a multiple of 10, or a division of 10.

NAMES OF DECIMAL PLACES

0.00001	Hundred thousandths
0.0001	Ten thousandths
0.001	Thousandths
0.01	Hundredths
0.1	Tenths
1.	Unit (whole numbers)
10	Tens
100	Hundreds
1000	Thousands
10,000	Ten thousands
100,000	Hundred thousands

RULE 1: A decimal point found to the left of a number means that the number is a *fraction* of a whole number.

EXAMPLE: 0.1—also called "point one"—is $\frac{1}{10}$ of the whole number 1.

HINT: Place a zero to the left of the decimal point to prevent mistaking ".1" for "1."

Correct placement of decimal points in drug dosages is *critical* (see The Joint Committee's [TJC's] Official "Do No Use" list, 2018).

TJC's Official "Do Not Use" List

DO NOT USE	POTENTIAL PROBLEM	USE INSTEAD
U, u (unit)	Mistaken for "0" (zero), the number "4" (four) or "cc"	Write "unit"
IU (International Unit)	Mistaken for IV (intravenous) or the number 10 (ten)	Write "International Unit"
Q.D., QD, q.d., qd (daily)	Mistaken for each other	Write "daily"
Q.O.D., QOD, q.o.d, qod (every other day)	Period after the Q mistaken for "I" and the "O" mistaken for "I"	Write "every other day"
Trailing zero (X.0 mg)*	Decimal point is missed	Write X mg
Lack of leading zero (.X mg)		Write 0.X mg
MS	Can mean morphine sulfate or magnesium sulfate	Write "morphine sulfate"
MSO_4 and $MgSO_4$	Confused for one another	Write "magnesium sulfate"

*From The Joint Commission: Official "do not use" list, 2017. Retrieved from *https://www.jointcommission.org/facts_about_do_not_use_list/*

RULE 2: A decimal point found *after* (to the right of) a number means that it is a whole number.

EXAMPLE: 5. = 5

RULE 3: A number *without* a decimal point is understood to have an "invisible" decimal point after it.

EXAMPLE: 2 = 2.

HINT: Do not place a zero to the right of the decimal point to prevent mistaking "2.0" for "20"
Correct placement of decimal points in drug dosages is *critical.* Decimals points should not be placed after a whole number.

ADDING DECIMALS

RULE 1: Align the decimal point of each decimal fraction in a column.
RULE 2: Add.
PROBLEM: Add 3.34 and 0.6.

EXAMPLE:

$$\begin{array}{r} 3.34 \\ +\ 0.6 \\ \hline 3.94 \end{array}$$

Align decimal point in column; add

↑ Make sure that the decimal point is aligned properly in the answer.

SUBTRACTING DECIMALS

RULE 1: Align the decimal points of each decimal fraction in a column.
RULE 2: Subtract.
PROBLEM: Subtract 7.45 from 15.

EXAMPLE:

$$\begin{array}{r} 15.00 \\ -\ 7.45 \\ \hline 7.55 \end{array}$$

Align decimal point in column; subtract

↑ Make sure that the decimal point is aligned properly in the answer.

MULTIPLYING DECIMALS

RULE 1: Multiply. You do not have to align decimal points in the problem.
RULE 2: To determine the location of the decimal point in the answer, note how many numbers are found to the right of the decimal points in all the numbers multiplied.

EXAMPLE:

$$\begin{array}{r} 5.50 \\ \times\ 2.15 \\ \hline 27\,50 \\ 55\,0 \\ 11\,00 \\ \hline 11.8250\,x \end{array}$$

(There are two numbers found after the decimal points on the top and two on the bottom.)

$x = 11.8250$ or 12 (rounded)

NOTE: A small "x" hereafter indicates the unexpressed decimal after a whole number or a decimal point that has been moved from one place to another.

DIVIDING DECIMALS

RULE 1: Change a decimal fraction in the divisor to a whole number by moving the decimal point *all* the way to the right.

PROBLEM: Divide 2.5 by 1.5.

EXAMPLE: 1. (divisor) $1.5\overline{)2.5}$ (dividend)

2. $1.5x\overline{)2.5}$ $15\overline{)2.5}$

RULE 2: Move the decimal point in the dividend the *same number of places moved in the divisor.*

EXAMPLE: $1.5x\overline{)2.5x}$ The decimal point in the divisor is unexpressed after it is moved.

RULE 3: Place the decimal point in the answer directly over the decimal point in the dividend after moving the decimal point in the dividend.

EXAMPLE: $15\overline{)25}$

RULE 4: If a decimal point is in the divisor but not in the dividend (as in $0.5\overline{)15}$), move it the same number of places as the divisor. Remember that there is an unexpressed decimal point at the right of all whole numbers.

EXAMPLE: $0.5x\overline{)15.x}$ $5\overline{)150}$

RULE 5: If the dividend contains a decimal fraction and the divisor does not, leave the divisor as it is.

EXAMPLE: $5\overline{)2.5}$ would remain unchanged.

CHANGING FRACTIONS TO DECIMALS

RULE 1: Divide the numerator (the top number) by the denominator (the bottom number).

PROBLEM: Change $\frac{3}{4}$ to a decimal fraction.

EXAMPLE: $\frac{3}{4} = 4\overset{0.75}{\overline{)3.00}}$ ANSWER: 0.75

CHANGING A DECIMAL FRACTION TO A COMMON FRACTION

Decimal fractions are based on 10s, multiples of 10, and divisions by 10. The position or place of the decimal point indicates the denominator.

RULE 1: To change a decimal fraction to a common fraction, give the decimal fraction a denominator according to the position of the decimal point in the decimal fraction.

PROBLEM: Change 0.1 to a common fraction.

EXAMPLE: $\frac{0.1}{10}$ (The decimal point is in the "tens" place; 10 is the denominator.)

Now that the denominator is 10, place the 1 over it to make a common fraction.

$$\frac{1}{10}$$

PERCENTAGES

The word **percent** and its symbol, %, mean "hundredths." A hundredth is a fraction of a whole number; therefore a number followed by % is a *fraction* (such a fraction is called a "percentage"). The denominator of the fraction is understood to be 100.

EXAMPLE: 25% is the same as $\frac{25}{100}$.

Reduce $\frac{25}{100}$ to $\frac{1}{4}$.

CHANGING A PERCENTAGE TO A DECIMAL FRACTION

RULE 1: Remove the percent sign; move the decimal point two places to the left to indicate "hundredths."

PROBLEM: Change 25% to a decimal fraction.

ANSWER: 0.25

CHANGING A FRACTION TO A PERCENTAGE

RULE 1: Change a fraction to a percentage by dividing the numerator by the denominator.
RULE 2: Multiply the answer by 100.
RULE 3: Label the answer with the percent symbol.

EXAMPLE:

$$\begin{array}{r} 100 \\ \times 0.75 \\ \hline 500 \\ 700 \\ \hline 75.00x \end{array}$$

(There are two decimal places in this problem; move the decimal point in the answer two places to the left)

75% Therefore $\frac{3}{4} = 75\%$

MULTIPLYING BY PERCENTAGE

RULE 1: Change percentage to a decimal (move decimal point two places to the left).
RULE 2: Multiply.

PROBLEM: Multiply 80 by 7.5%.

EXAMPLE: 7.5% is .075.

ANSWER: 6

RATIOS

Ratio is the relationship of one number or quantity to another number or quantity. Numbers of a ratio are separated by a colon. A ratio is also a fraction. The value of a ratio is not changed if both terms are multiplied or divided by the same number.

EXAMPLE: 2:4 is the same as 1:2 or 4:8.

PROBLEM: Write numbers as ratios, and express them all in the same units.

EXAMPLE: Express 1 L, 2 oz, and 30 mL all in the same way: 1000 mL:60 mL:30 mL.

PROBLEM: Write a fraction as a ratio.

EXAMPLE: $\frac{1}{25} = 1:25 \quad \frac{3}{4} = 3:4 \quad \frac{1}{25} = 1:25 \quad \frac{3}{4} = 3:4$

Ratio is an important concept that is used in the following methods of calculating dosages.

PROPORTIONS

Proportion is a relationship between two ratios of equal value.

EXAMPLE: 1 is to 2 as 4 is to 8, or 1:2 = 4:8.

Means are the inner terms of the proportion. **Extremes** are the outer terms of the proportion.

EXAMPLE: 1:2 = 4:8 (means: 2 and 4) 1:2 = 4:8 (extremes: 1 and 8)

Set up the left side, or first ratio, of the proportion as the "known" side by using information that is known or given. Examples of known information are as follows:

An equivalent such as 60 milligrams = 1 grain (60 mg: 1 gr)
A physician's medication or IV order, such as "give 1000 mL in 8 hr" (1000 mL:8 hr)
A drug dosage on hand or available, such as information on a drug label that reads "50 mg/mL" (50 mg:1 mL)

PROBLEM: The physician orders Demerol, 25 mg q 3–4 h, as needed (prn) for pain. On hand is a vial labeled "50 mg/1 mL."

RULE 1: Set up the known side.

EXAMPLE: 50 mg:1 (quantity given on the label)

RULE 2: Set up the unknown side. Use x for what the equation asks, such as "How many milliliters are needed to give 25 mg?"

EXAMPLE:

KNOWN		UNKNOWN
50 mg:1 mL	=	25 mg:x mL

RULE 3: Set up the units, such as mg and mL, in the *same position on each side* of the problem.

EXAMPLE: _______ mg:_______ mL = _______ mg:_______ mL

RULE 4: Multiply the means.

RULE 5: Multiply the extremes.

PROBLEM: 50 mg:1 mL = 25 mg:x mL

EXAMPLE: Multiply the means.

50 mg : 1 mL = 25 mg : x mL
= 25

Multiply the extremes.

$$50\text{ mg} : 1\text{ mL} = 25\text{ mg} : x\text{ mL}$$
$$= 50x$$

Express the proportion.

$$50x = 25$$

RULE 6: Solve for x (divide the number with the x into the number on the opposite side of the problem).

EXAMPLE: $50\text{ mg} : 1\text{ mL} = 25\text{ mg} : x\text{ mL}$

$$50x = 25 = 50\overline{)25.0}\ \ (0.5)$$
$$x = 0.5$$

RULE 7: Label the answer with the unit of measurement that accompanies the x in the problem.

EXAMPLE: $50\text{ mg} : 1\text{ mL} = 25\text{ mg} : x\text{ mL}$

$$50x = 25$$
$$x = 0.5\text{ mL}$$

Review of Proportion Method

1. Set up problems in the *same order* on both sides.
2. Multiply the means; then multiply the extremes.
3. The number multiplied with the x is always that number with the x to the right of it.

   EXAMPLE: 2 mg:1 mL = 5 mg:x mL
4. Divide the number with the x into the number on the other side of the problem.
5. Label the problem by determining which unit of measurement is associated with the x in the proportion.

$$\frac{\text{Desired dosage}}{\text{Available dose}} \times \text{Amount}$$

Many nurses use the following method of solving dosage problems:

RULE 1: Place the dose that the physician wants given over the dose that is available (on hand).

PROBLEM: The physician orders 40 mg of furosemide (Lasix). An ampule (small glass container that usually contains a single dose of a solution) of furosemide labeled "Lasix 20 mg/mL" is available.

EXAMPLE: $\frac{\text{(Desired dosage) } 40\text{ mg}}{\text{(Available dose) } 20\text{ mg}} \times \frac{1\text{ mL}}{1} = \frac{40}{20}$

$$= 40 \div 20 = 2\text{ mL}$$

PROBLEM: The physician orders 15 mg of diazepam (Valium). Valium tablets that contain 5 mg/tablet are available.

EXAMPLE:

$$\frac{\text{(Desired dosage) } 15\text{ mg}}{\text{(Available dose) } 15\text{ mg}} \times \frac{1\text{ tab}}{x\text{ tab}} = \frac{15}{5x} = x$$
$$= 15 \div 5 = 3\text{ tabs}$$

DIMENSIONAL ANALYSIS[a]

In the **dimensional analysis** method (also called *factor labeling* or the *label factor method*), dosages are calculated with the use of the following three factors:

1. *Drug label factor:* The form in which the drug dose is delivered, or the vehicle *(V)*, with the equivalence in units on hand *(H)*; for example, 1 capsule *(V)* = 500 mg *(H)*.
2. *Conversion factor (C):* It helps to memorize the following common conversions (see the section on the apothecary system with its abbreviations, for a discussion of grains *[gr]*):

   1 g = 1000 mg   1 g = 15 gr
   1000 mg = 15 gr   1 gr = 60 mg
3. Drug order factor: The dosage desired (D).

These three factors are set up in an equation that allows the units to be canceled, and then you can calculate the correct units for delivery.

$$V = \frac{V\text{ (vehicle)}}{H\text{ (on hand)}} \times \frac{C\,(H)}{C\,(D)} \times \frac{D\text{ (desired)}}{1}$$

(drug label) (conversion factor) (drug order)

With dimensional analysis, the conversion factor is built into the equation and is included when the units of measurement of the drug order and drug container differ. If the two are of the same units of measurement, the conversion factor is eliminated from the equation.

EXAMPLE: Order calls for acetaminophen (Tylenol) gr xv, PO, prn (15 grains, by mouth, as needed)

AVAILABLE:

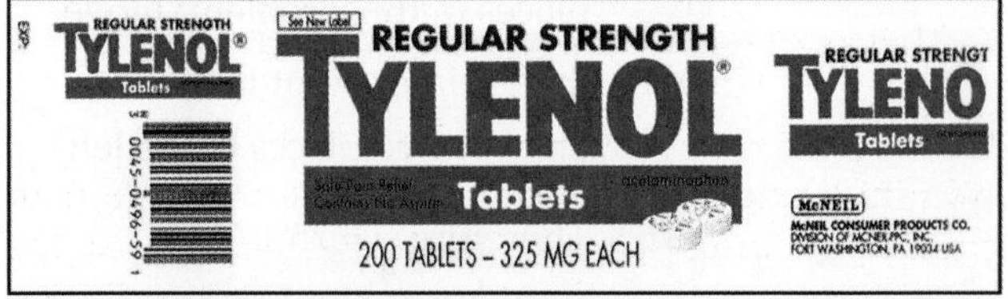

Factors: 325 mg = 1 tablet (from drug label)
15 gr/1 (from drug order)
Conversion factor: 1000 mg = 15 gr
How many tablets should be given?

$$\text{Tab} = \frac{\text{gr}}{\text{x}} \times \frac{\text{mg}}{\text{gr}} \times \frac{\text{tab}}{\text{mg}}$$

$$\text{Tab} = \frac{15\ \cancel{\text{gr}}}{\text{x}} \times \frac{1000\ \cancel{\text{mg}}}{15\ \cancel{\text{gr}}} \times \frac{1\text{ tab}}{325\ \cancel{\text{mg}}} = \frac{15{,}000}{4875} =$$

$$\text{Tab} = 3.07$$
$$= 3\text{ tabs}$$

[a]This section is reprinted from Kee JL, Hayes ER: *Pharmacology: A nursing process approach*, ed 7, St. Louis, 2012, Saunders.

Box 17.1 Nursing Responsibilities in Solving Dosage Problems

- Check whether the answer is reasonable.
- Do not allow for any errors in calculating dosages.
- Recheck calculations.
- Reduce distractions while working problems.
- Work problems systematically and carefully.
- Perform dosage calculations independently; then ask another nurse to perform the same dosage calculation problem, and check answers.

Box 17.1 lists the nurse's responsibilities in solving dosage problems accurately.

CALCULATING MEDICATIONS USING THE MILLIGRAM/KILOGRAM METHOD

Some medication dosages are based on the patient's weight. The method of calculation is used most commonly for dosages of medications for infants and children, but it can be used for a patient of any age. When using this method, convert the patient's weight to kilograms if the weight is measured or recorded in pounds (lb). Refer to the following example when using this method of dosage calculation:

Example: A medication order specifies administering cefazolin, 50 mg/kg, divided into four equal doses.

If the child weighs 95 lb, first convert the weight to kilograms:

95 lb/2.2 = 43.18 kg; then multiply the weight in kilograms by the milligrams:

50 mg × 43.18 kg = 2159 mg; then divide by the number of doses to be administered:

2159 kg/4 (four equal doses) = 539.75 mg

PEDIATRIC DOSAGE CONSIDERATIONS

Administering the correct dosages of medication to children requires caution. There are factors that the health care provider should consider when ordering medication for a child: age, weight, body surface area, and the ability of the child to absorb, metabolize, and excrete medication. It is the health care provider's responsibility to provide medication orders and specify dosages for a pediatric patient, but the nurse must be able to recognize appropriate medication dosages and orders.

There are several different ways to determine appropriate pediatric doses, but this discussion focuses on how to use the body surface area and a nomogram.

Young's Rule

Young's rule is a method of calculating the appropriate dose of a drug for a child 2 years of age or older:

$$\frac{\text{Age of child}}{\text{Age of child} + 12} \times \text{Average adult dose} = \text{Child's dose}$$

This rule applies to children up to the age of 12.

PROBLEM: The average adult dose of a medication is 50 mg. What is an appropriate dose of this medication for an 8-year-old child?

ANSWER: 20 mg is an appropriate dose.

Clark's Rule

Clark's rule is another method of calculating the appropriate dosage of a drug for a child. In this rule, the child's weight is used to determine dosage:

$$\frac{\text{Weight of child in pounds}}{150} \times \text{Average adult dose} = \text{Child's dose}$$

PROBLEM: The average adult dose of a medication is 25 mg. What is an appropriate dose of this medication for a child who weighs 40 lb?

EXAMPLE:

$$\frac{40\text{ lb}}{150} \times 25\text{ mg} = \frac{40}{150} \times \frac{25}{1} = \frac{1000}{150} = 150\overline{)1000.00}$$

quotient 6.66; 900, 1000, 900, 1000

$$= 6.7\text{ mg or } 7\text{ mg}$$

ANSWER: 6.7 or 7 mg is an appropriate dose.

Fried's Rule

Fried's rule is used to calculate appropriate dosages for infants younger than 2 years:

$$\frac{\text{Age in months}}{150} \times \text{Average adult dose} = \text{Child's dose}$$

PROBLEM: The average adult dose of a medication is 25 mg. What is an appropriate dose of this medication for a child who is 22 months of age?

EXAMPLE:

$$\frac{22}{150} \times 25\text{ mg} = \frac{550}{150} = 150\overline{)550.00} = 3.7\text{ or } 4\text{ mg}$$

quotient 3.66; 450, 1000, 900, 1000

ANSWER: 3.7 or 4 mg is an appropriate dose.

Estimating Body Surface Area in Children

Body surface area is defined as the total area exposed to the outside environment. For pediatric patients of average size, it is acceptable to estimate body surface area with the scales shown in Fig. 17.1. Match the child's weight to the corresponding surface area. Lay a straight edge on the correct height and weight points for the pediatric patient (as on the right side of Fig. 17.1) and

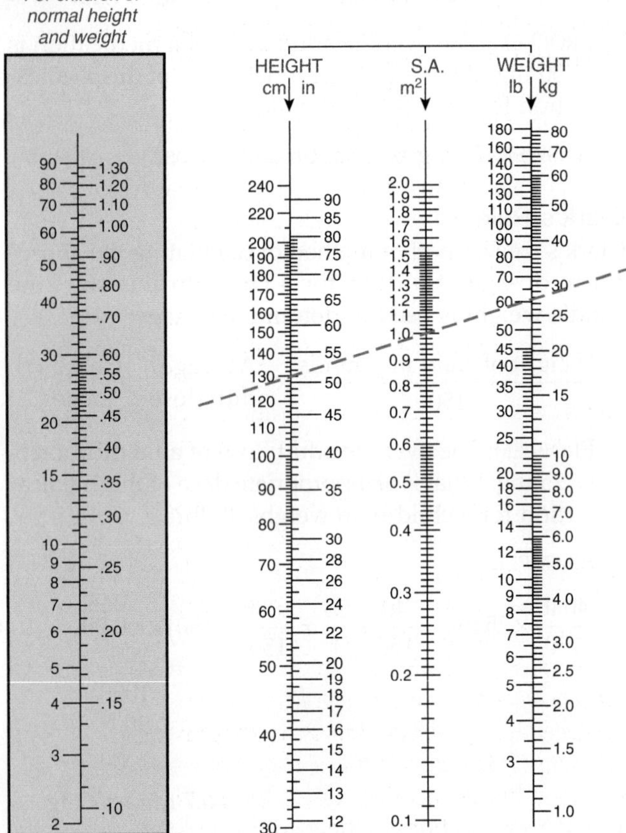

Fig. 17.1 Estimating body surface area *(S.A.)* in children. (From Behrman RE, Kliegman RM: *Nelson's textbook of pediatrics*, ed 18, Philadelphia, 2007, Saunders.)

find the point where it intersects on the surface area scale at center.

PROBLEM: Trey, an 8-year-old, weighs 60 lb and is 51 inches tall. His body surface area (as determined with the nomogram in Fig. 17.1) is 1.0. If an adult dose is 50 mg, how many milligrams should Trey receive?

EXAMPLE: Use the following formula:

$$\frac{\text{Child's body surface area}}{1.73} \text{ Adult dose} = \text{Child's dose}$$

ANSWER: 29 mg is appropriate for a child of Trey's height and weight.

PRINCIPLES AND PRACTICE OF MEDICATION ADMINISTRATION

PHARMACOLOGY

Pharmacology is the study of drugs (medications) and their action on the living body. Substances derived from plants and animals, from vitamins and minerals, and from synthetic (artificial) sources can be used as drugs in the treatment and prevention of disease. The terms *drug* and *medication* often are used interchangeably. Drugs are used to restore and maintain the healthy functioning of body tissues, organs, and systems and in diagnostic procedures.

Box 17.2 Terms Used With Dosages

Minimal dose: The smallest amount of a drug that produces a therapeutic effect
Maximal dose: The largest amount of a drug that it is possible to give safely
Toxic dose: The amount of a drug that produces signs and symptoms of poisoning
Lethal dose: The amount of a drug that causes death

The action of any drug on the body is a complicated process. This process begins with the pharmaceutical phase: from the manufacturing of the drug until the absorption of the drug in the patient's body. Absorption occurs when the active ingredient of the drug enters the body fluids.

The pharmacokinetic phase involves the movement of the drug's active ingredients from the body fluids into the patient's system and to the site where the intended action of the drug takes place.

In the pharmacodynamic phase, the drug's active ingredient interacts with the intended body tissues. The body's cells respond to the action of the drug and change as the drug is metabolized.

The liver is the main organ that inactivates and metabolizes drugs. The kidneys are the principal organs that eliminate the metabolites of drugs from the body. A **metabolite** is a substance produced by metabolic action, which results in the breakdown of the drug.

The nurse needs to understand the process of drug action in and elimination from the body because each patient is affected differently by the medications prescribed. It is necessary to assess and consider each patient's hepatic (liver) and renal (kidney) functions, because decreased hepatic or renal function has the potential to prolong the length of time a drug stays in the body and may continue to be active.

Drugs that are not excreted adequately in the urine, feces, sweat, tears, breast milk (in lactating mothers), and exhaled air build up in the patient's body. A drug that builds up in the body is said to have a **cumulative** (increasing by increments) effect, which sometimes leads to toxic (harmful) or even lethal (deadly) outcomes for the patient (Box 17.2).

Drug Dosage

Dosage is the schedule of administration (amount and frequency) of a drug prescribed for the patient by the health care provider. The health care provider's order includes information regarding the medication to be administered to the patient, including drug name, dosage, and route of administration. The order would read, "Give 100 mg Dilantin PO tid." A *dose* of medicine refers to a single administration of a drug. The dose ordered in the example is thus 100 mg. The nurse administers a 100-mg dose (one capsule) of phenytoin

Box 17.3 Terms Used With Medication Orders

Stat: Medications ordered to be administered stat are those that are planned to manage an emergency patient condition. Stat orders have the highest priority ranking. They are to be completed before other orders. The time of actual administration must be documented. A stat order is a one-time-only dose.
Now: Now orders are high in priority but should be completed after stat orders.
One time only: In these orders, a medication is to be administered as a single dose.
prn (give as necessary): The patient is permitted to request prn medication, or the nurse may offer a prn medication; prn medication orders must specify a definite time interval between permitted repeat administrations.

(Dilantin) three times a day; the total daily dosage is thus 300 mg (given in divided doses by mouth, or *per os* [PO]). It is important for the nurse to be familiar with **therapeutic** (beneficial) dosages of frequently used drugs to administer doses of medication competently to patients (Box 17.3). Look up any unfamiliar medications in an approved resource before administering the medication.

Drug Actions and Interactions

Medications produce two general types of actions in a patient's body: local and systemic. A local action by a drug produces an effect only in the area where the drug has been placed. A systemic action affects the entire body, because the drug enters the patient's systemic circulation.

When one drug alters the action of another drug, it is called a **drug interaction** (a modification of the effect of a drug when administered with another drug). When two or more drugs are given together, the combined actions of the drugs sometimes produce an effect totally different from the expected action of either drug. These effects may benefit or harm the patient. When one drug increases the action or the effect of another drug, it is called **potentiation** of the drug, or *synergism.* Drug combinations may be administered with the express purpose of boosting the action of the administered drugs. **Compatibility** is the quality or state of harmonious coexistence. Drug compatibility is the ability to administer medications together easily without any difficulty for the patient. Compatibility charts provide quick reference for the nurse to determine whether it is acceptable to administer one drug along with another drug in the same syringe or in an IV infusion.

Some drugs should not be given together because the medications do not combine well chemically or physically. This problem is referred to as drug *incompatibility.* Suspect drug incompatibility when two drugs are mixed together and the solution changes color, becomes cloudy, or forms a precipitate (a reaction in which a new solid mass is formed). Drug interactions are more likely to occur with drugs that are especially potent (strong), such as digitalis. The cardiotonics (drugs that slow and strengthen the heart), antihypertensives (drugs that lower blood pressure), hypoglycemic agents (oral medications that lower blood glucose level), insulin (injectable medication that lowers blood glucose level), and heparin (medication that decreases the clotting of blood) are common powerful agents; be familiar with these drugs before administering them. With drug interactions, the medication may increase or decrease the action of one or more other medications. Sometimes the medications may create an adverse reaction that is not normally associated with either drug. Drug interactions are often the result of drug incompatibilities that alter how the medication is absorbed, distributed, metabolized, or excreted. Drug interactions may produce adverse effects in the patient, which may lead to reduced patient compliance and prolonged hospitalization. During the assessment of the patient, the nurse is responsible for monitoring the patient for occurrence of drug interactions and adverse reactions to medications. Assess the patient for changes in level of consciousness, slurred speech, ataxia, and changes in the patient's vital signs. Listen to what the patient says about the effects of the medication. The LPN/LVN should report any adverse reactions to the medication or possible drug interactions to the registered nurse (RN) and document these findings objectively. Health care providers depend on the ongoing nursing assessment of each patient's response to drug therapy.

The nurse must be knowledgeable about agonistic and antagonistic effects associated with medications. A drug that produces a predictable response at the intended site of action is called an **agonist.** An **antagonist** is a drug that blocks the action of another drug. Antagonistic drugs are used to counteract the effects of a previously given drug. A common antagonist prescribed is naloxone hydrochloride (Narcan). It is given when a person has received too much of an opioid medication, such as morphine sulfate. Too much morphine sulfate may produce life-threatening depression of the respiratory and central nervous systems. Naloxone blocks the action of the opioid. Remember that each patient may respond differently to medications. Assess the patient for the development of an idiosyncratic reaction. An **idiosyncratic** reaction to a drug results from the individual's unique hypersensitivity to it. It is an unexpected response to a medication. For example, a patient takes a medication prescribed to help reduce anxiety, but the patient becomes more agitated and restless instead. These manifestations are consistent with an idiosyncratic reaction. It is important to monitor all patients who are receiving medication for signs of overdose, **toxicity** (dangerous buildup of a substance), and unexpected drug reactions.

Some patients may have had hypersensitivity reactions or allergic reactions to drugs. If possible, assess the patient's drug history before administering medication to the patient. For example, the following questions may be helpful to ask the patient: Have you taken the drug before? Do you have any known allergies to medications? If you determine the patient has had a reaction to that medication, withhold the drug and report this information to the RN. Also notify the patient's health care provider.

A reduced response to a drug over time is called drug **tolerance.** The patient who has developed tolerance to a drug requires a larger dose of the drug to achieve the same effect that a smaller therapeutic dose once produced. Drug tolerance either is acquired from taking increasing dosages of the drug over time or may result from genetic factors that are unique to the individual.

It is essential to monitor each patient's reaction to drug therapy, particularly when the patient receives a medication for the first time. To establish baseline information, the patient should be assessed before and after a new medication is started. Any changes in mental or physical status should be reported to the RN. Mental or physical changes that occur after administration of a medication could represent an **adverse drug reaction** (a harmful, unintended reaction to a drug administered at a normal dosage), drug hypersensitivity, or intolerance to the drug.

Drug administration is a tremendous nursing responsibility. Never give any medication that you are not familiar with to a patient without first accessing information about it from an approved facility resource (such as the pharmacy department, a current drug handbook, or an online resource). Use the resource to determine the therapeutic dosage, indications for use of the drug, *contraindications* (conditions in which the drug should not be used), side effects, available formulations and routes of administration, generic and trade names, and information regarding how to manage overdoses. The following factors may affect how patients respond to medication:

- *Age:* Very young and very old people generally react more acutely to drugs than do other people. Older adults tend to have a higher ratio of fat tissue to muscle tissue, and the higher fat percentage typically affects how the fat-soluble medication is distributed and stored. Drug action is likely to be prolonged in older adults, because renal and hepatic function often is diminished with age (Table 17.1). In very young children, liver and kidney function is not fully developed; as a result, metabolism or excretion of medications may be inefficient.
- *Weight:* Overweight people sometimes require more medication or higher drug dosages than do patients who are of average weight. Patients who are underweight may require lower drug dosages. Body surface area, height, and weight often are used to help determine drug dosages in children.
- *Gender:* Women tend to have a higher percentage of body fat than men. Because some drugs are fat soluble, women with a high body fat percentage tend to accumulate fat-soluble drugs in their bodies. Advise pregnant and lactating women that the substances taken during pregnancy may have the capacity to pass through the placenta and adversely affect the fetus. It is also possible for drugs to pass to infants through breast milk.
- *Ethnicity:* There are slight differences in the responses between certain ethnic groups regarding the effects of certain drugs on their systems. The differences may be in part related to differences in the drug metabolism enzymes in the liver between some races. Examples include the variations in sensitivity (increased or reduced) of African Americans to certain classes of antihypertensive medications and the increased difficulty controlling asthma in whites who have certain genetic makeups (Belle and Singh, 2008).
- *Physical condition:* Disease processes may alter medication dosage requirements, particularly in patients with renal, hepatic, cardiovascular, and gastrointestinal (GI) disorders.
- *Psychological status:* Stress, emotional conflict, anxiety, and fear have the capacity to alter the patient's response to drug therapy. Help increase the patient's compliance with the medication regimen with adequate education about the medication. Your skill set, actions, and attitudes regarding drug administration can affect the patient's response to drug therapy as well.
- *Environmental temperature:* The patient may metabolize a drug more quickly when the patient is in a warm environment and may metabolize a medication more slowly when in a cold environment.
- *Amount of food in the stomach:* A medication taken on an empty stomach tends to reach the bloodstream faster than a medication taken on a full stomach. Irritating drugs are administered after or with meals so that they produce fewer GI side effects, such as nausea.
- *Route of administration:* The route that the medication is given influences the onset, intensity, and duration of a drug. A medication that is administered through an IV route or injected into the patient's muscle works more quickly than medications given by mouth.

Stay current regarding the basics of drug actions, how medication orders are written, how to interpret them, how the orders are received, and how they are transcribed. Always follow the basic practices and principles of safe medication administration. High personal and professional standards protect the patient and help avoid medication errors.

MEDICATION ORDERS

The nurse is legally and ethically responsible for ensuring that the patient receives the correct medication that has been ordered by the health care provider. Health care providers may give the nurse medication orders during patient admissions, during morning and evening rounds, after surgery, and any other time throughout the day

Table 17.1 Influence of Aging on Drug Actions in Older Adults

AGE-RELATED PHYSIOLOGIC CHANGE	EFFECT ON DRUG ACTION AND PATIENT RESPONSE	NURSING INTERVENTIONS
Gastrointestinal Tract		
Oral Cavity		
Loss of elasticity in oral mucosa, which becomes dry and easily abraded	Difficulty in swallowing tablets or capsules; sensitivity to drugs that cause dryness of mouth, which increases susceptibility to gum disease and dental caries	Have patient rinse oral cavity frequently with clear tepid water, floss daily, and brush teeth and gums gently. Recommend synthetic saliva substitute.
Esophagus		
Delayed esophageal clearance because of weakened contractions and failure of lower esophageal sphincter to relax	Difficulty in swallowing large tablets or capsules; tissue erosion caused by drugs such as aspirin and uncoated potassium chloride	Position patient upright. Administer full glass of liquid with drug. Crush tablets and mix with food (if gastric pH does not affect absorption).
Stomach		
Decrease in gastric acidity and peristalsis	Irritation from highly acidic drugs (e.g., aspirin)	Have patient drink full glass of water and take medication with nonfat snack to reduce gastric distress.
Large Intestine		
Reduced colon muscle tone; loss of defecation reflex; decreased intestinal blood flow	Slowing of drug excretion; overuse and abuse of laxatives by patient; delayed drug absorption	Provide normal fluid intake. Instruct patient to eat bulk-forming foods and to avoid use of constipating drugs.
Skin and Vascular System		
Reduced subcutaneous skinfold thickness in extremities (less body fat); reduced elasticity in skin and vascular system; increased fragility of blood vessels	Tendency for bleeding after injections	Avoid using veins in hands for intravenous (IV) injections. Apply pressure to injection sites after administration. Observe injection sites for bleeding.
Liver		
Reduced liver size; decline in hepatic blood flow	Longer biotransformation time; prolonged duration of drug action; greater risk for drug sensitivity and toxicity	Monitor for signs and symptoms of liver impairment (jaundice, pruritus, dark urine). Monitor blood chemistry values for hepatic toxicity.
Kidneys		
Reduced glomerular filtration; decreased tubular function and renal blood flow	Risk of drug accumulation and toxicity	Prevent urinary retention (keep catheters flowing freely and observe frequency of urination). Monitor for signs and symptoms of renal impairment (reduced output and difficulty in urinating). Provide normal fluid intake. Monitor blood urea nitrogen (BUN) and serum creatinine levels.

or night as needed. As soon as possible after a health care provider writes an order, read and interpret the order. Within acute care settings, the medication order commonly is shared electronically with the pharmacy department so that the order may be entered accurately into the computerized system. Because of the possibility of inaccurately interpreting the handwritten medication order, more health care facilities are now requesting health care providers to enter medication orders into computers. If you do need to read the health care provider's handwriting and it is illegible, ask another nurse or staff member to help interpret the order. If unsure about what the order states, contact the health care provider for clarification.

Drug Distribution Systems

There are various methods used for storing and distributing medications in health care settings. Many health care facilities have designated areas for storing medications. Medications that are stored on a patient care unit are referred to as *floor stock* because they are available on the unit and not stored solely in the pharmacy department. Areas that are used to store medications should remain locked when unattended.

In some long-term care facilities and hospitals, the unit-dose system is used to store and dispense medications. The *unit-dose system* typically is used with a portable medication cart that contains drawers. A *unit dose* is the ordered amount of medication that the patient is supposed to receive at a prescribed time. The medication cart holds the unit doses for each patient. The nurse transports the medication cart from room to room to administer the medication at designated times. The medication cart is locked when not attended. In some institutions, there is a locked cabinet in each patient's room where their medications are stored.

Computer-controlled dispensing systems are a combination of unit-dose and floor stock systems. These machines contain various medications that are placed in individual compartments. The machine commonly is stocked by the pharmacy department with medications that are prescribed commonly for patients on that unit. The nurse uses a computer to choose the medication to remove. The nurse is assigned a security code that allows access to the medications specifically prescribed for an individual patient. The system's computer records medications removed and can be used to assist the health care facility with charging the patient for medications that were administered to the patient (Fig. 17.2).

Regardless of the type of system used to store and dispense medications, it is the nurse's responsibility to properly store medications according to the policies and procedures of the health care facility where the nurse is working. The storage instructions must be followed for each medication. The chemical properties of some medications may necessitate refrigeration or storage in cool or even reduced-lighting environments.

Medications may be referred to by several different names. The two most common names for medications are the trade name and the generic name. The trade name is the brand name given to it by the manufacturer for use especially by consumers and health care providers.

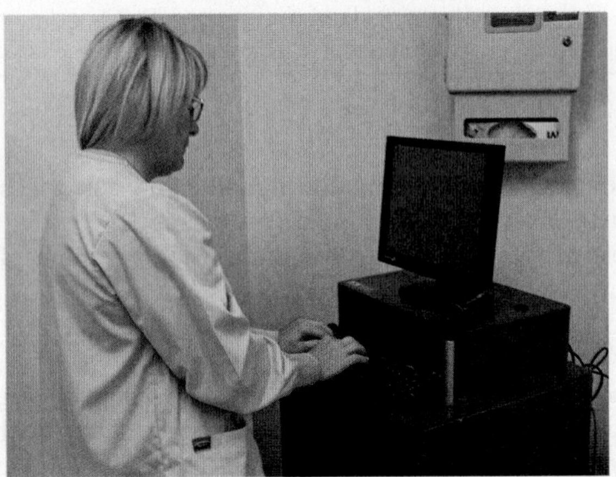

Fig. 17.2 Nurse using computer-controlled dispensing system.

On the packaging, this name often is followed by the symbol "®." The trade name is usually short, readily recognized, easy to spell, and easy to pronounce, such as "Lasix." The first letter is capitalized. The generic name is usually longer, may refer to the chemical composition of the medication, and is not capitalized. It often is written after the trade name and is listed in parentheses. Medications may be marketed under either their generic or trade names; for example, the generic name for Lasix is "furosemide" (US Food and Drug Administration, 2009). Generic medications traditionally cost less than their more easily recognized trade (brand) names, but the generic medications have the same ingredients, potency, dosage, quality, and purity of brand-name medications. The US Food and Drug Administration requires testing for all approved medications.

Knowledge regarding suffixes (an appendage at the end of a word or phrase to form a commonality) and the category of medications associated with specific suffixes is helpful to the nurse. The suffixes provide information about the classification and uses of medications. For instance, the suffix "-semide," as in "furosemide" and "torsemide," indicates that these medications are loop diuretics.

Ensure that the medication that was ordered by the health care provider is administered correctly. If you have any questions regarding the medication for the patient, consult resources available for the facility nurses such as the pharmacy department, drug reference book, or online resources.

Ensure that the health care provider's order includes the following:

- Patient's name (on the health care provider's order sheet)
- Patient's date of birth
- Date and time of the order (usually on the left side of the order sheet), written by the health care provider
- Name of drug (may be brand name or generic name, or both)
- Dosage of the drug, including dose size and frequency (e.g., "650 mg q 4 hr prn" [i.e., every 4 hours as needed])
- Route of administration, as prescribed by the health care provider
- Signature of the health care provider
- Any special instructions regarding any aspect of administering the drug (e.g., "650 mg q 4 hr if temperature >101°F")

Controlled Substances

Opioids, barbiturates, and other controlled medications that have a high possibility for abuse, addiction, or theft are kept in a secured area. In facilities where computerized systems are not used, special keys must be used to obtain these types of medications for patients when they are ordered. The special keys, called "narcotic keys," are kept by designated nurses each shift. The narcotic keys are used to unlock the storage container where the controlled substances are stored. The nurse usually must use a double-locking system with two separate keys. It is the nurse's responsibility to ensure that each controlled drug used during that shift is logged in a narcotic log book. At the end of each shift, controlled drugs in the storage container are counted carefully by a designated nurse from the outgoing shift and by a nurse from the incoming shift. The number of drugs given, according to the log book, and the actual number of medications contained in the storage container should be reviewed for accuracy. The outgoing staff should not be dismissed until the narcotic count is done and verified. If the count is incorrect and medication is missing, it is necessary to find the error or identify the issue before anyone is dismissed from the facility.

Many agencies now use computerized systems for medication access and distribution. Computerized storage has eliminated the need to perform the narcotic count at the end of each shift. Discrepancies with narcotic counts can be identified more readily with computerized systems. Counts of controlled substances are performed each time pharmacy staff members restock medications. Nurses are required to count before the removal of controlled substances from these types of computerized machines.

Medications are available in specific dosages. The dosage order may necessitate the use of only a portion of the available medication; thus the nurse must dispose of ("waste") it. When disposing of a controlled substance, the nurse must have a witness that is a licensed member of the nursing team. The witness and the nurse wasting the medication are required to document the information in accordance with the health care facility's policy and procedure (via computerized documentation or log book) to indicate that the medication was wasted (Box 17.4).

Box 17.4 Guidelines for Safe Administration and Storage of Opioids and Other Controlled Substances

- All opioids and other controlled substances must be stored in a locked, secure cabinet, computerized medication dispenser, or secure medication storage container, per facility policy.
- Nurses must use keys to unlock secured medication storage containers or sign in to a computerized medication dispenser to remove controlled substances.
- The controlled substances are counted per facility policy. In some long-term care facilities, the controlled medications may be counted at each change of shift. Other acute care agencies may require the pharmacy counts during restocking of the controlled substances within the computerized medication system. Also, each nurse who removes a controlled substance is required to count the remaining medication at the time that a controlled medication is removed.
- Discrepancies in opioid counts must be reported immediately.
- In some long-term care facilities, the paper inventory record is used to document the patient's name, birth date, room number, date, time of drug administration, name of drug, dosage, and signature of nurse dispensing the drug.
- This form provides an accurate, ongoing count of opioids and other controlled substances used and remaining.
- If only one part of a premeasured dosage of a controlled substance is given, a second nurse witnesses disposal of the unused portion and documents such on the record form or in the computer, per facility policy.

Types of Orders

Standing orders. Standing orders are those that already are created by a health care provider for his or her patients who are admitted to a particular unit. The nurse may enact the orders without having to contact the health care provider to request orders. The orders are accessible to the nurses on the unit via computer or on paper. Know how to locate the orders and enact the orders. Standing orders can make the admission process easier and more efficient for the patient and the nurse. Know when to question an order because it is not applicable or appropriate for a specific patient. Questions or concerns about the orders must be clarified with the health care provider.

Verbal or telephone orders. Ideally, medication orders should be written by the health care provider on the patient's order sheet. Situations may arise in which the provider is not able to write the orders. In this case, a verbal order may be given to the LPN/LVN or RN directly or over the phone. Follow the health care facility's policy when taking verbal or telephone orders. Verbal orders should be transcribed or entered into a computer, per facility policy. The health care provider should sign (or electronically sign) the order as soon as possible. Be careful when taking verbal orders. If anything about the order is unclear or confusing, do not hesitate to clarify the information with the health care provider. When receiving a verbal order, always repeat the order to the health care provider to ensure that it is correct.

SIX "RIGHTS" OF MEDICATION ADMINISTRATION

Use each step of the nursing process when carrying out responsibilities pertaining to medication administration. Medications are administered in a variety of ways. Regardless of the route by which a drug enters the body, the same practices and principles of medication administration apply.

Proper and accurate medication administration can be achieved by following the six "rights" of medication administration (Box 17.5), performing the three label checks (to be described), using standard precautions, practicing good hand hygiene, and using aseptic technique.

1. Right Medication

The Joint Commission requires nurses to reconcile the patient's medication record with the medications the patient reports taking, to verify that the patient is receiving the correct medications. Obtain a list of medications that the patient was taking at home and review it with the patient and/or family to make sure the information is correct. Document the information about these medications to share with the health care provider. The health care provider may wish to reorder the patient's home medications when the patient is admitted to the hospital. It is essential that the patient receives the correct medications. When the patient is transferred to another health care setting or discharged home, verify again the list of medications that the patient should take after discharge.

Make sure the drug to be given is the correct drug, and perform the three label checks: checking the label on the drug's container three times—before, during, and after preparation. Take the medication to the patient's bedside in its original packaging, and open the packaging immediately before administering the dose (Box 17.6).

Never give a medication that another person has prepared, and *never* prepare or use a medication that is not labeled. In both cases, it is impossible to know for sure which medication was prepared or which medication was in the unlabeled container.

If you have any questions regarding the medication, check the health care provider's order to verify information about a medication order. Become familiar with generic and trade names of frequently used medications.

Box 17.5 Six "Rights" of Medication Administration

1. Right medication
2. Right dose
3. Right time
4. Right route
5. Right patient
6. Right documentation

Box 17.6 Three Label Checks of Medication Administration

1. Check the label when taking the medication from where it has been stored.
2. Check the label before removing the medication from its container.
3. Check the label before discarding or replacing the medication container and before giving the medication to the patient.

2. Right Dose

If there is a question regarding a medication dose, check the health care provider's order. Always check the label on the container to determine how the medication is supplied. For example, a medication may be supplied as 10 mg per 1 mL or 325 mg per tablet. Consult with another nurse to check any calculations or to clarify a dosage. Some computerized medication documentation systems require that another nurse document along with the nurse preparing and administering the dose (such as with insulin), to ensure that it is the correct dose.

The chance of an error during the process of administering medication increases when a medication is prepared from a dose formulation other than what has been ordered. Always compare the calculation of a dose with a second nurse who has calculated the dose independently. It is especially important to double-check a peer's calculation if it is an unusual or uncommonly performed calculation on that unit or if the calculation involves a dosage of a potentially toxic medication. Always use the correct type of measuring devices while preparing medications.

The assessment must include consideration to the appropriateness of the prescribed dose. Consider several questions: Is the dose appropriate related to the age of the patient, the diagnosis of the patient's condition, and the sex of the patient? Look at the number of tablets that constitute the dose or the number of milliliters that make up the dose. Does the number of tablets or the number of milliliters in the syringe look and sound reasonable? It is important to double-check the decimal place in the dosage ordered and the calculations: a decimal in the wrong place could produce a toxic or lethal patient outcome.

3. Right Time

The nurse is responsible for administering the medication at the right time. Many health care facilities use a standardized schedule for medication administration. Refer to the facility's policy regarding the timing of medications that are given routinely. Table 17.2 lists commonly used abbreviations.

Table 17.2 Commonly Used Abbreviations

ABBREVIATION (LATIN TERM)	MEANING	EXAMPLE
bid (bis in die)	Two times a day	0900 and 1700 hr
tid (ter in die)	Three times a day	0900, 1300, and 1700 hr
qid (quater in die)	Four times a day	0800, 1200, 1600, and 2000 hr
ac (ante cibum)	Before meals	Varies with hospital or unit
pc (post cibum)	After meals	Varies with hospital or unit

Medications should be administered within 30 minutes of their scheduled time: usually no earlier than 30 minutes beforehand and no later than 30 minutes afterward. Follow the health care facility's policies and procedures regarding timing of medication. Some long-term care facilities allow administration as long as 60 minutes before or 60 minutes after the scheduled time. As-needed (prn) medications may not be administered before the time intervals ordered by the prescriber. The date that the order was written should be reviewed to ensure that administration of the drug, the IV infusion, or the blood product is started and given on the right day and at the right time.

4. Right Route

The route chosen for administering a drug depends on the drug's properties and desired effect and the patient's physical and mental condition. It is necessary to specify the route of administration on all prescribed medication orders. If the route of administration is not noted on the medication order, contact the prescriber immediately. The nurse may be involved in judging the best route for a drug to be given. If an injection is prescribed, only special sterile solutions called *parenteral medications* are acceptable to use. Parenteral medications are labeled "for injectable use only." Serious complications may result if a liquid intended for oral use is injected. When the medication preparation is parenteral (intramuscular [IM], subcutaneous [subcut], intradermal [ID], or intravenous [IV]), the nurse must inject the medication into the appropriate type of body tissue.

5. Right Patient

Give the right medication to the right patient. Prevent medication errors by systematically identifying the patient before administering medication. There are several ways to do this; follow the facility's policy. Check the patient's identification bracelet to validate his or her name and date of birth, and then ask the patient his or her name and date of birth. Some facilities employ the use of a portable cart with a laptop computer that the nurse uses to verify medications. The nurse scans a barcode located on the patient's identification bracelet to ensure that the right patient is receiving the right medication.

An unconscious or confused patient may be unable to provide self-identification. A family member or visitor may be at the bedside, but do not rely solely on others to identify the patient. Check the identification bracelet on all patients. Review allergies before medication administration. In long-term care facilities, residents may not be required to wear identification bracelets or may be confused or unable to communicate their identity. Long-term care facility patients traditionally have numerous health concerns and as a result take large quantities of medications. This presents a unique safety challenge for the nurse who is assigned to complete the administration of medications. Follow facility policy to ensure proper identification of patients.

6. Right Documentation

Document the medication administration appropriately to help reduce medication errors (Fig. 17.3). Make a notation of the medication administration on the patient's chart or in the computer *immediately* after administering the drug. The policy of the health care facility may require that the documentation of injected (subcutaneous, intradermal, intramuscular) medications also include the site of the injection. In the medication administration record (MAR), whether a chart or in a computer, identify the drug given, the dosage, and the time the medication actually was given (not the time it was supposed to be given). In areas where immunizations are given, policy typically requires the nurse to note the lot number listed on the vial, the manufacturer of the vaccine, and the expiration date of the vaccine. The nursing assessment must include a description of any response the patient has to the medications or their administration. Examples of information to include may involve any complaints, adverse effects, and therapeutic effects. This information may have to be shared with the RN and the health care provider. It is not appropriate to document the administration of a medication until after the medication is given (see Box 17.8 and the Safety Alert box).

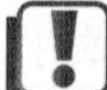 Safety Alert

The Joint Commission's "Do Not Use" List of Abbreviations

Each health care facility is obliged to develop and adhere to a "Do Not Use" list of abbreviations, acronyms, and symbols that must include those banned by The Joint Commission (2018). These abbreviations are not to be used during documentation. Each health care facility is permitted to add its own entries to the list of banned abbreviations. The Joint Commission's banned abbreviations must not appear in any documentation, including preprinted forms and computer documentation systems (see Appendix A).

If the six "rights" of medication administration are followed, it is not possible to give medication prepared by another nurse. It is impossible to assume that all the "rights" are followed unless the person who prepares the medication is the one who administers it.

To reduce the chance of making a medication error, follow the health care facility's policies and procedures and use common sense. If you do make an error, be honest when reporting the issue and perform prompt follow-up activities as directed by the RN and health care provider (Boxes 17.7 and 17.8).

IMPORTANT CONSIDERATIONS OF MEDICATION ADMINISTRATION

While handling equipment during medication administration, follow the principles of clean and sterile technique as applicable. Wash hands before and after caring for each patient. Keep work spaces and equipment clean

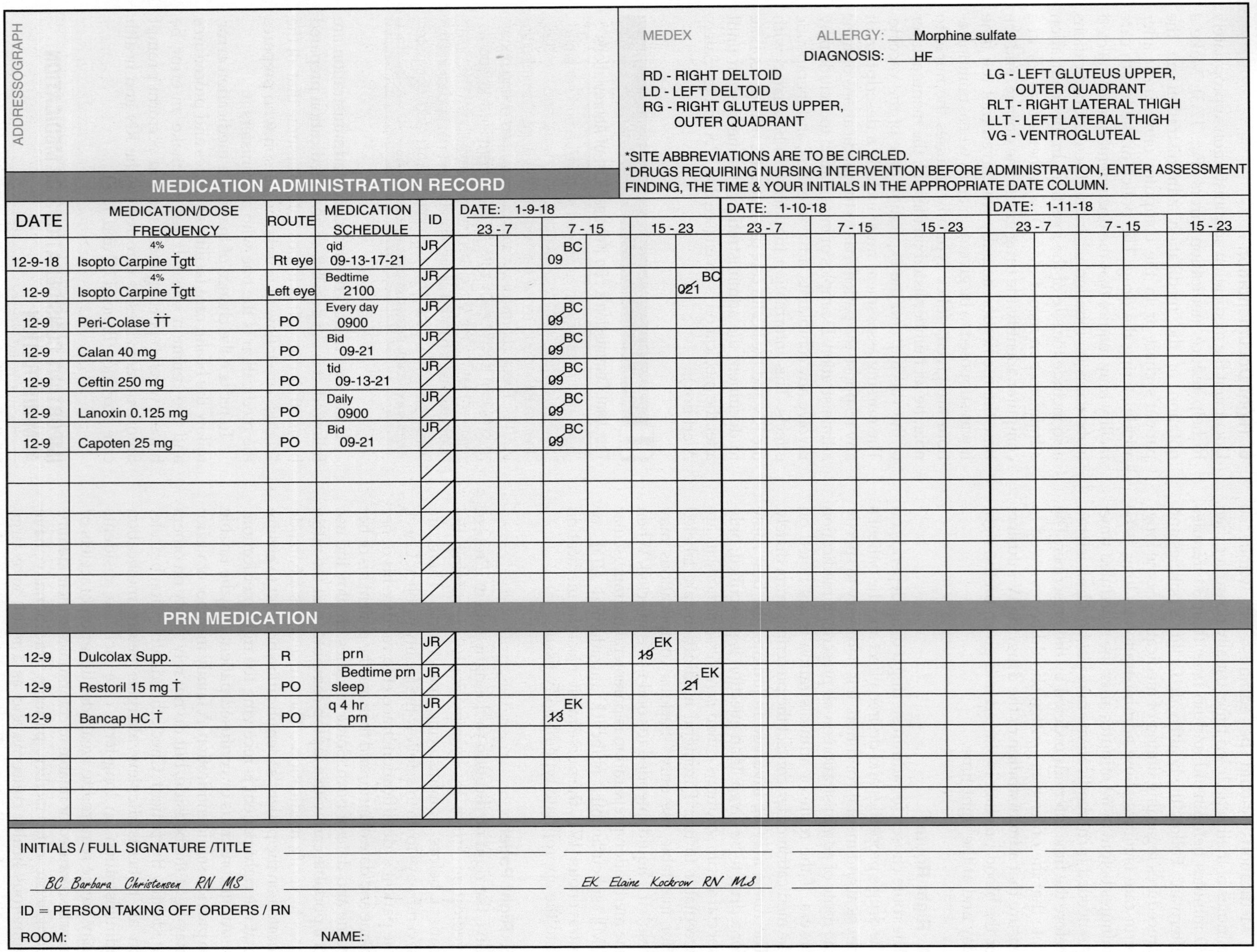

ADDRESSOGRAPH

MEDEX

ALLERGY: Morphine sulfate

DIAGNOSIS: HF

RD - RIGHT DELTOID
LD - LEFT DELTOID
RG - RIGHT GLUTEUS UPPER, OUTER QUADRANT
LG - LEFT GLUTEUS UPPER, OUTER QUADRANT
RLT - RIGHT LATERAL THIGH
LLT - LEFT LATERAL THIGH
VG - VENTROGLUTEAL

*SITE ABBREVIATIONS ARE TO BE CIRCLED.
*DRUGS REQUIRING NURSING INTERVENTION BEFORE ADMINISTRATION, ENTER ASSESSMENT FINDING, THE TIME & YOUR INITIALS IN THE APPROPRIATE DATE COLUMN.

MEDICATION ADMINISTRATION RECORD

DATE	MEDICATION/DOSE FREQUENCY	ROUTE	MEDICATION SCHEDULE	ID	DATE: 1-9-18 23 - 7	7 - 15	15 - 23	DATE: 1-10-18 23 - 7	7 - 15	15 - 23	DATE: 1-11-18 23 - 7	7 - 15	15 - 23
12-9-18	Isopto Carpine 4% Ṫgtt	Rt eye	qid 09-13-17-21	JR		09 BC							
12-9	Isopto Carpine 4% Ṫgtt	Left eye	Bedtime 2100	JR			021 BC						
12-9	Peri-Colase ṪṪ	PO	Every day 0900	JR		09 BC							
12-9	Calan 40 mg	PO	Bid 09-21	JR		09 BC							
12-9	Ceftin 250 mg	PO	tid 09-13-21	JR		09 BC							
12-9	Lanoxin 0.125 mg	PO	Daily 0900	JR		09 BC							
12-9	Capoten 25 mg	PO	Bid 09-21	JR		09 BC							
PRN MEDICATION													
12-9	Dulcolax Supp.	R	prn	JR			19 EK						
12-9	Restoril 15 mg Ṫ	PO	Bedtime prn sleep	JR			21 EK						
12-9	Bancap HC Ṫ	PO	q 4 hr prn	JR		13 EK							

INITIALS / FULL SIGNATURE /TITLE

BC Barbara Christensen RN MS

EK Elaine Kockrow RN MS

ID = PERSON TAKING OFF ORDERS / RN

ROOM: NAME:

A

Fig. 17.3 A, Medication administration record.

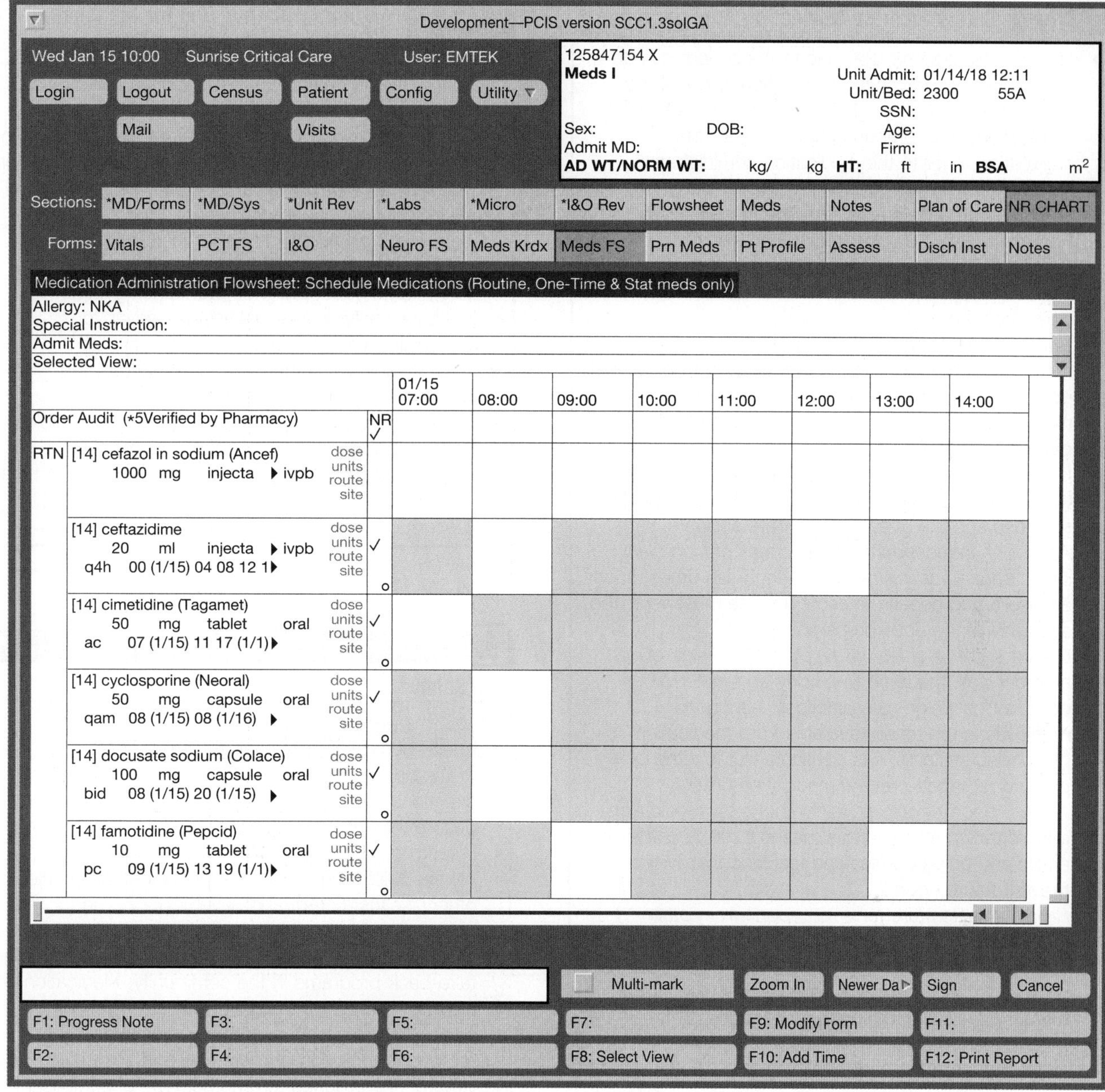

Fig. 17.3, cont'd B, Computerized list of ordered medications. (B, Courtesy Barnes-Jewish Hospital, St. Louis, Missouri. In Elkin MK, Perry AG, Potter PA: *Nursing interventions and clinical skills*, ed 4, St. Louis, 2008, Mosby.)

and organized, and work with the health care facility to establish practices that keep staff members and patients safe. Do not take shortcuts, and never deviate from principles that are effective. Follow these guidelines:

1. If you did not pour it, do not give it.
2. If you gave it, chart it.
3. Do not chart for someone else or have someone else chart for you.
4. Do not transport or accept a container that is not labeled.
5. Do not put down an unlabeled syringe; keep it in your hand or label it before you put it down.
6. If given a verbal order, write it down, and then repeat the order to the health care provider.
7. If you make an error, report it to the charge nurse or supervisor and health care provider. An incident report also should be completed.
8. Never leave a medication tray or cart unattended or unlocked.
9. Do not leave a medication with a patient or family member. Watch the patient take and swallow the medication.
10. Monitor the patient's response to the medication.
11. Chart immediately after giving medication.
12. If a patient refuses medication even after you have performed patient education regarding the medication, do not attempt to force the patient to take it; document "Refused _______ medication because of [state reason patient refused medication]."
13. If you choose to omit a dose based on nursing judgment, request that an RN or another nurse in charge help make the decision. If the medication is omitted, the reason for the omission must be documented. Be objective and exact in charting. Report

Box 17.7 Safety Tips for Medication Administration

- *Listen to the patient.* Listening to the patient can be a mechanism for preventing medication errors. If the patient says that he or she does not take a certain medication when preparing to administer the medication, refer to the medication administration record to ensure an error has not been made.
- *Rely on pharmacists as a resource to prevent errors.* Pharmacists can provide information about medications, including mechanism of action, interactions, compatibility concerns, side effects, and correct dosages.
- *Unit-dose packages.* Prepare only one patient's medications at a time, and leave drugs in their labeled packages. This allows for identification of the medication name before it is administered to the patient.
- *Keep calculations to a minimum.* If calculating a drug dosage, ask another nurse to independently calculate the dose and the rate, and compare answers.
- *Ask for an independent double-check of high-alert drugs before administration.* For high-risk drugs, such as insulin and heparin, a second nurse must verify the accuracy of the dose prepared.
- *Do not sacrifice safety for timeliness.* Outside of emergencies, the need to quickly administer drugs does not outweigh safe practices. Although medications are readily available from medication dispensing systems, it is advisable to allow the pharmacist time to review medication orders.
- *Always report errors.* Incident reports for medication administration errors offer a means to track common errors and guide policies and teaching that will help prevent future errors.
- *Review the literature for error reports from other facilities.* Review of medication error literature is a common practice among quality improvement teams within a facility. A high volume of errors with similar themes may signal the need for review and modification of current medication practices.

Modified from Institute for Safe Medication Practices: *www.ismp.org*.

the decision to the health care provider (see the Home Care Considerations box).

ROUTES OF ADMINISTRATION

Drugs enter the body through three general routes: enteral, percutaneous, and parenteral. The drugs that enter the body by these routes come in various forms, or formulations. In addition to these most common routes, medications may also be administered vaginally and through the anus.

ENTERAL ADMINISTRATION

Drugs that enter through the **enteral** routes (i.e., are absorbed within the GI tract) are given in these forms:

1. *Powders:* Often mixed with a liquid (diluent) before administration

Box 17.8 Additional Safety Tips for Medication Administration

- Follow the six "rights" of medication administration (see Box 17.5).
- Be sure to read labels at least three times (comparing medication administration record with label): (1) when you remove the drug from where it has been stored, (2) before you take it to a patient's room, and (3) before you administer the drug (see Box 17.6).
- Use at least three patient identifiers when possible (e.g., name band, patient's pronouncing name, patient's verifying date of birth) whenever you administer a medication.
- Do not allow any other activity to interrupt the administration of medication to a patient.
- If the health care provider's handwriting is illegible, clarify the order with the health care provider.
- Question orders for unusually large or unusually small doses.
- Document all medications as soon as you give them.

Data from Perry AG, Potter PA, Elkin MK: *Nursing interventions and clinical skills,* ed 5, St. Louis, 2012, Mosby.

Home Care Considerations

Drug Safety

Instruct the patient to do the following:

- Keep each drug in its original labeled container.
- Protect drugs from exposure to heat and light, per directions from manufacturer of the medication.
- Ensure that labels are legible.
- Discard outdated medications.
- Always finish the course of a prescribed drug unless otherwise instructed, and never save a drug for future illnesses.
- The very best way to dispose of drugs is via medicine take-back programs in the community. Medications that are flushed down a sink or toilet may end up in the general drinking water. Some medications can be removed from original containers and mixed with kitty litter, coffee grounds, or another type of unpleasant substance. This would deter animals or other people who may go through the trash from taking the medications.
- Never give a family member or friend a drug prescribed for another person.
- Refrigerate drugs as directed.
- Read labels carefully and follow instructions.
- Notify health care provider of any side effects.

2. *Pills:* Round, solid drug form that must break down into solution form (dissolution) in the stomach
3. *Tablets:* Round, spherical, or other-shaped forms that dissolve in the stomach
   a. *Scored* tablets are indented to allow tablet to be broken in half.
   b. **Enteric-coated** tablets are encased by a coated shell that keeps the tablet from being absorbed in the stomach; absorption takes place in the intestines. *Enteric* pertains to the small intestine.

c. *Capsules* are powders or pellets enclosed in a gelatin-like, elongated, spherical form; the medications are encapsulated because (1) the substance is bad tasting or (2) the substance is a spansule with time-release pellets to delay the action of the drug.
d. *Lozenges,* or *troches,* are sweet mucilage types of tablets that dissolve in the mouth to release medication.

4. *Liquids and suspensions:* Solid particles and liquid that the nurse must shake to allow for the dispersion of solid particles throughout the liquid portion before they can be absorbed by the body
5. *Suppositories:* Drugs mixed with a lubricated substance molded to insert into body cavities such as the rectum, vagina, urethra; absorption occurs after substance melts at body temperature

The following are terms used to describe how medications are administered enterally:

- *PO:* By mouth (oral)
- *Enema:* By rectum
- *Suppository:* By rectum, vagina, or urethra
- *Tubal:* By nasogastric, gastrostomy, or jejunostomy tube

Preparation of Tablets, Pills, and Capsules

Medications in tablet, pill, and capsule form enter the GI tract and are absorbed more slowly into the bloodstream than those taken by any other route. The slow absorption rate makes the PO route safer. Some PO medications are irritating to the patient's GI tract. Also, larger tablets may be difficult for some patients to swallow (Skill 17.1).

Skill 17.1 Administering Tablets, Pills, and Capsules

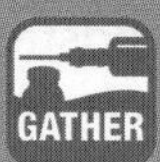

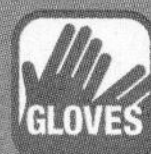

NURSING ACTION *(RATIONALE)*

1. Follow the six "rights" of medication administration (see Box 17.5). *(Prevents medication errors.)*
2. Perform the three label checks (see Box 17.6). *(Prevents medication errors.)*
3. Follow standard precautions. *(Prevents spread of microorganisms.)*
4. Perform hand hygiene. *(Prevents spread of microorganisms.)*
5. If using a unit-dose package, place unopened medication package in medicine cup. *(Prevents medication errors.)*

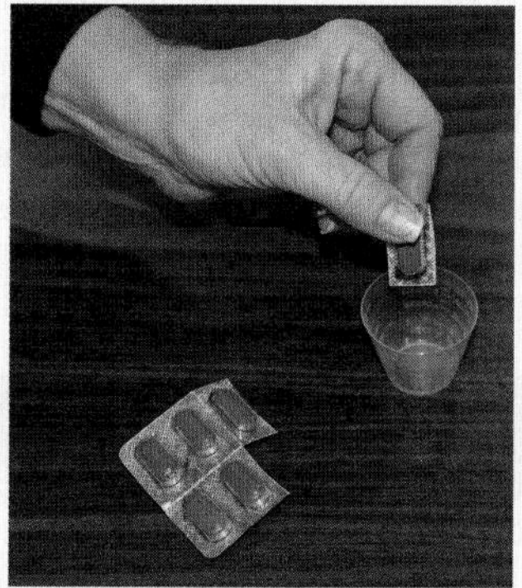

6. If using a multidose bottle, pour tablet, without touching it, into cap of bottle. *(Prevents contamination.)*
7. Pour tablet from cap into medicine cup.
8. If pouring from multidose bottle and patient is to receive several tablets, use a separate cup for medications such as digitalis, and label this cup with the name of the medication. If the patient's pulse is less than 60 bpm, withhold the medication and report this action to the RN and the health care provider. *(Placing digitalis in a separate cup marked with the medication's name allows easy identification.)*
9. If a tablet must be broken in half to administer half the dose, use gloved hands or a cutting device. Break the tablet along the scored line located along the center of the tablet. Depending on the health care facility's policy, the remainder of the tablet should either be disposed of or saved in its original container.
10. If a patient has difficulty swallowing, use a mortar and pestle or other pill-crushing device. The crushed medication often is mixed with applesauce, yogurt, or some other soft food item. Ask the patient his or her preference regarding in what to place the medication. Remember that it is not appropriate to crush drugs that are capsules, enteric coated, long acting, or slow release. These types of drugs are developed to prevent stomach irritation, or the medication may be destroyed by gastric acids. Some medications are not meant to be crushed because crushing increases the absorption rate, and the medication is meant to be released and absorbed slowly. If the medication label specifies "extended release," "sustained release," "XL," "SR," or "CD," then the medication should not be crushed.
11. Any medications dropped during the medication pass must be disposed of according to facility policy. *(Prevents contaminated medications from being administered to patient.)*
12. Transport medication to patient's room.

Continued

Skill 17.1 Administering Tablets, Pills, and Capsules—cont'd

13. Identify patient by checking identification bracelet and per facility policy. *(Prevents medication errors.)*
14. Explain procedure to patient.
15. Document administration of medication on medication administration record (MAR) with time, date, and name or with computerized documentation.
16. Return at an appropriate time to assess patient's response to medication. *(Enables you to determine effectiveness of medication and any occurrence of adverse reactions. Some medication routes act more quickly than other routes.)*
17. Document side effects and therapeutic responses per facility policy.

If the LPN/LVN makes an error in administering medication, it should be reported immediately to the RN. The facility may require the nurse to fill out an incident report to document the error. Do not hesitate to report an error, because prompt intervention may help prevent patient complications related to the error.

Preparation of Liquid Medications

Liquid medication is the formulation often chosen for children; for patients who are not able to swallow tablets, pills, or capsules; and for older adult patients. It is possible to give liquids PO or via a nasogastric, gastrostomy, or jejunostomy tube.

Never give PO liquids to unconscious patients because they could aspirate (inhale) the medication into the respiratory tract.

Some liquid medications (such as cough medicine) are not to be followed with water, and some medications (iron) tend to stain the teeth. Inspect the medication's label (Skill 17.2) for instructions before administering.

Tubal Medications

Nasogastric (NG) tubes that are used to provide nutrition directly into the stomach are used to administer liquid medications to unconscious patients, dysphagic patients (patients who have difficulty swallowing), and those who are too ill to eat. It is also possible to use a gastrostomy tube (placed through the abdominal wall and into the stomach) or jejunostomy tube (placed through the abdominal wall and into the jejunum) in the same manner as the NG tube.

Many tubal medicines come in liquid form. Some that do not, such as those available only as solid tablets, may have to be **pulverized** (crushed to a powder) with the use of crushing device for some patients. Mix the crushed tablet with 30 mL of water, and administer the mixture through the tube. It is also possible to open capsules, mix the contents with 30 mL of water, and administer this mixture through a tube (Skill 17.3). However, not all tablets are safe to be crushed (e.g., enteric coated), and not all capsules are safe to be opened (e.g., medications that are time released). Doing so creates the risk of toxic effects (see Skill 17.1, Step 10). Check the correct clinical pharmacology reference or the *Physician's Desk Reference* to verify the safety of pulverizing specific tablets or opening specific capsules.

OTHER METHODS OF MEDICATION ADMINISTRATION

Suppositories

A suppository is a cone-, egg-, or spindle-shaped medication made for insertion into the rectum, vagina, or urethra. Suppositories dissolve at body temperature and are absorbed directly into the bloodstream. Suppositories are useful for infants, patients who cannot take oral preparations, and patients who are experiencing nausea or are vomiting (Skill 17.4).

Suppositories should be stored in a cool place so that they do not melt. They often are stored in a refrigerator.

Vaginal Irrigation and Medication Administration

Internal vaginal irrigation, or douching, usually is avoided medically unless as a preparation for surgery. Secretions from the vaginal membranes protect the vaginal area from infection, and so it is desirable *not* to wash these protective agents away. The health care provider orders the type of solution to use, such as saline, sterile water, or medicated solutions and how often to perform the procedure. Commercially prepared douches are also available for one-time use, but the patient should be advised that it is not recommended to douche routinely, even at home (Skill 17.5 and the Coordinated Care box on vaginal irrigation). In addition, female patients may develop vaginal infections, which necessitate topical application of antiinfective agents.

 Coordinated Care

Delegation

Vaginal Irrigation

- The task of administering a vaginal irrigation can be delegated to unlicensed assistive personnel (UAP) in some settings (check facility policy), unless the irrigation consists of medication administration. Initial patient evaluation requires the critical thinking of a nurse, and delegation of medical administration is inappropriate.
- Vaginal medications are available in foam, jelly, cream, and suppository forms. Excessive use of medicated douches can lead to irritation of the vaginal mucosa, and their use should be avoided (see Skill 17.5).

Text continued on p. 449

Skill 17.2 Administering Liquid Medications

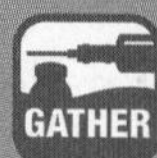
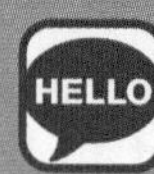

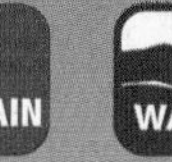
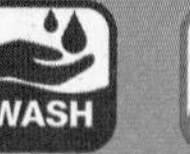
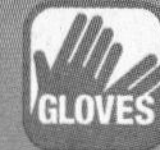

NURSING ACTION *(RATIONALE)*

1. Follow the six "rights" of medication administration (see Box 17.5). *(Prevents medication errors.)*
2. Perform the three label checks (see Box 17.6). *(Prevents medication errors.)*
3. Follow standard precautions. *(Prevents spread of microorganisms.)*
4. Perform hand hygiene. *(Prevents spread of microorganisms.)*
5. Remove liquid preparation from patient's drug box, bin, medication cabinet, or computerized medication dispenser.
6. Check dose/milliliter and total volume of medication in container.
7. Calculate dosage; if the dose ordered is different from the dose/milliliter stated on the label, calculate correct dose; if ordered medication is labeled according to a different measurement system, convert by using appropriate equivalent. Work calculation on paper.
8. Check calculations with another nurse. *(Helps prevent errors.)*
9. Obtain medicine cup that is **graduated** (has markings indicating marked amount; total volume of cup is 30 mL, or 1 oz) or appropriate graduated syringe. *(For accuracy.)*
10. Face label of bottle toward palm of hand *(to avoid soiling label)*; if label becomes soiled, return the bottle to the pharmacy. Do not give medication if label is unreadable. *(Maintains accuracy and prevents errors.)*
11. Place medicine cup on flat surface to pour while you watch at eye level, or hold medication cup up at eye level while you pour. *(Maintains accuracy.)*
12. Place cap of bottle with inner rim up to prevent contaminating inside of cap. *(To prevent contaminating remaining contents of bottle.)*
13. Read dosage amount at lowest level of **meniscus** (curve formed by liquid's upper surface). *(For accuracy.)* This can be achieved by holding the medicine cup or sitting it on a flat surface.

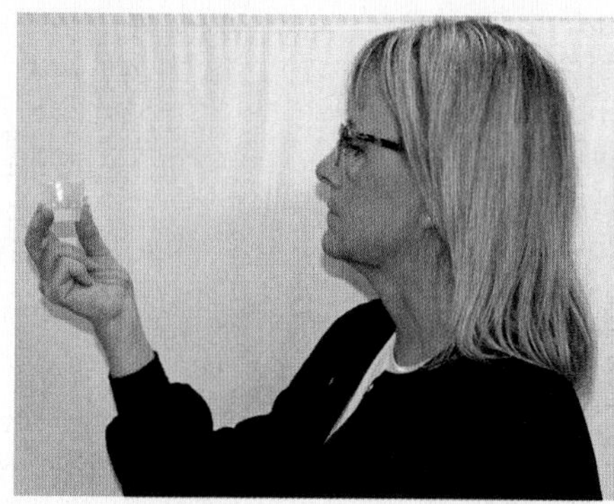

14. Transport medication to patient's room.
15. Identify patient by checking identification bracelet and per facility policy. *(Prevents medication errors.)*
16. Explain procedure to patient.
17. Document administration on medication administration record, whether on paper copy or with computer. Note time, date, and medication name.
18. Return at appropriate time to assess patient's response to medication. *(Enables you to determine effectiveness of medication and any occurrence of adverse reactions.)*
19. Document assessment findings in nursing notes.

Skill 17.3 Administering Medications Through Nasogastric Tubing

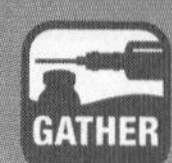
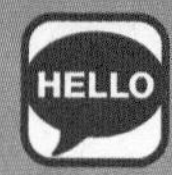

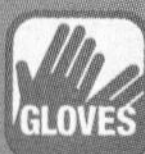

NURSING ACTION *(RATIONALE)*

1. Follow the six "rights" of medication administration (see Box 17.5). *(Prevents medication errors.)*
2. Perform the three label checks (see Box 17.6). *(Prevents medication errors.)*
3. Follow standard precautions. *(Prevents spread of microorganisms.)*
4. Perform hand hygiene. *(Prevents spread of microorganisms.)*
5. Prepare medication by using the same procedure as for liquid medications.

Continued

Skill 17.3 Administering Medications Through Nasogastric Tubing—cont'd

6. Gather equipment. *(Organizes procedure.)*
   - Disposable gloves
   - 10- to 20-mL syringe
   - One or more towels
   - Stethoscope
   - Bulb or Asepto syringe
   - Tap water
7. Transport equipment and medication to patient's room.
8. Identify patient by checking identification bracelet and per facility policy. *(Prevents medication errors.)*
9. Explain procedure; answer questions that patient may have about the procedure. *(Establishes trust.)*
10. Place patient in high Fowler's position.
11. Put towel or towels over patient's chest and abdomen. *(Protects clothing and bed linens.)*
12. Don clean gloves. *(Reduces spread of microorganisms.)*
13. Check and recheck placement and patency of tube per facility policy (see also Chapter 15, Skill 15.5, Step 24). *(Ensures that tube is in the stomach and not in the respiratory tract.)* The following are several methods that may be used to check for accurate placement of a nasogastric (NG) tube:
    a. *Method A:* Attach piston or Asepto syringe to end of NG tube. Pull plunger back or release suction of bulb syringe to aspirate stomach contents. If stomach contents are seen, instill 10 to 20 mL of water before medication administration to clear tube; proceed with administration of medication. Because of the difficulty in withdrawing fluid from small-bore feeding tubes, nurses often rely incorrectly on the auscultatory method to confirm NG feeding tube placement. Monitor the patient for signs and symptoms of tube displacement.

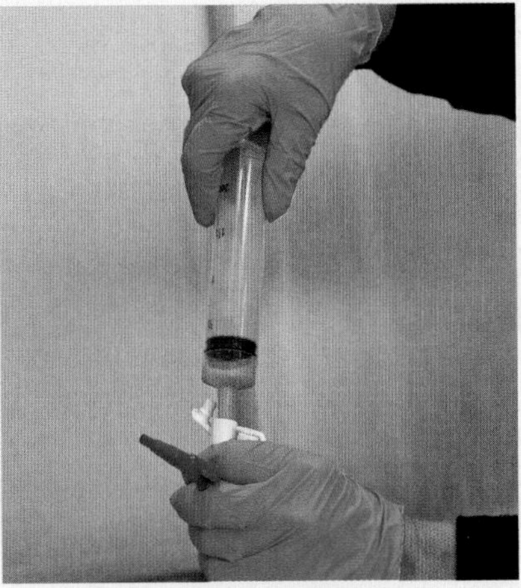

    b. *Method B:* Place stethoscope over patient's stomach. Push 10 mL of air through NG tube with syringe. *(The rush of air is heard in stomach with stethoscope if tube is in stomach.)* Proceed with medication. (This method is still sometimes used at the patient's bedside to check placement, but some studies indicate that this is not a reliable method. Sounds created by instillation of air may be transmitted from the pleural space to the upper abdomen, giving a false impression of accurate placement. Follow facility policy.)
    c. *Method C:* Some facilities are using the litmus test instead of the auscultatory (air-instillation) method. Measure pH of aspirate with color-coded pH paper. The reference numbers associated with specific colors are whole numbers and range from 1 to 11. Gastric aspirates are acidic with pH values of 5 or less.
14. Clamp enteral tube with rubber-tipped hemostats, with another clamping device, or by bending tubing in one hand, per facility policy. *(Prevents leakage of fluid from tube.)*
15. Attach syringe to end of tube (with plunger out of syringe).
16. Pour medication into syringe.

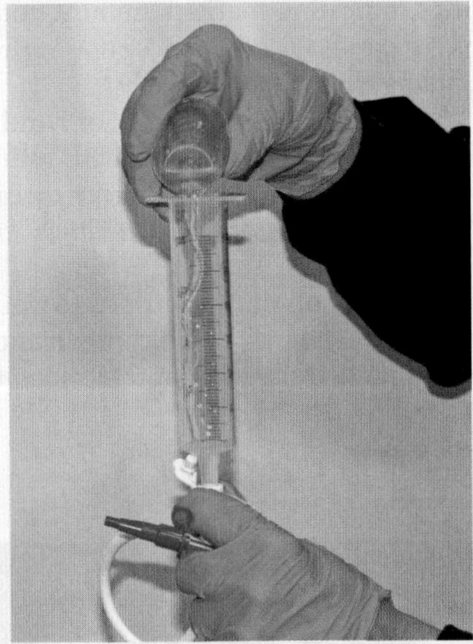

17. Unclamp tubing to allow medication to slowly flow by gravity.
18. Follow medication with 30 to 50 mL of water or per health care provider's order. *(Flushes the medication into stomach. Water is essential to enhance absorption of medication and is used to clean and maintain patency of NG tube.)*
19. Clamp tubing: secure tube after medication is given.

Skill 17.3 Administering Medications Through Nasogastric Tubing—cont'd

20. If NG tube is attached to suction, do not reconnect suction for 30 minutes or per facility policy. *(The medication will then have time to become absorbed because it will not be aspirated through tube.)*
21. Remove towel or towels from patient.
22. Remove gloves.
23. Leave patient in comfortable position.
24. Gather equipment; clean up patient and area.
25. Perform hand hygiene. *(Prevents spread of microorganisms.)*
26. Document administration of NG medication. Remember to document the amount of fluid used for medication administration as intake on the intake and output (I&O) sheet or per computerized documentation. *(Ensures accurate I&O measurement.)*
27. Return to assess patient's response to medication. *(Enables you to determine effectiveness of medication and any occurrence of adverse reactions.)*
28. Document assessment findings in nursing notes.

Skill 17.4 Administering Rectal Suppositories

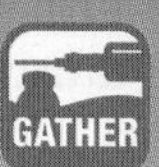

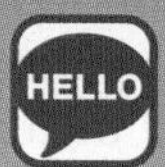

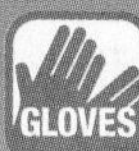

NURSING ACTION *(RATIONALE)*

1. Follow the six "rights" of medication administration (see Box 17.5). *(Prevents medication errors.)*
2. Perform the three label checks (see Box 17.6). *(Prevents medication errors.)* Ensure that the patient does not have any contraindications for giving the type of medication in a suppository form.
3. Follow standard precautions. *(Prevents spread of microorganisms.)*
4. Gather equipment. *(Organizes procedure.)*
   - Gloves
   - Lubricant
   - Suppository
   - Souffle cup
5. Perform hand hygiene. *(Prevents spread of microorganisms.)*
6. Obtain suppository from refrigerator or from patient's medication bin.
7. Place unopened suppository into medicine cup or **souffle cup** (ungraduated disposable paper cup).
8. Introduce yourself; explain procedure to patient. *(Enlists patient's cooperation and establishes trust.)*
9. Identify patient by checking identification bracelet and per facility policy. *(Prevents medication errors.)*
10. Provide privacy.
11. Don clean gloves. *(Protects you from fecal material and reduces the spread of microorganisms.)*
12. Position patient in Sims' position (on left side with upper leg flexed at knee). *(Position exposes anus and helps patient to relax external anal sphincter. Left-side positioning lessens the likelihood that the suppository or feces will be expelled.)*
13. Unwrap suppository.
14. Maintain privacy; expose patient's buttocks.
15. Assess anus externally and gently palpate rectal vault as needed. *(Enables you to determine presence of active rectal bleeding, as well as to note whether rectum contains feces, which potentially cause problems with suppository placement.)* Do not palpate a patient's rectum after rectal surgery. If a patient has hemorrhoids, always use a generous amount of a lubricating gel and gently manipulate the tissues to visualize the anus for insertion of the suppository.
16. Apply water-soluble lubricant to tapered end of suppository. *(Lubrication reduces friction as suppository enters rectal area.)*
17. Ask patient to take deep breath; insert tapered end of suppository beyond internal anal sphincter. Insert suppository as patient exhales to relax anal sphincter. *(Forcing suppository through constricted sphincter causes discomfort.)*
18. Ask patient to retain suppository as long as possible. *(This allows the medication to completely dissolve and absorb through mucous membranes of rectum into capillaries of systemic circulatory system.)* Hold the patient's buttocks together to help patient retain suppository. *(Provides sufficient time for the effects of the suppository to reach the maximum effectiveness.)*
19. Discard gloves.
20. Perform hand hygiene. *(Reduces spread of microorganisms.)*
21. Help patient assume a comfortable position.
22. Document administration of suppository per facility policy.
23. Return to assess patient's response to medication. *(Enables you to determine effectiveness of medication and any occurrence of adverse reactions.)*
24. Document assessment findings in nursing notes.

Skill 17.5 Performing a Vaginal Irrigation or Douche

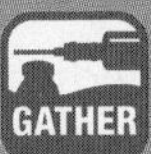

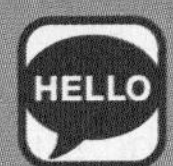

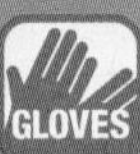

NURSING ACTION *(RATIONALE)*

1. Refer to Standard Steps 1 to 9.
2. Assemble equipment:
   - Bath blanket
   - Bedpan and tissues
   - Clean gloves
   - Douche kit
   - Drape
   - Ordered solution (1000 to 1500 mL at body temperature or commercially prepared solutions in smaller amounts)
   - Solution container, tubing, and nozzle
   - Wash basin, washcloths, and towel (disposable washcloths are acceptable)
   - Waterproof pad
3. Assist patient to the supine position with legs abducted slightly. *(Position allows for easy access to and good exposure of vaginal orifice.)*
4. Prepare patient:
   a. Drape patient's abdomen and lower extremities with blanket. *(Minimizes patient's embarrassment.)*
   b. Position patient on bedpan with waterproof pad underneath. *(Allows hips to be higher than shoulders so that solution will reach posterior vagina and distend the vaginal wall, ensuring that solution reaches between the folds of the vagina. Bedpan collects solution, and pad protects bed linens.)*
   c. Be certain vaginal orifice is well illuminated. *(Ensures visualization of external genitalia for proper insertion.)*
5. Evaluate for the following. *(Findings provide baseline to monitor effect of therapy.)*
   a. Condition of external genitalia and vaginal canal
   b. Symptoms of pruritus, burning sensation, or discomfort
   c. Possible vaginal discharge and odor; perineal care is sometimes necessary before the douche is administered. *(A thick, white, patchy, curdlike discharge clinging to the vaginal walls is a sign of yeast infection, a common female disorder.)*
   d. Signs of inflammation, erythema, or edema in the perineal area
6. Prepare equipment. *(Organizes procedure.)* Ensure solution is at body temperature. *(Prevents burning the delicate mucosa of the vagina.)*
7. Perform hand hygiene, and don clean gloves. *(Prevents spread of microorganisms.)*
8. Allow some solution to drain down the tubing out through the nozzle into bedpan. *(Removes air from tubing and moistens nozzle.)* Gently retract labial folds and maintain position. Direct nozzle toward the sacrum, following the floor of the vagina. *(Allows correct position of nozzle.)*
9. Raise the container approximately 12 to 20 inches (30 to 50 cm) above level of vagina, and insert nozzle 3 to 4 inches (7 to 10 cm). Allow solution to flow while nozzle is inserted and rotated. Instruct patient to tighten perineal muscles as if to suppress urination and then relax. Have patient repeat this maneuver four or five times during procedure. Administer all of the solution. *(Allowing solution to flow during insertion moistens the vaginal orifice, thus reducing friction. Rotating the nozzle allows irrigation of all areas in the vagina. Periodic contracting and relaxing of perineal muscles allows solution to flow between rugae.)*
10. Withdraw nozzle, raise head of bed, and assist patient to a comfortable position while she remains on the bedpan. *(The remaining solution drains by gravity. The bedpan collects solution.)*
11. Refer to Standard Steps 10 to 17.
12. Allow patient to remain on bedpan for approximately 10 minutes; then don clean gloves, remove bedpan, and observe results. Dispose of returned solution in proper manner (know facility policy). Cleanse patient or allow patient to cleanse herself with basin of warm water, towel, and washcloth. Assist patient to a comfortable position. Remove gloves, discard them in proper receptacle, and perform hand hygiene. *(Reduces spread of microorganisms and provides for patient comfort.)*
13. Document the following. *(Verifies performance of procedure and ensures continuity of care.)*
    - Date and time
    - Type, amount, and temperature of solution
    - Evaluation of external genitalia and vagina *(Documented description provides baseline to determine change in patient's condition.)*
    - Patient's response to procedure
    - Patient teaching
14. Report unusual findings.

PERCUTANEOUS ADMINISTRATION

Dosage forms used with the **percutaneous** route (through the skin or mucous membranes) include lotions, ointments, creams, and powders.

The percutaneous routes are as follows:

1. *Topical:* applied to the skin
2. *Instillation:*
   a. Applied to the mucous membranes of the mouth
      (1) **Sublingual** (under the tongue)
      (2) **Buccal** (in the cheek)
   b. Applied to the mucous membranes of eye, ear, nose, and vagina
3. *Inhalation:* aerosolized liquids, gases

The percutaneous routes are routes by which medications are absorbed through the skin or the mucous membranes. Most percutaneous medications produce a local action, but some also produce a systemic action.

The percutaneous routes include **topical applications** (applied to the skin), instillations, and inhalations. Absorption is rapid. Topical medications include ointments, creams, powders, lotions, and transdermal patches.

Ointments

An ointment is an oil-based semisolid medication; the nurse applies it to the skin or a mucous membrane. When nitroglycerin is applied topically, its effect lasts longer than that of the tablet form of nitroglycerin that is administered sublingually.

Creams

Creams are semisolid, nongreasy emulsions that contain medication for external application. The nurse gently rubs creams into the area. Certain creams are prescription medications, and it is necessary to follow directions for application carefully to prevent overdosage.

Lotions

Lotions are generally aqueous preparations that are used as soothing agents to relieve pruritus or protect the skin, cleanse the skin, or act as astringents. Lotions contain suspended particles that are dispersed throughout the solution by gentle shaking of the bottle before application. Gently pat (do not rub) lotions onto the skin; they can be removed with soap and water (Skill 17.6).

Transdermal Patches (Topical Disk)

Adhesive-backed medicated patches are applied to the skin and provide sustained, continuous release of medication over several hours or days. Examples of medications used in transdermal patches are analgesics, nitroglycerin, nicotine, and estrogen. Choose a clean, dry area of the body. It should not be placed over an area where the skin is impaired, an area with body hair, or an area that is oily. If the skin is impaired, more medication may be absorbed. If the skin has hair or is very oily, the transdermal patch does not stick well (Fig. 17.4).

Skills for Sensory Disorders

Eyedrops and eye ointments. Eyedrops and ointments are sterile. Ensure that the *ophthalmic* (eye) preparations are administered when at room temperature and that they remain sterile by not touching the dropper or the tube of ointment to the eye. Check the container to ensure that the medication is marked "for ophthalmic use." Eyedrops and ophthalmic ointments are prescribed for only one patient and are not meant to be shared between patients (Skill 17.7).

Eardrops. Containers of solutions to be used as eardrops are labeled *otic.* The eardrops should be at room temperature when applied. The eardrops are prescribed for only one patient and are not meant to be shared between patients (Skill 17.8).

Nose drops. Nose drops are for individual use only (Skill 17.9).

Nasal sprays. Because nasal sprays are absorbed quickly, less medication is used and wasted when the nurse administers them in this manner. Nasal sprays are for individual use only (Skill 17.10).

Irrigations

Eye irrigations. **Irrigations** involve a gentle washing of an area with a stream of solution delivered through a syringe. Irrigations of the eye usually are performed to relieve local inflammation of the conjunctiva, to apply antiseptic solution, or to flush out exudate or caustic or irritating solutions. In most cases, warm normal saline and a small syringe or eyedropper are used to instill a few hundred milliliters of solution. Plain water is also acceptable, especially in an emergency situation. Always perform irrigation from the inner to the outer canthus to lessen the chances that contaminants will be absorbed through the nasolacrimal duct (Skill 17.11 and the Patient Teaching box on eye care). Never allow the syringe tip to touch the eye. When caustic chemicals enter the eye, make sure to gently flush the eye continuously for at least 15 minutes with tap water to prevent burning of the cornea, and then refer the patient immediately to a health care provider.

Performing eye irrigation requires the skill and knowledge of a nurse. Delegation of this task to UAP is inappropriate.

In the home, a family member or the patient may perform eye irrigation with an eye cup. These cups are made of plastic or glass and are available in most drugstores. Instruct the patient about proper cleaning of the cup between uses and about the need to check for chips in the glass.

If copious amounts of irrigation solution are needed, it is possible to use intravenous (IV) tubing and a bag of

Text continued on p. 455

Skill 17.6 Applying Topical Agents

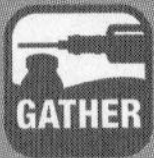

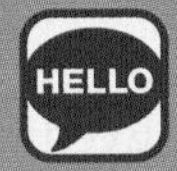

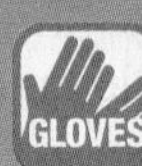

NURSING ACTION *(RATIONALE)*

1. Follow the six "rights" of medication administration (see Box 17.5). *(Prevents medication errors.)*
2. Perform the three label checks (see Box 17.6). *(Prevents medication errors.)*
3. Follow standard precautions. *(Reduces spread of microorganisms.)*
4. Gather equipment. *(Organizes procedure.)*
   - Gloves
   - Medication
   - Washing materials
5. Perform hand hygiene. *(Reduces spread of microorganisms.)*
6. Transport medication to patient's room.
7. Identify patient by checking identification bracelet and per facility policy. *(Prevents medication errors.)*
8. Introduce yourself; explain procedure to patient. *(Establishes trust.)*
9. Provide privacy; place patient in comfortable position that allows exposure of selected site.
10. Don gloves. *(Reduces spread of microorganisms and prevents absorption of topical agent into your skin.)*
11. Read prescription instructions carefully. *(For accuracy.)*
12. Prepare medicinal agent (ointments, creams, and lotions sometimes have to be squeezed or removed with a tongue blade, depending on preparation used).
13. Wash affected area, removing debris, encrustations, and previous medications. *(Removal of debris enhances penetration of topical drug through skin. Cleansing removes microorganisms resident in remaining debris.)* Area should be allowed to dry. *(Allows for better adherence to the skin.)*
14. With gloves on, apply medication lotion, ointment, or cream via paper, or apply medication patch (see Fig. 17.4) directly to skin. When using medication patches, be certain to remove old patch and remove plastic from disk of the new patch before applying to skin. Patches must be disposed of by folding it upon itself and following facility policy for disposal. *(Essential for absorption of medication. Do not massage medication into skin; this can cause a bolus of medication to be administered. Patches are folded upon themselves to prevent others from absorbing the medication. Some facilities may have special instructions for disposal of narcotic pain medication patches.)*
15. Remove gloves.
16. Leave patient in comfortable position.
17. Answer patient's questions and teach patient to perform self-applications if appropriate.
18. Clean work area.
19. Wash hands. *(Reduces spread of microorganisms.)*
20. Document administration per facility policy on paper copy of medication administration record or with computerized documentation system.
21. Return to assess patient's response to medication. *(Enables you to determine effectiveness of medication and any occurrence of adverse reactions.)*
22. Document assessment findings in nursing notes.

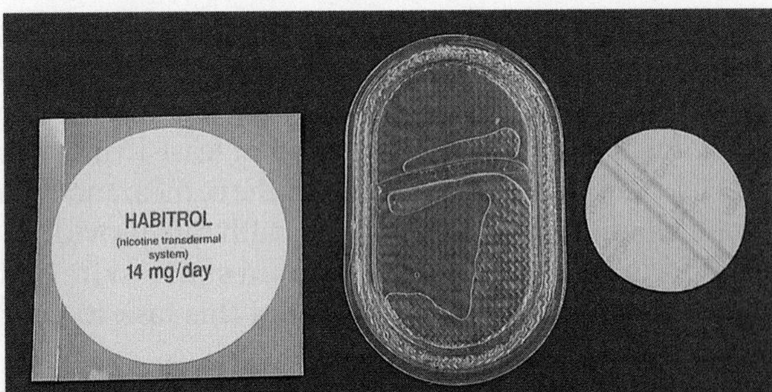

Fig. 17.4 Various medications are available as transdermal patches.

Patient Teaching

Eye Care

- Use a calm, confident, soft voice when talking with patient, and reinforce the importance of the procedure.
- Remove the patient's contact lenses if possible before beginning irrigation or applying a compress.
- Reassure patient that the eye can be closed periodically and that no object will touch the eye.
- Ask patient to report any pain or foreign body sensation in the eye after irrigation, as well as any excessive tearing or photophobia.
- Have the patient close the eye to avoid movement, and report to the health care provider at once if any symptoms of irritation or infection occur.
- If a patient needs continuing eye irrigations at home but is unable to perform them, teach a responsible family member or caregiver.
- If the patient's field of vision is limited, the home environment should be evaluated, and special safety precautions should be taken.

Skill 17.7 Administering Eyedrops and Eye Ointments

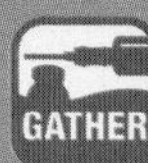

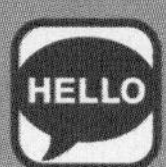

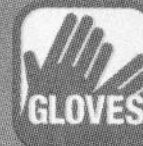

NURSING ACTION *(RATIONALE)*

1. Follow the six "rights" of medication administration (see Box 17.5). *(Prevents medication errors.)*
2. Perform the three label checks (see Box 17.6). *(Prevents medication errors.)*
3. Follow standard precautions. *(Prevents spread of microorganisms.)*
4. Gather equipment. *(Organizes procedure.)*
   - Cotton ball or tissue
   - Eyedrops
   - Gloves
   - Sterile saline
5. Perform hand hygiene. *(Prevents spread of microorganisms.)*
6. Confirm medication is ophthalmic preparation. Transport medication to patient's room.
7. Identify patient by checking identification bracelet and asking patient's name and birth date. *(Prevents medication errors.)*
8. Introduce yourself; explain procedure. *(Establishes trust.)*
9. Provide privacy; position back of patient's head on pillow; direct patient's face upward toward ceiling.
10. Determine which eye is to receive the medication or whether both eyes should.
11. Don gloves. *(Reduces spread of microorganisms.)*
12. Remove exudate; clean eye as needed with sterile solution of saline or water; use cotton balls to wipe away exudate; use one cotton ball per stroke, wiping from inner canthus outward. *(Cleansing eye from inner to outer canthus avoids introducing microorganisms into lacrimal ducts. Soaking allows easy removal of dried exudate that harbors microorganisms.)*
13. To apply drops:
    a. Expose lower conjunctival sac by having patient look upward while gentle traction is applied to lower eyelid.

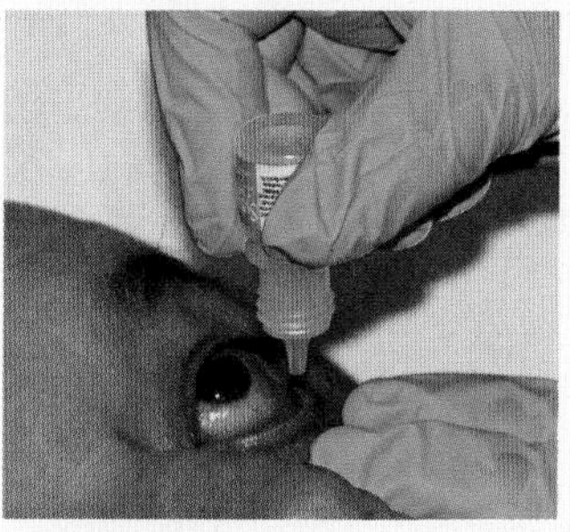

    b. Put prescribed number of drops into conjunctival sac, not onto eyeball. *(Therapeutic effect of drug is obtained only when drops enter sac.)*
    c. Conjunctival sac normally holds one or two drops. *(Applying drops to conjunctival sac provides even distribution of medicine across eye.)*
    d. Use tissue to apply gentle pressure above bone at inner corner of eyelid for 1 to 2 minutes. *(Minimizes absorption into circulatory system.)*
    e. Apply sterile dressing, if it is ordered.
14. To apply ointment:
    a. Expose lower conjunctival sac by having patient look upward while gentle traction is applied to lower eyelid.

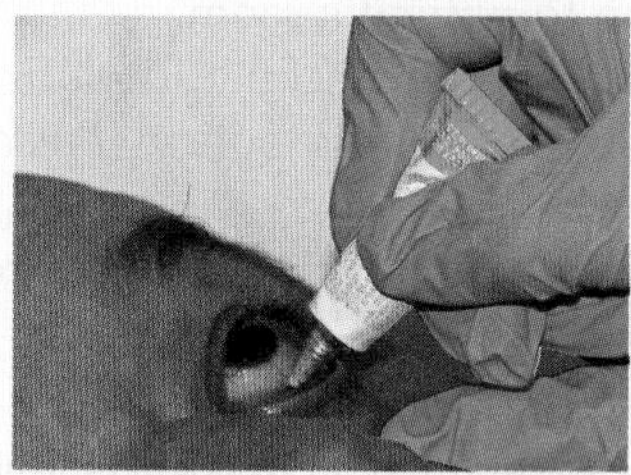

    b. Squeeze ointment into lower conjunctival sac.
    c. Ask patient to close eye and move it around in circular motion. *(Spreads medication evenly.)*
    d. Apply sterile dressing, if it is ordered.
15. After applying drops or ointment to an eye, leave patient in comfortable position; clean up the work area.
16. Remove gloves and wash hands. *(Reduces spread of microorganisms.)*
17. Answer patient's questions and, if appropriate, teach patient to perform self-care.
18. Record administration of medications per facility policy.
19. Return to assess patient's response to medication. *(Enables you to determine effectiveness of medication and any occurrence of adverse reactions.)*
20. Document assessment findings in nursing notes.

Skill 17.8 Administering Eardrops

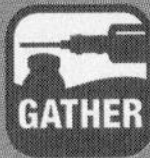

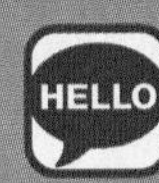

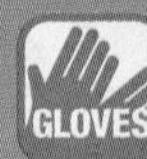

NURSING ACTION *(RATIONALE)*

1. Follow the six "rights" of medication administration (see Box 17.5). *(Prevents medication errors.)*
2. Perform the three label checks (see Box 17.6). *(Prevents medication errors.)*
3. Follow standard precautions. *(Prevents spread of microorganisms.)*
4. Gather equipment. *(Organizes procedure.)*
   - Eardrops
   - Gloves
   - Cotton ball
5. Perform hand hygiene. *(Prevents spread of microorganisms.)*
6. Confirm medication is otic preparation. Transport medication to patient's room.
7. Identify patient by checking identification bracelet and per facility policy. *(Prevents medication errors.)*
8. Introduce yourself; explain procedure. *(Establishes trust.)*
9. Provide privacy.
10. Determine which ear is to receive the medication; position patient with affected ear upward.
11. Don gloves. *(Reduces spread of microorganisms.)*
12. Remove external exudate from ear; it is necessary to obtain an order for irrigating the ear. *(Drainage harbors microorganisms and sometimes impedes distribution of medication into the canal.)*
13. Draw medication into dropper.
14. Instill drops:
    a. *For adults and for children older than 3 years:* Turn head with affected side up; pull earlobe upward and back to straighten external auditory canal; instill drops without touching ear with dropper. *(Straightening of ear canal provides direct access to deeper external structures.)*

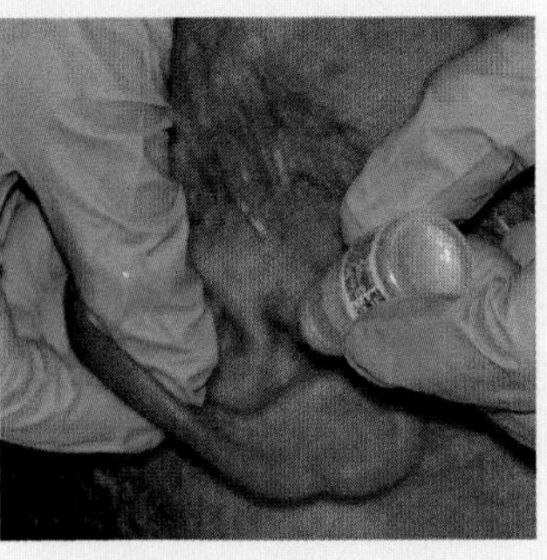

    b. *For children younger than 3 years:* Turn head with affected side up; pull earlobe downward and back; instill drops without touching ear with dropper. *(Straightening of ear canal provides direct access to deeper external structures.)*

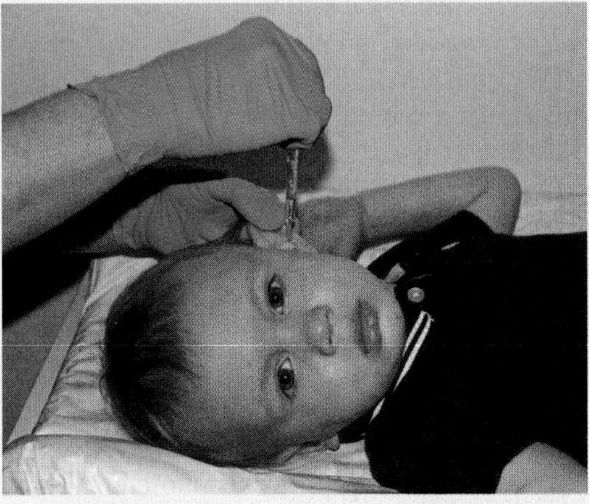

15. Tell patient to remain in same position for 5 to 10 minutes to allow medication to drain into ear by gravity. *(To promote distribution of drops in ear canal.)*
16. Place a cotton ball loosely into ear as needed. *(Prevents escape of medication when patient sits or stands.)*
17. Remove gloves.
18. Leave patient in comfortable position; clean work area.
19. Answer patient's questions and, if appropriate, teach patient self-care.
20. Perform hand hygiene. *(Reduces spread of microorganisms.)*
21. Record administration of medications per facility policy.
22. Return to assess patient's response to medication. *(Enables you to determine effectiveness of medication and any occurrence of adverse reactions.)*
23. Document assessment findings in nursing notes.

Skill 17.9 Administering Nose Drops

 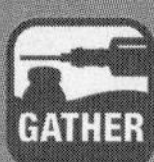 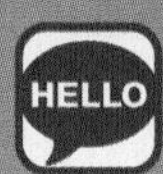 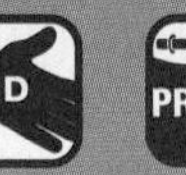   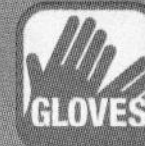

NURSING ACTION *(RATIONALE)*

1. Follow the six "rights" of medication administration (see Box 17.5). *(Prevents medication errors.)*

2. Perform the three label checks (see Box 17.6). *(Prevents medication errors.)*

3. Follow standard precautions. *(Prevents spread of microorganisms.)*

4. Gather equipment. *(Organizes procedure.)*
- Nose drops
- Gloves
- Tissues

5. Perform hand hygiene. *(Prevents spread of microorganisms.)*

6. Confirm medication is nasal preparation. Transport medication to patient's room.

7. Identify patient by checking identification bracelet and per facility policy. *(Prevents medication errors.)*

8. Introduce yourself; explain procedure. *(Establishes trust.)*

9. Provide privacy.

10. Don gloves. *(Reduces spread of microorganisms.)*

11. If patient is an adult or older child, ask patient to clear nose of accumulations by blowing gently into tissue. *(Allows absorption of medication.)*

12. Determine which nostril is to receive the medication or whether both nostrils should.

13. Position patient:

a. *Adult or older child:* Have patient lie down, hanging head backward over edge of bed (if condition permits) or with pillow under shoulders to hyperextend the neck if patient can tolerate it. *(Promotes absorption of medication.)*

b. *Younger child:* Position child on bed with head backward and downward. *(Promotes absorption of medication.)*

c. *Infant:* Hold infant with head backward and downward. *(Promotes absorption of medication.)*

14. After drawing medication into dropper, instill medication while holding dropper above (not touching) nostril being treated.

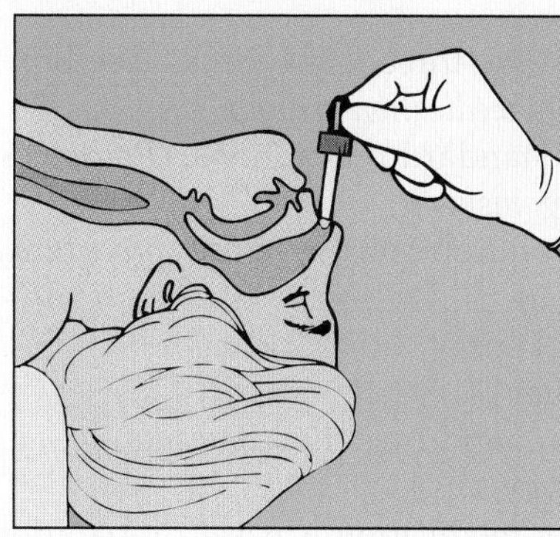

15. If orders specify treatment in both nostrils, repeat procedure to instill drops in other nostril.

16. Tell patient to hold position for a few minutes. *(Allows medication to remain in place.)*

17. Remove gloves.

18. Tell patient to refrain from blowing nose immediately after instillation. *(Prevents removal of medication.)*

19. Offer tissues for later use.

20. Leave patient in comfortable position; clean work area.

21. Answer patient's questions and, if appropriate, teach patient self-care.

22. Perform hand hygiene. *(Reduces spread of microorganisms.)*

23. Record administration of medications per facility policy.

24. Return to assess patient's response to medication. *(Enables you to determine effectiveness of medication and any occurrence of adverse reactions.)*

25. Document assessment findings in nursing notes.

Step 14 figure from Clayton BD, Willihnganz M: *Basic pharmacology for nurses*, ed 17, St. Louis, 2017, Elsevier.

Skill 17.10 Administering Nasal Sprays

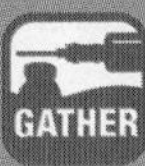

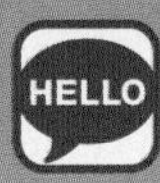

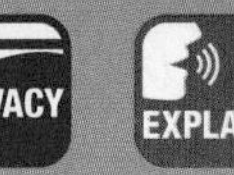

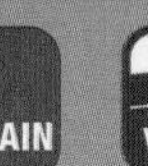

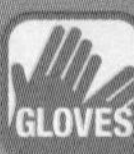

NURSING ACTION *(RATIONALE)*

1. Follow the six "rights" of medication administration (see Box 17.5). *(Prevents medication errors.)*
2. Perform the three label checks (see Box 17.6). *(Prevents medication errors.)*
3. Follow standard precautions. *(Prevents spread of microorganisms.)*
4. Gather equipment. *(Organizes procedure.)*
   - Gloves
   - Nasal spray
   - Tissues
5. Perform hand hygiene. *(Prevents spread of microorganisms.)*
6. Confirm medication is nasal preparation. Transport medication to patient.
7. Determine which nostril is to receive the medication or whether both should.
8. Identify patient by checking identification bracelet and per facility policy. *(Prevents medication errors.)*
9. Introduce yourself; explain procedure. *(Establishes trust.)*
10. Provide privacy; position patient upright.
11. Don gloves. *(Reduces spread of microorganisms.)*
12. Have patient gently blow nose, if capable, to clear nasal passages of accumulations. *(Promotes absorption of medication.)*
13. Compress one nostril.
14. Shake bottle while holding it upright. *(To mix solution.)*
15. Insert tip of spray bottle into patient's patent nostril.
16. Instruct patient to inhale through the nose; while patient inhales, squeeze bottle.
17. If orders specify treatment in both nostrils, repeat procedure for other nostril.
18. Tell patient to refrain from blowing nose for a few minutes; offer tissues for later use. *(Promotes absorption of medication.)*
19. Answer patient's questions and, if appropriate, teach self-administration.
20. Remove gloves and wash hands. *(Reduces spread of microorganisms.)*
21. Record administration of medications per facility policy.
22. Return to assess patient's response to medication. *(Enables you to determine effectiveness of medication and any occurrence of adverse reactions.)*
23. Document assessment findings in nursing notes.

Skill 17.11 Eye Irrigation

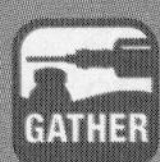

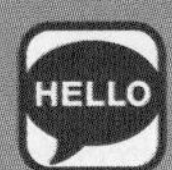

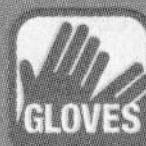

NURSING ACTION *(RATIONALE)*

1. Refer to Standard Steps 1 to 9.
2. Assemble equipment:
   - Aseptic syringe, small bulb syringe, or plastic squeeze bottle
   - Clean gloves (mask and protective eyewear are also recommended if splashing is anticipated)
   - Cotton balls
   - Cotton-tipped applicators
   - Curved emesis basin
   - Gauze
   - Moisture-proof towel or pad
   - Sterile basin for solution
   - Warm irrigation solution as prescribed (volume depends on purpose; 200 to 500 mL)
3. Determine condition of both eyes. *(Provides baseline data to help determine change after irrigation.)*
4. Position patient with affected eye down. *(Prevents solution and contaminants from flowing into other eye.)*
5. Place moisture-proof towel or pad under patient's head. *(Prevents soiling of bed linens.)*
6. Place an emesis basin at side of face. *(Collects irrigating solution.)*
7. Don gloves. *(Reduces spread of microorganisms and protects the patient and the nurse.)*
8. Check that the irrigating solution is the correct temperature. *(Using solutions at body temperature prevents adverse reactions.)* Pour a small amount of irrigating solution into sterile basin.

Skill 17.11 Eye Irrigation—cont'd

9. Using the thumb and index finger of the nondominant hand, separate the patient's eyelids. *(Retraction minimizes blinking and allows irrigation of conjunctiva. It also exposes eyeball and facilitates procedure.)* Never rest fingers on the eyeball but on the bone structure above and below the eye. *(Prevents placing direct pressure on the eyeball and causing damage.)*
10. Gently direct the irrigating solution along the conjunctiva from the inner to the outer canthus (see illustration). *(Follows the normal directional flow of tears and washes contaminants out of the eye.)* Use a plastic squeeze bottle unless very large amounts of solutions are needed. Sometimes a medicine dropper is sufficient or a cotton ball or a folded gauze saturated with the irrigating solution is used (depends on condition of the eye and health care provider's order).

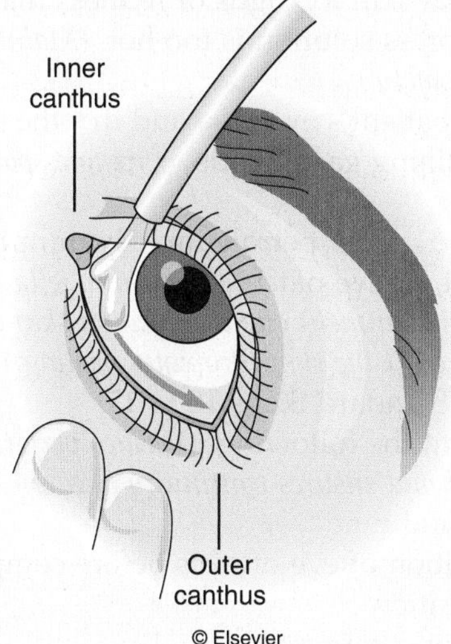

11. Ask the patient to blink occasionally to aid in moving particles toward the conjunctival sac and out of the eye.
12. Avoid directing a forceful stream onto the eyeball. *(Reduces spread of microorganisms and decreases the risk of damage to the delicate eye structure.)*
13. Avoid touching any part of the eye with irrigation equipment. *(Prevents trauma and infection to the eye.)*
14. Gently dry the eyelids with cotton balls or a soft towel. *(Avoids force that could damage the eye structure.)*
15. Refer to Standard Steps 10 to 17.
16. Document the following. *(Verifies performance of procedure and ensures continuity of care.)*
    - Date and time of irrigation
    - Condition of eye or eyes before irrigation
    - Type of solution
    - Amount of solution
    - Duration
    - Characteristics of drainage
    - Condition of eye or eyes after irrigation
    - Patient's response
    - Patient teaching (see the Patient Teaching box on eye care)

solution connected to a Morgan therapeutic lens for the irrigation. Connected to irrigation tubing, a Morgan lens enables continuous lavage of the eye and also can be used to instill medication if needed. An adapter is used to connect the lens to the IV tubing and the solution container, and the lens is inserted into the eye. To insert the device, ask the patient to look down as the lens is inserted under the upper eyelid. Then ask the patient to look up as the lower eyelid is retracted and released over the lens. Start the irrigation at the prescribed flow rate.

Eye compresses. *Compresses* (warmed, moist cloths used to reduce inflammation) frequently are used on the eyes to help temporarily relieve discomfort caused by irritation, inflammation, or infection. Skill 17.12 provides directions on how to apply a warm, moist eye compress safely.

Ear irrigations. Ear irrigations cleanse the external auditory canal of excess cerumen or exudate from a lesion or wound. Use a small syringe and solution at body temperature to prevent discomfort and severe vertigo in the patient. Be careful not to irritate the canal's sensitive skin lining by pulling the auricle excessively or introducing the tip of the irrigating syringe into the canal. Never occlude the auditory canal with the syringe tip; this could introduce fluid into the ear if excess pressure is applied and may cause the tympanic membrane to rupture. A slow, gentle irrigation works best (Skill 17.13 and the Patient Teaching box on ear care). Ear irrigations should not be attempted, however, when the obstruction is caused by a vegetable foreign body such as a bean: vegetables tend to attract and absorb moisture and will swell, causing intense pain and complicating removal of the object. This procedure also

Skill 17.12 Warm, Moist Eye Compresses

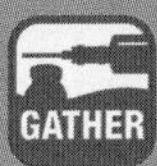

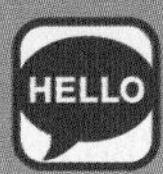

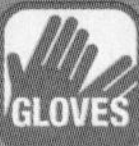

NURSING ACTION *(RATIONALE)*

1. Refer to Standard Steps 1 to 9.
2. Assemble equipment (use separate equipment for bilateral eye infections):
   - Basin of hot water
   - Prescribed solution, usually sterile water or normal saline solution
   - Sterile 4- × 4-inch gauze pads
   - Sterile basin for sterile solution
   - Sterile gloves, one pair for each eye treated
   - Sterile petroleum jelly or ophthalmic ointment and, if ordered, eye patch
   - Towels, waterproof pad, or both
3. Evaluate condition of both eyes. *(Provides baseline data to determine change after therapy.)*
4. Assist patient to a comfortable position. When applying hot compresses have the patient sit, if possible, and support patient's head with a pillow. Turn patient's head slightly to the unaffected side. *(This position helps hold the compress in place.)*
5. Place the towel or waterproof pad under patient's head. *(Protects bed linens.)*
6. Use sterile technique when infection or ulceration is present; clean technique is acceptable for all other applications. *(Reduces transmission of microorganisms.)*
7. Change gloves, dispose of in proper receptacle, and perform hand hygiene before treating each eye. *(Prevents transmission of microorganisms from one eye to the other.)*
8. Do not allow temperature of compresses to exceed 120°F (49°C). Heat solution by placing the uncapped bottle of solution in a basin of hot water. Pour the warmed solution into a sterile bowl, filling it halfway. Place sterile gauze pads in the bowl. *(Temperatures exceeding 120°F [49°C] may burn the delicate eye structures and the surrounding skin.)*
9. Take two 4- × 4-inch gauze pads from the basin. Squeeze out excess moisture. *(Prevents excess moisture from dribbling over the patient.)*
10. Instruct the patient to close the eyes. Gently apply the pads, one on top of the other, to the affected eye. Do not exert pressure on eyelids. If the patient complains that the compress is too hot, remove it immediately. *(Promotes patient's safety and prevents skin damage.)*
11. Change compress every few minutes, as necessary, for the prescribed length of time, usually 10 to 20 minutes. *(Maintains consistent temperature for the duration of therapy.)*
12. If sterility is not necessary, it is possible to apply moist heat by means of a clean washcloth. *(Clean technique is sufficient if infection or open areas are not present.)*
13. After removing each compress, check the periorbital skin for signs of redness that indicate the compress solution is too hot. *(Maintains patient's safety.)*
14. Cleanse patient's eye area and dry the skin with the remaining gauze pads. *(Promotes patient comfort.)*
15. If ordered, apply petroleum jelly or ophthalmic ointment, or eye patch. *(Petroleum jelly or ophthalmic ointment often is used on skin around the eyes to protect the skin. Promotes healing.)*
16. Refer to Standard Steps 10 to 17.
17. Document the following. *(Verifies performance of procedure and ensures continuity of care.)*
    - Date and time
    - Condition of eye or eyes before compress application
    - Type of compress
    - Temperature of solution
    - Duration of application
    - Condition of eye or eyes after treatment
    - Application of ointment, dressing, or eye patch
    - Patient's response
    - Patient teaching (see the Patient Teaching box on eye care)

is contraindicated if the patient has a cold, an elevated temperature, an ear infection, or an injured or ruptured tympanic membrane.

Performing ear irrigation on the external ear requires the skill and knowledge of a nurse. Delegation of this task to UAP is inappropriate.

Nasal irrigations. Irrigation of the nasal passages is performed for several reasons. It soothes inflamed mucous membranes and washes away dried mucus, secretions, or any foreign matter present, all of which may cause obstruction of sinus drainage and airflow through the nares and may lead to development of headache,

Skill 17.13 Ear Irrigation

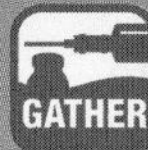

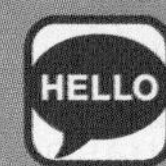

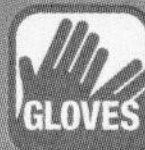

NURSING ACTION *(RATIONALE)*

1. Refer to Standard Steps 1 to 9.
2. Assemble equipment:
   - Asepto or small-bulb syringe
   - Clean gloves (mask and protective eyewear are also recommended if splashing is anticipated)
   - Cotton balls
   - Cotton-tipped applicator
   - Curved emesis basin
   - Otoscope
   - Sterile basin for solution
   - Towel or moisture-proof pad
   - Warm irrigating solution prescribed (volume depends on purpose)
3. Advise patient of possible sensations involved: vertigo, fullness, and warmth. *(Prepares patient to prevent sudden movement during procedure.)*
4. Evaluate condition of external ear structures and canal for erythema, edema, and exudate.
5. Assist patient to either a side-lying or sitting position with affected ear tilted downward and position emesis basin under ear. Patient may help hold basin if able. *(Irrigating solution will flow from auditory canal into the basin. Having patient hold basin increases participation and compliance.)*

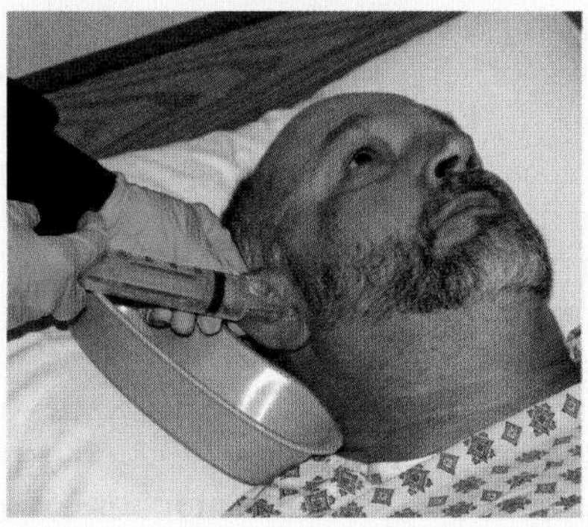

6. Place towel under patient's shoulder just under ear and emesis basin. If patient is sitting during procedure, place towel over patient's clothing. *(Prevents soiling of bed linens and of patient's clothing.)*
7. Inspect auditory canal for any accumulation of cerumen or debris. Remove what can be seen with the naked eye or the otoscope by using cotton or the applicator and solution (do not force cerumen into the canal). *(Cleanses the canal before irrigation.)*
8. Make sure irrigation solution is the proper temperature (body temperature: 98.6°F [37°C]). Test temperature of solution by sprinkling a few drops of solution on inner wrist. Fill irrigating device with appropriate volume. *(Irrigating solution at body temperature minimizes vertigo and discomfort and prevents damage to the ear.)*
9. Straighten auditory canal for introduction of solution. In infants, gently pull auricle (or pinna) down and back. In adults, gently pull auricle up and back. *(Facilitates entrance and flow of irrigating solution into ear canal.)*
10. With tip of syringe just above ear canal, irrigate gently by creating steady flow of solution against roof of canal. *(Flow of solution drains safely out of the canal while loosening debris.)* Do not occlude canal with tip of syringe. *(Occlusion of canal with syringe causes pressure against tympanic membrane during irrigation and could damage the tympanic membrane.)*

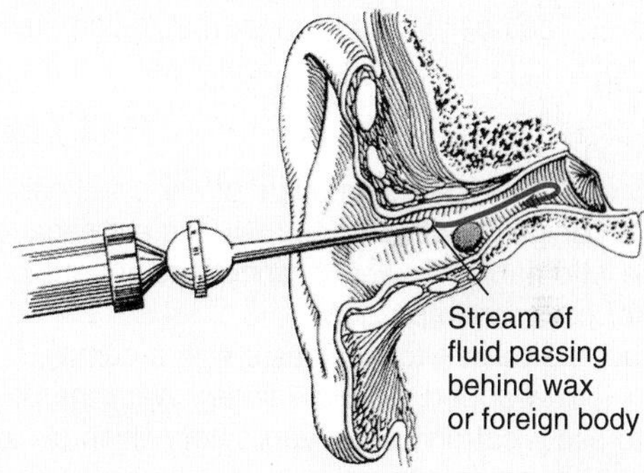

11. Continue irrigation until all debris has been removed or all solution has been used. Check auditory canal with otoscope. *(Helps determine whether purpose of irrigation has been accomplished: to cleanse canal, instill antiseptic, or provide local heat.)*
12. Check patient for vertigo or nausea throughout procedure. Onset of symptoms may make it necessary to halt the procedure temporarily. *(Irrigating solution may cause irritation of the ear canal, which produces vertigo and nausea.)*
13. Dry auricle and apply cotton ball loosely to auditory meatus. *(Promotes comfort. Cotton ball collects drainage.)*
14. Position patient with affected ear down for 10 minutes. *(Allows solution remaining in auditory canal to drain.)*
15. Refer to Standard Steps 10 to 17.

Continued

Skill 17.13 Ear Irrigation—cont'd

16. Ten minutes after irrigation, return to patient to remove cotton ball and check exudate. Determine patient's level of comfort, and permit patient to resume normal level of activity when ready. *(Increase in exudate or onset of pain indicates possible injury to tympanic membrane. Aids in determining patient's tolerance of procedure.)*
17. Document the following. *(Verifies performance of procedure and ensures continuity of care.)*
    - Date and time
    - Type, temperature, and volume of solution used
    - Character and amount of exudate
    - Condition of the ear canal before and after irrigation
    - Patient's response to irrigation
    - Patient teaching (see the Patient Teaching box on ear care)

Patient Teaching

Ear Care

- Talk in a confident, calm voice to help patient relax. Explain the procedure in terms that the patient will understand, and instruct the patient to inform the nurse if he or she feels any pain or discomfort.
- Advise the patient not to make any sudden moves, to prevent trauma to the ear during irrigation.
- Older adults often require ongoing ear care for cerumen removal. The health care provider may recommend use of a softening agent such as slightly warmed mineral oil (0.5 to 1 mL), twice daily for several days before the irrigation.
- Older adults with large amounts of ear canal hair, those with a benign growth that narrows the ear canal, and those who habitually wear hearing aids are at higher risk for cerumen impaction.
- Instruct the patient to clean ears with a damp washcloth wrapped around a finger. Warn the patient not to use a cotton-tipped applicator (which could rupture the eardrum).
- If patient uses a wax softener, instruct that these are softening products only and will not remove a cerumen impaction.
- Instruct patient to report the following signs and symptoms to the health care provider right away because these may indicate a cerumen impaction:
    - Crackling noise in the ear
    - Decrease in hearing
    - Pain
    - Tinnitus (ringing in the ear)

unpleasant odors, and infection. Nasal irrigation can be done with a specially designed (sometimes electronic) device, with a Neti pot, or with a bulb syringe. If the irrigation is meant to provide medication to the nares, the knowledge and skill of a nurse are required. If the irrigation is meant to remove dried mucus or secretions, it may be possible to delegate the task to UAP. Check facility policy.

Patients with acute or chronic nasal conditions, such as rhinitis or sinusitis, and patients who inhale allergens and toxins (e.g., coal dust, paint fumes, sawdust, pesticides) often benefit from nasal irrigations. Sometimes the health care provider orders nasal irrigations after nasal surgery to enhance healing by removing debris and stimulating repair of the mucosal membranes.

Advanced destruction of the sinuses, foreign bodies in the nasal passages, and frequent nosebleeds are contraindications to nasal irrigation because irrigation may damage the nasal mucosa or push foreign bodies farther into the nasal cavity. Some health care providers may order nasal irrigation for such patients because they may benefit from the irrigation even if contraindications exist (Skill 17.14).

Administering Medications by Inhalation

Some drugs can be absorbed through the mucous membranes of the respiratory tract. Most often, they produce a localized effect within the respiratory tract; sometimes they produce a systemic effect.

Respiratory therapy departments use the inhalation route routinely to administer medications, as do anesthesiologists and nurse anesthetists.

The nurse's participation in inhalation therapy usually involves helping patients use metered-dose inhalers (MDIs) that contain bronchodilators or corticosteroids. Not all facilities employ a respiratory therapy department, so the nurse in these facilities may need to administer other types of medications via the respiratory route. Read and follow directions for use of these inhalers, because methods of use may vary among manufacturers.

Drugs administered with handheld inhalers are dispersed through an aerosol spray, mist, or powder that penetrates lung airways. The alveolar-capillary network absorbs medications rapidly. The purpose of most MDIs is to produce local effects such as bronchodilation or reduced inflammation. Some medications have the capacity to create systemic side effects, such as an increased heart rate or increased blood pressure.

Skill 17.14 Performing a Nasal Irrigation

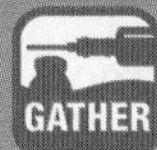

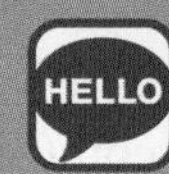

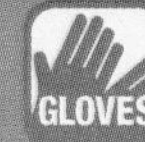

NURSING ACTION *(RATIONALE)*

1. Refer to Standard Steps 1 to 9.
2. Assemble equipment and supplies: *(Organizes procedure.)*
   - Apron or towels
   - Bath basin or sink
   - Bulb syringe or oral irrigation device
   - Facial tissues
   - Gloves
   - Hypertonic saline solution (500 to 1000 mL)
   - Irrigating device (prefilled kits are available at most pharmacies)
   - Plastic sheet
   - Rigid or flexible disposable irrigation tip (single use only)
3. Describe sensations that patient is likely to experience (e.g., feelings of fullness in the sinuses, warmth, and wetness). *(Helps relieve patient's anxiety and prepares patient to prevent sudden movement during procedure.)*
4. Evaluate nasal cavities and any nasal discharge. *(Provides baseline for evaluation after procedure.)*
5. Remove gloves used for evaluation of nasal cavity, dispose of appropriately, and perform hand hygiene. *(Prevents spread of microorganisms and protects patient and nurse.)*
6. Assemble and prepare equipment:
   - Warm saline solution (105°F [40.5°C]). *(A warm solution is comfortable and promotes healing. Keeping the solution at the appropriate temperature will prevent damage to the nasal cavity.)*
   - If an electrical device is to be used, plug instrument into an outlet near the patient, and run approximately 240 mL of the saline solution through the tubing. *(Facilitates procedure, rinses any residual solution from the tubing, and warms the tubing.)*
   - If a bulb syringe is to be used, fill bulb with warmed solution and then expel it. *(Rinses any residual solution from previous irrigation and warms the bulb.)*
7. Don disposable gloves. *(Reduces spread of microorganisms and protects patient and nurse.)*
8. Assist patient to sit upright close to equipment with the head bent forward over the collecting receptacle (basin or sink). The nose and the ear should be on the same plane vertically. Do not tilt the head back. *(The patient is less likely to breathe in the solution when holding the head in this position. This position will also keep solution from entering the eustachian tube.)* Provide towels to collect any excess moisture. *(Helps keep patient dry and provides comfort.)*
9. Instruct patient to keep the mouth open and to breathe rhythmically through the mouth during the procedure. *(This causes the soft palate to seal the throat, allowing the solution to flow out the other nostril and bring any discharge with it.)*
10. Instruct patient to neither speak nor swallow during the procedure. *(This prevents forcing any infectious material into the eustachian tube or sinuses.)*
11. If the patient reports the need to sneeze or cough, remove the irrigating device tip from the patient's nares. *(Helps prevent injury to the nasal mucosa.)*
12. Perform procedure.
    a. If a commercial kit is to be used, follow directions on package.
    b. If an electrical irrigating device is to be used, insert the tip about ½ to 1 inch (1 to 3 cm) into the patient's nostril, and turn on the irrigating device. Begin with a low pressure setting, increasing pressure as needed. *(A gentle stream of solution helps prevent material in the nose from being forced into the sinuses or eustachian tube and causing an infection.)* Insert the irrigation tip far enough into the patient's nostril to ensure that the irrigating solution cleans the nasal membranes before draining out. Irrigate both nostrils.
    c. If a bulb syringe is to be used:
       (1) Fill bulb with warm saline solution, and insert tip about ½ to 1 inch (1 to 3 cm) into the patient's nostril. *(Allows the procedure to be effective without causing damage to the nasal mucosa.)*
       (2) Squeeze bulb until a gentle stream of warm solution washes through the nose. Avoid forceful squeezing. Alternate nostrils until the returned solution is clear. *(A gentle squeeze helps prevent debris from the nasal passages from being forced up into the sinuses or eustachian tube and causing an infection.)*
13. Inspect returned solution for the following. *(Indicates symptoms of infection that need to be reported to the health care provider.)*
    - Blood
    - Color
    - Necrotic material
    - Viscosity
    - Volume

Continued

Skill 17.14 Performing a Nasal Irrigation—cont'd

14. Provide the patient with tissues. *(Helps contain secretions.)* Wait a few minutes after the procedure, and then ask the patient to blow the nose gently from both nostrils at once. *(Waiting allows for more thorough cleansing of mucous membranes. Gently blowing prevents fluid or pressure buildup in the sinuses and helps loosen and expel any crusted secretions and mucus.)*

15. Clean irrigating equipment with soap and water, and disinfect it according to facility policy. Rinse, dry, and properly store equipment. *(Prevents spread of microorganisms and prepares supplies for the next time the procedure is performed.)*

16. Refer to Standard Steps 10 to 17.

17. Document the following. *(Verifies performance of procedure and ensures continuity of care.)*
- Date and time
- Duration of procedure
- Type of solution used (formula of ingredients used)
- Amount and temperature of solution used
- Appearance and amount of returned solution
- Evaluation of patient's comfort level and ease of breathing before and after procedure
- Patient teaching; to teach irrigations at home, include the following points:
  - **(a)** Fill a clean 1-L plastic bottle with bottled or distilled water.
  - **(b)** Add 1 teaspoon of noniodized salt. *(Some health care providers also order addition of 1 tsp of baking soda.)*
  - **(c)** Hold patient's head over the sink. Do not tilt head back.
  - **(d)** Introduce the irrigating device approximately one finger width into the nasal cavity.

18. After irrigation, rinse equipment well to remove debris. Follow cleaning directions that accompany electrical device or equipment (other than the bulb syringe). Store clean equipment in clean, dry container.

Many patients who routinely receive drugs by inhalation suffer from chronic respiratory disease such as asthma, emphysema, or chronic bronchitis. Some patients have acute respiratory problems and require inhaled medications until their condition improves. Medications given by inhalation help provide these patients with better air flow through their airways. Because these patients depend on medications for disease control, they need to learn about them and the ways to administer them safely. Educate the patient about the importance of taking these types of medications and the correct way to administer the medications whenever this type of learning is needed.

An MDI delivers a measured dose of drug with each push of a canister. Approximately 5 to 10 pounds of pressure are necessary to activate the aerosol. Hand strength may diminish with age and from chronic diseases that may affect an older patient, such as arthritis, chronic respiratory disease, or heart disease. A three-point or lateral hand position is effective in activating this type of canister. Some patients need to use two hands to administer the medication, or they may use an adapted inhaler device.

Proper administration of an MDI necessitates coordination during the breathing cycle. Some patients who have difficulty with this coordination do not depress the canister at the appropriate time. The medication must be administered at the beginning of an inhalation. The patient who cannot coordinate the medication with the inhalation cannot receive a full dose. A device has been created for such patients to help them receive a full dose. The device is called a *spacer (AeroChamber)*. It fits onto the MDI and improves a patient's ability to deliver a proper dose of medication. Provide the following instructions to the patient who is using an MDI:
- Do not inhale too quickly.
- Do not hold the inhaler upside down or sideways during administration.
- Do not depress the canister more than once during one inhalation.
- Remain in an upright position during administration of the medicine.

Assess the patient's ability to hold and manipulate the inhaler and depress the canister (Skill 17.15).

Sublingual Administration

For sublingual administration of a drug (usually in tablet form), the tablet is placed beneath the tongue and held there until the tablet dissolves and is absorbed into the patient's circulation. It also may be acceptable to squeeze liquid out of a capsule if it is ordered by sublingual route. Instruct the patient not to eat, drink, or smoke while the tablet is dissolving under the patient's tongue. After dissolution, the active ingredient is absorbed rapidly into the bloodstream. Drugs given by the sublingual route bypass the liver, which reduces the time it takes for the drug to produce its desired action.

Nitroglycerin is a common type of sublingual medication. In long-term care facilities, it may be left at the bedside so that the patient is able to take it *ad lib* (as desired) if ordered this way by the health care provider. Instruct the patient to notify a nurse of any usage of

Skill 17.15 Administering Metered-Dose Inhaler

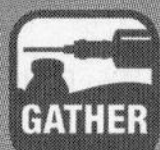

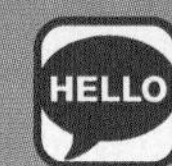

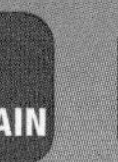

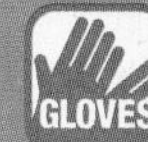

NURSING ACTION *(RATIONALE)*

1. Follow the six "rights" of medication administration (see Box 17.5). *(Prevents medication errors.)*
2. Perform the three label checks (see Box 17.6). *(Prevents medication errors.)*
3. Follow standard procedures. *(Prevents spread of microorganisms.)*
4. Gather equipment. *(Organizes procedure.)*
   - Canister
   - Gloves
   - Inhaler
   - Spacer device
5. Perform hand hygiene. *(Prevents spread of microorganisms.)*
6. Transport medications to patient's room.
7. Identify patient by checking identification bracelet and per facility policy. *(Prevents medication errors.)*
8. Introduce yourself; explain procedure. *(Establishes trust.)*
9. Provide privacy.
10. Don gloves. *(Reduces spread of microorganisms.)*
11. Allow patient opportunity to manipulate inhaler, canister, and spacer device (e.g., AeroChamber). Explain and demonstrate how canister fits into inhaler. *(Patient needs to be familiar with how to assemble and use equipment.)*
12. Explain what metered dose is and warn patient about overuse of inhaler, including drug side effects. *(Patient needs to know the dangers of excessive inhalations because of risk of serious side effects. If drug is received in recommended doses, side effects are minimal.)*
13. Remove mouthpiece cover from inhaler. Shake inhaler well. *(Ensures mixing of medication in canister.)*
14. Position inhaler:
    a. *Without AeroChamber (spacer):* Have patient open lips and place inhaler ½ to 1 inch (1 to 2 cm) from mouth with opening toward back of pharynx. Lips will not touch inhaler. *(Prevents rapid influx of inhaled medication and subsequent airway irritation. Positioning the mouthpiece 1 to 2 cm from the mouth is considered the best way to deliver the medication without a spacer.)*

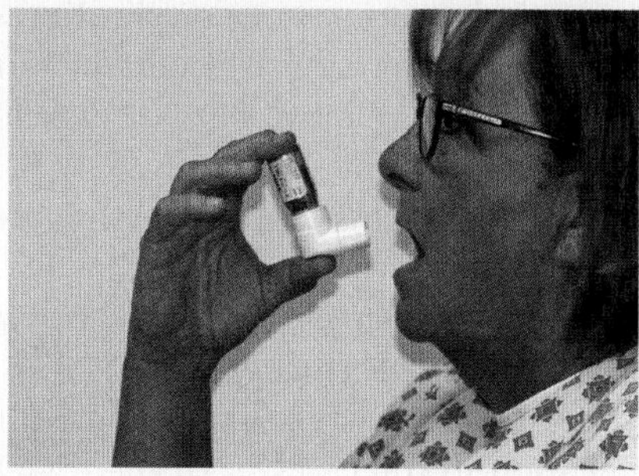

    b. *With AeroChamber (spacer):* Have patient exhale fully and then grasp mouthpiece with teeth and lips while holding inhaler with thumb at the mouthpiece and fingers at the top. *(Spacers are recommended because the device allows particles of the medication to "ride" the breath into the airways rather than hit the back of the pharynx.)*

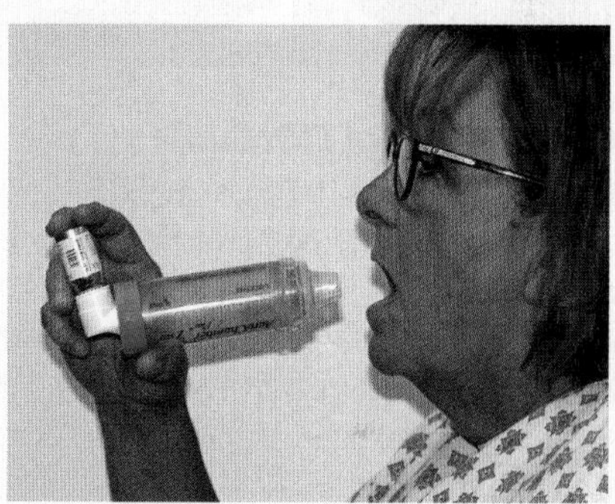

15. Instruct patient to press down on inhaler to release medication while inhaling slowly and deeply through mouth.
16. Instruct patient to breathe in slowly for 2 to 3 seconds and to hold breath for approximately 10 seconds. *(Holding breath allows tiny drops of aerosol spray to reach deeper branches of airway.)*
17. Instruct patient to exhale through pursed lips.
18. Instruct patient to wait 2 to 5 minutes between puffs. More than one puff is usually prescribed. *(First inhalation opens airways and reduces inflammation. Second or third inhalation penetrates more deeply into airways.)*
19. If more than one type of inhaled medication is prescribed, wait 5 to 10 minutes between inhalations or as ordered by health care provider. *(Drug administration is prescribed at intervals during day to promote bronchodilation and keep side effects to a minimum.)*

Continued

Skill 17.15 Administering Metered-Dose Inhaler—cont'd

20. Explain that patient will sometimes feel gagging sensation in throat caused by droplets of medication on pharynx or tongue.
21. Instruct patient in removing medication canister and cleaning inhaler in warm water. *(To remove residue that can interfere with proper distribution of medication.)*
22. Instruct patient to rinse mouth with water and spit.
23. *Evidence-based practice for patient to determine when the metered-dose inhaler (MDI) is empty:* In the past, patients were taught to determine the remainder of medication in the canister of their MDI by floating it in water. This method was found to be inaccurate because of the variety of canister sizes and designs. Patients used different methods to try to determine whether a canister was empty and tended to use the medication canister much longer than its intended duration. Rubin and Bollinger (2005) recommended that when MDIs do not have built-in dose counters, it is best to instruct the patient in how to count doses still available in the canister by calculating the number of puffs used per day to calculate the number of days to expect the inhaler to last.

Skill 17.16 Administering Sublingual Medications

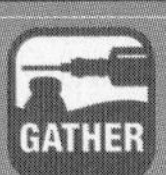

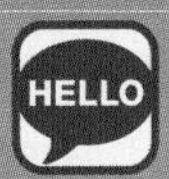

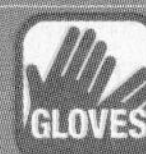

NURSING ACTION *(RATIONALE)*

1. Follow the six "rights" of medication administration (see Box 17.5). *(Prevents medication errors.)*
2. Perform the three label checks (see Box 17.6). *(Prevents medication errors.)*
3. Follow standard precautions. *(Prevents spread of microorganisms.)*
4. Perform hand hygiene. *(Prevents spread of microorganisms.)*
5. Transport drug to patient's room and identify patient by checking identification bracelet and per facility policy. *(Prevents medication errors.)*
6. Don gloves and place tablet under patient's tongue. *(Reduces spread of microorganisms and prevents absorption of medication into your skin.)*
7. Do not give patient water immediately afterward. *(Water reduces absorption of medication.)*
8. Instruct patient not to swallow tablet but to let it dissolve. *(Swallowing reduces absorption of medication.)*
9. Teach patient how to place medication under tongue when self-administering. Instruct patient to let it dissolve.
10. Remove gloves and wash hands. *(Reduces spread of microorganisms.)*
11. Record sublingual administration of medications per facility policy.
12. Return to assess patient's response to medication. *(Enables you to determine effectiveness of medication and any occurrence of adverse reactions.)*
13. Document assessment findings in nursing notes.

nitroglycerin and its effect so that the time the medication was administered can be documented accurately and any associated effect of the drug can be noted. Follow the same procedure to prepare the administration of sublingual tablets as for solid formulations of oral medication, with the exceptions noted in Skill 17.16.

Buccal Administration

For buccal administration of a drug, a tablet is placed between the cheek and the teeth or between the cheek and the gums. It is left there until it dissolves. Absorption into the capillaries of the mucous membranes of the cheek provides rapid onset of the drug's active ingredient because of its direct entry into the systemic circulation.

Use the same procedure for buccal administration as for solid formulations of oral medication (Skill 17.17).

PARENTERAL ADMINISTRATION

The **parenteral** routes are those other than the digestive system route. These usually are given with a needle and syringe. The dosage forms are liquids that are contained in the following:

- *Ampules:* Ampules are glass containers accessed by snapping off the top part of the ampule with a collar (shown in Skill 17.18, Step 10b[2]), gauze, or alcohol

Skill 17.17 Administering Buccal Medications

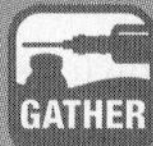

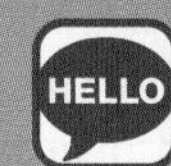

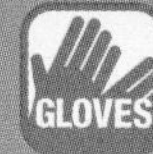

NURSING ACTION *(RATIONALE)*

1. Follow the six "rights" of medication administration (see Box 17.5). *(Prevents medication errors.)*
2. Perform the three label checks (see Box 17.6). *(Prevents medication errors.)*
3. Follow standard precautions. *(Prevents spread of microorganisms.)*
4. Perform hand hygiene. *(Prevents spread of microorganisms.)*
5. Transport drug to patient's room and identify patient by checking identification bracelet and per facility policy. *(Prevents medication errors.)*
6. Don gloves and place medication between patient's cheek and gum. *(Prevents spread of microorganisms.)*
7. Do not give patient water immediately afterward. *(Reduces absorption of medication.)*
8. Instruct patient not to swallow tablet but to let it dissolve.
9. Teach patient how to place medication between gum and cheek when self-administering.
10. Remove gloves and wash hands. *(Reduces spread of microorganisms.)*
11. Record buccal administration of medications per facility policy.
12. Return to assess patient's response to medication. *(Enables you to determine effectiveness of medication and any occurrence of adverse reactions.)*
13. Document assessment findings in nursing notes.

Skill 17.18 Preparing Parenteral Medications

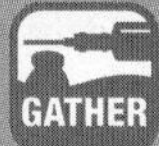

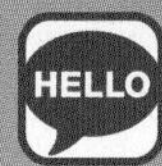

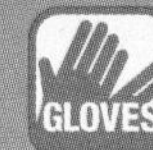

NURSING ACTION *(RATIONALE)*

1. Follow the six "rights" of medication administration (see Box 17.5). *(Prevents medication errors.)*
2. Perform the three label checks (see Box 17.6). *(Prevents medication errors.)*
3. Follow standard precautions. *(Prevents spread of microorganisms.)*
4. Perform hand hygiene before handling equipment, and prepare medication in clean area. *(Prevents spread of microorganisms.)*
5. Maintain sterility of sterile parts of syringe and needle. Use aseptic technique throughout preparation. *(Prevents contamination.)*
6. Compare drug and dosage ordered with drug and dose on hand; check expiration date, dose/milliliter, and total volume of solution in vial or ampule. Look for contaminants such as solutes present in the solution or defects in vial or ampule.
7. Calculate drug dosage, and check calculations with another nurse. *(Prevents drug errors.)*
8. Check compatibility chart, consult pharmacy department, or consult facility resource if you are mixing two medications. *(It is essential that any medications mixed are compatible.)*
9. Don gloves. *(Prevents spread of microorganisms.)*
10. Prepare medication syringe:
    a. Withdrawing medication from a vial:
        (1) Remove cap from top of vial; wipe rubber stopper briskly with alcohol sponge and allow alcohol to dry. *(It is necessary to swab seals before drawing up medication, to ensure that the rubber stopper of the vial is sterile.)*
        (2) Pull plunger of syringe back to aspirate air into syringe equal to amount of drug to be withdrawn. *(It is necessary to inject air into the vial to prevent buildup of negative pressure in vial when you attempt to aspirate medication.)*
        (3) Insert needle into inverted vial; inject air and withdraw volume of solution to be given. Keep needle within solution. *(Prevents aspiration of air into syringe.)*
        (4) Push plunger gently to disperse solution to tip of needle. Remove air bubbles by gently tapping syringe.
    b. Withdrawing medication from an ampule:
        (1) Tap the top of ampule to move solution from top of ampule to bottom of ampule.

Continued

Skill 17.18 Preparing Parenteral Medications—cont'd

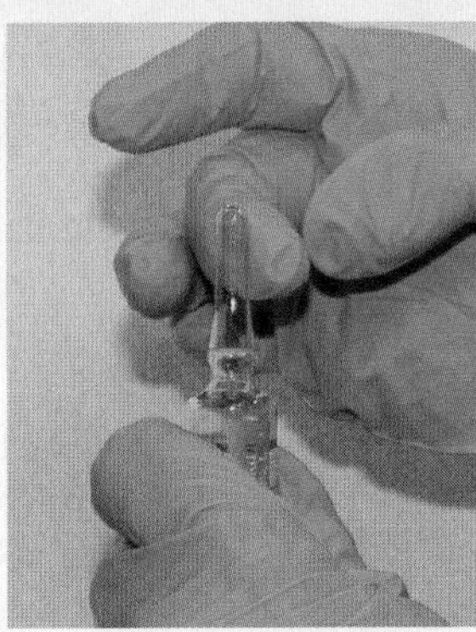

(2) Cover neck of ampule with an alcohol pad or 2- × 2-inch gauze pad; break off top of ampule; deposit top of glass ampule in sharps container. *(Prevents injury.)*

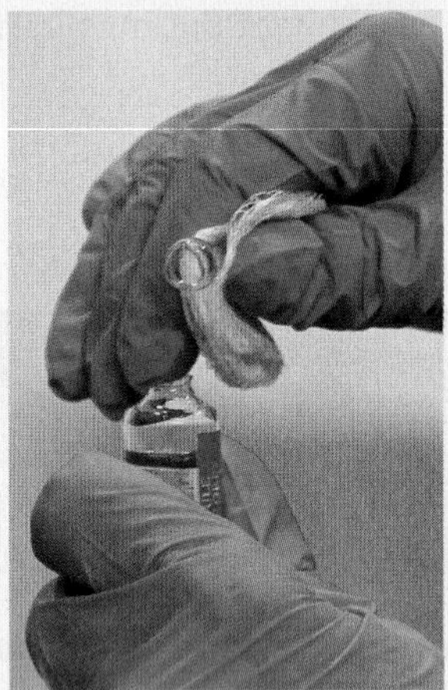

(3) Use a filter needle to aspirate medication from ampule. *(Filter or aspiration needles catch particles of glass that may be in the solution from the broken ampule.)*
(4) Insert filter needle into open neck of ampule; invert ampule to withdraw correct dose.
(5) Replace filter needle with needle appropriate for purpose and viscosity of solution.
(6) Push plunger gently until the plunger measures the correct dose.

c. Reconstituting a powdered dosage form:
(1) Follow instructions on manufacturer's box and drug insert. The instructions specify the type and the amount of diluent to use (e.g., the directions may direct the nurse to add 10 mL of bacteriostatic saline to prepare a solution of 500 mg/mL).
(2) Remove the protective cap from diluent, cleanse vial top with alcohol pad, and allow the alcohol to dry. Withdraw diluent by using sterile technique.
(3) Withdraw needle from diluent vial.
(4) Inject diluent into vial of powdered drug; remove syringe and needle. Gently shake and tap vial. *(Dissolves powder into solution.)*
(5) If necessary, label vial of solution with the following, if to be used for more than one dose:
(a) Date and time mixed
(b) Name of person who mixed drug and diluent
(c) Dose/milliliter obtained (concentration)
(d) Amount and type of diluent used
(6) Withdraw correct dose; facility policy may suggest to change needle and replace with a new needle of appropriate gauge and length for administering the medication to the patient. *(It is necessary to exchange the needle with the needle for injection into patient's tissue. Needles become dull as they enter the rubber stopper. Changing needles also prevents tracking of medication through patient's tissues, reducing the pain that may be associated with the injection.)*

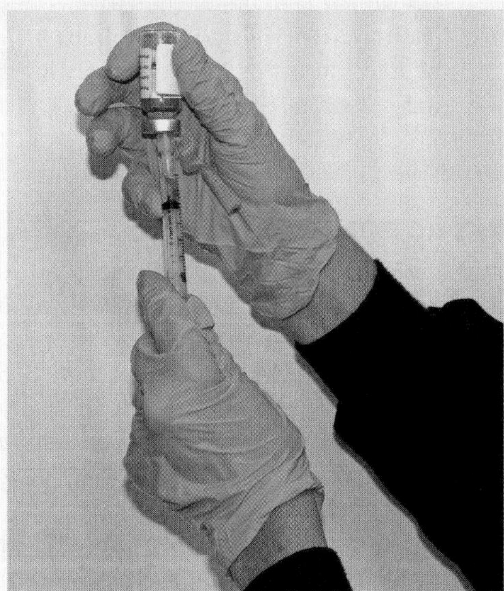

d. Placing two medications into one syringe (insulin example used):
(1) Check compatibility of the two drugs by using compatibility chart, calling pharmacy department, or using facility-provided resource.
(2) Check and compare label of each drug ordered with label of each drug on hand.
(3) Compare each label with medication order.
(4) Roll vials of long- and intermediate-acting insulin between the palms. *(Resuspends insulin.)* Do not shake any insulin. *(Causes air bubbles.)* NOTE: Do *not* mix long-acting insulin glargine (Lantus)

Skill 17.18 Preparing Parenteral Medications—cont'd

with any other kind of insulin. *(Lantus cannot be mixed with other kinds of insulin.)*

(5) Briskly wipe tops of both vials with separate alcohol swabs and allow to dry. *(Prevents contamination.)*

(6) Pull back plunger of syringe to amount equal to volume of longer-acting insulin to be given. *(Prevents buildup of negative pressure.)*

(7) Insert needle and inject air into vial of longer-acting insulin.

(8) Withdraw needle from vial without having removed insulin.

(9) Pull back plunger of syringe to amount equal to volume of shorter acting (regular or rapid-acting) insulin to be given.

(10) Insert needle through rubber stopper of second vial; inject air into vial.

(11) Invert vial; withdraw volume of shorter acting (regular or rapid-acting) insulin first. *(Prevents contamination of regular or rapid-acting insulin by intermediate or long-acting insulin.)*

(12) Check dosage in syringe against medication order, as well as with another nurse. *(Prevents dose error.)*

(13) Wipe rubber stopper of longer-acting insulin; insert needle of the syringe containing shorter or rapid-acting insulin, and withdraw ordered dose of longer acting insulin. Check dose in syringe against medication order with second nurse. *(Prevents dose error.)*

(14) Remove needle or syringe from vial.

(15) Check labels of both vials against medication order. *(Ensures accuracy.)*

(16) Pull plunger back enough to allow space in barrel of syringe for insulin to be gently mixed. Mix by tilting syringe back and forth; remove air. Administer mixtures of insulin within 5 minutes of preparation. *(Regular insulin binds with NPH insulin and the action of regular insulin is reduced.)*

11. Identify patient by checking identification bracelet and per facility policy. *(Prevents medication errors.)*

12. Don gloves. *(Prevents spread of microorganisms.)*

13. Prepare injection site and inject according to prescribed route and method (see Skills 17.14 through 17.17).

swab. They are intended for a single unit-dose use. Some facilities recommend the use of filter needles to prevent particles of glass from the ampule from being aspirated into the syringe barrel.

- *Vials:* Vials are glass containers sealed with a metal cap, with a rubber diaphragm in the middle of the cap. The vial may contain a single dose, or it may be used to provide multiple doses for several patients.

Large volumes of fluids meant to be infused through an IV line are placed in glass or plastic containers, such as IV fluid bags. IV fluid bags or bottles range in capacity from 50 to 1000 mL.

The parenteral routes are as follows:

- *ID:* intradermal (within the dermis)
- *IM:* intramuscular (within the muscle)
- *IV:* intravenous (within the vein)
- *Subcut:* subcutaneous (under the dermis; in fatty tissue)

Parenteral routes are used for the following reasons:

- Some medications, such as insulin, are altered or destroyed by the secretions found in the GI tract.
- Some patients—such as those who are (1) intubated, (2) severely dysphagic (unable to swallow effectively), or (3) experiencing shock, nausea, or vomiting—are unable to take medications by mouth.
- The parenteral route produces a more rapid onset of action than does the oral route.
- The duration of the action of medications that are administered through the parenteral route is commonly shorter than that of medications administered orally.
- Smaller doses of parenteral drugs can be administered because active drug ingredients are not reduced by the action of the GI tract and liver.
- IV administration of a drug can be regulated closely. Immediate entry into the bloodstream produces a very rapid response.

Always perform hand hygiene before selecting and handling syringes, needles, and other equipment. Use aseptic technique during the preparation and administration of parenteral medications because during the injection, the penetration of the skin creates a portal of entry into the body by pathogenic organisms.

Administer parenteral medication skillfully and accurately. Exact dosages are essential, as is selection of the proper site for the injection.

Equipment

Syringes. A syringe consists of a barrel, a plunger, and a tip (Fig. 17.5). The outside barrel is calibrated in milliliters, insulin units, and in some agencies, heparin units.

Barrel sizes commonly range from 0.5 to 50 mL. The outside of the barrel is not sterile, but the inside is. The

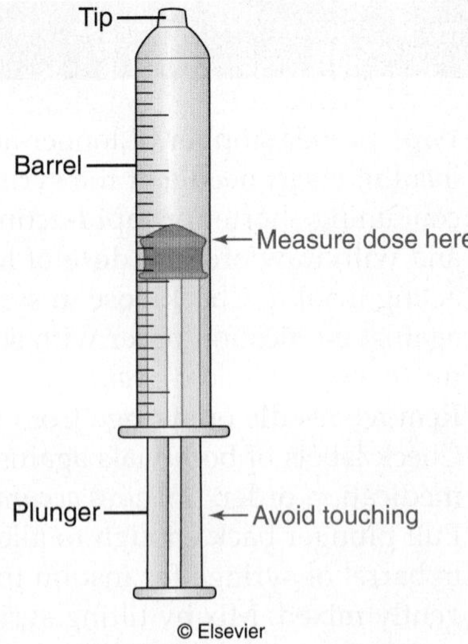

Fig. 17.5 Parts of a syringe.

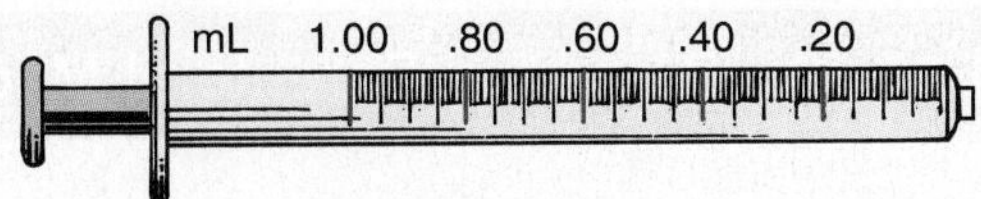

Fig. 17.6 Tuberculin syringe calibration. Tuberculin syringe is marked in 0.01 increments (hundredths) for doses of less than 1 mL. (From Clayton BD, Willihnganz M: *Basic pharmacology for nurses*, ed 17, St. Louis, 2017, Elsevier.)

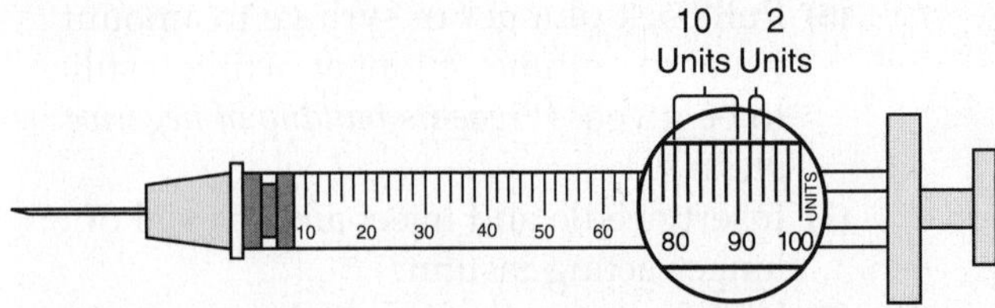

Fig. 17.7 Calibration of U100 insulin syringe. (From Clayton BD, Willihnganz M: *Basic pharmacology for nurses*, ed 17, St. Louis, 2017, Elsevier.)

tip of the barrel is either the plain slip tip or the Luer-Lok type. The needle slips directly onto the slip tip barrel tip, whereas it is necessary to turn the Luer-Lok needle to the right as the nurse attaches it onto the barrel.

The plunger that is located inside of the barrel is also sterile; avoid touching the plunger anywhere except the tip. Manipulate the plunger to draw up and inject medication with the syringe. The plunger has a rubber stopper on the end that is inside the barrel. Read the volume of a medication at the area of the rubber stopper nearest the needle (see Fig. 17.5, *bottom*).

The most commonly used syringe sizes are 0.5 mL (insulin syringe), 1 mL (tuberculin syringe and insulin syringe), 3 mL, and 5 mL.

Tuberculin syringe. The tuberculin syringe (Fig. 17.6) holds a total volume of 1 mL. It is used to give volumes of medication of 1 mL or less, such as for giving small doses of epinephrine, intradermal skin tests, and subcutaneous medication.

The tuberculin syringe is measured in milliliters. The long lines represent 0.1 ($\frac{1}{10}$) mL, the shorter lines represent 0.05 ($\frac{5}{100}$) mL, and the shortest lines represent 0.01 ($\frac{1}{100}$) mL.

Insulin syringe. Use the insulin syringe only for insulin because it is calibrated in units with which insulin is measured (Fig. 17.7). Most insulin is made in the concentration of U100. The U100 syringe holds 100 units of insulin per 1 mL. The U50 syringe holds 50 units of insulin per 0.5 mL. There is also a U30 syringe in 0.3-mL size. The unit scale on the barrel of the syringe usually differs with syringe size. The 1-mL syringe usually is marked in 2-unit increments. The 0.5-mL syringe is marked in 1-unit increments. The 0.3-mL syringe is marked in either 1- or 0.5-unit increments and is preferred for use in patients who require small doses of insulin. Check all insulin dosages with another nurse before administering the medication to the patient. Both nurses must verify and document the insulin dose to be administered to the patient.

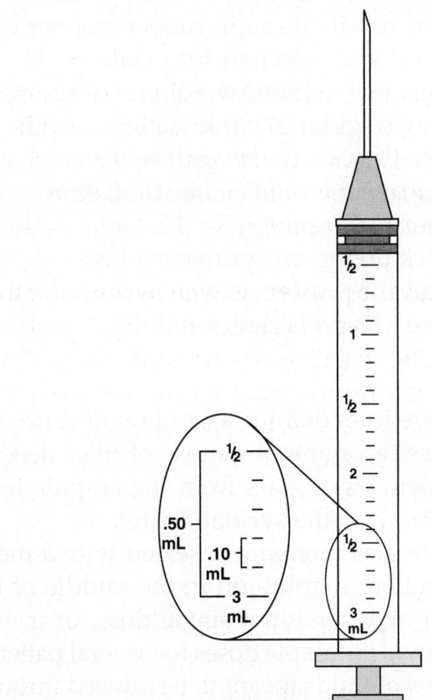

Fig. 17.8 Reading the calibrations of a 3-mL syringe.

3-mL syringe. The 3-mL syringe is chosen for giving volumes of medication of 1 to 3 mL (Fig. 17.8). It is used for most IM injections. The 3-mL syringe is calibrated in milliliters or cubic centimeters (cc), which are equivalent units. The short lines represent 0.1 mL; the longer lines represent 0.5 mL.

Select syringes based on the volume of medication to be given (Fig. 17.9A to C).

Safety-Glide syringes. Safety-Glide syringes are used to prevent needlesticks (see Fig. 17.9C). Many hospitals and long-term care facilities use syringes with safety glides or some sort of safety feature to protect personnel from needlestick injuries.

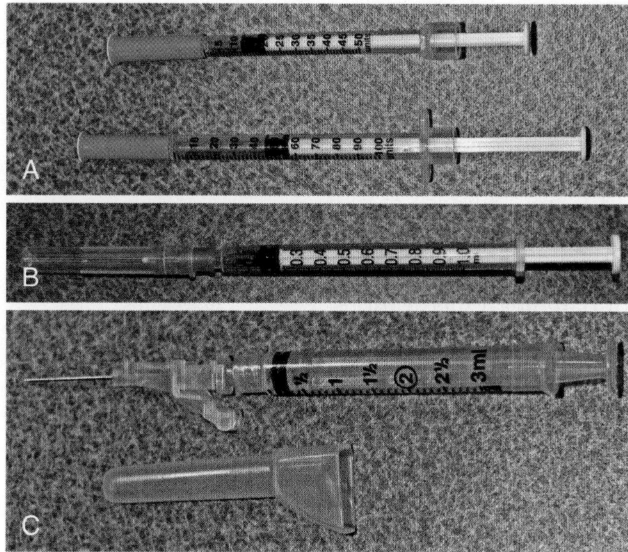

Fig. 17.9 Types of syringes. A, Insulin syringes: U-50 *(top)* and U-100 *(bottom)*. B, Tuberculin syringe. C, Safety 3-mL syringe.

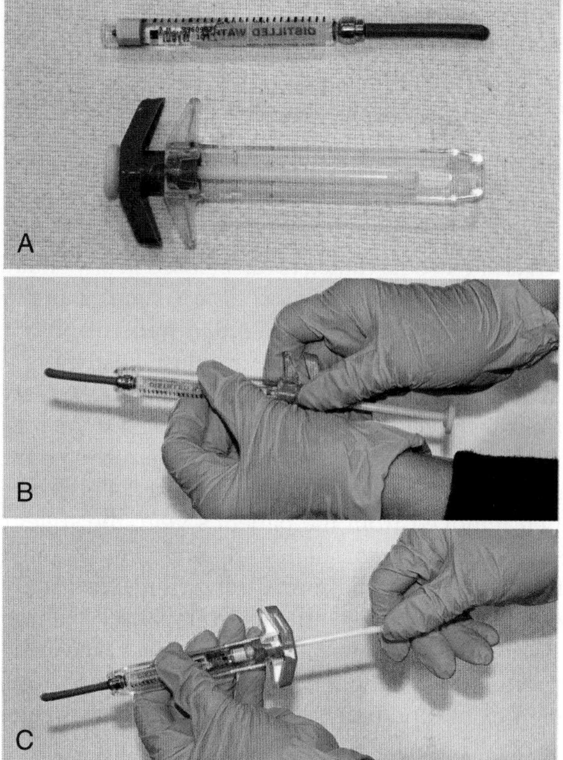

Fig. 17.10 A, Carpuject syringe and prefilled sterile cartridge with needle. B, Assembling the Carpuject. C, Cartridge slides into syringe barrel, turns, and locks at needle end. Plunger then screws into cartridge end.

Disposable injection units. Disposable, single-dose, prefilled syringes are available for some medications such as morphine sulfate or enoxaparin sodium (Lovenox). Calculate the dose needed for the patient and expel any unneeded portion of the contents before administering.

The Tubex and Carpuject injection systems include reusable plastic or metal syringes that hold prefilled, disposable, sterile cartridge-needle units (Fig. 17.10). Slip the cartridge into the mechanism, secure it (per package directions), and check for air bubbles. Advance the plunger to get rid of air bubbles, to obtain the correct dosage, and then to inject the medication, as with a regular syringe.

Needles. The parts of a needle are the hub, the shaft, and the beveled tip (Fig. 17.11). The opening at the needle's beveled tip reveals the **lumen** (the inside of the hollow shaft). The diameter of the lumen determines the **gauge** (a standard or scale of measurement) of the needle (Fig. 17.12). The smaller the gauge of the needle, the larger the diameter; thus an 18-gauge needle has a much larger diameter than a 25-gauge needle. Needle gauge selection is based on the viscosity (thickness) of the medication: the thicker the medication, the smaller the gauge (the larger the lumen) required. A 20- to 22-gauge needle is usually adequate for most nonviscous IM injections. A 16- to 18-gauge needle is appropriate for blood administration, emergency IV routes, and surgical cases. A 25- to 26-gauge needle is used frequently for infants and children and for intradermal injections, and 27- to 28-gauge needles are available for subcutaneous injections. Insulin-syringe needles are typically 29- and 30-gauge.

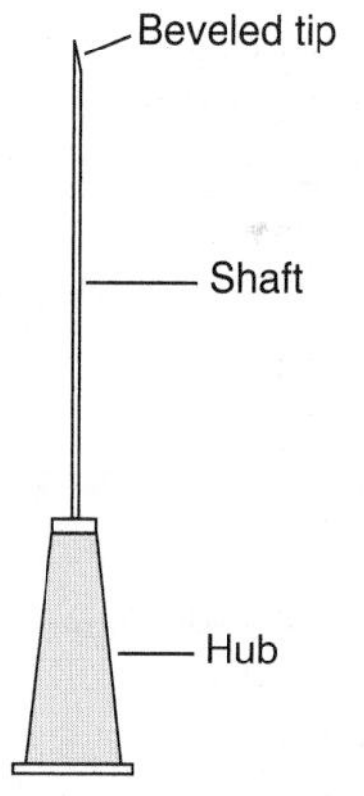

Fig. 17.11 Parts of a needle. (From Clayton BD, Willihnganz M: *Basic pharmacology for nurses*, ed 17, St. Louis, 2017, Elsevier.)

Needle length. Select the needle length according to the depth of the tissue into which you need to inject the medication. Intradermal injections require only ⅜- to ⅝-inch needle length, whereas an IM injection often requires 1- to 1½-inch needle length, depending on the amount of muscle tissue the patient has. Needle length for subcutaneous injections is usually ½ to ⅝ inch, depending on the depth of the tissue where the injection is to be administered (see Fig. 17.12). Insulin-syringe needles are available in a standard ½-inch length and a 5⁄16-inch length. The shorter needle tends to be less intimidating, and many patients with diabetes perceive it to be less painful than standard-length needles.

Intravenous needles. Two items made especially for IV use are the over-the-needle catheter and the winged-type (or butterfly) needle (Fig. 17.13 A and B).

The wing-tipped (butterfly) needle is useful in administering IV fluids on a short-term basis. The nurse may use it in pediatric cases, in which veins are sometimes hard to find except in the scalp. Wing-tipped needles are easy to put in, but some health care providers prefer over-the-needle catheters. Butterfly infusion sets require that the stainless steel needle remain in the patient's vein.

Over-the-needle catheters can be used in any situation in which an IV infusion is necessary, such as an emergency situation, surgery, and blood transfusions.

Over-the-needle catheters are plastic catheters that fit over a stainless steel needle called a *stylet*. A stylet is a sharp, bevel-tipped metal guide used to pierce the skin and vein. Once the stylet and the catheter are in the vein, blood return occurs, and the stylet is removed. When removed from the patient's vein, the stylet can be activated or manipulated in some way to make it safer, to reduce needlesticks during IV needle insertion. The plastic catheter is left in the vein, and IV tubing or an IV lock may be attached to the catheter. The catheter is preferred over the wing-tipped needle because it is more flexible and better withstands patient movement (see Fig. 17.13A).

Wing-tipped needles and over-the-needle catheters cannot be left in place indefinitely. Assess them every shift for patency, intactness, and the development of any complications. Follow the health care facility's policies regarding how long an IV catheter or needle may be left in place. If phlebitis or infiltration occurs at the IV insertion site, discontinue the infusion.

A physician may insert a central line. There are several different types of central lines. They are used for IV administration of a fluid that may be given over a long period of time, such as total parenteral nutrition, chemotherapy, or antibiotics. See Skill 17.18 for preparation of parenteral medications.

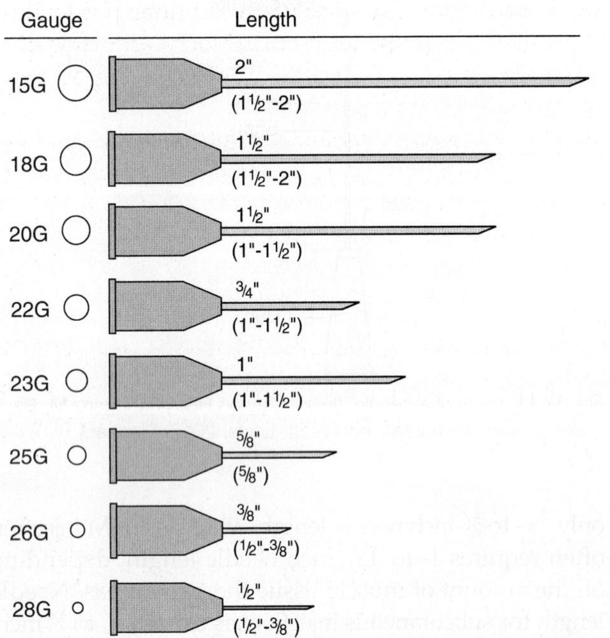

Fig. 17.12 Needle length and gauge. (From Clayton BD, Willihnganz M: *Basic pharmacology for nurses*, ed 17, St. Louis, 2017, Elsevier.)

Needleless devices. Each year, many people suffer from accidental needlesticks and sharps injuries in health care settings. These injuries commonly occur when nurses attempt to recap needles, manipulate needles, or come into contact with stray needles left at a patient's bedside. The risk of exposure to bloodborne pathogens in health care workers led to the development of needleless devices, or special needle safety devices due to the 1999–2000 Needlestick Safety and Prevention Act (ANA, n.d.).

Special syringes are designed with a sheath or guard that can cover the needle after it is withdrawn from the skin (see Fig. 17.9C). The safety aspect of the device commonly is required to be activated by the nurse, and the needle is covered immediately, which reduces the chance of a needlestick injury. The syringe and sheath are disposed of together in a receptacle designed for disposal of sharp items. The Centers for Disease Control and Prevention (CDC) and OSHA have mandated that health care agencies use safer medical devices (sharps disposal containers, self-sheathing needles) that eliminate or reduce exposures to bloodborne pathogen within the workplace.

IV tubing and access ports have been developed for use with Luer-Lok–tipped syringes to reduce the occurrence of injuries during medication delivery.

Intramuscular Injections

An IM injection involves inserting a needle into the muscle tissue to administer medication (Skill 17.19). Because muscle tissue has a large blood supply, IM medication is absorbed faster than medication administered subcutaneously. The most commonly used sites are the ventrogluteal area, the vastus lateralis of the thigh, and the deltoid muscle of the arm.

When selecting an IM site, ensure that the site is free of pain, infection, necrosis, ecchymosis, and abrasions. Additional important factors to consider are the location of underlying bones, nerves, and major blood vessels, as well as the amount of solution to be injected. Each

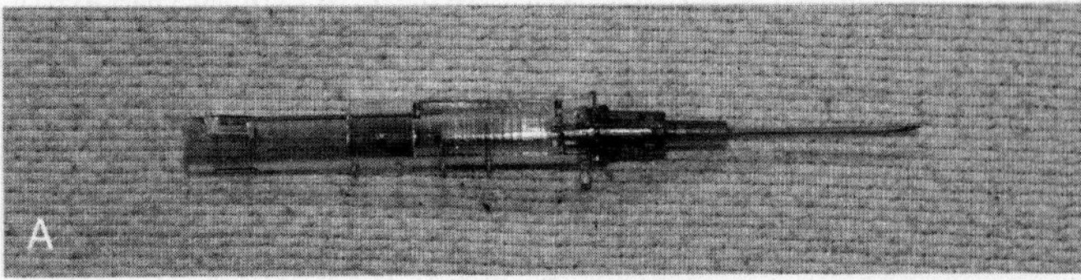

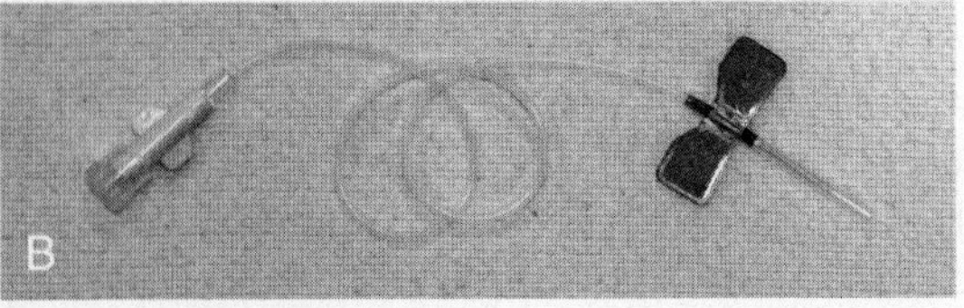

Fig. 17.13 A, Over-the-needle catheter. B, Winged-tip (butterfly) needle.

Skill 17.19 Giving an Intramuscular Injection

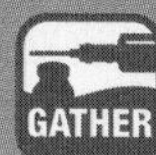

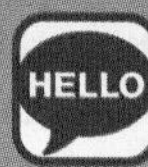

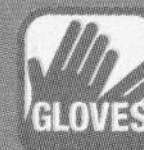

NURSING ACTION *(RATIONALE)*

1. Follow the six "rights" of medication administration (see Box 17.5). *(Prevents medication errors.)*
2. Perform the three label checks (see Box 17.6). *(Prevents medication errors.)*
3. Follow standard precautions. *(Prevents spread of microorganisms.)*
4. Perform hand hygiene. *(Prevents spread of microorganisms.)*
5. Prepare medication according to standard procedure for injectables (see Skill 17.13).
6. Don gloves. *(Prevents spread of microorganisms.)*
7. Identify patient by checking identification bracelet and per facility policy. *(Prevents medication errors.)* Explain the procedure.
8. Select and expose site (according to intramuscular [IM] site selection procedure); provide privacy.
9. Clean skin with alcohol swab (from center outward), spread skin tight with thumb and index finger; allow site to dry. *(Mechanical and chemical action removes microorganisms.)*
10. Ask patient to take a deep breath and to exhale slowly to relax muscle as needle is inserted. *(Lessens pain from injection.)*
11. Insert needle at a 90-degree angle quickly in a dartlike motion. *(Quickness reduces discomfort. A quick, dartlike insertion followed by slow injection of the medication is much less painful to the patient.)*
12. Maintain needle's position in muscle; gently aspirate (pull back plunger) to be certain needle is in muscle (and not in a vein or an artery).
    a. If blood is seen, needle is in a vein or an artery. Withdraw needle and discard medication; prepare new medication (see Skill 17.13). Select another site for new attempt and begin again from Step 8.
13. Slowly inject medication into muscle to lessen discomfort. *(A slow, steady injection rate of medication promotes comfort and minimizes tissue damage.)*
14. Withdraw needle quickly without bending or twisting it. *(Minimizes tissue injury.)*
15. Apply gentle pressure with gauze (2- × 2-inch) to stop any bleeding. *(Massaging site can cause tissue irritation.)*
16. Do not recap needle; activate safety feature of needle and discard directly into sharps container. *(Prevents needlesticks.)*
17. Remove gloves and wash hands. *(Prevents spread of microorganisms.)*
18. Record administration of medications per facility policy. Chart site used and amount and type of medication (e.g., "meperidine [Demerol], 50 mg, given IM left ventrogluteal").
19. Return to assess patient's response to medication. *(Enables you to determine effectiveness of medication and any occurrence of adverse reactions.)*
20. Document assessment findings in nursing notes.

anatomic site has advantages and disadvantages. In the past, the dorsogluteal muscle site was used frequently. Because of its proximity to the sciatic nerve and superior gluteal artery, this muscle is no longer recommended as a preferred injection site. Damage to the sciatic nerve may occur as a result of accidentally hitting the nerve during the administration of an IM injection at this site.

The ventrogluteal site is preferred for IM injections. The advantages of this site are that (1) it provides the greatest thickness of gluteal muscle, (2) fewer nerves and blood vessels penetrate this site, and (3) it has the most consistent and thinnest layer of adipose tissue covering it. Develop skill in finding the proper location for giving an IM injection by palpating anatomic landmarks correctly and being knowledgeable about the location of underlying nerves and blood vessels (Boxes 17.9 and 17.10).

Intramuscular injections for analgesia are given much less often than they were previously because of the more common use of patient-controlled analgesia (PCA) and patient-controlled epidural that are used to help control patients' pain. IM injections are more painful than the use of PCA.

Site selection

Ventrogluteal site. The gluteal sites are the ventrogluteal and the dorsogluteal. The *ventrogluteal site* (Fig. 17.14) is located by means of three landmarks: the greater trochanter, the anterior iliac spine, and the iliac crest (the hip bone). Place the palm of your hand on the lateral portion of the patient's greater trochanter and your index (pointer) finger on the patient's anterior superior iliac spine (your left hand on the patient's right hip or your right hand on the patient's left hip); then extend the middle finger toward the iliac crest. Inject medication into the V formed by the index and middle fingers. You may place the patient in a side-lying position, with muscle relaxation promoted by flexing of the upper leg.

Box 17.9 Characteristics of Intramuscular Sites

VASTUS LATERALIS MUSCLE

- Drug absorption at this site is rapid.
- It is the preferred site for administration of immunizations to infants younger than 12 months.[a] This site is also is used in adults.
- This large, developed muscle lacks major nerves and blood vessels and is the most fully developed muscle in the newborn.

VENTROGLUTEAL MUSCLE

- This complex consists of the gluteus medius and the gluteus minimus muscles.
- It is situated deep and away from major nerves and blood vessels.
- The ventrogluteal site is preferred over other gluteal muscles because it is not associated with injuries such as fibrosis, nerve damage, abscess, tissue necrosis, muscle contraction, gangrene, and pain, as are other intramuscular sites.[a]
- It is the preferred injection site for infants, children, and adults.

DORSOGLUTEAL MUSCLE

- There is risk of striking the underlying sciatic nerve, the greater trochanter, or major blood vessels if the site is not landmarked correctly.
- This muscle is no longer considered a preferred intramuscular site according to many sources.[a]

DELTOID MUSCLE

- This site is easily accessible, but the muscle is not well developed in most patients.
- It is used only for small volumes (0.5 to 1 mL) of medication and is the preferred site for administration of routine immunizations in toddlers, older children, and adults.[a]
- Hepatitis B vaccine is given primarily in the deltoid.[b]
- Avoid using the deltoid muscle in infants or in children with underdeveloped muscles.

[a]Modified from Nicoll LH, Hesby A: Intramuscular injection: An integrative research review and guideline for evidence-based practice, *Appl Nurs Res* 15(3):149–162, 2002.
[b]Modified from Perry AG, Potter PA, Elkin MK: *Nursing interventions and clinical skills*, ed 5, St. Louis, 2012, Mosby.

Vastus lateralis muscle. The vastus lateralis muscle (Fig. 17.15) is the preferred site for children younger than 3 years of age because it is free of nerves and blood vessels. It is also used in adults. This muscle is located on the anterior lateral thigh. The patient may be placed in a supine or sitting position. Place one hand above the patient's knee and one hand below the greater trochanter. Give the IM injection in the area between your two hands.

Deltoid muscle. The deltoid muscle (Fig. 17.16) of the upper arm is a relatively small area. Position the patient in a sitting, standing, prone, or supine position. Ask the patient to relax his or her arm during the injection to help decrease discomfort.

The landmark for locating the proper area for this injection site is the acromion process of the scapula. Place a finger on the acromion process and move down three more fingerbreadths. The injection site is the center

Box 17.10 Locating Sites for Intramuscular Injections

VENTROGLUTEAL SITE

1. Position patient on either side, with knee of upper leg bent and upper leg slightly ahead of the bottom leg. It is also acceptable for the patient to remain supine, lie on side, or lie on abdomen. Instruct patient to relax muscles where you are placing injection.
2. Palpate the greater trochanter at the head of the femur and the anterior superior iliac spine. To locate the proper site, use your left hand when the patient lies on the left side and your right hand when the patient lies on the right side.
3. Using your right hand for the left hip and your left hand for the right hip, place the heel of your hand over the greater trochanter of the patient's hip. Point your thumb toward the patient's groin, point your index finger toward the anterior superior iliac spine, and extend your middle finger back along the iliac crest toward the buttock as far as possible (NOTE: A "V" is formed between the index and middle finger) (see Fig. 17.15).
4. The injection site is the center of the triangle formed by your index and middle fingers.
5. Spread skin taut to give injection. Use your dominant hand to give injection (see Fig. 17.15).

VASTUS LATERALIS SITE

1. Position patient lying supine or sitting with site well exposed. If patient is supine, have patient flex knee on side where medication will be given.
2. Use the greater trochanter and the knee as landmarks for injection site. Place one hand above the knee and one hand below the greater trochanter of the femur.
3. Locate the middle third of the muscle, the midline of the anterior thigh, and the midline of the thigh's lateral (outer) side.
4. The injection site is located within a rectangle formed by these boundaries (see Fig. 17.16).

DELTOID SITE

1. Position patient sitting or lying down. Expose the upper arm and shoulder; remove any tight-fitting sleeves, rather than rolling them up.
2. Ask patient to relax the arm at the side with the elbow flexed. Instruct patient to place the forearm across the abdomen or the chest.
3. Palpate the lower edge of the acromion process, which forms the base of a triangle in line with the midpoint of the lateral aspect of the upper arm (see Fig. 17.18).
4. Place four fingers across the deltoid muscle, with the top finger along the acromion process.
5. The injection site is in the center of the triangle, about 3 to 5 cm (1 to 2 inches) below the acromion process (see Fig. 17.18).

From Perry AG, Potter PA, Elkin MK: *Nursing interventions and clinical skills*, ed 5, St. Louis, 2012, Mosby.

of the muscle, about 3 to 5 cm (1 to 2 inches) below the acromion process.

Z-track method. Use the Z-track method for injecting medications that may be irritating to the tissues. In Z-track IM administration, the medication is sealed deep

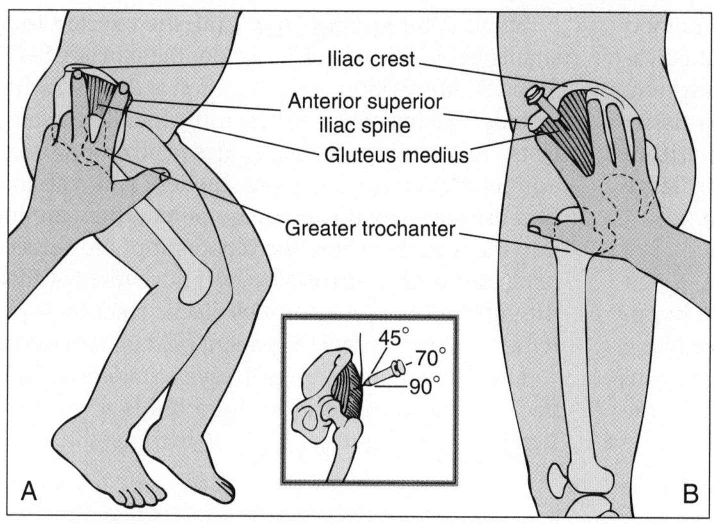

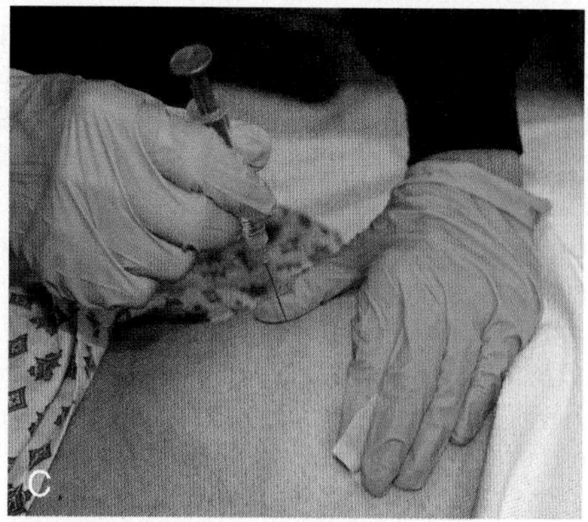

Fig. 17.14 Ventrogluteal site. A, In a child or an infant. B, In an adult. C, Locating ventrogluteal site for intramuscular injection. (A, From Clayton BD, Willihnganz M: *Basic pharmacology for nurses,* ed 17, St. Louis, 2017, Elsevier.)

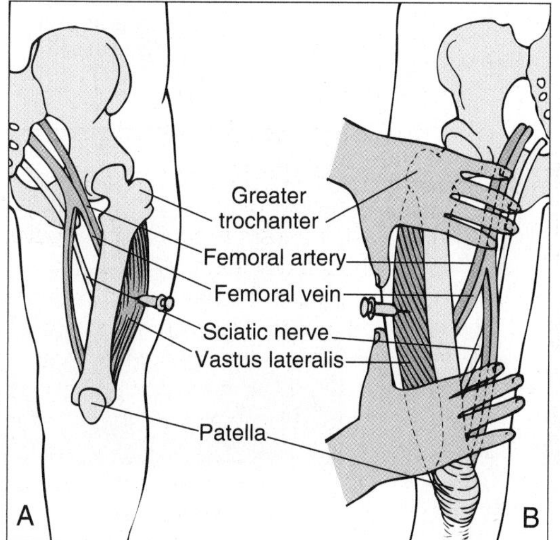

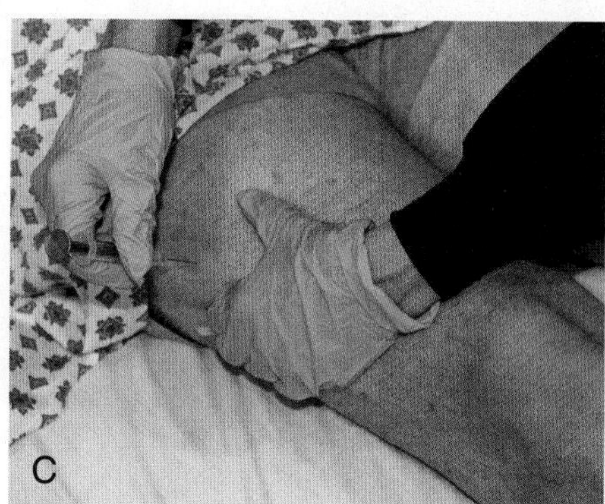

Fig. 17.15 Vastus lateralis muscle site. A, In a child or an infant. B, In an adult. C, Giving intramuscular injection in vastus lateralis site in an adult. (A, From Clayton BD, Willihnganz M: *Basic pharmacology for nurses,* ed 17, St. Louis, 2017, Elsevier.)

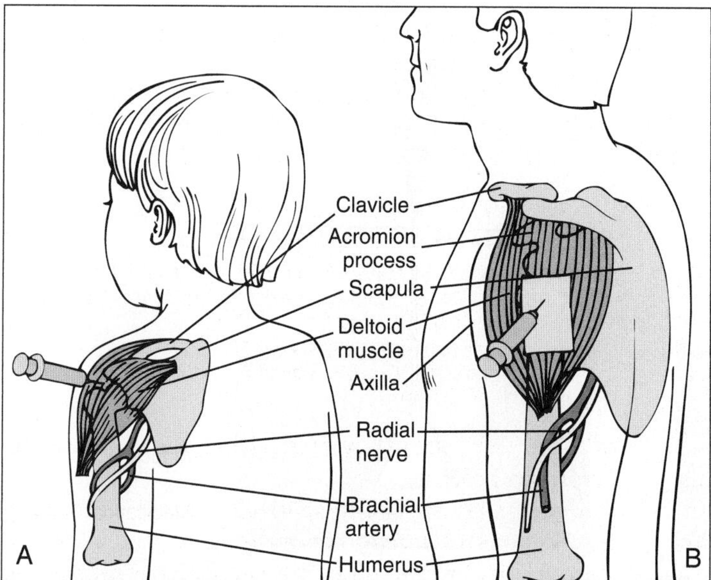

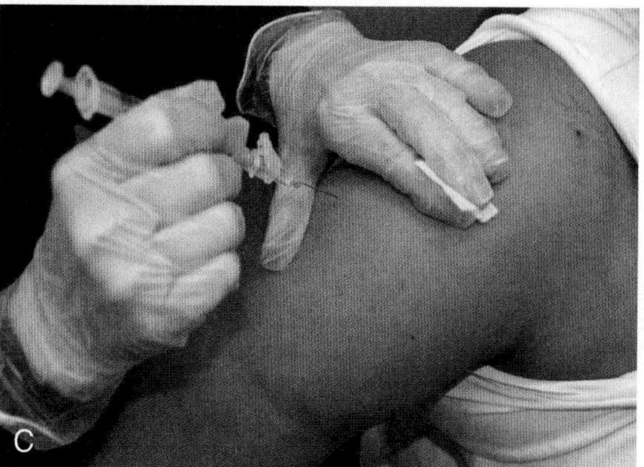

Fig. 17.16 Deltoid muscle site. A, In a child or an infant. B, In an adult. C, Giving intramuscular injection in deltoid site. (A and B, From Clayton BD, Willihnganz M: *Basic pharmacology for nurses,* ed 17, St. Louis, 2017, Elsevier.)

within muscle tissue (see Skill 17.19). The Z-track method reduces the chance of staining or tracking of the medication back into the tissue as the needle is withdrawn. The Z-track method of IM injection also keeps tissue irritation to a minimum by sealing the drug within muscle tissues (Fig. 17.17). Select an IM site in large muscles, such as those in the ventrogluteal site.

Intradermal Injections

An intradermal injection is the introduction of a hypodermic needle into the dermis for the purpose of instilling a substance such as a serum, vaccine, or skin test agent (Fig. 17.18 and see Skill 17.19). Do not aspirate from the site when performing an intradermal injection.

Small volumes such as 0.1 mL are injected to form a small bubble-like wheal just under the skin (see Skill 17.19, Step 11). Absorption in this location is slow, which makes intradermal injection the best route for allergy sensitivity tests, tuberculin screening, desensitization injections, administration of local anesthetics, and vaccinations. Because these medications are potent, they are injected into the dermis, where the blood supply is reduced and drug absorption occurs slowly. If the patient is allergic to the substance, a severe anaphylactic reaction is possible if the substance enters the patient's circulation too rapidly.

Use a tuberculin syringe to give intradermal injections, because the tuberculin syringe holds a maximum of 1 mL. Use a 25-gauge, ⅜- to ⅝-inch needle.

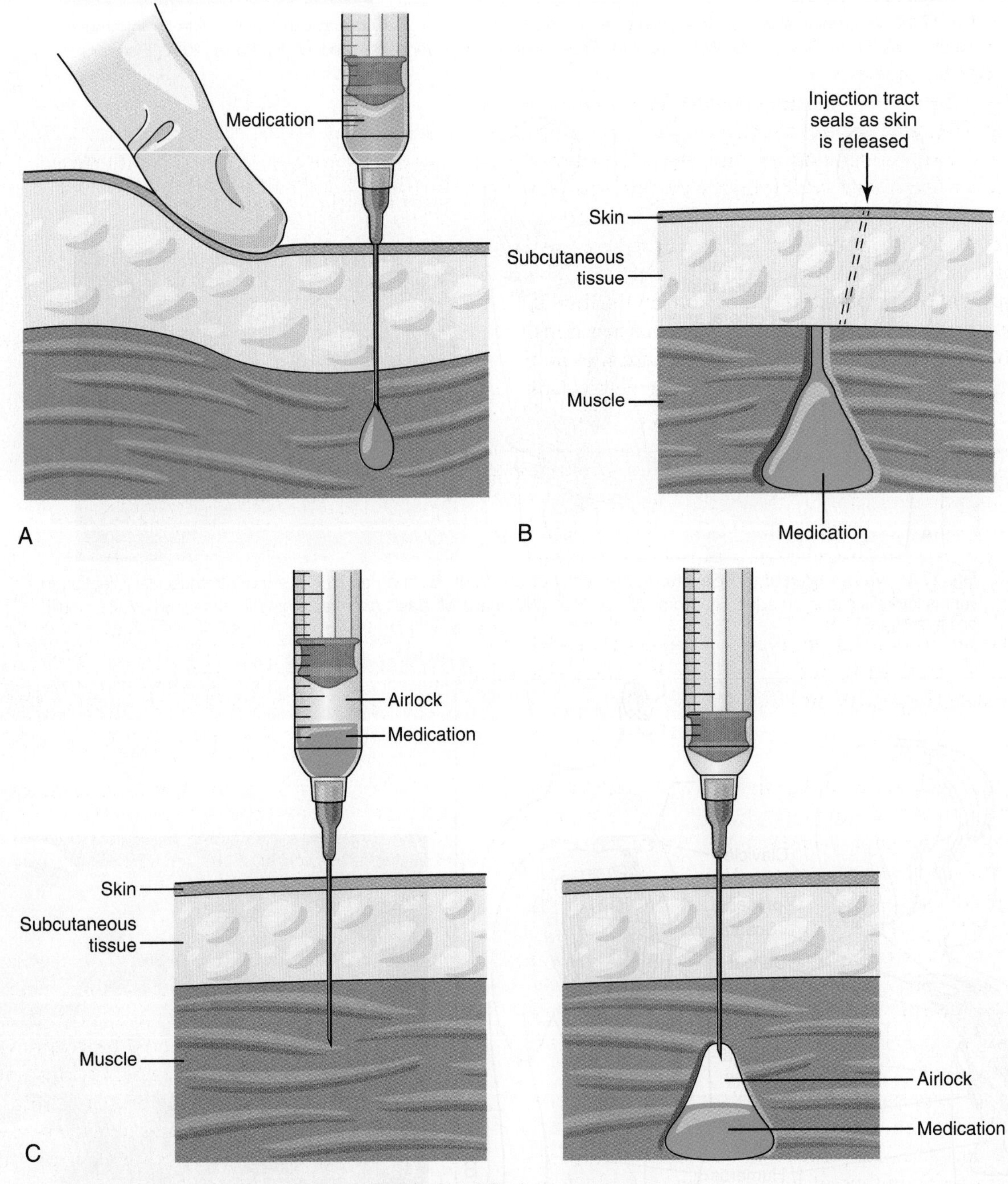

Fig. 17.17 Z-track method. A, Injection. B, Using an air lock. C, Administering IM injection by air lock technique.

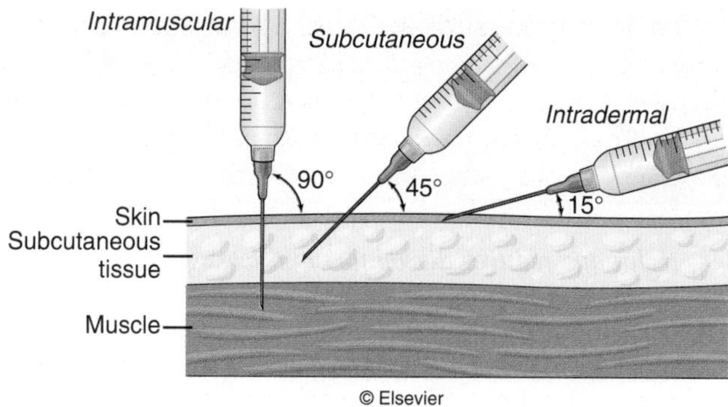

Fig. 17.18 Angles of insertion for intramuscular (90 degrees), subcutaneous (45 degrees), and intradermal (15 degrees) injections.

Use the upper chest, the inner aspect of the lower arm, or the scapular area for intradermal injections (see Skill 17.19).

Subcutaneous Injections

Administer insulin, heparin, enoxaparin (Lovenox), dalteparin (Fragmin), epoetin alfa (Epogen), and filgrastim (Neupogen) by the subcutaneous route. Inject these types of medications into the loose connective tissue between the dermis and the muscle layer. Because subcutaneous tissue is not as richly supplied with blood as the muscles, drug absorption is slower than with IM injections. The outer aspect of the upper arms, the abdomen, the thighs, and the scapula are sites used for subcutaneous injections. Inject no more than 1 mL of solution into these sites and always carefully document the injection. With medications that must be given routinely, rotate injection sites to help prevent tissue damage.

Subcutaneous injections should be given at a 45-degree angle if the patient is thin or at a 90-degree angle if the patient has ample subcutaneous tissue. Use your own clinical judgment in selecting sites for injection and in determining the angle of injection. Select a needle length so that the medication will be injected into subcutaneous tissue and not muscle tissue. Typically the usual needle length is ½ to ⅝ inch, and a 25-gauge needle is the one of choice (Fig. 17.19 and Skills 17.20 to 17.22).

Intravenous Therapy

Advances in technology of IV equipment enable nurses and health care providers to deliver IV fluids and medications more safely. The IV route (1) provides fluid and electrolyte maintenance, restoration, and replacement; (2) administers medications and sterilized nutrition (such as total parenteral nutrition through a central line); (3) administers blood and blood products; (4) administers chemotherapy to patients who are being treated for cancer; (5) administers patient-controlled analgesics; and (6) keeps a vein open for quick access.

Methods of intravenous administration. IV medications are possible to administer by several methods.

Intravenous push. Administer the medication directly into a vein or by means of a heparin or saline lock or port of an existing IV tubing set.

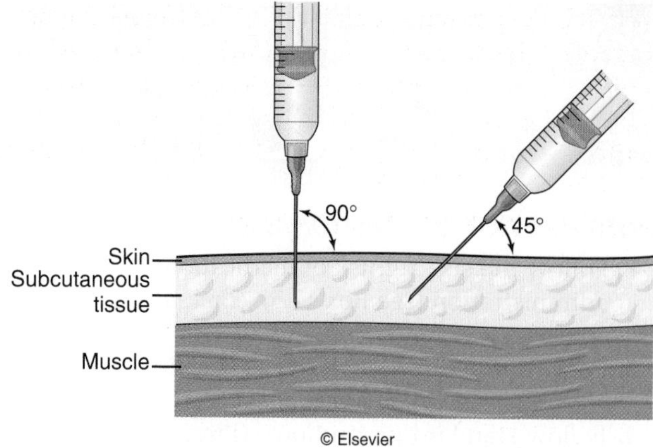

Fig. 17.19 Subcutaneous injection. Angle and needle length depend on thickness of the skinfold.

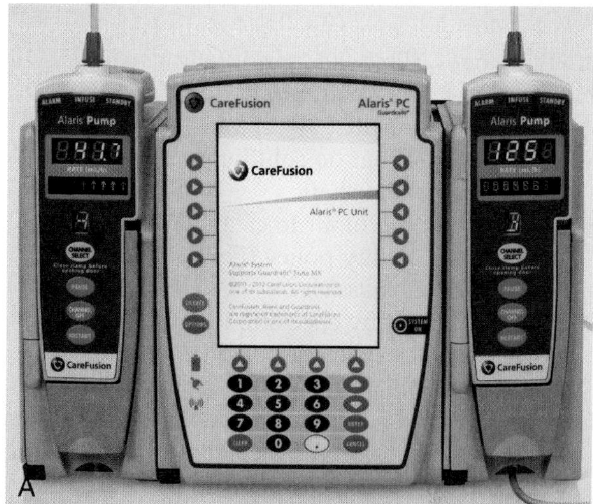

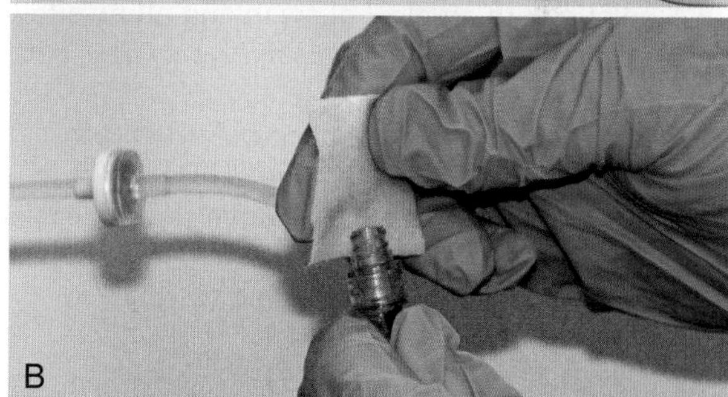

Fig. 17.20 Intravenous (IV) therapy. A, IV electronic infusion pump. B, Cleaning injection port with alcohol swab before medication administration via IV push. Injection port of IV tubing is used for drug infusion. (A, The Alaris System images are © 2014 CareFusion Corporation; Used with permission.)

Intermittent venous access device. An **intermittent venous access device** (commonly called a *saline lock,* previously called a *heparin [hep] lock*) is an IV infusion device with male adapters covered by diaphragms for the administration of intermittent infusions and as an access site for emergency drug infusion (Fig. 17.20). Intermittent venous access devices provide ready access for IV antibiotic therapy and other IV drug therapies without causing the unnecessary pain of a restick with every dose. Refer to the nursing practice act in the state

Skill 17.20 Giving a Z-Track Injection

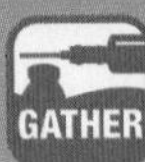

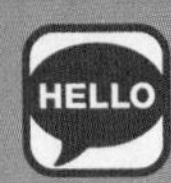

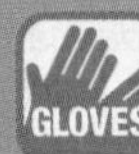

NURSING ACTION *(RATIONALE)*

1. Follow the six "rights" of medication administration (see Box 17.5). *(Prevents medication errors.)*
2. Perform the three label checks (see Box 17.6). *(Prevents medication errors.)*
3. Follow standard precautions. *(Prevents spread of microorganisms.)*
4. Perform hand hygiene. *(Prevents spread of microorganisms.)*
5. Prepare medication according to standard procedure for injectables (see Skill 17.13).
6. Don gloves. *(Prevents spread of microorganisms.)*
7. Use one needle to withdraw dose from container. Use another needle (1½ to 2 inches) to inject medication so that no solution remains on the outside of needle shaft.
8. Draw up 0.2 mL of air to create an air lock if advised per facility policy *(Further locks medication into muscle).*
9. Identify patient by checking identification bracelet and per facility policy. *(Prevents medication errors.)*
10. Provide privacy. Expose and locate ventrogluteal site according to intramuscular (IM) site selection procedure.
11. Clean site with an alcohol swab and allow site to dry. *(Mechanical and chemical action removes microorganisms.)*
12. Ask the patient to take a deep breath and to slowly exhale. *(Relaxes the muscle.)* Pull skin tightly in a lateral direction (move skin at least 1 to 1½ inches laterally) to one side. Hold the skin taut with the nondominant hand. *(Z-track technique reduces discomfort and leakage of medication into tissue.)*
13. Insert needle at a 90-degree angle; aspirate. *(It is necessary to insert a needle at 90-degree angle for it to enter muscle.)*
    a. If blood is seen, needle is in a vein or artery. Withdraw needle and discard medication; prepare new medication (see Skill 17.13). Select another site for new attempt and begin again from Step 13.
    b. If no blood is seen, inject medication and air slowly; wait 10 seconds to allow the medication to disperse slowly.
14. Withdraw needle quickly. Allow skin to return to its normal position, which leaves a zigzag path that seals the needle track wherever tissue planes slide across each other. *(The drug is not able to escape from the muscle tissue.)* (See Fig. 17.18.)
15. Place a 2- × 2-inch gauze pad or bandage on the injection site as needed.
16. Do not massage site. *(Massaging sometimes causes tissue irritation.)*
17. Do not recap needle; activate safety feature of needle and discard directly into sharps container. *(Prevents needlesticks.)*
18. Remove gloves and wash hands. *(Prevents spread of microorganisms.)*
19. Record administration of medications per facility policy. Chart site used, Z-track method used, and amount and type of medication given.
20. Return to assess patient's response to medication. *(Determines effectiveness of medication and occurrence of adverse reactions.)*
21. Document assessment findings in nursing notes.

where you are employed to determine the role of the LPN/LVN in administering IV medication.

Intermittent venous access devices attach onto a needleless hub. Once attached, the intermittent venous access device is filled with the anticoagulant heparin or normal saline. This keeps the vein open and makes it possible to administer IV medication at intervals without the need for a continuous infusion of fluid to ensure patency.

Intermittent infusion (or piggyback). IV piggybacks are drug infusions that are given at intervals, such as every 6 hours (q 6 hr). It is possible to connect them either to heparin or saline locks or to the injection port of the IV tubing (Fig. 17.20B). Once the medication has been infused, remove the piggyback device from the heparin or saline lock or IV tubing and flush the lock with heparin or saline. This is a common way to administer antibiotics.

Continuous infusions. Medication is added to a bag of IV fluid and infuses with the IV fluid.

Electronic IV pumps. Pumps regulate the flow rate of IV infusions.

Patient-controlled analgesia. **Patient-controlled analgesia (PCA)** is a drug-delivery system that dispenses a preset IV dose of an opioid analgesic into a patient's vein when the patient pushes a button that is connected to

Skill 17.21 Giving an Intradermal Injection

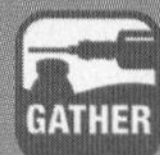

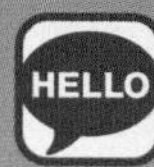

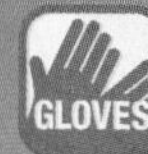

NURSING ACTION *(RATIONALE)*

1. Follow the six "rights" of medication administration (see Box 17.5). *(Prevents medication errors.)*
2. Perform the three label checks (see Box 17.6). *(Prevents medication errors.)*
3. Follow standard precautions. *(Prevents spread of microorganisms.)*
4. Perform hand hygiene. *(Prevents spread of microorganisms.)*
5. Prepare medication according to standard procedure for injectables (see Skill 17.13).
6. Don gloves. *(Prevents spread of microorganisms.)*
7. Identify patient by checking identification bracelet and per facility policy. *(Prevents medication errors.)*
8. Select arm and expose inner aspect of forearm.
9. Clean site gently with alcohol swab from center outward; let dry. *(Mechanical and chemical action removes microorganisms.)*
10. Two injections are made if test is for sensitivity. *(One injection is a control test with sterile water or bacteriostatic saline; the other is test substance.)* Insert a 25-gauge needle with bevel up directly under skin. Advance needle through epidermis to approximately ⅛ inch (3 mm) below the skin surface. You will be able to see the needle tip through the skin.
11. Make a small, bubble-like wheal with test solution. *(Creation of bleb shows placement of needle is correct.)* Insert needle at approximately a 15-degree angle. Do not inject into subcutaneous tissue. Inject control of saline into another site for comparison with test substance after designated time interval.
12. Do not massage site. *(Massage will most likely disperse medication into underlying tissue layers and alter test results.)*
13. Draw a circle around skin test with a marker; label area with time, date, and name of test. Another method is to make a diagram in patient's chart to indicate location of site. *(Facilitates assessment of site and reading of test results.)*
14. Remove gloves and wash hands. *(Prevents spread of microorganisms.)*
15. Record administration of medications per facility policy.
16. After the appropriate amount of time for the specific type of test has passed, note the presence of an indurated (hardened) erythematous area, measure indurated area, and record results in millimeters with metric ruler.
17. Compare control bleb with agent bleb; document results in chart.
18. Return to assess patient's response to medication. *(Enables you to determine effectiveness of medication and any occurrence of adverse reactions.)*
19. Document assessment findings in nursing notes.

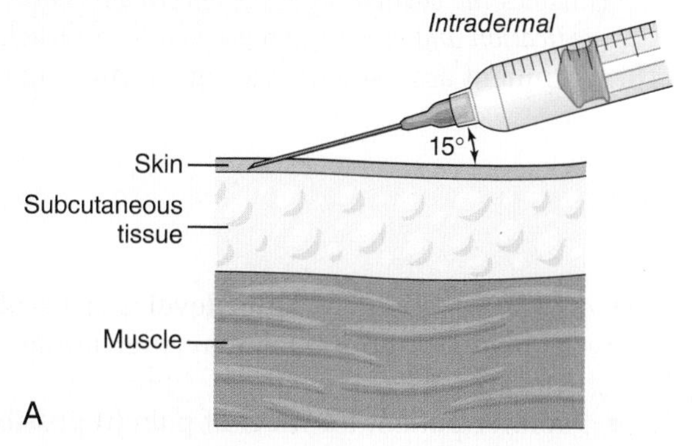

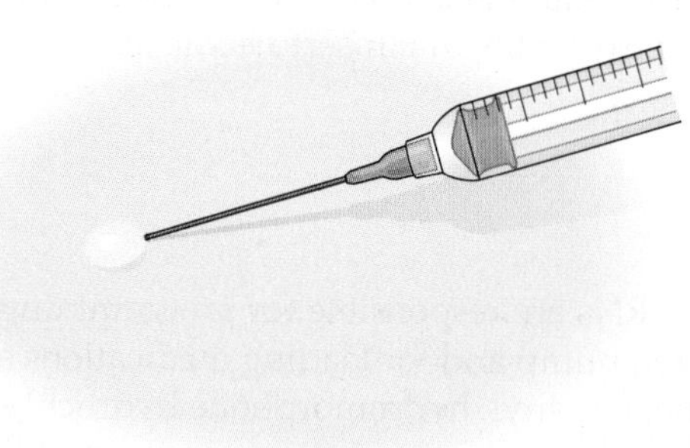

Step 11B figure from Elkin MK, Perry AG, Potter PA: *Nursing interventions and clinical skills,* ed 4, St. Louis, 2008, Mosby.

the PCA system via a cord (Fig. 17.21). The medication is administered by a programmable pump controlled by the patient. The RN programs the pump according to the health care provider's order, which specifies the amount of an opioid the patient receives per dose. The pump also controls the total amount of drug that it is possible for the patient to receive over a specific period. A lockout interval device automatically inactivates the system if a patient tries to press the button to receive another dose before the specified amount of time has passed.

Skill 17.22 Giving a Subcutaneous Injection

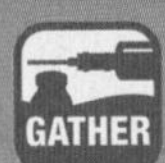

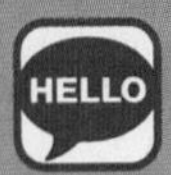

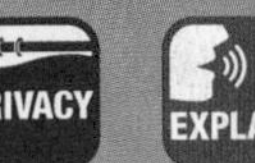

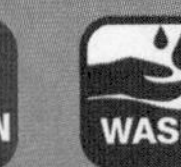

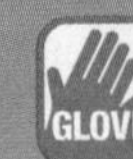

GLOVES

NURSING ACTION *(RATIONALE)*

1. Follow the six "rights" of medication administration (see Box 17.5). *(Prevents medication errors.)*
2. Perform the three label checks (see Box 17.6). *(Prevents medication errors.)*
3. Follow standard precautions. *(Prevents spread of microorganisms.)*
4. Perform hand hygiene. *(Prevents spread of microorganisms.)*
5. Prepare medication according to standard procedure for injectables (see Skill 17.13).
6. Don gloves. *(Prevents spread of microorganisms.)*
7. Identify patient by checking identification bracelet and per facility policy. *(Prevents medication errors.)*
8. Select and expose site (check which site was used previously, and choose a different site). The abdomen is the usual preferred site when administering heparin, enoxaparin (Lovenox), or dalteparin (Fragmin).
9. Clean site with an alcohol swab from center outward in circular motion; let dry. *(Mechanical and chemical action removes microorganisms.)*
10. Perform injection:
    a. Thin patient or child: Grasp and press together skin of selected site so that it forms roll between fingers. Insert needle at 45-degree angle. *(Angle ensures that medication reaches subcutaneous tissue rather than muscle.)* Inject medication slowly. *(Slow injection reduces pain and trauma.)*
    b. Average-size or obese patient: Grasp and press together skin of selected site so that it forms roll between fingers. Insert needle at a 90-degree angle. Inject medication slowly. *(Slow injection reduces pain and trauma.)*

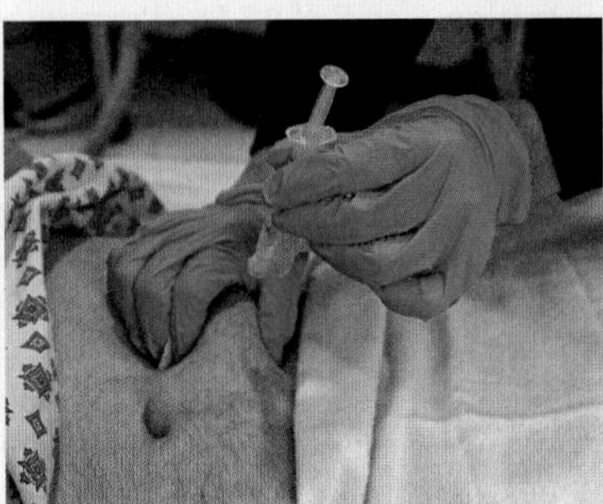

11. Withdraw needle quickly, and apply an antiseptic swab or a 2- × 2-inch gauze sponge. Supporting skin around injection site keeps discomfort to a minimum during withdrawal. Do not massage the site when administering insulin *(alters absorption rate)*, heparin, enoxaparin (Lovenox), or dalteparin (Fragmin). *(Massage will increase local bleeding, and ecchymosis will occur.)*
12. Do not recap needle; activate safety feature of needle and discard directly into sharps container. *(Prevents needlesticks.)*
13. Remove gloves and wash hands. *(Prevents spread of microorganisms.)*
14. Record administration of medications per facility policy. Chart site used and the amount and type of medication.
15. Return to assess patient's response to medication. *(Enables the evaluation of the effectiveness of medication and any occurrence of adverse reactions.)*
16. Document assessment findings in nursing notes.

Typically, RNs are responsible for programming the computerized pump and for loading medications such as morphine, fentanyl, hydromorphone hydrochloride (Dilaudid), or buprenorphine (Buprenex) into it. The LPN/LVN may perform the following activities (again, refer to the state's nursing practice act):

- Instruct patients to press button when analgesia is needed. (Ask patients to demonstrate or verbalize understanding.) Reassure them that they will not receive too much medication because of the lockout mechanism.
- Maintain PCA therapy:
    - Monitor number of doses received by patient.
    - Monitor patient for the development of clinical manifestations that may indicate an opiate overdose.
    - Monitor patient for relief of pain (if possible, use pain assessment scale).
    - Document total volume infused and remaining volume of analgesic left every shift.
    - Monitor accuracy of infusion; make certain that the opioid antagonist naloxone (Narcan) is readily available in case of opiate overdose.
- Educate visitors and family members regarding the importance of allowing the patient to push the button to self-administer doses.

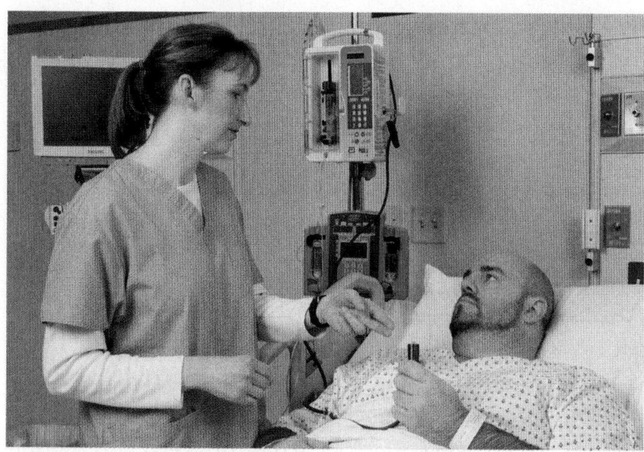

Fig. 17.21 Patient-controlled analgesia (PCA) infusion pump. The patient presses the button on a cord connected to the PCA pump. (From Perry AG, Potter PA, Ostendorf WR, et al: *Clinical nursing skills and techniques*, ed 9, St. Louis, 2018, Elsevier.)

Two RNs are needed to verify the PCA pump settings with the order. These nurses perform the six "rights" of medication administration and program the dose volume limits, lockout interval and frequency, and 4-hour limit. The LPN/LVN should refer to the state nursing practice act and the facility policy regarding his or her responsibilities.

PCA medication infusion is considered by many patients to provide more pain relief with less medication. Also, the patient has more control over medication administration, which often helps lessen the patient's anxiety and pain. The PCA is an effective and efficient method for administration of analgesic medications. Special PCA order sheets are used by the health care provider to specify the following:

1. Type and strength of medication
   EXAMPLE: Morphine sulfate, 1 mg/mL
2. Loading dose (an optional larger-than-usual dose to give initial pain relief)
   EXAMPLE: Range is 1 to 5 mL; usual is 1 to 2 mL
3. Maintenance dose (dose dispensed each time patient presses control button)
   EXAMPLE: Range is 0.1 to 5 mL; usual is 0.5 to 1 mL
4. Lockout interval (minimum time between doses)
   EXAMPLE: Range is 5 to 99 minutes; usual is 6 to 15 minutes
5. 4-hour limit (maximum volume delivered in 4 hours)
   EXAMPLE: Range is 5 to 30 mL in 5-mL increments; usual is 10 to 20 mL

Volumetric chambers. A volumetric chamber consists of IV tubing with a chamber that holds a prescribed amount of fluid; it is separate from the drip chamber. Medication such as oxytocin (Pitocin) or lidocaine can be added to the fluid in the chamber. The delivery of the medication to the patient can be controlled carefully when this method is used.

Nursing responsibility. The health care provider orders the type of IV fluid, the infusion rate, and sometimes the length of time that the infusion is to run. Ensure that the ordered type and amount of fluid is started and that the fluid is regulated to be infused at the appropriate rate. The use of an electronic infusion pump eliminates the need to count drops. In the absence of an infusion pump, regulate the IV infusion by knowing the number of drops per minute that it will take for the entire volume of fluid to infuse over the specified time ordered by the health care provider.

To find the number of drops per minute (the *drip rate*), know which type of IV tubing will be used with the infusion. Look on the IV tubing box for the **drip factor** (an apparatus that is used to deliver measured amounts of IV solutions of specific flow rates that are based on the size of drops of the solution). The box indicates whether the IV tubing is calibrated to deliver macrodrops or microdrops. To calculate IV flow rates, change milliliters to drops; for that, you need to know the drip factor. Macrodrop sets deliver 10, 15, or 20 drops per 1 mL of fluid; microdrop, or minidrop, sets deliver 60 drops per 1 mL of fluid.

EXAMPLE 1: The health care provider orders 1000 mL of 5% dextrose (D_5) in ½ normal saline (NS) with 20 mEq KCl to be infused over an 8-hour period. The nurse is using a microdrop set (60 drops per 1 mL of fluid). Use the following formula to determine how many drops will drip each minute.

First, convert number of milliliters per hour:

Then, place the information into the following formula:

$$\frac{\text{Drip rate (mL/hr)}}{\text{60 minutes}} \times \text{drip factor} = \text{drops per minute}$$

$$\frac{\text{125 mL/hr}}{\text{60 minutes}} \times 60 = 124.9 \text{ drops (gtt) per minute}$$

"Drops" is also written as "gtt."

ANSWER: 125 gtt/min

EXAMPLE 2: The health care provider orders 1000 mL D_5 in ½ NS to be infused over a 4-hour period. The drip factor on the box is 10 drops per 1 mL of fluid. To get the rate of milliliters per hour, divide the amount to infuse (1000 mL) by the time (4 hours). Place the information into the formula listed above.

$$\frac{\text{1000 mL}}{\text{4 hours}} = \text{250 mL/hour}$$

$$\frac{\text{250 mL/hour}}{\text{60 minutes}} \times 10 = 41.66 \text{ drops (gtt)/minute}$$

ANSWER: 42 gtt/min

Infusion pumps also have the capacity to record the volume of the fluid infused. An infusion pump is designed to deliver a measured amount of fluid over a period (e.g., milliliters per hour). The pump has a drop sensor and an alarm that will sound if drops are not detected at the appropriate rate. There are also alarms to alert the nurse regarding increased system pressure that can occur with an infiltration (IV fluid seeping into the tissue instead of the vascular space). An accurate measurement of intake of all IV therapy is recorded.

Monitoring intravenous therapy. Check the infusion and the IV site at least every hour, or per facility policy, to ensure that the IV infusion is continuing without any difficulty. If there is a problem with the site, discontinue using it, select a new IV site, and perform another venipuncture. Refer to the state nursing practice act and refer to the facility's policy to determine the responsibilities of the LPN/LVN regarding the IV infusion.

Monitor the IV site for the development of problems. Assess for erythema, wetness, and edema. Inflammation, erythema, warmth, and pain often signify the onset of phlebitis (inflamed vein), and edema, coolness to touch, pallor, and pain indicate a possible infiltration of fluid into the tissue. Report these conditions to the RN and discontinue the IV infusion. Assess and document the degree of infiltration as evidenced by the level of discomfort, swelling, and erythema. Worsening of the site condition requires reporting to the RN and possibly the primary care provider. In addition, report the following:

- A patient with sudden onset of chills, fever, headache, nausea, and vomiting
- An anxious, dyspneic patient with a weak and rapid pulse

These factors sometimes indicate complications of IV therapy that necessitate immediate medical intervention.

Allergic reactions are possible as a result of IV medication administration. Reactions range from a mild rash to **anaphylactic shock** (a severe, life-threatening hypersensitivity reaction). Signs and symptoms may appear suddenly or at some point after the administration of the medication. Report if any of the following occurs:

- Respiratory distress from bronchospasms, manifested by restlessness, dyspnea, wheezing, and cyanosis (bluish coloration of the skin)
- Skin reactions such as pruritus (itching) or urticaria (hives)
- Signs of circulatory collapse, such as rapidly falling blood pressure, weak and rapid (thready) pulse, or vertigo
- GI signs and symptoms such as nausea, vomiting, and diarrhea
- Change in mental status

Anaphylactic shock necessitates immediate intervention. The LPN/LVN should notify the RN immediately if the patient develops clinical manifestations of an allergic reaction.

❖ NURSING PROCESS

The role of the LPN/LVN in the nursing process as stated is that the LPN/LVN will:

- Act in accordance with the state's nurse practice act
- Act in accordance with the facility's policies and procedures
- Participate in planning care for patients based on patient needs
- Review patient's plan of care and recommend revisions as needed
- Review and follow defined prioritization for patient care
- Use clinical pathways, care maps, or care plans to guide and review patient care

◆ ASSESSMENT

The nurse assesses many factors to determine the need for and potential response to drug therapy. These factors include the patient's medical history, diet, and allergy history. Assess the patient's current physical and mental status. Poor coordination and musculoskeletal problems may sometimes interfere with the patient's ability to prepare doses and take medications correctly. Consider the patient's knowledge and understanding of drug therapy. Know as much as possible about each drug given, including normal dosages, purpose, action, routes, side effects, and interaction with other drugs.

◆ PATIENT PROBLEM

Use assessment findings to determine actual or potential problems with drug therapy. Potential patient problems may include the following:

- *Anxiousness*
- *Potential for Unsafe Health Behaviors*
- *Potential for Harm or Damage to Body*
- *Insufficient Knowledge (specify)*
- *Compromised Physical Mobility*
- *Noncooperation or Nonconformity: Drug Regimen*

◆ EXPECTED OUTCOMES AND PLANNING

The plan of care should be focused on the safe administration of drugs. Use the time during drug administration to teach patients about their medications. Collaboration with the patient's family and significant others about drug regimens after discharge is necessary.

The plan of care is likely to include the following goal and outcome:

Goal: Patient and family understand the importance of the medication and how and when to administer the medication.

Outcome: Patient and family describe information about the drug, dosage, schedule, purpose, and adverse effects.

◆ IMPLEMENTATION

Identify factors that have the potential to improve or diminish a patient's health and well-being. Physical limitations, economic status, cultural beliefs, values, and habits tend to influence a patient's compliance with medication schedules. The nurse is responsible for knowing about medications and their potential adverse effects on the patient, especially if the patient has multiple prescriptions. The capabilities and limitations of older adult patients are especially important considerations (see the Lifespan Considerations box for older adults).

◆ EVALUATION

Use evaluative measures to determine whether patient outcomes were met. Always be prepared to revise the care plan on the basis of the evaluation findings.

Goal: Patient and family understand drug therapy.
Evaluative measure: Ask patient or family to describe purpose, dosage, and adverse effects of each prescribed medication.

Lifespan Considerations

Older Adults

Medications and Aging

- All phases of pharmacokinetics are affected by aging. When the nurse has an option or is required to use clinical judgment regarding a patient's dose (e.g., an order of pain medication may note that the patient may receive 1 or 2 tablets), give older people the lowest dosages of medication necessary to achieve the desired therapeutic results.
- Dry mouth often contributes to difficulty swallowing medications. Sipping water before attempting to swallow the medication or covering the medication with a moist food such as applesauce tends to facilitate swallowing.
- It is necessary to take more precautions when parenteral medication is administered to older adults because of a decreased amount of muscle and subcutaneous tissue. Examine sites for suitability and rotate them with each use. Carefully select needles of the proper length on the basis of the selected site and a tissue assessment of the individual.
- Because of decreased tolerance to intravenous (IV) medications, it is necessary to carefully assess the older adult for toxicity.
- Polypharmacy (the use of excessive numbers of different medications) is a common problem for older adults. Each medication taken increases the risk of interactions or toxicity. It is best if the older patient has only one primary health care provider who manages the patient's medications. Educate older adults to refrain from taking any medication unless it is approved by the health care provider.
- Teach the older person to keep accurate and current records of all prescription and over-the-counter medications and to present this list each time he or she seeks medical attention.
- Because of decreased renal, cardiac, and hepatic functioning, the older adult is at greater risk of becoming adversely and even fatally affected by medications. Also, hospitalized older adults often have one or more chronic illnesses for which they take multiple medications.
- Monitor the patient for signs and symptoms of decreased drug excretion, cumulative effects of drugs, drug potentiation, and drug incompatibilities. Frequent assessments and careful, thoughtful monitoring of the older patient aid in the prevention of medication-related complications.
- Some older adults do not hear, see, communicate, or move about as well as younger patients. Some also are disoriented and perhaps even more so at night. When administering medications to older patients, take time to carefully assess their level of consciousness beforehand and afterward.
- Carefully evaluate the list of medications prescribed for each patient, and ascertain whether there have been any incompatibilities or incorrect dosages or whether any medications are possibly adversely affecting the patient.
- The prevention of drug-related problems is the combined responsibility of the nurse, the health care provider, the pharmacist, and others who care for the patient. Effective communication between the health care team, the patient, and the patient's family is necessary to administer medication safely and effectively to the older adult.

Get Ready for the NCLEX® Examination!

Key Points

- Calculate drug dosages accurately to administer medication safely to each patient.
- To reduce the chance of making a medication error, verify the correct dosage calculation with another nurse and reduce distractions while calculating dosages.
- The metric system is the preferred system of weights and measures; it is more accurate and easier to use in calculating dosage problems.
- When calculating dosages, always use the same units of measurement in the problem to avoid errors; if different units are used, convert them to one type of unit.
- Age, weight, body surface area, and the ability of the body to absorb, metabolize, and excrete medication are necessary to consider when medications are administered to a child.
- Be knowledgeable about the body surface area method for calculating children's dosages.
- When preparing medications, check the medication container label against the medication administration record or computer three times.
- The six "rights" of medication administration ensure accurate preparation and administration of medication dosages.
- Administer only those medications that you prepare.

- Never administer medication without accurately identifying the patient by patient's name and birth date. Follow facility policy if the patient is unable to identify himself or herself.
- Chart medications immediately after administration.
- Never leave a prepared medication unattended.
- Failure to select injection sites by anatomic landmarks poses the risk of tissue, bone, or nerve damage.
- Nurses are ethically and legally responsible for ensuring that the patient receives the correct medication ordered by the health care provider.
- Each medication order is required to include the patient's name and date of birth; order; date; medication name, dosage, route, and frequency of administration; and health care provider's signature.
- Always have a second nurse witness the "wasting" (disposal of unused portions) of a controlled substance or medication; both nurses must sign the log book or document via facility policy to indicate that the medication was wasted.
- Medications enter the body through oral, sublingual, buccal, parenteral, percutaneous, inhalation, and topical (skin and mucous membranes) routes.
- Irrigations of the eye are used to relieve local inflammation of the conjunctiva, to apply antiseptic solution, or to flush out exudate or caustic or irritating solutions.
- Using a small syringe and solution at body temperature, the nurse can clean a patient's external auditory canal of excess cerumen or exudate from a lesion or inflamed area.
- Internal vaginal irrigation, or douching, should not be performed routinely because it tends to wash away protective agents.
- Medications administered parenterally are absorbed more quickly than are medications administered by other routes.
- The Z-track method for intramuscular injection minimizes irritation by sealing the medication in muscle tissue.
- Intramuscular injections for analgesia are given less frequently currently because of the use of PCA and patient-controlled epidural pumps.
- The nurse may give intradermal injections for skin testing (e.g., tuberculin screening and allergy tests).
- Because of decreased renal, cardiac, or hepatic functioning, the older adult is at greater risk of becoming adversely and possibly fatally affected by medications.

Additional Learning Resources

SG Go to your Study Guide for additional learning activities to help you master this chapter content.

evolve Be sure to visit the Evolve site at *http://evolve.elsevier.com/Cooper/foundationsadult/* for additional online resources.

Review Questions for the NCLEX® Examination

Work the following problems. Use the proportion method, dimensional analysis, or desired dose/available dose formula, frequently used equivalents, and the big-to-small rule.

1. The health care provider has ordered 0.5 g of ceftriaxone (Rocephin). The nurse has available a vial labeled "250 mg/mL." How many milliliters will the nurse give the patient?
 1. 2 mL
 2. 0.2 mL
 3. 0.05 mL
 4. 0.5 mL

2. Digoxin (Lanoxin), 0.125 mg, is ordered. On hand is Lanoxin, 0.5 mg/mL. How many milliliters will the nurse give?
 1. 3 mL
 2. 0.25 mL
 3. 2.5 mL
 4. 0.025 mL

3. The pediatrician has requested the pediatric patient's weight in kilograms. The scales say that the patient weighs 30 lb. How many kilograms will be reported to the health care provider?
 1. 20.6 kg
 2. 15 kg
 3. 13.6 kg
 4. 66 kg

4. Ordered is 1 L of D_5 ½ NS to run over 8 hours. The drip factor stated on the IV tubing is 15 gtt/mL. How many milliliters will be infused every hour?
 1. 100 mL/h
 2. 125 mL/h
 3. 150 mL/h
 4. 175 mL/h

5. An IV infusion of 1 L of D_5 ½ NS is to run at 150 mL/h. How long will this infusion run?
 1. 6 hours
 2. 6.7 hours
 3. 7.5 hours
 4. 8 hours

6. Which intramuscular injection site is no longer recommended for use because of the nearness of the sciatic nerve to the muscle and potential for permanent or partial paralysis of the involved leg?
 1. Ventrogluteal site
 2. Deltoid site
 3. Vastus lateralis site
 4. Dorsogluteal site

7. The average dose of a medication is 0.4 mg (gr 1/150) for an adult. What is the dosage for a 12-year-old?
 1. 2 mg
 2. 0.002 mg
 3. 0.02 mg
 4. 0.2 mg

8. An adult dose of diazepam (Valium) is 5 mg. Which dose is appropriate for a child who weighs 27 kg?
 1. 2 mg
 2. 1.5 mg
 3. 3 mg
 4. 2.5 mg

9. A 71-year-old patient is receiving the following medications: carvedilol tablet for hypertension, furosemide tablet heart failure, paroxetine tablet for anxiety, and guaifenesin cough syrup for a productive cough. He is to receive his medications at 8 a.m. daily. Which medication will be given last?
1. furosemide tablet
2. carvedilol tablet
3. guaifenesin cough syrup
4. paroxetine tablet

10. The LPN is asked by an RN to take an unlabeled container of solution to the operating room. What is the LPN's best response?
1. "Of course, I'll take it right away!"
2. "What is in the container?"
3. "I will have the orderly take it."
4. "I am not permitted to transport an unlabeled container."

11. After a possible exposure to tuberculosis, a 25-year-old health worker receives a tuberculin skin test. What type of injection is this?
1. Intramuscular
2. Intradermal
3. Subcutaneous
4. Intravenous

12. Insulin is to be given to a 55-year-old patient with diabetes who weighs 275 lb (125 kg) and measures 72 inches (183 cm) tall. His insulin is to be given via subcutaneous injection. What angle is acceptable for the injection?
1. 45 degrees
2. 90 degrees
3. 15 degrees only
4. 35 degrees only

13. The nurse is deciding on the angle used in delivering subcutaneous heparin. What factor will determine the angle to be used for the injection? *(Select all that apply.)*
1. The amount of solution in the syringe
2. The length of the needle
3. The gauge of the needle
4. The amount of subcutaneous tissue of the patient
5. The size of the bevel of the needle

14. The patient complains of nausea after having a total abdominal hysterectomy. The nurse prepares an injection of promethazine (Phenergan), 25 mg, for IM injection. What needle length is most appropriate for selection?
1. ⅜ inch
2. ⅝ inch
3. 1 to 1½ inches
4. 2 to 2½ inches

15. A 6-month-old is to be immunized for diphtheria, tetanus, and pertussis. His IM injection will be given in which muscle?
1. Deltoid
2. Ventrogluteal
3. Gluteus maximus
4. Vastus lateralis

16. The LPN/LVN is administering 8 a.m. medications in an acute care hospital. What is the acceptable time range for the nurse to administer these medications?
1. 0800 to 1000
2. 0700 to 0900
3. 0800 to 0830
4. 0730 to 0830

17. While administering routine medications to a patient at 1200 hours, the nurse realizes he has made a medication error. What is the nurse's priority action?
1. Notify the health care provider.
2. Call the supervisor.
3. Complete an incident report.
4. Assess the patient.

18. Prescribed medications are prepared and administered during which phase of the nursing process?
1. Assessment
2. Planning
3. Implementation
4. Evaluation

19. A patient hospitalized with newly diagnosed hypertension is taking enalapril (Vasotec), 5 mg PO bid, to lower his blood pressure. His next dose is at 0900. When taking his vital signs, the nurse discovers the patient's blood pressure is 90/42. What should the nurse do?
1. Withhold the medication and inform the health care provider of the change in the patient's blood pressure.
2. Give the medication on time (the blood pressure is within normal limits).
3. Ask the patient how he is feeling; if he is not having adverse signs or symptoms of low blood pressure, give him the medication.
4. Give half the dose ordered.

20. Which action would be correct when a patient's ear is irrigated?
1. Straighten the ear canal and irrigate with a large-tipped bulb syringe.
2. Direct the solution to the middle of the canal to avoid damaging the ear.
3. Use a solution that is body temperature and have the patient hold a basin under the ear while the solution is directed toward the top of the canal.
4. Repeat the irrigation with hotter water.

21. The nurse performing eye irrigation should perform which procedure?
1. Have the patient tip her head up, and run the irrigation fluid over the open eye.
2. Direct the irrigating fluid from the inner to the outer canthus.
3. Do not allow the patient to blink.
4. Place the irrigating syringe directly onto the corner of the eye and allow the fluid to move across the eye.
5. Position the patient with the effected eye down.

18 Fluids and Electrolytes

http://evolve.elsevier.com/Cooper/foundationsadult/

Objectives

1. Discuss how very young, very old, and obese patients are at risk for fluid volume deficit.
2. List, describe, and compare the body fluid compartments.
3. Discuss how homeostasis is maintained.
4. Describe the thirst mechanism.
5. Discuss active and passive transport processes, and give an example of each.
6. Describe the cause and effect of deficits and excesses of sodium, potassium, chloride, calcium, magnesium, phosphorus, and bicarbonate.
7. Differentiate among the roles of the buffers, the lungs, and the kidneys in maintaining acid-base balance.
8. Compare and contrast the four primary types of acid-base imbalances.
9. Discuss the role of the nursing process in maintaining fluid, electrolyte, and acid-base balances.
10. Summarize the nurse's responsibilities for the patient receiving intravenous therapy and related procedures.
11. Discuss complications of intravenous therapy.
12. Explain the nurse's responsibility in the administration of blood transfusion therapy.
13. Describe the complications of blood therapy.

Key Terms

acid-base balance (ĂS-ĭd BĀS BĂL-ĭns, p. 494)
active transport (ĂK-tĭv TRĂNZ-pŏrt, p. 487)
adenosine triphosphate (ATP) (ă-DĔN-ŏ-sēn trī-FŎS-fāt, p. 485)
anions (ĂN-ī-ŏnz, p. 487)
autologous blood transfusions (ăw-TŎL-ă-gŭs BLŬD trănz-FYŪ-zhŭn, p. 516)
bicarbonate (bī-KĂHR-bō-nāt, p. 494)
blood buffers (BLŬD BŬF-ŭrz, p. 495)
calcium (KĂL-sē-ŭm, p. 491)
cations (KĂT-ī-ŏnz, p. 487)
chevron (SHĔV-rŏn, p. 510)
chloride (KLŎR-īd, p. 490)
diffusion (dĭf-YŪ-zhĭn, p. 485)
electrolyte (ĕ-LĔK-trō-līt, p. 487)
extracellular (ĕks-tră-SĔL-yū-lăr, p. 483)
filtration (fĭl-TRĀ-shĭn, p. 487)
glomerular filtration rate (GFR) (glŏ-MĔR-yū-lŭr fĭl-TRĀ-shĭn RĀT, p. 484)
homeostasis (hō-mē-ō-STĀ-sĭs, p. 484)
hydrostatic pressure (hī-drō-STĂT-ĭk PRĔSH-ŭr, p. 487)
hypertonic (hī-pŭr-TŎN-ĭk, p. 486)
hypotonic (hī-pō-TŎN-ĭk, p. 487)
induration (ĭn-dū-RĀ-shŭn, p. 507)
infiltration (ĭn-fĭl-TRĀ-shŭn, p. 508)
interstitial (ĭn-tŭr-STĬSH-ăl, p. 483)
intracellular (ĭn-tră-SĔL-yū-lăr, p. 483)
intravascular (ĭn-tră-VĂS-cyū-lăr, p. 484)
intravenous (IV) (ĭn-tră-VĒ-nŭs, p. 498)
ions (Ī-ŏnz, p. 487)
isotonic (ī-sō-TŎN-ĭk, p. 486)
magnesium (măg-NĒ-zē-ŭm, p. 493)
milliequivalent (mEq) (mĭl-ē-ĕ-KWĬV-ă-lĕnt, p. 487)
osmosis (ŏz-MŌ-sĭs, p. 486)
passive transport (PĂS-ĭv TRĂNZ-pŏrt, p. 485)
patent (PĀ-tĕnt, p. 510)
peripheral (pĕ-RĬF-ŭr-ăl, p. 505)
phosphorus (FŎS-fŭ-rŭs, p. 493)
potassium (pŏ-TĂS-ē-ŭm, p. 488)
sodium (SŌ-dē-ŭm, p. 487)
venipuncture (VĔN-ĭ-pŭnk-chŭr, p. 500)

This chapter discusses fluids and electrolytes and acid-base balance. The body's fluid, electrolyte, and acid-base balance must be maintained to keep body systems healthy and functioning properly. These are maintained by water intake and output, distribution of electrolytes in the body, and the regulation of the renal and pulmonary systems.

FLUIDS (WATER)

Water has many functions in the body. It is necessary to carry nutrients to the body cells and waste products from the cells. Once inside the cells, water provides a medium in which chemical reactions, or metabolism, occur. Water also acts as a lubricant for tissues, aids in

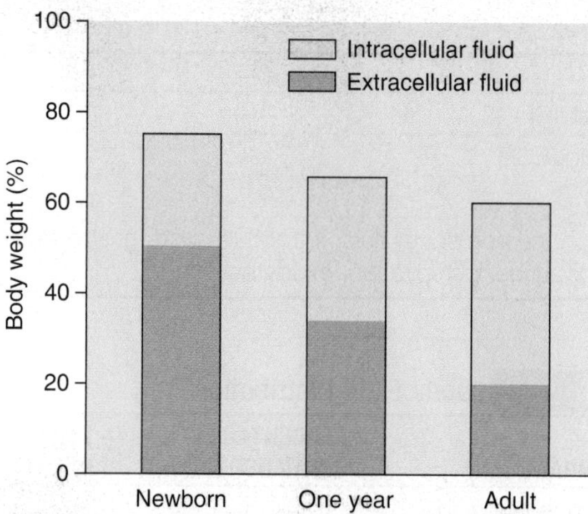

Fig. 18.1 In the newborn, more than half of total body fluid is extracellular. As the child grows, proportions gradually reach adult levels. (From Monahan F, Sands JK, Neighbors M, et al: *Phipps' medical-surgical nursing: Health and illness perspectives*, ed 8, St. Louis, 2007, Mosby.)

the maintenance of acid-base balance, and assists in heat regulation by evaporation.

Water is the largest component of the body. It makes up from 50% to 80% of total body weight, depending on age, sex, and body fat. This percentage depends on several factors and varies by individual. Between 70% and 80% of a newborn's body weight is water. That percentage increases in a premature infant to as high as 90%. As the infant ages, that percentage steadily decreases, and by 12 years of age, the ratio of water to body weight approaches that of an adult. The percentage of water in the adult body is 50% to 60%, and in the older adult, it drops to 45% to 55%.

In addition to age, fat also plays a role in the amount of water found in the body. Fat contains relatively little water in comparison to muscle. Women have proportionately more body fat than do men and thereby have less body fluid than do men. Individuals having more body weight, as in obesity, have smaller percentages of body water. Similarly, the more obese an individual is, the smaller the percentage of body water. Older adults and obese populations are at a greater risk for complications resulting from dehydration because of the reduced fluid reserve in their bodies (see the Lifespan Considerations box). Infants are also at higher risk for dehydration because more than half of an infant's body fluid is found outside the cells (**extracellular**) (Fig. 18.1). Extracellular fluid is lost from the body more rapidly than **intracellular** fluid (fluid inside the cells). A loss of 10% of body fluid is serious in an adult, and a 20% loss is fatal. In an infant, the percentages are even more significant: a 5% loss is serious, a 10% loss is very serious, and a 15% or more loss can be fatal.

FLUID COMPARTMENTS

Body fluids are found in two compartments in the body: inside the cells (intracellular) and outside the cells (extracellular). However, *compartment* is an abstract term because rather than being contained in a compartment, in a specific area, the fluids are in constant motion throughout the body to carry out their functions. Although each compartment is specific in its location and functions, there is constant interaction between them.

The intracellular fluid compartment is the larger of the two compartments, making up 66% of the body's fluid. It is composed of all the fluid inside the cells within the body and contains dissolved particles, called *solutes*.

The extracellular fluid compartment contains any fluid outside the cells. It contains large amounts of oxygen and carbon dioxide, as well as glucose, amino acids, fatty acids, sodium, calcium, chloride, and bicarbonate. The extracellular compartment is divided further into the interstitial and the intravascular fluid compartments (Fig. 18.2).

Interstitial fluid is found between the cells or in the tissues. It accounts for approximately 27% of the fluid in

Lifespan Considerations

Older Adults

Dehydration

Older adults are at increased risk of dehydration because of several factors. Keep the following factors in mind when considering dehydration in an older adult:

- Fat replaces lean muscle as aging progresses, leading to a decrease in total body fluid.
- The aging kidney is less able to concentrate urine, so more fluid is lost.
- Decreases in mobility and a diminished sense of thirst often result in decreased fluid intake.
- Incontinent older individuals sometimes restrict fluid intake to reduce the frequency of urination and incontinence.
- To compensate for changes in taste, older adults often put excess salt on their food, which results in electrolyte and fluid imbalances.
- Physiologic changes in the skin and mucous membranes decrease their reliability as indicators of dehydration.
- Mild disorientation may be the first indication of dehydration.
- Signs and symptoms of dehydration include thirst, dry mucous membranes, increased heart rate, decreased blood pressure, poor skin turgor, and flat neck veins.
- Dehydration increases the risk of orthostatic hypotension.
- Decreased fluid intake increases the likelihood of constipation.
- Because the aging kidney is less efficient at excretion, giving intravenous (IV) infusions or supplements containing sodium or potassium increases the risk of electrolyte imbalance.
- Monitor the complete blood cell count carefully to detect changes in the hematocrit as it relates to hemoglobin. Decreased plasma volume elevates the hematocrit, whereas the hemoglobin level remains constant.

Table 18.1 Body Fluid Distribution

COMPARTMENT	DESCRIPTION	FLUID
Intracellular	Fluid within cells	Intracellular fluid (ICF)
Extracellular	Fluid outside cells	Extracellular fluid (ECF)
Intravascular	Fluid within blood vessels	Plasma
Interstitial	Fluid in tissues (between cells or in body spaces)	Examples: lymph, cerebrospinal fluid, intraocular fluid, gastrointestinal (GI) secretions, urine, perspiration, exudates

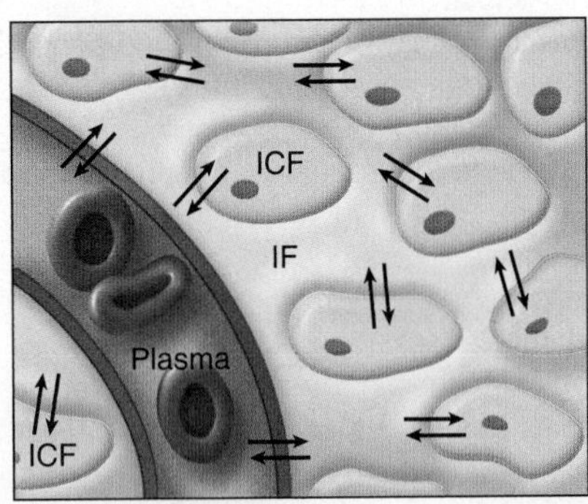

Fig. 18.2 Major fluid compartments. Intracellular fluid *(ICF)* is fluid within cells. Extracellular fluid is fluid outside of cells. The extracellular fluid also includes interstitial fluid *(IF)*, which surrounds the cells, and plasma, the fluid component of blood. Fluid continually moves between the major compartments. (From Patton KT, Thibodeau GA: *The human body in health and disease*, ed 6, St. Louis, 2014, Mosby.)

Table 18.2 Body Fluid Distribution

COMPARTMENT	PERCENTAGE OF TOTAL BODY FLUID	FLUID VOLUME (L)
Extracellular fluid		
Interstitial fluid	27	11.2
Intravascular fluid (plasma)	7	2.8
Intracellular fluid	66	42.0

Table 18.3 Normal Fluid Intake and Output in an Adult Eating 2500 Calories Per Day (Approximate Statistics)

TYPE OF CONTENT	GAIN (mL)	ROUTE	AMOUNT OF LOSS (mL)
Water in food	1000	Skin	500
Water from oxidation	300	Lungs	350
Water as liquid	1200	Feces	150
		Kidney	1500
Total	2500	Total	2500

the body. Examples of interstitial fluid include lymph, cerebrospinal fluid, and gastrointestinal (GI) secretions.

Intravascular fluid is the plasma within the vessels. This fluid contains serum, protein, and other substances necessary to sustain life. This fluid is usually what carries the nutrients and waste products between cells and tissues. It makes up the remaining 7% of fluid volume.

The intracellular and extracellular fluid compartments are separated by a semipermeable membrane. This membrane allows for a constant flow as nutrients are taken into the cell and waste products are carried out (Tables 18.1 and 18.2).

INTAKE AND OUTPUT

As water moves through all parts of the body, it constantly is being lost and must be replaced. Fluid leaves the body through the kidneys, the lungs, the skin, and the GI tract. **Homeostasis** is the process of keeping body fluids in balance. The body is equipped with several homeostatic mechanisms to keep the composition and volume of body fluid within narrow limits of normal. The average adult fluid intake is approximately 2200 to 2700 mL/day. Oral intake of fluids should be approximately 1100 to 1400 mL/day; solid foods contribute approximately 800 to 1000 mL/day; and fluid produced from cellular metabolism provides approximately 300 mL/day (Table 18.3).

Fluid intake is regulated mainly through the thirst mechanism. Receptors in the hypothalamus called *osmoreceptors* measure the concentration of the blood. When the number of particles (solutes) in the blood is higher than normal, the sensation of thirst is present, and the person drinks to satisfy that sensation. Anyone who is unable to respond to or perceive the thirst mechanism is at increased risk for dehydration and may require fluids administered by way of tube feedings, IV infusion, or total parenteral nutrition (TPN).

Fluid loss from the body is considered either sensible (measurable) or insensible (not measurable). Sensible losses are seen in urine, feces, vomiting, and wound drainage. Insensible fluid losses include those from perspiration and expiration. Because it is difficult to measure insensible fluid losses accurately, approximations are acceptable. However, because measurement of sensible losses is possible, it is very important to keep accurate records of fluid intake and output to help determine a patient's fluid needs.

The kidneys play an extremely important role in fluid balance. If the kidneys are not functioning properly, the body has great difficulty regulating fluid balance. The nephrons are the functioning units of the kidneys, and they filter blood at a rate of 125 mL/min, or about 180 L/day. This is called the **glomerular filtration rate (GFR)** and leads to an output of 1 to 2 L (1000 to 2000 mL) of urine per day. The nephrons reabsorb the remaining fluid based on bodily needs. If the body loses even 1% to 2% of its fluid, the kidneys conserve fluid by reabsorbing more water from the renal filtrate, which results in less water excreted and more concentrated urine. To effectively eliminate waste products from the body, the kidneys must excrete a minimum of 30 mL/h of urine. In the presence of fluid excesses, the kidneys react by excreting more dilute urine, thus ridding the body of excess fluid and conserving electrolytes.

One simple and accurate way to determine water balance is by weighing the patient under controlled conditions: for example, at the same time of day, with the same amount of clothing, and when attached to the same equipment, such as electrodes, IV tubing, braces, or splints. It is important to empty all drainage bags before the patient is weighed to get an accurate measurement. One liter of fluid equals 2.2 pounds (1 kg); therefore a weight change of 2.2 pounds reflects a loss or gain of 1 L of body fluid (Skill 18.1).

Urine specific gravity is a measurement of urine concentration. It is also a good indicator of fluid balance. A urine specific gravity value of more than 1.030 indicates that the urine is concentrated, as in conditions of dehydration, whereas a measurement of less than 1.003 to 1.000 indicates that the urine is dilute, as in conditions of overhydration.

MOVEMENT OF FLUID AND ELECTROLYTES

In a healthy person, body fluids are constantly in motion. This constant motion is what helps balance the fluids inside and outside the cells. The extracellular fluid transports nutrients to the cells and carries waste products away from them by way of the capillary bed. Movement of substances through the capillary bed depends on cell membrane permeability. Passage of substances across the cell membrane is accomplished in one of two ways: passive transport or active transport.

As implied by their name, active transport processes necessitate the expenditure of energy by the cell, and passive transport processes do not. The energy required for active transport processes is obtained from a chemical substance called **adenosine triphosphate (ATP).** ATP is produced in the mitochondria of cells from nutrients and is capable of releasing energy that enables the cell to work. For active transport processes to occur, the breakdown of ATP and the use of the related energy are required.

Two simple points to remember about active and passive transport are that (1) passive transport processes do not require cellular energy and (2) active transport processes do require cellular energy.

PASSIVE TRANSPORT

The primary **passive transport** processes that move substances through the cell membranes include the following:

- Diffusion
- Osmosis
- Filtration

DIFFUSION

Diffusion is the natural tendency of a substance to move from an area of higher concentration to one of lower

Skill 18.1 Measuring Intake and Output

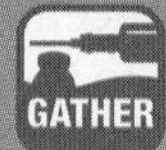

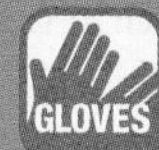

NURSING ACTION *(RATIONALE)*

1. Identify patient. *(Ensures accuracy.)*
2. Explain procedure. *(Enlists patient's cooperation and promotes patient participation.)*
3. Instruct patient to inform staff of all oral intake. Provide a marked intake and output (I&O) container. *(Facilitates accuracy of I&O measurement.)*
4. Instruct patient not to empty any output collection receptacles and to notify the nurse after elimination. *(Contributes to accuracy of I&O measurement.)*
5. Alert all staff and remind patient of need to measure I&O. *(Promotes compliance and accuracy.)*
6. Measure and record all fluids taken orally, gastric tube feedings, and all fluids administered parenterally. *(Helps ensure accurate measurement of intake.)*
7. Wash hands and don gloves. *(Prevents transmission of microorganisms.)*
8. Measure and record output in Foley drainage system, diarrhea stools, nasogastric suction, emesis, ileostomy, and surgical wound receptacles such as Davol, Jackson-Pratt, and Hemovac drains. Measure and record output from chest tube drainage in water-sealed container by marking with felt-tip pen. *(Ensures accurate measurement and proper disposal of output.)*
9. Remove gloves and wash hands. *(Prevents cross-contamination.)*
10. Compute I&O, and document it on patient's record. *(Ensures accurate documentation of total I&O.)*

Table 18.4 **Passive Transport Processes**

PROCESS	DESCRIPTION	EXAMPLES
Diffusion	Movement of particles through a membrane from an area of high concentration to an area of low concentration—that is, down the concentration gradient	Movement of carbon dioxide out of all cells; movement of sodium ions into nerve cells as they conduct an impulse
Osmosis	Diffusion of water through a selectively permeable membrane in the presence of at least one impermeable solute	Diffusion of water molecules into and out of cells to correct imbalances in water concentration
Filtration	Movement of water and small solute particles, but not larger particles, through a filtration membrane; movement occurs from area of high pressure to area of low pressure	In the kidney, movement of water and small solutes from blood vessels but lack of movement by blood proteins and blood cells; begins the formation of urine

From Patton KT, Thibodeau GA: *Structure and function of the body*, ed 15, St. Louis, 2016, Elsevier.

concentration (Table 18.4). This eventually results in an equal distribution of solutes within the two areas. A concentration gradient is generally the stimulus for this migration or movement of molecules. A concentration gradient is the situation in which molecules become more numerous in one area of a solution. The process of diffusion occurs when the molecules move from this area of higher concentration to an area less concentrated. This results in a more even distribution of particles.

The exchange of oxygen and carbon dioxide occurs by diffusion. On inspiration, more oxygen molecules are brought into the lungs than carbon dioxide molecules. Because of this, diffusion occurs: the oxygen molecules move through the cell membranes into the capillary bed and are taken to all body tissues. At the same time, the capillary bed has more carbon dioxide molecules than oxygen molecules, and the carbon dioxide diffuses into the alveoli of the lungs to be eliminated on exhalation.

Facilitated diffusion, or carrier-mediated diffusion, is the process by which material combines with carriers to cross the cell membrane. Facilitated diffusion enables amino acids and glucose to cross the cell membrane into the cells.

OSMOSIS

Osmosis is the movement of water across a semipermeable membrane, from an area of lower concentration to an area of higher concentration (see Table 18.4). In other words, two different solutions are separated by a membrane through which they cannot pass. One side of the membrane has more particles than the other side in relationship to the water. Because of this inequality of particles, water moves through the membrane from the area of low particle concentration to the area of high particle concentration until the solutions are of equal concentration. When the solutions reach equal concentration, they are said to be *isotonic.*

The red blood cells offer an example of the osmotic process in the body; if extracellular fluid is more concentrated (has more particles) than intracellular fluid, the fluid from inside the cell moves out to the extracellular fluid, causing the red blood cell to shrink. If the fluid among the compartments is in equilibrium, fluid enters and leaves the cell at the same rate and the cell size does not change. Another example of osmosis arises when extracellular fluid is less concentrated (has fewer particles) than the fluid in the red blood cells. Fluid then moves into the cell to even out the solutions and causes the cell to enlarge. It is possible for the cell to rupture if too much fluid moves into it.

Solutions in the body are classified according to the electrolyte (particle) concentration. Solutions that have the same concentration of electrolytes as body fluids are said to be *isotonic,* solutions that have higher concentrations of electrolytes than body fluids are considered *hypertonic,* and those with fewer electrolytes than body fluids are *hypotonic.* The concentration of the solution causes the cells of the body to react the same way the red blood cell does. **Hypertonic** solutions pull fluid from the cells; **isotonic** solutions expand the body's fluid volume without causing a fluid shift from one compartment to another; and **hypotonic** solutions move into the cells, causing them to enlarge. Each of these actions occurs through osmosis.

FILTRATION

Filtration is the transfer of water and dissolved substances from an area of higher pressure to an area of lower pressure. The force behind filtration is called **hydrostatic pressure**, which is the force of fluid pressing outward on a vessel wall (see Table 18.4). An example of filtration is the passage of water and electrolytes from the arterial capillary bed to the interstitial fluid. In this example, hydrostatic pressure is created by the pumping action of the heart. At the arterial end of the capillary, the hydrostatic pressure is greater than the pressure within the capillary; this forces water and electrolytes out of the capillary and into the interstitial fluid.

ACTIVE TRANSPORT

The fluid movements discussed to this point necessitate no energy expenditure by the body; they are examples of passive transport. **Active transport** is the process of moving molecules, against pressure, through a membrane with the use of "carriers" and energy from the cell. Active transport carriers are also referred to as *pumps.*

Just as with facilitated diffusion, active transport requires a carrier to move the particles from the outside of the cell to the inside. In active transport, the particles are moving against pressure and require energy to move into the cell.

The sodium-potassium pump is an example of active transport. The sodium-potassium pump is the body's way of maintaining the sodium-potassium balance. Sodium is found mostly on the outside of the cell; potassium is found mainly inside the cell. Both can flow freely through the cell membrane, and if there were no control of this flow, eventually the amount of sodium in the cell would increase and cause the cell to enlarge and burst.

To help prevent this, the sodium-potassium pump transports sodium out of the cell and pulls potassium back into the cell. Excessive sodium inside the cell can be hazardous just as excess potassium outside the cell can be hazardous. Maintaining the proper balance is one essential component of maintaining fluid balance within the body.

ELECTROLYTES

An **electrolyte** is a substance that develops an electrical charge when it dissolves in water. These electrically charged particles are called **ions.** Ions develop either a positive or negative electrical charge. Ions with a positive charge are called **cations.** Ions with a negative charge are called **anions.**

Cations within the body include:

- Sodium (Na^+)
- Potassium (K^+)
- Calcium (Ca^{2+})
- Magnesium (Mg^{2+})

The anions found in the body are as follows:

- Chloride (Cl^-)
- Bicarbonate (HCO_3^-)
- Sulfate (SO_4^-)
- Hydrogen phosphate (HPO_4^-)

A balance exists among the electrolytes. For this balance to occur, a negatively charged anion must be present for each positively charged cation. In all fluid compartments in the body, the cations and anions combine to balance one another and keep the body in homeostasis.

Electrolytes are measured in milliequivalents. A **milliequivalent (mEq)** is a measure of the chemical activity of an ion. The chemical activity of an electrolyte is compared with the chemical activity of hydrogen. One milliequivalent of any electrolyte has the same chemical activity as 1 mEq of hydrogen. In each fluid compartment in the body, the cations and anions balance each other with their chemical activity to maintain electrical neutrality, which again keeps the body in homeostasis.

Although the electrolytes move freely among the fluid compartments, each has a primary location. For example, sodium is the primary extracellular electrolyte, whereas potassium is the primary intracellular electrolyte. The healthy body maintains homeostasis by correcting any excesses or deficiencies of the electrolytes.

Sodium

Sodium is the most abundant electrolyte in the body. It is the major extracellular electrolyte, although a small amount is found in the intracellular fluid. Sodium has many functions in the body, one of which is to regulate the body's fluid volumes. It does this mainly through osmotic pressure, because water follows the sodium throughout the body. Sodium helps regulate the contractility of muscular activity, especially in the heart, and helps maintain neuromuscular irritability to improve nerve impulse conduction. It is also necessary for maintaining acid-base balance.

The major source of all electrolytes is the diet; sodium is no exception. However, sodium, unlike the other electrolytes, usually is consumed in excessive amounts by most Americans. Sodium can be found in cheese, table salt, seafood, processed meat, canned vegetables, canned soups, ketchup, and snack foods, such as pretzels and potato chips.

The kidneys are the primary excretion route for sodium. Many electrolytes, such as sodium, not only pass into and out of the body but also move back and forth between several body fluids. Fig. 18.3 shows the large volumes of sodium-containing internal secretions that are produced each day. During a 24-hour period, more than 8 L of fluid containing 1000 to 1300 mEq of sodium are poured into the digestive system. This sodium, along with most of that contained in the diet, is reabsorbed almost completely. The normal blood level of sodium is 135 to 145 mEq/L.

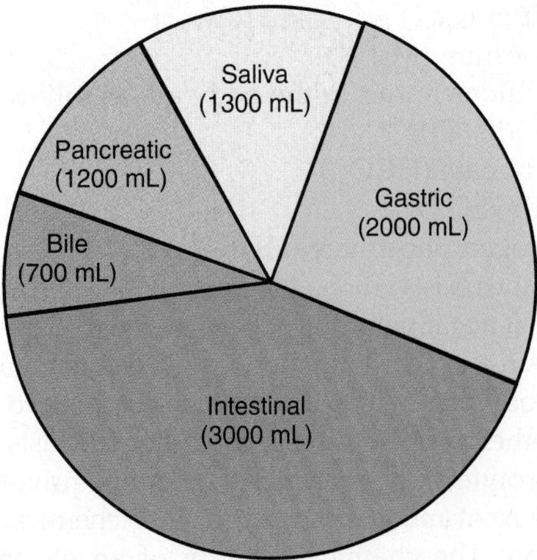

Fig. 18.3 Sodium-containing internal secretions produced every day. (Redrawn from Long BC, Phipps WJ, Cassmeyer VL: *Medical-surgical nursing: A nursing process approach,* ed 3, St. Louis, 1993, Mosby.)

Hyponatremia. *Hyponatremia* is the state in which the concentration of sodium in the blood is less than normal. This happens when there is a sodium loss, such as with vomiting or diarrhea, or an excessive intake of water that dilutes the sodium excessively (Box 18.1). Hyponatremia occurs when the sodium level in the extracellular fluid drops to less than 135 mEq/L.

When a deficiency results from sodium loss, the body attempts to compensate by decreasing water excretion. The signs and symptoms of hyponatremia depend on the cause and on how rapid and severe the sodium loss is. As sodium levels decrease in the extracellular fluid, water is pulled into the cells, which causes them to become edematous. As the fluid moves into the cells, potassium is shifted out and the patient is likely to have a potassium imbalance as well. The patient may experience weakness, anorexia, muscle cramps, confusion, fatigue, headache, edema, and seizures. Treatment for hyponatremia includes sodium replacement and water restrictions.

Hypernatremia. *Hypernatremia* is when the concentration of sodium is greater than normal and exceeds 145 mEq/L. It is caused by an excess of sodium or a decrease in body water (Box 18.2). The body attempts to correct the imbalance by conserving water through renal reabsorption.

Hypernatremia causes fluid to shift from the cells to the interstitial spaces, which results in cellular dehydration and an interruption in cellular processes. Again, a potassium imbalance frequently occurs because potassium is excreted. Treatment for hypernatremia is to lower the sodium levels gradually by decreasing sodium intake or by increasing water in the body.

Potassium

Potassium (K^+) is found primarily in the intracellular fluid and is the major intracellular cation. However, some potassium is present in the extracellular compartments. Of the body's potassium, 98% is inside the cells and 2% is in the extracellular fluid.

The main function of potassium is regulation of water and electrolyte content within the cell. Along with sodium and calcium, it promotes transmission of nerve

Box 18.1 Hyponatremia: Causes, Signs and Symptoms, and Nursing Interventions

CAUSES

- Ascites
- Burns
- Diaphoresis
- Diarrhea
- Fistulas
- GI or biliary drainage via nasogastric tube or T tube
- Inadequate sodium intake
- Large open lesions (burns)
- Lengthy hydrotherapy
- Loss of GI fluids
- Loss through skin
- Massive edema
- Shifting of body fluids
- Small bowel obstruction
- Vomiting

SIGNS AND SYMPTOMS

- Abdominal cramps
- Apathy
- Apprehension
- Fatigue[a]
- Headache[a]
- Irritability
- Muscle weakness, muscle twitching, tremors
- Nausea and vomiting
- Postural hypotension[a]

SEVERE OR PROLONGED SODIUM DEFICIT

- Altered level of consciousness (lethargy, confusion)[b]
- Coma
- Seizures
- Shock

NURSING INTERVENTIONS

- Monitor and record vital signs, especially blood pressure and pulse.
- Monitor intake and output if patient is receiving diuretic medications.
- Monitor neurologic status frequently; report any change in level of consciousness.
- Monitor skin turgor at least every 8 hours.
- Observe for abnormal fluid losses from gastrointestinal system, kidneys, or skin.
- Replace fluid loss with fluids containing sodium, not with plain water.
- Restrict fluid intake as ordered. This is primary treatment for dilutional hyponatremia; post a sign about fluid restriction in the patient's room.
- Weigh patient daily.

[a]Most common signs and symptoms.
[b]Altered level of consciousness usually accompanies a serum sodium level lower than 125 mEq/L and indicates that the patient's condition is deteriorating.
GI, Gastrointestinal.

Box 18.2 Hypernatremia: Causes, Signs and Symptoms, and Nursing Interventions

CAUSES
- Abnormally large intake of sodium
- Consumption of antacids containing sodium
- Dairy products in large amounts
- Loss of more water than sodium from the body
- Overuse of table salt
- Prepared foods: frozen, canned, smoked
- Taking too many salt tablets
- Too-rapid infusion of intravenous saline solution

SIGNS AND SYMPTOMS
- Dry mucous membranes with tenacious (thick) mucus
- Firm, rubbery tissue turgor
- Low urinary output
- Restlessness, agitation, confusion, flushed skin

SEVERE OR PROLONGED SODIUM EXCESS
- Death
- Manic excitement
- Tachycardia

NURSING INTERVENTIONS
- Decrease sodium intake in patient's diet
- Monitor and record vital signs, especially blood pressure and pulse
- Monitor for increased respiratory rate
- Monitor intake and output
- Monitor serum sodium level
- Monitor water loss from fever, infection
- Provide a safe environment for a confused or agitated patient
- Weigh patient daily to check for body fluid loss

impulses and skeletal muscle function. Potassium assists in the cellular metabolism of carbohydrates and proteins and helps control the hydrogen ion concentration. When potassium moves out of the cell, sodium and hydrogen ions move in. The result is the regulation of acid-base balance.

A well-balanced diet usually provides adequate potassium. Approximately 65 mEq of potassium is required each day to maintain the normal blood serum level of 3.5 to 5.0 mEq/L. Potassium is distributed in natural foods. Good sources of potassium include fruits, such as oranges, bananas, apricots, and cantaloupe; legumes; leafy vegetables; potatoes; mushrooms; tomatoes; carrots; and meat (Box 18.3).

Potassium is excreted through the kidneys (80% to 90%) and in the feces and perspiration (10% to 20%). In the kidneys, sodium and potassium seem to pair off against each other, and the kidneys prefer to conserve sodium, even when both electrolytes are depleted. Therefore any condition that causes a decrease in urinary output also causes potassium retention and the potential for life-threatening consequences. Too little or too much potassium affects the heart muscle and has the potential to result in a deadly disturbance in cardiac rhythm (dysrhythmia).

Box 18.3 Foods Rich in Potassium

FRUITS (INCLUDING JUICES)
- Apricots, bananas, cantaloupe, dried fruits (e.g., figs, dates, raisins), grapefruit, honeydew, melon, oranges

PROTEIN FOODS
- Beef, chicken, liver, milk, nuts, peanut butter, pork, veal, turkey

VEGETABLES
- Asparagus, broccoli, cabbage, carrots, celery, dried beans, dried peas, mushrooms, potatoes (especially skins), spinach, squash, tomatoes

BEVERAGES
- Cocoa, cola drinks, fruit and vegetable juices

Hypokalemia. *Hypokalemia* is a decrease in the body's potassium level to less than 3.5 mEq/L. Because the normal range for a serum potassium level is narrow, a slight decrease has profound consequences. The major cause of potassium loss is renal excretion (Box 18.4). The kidneys do not conserve potassium, and they excrete it even when the body needs the potassium. Intestinal fluids contain large amounts of potassium; therefore, with excessive GI losses from gastric suctioning or prolonged vomiting, potassium levels tend to become depleted. Severe diarrhea, fistulas, ileostomy, and excessive diaphoresis also can result in potassium loss, as does the use of diuretics, such as thiazides or furosemide (Lasix). Strenuous exercise and any conditions that cause injury to the cells cause the release of potassium from the cells into the interstitial spaces and ultimately to the kidneys. If renal function is normal, the potassium is excreted, which causes a deficiency in potassium. Hypokalemia has the capacity to affect skeletal and cardiac function. The resulting muscle weakness can cause life-threatening cardiac conduction abnormalities. Treatment of hypokalemia involves replacing the potassium, possibly with IV potassium supplements, and monitoring kidney and cardiac function until the potassium levels become normal again.

Hyperkalemia. An increase in the body's serum potassium level greater than 5 mEq/L is known as *hyperkalemia.* The major cause of potassium excess is renal disease, in which potassium is not excreted adequately (Box 18.5). When tissue damage occurs, potassium is released from the cells. If kidney output also is reduced, the result is an elevation in the potassium level.

Excessive intake of foods high in potassium, especially with decreased urine output, also may cause an increase in the serum potassium level, as does excessive use of salt substitutes (most of which use potassium as a substitute for sodium); potassium supplements (oral or IV); and drugs, such as beta blockers (which inhibit potassium shifts into cells), potassium-sparing diuretics (e.g., spironolactone), chemotherapy (which causes death or lysis of cells with release of high levels of intracellular

Box 18.4 Hypokalemia: Causes, Signs and Symptoms, and Nursing Interventions

CAUSES
- Conditions causing very large urine output
- Decreased potassium intake
- GI losses (vomiting, diarrhea, GI suctioning)
- Ileostomy
- Increased aldosterone activity
- Increased potassium loss
- Loss from cells, as in trauma, burns, fistulas
- Metabolic alkalosis
- Potassium shift into cells
- Potassium-losing diuretics
- Skin losses, diaphoresis
- Treatment of acidosis
- Villous adenoma (tumor of the intestine that produces potassium-containing mucus)

SIGNS AND SYMPTOMS
- Cardiac dysrhythmias; weak, irregular pulse
- Decreased bowel sounds, cramps, constipation, anorexia, nausea, vomiting[a]
- Diminished deep tendon reflexes, lethargy, confusion; paralysis involving the respiratory muscles; coma
- Electrocardiographic changes
- Orthostatic hypotension
- Paresthesia, hyporeflexia
- Polyuria
- Skeletal muscle weakness (especially in lower extremities), leg cramps[a]

SEVERE OR PROLONGED POTASSIUM DEFICIT
- Cardiac or respiratory arrest
- Flaccid paralysis
- Kidney damage
- Paralytic ileus

NURSING INTERVENTIONS
- Administer potassium chloride (KCl) supplement as prescribed by the health care provider (oral or IV).[b]
- Carefully assess patients who are taking digitalis glycosides, especially if they also are taking a diuretic. The low potassium levels could potentiate the action of the digitalis glycoside and cause digitalis toxicity.
- Encourage increased intake of foods high in potassium.
- Monitor bowel sounds.
- Monitor I&O (about 40 mEq of potassium is lost in each liter of urine; diuresis has potential to put the patient at risk for potassium loss).
- Monitor laboratory findings relating to kidney function. If renal function is impaired, there is a significant risk for hyperkalemia.
- Monitor serum potassium level.
- Monitor telemetric values.

[a]Most common signs and symptoms.
[b]It is necessary to administer IV potassium with care to prevent serious complications; always dilute IV potassium and administer it by means of an infusion controller. IV potassium never should be given as an IV "push."
GI, Gastrointestinal; *I&O*, intake and output; *IV*, intravenous.

potassium into the blood), angiotensin-converting enzyme inhibitors, nonsteroidal antiinflammatory drugs, and aminoglycosides.

Although hyperkalemia is less common than hypokalemia, it is often more dangerous because overstimulation of the cardiac muscle can cause cardiac arrest. A serum potassium level of 7 mEq/L or greater carries the risk of serious cardiac dysrhythmias. Treatment is aimed at lowering the potassium levels and correcting the underlying cause, if possible. Treatment could involve restricting potassium intake, giving IV calcium gluconate to decrease the effects of the high potassium levels on the heart, giving sodium bicarbonate or insulin in a glucose solution to shift the potassium back into the cell, or by giving sodium polystyrene sulfonate (Kayexalate) orally or rectally. Kayexalate binds with the potassium to remove it from the system by way of the GI tract.

Chloride

Chloride (Cl^-) is an extracellular anion that is rarely present alone. Chloride usually is bound to another ion, such as sodium or potassium. Chloride can diffuse quickly between the intracellular and extracellular compartments and combines easily with sodium to form sodium chloride or, less often, with potassium to form potassium chloride. The normal blood level of chloride is 96 to 106 mEq/L.

Chloride is necessary for the formation of hydrochloric acid in gastric secretions, and it is necessary in the regulation of the osmotic pressure between the body's fluid compartments. It also assists in the regulation of acid-base balance.

Foods containing sodium also contain chloride: cheese, table salt, seafood, processed meat, canned vegetables, canned soups, ketchup, and snack foods, such as pretzels and potato chips. The main route of excretion for chloride is through the kidneys.

Hypochloremia. *Hypochloremia* usually occurs when chloride levels fall below 96 mEq/L in association with sodium loss because sodium and chloride are frequently paired. Vomiting, diarrhea, gastric suctioning, and acute infections all cause a loss of both sodium and chloride. Symptoms of hypochloremia include depressed respirations, tetany, and alkalosis. Treatment involves alleviating the underlying cause and replacing the chloride with sodium chloride IV solutions.

Hyperchloremia. *Hyperchloremia* is rare; it can occur when bicarbonate levels fall and metabolic acidosis occurs. The increase in chloride anions represents an attempt to compensate and maintain equal numbers with the cations in the body fluid. Because chloride imbalances rarely occur independently of other electrolyte imbalances, there are no specific signs and symptoms to identify a chloride imbalance. However, symptoms of acidosis may indicate high chloride levels.

Box 18.5 Hyperkalemia: Causes, Signs and Symptoms, and Nursing Interventions

CAUSES
- Adrenal insufficiency
- Aminoglycosides
- Angiotensin-converting enzyme inhibitors
- Beta blockers
- Entrance of potassium into the bloodstream from injured cells with extensive trauma (shift of potassium out of the cells into extracellular fluid)
- Excessive use of salt substitutes
- Infusion of large volume of blood nearing expiration date
- Metabolic acidosis
- Nonsteroidal antiinflammatory drugs
- Potassium intake (parenteral or oral) in excess of kidney's ability to excrete
- Potassium-sparing diuretics
- Renal failure
- Tumor lysis syndrome after chemotherapy

SIGNS AND SYMPTOMS[a]
- Cardiac dysrhythmias[b]
- Diarrhea, colic[b]
- ECG changes
- Hypotension
- Irregular pulse rate
- Irritability
- Nausea, vomiting[b]
- Numbness, tingling
- Paresthesias
- Skeletal muscle weakness, especially of lower extremities

SEVERE OR PROLONGED POTASSIUM EXCESS
- Anuria
- Cardiac arrest[b] (serious dysrhythmias become especially dangerous when the serum potassium level reaches 7 mEq/L or more)
- Flaccid paralysis
- Signs and symptoms similar to those of hypokalemia (from prolonged potassium excess)

NURSING INTERVENTIONS[c]
- Administer loop diuretics.
- Administer sodium polystyrene sulfonate (Kayexalate) as prescribed by the health care provider (Kayexalate can be given orally, through a nasogastric tube, or as a retention enema); keep in mind that Kayexalate can sometimes cause serum sodium level to rise; monitor for congestive heart failure.
- Assess vital signs.
- Decrease intake of foods high in potassium.
- Decrease or stop medications associated with high potassium level.
- Monitor bowel sounds, as well as number and character of bowel movements.
- Monitor I&O (report an output of less than 30 mL/h; an inability to excrete potassium in the urine can potentially lead to dangerously high potassium level).
- Monitor serum potassium level.
- Monitor telemetric values to detect dysrhythmias.
- Monitor underlying disorders that may lead to high potassium level.

[a]Signs and symptoms are often nonspecific; serum potassium level and ECG tracings are often the best clinical indicators.
[b]Most common signs and symptoms.
[c]Hemodialysis may be necessary for treating acute symptomatic hyperkalemia.
NOTE: Hyperkalemia may be the most dangerous of the electrolyte disorders.
ECG, Electrocardiogram; *I&O*, intake and output.

Calcium

Calcium (Ca^{2+}) is a positively charged ion found mainly in the bones and teeth. Of all the calcium in the body, 99% is concentrated in the bones and the teeth, where it is essentially inactive until the calcium levels in the blood fall. At that time, calcium is released from the bones to raise the serum calcium level. The remaining 1% of calcium is found in the soft tissue and the extracellular fluid. Regulation of the calcium level in the body is based on the deposition and resorption of bone, the amount of calcium absorbed from the GI tract, and the amount excreted in the urine and feces.

Vitamin D, calcitonin, and parathyroid hormone (parathormone) increase absorption and utilization of calcium; phytic acid and oxalic acid, found naturally in some plants, bind to calcium and inhibit its absorption. The normal ionized calcium level should be 4.5 to 5.6 mEq/dL. Total calcium levels may vary with the amount of albumin in the system; therefore an ionized level is a more reliable indicator of calcium in the body. Calcium is required for the formation and maintenance of strong bones and teeth and the prevention of osteoporosis. It is also necessary for normal blood clotting. Calcium has a depressing or sedative effect on neuromuscular irritability and thus promotes normal transmission of nerve impulses; it also helps regulate normal muscle contraction and relaxation. It helps hold body cells together by establishing the thickness and strength of cell membranes. One of its most important functions is to act as an enzyme activator for chemical reactions in the body.

The best food sources of calcium are milk and cheese. Other sources include beans, nuts, cauliflower, lettuce, and egg yolks. Prevention of osteoporosis focuses on adequate calcium intake. Premenopausal women and postmenopausal women who are taking estrogen need at least 1000 mg of calcium per day and postmenopausal women who are not taking supplemental estrogen need about 1500 mg of calcium per day. Calcium needs in children vary, depending on their age and physiologic needs. However, during times of growth—the first year of life, puberty, and adolescence—calcium needs are increased. Calcium is removed from the body in the urine and feces.

Hypocalcemia. *Hypocalcemia* develops when the serum level of calcium falls below 4.5 mg/dL. Possible deficiencies arise from a variety of problems (Box 18.6).

Box 18.6 Hypocalcemia: Causes, Signs and Symptoms, and Nursing Interventions

CAUSES
- Alkalosis
- Anticonvulsants, such as phenobarbital and phenytoin (Dilantin)
- Chronic renal failure
- Deficiency of parathyroid hormone or vitamin D
- Dietary deficiency of calcium and vitamin D
- Disease of small bowel; malabsorption
- Diuretics (Lasix, Edecrin)
- Draining intestinal fistulas
- Excess alcohol intake
- Excess binding of calcium ions
- Excessive nasogastric suctioning
- Increased magnesium
- Injury or disease of parathyroid gland
- Large amount of citrated blood
- Low serum albumin levels
- Pancreatic disease
- Severe burns
- Severe diarrhea
- Thyroid surgery (surgical removal of parathyroid glands, removal of parathyroid tumor)

SIGNS AND SYMPTOMS
- Anxiety, confusion, irritability
- Calcium deposits in body tissues
- Cardiac dysrhythmias, cardiac arrest
- Diarrhea[a]
- Diminished response to digitalis glycosides
- Hyperactive deep tendon reflexes
- Laryngeal spasms
- Muscle spasm of feet and hands[a]
- Nausea, vomiting[a]
- Osteoporosis, pathologic fractures
- Tetany (note positive Trousseau or Chvostek sign [see Fig. 18.4])
- Tingling sensation around nose, mouth, ears, fingers, and toes[a]
- Twitching

NURSING INTERVENTIONS
- Administer calcium and vitamin D as prescribed by the health care provider[b]
- Encourage intake of a diet high in calcium-rich foods, vitamin D, and protein
- For acute hypocalcemia, keep a tracheotomy tray and resuscitation bag at bedside in case of laryngeal spasms
- Monitor electrocardiogram
- Monitor I&O
- Monitor pertinent laboratory values, including those of calcium, albumin, and magnesium
- Monitor treatment of underlying causes
- Monitor vital signs; especially monitor respiratory status, including rate, depth, and rhythm; be alert for stridor, dyspnea, or crowing (laryngeal spasms)

[a]Most common signs and symptoms.
[b]Acute hypocalcemia necessitates intravenous administration of either calcium gluconate or calcium chloride.
I&O, Intake and output.

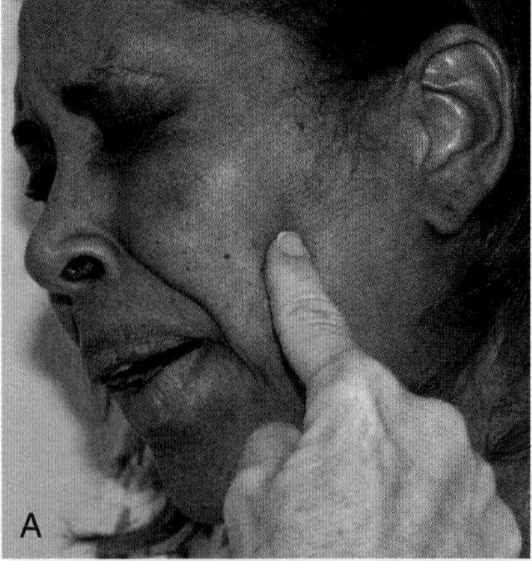

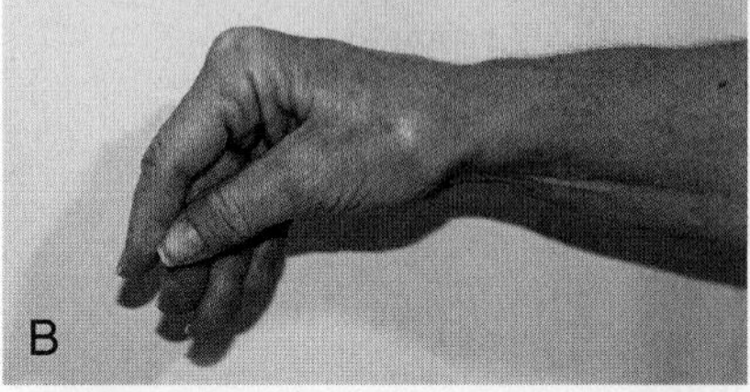

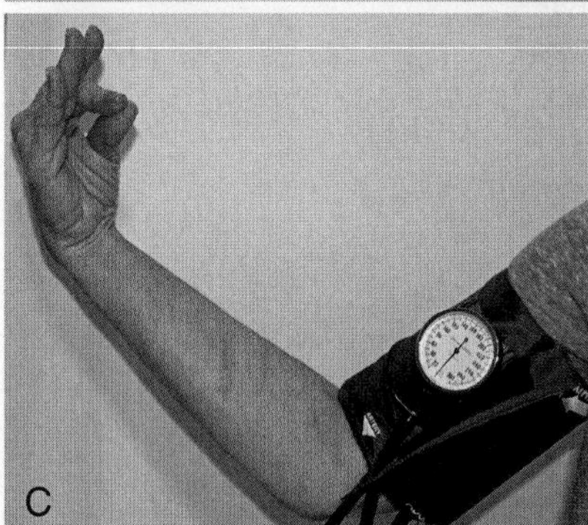

Fig. 18.4 Tests for hypocalcemia. A, The Chvostek sign is a contraction of facial muscles in response to a light tap over the facial nerve in front of the ear. B, The Trousseau sign is a carpal spasm induced by inflation of a blood pressure cuff (C) above the systolic pressure for a few minutes.

Symptoms of hypocalcemia involve neuromuscular irritation and increased excitability, manifested by hyperactive deep tendon reflexes and seizures. As neuromuscular signs and symptoms increase, tetany is also possible. Tetany is a condition characterized by excessive muscle cramps, laryngeal spasms, stridor, carpal spasms (Trousseau sign), pedal spasms, and contraction of facial muscles (Chvostek sign) (Fig. 18.4). Treatment involves replacing calcium with IV calcium gluconate and 1000-mg of oral calcium supplements daily. If the low calcium level is related to decreased levels of parathyroid hormone, it also is necessary to replace that.

Hypercalcemia. *Hypercalcemia* occurs when calcium levels exceed 5.6 mEq/L. It may occur when calcium stored in the bone enters the circulation: for example, in patients who are immobilized (Box 18.7). Excessive intake of calcium or vitamin D also causes hypercalcemia.

Box 18.7 Hypercalcemia: Causes, Signs and Symptoms, and Nursing Interventions

CAUSES
- Movement of calcium from bone to circulation
- Immobilization
- Metastatic bone cancer
- Multiple myeloma
- Excess intake of supplemental calcium
- Excess intake of dietary calcium
- Excess intake of antacids containing calcium
- Increased absorption of calcium
- Increased levels of parathyroid hormone
- Increased levels of vitamin D

SIGNS AND SYMPTOMS
- Anorexia, nausea, vomiting
- Behavioral changes, including confusion
- Thirst, polyuria[a]
- Renal calculi
- Decreased deep tendon reflexes
- Constipation
- Paralytic ileus
- Lethargy, coma
- Cardiac dysrhythmias, cardiac arrest
- Hypertension
- Decreased muscle tone[a]
- Decreased GI motility
- Bone pain

NURSING INTERVENTIONS[b]
- Administer diuretics as ordered by the health care provider
- Encourage patient to drink 3000 to 4000 L of fluids per day
- Monitor I&O

[a]Most common signs and symptoms.
[b]In life-threatening hypercalcemia, measures to increase calcium secretion sometimes include hemodialysis or peritoneal dialysis.
GI, Gastrointestinal; *I&O*, intake and output.

Symptoms of hypercalcemia are neuromuscular activity depression and the formation of renal calculi as a result of the excretion of high levels of calcium by the kidneys.

Phosphorus

Phosphorus is a mineral that makes up about 1% of a person's total body weight. It is present in every cell of the body, but it is found mostly in the bones and teeth, with calcium. Phosphorus and calcium have an inverse relationship; an increase in one causes a decrease in the other. As blood calcium levels increase, a decrease in phosphorus levels is necessary, and vice versa. Most phosphorus is found combined with calcium in bones and teeth, but it also can be found in muscles and nerve tissue. Normal values range from 2.4 to 4.1 mEq/dL.

Along with calcium, phosphorus contributes to the support and maintenance of bones and teeth. It is a component of DNA and RNA, and it is an essential component of phospholipids, which are structural components of cell membranes. Phosphorous compounds are used as a buffer system to maintain the pH of the blood, and phosphorus promotes the effectiveness of many of the B vitamins. Phosphorus also assists in normal nerve and muscle activity and is needed in carbohydrate metabolism. Foods especially high in phosphorus include beef, pork, fish, poultry, milk products, and legumes. As with calcium, an adequate intake of vitamin D is necessary for absorption of phosphorus. The kidneys are responsible for approximately 90% of the excretion of phosphorus. The remainder is excreted in the feces.

Hypophosphatemia. Because a generous amount of phosphorus is present in many foods, a deficiency seldom occurs. However, *hypophosphatemia* is possible as a result of a dietary insufficiency, impaired kidney function, or maldistribution of phosphorus. Low phosphorus levels have been associated with muscle weakness, especially of the respiratory muscles; with bone and joint pain; and with disorientation and confusion. Treatment involves replacing the phosphorus with oral or IV supplementation and monitoring the patient.

Hyperphosphatemia. *Hyperphosphatemia,* also a rarity, occurs most commonly as a result of renal insufficiency but can occur with an increased intake of phosphate or vitamin D. Signs and symptoms include tetany, numbness and tingling sensation around the mouth, and muscle spasms. Restricting phosphorus intake and treating the underlying cause will bring phosphorus levels down. However, phosphate-binding gels such as aluminum hydroxide (Amphojel) and IV calcium supplementation may be needed.

Magnesium

Magnesium (Mg^{2+}) is the fourth most abundant mineral in the body and the second most abundant cation in the intracellular fluid. Only small amounts of magnesium are found in the blood, but it is important in maintaining normal body function. The majority (60%) of magnesium is found in the bone, with lesser amounts in the muscle and soft tissue; only 1% is in the extracellular fluid, mostly in the cerebrospinal fluid.

The importance of magnesium as an electrolyte was not recognized widely until recently. It is now recognized as a cofactor in the activation of many enzymes. It also promotes regulation of serum calcium, phosphate, and potassium levels and is essential for integrity of nerve tissue, skeletal muscle, and cardiac functioning. Magnesium also may enhance the effectiveness of treatment for asthma, depression, diabetes, hypertension, cardiac arrhythmias, migraine headaches, fibromyalgia, osteoporosis, and restless leg syndrome. Normal blood values are 1.5 to 2.5 mEq/L.

Magnesium is another electrolyte commonly distributed in foods. Whole grains, fruits, green vegetables, meat, fish, legumes, and dairy products are dietary sources. It is a good idea to take a multivitamin containing B-complex vitamins along with magnesium-rich foods. The level of vitamin B_6 in the body determines how much magnesium is absorbed into the cells. The major route of magnesium excretion is through the kidneys, in which the amount of magnesium is correlated with the amount of potassium excreted. The kidneys do not conserve potassium, but they do conserve magnesium; therefore, if a magnesium deficiency develops, the body conserves magnesium at the expense of excreting potassium.

Hypomagnesemia. *Hypomagnesemia* develops when blood levels fall to less than 1.5 mEq/L. A decrease in magnesium also is associated with decreased potassium levels because the kidneys tend to conserve magnesium by excreting more potassium. Hypomagnesemia causes symptoms of increased neuromuscular irritability similar to those observed with hypocalcemia (Box 18.8): tremors, cramping, numbness, and tingling sensation in the hands and feet, disorientation, confusion, tetany and seizures. The major causes of low magnesium levels are increased excretion by the kidneys, impaired absorption from the GI tract, and prolonged malnutrition. Oral or IV magnesium is given to treat hypomagnesemia.

Hypermagnesemia. *Hypermagnesemia* develops when magnesium blood levels exceed 2.5 mEq/L. It rarely occurs when kidney function is normal, but in the presence of impaired renal function, excess magnesium administration, and diabetic ketoacidosis with severe water loss, it may develop (Box 18.9). An excess of magnesium severely restricts nerve and muscle activity and causes respiratory depression, hypotension, and, potentially, cardiac arrest. Treatment involves decreasing the patient's intake of magnesium while supporting cardiac and respiratory function. Dialysis may be necessary to remove excess amounts from the blood.

Box 18.8 Hypomagnesemia: Causes, Signs and Symptoms, and Nursing Interventions

CAUSES
- Alcoholism
- Conditions causing large losses of urine
- Decreased intake
- Diarrhea
- Draining intestinal fistulas
- Hypercalcemia
- Impaired absorption from GI tract
- Prolonged IV feedings without magnesium supplementation
- Prolonged malnutrition
- Starvation

SIGNS AND SYMPTOMS
- Agitation, depression, confusion
- Anorexia
- Ataxia
- Cardiac dysrhythmias
- Cramps, spasticity
- Dysphagia
- Hyperactive deep tendon reflexes
- Hypotension
- Mental changes[a]
- Nausea and vomiting
- Paresthesia[a]
- Seizures
- Tachycardia
- Tetany
- Tremors

NURSING INTERVENTIONS
- Administer magnesium supplements as prescribed by the health care provider
- Assess dysphagia
- Assess neuromuscular status
- Increase patient's intake of magnesium-rich foods
- Institute seizure precautions
- Monitor electrocardiogram
- Monitor I&O
- Monitor respiratory status
- Monitor vital signs

[a]Most common signs and symptoms.
GI, Gastrointestinal; *I&O*, intake and output.

Bicarbonate

Bicarbonate (HCO_3^-) is one of the main anions in the extracellular fluid. It is an alkaline electrolyte whose major function is the regulation of acid-base balance. Bicarbonate acts as a buffer to neutralize acids in the body and maintain the 20:1 ratio of bicarbonate to carbonic acid needed to keep the body in homeostasis (discussed in the next section). The normal bicarbonate level is 22 to 24 mEq/L. The kidneys selectively regulate the amount of bicarbonate retained or excreted based on need.

ACID-BASE BALANCE

Acid-base balance (also called *acid-alkaline balance*) refers to the homeostasis of the hydrogen ion (H^-) concentration in the body fluids. A solution with a high number of hydrogen ions is an acid, and a solution with a low number of hydrogen ions is an alkaline, or base. The hydrogen ion concentration is determined by the ratio of carbonic acid (H_2CO_3) to bicarbonate (HCO_3^-) in the extracellular fluid. The ratio needed for homeostasis is 1 part carbonic acid to 20 parts bicarbonate. The symbol used to indicate hydrogen ion balance is pH. A pH value is actually the hydrogen ion concentration in the body. A sample of arterial blood is used to determine the body's pH.

Arterial blood gas levels reveal whether the blood is acid, neutral, or alkaline. An inverse relationship exists between hydrogen ion concentration and the pH level: as the number of hydrogen ions increases, the acidity of the solution increases and the pH decreases. The opposite happens with alkalinity: the number of hydrogen ions decreases and the pH increases. A pH of less

Box 18.9 Hypermagnesemia: Causes, Signs and Symptoms, and Nursing Interventions

CAUSES
- Diabetic ketoacidosis with severe water loss
- Renal failure

SIGNS AND SYMPTOMS
- Heat
- Hypotension[a]
- Loss of deep tendon reflexes
- Nausea and vomiting
- Respiratory depression
- Thirst
- Vasodilation[a]

PROLONGED OR SEVERE EXCESS
- Cardiac arrest
- Coma

NURSING INTERVENTIONS
- Administer diuretics as prescribed by the health care provider
- Decrease patient's intake of foods or medications high in magnesium
- Encourage frequent urination
- Monitor I&O

[a]Most common signs and symptoms.
I&O, Intake and output.

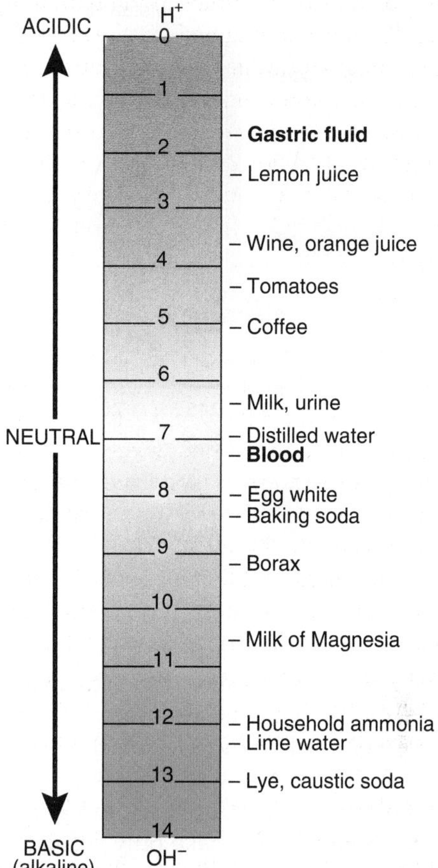

Fig. 18.5 The pH scale. A pH of 7 is considered neutral. Values toward the top (less than 7) are acidic (the lower the number, the more acidic). Values toward the bottom (greater than 7) are basic, or alkaline (the higher the number, the more basic). Representative fluids and their approximate pHs are listed at the side. (From Thibodeau GA, Patton KT: *The human body in health and disease,* ed 4, St. Louis, 2005, Mosby.)

than 7.35 is acid. A pH of greater than 7.45 is alkaline. The normal pH of arterial blood is approximately 7.45, whereas the normal pH of venous blood and interstitial fluid is approximately 7.35. Between 7.35 and 7.45 is considered normal blood pH. A pH lower than 6.8 or higher than 7.8 is usually fatal (Fig. 18.5).

Two types of disturbances can cause a pH imbalance. One imbalance arises from an increase or a decrease in the base substance bicarbonate. The other imbalance results from an increase or decrease in carbonic acid, the acid substance. The body's metabolism affects the base portion of balance, and so a bicarbonate imbalance causes metabolic acidosis or alkalosis. The body's respiratory system affects the acid side of the balance, and so a carbonic acid imbalance causes respiratory acidosis or alkalosis. Fig. 18.6 depicts the relationship between pH and the ratio of bicarbonate to carbonic acid.

The body has three systems that work to keep the pH in the narrow range of normal: the blood buffers, the respiratory system, and the kidneys. These systems are working constantly to maintain a normal pH.

BLOOD BUFFERS

Blood buffers (also called *physiologic buffers*) consist of either a weak acid and its base salt or a weak base and its acid salt. These buffers include the bicarbonate/carbonic acid buffering system, the intracellular protein buffers, and the phosphate buffers in the bone. Of these, the bicarbonate/carbonic acid system is the most important. It is responsible for buffering blood and interstitial fluid and decreasing the strength of potentially damaging acids and bases. Think of these blood buffers as chemical sponges. They circulate throughout the body in pairs, neutralizing excess acids or bases by contributing or accepting hydrogen ions. One buffer takes away a hydrogen ion if the fluid is too acid; the other adds a hydrogen ion if the solution is too alkaline. They work within a fraction of a second to prevent an excessive change in the hydrogen ion concentration. The kidneys assist the bicarbonate buffer system in regulating production of bicarbonate.

RESPIRATORY SYSTEM

Once the blood buffer systems are exhausted, the body calls on the second line of defense, the lungs, to help balance the hydrogen concentration in the body. By speeding up or slowing down respirations, the lungs have the capacity to increase or decrease the amount of carbon dioxide in the blood. Carbon dioxide is a potential acid. When it is dissolved in water, it becomes carbonic acid. Removing carbon dioxide from the blood

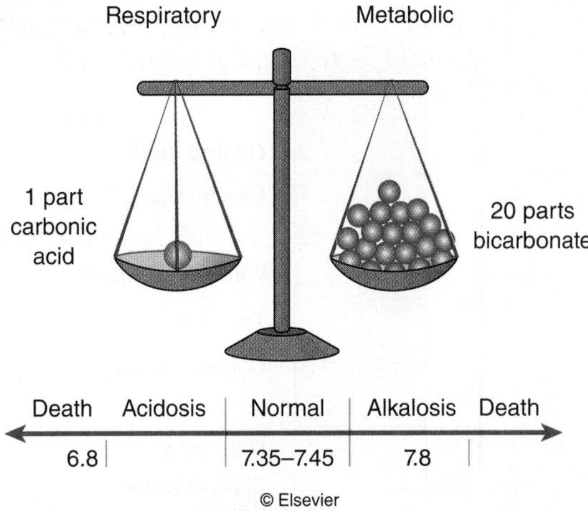

Fig. 18.6 Relationship between pH and the ratio of bicarbonate to carbonic acid. The normal plasma range is 7.35 to 7.45. A normal pH is maintained by a ratio of 1 part carbonic acid to 20 parts bicarbonate.

lowers the carbonic acid level and raises pH to make the environment more alkaline. When there is too much alkaline in the system, the respiratory system slows down and retains carbon dioxide, which results in lower pH (acidosis). This buffering system takes 1 to 2 minutes to adjust the acid-base balance back to a normal range, whereas the blood buffers take only seconds to work. Even though the respiratory system is slower than the blood buffers, it is still just as efficient; the lungs can eliminate large amounts of acid (in the form of carbon dioxide) from the body and keep just enough carbon dioxide to maintain a normal pH level. If the pH drops suddenly, the respiratory system can return the pH to near normal within 1 minute. Chemoreceptors in the medulla of the brainstem provide the stimulus to increase respirations; however, as the hydrogen ion concentration approaches normal, the stimulus is lost, and the blood buffers make the remaining adjustments needed to return the level to normal.

KIDNEYS

The third line of defense in regulating hydrogen ions is the kidneys. They regulate pH by excreting acids or bases as needed. In the state of acidosis, the kidneys excrete hydrogen in urine and retain bicarbonate. In the state of alkalosis, the kidneys excrete bicarbonate and retain hydrogen. Normal urine pH tends to be more acidic, not necessarily because the body is in a constant state of acidosis and is attempting to compensate, but because the body produces excess acids in the metabolic processes and must eliminate them constantly in the urine.

The kidneys are the slowest of the systems to balance the hydrogen concentration in the body; it may take several hours or several days for the kidneys to compensate, but they are efficient enough to return the pH to exactly normal. The three systems work closely together to maintain a normal hydrogen ion concentration. The blood buffers are immediate and continuous in contributing or accepting hydrogen ions. The respiratory system has the capacity to come into play within minutes, regulating the carbon dioxide level in the blood and thus controlling carbonic acid. Although the kidneys work more slowly than the other two systems, they are still able to eliminate either hydrogen ions or bicarbonate ions, which means they can either increase or decrease pH.

Table 18.5 Acid-Base Imbalances and Compensatory Mechanisms

ACID-BASE IMBALANCE	MODE OF COMPENSATION
Respiratory acidosis	Kidneys retain increased amounts of HCO_3^- to increase pH
Respiratory alkalosis	Kidneys excrete increased amounts of HCO_3^- to lower pH
Metabolic acidosis	Lungs excrete CO_2 to raise pH
Metabolic alkalosis	Lungs retain CO_2 to lower pH

From Pagana K, Pagana T: *Mosby's diagnostic and laboratory test reference*, ed 11, St. Louis, 2013, Mosby.

TYPES OF ACID-BASE IMBALANCE

If the regulatory systems fail, one of four major acid-base imbalances may occur. An acid-base imbalance results in either acidosis (when blood pH is less than 7.35) or alkalosis (when blood pH is greater than 7.45). Because the lungs and the kidneys are the two major organs responsible for regulation of the acid and base substances in the body, acid-base imbalances probably are caused by an imbalance in the function of the lungs, the kidneys, or both. Many diseases create a potential for acid-base imbalances. Diseases and other conditions that predispose a patient to these imbalances include diabetes mellitus, chronic obstructive pulmonary disease, end-stage renal disease, severe vomiting, and diarrhea.

There are four primary types of acid-base imbalances: respiratory acidosis, respiratory alkalosis, metabolic acidosis, and metabolic alkalosis (Table 18.5).

RESPIRATORY ACIDOSIS

Any condition that impairs normal ventilation and prevents the respiratory system from eliminating the appropriate amount of carbon dioxide causes respiratory acidosis (Box 18.10). Carbon dioxide is retained, and the level of carbonic acid in the blood increases. As pH falls and the normal 20:1 ratio of bicarbonate to carbonic acid ratio is upset, the partial pressure of carbon dioxide (PCO_2) increases. The body then attempts to eliminate the excess carbon dioxide by increasing respirations. The activity of the central nervous system also is depressed, and the patient becomes lethargic and confused. The heart rate increases, and the patient also may experience palpitations and dizziness. The kidneys attempt to compensate by retaining the base substance bicarbonate and eliminating hydrogen. However, because

Box 18.10 Respiratory Acidosis: Causes, Common Clinical Signs and Symptoms, and Laboratory Data

CAUSES
- Airway obstruction
- Atelectasis
- Barbiturate or sedative overdose
- Compromise in any of the three essential parts of breathing: ventilation, perfusion, or diffusion
- COPD
- Cystic fibrosis
- Drowning
- Head injuries
- Obesity
- Paralysis of respiratory muscles (Guillain-Barré syndrome, poliomyelitis, myasthenia gravis)
- Pneumonia
- Respiratory failure
- Stroke (cardiovascular accident)
- Traumatic injuries to the thorax (flail chest)

COMMON CLINICAL SIGNS AND SYMPTOMS
Central Nervous System
- Coma
- Decreased deep tendon reflexes
- Decreasing level of consciousness
- Disorientation
- Dizziness
- Lethargy
- Occipital headache
- Seizures

Cardiopulmonary System
- Cardiac dysrhythmias
- Dyspnea
- Hypotension
- Tachycardia

Musculoskeletal System
- Tremors
- Weakness

LABORATORY DATA
- HCO_3^- normal in early respiratory acidosis
- K^+ <5 mEq/L
- O_2 saturation normal or <95%, depending on severity of acidosis
- $PaCO_2$ >45 mm Hg (unless the patient has COPD)
- PaO_2 normal or <80 mm Hg, depending on severity of acidosis
- pH <7.35

COPD, Chronic obstructive pulmonary disease; *$PaCO_2$*, partial pressure of arterial carbon dioxide; *PaO_2*, partial pressure of arterial oxygen.

the renal system is a slow system, compensation may not occur for 24 hours or more.

Treatment for respiratory acidosis is aimed at improving ventilation. To do this, the underlying cause of the respiratory acidosis must be found and treated while support is given to the patient's respiratory efforts. Intermittent positive-pressure breathing (IPPB) or continuous positive airway pressure (CPAP) may be used to promote exhalation of carbon dioxide; antibiotics may be administered for any respiratory infection; adequate hydration (2 to 3 L/day) helps liquefy and aids in the removal of secretions; and bronchodilators may help reduce bronchial spasms. Intubation and mechanical ventilation also may be necessary.

Box 18.11 Respiratory Alkalosis: Causes, Common Clinical Signs and Symptoms, and Laboratory Data

CAUSES
- Anemia
- Asthma
- Disorders of the central nervous system (head injuries, infections)
- Drugs (aspirin overdose)
- Hypermetabolic states
- Hyperventilation (caused by hypoxia, pulmonary emboli, anxiety, fear, pain, exercise, fever)
- Inappropriate mechanical ventilator settings
- Pneumonia

COMMON CLINICAL SIGNS AND SYMPTOMS
Central Nervous System
- Anxious appearance
- Confusion
- Dizziness
- Fainting
- Irritability
- Seizures
- Tingling sensation in the extremities

Cardiopulmonary System
- Cardiac dysrhythmias
- Tachypnea

Musculoskeletal System
- Muscle weakness
- Tetany

LABORATORY DATA
- HCO_3^- levels may be normal but are more likely to be below 21 as the $PaCO_2$ levels fall.
- K^+ <3.5 mEq/L
- O_2 saturation normal
- $PaCO_2$ <35 mm Hg
- PaO_2 normal
- pH ≥7.45

$PaCO_2$, Partial pressure of arterial carbon dioxide; *PaO_2*, partial pressure of arterial oxygen.

RESPIRATORY ALKALOSIS

Respiratory alkalosis is caused most frequently by hyperventilation secondary to anxiety, adult respiratory distress syndrome, congestive heart failure, head trauma, severe blood loss, or pneumonia (Box 18.11). Increased respiratory rate, depth, or both have the potential to cause the loss of excessive amounts of carbon dioxide, which results in a low carbonic acid level in the blood. The pH then increases because of the decrease in carbonic acid, and respiratory alkalosis results. The kidneys attempt to compensate by conserving hydrogen ions and excreting bicarbonate ions, but, as mentioned previously, the renal system is slow, and the compensation may not occur for 24 hours or more.

Symptoms include lightheadedness, numbness and tingling sensation in extremities, tinnitus, blurred vision, increased heart rate, and irritability. In extreme cases, confusion, seizure activity, and loss of consciousness may occur.

Treatment for respiratory alkalosis involves treating the underlying cause. If the cause is anxiety, it helps to make the patient aware of the abnormal breathing pattern and instruct the patient to breathe slowly to retain and accumulate carbon dioxide in the body. Breathing into a paper bag may also help. If these fail, it may be necessary to sedate the patient.

METABOLIC ACIDOSIS

Metabolic acidosis occurs as a result of a gain of hydrogen ions or a loss of bicarbonate (Box 18.12). This then causes the pH of the blood to fall and acidosis develops. Because metabolic acidosis is a problem involving the kidneys, the other compensatory system—the lungs—attempts to compensate by increasing the respiratory rate and eliminating more carbon dioxide. This results in hyperventilation. In the extracellular fluid, there is also an exchange of potassium and hydrogen. Potassium ions move out of the cell, and hydrogen ions move into the cell. This is a means to reduce the concentration of hydrogen in the extracellular fluid and compensate for the acidosis that has developed. Causes of metabolic acidosis include diabetic ketoacidosis from ketone accumulation, increased levels of lactic acid (as seen in shock), starvation, severe diarrhea (dehydration), and renal failure.

Symptoms of metabolic acidosis may vary, depending on the underlying cause and severity. Common symptoms include a change in the patient's level of consciousness, headache, vomiting, diarrhea, anorexia, and cardiac dysrhythmias. Administration of sodium bicarbonate is the usual treatment for acidosis, but the underlying cause must be treated as well. Mechanical ventilation may be necessary if the metabolic acidosis is severe and the patient is comatose.

Box 18.12 Metabolic Acidosis: Causes, Common Clinical Signs and Symptoms, and Laboratory Data

CAUSES

- Dehydration
- Diabetic ketoacidosis
- Drugs (methanol, ethanol, formic acid, paraldehyde, aspirin)
- Lactic acidosis
- Renal failure
- Renal tubular acidosis
- Severe diarrhea
- Shock
- Starvation

COMMON CLINICAL SIGNS AND SYMPTOMS

Central Nervous System

- Coma
- Decreasing level of consciousness
- Headache
- Lethargy

Cardiopulmonary System

- Dysrhythmias
- Kussmaul respirations (deep, rapid respirations)
- Warm, flushed skin

Gastrointestinal System

- Abdominal pain
- Anorexia
- Diarrhea
- Nausea
- Vomiting

Musculoskeletal System

- Weakness

LABORATORY DATA

- HCO_3^- <22 mEq/L
- K^+ >5 mEq/L
- O_2 saturation normal
- $PaCO_2$ normal or <35 mm Hg if lungs are compensating
- PaO_2 normal or <80 mm Hg if lungs are compensating
- pH <7.35

$PaCO_2$, Partial pressure of arterial carbon dioxide; *PaO_2*, partial pressure of arterial oxygen.

METABOLIC ALKALOSIS

Metabolic alkalosis results when a significant amount of acid is lost from the body or the bicarbonate level increases (Box 18.13). The most common causes of metabolic alkalosis are vomiting gastric content (normally high in acid) and prolonged gastric suction. Metabolic alkalosis is also possible in patients who ingest excessive amounts of alkaline agents, such as bicarbonate-containing antacids. Metabolic alkalosis often develops in the presence of renal failure as well. In this situation, the renal system is not able to correct the imbalance, and compensation is left to the respiratory system. The respiratory system responds by causing hypoventilation. Metabolic alkalosis depresses the central nervous system, which results in headaches, irritability, lethargy, changes in level of consciousness, and confusion. Changes in heart rate; slow, shallow respirations; nausea and vomiting; and numbness in the extremities may also be present. As with the other acid-base imbalances, treatment is aimed at treating the underlying cause.

INTRAVENOUS THERAPY

The body's fluid and electrolyte balance must be maintained to keep all body systems healthy and functioning properly. When there is an imbalance either in fluid intake and output or in electrolyte concentration, complications can arise. To help prevent these complications, the health care provider may order **intravenous (IV)** therapy (infusion of medication or other liquid therapeutic agents).

IV therapy may be ordered for many reasons. It may be needed to maintain fluid volume if a patient is not

Box 18.13 Metabolic Alkalosis: Causes, Common Clinical Signs and Symptoms, and Laboratory Data

CAUSES

- Cushing's disease
- Drugs (steroids, sodium bicarbonate, diuretics); overdose of baking soda, excessive use of antacids such as Mylanta
- Electrolyte disturbance
- Excessive vomiting
- Hyperaldosteronism
- Prolonged gastric suctioning

COMMON CLINICAL SIGNS AND SYMPTOMS

Central Nervous System

- Decreases in level of consciousness
- Headache
- Irritability
- Lethargy
- Seizures

Cardiopulmonary System

- Atrial tachycardia
- Cardiac dysrhythmias (related to hypokalemia)
- Slow, shallow respirations with periods of apnea

Gastrointestinal System

- Anorexia
- Nausea
- Vomiting

Musculoskeletal System

- Hypertonicity of muscles, muscle cramps
- Numbness and tingling sensation in extremities
- Tetany
- Tremors

LABORATORY DATA

- HCO_3^- >26 mEq/L
- K^+ <3.5 mEq/L
- O_2 saturation normal
- $PaCO_2$ normal or >45 mm Hg if lungs are compensating
- PaO_2 normal
- pH >7.45

$PaCO_2$, Partial pressure of arterial carbon dioxide; *PaO_2*, partial pressure of arterial oxygen.

taking in fluid or nutrients orally, or it can be used as replacement for fluid lost through prolonged nausea or vomiting. It also can be used to give medications, blood, or blood products and to provide the patient with nutritional support. The IV route provides faster absorption and more rapid distribution of medications, solutions, or nutrients and can be used for either long-term or short-term applications.

Each state's nurse practice act determines the legal guidelines for IV administration, and facility policy further defines the LPN/LVN's role in the administration of IV medications, fluids, blood, or blood products. Only specially trained nurses who meet the legal qualifications and facility guidelines should be involved in IV administration (see the Coordinated Care box on IV therapy).

Coordinated Care

Collaboration

Intravenous Therapy

- The skills of basic intravenous (IV) needle insertion, adjusting IV flow rate, administering IV medications, and maintaining an IV site require the knowledge of a nurse. Many states include this skill in the scope of practice for LPNs/LVNs. Delegation of these tasks to unlicensed assistive personnel (UAP) is inappropriate.
- It is acceptable for UAP to inform the nurse when a fluid container is almost empty, when the patient complains of any discomfort at the IV site, and when an electronic controlling device sounds an alarm.
- In the clinical setting, the registered nurse (RN) is responsible for supervising infusion therapy and may delegate the task of IV insertion, adjusting IV flow rate, administering IV medications, and maintaining an IV site to the LPN/LVN if those tasks are within the LPN/LVN's scope of practice for that state.

The insertion of an IV catheter involves several steps (Skill 18.2 and Figs. 18.7 and 18.8). Before inserting an IV needle, always check the health care provider's order. It should indicate the solution type, as well as any medication that may have to be added to the solution, the volume to be infused, the rate of infusion, and the duration of infusion. Next, assemble and ready the equipment. Over-the-needle catheters are the most commonly used IV catheters today. They have a metal needle extending past the tip of a soft catheter. After the venipuncture, withdraw the needle and leave just the soft catheter in place (Box 18.14 and see Skill 18.2). Select a venipuncture needle and catheter according to the solution to be infused and the size and condition of the patient's veins. Choose a catheter that is smaller than the vein but large enough for the solution to flow through it without clogging it. A 20-, 21-, or 22-gauge catheter is acceptable for an adult patient who is receiving only fluids or medications (or both). If administering blood, use a catheter with a larger lumen (18- or 22-gauge). Many patients who require IV hydration have such low blood volume that only the smaller gauge IV catheters suffice for venipuncture.

Next, select tubing based on the patient's needs and the type of infusion to be initiated. Remove the tubing from the sterile packaging and inspect it for kinks. Ensure that the roller or slide clamp is functional and closed (Fig. 18.9A). Remove the correct solution from the sterile packaging and inspect it for expiration date, leaks, or contamination, then invert it to allow easy access to the tubing insertion port. Remove the insertion port cover (see Fig. 18.9B), remove the cover from the tubing spike, and insert the spike into the port until the plastic diaphragm covering the port is pierced (see Fig. 18.9C). Hold the fluid bag upright and gently squeeze the tubing

Text continued on p. 504

Skill 18.2 Initiating Intravenous Therapy

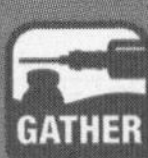

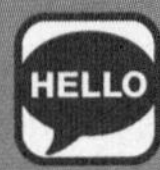

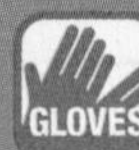

NURSING ACTION *(RATIONALE)*

1. Refer to Standard Steps 1 to 9.
2. Assemble equipment:
   - Clean gloves
   - Intravenous infusion tray or kit containing tourniquet, alcohol swab, povidone-iodine (Betadine) or chlorhexidine (follow facility policy regarding cleaning agent), angiocatheter, tubing, adhesive tape, and sterile dressing
   - Solution to be infused
3. Identify appropriate **venipuncture** (access of a vein with a needle for the purpose of starting an IV or withdrawing a blood sample) sites (see Fig. 18.7). *(Choosing an appropriate venipuncture site allows for patient movement and comfort. LPN/LVNs may start an IV infusion in only certain areas of the arm in some states; make sure the chosen site is in an allowable site.)*
4. Apply tourniquet. Tourniquet should be tight enough to impede venous return but not occlude arterial flow (see Fig. 18.8A). *(Facilitates observation and puncture of vein.)*
5. Select venipuncture site (see Fig. 18.8A).
   a. Use the most distal site in the nondominant arm, or on the nonoperative side, if possible.
   b. Avoid areas that are painful on palpation, bruised, swollen, or traumatized.
   c. In the nondominant arm, select a vein large enough for catheter placement.
   d. Choose a site that will not interfere with planned procedures or the patient's activities of daily living.
      (1) Palpate the vein by pressing downward and noting the resistant, soft, bouncy feeling as pressure is released. *(Softness and bounciness of the vein indicate that the vein is healthy.)*
      (2) Instruct the patient to open and close the fist several times, lower the patient's arm, and rub or stroke the patient's arm. *(Promote venous distention.)*
      (3) Avoid sites distal to previous venipuncture sites, hardened cordlike veins, infiltrated sites or phlebitic vessels, and bruised areas. *(In such sites, infiltration tends to occur with new IV lines, and excessive vessel damage may result.)*
      (4) Avoid vessels in an extremity with compromised circulation, as in cases of mastectomy, dialysis graft, or paralysis. *(Venous alterations increase risk of complications such as infiltration.)*
6. Release tourniquet. *(Never leave tourniquet on for longer than 1 minute, to decrease the risk for vein damage.)*
7. Cleanse site with alcohol swab or other cleaning agent, using friction (see Fig. 18.8B). Cleanse in clean-to-dirty direction, starting at selected insertion site and working outward, creating concentric circles. Use alcohol first and then chlorhexidine or povidone-iodine. Allow to dry. *(Removes microorganisms from puncture site. Make sure to follow facility policy regarding cleaning agent.)*
8. Stretch skin taut, and stabilize vein with nondominant hand (see Fig. 18.8C). *(Prevents vein from moving during procedure.)*
9. Insert the catheter:
   a. Using an over-the-needle catheter with safety device:
      (1) Hold the over-the-needle catheter with bevel up between index finger and thumb, and pierce skin above and slightly to side of vein at 30-degree angle (indirect method). *(Allows needle to enter smoothly through skin and approach vein wall.)*

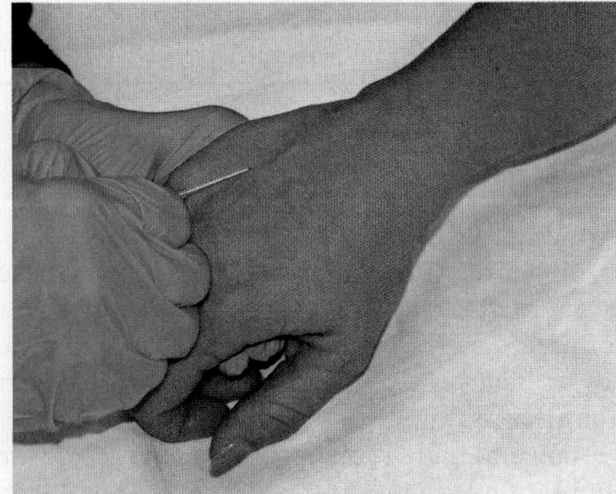

      (2) Lower angle to 10 degrees and enter vein wall. Slight resistance and "pop" sensation accompany entry into vein. *(Reduces risk of going completely through vein and enhances placement within vein.)*

Skill 18.2 Initiating Intravenous Therapy—cont'd

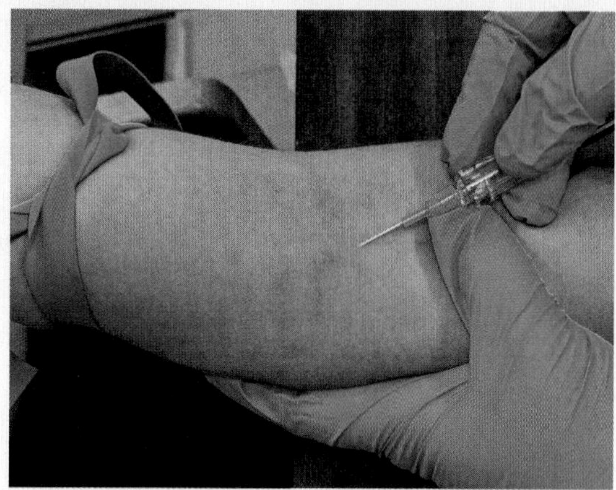

(3) Once the "pop" is felt, watch for blood return in flashback chamber. *(Confirms placement within vein.)*

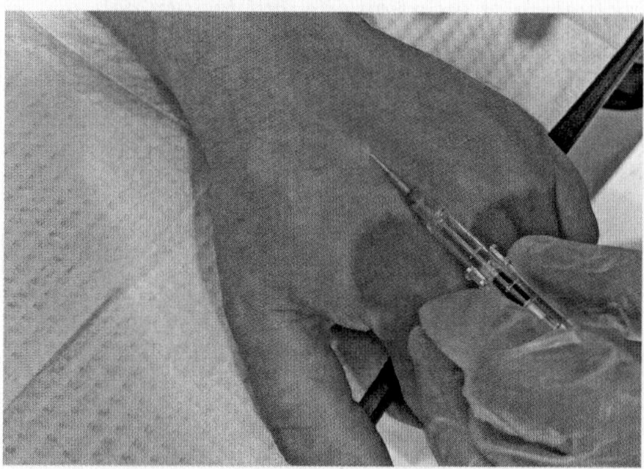

(4) Advance catheter and stylet ¼ inch into vein, and then loosen stylet. Advance catheter over the needle into vein until hub rests at venipuncture site. Do not reinsert the stylet once it is loosened. *(Advancing the catheter and stylet ensures catheter is completely through vessel wall and into vein lumen. Threading catheter to hub reduces the risk of introducing infectious organisms along the catheter length. Reinserting the stylet has potential to cause damage to the catheter and formation of a catheter embolus.)*

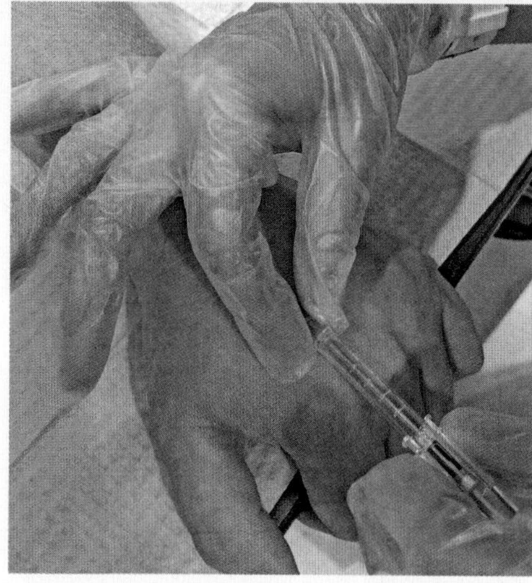

(5) Release tourniquet. *(Decreases potential for vein rupture and allows for venous flow.)*

(6) Stabilize the catheter. Apply gentle but firm pressure with the index finger of nondominant hand 1¼ inches (3 cm) above insertion site, and retract stylet from over-the-needle catheter. Do not recap the stylet. For safety, slide the catheter off the stylet while gliding the protective guard over the stylet. A click indicates the device is locked. *(Stabilizing catheter prevents accidental withdrawal or dislodgment. Applying gentle pressure above insertion site decreases flow of blood and prevents blood loss through open catheter hub. Immediately covering stylet with protective guard prevents accidental needle sticks.)*

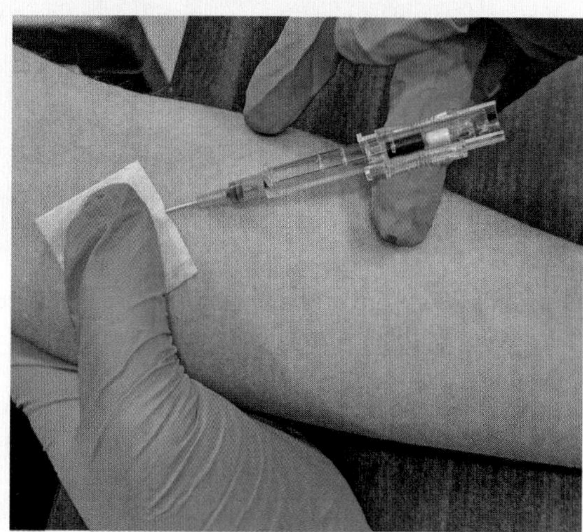

Continued

Skill 18.2 Initiating Intravenous Therapy—cont'd

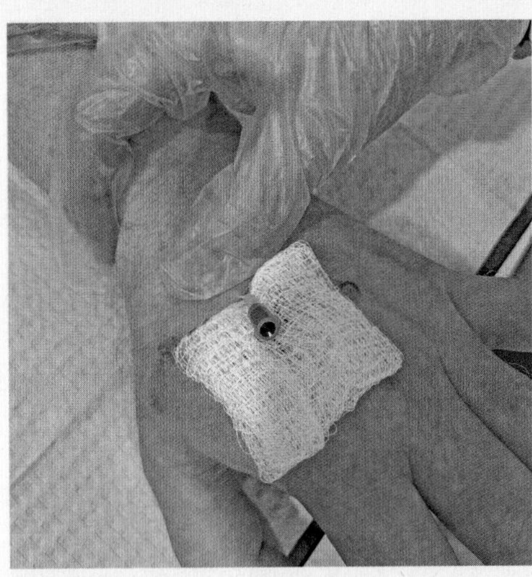

10. Attach sterile end of primed tubing to catheter hub. *(Helps prevent backflow, connects fluid source to venous access, and maintains sterility of system.)*
11. Stabilizing insertion site, slowly open roller or slide clamp to begin intravenous infusion of solution. *(Keeps catheter in place, initiates infusion, and helps prevent clotting of blood in catheter.)*
12. Secure catheter, in accordance with facility policy (see illustration). *(Prevents unintentional dislodging of catheter from vein. Infusion Nurses Society [INS; 2011] guidelines suggest not using chevron method of securing catheter in place as it increases risk of infection. Instead, an IV stabilization device is recommended.)* Apply dressing recommended by facility policy. *(Prevents infection. Transparent dressings allow easier evaluation of insertion site, but facility policy should be followed.)*

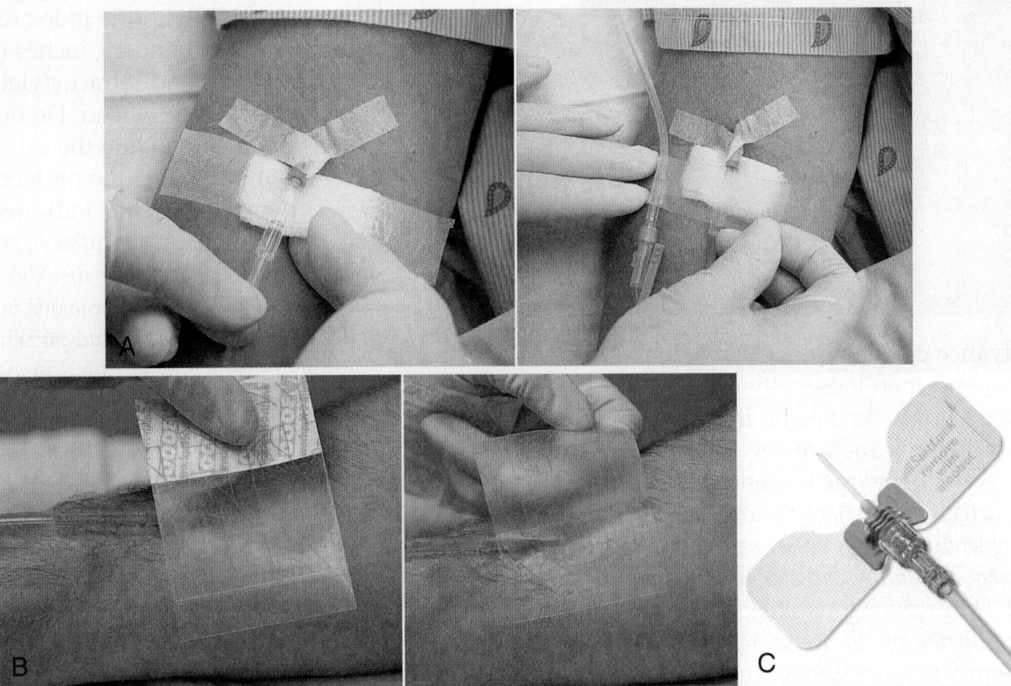

13. Label site and tubing according to facility policy. *(Serves as reminder to change site and tubing at appropriate intervals.)*
14. Adjust solution flow rate according to accurate rate calculations or IV pump rate according to health care provider orders (see Chapter 17). *(Ensures patient receives appropriate amount of solution in the prescribed amount of time.)*
15. Refer to Standard Steps 10 to 17.
16. Document the following on appropriate facility form:
    - Date and time of insertion
    - Type of fluid
    - Insertion site
    - Size and type of catheter or needle
    - Number of attempts made
    - Flow rate
    - Patient's response
    - Patient teaching (see the Patient Teaching box and Lifespan Considerations for older adults box on intravenous therapy)
17. Immediately report to health care provider any adverse conditions or reactions such as pulmonary congestion, shock, or thrombophlebitis.

Illustration for step 12 from Potter PA, Perry AG: *Fundamentals of nursing: Concepts, process, and practice,* ed 7, St. Louis, 2009, Mosby. Step 12C figure copyright Bard Access Systems.

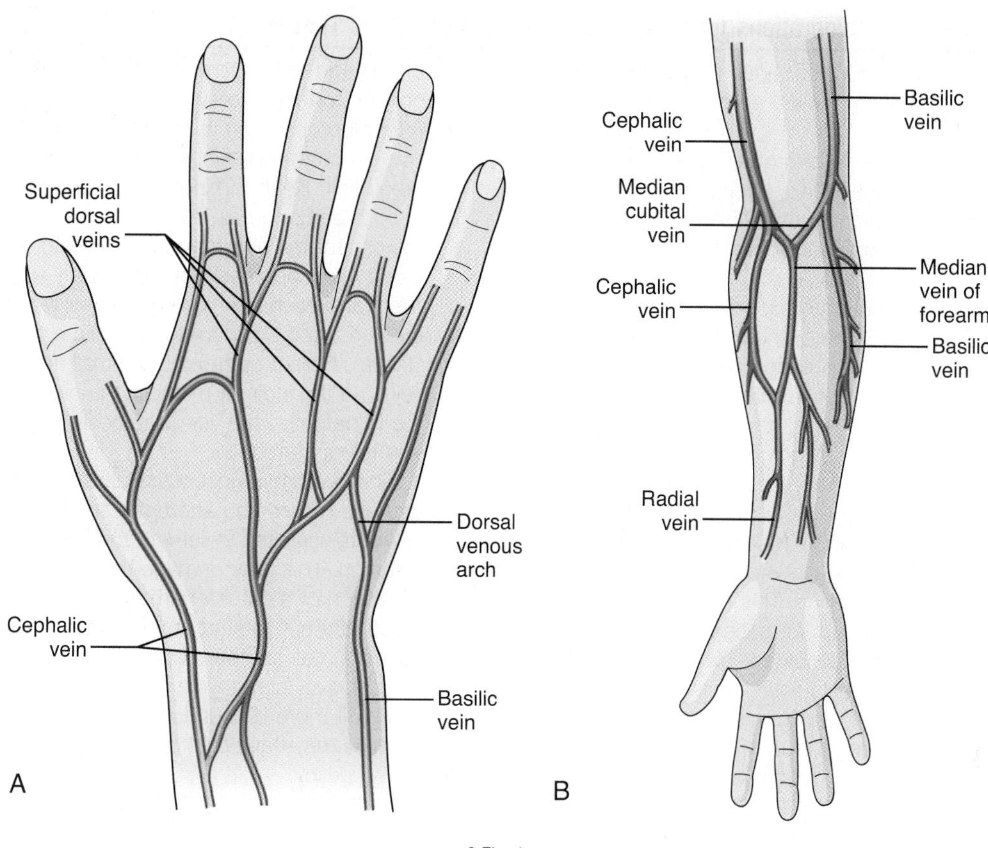

Fig. 18.7 Common intravenous sites. A, Dorsal surface of the hand. B, Inner arm.

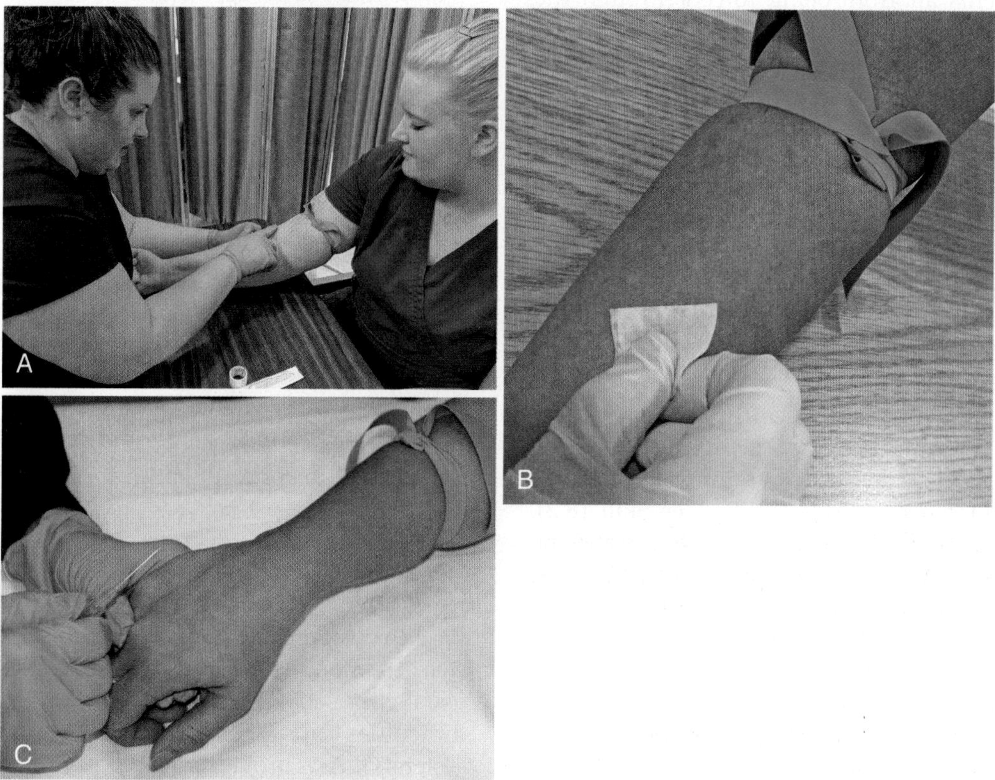

Fig. 18.8 A, Applying tourniquet and selecting site. B, Cleansing skin for venipuncture. C, Pulling skin taut as catheter is inserted.

Box 18.14 Special Considerations for Patients Receiving Intravenous Therapy

- Very young children and older adult patients have fragile veins; avoid using sites that are easily moved or bumped.
- Venipuncture is problematic in obese patients because of difficulty in locating superficial veins.
- Avoid using any extremity with circulatory or neurologic impairment, or the dominant extremity, whenever possible.
- When the need to administer blood or blood components is anticipated or the IV is in a patient preoperatively, use a large-gauge (16- or 18-gauge) catheter that will accommodate faster infusions or thicker solutions.
- Critically ill patients at all stages of life require more frequent monitoring to check for complications related to IV therapy.
- When solution has less than 100 mL remaining, have new bag of solution at patient's bedside so that it is readily available for changing. This reduces the risk of air entering the tubing and the patient's vein.
- In patients with fragile or engorged veins, avoid the use of tourniquets. In such patients, tourniquets increase the chance of excessive vein wall damage and hematoma formation. Consider using instead a blood pressure cuff to exert even, gentle pressure on the vessel.
- Encourage the patient to ask questions, and provide honest, forthright answers in a calm, reassuring manner.
- After all preparation is complete and immediately before you puncture the skin, inform the patient that there will be a stick. Keep reminding the patient to take slow, deep breaths to help the patient calm down. Distract the patient by talking about other subjects if necessary.
- Use a direct approach for large, easily seen veins. In the direct approach to IV insertion, the skin and the vein wall are punctured simultaneously with the catheter.
- Use an indirect approach for small, fragile, or deeper veins. In the indirect method, the skin is punctured with the IV catheter, the vein is relocated, and then the vein wall is punctured.
- If venipuncture is unsuccessful, always obtain a new catheter before you attempt a second venipuncture. Never reinsert the stylet into the catheter during insertion. This may damage the catheter and cause formation of a catheter embolism.
- If you attempt to start an IV infusion two times without success, call another nurse for assistance. The patient's anxiety level increases with multiple attempts, and this makes it more difficult to access the vein. Some facilities may have different policies regarding this. Know facility policy.

drip chamber to fill it partially (one-third to one-half) with fluid. Open the roller or slide clamp slowly to enable the flow of the solution down the tubing. This priming prevents air from being forced through the tubing into the patient's circulatory system, which would create an air embolus. As the fluid fills the tubing, invert injection ports to fill them with fluid as well.

After preparing the equipment, enter the patient's room and explain the procedure to the patient. Allow time for the patient to ask questions and to clarify any misunderstandings. Next, evaluate the patient's veins. Select a vein in the nondominant arm, if possible. Starting low and working up the arm, look for a soft, bouncy vein large enough to accommodate the solution or medication ordered. Using alcohol, povidone-iodine, or a solution preferred by the facility, cleanse the intended puncture site. Once the site is cleaned, perform the venipuncture and secures the catheter. Begin the infusion at the prescribed infusion rate, and watch the site for redness or swelling (see Skill 18.2). Because venipuncture is an invasive procedure and the pierced skin is no longer a barrier to microorganisms, follow strict aseptic technique when performing this procedure.

When the venipuncture is complete and the infusion is running, instruct the patient on limitations related to the IV infusion and the patient's responsibilities regarding the infusion (see the Patient Teaching and Lifespan Considerations for older adults boxes on IV therapy). Answer any questions the patient may have.

Patient Teaching

Intravenous Therapy

- If intravenous (IV) apparatus is positional, instruct patient in how to position arm properly to maintain flow.
- Instruct patient to wear clothes with wide sleeves.
- Instruct patient about signs and symptoms of infiltration, phlebitis, and inflammation, such as redness, swelling, or discomfort at site.
- Instruct patient to inform the nurse if flow slows or stops, if blood is seen in the tubing or if the site becomes red, swollen, tender, or warm.
- Instruct patient how to ambulate with IV pole or stand.
- Instruct patient not to silence any IV pump alarms.
- Teach patient that to wash, it is best to take tub baths, but showering may be allowed. If a patient chooses to shower, the patient will have to have the IV site completely covered to ensure that it does not get wet.
- Teach the importance of not changing the flow rate, not lying on the tubing, and not allowing the tubing to kink.

CENTRAL VENOUS ACCESS DEVICES

When IV therapy is needed over a long term (several weeks or months), a central venous access device (CVAD) usually is used. CVADs were developed to address the difficulties caused by repeated access to the venous system. CVADs provide safer access to the venous system and avoid the dangers of multiple venipunctures, such as vein sclerosis (hardening), bruising, infection, and

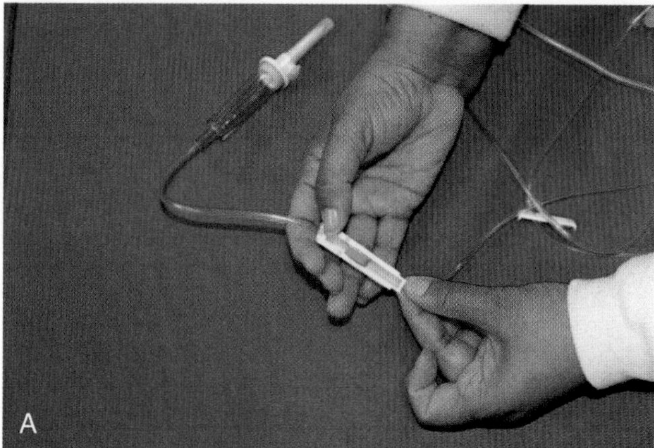

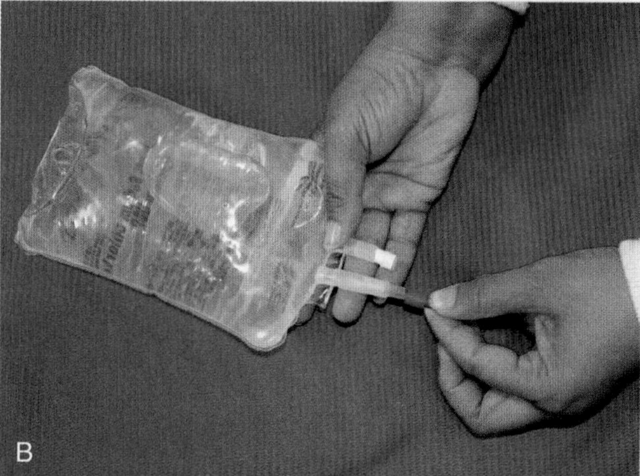

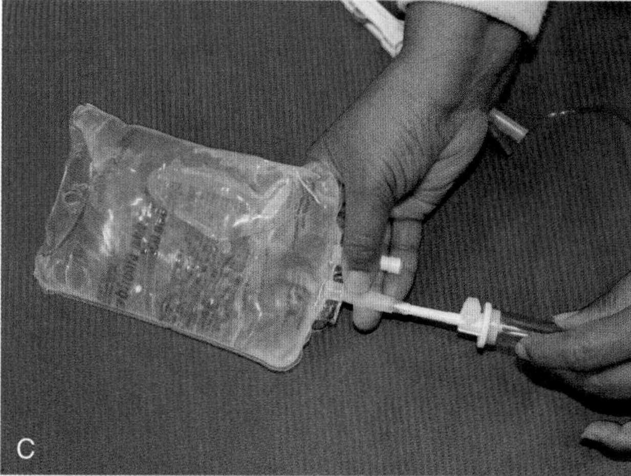

Fig. 18.9 A, Closing valve. B, Removing insertion port cover. C, Inserting spike.

pain. They are used mainly to administer various fluids, including chemotherapy and parenteral nutrition; to obtain blood samples on patients requiring daily laboratory tests; and for hemodialysis.

Various catheters and ports are used for patients requiring long-term IV therapy; therefore nurses must be familiar with these devices. The three categories of CVADs currently used are tunneled central venous catheters (CVCs), percutaneous CVCs, and implanted infusion ports. Common brand names for the various catheters used include Hickman, Groshong, Raaf, and Port-a-Cath. Percutaneous CVC insertion can be performed at the patient's bedside, whereas tunneled CVCs are inserted in the operating room with the use of local or general anesthetic. Both are inserted into a large vein; the percutaneous CVC is inserted through the cephalic or basilic veins in the arm and then advanced into the superior vena cava, and the tunneled CVC is tunneled through the subcutaneous tissue into the subclavian vein and into the superior vena cava (Fig. 18.10). The advantage of both types of CVC is that they produce less chance of irritation, inflammation, and vessel sclerosis.

Depending on the type of catheter, the device may have single, double, or triple lumens and is left in place as long as needed according to the manufacturer's guidelines (Fig. 18.11).

Implanted infusion ports are CVCs that are implanted surgically, with the use of local anesthetic, into the subcutaneous tissue in the area of the intraclavicular fossa. The catheter is inserted into a large vessel, as are the other CVCs, and threaded into the superior vena cava (Fig. 18.12). The body of the port is then left in the subcutaneous tissue for easy access (see Fig. 18.12B and C). The port placement is possible to palpate and is accessed with either a 90-degree angle or straight Huber needle directly through the skin (see Fig. 18.12A); to keep the port viable, it is necessary to heparinize the port every 4 weeks. The two most common complications of implanted CVCs are infection and occlusion of the catheter cannula. These complications are usually preventable by appropriate dressing changes and heparinization of the ports. It is necessary to teach patients how to care for their devices in the home setting so that they can start and discontinue infusions, heparinize their devices, and perform dressing changes appropriately.

PERIPHERALLY INSERTED CENTRAL CATHETERS

Peripherally inserted central catheters (PICCs) are an alternative to CVCs for patients requiring IV access beyond the length of time that **peripheral** (distal from the heart) IV lines can be maintained, usually between 7 days and 3 months. PICCs are inserted by specially trained registered nurses (if permitted by the state nurse practice act) or by the health care provider. They are inserted into the cephalic or basilic vein in the upper arm and threaded into the subclavian vein. The PICC may be left in place for extended periods as long as there are no problems with the device and complications do not occur.

PICCs pose less risk of pneumothorax, hemothorax, and air embolisms than do CVCs, are less expensive to maintain than are CVCs, and pose less risk of phlebitis and infiltration than do peripheral lines. Problems associated with PICCs include clotting, leaking from the catheter, migration of the catheter, infection, and catheter breakage.

Lifespan Considerations

Older Adults

Intravenous Therapy

- Changes in cardiac and renal function related to the aging process or chronic conditions create the need for extreme accuracy in flow control and thus necessitate the use of electronic infusion devices (see Chapter 17).
- Fragility of veins in older adult patients increases the risk of infiltration. Monitor infusion site carefully and frequently.
- Fragile skin necessitates the use of nonporous tapes and skin protectant solutions.
- Older adults are more prone to fluid imbalances, and all infusions must be monitored carefully to prevent fluid volume overload.
- Visual and hearing deficits pose challenges to patient education. Face the patient, and speak clearly and calmly.
- Short-term memory loss, depression, and confusion sometimes lead patients to remove the IV catheter or change their attitude or decisions about care. An adult patient who is competent and is taught properly about the benefits and risks of IV therapy has the right to refuse it. Decisions made by competent patients to refuse treatment must be honored as legally binding.
- Because of fragility of veins, use extra care in injecting medication boluses.
- If the patient is not able to tolerate the infusion of whole blood or red blood cells in 4 hours, it may be necessary for the blood bank to split the unit into two bags. Make sure to refrigerate the second bag during the infusion of the first.
- In older adults, use the smallest gauge catheter or needle possible (e.g., 24- to 26-gauge). This is less traumatizing to the vein and allows better blood flow to provide increased hemodilution of the IV fluids or medications.
- Avoid the back of an older adult's hand or the dominant arm for venipuncture because the resulting pain or disability at these sites greatly interferes with the patient's independence.
- If an older adult has fragile skin and veins, a tourniquet may cause rupture of veins, bruising, or both. Opt to perform the venipuncture without the use of a tourniquet, or use a blood pressure cuff to provide enough pressure for vein dilation.
- When an older adult has lost subcutaneous tissue, the veins lose stability and may roll away from the needle. To stabilize the vein, apply traction to the skin below the projected insertion site.
- Using an angle of 5 to 15 degrees on insertion is helpful because an older adult's veins are more superficial.
- In an older person with fragile skin, prevent skin tears by minimizing the amount of tape used.

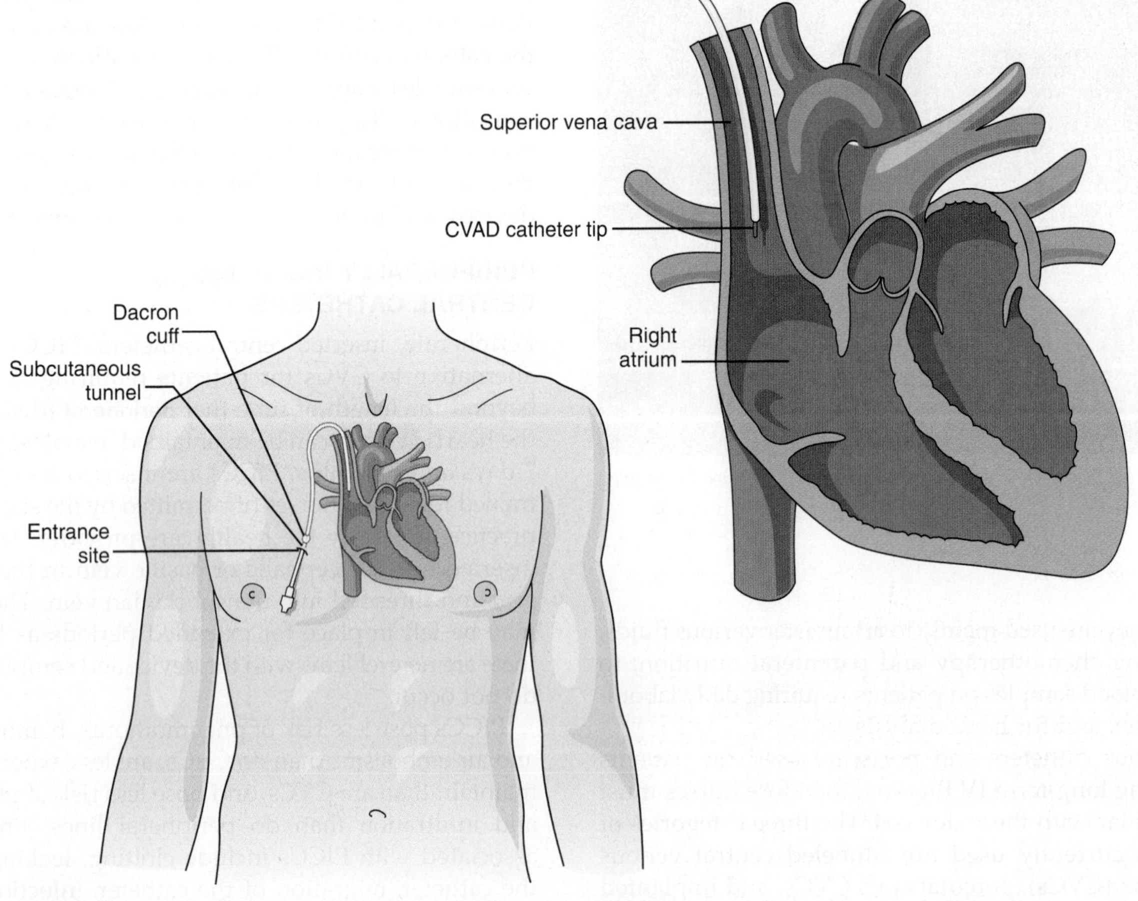

Fig. 18.10 Small-gauge tunneled catheter in its place, threaded into superior vena cava. *CVAD,* central venous access device.

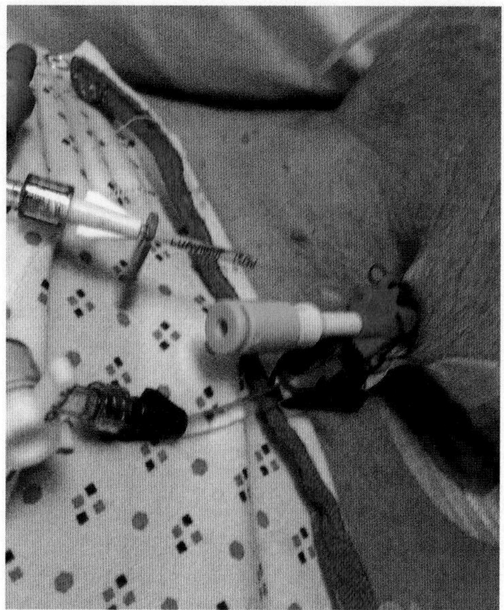

Fig. 18.11 Triple-lumen central venous access device (CVAD) placed in jugular vein.

PICCs come with single or double lumens ranging in diameter from 16- to 24-gauge and in length from 40 to 65 cm (16 to 26 inches).

INTRAVENOUS MONITORING

To keep the IV site intact and infusing without problems, the site must be monitored frequently. Each facility specifies how often IV sites should be monitored; it may be hourly, every 2 hours, or even every 4 hours.

When monitoring an IV site, establish a routine beginning at the solution container and ending at the site. Check the flow rate against the health care provider's order. Check tubing for kinks or obstructions and check the position of the patient's hand or arm. If the extremity is flexed, the vein may become occluded; remind patients to keep extremities extended. Inspect and palpate the site for edema, erythema, **induration** (hardness), heat, and discomfort. A burning sensation often means that the solution is irritating the vein; the infusion rate should be slowed, and monitoring should

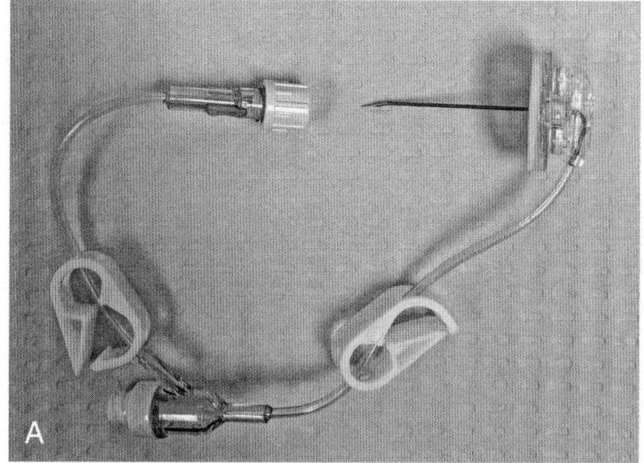

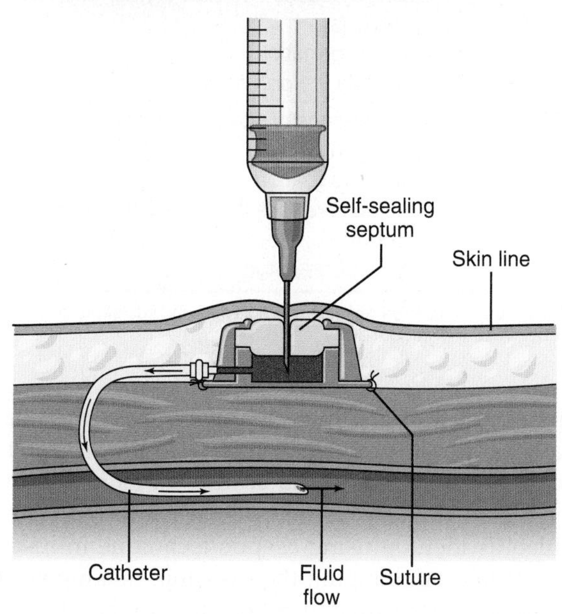

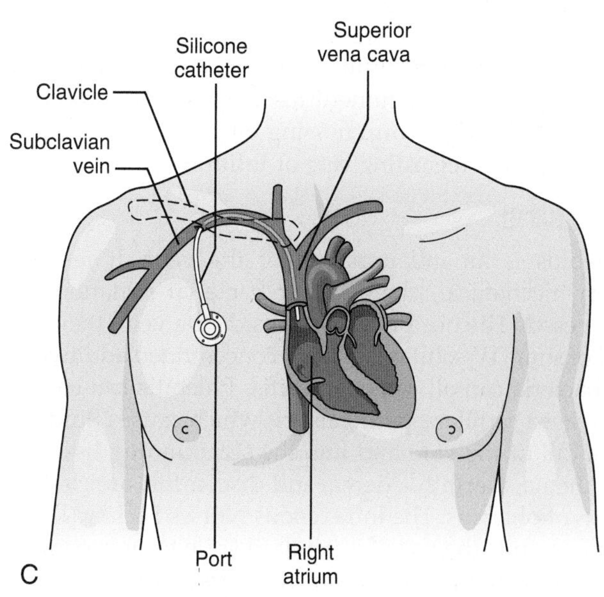

Fig. 18.12 Implantation of infusion ports. A, Infusion set. B, Cross-section illustration of implantable port, showing access of the port with the Huber needle. C, Implanted port and catheter.

continue. Compare the hand or arm with the opposite hand or arm if the site seems edematous. Edema often indicates that infiltration has occurred.

If the patient is dehydrated, in shock, or critically ill, a slow infusion rate does not provide the cardiovascular system with enough fluid. In contrast, an infusion rate that is too rapid may place too much fluid into the circulation and overload the cardiovascular, neurologic, and urinary systems. Fluid volume overload can be fatal in certain patients; to prevent overload, monitor for symptoms such as dyspnea; a rapid, weak pulse; cough; disorientation; increased or decreased blood pressure; crackles; pitting edema; weight gain; and decreased urine output. If fluid volume overload is suspected, slow the infusion rate immediately and notify the charge nurse or health care provider. Check the volume infused by comparing the bag contents with the pump readout to ensure pump accuracy.

INFILTRATION

Infiltration is the seepage of a nonirritating solution or medication into tissue surrounding the vessel. It is one of the most common complications of IV therapy and is caused by dislodgment of the IV cannula from the vein (going through vein, pulling out of vein), by phlebitis, or by excessive movement of the cannula in the vein.

If edema is detected at the insertion site, loosen the tape over the site and observe the site for a short time. Edema that does not subside generally indicates that the catheter is out of the vein and infiltration has occurred. Discomfort, burning sensation, blanching, or coolness around the site are other possible indications of infiltration. The drip rate on gravity-flow IV lines also may decrease when an infiltration occurs. If fluid seeps into the tissue, and infiltration is confirmed, discontinue the infusion and access another site to continue therapy, preferably in the opposite extremity. Monitor the site of the infiltration; fluid usually reabsorbs within 24 hours. Document the degree of infiltration (Table 18.6) and perform nursing interventions. Follow agency policy regarding care of infiltration.

PHLEBITIS

Phlebitis is an inflammation of the vein. It results from mechanical, chemical, or bacterial irritation of the vessel. The needle moving inside the vein, the low pH of some IV solutions, highly concentrated additives, or bacteria can all cause phlebitis. Phlebitis can cause increased capillary permeability, which causes fluid to leak out of the vein and into the surrounding tissues. Erythema, warmth, edema, and discomfort are classic signs of phlebitis. The Intravenous Nurses Society (INS) recommends the use of a standard scale for measuring the degree of phlebitis (Infusion Nurses Society, 2011) (Table 18.7).

Prevention is the best treatment of phlebitis. To help prevent vein irritation and trauma, it is important to use large veins for hypertonic solutions, to use the smallest gauge cannula possible for the solution, to rotate IV sites every 72 hours, and to use CVCs or PICCs for long-term therapy. Some other ways to help prevent phlebitis include using aseptic technique in inserting the IV line or changing the dressing; making sure the IV catheter is secured appropriately so that it does not move; changing the IV solution, tubing, and dressings as appropriate; and decreasing the irritation of

Table 18.6 Infiltration Scale

GRADE	CLINICAL CRITERIA
0	No symptoms
1	Skin blanching Edema less than 1 inch in any direction Coolness to touch Presence or absence of pain
2	Skin blanching Edema 1 to 6 inches in any direction Coolness to touch Presence or absence of pain
3	Skin blanching, translucence Gross edema greater than 6 inches in any direction Coolness to touch Mild to moderate pain Possible numbness
4	Skin blanching, translucence Gross edema greater than 6 inches in any direction Deep pitting tissue edema Circulatory impairment Moderate to severe pain Infiltration of any amount of blood product, irritant, or vesicant

From Infusion Nurses Society: Infusion nursing standards of practice, *J Intraven Nurs* 34(1S):S65, 2011.

Table 18.7 Phlebitis Scale

GRADE	CLINICAL CRITERIA
0	No clinical symptoms
1	Erythema at access site with or without pain
2	Pain at access site with erythema and/or edema
3	Pain at access site with erythema and/or edema Streak formation Palpable venous cord
4	Pain at access site with erythema and/or edema Streak formation Palpable venous cord greater than 1 inch in length Purulent drainage

From Infusion Nurses Society: Infusion nursing standards of practice, *J Intraven Nurs* 34(1S):S65, 2011.

medications/solutions by diluting them or slowing the rate. Using in-line filters to remove air, bacteria, and particulate matter also aids in preventing phlebitis. If phlebitis symptoms appear, notify the health care provider, discontinue the IV infusion, and, using new IV tubing and fluids, restart it in the opposite extremity, if possible. Cold compresses applied within the first hour after phlebitis is found may help decrease complications; applying warm compresses to the inflamed area lessens discomfort. Document symptoms present, phlebitis rating, nursing interventions, and the patient's response to interventions.

SEPTICEMIA

Septicemia occurs when microorganisms enter the blood. It may occur as a result of IV therapy when poor aseptic technique or contaminated equipment is used during IV line insertion and pathogens are introduced into the bloodstream. The use of sterile technique reduces the potential for introduction of pathogenic organisms. Signs and symptoms of septicemia include fever, chills, lethargy, pain, headache, nausea, vomiting, and diarrhea. If septicemia is suspected, notify the health care provider, discontinue the IV infusion, and, using new IV tubing and fluids, restart it in the opposite extremity, if possible. The discontinued IV catheter, tubing, and solution should be saved for possible culture (in accordance with the agency's policy and health care provider's orders). If an antibiotic is ordered, it should be started after cultures have been obtained. Monitor the patient closely and document symptoms present, nursing interventions, and the patient's response to interventions.

MAINTAINING AN INTRAVENOUS SITE

Complications sometimes occur with peripheral IV infusions. Infiltration of the site, phlebitis of the vessel, and local or systemic infections are possible. Appropriate management of IV sites helps prevent or minimize these complications (Skill 18.3).

Text continued on p. 515

Skill 18.3 Maintaining an Intravenous Site

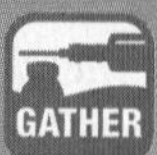

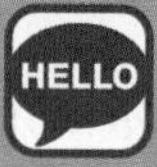

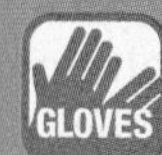

NURSING ACTION *(RATIONALE)*

Changing a Peripheral Intravenous Dressing

1. Refer to Standard Steps 1 to 9.
2. Assemble equipment:
   - Adhesive remover (optional)
   - Antiseptic swabs, alcohol, povidone-iodine, chlorhexidine
   - Arm board, hand board, or housing device (optional)
   - Clean gloves
   - Intravenous (IV) catheter stabilization device
   - Skin protectant solution (optional)
   - Strips of precut tape (if chevron method of securing IV catheter is to be used, tape should be sterile)
   - Transparent dressing or sterile 2- × 2-inch gauze pads
3. Site evaluation:
   a. Determine when the dressing was last changed by checking the dressing label. *(Labeling provides instant identification for determining status of the site.)*
   b. Observe current dressing for moisture, and determine whether moisture is leakage from the puncture site or from an external source. *(Determines urgency of the dressing change. Change soiled dressing immediately.)*
   c. Observe IV system for proper functioning or complications (tubing or catheter kinks).
   d. Apply clean gloves, and palpate the catheter site through the intact dressing to elicit any complaints of tenderness, pain, or burning sensation. *(These signs are indicative of phlebitis.)*
   e. Inspect catheter site for edema, erythema, drainage, or blanching. *(These signs are indicative of phlebitis or infiltration.)*
4. Remove any overlying tape. Then remove transparent membrane dressing by picking up one corner and pulling the side laterally while holding catheter hub. Repeat for other side. *(Technique minimizes discomfort during tape removal.)*

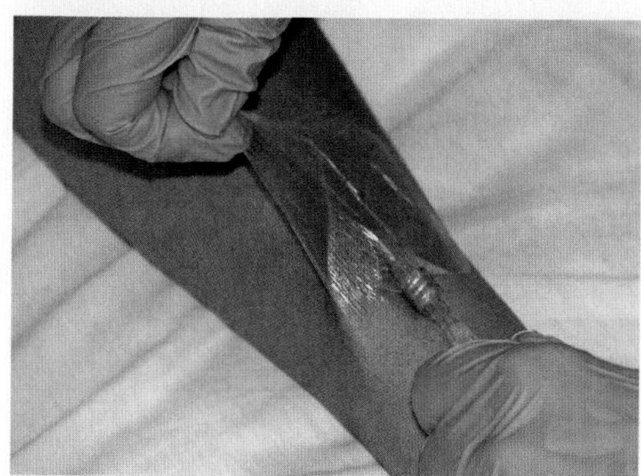

Continued

Skill 18.3 Maintaining an Intravenous Site—cont'd

a. Alternative is to remove gauze dressing and tape from site one layer at a time by pulling toward the insertion site. Tape securing catheter to skin should be left intact. *(Leaving the catheter secured prevents its accidental dislodgment and puncturing of the blood vessel.)*

5. Observe insertion site for redness, erythema, edema, exudate, pallor, or pain. If any of these is present, discontinue infusion. *(These signs are indicative of phlebitis or infiltration. Notify health care provider, and restart infusion in opposite extremity.)*

6. If IV solution is infusing properly, gently remove tape securing catheter. Leave IV stabilization device in place (if one is used), or stabilize catheter with one hand. Remove adhesive residue with adhesive remover, if necessary. *(Prevents catheter from dislodging while site is cleaned and dressing is being changed.)*

7. If appropriate according to facility policy, clean insertion site with antiseptic swab. Using circular motion, start at insertion site and work outward in concentric circles. Allow antiseptic solution to dry completely. *(Allow antimicrobial solutions to air-dry completely, which effectively reduces microbial counts. If antiseptic agents are used in combination, allow each to air-dry separately.)* Option: Apply skin protectant solution (SKIN PREP Protective Barrier Wipe or 3M Cavilon No Sting Barrier Film) to the area where the tape or dressing will be applied. Allow skin protectant solution to dry.

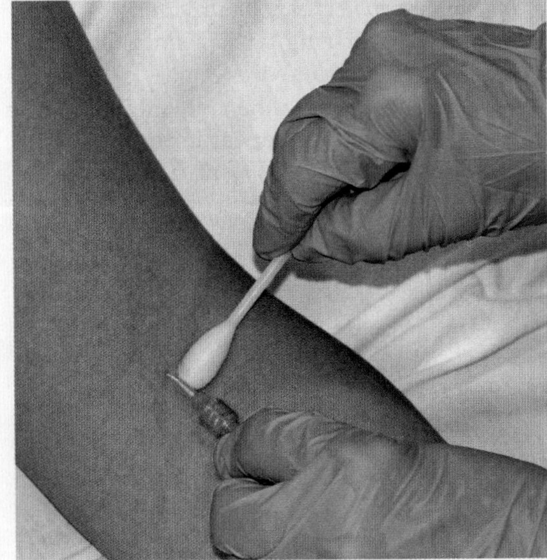

8. Apply dressing.
   a. Transparent dressing:
      (1) Place transparent dressing over venipuncture site by smoothing dressing over IV site and catheter up to the hub (refer to manufacturer's directions). Do not completely cover the catheter hub or tubing junction with the dressing.
   b. Gauze dressing:
      (1) If IV stabilization device is not used to secure catheter, use **chevron** method (crossing the tape over the catheter) to stabilize catheter. Place single 4-inch (10-cm) strip of sterile ½-inch (1.5 cm) nonallergenic tape under peripheral catheter hub with sticky side up. Crisscross tape over catheter hub to anchor it to skin. *(Chevron method secures catheter to skin.)* Do not cover insertion site. If a second piece of sterile tape is desired, place it across catheter at hub.
      (2) Place sterile 2- × 2-inch gauze over venipuncture site and catheter hub. Secure all edges with tape. Do not cover the connection between IV tubing and catheter hub with the dressing. *(Use occlusive gauze dressings to prevent airflow. Access to catheter hub is needed in an emergency; therefore, when tubing is changed, hub should not be covered.)*

9. Fold 2- × 2-inch gauze in half, and cover with tape 1 inch (2.5 cm) wide extending about an inch (2.5 cm) from each side of gauze. Place under the tubing and catheter hub junction. *(Placing 2- × 2-inch gauze under the catheter hub and tubing decreases skin irritation.)* When a transparent dressing is used, avoid placing tape directly over dressing. *(Tape application loosens transparent dressings.)*

10. Label the dressing with date and time of insertion, date and time of dressing change, gauge and length of catheter, and name of nurse (see illustration in Step 4). *(Allows easy recognition of type of device and time interval for site rotation.)* Option: Apply armboard, hand board, or commercial housing device if venipuncture site or dressing is affected by the motion of the elbow or wrist. *(Reduces the risk of phlebitis and infiltration from motion of the joint.)*

11. Discard used supplies, remove gloves, and perform hand hygiene.

12. Document and report the following:
    - Time dressing was changed
    - Reason for dressing change
    - Type of dressing material used
    - Condition of venipuncture site
    - Treatment of venipuncture site (if any)
    - Tubing is **patent** (tubing is open and not occluded)

13. Refer to Standard Steps 10 to 17.

Skill 18.3 Maintaining an Intravenous Site—cont'd

Changing Infusion Tubing

1. Refer to Standard Steps 1 to 9.
2. Assemble equipment:
   a. Continuous infusion:
      - Infusion tubing as appropriate: microdrop (delivers 60 drops [gtt] per milliliter and is used for slow infusions in patients susceptible to fluid volume overload) or macrodrip (delivers 10 to 15 drops [gtt] per milliliter and is used for rapid infusions)
      - Filter and extension tubing if necessary *(Patients sometimes require IV extension tubing to increase mobility, decrease manipulation and potential contamination at insertion site, or facilitate changes in position.)*
      - Tubing label
   b. Intermittent use saline or heparin lock:
      - 5-mL syringe filled with normal saline or heparin flush solution (check facility policy)
      - Clean gloves
      - Injection cap or as-needed (prn) adapter
      - Loop or short extension tubing (if necessary)
      - Sterile 2- × 2-inch gauze pads
      - Additional dressing supplies as needed if application of new IV dressing is required (see earlier Changing a Peripheral Intravenous Dressing section, Steps 4 to 7)
3. Evaluation of equipment:
   a. Determine when new infusion set is needed (e.g., according to facility policy or label, or after contamination or puncture of infusion tubing).
   b. Observe for occlusion in tubing such as kinking, drug or mineral precipitate, or blood. *(Infusion of incompatible medication potentially leads to precipitate formation and occlusion of tubing. Blood may flow from the vein into the tubing and will adhere to tubing. Infusion of viscous blood components sometimes causes adherence to walls of tubing and results in occlusion.)*
   c. Determine patient's need for continued IV infusion. *(If the health care provider has discontinued the IV infusion or the nurse anticipates that the IV infusion will be discontinued, it is advisable to wait to change tubing so as not to increase costs. Call the health care provider for further orders. If the tubing has been contaminated or punctured, however, change the tubing immediately.)*
4. Open new infusion set, and connect add-on pieces such as filters or extension tubing. *(Use add-ons only if absolutely necessary to decrease the risk of contamination and infection.)* Keep protective covering over spike and distal adapter. *(Protective covers reduce entrance of microorganisms.)* Secure each junction with a Luer-Lok, clasping device, or threaded device. Avoid the use of tape.
5. If catheter hub is not visible, remove IV dressing as directed in Changing a Peripheral Intravenous Dressing section, Steps 3 and 4. Do not remove tape securing catheter to skin. If transparent dressing must be removed, place small piece of sterile tape across hub to temporarily anchor catheter during disconnection. *(Keeping catheter secured decreases risk of dislodging catheter.)*
6. For existing continuous infusion *(Infusion bag and tubing should be changed at the same time whenever possible to decrease risk of contamination)*:
   a. Close roller clamp on new tubing.
   b. Slow rate of infusion to keep vein open (KVO) on existing IV by regulating roller clamp on old tubing.
   c. Compress and fill drip chamber of old tubing.
7. Remove IV container from pole, invert container, and remove old tubing from solution. Carefully hold container while hanging or taping the drip chamber on IV pole 36 inches (90 cm) above IV site. *(Fluid in drip chamber will run slowly to keep catheter patent.)*
8. Place insertion spike of new tubing into old fluid container opening. Hang container on IV pole, compress and release drip chamber on new tubing, and fill drip chamber one-third to one-half full.

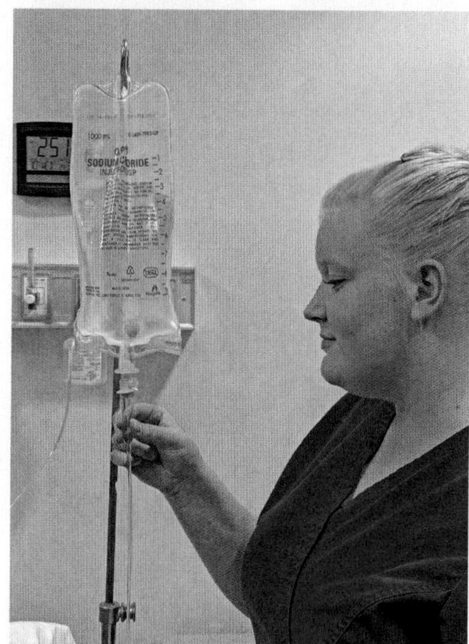

Continued

Skill 18.3 Maintaining an Intravenous Site—cont'd

9. Slowly open roller clamp, remove protective cap from adapter (if necessary), and flush new tubing with solution. Stop infusion and replace cap. *(Slow flushing of solution into tubing reduces formation of air bubbles in tubing.)*
10. Turn roller clamp on old tubing to "off" position. Option: Place 2- × 2-inch gauze under catheter hub. *(Prevents tubing from accidentally contacting skin and collects blood that may leak from catheter hub.)*
11. Stabilize hub of catheter, and apply pressure over vein just above catheter tip (at least 1½ inches above insertion site). Gently disconnect old tubing from catheter hub, and quickly insert adapter of new tubing into catheter hub. *(Minimizes loss of blood as tubing is changed.)*

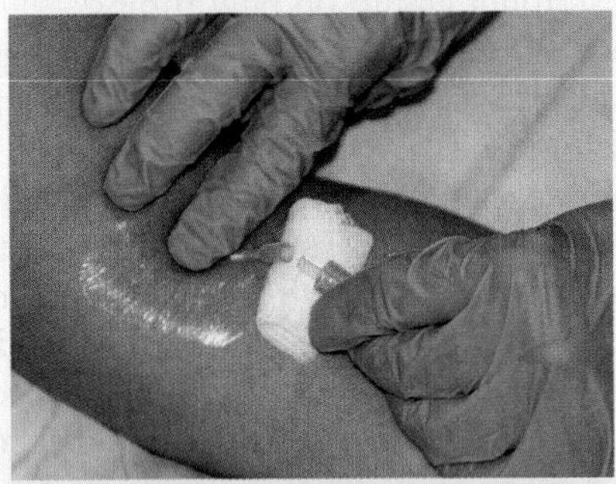

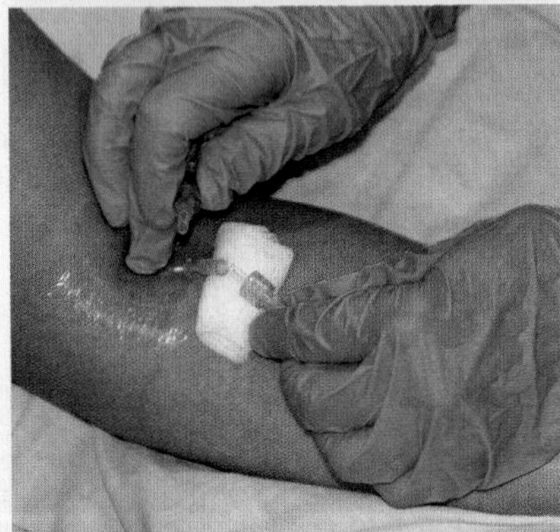

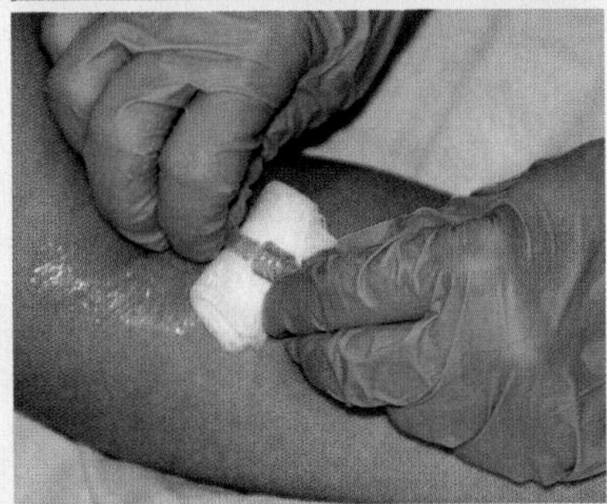

12. Open roller clamp on new tubing, allowing solution to run rapidly for 30 to 60 seconds, and then regulate IV drip according to health care provider's orders. *(Clears catheter of any blood in lumen, preventing occlusion.)*

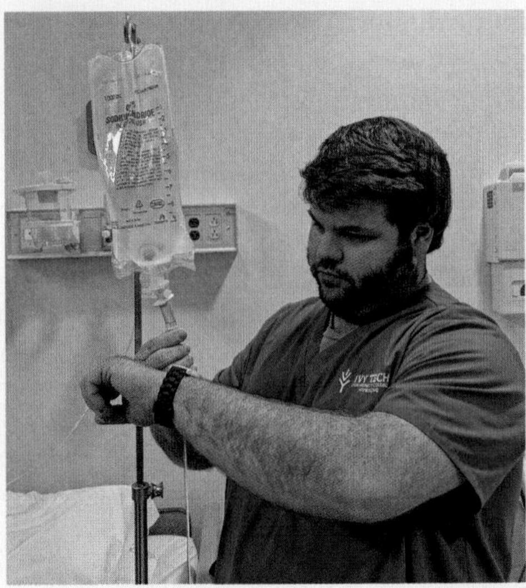

13. Attach a piece of tape or a preprinted label with date and time of tubing change onto tubing below the drip chamber. *(Provides reference to determine next time for tubing change.)*
14. Remove and discard 2- × 2-inch gauze (if used) and old IV tubing. If necessary, apply new dressing. Dispose of gloves.
15. Form a loop of tubing, and secure it to patient's arm with a strip of tape. *(Prevents accidental pulling against site and catheter movement.)*
16. Document and report the following:
    - Time tubing was changed
    - Rate of infusion

    A special IV flow sheet may be used to record tubing changes. Check facility policy.
17. Refer to Standard Steps 10 to 17.

Changing Solution Container

1. Refer to Standard Steps 1 to 9.
2. Assemble equipment:
    - Bottle or bag of IV solution as ordered by health care provider
    - Pen
    - Time tape
3. Determine need to change solution container:
    a. Check health care provider's orders. *(Ensures that correct solution will be used and that the order is complete.)*
    b. If order is written for KVO, contact health care provider for clarification of the rate of infusion. Note date and time when solution was last changed. *(Orders for KVO do not provide complete information and have potential to result in fluid overload or deficit and in electrolyte imbalance. A KVO order is required to contain a specific infusion rate; check facility policy.)*
    c. Verify patient's identification. *(Ensures right patient receives ordered IV fluid.)*

Skill 18.3 Maintaining an Intravenous Site—cont'd

d. Determine the compatibility of all IV fluids and additives by consulting appropriate literature or the pharmacy. *(Precipitates caused by incompatible medications could slow infusion or occlude catheter.)*
e. Determine patient's understanding of need for continuing IV therapy. *(Allows patient's questions to be answered and increases compliance.)*
f. Assess patency of current IV access site. Check for blood return and free flow of infusion.

4. Prepare next solution at least 1 hour before it is needed. If it is prepared in pharmacy, be sure it has been delivered to the patient's location. Check that the solution is correct and properly labeled. *(Ensures no disruption in fluid therapy to patient.)* Check solution expiration date. Observe for precipitate and discoloration. *(Prevents infusion of contaminated or outdated solution.)*
5. Change solution when fluid remains only in neck of container or when new type of solution has been ordered. *(Prevents air in tubing and waste of solution.)*
6. Move roller clamp to stop flow rate, and remove old IV fluid container from IV pole.
7. Invert old container and quickly remove spike, keeping it sterile. Remove protective cover from new fluid container. Without touching tip of spike, insert it into new bag or bottle. *(Ensures sterility of solution.)*
8. Hang new bag or bottle of solution on IV pole.
9. Check for air in tubing. If bubbles form, it is possible to remove them by closing the roller clamp, stretching the tubing downward, and tapping the tubing with the fingers (the bubbles rise in the tubing to the drip chamber). For larger amounts of air, swab port with antiseptic swab, allow to dry, and connect a syringe to an injection port below the air and aspirate the air into the syringe. *(Infusion of large amounts of air in tubing potentially results in air embolus, which is sometimes fatal.)* Reassure patient that small air bubbles are harmless.
10. Make sure drip chamber is one-third to one-half full. If drip chamber is too full, invert solution container and squeeze solution from the drip chamber back into the solution container. Replace container on IV pole. *(If chamber is completely filled, the drip rate cannot be observed.)*
11. Regulate flow to prescribed rate.
12. Place label on the side of container. Label should contain time hung, approximate time of completion, any medication added, and patient identification. If plastic bags are to be used, mark only on the label and not on the container. *(Allows accurate determination of next solution change and medication infusion.)*
13. Document and report the following:
    - Amount and type of fluid infused
    - Amount and type of new fluid
    - Patency of system

    A special IV flow sheet may be used to record parenteral fluids.
14. Refer to Standard Steps 10 to 17.

Discontinuing Intravenous Medications

1. Refer to Standard Steps 1 to 9.
2. Assemble equipment:
    - 5- or 10-mL syringe filled with normal saline, heparin flush solution, or both (depending on facility policy)
    - Antiseptic swabs
    - Clean gloves
    - Injection cap replacement (if needed)
    - Sterile cap or cover for infusion tubing
3. Evaluation:
    a. Observe fluid container for complete infusion of all medications.
    b. Review health care provider's order to determine whether blood samples are required after medication infusion. *(Monitoring of serum concentration of some IV medications is necessary to prevent reaching toxic levels. Dosage adjustment or alterations of timing for next dose are sometimes required.)*
    c. Monitor patient's response to medications. *(Enables evaluation of medication's effects.)*
4. Move roller clamp on infusion tubing to the "off" position. *(Prevents air from entering vein and prevents medication from leaking from tubing.)*
5. Disconnect medication delivery tubing from injection port, and replace with a sterile cap or cover. *(Infusion tubing can be reused with next ordered medication if it is not contaminated.)*
6. If the tubing has a needle or needleless adapter on the infusion tubing, remove and discard it appropriately, and replace with a sterile cap or cover as indicated. *(If tubing is to be reused, the tubing must remain sterile. If tubing spike, connector end, fluid pathway, or fluid container is contaminated, a new tubing set or fluid container is required.)*
7. Cleanse injection port or as-needed (prn) adapter on main IV tubing with antiseptic swab. *(Ensures sterility of port.)*

Continued

Skill 18.3 Maintaining an Intravenous Site—cont'd

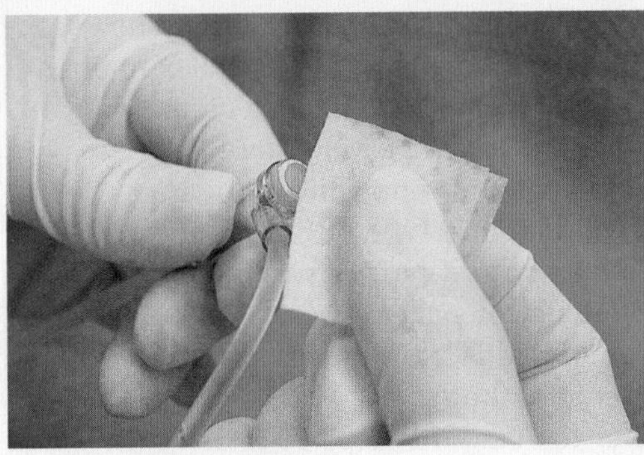

8. For intermittent medication piggybacked into a continuous infusion, attach 5-mL saline-filled syringe to injection port, and flush the line gently. Regulate fluid flow of the continuous infusion as ordered. *(Saline flush prevents incompatible medications from coming into contact in the infusion tubing. There is no way to know how much pressure is exerted inside catheter lumen. A 5-mL syringe generates less pressure than a 3-mL syringe. Do not force irrigation if resistance is felt.)*
9. For intermittent medications through a saline or heparin lock, attach saline-filled 5- to 10-mL syringe to injection port and flush catheter gently, or attach syringe filled with heparin flush solution to injection port and flush gently, if necessary (check facility policy). Attach sterile injection port cover if necessary. *(Flushing with 3 to 10 mL of saline after each medication is crucial. Volume of flush depends on lumen size, catheter length, and medication infused.)*
   a. Approach flushing of any IV catheter carefully. If resistance is met, assess for mechanical causes (e.g., closed clamps, kinked tubing, and the position of extremity). Never force flushing. *(Fibrin formation, drug precipitates, and blood clots sometimes occlude catheter lumen. Forceful flushing against these occlusions has the potential to cause embolus formation and catheter damage.)*
10. Prepare patient for blood testing after medication infusion if necessary.
11. Document and report the following:
    - Time that medication is discontinued
    - How tubing or catheter (or both) is flushed
    - Amount and type of flush solution
    - Condition of site
    - If facility policy requires it, use special IV flow sheet to document IV interventions.
12. Refer to Standard Steps 10 to 17.

Discontinuing Peripheral IV Access

1. Refer to Standard Steps 1 to 9.
2. Assemble equipment:
   - Antiseptic swab
   - Clean gloves
   - Sterile 2- × 2-inch or 4- × 4-inch gauze pad
   - Tape
3. Site evaluation:
   a. Observe existing IV site for signs and symptoms of infection, infiltration, or phlebitis. *(Indications of need to discontinue IV infusion.)*
   b. Review health care provider's orders for discontinuation of IV therapy. *(The health care provider's order is required to discontinue IV therapy.*
   c. Determine patient's understanding of the need for removal of peripheral IV catheter. *(Increases patient's knowledge and cooperation.)*
4. Explain procedure to patient. *(Minimizes patient's anxiety and discomfort.)*
5. Turn IV tubing roller clamp to "off" position. Remove tape securing tubing.
6. Remove IV site dressing and tape while stabilizing catheter. *(Movement of catheter will cause discomfort. Never use scissors to remove the tape or dressing because it is possible to accidentally cut the catheter.)*
7. With dry gauze held over site, apply light pressure and withdraw the catheter, using a slow steady movement, keeping the hub parallel to the skin. *(Changing the angle of the catheter inside the vein sometimes causes additional vein irritation, increasing the risk of postinfusion phlebitis.)*

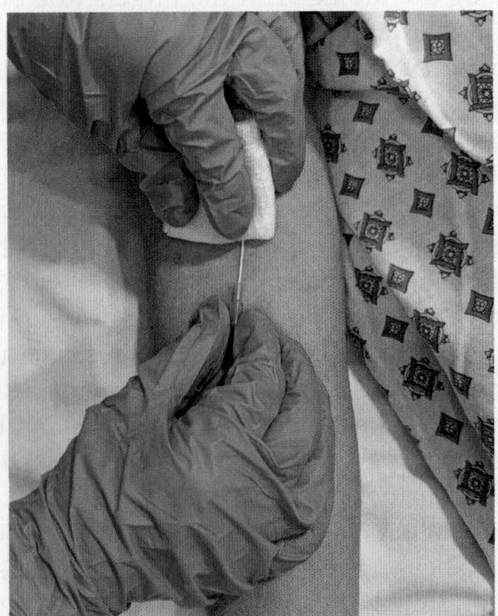

Skill 18.3 Maintaining an Intravenous Site—cont'd

8. Apply pressure to the site for 2 to 3 minutes, using a dry, sterile gauze pad. Secure the tape over the gauze snugly. *(Subcutaneous hematoma is a common complication. Applying tape snugly acts as a pressure dressing to stop bleeding and hematoma formation.)*
9. Inspect the catheter for intactness, noting tip integrity and length. *(Tips of catheters sometimes break off, causing an embolus, which is an emergency situation. Notify health care provider if tip is broken.)*
10. Discard used supplies.
11. Remove and discard gloves, and perform hand hygiene.
12. Instruct patient to report any erythema, pain, drainage, or edema that occurs after catheter removal. *(Postinfusion phlebitis sometimes occurs within 48 to 96 hours after catheter removal.)*
13. Document and record the following:
    - Time peripheral IV infusion was discontinued
    - Condition of site
    - Gauge and length of catheter
    - Whether catheter is intact
14. Refer to Standard Steps 10 to 17.

Keeping the IV insertion site covered and dry helps prevent the introduction of microorganisms and reduces the possibility of infection. Most often, a gauze dressing or a transparent dressing is used to cover the insertion site. Transparent dressings make visualization of the site easier and keep the site dry. Gauze dressings do not allow visualization of the site and can become soiled or damp; therefore their use is limited. No matter which dressing is used, it is important to change the dressing according to facility policy, usually every 48 to 72 hours, and whenever a dressing becomes wet, soiled, or loose.

It is also necessary to change the IV solution container and tubing at appropriate intervals to prevent complications. There are several types of IV solution containers, including plastic and glass. These containers must be changed according to the type of solution, the type of container, and the rate at which the IV is infusing. The INS (Infusion Nurses Society, 2011) recommends changing the solution container every 24 hours or sooner if the solution has been infused completely. Most facilities follow this recommendation or have even stricter guidelines.

The INS guidelines (Infusion Nurses Society, 2011) recommend changing tubing every 72 to 96 hours for continuous infusions and every 24 hours for intermittent infusions or infusions through an injection or access port. Some facilities have a stricter policy and may require changing tubing on continuous infusions every 48 hours; thus be aware of and follow facility policy.

If possible, the IV solution container, the tubing, and the dressing should be changed at the same time. This reduces the risk of introducing bacteria into the system and cuts down on infections at the site. Never disconnect the tubing when assisting with a gown or clothing change. Instead, the IV solution container and tubing should be threaded through the sleeve of the patient's garment. If the patient is allowed to shower, make sure the IV insertion site and dressing are protected with a water-resistant covering. Inspect the dressing and site after the shower, and change the dressing if it becomes wet or loose. Box 18.15 lists patient problem statements for the patient receiving IV therapy.

Box 18.15 Patient Problem Statements for the Patient Receiving Intravenous Therapy

Compromised Skin Integrity:
- Related to invasive procedure

Insufficient Knowledge:
- Related to lack of exposure to information

Potential for Inadequate Fluid Volume:
- Related to alterations in regulatory mechanisms of hydration
- Related to fluid and electrolyte imbalance

Potential for Infection:
- Related to break in skin integrity

Potential for Injury:
- Related to adverse effects of intravenous (IV) therapy
- Related to presence of IV catheter acting as a foreign body
- Related to IV medications

BLOOD TRANSFUSION THERAPY

Any time a patient has a problem with the amount of blood circulating in the body or with any of the blood components, the health care provider may order a blood transfusion. Most often, a blood or blood component transfusion is ordered to replace blood volume, to preserve oxygen-carrying capacity, or to increase coagulation capabilities. It is up to the health care provider to determine the type of transfusion and how many units are to be transfused.

In some states, the administration of blood and blood components is included within the scope of practice for the LPN/LVN, and in others the LPN/LVN may be responsible only for measuring baseline vital signs and monitoring the transfusion. Therefore it is important to be aware of the LPN/LVN's scope of practice and facility policy when dealing with blood or blood component transfusions.

The fear of human immunodeficiency virus (HIV) infection has led some patients to refuse transfusions of blood or blood products. The testing procedures implemented to screen donated blood have reduced the incidence of transmission of HIV dramatically resulting a safer supply for transfusion. Most often, health care providers use the patient's hemoglobin level as a guideline to determine when a transfusion is necessary, but current recommendations from the American Association of Blood Banks (AABB) suggest that blood transfusions should be given only when clinically necessary to lower health care costs and decrease the risk of bloodborne infections (Choosing Wisely, 2014).

Individuals who have concerns about receiving another person's blood may donate their own blood before anticipated surgery to be infused during their hospitalization (autologous blood transfusion). **Autologous blood transfusions** also can be given with blood lost during surgery or after traumatic injury. Health care providers may suction a patient's lost blood into a canister, filter it, and then return it to the patient to allay fears that the patient may have regarding donated blood.

For religious reasons, some patients do not accept blood transfusions. In these situations, plasma expanders may be used instead of a blood transfusion.

INITIATING A BLOOD TRANSFUSION

Before a blood transfusion, a type and cross-matching test is done to match the donor's blood type with the recipient's blood type. A transfusion of incompatible blood can be fatal. Facilities require very strict identification and labeling procedures for transfusions.

Caring for a patient receiving a blood transfusion is the responsibility of the nurse (see the Coordinated Care box on blood transfusions). Before the initiation of a blood transfusion, the patient must be educated about the need for the transfusion, alternatives to transfusion, and risks of transfusions, as well as measures that are implemented to ensure a safe blood supply. Some facilities also require an informed consent to be signed; know facility policy.

Vital sign measurements are recorded before the transfusion and at regular intervals throughout and after the procedure to detect or prevent transfusion reactions. Transfusion reactions are possible at any time during or even after a blood transfusion, but they usually occur within the first 15 minutes.

The health care provider's order specifies the rate of the blood infusion. Each unit of blood should be infused within 2 to 4 hours. The risk of blood cell damage and infection increases after that time. Each facility has a specific policy regarding disposal of used blood bags or any blood remaining in the bag after 4 hours. It is essential to follow the protocol for discarding or returning the container to the blood bank whenever a unit of blood is infused.

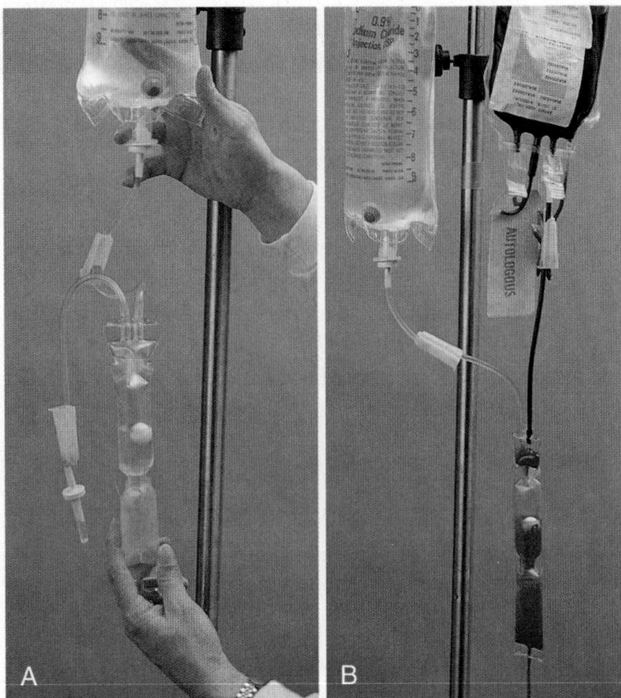

Fig. 18.13 A, Opened blood administration set and tubing primed with 0.9% normal saline. Note that the filter is filled completely with the saline. B, Attached blood product to the 0.9% normal saline. Note the clamp is closed on the saline and the clamp is opened above the filter to the blood product.

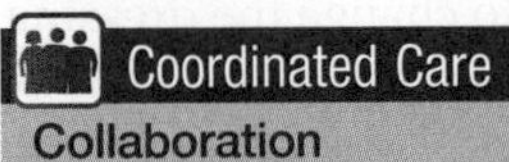

Coordinated Care

Collaboration

Blood Transfusions

- The skill of transfusing blood and blood products requires the critical thinking and knowledge of a nurse. In some states, the administration of blood and blood components is included within the scope of practice for the LPN/LVN; in some states it is not. Be aware of the scope of practice for the LPN/LVN, as well as facility policy.
- Tasks that may be delegated to an unlicensed assistive personnel (UAP) include measuring vital signs, collecting equipment, and instituting patient comfort measures. The primary responsibility for donor and recipient identification, infusing the unit within the required time, and monitoring outcomes remains with the nurse. (It is generally a registered nurse's responsibility.)

When a blood transfusion is begun, a primary IV infusion of 0.9% or 0.45% normal saline is started with a Y administration set (Fig. 18.13). An IV solution containing dextrose should not be used when blood is administered. Dextrose in the solution causes the blood to lyse or be destroyed. When the tubing is primed, the blood filter must be filled completely with saline solution. This prevents debris buildup within the filter and allows the blood to flow without interruption. The blood administration tubing then can be attached to a low port on an existing IV line, or it can be used with a resealable intermittent lock device.

Inspect the blood or blood product bag for signs of leakage or unusual appearance, including bubbles or purplish color. Report these signs immediately because they could indicate the presence of contamination, and the product should be returned to the laboratory or blood bank. After the donated blood and the patient have been properly identified, the blood is added to the appropriate section of the Y tubing, and the rate is set according to the health care provider's order. Make sure to close the roller clamp to the normal saline before opening the roller clamp to the blood. This prevents blood from backing up into the normal saline solution.

Remain with the patient for the first 15 to 20 minutes of the transfusion to monitor for reactions. The transfusion should be started slowly and vital signs monitored frequently according to facility policy. Any complaint of discomfort could indicate a possible reaction and should be addressed immediately.

At the completion of the blood transfusion, the IV tubing should be flushed with the normal saline solution. If more than one unit of blood is ordered, use fresh tubing; do not reuse tubing. This prevents blood from the separate units from mixing within the tubing and prevents clotting. Always refer to agency policy for specific instructions on tubing changes for blood products.

BLOOD TRANSFUSION REACTIONS

Infusing blood that is not compatible with the patient's blood type can lead to a transfusion reaction. A transfusion reaction can be life threatening and is considered an emergency. Therefore close monitoring is crucial to determine the patient's tolerance to the infusing blood. Patients experiencing transfusion reactions frequently say they are "not feeling right" or have a sense of impending doom. They sometimes have chills, fever, low back pain, pruritus (itching), hypotension, nausea and vomiting, decreased urine output, back pain, chest pain, wheezing, and dyspnea. If the patient is unconscious and unable to indicate symptoms, closely assess vital signs, urine output, and skin appearance. If you suspect a transfusion reaction, stop the infusion immediately. Keep the vein open with the normal saline solution, and notify the health care provider and the blood bank. Keep the remaining blood product and bag and send them to the pharmacy, the laboratory, or the blood bank (depending on facility policy) so that they can be checked for infectious agents and cross-matching problems. Also, document the incident on the appropriate "blood transfusion reaction" form, and be prepared to collect blood and urine specimens from the patient. Monitor the patient's vital signs and urine output every 15 minutes; medications to treat the presenting symptoms may be necessary. Because a transfusion reaction tends to be frightening, reassure and support the patient and family.

Although a transfusion reaction normally occurs within the first 15 minutes, it is possible at any time during or after the infusion process. There are several types of blood transfusion reactions, including hemolytic, nonhemolytic, allergic, and anaphylactic reactions. Most often these reactions occur within the first 60 to 90 minutes after the transfusion has been started and are caused by an incompatibility between the patient's blood and some component of the donated blood. Another type of transfusion reaction is the delayed reaction, which may occur days to weeks later. This type of reaction occurs in patients who have developed antibodies to the blood from a previous transfusion and results in hemolysis of the patient's blood. Circulatory overload is another complication of a blood transfusion and may be considered yet another form of a transfusion reaction. With circulatory overload, the patient is unable to handle the additional fluid from the transfusion and develops a cough, frothy sputum, and cyanosis, and the blood pressure drops. This can occur any time during and for several hours after the transfusion. To prevent this in susceptible patients, the rate of infusion should be slowed, and the patient should be monitored closely for symptoms. Box 18.16 lists further precautions in giving blood transfusions.

❖ NURSING PROCESS

The role of the LPN/LVN in the nursing process involves the following:

- Participating in planning care for patients based on patient needs
- Reviewing the patient's plan of care and recommending revisions as needed
- Reviewing and following defined prioritization for patient care
- Using clinical pathways, care maps, or care plans to guide and review patient care

◆ DATA COLLECTION

When collecting data on fluid, electrolyte, and acid-base balances, know whether the patient is at risk for imbalances, be aware of the presence of any alterations, and know the extent to which body systems are involved. Data collection helps the nurse anticipate the patient's needs for nursing interventions and helps determine the effectiveness of therapies and any adverse reactions to them.

Data collection for patients with fluid, electrolyte, or acid-base imbalances should include physical examination, including measurements of vital signs, height, and weight, as well as neurologic function; intake and output measures; results of laboratory studies; patient's past and present medical history, with notes about renal, endocrine, or respiratory disease; and a complete medication history, including over-the-counter medications and herbal supplements.

Box 18.16 Blood Transfusion Precautions

- Make sure IV catheters for blood transfusions are of appropriate size in relation to the size of the vessel.
- One unit of blood is released from the blood bank at a time. Before administration, each unit of blood and recipient information must be verified by two nurses according to facility policy.
- Completely prime blood transfusion filters with saline to prevent collection of debris in a partially primed filter. Saline reduces the viscosity of red blood cells by diluting them and thus flushes blood from the tubing (see Fig. 18.13A).
- In the event of a blood transfusion reaction, stop the blood infusion and remove the Y tubing from the main IV tubing or intermittent use device. Infuse normal saline slowly through the IV line. This prevents any more of the transfusing blood from entering the patient and keeps the vein open.
- A transfusion reaction produces a hemolytic reaction that causes red blood cells to appear in the urine. Therefore it is important that the patient voids or the catheter drainage device is emptied before the transfusion is started so that if a reaction occurs, a fresh urine sample is available to test for red blood cells.
- A registered nurse (RN) regulates the flow rate so that only 10 to 24 mL of product infuses during the first 15 minutes, and the RN remains with the patient during this time. If a reaction occurs, only a small amount of incompatible blood product will have been administered to the patient at this slow rate.
- An alteration in the vital signs from baseline values indicates the possibility that a transfusion reaction has occurred.
- An RN is required to hang the blood, but an LPN/LVN is permitted to verify type with the RN in some facilities. The RN is required to sit with the patient for the first 15 to 30 minutes of transfusion.
- If the nurse believes that a transfusion reaction is occurring, the following steps should be implemented:
  1. Stop the transfusion *immediately*.
  2. Infuse 0.9% normal saline directly into the vein with new tubing to prevent any more incompatible blood from being infused into the patient.
  3. Notify the health care provider.
  4. Monitor the patient's signs and symptoms of reaction continuously, and check vital signs every 5 minutes.
  5. Anticipate the health care provider's order of emergency drugs such as antihistamines, vasopressors, IV fluids, and steroids to counteract and treat the symptoms present.
  6. Cardiac and respiratory arrest may develop, so prepare to perform CPR if necessary.
  7. Collect a urine specimen and send it to the laboratory to check for red blood cells from a hemolytic reaction.
  8. Do not discard the blood container, the tubing, the labels, or the transfusion record. These items must be sent to the laboratory, the pharmacy, or the blood bank as outlined by agency policy for review.
  9. On the appropriate forms, document the events that occurred during the transfusion reaction.

CPR, Cardiopulmonary resuscitation; *IV*, intravenous.

◆ PATIENT PROBLEMS

It is particularly important that the registered nurse (RN) choosing patient problem statements for alterations in fluid, electrolyte, and acid-base balances be skilled in critical thinking to choose appropriate patient problem statements. Some of the following patient problem statements may be appropriate for the patient with a fluid, electrolyte, or acid-base alteration:

- *Compromised Blood Flow to Tissue*
- *Compromised Oral Mucous Membrane*
- *Compromised Tissue Integrity*
- *Fluid Volume Overload*
- *Inability to Maintain Adequate Breathing Pattern*
- *Inadequate Fluid Volume*
- *Inefficient Oxygenation*
- *Insufficient Cardiac Output*
- *Insufficient Nutrition*
- *Potential for Compromised Skin Integrity*
- *Potential for Inadequate Fluid Volume*

The data collected to establish the potential for or the actual presence of a specific patient problem in these areas are often subtle. Patterns and trends emerge only when the nurse consciously looks for them because many body systems are involved. For example, relevant data for the patient problem statement of inadequate fluid volume may include the presence of insufficient oral intake, weight loss, dry skin and mucous membranes, inelastic skin turgor, decreased blood pressure, and increased heart rate. The serum sodium level may be elevated. The urine may be dark, with an elevated specific gravity. In some cases, the volume of the urine has been decreasing over a period of days. The omission of any of these data leads the nurse to formulate an incomplete assessment of the patient's condition and perhaps result in an incorrect patient problem statement.

In addition to the accurate clustering of data, the RN must identify the related factor for the patient problem statement to plan appropriate nursing interventions. For example, for the patient problem statement of *Inadequate Fluid Volume*, the related factor is sometimes diarrhea and sometimes vomiting or difficulty swallowing. This patient problem statement is not assigned if the patient is receiving nothing by mouth (NPO) as part of the treatment regimen. If the related factor is diarrhea, administer ordered antidiarrheal medication and provide oral fluids that contain electrolytes and glucose. Teach the patient to use careful hand washing and to avoid dairy products. In contrast, if the related factor is vomiting, administer antiemetics, remove sights and odors that have the potential to induce nausea, and provide a small amount of fluids containing electrolytes. If the related factor is difficulty swallowing, attempt to ensure that the patient is fully alert; position the patient in a high Fowler's position when possible during times of intake; provide foods and fluids with a soft, pureed, or thickened consistency; provide small amounts with each mouthful; and investigate the need for enteral or total parenteral nutrition.

◆ EXPECTED OUTCOMES AND PLANNING

The first step in the planning process is setting priorities. Many patient problem statements in the areas of fluid, electrolyte, and acid-base balance represent high-priority patient problems. The consequences are potentially serious, even life threatening (e.g., seizures, dysrhythmias, or coma).

During the planning process, the LPN/LVN works with the RN to formulate nursing interventions to prevent or treat fluid, electrolyte, and acid-base imbalances. It is important to collaborate with the patient and the family during this part of the planning processes. The family is helpful in identifying the subtle changes in behavior associated with these imbalances, such as anxiety, confusion, or irritability. During the planning process, remember that the patient and the family need to know preventive measures, signs and symptoms to report, and measures that are possible to implement if an imbalance occurs. When medications, special diets, or oral or IV fluids are administered in the home, the patient and the family need careful teaching to be able to perform these interventions safely. Consider the patient's preferences and resources during each step of the planning process (e.g., if the patient needs to be encouraged to increase oral intake, determine the patient's favorite beverages and incorporate them into the plan of care). In the hospital, anticipate the needs of the patient and family for specific information, and initiate teaching before discharge so that they will be ready for these procedures. Inform the home health nurse of discharge preparations because the home health nurse will continue the teaching plan and evaluate the effectiveness of the home interventions.

The nurse also works closely with other members of the health care team, such as the health care provider, the dietitian, and the physical therapist. For example, when the nurse collects new data that suggest that the patient is developing a fluid, electrolyte, or acid-base imbalance, the nurse consults with the health care provider to determine the need for dietary, pharmacologic, IV fluid, or other therapy. The nurse's responsibilities also include ongoing monitoring of the patient's fluid, electrolyte, and acid-base status to determine the safety of implementing the health care provider's and nursing orders and any need for a change in the plan of care. For example, perhaps the health care provider orders an oral potassium supplement to be given to the patient three times each day. Before administering the first dose each day, the nurse must verify that the serum potassium level is normal and that the urine output is adequate. If the serum level is elevated or if the urine output has decreased, the dose of potassium must be withheld, and the health care provider must be consulted.

After priority setting and collaboration with the patient, family, and health care team, the nurse should assist with the development of a care plan that is individualized according to the patient's acute or chronic fluid, electrolyte, or acid-base status.

◆ GOAL

The patient's fluid, electrolyte, and acid-base balances will be restored and maintained.

◆ OUTCOMES

- The patient's vital signs will return to baseline normal.
- The patient will have normal skin turgor.
- The patient will have moist oral mucous membranes.
- The patient's weight will be stable at baseline normal.
- The patient will have no edema.
- The patient will have clear breath sounds.
- The patient's serum and urine electrolyte and chemistry results and arterial blood gas values will be within normal limits.
- The patient's urine output will equal intake.

◆ IMPLEMENTATION

Prevention of fluid, electrolyte, and acid-base imbalances is important. When imbalances occur, remove or treat the cause of the imbalance if possible. Other nursing interventions aim at correcting the imbalances.

When a patient's fluid volume is depleted, it is possible to replace fluids and electrolytes orally, with IV administration of fluids and blood components, or through total parenteral nutrition if the fluid deficit is caused by malnutrition. For patients with fluid volume excess, implement measures to reduce fluids, such as fluid intake restrictions, reduced sodium intake, and use of diuretics. When the patient has an electrolyte imbalance, provide an appropriate diet and administers supplements when they are ordered. For patients with acid-base imbalances, initiate such measures as reducing anxiety, improving pulmonary function, controlling the loss of GI content, or ensuring the control of conditions such as diabetes mellitus or renal failure.

◆ EVALUATION

Evaluate the interventions by comparing the patient's responses to the expected outcomes of the established goals. Be prepared to revise the plan of care based on the evaluation findings.

◆ GOAL

Patient's fluid and electrolyte balances will be restored and maintained.

◆ EVALUATIVE MEASURES

- Obtain daily weight and monitor.
- Obtain patient's vital signs.
- Measure all routes of intake and output.
- Auscultate for adventitious lung sounds.
- Check oral mucous membranes for dryness or moistness.
- Check tissue turgor for tenting or edema.
- Monitor serum electrolyte levels.

The patient's status and the effectiveness of the nursing care must be evaluated continuously, and the care plan must be modified as needed. If any of the measures identified have not been effective, it is important to collaborate with other health care team members to determine the changes needed to improve the patient's status.

Get Ready for the NCLEX® Examination!

Key Points

- Water is the primary fluid in the body.
- The two fluid compartments in the body are the intracellular and extracellular compartments. The extracellular compartment includes the interstitial and intravascular areas.
- Homeostasis must be maintained to maintain health.
- Fluid movement takes place by means of three passive transport systems—diffusion, osmosis, and filtration—and one active transport system, in which ATP is used for energy.
- Electrolytes are chemical compounds that carry either a positive or negative charge. Positive ions are called *cations;* negative ions are called *anions.* To maintain homeostasis, it is necessary for the cations and the anions to balance each other in the body fluids.
- Sodium is the major extracellular cation in the body. Water follows sodium as it moves from one fluid compartment to another.
- Potassium is the major intracellular cation in the body. Imbalances in potassium, either high or low levels, have the potential to cause life-threatening cardiac conditions.
- Arterial blood has a normal pH range of 7.35 to 7.45. A pH lower than 7.35 is considered abnormally acidic; a pH higher than 7.45 is considered abnormally alkaline. A pH lower than 6.8 or higher than 7.8 can be fatal.
- The four types of acid-base imbalance are respiratory acidosis, respiratory alkalosis, metabolic acidosis, and metabolic alkalosis.
- Any process that interferes with normal ventilation and causes a decrease or an increase in the excretion of acids in the body poses the risk of causing respiratory acidosis or respiratory alkalosis.
- Any process that interferes with normal production or excretion of hydrogen ions poses the risk of causing metabolic acidosis or metabolic alkalosis.
- Respiratory acidosis or alkalosis results when the lungs fail to regulate the carbonic acid concentration in the blood. Metabolic acidosis or alkalosis results when the kidneys fail to regulate the bicarbonate concentration in the blood.
- If the lungs are unable to correct respiratory acidosis, the kidneys respond to correct the imbalance. If the kidneys are unable to correct metabolic acidosis, the lungs respond to correct the imbalance.
- The nurse practice act of each state legally defines the nurse's qualification for and scope of practice in administering parenteral therapy and inserting nasogastric tubes.
- Any nurse administering IV therapies must have knowledge of the complications that can occur during therapy and of the nursing interventions associated with these complications.
- IV therapy poses the risk of infiltration, phlebitis, infection at the IV site or systemic infection, fluid volume excess, and bleeding at the IV site.
- By following strict guidelines when administering blood or blood products and by being aware of the symptoms of transfusion reactions, the nurse can identify more quickly a reaction to a transfusion.

Additional Learning Resources

SG Go to your Study Guide for additional learning activities to help you master this chapter content.

evolve Be sure to visit the Evolve site at *http://evolve.elsevier.com/Cooper/foundationsadult/* for additional online resources.

Review Questions for the NCLEX® Examination

1. A 66-year-old patient has recently been experiencing excessive edema in his feet. The nurse discusses with the patient the dietary changes that may be causing the water retention in association with the patient's edema. Which electrolyte has the greatest influence on water balance in the body?
   1. Sodium (Na^+)
   2. Potassium (K^+)
   3. Chloride (Cl^-)
   4. Calcium (Ca^{2+})
2. Which regulatory system is the body's second line of defense in keeping the pH within normal limits?
   1. Blood buffers
   2. Respiratory system
   3. Renal system
   4. Blood pressure

3. A patient is concerned about giving her family adequate amounts of potassium in their diet. She asks the nurse to help plan a meal containing foods with potassium. Which dietary selections contain foods with the most potassium?
   1. Baked chicken, green salad, and fresh fruit plate
   2. Macaroni and cheese, cornbread, and gelatin
   3. Tacos, chips and salsa, and ice cream
   4. Seafood plate, marinated vegetables, cake
4. What is the primary major route of excretion of sodium by the body?
   1. Via the skin
   2. Via the lungs
   3. Via the kidneys
   4. Via the feces
5. The movement of water from an area of lower concentration to an area of higher concentration occurs through which of the following?
   1. Diffusion
   2. Filtration
   3. Active transport
   4. Osmosis
6. What is the largest fluid compartment in the body?
   1. Intracellular
   2. Extracellular
   3. Interstitial
   4. Intravascular
7. Passive transport includes what physiologic processes? *(Select all that apply.)*
   1. Osmosis
   2. Diffusion
   3. Filtration
   4. Sodium-potassium pump
   5. Compensatory metabolic acidosis
8. Which abbreviation is used to indicate hydrogen ion concentration in the body?
   1. mEq
   2. ATP
   3. pH
   4. mL
9. Potential causes of hypocalcemia may include which conditions? *(Select all that apply.)*
   1. Vitamin D deficiency
   2. Diuretic use
   3. Injury of the thyroid gland
   4. Severe burns
   5. Renal failure
10. The nurse is reviewing the daily weight recordings of an assigned patient who is receiving diuretic therapy. The nurse notes a weight decrease of 2 kg (4.4 lb). This will be reflected by a loss or gain of _______ body fluid.
11. When the body senses hypoxemia or hypercapnia, the chemoreceptors in the medulla of the brainstem will have what response?
    1. Slowing the respiratory rate
    2. Decreasing the heart rate
    3. Increasing the depth and rate of respirations
    4. Lowering the blood pressure
12. The nurse is caring for a patient with severe hyperkalemia. What actions should be included in the plan of care for the shift? *(Select all that apply.)*
    1. Monitor serum potassium levels.
    2. Administer Kayexalate as prescribed by the health care provider.
    3. Report a urinary output less than 30 mL/h.
    4. Monitor vital signs every 12 hours.
    5. Restrict fluid intake.
13. In acute respiratory acidosis, the renal compensatory mechanisms begin to operate within how many hours?
    1. 6
    2. 12
    3. 24
    4. 48
14. Normal daily water intake and output (I&O) is approximately how many milliliters?
    1. 1500
    2. 2500
    3. 3500
    4. 6500
15. How many milliliters of urine per hour must the kidneys secrete to eliminate waste products from the body?
    1. 30
    2. 60
    3. 20
    4. 100
16. The normal pH of blood is approximately _______.
17. Which statement best describes the risk of fluid and electrolyte imbalances in the older adult?
    1. Most older adults can maintain fluid and electrolyte balance just as well as younger adults.
    2. Older adults have unlimited reserves to maintain fluid balance when abnormal losses occur.
    3. Body water increases with age, which puts the older adult at risk for fluid volume excess.
    4. Physiologic changes in the skin and mucous membranes decrease their reliability as indicators of dehydration.
18. The nurse is assigned a patient with a potassium imbalance. What assessment is most critical for this patient?
    1. Auscultate bowel sounds.
    2. Evaluate muscle strength.
    3. Monitor heart rate and rhythm.
    4. Assess reflexes.
19. The patient's potassium level is 5.2. When the nurse discusses dietary selections, the patient should be instructed to limit intake of what food items? *(Select all that apply.)*
    1. Orange juice
    2. Bananas
    3. Apples
    4. Tomatoes
    5. Red meat
20. Fluid balance is maintained in the body by which of the following systems? *(Select all that apply.)*
    1. Cardiac
    2. Respiratory
    3. Renal
    4. Hepatic
    5. Immune

21. A central line is preferred over a peripheral IV line under which conditions? *(Select all that apply.)*
1. When irritating IV fluids are given
2. In an infant
3. When short-term IV therapy is required
4. When the patient has poor peripheral veins
5. When the patient is to receive chemotherapy

22. The nurse is assisting to prepare a nursing care plan for a patient with continuous IV infusions. What is the goal of IV therapy?
1. Promote and maintain fluid and electrolyte balance.
2. Promote drug blood levels when the patient is able to take liquid medication by mouth.
3. Promote oxygen and carbon dioxide homeostasis.
4. Balance plasma acidity levels.

23. The nurse is checking IV sites carefully for signs of infiltration. Which symptoms indicate infiltration at the IV site?
1. Burning sensation, pain, and puffiness at the site
2. Pain, heat, and puffiness at the site
3. Burning sensation and numbness at the site
4. Red streak up the arm

24. The nurse is assessing the IV site. If redness, swelling, and warmth are noted, what is likely indicated?
1. Infiltration and air embolus
2. Inflammation and possible phlebitis
3. Blood loss and hemorrhage
4. Embolus from the former catheter

25. An older adult patient is evaluated by the nurse for signs of fluid volume excess in association with IV therapy. Which symptom would indicate fluid volume excess in an elderly patient?
1. Redness, warmth, and drainage of fluid at the IV site
2. Decreased pulse and low urine output
3. Complaints of shortness of breath and bounding pulse
4. Puffiness of face, dyspnea, and decreased blood pressure

26. A patient's IV has infiltrated. When selecting a site for a new IV line, the nurse should perform which of the following?
1. Choose an area proximal to the current site.
2. Look for hard, cordlike veins.
3. Use sites distal from the current site.
4. Select the patient's dominant arm.

27. A patient complains of a headache, nausea, and vomiting during a blood transfusion. Which action is necessary for the nurse to take immediately?
1. Check the vital signs.
2. Stop the blood transfusion.
3. Slow down the rate of blood flow.
4. Notify the health care provider and the blood bank personnel.
5. Flush the IV line with normal saline.

28. Which nursing intervention is the most important in preventing the introduction of microorganisms to the patient when an IV infusion is initiated?
1. Hand hygiene
2. Checking the identification of the patient
3. Ensuring the six rights of medication administration
4. Carefully checking the order for the correct IV solution

29. The nurse demonstrates knowledge by choosing which needle gauge when starting a rapid transfusion of whole blood?
1. 14- to 16-gauge
2. 18- to 22-gauge
3. 22- to 24-gauge
4. 26- to 28-gauge

30. It has been 15 minutes since a blood infusion was initiated. What is most indicative that the patient is experiencing a blood transfusion reaction?
1. The patient's blood pressure decreases.
2. The patient feels an urgent need to void.
3. The patient's skin is pale at the infusion site.
4. Localized edema is noticed at the infusion site.

Nutritional Concepts and Related Therapies

19

http://evolve.elsevier.com/Cooper/foundationsadult/

Objectives

1. Discuss the role of the nurse in promoting good nutrition.
2. Explain the use of diet planning guides in medical nutrition therapy.
3. List the six classes of essential nutrients, and identify those that provide energy.
4. List the functions and food sources of protein, carbohydrates, and fats.
5. List food sources and possible health benefits of dietary fiber.
6. Distinguish between saturated, unsaturated, and *trans* fats and cholesterol; identify current recommendations for dietary intake of fats and cholesterol.
7. Discuss key vitamins and minerals, their role in health, and their food sources.
8. Discuss changes in nutrient needs throughout the life cycle, and suggest ideas to ensure adequate nutrition during each stage of life.
9. Identify the effects of common medications on nutritional status.
10. Identify standard hospital diets and modifications for texture, consistency, and meal frequency.
11. List medical and surgical conditions that require a high-kilocalorie and high-protein diet, and suggest ways to increase kilocalories and protein in the diet.
12. Define obesity, and list components of an effective weight management program.
13. Describe dietary management of type 1 and type 2 diabetes mellitus.
14. Describe fat-modified diets and list conditions requiring a fat-modified diet.
15. Identify medical and surgical conditions necessitating modifications in sodium, potassium, protein, or fluid intake, and describe the dietary adjustments necessary in these conditions.
16. Define enteral nutrition and parenteral nutrition, and list medical and surgical conditions in which nutritional support is often indicated.

Key Terms

amino acids (ă-MĒ-nō ĂS-ĭdz, p. 531)
anabolism (ă-NĂB-ŏ-lĭzm, p. 531)
basal metabolic rate (BMR) (BĀ-săl mĕt-ă-BŎL-ĭk rāt, p. 548)
body mass index (BMI) (BŎD-ē MĂS ĬN-dĕks, p. 548)
catabolism (kă-TĂB-ŏ-lĭsm, p. 531)
cholesterol (kŏ-LĔS-tŭr-ŏl, p. 530)
dietary fiber (DĪ-ĕ-tăr-ē FĪ-bŭr, p. 528)
dumping syndrome (DŬMP-ĭng SĬN-drōm, p. 552)
enteral nutrition (ĔN-tŭr-ăl nū-TRĬ-shŭn, p. 557)
essential nutrients (ē-SĔN-chŭl NŪ-trē-ŭnts, p. 526)
glycogen (GLĪ-kŏ-jĕn, p. 528)
hydrogenation (hī-drŏ-jĕn-Ā-shŭn, p. 529)
kilocalorie (kcal) (kĭl-ō-KĂL-ō-rē, p. 526)
lipids (LĬ-pĭdz, p. 529)
lipoproteins (lī-pō-PRŌ-tēnz, p. 530)
medical nutrition therapy (MĔD-ĭ-kŭl nū-TRĬSH-ŭn THĔR-ŭ-pē, p. 546)
nitrogen balance (NĪ-trŭ-jŭn BĂL-ŭns, p. 531)
nutrient (NŪ-trē-ŭnt, p. 526)
nutrient-dense foods (NŪ-trē-ŭnt–DĔNS FŪDZ, p. 540)
obesity (ō-BĒ-sĭt-ē, p. 548)
parenteral nutrition (pă-RĔN-tŭr-ăl nū-TRĬSH-ŭn, p. 565)
pernicious anemia (pŭr-NĬSH-ŭs ă-NĒ-mē-ă, p. 535)
residue (RĔZ-ĭ-dū, p. 547)
satiety (să-TĪ-ĕ-tē, p. 529)
therapeutic diet (thĕr-ŭ-PYŪ-tĭk DĪ-ĭt, p. 546)
total parenteral nutrition (TPN) (TŌ-tŭl pă-RĔN-tŭr-ăl nū-TRĬSH-ŭn, p. 565)
tube feeding (TŪB FĒD-ĭng, p. 557)
vegan (VĒ-găn, p. 531)

Nutrition is the sum of all processes involved in taking in nutrients and using them to maintain body tissue and provide energy. It is one of the foundations for life. Over the past century, tremendous progress has been made to improve the general level of health in all people, and health care providers have come to realize that good nutrition is essential for optimal health throughout all stages of life. Eating the right kinds and amounts of food and following good dietary habits throughout the entire life means a healthier body and mind, greater vitality and energy, and greater resistance to disease. Nurses must always consider the patient's nutritional state and evaluate the patient's nutritional history to plan quality patient care.

ROLE OF THE NURSE IN PROMOTING NUTRITION

Because the nurse spends a considerable amount of time caring for patients, patients look to the nurse as a source of health information. The licensed practical nurse (LPN/LVN) may be responsible for assisting a patient to eat, for recording a patient's intake, for observing a patient for signs of poor nutrition, and for communicating any dietary concerns to the health care provider, dietitian, or other members of the health care team. Therefore nurses must have a basic knowledge of nutrition and help patients understand the importance of their diets to encourage compliance.

BASIC NUTRITION

DIET PLANNING GUIDES

To help people maintain optimal nutrition, most of the developed countries of the world have adopted nutrition standards. These standards are guidelines describing how good dietary habits can promote health and reduce the risk for major chronic diseases.

Over the years, these nutritional guidelines have changed in accordance with the growing knowledge of how nutrition affects health. The guidelines started as a farmers' bulletin more than 100 years ago and then evolved to the Basic 7, the Basic Four, the Food Guide Pyramid, MyPyramid, and currently MyPlate.

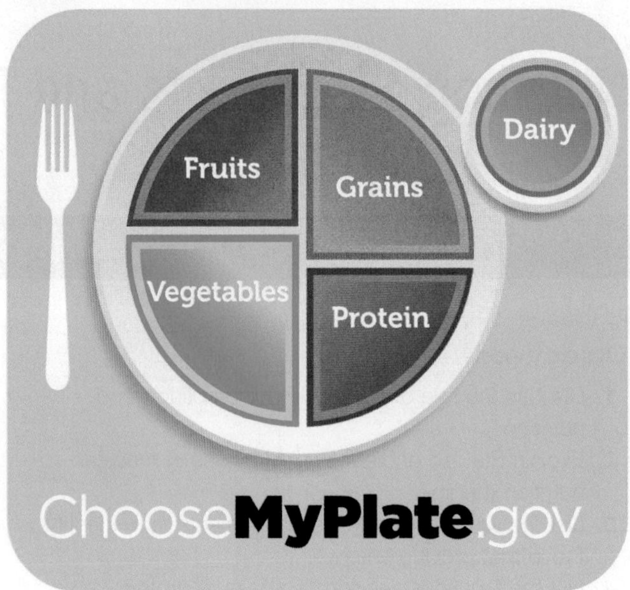

Fig. 19.1 MyPlate. (From the US Department of Agriculture, *www.ChooseMyPlate.gov*.)

MyPlate

MyPlate (Fig. 19.1) was developed in the United States by the US Department of Agriculture (USDA) and introduced in 2011. MyPlate is an image of a round plate divided into four different color sections. The colored areas show people how much they should eat from three of the four food groups: vegetables and fruits, grains, and proteins. A smaller circle next to the plate represents the fourth food group, dairy. Along with the image, the USDA suggests that people balance calories by reducing portions; increase intake of fruits, vegetables, and whole grains; and reduce the amount of sodium and sugary foods in the diet.

By developing this simple, visually graphic image and combining it with a few easy rules, the USDA hoped to eliminate the confusion that existed with previous guidelines and help people make better food choices (Box 19.1).

Dietary Guidelines for Americans

The US Department of Health and Human Services and the USDA have developed dietary guidelines for the US population. The *Dietary Guidelines for Americans 2015–2020* (USDHHS and USDA, 2015) is the most current of these guidelines; it focuses on healthy eating patterns as a whole rather than on individual nutrients or foods. The recommendations are intended to help people choose an overall healthy diet. These guidelines emphasize balancing calories with activity to manage weight; consuming a variety of fruits, vegetables, and whole grains; increasing fat-free or low-fat dairy products, lean meats and seafood; and consuming less sodium, saturated fat, *trans* fat, cholesterol, added sugars, and refined grains.

The *Dietary Guidelines for Americans 2015–2020* (USDHHS and USDA, 2015) is used to form the US federal nutrition policy and directly affects federal nutrition programs such as food stamps, school breakfast and lunch programs, and the Special Supplemental Nutrition Program for Women, Infants, and Children (WIC).

The government developed these guidelines to address the importance of adequate nutrition, as well as the prevention of overnutrition and chronic disease. They are intended for healthy children (aged 2 years and older) and adults of any age (Box 19.2).

Dietary Reference Intakes

Dietary reference intake (DRI) refers to a set of nutrient-based values for evaluating and planning diets. The DRIs replace and expand on the recommended dietary allowances (RDAs), which have been used for more than 50 years in the United States. The DRIs are a combination of the RDAs, adequate intake, tolerable upper intake level, and the estimated average requirement of each nutrient. The purpose of DRIs is to help individuals optimize their health, prevent disease, and avoid consuming too much of a nutrient. For more information

Box 19.1 Choose MyPlate: 10 Tips to a Great Plate

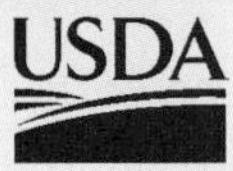

United States Department of Agriculture

10 tips Nutrition Education Series

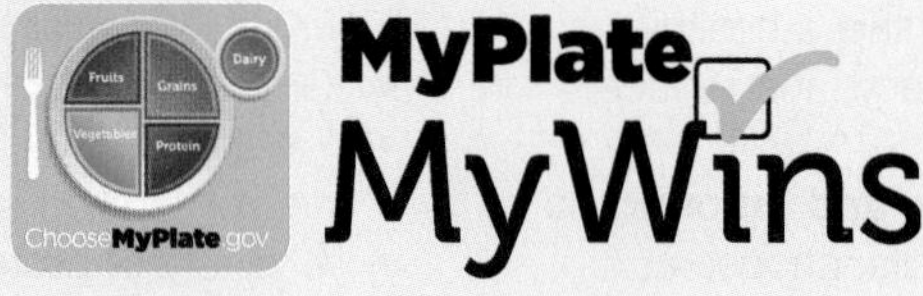

Based on the Dietary Guidelines for Americans

Build a healthy meal

Each meal is a building block in your healthy eating style. Make sure to include all the food groups throughout the day. Make fruits, vegetables, grains, dairy, and protein foods part of your daily meals and snacks. Also, limit added sugars, saturated fat, and sodium. Use the MyPlate Daily Checklist and the tips below to meet your needs throughout the day.

1 Make half your plate veggies and fruits
Vegetables and fruits are full of nutrients that support good health. Choose fruits and red, orange, and dark-green vegetables such as tomatoes, sweet potatoes, and broccoli.

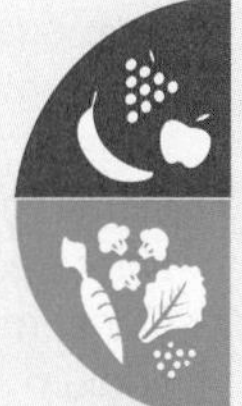

2 Include whole grains
Aim to make at least half your grains whole grains. Look for the words "100% whole grain" or "100% whole wheat" on the food label. Whole grains provide more nutrients, like fiber, than refined grains.

3 Don't forget the dairy
Complete your meal with a cup of fat-free or low-fat milk. You will get the same amount of calcium and other essential nutrients as whole milk but fewer calories. Don't drink milk? Try a soy beverage (soymilk) as your drink or include low-fat yogurt in your meal or snack.

4 Add lean protein
Choose protein foods such as lean beef, pork, chicken, or turkey, and eggs, nuts, beans, or tofu. Twice a week, make seafood the protein on your plate.

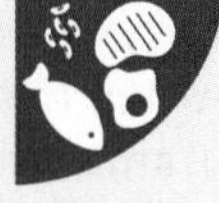

5 Avoid extra fat
Using heavy gravies or sauces will add fat and calories to otherwise healthy choices. Try steamed broccoli with a sprinkling of low-fat parmesan cheese or a squeeze of lemon.

6 Get creative in the kitchen
Whether you are making a sandwich, a stir-fry, or a casserole, find ways to make them healthier. Try using less meat and cheese, which can be higher in saturated fat and sodium, and adding in more veggies that add new flavors and textures to your meals.

7 Take control of your food
Eat at home more often so you know exactly what you are eating. If you eat out, check and compare the nutrition information. Choose options that are lower in calories, saturated fat, and sodium.

8 Try new foods
Keep it interesting by picking out new foods you've never tried before, like mango, lentils, quinoa, kale, or sardines. You may find a new favorite! Trade fun and tasty recipes with friends or find them online.

9 Satisfy your sweet tooth in a healthy way
Indulge in a naturally sweet dessert dish—fruit! Serve a fresh fruit salad or a fruit parfait made with yogurt. For a hot dessert, bake apples and top with cinnamon.

10 Everything you eat and drink matters
The right mix of foods in your meals and snacks can help you be healthier now and into the future. Turn small changes in how you eat into your MyPlate, MyWins.

Center for Nutrition Policy and Promotion
USDA is an equal opportunity provider, employer, and lender.

Go to ChooseMyPlate.gov for more information.

DG TipSheet No. 7
June 2011
Revised October 2016

From USDA: MyPlate. Retrieved from *www.choosemyplate.gov/food-groups/downloads/TenTips/DGTipsheet1ChooseMyPlate.pdf*.

Box 19.2 2015–2020 Dietary Guidelines for Americans

THE GUIDELINES

1. **Follow a healthy eating pattern across the lifespan.** All food and beverage choices matter. Choose a healthy eating pattern at an appropriate calorie level to help achieve and maintain a healthy body weight, support nutrient adequacy, and reduce the risk of chronic disease.
2. **Focus on variety, nutrient density, and amount.** To meet nutrient needs within calorie limits, choose a variety of nutrient-dense foods across and within all food groups in recommended amounts.
3. **Limit calories from added sugars and saturated fats and reduce sodium intake.** Consume an eating pattern low in added sugars, saturated fats, and sodium. Cut back on foods and beverages higher in these components to amounts that fit within healthy eating patterns.
4. **Shift to healthier food and beverage choices.** Choose nutrient-dense foods and beverages across and within all food groups in place of less healthy choices. Consider cultural and personal preferences to make these shifts easier to accomplish and maintain.
5. **Support healthy eating patterns for all.** Everyone has a role in helping to create and support healthy eating patterns in multiple settings nationwide, from home to school to work to communities.

KEY RECOMMENDATIONS

Consume a healthy eating pattern that accounts for all foods and beverages within an appropriate calorie level.

A healthy eating pattern includes:

- A variety of vegetables from all of the subgroups—dark green, red and orange, legumes (beans and peas), starchy, and other
- Fruits, especially whole fruits
- Grains, at least half of which are whole grains
- Fat-free or low-fat dairy, including milk, yogurt, cheese, and/or fortified soy beverages
- A variety of protein foods, including seafood, lean meats and poultry, eggs, legumes (beans and peas), and nuts, seeds, and soy products
- Oils

A healthy eating pattern limits:

- Saturated fats and *trans* fats, added sugars, and sodium

Key recommendations that are quantitative are provided for several components of the diet that should be limited. These components are of particular public health concern in the United States, and the specified limits can help individuals achieve healthy eating patterns within calorie limits:

- Consume less than 10% of calories per day from added sugars
- Consume less than 10% of calories per day from saturated fats
- Consume less than 2300 milligrams (mg) per day of sodium
- If alcohol is consumed, it should be consumed in moderation—up to one drink per day for women and up to two drinks per day for men—and only by adults of legal drinking age.

on DRIs and *Dietary Guidelines for Americans,* visit the USDA website at *www.nutrition.gov/smart-nutrition-101.*

Nutrition Facts Label

Because of heightened awareness of nutrition, Americans are learning to pick healthier foods and are demanding that more healthy foods be made available in restaurants. To assist with this, the FDA has mandated that Nutrition Facts labels be included on all packaged foods and that restaurants make this information available to their patrons.

The FDA currently requires that the product's ingredients be listed on the label in descending order by weight. That means that there is more of the first ingredient listed on the label, based on weight, and the rest of the ingredients listed are less prevalent in the product.

The label (see Fig. 19.3) currently also must list calories from fat, total amount of fat, saturated fat, *trans* fats, and cholesterol. It also must include the amount of proteins, carbohydrates, sodium, vitamins A and C, calcium, and iron.

In May 2016 the FDA finalized a new Nutrition Facts label for packaged foods. This new label simplifies making informed food choices that support a healthy diet. The updated label has a new design and reflects current scientific information, including the link between diet and chronic diseases (see Fig. 19.3).

ESSENTIAL NUTRIENTS

Basic Functions

A **nutrient** is a chemical compound or element necessary for good health that is found in food. **Essential nutrients** are nutrients that the body cannot make in the amounts essential for good health; therefore it is necessary to obtain these nutrients through the diet or from other sources. There are six classes of essential nutrients: carbohydrates, fats, proteins, vitamins, minerals, and water. Each is necessary for life. Three major functions of nutrients include (1) providing energy, (2) building and repairing tissue, and (3) regulating body processes.

Providing energy. A **kilocalorie (kcal)** is a measurement of energy, much as a pound is a measurement of weight. If a certain food has X number of kilocalories, it provides that amount of energy. The more kilocalories a food has, the more energy it provides. Of the six essential nutrients, three provide energy: carbohydrates, fats, and proteins. Vitamins, minerals, and water do not provide energy but are nonetheless essential nutrients. Carbohydrates and protein provide approximately 4 kcal/g, whereas fat provides 9 kcal/g. Nutrition experts recommend obtaining about 45% to 65% of daily kilocalories from carbohydrates, 20% to 35% from fat, and 10% to 35% from protein. This distribution is called the *caloric distribution* of the diet.

Building and repairing tissue. Many nutrients are necessary for building and repairing tissue, but the nutrient that plays the biggest role is protein. It contains the amino acids that the body uses to build and repair tissue. Calcium and phosphorus, both minerals, are necessary nutrients in bone structure, and iron, another mineral, makes up a large part of the hemoglobin in red blood cells. Fat also plays a role in building and repairing tissues; it is found in all cell walls.

Regulating body processes. *Metabolism* is the combination of all chemical processes that take place in living organisms. It is a continuous process of building and breaking down tissues. Nutrients play various roles in metabolism and thereby help regulate certain body processes. For example, the presence of carbohydrates is required for fat to be used correctly and completely. The B vitamins are necessary for the body to derive energy from foods. Water is an integral part of almost all chemical reactions in the body. By studying how the body uses nutrients, researchers have found out two important facts: (1) individual nutrients have many functions in the body, and (2) no nutrient works alone.

Table 19.1 Summary of Carbohydrate Classification

CHEMICAL CLASS	CLASS MEMBERS	DIETARY SOURCES
Simple Carbohydrate		
Monosaccharides	Glucose	Dextrose, corn syrup
	Fructose	Fruits, honey, high-fructose corn syrup
	Galactose	Milk (only found in lactose)
Disaccharides	Sucrose	Table sugar, sugarcane, beet sugar, powdered and brown sugar, fruits
	Lactose	Milk
	Maltose	Malted grain products
Complex Carbohydrate		
Polysaccharides	Starch	Grains and grain products (e.g., cereals, breads, crackers, pasta, rice, legumes, corn, potatoes, vegetables)
	Glycogen	No significant dietary source (storage form of carbohydrate in animal tissue)
	Dietary fiber	Whole grains, legumes, fruits, vegetables, nuts, seeds

Carbohydrates

Carbohydrates (CHO) are organic compounds containing carbon, hydrogen, and oxygen. The main function of carbohydrates is to provide energy. However, they also are needed in adequate amounts to keep protein from being used as an energy source. Carbohydrates are classified as either simple or complex according to the number of sugar units they contain (Table 19.1).

Simple carbohydrates. Carbohydrates are made of molecular units called *saccharides*, or sugar units. The simple carbohydrates (often called *simple sugars*) include the monosaccharides and the disaccharides. Monosaccharides have only one sugar unit. They require no digestion and are absorbed directly into the blood. Fructose, the sugar found naturally in fruits, is a monosaccharide. Another important monosaccharide is glucose. Glucose often is called "blood glucose" because it is the major form of saccharides, or sugar, in the blood.

Disaccharides are made up of two sugar units bonded together. Once taken into the body, disaccharides are reduced by hydrolysis into monosaccharides before being absorbed. Table sugar (sucrose) and the sugar found naturally in milk (lactose) are examples of disaccharides (see Table 19.1).

Simple carbohydrates are part of a healthy diet. However, in the United States, refined sugar consumption is high and is contributing to an increase in obesity. Table sugar and sweeteners such as honey and corn syrup are high in kilocalories, have low nutritive value, and contribute to dental caries (cavities). DRIs relating to carbohydrates indicate that 45% to 65% of an adult's total calorie intake should be in the form of carbohydrates and that added sugars should be limited to no more than 8% (approximately 40 g) of the total number of calories consumed daily. Simple sugars are found naturally in many nutritious foods such as milk and fruit and should not be excluded from the diet. Encourage people to use moderation in their consumption of added sugars, sweets, and soft drinks.

Complex carbohydrates. Complex carbohydrates are termed *polysaccharides* because they are made of long chains of glucose (sugar) units. The three types of complex carbohydrates, or polysaccharides, include starch, glycogen, and dietary fiber. Starch is found in many plant foods such as grains, legumes, and vegetables, particularly starchy vegetables such as corn and potatoes. It also is found in small amounts in some fruits. All carbohydrates, including complex carbohydrates, break down into simple sugars when they are digested, but because starch is a larger, more complex molecule, it breaks down more slowly and provides energy over a longer period.

Glycogen, also called *animal starch,* is the stored form of carbohydrates. It is made from simple sugars and stored mainly in the liver and in muscles. It is used when the body's blood glucose level is low.

Dietary fiber refers to foods that humans cannot break down (digest). It is found mostly in plants and, like polysaccharides, is made of long chains of glucose units. Most of the fiber consumed eventually is excreted in the feces and has no nutritive value. Fiber does provide roughage, or bulk, which is important for health maintenance. It can lower cholesterol and blood glucose levels and assist in weight loss. Dietary fiber is classified based on its ability to dissolve in water. Both types of fiber, soluble and insoluble, provide a variety of health benefits and should be included in a healthy diet.

Insoluble fiber is found in wheat bran, vegetables, whole grains, and some fibrous fruits. Insoluble fiber softens stools, speeds transit of foods through the digestive tract, and reduces pressure in the colon. Thus it may help relieve constipation and reduce the risk of certain gastrointestinal (GI) disorders such as diverticulosis or hemorrhoids.

Water-soluble fiber is found in fruits, oats, barley, and legumes. It binds with bile acids and cholesterol in the digestive tract to prevent their absorption. This helps lower cholesterol levels and reduces the risk of cardiovascular disease. *Soluble fiber* attracts water and turns to gel during digestion, thus slowing digestion. This provides a feeling of fullness and may aid in weight loss (Fig. 19.2).

Daily requirements. Many health organizations have recommended increasing the intake of complex carbohydrates and dietary fiber. Current DRI recommendations are that 45% to 65% of total calories should come from carbohydrates. Fiber intake should be between 25 and 38 g/day, depending on age and gender. The *Dietary Guidelines for Americans* (USDHHS and USDA, 2015) and the MyPlate guide recommend increasing fruit and vegetable intake and consuming at least half of all grains as whole grains, not refined grains. Health care providers should encourage patients to choose carbohydrates and fiber closer to the whole state rather than in a refined or processed state to increase the nutritive value of the diet.

Although eating enough fiber is important in a healthy diet, there may be hazards to consuming too much fiber. Sudden increases in fiber can cause bloating, gas, and constipation. This can be avoided by slowly increasing fiber content in the diet and by adding at least 8 glasses of water a day. In addition, too much fiber can interfere with mineral absorption, which can lead to problems such as osteoporosis and anemia. It is suggested that adequate fiber be obtained by eating appropriate amounts of fruits and vegetables rather than adding fiber supplements. For more specific information concerning the fiber content of selected foods, check the Nutrition Facts label of that food (Fig. 19.3).

Digestion and metabolism of carbohydrates. Digestion of carbohydrates begins in the mouth with mechanical digestion. Chewing breaks up the food (carbohydrates) into small pieces so that it can be swallowed. In the stomach, mechanical digestion continues so that the pieces are broken down into even smaller parts and combined with gastric secretions. Once the pieces are in the small intestine, chemical digestion begins in full force. Enzymes from the intestinal wall and the pancreas aid in digesting the carbohydrates.

All carbohydrates except fiber are broken down in the digestive tract into monosaccharides (single-sugar

Soluble Fiber	Insoluble Fiber
Oat bran, barley, nuts, seeds, citrus, apples, strawberries, and many vegetables	Whole wheat and grains, vegetables and wheat bran

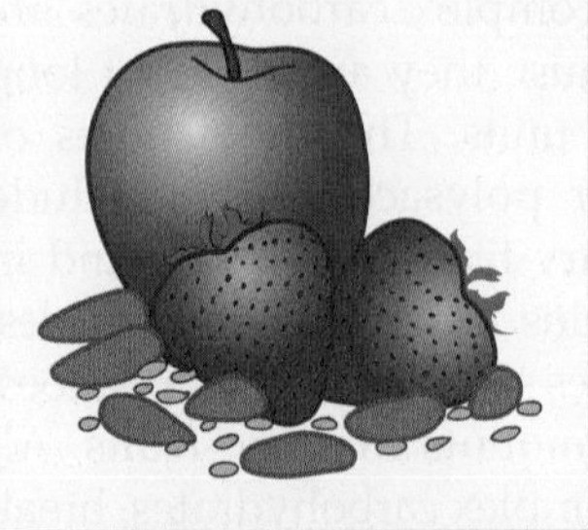

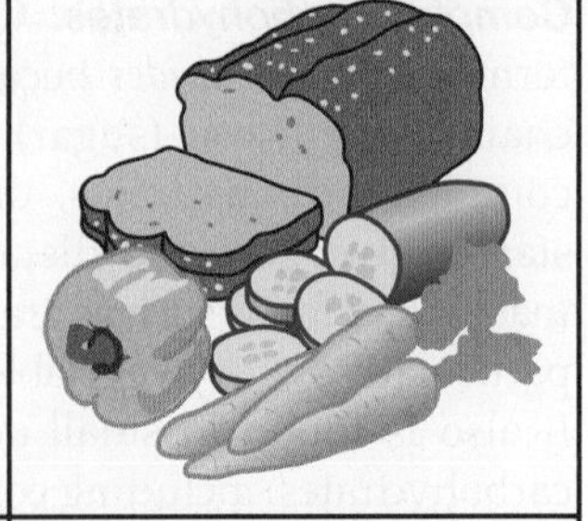

Fig. 19.2 Examples of sources of soluble and insoluble fiber.

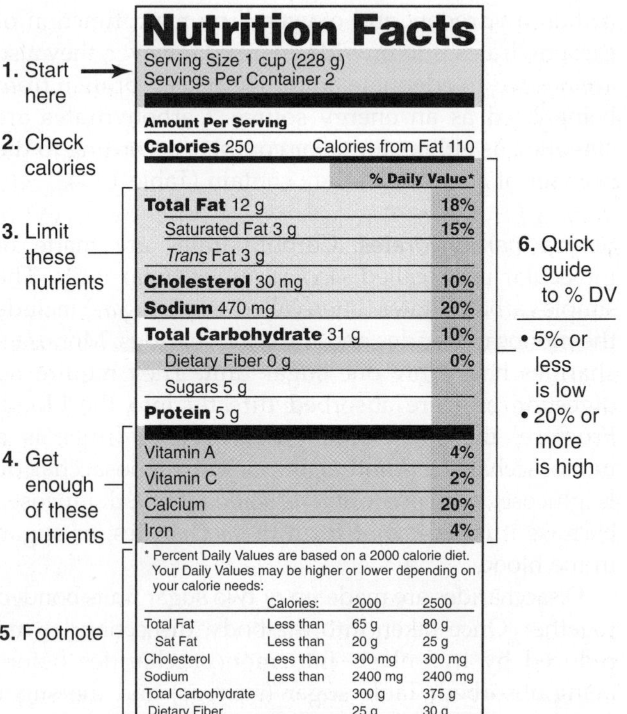

Fig. 19.3 Example of Nutrition Facts label. The food label provides a variety of information. Using the numbers listed provided a means to review and understand the information listed. (From https://www.fda.gov/Food/GuidanceRegulation/GuidanceDocumentsRegulatoryInformation/LabelingNutrition/ucm385663.htm.)

units) before they are absorbed and eventually converted to glucose. Glucose circulates in the bloodstream and is used by the cells for energy.

When the body's energy needs are met, the extra carbohydrates are converted to glycogen, which is stored in the liver and muscles until it is needed. Once glycogen stores in the liver and muscles are full, the body converts the remaining carbohydrates to fat and stores them as adipose tissue.

Fats (Lipids)

Lipids are organic substances of a fatty nature that are insoluble in water and necessary for good health. Fats and cholesterol are lipids.

Lipids perform many functions in the body. They provide the most concentrated source of energy of all the nutrients (9 kcal/g) and can be used either directly from the fat in foods or from adipose tissue, the body's stored form of fat. As *adipose tissue,* fat helps insulate the body from temperature extremes and acts as a cushion to protect organs and other tissues from being bumped or jarred. Fat is also a component of all cell membranes.

Dietary fat provides **satiety,** a feeling of fullness and satisfaction from food. It adds flavor and aroma to foods and provides the body with the essential fatty acids linoleic acid and linolenic acid. Dietary fat also carries the fat-soluble vitamins: A, D, E, and K.

Like carbohydrates, lipids are composed of carbon, hydrogen, and oxygen. Unlike carbohydrates, lipids contain fatty acids and glycerol. Because of this, lipids also may be called *glycerides* or, more specifically, *triglycerides* because most of the fat in the body is a combination of three fatty acids that combine with one glycerol unit.

Fatty acids, the building blocks of fat, are classified as either saturated or unsaturated. All fats and oils contain a combination of saturated and unsaturated fatty acids in various proportions.

Saturated fatty acids. A saturated fatty acid is one whose chemical bonds are filled completely, or saturated, with hydrogen. Saturated fats are generally of animal origin and are solid at room temperature. Because the chemical bond in saturated fats is so strong, they tend to take a long time to spoil, or become rancid, which allows them to have a long shelf life. Food sources of saturated fatty acids can be found in Table 19.2.

Saturated fats, although an important part of a healthy diet, tend to increase blood cholesterol levels, thus increasing the risk for atherosclerosis (the buildup of fatty deposits on the artery walls) and heart disease. In response to the effects of saturated fats the American Heart Association recommends that they be limited to only 5% to 6% of the dietary intake.

Unsaturated fatty acids. An unsaturated fatty acid has one or more places on its chemical chain in which hydrogen is missing. These are called *points of unsaturation.* A fatty acid with only one point of unsaturation is called a *monounsaturated fatty acid.* Fatty acids with two or more points of unsaturation are termed *polyunsaturated.* Most unsaturated fats are from plant sources and are liquid at room temperature. Sources of monounsaturated fats and polyunsaturated fats are listed in Table 19.2. Unsaturated fats, especially monounsaturated fats, are thought to lower low-density lipoprotein cholesterol, especially when combined with lower intake of saturated fat and *trans* fat.

Table 19.2 Food Sources of Fatty Acids

FATTY ACID CLASS	FOODS CONTRIBUTING SIGNIFICANT AMOUNTS TO THE DIET
Saturated	Coconut, palm, and palm kernel oils (tropical oils) Fat in and on meats and poultry Egg yolk Butter, cream, milk fat Cocoa butter Olive oil, olives
Monounsaturated	Canola oil Peanuts and peanut oil Most other nuts Avocados
Polyunsaturated	Safflower oil Sunflower oil Cottonseed oil Soybean oil Corn oil Most fish oil
Trans	Partially hydrogenated plant and fish oils Stick margarines, shortening Commercial fats used for frying, baking

Hydrogenated fats. **Hydrogenation** is a process in which hydrogen is added to a fat of vegetable origin (unsaturated) to make it more saturated or solid. This then makes the oil more stable and less susceptible to becoming rancid. When only some of the hydrogen has been replaced, the oil is considered partially hydrogenated. Most vegetable spreads, such as corn oil margarine, have been hydrogenated to some extent.

Trans *fatty acids.* *Trans* fatty acids are unsaturated fatty acids that have been completely hydrogenated. Synthetic *trans* fatty acids are produced during hydrogenation and can be found in some deep-fried restaurant foods; packaged cookies, crackers, and other baked goods; some margarines; and shortening. Naturally occurring *trans* fatty acids are found in smaller amounts in dairy products and some meats. *Trans* fatty acids in the diet are similar to saturated fats and tend to increase blood cholesterol levels. Therefore they also should be used sparingly in a healthy diet.

The American Heart Association recommends healthy individuals older than 2 years old obtain 25% to 35% of their total calories from fat, with less than 5% to 6% of total calories from saturated fats and less than 1% of total calories from *trans* fatty acids.

Cholesterol. **Cholesterol** is a lipid belonging to a class of chemical substances called *sterols*. Cholesterol is a building block for cell membranes and for hormones, such as estrogen and testosterone. It is synthesized in the liver and is found in foods of animal origin. Plant foods and oils do not contain cholesterol. In fact, plant sterols sometimes decrease cholesterol levels in the blood. The amounts of *dietary cholesterol* (the cholesterol found in foods) are highest in organ meats and egg yolks. Dietary cholesterol is also present in smaller but significant amounts in seafood, meats, poultry, and dairy products. Low-fat dairy products have less cholesterol than their higher-fat counterparts. The recommended intake of dietary cholesterol is an average of no more than 300 mg/day. Decreasing the intake of animal fats helps decrease the amount of dietary cholesterol consumed.

Digestion and metabolism of fat. For fat to be digested, it must be emulsified, or broken into smaller globules. Bile, a secretion of the liver, is necessary to emulsify fat. Bile is stored in the gallbladder and dispensed into the duodenum when fat is present. Once fats are emulsified, the body can break them down and absorb them.

After absorption, lipids are packaged as lipoproteins. **Lipoproteins** are molecules made of lipids surrounded by protein. They facilitate the transport of lipids in the bloodstream. The human body makes four types of lipoproteins; chylomicrons, high-density lipoproteins (HDLs), low-density lipoproteins (LDLs), and very low–density lipoproteins (VLDLs). The amounts of fat and protein in each of these lipoproteins vary. The higher the protein content of the lipoprotein, the greater the density. The type and amount of lipoproteins in the blood can protect the body from, or predispose it to, heart disease. LDLs and HDLs are important in the study of cardiovascular disease. Both of these lipoproteins carry cholesterol in the bloodstream. It appears that the cholesterol found in LDLs increases the risk of atherosclerosis by contributing to plaque buildup on the artery walls. In contrast, HDLs seem to have the opposite effect. HDLs transport cholesterol from the bloodstream to the liver to be degraded and excreted. LDLs sometimes are referred to as carrying "bad" cholesterol, whereas HDLs are referred to as carrying "good" cholesterol.

The National Institutes of Health (NIH) recommend that total serum cholesterol levels stay below 180 mg/dL. Therefore teaching should be aimed at reducing LDL levels and increasing or maintaining HDL levels.

Table 19.3 Classification of LDL, Total, and HDL Cholesterol

LDL Cholesterol	
<100 mg/dL	Optimal
100–129 mg/dL	Near or above optimal
130–159 mg/dL	Borderline high
160–189 mg/dL	High
≥190 mg/dL	Very high
Total Cholesterol	
<200 mg/dL	Desirable
200–239 mg/dL	Borderline high
≥240 mg/dL	High
HDL Cholesterol	
<40 mg/dL for men; <50 mg/dL for women	Low

HDL, High-density lipoprotein; *LDL*, low-density lipoprotein.
Data from National Cholesterol Education Program: *ATP III executive summary*, 2001, rev. 2004; Toth PP: The "good cholesterol": High-density lipoprotein. *Circulation* 111:e89, 2005.

Table 19.3 classifies the blood cholesterol values used to determine health risk. To lower cholesterol levels and maintain a healthy diet, the *Dietary Guidelines for Americans* (USDHHS and USDA, 2015) recommend increasing the amount of seafood consumed to reduce the amount of cholesterol-containing meat and poultry and to replace foods containing higher solid fats with ones that contain unsaturated fats. The guidelines also recommend using oils instead of solid fats when possible.

Protein

Protein is another nutrient vital to the human body. Proteins provide the building blocks for blood and bone, and they are a structural part of every cell. The human body contains thousands of different proteins, all of which are essential for tissue growth, repair, and wound healing. Collagen, a vital connective tissue, is made of protein. Some hormones, including thyroxine and insulin, are proteins. Enzymes are proteins produced by living cells. They cause chemical reactions within the body without being changed in the process. They are necessary for digestion and metabolism. The plasma proteins aid in fluid balance within the body. Albumin, a plasma protein, attracts water and has the capacity to pull fluid from one body compartment to another. Hemoglobin, a protein in the red blood cells, carries oxygen throughout the body. Immunoglobulins (antibodies) are also proteins, which emphasizes the role of protein in immune function.

If necessary, the body can use protein for energy. It supplies 4 kcal/g. However, if the body uses protein as an energy source, it is no longer available for any other function; thus proteins responsible for the building and repairing of tissues cannot perform their usual function.

Carbohydrates, fat, and protein contain carbon, hydrogen, and oxygen, but protein is unique in that it also contains nitrogen. All these elements—carbon, hydrogen, oxygen, and nitrogen—combine in specific ways to form amino acids. **Amino acids** are the building blocks of protein. Approximately 20 amino acids have been identified as important to the body's metabolism, but only 9 of them are considered indispensable *(essential) amino acids;* because the body does not make them in sufficient quantity to sustain health, it is necessary to obtain them from the diet. The body can manufacture adequate amounts of the other amino acids from the indispensable (essential) amino acids.

The recommendation is for 10% to 35% of total daily calories to come from protein. The DRI for protein in healthy adults is 0.8 g/kg of body weight per day. However, keep in mind that severe illness or stress can increase the need for protein.

Complete proteins. Food proteins are classified according to the number and kind of amino acids they contain. A complete protein is one that contains all nine essential amino acids in sufficient quantity and ratio for the body's needs. Complete proteins are generally of animal origin and are found in foods such as meat, poultry, fish, milk, cheese, eggs, and soy products.

Incomplete proteins. Incomplete proteins are those that are lacking in one or more of the essential amino acids. Incomplete proteins are of plant origin. This includes the protein in grains, legumes, nuts, and seeds. Even though the proteins in these foods are considered incomplete, these foods should not be avoided. By combining a variety of incomplete proteins in the diet, the body can obtain the necessary balance of the essential amino acids.

Vegetarian diets. For vegetarians and other people who choose to limit their intake of animal foods, obtaining sufficient amounts of protein may be challenging. Depending on the beliefs of the person following a vegetarian diet, the diet may vary, and the amount of protein may or may not be adequate to meet the body's needs. There is no single vegetarian diet. A vegetarian diet is made up of mainly plant foods. Some vegetarian diets include dairy products or eggs, or both, as well. Legumes play an important role in vegetarian diets. Legumes are plants that have nitrogen-fixing bacteria in their roots. These nitrogen-fixing bacteria lock nitrogen into the plant's structure, thereby increasing its protein content. Legumes contain two to three times as much protein as most vegetables. Most vegetarian diets supply sufficient protein if a variety of allowed foods are eaten throughout the day. However, the strictest vegetarian diet, the **vegan** diet, excludes all animal products, and more planning is required to obtain sufficient protein. To offset this deficit, vegans consume soybeans, soy milk, and other soy products to enhance protein intake. Strict vegetarians also need to include a reliable source of vitamin B_{12} in the diet, because vitamin B_{12} is found exclusively in animal foods.

Studies of vegetarians indicate that they, because of their dietary choices, may be at lower risk for various chronic diseases such as coronary artery disease, colon cancer, obesity, and type 2 diabetes.

Digestion and metabolism of protein. Protein-containing foods are the body's only external source of nitrogen. Once a protein-containing food is eaten, the nitrogen is removed from the amino acid, and some of it is excreted as urea nitrogen in the urine. The nitrogen that is not excreted is then used to make other amino acids. **Nitrogen balance,** or nitrogen equilibrium, is achieved when the amount of nitrogen (protein) taken in is equal to the amount of nitrogen excreted in the urine. Although a healthy adult is generally in a state of nitrogen balance, under certain circumstances nitrogen balance may be either positive or negative.

Positive nitrogen balance. A positive nitrogen balance exists when more nitrogen is taken in than is excreted. In this situation, the body is building more tissue (**anabolism**) than it is breaking down. This is seen during periods of growth, such as infancy, childhood, adolescence, and pregnancy.

Negative nitrogen balance. A negative nitrogen balance exists when less nitrogen is being consumed than is being excreted. This condition occurs when insufficient protein is being taken in and the body is breaking down more tissue (**catabolism**) than it is building. Nitrogen balance is negative in states of undernutrition, illness, and trauma. Skipping protein food for one day is not likely to create a negative nitrogen balance, so noticeable physical signs are not likely to occur. In contrast, prolonged negative nitrogen balance eventually can cause atrophy of muscles, as well as poor functioning of all body systems.

When protein is consumed in amounts greater than the body needs, the amino acids are changed chemically, converted to fat, and stored as adipose tissue. Therefore more dietary protein does not necessarily make more muscle; it may create more adipose tissue.

Excess dietary protein is sometimes unhealthy. Usually high-protein diets are also high in saturated fats, which increase the risk for cardiovascular disease. High-protein diets also tend to cause excretion of more calcium, thereby increasing the risk for osteoporosis. Too much dietary protein also places an excessive burden on the kidneys, which could possibly lead to renal insufficiency or renal failure.

Protein energy malnutrition. When there is a lack of energy or protein intake, protein energy malnutrition (PEM) may result. PEM is fairly common in children and adults in developing countries, and malnutrition is associated with more than half the deaths of children

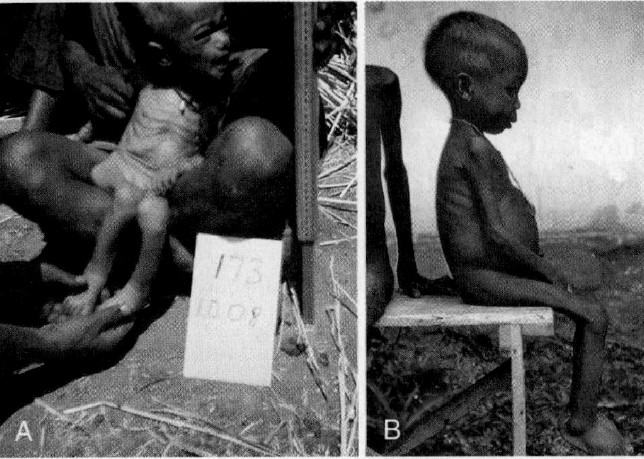

Fig. 19.4 Protein energy malnutrition. A, Marasmus. B, Kwashiorkor. (Courtesy Centers for Disease Control and Prevention.)

younger than 5 years worldwide. In developed countries, PEM is found most often in hospital settings, usually is associated with disease, and is more common in older adults. Two types of PEM exist: marasmus and kwashiorkor.

Marasmus is a protein deficiency that affects people of all ages. It involves a deficiency of protein, as well as of all other energy-providing foods. It is a chronic condition characterized by wasting of body tissues. As the disease progresses, subcutaneous fat stores and then muscle stores are depleted, leaving the victim with a "skin-and-bones" appearance (Fig. 19.4A).

Kwashiorkor occurs as a result of severe protein restriction in the presence of other calories. It occurs most often in children in developing countries, with onset at approximately the time the child is weaned from breastfeeding. Kwashiorkor is characterized by edema in the feet, legs, and often in the face and hands (see Fig. 19.4B). There also may be swelling in the abdomen. This swelling of the abdomen is due to ascites related to hypoalbuminemia and the resulting low oncotic pressure, as well as an enlarged fatty liver. As a result of the abdominal swelling, the child sometimes appears "fat," and the parents regard the child as well fed.

PEM usually is accompanied by multiple nutrient deficiencies and can lead to stunted growth and impaired cognitive development in children, reduced mental and physical capacity, and lowered resistance to infections.

Vitamins

Vitamins are organic compounds that are essential in small quantities for normal metabolism and for growth and maintenance of the body. Organic compounds are derived from living matter and contain carbon. Vitamins themselves are not sources of energy; they work in conjunction with other nutrients in the body to regulate many processes, including energy production. Because the amount of vitamins needed by the body is so small, they sometimes are referred to as *micronutrients*.

Many compounds, including vitamins, are susceptible to destruction by heat, light, and exposure to air. Therefore some of the vitamin content may be lost when foods are prepared or stored, resulting in value of the nutrient being lessened (Box 19.3).

Box 19.3 Methods of Preserving the Nutrient Content of Foods

- Avoid very high temperatures, long cooking times, and keeping foods hot for an extended time, as in a buffet line.
- Expose food to as little air as possible; keep prepared vegetables, fruits, and juices covered and airtight; cut and manipulate food as little as possible; and keep lids on pans while cooking.
- Expose food to as little water as possible; steam, microwave, stir-fry, or bake rather than boil.
- Keep and use the cooking water.
- Keep milk in opaque containers.
- Store fruits and vegetables cold.
- Use foods in whole form whenever possible.

Vitamins have many functions in the body, and those functions are specific to each vitamin. One vitamin cannot perform the functions of another. If an insufficient amount of vitamin C is taken in, the deficiency cannot be corrected by vitamin D.

Vitamins are classified by whether they are soluble in fat or soluble in water. Vitamins A, D, E, and K are fat soluble. Fat-soluble vitamins are absorbed from the intestine in the same way as fats, and, like fats, they can be stored in the body. Because of this storage capacity, excessive intake of fat-soluble vitamins, especially A and D, can lead to toxicity and death.

The water-soluble vitamins are those that dissolve in water and include the B vitamins and vitamin C. The body is not readily able to store these vitamins because they are water soluble, and excesses generally are excreted in the urine. Daily intake of these vitamins is necessary because body reserves are minimal. Table 19.4 lists all the vitamins with their food sources, their functions, and symptoms of deficiency and toxicity.

Antioxidant vitamins. Certain vitamins have attracted public interest and are of interest to health care professionals in the treatment of some diseases. These vitamins, E, C, and A (in the previtamin form, discussed later), have been found to delay or prevent the destruction or breakdown of cell membranes in the presence of oxygen (antioxidants) and thereby reduce the risk of developing certain cancers, inflammatory diseases, Alzheimer's disease, and heart disease. The link between these vitamins and disease has led to recommendations to increase intake of foods high in vitamins. Thus a focus on eating more fruits and vegetables is the current recommendation to delay or prevent these diseases.

Vitamin C. Vitamin C, or ascorbic acid, has many functions in the body. It contributes to the healing of wounds, burns, and fractures; it serves as an antioxidant;

Table 19.4 Vitamins

FOOD SOURCES	FUNCTION	SIGNS AND SYMPTOMS: DEFICIENCY	SIGNS AND SYMPTOMS: TOXICITY
Vitamin A[a]			
Egg yolks, liver, milk Carrots, winter squash, sweet potatoes, spinach, collards, kale, broccoli, apricots, cantaloupe	Vision, epithelial tissue integrity, growth, reproduction, embryonic development, immune function	Night blindness, xerophthalmia, increased susceptibility to infections, follicular hyperkeratosis	Fatigue, headache, nausea, vomiting, blurred vision, liver abnormalities, bone and skin change
Vitamin B_1 (thiamine)			
Unrefined whole grains, enriched and fortified grains and cereals, liver, pork, legumes, nuts	Carbohydrate metabolism	Beriberi: mental confusion, anorexia, muscle weakness and wasting, found in association with chronic alcoholism	None exhibited
Vitamin B_2 (riboflavin)			
Milk, meats, poultry, fish, enriched and fortified grains and cereals	General metabolism	Ariboflavinosis: sore throat, cheilosis (a disorder of the lips and mouth characterized by scales and fissures), glossitis, dermatitis	None exhibited
Vitamin B_3 (niacin)			
Meat, poultry, enriched and fortified grains and cereals (high-protein foods that contain tryptophan)	General metabolism	Pellagra: dermatitis, constipation or diarrhea, dementia, depression	Nausea, vomiting, flushing, pruritus (itching) of the skin, abnormal liver function
Vitamin B_5 (pantothenic acid)			
Widespread in foods; abundant in animal tissue, whole grains, and legumes	General metabolism	Listlessness and fatigue (rare)	Diarrhea and water retention
Vitamin B_6 (pyridoxine)			
Meat, poultry, fish, eggs, brown rice, wheat, oats, soybeans	Amino acid metabolism, general metabolism	Anemia, convulsions, dermatitis, depression, confusion	Peripheral neuropathy, irregular muscle coordination
Vitamin B_7 (biotin)			
Liver, egg yolks, soy flour, cereals, yeast (synthesis by intestinal bacteria)	General metabolism	Dermatitis, conjunctivitis, alopecia, depression (rare)	None exhibited
Vitamin B_9 (folic acid)			
Liver, green leafy vegetables, legumes, fruits, enriched grain products	Nucleic acid synthesis, amino acid metabolism	Macrocytic (large-cell) anemia, elevated homocysteine level	Sometimes masks vitamin B_{12} deficiency; interferes with the anticonvulsant drug phenytoin (Dilantin)
Vitamin B_{12} (cyanocobalamin)			
Animal products (meat, fish, poultry, milk, dairy products, eggs)	Synthesis of new cells, maintenance of nerve cells	Pernicious anemia: macrocytic megaloblastic anemia	None exhibited
Vitamin C (ascorbic acid)			
Citrus fruits and juices, strawberries, kiwi fruit, melons, broccoli, peppers, tomatoes, potatoes, fortified beverages	Antioxidant; wound healing, tissue growth and maintenance, proper immune function, absorption of iron	Scurvy: gingivitis, bleeding gums, easy bruising, increased infections, poor wound healing, rough skin, joint pain, muscle atrophy, fatigue	Abdominal cramps and diarrhea

Continued

Table 19.4 **Vitamins—cont'd**

		SIGNS AND SYMPTOMS	
FOOD SOURCES	**FUNCTION**	**DEFICIENCY**	**TOXICITY**
Vitamin D (calciferol)			
Fortified milk, fortified margarine, egg yolks, liver, fish oils Sunlight on skin	Maintenance of blood calcium and phosphorus balance	Rickets (children): abnormal shape and structure of bones Osteomalacia (adults): weakening and softening of bones	Calcification of soft tissues
Vitamin E (alpha-tocopherol)			
Vegetable oils, dark green, leafy vegetables, wheat germ, nuts	Antioxidant; protection of cell membranes	Peripheral neuropathy, ataxia, skeletal myopathy, retinopathy, and impairment of the immune response	Increased tendency to hemorrhage
Vitamin K			
Green, leafy vegetables, milk, dairy products, liver, meat, egg yolks, green tea (synthesis by intestinal bacteria)	Formation of blood clotting factors	Increased prothrombin time; in severe cases, hemorrhaging	None exhibited
Choline[b]			
Richest sources are liver, kidney, wheat germ, brewer's yeast, and egg yolks	Maintenance of cell membranes, memory retention, muscle control, lipid metabolism	Liver damage	Hypotension, sweating, diarrhea, fishy body odor

US Department of Health and Human Services. Vitamin E Fact Sheet for Health Professionals. March 2, 2018. Retrieved from https://ods.od.nih.gov/factsheets/VitaminE-HealthProfessional.
[a]Beta-carotene is a previtamin; it is converted to vitamin A in the body.
[b]Choline is an essential nutrient that works with folate in preventing neural tube defects and plays a role in cell functions and nerve communication.

and it is necessary for adrenal gland function. It also enhances the absorption of iron and is needed to convert folic acid, a B vitamin, to its active form. Vitamin C supplementation has become a common practice because of claims that it helps prevent the common cold and prevents or cures cancer. Although it is true that adequate vitamin C is necessary for proper immune function, large supplemental doses of the vitamin have not been shown consistently and conclusively to be of greater value than what can be obtained solely through diet. The adult DRI for vitamin C is 90 mg/day for men and 75 mg/day for women. The National Institutes of Health's Office of Dietary Supplements suggests an additional 35 mg/day for those who smoke cigarettes because cigarette smoke increases oxidative stress. The DRI recommended a vitamin C intake upper limit of 2 g/day for adults (USDHHS, NIH, 2018g). Intakes above this level pose the risk of causing diarrhea and GI disturbances and cause the body to store too much iron, which results in tissue damage. It is easy to meet the DRI recommendations by increasing intake of citrus fruits; green, leafy and yellow vegetables; and other foods containing vitamin C (Table 19.5). A deficiency of vitamin C can result in bleeding in the bones and joints, easy bone fracture, poor wound healing, and anemia.

B-complex vitamins. There are several different B vitamins. All are water soluble, and all are necessary for proper metabolism. Of all the B-complex vitamins, three are especially important.

Niacin. Niacin (vitamin B_3) is important in the production of energy from glucose and is involved in the repair of DNA. The body can produce some niacin if tryptophan is present. Niacin is measured in niacin equivalents. The DRI for niacin is 16 mg niacin equivalents/day for men and 14 mg niacin equivalents/day for women. This requirement is obtained easily by eating meat, poultry, fish, peanuts, or enriched whole grain breads and cereals. Niacin deficiency is rare, and there is usually no risk for toxicity except with excess vitamin supplementation.

Folate (folic acid). Folate is a water-soluble B vitamin that is the natural form found in foods such as spinach, lentils, and garbanzo beans. Folic acid is the synthetic form of the vitamin. Folic acid can be found in dietary supplements and in foods that are fortified with the vitamin. Both forms work the same in the body, but the synthetic form is easier for the body to absorb. Folic acid (vitamin B_9) is necessary for the formation of DNA and proper cell division. A deficiency can lead to megaloblastic anemia (see *Adult Health Nursing,* Chapter

Table 19.5 Vitamin C Content of Selected Foods[a]

FOOD	SERVING SIZE	VITAMIN C CONTENT (mg)
Orange juice, fresh squeezed	1 cup	124
Strawberries, whole	1 cup	98
Orange juice from concentrate	1 cup	97
Green pepper	1	96
Orange	1 medium	96
Grapefruit juice from concentrate	1 cup	83
Broccoli, cooked	½ cup	74
Brussels sprouts, cooked	½ cup	71
Kiwi	1 medium	71
Cantaloupe	1 cup	59
Cauliflower, cooked	1 cup	55
Tomato juice	1 cup	45
Grapefruit, pink	½ medium	38
Tomato	1 medium	23
Watermelon	1 wedge	23
Potato, baked	1	20
Spinach, cooked	½ cup	18

[a]The adult recommended daily allowances (RDAs) for vitamin C are 90 mg/day for men and 75 mg/day for women.
Data from US Department of Agriculture: *USDA national nutrient database for standard reference, release 22. Vitamin C.* Retrieved from *www.ars.usda.gov/SP2UserFiles/Place/12354500/Data/SR22/nutrlist/sr22w401.pdf.*

7). Adequate folic acid intake before and during pregnancy has been found to reduce the risk of neural tube defects (defects of the brain, spine, or spinal cord) in the infant. The recommendation for women who are capable of becoming pregnant is 400 mcg/day from fortified foods or a supplement in addition to the folic acid found in a varied diet containing green, leafy vegetables; beets; oranges; and kidney beans (USDHHS, NIH, 2018b).

Vitamin B_{12}. Cyanocobalamin (vitamin B_{12}) plays an essential part in the production of hemoglobin and myelin. To absorb vitamin B_{12}, a protein secreted by the stomach is required. This protein is called *intrinsic factor* and is produced in the lower portion of the stomach. When the intrinsic factor is missing—for example, after stomach excision or resection—vitamin B_{12} cannot be absorbed, and **pernicious anemia** (a progressive macrocytic megaloblastic anemia) develops. Treatment of pernicious anemia consists of vitamin B_{12} injections for a lifetime. Oral vitamin B_{12} supplementation is ineffective because of the lack of intrinsic factor. Because vitamin B_{12} is found primarily in foods of animal origin, people who follow a strict vegetarian diet (vegans) do not always receive adequate vitamin B_{12} from food and are likely to benefit from an oral supplement. People older than 50 years also tend to have difficulty absorbing vitamin B_{12} from foods because of low stomach acid secretion; therefore oral supplementation of vitamin B_{12} is recommended for them as well. It is recommended that individuals older than 50 receive most of their vitamin B_{12} from fortified foods or supplements containing vitamin B_{12} (NIH, Office of Dietary Supplements 2018f).

The DRI for vitamin B_{12} in adults is 2.4 mcg/day. This can be obtained easily from eating animal products such as lean meat, liver, seafood, eggs, and dairy products.

Vitamin A. Vitamin A, an antioxidant and a fat-soluble vitamin, is available in two forms: retinol (preformed) and carotene (provitamin). A preformed vitamin (retinol) is in a complete state when it is eaten, and it can be used immediately by the body. A provitamin (carotene) must be converted in the body to a form that can be used. Both forms of vitamin A are important for maintaining vision, as well as for skin and bone growth. The DRI for vitamin A is 700 mcg for women and 900 mcg for men (USDHHS, 2018). Most people consume vitamin A in the form of beta-carotene, found in bright yellow and orange fruits, carrots, pumpkin, and dark green, leafy vegetables. The liver contains about 90% of the body's stored vitamin A.

Vitamin D. Vitamin D promotes the absorption of calcium and phosphorus, which in turn promote bone and tooth health. It can be found in most fortified dairy products, in yeast, and in fish liver oils. The body also synthesizes vitamin D when the skin is exposed to sunlight. Because vitamin D is a fat-soluble vitamin and can be stored in the body, excess intake can cause GI upset, muscular weakness, and, in extreme cases, calcium deposits in the kidneys, lungs, brain, or heart. Vitamin D deficiency can lead to brittle bones (osteoporosis) and may be of concern for some older adult patients in long-term care facilities. A patient in long-term care who is confined indoors and does not drink milk or consume milk products is likely to be at risk for obtaining inadequate amounts of vitamin D. The DRI for vitamin D for adults up to 70 years of age is 15 mcg/day. After the age of 70, the DRI is 20 mcg/day (USDHHS, NIH, 2018h).

Vitamin K. Vitamin K plays a role in blood clotting. It is important in maintaining four of the eleven clotting factors found in the blood. There are two forms of vitamin K: one is present in green, leafy vegetables, and the other is made by intestinal bacteria. Because of the effect that vitamin K has on clotting, patients who are taking antiplatelet drugs or anticoagulants should consume consistent amounts of vitamin K from day to day. Large fluctuations in vitamin K intake have the potential to alter the effects of the anticoagulant drug. The DRI for vitamin K is 120 mcg/day for adult males and 90 mcg/day for adult females (USDHHS, NIH, 2018i).

Minerals

Minerals differ from vitamins: they are inorganic, and they are single elements rather than compounds. Minerals are also similar to vitamins: they help regulate bodily functions without providing energy and are essential to good health.

Minerals are classified as either major minerals or trace minerals. Major minerals are those needed in amounts greater than 100 mg/day (National Academies of Sciences, Engineering, and Medicine, n.d.). They include calcium, phosphorus, magnesium, sulfur, sodium, potassium, and chloride. The trace minerals are needed in much smaller amounts (less than 100 mg/day); they include iron, zinc, iodine, selenium, copper, manganese, fluoride, chromium, and molybdenum. Other trace minerals thought to be essential, but of which less is known, include arsenic, boron, nickel, and silicon. Table 19.6 lists the minerals with a summary of their food sources and function, as well as symptoms of deficiency and toxicity.

Calcium. Calcium has several functions in the body. It is important in the formation of bones and teeth; it plays a role in blood clotting; and it plays a role in the transmission of nerve impulses and muscle action. It is also important for metabolic reactions throughout the body. Because of these functions, calcium is necessary to protect against osteoporosis. *Osteoporosis* is an abnormal reduction in bone density that leads to bone pain, fractures, loss of stature, and deformities such as kyphosis (hunched back). In the United States, 1.5 million bone fractures are attributed to this bone disease annually. Women are affected more than men. Many hip fractures are the result of osteoporosis. Besides pain,

Table 19.6 Minerals

		SIGNS AND SYMPTOMS	
FOOD SOURCES	**FUNCTION**	**DEFICIENCY**	**TOXICITY**
Calcium			
Milk, cheese, milk products, green, leafy vegetables, broccoli, legumes, fish with bones, fortified cereals	Formation and maintenance of bones and teeth, blood clotting, nerve conduction, muscle contraction	Osteoporosis (adults): weak, more porous bones Stunted growth in children	Constipation; increased risk for urinary stone formation in men; reduced absorption of iron and zinc
Chloride			
Salt, processed foods, water supply	Fluid and acid-base balance	Metabolic alkalosis	None exhibited
Chromium			
Whole grains, liver, nuts, cheese	Maintenance of normal glucose metabolism	Impaired glucose tolerance, diabetes-like symptoms	None exhibited
Copper			
Organ meats, seafood, nuts, seeds, whole grains, cocoa	Necessary for utilization of iron	Anemia, vascular skeletal problems	Nausea, vomiting, liver damage
Fluoride			
Water supply, plants grown in fluoride-rich soil	Increases tooth resistance to decay, stimulates new bone formation	Increased susceptibility to tooth decay	Fluorosis: mottled tooth enamel, altered bone health
Iodine			
Iodized salt, seafood, plants grown in iodine-rich soil	Part of thyroxin, which helps regulate metabolism, growth, and development	Goiter: enlarged thyroid gland, weight gain, skin and hair changes Cretinism: mental and physical retardation of fetus	Enlarged thyroid gland
Iron			
Clams, liver, oysters, meat, poultry, fish, legumes, whole and enriched grains, fortified cereals	Part of hemoglobin and myoglobin; necessary for oxygen transport and use in the body; part of some enzymes; energy metabolism	Microcytic, hypochromic anemia: fatigue, weakness, headache, apathy, pale skin, decreased immune function Children: reduced attention span, decreased ability to learn	Tissue damage, constipation, decreased zinc absorption Accidental poisoning in children: nausea, vomiting, diarrhea, rapid heartbeat, weak pulse, dizziness, shock, disorientation

Table 19.6 **Minerals—cont'd**

FOOD SOURCES	FUNCTION	SIGNS AND SYMPTOMS	
		DEFICIENCY	TOXICITY
Magnesium			
Nuts, legumes, whole grains, green leafy vegetables, fortified cereals	Bone mineralization, muscle contraction and relaxation, general metabolism, blood pressure regulation	Nausea, muscle weakness, confusion, tetany (rare, usually caused by other disease states)	Diarrhea
Manganese			
Widely distributed in food; richest in whole grains, cereals, fruits, vegetables	General metabolism, formation of bone	Dermatitis, reduced bone mineralization, altered lipid and carbohydrate metabolism	Central nervous system abnormalities
Phosphorus			
Milk, meat, poultry, fish, grains, food additives; found in almost all foods	Essential component of bone, energy metabolism, acid-base balance	Rare, but sometimes occurs in patients using aluminum hydroxide antacids	Calcification of nonskeletal tissues
Potassium			
Sweet potatoes, fruits, vegetables, fresh meat, legumes, milk	Nerve conduction; muscle contraction, including the heart; fluid and acid-base balance	Severe: cardiac dysrhythmias, muscle weakness, glucose intolerance Moderate: increased blood pressure, risk of kidney stones, increased bone turnover	Cardiac arrest
Selenium			
Meat, poultry, fish, bread, grains, seeds	Antioxidant	Cardiomyopathy	Nail and hair changes, nausea, diarrhea, skin rash, garlic breath odor, fatigue
Sodium			
Salt, processed foods, small amounts in whole unprocessed foods	Fluid and acid-base balance, nerve conduction, muscle contraction	Cramps, mental confusion, apathy, appetite loss (usually secondary to diarrhea or disease)	Hypertension in susceptible individuals, increased calcium excretion
Sulfur			
All foods containing protein	Essential constituent of proteins, metabolism	None exhibited except in severe protein deficiency (problems with cartilage, tendons, and ligaments)	None exhibited
Zinc			
Red meat, liver, eggs, seafood, cereal, whole grains, legumes	Part of many enzymes involved in metabolism	Loss of appetite, growth retardation, skin changes, immune system dysfunction	Impaired immune response, impaired copper status, reduced HDL cholesterol level

HDL, High-density lipoprotein.

hip fractures often result in dramatic lifestyle changes, disability, and loss of independence. An estimated 12% to 20% of people with hip fractures die from complications within 1 year of the fracture (Centers for Disease Control and Prevention, 2013).

The causes of osteoporosis are multiple. Peak bone mass is determined not only by calcium intake but also by genetic influences, gender, hormone levels, physical activity, and dietary intake of vitamin D, fluoride, and other trace minerals. In the United States, diets high in sodium and protein and low in potassium appear to contribute to osteoporosis by increasing the amount of calcium that is excreted in the urine. Growth and mineralization of bone occur from birth until early adulthood. Peak bone mass is achieved between 19 and 30 years of age. A higher peak bone mass in young adulthood lowers the risk of bone fractures later in life. In women, menopause greatly accelerates the rate of bone loss. Therefore calcium intake in childhood, adolescence, and young adulthood is important.

The recommended intakes of calcium are similar for men and women, but it varies across age groups. The requirement for older children and adolescents is set at 1300 mg/day (USDHHS, NIH, 2017). The suggested intake for adults is 1000 mg/day up to age 50 and 1200 mg/day for adults 51 years of age and older. No increases in calcium intake are recommended during pregnancy and lactation, because additional dietary calcium does not appear to have any influence on the changes seen in maternal bone mass during pregnancy and lactation. The calcium recommendation for patients with osteoporosis is 1500 mg/day.

The amount of calcium recommended for good health is often difficult to achieve from diet alone, and many foods, such as orange juice and breakfast cereals, have been fortified with calcium. It is also possible to take calcium supplements, but they should never be allowed to replace calcium-rich foods in the diet. Foods provide not only calcium but also other nutrients that are beneficial in disease prevention (Table 19.7).

Calcium absorption and excretion may be affected by physiologic circumstances and dietary factors. Box 19.4 discusses factors that influence calcium absorption and excretion.

Sodium. In the body, sodium functions as an *electrolyte* (a compound that can conduct an electrical current). Sodium is needed in very small amounts for good health and is found naturally in almost all foods. Therefore dietary sodium deficiency is extremely rare in the United States. Of greater concern is that excess sodium has the potential to be detrimental to health. Salt (sodium chloride) is the largest contributor of sodium in the diet and, if eaten in large quantities, can cause hypertension and edema. Approximately 65 million, or 31%, of American adults suffer from hypertension. DRIs for sodium suggest that intake of 1500 mg/day is adequate for healthy adults younger than 50, 1300 mg is adequate for adults between 50 and 70 years of age, and 1200 mg is adequate for adults older than 70 (USDHHS and USDA, 2015). The upper limit of intake is set at 2300 mg/day. Most adults in the United States consume approximately 3400 mg of sodium per day. Because sodium may be lost with heavy sweating, diarrhea, vomiting, renal disease, and cystic fibrosis, it is important to monitor sodium levels in individuals presenting with any of these symptoms or diseases.

Potassium. Potassium, also an electrolyte, is needed for conduction of nerve impulses and the contraction of muscles, including the heart muscle. It helps maintain acid-base balance and is required for conversion of glucose to glycogen. It also plays a role in energy production and insulin release from the pancreas. A severe deficiency of potassium can lead to hypokalemia (blood potassium level less than 3.5 mmol/L), which is a life-threatening state. Individuals taking potassium-wasting diuretics and chronic laxative users also may be at risk for developing hypokalemia and need to achieve adequate potassium intake through diet or supplementation, or both. Excessive intake of potassium is also a problem and can lead to hyperkalemia (blood potassium levels above 5.0 mmol/L). This can result in renal failure, adrenal failure, and cardiac arrest.

The DRIs for potassium suggest that intake of 4700 mg/day is adequate for all adults (USDHHS, NIH, 2018d). At present, most Americans consume much less

Table 19.7 Calcium Content of Selected Foods

FOOD	SERVING SIZE	CALCIUM CONTENT (mg)
Sardines	3 oz	371
American cheese	1 oz	348
Cheddar cheese	1 oz	306
Milk	1 cup	291–316
Yogurt	1 cup	274–415
Tofu (processed with calcium)	3 oz	225
Ice cream	1 cup	176
Salmon with bones (canned)	1 oz	167
Processed cheese	1 oz	159–199
Collard greens (cooked)	1 cup	148–357
Broccoli (cooked)	1 cup	94–177
Cottage cheese	½ cup	77

Box 19.4 Factors Affecting Calcium Absorption and Excretion

FACTORS THAT IMPROVE CALCIUM ABSORPTION FROM THE GASTROINTESTINAL TRACT

- Acidic conditions in the stomach (presence of food in the stomach increases stomach acid secretion)
- Increased physiologic need (e.g., infancy, childhood, adolescence, pregnancy)
- Small doses (less than 500 mg) of calcium are better absorbed than large doses

FACTORS THAT DECREASE CALCIUM ABSORPTION FROM THE GASTROINTESTINAL TRACT

- Calcium absorption decreases with age
- Calcium is poorly absorbed from foods rich in oxalic or phytic acids (spinach, sweet potatoes, rhubarb, beans, seeds, nuts, grains)

DIETARY FACTORS THAT INCREASE EXCRETION (LOSS) OF CALCIUM IN URINE

- Caffeine
- High-protein diets
- High-sodium diets
- Low-potassium diets

than this. Studies indicate that a moderate potassium deficiency (in the absence of hypokalemia) may lead to increased blood pressure, increased risk of kidney stones, and increased bone loss. Therefore adequate potassium intake is necessary to prevent these health risks.

Potassium is found naturally in many foods, especially fruits, vegetables, and milk. Plant forms of potassium are water soluble; therefore much of the potassium may be lost during food processing. Processed foods almost always have added salt or other sources of sodium. Therefore eating more foods in their natural states and reducing the amount of processed foods help reduce sodium intake and increase potassium intake. Potassium supplementation is not recommended, except when prescribed by a health care provider, because the risk of toxicity and cardiac arrest is high.

Iron. Iron is an essential part of hemoglobin, myoglobin, and many enzymes throughout the body. Hemoglobin is part of the red blood cell and carries oxygen to the cells. Myoglobin is similar to hemoglobin but is found in the muscle tissue and is responsible for storing oxygen in the muscle. A lack of iron in the body can cause iron-deficiency anemia.

Iron-deficiency anemia seems to be the most prevalent nutritional problem in the world, and it may result not only from inadequate iron in the diet but also excessive blood loss, absorption problems, and hemoglobin production problems. A deficiency of iron limits oxygen delivery to the cells, which results in fatigue, weakness, headaches, pallor of skin and mucous membranes, poor work performance, and decreased immune function. In children, iron deficiency has been associated with a short attention span, irritability, and a reduced ability to learn.

Children aged 6 months to 4 years, adolescents, menstruating women, and pregnant women are at greatest risk for iron-deficiency anemia. Dietary requirements are higher for women than for men because of the monthly blood loss during menstruation. Iron DRIs are set at 15 mg/day for adolescent girls and 18 mg/day for premenopausal adult women (USDHHS, 2018). For postmenopausal women, men, and children, the DRI is 8 mg/day of iron. Pregnant women have an iron requirement set at 27 mg/day. Because this requirement is so high, it is almost impossible to obtain it through diet alone, and supplementation is required.

Food sources of iron include meat (especially organ meats), poultry, fish, whole grains, and soy foods, as well as fortified and enriched grain products. Dietary iron is found in two forms: heme and nonheme. Heme iron is found in animal tissues (meats, poultry, and fish) and is absorbed well. The iron in plant products and iron supplements is nonheme iron. Nonheme iron is not absorbed well from the GI tract and therefore may not be as available as heme forms of iron. Iron absorption from the GI tract may be enhanced or inhibited by certain dietary factors. For example, taking vitamin C with iron supplements may enhance the absorption, whereas consuming iron along with fiber and coffee may inhibit absorption (Box 19.5).

Box 19.5 Factors Affecting Iron Absorption

FACTORS THAT ENHANCE IRON ABSORPTION

- Meat, fish, and poultry (MFP) have a factor (sometimes called the *MFP factor*) that enhances iron absorption
- Vitamin C (ascorbic acid), when eaten in the same meal with iron-containing foods

FACTORS THAT INHIBIT IRON ABSORPTION

- Bran and some fibers that contain phytates bind iron in the gastrointestinal tract, so it is not absorbed
- Calcium in milk and supplement form
- Polyphenols, which are compounds found in coffee, tea, and red wine
- Some medications such as antacids
- Vegetable proteins, especially soy protein

Even though iron is a necessary mineral, overdoses can be toxic and even fatal. Iron poisoning is seen each year in children who ingest overdoses of iron-containing vitamin and mineral supplements. Immediate medical attention is necessary if a child ingests large amounts of iron-containing supplements.

Chromium. *Chromium* is necessary for glucose metabolism and seems to work with insulin in regulating blood glucose levels. Adequate intake of chromium is thought to help patients suffering from type 2 diabetes mellitus; however, some studies have revealed that the value of chromium supplements for patients with diabetes is inconclusive and controversial and more studies are needed.

The average healthy adult (19 to 50 years old) requires only 25 mcg/day (women) to 35 mcg/day (men), so it is possible to obtain adequate chromium through diet alone (USDHHS, NIH, 2018a). Good sources of chromium include whole grains, cheese, liver, eggs, peas, apples, and nuts.

Vitamin and mineral supplementation. Many Americans are interested in vitamin and mineral supplementation. There have been claims that these nutrients help reduce stress, prevent colds, increase sexuality, increase energy, improve physical performance, and reduce the risk for certain diseases. Many people believe that if some is good, more is better. The truth is that for most people, vitamins and minerals are obtained best from a balanced, varied diet. Except in certain cases, supplementation is not necessary. For people who like to use a supplement as "insurance" against an imperfect diet, a simple multivitamin and mineral supplement should suffice.

It is best to avoid large doses, or megadoses, of nutrients and to avoid taking numerous types of supplements, except for therapeutic purposes. All medications, including vitamins and minerals, should be taken under the supervision of a health care provider.

Water

Water is the nutrient most vital to life; humans can survive longer without food than they can without water. Lack of this nutrient brings about detrimental changes in the body more rapidly than lack of any other. Water makes up approximately 60% of adult body weight and 80% of infant weight and performs many functions in the body. It provides form and structure to body tissues, acts as a solvent, and is necessary for most of the body's chemical processes. Water transports nutrients and other substances throughout the body by way of the blood, body secretions, and tissue fluids; it lubricates and protects moving parts of the body, such as joints; it aids in digestion; and it is necessary for regulating body temperature. If fluid needs are not met, in relation to inadequate intake or through abnormal losses such as vomiting, hemorrhage, burns, or an increase in perspiration or urination, dehydration results. Severe dehydration (more than 10% of body weight lost) could become a life-threatening situation. Signs of dehydration include poor skin turgor; flushed, dry skin; dry mouth; cracked, dry lips; decreased urine output; irritability; and disorientation. Dehydration in infants is evidenced by sunken fontanels, a decrease in the number of wet diapers, and no tears when the child cries.

About 80% of total water intake comes from drinking water and other beverages, and 20% comes from the water contained in foods. The need for water varies, depending on factors such as body size, age, activity level, metabolic needs, and temperature, and so it is not possible to give a specific recommendation; however, a suggested daily intake of 9 cups (women) to 13 cups (men) of fluids from drinking water and other beverages is adequate for most adults. Pregnant and lactating women have increased water needs (up to 3 L/day). Infants tend to be at greater risk for dehydration because they have a higher percentage of body water and are more susceptible to greater skin losses of water. In young infants, breast milk and formula normally provide adequate fluid, but extra fluids may be needed in warmer weather. Older adults have decreased sensitivity to thirst and are also at greater risk for dehydration. Young infants and older adults require special attention to make certain that their fluid needs are met and to avoid dehydration.

LIFE CYCLE NUTRITION

PREGNANCY AND LACTATION

Nutrient needs are greater during periods of intensive growth, such as pregnancy and infancy, than at any other time during the life cycle.

Optimal nutrition during pregnancy reduces the risk of complications, premature deliveries, and low birth weight. Even the mother's nutrition before conception plays a role in the outcome of a pregnancy. Women of childbearing age should be encouraged to consume a healthy diet and use care in the consumption of alcohol and caffeine. The focus of maternal education regarding nutrition should be expanded to include preconceptional, as well as prenatal, nutrition. Many women are unaware of their pregnancy during the first weeks after conception, and most women do not attend prenatal information classes until the later months of their pregnancy. Therefore it is important to provide information before conception or within the first few weeks of pregnancy. During these early weeks of pregnancy, adequate folic acid is thought to reduce significantly the risk of neural tube defects, such as spina bifida, in the infant. For this reason, women of childbearing age should be advised to consume adequate amounts of folate from fortified foods in addition to natural food sources.

To consume enough nutrients for mother and fetus, pregnant women should increase their caloric intake by about 300 kcal/day during the first trimester, 340 kcal/day during the second trimester, and 450 to 500 kcal/day during the third trimester of pregnancy. These additional calories should be from **nutrient-dense foods** (foods that contain large amounts of nutrients in relation to kilocalories). For a detailed discussion on nutrient needs during pregnancy and sample menus for pregnancy, see Tables 19.8 and 19.9.

Concerns in Pregnancy

Weight gain. Weight gain in pregnancy is important. Recommended weight gain varies based on a woman's prepregnancy weight. Optimal weight gain for the average woman is 25 to 35 pounds. Underweight women should gain between 28 and 40 pounds, whereas overweight women should gain only between 15 and 25 pounds. Encourage pregnant young adolescents to strive for higher weight gain to maintain their health, as well as that of the fetus.

Intentional weight loss should not be attempted during pregnancy. Mothers who do not gain adequate weight during pregnancy risk giving birth to a low–birth weight (LBW) infant (weighing less than 5.5 pounds). These babies are at greater risk for complications during and after birth.

Discomforts and complications. Many women experience discomforts during pregnancy. Common among these are nausea and vomiting, often referred to as "morning sickness." There are many ways to alleviate the nausea and vomiting associated with pregnancy. Mild nausea and vomiting, as well as other discomforts, often can be alleviated with safe and simple dietary alterations (Box 19.6). However, women should be advised to discuss any concerns they may have with their health care provider.

Table 19.8 Nutrient Needs During Pregnancy and Lactation

AMOUNT (DIETARY REFERENCE INTAKES)				
NONPREGNANT ADULT	PREGNANCY	LACTATION	REASONS FOR INCREASED NUTRIENT NEED DURING PREGNANCY	FOOD SOURCES
Protein				
46–50 g	60 g	65 g	Rapid fetal tissue growth Amniotic fluid Placental growth and development Maternal tissue growth: uterus, breasts Increased maternal circulating blood volume: • Hemoglobin increase • Plasma protein increase Maternal storage reserves for labor, delivery, and lactation	Milk, cheese, eggs, meat, grains, legumes, nuts, soy products
Calories[a]				
2200	2500	2700	Increased basal metabolic rate, energy needs Protein sparing	See individual foods
Minerals				
Calcium[b]				
1000 mg	1000 mg[b]	1000 mg[b]	Fetal skeleton formation Fetal tooth bud formation Increased maternal calcium metabolism Maternal blood pressure control	Milk, yogurt, cheese, fortified soy milk, dark green, leafy vegetables
Iron				
18 mg	27 mg	9 mg	Increased maternal circulating blood volume, increased hemoglobin Fetal liver iron storage High iron cost during pregnancy	Liver, meats, eggs, whole or enriched grain, leafy vegetables, nuts, legumes, dried fruits, fortified cereals
Iodine				
150 mcg	220 mcg	290 mcg	Increased basal metabolic rate Increased thyroxine production	Iodized salt
Magnesium				
310 mg	350 mg	310 mg	Coenzyme in energy and protein metabolism Enzyme activator Tissue growth, cell metabolism Muscle action	Nuts, soybeans, cocoa, seafood, whole grains, dried beans and peas
Vitamins				
Vitamin B_6 (Pyridoxine)				
1.3 mg	1.9 mg	2 mg	Coenzyme in protein metabolism Increased fetal growth requirement	Milk, wheat, corn, liver, meat
Folic Acid				
400 mcg	600 mcg	500 mcg	Increased red blood cells Prevention of macrocytic anemia Prevention of neural tube defects	Green leafy vegetables, oranges, artichokes, broccoli, asparagus, liver, fortified grain products
Vitamin C				
75 mg	85 mg	120 mg	Tissue formation and integrity Formation of connective tissue Enhanced iron absorption	Citrus fruits, strawberries, broccoli, tomatoes, raw green, leafy vegetables
Vitamin A				
700 mcg	770 mcg	1300 mcg	Vitamin content in breast milk Embryonic development Breast milk production	Milk, egg yolks, organ meats, deep orange and green fruits and vegetables

[a]Provision of adequate nonprotein calories so that protein is available for tissue synthesis and maintenance rather than used for energy needs.
[b]Calcium absorption increases during pregnancy and lactation, so no additional dietary calcium is advised.

Table 19.9 Sample Menus for Diet During Pregnancy

MENU 1	MENU 2
Breakfast	
1 cup high-fiber ready-to-eat cereal 1 slice wheat toast 1 tsp vegetable oil spread 1 banana 1 cup 1% or skim milk	2 eggs, scrambled in 1 tsp vegetable oil with ½ cup chopped onion, pepper, mushroom, tomato, 1½ oz shredded cheese 1 bran muffin 1 tbsp vegetable oil spread 6 oz orange juice
Snack	
1 apple 2 tbsp peanut butter	½ cup mixed nuts and dried fruit
Lunch	
2 oz turkey on 2 slices wheat bread 1 tsp mayonnaise 1 cup spinach salad 6 whole-grain crackers 1 cup skim or 1% milk	1 cup black bean and vegetable soup 2 slices corn bread 1 tbsp vegetable oil spread 2 tsp honey 1 cup fresh strawberries 1 cup skim or 1% milk
Snack	
½ cantaloupe with ½ cup low-fat cottage cheese	3 cups popcorn
Dinner	
Pork-vegetable stir-fry: 3 oz lean pork 1½ cups fresh vegetables 2 tsp olive oil Seasonings 1 cup steamed brown rice Water	4 oz grilled chicken breast 1 baked potato 2 tbsp sour cream and chives 1 cup steamed broccoli ½ cup pasta salad with vinegar and oil dressing 1 dinner roll 1 tsp vegetable oil spread Water
Snack	
2 oatmeal raisin cookies 1 cup 1% or skim milk	1 cup low-fat yogurt topped with ⅓ cup granola
Approximate Number of Servings Provided per Menu	
Grain group	8
Fruit group	3
Vegetable group	4
Dairy group	3
Meat group	6 oz
Fats, oils, and sweets	5–6

Occasionally, pregnancy brings about medical conditions that pose potential dangers for the mother and the fetus. Hypertensive disorders of pregnancy include chronic hypertension, preeclampsia, eclampsia, and gestational hypertension. These disorders are the second leading cause of maternal death in the United States and contribute significantly to stillbirths and neonatal complications. Proper nutrition is vital before and throughout pregnancy and may help in the management of blood pressure during pregnancy. A diet rich in fruits, vegetables, and milk products, as well as in adequate protein, and moderate sodium intake should be encouraged.

Box 19.6 Nutritional Suggestions to Relieve Some Discomforts of Pregnancy

NAUSEA, VOMITING, GASTRIC DISTRESS

- Allow time after eating before lying down or going to bed to prevent epigastric distress.
- Avoid high-fat or fried foods in excess.
- Avoid letting the stomach become empty.
- Consume five or six small meals that include protein each day.
- Drink plenty of fluids during the day; however, drink liquids before or after meals to avoid feeling too full.
- Limit consumption of foods with strong odors during times of nausea. Avoid odors that bother the patient.
- To reduce nausea, eat soda crackers or other dry grain products before getting out of bed.

CONSTIPATION

- Drink plenty of fluids, especially water.
- Include fiber-rich foods at each meal.
- Include moderate daily exercise.

Controlling blood glucose levels during pregnancy is very difficult. Hypoglycemia is common in the first trimester because of low glucose levels, increased insulin production, and nausea and vomiting. During the latter two trimesters, insulin resistance is common, and so the woman may be more likely to experience hyperglycemia. With the incidence of diabetes on the rise in the United States, it is important to make sure all women undergo screening for gestational diabetes during pregnancy. For women with preexisting diabetes, achieving good blood glucose control before and during pregnancy is important. Gestational diabetes often is controlled through nutrition therapy and moderate exercise, but for women who are unable to achieve glycemic control, insulin therapy is often necessary.

Anemia is another common nutritional problem in pregnancy; iron-deficiency anemia and folic acid–deficiency anemia are possible. An adequate diet that includes meats, poultry, fish, vegetables (especially green, leafy vegetables), and a variety of fruits should be consumed, along with a prenatal supplement containing iron and folic acid.

Practices to avoid. During pregnancy, there are several things a woman should avoid in her diet. Alcohol, caffeine, and nicotine are three of the more important substances to avoid. Alcohol contributes to an increased risk for mental and physical disabilities in the fetus, and if the mother consumes large amounts of alcohol during pregnancy, *fetal alcohol syndrome* could develop. Fetal alcohol syndrome is characterized by physical deformities, learning disabilities, and behavioral problems. No safe level of alcohol consumption during pregnancy has been determined, and most nutrition experts favor total abstinence. The American Medical Association recommends that women of childbearing age abstain from drinking alcohol as soon as they plan to become pregnant.

High caffeine consumption may be a problem and is associated with delayed conception, increased risk of spontaneous abortion, and low birth weight. The March of Dimes (2015) recommends that women who are pregnant should not consume more than 200 mg of caffeine per day (one 12-ounce cup) to avoid decreased blood flow to the fetus and the complications that could occur (March of Dimes, 2015).

Nicotine in tobacco smoke also should be avoided during pregnancy. Studies have shown that smoking decreases blood supply to the fetus. This can cause premature birth and low birth weight. Birth defects such as cleft palate or cleft lip are also more common in babies born to mothers who have smoked during pregnancy.

Taking drugs of any kind during pregnancy should be avoided unless done under the direct supervision of a health care provider. Advise women to avoid all drugs, including over-the-counter medications and herbal or botanical supplements, until they have consulted their health care provider.

Another dietary concern for pregnant women is the intake of mercury. High mercury intake during pregnancy can cause fetal brain damage, as well as hearing and vision problems in the baby after birth. Pregnant women should be advised to avoid such foods as shark, swordfish, and king mackerel because of the high mercury content.

Lactation

During lactation, a woman should follow a diet similar to that followed during pregnancy. Kilocalorie needs and many nutrient needs are higher than during pregnancy (see Table 19.8). Lactating women should increase their caloric intake by 500 kcal/day more than their prepregnancy intake. These calories should come from foods that are going to provide the lactating woman with increased protein, calcium, phosphorus, and iron, as well as vitamins and minerals. Fluid needs are increased during lactation and should be obtained through the consumption of water, milk, juices, and other nutritious beverages. Advise moderation in any consumption of coffee, tea, and alcohol, because caffeine and alcohol can enter the breast milk and affect the infant.

During lactation, adequate fluid and nutrient intake is important to maintain the quantity and quality of breast milk. Poor kilocalorie and nutrient intake causes a decrease in the quantity of milk produced, as well as in the nutritional quality of the breast milk. Therefore it is essential for the lactating mother to be nourished properly to ensure that lactation continues and milk supply is adequate.

INFANCY

The time from birth to 1 year of age is one of rapid growth and development. The infant's birth weight doubles by 6 months and triples by 1 year of age. Nutrition plays an important part in this rapid growth.

Breast milk or iron-fortified infant formula is recommended for the entire first year of life. Breast milk contains antibodies and easily digested fats. This composition tends to lead to a lower incidence of infections in breast-fed infants and fewer episodes of GI upset. Regular cow's milk (whole, low-fat, or skim) should be avoided during the first year of life. Introduction of regular cow's milk before 1 year of age could lead to iron-deficiency anemia and increase the risk for developing milk allergies later in life. Also, the fat in cow's milk is more difficult for the infant to digest and could cause GI disturbances. The large amounts of protein, sodium, and potassium found in cow's milk also could overwhelm the infant's system and cause damage to the kidneys. Acceptable alternatives to cow's milk during the first year of life are breast milk and iron-fortified infant formula. Whole milk is acceptable after the first year, but skim and low-fat milk are inappropriate until the child is 2 years of age because the fat content is insufficient. In the first 6 months, water, juice, and other solid foods are generally unnecessary for infants. In most cases, breast milk or formula provides adequate nutrition for about the first 4 to 6 months. At approximately 4 to 6 months of age, depending on the infant's development, it is possible to introduce solid foods into the diet. Solid feedings usually are initiated with iron-fortified rice cereal, because rice cereal is less allergenic than most other foods. Infants should start with 1 to 2 teaspoons, and the amount is increased gradually. Fruits are added next, then vegetables, and then meats. Single-ingredient foods should be introduced one at a time at weekly intervals. This allows sufficient time to detect any food-related allergies. If the family has a history of food allergies, it is generally best to withhold wheat cereal, wheat products, and egg whites until the child is 1 year of age. Infants younger than 12 months of age also should never be given honey, especially wild honey, because of the potential for botulism. Wild honey is a potential source of *Clostridium botulinum* spores and easily can cause botulism in the infant.

Most commercially prepared baby foods in the United States are nutritious, safe, and of high quality. However, it is important to read labels and use foods without added salt, sugar, or honey. If baby foods are prepared at home, it is important to take care to reduce the risk of foodborne illness by having a sanitary preparation area and proper storage conditions.

There is no nutritional benefit to feeding juice to infants younger than 6 months. Offering juice before solid foods are introduced into the diet may cause the infant to prefer juice over breast milk or infant formula and tends to reduce the intake of important nutrients such as protein, fat, vitamins, and minerals.

It is important to remind parents that once the baby develops teeth, the nighttime feeding should be limited to water, and breastfeeding mothers should not allow the infant to nurse continuously throughout the night. Prolonged exposure of the teeth to formula or breast milk is a major contributing factor to dental caries.

CHILDHOOD

At approximately 1 year of age, appetite generally tapers off, and the growth rate slows. Children still need adequate nutrition, although nutrient needs relative to weight are generally less than in infancy. The website *www.ChooseMyPlate.gov* offers an appropriate guide for children's diets (see Fig. 19.1). Younger children typically need smaller serving sizes than adults, and as a child grows, serving sizes should increase. By the toddler years, the child's digestive system should be able to handle all the nutrients found in the normal family diet, and by school age, the child's taste preferences should be emerging. Most children prefer simple, plain foods and will eat what they need if they are not coaxed, nagged, bribed, rewarded, or influenced by television commercials. Childhood is a critical time for instilling good dietary habits. It is also a time for children to test their independence. Food is often a source of contention at mealtime, with the parents resorting to coaxing to get the child to eat or arguing with the child to gain compliance. Often the more pressure that is placed on the child at mealtime, the more negative the experience (see the Health Promotion box on fostering good dietary habits in children). Caregivers must supervise children's eating habits carefully and offer nutritious meals and snacks, but they also must allow the child the freedom to decide what and how much to eat.

 Health Promotion

Ways to Encourage Good Dietary Habits in Children

- Encourage children to be physically active.
- Encourage children to eat meals and snacks at regular times and at the table. By having set eating times, children learn that they cannot eat continually all day.
- Encourage children to help with food selection and preparation.
- Give small servings, or teach children how to serve themselves small servings. Then let them have seconds if they are still hungry.
- Keep nutritious snacks available, such as fruits, cheese, crackers, raw vegetables, and bread. Most children need to snack.
- Limit sweets, and do not use sweets and foods as rewards or bribes.
- Offer a variety of foods from all food groups, and allow children a choice of food, within reason.
- Offer new foods, but do not force children to eat foods they dislike. If the child will not eat a new food, quietly remove the food and offer it again at another time.
- Remember that physical growth and appetite come in spurts. Do not force children to eat more than they want to eat.
- Set a good example by practicing sound dietary and exercise habits.
- Try to make meals relaxed and enjoyable. Children need time to eat, and mealtimes should be a positive experience.

ADOLESCENCE

Puberty is another time in the child's life when growth is very rapid and nutrition becomes more important for proper development. Even though adolescents may understand good nutrition concepts, they may not relate this understanding to their own dietary habits. They usually react more readily to nutritional teaching if it applies to them directly. Adolescents may be more likely to practice good nutrition if they consider factors such as how nutrition helps skin (facial appearance), strength (for any athlete), and the ability to concentrate in school. Because of the accelerated growth rate and participation in sports, adolescents may need more food to supply their energy requirements. Because adolescents are seeking to establish their independence, their food choices are sometimes not wise ones and tend to be influenced by peer preference rather than by parental advice. Their diets often are filled with kilocalorie-rich and nutrient-poor snack foods. The era of fast food has given the adolescent access to high-calorie, nutritionally unbalanced meals. Too many fast food meals and too much snacking on empty calorie foods can lead to nutritional deficiencies. Common dietary inadequacies in adolescence include iron and calcium deficiencies (particularly in girls) and deficiencies in vitamins A and C and folic acid. Iron needs increase with the onset of menstruation in girls, and anemia is a common problem. When good nutritional habits have been established earlier in life, adolescent nutrition is likely to be better balanced than in cases in which nutritional teaching has been insufficient. Being part of a family that practices sound nutrition ensures that occasional lapses into sweets, fast foods, and other peer group food preferences do not create serious deficiencies.

Another nutritional factor to consider is that during adolescence, many teenagers experiment with alcohol and drugs, and these substances may have detrimental effects on their nutritional status as well.

Obesity in young people is a common problem in the United States. These years are a time of growth, and although obesity is not ideal, restrictive diets sometimes cause harm by suppressing development and can even lead to eating disorders. Adolescents should be encouraged to develop healthy eating habits and to use moderation when they consume soft drinks and sugar- and fat-laden snack foods. Adequate physical activity should be emphasized and television viewing and computer usage limited, along with other sedentary activities. Remind the adolescent that it is best to attempt weight-reduction diets only under the advice of a health care provider and with the guidance of a dietitian.

ADULTHOOD

During adulthood, nutrient needs change little in comparison with those of the adolescent. However, basal metabolic rate gradually slows, and the caloric needs decrease. At the same time, the activity level of many adults tends to decrease. The combined effects of decreased energy (caloric) needs and reduced physical activity often result in weight gain. As adults advance in years, it is important to remind them to eat nutrient-dense foods so that they can maintain adequate nutrition with fewer kilocalories and to maintain an active lifestyle.

Aging is associated with increased health concerns. Older adults suffer from conditions such as heart disease, arthritis, osteoporosis, diabetes, kidney disease, and other disorders with increased frequency. Special conditions may warrant differing nutrient needs that may vary greatly from individual to individual (see the Lifespan Considerations box for older adults). It is important to educate each patient about his or her dietary needs and explain the importance of any restrictions.

Nutritional Concerns of Adults in Long-Term Care Facilities

Malnutrition is a common problem among residents in long-term care facilities and profoundly influences physical health and quality of life. Poor nutritional status in these residents is related to several factors:

- Residents of long-term care facilities may experience cognitive or physical impairment, disease processes, and emotional disturbances, all of which affect nutritional intake and status.
- Many residents in the long-term care environment need some assistance or encouragement with eating and drinking. All care providers within the facility must be educated and trained to ensure that residents are able to obtain the nutrients needed.
- Restricted diets may be prescribed for residents of long-term care facilities. Common modifications include sodium and fat restrictions. Diabetic features may be instituted for groups of residents. Dietary restrictions can affect the palatability of the food and thereby hinder nutritional intake.
- Inadequate fluid intake and dehydration are sometimes secondary to decreased thirst sensation, decreased independence, dysphagia (difficulty swallowing), and incontinence.
- *Pressure injuries* may occur in nonambulatory residents, increasing kilocalorie, protein, and nutrient needs.

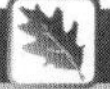

Lifespan Considerations

Older Adults

Aging and Nutrition

- Aging often affects the eating process. Changes in dentition, decreased saliva production, and alterations in swallowing have the potential to affect nutrient intake. It is sometimes necessary to adjust food consistency to facilitate food intake. Chopped, ground, pureed, and liquid diets tend to be less appealing to older people; serve them in as palatable a manner as possible.
- The aroma and taste of foods sometimes are affected by normal changes of aging. In addition, many older adults are on special diets that restrict the use of salt, sugars, and fats. This could lead to inadequate nutrient intake. The use of flavorings, seasonings, and spices to enhance flavor and aroma is often helpful.
- Older adults experience changes in digestive secretions, gastrointestinal mucosa, and enzyme production. This affects how food is digested, absorbed, and excreted. Water, dietary fiber, and adequate physical activity play an important role in preventing constipation in older adults.
- Aging often leads to loss of muscle mass, thereby reducing basal metabolic rate. Kilocalorie needs may decrease approximately 5% for each decade between ages 55 and 75 and 7% for each decade after age 75 depending on the activity level.
- Older adults may have a greater need for certain nutrients, including protein, riboflavin, vitamin B_6, folic acid, vitamin B_{12}, vitamin D, and calcium. A multivitamin and mineral supplement supplying 100% of the RDA is often beneficial for individuals with a low kilocalorie intake or during periods of poor intake. In addition, many older adults do not need as much vitamin A as do younger adults. Advise patients not to consume large doses of any nutrient unless they do so under a health care provider's supervision.
- Many older adults take numerous medications. Many medications tend to affect nutritional status. Be aware of drug-nutrient interactions and side effects that have the potential to influence dietary intake.
- Because of illness, restricted mobility, or financial limitations, or a combination of these, some older adults have difficulty obtaining and preparing nutritious food.
- Age-related social and mental changes such as forgetfulness, loneliness, and apathy are likely to affect the eating habits of older adults.
- Chronic medical conditions often necessitate the use of therapeutic diets. The most common such conditions in older adults include diabetes mellitus, cardiovascular disease, renal insufficiency, osteoporosis, diverticulosis, anemia, and lactose intolerance. Older adults who have long-standing dietary preferences and eating habits often find diet modification difficult. Always determine individual needs and situations before deciding the most appropriate nutrition therapy.

All members of the health care team must work together to coordinate care to ensure that the nutritional needs of the facility residents are met. Concerns must be identified quickly and treatment planned to ensure that nutritional compromise does not occur.

Offering familiar foods and incorporating cultural needs within the prescribed diet is important. Long-term care facilities have begun to embrace these principles in their dietary offerings. The more liberalized diet has mild restrictions on salt, fat, and concentrated sweets but avoids severe restrictions when possible. These dietary policies promote a sense of control and independence. Liquid nutritional supplements may help increase kilocalorie, protein, and nutrient intake if the resident's intake is less than optimal; however, these supplements should not be used as a substitute for regular food.

Fluids should be offered to residents at all meals and between meals to ensure adequate intake. It is important for health care providers to watch for signs of dehydration in long-term care residents and to correct any deficits quickly.

Family involvement and socialization at mealtime may help increase residents' dietary intake; encourage it whenever possible.

Nutrient-Drug Interactions

Many older adults take many prescription medications daily to manage medical conditions or disease states. They may be taking over-the-counter medications as well and not realize the consequences to their nutritional state; many medications have the capacity to affect a person's nutritional status adversely.

Medications have the potential to either increase or decrease appetite or the ability to eat. In many instances, they also affect the absorption, metabolism, and excretion of some nutrients. Conversely, food intake and vitamin or mineral supplementation may affect the absorption, distribution, metabolism, and action of some medications (Table 19.10).

Caffeine. Caffeine is a central nervous system stimulant and a diuretic. It has potential to cause nervousness, irritability, anxiety, insomnia, and heart dysrhythmias and palpitations. It also tends to affect blood pressure, circulation, and gastric acid secretion. Caffeine tolerance may lessen with aging. Older adults should be encouraged to use moderation in their intake of caffeine, as well as to be aware of its possible effects, which may resemble an anxiety attack. Reducing caffeine intake often can alleviate the symptoms of an anxiety attack and possibly prevent the need for another drug to relieve anxiety.

Table 19.10 Common Medications and Their Effect on Nutrition

DRUG TYPE	POSSIBLE DIETARY SIGNIFICANCE
Antacids	Reduced phosphorus, vitamin A, and iron absorption
Antibiotics	Reduced absorption as a result of vomiting, and increased excretion of multiple nutrients as a result of diarrhea Long-term therapy: may decrease vitamin K synthesis
Anticoagulants (e.g., warfarin)	Counteracted by vitamin K; consistent intake of vitamin K is essential Avoid high-dose supplements of vitamins A and E
Antihypertensives	Vitamin B_6 depletion; vitamin B_6 (hydralazine) supplementation is encouraged for patients with marginal diets
Aspirin	In long-term therapy: increased excretion of and decreased serum levels of ascorbic acid (vitamin C); with possible GI bleeding, loss of iron; vitamin K depletion Encourage diet rich in vitamin C
Diuretics (e.g., furosemide, chlorothiazide, hydrochlorothiazide)	Increased electrolyte excretion, leading to potassium, magnesium, and calcium depletion Potassium-rich diet is encouraged May necessitate potassium supplements
Diuretics (spironolactone)	Decreased potassium excretion; avoid supplements and salt substitutes
Laxatives	Decreased absorption of calcium, potassium, fat-soluble vitamins (especially vitamin D) Encourage fiber- and fluid-rich diets Encourage physical activity (may reduce the need for laxatives)

GI, Gastrointestinal.

MEDICAL NUTRITION THERAPY AND THERAPEUTIC DIETS

Medical nutrition therapy is the use of specific nutritional variations to build good health. It may involve simply modifying a nutritionally inadequate diet so that it becomes nutritionally adequate, or it may involve changing the texture or calorie content of the diet. A diet used as a medical treatment is called a **therapeutic diet.** Modifying a diet usually means adding or taking away specific nutrients or calories in a diet or changing the consistency of a diet, such as a pureed or soft diet. If a patient needs a special diet, the health care provider prescribes the diet, and it is up to the nurse to ensure that the patient understands and follows the diet, as well as to record how the patient reacts to it. When therapeutic diets are considered, it is important to account for the patient's cultural and religious preferences to increase compliance with the diet (see the Cultural Considerations box on nutrition).

Cultural Considerations

Culture and Nutrition

There is much to consider in dealing with patients of varied cultural, social, or religious backgrounds:

- Food habits are among the oldest and most deeply rooted aspects of many cultures.
- Food plays an important role in quality of life. The loss of culturally related foods during hospitalization or long-term care has great potential to affect the patient emotionally and physically.
- Never make assumptions. Be specific when asking questions regarding the patient's dietary preferences. Ask patients to provide a list of foods they like and dislike.
- The patient is likely to need help in marking the menu if he or she speaks another language or is unfamiliar with foods on the menu. Pictures of food are often helpful when there is a language barrier.
- Communication between the nursing staff and nutrition services is key to maintaining an adequate diet for the patient. Inform nutrition services if poor intake is noted so that the diet can be adjusted.
- Patients often have strong beliefs regarding certain foods or food combinations. Unless these beliefs are harmful to the patient, try to respect the patient's beliefs.
- In long-term care facilities, it is important to make every effort to work with the patient or family to provide special foods for observance of holidays, festivals, and other occasions.
- Occasionally, the family of a patient is permitted (with the health care provider's approval) to bring in food for the patient if the facility is unable to provide that food. Take special care to ensure food safety.

CONSISTENCY, TEXTURE, AND FREQUENCY MODIFICATIONS

The term *therapeutic diet* often is associated with nutrient-modified diets, such as low-fat or low-sodium diets. Modifications in textures, consistencies, and meal frequency, however, are also therapeutic in some cases. Most hospitals have standard diets based on consistency; these may include liquid, soft, and regular diets.

Liquid Diets

There are two types of liquid diets: clear liquid and full liquid. The clear liquid diet is nonirritating and consists of liquids that are easily digested and absorbed and leave little **residue**, or waste, in the GI tract. Because of that, very little stool is formed on a liquid diet. The clear liquid diet typically is used before diagnostic tests, particularly tests on the GI tract, and before surgery. It frequently is used postoperatively until peristalsis returns and sometimes is used during episodes of vomiting or diarrhea. The clear liquid diet is low in kilocalories, protein, and most nutrients. It is to be used temporarily, preferably for 2 to 3 days or less. Foods on a clear liquid diet include any type of liquid that you can see through, such as apple juice or white grape juice, fat-free broth or bouillon, plain gelatin, tea, or black coffee. When patients are on a clear liquid diet, they usually are given small meals more frequently, usually every 2 to 3 hours (Box 19.7).

Box 19.7 Foods Included in Liquid Diets

CLEAR LIQUIDS

- Bouillon
- Fat-free broth
- Gelatin
- Ginger ale, lemon-lime soda
- Popsicles
- Tea, coffee
- White grape, apple, cranberry juice

FULL LIQUIDS

- All clear liquids
- Custard
- Fruit and vegetable juices
- Ice cream, sherbet
- Milk, milk shakes
- Puddings
- Strained cereals
- Strained soups
- Supplemental formulas

The full liquid diet is used as a transition diet after a clear liquid diet. It is more nutritionally complete than a clear liquid diet but still is lacking in some nutrients, such as iron, zinc, and fiber. A liquid dietary supplement, or vitamins, may be added to increase the nutritive value of the diet. This diet, too, is best used only temporarily. Examples of foods on a full liquid diet include ice cream, creamy soups, gelatin, pudding, milk, and juices.

Soft and Low-Residue Diets

Soft diets often are an intermediate step when a patient is progressing from a liquid to a regular diet. Soft diets and low-residue diets also are used for many people with conditions affecting the GI tract, such as acute diverticulitis, inflammatory bowel disease, gastritis, and esophageal varices, and during periods of indigestion or diarrhea.

A soft diet is generally low in fiber and is similar to a regular diet. It includes foods from all food groups, including meat, fish, poultry, eggs, milk, grains, fruits, and vegetables, but foods with strong spices are avoided. Mechanical soft diets often are ordered for patients who have difficulty chewing or swallowing. All meats are ground, and fruits and vegetables are cooked and pureed. This diet is nutritionally adequate, but supplements may be added.

The low-residue diet is similar to the soft diet but also includes restrictions on milk and milk products, because they leave more residue in the colon. If milk is omitted, the patient needs to get adequate calcium from other sources.

High-Fiber Diets

The high-fiber diet is a variation of the regular diet and sometimes is used therapeutically. High-fiber diets often are used in the treatment of constipation. With adequate fluids, fiber has the capacity to reduce constipation in young patients, as well as in older adults, which helps reduce or eliminate the need for laxatives. A high-fiber diet also is recommended for patients with diverticulosis and often helps lessen the severity of symptoms and inflammation (diverticulitis).

Patient instructions concerning high-fiber diets should include recommendations promoting higher fiber options such as whole grains. Fiber intake should be increased gradually to prevent excess gas formation. Fresh cooked or raw fruits and vegetables are preferred over processed foods, which have lesser nutritional values and contain high levels of sodium and other preservatives.

KILOCALORIE MODIFICATIONS

The body requires a specific amount of energy each day to carry out its tasks. This energy comes from the intake of food and fluids. The body uses this energy to maintain necessary, involuntary body functions, also called **basal metabolic rate (BMR),** to digest nutrients, or diet-induced thermogenesis, and for physical activity. When energy intake equals energy output, the body is in zero energy balance, or equilibrium. During zero energy balance, weight remains constant. If energy intake exceeds energy output, the energy balance becomes positive. Positive energy balance results in weight gain. Conversely, if energy intake is less than energy output, the energy balance becomes negative, leading to weight loss.

High-Kilocalorie and High-Protein Diets

During times of physiologic stress—such as after surgery, during sepsis, or in the presence of bone fractures, burns, or pressure injuries—the body's energy and protein needs are increased. Medical trauma has the potential to increase the BMR greatly. Therefore, if energy needs are not met by diet, the patient loses protein stores and weight, and energy balance and nitrogen balance become negative.

In addition to the increased energy and protein needs, many patients with trauma and cancer suffer from *anorexia,* or lack of appetite. This adds to the already difficult task of maintaining adequate nutrition. High-kilocalorie and high-protein diets provide increased amounts of kilocalories and protein in small volumes and are used to help the compromised patient maintain adequate nutritional intake. Suggestions to help increase intake of kilocalories and protein are listed in Box 19.8.

Box 19.8 Suggestions for Increasing Kilocalories and Protein

- Add cheese to casseroles, soups, and sauces.
- Add nuts and dried fruits to cereals, breads, or desserts.
- Add powdered milk or protein powder to milkshakes, beverages, soups, puddings, and cooked cereals.
- Add sugar to foods when reasonable (this adds only kilocalories).
- Encourage the patient to eat high-calorie foods first and eat the low-calorie foods if still hungry.
- Have snacks available at all times.
- Spread peanut butter on crackers, fruit, or celery.
- Use extra meat, chicken, or fish in casseroles and soups.
- Use generous amounts of calorie-dense foods such as butter, vegetable oils, mayonnaise, cream cheese, sour cream, and cream in recipes, as spreads, or as dips.

When a patient is suffering from anorexia, the appearance of the food and how it is served may be the deciding factors in whether the patient eats it. Therefore it is important to maintain a positive attitude and provide encouragement when serving meals. Make meals as attractive as possible, and serve beverages, especially liquid nutritional supplements, in glasses, not cans. Make sure to serve meals promptly and at the correct temperature. Refrigerate snacks and supplements if necessary.

Obesity. The prevalence of obesity has reached epidemic proportions in the United States, and obesity is a growing health concern in developed and developing countries. In the United States, nearly 38% of adults and more than 17% of children and adolescents are obese. Obesity increases the risk for many diseases and health conditions, including hypertension, coronary heart disease, stroke, type 2 diabetes, dyslipidemias, osteoarthritis, gallbladder disease, some cancers, and sleep apnea. In addition to physical health risks, people who are obese often suffer from social prejudice and psychological issues related to their disease. Obesity dramatically affects quality of life and reduces average life expectancy.

Measurement of obesity. **Obesity** is defined as an excess of adipose tissue or body fat above the level considered healthy. **Body mass index (BMI)** is a number calculated from a person's weight and height (USDHHS, NIH, NHLBI, n.d.a). It provides an indicator of body fat and is used to screen for health problems related to weight. BMI accounts for total body weight and not just fat; some researchers say that this method is therefore not as accurate. Nonetheless, the BMI is recognized by many health care providers as the standard that defines overweight and obesity. BMI is determined by dividing body weight (in kilograms) by height (in meters squared). Fig. 19.5 lists the BMIs for various heights and weights. In general, if the BMI is below 18.5, the person is considered underweight; a BMI between 18.5 and 24.9 is considered within the "normal" range; if the BMI falls between 25 and 29.9, the person is considered overweight; and people with BMIs of 30 or greater are considered obese. To evaluate health status, it is important to consider *body composition* (the percentages of weight that comprise body fat versus lean tissue) as well as BMI. The location and amount of body fat in combination with BMI are sometimes better predictors of health risk than is BMI alone. Excess body fat in the upper body and the abdominal area in particular (central adiposity) increases the risk of cardiovascular disease and diabetes, whereas excess weight in the hips and the lower body poses a lesser risk.

Etiology of obesity. Obesity is caused by the chronic energy imbalance that results when more energy is consumed than expended. It is a complex disease, and much remains to be learned regarding its cause. Most experts agree that genetic, environmental, and behavioral factors contribute to obesity. The body has a powerful and multifaceted system that regulates energy intake and expenditure. Genetic, hormonal, and metabolic factors combine to control and regulate appetite and energy metabolism. Many obese individuals have a probable predisposition toward obesity that is precipitated by the environment in which they live and the lifestyle choices they make based on that environment.

Sedentary lifestyles are common in the United States. Only half of adults achieve the recommended amount of physical activity each day, and 25% report no leisure-time physical activity at all. Today's workforce has fewer positions requiring significant physical activity. Many workers spend their entire workday seated behind a desk. Some schools have cut physical education classes and recess time, so children are less physically active at school. Adults and children spend increasing amounts of time engaged in electronic entertainment with the television, computer, or handheld electronic devices. The typical American diet is also a factor in the cause of obesity. Because the food supply is abundant, it is easier to overeat. Food is readily available at any time of day, and it is possible to eat almost anywhere. High-fat, high-calorie prepackaged foods and sugar-laden soft drinks are readily accessible, and restaurants and supermarkets serve increasingly larger portions and package sizes. More people are consuming meals and snacks on the run, in the car, or in front of the computer or television and do not get much satiety, or satisfaction, from the food they eat.

Treatment of obesity. Obesity should be treated as a complex, chronic, relapsing disease. It is necessary to treat the obese person with empathy and without prejudice. Effective therapy requires a lifelong commitment to healthy lifestyle behaviors and addresses the medical and the psychosocial aspects of the disease. The goal of obesity treatment should be to achieve weight management, not just weight loss. That means the person should achieve the best weight possible in the context of overall health. For many people, the ideal weight goals suggested on charts and tables are impossible to realize. Patients need to set realistic, achievable goals that they can maintain. Even a modest weight loss of 5% to 15% of body weight often reduces obesity-related health risks significantly.

A sound weight management program requires hard work and strong individual motivation. Weight management must be something the patient is able to follow; it must focus not only on reducing energy intake but also on changing the patient's dietary and exercise habits. In general, a good diet should provide no fewer than 1200 kcal/day. When the diet provides less than 1500 kcal/day, a multivitamin and mineral supplement is recommended. Caution patients against the use of very low calorie and semistarvation diets unless they are under the strict care of a health care provider.

Physical activity is an integral part of any weight loss effort and is critical for weight maintenance after initial loss. Recommend the inclusion of physical activity most days of the week for the prescribed amount of time for initial weight loss, and encourage physical activity for weight maintenance. Increasing physical activity may seem daunting to patients who have previously been inactive, but encourage a gradual increase of physical activity until the goal is achieved. It may be necessary to exert the proper amount of physical activity in shorter increments throughout the day rather than in one long session. Recreational activities such as sports and gardening count toward the physical activity total. Aerobic (oxygen-using) exercises such as brisk walking, jogging, cycling, cross-country skiing, and cross-training appear to be most helpful in decreasing body fat. Resistance training (weight lifting, calisthenics) is also beneficial to maintain lean body mass and bone density. BMR decreases when muscle mass is lost; therefore resistance training tends to help prevent a reduction of BMR. As with the diet, encourage people to find a physical activity that they enjoy and are able to continue. Exercise does not have to be extreme; in fact, moderate-intensity exercise is more sustainable and carries less risk of injury.

Effective psychological interventions in the treatment of obesity foster a more healthy attitude about eating and body image. This usually includes counseling about self-esteem, body image, body acceptance, and coping with societal pressures. Patients often need to practice mindfulness and body awareness, learning to sense feelings of fullness by responding to internal rather than external cues. Through this process, many patients can reduce their focus on weight loss and food and establish a more constructive focus on life and good

	Normal						Overweight					Obese										Extreme Obesity														
BMI	19	20	21	22	23	24	25	26	27	28	29	30	31	32	33	34	35	36	37	38	39	40	41	42	43	44	45	46	47	48	49	50	51	52	53	54
Height (inches)	Body Weight (pounds)																																			
58	91	96	100	105	110	115	119	124	129	134	138	143	148	153	158	162	167	172	177	181	186	191	196	201	205	210	215	220	224	229	234	239	244	248	253	258
59	94	99	104	109	114	119	124	128	133	138	143	148	153	158	163	168	173	178	183	188	193	198	203	208	212	217	222	227	232	237	242	247	252	257	262	267
60	97	102	107	112	118	123	128	133	138	143	148	153	158	163	168	174	179	184	189	194	199	204	209	215	220	225	230	235	240	245	250	255	261	266	271	276
61	100	106	111	116	122	127	132	137	143	148	153	158	164	169	174	180	185	190	195	201	206	211	217	222	227	232	238	243	248	254	259	264	269	275	280	285
62	104	109	115	120	126	131	136	142	147	153	158	164	169	175	180	186	191	196	202	207	213	218	224	229	235	240	246	251	256	262	267	273	278	284	289	295
63	107	113	118	124	130	135	141	146	152	158	163	169	175	180	186	191	197	203	208	214	220	225	231	237	242	248	254	259	265	270	278	282	287	293	299	304
64	110	116	122	128	134	140	145	151	157	163	169	174	180	186	192	197	204	209	215	221	227	232	238	244	250	256	262	267	273	279	285	291	296	302	308	314
65	114	120	126	132	138	144	150	156	162	168	174	180	186	192	198	204	210	216	222	228	234	240	246	252	258	264	270	276	282	288	294	300	306	312	318	324
66	118	124	130	136	142	148	155	161	167	173	179	186	192	198	204	210	216	223	229	235	241	247	253	260	266	272	278	284	291	297	303	309	315	322	328	334
67	121	127	134	140	146	153	159	166	172	178	185	191	198	204	211	217	223	230	236	242	249	255	261	268	274	280	287	293	299	306	312	319	325	331	338	344
68	125	131	138	144	151	158	164	171	177	184	190	197	203	210	216	223	230	236	243	249	256	262	269	276	282	289	295	302	308	315	322	328	335	341	348	354
69	128	135	142	149	155	162	169	176	182	189	196	203	209	216	223	230	236	243	250	257	263	270	277	284	291	297	304	311	318	324	331	338	345	351	358	365
70	132	139	146	153	160	167	174	181	188	195	202	209	216	222	229	236	243	250	257	264	271	278	285	292	299	306	313	320	327	334	341	348	355	362	369	376
71	136	143	150	157	165	172	179	186	193	200	208	215	222	229	236	243	250	257	265	272	279	286	293	301	308	315	322	329	338	343	351	358	365	372	379	386
72	140	147	154	162	169	177	184	191	199	206	213	221	228	235	242	250	258	265	272	279	287	294	302	309	316	324	331	338	346	353	361	368	375	383	390	397
73	144	151	159	166	174	182	189	197	204	212	219	227	235	242	250	257	265	272	280	288	295	302	310	318	325	333	340	348	355	363	371	378	386	393	401	408
74	148	155	163	171	179	186	194	202	210	218	225	233	241	249	256	264	272	280	287	295	303	311	319	326	334	342	350	358	365	373	381	389	396	404	412	420
75	152	160	168	176	184	192	200	208	216	224	232	240	248	256	264	272	279	287	295	303	311	319	327	335	343	351	359	367	375	383	391	399	407	415	423	431
76	156	164	172	180	189	197	205	213	221	230	238	246	254	263	271	279	287	295	304	312	320	328	336	344	353	361	369	377	385	394	402	410	418	426	435	443

Fig. 19.5 Body mass index. (Data from National Institutes of Health [NIH]: *Body mass index table 1*, n.d. From *https://www.nhlbi.nih.gov/health/educational/lose_wt/BMI/bmi_tbl.htm*.)

health. A support system—consisting of family, friends, or a support group—is also beneficial.

Bariatric surgery for the treatment of obesity has become common. Candidates for bariatric surgery are usually morbidly obese (BMI ≥ 40) or have a BMI of 35 or higher with other medical conditions such as cardiovascular disease or type 2 diabetes. Patients achieve substantial weight loss after bariatric surgery, and if diet and exercise recommendations are followed, do not regain the weight. Patients with weight-related disorders such as preexisting diabetes, hyperlipidemia, hypertension, or sleep apnea also may experience substantial improvement in these conditions. In addition, mortality rates among surgically treated obese patients appear to be lower than in those who receive treatment with traditional methods. For most patients, the benefits of bariatric surgery outweigh the risks; however, as with any major surgery, risks do exist and include nutrition-related complications such as nutrient deficiencies, dumping syndrome, and diarrhea. Because patients can eat only small amounts of food after bariatric surgery, the health care provider usually prescribes a multivitamin and mineral supplement, along with other nutritional supplements as needed. The most common nutritional deficiencies after bariatric surgery include those of iron, folic acid, and vitamin B_{12}. After bariatric surgery, it is important to encourage the patient to eat small portion sizes, to eat slowly, and to chew foods completely. They also should consume beverages and food at separate times and avoid foods that are poorly tolerated. It is also important to encourage adequate amounts of physical activity to help maintain the weight loss (USDHHS, NIH, NIDDK, n.d.a).

Pharmacologic therapy involves the use of prescription drugs or over-the-counter medications to treat obesity. If patients use weight-loss drugs, it is important to make these drugs part of a comprehensive program along with diet therapy and physical activity. Over-the-counter medications sometimes help suppress appetite; however, the effect is usually temporary.

CARBOHYDRATE-MODIFIED DIETS

Diabetes Mellitus

Carbohydrate-modified diets are used most often in the treatment of diabetes mellitus. Diabetes mellitus is a disease in which the body does not produce or properly use insulin. Insulin is a hormone that is needed to convert sugar, starches, and other food into the energy needed for daily life. The cause of diabetes is unknown, although genetics and environmental factors such as obesity and lack of exercise appear to play a role.

There are two major types of diabetes mellitus. Type 1 diabetes mellitus, most often diagnosed in children and young adults, is a disease in which the body does not produce any insulin (hormone produced by the pancreas needed to use glucose). People with type 1 diabetes are required to take insulin therapy for life. Type 1 diabetes accounts for approximately 5% of diabetes cases (American Diabetes Association, n.d.b). Type 2 diabetes mellitus is a metabolic disorder resulting from the body's inability to make enough or properly use insulin. It is the most common form of the disease and accounts for about 95% of diabetes cases (American Diabetes Association, n.d.a). Because of the increasing number of older Americans and a higher incidence of obesity and sedentary lifestyles, the number of people in whom type 2 diabetes is diagnosed has increased dramatically.

Nutrition therapy for diabetes mellitus. Diabetes is a disease that directly involves how well the body uses the nutrients consumed. Because of that, nutrition plays a major role in the treatment of diabetes. Overall, the goals for people with diabetes are the control and prevention of complications. Therefore normal nutrition and dietary modification to control blood glucose and lipid levels are extremely important. Educating the patient on the proper diet is important so that the patient can make changes in food and exercise habits to improve metabolic control.

Achieving nutrition-related goals necessitates a coordinated effort by a health care team that includes the patient's health care provider, the nurse, the diabetic educator, the registered dietitian, the patient, and the patient's family. It is necessary to individualize nutrition therapy for each patient with diabetes; standardized preprinted diet sheets should be avoided. All patients with diabetes need the opportunity to develop a realistic and achievable eating plan to which they will adhere. Lifestyle, current eating and exercise patterns, caloric and nutrient needs, the presence of other diseases, and the use of insulin or oral antidiabetic medication are necessary considerations in developing an eating plan for a patient with diabetes.

Nutrition recommendations for a healthy lifestyle are important for all people; what differs for those with diabetes is the need to monitor more closely and control carbohydrate intake. The patient with diabetes must coordinate the timing of meals and snacks and administration of insulin or oral diabetic medications with exercise. Consistent meal timing, approximately every 4 to 5 hours, and consistent carbohydrate content are important to stress during patient teaching. Advise inclusion in the diet of foods containing carbohydrates from whole grains, fruits, vegetables, and low-fat milk. The amount of dietary carbohydrate intake should be based on individual needs as outlined in the MyPlate dietary guidelines, as well as the *Dietary Guidelines for Americans* (USDA and USDHHS, 2015). The *total amount* of carbohydrate in meals and snacks is more important than the source or type of carbohydrate. Patients with diabetes should be encouraged to consume a variety of fiber-containing foods, but there is no reason to recommend a greater amount of fiber than any person in the general population would consume.

People with diabetes also should limit the amount of fat in their diet to control blood lipid levels. It is recommended that saturated fat be limited to less than 5% to 6% of calories and dietary cholesterol to less than 200 mg/day (AHA, 2017). In addition, *trans* fatty acids should be kept to a minimum. Evidence suggests that the use of monounsaturated fats in place of some carbohydrates often helps lower blood triglyceride levels and improves glycemic control as well. Two or more servings of fish per week (except commercially fried filets) are recommended (USDHHS, 2005).

Type 1 diabetes mellitus. Because most patients with type 1 diabetes are still in childhood or adolescence at the time of diagnosis, it is necessary for the eating plan to provide adequate kilocalories for normal growth and development and to be as flexible as possible. It is also important to balance carbohydrate intake with insulin administration and exercise. Initially, consistent timing and consistent content of meals and snacks are essential to determine insulin requirements. Patients are then able to monitor blood glucose levels and learn to adjust insulin dosages according to blood glucose patterns.

Type 2 diabetes mellitus. The primary goals of nutrition therapy for type 2 diabetes are to achieve and maintain desirable weight, normal blood cholesterol concentration, and normal blood glucose levels. Because many people with type 2 diabetes are overweight and insulin resistant, it is helpful to encourage lifestyle changes that result in reduced energy intake and increased physical activity. Mild to moderate weight loss (5% to 7% of starting weight) has been shown to improve metabolic control, even if desirable weight is not achieved. Increased physical activity can aid in weight reduction, improve blood glucose levels, decrease insulin resistance, and reduce cardiovascular risk factors.

Meal planning approaches. Even though patients with diabetes must monitor the carbohydrate and fat content of their diet, they do not need to buy special foods. Many meal planning tools are available for them to use with foods normally available.

Exchange lists have been used for many years and sometimes still are used in diabetic meal planning. They are complicated and may be overwhelming for some patients. In an exchange list, foods are divided into groups on the basis of carbohydrate, protein, and fat content. Typically, the patient receives instructions to include a certain number of servings from each food group at a particular meal or snack. By identifying correct serving sizes and the nutrient components of food groups, patients are able to better control their carbohydrate, fat, and kilocalorie intake throughout the day (Table 19.11).

Carbohydrate counting is a meal planning approach that focuses on the total amount of carbohydrates eaten at meals and snacks. For some patients with diabetes, this approach is much simpler than exchange lists. It focuses on just one nutrient, and patients can see a direct correlation between carbohydrate intake and the blood glucose level, which makes it easier for them to comply with the recommended eating plan. For others, carbohydrate counting can be difficult because of the weighing and measuring of the food and the need to calculate the grams of carbohydrates consumed. Protein and fat are not counted with this type of meal planning, but the patient should be encouraged to eat the same amount of protein each day and choose foods that are low in fat.

Other nutritional considerations. If a person taking insulin fails to consume adequate carbohydrates, the blood glucose level may drop, causing hypoglycemia (low blood glucose level). Symptoms of hypoglycemia include headache, disorientation, weakness, perspiration, shallow breathing, nervousness, visual disturbances, and vertigo, and sometimes the individual may become unconscious. It is necessary to treat hypoglycemia with immediate administration of glucose or any carbohydrate that contains glucose. A good strategy for patients to practice is the 15-15 rule: take 15 g of carbohydrate, wait 15 minutes, and test blood glucose to see whether the response to the carbohydrate is adequate. If the patient becomes unconscious, intravenous administration of glucose is essential.

Acute illness increases the risk of diabetic ketoacidosis in patients with type 1 diabetes and increases the risk for hyperosmolar hyperglycemic nonketotic syndrome in patients with type 2 diabetes. During acute illness, it is important for the patient to continue taking insulin and carefully monitoring blood glucose levels. Encourage the patient to drink adequate amounts of fluids and to ingest carbohydrates, especially if the blood glucose level falls below normal levels. Beverages such as juices and punch, popsicles, flavored gelatin, crackers, puddings, and ice cream contain carbohydrates and tend to be more palatable to sick people.

For people with diabetes, the guidelines for alcohol use are the same as for the general population. If individuals choose to drink alcohol, teach them to limit intake: one drink per day for women and two drinks per day for men. Because alcohol increases the risk of hypoglycemia, consuming it with food is best.

Dumping Syndrome

Dumping syndrome is possible after surgery in which a portion or all of the stomach is removed (partial or total gastrectomy) or after bariatric surgery for weight reduction. Dumping syndrome can occur when the contents of the stomach empty too quickly into the small intestine. The partially digested food draws excess fluid into the small intestine, which causes nausea, cramping, diarrhea, sweating, lightheadedness, and palpitations.

Table 19.11 Example of an Exchange List

FOOD	SERVING SIZE
Grains	
Bagel	1/4 large bagel (1 oz)
Breads	
White, whole-grain, French, Italian, pumpernickel, rye, sourdough, unfrosted raisin or cinnamon	1 slice (1 oz)
Reduced calorie, light	2 slices (1 1/2 oz)
Cornbread	1 3/4-inch cube (1 1/2 oz)
Hot dog bun or hamburger bun	1/2 bun (3/4 oz)
Roll, plain	1 small roll (1 oz)
Stuffing, bread	1/3 cup
Crackers	
Animal	8 crackers
Graham, 2 1/2 inch square	3 squares
Oyster	20 crackers
Round, butter-type	6 crackers
Saltine-type	6 crackers
Granola or snack bar	1 bar (3/4 oz)
Matzoh, all shapes and sizes	3/4 oz
Pancake	1 pancake (4 inches across, 1/4 inch thick)
Waffle	1 waffle (4-inch square or 4 inches across)

FOOD	SERVING SIZE
Vegetable	
Hominy	3/4 cup
Marinara, pasta or spaghetti sauce	1/2 cup
Mixed vegetables with corn or peas	1 cup
Parsnips	1/2 cup
Peas, green	1/2 cup
Potato	
Baked with skin	1/4 large potato (3 oz)
Boiled, all kinds	1/2 cup or 1/2 medium potato
Mashed with milk and fat	1/2 cup
French-fried (oven baked)	1 cup (2 oz)
Squash, winter (acorn or butternut)	1 cup
Yam or sweet potato, plain	1/2 cup (3 1/2 oz)
Snacks	
Popcorn	
No fat added	3 cups
With butter added	3 cups
Pretzels	3/4 oz
Rice cakes	2 cakes (4 inches across)
Snack chips	
Baked (potato, pita)	About 8 chips (3/4 oz)
Regular (tortilla, potato)	About 13 chips (1 oz)

The Food Lists are the basis of a meal planning system designed by a committee of the American Diabetes Association and The Academy of Nutrition and Dietetics. Although designed primarily for people with diabetes and others who must follow special diets, the Food Lists are based on principles of good nutrition that apply to everyone.

These signs and symptoms usually occur shortly after meals or after the consumption of too much simple or refined sugar.

Diet therapy is aimed at slowing gastric emptying and distributing the amount of gastric contents in the bowel over time. This involves giving small, frequent meals that are higher in protein and fat and lower in carbohydrates. The patient is encouraged to avoid concentrated sweets and to drink fluids 30 to 60 minutes before or after a meal. Having the patient lie down for 30 to 60 minutes after a meal also may help slow stomach emptying. The dumping syndrome diet is, in some cases, needed only temporarily until the body adjusts to the changes caused by surgery.

Lactose Intolerance

Lactose intolerance occurs when there is a lack of the digestive enzyme *lactase.* In the absence of lactase, the GI tract is unable to break down lactose, the milk sugar. This condition is hereditary; the incidence of this disorder is increased among African Americans, Hispanics, Asian Americans, and Native Americans. Lactose intolerance is not the same condition as an allergy to cow's milk. Symptoms usually occur 30 minutes to 2 hours after ingestion of milk products and include nausea, cramps, a bloated feeling, flatulence, and diarrhea.

The diet for lactose intolerance excludes milk and milk products, such as ice cream, puddings, cheese, and powdered milk. Affected patients often need to avoid foods with milk added, such as biscuit or muffin mixes, some soups, and other prepared foods. In addition, many processed foods—such as waffles, pancakes, and processed meats—contain lactose. Dietary counseling should include alternative sources of calcium and potential recommendations for supplementation.

When there is a deficiency rather than a total absence of lactase, patients are often able to tolerate small amounts of milk products, especially yogurt and cheese. Several lactase enzyme–containing preparations are also available to take before consuming dairy products, and many grocery stores now carry lactose-free milks and milk products.

FAT-MODIFIED DIETS

Research has shown that modifying the amount of fat in the diet may reduce the risk of heart and vascular disease by about 14% and that the risk for some cancers can be reduced as well.

Low-Fat Diets

A low-fat diet has limited amounts of total fat, saturated fat, and *trans* fatty acids. This type of diet is needed for the prevention and treatment of *atherosclerosis* (a disorder characterized by buildup of cholesterol and lipids on the artery walls), heart disease, and *hyperlipidemia* (elevated levels of blood lipids).

To help Americans reduce the risk of cardiovascular disease, the American Heart Association has recommended dietary guidelines for the general population to decrease the amount of fat in the diet. The National Cholesterol Education Program has also developed the Therapeutic Lifestyle Changes (TLC) diet to help decrease the amount of fat and cholesterol ingested (Table 19.12) (USDHHS, 2005).

Many patients have a difficult time complying with a low-fat diet because they think the required foods lack flavor and are not as satisfying. Even though they need to reduce saturated and *trans* fatty acids in the diet, patients are still able to choose low-fat foods from all the food groups. Encourage them to choose low-fat dairy products, lean meats, skinless poultry, and fish. Advise limiting eggs to four or fewer per week and limiting organ meats, such as liver, to one serving or less per week. Limits are also necessary on added fats, such as butter, stick margarine, mayonnaise, cream, and sour cream.

The inclusion of monounsaturated fats and omega-3 fatty acids in the diet often helps lower blood cholesterol and triglyceride levels. Therefore encourage patients to substitute unsaturated fatty acids in the diet instead of saturated and *trans* fatty acids. Teach patients to identify food sources of these fats, such as fish, olive oil, canola oil, peanut oil, flaxseed oil, soy products, and nuts.

Keep in mind that fat possesses many good qualities and offers much pleasure when eaten. Many Americans tend to rebel against a low-fat diet because they believe it is necessary to eliminate all fatty foods. Choosing a low-fat and low-cholesterol diet does not mean "never eat cheese because it contains fat" or "never eat egg yolks because they contain cholesterol." It is the *total* amount of fat, saturated fat, and cholesterol that matters. Besides, foods such as cheese and egg yolks contribute nutrients necessary to the diet, and sometimes eliminating all high-fat foods compromises the diet's overall nutritional value. Therefore rather than totally eliminating high-fat foods, patients should be encouraged to use moderation. They should balance high-fat foods with other foods that contain less fat and cholesterol. By adhering to balance, variety, and moderation, patients are still able to enjoy some of their favorite foods while following a healthy, fat-controlled diet.

Fat-Controlled Diets

The fat-controlled diet is used to treat symptoms of diarrhea, steatorrhea, and flatulence or to treat diseases of the hepatobiliary tract, pancreas, intestinal mucosa, and the lymphatic system, as well as malabsorption syndromes.

These diets sometimes restrict fat to as little as 25 g/day depending on the severity of the symptoms. With this severe fat restriction, no visible fats (e.g., butter, cream, oil) are allowed. Only nonfat dairy products and lean meat, fish, and poultry (no more than 5 oz/day) are allowed. It is important to encourage adequate consumption of grains, cereals, fruits, and vegetables. Vitamin and mineral supplementation also may be necessary to offset the nutrient deficiencies caused by prolonged or excessive diarrhea or steatorrhea.

Metabolic Syndrome

Metabolic syndrome is a name for a group of metabolic risk factors that occur together and increase the risk for coronary artery disease, stroke, and type 2 diabetes. These risk factors include abdominal obesity, dyslipidemia, elevated blood pressure, and insulin resistance. The most important of these risk factors appears to be abdominal obesity (waist circumference of 40 inches or more in men and 35 inches or more in women) and insulin resistance (fasting blood glucose level of 100 mg/dL or higher). The prevalence of metabolic syndrome has increased dramatically; 50 million cases have been estimated in the United States. For affected patients without established diabetes, metabolic syndrome doubles the risk of developing atherosclerotic cardiovascular disease (ASCVD); for those with diabetes, the risk is increased fivefold. Thus the early diagnosis and treatment of metabolic syndrome is likely to help reduce the incidence of ASCVD.

The goal of treatment for metabolic syndrome is to reduce the risk for heart disease and diabetes. Lifestyle changes usually are initiated first in the treatment of metabolic syndrome. Lifestyle changes include cessation of cigarette smoking, weight loss in overweight or obese individuals, increased physical activity, and a fat-controlled diet. Depending upon the severity of risk factors and the patient's response to the therapeutic lifestyle changes, more aggressive treatments or medications may be needed.

PROTEIN-, ELECTROLYTE-, AND FLUID-MODIFIED DIETS

Protein-Restricted Diets

In disease states, increased protein intake often is needed to facilitate healing. However, in the presence of defects in protein metabolism or excretion, it is best to reduce or at least control protein intake. Two such conditions, chronic renal failure and cirrhosis of the liver, sometimes necessitate protein restrictions.

In renal failure, the kidneys are unable to excrete protein waste products. These waste products build up in the bloodstream, leading to a condition known as *azotemia*. If a patient is experiencing renal failure, a modest protein restriction may delay the need for

Table 19.12 **Guidelines for Following the Therapeutic Lifestyle Changes (TLC) Diet**

FOOD GROUPS	CHOOSE ...	GO EASY ON ...
Meat, Poultry, and Fish		
<5 oz/day; 2 servings of fish/week	• Lean fresh meats, extra-lean ground beef, and lean deli meats[a] • Poultry without the skin, ground turkey made from white meat • Fish and shellfish	• Meats with visible fat and marbling • Regular ground beef • Processed meats: sausage, bacon, frankfurters, cold cuts • Organ meats • Duck and goose • Deep-fried meats, poultry, or fish • Shellfish (some are high in cholesterol; use moderate portions)
Eggs		
<2 egg yolks/week	• Eggs (limit yolks to 2/wk; substitute 2 egg whites for 1 egg in recipes)	
Dry Beans and Nuts		
	• Dry beans and peas, fat-free refried beans, tofu • Nuts[a] (in moderation)	
Milk, Yogurt, and Cheese		
2–3 servings/day	• Fat-free (skim) or 1% milk, buttermilk, soy milk • Fat-free or reduced-fat cheeses[a] (3 g of fat or less per oz) • Low-fat or nonfat cottage cheese[a] • Low-fat or fat-free yogurt	• Whole or 2% milk, half-and-half • Whole-milk yogurt • Full-fat cheese with more than 3 g fat per oz
Fruits and Vegetables		
5 or more servings/day	• Fresh, frozen, canned, or dried fruits and vegetables • Add more vegetables to meat dishes, casseroles, or soups • Keep fresh fruits and vegetables readily available for snacks • Use fruit as dessert	• Vegetables with high-calorie sauces • Fruits with added sugar • Deep-fried vegetables (including French fries) • Limit juices, instead choosing whole fruits and vegetables for more fiber
Breads, Cereals, Rice, Pasta, and Other Grains		
6 or more servings/day depending on energy needs	• Breads, bread products, and cereals made from whole grains such as whole wheat, buckwheat, bulgur (cracked wheat), oats, rye, millet, quinoa, bran • Brown rice, wild rice • Whole-grain pastas • Popcorn	• White breads and products made with refined grains that are lower in fiber (check label) • Baked goods made with added fat and eggs, such as muffins, biscuits, croissants, and butter rolls
Fats and Oils		
Limited total amount; replace saturated fats with unsaturated fats; read labels to identify saturated and *trans* fat content	• Liquid vegetable oils (canola, corn, olive, peanut, safflower, sesame, soybean, and sunflower) • Margarines with liquid vegetable oils as first ingredient (soft tub, liquid, or vegetable oil spreads) • Light or nonfat mayonnaise and salad dressing • Reduced-fat sour cream, cream cheese, and whipped toppings	• Butter, lard, fatback, bacon drippings • Margarines with hydrogenated or partially hydrogenated oil as the first ingredient (read label for *trans* fat) • Solid shortening • Coconut milk; coconut, palm and palm-kernel oils • Full-fat sour cream, cream cheese, whipped cream
Sweets, Snacks, Condiments		
To be used occasionally on basis of caloric needs	• Low-fat ice cream, frozen yogurt, sorbet, sherbet, or low-fat puddings • Angel food cake; low-fat brownies • Fat-free or low-fat cookies such as animal crackers, vanilla wafers, gingersnaps, graham crackers • Whole-grain snack crackers[a]	• Regular ice cream; pudding made with whole or 2% milk • Doughnuts and pastries • Pie, regular cakes, and cookies • Snack crackers with high fat content

[a]Sometimes contain high levels of sodium.
Modified from US Department of Health and Human Services: *Lowering your cholesterol with TLC.* Retrieved from *www.nhlbi.nih.gov/health/public/heart/chol/chol_tlc.pdf.*

dialysis. Protein restriction in renal failure involves limiting the total amount of protein consumed and emphasizing the use of high-quality proteins. High-quality proteins are complete proteins found in eggs, meat, poultry, fish, and milk products. Incomplete proteins, those found in plant products such as dried beans and whole grains, contribute to azotemia and must be limited. Once a patient has been placed on renal dialysis, protein needs are greater than for the normal population; however, the dietary emphasis is still on complete proteins.

Cirrhosis is a chronic degenerative disease of the liver in which scar tissue develops and hinders the liver's effectiveness in removing ammonia. The ammonia then builds up in the bloodstream and, if not controlled, can lead to hepatic coma, brain damage, and death. In the presence of cirrhosis, protein intake initially should be at or above the DRI to facilitate healing and tissue regeneration. However, if blood ammonia levels become elevated, a low-protein diet is recommended. Special nutritional support formulas with modified protein content have been developed for use by patients with renal failure and cirrhosis to lower the protein content of the diet.

Sodium-Restricted Diets

Sodium-restricted diets may be used for a variety of medical conditions; however, they are used most often in the treatment of hypertension or heart failure. In 2001 the National Institutes of Health and the National Heart, Lung, and Blood Institute developed the Dietary Approaches to Stop Hypertension (DASH) diet. This diet quickly became popular among health care providers because it was shown to effectively lower blood pressure by limiting sodium intake to either 1500 to 2400 mg/day. The DASH diet also emphasizes the inclusion of fruit and vegetables, as well as low-fat or nonfat milk products (Box 19.9) (National Heart, Lung, and Blood Institute, n.d.).

Sodium-restricted diets also may be used in cases of water retention or edema, especially in the presence of heart failure. With congestive heart failure, a decrease in sodium intake is necessary to alleviate pulmonary and peripheral edema and reduce the workload of the heart. Some other conditions that may warrant a sodium-restricted diet include myocardial infarction, cirrhosis accompanied by ascites, and chronic renal failure.

Sodium-restricted diets vary in degree. The no-added-salt diet is the least restrictive, allowing 2000 to 3000 mg/day of sodium. This diet allows the use of most foods with the exception of highly salted snack foods and prepared foods. Patients following this diet must read nutrition labels to determine the sodium content of food products and then decide which foods are appropriate for their diet. Encourage patients to limit the amount of salt in cooking or at the table (Box 19.10). Other sodium-restricted diets may allow as much as 2000 mg/day or as little as 500 mg/day of sodium.

Box 19.9 Daily and Weekly DASH Eating Plan Goals for a 2000-Calorie-a-Day Diet

FOOD GROUP	DAILY SERVINGS
Grains	6–8
Meats, poultry, and fish	6 or less
Vegetables	4–5
Fruit	4–5
Low-fat or fat-free dairy products	2–3
Fats and oils	2–3
Sodium	2300 mg[a]
	WEEKLY SERVINGS
Nuts, seeds, dry beans, and peas	4–5
Sweets	5 or less

[a]1500 milligrams (mg) sodium lowers blood pressure even further than 2300 mg sodium daily.
From National Institutes of Health: DASH eating plan, 2015. Retrieved from *https://www.nhlbi.nih.gov/health/health-topics/topics/dash*.

Box 19.10 What to Limit in Sodium-Restricted Diets

- Canned vegetables (fresh and frozen are lower in sodium)
- Commercial mixes such as pasta, stuffing, muffins, and potatoes
- Leavening agents such as baking soda and baking powder
- Processed cheeses
- Regular canned soups, broths, and bouillon
- Salt in cooking or at the table
- Salt-preserved foods, such as smoked or cured meats or pickled foods
- Salty snack foods such as pretzels, popcorn, and chips
- Spices and condiments that contain sodium, such as soy sauce, barbeque sauce, Worcestershire and steak sauces, meat tenderizers, monosodium glutamate (MSG), spice salts, and salad dressings

NOTE: In general, the more processed or "instant" a food is, the more sodium it contains.

Potassium-Modified Diets

Potassium plays many important roles in the body, and a lack of, or an increase in the amounts of, potassium can cause a variety of problems. Increased intake of potassium may help with blood pressure control when it is in direct proportion to sodium intake. The American Heart Association and proponents of the DASH diet encourage balanced sodium/potassium intake in a diet that emphasizes fruits, vegetables, and low-fat dairy products. This diet is rich in potassium, magnesium, and calcium and helps reduce blood pressure in many cases. People taking potassium-wasting diuretics may need larger amounts of potassium in their diet or potassium supplements to offset the loss of potassium.

In end-stage renal disease and other kidney disease, it is sometimes necessary to restrict potassium intake to as little as 2000 mg/day. During renal failure, potassium is retained, which leads to a buildup of potassium in the bloodstream. If dietary intake is not controlled, blood potassium levels potentially can increase to the point of causing dysrhythmias and sudden cardiac arrest.

Fluid-Modified Diets

Fluid is a big part of the diet and can be found in many foods. Of course, all beverages add fluid to the diet, as do gelatins, ice cream, sherbet, puddings, popsicles, fruit ices, and soups. In good health, most adults need between 2 and 3 L of water a day to maintain hydration; in the presence of certain illnesses, however, the patient's water intake may be restricted.

During end-stage renal disease and other kidney disease with low urine output, fluid is restricted to 500 to 750 mL/day (approximately 2 to 3 cups) plus an amount equal to any daily urine output. Fluid restrictions are also common during congestive heart failure, directly after a myocardial infarction, in hepatic coma, or in the presence of ascites.

In the hospital, fluid restrictions often are divided between the nursing and the dietary departments. For example, if a patient has a 1000-mL fluid restriction, the dietary department sometimes is allowed to provide the patient with 600 mL/day, and the nursing department gives 400 mL/day. The amount of fluid allowed for nursing depends on the patient's intravenous (IV) and medication needs.

Although patients have fluid restrictions, they often experience excessive thirst. Some suggestions to help alleviate thirst include rinsing the mouth with cold mouthwash, putting lemon into cold water to make it more refreshing, freezing fluid so that it takes longer to consume, eating cold fruits and raw vegetables, chewing gum, sucking on breath mints or hard candies (in moderation), brushing teeth often, and limiting sodium intake (see the Patient Teaching box on fluid restrictions).

 Patient Teaching

Fluid Restrictions

The health care provider and dietitian determine the exact fluid restriction. The nurse must teach and reinforce the fluid restriction by

- Explaining the rationale for the fluid restriction
- Indicating whether the restriction is temporary or permanent
- Identifying the various sources of fluid intake (e.g., intravenous fluids; fluid with medications; fluid in foods such as soup, ice cream, or gelatin)
- Teaching what "mL" represents and comparing it with measures with which the patient is familiar; for example, "You are allowed 1000 mL of fluid per day; this is about the same as 1 quart, or 4 cups"
- Showing patients the volume of fluid they are allowed
- Suggesting ways to alleviate thirst without drinking fluids
- Discussing the consequences of overconsumption of fluids

Increased fluid intake is a common dietary treatment for renal calculi (kidney stones) and urinary tract infection. Additional fluid helps dilute the urine and increase urinary output. Fluid needs are also higher during periods of diarrhea, vomiting, or malabsorption, as in inflammatory bowel disease. To prevent dehydration, the patient needs to replace fluids that are lost.

Patients with burn injuries lose a large amount of fluids from the wounds. Immediately after a severe burn, fluids, electrolytes, and protein are given intravenously rather than orally, because burn-injured patients experience a temporary loss of bowel function. Once bowel activity resumes, adequate fluids are a necessary part of dietary treatment. Burn-injured victims also require large amounts of protein, kilocalories, and certain vitamins and minerals.

Most conditions necessitating medical nutrition therapy involve combinations of therapeutic diets. To summarize, Table 19.13 lists different medical conditions and the diets commonly prescribed.

NUTRITIONAL SUPPORT

Occasionally a patient is unable to consume an oral diet. In these instances, alternative feeding methods are available in the form of tube feedings or IV feedings.

TUBE FEEDINGS

A **tube feeding** is the administration of nutritionally balanced, liquefied foods or formula through a tube inserted into the stomach, the duodenum, or the jejunum by way of a nasogastric tube or an ostomy. The feeding sometimes is referred to as **enteral nutrition** (administration of nutrients into the GI tract). Tube feedings typically are indicated when a patient is unable to chew or swallow, such as after oral surgery or facial trauma; when a patient has no appetite or refuses to eat; in times of great nutritional need, such as in the patient suffering burns or trauma; in comatose patients; or during periods of moderate malabsorption or diarrhea.

Tube feedings are used only when all or part of the GI tract is functioning. Tube feedings can be administered by way of a nasogastric tube, a tube that is passed through the nose and into the stomach (Fig. 19.6). If regurgitation is common or the amount of gastric residual is high, a nasojejunal or nasoduodenal tube (a tube that is passed through the nose and into the jejunum or the duodenum) sometimes is used to reduce the risk of aspiration.

In cases in which long-term tube feedings are necessary, as in a patient with a gastrectomy or intestinal resection or in a patient with an upper GI obstruction, feeding ostomies sometimes are employed. Feeding ostomies are surgical openings through which a feeding tube is passed. It is possible to make ostomies into the esophagus (esophagostomy), the stomach (gastrostomy), or the jejunum (jejunostomy) (see Fig. 19.6). Ostomy feedings do not have to be continuous and sometimes

Table 19.13 Summary of Diet Modifications

CONDITION	POSSIBLE DIET MODIFICATIONS
Acquired immunodeficiency syndrome (AIDS)	High calorie and high protein; increased fluid intake; mechanical soft diet; possible tube feeding or total parenteral nutrition (TPN)
Atherosclerosis	Low fat and cholesterol; avoid *trans* fatty acids; high fiber; increase fruits, vegetables and whole grain products; low calorie or sodium restrictions if necessary
Burns	High calorie and high protein; increased fluid intake; increased vitamins and minerals
Cancer	High calorie and high protein, depending on the type of cancer, dietary adjustments are made on the basis of symptoms; increased vitamins and minerals; increased fluids; possible tube feeding or TPN
Cirrhosis, hepatic coma	Protein restricted; possible sodium, fat, and fluid restriction; no alcohol; vitamin and mineral supplementation; mechanical soft diet
Congestive heart failure	Sodium restricted; fluid restricted; small, frequent feedings; soft diet; possible calorie restriction; avoid or limit alcohol
Constipation	High fiber; increased fluid intake; increased natural laxative fruits
Cystic fibrosis	High calorie, fat, and protein; increased sodium intake; vitamin and mineral supplementation, enzyme replacement therapy; possible tube feeding or TPN
Diabetes mellitus	Carbohydrate counting and Food Exchange System to meet individual needs; fat controlled; high fiber; planned consistent meals
Diverticular disease	Increased fiber and fluid; avoid foods that cause discomfort
Dumping syndrome	Carbohydrate restricted; no concentrated sweets; small, frequent feedings
Gallbladder disease	Low fat; when necessary, calorie-restricted; small frequent meals
Gastritis	Low fat and/or acidic foods; avoid foods that increase symptoms
Gastroesophageal reflux disease (GERD)	Calorie restrictions to decrease weight; low fat and/or acidic foods; avoid lying down after meals; don't eat within 3 hours of going to bed and sleep with head of bed elevated
Hepatitis	High protein, high carbohydrate, moderate fat; tube feedings or TPN may be necessary
Hiatal hernia	Small, frequent feedings; calorie restrictions to decrease weight; avoid lying down after meals; don't eat within 3 hours of going to bed and sleep with head of bed elevated
Hyperlipidemia	Low cholesterol and saturated *trans* fats; high fiber
Hypertension	Restricted calorie to decrease weight; sodium restrictions; DASH diet; vitamin/mineral supplementation esp. calcium, potassium and magnesium; increased fiber
Hypoglycemia	Carbohydrate counting and Food Exchange System to meet individual needs; fat controlled; high fiber; consistent meals
Inflammatory bowel disease	Consistent diet; avoid fructose, lactose, sorbitol, caffeine and alcohol; avoid gas forming foods; increased fiber; fluid and electrolyte replacement; vitamin and mineral supplementation
Lactose intolerance	Lactose restricted
Myocardial infarction (heart attack)	Low calorie initially then advanced to meet energy needs; small, frequent meals; soft diet; low fat and sodium; possible fluid restrictions
Nausea and vomiting	Small, frequent feedings; low fat; bland, soft, dry foods; increase fluid intake slowly
Obesity	Calorie restricted; fat controlled; high fiber
Oral disorders	
Broken jaw or oral surgery	Mechanical soft or liquid diet; small, frequent meals
Dental caries, periodontal disease, ill-fitting dentures, missing teeth	Mechanical soft diet
Dry mouth	Mechanical soft diet; increased fluid intake
Dysphagia (difficulty swallowing)	Individualize diet; mechanical soft diet; possible enteral feeding
Ulcers of mouth or gums	Mechanical soft diet; limited acidic and spicy foods
Pancreatitis	Low fat; small, frequent feedings; increased fluids; possible enteral feedings or TPN

Table 19.13 Summary of Diet Modifications—cont'd

CONDITION	POSSIBLE DIET MODIFICATIONS
Renal calculi (kidney stones)	Depends on type of calculi
Calcium oxalate	Low animal protein and sodium intake; increase fiber; maintain calcium intake; avoid high doses of vitamin C; increase fluid intake
Calcium phosphate	Decrease phosphorus intake; increase fluid intake
Uric acid	Low animal protein and purine intake; increase fluid intake
Cystine	Low sodium; avoid excess protein; increase fluid intake
Renal failure	
Acute	Protein restricted; high calorie; sodium and potassium controlled based on individual losses; vitamin/mineral supplementation possible; phosphate and calcium maintained based on body weight; possible fluid restrictions
Chronic	Limited protein; low sodium, potassium, phosphorus and calcium; vitamin and mineral supplementation; fluid intake balanced with output but not necessarily restricted
Underweight	High calorie; high protein; high carbohydrate; moderate fat; vitamin/mineral supplementation
Wound healing, pressure injuries	High protein, increased carbohydrate and fat intake; increased fluid intake; increased vitamins (especially vitamin C) and minerals (especially zinc and iron)

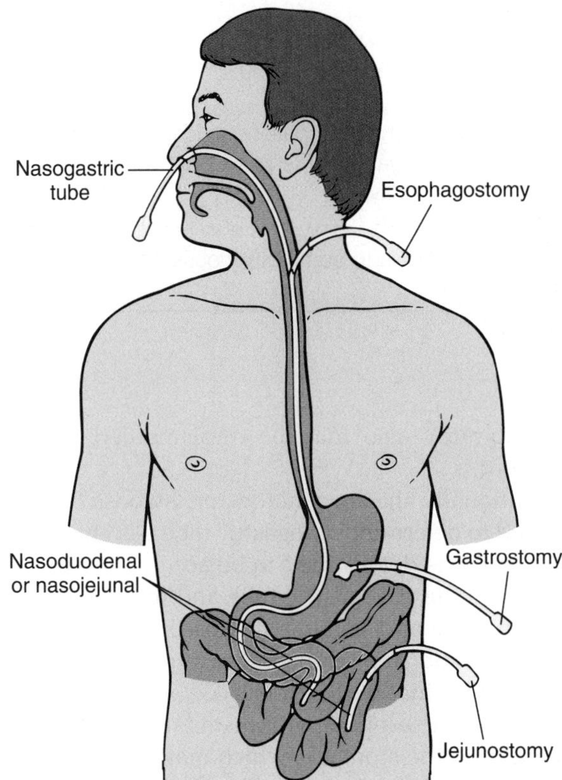

Fig. 19.6 Tube feeding sites.

are given intermittently, thus permitting more freedom of movement.

Tube feedings given on a continuous basis usually are administered through a continuous-drip pump that administers the formula slowly over 16 to 24 hours. In intermittent feedings, a specific volume of formula is administered over a short time, usually about 20 to 30 minutes. This type of intermittent feeding usually is done four to six times daily. Bolus feedings (in which a 4- to 6-hour volume of formula is administered in a matter of minutes) also may be given, but most patients tolerate them poorly.

Tube feedings, although necessary in some circumstances, are not without complications, and it is necessary to monitor them closely. Distention, diarrhea, and nausea may indicate that the formula strength, volume, or rate is too great. Dumping syndrome is also possible with rapid and concentrated formula delivery. Other complications that can arise include diarrhea; contamination of formula; infection; aspiration; overhydration or dehydration; electrolyte and glucose abnormalities; and disturbances in the levels of other nutrients. The development of liver abnormalities also may occur (Table 19.14). See the Home Care Considerations box for patients receiving home enteral feeding.

Home Care Considerations

Patients Receiving Enteral Feeding

- Teach the patient or primary caregiver (1) to verify correct placement of the tube before administering formula; (2) the method of gastrointestinal (GI) fluid pH measurement and the expected range; (3) *not* to administer a feeding if there is any doubt concerning tube placement; and (4) to administer feedings at room temperature.
- Teach the patient to report any adverse signs and symptoms, such as diarrhea, abdominal cramps, nausea and vomiting, or respiratory distress.
- Teach the patient to care for the gastrostomy or jejunostomy tube site and about adverse signs and symptoms to report (such as drainage, redness, swelling, or tube displacement).

Table 19.14 Common Problems and Nursing Interventions Associated With Administering Tube Feedings

PROBLEM	NURSING INTERVENTION
Abdominal distention	Abdominal distention commonly occurs when the stomach empties too slowly. Omit the nourishment if the amount aspirated from the stomach before feeding is 100–150 mL. In some instances, the health care provider orders the feedings to be stopped, at least temporarily.
Acute otitis media	Otitis media is possible when the nasogastric tube presses against the eustachian tube, which causes obstruction and edema. It is best prevented by turning the patient from side to side frequently, at least q 2 hr, and by using as small a nasogastric tube as possible.
Aspiration	Aspiration is best prevented by ensuring that the tube is in the stomach before the nourishment is introduced and by keeping the head of the patient's bed elevated between 30 and 45 degrees. Suction of the mouth and throat sometimes is necessary when regurgitation and vomiting occur.
Clogged tube	Occlusion of the tube is prevented by keeping a constant flow rate when nourishment is given continuously and by flushing the tube well after single feedings. It is acceptable to gently irrigate the tube after obtaining a medical order. If irrigation does not relieve the obstruction, sometimes it is necessary to remove and replace the tube.
Diarrhea	Diarrhea commonly is caused by introducing nourishment too rapidly or using formula or nourishment that is too concentrated. The usual care is to decrease the strength of the nourishment and administer it more slowly. An antidiarrheal drug sometimes is ordered.
High electrolyte blood levels	High electrolyte blood levels are usually the result of the patient's receiving insufficient fluids. Water usually is offered through the tube at a rate of 100 mL q 4–6 hr (exact amount varies according to health care provider's order).
Irritation of nasal and palate tissues	Tissue irritation occurs as a result of pressure on tissues by the nasogastric tube. Some procedures include removal of the tube a few inches every day, coating of the tube with an antibiotic ointment, and then reinsertion.
Irritation of oral mucous membranes	Oral mucous membranes often become dry and irritated when the patient is unable to take nourishment by mouth and is receiving nourishment by gavage. Frequent oral hygiene helps prevent this problem; administer it at least four times a day.
Nausea	Nausea commonly is caused by introducing nourishment too rapidly. It is also possible that the formula of the nourishment is unsatisfactory. Usual care is to administer nourishment more slowly and possibly change the formula.

Nasogastric Tube Feedings

When a nasogastric tube is used for enteral nutrition or medication administration, it is important to check for placement of the tube before administering medication or tube feedings. An improperly placed feeding tube can cause complications such as aspiration pneumonia, pneumothorax, and peritonitis, all of which can be avoided simply by checking placement of the tube before giving any medication or feeding.

The most dependable means of checking tube placement is through radiologic confirmation. Chest radiographs are considered the standard of care, especially for confirming placement of small-diameter tubes. Unfortunately, not all institutions have policies mandating this method. X-ray studies also are not performed usually for large-diameter nasogastric and nasointestinal tubes, because most clinicians believe that the tubes are less likely to enter the lung undetected. The next best method for confirming feeding tube placement is through pH measurement. By testing the pH of fluid aspirated from a newly inserted feeding tube, it is possible to make reasonable assumptions about the tube's location. Visual inspection of gastric fluid aspirated also may be implemented to verify placement.

Traditionally, the auscultatory, or "swoosh," method was used to determine nasogastric tube placement. Tube placement was determined to be accurate by pushing air through the nasogastric tube and into the stomach with a syringe and using a stethoscope to listen for a gurgling sound over the epigastric region. However, air in a tube inadvertently placed in the lungs, the pharynx, or the esophagus transmits sound similar to that entering the stomach, which makes the reliability of this method questionable. Therefore it is not a good method to use solely to verify tube placement.

Many potential complications are possible with administration of tube feedings, and the cost of managing those complications or infections is high. It is important to use proper technique when administering enteral feedings and to maintain the cleanliness of the equipment. Skill 19.1 describes the administration of enteral feedings through a nasogastric tube, and Skill 19.2 describes the administration of enteral feedings via a gastrostomy or jejunostomy tube. Using good

Text continued on p. 565

Skill 19.1 Administering Nasogastric Tube Feedings

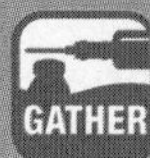

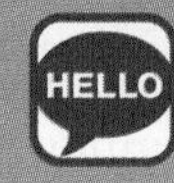

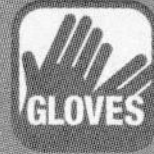

NURSING ACTION *(RATIONALE)*

1. Check health care provider's order. *(Verification of order is needed to determine formula type, rate, route, and frequency of feedings.)*
2. Introduce self. *(Decreases patient's anxiety.)*
3. Identify patient. *(Use two identifiers [name/birth date] to ensure that procedure is performed on the correct patient.)*
4. Explain procedure and reason it is being done in terms that the patient will understand. *(Decreases patient's anxiety and prepares the patient for the procedure.)*
5. Allow time for the patient to ask questions. *(May increase patient cooperation.)*
6. Determine the need for and provide patient teaching during procedure. *(Reduces patient anxiety and increases patient's knowledge of procedure. May also increase compliance.)*
7. Determine whether there is abdominal distention or tenderness. *(Absence of bowel sounds indicates inability of the GI tract to digest or absorb nutrients, and feeding should be withheld.)*
8. Listen for bowel sounds before each feeding. *(Action also provides baseline information for later comparisons.)*
9. Assemble equipment. *(Having appropriate equipment assembled may help the procedure move more smoothly and help gain patient's trust.)*
   - 30- to 60-mL syringe
   - Testing equipment (Some facilities require glucose testing before feedings.)
   - Disposable feeding bag
   - Gloves
   - Infusion pump (for intestinal feedings)
   - Prescribed enteral feeding formula
   - Stethoscope and pH indicator strips
10. Wash hands and don clean gloves according to agency policy and guidelines from CDC and OSHA. *(Reduces spread of microorganisms and protects the patient and the nurse.)*
11. Close door or pull privacy curtain. *(Maintains patient's privacy.)*
12. Raise bed to comfortable working height; lower side rail on side nearest the nurse. *(Raising bed promotes proper body mechanics in the patient and prevents muscle strain in the caregiver.)*
13. Elevate head of bed (Fowler's position). *(Elevating head of bed decreases risk of aspiration during feeding.)*
14. Establish tube placement/check for residual. *(Indicates accurate tube placement and gastric emptying.)*
    a. Aspirate gastric contents with syringe. *(Gastric secretions are usually green, brown, or tan.)*

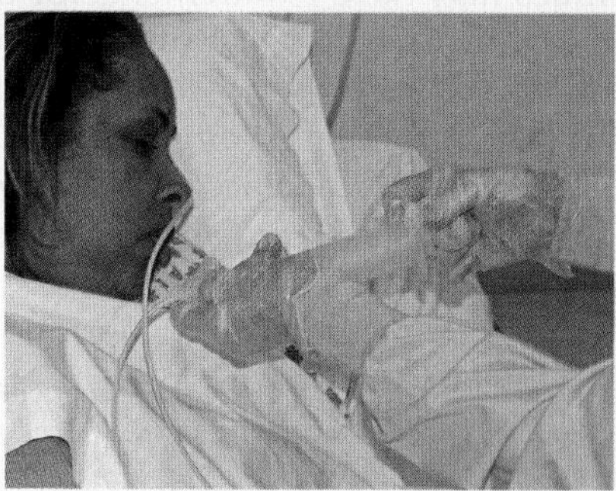

    b. Place drop of gastric contents on pH paper. *(Gastric contents normally have a pH range of 0 to 4.)*

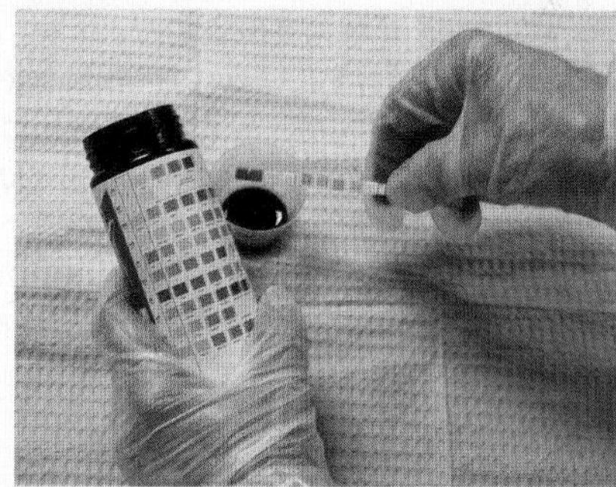

    c. If aspiration cannot be done, suspect that tube is occluded or kinked. Attempt to flush with 30 mL tap water. *(Flushing may dislodge any obstruction if present.)*
    d. If flushing cannot be done, check nasal cavity or back of throat (if tube is inserted nasally). Check for kinking. *(If no kinking is seen, inability to flush may indicate tube is no longer in the correct location.)*
15. Replace gastric contents. If residual amount is greater than 150 mL, check orders for further direction. *(Prevents fluid and electrolyte imbalances.)* May need to notify health care provider of excess residual. Feeding may be withheld 1 h and then started at slower rate.
16. Prepare formula for feeding. Check expiration date to make sure formula has not expired.
    a. Before pouring from can, check expiration date, and wipe off top of can. *(Wiping off top of can prevent debris from entering the formula when it is poured.)*

Continued

Skill 19.1 Administering Nasogastric Tube Feedings—cont'd

b. Before using premixed base, check date and time, as well as correct strength of formula. Check temperature. *(Some patients cannot handle full-strength formula, and it must be diluted before feeding.)* Check agency policy. Facilities may have requirements for the temperature and storage of the solutions.

17. Administer feeding.

a. Bolus or intermittent feedings:

(1) Kink or pinch feeding tube. *(Prevents leakage and air from entering patient's stomach.)*

(2) Remove plunger from syringe and insert syringe tip into feeding tube. Release feeding tube. *(Allows formula to be poured into syringe, and allows free flow of formula through the tube.)*

(3) Fill syringe with formula. Keep syringe 18 inches or less above site. *(Keeping the syringe low prevents too rapid an infusion of formula and is better tolerated.)*

(4) Flush tube with 30–60 mL tap water (or prescribed amount/solution) when feeding is completed. *(Prevents tube from clogging with thick formula.)*

(5) Remove syringe and cap or plug tube. *(Prevents leakage of gastric contents between feedings.)*

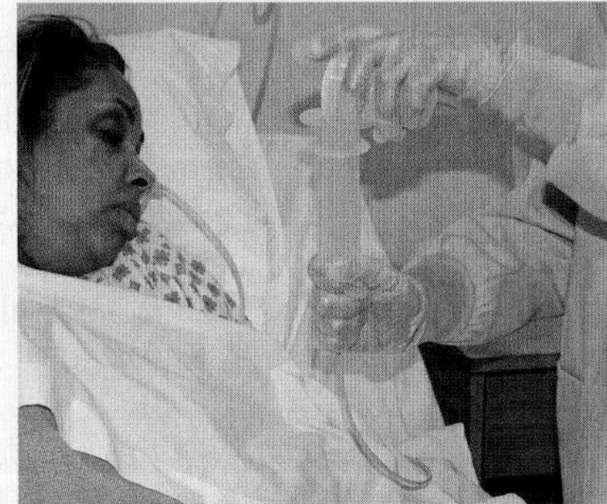

b. Continuous drip method:

(1) Assemble gavage bag and tubing. *(Gavage bag allows larger amounts of formula to be given.)*

(2) Verify tube placement and residual. *(Ensures feeding is delivered to stomach.)*

(3) Clamp tubing, and attach gavage bag. *(Clamping prevents unwanted leakage of formula.)*

(4) Fill gavage bag with appropriate type and amount of formula. *(Verify formula type and amount before starting feeding.)*

(5) Unclamp and prime tubing, and then reclamp. *(Eliminates air from tubing and helps prevent gas formation.)*

(6) Label gavage bag with date, time, initials, formula type and strength, and amount of formula. *(Communicates essential information to all staff.)*

(7) Kink feeding tube and uncap; secure gavage tubing to feeding tube. *(Kinking tubing prevents leakage of gastric contents.)*

(8) Set rate by adjusting roller clamp on tubing. *(Set to infuse ordered amount of feeding in appropriate amount of time.)*

(9) Flush tube with 30–60 mL tap water (or prescribed amount/solution) when feeding is completed. *(Prevents clogging of the feeding tube by thick formula.)*

(10) Kink feeding tube, remove gavage tubing, and recap feeding tube. *(Prevents leakage of gastric contents between feedings.)*

(11) Place cap on end of gavage tubing. *(Protects gavage tubing from contamination between feedings.)*

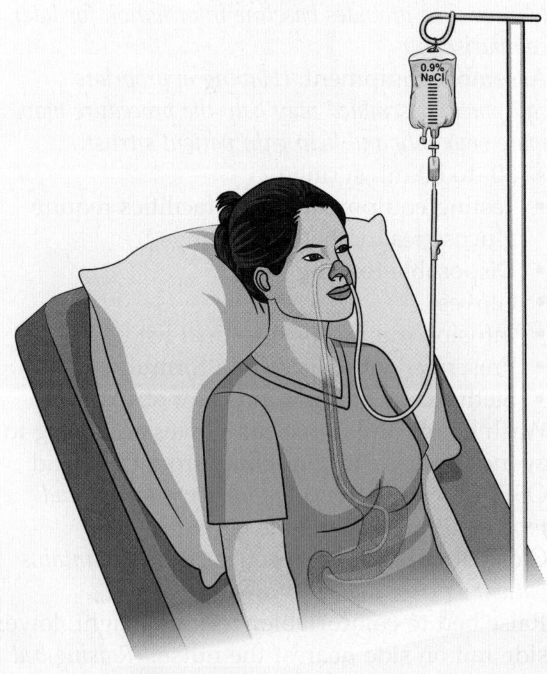

Skill 19.1 Administering Nasogastric Tube Feedings—cont'd

c. Feeding via infusion pump:

(1) Verify feeding tube placement and residual. *(Ensures feeding is delivered to stomach and it is emptying appropriately.)*

(2) Prepare administration set with correct type and amount of formula. *(Use only enough formula for 8 hr to prevent spoiling.)*

(3) Clamp gavage tubing, spike bag, unclamp and prime tubing, and reclamp tubing. *(Prevents air from entering stomach and causing gas formation.)*

(4) Label bag with date, time, initials, and formula type and strength. *(Enhances communication between caregivers.)*

(5) Hang tube feeding set on IV pole with infusion pump. Connect tubing to pump and set rate. *(Make sure to check facility policy for pump type and use.)*

(6) Kink end of feeding tube, remove cap, and attach infusion tubing. *(Kinking the feeding tube prevents air from entering stomach and leakage of gastric contents.)*

(7) Open roller clamp on tubing, and turn on infusion pump. *(Pump will sound alarm if roller clamp is not open.)*

(8) Check residual q 4 hr. *(Ensures that tubing has not been dislodged.)*

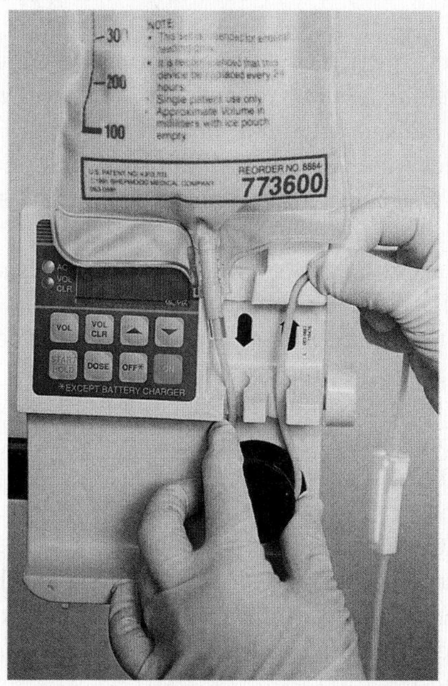

18. Flush tube with 30–60 mL water (or ordered solution) after a bolus feeding or q 4–8 hr during continuous feeding. *(Prevents clogging of the tube by thick formula or gastric secretions. Water replacement is needed to help maintain fluid volume.)*

19. Clean equipment appropriately after use. *(Helps prevent bacterial growth and allows for reuse of equipment. Most facilities require replacing equipment q 24 hr.)*

20. Make sure patient is comfortable, and educate about symptoms to report. Make sure call light is within patient's reach. *(Cramping and diarrhea must be reported as this may signal the infusion is being administered too rapidly or the patient is not tolerating it.)*

21. Raise side rails and lower bed to lowest position. *(Promotes safety. Be aware of facility policy regarding side rail use.)*

22. Remove gloves, dispose of used supplies, and wash hands. *(Reduces spread of microorganisms.)*

23. Document the following. *(All treatments and patient's response must be documented.)*
- Verification of tube placement/residual
- Type and amount of feeding
- Rate of feeding (if applicable)
- How feeding tube flushed
- Patient's tolerance of feeding
- Any adverse effects of feeding
- Patient education

24. Monitor weight and laboratory values daily. *(Improving laboratory values and weight gain are indications of improved nutritional status.)*

25. Observe patient for shortness of breath, low oxygenation saturation, vomiting, or color changes. *(Could indicate aspiration or intolerance of feeding.)*

CDC, Centers for Disease Control and Prevention; *GI*, gastrointestinal; *IV*, intravenous; *OSHA*, Occupational Safety and Health Administration.
Figure for Step 17c(8) from Potter PA, Perry AG: *Essentials for nursing practice*, ed 8, St. Louis, 2015, Mosby.

Skill 19.2 Administering Enteral Feedings via Gastrostomy or Jejunostomy

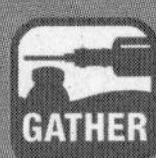

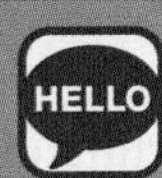

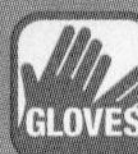

Observe all guidelines for nasogastric tube feedings. Follow Skill 19.1 to verify tube placement; then continue with the following steps.

NURSING ACTION *(RATIONALE)*

1. Verify tube placement. *(Indicates accurate tube placement and gastric emptying.)*
   a. Gastrostomy tube:
      (1) Aspirate gastric secretions. *(Gastric secretions are usually green, brown, or tan.)*
      (2) Check appearance and pH. *(Gastric contents have a pH range of 0–4.)*
      (3) Return contents to stomach. *(Prevents fluid and electrolyte imbalances.)*
      (4) Note amount of residual. *(May need to notify health care provider if residual is excessive.)*
   b. Jejunostomy tube:
      (1) Aspirate intestinal secretions. *(Intestinal contents are medium to deep golden or bile stained.)*
      (2) Observe appearance and amount (usually 10 mL or less).
      (3) Check pH. *(Intestinal contents have a pH of 7 or greater.)*
2. Flush tube with 30 mL tap water. *(Clears tube of any remaining formula or obstructions.)*
3. Initiate feedings.
   a. Syringe feedings *(Initial feeding may be via syringe to determine patient's tolerance.)*
      (1) Pinch proximal end of tube.
      (2) Remove plunger, and attach syringe to end of tube.
      (3) Fill syringe with formula and allow it to empty gradually. *(Too rapid an infusion may cause complications.)*
      (4) Refill until appropriate amount has been delivered.
   b. Continuous drip method *(Feedings are usually given continuously via pump to ensure proper absorption.)*
      (1) Fill feeding container with enough formula for 8 h of feeding. *(More than 8 h worth of formula may spoil.)*
      (2) Hang container on IV pole and prime tubing. *(Excess air in the GI tract can cause gas formation and patient discomfort.)*
      (3) Thread tubing on pump.
      (4) Connect tubing to end of feeding tube.
      (5) Begin infusion at prescribed rate.
4. Evaluate skin around tube exit site. *(Redness, swelling, drainage, or foul odor could indicate infection and must be reported to the health care provider.)*
5. Clean skin around tube. *(Helps prevent infection. Dressings may or may not be ordered.)*
6. Dispose of supplies. Wash hands. *(Prevents transmission of microorganisms.)*
7. Monitor fingerstick blood glucose levels q 4–6 h until maximum administration rate is reached and maintained for 24 h. *(Enteral feeding formulas may increase blood glucose levels.)*
8. Monitor intake and output q 24 h. *(Indicators of fluid balance or fluid volume excess.)*
9. Weigh patient daily until tolerance is established; then weigh three times a week. *(Weight gain is a good indicator of improved nutritional status. A sudden gain of 2 lb in 24 h may indicate fluid volume excess.)*
10. Observe return of normal laboratory values. *(Improving albumin, transferrin, and prealbumin levels indicate improved nutritional status.)*
11. Inspect tube site for signs of pressure. *(Enteral tubes may cause pressure areas on patient's skin especially if they are tucked into clothing.)*
12. Document the following. *(All treatments and patient's response must be documented.)*
    - Verification of tube placement/residual
    - Type and amount of feeding
    - Rate of feeding (if applicable)
    - How feeding tube is flushed
    - Patient's tolerance of feeding
    - Any adverse effects of feeding
    - Patient education
13. Observe patient for shortness of breath, low oxygenation saturation, vomiting, or color changes. *(Could indicate aspiration or intolerance of feeding.)*

hand hygiene technique and clean equipment and hanging formula only for the recommended time to prevent spoiling are crucial steps to avoid contamination of the system and subsequent infection in the patient.

PARENTERAL NUTRITION

Parenteral nutrition, or *hyperalimentation,* is the term used to describe intravenous feedings. Parenteral nutrition can be given in several ways: through peripheral veins, such as those in the arms or the legs, and through a large central vein. When the nurse administers parenteral nutrition through peripheral veins, it is called *peripheral parenteral nutrition (PPN).* If it is given through a large central vein, it is called **total parenteral nutrition (TPN).**

TPN usually refers to the administration of a hypertonic solution into the superior vena cava by way of a catheter threaded through either the subclavian vein or the internal jugular vein (Fig. 19.7). TPN and PPN formulas generally are composed of glucose, amino acids, vitamins, minerals, and electrolytes in amounts individualized for the patient. Fat, in the form of triglycerides, also can be given as a supplement to the main formula, but it is administered separately through a Y-connector tube or into a peripheral vein.

Parenteral nutrition is indicated for patients with a nonfunctioning or dysfunctional GI tract, those needing 3000 kcal/day or less, those needing supplementation to an oral diet, and those requiring short-term therapy (less than 3 weeks). When IV nutrition is necessary, PPN should be considered the first choice of administration because it carries less risk of complications, necessitates less monitoring, and costs less than administration by the central venous route. TPN is indicated for patients needing a highly concentrated formula, such as those who need more kilocalories than can be administered peripherally or those requiring fluid restrictions. A concentrated formula delivers more kilocalories and nutrients in a smaller volume. Other candidates for TPN include patients who have to receive IV feedings for more than 3 weeks and those with unsuitable or unavailable peripheral veins.

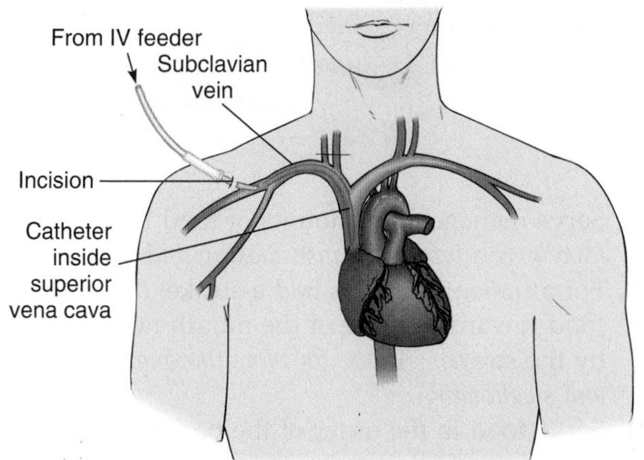

Fig. 19.7 Central venous catheter placement during administration of parenteral nutrition.

TPN necessitates surgical placement of a catheter in one of the central veins to establish central venous access. This imposes significant risks on the patient, including sepsis, pneumothorax, hemothorax, phlebitis, and thrombosis. It is necessary to maintain catheter site asepsis and keep feeding solutions sterile. Constant monitoring of the clinical status of the patient is essential.

Some patients receiving TPN experience fluid and electrolyte imbalances, hyperglycemia or hypoglycemia, metabolic disturbances, and bone disorders such as osteomalacia (softening of the bones). For this reason, monitor blood chemistry values frequently and check the blood glucose level several times each day. Administration of regular insulin on a sliding scale may be necessary to maintain blood glucose levels below 200 mg/dL.

FEEDING THE PATIENT

Patients who are weak, are paralyzed, have a cast, or have some other form of physical or neurologic limitation may not be able to feed themselves or may need assistance with feeding. It may be the responsibility of the nurse or the unlicensed assistive personnel to assist these patients with meals.

In assisting patients to eat, it is necessary to create a relaxed mood so that patients do not feel rushed. It is also important to allow them time for their usual before-meal rituals. Many people pray before eating; others need to wash their hands and face. Provide the time and privacy for the patient's usual routine. This demonstrates caring and respect for the patient. Before feeding, ask the patient in which order he or she wants food and fluids offered. Also make sure the temperature of the food is not too hot to burn the patient. When feeding a patient, use a spoon because spoons are less likely than forks to cause injury. Give the patient small bites, and allow for chewing and swallowing the food without being rushed.

Patients who are not able to feed themselves sometimes believe they are losing control over their lives and feel angry, humiliated, and embarrassed. Some of them do not like depending on others. Some may be depressed and resentful, and others may refuse to eat. Allow these patients to try to feed themselves as much as possible, and offer assistance as needed. Make sure they do not exceed activity limits ordered by the health care provider, but provide them positive reinforcement and support.

Many visually impaired patients are keenly aware of food aromas. Often they can identify foods being served. Always tell a visually impaired patient what foods and fluids are on the tray and indicate their location on the tray by referring to the numbers on a clock (Fig. 19.8). When feeding a visually impaired

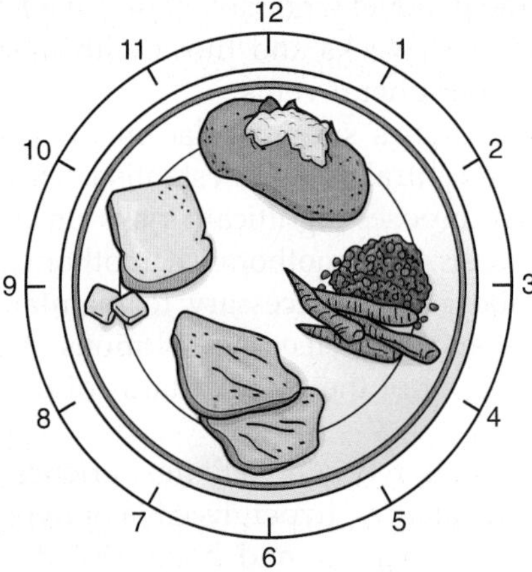

Fig. 19.8 For the visually impaired patient: "The potato is at the 12 o'clock position." (From Sorrentino SA, Remmert LN: *Mosby's textbook for nursing assistants*, ed 9, St. Louis, 2017, Mosby.)

patient, identify what food or fluid is offered before placing the food or drink in the patient's mouth.

Meals have always been a social activity, and many patients may not have family or friends visiting at mealtime. Therefore engage the patient in pleasant conversation while giving the patient enough time to chew and swallow food. Also, sit facing the patient. Sitting is more relaxing and demonstrates to the patient unhurried care and support from the staff. Standing communicates nonverbally that the staff does not have time and that they really are not interested in the patient. Facing the patient allows the nurse to see how well the patient is eating and whether the patient has problems swallowing. Skill 19.3 describes techniques to use in assisting patients with eating.

Skill 19.3 Assisting Patients With Eating

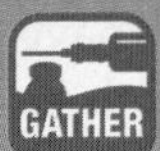

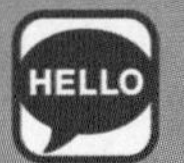

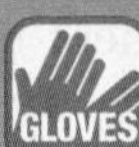

NURSING ACTION *(RATIONALE)*

1. Complete or delay care that will interfere with eating. *(It is best to serve food at its appropriate temperature.)*
2. Provide a period of rest or quiet before meals. *(A tired or excited patient is usually in no mood to eat.)*
3. Offer the patient a bedpan or urinal before mealtime. *(Having to urinate may decrease the patient's appetite.)*
4. Provide the patient with an opportunity for hand washing, and offer mouth care before the meal. *(Freshening up before a meal may increase appetite.)*
5. Remove soiled articles or clutter from room. *(An unattractive environment may decrease the desire to eat.)*
6. Make the patient comfortable for eating; give pain medication at least 30 minutes before a meal. *(Patients can enjoy their food more if they are comfortable.)*
7. Raise the head of the bed to a sitting position. *(Sitting or semi-sitting position makes swallowing easier.)*
8. Cover the patient's upper chest with a napkin or some form of clothing protector. *(Prevents soiling of patient's clothes or gown.)*
9. Sit beside the patient to assist with feeding. *(Sitting is more relaxing and can decrease anxiety in patients, thus encouraging them to eat better.)*
10. Encourage patients to feed themselves as much as possible. *(Encourages independence and maintains patient's dignity.)*
11. Provide a flexible straw for patients who are unable to use a cup or glass. *(Helps direct liquids into patient's mouth and allows him or her to set the pace and amount taken.)*

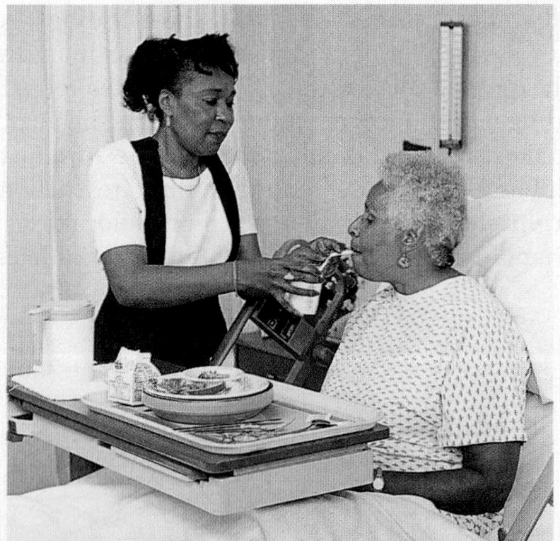

12. Serve manageable amounts of food in each bite. *(Too large a bite may cause choking and aspiration.)*
13. For a patient who has had a stroke, direct the food toward the side of the mouth not affected by the stroke. *(Allows for more thorough chewing and swallowing.)*
14. Serve food in the order of the patient's preference. *(Allows patients to eat in the manner in which they are accustomed.)*

Skill 19.3 Assisting Patients With Eating—cont'd

15. Give the patient time to chew and swallow food. *(Allows for more relaxed atmosphere and prevents choking and aspiration.)*
16. Modify utensils and texture of food if the patient has to remain flat while eating. *(A flat position decreases the patient's ability to control food in the mouth and increases the risk of choking and aspiration.)* Use a training cup or a large syringe with flexible rubber tube. Puree or grind foods.
17. During the feeding, do not leave the patient until he or she has finished eating. Do not interrupt the meal. *(Delays or interruptions may cause food to cool or warm and become less appealing. Patients may not begin eating again if interrupted.)*
18. Carry on pleasant conversation with patient during the meal. *(Eating is a social event and should be pleasant. A pleasant atmosphere may enhance appetite.)*
19. Remove the tray from the patient's room as soon as the meal is completed. *(Having to look at or smell food that has been sitting may cause the patient to become nauseated or to vomit.)*

Keep in mind that odors, unpleasant equipment, an uncomfortable position, the need for oral hygiene, the need to void, and the presence of pain may affect appetite. To improve a patient's appetite, remove any offensive odors or equipment and offer to help the patient void or wash before meals. Also, check for pain and offer pain medication at least 30 minutes before a meal. It is also important to serve the meal as quickly as possible so that the food is at the correct temperature and more appetizing to the patient.

Get Ready for the NCLEX® Examination!

Key Points

- Nurses play an important role in promoting good nutrition.
- Nutrients are necessary for the proper functioning of all life processes in the body.
- Food planning guides are available to help plan and determine the nutritional adequacy of diets.
- Essential nutrients include protein, carbohydrates, fat, vitamins, minerals, and water.
- Deficiencies or excesses of nutrients often lead to disease or dysfunction of various body systems.
- For healthy Americans, a well-planned diet can provide adequate nutrition without supplementation.
- Nutrient needs change throughout the life cycle, and people must adjust their diet to meet those needs.
- Medications may affect nutritional status. Be aware of drug-nutrient interactions.
- Medical nutrition therapy involves using diet in the treatment of disease or injury.
- Diets often are altered in consistency or frequency when GI function precludes the use of a regular diet.
- Kilocalorie modifications are used when patients need to gain or lose weight. High-kilocalorie and high-protein diets may be necessary for weight maintenance in patients with increased metabolic needs.
- Obesity is a complex disorder; individualized treatment is necessary, and treatment involves a healthy diet combined with physical activity and psychological counseling.
- The eating disorders anorexia nervosa, bulimia nervosa, and binge eating necessitate multidisciplinary treatment efforts, including nutritional, family, and psychological therapy. Place an emphasis on the prevention of these disorders in youth by promoting good health and the value of individuality.
- Carbohydrate-controlled, fat-controlled, high-fiber diets are used in the treatment of diabetes mellitus.
- Fat-controlled and low-fat diets emphasize reduction of total fat, saturated fat, and *trans* fatty acids. They are used in the treatment of a variety of diseases, including heart disease, atherosclerosis, obesity, diabetes, metabolic syndrome, malabsorption syndromes, and gallbladder disease.
- Sodium-restricted diets are used to treat hypertension, congestive heart failure, and renal disease. They also are used sometimes when edema is present.
- Protein- and electrolyte-modified diets are used to treat renal disease and cirrhosis.
- Fluid restrictions are necessary when urine output is decreased, when edema is present, or during heart failure. Adequate fluid is necessary to prevent dehydration, particularly in older adults.
- Nutritional support (tube feedings or parenteral nutrition) is often necessary when oral intake is impossible or inadequate. GI function usually indicates which type of feeding is appropriate.
- In feeding a patient or resident, ask about the preferred order in which to offer foods and fluids, and allow sufficient time for the patient to chew and swallow the food.
- Remove any offensive odors or equipment, offer pain medication before a meal, and then serve meals promptly to maintain appropriate temperature and increase nutritional intake.

Additional Learning Resources

SG Go to your Study Guide for additional learning activities to help you master this chapter content.

evolve Be sure to visit the Evolve site at *http://evolve.elsevier.com/Cooper/foundationsadult/* for additional online resources.

Review Questions for the NCLEX® Examination

1. A healthy 35-year-old patient wishes to lose weight because her BMI is 27. Which suggestion would be most appropriate for her?
   1. This BMI is too low for good health; the patient needs to supplement the diet to increase weight.
   2. This is an acceptable BMI, and it is best to maintain weight at this level for continued good health.
   3. Appropriate weight loss is possible with a healthy, reduced-calorie diet and incorporating at least 30 minutes of physical activity into each day.
   4. This BMI is elevated to the point that treatments, such as surgery, are necessary.
2. A patient takes medication for hypertension and asks whether there is anything else he can do to help to reduce his blood pressure. What is the best nursing response?
   1. "A low-fat, low-cholesterol diet with only a limited amount of simple sugars will have the greatest effect on your blood pressure."
   2. "A salt-free diet will have the greatest effect on your blood pressure. Do not add salt in your cooking or at the table."
   3. "Adequate calcium and potassium intake, as well as lower sodium intake, offers some possibility of helping your blood pressure. Eat plenty of fruits, vegetables, and low-fat milk products."
   4. "Discontinue the use of processed foods, and buy only natural foods. That way, you will have less sodium in your diet."
3. A patient with cancer has anorexia and weight loss. Which suggestion is most likely to help him increase intake and prevent weight loss?
   1. Encourage the patient to eat double portions at each meal.
   2. Suggest that the patient snack often on high-calorie foods.
   3. Encourage the patient to eat the low-calorie foods first.
   4. Suggest to the patient that he decrease his amount of exercise.
4. Which dietary recommendation should the nurse include in the discharge instructions for a client who has been diagnosed with coronary artery disease?
   1. Limit intake of whole grains.
   2. Limit intake of tuna.
   3. Limit intake of soybean products.
   4. Limit intake of egg yolks.
5. The nurse is reviewing a patient's dietary intake. Which patient behavior reflects compliance with a 2-g sodium-restricted diet?
   1. Using only the two packets of salt found on the meal tray
   2. Limiting milk to 1 cup per day
   3. Avoiding use of salt in cooking
   4. Using salt-free butter with meals
6. A patient with iron-deficiency anemia started taking iron supplements. What recommendation can the nurse give the patient to increase iron absorption?
   1. Drink milk or take calcium supplements at the same time as eating iron-rich foods.
   2. Take iron supplements with coffee, tea, or red wine.
   3. Consume vitamin C–rich foods at the same meal with iron-containing foods.
   4. Take iron supplements with a high-fiber bran cereal.
7. The nurse determines that a hypertensive patient understands the DASH diet when the patient chooses which items from a sample menu used in dietary teaching?
   1. Caesar salad, bread sticks, and frozen yogurt
   2. Grilled chicken sandwich, strawberries, and lettuce salad
   3. Grilled cheese sandwich, canned pineapple, and brownie
   4. Chicken and vegetable stir fry, rice, and egg roll
8. A patient planning for pregnancy has heard that some experts recommend folic acid supplements for women of childbearing age. The patient understands the need for this recommendation by making which statement?
   1. "Folic acid may help prevent neural tube defects in my baby."
   2. "Folic acid provides me with extra calories to make new cells."
   3. "It is impossible for me to receive adequate amounts of folic acid in my diet."
   4. "Folic acid will help me to increase iron absorption in my diet."
9. While the nurse is completing discharge teaching for a patient with elevated cholesterol levels, the patient asks how to distinguish between an unsaturated fat and a saturated fat. Which statement is most accurate?
   1. Saturated fats are generally from plant sources and are solid at room temperature.
   2. In unsaturated fats the hydrogen bonds are full.
   3. Saturated fats are missing hydrogen at points of unsaturation.
   4. Unsaturated fats are generally from plant sources and are liquid at room temperature.

10. A nurse is caring for a patient recently diagnosed with type 2 diabetes. The patient asks the nurse to tell her about the dietary changes she will need to make. Which actions are appropriate and within the scope of practice for a nurse?
    1. Review the patient's chart, and recommend a calorie and carbohydrate intake that is based on blood glucose and lipid values.
    2. Discuss the rationale for and the general principles of the diabetic diet with the patient, and then communicate the patient's concerns to the registered dietitian and health care provider.
    3. Locate the health care provider's diet order in the medical chart, and then obtain a preprinted diet sheet showing the exchange lists for meal planning and a menu pattern based on the prescribed calorie level.
    4. Decline to comment on the diet because the nurse is not a trained professional in the area of nutrition; refer all questions to a registered dietitian.
11. A 40-year-old patient recently received a diagnosis of type 2 diabetes. He is in the hospital for tests and is receiving a diabetic diet. His wife expresses concern because she notices cookies on his lunch tray. Which response best describes current recommendations for the use of concentrated sweets in the diabetic diet?
    1. "Sugars and sweets are permitted in moderation in the diabetic diet. The important thing is that the total carbohydrate content of the meal is controlled and balanced with your husband's medication and nutrient needs."
    2. "I can understand your concern. Sugars are more rapidly absorbed and have the capacity to raise blood glucose levels more quickly than other carbohydrates. I will check with the kitchen and see if your husband received the wrong tray."
    3. "I am sure that if the cookies were on the meal tray, they must be allowed in the diet. They are probably low in sugar. There is likely no need for concern."
    4. "Sugar is used to treat hypoglycemia or low blood sugar. Perhaps your husband had a low blood sugar reading before breakfast, and the dietitian sent up the cookies to give him some extra sugar on his lunch meal tray."
12. The health care provider has recommended that a patient increase the amount of fiber in her diet to help control her blood cholesterol levels. Which guidelines are most appropriate for increasing water-soluble fiber in the diet?
    1. Choose a daily fiber supplement that contains no artificial additives and preservatives; follow the instructions on the container, and be sure to drink plenty of water.
    2. Choose foods that are closer to their whole state rather than refined or processed, including more fruits, oats, and legumes to increase soluble fiber; and drink plenty of water.
    3. Choose more vegetables, vegetable juices, whole wheat, and whole wheat products to increase soluble fiber; and drink plenty of water.
    4. Choose more fruit juices to provide fluid and fiber, and include iron-fortified breakfast cereals to enhance the absorption of fiber from the fruit juice.
13. A patient is controlling his blood cholesterol through diet. He is familiar with food sources of saturated fat and cholesterol but is confused about *trans* fatty acids. The nurse should explain that which group of foods contributes the most *trans* fatty acids?
    1. Butter, cream, fats in meats, and tropical oils such as palm and coconut oils
    2. Fish oils, nuts and seeds, and vegetable oils such as olive oil and canola oil
    3. Stick margarines, shortening, deep-fried restaurant foods, and commercially prepared baked goods
    4. Liquid margarines, vegetable oil spreads, and vegetable oils such as corn, soybean, and cottonseed
14. A patient with a family history of osteoporosis is taking calcium supplements to help reduce her risk of developing osteoporosis. What recommendations can be made to prevent the development of reduced calcium balance? *(Select all that apply.)*
    1. Taking small doses of calcium throughout the day rather than one large dose
    2. Choosing plenty of milk products, and avoiding excess caffeine intake
    3. Consuming a high-protein diet
    4. Consuming a diet that has moderate levels of sodium
    5. Increasing potassium intake
15. Which patient comment indicates to the nurse that more teaching is needed for the patient experiencing dumping syndrome after gastric surgery?
    1. "I should eat six small meals per day."
    2. "I should not drink fluids with my meals."
    3. "I should use honey or jelly instead of butter."
    4. "I should lie down for 30 to 60 minutes after eating."
16. A 14-year-old trauma patient has just been started on nasogastric tube feedings. Shortly after the formula begins, the patient complains of nausea and abdominal cramps. What is the appropriate nursing action?
    1. Check the formula rate, strength, or volume; any of these could possibly be too high.
    2. Nothing; these are normal symptoms with tube feedings.
    3. Stop the infusion immediately; these are symptoms of aspiration.
    4. Stop the infusion because the feeding tube is emptying into the lung rather than the stomach.
17. A patient in the early stages of pregnancy is experiencing some nausea and vomiting. Which suggestions would be appropriate for the nurse to recommend? *(Select all that apply.)*
    1. Limit foods with strong odors, and avoid food odors that bother you.
    2. Avoid foods with a high fat content.
    3. Try consuming five or six smaller meals each day, and include a source of protein in each meal.
    4. Try not to let your stomach get completely empty. Eat before you are overly hungry.
    5. Increase carbonated beverage intake.

20 Complementary and Alternative Therapies

http://evolve.elsevier.com/Cooper/foundationsadult/

Objectives

1. Differentiate between complementary and alternative therapies.
2. Describe the practice of holistic nursing.
3. Explain why a good health history is important for a patient who is using complementary and alternative therapies.
4. Describe how herbs differ from pharmaceuticals.
5. Describe safe and unsafe herbal therapies.
6. Explain the scope of practice of chiropractic therapy.
7. Explain the difference between acupuncture and acupressure.
8. Describe the principles behind acupuncture and acupressure.
9. Identify conditions whose presence may contraindicate use of therapeutic massage.
10. Explain the use of essential oils in aromatherapy.
11. Explain the theory behind reflexology.
12. Discuss animal-assisted therapy.
13. Discuss the therapeutic results of yoga, t'ai chi, and energy field therapies.
14. Describe the purpose and principles of biofeedback.
15. Discuss the risks and benefits of marijuana used as complementary or alternative medicine.

Key Terms

acupressure (ĂK-yū-prĕsh-ŭr, p. 577)
acupuncture (ĂK-yū-pŭnk-chŭr, p. 577)
allopathic medicine (ăl-ō-PĂTH-ĭk MĔ-dĭ-sĭn, p. 570)
alternative therapies (ŭl-TĔR-nă-tĭv THĔR-ŭh-pēz, p. 570)
aromatherapy (ŭh-RŌM-ŭ-THĔR-ŭh-pē, p. 580)
biofeedback (bī-ō-fēd-băk, p. 584)
cannabidiol (kă-nĭ-bĭ-DĪ-ōl, p. 585)
cannabinoid (kă-NĂ-bĭ-noid, p. 585)
chiropractic therapy (kī-rō-PRĂK-tĭk, p. 577)
complementary therapies (kōm-plĭ-MĔN-tŭ-rē THĔR-ŭh-pēz, p. 570)
focusing (FŌ-kŭs-ĭng, p. 582)
herbal therapy (ĔR-bŭl THĔR-ŭh-pē, p. 571)
holistic nursing (hō-LĬS-tĭk, p. 571)
imagery (ĬM-ĭj-rē, p. 581)
meridians (mĕ-RĬD-ē-ănz, p. 577)
passivity (păs-ĬV-ŭ-tē, p. 582)
pharmaceuticals (făhr-mă-SŪ-tĭ-kălz, p. 571)
Qi (CHĒ, p. 577)
receptivity (rē-sĕp-TĬV-ŭ-tē, p. 582)
reflexology (rē-flĕks-ŎL-ŭh-jē, p. 580)
Reiki (RĀ-kē, p. 577)
relaxation (rē-lăks-Ā-shŭn, p. 581)
Taiji or t'ai chi (tī JĒ, p. 584)
tetrahydrocannabinol (tĕ-trŭ-HĪ-drŭ-kă-NĂ-bĭ-nŭl, p. 585)
therapeutic massage (thĕr-ŭ-PYŪ-tĭk mŭ-SŎZH, p. 579)
yoga (YŌ-gŭh, p. 583)

More and more people are considering the use of complementary therapies to help restore and maintain health. This chapter discusses the use of these therapies, which are referred to frequently as either complementary or alternative medicine (CAM) therapies.

Complementary therapies are treatments used in addition to conventional health care regimens recommended by a person's health care provider. As the name implies, complementary therapies do not substitute for but rather complement the conventional treatment plan. Complementary therapies include exercise, massage, reflexology, prayer, biofeedback, creative therapies (art, music, or dance therapy), guided imagery, acupuncture, relaxation strategies, chiropractic therapy, therapeutic touch, and herbalism.

Alternative therapies, on the other hand, often include the same interventions as complementary therapies but frequently become the primary treatment modality that replaces **allopathic medicine** (traditional or conventional Western medicine).

The number of patients seeking unconventional treatments has risen considerably over the past few years. According to data collected in the 2012 National Health and Nutrition Examination Survey (NHANES), one-third of American adults use some form of CAM each year (Clark et al, 2015). In large part, CAM is popular because of (1) the perception that the treatments offered by the medical profession do not provide relief for a variety of common illnesses; (2) the increasing interest of patients in becoming more educated about their health and the need to take a more active role in their treatment; (3) the increased number of articles in journals such as *Annals of Behavioral Medicine, Alternative Therapies in Health and Medicine,* and *Journal of Alternative and Complementary Medicine,* as well as coverage of CAM therapies in respected general medical journals; (4) programs seen on television; and (5) the attraction to a holistic approach to health care that incorporates the mind, the body, and the spirit.

People may turn to alternative therapies because they believe them to be less invasive and gentler than allopathic or traditional medicine and perceive them to incorporate a more holistic approach. Prevention is fundamental to most of the CAM therapies. They usually are not used as an immediate cure for an illness or acute injury but provide an ongoing method of maintaining optimal health. Practitioners often recommend lifestyle changes and encourage patients to follow health practices on a daily basis, thereby improving their overall health. Some practitioners incorporate therapies from a variety of treatments to provide *holistic* care for the patient.

In contrast, the strength of allopathic medicine is its effectiveness in treating certain physical ailments (e.g., bacterial infections, structural abnormalities, acute emergencies). In general, it focuses less on preventing disease, decreasing stress-induced illnesses, managing chronic disease, and caring for the emotional and spiritual needs of individuals.

Complementary and alternative therapies vary in the degree to which they are compatible with allopathic or conventional medicine. Many of the complementary therapies, such as acupuncture, make use of diagnostic and therapeutic methods specific to their field, whereas others, such as guided imagery, are essentially adjunctive in nature. For example, chiropractic practitioners frequently use diagnostic terminology and methods similar to those used by allopathic or conventional practitioners. They base interventions on conventional pathophysiology, anatomy, and kinesiology but at the same time explore mind-body connections that they believe drive the physiologic condition. Some alternative therapies, however, are not supported by scientific data, and some conflict with or even contradict traditional, scientifically based medical practices.

Most patients using CAM therapies do so in conjunction with traditional medicine. Rarely do patients choose to make the alternative health care provider the only source of health care. Patients are often hesitant to talk to an allopathic health care provider about any treatment they are receiving other than that prescribed by a provider with a medical degree. It is estimated that almost half of all health care consumers in the United States take some form of herbal or natural product supplement alone or in combination with conventional medicines but rarely report this practice to their health care providers.

However, it is important to obtain as clear a view as possible of all efforts a patient is making to improve or maintain health. Although many alternative therapies do not interfere with therapies prescribed by a health care provider, some pose the risk of serious interactions. When obtaining a health history from a patient, carefully assess the patient's use of any other therapies that may interact with traditional medical care. Project an open, nonjudgmental attitude when obtaining a health history so that the patient feels comfortable providing all information about any therapies he or she currently is receiving.

Reimbursement by insurance companies is becoming more common for several of these treatments. Chiropractic treatments and massage may be covered by policies if ordered by a health care provider. Acupuncture also is covered under some policies. Insurance companies are beginning to see the value of preventive measures, as well as that of treatment for acute injury or illness. From a risk management perspective, many of the alternative therapies are attractive because they work to maintain health, as well as restore it. **Holistic nursing** addresses and treats the mind-body-spirit of the patient. Nurses use holistic nursing interventions such as relaxation therapy, guided imagery, music therapy, simple touch, massage, and prayer. Such interventions affect the whole person (mind-body-spirit) and are effective, economical, noninvasive, nonpharmacologic complements to medical care. Holistic interventions can be used to augment standard treatments, to replace interventions that are ineffective or debilitating, and to promote or maintain health. The American Holistic Nurses Association *(www.ahna.org)* maintains standards of holistic nursing practice, which define and establish the scope of holistic practice and describe the level of care expected from a holistic nurse.

The Office of Alternative Medicine (now the National Center for Complementary and Integrative Health [NCCIH]) was established in 1992 as part of the National Institutes of Health. *The mission of NCCIH is to define, through rigorous scientific investigation, the usefulness and safety of complementary and integrative health interventions and their roles in improving health and health care* (NCCIH, 2016).

HERBAL THERAPY

The use of **herbal therapy** as medical treatment began thousands of years ago. Neanderthal gravesites have been found that have the remains of plants surrounding the body. Herbalists were consulted by and worked in conjunction with medical physicians until the 1930s, when the last accredited herbal schools closed. In the meantime, the number of **pharmaceuticals,** or drugs, was increasing and their use becoming commonplace. Nonetheless, many of those drugs, as well as medications in use today, originated in herbs. An example is digitalis, which comes from the finger-shaped foxglove herb. Used in the treatment of heart failure, it commonly is prescribed by health care providers. Interest in the use of herbs and natural supplements to treat illness and maintain health has increased among the general population.

Herbs differ from pharmaceuticals—even those that are plant based—in several ways. An herbal preparation usually includes an unpurified extract of the whole plant. One herb may be used for a variety of purposes, and its action is usually gentler than those of pharmaceuticals. Pharmaceuticals that are derived from herbs include only the active part, and the rest of the plant is separated out and discarded; thus the pharmaceutical is likely to be more potent and to incur more adverse effects. There are several herbal medicine handbooks and websites that list adverse effects for each herbal preparation.

Herbal medicines have not undergone the same rigorous study as have pharmaceuticals. The majority have not received approval in the United States for use as drugs. For this reason, many herbal medicines are sold as foods or food supplements in health food stores and through private companies. The Dietary Supplement Health and Education Act, passed in 1994, now allows for herbs to be sold as dietary supplements as long as no health claims are written on their labels.

Herbal products are not viewed as drugs, which reduces the level of accountability for their manufacturers compared with that required of pharmaceutical companies. Herb manufacturers are not required by law to demonstrate the safety, the efficacy, or the quality of their products. Herb manufacturing remains unregulated and is likely to continue to be so in the current political and economic climate. Some manufacturers voluntarily adhere to so-called "good manufacturing practices" and make every effort to produce a quality product; others do not. However, nothing guarantees that the active chemical constituents in an herbal product remain constant from manufacturer to manufacturer. Chemical analysis of samples labeled as the same herbal product but purchased from various suppliers or outlets has revealed wide variations in potency, quality, and chemical content. In contrast to prescription drugs, no standardized dosages have been established for most herbs, and few manufacturers produce the standardized preparations of predictable and consistent strength that make an herbal regimen possible to follow.

Herbal therapy is based on a different philosophy than conventional drug therapy. The goal of herbal therapy is to restore balance within the individual by facilitating the person's self-healing capacity. Drug therapy, on the other hand, is aimed at the treatment of specific diseases or symptoms. Herbal therapy also is prescribed on an individual basis, with unique herbal concoctions tailored for each person.

Many herbs are potentially toxic if used incorrectly. Some herbs are safe and effective when used topically in the amount specified but are highly toxic if taken internally. Many of the toxic effects of herbs have yet to be determined because of insufficient research and because no law requires reporting of adverse effects from herbal products (Table 20.1).

With these cautions in mind, remember that many herbs may produce beneficial effects when used as directed. Research continues to confirm the efficacy of many popular herbs, echinacea and ginkgo, for example.

There is much confusion and misinformation regarding herbal medicine. Herbal medicine has yet to be subjected to the same level of scientific scrutiny as traditional medical treatments. As a result, it has not yet gained wide acceptance by mainstream medicine. Because herb use is not widely accepted or understood by mainstream medical caregivers, patients often do not disclose their use of herbs to their health care

Table 20.1 Commonly Used Herbs

HERB	USES	CONSIDERATIONS
Asian ginseng (Panax ginseng)	Improves overall health and well-being Atherosclerosis, bleeding disorders, colitis, diabetes, depressant cancer	Do not administer to pregnant or breast-feeding patients. Do not administer to patients with cardiovascular disease, hypertension, diabetes, or concurrent therapy. Patients taking anticoagulants should avoid use because it can prolong clotting. Avoid giving to patients who are taking CNS stimulants, estrogen, furosemide, ibuprofen, caffeine, or drugs metabolized by CYP3H4. Drug and herb interactions are possible with agents that inhibit monoamine oxidase (phenelzine, St. John's wort, selegiline).
Aloe vera *(Aloe ferox, Aloe barbadensis)*	Burns, skin irritation Has laxative properties	Internal use produces a cathartic action and has resulted in painful cramps, electrolyte imbalance, hemorrhagic diarrhea, and kidney damage. Drug interactions exist with antidysrhythmics, cardiac glycosides (e.g., digoxin), antidiabetics, beta blockers, steroids, diuretics, and disulfiram. Herb interactions exist with licorice.

Table 20.1 Commonly Used Herbs—cont'd

HERB	USES	CONSIDERATIONS
Cayenne (*Capsicum* sp.)	General cardiovascular health: reduces cholesterol level; topical application produces analgesia, controls bleeding	Topical application as a counterirritant produces a "heat" sensation. Repeated applications produce analgesia that results from neuronal depletion of substance P (a mediator of pain transmission between peripheral nerves and spinal cord). Burning and pruritus diminish with continued use. Drug interactions exist with ACE inhibitors, heparin, ASA, disulfiram, and theophylline. Herb interactions exist with feverfew, garlic, ginger, and ginseng.
Comfrey *(Symphytum officinale)*	Cell proliferant, stimulates quick healing of strains and slow-healing wounds (for external use only)	When used internally, comfrey is potentially harmful: there are reports of liver toxicity. Some preparations contain significant levels of alcohol; they should be used with caution. Monitor patients for abdominal distention, nausea, abdominal pain, and elevated liver function test results. Limit use to 4–6 wk/yr to prevent exposure to large amounts of toxic alkaloids.
Echinacea *(Echinacea purpurea, E. angustifolia, E. pallida)*	Stimulates immune function; excellent blood cleanser; upper respiratory infections; wound healing	Activity has been shown against influenza, herpes, and *Candida* infections. Adverse reactions include fever, taste disturbance, gastrointestinal disturbances, nausea and vomiting, diuresis, photosensitivity. Patients with ragweed allergies should avoid use. Prolonged use potentially leads to overstimulation of the immune system and possible immune suppression. Drug interactions are possible with protease inhibitors, disulfiram, metronidazole, immunosuppressants, cyclosporine, methotrexate, prednisone, alcohol, warfarin, digoxin, contraceptives, SSRIs, and MAOIs.
Evening primrose oil *(Oenothera biennis)*	Premenstrual syndrome, attention-deficit hyperactivity disorder, cardiovascular problems, hot flashes, mastalgia	Use of the oil occasionally unmasks previously undiagnosed epilepsy, especially when taken with a drug that treats depression or schizophrenia. Herb should be taken with food to decrease adverse gastrointestinal reaction. Use is contraindicated in patients with an allergy to evening primrose oil and those who are pregnant or breast-feeding. Do not give to patients with a history of epilepsy or who are taking a tricyclic antidepressant, phenothiazine, or another drug that lowers the seizure threshold.
Ginger *(Zingiber officinale)*	Nausea, vomiting, motion sickness, appetite improvement, impotence, liver toxicity, burns	Overdose possibly produces CNS depression and dysrhythmias. Ginger sometimes enhances the effect of anticoagulants. Pregnant patients should not take large doses because the teratogenic potential is largely unstudied. No consensus exists regarding dosage or monitoring. Drug interactions are possible with antacids, histamine H_2 receptor blockers, proton pump inhibitors, anticoagulants, barbiturates, disulfiram, and metronidazole.
Ginkgo, maidenhair tree *(Ginkgo biloba)*	Improves memory, increases circulation to the extremities and the brain	Studies have shown that ginkgo produces arterial and venous vasoactive changes that increase tissue perfusion and cerebral blood flow. Adverse reactions include dizziness, headache, subarachnoid and subdural hemorrhage, and cardiac insufficiency. There have been reports of seizures in children and bleeding complications. Potential drug interactions exist with antiplatelet therapy, anticoagulants, anticonvulsants, bupropion, tricyclic antidepressants, disulfiram, metronidazole, MAOIs, SSRIs, and trazodone. Herb interactions include garlic.
Goldenseal *(Hydrastis canadensis)*	Antibiotic and antiseptic, especially effective on mucous membranes, urinary tract infection, diarrhea, and hemorrhoids Digestive aid and expectorant	This herb increases hypoglycemic effects in patients using insulin. Possible effects of this herb include reducing effects of anticoagulants; reducing or enhancing hypotensive effects of antihypertensives; interfering with or enhancing cardiac effects of beta blockers, calcium channel blockers, and digoxin; enhancing sedative effects of CNS depressants; and enhancing sedative effects of alcohol. Do not give to children.

Continued

Table 20.1 **Commonly Used Herbs—cont'd**

HERB	USES	CONSIDERATIONS
Kava (kava-kava) *(Piper methysticum)*	Anxiety, stress, and restlessness, insomnia, wound healing	Kava does not appear to cause physiologic dependence. Expect enhanced sedative effects if combined with other CNS depressants (alcohol, benzodiazepines, and opioid analgesics). Heavy use sometimes causes nutritional deficiencies, skin dermopathy, blood dyscrasias, pulmonary hypertension, cirrhosis, liver failure, hepatitis, and dopamine antagonism. It is generally well tolerated except in high doses or with long-term use. Patients should not use kava when ingesting alcohol or during pregnancy and breast-feeding, and it should not be given to children younger than 12 yr. Drug interactions may exist with antiplatelet medications, MAOIs, drugs metabolized in cytochrome P-450 system, hepatotoxic drugs, and levodopa.
Lavender *(Lavandula officinalis)*	Antiseptic, antidepressant, sedative, relaxation, minor cuts, psoriasis, fragrance	Lavender is used for its calming mild sedative effect. Add to warm bath water if desired to aid in relaxation. Orally it sometimes is used as a tea to calm a "nervous stomach." Monitor patient closely for oversedation because it will possibly potentiate actions of other sedative drugs. It possibly potentiates CNS depressant effects of alcohol. Avoid giving to patients who are pregnant or breast-feeding. Some patients are allergic to lavender-containing perfumes. Do not confuse true lavender oil with lavandin or spiked lavender oil; the latter two contain high enough levels of camphor to elicit neurotoxicity. Excessive inhalation of the oil sometimes leads to vertigo, nausea, and syncope. Tell patients to avoid hazardous activities until lavender's full effects are known.
St. John's wort *(Hypericum perforatum)*	Mild to moderate depression, anxiety, viral infection, insomnia, premenstrual syndrome, topical myalgia, inflammation	There are numerous case reports and clinical trials evaluating the efficacy and safety of St. John's wort. Most trials contain design flaws, but overall results suggest that St. John's wort is sometimes beneficial for mild to moderate depression. Adverse reactions, which are uncommon, include photosensitivity, constipation, vertigo, dry mouth, restlessness, and sleep disturbance. Patients should avoid concurrent use with MAOIs, alcoholic beverages, opioids, prescription antidepressants, sympathomimetics, and foods such as chocolate, aged cheeses, and beer. Do not give to patients who are pregnant or breast-feeding. Do not give to children. Drug interactions include amiodarone, amitriptyline, chemotherapy drugs, cyclosporine, digoxin, drugs metabolized in cytochrome P-450 system, contraceptives (oral), protease inhibitors, theophylline and warfarin, SSRIs, reserpine, and nonnucleoside reverse transcriptase inhibitors.
Tea tree oil *(Melaleuca alternifolia)*	Skin irritations, acne, athlete's foot Topical antiseptic, antifungal, inhalation for respiratory disorders	Do not give in combination with drugs that affect histamine release. Do not apply to dry skin, cracked or broken skin, open wounds, or areas affected by rash that is not fungal. It should not be used internally because of systemic toxicity. Administer externally only after dilution, especially for patients with sensitive skin. Do not apply around nose, eyes, and mouth because it sometimes causes burns or pruritus in tender areas. Use the pure oil only under close supervision by a health care provider.
Valerian *(Valeriana officinalis)*	Insomnia, hyperactivity, stress, anxiety	Valerian causes addictive effects in some patients taking barbiturates. It possibly potentiates (1) sedative effects of catnip, hops, kona, kava, and passionflower and (2) the sedative effects of alcohol. Do not give to patients who are pregnant or breast-feeding. Evidence of toxicity includes difficulty walking, hypothermia, and increased muscle relaxation. Possible adverse reactions include hepatotoxic effects upon withdrawal.

ACE, Angiotensin-converting enzyme; *ASA,* acetylsalicylic acid (aspirin); *CNS,* central nervous system; *MAOI,* monoamine oxidase inhibitor; *SSRI,* selective serotonin reuptake inhibitor.

provider. Many use prescription drugs concurrently with herbal remedies and face possible health risks as a result of adverse interactions. A well-informed, nonjudgmental care provider is most likely to gain the patient's trust and obtain not only a more accurate view of the patient's herb use but also an opportunity to provide valuable information about herb safety issues (see the Patient Teaching box).

Reduced insurance coverage, constraints on access to care, and increased costs of prescriptions and services are the norm in the current health care climate. People are living longer, and chronic diseases—arthritis, diabetes, cancer, Alzheimer's disease, human immunodeficiency virus (HIV) infection, and acquired immunodeficiency syndrome (AIDS)—are on the rise. Many conventional prescription drugs used to treat these conditions are expensive, and because at least a portion of the cost often is not reimbursed by insurance carriers, consumers are paying more out of pocket for them. People are becoming increasingly interested in preventive strategies and holistic approaches to health, such as eating a nutritionally sound diet, maintaining fitness, and reducing stress. According to the NCCIH, Americans spend almost one-third as much money out of pocket on visits to alternative practitioners as they do on visits to physicians (NCCIH, 2016).

The nurse assists patients in making educated decisions about their health; there is no reason to exclude the use of herbs. Most patients receive information about herbs from the media and the Internet, sources whose claims do not always coincide with results of clinical studies. Teach patients that before taking any herbal product, it is best to review it with a health care provider, pharmacist, or certified herbalist.

Treatment is provided in a variety of ways. It is possible to take dried herbs orally in capsule or tablet form. Tinctures are made by placing herbs in alcohol or vinegar and allowed to sit until the liquid absorbs the

 Patient Teaching

Using Complementary and Alternative Therapies

HERBAL PREPARATIONS

- Inform your primary care provider of any drugs you use, including herbal remedies, so that all agents—whether "nutraceutical" or pharmaceutical—will be considered in the plan of care.
- Use herbal preparations according to package or health care provider's direction.
- Stop taking the herb and notify your primary care provider if adverse effects or side effects occur.
- "Natural" does not mean safe. Seek objective and scientifically based sources of information. Use caution when evaluating the claims made by herb manufacturers.
- Avoid using combinations of herbs.
- Use only products that are standardized and known to contain a specific amount of active ingredients.
- Select herbal products carefully, buying only those that list the following information on the package: herb's common and scientific names, name and address of the manufacturer, batch or lot number, expiration date, dosage and administration guidelines, potential side effects, and details of how quality is ensured.
- Avoid using herbs and spices for at least 2 weeks before any surgery.
- Bear in mind that patients who self-prescribe medications may have serious underlying physiologic or psychological conditions that necessitate attention. Learn to devise a health regimen that best suits your needs, regardless of whether herbs are used.
- Herb-drug interactions do occur, as do herb-herb interactions, and they pose serious risks; therefore it is best to let the primary care provider determine the safety of combining herbs and drugs.
- Purchase herbal products that have been standardized: that is, products for which the effects are known for a given dosage and for which the manufacturer ensures consistency from batch to batch.
- Buy from reputable sources. Ask the primary health care provider for assistance in determining where to purchase herbs.
- Avoid herbs during pregnancy and lactation or when attempting to become pregnant.
- Neither the safety nor the efficacy of herbs has been documented conclusively in scientific literature.
- It is in your best interest to undergo a complete medical evaluation before self-medicating with supplements: whether to treat specific symptoms of an illness or as a preventive measure.
- Do not use herbs in dosages larger than recommended or for more than several weeks (unless approved by the health care provider).
- Keep all herbs out of the reach of children and pets.

YOGA AND REFLEXOLOGY

- Consult your health care provider before starting a yoga program, because some yoga postures are stressful to people with certain health problems (muscle injury is possible if the positions are not performed correctly or if the body is forced into certain positions).
- When practicing yoga, try different positions cautiously; few people can perform all the movements in the beginning. Yoga requires regular practice to be effective.
- Postpone reflexology treatment if your feet have cuts, boils, bruises, or other injuries.
- Check with your health care provider before trying reflexology if you have diabetes, peripheral vascular disease, or other vascular problems in the legs, such as thrombosis or phlebitis.
- Many people who claim to perform reflexology actually are performing a simple foot massage; make sure the therapist has been trained in reflexology.

Table 20.2 Common Essential Oils and Their Uses

ESSENTIAL OIL	USE	CONSIDERATIONS
Chamomile	Pain, gastrointestinal spasms, stress, insomnia	Chamomile oil has theoretic potential to decrease absorption of certain antispasmodic medications. Excessive anticoagulation is possible when it is used with other anticoagulants. Avoid giving to pregnant patients because of potential abortifacient and teratogenic effects. Instruct patients with atopic eczema to avoid use because of potential allergic reactions.
Eucalyptus	Respiratory problems	Eucalyptus oil sometimes causes nausea, vomiting, diarrhea, and asthma-like attacks. It may enhance the effects of hypoglycemic agents. The oil has potential to affect the action of any drug that the liver metabolizes, so monitor patients for effect and toxic reaction. It decreases blood glucose levels; monitor patients for effect. Do not use with herbs that cause hypoglycemia such as basil, glucomannan, or Queen Anne's lace. When applied to an infant's or child's face, it sometimes causes severe bronchial spasm. Do not give to patients who are pregnant or breast-feeding or to patients who have liver disease or intestinal tract inflammation.
Lavender	Insomnia, stress, depression	Lavender oil possibly causes CNS depression, confusion, vertigo, syncope, drowsiness, headache, neurotoxicity, hypotension, nausea, vomiting, constipation, and respiratory depression. It may potentiate the effects of sedative drugs, so monitor patient closely for oversedation. It also possibly potentiates CNS depressant effects of alcohol, so it should not be used with alcohol. Massaging with diluted oil is unlikely to be toxic. Do not give to pregnant or breast-feeding patients. Do not confuse true lavender oil with lavandin or spike lavender oil; the latter two contain high enough levels of camphor to elicit neurotoxicity.
Lemon	Colds and flu, mental stimulation Diuretic, antiinflammatory	Patients who are pregnant or breast-feeding should avoid oral ingestion of expressed oil. Do not give to patients who are hypersensitive to members of the citrus family. Skin reactions of photodermatotoxicity from expressed oil are possible.
Peppermint	Acne, stomach upset General stimulant	Patients with gastroesophageal reflux disease should avoid peppermint oil because it sometimes exacerbates the disease. Do not give peppermint teas and mentholated ointment to infants and small children. Menthol sometimes causes sensitization and allergic reactions. Advise patients not to apply to broken skin. Internal use of peppermint other than for flavoring is not recommended.
Rosemary	Internally: mental stimulant; alleviating stress, circulatory problems Externally: myalgias, neuralgia, pruritus, migraines	Rosemary oil promotes menstrual flow, induces abortions (do not give to pregnant patients); and relieves headache, liver, and gallbladder complaints and blood pressure problems. In high doses, it sometimes causes seizures. Asthma can result from repeated occupational exposure. The oil also sometimes causes contact dermatitis and photodermatosensitivity. Encourage patients to take precautions and use sunscreen. Avoid use with herbal products containing alcohol. Do not give to pregnant or breast-feeding patients, children, or patients with seizure disorders. Bronchospasm and glottal spasm have been reported in children.
Tea tree	Antiseptic Skin irritations, viral illness, respiratory infection	Topical applications have not shown to be toxic, but ingesting the oil possibly will produce CNS depression and gastrointestinal irritation. Its antimicrobial activity has been well documented, but only anecdotal evidence exists for its efficacy in treating skin maladies. Advise patients of various product concentrations. It is probably best for patients with propensity for contact dermatitis to avoid the use of tea tree oil.

CNS, Central nervous system.

properties of the herb. The liquid then is strained and used. Teas made of an infusion of herbs and hot water are consumed, or a moist compress is made from the tea and applied to the affected area. Topical application of herbs is also possible by making a salve or ointment (Table 20.2).

Thousands of herbs are available. Table 20.1 lists some of the most common herbs and their uses. Remind patients to take care to use herbs from only a reliable source. Before a patient uses any fresh herbs, it is best to obtain exact identification from a trained professional. The patient always should know exactly what any herb is and what its actions are before using it.

Many herbs interact with various medications. For example, the combination of valerian and barbiturates probably causes excessive sedation. Ginseng is likely to interfere with the actions of digoxin. Advise against taking St. John's wort concurrently with antidepressant medications. Screen patients carefully in regard to herbal use and possible interactions with other medications.

CHIROPRACTIC THERAPY

Chiropractic therapy has been in existence since the late 1800s. Doctors of chiropractic medicine undergo extensive training in manipulation of the musculoskeletal system. Although chiropractic therapy has been criticized severely, it currently is considered an acceptable treatment for certain disorders, including back pain and headaches. Many insurance companies provide coverage for chiropractic therapy care.

This form of therapy is based on a holistic belief in the body's capacity to take care of itself. The chiropractor adjusts the joints of the body by gentle manipulation to put an area of disturbed structural integrity, usually the vertebrae, back in proper alignment. When properly performed, this treatment does not cause pain to the patient. Often patients seek treatment from a medical physician for an acute injury or illness and use chiropractic care on a routine basis. If distress is acute, visits sometimes are recommended several times a week or daily, but monthly visits to keep the patient at a maximal level of health are typical.

The chiropractor often uses x-rays to assist with diagnosis. Chiropractors do not prescribe medications as part of the treatment. Other treatments, such as hot and cold packs, are sometimes used during the course of chiropractic treatment. Chiropractors often consider lifestyle changes and nutritional supplements to help keep the patient functioning well without recurrence of the injury. Various suggested exercises often play a role in treatment.

LIMITATIONS OF CHIROPRACTIC THERAPY

It is unwise to treat certain diseases or joint conditions with manipulation. Contraindications to chiropractic therapy include acute myelopathy, fractures, dislocations, rheumatoid arthritis, and osteoporosis. If a malignancy is suspected or determined through diagnostic testing, the patient is referred to a health care provider for further evaluation and treatment. Bone and joint infections also necessitate pharmaceutical or surgical intervention. Care must be taken not to compromise the structural integrity of the bone, which is possible if excessive force is used.

ACUPUNCTURE AND ACUPRESSURE

Acupuncture and acupressure are therapies that are based on the belief that there is a form of energy, or **Qi** (life force), that flows through the body along **meridians** (channels of energy). The human body has 12 meridians. These meridians can become blocked, thus causing illness or discomfort. Therapy involves stimulating the channels at specific points to open them and allow the Qi to flow freely. Pain is understood to result primarily from stagnant or blocked Qi, and opening up the dam in the flow of energy through a meridian relieves the pain (Fig. 20.1).

Acupuncture is a method of stimulating certain points (acupoints) on the body by the insertion of special needles to modify the perception of pain, normalize physiologic functions, or treat or prevent disease. Fine needles inserted at specific points open the meridians. These needles are sterile and extremely thin, much smaller than the needles used for insulin injection; each one is for one-time-use only. Acupuncturists usually insert the needles only a few millimeters. When all the needles are in place, the needles are stimulated manually, electrically, or with heat (Fig. 20.2). After the needles have been in place for about 20 minutes, the acupuncturist removes and discards them. There is usually little discomfort while the needles are inserted, and most patients state that they feel no distress at all.

Acupuncture is the primary treatment modality used by health care providers of Chinese medicine. Many allopathic or conventional Western health care providers also are being trained and certified in acupuncture. Many states now have regulations and licensure requirements to practice as an acupuncturist.

The most common problems for which acupuncture is used include low back pain, myofascial pain, simple and migraine headaches, sciatica, shoulder pain, tennis elbow, osteoarthritis, whiplash, and musculoskeletal sprains. Other problems that have been treated successfully include sinusitis, gastrointestinal disorders, bladder leakage, premenstrual symptoms, neurologic disorders, chronic pulmonary disease (including asthma), hypertension, smoking and other addictions, and clinical depression.

Acupressure entails the use of gentle pressure at similar points on the body (Fig. 20.3). Pressure sometimes is applied with a finger and sometimes with a small, blunt object. Acupressure is used primarily for prevention and relief of symptoms of muscle tension. Acupressure reduces tension, increases circulation, and enables the body to relax deeply. By relieving stress, acupressure increases resistance to disease and promotes wellness. Acupressure is beneficial in situations of discomfort and promotes the ability to rest or sleep.

With acupuncture and acupressure, several treatments are usually necessary to achieve the desired results. These methods are properly performed only by a professional with appropriate training.

HEALING TOUCH, THERAPEUTIC TOUCH, AND REIKI

Energy field therapies go by many names. Healing touch, therapeutic touch, and **Reiki** are probably the most popular methods taught in the United States. These

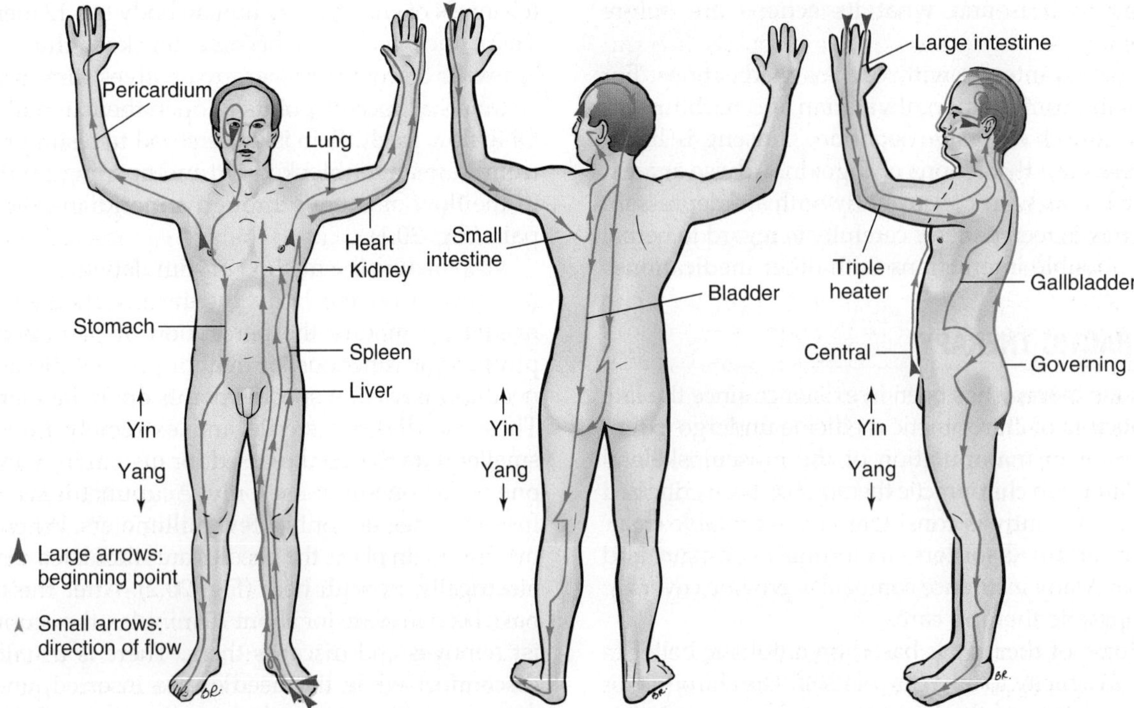

Fig. 20.1 Meridians of the human body. (From Fritz S: *Mosby's fundamentals of therapeutic massage*, ed 6, St. Louis, 2017, Elsevier.)

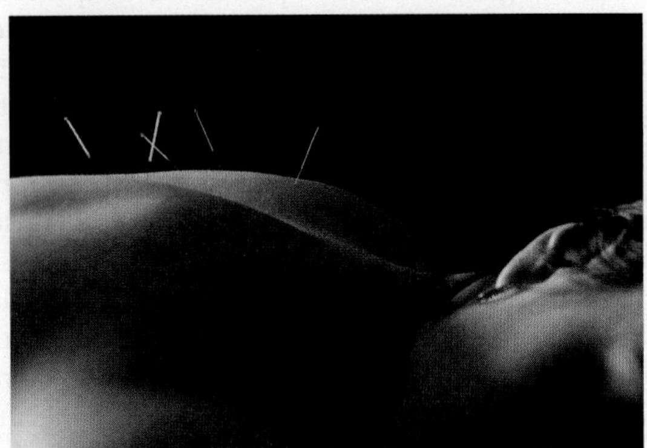

Fig. 20.2 Acupuncture uses fine needles inserted at specific points to open the meridians. (Copyright 1999–2012 Thinkstock. All rights reserved.)

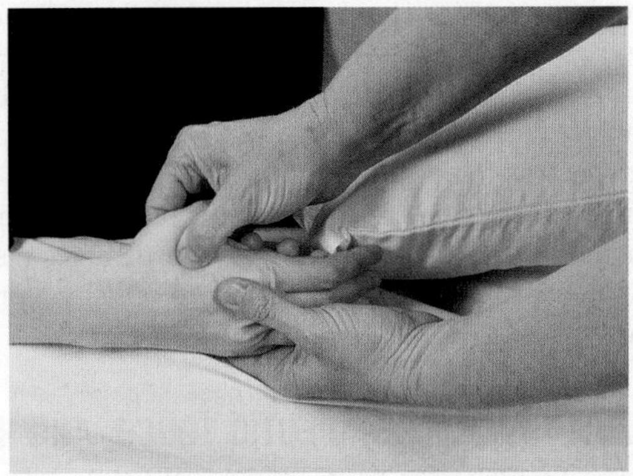

Fig. 20.3 Acupressure. (From Fritz S: *Clinical massage in the healthcare setting*, St. Louis, 2008, Mosby.)

therapies use the human energy field to interact with another person's energy field.

Practitioners of energy field therapies have similar general procedures. Verbal consent is established, and the person is informed he or she may end the session at any point. It is not appropriate to attempt to persuade a person who does not want the therapy to accept it. The practitioner quiets his or her own mind. Then he or she "sets the intention," which means focusing on the goal of the process. This is usually pain relief, relaxation, or healing. It may be given as part of end-of-life care to assist with a peaceful transition.

The person performing the energy field therapy often assesses the energy field. There are several methods for assessment. Often this information is felt in the practitioner's hands while moving the hands several inches away from the body. Intuition is not only valued but also encouraged as an assessment tool. The hands are held over the body or rested gently on the body in the areas where the practitioner feels it is needed. Sometimes this is a structured sequence of positions, but intuition may direct part or all of the intervention. There is no manipulation of the physical body. Ending the session is an important part of the process. Unless there is a contraindication (situation or condition where it could be harmful), both participants benefit from increasing water intake for the day. It is believed that energy field therapies improve the flow of energy through the body. Once the session ends, the improved flow of energy through the body continues to improve the mind, the body, and the spirit.

The experience of the person receiving the energy field therapy varies. A sense of relaxation during and after the procedure is common. Physical sensations are not uncommon. The sensations may be similar to or different from those experienced by the practitioner. It is not necessary for either participant to have physical sensations or intuition for the session to be successful. Most therapies recognize the interaction does not consist of one person who "gives" and the other person who "takes." Both participants benefit from quieting the mind and allowing the energy to flow through each of them. Novice practitioners may focus on the steps and neglect humility and love as key aspects of the process. A practitioner who has excessive fatigue or discomfort after the procedure must remember the person receiving the treatment is not responsible for any unpleasant sensations experienced by the facilitator. It is the responsibility of the person offering the energy field therapy to be mindful of his or her own energy during the process.

The development of the energy field practitioner is ongoing. With practice, skills and intuition improve. It is a personal journey that may lead to a greater sense of purpose and connectedness. Just as love is not exclusive to religious beliefs, energy field therapies are not religious practices, nor are they atheistic practices. Prayer may be included to the extent that it is acceptable to the practitioner and the person receiving the treatment.

THERAPEUTIC MASSAGE

Nurses have used massage to relax patients and help prevent impairment of skin integrity in the patient confined to bed. The effects are physical and psychological (see the Lifespan Considerations for older adults box). **Therapeutic massage** is massage performed by trained professionals to manipulate the soft tissues of the body and assist with healing (Nursing Care Plan 20.1). There are various types of massage designed to heal or prevent injury. Some massage is relaxing, and other forms are energizing.

A health profile should be reviewed before the initial massage. Certain medical conditions contraindicate massage. These conditions include acute back pain, phlebitis, and thrombosis. Areas with bruises or swellings should be evaluated by a physician before massage. Infectious skin diseases are also conditions in which massage is contraindicated. Abdominal massage in pregnant women is controversial. Some practitioners receive special training in pregnancy massage. Other massage therapists do not perform massage during pregnancy. They may fear adverse effects, or they may want to avoid any suspicion that massage has contributed to unwanted outcomes.

Massage is conducted in a warm, relaxing atmosphere (Fig. 20.4). A session lasts approximately an hour. A whole-body massage sometimes is performed, with extra attention to the affected area. Oils or lotions often

Nursing Care Plan 20.1 Using Complementary and Alternative Therapies in Treatment

Ms. L., 40 years old, underwent an abdominal hysterectomy 2 days ago. The nurse finds her awake at midnight. Ms. L. voices concern about how long she will be in the hospital because she has four children, ages 4 to 15 years, at home and she is worried how well her family is managing without her. She also states that she has abdominal pain at the incision site that she rates at 5 on a scale of 0 to 10. Her vital signs are normal. Hydrocodone, 1 or 2 tablets q 4 hr prn for pain, is ordered, but she does not want to take any more drugs. She wonders if there is anything else she can do to decrease her anxiety and pain.

PATIENT PROBLEMS

Anxiousness, level 2, related to hospitalization
Recent Onset of Pain, related to surgical procedures

Patient Goals and Expected Outcomes	Nursing Interventions	Evaluation
Patient will state that anxiety is reduced to an acceptable level Patient will state that pain rating is 1 to 2 on a scale of 0 to 10	Explain the procedure for therapeutic massage. Position the patient comfortably. Reduce noise, lighting, and distractions. Perform therapeutic massage. Make patient comfortable after procedure by proper positioning, freshening linens, darkening the room, and providing a quiet environment.	Patient states that feelings of anxiety are reduced, and pain rating is now 2 on a scale of 0 to 10.

CRITICAL THINKING QUESTIONS

1. Ms. L. complains of feeling fatigued and tense. List some nonpharmacologic methods of bringing about a state of physical and mental tranquility that may be helpful. Why may each of these methods be helpful for Ms. L.?
2. Ms. L. turns on her light and is crying. She complains of feeling helpless and inadequate to assume responsibility for her children and husband when she is discharged. What are some therapeutic interventions that will promote her feelings of stability and validation of her anxiety?

Lifespan Considerations

Older Adults

Focus on Touch

- Touch is a primal need, as necessary as food, growth, or shelter. Think of touch as a nutrient transmitted through the skin. "Skin hunger," or "poverty of touch," has been described as a form of malnutrition that has reached epidemic proportions in the United States, especially among older adults.
- Older adults need touch as much as or more than any other age group. However, skin hunger is often acute among older adults. It is an unfortunate irony that older adults often have fewer family members or friends to touch them just at the time in life when there is greatest need to use simple touch to enhance communication or when other senses sometimes are reduced in acuity.
- Simple touch helps older adult patients feel more connected to and accepted by those around them and to their environment. Self-esteem and sense of worth are enhanced.
- A nurse who reacts adversely to the skin changes of older adults may find it difficult to touch an older patient. Such reluctance communicates a negative message to older adults.
- A truly holistic nursing approach to the care of older adults also includes the caregivers, who often experience poor health or have neglected their own health and find themselves challenged by their own psychosocial issues as they relate to the caregiving experience, feel the effects of multiple stressors, or feel spiritual distress.

Adapted from Potter PA, Perry AG, Stockert PA, et al: *Fundamentals of nursing: Concepts, process, and practice*, ed 8, St. Louis, 2013, Mosby.

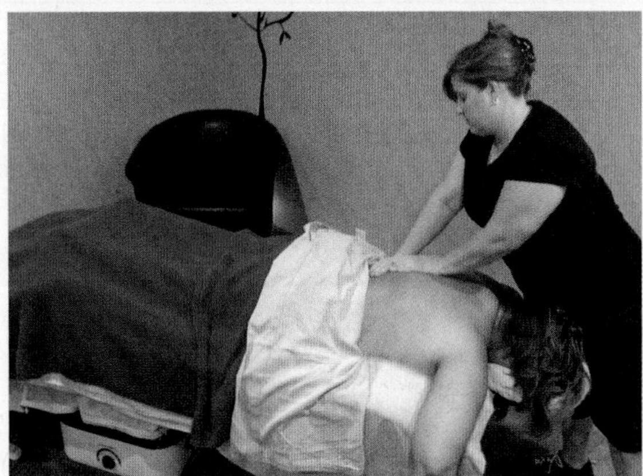

Fig. 20.4 Massage therapy is used to relieve tension.

are used during the massage; ensure the patient is not allergic to them before their use.

AROMATHERAPY

Aromatherapy entails the use of pure essential oils, produced from plants, to provide health benefits. The oils are formulated for inhalation or are applied topically.

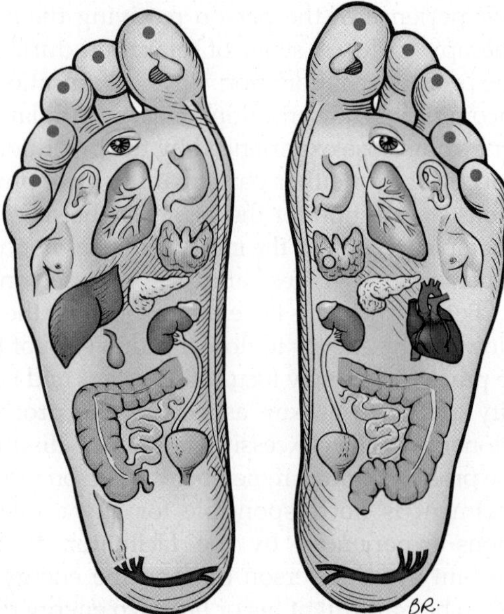

Fig. 20.5 Reflexology. Foot chart shows areas that correspond to organs and systems of the body. (From Fritz S: *Mosby's fundamentals of therapeutic massage*, ed 6, St. Louis, 2017, Elsevier.)

Sometimes the scent is dispersed into the air through the use of candles or oil dispersers. Aromatic oils often are used during massage. Bathing provides a good modality for aromatherapy when oil is added to the water. On occasion, essential oils are taken orally in small amounts but only when prescribed by a qualified health care professional.

Many scents are used for their psychological effects. Different scents are thought to evoke different responses in the body as well. Nurses know that certain odors in a clinical setting have the potential to cause nausea or vomiting. Aromatherapy is based on similar principles: specific scents are thought to relax or stimulate, improve digestion, increase hormone production, reduce nausea, and improve circulation or memory. Table 20.2 presents some common essences and their uses.

Patients with asthma sometimes develop exaggerated symptoms from certain aromatic essences. Do not use essential oils on the skin of a patient with atopic eczema.

REFLEXOLOGY

Reflexology is based on the premise that it is possible to exert an effect on the entire body by applying pressure to specific areas on the feet, hands, and ears with the thumbs. The theory underlying reflexology is that these areas correspond to organs and systems of the body. Reflexologists use foot charts to guide them as they apply pressure to specific areas (Fig. 20.5). The manipulation of specific reflexes removes stress, enabling the release of disharmonies by a physiologic change in the body. With stress removed and circulation improved, the body is allowed to return to a state of homeostasis.

When reflexology is performed, the patient is assisted into a comfortable position, either lying or sitting. The feet are exposed so that the practitioner is able to perform specific massage movements and techniques on the feet. Treatments typically last up to 1 hour. Most people consider treatments to be very relaxing.

Reflexologists believe that treatment has the capacity to interfere with other medical or alternative treatment; therefore it is important that the patient informs the practitioner of any other treatments being received. Reflexology generally is considered safe for people of all ages, although very vigorous pressure may cause discomfort for some people. Lighter pressure should be used on corresponding reflex areas on people with cardiac problems, blood problems, high blood pressure, epilepsy, and diabetes. Extreme caution should be used in performing reflexology on patients with diabetes who use artificial insulin. Overstimulation of the corresponding reflexes can cause the pancreas to produce increased amounts of insulin, resulting in a decreased need of artificial insulin.

Reflexology demonstrates the following four main benefits:

1. Relaxes the body and removes stress
2. Enhances the circulation
3. Assists the body in normalizing metabolism naturally
4. Complements all other healing modalities

When the reflexes are stimulated through the process of reflexology, the body's natural electrical energy works along the nervous system pathways and meridian lines to clear any blockages along those lines and in the corresponding zones. A treatment seems to break up deposits (felt as a sandy or gritty area under the skin) that interfere with this natural flow of the body's energy. Reflexologists are not qualified to diagnose medical conditions.

MAGNET THERAPY

Early research on the use of magnets showed promise as a treatment for pain. However, larger studies failed to demonstrate a clear benefit. Magnet therapy has been marketed in a variety of products, including jewelry, shoe inserts, and mattress toppers. Most users of magnet therapy have neither beneficial nor detrimental effects. However, it is contraindicated in patients with metal devices such as defibrillators, pacemakers, cochlear implants, and insulin pumps (NCCIH, 2017).

IMAGERY

In **imagery,** or visualization techniques, the conscious mind is used to create mental images to evoke physical changes in the body, create a sense of improved well-being, and enhance self-awareness. Imagery frequently is combined with some form of relaxation training to facilitate the effect of the relaxation technique. Imagery is sometimes self-directed, whereby the individual creates his or her own mental images; and sometimes the process is guided, whereby a health care professional leads the individual through a particular scenario. Here is a sample scenario of guided imagery with the professional as the guide:

> First direct the patient to begin slow abdominal breathing while focusing on the rhythm of breathing. Then instruct the patient to visualize ocean waves coming to shore with each inspiration and receding with each expiration. Next instruct the patient to take notice of the smells, the sounds, and the temperatures that he or she is experiencing. As the imagery session progresses, perhaps instruct the patient to visualize warmth entering the body during inspiration and tension leaving the body during expiration.

The professional works in this manner but individualizes imagery scenarios for each patient or leaves them to the patient to develop.

Imagery has the power to evoke significant psychophysiologic responses, such as alterations in immune function. Many imagery techniques involve visual imagery, but they also sometimes include the auditory, proprioceptive, gustatory, and olfactory senses. For example, visualize slicing a lemon in half and squeezing the lemon juice under your tongue. This visualization produces increased salivation as effectively as the actual event. People typically respond to the environment according to the way it is perceived. The body has a physiologic response (salivating) to the visualization of an event that did not actually happen (the lemon slicing and juice tasting). As a result, an individual learns to regulate the body's responses to environmental stimuli by appropriately regulating expectations and perceptions. Imagery has applications in a number of patient populations. Imagery has been used to visualize the destruction of cancer cells by cells of the immune system, to control or relieve pain, and to achieve calmness and serenity (University of Michigan Health System, 2017).

RELAXATION THERAPY

Relaxation is the state of a generalized decrease in cognitive, physiologic, or behavioral arousal. Relaxation also is defined as the act or process of arousal reduction. The process of relaxation elongates the muscle fibers and reduces the neural impulses sent to the brain and thus decreases the activity of the brain and other body systems. The relaxation response is characterized by decreased heart and respiratory rates, blood pressure, and oxygen consumption and increased alpha-wave brain activity and peripheral skin temperature. The relaxation response can be obtained through a variety of techniques that incorporate a repetitive mental focus and the adoption of a calm, peaceful attitude. Teaching strategies for relaxation exercises are listed in Box 20.1.

Relaxation training involves developing cognitive skills that help people reduce the negative ways in which they respond to situations and their environment. The

Box 20.1 Relaxation Strategies

RHYTHMIC BREATHING[a]

1. Provide a quiet environment.
2. Help the patient get comfortable by elevating the legs with the knees bent (relaxing the leg, back, and abdominal muscles).
3. Instruct the patient to close eyes and to breathe in and out slowly; say rhythmically, "Breathe in, 2, 3, 4; breathe out, 2, 3, 4."
4. Once rhythmic breathing is established, instruct patient to listen to your voice, and with a low and steady voice, instruct patient to do the following:
   a. Breathe in and out slowly and deeply.
   b. Try to breathe from the abdomen.
   c. Feel more relaxed with each exhalation.
   d. Try to identify your own special feeling of relaxation (e.g., light and weightless or very heavy).
   e. While you are breathing, let your imagination take you to a place you remember as peaceful and pleasant; look around, listen to the sounds, feel the air, notice the smells.
   f. When you are ready to end this relaxation exercise, count silently from 1 to 3; on 1, move your lower body; on 2, move your upper body; on 3, breathe in deeply, open your eyes, and while breathing out slowly, say silently, "I am relaxed and alert." Stretch as if just waking up.

PROGRESSIVE RELAXATION

1. Follow steps 1, 2, and 3 of rhythmic breathing.
2. Once patient is breathing slowly and comfortably, instruct patient to tighten and relax an ordered succession of muscle groups, tensing them and then relaxing them, leaving each part feeling relaxed.
3. Instruct patient to begin by tensing and then relaxing the calves, then the knees, and so on.

RELAXATION BY SENSORY PACING

1. Follow steps 1 and 2 of rhythmic breathing.
2. Instruct patient to slowly repeat and finish either in a low voice or to self each of the following sentences:
   a. "Now I am aware of seeing ..."
   b. "Now I am aware of feeling ..."
   c. "Now I am aware of hearing ..."
3. Instruct patient to repeat and complete each sentence four times, then three times, then twice, and finally once.
4. Instruct patient to allow the eyes to close when they feel heavy.

RELAXATION BY COLOR EXCHANGE

1. Follow steps 1, 2, and 3 of rhythmic breathing.
2. Instruct patient to notice any tension, tightness, aches, or pains in the body and to give that sensation the first color that comes to mind.
3. Instruct patient to breathe in pure white light from the universe and send the light to the tense or painful place in the body, letting the white light surround the color of the discomfort.
4. Instruct patient to exhale the color of the discomfort and let the white light take its place.
5. Instruct patient to continue breathing in the white light and exhaling the color of the discomfort, allowing the white light to fill the entire body and bring about a sense of peace, well-being, and energy.

MODIFIED AUTOGENIC RELAXATION

1. Follow steps 1, 2, and 3 of rhythmic breathing.
2. Instruct patient to repeat each of the following phrases to oneself four times, saying the first part of the phrase while breathing in for 2 to 3 seconds, then holding the breath for 2 to 3 seconds, and then saying the last part of the phrase while breathing out for 2 to 3 seconds.

BREATHING IN	BREATHING OUT
I am	relaxed.
My arms and legs	are heavy and warm.
My heartbeat	is calm and regular.
My breathing	is free and easy.
My abdomen	is loose and warm.
My forehead	is cool.
My mind	is quiet and still.

RELAXING WITH MUSIC

1. Provide patient with an MP3 player or other listening device and headset.
2. Ask patient to select a favorite choice of slow, quiet music.
3. Instruct patient to get into a comfortable position (either sitting or lying down but with arms and legs uncrossed) and to close eyes and listen to the music through the headset.
4. Instruct patient to imagine floating or drifting with the music while listening.

[a]In conditioning a relaxation response, a "signal breath" involving deep inhalation through the nose and forceful exhalation through the mouth is the key. The signal breath precedes and follows each run through the exercise.

cognitive skills include **focusing** (the ability to identify, differentiate, keep attention on, and return attention to simple stimuli for an extended period), **passivity** (the ability to stop unnecessary goal-directed and analytic activity), and **receptivity** (the ability to tolerate and accept experiences that are sometimes uncertain, unfamiliar, or paradoxical). In addition, the individual performs cognitive restructuring, during which he or she replaces negative thoughts with positive ones. The long-term goal of relaxation therapy is for the person to continually monitor the self for indicators of tension and to consciously let go and release the tension contained in various body parts.

ANIMAL-ASSISTED THERAPY

Animal-assisted therapy (AAT) involves the use of trained animals to enhance an individual's physical, emotional, and social well-being (Fig. 20.6). This method improves self-esteem, reduces anxiety, and facilitates

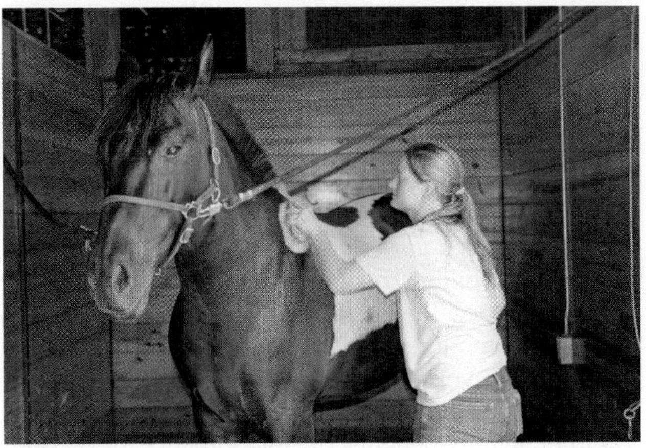

Fig. 20.6 Animal-assisted therapy. Caring for an animal is one aspect of animal-assisted therapy.

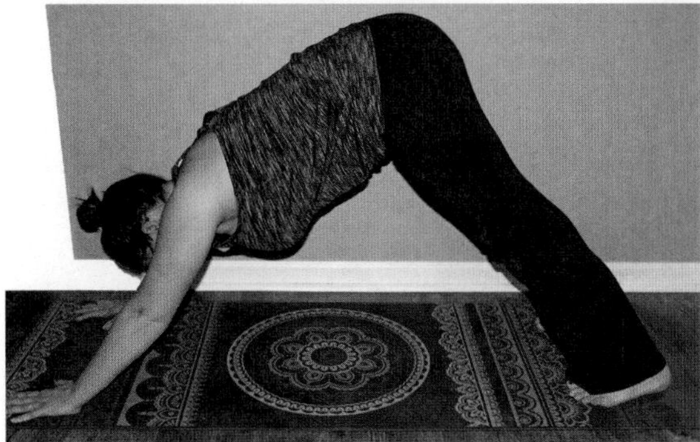

Fig. 20.7 Yoga is useful in achieving control of the body through correct posture and breathing, control of the emotions and the mind, and meditation and contemplation.

healing. AAT began in the 1940s, when an army corporal brought his Yorkshire terrier to a hospital to cheer wounded soldiers. The response was so positive that the dog continued to comfort others for 12 more years.

Research has concluded that animals have a calming effect, reducing blood pressure and anxiety. They tend to decrease loneliness and bring out positive social characteristics. Health care practitioners at many hospitals and nursing homes use AAT programs to help decrease feelings of depression and isolation in their patients, as well as stimulating mental activity through interaction with the animals.

Many different types of animals are used in AAT, from dogs and cats to horses and dolphins. Safety is always a consideration when working with any type of animal. AAT professionals and volunteer handlers must ensure that the animal has been trained adequately and is in good health, with all necessary vaccinations. Patient allergies and autoimmunity issues necessitate consideration before implementation of AAT. Clearance by a health care provider should be obtained if there is any question regarding the patient's safety. Not all animals used in AAT are service animals. Service animals must meet specific criteria, but they are protected legally under the Americans with Disabilities Act (ADA).

AAT is a complementary intervention that is continuing to gain popularity in the medical setting. It can be an effective treatment, or part of one, for a long list of disorders (Mayo Foundation for Medical Education and Research, 2016).

YOGA

The word *yoga* means "yoke," or union of the personal self with the divine source. Yoga is a healing system of therapy and practice. It is a combination of breathing exercises, physical postures, and meditation that has been practiced for more than 5000 years. **Yoga** has emerged as a therapeutic treatment and now is being recognized by Western medical practice. As scientific research increasingly verifies the importance of the integration of the whole person in healing disease, the medical community no longer can ignore the efficacy of yoga's body-mind connection.

With consistent and earnest practice, change and personal transformation take place on numerous levels. Typically, these changes include improved health and energy, reduced stress, feelings of well-being, and the healing of disease. What perhaps started as a search for increased flexibility and stress reduction slowly enlarged to a greater understanding of the self, emotional growth, and spiritual awakening.

There are more than 100 different schools of yoga. Hatha yoga is the most familiar type in the United States. However, all systems recognize the validity of certain basic principles, including control of the body through correct posture and breathing, control of the emotions and the mind, and meditation and contemplation (Fig. 20.7).

The regular practice of yoga offers the potential to tone the muscles that balance all parts of the body, including internal organs, heart, lungs, glands, and nerves. It increases flexibility of the spine and therefore helps treat chronic back problems. It is beneficial for the nervous system, promoting deep relaxation and reduction of stress. Although the risk of injury from yoga is very small, a possibility of injury exists. Some poses may have to be modified. The participant and the instructor must be accepting of the participant's limits and present level of skill. As with most forms of exercise, the participant should not try to do too much too quickly.

Patients with glaucoma should not do inverted poses, such as downward facing dog. Head-down yoga poses cause a temporary, but significant, increase in pressure within the eye. The short period of time when the eye pressure is increased is not thought to be harmful to most people. However, patients with the eye disease glaucoma have a higher risk for optic nerve damage because of increases in eye pressure (American Optometric Association, 2016).

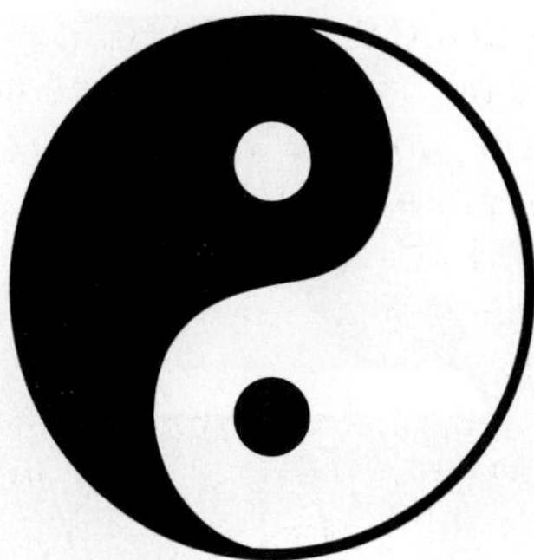

Fig. 20.8 The t'ai chi diagram.

TAIJI

Taiji (also called **t'ai chi**) originally was developed as a martial art in 17th-century China. Origins of the art are debated by proponents of various styles, but nearly all agree that the art was a fusion of existing martial arts practices with Daoist philosophical concepts, traditional Chinese medicine, and qigong theory and practice. The meaning of Taiji (Fig. 20.8) was described by Yang and colleagues (2008):

> The word Taiji is an ancient Daoist philosophical term symbolizing the interaction of yin and yang, which are opposite manifestations of the same forces in nature. The dynamic interaction of yin and yang, underlying the relation and changing nature of all things, is epitomized in the famous "Taiji Diagram."

A fundamental principle of Taijiquan is the relationship between seemingly opposite forces. It is helpful to think of yin and yang as complementary opposites: each necessarily relies upon, and "gives birth" to, the other. In Taiji practice, emphasis is placed on relaxing the body and calming and focusing the mind. Taiji form movement is performed slowly; the intention, mechanics, accuracy, and precision of the motion are accentuated. By practicing in accordance with Taiji principles of softness and slowness, the person paradoxically begins to experience a quality of hardness, strength, and efficiency of movement that are significantly different from that of ordinary natural ability (Yang et al, 2008).

The Taiji training system includes form movement, static and dynamic qigong exercises, and two-person balance and reaction training called "push-hands." Form movement typically is performed slowly with relaxed body and calm and focused mind and thus is referred to as a "moving meditation." Static standing and sitting meditation exercises are practiced as fundamental qigong exercises. Lying-down meditation is another qigong practice that is an effective relaxation and stretching exercise. In its complete form, Taiji is a holistic art that emphasizes mind-body integration, physical and mental balance, and spiritual development. Practice of the art is direct exercise of central and peripheral nervous system function.

Taiji practice originally was intended to improve the variables of fundamental skills, including balance, strength, flexibility, coordination, agility, reaction time, sensitivity or awareness, and confidence. Although essential for self-defense, these variables are, at the same time, fundamentally health issues. Because the intensity (e.g., range of motion and height of stance) of any Taiji form sequence is varied easily to suit the individual's physical capabilities, people of all physical abilities are able to practice Taiji. It is especially well suited as a low- to medium-intensity exercise for older adults. Those unable to learn or perform movements do well to begin with the static qigong exercises.

Other health benefits of Taiji practice have been recognized in China for a long time and are receiving more attention in Europe and the Americas. Research articles and studies are increasing as interest grows about these concepts. Health benefits documented in these studies include significant improvements in balance, leg strength, cardiorespiratory function, range of motion and treatment of arthritic symptoms, self-efficacy, sleep quality, prevention of osteoporosis, and immune function. Other health benefits, not yet studied in Europe and the Americas but appreciated in China, include improvements in bowel function, general strengthening of the immune system, and improvements in cognitive function (attention, concentration, learning, and memory) (Yang et al, 2008).

BIOFEEDBACK

Biofeedback is a noninvasive method that an individual can employ to learn control of the body to manage certain conditions. It may be considered when other therapies have not been successful or in conjunction with other treatments. Health concerns such as anxiety, stress, irritable bowel syndrome, and asthma may be managed through biofeedback. Monitoring equipment is used to measure vital signs and muscle tension. The messages are sent back to the individual. These responses are conveyed to the patient through auditory, visual, physical, or physiologic signals, or a combination of these (Mayo Clinic, 2012). Once the messages are sent to the patient, there is opportunity to control the body and manage the disorders. One key advantage of biofeedback is the increased awareness achieved by the patient about physiologic functions and influencing factors of these functions.

Another advantage of biofeedback is the reduction of the stress response. Biofeedback has been found to be beneficial in the treatment of disorders such as migraine headaches, pain, and urinary tract and gastrointestinal tract disorders. Commitment of the patient to the program determines a successful outcome.

Although biofeedback is considered noninvasive, precautions with the therapy are necessary in connection with repressed emotions or feelings that may surface during the relaxation or biofeedback sessions. It is important for the health care provider to be aware of these precautions so that proper psychologic support is available at the time of the sessions or proper referral is made.

MARIJUANA AND CANNABINOIDS

Cannabis (marijuana) and its chemical compounds are receiving renewed interest as a potential treatment for a variety of health conditions. Marijuana is the common name for cannabis that can be used as a drug. Therapeutic use of marijuana is controversial. Over half the states have some form of medical marijuana laws. Marijuana remains federally banned and is designated as a schedule I drug in the United States. Schedule I drugs are drugs with no currently accepted medical use and have the highest potential for abuse. States that legalize marijuana are doing so in conflict with the current Drug Enforcement Agency's (DEA's) classification of marijuana as a schedule I drug. A petition to reschedule marijuana was denied in August of 2016. The head of the DEA, Chuck Rosenberg, told National Public Radio that "marijuana is not as dangerous as heroin, for instance…clearly not as dangerous. But this decision isn't based on danger. This decision is based on whether marijuana, as determined by the FDA, is a safe and effective medicine … and it's not." He said the DEA supports scientific research of marijuana and could change its mind based on the findings of the research. The DEA declined to reschedule marijuana but has loosened restrictions on who may cultivate marijuana for research purposes (Johnson, 2016).

Cannabinoids are compounds found in marijuana that attach to cannabinoid receptors in the body. There are more than 60 cannabinoids unique to marijuana. **Tetrahydrocannabinol** (THC) is the most well-known cannabinoid. THC is psychoactive and may cause euphoria, paranoia, drowsiness, and increased hunger. This chemical causes the "high" that is responsible for the abuse potential of the drug. Therapeutically, THC is used to treat nausea, pain, and weight loss in patients with cancer and human immunodeficiency virus (HIV). Because of breeding techniques, **cannabidiol** (CBD), THC, and other cannabinoids are present at highly variable levels in marijuana. CBD has no psychoactive properties and inhibits the psychoactive properties of THC. In states where marijuana is available, consumers may select strains based on the THC to CBD content. Strains with a high CBD content are being used for a variety of neurologic disorders. Parents may seek out marijuana with high CBD content as a treatment for their children with life-threatening seizures that are not responsive to allopathic medicine. Several states have legalized CBD preparations, while maintaining marijuana as an illegal drug.

Three species of cannabis have been identified. *Cannabis sativa* is used for industrial purposes, therapeutic uses, and as a recreational drug. *Cannabis indica* tends to have more CBD content, but THC is present as well. Selective breeding of *C. indica* has resulted in strains with higher CBD content. *Cannabis ruderalis* may be used as an herbal treatment but is not used as a recreational drug. Hybrids and selective breeding have led to further variation of components for therapeutic and recreational purposes.

Supporters of rescheduling marijuana point out that marijuana is a schedule I drug, like LSD and heroin. They would like to see marijuana reclassified as a schedule II drug, like narcotics used for pain control, such as morphine, hydromorphone, oxycodone, and fentanyl. Schedule II drugs have high potential for abuse but also have an accepted medical use. There is no known "lethal dose" of marijuana (Leafscience.com, 2014). Many schedule II drugs used for pain control may lead to severe respiratory depression, whereas marijuana does not. Concentrated THC preparations potentially may cause changes in blood pressure and heart rate but there is almost no risk of heart attack. The risk of heart attack from using marijuana is estimated to be comparable to the risk caused by air pollution (Russo, 2015).

Selective breeding may lead to new treatments for a variety of conditions, such as depression, anxiety, dementia, drug addiction, nausea, and pain (Russo and Hohmann, 2013). Marijuana and specific **cannabinoids** may be used for a variety of psychological, neurologic, and inflammatory conditions. Research into the treatment of cancer has had conflicting results. THC and synthetic THC may be used to treat the side effects of cancer treatment. Synthetic THC, dronabinol, is US Food and Drug Administration (FDA) approved for the treatment of nausea, vomiting, and anorexia in patients with cancer and AIDS. It is available in the trade names of Marinol and Syndros. They have been designated schedule III drugs. There is ongoing research into medical uses of synthetic marijuana derivatives. These should not be confused with non–FDA-approved products marketed as "synthetic marijuana" in an effort to bypass FDA regulations. These often are sold online or in gas stations under many names, including Spice, K2, Herbal Incense, and synthetic marijuana. These have variable synthetic compounds that may or may not resemble those in marijuana. These drugs do not have FDA approval and can be lethal. Once these drugs were identified as dangerous substances, they were banned, but there have been similar drugs marketed with new names. Patients should be warned not to use over-the-counter products marketed as synthetic versions of marijuana.

Marijuana and cannabinoids are in a unique position as potential herbal or dietary treatments (Russo, Mead, and Sulak, 2015), medications as well as potentially addictive substances that may necessitate treatment. Marijuana has abuse potential but also may be a less addictive form of pain management. It may be used in place of more addictive medications or even in the treatment of addiction. The large number of cannabinoids and other natural components complicate the regulation of the drug. Although pharmaceutical companies often look at the individual components of the drug, others believe selective breeding of the whole plant has more therapeutic uses (Russo and Hohmann, 2013).

Several states and the District of Columbia have passed laws that permit some form of medical or recreational marijuana use. Arguments for legalization of marijuana often point out that legalization can improve state finances through tax revenue. States that have recreational marijuana also have had a new form of tourism, called "weed tourism." The recreational use of marijuana has been called a "gateway drug" for decades. Opponents believe that easy access to marijuana may result in increased use of more dangerous and addictive drugs. Several states permit the use of only CBD oil. Other states have decriminalized marijuana. Decriminalizing marijuana is not the same as legalizing marijuana, but patients may be more likely to self-medicate where there are fewer consequences.

Patients that use marijuana as CAM need to stay informed of the rapidly changing state laws that restrict obtaining, cultivating, and possessing marijuana. Parents providing marijuana for their minor children may have additional legal consequences. State laws vary, and the individual is held to the law of the state they are in, regardless of residence. Even in states where marijuana is legal, employees may be terminated for obtaining a medical marijuana card or evidence of marijuana use. With these considerations in mind, patients should be encouraged to exhaust medical options before attempting to use marijuana to treat symptoms.

Nurses must be aware of the complexities of marijuana and cannabinoids as CAM. Patients may think that marijuana is safe or unsafe based on state and federal laws governing its use. The legal status of a drug does not determine its safety. Alcohol and tobacco abuse are legal, but clearly each has negative health consequences. Particularly concerning is the marketing of dangerous substances as legal alternatives to marijuana. Some state laws may require a physician to prescribe and monitor medical marijuana. However, the appropriate cannabis strain, dose, frequency, and route often are determined by providers without medical training. Plant quality, chemical components, and contamination concerns are similar to those seen with herbal treatments. Although there is no known toxic dose of marijuana, intoxication can lead to death or injury because of impaired judgment and inability to operate a vehicle safely. Concentrates of the psychoactive portion of cannabis, THC, can cause concerning changes in vital signs. Factors that may affect the response and side effects include previous marijuana use, the amount taken, the route (smoking, vaping, ingesting, applying topically or instilling eye drops), and the levels of specific cannabinoids (Russo, 2015).

The American Cannabis Nurses Association (ACNA) is a professional nursing organization that is a resource for nurses wanting to learn more about cannabinoid therapeutics. The ACNA's mission is *"to advance excellence in cannabis nursing practice through advocacy, collaboration, education, research and policy development"* (ACNA, n.d.). The Medical Cannabis Institute (TMCI) aims to *"educate a growing global community of healthcare professionals, caregivers and patients who want to learn about the science and clinical data behind medical cannabis"* (TMCI, 2018). The ACNA and TMCI offer online curriculums for nurses and other health care professionals wanting objective, scientific information. Patients Out of Time offers

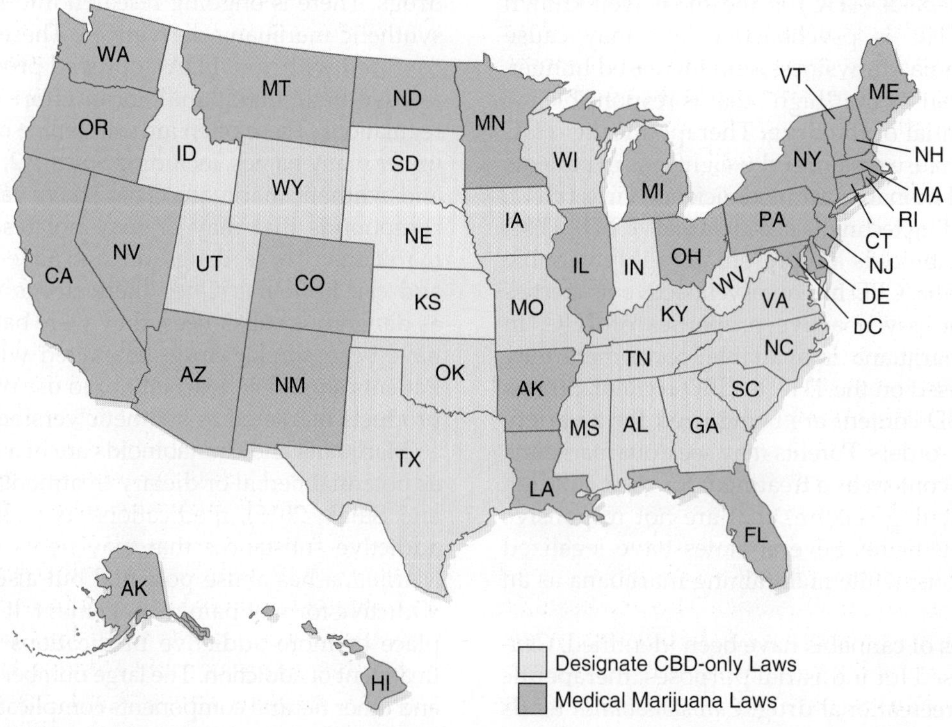

(From The National Organization for the Reform of Marijuana Laws—NORML, *www.norml.org/laws.*)

conferences and resources for patients and health care providers *(http://patientsoutoftime.org)* (ACNA, n.d.).

INTEGRATIVE MEDICINE AND THE NURSING ROLE

The interest in CAM therapies has increased significantly since 1990. The majority of people using and seeking information about CAM are well educated and have a strong desire to participate actively in the decision making about their health care. This interest is increased not only among health care consumers but also among allopathic health care providers who have increasing concerns that current Western medicine is not meeting the needs of their patients. Many allopathic health care providers do not refer their patients for CAM, because they are not familiar with the therapies and have had little, if any, education and training in CAM. Many health care providers have reservations about CAM, because its modalities have not been tested appropriately in clinical trials with strict controls for the other factors that have the capacity to influence the outcomes. Many studies related to CAM have involved small numbers of subjects and were not well controlled. More research is needed to establish evidence-based practice and to validate the effectiveness of CAM therapies (Potter, Perry, and Stockert, 2013).

In North America and the United Kingdom, many professional groups are exploring the use of CAM and facilitating and monitoring research in this area. Proposals put forth by several of these groups include assessing the need of the public for CAM therapies, incorporating CAM educational components into the curriculum from all health care programs, providing appropriate information to the public, and encouraging and facilitating communication between CAM practitioners from various backgrounds and geographic locations. If CAM therapies are to be accepted and integrated into the Western medical approach, they must be subjected to more rigorous research—an undertaking that perhaps will worry some practitioners but also will refine and improve the therapies. Integrating CAM therapies to promote a more holistic approach to health care is beneficial to all parties. These health interventions promote patient participation, thus potentially preventing illness or chronic disease processes and ultimately leading to reduced reliance solely on surgery and drug therapy. Integrative medicine, a health care strategy that is gaining popularity, involves an interdisciplinary, multiple-professional treatment group that a patient consults as a cooperative entity, instead of seeking care from one type of health care provider at a time. Patients have the option to choose the kind of professional they think would benefit their health problem, and the professionals of different types and specialties also refer to and consult among one another. This represents a pluralistic and truly complementary health care system in which alternative and allopathic health care providers work together to improve the well-being of their patients. Although this is not the reality in the majority of settings, this approach of open communication and practice between allopathic and alternative health care providers has great potential to benefit a large number of patients (see the Lifespan Considerations box on complementary and alternative therapy for older adults). Patients likely to benefit from these groups are those who have chronic health problems that historically have been difficult to treat with traditional allopathic medicine, such as fibromyalgia or chronic fatigue syndrome.

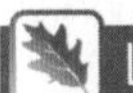

Lifespan Considerations

Older Adults

Complementary and Alternative Therapy

- Use essential oils with caution. Older adult patients are usually more sensitive to essential oils and thus require smaller amounts and less concentrated forms of the essence.
- Advise older adult patients to take herbal treatments only under professional supervision.
- Older adults typically achieve positive results from regular exercise and weight-lifting, including increased physical strength and flexibility and improved mental status in areas such as memory and depression. It is necessary to adapt the exercise regimen to each patient's physical condition.
- In massage therapy, a lighter pressure is necessary; other modifications for body status of an older adult patient also may be needed.
- Magnet therapy has not been shown to be effective, and the use of magnets interferes with pacemaker functions.

The integrative medicine approach is consistent with the holistic approach that nurses are taught to practice. Nurses have the potential for becoming essential participants in this type of health care model. Many nurses already practice forms of CAM by offering relaxation, imagery, and massage to their patients. Nurses need a good knowledge of CAM therapies to make appropriate recommendations to allopathic primary care providers about potentially useful therapies. They should be prepared to advise patients regarding when to seek conventional therapy and when CAM therapy is appropriate (see the Patient Teaching box on using complementary and alternative therapies). For example, if a patient complains of right lower abdominal pain, nausea, and vomiting, the nurse should suspect appendicitis and recommend assessment by an allopathic health care provider. However, if the patient has a chronic gastrointestinal disorder and irritable bowel syndrome has been diagnosed, it is possible that the patient will benefit from relaxation and herbal therapy. Nurses must be aware of their state's nurse practice act with regard to complementary therapies and practice accordingly within the scope of these laws.

Nurses work closely with their patients and are in the unique position of becoming familiar with the patient's religious and cultural viewpoints (see the Cultural Considerations box) and existential issues.

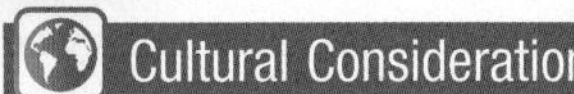

Cultural Considerations

Providing Culturally Appropriate Complementary and Alternative Therapy

- Avoid using the term *alternative therapy;* patients may not consider their practices to be alternative at all. For some Chinese Americans, for example, treatments such as acupuncture and use of herbal preparations are grounded in their culture and passed down from generation to generation. They may consider Western medicine to be the alternative.
- Acupuncture originated in China approximately 4000 to 5000 years ago, but very little acupuncture was performed in the United States outside of Chinese immigrant communities until the 1970s.
- Yoga began in India more than 6000 years ago.
- Members of some cultures often have more faith in an alternative or traditional care practitioner than in a conventional Western health care provider. Respect the patient's beliefs and look for ways to combine therapies when there are no contraindications.
- Regardless of your personal faith in another type of care, be sensitive to cultural differences (e.g., ethnic, racial, gender). Question the patient appropriately and support the patient's choices as needed.
- Show respect for the cultural differences by honoring the patient's culturally based health beliefs.
- Ask permission before touching the patient. Determine the meaning of touch and which body areas are considered touchable. Acceptability of touch varies from culture to culture.
- To provide culturally appropriate and competent alternative and complementary therapies, remember that each individual is culturally unique and is the product of a mixture of past experiences, cultural beliefs, and cultural norms.

See Chapter 6 for further discussion of cultural considerations.

The nurse is in a good position to determine which CAM therapies are aligned most appropriately with these beliefs and to offer recommendations accordingly.

Increased awareness of complementary and alternative therapies means that many patients whom you encounter already have had experience with or are amenable to investigating these therapies. In making choices concerning their health care, patients tend to be receptive to holistic interventions and often seek guidance in exploring various options (Potter, Perry, and Stockert, 2013). Therefore be knowledgeable about the multiple CAM therapies available and the use of these therapies by patients. Keep abreast of the current research in this area to provide accurate information not only to patients but also to other health care providers.

Get Ready for the NCLEX® Examination!

Key Points

- Complementary and alternative therapies are used to restore or maintain health.
- Patients tend to think of CAM therapies as gentler and less invasive than traditional medical treatments.
- Patients are often hesitant to tell a health care provider about CAM therapies they are using.
- Herbs used for treatment are formulated in many ways for consumption and use: as dried herbs in capsules or tablets, tinctures, teas, compresses, salves, or ointments.
- Some herbs interfere with the actions of medications. A thorough health history is important.
- Chiropractic treatment achieves its effects through manipulation of the musculoskeletal system. Gentle manipulation puts the vertebrae in proper alignment.
- In acupuncture and acupressure, needles or pressure is applied to specific points on the body. The points correspond to meridians that flow through the body.
- Energy field therapies have benefits for the practitioner and the recipient. Energy field therapies can reduce pain and increase relaxation. Practice fosters intuition, skills, and connectedness.
- Energy field therapies do not require physical touch. Touch may be used, but there is no manipulation of the physical body.
- In its complete form, Taiji (t'ai chi) is a holistic art that emphasizes mind-body integration, physical and mental balance, and spiritual development.
- Therapeutic massage is used to promote healing and prevent injury. Contraindications include a history of phlebitis or thrombosis of the extremities.
- In aromatherapy, essential oils are used to provide health benefits. Inhalation is the most common method of using the oils.
- Pressure to the feet in the form of massage is performed in reflexology.
- Reflexology is a focused pressure technique; it is based on the premise that the feet are divided into zones or reflex areas that correspond to all organs, glands, and systems of the body.
- Regular practice of yoga potentially tones the muscles that balance all parts of the body—including internal organs, heart, lungs, glands, and nerves—and controls the emotions and mind.
- There has been an increase in state laws legalizing the use of marijuana for medicinal as well as recreational use. Marijuana remains federally banned.

- Cannabis (marijuana plant) has been bred to increase or decrease specific cannabinoids for therapeutic use.
- Patients considering self-medicating with marijuana should be encouraged to exhaust traditional medical options first.
- Although some CAM therapies have been researched and the findings published in professional journals, others lack scientific proof. However, those that lack scientific proof need not be discarded because many patients report positive outcomes from these therapies.

Additional Learning Resources

SG Go to your Study Guide for additional learning activities to help you master this chapter content.

evolve Be sure to visit the Evolve site at *http://evolve.elsevier.com/Cooper/foundationsadult/* for additional online resources.

Review Questions for the NCLEX® Examination

1. Among alternative therapies, acupressure may be most effective with which patient?
   1. A patient who is restless and anxious
   2. A patient in whom ulcerative colitis has been diagnosed
   3. A pregnant patient
   4. A patient with mental health concerns
2. The nurse is preparing a presentation on alternative therapies for a community group. Which statement should be included in the presentation?
   1. Herbal therapies are approved by the US Food and Drug Administration under the Food, Drug, and Cosmetic Act.
   2. Herbal therapies are sold as medicines in most stores because they lack major side effects.
   3. Herbal therapies may be packaged as dietary supplements if they are without health claims.
   4. Herbal therapies are consistent in their standards for concentrations of major ingredients and additives.
3. A patient asks about different herbal therapies that may promote physical endurance and reduce stress. Which herb promotes physical endurance and reduces stress?
   1. Ginseng
   2. Ginger
   3. Echinacea
   4. Chamomile
4. When assessing a patient's use of alternative therapies, the nurse should ask which question?
   1. "What herbal supplements have you taken?"
   2. "Have you ever used relaxation therapy?"
   3. "What types of activities or remedies do you use when you do not feel well?"
   4. "Do you use holistic treatments?"
5. A patient questions the nurse about the use of complementary and alternative medicine. Which statement made by the nurse is correct regarding complementary and alternative medicine?
   1. One-third of the US population uses one or more forms of alternative therapy.
   2. Decreasing amounts of insurance coverage are available to meet the needs of alternative therapies.
   3. Discussion of alternative therapies is still not provided in traditional medical journals.
   4. Integration of alternative therapies is regulated by state and national agencies.
6. A patient receiving chemotherapy is implementing relaxation therapy in conjunction with medical protocol. Which benefit can this patient gain from relaxation therapy?
   1. Decreased receptivity
   2. Decreased peripheral skin temperature
   3. Decreased oxygen consumption
   4. Decreased α-wave brain activity
7. The nurse is preparing to administer medications to a patient taking several herbal preparations. Which factor makes accurate administration of precise dosages of herbs difficult?
   1. The fact that multiple clinical trials are under way
   2. Availability in many different forms
   3. Infrequent usage by consumers
   4. Excessive standardization by international organizations
8. A nurse is educating patients at a health care clinic about the use of herbs as a complementary therapy. Which instruction should be included in education about safe herbal product usage? *(Select all that apply.)*
   1. "Combine several herbs to maximize the benefits."
   2. "Believe all claims made by the manufacturer."
   3. "Discontinue using herbs if side effects develop."
   4. "Inform your primary care provider of all herbal products you use."
   5. "Drug interactions may exist with antiplatelet medications."
9. Patients at an integrative health care center are learning about various types of complementary and alternative health care methods. What is a method of stimulating certain points on the body by the insertion of special needles to modify the perception of pain, normalize physiologic functions, or treat or prevent disease?
   1. Acupressure
   2. Magnet therapy
   3. Acupuncture
   4. Chiropractic therapy

10. A patient has reported to the ambulatory care clinic. During the collection of data, the patient reports using reflexology on a weekly basis. What is a contraindication to the use of reflexology? *(Select all that apply.)*
   1. Taking chemotherapy for cancer
   2. History of hypertension
   3. Pregnancy
   4. Epilepsy
   5. History of cardiac disease
11. The patient reports a reduction in pain and spasms since taking marijuana daily for her multiple sclerosis. What side effect is the nurse most likely to assess?
   1. Decreased respiratory rate
   2. Increased appetite
   3. Nausea
   4. Rash
12. _______ *(fill in the blank)* nursing addresses and treats the mind, body, and spirit.
13. Which statement about complementary and alternative medicine (CAM) therapies is most correct?
   1. The patient is actively involved in the treatment.
   2. The patient becomes a total believer in what is being taught.
   3. The patient becomes increasingly submissive to the practitioner.
   4. The patient becomes less competent in his or her own care.
14. A patient is taking the herb comfrey on a daily basis for its wound-healing properties. What information is important for the nurse to tell this patient?
   1. Comfrey should be taken internally.
   2. Comfrey may cause cancer.
   3. Comfrey can be used only externally.
   4. Comfrey is a known antiseptic.
15. When the nurse reviews the patient's medical diagnoses, which condition would be a cause for concern with regard to chiropractic treatments? *(Select all that apply.)*
   1. Acute myelopathy
   2. Vertigo
   3. Osteoporosis
   4. Hypertension
   5. Rheumatoid arthritis
16. The nurse is caring for a patient on the acute care unit. The patient reports that he takes St. John's wort for mild depression. When the nurse reviews the patient's dietary selections, which choice indicates the need for further teaching? *(Select all that apply.)*
   1. Foods high in salt or sodium
   2. Milk products
   3. Anything containing barley, such as beer
   4. Aged cheese
   5. Red wine

Pain Management, Comfort, Rest, and Sleep

21

http://evolve.elsevier.com/Cooper/foundationsadult/

Objectives

1. Define the key terms.
2. List 10 possible causes of discomfort.
3. Discuss McCaffery and Pasero's description of pain.
4. Describe the use of gate control theory to guide selection of nursing interventions for pain relief.
5. Identify subjective and objective data in pain assessment.
6. Discuss the concept of pain assessment as the fifth vital sign.
7. Discuss the synergistic impact of fatigue, sleep disturbance, and depression on the perception of pain.
8. Analyze several scales used to identify intensity of pain.
9. Discuss pain mechanisms affected by each analgesic group.
10. Discuss the role of the nurse in controlling pain.
11. List several methods for pain control.
12. Discuss the differences and similarities between sleep and rest.
13. Outline nursing interventions that promote rest and sleep.
14. Discuss the sleep cycle, differentiating between non–rapid eye movement (NREM) and rapid eye movement (REM) sleep.
15. List six signs and symptoms of sleep deprivation.
16. Identify two nursing diagnoses related to sleep problems.

Key Terms

acute pain (ă-KYŪT PĀN, p. 593)
chronic pain (KRŎN-ĭk PĀN, p. 593)
endorphins (ĕn-DŎR-fĭnz, p. 593)
gate control theory (GĀT kŏn-trōl THĒ-ŏ-rē, p. 593)
non–rapid eye movement (NREM) (NŎN-răp-ĭd Ī MŪV-mĕnt, p. 608)
noxious (NŎK-shŭs, p. 592)
patient-controlled analgesia (PCA) (PĀ-shĕnt kŏn-TRŌLD ăn-ăl-JĒ-zē-ă, p. 600)
rapid eye movement (REM) (RĂP-ĭd Ī MŪV-mĕnt, p. 608)
referred pain (rē-FŬRD PĀN, p. 593)
synergistic (sĭn-ŭr-JĬS-tĭk, p. 593)
transcutaneous electric nerve stimulation (TENS) (trăns-kyū-TĀ-nē-ŭs ē-LĔK-trĭk NŬRV stĭm-ū-LĀ-shŭn, p. 595)
visual analog scale (VĬZH-ū-ăl ĂN-ă-lŏg SKĀL, p. 604)

One of the greatest challenges in nursing is to provide comfort to the patient. To comfort means to give strength and hope, to cheer, and to ease the grief, pain, or trouble of another. Promoting physical and psychological comfort is a vital aspect of nursing care. Many health care providers refer to pain as the fifth vital sign and recommend its assessment and management in much the same manner the traditional vital signs are regarded.

Many factors contribute to a patient's lack of comfort, which manifests in many forms, including the following:

- Anxiety
- Constipation
- Constricting edema
- Depression
- Diaphoresis
- Diarrhea
- Distention
- Dry mouth
- Dyspnea
- Fatigue
- Fear
- Flatus
- Grief
- Headache
- Hopelessness
- Hyperthermia
- Hypothermia
- Hypoxia
- Incontinence
- Muscle cramping
- Nausea
- Pain
- Powerlessness
- Pruritus
- Sadness
- Singultus
- Thirst
- Urinary retention
- Vomiting

Explore the patient's concept of what constitutes comfort. Actively listening to the patient is helpful for planning nursing interventions. Knowing the possible elements of patient discomfort allows for recognition of discomfort signals even when the patient is not able to verbalize, as in the case of a patient who is aphasic or one who is semicomatose. Be diligent in efforts and pursue all the methods to relieve patients' discomfort.

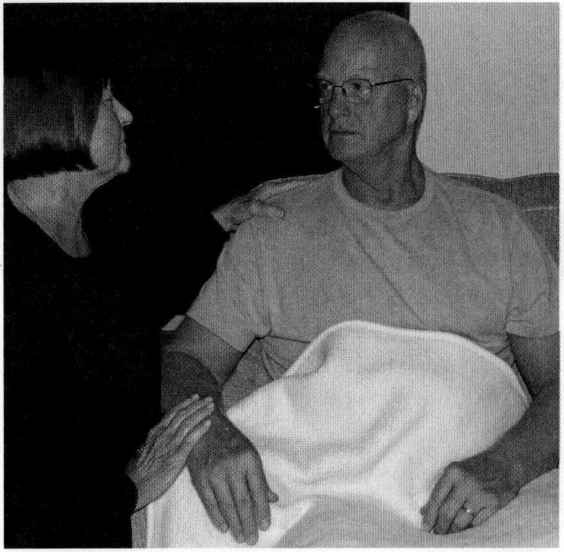

Fig. 21.1 Eye contact and gentle touch promote comfort and well-being.

If interventions are not successful, seek and apply alternative interventions.

Regardless of age, patients typically receive comfort and a sense of well-being from gentle touch and eye contact (Fig. 21.1).

Box 21.1 Behavioral Characteristics of Patients in Pain

The patient with pain exhibits the following behaviors:

- Is self-protective; guards (places hands over) the painful area
- Has narrowed focus; cannot think of anything but the pain, has reduced attention span
- May withdraw from social contact, may avoid conversation or social contacts
- Has impaired thought processes
- Demonstrates distraction behavior, which includes moaning, rocking, crying, pacing, restlessness, or seeking out different activities or possibly other people
- Presents facial mask of pain; eyes appear dull or lusterless, fixed or rapidly changing facial movements, grimacing, teeth clenching, lip biting, or jaw tightening
- Experiences alterations in muscle tone, ranging from flaccidity to rigidity
- Exhibits diaphoresis, changes in blood pressure and pulse rate, pupillary dilation, and increased or decreased rate of respiration
- Sometimes demonstrates no outward expression of pain. Remember that lack of pain expression does not mean lack of pain. There is no specific "picture" of a patient in pain.

PAIN

NATURE OF PAIN

Pain is a complex, abstract, personal subjective experience. It is an unpleasant sensation caused by **noxious** (injurious to physical health) stimulation of the sensory nerve endings. Pain serves as a warning to the body: it often occurs with actual or potential tissue damage. Pain is often a cardinal symptom of inflammation and is valuable in the diagnosis of many disorders and conditions. Pain also may occur when there is no tissue damage, such as the emotional pain of grief at the death of a loved one or the pain of migraine headaches. Pain causes fatigue and decreases the patient's ability to cope physically, emotionally, and mentally. Pain has the potential to be totally debilitating and is one of the most common reasons that patients seek out a health care provider.

Pain is subjective; the interpretation and significance of pain depend on an individual's learned experiences and involve psychosocial and cultural factors. The defining characteristic of pain is the verbal or nonverbal communication by the patient of the presence of pain (Box 21.1). McCaffery and Pasero's (2003) description of pain is a practical one: "Pain is whatever the experiencing person says it is, existing whenever he says it does." According to McCaffery and Pasero's description, nurses are obliged to believe every patient who says he or she has pain.

Only the person with pain, and not the health care provider, is the expert about that pain: its onset, duration, location, intensity, quality, and pattern, as well as the degree of pain relief obtained from therapy. Many patients do not recognize that health care providers are not able to tell how much pain the patients are experiencing. Individuals experiencing pain may not know how best to report their pain and its defining characteristics. Help the patient to recognize his or her expertise about the pain and to use that expertise in partnership with health care providers to obtain better pain management. Empowering the patient to be an active partner in reporting information about the pain is an important nursing skill.

DEFINITIONS OF PAIN

The most widely accepted definition of pain, adopted by the International Association for the Study of Pain and the American Pain Society, is as follows: "Pain is an unpleasant sensory and emotional experience associated with actual or potential tissue damage, or described in terms of such damage" (McCaffery and Pasero, 2003). According to this definition, pain is a phenomenon with multiple components that makes an impact on a person's psychosocial and physical functioning. It acknowledges the complexity of the pain experience. Pain is not determined by tissue damage alone. In fact, no predictable relationship exists between identifiable tissue injury and the sensation of pain. The patient's description of pain may be disproportionate to the evidence of tissue damage. In times of high stress and trauma, patients sometimes describe pain as less severe than expected. Patients with chronic nonmalignant pain often describe pain for which little or no tissue damage can be found. Such pain possibly is caused by abnormalities in the neural processing of stimuli. The inability to identify tissue damage sufficient to explain the pain is not proof that the pain is of psychological origin.

TYPES OF PAIN

There are many types of pain: mild and severe; chronic and acute; intermittent and intractable (constant); burning, dull, and sharp; precisely and poorly localized; and referred. **Referred pain** is felt at a site other than the injured or diseased organ or part of the body. An example of referred pain is the pain of coronary artery insufficiency that sometimes is felt in the left shoulder, the left arm, or the jaw.

Acute pain is intense and of short duration, usually lasting less than 6 months. In general, acute pain provides a warning to the individual of actual or potential tissue damage. It creates an autonomic response that originates within the sympathetic nervous system, flooding the body with epinephrine and commonly referred to as the *fight-or-flight response*. Anxiety usually is associated with the pain. Because the pain is of short duration, health care providers are likely to prescribe opioids and other analgesics.

Chronic pain generally is characterized as pain lasting longer than 6 months. Sometimes the pain is continuous and sometimes it is intermittent; at times, it may be as intense as acute pain. Chronic pain does not serve as a warning of tissue damage in process; rather, it signals that such damage has occurred. Chronic pain may be linked to arthritis, back injuries, fibromyalgia, accidents, or neurologic conditions. In some instances, the root cause of the pain may be elusive and unidentifiable. The pain may be the result of an active condition or from damage left to a body structure such as a joint. Because of the prolonged time involved in chronic pain, many patients develop chronic low self-esteem, change in social identity, changes in role and social interaction, fatigue, sleep disturbance, and depression. Sufferers of chronic pain are also more likely to experience comorbid psychiatric conditions.

Fatigue, sleep disturbance, and depression may act in a type of **synergistic** relationship, in which the actions of two or more substances or organs achieve an effect that cannot be achieved by an individual substance or organ. The combination of fatigue, sleep disturbance, and depression has the potential to markedly change a person's perception of pain. Depression is associated with sleep disturbance, which in turn increases the intensity of the fatigue. As the pain continues unmanaged and unchecked, the patient becomes less aware of other events and begins to focus solely on his or her own body and mind. As the focus narrows further, it entraps the individual in a vicious cycle, making the pain difficult to treat. Pain-related disability, such as inability to perform activities of daily living, contributes to low self-esteem and social problems. Depression is common in patients with chronic pain. Results of a study conducted by researchers at the University of Michigan in Ann Arbor suggested a connection between pain and an increased risk for suicide. Pain types linked most heavily to suicide were psychogenic, back, and migraine (Lowry, 2013).

Because of the general differences between acute and chronic pain, some aspects of nursing interventions for these conditions often differ. Keep in mind that the patient's perception of pain, whether acute or chronic, is real, and use appropriate measures to relieve that pain.

THEORIES OF PAIN TRANSMISSION

Gate Control Theory

The **gate control theory** of pain suggests that pain impulses are regulated and even blocked by gating mechanisms located along the central nervous system (CNS). The proposed location of the gates is in the dorsal horn of the spinal cord. Pain and other sensations of the skin and muscles travel the same pathways through the large nerves in the spinal cord. If other cutaneous stimuli besides pain are transmitted, the "gate" through which the pain impulse must travel is blocked temporarily by the stimuli. The brain does not have the capacity to acknowledge the pain while it is interpreting the other stimuli. When gates are open, pain impulses flow freely (Fig. 21.2). When gates are closed, pain impulses become blocked. Partial openings sometimes occur. A bombardment of sensory impulses, such as those from the pressure of a back rub, the heat of a warm compress, or the cold from ice applications, causes the gates to close to painful stimuli. Some patients may be distracted from pain by removing the sensation of pain from their center of attention. Auditory or visual stimuli often distract patients and help make pain more tolerable.

Gating mechanisms also are subject to alteration by thoughts, feelings, and memories. The cerebral cortex and the thalamus have the capacity to influence whether pain impulses reach a person's conscious awareness. There is conscious control over how pain is perceived, and this helps explain the various ways people react and adjust to pain.

Endorphins

The body produces morphine-like substances called **endorphins** (potent polypeptides composed of many amino acids, found in the pituitary gland and other areas of the CNS). Stress and pain activate endorphins. Analgesia results when certain endorphins attach to opioid receptor sites in the brain and prevent the release of neurotransmitters, thereby inhibiting the transmission of pain impulses. People who feel less pain than do others from a similar injury have higher endorphin levels. Pain relief measures, such as transcutaneous electric nerve stimulation (TENS), acupuncture, and placebos, may cause the release of endorphins.

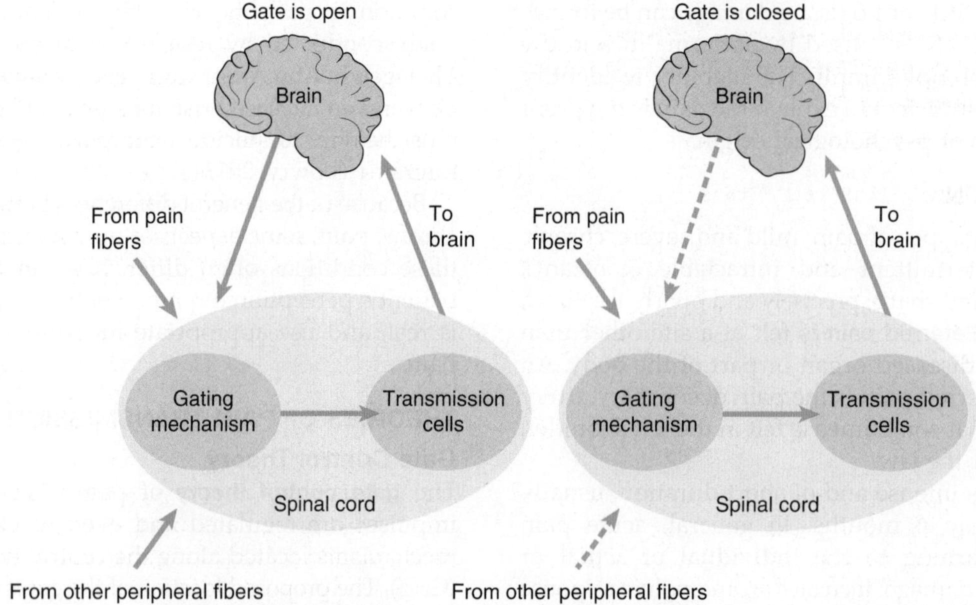

Fig. 21.2 Diagram depicting gate control theory.

CONTROLLING PAIN

Requirements of the Joint Commission for Pain Control

Assessing and managing pain have been primary nursing responsibilities for a long time. In the 1992 standards manual issued by The Joint Commission (TJC) (McCaffery and Pasero, 2003), effective pain management was stated as one of the rights of a dying patient. In 1994 TJC broadened this statement to cover all patients, stating, "The management of pain is appropriate for all patients, not just dying patients" (McCaffery and Pasero, 2003). TJC accreditation visits began to include a focus on what institutions were doing about pain management.

In 1997, under a grant from the Robert Wood Johnson Foundation, TJC began working collaboratively with institutions to create standards for pain assessment and treatment, with plans to conduct national quality improvement programs to help health care facilities meet these standards (McCaffery and Pasero, 2003). TJC now requires accredited facilities and organizations to develop policies and procedures that formalize this obligation (TJC, 2016).

The Joint Commission standards. Under the new TJC standards, health care providers are expected to be knowledgeable about pain assessment and management, and facilities are expected to develop policies and procedures supporting the appropriate use of analgesics and other pain control therapies. The standards do NOT require or mandate the use of medications to manage the pain. These pain standards require education for practitioners on pain assessment and management; respect to the patient's right to pain management; and assessment and management of the patient's pain.

Making Pain the Fifth Vital Sign

One simple strategy to increase accountability for pain control is for an institution to make pain intensity ratings a routine part of assessment and documentation of vital signs. This makes any presence of pain known and raises awareness of the problem of unmanaged pain. Thanks to the work of pain and palliative care associations, more attention is being paid to pain management, and many institutions have included pain assessment as a vital sign.

Giving pain assessment as much attention as that of other vital signs makes it more likely the pain will be treated properly. Vital signs are monitored to detect changes or trends that signal a need for further assessment, diagnosis, and treatment. Considering pain a vital sign—along with pulse, temperature, blood pressure, and respiration—ensures regular monitoring. Use of a pain rating scale allows patients to articulate their pain clearly and makes them more likely to receive proper treatment.

The essential message about pain assessment is this: ask patients about their pain, accept and respect what they say, intervene to relieve their pain, and ask them again about their pain. It is a circle of assessment, intervention, and reassessment. Without assessment of the patient with pain, none of the pain relief measures are useful. Approximately half the people who suffer moderate to severe pain continue to suffer, primarily because nurses fail to assess pain.

Comparing the pain scale (see discussion of *pain rating scales* later in this chapter) to the thermometer is a helpful way to open a discussion about reporting pain. Explain that just as an elevation in the temperature higher than 100°F (37.8°C) would be reported to the health care provider, so would a pain rating of 4 or greater on a

Pain Assessment Guide

Tell Me About Your Pain

H ow does your pain feel?

aching	throbbing	shooting
stabbing	gnawing	sharp
tender	burning	exhausting
tiring	penetrating	nagging
numb	miserable	unbearable
dull	radiating	squeezing
crampy	deep	pressure

Pain in other languages

Vietnamese	Spanish	French
dau	dolor	douleur

I ntensity (0–10)

If 0 is no pain and 10 is the worst pain imaginable, what is your pain now?
... in the last 24 hours?

L ocation

Where is your pain?

D uration

Is the pain always there?
Does the pain come and go? (Breakthrough Pain)
Do you have both types of pain?

A ggravating and Alleviating Factors

What makes the pain better?
What makes the pain worse?

How does pain affect

sleep	energy	relationships
appetite	activity	mood

Are you experiencing any other symptoms?

nausea/vomiting	itching	urinary retention
constipation	sleepiness/confusion	weakness

Things to check

vital signs, past medication history, knowledge of pain, and use of non-invasive techniques

Fig. 21.3 Pain assessment guide. (Courtesy Great Plains Regional Medical Center, North Platte, Nebraska.)

scale of 0 to 10. As with temperature, the higher the pain score is, the more concern and urgency are warranted (Fig. 21.3).

Unrelieved pain has harmful physical effects, such as increased oxygen demand, respiratory dysfunction, decreased gastrointestinal motility, confusion, and depressed immune response. Possible emotional consequences of unrelieved pain include anxiety, depression, irritability, and an inability to enjoy life. Neglected pain erodes a patient's trust in the health care system and possibly leads to setbacks and increased costs in treatment. Conversely, appropriate pain management typically results in quicker recoveries, shorter hospital stays, fewer readmissions, and improved quality of life.

Noninvasive Pain Relief Techniques

Pain is controlled most effectively through a combination of noninvasive pain relief measures and pharmacologic therapy. The purpose of noninvasive pain relief techniques, which are sometimes helpful even when used alone, is to decrease the patient's perception of pain and to improve the patient's sense of control. Useful noninvasive approaches include cutaneous stimulation (heat, cold, massage, and TENS), the removal of painful stimuli, distraction, relaxation, guided imagery, meditation, hypnosis, and biofeedback (Table 21.1). In guided imagery, the patient is encouraged to concentrate on an image that helps relieve pain or discomfort. For the best results, help the patient choose a scene that holds especially pleasant memories. Ask the patient where he or she feels the most relaxed, such as at a lake, in a forest, or in a meadow, and then encourage the patient to use sensory memories to make the image as realistic as possible.

Regardless of whether the gate control theory explains why these techniques are successful or whether they work by decreasing anxiety, they undoubtedly have many advantages for pain control. Most are inexpensive and easy to perform, have low risk and few side effects, and frequently do not require an order by the health care provider. The greatest advantage of these techniques is patients' ability to have some control over the treatment of their pain. Having options provides comfort and assurance to the patient. Although not everyone reacts successfully to these pain relief measures, it is worthwhile to attempt any of them before advancing to more invasive techniques.

Transcutaneous electric nerve stimulation. A special pain relief system, **transcutaneous electric nerve stimulation (TENS)**, entails the use of a pocket-sized, battery-operated device that provides a continuous, mild electric current to the skin via electrodes attached to a stimulator by flexible wires (Fig. 21.4). The electric current is adjustable. Like other forms of cutaneous stimulation, TENS is thought to work by stimulating large nerve fibers to "close the gate" in the spinal cord, thus blocking transmission of pain impulses. In addition, TENS is hypothesized to stimulate endorphin production.

TENS is used typically for patients suffering postoperative or chronic pain. It is customary to place the electrodes on or near the painful site. Be alert to the possibility that a TENS unit can interfere with the function of a cardiac pacemaker device.

Invasive Pain Relief Techniques

Invasive means anything that enters the body. Examples of invasive techniques are nerve blocks, epidural analgesics, neurosurgical procedures, and acupuncture. Certain invasive techniques offer relief for many patients with pain. However, careful patient selection and proper technique are essential because the costs and risks are potentially high.

Table 21.1 Nonpharmacologic Interventions for Pain[a]

INTERVENTIONS	COMMENTS
Physical	
Deep tissue massage	Used to reduce muscle tension and spasms. Effective for mild to moderate discomfort. May be of varying intensity.
Exercise	Physical activity can strengthen core muscles and stabilize the spine to aid in the reduction of discomfort.
Transcutaneous electric nerve stimulation (TENS)	Effective in reducing mild to moderate pain by stimulating the skin with mild electric current. Electrodes are placed over or near the site of pain. Requires special equipment.
Heat or cold application	Selection of heat versus cold varies with the type, location of the pain, and duration of the pain. Moist heat relieves stiffness of arthritis and relaxes muscles. Cold applications reduce acute pain associated with inflammation from arthritis or from acute injury.
Flotation therapy	Involves a flotation period in a chamber of water and Epsom salts (magnesium sulfate), which are absorbed through the skin. Benefits included a near zero gravity state achieved with flotation in water. Magnesium sulfate is linked to reduced musculoskeletal pain.
Acupuncture	Involves the insertion of fine, thin needles into the skin. Researchers believe it works by counteracting imbalances in the body's energy flow. This should be undertaken only by a trained professional.
Psychological and Cognitive	
Music	Music can promote relaxation and reduce anxiety. It can be used in the postoperative period to manage chronic pain and in labor and delivery. Studies have shown that postoperative pain may be reduced by 50% using music.
Biofeedback	Reduces mild to moderate pain and operative site muscle tension. Requires patient to have high level of cognitive function. Requires skilled personnel and special equipment.
Imagery	Reduces mild to moderate pain. The patient is encouraged to focus internally on positive memories or environments. Some patients may require assistance to relax and focus on attention away from the pain.
Humor	Reduces mild to moderate pain. Humor and laughter increase oxygenation and circulation. Rest and sleep also can be improved in the periods after laughter.
Education	Effective for reduction of all types of pain. Should include sensory and procedural information and instruction aimed at reducing activity-related pain.

[a]Should be used with analgesic medication.

Medication for Pain Management

Analgesics often provide effective pain relief. Members of the health care team frequently have misconceptions about the dangers and effects of analgesics. Undertreatment of pain and administration of analgesics in amounts less than what are prescribed may occur because of misunderstandings or insufficient knowledge of pharmacologic principles, concerns about addiction, and anxiety over administering too large a dose of an opioid analgesic. Because of such uncertainties, the patient's pain is only reduced, not relieved. Make sure you understand the medications available for pain relief and their effects.

Nonopioid analgesics. Acetaminophen and nonsteroidal antiinflammatory drugs (NSAIDs)—the nonopioid analgesics—are the most widely available and frequently used analgesic group. Acetaminophen may block pain impulses peripherally that occur in response to inhibition of prostaglandin synthesis, primarily in the CNS. Nonopioid analgesics are used primarily for mild to moderate pain but sometimes also are used to relieve certain types of severe pain. Some NSAIDs are available without a prescription, such as aspirin, ibuprofen (Advil, Nuprin, Motrin), and naproxen sodium (Aleve). Aspirin blocks pain impulses in the CNS and reduces inflammation.

The maximum recommended dosage of acetaminophen is 4000 mg (4 g) in 24 hours. Its toxic side effect, a basic consideration in all analgesic regimens, is hepatotoxicity. Patient responses to NSAIDs vary, so if one is ineffective, try another. Their mechanisms of action appear to be different enough to warrant changing NSAIDs until the best one for the patient is identified. All NSAIDs pose the risk of gastrointestinal bleeding.

Opioid analgesics. Opioids such as morphine, meperidine (Demerol), hydromorphone (Dilaudid), and fentanyl (Actiq, Duragesic) act on higher centers of the brain to modify perception and reaction to pain. Opioids decrease the perception of pain by binding to pain receptor sites in the CNS.

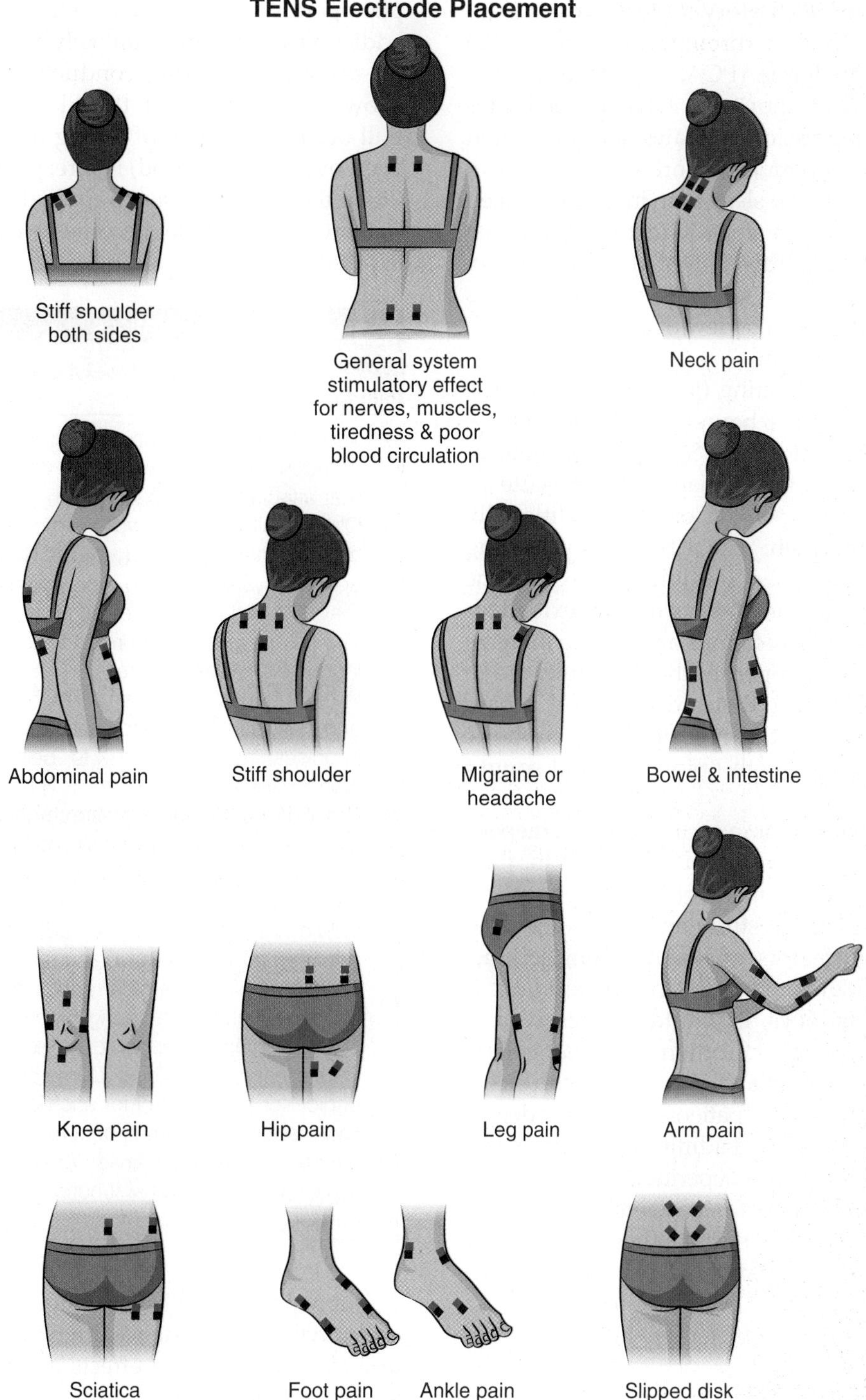

Fig. 21.4 Transcutaneous electric nerve stimulation (TENS).

Opioid analgesics are the cornerstone for managing moderate to severe acute pain. Morphine is the standard agent in opioid therapy, but other opiates, such as hydromorphone, levorphanol, oxycodone, and fentanyl, are ordered as substitutes if the patient has an unusual reaction or allergy to morphine. Morphine is a highly effective drug; however, its use in the presence of compromised renal function must be monitored carefully.

The danger of morphine and other opioid analgesics is their potential to cause depression of vital nervous system functions. Of most significance is that opiates cause respiratory depression by depressing the respiratory center within the brainstem. The rate and regularity of respirations diminish under the influence of opiates. Instances of clinically significant or death-inducing scenarios when opiates are administered are less than 1%. However, opiate use in the unmonitored drug-addicted population is associated with less favorable outcomes. Not all opiates have the same degree of respiratory impact. In addition the route of administration affects the influences on the respiratory system. Administering opiates via epidural or through intravenous (IV) patient-controlled analgesia (PCA, explained later in this chapter) has been shown to have fewer issues with respiratory depression. Opiates are associated with changes in sleep patterns. More time is spent in rapid eye movement (REM) sleep than in the deep sleep stage. This warrants further study to identify additional information concerning this potential complication. Predicting the potential for respiratory complications is not always possible, but a review of a patient's health history may provide insight.

Opiates may be short acting (lasting 3 to 6 hours), long acting (lasting at least 8 hours), or extended release (providing 24-hour pain relief). Short-acting medications are used best for the management of acute or breakthrough pain. Long-acting opiates traditionally are used on chronic pain. The US Food and Drug Administration has released Targiniq ER (oxycodone hydrochloride and naloxone hydrochloride extended-release tablets). These medications are used to manage severe pain. They have properties that hopefully aid in deterring abuses. Although they are successful in pain control, they have properties that block the euphoric feelings often associated with opioid use and sought out by addicts.

Because of its potential for inducing seizures, meperidine (Demerol) is no longer the drug of choice for pain management. The active metabolite in meperidine, normeperidine, is a CNS stimulant and sometimes produces irritability, tremors, muscle twitching, jerking, agitation, and seizures. Because normeperidine is eliminated by the kidneys, it should not be given to patients with decreased renal function. It is a particularly poor choice in older adults and in patients with sickle cell disease because most such patients have some degree of renal insufficiency. Repeated administration increases the risk of accumulation of normeperidine, so meperidine generally is not prescribed for patients who require long-term opioid treatment, such as those with cancer or chronic nonmalignant pain. The effects of normeperidine have been observed even in young, otherwise healthy patients given sufficiently high doses of meperidine postoperatively.

Meperidine administration is contraindicated in patients receiving monoamine oxidase inhibitors and in patients with untreated hypothyroidism, Addison's disease, benign prostatic hypertrophy, or urethral stricture. Meperidine is more likely than other opioid drugs to cause delirium in postoperative patients of all ages, especially if given epidurally or intravenously. The logic of using meperidine for any type of pain management, by any route of administration, is questionable. There are opioid choices that are clearly safer (see the Lifespan Considerations box on pain control in older adults).

Tolerance and addiction. Opioid tolerance and physiologic dependence are unusual with short-term postoperative use, and psychological dependence and addiction are extremely unlikely after a course of opiates for acute pain. Studies conducted over 20 years have shown uniformly that the likelihood that addiction will occur as a result of taking opioids for pain relief, even over a long period, is rare: probably less than 1%. Often the term *addiction* is applied inappropriately to a patient, and the label becomes a barrier to pain relief for that person.

Lifespan Considerations

Older Adults

Pain Control

- The effects of aging on the pain process sometimes are compounded in an older adult who has a chronic illness that affects the nervous system.
- Older adults who are well instructed in use of pain measurement tools and without diseases affecting the nervous system tend to report pain intensity similar to that reported by younger persons.
- The risk for gastric and renal toxicity from NSAIDs is increased in older adults.
- In older adults, changes in peripheral vascular function and skin, as well as decreased transmission of pain impulses, increase the risk for being unable to sense pain.
- Older age is associated with chronic health problems, increased risk for musculoskeletal pain, depression, and limitations in activities of daily living.
- Increased pain intensity has been noted in older individuals, particularly when adequate treatment is not provided for chronic and recurrent pain.
- Treatment of pain in older adults is as likely to be successful as that in younger persons.
- Because many older adults have some degree of renal insufficiency, meperidine (Demerol) is a particularly poor choice for pain control for such patients.
- Older adults sometimes become susceptible to side effects of opioids because of changes in serum proteins, liver and renal function, and a reduction in cardiac output.

Many patients will exhibit signs of physical tolerance and physical dependence after 1 to 4 weeks of regular opioid therapy. These effects are not abnormal. They should not be confused with addiction.

A helpful rule is that relief of severe pain requires a greater amount of analgesic; remembering this helps overcome any fear of overtreating patients' pain. Dosages at the upper end of normally prescribed ranges are usually safe. Administering a low dose that proves to be ineffective causes the patient to suffer until the required time interval has passed for another dose to be given.

Preventing and managing opioid-induced constipation. Opioids often delay gastric emptying, slow bowel motility, and decrease peristalsis. They also tend to reduce secretions from the colonic mucosa. The result is slow-moving, hard stool that is difficult to pass. At its worst, gastrointestinal dysfunction can result in ileus, fecal impaction, and obstruction.

Constipation is the most common side effect of opioids and the only one for which individuals do not develop tolerance. Thus it necessitates a preventive approach, regular assessment, and aggressive management. Factors contributing to constipation in patients who take opioids include advanced age, immobility, abdominal disease, and concurrent medications that also may have constipating side effects. Patients prescribed opioid analgesics also may be prescribed a stool softener with a mild peristaltic stimulant.

Instruct the patient in proper diet, fluids, and exercise, and provide for the patient's privacy and convenience. Keep in mind, however, that these aspects of bowel management are important but usually insufficient on their own to prevent opioid-induced constipation. Bulk laxatives, natural roughage, and large amounts of fluid are sometimes unpalatable and ineffective. In addition, if fluid intake is inadequate, bulk laxatives, such as psyllium (Metamucil), sometimes cause fecal impaction and obstruction. Stool softeners alone are inadequate.

Pain mechanisms affected by each analgesic group. It is useful and clinically relevant to distinguish among analgesics that relieve pain by different mechanisms. Because different analgesics relieve pain in different ways, it is sometimes logical to combine analgesics from different groups to relieve one specific type of pain or to relieve different types of pain occurring in the same patient.

Following is a brief description of selected mechanisms of action thought to be unique to each analgesic group.

- *Nonopioids* (acetylsalicylic acid [aspirin], acetaminophen, and NSAIDs). The analgesia produced by acetaminophen (Tylenol) appears to be related to the inhibition of prostaglandins that may serve as mediators of pain and fever, primarily in the CNS, but they also may block pain impulses peripherally. Aspirin blocks pain impulses in the CNS and reduces inflammation by inhibition of prostaglandin synthesis. NSAIDs such as tramadol (Ultram), ibuprofen (Motrin), naproxen (Aleve), ketorolac tromethamine (Toradol), and celecoxib (Celebrex) also work in the CNS, but their better characterized actions are peripheral (at the site of injury), where they are thought to exert analgesic effects through the inhibition of prostaglandin production. Prostaglandin is an inflammatory mediator, released when cells are damaged, that sensitizes nerves that carry information about pain. By inhibiting prostaglandin release, these drugs diminish transmission of pain stimuli.
- *Opioids.* Opioids relieve pain mainly by action in the CNS, binding to opioid receptor sites in the brain and the spinal cord. There are multiple opioid receptor sites. When a drug binds to any of these sites, pain relief occurs. When a drug attaches to these opioid receptor sites as an antagonist, pain relief and other effects are blocked. A well-known opioid antagonist is naloxone (Narcan), which antagonizes (blocks or reverses) the action of all opioids.
- *Adjuvant analgesics.* It is not possible to identify any one mechanism of action for pain relief for this analgesic group. This group is composed of diverse classes of drugs that relieve pain by a variety of mechanisms, many of which are not understood. For example, certain antidepressants appear to relieve pain by blocking the reuptake of serotonin, which results in the presence of greater amounts of serotonin. Orally formulated local anesthetics such as mexiletine (Mexitil) and certain anticonvulsants such as carbamazepine (Tegretol) are sodium channel–blocking agents, and this is perhaps part of the mechanism underlying their ability to relieve certain types of pain. Neuropathic pain is difficult to treat. Gabapentin (Neurontin), an anticonvulsant, binds to the neocortex and is used in the treatment of chronic neuropathic pain. Duloxetine (Cymbalta), an antidepressant, is used for control of the pain associated with diabetic neuropathy, as is pregabaline (Lyrica), an anticonvulsant.

Administration routes for analgesics. Learn the most effective analgesic and means of administration for the patient's specific need. It takes skill to determine the most effective method of administration.

The IV route is best for administration of opioid analgesics after major surgery. This route provides a rapid onset of pain relief and best manages escalating pain. The most appropriate opioids for pain relief for rapidly escalating, severe pain include morphine, hydromorphone, and fentanyl. For rapid onset of analgesia to treat escalating pain, these drugs should be administered via the IV route. They are suitable for bolus administration and continuous infusion, including PCA. The ability to obtain a dose when it is needed places the patient in control and eliminates the wait for medication administration.

Intramuscular (IM) administration of opioids is associated with wide fluctuations in absorption, including delayed absorption in postoperative patients; thus it is an ineffective and potentially dangerous method of managing pain. Furthermore, repeated IM injections are often painful and traumatic, which deters patients from requesting medications for relief of pain; they also have the potential to cause fibrosis of muscle and soft tissue, as well as sterile abscesses. Therefore the IM route, especially repeated IM administration, generally should be avoided.

The oral route is often the optimal route, especially for chronic pain treatment, because of its convenience, its flexibility, and the relatively steady blood levels produced. However, the IV route is usually necessary when a quick onset of analgesia is desired or when the patient is unable to take oral medication. When the

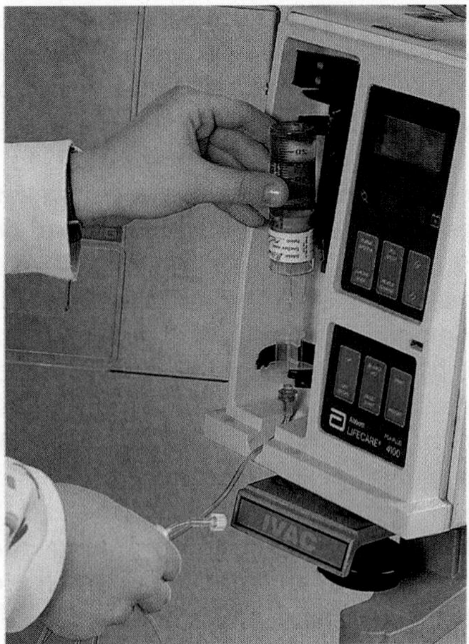

Fig. 21.5 Patient-controlled analgesia (PCA) pump with syringe chamber. (From Potter PA, Perry AG: *Basic nursing*, ed 7, St. Louis, 2011, Mosby.)

pain is under control, the regimen then may be changed to oral administration of the analgesic. Oral administration is convenient and inexpensive. Its use is appropriate as soon as the patient can tolerate oral intake and is the mainstay of pain management for ambulatory surgical patients.

Patient-controlled analgesia. A drug delivery system called **patient-controlled analgesia (PCA)** allows patients to self-administer analgesics whenever needed. The PCA device is a portable, computerized pump with a chamber for a syringe (Fig. 21.5). The pump delivers a small, preset dose of IV medication, usually morphine, meperidine, hydromorphone, or fentanyl. To receive a dose, the patient pushes a button on a cord attached to the pump. A timer prevents the system from delivering more than a specified number of doses every hour, to prevent overdose. Each dose may be as low as 1 mL or 1 mg of morphine every 6 to 12 minutes. It has a locked safety system that prevents tampering.

PCA is based on the idea that only the patient can feel the pain and only the patient knows how much analgesic will relieve it. By allowing patients to determine the need for doses, PCA addresses the significant variations in analgesic requirements between individuals.

Analgesia is more effective when the patient, rather than the nurse or the health care provider, is in control. PCA is similar to responsive prn dosing in that it requires patients to recognize that they are experiencing pain and to request analgesia (e.g., by pressing a button on a pump to deliver a PCA bolus). The difference between prn administration and PCA is that with PCA, the patient rather than a nurse administers the analgesic; thus the delay in waiting for a nurse's response to the request for analgesia is eliminated. Remind patients to "stay on top of pain" to maintain a steady analgesic level and self-administer a dose before pain is severe and out of control.

PCA has been used to manage all types of acute pain, although less often for cancer pain because most cancer pain is manageable with orally administered opioids. To be a candidate for PCA, a patient must be alert, oriented, and able to follow simple directions. Patient preparation and teaching are critical in the safe and effective use of PCA (see the Patient Teaching box).

Patient Teaching

Preparation for Patient-Controlled Analgesia

- Teach the use of patient-controlled analgesia (PCA) before surgery so that patients will know how to use it after awakening from anesthesia. (Confused and unresponsive patients, patients with neurologic disease, patients with impaired renal or pulmonary function, and those unable to press the delivery button are not candidates for PCA.)
- Instruct patients on the purpose of PCA, operating instructions, lockout intervals, expected pain relief, precautions, and potential side effects, emphasizing that the patient controls medication delivery.
- Explain that the pump prevents overdose.
- Tell family members and friends not to operate the PCA device for the patient.
- Ask the patient to demonstrate use of the PCA delivery button.

Older adult patients and those with respiratory compromise or hypovolemia are typically at high risk for respiratory complications with IV opioids of any type. They and patients with significant impairment of renal or hepatic function probably will be determined unsuitable candidates to use PCA.

If someone other than the patient pushes the button on a PCA pump, even at the patient's request, it is termed *PCA by proxy*. Proxy administration of opioids leads to possible oversedation and opioid toxicity. PCA is for patient use only, and nurses, other patients, and visitors must be reminded not to push the button.

Although patients with pain often self-administer their oral analgesics, the term *patient-controlled analgesia* is applied usually when opioids are administered by the IV and epidural routes. Typically, a special infusion pump is used to deliver PCA by these routes. In this context, PCA refers to the bolus dose that the patient controls when pressing a button on or attached to the pump. PCA is delivered by one of two modes: PCA bolus doses with a continuous infusion (also called a *basal rate*) or PCA bolus doses alone.

When caring for the patient who uses the PCA delivery system, assess the IV site and the PCA device for proper functioning and correct drug dosing. Closely monitor vital signs for signs of respiratory depression. Evaluate the patient's level of orientation for signs of oversedation. Record the amount of medication being used every shift or per agency policy.

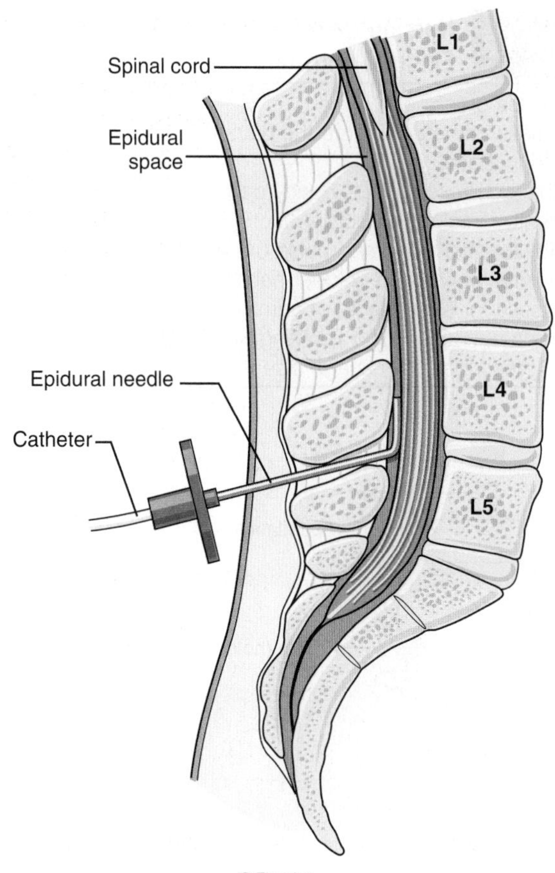

Fig. 21.6 Epidural catheter placement.

Epidural analgesia. Another method of delivery of analgesia is the insertion of an epidural catheter and the infusion of opiates into the epidural space. Containing blood vessels, fat, and nerves, the epidural space is a "potential" space (there is no free-flowing fluid in it) between the walls of the vertebral canal and the dura mater of the spinal cord. It surrounds the spinal meninges and extends from the foramen magnum to the sacral hiatus. The epidural medication diffuses slowly from the epidural space across the dura and arachnoid membranes into the cerebrospinal fluid (Fig. 21.6). Epidural administration of opioids brings the drug close to the action site (opioid receptors); therefore, in comparison with systemic administration, relatively small doses are effective. Because of the vasculature in the epidural space, the drug also is absorbed systemically. There are three methods of administering epidural analgesia: by bolus doses, by continuous infusion, and by patient-controlled epidural analgesia.

The epidural route of administration is an appropriate first-line route for moderate to severe acute pain expected to last for at least 24 hours. The pain relief and improvement in functional outcomes after major surgery are superior in patients who receive epidural analgesia in comparison with patients who receive traditional postoperative pain management therapies administered by IV push or intramuscularly. Epidural medications have a rapid onset: relief is experienced within 15 minutes. Drugs used for epidural analgesia are morphine, fentanyl, and hydromorphone. The epidural opioids have side effects, including urinary retention, postural hypotension, pruritus, nausea, vomiting, and respiratory depression. Epidural analgesia is beneficial for controlling acute pain during labor and for relieving chronic pain, such as that seen in patients with advanced cancer (Box 21.2).

The insertion and maintenance of the epidural catheter for the infusion are invasive techniques that are the responsibility of the anesthetist or the anesthesiologist. Nursing staff members are responsible for monitoring the patient's level of consciousness, pain intensity, respiratory rate, and the infusion rate and volume on the pump. Monitor respiratory rate, pulse, blood pressure, and oxygen saturation levels every 15 minutes during infusion. Because hypotension may occur, an IV infusion is initiated before the administration of the epidural medications. Examine the dressing site for signs of infection or leakage of medication around the catheter (Table 21.2).

There are complications associated with epidural therapies. These complications include infection, bleeding at the site, nerve damage, and seizures. Less frequently, respiratory complications may result.

Elastomeric Pumps

Elastomeric pumps or "pain balls" are used to administer local anesthetic medications (Fig. 21.7). The medication, located inside of a ball, is administered through a small catheter that has been placed beneath the skin during a surgical procedure. The medication is intended as a supplement to the regularly prescribed narcotic postoperative pain medications. Dosages of the medication may be set to provide a continuous administration, or it may allow for patient-necessitated adjustments to the dosage or even allow demand bolus administrations in the event of breakthrough pain. As the medication is dispensed, the ball gradually begins to soften and eventually appeared "collapsed" or smaller. The longevity of a device varies by the size of the device employed and the dosage prescribed. The average time for a single pump to be in use is 2 to 5 days. When a device is empty, it is removed easily by the patient or a caregiver in the home. The device is small and portable and can be secured to clothing. Patients using the pumps may demonstrate a reduced intake of narcotic analgesics. If smaller doses of narcotics are used, their related side effects such as nausea, vomiting, and constipation also may be lessened.

Responsibility of the Nurse in Pain Control

The founding principle of effective pain management is Meinhart and McCaffery's statement that "the failure to treat pain is inhumane and constitutes professional negligence" (Meinhart and McCaffery, 1983). Every patient has the right to be free of pain; it is the nurse's

Box 21.2 Nursing Principles for Administering Analgesics

KNOW THE PATIENT'S PREVIOUS RESPONSE TO ANALGESICS
- Assess past history of analgesic use. Include the patient's success with the medications.
- Determine what medications have been used in the past and their degree of effectiveness.
- Determine whether the patient has allergies.

SELECT PROPER MEDICATIONS WHEN MORE THAN ONE IS ORDERED
- Use NSAIDs or milder opioids for mild to moderate pain.
- The concurrent use of opioids and NSAIDs often provides far more effective analgesia than use of an agent from either drug class alone.
- Use of NSAIDs can help reduce opioid side effects.
- In older adults, avoid combinations of opioids.
- Remember that morphine and hydromorphone are the opioids of choice for long-term management of severe pain.
- Know that injectable medications act more quickly, often relieving severe, acute pain within 1 hour, and that oral medication sometimes takes as long as 2 hours to take effect.
- For longer, more sustained relief in connection with chronic pain, give an oral drug.

KNOW THE OPTIMAL DOSAGE
- Remember that doses at the upper end of normal generally are needed for severe pain.
- Ask patient to rate pain before analgesic administration and after to determine level of effectiveness.
- Consult with members of the health care team about dosage adjustments.

DETERMINE THE RIGHT TIME AND INTERVAL FOR ADMINISTRATION
- Use an appropriate pain scale for more accurate pain assessment.
- Administer analgesics as soon as pain occurs and before it increases in severity.
- Premedicate patient if interventions or activities are planned that may cause increased discomfort.
- Do not give analgesics only on as-needed schedules. An around-the-clock administration schedule is best.
- Know the average duration of action for a drug, and time the administration so that the peak effect occurs when the pain is most intense.

CHOOSE THE RIGHT ROUTE
- Intravenous and oral routes are preferred.
- Intramuscular and subcutaneous administrations are best avoided because these routes are frequently painful and absorption is not reliable. Intramuscular injections have the potential to cause fibrosis of muscle and soft tissue and sterile abscesses.

NSAIDs, Nonsteroidal antiinflammatory drugs.

Table 21.2 Nursing Care for Patients With Epidural Infusions

- Assess dressing.
- Assess catheter. Ensure the catheter remains unkinked and in place.
- Change dressing per agency policy.
- Monitor intake and output.
- Monitor vital signs and pulse oximetry.
- Monitor bowel and bladder habits.
- Assess for side effects of administration including pruritus, nausea, and vomiting. Administer medications as prescribed to manage side effects.

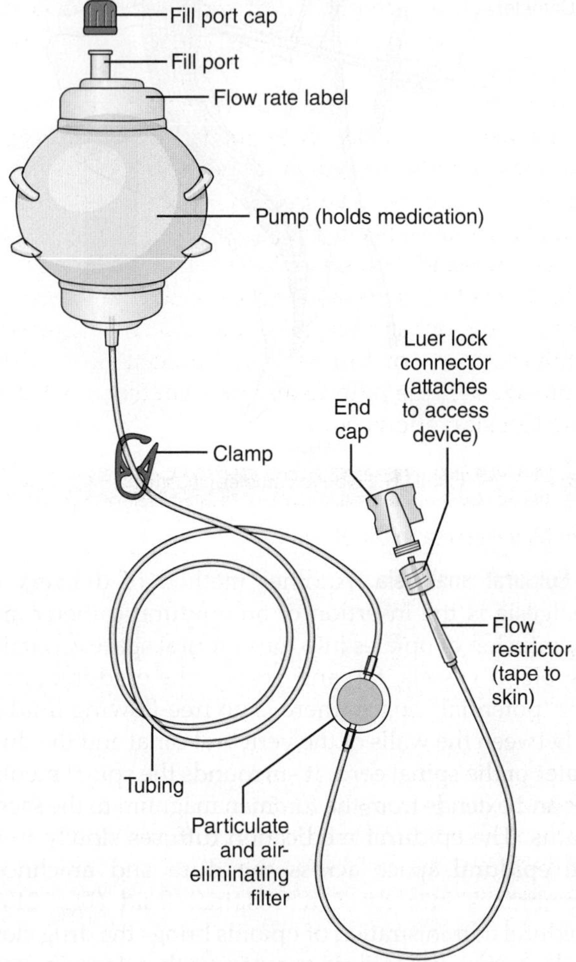

Fig. 21.7 Elastometric pump.

responsibility to do everything possible to alleviate the patient's pain.

Assist the patient in pain relief by telling the patient, "I believe that you are in pain, and I will assist you in whatever way I can to reduce or relieve your pain." This reduces the patient's anxiety level. Patients should not be expected to convince the health care team that the pain experienced is real. Pain management interventions begin as soon as the patient states that she or he is in pain.

Encourage the patient to be an active participant in the plan of care. It is important for the patient to report pain promptly as it occurs. Teach the patient not to wait until the pain is intolerable to seek medications. Assess for nonverbal expressions of pain. If any pain-producing procedure or activity is scheduled, such as ambulating, coughing, or a dressing change, give an analgesic beforehand. Administer the medications to achieve the peak effect during the patient's most active time.

Pain control requires nurses to have a strong advocacy role. Nurses must clarify concerns, answer questions, and supply information needed by the patient. Collaboration with the health care provider is needed to ensure that the appropriate analgesics are being used. Effective patient advocacy requires time, patience, and courage. Good listening skills are essential. Ask the patient how he or she is feeling, and attentively wait to hear the answer.

The ultimate goal of pain management is to provide pain relief and enable the patient to carry on with activities of daily living in as comfortable a manner as possible. If pain is to be prevented or managed well, all members of the health care team caring for the patient must understand the pain management plan. Assessment of the patient's pain is ongoing and is documented with each assessment and reassessment. There is increasing emphasis on combining psychosocial and drug approaches in the pain treatment plan (see the Home Care Considerations box).

Home Care Considerations

Pain Management in the Home

- In current practice, nurses recognize the need to include the patient and family in planning and implementing effective pain management strategies.
- With so much care being given in clinics, physicians' offices, and patients' homes rather than in hospitals, the need for patients and families to be well informed has become even more important.
- Explain the pain management program that is likely to be used in the patient's home.
- Discuss and have the patient practice pain management techniques to use in the home.
- Home health care and hospice patients are assessed for pain at every visit. Instruct patients to notify a home health or hospice nurse at any time of unrelieved pain.

Pain management is a challenge that every nurse must face, regardless of the practice setting. In fact, the nurse's role in pain management is probably more important than that of any other member of the health care team (Nursing Care Plan 21.1).

Nursing Assessment of Pain

Collection of subjective data. Because pain is a subjective experience, you must become a well-versed and competent practitioner of the art of pain assessment. Obtaining accurate information from the patient concerning the pain, including characteristics and description of the pain, is critical. Characteristics worth noting include the site, the severity, the duration, and the location of pain. When documenting the presence of pain, describe the specific location and intensity. Charting "patient complains of pain" provides no useful information. Ask the patient what relieves the pain, what actions cause the pain to be worse, and what does not relieve the pain. Sociocultural information is beneficial. Identify normal coping mechanisms used by the patient and close family members. Determine how the pain is interpreted by those close to the patient (see the Cultural Considerations box). If medications are taken for relief of pain, the name, the dosage, the frequency, and the effect of the drugs must be determined.

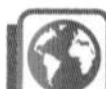

Cultural Considerations

Pain Management

- The primary strategy for working with a patient in pain who is from a different culture is to establish a relationship by listening, showing respect, and allowing the patient to help develop and choose treatment options.
- To further increase cultural sensitivity, cultivate rapport with the patient and family, maintain an open attitude, and remain flexible.
- Understanding cultural background and personal characteristics aids in the accuracy of the pain assessment and its meaning to the patient.
- It may be difficult to understand some non-Western pain remedies, so it is important that the patient feels free to ask for what is needed.
- Respect the patient's attitudes and beliefs about pain, as well as preferred treatment options, even if these conflict with your personal beliefs about pain treatment.
- During the assessment process, explore how the patient feels about combining therapies so that the patient is made familiar with a range of pain treatment options.
- Traditional Latino men believe that men are supposed to endure pain without complaining and that alleviating it would be "unmanly" and demeaning in the eyes of their children.
- Chinese people may avoid eye contact, making pain assessment more difficult.
- Italian, Jewish, African American, and Spanish-speaking people often smile readily and use facial expressions and gestures to communicate pain or displeasure.
- Irish, English, and northern European people tend to show fewer facial expressions and are less responsive, especially to strangers such as professional caregivers.

Data collection is dictated largely by the patient's condition. If the patient is critically ill or in excruciating pain, limit questions to key items needed to proceed with the plan of care.

Try to have patients use their own words to describe the pain because the terms they use often provide clues about the cause of the pain. For example, patients who experience chest pain during a myocardial infarction

Nursing Care Plan 21.1 The Patient With Chronic Pain

The nurse is caring for Mr. J., a 45-year-old male patient with a 15-year history of severe, crippling rheumatoid arthritis. He has had numerous joint replacements, has lost 40 lb (18.18 kg) in the past year, and has developed corneal ulcers from the presence of Sjögren's syndrome. He is in constant chronic pain and has limited mobility. He states that he has difficulty accomplishing activities of daily living (ADLs).

PATIENT PROBLEM

Prolonged Pain, related to joint and muscle inflammation and degeneration manifested by complaints of pain, anorexia, narrow focus of interest, fatigue, guarded movement, changes in sleep pattern, and social withdrawal

Patient Goals and Expected Outcomes	Nursing Interventions	Evaluation
Patient or family (or both) will verbalize a reduction in anxiety and pain when using relaxation, massage, cutaneous stimulation, and analgesics within 1 h after initiation of pain relief measures	Encourage patient to report pain or discomfort location, intensity, and duration with the use of the pain scale. Teach relaxation exercises. Perform massage to relieve pain and to enhance communication. Administer analgesics and apply cold or heat applications as ordered. Maintain transcutaneous electric nerve stimulation (TENS) as ordered. Encourage relaxation by teaching use of guided imagery.	Patient indicates improved pain relief within 1 h of implementation of pain management techniques. Patient reports pain level reduced to 4 on a scale of 0 to 10.

PATIENT PROBLEM

Prolonged Low Self-Esteem, related to inability to work, carry out ADLs, and with body image changes, manifested by preoccupation with body changes, verbalization of powerlessness, expressions of guilt, and self-negating verbalizations

Patient Goals and Expected Outcomes	Nursing Interventions	Evaluation
Patient will verbalize understanding of changes in body image caused by disease process and will begin to exhibit increased confidence in dealing with self-esteem within 1 week	Encourage verbalization about fears and anxiety; listen attentively. Deal with behavioral changes, denial, powerlessness, anxiety, and dependence. Be supportive in setting goals. Encourage independence, and give praise for tasks accomplished. Modify environment, and allow time for patient to accomplish goals.	Patient states improved feeling of self-esteem within 1 week of implementation of techniques outlined.

CRITICAL THINKING QUESTIONS

1. During the morning ADLs, Mr. J. states, "I feel so useless. I can't even place the urinal for myself." What would be the nurse's most therapeutic response?
2. What would be the most useful nursing intervention to achieve the goal of reduced pain during Mr. J.'s assisted ambulation?
3. Which comfort measures could the nurse perform to ensure that the patient has several hours of restorative sleep?
4. Mr. J. complains of his eyes burning and feeling dry and the lights annoying him. What measures are most likely to help relieve his symptoms?

frequently describe the pain as a pressure or as if someone were squeezing the chest.

Several studies have been focused on the development of tools to assess the patient's pain perception specifically. Pain is a subjective experience, and nurses face difficulty when attempting to measure and evaluate this experience for the patient. Pain rating scales aid with this assessment.

Pain rating scales. Visual analog scales and numeric scales are used commonly to qualify the intensity of the pain experience (Fig. 21.8).

With the **visual analog scale,** the patient marks a spot on a horizontal line to indicate pain intensity (intensity increases as the line moves from left to right). The most frequently used numeric scale is 0 to 10; the patient chooses the pain rating, with 0 being no pain and 10 being the worst pain imaginable. A visual scale with numeric ratings combines both, providing a description and facial expressions with assigned numbers from 0 to 10 (see Fig. 30.8). For clinical assessment, any of these scales is adequate and appropriate. The same scale always must be used with the same patient. All personnel in a given health care setting also must use the same scale.

A good pain scale is easy to use and not time consuming. If a patient can read and understand a scale easily, the description of pain is more accurate. If the patient wears a hearing aid or glasses, be sure they are

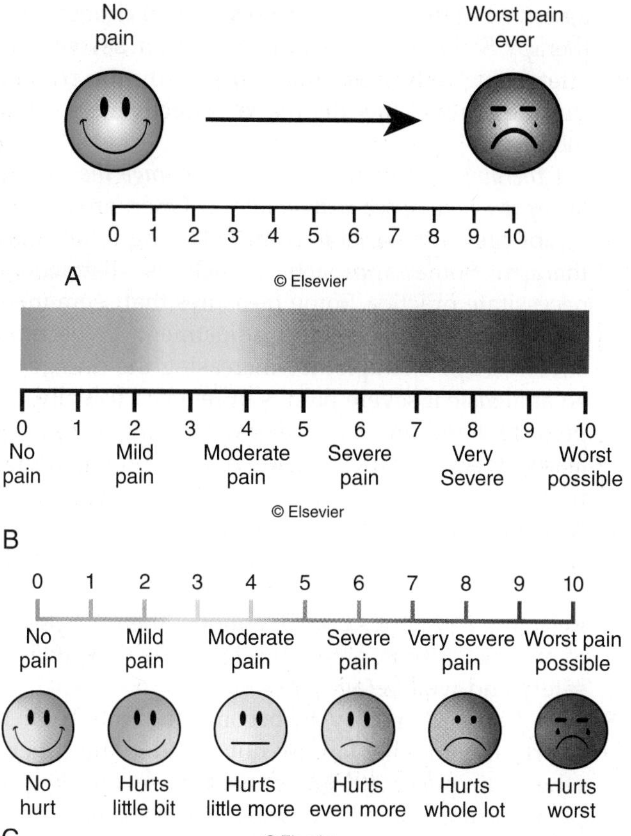

Fig. 21.8 Sample pain scales. A, Visual analog. B, Numeric. C, Verbal descriptive.

worn when the patient is answering pain assessment questions or marking a pain scale. Several pain scales have been developed to assess pain in children. Wong and Baker developed the FACES pain rating scale (see Fig. 30.8). Most patients require a pain level of 4 or less to function well.

Collection of objective data. Carefully observe the patient. Possible objective signs are tachycardia, increased rate and depth of respirations, diaphoresis, increased systolic or diastolic blood pressure, pallor, dilated pupils, and increased muscle tension. Some patients complain of nausea or weakness (Box 21.3). Other patients have a subjective complaint of pain with no observable objective signs.

If the pain is chronic or less severe, the physiologic changes are likely to be less prominent. Changes in facial expressions, such as frowning or gritting teeth, may be exhibited. Some people clench their fists and withdraw from social activities when in pain. Others complain bitterly, cry, moan, toss about in bed, assume a fetal position, or clutch at the affected body part. Pacing may be performed by some patients if their energy level allows. The amount of attention desired by a patient in pain varies; some patients in pain want someone in constant attendance, whereas others want to be left alone.

Box 21.3 Objective Signs of Pain

PHYSIOLOGIC SIGNS

- *Pulse:* Increased rate
- *Respirations:* Increased depth and frequency
- *Blood pressure:* Increased systolic and diastolic
- The body seeks equilibrium. In an hour or less, vital signs usually return to what they were previously, even if the patient is still in severe pain. Continuous severe pain sometimes causes vital signs to increase again from time to time, but they rarely remain elevated.
- Diaphoresis, pallor
- Dilated pupils
- Muscle tension (face, body)
- Nausea and vomiting (if pain is severe)

BEHAVIORAL SIGNS

- Rigid body position
- Restlessness
- Frowning
- Grimacing
- Clenched teeth
- Clenched fists
- Crying
- Moaning

Be unbiased and nonjudgmental when gathering objective data; consider that the patient is doing the best he or she can do at the given moment. The priority intervention is to relieve or decrease the pain. Remember that pain is what the patient says it is. Do not expect the patient to behave in any set manner when in pain.

Nursing Interventions

The following measures are performed to assist in pain control and comfort (see the Health Promotion box):

- Tighten wrinkled bed linens.
- Reposition drainage tubes or other objects on which patient is lying.
- Place warm bath blankets if the patient is cold.
- Loosen constricting bandages.
- Change moist dressings.
- Check tape to prevent pulling on skin.
- Position patient in anatomic alignment.
- Check temperature of hot and cold applications, including bath water.
- Lift—do not pull—patient up in bed; handle gently.
- Position patient correctly on bedpan.
- Avoid exposing skin or mucous membranes to irritants (e.g., diarrheal stool or wound drainage).
- Prevent urinary retention by ensuring patency of Foley catheter.
- Prevent constipation by encouraging appropriate fluid intake, diet, and exercise and by administering prescribed stool softeners.

Guidelines for individualizing pain therapy. When you provide pain relief measures, choose therapies suited to the patient's unique pain experience. McCaffery (2002)

 Health Promotion

Promoting Comfort

- Measures that promote a sense of well-being to minimize or avoid discomfort include warm baths, thorough personal hygiene, and adequate rest.
- Pain has the potential to disable and immobilize a person enough to impair the ability to perform self-care activities. This results in social isolation, depression, and changes in self-concept. Help patients and families learn to discuss their feelings about the loss of function and to find ways to cope with pain and the lifestyle it imposes.
- When a patient has chronic, disabling pain, instruct family members on proper positioning techniques and methods of assisting the patient with ambulation.
- Nonpharmacologic or complementary therapies used for pain relief include massage, guided imagery, music, biofeedback, meditation, hypnosis, exercise, therapeutic touch, acupuncture, and relaxation techniques.

suggested the following guidelines for individualizing pain therapy:

1. *Use different types of pain relief measures.* Using more than one therapy has an additive effect in reducing pain. In addition, the character of pain often changes throughout the day, which necessitates the use of several different therapies. A combination of physical and psychological approaches (e.g., analgesics or antidepressants and relaxation) helps control all components of the pain experience.
2. *Provide pain relief measures before pain becomes severe.* It is easier to prevent severe pain than to relieve it. Giving an analgesic 30 to 40 minutes before a patient must walk or perform an activity is an example of controlling pain early. Implement prn medications around the clock to control moderately severe to severe pain effectively. Waiting for the patient or the family to request analgesics results in delays in administration and inadequate pain control.
3. *Use measures the patient believes are effective.* The patient is the expert on the pain and probably has realistic ideas about what measures to use (e.g., rubbing lotion on an edematous finger) and when to use them.
4. *Consider the patient's ability or willingness to participate in pain relief measures.* Some patients are not able to assist actively with pain therapy because of fatigue, sedation, or altered levels of consciousness. However, some variations of pain relief measures require little effort, such as relaxation exercises in bed or listening to music as a distraction. You will not relieve pain by forcing an unwilling patient to participate in therapy. The depressed patient with chronic pain has little motivation to participate.
5. *Choose pain relief measures appropriate to the severity of the pain as reflected by the patient's behavior.* It would be poor judgment to administer a potent opioid to a patient who is displaying only mild pain. Carefully assess what the patient says before you choose pain therapy. Some patients acquire relief from severe pain after using only mild analgesics. Only the patient can determine the degree of effectiveness of a therapy.
6. *If a therapy is ineffective at first, encourage the patient to try it again before abandoning it.* Often anxiety or doubt prevents patients from obtaining relief from therapy. Some approaches, such as distraction, necessitate practice. Some measures that seem ineffective merely necessitate adjustment to become effective. For example, try increasing the dosage of an analgesic if severe pain is unrelieved initially. Be persistent and understanding in helping the patient learn to use measures that do not afford immediate relief.
7. *Keep an open mind about what has potential to relieve pain.* New ways to control pain sometimes are found. Much remains to be learned about the pain experience. Rejecting a patient's unconventional therapies leads to mistrust. Monitor therapies to ensure the patient's safety and well-being.
8. *Keep trying.* It is easy to become frustrated when efforts at pain relief fail. Do not abandon the patient when pain persists. Some patients in severe chronic pain who are ignored choose suicide as an alternative. If the patient obtains no relief, reassess the situation and consider whether alternative therapies are needed.
9. *Protect the patient.* Pain therapy that causes more distress than the pain is misguided and inappropriate. Always observe the response to therapy. Any pain relief measure poses a risk of side effects, such as fatigue, anxiety, or additional pain. The goal is to relieve pain without disabling the patient mentally, emotionally, or physically. It is important to maintain safety of the patient and environment.

SLEEP AND REST

A patient at rest feels mentally relaxed, free from worry, and physically calm. A patient at rest is free from physical or mental exertion. Everyone has his or her own method of obtaining rest and is usually able to adjust to new environments or conditions that affect the ability to rest.

Rest is important in healing the body of physical and psychological illness. Patients often are prescribed bed rest. This treatment confines patients to bed to decrease physical or psychological demands on the body. Bed rest does not necessarily mean that a patient is resting. Emotional or metabolic stressors naturally cause the patient to be restless.

Sleep is a state of rest that occurs for a sustained period. The reduced consciousness during sleep provides time for repair and recovery of body systems for the next period of wakefulness. The theory that sleep is associated with healing suggests that achieving optimal

Box 21.4 Factors Affecting Sleep

PHYSICAL ILLNESS

- Pain and physical discomfort result in difficulty falling or staying asleep.
- Chronic pain sometimes has a circadian rhythm, including increasing in intensity at night, thus disrupting sleep.
- Illness frequently forces patients to sleep in positions to which they are unaccustomed.
- Respiratory diseases interfere with the rhythm of breathing and sometimes oblige a person to assume a certain position to be able to breathe easily. Both factors can disturb sleep.
- A patient with heart disease may be afraid to go to sleep at night.
- Hypertension causes early morning awakening and fatigue.
- Nocturia and restless legs syndrome disrupt sleep, causing the patient to awaken and have trouble going back to sleep during the night.
- Conditions that increase intracranial pressure or alter central nervous system physiology alter sleep patterns and sometimes cause excessive daytime sleepiness.

ANXIETY AND DEPRESSION

- As anxiety and depression increase, so does lack of sleep; as amount of sleep decreases, anxiety and depression increase.
- Bereaved people may experience sleep problems related to fear of intruders, loneliness, and the dreams or nightmares that occur involving the lost loved one.

DRUGS AND SUBSTANCES

- Various drugs and substances affect the pattern and the quality of sleep.
- Hypnotic medications interfere with reaching deeper sleep stages, provide only a temporary (1-week) increase in quality of sleep, and eventually cause a "hangover" feeling during the day. Hypnotic drugs often worsen sleep apnea in older adults.
- Older adults often take several drugs, the combined effects of which disrupt sleep.
- L-Tryptophan, a protein found in foods such as milk, cheese, and meats, frequently helps induce sleep.

LIFESTYLE

- Daily routines such as work shifts influence sleep patterns; changing routines, as with rotating shifts, disrupt these patterns. Only after several weeks of working a night shift does an individual's biologic clock adjust.
- Performing unaccustomed heavy work, late-night social activities, and changing evening mealtimes are activities that can disrupt sleep.

SLEEP PATTERNS

- Sleep patterns include starting time and duration of sleep. The most significant cause of daytime sleepiness is inadequate or abnormal sleep at night.
- Everyone has an increased tendency to feel sleepy from 2 a.m. to 7 a.m.
- When sleep patterns are disrupted, the natural tendency to sleep at certain times increases.
- Sleep patterns influence future attempts to fall asleep because of changes in circadian rhythm. Sleeping 1 hour later results in falling asleep 1 hour later the next night.

STRESS

- Stress resulting from personal problems or situational crises causes tension and at times cause a person to try too hard to fall asleep, to awaken frequently, or to oversleep.
- Stress causes release of corticosteroids and adrenalin, which leads to catabolism and sleeplessness.
- Patients with advanced cancer or chronic illness often are afraid to go to sleep for fear they might die.
- The stress of losses such as retirement or death of a loved one sometimes causes older adults to suffer delays in falling asleep, earlier REM (rapid eye movement) sleep, frequent awakening, increased total bedtime, and feelings of sleeping poorly.

ENVIRONMENT

- Environmental factors influence the ability to fall and remain asleep. Significant factors include ventilation, lighting, type of bed, sound level, and the presence or absence of a bed partner.
- In hospitals, unfamiliar noises and higher noise levels such as that created by wall suction, opening packages, ringing alarms, and flushing toilets can cause sleep deprivation.
- Intensive care units have high noise levels.

EXERCISE AND FATIGUE

- Exercise and fatigue in moderation usually facilitate restful sleep, but excess fatigue from exhausting or stressful work typically make falling asleep difficult.
- Performing exercise 2 hours before bedtime allows the body to cool down and promotes relaxation.

NUTRITION

- Weight gain causes longer sleep periods with fewer interruptions and later awakening.
- Weight loss sometimes causes reduction in total time spent asleep along with broken sleep and earlier awakening.

sleep quality is important for patients' recovery. Sleep restores a person's energy and feeling of well-being.

The routines of health care facilities easily disrupt the rest and sleep habits of patients (Box 21.4). The extent of the change depends on the gravity of the illness, as well as the environment in which the patient is placed. Remain aware of the patient's need for rest. Without it, the patient becomes fatigued and irritable and has a decreased ability to cope with stressors (see the Lifespan Considerations for Older Adults box).

Lifespan Considerations

Older Adults

Sleep

- Older adults require about the same amount of sleep as younger people but are more likely to achieve it in separate episodes; they take more daytime naps and get less sleep at night.
- The sleep of an older adult is less deep. This increases the risk of early awakening and complaints of sleep disturbance.
- Sleep is likely to be disturbed in older adults with chronic health problems such as arthritis, heart failure, and chronic obstructive pulmonary disease. Adequate pain control and positioning facilitate breathing and help promote rest and sleep.
- Many older adults take medications such as diuretics and theophylline that are likely to disturb sleep. Carefully assess time of administration and the effect on sleep, and modify the schedule when possible.
- Insufficient sleep may lead to memory and personality changes in older adults.
- Include nonpharmacologic comfort measures among nursing interventions to promote rest and sleep.

PHYSIOLOGY OF SLEEP

Sleep is a cyclic physiologic process that alternates with longer periods of wakefulness. The sleep-wake cycle influences and regulates body functions and behavioral responses. The influence of sleep is not limited to physiologic functions. Sleep and rest have an impact on memory, mood, and cognitive performance.

People experience cyclic rhythms as part of everyday life. The most familiar rhythm is the 24-hour day-night cycle known as the *diurnal* or *circadian rhythm.* All circadian rhythms, including the sleep-wake cycle, are affected by light and temperature and external factors such as social activities and environmental stressors. Each person has a biologic clock that synchronizes sleep cycles. Some people can fall asleep at 8 p.m., whereas others go to bed at midnight or early in the morning. Different people also function best at different times of the day.

The biologic rhythm of sleep frequently becomes synchronized with other body functions. Normal variations in body temperature, for example, are correlated with sleep patterns. When the sleep-wake cycle is disrupted (e.g., by working rotating shifts), other physiologic functions typically change as well.

Box 21.5 Stages of Sleep

NON–RAPID EYE MOVEMENT (NREM) SLEEP

Stage 1

- Lightest level of sleep
- Lasts a few minutes
- Decreased physiologic activity, beginning with a gradual fall in vital signs and metabolism
- Person is easily aroused by sensory stimuli such as noise
- If person awakes, feels as though daydreaming has occurred
- Reduction in autonomic activities (e.g., heart rate)

Stage 2

- Period of sound sleep
- Lasts 10 to 20 minutes
- Relaxation progresses
- Arousal is still easy
- Body functions are still slowing

Stage 3

- Initial stage of deep sleep
- Lasts 15 to 30 minutes
- Arousal is difficult, movement is rare
- Muscles are completely relaxed
- Vital signs decline but remain regular
- Hormonal response includes secretion of growth hormone

Stage 4

- Deepest stage of sleep
- Lasts approximately 15 to 30 minutes
- Arousal is very difficult
- If sleep loss has occurred, sleeper spends most of night in this stage
- Restores and rests the body
- Vital signs are significantly lower than during waking hours
- Sleepwalking and enuresis are possible
- Hormonal response continues

RAPID EYE MOVEMENT (REM) SLEEP

- Stage of vivid, full-color dreaming consistent with sensory experiences (less vivid dreaming sometimes occurs in other stages)
- First occurs approximately 90 minutes after sleep has begun, thereafter occurs at end of each NREM cycle
- Duration increasing with each cycle and averaging 20 minutes
- Typified by autonomic response of rapidly moving eyes, fluctuating heart and respiratory rates, and increased or fluctuating blood pressure
- Loss of skeletal muscle tone
- Responsible for mental restoration
- Stage in which sleeper is most difficult to arouse

SLEEP CYCLE

Sleep involves two phases: **rapid eye movement (REM)** and **non–rapid eye movement (NREM)** (Box 21.5). NREM sleep is further divided into four stages through which a sleeper progresses during a typical sleeping cycle. The sleeping stages are highly individualized (Fig. 21.9).

Normally an adult's routine sleep pattern begins with a presleep period, during which the person is aware only of a gradually developing drowsiness. This period normally lasts 10 to 30 minutes, but if a person has difficulty falling asleep, it can last an hour or longer.

As adults fall asleep, they progress through the four stages of NREM sleep. At the end of the fourth stage, they come out of a deep sleep, go back to stage 2, and then enter a period of REM sleep. A person reaches

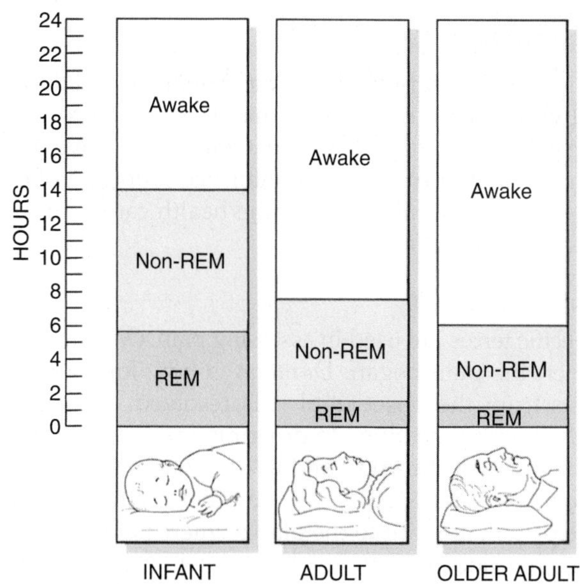

Fig. 21.9 Sleep-wake cycles across the life span. *Infants:* Approximately 40% of total sleep time is spent in rapid eye movement (REM) sleep. *Adults:* 20% of total sleep time is spent in REM sleep. *Older adults:* Total sleep time is slightly reduced; REM sleep continues to make up 20% of total sleep time.

REM sleep in about 90 minutes (average). Each person differs, but a typical night's sleep consists of four to six such cycles.

Dreams occur during the NREM and REM stages. The dream of REM sleep is believed to be functionally important, more vivid, and elaborate, allowing a person to clarify emotions and prepare the mind for events of the next day.

NREM sleep provides a period of body maintenance. This stage of sleep has been attributed to wound healing, immune functions, hormone release, and muscle restoration. A person's biologic functions slow during NREM sleep. For example, a healthy adult has a heart rate of 70 to 80 beats per minute during the day; however, during sleep the heart beats at 60 beats per minute or less. Respiration rate and blood pressure also decrease during sleep. It is very difficult to arouse the sleeper in REM sleep.

REM sleep is important for brain and cognitive restoration. During REM sleep, there are changes in cerebral blood flow and increases in cortical activity, oxygen consumption, and epinephrine release, which are beneficial to memory storage and learning.

SLEEP DEPRIVATION

The amount of sleep needed varies by age and health condition. Infants need the most: 16 hours. Teens require 9 hours and adults 8 hours per night. Sleep deprivation is a problem many patients experience as a result of hospitalization. Sleep deprivation involves decreases in the amount, the quality, and the consistency of sleep. When sleep is interrupted or fragmented, changes in the normal sequence of sleep stages occur, and cycles are not completed. Cumulative deprivation gradually develops. Sleep deprivation has been tied to hypertension, diabetes, heart disease, and stroke.

> **Safety Alert**
>
> **Daytime Sleepiness**
>
> - Safety precautions are important for patients and residents who awaken during the night to use the bathroom and for those with excessive daytime sleepiness.
> - Set beds lower to the floor to lessen the chance that the patient or resident will fall when first standing.
> - Some patients and residents who experience daytime sleepiness fall asleep while sitting up in a chair or wheelchair. Position the person so that he or she will not fall out of the chair while sleeping.

Patients with sleep deprivation experience a variety of physiologic and psychological signs and symptoms. Possible physiologic signs and symptoms include hand tremors, decreased reflexes, slowed response time, reduction in word memory, decreased reasoning and judgment, and cardiac dysrhythmias. Possible psychological signs and symptoms include mood swings, disorientation, irritability, decreased motivation, fatigue, sleepiness, and hyperexcitability.

PROMOTING REST AND SLEEP

Determine the patient's usual rest and sleep patterns, decide whether they are sufficient, and note why the patient is not getting sufficient rest. Work with the patient and the family to develop a plan to provide for more rest. A typical plan includes limiting interruptions during the night for vital sign checks and other procedures, providing a quiet environment with a comfortable room temperature, limiting the number of visitors and the duration of visits, and carrying out all procedures within a given time frame (see the Coordinated Care box).

> **Coordinated Care**
>
> **Supervision**
>
> **Promoting Sleep**
>
> - Encourage nursing assistants to provide for patients or residents a quiet, undisturbed environment that causes the least interference with sleep.
> - Instruct the nursing assistant to provide comfort measures such as toileting, a back rub, and a comfortable bed to help the patient or resident prepare for sleep.
> - Communicate to the nursing assistant that it is essential to keep excessive noise from conversation or equipment to a minimum because this disturbs residents or patients who already are having difficulty sleeping.

In preparing the patient for sleep, wash the patient's back if the patient is on bed rest, gently massage it, change the linens, make certain the patient is warm enough, offer an uncaffeinated beverage such as milk (if allowed), change soiled dressings, and give the patient an opportunity to void.

Decrease environmental stimuli by dimming the lights and decreasing the noise level. Direct the patient to assume a comfortable position, and assist if needed. A night light is a necessity for promotion of safety for the older adult. Administer a sleeping medication or analgesic as ordered if the patient cannot sleep (see Box 21.4).

Patient problems and interventions for the patient with sleep disturbance include but are not limited to the following:

Patient Problem	Nursing Interventions
Ineffective Sleep Pattern, related to illness and psychological stress manifested by change in behavior, increased irritability, listlessness, and verbal complaints of not feeling well rested	Encourage patient to ambulate in the early evening, if permitted Provide glass of milk 30 min before patient's bedtime unless contraindicated Perform all necessary procedures before 9 p.m. to ensure uninterrupted sleep Massage patient's back, freshen linens, reduce noise, and dim lights Administer hypnotic as prescribed
Ineffective Thought Processes, related to sleep deprivation manifested by slower reaction time, altered attention span, and disorientation	Maintain periods of uninterrupted rest Provide safe environment Close door to patient room Orient patient to reality Administer analgesic or sedative (or both) about 30 min before patient's bedtime, if ordered

NURSING PROCESS FOR PAIN MANAGEMENT, COMFORT, REST, AND SLEEP

The role of the licensed practical nurse/licensed vocational nurse (LPN/LVN) in the nursing process is that the LPN/LVN will:

- Participate in planning care for patients based on patient needs
- Review patient's plan of care and recommend revisions as needed
- Review and follow defined prioritization for patient care
- Use clinical pathways, care maps, or care plans to guide and review patient care

ASSESSMENT

Pain assessment is one of the most frequent and difficult activities that a nurse performs. It is crucial to assess the pain experience from the patient's perspective. Make sure patients are aware that informed reporting of pain is valuable and necessary if the health care team is to manage pain effectively.

TERMINOLOGY

Specific terms are used in assessing pain. *Onset* indicates when the pain began. *Duration* is how long the pain lasts from the onset until it is resolved. Pain also is classified by location. To determine pain location, use a drawing of the body and ask the patient to mark all the areas where pain is felt. Another method is to ask the patient to point to the places where pain is felt, and you then document those places either on a body outline or descriptively in the medical record and on the care plan. Remind the patient to report new pain sites, because they may signal complications.

Severity indicates whether the pain is mild, moderate, or intense. Sample pain scales are useful to assist in assessing pain (see Fig. 21.8). Terms the patient uses to describe the pain, such as "sharp," "stabbing," "dull," or "throbbing," provide more information.

Many patients experiencing acute pain exhibit a rise in pulse rate and blood pressure, diaphoresis, and dilated pupils.

PATIENT PROBLEM

An accurate patient problem statement of the patient with pain enables you to plan and implement relief measures effectively. The following patient problem statements are associated directly with the care of patients with pain:

- *Recent Onset of Pain*
- *Prolonged Pain*

Other possible patient problem statements that are appropriate when pain affects other aspects of a patient's life include the following:

- *Inability to Tolerate Activity*
- *Anxiousness*
- *Distorted Body Image*
- *Excessive Demand on Primary Caregiver*
- *Infrequent or Difficult Bowel Elimination*
- *Impaired Coping*
- *Impaired Family Coping*
- *Risk for Contractures or Muscle Atrophy*
- *Impaired Family Processes*
- *Lethargy or Malaise*
- *Fearfulness*
- *Grief*
- *Despair*
- *Insufficient Knowledge (specify)*
- *Compromised Physical Mobility*
- *Insufficient Nutrition*
- *Helplessness*

- *Impaired Role Functioning*
- *Inability to Bathe Self*
- *Inability to Toilet Self*
- *Impaired Sexual Function*
- *Deficient Sleep*
- *Ineffective Sleep Pattern*
- *Compromised Social Interaction*
- *Social Seclusion*

The extensiveness of the list alerts you to the numerous problems that may develop because of pain.

◆ EXPECTED OUTCOMES AND PLANNING

When participating in the development of the plan of care, you establish priorities based on the patient's level of pain and its effect on the patient's condition. You and the patient set realistic expectations for pain relief and discuss the degree of pain relief to expect. Typical patient-centered goals and outcomes include the following:

Goal 1: Patient attains a sense of well-being and improved comfort within 1 hour.

Outcome: Patient nonverbally (facial expression, tone of voice) demonstrates improved relief from pain within 1 hour.

Goal 2: Patient regains ability to perform self-care independently within 24 hours.

Outcome: Patient bathes and grooms self without hesitancy or restriction within 24 hours.

◆ IMPLEMENTATION

Establish a trusting nurse-patient relationship so that the patient believes that relief measures will be beneficial. You help accomplish this when you see the patient in a holistic manner, listen attentively to concerns, attend promptly to the patient's needs, and respect any response to pain. In a successful nurse-patient relationship, the nurse understands that the patient is the expert on his or her own pain and its relief.

You probably will teach various measures to help the patient and the family deal with pain. Comfort measures sometimes avert the need for analgesics. Some measures are appropriate positioning and alignment in bed, washing and massaging the back, and ambulation, unless contraindicated.

Try teaching distraction and relaxation techniques to the patient. Sometimes distraction and relaxation do not help control the patient's pain, so it is necessary to use analgesic medications.

Nursing interventions that promote the establishment of an effective relationship with the person who is experiencing pain and with the family should include the following:

- *Believe the patient.* The patient needs to be able to trust the nurse and to recognize that the reports of pain are valid. Convey this message verbally to the patient by saying, "I know you are in pain."
- *Clarify responsibilities in pain relief.* Discuss what actions are going to be taken to manage the pain. Clarify the roles of the patient and family in the interaction.
- *Respect the patient's response to pain.* Accept the right of the patient to respond to the pain in the necessary manner. The family also needs help in this area. Sometimes the patient needs help accepting the response to the pain, if the behavior is not as expected by the patient and family.
- *Confer with the patient.* Encourage the patient to use coping techniques that have been effective in the past. Assist the patient and the family in using personal resources more effectively. Help the patient and the family to participate actively in setting goals for pain relief.
- *Explore the pain with the patient.* Find out what the pain means to the patient and the family.
- *Be with the patient often.* Act as a buffer for the patient and the family during difficult times. The physical presence of the nurse reassures or distracts the patient at times and offers comfort at others, thus relieving the pain (McCaffery and Pasero, 2003).

◆ EVALUATION

Effective communication between the nurse and the patient is essential in achieving pain control. Continuous evaluation allows you to determine whether new or revised therapies are required. Refer to the goals and outcomes identified when you plan care, and perform evaluative measures to determine whether the goals have been reached. Examples of goals and evaluative measures include the following:

Goal 1: Patient obtains a sense of well-being and improved pain relief within 1 hour.

Evaluative measure: Ask the patient to rate the pain on a scale of 0 to 10, 10 being the most severe. Observe the patient's facial expressions and body movement, noting whether there is freedom of movement.

Goal 2: Patient regains ability to perform self-care independently within 24 hours.

Evaluative measure: Observe patient performing activities of daily living.

Get Ready for the NCLEX® Examination!

Key Points

- McCaffery and Pasero (2003) provided a realistic description of pain: “Pain is whatever the experiencing person says it is, existing whenever he says it does.”
- Pain is largely a subjective experience.
- Pain is often a protective mechanism that warns of tissue injury.
- A nurse’s bias and misconception of pain potentially results in ineffective control of the patient’s pain.
- Pain scales are used to evaluate objectively pain intensity and the effectiveness of pain therapies.
- Considering pain the fifth vital sign helps ensure that pain is monitored on a regular basis.
- Individualize pain therapy by working closely with the patient, using assessment findings, and trying a variety of therapies.
- Patient-controlled analgesic devices and epidural analgesia give pain control with low risk of overdose.
- Nursing implications for administering epidural analgesia include closely monitoring for respiratory depression.
- Appropriate pain management has the potential to bring about quicker recoveries, shorter hospital stays, fewer readmissions, and improved quality of life.
- Constipation is the most common opioid side effect and the only one for which the individual does not develop tolerance.
- Fatigue, sleep disturbance, and depression act in a type of synergistic relationship that can change a person’s perception of pain markedly.
- The circadian rhythm is the 24-hour, day-night cycle known also as the diurnal rhythm.

Additional Learning Resources

SG Go to your Study Guide for additional learning activities to help you master this chapter content.

evolve Be sure to visit the Evolve site at *http://evolve.elsevier.com/Cooper/foundationsadult/* for additional online resources.

Review Questions for the NCLEX® Examination

1. After surgery for a total knee replacement, a patient was given an epidural catheter for fentanyl epidural analgesia. What is the most important nursing intervention?
   1. Administer additional analgesic medications as needed.
   2. Change the epidural dressing every shift.
   3. Assess respiratory rate.
   4. Encourage ambulation.
2. A 52-year-old patient admitted for deep vein thrombosis of the left internal iliac vein complains of excruciating pain in his left leg. What is the most appropriate response by the nurse?
   1. “Pain is what you say it is; I will assist you in whatever way I can.”
   2. “Your pain is an unpleasant sensation caused by inflammation of the vein and difficult to control.”
   3. “Your pain is one of the cardinal signs of inflammation.”
   4. “I know you are in pain, but it is important that we guard against possible addiction to opioids.”
3. A 63-year-old patient underwent a lower anterior bowel resection yesterday. What common central nervous system analgesic is prescribed often to control pain?
   1. Aspirin
   2. Acetaminophen (Tylenol)
   3. Morphine
   4. Ibuprofen (Motrin)
4. What drug delivery system is used to control pain via a portable computerized pump with a chamber for a syringe?
   1. Patient-controlled analgesia
   2. Transcutaneous electric nerve stimulation
   3. A venous access device
   4. An intrathecal delivery system
5. The nursing student is discussing the gate control theory of pain. Which statement by the student indicates the need for further instruction? *(Select all that apply.)*
   1. “The gates of the pain pathways can be opened with therapeutic massage and heat treatments.”
   2. “Pain has exclusive use of the pathways ahead of other stimuli, according to the theory.”
   3. “Distraction is beneficial in pain management, according to the theory.”
   4. “Pain is a manifestation of an intricate chain of electrochemical events.”
   5. “Memories and feelings may alter gating mechanisms.”
6. A patient admitted with severe cellulitis of the left breast states, “I have a severe burning pain, and it feels like my breast is on fire.” She rates her pain as 7 on the 0-to-10 pain assessment scale. How would this collection of data by the nurse in assessing the patient’s pain be classified?
   1. Deductive
   2. Speculative
   3. Objective
   4. Subjective
7. The nurse listens attentively while the patient describes her angina pectoris pain as radiating down her left inner arm to the little finger and upward to the jaw and the shoulder. What term is used to classify this type of pain?
   1. Precisely localized
   2. Referred
   3. Intermittent
   4. Chronic

8. The nurse is assessing the patient's description of his back pain. He states that it is "immobilizing, intense, and on a scale of 0 to 10, it is an 8." What type of pain assessment scale is the patient using?
   1. Visual analog
   2. Categorical
   3. Functional
   4. Numeric
9. The nurse is caring for two patients with similar injuries. One patient expresses severe pain, and the other reports feeling fine with low levels of pain. Which statement is most correct?
   1. The patient having more intense reports of pain has dysfunctional endorphins.
   2. The patient having lesser levels of pain has a higher level of endorphins.
   3. The patient experiencing intense pain has lower levels of endorphins.
   4. The patient having elevated levels of pain has an alteration in recognition of endorphins by the hypothalamus of the brain.
10. A patient was admitted to the orthopedic section for acute back pain. The health care provider is planning to use cutaneous stimulation management. Which is an example of this pain control method?
    1. Epidural analgesia
    2. Transcutaneous electric nerve stimulation (TENS)
    3. Nonsteroidal antiinflammatory drugs (NSAIDs)
    4. Patient-controlled analgesia
11. What statement concerning unrelieved pain is most correct?
    1. Unrelieved pain is a normal expectation after major surgery.
    2. Patients with cancer diagnoses can expect to experience unrelieved pain.
    3. Physiologic and psychological complications can result from unrelieved pain.
    4. Although unrelieved pain is stressful and annoying, it is not as important as other physical care needs.
12. What is the priority responsibility of the nurse related to pain?
    1. Leave the patient alone to rest.
    2. Help the patient appear to not be in pain.
    3. Believe what the patient says about pain.
    4. Assume responsibility for eliminating the patient's pain.
13. Research indicates that the risk of clinically significant opioid-induced respiratory depression is
    1. less than 1%.
    2. 5%.
    3. 20%.
    4. 30%.
14. Which route is most appropriate for treating rapidly escalating severe pain?
    1. Oral
    2. Intramuscular (IM)
    3. Intravenous (IV)
    4. Transdermal
15. Which opioid is no longer a drug of choice for managing pain because of its toxic complications, such as causing seizures?
    1. Codeine
    2. Morphine
    3. Meperidine
    4. Fentanyl
16. The nurse has recommended the patient consider music therapy to manage pain after an upcoming surgery. What information should be provided to the patient? *(Select all that apply.)*
    1. Music therapy works best when selections are instrumental instead of songs containing words.
    2. Music therapy is successful for at least 50% of people who try it.
    3. Music therapy promotes relaxation and takes the focus away from the pain being experienced.
    4. Music therapy is easily a self-directed means of pain management.
    5. Music therapy's success is limited to postoperative pain.
17. A patient has been prescribed acetaminophen to manage pain after a sports injury. What information can be included in the discussion about this medication with the patient? *(Select all that apply.)*
    1. This medication is limited to the management of mild pain.
    2. The dosage of acetaminophen should be limited to 4000 mg in a 24-hour period.
    3. Acetaminophen is associated with gastrointestinal upset.
    4. Excessive dosages are associated with hepatotoxicity.
    5. Acetaminophen works by blocking pain impulses.

22 Surgical Wound Care

http://evolve.elsevier.com/Cooper/foundationsadult/

Objectives

1. Discuss the body's response during each stage of wound healing.
2. Discuss the role of nutrition in wound healing.
3. Identify common complications of wound healing.
4. Differentiate between healing by primary intention and healing by secondary intention.
5. Discuss the classification of wounds according to the Centers for Disease Control and Prevention.
6. Discuss the factors that impair wound healing and the interventions for each type of wound.
7. Explain procedure for applying dry dressings and wet-to-dry dressings.
8. Discuss dehiscence and evisceration and the nursing care they involve.
9. Identify the procedure for removing sutures and staples.
10. Discuss care of the patient with a wound drainage system: Hemovac or Davol suction or T-tube drainage.
11. Identify the procedure for performing sterile wound irrigation.
12. Identify the nursing interventions for the patient with vacuum-assisted closure of a wound.
13. Describe the purposes of bandages and binders and the precautions taken when applying them.
14. List nursing diagnoses associated with wound care.

Key Terms

bandage (p. 638)
binder (p. 638)
dehiscence (dē-HĬS-ĕns, p. 642)
drainage (p. 633)
evisceration (ē-vĭs-ŭr-Ā-shŭn, p. 642)
exudate (ĔKS-ū-dāt, p. 616)
granulation (grăn-ū-LĀ-shŭn, p. 616)
incision (ĭn-SĬZH-ŭn, p. 615)
infectious process (p. 619)
inflammatory response (p. 619)
irrigation (p. 625)
primary intention (p. 616)
puncture (p. 615)
purulent (PYŪ-rū-lĕnt, p. 616)
sanguineous (săng-GWĬN-ē-ŭs, p. 619)
secondary intention (p. 616)
serosanguineous (SĒR-ō-săng-GWĬN-ē-ŭs, p. 619)
serous (SĒR-ŭs, p. 619)
T tube (p. 633)
tertiary intention (TŬR-shē-ăr-ē, p. 616)
vacuum-assisted closure (p. 633)
wound (p. 614)

The term **wound** refers to any injury to the body's tissues that involves a break in the skin. Injury results in either an open or a closed wound. This break in the integrity of the integument results in a potential compromise to the individual's defensive barriers against outside pathogens. Prompt assessment and interventions to reduce the potentially negative impact of the skin's breech are important. Stressors to the individual affect the efficiency of wound healing. Healing is affected by age, nutritional status, physical well-being, and medication therapies. Social factors, including smoking, can impair wound healing. Alterations in health, including diabetes, cancer, and heart disease, slow the body's ability to heal. Stress and strain (nausea, vomiting, abdominal distention, coughing, respiratory efforts) place tension against a surgical incision, especially an abdominal incision. During this phase, the abdominal muscles contract and cause intraabdominal pressure; if the incisional area is weak, dehiscence is possible. Other factors that have the capacity to affect wound healing include preoperative skin preparation, type of surgical procedure, environment within the surgical suite, and postoperative wound care.

WOUND CLASSIFICATION

Wound classifications are determined based on a series of factors that include cause, the severity of injury, the amount of contamination, and size. An understanding of the causative factors of a wound is vital to determination of the proper treatment plan. Obtain a complete history, including what caused the wound and any underlying disease process.

In planned surgery, the surgeon makes a wound by **incision** (a cut produced surgically by a sharp instrument that creates an opening into an organ or space in the body) or **puncture** (stab wound for a drainage system); the surgical wound usually is closed or managed (e.g., a drain inserted, a stoma created) in the final stage of the procedure. By contrast, in traumatic injury (e.g., from a knife stabbing) and unplanned or emergency surgeries, the practitioner brings wound edges together to aid healing. Unless a "dirty surgery" is performed (e.g., a perforated bowel, ruptured appendix), a surgical incision is cleaner and easier to repair than a traumatic wound.

Surgical wounds are classified based on the level of contamination. The Centers for Disease Control and Prevention (CDC) has classified wounds by the level and type of contamination. Levels range from class I (clean) to class IV (dirty, infected). The Association of Perioperative Registered Nurses developed a decision tree to assist in classification of the stage of the surgical wound (Fig. 22.1).

The risk for infection in a clean surgical wound is less than 5%. The risk for other wound types increases based on the type of contamination that may be introduced. Contamination may result from the presence of gastrointestinal (GI) matter, such as feces, which contain *Escherichia coli* from the colon or from environmental conditions at the time of injury preceding the surgical intervention. Wounds that are contaminated, such as

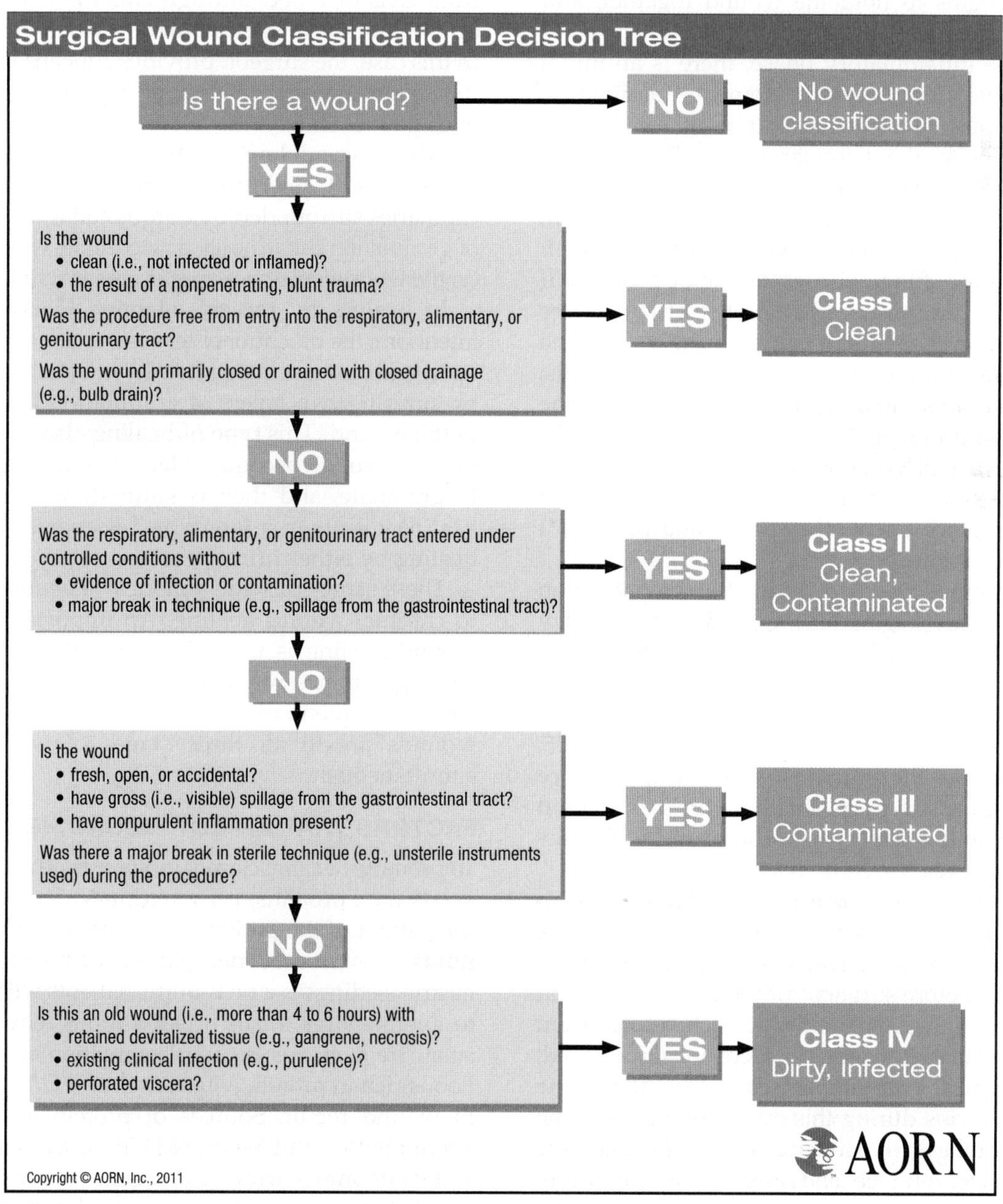

Fig. 22.1 Surgical wound classification decision tree. (Reprinted with permission from AORN.org. Copyright 2015 AORN, Inc., 2170 Parker Road, Suite 400, Denver, CO 80231. All rights reserved.)

those with gangrene, have a significantly elevated risk of infection, nearing 27%.

WOUND HEALING

The healing process begins immediately after an injury and sometimes continues for a year or longer. Although the healing process follows the same pattern, the type of wound and tissue, the wound's severity, and the overall condition of the patient influence the overall process. Wound healing follows four phases: hemostasis, inflammatory phase, reconstruction, and maturation.

PHASES OF WOUND HEALING

Hemostasis (termination of bleeding) begins as soon as the injury occurs. As blood platelets adhere to the walls of the injured vessel, a clot begins to form. Fibrin in the clot begins to hold the wound together, and bleeding subsides.

During the inflammatory phase, there is an initial increase in the flow of blood elements (antibodies, electrolytes, plasma proteins) and water out of the blood vessel into the vascular space. This process causes the cardinal signs and symptoms of inflammation: erythema (redness), heat, edema (swelling), pain, and tissue dysfunction. Leukocytes appear and begin to engulf bacteria, fungi, viruses, and toxic proteins. If an infection is not present, the number of leukocytes decreases. During the inflammatory phase, cells in the injured tissue migrate, divide, and form new cells. Slowly, blood clots dissolve and the wound fills; the sides of the wound usually meet in 24 to 48 hours. As the inflammatory phase ends, new cells and capillaries fill in the wound from the underlying tissue to the skin surface. This process seals the wound and protects it from contamination.

Collagen formation occurs during the reconstruction phase. This phase begins on the third or fourth day after injury and lasts for 2 to 3 weeks. Fibroblasts produce collagen, a gluelike protein substance that adds tensile strength to the wound and the tissue. Collagen formation increases rapidly between postoperative days 5 and 25. During this phase, the wound takes on the appearance of an irregular, raised, purplish, immature scar. Wound dehiscence most frequently occurs during the reconstruction phase.

Approximately 3 weeks after surgery, fibroblasts begin to exit the wound. The wound continues to gain strength, although healed wounds rarely return to the strength the tissue had before surgery. Although tissue heals at varying speeds, internal wounds (stomach, colon) regain strength faster than skin wounds. Occasionally a keloid, an overgrowth of collagenous scar tissue at the site of a wound, forms during this maturation phase. The keloid's color ranges from red to pink to white. This new tissue is elevated, rounded, and firm. African Americans, dark-complexioned whites, and young women have the highest incidence of keloid formation.

PROCESS OF WOUND HEALING

The process of wound healing occurs by primary intention (primary union), secondary intention (granulation), or tertiary (third) intention (Fig. 22.2). Wounds in which skin edges are close together and little tissue is lost, such as those made surgically, heal by **primary intention;** minimal scarring results. Closure can be by sutures, staples, skin glue, or Steri-Strips. Primary intention healing begins during the inflammatory phase of healing; in surgery, this is usually during closure of the wound.

Healing by **secondary intention,** when a wound must granulate during healing, occurs when skin edges are not close together (approximated) or when pus has formed. Some wounds develop a **purulent** (producing or containing pus) **exudate** (fluid, cells, or other substances that have been slowly exuded, or discharged, from cells or blood through small pores or breaks in cell membranes) when injured or diseased tissue dies. In this case, the surgeon provides a means for its release through a drainage system or by packing the wound with gauze. Slowly, the necrotized tissue decomposes and escapes, and the cavity begins to fill with **granulation** tissue, or soft, pink, fleshy projections that consist of capillaries surrounded by fibrous collagen. The amount of granulation tissue necessary to fill the wound depends on the wound's size; scarring is greater in a large wound.

In healing by **tertiary intention** (delayed primary intention), the practitioner leaves a contaminated wound open and closes it later, after the infection is controlled, by suturing two layers of granulation tissue together in the wound. This type of healing also occurs when a primary wound becomes infected, is opened, is allowed to granulate, and then is sutured. Tertiary intention healing results in a larger and deeper scar than does healing by either primary or secondary intention.

These stages provide a model for acute (as opposed to chronic) wound healing. An important concept in wound healing is that the stages of wound healing, although progressive, do not necessarily occur in a linear (strictly sequential) fashion. Some normally healing wounds are in all three stages of wound healing simultaneously.

FACTORS THAT AFFECT WOUND HEALING

To promote healing, closely monitor fluid and nutritional needs (i.e., proteins, carbohydrates, fats, vitamins) of the patient. If the patient is not able to tolerate food or fluids, provision of total parenteral nutrition or nasogastric feedings is a possibility. Patients who are unable to tolerate large meals or solid foods may need to eat small, frequent meals. Supplementation may be needed. Foods rich in protein, vitamins A and C, and zinc assist in wound repair. Sources of protein include meats, peanut butter, and legumes. Dark, leafy vegetables and yellow or orange fruits and vegetables provide vitamin A. Strawberries, tomatoes, spinach, and cruciferous vegetables, including broccoli, cauliflower, and cabbage,

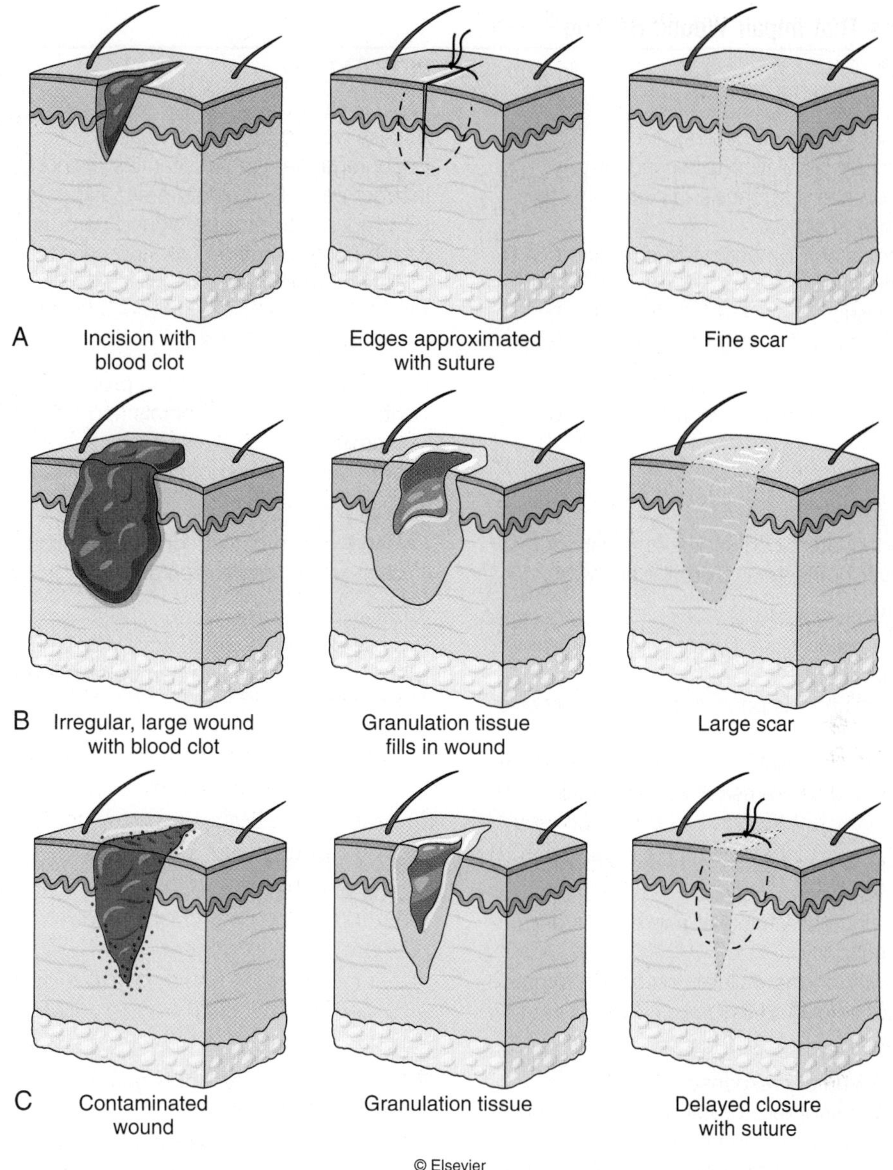

Fig. 22.2 Types of wound healing. A, Primary intention. B, Secondary intention. C, Tertiary intention.

are rich sources of vitamin C. Zinc may be obtained from fortified cereals, red meat, and seafood. Offer fluids, when tolerated, on an hourly basis. Unless contraindications exist, encourage an intake of 2000 to 2400 mL in 24 hours. As the patient progresses from clear to full liquids, provide fluids the patient enjoys. Until the patient's hydration level is stable (usually 48 to 72 hours), monitor the patient's intake and output (I&O).

Assist the patient to achieve a balance between rest as a means to facilitate healing and activity to decrease venous stasis. The location and size of the incision influence the patient's movements. Take care to avoid strain on the suture line. When the patient is confined to bed, provide instruction about the best means to move in bed, moving one body section at a time—head, chest, hips, and legs. To sit up, the patient should roll to the side and, with the elbow as a lever, push to a sitting position; this reduces the stress placed on the incision. If coughing occurs, apply a pillow, rolled bath blanket, or the palms of the hands to the incisional area to lessen intraabdominal pressure; this technique is called *splinting*. Limiting of visitors sometimes may be necessary if the patient tires too easily.

Preexisting conditions, such as malnourishment, and chronic diseases (arthritis, diabetes mellitus, hypertension) add stress to the recovering body and necessitate ongoing monitoring (Table 22.1).

SURGICAL WOUND

The selection of the site for the surgical wound is based on the tissue and the organs involved, the nature of the injury or disease process, the presence of inflammation or infection, and the strength of the site. If a surgical procedure calls for a drainage system, the positioning of the drain also influences the placement

Table 22.1 **Factors That Impair Wound Healing**

PHYSIOLOGIC EFFECTS	INTERVENTIONS
Age	
Aging alters all phases of wound healing. Vascular changes impair circulation to wound site. Reduced liver function alters synthesis of clotting factors. Inflammatory response is slowed. Formation of antibodies and lymphocytes is reduced. Collagen tissue is less pliable. Scar tissue is less elastic.	Assess wound for rate of healing. Encourage diet high in vitamins A and C, protein, and zinc. Instruct patient on safety precautions to prevent injuries. Be prepared to provide wound care for longer period. Teach home caregivers wound care techniques (see the Patient Teaching box).
Malnutrition	
All phases of wound healing are impaired. Stress from burns or severe trauma increases nutritional requirements.	Provide balanced diet rich in protein, carbohydrates, lipids, vitamins A and C, minerals (e.g., zinc, copper), and B vitamins. Provide adequate amounts of calories and fluids.
Obesity	
Fatty tissue lacks adequate blood supply to resist bacterial infection and deliver nutrients and cellular elements.	Observe obese patient for signs of wound infection, dehiscence, and evisceration.
Impaired Oxygenation	
Low arterial oxygen tension alters synthesis of collagen and formation of epithelial cells. If local circulating blood flow is poor, tissues fail to receive needed oxygen. Decreased hemoglobin (anemia) reduces arterial oxygen levels in capillaries and interferes with tissue repair.	Provide diet adequate in iron, vitamin B, and folic acid. Monitor hematocrit and hemoglobin levels of patients with wounds.
Smoking	
Smoking reduces amount of functional hemoglobin in blood, thus decreasing tissue oxygenation. Smoking sometimes increases platelet aggregation and causes hypercoagulability. Smoking interferes with normal cellular mechanisms that promote release of oxygen to tissues.	Discourage patient from smoking by explaining its effects on wound healing.
Drugs	
Steroids reduce inflammatory response. Antiinflammatory drugs suppress protein synthesis, wound contraction, epithelialization, and inflammation. Prolonged antibiotic use increases risk of superinfection. Chemotherapeutic drugs often depress bone marrow function, number of leukocytes, and inflammatory response.	Carefully observe patient; signs of inflammation are not always obvious. Vitamin A has the capacity to counteract effects of steroids.
Diabetes Mellitus	
Chronic disease causes small blood vessel disease that impairs tissue perfusion. Diabetes causes hemoglobin to have greater affinity for oxygen, so it fails to release oxygen to tissues. Hyperglycemia alters ability of leukocytes to perform phagocytosis and supports overgrowth of fungal and yeast infections.	Instruct patient to take preventive measures to avoid cuts or breaks in skin. Provide preventive foot care. Control blood sugar to reduce the physiologic changes associated with diabetes.
Radiation	
Fibrosis and vascular scarring eventually develop in irradiated skin layers. Tissues become fragile and poorly oxygenated.	Closely observe patients who have had surgery for wound complications.
Wound Stress	
Vomiting, abdominal distention, and respiratory effort sometimes stress suture line and potentially disrupt wound layer. Sudden, unexpected tension on incision inhibits formation of endothelial cell and collagen networks.	Control nausea with ordered antiemetics. Keep nasogastric tubes patent and draining to prevent accumulation of secretions. Instruct patient to splint abdominal wound during coughing.

of the incision. The surgeon's goal is to enter the cavity involved and repair the injured or diseased area as quickly and with the least trauma possible. To facilitate the surgery, patients often are placed in positions that add stress to the tissue. Retraction instruments often are used during procedures and compound the inflammation experienced after the surgical procedure. Pain after surgery thus results at times from strained muscles and ligaments and from the surgical process.

Many options are available to the surgeon for closing the surgical incision. Common closures are sutures, staples, adhesive skin closure strips, butterfly strips, and transparent sprays and films. A binder or bandage helps support the incision or secure dressings and makes use of adhesive materials unnecessary. A protective dressing often is used to cover the surgical wound for the first 24 hours. It is removed the day after surgery by the surgeon. After surgery, inspect the dressing hourly during the first 4 hours after the procedure. Then inspect dressings every 2 to 4 hours for the first 24 hours. On the day of surgery, most wounds produce either **sanguineous** (composed of or pertaining to blood) or **serosanguineous** (thin and red, composed of serum and blood) exudate. Later, as the exudate subsides, it becomes **serous** (thin and watery, composed of the serum portion of blood) (Table 22.2). Because pressure to wounds retards bleeding, the general practice is to keep surgical wounds covered with a gauze dressing. To prevent undetected hemorrhaging, inspect the dressing or incisional area and the area under the patient. Exudate follows the flow of gravity; therefore, depending on the contour of the body, the dressing sometimes remains dry even though blood or exudate is flowing away, under the body.

The extent of the **inflammatory response** (a tissue reaction to injury) depends on the level of injury inflicted, the size of the area involved, and the physical condition of the patient. Gradually, fluid from the cells and leukocytes collects along the vessel walls and fibrin walls off the injury and provides a matrix along which new cells form. Leukocytes perform one of their important functions, phagocytosis (a process by which certain cells engulf and dispose of microorganisms and cell debris), by surrounding, engulfing, and digesting exudate from the injured cell. The leukocyte becomes the body's vacuum cleaner by removing its debris. Evidence of leukocyte action is given through changes in the white blood cell (WBC) count. An **infectious process** (a condition caused by the invasion of the body by pathogenic microorganisms) usually is evidenced by an elevated WBC count.

Table 22.2 Types of Wound Drainage

TYPE	APPEARANCE
A. Serous	Clear, watery plasma
B. Purulent	Thick, yellow, green, tan, or brown
C. Serosanguineous	Pale, red, watery: mixture of serous and sanguineous
D. Sanguineous	Bright red: indicates active bleeding

A, From Perry AG, Potter PA: *Clinical nursing skills & techniques*, ed 9, St. Louis, 2018, Elsevier.

STANDARD STEPS IN WOUND CARE

All nursing skills include certain basic steps for the safety and well-being of the patient and the nurse. To save space and minimize repetition, instructions for these steps are not included in the description of each skill, unless clarification of their application for that skill is necessary. Remember the following essential steps and follow them precisely to deliver appropriate and responsible nursing interventions. The rationale for the skills follows each step in parentheses.

Before performing the skill:

1. Refer to the medical record, care plan, or Kardex for special interventions. *(Provides basis for care. Many nursing interventions require orders from the health care provider. Verification is ensured when the medical record is reviewed.)*
2. Provide an introduction to the patient; include name and title or role. *(Decreases patient anxiety.)*
3. Identify patients by checking armband and requesting that patients state their names. *(Identifies correct patient for procedure.)*
4. Explain the procedure and the reason for the procedure in terms the patient is able to understand; give the patient time to ask questions. Advise the

patient of any potential unpleasantness that will be experienced. *(Seeks cooperation, decreases patient's anxiety, and prepares patient. Also helps determine whether procedure is still appropriate.)*

5. Assess need for and provide patient teaching during procedure. *(Promotes patient's independence.)*
6. Assess patient. Each skill has an assessment section that includes specific data. *(Provides baseline information for later comparisons.)*
7. Perform hand hygiene and don clean gloves according to agency policy and guidelines from the CDC and the Occupational Safety and Health Administration (OSHA) (see Chapter 7). *(Reduces the spread of microorganisms.)*
8. Assemble equipment and complete necessary charges. *(Organizes procedure. Some equipment is reusable and is kept at the bedside. Some of the equipment is disposable and charged to the patient as used. Know agency policy. Specific equipment is listed for each skill.)*
9. Prepare patient for intervention:
   a. Close door or pull privacy curtain. *(Provides privacy and promotes patient's comfort.)*
   b. Raise bed to comfortable working height; lower side rail on side nearest you. *(Promotes proper body mechanics by minimizing muscle strain on caregivers and preventing injury and fatigue.)*
   c. Position and drape patient as necessary. *(Respect for privacy is basic for preserving human dignity. Patients have the right to privacy. Specific positions are included in each skill.)*

During the skill:

10. Promote patient involvement as possible. *(Participation encourages patient motivation and cooperation.)*
11. Assess patient's tolerance, being alert for signs and symptoms of discomfort and fatigue. Inability to tolerate a procedure is described in the nursing notes. *(Patient's ability to tolerate interventions varies depending on severity of illness and disability. Nurses need to use judgment in providing the opportunity for rest and comfort measures.)*

Completion of procedure:

12. Assist patient to a position of comfort and place needed items within easy reach. Be certain patient has a means to call for assistance and knows how to use it. *(Promotes safety; patients who attempt to reach items that are not close risk falling or injury.)*
13. Raise the side rails and lower the bed to the lowest position. *(This reduces the risk of patients getting out of bed unattended. With use of best nursing judgment, allow alert, cooperative patients to have the side rails down during daytime hours without the risk of injury.)*
14. Remove gloves (see Skill 22.3, Step 6) and all protective barriers, such as gown, goggles, and masks, if worn. Store or remove and dispose of soiled supplies and equipment according to agency policy and guidelines from the CDC and OSHA (see Chapter 17). *(Reduces spread of microorganisms, cleans environment, and enhances patient comfort.)*
15. Perform hand hygiene after patient contact and after removing gloves (see Chapter 7). *(Wearing gloves does not eliminate the need to wash hands. Hand hygiene is the most important technique in prevention and control of the spread of microorganisms.)*
16. Document patient's response, expected or unexpected outcomes, and patient teaching. *(Timely and proper documentation records patient progress and promotes continuity of care. Recording also fulfills legal responsibility of nurse.)* Specific notes for documentation are included in each skill.
17. Report any unexpected outcomes. (Additional therapies may be necessary.) Specific notes for reporting are included in each skill.

CARE OF THE INCISION

Surgical wounds, because they are created under aseptic conditions, generally heal well and quickly. For prevention of trauma until epithelialization occurs, and for keeping bleeding and exposure to bacteria to a minimum, the wound usually is covered at least initially by a dressing. Dressings over closed wounds usually are removed by the second or third day.

Incision coverings take the form of gauze, semiocclusive, or occlusive dressings (Fig. 22.3). Gauze dressings permit air to reach the wound; semiocclusive dressings permit oxygen but not air impurities to pass; and occlusive dressings permit neither air nor oxygen to pass. Occlusive and semiocclusive dressings are thought to promote healing by keeping wounds moist (yet sterile), so epithelial cells are able to slide more easily over the surface of the wound during epithelialization. Tape, ties, bandages, or cloth binders sometimes may be used to secure a dressing over a wound site. The selection depends on the wound size, the location, the presence

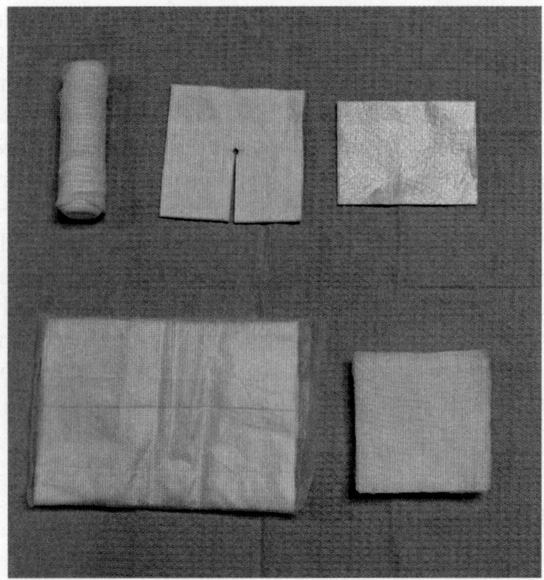

Fig. 22.3 Types of dressings. *Clockwise, from top left:* Rolled gauze, drain dressing, Telfa non-adherent dressing, flat gauze 4 × 4, ABD.

Box 22.1 How to Make Montgomery Straps

Use of Montgomery straps to secure dressings helps prevent tape irritation of skin when dressings require frequent changing (see the figure for Step 14 in Skill 22.1). If ready-made Montgomery straps are not available, follow these steps to make them:

1. Cut several strips of 3-inch–wide (7.6 cm) hypoallergenic tape. The number of strips of tape and the length of the tape depend on the size of the dressing for the wound.
2. Fold each strip 2 to 3 inches (5.08 to 7.62 cm) back on itself (sticky sides together) to form a nonadhesive tab. Small holes should be made to allow for straps to be used to lace the Montgomery straps to secure the dressing.
3. Clean the patient's skin to prevent irritation. After the skin dries, apply skin protectant. Apply the Montgomery straps with the sticky side on the skin on either side of the dressing. Thread a separate piece of gauze tie, umbilical tape, or twill tape (about 12 inches [30.5 cm]) through each pair of holes in the straps, and tie each strip similar to tying a shoelace.
4. Repeat this procedure for each of the Montgomery straps needed.
5. The straps can be left in place for several days unless they become soiled.

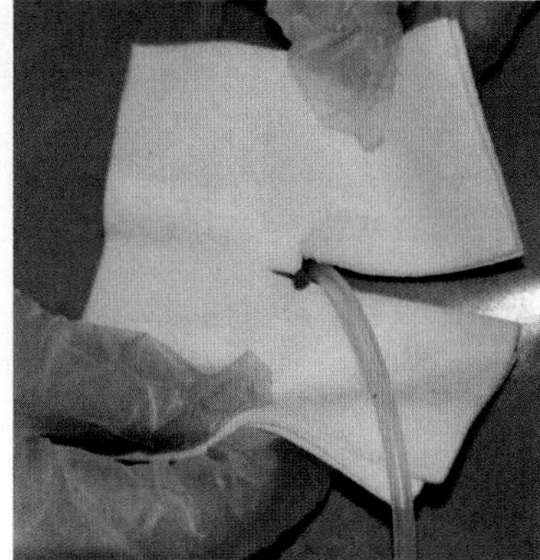

Fig. 22.4 Applying a drain dressing.

Box 22.2 Health Care–Associated Wound Infections

- Health care–associated infections are a continual threat to patients, especially the patient after surgery.
- Virulence of the bacterial contamination and resistance of the patient are two major factors in determining whether a wound becomes infected.
- Because wound infections usually have an incubation period of 4 to 6 days, some patients are discharged before problems are noted.
- Patient teaching includes ongoing observations to determine whether medical treatment is necessary.
- Exudate and drainage are signs of healing, but accurate assessments sometimes provide signals of potential complications of wound healing.

of drainage, the frequency of dressing changes, and the patient's level of activity. Montgomery straps, which remain in place around the wound while permitting the dressing over the wound to be changed, are one possibility; they reduce the need for frequent removal and reapplication of tape, which can cause considerable skin irritation (Box 22.1). If an occlusive dressing is used, place tape strips on all sides of the dressing. Otherwise, place the tape strips several inches apart to make the wound accessible to atmospheric oxygen.

The surgeon may leave sutured, clean wounds undressed after surgery or may use loose dressings. These methods allow atmospheric oxygen to circulate above the wound, aiding in the healing process. In many cases, if a dressing has been used for closed wounds, it is removed within 24 hours after surgery to allow air circulation. Within 24 hours, enough fibrin usually has been produced at the wound site to stop the entry of microorganisms. Refer to agency policy and the health care provider's or surgeon's preference. In many cases, the surgeon does the initial dressing change.

A dry dressing (as opposed to wet-to-dry, semiocclusive, or occlusive dressings) is often the choice for management of a wound with little exudate or drainage, such as abrasions and nondraining postoperative incisions. In addition to keeping initial bleeding to a minimum, the dressing protects the wound from injury, prevents introduction of bacteria, reduces discomfort, and speeds healing. A dry dressing also prevents deeper tissues from drying out by keeping the wound surface moist (*www.woundsource.com* is a helpful resource). The dry dressing does not debride the wound. If a dry dressing adheres to a wound, moisten the dressing with sterile normal saline solution or sterile water before removing the gauze. Moistening the dressing in this manner decreases the adherence of the dressing to the wound and reduces the risk of further trauma to the wound (Skill 22.1).

Dressing removal may be stressful to the patient. Provide instruction about what will be experienced during the procedure. If you anticipate the dressing removal to be painful, provide analgesic at least 30 minutes before exposing a wound. If underlying drains are present, take care not to remove or displace them accidentally during dressing removal (Fig. 22.4).

Follow sterile technique whenever handling the wound or the dressing (see Chapter 17 for principles of sterile technique). *Asepsis* (absence of germs) not only protects the nurse from wound drainage but also decreases the introduction of *pathogenic* (capable of producing disease) organisms into the wound. Use of sterile asepsis lessens the chance of the patient acquiring a health care–associated infection (Box 22.2). Use standard precautions (see Chapter 17) when handling body secretions. Good hand hygiene technique and the use of sterile aseptic procedures are essential when providing surgical wound care. Wear a gown, mask,

Skill 22.1 Changing a Sterile Dry Dressing

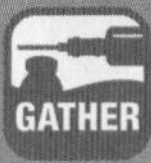

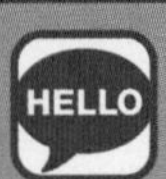

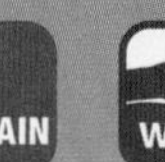

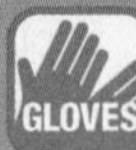

NURSING ACTION *(RATIONALE)*

1. See the section "Standard Steps in Wound Care," Steps 1 to 9.
2. Assemble equipment:
   - Clean gloves
   - Sterile gloves
   - Refuse container
   - Dressing set
   - Sterile normal saline solution (if indicated)
   - Antiseptic swabs
   - Ointment, if ordered
   - Sterile 4 × 4 gauze squares
   - Nonadherent dressing
   - Fluff-dried or loose gauze
   - Sterile abdominal pads
   - Barrier drape (optional)
   - Tape (e.g., paper or micropore), Montgomery straps (see Box 22.1), or binder
   - Adhesive remover (optional)
   - Protective apparel (gown, goggles, mask [optional])
   - Disposable measuring device to accurately assess wound size and amount of drainage
3. Place refuse container in convenient location away from sterile field. *(Prevents need to reach across sterile field and thus prevents contamination.)*
4. Set up sterile field. *(Maintains asepsis during procedure and organizes approach to procedure.)*
   a. Open sterile dressings.
   b. Use barrier drape as needed.
   c. Open sterile gloves.
   d. Open dressing set, if needed.
   e. Prepare antiseptic swabs.
5. Loosen tape by gently removing toward incision and gently using thumb to retract skin away from tape (countertraction). *(Minimizes tissue trauma and decreases patient discomfort.)*
6. Don clean gloves, remove dressing, and discard. If drains are present, remove dressings one layer at a time. *(Prevents accidental removal of drain.)*
7. Assess status of wound and wound drainage. *(Provides evaluation of healing process and collection of data for accurate documentation.)*
8. Remove gloves; discard. Wash hands and don sterile gloves. *(Prevents spread of microorganisms and maintains surgical asepsis.)*
9. Cleanse wound and surrounding area with antiseptic swab, starting from incision and moving outward, using one stroke per swab. Discard swabs. *(Aids in removing bacteria from wound areas. Prevents contaminating previously cleaned area.)*

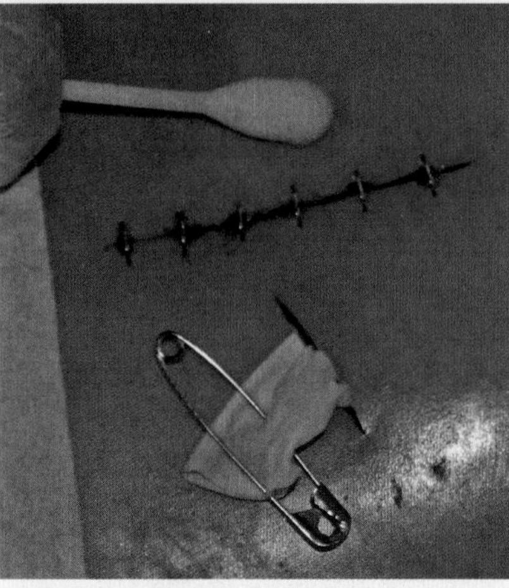

10. Use sterile gauze to dry in same manner, or allow antiseptic to air dry. *(Drying reduces excess moisture that eventually could harbor microorganisms.)*
11. Cleanse drain site if applicable. *(Helps to remove bacteria or prevent bacteria from entering wound area.)*

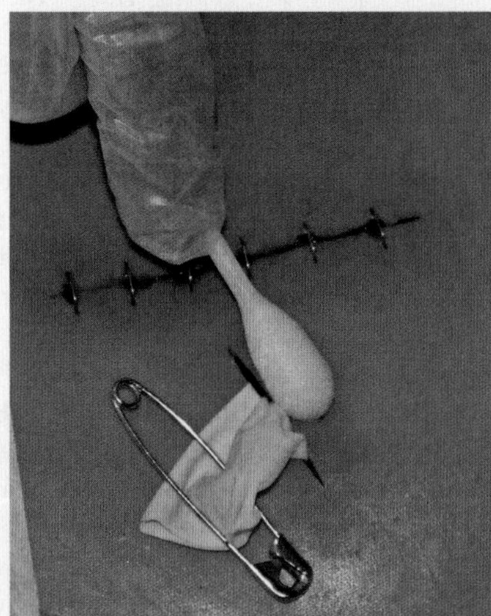

12. Apply antibiotic ointment, if ordered, using same techniques as for cleansing. *(Helps reduce growth of microorganisms.)*
13. Cover wound with appropriately sized dry sterile dressing and use drain dressing, if applicable (see Fig. 22.4). *(Protects wound and skin around drain site from skin impairment.)*
14. Secure dressing with tape, Montgomery straps, or binder. Some facilities use a skin preparation at tape sites to protect skin from irritation. Consider use of Montgomery straps when dressings require frequent changing to prevent

Skill 22.1 Changing a Sterile Dry Dressing—cont'd

tape irritation of skin (see Box 22.1). *(Supports wound and ensures placement and stability of dressings.)*

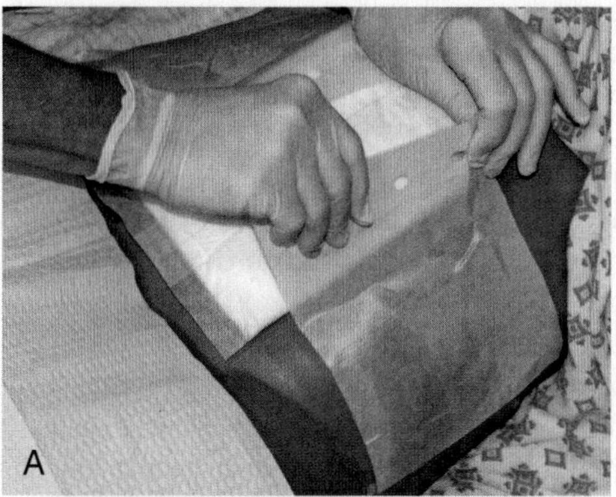
A

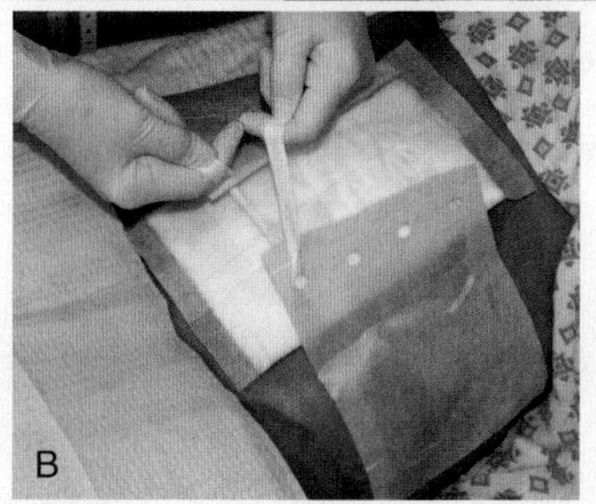
B

15. See the section "Standard Steps in Wound Care," Steps 10 to 17.
16. Document: *(Records patient's progress and therapy provided.)*
    - Location
    - Status of wound
    - Description of exudate or drainage (see Table 22.2)
    - Dressings applied
    - Any changes
    - Patient's response to procedure
    - Patient teaching (see the Patient Teaching box)
17. Report to health care provider any unexpected appearance of wound or drainage or accidental removal of drain within an hour. *(Unless patient shows evidence of wound dehiscence, notification of the health care provider of unexpected findings within an hour is adequate.)*

and protective goggles if soiling or splashing of wound exudate is anticipated.

WET-TO-DRY DRESSING

The wet-to-dry dressing is a type of wound management that frequently was used in the past. Some health care providers still order wet-to-dry dressings in certain circumstances. These dressings are most appropriate for wounds that do not have significant amounts of ischemic or necrotic tissue or large amounts of drainage or exudate (Skill 22.2). Traditionally, the purpose of wet-to-dry dressings was either to keep the wound bed moist or to provide mechanical débridement. Recent studies have called this practice into question, and some health care providers are starting to reconsider their use because during the débridement process granulation tissue often is damaged as the dressing is removed.

Commonly used wetting agents include normal saline solution and lactated Ringer's solution, isotonic solutions that aid in mechanical débridement. Acetic acid is effective against *Pseudomonas aeruginosa* but is toxic to fibroblasts in standard dilutions. Sodium hypochlorite solution (Dakin's) sometimes is used to facilitate débridement in a wound with necrotic debris and is an effective deodorizing solution. Povidone-iodine, usually one-quarter to one-half strength, is a rapid-acting antimicrobial agent for cleansing intact skin. In wounds, the solution is toxic to fibroblasts and has questionable efficacy in infected wounds. Other antibiotic solutions may be ordered, although their use is controversial. The containers of the wetting solutions should be labeled clearly with the date and time of opening. They should be discarded 24 hours after opening and replaced with fresh solution, because they can harbor microorganism growth.

ALTERNATIVES TO WET-TO-DRY DRESSING

The alternatives to wet-to-dry dressings include hydrogel gauze, hydrogel silver gauze, honey gauze, cadexomer iodine gel with high-ply gauze, hydrocolloid dressings, hydrogel dressing, and collagen dressings. The hydrocolloid dressing can be used for extra dry wound sites. The hydrocolloid dressing creates an airtight bond with the skin to prevent impermeable bacteria penetration. The hydrogel dressing works with many types of wounds by providing hydration to the wound and preventing spread of infection. The collagen dressing helps improve

Skill 22.2 Changing a Wet-to-Dry Dressing

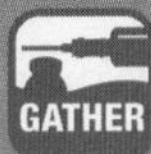

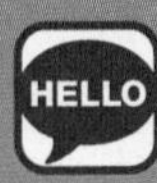

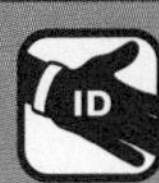

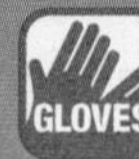

NURSING ACTION *(RATIONALE)*

1. See the section "Standard Steps in Wound Care," Steps 1 to 9.
2. Assemble equipment:
   - Barrier drape
   - Sterile dressing
   - Gauze
   - Sterile basin
   - Sterile solution
   - Antiseptic swabs
   - Instrument set, if needed
   - Clean gloves
   - Sterile gloves
   - Refuse container
   - Tape or Montgomery straps
   - Waterproof pad
3. Place waterproof pad appropriately. *(Prevents soiling of bed or linens.)*
4. Place refuse container appropriately. *(Prevents need to reach across sterile field and thus prevents contamination.)*
5. Set up sterile field. *(Maintains sterile technique during procedure and organizes approach to procedure.)*
   a. Open barrier drape.
   b. Add sterile dressing and gauze.
   c. Add sterile basin.
   d. Pour sterile solution into basin.
   e. Add instrument set, if needed.
   f. Add antiseptic swabs.
6. Loosen tape by gently removing toward incision and, using thumb, gently retracting the skin away from tape (countertraction). *(Minimizes tissue trauma. Decreases patient discomfort.)*
7. Don clean gloves. Remove dressing and discard. Do not moisten dressings to remove because this interferes with the débriding process. To be considerate of patient, provide analgesic medication at least 20 to 30 minutes before the procedure. *(Protects you from microorganisms. Prevents contamination of wound from soiled dressing and promotes patient comfort.)*
8. Assess status of wound and wound exudate or drainage on dressing (see Table 22.2). *(Provides evaluation of healing process and collection of data for accurate documentation.)*
9. Remove gloves; discard. Perform hand hygiene and don sterile gloves. *(Reduces spread of microorganisms and maintains surgical asepsis.)*
10. Cleanse wound and surrounding area with antiseptic swab, starting from incision and moving outward, using one stroke per swab. Discard swabs. *(Removes old drainage and bacteria from skin area.)*
11. Place gauze into basin. *(Wets gauze with solution.)*
12. Wring excess solution from dressing, leaving it slightly moist. *(Prevents growth of bacteria caused by dressing that is too wet.)*
13. Apply moist gauze dressing as a single layer directly onto wound surface. If wound is deep, gently pack gauze into wound with forceps until all wound surfaces are in contact with moist gauze. *(Allows solution to contact wound, which makes it effective. Moist gauze absorbs drainage and adheres to debris.)*

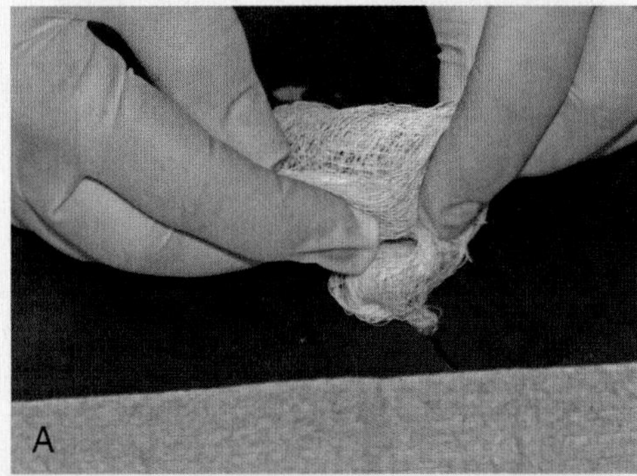
A

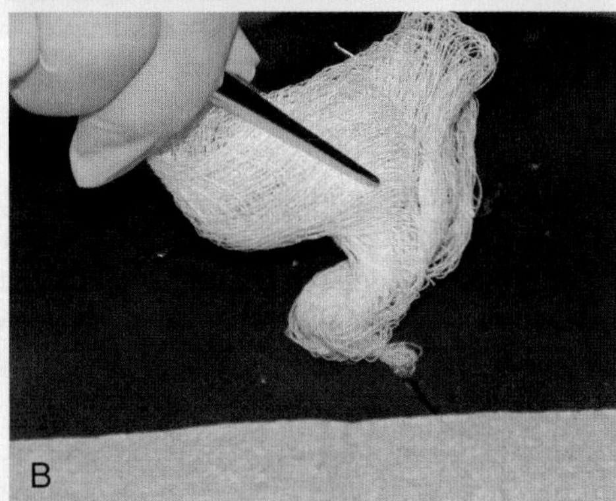
B

14. Apply dry dressing over wet gauze. *(Pulls moisture from the wound and allows for absorption of excess moisture.)*
15. Cover with additional dressing as needed. *(Protects wound from bacteria.)*
16. Secure with tape or Montgomery straps. *(Secures dressings in place.)*
17. See the section "Standard Steps in Wound Care," Steps 10 to 17.

Skill 22.2 Changing a Wet-to-Dry Dressing—cont'd

18. Document: *(Records patient's progress and therapy provided.)*
- Wound status
- Description of exudate or drainage (see Table 22.2)
- Dressings applied
- Patient's response to procedure
- Patient teaching (see the Patient Teaching box)

19. Discuss change in dressing procedure with the health care provider as wound surface becomes clean and granulation tissue is evident. *(Promotes anticipated wound healing.)*

20. Be aware this type of dressing is not widely used.

the movement of keratinocytes and fibroblasts to wound site to promote wound healing.

TRANSPARENT DRESSINGS

Thin, self-adhesive transparent film dressings (e.g., Op-site, Tegaderm) belong in the semiocclusive or occlusive categories. As a synthetic permeable (capable of allowing the passage of fluids or substances in solution) membrane, this dressing acts as a temporary second skin. It has several advantages. It adheres to undamaged skin to contain exudate and minimize wound contamination. It also is a barrier to external fluids and bacteria yet still allows the wound to breathe. It promotes a moist environment that speeds epithelial cell growth. This dressing type allows for wound assessment without removal of the protective film. Underlying tissue is protected against disruption caused by dressing removal. Film type dressings are beneficial for skin tears and over IV sites. Transparent dressings are available with and without adhesive borders. These dressings can stay in place up to 7 days, if complete occlusion is maintained. Transparent dressings are not absorbent, so they should not be used on draining wounds.

For best results, use these dressings on clean, débrided wounds that are not bleeding actively. The film is ideal for small, superficial wounds and as a dressing over an intravenous catheter site. Apply it so that no wrinkles form, but do not stretch it over the skin. Another option in some cases is to use it over another, smaller dressing (e.g., Telfa) cut to fit the area of the wound. Impregnated gauzes are more popular. Topical medications can be applied over nonadhesive transparent dressings without disturbing the dressing. Nonadhesive transparent dressings fall off as the wound heals. Saline solution can be used to moisten dressings that may be adhering or stuck to the wound bed. Showering and bathing are permitted with the health care provider's approval.

See Skill 22.3 for applying a transparent dressing.

IRRIGATIONS

Irrigation is gentle washing of an area with a stream of solution delivered through an irrigating syringe. The benefits of wound irrigation include cleansing and medication administration. Isotonic solutions are indicated for wound irrigation. Solutions for irrigation include topical cleansers, antibiotics, antifungals, antiseptics, and anesthetics. The most common wound irrigant is normal saline solution. Principles of basic wound irrigation include the following:

1. Cleanse in a direction from the least contaminated area to the most contaminated.
2. When irrigating, be sure all the solution flows from the least contaminated to the most contaminated area.

Wound irrigations promote wound healing by removing debris from the wound surface, decreasing bacterial counts, and loosening and removing eschar (a black, leathery crust). Nonsurgical indications include management of pressure injuries (see Chapter 9). Meticulous hand hygiene and proper infection control procedure before and after removal of soiled dressings, coupled with proper irrigation procedures, limit the risk of health care–associated infection. Perform basic wound cleansing by applying antiseptic solutions with sterile gauze or with irrigation. Skin cleansing in the area of the suture line or the drain site is indicated when an excessive amount of drainage occurs. The presence of wound exudate is an expected stage of epithelial cell growth.

When performing irrigation (Skill 22.4), be sure to provide for patient comfort; irrigation has potential to cause pain. Patients often must be medicated before the procedure is performed. Gentleness is important in performing any type of irrigation to prevent tissue damage and pain.

Wound irrigation may be performed with syringes, pressure canisters, whirlpool agitators, and hose sprayers. Guidelines from the Agency for Health Care Policy and Research (AHCPR) recommend pressures for irrigation that are 4 to 15 psi. Wound trauma and reintroduction of bacteria into the wound may result with pressures higher than 15 psi. Use sterile technique or clean technique for wound cleansing and irrigation. Introduce the cleansing solution directly into the wound with a syringe, syringe and catheter, shower, or whirlpool. When using a syringe, keep the tip 1 inch (2.5 cm) above the wound or area being cleansed. This prevents contamination of the syringe. Careful attention to placement of the syringe also prevents unsafe pressure of the

Skill 22.3 Applying a Transparent Dressing

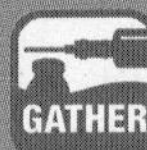

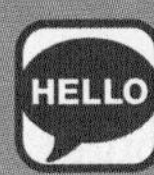

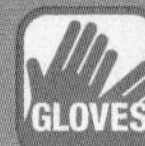

NURSING ACTION *(RATIONALE)*

1. See the section "Standard Steps in Wound Care," Steps 1 to 9.
2. Assemble equipment:
   - Clean disposable gloves
   - Sterile gloves (optional)
   - Sterile dressing set (scissors and forceps; optional)
   - Sterile saline solution or wound cleanser (as ordered)
   - Transparent dressings (size as needed and sterile 2 × 2 gauze pad)
   - Refuse container (waterproof bag)
3. Position refuse container within easy reach of work area. *(Helps prevent spread of microorganisms.)*
4. Don clean gloves. *(Protects you from patient's body fluids.)*
5. Remove old dressings by pulling back slowly across dressing in direction of hair growth and toward the center. *(Reduces excoriation, pain, and irritation of skin after dressing removal.)*
6. Remove disposable gloves by pulling them inside out over soiled dressings, and dispose of them in refuse container. *(Provides containment of soiled dressings and prevents contact of the hands with drainage.)*

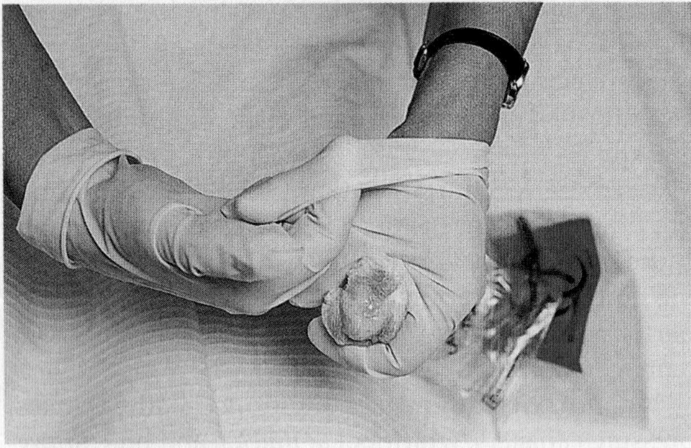

7. Inspect wound for color, odor, and drainage or exudates. Measure if indicated. *(Appearance indicates status of wound healing.)*
8. Clean area gently, swabbing toward area of most exudate, or spray with cleanser; know agency policy and physician's order. *(Reduces transmission from contaminated area to cleaner site.)*
9. Reapply sterile or clean gloves as indicated. *(Prevents risk of exposure to body fluids if present.)*
10. Dry skin around wound thoroughly with sterile gauze. Be sure skin surface is dry. *(Transparent dressings with adhesive backing do not adhere to damp surface.)*
11. Apply transparent dressing according to manufacturer's direction.
    a. Remove paper backing, taking care not to allow adhesive areas to touch each other. *(Often results in wrinkles and becomes impossible to use.)* NOTE: Chevrons of tape (wrapped around the needle head) are no longer widely used because the tape is not sterile and may cause infection.
    b. Place film smoothly over wound without stretching.

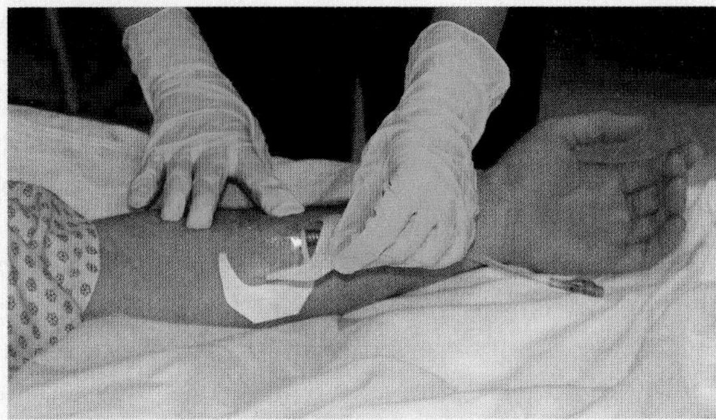

    c. Label with date, initials, and time, as agency policy requires. *(Communicates information to oncoming caregiver.)*

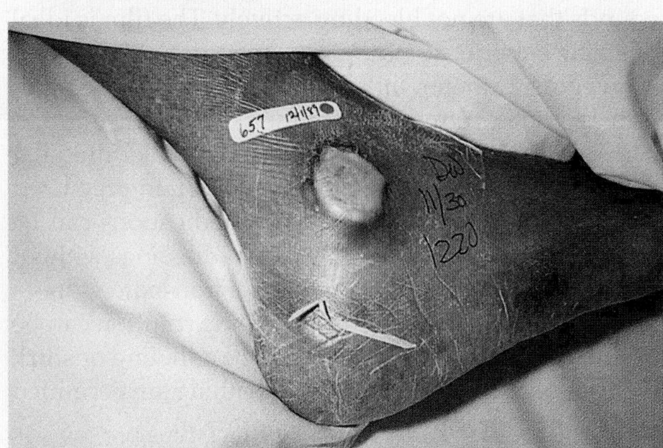

Skill 22.3 Applying a Transparent Dressing—cont'd

12. Remove gloves, discard them in refuse container, and wash hands. *(Prevents transmission of microorganisms.)*
13. See the section "Standard Steps in Wound Care," Steps 10 to 17.
14. Document: *(Records care given and progress of wound.)*
    - Wound status
    - Description of exudate or drainage
    - Dressing applied
    - Patient's response to procedure
    - Patient teaching
15. Report any unexpected appearance of the wound or exudates. *(Further treatment may be necessary.)*

Step 6 from Potter PA, Perry AG, Stockert P, et al: *Fundamentals of nursing: Concepts, process, and practice*, ed 8, St. Louis, 2013, Mosby; Step 11c from Potter PA, Perry AG, Stockert P, et al: *Fundamentals of nursing: Concepts, process, and practice*, ed 9, St. Louis, 2016, Mosby.

Skill 22.4 Performing a Sterile Irrigation

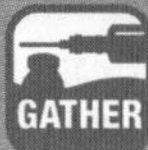

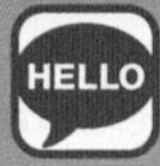

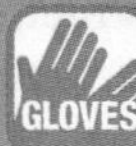

NURSING ACTION *(RATIONALE)*

1. See the section "Standard Steps in Wound Care," Steps 1 to 9.
2. Assemble equipment:
    - Refuse container
    - Clean gloves
    - Sterile gloves
    - Dressing set
    - Antiseptic swabs
    - Sterile basin
    - Warmed, sterile irrigation solution (200 to 1000 mL)
    - Irrigation syringe or spray bottle or soft catheter for deep wounds
    - Clean basin
    - Waterproof pad
    - Sterile dressings
    - Gown and goggles (optional)
    - Tape, gauze, and elastic bandage, if appropriate
    - Mask (optional)
3. Position waterproof pad appropriately. *(Protects patient and bed linens from contaminated fluids.)*
4. Place refuse container in convenient location away from sterile field. *(Prevents need to reach across sterile field and thus prevents contamination.)*
5. Set up sterile field. *(Maintains asepsis during procedure and organizes approach to procedure.)*
    a. Set up sterile basin.
    b. Add sterile, warmed irrigation solution to basin.
    c. Add antiseptic swabs.
    d. Open sterile gloves.
    e. Add dressing set (optional).
    f. Add sterile syringe and catheter if necessary.
    g. Add disposable measuring device.
6. Don gown and goggles if potential for splashing exists. *(Provides protection from body fluids.)*
7. Don clean gloves and remove dressing. Discard dressing in refuse container. *(Provides protection from pathogens and prevents wound contamination from soiled dressing.)*
8. Remove gloves, discard into proper receptacle, and wash hands. *(Reduces transmission of microorganisms.)*
9. Assess status of wound and exudate or drainage on dressing (see Table 22.2). *(Provides evaluation of healing process and collection of data for accurate documentation.)*
10. Place collection basin appropriately. *(Collects contaminated solution.)*

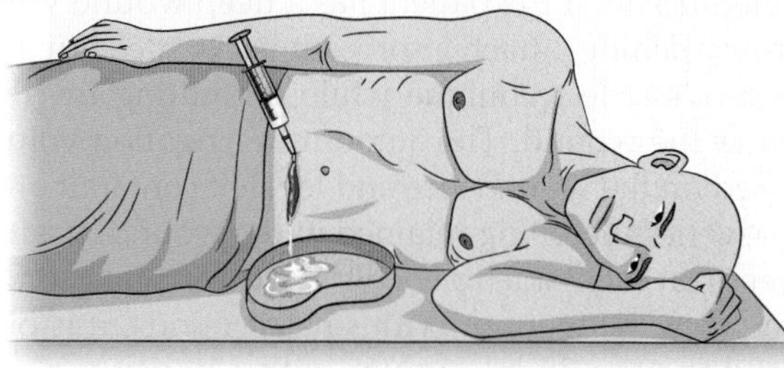

11. Perform hand hygiene and don sterile gloves. *(Maintains asepsis.)*
12. Cleanse area around wound with antiseptic swabs. *(Removes bacteria and drainage.)*
13. Fill irrigating syringe with solution. Attach soft catheter if irrigating a deep wound with small opening. *(Allows for direct flow of solution into wound.)* Use a 19-gauge needle (or angiocatheter) with a 35-mL syringe to clean most pressure ulcers, especially deep ulcers.

Continued

Skill 22.4 Performing a Sterile Irrigation—cont'd

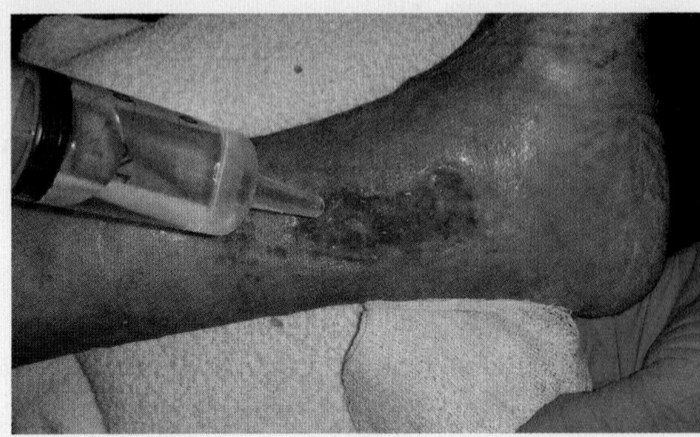

14. Instill solution gently into wound, holding syringe approximately 1 inch (2.54 cm) above wound. If using catheter, gently insert into wound opening until slight resistance is met, pull back, and gently instill solution. *(Minimizes tissue trauma, irritation, and bleeding.)*

15. Allow solution to flow from clean area of wound to dirty area. Position patient to facilitate drainage. *(Prevents contamination of clean tissue by exudate.)*

16. Pinch off catheter during withdrawal from wound. *(Avoids aspiration of contaminating fluid into syringe.)*

17. Refill syringe and continue irrigation until solution returns clear. *(Thoroughly cleanses wound.)*

18. Blot wound edges with sterile gauze. *(Prevents tissue damage from excess moisture.)*

19. Dress wound again, if applicable. *(Protects wound from injury and microorganisms and provides for patient comfort.)*

20. See the section "Standard Steps in Wound Care," Steps 10 to 17.

21. Document: *(Records care given and progress of wound.)*
- Status of wound
- Performance of wound irrigation
- Solution used
- Character of exudate and drainage
- Patient's response to procedure
- Patient teaching (see the Patient Teaching box)

22. Report immediately to the health care provider any evidence of fresh bleeding, sharp increase in pain, retention of irrigant, or signs of shock. *(These are signs of tissue damage and fistula or sinus tract development. Shock phenomena sometimes indicate internal bleeding or tissue damage.)*

flowing solution. Ensure that the flow of irrigant moves from the area being cleansed to an area that is distal to and lower than the wound area. In wound care, the area being cleansed is considered clean, and the surrounding skin surfaces are considered contaminated without respect to whether the wound is infected. Within the wound, direct the flow from healthy tissue toward infected tissue. If the patient has a deep wound with a narrow opening, attach a soft catheter to the syringe to maintain sterile technique while permitting the fluid to enter the wound. The amount of irrigation volume is based on the wound size and level of contamination. To prevent fluid being retained in the wound, position patients on their side to encourage the irrigant to flow away from the wound. With small wounds, it is often helpful to use a 35-mL syringe with a 19-gauge needle attached to obtain optimal pressure for cleansing with minimal risk of tissue injury.

Ambulatory or home patients are sometimes able to avail themselves of a handheld shower for wound cleansing, holding the shower spray approximately 12 inches (30.48 cm) from the wound. If the force of the spray results in too much pressure for comfort, suggest that the patient tie a clean washcloth around the shower head to disperse the force. During the procedure, protect the surrounding area and assisting care providers from splashing from the wound. An alternative means of irrigating wounds in acute care areas is the shower table, frequently used for cleansing in burn and trauma wound care units. For patients who need cleansing but cannot tolerate the methods mentioned earlier, the whirlpool is useful. Physical therapists often perform or assist with performing the whirlpool procedure and then help apply dressings.

COMPLICATIONS OF WOUND HEALING

Impaired wound healing, regardless of the cause, requires accurate observation and ongoing interventions. Because wound complications are potentially life threatening, it is vital throughout the patient's recovery phase to monitor signs and symptoms and assess their severity (Table 22.3).

Wound bleeding potentially indicates a slipped suture, dislodged clot, coagulation problem, or trauma to blood vessels or tissue. To help detect increased drainage and color changes, inspect the wound and dressing. The dressing should be marked with the time and initials of the nurse making the observation. Initial surgical dressings may require reinforcement if they become soiled. If hemorrhage results internally, the dressing sometimes remains dry while the abdominal cavity collects blood. Be attuned to the less obvious signs of internal bleeding, including restlessness; rapid, thready pulse; decreased blood pressure; decreased urinary output; and cool, clammy skin. Monitoring vital signs,

Table 22.3 Terms Associated With Wound Complications

TERM	DEFINITION
Abscess	Cavity that contains pus and is surrounded by inflamed tissue, formed as a result of suppuration in a localized infection
Adhesion	Band of scar tissue that binds two anatomic surfaces normally separated; most commonly found in the abdomen
Cellulitis	Infection of the skin characterized by heat, pain, erythema, and edema
Dehiscence	Separation of a surgical incision or rupture of a wound closure
Evisceration	Protrusion of an internal organ through a wound or surgical incision
Extravasation	Passage or escape into the tissues; usually of blood, serum, or lymph
Hematoma	Collection of extravasated blood trapped in the tissues or in an organ that results from incomplete hemostasis after surgery or injury

intake and output (I&O), skin condition, wound site, and overall patient response facilitates the timely identification of hemorrhage and hypovolemic shock. Internal abdominal bleeding, if allowed to continue, causes the abdomen to become rigid and distended. If hemorrhage is not detected and stopped, hypovolemic shock possibly causes the circulatory system to collapse, causing death.

When wound layers separate, resulting in dehiscence, some patients report that something has given way (refer to *Adult Health Nursing*, Chapter 2). Sometimes this feeling is brought on by periods of sneezing, coughing, or vomiting. Evidence of serosanguineous drainage on the dressing is an important sign to assess because dehiscence sometimes is preceded by serosanguineous drainage. If the wound is not covered and dehiscence occurs, the patient remains in bed and receives nothing by mouth (NPO). Tell the patient not to cough; place a warm, moist sterile dressing over the area until the physician evaluates the site; and provide reassurance. When a skin suture breaks and dehiscence occurs, the wound may be closed effectively with Steri-Strips or a butterfly strip. Dehiscence most frequently occurs between postoperative days 5 and 12. Because most patients have been dismissed from the hospital by day 12, include in patient teaching how to recognize dehiscence and what care to provide.

If an evisceration (when internal organs protrude through opened incision) follows the dehiscence, the patient is to remain in bed in a low Fowler's position, with the knees flexed to reduce pressure on the wound. Keep the patient on NPO status, and cover the wound and contents with warm, sterile saline solution dressings.

Box 22.3 Responding to Wound Evisceration

If a patient's wound eviscerates, prompt action is needed to reduce further complications.

1. Remain with the patient and either notify the health care provider or ask a coworker to notify the health care provider. Wound evisceration is considered a medical emergency.
2. Place the patient into a low Fowler's position with the knees slightly flexed. This position helps relieve pressure on the wound. This will prevent further dehiscence of the wound edges and reduces the risk of further evisceration.
3. The protruding organ is covered with a sterile dressing moistened with sterile normal saline solution. This keeps the eviscerated organ moist and helps prevent microorganisms from entering the wound.
4. Monitor the patient closely and assess vital signs and pulse oximetry readings to determine if the patient is exhibiting signs of shock.
5. Make sure the patient remains NPO (nothing by mouth), because the patient will need surgical correction of the evisceration.
6. Reassure the patient and family, because the occurrence of a wound evisceration is often frightening.

Modified from Harkreader H, Hogan MA, Thobaben M: *Fundamentals of nursing*, ed 3, Philadelphia, 2007, Saunders.

Notify the surgeon immediately (Box 22.3). Provide emotional support and explain to the patient what has happened and what can be expected in the next phase of care.

Wound infection, or wound sepsis, results when the wound becomes contaminated. The CDC labels a wound infected when it contains purulent (pus) drainage. A patient with an infected wound displays a fever, tenderness and pain at the wound site, edema, and an elevated WBC count. Purulent drainage has an odor and is brown, yellow, or green, depending on the pathogen. Culture of the exudate from an infected wound confirms the presence of the pathogenic organism, then the appropriate medical therapy is ordered (see Chapter 23).

STAPLE AND SUTURE REMOVAL

Institutional policy determines whether only the health care provider or the health care provider and the nurse may remove sutures and staples. Always obtain the health care provider's written order before implementing either skill. The time of removal is based on the stage of incisional healing and the extent of surgery.

Sutures and staples generally are removed in 7 to 10 days after surgery, or sooner, if healing is adequate. Sometimes one suture or staple comes out at a time, and sometimes removal is in two phases. First, every other suture or staple is removed and replaced with a Steri-Strip, then the remaining sutures or staples are removed

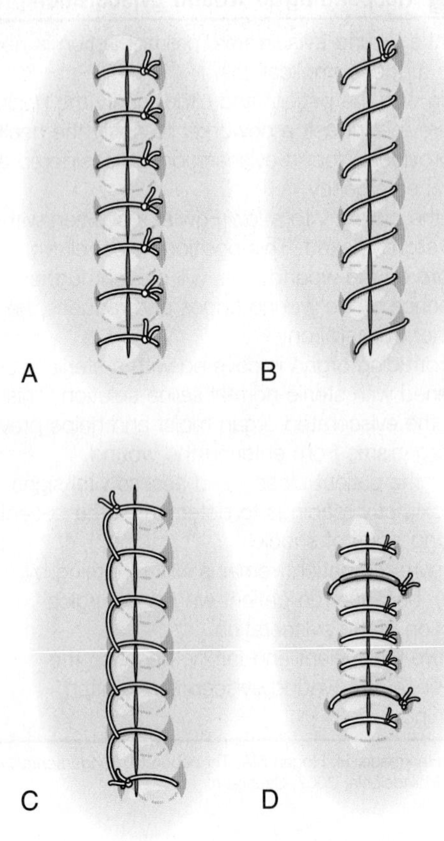

Fig. 22.5 Sutures. A, Interrupted, or separate, sutures. B, Continuous suture. C, Blanket continuous suture. D, Retention suture covered with rubber tubing to provide greater strength.

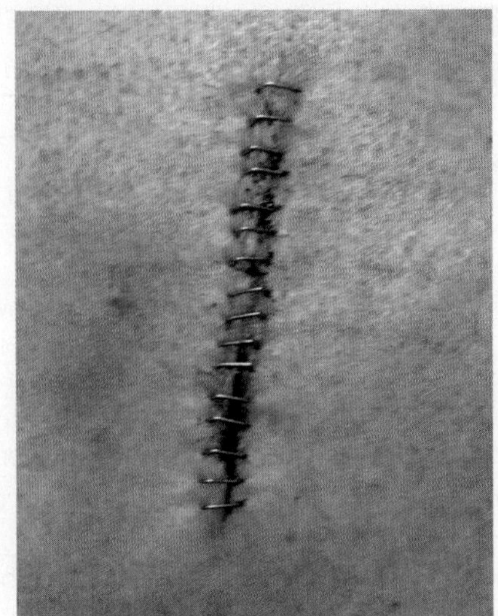

Fig. 22.6 Wound closure with staples.

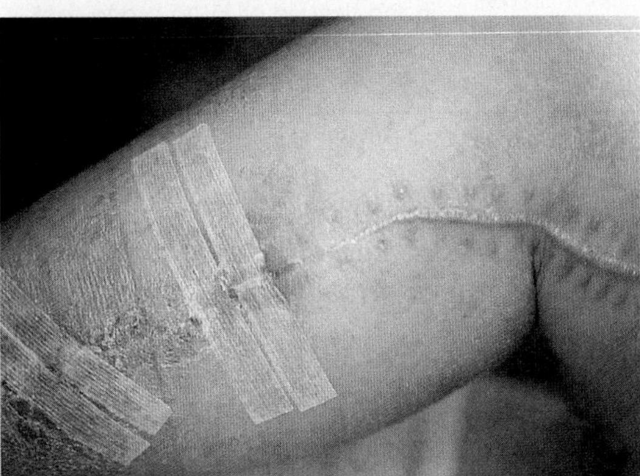

Fig. 22.7 Steri-Strips placed over incision for closure. (From Potter PA, Perry AG: *Essentials for nursing practice*, ed 8, St. Louis, 2015, Mosby.)

in the same fashion. The health care provider determines the timing and method and orders the removal.

Sutures are threads of wire or other material (silk, steel, cotton, linen, or nylon) used to sew body tissues together. Sutures are placed within tissue layers in deep wounds and superficially as the final means for wound closure. The deeper sutures usually are made of an absorbable material that disappears in several days. Many kinds of sutures are used: interrupted or separate sutures, continuous sutures, blanket sutures, and retention sutures covered with rubber tubing to provide greater strength (used primarily in obese patients who have had abdominal surgery). The cosmetic result of these latter sutures is often not as desirable as that obtained with finer suture material (Fig. 22.5).

Staples are made of stainless steel wire, are quick to use, and provide ample strength. They are popular for skin closure of abdominal incisions and orthopedic surgery when appearance of the incision is not critical (Fig. 22.6). The time of removal is based on the stage of incisional healing and the extent of surgery. Sutures and staples generally are removed within 7 to 10 days after surgery if healing is adequate. Retention sutures are left in place longer (22 days or more). Leaving sutures in too long makes removal more difficult and increases the risk of infection. Removal of staples requires a sterile staple extractor and maintenance of aseptic technique (Skill 22.5). After the suture removal is complete, inspect the area to ensure all the sutures or staples have been removed.

Remove every other suture or staple first and replace each with an adhesive closure strip (Fig. 22.7); if the incision remains securely closed, remove the rest with the same process. If any sign of suture line separation is evident during the removal process, leave the remaining sutures in place, document a description, and report it to the health care provider. In some cases, these sutures are left in place and removed several days to a week later.

The patient's history of wound healing, the site of the wound, the tissues involved, and the purpose of the sutures determine the selection of the suture material. For example, a patient with repeated abdominal surgeries often needs wire sutures for greater strength to promote wound closure.

Skill 22.5 Removing Staples or Sutures (Applying Steri-Strips)

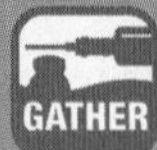

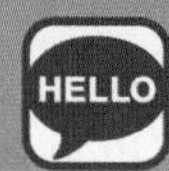

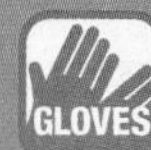

NURSING ACTION *(RATIONALE)*

1. See the section "Standard Steps in Wound Care," Steps 1 to 9.
2. Assemble equipment:
   - Refuse container
   - Clean gloves
   - Sterile gloves (optional)
   - Sterile sutures or staple removal set
   - Antiseptic swabs
   - Appropriate sterile dressings, including butterfly or adhesive Steri-Strips
   - Compound benzoin tincture or other skin protectant such as Skin Prep
3. Place refuse container in convenient location away from sterile field. *(Prevents need to reach across sterile field and thus prevents contamination.)*
4. Set up sterile field. *(Maintains asepsis during procedure and organizes approach to procedure.)*
   a. Open suture or staple set.
   b. Open sterile dressings (use sterile barrier if necessary for sterile field).
5. Remove dressing and soiled gloves. Discard into plastic refuse bag. (Use bag as needed for additional refuse.) *(Protects you from microorganisms and prevents contamination from soiled dressing.)*
6. Assess status of wound and drainage on dressing. *(Allows determination of alterations in healing process and collection of data for accurate documentation.)*
7. Perform hand hygiene and don sterile gloves. *(Allows for safe handling of sterile equipment.)*
8. Cleanse area with antiseptic swabs, starting from incision outward, using one stroke per swab. *(Removes bacteria from wound area.)*

STAPLE REMOVAL

On removal of sutures, the health care provider removes one to three sutures at a time and applies Steri-Strips in their place. This action is repeated until all sutures are removed and Steri-Strips applied.

9. Prepare patient for pulling sensation and site tenderness during removal. Place staple remover under staple while slowly closing the ends of the staple remover together. Squeeze the center of the staple with the tips, freeing the staple from the skin. *(Prevents putting excess pressure on suture line and secures removal of each staple.)*

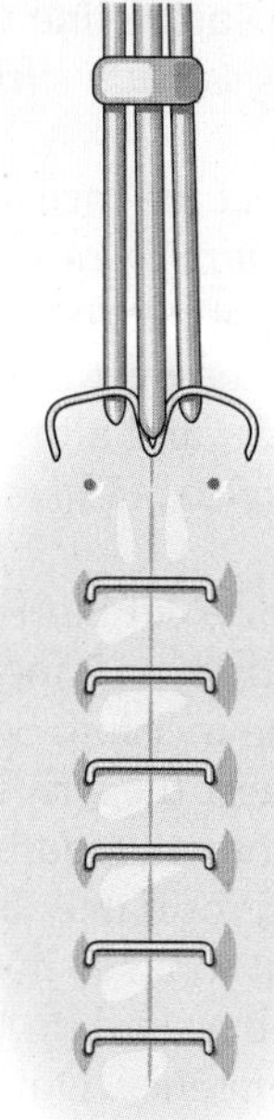

10. Release handles and discard staple in refuse container. *(Prevents contamination of sterile field with used staple.)*
11. Repeat Steps 9 and 10 until all staples have been removed. *(Permits complete removal of all staples.)* Every other staple may be removed and Steri-Strips applied, or two or three staples removed at a time and Steri-Strips applied until all staples have been removed and Steri-Strips applied.
12. Count number of staples removed. *(Provides count for documentation.)*

SPECIAL CONSIDERATIONS FOR SUTURE AND STAPLE REMOVAL

- Wire sutures are removed by the nurse or primary care provider.
- Limit amount of dressing supplies, because either a light dressing or no dressing is needed after suture or staple removal.
- Notify health care provider immediately if inadequate wound healing is noted; discontinue removal of staples.
- It is common to see wounds closed with Steri-Strips, or sterile tape applied along both sides of a wound to keep the edges approximated and closed (see Fig. 22.7).

Continued

Skill 22.5 Removing Staples or Sutures (Applying Steri-Strips)—cont'd

INTERVENTIONS TO FOLLOW WHEN APPLYING STERI-STRIPS

13. Prepare incision for Steri-Strip application.
  a. Gently cleanse suture line with antiseptic swab. *(Removes as much surface bacteria as possible.)*
  b. Carefully inspect the incision. *(Ensures that all sutures have been removed.)*
  c. Apply tincture of benzoin to the skin on each side of suture line over an area 1½ to 2 inches (4 to 5 cm) wide, and allow to dry a few minutes until tacky. *(Makes Steri-Strips adhere more securely.)*
  d. When skin is dry, cut Steri-Strips to allow strips to extend 1½ to 2 inches (4 to 5 cm) on each side of the incision. Some health care providers request the strips be placed side by side, whereas others request they be spaced evenly and appropriately apart (see Fig. 22.6).
  e. Instruct patient to take showers rather than soak in bathtub according to health care provider's preference. During showering, the patient should be advised to engage in positions that limit direct contact by the water spray with the Steri-Strips. Steri-Strips are not removed and are allowed to loosen and peel off gradually over the course of 3 to 5 days. Strip edges that begin to peel away from the skin may be clipped off.

14. Assess healing status of wound. *(Determines need for butterfly or Steri-Strip skin closures.)*
  a. Cleanse area with antiseptic swabs. *(Decreases the risk of infection.)*

REMOVAL OF INTERRUPTED SUTURES
(see Fig. 22.5A)

15. Each suture has a knot. Each interrupted suture is secured with its own knot. Knots are lined up on the same side of incision.

16. Grasp and elevate knotted end of suture with hemostat or forceps. *(Exposes the knot and ensures removal of suture and maintains skin integrity.)*

17. Snip suture at skin level on opposite side, proximal to knot. *(Releases suture.)*

18. Gently remove entire suture with forceps and discard on sterile gauze. *(Prevents contaminating sterile field with used materials.)*

19. Repeat Steps 16 to 18 until all sutures have been removed. *(Ensures removal of all sutures.)*

REMOVAL OF CONTINUOUS SUTURES
(see Fig. 22.5)

20. To remove continuous sutures:
  a. Snip suture close to skin surface at end distal to knot.
  b. Snip second suture on same side.
  c. Grasp knot and gently pull with continuous smooth action, removing suture from beneath the skin. Place suture on gauze.
  d. Grasp and lift next suture, and snip with tip of scissors close to skin.
  e. Grasp suture and gently remove loop of suture. Never pull the contaminated suture through tissue.
  f. Repeat these steps until the end knot is reached. Cut the last one and remove it by grasping and pulling the knot.

REMOVAL OF BLANKET CONTINUOUS SUTURE
(see Fig. 22.5C)

21. To remove blanket continuous sutures:
  a. Cut the suture opposite the looped blanket edge.
  b. Remove each suture by grasping at the looped end.

22. Apply sterile dressing or leave open to air as ordered. (Dressing is often needed only if patient's clothing will irritate wound area.) *(Protects wound and facilitates healing process.)*

23. See the section "Standard Steps in Wound Care," Steps 10 to 17.

24. Document: *(Records care given and progress of wound.)*
- Number of staples or sutures removed
- Condition of staple or suture line
- Patient's response
- Dressings applied, if necessary
- Patient teaching (see the Patient Teaching box)

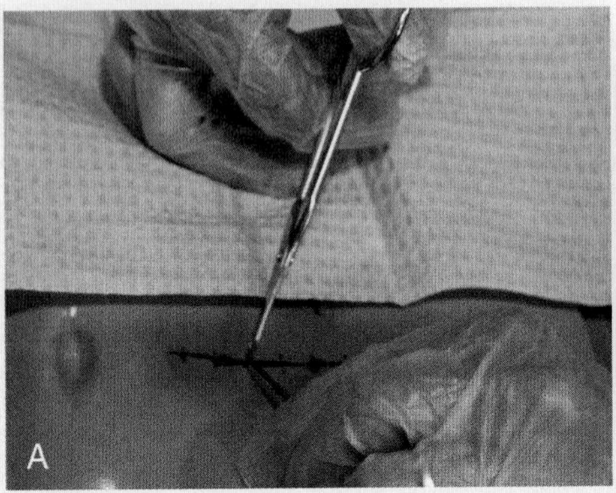

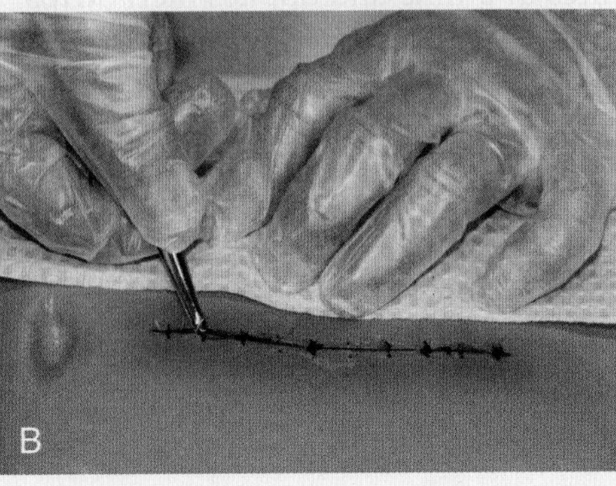

EXUDATE AND DRAINAGE

Exudate is fluid, cells, or other substances that have leaked slowly from cells or blood vessels through small pores or breaks in cell membrane. **Drainage** is the removal of fluids from a body cavity, wound, or other source of discharge by one or more methods; it may occur passively on its own or with mechanical assistance (see the section "Drainage Systems").

Exudate and drainage are described as serous, sanguineous, or serosanguineous. Serous exudate or drainage is a clear, watery fluid that has been separated from its solid elements (e.g., the exudate from a blister). Serous fluid has the characteristics of serum. Serum is the clear, thin, sticky fluid portion of blood that remains after coagulation. In contrast, sanguineous exudate or drainage is fluid that contains blood. Thus serosanguineous exudate or drainage is thin and red (usually described as pink), because it is composed of serum and blood. If the tissue is infected, exudate or drainage is likely to be purulent or brown-green. Exudate or drainage from specific organs has its own color (e.g., bile from the liver and gallbladder is green or green-brown).

The type and the amount of exudate or drainage produced depend on the tissue and organs involved. Treat exudate or drainage in quantities greater than 300 mL in the first 24 hours as abnormal, and report it immediately. When patients first ambulate, a slight increase of exudate or drainage sometimes occurs. If sanguineous exudate or drainage continues, small blood vessels possibly may be oozing.

Not all surgical wounds drain. If exudate or drainage does occur, accurate assessments are vital. The following exudate and drainage characteristics are important to note and chart: color, amount, consistency (thick or thin), and odor. If the exudate or drainage has a pungent or strong odor, infection is likely. Perform a wound culture (see Chapter 23). Exudate most likely is contained either in a drainage system or on a dressing. If a dressing is used, you can monitor the amount of exudate or drainage (such as from a Penrose drain) by weighing the soiled dressing (1 g of exudate or drainage equals 1 mL), by circling and dating the drainage area and comparing the circled area with later observations, or by reporting the number and the type of dressings used and saturated over a specific interval. Until the surgeon orders a dressing change, never remove the soiled dressings, only reinforce them.

DRAINAGE SYSTEMS

Frequently, surgical procedures are performed to remove or repair organs that lie within the body (e.g., gallbladder removal). In these cases, a mechanism is needed to assist gravity in removal of exudate from the cavity. If a gastrectomy is performed with an upper abdominal midline incision, fluid collects and remains at the surgical site. To facilitate drainage, the surgeon makes a secondary incision, or stab wound, close to the surgical incision. The site for the stab wound is planned deliberately. The surgeon's intent is to drain exudate away from the incision, not toward it. If the exudate enters the surgical incision, contamination and infection are likely to follow.

Several methods are available to facilitate the flow of exudate away from the wound site. *Closed drainage* is a system of tubing or other apparatus attached to the body to remove fluid in an airtight circuit that prevents environmental contaminants from entering the wound or cavity. *Open drainage* passes through an open-ended tube into a receptacle or out onto the dressing. *Suction drainage* uses a pump or other mechanical device to help extract a fluid (Skill 22.6).

Gentle suction is needed in some surgeries to help gravity move the exudate. A drainage system is chosen to fit the area to be drained and according to the type of exudate and amount of drainage expected. A rubber or plastic drain sometimes is used to remove exudate from the wound and bring it out through the skin onto a dressing (open drainage system); sometimes it is positioned through the surgical incision or stab wound. The Penrose drain commonly serves this purpose. When it is inserted, a sterile safety pin is placed through the drain to keep it from sliding into the wound. When the surgeon wants a gentle vacuum, a closed drainage system can be used. The portable vacuum container (e.g., Hemovac) is an expandable unit connected by tubes to the drainage site (see Skill 22.6). As the unit creates gentle suction, exudate collects in the drainage receptacle. The Jackson-Pratt evacuator is another type of closed drainage system that uses a bulb to provide the needed vacuum (Figs. 22.8 and 22.9).

T-Tube Drainage System

After surgical removal of the gallbladder (an open cholecystectomy), the bile duct often is inflamed and edematous. The health care provider frequently inserts a drainage tube into the duct to maintain a free flow of bile until edema subsides. This tube is called a **T tube.** The long end of the T tube exits through the abdominal incision or through a separate surgical wound (Fig. 22.10). The tube drains by gravity into a closed drainage system. The collection bag is emptied and measured every shift or as necessary (Box 22.4).

Wound Vacuum-Assisted Closure

Negative-pressure wound therapy may be beneficial in the management of some surgical wounds. The treatment uses a machine commonly referred to as a **vacuum-assisted closure** device (wound VAC). The wound VAC functions by applying negative pressure to wounds. Healing of the wound is facilitated by increased blood flow, improved or increased fluid drainage, and enhanced wound closure as the pressure draws the edges of the wound together. VAC accelerates wound healing by promoting the formation of granulation tissue, collagen, fibroblasts, and inflammatory cells to close

Skill 22.6 Maintaining Hemovac or Davol Suction and T-Tube Drainage

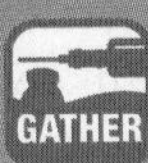

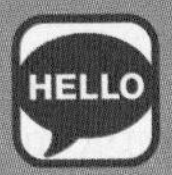

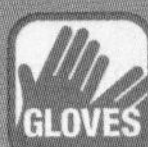

NURSING ACTION *(RATIONALE)*

1. See the section "Standard Steps in Wound Care," Steps 1 to 9.
2. Assemble equipment:
   - Clean gloves
   - Alcohol pads
   - Swabs
   - Calibrated drainage receptacle
   - Moisture-proof padding (optional)
3. Examine drainage system (pump and tubing) for seal, patency, and stability (see Figs. 22.8 and 22.9). If not working, notify head nurse or health care provider. *(Maintains efficiency of system.)*
4. Don goggles, if appropriate. *(Protects eyes from contaminants.)*
5. Remove Hemovac or Davol plug labeled "pouring spout." *(Permits accurate measuring of drainage.)*
   a. Empty drainage into measuring device.
   b. When emptying Hemovac, compress device by pushing top and bottom together with your hands.
6. Hold pump of Hemovac tightly compressed and reinsert plug to reestablish closed drainage system. When caring for a Davol, reestablish suction by pumping bulb until balloon is inflated completely. Recap drainage port. For Hemovac and Davol, keep plug out of drainage stream; hold the plug by stem. *(Maintains unit sterility.)*

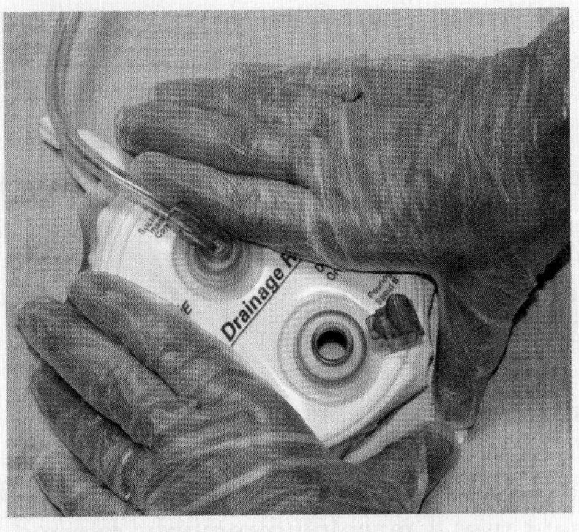

7. Observe the drainage for color, consistency, and odor. *(Provides basis for documentation.)*
8. Measure and record amount of drainage; rinse measuring container. *(Provides basis for documentation.)*
9. Position drainage system on bed, and secure system. *(Maintains efficiency of system.)*
10. Dispose of drainage and rinse container. Remove gloves and wash hands. *(Reduces spread of microorganisms.)*
11. If specimen is ordered, send to laboratory. (If dressing change is necessary, do it at this time.) *(Provides continuity of care.)*
12. Observe Davol or Hemovac every 2 to 4 hours. *(Ascertains integrity of suction.)* Measure drainage every 8 hours or as ordered. *(Recording an accurate output of drainage is necessary so that the health care provider can determine any change in the amount or the character of wound drainage.)*
13. See the section "Standard Steps in Wound Care," Steps 10 to 17.
14. Document: *(Records care given and progress of wound.)*
    - Time of procedure
    - Amount of drainage
    - Characteristics of drainage
    - Patient response
    - Suction reestablished
    - Patient teaching (see the Patient Teaching box)
15. Report any abnormal characteristics of drainage (see Table 22.2).

A drainage system requires close monitoring. In addition to noting the color, the consistency, and the amount of drainage, check the tube's patency. Do not allow a tube to become kinked or occluded; if blood clots or exudate have slowed drainage, record this and report it.

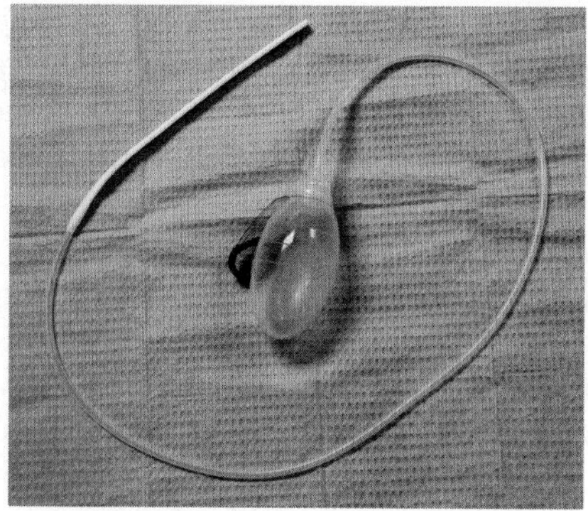

Fig. 22.8 Jackson-Pratt drains have wide, flat areas that must be brought through the stab wound with great force.

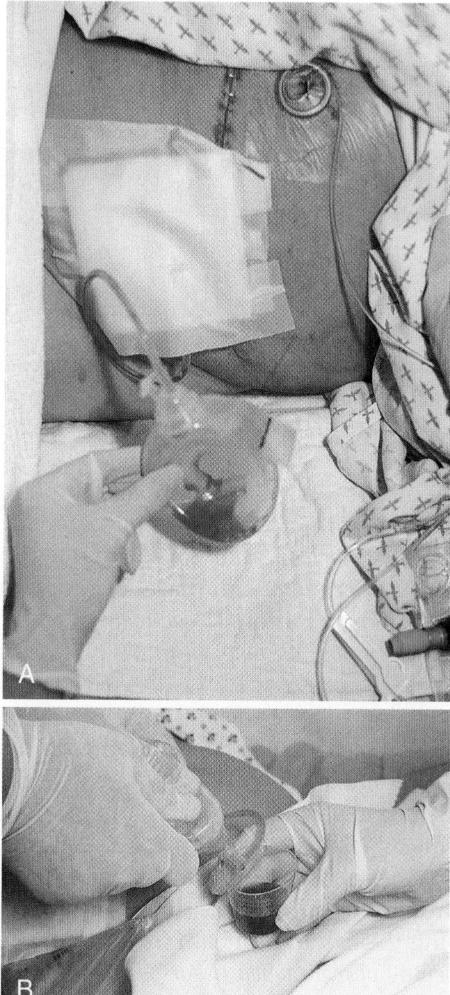

Fig. 22.9 Jackson-Pratt drainage device. A, Drainage tubes and reservoir. B, Emptying drainage reservoir. (From Perry AG, Potter PA, Ostendorf W, et al: *Clinical nursing skills and techniques*, ed 9, St. Louis, 2018, Elsevier.)

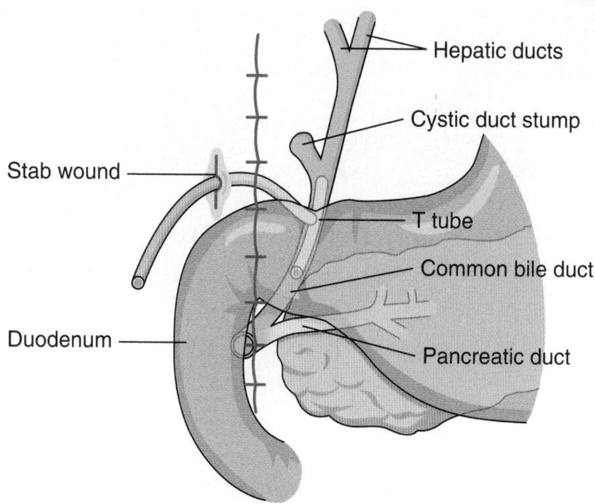

Fig. 22.10 T tube. (From Beare PG, Myers JL: *Adult health nursing*, ed 3, St. Louis, 1998, Mosby.)

Box 22.4 Care of the T-Tube Drainage System

Nursing interventions for the patient with bile drainage include the following:

- Make sure specific measures or techniques for dressing change are in the nursing care plan to provide continuity of care.
- Assess the patency of the drainage tube frequently, preventing twists or kinks to ensure appropriate, continuous drainage.
- Keep the collection receptacle below the level of the wound or common bile duct to ensure appropriate drainage.
- Keep the receptacle compressed, and frequently monitor it to maintain a vacuum. (Many T-tube drainage systems use drainage by gravity only.)
- Protect the skin surrounding the wound from bile drainage to prevent tissue damage.
- Assess excessive bile leakage from the wound because it may indicate occlusion of drainage tube.
- Assess for normal bile drainage: amount varies from 250 to 500 mL/24 h, with color normally greenish brown, thick, and slightly blood tinged in the first 24 hours.
- Consider the use of Montgomery straps when the dressing requires frequent changing, to prevent tape from impairing skin integrity (see Box 22.1 and Skill 22.1, Step 14).
- Assess the need for patient teaching during the dressing change and wound care.
- Secure the vacuum unit to the patient's gown with a safety pin, avoiding tension on the tubing.
- Record the amount of drainage on the intake and output (I&O) sheet to provide an accurate I&O record.

completely or improve the condition of a wound in preparation for a skin graft. The use of negative pressure removes fluid from the area surrounding the wound, thus reducing local or peripheral edema and improving circulation to the area (Fig. 22.11). In addition, after 3 or 4 days of therapy, bacterial counts in the wound drop.

Wound VAC is used to treat acute wounds (such as traumatic wounds, flaps, and grafts) and chronic wounds. The schedule for changing wound VAC dressings varies. An infected wound sometimes calls for a dressing change every 24 hours, whereas dressing changes three times a week suffice for a clean wound.

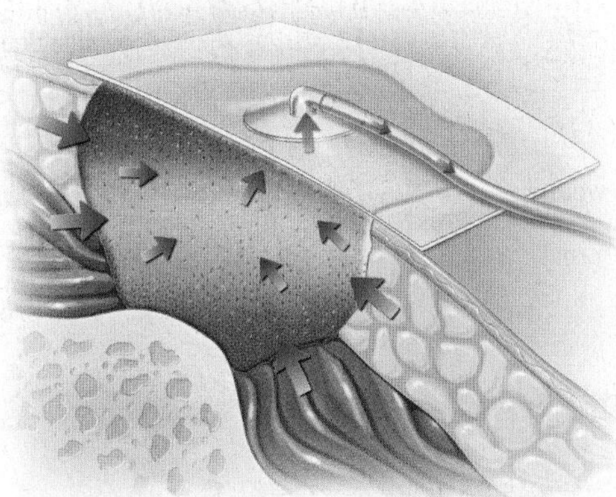

Fig. 22.11 Wound VAC system uses negative pressure to remove fluid from area surrounding the wound, reducing edema and improving circulation to the area. (Courtesy Kinetic Concepts, Inc. [KCI], San Antonio, Texas.)

During dressing changes, care must be taken to remove all sponges and remnants. Retained materials left on the wound may cause delays in healing and abscess formation. As the wound heals, the wound base becomes redder and granulation tissue lines its surface. The wound has a granulated appearance. Last, the surface area of the wound changes size, either increasing or decreasing depending on wound location and the amount of drainage removed by the wound VAC system. As the wound heals, paler areas in the wound often develop. This indicates an increase in fibrous tissue. The wound has to be assessed for location, appearance, and size. This provides information regarding status of wound healing, presence of complications, and the proper type of supplies and assistance needed to apply the new transparent dressing (Skill 22.7).

Skill 22.7 Wound Vacuum-Assisted Closure

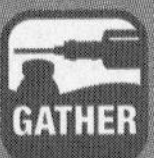

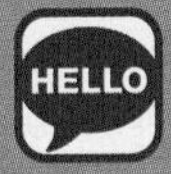

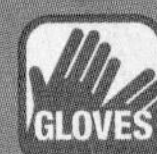

NURSING ACTION *(RATIONALE)*

1. See the section "Standard Steps in Wound Care," Steps 1 to 9.
2. Assemble equipment:
   - VAC system (requires health care provider's order)
   - VAC foam dressing
   - Tubing for connection between VAC system and VAC dressing
   - Gloves, clean and sterile
   - Scissors (sterile)
   - SKIN-PREP or skin barrier
   - Moist washcloth
   - Plastic or waterproof refuse bag
   - Linen bag

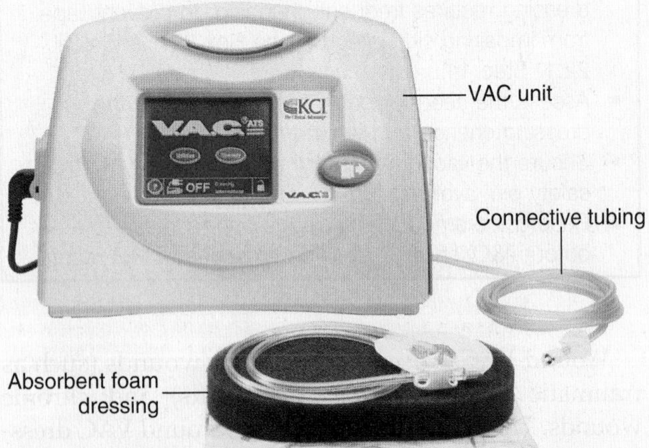

3. Position patient comfortably and drape to expose only wound site. Instruct patient not to touch wound or sterile supplies. *(Maintaining patient comfort assists in completing skill smoothly. Draping provides access to wound while keeping exposure to a minimum.)*
4. Place disposable waterproof bag within reach of work area with top folded to make a cuff. *(Facilitates safe disposal of soiled dressings.)*
5. When VAC system is in place, begin by pushing therapy on-off button. *(Deactivates therapy and allows for proper drainage of fluid in drainage tubing.)*
   a. Keeping tube connected to VAC system, disconnect tubes from each other to drain fluids into canister.
   b. Before lowering, tighten clamp on canister tube.
6. With dressing tube unclamped, introduce 10 to 30 mL of normal saline solution, if ordered, into tubing to soak underneath foam. *(Facilitates loosening of foam when tissue adheres to foam.)*
7. Gently stretch transparent film horizontally and slowly pull up from the skin. *(Reduces stress on wound edges and reduces irritation and discomfort.)*
8. Remove old VAC system dressing, observing appearance and drainage on dressing. Use caution to prevent tension on any drains that are present. Discard dressing and remove gloves. Perform hand hygiene. *(Determines dressings needed for replacement. Prevents accidental removal of drains that are sometimes sutured in place and sometimes not.)*

Skill 22.7 Wound Vacuum-Assisted Closure—cont'd

9. Apply sterile or clean gloves. Irrigate the wound (see Skill 22.4) with normal saline solution or other solution ordered by the health care provider. Gently blot to dry. (If this is a new surgical wound, sterile technique may be ordered. Chronic wounds often require clean technique.) *(Irrigation removes wound debris.)*

10. Measure wound as ordered: at baseline, at first dressing change, weekly, and at discharge from therapy. Remove and discard gloves. (Wound cultures sometimes are ordered on a routine basis. However, when drainage looks purulent, change is seen in amount or color, or drainage has a foul odor, obtain wound cultures even when they are not scheduled for that dressing change.) *(Objectively documents wound healing process in response to negative-pressure wound therapy.)*

11. Depending on the type of wound, apply sterile gloves or new clean gloves. *(Fresh sterile wounds require sterile gloves. Chronic wounds often require clean technique.)* Do not use the same gloves worn to remove old dressing. *(Cross-contamination is a possible result.)*

12. Prepare VAC foam.

a. Select appropriate foam.

b. With sterile scissors, cut foam to wound size. Proper size of foam dressing helps maintain negative pressure to entire wound. Dressing must be cut to fit the size and shape of the wound, including tunnels and undermined areas. *(Black polyurethane [PU] foam has larger pores and is most effective in stimulating granulation tissue and wound contraction. White polyvinyl alcohol [PVA] soft foam is denser, with smaller pores; use it when the growth of granulation tissue must be restricted.)*

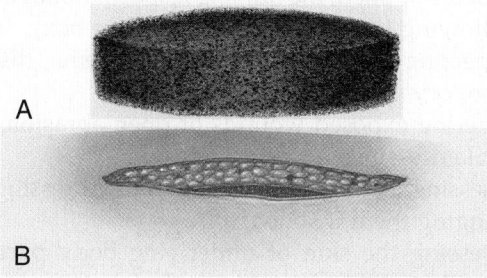

13. Gently place foam in wound, ensuring that the foam is in contact with entire wound base, margins, and tunneled and undermined areas. *(Maintains negative pressure to entire wound. Edges of the foam dressing must be in direct contact with the patient's skin.)*

14. Apply wrinkle-free transparent dressing over foam and secure tubing to the unit. (For deep wounds, regularly reposition tubing to minimize pressure on wound edges. In addition, frequent repositioning of patients with restricted mobility or sensation is important so that they do not lie on the tubing and cause further impairment of skin integrity.) *(Connects the negative pressure from the VAC system to the wound foam.)*

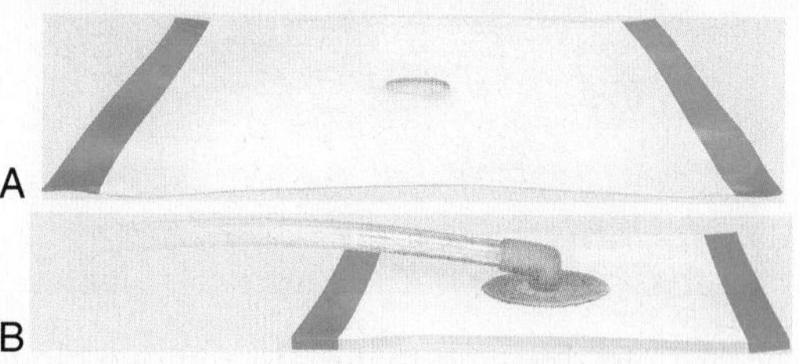

15. Apply skin protectant, such as SKIN-PREP or Stomahesive to skin around the wound. *(Protects periwound skin from injury that sometimes results from the occlusive dressing.)*

16. Apply wound VAC dressing. *(Ensures that the wound is covered properly and a negative pressure seal can be achieved.)*

a. Cover with VAC foam, keeping margin of 1 to 2 inches (3 to 5 cm) of surrounding healthy tissue. Apply wrinkle-free transparent dressing. *(Excessive tension has the potential to compress foam dressing and impede wound healing. Excessive tension also produces a shear force on periwound area.)*

b. Secure tubing to transparent film, aligning drainage holes to ensure an occlusive seal. **Do not apply tension to drape and tubing.**

17. Secure tubing several inches away from the dressing. *(Prevents pull on the primary dressing, which can cause leaks in the negative-pressure system.)*

18. Once wound is completely covered, connect the tubing from the dressing to the tubing from the canister and the VAC system. *(Administration of intermittent or continuous negative pressure between 5 and 200 mm Hg is acceptable, according to health care provider's order and patient comfort. The average is 125 mm Hg.)*

a. Remove canister from sterile packaging, and push into VAC system until a click is heard. NOTE: An alarm sounds if the canister is not properly engaged.

b. Connect the dressing tubing to the canister tubing. Be sure both clamps are open.

c. Place VAC system on a level surface, or hang from the foot of the bed. NOTE: The VAC system alarms and deactivates therapy if the unit is tilted beyond 45 degrees.

Continued

Skill 22.7 Wound Vacuum-Assisted Closure—cont'd

d. Press green-lit power button, and set pressure as ordered.

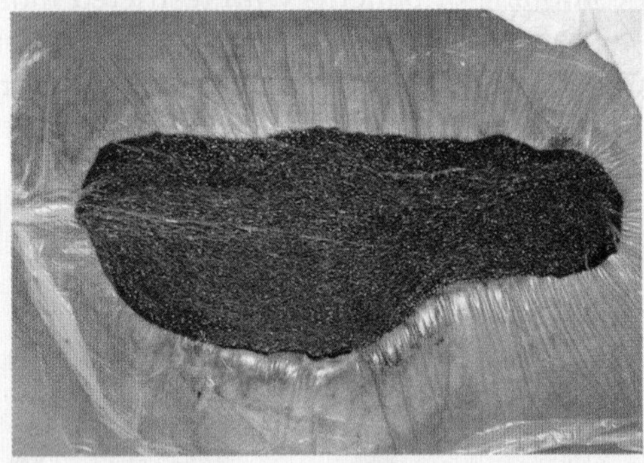

19. Discard old dressing materials, remove gloves, and perform hand hygiene. *(Reduces transmission of microorganisms.)*

20. Inspect wound VAC system to verify that negative pressure is achieved. *(Negative pressure is achieved when an airtight seal is achieved.)*
  a. Verify that display screen reads "THERAPY ON."
  b. Be sure clamps are open and tubing is patent.
  c. Identify air leaks by listening with stethoscope or by moving hand around edges of wound while applying light pressure.
  d. If a leak is present, use strips of transparent film to patch the edges of the wound.

21. See the section "Standard Steps in Wound Care," Steps 10 to 17.

22. Document: *(Records care given and progress of wound.)*
- Appearance of wound color; characteristics of any drainage. Compare wound with baseline wound assessment
- Presence of wound healing augmentation such as wound VAC
- Response to dressing change
- Record date and time of dressing change on new dressing

23. Report immediately to the health care provider:
- Bright, brick-red bleeding
- Evidence of poor wound healing
- Evisceration
- Dehiscence
- Possible wound infection *(These signs are abnormal and necessitate immediate interventions.)*

Figures courtesy Kinetic Concepts, Inc. (KCI), San Antonio, Texas.

Assess the patient's comfort level with use of a scale of 0 to 10. This determines effectiveness of comfort control measures before, during, and after dressing change. Determine the patient's knowledge of the purpose of the dressing change because this determines the level of support and explanation required. Focus on the expected outcomes of preventing infection, promoting healing, control of pain, and patient and family education.

BANDAGES AND BINDERS

A **bandage** is a strip or roll of cloth or other material that can be wound around a part of the body in a variety of ways for multiple purposes. Bandages are available in rolls of various widths and materials, including gauze, elasticized knit, elastic webbing, flannel, and muslin. Gauze bandages are lightweight and inexpensive, mold easily around contours of the body, and permit air circulation that helps prevent skin maceration (the softening and breaking down of skin from prolonged exposure to moisture). Elastic bandages conform well to body parts but also can be used to exert pressure over a body part. Flannel and muslin bandages are thicker than gauze and thus stronger for supporting or applying pressure. A flannel bandage also insulates to provide warmth.

A **binder** is a bandage that is made of large pieces of material to fit a specific body part (e.g., an abdominal binder or a breast binder). Most binders are made of elastic, cotton, muslin, or flannel.

Correctly applied bandages and binders do not cause injury to underlying and nearby body parts or create discomfort for the patient (Skills 22.8 and 22.9; Table 22.4). For example, a chest binder must not be tight enough to restrict chest wall expansion. Before a bandage or binder is applied, the nursing responsibilities include the following (see the Coordinated Care box):

- Inspecting the skin for abrasions, edema, discoloration, or exposed wound edges
- Covering exposed wounds or open abrasions with sterile dressings
- Assessing the condition of underlying dressings and changing them if soiled
- Assessing the skin of underlying body parts and parts that will be distal to the bandage for signs of circulatory impairment (coolness, pallor or cyanosis, diminished or absent pulses, numbness, and tingling) to provide a means for comparing changes in circulation after bandage application

After a bandage is applied, assess, document, and immediately report changes in circulation, skin integrity, comfort level, and body function, such as ventilation or movement. When applying a bandage, loosen or

Skill 22.8 Applying a Bandage

 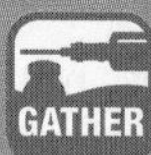 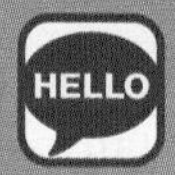   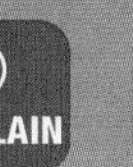  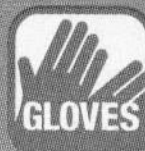

NURSING ACTION *(RATIONALE)*

1. See the section "Standard Steps in Wound Care," Steps 1 to 9.
2. Assemble equipment:
   - Correct width and number of bandages
   - Safety pins, fasteners, or tape
   - Gloves, if wound drainage is present
3. Ensure that skin and dressing are clean and dry. *(Allows bandages to be applied to clean, dry areas to prevent further impaired skin integrity.)*
4. Separate any adjacent skin surfaces. *(Prevents irritation and impairment of skin integrity.)*
5. Align part to be bandaged, providing slight flexion as appropriate and not contraindicated. *(Promotes comfort and functional use.)*
6. Apply bandage from distal to proximal part. *(Encourages return of venous blood flow to heart.)*
7. Apply bandage with even distribution of pressure. *(Maintains uniform bandage tension, prevents impairment of circulation.)*
   a. For the circular bandage, see Table 22.4.
   b. For the spiral bandage, see Table 22.4.
   c. For the spiral-reverse bandage, see Table 22.4.
   d. For the recurrent (stump) bandage, see Table 22.4.
   e. For the figure-of-8 bandage, see Table 22.4.
   f. Secure first bandage before applying additional rolls. Apply additional rolls without leaving any uncovered areas. *(Prevents wrinkling or loose ends.)*
8. Assess tension of bandage and circulation of extremity. *(Ensures that bandage is applied appropriately.)*
9. See the section "Standard Steps in Wound Care," Steps 10 to 17.
10. Document. *(Records care given and application of binder.)*

Skill 22.9 Applying a Triangular Binder (Sling), T-Binder, and Abdominal Binder

 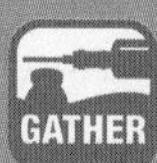 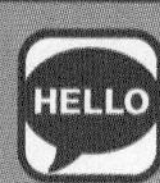     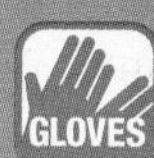

NURSING ACTION *(RATIONALE)*

1. See the section "Standard Steps in Wound Care," Steps 1 to 9.
2. Assemble equipment:
   - Binder
   - Safety pins
   - Washcloth
   - Towel
   - Soap
   - Water
   - Cotton or gauze pad
   - Pain medication, if indicated
   - Dressing, as necessary
3. Change dressing if appropriate; cleanse skin if needed. *(Prepares underlying skin surfaces for binder application.)*
4. Separate skin surfaces or pad bony prominences. *(Protects skin surfaces from contact, preventing irritation and impairment of skin integrity.)*
5. Apply binder.
   a. Triangular binder (sling)
      (1) Have patient flex arm at approximately 80-degree angle, depending on purpose of binder. *(Allows proper angle for application.)*
      (2) Place end of triangular binder over shoulder of the uninjured side, anterior to posterior. *(Places point of triangle under patient's elbow of injured arm.)*

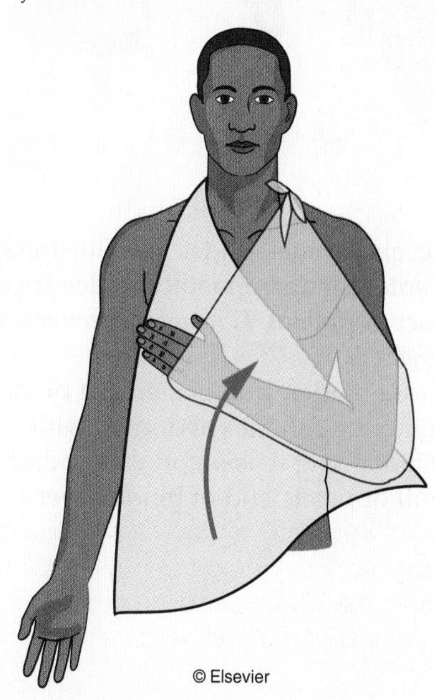

Continued

Skill 22.9 Applying a Triangular Binder (Sling), T-Binder, and Abdominal Binder—cont'd

(3) Grasp other end of binder and bring it up and over injured arm to shoulder of injured arm. *(Supports the impaired arm.)*

(4) Use square knot to tie two ends together at lateral area of neck on uninjured side. *(Prevents slippage to knot. Prevents wear on bony prominences.)*

(5) Support wrist well with binder; do not allow it to extend over end of binder. *(Maintains body alignment. Prevents circulation impairment.)*

(6) Fold third triangle end neatly around elbow and secure with safety pins. *(Secures binder. Prevents arm from slipping out.)*

b. T-binder

(1) Using appropriate binder, place the waistband smoothly under patient's waist; patient should be positioned lying supine; tails should be under patient. *(Allows use of appropriate binder; single tail for female patients and two tails for male patients.)*

(2) Secure two ends of waistband together with safety pin. *(Allows securing at the waist.)*

(3) Single tail: bring the tail up between legs to secure dressing in place. Two tails: bring tails up one on each side of penis or large dressing. *(Secures dressing, pad, or other item without causing pressure on the genitalia.)*

(4) Bring tails under and over waistband; secure with safety pins.

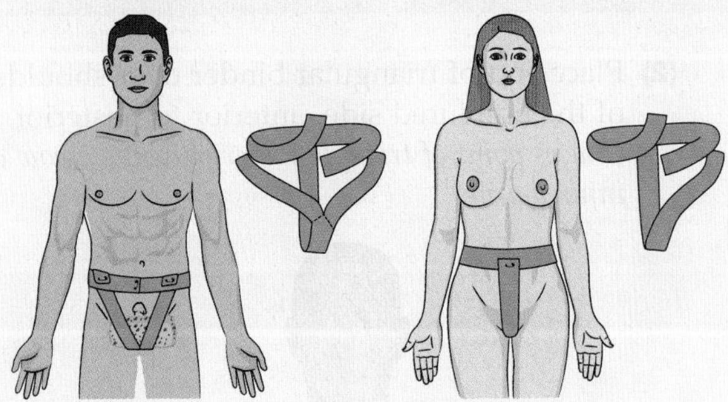

© Elsevier

c. Elastic abdominal binder (see illustration)

(1) Center binder smoothly under appropriate part of patient. *(Promotes effectiveness of binder.)*

(2) Close binder: pull one end of binder over center of patient's abdomen while maintaining tension on that end of binder; pull opposite end of binder over center and secure with Velcro closure tabs, metal fasteners, or horizontally placed safety pins. *(Provides continuous wound support and comfort.)*

(3) Observe patient's respiratory status. *(Abdominal binders that are too tight often interfere with respirations.)*

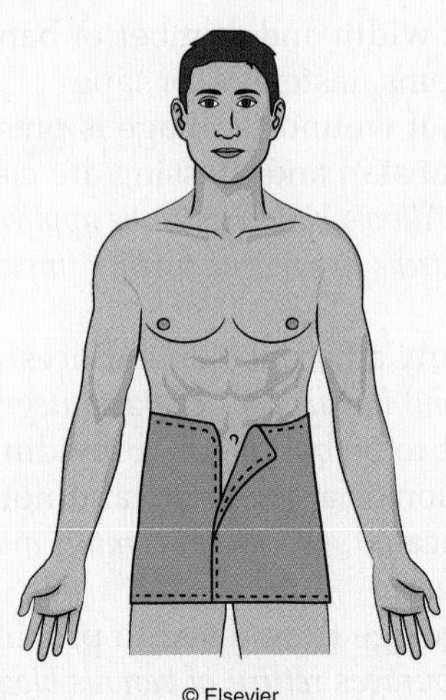

© Elsevier

d. For postsurgical application of abdominal binders, proceed upward from bottom (except for a patient after cesarean delivery) to minimize pull on the suture line.

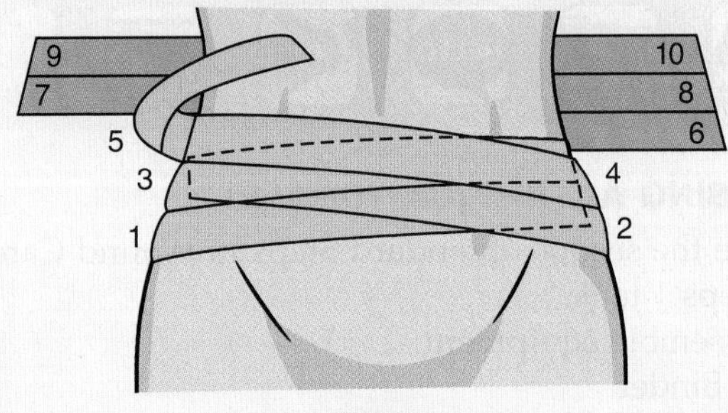

© Elsevier

6. Note comfort level of patient. Smooth out binder to prevent wrinkles. Adjust binder as necessary. *(Promotes comfort and chest expansion.)*

7. See the section "Standard Steps in Wound Care," Steps 10 to 17.

8. Document: *(Records care given and application of binder.)*

- Time of application
- Type of binder
- Patient's response
- Patient teaching (see the Patient Teaching box on wound care)

Table 22.4 Basic Bandage Turns

BASIC BANDAGE TURNS	USE
Circular	
1. Unroll 3 to 4 inches (7.62 to 10.16 cm) of bandage from back of roll. 2. Place flat bandage surface on anterior surface of portion of body to be covered and hold end in place with thumb of nondominant hand. 3. Continue rolling bandage around same area until two overlapping layers of bandage cover part. Remove excess bandage roll. 4. Secure end of bandage with safety pin or clip if it is attached to end of bandage. If end of bandage has raw edge, fold ½ to 1 inch (1.27 to 2.54 cm) under before securing bandage. Gauze bandage is possible to secure with strip of adhesive tape.	Circular turns are used to cover small body regions such as a digit or wrist and are used to anchor bandaging materials. 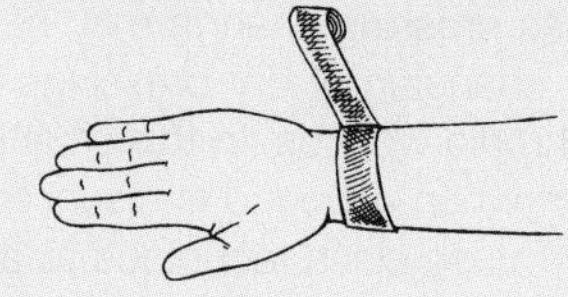
Spiral	
1. Anchor bandage at distal end of body part with two circular turns (note Steps 1 through 3, Circular). 2. Advance bandage on ascending angle, overlapping each preceding turn by half to two-thirds the width of bandage roll until proximal border of area is covered. 3. Secure end of bandage.	Used to cover cylindric body parts, where contour of part does not vary significantly in size (e.g., slender wrist and forearm). 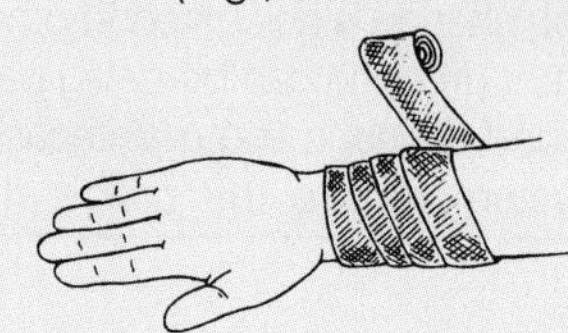
Spiral-Reverse	
1. Anchor bandage at distal border of area to be covered (use one to three circular turns). 2. Advance bandage on ascending angle of approximately 30 degrees. 3. Halfway through each turn fold bandage toward you and continue around part in downward stroke. 4. Continue advancing bandage as in Steps 2 and 3 until desired proximal point is reached. Secure bandage.	Used to cover inverted cone-shaped body parts such as calf or thigh. 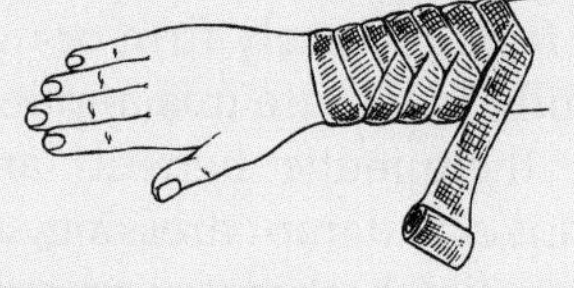
Figure-of-8	
1. Anchor bandage at center of joint (see Steps 1 through 3, Circular). 2. Ascend obliquely around upper half of circular turn above joint followed by turn that descends obliquely below joint. 3. Continue in same manner, overlapping half of previous turn until desired immobilization is attained. 4. Be certain to cover the joint with bandage to prevent fluid shift to those tissues and subsequent impaired circulation. 5. Secure end of bandage.	Used to cover joints and provide immobilization. Outer surface of fabric is against skin during ascending application of bandage. Each reverse turn places alternate side of bandage toward skin. 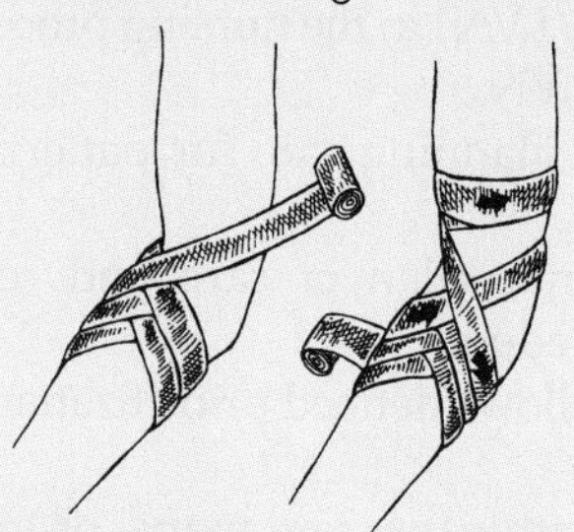
Recurrent	
1. Anchor bandage with two circular turns (see Steps 1 through 3, Circular) at proximal ends of body part to be covered. 2. Make reverse turn at center front, and advance fabric over distal end of the body part to center back, forming covering perpendicular to first circular turns. 3. Make reverse turn at back and bring bandage forward, overlapping one-half of perpendicular bandage on one side. Make reverse turn at front and overlap opposite side of center, continuing on to back. Repeat these steps, overlapping each previous strip of bandage until entire area is covered. 4. Anchor bandage with two circular turns. 5. Secure end of bandage.	Provides caplike coverage for scalp or amputation stump. 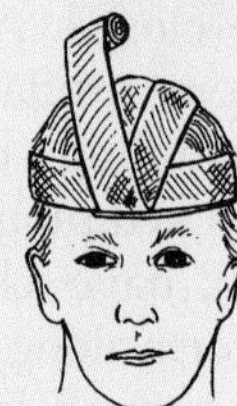 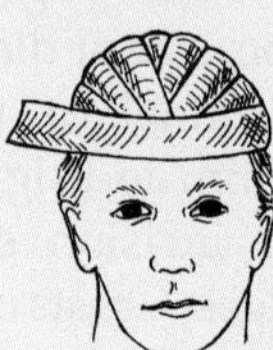

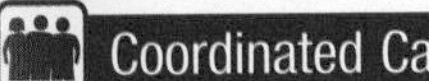

Coordinated Care

Delegation

Dressing Changes

Check institutional policy and the state's nurse practice act regarding which wound care interventions can be delegated to unlicensed assistive personnel (UAP). In some states, aspects of wound care such as dressing change may be delegated. This may include the changing of dry dressings with use of clean technique for chronic wounds. In this situation, instruct staff on what to report when a wound is cleansed. The UAP also must know how to use clean technique to avoid cross-contamination. All wound assessment—the care of acute new wounds and those that require sterile technique for dressing changes—generally remains within the domain of professional nursing practice. The assessment of the wound requires the critical thinking and knowledge application unique to a nurse even when the dressing change is delegated to others. The skill of applying a transparent dressing can be delegated to a UAP.

Assessment of wound drainage and maintenance of drains and the drainage system require the critical thinking and knowledge application unique to a nurse. Delegation to a UAP is often appropriate for emptying a closed drainage container, measuring the amount of drainage, and reporting the amount on the patient's intake and output (I&O) record.

The skill of suture removal requires the critical thinking and knowledge application unique to the nurse. For this skill, delegation is inappropriate.

The skills of applying a binder (abdominal or breast) can be delegated to UAP. However, it is the responsibility of the nurse to assess the patient's ability to breathe deeply, cough effectively, and move independently before and after binder application. The nurse is also responsible for assessing the patient's skin for irritation or abrasion, the underlying wound, and patient's level of comfort.

The skill of applying the wound vacuum-assisted closure (VAC) is inappropriate to delegate because of the unique knowledge necessary for application.

readjust it as necessary. Obtain the health care provider's order before loosening or removing a bandage the health care provider applied. Explain to the patient that any bandage or binder feels relatively firm or tight. Assess any bandage carefully to be sure it is applied properly and is providing therapeutic benefit, and replace soiled bandages. Like a damp dressing, a bandage or binder is a potential harbor for microorganisms (Box 22.5).

❖ NURSING PROCESS

The role of the licensed practical nurse/licensed vocational nurse (LPN/LVN) in the nursing process as stated is that the LPN/LVN

- Participates in planning care for patients based on patient needs
- Reviews patient's plan of care and recommends revisions as needed
- Reviews and follows defined prioritization for patient care
- Uses clinical pathways, care maps, or care plans to guide and review patient care

◆ ASSESSMENT

Note whether wound edges are closed. Assessment consists of location, size or dimensions, exudates, wound bed or edges, tunnel or undermining, periwound characteristics, pain, and signs and symptoms of infection. A surgical incision should have clean, well-approximated edges. Crusts often form along the wound edges from exudate. A puncture wound is usually a small, circular wound with the edges coming together toward the center. If a wound is open, separate the wound edges and inspect the condition of underlying tissue such as adipose and connective tissue. Also look for complications such as **dehiscence** (separation of surgical incision or rupture of wound closure, typically an abdominal incision) and **evisceration** (the protrusion of an internal organ through a wound or surgical incision, especially in the abdominal wall). The outer edges of a wound normally appear inflamed for the first 2 to 3 days, but this slowly disappears. Within 7 to 10 days, a normally healing wound fills with epithelial cells and edges close. If infection develops, the wound edges become brightly erythematous and edematous.

If a closed wound is covered by a dressing, observe the dressing but do not change it until an order is issued. If a dressing becomes saturated with exudate before the order is given, reinforce the dressing over the incisional area by placing sterile gauze on top of the original dressing and anchoring it securely. Record and report any dressing that is reinforced. Observe and document the amount of exudate and the dressings applied.

◆ PATIENT PROBLEMS

After completing an assessment of the patient's wound, identify patient problem statements that direct supportive and preventive care. Existence of a wound clearly indicates the following patient problem:

- *Compromised Skin Integrity*

This patient problem statement leads to initiation of interventions that promote the healing process.

Some patients are at risk for poor wound healing because of preexisting conditions that impair healing (see Table 22.1). Thus, even though the patient's wound appears normal, it is important to identify patient problem statements that direct nursing interventions toward support of wound repair, such as the following:

- *Insufficient Nutrition*
- *Compromised Blood Flow to Tissue*

Box 22.5 Guidelines for Applying a Bandage or Binder

1. Position body part to be bandaged in comfortable position of normal anatomic alignment. Bandages cause restriction in movement. Immobilization in position of normal functioning reduces risk of deformity or injury.
2. Prevent friction between and against skin surfaces by applying gauze or cotton padding. Skin surfaces in contact with each other (e.g., between toes, under breasts) are likely to rub against each other and cause abrasion or chafing. Bandages over body prominences often rub against skin and cause impairment of skin integrity.
3. Apply bandages securely to prevent slippage during movement. Friction between bandage and skin can cause impairment of skin integrity.
4. When bandaging extremities, apply bandage first at the distal end and progress toward the trunk (heart).
5. Gradual application of pressure from the distal toward the proximal portion of the extremity promotes venous return and keeps the risk of edema or circulatory impairment to a minimum.
6. Apply bandages firmly, with equal tension exerted over each turn or layer. Avoid excess overlapping of bandage layers. (Approximately one-third to one-half of previous layer should be covered by successive layers.) Proper application prevents unequal pressure distribution over bandaged body part. Localized pressure causes circulatory impairment.
7. Position pins, knots, or ties away from wound or sensitive skin areas. These materials potentially exert localized pressure and cause irritation.
8. Remove and reapply an elastic bandage at least once every 8 hours unless otherwise directed by health care provider.
9. Remove elastic bandage whenever necessary to readjust wrinkles, looseness, or tightness; because of patient discomfort; or when you note signs and symptoms of nerve or vascular impairment.
10. Apply bandages to the lower extremities before the patient sits or stands (i.e., with patient lying down).
11. Use increasingly wider bandages as size of area to be covered increases.
12. Use adhesive tape rather than loose clips or pins to fasten bandages on small child or infant. Safety pins are more effective than clips and do not fall out of bandage. Many facilities prefer tape for safety and maintenance of skin integrity.
13. Patients with tubes or drains who have binders need frequent assessment to ensure patency of tubes for drainage.

The nature of a wound can cause problems unrelated to wound healing. Pain and impaired mobility can affect a patient's eventual recovery. For example, a large abdominal incision can cause enough pain to interfere with the patient's ability to turn in bed effectively (Box 22.6).

Box 22.6 Patient Problems Related to Wound Healing

- *Inability to Maintain Adequate Breathing Pattern, related to:*
  - *Pain from abdominal or thoracic incision*
- *Potential for Infection, related to:*
  - *Malnutrition*
  - *Tissue loss and increased environmental exposure*
- *Compromised Physical Mobility, related to:*
  - *Pain of surgical wound or site of surgery (e.g., joint replacement)*
- *Insufficient Nutrition, related to:*
  - *Inability to ingest or tolerate food*
  - *Inability to accommodate the increased calories needed to promote wound healing*
- *Recent Onset of Pain, related to:*
  - *Surgical incision*
- *Impaired Self-Esteem due to Current Situation, related to:*
  - *Perception of scars*
  - *Perception of surgical drains*
  - *Reaction to surgically removed body part*
- *Compromised Skin Integrity, related to:*
  - *Surgical incision*
  - *Pressure*
  - *Chemical injury*
  - *Secretions and excretions*
- *Potential for Compromised Skin Integrity, related to:*
  - *Physical immobilization*
  - *Exposure to secretions*

◆ EXPECTED OUTCOMES AND PLANNING

Establish a plan of care based on the patient's health care needs. These needs are identified during the assessment phase of the nursing process. Next, form the nursing diagnostic statement and devise the plan of care. Consider the patient's plan of care for discharge, because patients are discharged earlier than in the past (see the Home Care Considerations box). Incorporate patient and family teaching into the patient's plan of care (see the Patient Teaching box). Consider special needs of the older adult when performing wound care (see the Cultural Considerations and Lifespan Considerations for older adults boxes).

Goals such as the following are developed for the patient based on the patient problem. Expected outcomes are based on the goals of care.

Goal 1: Patient's wound heals without complications.

Outcome 1: Patient's wound is free of infection; edges are approximated.

Goal 2: Patient has minimal pain.

Outcome 2: Patient reports minimal discomfort.

◆ IMPLEMENTATION

While performing wound care, observe the wound for signs and symptoms of infection. Be certain sterile technique is used when gloving, handling sterile equipment and dressings, performing procedures that involve

Home Care Considerations

Wound Care

- Demonstrate wound care and provide time for return demonstration.
- Explain need for specialized supplies such as irrigating solutions and dressings and need to maintain sterile asepsis when performing care.
- Instruct where and how to obtain additional supplies.
- Instruct about signs of improper wound healing and wound infections.
- Explain why wound is being allowed to heal by secondary intention.
- Assess understanding of need for the methods of wound care.
- Teach primary caregiver and patient how to maintain clean technique when changing dressings. Wear clean gloves, and perform hand hygiene after procedure. Use of clean dressings is permitted in the home environment.
- Be certain patient knows when and what signs and symptoms to report to health care provider or primary caregiver.
- Assess extent of wound or incision in relation to patient's level of activity to determine type of dressing that will achieve desired purpose.
- Assess area where procedure will be performed for adequate lighting and running water. Determine whether there is a table or cabinet on which sterile supplies may be placed with reasonable security.
- A bedroom or bathroom is usually ideal for procedure.
- Cleansing wound in the shower is acceptable if approved by health care provider.
- If drainage system is present, explain how system operates.
- Explain importance of drainage system.
- Demonstrate procedure for emptying the drainage chamber and how to reseal it without contaminating unit.
- Be sure the drain is protected from the disoriented patient, who may pull it out.
- Teach proper application and care of binder.

Patient Teaching

Wound Care

- Assist patient to accept the surgical wound by stating the progress of the wound and how healing is occurring.
- Teach importance of early ambulation after surgery.
- Teach importance of a nutritious diet in wound healing.
- Explain that dressings perhaps will be required at home and how to purchase what will be needed. Inform of home health services if needed or per health care provider's order.
- Wounds out of patient's reach and vision necessitate assistance by a family member or other caregiver.
- Explain expected wound appearance, what should be reported, and risks of improper wound care.
- After demonstrating wound care, allow the patient or the family member to perform wound care with supervision.
- Teach the importance of keeping dressings, sutures, and staples dry and clean.
- Explain the importance of washing hands before and after dressing changes.
- Teach signs and symptoms of infection.
- Instruct the patient to notify the health care provider if signs of wound infection appear.
- Follow health care provider's instructions for limiting activity.
- Provide written instructions in addition to verbal ones.
- Allow time for patient's questions.
- If drainage system is present:
  - Explain purpose of drainage system.
  - Explain importance of measuring output.
  - Instruct to keep Hemovac or Davol tubing clipped or pinned to clothing to prevent accidental dislodgement.
  - Teach what to do if the drain accidentally comes out.
- If binder is present, teach function of the binder.
- Teach to report if binder is loose or causing pain or discomfort.
- Teach to report any breathing restrictions if binder is too tight.

care of the open wound, and caring for wound drainage systems. Documentation of wound care is required to include the appearance of the wound, presence of drains and drainage or exudate, medication or solutions used in wound care, type of dressings applied, and patient response to the procedure. Report any variation from normal healing. Include specific interventions or techniques of dressing changes in the nursing care plan to provide continuity of care.

◆ EVALUATION

Evaluate wound healing with each dressing change, after application of heat and cold therapies, after wound irrigation, and after stress to the wound site.

Determine whether expected outcomes have been met. Take the following evaluative measures: assess condition of the wound, ask whether patient notes discomfort during procedure, and inspect condition of dressings at least every shift. Note the following examples:

Goal 1: Patient's wound heals without complications.

Evaluative measure: Assess the wound and dressing for odor, exudate, separation, color, and edema.

Goal 2: Patient has minimal pain; rates pain at 3 on a scale of 1 to 10.

Evaluative measures: Compare dosage and frequency of pain medication delivered over recovery period. Request patient to rate pain on a scale of 0 to 10, with 10 being the most pain and 0 being no pain.

 Cultural Considerations

Wound Care

Detection of cyanosis and other changes in skin color in patients is an important clinical skill. This detection can become a challenge in patients with dark skin. Cyanosis is defined as a slightly blue-gray, slatelike, or dark purple discoloration of the skin that results from a reduction of at least 5 g of hemoglobin in arterial blood. Color differentiation of cyanosis varies according to skin pigmentation. In patients with dark skin, you need to know the individual's baseline skin tone. Do not confuse the normal hyperpigmentation of Mongolian spots that may be seen on the sacrum of African American, Native American, and Asian American patients as cyanosis. Observe the patient's skin in daylight without glare.

Keep in mind the following points:

- Cyanosis is difficult but possible to detect in a patient with dark skin.
- Be aware of situations that produce changes in skin tone.
- Examine body sites with the least melanin (mucous membranes) for underlying color identification.
- The pigmented skin should be assessed for specific color changes in skin tone.

 Lifespan Considerations

Older Adults

Wound Care

- Assess ability of the older adult to perform self-care, to reach the wound, and to manipulate the wound dressings.
- The skin of older adults is fragile and sometimes does not tolerate adhesives. Frequent dressing changes should be avoided. Assess for tape allergies. Use paper tape.
- Decrease extraneous noises as much as possible to alleviate or prevent patient anxiety.
- Increase time allowed for the skills and allow time for repetition of teaching.
- Slow the pace.
- Give small amounts of information at a time.
- Older patients learn better by doing and using multiple senses than by reading instructions.
- The increased fragility of the skin of the older adult sometimes contraindicates the use of a binder. Assess skin thoroughly before any binder application.
- Observe underlying skin of the older adult more frequently.
- Patient needs two binders because binders are washable and must be "line dried." Thus the patient has one to wear while the other is being washed and dried.
- Older adults often need reassurance about the suture removal procedure. Assess mental status for comprehension of the procedure.
- Older skin is frequently at higher risk for dehiscence after sutures are removed.
- Be aware that patients need additional fluid intake to prevent dehydration.
- Certain measures are sometimes necessary to prevent a confused patient from pulling out the drain.
- Compensate for any auditory, visual, or cognitive impairment the patient has when performing a dressing change.
- A decrease in sensory receptors causes a decrease in pain sensation.

Get Ready for the NCLEX® Examination!

Key Points

- Wounds are described as open or closed. Care of the open wound is determined by the extent of the wound.
- Maintenance of sterile technique is essential when providing care for an open wound.
- Size, description of appearance, amount and type of exudate, presence of drains, integrity of wound closures, and pain level are included in a proper wound assessment.
- The wet-to-dry dressing can be used to débride mechanically a wound of necrotic tissue or wound exudate.
- Do not moisten the wet-to-dry dressing before removing it, because this defeats the goal of débriding the wound.
- Wound drains remove secretions within tissue layers to promote wound closure.
- A drainage system requires close monitoring. In addition to noting color, consistency, and amount of drainage, checking the tube patency is important.
- After a bandage or binder is applied, assess, document, and immediately report changes in circulation, skin integrity, comfort level, and body function, such as ventilation or mobility.

- Remove dressings gently to prevent further injury to the wound. Dispose of used dressings appropriately to prevent cross-contamination.
- The type of suture securing a wound influences the method of suture removal.
- Wound care involves cleaning wounds, changing dressings, maintaining drains, irrigating, inserting packing, applying heat and cold treatments, and applying bandages and binders.
- Major types of wound exudate are serous, purulent, and sanguineous. The main complications of wound healing are hemorrhage, infection, dehiscence, and evisceration.
- Major nursing responsibilities related to wound care include preventing infection, preventing further tissue damage, preventing hemorrhage, promoting healing, and preventing skin excoriation around draining wounds.
- Wound assessment requires a description of the appearance of the wound base, the wound's size, the presence of exudates, and the periwound skin condition.
- When cleansing wounds or drain sites, clean from the least to the most contaminated area, away from the wound edges.
- Physical stress from vomiting, coughing, or sudden muscular contraction could cause separation of wound edges or dehiscence.
- Apply bandages and binders in a manner that does not impair circulation or irritate the skin.

Additional Learning Resources

SG Go to your Study Guide for additional learning activities to help you master this chapter content.

evolve Be sure to visit the Evolve site at *http://evolve.elsevier.com/Cooper/foundationsadult/* for additional online resources.

Review Questions for the NCLEX® Examination

1. The patient has just returned from the postanesthesia care (PAC) unit. During report, the nurse is told that the patient has a Penrose drain in the left lower quadrant (LLQ). The patient asks why the drain is being used. What response by the nurse is most accurate?
   1. "The drain allows for the postoperative instillation of wound irrigation fluid."
   2. "The drain is used to reduce infection in the postoperative period."
   3. "Penrose drains are used to drain body fluids from the area surrounding the wound by suction."
   4. "Gravity is used to drain fluid from the area around the wound with the Penrose drain."
2. The nurse finds that the patient's incision has eviscerated. What action should the nurse take? *(Select all that apply.)*
   1. Place the patient in high Fowler's position.
   2. Give the patient fluids to prevent shock.
   3. Do not allow the patient to get out of bed.
   4. Replace dressings with sterile fluffy pads.
   5. Apply warm, moist sterile dressings.
3. The health care provider has ordered the patient's wound be irrigated. What is the primary rationale for this procedure?
   1. To remove debris from the wound
   2. To decrease scar formation
   3. To improve circulation from the wound
   4. To decrease irritation from wound drainage
4. What is the best indicator that a wound has become infected?
   1. Palpation of the wound reveals excess fluid under its edges.
   2. Wound cultures are positive.
   3. Purulent drainage is coming from the wound area.
   4. The wound has a distinct odor.
5. Which nursing entry is the most complete in its description of a wound?
   1. Wound appears to be healing well, dressing dry and intact
   2. Wound well approximated with minimal drainage
   3. Drainage size of quarter; wound pink; 4 × 4 applied
   4. Incisional edges approximated without erythema or exudate; two 4 × 4s applied
6. Which statement is correct in regard to the use of an abdominal binder?
   1. It replaces the need for underlying dressings.
   2. It should be kept loose for patient comfort.
   3. The patient has to be sitting or standing when it is applied.
   4. The patient must have adequate ventilatory capacity.
7. What is the first step when packing a wound?
   1. Assess its size, shape, and depth.
   2. Prepare a sterile field.
   3. Select gauze packing material.
   4. Irrigate the wound.
8. What is the correct procedure for the wet-to-dry dressing method?
   1. Place dry gauze into the wound and remove it when it is wet.
   2. Medicate the patient for pain after you change the dressing.
   3. Complete this type of dressing change just once a day.
   4. Place moist gauze into the wound and remove it when it is dry.
9. Which phrase best describes serous drainage?
   1. Fresh bleeding
   2. Thick and yellow
   3. Clear, watery plasma
   4. Beige to brown and foul smelling

10. The health care provider has ordered an abdominal binder placed around a surgical patient with a new abdominal wound. What is the likely indication for this intervention?
    1. Collection of wound drainage
    2. Reduction of abdominal swelling
    3. Reduction of stress on the abdominal incision
    4. Stimulation of peristalsis from direct pressure
11. What are the traditional purposes of a wet-to-dry dressing? *(Select all that apply.)*
    1. Débridement
    2. Cooling
    3. Comfort
    4. Prevent infection
    5. Maintenance of moisture at the wound bed
12. What action should the nurse implement to reduce surgical wound infection? *(Select all that apply.)*
    1. Adhering to the principles of hand hygiene
    2. Cleansing the incision from the least contaminated to the most contaminated area
    3. Leaving the incision open to the air
    4. Changing the dressing using sterile technique
    5. Ensuring the patient is consuming an adequate diet
13. The student nurse is changing a patient's dressing. What action indicates the need for further education? *(Select all that apply.)*
    1. Enclose the soiled dressing within a latex glove.
    2. Clean the wound in circles toward the incision.
    3. Free the tape by pulling it away from the incision.
    4. Remove the soiled dressing with sterile gloves.
    5. Apply the clean dressing with clean gloves.
14. When the drainage in a Hemovac reservoir is emptied, which nursing action is essential for reestablishing the negative pressure within this drainage device?
    1. Fill the reservoir with sterile normal saline solution.
    2. Secure the reservoir to the skin near the wound.
    3. Compress the reservoir and close the vent.
    4. Open the vent, allowing the reservoir to fill with air.
15. Which patient is more at risk for wound dehiscence?
    1. The patient who smokes
    2. The patient who is obese
    3. The patient with a history of peripheral vascular disease
    4. The patient who is immunocompromised
16. The student nurse is correct when indicating which drain as providing suction-assisted drainage?
    1. Jackson-Pratt
    2. Hemovac
    3. Penrose
    4. Wound VAC system
    5. T-tube system
17. The health care provider has ordered all sutures on a patient with an abdominal hysterectomy be removed on the 5th postoperative day and Steri-Strips applied. During suture removal, the nurse notices the incision edges are slightly separating. What is the best action by the nurse?
    1. Continue removing the sutures and apply the Steri-Strips.
    2. Stop the suture removal and contact the health care provider immediately.
    3. Continue removing the sutures and applying the Steri-Strips, then cover the incision with a dry sterile dressing.
    4. Stop the suture removal, apply Steri-Strips where sutures already have been removed, and notify the health care provider.
18. When providing care to a patient with a Hemovac drain, what actions are included in the plan of care?
    1. Record the appearance of the drainage in the nursing progress notes and include the amount in the fluid output calculations.
    2. Clamp the tubing during patient ambulation and activity to prevent excess drainage during these times.
    3. Empty the bulb drainage receptacle when it is one-fourth full.
    4. Pin the bulb above the insertion site to assist in proper drainage of exudate.
19. During assessment of a patient after abdominal surgery, the nurse suspects internal hemorrhaging based on which finding?
    1. The dressing is saturated with bright red sanguineous drainage, and the patient has an increased urinary output.
    2. The dressing is dry and intact, the patient's blood pressure has decreased, and pulse and respirations have increased.
    3. The dressing is saturated with serosanguineous drainage, and the patient is diaphoretic with a decrease in pulse and respirations.
    4. The dressing is dry and intact, and the patient reports shortness of breath and has an elevated temperature.

23 Specimen Collection and Diagnostic Testing

http://evolve.elsevier.com/Cooper/foundationsadult/

Objectives

1. Describe the necessary documentation of the patient's condition before, during, and after a laboratory or diagnostic test.
2. Discuss nursing interventions necessary to properly prepare a patient who is to have a diagnostic examination.
3. Discuss patient teaching for diagnostic testing.
4. Describe the role of the nurse in procedures for specimen collection.
5. Discuss guidelines for specimen collection.
6. Explain the rationales for collection of each specimen listed.
7. State appropriate labeling for a collected specimen.
8. List the proper steps for obtaining urine specimens.
9. List the proper steps for teaching blood glucose self-monitoring.
10. Discuss the procedure for obtaining stool specimens.
11. State the correct procedures for collecting a sputum specimen.
12. Identify the procedure for performing a phlebotomy.
13. Identify the procedure for performing electrocardiography.

Key Terms

culture (KŬL-chŭr, p. 673)
cytology (sī-TŎL-ō-jē, p. 673)
electrocardiogram (ECG) (ē-lĕk-trō-KĂR-dē-ō-grăm, p. 683)
expectorate (ĕks-PĔK-tō-rāt, p. 673)
fixative (FĬKS-ŭ-tĭv, p. 660)
Hemoccult (HĒ-mō-kŭlt, p. 673)
midstream urine specimen (p. 667)
occult (ō-KŬLT, p. 673)
residual urine (p. 667)
sensitivity (SĔN-sĭ-TĬV-ĭ-tē, p. 673)
specimen (SPĔS-ĭ-mĭn, p. 667)
tourniquet (TŪR-nĭ-kĕt, p. 682)
Vacutainer (VĂC-yū-tā-nŭr, p. 680)
venipuncture (VĔN-ĭ-pŭnk-chŭr, p. 680)

DIAGNOSTIC EXAMINATION

Diagnostic examination is performed by a health care provider, sometimes at the patient's bedside and sometimes in a room specially equipped for therapeutic or diagnostic purposes. The nurse is responsible for assessing the patient's knowledge of the procedure and preparing the patient for it; assisting the health care provider with the procedure; and caring for the patient after tests are completed. The nurse's knowledge and organization of the procedure ensure that it is carried out smoothly.

Patients have fundamental rights and protections during their care. One of the patient's most important rights is informed consent, which requires that the patient, parent, or guardian (or legally designated health care power of attorney if the patient is legally incompetent) fully understands what will be done during a test, surgery, or any medical procedure and understands its risks and implications *before* legally consenting to it.

Explaining a procedure, the method by which it will be performed, and its potential benefits and risks are primarily the health care provider's responsibility. Reinforcement of the health care provider's explanation is a role of the nurse. Be prepared to answer any questions the patient has and to clarify the requirements for the examination, such as whether nothing is permitted to be taken by mouth (NPO) after midnight or whether breakfast will be withheld until the examination is completed. The patient needs to know whether a special room or equipment is required for the test, as well as whether any medications are needed before or during the test. An informed patient is better prepared to participate in the testing process as required by the examination (Skill 23.1 and the Patient Teaching box). The nurse is responsible for knowing the guidelines for and the potential complications of diagnostic examinations (Boxes 23.1 and 23.2, Table 23.1).

Consent for treatment upon admission at the health care facility encompasses most diagnostic tests and

Skill 23.1 Preparing the Patient for Diagnostic Examination

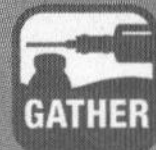

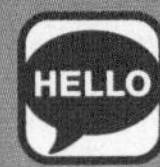

PRIVACY

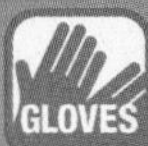

NURSING ACTION *(RATIONALE)*

1. Refer to the health care provider's order.
2. Ensure that informed consent has been obtained when necessary. For most invasive diagnostic tests a signed informed consent form is required. The health care provider is ultimately responsible for disclosure, but the nurse also must be aware of agency policies regarding consent forms and ensure that informed consent is obtained before the procedure. *(Ensures that legal implications of diagnostic procedures are taken into consideration.)*
3. Assemble equipment and supplies. *(Organizes procedure.)*
4. Introduce self. *(Decreases patient's anxiety.)*
5. Identify patient. *(Ensures procedure is performed with correct patient.)*
6. Explain procedure. Assess patient's understanding of procedure and purpose. If contrast dye is to be used, assess patient for allergies (see Box 23.2). *(Promotes understanding and cooperation.)*
7. Prepare patient for procedure. *(Facilitates procedure.)*
   a. Transport patient to examining room, if necessary. Maintain safety precautions. *(Facilitates procedure; some facilities have special examination rooms, but frequently procedures are performed at the patient's bedside.)*
   b. Close door and pull curtains. *(Provides privacy.)*
   c. Raise bed or arrange examination table to convenient height. *(Promotes proper body mechanics.)*
   d. Drape patient for procedure, if necessary. *(Prevents unnecessary exposure of patient.)* (See Table 23.1.)
8. Perform hand hygiene and don clean gloves according to agency policy and guidelines from the Centers for Disease Control and Prevention (CDC) and Occupational Safety and Health Administration (OSHA). *(Reduces spread of microorganisms.)*
9. Assist health care provider with procedure. *(Provides help to the health care provider while providing support to patient.)*
10. Answer patient's questions. *(Provides for patient's security and emotional support.)*
11. Label specimen according to agency policy (see Box 23.5): patient's name and age, room number, health care provider, date and time, type of specimen, and collector's initials. Most facility policies recommend inserting the specimen (in container) into a biohazard bag for transport to laboratory. Deliver specimen to laboratory promptly. *(Prevents loss and potential delays in obtaining results. Biohazard bag further prevents contamination from specimen.)*

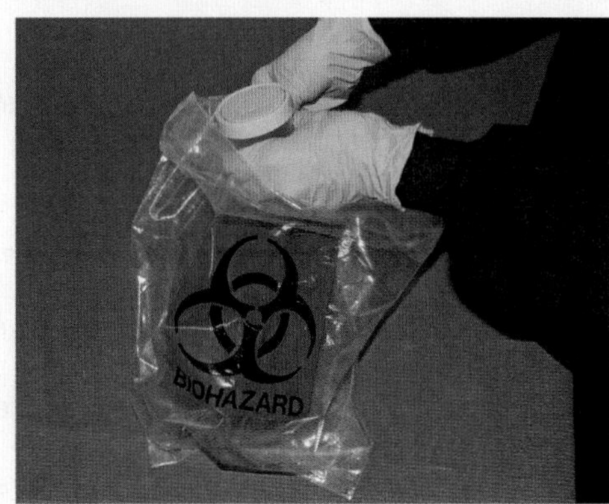

12. Document procedure. *(Communicates performed procedure and patient's response.)*
    - Type of procedure
    - Time
    - Specimen obtained
    - Sent to laboratory with requisition
    - Patient's response
13. Provide patient teaching (see the Patient Teaching box).

procedures. Some tests, however, do require the completion of additional consents. Traditionally, human immunodeficiency virus (HIV) testing and invasive procedures belong to this category. Written consent is not always necessary for an individual test if it is considered noninvasive; informed verbal consent is adequate in many cases. The patient retains the legal right to withdraw consent—verbal or written—at any time and for any reason and to refuse care or treatment.

Nursing responsibilities include anticipating the needs of the health care provider who performs the procedure,

Box 23.1 General Guidelines for Diagnostic Examination

(Rationales are provided in parentheses.)

- Know the patient's baseline vital signs. Some diagnostic tests are invasive procedures and have associated complications. *(Changes from baseline vital signs provide early physiologic data about potential complications.)*
- Assess for the presence of tattoos. Older body art may have been prepared with dyes containing metal-based components. This may present issues with CT and MRI such as burning or skin irritation. Report findings to health care provider.
- Know the patient's level of education. The nurse is required to teach the patient about diagnostic tests. *(Knowing the patient's educational background enables the development of an individualized teaching plan.)*
- Determine the patient's awareness of actual or potential medical diagnoses. *(Provides data about the patient's knowledge and perception of medical diagnoses.)*
- Perform a thorough nursing assessment, including assessment of the patient's cultural background. *(Reveals abnormal findings, which can indicate or contraindicate a diagnostic test.)*
- Determine the patient's previous experience with diagnostic testing. *(Patients who have had smooth, uncomplicated diagnostic tests are usually less anxious about a test. If a patient has had a complication from a diagnostic test, it is possible that the patient will require more pre-procedure education and support.)*
- Most agencies adhere to standard precautions; know agency policy. *(Some facilities have policies that require all specimen containers of body substances to be placed in biohazard bags for transportation to various laboratories. Attach requisitions to specimen container.)*
- Know normal values of the test being performed and causes of deviations from these normal values. (Be aware that some deviations from normal values occur as a result of medications or dietary intake.) *(Allows notification of the prescribing health care provider of end results in a timely manner.)*
- Refer to the policy manual for the facility's instructions for collection of each specimen during diagnostic examinations (see Table 23.1).
- Many factors have the potential to contribute to dysrhythmias in association with diagnostic examinations, including medications such as digitalis and quinidine, hypertrophy of cardiac muscle, alcohol, thyroid dysfunction, coffee, tea, tobacco, electrolyte imbalances, edema, acid-base imbalances, and myocardial ischemia. *(Patients with dysrhythmias are at risk for cardiac arrest. Be familiar with crash cart location, and be knowledgeable about emergency equipment, medications, and cardiopulmonary resuscitation [CPR].)*

Box 23.2 Patient Evaluation for Iodine Dye Allergies

- Many types of contrast media are used in radiographic studies: for example, organic iodine and iodized oils.
- Possible allergic reactions to iodinated dye vary from mild flushing, itching, and urticaria (hives) to severe, life-threatening *anaphylaxis* (an exaggerated life-threatening hypersensitivity reaction to a previous encountered antigen; evidenced by respiratory distress, drop in blood pressure, shock, or a combination of these). In the unusual event of anaphylaxis, treatment consists of administration of drugs such as diphenhydramine (Benadryl), steroids, and epinephrine. Always have oxygen and endotracheal equipment on hand for immediate use.
- Always assess the patient for allergies to the iodine dye before its administration. Inform the radiologist if an allergy is suspected. Patients who are allergic to shellfish are likely allergic to iodine-based dyes, because shellfish contain iodine. Non–iodine-based dyes often are used for these patients, or they are pretreated for the likelihood of an allergic reaction. The radiologist is likely to prescribe a diphenhydramine and steroid preparation to be administered before testing. Usually, hypoallergenic contrast media is used during the test.[a]
- After the x-ray procedure, evaluate the patient for delayed reaction to dye (dyspnea, rashes, tachycardia, urticaria). This usually occurs within 2 to 6 hours after the test. Treat with antihistamines or steroids, according to the health care provider's order.

[a]The American College of Radiology recommends that patients who have a prior documented reaction to contrast material be given a different contrast agent in combination with a premedication regimen if it is not possible to avoid using a contrast medium.

having the proper supplies ready, and assisting the patient through the procedure. The patient should be kept apprised of the procedural details. Certain procedures may cause discomfort. Providing support and information to these patients is key to their tolerance of the procedures. Nurses should take special care with older adults during specimen collection and diagnostic examination (see the Lifespan Considerations for Older Adults box) and be aware that sociocultural variations often affect a patient's response and willingness to participate in various diagnostic procedures (see the Cultural Considerations box).

When patients have questions about diagnostic examinations, consult the agency's procedural manual or the designated department involved. Maintain confidentiality when disclosing results from testing and diagnostic procedures. Health care agencies are required to have and to follow policies regarding confidentiality of these records.

Text continued on p. 666

Table 23.1 Nursing Interventions for Diagnostic Examinations

BEFORE EXAMINATION	AFTER EXAMINATION
Abdominal Scan[a]	
Order prescribed test per facility policy. Explain procedure. Obtain informed consent, if required by facility. Assess laboratory results for kidney function. If contrast medium is to be used, instruct patient to maintain NPO status for 4 h before examination. Assess patient for allergies to dye or shellfish; it is possible to perform the abdominal scan with or without the dye. Assess patient for claustrophobia. Patients who are mildly claustrophobic often benefit from premedication with antianxiety drugs. Some patients experience mild nausea from the contrast medium; provide emesis basin. Advise patient that he or she may experience a salty taste, flushing, and a sensation of warmth when dye is injected.	Evaluate patient for delayed reaction to dye (see Box 23.2). Encourage oral intake of fluids. Report results. Diarrhea is possible.
Amniocentesis	
Explain procedure. Encourage patient's verbalization of concerns. Obtain written consent from patient. Monitor fetal heart tones. No fluid or food restrictions are necessary. Monitor mother's blood pressure. Follow instructions regarding emptying the bladder, which depend on gestational age. • Before 20 wk of gestation, it is necessary to keep the bladder full to support the uterus. • After 20 wk, the bladder typically is emptied to minimize the chance of puncture. • After 20 wk gestation, the health care provider may order external fetal monitoring for 30-60 min before and after the procedure. NOTE: The location of the placenta is determined by ultrasonography before the study to enable selection of a site that will help prevent placental puncture.	Monitor fetal heart tones. If patient complains of vertigo or nausea, allow her to rest on her left side for several minutes before leaving examination room; assess her vital signs. If any fluid loss or temperature elevation, abdominal pain or cramping, or fetal hyperactivity or unusual fetal lethargy occurs, instruct patient to notify her health care provider. Instruct patient to contact her health care provider to obtain results (usually after 2 wk). For women who have Rh-negative blood and are not sensitized, administer RhoGAM because of the risk of immunization from the fetal blood. Observe puncture site for bleeding.
Arteriography	
Explain procedure. Obtain written consent. Advise patient that he or she may experience flushing and a sensation of warmth when dye is injected. Assess allergies to dye. Assess whether patient has been taking anticoagulants. Keep patient on NPO status for 2–8 h. Mark site of peripheral pulses with a pen (this enables assessment after the procedure). Document the diminished or absent peripheral pulses. Administer medications as ordered. Ensure that the appropriate coagulation studies have been done and results are within normal range. For cerebral arteriography, perform baseline neurologic assessment to compare subsequent assessment findings. Instruct patient to remove and safely store all dental prostheses and all valuables before study. Instruct patient to void before study. Inform the patient that bladder distention will possibly cause some discomfort during study.	Keep patient on bed rest for 8 h or as ordered by the health care provider. Monitor vital signs and observe for bleeding at puncture site. Assess peripheral arterial pulse at premarked site. If cerebral arteriography has been done, perform neurologic assessment. Maintain pressure at the puncture site. Perform neurovascular assessment on patient's lower extremities; compare the involved extremity with the uninvolved extremity. Administer analgesic as indicated; notify health care provider if patient has severe, continuous pain. Have patient drink fluids to prevent dehydration. Evaluate patient for delayed allergic reaction to the dye (see Box 23.2). If patient has continuous, severe pain, notify health care provider.

[a]Showing a picture of the x-ray machine (used for scans and MRI) and encouraging the patient to verbalize concerns regarding claustrophobia help reduce anxiety. Most patients who are mildly claustrophobic are able to tolerate these studies after appropriate premedication with antianxiety medications. Most of these tests require lying still on a hard table and peripheral venipuncture, which sometimes cause mild discomfort. Mild nausea is a common sensation when contrast dye is used; have an emesis basin readily available. Some patients experience a salty taste, flushing, and a sensation of warmth during the dye injection. Encourage patients who receive dye injections to increase their fluid intake, because the dye is excreted by the kidneys and causes diuresis. Assure patients that they will be draped sufficiently to prevent unnecessary exposure.

NPO, nothing by mouth.

Continued

Table 23.1 Nursing Interventions for Diagnostic Examinations—cont'd

BEFORE EXAMINATION	AFTER EXAMINATION
Barium Enema	
Order prescribed test per facility policy. Provide needed emotional support. Instruct patient to maintain NPO status after midnight (some facilities allow liquids for breakfast). Assist patient with bowel preparation, which varies among facilities. (In elderly patients, this preparation is sometimes exhausting and even causes severe dehydration in some.) A typical day before preparation: Instruct patient to have clear liquid for lunch and supper (no dairy products). Have patient drink one glass of water or clear liquid every hour for 8–10 h. Administer a cathartic as prescribed. Keep patient on NPO status after midnight. Day of examination: Keep patient on NPO status. Administer a suppository or cleansing enema as prescribed. Pediatric patients have specific bowel preparations. Patients with an ileostomy or colostomy have special preparations. Determine whether the bowel is cleansed adequately. When fecal return is similar to clear water, preparation is adequate; if large, solid fecal waste is still being evacuated, preparation is inadequate. Notify radiologist, who, in some cases, will want to extend bowel preparation.	Allow patient to resume regular diet as soon as examination is completed. Encourage fluid intake. Monitor stools; barium sometimes causes constipation. Administer laxative after examination per facility protocol. Allow time for rest. Be aware of dehydration and electrolyte abnormalities. Inform patient that the stools will be white; when all the barium is expelled, the stool will return to normal color.
Barium Swallow	
Order prescribed test per facility policy. Obtain consent if required by facility or agency. Explain procedure. Instruct patient to maintain NPO status for at least 8 h (usually NPO after midnight). Assess patient's ability to swallow (if patient tends to aspirate, inform the radiologist). Accompany hospitalized patient to radiology department if vital signs are not stable and the test is to be performed.	Inform the patient of the need to evacuate all the barium. Advise patient that at first the stools are white but will return to normal color when evacuation is completed. NOTE: Laxatives sometimes are ordered to facilitate evacuation of barium.
Blood Chemistry Test	
Order prescribed test per facility policy. Instruct patient to maintain NPO status (as indicated). Water is permitted. Explain procedure. Prohibit smoking as per agency policy. Prohibit alcohol intake for 24 h before test. Indicate to patient that dietary intake at least 2 wk before testing will affect results.	Observe site for bleeding. Apply pressure as indicated. Ensure that patient's meal is served after test is completed. Report results. Instruct patients with high levels regarding a low-cholesterol diet, exercise, and appropriate body weight.
Body Scan[a]	
Order prescribed test per facility policy. Explain procedure. Specific anatomic locations will dictate particular interventions.	See specific anatomic locations for particular interventions.

[a]Showing a picture of the x-ray machine (used for scans and MRI) and encouraging the patient to verbalize concerns regarding claustrophobia help reduce anxiety. Most patients who are mildly claustrophobic are able to tolerate these studies after appropriate premedication with antianxiety medications. Most of these tests require lying still on a hard table and peripheral venipuncture, which sometimes cause mild discomfort. Mild nausea is a common sensation when contrast dye is used; have an emesis basin readily available. Some patients experience a salty taste, flushing, and a sensation of warmth during the dye injection. Encourage patients who receive dye injections to increase their fluid intake, because the dye is excreted by the kidneys and causes diuresis. Assure patients that they will be draped sufficiently to prevent unnecessary exposure.

Table 23.1 **Nursing Interventions for Diagnostic Examinations—cont'd**

BEFORE EXAMINATION	AFTER EXAMINATION
Bone Marrow Aspiration	
Order prescribed test per facility policy. Explain procedure. Assess coagulation study results and inform health care provider of any abnormalities. Obtain written consent. Advise patient that the procedure may cause discomfort or a feeling of pressure, but this feeling will be brief. Assist in obtaining specimens. Provide needed emotional support. Obtain order for sedative, as necessary. Remind patient to remain very still throughout procedure.	Apply pressure to puncture site. Apply adhesive dressing. Observe the puncture site for bleeding. Monitor patient for signs and symptoms of shock (e.g., increased pulse rate, decreased blood pressure) and for pain. Allow patient to resume normal activity 30–60 min after examination. Some patients need mild analgesics for tenderness at the puncture site for several days after this procedure. Instruct patient to notify health care provider if any tenderness persists or erythema occurs, because these indicate possible infection.
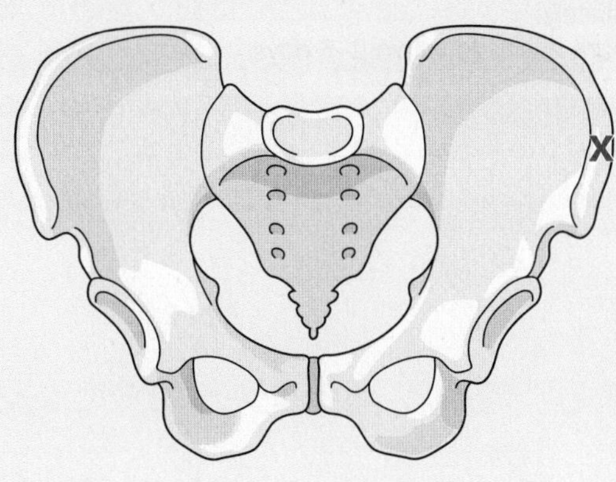	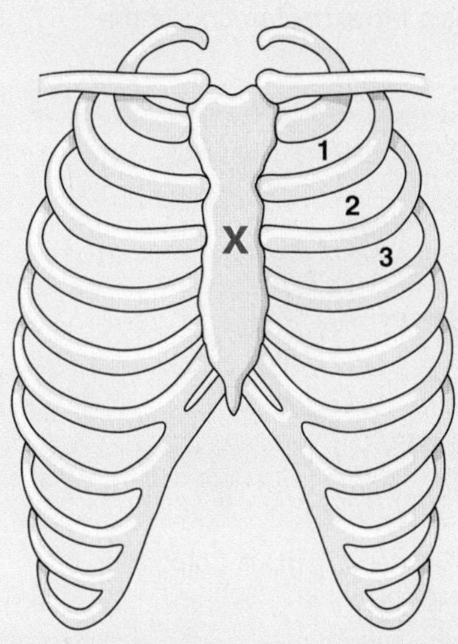 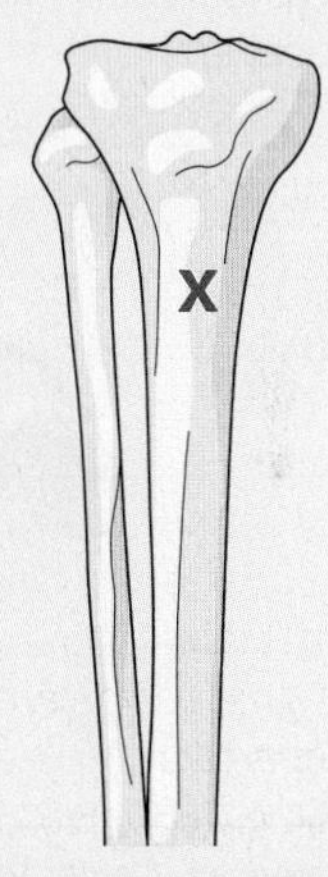
Bone Scan[a]	
Order prescribed test per facility policy. Explain procedure. Instruct patient to remove dental prosthetics, jewelry, and any metal objects. Encourage patient to drink several glasses of water. Tell the patient the injection causes slight discomfort. No fasting or sedation is required. Have patient void before examination. Assure patient that he or she will not be exposed to large amounts of radioactivity because only tracer doses of the isotope are used. Tell the patient the injection causes slight discomfort; no fasting or sedation is required.	Because only tracer doses of radioisotopes are used, no precautions must be taken to prevent radioactive exposure of other personnel or family members. Observe injection site for erythema or edema; if hematoma forms, apply warm soaks to the area to relieve pain. Assure patient that the radioactive substance is usually excreted from the body within 6–24 h. (To assess for allergic reaction, see Box 23.2.) Encourage fluid intake.
Brain Scan[a]	
Order prescribed test per facility policy. Obtain informed consent. Keep patient on NPO status for 4 h before examination if contrast dye is to be used. Instruct patient not to wear wig, hairpins, clips, or partial denture plates. Observe patient for iodine allergies. If sedation is ordered, administer sedative. Inform patient that a clicking noise will be heard as the scanner moves.	Assess patient for iodine allergies (see Box 23.2). Encourage fluid intake. Report results.

[a]Showing a picture of the x-ray machine (used for scans and MRI) and encouraging the patient to verbalize concerns regarding claustrophobia help reduce anxiety. Most patients who are mildly claustrophobic are able to tolerate these studies after appropriate premedication with antianxiety medications. Most of these tests require lying still on a hard table and peripheral venipuncture, which sometimes cause mild discomfort. Mild nausea is a common sensation when contrast dye is used; have an emesis basin readily available. Some patients experience a salty taste, flushing, and a sensation of warmth during the dye injection. Encourage patients who receive dye injections to increase their fluid intake, because the dye is excreted by the kidneys and causes diuresis. Assure patients that they will be draped sufficiently to prevent unnecessary exposure.

Continued

Table 23.1 Nursing Interventions for Diagnostic Examinations—cont'd

BEFORE EXAMINATION	AFTER EXAMINATION
Bronchoscopy	
Order prescribed test per facility policy. Explain procedure. Obtain informed consent before patient is premedicated. Instruct patient to maintain NPO status after midnight (4–8 h). Administer preoperative medication as ordered. Instruct patient to remove and safely store contact lenses, dentures, and glasses. Reassure patient that he or she will be able to breathe during procedure. Instruct patient to perform good mouth care to minimize risk of introducing bacteria into the lungs during procedure. Instruct patient not to swallow the local anesthetic sprayed into the throat. Provide a basin for expectoration of the lidocaine. 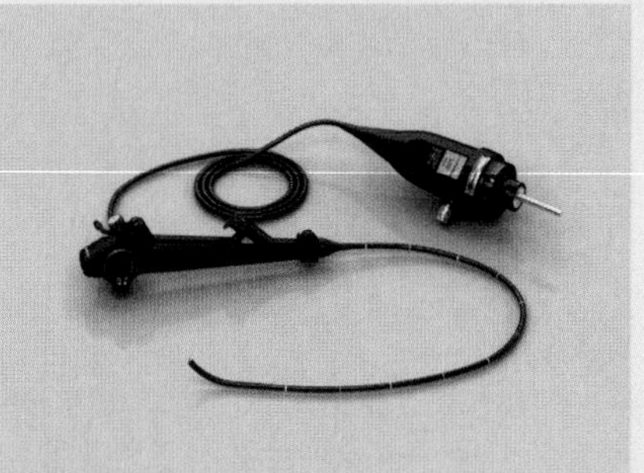 Flexible fiberoptic bronchoscope. (Courtesy Olympus Corporation of the Americas, Center Valley, Pennsylvania.)	If an anesthetic has been sprayed on the throat, do not allow the patient to eat or drink until the gag reflex returns (2–4 h). Ask patient to open mouth, and hold tongue down with tongue blade. Touch back of pharynx on each side with applicator stick. Observe any sputum for blood; small amounts are normal. Monitor vital signs frequently. Observe for impaired respirations. Observe closely until no effects of anesthesia remain. If patient complains of sore throat, provide warm saline gargles and lozenges as desired. If a tumor is suspected, collect a postbronchoscopy sputum sample for cytologic determination. Inform patient to report bronchospasms or laryngospasms immediately. Reports are available within 2–7 days.
Cardiac Catheterization	
Explain procedure. Obtain written consent. Provide needed emotional support. Instruct patient to maintain NPO status for 4–8 h. Determine whether patient has any dye allergies (see Box 23.2). Administer premedications as ordered. Prepare catheter insertion site by shaving and preparing the skin. Mark the site of the patient's peripheral pulses with a pen to facilitate postprocedure assessment. Instruct patient to void before going to the catheterization laboratory. Instruct patient to remove and safely store all valuables and dental prostheses. Obtain IV access for delivery of IV fluids and cardiac drugs, if necessary.	Monitor vital signs. Observe catheter site for bleeding; apply pressure as necessary. Encourage rest (4–8 h). Encourage fluids; monitor urinary output. Keep affected extremity extended and immobilized to decrease bleeding. Assess the patient's pulses in both extremities. Compare pulses with preprocedure marking and assessment findings. Instruct the patient that the test data will be reviewed by the cardiologist and the results will be available in 1–2 days. Perform serial neurovascular assessment on the patient's involved extremity; compare with uninvolved extremity. Instruct the patient to report any sign of numbness, tingling, pain, or loss of function in the involved extremity immediately.
Chest Radiography	
Prepare requisition form. Explain procedure; no fasting is required. Be certain that patient's gown has no snaps or pins and that the patient is not wearing a bra. Instruct patient to remove all metal objects (necklaces, pins). Tell patient that he or she will be asked to take a deep breath and to hold it while the x-ray images are taken.	Report results. NOTE: No special care is required after the procedure.

IV, Intravenous.

Table 23.1 Nursing Interventions for Diagnostic Examinations—cont'd

BEFORE EXAMINATION	AFTER EXAMINATION
Colonoscopy	
Order prescribed test per facility policy. Explain procedure. Obtain written consent. Assist with the bowel preparation. The bowel preparation ordered depends on the health care provider's preference. Avoid oral bowel preparation in patients with upper gastrointestinal obstruction or suspected acute diverticulitis or following recent bowel surgery. Assure patient that he or she will be draped appropriately to prevent unnecessary embarrassment. Administer appropriate preprocedure sedation as ordered. Record results from cathartics and enemas. Determine whether the bowel is cleansed adequately. When fecal return is similar to clear water, preparation is adequate; if large, solid fecal waste still is being evacuated, preparation is inadequate. Notify health care provider who will be performing the colonoscopy, who will in some cases want to extend the bowel preparation.	Observe for abdominal pain, tenderness, and bleeding or gas pains from air in the bowel. Examine stools for gross blood. Offer normal diet if no bowel perforation exists. Suggest a warm bath for relaxation. Allow time for rest. Monitor patient until the effects of the medications have diminished. Assess patient's vital signs. Watch for decrease in blood pressure with an increase in pulse rate as an indication of hemorrhage. Notify health care provider if patient develops increased pain or significant gastrointestinal bleeding. Examine abdomen for evidence of colon perforation (abdominal distention and tenderness). Encourage patient to drink a lot of fluids when intake is allowed. This will make up for the dehydration from the bowel preparation.
Complete Blood Cell (CBC) Count (See Skill 23.13)	
Order prescribed test per facility policy. Explain procedure.	Observe site for bleeding. Report results.
Computed Tomography (CT)[a]	
Explain procedure. Obtain informed consent if required. Assess for allergies to iodine (see Box 23.2). Inform patient that it is necessary to remove wigs, hairpins or clips, and dental prostheses if scan will include head. Maintain NPO status 4 h before oral contrast medium is administered, except in emergencies. See specific anatomic locations for particular interventions.	Encourage patient to drink fluids to prevent renal complications and to promote excretion of dye. See specific anatomic locations for particular interventions. 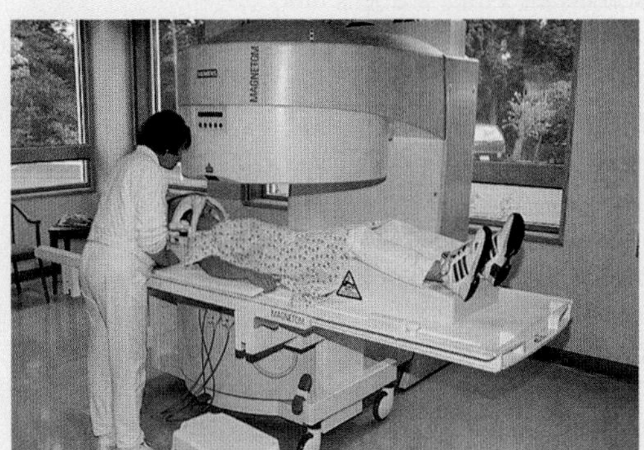 Machinery for computed tomography (CT). (From Elkin MK, Perry AG, Potter PA: *Nursing interventions and clinical skills*, ed 4, St. Louis, 2008, Mosby.)
Cystoscopy	
Explain procedure. Instruct patient to lie still during the procedure. Obtain written consent. Administer enemas as ordered, and record results. If local anesthesia is used, liquid breakfast is sometimes allowed. If general anesthesia is used, keep patient on NPO status after midnight on day of test. Administer premedications as ordered. Insert a Foley catheter if ordered.	For at least 24 h after procedure, assess patient's ability to void; urinary retention sometimes occurs secondary to edema caused by instrumentation. Record urine color; if it is bright red, report to health care provider. Suggest warm sitz baths for relaxation. Encourage fluid intake to maintain a constant flow of urine. Observe vital signs; watch for decrease in blood pressure and increase in pulse, which indicate possible hemorrhage.

[a]Showing a picture of the x-ray machine (used for scans and MRI) and encouraging the patient to verbalize concerns regarding claustrophobia help reduce anxiety. Most patients who are mildly claustrophobic are able to tolerate these studies after appropriate premedication with antianxiety medications. Most of these tests require lying still on a hard table and peripheral venipuncture, which sometimes cause mild discomfort. Mild nausea is a common sensation when contrast dye is used; have an emesis basin readily available. Some patients experience a salty taste, flushing, and a sensation of warmth during the dye injection. Encourage patients who receive dye injections to increase their fluid intake, because the dye is excreted by the kidneys and causes diuresis. Assure patients that they will be draped sufficiently to prevent unnecessary exposure.

Continued

Table 23.1 Nursing Interventions for Diagnostic Examinations—cont'd

BEFORE EXAMINATION	AFTER EXAMINATION
	Observe for hemorrhage and for sepsis. Administer antibiotic as ordered. Instruct patient not to walk or stand alone immediately after legs have been removed from stirrups. The orthostatic hypotension that sometimes results from standing erect has the potential to cause vertigo or syncope. Mild analgesics sometimes are ordered for back pain, bladder spasms, and burning on urination. Antibiotics occasionally are ordered, to be taken 1 day before and 3 days after procedure. Encourage patient to prevent constipation. (Increases in intraabdominal pressure have the capacity to initiate severe lower urologic bleeding.) Postprocedure irrigation sometimes is ordered. If catheter remains in, provide catheter care instructions.
Echocardiography	
Order prescribed test per facility policy. Review pertinent patient history. Explain procedure; it is a painless study. Answer questions. NOTE: This procedure usually takes 45 min.	Remove the gel from the patient's chest wall with a tissue. Inform patient that the results will be available in a few hours after the health care provider has interpreted the findings.
Electrocardiography (See Skill 23.14)	
Order prescribed test per facility policy. Review all medications the patient is taking. Explain procedure. No food or fluid restriction is necessary. Expose only the patient's chest and arms. Keep the abdomen and thighs adequately covered. Assure the patient that they will not feel anything during this procedure.	Remove electrodes and gel from patient's skin with a tissue. If patient experiences chest pain during the study, indicate this on the ECG strip or request slip (it is possible that the pain will correspond to a dysrhythmia on the ECG tracing).
Electroencephalography (EEG)	
Order prescribed test per facility policy. Explain procedure. Make sure patient's hair is clean; administer shampoo as necessary; do not use any oils, sprays, or lotions. Confer with health care provider regarding the need to discontinue any medications before examination. Do not administer sedatives or hypnotics, unless ordered. Encourage food intake, but instruct patient to eliminate coffee, tea, and colas. Explain need to patient of remaining still during test; even blinking will create interference. If sleeping time is to be shortened the night before the test, instruct patient accordingly.	Assist the patient in removing the electrode paste with acetone or witch hazel. Shampoo patient's hair. Ensure safety precautions until no effects of the sedatives remain; keep side rails up. Ensure that the patient who has had sleep EEG does not have to drive home alone.
Endoscopy and Gastroscopy	
Order prescribed test per facility policy. Administer premedication, if ordered. Explain procedure. Obtain written consent before administering medication. Keep patient on NPO status after midnight. Provide emotional support.	Perform oral hygiene measures. If an anesthetic has been sprayed on the throat, do not allow the patient to eat or drink until the gag reflex returns (2–4 h). Ask patient to open mouth, and hold patient's tongue down with tongue blade. Touch back of pharynx on each side with applicator stick.

Table 23.1 Nursing Interventions for Diagnostic Examinations—cont'd

BEFORE EXAMINATION	AFTER EXAMINATION
Remove and safely store patient's dentures and eyewear. Perform oral hygiene measures, because the tube will pass through the mouth. Reassure the patient that the procedure is not painful. In most of these procedures, conscious sedation is used, which is the administration of central nervous system depressant drugs or analgesics to supplement topical, local, or regional anesthesia during surgical or diagnostic procedures. It is used most often to supplement analgesia, relieve anxiety, or provide amnesia for the event. Consciousness is depressed, and some patients fall asleep but are not unconscious. Patients "wake up" in 20–30 min with no memory and no sense of the passage of time. If the patient's throat is to be sprayed with an anesthetic, caution patient that he or she will not be able to speak during the examination, but respiration will not be affected. Check the patient for gag reflex. Instruct the patient not to bite down on the endoscope.	If conscious sedation has been used, monitor patient carefully, because oversedation or adverse response to sedation has the potential to result in life-threatening complications, such as hypotension, loss of airway reflexes, inability to maintain patent airway, hypoventilation, and apnea. Explain that drinking cool fluids and gargling helps relieve some soreness. Observe the patient for bleeding, fever, abdominal pain, dysphagia, and dyspnea. Notify health care provider immediately if these occur. Monitor vital signs. Observe safety precautions until no effects of the sedatives remain. Inform patient that it is normal to have some bloating, belching, and flatulence after the procedure. 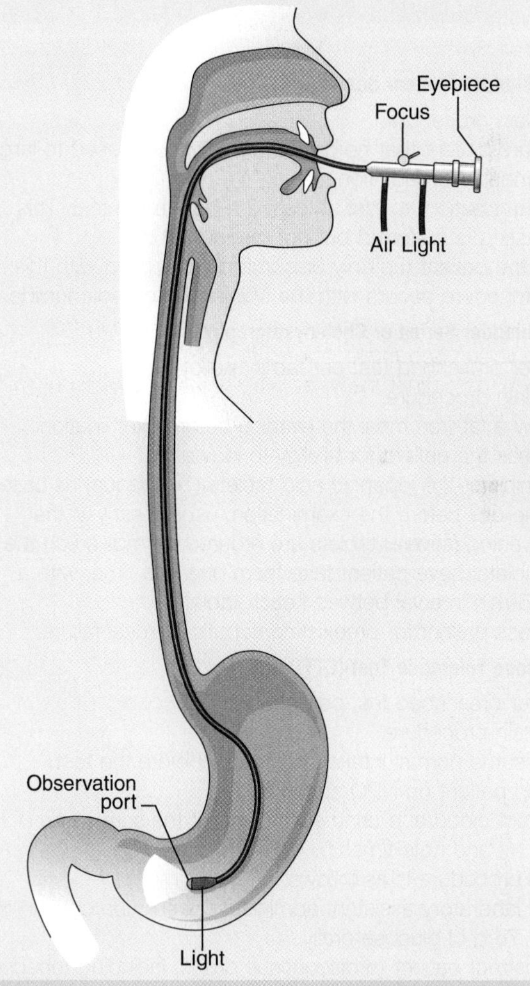
Exercise Tolerance Test (Treadmill)	
Explain procedure. Keep patient on NPO status for 4 h before the test, except for water, unless medications are otherwise ordered. Never withhold heart medications. Instruct patient not to smoke. Instruct patient to wear suitable clothing; slippers are not acceptable.	Have patient resume diet as usual. Have patient resume medication regimen. Have patient rest supine for several hours after examination. Instruct patient not to shower immediately after examination. Monitor and record vital signs until recordings and values return to pretest levels. Remove electrodes and paste or gel from patient's skin.

Continued

Table 23.1 Nursing Interventions for Diagnostic Examinations—cont'd

BEFORE EXAMINATION	AFTER EXAMINATION
Inform patient about the risks of the test, and obtain informed consent. Inform patient of any medications that must be discontinued before testing. Record patient's vital signs for baseline values. Apply and secure appropriate electrodes. Obtain a pretest ECG.	
Femoral Angiography (See Arteriography)	
Provide emotional support. Observe patient for allergies to iodine dye (see Box 23.2). Obtain written consent. Keep patient on NPO status after midnight.	Observe catheter insertion site for inflammation, hemorrhage, or hematoma, and observe for absence of peripheral pulses. Observe the involved extremity for numbness, tingling, pain, or loss of function. Monitor vital signs. Apply cold compresses to the puncture site as needed to reduce discomfort and edema. If patient complains of continuous, severe pain, notify health care provider.
Gallbladder Nuclear Scanning[b]	
Explain procedure. Assure patient that he or she will not be exposed to large amounts of radiation. Instruct patient to fast at least 2 h before the test. This fasting is preferred but not mandatory. Tell the patient the only discomfort associated with this procedure occurs with the IV injection of radionuclide.	Obtain a meal for the patient if indicated.
Gallbladder Series or Cholecystography	
Order prescribed test per facility policy. Explain procedure. Allow a fat-free meal the evening before examination. Assess the patient for allergy to iodine. Administer the iopanoic acid tablets (Telepaque) as ordered the day before the examination, usually early in the evening (several tablets are ordered; do not crush the tablets; have patient take them one at a time, with a 15-min interval between each tablet). Assess patient for preexisting hepatic or renal failure.	Monitor patient for side effects to the tablets, such as nausea, vomiting, diarrhea, abdominal pain, rash, and anaphylaxis. (If diarrhea develops before the examination, it is possible that the radiopaque dye will not be absorbed and, as a result, the gallbladder will not be visualized.) Instruct patient to resume usual diet as soon as series is completed. No other postprocedure care is necessary.
Glucose Tolerance Test (GTT)	
Order prescribed test per facility policy. Explain procedure. Consume normal intake in the days before the test. Keep patient on NPO status for 8 h. Collect blood and urine specimens at the same time (1 h, 3 h), and note times.[c] The procedure is as follows: A laboratory assistant administers a solution containing 75 g of glucose orally. Instruct patient to discontinue drugs, including tobacco, that have potential to interfere with test results. Consult health care provider. If necessary, give patient written instructions concerning the test requirements. Obtain patient's weight to determine the appropriate loading dose.	Mark on the tube the times specimens are collected. Send all specimens promptly to the laboratory. Observe venipuncture site for bleeding; apply pressure as necessary. Make certain patient receives meal when test is completed. Report results. An elevated blood glucose level at the 2-h point usually indicates some disorder of carbohydrate metabolism; depending on how elevated the blood glucose level is, glucose may be present in the urine. Administer insulin or oral hypoglycemic, if ordered.

[b]Gallbladder nuclear scanning has replaced the gallbladder series.
[c]Specific collection times depend on health care provider's orders.

Table 23.1 Nursing Interventions for Diagnostic Examinations—cont'd

BEFORE EXAMINATION	AFTER EXAMINATION
Hematest of Stools (Guaiac): Hemoccult Slide Test (See Skill 23.7)	
Explain procedure. Assist patient in obtaining specimens. There are many options for type of procedural materials (cards, tissue wipes, test paper). Tests often are permitted to be done at home with cards (Hemoccult) that can be mailed when the specimen is collected. Inform patient of the need for obtaining multiple specimens on separate days to increase test accuracy. Document specimens as sent to laboratory. Instruct patient not to eat foods that may affect the test for at least 3 days before the test. Foods include red meat, cantaloupe, uncooked broccoli, and turnips. Medications that can affect the test results include vitamin C, aspirin, and NSAID medications and should be held in the days preceding the test if approved of by the health care provider. Instruct patient not to mix urine with the stool specimen. Some laboratories recommend a high-residue diet to increase abrasive effect of stool. Note on laboratory slip any anticoagulants or medications the patient is taking. Be gentle when obtaining stool by digital rectal examination. Traumatic digital examination can cause a false-positive result, especially in patients with prior anorectal disease such as hemorrhoids.	No specific follow-up care is necessary. Read results and inform patient. If test results are positive, ascertain whether the patient violated any of the preparation recommendations.
Intravenous Pyelography (IVP) or Intravenous Urography (IUG)	
Order prescribed test per facility policy. Be certain IVP is done before any barium studies. Explain procedure to patient. Check for allergies to iodine and shellfish (the intravenous dye contains iodine). Administer cathartics or laxatives as ordered (children and infants are not given cathartics or laxatives). Keep patient on NPO status after midnight (if an IV solution is infusing, ask whether health care provider wishes to decrease infusion to keep-open rate to prevent hydration; for IVP, fluid restriction is necessary for the dye to be taken up by the kidneys). Some facilities prefer abstinence from solid food for 8 h before testing; some allow a clear liquid breakfast on test day. Assess the patient's blood urea nitrogen (BUN) and creatinine levels. (Renal function that is already abnormal sometimes deteriorates further as a result of the dye injection.) Give patient an enema or suppository on the morning of study, if ordered. NOTE: Indicate specific fasting times for older adults and debilitated patients.	Observe for anaphylaxis (respiratory distress, shock, and drop in blood pressure) (see Box 23.2). Allow patient normal diet. Encourage fluid intake to help eliminate any dye left in body and counteract any fluid depletion. Encourage patient to ambulate with assistance unless contraindicated. Some patients will be weak because of the fasting and catharsis necessary for test preparation. Assess urinary output (a decreased output indicates possible renal failure).
Kidney, Ureter, and Bladder X-Ray Study (KUB, Flat Plate of the Abdomen)	
Order prescribed test per facility policy. Explain procedure; no GI contrast media will be used. No fasting or sedation is required. Schedule this study before any barium studies. Ensure all radiopaque clothing has been removed.	No specific follow-up. Report results to health care provider. Schedule IVP or gastrointestinal studies after completion of the KUB.

GI, Gastrointestinal.

Continued

Table 23.1 Nursing Interventions for Diagnostic Examinations—cont'd

BEFORE EXAMINATION	AFTER EXAMINATION
Liver Biopsy	
Explain procedure. Obtain written consent. Assess blood coagulation profile; it must be normal for study to proceed. Keep patient on NPO status after midnight before examination. Assist health care provider. Send specimens to laboratory promptly. Have specimen placed in proper **fixative** (any substance used to preserve gross or histologic specimens of tissue for later examination); usually 10% formalin is used, but confirm with laboratory or pathologist. If liver specimen is for detection of lymphoma, saline solution is used. Administer any sedative medications as ordered. 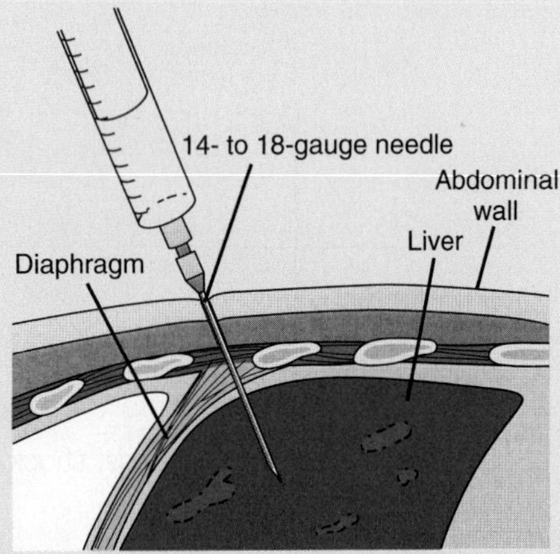 Liver biopsy: Percutaneous liver biopsy requires the patient's cooperation. The patient has to be able to lie quietly and hold his or her breath after exhaling. (From Pagana KD, Pagana TJ: *Mosby's diagnostic and laboratory test reference*, ed 12, St. Louis, 2015, Mosby.)	Keep patient on bed rest for 24 h. Keep patient on right side for about 1–2 h immediately after the procedure. (In this position, the liver capsule is compressed against the chest wall, thereby decreasing the risk of hemorrhage or bile leak.) Observe for hemorrhage. Apply pressure dressing. Monitor vital signs frequently for evidence of hemorrhage (i.e., increased pulse and decreased blood pressure) and for peritonitis (i.e., increased temperature). Observe biopsy site. Tell patient to avoid coughing or straining, which tend to increase intraabdominal pressure. Instruct patient to avoid strenuous activities and heavy lifting for 1–2 wk. Evaluate the rate, rhythm, and depth of respirations. Assess breath sounds. Report chest pain and signs of dyspnea, cyanosis, and restlessness (indicate possible pneumothorax).
Lumbar Puncture (Spinal Tap)	
Explain procedure. Obtain written consent. Have patient empty bladder and bowel. No fasting or sedation is required before procedure. Provide necessary equipment. Assist patient in assuming appropriate position. Hold manometer straight, if requested. Label and number specimen containers. Perform baseline neurologic assessment of the legs by assessing patient's strength, sensation, and movement. Explain to patient that it is necessary to lie very still throughout procedure (movement has potential to cause injury). Encourage patient to relax and take deep, slow breaths with mouth open.	Apply digital pressure and an adhesive dressing to the puncture site. Notify health care provider if any unusual findings from puncture site occur. Encourage fluids (using a drinking straw so that patient can keep head flat). Usually patient is kept in the supine position with the head of the bed elevated no more than 30 degrees until activity is changed by the health care provider to prevent discomfort from potential postpuncture spinal headache. Allow patient to turn from side to side as long as head is not raised. Transport specimens to laboratory immediately (refrigeration will alter test results). A delay between collection time and testing can result in invalid results, especially cell counts. Instruct patient to report any abnormalities such as numbness and tingling in the legs. Assess patient for numbness, tingling, and movement of the extremities; pain at the injection site; drainage of blood or CSF at the injection site; and the ability to void. Notify health care provider of any unusual findings.

CSF, Cerebrospinal fluid.

Table 23.1 Nursing Interventions for Diagnostic Examinations—cont'd

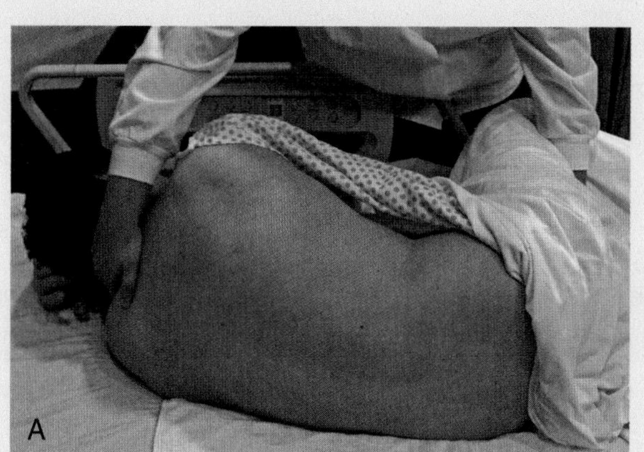
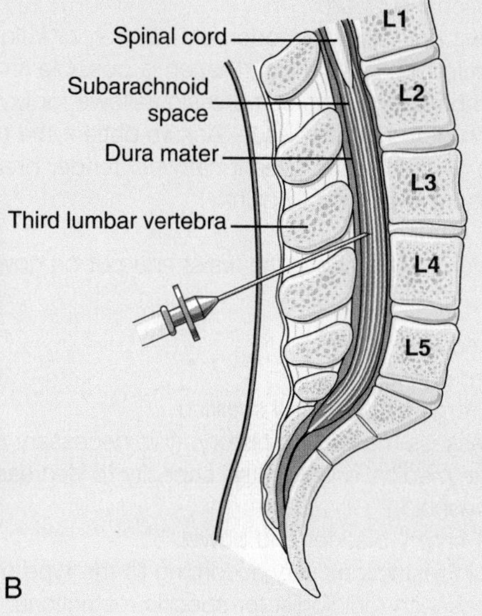

Position of patient (A) and site of needle insertion (B) for lumbar puncture.

BEFORE EXAMINATION	AFTER EXAMINATION
Lung Scan[a]	
Order prescribed test per facility policy. Obtain informed consent if required by facility. Explain procedure. Observe the patient for allergies to iodine (see Box 23.2). Keep patient on NPO status for 4 h before test if contrast medium is administered. Have a recent chest radiograph available. Remove jewelry around the chest area.	Apply pressure to venipuncture site. Encourage fluid intake. No radiation precautions are necessary. Encourage patients who received dye injection to increase fluid intake because the dye causes diuresis.
Magnetic Resonance Imaging (MRI), Nuclear Magnetic Resonance Imaging (NMRI)[a]	
Order prescribed test per facility policy. Explain procedure. Obtain informed consent. Assess the patient for any contraindications to testing (e.g., aneurysm clips, plates, pacemaker, spinal cord stimulator, and shrapnel). Instruct patient to remove all metal objects: dentures, partial dentures, jewelry, hairpins, and belts; provide safe storage. Inform patient of the need to remain motionless during the test. Have patient empty bladder for comfort. Encourage adults to read or talk to pediatric patients in scanning room. Some patients experience claustrophobia; antianxiety medications are often helpful. Explain that during the procedure, patient will hear a thumping sound. (Earplugs are available if the patient wishes to use them.) There are no food or fluid restrictions.	No postprocedure care is necessary. Patient is permitted to drive without assistance after procedure. 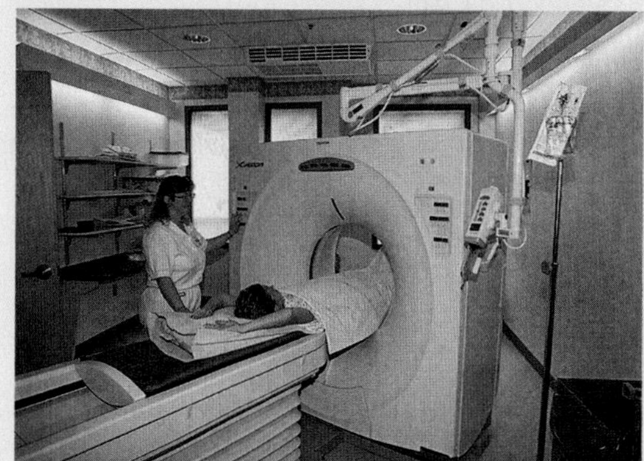 Assisting with magnetic resonance imaging (MRI). (From Elkin MK, Perry AG, Potter PA: *Nursing interventions and clinical skills*, ed 4, St. Louis, 2008, Mosby.)
Mammography	
Order prescribed test per facility policy. Explain procedure. If patient is embarrassed by the procedure, ask patient to verbalize her feelings.	Explain how to obtain test results. Instruct patient on breast self-examination.

[a]Showing a picture of the x-ray machine (used for scans and MRI) and encouraging the patient to verbalize concerns regarding claustrophobia help reduce anxiety. Most patients who are mildly claustrophobic are able to tolerate these studies after appropriate premedication with antianxiety medications. Most of these tests require lying still on a hard table and peripheral venipuncture, which sometimes cause mild discomfort. Mild nausea is a common sensation when contrast dye is used; have an emesis basin readily available. Some patients experience a salty taste, flushing, and a sensation of warmth during the dye injection. Encourage patients who receive dye injections to increase their fluid intake, because the dye is excreted by the kidneys and causes diuresis. Assure patients that they will be draped sufficiently to prevent unnecessary exposure.

Continued

Table 23.1 Nursing Interventions for Diagnostic Examinations—cont'd

BEFORE EXAMINATION	AFTER EXAMINATION
Provide emotional support. Instruct patient not to wear deodorant, powder, or lotion. Some discomfort during the examination is possible (from breast compression). This compression allows for better visualization of the breast tissue. Assure patient the breast will not be harmed. If the patient has very tender breasts, this procedure is potentially painful. No fasting is required. Patient should disrobe above the waist and put on gown.	
Myelography	
Explain procedure. Obtain written consent. Assess for allergies to dye and shellfish. Obtain and assess medication history. (It is necessary to avoid some medications with the capacity to decrease seizure threshold.) Have patient empty bladder and bowel. Food and fluid restrictions vary according to the type of dye used. Check with radiologist for specific restrictions. Instruct patient to lie very still during procedure. Inform patient that he or she will be tilted into an up-and-down position on the table so that the dye can fill the spinal canal properly and provide adequate visualization in the desired area.	If necessary, assist with proper positioning, as prescribed by the health care provider. Usually, the patient is on bed rest for several hours. The head position varies with the dye used. (Examples: Elevate the head after using oil-based and water-soluble agents. After an air-contrast study, position the head lower than the rest of the body.) Observe the patient for fever, stiff neck, occipital headache, or photophobia, which are signs and symptoms of meningeal irritation. Monitor vital signs. Monitor ability to void. Encourage fluids so that patient does not get dehydrated; dehydration will result in a severe headache. Observe for seizure activity, which some types of dye potentially cause.
Paracentesis	
Explain procedure. Obtain written consent. Provide emotional support. Obtain equipment. Assist health care provider. No fasting or sedation is necessary. Have patient urinate before the test (helps prevent accidental bladder trauma). Measure abdominal girth. Measure patient's weight. Measure baseline vital signs. Although local anesthetics eliminate pain at insertion site, tell patient that he or she will feel a pressure-like pain as the needle is inserted. 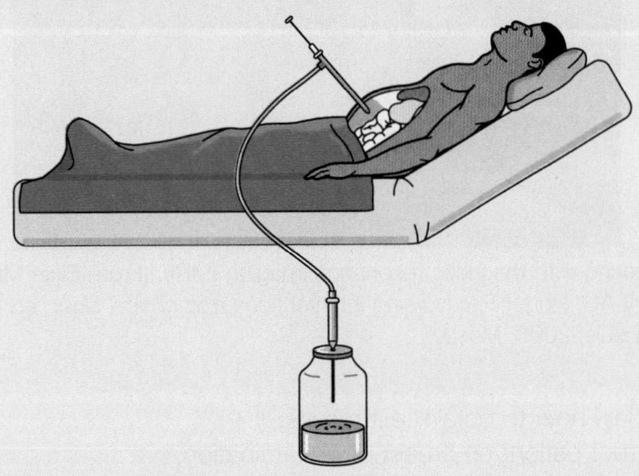 Paracentesis. A catheter is placed through the skin and the abdominal muscle wall into the peritoneal cavity that contains free fluid. (From Pagana KD, Pagana TJ: *Mosby's diagnostic and laboratory test reference*, ed 12, St. Louis, 2015, Mosby.)	Observe for syncope. Monitor vital signs. Encourage a period of rest after examination. Send specimen to laboratory for examination, if requested. (It is necessary to perform all laboratory tests immediately to ensure accuracy of results. Label all specimen containers appropriately.) Observe puncture site for bleeding, continued drainage, or signs of inflammation. Measure abdominal girth and weight of the patient, and compare measurements with baseline values. Observe for signs of hypotension if a large volume of fluid was removed. Record any recent antibiotic therapy on requisition slip. Monitor serum protein and electrolyte levels, especially sodium (protein content of ascitic fluid is high). Occasionally, fluid continues to leak from the needle tract. It is possible to stop this with a suture. If the suture is unsuccessful, apply a collection bag to the skin to allow for measurement of volume of fluid and treatment of fluid loss.

Table 23.1 Nursing Interventions for Diagnostic Examinations—cont'd

BEFORE EXAMINATION	AFTER EXAMINATION
Positron Emission Tomography (PET)	
Order prescribed test per facility policy. Obtain informed consent. Instruct patient not to have alcohol, caffeine, tobacco, sedatives, or tranquilizers for 24 h before examination; no other restrictions are necessary. Have patient empty bladder before examination. Explain procedure (because many patients have not heard of this study, they are often anxious and require emotional support). Excessive anxiety has the capacity to affect brain function evaluation. Inform patient that two IV lines probably will be inserted: one for infusion of the isotope and the other for serial blood samples. Instruct patients with diabetes to take their pretest dose of insulin at a meal 3–4 h before the test. High glucose levels potentially will decrease accuracy and invalidate results of PET scans. Inform patient that the only discomfort associated with this study is the insertion of the two IV lines.	Instruct patient to change position slowly from lying to standing to prevent postural hypotension. Encourage patient to drink fluids and urinate frequently to aid in removal of the radioisotope from the bladder. Report results.
Proctoscopy and Sigmoidoscopy	
Order prescribed test per facility policy. Explain procedure. Provide emotional support. Obtain written consent. Allow patient a light breakfast on day of examination. Administer enemas as ordered and record results. In most cases, two Fleet enemas are sufficient. Ensure patient is draped properly to prevent unnecessary embarrassment. Inform patient that he or she will feel discomfort and the urge to defecate as the proctoscope or sigmoidoscope is inserted. 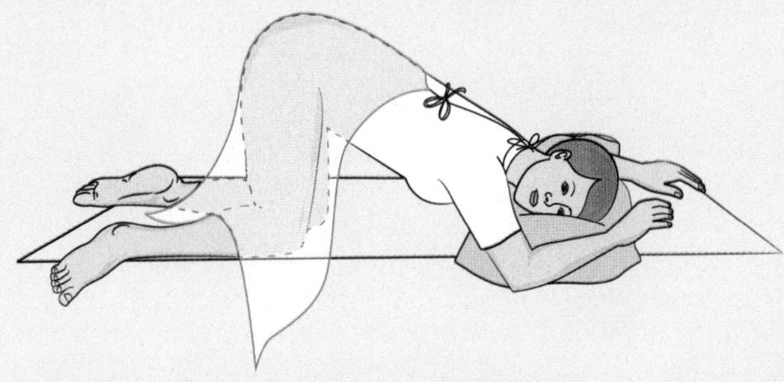 Position for proctoscopy.	Observe the patient for fever, rectal bleeding, abdominal distention, unusual complaints of pain, and increased tenderness. Inform patient that because air has been insufflated into the bowel during the procedure, he or she may have flatulence or gas pains. Ambulation often helps. If biopsy samples have been taken, slight rectal bleeding is possible. Instruct patient to report increasing abdominal pain (indicates possible bowel perforation). Fever and chills are further indications of a possible bowel perforation. Inform patient that frequent bloody bowel movements possibly indicate poor hemostasis if biopsy or polypectomy was performed. Observe for abdominal bloating and inability to pass flatus, which indicates possible colon obstruction, if a neoplasm was identified.
Renal Angiography	
Explain procedure. Answer questions. Obtain written consent. Determine whether patient has been taking anticoagulants. Assess patient for allergy to iodine dye (see Box 23.2). Keep patient on NPO status at least 2–8 h before testing. Administer cathartics as ordered. Administer premedications. Advise patient that he or she may experience flushing and a sensation of warmth when dye is injected. Mark the site of the peripheral pulses with a pen (allows for postprocedure assessment).	Observe arterial puncture site frequently; apply pressure dressings. Monitor the extremity for adequate circulation. Monitor pedal pulses and vital signs frequently. Keep patient on bed rest for about 8 h (this will allow for complete sealing of the arterial puncture site). Inform patient that cold compresses to puncture site will help reduce discomfort and edema. Encourage intake of fluids. Assess peripheral arterial pulse in the extremity used for vascular access and compare with preprocedure baseline values.

Continued

Table 23.1 Nursing Interventions for Diagnostic Examinations—cont'd

BEFORE EXAMINATION	AFTER EXAMINATION
Document abnormalities in peripheral pulses. Ensure that the appropriate coagulation studies have been performed and results are normal. Remove and safely store all valuables and dental prostheses. Have patient void (the dye sometimes acts as a diuretic). Inform patient that bladder distention sometimes causes some discomfort during the study.	Maintain pressure at the puncture site with 1- to 2-lb sandbag or IV bag. Assess extremities for signs of reduction in blood supply (i.e., absence of pulses, numbness, pallor, tingling pain, loss of sensory or motor function). Note and compare the color and temperature of the involved extremity with those of the uninvolved extremity. Notify health care provider if there is severe, continuous pain. Encourage fluids to prevent dehydration caused by diuretic action of the dye. Evaluate for delayed reaction to dye. Administer mild analgesics for minor discomfort at arterial puncture site.
Thoracentesis	
Explain procedure. Obtain written consent. Obtain equipment. Assist patient in assuming the appropriate position (usually sitting). Offer emotional support. No fasting or sedation is necessary. Advise patient to keep movement or coughing to a minimum to prevent the needle from causing damage to the lung or the pleura during procedure. Administer cough suppressant if patient has troublesome cough. A radiograph or ultrasound scan often is used to assist in location of the fluid. Fluoroscopy may also be used. Inform patient that although local anesthetics eliminate pain at the insertion site, a pressure-like pain is possible when the pleura is entered and the fluid is removed. 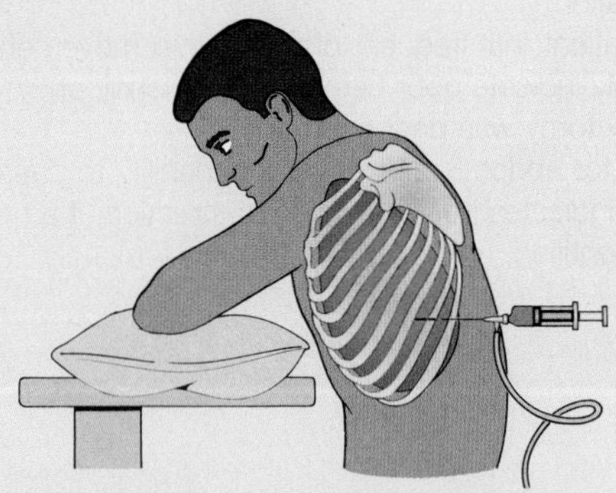 Patient positioning for thoracentesis. (From Beare PG, Myers JL: *Adult health nursing*, ed 3, St. Louis, 1998, Mosby.)	Monitor vital signs. Monitor patient for coughing or for hemoptysis, which indicates possible trauma to the lung. If patient has no complaints of dyspnea, he or she may resume normal activity in an hour. Place small dressing over needle site. Usually, you will turn patient on the unaffected side for 1 h to allow the puncture site to seal. Label specimen containers appropriately and send promptly to the laboratory. Obtain chest radiograph, if ordered, to assess for pneumothorax. Assess patient for signs and symptoms of subcutaneous emphysema or infection (e.g., tachypnea, dyspnea, diminished breath sounds, anxiety, restlessness, fever). Assess patient's lungs for diminished breath sounds, which are a sign of possible pneumothorax.
Ultrasonography or Sonography[a]	
Order prescribed test per facility policy. Explain procedure. If a pelvic sonogram is ordered, the patient needs a full bladder. If a gallbladder sonogram is ordered, keep patient on NPO status. For other sonograms, no fasting or sedation is needed. Obtain a signed consent form, if required.	Because this procedure is noninvasive, no specific follow-up care is needed. Patient should resume usual diet after examination. Remove the lubricant from the patient's skin. Encourage voiding.

[a]Showing a picture of the x-ray machine (used for scans and MRI) and encouraging the patient to verbalize concerns regarding claustrophobia help reduce anxiety. Most patients who are mildly claustrophobic are able to tolerate these studies after appropriate premedication with antianxiety medications. Most of these tests require lying still on a hard table and peripheral venipuncture, which sometimes cause mild discomfort. Mild nausea is a common sensation when contrast dye is used; have an emesis basin readily available. Some patients experience a salty taste, flushing, and a sensation of warmth during the dye injection. Encourage patients who receive dye injections to increase their fluid intake, because the dye is excreted by the kidneys and causes diuresis. Assure patients that they will be draped sufficiently to prevent unnecessary exposure.

Table 23.1 Nursing Interventions for Diagnostic Examinations—cont'd

BEFORE EXAMINATION	AFTER EXAMINATION
Upper Gastrointestinal Series	
Prepare requisition form. Explain procedure, and answer questions. Offer emotional support; the test will not cause discomfort. Keep patient on NPO status for at least 8 h before examination. Advise patient of potential discomfort from lying on the hard table and possible sensation of bloating or nausea during the test.	Permit patient to eat as soon as series is completed, unless food is contraindicated. Encourage intake of fluids. Administer barium liquid or per hospital protocol. Inform patient that if diatrizoate (Gastrografin) was used as contrast medium, significant diarrhea is possible. Monitor stools to make certain all of the barium has been eliminated. Initial stools will be chalky in appearance. The stools usually return to normal color after complete expulsion of the barium, which sometimes takes as long as a day and a half.
Urinalysis (UA)	
Order prescribed test per facility policy. Explain purpose and specific method of urine collection. Wash patient's perineal area, if soiled. If patient is menstruating, note this on requisition form. Use midstream urine collection guidelines (see Skill 23.2).	Take specimen to laboratory promptly. If it is not processed immediately, refrigerate specimen. If 24-h urine collection is requested, refrigerate specimen or preserve with formalin when collected. It is necessary to perform examination for casts on fresh urine specimens.

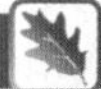

Lifespan Considerations

Older Adults

Specimen Collection and Diagnostic Tests

- Because of the degree of agility necessary to collect a midstream specimen, greater assistance from the nurse or catheterization of the older person is sometimes necessary. It is important to explain the purpose of the procedure and provide privacy during specimen collection.
- The use of medications (such as hypnotics and opioids) to reduce pain and anxiety during a procedure may impair respiratory and renal functioning. Monitoring vital signs and intake and output is necessary.
- Decreased peripheral circulation sometimes makes it difficult to collect a specimen for blood glucose determination. Wrapping the hand in a warm, moist washcloth or massaging the hand for a few minutes may facilitate the procedure.
- Changes in blood vessels make venipuncture more difficult in many older adults. Repeated sticks to obtain blood samples pose the risk of causing emotional and physical trauma to the older adult. Care should be taken to avoid multiple venipunctures.
- Collect stool specimens from older adults by using a bedpan or specimen pan in the toilet or commode.
- Assessment of certain specimens involves comparing results to a color chart. Older adults may have difficulty reading the color chart.
- Many older adults need a written reminder placed on the bathroom mirror to collect all urine samples during a 24-hour specimen collection.
- When obtaining a specimen through venipuncture, remember that some older adults do not need a tourniquet for this procedure.
- Older adults have fragile veins that are traumatized easily during venipuncture.
- If multiple procedures are necessary, schedule adequate rest time between tests.
- Restlessness after a procedure in an older adult possibly indicates hypoxia or pain. Assess the patient thoroughly for the cause.
- Many older adult patients take multiple medications. Keep in mind that alterations in administration schedules are sometimes necessary because NPO status may be required for certain diagnostic tests.
- In older adults, slight variations in vital signs or in behavior often indicate impending problems; therefore skilled observations are critical.
- Be aware that NPO status in an older adult patient may result in dehydration.
- Many older adults have difficulty assuming various positions needed for specimen collection. Give assistance before and during procedure.
- If a patient is confused, it is sometimes useful for an assistant to comfort the patient.
- Older adults are at greater risk for skin impairment. Assess skin integrity of a patient after he or she has lain on the examination table.
- Older adults often need additional clothing, slippers, and extra blankets to keep them warm in waiting rooms and examination rooms.

Cultural Considerations

Diagnostic Testing

- If the patient's language skills are inadequate for communication, assistance from interpreters, word signs, or charts may be necessary.
- A patient who is modest and self-conscious about the body will need psychological preparation before some procedures and tests.
- Patients may fear medical facilities because of language barriers, unfamiliarity with the facilities, or inadequate understanding of illness and treatment regimen. As a result, they may not comply with medical regimens.
- Be aware that diverse age groups and sociocultural groups typically use different words to describe urine and stool.
- Avoid cultural conflicts by communicating with the patient and respecting the ethnicity and individuality of each patient.

Patient Teaching

Specimen Collection and Diagnostic Tests

- Explain importance of collecting specimens on time and in the correct amount.
- Explain importance of specimen collection (why it is performed).
- Explain appropriate hand hygiene, and instruct patient to perform it before and after specimen collection.
- Explain proper procedure for obtaining each specimen and preparing for each diagnostic examination.
- Some specimen collection is completed outside the health care facility. Make certain patient understands how to complete the collection. Ask patient to perform return demonstration of obtaining a specimen. Example: Skin puncture for measuring blood glucose level
- If dietary restrictions are required, explain importance of adhering to direction. Example: A meat-free diet often is ordered before a stool specimen for occult blood.
- Explain results of test when applicable. Example: Complete blood cell count
- Explain normal laboratory values when appropriate. Example: Blood glucose levels desired
- Explain when to notify health care provider. Example: Elevated blood glucose level
- Advise patient to perform oral hygiene after sputum collection as a comfort measure.
- Explain the importance of drinking fluids to decrease thickness of mucus (this is helpful before sputum collection).
- Ensure that patient understands the importance of obtaining an uncontaminated specimen.
- Allow time for patient questions and provide answers.
- Instruct patient to check with the primary health care provider about taking, or readjusting the time schedule for, prescribed medications on the day of the test or examination.

Box 23.3 Preventing Inaccuracy in Examination and Test Procedures

Many factors have the capacity to interfere with examinations and tests and potentially can alter the accuracy of or even nullify their results:

- Drug interactions
- Insufficient bowel cleansing
- Failure to maintain fasting requirements
- Inadequate diet preparation
- Incompleteness or absence of test requisition
- Specimen not delivered on schedule
- Inappropriate specimen amount
- Contamination of sterile specimen
- Absence of required informed consent

SPECIMEN COLLECTION

The nurse is often responsible for collecting specimens that have been ordered. Laboratory examination of specimens of urine, stool, sputum, blood, and wound drainage provides important information about body functioning and contributes to the assessment of the patient's health status. Laboratory test results often facilitate the diagnosis of health care problems, provide information about the stage and activity of a disease process, and measure the response to therapy.

Patients often experience embarrassment or discomfort when giving a sample of body excretions or secretions. Most people believe excretions should be handled discreetly; affording the patient privacy is helpful in achieving comfort during the sample collection. Anxiety also is provoked by the invasive nature of some collection procedures, as is the fear of what the test results will reveal. Patients given a clear explanation about the purpose of the specimen and how it is to be obtained will be more cooperative in its collection. With proper instruction, many patients can obtain their own specimens of urine, stool, and sputum, thus minimizing embarrassment. Often the success of specimen collection depends on cooperation.

GUIDELINES FOR SPECIMEN COLLECTION

Laboratory tests are often expensive. Help prevent unnecessary costs by using the correct procedures for obtaining and processing specimens (Box 23.3). When a patient has questions about laboratory tests, consult the agency's procedure manual or call the laboratory.

It is the nurse's responsibility to notify the prescribing health care provider when results of laboratory and diagnostic studies deviate from the norm and intervention is necessary. Each health care facility has its own policy and procedure manuals. These manuals (often in electronic form) contain routine orders for each diagnostic test. The manuals are a valuable resource that prevents the nurse from overlooking critical patient preparation information or the need to take action or notify the prescribing health care provider of results.

Remembering the meaning of root words, prefixes, and suffixes helps in identifying test names. Knowing the following suffixes is useful:

-ography	Procedure in which an image is produced (e.g., mammography)
-ogram	Actual image or results of a test (e.g., mammogram)
-oscopy	Procedure in which body structures are visualized (e.g., colonoscopy)
-centesis	Procedure involving puncture of a body cavity (e.g., thoracentesis)

Box 23.4 lists general guidelines for specimen collection.

COLLECTING A MIDSTREAM URINE SPECIMEN

There are several methods for collecting a urine **specimen** (a small sample of something, intended to show the nature of the whole) for urinalysis, one of the most commonly ordered diagnostic tests. Typically, the urinalysis consists of several tests, including determination of pH, specific gravity, and the presence of any protein, glucose, ketones, blood, and white blood cells (WBCs). In addition, a urine specimen sometimes is ordered for a culture and sensitivity test, which is used to diagnose and treat urinary tract infections. The nurse's responsibilities are to collect and label the urine sample, to ensure its safe delivery to the laboratory, and to assess the results. The nurse also explains the collection procedure to the patient and, if appropriate, notifies the health care provider of the results.

It is necessary that the patient is aware of the upcoming test and knows to contact the nurse before the next voiding. The nurse may instruct the patient to drink extra water to assist voiding, to avoid putting toilet tissue in the specimen container, and to prevent fecal matter from coming in contact with the urine specimen. A **midstream urine specimen** is collected to perform a culture and sensitivity. Urine is collected after voiding is initiated (midstream) and before voiding is completed (Skill 23.2). A midstream specimen is the cleanest part of the voided specimen and is collected in a sterile container.

Box 23.4 General Guidelines for Specimen Collections

- Consider the patient's needs and his or her ability to participate in specimen collection procedures.
- Recognize that collection of a specimen sometimes provokes anxiety, embarrassment, or discomfort.
- Provide support for patients who are fearful about the results of a specimen examination.
- Recognize that children require a clear explanation of procedures and often benefit from the support of parents or family members.
- Obtain specimens in accordance with specific prerequisite conditions (e.g., fasting, nothing-by-mouth [NPO] status) as required.
- Wear gloves when collecting specimens of blood or other body fluids, because it is not possible to identify everyone infected with bloodborne pathogens such as human immunodeficiency virus (HIV), hepatitis B, or other pathogens.
- Remove gloves, discard them in proper receptacle, and immediately perform hand hygiene; similarly cleanse other skin surfaces thoroughly if contaminated with blood or body fluids.
- Collect specimens in designated containers, at the correct time, in the appropriate amount.
- Properly label all specimens with the patient's identification; complete laboratory requisition form as necessary (see Box 23.5).
- Most specimens are transported to the laboratory in a separate biohazard bag (see illustration for Skill 23.1, Step 11).
- Deliver specimens to the laboratory within the recommended time, or ensure that they are stored properly for later transport.
- Use aseptic technique in all collections to prevent contamination, which has the potential to render test results inaccurate.
- Transport specimens under special conditions (e.g., iced specimens or special containers with preservatives) as required.

COLLECTING A STERILE URINE SPECIMEN

A sterile urine specimen may be collected by inserting a straight catheter into the urinary bladder to remove urine or by obtaining a specimen from the port of an indwelling catheter with the use of sterile technique. Never use urine from a dependent drainage bag for a specimen. This urine may be contaminated and the test results inaccurate. It is possible to measure **residual urine** (urine left in the bladder after voiding) at the time of catheterization.

Catheterization is performed within 10 minutes after the patient voids. More than 50 mL of urine remaining in the bladder is considered residual urine, and the patient may require insertion of an indwelling catheter.

Prepare the patient by explaining which type of urine specimen will be collected. Relieve any anxiety by assuring the patient that there will be minimal or no discomfort if the patient remains relaxed and that he or she will experience only a sensation of mild pressure as the catheter is inserted and no discomfort or sensation when urine is collected from the catheter port. See Chapter 15 and Skill 15.1 for insertion of a sterile urinary catheter.

If a urinary catheter is already in place, a sterile urine specimen may be obtained from the port of the urinary drainage system. With this approach, the sterility of the urinary drainage system is not compromised (Skill 23.3).

COLLECTING A 24-HOUR URINE SPECIMEN

Tests of renal function and urine composition, such as measurements of levels of adrenocortical steroids, hormones, protein, and creatinine clearance, necessitate a 24-hour collection of urine. The licensed practical nurse/licensed vocational nurse (LPN/LVN) must follow carefully the procedure for ensuring accurate performance

Skill 23.2 Collecting a Midstream Urine Specimen

CHECK
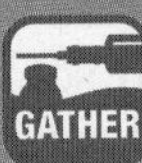
GATHER
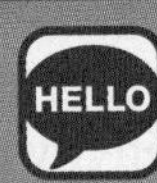
HELLO

ID

PRIVACY
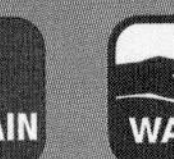
EXPLAIN
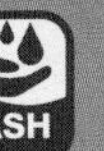
WASH
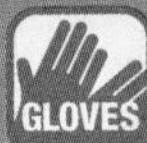
GLOVES

NURSING ACTION *(RATIONALE)*

1. Refer to the health care provider's order. *(Provides basis for care.)*
2. Assemble supplies (see illustration). *(Organizes procedure.)*
   - Antiseptic wipes
   - Sterile specimen container with label
   - Nonsterile gloves
   - Additional PPE if indicated
   - Biohazard bag
   - Requisition slip

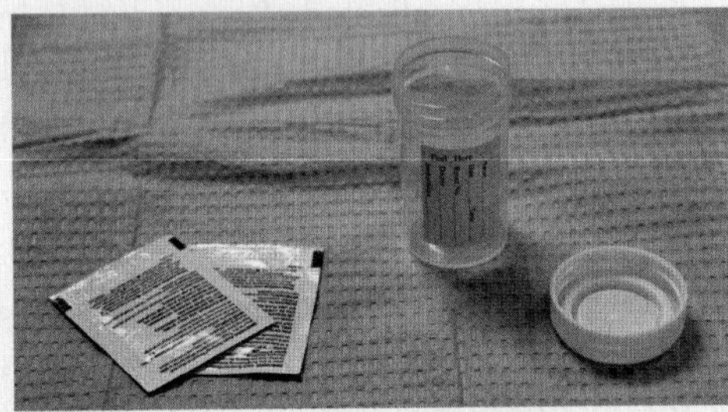

3. Introduce self. *(Decreases patient's anxiety.)*
4. Identify patient. *(Ensures procedure is performed with correct patient.)*
5. Explain procedure. Assess patient's understanding of procedure. *(Decreases patient's anxiety, promotes patient's cooperation, and ensures accuracy.)*
6. Prepare patient for procedure. *(Facilitates procedure.)*
   a. Close door and pull curtain. *(Provides privacy.)*
   b. Varying degrees of assistance are required by patients who are seriously ill, have difficulty standing, or are disoriented. Some patients need assistance in the bathroom, whereas others require a bedpan or urinal in bed. Older patients may have difficulty maintaining balance and raising or lowering toilet seats.
7. Perform hand hygiene and don nonsterile gloves. *(Reduces spread of microorganisms.)*
8. Allow the patient to cleanse self with the antiseptic wipes if the patient is able; instruct female patients to separate the labia well and cleanse the perineum in an anterior-to-posterior direction. Instruct male patients to cleanse in a circular motion from the meatus outward; if the penis is uncircumcised, the foreskin should be retracted. If the patient is unable to cleanse the area, provide assistance. *(Provides a cleaner specimen and prevents organisms at or near the meatus from being washed into the specimen. Cleansing from anterior to posterior aspect prevents microorganisms from the anus from entering through the urinary meatus.)*
9. Guide female patients to straddle bedpan or toilet, if possible, to allow for labial spreading and to keep the labia separated during voiding. Request that patient (1) begin by voiding about 30 mL into the toilet, and then position the sterile specimen container, making sure the sides of the labia do not touch the container or each other; (2) without stopping flow, void a small amount into specimen cup; (3) remove cup and, without stopping flow, finish voiding into toilet. *(Collects midstream urine specimen appropriately. The first 30 mL, containing the organisms washed away from the meatus, is discarded.)*
10. Secure lid on container without touching the inside of the lid. *(Prevents spillage and contamination.)*
11. Remove gloves, discard them in proper receptacle, and perform hand hygiene. *(Reduces spread of microorganisms.)*
12. Cleanse and return toilet seat collector, or empty and flush bedpan or urinal if any of these are in use. *(Prepares equipment for next use.)*
13. Label specimen appropriately. Place in biohazard bag for transport to laboratory (see illustration for Skill 23.1, Step 11). *(Ensures proper identification of specimen; ensures accuracy of results; prevents loss and potential delays in obtaining results.)* Follow agency policy (see Box 23.5).
14. Ensure prompt delivery to laboratory with proper requisition slip (many facilities mandate delivery within 1 hour). *(Ensures a fresh specimen for testing and prevents loss of specimen.)*
15. Document procedure. *(Provides communication of procedure and patient's response.)*
    - Time
    - Type of specimen collected
    - Sent to laboratory with requisition
    - Patient's response (if appropriate)
16. Provide patient teaching (see the Patient Teaching box on specimen collection and diagnostic tests).

PPE, Personal protective equipment.

Skill 23.3 Collecting a Sterile Urine Specimen via Catheter Port

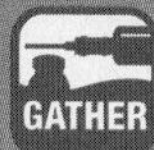

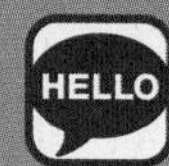

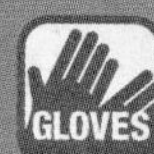

GLOVES

NURSING ACTION *(RATIONALE)*

1. Refer to the health care provider's order. *(Provides basis for care.)*
2. Assemble supplies. *(Organizes procedure.)*
   - Nonsterile gloves
   - Sterile specimen container with label
   - Clamp or rubber band
   - Sterile syringe and needle
   - Alcohol preparation
   - Requisition slip
   - Biohazard bag
   - Additional PPE if indicated
3. Introduce self. *(Decreases patient's anxiety.)*
4. Identify patient. *(Ensures procedure is performed with correct patient.)*
5. Explain procedure. *(Promotes cooperation and decreases patient's anxiety.)*
6. Perform hand hygiene and don nonsterile gloves. *(Reduces spread of microorganisms.)*
7. Catheter port collection:
   a. Clamp just below catheter port for about 30 minutes. *(Allows for urine to collect for removal.)*

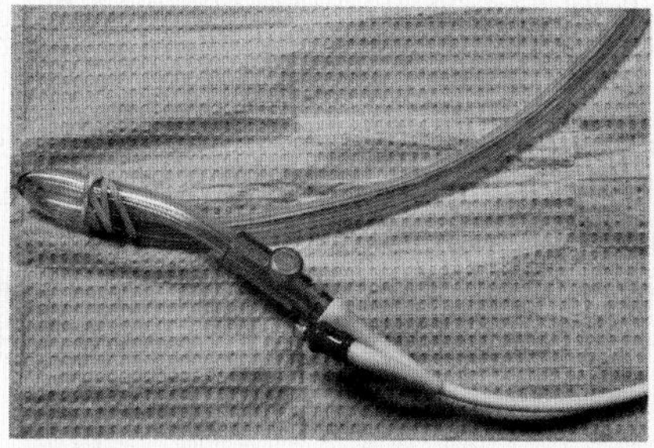

   b. Return in 30 minutes; clean port with alcohol preparation. *(Prevents needle puncture from causing contamination.)*
   c. Insert needle into port at 30-degree angle and withdraw 5–10 mL of urine for a specimen. *(Inserting needle at an angle prevents puncturing opposite side of tubing. Provides for specimen.)*
   d. Place urine in sterile specimen cup. *(Keeps specimen sterile.)*
   e. Unclamp catheter. *(Allows continuous urine flow to resume.)*
   f. Label specimen and place in biohazard bag for transport to laboratory (see illustration for Skill 23.1, Step 11, and Box 23.5) and send to laboratory with requisition. *(Ensures proper identification of specimen; ensures accuracy of results; prevents loss and potential delays in obtaining results.)*
8. Remove gloves, discard them in proper receptacle, and perform hand hygiene. *(Reduces spread of microorganisms.)*
9. Document procedure and observations (see Skill 23.2, Step 15). *(Records procedure and patient's response.)*

PPE, Personal protective equipment.

of the test. Some tests require collecting the entire volume of urine from a 24-hour period (Skill 23.4). If urine is discarded accidentally or contaminated or if the patient is incontinent, the prescribing health care provider must order an indwelling catheter.

MEASURING BLOOD GLUCOSE LEVELS

Using a meter to measure the blood glucose of a patient with diabetes provides more meaningful data than testing urine for the presence of glucose. The patient easily may perform skin puncture at home (Skill 23.5).

COLLECTING A STOOL SPECIMEN

Stool specimens are collected and examined for a variety of reasons, including the following: to determine the presence of infection or blood; to observe the amount, color, and consistency of the stool; to determine the presence of fats; or to identify parasites, ova, and bacteria. The LPN/LVN collects the feces, labels the specimen appropriately, and sends the specimen and the laboratory request to the laboratory. When stool is to be examined for parasites, it must be taken immediately to the laboratory for parasites to be examined under the microscope while they are alive. It is also possible to collect a stool specimen from a colostomy or an ileostomy.

Inform the patient that a stool specimen is needed, then carry out collection in a manner that does not cause stress or make the patient feel hurried or embarrassed. Arrange supplies if the patient is to collect the stool. When a stool specimen is to be obtained, place the specimen hat toward the back of the toilet or commode. When a urine specimen is to be obtained, place the specimen hat toward the front (Fig. 23.1). If urine and stool specimens are to be collected, use two

Skill 23.4 Collecting a 24-Hour Urine Specimen

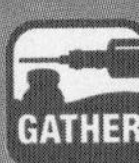

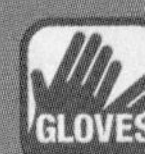

NURSING ACTION *(RATIONALE)*

1. Refer to the health care provider's order. *(Provides basis for care.)*
2. Assemble supplies and equipment. *(Organizes procedure.)*
   - Specimen hat for bedpan, commode, or toilet; or urinal
   - Specimen container, including preservative of agency's choice, and label
   - Nonsterile gloves
   - Additional PPE if indicated
   - Requisition
3. Introduce self. *(Decreases patient's anxiety.)*
4. Identify patient. *(Ensures procedure is performed with correct patient.)*
5. Explain procedure. *(Promotes cooperation and decreases anxiety.)*
   a. Stress importance of collecting all urine for a 24-hour period. *(Ensures validity of results of a 24-hour kidney function test.)*
   b. Instruct patient not to allow tissue or fecal material to touch specimen or enter container. *(Contaminates specimen.)*
6. Post signs on bathroom door and near patient's bed to alert staff and patient to save all urine.
7. Perform hand hygiene and don nonsterile gloves according to agency policy and guidelines from the CDC and OSHA each time a specimen is collected and transferred to the large collection container. *(Reduces spread of microorganisms.)*
8. Have patient void just before the 24-hour specimen collection is to begin; discard this urine. *(This urine was formed in urinary system before the study began.)*
9. Place labeled container on ice if required. (Some agencies require refrigeration of all specimens. Others advocate that the urine container be placed on ice. For some collection procedures, refrigeration is not always necessary, or a preservative may be used in 24-hour specimen collection device.) *(Keeps the specimen cool, which decreases decomposition and odor.)*
10. Save all urine for the 24-hour period; place each voided specimen into the larger container. *(It is essential to save all urine; otherwise results will be altered.)*
11. Instruct patient to void a few minutes before end of 24 hours; this urine is part of the 24-hour specimen. *(This will empty bladder before the end of testing.)*
12. Send collection to laboratory promptly; be certain label includes date and time specimen started (see Box 23.5). If more than one container is necessary, make certain both are labeled and numbered. If patient is menstruating, be certain to note this on the requisition slip. *(Ensures proper identification of specimen; ensures accuracy of results; prevents loss and potential delays in obtaining results.)*
13. Document procedure and observations (see Skill 23.2, Step 15). *(Communicates the patient care administered.)*
14. Perform patient teaching (see the Patient Teaching box on specimen collection and diagnostic tests).

CDC, Centers for Disease Control and Prevention; *OSHA*, Occupational Safety and Health Administration; *PPE*, personal protective equipment.

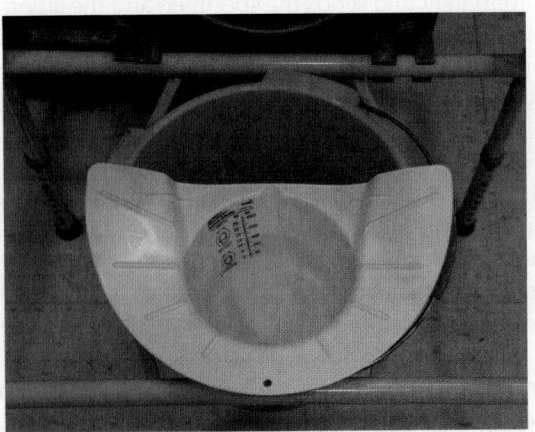

Fig. 23.1 Specimen "hat."

specimen hats: one placed at the front and one placed toward the back of the toilet or commode. A bedpan may be used to collect a stool specimen if the patient is cautioned not to void in the bedpan, which would compromise the stool specimen. The LPN/LVN must understand why the stool specimen is being collected to choose the appropriate supplies. If the stool specimen is for ova and parasites, an appropriate container with a special solution must be obtained (Skill 23.6).

DETERMINING THE PRESENCE OF OCCULT BLOOD IN STOOL (GUAIAC)

The presence of blood in body waste is abnormal. Bright red blood in the stool indicates that the blood is fresh

Skill 23.5 Measuring Blood Glucose Levels

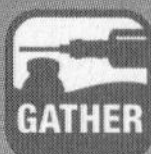

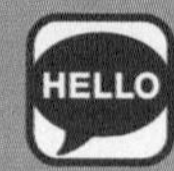

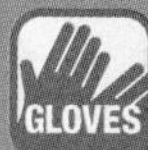

NURSING ACTION *(RATIONALE)*

1. Refer to the health care provider's order. *(Provides basis for care.)*
2. Assemble supplies. *(Organizes procedure.)*
   - Sterile lancet
   - Automatic lancing device
   - Alcohol swab or soap and water (see Step 10)
   - Blood glucose meter
   - Testing strips for meter
   - Cotton balls
   - Nonsterile gloves
3. Introduce self. *(Decreases patient's anxiety.)*
4. Identify patient. *(Ensures procedure is performed with correct patient.)*
5. Explain procedure to patient. *(Promotes cooperation and decreases patient's anxiety.)*
6. Perform hand hygiene and don nonsterile gloves according to agency policy and guidelines from the CDC and OSHA. *(Reduces spread of microorganisms.)*
7. Remove cap from lancet by using sterile technique. *(Maintains sterility of point.)*
8. Place lancet into automatic lancing device according to instructions in operating manual. *(Allows proper puncture of skin.)*
9. Select site on side of any fingertip (for infant, use heel). *(The side of the finger is less responsive to pain from puncture than are other sites.)*
10. Wipe selected site with alcohol swab and discard swab. *(Prepares site. Some manuals now specify washing hands with soap and water—no alcohol because it alters the test strip and dries the skin.)*
11. Ask patient to hold arm at side 30 seconds. *(Increases blood flow to site and allows site to dry.)*
12. Gently squeeze patient's fingertip with thumb of same hand. *(Increases blood supply to site.)*
13. Hold lancing device. *(Provides easy access to device.)*
14. Place trigger platform of lancing device on side of finger and press. *(Activates lancing mechanism.)*

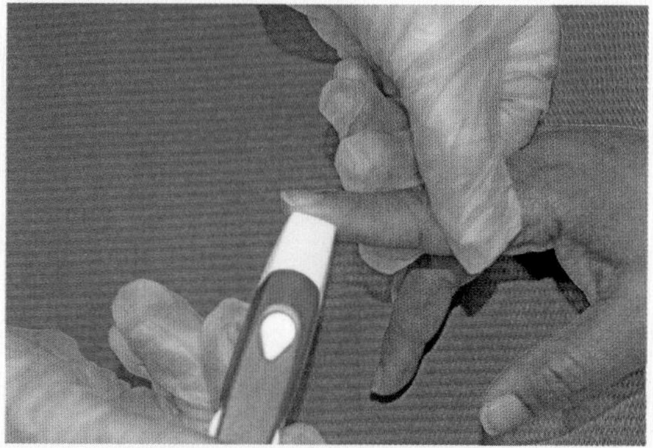

15. Stroke finger with downward motion; using cotton ball, wipe off first drop of blood that appears (if recommended by glucose meter manufacturer) and continue stroking. *(Produces enough blood to cover test pad on test strip; producing and wiping first drop removes surface contaminants.)*
16. While holding strip level, touch new drop of blood on finger to test pad. Do not allow finger (skin) to touch the test pad. Apply pressure to puncture site using cotton ball. *(Causes blood to cover test pad without smearing and prevents alteration of test results.)*

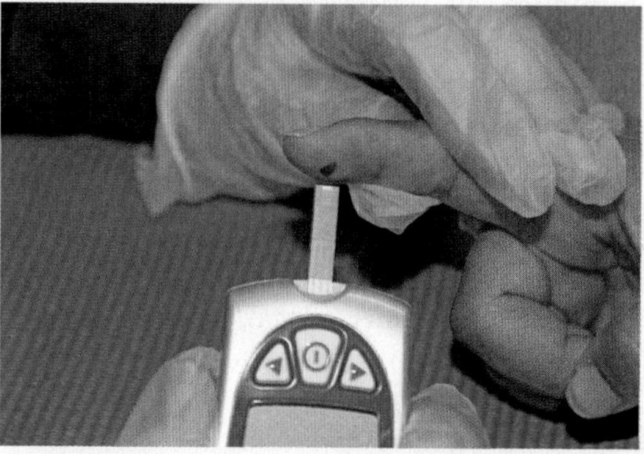

17. Begin timing as recommended by glucose meter instructions. Wait for numeric readout. *(Ensures test accuracy.)*
18. Remove lancet from device and discard. *(Prevents accidental needlestick injury.)*
19. Remove gloves, discard them in proper receptacle, and perform hand hygiene. *(Reduces spread of microorganisms.)*
20. Document procedure and observations (see Skill 23.2, Step 15). *(Communicates patient care administered.)*
21. Perform patient teaching (see the Patient Teaching box on specimen collection and diagnostic tests).

Skill 23.6 Collecting a Stool Specimen

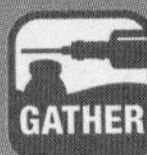

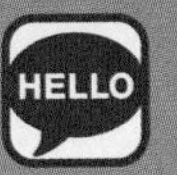

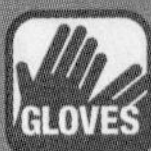

NURSING ACTION *(RATIONALE)*

1. Refer to the health care provider's order. *(Provides basis for care.)*
2. Assemble supplies. *(Organizes procedure.)*
   - Stool specimen cup or container
   - Nonsterile gloves
   - Additional PPE if indicated
   - Bedpan, specimen device, or commode
   - Tongue depressor
   - Specimen container label
   - Laboratory requisition
   - Biohazard bag
3. Introduce self. *(Decreases patient's anxiety.)*
4. Identify patient. *(Ensures procedure is performed with correct patient.)*
5. Explain procedure to patient; make certain patient understands what is expected. *(Promotes cooperation and decreases anxiety.)*
6. Perform hand hygiene and don nonsterile gloves according to agency policy and guidelines from the CDC and OSHA. *(Prevents transmission of microorganisms.)*
7. Assist patient to bathroom when necessary. *(Provides patient safety.)*
8. Ask patient to defecate into commode, specimen device, or bedpan, preventing urine from entering specimen. *(Prevents contamination of specimen.)*

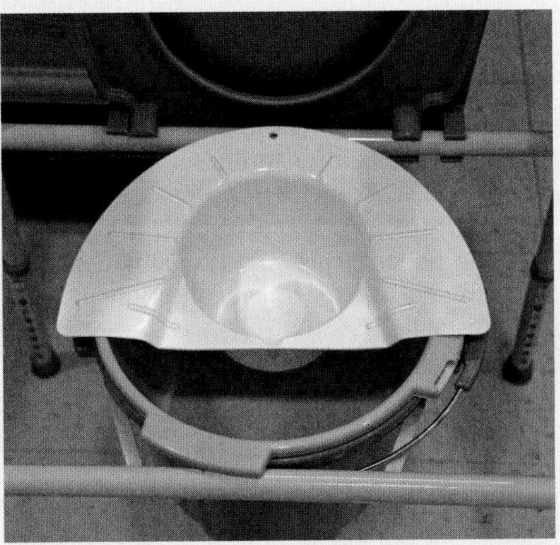

9. Transfer stool to specimen cup with use of a tongue blade, and close the lid securely. *(Protects specimen.)*

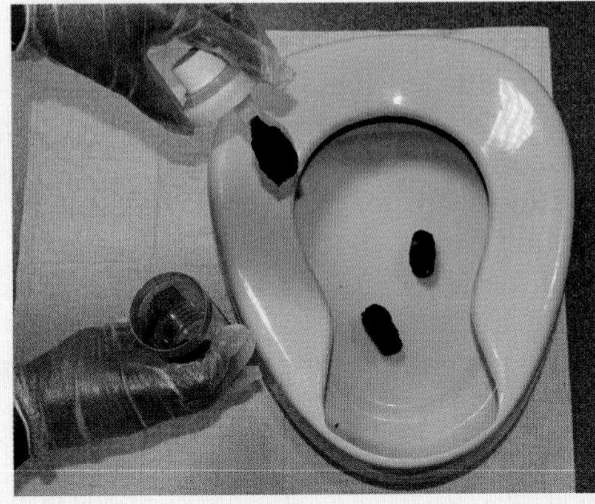

10. Remove gloves, discard them in proper receptacle, and perform hand hygiene. *(Reduces spread of microorganisms.)*
11. Attach requisition slip, enclose in a biohazard bag (see illustration for Skill 23.1, Step 11), label the bag (see Box 23.5), and send specimen to laboratory (it is necessary to take specimens for ova and parasites to the laboratory stat; it is acceptable to keep other stool specimens at room temperature). *(Ensures proper identification of specimen; ensures accuracy of results; prevents loss and potential delays in obtaining results.)*
12. Assist patient to bed. *(Provides for patient safety and comfort.)*
13. Document procedure and observations (see Skill 23.2, Step 15). *(Communicates care administered.)*
14. Perform patient teaching (see the Patient Teaching box).

CDC, Centers for Disease Control and Prevention; *OSHA*, Occupational Safety and Health Administration; *PPE*, personal protective equipment.

Box 23.5 Correct Labeling Information

- Patient's full name (last name, first name, and middle name or initial)
- Patient's identification number, bed number, room number, and medical record number
- Patient's age, sex (male or female)
- Health care provider's name
- Date and time of specimen collection
- Collector's name or initials
- Test ordered
- Most facilities have an electronic health record (EHR) label containing necessary information.

and that the site of bleeding is in the lower gastrointestinal (GI) tract. In contrast, black, tarry feces indicate the presence of old blood and that the site of bleeding is higher in the GI tract. When blood is present in the stool but not visible without the use of a microscope, it is referred to as **occult** (hidden). A **Hemoccult** test detects occult blood in feces (Skill 23.7).

Instruct the patient on how many stool specimens are ordered by the health care provider and how to collect a stool specimen. Then label the Hemoccult card appropriately (Box 23.5) and send it to the laboratory. Some facilities permit nursing staff to perform reagent testing without sending the Hemoccult card to the laboratory.

DETERMINING THE PRESENCE OF OCCULT BLOOD IN GASTRIC SECRETIONS OR EMESIS (GASTROCCULT TEST)

This test determines bleeding in the esophagus, the stomach, the small intestine, or the large intestine. The test confirms the suspected presence of blood when gastric contents have red or black coloration or when emesis or the product of nasogastric (NG) suction has a coffee-grounds appearance (Skill 23.8) (see Chapter 15, Skill 15.5 for insertion of nasogastric tube).

COLLECTING A SPUTUM SPECIMEN

Sputum is secretion from the lungs. It contains mucus, cellular debris, microorganisms, or some combination of these, and it sometimes contains blood or pus. A sputum specimen must be obtained from deep in the bronchial tree. Expectoration of throat and mouth secretions is not to be used as a sputum specimen, because saliva with food particles does not produce desired results. Early morning is the best time to collect a sputum specimen, because the patient has not yet cleared the respiratory passages. Many tests are possible to perform on sputum, such as **culture** (a laboratory test involving cultivation of microorganisms or cells in a special growth medium) and **sensitivity** (a laboratory method of determining the effectiveness of antibiotics, usually performed in conjunction with culture); cytologic analysis (**cytology** is the study of cells, including their formation, origin, structure, function, biochemical activities, and pathologic processes); and examination and testing for acid-fast bacillus (the organism responsible for tuberculosis of the lung).

Collecting a Sputum Specimen by Suction

Some patients are not able to **expectorate** (eject mucus, sputum, or fluids from trachea and lungs by coughing or spitting) a sputum specimen, and nasotracheal suctioning is required to obtain a sputum specimen. Suctioning sometimes provokes coughing, which has potential to induce vomiting and constriction of pharyngeal, laryngeal, or bronchial muscles. In some cases, suctioning also causes direct stimulation of vagal nerve fibers, which results in cardiac dysrhythmias and increased intracranial pressure (Skill 23.9).

Closed-method collection containers, such as a Lukens specimen container, protect the nurse from contamination with body fluids. Explain the procedure and prepare the patient for the test. Provide instructions to the patient the night before the test to drink extra fluids, which helps loosen secretions and makes expectoration for the specimen easier. Instruct the patient that it is not possible to use saliva as a specimen. Saliva is clear, whereas sputum is thick, sometimes colored, and tenacious (sticky) (Skill 23.10).

OBTAINING A WOUND CULTURE

If the LPN/LVN detects purulent or suspect-looking exudate or drainage, the health care provider will probably order a wound culture. The patient should be assessed for fever, chills, malaise, and elevated WBC count, which indicate a possible systemic infection. It is not possible to confirm or treat infection accurately without results from a wound culture. Assess pain at the wound site with the use of a pain scale, such as a scale of 0 to 10 in which 0 indicates no pain and 10 indicates the worst pain imaginable by the patient. If a patient requires an analgesic before a dressing change, give this medication 30 minutes before the dressing change so that the analgesic effect peaks when the procedure is performed. Determine when the dressing change is scheduled, because this is the ideal time to obtain a wound culture as part of the procedure (see Chapter 22).

A wound culture sample should not be collected from old drainage, because resident colonies of bacteria grow in exudate. Obtain the specimen from inside the wound. Aerobic organisms grow in superficial wounds exposed to the air, and anaerobic organisms tend to grow within body cavities. To collect an aerobic specimen, insert a sterile swab from the Culturette tube (Fig. 23.2) into wound secretions. Then return the swab to the Culturette tube, cap the tube, and crush the inner ampule so that the medium for organism growth coats the swab tip (Fig. 23.3). Immediately send the labeled specimen to the laboratory with a requisition slip. To collect an anaerobic specimen deep in a body cavity, use a sterile syringe tip to aspirate visible drainage from the inner wound; expel any air from the syringe and inject the

Text continued on p. 678

Skill 23.7 Determining the Presence of Occult Blood in Stool

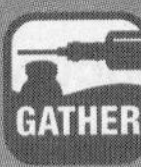

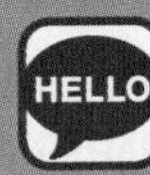

NURSING ACTION *(RATIONALE)*

1. Refer to the health care provider's order. *(Provides basis for care.)*
2. Assemble supplies. *(Organizes procedure.)*
   - Nonsterile gloves
   - Additional PPE if indicated
   - Clean bedpan or specimen device for commode
   - Hemoccult card
   - Wooden applicator
   - Hemoccult developer
   - Laboratory requisition
   - Biohazard bag
3. Introduce self. *(Decreases patient's anxiety.)*
4. Identify patient. *(Ensures procedure is performed with correct patient.)*
5. Explain procedure. *(Promotes cooperation and decreases patient's anxiety. It is advisable to label card before gathering specimen to prevent contamination.)*
6. Perform hand hygiene and don nonsterile gloves according to agency policy and guidelines from the CDC and OSHA. *(Reduces spread of microorganisms.)*
7. Collect stool specimen. (See Skill 23.6, Steps 8 and 9.) *(Provides stool for Hemoccult test.)*
8. Follow steps on Hemoccult slide test:
   a. Open flap. *(Begins test.)*

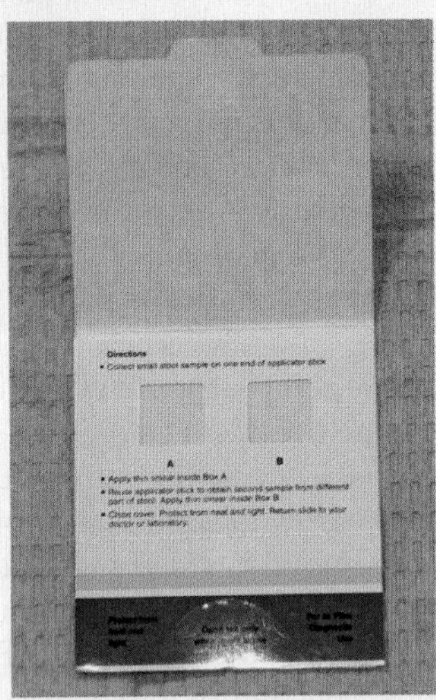

   b. Use one end of tongue blade to gather stool, and smear very small amount of stool in box A. *(Prepares slide.)*

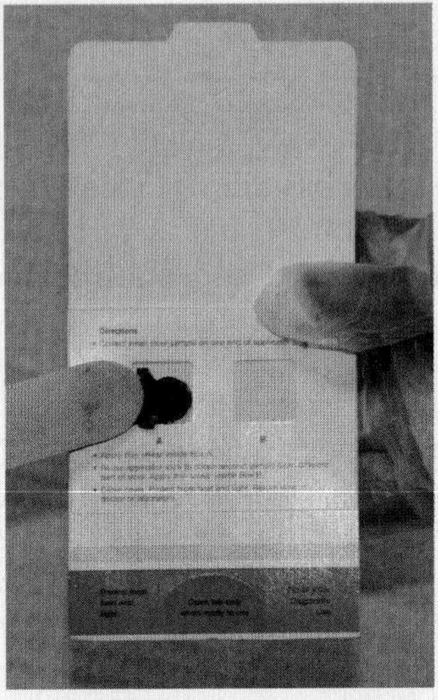

   c. Use other end of tongue blade to gather from another part of stool, and smear very small amount in box B. *(Prepares second slide.)*
   d. Close card and label, if you have not already done so (see Box 23.5). *(Ensures accuracy in identification of specimen.*
   e. Enclose specimen in biohazard bag and send to laboratory with requisition slip. *(Ensures proper identification.)*
   f. If testing is to be performed on the nursing unit, follow directions on the Hemoccult card. Document findings of occult blood in stool and results of quality control area.
9. Remove gloves, discard them in proper receptacle, and perform hand hygiene. *(Reduces spread of microorganisms.)*
10. Document procedure and observations (see Skill 23.2, Step 15). *(Communicates collection of stool specimen.)*
11. Perform patient teaching (see the Patient Teaching box).

CDC, Centers for Disease Control and Prevention; *OSHA*, Occupational Safety and Health Administration; *PPE*, personal protective equipment.

Skill 23.8 Collecting Gastric Secretions or Emesis Specimen

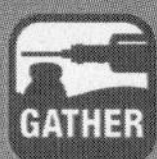

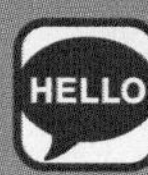

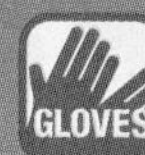

NURSING ACTION *(RATIONALE)*

1. Refer to the health care provider's order. *(Provides basis for care.)*
2. Assemble supplies. *(Organizes procedure.)*
   - Nonsterile gloves
   - Additional PPE if indicated
   - Facial tissues
   - Emesis basin
   - Wooden applicator
   - Bulb syringe (60 mL) or catheter-tip syringe
   - Gastroccult test
   - Cardboard slide
   - Gastroccult developing solution
   - Laboratory requisition
   - Biohazard bag
3. Introduce self. *(Decreases patient's anxiety.)*
4. Identify patient. *(Ensures procedure is performed with correct patient.)*
5. Explain procedure. *(Promotes cooperation and decreases patient's anxiety.)*
6. It is advisable to label card before obtaining specimen to prevent contamination.
7. Perform hand hygiene and don nonsterile gloves according to agency policy and guidelines from the CDC and OSHA. *(Prevents transmission of microorganisms.)*
8. To obtain specimen of gastric contents through nasogastric (NG) or nasoenteral tube, position patient in high Fowler's position in bed or chair. *(Keeps risk of aspiration of gastric contents to a minimum. Position relieves pressure on abdominal organs. If patient is nauseated, flat position in bed or one in which the patient is not able to sit straight sometimes causes abdominal discomfort.)*
9. Verify NG tube placement (see Chapter 15). *(Ensures aspiration of gastric contents.)*
10. Collect gastric contents via NG or nasoenteral tube (see Chapter 15). (Only a small amount of specimen is needed for pH and occult blood testing.)
    a. Disconnect tube from suction or gravity drainage.
    b. Attach bulb syringe or catheter-tip syringe.
    c. Aspirate 5–10 mL.
    d. Obtain sample of emesis with a 3-mL syringe or wooden applicator.
    e. Using applicator or syringe, apply 1 drop of gastric sample to test area of Gastroccult test slide. *(Sample must cover test paper for test reaction to occur.)*
    f. Follow directions on the Gastroccult card.
11. Close card and label, if you have not already done so (see Box 23.5). *(Ensures accuracy in identification of specimen.)*
12. Enclose specimen in biohazard bag and send to laboratory with requisition slip (see illustration for Skill 23.1, Step 11). *(Ensures proper identification.)*
13. Reconnect NG tube to drainage system, suction, or clamp as ordered. *(NG tube serves to decompress abdomen by promoting drainage. Clamping sometimes is ordered to determine tolerance to stomach filling.)*
14. Dispose of equipment; remove gloves and discard them in proper receptacle; and perform hand hygiene. *(Reduces spread of microorganisms.)*
15. Document procedure and observations. *(Communicates collection of specimen and completion of test.)*
16. Perform patient teaching (see the Patient Teaching box).

CDC, Centers for Disease Control and Prevention; *OSHA*, Occupational Safety and Health Administration; *PPE*, personal protective equipment.

Skill 23.9 Collecting a Sputum Specimen by Suction

 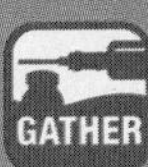 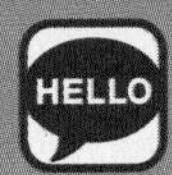 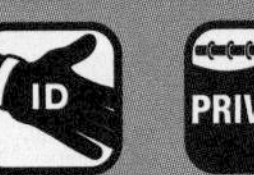   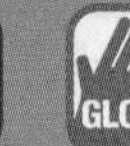

NURSING ACTION *(RATIONALE)*

1. Refer to the health care provider's order. *(Provides basis for care.)*
2. Assemble supplies. *(Organizes procedure.)*
   - Suction device (wall or portable)
   - Sterile suction catheter (size 14, 16, or 18) *(Use of a catheter that is too large causes trauma to nasal mucosa.)*
   - Sterile gloves
   - Sterile saline or container
   - In-line specimen container (sputum trap)
   - Oxygen therapy equipment, if indicated
   - Protective eyewear and other PPE as appropriate (to protect from sputum drops/particles)
   - Laboratory requisition
   - Biohazard bag
3. Introduce self. *(Decreases patient's anxiety.)*
4. Identify patient. *(Ensures procedure is performed with correct patient.)*
5. Explain procedure. Encourage patient to breathe normally to prevent hyperventilation. *(Promotes cooperation and decreases patient's anxiety.)*
6. Assess patient.
   a. Determine when patient last ate a meal. *(It is best to obtain the specimen 1–2 hours after a meal or 1 hour before to minimize gagging, which can cause vomiting and aspiration.)*
   b. Assess patient's respiratory status: rate, depth, pattern, lung sounds, and color. *(Changes in respirations indicate the possible presence of secretions in the tracheobronchial tree and potential need for supplementary oxygen.)*
   c. Assess patient's anxiety level. *(Procedure usually is contraindicated if patient is not able to cooperate or remain still during procedure.)*
7. Arrange equipment and prepare necessary charges. *(Facilitates procedure and facilitates proper billing.)*
8. Position patient for procedure.
   a. Close door or pull curtains. *(Provides privacy.)*
   b. The higher semi-Fowler's position is recommended. *(Promotes full lung expansion and facilitates ability to cough.)*
   c. Prepare suction machine or device and ensure that it is functioning properly. *(Adequate amount of suction is necessary to aspirate sputum.)*
   d. Drape patient as necessary. *(Prevents unnecessary exposure.)*
   e. Adjust bed to appropriate height and lower side rail. *(Promotes proper body mechanics and facilitates procedure.)*
9. Perform hand hygiene. *(Reduces spread of microorganisms.)*
10. Connect suction tube to adapter on sputum trap. *(Facilitates procedure.)*
11. Prelubricate tip of catheter with sterile water.
12. Apply sterile glove to dominant hand. *(Allows handling of suction catheter without introducing microorganisms into the tracheobronchial tree, which is a sterile body cavity.)*
13. Administer 100% oxygen to the patient for 1 minute, if necessary. *(Use caution if patient has chronic obstructive pulmonary disease [COPD], because 100% oxygen has the capacity to depress respiratory effort.)*
14. Using gloved hand, connect sterile suction catheter rubber tubing on sputum trap. *(Aspirated sputum will go directly to trap instead of to suction tubing.)*
15. Gently insert tip of suction catheter prelubricated with sterile water through nasopharynx, endotracheal tube, or tracheostomy without applying suction. *(Minimizes trauma to airway as catheter is inserted. Lubrication allows for easier insertion.)*

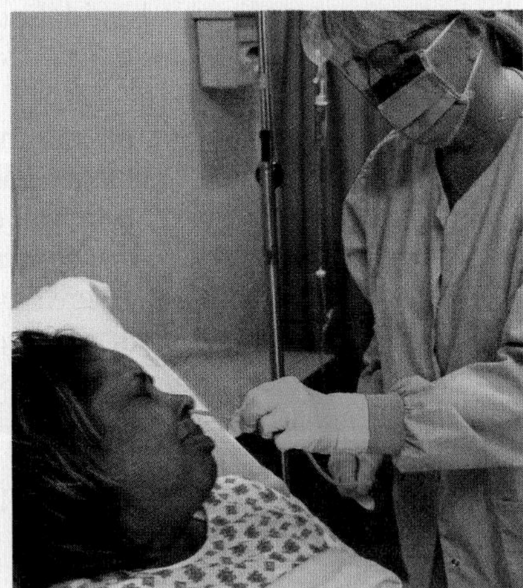

16. Warn patient to expect to cough, and gently and quickly advance catheter into trachea. *(Triggers cough reflex.)*
17. As patient coughs, apply suction for 5–10 seconds, collecting 2–10 mL of sputum. *(Suctioning longer than 10 seconds risks causing hypoxia and mucosal damage.)*
18. Release suction and remove catheter, and then turn off suction. *(Releasing suction prevents unnecessary trauma to mucosa as the catheter is withdrawn.)*

Skill 23.9 Collecting a Sputum Specimen by Suction—cont'd

19. Detach catheter from specimen trap, and dispose of catheter into appropriate receptacle. Connect rubber tubing on sputum trap to plastic adapter. *(Aids in keeping specimen intact.)*

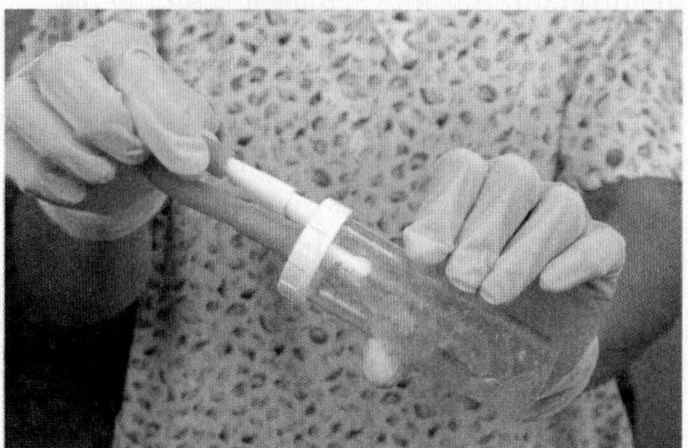

Step 19 from Perry AG, Potter PA, Elkin MK: *Nursing interventions and clinical skills*, ed 5, St. Louis, 2012, Mosby.

20. If any sputum is present on outside of container, wash it off with disinfectant. *(Prevents spread of infection to persons handling specimen.)*

21. Offer patient tissues after suctioning. Dispose of tissues in emesis basin or trash container. Remove gloves, and discard them in proper receptacle. *(Reduces spread of microorganisms.)*

22. Securely attach properly completed identification label and laboratory requisition to side of specimen container (not the lid). *(Ensures proper identification of specimen; ensures accuracy of results; prevents loss and potential delays in obtaining results.)*

23. Enclose specimen in a biohazard bag (see illustration for Skill 23.1, Step 11). Send specimen immediately to laboratory. *(Bacteria multiply quickly. Prompt analysis of specimen is necessary for accurate results.)*

24. Offer patient mouth care; assist patient to a comfortable position, and place needed items within easy reach. *(Ensures patient's comfort and well-being.)*

25. Raise side rail, and lower bed to lowest position. *(Ensures patient's safety.)*

26. Store, remove, or dispose of supplies and equipment as appropriate. *(Ensures equipment is available for next use.)*

27. Document procedure. *(Provides communication that procedure was carried out and patient's response.)*
- Method used to obtain specimen
- Date and time collected
- Type of test ordered and how specimen was transported to the laboratory
- Characteristics of sputum specimen
- Patient's oxygenation and respiratory status

28. Perform patient teaching (see the Patient Teaching box).

PPE, Personal protective equipment.

Skill 23.10 Collecting a Sputum Specimen by Expectoration

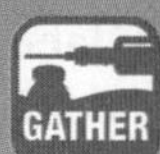

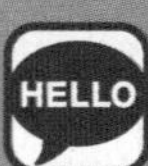

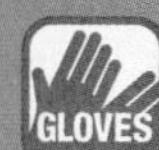

NURSING ACTION *(RATIONALE)*

1. Refer to the health care provider's order. *(Provides basis for care.)*
2. Assemble supplies. *(Organizes procedure.)*
   - Sterile sputum collector
   - Tissues
   - Label for specimen
   - Laboratory requisition
   - Nonsterile gloves
   - Additional PPE if indicated
   - Biohazard bag
3. Introduce self. *(Decreases patient's anxiety.)*
4. Identify patient. *(Ensures procedure is performed with correct patient.)*
5. Explain procedure. *(Promotes cooperation and decreases patient's anxiety.)*
6. Perform hand hygiene and don nonsterile gloves according to agency policy and guidelines from the CDC and OSHA. *(Prevents transmission of microorganisms.)*
7. Position patient in Fowler's position. *(Helps with coughing.)*
8. Instruct patient to take three breaths and force cough into sterile container. *(Helps patient expectorate mucus.)* (Be prepared to obtain the specimen by nasotracheal suctioning if patient is not able to cough.)

Continued

Skill 23.10 Collecting a Sputum Specimen by Expectoration—cont'd

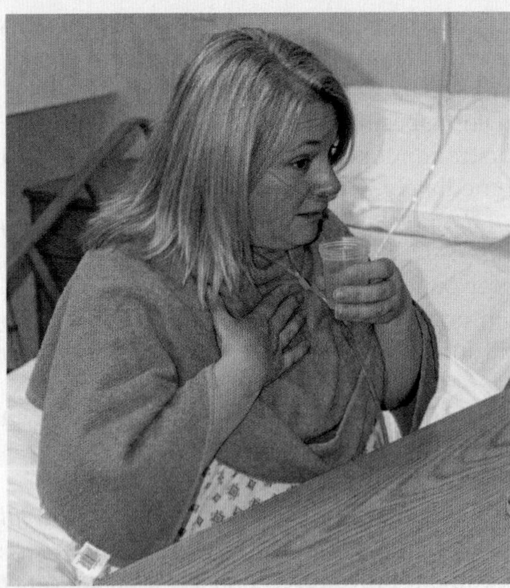

9. Label specimen container (see Box 23.5). *(Ensures proper identification of specimen; ensures accuracy of results; prevents loss and potential delays in obtaining results.)*

10. Enclose specimen in biohazard bag and attach laboratory requisition. Immediately send specimen to laboratory. If any sputum is present on outside of container, wash it off with disinfectant. *(Ensures specimen is sent to the laboratory. Bacteria multiply quickly. Prompt analysis of specimens is necessary for accurate results. Removing sputum from outside of container prevents spread of infection to anyone handling specimen.)*
11. Remove gloves, discard them in proper receptacle, and perform hand hygiene. *(Reduces spread of microorganisms.)*
12. Document procedure and observations (see Skill 23.2, Step 15). *(Communicates care administered.)*
13. Perform patient teaching (see the Patient Teaching box).

CDC, Centers for Disease Control and Prevention; *OSHA,* Occupational Safety and Health Administration; *PPE,* personal protective equipment.

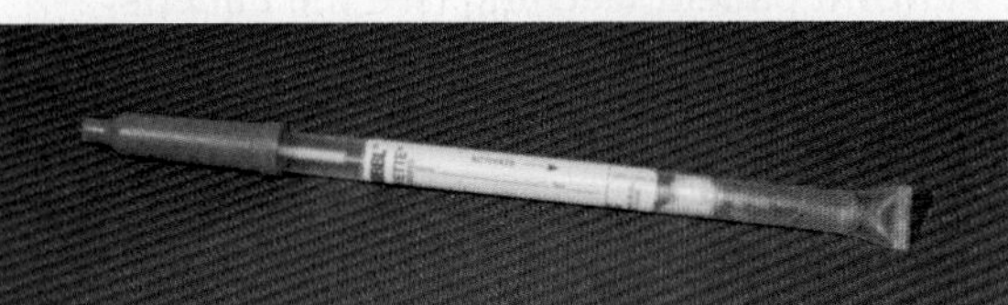

Fig. 23.2 Wound culture tube.

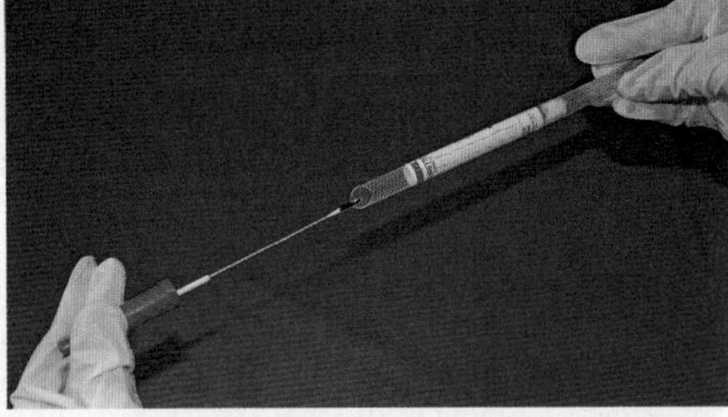

Fig. 23.3 Aerobic culture tube.

syringe contents into a special vacuum container with culture medium. In some facilities, place a cork over the needle to prevent entrance of air and then send the syringe to the laboratory with a requisition slip.

COLLECTING SPECIMENS FROM THE NOSE AND THROAT

When a patient has signs and symptoms of upper respiratory or sinus infection, a nose or throat culture is a simple diagnostic tool often used to determine the nature of the patient's problem. A nose culture also is performed to detect methicillin-resistant *Staphylococcus aureus* (MRSA). The laboratory staff places the specimen on a culture medium to determine whether pathogenic microorganisms will grow. Regardless of what body fluids are cultured, certain principles apply. It is necessary to obtain culture specimens before antibiotic therapy is started because the antibiotics have the capacity to interrupt the organism's growth in the laboratory. If the patient is receiving antibiotics, notify the laboratory and communicate specifically what antibiotics the patient is receiving.

Collection of nose and throat specimens sometimes causes the patient discomfort owing to heightened sensitivity of the mucosal membranes. Collection of a throat specimen often causes gagging, and so it is important to collect a throat culture before or at least 1 hour after mealtime to lessen the chance of inducing vomiting. To keep the patient's anxiety and discomfort to a minimum, make certain the patient clearly understands how each specimen is to be collected (Skills 23.11 and 23.12).

When collecting nose and throat specimens, perform the following:

- Assess the condition of and drainage from nasal mucosa and sinuses. *(Reveals physical signs that indicate possible infection or allergic irritation.)*

Skill 23.11 Obtaining a Throat Specimen

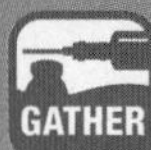

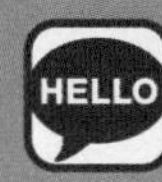

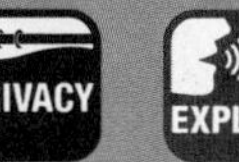

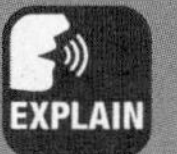

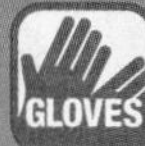

NURSING ACTION *(RATIONALE)*

1. Refer to the health care provider's order. *(Provides basis of care.)*
2. Assemble supplies. *(Organizes procedure.)*
   - Nonsterile gloves
   - Additional PPE if indicated
   - Swab and culture tube
   - Nasal speculum (optional)
   - Tongue blades
   - Penlight
   - Emesis basin or clean container (optional)
   - Facial tissues
   - Label (completed)
   - Laboratory requisition
   - Biohazard bag
3. Introduce self. *(Decreases patient's anxiety.)*
4. Identify patient. *(Ensures procedure is performed with correct patient.)*
5. Explain procedure to patient; make certain patient understands what is expected. *(Promotes cooperation and decreases anxiety.)*
6. Perform hand hygiene and don nonsterile gloves according to agency's policy and guidelines from the CDC and OSHA. *(Prevents transmission of microorganisms.)*
7. Instruct patient to tilt head backward. For patients in bed, place pillow behind shoulders. *(Facilitates visualization of pharynx.)*
8. Ask patient to open mouth and say "ah." *(Enables exposure of pharynx, relaxes throat muscles, and minimizes gag reflex.)*
9. Have swab ready for use. Loosen top of swab from culture tube for easy removal. *(Most commercially prepared tubes have a top that fits securely over end of swab, which allows touching of the outer top without contaminating swab stick.)*
10. If pharynx is not visualized, depress tongue with tongue blade and note inflamed areas of pharynx or tonsils. Depress anterior third of tongue only (illuminate with penlight as needed). *(It is necessary to visualize area to be swabbed. Placement of tongue blade along back of tongue is more likely to initiate gag reflex.)*
11. Insert swab without touching lips, teeth, tongue, or cheeks. *(Touching lips or oral mucosal structures potentially contaminates swab with resident bacteria.)*
12. Gently but quickly swab tonsillar area from side to side, making contact with inflamed or purulent sites. *(These areas contain the most microorganisms.)*
13. Carefully withdraw swab without striking oral structures. Immediately place swab securely in culture tube. Crush ampule at bottom of tube to release culture medium, and push tip of swab into liquid medium. *(Retains microorganisms within culture tube. Placing tip in culture medium maintains life of bacteria for testing.)*
14. Securely attach properly completed label and requisition slip to side of specimen container (not lid). *(Ensures proper identification of specimen; ensures accuracy of results; prevents loss and potential delays in obtaining results.)*
15. Enclose in a biohazard bag (see illustration for Skill 23.1, Step 11). *(Complies with guidelines from the CDC and OSHA.)*
16. Send specimen immediately to laboratory or refrigerate. *(Leaving specimen at room temperature permits bacterial content to increase.)*
17. Remove gloves, discard them in a proper receptacle, and perform hand hygiene. *(Prevents spread of microorganisms.)*
18. Document procedure. *(Communicates that procedure was completed.)*
    - Date and time collected
    - Type of specimen
    - Fact that specimen sent to laboratory with requisition slip
    - Patient response (if appropriate)
19. Perform patient teaching (see the Patient Teaching box).

CDC, Centers for Disease Control and Prevention; *OSHA*, Occupational Safety and Health Administration; *PPE*, personal protective equipment.

- Determine whether patient has experienced postnasal drip, sinus headache or tenderness, nasal congestion, or sore throat. *(Further clarifies nature of problem.)*
- Assess the condition of posterior pharynx (see Chapter 13).
- Assess for systemic indications of infection, including fever, chills, and malaise.
- Do not let the culture swab come in contact with the buccal mucosa, tongue, or teeth, because such contact contaminates the specimen.

COLLECTING A BLOOD SPECIMEN (VENIPUNCTURE) AND BLOOD FOR CULTURE

Veins are a primary source of blood for laboratory testing, as well as routes for intravenous (IV) fluids or

Skill 23.12 Obtaining a Nose Culture

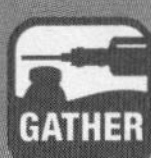

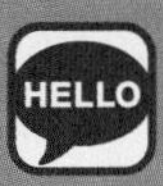

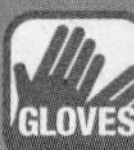

NURSING ACTION *(RATIONALE)*

1 to 6. Refer to Steps 1 to 6 of Skill 23.11.

7. Ask patient to blow nose, and then check nostrils for patency with penlight. Select nostril with greatest patency. *(Clears nasal passage of mucus that contains resident bacteria.)*

8. Ask patient to tilt head back. Patients in bed should have a pillow behind the shoulders.

9. Gently insert nasal speculum in one nostril (optional). Carefully pass swab into nostril until it reaches portion of mucosa that is inflamed or contains exudate. Rotate swab quickly. NOTE: If nasopharyngeal culture is to be obtained, use a special swab on a flexible wire that is able to flex downward to reach nasopharynx. *(It is necessary that swab remain sterile until it reaches area to be cultured. Rotating swab covers all surfaces where exudate is present.)*

10. With dominant hand, remove swab without touching sides of speculum or nasal canal. *(Prevents contamination by resident bacteria.)*

11. With nondominant hand, carefully remove nasal speculum (if used) and place in basin. Offer patient facial tissue. *(Removing speculum carefully prevents trauma to nasal mucosa; offering patient facial tissue provides comfort.)*

12. Immediately place swab securely in culture tube. *(Prevents contamination and spillage of specimen.)*

13. Crush ampule at bottom of tube to release culture medium. Push tip of swab into liquid medium. *(Placing tip in culture medium maintains life of bacteria for testing.)*

14. Discard supplies into proper receptacle. *(Prevents transmission of microorganisms.)*

15. Send culture tube to laboratory with completed requisition and attached label not attached to the lid of the container (see Box 23.5). Enclose in a biohazard bag. *(Ensures proper identification of specimen; ensures accuracy of results; prevents loss and potential delays in obtaining results.)*

16. Remove gloves, discard them in proper receptacle, and perform hand hygiene. *(Reduces spread of microorganisms.)*

17. Document procedure. *(Ensures procedure was completed.)*

18. Perform patient teaching (see the Patient Teaching box).

blood replacement; therefore maintaining their integrity is essential. Acquire and maintain skill in venipuncture, if allowed by facility policy or state's nurse practice act, to prevent unnecessary injury to veins.

Venipuncture may cause discomfort and anxiety in the patient. A calm approach and skilled technique help limit anxiety. Children may benefit from being able to have access to a comforting stuffed toy or parental presence.

Blood tests, one of the most commonly used diagnostic aids in the care and evaluation of patients, typically yield valuable information about nutritional, hematologic, metabolic, immune, and biochemical status. Tests allow health care providers to screen patients carefully for early signs of physical alterations, plot the course of existing disease, and monitor responses to therapies.

Nurses are sometimes responsible for collecting blood specimens; however, many facilities have specially trained technicians (phlebotomists) whose sole responsibility is to draw blood. Be familiar with facility policies and procedures and the state's nurse practice act regarding guidelines for collecting blood samples.

Venipuncture, the most common method, involves inserting a hollow-bore needle into the lumen of a large vein to obtain a specimen. In some cases, a needle and syringe are used, and in others, a special **Vacutainer** tube is used to collect multiple blood samples.

Assess the patient for special conditions that will affect the test procedure or results. With some tests, certain preparations are necessary to obtain accurate measurements, such as NPO status. A variety of factors put the patient undergoing venipuncture at risk, including anticoagulant therapy, low platelet count, bleeding disorders, presence of arteriovenous shunt or fistula, and having had breast or axillary surgery performed on that side. Abnormal clotting abilities, medications, and compromised circulation tend to impair blood flow. Assess the patient's ability to cooperate with the procedure; some patients need assistance from another health care team member (e.g., when the procedure appears threatening to the patient).

A health care provider's order is required for tests. Before collecting the specimen, review the order to ensure that the specimens and amount for all the tests to be performed are correct, eliminating the need for multiple blood draws. Older adults have fragile veins that are traumatized easily during venipuncture. Sometimes an application of a warm compress helps with sample collection. Using a small-bore catheter is another helpful strategy.

In the home care setting, it may be helpful to use a blood pressure cuff, rather than a tourniquet, when performing the venipuncture. Ask the patient if persistent or recurrent bleeding or expanding hematoma occurs at venipuncture site, and if so, notify the primary health care provider.

Children are often afraid of needles and the loss of blood. Explain the procedure and tell children that they have a lot of blood and that their bodies constantly make blood. Provide honest patient teaching for the pediatric patient. Fabrications and mistruths may damage the nurse-patient relationship irrevocably. Ask a parent or another staff member to hold and comfort the child. Toys or books may distract the child. Keep the needle out of the child's sight for as long as possible. Perform the venipuncture and collection of the blood quickly, and an adhesive bandage should be placed over the site.

The bloodborne pathogens standard of the Occupational Safety and Health Administration (OSHA) requires employers to protect workers from any occupational exposure that is related to bloodborne pathogens. The standard also requires that employers have a written Exposure Control Plan in place (OSHA, n.d.). As a result, phlebotomy equipment includes needle safety devices. Using standard precautions and appropriate personal protective equipment helps protect skin and mucous membranes from contact with blood; however, most barriers are penetrated easily by needles. Safety devices and features protect health care workers as follows:

- Provide a barrier between the hands and the needle after use
- Allow or require the worker's hands to remain behind the needle at all times
- Are simple to operate and necessitate little training to use effectively

A less invasive method of collecting a blood specimen is called a *capillary puncture.* It is used commonly to collect blood specimens from newborns and for glucose monitoring in all patients. The procedure usually is performed by puncturing a vascular area on a finger, toe, or heel with a lancet, although sometimes a sterile needle is used instead.

Even when safety needles are used, never recap needles, and always discard them carefully in puncture-resistant containers close to the patient (Fig. 23.4). A significant exposure occurs when a deep puncture is caused by a needle that has been used to collect blood. All needlestick injuries must be reported. Not all needlestick injuries are preventable; however, the use of needles with safety features has decreased substantially the risk of exposure to bloodborne pathogens for health care workers.

Blood culture, a specific blood test used to detect the presence of bacteria in the blood (bacteremia), requires

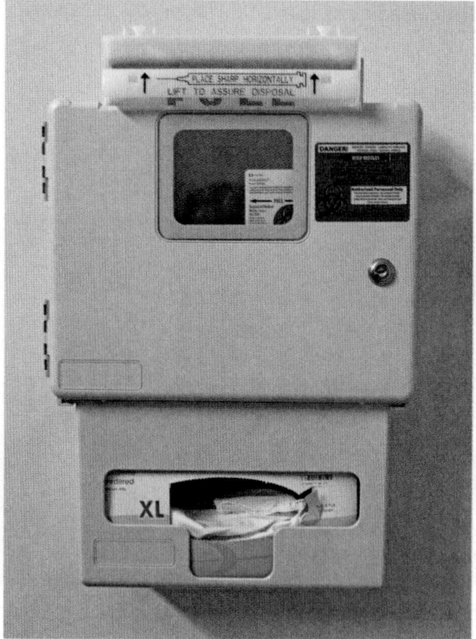

Fig. 23.4 Safety container for used needles and other sharps.

a special phlebotomy technique. Specimens for cultures are drawn when the symptoms of fever and chills that often accompany bacteremia are present. It is important to draw at least two culture specimens, one each from a different site. The venipuncture sites are prepared thoroughly according to agency policy before the collection of the blood specimens. The diagnosis of bacteremia is confirmed when both cultures grow an infecting agent. If only one culture produces bacteria, the assumption is that the bacteria were skin contaminants rather than the infecting agent. Because culture specimens obtained through an IV catheter frequently are contaminated, do not perform tests on them unless catheter sepsis is suspected. Blood culture specimens always are drawn before antibiotic therapy is started, because the antibiotic usually interferes with the organism's growth in the laboratory.

Collection Methods

Several collection methods are available. Using a syringe and attached needle is one method. Another is the use of a Vacutainer. With the syringe method, blood is drawn into the barrel by pulling back on the plunger. After the blood is collected, it is transferred to a test tube.

The Vacutainer system has a needle, a holder for the needle and tube, and one or more evacuated tubes with rubber stoppers (Fig. 23.5A). In evacuated tubes, air is removed, which creates a vacuum. When a vein is punctured, blood flows into the tube (see Fig. 23.5B). After a tube fills, it is removed from the holder, and a new tube is attached without withdrawal of the needle from the vein. The Vacutainer system thus allows the collection of multiple blood specimens with one venipuncture.

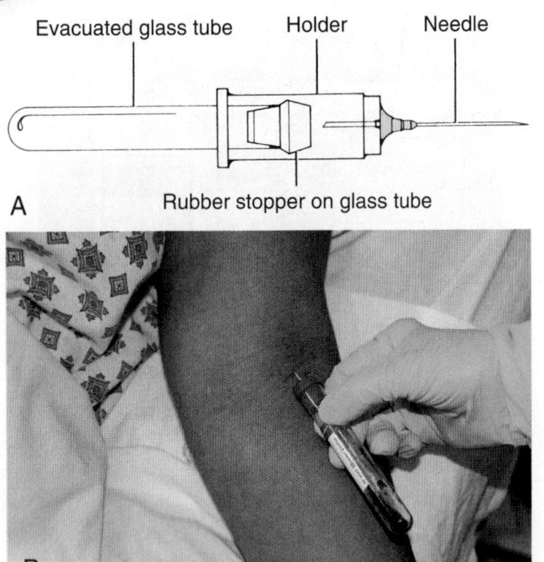

Fig. 23.5 Vacutainer method of collecting blood. A, Parts of the Vacutainer. B, Blood collection in a Vacutainer tube. (A from Zakus SM: *Clinical procedures for medical assistants*, ed 3, St. Louis, 1995, Mosby.)

Collection Tubes

Types of collection tubes. Blood collection tubes come in different sizes. The blood tests ordered determine the amount of blood needed. Some tests require additives that are added to the collection tube and mix with the blood. Some additives preserve the blood until testing; others aid in separating the blood cells from the plasma for testing. In the Vacutainer system, the tubes contain the necessary additives. The rubber stoppers are color coded. Red, lavender, blue, green, gray, and yellow are common colors. The color coding signals the type of additive, the amount of blood to collect, and the recommended blood tests to perform on the sample. Color coding sometimes varies, and so agency procedures must be followed. After the collection tubes are selected, they are placed in order of use. The order is important for preventing tube contamination. Different tubes have different additives. The additive from one tube should not be transferred inadvertently to another through use in the wrong order. Agency policy should be followed for the order in which to collect blood specimens.

Labeling collection tubes. After collection is completed and before the blood specimens are sent to the laboratory, the collection tube is labeled with the patient's identifying information (Fig. 23.6). Labeling is necessary to make sure that the right tests are done for the right patient. When wrong test results are reported for the patient, the wrong treatment will be given, and the patient is at risk for serious harm. Box 23.5 discusses a patient's identifying information. Labels generally are generated using data stored in the patient's electronic health record (EHR).

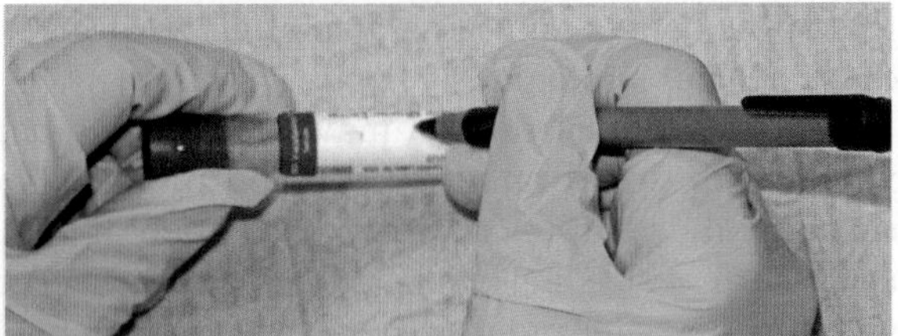

Fig. 23.6 Labeling the blood collection tube.

Selecting a Venipuncture Site

The basilic and cephalic veins in the antecubital space are the most common venipuncture sites (Fig. 23.7). These veins are large and near the skin surface. Hand veins offer alternative sites.

Select the arm to be used before selecting the vein. An arm on the side of a mastectomy, with a paralysis, with a hemodialysis access site, or with an IV site should not be used. An arm with existing hematomas or skin impairment also should be avoided.

A tourniquet is applied to the arm when the vein selection process begins (Fig. 23.8A). A **tourniquet** is a constricting device traditionally applied to control bleeding. It prevents arterial blood flow to the part below the tourniquet and prevents venous blood from returning to the heart. The veins fill with blood and distend, which makes them firmer and easier to see and palpate (see Fig. 23.8B); thus the tourniquet is useful for venipuncture.

The tourniquet is removed after the blood specimen is collected but before the needle is withdrawn from the vein. The tourniquet is applied 2 to 4 inches (5.08 to 10.16 cm) above the elbow. One end is crossed tightly over the other, and then the upper end is tucked under the band to form a half bow (see Fig. 23.8A). This allows for quick release.

When used for obtaining a venous specimen, tourniquets prevent venous blood flow but not arterial blood flow. Make sure the tourniquet is tight enough that the veins distend; however, the radial pulse should be palpable. If the radial pulse is not detected, release and reapply the tourniquet. The tourniquet should be in place for no longer than 1 to 2 minutes.

To select a vein in the antecubital space, a tourniquet is applied 2 to 4 inches (5.08 to 10.16 cm) above the elbow. The patient is asked to open and close the fist. While the patient's fist is closed, look and palpate for a vein. A vein that is suitable for venipuncture is straight, feels full and firm, and is elastic and springs back after palpation (see Fig. 23.8B). Veins with the following characteristics are avoided:

- Small and narrow veins are usually fragile.
- Weak veins are soft and do not rebound.
- Sclerosed veins are hard and rigid.
- Veins that are easy to roll when palpated are often difficult to pierce successfully with the needle.

Perform the venipuncture (Skill 23.13). After the needle is withdrawn from the vein, apply pressure to the site to

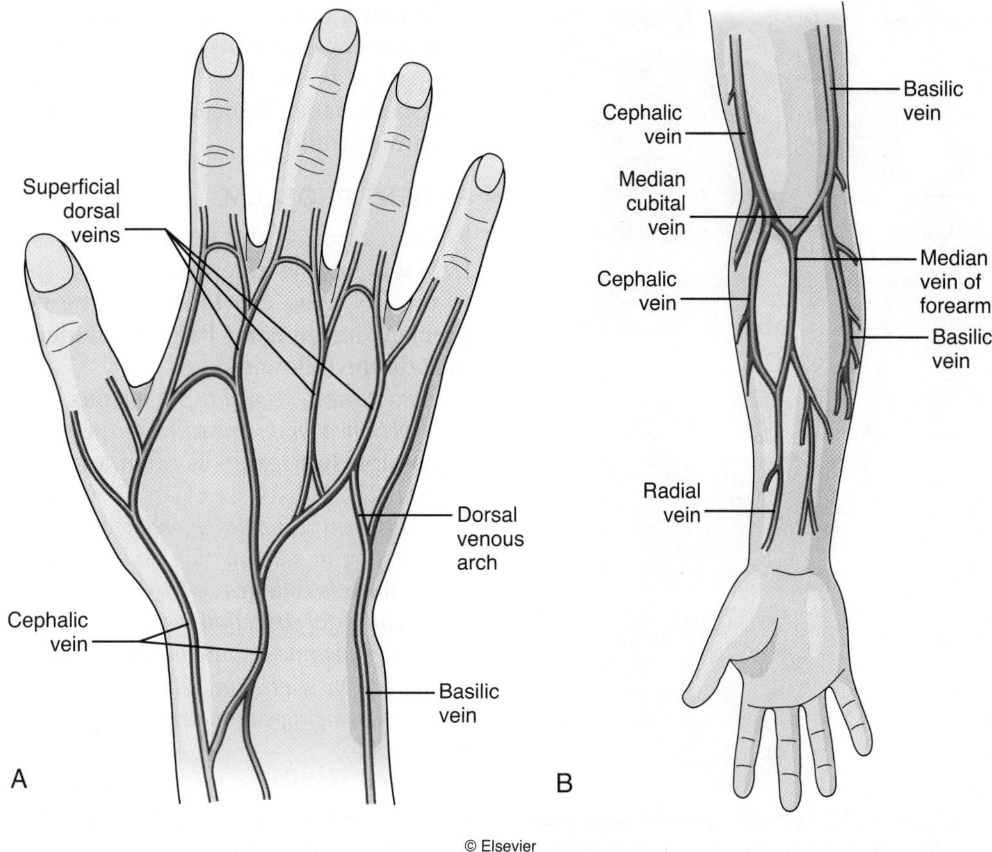

Fig. 23.7 Venipuncture sites. A, Inner arm. B, Dorsal surface of hand.

prevent bleeding. The patient should not bend the arm, because this may cause the formation of a hematoma.

See the Home Care Considerations and Coordinated Care boxes.

ELECTROCARDIOGRAPHY

Electrocardiography may be performed by nurses or by technicians specifically trained for this test. The **electrocardiogram (ECG)** is a graphic representation of electrical impulses generated by the heart during a cardiac cycle; it identifies abnormalities that interfere with electrical conduction through cardiac tissue. This procedure usually is done at the patient's bedside, but sometimes it is done in a specially equipped laboratory.

The patient is assessed for knowledge level of the procedure; ability to understand and follow directions (this procedure requires patient to follow directions closely and assume proper positioning); ability to assume proper position; and vital signs (baseline) for comparison with postprocedure vital signs.

If the patient has large amounts of hair, it is sometimes necessary to clip or shave the hair at the lead placement site. This promotes adherence of the leads (electrodes) to the chest and on the extremity. Skill 23.14 describes how the ECG is obtained.

❖ NURSING PROCESS FOR SPECIMEN COLLECTION AND DIAGNOSTIC TESTING

The role of the LPN/LVN in the nursing process is that the LPN/LVN will

- Participate in planning care for patients based on patient needs
- Review patient's plan of care and recommend revisions as needed
- Review and follow defined prioritization for patient care
- Use clinical pathways, care maps, or care plans to guide and review patient care

◆ ASSESSMENT

Do the following in regard to specimen collection and diagnostic testing:

- Assess patient's knowledge of procedure to determine level of health teaching required.
- Observe verbal and nonverbal behavior to determine patient's anxiety.
- Determine patient's ability to understand and follow directions.
- Evaluate patient's ability to assume position required for procedure and ability to remain in that position.

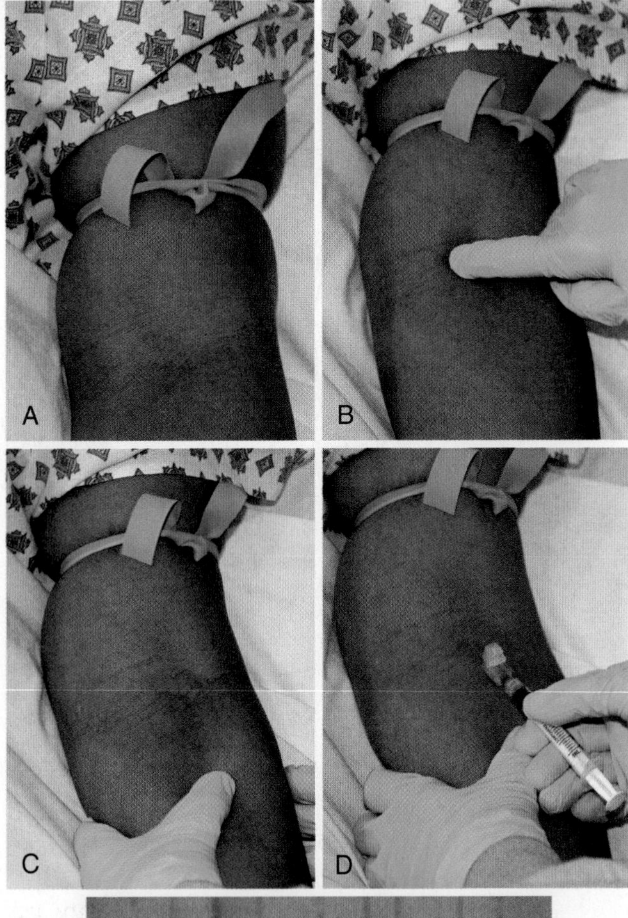

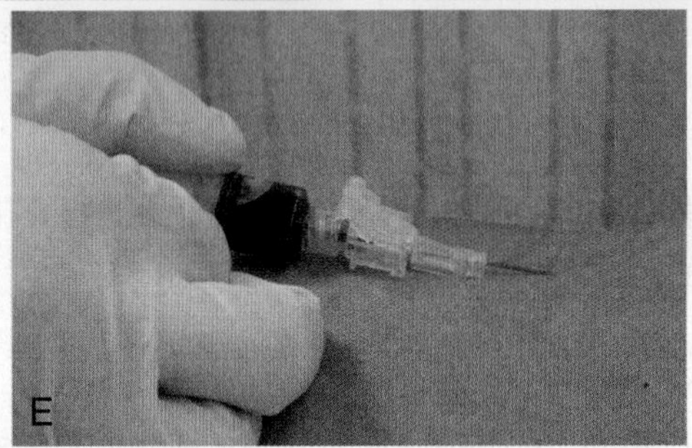

Fig. 23.8 Venipuncture. A, Applying tourniquet to select a venipuncture site. B, Palpating a vein. C, Pulling the skin taut over the venipuncture site. D, Inserting a double-ended needle into the vein. E, Pulling back on the plunger to withdraw blood; note safety feature. (E from Elkin MK, Perry AG, Potter PA: *Nursing interventions and clinical skills*, ed 4, St. Louis, 2008, Mosby.)

- Determine whether patient is allergic to antiseptics, anesthetic solutions, or any of the dyes that will possibly be used.
- Assess patient's need for preprocedure analgesic administration.

◆ PATIENT PROBLEM

With an accurate and thorough assessment, the LPN/LVN will be able to report patient assessment findings to the RN, who can formulate the necessary patient problem statements. Patient problems are likely to include the following:

- *Anxiousness, related to the manner in which a specimen is obtained or a procedure is performed.* Fear of the possible test results is often a factor (Nursing Care Plan 23.1).
- *Insufficient Knowledge, related to the purpose of the collection or examination and the manner in which the specimen is collected or the test is performed.*
- *Potential for Infection, related to the patient's skin or tissue impairment (broken during a diagnostic procedure).*
- *Recent Onset of Pain, related to invasive diagnostic test (when some type of instrument is inserted into a part of the body).*

Patient problems related to optimal oxygenation during diagnostic procedures involving the airway include the following:

- *Inefficient Oxygenation*
- *Inability to Maintain Adequate Breathing Pattern*
- *Potential for Aspiration Into Airway*
- *Inability to Clear Airway, related to collection of sputum specimen by sneezing and coughing or related to collection of sputum specimen by suctioning*

◆ EXPECTED OUTCOMES AND PLANNING

Identify goals and outcomes of care, and set priorities for the plan of care that is likely to result in goal achievement. Expected outcomes focus on the collection of an uncontaminated specimen by the health care personnel or the patient and the patient's understanding of the purpose of the examination that requires the specimen.

Text continued on p. 692

Skill 23.13 Performing the Venipuncture

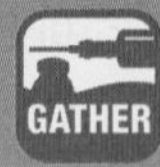

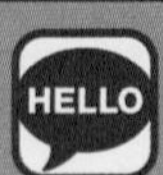

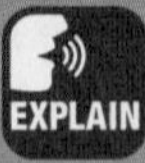

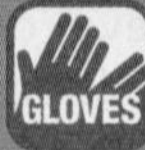

NURSING ACTION *(RATIONALE)*

1. Refer to the health care provider's order. *(A health care provider's order is necessary.)*
2. Assemble supplies. *(Organizes procedure.)*
   - Alcohol or antiseptic swab (check agency policy for specific antiseptic solution)
   - Nonsterile gloves
   - Additional PPE if indicated
   - Small pillow or folded towel
   - Rubber tourniquet
   - Sterile 2 × 2 gauze pads
   - Bandage or adhesive tape
   - Appropriate blood tubes, culture bottles
   - Identification labels

Skill 23.13 Performing the Venipuncture—cont'd

- Laboratory requisition
- Biohazard bag for delivery of specimen to laboratory (or container as specified by agency)

a. Syringe method:
  (1) Sterile needles (20- to 21-gauge for adults, 23- to 25-gauge for children, 23- to 25-gauge butterfly for older adults)
  (2) Sterile syringe of appropriate size

b. Vacuum tube method:
  (1) Vacuum tube with needle holder
  (2) Sterile double-ended needles (20- to 21-gauge for adults, 23- to 25-gauge for children)

3. Introduce self. *(Decreases patient's anxiety.)*

4. Identify patient. *(Ensures procedure is performed with correct patient.)*

5. Explain procedure, including the reason it is being done. *(Promotes patient's cooperation and decreases patient's anxiety.)*

6. Assess patient. *(To determine whether test is still appropriate.)*

7. Arrange equipment and complete necessary charges. *(Facilitates procedure and facilitates proper billing.)*

8. Prepare patient for procedure.
  a. Close door or pull curtain. *(Provides privacy.)*
  b. Assist patient into supine or semi-Fowler's position with arms extended to form straight line from shoulders to wrists. Place small pillow or towel under upper arms. *(Helps stabilize extremity. Supported position in bed reduces chance of injury to patient if fainting occurs.)*
  c. Adjust bed to appropriate height, and lower nearest side rail. *(Promotes proper body mechanics and facilitates procedure.)*
  d. Drape patient. *(Prevents unnecessary exposure.)*

9. Perform hand hygiene and don nonsterile gloves according to agency policy and guidelines from the CDC and OSHA. *(Reduces exposure to bloodborne pathogens.)*

10. Apply tourniquet 2 to 4 inches (5.08 to 10.16 cm) above puncture site (see Fig. 23.8A). *(Causes vein to distend for easier visibility.)*

11. Palpate distal pulse. If pulse is not palpable, reapply tourniquet more loosely. *(If too tight, tourniquet will impede arterial blood flow.)*

12. Keep tourniquet on patient no longer than 1–2 minutes. If tourniquet is left on arm too long, remove and assess other extremity or wait 60 seconds before reapplying. *(Prolonged time has potential to alter test results and cause pain and venous stasis.)*

13. Ask patient to open and close fist several times, finally leaving fist clenched. Patient should avoid vigorous opening and closing of fist, which sometimes causes erroneous laboratory results. *(Facilitates distention of veins by forcing blood up from distal veins.)*

14. Quickly inspect extremity for best venipuncture site, looking for straight, prominent vein without swelling or hematoma. *(Straight and intact veins are easiest to puncture.)*

15. Palpate selected vein with fingers. Note whether vein is firm and rebounds when palpated or whether vein feels rigid and cordlike and rolls when palpated (see Fig. 23.8B). *(Patent, healthy vein is elastic and rebounds on palpation. Thrombosed vein is rigid, rolls easily, and is difficult to puncture.)*

16. Select venipuncture site (see Fig. 23.8). *(Prevents discomfort to patient and ensures accuracy of test results.)*

17. Obtain blood sample.
  a. Syringe method:
    (1) Use syringe with appropriate needle securely attached. *(Ensures needle will not dislodge from syringe during venipuncture.)*
    (2) Cleanse venipuncture site with alcohol swab, moving in circular motion outward from site for approximately 2 inches (5 cm). Allow to dry. *(Antimicrobial agent cleans skin surface of resident bacteria so that organisms do not enter puncture site. Allowing alcohol to dry reduces "sting" of venipuncture.)*
    (3) Remove needle cover, and inform patient that a "stick" lasting only a few seconds will be felt. *(Patient has better control over anxiety when prepared for what to expect.)*
    (4) Place thumb or forefinger of nondominant hand 1 inch (2.5 cm) below site, and pull patient's skin taut (see Fig. 23.8C). *(Stabilizes vein and prevents rolling during needle insertion.)*
    (5) Hold syringe and needle at 15- to 30-degree angle from patient's arm with bevel up (see Fig. 23.8D). *(Reduces chance of penetrating both sides of vein during insertion. Keeping bevel up reduces vein trauma.)*
    (6) Slowly insert needle into vein (see Fig. 23.8D). *(Reduces chance of penetrating both sides of vein during insertion.)*
    (7) Hold syringe securely and pull back gently on plunger (see Fig. 23.8E). *(Holding syringe securely prevents needle from advancing. Pulling on plunger creates vacuum needed to draw blood into syringe.)*

Continued

Skill 23.13 Performing the Venipuncture—cont'd

(8) Look for blood return. *(If blood flow fails to appear, needle is not well seated in vein; withdraw needle and prepare for a second attempt.)* **NOTE:** No more than two attempts should be made by a single nurse in the same session and no more than four attempts total (Infusion Nurses Society, 2016).

(9) Obtain desired amount of blood, keeping needle stabilized. *(Test results are more accurate when required amount of blood is obtained. Some tests are not possible to perform without minimal blood requirement. Movement of needle increases discomfort.)*

(10) After specimen is obtained, release tourniquet. *(Reduces bleeding at site when needle is withdrawn.)*

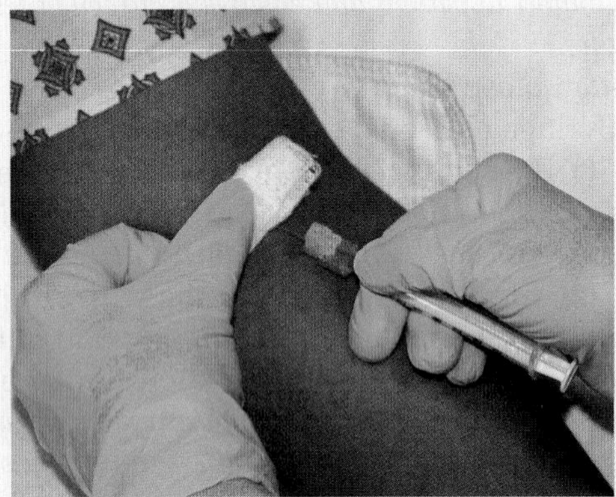

(11) Apply 2 × 2 gauze pad or alcohol swab over puncture site without applying pressure, and quickly but carefully withdraw needle from vein; apply pressure with gauze after removal of needle. *(Pressure over needle causes discomfort. Careful removal of needle keeps discomfort and vein trauma to a minimum.)*

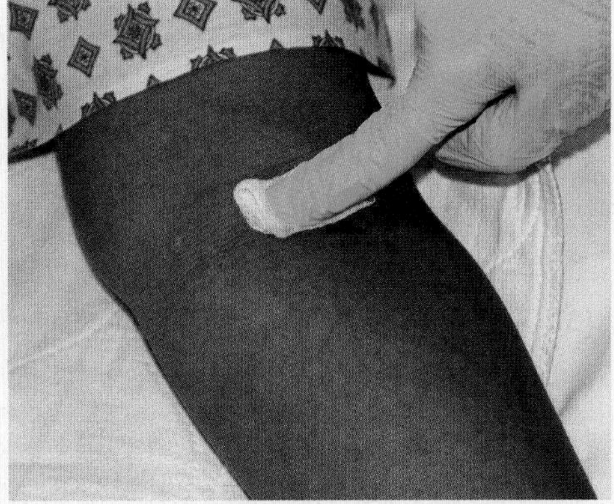

(12) Carefully transfer blood from syringe into vacuum tube.

(13) Without recapping, discard needle in proper receptacle. *(Reduces risk of needlestick injury.)*

(14) Remove gloves, discard them in proper receptacle, and perform hand hygiene. *(Reduces spread of microorganisms.)*

b. Vacuum tube method:

(1) Attach double-ended needle to vacuum tube or Vacutainer. (Long end of needle is used to puncture vein. Short end fits into blood tube.)

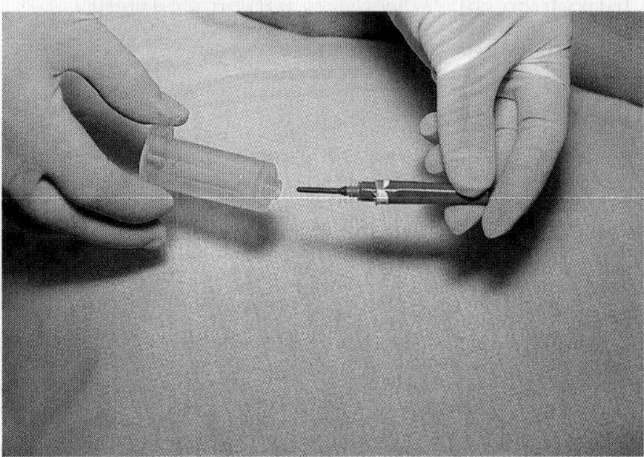

(2) Have proper blood specimen tube resting inside vacuum tube, but do not push onto needle and puncture rubber stopper. *(Causes loss of tube's vacuum.)*

(3) Cleanse venipuncture site with alcohol swab, moving in circular motion outward from site for approximately 2 inches (5 cm). *(Cleans skin surface of resident bacteria so that organisms do not enter through puncture site.)*

(4) Remove needle cover and inform patient that a "stick" lasting only a few seconds will be felt. *(Patient has better control over anxiety when prepared for what to expect.)*

(5) Place thumb or forefinger of nondominant hand 1 inch (2.5 cm) below site and pull patient's skin taut. Stretch skin down until vein is stabilized. *(Stabilizes vein and prevents rolling during needle insertion.)*

(6) Hold vacuum tube at 15- to 30-degree angle from arm with bevel up. *(Reduces chance of penetrating both sides of vein during insertion. Keeping bevel up causes less trauma to vein.)*

Skill 23.13 Performing the Venipuncture—cont'd

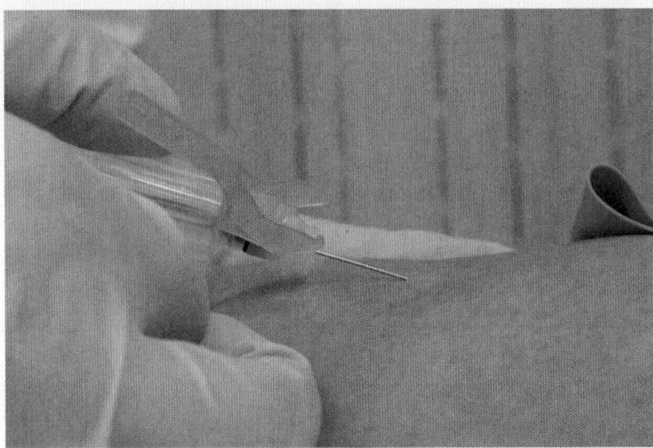
Steps 17b(1) and 17b(6) from Elkin MK, Perry AG, Potter PA: *Nursing interventions and clinical skills*, ed 4, St. Louis, 2008, Mosby.

(7) Slowly insert needle into vein (see Fig. 23.8D). *(Reduces chance of penetrating both sides of vein during insertion.)*

(8) Grasp vacuum tube securely so that you do not move it or advance needle in vein, and advance specimen tube into needle of holder. *(Pushing needle through stopper breaks vacuum and causes blood to flow into tube. If needle in vein advances, it is possible to puncture vein on other side.)*

(9) Note flow of blood into tube (normally fairly rapid). *(Failure of blood to appear indicates that vacuum in tube is lost or needle is not well seated in vein.)*

(10) After specimen tube is filled, grasp vacuum tube firmly and remove tube without allowing needle in vein to move in or out. Insert additional specimen tubes as needed, as described in Step 8. *(Prevents needle from advancing or dislodging. It is necessary to fill tube completely to keep additives in certain tubes in proper proportion to blood volume of tube. Invert tubes with additives as soon as possible to mix.)*

(11) While last tube is filling, release tourniquet. *(Reduces bleeding at site when needle is withdrawn.)*

(12) Apply 2 × 2 gauze pad over puncture site without applying pressure, and quickly but carefully withdraw needle from vein. *(Pressure over needle causes discomfort. Careful removal of needle keeps discomfort and vein trauma to a minimum.)*

(13) Remove gloves, discard them in proper receptacle, and perform hand hygiene. *(Reduces spread of microorganisms.)*

18. For blood obtained by syringe, transfer specimen to tubes.

a. Using one-handed technique, insert syringe needle through stopper of blood tube and allow vacuum to fill tube. Do not force blood into tube. *(Forcing blood into tube has the potential to cause hemolysis of red blood cells and invalidates test with tubes containing anticoagulants or additives. OSHA recommends one-handed technique to help prevent needlestick injury.)*

b. Alternative method is to remove needle from syringe and stopper from each test tube. Gently inject required amount of blood into each tube. Reapply stopper. *(Blood injected too quickly sometimes causes frothing or hemolysis of red blood cells. Stopper maintains sterility of specimen.)*

19. When obtaining blood for culture (it is necessary to obtain cultures from two sites):

a. Cleanse venipuncture sites with povidone-iodine or appropriate antiseptic. Allow to dry. *(Antimicrobial agent cleans skin surface so that organisms do not enter puncture site or contaminate culture.)*

b. Clean bottle tops of vacuum tubes or culture bottles with appropriate antiseptic (check agency policy). *(Ensures that specimen is sterile.)*

c. Collect 10 to 15 mL of venous blood by venipuncture from each venipuncture site.

d. Discard needle on syringe; replace with new sterile needle before injecting blood sample into culture bottles. *(Maintains sterile technique and prevents contamination of specimen.)*

e. If aerobic and anaerobic cultures are needed, inoculate anaerobic culture first. *(Anaerobic organisms often take longer to grow.)*

f. Mix medium gently after inoculation. *(Mixes medium and blood.)*

g. After venipuncture, apply 2 × 2 gauze pad over puncture site without applying pressure, and quickly but carefully withdraw needle from vein. *(Pressure over needle causes discomfort. Careful removal of needle keeps discomfort and vein trauma to a minimum.)*

20. For blood tubes containing additives, gently rotate tubes back and forth 8 to 10 times. *(It is necessary to mix additives with blood to prevent clotting. Shaking has potential to cause hemolysis of red blood cells, rendering test results inaccurate.)*

21. Inspect puncture site for bleeding, and apply adhesive tape with gauze. *(Keeps puncture site clean and controls any final oozing.)*

Continued

Skill 23.13 Performing the Venipuncture—cont'd

22. Check tubes for any sign of external contamination with blood. Decontaminate with alcohol if necessary. Remove gloves, discard them in proper receptacle, and perform hand hygiene. *(Prevents cross-contamination. Reduces risk of exposure to pathogens present in blood.)*

23. Securely attach properly completed identification label to each tube, affix proper requisition, place tubes in biohazard bag, and transport to laboratory promptly. *(Ensures proper identification of specimen; ensures accuracy of results; prevents loss and potential delays in obtaining results.)*

24. Remove gloves, discard them in proper receptacle, and perform hand hygiene. *(Prevents the spread of microorganisms.)*

25. Assist patient to a comfortable position, and place needed items within easy reach. *(Ensures patient's comfort and well-being.)*

26. Raise side rail, and lower bed to lowest position. *(Promotes patient safety.)*

27. Store, remove, or dispose of supplies and equipment as appropriate. *(Ensures equipment is available for next use.)*

28. Document procedure. *(Provides communication that the procedure was carried out and patient's response.)*
- Time
- Test performed
- Patient's response
- Any adverse findings (e.g., hematoma, prolonged bleeding, unusual pain)

CDC, Centers for Disease Control and Prevention; *OSHA*, Occupational Safety and Health Administration; *PPE*, personal protective equipment.

Skill 23.14 Performing Electrocardiography

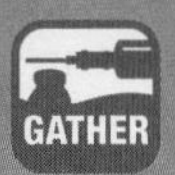

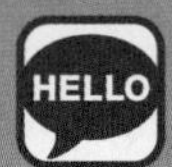

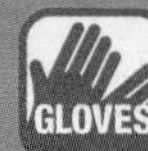

NURSING ACTION *(RATIONALE)*

1. Refer to the health care provider's order. *(Provides basis for care.)*
2. Assemble supplies. *(Organizes procedure.)*
   - Electrocardiogram (ECG) machine
   - Electropaste (gel)
   - ECG leads or electrodes
   - Alcohol wipes
   - Razor or clippers
   - Nonsterile gloves (optional)
3. Introduce self. *(Decreases patient's anxiety.)*
4. Identify patient. *(Ensures procedure is performed with correct patient.)*
5. Explain procedure. Include the reason it is being done in terms that the patient can understand. *(Promotes cooperation and decreases patient's anxiety; ensures accuracy.)*
6. Assess patient for chest pain, pulse, and respirations. *(Enables determination of whether the test is still appropriate.)*
7. Arrange equipment and complete necessary charges. *(Facilitates procedure and proper billing.)*
8. Prepare patient for procedure.
   - **a.** Close door or pull curtains. *(Provides privacy.)*
   - **b.** Usually supine is the preferred position. Arrange for patient's comfort. *(Promotes accuracy of test.)*
   - **c.** Drape patient as necessary. *(Prevents unnecessary embarrassment.)*
   - **d.** Adjust bed to appropriate height, and lower the nearest side rail. *(Promotes proper body mechanics and facilitates procedure.)*
   - **e.** Perform hand hygiene and don nonsterile gloves according to agency's policy and guidelines from the CDC and OSHA. *(Reduces spread of microorganisms.)*
9. Perform electrocardiography.
   - **a.** Cleanse and prepare skin (shave or clip hair, as necessary, after obtaining consent); wipe skin with alcohol. *(Promotes adherence of leads [electrodes] to chest or extremity.)*
   - **b.** Apply electrode paste and attach leads. *(Position of leads promotes proper display of ECG on paper.)*

Skill 23.14 Performing Electrocardiography—cont'd

For 12-Lead Electrocardiography

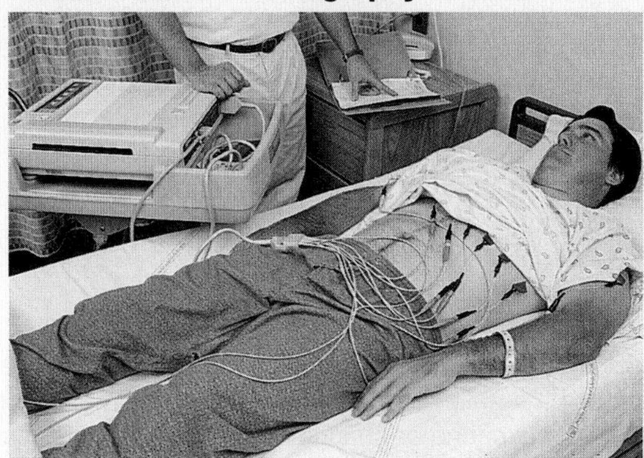

(1) Chest (precordial leads)
V_1: Fourth intercostal space (ICS) at right sternal border
V_2: Fourth ICS at left sternal border
V_3: Midway between V_2 and V_4
V_4: Fifth ICS at midclavicular line
V_5: Left anterior axillary line at level of V_4 horizontally
V_6: Left midaxillary line at level of V_4 horizontally

(2) Extremities: one at lower portion of each extremity:
$_aV_R$: Right wrist
$_aV_L$: Left wrist
$_aV_F$: Left ankle

c. Obtain tracing (it is possible to perform 12-lead electrocardiography without removing precordial leads). *(Transfers electrocardiac conduction on ECG tracing paper for subsequent analysis by cardiologist.)*

d. Disconnect leads; wipe excess electrode paste from patient's chest. *(Promotes comfort and hygiene.)*

e. Remove gloves, discard them in proper receptacle, and perform hand hygiene. *(Reduces spread of microorganisms.)*

f. Deliver ECG tracing to appropriate laboratory or nursing unit promptly. *(Provides for review of ECG by cardiologist.)*

10. Assist patient to a comfortable position, and place needed items within easy reach. *(Ensures patient's comfort and well-being.)*

11. Raise side rail, and lower bed to lowest position. *(Ensures patient's safety.)*

12. Store, remove, or dispose of supplies and equipment as appropriate. *(Ensures equipment is available for next use.)*

13. Document procedure. *(Provides communication that the procedure was carried out and patient's response.)*
- Time
- Test performed
- Patient's response
- Provide patient teaching (as appropriate)

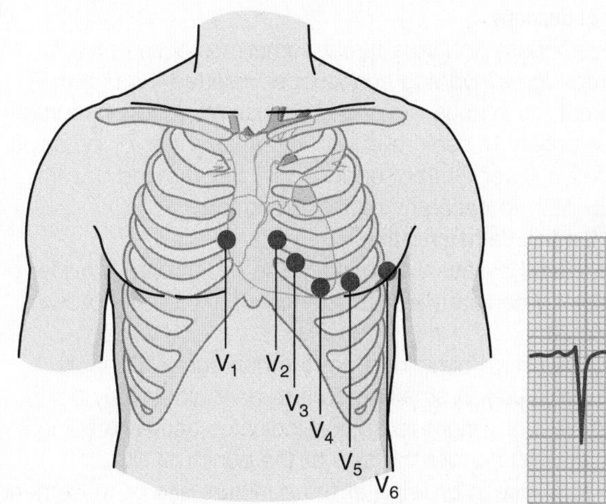

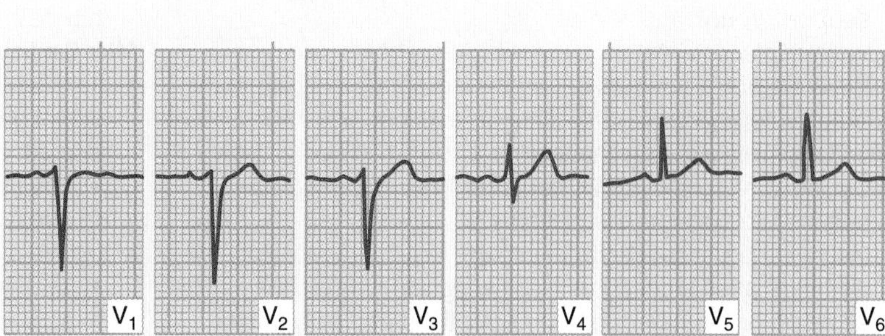

CDC, Centers for Disease Control and Prevention; *OSHA,* Occupational Safety and Health Administration.
Step 9 figure from Elkin MK, Perry AG, Potter PA: *Nursing interventions and clinical skills,* ed 4, St. Louis, 2008, Mosby.

Home Care Considerations

Specimen Collection and Diagnostic Examination

SPECIMEN

Urine

- It is best to collect urine specimens for culture and sensitivity in the laboratory setting rather than at home because the chance of bacterial growth is increased by the delay in testing. If a specimen is collected at home, the patient must refrigerate the specimen until time of transport to the laboratory and must keep the specimen on ice during transport.
- When obtaining a urine testing kit, the patient needs to know that all supplies except for the specimen container are usually included in the kit.
- Urine testing at home typically is performed with reagent strips.

Stool

- Frequently, patients are instructed to obtain stool specimens at home and then bring the specimen to the laboratory setting or health care provider's office.
- If a stool specimen is obtained for occult blood testing, the patient is asked to prepare the slide at home and return the slide to the laboratory or health care provider's office for testing.
- Instruct the patient obtaining a stool specimen at home to prevent the specimen from contact with the toilet bowl by using the specimen hat provided by the health care provider.
- Many older adults need assistance with the collection of stool specimens.

Sputum

- Instruct patients obtaining sputum specimens at home on proper specimen collection and the importance of returning the specimen to the laboratory in a timely manner.

Wound Drainage

- Teach proper technique for obtaining a wound specimen (e.g., hand hygiene) if the specimen is obtained in the patient's home.

Venipuncture

- In the home setting, a tourniquet is often not available; use a blood pressure cuff before venipuncture.

Blood Glucose Testing

- Encourage patients to attend meetings of a diabetic support group.
- Various glucose meters are available for home use.
- Patient teaching should be performed on the specific glucometer model that the patient purchases.

Other Specimens and Examinations

- Driving is restricted for 24 hours after procedures that necessitate conscious sedation.
- Instruct the patient not to make any legal decisions for 24 hours after procedures that necessitate conscious sedation or the use of other medications that may impair judgment.

POSTPROCEDURAL CONSIDERATIONS

After Intravenous Pyelography (IVP)

Discharge instructions typically include the following:

- The kidneys excrete the contrast medium. Instruct the patient to drink at least 24 ounces (720 mL) of water if this is not contraindicated by a current condition.
- Delayed allergic reaction from the contrast medium is possible as much as 24 hours after the procedure. Instruct patients to call the primary health care provider if they have such reactions. If the reaction is an emergency (facial swelling, especially around the eyes, lips, and mouth; difficulty breathing; difficulty swallowing; wheezing), the patient is to go immediately to the emergency department rather than contacting the primary health care provider.

After Lumbar Puncture

- Provide the patient with written instructions upon discharge after a lumbar puncture. Instructions include directing the patient to get immediate medical attention if a severe headache or change in level of consciousness occurs after the procedure.

After Paracentesis

- Instruct the patient to contact the health care provider if he or she develops a fever or experiences pain, swelling, or discharge from the puncture site. The patient should rest after this procedure because he or she may feel dizzy or light-headed related to the amount of fluid removed.

After Thoracentesis

- Give patients written instructions that include signs and symptoms of complications related to perforation of the spleen, liver, or lung. Signs and symptoms to be alert to include fever, leakage of fluid from the puncture site, difficulty breathing, or chest pain. Inform the patient that sometimes these signs and symptoms do not occur until several days after the procedure.

After Bronchoscopy

- Instruct patients experiencing fever, chest pain or discomfort, or respiratory symptoms such as dyspnea, wheezing, or hemoptysis to contact the health care provider or to seek medical attention immediately.
- Inform patients that throat discomfort is common and often is relieved with throat lozenges.

After Endoscopy

- Hoarseness and sore throat sometimes occur after procedures involving endoscopes inserted through the throat; as long as the gag reflex has returned, encourage the patient to seek relief with throat lozenges or ice chips.
- After a lower GI tract endoscopy, recommend a warm tub bath to ease any rectal discomfort.

After Cardiac Catheterization

- Instruct the patient to contact the health care provider or seek immediate medical attention if any of the following occurs:
  - Excessive bleeding from the puncture site (apply pressure). A small amount of dark blood may be present. Bright red blood indicates active bleeding.
  - Swelling under the skin at the puncture site.
  - Increase in bruising at the puncture site or movement of bruising down the extremity that was used for the procedure.
  - Increased or new sensation of pain at the puncture site or in the extremity used for the procedure.
  - Paleness, or if the extremity of the puncture site becomes pale or cold.
  - Redness or warmth at the puncture site.

 Coordinated Care

Collaboration

Specimen Collection

- The collection of urine specimens may be performed by unlicensed assistive personnel (UAP) who are familiar with aseptic and sterile technique and if allowed by the facility policy. UAP should be informed of when to collect a specimen and proper transport of the specimen. UAP are directed to immediately notify the nurse if appearance of urine a specimen is abnormal (e.g., presence of blood, cloudiness, or excess sediments).
- The collection of stool and emesis for testing may be performed by UAP. However, assessing the significance of test results requires skills of critical thinking and knowledge application that are unique to a nurse. Delegation of the analysis of test results to UAP is inappropriate. UAP are directed to notify the nurse immediately if results are positive so that testing can be repeated by the nurse.
- The skills used to obtain and test gastric secretions from an NG or nasoenteral tube require the critical thinking and knowledge application unique to a nurse. Delegation of these procedures to UAP is inappropriate.
- Obtaining and testing the blood glucose level after skin puncture can be performed by UAP who are certified to perform the procedure. It is necessary to assess the patient to determine whether his or her need for glucose monitoring is appropriate for delegation. If the patient's condition changes frequently, this procedure should not be delegated to UAP.
- Phlebotomy staff, registered nurses (RNs), and licensed practical nurses/licensed vocational nurses (LPNs/LVNs) are permitted to obtain venipuncture samples in accordance with agency policy and their state's nurse practice act. The LPN/LVN should consult agency policy to determine who is permitted to draw blood.
- The skills used to obtain throat, nasal, and nasopharyngeal cultures require the critical thinking and knowledge application unique to a nurse. Delegation of these procedures to UAP is inappropriate.
- Collection of expectorated sputum specimens can be performed by UAP. However, the skills used to collect a sputum specimen through sterile suction require the critical thinking and knowledge application unique to a nurse. Delegation of this procedure by suction to UAP is inappropriate.
- Obtaining a wound culture requires the critical thinking and knowledge application unique to a nurse. Delegation of this procedure to UAP is inappropriate.
- UAPs are permitted to transport stable patients to the testing department. Monitoring vital signs after the procedures is possible to delegate to a UAP, but assessment is not. Monitoring during intravenous conscious sedation (IVCS) requires the critical thinking and knowledge application unique to a nurse. Delegation of this task to UAP is inappropriate.
- Diagnostic studies requiring the use of a contrast medium subject patients to potentially life-threatening complications. Direct the UAP to notify the nurse immediately of any complications (e.g., allergic reactions, bleeding, respiratory distress, or coughing up blood).
- Electrocardiography often is performed by technicians specifically trained for this test. Nurses with advanced training often monitor patient electrocardiographic patterns continuously in an intensive care setting, in the emergency department, or on units where telemetry is used. It is acceptable for UAP to monitor the vital signs of stable patients. UAPs must notify the nurse immediately of complaints of chest pain or altered vital signs.

 Nursing Care Plan 23.1 **Specimen Collection or Diagnostic Examination**

This care plan has been adapted for the patient who is at risk for anxiousness with regard to diagnostic tests and examinations.

PATIENT PROBLEM

Potential for Anxiousness, related to intrusive diagnostic tests and procedures

Patient Goals and Expected Outcomes	Nursing Interventions and Rationale	Evaluation
Patient describes a reduction in the level of anxiety experienced	Acknowledge awareness of patient's anxiety. *(Acknowledgment of the patient's feelings validates the feelings and communicates acceptance of these feelings.)* Stay with the patient if this appears necessary. *(The presence of a trusted person is often helpful.)* Maintain a calm manner while interacting with patient. *(The patient's feeling of stability increases in a calm and nonthreatening atmosphere.)* Orient patient to environment, new experiences, or people. *(Orientation and awareness promote comfort and may decrease anxiety.)* Use simple language and brief statements when instructing patient about diagnostic procedures. *(When experiencing moderate to severe anxiety, patients are frequently unable to comprehend anything more than simple, clear, and brief instructions.)* Encourage patient to ask questions. Assist patient in identifying factors causing anxiety. *(Patient is possibly unaware of the relationship between emotional concerns and anxiety.)*	Patient states fewer feelings of anxiety. Patient states an understanding of the upcoming examination.

Continued

Nursing Care Plan 23.1 Specimen Collection or Diagnostic Examination—cont'd

CRITICAL THINKING QUESTIONS

1. The patient has been very quiet during his morning care. When you attempt a conversation, he is obviously not interested. What is a way for you to initiate a conversation to encourage him to relate his concerns over his upcoming bronchoscopy?
2. Your patient is scheduled for an intravenous pyelogram (IVP). During your preparation of this patient, he remarks he once had a reaction while eating shellfish. What will you probably do next?
3. The patient is obviously anxious about his upcoming magnetic resonance imaging (MRI) scan. He breaks out in a cold sweat and is breathing rapidly, and when assessing his pulse, you note tachycardia. How will you respond to this patient?

All Specimens

- Patient explains procedure for specimen collection before collection is attempted.
- Patient explains purpose of specimen analysis before collection is attempted.
- Patient verbalizes lack of fear of specimen collection and test results.

24-Hour Urine Collection

- All of patient's urine voided during the specified time is saved.

Urine and Stool Specimens

- Patient specimen is free of contaminants, including urine or toilet tissue in stool or toilet tissue in urine.

Sputum Specimen Obtained by Suction

- Patient maintains adequate oxygenation throughout procedure.

Wound Drainage Specimen

- Specimen is free of contaminants from skin.

Contrast Media Studies

- Patient explains the purpose and basic steps of the procedure before it begins.
- Patient assumes the correct position and remains still during the procedure.
- Patient does not experience postprocedure complications, such as flushing, pruritus, and urticaria; respiratory depression or decreased cardiovascular function; diminished or absent peripheral pulses; hypotension and tachycardia; or decreased or absent urinary output.

Nuclear Imaging Studies (Scans)

- Patient expresses fear and anxieties related to testing and results.
- Patient does not experience postprocedure complications such as hematoma, erythema, or edema at injection site.

◆ IMPLEMENTATION

Implementation includes performing preexamination and postexamination responsibilities that will assist a patient to achieve an optimal state of health (see Table 23.1).

If patient is discharged home, teach home care instructions (see the Home Care Considerations box on specimen collection and diagnostic examination).

◆ EVALUATION

Evaluation involves observing for a patient's response to determine whether goals and outcomes have been met.

1. Ask patient to state purpose and explain steps of the procedure before it is started.
2. Ask whether patient has questions or concerns about the procedure before it begins and later about test results. Assess nonverbal behaviors of anxiety before, during, and after procedure.
3. Ask patient to demonstrate body position required for procedure. Assess patient's body position throughout procedure, and assist to maintain position as necessary.
4. Ask patient to describe level of comfort during and after procedure.
5. Assess patient's respiratory status (rate, rhythm, and depth of respirations; symmetry of chest movement) during and after abdominal paracentesis, thoracentesis, and bronchoscopy.
6. Compare patient's heart rate and blood pressure during and after procedure with preprocedure baseline values. (Check hospital policy; sometimes performed as often as every 15 minutes, typically for a period of 2 hours.)
7. Inspect dressing over puncture site for drainage every hour after the procedure until patient's condition is stable.
8. Assess patient for postprocedure complications.
   a. Assess patient for a decrease in blood pressure and tachycardia (could signify hemorrhage or allergic reaction to dye [see Box 23.2]).
   b. Assess patient for flushing, itching, and urticaria (could signify allergic reaction to dye [see Box 23.2]).
   c. Assess the patient's respiratory status for sudden, severe shortness of breath (signifies possible laryngospasm and bronchospasm).
   d. Assess patient for abdominal pain, fever, and bleeding (signify possible perforation of abdominal structures).

e. Assess patient for low oxygen saturation; rate and depth of respirations; cyanosis or mottled skin; hypotension; changes in heart rate or rhythm (usually bradycardia); decreased or nonpalpable peripheral pulses; decreased or absent reflexes; and changes in level of consciousness related to conscious sedation.

9. Ask patient to describe postprocedure positioning and activity restriction for lumbar puncture, liver biopsy, and thoracentesis.

Get Ready for the NCLEX® Examination!

Key Points

- Laboratory examinations of specimens of urine, stool, sputum, blood, and wound drainage provide important information about body functioning and contribute to the assessment of health status.
- Patients who are given a clear explanation about the purpose of the specimen and how it is obtained will be more cooperative during its collection.
- Prepare properly to ensure that the patient is ready for the test and to prevent prolonging the hospital stay because of inadequate test preparations.
- Most people prefer that excretions be handled discreetly; therefore it is important to provide the patient with as much comfort and privacy as possible.
- Health care professionals are obliged to take into consideration the patient's age and socioeconomic, cultural, and educational background when discussing and collecting laboratory specimens.
- Wear gloves when collecting specimens of blood or other body fluids to prevent spread of bloodborne pathogens such as human immunodeficiency virus (HIV), hepatitis B, and other pathogens.
- Collect specimens in proper containers at the correct time and in the appropriate amount.
- Label all specimens properly with the patient's identification, and complete laboratory requisition as necessary.
- Most invasive diagnostic tests require a signed informed consent.
- Wound cultures identify aerobic and anaerobic organisms.
- Some diagnostic tests can be performed at the patient's bedside; the nurse's responsibility in this case includes caring for the patient and assisting the health care provider.
- After diagnostic testing, provide care and teach the patient what to expect, including the outcomes or side effects of the test.

Additional Learning Resources

SG Go to your Study Guide for additional learning activities to help you master this chapter content.

evolve Be sure to visit the Evolve site at *http://evolve.elsevier.com/Cooper/foundationsadult/* for additional online resources.

Review Questions for the NCLEX® Examination

1. A 64-year-old patient who has newly diagnosed diabetes mellitus has been learning how to perform her own blood glucose monitoring. The patient has impaired circulation. What action can help to improve the specimen collection process?
   1. Use a tourniquet on the finger to be used in the specimen collection.
   2. Apply a cool, damp cloth to the finger to be used in the specimen collection.
   3. Massage the hand before performing the specimen collection.
   4. Elevate the hand before the specimen collection.
2. A sputum specimen has been ordered for a patient admitted with possible pneumonia of the right lower lobe. Which is the best method for the nurse to use with a patient who cannot expectorate sputum on their own?
   1. Pharyngeal suctioning
   2. Nasotracheal suctioning
   3. Oropharyngeal suctioning
   4. Tracheal suctioning
3. The health care provider has ordered a stool specimen for blood that it is not possible to see with the naked eye. What does this examination detect?
   1. Profuse bleeding
   2. Gross blood
   3. Obscure blood
   4. Occult blood
4. A 46-year-old patient is seen by the health care provider for recurrent symptoms of cystitis. The patient is to provide samples for urine culture and sensitivity. Which is the best answer that the nurse can give to the patient when asked why the urine culture study has been ordered?
   1. To identify the organism causing the infection
   2. To determine the presence of malignant cells
   3. To analyze the elements present in the urine
   4. To localize the site of the inflammatory process
5. Rank order the instructions that would be given to the patient who is to collect a 24-hour urine specimen.
   1. Place the collection container on ice.
   2. Discard the first voided specimen and then collect the total volume of each void.
   3. Explain the importance of collecting all voiding.
   4. Instruct the patient not to allow toilet tissue or stool to enter the collection container.
   5. Collect each void in a urine hat and add to the larger collection container.

6. A patient has an indwelling urinary catheter. A sterile urine specimen has been ordered for culture and sensitivity. Which is the best method for the nurse to collect the urine specimen?
   1. Obtain 60 mL of urine from the collection bag.
   2. Remove the current catheter, have the patient void, and then recatheterize.
   3. Disconnect the tubing from the catheter and drain 2 mL of urine.
   4. Aspirate 10 mL of urine with a sterile syringe from the tubing port after cleaning with alcohol.
7. A patient performing a fingerstick for blood glucose determination asks why the side of the fingertip is advised as the preferred site. Which is the best answer that the nurse will give to the patient?
   1. The blood supply is greater in this area.
   2. It is easier for the self-determination method.
   3. The side of the finger is less responsive to pain than other sites.
   4. It leaves more room for other site selection.
8. A patient is scheduled for a barium enema study. Which instructions will the patient be given? *(Select all that apply.)*
   1. Maintain NPO status after midnight before the examination.
   2. Ingest the strong laxative ordered as instructed before the procedure.
   3. Take radiographic dye tablets the evening before the examination.
   4. Monitor bowel movements after the procedure.
   5. Increase fluid intake after the procedure.
9. On evaluation of the patient after a venipuncture, the nurse recognizes which finding to be unexpected? *(Select all that apply.)*
   1. The patient's heart rate is 80 and regular.
   2. A large lump is noted under the skin at the venipuncture site.
   3. The patient complains of a stinging sensation when the needle is inserted.
   4. A small amount of blood is noted on the bandage over the venipuncture site.
   5. The patient reports a tingling sensation down the arm used for the venipuncture.
10. When obtaining a residual urine specimen, the nurse knows that it is important to catheterize the patient after the patient voids within which time frame?
    1. 10 minutes
    2. 30 minutes
    3. 50 minutes
    4. 90 minutes
11. The nurse has just received an order for electrocardiography. Arrange the following steps in the order that the nurse would perform them.
    1. Perform hand hygiene and don clean gloves.
    2. Obtain the tracing.
    3. Position the patient lying supine.
    4. Raise the side rail, and lower the bed to the lowest position.
    5. Shave or clip hair if necessary.
    6. Attach the leads to the patient.
12. Rank order the following instructions that the nurse would tell a female patient who needed to obtain a midstream urine specimen.
    1. Start voiding directly into the toilet.
    2. Discard the last of the stream of urine into the stool.
    3. Perform hand hygiene before obtaining the specimen.
    4. Clean the perineum by wiping from front to back.
    5. Collect a small amount of urine in the container.
13. Which nursing action is essential before a chest radiograph is obtained?
    1. Make certain the patient does not eat or drink.
    2. Remove the patient's metal necklace.
    3. Have the patient swallow contrast medium.
    4. Administer a dose of medication for pain relief.
14. A nursing student asks the nurse to explain the difference in testing between a midstream urine specimen and a urinalysis. Which explanation would answer the nursing student's question? *(Select all that apply.)*
    1. The midstream specimen is used to determine the culture and sensitivity of the urine specimen.
    2. The midstream specimen is used to measure the specific gravity of the urine.
    3. The midstream specimen is used to determine the presence of glucose and ketones in the urine.
    4. The midstream specimen is used to check the urine for the presence of white blood cells (WBCs).
    5. The midstream specimen is the cleanest portion of the urine specimen.
15. In the assessment of a patient's urine sample, what will the nurse consider an abnormal finding? *(Select all that apply.)*
    1. Clear, straw color
    2. A few mucus flecks
    3. Bloody mucus
    4. A slight aromatic odor
    5. Dark amber color with sediment
16. When is the best time to collect a sputum sample from a patient?
    1. After episodes of coughing
    2. In the morning upon awakening
    3. Immediately after respiratory treatments
    4. Before initiation of oxygen therapy
17. Because of loss of subcutaneous tissue and skin elasticity in older adults, which step of the venipuncture procedure will the nurse sometimes eliminate?
    1. Application of the tourniquet before venipuncture
    2. Applying pressure to the venipuncture site after the procedure
    3. Cleansing of the intended venipuncture site with a topical antiseptic
    4. Placement of a small dressing to the venipuncture site after the procedure

Lifespan Development

24

http://evolve.elsevier.com/Cooper/foundationsadult/

Objectives

1. Differentiate among the types of family patterns and their functions in society.
2. Describe different types of stresses that commonly affect today's families.
3. Describe Piaget's four stages of cognitive development.
4. Describe the physical characteristics at each stage of the life cycle.
5. List the psychosocial changes at the different stages of development.
6. Describe the normal age-related changes that affect the major body systems.
7. Discuss the effect of the aging process on personality, intelligence, learning, and memory.
8. Discuss Erikson's stages of psychosocial development.
9. Describe the cognitive changes that occur in the early childhood period.
10. Discuss the developmental tasks of the adolescent period.
11. List the developmental tasks for early adulthood.
12. Describe the developmental tasks for middle adulthood.
13. Define aging.
14. Discuss theories of aging.

Key Terms

adoptive family (p. 699)
ageism (ĀG-ĭzm, p. 725)
autocratic family pattern (ăw-tō-KRĂ-tĭk FĂ-mĭ-lē PĂ-tĕrn, p. 700)
blended (reconstituted) family (rē-KŎN-stĭ-tū-tĕd, p. 699)
cephalocaudal (sĕf-ă-lō-KŎ-dăl, p. 697)
chromosomes (KRŌ-mō-sōmz, p. 697)
cohabitation (kō-hăb-ĭ-TĀ-shŭn, p. 699)
conception (fertilization) (kŏn-CĔP-shŭn; fĕr-tĭ-lī-ZA-shŭn, p. 697)
concrete operational phase (KŎN-krēt ŏp-ĕr-Ā-shŭn-ăl FĀZ, p. 715)
democratic family pattern (dĕm-ō-KRĂ-tĭc, p. 700)
depression (dĕ-PRĔ-shŭn, p. 720)
development (dĕ-VĔL-ŏp-mĕnt, p. 697)
disengagement stage (dĭs-ĕn-GĀG-mĕnt STĀG, p. 702)
engagement or commitment stage (kŏ-MĬT-mĕnt, p. 700)
establishment stage (ĕs-TĂB-lĭsh-mĕnt, p. 700)
expectant stage (ĕks-PĔC-tănt, p. 701)
extended family (ĕks-TĔN-dĕd, p. 698)
formal operational thought stage (FŌR-măl ŏp-ĕr-Ā-shŭn-ăl THŎT, p. 718)
foster family (FŎS-tĕr, p. 700)
grandfamilies (GRĂND-fă-mĭ-lēz, p. 699)
growth (GRŌTH, p. 697)
homosexual family (hō-mō-SĔK-shū-ăl, p. 699)
infant mortality rate (p. 696)
life expectancy (LĪF ĕk-SPĔC-tăn-cē, p. 696)
matriarchal family pattern (mā-trē-ĂR-kăl, p. 700)
nuclear family (NŪ-clē-ăr, p. 698)
parenthood stage (PĂR-ĕnt-hūd, p. 701)
patriarchal family pattern (pā-trē-ĂR-kăl, p. 700)
preoperational thought stage (prē-ŏp-ĕr-Ā-shŭn-ăl, p. 710)
presbycusis (prĕz-bē-KYŪ-sĭs, p. 722)
presbyopia (prĕz-bē-Ō-pē-ă, p. 722)
proximodistal (prŏk-sĭ-mŏ-DĬS-tăl, p. 697)
schema (SKĒ-mă, p. 706)
school violence (SKŪL VĪ-ō-lĕnz, p. 717)
senescence stage (sĕ-NĔS-ăns, p. 702)
sensorimotor stage (sĕn-sŏ-rē-MŌ-tŏr, p. 706)
single-parent family (p. 699)
social contract family (SŌ-shăl KŎN-trăkt, p. 699)
surrogacy (SŪR-rŏ-gă-cē, p. 701)
teratogen (tĕ-RĂ-tō-jĕn, p. 697)
transgender family (p. 699)
zygote (ZĪ-gōt, p. 697)

Table 24.1 *Healthy People 2020* Health Indicators

LEADING HEALTH INDICATORS	GOAL OF TAKING ACTION
Access to health services	Improve access to comprehensive, quality health services
Clinical preventive services	Aid in weight control Enhance well-being
Environmental quality	Promote health for all through a healthy environment
Injury and violence	Prevent unintentional injuries and violence, and reduce their consequences
Maternal, infant, and child health	Improve the health and well-being of women, infants, children, and families
Mental health	Improve mental health through prevention and by ensuring access to appropriate, quality mental health services
Nutrition, physical activity, and obesity	Promote health and reduce chronic disease risk by consuming a healthy diet as well as achieving and maintaining a healthy body weight
Oral health	Prevent and control oral and craniofacial diseases, conditions, and injuries, and improve access to preventative services and dental care
Reproductive and sexual health	Promote healthy sexual behaviors, strengthen community capacity, and increase access to quality services to prevent sexually transmitted diseases and their complications
Social determinants	Create social and physical environments that promote good health for all
Substance abuse	Reduce substance abuse to protect the health, safety, and quality of life for all, especially children
Tobacco	Reduce illness, disability, and death related to tobacco use and secondhand smoke exposure

From US Department of Health and Human Services: *Healthy People 2020*, Washington, DC, 2010, US Department of Health and Human Services.

The United States is in an era of increasing interest in health and well-being. Many improvements have contributed to better health and longer life. Improved sanitation, medications, immunizations, exercise, and nutrition help people stay healthy and live longer. In the coming decades, an increasing portion of the population will occupy the category of "older adult." Many factors have been identified as predictors of longevity, including health, happiness, avoidance of tobacco products, and job satisfaction. The exact number of years a person will live is not possible to predict, but estimations can be made. This estimate is referred to as the life expectancy.

Life expectancy is the number of years an individual probably will live, based on the average for others with similar characteristics. Life expectancy in the United States in the beginning of the 20th century was 47.3 years. This has increased in the past 100 years. The average life expectancy for 2015 in the United States is 79.3 years, with women's life expectancy being longer than men's life expectancy. Despite the increases in longevity, room for improvement still exists. Many countries have life expectancies greater than that of the United States, such as the 2015 life expectancy in Japan with 83.7 years and Australia with 82.8 years (World Health Organization, 2016).

Within the United States, life expectancy differs with population groups. For example, females outlive males by an average of 5 years. Those with household incomes of greater than $25,000 live 3 to 7 years longer, depending on gender and race, than those in households with incomes of less than $10,000.

Infant mortality rate refers to the number of deaths before age 1 year. This number affects overall life expectancy statistics. The infant mortality rate for African Americans is more than double that for white infants. Education and access to preventive health care is needed for pregnant women of all ages and races.

Other factors also influence the life expectancy for different groups, and *Healthy People 2020* has created national objectives to achieve their vision of "a society in which all people live long, healthy lives" (US Department of Health and Human Services, Office of Disease Prevention and Health Promotion, 2014). To motivate action toward change and progress, *Healthy People 2020* is organized around a list of 12 leading health indicators (Table 24.1).

According to *Healthy People 2020*, the four overarching goals for the population during the next 10 years are (1) to attain high-quality, longer lives free of preventable disease, disability, injury, and premature death; (2) to achieve health equity, eliminate disparities, and improve the health of all groups; (3) to create social and physical environments that promote good health for all; and (4) to promote quality of life, healthy development, and healthy behaviors across all life stages (US Department of Health and Human Services, Office of Disease Prevention and Health Promotion, 2014).

HEALTH PROMOTION ACROSS THE LIFESPAN

Development is a lifelong process that begins at conception, the beginning of pregnancy, and ends with death. Middle adulthood and late adulthood have been recognized recently as having equal importance as the earlier stages of development. Development is influenced by a series of interacting events, including personal behaviors, genetics, and the environment. An individual's experiences affect his or her future development. Lifespan development studies examine the changes in the life cycle of an individual and the impact of these factors on the growth and development of individuals.

Lifespan development comprises eight stages. Their approximate ages are as follows:

- Infancy: birth to 1 year
- Toddler: 1 to 3 years
- Preschool: 3 to 5 years
- School age: 6 to 12 years
- Adolescence: 13 to 19 years
- Early adulthood: 20 to 40 years
- Middle adulthood: 40 to 65 years
- Late adulthood: 65 years and over

Each stage of the lifespan is unique and has certain distinguishable features. Not all people experience the same milestones during the ages listed. Some may have delayed development or accelerated achievement of skills or behaviors. The guidelines are generalized. The goal of studying the lifespan is to enable better understanding and improved interaction and communication with individuals at various stages of development. In particular, given the significant growth of the population in the older age group, we must become more aware of the unique characteristics, needs, and problems of the older adult.

GROWTH AND DEVELOPMENT

Living beings undergo continuous changes throughout the lifespan. Some changes are physical, such as the replacement of cells, tissues, and fluids. Other changes involve cognition, communication, emotions, behavior, and feelings.

Growth refers to an increase in size and may involve the entire being or parts within. **Development** refers to function and the gradual process of change and differentiation, from simple to complex. Development proceeds as an orderly, sequential series of changes. Two directional terms important to understanding growth and development are *cephalocaudal* and *proximodistal.* **Cephalocaudal** is defined as growth and development that proceeds from the head toward the feet. The infant's head is large as compared with the rest of its body; gradually the body catches up. **Proximodistal** refers to growth and development that originates in the center of the body and moves toward the outside. For example, the infant gains control of the shoulders before developing control of the hands and fingers.

The principles of growth and development may be summarized as follows:

- Growth and development proceed at a highly individualized rate that varies from person to person. Do not expect two people to react in the same manner to the same stimuli.
- Growth and development are continuous and interdependent processes characterized by spurts of growth and periods of rest.
- Growth and development proceed from the simple to the complex in a predictable sequence of progressive changes.
- Growth and development vary for specific structures at specific times. In other words, not all organs grow and develop at the same rate; for example, the ovaries in the female and the testes in the male do not mature until puberty.
- Growth and development are a total process that involves the whole person. The person grows physically, socially, mentally, and emotionally. Types of growth are interrelated.

PATTERNS OF GROWTH

Growth patterns appear to be controlled genetically. Nutrition, heredity, and environment play an important role in the patterns as well. The blueprint for all inherited traits is contained in the **chromosomes** (threadlike structures in the nucleus of a cell that function in the transmission of genetic information). At conception, the individual is endowed with a complex set of biologic potential that involves characteristics such as height; skin, hair, and eye color; and talents and interests. Only identical twins have the same combinations of chromosomes (karyotype). The process of division, transmission, and mixing of chromosomes accounts for the variations in distinctive family traits or, in contrast, their continuity.

BEGINNINGS

Development begins with **conception (fertilization),** or the union of the sperm and ovum, which combines the genetic material of both parents. This combination of genetic material and environmental influences produces the unique individual.

After fertilization, the **zygote** (the developing ovum from the time it is fertilized until, as a blastocyst, it is implanted in the uterus) contains 23 pairs of chromosomes, for a total of 46 chromosomes. One of each pair has been contributed by the mother and one by the father. The sex chromosomes, one of the chromosome pairs, determine the gender of the baby. The ovum always carries an X chromosome, whereas the sperm sometimes carries an X and sometimes a Y chromosome. The presence of a Y chromosome in the sperm that fertilizes the ovum means that the baby will be male; if the fertilizing sperm has an X chromosome, the baby will be a female.

In some instances, environmental factors also play a role in contributing to certain diseases or defects in the unborn. A **teratogen** is a substance, agent, or process that interferes with normal prenatal development, causing the formation of one or more developmental abnormalities in the fetus. Drugs, alcohol, viruses, and cigarette smoke are just a few of the known harmful substances that are best avoided during pregnancy. A possible 5% to 25% of unfavorable outcomes in all pregnancies are estimated to be attributable to smoking. Smoking also may increase the incidence of low–birth weight babies.

Ethical Considerations

The transmission of certain abnormalities is determined genetically. Examples of such inherited disorders include Tay-Sachs disease, sickle cell disease, phenylketonuria, and spina bifida. Genetic testing provides prospective parents with information about whether they are carriers of genes associated with certain inherited diseases. Genetic testing may be suggested for couples based on several factors, including age, medical history, and ethnicity. Test results can provide families information to use for future decision making. Decisions may be difficult for families, and supportive services should be made available. A genetic counselor can review the test results and provide information regarding the likelihood of genes being passed on to a child.

FAMILY

The family is the basic unit of society. Families are composed of two or more individuals united by marriage, blood, adoption, emotional bonds, and social roles. The individuals of the family share emotional ties that usually persist over their entire lifetime (see the Cultural Considerations box).

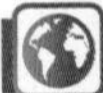 Cultural Considerations

Family and Culture

- Know the patient's family and kinship.
- Understand the values, flow of authority, and decision-making patterns within the family.
- Understand different gender roles.
- Listen carefully to direct verbal and indirect nonverbal cultural cues.
- Be aware of common foods and eating rituals.
- Recognize that religious beliefs are likely to affect a person's response to health, illness, birth, and death.

Signs of several significant changes in American families are evident today. The factors that have contributed to the changed family are listed in Box 24.1. As a result of these influences, family roles and lifestyles have changed to meet society's needs.

Box 24.1 Changes That Have Affected Modern Families

- Economic changes, which resulted in an increase in the number of women in the workforce
- The feminist movement
- More effective birth control
- Legalization of abortion
- Postponement of marriage and childbearing
- Increase in divorce rate

TYPES OF FAMILIES

Regardless of the type of family, certain basic functions are inherent to the family unit. These basic functions include protection, nurturance, education, sustenance, and socialization. Ideally, unconditional affection, acceptance, and companionship are guaranteed to each family member. The family attempts to meet the individual's needs for growth and development, which helps support personal fulfillment and strengthen self-esteem.

The family is the first socializing agent for teaching children society's expectations and limitations. As a part of that socialization, the family is responsible for ensuring that the child receives a formal education. The family is also responsible for instilling morals, values, and ideals into the children. These roles and functions of families are not necessarily stable or constant but are vulnerable to change. For example, the birth of a baby or the death of a family member makes rearrangement of family roles and structures necessary. See Box 24.2 for types of families.

Nuclear Family

Historically, the nuclear family was considered the normal family composition. The **nuclear family** is a family unit that consists of parents and their biologic offspring. This family type had gender-based roles assigned to its members but has been less prevalent in the United States for many decades. Currently, only 46% of children in the United States younger than 18 years of age live in a home that consists of a married mother and father who are in their first marriage. This number is significantly different from years past; greater than 70% of children who fit that description were living in nuclear families in the 1970s. Regardless of the various reasons for this declining number, the fact is that the so-called "normal family" is no longer the norm (Livingston, 2014).

The modern-day nuclear family usually consists of a husband and wife with or without children living in an independent household setting. In the past, one parent, usually the father, was the primary source of income. Today, these roles have been redefined in their structure and function. In many families, both parents work and share equally in the financial support and the roles and responsibilities of the family unit.

Extended Family

The **extended family** consists of the nuclear or traditional family and additional family such as grandparents, grandchildren, aunts, and uncles who live in the same household. A sharing of support, roles, and

Box 24.2 Types of Families

NUCLEAR
- Consists of married man and woman and their children
- Lives in independent household

EXTENDED
- Consists of nuclear plus additional family members living in same household
- Provides a sharing of responsibilities

SINGLE-PARENT
- Occurs by divorce, death, separation, abandonment, or choice
- More common in recent years
- Typically, one adult performs roles of two people

BLENDED (RECONSTITUTED)
- Occurs when adults from previous marriages remarry and combine children within new household

SOCIAL CONTRACT AND COHABITATION
- Made up of man and woman living together without legal commitment but sharing roles and responsibilities

HOMOSEXUAL
- Involves homosexual partners living together with shared responsibilities

ADOPTIVE
- Consists of usually traditional nuclear family members, husband, wife, and adoptive child

GRANDFAMILIES
- Children living in households headed by their grandparents
- Biologic parents may or may not be involved in the child's care

FOSTER
- Responsible for care, supervision, and nurturing of children in their charge

responsibilities is common to this family structure. This family type constitutes the basic family structure in many societies.

Single-Parent Family

The **single-parent family** exists today by choice or as the result of death, divorce, separation, or abandonment. More than 40% of single-parent families are the result of divorce. The head of the household may be male or female. This type of family unit also results when an unwed parent lives alone or a single person adopts a child. The single parent has the sole responsibility of carrying out the functions that typically are shared by two members.

Blended (Reconstituted) Family

The **blended (reconstituted) family** (also called the stepfamily) is formed when adults remarry and bring together children from previous marriages. It is estimated that 15% of children are living in a household with two parents who are in a remarriage. Unlike the steady decline of the nuclear family, the percentage of blended families has stayed fairly consistent over the years. This type of family potentially presents many types of stresses. Losses resulting from death or divorce sometimes cause adults and children to be fearful of love and trust. Children may have loyalties to one parent, which results in difficulties achieving a bond with the new stepparent. Jealousies may arise as efforts are made to unite the stepchildren into a single family (Livingston, 2014).

Social Contract Family and Cohabitation

The **social contract family** style also is referred to as **cohabitation.** It involves an unmarried couple living together and sharing roles and responsibilities.

Homosexual Family

The **homosexual family** comprises a same-sex couple. Homosexual adults form family units. The members share bonds of emotional commitment and roles of child rearing. Many of these family structures consist of biologic, adopted, or foster children. Regardless of the specific family structure, all families share common parenting concerns and responsibilities.

Transgender Family

The **transgender family** may consist of one or more parents who have had a gender reassignment or are gender nonconforming. Current surveys have found that between 25% to 50% of transgender people are parents and that they have generally good relationships with their children. Like the other types of family units, transgender families share the same parenting concerns and responsibilities of raising children (Stotzer, et al, 2014).

Adoptive Family

The **adoptive family** is a family unit with adopted children. Each year, approximately 120,000 children are adopted in the United States (AACAP, 2015). Adoption may be time consuming, anxiety provoking, and expensive. The couples who adopt children may have experienced years of infertility and related treatments. Families created by adoption achieve the same fulfillment associated with parenting as those families created by natural procreation.

Grandfamilies

Grandfamilies refer to families with children under the age of 18 years who live with or in the custody of grandparents. This group represents a growing demographic. Research shows that parental substance abuse is one of the most common reasons grandfamilies are becoming more prevalent. In 2014 of all the children removed from their homes because of parental substance abuse, more than one-third of them were placed with relatives. The number of children in foster care being raised by relatives because of alcohol and drug abuse has increased from 33% in 2008 to just more than 40% in 2014. Unfortunately, 21% of these families live below the poverty line and have to deal with various other stressors, which may include their own mental health issues stemming from shame or guilt about their adult child's inability to parent and their substance abuse disorder, social isolation, and depression. Research confirms that, although it presents a challenging situation, children have more stable and safe childhoods when raised by grandparents and other relatives than when they are placed with nonrelatives. Other reasons grandfamilies are formed include substance abuse, mental illness, military deployment, incarceration, and parental death (Generations United, 2016).

Foster Family

The **foster family** results when the biologic parents are unable or unwilling to provide adequate, safe care for their children. Children placed in foster care typically are placed there by the court system. The reasons for placement traditionally involve abuse or neglect. Individual circumstances determine the amount of time for the placement. Ideally, the parents can achieve stability and are allowed to again care for their children, thus protecting the parental bond. The number of US children living in foster care has decreased significantly in recent years. In 2002 more than 500,000 children were in foster care; in 2012 the number was substantially less at fewer than 400,000 children in foster care. The actual percentage declined by 23.7% from 2002 to 2012 (US Department of Health and Human Services, Administration for Children and Families, Administration on Children, Youth and Families, 2013). Although there has been a national decline in the number of children entering the foster care system, unfortunately, many children will never return to the care of their biologic parents; they face living in the foster care system until they "age out" as they reach legal adulthood.

FAMILY PATTERNS

Family patterns refer to the way in which family members relate to one another. Examples of family patterns include autocratic, patriarchal, matriarchal, and democratic patterns. Researchers have identified 12 qualities common to all functional families, listed in Box 24.3.

In the **autocratic family pattern,** the relationships are unequal. The parents attempt to control the children with strict rigid rules and expectations. This family pattern is least open to outside influence.

In the **patriarchal family pattern,** the adult male (or males of the family) usually assumes the dominant role. The adult male member functions in the work role, is responsible for control of finances, and makes most decisions.

Box 24.3 Qualities of Functional Families

- Sense of commitment toward promoting the members' well-being
- Sense of appreciation and encouragement for tasks accomplished
- Directed effort toward spending quality time with individual members
- Sense of purpose that encourages progress during good or difficult times
- Sense of harmony between members of the family
- Effective communication between individuals
- Established values, rules, and beliefs
- Variety of different coping techniques to enhance functioning
- Use of effective problem-solving measures and the use of a variety of options
- Positive outlook
- Ability to be flexible and adapt to changes
- Use of varied resources to facilitate coping skills

In the **matriarchal family pattern** (also known as the matrifocal family), the adult female (or females of the family) assumes primary dominance in areas of child care and homemaking and in financial decision making. In some families of this type, an older female relative provides child care so that the mother of the children is free to work outside of the home.

In the **democratic family pattern,** the adult members function as equals. As is often true in other types of families, children are treated with respect and recognized as individuals. This style encourages joint decision making, and it recognizes and supports the uniqueness of each individual member. This family pattern favors negotiation, compromise, and growth.

STAGES OF FAMILY DEVELOPMENT

Engagement or Commitment Stage

The **engagement or commitment stage** begins when the couple acknowledges to themselves and others that they are considering marriage. At this time, opposition or support is evident from friends and parents. Wedding plans are arranged. Housing, work, and furnishings are some of the items on the agenda that require discussion and exploration.

Establishment Stage

The **establishment stage** extends from the wedding up until the birth of the first child. During this phase, one of the important tasks is the adjustment from the single, independent state to the married, interdependent state. The challenges that face the newly married couple include learning to live with another person and together managing two-person decision making, conflict resolution, and communication. The relationship established with the couple's parents and families can enhance the cohesiveness or weaken the couple's ties. To the average young adult, marriage is an important serious change that requires major adjustments. A good marriage does

Table 24.2 Erickson's Stages of Psychosocial Development

STAGE	APPROXIMATE AGE (YEARS)	DEVELOPMENTAL TASK	OUTCOMES
1. Infancy	Birth to 1	Basic trust vs mistrust	Infants learn to either trust or not trust that significant others will properly care for their basic needs, including nourishment, sucking, warmth, cleanliness, and physical contact.
2. Toddler	1 to 3	Autonomy vs shame and doubt	Children learn to be either self-sufficient in many activities (including toileting, feeding, walking, and talking) or doubt their own abilities.
3. Preschool	4 to 6	Initiative vs guilt	Children want to undertake many adult-like activities, sometimes going beyond the limits set by parents and feeling guilty because of it.
4. School age	7 to 11	Industry vs inferiority	Children eagerly learn to be competent and productive or feel inferior and unable to do any task well.
5. Adolescence	12 to 19	Identity vs role confusion	Adolescents try to figure out their personal identity. They establish sexual, ethnic, and career identities or are confused about what future roles to play.
6. Young adulthood	20 to 44	Intimacy vs isolation	Young adults seek companionship and love with another person or become isolated from others.
7. Middle adulthood	45 to 65	Generativity vs stagnation	Middle-aged adults are productive, performing meaningful work and raising a family, or become stagnant and inactive.
8. Late adulthood	65+	Ego integrity vs despair	Older adults try to make sense out of their lives, either seeing life as meaningful and whole or despairing at goals never reached and questions never answered.

not just happen; both parties must work at and contribute to a marriage for success. Commitment, goals, and respect for each other require equal time and energy. Success at marriage satisfies Erikson's task of intimacy (Table 24.2 and see Psychosocial Development in the Early Adulthood section) and helps fulfill the individual's need for love and belonging (Fig. 24.1).

Expectant Stage

The **expectant stage** begins with conception and continues through the pregnancy. One of the most important decisions of a person's life is that of starting a family. Many people describe becoming a parent as one of the most challenging, and most rewarding, roles in their life. Pregnancy requires physiologic and psychological adjustments. Many important decisions must be considered during pregnancy, including childbirth methods, continuation or modification of employment, child care, and feeding methods. The desired outcome of pregnancy is that a bond or attachment is established between the parents and the new baby.

Ethical considerations. The agreement a woman makes to be artificially inseminated, voluntarily or for a fee, to bear a child, and then relinquish the parenting rights to the baby's natural father or another couple is called **surrogacy.** Presently, no national laws exist regarding surrogacy, and state laws vary. A surrogacy can cost $100,000 or more with added costs, including medical expenses and health insurance, and often insurance companies do not cover surrogacy expenses.

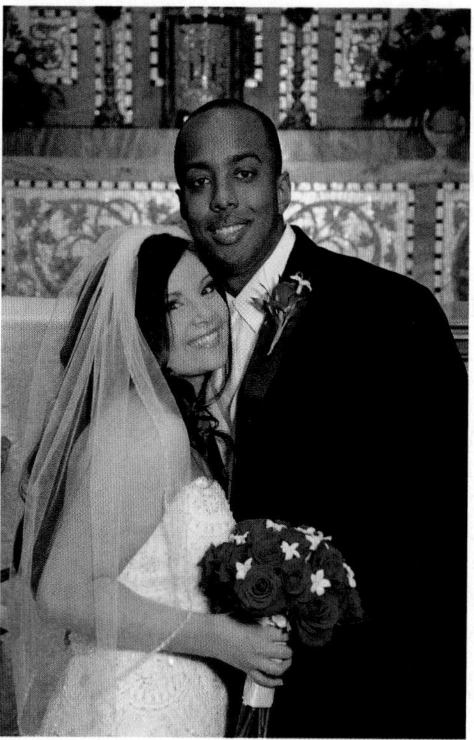

Fig. 24.1 Establishment stage: the newly married couple.

Parenthood Stage

The **parenthood stage** begins at the birth or adoption of the first child. The transition to parenthood is a major event. Even couples with good preparation express a great deal of anxiety associated with the onset of this new role. One of the most frequently described problems is lack of time: less free time, less sleep time, less time together, and less intimate sexual time. Compounding the lack of time is the stress of parenting and the self-doubt about ability and competency in this new role.

Disengagement stage of parenthood. The **disengagement stage** of parenthood is that period of family life when the grown children depart from the home. The role of parenting changes during this phase of the life cycle. The departure of children does not end the role of parenting. Although grown children perhaps do not live with their parents, they usually continue to need emotional guidance and some financial support. Many grown children return to living at home for financial reasons. Regardless, during the disengagement stage, couples or the single parent need to redefine personal roles and structure time so that there is a sense of usefulness, accomplishment, and self-fulfillment.

Senescence Stage

The **senescence stage** is the last stage of the life cycle and requires the individual to cope with a large range of changes. For the older adult, the family unit continues to be a major source of satisfaction and pleasure. Most older adults prefer to live independently. The greater life expectancy for women means that older women commonly outlive their spouses and continue life alone. Most older adults have regular contact with other family members. The grandparenting role requires new adaptations, such as a change in one's roles and sense of identity. In the past, grandparents often lived with their extended families because they had to, not necessarily because they wanted to. Grandparents today are independent. Grandparents want close, stable, emotionally satisfying family ties. Simultaneously, they tend to want an independent life, away from kin. They want to see and love their grandchildren but not be responsible for them.

CAUSES OF FAMILY STRESS

Various stressors affect the family unit. Chronic illness, abuse, and divorce are some of the most common factors. Stress, when it occurs, affects everyone, at all ages. Like adults, children often have feelings of stress. Stress in childhood results from either internal or external pressures or from a combination of both. At very early ages, stress sometimes results when the infant's needs are not met. Toddlers often perceive stress when they are separated from their mothers. School-age children sometimes feel stress from pressures in school or from parental expectations. Even social interactions at this stage have the potential to be somewhat difficult and stressful. Parents need to observe and listen to their children and be watchful for signs of stress (Box 24.4). They must be ready to help their children deal with stress. One way to help is to anticipate what holds stress potential and to prepare children ahead of time. For example, if the child is starting a new school, the parents should talk about it before the day of the event and allow children to express their feelings. Children must know that having uneasy feelings is all right. Children need to have someone validate their feelings. Talking about what is causing the child's uneasy feelings helps minimize the child's discomfort and helps bring about possible solutions.

Box 24.4 Common Signs of Stress in Children

- Mood swings
- Acting-out behavior
- Change in eating or sleeping patterns
- Frequent stomachaches, headaches, or other unexplained somatic symptoms
- Excessive clinging to parents
- Thumb-sucking
- Bedwetting
- Return to behavior typical of an earlier stage of development

Chronic Illness

Chronic physical or emotional illness of the parent or the child affects all family members. Factors such as financial resources, family stability, and the adequacy of the support system determine an individual's ability to cope with a family member's chronic illness.

Working Mothers

Alternative family patterns are more common, and today's families often experience change and must adjust to new circumstances. Changes to the family's composition and economic factors have resulted in more women in the labor force. Working mothers are considered common today. Aside from the financial rewards, many believe that working mothers create a wider range of valid role models for young children. Many working mothers compensate for the time they are not with their child by establishing quality time during their limited at-home time. Some fathers opt to assume primary child care responsibilities. Certainly, when both parents work outside the home, caregiving arrangements must be considered. Child care is sometimes available; some of the various forms include in-home care by a relative or paid caregiver and out-of-home care in an organized or group setting. The federal government and most states have regulations that control and regulate staff size and safety issues concerning daycare centers. Optimal qualities in a daycare center include the following: a balance of age-appropriate educational structure and an open environment, ample space with a variety of materials and activities, small class size with appropriate staff-to-child ratio, an environment that fosters active staff involvement, positive encouragement, and high-quality care in a safe and healthy environment.

Abuse

Abuse refers to physical, emotional, financial, and verbal abuse, sexual assault, and neglect. Approximately 700,000 American children are victims of child abuse each year; in 2014 more than 1500 children died from abuse and neglect in the United States (National Children's Alliance, 2014). Children younger than 1 year of age have the highest rate of victimization, and the abuser is most commonly a parent. Certain objective and measurable factors are related to family violence. They include financial strain, social isolation, low self-esteem, and history of abuse. The presence of several of these risk factors raises the risk that an individual will resort to abuse. The following are some common characteristics of parents who abuse their children: they were abused themselves as children; they are often loners; they are harsh, strict, and punitive; they have unreasonable expectations; and they are immature, lack self-control, and have low self-esteem. Early recognition, prompt reporting, and preventive measures are called for to help detect and end all forms of abuse and neglect.

Divorce

Divorce is widespread; it continues to affect more than 1 million children annually. The effects of divorce on children are varied and complex. One of the factors is the age of the child at the time of the divorce. Younger children often feel abandoned and believe they are no longer loved by both parents. Other factors that sometimes affect the child are the bitterness and conflict surrounding the divorce, the child's prior relationship with the absent parent, the effects of the divorce on the custodial parent, and the postdivorce relationship of the parents. Many children have reconciliation fantasies for extended periods after the divorce is finalized. Changes in one parent's status create changes in emotional milieu, family role, finances, lifestyle, and the neighborhood to which the child has lived in prior to the divorce (Box 24.5).

STAGES OF GROWTH AND DEVELOPMENT

The following sections discuss development by age group. Fully appreciating the scope of human growth and development involves examining a few aspects of development across a larger spectrum.

Box 24.5 Tips for Divorcing Parents

- Encourage children to talk about their feelings.
- Do not use children as pawns or "go-betweens."
- Never speak negatively about ex-spouse in front of children.
- Seek professional help if children need additional support.
- Reassure children that the divorce is not their fault.

PSYCHOSOCIAL DEVELOPMENT

Erik Erikson, an American psychoanalyst, viewed the life cycle as a series of developmental stages, each accompanied by a developmental task or challenge. Table 24.2 provides an overview of Erikson's stages of psychosocial development. Many of the subsections that follow include stage-appropriate characterization according to Erikson's framework.

COGNITIVE AND INTELLECTUAL DEVELOPMENT

Swiss theorist Jean Piaget's stages of cognitive development are outlined in Box 24.6.

COMMUNICATION AND LANGUAGE

Humans have an innate capacity to learn language. They are born with the mechanism and the capacity to develop speech and language skills. During infancy, the unique ability of the brain to sort out basic sounds and to extract from sentences the most meaningful elements becomes apparent. During early childhood, the brain's language-acquisition ability becomes even more sophisticated. Parents and other caregivers have an enormous potential to influence the infant's intellectual and language development. Infants do not speak spontaneously. Interaction with the environment provides a means for them to acquire these skills. Speech requires intact physiologic functioning of: (1) the respiratory system; (2) the speech control centers in the cerebral cortex; and (3) the articulation and resonance structures of the mouth and nasal cavities. In addition, acquisition of language requires: (1) an intact and discriminating auditory apparatus; (2) intelligence; (3) a need to communicate; and (4) stimulation. The rate of speech development varies from child to child and is related directly to neurologic competence and intellectual development. All children go through the same sequence of stages in language and speech development in early childhood unless abnormal conditions are present (Table 24.3).

The basic sequence of language is as follows:

- *At 3 months, babbling.* When infants babble, they typically explore all the possible sounds they can make by enhancing the force of the air stream as it passes their vocal cords and by varying the positions of their tongue and mouth.
- *At 1 year, recognition of words.* Between ages 1 and 2 years, infants generally acquire the ability to produce holo phrases (one-word sentences that convey a complete message ["up"]). Infants learn to expand their holo phrases by attaching them back-to-back to other nouns or verbs. They thus form two-word sentences ("mommy milk," "daddy come"). Early speech often is referred to as telegraphic speech because, as in telegram messages, the articles, pronouns, prepositions, and conjunctions are omitted. In organizing and coding language, infants acquire an understanding of the most meaningful units of

Box 24.6 Piaget's Stages of Cognitive Development

SENSORIMOTOR: BIRTH TO 2 YEARS
- Uses senses and motor abilities to understand the world and coordinates sensorimotor skills; this period begins with reflexes
- Develops schema
- Begins to interact with environment
- Learns that an object still exists when it is out of sight (object permanence) and begins to remember and imagine experiences (mental representation)
- Develops thinking and goal-directed behavior

PREOPERATIONAL THOUGHT: 2 TO 7 YEARS
- Develops egocentric thinking (understands the world from only one perspective—that of the self)
- Uses trial and error to discover new traits and characteristics
- Conceptualizes time in present terms only
- Uses symbols to represent objects
- Develops more logical, intuitive thinking
- Centers or focuses on a single aspect of an object, producing some distortion of reality
- Gains in imaginative ability
- Gradually begins to "decenter" (becomes less egocentric and understands other points of view)

CONCRETE OPERATIONAL THOUGHT: 7 TO 11 YEARS
- Understands and applies logical operations or principles to help interpret specific experiences or perceptions
- Has more realistic views; better understands other viewpoints
- Improves use of memory
- Focuses on more than one task; develops logical, socialized thoughts
- Recognizes cause-and-effect relationships
- Learns to identify behavior outcome
- Understands basic ideas of conversation, number classification, and other concrete ideas

FORMAL OPERATIONAL THOUGHT: 12+ YEARS
- Uses a systematic, scientific problem-solving approach
- Recognizes past, present, and future
- Is able to think about abstractions and hypothetical concepts and is able to move in thought "from the real to the possible"
- Becomes more interested in ethics, politics, and all social and moral issues as ability to take a broader and more theoretic approach to experience increases

speech. No one teaches infants to use nouns and verbs first. They learn this sequence on their own.

- *At preschool age, acquisition of structure of native language.* The language explosion that occurs during the preschool years is most obvious in the growth of vocabulary, from 50 words at 18 months to 200 words at age 2 years to between 8000 and 14,000 words at age 6 years. From ages 2 to 6 years, the average child learns between 6 and 10 words per day. Preschoolers have an outstanding ability to learn language. Most researchers regard early childhood as a crucial period for language learning.
- *At 6 years, ability to speak and understand new words and sentences.* Even compared with the preschool years, language development from 6 years on is remarkable, albeit much more subtle, as children consciously come to understand more about the many ways language can be used. This understanding gives them greater control in their comprehension and use of language and, in turn, enhances the range of their cognitive powers generally.

A common rule of thumb about the evolution of early speech acquisition is that the number of words in an average response usually corresponds to the chronologic age of the child. For example, a 2-year-old may say, "Me do"; a 3-year-old may add a word, "Me do it"; and a 4-year-old may say, "Let me do it."

Girls advance more rapidly in language development than do boys. Firstborn children develop language earlier than do later-born children, and children of multiple births (twins, triplets) develop language later than children of single births.

INFANCY: 1 TO 12 MONTHS

Physical Characteristics

An infant's physical development happens so rapidly that size, shape, and skills seem to change daily (see Chapter 28 for discussion of the newborn). Growth, which proceeds in a cephalocaudal and proximodistal sequence, is rapid during the first 6 months of life. Infants are expected to gain about 1½ pounds (3.3 kg) per month until 5 months, and infants usually double their birth weight by 4 to 6 months. By the time the baby is 1 year of age, the birth weight has tripled (average weight is 21½ pounds, or 47.3 kg). Most of the weight gain in the first months of life is in the form of fat, which provides insulation and a source of nourishment to draw on if teething or other problems decrease food intake for a few days. After 8 months, weight gain includes more bone and muscle.

Height (length) increases by about 1 inch (2.54 cm) per month for the first 6 months. By 12 months of age, the infant's birth length has increased about 50%; the typical length is 30 inches (75 cm).

Vital signs. Infants are subject to wide variations in body temperature related to activity levels and state of health. Apical rates slow in infancy. At 2 months, the average apical rate is about 120 beats per minute. Count the apical pulse for a full minute, noting variations in rate, volume, and rhythm. Respiratory rates also decrease during infancy; these rates are related to activity level. Average resting respiratory rate for the 12-month-old is about 30 breaths per minute. Blood pressure readings gradually increase to 90/60 mm Hg at 12 months.

Dentition. Teething begins at about 5 to 6 months of age. Signs of teething—irritability, edematous red gums,

Table 24.3 Normal Language and Speech Development During Early Childhood

AGE (YEARS)	NORMAL LANGUAGE DEVELOPMENT	NORMAL SPEECH DEVELOPMENT	INTELLIGIBILITY
1	Says two or three words with meaning Imitates sounds of animals	Omission of most final and some initial consonants Substitution of consonants *m, w, p, b, k, g, n, t, d,* and *h* for more difficult sounds Use of unintelligible jargon peaks at age 18 mo	Usually no more than 25% intelligible to unfamiliar listener
2	Uses two-word or three-word phrases in context Has vocabulary of about 300 words and uses "I," "me," and "you"	Use of consonants *m, w, p, b, k, g, n, t, d,* and *h* with vowels, but inconsistently and with much substitution Omission of final consonants Articulation lags behind vocabulary	At age 2 yr, 65% intelligible in context
3	Says four-word or five-word sentences Has vocabulary of about 900 words Uses "who," "what," and "where" in asking questions Uses plurals, pronouns, and prepositions	Mastery of *b, t, d, k,* and *g; r* and *l* may still be unclear; omission or substitution for *w* Repetitions and hesitations common	At age 3 yr, 70% to 80% clear
4 to 5	Has vocabulary of 1500 to 2100 words Able to use most grammatical forms correctly, such as past tense of verb with "yesterday" Uses complete sentences with nouns, verbs, prepositions, adjectives, adverbs, and conjunctions	Mastery of *f* and *v;* possible distortion of *r, l, s, z, sh, ch, y,* and *th* Little or no omission of initial or last consonant	Speech is totally intelligible, although some are still imperfect
6 to 7	Has vocabulary of 3000 words Comprehends "if," "because," and "why"	Mastery of *r, l,* and *th;* possible continuing distortion of *s, z, sh, ch,* and *j* (usually mastered by age 7½ to 8 yr)	Speech is totally intelligible

Box 24.7 Primary Dentition Schedule

6 months: Teething begins with eruption of two lower central incisors
7 months: Eruption of upper central incisors
9 months: Eruption of upper lateral incisors
11 months: Eruption of lower lateral incisors
12 months: Approximately 6 to 8 teeth present
24 months: Approximately 16 teeth present
30 months: Completion of primary dentition; 20 teeth present

excessive drooling, and change in stooling—begin 3 to 4 weeks before the appearance of the tooth (Box 24.7). Dental decay can begin at any time after tooth development. Oral hygiene for the young infant consists of offering sips of clear water and wiping and massaging the infant's gums. The American Academy of Pediatric Dentistry (n.d.) recommends that children have their first dental visit when the first tooth appears but no later than the child's first birthday.

Advise parents to begin toothbrushing after the first teeth appear; this element of dental hygiene is important to continue throughout the lifespan. In areas without added fluoride in the water, recommend the use of fluoride toothpaste. To prevent bottle-mouth syndrome, instruct caregivers to avoid putting anything but water in the infant's night bottle. Sugar in milk, formula, and juice causes severe decay and destruction of the tooth enamel. Also, instruct all caregivers not to prop up the bottle and then leave the child alone with it, because this practice potentially leads to aspiration. Furthermore, holding the infant during feeding provides warmth, comfort, and bonding, all vital factors in providing a feeling of love and security.

Motor Development

At 2 months, the infant can hold the head up while in the prone position. By 4 months, the infant can hold the head up steadily to a 90-degree angle while in the prone position. At 6 months, most infants can balance the head well. By the end of the 7 months, infants have acquired the ability to sit up steadily without support.

Locomotion. Crawling, an early form of movement, is a motion made with the infant's abdomen touching the floor (Fig. 24.2E). A more advanced form of locomotion is creeping. The infant accomplishes this by resting the weight on the hands and knees. Infants sometimes crawl

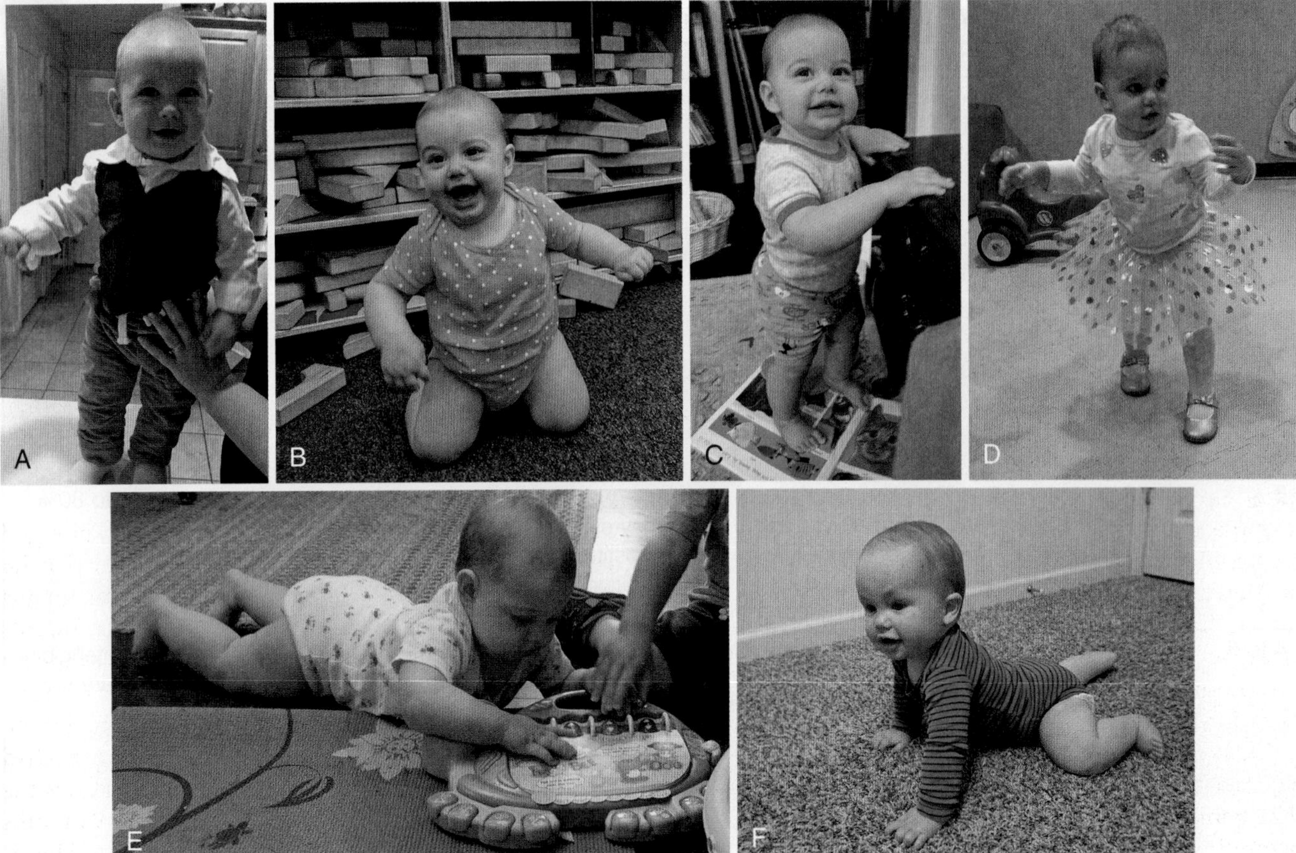

Fig. 24.2 Development of locomotion. A, Infant bears full weight on feet by 7 months. B, Infant can maneuver from sitting to kneeling position. C, Infant can stand holding on to furniture at 9 months. D, While standing, infant takes deliberate step at 10 months. E, Infant crawls with abdomen on floor and pulls self forward, and then, F, creeps on hands and knees at 9 months.

at 7 months and creep at about 9 months. Creeping appears after age 9 months in most children (Fig. 24.2F). Standing with support and walking follow at about 8 months to 15 months (Fig. 24.2D).

Psychosocial Development

Erikson defined the task of the infant as basic trust versus mistrust. The responsiveness of others to the needs of the infant helps establish the basis of trust. Infants obtain gratification when their basic needs are fulfilled. Infants whose needs are not met develop a sense of dissatisfaction or mistrust. (See Table 24.2 for an overview of Erikson's stages of psychosocial development.)

Cognitive and Intellectual Development

During this stage, the infant uses the senses to learn about self and environment. The infant learns with exploration of objects and events and with interaction. Piaget describes the infant as being in the sensorimotor stage of cognitive development.

In the **sensorimotor stage**, an infant's knowledge comes about primarily through sensory impressions and motor activities. Behavior is completely reflective. The infant develops an image or **schema** (an innate knowledge structure that allows a child to mentally organize ways to behave in the immediate environment) and assimilates and interprets the information. Infants learn by encountering and responding to stimulation from the environment. As the infant interacts with the environment, changes occur in mental structure and in development of thinking ability. During the first 1 to 4 months, the infant follows objects visually with the eyes and auditorily with the ears. By 4 months of age, infants become notably better at using both eyes together, which makes them more astute observers. From 4 to 8 months of age, the infant begins to recognize and imitate. Reaching and grasping are improved skills.

By age 3 months, most infants respond differently to their parents or primary caregiver than they do to other people. By age 4 months, many infants can identify the voices of the most familiar people in their lives. Smiling occurs in response to different people and events. At the sight of their parents or primary caregivers, infants smile and begin to vocalize.

Studies in children ages 15 to 30 months who had good attachment relationships showed that they experienced a predictable behavior pattern after separation, known as separation anxiety. Beginning at approximately 8 months of age, infants show this anxiety when they are separated from their primary caregiver. They develop shyness and a fear of strangers. The infant may cling and protest any separation from the primary caregiver. By age 9 months, most children show alarm at the presence of a stranger.

Health Promotion

Nutrition. Human breast milk and commercially prepared formula are options that meet the nutritional needs of the infant. Although today's excellent infant formulas approximate human milk, breast milk is still almost always the best food for newborns. It has been called the "ultimate health food" because it offers so many benefits. However, infants who are fed with properly prepared formula and raised with love also grow up healthy and well adjusted. Breast milk or formula is the only food most babies need until they are about 4 to 6 months of age. The American Academy of Pediatrics (2012) recommends exclusive breast-feeding for the first 6 months of a baby's life. After 6 months breastfeeding should be continued for the first year of life, or longer if desired by the mother, while foods are introduced.

Most experts agree that newborns should be fed on a demand schedule. Early in life, this practice may mean that babies are fed as often as every 2 hours. In the beginning, nursing mothers often start nursing for 10 to 15 minutes on each breast and then lengthen the feeding time as demanded by the infant. When infants suckle more slowly or appear uninterested in either the breast or the bottle, it is a good indication that they have had enough. The baby should have four to six wet diapers per day by the fourth day after birth. A baby who is breast-feeding should have at least two to three seedy stools each day. Breast milk is digested readily by the baby, which may result in a bowel movement shortly after each feeding. Signs of underfeeding include lack of satisfaction; a cranky, fussy baby; little weight gain; and persistent wrinkling of the skin. Signs of overfeeding include vomiting after feeding and frequent watery stools. Full-term infants have enough stored iron to last for at least the first 5 to 6 months of life. After this time, iron supplements or food sources are options to replenish the diminishing supply. Certain foods are best avoided in the first 6 months of life. Those foods include citrus fruits, egg whites, and wheat flour, all of which are identified frequently as allergy-producing substances.

Much controversy exists regarding the best time to introduce solid foods into the infant diet. Many physicians believe that very early introduction of solids leads to a variety of problems. A description of how to first introduce these foods into the infant diet is simpler than the decision of when to introduce solid food. The rules for solid foods include the following:

- Introduce only one new food at a time, allowing several days between new foods, which provides an opportunity to recognize allergies.
- Introduce cereals first, fruits and vegetables next, and meats last.
- Avoid mixing foods to allow the infant to develop interest in different foods and tastes.

Never leave infants alone while they are eating, because infants choke easily. Avoid giving older infants round, hard foods that can get caught in the throat easily. Foods that have high potential to cause choking include popcorn, grapes, raisins, hot dogs, and chicken nuggets.

This period often is an excellent time to look at the type of foods the whole family is eating. Limiting the amount of sodium, fats, and sugar in the family diet is best. Lifelong eating habits are established early on, in these toddler years. The entire family should be offered plenty of fresh fruits, vegetables, lean meats, and whole grains.

In warmer weather, febrile conditions, prolonged vomiting, and diarrhea place infants at higher risk for dehydration because of their small fluid volume. Infants must receive adequate breast milk or formula. Infants do not need additional fluids during the first 4 months of life. Excessive intake of water can cause water intoxication, failure to thrive, and hyponatremia in the infant. By age 8 to 9 months, most babies master eating mashed or junior foods. Self-feeding of finger foods allows the infant further opportunity for exploration. By 9 months of age, the process of weaning should begin. This is usually a gradual process, with a training cup substituted for one bottle at a time, usually starting with the lunchtime feeding.

Sleep, play activity, and safety. Newborns and infants sleep 18 out of 24 hours. These sleep periods usually consist of short, naplike periods. Infants are normally restless and make noises during these periods. Toward the end of the first 3 months, definite sleep patterns emerge, and nap and wake periods clearly are established. By the end of the first year, infants usually sleep 12 hours at night and take one nap during the day. Persistent crying during usual sleep or nap periods often signals discomfort or illness and calls for investigation.

A concern for parents of young infants is sudden infant death syndrome (SIDS). This disorder produces sudden, abrupt death with no identifiable warning signs. Formerly known as crib death, its incidence seems to peak 2 to 3 months after birth. Steps to reduce the incidence of SIDS are outlined in the Safety Alert box.

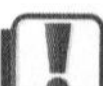

Safety Alert

Steps to Reduce the Incidence of Sudden Infant Death Syndrome

1. Back to sleep: place infants on their back to sleep.
2. Avoid exposure to cigarette smoke.
3. Avoid use of soft bedding or pillows.
4. Keep room well ventilated.
5. Breast-feed if possible.
6. Maintain regular medical checkups for infants.

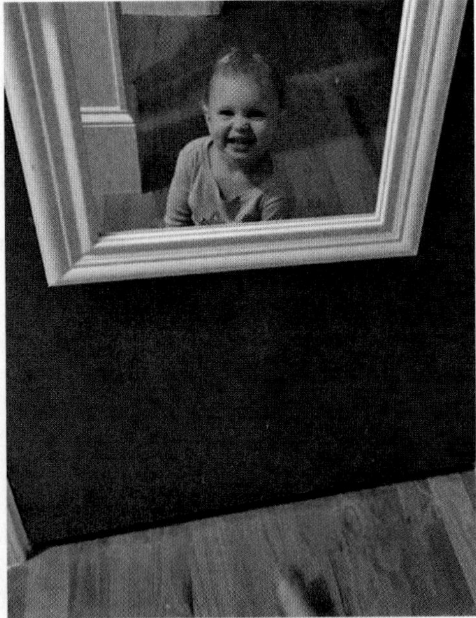

Fig. 24.3 Nine-month-old infant enjoying own image in a mirror.

Play is important for learning. Play that captures the pleasures of using the senses and motor abilities is called sensorimotor play (Fig. 24.3). Early play items include turning mobiles, mirrors, colorful shapes, and toys of different textures. As hand coordination improves, other items, such as rattles and shapes, become useful play objects. Toward the end of the first year, stacking items, blocks, and puzzles encourage developing motor skills. Music is useful to soothe the infant or to stimulate awareness of sounds and rhythms. Play style during infancy is described as solitary play, which means that the infant plays alone and does not interact with or need other children to play. Allowing adequate freedom of movement helps enhance good development of muscles and bones. Young infants need room to stretch and kick. Care should be taken to prevent injury during this early stage of development. Do not push children to sit or walk before adequate muscle strength is achieved.

Accidents are the leading cause of injury and death in infants and young children. Safety precautions are essential to institute immediately at the birth of the child (Fig. 24.4). The Safety Alert box lists safety rules for infants and young children.

Infancy is also a time of daily changes. Goals for the developmental tasks of infancy are shown in Box 24.8.

TODDLER: 1 TO 3 YEARS

Physical Characteristics

Rate of growth in the toddler years is slower than in infancy but follows the same general principles. It is orderly. It proceeds from head to foot, from the center outward, and from general to specific movements.

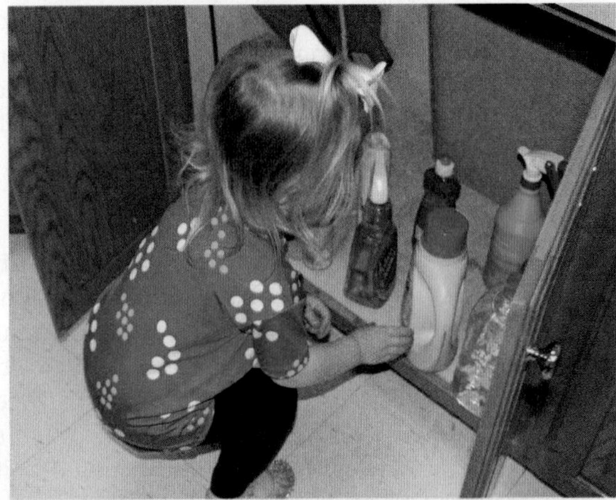

Fig. 24.4 Children are most likely to ingest substances that are on their level, such as cleaning agents stored under sinks, rat poison, plants, and diaper pail deodorants.

Box 24.8 Developmental Tasks of Infancy

- Establishes trusting, meaningful relationships
- Recognizes primary caregiver
- Develops attachment behavior
- Learns to recognize objects
- Develops exploration skills
- Develops communication skills by beginning vocalization, learning nonverbal communication techniques, and imitating simple vocalizations
- Develops muscular control, eye-hand coordination, and object manipulation
- Develops mobility: crawling, creeping, cruising, walking
- Establishes patterns of living: eating, sleeping, elimination habits
- Begins to develop independent living skills: self-feeding, walking, undressing, communication of needs

One of the most striking changes from infancy is the upright stance of the toddler. The chubby look of infancy is gone by 12 to 15 months. In the beginning of this stage, the toddler's body proportions result in a top-heavy appearance. By the end of this period, however, rapid growth of the extremities and slowed growth in the trunk produce a more proportionate body appearance (Fig. 24.5). An exaggerated lumbar lordosis (convex lumbar curve) and protruding abdomen produce a potbelly appearance, which disappears as the abdominal muscles strengthen. By age 2½ years, all 20 deciduous teeth are present. Advise parents to begin routine dental examinations and tooth brushing during this period.

Vital signs. During the toddler period, the pulse ranges from 90 to 120 beats per minute. Blood pressure averages 80 to 100 mm Hg systolic and 64 mm Hg diastolic. Body

Safety Alert

Safety Rules for Infants and Young Children

- Never leave an unsupervised infant on an elevated surface.
- Never leave an infant unattended in a high chair, stroller, walker, or any other device.
- Secure stairways and exits.
- Keep crib sides up and set mattress at lowest setting.
- Never leave infants or young children unattended in a bath for even a few seconds.
- Keep windows locked and secured with child guards.
- Never use plastic bags or coverings on mattresses or near infant's playthings.
- Avoid the use of pillows with small infants.
- Infant cribs must meet US Consumer Product Safety regulations to prevent strangulation between crib bars.
- Remove wires and dangling electric cords from the crawling child's reach. Cover outlets with protective caps.
- Inspect all toys carefully for long strings and small removable parts.
- Use pacifiers that have one-piece construction.
- Do not allow children to play with balloons.
- Avoid giving infants and young children hard candies, nuts, popcorn, and other foods that are easily aspirated.
- Lock all poisons and medicines out of the reach of infants and young children (see Fig. 24.4).
- Avoid drinking hot fluids while holding an infant.
- Check temperature of foods and formula before feeding.
- Turn pot handles toward back of stove and remove burner knobs if within child's reach.
- Avoid smoking near infants and children to prevent burns and smoke inhalation.
- Keep infants and children away from hot surfaces, stoves, fireplaces, and barbecues.
- Use flame-retardant sleepwear.
- Never say that medication is candy to facilitate administration.
- Keep poison control hotline phone number accessible.
- Keep plants out of child's reach.
- Use plastic rather than glass eating and drinking utensils.
- Inspect toys and household items for sharp points.
- Inspect for chipped lead-based paint on surfaces painted before 1978 (production of lead paint for consumer use was banned in 1978).
- Keep knives and forks away from young children.
- Supervise infants and children playing around animals and pets.
- Teach children early about street dangers and supervise their play.
- Instruct children to never go anywhere with strangers.
- Teach young children the use of the telephone for emergencies.
- Instruct children that others should not touch their "private" body parts and to report happenings if they occur. Accept the child's story unless you can prove otherwise.
- Always use safety seats and restraints when transporting infants and young children.

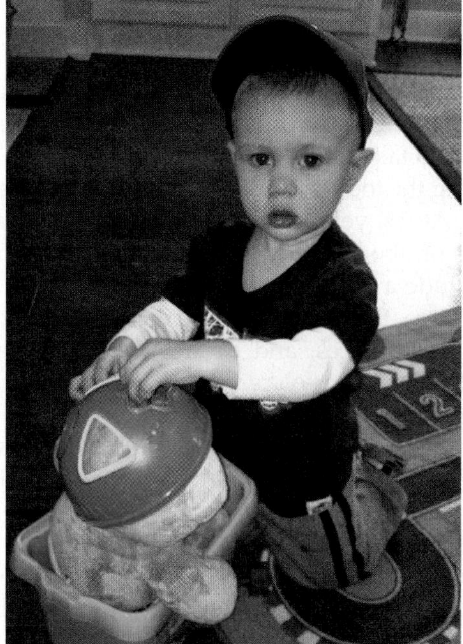

Fig. 24.5 The toddler with proportionate body appearance.

temperature ranges between 98° and 99°F (36.6° and 37.2°C). Respiration slows to 20 to 30 breaths per minute.

Neuromuscular Development

Many gross motor skills emerge in this period, including walking, climbing stairs (2 years), and hopping (3 years). The toddler develops running, pulling, and holding-on-tight skills, exploring the world in ways previously impossible. This time is also when the toddler begins acquiring fine motor skills, such as beginning to scribble (2 years) and copying a circle (3 years).

Toilet training. Children do not reach the physiologic or psychological maturity necessary to begin toilet training until 18 to 24 months of age. Children need to reach maturity to have neuromuscular control, the cognitive ability to understand what is expected of them, and the language skills to express their needs. Bowel control is achieved first. Bladder control begins at the same time but takes longer to achieve. Nighttime control usually is achieved after daytime control is established.

Advise parents and caregivers to expect setbacks and accidents, particularly during times of stress or illness. Deemphasize accidents; never make the child feel inadequate. Praise success and ignore accidents. If praise is given for toileting successes and accidents are cleaned up without negativism, the toddler gains a sense of self-control, inner goodness, and pride. However, if the toddler is punished and made to feel foolish, a sense of shame develops. If the toddler is kept in diapers and given no opportunities to control the urges, a sense of doubt is fostered. Feelings of shame and doubt are not healthy personality attributes.

Psychosocial Development

The toddler is an uninhibited, energetic little person who always seeks attention, approval, and achievement of personal goals. Sometimes the toddler is cuddly and loving; at other times, the toddler may bite, hit, or pinch. The toddler only slowly realizes that everything desired is not attainable and that some behaviors annoy others. The toddler tries to be independent yet becomes easily frightened and runs to the caregiver for protection, security, reassurance, and approval.

Erikson sees the toddler as struggling with autonomy (self-control) in opposition to shame and doubt. With newfound skills of independence, walking, talking, self-feeding, and beginning toilet training, the toddler is struggling to be independent. Characteristic of this search for autonomy is the toddler's use of the word "no," which gives a sense of control. The toddler possesses endless energy yet often falls asleep almost while still in motion. As toddlers struggle for independence, they frequently display possessiveness and a desire to have things go their way. Ritualistic behavior and repetitive rituals are self-consoling behaviors at this stage. Toddlers enjoy the same story, the same routine, and the same foods at each meal. Rituals decrease their anxiety by helping them know what to expect. When health care providers follow a hospitalized child's usual rituals, the toddler feels safer and more secure in the strange environment.

Temper tantrums are common and are the result of frustration. A combination of wanting things "my way," the inability to communicate feelings, and the lack of impulse control are perhaps behind outbursts of temper. This type of negativism is best ignored unless the child or others are in danger of harm.

Toddlers need many experiences of being able to choose among alternatives (to play inside or outside, to wear green pants or red pants). However, advise caregivers to make use of questions and offer alternatives for children only in situations in which either choice is acceptable. When a particular behavior is necessary (such as going to bed, holding hands to cross a street, letting go of another child's hair), it is better not to offer a choice. Erikson stressed that young children do not have the wisdom to know what behaviors are acceptable or unacceptable, healthy or unhealthy.

Box 24.9 Basic Principles of Discipline

- *Consistency:* Apply rules uniformly.
- *Follow-through:* Say and do what you mean.
- *Positive modeling:* Practice role model–approved behavior.
- *Promptness:* Administer any punishment in a nonhostile manner immediately after incident occurs.
- *Trust:* Express trust in the child.
- *Prevention:* Remove temptation.
- *Reinforcement:* Offer positive reinforcement for acceptable behavior.

Discipline is a necessary means of teaching limit setting and impulse control. Basic principles of discipline are listed in Box 24.9. Toddlers seek attention, approval, and love as they struggle for independence.

Cognitive and Intellectual Development

The period from 12 to 24 months of age completes the last phase of sensorimotor development, in which the toddler's knowledge of the world comes about primarily through sensory impressions and motor activities. The period of early childhood is the **preoperational thought stage.** (When the child focuses on the use of language as a tool to meet needs, the child has the emerging ability to think.) The child uses trial and error to discover new traits and characteristics. According to Piaget, this stage extends from 2 to 7 years of age.

Toddlers constantly are absorbing new ideas, widening their cognitive world, and expanding memory. Activities can be connected to past events or memories. The toddler's concept of time is limited to the present. The child's thinking is egocentric at this stage. Toddlers are often demanding, wanting things to go their way.

Communication and Language

The cognitive and language development of toddlers makes it possible for them to express their wishes. Commonly used words at this age are "no" and "me." Toddlers use these words in an attempt to exert their will and to take on new challenges.

During the toddler period, the child identifies objects by use. At 2½ years of age, the toddler's vocabulary consists of about 450 words and two-word sentences that include a noun and verb (e.g., "Me run."). By 3½ years of age, the child is able to answer questions and use brief sentences, and even recite television commercials. The 3-year-old's vocabulary is approximately 900 words. Regular reading to children by parents and caregivers can increase the size of the children's vocabularies greatly. This activity also promotes bonding.

Health Promotion

Nutrition. Good nutrition requires that the toddler's daily diet consist of one serving from the meat group; two or more servings of vegetables; and at least two servings of fruit, cereal, or breads. The US Department of Agriculture's guidelines *(www.choosemyplate.gov)* should be followed. The toddler needs 2 cups of food from the dairy group per day. Too few solid foods can lead to iron deficiency; many times this is the result of consuming too much milk (more than 24 oz/day), which causes the toddler's stomach to feel full and result in a decreased appetite. Most children are more likely to eat foods with which they are familiar; therefore gradual introduction of new foods is advisable. Bite-sized pieces, finger foods, and smaller portions are generally more acceptable. Foods with a high risk for choking, such as hot dogs, grapes, carrots, and small candies, should not be given to toddlers. In the past experts suggested to avoid the early introduction of foods known to be common allergens, such as eggs, wheat, nuts, and cow's milk. Newer research is indicating that early introduction, around six months of age, actually helps prevent allergies to these foods from developing (Chin, Chan, and Goldman, 2014). There is ongoing research regarding food allergens and when to introduce these foods to children, so parents should always be referred to their pediatrician or health care provider to determine what is best for their child. Idiosyncratic eating patterns are common at this stage. Toddlers can be picky eaters and often are too busy playing to stop and eat. Parents should be encouraged to provide frequent, smaller, and nutritious meals throughout the day. Toddlers need less food per unit of body weight than they did during infancy. A general guideline for serving size is 1 tablespoon of each solid food for each year of age. Parents must be informed that during illness, brief periods of anorexia are usually not serious. Examples of nutritious finger foods that are safe and easy to eat on the run include ripe fruits such as bananas, pears, melons, and avocados; cooked vegetables including squash and sweet potatoes; shredded cheese is another good option.

Sleep, play activity, and safety. Toddlers expend a high level of energy in daily growth, play, and exploration. Adequate rest and sleep are essential for maintaining optimal wellness. The toddler needs 12 hours of sleep each night plus a daytime nap. Suggestions helpful in promoting healthy sleeping patterns include limiting stimulation before sleep time, using quiet-time activities before sleep, allowing a favorite bedtime toy, telling a specified number of stories, and establishing and maintaining bedtime rituals. Box 24.10 lists guidelines for bedtime preparation.

Play improves muscle coordination, balance, and muscle strength. The toddler's play style, described as parallel play (Fig. 24.6), refers to the need that toddlers have to play along with, but not directly with, their peers. Unable to share and interact with their peers at this stage, they play side by side with similar toys in similar ways, but without interacting. Toddlers thrive on activities that allow them to move. Running, jumping, and climbing activities help toddlers to develop bones and muscles. This age group's natural curiosity about how things work encourages them to explore. Play groups help encourage the shy or reluctant child to participate and try new activities. The developmental tasks of toddlers are summarized in Box 24.11.

More than half of all childhood deaths are caused by accidents, many of which are motor vehicle accidents. About 90% of the accidents that occur in the home are believed to be preventable. Prevention methods must include supervision and education.

PRESCHOOL: 3 TO 5 YEARS

Physical Characteristics

Physical development during early childhood occurs on many fronts. The most obvious are the striking

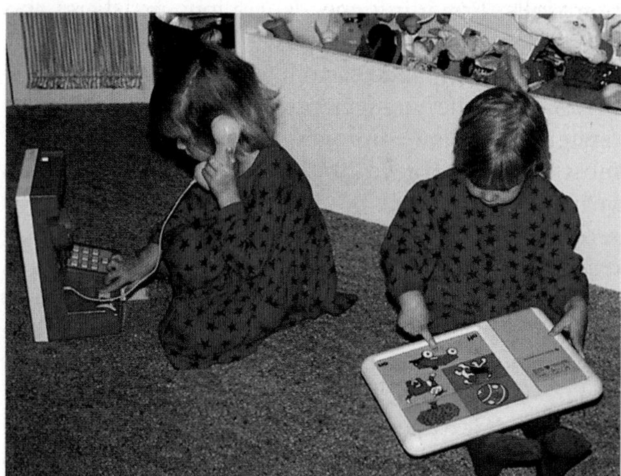

Fig. 24.6 Parallel play. (From Hockenberry MJ, Wilson D, Winkelstein ML, et al: *Wong's nursing care of infants and children,* ed 8, St. Louis, 2007, Mosby.)

Box 24.10 Guidelines for Bedtime Preparation

- Reduce activity level before bedtime.
- Establish a simple ritual (e.g., bathroom, story time, goodnight song).
- Make bedtime a pleasurable experience.
- Familiarize children with a nightly routine.
- Reassure children that they are not alone.
- Use a night-light.
- Expect disruptions or setbacks during and after illness and stress or after stimulating activities.

Box 24.11 Developmental Tasks of the Toddler

- Recognizes self as a separate person; tolerates separation from primary caregiver, expresses own ideas and needs
- Develops increased attention span
- Begins to develop communication skills
- Begins to develop self-control skills
- Masters toilet-training basics
- Achieves independent mobility
- Develops independent skills of daily living: feeding, dressing, toileting, and managing simple tasks

changes in size and shape; and the most important—maturation of the nervous system and mastery of motor skills—are the least obvious.

Growth during the preschool period tends to be slow and steady. The preschooler looks taller and thinner than at earlier stages as the toddler's lordosis and protuberant abdomen are left behind (the abdominal muscles strengthen, and the child loses the potbelly appearance). Average weight gain is less than 5 pounds (11 kg) per year. Linear growth is about 2 to 2½ inches (5.08 to 6.35 cm) per year. Height of the 4-year-old is usually double the birth length. The gait of the preschooler becomes steadier. The preschooler is more capable of focusing and refining activities, and the body grows slimmer, stronger, and less top heavy. Because of these developments, gross motor skills (large body movements such as running, climbing, jumping, and throwing) improve dramatically. Tasks such as tying shoelaces, cutting food with a knife and fork, and putting together a puzzle prove more difficult because of the preschooler's undeveloped fine motor skills (skills that involve small body movements); these are much harder for them to master than gross motor skills. Development of fine motor skills is important to encourage. The scribbling of the young child is comparable with the babbling of the infant. Both are ways to obtain practice with the means to later mastery of essential communication skills. Providing pencils, crayons, markers, and paper is as important as providing things to climb, objects to throw, and places to run.

Vision in the younger preschooler is described as farsighted. Vision improves during this period, and most children achieve 20/30 visual accuracy by age 4 years. A yearly check of preschool children's vision is recommended. Sometimes amblyopia, a condition commonly known as lazy eye, is detected during a simple eye examination. Corrective measures, such as patching the good eye, usually strengthen the lazy eye and are necessary to prevent blindness.

Vital signs. Heart rate for the preschooler ranges between 70 and 110 beats per minute. Respiratory rate slows to about 23 breaths per minute at rest. Blood pressure averages 110/60 mm Hg. Temperature ranges from 97° to 99°F (36.1° to 37.2°C), depending on the method used for measurement.

Psychosocial Development

First, children learn to function independently; they subsequently use imagination to explore new experiences creatively. Erikson describes the task of the preschooler in terms of initiative versus guilt. Preschoolers search for and create fantasies about the different kinds of people they would like to become. They pretend to be grown up and try out a variety of roles (Figs. 24.7 and 24.8). During the preschool period, the child's superego (conscience) functions as a censor of behavior. The dilemma of the preschooler, according to Erikson, is to test initiative without creating an overwhelming sense of guilt. Typical development of the preschooler includes gender identification. At this time, the child commonly stereotypes roles and shows marked interest in sexual differences. Strong sibling bonding is established (Fig. 24.9).

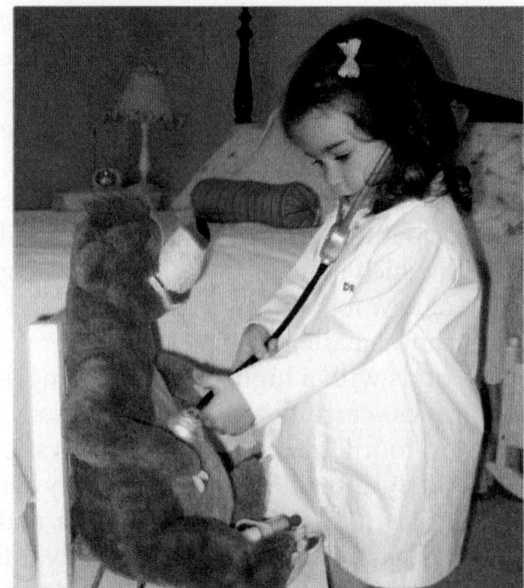

Fig. 24.7 Trying out new roles. (From Hockenberry MJ, Wilson D: *Wong's nursing care of infants and children*, ed 10, St. Louis, 2015, Mosby.)

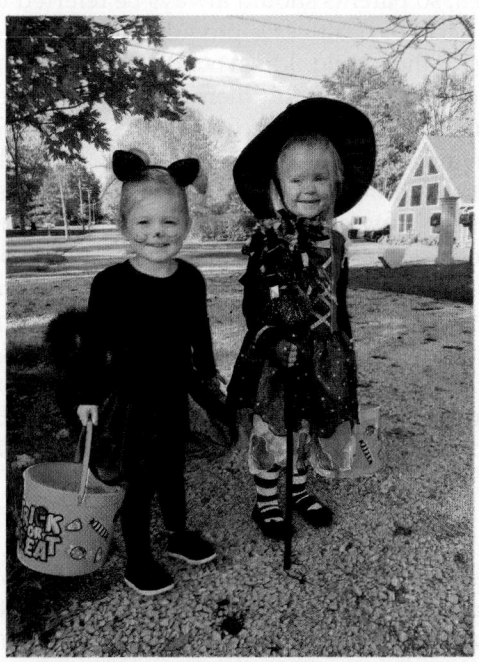

Fig. 24.8 Young children enjoy dressing up.

Cognitive and Intellectual Development

According to Piaget, the preschool child is at the preoperational stage of cognitive development. Preschoolers use symbols to represent objects. They use trial and error to discover and adopt new traits and characteristics. Between ages 4 and 7 years, intuitive thinking develops, and the child begins to think logically. Children in the

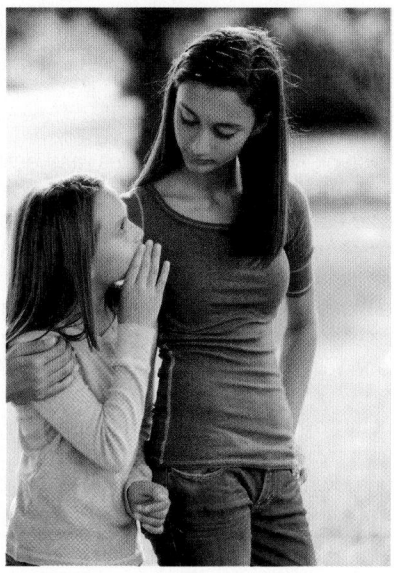

Fig. 24.9 Siblings establishing a bond. (Copyright Thinkstock Photos.)

preoperational stage see the world from their own viewpoint. They see things as absolutes, in terms of white and black and either good or bad.

During the preschool stage, time is associated with weekly and seasonal events. Magical thoughts are typical of the child of this age, who believes that wishes have the power to make things happen. As a result, the preschool child sometimes feels powerful—and responsible—for events that occur. Because of the belief that a wish has caused serious harm or even death to a loved one, the preschooler at times feels guilty. The occasional "white lies" or untruths of this period usually reflect some of the child's fantasies. During this stage of development, the child needs trustworthy guidance to distinguish truth from fantasy. At this stage, the child is more vulnerable to certain fears, probably fallout from the typically vivid imagination. Excessive exposure to inappropriate television content and other media has the potential to further distort reality testing. Common fears that manifest at this stage include fear of thunder, lightning, the dark, pain, abandonment, and monsters.

Communication and Language

By age 3 years, children are able to carry on a conversation. Pronunciation problems continue into the school years. Language becomes more adult-like. If the child is not talking by age 3 years, evaluation by a physician for possible hearing loss or other pathologic speech disturbances is necessary. Advise parents to continue to read to their child to help expand language ability and comprehension and to continue to foster positive child-caregiver relationships.

Health Promotion

Nutrition. Because body systems and muscles still are growing steadily, the preschool child continues to need high levels of protein. Dietary calcium and phosphorus are important to toddlers and preschool children because of the increasing mineralization of their teeth and bones. Food habits, likes, dislikes, and appetites vary greatly from child to child. Some physicians recommend supplementary vitamins. Vitamins, like any other medication, are not intended and do not have the capacity to take the place of good eating habits (see Chapter 19).

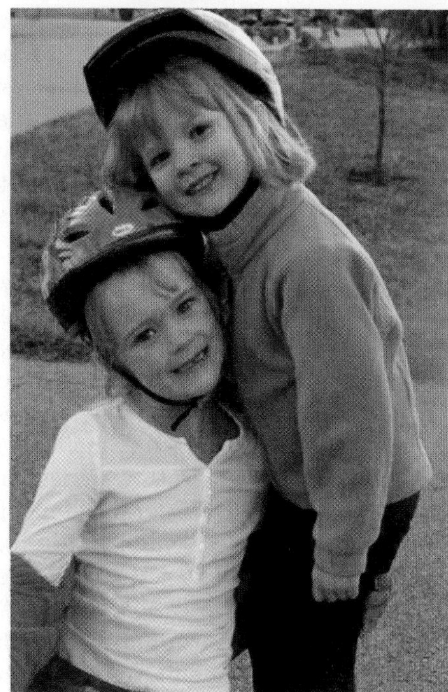

Fig. 24.10 Playmates.

A body mass index (BMI) at or above the 85th percentile and lower than the 95th percentile for children of the same gender and age is considered overweight. A BMI at or above the 95% percentile for children of the same gender and age is considered obese (CDC, 2015). Most cultures hold strong views regarding obesity, which results in emotional consequences for an obese child. Control of weight is an important parental concern, because it helps prevent serious health issues later in life. Overweight infants are more likely to become overweight later in life. Genetic factors may predispose individuals to obesity; additionally, children often adopt the eating habits of parents. Make suggestions to parents of ways to help with their children's weight control: model good eating behaviors, provide healthy food, and encourage physical activity.

Sleep, play activity, and safety. Preschoolers often resist nap periods but still need 11 to 12 hours of sleep at night. Rest periods offered during the day enable children to reenergize and carry out the rest of their daily activities.

Play style for the preschool child becomes cooperative. The child begins to share, take turns, and interact with playmates (Fig. 24.10). Preschoolers enjoy pretending to carry out activities such as cooking, shopping, and driving. Through dramatic play, the child tries on different roles and identifies with adult models. Not only is it fun for two or more children to cooperate in creating their own scenario but it also helps their social development to try out social roles, express their fears and fantasies, and learn to cooperate. Experiences with imaginary playmates are not uncommon in this age group. Children often feel a sense of control over what happens in their "imaginary world" and slowly learn to deal with reality through practice and experimentation.

Children during the preschool period are becoming more coordinated and want to begin participating in more organized games. By age 4 to 5 years, children learn to ride a bicycle with training wheels. They need guidance because they have difficulty maneuvering the bicycle, and their judgment and awareness of safety issues is limited (see the Safety Alert box for safety and injury prevention tips for preschool children). Swimming, skating, and dancing are activities that children in this age group often begin to learn and enjoy. Activities of this nature should be fun for the child. It is not beneficial or appropriate for children to be pressured to participate in activities that they do not like or enjoy. Also advise parents and caregivers to space activities so that children are not overstressed by having too many lessons, practices, or games.

Safety Alert

Safety Tips and Injury Prevention for Preschool Children

- Use proper equipment that fits the child.
- Never leave children alone in pools of water. Teach children not to touch or go near pool drains.
- Inspect protective equipment, such as bicycle helmets, for potential hazards.
- Use protective sunscreen.

All the safety precautions described previously apply to the preschool child and the infant and toddler (see the Safety Alert box). Instruct parents and caregivers to teach preschool children their full names, addresses, and telephone numbers. Children need to know how to use the phone in case of an emergency.

Discipline and limit setting are needed and are as important to the child as are love and security. Necessary guidance includes offering alternative ways of expressing feelings and meeting needs (Box 24.12).

The preschool period is a time of learning to function independently and exploring the imagination. Box 24.13 shows the developmental tasks of preschoolers.

SCHOOL AGE: 6 TO 12 YEARS

Physical Characteristics

During the school-age period, the growth pattern is usually gradual and subtle. The most obvious growth is in the long bones of the extremities and in the development of the facial bones. As a result of this bone growth, some children report "growing pains," particularly at night. Persistent pains call for evaluation by a physician to rule out any underlying pathologic condition. From ages 6 to 12 years, height and weight increase by about 2 inches and 4½ to 6½ pounds per year for boys and girls.

Motor skills in boys and girls develop with some differences; boys often become stronger, and girls more graceful and accurate.

The child's posture becomes straighter. The causes of poor posture range from fatigue to emotional states or even minor skeletal defects. Ensure that school-age children are screened routinely for scoliosis (abnormal lateral curvature of the spine). Muscle mass and strength gradually increase, and the body loses the "baby fat" appearance of earlier childhood. Gross motor and fine motor development continue to be refined during the school-age years.

Vision improves, and most children have 20/20 vision at this stage. Regular vision testing is advisable throughout the school years.

Box 24.12 Steps for Discipline and Limit Setting

- Define acceptable as opposed to unacceptable behaviors.
- Set limits: "I will not let you hurt anyone."
- Be consistent: keep the same rules, and enforce them reliably.
- Recognize escalating emotions and intervene: "I can see you are upset; let's go over there and sit down."
- Suggest "time out."
- Choose punishment that "fits" wrongdoing, and enact it in a timely way (and in a nonhostile manner).
- Praise and reinforce positive behavior: "I like the way you…"
- Always start over with a clean slate.
- Stay calm; avoid arguing.
- Avoid putdowns: "You are acting like a bad boy."
- Remember to listen to the child.

Box 24.13 Developmental Tasks of Preschoolers

- Develops stronger sense of self; is able to express own needs, ideas, and feelings; has capacity to postpone immediate gratification
- Attains greater attention span; listens more attentively
- Develops and refines gross motor skills and fine motor skills
- Recognizes gender identification
- Begins to work and play more cooperatively with others
- Improves communication skills
- Develops self-control skills; learns socially acceptable ways of expressing anger, frustration, and disappointment; obeys simple rules; develops self-awareness and sense of self-protection
- Seeks information, asks questions, learns values and beliefs of the family

Vital signs. Heart and respiratory rate steadily decrease, whereas blood pressure increases. Normal pulse rate is between 55 and 90 per minute, respiratory rate is 22 to 24 per minute, and blood pressure is 110/65 mm Hg.

Dentition. By age 6 years, the child begins to lose the deciduous teeth. Permanent teeth develop rapidly. Dental checkups should continue every 6 months throughout childhood.

Psychosocial Development

Entrance into school challenges the child and creates demands for new social and cognitive skills. The child becomes more independent and participates in a broader world of peers and new experiences. School-age children become increasingly aware of rules and socialization skills and expectations. The beginning abilities to compromise and compete are challenges faced in this age group.

Erikson identified the task of the school-age years as industry versus inferiority. After the child realizes that "there is no workable future within the womb of his family," says Erikson, the school-age child "becomes ready to apply himself to given skills and tasks." Children develop their own goals and direct their efforts toward mastery of these goals. As children discover their talents and accomplishments, they gain self-confidence and a sense of purpose. During these years, the child learns to work and masters skills that produce satisfaction as the result of that work. Successful mastery of learning in school leads to strengthening and stabilizing the child's sense of self. According to Erikson, as children busily try to master the skills valued in their culture, they develop views of themselves as either competent or incompetent—as either industrious and productive or inferior and inadequate.

Input from the outside is a key influence on which direction the child's self-concept will take. If the environment inadequately supports a child's pursuits, the stage perhaps is set for the development of feelings of inferiority and the lack of self-confidence. The good school setting is a pleasant, comfortable environment. Teachers and caregivers need to use praise, encouragement, and rewards to reinforce the school-age child's efforts positively. Teachers also must be positive role models. School helps the child learn new routines and establish important social relationships (Fig. 24.11). However, the school climate can be affected negatively by bullying. Bullying can take on many forms, including physical (hitting, tripping), verbal (name calling, teasing), relational (spreading rumors, excluding), and cyber (e-mail, text messaging). CDC defines bullying as "any unwanted aggressive behavior(s) by another youth or group of youths who are not siblings or current dating partners that involves an observed or perceived power imbalance and is repeated multiple times or is highly likely to be repeated" (2016). In 2015 20% of high school students reported they had been bullied on school property. Bullying can lead to physical injury as well as depression, anxiety, sleep difficulties, and even death. One way to prevent bullying is for schools to have a consistently enforced antibullying policy (CDC, 2016).

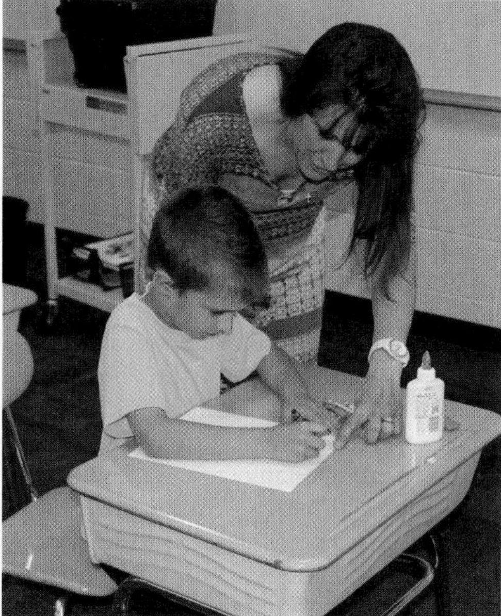

Fig. 24.11 School represents an important change in a child's life, and teachers exert a significant influence on the child.

Cognitive and Intellectual Development

According to Piaget, children in the school years move into the **concrete operational phase.** During this phase, thoughts become increasingly logical and coherent so that the child is able to classify, sort, and organize facts while still being incapable of generalizing or dealing with abstractions. Children have the capacity to think rationally about almost any specific and concrete perception. Between ages 7 and 11 years, children usually come to understand logical principles—again, as long as the principles can be applied to concrete, specific cases. They distinguish purpose from behavior and outcome and are able to focus on more than one aspect of a task. Children in this age group have begun to develop logical socialized thought. They view the world more realistically than they did at younger ages, and they are capable of understanding the views of others. Movement is away from fantasy as the child realizes that a physical cause is behind an event. The child's developing cognitive skills serve as a motivator for learning how to work. A supportive learning environment often enhances the child's approach to problem solving and helps lead to success.

The school-age child experiences gradual and subtle growth changes while learning new social and cognitive skills. Box 24.14 contains a list of the developmental tasks of the school-age child.

Communication and Language

Most 6-year-olds have a good command of sentence structure. The child's vocabulary has become more

Box 24.14 Developmental Tasks of the School-Age Child

- Develops a sense of belonging with family, peers
- Develops work habits and learns to organize, set, and reach goals; evaluate work; and accept criticism
- Learns competence in reading, writing, calculation, grammar, and communication
- Refines fine-motor and gross-motor coordination

extensive and includes slang and swear words, which many children enjoy using for the effect they create. Fine motor development continues and, combined with growth in cognitive and communication skills, produces refinements in written-language and musical abilities. By age 7 years, the hands of the child have become steadier. Printing becomes clearer and smaller. Between ages 8 and 10 years, the hand becomes more efficient, which enables the child to write rather than print. The 10- to 12-year-old child has the capacity to accomplish complex, intricate, fine-quality handcrafts and sometimes begins piano, violin, or guitar lessons.

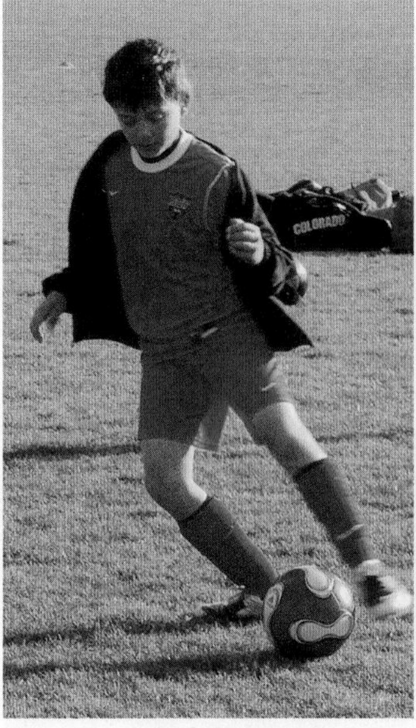

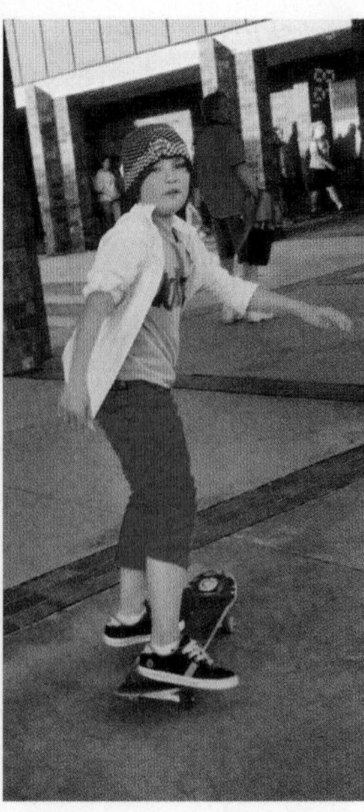

Fig. 24.12 Activities engaged in by school-age children, such as soccer and skateboarding, vary according to the child's interest and opportunity.

Health Promotion

Nutrition. Total metabolic needs are determined by the energy expenditure of each individual child. The sedentary, quiet child who prefers fine motor activities needs fewer calories than the child who is more oriented to athletics or is more physically active. The recommended daily intake of food is listed at the ChooseMyPlate website *(www.choosemyplate.gov)*.

Building on toddler-age and preschool-age foundations, strong dietary habits and food preferences are established during the school-age period. Cultural influences, family habits, and peer pressure are critical factors in how a child's food habits develop. Obesity during this period is correlated closely with obesity in adult years; therefore the child's weight must be maintained within normal limits. In middle childhood, obese children are teased, picked on, and rejected. They know they are overweight, and they often hate themselves for it. Obese children usually have fewer friends than other children. The best way to get children to lose weight is to increase their physical activity. Indeed, inactivity is possibly as responsible for childhood obesity as overeating. Diets high in saturated fat increase a child's risk for high blood cholesterol and earlier occurrence of heart disease unless steps are taken to lower these levels.

Sleep, play activity, and safety. Fatigue, irritability, inattention, and poor learning are often signs of inadequate sleep. The 6-year-old needs about 12 hours of sleep at night. By 12 years of age, the child usually needs about 10 hours of sleep. Some children have frequent nightmares that disrupt their sleep. Stress, violence on television, and overtiredness may contribute to a child's nightmares. Relaxation techniques such as quiet music, story time, and bathing often help the child relax before sleep.

School-age children need adequate exercise to enhance muscle development, coordination, balance, and strength. In addition, music, craft projects, board games, appropriate television, and video games are all enjoyed by the school-age child. Privacy and a place for their belongings are important at this age. The school-age child is often a willing worker and enjoys being paid for small jobs. Collection and hoarding of "treasures" among their belongings are a part of this stage of development.

Many children during the school years become involved with competitive or team sports (Fig. 24.12). Children of this age show interest and loyalty to peers of the same gender. They learn to follow the rules of games. Some may benefit from team competitiveness and use it to motivate themselves to excel. Others shy away from competition and become disinterested or develop feelings of inadequacy and disappointment.

Accidents are still the leading cause of death in this age group. Impulsiveness, poor judgment, curiosity, and incomplete control over motor coordination are some of the factors that increase the school-age child's risk of accidents.

Television often exerts a powerful influence on a child's development, and children are watching an average of 4 hours of television daily (AACAP, 2014). One concern about television today is the increased amount of violence it portrays. Many believe that, although not the cause of aggressive behavior, a good deal of available television content offers the child a potent model for aggressive behavior and is a significant factor in the development of aggressive behavior. Suggest ways for parents to help reduce the negative influence of television: (1) limit the amount of time children watch television; (2) screen programs for content and age appropriateness; and (3) watch programs with children and discuss the content.

Preventing school violence is another critical issue these days. **School violence** is defined as anything that physically or psychologically injures schoolchildren or damages school property. Today, school violence seems to have increased in many locations. Two factors that possibly are contributing to this increase are an increased availability of weapons and a breakdown of communication. Experts agree that children need resources to help them deal with the daily stressors that they face. Many children today spend less time with parents and more time in front of a television and on the Internet watching or playing violent shows and games. Parents must be aware of the effects of television violence on children. Children who view violent acts are more likely to show aggression but are also fearful that something bad will happen to them. Children need to feel comfortable discussing their feelings and concerns with parents and teachers and must be able to use these discussions to learn how to recognize whether they are in danger and whether others are exhibiting signs of troubled behavior. Encourage parents to ask questions about their child's feelings and their school activities daily. If children have difficulty talking to parents or answering their questions, advise parents to seek professional help. A key responsibility of parents is to stay involved and be active participants in their child's daily affairs.

Children need to be taught constructive ways to handle their impulses; otherwise they are more likely to resort to unacceptable ways of channeling their feelings. One possibility is that they will look for revenge, which perhaps makes them feel in control and powerful. Although many children have access to weapons, most of them do not engage in violent behavior. However, we need to work to inhibit violent tendencies and to look for ways to prevent the few who do act out their feelings in violent ways from causing harm to others (see school safety tips in the Safety Alert box). The first step in preventing a tragedy is recognizing the behavioral tendencies that have the potential to lead to violence or other problem behavior. Give children the guidance and encouragement they need to recognize and report the signs of troubled behavior if they notice them in a friend or classmate without feeling that they have deceived the other person or let the other person down (Box 24.15).

Safety Alert

Safety in Schools

- Secure weapons in homes.
- Develop a zero-tolerance program with school officials.
- Work with a parent-teacher association (PTA) to make schools safe.
- Determine with school officials an emergency and security plan.
- Maintain open lines of communication between child and parent and school officials.

Box 24.15 Common Signs of Troubled Childhood Behavior

- Problems getting along with peers
- Difficulty accepting authority and resistance to direction
- Outbursts of uncontrolled behavior
- Bullying tendencies
- Frequent victimizing or teasing
- Social isolation
- Poor school performance
- Violence to pets or other living creatures
- Preoccupation with weapons
- Verbal expression of threatening behavior or revenge

Gun safety is necessary regardless of opinions about gun ownership. Gun enthusiasts, collectors, and law enforcement agents are obliged to ensure the safety of others. Most children and many adults have a fascination with guns. Even when children and adults are taught gun safety, some exhibit unsafe behavior when the opportunity arises. Even toy guns create the potential for dangerous situations. Parents and individuals with weapons in the home must take adequate steps to prevent accidents and injury from their weapons. Knowledge of how to handle a gun is not sufficient to protect the owner's family and others from injury. Ammunition must be removed from firearms, and guns must be locked away securely and apart from ammunition, which is kept secured in another, separate locked area. In addition, and most important, children of all ages must be taught what to do if they find a gun (see gun safety rules in the Safety Alert box).

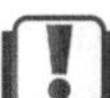

Safety Alert

Gun Safety Rules

FOR CHILDREN

- Stop and **DO NOT TOUCH** any gun, real or toy.
- Leave the area if a gun is found.
- Report any gun to an adult.

FOR ADULTS

- Never store ammunition with the gun.
- Keep the gun in a locked location out of reach of children.
- Lock the ammunition in a separate location from the gun.
- Lock gun-cleaning supplies, which are often poisonous.

ADOLESCENCE: 12 TO 19 YEARS

Physical Characteristics

The term *adolescence* covers the transition period from childhood to adulthood. Adolescence begins at puberty; accompanying the pubertal changes are corresponding changes in the personality. *Puberty,* the period of life at which the ability to reproduce begins, entails the maturation of the reproductive system, including all the primary and secondary sexual developmental changes. Primary changes occur in the organs related to reproduction (ovaries, breasts, uterus, testes, and penis). Secondary sexual changes occur in other parts of the body (development of pubic and facial hair, voice changes, and fat deposits). Adolescence literally means "to grow into maturity" and generally is regarded as the psychological, social, and maturational process initiated by pubertal changes.

Adolescence is characterized as the second major period of rapid growth. Females grow 2 to 8 inches (5 to 20 cm), whereas males grow 4 to 12 inches (10 to 30 cm). During this adolescent period, females gain 15 to 55 pounds (7 to 25 kg), and males gain 15 to 65 pounds (7 to 30 kg). Females develop more body fat, and males develop more muscle tissue. After puberty, men average 50% muscle and 16% fat, whereas women average 40% muscle and 27% fat. Muscle strength and muscle mass increase in the male, which causes the average male to have more muscle strength. Exercise facilitates the size, strength, and endurance of each adolescent.

In the female, menarche (the first menstrual period) signals the beginning of adolescence; sperm production signals the beginning of adolescence in the male. Girls develop larger breasts, a narrower waist, wider hips, and a lower center of gravity. Boys develop broader shoulders, narrower hips, and larger limbs. Boys and girls experience voice changes. Girls' voices become fuller and richer because of the lengthening of their vocal cords. Boys' voices become lower and louder. The deeper male voice results from enlargement of the larynx (the Adam's apple) and lengthening of the vocal cords.

Sexual interests increase markedly in vigor and intensity and usually focus on members of the opposite sex. New problems arise as adolescents find social disapproval and prohibitions arising in their own conscience that conflict with intense sexual drives.

Vital signs. Average pulse rate is 70 beats per minute. Respiratory rate averages 20 breaths per minute. Blood pressure increases to 120/70 mm Hg.

Psychosocial Development

Exactly when adolescence begins is different in each person. Some enter adolescence at an early age; others develop later. Regardless of the exact age of onset, the nearing of this stage is evident by recognizing the onset of distinct behavioral changes. A mother may notice that her 11-year-old daughter has become tight-lipped about school and activities, no longer wanting her mother's opinion or listening ear. Her daughter is now spending most of her time at home in her room with the door closed. A father may delight in his son's musical talents and his band's energy and success, although the two may argue over the taste of their lyrics and the decibel level.

The period of adolescence frequently is described as difficult and involving a stormy search for oneself.

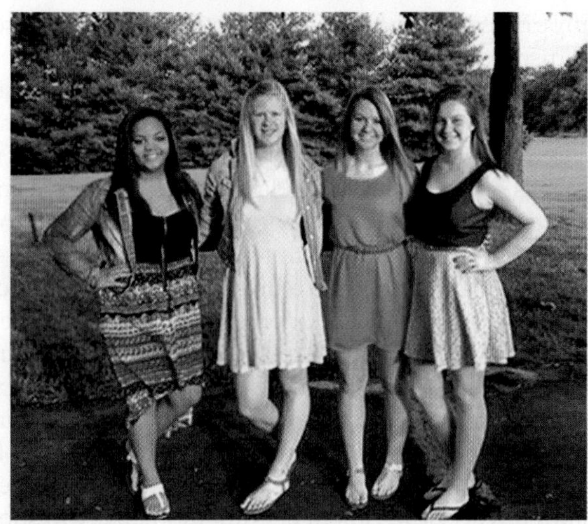

Fig. 24.13 The peer group provides the adolescent with a sense of belonging.

Confronting every adolescent are a changing body, sexual demands, responsibilities, expectations, and questions about values and beliefs. The search for identity amid a world of social pressures creates a painful struggle.

Erikson described the developmental task of adolescence as establishing a sense of identity. He proposed the conflict of identity versus role confusion as characteristic of adolescence. The search for a sense of identity, he believed, reaches crisis proportions at this time. Not only does the adolescent need to adjust to a sexually mature body but also all previous conflicts (trust versus mistrust, autonomy versus doubt, initiative versus guilt, and industry versus inferiority) must be resolved yet again in light of the newly sensuous self. The period of adolescence requires major reorganization of the personality, resolution of childhood insecurities, and acceptance of adult responsibilities. The value of peers is usually significant to the adolescent (Fig. 24.13). Peers influence preferences of dress, speech, and leisure activities. The peer group is often the milieu to learn and test developing interpersonal skills. Many adolescents use conforming behavior to win praise and acceptance by peers. If handled properly, adolescence is often a great period of accomplishment and creativity (Box 24.16).

Cognitive Development

According to Piaget, an individual's cognitive function reaches maturity during adolescence. Piaget describes this stage as the **formal operational thought stage**. This is a higher process that permits abstract reasoning and systematic, scientific problem solving. Adolescents become capable of reasoning and formal logic. At this time, thoughts may be influenced more by logical principles than by personal perceptions and experiences. The adolescent thinks beyond the present. Without having to focus exclusively on the immediate situation, the adolescent can imagine the possible: a sequence of

Box 24.16 Parenting Tips During Adolescence

- Educate yourself and your adolescent.
- Maintain open communication.
- Choose your battles.
- Set realistic expectations.
- Set good examples for behavior.
- Honor individuality.
- Respect privacy.
- Try to remember your own experiences during this stage.
- Set appropriate rules and regulations.
- Be consistent.
- Stay involved; meet your child's friends and acquaintances.
- Be active in school and after-school activities.

events that may occur, such as college and occupational possibilities; how things may change in the future, such as relationships with parents; and the possible consequences of actions he or she is considering, such as dropping out of school.

Moral Development

As children move through the stages of cognition and logical thinking, they also progress through stages of moral development. As with other developmental processes, moral development approaches or achieves adult levels during adolescence.

In some ways, adolescence is an uncomfortable in-between phase. Old principles are challenged, but new and independent values do not emerge immediately. As a consequence, young people search for a moral code that preserves their personal integrity and guides their behavior, especially in the face of strong pressure to violate the old values. They face many decisions involving moral dilemmas. They need to internalize gradually a set of principles that provides them with the resources to evaluate the demands of a situation and to plan a course of action consistent with their ideals.

Health Promotion

Nutrition. The rate of body growth and the adolescent's increased basal metabolic rate require an increase in the individual's caloric needs. At peak growth, females may need as much as 2600 calories per day and males as much as 3600 calories per day. Many factors affect the individual's dietary habits, including cultural background, family habits, work schedules, school, concern about weight gain, peer influence, and lack of knowledge concerning correct food choices. Of particular concern are eating disorders. Anorexia nervosa and bulimia are on the rise in young women. Parents should be educated about the warning signs, because these disorders can be fatal. Protein needs are increased as a consequence of the rapid growth of this period. Advise adolescents to obtain 12% to 16% of their total daily food intake from protein.

The adolescent diet is most likely to be deficient in calcium, iron, and zinc. The need for these minerals during the period of rapid growth is increased substantially—calcium for skeletal growth; iron for expansion of muscle mass and blood volume, soft tissue growth, and the rapid growth demands of the expanding red blood cell mass; and zinc for the generation of skeletal and muscle tissue. Adolescent boys have greater muscle mass, but adolescent girls have an additional iron loss from menstruation. Consequently, the need for iron is equivalent in both sexes.

Increased amounts of milk usually are required to supplement the average diet to ensure an adequate calcium intake during this time.

The adolescent is advised to follow the guidelines at the ChooseMyPlate website (see Chapter 19).

Sleep, play activity, and safety. The adolescent needs to pace activities to allow for adequate rest. The adolescent often requires increased hours of sleep to restore energy levels. During puberty and adolescence, caution must be taken to prevent injuries related to exercise and sports. Injuries sometimes occur in connection with the adolescent's growth spurt. Growth spurts cause the bones to grow more quickly than the muscles and tendons, which causes the muscles and tendons to become short and tight. Sports-related injuries may result from these factors. Teaching youngsters to perform appropriate warm-up and stretching exercises before starting any strenuous sport can lessen the risk of injury (see sports-related safety tips in the Safety Alert box). Participating in organized sports at this age helps adolescents learn to work with others, meet challenges, and set personal goals. Parents have an opportunity to encourage children to exercise by setting an example and practicing good, healthy behaviors for themselves. Having parents involved on the sidelines supporting their adolescent's efforts potentially enhances self-esteem.

Safety Alert

Sports-Related Safety Tips

- Use safety helmets.
- Use properly fitting equipment.
- Play on properly maintained surfaces.
- Perform warm-up exercises before sports practice.
- Avoid overuse of muscles.
- Insist on adequate supervision.
- Obtain proper training.
- Treat existing injuries and prevent reinjury.

Accident prevention is vital during this stage of development. The greatest number of deaths in this age group is due to accidents. Adolescents are known to participate in more risk-taking behaviors; therefore driver's education, water safety training, education about safe sex practices, and drug education are necessary to inform adolescents of the risks and dangers inherent in these activities. The Safety Alert box lists safe sex practices that are crucial to emphasize early in adolescence, with special emphasis on abstinence.

Safety Alert

Guidelines for Practice of Safe Sex

- The safest sexual practice is abstinence.
- Be familiar with your sexual partners. Ask about their sexual lifestyle before you engage in sexual relations.
- Avoid engaging in sexual relations with intravenous drug users or with individuals who have had multiple sex partners.
- Use a latex condom as the best type of protection from infection.
- Condoms should be inspected for tears before use. Avoid lengthy storage and exposure to excessive heat.
- Fit the condom over the erect penis, leaving a small space at the end for the collection of semen.
- Hold the upper end of the condom when withdrawing from the vagina to prevent slippage.
- Avoid sexual relations with individuals who have genital lesions or unusual drainage.
- Be aware that the risk of human immunodeficiency virus (HIV) infection is increased with oral sexual practices. Anal intercourse requires additional education for safe practice.

Emotional health. Adolescence is, as described previously, a period of maturation that covers the transition from childhood to adulthood (Box 24.17). In part as a result of the complexity of the tasks that face them, adolescents experience different moods. At times they are outgoing and gregarious and active participants in family matters. They offer their opinions and seem to ignore others. There are also times when they are moody and loners who seem not to want any part of family activities. Such mood swings generally occur at this stage. Families should recognize and distinguish normal moodiness from signs of depression. **Depression** is defined as a mood disturbance characterized by feelings of sadness, despair, and hopelessness. People who are depressed are often unable to improve their condition without help from professional therapy. Teach parents, teachers, and health care workers to recognize the common signs of depression. Early detection and intervention are crucial when dealing with depression because this leads to higher success rates. Untreated depression can lead to suicide (Box 24.18). Advise parents to seek professional help if their child expresses feelings of marked depression. All threats must be taken seriously, and it is imperative to be alert to sudden changes in behavior, such as a change from extreme sadness to manic behavior. This mood swing potentially signals a decision to carry out the person's suicide plan.

EARLY ADULTHOOD: 20 TO 40 YEARS

The transition to adulthood in the United States is marked by events such as taking on financial responsibilities, making career choices, beginning social relationships, entering marriage, and becoming a parent. All the challenges and accomplishments of the earlier developmental stages have helped prepare the individual for the responsibilities of adult maturity. Fantasies of what adulthood entails usually give way to more realistic expectations and hopes.

Early adulthood, the period of optimal physical condition, is marked by momentous changes in lifestyle. Box 24.19 contains a list of the developmental tasks of early adulthood.

Box 24.17 Developmental Tasks of the Adolescent

- Recognizes individuality
- Accepts strengths and weaknesses
- Develops own value system
- Assumes responsibility for own behavior
- Develops philosophy of life
- Adapts to somatic changes (changes that affect the body)
- Acquires skills necessary for adult living
- Refines social skills
- Develops independent living skills

Box 24.18 Signs of Depression and Indicators of Suicide Risk

- Change in appetite
- Change in mood (sadness, hopelessness)
- Inability to concentrate
- Loss of interest in activities
- Change in sleep habits (either always sleeping or unable to sleep)
- Talk of suicide
- Preoccupation with death or dying
- Giving away of possessions

Box 24.19 Developmental Tasks of Early Adulthood

- Achieves financial and social independence
- Maximizes personal worth and identity
- Develops meaningful and satisfying social relationships
- Assumes responsibilities and independent decision making
- Learns to balance personal needs and societal expectations
- Accepts self and others
- Distinguishes physical attraction from love and permanent commitment
- Decides on a marriage, career, and children

Physical Characteristics

The body during early adult years is at its optimal level of functioning. The typical young adult is a fine physical specimen. During the middle 20s, most body functions are fully developed, and muscular strength, energy, and endurance are now at their peak.

Physical appearance is influenced by heredity, environment, and general state of wellness. Females usually reach their maximal height at about 16 to 17 years of age. Males continue to grow until 18 to 20 years of age. Between ages 30 and 45 years, height is stable, and then it begins to decline because of settling of spinal disks. Often an increase in fatty tissue causes weight gain, a decrease in muscle strength, and a stabilization of reaction time. The senses are also at their sharpest during young adulthood. Visual acuity is keenest at about age 20 years and does not begin to decline until about age 40 years.

Psychosocial Development

Dual-career families have emerged based on current economic realities and women's interest in pursuing careers. The feminist movement has resulted in many positive social changes. The home and the workplace show the effects of these changes and the dual-career lifestyle.

Another important option for this age group is the decision to start a family (Fig. 24.14). If procreation is the choice, a subsequent issue is how many children to have. Further consideration is given to financial means, safety, family support, housing, the relationship to members of the extended family, and the roles and responsibilities of the nuclear family unit. Young adults who establish a family need to have open communication about self-development, which includes issues of dual careers, child-rearing practices, and domestic duties within the home.

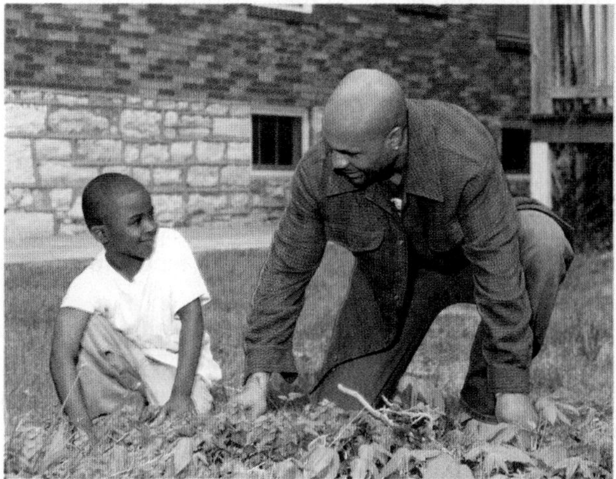

Fig. 24.14 Father and child bonding. (From Sorrentino SA, Remmert LN: *Mosby's textbook for nursing assistants*, ed 8, St. Louis, 2012, Saunders.)

Family development and harmony are important goals for many young adults. Although family size and structure have undergone dramatic changes in the past decades, concerns about individual members' health and safety continue to form a primary focus within the family as a unit. Family life is influenced by the characteristics of individual family members. Typically, healthy family adjustment is associated with the age of the individuals, job security, the family's and the individuals' places in the community, and healthy patterns of living (good nutrition, personal cleanliness, physical fitness). Therefore the physical and mental health of one family member affects all family members.

Erikson identified early intimacy versus isolation as the developmental task of adulthood. Intimacy is the ability to develop one's deepest hopes and concerns in connection to another person. One aspect of intimacy is the capacity to accept the closeness of another person. Intimacy leads to commitment, sharing, and compromise. The "virtue" that develops in young adulthood is the virtue of love, or the mutuality of devotion between partners who have chosen to share their lives. As young adults resolve conflicting demands of intimacy, competitiveness, and distance, they develop an ethical sense, which Erikson considers the mark of the adult. The opposite of intimacy, the distancing of oneself from intimate relationships, is the negative resolution of the task of this life stage and leads to isolation and self-absorption.

Cognitive Development

Piaget saw adulthood as actively developing the formal operational approach to learning and problem solving. He believed that the same cognitive operations apply throughout adulthood to a larger, more expansive list of experiences. Adults tend to think in an integrative way.

Health Promotion

Nutrition. Fewer total numbers of calories are needed compared with the amount needed in adolescence because the adult has completed biophysical growth. Calories are needed to maintain body functioning for cell replacement and repair and for provision of energy. Calorie needs vary based on age, gender, size, physical activity, metabolism, and levels of stress.

Diet plays an important role, as it does throughout the developmental stages. Heart disease and cancer are major concerns in the adult years. Proper diet and exercise often have a decisive impact on the control of heart disease, which is caused by increased cholesterol deposits occluding the walls of blood vessels. Likewise, low-fat, high-fiber, and low-cholesterol diets are recommended as preventive measures against cancers of the breast, the stomach, and the intestine. Other lifestyle habits such as the use of tobacco, drugs, and alcohol affect the adult's health status (see the Health Promotion box).

 Health Promotion

Recommendations for a Healthy Lifestyle

- Follow the guidelines at *www.choosemyplate.gov*.
- Drink adequate fluids.
- Avoid smoking and drugs.
- Consume little or no alcohol.
- Maintain optimal weight.
- Participate in a scheduled program of daily exercise.
- Obtain adequate restorative sleep.
- Practice stress reduction.
- Enjoy leisure activities.

Rest and sleep. Most adults function well with 7 to 9 hours of restorative sleep. Adults commonly do not schedule daytime rest opportunities to prevent fatigue; however, they can increase their productivity by obtaining adequate rest during the day. Adequate rest is essential for the pregnant woman to ensure her health and that of her unborn baby.

Physical Activity

In the past few decades, attention to physical fitness has become more popular, with benefit to general welfare. Regular, paced exercise increases heart and lung capacity, lowers blood pressure, helps control weight, enhances body function, and improves emotional health.

By adulthood, men and women have reached their sexual maturity. Sexual drive continues for men and women throughout adulthood.

Physical and dental examinations. Annual physicals are recommended. A routine testicular examination for the male and an annual Papanicolaou (Pap) smear for the female are essential for early detection of cancer. The American Cancer Society recommends that women have a mammogram yearly starting between the age of 40 to 44 years. From the ages of 45 to 54 years mammograms should be performed yearly. At age 55 and older the health care provider and patient should determine whether to continue yearly mammograms or switch to every other year (ACS, 2017). According to the American Cancer Society (2016), beginning at age 50 men should talk to their health care provider about pros and cons of prostate cancer screening so that they can decide if testing is the right choice for them. African Americans or those with a father or brother who had prostate cancer before age 65 should have this talk with a health care provider starting at age 45. Testing includes a prostate-specific antigen (PSA) blood test with or without a digital rectal examination (DRE). The frequency of retesting depends on the person's PSA level. Routine dental examinations should be scheduled for adults every 6 months. Eye examinations are necessary every 2 years unless otherwise indicated.

Safety. Accidents are the leading cause of disability and death in this age group. Injuries commonly result from work, vehicle, and sports accidents and from violence.

MIDDLE ADULTHOOD: 40 TO 65 YEARS

The middle adulthood period is designated arbitrarily as occurring between 40 and 65 years of age. Most individuals of this age group enjoy a healthy body. Some changes result in a gradual shift of balance away from peak performance. The extent of these changes is related directly to diet, heredity, exercise, rest, mental outlook, stress, and disease.

Physical Characteristics

Bone mass decreases as skeletal growth cells are depleted. This bone loss leads to an increased risk of osteoporosis. Women lose calcium from bone tissue after menopause. Men also lose calcium from bones but at a more gradual rate than women, and their risk of osteoporosis is lower. Slight changes in height continue to occur as a result of the compression of the spinal vertebrae and the hardening of collagen fibers. A decrease in muscle fibers results in a reduction of muscle mass. Heredity, nutrition, and exercise patterns account for much of the individual variation commonly seen. Changes in muscle strength are perhaps related more to level of activity than to age. A redistribution of body weight leads to changes in body shape and contour. A decrease in basal metabolism and less activity often necessitate calorie reductions to prevent weight gain.

Basic neurologic functioning remains at a high level during this age period.

Noticeable changes in vision occur as a result of **presbyopia** (a defect in vision in advancing age that involves loss of accommodation or the recession of the near point caused by loss of elasticity of the crystalline lens and the ensuing change in close vision).

Other sensory changes may include **presbycusis** (a normal progressive, age-associated loss of hearing acuity, speech intelligibility, auditory threshold, and pitch). These changes usually begin around age 40 years and occur more commonly in men than in women.

One of the most noticeable changes that occurs during this period is in the appearance of the individual's skin. A decrease in the elastic fibers and a slight loss of subcutaneous tissue give skin a looser, more wrinkled appearance. Hair color often changes with age with the onset of graying. Graying usually begins at the temples. Hair growth and distribution sometimes change during the middle adult years. Scalp hair tends to become thinner.

A higher incidence of periodontal (gum) disease is seen in the middle adult years. Preventive treatment programs that include fluoride usage, regular flossing, and dental cleaning are important.

Hormonal changes include the woman's declining production of estrogen and progesterone. Menopause (female climacteric) is a gradual process that takes about 5 years to complete. A woman's perception of menopause is likely to be affected by her perceptions of her general health. The period of menopausal transition is known as perimenopause. During this process, the functions of the ovaries diminish and eventually cease. Noticeable signs and symptoms of menopause typically include irregular menstrual periods, flow changes, excess fluid retention, breast tenderness, hot flashes (feeling "hot," flushing, and blushing), palpitations, night sweats, and irritability or mood swings. Some women have very few signs or symptoms related to menopause. Some women receive small doses of estrogen aimed at relieving the complications of decreased estrogen levels. Some investigators suggest that hormone replacement therapy (HRT) offers a way to reduce osteoporosis and the risk of atherosclerosis and heart disease; however, HRT also is feared to increase the risk of stroke, endometrial cancer, and breast disease and to raise blood pressure. Therefore the risks and the benefits of this treatment must be evaluated on an individual basis. The woman can continue to experience positive, satisfying sexuality and sexual responses throughout her middle adult years. With any fears of pregnancy now out of the picture, many women enjoy a period of enhanced sexuality.

Possible evidence of the male climacteric includes decreased libido (sex drive), loss of body hair, and delayed erection. Men do not lose the ability to reproduce during the middle adult years. Changes in male sexual function often are related more to psychological than physiologic occurrences. A man's actual capacity to function sexually often has more to do with self-perception and mental outlook and less with the changes he experiences in body appearance, including weight gain, hair loss, and decreased muscle strength. These changes cause some men to go through what is described as a "midlife crisis." During this time, many people may engage in extramarital affairs, often leading to divorce. Many men are unaffected by the physiologic and psychological occurrences of the climacteric.

Psychosocial Development

According to Erikson, the developmental task of middle age is generativity versus stagnation, which means accepting responsibility for and offering guidance to the next generation. Generativity encompasses productivity, continuity, and creativity (Fig. 24.15). If this developmental task is not met, people become stagnant—inactive or lifeless. The middle adult years are a time for vocational, interpersonal, and personal fulfillment. The impulse to foster development of the young is not limited to guiding one's own children and does not cease with their maturation. Many middle-aged adults enjoyably express this desire through activities such as teaching and mentorship, a mutually fulfilling relationship that satisfies a younger protégé's need for guidance along with an older person's need for generativity. Resumption of education, career growth or changes, reentry into the workforce, and involvement with community activities create a multitude of possibilities for personal growth and satisfaction during the middle adult years. Box 24.20 contains a list of the developmental tasks of middle adulthood.

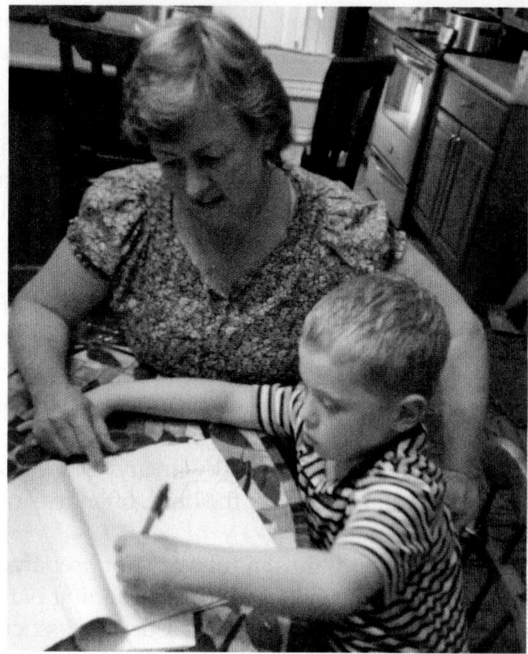

Fig. 24.15 According to Erikson, generativity is the developmental task of middle adulthood. Nurturing and guiding the younger generation is a task people accomplish with their own children or with other children and adolescents in their family and community.

Box 24.20 Developmental Tasks of Middle Adulthood

- Balances goals and realities and redirects energies as necessary
- Extends caring and concern beyond immediate family (to neighborhood, community, society)
- Develops career and job satisfaction
- Adapts to physical changes
- Establishes new roles and relationships with spouse, children, grandchildren, and parents

Family roles change during this stage. Children are sometimes present in the home. For most caregivers, a significant change in their lives occurs with the end of daily, active responsibility for children. Relationships between spouses change, and the couple often has to regain familiarity with each other. For many, this offers the opportunity for new or renewed companionship. Survival of the marriage after children leave home possibly depends on the growth, the maturity, and the commitment of each partner. Most women with an "empty nest" look forward to their emancipation from parenting duties, seeing it as an occasion to develop further their personal and social roles.

The role of grandparenting often begins at this developmental stage. Because it often does not have the constraints and responsibilities of childrearing, grandparenting becomes a rich and rewarding experience for many middle-aged adults. The past few decades have probably been the best time ever to be an American grandparent and to enjoy grandparenting as a joyful experience. Grandparents now have the longest, healthiest lifespans ever recorded, the best social services, and the most independence. Many still hover just above the poverty line, and some are below it; however, many grandparents are prosperous. Many of today's grandparents have lots of grandchildren to enjoy. Many American grandparents are not involved in the upbringing and disciplining of their grandchildren, preferring a "norm of noninterference." Grandparents often refrain from giving their grown children childrearing instruction, even when they do not like something they see going on with their grandchildren. Most contemporary grandparents value their independence; many are unwilling to exchange their hard-won and long-awaited lifestyles for another round of the hard, often frustrating work of raising children.

On the other hand, most adults are not prepared for the increased responsibility of caring for aging parents. Economic stress and emotional pressure are associated with the role reversal sometimes known as "parenting the parent." Studies have indicated that a midlife daughter is most likely to be involved in elder care with her parents and her husband's parents.

Health Promotion

Nutrition. Many adult active lifestyles slow in their middle adult years; therefore they need fewer calories than they did in their teenage years and 20s. The Centers for Disease Control and Prevention (CDC) reports that 69% of Americans over age 20 years are overweight or obese, which is defined as being 20% over the desirable weight for one's gender, height, and body build. Inadequate calorie intake, or undernutrition, is also becoming more common. In some cases, this is the result of poverty; however, in many cases, it is a result of self-imposed dieting.

Positive lifestyles with regular exercise are important to maintain healthy joints and bones. Activities that are stress reducing, such as walking, swimming, golf, and tennis, also have the potential to enhance calcium utilization. Premenopausal women need to obtain about 1000 mg of dietary calcium per day, whereas postmenopausal women need 1200 mg of calcium to prevent osteoporosis if they are not taking a hormone replacement with estrogen (NIH, 2016). A good diet with supplemental vitamins and minerals combined with regular exercise often helps lessen the effects of menopause.

The diet also should be rich in phosphorus and magnesium. A diet rich in green, leafy vegetables, fresh fruits, whole-grain cereals or breads, and dairy products helps support healthy bones. A reduced intake of fat is recommended; most of it should come from unsaturated fats such as soy, sunflower, corn, or safflower oil. High blood levels of saturated fats and cholesterol contribute to atherosclerosis, coronary heart disease, and cancer.

Box 24.21 Developmental Tasks of Late Adulthood

- Accepts own life
- Recognizes accomplishments
- Finds satisfaction with new roles, relationships, and leisure time
- Maximizes independence and maintains high level of involvement
- Accepts own mortality and prepares for death

Physical and dental examinations. The person in middle adulthood needs an annual physical examination and biannual dental examinations. Preventive American Cancer Society guidelines should be followed.

Sleep and rest. The adult in this age group sleeps less and experiences more nighttime awakenings than does the younger adult. In somewhat circular fashion, the subsequent need for additional daytime rest sometimes lessens the number of nighttime hours of sleep necessary.

LATE ADULTHOOD: 65 YEARS AND OLDER

Older adults represent a rapidly growing segment of the population, and everyone should prepare for and understand the aging process (Box 24.21). There are many approaches to examining the experience of growing old. Aging is a normal condition of human existence and has been studied from sociologic, physiologic, and psychological perspectives. Throughout the lifespan, all these aspects of the human experience are interrelated. Gerontologists, who study the older adult and the aging process, note that many 70-year-olds today act and think as 50-year-olds did as recently as the 1960s.

The fact remains that everyone ages. The physiologic changes are not universal, however, or even necessarily inevitable, and the changes are often amenable to many interventions and treatments. An individual's adjustment to aging is a uniquely complex process. How an individual responds to the age-related changes visible in the mirror has much to do with the person's self-esteem. Successful aging depends on the individual's capacity to cope and ability to change. The process of aging affects the individual, the family, and society at large (see the Lifespan Considerations for Older Adults box).

The sociologically relevant issues of aging have to do with work, retirement, social security, and health care. As more and more people reach late adulthood, society must recognize and value these individuals' knowledge, skills, and contributions. Arrangements and plans for the future that are addressed and encouraged in the early adult years help prepare, support, and enhance adjustments once they are necessary. Implementation of flexible services and financial assistance programs helps people fulfill their goals.

The response to getting older often is also related to lifelong health habits, diet, and exercise patterns. Family,

Lifespan Considerations
Older Adults

Effects of Aging on Older Adults

- With increased emphasis on wellness and preventive care, today's older adults are living longer, healthier lives. However, longer lifespans result in an increased presence of chronic and degenerative disorders.
- Each generation has its own central life tasks to complete. As life expectancy grows, more generations coexist, and the needs of one age group sometimes come into conflict with those of others. This increases intergenerational stress and typically causes alterations in family dynamics.
- Changes in roles and relationships present major developmental challenges to older adults.
- Health care needs of the aging population place increased demands on the health care delivery system.
- The cost of care for the older adult population is a major societal concern. This cost is likely to have a significant impact on the amount and the type of health care coverage provided by insurance companies and the government.
- Older adults are a politically active group, and as their numbers increase, they are having an impact on all aspects of society, including the entertainment, travel, and housing industries.
- Although some older adults are poor, as a group they generally have more income than younger individuals and therefore have a significant effect on the economy.

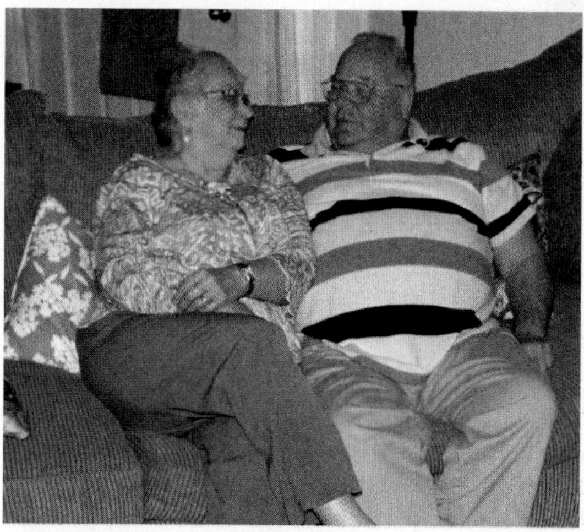

Fig. 24.16 According to Erikson, generativity versus stagnation is the developmental task of older adulthood. A loving relationship with a spouse is an example of a positive influence during this stage of life.

love, friendships, and intimate relationships are additional factors important to survival and well-being (Fig. 24.16). These relationships are crucial to people's happiness whatever the age. Love relationships vary in intensity and meaning in adulthood. Early on, these relationships usually have an intense physical basis, which leads to intimacy, respect, and commitment. Although intense sexual drive decreases with age, sexual behavior remains an important part of many adult relationships.

Box 24.22 Your Beliefs on Aging

TRUE OR FALSE?

___ 1. All older people become senile.
___ 2. Most older people live in a nursing home or other institutional setting.
___ 3. Most older people are isolated from their families.
___ 4. Most older people have no interest in or capacity for sexual relationships.
___ 5. Older workers are less productive than younger workers.
___ 6. Intelligence declines in old age.
___ 7. Older people do better to cease exercising and just rest.
___ 8. Marked personality changes occur in the older person.
___ 9. Older people naturally become inflexible and demanding.

NOTE: All of these statements are false.

Ageism

Ageism, a form of discrimination and prejudice against the older adult, is an unfortunate reality. Like racism and sexism, ageism prevents people from being as happy and productive as they otherwise can be. It is passed on from generation to generation by the process of socialization. Society must relinquish old stereotypes about the older adult and learn to affirm the positive aspects of aging. It is a mistake to view aging only as a decline; it involves growth as well. Box 24.22 provides a brief list of true-false statements that helps clarify beliefs on aging.

The number of older people has grown steadily over the past century and will continue to do so. In 2014 there were 46 million people in the United States 65 years of age or older. That number is expected to more than double by the year 2060 to 98 million (Mather, 2015).

Every year another group of adults reaches late adulthood. Late adulthood is defined as age 65 years and older. It can be subdivided further into "young older adult" (ages 65 to 74 years), "middle older adult" (ages 75 to 84 years), and "old older adult" (older than age 85 years). This population is changing constantly as new individuals enter the group and others leave through death. Each person has a unique personal history that reflects many influences. Box 24.23 lists keys to successful aging. The fastest growing segment of the US population is the group aged 85 years and older.

Biologic Theories of Aging

For centuries, humanity has been fascinated with the concept of aging. Many theories have attempted to define the causes of aging and to develop measures to halt or

Box 24.23 Keys to Successful Aging

- Practice pleasurable activities.
- View life as meaningful.
- Maintain a positive self-image.
- Accept responsibility for the past.
- Be optimistic.
- Remain motivated to maintain or expand intellectual capacity.
- Participate in a planned exercise program.

postpone the aging process. One of the earliest theories of aging, generated by Hippocrates, speculated that aging was an irreversible natural event caused by a decrease in body heat. Later, Galen supported this concept and claimed that aging was a lifelong process rather than an event that occurred at the end of the lifespan. Leonardo da Vinci, among the first to attempt to identify the physical changes associated with aging, performed autopsies to compare old men and young children. In the period after 1900, only a few scientists focused on aging as their main interest. Finally, in the past 30 years, we have begun to see a renewed interest in researching the causes of the aging process. Recent theories focus on the roles of autoimmunity, free radicals (compounds with an extra electron or protein), wear and tear, and biologic programming, among others. The only definitive conclusion, however, is that aging is a slow, continuous, complex process that probably involves intrinsic and extrinsic factors.

Autoimmunity theory. The autoimmunity theory states that with aging, the body becomes less able to recognize or tolerate the "self." As a result, the immune system produces antibodies that act against the self. This theory is supported by the increased accumulation of lymphocytes, plasma cells found in the tissues of healthy older people.

The primary organs of the immune system (thymus and bone marrow) are believed to be affected by the aging process. With aging, the thymus decreases in size and weight and becomes less able to produce T cells. The bone marrow stem cells also show reduced efficiency in performing certain functions. As immune system function decreases, the risk of development of infection and cancer increases.

Free radical theory. Free radicals are highly reactive cellular components derived from unstable atoms or molecules. Free radicals have a reduced cellular efficiency and cause cellular waste to accumulate. Some free radicals are produced by radiation, heat, and oxidation. The presence of free radicals possibly accelerates aging and results in the death of an organism. Lipofuscin is a pigmented material that accumulates in many organs as a part of aging. This accumulation interferes with the diffusion and transportation of essential metabolites and perhaps also contributes to the aging process.

Wear-and-tear theory. According to the wear-and-tear theory, age is not based on chronologic age but is determined by the amount of wear and tear experienced. Many believe that the structural and functional changes associated with growing old are accelerated by abuse of the body.

Genetic theory. Similar life expectancies within families lend support to the idea of a hereditary basis for aging. After all, our hair color and height are determined by our genes, so it could be that our lifespan also is determined by our genes. Scientists have been studying short-lived animals to identify longevity genes and manipulate them to study how those changes affect the animal's lifespan. Studying the genetics of aging is complex and requires much more research to fully understand; however, it is not expected that one gene solely determines the lifespan for a human, but rather several genes affect the process of aging (Stibich, 2018).

Psychological Theories of Aging

Disengagement theory. According to supporters of the disengagement theory of aging, a natural withdrawal, or disengagement, between the individual and society is best. This withdrawal is initiated either by the individual or by others in society. Adherents to this belief suggest that such withdrawal prevents older adults from experiencing frustration when they can no longer function adequately and allows a younger member of society to fulfill the now-empty role. They characterize this process as a normal, inevitable, universal process. Two major criticisms of the disengagement theory are as follows:

- It does not allow for the many active, functional older adults.
- The process is not seen in all cultural groups; it is therefore not universal.

Activity theory. According to this theory, the older person who is more active socially is more likely to adjust well to aging. Older adults with more social involvement have higher morale and better life satisfaction and personal adjustment. The number and the quality of the activities are important. People who give up activities or roles should be advised to find replacements. Meaningful activities that involve close personal contact with others are extremely important. Activities of this nature reinforce self-concept, which in turn is associated with a higher life satisfaction.

Continuity theory. Supporters of this theory suggest that the critical factors in adjustment to old age are the coping abilities developed previously in life and an ability to maintain previous roles and activities. Knowledge and understanding of a person's personality type are often useful in predicting response to the aging process. People who were never highly involved in society are likely to maintain the same mild level of involvement in old age. On the other hand, individuals who were highly involved and actively engaged with society need to remain active and involved with similar intensity. Supporters of the continuity theory contend that adjustment to the aging process is eased by maintaining roles and interests similar to those developed earlier in life.

Physical Characteristics

Aging is a complex process that affects cells, tissues, and organs. Like growth and development, aging occurs at a highly individualized rate. A gradual reduction in the number of aging cells and a change in the composition of aging cells occur. A slow increase in body weight usually is seen until 45 to 50 years of age, and then a gradual decline begins. Body fat content and distribution differ in men and women. The accumulation of adipose tissue in females typically is found over the chest, the waist, the hips, and the thighs. Adipose tissue in the male is deposited mostly in the waist, the chest, and the lower abdomen.

Loss of height begins after age 50 years. Most of the noticeable decrease in trunk length is a result of the increase in spinal curvature caused by a slight thinning of the intervertebral disks. In addition to the shortening of the spine, certain abnormal postures and contours are noted. Kyphosis, an exaggeration of the thoracic curvature, may increase with aging. This sometimes leads to a barrel-chest appearance, which possibly affects the position of the diaphragm and reduces the effectiveness of inspiration. These and other postural changes have the potential to affect body posture, mobility, gait, and respiratory efficiency.

Common age-related changes specific to each body system are listed in Table 24.4, along with suggested nursing interventions to minimize the effect of these changes.

Psychosocial Development

Years of living along with successes, failures, strengths, weaknesses, and all the early experiences influence the emotional stability of older adults. Despite the physiologic changes associated with the aging process, the older years should be viewed as a time of satisfaction and pleasure. Many older adults choose to work after age 65 years. These activities provide interest, intellectual stimulation, and added income (Fig. 24.17). Older people need to recognize their changing capabilities and begin a process of adjustment.

Erikson described the challenge of late adulthood as ego integrity versus a sense of despair. The task here is to evaluate one's life and accomplishments and find satisfaction and meaning in life. The process of reminiscing with others often further validates the meaning and importance of the individual's life. Those who can believe that their lives have been well spent and are

Table 24.4 Common Age-Related Changes

SYSTEM	NORMAL CHANGES	SUGGESTED NURSING INTERVENTIONS
Musculoskeletal System		
Bones, muscles, joints, and connective tissue	Mineral salts move from bones to blood, making bones more porous; tendons, ligaments less elastic; increase in joint stiffness with less range of motion; varying degrees of increase of flexion at wrists, hips, knees, producing less joint mobility, agility, and endurance; thinning of vertebral disks	Maintain mobility. Encourage exercise (with physician's guidance). Encourage passive and active exercises. Avoid fatigue. Use assistive aids when indicated.
Nervous System		
	Fewer, smaller neurons (nerve cells), slowed reaction time, decrease in tactile sensitivity, decrease in pain perception, altered motor coordination	Allow adequate time to complete activities. Be alert to danger of and prevent burning and chilling related to diminished sensitivity. Encourage position changes; inspect skin daily.
Special Senses		
Taste and smell	Decline in taste and smell perception	Use smoke detectors. Serve attractive, colorful food.
Vision	Decreased tear production, increase in lens density; presbyopia (farsightedness; loss of elasticity of lens); yellowing of lens; slowing of accommodation (reaction to changes in light and distance); narrowing of visual field; decrease in depth perception	Encourage annual eye examinations. Use more diffuse lighting. Use bright colors (red, yellow). Place articles within visual field. Use night-lights.
Hearing	Presbycusis (increased difficulty hearing high-pitched sounds); increase in degenerative changes within ear structure; increase in buildup of wax production	Speak slowly, clearly. Face individual. Do not shout. Speak in lower tones. Control background noise. Encourage use of hearing aids if available.

Continued

Table 24.4 Common Age-Related Changes—cont'd

SYSTEM	NORMAL CHANGES	SUGGESTED NURSING INTERVENTIONS
Respiratory System		
Ribcage	Increase in calcification of thorax; respiratory muscles weaken, producing diminished respiratory efficiency; maximum breathing capacity reduced; more susceptible to respiratory infection; easily fatigued	Allow for rest periods. Encourage coughing and deep breathing.
Lungs	Alveoli (air sacs) thinner, smaller, with decreased alveolar surface for gaseous exchange; decreased cough reflex action; decreased ciliary action, reduced maximum breathing capacity	Maintain adequate exercise and nutrition. Encourage regular physical examinations. Avoid overexertion and allow for rest between activities. Discourage smoking. Obtain streptococcal pneumonia (pneumococcal) vaccine.
Cardiovascular System		
	Fewer blood cells produced; loss of elasticity and narrowing of blood vessels, with an increase in blood pressure; valves thicker, more rigid; heart needs more time to return to resting state; decreased cardiac output	Encourage regular, paced exercise with adequate rest periods. Maintain low-fat, low-sodium diet. Obtain regular physician examinations.
Integumentary System		
Skin	Paler, thinner, irregularly pigmented; decrease in moisture; decrease in sweat and sebaceous gland activity; less elastic, more wrinkling; loss of subcutaneous fat; skin more fragile and prone to injury	Inspect skin for impairment or signs of pressure. Change position frequently. Wash with water and mild soap as needed. Rinse thoroughly and pat skin dry. Use lotions to replenish moisture. To maintain body warmth, provide adequate clothing.
Reproductive System		
Female	Fallopian tubes atrophy and shorten; ovaries smaller, thinner; uterus, cervix smaller; vagina less elastic, more alkaline, drier; reproductive capacity ceases	Suggest use of vaginal lubricants if indicated. Instruct person to have annual mammogram and vaginal examination with Papanicolaou test.
Male	Increased size of prostate; decreased testosterone levels; decreased circulation, and decreased rate and force of ejaculation	Instruct person to have annual prostate examination and prostate-specific antigen (PSA) test.
Endocrine System		
	Slowing of thyroid gland activity; decreased basal metabolic rate; decreased hormone production that affects other systems	Recommend annual physical examination with thyroid function testing.
Urinary System		
	Fewer cells in kidney, decreased renal blood flow; less effective filtration; decreased bladder elasticity and capacity; need for more frequent voiding	Observe for signs of urinary tract infections. Observe closely for adverse drug reactions. Observe male for signs of benign prostatic hypertrophy causing impairment of urinary flow.
Hair		
	Increase in graying; balding and changes in thickness of hair occur; changes in distribution of body hair	
Nails		
	More fragile, brittle; appear dull, opaque yellow or gray in color; toenails thicken	Have toenails trimmed by podiatrist as indicated.
Gastrointestinal System		
	Decreased saliva production; decreased chewing efficiency; decreased esophageal motility; total capacity of stomach reduced; decreased gastric enzyme secretion; liver smaller; less absorption of nutrients; slowing of peristalsis	Ensure adequate fluid intake. Encourage annual dental checkups. Offer five or six small daily meals, rather than three large ones. Assess for indigestion. Encourage regular toileting habits.

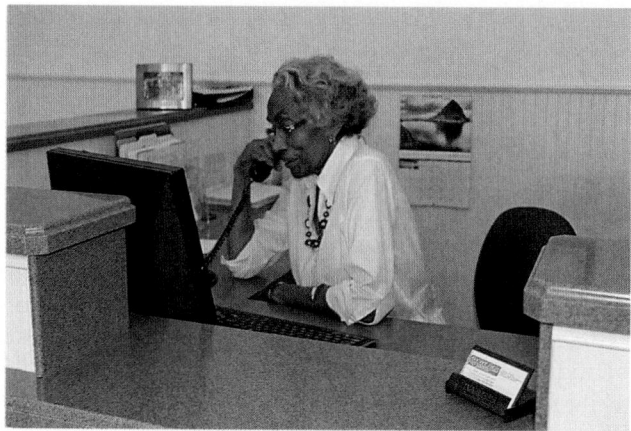

Fig. 24.17 Many older people continue to work and learn after the traditional retirement age.

satisfied with their decisions and achievements have mastered this task of integrity. This allows the person to continue life with a sense of dignity and peacefulness. Adults who are dissatisfied with their accomplishments often experience conflict and despair. Dissatisfaction contributes to a feeling of restlessness and a sense of panic that time is "running out." Often the individual feels the need for more time and a chance to do things over again differently.

Many other factors also affect the older adult's adjustment to this stage of life. Retirement is a major adjustment for the older adult. Health and financial resources are critical elements in determination of life satisfaction after retirement. Generally speaking, society is relatively unprepared for the phenomenon known as retirement. Retirement creates many changes—some welcome, some not. Examples are changes in roles, self-esteem, support systems, life patterns, and leisure time. Retirement brings more time to spend as one wishes; therefore individuals need to plan and discuss their hopes and expectations for the retirement period. Planning for retirement helps identify activities that will be meaningful and promote self-esteem and a sense of usefulness to oneself and society.

Family Roles

For many individuals, the older years become a time to explore feelings about parenting and grandparenting. Grandparenting today, as discussed previously, is often very different from the role of grandparenting three or four decades ago. Today's grandparent often works and remains highly active. For some grandparents, caring for grandchildren has become a full-time responsibility that leads to multiple stresses. Raising grandchildren has the potential to create financial stress, cause a decrease in living space, and limit roles. Events that affect children such as divorce, abandonment, unemployment, death or illness, and incarceration are some of the factors that have contributed to the increased numbers of grandparents raising grandchildren on a full-time basis. Support groups, community resources, and other organizations are some of the resources that assist grandparents in their grandparenting roles.

During this stage, couples may need to adjust to increased time together; couples often enjoy the increase in companionship and closeness. Maintaining old friendships and exploring ways to form new ones, along with continuing strong family ties, are means to help soften the losses that frequently are experienced during this period.

The death of a spouse is traumatic at any age. In the older years, widowhood is more common for women than men. Children and a strong social network often play important roles in supporting the surviving spouse. The experience of being widowed goes beyond ending a partnership. Role changes, changes in lifestyle, and access to fewer financial resources are just some of the adjustments that are called for when a spouse dies. Some older people find remarriage to be a solution to the challenge of being widowed and discover the companionship, love, and security they seek.

Cognitive and Intellectual Development

Evidence suggests that older adults in good health and in nurturing environments have the capacity to maintain or increase their level of functioning, particularly in their areas of interest or specialization. Several factors are important to continued cognitive functioning: level of education, work roles, personality, health, lifestyle, and the relevancy or associated meaning of the tasks one is called on to perform. Some "practical" abilities may decline with age, whereas others may remain stable or improve with age.

Memory. Some older adults notice changes in memory. Such benign forgetfulness is far more common than the forgetfulness associated with Alzheimer's disease. As adults advance in years, there appears to be a greater loss of recent memory over remote memory. An older individual perhaps forgets what was served for breakfast 2 hours earlier and yet may remember in great detail the events of a wedding many decades ago. Older people are slower than younger people but often are more accurate in what they remember and do. Many people believe that this is deliberate: the older person is more willing to sacrifice speed for accuracy.

Health Promotion

Health promotion rests on the belief that individuals can have a strong influence on their health status. Environment, social patterns, diet, exercise, and personal habits are factors that determine a person's state of health. Health care workers must clarify the common misconceptions about health and aging. It is essential to emphasize that people of all ages can benefit from living a healthy lifestyle, even in the later years (see the Health Promotion box on the benefits of exercise).

 Health Promotion

Benefits of Exercise in the Older Adult

- Maintains or improves cardiovascular fitness
- Prevents or reduces intensity of chronic diseases, such as coronary artery disease, congestive heart failure, hypertension, osteoarthritis, osteoporosis, diabetes, obesity, and chronic obstructive lung disease
- Prevents many falls and fractures
- Improves muscle strength, flexibility, and balance
- Enhances self-care abilities and promotes independent activities
- Encourages social contact
- Decreases anxiety, depression, and insomnia

Advise older adults to receive pneumococcal and influenza vaccines yearly. Individuals who have compromised immune systems, who have a history of an allergy to eggs or egg products, or who have had a severe reaction to a previous vaccine should check with their physician before immunization.

Nutrition. Adequate nutrition plays a significant role in health maintenance and contributes to the older person's quality of life. Activities related to food and diet include transportation for food purchase, meal planning, and meal preparation. The task of providing older individuals with assistance for these activities often falls to family members. Older adults need a diet of foods of higher quality and lower quantity that provide the basic necessary nutrients. Although caloric needs are individualized, older adults are generally less active and have more adipose tissue and less body mass and therefore often need less daily caloric intake. Diets that are low in saturated fats and carbohydrates and high in fiber usually are recommended. Common threats to the adequacy of the older adult's diet are poor oral health, lack of appetite, food intolerances, and constipation. Proper nutritional assessment and counseling help identify problems and useful interventions. To ensure dietary compliance, take long-standing habits and cultural influences into consideration when introducing any dietary changes.

Various psychosocial factors also have the potential to affect the older person's diet. The choice of foods purchased and included in the diet sometimes is the result of economic factors. Loneliness also contributes to inadequate dietary intake for some people. If people are not able to shop for and prepare meals, their diets are likely to become less than desirable. Another crucial component in the older person's diet is adequate fluid intake. Advise older adults to maintain a minimum daily intake of 1500 mL/day. Often an older person avoids fluids out of a fear of incontinence and a lack of thirst.

Activity. Throughout the lifespan, evenly paced, satisfying exercise is crucial to general well-being. Exercise has benefits for cardiovascular functioning, lowering blood pressure while enhancing oxygen utilization, and maintaining joint mobility. Exercise to the point of exhaustion is misguided; always recommend a rest period after exercise to recuperate and restore the body to its maximum level of functioning (see the Health Promotion box for benefits of exercise).

Sleep. Older individuals need more rest but less actual sleep. The incidence of accidents that occur during nighttime awakenings is increased, and safety concerns must be handled. Use of night-lights and reduced excess furniture and clutter are some methods of decreasing the risk of nighttime injury. Sleep for the older person often is affected by medications, alcohol, caffeine, stress, and environmental noise and temperature.

Safety. Most accidents are preventable (see safety tips for the older adult in the Safety Alert box). The key to prevention is knowledge and recognition of and attention to the factors that contribute to the increased risk for accident or injury. Diminished sight and changes in posture or balance sometimes expose the older person to the risk of falls. A single fall has the potential to produce an injury that necessitates a long period of immobilization, thus diminishing the person's independence and self-esteem.

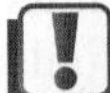 Safety Alert

Safety Tips for the Older Adult

- Minimize clutter and excess furniture in rooms and hallways.
- Remove scatter rugs.
- Use handrails on stairs.
- Install grab bars in showers and bathrooms.
- Use night-lights.
- Get up slowly from a lying-flat position.
- Use caution in going from well-lighted areas to darkened areas or vice versa.
- If self-medicating, use dispensing aids to decrease the risk of error.
- Wear properly fitting shoes and clothing.
- Allow enough time; do not rush or hurry.

Get Ready for the NCLEX® Examination!

Key Points

- Development is a lifelong process that begins at conception and ends at death.
- All types of families serve similar basic functions: protection, nurturance, education, sustenance, and socialization of their members.
- Growth patterns suggest rapid growth during infancy, continued growth during toddler and preschool years, and slowed but steady growth during the school years, followed by a rapid surge of growth during puberty and adolescence.
- Erikson identified a central task that must be resolved at each stage of the lifespan: infancy, toddler, preschool, school age, adolescence, early adulthood, middle adulthood, and late adulthood.
- Piaget focused on the concept of cognitive development beginning in infancy and continuing throughout the childhood years.
- Accidental injuries are a major cause of death during infancy, childhood, and adolescence.
- Consistent discipline and supervision are needed throughout childhood.
- Peer relationships become significant at school age.
- Adolescence is the transitional period between childhood and adulthood.
- Adulthood is marked by significant events: career decisions, marriage, new social relationships, and financial concerns.
- Certain physical changes become evident during middle age, including graying of hair and vision changes.
- Menopause and hormonal changes characterize the reproductive changes of the middle-age female.
- Roles undergo change during middle adulthood, including nuclear family roles, relationships with grown children, grandparenting, and possibly career changes.
- Late adulthood is marked by a gradual slowing of the body's functioning.
- Several significant physical changes become evident in the older adult.
- Family changes and an increased awareness of one's mortality are common adjustments called for by the aging process.
- Life review and acceptance of one's strengths and weaknesses are necessary aspects of the aging process.
- Several theories attempt to explain aging; however, no one theory is accepted universally.
- Aging, like growth, is a highly individualized process.

Additional Learning Resources

SG Go to your Study Guide for additional learning activities to help you master this chapter content.

evolve Be sure to visit the Evolve site at *http://evolve.elsevier.com/Cooper/foundationsadult/* for additional online resources.

Review Questions for the NCLEX® Examination

1. The nurse is aware that the first socializing agent for the child is:
   1. daycare.
   2. family.
   3. school.
   4. play groups.
2. The nurse is educating a group of preschool teachers about psychosocial development for their population. The nurse is correct when stating a 4-year-old child is working on achieving which of Erikson's developmental tasks?
   1. Trust versus mistrust
   2. Industry versus inferiority
   3. Autonomy versus shame and doubt
   4. Initiative versus guilt
3. The student nurse is preparing for a clinical day at a local long-term care facility. The student has a correct understanding of the theories of aging when she/he makes which statement? *(Select all that apply.)*
   1. "Free radicals improve cellular efficiency and delay the aging process."
   2. "With aging the body becomes less able to recognize itself and produces antibodies that act against the self."
   3. "Free radicals cause an accumulation of cellular waste that may accelerate the aging process."
   4. "Abuse of the body can accelerate functional and structural changes associated with growing old."
   5. "The immune system function increases which reduces the risk for infection as people age."
4. An 8-year-old loves to draw and do craft projects. The nurse understands that the child's need for praise and encouragement for the work efforts demonstrates the development of which of Erikson's tasks?
   1. Autonomy
   2. Initiative
   3. Industry
   4. Identity
5. The school nurse is preparing a presentation for the high school football team. The nurse should include that peak physical strength and endurance occurs during what period of life?
   1. Adolescence
   2. Early adulthood
   3. Middle adulthood
   4. Late adulthood
6. The nurse is completing the assessment of an 8-month-old infant at a well child visit. The nurse notes that the child has good head control and can now sit up unsupported. What term accurately describes this sequence of growth and development?
   1. Integrated
   2. Proximodistal
   3. Cephalocaudal
   4. Differential

7. The nurse is discussing stressors that are common for children when their parents remarry after a divorce. Which statement by the nurse indicates a need for further teaching? *(Select all that apply.)*
   1. Losses from a previous divorce can cause children to be fearful of love and trust.
   2. Children may have loyalties to the other parent.
   3. Jealousies may arise from the unity of stepchildren.
   4. There are no stressors to consider because the new marriage only concerns the parents, not the children.
8. A 5-year-old child is brought to the doctor's office for an annual well child visit by his grandmother. The student nurse knows which of the following is true regarding grandfamilies?
   1. Children have more stable childhoods when placed with nonrelative foster families.
   2. Finances are never a concern for grandfamilies.
   3. The number of children in foster care being raised by relatives because of substance abuse is increasing.
   4. If the grandparent is the primary caregiver for a child, the biologic parents are not involved in the child's life.
   5. As long as counseling is sought before a new marriage occurs the children will not experience any difficulties.
9. The parents of a 1-week-old infant are concerned that they are going to "spoil" their baby if they hold him too much. The nurse understands that according to Erikson, when infants are cuddled, fed, and loved, they develop which characteristic?
   1. Autonomy
   2. Trust
   3. Industry
   4. Identity
10. The nurse is observing a group of preschool children playing. What type of play is most common with this age group?
    1. Parallel play
    2. Imaginary play
    3. Organized, team play
    4. Cognitive play
11. The nurse understands that characteristics of the cognitive development for a 10-year-old child include which concepts? *(Select all that apply.)*
    1. Better understands other viewpoints
    2. Recognizes cause-and-effect relationships
    3. Uses a systematic, scientific problem-solving approach
    4. Is able to think about abstractions and hypothetical concepts
    5. Understands basic ideas of conversation and number classification
12. The young adult struggles with which of Erikson's developmental tasks?
    1. Trust versus mistrust
    2. Identity versus confusion
    3. Generativity versus stagnation
    4. Intimacy versus isolation
13. A mother asks the nurse why her toddler always says "no" and has a negative attitude. The nurse assures the mother that such behavior is common in toddlers and helps the child meet which developmental task?
    1. Discipline
    2. Trust
    3. Independence
    4. Love
14. The nurse is explaining Piaget's preoperational thought stage of development to a mother. Which statements by the mother indicate that the teaching was effective? *(Select all that apply.)*
    1. "This stage of development will last from ages 2 through 7 years."
    2. "My child's thinking will be focused mainly on himself during this time."
    3. "My child will be able to use his imagination."
    4. "My child will use trial and error to discover new things."
    5. "My child will begin to show behaviors that embrace the feelings and needs of others."
15. A father is concerned that his 8-year-old son does not seem to be growing very quickly. The nurse reassures the father that growth during the school-age period can best be described in what manner?
    1. Irregular and slow
    2. Steady and slow
    3. Regular and fast
    4. Irregular and fast
16. The nurse is caring for a hospitalized 2-year-old child. What interventions are appropriate for inclusion in the plan of care? *(Select all that apply.)*
    1. Establish a routine.
    2. Offer choices when possible.
    3. Provide detailed explanations for care activities.
    4. Encourage parental involvement.
    5. Encourage play interaction with other older children also hospitalized on the care unit.
17. A 60-year-old female is being seen for her annual physical. She conveys to the nurse that she is concerned about losing her memory and intelligence as she enters her late adult years. Which statement by the nurse indicates a need for further teaching? *(Select all that apply.)*
    1. "Older adults have a greater loss of recent memory, rather than remote memory."
    2. "Benign forgetfulness is uncommon in older adults and indicates a need for further examination."
    3. Older adults may be slower to recall past memories but are more accurate in what they recall."
    4. Older adults in good health have the capacity to maintain or increase their cognitive function."
    5. The older adult often confuses recent memories and past memories.
18. Which statement by the older adult indicates that nutritional counseling was effective?
    1. "I need to eat more fats and proteins."
    2. "I need to eat less fiber."
    3. "I need to eat less saturated fats and carbohydrates."
    4. "I can take a supplement for all my nutritional needs."

19. The nurse is reviewing the assigned patients for the shift. One assigned patient is a 45-year-old man. When considering the needs of the patient, the nurse should recognize that the patient is in which developmental stage?
    1. Intimacy versus isolation
    2. Generativity versus stagnation
    3. Ego integrity versus despair
    4. Initiative versus guilt
20. Which developmental skill commonly is accomplished by the fourth month of life?
    1. Sitting up unsupported
    2. Holding head up at 90-degree angle
    3. Creeping
    4. Transferring objects from one hand to the other
21. A new parent asks how to introduce solid foods to the infant. Which statement indicates that teaching was effective?
    1. "I will introduce several foods at once to see what food my baby likes best."
    2. "I will start feeding my baby my favorite foods first."
    3. "I will introduce one new food at a time."
    4. "I will mix foods together to cover up tastes that he might not like."
22. When teaching a parenting class, the nurse explains that nighttime bottles should be avoided to help prevent which occurrence?
    1. Dental caries
    2. Dental malocclusion
    3. Otitis media
    4. Lactose intolerance
23. The father of 17-year-old boy is concerned because his son is questioning all of the family's morals and values. Which is true regarding the developmental tasks of an adolescent?
    1. Adolescents should achieve independence from their parents financially and socially.
    2. Adolescents learn to accept their own mortality and prepare for death.
    3. Adolescents question their own values and beliefs as they search for their own identity.
    4. Adolescents continue to deny responsibility for their behavior.

25 Loss, Grief, Dying, and Death

http://evolve.elsevier.com/Cooper/foundationsadult/

Objectives

1. Explain the role of loss in the grief reaction.
2. Describe the stages of dying.
3. Explain the concepts of euthanasia, do not resuscitate (DNR) orders, organ donations, fraudulent methods of treatment, and the Dying Person's Bill of Rights.
4. Describe techniques in assisting the dying patient to say goodbye.
5. Discuss the principles of palliative care.
6. Discuss nursing interventions for the dying patient.
7. List nursing interventions that may facilitate grieving in special circumstances (perinatal, pediatric, older adult, and suicide).
8. Identify the unique physical signs and symptoms of the patient who is near death.
9. Describe nursing responsibilities in care of the body after death.
10. Identify needs and discuss support for the grieving family.
11. Discuss support for the nurse who is experience grief after the loss of a patient.

Key Terms

advance directives (p. 750)
allow natural death (p. 750)
anticipatory grief (ăn-TĬS-ĭ-pă-TŌ-rē, p. 737)
autopsy (ĂW-tŏp-sē, p. 756)
bereavement (bĭ-RĒV-mĕnt, p. 736)
bereavement overload (p. 738)
complicated grieving (p. 739)
death (p. 734)
do-not-resuscitate (DNR) (p. 750)
durable powers of attorney (p. 750)
dysfunctional grieving (p. 739)
euthanasia (yū-thĕ-NĀ-zhă, p. 749)
grief (p. 734)
grief therapy (p. 735)
grief work (p. 734)
inquest (ĬN-kwĕst, p. 756)
living will (p. 750)
loss (p. 734)
maturational loss (măch-ŭ-RĀ-shŭn-ăl, p. 736)
morbidity (mōr-BĬ-dĭ-tē, p. 736)
mortality (mōr-TĂ-lĭ-tē, p. 735)
mortician (mōr-TĬ-shŭn, p. 756)
mourning (p. 736)
palliative care (PĂL-ē-ă-tĭv, p. 752)
postmortem care (pōst-MŌR-tĕm, p. 756)
situational loss (p. 736)
thanatology (thăn-ă-TŎL-ŏ-jē, p. 739)
unresolved grief (p. 739)

Life is a series of losses and gains. When any aspect of self is no longer available to a person, that person suffers a **loss.** Loss and **death** (cessation of life) are universal in the human experience, but they are unique events to the individual. Coping mechanisms determine a person's ability to face and accept loss. **Grief** is a pattern of physical and emotional responses to bereavement, separation, or loss. It is a natural response to loss. All losses have the possibility of triggering the grief process. The severity of the loss may vary, but the grief that accompanies it is real nonetheless.

Illness and hospitalization frequently cause loss, and nurses work with many patients who experience losses of different types. The nurse helps them understand and accept loss so that life can continue. The process of adapting to and mourning a loss is called **grief work.** After a loss, serious emotional, mental, and social problems may occur if a patient does not perform grief work.

Humans can anticipate death. This anticipation causes a variety of possible responses: anxiety, planning, denial, love, loneliness, achievement, or lack of achievement. Death affects dying patients and their families, significant others, friends, and caregivers. It can be an overwhelming experience. A person's style of dying reflects that person's style of living, and attitudes about death depend on a person's beliefs and emotional strengths.

Care of dying patients and their families can be one of the most challenging aspects of nursing care. Dying is the final stage of human growth and development; thus nurses must be as knowledgeable about the process of dying as they are about the process of birth. Because health care usually emphasizes the cure of disease and the promotion of health, health care providers often perceive the death of a patient as a form of failure. Health care personnel who care for dying patients often withdraw from patients emotionally while providing adequate physical care.

When nurses deal with grieving families and dying patients, they are confronted with their own **mortality** (the condition of being subject to death) and other distressing issues that accompany loss. Nurses can deliver quality of care to patients and families experiencing death if they understand the stages of the grief process and the task of dying.

CHANGES IN HEALTH CARE RELATED TO DYING AND DEATH

Before the 1950s, patients commonly died at home in their own beds with assistance only from their family. From the 1950s to the 1980s, the health care system became highly mechanized, and dying occurred mostly in institutions, often with sophisticated equipment attached to the dying individual to prolong life. When diagnosis-related groups (DRGs) came into play in the early 1980s, the trend changed again. Today, in general, the only patients placed in hospital beds are those who are considered at risk for medical complications or who need hospital recovery time after surgery or special procedures. This type of bed often is used in the home as well. Many recuperating or terminally ill patients are discharged to home, a convalescent center, or a nursing home. Nurses who provide care to the terminally ill patient in the home health care setting have felt the impact of this development. At home, these patients receive intravenous infusions and other technical and mechanical assistance. Nurses in health care facilities and homes are the health care providers most often available to the grieving family during the crisis of death.

HISTORICAL OVERVIEW

Discussions of the dynamics that surround grief, dying, and death are not new. In the 1960s pioneers in death and dying theory, such as Kübler-Ross and Glasser and Strauss, produced works that stimulated the health care industry. Dying and death became topics of research and seminars. In the 1970s hospices in the United States became recognized as health care delivery systems (see Chapter 40). **Grief therapy** (mental health treatment aimed at helping a patient deal with the pain of loss; a program that assists the bereaved to cope with a loss) continues to evolve as various theories on grief and loss are developed. Grief therapy helps the nurse meet the needs and plan the care for the dying patient.

On October 27, 1997, Oregon enacted the Death With Dignity Act, which allows terminally ill Oregonians to end their lives through the voluntary self-administration of lethal medications, expressly prescribed by a physician for that purpose. The Oregon Death With Dignity Act required the Oregon Health Authority to collect information about the patients and physicians who participate in the Act and publish an annual statistical report (The Oregon Death With Dignity Act, 1997). Since that time similar acts have been enacted in other states. At the date of this publication, states that have such acts include Washington (*Washington Death with Dignity Act*, 2008), Vermont (*Patient Choice and Control at the End of Life Act*, 2013), California (*End of Life Option Act*, 2015/2016), Colorado (*End of Life Options Act*, 2016), District of Columbia (*D.C. Death with Dignity Act*, 2016/2017), and Hawaii (*Our Care, Our Choice Act*, 2018/2019). The state of Montana does not actually have an act that supports physician-assisted suicide, but in 2009 the state's supreme court did not rule against any physician who has prescribed medication that allows voluntary self-administration of lethal medications.

Care providers have been learning to assist patients and families to exercise more control over their care. Individuals become involved by determining treatment options and choosing the setting, circumstances, and management of the dying process. Advance directives are upheld as legal documents in courts of law, and terminal health care is shifting away from hospital settings. Because of developments such as these, nurses continue to play a primary role in the care of the dying person at home and of the family experiencing loss.

When viewing death as a natural process, the nurse helps the patient die comfortably and with dignity. The eight domains established by the National Consensus Project for Quality Palliative Care (2013) are structure and process of care; physical aspects of care; psychological and psychiatric aspects of care; social aspects of care; spiritual, religious, and existential aspects of care; cultural aspects of care; care of patient at the end of life; and ethical and legal aspects. The structure and process of care involve a comprehensive interdisciplinary assessment that is used as a baseline for the development of a comprehensive, individualized care plan carried out through the nursing process. This individual plan of care involves coordination of care across settings with high-quality of communication between health care providers and the patient/family unit. The physical aspects of care focus on pain and symptom control and relief of suffering. The psychological and psychiatric aspects of care focus on stress, coping strategies, grieving processes, and treatment of psychiatric conditions. Nurses can provide support and education on the dying process, the grieving process, and the decision-making process by including the benefits and burdens of treatment. Social aspects of care focus on the patient and family structure of culture, values, beliefs, and strengths, which drives the patient's goals and treatment preferences.

Spiritual, religious, and existential aspects of care focus on those practices and rituals that bring the patient and family hope, meaning, purpose, comfort, and closure to the dying process. Cultural aspects of care convey a respect of the patient's and family's perceptions, preferences, and practices and tailor communication to the patient's and family's literacy level. Care of the patient at the end of life focuses on promoting care that will help the patient incorporate perceptions, preferences, and practices of spiritual, religious, and cultural needs to achieve a peaceful, dignified, and respectful death. Ethical and legal aspects of care can be followed by practicing within one's guidelines established by the governing board's code of ethics.

Not all losses are obvious or immediate. Obvious losses are such events as the death of a loved one, divorce, breakup of a relationship, or loss of a job. Not as obvious are the losses precipitated by illness, aging, birth of a child with defects, and changes in schools, jobs, or neighborhoods.

Some losses are actual, and some are perceived. An actual loss is identified easily, such as a woman who has a mastectomy. A perceived loss, such as the loss of confidence or when a woman who hopes to give birth to a female child delivers a male child instead, is less obvious. Perceived losses are overlooked or misunderstood easily, yet the associated process of grief follows the same sequence as with losses that are considered "real."

Another way to look at loss is to classify it as maturational, situational, or both. **Maturational loss** is a loss that results from normal life transitions. Examples include the loss of childhood dreams, the loss felt by an adolescent when a romance fails, and the loss felt when leaving the family home for college or marriage and establishing a home of one's own. Later, as individuals age, they may experience losses such as menopause and loss of hair, teeth, hearing, sight, and "youth." **Situational loss** is defined as a loss that occurs suddenly in response to a specific external event, such as the sudden death of a loved one. Loss of a job can lead to a loss of self-esteem. Such changes promote emotional growth and the development of coping skills. People use these skills later to cope with even more significant losses. Early experiences with loss can prepare the individual to deal with loss throughout the life cycle. Each person experiences loss as it individually affects him or her. Each loss is followed by a time of grieving.

Personal loss is any significant loss that necessitates adaptation through the grieving process. When something or someone can no longer be seen, felt, heard, known, or experienced, a sense of loss occurs. The type of loss influences the degree of stress it causes. For example, the loss of an object may not generate the same stress as the loss of a significant other. On the other hand, individuals respond to loss differently. In general, people expect the death of a family member to cause more stress than the loss of a pet. For an older person living alone, however, the death of a pet that has been a constant companion can cause more emotional stress than that of a cousin who had not been seen in years.

Box 25.1 Factors That Influence the Experience of Loss

- Childhood experiences
- Significance assigned to the loss
- Physical and emotional state
- Accumulated loss experience
- View of loss as crisis
- Duration and timing
- Abruptness or suddenness
- Financial impact
- Availability of resources
- Cultural factors
- Personal attributes
- Coping mechanisms
- Relationship with the lost person or object

Therefore recognize how highly individualized each person's interpretation of a loss is, whatever type of loss it may be. Loss is a complex phenomenon influenced by many factors (Box 25.1). It threatens self-concept, self-esteem, security, and sense of worth. Recognize the meaning of each loss to a patient and its impact on physical and psychological functioning.

GRIEF

Grief is the subjective response to actual or anticipated loss. It is a natural, normal, and universal part of human experience. **Bereavement** is defined as a common depressed reaction to the death of a loved one. **Mourning** (reaction activated by a person to assist in overcoming a great personal loss) refers to culturally defined patterns for the expression of grief. Mourning patterns include funerals, wakes, memorials, black dress, and defined time of social withdrawal.

Grief involves thoughts, feelings, and behaviors. Many examples of increased **morbidity** (an illness or an abnormal condition), physical and mental, are seen after significant losses. For example, an increase is found in the breakup of marriages and other significant relationships after the loss of a child or when one partner suffers a loss of a body part or function.

When allowed to operate normally, grief has a useful function. Grief is not an episode. It is a process, sometimes one that goes on forever (e.g., parents grieving for a child). On the other hand, the grieving process can lead to resolution of the hurt and the reestablishment of one's life. Still, the emotional pain involved in grief comes and goes with a person's life experiences. Many years after a loss, something reminds the person of the loss and the associated feelings return. The reminder may be an encounter with smells, places, foods, dates, holidays, clothing, or other people.

The grieving person may try a variety of strategies to cope. The following tasks facilitate the passage from grief to closure:

- Accepting the reality of the loss
- Experiencing the pain of grief
- Adjusting to an environment that no longer includes the lost person, object, or aspect of self
- Reinvesting emotional energy into new relationships

The successful completion of these tasks leads to healthy adjustment to loss. These tasks are not sequential. In fact, grieving people often work on all four tasks simultaneously or place priority on only one or two. One of the nurse's roles is to assist patients and families in working through these tasks. Unresolved grief can result if the tasks are not completed and can lead to incomplete relationships and health problems.

In the past, society discouraged the open display of emotions such as grief. Unhappy children were told not to cry when playmates moved away, awkward adolescents were told not to be embarrassed about sudden growth spurts, and dying people were told to remain calm and dignified. Changes in attitudes, beliefs, and values have promoted more open expressions of grief. For example, nurses learn to seek support from peers and to express their concerns about dealing with terminally ill patients. Similarly, family members seek support from caregivers to express anger over loss. Grieving leads to new understandings that promote growth if a person can be open and obtains encouragement and adequate support from others.

Sometimes losses such as physical disfigurement or the death of close friends stimulate behaviors and feelings associated with the grieving process. These behaviors and feelings also occur when individuals face their own death. A patient who is dying is undergoing loss and the impact of the family's grief. Some patients feel that their families do not need any other problems and cannot cope with additional concerns. The dying patient in this situation sometimes depends extensively on the nurse, and identification of sources of support becomes a major task (Fig. 25.1).

Loss, through death or otherwise, is somewhat easier to cope with if it is expected. Sometimes the diagnosis of terminal illness allows a period of **anticipatory grief** (to expect, await, or prepare for the loss of a family member or significant other) when the dying person and the mourners can cry together and enjoy their mutual affection. Time for anticipation does not ease the pain of loss necessarily because attachment often is strengthened during the period of anticipatory grief. However, sometimes the emotions expressed at this time make the loss less conflicted than when such exchanges never occur. When individuals achieve an awareness of mortality, this maturity often leads them to anticipate eventual grief. They make a special effort to express affection and appreciation of their older adult relatives, even without evidence of impending death.

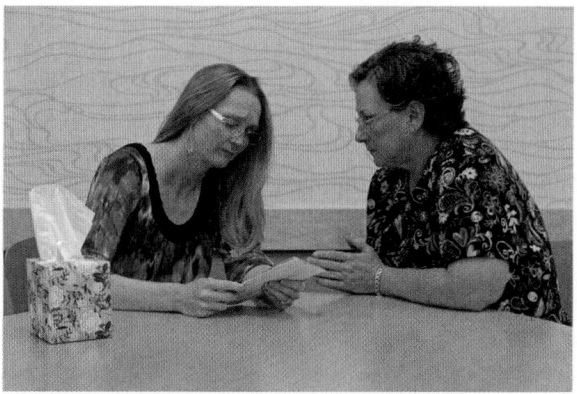

Fig. 25.1 Nurses assist family members in finding resources to help with the grieving process.

The sudden death of someone who is not "supposed to" die (sometimes referred to as "out-of-sequence" death) is the most difficult grief to bear. The clearest example is the death of a child, especially one who has lived long enough to have a distinct personality and position in the family. If the death is a violent and sudden one, the loss is particularly devastating. Parents and siblings often are wracked by powerful and personal emotions of guilt, denial, and anger, as well as sorrow. One protective impulse is to blame someone—perhaps oneself for not having been more careful or more loving, perhaps a spouse, and perhaps even the dead child.

Blame and guilt may destroy a family just when family members need one another most. The Compassionate Friends, a national self-help support organization that assists families after the death of a child, finds that many married couples are driven apart by their separate reactions to the death. Perhaps one parent needs to talk about the death, whereas the other cannot bear to hear the child's name. Siblings suffer, too—partly because parents are so involved in their own grief that the surviving children are deprived of attention, and partly because a child's grief may follow a different course from that of adults. Denial and regression are common at first, with sorrow and acceptance coming much later than for adults. Each family member should try to understand and accept the many possible individual forms and paces of mourning that may be exhibited by others. Children, in particular, need to know that all questions and feelings are acceptable.

SENSE OF PRESENCE

Individuals who have experienced a loss sometimes have a nonthreatening, comforting perception that the deceased is present. Such perceptions, known as *sense of presence*, vary from general feelings of the deceased's presence to actual sensory experiences. Sometimes these sensory experiences manifest as dreams or conversations; sometimes they involve the senses and include visions, hallucinations, or the perception of voices, smells, or touch. This is a part of the mourning process that occurs because of the bond that continues between the bereaved loved ones and the deceased. Searching allows the individual to see the deceased as safe, comfortable, and at peace. Sense of presence is known to occur during the grief process and beyond.

GRIEF ATTACKS

The involuntary and unexpected reappearance of emotions and behaviors associated with grief is known as a *grief attack.* These attacks can occur in response to a variety of triggers. Eating at a restaurant or eating a certain food that triggers a memory of the deceased loved one may cause a grief attack. At other times a memory about the deceased may enter the loved one's mind and cause an attack for no particular reason. Hearing about the death of someone or reading a book that depicts a similar death as the loved one could also trigger a grief attack.

When a loved one dies, the hurt of their loss does not typically ever disappear. Time does seem to help most people with coping with the loss in a way that does not bring sadness as frequently as it once did. Generally, after some time, the sadness is replaced with fond memories of the loved one except during special occasions such as birthdays or holidays.

NURSES' GRIEF

The universality of the loss experience often leads nurses who work with the terminally ill and the bereaved to develop a heightened empathy for their patients. Identifying with patients and sharing the impact of the loss are likely to help the nurse prepare for the death experience. On the other hand, the nurse's role in supporting grieving patients and families can become complicated when nurses experience grief themselves, especially when working with dying patients. Nurses should not allow their grief to overshadow the care of patients and families. Nurses who are not aware of their own grief issues have more difficulty relating to patients as unique individuals. An example is a dying patient who reminds the nurse of a beloved grandparent, and the nurse becomes too emotionally involved. Other tasks and abilities that may be useful to the nurse working with dying patients include coming to grips with and understanding the grief process, appreciating the experience of the dying patient, using effective listening skills, acknowledging personal limits, and knowing when there is a need to get away and take care of one's self. Recognizing the need to grieve assists the nurse in moving through this process.

Nurses who experience multiple losses during work and fail to process them adequately run the risk of **bereavement overload** (before an initial loss is resolved, it is compounded by an additional loss). Frustration, anger, guilt, sadness, helplessness, anxiety, depression, and feelings of being overwhelmed are common. Self-care is critical to survival. Practice self-care and take the time to work through the grief process and mourn losses (Box 25.2). Unrelieved grief and stress can lead to diminished well-being and inability to care for others (Fig. 25.2). Develop an ongoing personal support system when working in areas where a high number of deaths occur. Opportunities for energy renewal and mutual support foster a sense of closure for each experience. When the stresses of the job exceed its rewards and the support of peers is lacking, the result is burnout. (See Chapter 41 for further discussion of burnout.)

Box 25.2 Survival Strategies for Nurses

- Identify personal spiritual beliefs.
- Take regular breaks or "time-outs" from the patient care area; consider rotating out of high-stress areas.
- Identify specific patients who are the most stressful so that stress can be anticipated.
- Trade patients or ask for special assistance in working in stressful situations.
- Acknowledge physical needs as key factors in stress reduction.
- Integrate decompression routines into daily life (e.g., before leaving the work area and going home, take a moment to review the day and set it aside).
- Engage in life-affirming activities (e.g., spend time with loved ones and friends).
- View losses as an opportunity to reevaluate and grow.
- Avoid the "rescuer" or "savior" complex; recognize limits.
- Recognize the need for support and do not hesitate to ask for it.
- Say "I choose" rather than "I should."
- Develop the skills of setting limits and feeling OK about saying no.
- Laugh and play in the face of tragedy without guilt.
- Seek consultation on a regular basis.

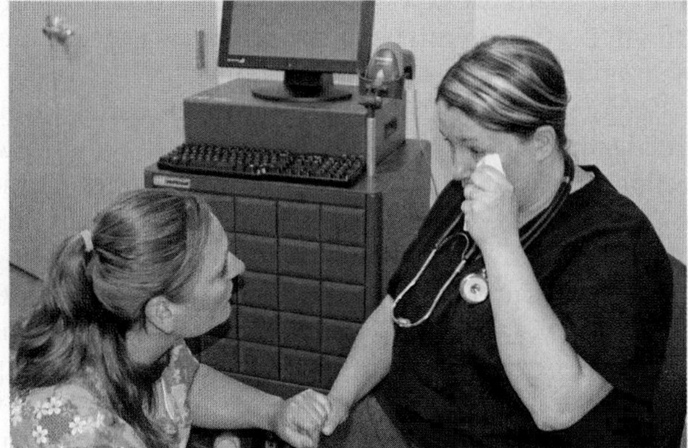

Fig. 25.2 Nurses benefit from support of colleagues during their time of loss.

The nurse, who is always giving, eventually realizes that receiving is also necessary to be effective. Nursing is a job with increasingly high demands. Nurses need the ability to modify their role, acquire new ones compatible with new trends in health care delivery, and permit ethical decision making about allocation of resources. Understanding the impact of work allows improved use of problem-solving techniques to guide choices and prevent dysfunctional responses to loss.

Being informed and current, practicing within the legal parameters of professional responsibilities, and using current trends in health care promote competence in many fields, including the expertise of caring for the dying patient.

Box 25.3 Theories of Grief and Mourning

KÜBLER-ROSS'S STAGES OF DYING

A behavior-oriented theory that includes five stages:

- *Denial:* Individual acts as though nothing has happened and may refuse to believe or understand loss has occurred.
- *Anger:* Individual resists the loss and may strike out at everyone and everything.
- *Bargaining:* Individual postpones awareness of reality of the loss and may try to deal in a subtle or overt way as though the loss can be prevented.
- *Depression:* Individual feels overwhelmingly lonely and withdraws from interpersonal interaction.
- *Acceptance:* Individual accepts the loss and looks to the future.

BOWLBY'S PHASES OF MOURNING

A behavioral theory that includes four phases:

- *Numbing:* Individual describes phase as feeling "stunned" or "unreal." It is a period of intense emotion that serves to protect the body from consequences of loss and lasts from a few hours to a week or more.
- *Yearning and searching:* Phase arouses acute distress in most people. Painful phase is characterized by physical symptoms such as tightness in the chest and throat, shortness of breath, a feeling of weakness, and lethargy, insomnia, and anorexia. Phase may last for months or years.
- *Disorganization and despair:* Individual endlessly examines how and why the loss occurred. It is a common time for person to express anger. Gradually phase gives way to an acceptance that loss is permanent.
- *Reorganization:* Individual begins to accept unaccustomed roles, acquire new skills, and build new relationships. Phase may last a year or more. Individual needs support to unlink self from the lost relationships.

WORDEN'S TASKS OF MOURNING

A behavioral theory that indicates four tasks:

- *Accept reality of loss:* There is always some period of disbelief and surprise over a loss. This task involves processes needed to accept that the person or object is gone and will not return.
- *Work through pain and grief:* Emotional pain comes as a natural part of loss. Individuals who deny or shut off the pain prolong their grief.
- *Adjust to environment in which the deceased is missing:* Individual does not realize full impact of loss for at least 3 months. At this point, friends and associates stop calling, and the person is left prey to loneliness. Often the individual must take on roles formerly filled by the deceased.
- *Emotionally relocate the deceased and move on with life:* Individual does not forget the deceased or give up the relationship with the deceased. The deceased, however, must take a new, less prominent, place in a person's emotional life. People dealing with this task fear they will forget their loved one.

From Perry A, Potter P, Ostendorf W: *Clinical nursing skills and techniques,* ed 8, St. Louis, 2014, Mosby.

STAGES OF GRIEF AND DYING

There is no right or wrong way to grieve. The concepts and theories of grief are only tools for the nurse to use to anticipate potential needs of patients and families and to plan interventions to help patients understand their grief while trying to deal with it. It is a mistake, and possibly harmful, to expect patients to progress in some specific manner over a specified time. The nurse's role is to assess grieving behaviors, recognize the influence of grief on behavior, and provide empathic support.

Thanatology (the study of dying and death) has sparked much interest since the 1970s. See Box 25.3 for more information on theories of grief and mourning.

Table 25.1 describes some of the concepts of death and dying typically held by specific age groups. With knowledge of these developmental stages, the nurse can better understand a patient's responses to a life-threatening situation and the grief responses of individuals after a loss.

COMPLICATED GRIEF

Bereavement is a state of great risk physically, emotionally, and socially. For this reason, the importance of grief work cannot be overstated.

Various theorists have described behaviors indicative of unresolved grief. As the term indicates, **unresolved grief** signifies some disturbance of the normal progression toward resolution. **Complicated grieving** (unresolved grief or complicated mourning; also called **dysfunctional grieving**) is a delayed or exaggerated response to a perceived, actual, or potential loss. Complicated grieving occurs when individuals: (1) get "stuck" in the grief process and become depressed; (2) are unable to express feelings; (3) cannot find anyone in their daily life who acts as the listener they need; (4) suffer a loss that stirs up other, unresolved losses and causes them to explore long-standing feelings or emotional concerns; or (5) lack the reassurance and support to trust the grief process and fail to believe that they can work through the loss. A surviving spouse who seeks additional support for many years after the loss of a significant other (Box 25.4) provides one example. The more signs, symptoms, and behaviors the mourner has, the stronger the likelihood of unresolved grief (Nursing Care Plan 25.1). These individuals must be recognized and referred for appropriate counseling or treatment (see Fig. 25.1).

SUPPORTIVE CARE DURING THE DYING AND GRIEVING PROCESS

Assessment

To give compassionate nursing care and support to the family and the patient during the grieving and dying process, consider the five aspects of human functioning:

Table 25.1 Age-Related Influences on the Concept of Death

Infancy to 5 yr	• Does not understand concept of death • Infant's sense of separation forms basis for later understanding of loss and death • Believes death is reversible, a temporary departure, or sleep
5 to 9 yr	• Understands that death is final • Believes own death can be avoided • Associates death with aggression or violence • Believes wishes or unrelated actions can be responsible for death
9 to 12 yr	• Understands death as the inevitable end of life • Begins to understand own mortality • Concept of death expressed as interest in afterlife or as fear of death
12 to 18 yr	• Fears a lingering death • May fantasize that death can be defied, acting out defiance through reckless behaviors (e.g., dangerous driving, substance abuse) • Seldom thinks about death, but views it in religious and philosophic terms • May seem to reach "adult" perception of death but is emotionally unable to accept it
18 to 45 yr	• Has attitude toward death influenced by religious and cultural beliefs
45 to 65 yr	• Accepts own mortality • Encounters death of parents and some peers • Experiences peaks of death anxiety • Death anxiety diminishes with emotional well-being
65+ yr	• Fears prolonged illness • Encounters death of family members and peers • Sees death as having multiple meanings (e.g., freedom from pain, reunion with already deceased family members)

Box 25.4 Complicated Grief

When a person has difficulty progressing through the normal stages of grieving, bereavement becomes complicated. In these cases, bereavement appears to "go wrong," and loss never resolves, which threatens a person's relationships with others. Complicated grief includes four types:

- *Chronic grief:* Active acute mourning characterized by normal grief reactions that do not decrease but persist over long periods. People verbalize an inability to "get past" the grief.
- *Delayed grief:* Characterized by normal grief reactions that are suppressed or postponed. The survivor consciously or unconsciously avoids the pain of the loss. Active grieving is held back, only to resurface later, usually in response to a trivial loss or upset. For example, a wife only grieves a few weeks after the death of her spouse, only to become hysterical and sad a year later when she loses her car keys. The extreme sadness is a delayed response to the death of her husband.
- *Exaggerated grief:* People become overwhelmed by grief, and they cannot function. This is reflected in the form of severe phobias or self-destructive behaviors such as alcoholism, substance abuse, or suicide.
- *Masked grief:* Survivors are not aware that behaviors that interfere with normal functioning are a result of their loss. For example, a person who has lost a pet has changes in sleeping or eating patterns develop.

From Perry A, Potter P, Ostendorf W: *Clinical nursing skills and techniques*, ed 8, St. Louis, 2014, Mosby.

physical, emotional, intellectual, sociocultural, and spiritual. Assess each area, using the nursing process, to fully understand the patient's needs and provide appropriate interventions.

Physical assessment. While interviewing and observing the patient, assess such areas as sleeping patterns, body image, activities of daily living (ADLs), mobility, general health, medication use, and pain. Additional areas of concern include the basic needs of nutrition, elimination, oxygenation, activity, rest, sleep, and safety (Nursing Care Plan 25.2).

Interventions should target: (1) energy conservation; (2) pain-reduction techniques; (3) comfort measures; (4) promotion of sleep and rest; and (5) increasing self-esteem through body image acceptance.

Emotional assessment. Preparation for death is an endeavor filled with anxiety and fear for most people. Assess the patient's and the family's level of anxiety, guilt, anger, and acceptance. Major fears of the dying patient include fears of abandonment (fear of dying alone), loss of control, pain and discomfort, and the unknown.

Nurses intervene appropriately when they can accept the patient's and the family's feelings, whatever they may be. Offer encouragement and support and give the patient "permission to die" by assisting the patient in saying goodbye.

 Nursing Care Plan 25.1 **The Patient Experiencing Complicated Grieving (Unresolved Grief)**

Ms. S. is 78 years old and is being admitted for weakness, chronic fatigue, anorexia, and weight loss. Her nursing history reveals that Ms. S. refuses to care for herself, has stopped participating in her church activities, and is unable to discuss the deceased without crying. The social history of Ms. S. reveals that her only child, a daughter, died unexpectedly at age 47. Her husband of 50 years died 1 year later. Ms. S. is accompanied by her grandchildren, who offer support and concern. The nursing assessment reveals that Ms. S. lacks resolution of previous grieving response and is experiencing bereavement overload.

PATIENT PROBLEM

Complex Grief, related to bereavement overload, as a result of death of daughter and husband, manifested by refusing to care for self, abstaining from participation in church activities, the inability to discuss the deceased without crying, alterations in eating habits, and interference with performance of activities of daily living (ADLs)

Patient Goals and Expected Outcomes	Nursing Interventions
Patient will establish new and meaningful relationships and interests Patient will engage in constructive, meaningful lifestyle (precrisis level of functioning) Patient will relate realistically to the pleasures and the disappointments of the lost relationships Patient will participate in decision making and cooperate with recommended treatment within 2 wk	Establish trust and positive regard by creating an atmosphere of sharing. Offer privacy and security. Identify significance of multiple losses. Promote resolution of the grieving process. Discuss ambivalence. Assess stage of grief and support patient's expressions of grief. Use active listening. Facilitate discussion of positive and negative aspects of loss. Provide opportunities for social interaction, especially with those who have coped with similar losses. Teach patient and significant others about the grieving process. Assure patient that feelings are normal. Expect patient to meet responsibilities and give positive reinforcement. Help patient identify ways to adapt lifestyle to accommodate loss. Explore ways to assist patient to make new emotional investments. If you become uncomfortable with your unresolved feelings of loss, contact another nurse to counsel the patient.

CRITICAL THINKING QUESTIONS

1. Ms. S. is admitted to the medical unit for severe weakness, weight loss, and chronic depression. She is reluctant to get out of bed to dress and have meals. How can the nurse facilitate progression through the grieving process?
2. Ms. S. appears thin, with poor tissue turgor. How can the nurse and dietitian encourage improvement of her nutritional status?
3. The nursing assessment for Ms. S. revealed a flat affect, little verbalization, and poor personal hygiene. Which therapeutic nursing interventions can help achieve patient goals and expected outcomes?

From Moorhead S, Johnson M, Maas M, & Swanson E: *Nursing outcome classification (NOC)*, ed 5, St. Louis, 2013, Mosby.

 Nursing Care Plan 25.2 **The Patient Facing Death**

Ms. B. is 68 years old and has been admitted to the hospital for weakness and debilitation caused by widespread metastatic cancer of the colon. She reports pain and is anxious to return home. Ms. B. and her family are aware of her terminal prognosis. The nursing history identified that Ms. B.: (1) is unable to care for herself because of severe weakness; (2) has chronic pain; (3) has a decreased appetite; (4) appears anxious and wants to be home with her family; and (5) is grieving the loss of her health and expresses fears regarding her death.

PATIENT PROBLEM

Prolonged Pain, related to disease progression

Continued

Nursing Care Plan 25.2 The Patient Facing Death—cont'd

Patient Goals and Expected Outcomes	Nursing Interventions	Evaluation
Patient will verbalize moderate comfort and decreased pain while receiving analgesics and other comfort measures	Position patient comfortably; change position gradually and unhurriedly. Provide pain-relief measures patient prefers (e.g., relaxation therapy, diversion, and distraction). Give analgesics as ordered. Evaluate pain for intensity and quality. Know that pain is what patient says it is. Observe patient's freedom of movement. Ask patient to rate pain on a scale of 1 to 10 and compare with baseline data. Use after nursing therapies are administered. Use combinations of analgesics or other therapies as patient's needs change. Provide frequent rest periods in a quiet environment. Time and pace nursing activities to conserve patient's energy. Minimize irritants through skin care, including daily baths, lubrication of skin, frequent repositioning, and dry, clean bed linens.	Patient states pain is relieved or decreased in intensity within 30 min to 1 h after administration of medication 75% of the time.

PATIENT PROBLEM

Inability to Bathe Self, Dress Self, Toilet Self, or Feed Self, related to advanced disease

Patient Goals and Expected Outcomes	Nursing Interventions	Evaluation
Patient will carry out ADLs at highest ability with nurse's assistance as necessary	Assist with ADLs but allow patient and family to assist when able. Provide sufficient time for ADLs. Include patient in determining care routine. Provide frequent oral care q 2–4 hr. Use soft toothbrushes or foam swabs for frequent mouth care. Apply a light film of petroleum jelly to lips and tongue. Remove crusts from eyelid margins and provide eye care. Reduce corneal drying with artificial tears. Protect skin from irritation and breakdown using absorbent pads and clean linen.	Patient indicates satisfaction with level of personal hygiene achieved.

PATIENT PROBLEM

Insufficient Nutrition, related to disease progression

Patient Goals and Expected Outcomes	Nursing Interventions	Evaluation
The patient will be able to consume 50% of her meals	Maintain and document food intake. Confer with dietitian to increase kilocalories and protein intake and discuss patient's nutritional needs. Assist with frequent oral hygiene. Assist with environmental control (temperature, appearance, odors). Identify food preferences and provide the preferences as often as possible. Suggest that smaller portions may be more palatable. Allow home-cooked meals, as preferred by patient (gives family a chance to participate). Provide relief of thirst by using ice chips, sips of fluids, or moist cloth to lips.	Patient has maintained weight for 2 wk or demonstrates weight gain weekly.

CRITICAL THINKING QUESTIONS

1. Ms. B. reports severe bone pain and nausea. She appears cachexic and extremely weak. What are some nursing interventions to decrease Ms. B.'s symptoms?
2. Ms. B. says, "I want to go home to die. I don't want to stay in the hospital. All I want to do is go home and be with my family." How can the hospice team most beneficially assist Ms. B.?
3. When the nurse enters Ms. B.'s room to begin ADLs, she notes the patient's extreme fatigue and lethargy. What are some nursing interventions to conserve Ms. B.'s strength?

From Moorhead S, Johnson M, Maas M, & Swanson E: *Nursing outcome classification (NOC)*, ed 5, St. Louis, 2013, Mosby.

Intellectual assessment. Intellectual assessment includes an evaluation of the patient's and the family's educational level, their knowledge and abilities, and the expectations they have in regard to how and when death will occur. Some aspects of functioning in the intellectual dimension frequently are altered during the dying process because of physiologic changes, medications, the patient's emotional state, and the disease process. Remaining alert to these changes allows for the avoidance of problems if the patient's memory or sensations are decreased.

In most cases, interventions are directed toward patient and family education and support. Keeping everyone informed of procedures, changes in the patient's condition, and hospital policies can allow the patient and family to make well-informed and satisfactory decisions.

Sociocultural assessment. The assessment of the patient's and the family's support systems is valuable. Assessment helps to ascertain whether family members want to assist in the patient's daily care. Not only does this lessen the family's sense of loss of control but it also helps clarify what tasks the family will do and what will be done by nursing staff. If these needs and desires are not clear, distrust and hostility between family and nursing staff can result. Each family and each member in that family are unique in what they wish to do. Never assume that families want to deliver daily care. Many do, but others do not, and they need the opportunity to make that choice (Box 25.5).

Family members need support to get through the dying and death of their loved one. It is also beneficial for family members and loved ones to provide support for one another; encourage this mutual support. Recognize the value of family members as resources and assist them in working with the dying person.

In the home, the family becomes closely involved in the patient's care (see Chapters 37 and 40). A terminal illness places heavy demands on social and financial resources. The emotional strain often disrupts normal communication channels. Sometimes the family becomes afraid to interact with the patient.

When families choose to take the patient home for care, be sure that they are well prepared before discharge for what they need to know. Arrange for hospice services to assist the family, if they are receptive. Emphasize continuity of care and constant availability for when the patient has an emotional or physical crisis and needs ongoing support.

During the social assessment, learn whom the patient considers to be the most supportive person in his or her life. It may be a friend, coworker, or fellow church member. Help this person to become a part of the patient's supportive network and be included in planning the patient's care. Encourage these social support people to become involved, and at the same time, maintain and promote the patient's independence whenever possible.

Box 25.5 Suggestions for Involving the Family in the Care of the Dying Patient

- The thanatologic philosophy dictates that family members are free to choose if and when they wish to be with the patient who is dying. Do not raise a barrier because of "visitation hours."
- Allow young children to visit a dying patient when the patient is able to communicate.
- Be willing to listen to family members' complaints about the patient's care and to their feelings about the patient.
- Help family members learn to interact with the dying patient (e.g., using attentive listening, avoiding false reassurances, conducting conversations about normal family activities or problems).
- Allow family members to help with as much or as little patient care as they desire.
- When the family becomes fatigued with care activities, relieve them from their duties so that they can get the rest and support they need. Refer them to resources for meals and lodging.
- Support the act of shared grieving among patient and family. Provide privacy when preferred. Do not discourage open expression of grief between family and patient.
- As the time of death approaches, assist family members to stay in communication with the dying patient through short visits, caring silence, touch, and telling the patient of their love for him or her.
- After death, assist the family with decision making, such as selection of a mortician, transportation of family members, and collection of the patient's belongings.

Spiritual assessment. Assess the spiritual dimension by gaining insight into the patient's philosophy of life, spirituality, and religious resources. Find out what significance the rituals of the particular faith group have for the patient in dealing with death. Assess your own feelings related to death and dying experiences. It is equally important to avoid judging others and avoid attempting to interpret and analyze the spiritual aspect of death and dying. Create an atmosphere of openness to discuss the patient's spiritual concerns.

Interventions in this area come from clergy, friends, family, health care providers, and significant others. Support of the patient's and the family's belief systems and values is important (see Chapter 6).

One aspect of this belief system is hope. Hope can take many forms. The challenge is to assist the patient and the family to identify those hopes that are most important to them to help them to cope.

Hope can be considered a life force that is multidimensional (taking many forms) and fluid. Hope is the common thread identified in all stages of grief. It is characterized by confidence, even though the hopeful individual does not necessarily expect to achieve a specific goal. Hope does not comprise a single act but is a complex series of changing thoughts, feelings, and actions. Many sources report a significant relationship between the level of hope and the level of coping. In addition, the strength of religious connections and the performance of family role responsibilities are related significantly to the variables of hope and coping.

Hope is difficult to maintain during the dying process. As the patient's condition deteriorates, the nurse's challenge becomes one of assisting the patient and family in translating their hope for a cure into realistic hopes that are focused on short-term, achievable goals. These may be the hope for a comfortable and pain-free life or the desire to live long enough to participate in some important family event, such as the wedding of a child. A total lack of hope exhausts the human spirit. When hope is relinquished, death follows rapidly.

Shock and Denial

Shock and denial are common reactions that occur during the grieving process. Nurses can be a great source of support during the time of experiencing these reactions. Nursing responsibilities often include providing guidance and understanding and answering questions that loved ones have when in shock or denial. The nurse frequently spends time with the family while dealing with shock and denial and may offer further support through counselors, clergy, or various support groups. See Box 25.6 for tips on breaking bad news to the family or patient.

Box 25.6 Breaking Bad News

Generally, the health care provider delivers any unexpected bad news, but occasionally, nurses must give families the news of a death. Accompany the health care provider who is approaching a family with unexpected or traumatic news, especially when it involves a death, and remain with the family after the health care provider leaves. When you must deliver bad news, use the following guidelines:

- Determine the relationship of family members with whom you will be talking and their role in the patient's care and daily life. Be sensitive to cultural influences within family structure and roles. Ascertain family dynamics so that the appropriate people receive the information from a health professional.
- Plan words ahead, organize thoughts, and have all the facts and the answers to questions that can be predicted.
- Provide privacy, and establish rapport. If other team members already have developed such rapport, include them in the meeting with the family.
- Introduce personnel, and identify nurses involved in the care of the patient.
- Create an environment that allows time for the presentation of information and discussion of the meaning and consequences of the information. Turn off pager or cellular phone, sit down, maintain eye contact, and listen attentively.
- Determine what the family already knows and what the individuals want to know. Do not make assumptions about the extent of information or details desired by family members.
- Use language that is unambiguous; avoid medical terms and acronyms. Use basic terms to discuss medical situations and interventions. Present information at a level commensurate with the educational level of the participating family members. Use medical personnel as interpreters, if needed, rather than having a family member interpret facts and medical information to other family members.
- Assess nonverbal body language and indicators of emotional status.
- Continually assess and reassess family members' understanding of information being presented and discussed. State information repeatedly until it is heard and understood by families who are in shock or numb from the related events.
- Bring in clergy who can support and remain with families after the formal discussion of facts has concluded, if the family desires. Seek nursing supervisor assistance when needed to further assist family members as indicated (see Fig. 25.1).
- Confirm that safe transportation is available when the family is ready to leave. Escort them to the car in which they will drive away from the facility. A last measure of respect for the deceased person is conveyed when a staff member accompanies the family as they exit the place where a loved one has died.

From Harkreader H, Hogan MA, Thobaben M: *Fundamentals of nursing: Care and clinical judgment,* ed 3, St. Louis, 2007, Mosby.

NURSING PROCESS IN LOSS AND GRIEF

The role of the licensed practical nurse/licensed vocational nurse (LPN/LVN) in the nursing process as stated is that the LPN/LVN will:

- Participate in planning care for patients based on patient needs.
- Review the patient's plan of care and recommend revisions as needed.
- Review and follow defined prioritization for patient care.
- Use clinical pathways, care maps, or care plans to guide and review patient care.

By completing the assessment, diagnosis, planning, outcomes identification, implementation, and evaluation, the LPN/LVN can develop a nursing care plan.

ASSESSMENT

Begin care of the grieving patient by collecting subjective and objective data about the meaning of loss to the patient and family or significant others. Interview the patient and family, observing their responses and behavior. Do not try to assess how the patient *should be* reacting but rather how the patient *is* reacting. Some behaviors or phases occur in sequence. In contrast, sometimes behaviors or phases in the death and dying process may be skipped, omitted, or experienced in a different order. Many variables affect grief. Assessment of these variables gives the nurse a broad database with which to individualize care. When nurses provide care to patients from other backgrounds, they should perform the assessment attentively and listen for clues to beliefs and practices regarding health and illness.

Interpretation of a loss varies greatly with a person's cultural and ethnic background. Many sources note that ethnicity is related strongly to attitudes toward life-sustaining treatments during terminal illness. The form the expression of grief takes generally is linked to cultural background and family practices. Culturally determined traditions often dictate how a family support system is to behave. For example, in the Western tradition, the grieving process is usually personal and private, with individuals showing emotional restraint. The ceremonies that surround a person's death offer time and a means for grief resolution and reminiscing. In Eastern nations, respect for the dead may be shown with louder verbal expression and physical demonstration of grief for a specified period. Despite these general tendencies, however, members of the same ethnocultural background often respond differently to loss and death.

◆ PATIENT PROBLEM

After thorough and thoughtful data collection, identify patient problems related to the patient's clinical situation. Formulate an individualized patient problem statement by noting and analyzing any clustering of patient or family behaviors, actual or potential losses, and data involving the loss (Box 25.7).

The mere presence of one or two defining characteristics is usually insufficient to identify a patient problem accurately. Be vigilant and do not overlook competing patient problems. For example, if a patient who is dying manifests an increase in crying or tearfulness, displays of anger, and frequent nightmares, consider several possible patient problem statements, because these characteristics are common to more than one patient problem. Among the choices are *Recent Onset of Pain, Impaired Coping,* and *Impaired Belief System.* Until you examine all the available data and inquire about the presence of other behaviors and symptoms, you are unable to determine a correct patient problem with any accuracy.

For selection of appropriate interventions for the patient's care, identification of the relevant context, or the related factor, is also necessary. For example, *Dysfunctional Grief related to loss of physical function* necessitates different interventions than *Dysfunctional Grief related to the loss of a job.*

For the patient who is seriously ill, several patient problems are possible. Addressing all of these complex problems simultaneously is impossible. On any given day or at any one time, two or three problem areas demand the nurse's attention. These priorities shift according to the patient's condition, so reevaluate and restate priorities constantly.

Box 25.7 Patient Problem Statements Related to Grieving

Grief, related to:
- *Potential loss of significant other*
- *Potential loss of physiopsychosocial well-being*

Complex Grief or Potential for Complex Grief, related to:
- *Actual or potential object loss*
- *Absence of anticipatory grieving*
- *Lack of resolution of previous grieving response*
- *Loss of significant other*
- *Thwarted grieving response to a loss*

Fear of Dying/Death, related to:
- *Anticipation of pain, suffering, and impact of death on others*
- *Confronting the reality of terminal disease*
- *Discussions on the topic of death*
- *Uncertainty about the after-life following death*

Insufficient Nutrition, related to:
- *Depressed grief response*
- *Loss of significant other*
- *Change in social status*
- *Situational transition or crisis*

Impaired family processes related to:
- *Situational transition or crisis*

Despair, related to:
- *Failing or deteriorating physiologic condition*

Impaired Belief System or Potential for Impaired Belief System, related to:
- *Separation from religious and cultural ties*
- *Situational transition or crisis*

Potential for Impaired Human Dignity, related to:
Compromised maintenance of health
Impaired decision-making ability

In addition to a patient problem related directly to grief, other health problems common to grieving also are likely to be diagnosed, such as *Anxiousness* or *Insufficient Nutrition*. In these situations, focus the interventions on supporting or resolving grief before attempting to solve the other problems. For example, if the patient continues to have loss of appetite related to severe anxiousness, simply improving the nutritional value and variety of available foods has little impact on nutritional status.

◆ EXPECTED OUTCOMES AND PLANNING

Nursing interventions should be planned to meet the physiologic, emotional, developmental, and spiritual needs of the grieving patient. Draw on resources among the patient's friends and family, clergy, support groups, and legal consultants and focus on achieving specific goals and outcomes that relate to the identified patient problem statement.

The following are examples of possible goals and outcomes:

Goal 1: Patient will actively participate in grief work.
Outcome: Patient expresses thoughts and feelings related to loss.
Goal 2: Patient will verbalize finding meaning in life.
Outcome: Patient verbalizes future goals and plans.

In developing a comprehensive plan to help patients deal with loss and grief, use other professionals within the health care team and in the greater community as resources. Suggesting consultation with other professionals or providing resources contributes to the patient's well-being. These external resources should be incorporated into the plan of care. Patients may have concerns about financial matters or the making or revising of a will; the best intervention for them may be referral to legal aid or to a private attorney. Also remember to treat each patient and family as unique, and recognize that their needs, fears, hopes, expectations, and concerns change throughout the illness.

◆ IMPLEMENTATION

Nursing care of the terminally ill patient is often demanding and stressful. It is important to recognize the value of family members as resources and assist them in working with the dying patient (see Box 25.5 and the Patient Teaching box on the dying patient and family). Also, consider any special needs of the older adult (see the Lifespan Considerations for Older Adults box).

Patient Teaching

Dying Patient and Family

- Describe and demonstrate feeding techniques and selection of foods to facilitate ease of chewing and swallowing.
- Demonstrate bathing, mouth care, and other hygiene measures and allow the family to perform a return demonstration.
- Show a video on simple transfer techniques to prevent injury to themselves and the patient; help family members practice.
- Teach the family to recognize the signs and symptoms to expect as the patient's condition worsens and provide information on whom to call in an emergency.
- Discuss ways to support the dying person and listen to needs and fears.
- Solicit questions from the family and provide information as needed.
- Provide teaching, information, and encouragement in the use of creative outlets for expressing feelings and communicating with others. Encourage the use of tape-recorded messages, drawings, writings, imagery, music, and poetry. (This also assists patients and families in creating memories that can be comforting later.)
- Inform the patient and family of relaxation techniques.
- Observe the family and patient interacting with effective communication skills.

Lifespan Considerations

Older Adults

Dying and Death

- Many older adults have long-standing religious beliefs that are likely to influence their response to death and dying. Be sure spiritual counselors are available.
- Many older adults have come to accept death; others remain in earlier stages. Sometimes verbalization of the "wish to die" indicates acceptance and sometimes it indicates depression.
- Some older adults feel free to discuss death; others avoid this topic. Encourage patients to discuss their feelings by giving permission and making yourself available to the bereaved.
- The older person may experience many losses that result in a grief response. These include loss of job, possessions, home, friends, spouse, and autonomy. The older adult often needs emotional support to cope with grief.
- Loss of a spouse in older adulthood is highly likely to result in relocation. This increases the stress level of an already grieving older person and the risk of new health problems or an exacerbation of existing illness.
- Many older adults have instituted advance directives regarding their wishes in case of terminal illness.
- Older adults have the right to a dignified death.
- When caring for an older patient who is dying, it is important to prevent feelings of loneliness and abandonment and to maintain the patient's self-esteem. This can be achieved by ensuring that attentive care is given: speak directly to the patient, ensure that pain control measures are effective, and keep the room environment pleasant.
- The older adult often feels a loss of control; therefore the nurse should offer choices to the patient regarding care. Family members are often unaware that the dying older adult seeks their permission to die. Educate family members about this need and allow family members to be with the dying patient at any time.
- Comorbidity (more than one disease process) is common among older adults.
- Uncertainty of the prognosis of chronic illnesses can make treatment decisions difficult.
- Geriatric pharmacology and awareness of multiple drug interactions is vital.
- The most frequent symptoms experienced by the dying older adult are pain, respiratory distress, and confusion.
- Older adults often have experienced numerous losses, which affects their reactions to subsequent losses.

Data from Perry A, Potter P, Ostendorf W: *Clinical nursing skills and techniques*, ed 8, St. Louis, 2014, Mosby; and Ebersole P, Touhy TA, Hess P, et al: *Toward healthy aging: Human needs and nursing response*, ed 9, St. Louis, 2016, Mosby.

A return to full functioning is not an expected outcome for a terminally ill patient or even a person who experiences significant disability or other loss of function. Always have the goal of enabling the patient to return to optimal physical and emotional functioning. This does not mean that the patient and family do not experience sadness or other disturbing emotions but that they adapt and cope effectively with the stressors in their life. Use a variety of techniques and interventions to assist patients to function optimally under severe stress; to make effective decisions regarding their care; and to cope with disappointment, frustration, and other emotions caused by their illness.

◆ EVALUATION

Refer to the goals and outcomes identified when planning care, and perform measures designed to evaluate the achievement of those goals.

Goal 1: Patient will actively participate in grief work.

Evaluative measures:

- Patient observed discussing loss with significant other.
- Patient demonstrates progress in dealing with stages of grief at his or her own pace.
- Patient participates in self-care, ADLs, and family conversations.

Goal 2: Patient will verbalize finding meaning in life.

Evaluative measures:

- Patient indicates to the health care team or family that he or she finds "peace" in meditation.
- Patient verbalizes goals and plans.
- Patient verbalizes progress in resolution of grief.

The patient expects individualization of care, including comfort, dignity, and cooperation, to maximize quality of life. The success of the evaluation depends partially on the bond you form with the patient. Unless the patient can trust you fully, he or she is not likely to share personal desires. Once you establish rapport, be ever vigilant to avoid problems that threaten it.

The following questions validate the achievement of the nursing interventions:

- "Am I meeting your expectations while providing your care?"
- "Would you like me to assist you in a different manner?"
- "Do you have a specific request that I can use in your care at this time?"
- "Is there another problem that we are overlooking or that you feel is of higher priority?"
- "Are we dealing with your problems in a timely manner?"

Through communication and assessment, continue to evaluate whether the outcome criteria have been satisfied. Use this process to judge the extent to which the goals that were chosen initially have been accomplished. Often evaluation of how well the patient's needs have been met is easy, but ascertaining the same for the family may prove to be more difficult.

SPECIAL SUPPORTIVE CARE

Often death occurs outside the realm of serious illness, injury, or aging. Perinatal, pediatric, suicidal, and older adult deaths are some examples that warrant special consideration.

PERINATAL DEATH

The death of a child often is viewed as one of the most devastating losses that can occur in a family. If the death of the child occurs before, during, or shortly after birth, it is called perinatal death.

Give special consideration to permitting the parents and family to grieve adequately. Loved ones have few or no memories about the child to hold on to, and "acting as though it never happened" places parents in jeopardy of living with unresolved grief. When possible, enable the parents to see, touch, and hold the infant so that they can face the reality of the situation and resolve their grief. Listen attentively, and allow the parents to express their feelings over their loss. Refer to the baby as "your baby," "your son," or "your daughter," or use the given name, to reinforce that the baby was a unique individual who was loved and will be missed. Support the usual cultural rituals after death for the baby, such as a funeral or memorial service.

Some agencies give a lock of the baby's hair, a blanket the baby was wrapped in, or an identification bracelet to the parents. In some cases, parents have refused these items, only to express a desire for these mementos later. Most agencies hold these items until a time when the parents may desire the objects. A disposable camera may even be provided to the family. Agencies also often acknowledge the first-year anniversary of the infant's death.

Other agencies provide angel boxes, which are decorated or painted memorial boxes containing some mementos for the bereaved parents. Suggested items for the angel boxes are booklets on loss and coping with a loss, a wooden angel, a crocheted angel that was touched by the newborn or used during the pictures, a quilt or crocheted blanket, a lock of hair of the newborn if the hair is long enough, footprints and handprints, a clay imprint of the foot, seeds to plant in remembrance of the infant, and the digital camera card with pictures of the infant.

The Angel Gown program provides comfort to the bereaved families through the gift of a beautiful custom-made gown or vest for final photos and for burial services along with support resources and mentoring programs for the family (NICU Helping Hands, n.d.). The custom-made gown or vest is made from wedding and pastel bridesmaid dresses that were donated to the organization. "Now I Lay Me Down to Sleep" provides a specially trained photographer to take pictures of the infant and family for free (Now I Lay Me Down to Sleep, n.d.). Each agency handles the death of an infant in a specific way; please check with your facility for the nursing practices being used.

PEDIATRIC DEATH

The nurse caring for children faced with death needs special skills. Be aware of how children view or understand death, their own and that of others. These children are usually aware that they are going to die. They often try to protect their parents. They need to be told the truth in language they can understand and be allowed to share fears, feelings, and opinions (see the Lifespan Considerations for Infants and Children box).

Most of all, children, like adults, need reassurance from their nurse, health care provider, and family that

Lifespan Considerations

Infants and Children

A Child's Understanding of Death

A child's reaction to and understanding of death and dying depends on the developmental stage of the child and parental values and beliefs, culture, and religious orientation. The first way to help children develop a positive attitude toward death is to counsel parents. Parents need to understand a child's age-specific understanding of death and the normal reactions of a child to death. Parents may use "small deaths"—of a pet, for example—to help children become familiar and comfortable with a loss.

When death occurs in a family, parents often try to shield children from the loss. They fear the child will not be able to cope with the grief. However, allowing children to feel emotions appropriate to events prepares them for more traumatic experiences later in life. The child's developmental level determines the proper amount and type of detailed information to discuss with the child.

When a child is dying, parents and siblings often feel considerable anger and resentment. The death of a child usually is seen as unfair. Some parents' inclination is to withhold information about the illness from the dying child. Even young children, however, often perceive that something is wrong with them because of the changes in behavior they see in parents. Work together with parents to plan their child's care, and determine the level of participation they desire. Do not attempt to assume a parental role or relinquish important nursing responsibilities. Parents and children need to know specifics about the plan of therapy and the normalcy of their reaction to the loss. Friends and relatives commonly avoid contact with the dying child and family because of fear over the child's illness. Parents must decide whether they wish to maintain contact with significant others. Such a resource frequently proves valuable.

The following are basic guidelines to follow while providing care for a child who is dying or experiencing the death of a loved one:

- Allow young children to visit a dying parent or grandparent if all parties consent. (Some dying patients have strong feelings about possibly traumatizing children during this transition.)
- Ascertain the child's understanding and experience of death. Developmental theories regarding children's concepts of death are based on cognitive stage of development.
- Respect the family's wishes for how and what to tell children about serious illness, dying, and death. If the parents wish to be honest with the child, straightforward, yet caring, explanations are important.
- Use of play therapy or drawing may help a child express emotions, fears, and understanding about death.
- Answer parents' questions with specific details, taking into consideration the family's cultural background and knowledge level.
- Parents should be allowed to stay with the child at any time of day or night.
- Explain signs and symptoms of approaching death.
- Reassure parents that everything possible was done for the child.
- When possible, the topic of organ donation should be approached with the family before the death of the child. Many families appreciate this topic being brought to their attention because they would not think of it on their own. Many find it comforting to know they can help others.
- Make every effort to arrange for family members, especially parents, to be with the child at the time of death, if they wish to be present. For many, viewing the body is a sign of closure, an opportunity to finish their goodbyes.
- Treat the family and child as a unit. Encourage parents to stay with the child and participate in care as much as desired or possible.
- Understand that decisions to end treatment can be more difficult when children are involved.

Data from Perry A, Potter P, Ostendorf W: *Clinical nursing skills and techniques,* ed 8, St. Louis, 2014, Mosby; and Hockenberry M, Wilson D: *Wong's essentials of pediatric nursing,* ed 9, St. Louis, 2013, Mosby.

they will not suffer or be abandoned and left alone. A letter written by a 13-year-old boy who died of leukemia beautifully summarizes the needs of the dying child. This letter was written to the editor of a newspaper in the 1970s and published in a column written by Saul Kapel, MD (1974):

> I am a 13-year-old boy. I am dying. I write this to you who are and will become nurses and doctors in the hope that by sharing my feelings with you, you may someday be better able to help those who share my experience.
>
> But no one likes to talk about such things. In fact, no one likes to talk much at all. Doctoring and nursing must be advancing, but I wish it would hurry. The dying person is not yet seen as a person and thus cannot be communicated with as such. He is a symbol of what every human fears and what we each know….
>
> But for me, fear is today and dying now. You slip in and out of my room, give me medication and check my blood pressure. Is it because you are insecure or just a human being that I sense your fright? Why are you afraid?
>
> I am the one who is dying. I know you feel insecure, don't know what to say, don't know what to do. But please believe me, if you care, you can't go wrong. Just admit that you care. This is really what we search for. We may ask for whys and wherefores, but we really don't want answers.
>
> Don't run away. Wait. All I want to know is that there will be someone to hold my hand when I need it. I'm afraid. Death may be routine to you, but it is new to me. You may not see me as unique, but I've never died before. To me once is unique.
>
> You whisper about my youth, but when one is dying, is he really so young anymore? I have lots I wish we could

> talk about. It really would not take much of your time, because you are in here quite a bit anyway.
>
> If only we could be honest—both admit of our fears, touch one another. If you really care, would you lose so much of your professionalism if you even cried with me just person to person? Then it might not be so hard to die in a hospital with friends and relatives close by.

This heartrending essay describes the need of a child for honest and caring communication. Parents and loved ones have much difficulty in accepting the reality of a child's impending death. The death of a child is an "out-of-sequence" death and therefore is often more difficult to accept. Parents often harbor extreme guilt. They may express hostility and anger toward health care providers, God, or the world in general. Grandparents suffer a double grief—for themselves and for their son or daughter. Siblings also are affected extremely and need much support at this time. During the dying process and after a child's death, survivors often can derive benefit from supportive group therapy.

SUICIDE

There were 44,193 suicides according to 2017 statistics in the United States, an average of 121 each day. Suicide was the tenth leading cause of death for all ages (CDC, 2017). Survivors of someone who has committed suicide suffer grief in its many forms, in addition to profound guilt or shame. Sometimes they become obsessed with their failure to "see the signs." Rejection and lack of social and religious support is something survivors fear and, unfortunately, often experience. Suicide sometimes is not considered acceptable; many families of suicide victims are not given the same support from the church, community, or workplace as those whose loved ones have died from other causes. Because of the family's anger, fear, and shame, others may avoid reaching out to help. The grief of survivors is complicated and intense. Survivors may be at an increased risk for suicide themselves, and a grief counselor is frequently helpful.

GERONTOLOGIC DEATH

Older adults often are assumed to have some understanding and acceptance of the death process. This is not always true. Treat the older patient as an individual and assess the patient's needs in the same way as those of any individual facing a terminal illness (see the Lifespan Considerations for Older Adults box earlier in the chapter). The older person must be included in self-care and in decisions to undergo or refuse extensive therapeutic or resuscitative measures. Even when aggressive technological options are rejected, patients still need intensive nursing interventions and pain control measures. Sometimes families who suffer the loss of an older person accept the death, but they must experience the grieving process nonetheless.

Factors that influence grief in older adults include the following:

- Physical changes that accompany aging
- Loss of employment
- Loss of social respect
- Loss of relationships
- Loss of self-care capabilities
- Fear of loss of control
- Sense of fulfillment and contributions made
- Personality traits
- Feelings of self-worth
- Degree to which functional ability is retained

SUDDEN OR UNEXPECTED DEATH

Coping with a sudden, unexpected, or violent death, such as through accident, homicide, or sudden illness (e.g., myocardial infarction), is often difficult. Families experiencing this type of loss require a great deal of support. Often there is preoccupation with the final hours or minutes before death. There is "unfinished business," such as things left unsaid or undone. There are usually guilt feelings (e.g., "If only I had not let him go to the party, he would still be alive"). There may be involvement of law authorities, such as the police or coroner. Sometimes there is an obsessive need to understand or know why this has happened. Grief therapy and referral to support groups can be beneficial to those who are left behind from the death of a loved one.

ISSUES RELATED TO DYING AND DEATH

EUTHANASIA

Euthanasia (Greek for "easy death") is sometimes active, a deliberate action taken with the purpose of shortening life to end suffering or to carry out the wishes of a terminally ill patient. Passive euthanasia is permitting the death of a patient by withholding treatment that may extend life, such as medication, life-support systems, or feeding tubes. Active euthanasia is assisting in such a death.

Euthanasia raises many moral and ethical questions for society and for patients and their families. Technologies that can keep patients alive indefinitely after the brain has, for all practical purposes, stopped functioning are largely responsible for the change in attitudes in the past 25 years.

A 2015 Gallop Poll on values and beliefs asked the following two questions: When a person has a disease that cannot be cured, do you think doctors should be allowed by law to end the patient's life by some painless means if the patient and his or her family request it? When a person has a disease that cannot be cured and is living in severe pain, do you think doctors should or should not be allowed by law to assist the patient to commit suicide if the patient requests it? A total of 70% of 527 people answered yes to the first question and 68% of 527 people answered yes to the second question (ProCon.org, 2011).

DO-NOT-RESUSCITATE ORDER

It is proper for patients and families to retain control over decisions about withholding or withdrawing treatment. Death with dignity remains a concern for all. A joint decision for a **do-not-resuscitate (DNR)** decision made by the patient, the family, and the health care providers is best. Be sure the patient and family obtain an explanation of all facts regarding the patient's condition and all treatment options. DNR means only not to resuscitate. It does not mean to withhold any other care, such as hygiene, nutrition, fluids, or medications. The health care provider writes a "no code" or "do not resuscitate" order once a health care provider has documented in the progress notes the deterioration of the patient's condition and the decision by the health care provider and the patient not to administer cardiopulmonary resuscitation. Often the instructions regarding lifesaving treatment are written in the patient's living will or durable power of attorney. Check that the no-code or DNR order is written, not given verbally. In optimal circumstances, the health care provider regularly reviews DNR orders because of changes in the patient's condition. The nurse must be familiar with the institution's policies and procedures concerning DNR orders. Health care providers can list all specifics of DNR orders as a follow-up to the patient's living will. The patient may choose to allow some parts of resuscitative efforts, such as medication administration, but specifically prohibit chest compression or intubation for cardiac dysrhythmias or respiratory arrest. Thoroughly document in the patient's chart all DNR orders and the associated discussion with the patient and family.

With pediatric populations, the term **allow natural death** is more acceptable to parents. "Allow a natural death" acknowledges that one is going to die and forgoes aggressive treatment. Resources that can help patients and families decide what type of care they want to receive are "My Wishes" for children and "Five Wishes" for adults (Aging with Dignity, 2015). *PartingWishes.com* is a website where individuals can write wills, living wills, powers of attorney, funerals, and memorials.

ADVANCE DIRECTIVES

The two basic types of advance directives are **living wills** and **durable powers of attorney** for health care. Many patients have instituted one or both. **Advance directives** are signed and witnessed documents that provide specific instructions for health care treatment if a person is unable to make these decisions personally at the time they are needed. For more information on advance directives, see Chapter 2.

ORGAN DONATIONS

Legally competent people are free to donate their bodies or organs for medical use. Consent forms are available for this purpose. In many states, adults can request organ donation by signing the back of their driver's license. State laws determine whether a nurse is allowed to serve as a witness when individuals wish to give consent for the donation of organs, tissue, or the body. Be aware of the policies and procedures of your employing institution.

In most states (National Organ Transplantation Act, Public Law 98-507, 10-14, 1984), required request laws stipulate that at the time of a person's death, a qualified health care provider must ask family members to consider organ or tissue donation. Required request laws are the result of the shortage of suitable organs for transplant.

The Uniform Anatomical Gifts Act addresses many problems of organ donation and stipulates that the health care provider who certifies death shall not be involved in removal or transplantation of the organs. The National Organ Transplantation Act, which governs this area of medical and nursing practice, prohibits selling or purchasing organs. Organ and tissue donations remain voluntary.

Donations can include the following:

- Vital organs
  - Kidney
  - Heart
  - Lung
  - Liver
  - Pancreas
  - Small intestine
- Nonvital tissues
  - Cornea
  - Long bones
  - Skin
  - Middle ear bones
  - Saphenous and femoral veins
  - Heart valves

Vital organs are recovered after a patient is pronounced clinically dead or brain dead; circulatory and ventilatory support is maintained to perfuse the organs before removal. Additional information about organ and tissue donation can be found at *www.giftofhope.org/about_donation/faqs_about_donation.htm*.

RIGHTS OF DYING PATIENTS

Death with dignity is the goal in caring for the dying patient. The Dying Person's Bill of Rights (Box 25.8) is honored at hospitals and other health care agencies and is posted in prominent areas.

FRAUDULENT METHODS OF TREATMENT

Often the patient and family seek unconventional methods of treatment to prolong the patient's life. Such treatments may include special diets, enemas, unproven drugs, and machines or devices. The nurse may be asked to help patients and families sort out which treatments are real and which are fraudulent. Fraudulent treatments are those that are misrepresented, whether by concealment or nondisclosure of facts, for the purpose of

Box 25.8 The Dying Person's Bill of Rights

- I have the right to be treated as a living human being until I die.
- I have the right to maintain a sense of hopefulness, however changing its focus may be.
- I have the right to be cared for by those who can maintain a sense of hopefulness, however changing this might be.
- I have the right to express my feelings and emotions about my approaching death in my own way.
- I have the right to participate in decisions concerning my care.
- I have the right to expect continuing medical and nursing attention, even though "cure" goals must be changed to "comfort" goals.
- I have the right not to die alone.
- I have the right to be free from pain.
- I have the right to have my questions answered honestly.
- I have the right not to be deceived.
- I have the right to have help from and for my family in accepting my death.
- I have the right to die in peace and dignity.
- I have the right to retain my individuality and not be judged for my decisions that may be contrary to beliefs of others.
- I have the right to discuss and enlarge my religious and/or spiritual experiences, whatever these may mean to others.
- I have the right to expect that the sanctity of the human body will be respected after death.
- I have the right to be cared for by caring, sensitive, knowledgeable people who will attempt to understand my needs and will be able to gain some satisfaction in helping me face my death.

From Barbus A: The dying patient's bill of rights, *Am J Nurs* 75:99, 1975.

inducing another to use them. View with suspicion any treatment that does not offer the patient informed consent after providing information regarding options, results, and approvals from federal agencies.

DYING PATIENT

COMMUNICATING WITH THE DYING PATIENT

Express respect for the patient, offer realistic hope, and impart appropriate reassurance and support when using therapeutic communication. Supportive words without an accompanying supportive attitude are empty in meaning and fail to provide comfort. Verbal and nonverbal communication should be equivalent in message. Reassurance that is unrealistic or given merely to calm a patient does not work. Stating that "everything will be just fine" when this is untrue or uncertain only increases the patient's anxiety and violates trust in the nurse. Do not offer false reassurance. Limited reassurance that is consistent with the facts is far better.

Therapeutic communication also requires paying careful attention to what the patient expresses verbally and nonverbally. Always verify with the patient any interpretations or summaries of the patient's thoughts and feelings to ensure they are accurate and effective.

If patients prefer not to communicate at a particular time, accept and respect their wishes. Indicate a willingness to return at another time when the patient is feeling more comfortable. Be available to listen actively, without judgment, and with acceptance. Allow the patient to express emotions and feelings without fear.

Behavior that indicates listening to the patient is called "attending behavior." It includes appropriate eye contact, attentive body language, and verbally acknowledging that the nurse is listening by using terms such as "uh huh," "I understand what you are saying," or "go on." Demonstrate attentiveness in nonverbal and verbal ways. For instance, sit in a chair close to the patient's bed to reduce the physical distance and the emotional distance it implies. When appropriately used, touching is a highly effective means of communication. Later in the illness, when strength for or interest in verbal communication has dwindled, a patient derives benefit from being touched. Holding a hand, patting an arm, or gently wiping away a tear indicates attending behavior and concern and care.

Remember that you cannot "solve" the problem of dying, but you can have a positive impact on the dying patient's feelings and fears. Communicate openly and sensitively with the patient. This facilitates the expression of emotion and affirms that the patient is a living human who has your support and compassion.

One of the most important tasks of the bedside nurse is to empower patients and families to participate in the final act of living. Communicate reassurance, confidence, and support for the vulnerable patient and family by sustaining nursing assessment practices, continuing to communicate, and providing skilled physical care. The seasoned hand of a skilled professional supporting and guiding the patient can change the journey through dying and death from a frightening process to one of peace and comfort.

Other resources to summon during management of the dying patient depend on the patient's needs and wishes. Patients sometimes desire greater focus on spiritual needs; many request a visit by a clergyman or clergywoman or the performance of a religious ritual. You may be asked to assist in religious rituals such as prayer or reading of scripture. If you are uncomfortable with this task, ask another nurse who is comfortable assisting with the patient's needs or contact chaplain services. Other patients seek answers in nutritional approaches, miracles, and other sources of hope, although these often come with a high price tag. Support nontraditional therapies if they give the patient hope and do no harm (see Chapter 20). The nurse's primary role in the care of the dying patient is to explain realistic options without destroying hope. The attitude of the nurse and the patient makes the difference between the perceived success or failure of a dying experience.

ASSISTING THE PATIENT IN SAYING GOODBYE

One of the most difficult tasks a terminally ill patient faces is leaving loved ones behind. The patient who is aware of dying must say goodbye, whether in a verbal, nonverbal, concrete, or symbolic way. For their part, family members also must work through the process of acknowledging the impending parting. Goodbyes help them move toward the completion of unfinished business with the patient that otherwise could complicate their transition through the grieving process. The nurse's assistance in this area is important to the dying person and the family (see the Communication box).

 Communication

Counseling a Family Member

Family member: I can't go back in that room. He just lies there and stares. I don't know what to do or say.
Nurse: Being near someone who is dying can be uncomfortable.
Family member: It makes me so sad to see him like that. Do you think he knows I'm there?
Nurse: It's very possible that he does. Would you like me to go in with you?
Family member: Yes, please. I wonder if he can hear me?
Nurse: It must be very difficult for you not to be certain that he is hearing you. The last sense to go is hearing. If there is something you want to say to him, get close, take his hand, and speak directly to him. Most people in his condition can hear but are very weak and may not have the strength to respond.
Family member: I just feel like I am not able to do anything for him anymore.
Nurse: Just being there is letting him know that you care. That's something very important to any person.
Family member: I suppose you're right. I guess I'm ready to go in now.
Nurse: I'll be right here by your side.

First, provide a private, comfortable environment. Sometimes emotional expression becomes overwhelming for the patient, the family, or both; offer to remain present or nearby to help support the family member or loved one and the patient. Various ways are available to assist patients in saying their goodbyes, such as role playing, letter writing, or making audio or video recordings. Help patients focus on what they want to say. One way to facilitate this is to ask them to talk to their loved ones as if they were going to be separated for a long time. Encourage them to express those feelings and thoughts they most want their loved ones to know in their absence. Help the dying person to formulate appropriate letters or tape recordings by asking, "What would you want to say to your 6-year-old when the child is 12?" Often dying patients become depressed because they do not have a purpose in life. Working on tasks such as poems, letters, and recordings affords patients feelings of control and productivity in their last days.

PALLIATIVE CARE

People who face life-threatening illnesses can take advantage of many medical and technological advances to reverse the course of their disease or to prolong their lives. For patients with life-limiting illness, finding ways to help them approach their end of life becomes important. Such is the goal of **palliative care:** the prevention, relief, reduction, or soothing of symptoms of disease or disorders without affecting a cure. Palliative care allows patients to make more informed choices, achieve better alleviation of symptoms, and have more opportunity to work on issues of life closure. According to the World Health Organization, when delivering palliative care, the nurse does the following:

- Provides relief from pain and other distressing symptoms
- Affirms life and regards dying as a normal process
- Intends neither to hasten or postpone death
- Integrates the psychological and spiritual aspects of patient care
- Offers a support system to help patients live as actively as possible until death
- Offers a support system to help families cope during the patient's illness and their own bereavement
- Uses a team approach to address the needs of patients and their families, including bereavement counseling, if indicated
- Will enhance quality of life, and may also positively influence the course of illness
- Is applicable early in the course of illness, in conjunction with other therapies that are intended to prolong life, such as chemotherapy or radiation therapy, and includes those investigations needed to better understand and manage distressing clinical complications (WHO, n.d.)

Palliative care is a philosophy of total care. Palliative care is appropriate to deliver at any time and to patients of any age, with any diagnosis. Although it has particular relevance to the care of the terminally ill, it is not reserved for only the last few months of life. The approach to care usually involves an interdisciplinary team of health care providers, nurses, social workers, pastoral care professionals, physical and occupational therapists, and pharmacists. Massage therapists or music or art therapists who provide alternative therapies are also a part of the team. In the context of end of life, a palliative care approach ensures that a patient experiences a "good death," free of avoidable pain and suffering in accord with the patient's and family's wishes and reasonably consistent with clinical, cultural, and ethical standards.

One of the most important tasks for a nurse providing palliative care is to establish a caring relationship with patient and family. Furthermore, the symptom-control measures the nurse provides are important to help maintain the patient's dignity and self-esteem, prevent abandonment or isolation, and establish a

Box 25.9 Long-Term Care Considerations

- Less physician involvement means nurses have an important role in assessing and managing pain and symptom control.
- Challenges include providing privacy and autonomy for the patient and family, involving the family as much as possible or desired, individualizing care, keeping family members informed of changes, and making the environment as homelike as possible.
- The goal of a nursing facility is to provide a caring environment for those who are dying. However, many facilities sorely lack appropriate supportive care. Compassionate care allows family members to be present whenever they choose, day or night, and involves aggressive and appropriate symptom management.
- Nighttime is a time of least attention and a time of loneliness and pain. Night is also a time when people fear they will die alone and no one will know. If a friend or relative cannot stay with the patient, a mature sitter is an option. A volunteer from hospice may provide the same support. For those older adults who have developed a lifestyle around aloneness, solitude may be preferred. Be sensitive to the patient's preference.

Data from Perry A, Potter P, Ostendorf W: *Clinical nursing skills and techniques*, ed 8, St. Louis, 2014, Elsevier.

comfortable and peaceful environment for death to occur (Box 25.9).

PHYSICAL CARE

The nurse has an important responsibility in assisting patients to meet their physical needs. Providing adequate nutrition and maintaining elimination patterns are priorities for the dying patient (see Chapter 40). Keep the patient clean, dry, well groomed, odor free, and comfortable to decrease the chances of skin impairment and provide the patient with feelings of self-esteem and self-worth (see Chapter 9). Sometimes nurses provide care in a facility (see the Coordinated Care box) and sometimes in the patient's home (see the Home Care Considerations box).

Adjusting the environment to increase comfort and safety is paramount. Use side rails for safety and, when possible, to assist weak patients to adjust their own positions.

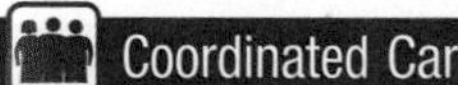

Coordinated Care

Collaboration

Caring for the Dying Patient

The task of supporting patients and families in grief should not be delegated to assistive personnel. A professional nurse has the responsibility for recognizing a patient's grief and knowing the appropriate communication and counseling strategies to use. Provide assistive personnel with information, assistance, and direction, including the following:

- Ask assistive personnel to inform the nurse when the patient expresses behaviors of grief (e.g., crying, anger, loss of appetite).
- Encourage assistive personnel to conduct conversations with patients but to inform the nurse when patients express needs or concerns.
- Ask assistive personnel to inform the nurse when family members arrive so that the nurse can meet with them and assess how they are coping.

A professional nurse is responsible for assessment of patient symptoms and a determination of which symptoms can be managed independently and which symptoms necessitate medical intervention. Certain symptom therapies can be delegated to assistive personnel, such as positioning and environmental controls, hygiene approaches, and hydration. Therapies such as administration of opioids, anxiolytics, and antidepressants require a nurse's intervention. The nurse provides assistive personnel with instruction and assistance regarding the following:

- When to notify the nurse if the patient's symptoms worsen or change in nature
- Potential adverse effects of pharmacologic agents and what to report to the nurse
- The need to maintain communication with dying patients who still retain the sense of hearing

Certain aspects of care of the body after death can be delegated to assistive personnel. Also, care after death can, in fact, begin before the actual death so that patients and families can preserve cultural practices. Check agency policy regarding which staff members are permitted to remove invasive tubes or lines. At the time of death, it may be best for the nurse and assistive personnel to work together in preparing the body (Skill 25.1).

- Inform other care providers of any preference the family may have because of cultural, religious, or ethnic beliefs that influence the routine procedures of caring for the patient's body.
- Reinforce the importance of handling the body with respect.

Modified from Perry A, Potter P, Ostendorf W: *Clinical nursing skills and techniques*, ed 8, St. Louis, 2014, Elsevier.

ASSESSMENTS AND INTERVENTIONS

Care of the dying patient has many facets. Of all the needs of the dying patient, the three most crucial are the need for love and affection, for the control of pain, and for the preservation of dignity and self-worth.

The patient near death continues to need meticulous nursing interventions. Because of the increased weakness and deterioration of the body, the patient's physical needs are important. One of the nurse's goals in end-of-life nursing goes beyond merely allaying the physical suffering of patients to the greatest extent possible. Ideally, the nurse also helps patients recognize and accept death as a reality of life so that they can undertake their last task in life with self-esteem and dignity. Work to prevent the abandonment by family, friends, and caregivers that is sometimes a part of the dying patient's experience. Ensuring support by others can help prevent a patient from being left to die alone. Be aware of the availability of the *No One Dies Alone program* in your employing institute. *No One Dies Alone* is a national volunteer program that will allow compassionate

Skill 25.1 Care of the Body After Death

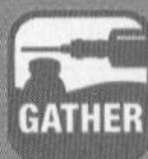

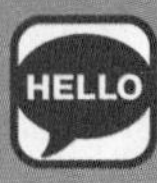

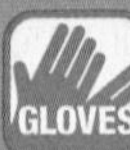

NURSING ACTION *(RATIONALE)*

1. Gather equipment. *(Organizes procedure.)*
   - Disposable gloves, gown, and other protective clothing
   - Plastic bag for hazardous waste disposal
   - Washbasin, washcloth, warm water, bath towel
   - Clean gown or disposable gown for body
   - Absorbent pads
   - Body bag or shroud kit (know agency policy)
   - Paper tape and gauze dressing
   - Suitable receptacle for patient's belongings and other items to be returned to family
   - Valuables envelope
   - Identification tags, as required by agency policy
2. Wash hands. *(Reduces spread of microorganisms.)*
3. Don clean gloves. *(Protects nurse from contamination.)*
4. Close patient's eyes and mouth if needed. *(Provides a more normal appearance.)* A rolled towel placed under the chin is helpful to keep the mouth closed.
5. Remove all tubing and other devices from patient's body.[a] *(Makes patient look more peaceful.)*
6. Place patient in supine position. *(Allows access for procedures.)* Elevate the head. *(Prevents discoloration.)* Do not place one hand on top of the other. *(This can lead to discoloration.)*
7. Replace soiled dressings with clean ones. *(Prevents odor.)*
8. Bathe patient as necessary. *(Reduces odor.)*
9. Brush or comb hair. *(Gives more normal appearance.)*
10. Apply clean gown. *(Prepares body for viewing.)*
11. Care for valuables and personal belongings. *(For legal considerations.)* If wedding band is to remain on the deceased, secure ring to finger with a small strip of tape over ring. *(Prevents loss and protects jewelry.)*
12. Allow family to view body and remain in room for as much time as needed. *(Provide emotional support if family wishes.)* A sheet or light blanket placed over the body with only the head and upper shoulders exposed maintains dignity and respect for the deceased. Remove unneeded equipment from the room. Provide soft lighting and offer chairs. *(Demonstrates respect for significant others.)*
13. After the family has left the room, attach identification per hospital policy. Attach special label if patient had a contagious disease. *(Protects those who handle the body.)*
14. Close door to room. *(Prevents exposure to patients and visitors.)*
15. Await arrival of ambulance or transfer to morgue. *(Out of respect for patient.)* (Some agencies use a shroud to enclose the body before transfer to the morgue.)

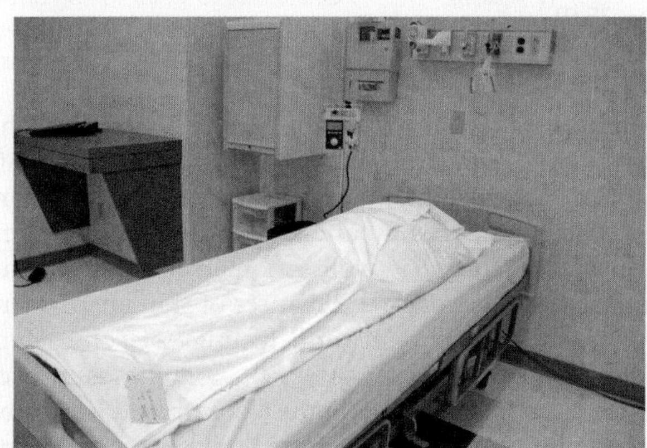

16. Document procedure and disposition of patient's body and of belongings and valuables. *(For legal purposes.)*

[a]Some situations require that all tubing remain in the body (e.g., when an autopsy is scheduled). Know agency policy.

companions to sit with the dying patient so that the patient will not die alone. During the dying process the compassionate companion can talk to the patient, hold the patient's hand, or just be a loving presence in the room (Eskanazi Health, 2016).

Assess the patient for impending death. Although patients may appear comatose, unconscious, or unresponsive, this appearance is often a result of extreme fatigue, and patients may be aware of activities that occur around them. Sometimes the patient may become restless and pick or pull at the bed linens. Remember that this is among the signs and symptoms of decreased oxygenation. Discoloration of arms and legs is a result of impaired circulation. Table 25.2 shows signs of approaching death as expressed in patient needs and the appropriate interventions.

Changes in vital signs are observed, including (1) slow, weak, and thready pulse; (2) lowered blood pressure; and (3) rapid, shallow, irregular, or abnormally slow respirations. Mouth breathing occurs, which leads to dry oral mucous membranes. The patient often has a detached look in the eyes. Diminished sensory and

Home Care Considerations

The Dying Patient

- The trend is toward more people choosing to die at home.
- The family needs to know who to call for help if symptom control is needed, what to do at the time of death, who must be notified, and how the body is to be transported.
- Knowledge of types of home care reimbursement is essential, including Medicare and Medicaid, and hospice benefits.
- Family members assume primary care responsibility, necessitating ongoing teaching and support. Educate family members about symptom management approaches and when to seek help.
- Volunteers may be needed to give family respite time.

Data from Perry A, Potter P, Ostendorf W: *Clinical nursing skills and techniques,* ed 8, St. Louis, 2014, Elsevier.

motor function is seen in the lower extremities, which progresses to the upper extremities. Touch sensation diminishes while pressure and pain sensations may remain intact. As death becomes imminent, the pupils become dilated and fixed, Cheyne-Stokes respirations occur, the pulse becomes increasingly weaker and more rapid, and the blood pressure continues to fall. Peripheral circulation diminishes. The skin is cool and clammy; profuse diaphoresis may occur. If mucus collects in the patient's throat, noisy respirations are heard. This sound is referred to as the *death rattle.* A period of peace may immediately precede the moment of death. The clinical signs of death are given in the following list:

1. Unreceptivity and unresponsiveness
2. No movement or breathing
3. No reflexes
4. Flat encephalogram
5. Absence of apical pulse
6. Cessation of respirations

Table 25.2 Needs and Interventions for the Patient Near Death

Patient Needs	Interventions
Discomfort	Provide thorough skin care, including daily baths, lubrication of skin, and dry clean bed linens to reduce irritants. Provide oral care at least q 2–4 hr. Use soft toothbrushes or foam swabs for frequent mouth care. Apply a light film of water soluble lubricant or lip balm to lips and tongue. Eye care removes crusts from eyelid margins. Artificial tears reduce corneal drying.
Fatigue	Help patient to identify values or desired tasks; then help patient to conserve energy for only those tasks. Promote frequent rest periods in a quiet environment. Time and pace nursing care activities.
Nausea	Administer antiemetics; provide oral care at least q 2–4 hr; offer clear liquid diet and ice chips; avoid liquids that increase stomach acidity such as coffee, milk, and juices with citric acid; and uncover food outside of the room to reduce strong odors.
Constipation	Give preventive care, which is most effective: increase fluid intake; include bran, whole-grain products, and fresh vegetables in diet; and encourage exercise. Administer prophylactic stool softeners. Assess for fecal impaction.
Diarrhea	Confer with health care provider to change medication, or get order for antidiarrheal medication, if possible. Provide low-residue diet.
Urinary incontinence	Protect skin from irritation or breakdown. Indwelling urinary catheter or condom catheters may be used.
Inadequate nutrition	Serve smaller portions and bland foods, which may be more palatable. Allow home-cooked meals, which may be preferred by patient and gives the family a chance to participate.
Dehydration	Remove factors that cause decreased intake; give antiemetics, and apply topical analgesics to oral lesions. Reduce discomfort from dehydration; give mouth care at least q 2–4 hr; and offer ice chips or moist cloth to lips.
Dyspnea, shortness of breath	Treat or control underlying cause. Maximize patient's oxygenation (e.g., position patient upright, provide supplemental oxygen, maintain a patent airway, and reduce anxiety or fear). Administer medications such as bronchodilators, inhaled steroids, or narcotics to suppress cough and ease breathing and apprehension.

From Potter PA, Perry AG, Stockert P, et al: *Fundamentals of nursing,* ed 8, St. Louis, 2013, Mosby.

INQUEST

An **inquest** is a legal inquiry into the cause or the manner of a death. When a death is the result of an accident, for example, an inquest is held into the circumstances of the accident to determine any blame. The inquest is conducted under the jurisdiction of a coroner or medical examiner. A *coroner* is a public official, not necessarily a health care provider appointed or elected to inquire into cause of death. A *medical examiner* is a trained health care provider and usually has advanced education in pathology or forensic medicine. Agency policy dictates who is responsible for reporting deaths to the coroner or medical examiner.

POSTMORTEM CARE

In most states, the health care provider is responsible for certifying a death in the medical record. The health care provider notes time of death and records a description of therapies or actions taken in the medical record. The health care provider may request permission from the family for the **autopsy** (examination performed after a person's death to confirm or determine the cause of death). Autopsies are required in circumstances of unusual death (e.g., violent trauma or unexpected death in the home).

Because of the therapeutic nurse-patient relationship, the nurse may be the best person to provide **postmortem care** (care for the patient's body after death). Keep in mind the need to care for the patient's body with dignity and sensitivity. Provide postmortem care as soon as possible after death to prevent tissue damage or disfigurement. If the family has requested organ donation, take immediate measures as appropriate. Know the state laws and the policies and procedures of the employing institution.

Prepare the body and the room to keep the stress of the experience to a minimum, after the patient has been pronounced dead by a health care provider or professional nurse and before the family views the body. Remove supplies and equipment from sight. Remove, clamp, or cut tubes that remain in the body to within 1 inch (2.5 cm) of the skin, and tape them in place. Care of tubes and specimens depends on agency policy and whether an autopsy will be performed. Never, however, remove tubes, dressings, drains, and other equipment that is in place on or in the patient when an autopsy is to be performed. Clear away soiled linen and other clutter. Use spray deodorizer to help eliminate unpleasant odors.

Prepare the body by making it look as natural and comfortable as possible. Place the body in the supine position with arms at the sides, palms down or across the abdomen (but not one hand over the other); this helps the **mortician** (person trained in the care of the dead) better prepare it for interment. Discoloration of the face can result if blood is allowed to pool; to prevent this, place a small pillow or folded towel under the head. The eyelids usually remain closed if gently held down for a few seconds. If not, a moistened cotton ball can hold them in place. Insert the patient's dentures to maintain normal facial features. A rolled-up towel under the chin keeps the mouth closed (see Skill 25.1). The Cultural Considerations box on care of the body after death presents culturally related attitudes toward preparation of the body. It should be noted that these are only common attitudes of the cultural groups listed. These are not necessarily the beliefs or practices of all members of these cultural groups.

Cultural Considerations

Care of the Body After Death

African Americans: Most families prefer that members of the health care team clean and prepare the loved one's body. Some may have misgivings about organ donation but may agree to an autopsy. Cremation usually is not done.

Chinese Americans: Some families may prefer to bathe the deceased themselves. Often they feel the body should remain intact; organ donation and autopsy are uncommon.

Filipino Americans: Some families may prefer to wash the body themselves and are likely to want time for all family members to say goodbye. The family may not permit organ donation or autopsy.

Hispanics or Latino Americans: Family members may want to help with care of the body and are likely to want to say goodbye. Organ donation and autopsy are uncommon.

Jews: The dying person may want to make a deathbed confession or desire prayers. Observant Jews usually oppose autopsies but may consider organ donation. The body must not be left unattended until burial; a family member may remain present while the body is prepared by nursing staff, during transport to and while in the morgue, and then to the funeral home.

Roman Catholics: The dying person may desire to receive the sacraments of Reconciliation and Anointing of the Sick within 30 days before death. The religion does not oppose autopsies or organ donation.

Muslims: When close to death, a devout Muslim may wish to recite the Islamic Creed with help from others. After death, the person's eyes and mouth should be closed and the limbs should be straightened.

Hindus: The dying person should be in a peaceful room if not at home. The patient or someone else should recite the Gita. Family members may prefer to wash the body and may feel that organ donation is an individual choice.

Buddhists: An ordained monk or nun should care for the dying person. After death, the body should be covered with a cotton sheet. The body should not be touched or manipulated. The eyes and the mouth should not be closed. No noise, talking, or crying is allowed. Buddhists consider organ donation to be an individual choice.

Data from Mazanec P, Tyler MK: Cultural considerations in end-of-life care, *Am J Nurs* 103(3):50, 2003; Giger JN: *Transcultural nursing: Assessment and interventions*, ed 6, St. Louis, 2013, Mosby; and Gift of Hope Organization: *Religious viewpoints*, 2003. Retrieved from *www.giftofhope.org/about_donation/religious_viewpoints_list.htm#c.*

Box 25.10 Documentation of End-of-Life Care

Documentation includes the following:
- Time of death and actions taken to prevent the death if applicable
- Who pronounced the death of the patient
- Any special preparation and type of donation, including time, staff, and company
- Who was called and who came to the hospital: donor organization, morgue, funeral home, chaplain, or individual family members making any decisions
- Personal articles left on the body and taped to skin or tubes left in
- Personal items given to the family and specific names and description of items
- Time of discharge and destination of the body
- Location of name tags on the body
- Special requests by the family
- Any other personal statements that may be needed to clarify the situation

At the time of death, make a notation of any valuables, such as watch, rings, or money, and secure these articles so that they may be delivered to the family according to agency policy. Documentation of all valuables and their disposition in the patient's medical record is required (Box 25.10).

Offer the family the opportunity to view the body. An often helpful suggestion is that this is an opportunity to say goodbye to their loved one, especially if they were not present at the time of death. If the family hesitates to view the body, let them think about it. If they decide not to view the body, accept their decision without judgment. If the family decides to view the body, assure them that they will not be alone if they prefer the nurse be present. Offer to accompany them, or ask to call on someone else to be present if they would like. Spend as much time as possible assisting the grieving family, and offer to contact other support services, such as social services and the spiritual adviser. (Many health care facilities employ a full-time chaplain who may be summoned in the event of death.) The family now becomes the patient.

DOCUMENTATION

Document the care given to the dying patient objectively, completely, legibly, and accurately. As death approaches, make frequent documentation, and include the signs of impending death as they occur. Recording who was present at the time of the patient's death is important. Continue documentation until the last entry, which states where and to whom the body was transferred (see Box 25.10).

GRIEVING FAMILY

SUPPORT

The needs of the grieving family and significant others deserve the nurse's caring, compassionate attention. Make every attempt to contact someone—family, clergy, or friends—to be with the grieving survivor if he or she is alone at the time of the loved one's death. Express words that convey sympathy. If appropriate, use a spontaneous touch, such as a hand on the arm or an embrace, as a comforting gesture. Answer any questions the family may have, and encourage them to view, touch, and talk to the deceased family member. Remain nonjudgmental as the family expresses feelings of anger, guilt, or unfairness. Help with the notification of the mortician and any individuals involved in the procurement of donated organs.

Informing others can be a major emotional step for family members. The nurse's presence and assistance in this area is very supportive. Direct family members to support groups and other referral agencies (churches, therapists, social workers); such connections expand the family's social network, foster relatedness, and decrease isolation.

Grief work helps an individual cope with the loss of a loved one. The use of counseling techniques in order to address symptoms related to suffering a loss is one way grief work can be achieved. Grief work includes:
- Adapting to life without their loved one
- Realizing the reality of the loss of the loved one
- Reinvesting in life while maintaining a healthy bond with the deceased loved one
- Dealing effectively with the emotional pain of the loss (Worden, 2009)

RESOLUTION OF GRIEF

Resolution of grief has begun when, after the loss, the grieving person or family can complete the following tasks:
- Have positive interactions with others
- Participate in support groups with others who are similarly bereaved to articulate loss together and offer companionship
- Establish goals, and work to achieve them
- Discuss the meaning of the loss and its effect on the survivor's life

People need support and understanding to deal with the grief that comes with the loss of a loved one. Months or years may elapse before an individual can complete grief work and begin the full process of resolution. The grief experienced by an individual depends on the energy expended in the relationship. Many believe that about a year must pass before the bereaved can begin to think of the deceased without feeling intense emotional pain.

Get Ready for the NCLEX® Examination!

Key Points

- Care of the dying patient has moved from the home to hospitals and back again in the past 50 years.
- Dr. Elizabeth Kübler-Ross has been instrumental in identifying the five stages of death and dying: denial, anger, bargaining, depression, and acceptance.
- Losses occur throughout the life cycle, provide the individual experience with loss, and promote emotional growth and development of coping skills.
- The effect a loss has on a person is individualized: duration, abruptness, extent, time required for treatment or replacement, and financial impact affect the sense of loss.
- Grief is not an episode but a process—an active, not a passive, process. It takes work and emotional energy. The grief experienced by an individual depends on the energy expended in the relationship.
- When people do not do "grief work" after any significant loss, they are at risk for emotional, mental, and social problems.
- The grief theory demonstrates that the normal grief process includes an onset, active grief work, and a resolution or reorganization of the survivors' lives after the loss.
- Nurses experience all the emotions of grief in response to not only their own losses but also the death of their patients.
- Assessment of whether family members are willing to be involved in a dying patient's care is mandatory before they are used as resources.
- The major concerns of the dying patient are (1) fear of abandonment (fear of dying alone); (2) fear of loss of control; (3) fear of pain and discomfort; and (4) fear of the unknown.
- Euthanasia is an ethical and legal issue faced by nurses. Oregon, Washington, Vermont, California, Colorado, District of Columbia, and Hawaii have a form of Death with Dignity Acts at the time of this publication.
- A do-not-resuscitate (DNR) order or allow natural death order means only that. It does not mean to withhold hygiene, hydration, nutrition, or medications.
- Patients who decide ahead of time what kind of care they want and communicate these decisions to others help to ensure they receive the extent of care they desire. These communications, called advance directives, most often involve the living will and the durable power of attorney.
- The Dying Person's Bill of Rights includes the elements characteristic of dying with dignity.
- Assisting a dying patient in saying goodbye is an intervention nurses can initiate.
- The physical care requirements of the dying patient are primarily nursing interventions. Providing adequate nutrition, elimination, hygiene, safety, and comfort is a nursing priority.
- Continuing to speak to and include patients in their care is essential, because as death approaches, the dying patient becomes weaker. Patients may appear comatose yet be aware of activities around them.
- Signs of impending death are (1) slow, thready, and weaker pulse; (2) lowered blood pressure; (3) rapid, shallow, irregular, or abnormally slow respirations; and (4) mottling of lower extremities.
- Postmortem care is the care administered to the body after death. Follow procedures including cleansing, positioning, and labeling the body.

Additional Learning Resources

SG Go to your Study Guide for additional learning activities to help you master this chapter content.

evolve Be sure to visit the Evolve site at *http://evolve.elsevier.com/Cooper/foundationsadult/* for additional online resources.

Review Questions for the NCLEX® Examination

1. A 77-year-old patient has been admitted with pneumonia. Her husband asks the nurse about the living will. Which statement is correct about living wills?
   1. Living wills allow the courts to decide when care can be given.
   2. Living wills allow individuals to express their wishes regarding care.
   3. Living wills are legally binding in all states.
   4. Living wills allow health care workers to withhold fluids and medications.
2. The patient's daughter remained at the bedside of her dying mother throughout the night. When her mother died the following morning, the daughter cried out angrily at the nurse and the physician. Which is the most appropriate action by the nurse?
   1. Explain that everything possible was done for her mother.
   2. Remain with the daughter and listen to what she is saying.
   3. Leave the daughter in privacy and allow her to work through her grief.
   4. Notify a clergyman and call other family members.
3. A newly licensed nurse is assigned to his first dying patient. When he is caring for a dying patient, what best prepares the nurse?
   1. Having completed a course dealing with death and dying
   2. Being able to control his own emotions about death
   3. Having experienced the death of a loved one
   4. Being aware of his own thoughts and feelings toward death

4. A nurse is assigned to a patient who recently was diagnosed with a terminal illness. While the nurse was assisting her with morning care, the patient asked about organ donation. Which nursing action is most appropriate?
   1. Assist her in obtaining the necessary information to make this decision.
   2. Have the patient first discuss the subject with her family.
   3. Suggest she delay making a decision at this time.
   4. Contact the physician so that consent can be obtained from the family.
5. Which statement describes a person experiencing anticipatory grief?
   1. A person faces the possibility of losing a loved one.
   2. A person has placed the death of a loved one in perspective.
   3. A person displays grief responses after a loved one's death.
   4. A person has difficulty making decisions after a loved one's death.
6. When talking with a patient what would be considered a therapeutic communication technique? *(Select all that apply.)*
   1. Stating, "I know just how you feel"
   2. Saying, "Her death was for the best"
   3. Never crying in front of family members
   4. Encouraging family members to share their feelings
   5. Sitting at the same level of the patient when conversing with them.
7. Which of the following helps family members make difficult decisions?
   1. Discussing autopsy and organ donation at the time of the loved one's death
   2. Addressing one matter at a time, giving them adequate time to discuss each issue
   3. Publicly discussing issues with other hospital staff
   4. Addressing all of the issues at once
8. Which comment is most likely to help grieving family members express themselves more easily? *(Select all that apply.)*
   1. "Tell me how you're feeling."
   2. "I know just how you feel."
   3. "Things will get better."
   4. "Time heals all wounds."
   5. "I hear you saying that you miss your loved one very much."
9. Which of the following is most therapeutic when talking with family members with an unresolved issue?
   1. Explain that they are simply experiencing normal anticipatory grief.
   2. Explain that they missed their chance to make amends and now it is too late.
   3. Encourage them to verbalize their thoughts and feelings to the loved one.
   4. Tell them not to worry, and explain that they are just going through the searching and yearning phase of bereavement.
10. Nurses care for all types of patients with various conditions, including those with a terminal illness. Which statement is true about terminal illnesses?
    1. Death from terminal illness is sudden and unexpected.
    2. Physicians know when death will occur.
    3. An illness is terminal when no reasonable hope of recovery exists.
    4. All severe injuries result in death.
11. After the death of a patient, the nurse leaves the room quickly; she is found sobbing in the utility room. Which action is the most supportive to the nurse?
    1. Sending the nurse home for the rest of the shift
    2. Reassigning the nurse to an area where it is unlikely a patient will die
    3. Sitting with her and allowing her to express herself
    4. Insisting that she perform postmortem care for the patient
12. What type of care allows a patient to make more informed choices, achieve better alleviation of symptoms, and have more opportunity to work on issues such as closure?
    1. Acute care
    2. Mourning care
    3. Palliative care
    4. Terminal care
13. A healthy 25-year-old who sustained a head injury during a motor vehicle accident is in the emergency department. The patient has no brain activity and is on life support. The family has expressed an interest in organ donation. What should the nurse know about organ donations?
    1. Organ donations can occur only if the patient has given prior consent.
    2. Vital organs, such as the heart and pancreas, must be harvested while the patient remains on the ventilator.
    3. Brain death can be reversed, so the family should be informed to take more time in making their decision.
    4. The attending physician must be present in the operating room during harvesting of the organs.
14. A bereaved widow of 3 months tells the nurse she has smelled her deceased husband's aftershave scent clearly as she sat in church recently. She questions if she might be "going crazy." What is the widow experiencing?
    1. Intrusive memories
    2. Dysfunctional or complicated grief
    3. Sense of presence
    4. Grief attacks

15. The adult children of a dying patient, who is alert and oriented, disagree on the patient's choice of a do-not-resuscitate order. The children ask the opinion of the nurse, who has cared for this patient over an extended period. How should the nurse respond to this question about the patient's dying request?
    1. Encourage the children to speak with the physician regarding their concerns.
    2. Remind the children that this is the wish of their parent.
    3. Ask the patient to speak with the children regarding their concerns.
    4. Listen to the children's concerns and encourage them to talk to their parent.
16. A nurse is preparing to care for a dying patient, and several family members are at the bedside. Select the therapeutic techniques that the nurse uses when communicating with the family. *(Select all that apply.)*
    1. Be honest and truthful and let the patient and family know that the nurse will not abandon them.
    2. Explain everything that is happening to all family members.
    3. Encourage expression of feelings, concerns, and fears.
    4. Extend touch and hold the patient's or family member's hand if appropriate.
    5. Make the decisions for the family.
    6. Discourage reminiscing.
17. The nurse is providing postmortem care for a patient. Which interventions are appropriate before allowing the family to visit? *(Select all that apply.)*
    1. Prepare the body to look as clean and natural as possible.
    2. Wear sterile gloves to provide postmortem care.
    3. Keep the sheet cover over the patient's face until the family is comfortably seated in the room.
    4. Remove the external tubes and drains if there is no autopsy required.
    5. Call the health care provider to obtain an order to release the body to the mortician.
18. The nurse is caring for a dying patient. What are clinical signs of death? *(Select all that apply.)*
    1. Slow, thready pulse
    2. Absence of apical pulse
    3. Cessation of respirations
    4. Cessation of bowel sounds
    5. Flat encephalogram
19. The nurse is conducting an assessment on the dying patient. Which statement by the patient would indicate the patient is experiencing the stage of acceptance by Kübler-Ross?
    1. "I am helping my spouse plan my obituary and funeral."
    2. "I can do anything I want. I plan to live forever."
    3. "I promise I will do better for my family if I just could live a few more weeks."
    4. "This cannot be happening. I did not do anything to deserve this condition."
20. A young mother has just given birth to a boy born with severe birth defects. She states, "I feel so sad, I wanted a normal child. I do not want to see the baby." Which type of loss is the mother experiencing?
    1. Anticipatory loss
    2. Complicated loss
    3. Maturational loss
    4. Situational loss
21. The community hospice nurse is conducting a follow-up visit with the family 3 months after the death of a loved one. Which statement by the family member indicates that she is experiencing grief?
    1. "I really miss Charlie; it is hard to accept that he is gone."
    2. "I realize that Charlie is gone; I am adjusting to sleeping alone."
    3. "I was able to go on a date with a friend I met a couple of weeks ago."
    4. "I believe that Charlie would want me to move on with my life and meet new people."
22. The dying patient asks to nurse to assist him to say goodbye to his son, who is 4 years old. Which suggestion by the nurse is age appropriate for the 4-year-old?
    1. We could do a role play.
    2. You could read him a poem.
    3. Tell him you are going on a trip to heaven.
    4. You could write him a letter that he can read when he gets older.
23. A teenager brought by ambulance to the Emergency Room from the scene of a motor vehicular accident is pronounced dead upon arrival. The family is notified of the death and request to see their child before the funeral home picks up the body. Which actions by the nurse are most respectful when caring for the patient and family during a sudden death? *(Select all that apply.)*
    1. Preparing the body to look as clean and natural as possible
    2. Encouraging the parents to discuss what caused the accident
    3. Allowing the parents to spend as much time as possible with the body
    4. Leaving the body uncovered while it is being transferred to a quiet room
    5. Rushing the parents to say goodbye because it's almost time for a shift change
    6. Offering to call the pastor of the family's church while the family is viewing the body

Health Promotion and Pregnancy

26

http://evolve.elsevier.com/Cooper/foundationsadult/

Objectives

1. Explain the physiology of conception.
2. Discuss the anatomic and physiologic alterations that occur during pregnancy.
3. Identify the components of antepartal assessment.
4. Differentiate among the presumptive, possible, and positive signs of pregnancy.
5. List the danger signs that might occur during pregnancy.
6. Describe nutritional requirements during pregnancy.
7. Discuss the common discomforts of pregnancy.
8. Discuss cultural practices and beliefs that may affect ongoing health care during pregnancy.
9. Identify nursing diagnoses relevant to care of the prenatal patient.

Key Terms

abortion (ă-BŎR-shĕn, p. 762)
amniocentesis (ăm-nē-ō-sĕn-TĒ-sĭs, p. 775)
antepartal (ăn-tē-PĂR-tăl, p. 777)
ballottement (bă-LŎT-mĕnt, p. 779)
blastocyst (BLĂS-tō-sĭst, p. 762)
chorionic villi (kō-rē-ŎN-ĭk VĬL-ī, p. 762)
chorionic villus sampling (p. 774)
crown-rump length (p. 773)
ectoderm (ĔK-tō-dĕrm, p. 763)
ectopic pregnancy (ĕk-TŎP-ĭk PRĔG-năn-sē, p. 762)
endoderm (ĔN-dō-dĕrm, p. 763)
flagellation (flăj-ĕ-LĀ-shŭn, p. 762)
fundus (fŭn-dŭs, p. 771)
Goodell's sign (p. 778)
gravida (GRĂV-ĭ-dă, p. 780)
Hëgar's sign (p. 778)
implantation (p. 762)
intrapartal (p. 777)
lanugo (lă-NŪ-gō, p. 771)
mesoderm (MĔZ-ō-dĕrm, p. 763)
morula (MŎR-ū-lă, p. 762)
nuchal translucency screening (p. 774)
para (p. 780)
perinatal (p. 777)
postpartal (p. 777)
prenatal (p. 777)
relaxin (p. 784)
teratogenic agents (tĕr-ă-tō-JĔN-ĭk Ā-gĕnts, p. 763)
trimesters (p. 777)
ultrasonography (ŭl-tră-sŏ-NŎG-ră-fē, p. 773)
villi (VĬL-ī, p. 762)
Wharton's jelly (p. 763)
zygote (ZĪ-gōt, p. 762)

Few experiences in life are as exciting and as challenging as childbearing. Profound and dramatic changes occur in a relatively short time. Childbearing is a challenge to the new mother, to the newly developing or changing family unit, to society, and to the nurse who assists in the childbearing process. The maternity nurse is in a unique position of providing care to the unborn.

The goal of maternity care is a healthy pregnancy with a physically safe and emotionally satisfying outcome for mother and infant. Consistent health supervision and surveillance are paramount. Many pregnant women and their families are unfamiliar with the changes that accompany pregnancy. The knowledgeable maternity nurse can help a pregnant woman recognize the relationship between her physical status and her care plan. Sharing information encourages the pregnant woman to participate in her own care, depending on her interest, need to know, and readiness to learn.

PHYSIOLOGY OF PREGNANCY

Understanding the physiologic changes of pregnancy begins with understanding the normal anatomy and physiology of the male and female reproductive systems. A review of the menstrual cycle and related hormonal activity is particularly important. Also important is recognition that specific cells (ova in the female and sperm in the male) carry genetic messages to their offspring. These cells are united to form a new individual with a unique genetic makeup.

FERTILIZATION

During sexual intercourse, sperm carried in the male's ejaculatory semen enter the female's vagina. By **flagellation** (whiplike movement), the sperm travel through the mucus of the cervical canal (if the mucus is receptive), enter the uterine chamber, and move into the ampulla, the outer third of the fallopian tube. If the timing is right, an ovum has been produced and is also within the ampulla of the tube; in such cases, fertilization may occur. Fertilization (also called *conception*) takes place when the sperm joins or fuses with the ovum. The fusion of the sperm into the ovum requires approximately 24 hours. Once fertilization has occurred, the new cell is referred to as a **zygote** (cell formed by the union of two reproductive cells) or a fertilized ovum. This cell carries 46 chromosomes (44 autosomes and 2 sex chromosomes). At the moment of fertilization, the sex of the zygote and all other genetic characteristics are determined and do not change.

IMPLANTATION

The zygote moves through the uterine tube via ciliary action and some irregular peristaltic activity. It takes 3 or 4 days to enter the uterine cavity. During this time, the zygote is in a phase of rapid cell division called *mitosis.* Further changes result in formation of a structure called the **morula** (developmental stage of the fertilized ovum in which a solid mass of cells resembles a mulberry), which develops into the **blastocyst** (the embryonic form; a spherical mass of cells with a central fluid-filled cavity surrounded by two layers of cells). Stem cells are derived from the inner cell mass of the blastocyst (Box 26.1). After the blastocyst is free in the uterine cavity for 1 or 2 days, the exposed cell walls of the blastocyst (called the *trophoblast*) secrete enzymes that can break down protein and penetrate cell membranes. These enzymes allow the blastocyst to enter the endometrium and implant. The action of the enzymes normally stops short of the myometrium but may cause slight bleeding in some individuals. This is called *implantation bleeding.* Although this bleeding is rarely more than spotting, it may confuse some women, who think that they had a very light and short menstrual cycle, when actually they are pregnant.

The condition of the uterine lining is critical for **implantation** (embedding of the fertilized ovum in the uterine mucosa) of the zygote. During the secretory phase of the menstrual cycle, the endometrium has an enriched vascular bed with enlarged blood vessels and an increased store of glycogen, which support development of the embryo if implantation occurs. Implantation usually occurs in the fundus of the uterus on either the anterior or the posterior surfaces. If uterine conditions are not suitable, implantation is unlikely to occur. If intrauterine vascular or hormonal conditions cannot sustain the implanted embryo, a spontaneous abortion occurs. **Abortion** is the medical term used to refer to the loss of a pregnancy before 20 weeks' gestation. Most spontaneous abortions occur during the first 8 weeks of pregnancy for these reasons. **Ectopic pregnancy** is a serious condition that refers to the implantation of the fertilized egg outside of the uterine cavity. These conditions are discussed further in Chapter 29.

During the first few weeks after implantation, primary **villi** (short vascular processes or protrusions that grow on certain membranous surfaces) appear. These villi use maternal blood vessels as a source of nourishment and oxygen for the developing embryo. The villi nourish the embryo from the time of implantation (about 2 weeks after conception) until the seventh or eighth week. Also during these first few weeks, the first stages of the **chorionic villi** (tiny vascular protrusions on the chorionic surface that project into the maternal blood sinuses of the uterus and help form the placenta) occur. Chorionic villi secrete human chorionic gonadotropin (HCG), a hormone that stimulates the continued production of progesterone and estrogen by the corpus luteum, which is the reason ovulation and menstruation cease during pregnancy. Primary villi also synthesize protein and glucose for approximately 12 weeks, until the fetus is developed adequately to meet its own needs. The chorionic villi become the fetal portion of the placenta.

Box 26.1 Stem Cells

Stem cells can divide for indefinite periods and can differentiate into the many different types of cells that make up an organism. Embryonic stem cells are derived from the blastocyst before it implants in the uterine wall. A zygote is described as *totipotent* because it has the potential to produce all the cells and tissues that compose an embryo and to support its in utero development. The term *pluripotent* is used to describe stem cells that generate cells derived from the three embryonic germ layers: endoderm, mesoderm, and ectoderm. The embryonic stem cell is pluripotent.

Human stem cells were derived and maintained for the first time in 1988 by Thomson and colleagues, with use of blastocysts donated by couples undergoing in vitro fertilization. Potential uses of human embryonic stem cells include transplant therapy, in which tissues damaged by disease or injury are replaced or restored, as in diabetes, Parkinson's disease, heart disease, and multiple sclerosis. Stem cell research raises ethical concerns related to the source of human embryonic stem cells (embryos left over from in vitro fertilization and aborted fetuses).

On May 9, 2009, President Obama lifted an 8-year ban on embryonic stem cell research, calling it "an important step in advancing the cause of science in America."

Data from National Institutes of Health: Stem cells: Scientific progress and future research directions, 2001, Department of Health and Human Services. Retrieved from *http://stemcells.nih.gov/info;* Hockenberry MJ, Wilson D: *Wong's maternal-child nursing care,* ed 8, St. Louis, 2007, Mosby; and Lite J: Obama ends embryonic stem cell research ban. Retrieved from *www.scientificamerican.com/blog/60-second-science/post.cfm?id=obama-ends-embryonic-stem-cell-rese-2009-03-09.*

EMBRYONIC AND FETAL DEVELOPMENT

Until the time of implantation (the germinal phase), the cell mass is referred to as the zygote. During this period, the fertilized ovum develops from the two original cells into a many-celled organism. When the growing mass of cells reaches about 32 cells, it is referred to as a morula. As the cells continue to divide, they separate into an inner group of cells and an outer group of cells. This stage is referred to as the blastocyst. The inner cells become the embryo. The zygote develops two separate and distinct cavities: the amniotic cavity and the yolk sac. The amniotic cavity has walls lined with the **ectoderm** (outer layer of embryonic tissue that gives rise to skin, nails, and hair) and is filled with amniotic fluid. The yolk sac is lined with the **endoderm** (the innermost of the cell layers, which develop into the lining of cavities and passages of the body and the covering of most internal organs). The yolk sac supplies nourishment until implantation. A third layer of primary cells, the **mesoderm** (embryonic middle layer of germ cells that gives rise to all types of muscles, connective tissue, bone marrow, blood, lymphoid tissue, and all epithelial tissue), is located between the two cavities. The embryo develops at the point at which these three layers meet, called the *trilaminar embryonic disk.*

The embryonic stage begins with implantation and encompasses approximately the first 8 weeks of pregnancy. During the embryonic stage, the three primary cell layers differentiate into tissue and layers, which form the placenta, embryonic membranes, and the embryo. Cell growth is rapid. A simple heart begins beating, and rudimentary (basic, initial, or primary) forms of all the major organs and systems develop. By the end of this stage, the embryo has acquired a human appearance. Starting with the ninth week, the embryo is referred to as the *fetus,* and the fetal stage begins. (See Chapter 32 and Fig. 32.1 for fetal circulation.)

Many structures develop simultaneously in the embryo; therefore, when an infant is born with one birth defect or abnormality, the physician checks for others that may be associated with the identified defect. During the early weeks of pregnancy, often before a woman even knows that she is pregnant, **teratogenic agents** (any drug, virus, or substance that can cause malformation of the fetus) can cause serious harm. For example, rubella, or German measles, is a known *teratogen* (a nongenetic factor that causes malformations and disease syndromes in utero). Although rubella is usually a mild childhood disease, at this stage of pregnancy, the virus can affect all of the germ layers and cause serious anomalies, such as cardiac defects, deafness, and cognitive impairment.

The prenatal calendar (Table 26.1) describes fetal development and maternal changes throughout pregnancy.

EMBRYONIC AND FETAL PHYSIOLOGY

Placenta

The *placenta* (Greek, "flat plate") is a disklike organ made up of about 20 sections called *cotyledons.* It is a unique structure, present only during pregnancy. The placenta becomes fully functioning by week 12. At full term, the placenta looks like a large red disk with a diameter of 8 inches (20 cm) and a thickness of 1 inch (2.5 cm). It normally weighs between 1 lb and 1 lb 5 oz (450 and 600 g). The bulk of the placenta is fetal in origin. The side attached to the uterine wall ("Dirty Duncan") appears dark red and has a rough surface; the cotyledons are apparent as distinct lobes with clefts or divisions between each lobe. Presentation of the Duncan side after delivery is associated with blood expulsion with the placenta. The fetal side is smooth and shiny ("Shiny Schultze"). It consists of the membranes of the amniotic sac that encases the fetus. A small gush of blood precedes the placenta when the Schultze side is presenting. On delivery, the placenta is assessed and the presenting side determined; then the placenta is examined for intactness. The findings are documented.

As mentioned, the placenta functions as an endocrine gland that secretes HCG and the steroidal hormones estrogen and progesterone, which maintain the pregnancy. In addition, the placenta is the site of the exchange of nutrients, oxygen, and waste products between the fetus and the maternal circulation. The placenta allows transfer of oxygen and nutrients through such processes as diffusion and active transport, and it also blocks the transfer of certain substances. This is called the placental barrier. Some viruses can cross the placental barrier, but most bacteria are too large to cross. Some drugs do not cross the placenta, but most do and can cause serious harm to the growing embryo or fetus. After delivery, the placenta is of no further use and is expelled.

Fetal Membranes

The amniotic sac is composed of two layers, both of which originate in the zygote. The outer layer, the *chorion,* attaches to the fetal portion of the placenta. The inner layer, the *amnion,* blends with the fetal umbilical cord. These membranes appear fragile, but in fact they are strong enough to contain the fetus and amniotic fluid even at full term.

Umbilical Cord

The umbilical cord joins the embryo to the placenta. It originates in the fetal portion of the placenta and normally is attached near the center. The cord is typically 20 to 22 inches (50 to 55 cm) long and less than 1 inch (2.5 cm) in diameter at the time of delivery. Umbilical cords can vary widely in appearance. The major part of the cord is a pale white, gelatinous-mucoid substance called **Wharton's jelly** (a gelatinous tissue that remains when the embryonic body stalk blends with the yolk sac within the umbilical cord). This substance prevents compression of the blood vessels and aids in insulating the vessels within the umbilical cord. The normal umbilical cord has two arteries and one vein that may give the cord a ropelike appearance. On occasion, the

Text continued on p. 771

Table 26.1 **Fetal Development and Maternal Events During Pregnancy and Drug Substances to Avoid**

WEEK 1	WEEK 2	WEEK 3	WEEK 4	WEEK 5	WEEK 6	WEEK 7	WEEK 8
Embryonic Development							
The ovum becomes fertilized, divides, and burrows into the uterus.	The embryonic disk (ectoderm, endoderm, mesoderm) is formed. These three primitive germ layers generate every organ and tissue in the infant's body.	The first body segments appear; they eventually form the primitive spine, brain, and spinal cord.	Heart, blood circulation, and digestive tract take shape. The embryo is now 0.2 inch long; the head is a third of its total length.	The heart starts to pump blood; limb buds appear. Major divisions of the brain can now be discerned.	Eyes begin to take shape; external ears develop from skin folds.	Development proceeds rapidly. The face is now complete, with eyes, nose, lips, and tongue—even primitive milk teeth. Tiny bones and muscles appear beneath the thin skin.	The embryo is now a little more than 1 inch long.
Maternal Events							
Ovaries increase production of the pregnancy-maintaining hormone, progesterone.	The first period is missed.	Placenta grows to cover $\frac{1}{15}$ of the uterine interior. Breasts may begin to feel tender. There is no weight gain.			Exchange of fetal and maternal metabolites across the placenta begins, yet the two circulations are completely separate.	No noticeable weight gain occurs.	The placenta now covers about one-third of the uterine lining.

Common Maternal Discomforts	Remedies
• Morning sickness occurs because increased hormonal activity slows down the digestive system, apparently to enhance the absorption of nutrients for the baby.	Eat a few dry crackers before rising. Eat frequent, small, low-fat meals during the day. Drink liquids.
• Fatigue is thought to be caused by a change in ovarian hormone production (progesterone and relaxin), the purpose of which is to relax pelvic ligaments, stimulate breast growth, and soften the cervix.	Exercise regularly and get plenty of sleep with frequent naps during the day.
• Urinary frequency is caused by the uterus compressing the bladder against the pelvic bones, thus reducing its capacity, and by hormonal changes that affect the water balance in the body.	Decrease pressure on the bladder at night by sleeping on the side.
Drug Substances to Avoid	**Acceptable Alternatives**
• Antiemetics: Most traditionally used antiemetic medications are avoided during pregnancy.	Doxylamine succinate (Diclegis) a prescribed medication to manage nausea and vomiting in pregnancy.
• Stimulants: amphetamines, excessive caffeine. *(Avoid throughout pregnancy.)*	

WEEK 9	WEEK 10	WEEK 11	WEEK 12	WEEK 13	WEEK 14	WEEK 15	WEEK 16
Embryonic and Fetal Development							
Genitalia are now well defined; the baby's sex is determined. Eyelids finish forming and seal shut. The embryo becomes a fetus.	The fetus assumes a more human shape as the lower body rapidly develops. Blood and bone cells form. The first movements begin.	Organs begin to function. The pancreas produces insulin; the kidneys produce urine.	The lungs have taken shape; primitive breathing motions begin. The swallowing reflex has been mastered as the fetus sucks its thumb while floating weightlessly in the amniotic fluid.		The musculoskeletal system has matured. The nervous system begins to exercise some control over the body; blood vessels rapidly develop.	With hands ready to grasp, the fetus, now weighing about 7 oz, kicks against the amniotic sac.	All organs and structures have been formed, and a period of growth begins.

Continued

Table 26.1 Fetal Development and Maternal Events During Pregnancy and Drug Substances to Avoid—cont'd

WEEK 9	WEEK 10	WEEK 11	WEEK 12	WEEK 13	WEEK 14	WEEK 15	WEEK 16
Maternal Events							
Maternal blood volume has increased 30%–40%.	Some women describe the sensation of these first movements as if something were blowing bubbles through a straw in their stomachs.	There is a 2- to 3-lb weight gain and a possible increase in perspiration.	The placenta has reached complete functional maturity, acting as the baby's lungs, kidneys, liver, and digestive and immune systems.		There is a 3- to 4-lb weight gain, and her belly begins to show.		Placenta begins producing the estrogen hormone.

Common Maternal Discomforts	Remedies
• Sleeplessness may result from the discomfort or anxieties of pregnancy.	Take warm shower before sleeping. Support body parts with pillows.
• Vaginal secretions are the result of an increased supply of blood and glucose to the vaginal mucosa. Severe pruritus, irritation, and malodor suggest infection. If infection is suspected, consult a professional.	Cleanse daily with warm water, keeping the area dry to prevent chafing. Apply yogurt for vulvar pruritus.
• Headaches may occur while her body adjusts to changes in blood volume and vascular tone. Emotional tension may also be a factor.	Change body positions slowly. Resting with a damp cloth on the forehead may help. Drink milk or eat a small snack to obtain some relief.
Drug Substances to Avoid	**Acceptable Alternatives**
• Tranquilizers, narcotics, antihistamines, alcohol, barbiturates *(Avoid throughout pregnancy.)*	None
• Vaginal antiinfectives may be employed in pregnancy but options such as metronidazole are avoided.	Nystatin, miconazole, and clortrimazole
• Avoid x-rays.	None
• Analgesics: salicylates (aspirin), phenacetin-caffeine, indomethacin (Indocin), tranquilizers. *(Avoid throughout pregnancy.)*	Acetaminophen

WEEK 17	WEEK 18	WEEK 19	WEEK 20	WEEK 21	WEEK 22	WEEK 23	WEEK 24
Fetal Development							
	An oily coating protects the fetus. Fine hair covers the body and keeps the oil on the skin.	Eyebrows, eyelashes, and head hair develop.	The fetus is now following a regular schedule of sleeping, turning, sucking, and kicking and has settled on a favorite position in the uterus.		The skeleton is developing rapidly as the bone-forming cells increase their activity.	Eyelids begin to open and close.	The fetus now weighs about 27 oz.
Maternal Events							
	There is a 3- to 4-lb weight gain. The fetal heartbeat can now be heard with an amplified stethoscope.	Breasts begin secreting colostrum in preparation for nursing.	Placenta reaches its largest size relative to fetus, covering half the uterine lining. The amniotic sac contains 400 mL of fluid.		There is a 3- to 4-lb weight gain.		The placenta becomes thicker rather than wider. Mother can now sense when baby is awake.

Continued

Table 26.1 Fetal Development and Maternal Events During Pregnancy and Drug Substances to Avoid—cont'd

WEEK 17	WEEK 18	WEEK 19	WEEK 20	WEEK 21	WEEK 22	WEEK 23	WEEK 24
Common Maternal Discomforts				**Remedies**			
• Faintness or dizziness occurs when standing suddenly, caused by reduced blood flow to the brain as the body adjusts to new circulatory patterns. Shortness of breath may occur.				Try to sit with feet up when possible; rise slowly and support yourself. Smelling salts, aromatic spirits of ammonia.			
• Varicose veins are often the result of rising blood pressure in the lower extremities. This is caused by the enlarged uterus cutting off blood flow back from the legs to the heart.				When sitting, rest legs on footstool with feet elevated; avoid pressure on lower thighs. Many women find support stockings helpful.			
• Allergies, such as hay fever, are a common problem.				Use air conditioning (with a clean filter) and wear a pollen mask to screen out allergens.			
• Skin changes such as darkened nipples, stretch marks, splotches on cheeks and forehead, acne, and redness on palms and soles are the result of increased hormone levels in the blood.				Be patient. Virtually all of these effects subside soon after childbirth. If nipples or abdomen itch, a lanolin-based cream or baby oil can provide relief.			
• Epistaxis sometimes occurs because of increased blood volume and nasal congestion.				Apply a little petroleum jelly in each nostril, which should stop the bleeding. Use a humidifier. Do not irritate nasal mucosa.			
Drug Substances to Avoid				**Acceptable Alternatives**			
• Tranquilizers, alcohol *(Avoid throughout pregnancy.)*				None			
• Traditionally antihistamines have been largely avoided in pregnancy.				Chlorpheniramine for congestion; pseudoephedrine or nasal spray for stuffy nose may be used occasionally, if necessary; calamine lotion for rashes.			
• Tetracycline (for acne) *(Avoid throughout pregnancy.)*				A mild soap can remove the excessive facial oil produced by acne.			
WEEK 25	**WEEK 26**	**WEEK 27**	**WEEK 28**	**WEEK 29**	**WEEK 30**	**WEEK 31**	**WEEK 32**
Fetal Development							
	To a certain extent, the fetus can now breathe, swallow, and regulate its body temperature, but it still depends greatly on maternal support.	A substance called surfactant forms in the lungs, preparing them to function independently after birth.	Fetus is two-thirds grown.	Fat deposits are building up beneath the skin to insulate the fetus against the abrupt change in temperature at birth.	The digestive tract and the lungs are now nearly fully matured, and the skin becomes less red and wrinkled.	The fetus has grown to about 14 inches.	

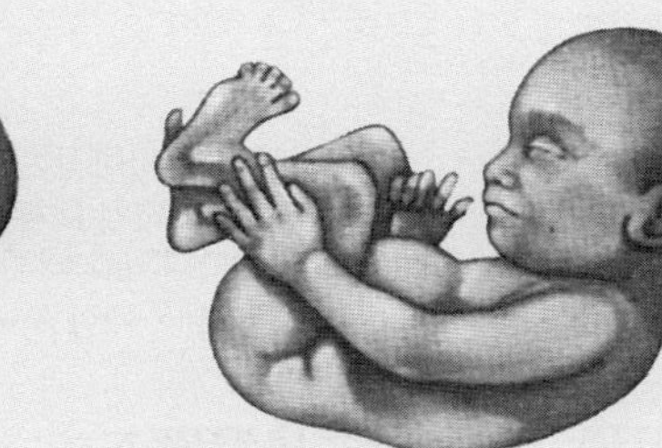

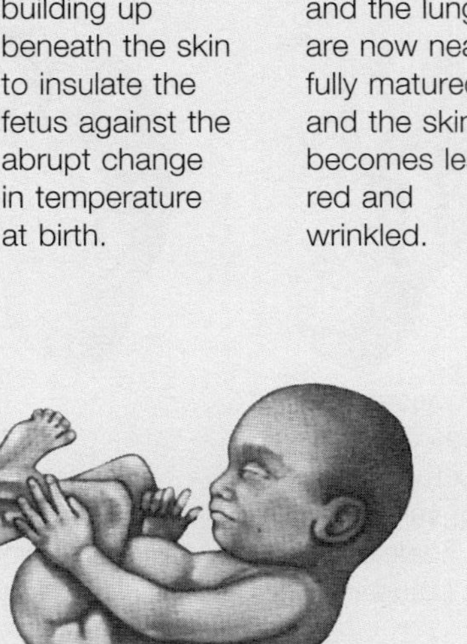

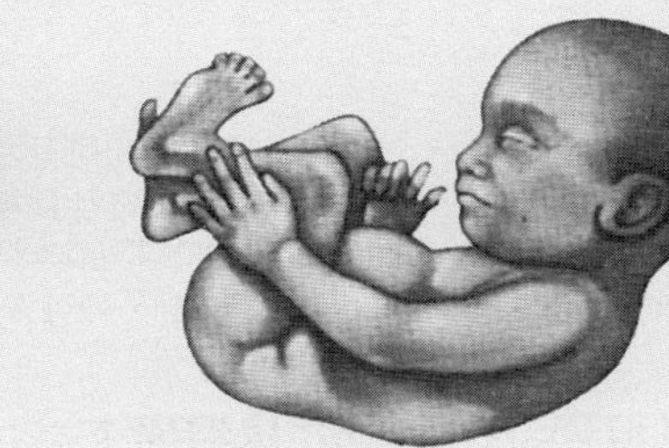

Maternal Events							
	There is a 3- to 4-lb weight gain.	Respiratory movements can be detected with ultrasound scan. Mother sometimes feels baby's breathing as "hiccups."	The volume of amniotic fluid decreases to make room for growing fetus.		There is a 3- to 5-lb weight gain.		

Common Maternal Discomforts	Remedies
• Leg and muscle cramps may be caused by fatigue, pressure exerted on the nerves by the uterus, or too little calcium or too much phosphorus in the diet.	Exercise regularly, especially walking. Elevate legs and flex toes when resting. Increase milk consumption.
• Pyrosis (heartburn) often occurs because the stomach emptying time is delayed, causing a burning sensation in the throat.	Drink milk between small, frequent meals. This problem disappears soon after the baby's birth.
• Edema of ankles occurs. The pressure of the uterus on the large veins returning blood to the heart may induce water retention.	Elevate legs, once or twice a day for an hour or so, level with the hips. Sleep on the left side.
• Constipation is another result of the decelerated digestive process. As food moves slowly through the intestines, more water is extracted, leaving the stool drier and harder.	Eat foods that contain roughage, such as raw fruits, vegetables, and cereals with bran. Drink liquids and exercise frequently.
• Mother may have trouble sleeping because of baby's activity.	Soak in a warm bath or sit on soft pillows to soothe the symptoms.
• Hemorrhoids may develop.	Dibucaine (Nupercainal) suppositories or cream, hydrocortisone (Anusol), benzocaine (Medicone)
Drug Substances to Avoid	**Acceptable Alternatives**
• Salicylates (aspirin), tranquilizers *(Avoid throughout pregnancy.)*	Calcium supplements with little or no phosphorus
• Antacids: calcium carbonate, magnesium trisilicate (Gaviscon), sodium bicarbonate (baking soda), cimetidine (Tagamet) *(Avoid throughout pregnancy.)*	Maalox, Mylanta (also for "gas")
• Most diuretics ("water pills") *(Avoid throughout pregnancy.)*	
• Laxatives: mineral oil, castor oil *(Avoid throughout pregnancy.)*	Metamucil, Senokot, teaspoon of Milk of Magnesia at bedtime

Continued

Table 26.1 Fetal Development and Maternal Events During Pregnancy and Drug Substances to Avoid—cont'd

WEEK 33	TO TERM	
Fetal Development		
Virtually the entire uterus is now occupied by the fetus, and its activity is restricted.	Maternal antibodies against measles, mumps, rubella, whooping cough, and scarlet fever are transferred to the baby, providing protection for about 6 mo until the infant's own immune system can take over.	
Maternal Events		
The placenta is nearly four times as thick as it was 20 wk before and weighs about 20 oz.	Preparing for birth, the fetus descends deeper into the mother's pelvis. There is a 3- to 5-lb weight gain.	In 9 mo, the miracle is complete; a single, microscopic fertilized cell has transformed into a 6 trillion–celled human.
Common Maternal Discomforts	**Remedies**	
• Backaches are often caused by muscles and ligaments relaxing in preparation for the stretching required in delivery and by the added off-center weight of the enlarged uterus.	Do back exercises, such as the "pelvic tilt," which can help strengthen back and abdominal muscles. Wear low-heeled shoes or flats; avoid heavy lifting.	
• Urinary frequency is caused (for the second time in pregnancy) by the uterus compressing the bladder against the pelvic bones, thus reducing its capacity.	Decrease pressure on the bladder at night by sleeping on your side. Urinate frequently.	
• Uterine contractions become perceptible as the cervix and lower uterine segment prepare for labor.		
Drug Substances to Avoid	**Acceptable Alternatives**	
• Analgesics: salicylates (aspirin), propoxyphene (Darvon), phenacetin-caffeine, indomethacin (Indocin), codeine *(Avoid throughout pregnancy.)*	Tylenol brand acetaminophen (occasional use)	

Figures from Lowdermilk DL, Perry SE: *Maternity and women's health care,* ed 9, St. Louis, 2007, Mosby.

cord has only two vessels, one artery and one vein. This phenomenon is seen in less than 3% of deliveries. It may be associated with fetal anomalies and requires follow-up. The vein carries oxygenated blood to the fetus; the arteries carry deoxygenated blood back to the placenta. The cord has no pain receptors, so cutting at the time of delivery does not cause pain.

Amniotic Fluid

Amniotic fluid surrounds the fetus in utero. It begins production early in the pregnancy and is present in increasing amounts. Approximately 30 mL (1 oz) are present at 10 to 12 weeks' gestation. The peak volume is noted around 34 weeks' gestation at approximately 800 to 1000 mL. The amniotic fluid has several important functions for the fetus. It acts as a cushion against mechanical injury; helps regulate fetal temperature; allows the developing embryo or fetus room for growth, which promotes musculoskeletal development; and provides for fetal lung development. The fluid is clear yellow with a slightly alkaline pH. Amniotic fluid contains albumin, urea, uric acid, creatinine, bilirubin, *lecithin* (phospholipids for fat metabolism), *sphingomyelin* (a compound of lipids and sphingosine, found in high concentrations in the brain and other tissues of the nervous system), fructose, fat, leukocytes, proteins, epithelial cells, enzymes, and strands of **lanugo** (downy, fine hair found on the fetus from 20 weeks' gestation until birth). Amniocentesis (discussed subsequently) can be done after the first trimester of pregnancy to aid in determination of fetal development, maturity, health, and gender.

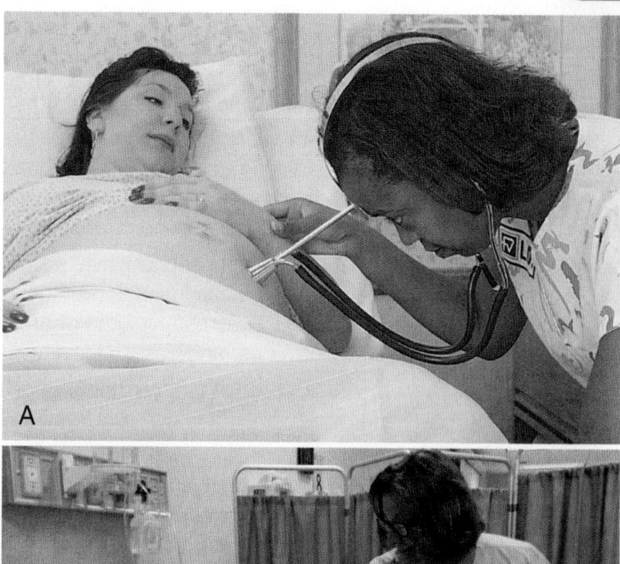

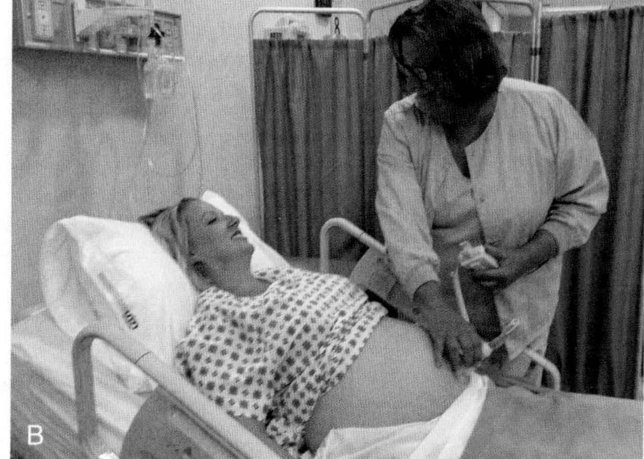

Fig. 26.1 Detecting fetal heartbeat. A, Fetoscope (18–20 wk). B, Doppler ultrasound stethoscope (12 wk). (A, From McKinney ES, James SR, Murray SS: *Maternal-child nursing*, ed 4, St. Louis, 2013, Saunders.)

ASSESSMENT OF FETAL WELL-BEING

A variety of technological and assessment tools can be used in evaluation of fetal well-being. These tools are used to evaluate maternal and fetal health problems, fetal congenital anomalies, and fetal growth and maturity (Table 26.2).

Fetal Heart Tones

The fetal heart shows activity by the seventh week of gestation. Practitioners can auscultate fetal heart tones between 10 and 12 weeks with Doppler scan (Fig. 26.1). To hear the fetal heart tones (FHTs), place the instrument in the midline, just above the symphysis pubis, and apply firm pressure. Some difficulty may be encountered in locating FHTs in obese women during the early stages. Offer the woman and her family the opportunity to listen to the FHTs. FHTs are to be assessed for a full minute. The rate and characteristics of the tones should be evaluated. FHTs are assessed at each of the expectant mother's visits for the remainder of the pregnancy.

Fundal Height

During the second trimester, the growing uterus rises from the pelvic cavity and becomes an abdominal organ. The top portion of the uterus is referred to as the **fundus.** The fundal height, or measurement of the height of the uterus above the symphysis pubis, is one indicator of fetal growth. McDonald's method is used commonly. The measurement also provides a gross estimate of the duration of pregnancy. When the fundal height is measured, the woman should be lying flat. Her bladder should be emptied. A paper tape measure or a pelvimeter may be used to measure fundal height. For increased reliability of the measurement, the same person should examine the pregnant woman at each of her prenatal visits. Often this is not possible, so a protocol should be established that specifies the measurement technique, including the woman's position on the examining table, the measuring device, and the method of measurement used (Fig. 26.2).

During the second and third trimesters (weeks 18 to 30), the height of the fundus in centimeters is approximately the same as the number of weeks of gestation. Some maternal characteristics may affect the accuracy of the measurement (Box 26.2). The measurement of fundal height may aid in identification of high-risk factors. A stable or decreased fundal height may indicate intrauterine growth restriction (IUGR); an excessive increase could indicate multifetal gestation or hydramnios (excessive amniotic fluid).

Human Chorionic Gonadotropin Levels

HCG is the hormone assessed in pregnancy tests. This hormone can be detected in urine and blood. Testing for

Table 26.2 Assessment Tools to Evaluate Fetal Well-Being

Diagnostic Test or Assessment Tool	Description and Purpose	Gestational Age
Transvaginal ultrasound	High-frequency sound waves visualize fetus to help determine gestational age, visualize number of fetuses and location of placenta, estimate volume of amniotic fluid, note presence of anomalies.	Performed up to the 12th week of pregnancy.
Abdominal ultrasound	High-frequency sound waves to visualize the fetus. Used to assess gestational age, number of fetuses, presentation of fetus, estimate volume of amniotic fluid, assess for anomalies, and assess location of placenta.	Performed throughout the pregnancy.
Maternal serum alpha-fetoprotein (AFP) screening	Assessment of four elements to assess for the potential probability of Down syndrome or neural tube defects.	Performed between 16 and 18 weeks' gestation.
Chorionic villus sampling (CVS)	Aspiration of small amount of tissue from the villi of the placenta. It may be performed transabdominally or transcervically.	Performed between 10 and 13 weeks' gestation.
Amniocentesis	Aspiration of small amount of amniotic fluid to reveal sex and chromosomal abnormalities, health status, and maturity of fetus.	May be performed as early as the 16th week of gestation and onward.
Nuchal translucency testing	Employs an ultrasound to assess the nuchal thickness of the fetus. Thicknesses greater than 2.5 mm are suspicious and may signal Down syndrome.	Performed between 10 and 13 weeks' gestation.
Nonstress test (NST)	Fetal movement and fetal heart rate recorded with external fetal monitors to evaluate the response of the fetal heart rate to fetal movement. The mother notes when movements are felt. This is reviewed in correlation to the fetal heart rates.	Performed from 28 weeks' gestation onward.
Contraction stress test (CST)	Contractions are simulated by nipple stimulation or the administration of oxytocin. The fetal heart rate is reviewed in relation to the contractions. Declines in heart rate at the midpoint or after of the contraction indicate the need for follow-up.	Performed after 32nd week of pregnancy with stimulation of uterine contractions.
Magnetic resonance imaging (MRI)	Noninvasive tool provides images of soft tissue. Vascular structures within the body may be seen without the use of iodinated contrast medium, without biologic risk. Interference from skeletal, fatty, or gas-filled structures is not a problem as it is in ultrasound scan.	May be performed throughout the pregnancy.
Biophysical profile (BPP)	Assesses the adequacy of the uterine environment to support the pregnancy. It applies a score to fetal breathing movements, fetal muscle tone, fetal movements, amniotic fluid volume, and an evaluation of the NST.	Normally performed after 32 weeks' gestation but can be considered as early as 24 weeks' gestation if fetal compromise is suggested.
Daily fetal movement count (DFMC; kick count)	Measurement of fetal movement as an indicator of fetal health. Advantages of the test include that it is simple, low cost, noninvasive, and fast. Instruct woman to count fetal movements for 1 hour two or three times daily. No exact number of movements has been identified as a "failing test." However, fewer than three fetal movements in a 1-hour period or the absence of fetal movements for 12 hour is an indication for further evaluation (see the Patient Teaching box on guidelines for counting fetal movements).	Daily fetal movement count can be done to evaluate the fetus in high-risk pregnancies for complications related to reduced oxygenation.

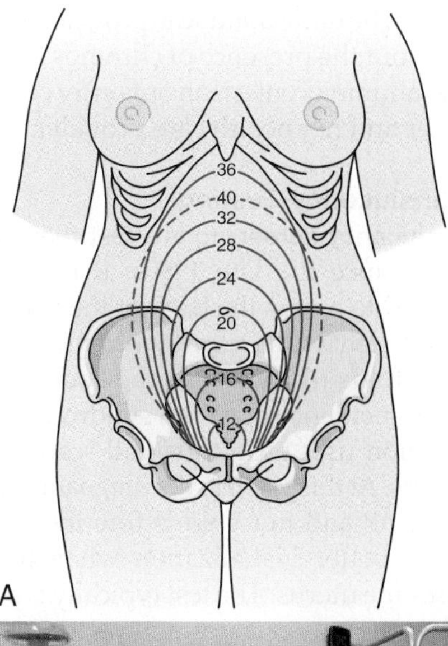

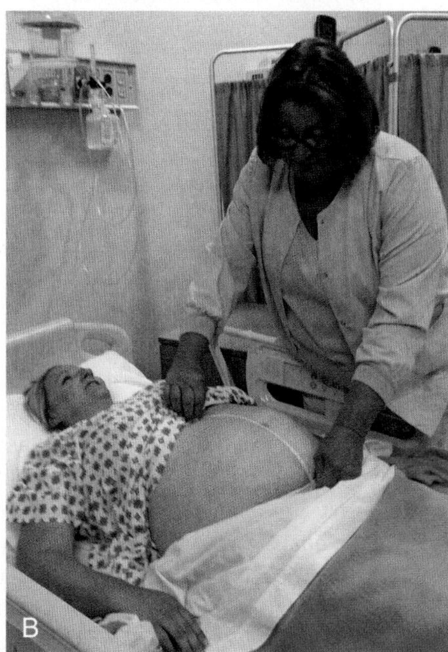

Fig. 26.2 A, Measurement of fundal height. B, McDonald's method.

Box 26.2 Factors That Influence Fundal Height Measurement

- Maternal position
- Maternal stature
- Maternal obesity
- Presence of uterine fibroids
- Elevations in amniotic fluid volume

Data from Davidson M, London M, Ladewig P: *Olds' maternal-newborn nursing and women's health across the lifespan,* ed 9, Upper Saddle River, NJ, 2010, Pearson.

HCG can be quantitative or qualitative. Quantitative testing considers the level or amount of the hormone in the specimen. Quantitative results are obtained from a blood specimen. Qualitative testing simply determines the presence or absence of a substance. Qualitative testing for HCG may be performed on the blood and the urine. During pregnancy, the levels of HCG may be used to assess the viability and gestation of the pregnancy. HCG levels that are less than anticipated for a specific point in gestation may signal a pregnancy that is no longer viable. Quantitative HCG levels may be reported every few days to determine whether they are rising as in a normally developing pregnancy or whether they are declining in a manner consistent with miscarriage.

Ultrasound Scan

During **ultrasonography,** high-frequency sound waves are used to visualize the fetus. Because soft tissue is visualized, this noninvasive tool can be used to determine gestational age, monitor fetal growth, determine the number of fetuses and the location of the placenta, estimate the volume of amniotic fluid, and detect anomalies. It also can be used in conjunction with invasive tests such as amniocentesis. The gestational age often determines the type of ultrasound scan performed. When used to determine the gestational age, the health care provider performs a series of measurements. In the first trimester, the fetal crown-rump length is used. **Crown-rump length** is the measurement from the top of the fetal head to the buttocks. This recording is correct within 2 to 5 days. As the pregnancy progresses and the fetal positioning changes, this becomes an ineffective means to measure gestational age. In the second trimester, the examiner measures fetal head circumference, biparietal diameter, and femur length to calculate gestational age. The degree of accuracy is 4 to 9 days. Estimation of fetal age in the third trimester is even less accurate because of a variety of interrelated factors that include genetics, gender differences, and maternal-related concerns (Behrman and Butler, 2007). During the first trimester, the transvaginal ultrasound scan may be used. The small distance between the probe, which is inserted vaginally, and the uterus makes the transvaginal ultrasound scan a prime tool for assessment of the early pregnancy (Gabbe, 2012) to confirm the presence and viability of the pregnancy.

After the first trimester, the abdominal ultrasound scan is preferred. It may be used singularly or in conjunction with other methods of maternal fetal assessment. Early in pregnancy, the mother is required to drink a quart of water and not void. This allows for the bladder to elevate the uterus for better viewing with the technology.

A growing number of nurses perform ultrasound scans and biophysical profiles (BPPs; a system of estimating current fetal status by analyzing five variables via ultrasound scan and nonstress testing). However, most nurses are involved primarily in counseling and educating women about the procedure (see the Patient Teaching box on ultrasound scan examination).

Maternal Serum Alpha-Fetoprotein Screening (Quadruple Marker Screening)

Maternal serum alpha-fetoprotein screening is referred to commonly as the quadruple marker screening. The assessment is a screening with results that provide a prediction for the occurrence of certain birth defects. The results do not provide a definitive diagnosis or

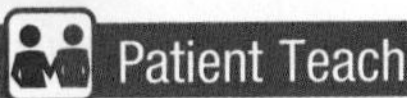

Patient Teaching

Preparing for Ultrasound Scan Examination

Inform the woman that she needs a full bladder for an abdominal ultrasound scan to allow better imaging of the fetus. Position her comfortably, with pillows under her head and knees, while the test is conducted. Apply ultrasonic gel to the abdomen and pass the scanner over it while images are reproduced. The woman and her partner can watch if they wish. The woman should not feel any discomfort.

For a transvaginal ultrasound scan, tell the woman that she may either be in a lithotomy position or have her pelvis elevated. These positions are optimal for imaging the pelvic structures. Introduce a transducer with a protective sheath covering into the vagina. If the woman wants to insert it herself, allow her to do so. The angle of the probe or the tilt of the table may be altered during the examination, but the procedure should not be painful.

presence of a disorder. Screening of the levels may be performed to identify the presence of chromosomal abnormalities, such as Down syndrome, or birth defects, such as neural tube defects. The factors assessed with the screening are alpha-fetoprotein, estriol levels, HCG, and inhibin A. Alpha-fetoprotein is a protein produced by the fetal yoke sac and liver. Serum testing should be done between 16 and 18 weeks of gestation. Elevated levels are suggestive of neural tube defects, whereas low levels may suggest a fetus with Down syndrome (trisomy 21). Screening results may be influenced by maternal age and weight, gestational age, and the presence of more than one fetus.

There are factors that may affect the reliability of the results. These include the maternal age, the presence of a multifetal pregnancy, and an incorrect recording of gestational age. Abnormal findings result in additional testing. Ultrasound scan may be performed to assess fetal structures. The ultrasound scan provides no definitive means to rule out the presence of chromosomal defects, which makes an amniocentesis an option for consideration by the mother and her health care provider.

Nuchal Translucency Testing

Nuchal translucency screening is a test that has grown in popularity since the late 1990s. It is a diagnostic procedure used to assess the back of the neck for characteristics consistent with Down syndrome. Fetuses with larger nuchal folds (thickness at the back of the neck) have a greater incidence of Down syndrome (Fig. 26.3). The examination uses an ultrasound scan to measure the nuchal folds. At this point in the pregnancy the patient is asked to drink and not void before the ultrasound. This provides better visualization when the urinary bladder raises the uterus. The test typically is performed between 11 and 12 weeks' gestation. Normal findings for a fetus at 11 weeks would be up to 2 mm. A finding of excessive nuchal folds is not a definitive diagnosis for Down syndrome but indicates the need for additional testing, such as an amniocentesis (US National Library of Medicine, 2012). Other conditions should be considered if findings show an excess in the nuchal region. They include trisomy 13, trisomy 18, Turner's syndrome, or congenital heart disorders (NIH, 2018a).

Chorionic Villus Sampling

Chorionic villus sampling (CVS) is a test to detect genetic disorders of the fetus. It usually is performed between 10 and 13 weeks of gestation and requires aspiration of a small amount of tissue from the chorion of the placenta. A primary advantage of the test is the ability to perform it at an early point in the pregnancy, which allows for preparation of the mother in the event of fetal abnormalities. The test may be performed vaginally or abdominally. There are minimal risks with the procedure,

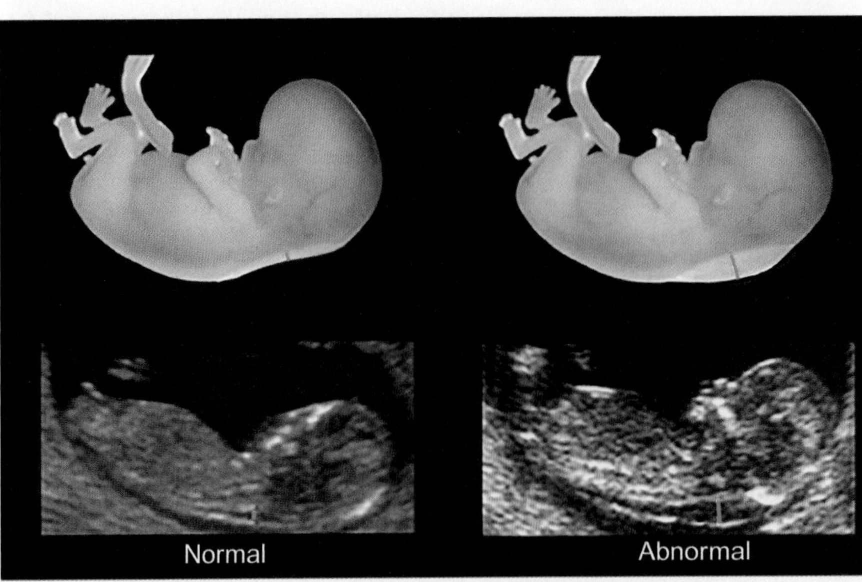

Fig. 26.3 Nuchal translucency testing. (Courtesy Dr. Greggory R. DeVore, Fetal Diagnostic Center, Pasadena, California. Reprinted with permission.)

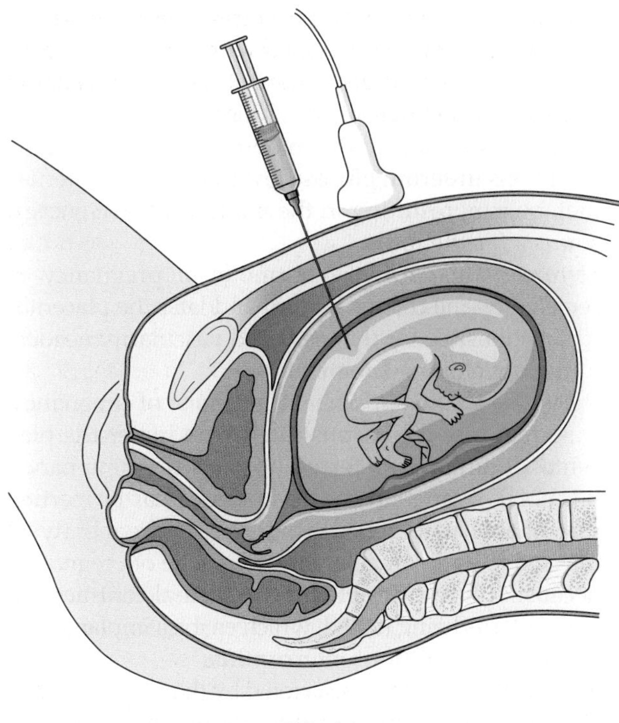

© Elsevier

Fig. 26.4 Transabdominal amniocentesis.

including Rh sensitization, infection, and miscarriage. At about 7%, the rate of pregnancy loss with CVS is slightly higher than with the amniocentesis.

Amniocentesis

Amniocentesis involves removal of a small amount of amniotic fluid with a needle passed through the abdominal wall (Fig. 26.4). This procedure is conducted in conjunction with abdominal ultrasound scan, which enables the physician to visualize the location of the fetus, the placenta, and a pocket of amniotic fluid. Laboratory examination of the amniotic fluid can reveal valuable information regarding genetic factors such as sex and chromosomal abnormalities, health status, and maturity of the fetus.

Early amniocentesis is performed at approximately the 16th week of pregnancy and is used to detect biochemical or chromosomal abnormalities. This is the earliest point at which there is adequate amniotic fluid for testing. Testing at this time allows the mother to consider termination of the pregnancy before the legal point of viability is reached. The fetus's ability to survive outside the uterus is known as *viability*. In the past several decades, the age of viability has decreased as a result of technological advances. A fetus as young as 22 to 25 weeks' gestation may survive outside of the mother's womb. Later in pregnancy, amniocentesis is used primarily to determine fetal lung maturity. It also may be performed to detect intrauterine infection and fetal distress and to assess fetal laboratory values.

Nonstress Test

The nonstress test (NST) is done to evaluate how the fetal heart rate responds to periods of fetal movement. It is indicated when a risk exists for placental insufficiency, such as pregnancy-induced hypertension, diabetes, postmaturity, maternal smoking, or inadequate maternal nutrition. It also may be done as a preventive screening tool for women who have had a past stillbirth. The test often is begun at 28 weeks' gestation and beyond. It may be ordered as a single test or repeated weekly or biweekly, depending on the mother's individual health history. With a baseline fetal heart rate of 120 to 160 bpm, the fetal heart rate normally accelerates at least 15 bpm for at least 15 seconds with fetal movement. Testing is done with external fetal monitors (see Chapter 27), with the tocotransducer recording fetal movement and the ultrasound transducer recording the fetal heart rate. A reactive result indicates a healthy fetus with findings of at least two fetal movements accompanied by two increases of 15 bpm in a 20-minute period. A nonreactive NST results when the fetal heart rate does not increase with fetal movements. This may indicate a compromised fetus and requires further evaluation with another NST, a BPP, or a contraction stress test.

Nursing responsibilities include explaining the procedure to the patient, assuring the patient that no discomfort is associated with the NST, encouraging the patient to verbalize her fears, ensuring the patient eats before the test to elevate serum glucose levels, requesting the patient empty her bladder and then assume a Sims position, applying the external fetal monitors to the patient's abdomen, observing for an increase in fetal heart rate with fetal movement, and stimulating fetal activity with external methods if the fetus remains quiet for more than 20 minutes.

Contraction Stress Test

The contraction stress test (CST) or oxytocin stress test uses external fetal monitoring and stimulation of contractions to evaluate how the fetal heart rate responds to the decreased oxygen supply during uterine contractions. Contractions are elicited with the administration of oxytocin or nipple stimulation. The desired response is termed negative, which means that no change in fetal heart rate occurs with the contractions. A positive test is noted when the fetal heart rate declines with the contractions. A drop in fetal heart rate indicates placental insufficiency and fetal hypoxia. Declines in fetal heart rates are identified by where in the cycle of the contraction they occur. Declines in the heart rate at or after the midpoint of the contraction are referred to as late decelerations. Late decelerations are considered an ominous sign. The fetus may be at risk during labor and need delivery via cesarean section.

Magnetic Resonance Imaging

Magnetic resonance imaging (MRI) is a noninvasive tool that can be used for obstetric and gynecologic diagnosis. As with computed tomographic (CT) scan, MRI provides excellent pictures of soft tissue. Unlike CT scan, ionizing radiation is not used; thus vascular structures within the body can be evaluated without injection of an iodinated contrast medium, thereby eliminating any known biologic risk. As with sonography, MRI is noninvasive and can provide images in multiple planes, but interference from skeletal, fatty, or gas-filled structures is not a problem. Also, imaging of deep pelvic structures does not depend on a full bladder. Although this procedure has many advantages, its complete safety has not been determined.

Biophysical Profile

The BPP assesses fetal status with evaluation of several factors (Table 26.3). These include the NST, fetal breathing movements, fetal muscle tone, fetal movements, and amniotic fluid volume. Each category is given a score of 0 or 2. A total score of 8 or more is reassuring; lower scores may warrant interruption of the pregnancy.

MATERNAL PHYSIOLOGY

HORMONAL CHANGES

During pregnancy, hormonal changes help to prepare the woman's body to accommodate the advancing pregnancy. Most pregnancy-related hormones initially are produced by the corpus luteum until the placenta begins to function adequately. Pregnancy-related hormones include the following:

- *HCG:* Initially secreted by the trophoplast in the developing pregnancy. It is responsible for stimulation of the corpus luteum to promote production of estrogen and progesterone until the placenta is functioning. HCG is the hormone assessed with a pregnancy test.
- *Human placental lactogen (HPL), also called human chorionic somatomammotropin:* This hormone promotes insulin resistance by the maternal cells resulting in elevations in serum glucose levels. It affects maternal metabolism, resulting in the maintenance of energy sources for the fetus.
- *Estrogen:* This primary hormone of pregnancy is secreted by the corpus luteum and later the placenta. It is responsible for the increased vascularity needed in the developing pregnancy.
- *Progesterone:* This important hormone of pregnancy is secreted by the corpus luteum and later the placenta. It often is referred to at the maintenance hormone of pregnancy. This hormone has properties that enable it to relax the organs. It frequently is referred to as the maintenance hormone of pregnancy because it is responsible for the normal contractility of the uterus being halted, which enables implantation to take place without interruption.
- *Relaxin:* This hormone is secreted by the corpus luteum and later the decidua of the uterine lining and the placenta. Relaxin is linked to the softening of the cervix and pubic symphysis in preparation for labor and delivery.

UTERUS

The uterus enlarges during pregnancy as a result of hormonal stimulus, which causes an increase in vascularity,

Table 26.3 Interpretation of Biophysical Profile Score Variables

Fetal Variable	Normal Behavior (Score = 2)	Abnormal Behavior (Score = 0)
Fetal breathing movements (FBMs)	Intermittent multiple episodes of more than 30-s duration, within 30-min BPS time frame. Hiccups count. With continuous FBM for 30 min, exclude fetal acidosis.	Continuous breathing without cessation. Completely absent breathing or no sustained episodes.
Body or limb movements	At least four discrete body movements in 30 min. Continuous active movement episodes count as a single movement. Includes fine motor movements, rolling movements, and so on, but not REM or mouthing movements.	Three or fewer body or limb movements in a 30-min observation period.
Fetal tone and posture	Demonstration of active extension with rapid return to flexion of fetal limbs and brisk repositioning or trunk rotation. Opening and closing of hand, mouth, kicking, and so on.	Low-velocity movement only. Incomplete flexion, flaccid extremity positions, abnormal fetal posture. Must score 0 when FM completely absent.
Cardiotocogram (CTG)	Normal mean variation (computerized FHR interpretation), accelerations associated with maternal palpation of FM (accelerations graded for gestation), 20-min CTG.	Fetal movement and accelerations not coupled. Insufficient accelerations, absent accelerations, or decelerated trace. Mean variation <20 on numeric analysis of CTG.
Amniotic fluid evaluation	At least one pocket >3 cm with no umbilical cord.	No cord-free pocket >2 cm or elements of subjectively reduced amniotic fluid volume deficit.

BPS, Biophysical profile score; *FHR,* fetal heart rate; *FM,* fetal movement; *REM,* rapid eye movement.
From Harman CR: Assessment of fetal health. In Creasy RK, Resnik R, Iams JD, editors: *Maternal-fetal medicine: Principles and practice,* ed 6, Philadelphia, 2008, Saunders.

hyperplasia (new muscle fiber and tissue), and hypertrophy (enlargement of existing fiber and tissue). The nonpregnant uterus is pear shaped and weighs approximately 2 oz (50 g). By the third trimester (the last 3 months of a 9-month pregnancy), it is egg shaped and has increased in weight to 2.2 lb (1000 g). At term, it can hold a fetus, a placenta, and amniotic fluid, totaling more than 8.5 lb (4000 g).

The consistency of the tissue changes also. Changes in the cervix and fundus, along with an altered position in the pelvis, are early signs of pregnancy. The uterus, which in a nonpregnant state is a pelvic organ, rises to the base of the rib cage. The superior aspect of the uterus (the fundus) is located at the level of the xiphoid process by the end of the third trimester.

BREASTS

Changes in the breasts during pregnancy are caused by hormonal stimulation. The changes include hypertrophy of the mammary glandular tissue and increased vascularization, pigmentation, size, and prominence of nipples and areolae. During the second trimester, the breasts begin to produce colostrum, often referred to as "premilk." The colostrum is produced actively from the second trimester to after delivery until the mother's milk comes in. This fluid is low in fat but high in carbohydrates and protein. It also contains valuable antibodies to provide protection to the newborn. The first newborn stool, meconium, is aided in passage by the laxative-like effects of the colostrum.

CYCLES OF PREGNANCY AND CHILDBIRTH

The maternity cycle, which is discussed in this and successive chapters, is divided into three distinct periods. The first portion of the cycle is called the **antepartal** period (from Latin root *ante,* "before," and *parere,* "to bring to bear") or **prenatal** period (from Latin root *pre-,* "before," and *natal,* "birth"). The antepartal period begins with conception and ends with the onset of labor.

The next portion of the cycle is referred to as the **intrapartal** period (from Latin *intra,* "within," and *parere,* "to bring to bear"). This period begins with the onset of labor and ends with delivery of the placenta. The same period sometimes is called the **perinatal** portion (from Latin *peri,* "around," and *natal,* "birth").

The final stage of the cycle is the **postpartal** period (from Latin *post,* "after," and *parere,* "to bring to bear"). This period starts after the delivery of the placenta and lasts for approximately 6 weeks or until the reproductive organs return to the prepregnancy state.

Pregnancy spans 9 months, approximately 40 weeks. Pregnancy is also divided into 3-month periods, or **trimesters.** The first trimester covers weeks 1 through 13; the second, weeks 14 through 26; and the third, weeks 27 through term gestation (38 to 40 weeks).

ANTEPARTAL ASSESSMENT

GENERAL PHYSICAL ASSESSMENT

Prenatal care and assessment should begin when pregnancy is planned or as soon as the first menstrual period is missed. Ideally, the woman has been receiving regular medical attention and already is known by the health care provider. Unfortunately, because of cost or frequent changes of residence, many people do not receive regular, routine health care. Some women seek the attention of a specialist, an obstetrician, a nurse practitioner, or a midwife during pregnancy.

On the first visit, *demographic* (the statistical and quantitative study of characteristics of the human population) data, such as age, occupation, and marital status, are obtained, along with insurance information. The basic information helps the primary care practitioner identify potential areas of concern. For example, an adolescent who is 15 years old, single, unemployed, and a high school dropout with no insurance presents a different set of concerns than a 25-year-old, married, college graduate with comprehensive health insurance.

A basic family and personal medical history is obtained. To anticipate any problems, the practitioner must be aware of any genetic diseases in either the mother's or the father's family. A family history that includes genetic diseases may concern the expectant parents until there are assurances that the baby is healthy. If serious genetic problems are known, couples may seek genetic counseling before they consider having children.

GENETIC COUNSELING

Rapid expansion in the identification, understanding, and diagnosis of genetic disease has only led to effective medical or surgical therapies for a small number of patients. For most genetic conditions, therapeutic or preventive measures are nonexistent or disappointingly limited. Consequently, the most useful means of reducing the incidence of these disorders is by preventing their transmission. As more becomes known about genetic disorders, more accurate predictions can be made about the probability of a couple passing a disorder to their offspring. At present, the best way to reduce the number of children born with genetic defects is for health professionals to provide families with genetic information and services.

Assessment begins with a personal medical history and a review of systems. Information is obtained about chronic diseases such as cardiac problems, hypertension, diabetes mellitus, and infectious diseases (e.g., rubella, acquired immunodeficiency syndrome, or other sexually transmitted infections). Any history of accidents or previous surgeries is documented. Significant findings in these areas may indicate the potential for problems and the need for early medical and nursing intervention. High-risk pregnancies are discussed in Chapter 29.

Box 26.3 Basic Prenatal Physical Examination

- Measurement of vital signs, height, and weight
- Assessment of heart, lungs, and reflexes
- General physical inspection of skin and mobility
- Laboratory studies (hemoglobin; hematocrit; serology tests for detection of syphilis, human immunodeficiency virus, and hepatitis virus; ABO and Rh factor; rubella titer)
- Routine urinalysis for glucose, protein, and ketones
- Pregnancy test if pregnancy has not been confirmed already

Assessment is made of lifestyle patterns, including recreational activities; nutrition and eating habits; use of prescription medications, street drugs, alcohol, or tobacco; and work exposure to hazardous conditions. Early detection and correction of problem situations can reduce hazards to the woman and prevent detrimental effects on the fetus.

A basic physical examination is completed (Box 26.3). These tests increase the data available and enable the primary care practitioner to plan comprehensive care.

OBSTETRIC ASSESSMENT

In addition to the general health history and physical examination, information is obtained about the woman's gynecologic, menstrual, and obstetric history. This includes the use of contraceptives and the regularity of the menstrual period, including frequency, duration, amount of flow, presence of pain, and any other significant comments. A review is made of any history of gynecologic surgery, vaginal discharge, or herpes infection. The physician may ask questions regarding exposure to diethylstilbestrol (DES), because daughters of women who took DES during pregnancy have an increased risk of spontaneous abortion caused by an incompetent cervix.

The number of pregnancies the patient has had and their outcomes are discussed. This includes the course of the pregnancy with special attention to any complications, the type of delivery (vaginal or cesarean), any complications during delivery, the use of forceps or other medical assistance, the type of anesthetic used, the condition of the newborn, and any complications of the postpartal period.

GYNECOLOGIC EXAMINATION

The gynecologic examination also is performed at this time. The nurse often is called on to prepare the necessary equipment and assist in this examination and to provide explanations and emotional support to the patient (Box 26.4).

Box 26.4 Gynecologic Examination

- Palpation and auscultation of the abdomen
- Visualization of the cervix and vagina
- Evaluation of the bony pelvis
- Palpation of the uterus externally or bimanually
- Examination of the vulva, the perineum, the anus, and the rectum
- Pap smear (done at the beginning of the examination)

DETERMINATION OF PREGNANCY

The woman may report to the physician after having suspected pregnancy and then taking a home pregnancy test to confirm suspicions. The initial visit to the health care provider includes a pregnancy test. After the entire history and physical examination have been done, the physician can determine with varying degrees of certainty whether she is pregnant.

PRESUMPTIVE SIGNS

The presumptive signs are indicators that a woman may be pregnant. They are subjective. These signs are those frequently attributed to pregnancy, but they also may indicate other conditions not related to pregnancy:

- Amenorrhea: Absence of menstruation
- Nausea and vomiting
- Frequent urination
- Breast changes: Swelling, tingling, and tenderness of the breasts are common during pregnancy, along with changes in pigmentation of the areolae. The sebaceous material secreted from the ducts of the glands to the skin of each areola lubricates and protects the breasts from infection and trauma during breast-feeding.
- Change in the shape of the abdomen
- Quickening: The subjective sensation of fetal movement first occurs at about 16 to 18 weeks of gestation in multigravida women. First-time mothers may not report these sensations until 18 to 20 weeks' gestation.
- Skin changes: Pigment changes, such as darkening of some areas of the body such as the areolae, may occur. Some women may experience chloasma (melasma).
- Chadwick's sign: During the pelvic examination, the physician may note that the vagina, the cervix, and sometimes the vulva have a violet or purplish discoloration. This change in color is the result of increased vascularity to the area.

PROBABLE SIGNS

The probable signs indicate a high likelihood that the woman is pregnant. These findings are objective and can be confirmed by an examiner. Still, these signs are not 100% reliable indicators:

- *Changes in the reproductive organs:* The uterus begins to grow early in the pregnancy. Enlargement of the uterus indicates a high probability of pregnancy, particularly if accompanied by changes in the consistency of the isthmus of the uterus (the segment between the fundus and the cervix). A softening of this segment is called **Hëgar's sign** (Fig. 26.5). This change and a softening or increased pliability of the cervix called **Goodell's sign** are seen most commonly

in pregnancy. **Ballottement,** which may be used at approximately 16 to 18 weeks of gestation, is a technique that involves palpating the uterus in such a way that the examiner feels the rebound of the floating fetus (Fig. 26.6).
- *Positive pregnancy test result:* Assessment of pregnancy may be done with either serum or urine testing. These tests measure the presence and or levels of HCG. A positive pregnancy test is not a definitive determination of pregnancy because other conditions may result in positive test results. Urine tests are readily available over the counter in stores. Reliability of these products depends on the technique used in collecting the urine specimen and performing the test. Tests administered by the primary care practitioner have a high level of reliability between 95% and 99%. The greatest advantages of pregnancy tests are that they can be administered early in pregnancy and are reasonably inexpensive. If the test results are positive and other indicators such as uterine changes are abnormal, the primary care provider may suspect complications such as an ectopic (outside the uterus) pregnancy or hydatidiform mole (abnormal growth of a fertilized ovum in which a large vascular mass, but no fetus, develops). Hydatidiform mole frequently results in a highly reactive pregnancy test, and the test may continue to indicate positive results even after surgical removal.

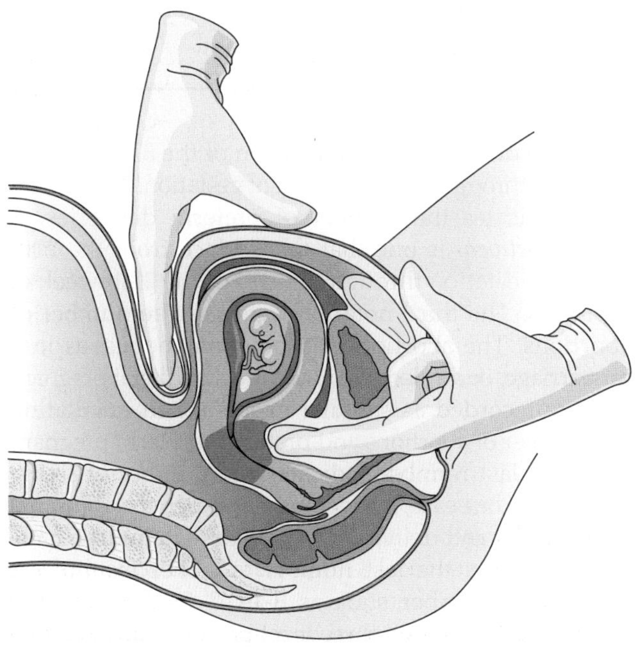

Fig. 26.5 Hëgar's sign. Bimanual examination for assessment of compressibility and softening of isthmus (lower uterine segment) while the cervix is still firm.

POSITIVE SIGNS

Positive signs are those that occur only with pregnancy and cannot be attributed to other physiologic occurrences. Positive signs definitively identify the presence of the fetus. The signs include palpation of the fetal outline, visualization of the pregnancy with ultrasound scan, and presence of a fetal heartbeat (Box 26.5).

DETERMINATION OF THE ESTIMATED DATE OF BIRTH

Normal human pregnancy, counting from the first day of the last menstrual period, is about 280 days, 40 weeks, 10 lunar months (28 days each), or slightly more than 9 calendar months.

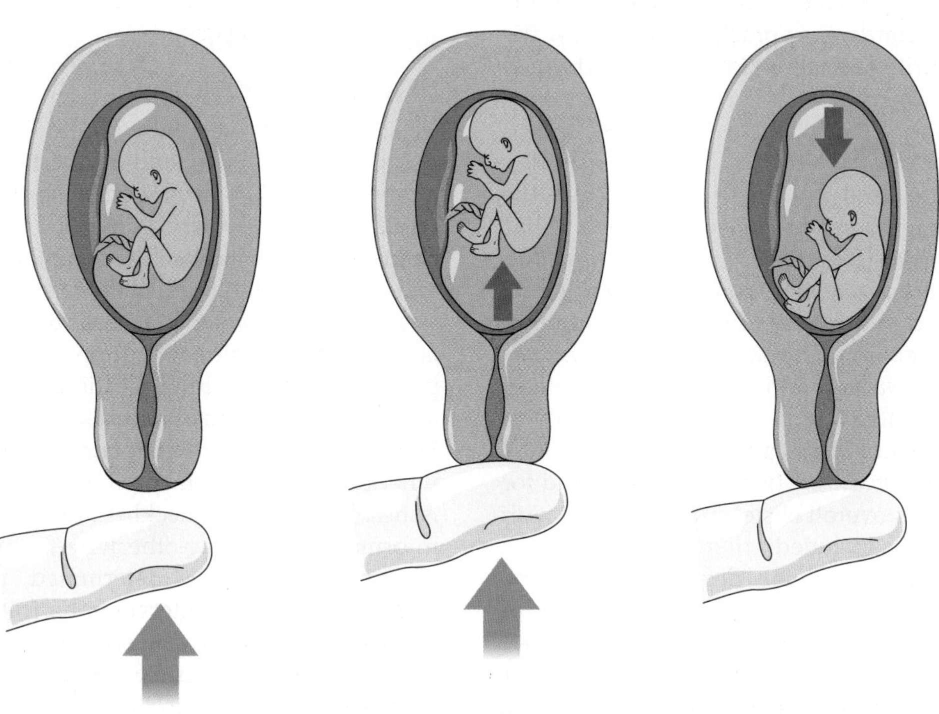

Fig. 26.6 Internal ballottement (18 weeks).

Box 26.5 Positive Signs of Pregnancy

- *Visualization:* The fetal skeleton seen on x-ray examination is a positive sign of pregnancy, but use of radiation generally is limited during pregnancy because of possible danger to the fetus. Ultrasound tracing of the fetus is also a positive indication of pregnancy.
- *Fetal movement:* Fetal movement may be detected by a trained observer (the primary care practitioner).
- *Auscultation of fetal heart tone:* Fetal heart activity can be detected with ultrasound scan at 6 weeks; tones are heard with Doppler at 10 to 12 weeks and with stethoscope at approximately 18 to 20 weeks.

Box 26.6 Defining Parity

FIVE-DIGIT SYSTEM: GTPAL
G: Gravidity
T: Term births
P: Preterm births
A: Abortions
L: Living children

FOUR-DIGIT SYSTEM: TPAL
T: Term births (also may be noted as F)
P: Preterm births
A: Abortions
L: Living children

The estimated date of delivery (EDD), often known as the "due date," involves calculations based on the woman's menstrual cycle. In the past, this date was referred to as the estimated date of confinement, or EDC. The term confinement is not used commonly today, because pregnancy and childbirth are seen as highly anticipated wellness-related experiences. The most common method is called *Nägele's rule.* To calculate, start with the first day of the woman's last normal menstrual period and count back 3 months, then add 7 days. For example, if the first day of the last menstrual period was June 14, counting back 3 months to March 14 and then adding 7 days would yield an EDB of March 21. Studies reveal that only a small percentage of infants actually are born on the date predicted; most deliveries, however, do occur within 10 days before or after the EDB.

If the woman does not keep a menstrual record, calculation of the EDB may be more difficult. The health care provider must then rely on observations such as quickening, estimation of fetal size with palpation, or ultrasound tests, all of which can be unreliable. If it is essential for the primary care practitioner to know the level of fetal maturity, specialized tests can be performed later in the pregnancy.

OBSTETRIC TERMINOLOGY

Specific terms are used in obstetrics to describe the number of times a woman has been pregnant and has given birth. **Gravida** (from the Latin root *gravidus,* "heavy") indicates a pregnant woman. Latin numeric prefixes are added to this term to indicate the number of pregnancies, such as *primigravida* (one), *nulligravida* (none), and *multigravida* (multiple). Similarly, prefixes are added to the Latin root **para** ("to bring forth") to indicate the number of births, such as *nullipara* (none), *primipara* (one), and *multipara* (multiple). Shorthand for noting the patient's overall obstetric status is GP with the correct numerals included.

A four-point or five-point description may be used to provide obstetric history. The four-part description, referred to as TPAL or FPAL, sometimes is used (Box 26.6). The first digit represents the total number of term pregnancies (or in the FPAL notation, full-term), including the present one. A *term pregnancy* is one that results in delivery after conclusion of the 37th week of gestation through the 42nd week of gestation. The second digit indicates the number of preterm deliveries. A *preterm delivery* is one that takes place from the 20th week of gestation through the end of the 37th week of gestation. The third notation indicates the number of abortions. The abortion may be spontaneous, as in a miscarriage, or an elective procedure. Multifetal pregnancies are recorded as singular events when calculating the number of abortions and preterm and term pregnancies. The last number indicates the number of living children. In one case, if a woman has experienced normal pregnancies and deliveries, but all of her children have died in a fire, the last number is 0. For example, a descriptive number such as 3-1-0-3 indicates that a woman has delivered three term pregnancies, had one preterm pregnancy and no abortions, and has three living children. The more detailed five-point method includes information about the total number of pregnancies a woman has had. It is denoted as GTPAL.

ANTEPARTAL CARE

HEALTH PROMOTION

Most pregnant women want to learn more about pregnancy, childbirth, and motherhood. Pregnancy is a time in life when most women see the importance of regular medical supervision and are willing to make changes in their habits. They think of their baby first and do everything that is best for the infant.

A checklist for antepartal needs throughout pregnancy is a valuable teaching tool. It provides the team of care providers with a communication tool to prevent gaps and to identify areas of repeated concerns for patients. Sharing the checklist with patients reassures them that other pregnant women and their families face the same issues. Reading the checklist also reminds patients of information they may otherwise forget (Box 26.7).

Once pregnancy is determined, prenatal care is instituted. Nursing interventions follow the nursing process: assessment, analysis, identification of patient problems, planning, implementation, and evaluation.

Pregnancy is an excellent time to establish good general health practices. Until they become pregnant,

Box 26.7 Trimester Checklist

- Schedule and events of visits
- Counseling for self-care
- Adaptations and discomforts
  - Dyspnea
  - Insomnia
  - Psychosocial responses and family dynamics
  - Gingivitis
  - Urinary frequency
  - Perineal discomfort and pressure
  - Braxton Hicks contractions
  - Leg cramps
  - Ankle edema
- Safety (balance)
- Exercise and rest
- Relaxation
- Nutrition
- Sexuality
- Personal hygiene
- Danger signs, general
- Danger signs, preterm labor
- Fetal growth and development
- Preparation for baby
  - Feeding method
  - Nipple preparation
- Preparation for labor
  - Recognition: false versus true
  - Prenatal classes
  - Control of discomfort
  - Hospital tour
  - Provision for other family members
- Preparation for homecoming
- Diagnostic tests (specify)
- Other

many women do not have regular physical examinations or Papanicolaou (Pap) smears and do not do home screening tests such as breast self-examination (BSE). The high motivation level makes this a good time to teach patients about health maintenance practices.

Early in pregnancy, the woman often begins to seek information and make choices regarding how and where she wishes to give birth. Information should be provided regarding the options available in her community (see Chapter 27).

Routine care during pregnancy begins with the initial examination and history, as previously described. Appointments are recommended once a month through the seventh month, once every 2 weeks for the next month, and then once every week until delivery. If any problems occur or the health care provider suspects anything unusual, such as a multiple pregnancy, the schedule of visits may be altered. Dental care should continue during pregnancy. Any major dental work, such as oral surgery or extractions, usually is delayed until after delivery.

Smoking during pregnancy can be dangerous to the developing fetus. Oxygen deprivation can lead to decreased intrauterine growth and low birth weight. Preterm delivery also is linked to maternal smoking. Drinking of alcoholic beverages during pregnancy also is contraindicated. Fetal alcohol syndrome is discussed in Chapter 29.

Ideally, women should avoid taking any medication or drugs during pregnancy. The use of over-the-counter drugs and prescription medications must be reviewed with the health care provider (Box 26.8). Most drugs can cross the placenta and are transmitted to the fetus. Street drugs, such as marijuana and cocaine, are dangerous to mother and fetus and must be avoided. Although complementary and alternative therapies may be used safely before pregnancy, certain elements may be dangerous to the developing fetus. To ensure safety, the nurse must be vigilant in assessing for their use and in subsequent reporting to the primary health care provider (Box 26.9).

Embryonic and fetal development is vulnerable to environmental teratogens. Many potentially dangerous chemicals are present in the home, yard, and workplace, including cleaning agents, paints, sprays, herbicides, and pesticides. The soil and water supply may be unsafe. Therefore the woman should: (1) read all labels for ingredients and proper use of product; (2) ensure adequate ventilation with clean air; (3) dispose of wastes appropriately; (4) wear gloves when handling chemicals and gardening; and (5) change job assignments or workplace as necessary.

Today many women continue to work throughout pregnancy. The work environment must be checked for chemicals and other hazards. The Occupational Safety and Health Administration has numerous guidelines for hazards in the workplace. Address working conditions such as lifting and standing or sitting for long periods. Encourage the woman to take frequent rest periods.

DANGER SIGNS DURING PREGNANCY

Although pregnancy involves many changes and normal discomforts, certain conditions signal the need for immediate medical attention (Box 26.10). Teach the pregnant woman these danger signs and how to monitor fetal movements (see the Patient Teaching box for guidelines for counting fetal movements). Stress the importance of contacting the primary care practitioner promptly if any of these signs are present.

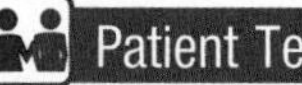

Patient Teaching

Guidelines for Counting Fetal Movements (Kick Counts)

- Kick count monitoring should begin at 28 weeks' gestation.
- The expectant mother should pick a time of day when she can sit or lie quietly. If deciding to lie down, a left side–lying position should be selected.
- Each fetal movement or kick should be counted. The goal is to experience 10 to 12 movements/kicks in a 1- to 2-hour period.

If an inadequate number of movements is felt, the health care provider should be notified.

Box 26.8 US Food and Drug Administration Drug Categories

The rational use of any medication requires a risk-versus-benefit assessment. Among the many risk factors that complicate assessment, pregnancy is one of the most perplexing. The US Food and Drug Administration has established five categories to indicate the potential of a systemically absorbed drug for causing birth defects. The key differences among the categories are the degree (reliability) of evidence and the risk:benefit ratio. Pregnancy category X is particularly notable; it is assigned to a drug if any data indicate the drug is a teratogen and the risk:benefit ratio does not support use of the drug. Category X drugs are contraindicated during pregnancy.

PREGNANCY CATEGORY AND DEFINITION

A: Adequate studies in pregnant women have not demonstrated a risk to the fetus in the first trimester of pregnancy, and no evidence of risk is found in later trimesters.

B: Animal studies have not demonstrated a risk to the fetus, but no adequate studies are found in pregnant women; or animal studies have shown an adverse effect, but adequate studies in pregnant women have not demonstrated a risk to the fetus during the first trimester of pregnancy, and no evidence of risk is found in later trimesters.

C: Animal studies have shown an adverse effect on the fetus, but no adequate studies are found in humans; the benefits from the use of the drug in pregnant women may be acceptable despite its potential risks; or no animal reproduction studies and no adequate studies in humans are found.

D: Evidence is seen of human fetal risk, but the potential benefits from the use of the drug in pregnant women may be acceptable despite its potential risks.

X: Studies in animals or humans demonstrate fetal abnormalities, or adverse reaction reports indicate evidence of fetal risk. The risk of use in a pregnant woman clearly outweighs any possible benefit.

NR: Not rated.

Regardless of the designated pregnancy category or presumed safety, no drug should be administered during pregnancy unless it is clearly needed and potential benefits outweigh potential risks.

Modified from Skidmore-Roth L: *Mosby's 2013 nursing drug reference*, ed 26, St. Louis, 2013, Mosby.

NUTRITIONAL AND METABOLIC HEALTH PATTERN

See Chapter 19 for information about basic nutrition and nutritional therapy for the life cycle, stages of pregnancy, and lactation.

Pica

Pica refers to craving and eating substances that are not normally considered edible. Pica may be associated by nutrient deficits such as iron or zinc. Some report the craving is due to a smell or need to experience a certain texture in their mouths (NIH, 2018b). It is seen more in lower socioeconomic groups and linked to certain cultural groups. Substances ingested may include clay, laundry starch, dirt, and chalk. Although the substances are not considered toxic, complications are associated with pica. Patients may experience constipation or other gastrointestinal ailments from the ingestion of the nonfood substances. Eating the craved items may reduce quality nutritional intake resulting in deficiencies. Problems that may occur as a result of pica include interference with iron absorption, constipation, and loss

Box 26.9 Complementary and Alternative Therapies Used in Pregnancy

MORNING SICKNESS AND HYPEREMESIS

- Acupuncture
- Acupressure
- Shiatzu
- Motion sickness bracelets (Sea Bands)
- Aromatherapy with lavender or rose scents
- Herbal remedies[a]
  - Lemon balm
  - Peppermint
  - Spearmint
  - Ginger root
  - Raspberry leaf
  - Fennel
  - Chamomile
  - Hops
  - Meadowsweet
  - Wild yam root

RELAXATION AND MUSCLE ACHE RELIEF

- Yoga
- Biofeedback
- Reflexology
- Therapeutic touch
- Massage

[a]Some herbs can cause miscarriage, preterm labor, or fetal or maternal injury. Pregnant women should discuss use in pregnancy and during lactation with the health care provider.

Data from Lowdermilk DL, Perry SE, Cashion K, et al: *Maternal and women's health care*, ed 10, St. Louis, 2012, Mosby; Edgren AR: Hyperemesis gravidarum. In *Gale encyclopedia of medicine*, 2008, The Gale Group, Inc.

Box 26.10 Danger Signs and Symptoms During Pregnancy

- Visual disturbances: diplopia (double vision), blurring, or spots
- Headaches: severe, sudden, or continuous
- Edema: swelling of the face, presacral area, or fingers
- Rapid weight gain in excess of normal gain for gestation
- Pain: severe abdominal or epigastric pain
- Signs of infection: fever, chills, diarrhea, changes in vaginal drainage, pain or burning with urination
- Vaginal bleeding (no matter how slight)
- Vaginal drainage (aside from normal mucus)
- Persistent vomiting
- Muscular irritability or convulsions
- Absence or decrease in fetal movement once felt

of important nutrients when normal caloric intake is replaced with the pica-related substances.

Common Discomforts

Many pregnant women experience some discomforts of the gastrointestinal tract during pregnancy. Some women have excessive salivation (ptyalism), presumably in response to the high levels of estrogen during pregnancy. Although it may be uncomfortable and awkward at times, ptyalism causes no serious problems and disappears late in pregnancy or after delivery. Teach the patient to try using astringent mouthwash, chewing gum, or sucking on hard candy to provide relief.

Nausea is common in the early stages of pregnancy. It typically occurs when the woman awakens in the morning, hence the name "morning sickness." However, it can occur at any time of the day. Nausea is thought to be caused by increased HCG levels and changes in carbohydrate metabolism. Mild nausea usually can be controlled by slowly eating a few soda crackers or dry toast before rising from bed. Other suggestions are eating smaller, more frequent meals and avoiding spicy or greasy food. Morning sickness rarely lasts beyond the fourth month. If it lasts longer, if it is more severe, and particularly if it involves vomiting, the health care provider should be contacted. The most severe form is called *hyperemesis gravidarum.* Its cause is not clear, but if left untreated, it can lead to dehydration, fluid and electrolyte imbalance, acid-base imbalance, altered kidney and cardiac function, and even fetal death. Hospitalization with close medical supervision, including intravenous therapy, may be necessary (see Chapter 29).

Pyrosis (heartburn) from gastric reflux into the esophagus can be caused by the increasing size of the fetus in the abdominal cavity, which displaces the stomach. Increased progesterone levels cause relaxation of the cardiac sphincter; decreased gastric mobility, which results in delayed stomach emptying time, also may contribute to the problem. Smaller, more frequent meals; decreased fat intake; low-sodium antacids; and avoidance of lying down after meals often give relief.

Skin Changes

Changes in pigmentation often occur during pregnancy as a result of increased amounts of melanocyte-stimulating hormone. The changes occur primarily in areas that already have greater pigmentation, such as the areolae, nipples, vulva, and perineal area. A darkening of a line from the midline of the abdomen from the pubis to the umbilicus may result and is called the *linea nigra.*

Chloasma, the mask of pregnancy, is an irregular darkening of the cheeks, forehead, and nose. These changes are often more obvious in women with darker hair and skin and may be worsened with sun exposure. This generally disappears or fades significantly soon after delivery.

Striae gravidarum, or stretch marks, are reddish, wavy streaks that can appear on the thighs, the abdomen, and the breasts. They are more common with distention but may occur even in relatively thin women. They usually fade after delivery. Because integumentary system changes vary greatly among women of different racial backgrounds, the color of a woman's skin along with any changes that may be attributed to pregnancy should be noted in the physical assessment.

Spider nevi (a branched growth of dilated capillaries on the skin) and *palmar erythema* (reddened palms) sometimes are seen. These conditions are caused by increased blood flow that results from high estrogen levels. Both usually disappear when the pregnancy ends.

Hair and nail growth frequently are accelerated during pregnancy, with *hirsutism* (excessive body hair in a masculine distribution pattern as a result of heredity, hormonal dysfunction, or medication) commonly reported. Oily skin and acne may occur in some women, whereas others report a clearing of their skin. This is usually temporary unless other physiologic problems are active.

Occasionally, decreased emptying of the gallbladder may result in subclinical jaundice, which causes generalized pruritus (itching). This and other concerns are noted in Table 26.4.

Changes in the Cardiovascular System

Maternal adjustments to pregnancy involve extensive anatomic and physiologic changes in the cardiovascular system. Changes can result in episodes of orthostatic hypotension. An increase of platelets and fibrinogen increases the woman's risk for blood clots. Cardiovascular adaptations protect the woman's normal physiologic functioning, meet the metabolic demands of pregnancy, and provide for fetal development and growth (Table 26.5).

Changes in the Respiratory System

Structural and ventilatory adaptations during pregnancy provide for maternal and fetal needs. Maternal oxygen requirements increase in response to the accelerated metabolic rate and the need to add to the tissue mass in the uterus and breasts. In addition, the fetus needs oxygen and a way to eliminate carbon dioxide. Elevation of estrogen causes the ligaments of the rib cage to relax, permitting increased chest expansion (Table 26.6).

Changes in the Musculoskeletal System

The gradually changing body and increasing weight of the pregnant woman cause noticeable alterations in her posture (Fig. 26.7) and the way she walks late in pregnancy. The great abdominal distention that gives the pelvis a forward tilt, decreased abdominal muscle tone, and increased weight bearing create a realignment of the spinal curvature. The woman's center of gravity shifts forward. Lordosis (an increase in the normal lumbosacral curve) develops. An increased curvature in the cervicodorsal region also is seen. The expectant mother also may be noted with an exaggerated anterior flexion of the head. This is done to promote balance.

Table 26.4 Discomforts and Concerns Related to Maternal Adaptations During the Third Trimester

Discomfort	Physiology	Teaching for Self-Care
Shortness of breath and dyspnea in 60% of pregnant women	Expansion of diaphragm limited by enlarging uterus; diaphragm elevated approximately 1.5 inches (4 cm); some relief after lightening (when the fetus settles lower in the true pelvis, leaving more space in the upper abdomen)	Good posture; sleep with extra pillow; avoid overloading stomach; stop smoking; refer to physician if symptoms worsen to rule out anemia, emphysema, and asthma
Insomnia (later weeks of pregnancy)	Fetal movements, muscular cramping, urinary frequency, shortness of breath, or other discomforts	Reassurance; conscious relaxation; back massage or effleurage (deep or gentle stroking); support of body parts with pillows; warm milk or shower before retiring
Psychosocial responses: mood swings, mixed feelings, increased anxiety	Hormonal and metabolic adaptations; feelings about impending labor, delivery, and parenthood	Reassurance and support from significant other and nurse; improved communication with partner, family, and others
Return of urinary frequency and urgency	Vascular engorgement and altered bladder function caused by hormones; bladder capacity reduced by enlarging uterus and fetal presenting part; lightening	Kegel exercises (see the Patient Teaching box on Kegel exercises); limit fluid intake before bedtime; reassurance; wear perineal pad; refer to health care provider for pain or burning sensation
Perineal discomfort and pressure	Pressure from enlarging uterus, especially when standing or walking; multifetal gestation	Rest, conscious relaxation, and good posture; maternity girdle; refer to physician for assessment and treatment if pain is present; rule out labor
Braxton Hicks contractions	Intensification of uterine contractions in preparation for work of labor	Reassurance; rest; change of position; practice breathing techniques when contractions are bothersome; effleurage; rule out labor
Leg cramps (gastrocnemius spasm), especially when reclining	Compression of nerves supplying lower extremities because of enlarging uterus; reduced level of diffusible serum calcium or elevation of serum phosphorus; aggravating factors: fatigue, poor peripheral circulation, pointing toes when stretching legs or when walking, drinking >1 quart (1 L) of milk per day; cause unclear	Assess lower extremities for redness, warmth, tenderness, or swelling; some facilities may use the Homan's sign; this assessment is presently under review by many medical professionals because it is not considered completely reliable, and concerns exist about the safety of the practice Heat may be used over affected muscle; stretch affected muscle until spasm relaxes
Ankle edema (nonpitting) to lower extremities	Edema aggravated by prolonged standing, sitting, poor posture, lack of exercise, constrictive clothing (e.g., garters), or hot weather	Ample fluid intake for "natural" diuretic effect; put on support stockings before rising; rest periodically with legs and hips elevated; exercise moderately; refer to physician if generalized edema develops (diuretics are contraindicated)

As the pregnancy advances, common symptoms include muscle aches and numbness. Enlarging breasts and a stoop-shouldered stance further accentuate the lumbar and dorsal curves. Walking is more difficult, and the pregnant woman's waddling gait is well known. The ligamentous and muscular structures of the middle and lower spine may be severely stressed. Pregnant women who gain excessive weight or who carry more than one fetus may experience overdistention. This excessive stress on the abdominal wall muscles may cause a separation (diastasis recti abdominis). Management of this condition is typically conservative, but severe cases may necessitate surgical repair.

Slight relaxation and increased mobility of the pelvic joints are normal during pregnancy. They are a result of the exaggerated elasticity and softening of the connective tissue caused by increased circulating steroid sex hormones, especially estrogen. **Relaxin,** an ovarian hormone, assists in the relaxation and softening. These adaptations permit enlargement of pelvic dimensions to facilitate labor and birth. The degree of relaxation varies, but considerable separation of the symphysis pubis and the instability of the sacroiliac joints may cause pain and difficulty in walking. Obesity and multifetal pregnancy tend to increase the pelvic instability.

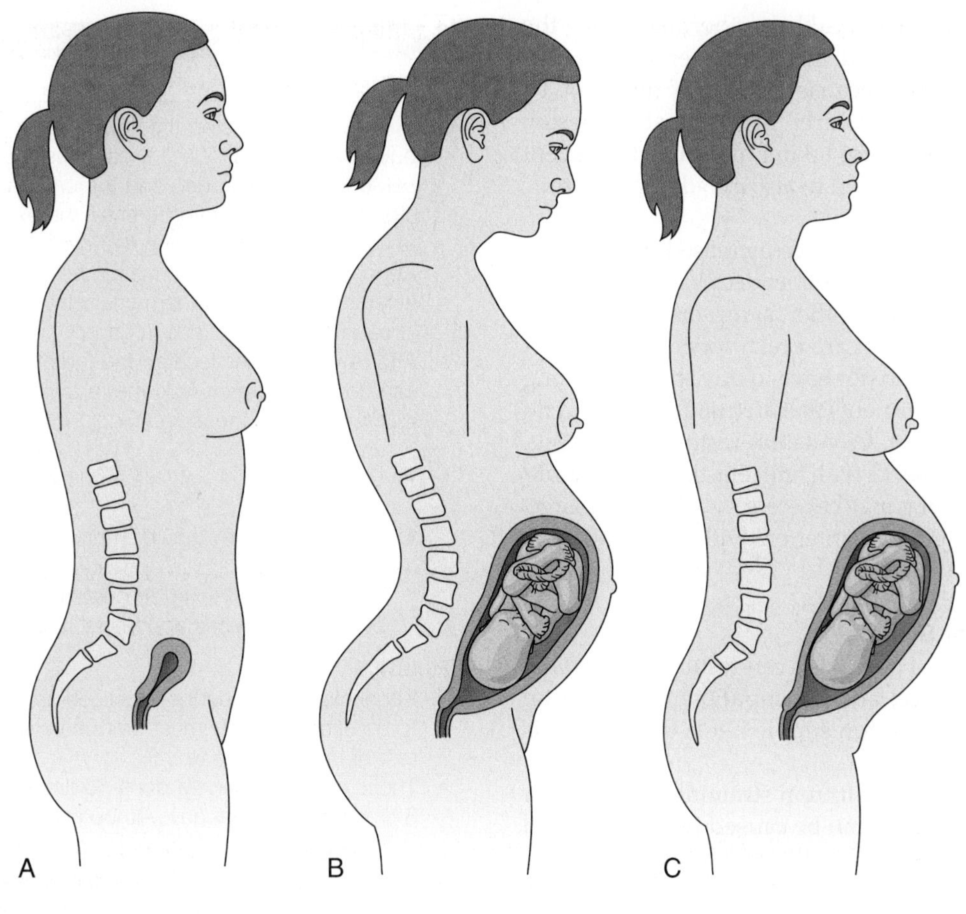

Fig. 26.7 Postural changes during pregnancy. A, Nonpregnant. B, Incorrect posture during pregnancy. C, Correct posture during pregnancy.

Table 26.5 Cardiovascular Changes in Pregnancy

Parameter	Change
Heart rate	Increases 10–15 bpm
Blood pressure	Remains at prepregnancy levels in first trimester (systolic) Slight decrease in second trimester (systolic and diastolic) Returns to prepregnancy levels in third trimester (diastolic)
Blood volume	Increases by 1500 mL or 40%–50% above prepregnancy level
Red blood cell mass	Increases 18%
Hemoglobin	Decreases
Hematocrit	Decreases
White blood cell count	Increases in second and third trimesters
Cardiac output	Increases 30%–50%

Modified from Lowdermilk DL, Perry SE, Cashion K, et al: *Maternal and women's health care,* ed 10, St. Louis, 2012, Mosby.

Table 26.6 Respiratory Changes in Pregnancy

Parameter	Change
Respiratory rate	Unchanged or slightly increased
Tidal volume	Increased 30%–40%
Vital capacity	Unchanged
Inspiratory capacity	Increased
Expiratory volume	Decreased
Total lung capacity	Unchanged to slightly decreased
Oxygen consumption	Increased 20%–40%

From Lowdermilk DL, Perry SE, Cashion K, et al: *Maternal and women's health care,* ed 10, St. Louis, 2012, Mosby.

Hygiene Practices

Bathing or showering during pregnancy should continue as part of routine hygiene. Increased perspiration is common, and good personal hygiene is important to prevent body odor. Tub bathing may become difficult in the later months of pregnancy because of changes in mobility and balance. Some primary care practitioners restrict tub baths in the last month because the cervix may have begun to dilate.

Most primary care practitioners recommend that women avoid hot tubs, sauna baths, and spas during pregnancy, because maternal hyperthermia during the first trimester may result in central nervous system defects of the fetus. Because a woman may not be aware she is pregnant early in the first trimester, those women who are not taking measures to prevent pregnancy are well advised to also avoid hyperthermic baths.

Pregnant women experience increased vaginal discharge. Douching is not recommended. Vaginal drainage that causes pruritus or other symptoms should be reported to the primary care practitioner.

Pregnant women do not have to buy special clothing but should choose garments that are comfortable and do not restrict movement. Circulation-restricting clothing, such as garters and socks with tight elastic bands, should be avoided. Larger bras may be necessary as breasts enlarge; a bra that is too tight may interfere with breathing.

ELIMINATION

Gastrointestinal System

Slowing of intestinal peristalsis can result in abdominal distention, flatulence, and constipation. Constipation also may be linked to iron supplements the woman is taking.

Hemorrhoids can result from straining as a result of constipation. They also can be caused by the enlarged uterus putting pressure on the pelvic blood vessels, slowing venous return from the lower extremities. Women with a history of cholelithiasis may experience problems with this as a result of an increased cholesterol level, which is common during pregnancy. Adequate fluid intake, dietary roughage, and exercise may help reduce problems related to constipation.

Urinary System

Frequency of urination is a common symptom of pregnancy. In the first trimester, this results from the enlarging uterus putting pressure on the bladder. Later, during the third trimester, the uterus moves back into the pelvic cavity in preparation for labor and delivery, again placing pressure on the urinary bladder. The increase in circulating blood volume results in increases in glomerular filtration rate (GFR). This causes an increase in urinary output. The stressors placed on the kidneys during pregnancy may result in protein and glucose to be detected in the urine samples. During the prenatal care period, the woman's urine is evaluated with a dipstick test to assess for the presence of glucose or protein. The patient can be taught Kegel exercises to help tone the muscles of the perineum and prevent stress incontinence (see the Patient Teaching box on Kegel exercises).

The ureter and kidneys may become dilated, particularly on the right side, as a result of placental progesterone and pressure from the enlarging uterus. Restricted circulation in the pelvis as the uterus enlarges increases the risk of bladder trauma and urinary tract infection.

 **Patient Teaching**

Kegel Exercises

- The muscles that stop the flow of urine are the pubococcygeal muscles. These muscles support the pelvic floor, the bladder, and the urethra. Attempts to stop the flow of urine or forestall the expulsion of gas aid the woman in targeting the involved muscles. Doing Kegel exercises during urination helps the woman know whether she is doing them correctly. If she can stop the stream of urine, her tone is good.
- After a woman has located the targeted muscles, she can do Kegel exercises in the following ways:
  - *Slow:* Tighten the muscle, hold it for a count of 3, and relax it.
  - *Quick:* Tighten the muscle, and relax it as rapidly as possible.
  - *Push out, pull in:* Pull up the entire pelvic floor as though trying to suck up water into the vagina. Then bear down as if trying to push the imaginary water out. This also uses abdominal muscles.

PRACTICE

- Kegel exercises must be practiced several times a day to be effective. They must be done every day for the rest of the woman's life.
- These exercises can be done 10 times in a row at least 3 times or more per day. Although some people recommend doing this as many as 100 times in a row, this only fatigues the pelvic floor muscles.
- A good time to practice is during trips to the bathroom, but additional practice at other times is even more beneficial.

Fatigue is reported commonly during pregnancy. The woman must pace herself and not overdo tiring activities.

ACTIVITY AND EXERCISE

Patients should continue normal activity throughout an uncomplicated pregnancy. If a woman regularly participates in a fitness program or sport, she probably can continue with most activities. This should be discussed with the health care provider. High-risk activities or those that require a great deal of balance and coordination are discouraged. Common sense is the best guide.

Changes in balance and posture occur as the fetus increases in size. To compensate for the shifting center of gravity, the lumbodorsal curve increases (lordosis), which may result in low backaches. Hormonal influence on pelvic bones, which results in joint relaxation, can lead to a waddling gait. Wearing footwear with low heels and using good body mechanics help reduce discomfort.

Leg cramps are common, perhaps related to pressure on the pelvic blood vessels and nerves or altered calcium and phosphorus balance. Dorsiflexion of the foot may help reduce these cramps. Dependent edema and varicose veins also may result from increasing intraabdominal pressure. Many women wear support hose to reduce edema; resting with legs elevated is also helpful.

Round ligament pain or tenderness in the lower abdomen is a result of stretching of the ligaments by the enlarging uterus. There is no way to prevent this, but use of good body mechanics reduces the discomfort.

Dyspnea (shortness of breath) may be experienced as the uterus enlarges and pushes the diaphragm upward, decreasing the size of the chest cavity. Avoiding large meals, which distend the stomach, and maintaining good posture help relieve this problem. Exercises often are recommended to help reduce discomfort and prepare for childbirth (Box 26.11).

REST AND SLEEP

Early in pregnancy, women experience increased fatigue. Napping is encouraged during this time. Left side-lying positioning is recommended to promote oxygenation. As the pregnancy progresses and the abdomen grows larger, the pregnant woman may have difficulty finding a position of comfort, particularly if she prefers to sleep in the prone position. The supine position is not recommended because the enlarged uterus may place excessive pressure on the aorta and vena cava. The pressure can result in vena cava syndrome (supine hypotensive syndrome). The woman may experience syncope and vertigo. The supine position also may result in decreased circulation for the fetus. A side-lying position is recommended (Fig. 26.8).

Encourage rest periods during the day with feet elevated. Placing pillows under the legs and abdomen promotes good body alignment and rest. Naps at intervals during the day can be helpful, but these are not always possible with busy lifestyles.

SEXUALITY AND REPRODUCTIVE SYSTEM

Breast Changes

Breast changes begin early in pregnancy. Many women report tingling and a feeling of fullness. Increased sensitivity is also common. Generally, the breasts grow

Box 26.11 Exercise Tips for Pregnant Women

- Consult your health care provider when you know or suspect you are pregnant. Discuss your medical and obstetric history, your current regimen, and the exercises you would like to continue throughout pregnancy.
- Seek help in determining an exercise routine that is well within your limit of tolerance, especially if you have not been exercising regularly.
- Consider decreasing weight-bearing exercises (jogging, running), and concentrate on non–weight-bearing activities such as swimming, cycling, or stretching. If you are a runner, you may wish to walk instead, starting in your 7th month.
- Avoid risky activities, such as surfing, mountain climbing, sky diving, and racquetball. Activities that require precise balance and coordination may be dangerous.
- Exercise regularly at least three times a week, as long as you are healthy, to improve muscle tone and increase or maintain your stamina. Sporadic exercises may put undue strain on your muscles.
- Limit activity to shorter intervals. Exercise for 10 to 15 minutes, rest for 2 to 3 minutes, then exercise for another 10 to 15 minutes.
- Decrease your exercise level as your pregnancy progresses. The normal alterations of advancing pregnancy, such as decreased cardiac reserve and increased respiratory effort, may produce physiologic stress if you exercise strenuously for a long time.
- Take your pulse every 10 to 15 minutes while you are exercising. If it is more than 140 bpm, slow down until it returns to a maximum of 90 bpm.
- Avoid becoming overheated for extended periods. It is best not to exercise for more than 35 minutes, especially in hot, humid weather. As your body temperature rises, the heat is transmitted to your fetus. Prolonged or repeated fetal temperature elevation may result in birth defects, especially during the first 3 months.
- Warm-up and stretching exercises prepare your joints for more strenuous exercise and lessen the likelihood of strain or injury to your joints.
- A cool-down period of mild activity after exercising helps bring your respiratory, heart, and metabolic rates back to normal and avoid pooling of blood in the exercise muscles.
- Rest for 10 minutes after exercising, lying on your left side. As the uterus grows, it puts pressure on a major vein carrying blood to your heart on the right side of your abdomen. Lying on your left side takes the pressure off and promotes return circulation from your extremities and muscles to your heart, increasing blood flow to your placenta and fetus.
- Drink two or three 8-oz glasses of water after you exercise to replace the body fluids you lost through perspiration. While exercising, drink water whenever you feel the need.
- Increase your caloric intake to replace the calories burned during exercise. Choose such high-protein foods as fish, cheese, eggs, or meat.
- Take your time. This is not the time to be competitive or train for activities that require long endurance.
- Wear a supportive bra. Your increased breast weight may cause changes in posture and put pressure on the ulnar nerve.
- Wear supportive shoes. As your uterus grows, your center of gravity shifts and you compensate by arching your back. These natural changes may make you feel off balance and more likely to fall.
- Stop exercising immediately if you experience shortness of breath, dizziness, numbness, tingling, abdominal pain, or vaginal bleeding, and consult your health care provider.

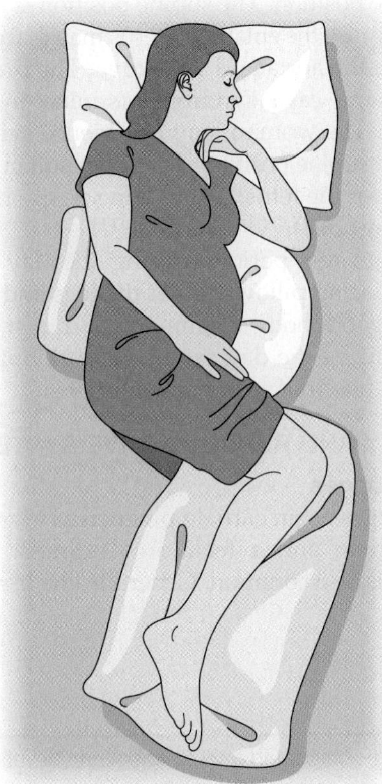

Fig. 26.8 During the third trimester, pillows that support the abdomen and back provide a comfortable position for rest.

in preparation for lactation. Nipples and areolae darken. Colostrum may be secreted by the nipples in second half of pregnancy. Supportive bras are recommended. If colostrum leakage is problematic, the woman should be encouraged to use breast pads.

Sexual Activity

Sexual desire is normal during pregnancy. The pregnant woman can have sexual relations unless contraindicated by other conditions. Complications during pregnancy, such as premature labor, bleeding, or rupture of membranes, necessitate that sexual activity be halted. Many factors have a strong influence on the frequency and type of sexual activity, including cultural, religious, and psychological influences. Partners must communicate their fears, concerns, and needs to each other. Many women experience a decrease in desire as a result of hormonal changes and discomfort. Change in body shape and body image also may cause concern. Discussion of various coital positions and sexual activity that does not include intercourse is appropriate. The health care provider may promote this discussion by introducing the topic during routine prenatal care.

Increased vaginal secretions are common during pregnancy. *Leukorrhea*, an increase in vaginal mucus, results from hormonal changes. If the discharge changes in color or odor, the physician should be informed at once.

Vaginal Bleeding

Vaginal bleeding at any time during pregnancy should be reported to the physician at once. Sexual activity should cease until the cause of the bleeding is determined and should be resumed only when the physician determines that no danger exists.

COPING AND STRESS TOLERANCE

Pregnancy is a developmental milestone. As with other significant developmental changes, anxiety is normal. All the physical and hormonal changes of pregnancy place additional stress on the woman. The woman and her partner normally have fears. They are concerned with the ability to cope with the pregnancy, the potential pain related to labor and delivery, and the health and well-being of the baby. Mood swings and ambivalence (conflicting emotions) are common as the woman works through her fears and comes to grips with the reality of pregnancy and how it will affect her life. During the early part of the pregnancy, the sudden hormonal changes combined with fatigue, nausea, and vomiting affect her concerns and ability to cope. As the pregnancy progresses, she will likely feel better and become increasingly able to adapt to the changes she experiences.

Women use problem-solving skills and methods of coping that worked in the past to adjust to this new situation. Provide support as this problem solving occurs and help the woman work through her unique situation. Explain the normal physiologic changes and discomforts. Listening and allowing the woman adequate time to verbalize her fears also may help reduce anxieties.

Roles, Relationships, and Adaptation

The expectant woman has generally held several roles in her life, such as child, student, employee, and wife. Pregnancy introduces a totally new role, that of mother. The woman often looks to her own life for role models and tends to seek guidance from family and friends. Culture has much to do with how she defines her role (Box 26.12).

Dynamics also change between the woman and the baby's father, particularly with the first pregnancy. The mother is no longer just a wife or girlfriend; she is also a mother. While she is coping with the role change to mother, he is coping with the role change to father (Box 26.13).

SELF-PERCEPTION AND SELF-CONCEPT

The rapid changes in body shape and size can lead to changes in self-image. Many women feel unattractive when they are pregnant. They also may feel a loss of control related to the changes taking place. They are no longer free to do as they please because all their actions may affect the growing fetus.

COGNITIVE AND PERCEPTUAL CHANGES

Although sensory changes are uncommon with pregnancy, blurred vision or diplopia (double vision) may

Box 26.12 Maternal Adaptation

Adaptation to the maternal role involves a complex social and cognitive learning process. Pregnancy functions as a rite of passage and indicates that physiologic maturity has been reached. Reva Rubin began studying maternal role adaptation in the 1960s. She described the developing tasks of pregnancy as accepting the pregnancy, identifying the role of mother, reordering the relationships between her mother and herself and between herself and her partner, establishing a relationship with the unborn child, and preparing for the birth experience.

Women who are prepared to accept a pregnancy seek medical validation early. When pregnancy is confirmed, a woman's emotional responses may range from delight to shock, disbelief, and despair. A general state of well-being predominates, but emotional lability is common. These rapid mood changes include increased irritability, explosions of tears and anger, and feelings of great joy and cheerfulness. Such changes are often attributed to hormonal changes.

Rubin describes changes in pregnancy as follows. The subjective experience of time and space changes during pregnancy; early in pregnancy, nothing seems to be happening, and the woman spends much time sleeping. With quickening (feelings of fetal movement) in the second trimester, there is a reduction of time and space, both geographic and social, as the woman turns her attention inward to her pregnancy. She examines or fosters relationships with her mother and other women who have been or are pregnant. With the third trimester, there is a slower pace and a sense that time is running out as the woman's activities are curtailed. A mother's positive reaction to her daughter's pregnancy signifies her acceptance of the grandchild and of her daughter. If the mother is supportive, the daughter has an opportunity to discuss pregnancy and labor and her feelings of joy or ambivalence with a knowledgeable and accepting woman.

The partner's emotional support is an important factor in successfully accomplishing the developmental tasks of pregnancy. Pregnant women express two major needs concerning their partner: feeling loved and valued and having the child accepted. The addition of a child changes forever the nature of the bond between partners. The partner can be a stabilizing influence, a good listener to expressions of doubts and fears, and a source of physical and emotional reassurance. The partner can also feel jealous of the unborn baby. Lesbian and unpartnered women have received little attention in the literature. Some suggest that a woman partner may be better able to understand and nurture her partner. An unpartnered woman may seek out her mother or other women friends to meet her dependence needs.

From Hockenberry MJ, Lowdermilk DL, et al: *Wong's maternal-child nursing care,* ed 8, St. Louis, 2007, Mosby.

Box 26.13 Paternal Adaptation

A man's emotional response to becoming a father, his concerns, and his informational needs change during the pregnancy. Men can experience three styles of involvement and one style of relative noninvolvement during pregnancy (May 1982). Men may be relatively uninvolved in pregnancy as observers, avoiding direct involvement in activities such as parent education classes and decisions about breastfeeding. Others are more involved and expressive, displaying a strong emotional response to pregnancy and a desire to be a full partner in the project. Some expectant fathers experience *couvade syndrome* and have pregnancy-like symptoms such as nausea, other gastrointestinal issues, and fatigue (couvade is a custom in some non-Western cultures in which a husband goes through mock pregnancy and labor). Some fathers adopt the instrumental style, performing tasks in their role as manager of the pregnancy. They feel responsible for the outcome of the pregnancy and are protective and supportive of their partners.

The father's beliefs and feelings about the ideal mother and father and his cultural expectation of appropriate behavior during pregnancy affect his response to his partner's need for him. One man may engage in nurturing behavior; another may feel lonely and alienated as the woman becomes physically and emotionally engrossed in the unborn child. The man may seek comfort and understanding outside the home or become interested in a new hobby or involved with his work. Some men view pregnancy as a proof of their masculinity and their dominant role. To others, pregnancy has no meaning in terms of responsibility to either mother or child. However, for most men, pregnancy is a time of preparation for the parental role, of fantasy or great pleasure, and of intense learning.

From Perry S, Hockenberry M, Lowdermilk D, et al: *Maternal-child nursing care,* ed 5, St. Louis, 2014, Mosby.

indicate problems with a hypertensive condition of pregnancy (see Chapter 28).

PREPARATION FOR CHILDBIRTH

Prenatal education is important. Most primary care practitioners give explanations during routine visits, but the time available is too brief to meet all of the average woman's needs. The nurse plays an important role in prenatal education. Provide pamphlets and referrals to community-based resources whenever possible. Libraries and bookstores also have many good books on prenatal care. Another source of information the expectant mother may consider are the special classes by hospitals and public health agencies to help the childbearing family understand and prepare for the demands of pregnancy, labor, the newborn, and parenthood. An increasing number of women seek information from Internet resources. Address the selection of reliable and safe online sites for obtaining information.

CHILDBIRTH PREPARATION CLASSES

Communities often have a variety of courses that complement one another and meet the differing needs of specific segments of the population (Fig. 26.9). Some classes are general, whereas others are targeted toward specific groups such as adolescents, those having cesarean or vaginal birth after cesarean delivery, siblings, or grandparents (Box 26.14).

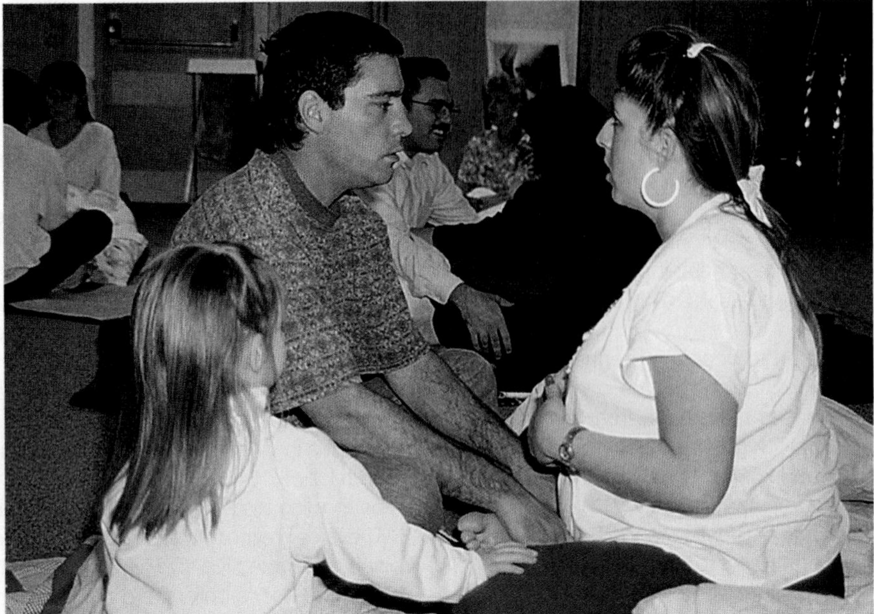

Fig. 26.9 Entire family participating in a childbirth preparation course. (From Lowdermilk DL, Perry SE: *Maternity and women's health care*, ed 10, St. Louis, 2016, Elsevier.)

Box 26.14 Topics Typically Discussed in Childbirth Preparation Classes

- A review of reproductive anatomy and physiology
- Physical and emotional changes commonly observed during pregnancy
- Fetal growth and development
- Nutrition
- Routine aspects of prenatal hygiene and exercise
- Danger signs during pregnancy
- Birth process, vaginal and cesarean
- Analgesia and anesthesia during labor and delivery
- Care of the newborn infant
- Selection of infant feeding methods
- Sibling preparation
- Changing family dynamics
- Postpartal exercises

Common methods of prepared childbirth include Dick-Read, which focuses on progressive relaxation techniques and avoidance of analgesics; Bradley, which stresses control of environmental factors, such as lighting, temperature, and noise, to provide a calm, supportive environment for childbirth; Leboyer, which uses a warm water bath to reduce the trauma of birth; and Lamaze, which uses breathing, distraction, and focusing techniques to control pain mentally and requires disciplined training throughout the pregnancy. The Patient Teaching box on safety during pregnancy provides activity and environmental guidelines.

CULTURAL VARIATIONS IN PRENATAL CARE

The practitioner must determine and explore cultural practices and beliefs with the patient (see the Cultural Considerations box; see Chapter 6 for further discussion of the cultural aspects of nursing).

 **Patient Teaching**

Safety During Pregnancy

Changes in the body as a result of pregnancy include relaxation of joints, alteration of the center of gravity, faintness, and discomfort. Problems with coordination and balance are common. Therefore the woman should follow these guidelines:

- Use good body mechanics.
- Use safety features on tools or vehicles (safety seatbelts, shoulder harnesses, headrests, goggles, helmets) as specified.
- Avoid activities that require coordination, balance, and concentration.
- Take rest periods; reschedule daily activities to meet rest and relaxation needs.

❖ NURSING PROCESS FOR NORMAL PREGNANCY

The role of the licensed practical nurse/licensed vocational nurse (LPN/LVN) in the nursing process as stated is that the LPN/LVN will:

- Participate in planning care for patients based on patient needs.
- Review patient's plan of care and recommend revisions as needed.
- Review and follow defined prioritization for patient care.
- Use clinical pathways, care maps, or care plans to guide and review patient care.

◆ ASSESSMENT

Assessment begins when the woman visits the physician's office or clinic during the early part of her pregnancy. The first visit includes obtaining demographic data, taking

Cultural Considerations

Pregnancy

- Many cultures and religions have customs that affect pregnant women. It is important not to generalize when giving care. Not all members of a cultural group behave in exactly the same way. Discuss beliefs with each individual to determine her unique cultural practices. If the practices do not cause harm, include them in planning care.
- Because of cultural and other factors—such as lack of money, lack of transportation, and poor communication on the part of health care providers—many women do not receive adequate prenatal care. Do not misinterpret the woman's behavior as uncaring, lazy, or ignorant.
- A concern for modesty can be a deterrent for prenatal care. Exposure of one's genitalia, especially to a male practitioner, is a significant breach of modesty. Thus many women prefer a midwife instead of a male practitioner. Health care providers frequently assume that women lose this sense of modesty during pregnancy and labor. Most women value and appreciate efforts to maintain their modesty.
- Almost all cultures advocate a socially harmonious and agreeable environment during pregnancy. Stressful relationships can hinder a successful outcome for the mother and baby.
- Extended family members may wish to accompany the pregnant woman to her prenatal care visits and during labor. To avoid discord, the nurse and other staff members must accommodate the situation in culturally prescribed ways.
- Some belief systems include magical thinking about events that may occur during pregnancy. Among Hispanics, it traditionally is thought that witnessing an eclipse of the moon may cause a cleft palate in the infant; exposure to an earthquake may result in preterm delivery or miscarriage, or cause a breech presentation if the earthquake was exceptionally strong. Some African Americans may warn a pregnant woman not to ridicule someone with an affliction or her child may be born with the same handicap. A widely held folk belief persists that raising one's arm above one's head or tying knots may cause the umbilical cord to wrap around the baby's neck and become knotted.
- Native people from some cultures of the American Southwest may wear amulets (charm, talisman, fetish, lucky piece), spirit medals, and beads to ward off evil.
- Pregnant Filipino women may be cautioned that any activity is dangerous, and others willingly take over their work. Inactivity is considered a protection for the mother and baby. The mother is encouraged to simply produce the succeeding generation. This behavior should not be misinterpreted as laziness or noncompliance.

a health history, and performing a general physical assessment and an obstetric assessment. The general assessment includes lifestyle patterns, body system examination, and laboratory screening of blood and urine. Also explore the woman's perceptions of her condition, cultural and ethnic influences, experiences with other caregivers, lifestyle, and patterns of coping. A symptom diary, in which the woman records emotions, behaviors, physical symptoms, diet, and exercise and rest patterns, is a useful diagnostic tool. The obstetric assessment includes a gynecologic and obstetric history and a gynecologic examination with Pap smear, if needed.

◆ PATIENT PROBLEM

Nursing assessment helps identify the needs of the pregnant patient. Care can be then based on these needs. Possible patient problems for a normal pregnancy include the following:

- *Deficient Sleep*
- *Distorted Body Image*
- *Fearfulness*
- *Impaired family processes*
- *Inability to Control Urination due to Physical Stress*
- *Inability to Tolerate Activity*
- *Infrequent or Difficult Bowel Elimination*
- *Insufficient Knowledge*
- *Insufficient Nutrition*
- *Lethargy or Malaise*
- *Potential for Compromised Parenting Skills*
- *Potential for Injury*

◆ EXPECTED OUTCOMES AND PLANNING

The care plan should focus on the pregnant patient's needs and the nurse's ability to address those needs effectively (Nursing Care Plan 26.1). Each patient has different needs, and care must be individualized accordingly.

The care plan focuses on goals and outcomes specific to the patient problem. Examples include the following:

Goal 1: Patient will use self-care behaviors to maintain optimal levels of wellness for herself and the fetus.

Outcome: Patient keeps all prenatal appointments, does not smoke or drink alcoholic beverages, and does not use other drugs unless prescribed by her physician.

Goal 2: Patient will become knowledgeable about needs and concerns experienced during each trimester.

Outcome: Patient keeps a symptom diary and discusses it on each visit to the primary caregiver. Patient attends prenatal classes regularly.

◆ IMPLEMENTATION

Nursing interventions during the prenatal period may include the following:

- Identify factors that may interfere with health maintenance.
- Provide information to the patient to promote health maintenance.
- Assess and counsel on nutritional habits and weight gain.
- Stress safety issues regarding risk of injury as the pregnancy progresses.
- Teach the importance of pacing activities.
- Review the importance of adequate fluid intake.
- Review patterns of elimination and any changes that have occurred.

Nursing Care Plan 26.1 The Patient With a Normal Pregnancy

Ms. P. is a 23-year-old gravida 1, para 0 at 30 weeks of gestation. She has gained 12 lb since the beginning of her pregnancy. She has a full-time job at an insurance company and plays tennis twice a week. She considers herself a vegan but reports she does eat some fish. She takes prenatal vitamins daily. She reports some constipation, although her bowel habits were normal before her pregnancy.

PATIENT PROBLEM

Insufficient Nutrition, related to dietary habits

Patient Goals and Expected Outcomes	Nursing Interventions	Evaluation
Patient will meet nutritional needs Patient will know about additional nutritional needs during pregnancy and how to fulfill them	Assess weight at regular intervals. Review the ChooseMyPlate guide. Provide information related to nutritional needs during pregnancy. Have patient keep dietary diary.	Patient meets her nutritional needs as evidenced by recommended weight gain. Patient displays knowledge of additional nutritional needs by eating a well-balanced diet as evidenced by dietary diary and appropriate weight gain.
	Encourage patient to drink 6–8 glasses of water daily to aid in bowel regularity.	Patient reports water intake of 6–8 glasses daily.

PATIENT PROBLEM

Potential for Compromised Parenting Skills or Ineffective Attachment, related to developmental stressors of pregnancy and to lack of knowledge and skill

Patient Goals and Expected Outcomes	Nursing Interventions	Evaluation
Patient will follow a lifestyle that is conducive to a positive pregnancy outcome	Discuss measures that promote a healthy pregnancy outcome, including nutrition, physical activity, rest, stress reduction, and lifestyle changes. Encourage patient to ask questions and express concerns.	The patient makes necessary lifestyle changes to promote a positive pregnancy outcome. Patient uses effective coping strategies regarding stressors of pregnancy.
Patient will express ability to cope with the changes and stressors of pregnancy	Provide encouragement for effective coping strategies used. Encourage patient to keep a symptom diary and bring it with her to each prenatal visit. Inform parents of community resources to assist and support them as needed. Help parents develop realistic expectations of newborn behaviors and demands. Assess parents' plans to incorporate the newborn into the family circle. Offer opportunity for demonstration of infant care skills, with return demonstration.	Patient keeps symptom diary and brings it to each prenatal visit; feels free to discuss concerns. Parents complete infant bathing, diapering, cord care, and feeding appropriately in return demonstration.

CRITICAL THINKING QUESTIONS

1. How should the nurse respond to Ms. P. if she expresses concern about her dietary practices and their effect on her baby? What suggestions can the nurse give her to ensure that her diet is adequate to support the pregnancy?
2. Ms. P. states that she is concerned about having to reduce her activity schedule, particularly tennis, which she enjoys. She is worried she will begin to resent her baby because of the need to alter her activities. How should the nurse respond to her concerns? What suggestions should the nurse give her?

- Teach ways to position body for sleep promotion and rest.
- Provide information on prenatal classes.
- Explain discomforts and danger signs.
- Encourage verbalization of fears and concerns.
- Incorporate patient's cultural values into the care plan.

See the Health Promotion box for self-care prenatal health maintenance measures.

◆ EVALUATION

Continually evaluate the success of the interventions. As the pregnancy progresses, the focus and interventions change. Refer to the goals and outcomes to determine whether the care plan was successful and the outcomes were met. Be assured that care has been effective when the woman reports improvements in the quality of her life, skill in self-care, and a positive self-concept and body image.

Health Promotion

Prenatal Health Maintenance Measures

Health maintenance is an important aspect of prenatal care. Patient participation in the care ensures prompt reporting of problematic responses to pregnancy. Patient responsibility for health maintenance is strengthened by a readiness to learn and by the nurse's understanding of maternal adaptations to the growth of the unborn child.

The expectant mother needs information about many topics. Be observant, listen, and know the typical concerns of expectant parents to anticipate what questions will be asked and to prompt mothers and their partners to discuss what is on their minds. Provide printed literature to supplement the individualized teaching; women often avidly read books and pamphlets related to their own experience. Read the literature before distributing it, and point out areas that may not correspond to local health care practices. Patients who receive conflicting advice or instruction may grow frustrated with members of the health care team and the care provided.

Topics to discuss with pregnant women may include the following:

EMPLOYMENT

- Employment of pregnant women usually has no adverse effects on pregnancy outcomes. Job discrimination that is based solely on pregnancy is illegal. However, some job environments pose a potential risk to the fetus (e.g., dry-cleaning plants, chemical laboratories, and parking garages).
- Discourage activities that require a good sense of balance, especially during the last half of pregnancy.
- Commonly, excessive fatigue is the deciding factor in the termination of employment.
- Women in sedentary jobs need to walk around at intervals and should neither sit nor stand in one position for long periods. Activity counters sluggish leg circulation, which can cause varices and thrombophlebitis. Women also should avoid crossing their legs at the knees because this fosters such conditions. Standing for long periods increases the risk of preterm labor.
- The pregnant woman's chair should provide adequate back support. Use of a footstool can prevent pressure on veins, relieve strain on varicosities, and reduce swelling of feet.

CLOTHING

- Comfortable, loose clothing is best. Washable fabrics (e.g., absorbent cottons) often are preferred. Maternity clothes may be purchased new or found in good condition at thrift shops or garage sales. Tight bras and belts, stretch pants, garters, tight-top knee socks, panty girdles, and other constrictive clothing should be avoided, because tight clothing over the perineum encourages vaginitis, and impaired circulation in the legs can cause varices.
- Maternity bras are constructed to accommodate the increased breast weight. These bras have drop-flaps over the nipples to facilitate breast-feeding. A good bra can help prevent neck and back discomfort.
- Elastic hose are comfortable and promote greater venous emptying in women with large varicose veins. Ideally, the supportive hose should be worn during waking hours.
- Comfortable shoes that provide firm support and promote good posture and balance are advisable. Tall high heels and platform shoes are not recommended because of the woman's changed center of gravity, which can cause her to lose balance. In addition, the woman's pelvis tilts forward in the third trimester, increasing her lumbar curve. The resulting leg aches and cramps are aggravated by shoes that do not provide good support.

TRAVEL

- Travel is not contraindicated for pregnant women at low risk, but those with high-risk pregnancies are advised to avoid long-distance travel after fetal viability has been reached, to avoid the economic and psychological consequences of delivering a preterm infant far from home.
- The second trimester is the ideal time for travel.
- Travel to areas where medical care is poor, water is untreated, and malaria is prevalent should be avoided if possible.
- Women who contemplate foreign travel should be aware that many health insurance carriers do not cover birth in a foreign setting or even hospitalization for preterm labor.
- Pregnant women who travel long distances should schedule periods of activity and rest. While sitting, women can practice deep breathing, foot circling, and alternately contracting and relaxing different muscle groups. They should avoid becoming fatigued.
- Although travel is not a cause of adverse outcomes, such as miscarriage or preterm labor, certain precautions are recommended while traveling in a car. The woman always should use automobile restraints, generally a combination lap belt and shoulder harness. The lap belt is worn low across the hip bones and as snug as is comfortable. The shoulder belt is worn above the pregnant uterus and below the neck to avoid chafing. The pregnant woman should sit upright and use the headrest to avoid a whiplash injury.
- Maternal death as a result of injury is the most common cause of fetal death. The next most common cause is placental separation. This occurs because body contours change in reaction to the force of a collision. The uterus as a muscular organ can adapt its shape to that of the body, but the placenta lacks the resiliency to change. At the impact of collision, placental separation can occur.
- Airline travel in large commercial jets usually poses little risk to the pregnant woman, but policies vary from airline to airline. The pregnant woman is advised to inquire about restrictions or recommendations from her carrier. Magnetometers (metal detectors) used at airport security checkpoints are not harmful to the fetus. Cabins of commercial airlines are maintained at 8% humidity, which may result in some water loss; hydration (with water) should be maintained under these conditions. Sitting in a cramped seat of an airliner for prolonged periods may increase the risk of superficial and deep thrombophlebitis. A pregnant woman is encouraged to take a 15-minute walk around the aircraft cabin during each hour of travel to minimize this risk.

Get Ready for the NCLEX® Examination!

Key Points

- Pregnancy is a normal process that involves many complex physiologic changes in the mother.
- Over a period of 280 days, two initial cells join and develop into a unique, viable human.
- Structures such as the placenta, membranes, the umbilical cord, and amniotic fluid protect and support the developing fetus. These structures are unique to pregnancy.
- All aspects of the mother's lifestyle potentially can affect her developing fetus.
- Many drugs and viruses can cross the placenta and present serious hazards to the developing embryo, particularly during the first trimester of pregnancy.
- Sophisticated diagnostic tests often are performed to identify genetic or developmental problems during pregnancy. Early identification of problems may influence a woman's decisions regarding a pregnancy.
- Although pregnancy is a normal process, regular and ongoing health care is important throughout pregnancy.
- At present, the best means of reducing the number of children born with genetic defects is for health professionals to provide families with genetic information and services.
- Many signs and symptoms of pregnancy are similar to those that are characteristic of other medical conditions. The positive signs of pregnancy are visualization of the fetus, fetal motion detected by a trained observer, and auscultation of fetal heart sounds.
- Every pregnant woman should be aware of the danger signs during pregnancy and contact her physician if any of them are present.
- The rational use of any medication requires a risk-versus-benefit assessment. Among the many risk factors that complicate assessment, pregnancy is one of the most perplexing.
- Nutritional needs change during pregnancy. To support normal growth and development of the fetus, the woman needs increased calories, minerals, and vitamins.
- Many discomforts may occur during pregnancy. Be aware of measures that can reduce these discomforts without harming the mother or the fetus.
- Pregnancy is a time of role adjustment for both prospective parents. All family members are affected by the addition of a new member.
- Adequate preparation enables the woman to become a knowledgeable participant in the entire childbearing process. Be aware of classes available in the community and the materials covered in these classes.
- The nurse and the patient are influenced by cultural and personal values and beliefs during the patient's pregnancy. Careful assessment is imperative.

Additional Learning Resources

SG Go to your Study Guide for additional learning activities to help you master this chapter content.

evolve Be sure to visit the Evolve site at *http://evolve.elsevier.com/Cooper/foundationsadult/* for additional online resources.

Review Questions for the NCLEX® Examination

1. A 25-year-old woman comes to the clinic and says she thinks she is pregnant. Her last period was July 20. Based on this fact, what is the expected date of delivery (EDD)?
   1. April 13
   2. April 27
   3. May 20
   4. March 27
2. The patient reports experiencing nausea, vomiting, and breast tenderness along with missing her period. These symptoms are considered to be what type of signs of pregnancy?
   1. Probable
   2. Positive
   3. Presumptive
   4. Possible
3. A pregnant patient is seen during her second trimester at the health care provider's office. She asks the nurse, "What can I do when my leg goes into a cramp?" The patient demonstrates understanding of the nurse's instruction regarding relief of leg cramps if she takes which action?
   1. Wiggles and points her toes during the cramp
   2. Applies cold compresses to the affected leg
   3. Extends her leg and dorsiflexes her foot during the cramp
   4. Avoids weight bearing on the affected leg during the cramp
4. A woman who is in her first trimester is talking with the nurse. The patient has inquired about the feelings she will have when she first feels her baby move. What information can be provided by the nurse?
   1. The movement will feel like cramps.
   2. The movement is rhythmic and called Goodell's sign.
   3. The movement is flutter-like and is called quickening.
   4. The movement is like a thud and is called Hëgar's sign.
5. While giving a health history to the nurse, the patient reports that she usually has a glass of wine with dinner. What is the safe level of alcohol intake for her during her pregnancy?
   1. No alcohol
   2. Wine only; one or two glasses daily with meals
   3. Up to 4 oz daily
   4. Beer or wine only after the first trimester

6. The nurse explains to the patient that she should contact her health care provider if she experiences any of the danger signs of pregnancy. Which symptoms are a danger sign during pregnancy? *(Select all that apply.)*
   1. Urinary frequency
   2. Severe headaches
   3. Dyspepsia
   4. Heartburn
   5. Diplopia
7. A test that may be done in late pregnancy to determine fetal well-being is the nonstress test. This test is based on which phenomenon?
   1. Fetal heart rate increases in connection with fetal movement.
   2. Braxton Hicks contractions cause an increase in fetal heart rate.
   3. Fetal heart rate slows in response to contractions.
   4. Fetal movement causes an increase in maternal heart rate.
8. Constipation is a frequent symptom as a pregnancy progresses. Which measures should be recommended to the gravid woman? *(Select all that apply.)*
   1. Drink six to eight glasses of water daily.
   2. Take an over-the-counter laxative.
   3. Take an iron supplement only every other day.
   4. Take mineral oil at bedtime.
   5. Increase dietary fiber intake.
9. At one of her prenatal visits, the patient is scheduled for a sonogram. Sonography can be used to assess which of the following? *(Select all that apply.)*
   1. Number of fetuses
   2. Gestational age of fetus
   3. Down syndrome
   4. Congenital anomalies
   5. Placement of the placenta
10. Which symptom is considered a first-trimester warning sign and should be reported immediately to the health care provider?
    1. Nausea with occasional vomiting
    2. Fatigue
    3. Urinary frequency
    4. Vaginal bleeding
11. A pregnant woman at 10 weeks of gestation jogs three or four times per week. She is concerned about the effect of exercise on the fetus. What information can be provided by the nurse?
    1. "You do not need to modify your exercising anytime during your pregnancy."
    2. "Stop exercising because it will harm the fetus."
    3. "You may find that you need to modify your exercising to walking later in your pregnancy, around the seventh month."
    4. "Jogging is too hard on your body; switch to walking now."
12. A woman at 23 weeks of gestation calls to tell the nurse she thinks she is leaking fluid from her vagina. What information should be included in the nurse's response to the patient?
    1. "As long as the baby is still moving around, there is nothing to worry about."
    2. "Come to the office right away."
    3. "Call me back in 2 hours, and tell me if there is any change in the leakage."
    4. "We can wait until your next appointment to check you."
13. A woman admitted in labor has an obstetric history that indicates that she has had four pregnancies and has 3 living children. One was born at 39 weeks of gestation, another at 34 of weeks of gestation, and another at 35 weeks of gestation. She had a miscarriage at 16 weeks gestation. What are her gravidity and parity with the TPAL system?
    1. 1-2-1-3
    2. 1-2-0-3
    3. 3-0-3-0
    4. 2-2-0-3
14. The nurse teaches a pregnant woman about the presumptive, probable, and positive signs of pregnancy. Which are positive signs of pregnancy? *(Select all that apply.)*
    1. A positive pregnancy test
    2. Fetal movement palpated by the primary caregiver
    3. Braxton Hicks contractions
    4. Nausea and vomiting
    5. Presence of fetal heart tones
15. A patient is scheduled for an ultrasound scan. She is at 22 weeks' gestation. The patient asks how they will be able to tell the gestational age of her fetus. When planning the response, the nurse correctly recognizes that which measurements will be used in this determination? *(Select all that apply.)*
    1. Abdominal circumference
    2. Biparietal diameter
    3. Quantity of amniotic fluid
    4. Femur length
    5. Crown rump length
16. An expectant father confides in the nurse that his pregnant wife (10 weeks of gestation) is driving him crazy. "One minute she seems happy, and the next minute she seems unhappy, and the next she is crying over nothing at all. Is there something wrong with her?" What is the most appropriate response by the nurse?
    1. "This is normal behavior and should begin to subside by the second trimester."
    2. "She may be having difficulty relating to the pregnancy. I will refer her to a counselor I know."
    3. "This is called emotional lability and is related to hormone changes and anxiety during pregnancy. The mood swings will subside as she adjusts to being pregnant."
    4. "You seem impatient with her. Perhaps this is precipitating her behavior."

17. When planning a diet with a pregnant woman, what should the nurse's initial action be?
    1. Review the woman's dietary intake.
    2. Teach the woman about the ChooseMyPlate guide.
    3. Caution the woman to avoid large doses of vitamins, especially those that are fat soluble.
    4. Instruct the woman to limit the intake of fatty foods.
18. A pregnant woman at 32 weeks of gestation reports feeling dizzy and lightheaded while her fundal height is being measured. Her skin is pale and moist. What should the nurse's initial action be?
    1. Assess the woman's blood pressure and pulse.
    2. Have the woman breathe into a paper bag.
    3. Raise the woman's legs.
    4. Turn the woman on her side.
19. When obtaining a reproductive health history from a female patient, what should the nurse do?
    1. Limit the time spent on exploration of intimate topics.
    2. Explain the purpose of questions asked and how they will be used.
    3. Avoid asking questions that may embarrass the patient.
    4. Use only acceptable medical terminology when referring to body parts and functions.
20. After admitting a new patient to the maternity unit, the nurse writes a care plan. This process of determining outcomes and interventions is which stage of the nursing process?
    1. Assessment
    2. Planning
    3. Implementation
    4. Evaluation

Fill in the Blank

Fill in the blank with the correct medical term.

21. ____________ Woman who is pregnant
22. ____________ Woman who is pregnant for the first time
23. ____________ Woman who has had two or more pregnancies
24. ____________ Capacity to live outside the uterus

Labor and Delivery

27

http://evolve.elsevier.com/Cooper/foundationsadult/

Objectives

1. Discuss birth planning.
2. Discuss birth setting choices.
3. Discuss the signs and symptoms of impending labor.
4. Distinguish between true and false labor.
5. Explain the five factors that affect the labor process.
6. Discuss cephalopelvic disproportion.
7. Describe the "powers" involved in labor and delivery.
8. Identify the mechanisms of labor.
9. Identify the stages of labor.
10. Describe the assessment for labor and delivery.
11. Identify nursing diagnoses relevant to the woman in labor.
12. Discuss nursing interventions related to labor and delivery.
13. Outline medical interventions related to labor and delivery.

Key Terms

amniotomy (ăm-nē-ŎT-ō-mē, p. 829)
attitude (p. 802)
Braxton Hicks contractions (p. 799)
cardinal movements of labor (p. 807)
cephalopelvic disproportion (sĕf-ă-lō-PĔL-vĭk dĭs-prō-PŌR-shŭn, p. 830)
descent (p. 807)
effacement (ĕ-FĀS-mĕnt, p. 799)
engagement (ĕn-GĀJ-mĕnt, p. 807)
episiotomy (ĕ-pĭs-ē-ŎT-ō-mē, p. 812)
expulsion (p. 809)
extension (p. 809)
external rotation (p. 809)
fetal lie (p. 802)
fetal position (p. 802)
fetal presentation (p. 802)
flexion (FLĔK-shŭn, p. 802)
hypoxia (hī-PŎK-sē-ă, p. 817)
internal rotation (p. 807)
lightening (p. 798)
meconium (mĕ-KŌ-nē-ŭm, p. 817)
oligohydramnios (ŏl-ĭ-gō-hī-DRĂM-nē-ŏs, p. 820)
oxytocin (ŏks-ē-TŌ-sĭn, p. 812)
restitution (p. 809)
surfactant (sŭr-FĂK-tănt, p. 817)
uterine inertia (YŪ-tĕr-ĭn ĭn-ĔR-shă, p. 829)

BIRTH PLANNING

Preparation of the mother and her partner for the birth of the baby ideally begins early in the pregnancy. Beginning teaching in the first trimester allows the family time to ask questions and retain information provided. The education provided should include information about the pregnancy-related changes the mother will experience, fetal development, labor, delivery, and the postpartum periods. Some health care providers and mothers initiate a birth plan. The plan begins as an outline of the options available for the mother and her baby for the labor, delivery, and postpartum periods. The mother then is encouraged to select preferred options. The mother must recognize that some desires in the plan cannot be satisfied. Inability to achieve all the elements may result from concern for the health and well-being of the mother and her baby or because of facility policies.

BIRTH SETTING CHOICES

The expectant mother should consider the location in which to give birth. Choices may be limited by the community of residence, the medical privileges and preferences of the selected practitioner, and the health of the mother and baby. The three primary options to consider are the hospital, birthing center, or home.

Hospitals

In previous generations home deliveries were considered commonplace. Technological advances, anesthesia options, and desires for the convenience of birthing in a facility have resulted in the movement of births to hospital settings. Today, the majority of births take place in hospital settings. Only 1.4% of births occur outside of a hospital (CDC, 2015). In 2013 more than 56,000 births occurred outside of the hospital. More than

60% of those deliveries took place in the home. The remaining deliveries were in a free-standing birthing center.

Birthing in a hospital has many advantages. The greatest is the availability of trained personnel in the event complications occur. Within the hospital facility, a variety of rooming options are available. Some facilities offer single-room LDRP (labor, delivery, recovery, postpartum) units. This type of arrangement allows for the labor, delivery, and birth to take place in a single location. After delivery, the new mother and her baby continue to be cared for in the same room by a single team of nurses. Some facilities have more traditional arrangements with LDR (labor, delivery, recovery) units. In the LDR setting, the mother is admitted to the labor suite and remains there until a specified time after birth. Then she is transferred to a postpartum care unit. The baby either is transferred to a nursery or remains with the mother.

Birthing Centers

A birthing center is a care facility focused on childbirth. The centers may be privately held or affiliated with an acute care hospital. Although still limited, the use of birthing centers has increased. Presently, less than 1% of births take place in birthing centers. The relationship with a hospital provides a degree of security should a complication arise and more invasive care be necessary. Birthing centers are family focused and are considered ideal only for those women with low-risk pregnancies. Complications of pregnancy or necessary cesarean section are factors that negate the woman's use of a birthing center. These facilities are viewed as desirable, because they allow the mother to experience labor and delivery in a more homelike setting. An emphasis is placed on the wishes of the woman and her partner. Typical room settings for birthing centers are LDRP rooms.

Home

Home births were common in the United States until the early 1900s. (Over the early decades of the 20th century, a shift toward hospital births took place.) Currently, women who want to have more control over their birth experience and desire reduced technology have led a renewed interest in home births. Giving birth at home is not an option for all women. It is intended for the healthy pregnant woman and fetus who have not experienced complications during the gestational period. Women who have experienced complications in previous pregnancies are also not likely candidates for home births. In a study of more than 16,000 women who planned home births only 11% were not successful and required transfer to a hospital facility. The most common reason was the failure of the labor to progress. The rates of cesarean section, augmentation, induction, and complications were lower than those found in hospital deliveries. Although most home births are attended by midwives, they also may be managed by a variety of medical professionals, including a physician, nurse, or physician's assistant (Cheyney, Bovbjerg, Everson et al, 2014).

NORMAL LABOR

ONSET

In most pregnancies, the uterus begins the process of labor once the fetus is matured and ready for birth. Although this process has been occurring throughout human history, researchers still are trying to discover the exact cause for the onset, or beginning, of labor. The theories fall into two main categories: those based on mechanical changes and those based on hormonal changes.

One mechanical theory involves uterine stretching. It is based on the principle that once a hollow-body organ reaches a certain state of distention, it spontaneously contracts and empties. For example, a full bladder empties by incontinence and a distended stomach empties by vomiting. The hypothesis is that when the uterus stretches to a certain size, it empties spontaneously. However, the wide variation of uterine size between different pregnancies in the same woman makes this a weak theory. For example, a woman may have one pregnancy in which she delivers a 6-pound baby at term. In her next pregnancy, she may again reach term but deliver twins, each weighing 6 pounds.

Several hormonal theories for the onset of labor are based on either an increase or a decrease in hormones. In some of the theories, the source of the hormones is the mother; in other theories, it is the fetus. Some of the more common (but still unproven) theories relating to hormones are (1) oxytocin stimulation; (2) progesterone withdrawal; (3) estrogen stimulation; and (4) fetal cortisol.

SIGNS OF IMPENDING LABOR

A series of signs may occur as labor is about to begin. Approximately 2 weeks before the onset of labor, the woman may notice that the fetus seems to have settled, or "dropped," into the pelvis. This is called **lightening** and is seen most often in nulliparas. Once lightening has occurred, the woman often notices that urinary frequency returns. She may be able to breathe more normally because the abdominal cavity has more space. Multiparas may not experience this change until they are in active labor.

Occasionally, a woman may have seepage or sudden outflow of fluid from the vagina. Although urine does not seep from the vagina, the close proximity of the urinary meatus may cause the woman to believe that it is amniotic fluid. Evaluation should be performed to determine what the fluid is. A simple test with nitrazine paper can distinguish between fluids (Box 27.1). The paper is moistened with the discharge from the

Box 27.1 Nitrazine Test for Rupture of Membranes

- Explain the procedure to the woman or the couple.
- Perform the procedure.
- Wash hands.
- Put on sterile gloves.
- Use nitrazine test paper, a dye-impregnated test paper for determination of pH (differentiates amniotic fluid, which is slightly alkaline, from urine and purulent material [pus], which are acidic).
- While wearing a sterile glove lubricated with water, place a piece of test paper on the cervical opening.
  or
- With a sterile, cotton-tipped applicator, dip deep into the vagina to pick up fluid; touch applicator to test paper. (Procedure may be done during speculum examination.)
- Read results:
  - Membranes probably intact: identifies vaginal and most body fluids that are acidic:
    Yellow, pH 5.0
    Olive-yellow, pH 5.5
    Olive-green, pH 6.0
  - Membranes probably ruptured: identifies amniotic fluid that is alkaline:
    Blue-green, pH 6.5
    Blue-gray, pH 7.0
    Deep blue, pH 7.5
- False test results are possible because of presence of bloody show, insufficient amniotic fluid, or semen.
- Provide pericare as needed.
- Remove gloves and wash hands.
- Document results (positive or negative).

unwashed area. If the paper reacts (turns blue), the discharge is probably amniotic fluid. If the test is nonreactive, the membranes are probably intact and the discharge is urine. The amniotic sac generally ruptures after labor has begun. If it ruptures before labor starts, medical attention is essential. If labor does not occur within a few hours of the rupture of the membranes, the physician usually attempts to start labor with administration of medication. Delivery should occur within 24 hours after membranes rupture. Prolonged rupture of membranes puts the woman and her fetus at risk for infection. Inability for delivery to take place within the specified time likely results in birth via cesarean section.

The amount of vaginal drainage typically increases as term approaches, and a blood-tinged mucus called *bloody show* may be observed. This mucus occludes the cervical os (the opening of the cervix) during pregnancy (mucous plug). The health care provider is likely to perform a vaginal examination during the last weeks of the pregnancy. Findings that the cervix has begun to soften, efface (thin), and open (dilate) are normal. Backache and contractions of the uterus, called **Braxton Hicks contractions** (irregular tightening of the pregnant uterus that begins in the first trimester and increases in frequency, duration, and intensity as pregnancy progresses), are common as the pregnancy approaches term. The severity of these contractions varies from mild to moderate. They remain irregular and do not dilate the cervix.

Table 27.1 Comparison of True and False Labor

TRUE LABOR	FALSE LABOR
Contractions follow a regular pattern.	Contractions rarely follow a pattern.
Contractions come closer together, are stronger, and tend to last longer.	Contractions vary in length and intensity.
Contractions get stronger with ambulation.	Contractions frequently stop with ambulation or position change.
Contractions seem to start in the lower back and then travel to the lower abdomen.	Contractions may be felt in the back but are noticed most often in the fundus.
Contractions usually are not stopped with controlled breathing, sedation, or other relaxation interventions.	Contractions eventually stop with relaxation interventions.
The cervix softens, effaces, and dilates.	The cervix may soften, but with little or no change in effacement or dilation.
The fetus continues descent into the pelvis.	No significant change in the fetal position occurs.

Some women notice a slight loss of weight (1 to 3 pounds) a few days before labor. Reports of nausea and diarrhea are not uncommon during this period. An energy burst often is experienced. Expectant mothers report cooking, cleaning, and preparing for the baby's arrival with renewed energy; this can be compared with the nesting behaviors noted in pregnant animals.

True labor is marked by the onset of regular, rhythmic contractions that cause progressive cervical dilation and **effacement** (thinning and shortening or obliteration of the cervix that occurs during late pregnancy, labor, or both).

FALSE LABOR VERSUS TRUE LABOR

Before the onset of true labor, many women may experience false labor. The discomforts of false labor do not promote the needed fetal descent and cervical changes that accompany true labor. The contractions experienced during this time often convince the woman that labor has begun. Fear of going to the hospital at the wrong time is common in expectant women. Explain how true and false labors differ (Table 27.1). The information should include an emphasis on the importance of seeking medical attention when any doubt exists.

LABOR AND DELIVERY

STANDARD PRECAUTIONS DURING CHILDBIRTH

During birth, nurses and other health care providers are exposed to a great deal of maternal and newborn blood and body fluids. Use standard precautions to avoid transmission of infection through contact with body fluids. The standard precautions applicable to childbirth include the following:

- Wash hands before donning gloves and after performing procedures and removing gloves.
- Wear gloves (clean or sterile, as appropriate) when performing procedures that require contact with the woman's genitalia and body fluids, including bloody show (e.g., during vaginal examination, amniotomy, hygienic care of the perineum, insertion of an internal scalp electrode and intrauterine pressure monitor, and catheterization).
- When assisting with a birth, wear a cover gown and a mask with a shield or protective eyewear. Cap and shoe covers are worn for cesarean birth but are optional for vaginal birth in a birthing room. The primary health care provider who is attending the birth should wear a sterile gown with a waterproof front and sleeves.
- Drape the woman with sterile towels and sheets as appropriate. Explain to the woman what can and cannot be touched.
- Help the woman's partner put on appropriate coverings for the type of birth, such as cap, mask, gown, and shoe covers. Show the partner where to stand and what can and cannot be touched.
- Wear gloves and gown when handling the newborn immediately after birth.
- Use an appropriate method to suction the newborn's airway, such as a bulb syringe, mechanical wall suction, or DeLee oral suction device.

PROCESS OF LABOR AND DELIVERY

To understand the complex process of labor and delivery, examine each of the factors involved. These factors are frequently called the five *Ps*:

- *Passageway:* The pelvis and soft tissues
- *Passenger:* The fetus
- *Powers:* Contractions
- *Position of mother:* Standing, walking, side lying, squatting, on hands and knees
- *Psyche:* Psychological response

Passageway

Pelvis. The superior portion of the pelvis (iliac segment of the innominate bones) supports the uterus and fetus during the late months of pregnancy. These bones aid in directing the fetus into the inferior (lower) portion of the pelvis, which is called the *true pelvis.* The two sections are divided by an imaginary line called the *linea terminalis,* or pelvic inlet.

The size and shape of the true pelvis are more important than those of the false pelvis, because the fetal head must be able to pass through this section of the pelvis for vaginal delivery to occur. Four different types of pelvis are recognized, each with a unique shape and characteristics (Table 27.2).

The true pelvis is divided further into three segments: the inlet; the cavity, or midpelvis; and the outlet (Fig. 27.1). The primary care practitioner can use several methods for evaluation of the size of the true pelvis:

Table 27.2 Comparison of Pelvic Types

CHARACTERISTIC	GYNECOID	ANDROID	ANTHROPOID	PLATYPELLOID
Percent of women	50%	23%	24%	3%
Brim	Slightly ovoid or transversely rounded Round	Heart-shaped, angulated Heart	Oval, wider anteroposteriorly Oval	Flattened anteroposteriorly, wide transversely Flat
Depth	Moderate	Deep	Deep	Shallow
Side walls	Straight	Convergent	Straight	Straight
Ischial spines	Blunt, somewhat widely separated	Prominent, narrow interspinous diameter	Prominent, often with narrow interspinous diameter	Blunted, widely separated
Sacrum	Deep, curved	Slightly curved, terminal portion often beaked	Slightly curved	Slightly curved
Subpubic arch	Wide	Narrow	Narrow	Wide
Usual mode of delivery	Vaginal • Spontaneous • Occiput anterior position	Cesarean Vaginal • Difficult, with forceps	Vaginal • With forceps or spontaneous • Occiput posterior or occiput anterior position	Vaginal • Spontaneous

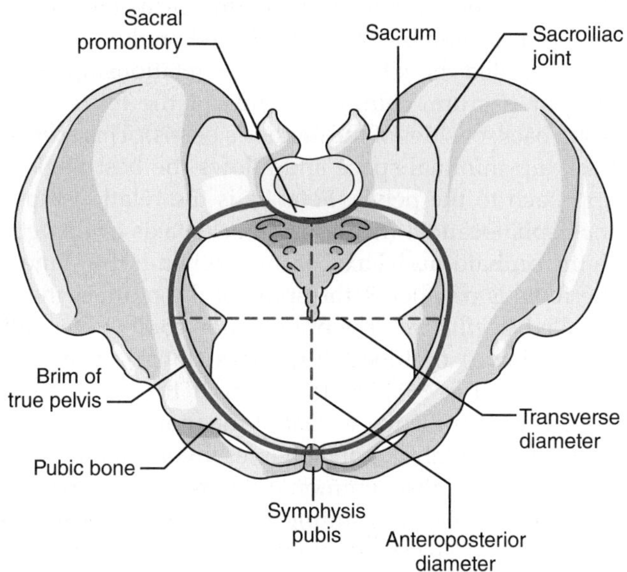

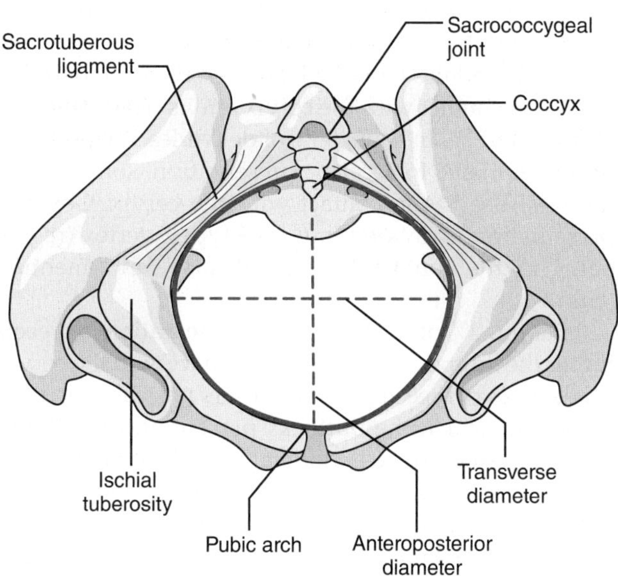

Fig. 27.1 Female pelvis. A, Pelvic brim (inlet, linea terminalis, or iliopectineal line) from above. B, Pelvic outlet from below.

- *Palpation:* Externally, the health care provider can use a pelvimeter to determine the distance between the ischial tuberosities. This measurement helps estimate the distance between the ischial spines, which otherwise can be obtained only with pelvic x-ray examination. Internally, additional bony prominences are evaluated to determine pelvic adequacy.
- *Pelvimetry:* With x-ray films from different views, the health care provider can measure accurately the bony prominences. This type of assessment may be done for a woman who is not currently pregnant but is seeking preconception care. The diagnostic measurement may be performed for women who have had an injury or known developmental problem, such as rickets.
- *Ultrasound scan:* Sound waves above the range of human hearing also can be used to estimate pelvic adequacy. Because ultrasound scanning does not involve the use of radiation, it generally is regarded as safe for the fetus. An ultrasound scan can show soft tissue and helps gather information regarding fetal growth, multiple pregnancy, placental location, and abnormal presentation that may complicate delivery.

Understand that adequacy of the pelvis is relative. For each delivery, a determination must be made whether the pelvis is adequate to allow passage of the fetus. Although certain measurements are considered "normal," the size and position of the fetus make each situation unique.

Soft tissues. During labor, the uterus, the cervix, the vagina, and the muscles of the perineum change in consistency and shape to allow passage of the fetus in the following ways:

- *Uterine tissues:* During labor, the walls of the upper section of the uterus have a thickened musculature that provides the force during contractions. The muscle walls of the lower section become thinner and act as a passive tube. Located between the two sections is a band of tissue, the physiologic retraction ring.
- *Cervical tissues:* As contractions of the muscular upper segment apply downward pressure, the uterine contents (fetal presenting part) efface and dilate the cervix.
- *Vagina:* In response to hormonal changes during pregnancy, the vagina undergoes many changes. Increased blood supply (vascularity), increased thickness of the mucosa, loosening of the connective tissue, and enlargement (hypertrophy) of smooth muscle cells make the vagina capable of stretching (dilating) to allow passage of the fetus.
- *Perineum:* The muscles of the pelvic floor are stretched and thinned by the pressure of the presenting part. The anus may appear dilated and bulging.

Passenger

Fetus. To be born, the fetus must be able to exit through the bony passageway just described. The fetal head is the largest part of the body. Delivery of the head is of the highest concern.

The bones of the fetal skull are not rigidly fused (joined), which allows the bony plates to move and overlap as they progress through the maternal pelvis. This reshaping of the skull bones in response to pressure against the maternal pelvis is called *molding.*

The major bones of the skull are the two frontal bones, the two parietal bones, the two temporal bones, and the occiput. They are joined by membranous spaces called *sutures.* Where sutures meet are larger membranous

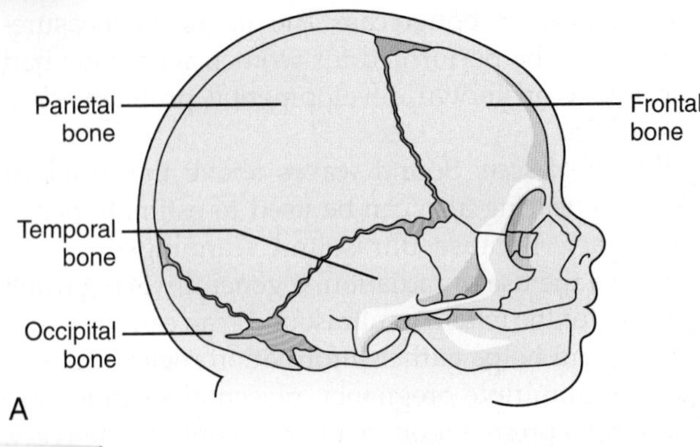

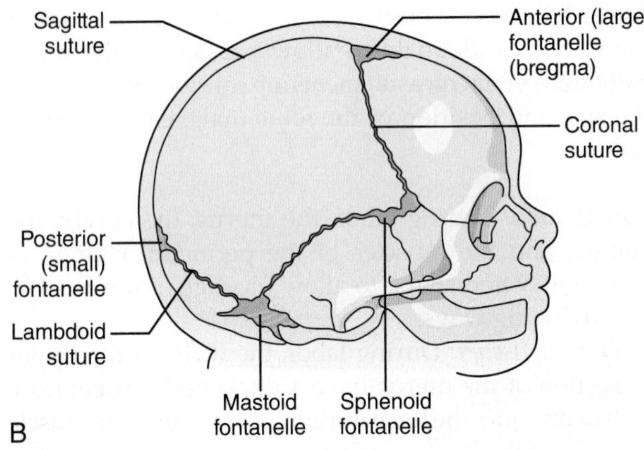

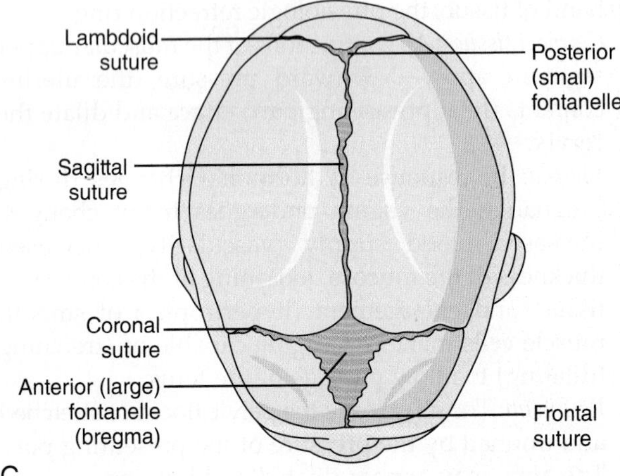

Fig. 27.2 Fetal head at term. A, Bones. B, Fontanelles. C, Sutures.

areas called *fontanelles* (Fig. 27.2). The anterior fontanel (bregma) is formed by four bones and thus tends to be larger and diamond shaped. The posterior fontanel is formed by three bones and is smaller and triangular. With palpation of the sutures and the fontanelles through the dilated cervix, the primary care practitioner can determine the presentation of the fetus during labor. The largest transverse diameter of the skull is the biparietal measurement. If this is too large, the skull may not be able to enter the mother's pelvis.

Fetal attitude. The relationship of fetal body parts to one another is called **attitude.** At term, the ideal attitude for the fetal body is **flexion.** The back is bowed outward, the chin is touching the sternum, the arms are crossed on the chest, and the thighs are flexed on the abdomen. This is called the **fetal position** (the relationship of the occiput, sacrum, chin, or scapula of the fetus to the front, back, or sides of the mother's pelvis). This attitude takes up minimal space and allows the best angle of approach to the pelvis. **Fetal lie** is the relationship of the cephalocaudal (head-to-buttocks) axis of the fetus to the cephalocaudal axis of the mother. If the spine of the fetus is parallel to the spine of the mother, the lie is called *longitudinal.* The presentation could be cephalic (head down) or breech (buttocks down). The lie is longitudinal in 99% of deliveries. If the spine of the fetus is perpendicular to that of the mother, it is called *transverse lie.* Only 1% of deliveries involve a transverse lie. This lie is most common in women who have had many pregnancies (resulting in weakened abdominal walls), maternal pelvic contracture, or placenta previa (see Chapter 28). While the fetus is small, it changes positions frequently. By term, the fetal lie seldom changes because space is limited.

Fetal presentation. **Fetal presentation** (that part of the fetus [head, face, breech, or shoulders] that first enters the pelvis and lies over the inlet) describes the part that will be in contact with the cervix and is determined by attitude and lie. In about 96% of deliveries, the presentation is cephalic. In cephalic presentation, some part of the fetal head is in contact with the cervix. Cephalic presentation is divided into four types: vertex (region between the fontanelles), brow, face, and mentum (chin).

In about 3% of deliveries, the presentation is breech. Either the buttocks or legs are in contact with the cervix. Three types of breech presentation are possible: complete breech, in which the buttocks present and the thighs are well flexed on the abdomen; frank breech, in which the buttocks present and the thighs are extended across the abdomen and chest; and footling breech, in which there is no flexion and one foot or two feet present. Breech presentations are more difficult to deliver vaginally. Attempts to deliver a breech presentation vaginally may result in fetal head entrapment. The fetal head is larger than the torso and may be unable to pass through the birth canal without difficulty. To decrease risks to the fetus, most breech births are delivered surgically (see the later section "Cesarean Delivery"). Vaginal deliveries of breech infants may be allowed if the fetus is preterm or the mother is multiparous.

In about 1% of deliveries, some other body part presents. These presentations occur when the fetus has been in a transverse lie. The shoulder, hand, elbow, and iliac crest are possible presenting parts. These cases also necessitate a cesarean birth.

Fetal position. Position is the relationship of the presenting fetal part to a quadrant of the maternal pelvis.

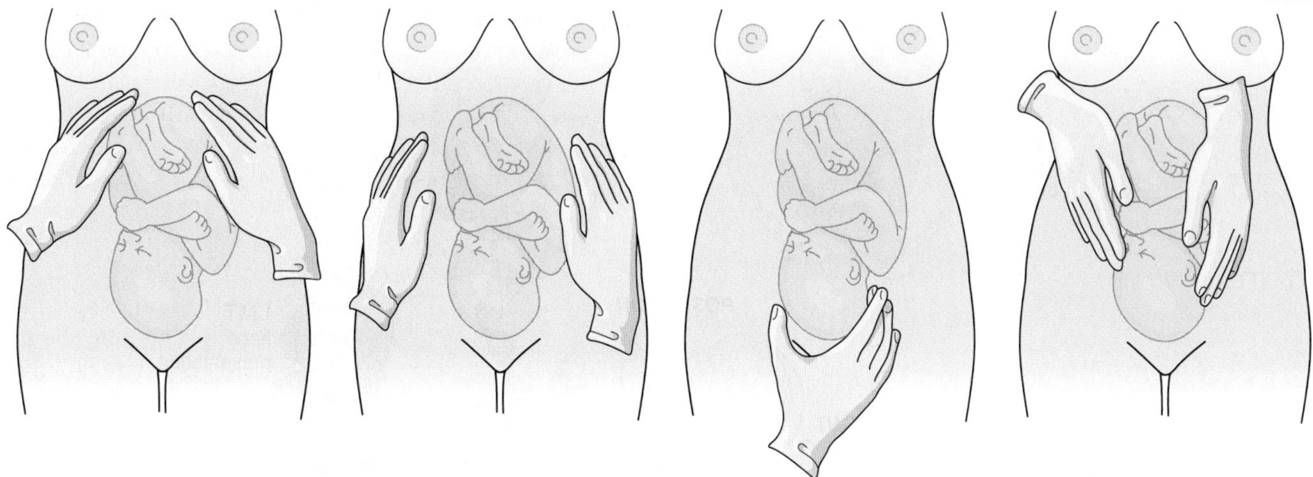

Fig. 27.3 Leopold's maneuvers. (From Lowdermilk DL, Perry SE, Cashion K, et al: *Maternity and women's health care*, ed 10, St. Louis, 2012, Mosby.)

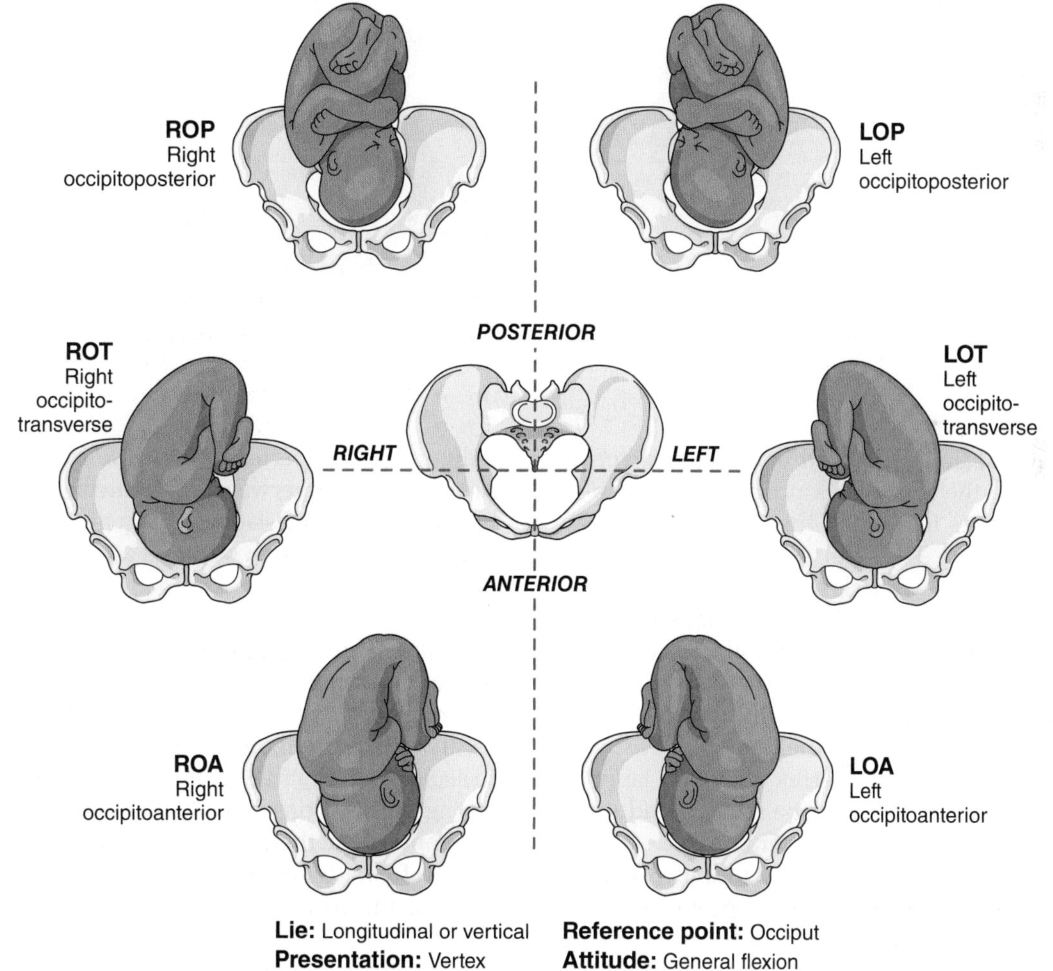

Fig. 27.4 Cephalic positions. Examples of fetal vertex (occiput) presentation in relation to front, back, and side of maternal pelvis.

Fetal position can be determined with abdominal inspection and palpation (Leopold's maneuvers) (Fig. 27.3), vaginal or rectal examination, auscultation of fetal heart tones, or ultrasound scan or x-ray examination. Once the position is determined, it is expressed in abbreviated form. For example, the most common position for delivery is left occiput anterior (LOA), in which the occiput of the fetus points toward the left anterior segment of the maternal pelvis. The right occiput anterior (ROA) position is the next most common position. Many combinations are possible (Figs. 27.4 and 27.5).

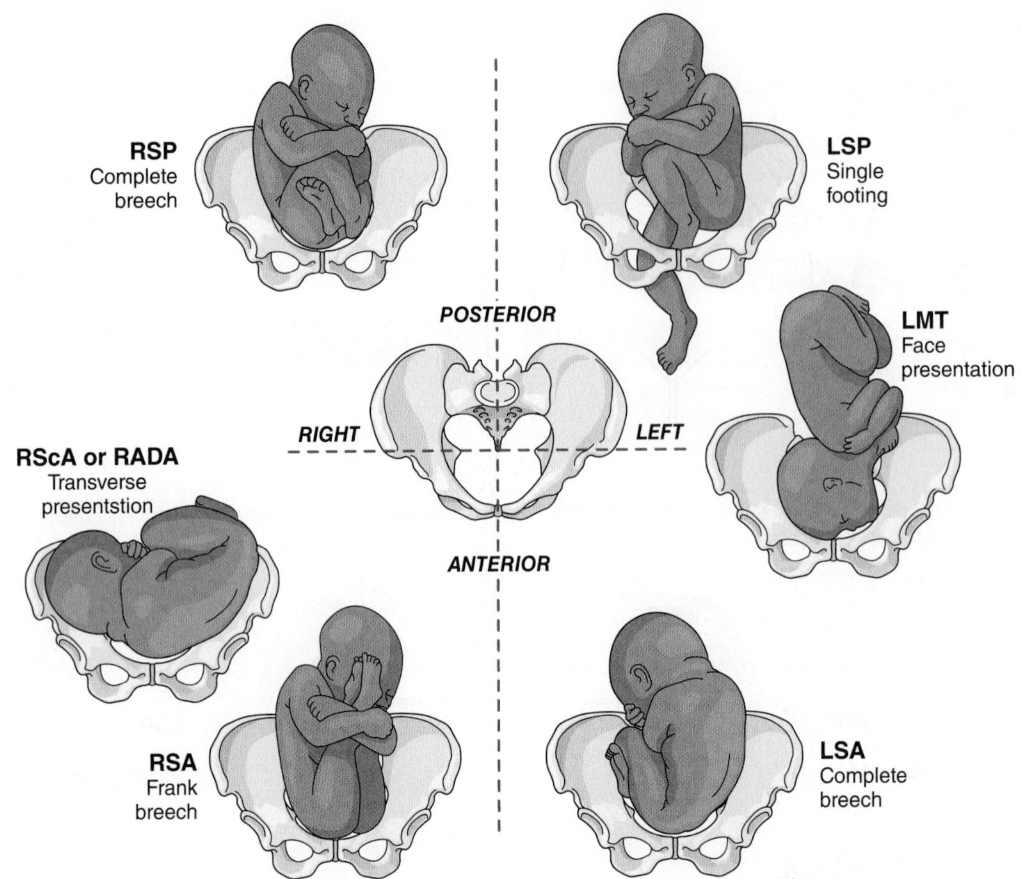

Fig. 27.5 Various presentations and positions. *LMT*, Left mentotransverse; *LSA*, left sacroanterior; *LSP*, left sacroposterior; *RADA*, right acromiodorsoanterior; *RSA*, right sacroanterior; *RScA*, right scapuloanterior; *RSP*, right sacroposterior.

A longitudinal lie, well-flexed attitude, and vertex presentation are the ideal. This position best enables the fetal skull bones to mold as they progress through the maternal pelvis. The fetal skull also provides a smooth, round surface, which is most effective in effacing and dilating the cervix. The smooth, regular shape also fills the cervix and prevents the umbilical cord from prolapsing, or coming before the fetus. Cord prolapse is dangerous because pressure on the vessels in the cord can restrict blood flow to the fetus.

If a part other than the vertex presents, labor is generally longer, more tiring to the mother, and more likely to necessitate surgical intervention.

Prompt recognition of a prolapsed umbilical cord is important because fetal hypoxia from prolonged cord compression (occlusion of blood flow to and from the fetus for more than 5 minutes) usually results in central nervous system damage or death of the fetus. The examiner can relieve pressure on the cord by putting a sterile gloved hand into the vagina and holding the presenting part off of the umbilical cord (Fig. 27.6A and B). The woman is assisted into a position such as a modified Sims (Fig. 27.6C), Trendelenburg, or knee-chest (Fig. 27.6D) position so that gravity keeps the pressure of the presenting part off of the cord. If the cervix is fully dilated, forceps-assisted or vacuum-assisted delivery can be performed for the fetus in a cephalic presentation; otherwise, a cesarean birth is likely. Nonreassuring fetal status, inadequate uterine relaxation, and bleeding also can occur as a result of a prolapsed umbilical cord.

Placenta. The placenta also is referred to as a passenger. After the fetus is delivered with strong uterine contractions, the placental attachment site is significantly smaller. This reduced size causes the placenta to separate from its attachment. Normally, the first few strong contractions 5 to 7 minutes after the birth of the baby shear the placenta from its base. A placenta is not freed easily from a flaccid (relaxed) uterus because the placental attachment site is not reduced in size.

Placental separation is indicated by the following signs (Fig. 27.7):

- A firmly contracting fundus
- A change in the uterus from discoid (disklike) to globular ovoid (egg-shaped) as the placenta moves to the lower segment
- A sudden gush of dark blood from the introitus (the entrance into the vagina)
- Apparent lengthening of the umbilical cord as the placenta gets closer to the introitus

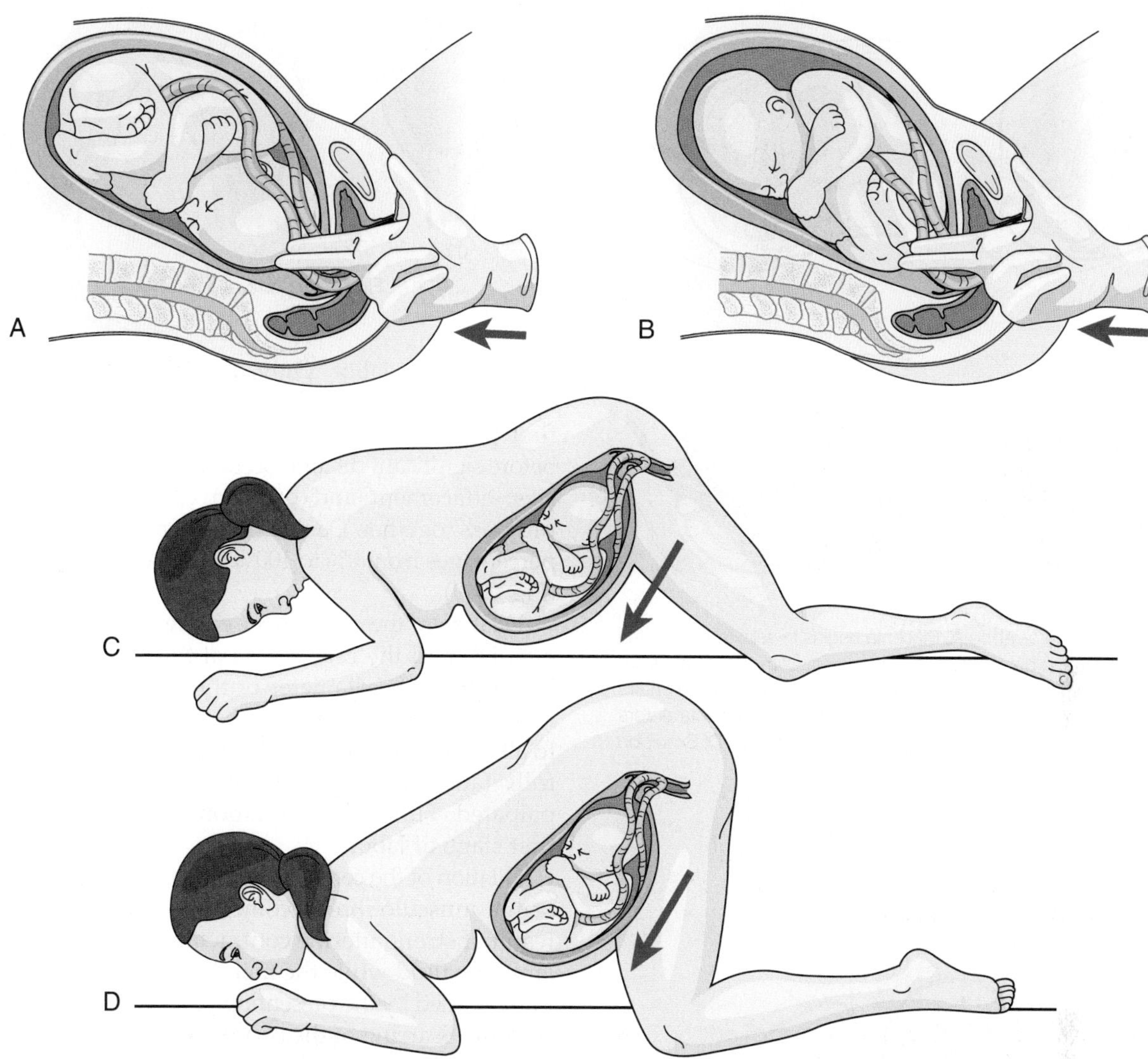

Fig. 27.6 *Arrows* indicate direction of pressure against presenting part to relieve compression of prolapsed umbilical cord. Pressure exerted by examiner's fingers in: A, vertex presentation; and B, breech presentation. C, Gravity relieves pressure when woman is in modified Sims position with hips elevated as high as possible without pillows. D, Knee-chest position.

- A vaginal fullness (the placenta) noted on vaginal or rectal examination or fetal membranes seen at the introitus

Whether the placenta shows its shiny fetal surface ("Shiny Schultze") or its dark, roughened maternal surface ("Dirty Duncan") is of no clinical significance. The delivery of the placenta completes the third stage of labor. This stage lasts 15 to 30 minutes or longer if the health care provider waits for the mother to express the placenta. When the delivery of the placenta is managed actively, it can take less than 5 minutes.

After the placenta (with its membranes) emerges, it is examined for intactness to be certain that no portion of it remains in the uterine cavity. The goal of this stage of labor is the prompt separation and expulsion of the placenta, achieved in the easiest and safest manner. If the fundus is not firm, stimulate the uterine muscle to regain tone and to expel any clots before measuring the distance from the umbilicus. Palpate the uterus gently only until it is firm; overstimulation causes uterine muscle fatigue and results in atonia (relaxation).

The uterus can contract only if it is free of intrauterine clots. Take care to avoid inversion of the uterus during expulsion of clots. To expel clots, place the hands as shown in Fig. 27.8, supporting the uterus from below with one hand. With the upper hand, apply firm pressure downward toward the vagina while observing the perineum for the number and size of expelled clots. While performing these assessments, teach the patient the rationale for the assessment and how to maintain uterine tone with self-palpation.

Powers

Involuntary and voluntary contractions combine to aid the fetus in movement through the birth canal and in expulsion from the mother. They are also responsible for delivery of the placenta. Involuntary uterine contractions, called primary powers, signal the beginning of labor. Once the cervix has dilated, the woman's voluntary

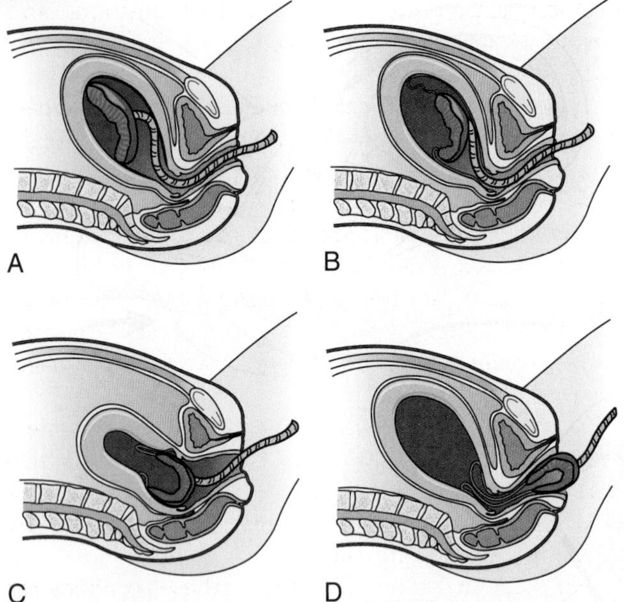

Fig. 27.7 Third stage of labor. A, Placenta begins to separate in central portion accompanied by retroplacental bleeding. Uterus changes from discoid to globular shape. B, Placenta completes separation and enters lower uterine segment. Uterus is globular shaped. C, Placenta enters vagina, cord is seen to lengthen, and bleeding may increase. D, Expulsion (delivery) of placenta and completion of third stage.

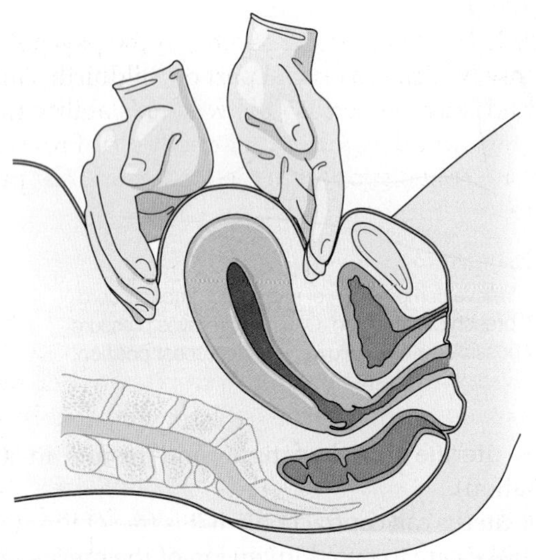

Fig. 27.8 Palpating fundus of uterus during first hour after delivery.

bearing-down efforts, called secondary powers, augment the force of the involuntary contractions.

Primary powers. The involuntary contractions originate at certain pacemaker points in the thickened muscle layers of the upper uterine segment. From the pacemaker points, contractions move downward over the uterus in waves, separated by short rest periods.

The primary powers are responsible for the effacement and dilation of the cervix and the descent of the fetus. Effacement is the shortening and thinning of the cervix during the first stage of labor. The cervix, normally 2 to 3 cm long and about 1 cm thick, is obliterated or "taken up" by shortening of the uterine muscle bundles

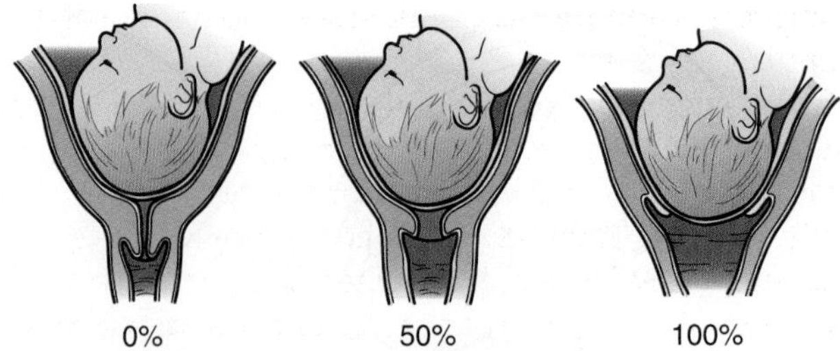

Fig. 27.9 Cervical effacement.

in advancing labor. Only a thin edge of the cervix can be palpated when effacement is complete. In a first pregnancy, effacement generally occurs at term before significant dilation occurs. In subsequent pregnancies, effacement and dilation of the cervix tend to progress together. Degree of effacement is expressed in percentages from 0% to 100% (e.g., a cervix 50% effaced) (Fig. 27.9).

Dilation of the cervix is the enlargement of the cervical opening and the cervical canal that occurs once labor has begun. The diameter of the cervix increases from less than 1 cm to full dilation (approximately 10 cm) to allow birth of a term fetus. When the cervix is dilated fully (and completely retracted), it can no longer be palpated. Full cervical dilation marks the end of the first stage of labor.

Dilation of the cervix occurs with the drawing upward of the musculofibrous components of the cervix as a result of strong uterine contractions. Pressure from the amniotic fluid while the membranes are intact and the force applied by the presenting part also promote cervical dilation. Scarring of the cervix as a result of prior infection or surgery may slow cervical dilation.

In the first and second stages of labor, increased intrauterine pressure caused by contractions places pressure on the descending fetus and the cervix. When the presenting part of the fetus reaches the perineal floor, mechanical stretching of the cervix occurs. Stretch receptors in the posterior vagina cause release of exogenous oxytocin, which triggers the maternal urge to bear down, or Ferguson's reflex.

Uterine contractions are involuntary and usually independent from external forces. For example, laboring women who are paraplegic have normal uterine contractions. Uterine contractions may temporarily become less frequent and intense when the woman receives narcotic analgesic medication or epidural analgesia early in labor. The relationship between prolonged labor and epidural analgesia is still under investigation.

Secondary powers. As soon as the presenting part reaches the pelvic floor, the contractions change in character and become expulsive. The woman experiences an involuntary urge to push. She uses secondary powers (bearing-down efforts) as she contracts her diaphragm and abdominal muscles and pushes. These bearing-down efforts result in increased intraabdominal pressure that compresses the uterus on all sides and increases the expulsive forces.

The secondary powers have no effect on cervical dilation, but they are important in expelling the infant from the uterus and vagina after the cervix is dilated fully. Pushing in the second stage is more effective, and the woman is less fatigued when she begins to push only after she has the urge to do so rather than beginning to push when she is fully dilated but does not yet have the urge to do so. The woman should not push before complete dilation. This can result in swelling or tearing of the cervix and ultimately may slow the birthing process.

The way a woman pushes in the second stage is much debated. Spontaneous bearing-down efforts, Valsalva's maneuver (closed glottis and prolonged bearing down), pushing, open glottis pushing, "mini" pushing, and forced methods of pushing have been investigated. Although no significant differences in length of second-stage labor have been found among these methods, fetal hypoxia and acidosis are associated with directed pushing. Continued study is needed to determine the effectiveness and safety of various pushing techniques in relation to maternal and fetal outcomes.

Position of the Woman in Labor

Maternal position affects the woman's anatomic and physiologic adaptations to labor. Frequent changes in position relieve fatigue, increase comfort, and improve circulation. Encourage a woman in labor to find the positions that are most comfortable for her (Fig. 27.10).

An upright position (e.g., walking, sitting, kneeling, or squatting) offers many advantages. Gravity can promote the descent of the fetus. Uterine contractions are generally stronger and more efficient in effacing and dilating the cervix, which results in shorter labor. An upright position is also beneficial for the mother's cardiac output, which normally increases during labor as uterine contractions return blood to the vascular bed. Increased cardiac output improves blood flow to the uteroplacental unit and the maternal kidneys. An upright position also helps reduce pressure on the descending aorta and ascending vena cava and prevents their compression. Compression of these vessels can compromise cardiac output and lead to supine hypotension and decreased placental perfusion. If the woman wishes to lie down, a lateral position is suggested.

The "all fours" position (on hands and knees) may be used to relieve backache if the fetus is in an occipitoposterior position. It also may assist in anterior rotation of the fetus.

The woman's preference may determine positioning for second-stage labor, but the decision also is affected by the condition of the woman or fetus, the environment, and the health care provider's confidence in assisting in a birth in a specific position. For physician-attended births in the United States, the lithotomy position is predominant. Alternative positions and position changes are practiced most commonly by nurse-midwives.

A woman in a semirecumbent position needs adequate body support to push effectively because her weight is on her sacrum, which moves the coccyx forward and causes a reduction in the pelvic outlet. In a sitting or squatting position, abdominal muscles work in greater synchrony with uterine contractions during bearing-down effort. Kneeling or squatting moves the uterus forward and straightens the long axis of the birth canal and can facilitate the second stage of labor by increasing the pelvic outlet.

Women can use the lateral position to help rotate a fetus that is in a posterior position. This position also may be used when less force is needed during bearing down, such as when the woman needs to control the speed of a precipitous birth.

No evidence shows that any of these positions for second-stage labor increases the need for operative techniques (e.g., forceps-assisted or vacuum-assisted birth, cesarean birth, and episiotomy) or causes perineal trauma. Also, no evidence shows that use of any of these positions adversely affects the newborn.

Psyche

The fifth *"P"* involves the psyche, or the psychological response, which is a crucial part of childbirth. Anxiety, fear, and fatigue decrease the woman's ability to cope with pain and the stressors of childbirth. Provision of information and support to the mother and her partner is imperative to her success.

MECHANISMS OF LABOR

As the fetus moves through the maternal pelvis, several maneuvers are necessary. These turns and adjustments are called the **cardinal movements of labor.** The mechanisms of labor in the vertex position are as follows.

Engagement occurs when the biparietal diameter of the fetal head crosses the pelvic inlet; the head is said to be fixed or engaged in the pelvis. In nulliparous women, this tends to occur early, often several days or weeks before labor begins. Multiparous women may not experience engagement until labor has started.

Descent is the downward progress of the presenting part. The amount of progress is measured by comparing the lowest point of the presenting part with the ischial spines. This is referred to as the *station* and is measured in centimeters above or below the level of the spines. For example, if the presenting part is even with the ischial spines, the station is 0; if the presenting part is 2 cm above the spines, the station is –2; if the presenting part is 2 cm below the ischial spines, the station is +2 (Fig. 27.11).

Internal rotation enables the fetal head to progress through the maternal pelvis. The largest diameter of the fetal head aligns with the largest diameter of the pelvis.

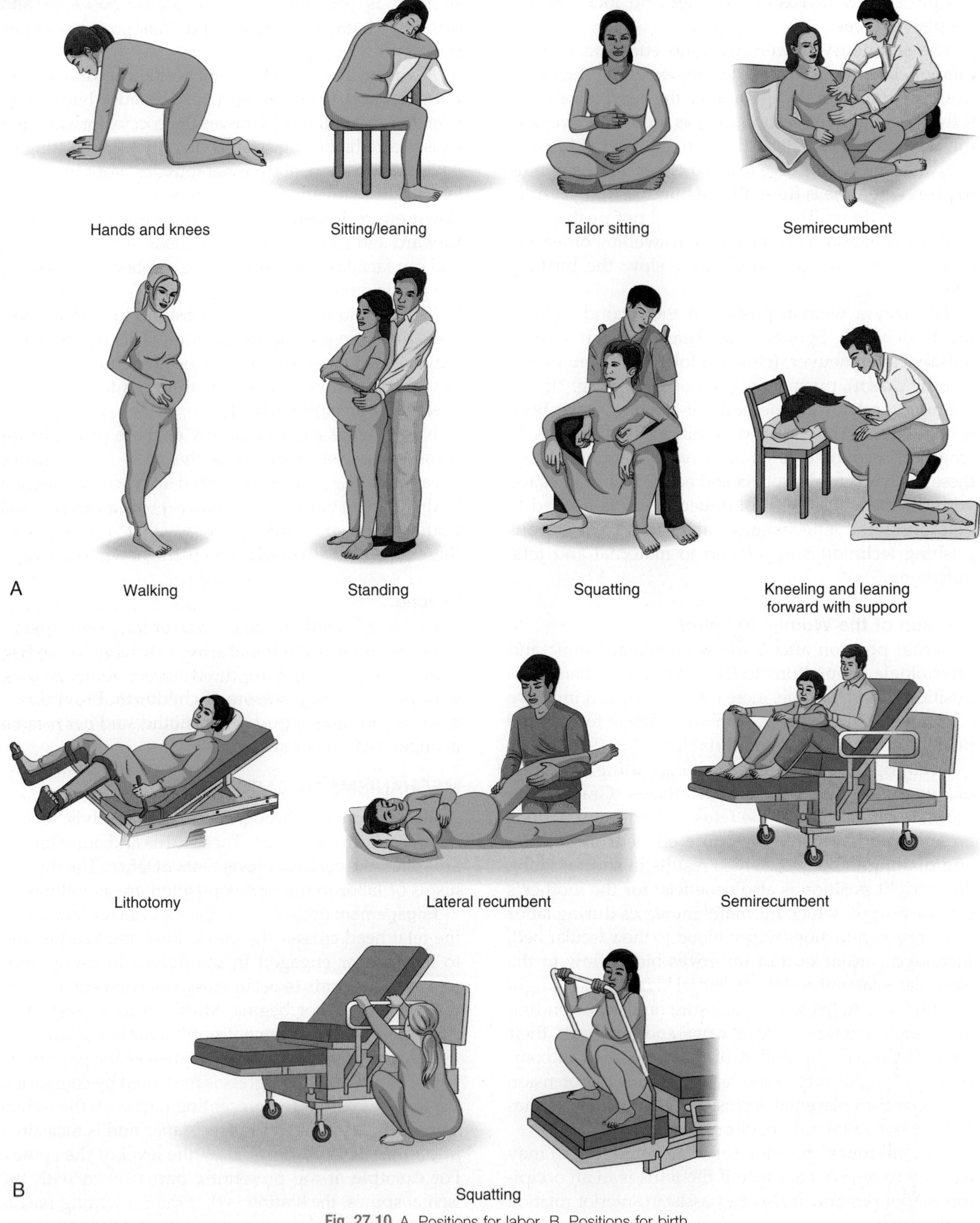

Fig. 27.10 A, Positions for labor. B, Positions for birth.

Extension occurs when the occiput passes under the symphysis pubis. This bony structure acts as a stable point and provides leverage, which enables the head to leave the pelvis. The actual delivery of the head is done by extension. As soon as the head is delivered, it moves to realign with the body and shoulders, referred to as **restitution** (Fig. 27.12).

External rotation occurs as the shoulders and body move through the birth canal, with the same maneuvers as the head. The shoulders are delivered similarly to the head, with the anterior shoulder pressing under the symphysis pubis, which again acts as a leverage point and assists in delivering the posterior shoulder. After the shoulders are delivered, the delivery ends with **expulsion**, in which the body of the infant leaves the pelvis. Delivery of the body occurs rapidly once the shoulders have been delivered (Fig. 27.13).

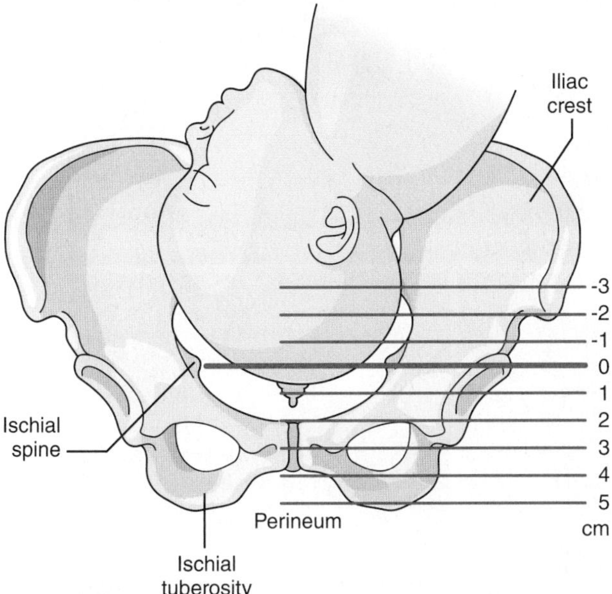

Fig. 27.11 Stations of presenting part, or degree of engagement. Location of the presenting part in relation to the level of ischial spines is designated station and indicates degree of advancement of the presenting part through pelvis. Stations are expressed in centimeters above (minus) and below (plus) the level of the ischial spines.

STAGES OF LABOR AND DELIVERY

First Stage: Dilation

The first stage begins with the onset of regular contractions and ends with complete dilation of the cervix (Fig. 27.14). This stage is generally the longest stage of labor; it averages 10 to 12 hours in nulliparas and 6 to 8 hours in multiparas. This stage often is divided into the following three phases:

1. *Latent phase* (0 to 3 cm dilation): Contractions occur 5 to 8 minutes apart and last 20 to 35 seconds. Dilation at this point is about the size of a penny. The woman generally is alert and talkative. The nulliparous woman may feel anxious about childbirth. This phase is ideal for teaching and establishing rapport. The nurse or a significant other may be the coach, reviewing techniques learned in prenatal classes. Pain tends to be mild and easily controlled. Backache is common. Many women, particularly multiparas, prefer to remain home during this stage. If the bag of waters has not ruptured, many women walk during this stage. Women should be advised that if the membranes rupture, they should seek care to be evaluated.
2. *Active phase* (4 to 7 cm dilation): Contractions occur at 3- to 5-minute intervals and last 40 to 60 seconds.

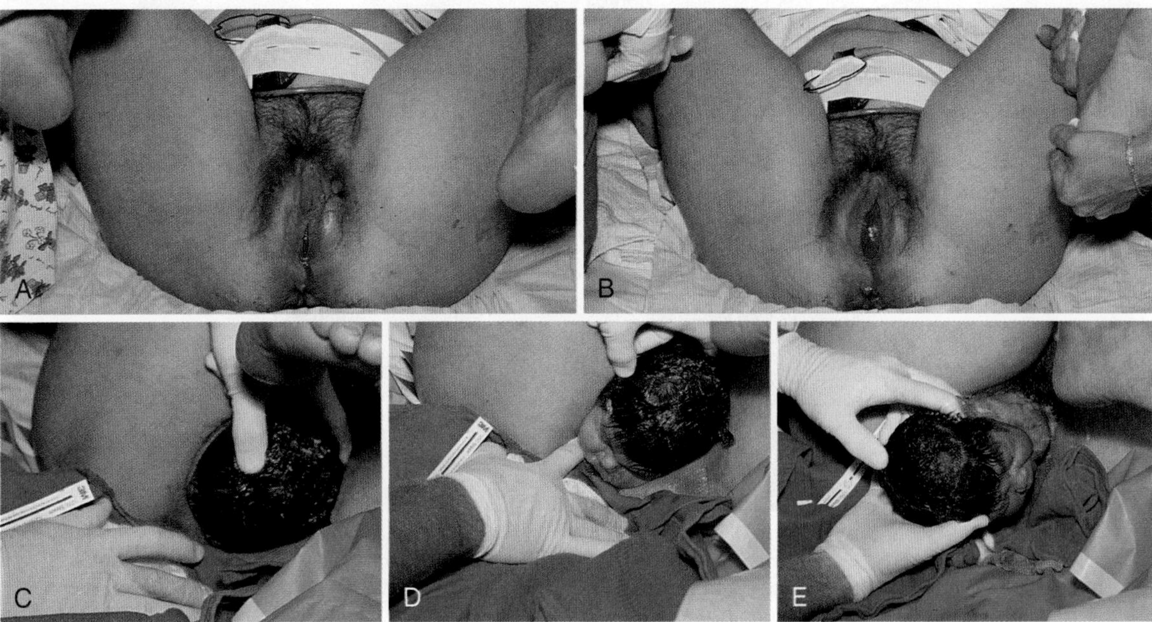

Fig. 27.12 Normal vaginal birth. A, Anteroposterior slit. Vertex visible during contraction. B, Oval opening. Vertex presenting. C, Crowning. D, Nurse-midwife using the Ritgen maneuver as head is born via extension. E, After nurse-midwife checks for nuchal cord, she supports head during external rotation and restitution. *Continued*

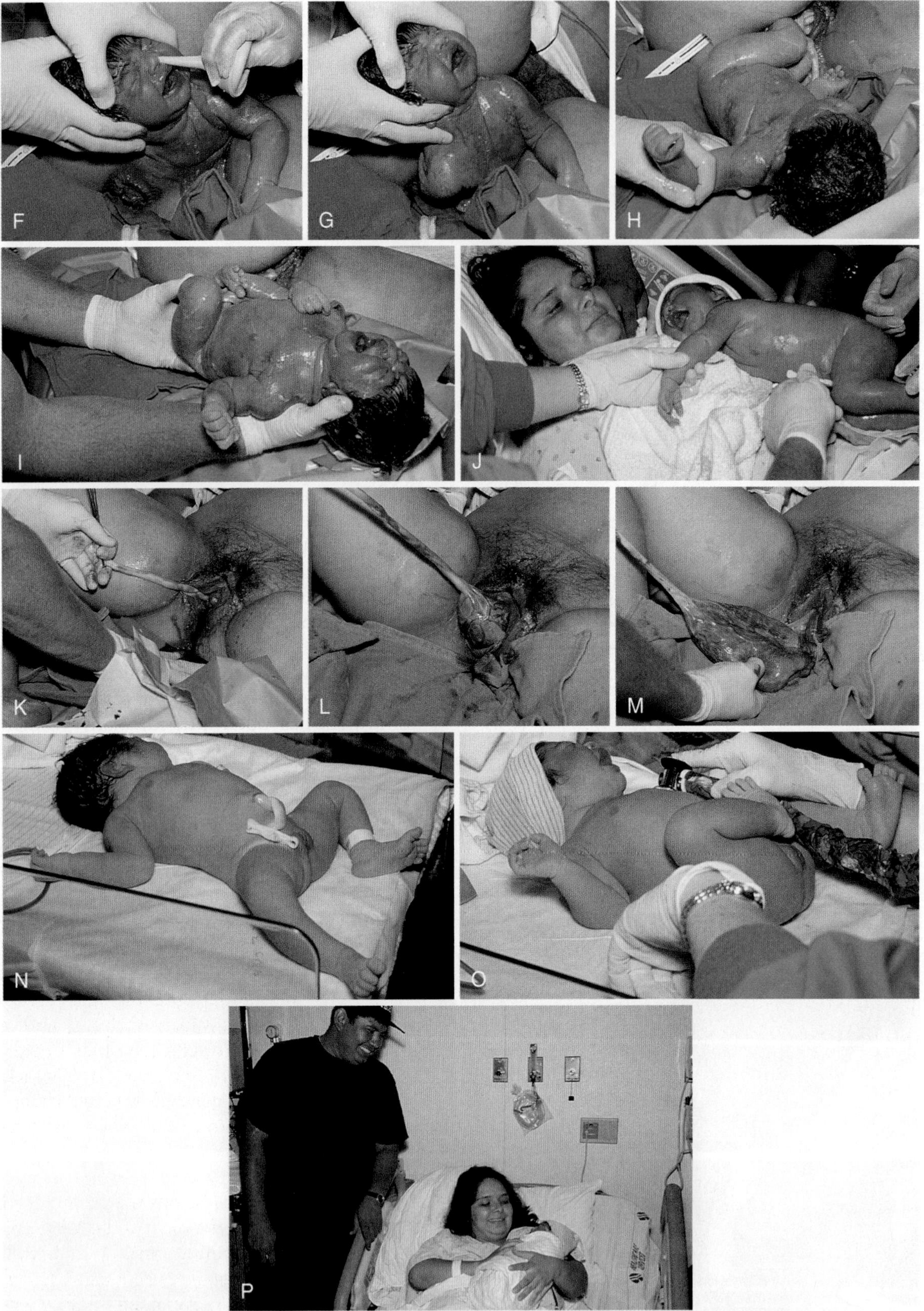

Fig. 27.12, cont'd F, Note the use of bulb syringe to suction mucus. G, Birth of posterior shoulder. H, Birth of newborn via slow expulsion. I and J, Second stage complete. Note that newborn is not completely pink yet. K, Note increased bleeding as placenta separates. L, Expulsion of placenta. M, Expulsion is complete, marking the end of the third stage. N, Newborn awaiting assessment. Note that color is almost completely pink. O, Newborn assessment under radiant warmer. P, Parents admiring their newborn. (Courtesy Michael S. Clement in Lowdermilk DL, Perry SE, Cashion K, et al: *Maternity and women's health care,* ed 10, St. Louis, 2012, Mosby.)

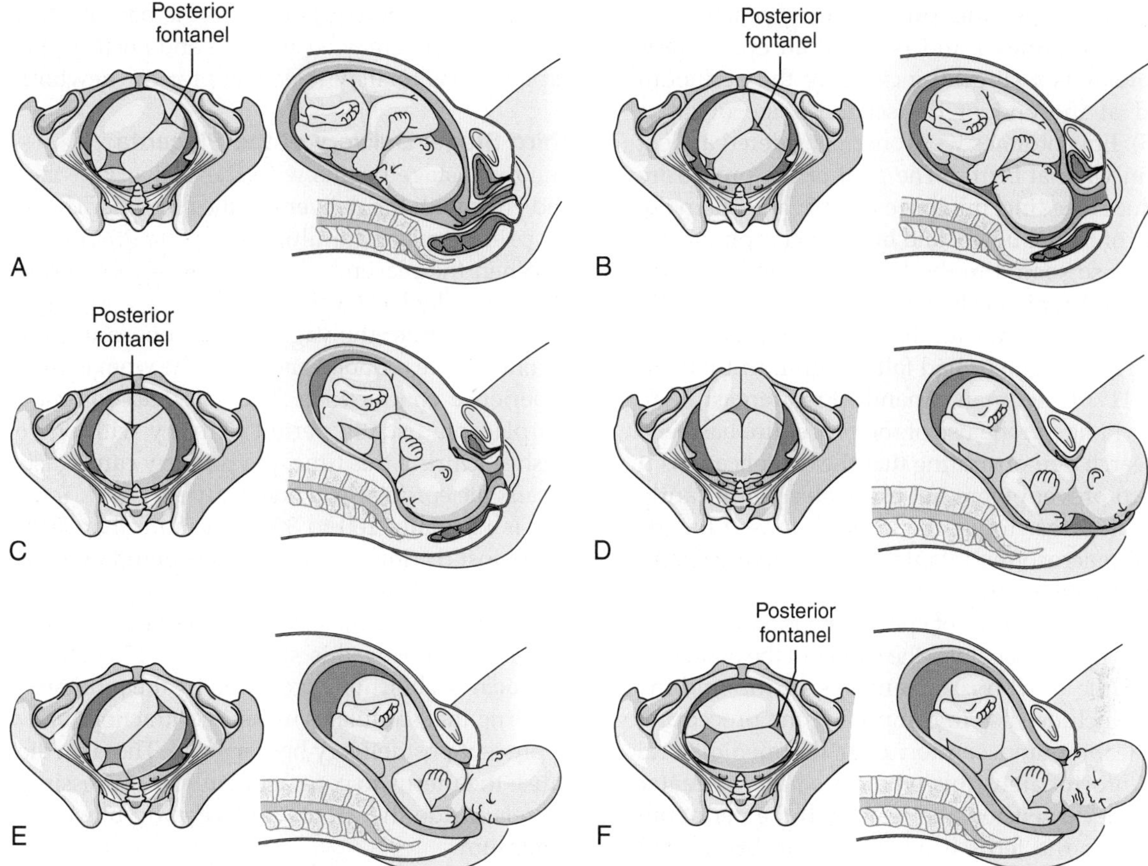

Fig. 27.13 Cardinal movements of labor in left occipitoanterior (LOA) presentation. A, Engagement and descent. B, Flexion. C, Internal rotation to OA. D, Extension. E, Restitution. F, External rotation.

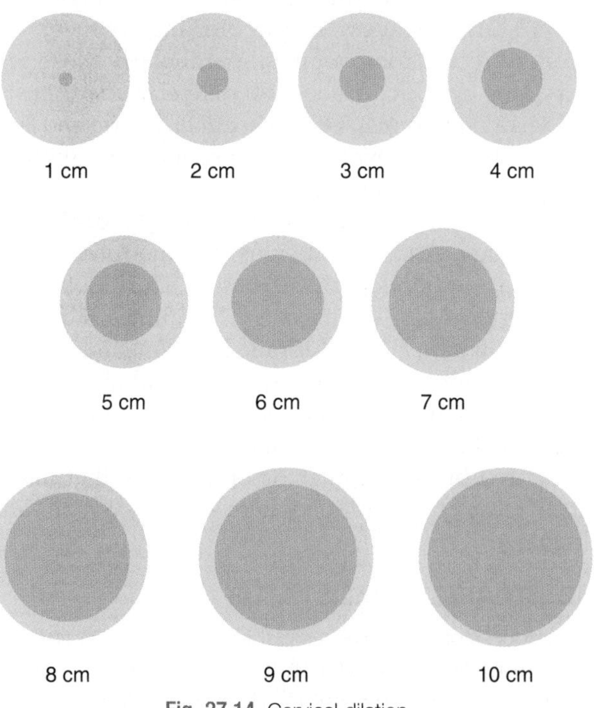

Fig. 27.14 Cervical dilation.

The woman becomes less talkative and focuses on breathing techniques learned during prenatal classes. If she has not learned breathing techniques already, teach them to her during labor. The intensity of the pain increases but still may be manageable without medication.

3. *Transitional phase* (8 to 10 cm dilation): Contractions occur at 2- to 3-minute intervals and last up to 90 seconds. The woman is focused deeply and may not wish to communicate with the nurse or significant other. She may be irritated easily by distractions. If the woman has not requested pain medication earlier, she may desire it at this time. Nausea is common.

Second Stage: Delivery of the Fetus

The second stage of labor begins with complete dilation at 10 cm and ends with the birth of the baby. This stage lasts an average of 30 minutes to 2 hours in nulliparas and 20 minutes to 90 minutes in multiparas. Contractions continue to last 80 to 90 seconds or slightly less.

Once the cervix is completely dilated, the woman usually feels the urge to push and is anxious to do so. Pushing is hard work, and the woman needs ongoing encouragement from the coach and the nurse. Resting between contractions, if possible, is important to conserve energy.

During this stage, the primary care practitioner may provide anesthesia and perform an episiotomy. The **episiotomy** is a surgical incision of the perineum performed at the end of the second stage of labor (Fig. 27.15). Episiotomies were once considered almost standard in vaginal births. The goal of the procedure was to reduce bleeding, minimize tearing, and aid in the prevention of future bowel and bladder complications. Episiotomy use soared in the 1970s with an incidence rate over 60%. A rapid decline started in the Cheyney. By the mid-Cheyney, the rate for the procedure was around 30%. In 2012 the number had fallen significantly to an estimated 11% (Friedman, Ananth, Prendergast et al, 2015). The change in the use of the procedure has been tied to research demonstrating that the complications it was used to prevent were not associated significantly with vaginal births. Today the incision is used for the delivery of macrosomic infants, rapid deliveries, and abnormal presentations.

The most common type of episiotomy is a midline, or median, incision that separates the tissues of the perineum at an anatomic junction. Advantages of the midline episiotomy include ease in completing the procedure, speed of healing, and comfort over the mediolateral incision. Unfortunately, this type does have a greater risk for further extension and tearing. If the perineum is too small or the fetus is anticipated to be large, a mediolateral incision, which involves cutting the muscle, is performed. This is generally more uncomfortable and is done only when necessary. Complications of an episiotomy include infection, blood loss, pain, and painful sexual intercourse.

Immediately after delivery, the baby's airway is established (see the section "Response of the Newborn to Birth") and the umbilical cord is clamped with two clamps and then severed between the clamps. If there are no complications, show the baby to the parents. Then either give the infant to the mother to hold or position the infant in a warming unit that allows for close observation and care. If any problems occur with the infant, administer care immediately. This emergency care may have to be performed in the delivery area.

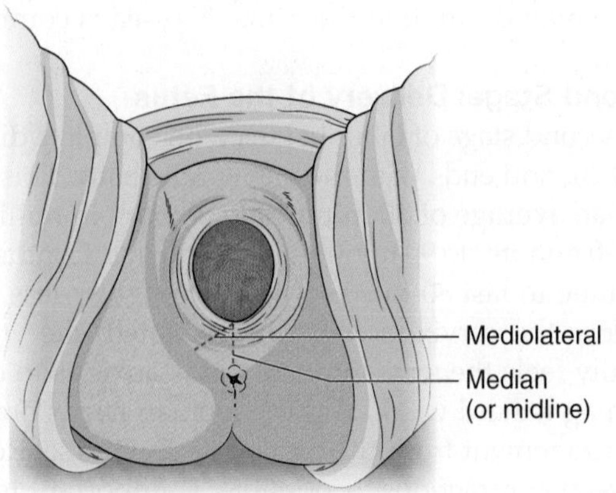

Fig. 27.15 Types of episiotomies.

Remain calm and supportive to the parents. Be aware that the parents may be alarmed and need support and explanations to allay their fears for the newborn.

Third Stage: Delivery of the Placenta

The third stage begins with the delivery of the infant and ends with the delivery of the placenta. The average for primiparas and multiparas is 5 to 20 minutes.

When the placenta detaches from the uterine wall, blood suddenly pours out of the vagina. The cord protruding from the vagina lengthens, and the uterus becomes more rounded and firm. The woman may again experience contractions. The size and consistency of the placenta usually permit delivery with one or two pushes. During this time, the primary care practitioner repairs the episiotomy if one was performed. Total blood loss is normally 200 to 300 mL; more than 500 mL of blood lost during delivery is considered excessive. An oxytocic medication, such as oxytocin (Pitocin) or methylergonovine maleate (Methergine), is administered commonly during this stage (Table 27.3). An *oxytocic* (**oxytocin** is a hormone produced by the pituitary gland) is a drug that stimulates uterine contractions and works to prevent postdelivery hemorrhage. These medications cause the uterus to contract firmly, compressing blood vessels inside the uterus and keeping blood loss to a minimum.

Fourth Stage: Stabilization

The time immediately after delivery is critical as the mother's body attempts to recover from the efforts of labor. Usually the mother is monitored closely for 2 to 4 hours after delivery in the birthing room or in a recovery room. Some women, particularly those who had a long or difficult labor and delivery, are exhausted and wish only to rest. Others seem euphoric and wish to talk about the experience or spend time with the baby and their significant other.

Monitor physiologic changes closely during the fourth stage. Assess vital signs, uterine tone, vaginal drainage, and the perineal tissue. During the first hour, perform assessments every 15 minutes. If observations are within normal limits, assessments are done every 30 minutes for the next hour. If all observations remain normal, the woman is transferred to a patient room for the remainder of her hospitalization (unless she is in a birthing center or in a facility that has an LDRP room configuration where she may remain until discharge).

MONITORING FETAL STATUS

The process of labor is stressful to the fetus, and continuous monitoring of the fetus is important during this time. Fetal heart rate (FHR) is a good indicator of the fetus's condition. The normal FHR range is 120 to 160 bpm. An increase or decrease of 30 bpm may indicate fetal distress and should be reported immediately (Box 27.2).

Table 27.3 **Medications for Normal Labor and Delivery**

GENERIC NAME (BRAND NAME)	ACTION	SIDE EFFECTS	NURSING IMPLICATIONS
butorphanol	Synthetic, centrally acting analgesic; provides relief of moderate to severe pain during labor	Drowsiness, sedation, headache, vertigo, dizziness, weakness, confusion, insomnia, nervousness, respiratory depression, change in blood pressure, palpitations, bradycardia, nausea, clammy skin, tingling, flushing and warmth, diaphoresis, skin rash, pruritus, increased urinary output Neonatal: respiratory depression, disorganized infant behavior, tendency for frequent crying	Monitor for respiratory depression; do not give if respiratory rate is <15 breaths/min; monitor vital signs; observe neonate for respiratory depression; observe safety precautions because of sedation and dizziness.
carboprost tromethamine (Hemabate)	Produces strong, prompt contractions of uterine smooth muscle; used in postpartum hemorrhage from uterine atony not managed with conventional methods	Headache, anxiety, weakness, arrhythmias, eye pain, nausea, vomiting, uterine rupture, backache, leg cramps, wheezing, fever, chills	It is used only by trained personnel in a hospital setting and may be injected into the uterus.
fentanyl citrate (Sublimaze): epidural	Binds with opiate receptors in the central nervous system, altering perception of and emotional response to pain through an unknown mechanism	Sedation, euphoria, vertigo, headache, confusion, anxiety, depression, seizures, blood pressure deviations, nausea, vomiting, respiratory depression	It is used occasionally. Monitor circulatory and respiratory status and urinary function. Monitor arterial oxygen saturation.
hydroxyzine (Vistaril)	Antianxiety antepartum and postpartum adjunctive therapy	Drowsiness, dry mouth, marked discomfort at IM injection site	It is used less frequently. Aspirate IM injection carefully to prevent inadvertent IV injection. Inject deeply into a large muscle mass. Observe for sedation.
magnesium sulfate	Decreases acetylcholine in motor nerve terminals, which is responsible for seizure prevention in preeclampsia and eclampsia	Diarrhea; side effects are related to magnesium levels: with >3 mg/dL, depressed central nervous system, blocked neuromuscular transmission that leads to anticonvulsant effects; with >5 mg/dL, depressed deep tendon reflexes; with >12.5 mg/dL, respiratory paralysis	Obtain vital signs q 15 min after IV dose; do not exceed 150 mg/min; monitor cardiac function; time contractions and monitor fetal heart rate; monitor intake and output (should remain ≥30 mL/h).
meperidine (Demerol)	Synthetic morphine-like compound that produces comparable analgesic effects and provides relief of moderate to severe pain	Pruritus, dizziness, sedation, weakness, euphoria, respiratory depression, hypotension, palpitations, bradycardia or tachycardia, dry mouth, nausea, constipation, oliguria, urinary retention Neonatal: respiratory depression	It is used less and less frequently. Monitor vital signs closely, especially respiratory rate, depth, and rhythm; encourage deep breathing and coughing to overcome respiratory depressant effects; assess patient's need for medication as needed; give IM or IV as ordered in smallest effective dose.

Continued

Table 27.3 Medications for Normal Labor and Delivery—cont'd

GENERIC NAME (BRAND NAME)	ACTION	SIDE EFFECTS	NURSING IMPLICATIONS
methylergonovine maleate (Methergine)	Stimulates uterine contraction, decreases bleeding	Headache, dizziness, nausea, vomiting, chest pain, palpitations, hypertension, tinnitus, sweating, rash	Monitor blood pressure, pulse, character, and amount of vaginal bleeding; monitor respiratory rate; give IM in deep muscle mass and IV only in emergency.
misoprostol (synthetic prostaglandin E; Cytotec)	Used most widely to prevent nonsteroidal antiinflammatory drug–induced gastric ulcer in patients at high risk	Headache, nausea, dyspepsia, vomiting, constipation, flatulence	Some physicians use it to induce labor, especially in the event of fetal death, administered vaginally in the posterior fornix. It is easier on the mother because labor and delivery can be over in as little as 45 min. To induce labor when fetal death has not occurred, administered vaginally into the posterior fornix.
nalbuphine hydrochloride	Binds with opiate receptors in the central nervous system, altering perception of and emotional response to pain through an unknown mechanism	Headache, sedation, vertigo, syncope, restlessness, crying, confusion, blood pressure variations, bradycardia, blurred vision, nausea and vomiting, urinary urgency, respiratory depression, asthma Neonatal: disorganized infant behavior, fussiness, refusal to nurse	Usually administer one or two doses and then begin an epidural. Monitor circulatory and respiratory status and bladder and bowel function; withhold dose and notify physician if respirations become shallow or fall below 12 breaths/min. Stool softeners may be ordered.
naloxone hydrochloride (Narcan)	Thought to displace previously administered narcotic-opioid analgesics from their receptors (competitive antagonism); indicated for use in known or suspected narcotic-induced respiratory depression in neonates (asphyxia neonatorum)	Tremors, seizures, blood pressure variations, nausea, vomiting Can cause seizure when used with street drugs (of which the health care worker is sometimes unaware)	It is not used as often as it once was. Respiratory rate increases within 1–2 min. Monitor respiratory depth and rate. Be prepared to provide oxygen, ventilation, and other resuscitation measures. Administer IV into umbilical vein. May be repeated q 2–3 min.
oxytocin (Pitocin)	Acts directly on myofibrils, producing uterine contractions; stimulates milk ejection by breasts	Anaphylaxis, postpartum hemorrhage, cardiac arrhythmias, nausea, vomiting, premature ventricular contractions, hypertension, convulsions Fetal: bradycardia, arrhythmias, jaundice, hypoxia, intracranial hemorrhage	Monitor intake and output ratio, contractions, fetal heart rate, blood pressure, pulse, and respirations.
promethazine hydrochloride	Prevents but does not reverse histamine-mediated responses; at high dosage, exhibits local anesthetic effects; used as adjunct to analgesics	Sedation, blood pressure deviations, blurred vision, nausea, vomiting, urine retention, seizures	It is used most of the time for postoperative cesarean delivery. Inject deep into large muscle mass. Often used as an adjunct to analgesics. It may be mixed with meperidine in the same syringe.

Table 27.3 Medications for Normal Labor and Delivery—cont'd

GENERIC NAME (BRAND NAME)	ACTION	SIDE EFFECTS	NURSING IMPLICATIONS
prostaglandin E (dinoprostone [Prepidil, Cervidil])	Stimulates uterine contractions like those seen in normal labor	Uterine contractile abnormalities, nausea, vomiting, diarrhea, back pain, warm feeling in vagina, fever Fetal: heart rate abnormalities, bradycardia	Use caution to prevent contact with skin; wash thoroughly after administration; bring to room temperature before administering; do not force warming process; have patient remain supine for 15–30 min after insertion.
ritodrine hydrochloride	Uterine beta$_2$-adrenergic receptor–stimulating effect, which reduces uterine contractions	Erythema, rash, dyspnea, hyperglycemia, headache, restlessness, anxiety, chills, tremor, nausea, vomiting, diarrhea, constipation, altered maternal and fetal heart rates	It is used less and less frequently. Monitor maternal and fetal heart tones during infusion; watch intensity and length of uterine contractions; monitor fluid intake to prevent overload; monitor blood glucose level in patients with diabetes.

IM, Intramuscularly, intramuscular; *IV,* intravenously, intravenous.

Box 27.2 Changes in Fetal Health Rate

NORMAL BASELINE RATE

- 120 to 160 bpm

TACHYCARDIA

- Moderate increase to 160 to 180 bpm
- Marked increase greater than 180 bpm; significant if variability is absent and late or variable decelerations (decreases in the speed or velocity of an object or reaction) are present

Nursing Interventions[a]

- Interventions depend on the cause.
- Reduce maternal fever with antipyretics as ordered and cooling measures.
- Oxygen at 8 to 10 L/min per face mask may be of some value.
- Carry out health care provider's orders to alleviate cause.

BRADYCARDIA

- Moderate decrease to 100 to 120 bpm
- Marked decrease to fewer than 100 bpm; significant if variability is decreased or absent or if late or variable decelerations are present

Nursing Interventions[a]

- Interventions depend on the cause.
- Intervention is not warranted in fetus with heart block diagnosed with electrocardiogram.
- Oxygen at 8 to 10 L/min per face mask may be of some value.
- Carry out health care provider's orders to alleviate cause.
- Scalp stimulation may be performed to determine whether the fetus is able to compensate physiologically for stress (fetal heart rate [FHR] accelerates).

VARIABILITY

- Measures the normal fluctuation of the FHR from the baseline
- Absent or minimal variability possibly indicative of fetal distress
- Variability classified as long-term variability (LTV) or short-term variability (STV)

DECELERATIONS

- Periodic decreases in the FHR in response to contractions; classified as early, late, or variable (Fig. 27.16)
- Early decelerations: caused by pressure on fetal skull; tend to be uniform; onset, shape, and recovery correspond to contractions
- Late decelerations: caused by decreased oxygen and blood flow to fetus through the placenta; noted at or after the peak of the contraction; may indicate fetal distress, particularly if associated with changes in baseline FHR and absence of variability
- Variable decelerations: caused by compression on the umbilical cord; occur randomly and onset may be sudden; FHR decreases below normal range

Nursing Interventions[a]

- Notify the primary caregiver immediately and initiate appropriate treatment when patient has a prolonged deceleration.

[a]See Box 27.3 for care of the woman being monitored electronically for fetal status during labor.

Auscultate the FHR with a fetoscope or a Doppler instrument every 15 to 30 minutes during the first stage of labor and every 5 minutes during the second stage. Also assess the FHR immediately after rupture of the membranes, particularly if the head is not engaged (i.e., not firmly settled into the pelvis).

Electronic Fetal Monitoring

Frequently, continuous electronic monitors, either internal or external, are applied for electronic fetal monitoring (EFM). Monitors can detect subtle changes of condition before they can be recognized with auscultation. The external, or indirect, mode uses external transducers on the maternal abdominal wall to assess FHR and uterine activity. An ultrasound transducer uses high-frequency sound waves to reflect movement of the fetal heart ventricles. A tocotransducer monitors uterine activity and records frequency and duration of contractions. A strip chart prints out FHR (upper part of the strip) and uterine activity (lower part of the strip) (Fig. 27.17A). External monitoring can be used in the antepartal and the intrapartal periods. It does not require rupture of membranes or cervical dilation; however, the tocotransducer cannot assess the intensity of contractions (Fig. 27.16). Maternal position can affect the accuracy of the recordings.

Internal monitoring uses a spiral electrode applied to the presenting part to monitor the FHR (Fig. 27.18). An intrauterine catheter is used to monitor frequency, duration, intensity, and resting tone of uterine contractions. This catheter is compressed during contractions, which places pressure on a strain gauge or pressure transducer. FHR and uterine pressure are reflected on a strip chart (Fig. 27.17B). Internal monitoring can be used only during the intrapartal period, because membranes must be ruptured and the cervix dilated 2 to 3 cm. Display of FHR and uterine activity is accurate regardless of maternal position. Box 27.3 lists guidelines

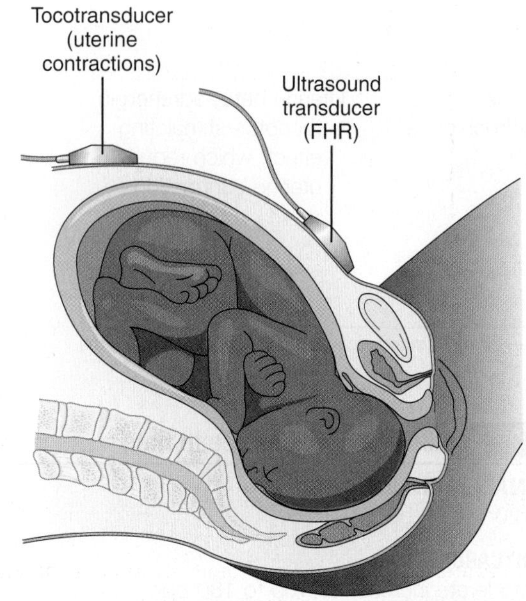

FIG. 27.16 Diagram of external noninvasive fetal monitoring with tocotransducer and ultrasound transducer, with ultrasound transducer placed below umbilicus and tocotransducer placed on uterine fundus position. *FHR*, Fetal heart rate.

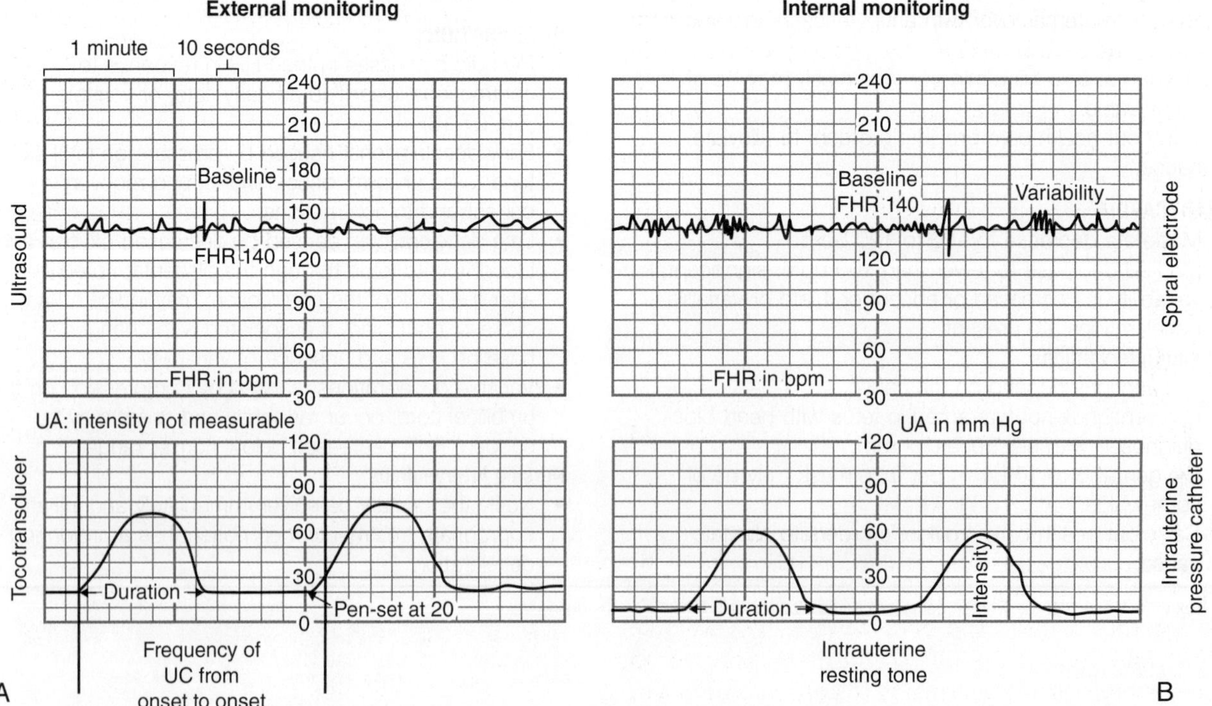

Fig. 27.17 Display of fetal heart rate *(FHR)* and uterine activity *(UA)* on chart paper. A, External mode with ultrasound transducer and tocotransducer as signal sources. B, Internal mode with spiral electrode and intrauterine catheter as signal sources.

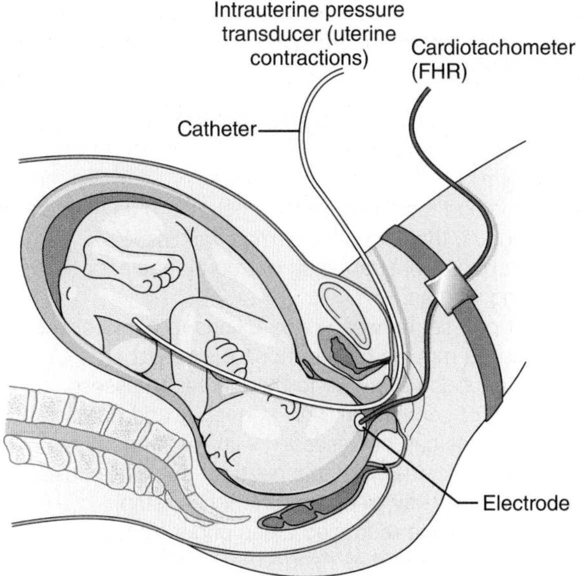

Fig. 27.18 Diagram of internal invasive fetal monitoring with intrauterine catheter and spiral electrode in place (membranes ruptured and cervix dilated). *FHR,* Fetal heart rate.

for care of the woman being monitored electronically for fetal status during labor.

FHR is monitored in relation to the contractions. A decrease in FHR occurs in response to the contractions and is called a *deceleration.* Decelerations can be early, late, or variable (Fig. 27.19 and see Box 27.2).

In the United States, electronic monitoring is used routinely for low-risk and high-risk labor.

Fetal Distress

Fetal distress from **hypoxia** (insufficient availability of oxygen to meet metabolic needs) is indicated with nonreassuring FHR patterns. These patterns can include a progressive increase or decrease in the baseline FHR, progressive decrease in baseline variability, tachycardia (more than 160 bpm), severe bradycardia (less than 100 bpm), persistent late decelerations, and severe variable decelerations with slow return to baseline. Another indication of fetal distress is greenish-stained amniotic fluid in a cephalic presentation. The color is a result of **meconium** (the infant's first stool, a viscid, sticky; dark greenish brown, almost black; sterile, odorless stool) being released from the fetal rectum in response to hypoxia (which increases intestinal activity and relaxes the anal sphincter). This color is referred to often as *meconium staining.* Table 27.4 describes characteristics of amniotic fluid.

Nurses who care for women during childbirth are legally responsible for correctly interpreting the FHR pattern, indicating appropriate nursing interventions based on that pattern, and documenting the outcome of those interventions. Notify the primary caregiver in a timely manner if an abnormal FHR pattern is detected. Initiate the institutional chain of command if health care providers disagree on the interpretation of the FHR pattern and the intervention necessitated.

RESPONSE OF THE NEWBORN TO BIRTH

The process of delivery is stressful to the newborn. Rapid adaptation from the intrauterine climate to that of extrauterine life is essential if the newborn is to survive.

The infant's physical condition is evaluated at birth. Most facilities use an evaluation guide called the *Apgar score* (Table 27.5). This scoring is done at 1 and 5 minutes of age. The score can range from 0 to 10, with 8 to 10 considered optimal. The criteria used include heart rate, respiratory effort, muscle tone, reflex irritability, and skin color. A low score indicates serious problems that may necessitate resuscitation. A high score indicates good condition, necessitating only routine care.

In utero, the fetus's need for oxygen was met by the mother. Once the umbilical cord is severed, the newborn must breathe to obtain oxygen. Fetal lungs must be mature enough that the alveoli can expand adequately. As the infant lungs begin to mature, they begin to produce increasing amounts of a substance called **surfactant**, which decreases surface tension within the alveoli and permits inflation. At the time of delivery, a combination of chemical, thermal, tactile, and mechanical changes initiates the first breath.

The airway must be cleared of fluids that are in the lungs. Some fluids are forced from the lungs as the thorax passes through the pelvis during delivery. Use a bulb syringe to remove excess fluid from the mouth and nasopharynx (Box 27.4). Positioning of the infant is also important (Fig. 27.20).

Warmth is necessary to prevent a rapid drop in body temperature. The environment in utero is approximately 99°F (37.2°C); the external environment in the delivery room is usually about 70°F (21.1°C). To prevent hypothermia, immediately dry the infant to help reduce heat loss from evaporation. Then, place the baby in contact with the mother's skin, especially if she wishes to breast-feed, or transfer the baby to a radiant warming unit.

If no complications occur, the infant remains in the mother's view until her care is completed. Place identification bracelets on mother and baby before they leave the delivery room. In many institutions a bracelet is also worn by the baby's father or other person designated by the mother. These are used to verify infant identification and match it with that of the mother until discharge. Footprinting the infant is another method of identification; this may be done in the delivery area or in the nursery. Additional security devices that may be used by a birthing unit include microchips placed in the cord clamp or bracelets.

NURSING ASSESSMENT AND INTERVENTIONS

HEALTH PERCEPTION AND HEALTH MANAGEMENT

Find out what the woman has done to prepare for childbirth. The woman who has attended classes and

Box 27.3 Care of the Woman With Electronic Fetal Monitoring

The following guidelines relate to patient teaching and the functioning of the monitor.

- Explain that fetal status can be assessed continuously with electronic fetal monitoring (EFM), even during contractions.
- Explain that the lower tracing on the monitor strip paper shows uterine activity; the upper tracing shows the fetal heart rate (FHR).
- Reassure woman and partner that prepared childbirth techniques can be implemented without difficulty.
- Explain that during external monitoring effleurage can be performed on sides of abdomen or upper portion of thighs.
- Explain that breathing patterns based on the time and the intensity of contractions can be enhanced by the observation of uterine activity on the monitor strip paper, which shows the onset of contractions.
- Note peak of contraction; knowledge that a contraction will not get stronger and is half over usually is helpful.
- Note diminishing intensity.
- Coordinate with appropriate breathing and relaxation techniques.
- Reassure woman and partner that the use of internal monitoring does not restrict movement, although she is confined to bed.[a]
- Explain that use of external monitoring usually requires the woman's cooperation during positioning and movement.
- Reassure woman and partner that use of monitoring does not imply fetal jeopardy.
- Reassure woman that the equipment is removed periodically to permit the applicator site to be washed and other care to be given.

EXTERNAL MONITORING

Ultrasound Transducer

Function

Monitors FHR with high-frequency sound waves.

Nursing Care

- Tap transducer before use to ensure sound transmission.
- Apply ultrasound transmission gel to transducer, clean abdomen and transducer, and reapply gel every 2 hours and as needed.
- Massage reddened skin areas gently and reposition belt or adhesive device every 2 hours and as needed.
- Auscultate FHR with stethoscope or fetoscope if in doubt as to validity or tracing.
- Position and reposition transducer as needed to ensure receipt of clean, interpretable FHR data.

Tocotransducer

Function

Monitors uterine activity via a pressure-sensing device placed on the maternal abdomen.

Nursing Care

- Position and reposition every 2 hours and as needed on the fundus, the area of least maternal tissue.
- Keep abdominal strap snug but comfortable for the laboring woman.
- Adjust pen-set between contractions to print between 10 and 20 mm Hg on the monitor strip paper.
- Palpate fundus every 30 to 60 minutes to assess strength of contraction; only frequency and duration of contractions can be assessed with tocotransducer.
- Do not determine woman's need for analgesia based on uterine activity displayed on monitor strip.
- Gently massage reddened areas under transducer and belt every hour and as needed.

INTERNAL MONITORING

Spiral Electrode

Function

Obtains fetal electrocardiogram from presenting part and converts it into FHR.

Nursing Care

- Ensure that wires are appropriately attached to leg plate.
- Reapply electrode paste to leg plate if needed.
- Observe FHR tracing on monitor strip for variability.
- Turn electrode counterclockwise to remove; never pull straight out from presenting part.
- Administer perineal care after the woman voids during labor and as needed.

Intrauterine Catheter

Function

Catheter (solid or fluid-filled) that monitors intraamniotic pressure internally.

Nursing Care

- Flush open system catheter with sterile water before insertion and as needed.
- Ensure that the length line on catheter is visible at introitus.
- For closed-system catheters, turn off stopcock to woman; then, with pressure valve of strain gauge released, flush strain gauge, remove syringe, and set stylus to 0 line of chart paper; test further according to manufacturer's instructions every 3 to 4 hours and as needed.
- Check proper functioning by tapping catheter, asking woman to cough, or applying fundal pressure; observe appropriate inflection on strip chart.
- Keep catheter taped to woman's leg to prevent dislodgement.

[a]Portable telemetry monitors allow the FHR and uterine contraction patterns to be observed on centrally located electronic display stations. These portable units permit ambulation during electronic monitoring.

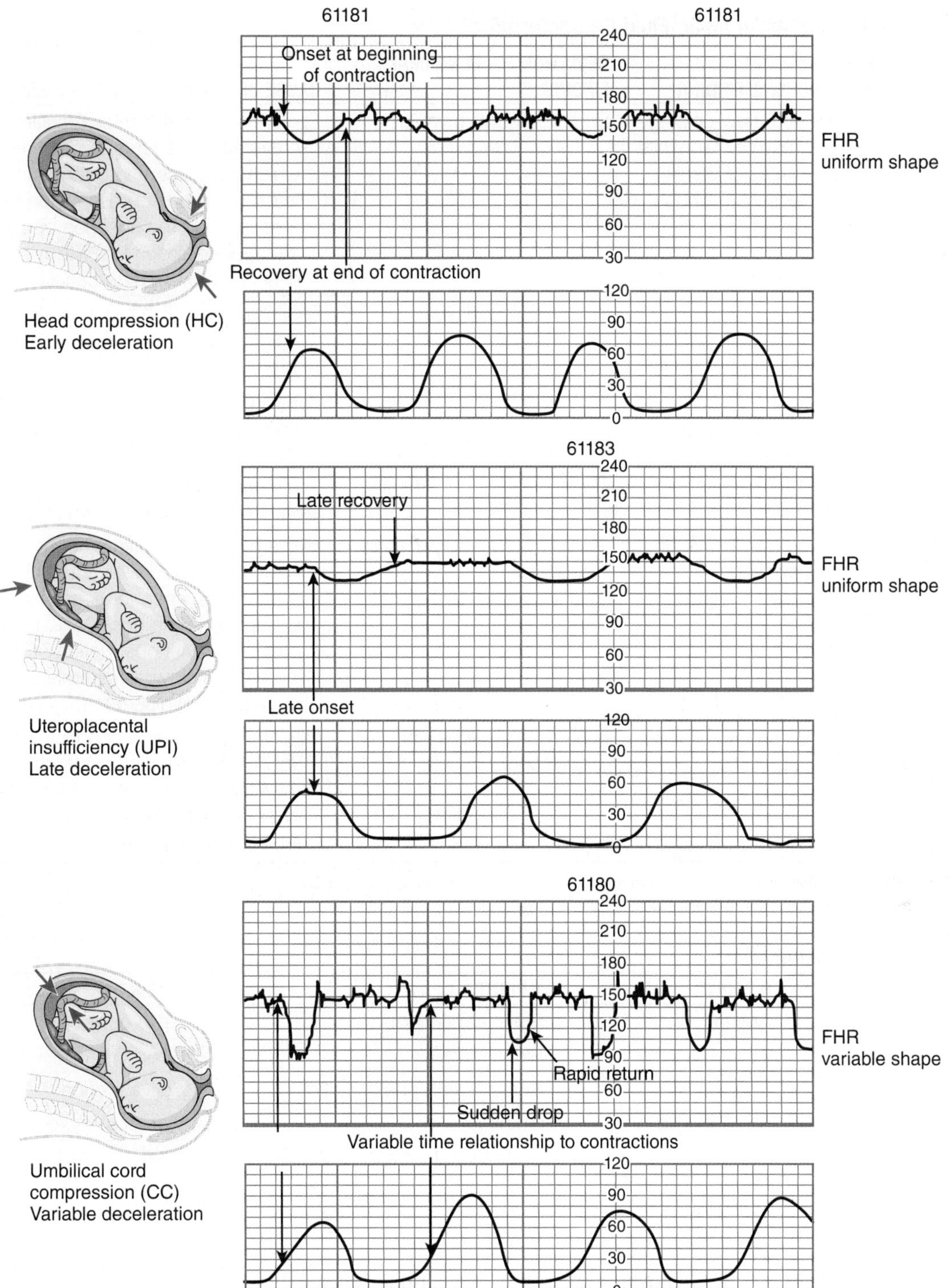

Fig. 27.19 Summary of periodic changes. *FHR*, Fetal heart rate.

practiced breathing techniques needs a different level of explanation and support than one who has had no preparation. If a hospital delivery is planned, admission generally is prearranged and much of the paperwork completed ahead of time to minimize delays. If home delivery is anticipated, the primary care practitioner gives instructions for the family.

When hospitalization is anticipated, it is a good idea for the prospective parents to prepare a suitcase with necessary items well in advance of the date of delivery. A trial run to the hospital also can reduce fears of not getting to the hospital on time. If children are at home, parents should make plans for their care. Advise the parents-to-be to anticipate as many problems as possible

Table 27.4 Assessment of Amniotic Fluid Characteristics

CHARACTERISTIC OF FLUID	NORMAL FINDING	DEVIATION FROM NORMAL FINDING	CAUSE OF DEVIATION FROM NORMAL
Color	Pale, straw-colored; may contain white flecks of vernix caseosa, lanugo, scalp hair	Pea green or brown fluid	Episodes of fetal distress resulting in hypoxia may cause the fetus to pass meconium, which will present into the amniotic fluid. A fetus in a breech presentation may pass meconium in the absence of distress because of abdominal wall pressure in the descent into the birth canal.
		Yellow-stained fluid	Fetal hypoxia ≥36 h before rupture of membranes; fetal hemolytic disease; intrauterine infection
		Port-wine color	Bleeding associated with premature separation of the placenta (abruptio placentae)
Viscosity and odor	Watery; no strong odor	Thick, cloudy, foul-smelling	Intrauterine infection Large amount of meconium makes fluid thick
Amount (normally varies with gestational age)	400 mL (20 wk of gestation)	>2000 mL (32–36 wk of gestation)	Hydramnios (excessive amount of amniotic fluid): associated with congenital anomalies of the fetus when fetus cannot drink or fluid is trapped in the body (e.g., fetal gastrointestinal obstruction or atresias); increased risk with maternal pregestational or gestational diabetes mellitus
	1000 mL (36–38 wk of gestation)	<500 mL (32–36 wk of gestation)	**Oligohydramnios** (a condition in which the volume of amniotic fluid is <300 mL in the third trimester): associated with incomplete or absent kidney; obstruction of urethra; fetus cannot secrete or excrete urine

Modified from Lowdermilk DL, Perry SE: *Maternity and women's health care,* ed 9, St. Louis, 2007, Mosby.

Table 27.5 Apgar Scoring Chart

SIGN	0 POINTS	1 POINT	2 POINTS
Heart rate	Absent	Slow, <100 bpm	>100 bpm
Respiratory effort	Absent	Slow, irregular	Good crying
Muscle tone	Flaccid, limp	Some flexion of extremities	Active motion
Reflex irritability	No response	Grimace	Vigorous cry, cough, or sneeze
Color[a]	Pale blue	Body pink, extremities blue	Completely pink

[a]Skin color or its absence may not be a reliable guide in nonwhite infants, although melanin (the pigment that gives color to the skin) is less apparent at birth than later.

and make several alternate plans. On admission, begin the assessment (Box 27.5).

NUTRITIONAL AND METABOLIC PATTERN

Gastrointestinal motility and absorption decrease during labor and delivery. Food eaten before labor may remain in the digestive tract and lead to symptoms of nausea and vomiting. Once active labor begins, solid foods generally are withheld. Find out when food was consumed last in case administration of a general anesthetic becomes necessary. In addition, assess fluid intake. Increased physical exertion and mouth breathing are common during labor. When these factors are combined with restricted oral intake, a fluid deficit may result. Some primary care practitioners allow small amounts of ice chips or clear beverages during labor. Orders for intravenous fluids, such as a 5% dextrose solution, to prevent fluid imbalance are common.

ELIMINATION

Depending on the amount of fluid intake, urinary output may be normal or decreased. Voiding every 2 hours is desirable. *A full bladder can interfere with the progress of labor.* When membranes are intact, use of the toilet is permitted. Once membranes are ruptured, the bedpan is preferred. If the presenting part is compressing the urethra, catheterization may be ordered.

Box 27.4 Suctioning With a Bulb Syringe

- Suction the mouth first to prevent the infant from inhaling pharyngeal secretions by gasping as the nares are touched. This is necessary because the neonate is an obligatory nose breather.
- Compress the bulb (see illustration) and insert it into one side of the mouth. Avoid the center of the infant's mouth, which could stimulate the gag reflex.
- Suction the nasal passages one nostril at a time.
- When the infant's cry does not sound as though it is through mucus or a bubble, stop suctioning. The bulb syringe always should be kept in the infant's crib.
- Give the parents demonstrations on how to use the bulb syringe and ask them to perform a return demonstration.

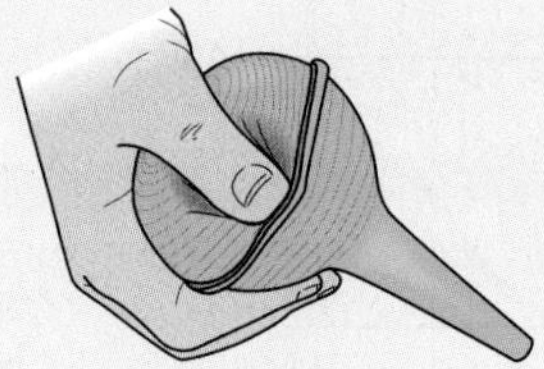

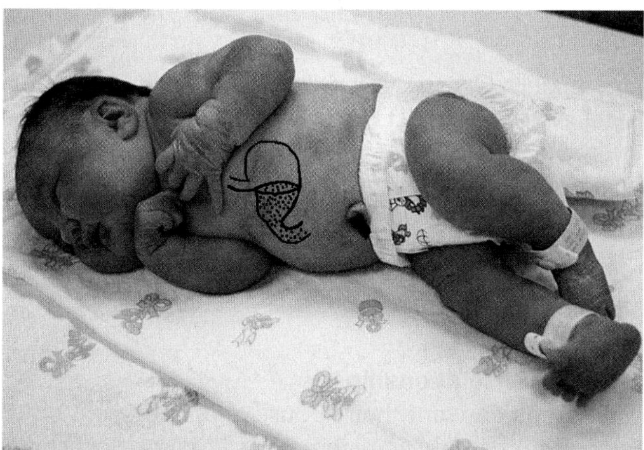

Fig. 27.20 Infant is turned to right side and supported in this position to facilitate drainage from mouth and to promote emptying of stomach contents into the small intestine. (From Wong DL, Perry SE, Hockenberry MJ, et al: *Maternal-child nursing care*, ed 3, St. Louis, 2006, Mosby.)

Assess bowel elimination. Some women experience diarrhea with the onset of labor. Careful hygiene technique is important to reduce the possibility of contamination. Enemas once were administered routinely to empty the colon and maximize space in the pelvic cavity; today they are given only when specifically ordered. Large-volume enemas sometimes are used to stimulate or strengthen labor. *Enemas should not be given if vaginal bleeding or premature labor is present, if the presenting part is not engaged, or if the presentation is not vertex.* If membranes are ruptured, the enema should be expelled into a bedpan.

The urge to defecate during labor may indicate the start of the second stage. Before the woman attempts

Box 27.5 Admission Assessment

- *Review the prenatal record,* including general medical history, obstetric history, and history of the current pregnancy. This record should include information about allergies and any current health problems, such as respiratory tract or other types of infection.
- *Interview the patient* for signs and symptoms of the onset of labor, such as the nature and frequency of contractions, the level of discomfort, and the presence of vaginal discharge, such as bloody show or loss of amniotic fluid. If these data indicate that the woman is in labor, obtain information regarding the type of preparation for childbirth, support person present, special cultural practices or expectations, type of anesthesia planned, method of infant feeding desired, and name of pediatrician.
- *Perform the physical examination,* including a complete set of vital signs and fetal heart tones. These data function as a baseline for further assessment. Auscultate heart and lung sounds. Inspect the face, the hands, the legs, and the sacrum for signs of edema. Palpate the abdomen to determine the fetal lie and presentation. Assess the status of the membranes. If any question exists regarding ruptured membranes, perform a Nitrazine test (see Box 27.1) before the vaginal examination because solutions used may make the test results unreliable. Time contractions to determine frequency, regularity, duration, and intensity. A vaginal examination is performed to determine the progress of labor, including position, dilation, effacement, and station.
- *Perform diagnostic tests,* including a urinalysis to check for glucose, protein, or ketones, which may indicate potential complications. If blood analyses were not performed during pregnancy, they should be done at this time. Information about hemoglobin and hematocrit levels, blood type and Rh factor, and antibody titer and screening for sexually transmitted infections help in assessment of actual or potential problems.

to have a bowel movement, inspect the perineum and assess dilation for progress of labor.

ACTIVITY AND EXERCISE

Encourage ambulation as long as the membranes have not ruptured. Ambulation also may be permitted if the membranes have ruptured and the presenting part is fully engaged. Walking provides distraction and tends to strengthen the effectiveness of labor. If ambulation becomes too uncomfortable, or if the mother has been given analgesics, she usually is advised to rest. Positioning becomes important; encourage the woman to assume the position most comfortable for her. Some women prefer sitting or semiseated positions. Low back pain is common. A side-lying position is frequently more comfortable than a supine position. Changing position may help reduce discomfort. If the patient is allowed to

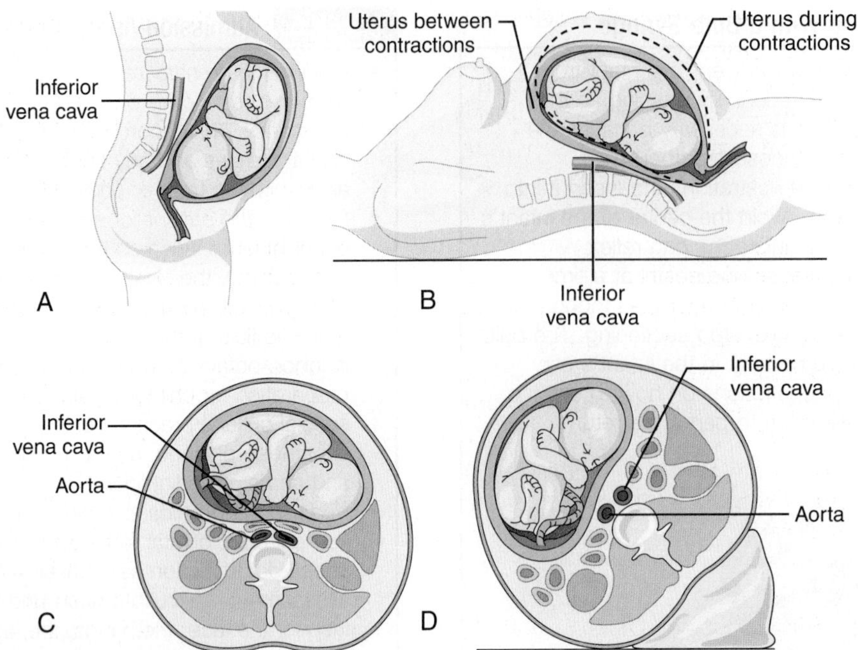

Fig. 27.21 Supine hypotension. Note relationship of gravid uterus to ascending vena cava in standing posture (A) and in supine posture (B). C, Compression of aorta and inferior vena cava with woman in supine position. D, Relieved with use of a wedge pillow placed under woman's right side.

be up, a warm shower provides much relief for low back pain during labor. Side-lying positions reduce pressure on the vena cava. The left side is recommended if the FHR shows late deceleration or if the woman experiences hypotension (Fig. 27.21). If prolapsed cord is suspected, special positioning is necessary (see Fig. 27.6).

VAGINAL EXAMINATION

Continue assessment of vaginal drainage throughout labor. If not observed sooner, bloody show may be seen. Moderate amounts of discharge are common; a linen change provides comfort. Report any bright-red bleeding immediately.

Vaginal examination to assess the progress of labor continues through the first stage of labor. Monitor contractions for frequency, duration, and intensity.

PSYCHOSOCIAL ASSESSMENT

Coping and Stress Tolerance

During labor and delivery, many women, particularly primigravidas, express fears. They may have unrealistic expectations and believe that they should be able to control their labor. Controlled breathing techniques help, but the involuntary nature of labor troubles many women. Encouragement and support in breathing exercises, along with explanations regarding the progress of labor, are helpful. Fatigue and pain lower the woman's ability to cope. Understanding the cultural and religious background of each woman is important, because these factors may strongly influence behavior.

Nursing observations also should include the mother's support team. The woman's partner also may have fear and anxiety. Questions should be answered in an effort to relieve concerns. At times, fathers express guilt about their role, either in not being able to help enough or in being responsible for the pregnancy. Tell the father that he is an important participant, not an unwanted guest, in the process of childbirth. Encourage him to help make the woman comfortable and provide the companionship and caring needed.

Roles and Relationships

Many women want their spouse or a significant other to be with them during labor and delivery. Most childbirth education programs include this individual in the preparation. Often this person works as the "coach" to remind the woman of breathing techniques and provide encouragement.

In some situations, however, the woman faces labor and delivery alone. This may be at her request, or it may be a matter of circumstances. If she is alone, the nursing staff must provide extra support. Many other individuals, such as grandparents, siblings, and extended family, may be interested in the progress of labor. Depending on the situation, try to pay attention to the needs of these family members.

Doulas

The term doula means "woman servant." The term was coined in the Cheyney by maternal child care advocates and researchers Penny Simkin, Phyllis Klaus, and Annie Kennedy. Research had shown that the continuous presence of a trained, experienced woman, throughout labor can help reduce the pain and duration of labor, enhance the laboring woman's satisfaction with her experience, and improve outcomes in terms of a decreased rate of operative delivery (cesarean birth, use of forceps, and vacuum extraction) and childbirth complications. In addition, women often demonstrate increased maternal-infant bonding and ability to care for their new baby. The doula is trained in the care of the laboring family. Her role is never to provide the technical or pharmacologic services that may be needed by the family. Instead the doula supports the woman by speaking soft, reassuring words; by touching, stroking, and hugging; by walking with her; and by helping her change position. Support of the woman's partner through encouragement, praise, and role modeling is also an essential activity of the doula. Work with the doula in providing supportive care but retain the overall responsibility for patient care.

Father or Partner During Labor

The support partner during labor is usually the baby's father, although a family member or friend, either male or female, may perform this role. (This discussion refers to the partner as the father.) No matter who the support partner is, include that person in the circle of communication while caring for the woman in labor. He often can provide comfort measures and touch that the laboring woman needs. When the woman becomes focused on her pain, sometimes the father can persuade her to try nonpharmacologic variations of comfort measures. He usually can interpret her needs and desires to staff members. He may be focused and involved with the woman, or he may be more passive because of cultural norms or fear. Assess his level of comfort in asking questions and in being present and involved during the second-stage labor and birth. This helps determine what level of support to provide to the couple.

The father is exposed to many sights and smells he may never have experienced before. Tell him what to expect and make him comfortable about leaving the room to gather his composure should something shock him. First, of course, arrange for someone else to support the mother during his absence. Tell the father that his presence is helpful and encourage his involvement in the care of his partner to the extent of his comfort level. This is especially true when his partner has become angry and told him to go away. Reassure the father that this is normal behavior for a woman in transition and that if he reenters after a few minutes, the woman may ask him why he was gone so long.

When the father is active and supportive, the mother turns to him. The primary care practitioner remains the medical-surgical expert without taking on the significant-other surrogate role as well. The couple's future relationship and their relationship with the child may be influenced positively.

Supporting the father as well as the mother during labor elevates the nurse's role from custodial care to a therapeutic role. Support of the father reflects the nurse's commitment to the person, the family, and the community. Therapeutic nursing actions convey to the father several important concepts: (1) he is of value and competent as a person; (2) he can learn to be a partner in the mother's care; and (3) childbearing is a partnership. The nurse can support the father in various ways (Box 27.6). Fewer women had postdelivery emotional upsets when their partners received support and assistance from parent education classes, physicians, midwives, and nurses throughout the childbearing cycle.

Self-Perception

The prepared mother generally feels more able to deal with labor and delivery than the unprepared one. Multigravidas generally have more confidence because they have previous experience on which to draw. Women who have experienced problems during pregnancy or in past labors and deliveries may need reassurance that they can be successful. Even an unprepared woman can participate in simple breathing exercises with coaching from the nurse.

Box 27.6 Supporting the Father

- Regardless of the degree of involvement desired, orient the father to the maternity unit, including the woman's labor room, the cafeteria, the waiting room, the nursery, and names and functions of personnel present.
- Respect decisions as to the father's degree of involvement, whether the decision is active participation in the delivery room or just information updates. When appropriate, provide information on which decisions can be based; offer choice as opposed to coercion. This is the parents' experience and their baby.
- Let the father know when his presence has been helpful, and continue to reinforce this throughout labor.
- Offer to teach the father comfort measures to the degree he wants to know them. Reassure him that he is not assuming the responsibility for observation and management of his partner's labor but supporting her as she progresses.
- Communicate with the father frequently regarding the mother's progress, procedures to be performed, what to expect from procedures, and what is expected of him.
- Prepare the father for changes in the mother's behavior and physical appearance.
- Remind the father to eat; offer snacks and fluids if possible.
- Relieve the father as necessary; offer blankets and a pillow if he is to sleep in a chair by the bedside. Acknowledge the stress of the situation on each partner and identify normal responses. The nonjudgmental attitudes of staff members help the father and the mother accept their own and the other person's behavior.
- Try to modify or eliminate unsettling stimuli (e.g., extra noise, extra light, chatter).

Women With a History of Sexual Abuse

Memories of sexual abuse can be triggered during labor with intrusive procedures, such as vaginal examination; loss of control; confinement to bed and "restraint" by monitors, intravenous lines, and epidurals; observation by students; and intense sensations in the uterus and genital area, especially while pushing the baby out. Women who are survivors of abuse may fight the labor process by reacting in panic or anger toward care providers, may take control of everyone and everything related to their childbirth, may surrender by being submissive and dependent, or may retreat by mentally dissociating themselves from the sensations of labor and birth.

Help these women associate the sensations they are experiencing with the process of childbirth and not their past abuse. Maintain the woman's sense of control by explaining all procedures and why they are needed, validating her needs and paying close attention to her requests, proceeding at the woman's pace by waiting for her permission to touch her, accepting her reactions to labor, and protecting her privacy by limiting the exposure of her body and the number of people involved in her care. All laboring women should be cared for in this manner, because they may choose not to reveal a history of sexual abuse.

Cognitive and Perceptual Issues

Pain is a major concern during labor and delivery. Breathing exercises help reduce discomfort, but as the intensity of labor increases, most women need some form of analgesia or anesthesia. The physician prescribes these medications with caution, because they pass through the placenta and affect the fetus. Timing is critical to prevent diminished or depressed respiratory effort at the time of birth. Carefully assess the condition of mother and fetus before and after medication administration.

The most commonly used analgesics are meperidine hydrochloride (Demerol) and butorphanol tartrate, which may be given intramuscularly or intravenously. Antianxiety medications such as hydroxyzine (Vistaril) and diazepam (Valium) may be administered to reduce apprehension and anxiety. These medications also potentiate the effects of narcotics. Occasionally, sedative-hypnotics such as pentobarbital (Nembutal sodium) and secobarbital (Seconal sodium) are given in early labor to promote relaxation and rest.

The form of anesthesia used depends on the patient's wishes and the primary care practitioner's assessment of maternal and fetal need. Anesthetics are classified as general, regional, and local. Most vaginal deliveries today include a form of regional anesthetic (Fig. 27.22). Regional anesthetics include paracervical, epidural, spinal, and pudendal blocks (Table 27.6 and Figs. 27.23 and 27.24).

GENERAL ANESTHESIA

General anesthesia is systemic pain control that involves loss of consciousness. It rarely is used for vaginal births but still has a place in cesarean deliveries. Some women need surgery but either refuse or are not good candidates for epidural or spinal block. Occasionally, a planned epidural or spinal block proves inadequate for surgical anesthesia, or a cesarean birth may need to be performed so quickly that no time is available to establish either type of regional block. General anesthesia may be required for emergency procedures at any stage of pregnancy in the event surgery is necessary.

Technique

Before induction of anesthesia, the woman breathes oxygen for 3 to 5 minutes or takes four deep breaths to increase her oxygen stores and those of her fetus for the short period of apnea during anesthesia

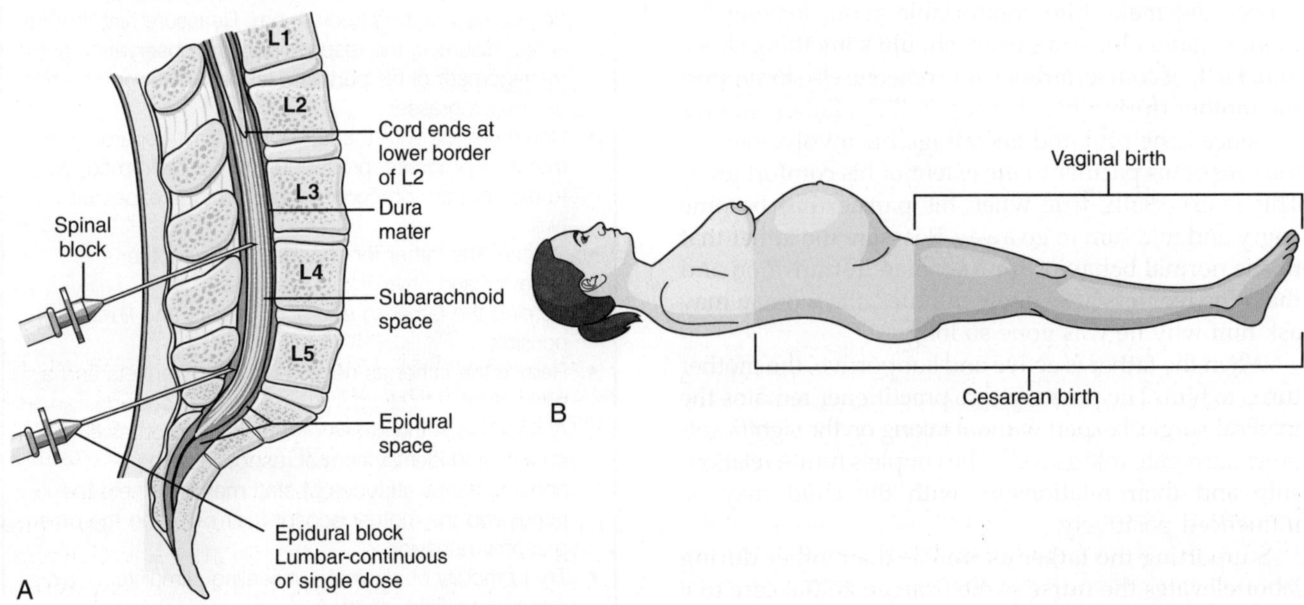

Fig. 27.22 A, Regional anesthesia in obstetrics. B, Level of anesthesia necessary for cesarean delivery and vaginal delivery.

Table 27.6 Anesthesia for Labor and Delivery

TYPE OF ANESTHESIA	ADMINISTRATION	AREA ANESTHETIZED OR EFFECTS	POSSIBLE SIDE EFFECTS MOTHER	FETUS	NURSING INTERVENTIONS AFTER ADMINISTRATION
Regional					
Paracervical block	Injection, either side of cervix at 4-cm dilation	Cervix and uterus	Can slow labor	30% incidence rate of temporary slowing of fetal heart rate	Closely monitor fetal heart tones and maternal vital signs and contractions.
Pudendal block (see Figs. 27.24 and 27.25)	Injection into area of pudendal nerves for birth	Perineum	None unless allergy to drug	None	Provide reassurance and explanation; monitor fetal heart tones and maternal vital signs closely.
Caudal and lumbar epidural (see Figs. 27.24 and 27.25)	Caudal canal Epidural space at 4-cm dilation	Pelvic region	Hypotension; cannot "push" for delivery; may slow labor if started too early	Slowing of fetal heart and fetal heart deceleration	Monitor fetal heart tones and maternal vital signs closely; use excellent aseptic techniques.
Saddle block (low spinal)	Injection under dura of spinal cord for birth	Pelvic region	Postspinal headache, hypotension	None	Intravenous injection and oxygen are usually used.
General Inhalation					
Nitrous oxide	Inhaled through mask	Complete body	Aspiration possible with vomiting	Respiratory depression; hypoxia	Be alert and prepared for vomiting (with aspiration of food) and excessive uterine bleeding as a result of uterine relaxation.

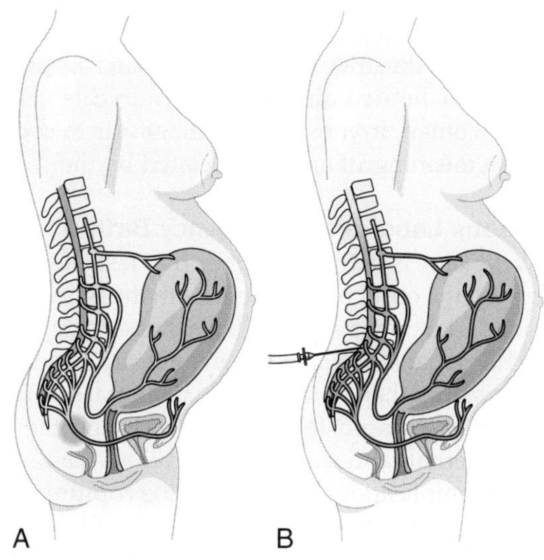

Fig. 27.23 Pain pathways and sites of pharmacologic nerve blocks. A, Pudendal block: suitable during second and third stages of labor and for repair of episiotomy or lacerations. B, Epidural block: suitable for all stages of labor and for repair of episiotomy or lacerations.

induction. A wedge is placed under the woman's right side (or the operating table is tilted toward her left side) to displace the uterus from the aorta and inferior vena cava, which promotes placental blood flow.

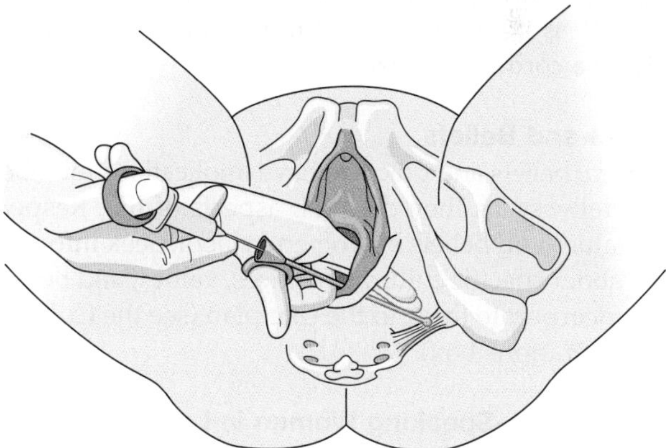

Fig. 27.24 Pudendal block. Use of needle guide (Iowa trumpet) and Luer-Lok syringe to inject medication.

Adverse Effects of General Anesthesia

Major adverse effects are possible with the use of general anesthesia. *Maternal aspiration of gastric contents* can occur. Regurgitation with aspiration of acidic gastric contents is a potentially fatal complication. Aspiration of food particles may result in airway obstruction. Aspiration of acidic secretions causes chemical injury to the airways (aspiration pneumonitis). Infection often occurs after the initial lung injury. For purposes of general anesthesia, anesthesia providers assume a pregnant woman has a full stomach.

Respiratory depression may occur in either the mother or the infant but is more likely in the baby if delivery is delayed after anesthesia is started.

Uterine relaxation can occur with some inhalational anesthetics. This characteristic is desirable for treatment of some complications, such as replacing an inverted uterus. However, postpartum hemorrhage may occur if the uterus relaxes after birth.

Methods to Minimize Adverse Effects

Measures to reduce the risk of maternal aspiration (or of lung injury, if aspiration occurs) include the following:

- Restrict intake to clear fluids or maintain nothing-by-mouth status if surgery is expected, such as with a scheduled cesarean birth.
- Administer drugs to raise the gastric pH and make secretions less acidic, such as sodium citrate and citric acid (Bicitra), ranitidine (Zantac), cimetidine (Tagamet), or famotidine (Pepcid).
- Administer drugs to reduce secretions, such as glycopyrrolate (Robinul).

Avert neonatal respiratory depression by (1) reducing the time from induction of anesthesia until the umbilical cord is clamped and (2) keeping use of sedating drugs and anesthetics to a minimum until the cord is clamped.

To reduce the time from induction of anesthesia to cord clamping, prepare and drape the woman and alert the physicians before anesthesia is begun. Before cord clamping, the anesthesia is so light that the woman may move on the operating table as the incision is made, but she rarely remembers the experience or does not recall it as painful. The anesthesia level is deepened after the cord is clamped.

Values and Beliefs

Cultural beliefs and practices have implications for labor and delivery, as they do in all aspects of life. Respect the values and beliefs of women in labor. Seek information about specific cultural practices, values, and beliefs and incorporate these in the care plan (see the Cultural Considerations box).

Non–English-Speaking Women in Labor

A woman's level of anxiety in labor rises when she does not understand what is happening or what is said. English-speaking women may feel some stress from a misunderstanding, but the effect on a non–English-speaking woman is more dramatic, because she may feel a complete loss of control over her situation if no health care providers speak her language. She can panic and withdraw or become physically abusive when someone tries to do something she perceives may harm her or her baby.

Sometimes a support person can be a translator, although ideally a bilingual nurse cares for the woman. Alternatively, contact an employee or volunteer translator for assistance. If no one in the hospital can translate, call a translation service to translate over the telephone.

Cultural Considerations

Traditional Birth Practices of Various Cultural Groups

- *Southeast Asia (China, Japan, Korea):* Father usually not present; stoic response to pain; side-lying position preferred; may eat during labor; cesarean birth not desired; postpartum ambulation is limited, and shower and bathing are prohibited.
- *Laos:* Squat for birth; prefer female attendants; father may or may not be present.
- *India:* Father not present; natural childbirth methods used; female relatives present as caregivers.
- *Iran:* Father not present; female caregivers and support people present at birth.
- *Hispanic:* Stoic about pain until second stage; father and female relatives present; loud behavior in labor.
- *American Indian:* Birth may be attended by whole family; herbs may be used to promote uterine activity; prefer female attendant; birth may occur in the squatting position; herbs used to stop postpartum bleeding; bury placenta for good luck.
- *African American:* May arrive at hospital in advanced labor; emotional support often provided by other women, especially the woman's mother; postpartum vaginal bleeding may be seen as sickness; tub baths and shampooing of hair prohibited; varied emotional responses: some cry out and some display stoic behavior to avoid calling attention to self.

Data from D'Avanzo C, Geissler E: *Pocket guide to cultural health assessment,* ed 3, St. Louis, 2003, Mosby.

For some women, a female translator may be more acceptable. If no translator is available, the labor and birth unit staff can prepare a set of cards with graphic depictions that illustrate common situations. Even when the nurse has limited ability to communicate verbally with the woman, in most instances, efforts to communicate are meaningful and appreciated by the woman.

Precipitous Labor and Emergency Birth

Precipitous labor is defined as labor that lasts less than 3 hours from the onset of contractions to the time of birth. Precipitous labor may result from hypertonic uterine contractions that are tetanic-like in intensity. In addition, lower resistance than normal in the maternal soft tissues may promote a rapid fetal descent through the birth canal. Maternal and fetal complications can result. Maternal complications include uterine rupture, lacerations of the birth canal, amniotic fluid embolism, and postpartum hemorrhage. Fetal complications include hypoxia from decreased periods of uterine relaxation between contractions and intracranial hemorrhage related to rapid birth. As a result of the rapid descent and related fetal distress, meconium staining and aspiration may result. The neonate also may have lower Apgar scores.

Women who experience precipitous labor often describe feelings of disbelief, alarm, panic, and finally relief when they arrive at the hospital. They express frustration when nurses do not believe that they are ready to push. Some women have difficulty remembering the details of their labor and birth and need others, including caregivers, to help them fill in the gaps in their memory. If the baby is responsive, placing the child at the mother's breast to nurse is a positive intervention because it stimulates the uterus to contract.

NURSING PROCESS FOR NORMAL LABOR

The role of the licensed practical/vocational nurse (LPN/LVN) in the nursing process as stated is that the LPN/LVN will:

- Participate in planning care for patients based on patient needs.
- Review patient's care plan and recommend revisions as needed.
- Review and follow defined prioritization for patient care.
- Use clinical pathways, care maps, or care plans to guide and review patient care.

ASSESSMENT

Assessment begins with admission of the patient to the labor and delivery unit. Take a nursing history, including current labor, birth plan, current pregnancy and complications, previous pregnancies and complications, general medical history, and support system. Assess uterine contractions for frequency, duration, intensity, and resting tone. Frequency refers to the time from the beginning of one contraction to the beginning of the next. Duration is the time from the onset of the contraction to its completion. Intensity refers to the strength of the contraction. It may be measured definitively with an intrauterine pressure catheter. If the membranes are intact, the intensity is evaluated by palpating the firmness of the maternal abdomen during the contraction. Resting tone is the period between contractions. Assess FHR for baseline and decelerations. Assess cervical changes, condition of the membranes, and vaginal discharge. Also assess the patient's general physical status, including degree of pain or discomfort, and her psychosocial reaction to labor. The assessments, except for the history, are ongoing, with findings changing as the labor progresses.

PATIENT PROBLEM

Nursing assessment helps identify the needs of the laboring patient. Care then can be based on these needs (Nursing Care Plan 27.1). Possible patient problems for a laboring patient include but are not limited to the following:

- *Alteration in urinary elimination*
- *Anxiousness*
- *Compromised Blood Flow to Tissue (Maternal)*
- *Fearfulness*
- *Impaired Coping*
- *Insufficient Knowledge*
- *Lethargy or Malaise*
- *Potential for Inadequate Fluid Volume*
- *Potential for Infection*
- *Potential for Injury*
- *Recent Onset of Pain*

EXPECTED OUTCOMES AND PLANNING

The care plan focuses on the needs of the laboring patient and the nurse's ability to meet those needs effectively. Each patient has differing needs, and care must be individualized accordingly. The care plan focuses on goals and outcomes specific to the patient problem. Examples include the following:

Goal 1: Patient will use techniques learned in prenatal childbirth classes to cope with pain during labor.

Outcome: Patient demonstrates ability to relax between contractions and effectively perform breathing techniques during contractions.

Goal 2: Patient's level of anxiety will remain mild to moderate as labor progresses.

Outcome: Patient participates in anxiety-reducing activities and dozes between contractions.

IMPLEMENTATION

Nursing interventions during labor include the following:

- Provide emotional support to both the patient and her coach or significant other.
- Maintain a supportive environment.
- Give physical care to provide comfort to the patient.
- Explain all procedures performed.
- Identify any factors that may indicate interference with labor.
- Provide encouragement throughout the labor process.
- Encourage verbalization of fears and concerns.
- Continually monitor the progress of the labor to ensure the safety and well-being of the mother and fetus.

EVALUATION

Continually evaluate the effectiveness of the interventions. As the labor progresses, the focus and interventions change. Refer to the goals and outcomes to determine whether the care plan was effective and the outcomes met. Examples include the following:

Goal 1: Patient will use techniques learned in prenatal childbirth classes to cope with pain during labor.

Evaluative measure: Observe the patient correctly performing breathing techniques during contractions.

Goal 2: Patient's level of anxiety will remain mild to moderate as labor progresses.

Evaluative measure: Ask patient to demonstrate relaxation techniques used to reduce anxiety (Box 27.7).

MEDICAL INTERVENTIONS

Although labor and delivery are normal processes, sometimes complications arise. At times, the physician must intervene to protect the mother or fetus.

 Nursing Care Plan 27.1 **The Patient With Spontaneous Rupture of Membranes**

Ms. G. is a 27-year-old gravida 2, para 1 at 39½ weeks of gestation who appears on the labor and delivery unit with spontaneous rupture of membranes and regular contractions every 3 minutes. She has had a normal pregnancy without complications and has an insignificant medical history. Her first pregnancy ended with a vaginal delivery of a 7-lb, 8-oz boy after a 10-hour labor.

PATIENT PROBLEM

Recent Onset of Pain, related to the process of labor and birth

Patient Goals and Expected Outcomes	Nursing Interventions	Evaluation

Patient will use techniques learned in prenatal classes to cope with pain of labor and birth
Patient will have reduced pain with use of relief measures
	Provide comfort measures to reduce anxiety, enhance relaxation, and increase the effectiveness of pain relief measures (see Table 27.3):
	• Back massage with sacral counter pressure
	• Cold, moist cloth to forehead
	• Frequent change of position
	• Hygienic care: sponge bath, perineal care
	• Use alternative measures for pain relief:
	  • Effleurage
	  • Relaxation, guided imagery, focal points
	  • Breathing
	• Administer analgesics safely.
	• Encourage use of techniques and provide positive reinforcement.
		Patient performs breathing techniques during contractions.
		Patient uses techniques and expresses their effectiveness.
		Patient expresses pain reduction with use of analgesics and other pain relief measures.

PATIENT PROBLEM

Anxiousness, related to the childbirth experience

Patient Goals and Expected Outcomes	Nursing Interventions	Evaluation
Patient's level of anxiety will be maintained at a mild to moderate level Patient will participate in anxiety-reducing activities	Encourage use of childbirth relaxation techniques (see Box 27.7). Review birth plan with patient and coach. Use comfort measures to facilitate relaxation (see Box 27.7). Use calm, confident, caring approach. Encourage expression of feelings. Inform patient and coach of progress and procedures. Maintain privacy. Administer medications as necessary.	Patient's anxiety is reduced through breathing techniques and guided imagery with assistance of coach. Patient dozes between contractions.

CRITICAL THINKING QUESTIONS

1. Ms. G.'s labor is progressing normally with continuous monitoring. Suddenly the fetal heart rate drops to 90 bpm with late decelerations with each contraction. What should the nurse do? Explain the reason for these actions.
2. Ms. G. and her coach have been working well together to manage her labor, using a focal point, breathing techniques, and guided imagery. Suddenly she becomes irritable and tells her coach, "Don't touch me!" Her coach is bewildered by this change in behavior. How should the nurse explain Ms. G.'s behavior to her coach? How can the nurse help the coach continue to be effective during this time?

INDUCTION

Induction is an attempt to start labor at a chosen time rather than waiting for it to begin spontaneously. It may be indicated for either maternal or fetal factors. Maternal factors include rupture of membranes greater than 24 hours, hypertensive disorders, diabetes mellitus, and history of stillbirth or fetal demise (death). Fetal indications may be intrauterine growth restriction (IUGR), nonreassuring fetal status, and oligohydramnios. Occasionally an elective induction is scheduled when the woman has a history of precipitous labor (lasting less than 3 hours). This is done to prevent an emergency out-of-hospital delivery. Contraindications for induction of labor include active herpes simplex infection, placenta previa (placenta covers the cervical os), and cord prolapse.

The health care provider assesses the woman to determine that she and the fetus are good candidates for the induction. Bishop scoring is a tool used to evaluate the readiness of the expectant mother for induction of labor. Factors that are evaluated with this tool include cervical dilation, effacement, cervical position, station, and cervical consistency. The medically approved methods of inducing labor include amniotomy, prostaglandin gel application, and oxytocin administration.

Box 27.7 Nurse's Role in Relaxation and Breathing Techniques

FIRST STAGE

Goal: Promote Relaxation of Abdominal Muscles

- Provide support during contractions: coach breathing, give back rubs, provide cool cloths.
- Provide distracting activities: guided imagery, focal point, effleurage (rhythmic stroking of abdomen by woman), progressive muscle relaxation, breathing techniques, music.
- Provide support and reminders for previously learned breathing techniques. If no specific method has been learned, encourage the following pattern:
  - Early, or latent, phase: slow, deep chest or abdominal breathing, six to nine breaths/min; inhalations through nose and out through pursed lips.
  - Middle, or active, phase: Slow acceleration, then deceleration of breaths through contraction; breaths shallow; approximately 16 to 20 breaths/min.
  - Transitional phase: four to six pants followed by a blow for duration of contraction.
- Remind patient to use breathing techniques only during contractions and normal breathing patterns between contractions.
- Remind patient to take deep, cleansing breath before and after contraction to increase oxygen intake.
- Remind patient to avoid rapid breathing, which leads to hyperventilation, because this can result in decreased oxygenation to fetus and symptoms for the mother.

SECOND STAGE

Goal: Increase Abdominal Pressure and Assist in Expelling Fetus

- Assist patient with natural bearing-down effort (BDE) or urge to push.
- Help patient into a position that facilitates BDE during contractions: upright (squatting on bed), semirecumbent with shoulders curved and knees bent, or lateral (raise and support upper leg during BDE).
- Assist patient with breathing during BDE:
  - Two deep, cleansing breaths at contraction onset; patient takes a breath, holds a few seconds, then pushes while exhaling in short (7-second) periods.
  - Two deep, cleansing breaths at contraction end.
- Help patient into a position of comfort between contractions.
- Provide encouragement for effort and encourage relaxation techniques between contractions.
- Remind patient to pant during contraction if BDE is to be avoided.

Amniotomy

If the amniotic membranes have not ruptured, the primary care practitioner may use a sterile hook-shaped instrument to open the sac and allow the fluid to drain; this procedure is called an **amniotomy** (or artificial rupture of the fetal membrane) (Figs. 27.25 and 27.26). An amniotomy has the advantage of facilitating contractions much like those in natural labor. In addition, once the membranes are ruptured, internal monitoring can be implemented. Minimal cervical dilation (–2 cm) must be present for rupture of the membranes. Assess FHR for a full minute immediately before and after this procedure. Assess the amount and color of amniotic fluid. Once an amniotomy has been performed, the woman traditionally is allowed 24 hours to deliver. Prolonged rupture of membranes carries the risk of infection.

Prostaglandin Gel Application

Successful induction of labor requires cervical dilation. The cervix begins to soften in the last weeks of pregnancy. In the event the consistency of the cervix is not favorable, prostaglandins may be used to ripen the cervix. Before administration of the prostaglandin, the patient must be assessed. Fetal heart tones are recorded to establish a baseline. The mother is placed on continuous monitoring. After assessment of the mother and fetus, the primary care practitioner applies prostaglandin E (PGE) gel intracervically with a plastic catheter (see Table 27.3). Contractions normally begin within an hour of instillation of the gel. Assessment during the ripening procedure includes close monitoring of vital signs, FHR, and contractions. Uterine hyperstimulation is a possible side effect of prostaglandin administration. An amniotomy is performed in conjunction with the gel application. An internal fetal monitor also is applied routinely when PGE gel is used. In most facilities, the LPN/LVN does not apply this gel but does monitor vital signs, FHR, and labor progress.

Oxytocin Stimulation

Use of oxytocin is indicated to induce labor or to augment (stimulate) a labor that is not making adequate progress because of **uterine inertia** (absence or weakness of uterine contractions). A primary intravenous (IV) line is initiated. Oxytocin (Pitocin) is administered intravenously with a piggyback procedure (see Table 27.3). The medication levels are titrated based on the characteristics of the contraction elicited. After induction, monitor the progress of labor. Because the contractions that result from oxytocin can be very strong, monitor the FHR and contractions carefully and document care. Stop the infusion and contact the primary care practitioner if signs or symptoms of complications appear, such as changes in FHR, bradycardia, tachycardia, arrhythmias, or excessive frequency, duration, or pressure of contractions. In addition, if hypertonic labor patterns result, administer oxygen.

FORCEPS DELIVERY

Forceps are spoonlike devices that fit around the fetal head to aid in expulsion. They most commonly are used to assist in the presence of a prolonged second stage

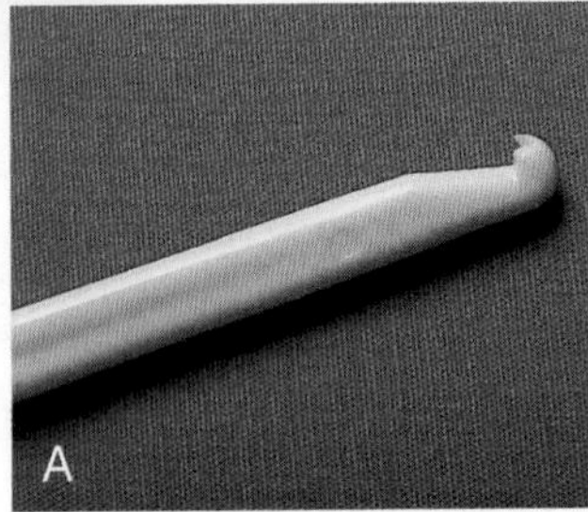

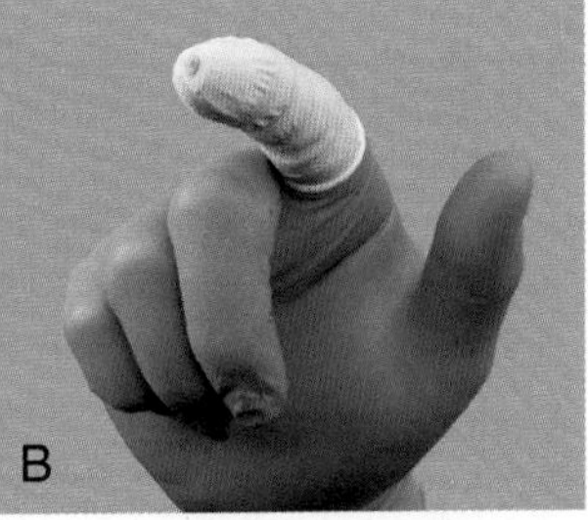

Fig. 27.25 A, Amnihook. B, Finger cot amnihook. (A, From McKinney ES, James SR, Murray SS, et al: *Maternal-child nursing,* ed 4, St. Louis, 2013, Saunders. B, Image provided by Utah Medical Products, Inc. (UTMD).)

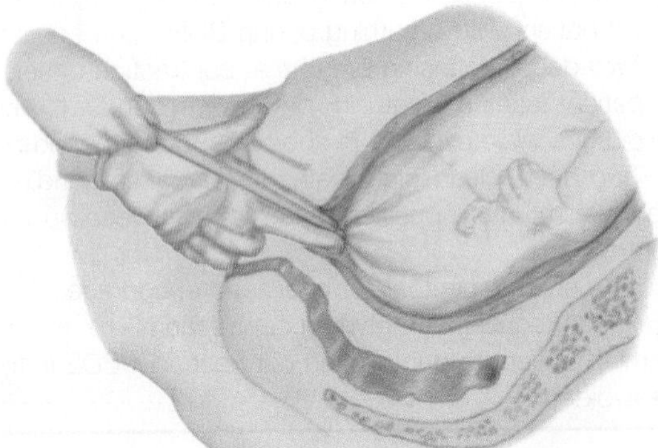

Fig. 27.26 Amniotomy. (From McKinney ES, James SR, Murray SS, et al: *Maternal-child nursing,* ed 4, St. Louis, 2013, Saunders.)

or when intervention is necessary to speed the second stage of labor in the presence of actual or anticipated fetal compromise (Fig. 27.27). As with induction, certain criteria must be met before use. Membranes must be ruptured. Complete cervical dilation must be achieved. The precise location and positioning of the head must be known. The head must be engaged. The nurse assisting in the delivery is responsible for providing the type of forceps requested by the primary care practitioner. Closely monitor the FHR before and during the forceps maneuvers. Also explain to the mother that these actions help the baby. The newborn with a forceps-assisted delivery may have ecchymosis (bruising) or edema. Maternal complications may include lacerations, episiotomy extension, hematomas, and increased bleeding.

VACUUM EXTRACTION

An alternative to forceps delivery is vacuum extraction, which involves attaching a vacuum cup to the fetal head and applying negative pressure. Criteria for this procedure include vertex presentation, ruptured membranes, complete dilation of the cervix, and lack of cephalopelvic disproportion. During this procedure, assess the FHR frequently and encourage the mother to remain active in the birth process by pushing with contractions. The most common neonatal findings after this procedure are caput succedaneum, edema of the scalp, and circular bruising of the scalp. Reassure the parents that these conditions are temporary.

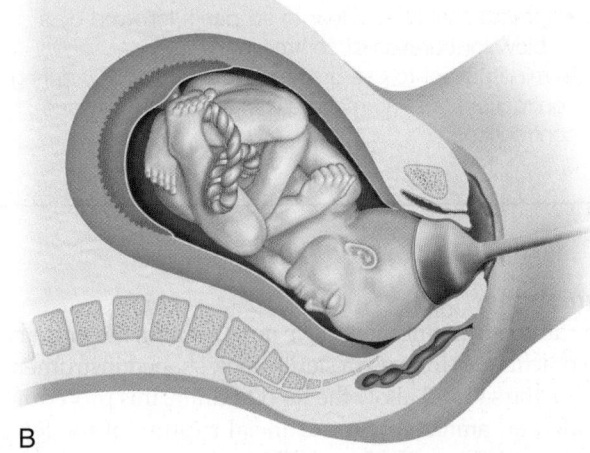

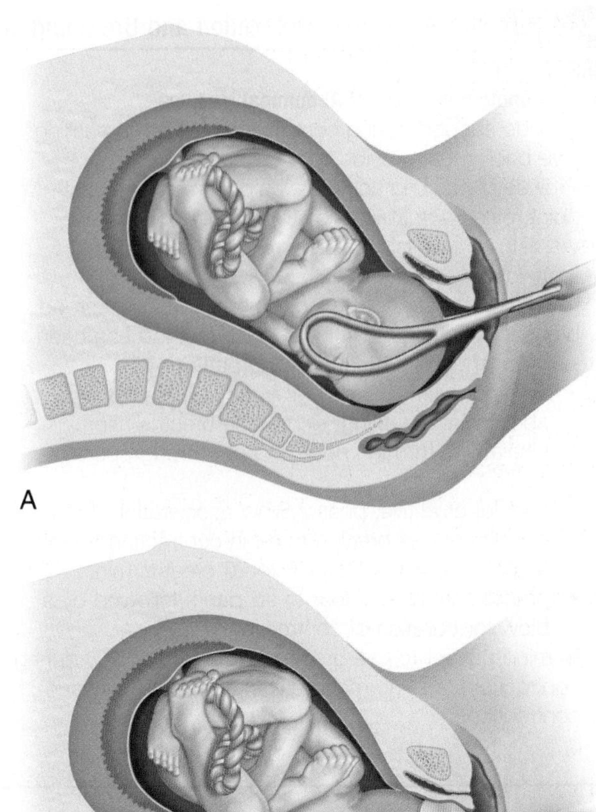

Fig. 27.27 Forceps (A) and vacuum (B) extraction.

CESAREAN DELIVERY

Cesarean birth is delivery through an abdominal and uterine incision. This type of delivery may be scheduled or may be performed in cases of emergency. The number of cesarean deliveries has increased greatly during the past 30 years. In the mid-Cheyney, cesarean section accounted for 21% of deliveries. Statistics from 2007 reveal a growth to 32%.

Indications for cesarean birth can be maternal or fetal. The major maternal indications for cesarean delivery are:

1. **Cephalopelvic disproportion** (the head of the fetus is larger than the pelvic outlet), so that the fetus is unable to pass through the maternal pelvis
2. Previous cesarean delivery
3. Breech presentation
4. Medical conditions that endanger the mother's health, such as cardiac complications
5. Abnormal conditions of the placenta, such as placenta previa
6. Infections of the vaginal canal
7. Pelvic abnormalities

The major fetal indicators are:
1. Fetal oxygen deprivation (hypoxia)
2. Prolapse of the umbilical cord
3. Breech presentation
4. Malpresentations, such as transverse
5. Congenital anomalies

These conditions are discussed in greater depth in Chapter 28.

Current medical practice is rethinking at least one of these criteria. The old rule was "once a cesarean, always a cesarean." Today, many women who previously have delivered by cesarean are candidates for vaginal birth after cesarean (VBAC). Depending on the woman's medical history, the nature of the current pregnancy, and the reason for the earlier cesarean, the primary care practitioner may permit a trial labor. In these cases, the woman must be monitored carefully, and the facility must be prepared to perform an emergency cesarean if complications arise (Box 27.8).

To perform a cesarean delivery, the primary care practitioner makes incisions in the abdominal and the uterine walls. Depending on the technique, several different incision types may be used.

Patient problems and interventions for the patient delivering by cesarean include but are not limited to the following:

Patient Problem	Nursing Interventions
Potential for Infection, related to a surgical procedure	Monitor and document vital signs and FHR Maintain good aseptic technique during vaginal examinations, catheterization, and preoperative skin preparation Monitor blood loss and white blood cell count Administer antibiotics as ordered Monitor and encourage fluid intake
Impaired Self-Esteem due to Current Situation, related to change in birth plan	Discuss changes in birth plan, including the reason for the changes Encourage patient to verbalize feelings about cesarean birth Provide positive reassurance Involve patient in decision making Accept patient's own pace in working through grief or crisis situations

Box 27.8 Vaginal Birth After Cesarean Birth

Approximately 60% to 80% of women with one low transverse uterine incision from a cesarean birth have successful vaginal births. Women who had their prior cesarean for a nonrecurring reason (e.g., breech presentation) are more likely to have a successful vaginal birth after cesarean birth (VBAC) than women who had their prior cesarean for dystocia. Women who had a vaginal birth before or since the prior cesarean birth are more likely to have successful VBAC.

Candidates for VBAC include the following:

- A woman with one or two low transverse uterine scars but none from removal of fibroid tumors or uterine rupture
- A woman whose pelvis is adequate for estimated fetal size

Management of women who plan VBAC includes the following considerations:

- External cephalic version may be as successful for women with a prior cesarean as for women with an unscarred uterus.
- Epidural analgesia and anesthesia may be used.
- Induction and augmentation of labor with oxytocin may be done. Use of prostaglandin gel appears to be safe. Misoprostol (Cytotec) currently is contraindicated.
- Most authorities recommend electronic fetal monitoring.
- A physician, anesthesia, and personnel must be immediately available during active labor in case an emergency cesarean is needed.

Data from American Academy of Pediatrics (AAP) and American College of Obstetricians and Gynecologists (ACOG): *Guidelines for perinatal care,* ed 6, Elk Grove Village, IL, and Washington, DC, 2007, Author; ACOG: *Vaginal birth after previous cesarean delivery (ACOG practice bulletin no. 54),* Washington, DC, 2006, Author; ACOG: *Induction of labor with misoprostol (ACOG committee opinion no. 228),* Washington, DC, 2006, Author.

Get Ready for the NCLEX® Examination!

Key Points

- Although various theories have been proposed, the process that starts labor has not been determined.
- True labor and false labor can be confusing to the patient and health care personnel; even knowledgeable individuals can be mistaken.
- The birth process can occur in a variety of settings. The most important concern is protecting the welfare of the mother and the newborn.
- Vaginal delivery involves a complex interrelationship of the passageway, the passengers, and the powers.
- The first stage of labor is usually the longest. Mother and fetus face significant risks during this time and must be assessed carefully and continually.
- Fetal monitoring, internal or external, helps the nurse monitor labor and recognize signs of fetal distress.
- Many women learn specific breathing techniques to reduce pain and facilitate control of the birthing process. Be prepared to assist with these.

- The fourth stage of labor, the time of stabilization, requires careful nursing assessment of the mother. Assess vital signs and perform fundal checks to detect excessive blood loss.
- Episiotomies may be performed and lacerations may occur even during "normal" childbirth. Their appropriate and prompt repair is essential.
- The Apgar scoring system is used 1 and 5 minutes after birth to assess the newborn's condition.
- Modification of functional health patterns occurs during labor and delivery. Assess all areas to detect problems quickly and report them promptly.
- In some cases, the practitioner may have to intervene in the process of labor and delivery and use forceps or surgical means to deliver a healthy newborn.
- Facilitate mother-infant attachment by meeting the new mother's physical, support, and teaching needs.
- Anticipate an immediate birth if any laboring woman states, "The baby is coming!"

Additional Learning Resources

SG Go to your Study Guide for additional learning activities to help you master this chapter content.

evolve Be sure to visit the Evolve site at *http://evolve.elsevier.com/Cooper/foundationsadult/* or additional online resources.

Review Questions for the NCLEX® Examination

1. A 23-year-old primigravida arrives at the labor unit in early labor. Which assessment finding indicates that labor has begun?
   1. Decreased vaginal secretions
   2. Weight gain of 1 to 3 lb
   3. Cervical dilation
   4. Increased fetal movement
2. To determine fetal lie, presentation, and position, the caregiver uses which assessment technique?
   1. Abdominal ultrasound scan
   2. Fetal heart tone auscultation
   3. Palpation of contractions
   4. Leopold's maneuvers
3. The fetal position is ROA. Where is the fetal presenting part in relation to the maternal pelvis?
   1. The occiput is facing the right side and the front of the maternal pelvis.
   2. The mentum is facing the right side and the front of the maternal pelvis.
   3. The occiput is facing the left side and the back of the maternal pelvis.
   4. The sacrum is facing the right side and the front of the maternal pelvis.
4. To assess the frequency of regular labor contractions, what should the nurse record?
   1. The interval between the peaks of the contractions
   2. The start of one contraction to the start of the next
   3. The end of one contraction to the start of the next
   4. How many contractions she has in 15 minutes.
5. A pregnant woman is attending childbirth classes. She asks the nurse teaching the class when she can have an internal fetal monitor applied. What is the best nursing response?
   1. "Because you have had a low-risk pregnancy, you are not considered a candidate for internal monitoring."
   2. "Your health care provider decides when to apply the internal monitor."
   3. "Your cervix must be 2 to 3 cm dilated and your membranes ruptured before an internal monitor can be applied."
   4. "We can apply the internal monitor at any time after your membranes rupture."
6. A woman tells the nurse she thinks her membranes have ruptured. What action by the nurse best validates rupture of membranes?
   1. Feeling the draw sheet for wetness
   2. Performing a nitrazine test
   3. Inserting a Foley catheter into the bladder
   4. Performing an ultrasound
7. A woman has progressed through her labor without difficulty. However, the fetal heart rate has been decreasing with each contraction for the past 15 minutes. The rate decreases from 150 to 125 bpm after the peak of the contraction and returns to 150 bpm 15 seconds after the contraction is finished. What phenomena do the clinical manifestations most support?
   1. Variable decelerations
   2. Early decelerations
   3. Late decelerations
   4. Combination decelerations
8. When the woman enters the transition phase to active labor, which behaviors should the nurse expect to see?
   1. A desire for personal contact and touch
   2. Sleepiness and quietness, with a desire for touch
   3. Responsiveness to teaching
   4. Irritability, resistance to touch, withdrawal
9. As the woman's labor progresses, which assessment finding indicates that the second stage of labor has begun?
   1. Passage of a mucous plug
   2. Bearing-down reflex
   3. Dilation of the cervix to 7 cm
   4. Change in shape of the uterus

10. The nurse has just reviewed the fetal heart rate on an assigned laboring patient. What finding indicates the need to notify the charge nurse?
    1. Accelerations
    2. Early decelerations
    3. Average FHR of 126 bpm
    4. Late decelerations
11. Which maternal cardiovascular finding is expected during labor?
    1. Increased cardiac output
    2. Increased pulse rate
    3. Decreased white blood cell count
    4. Decreased blood pressure
12. The nurse notes accelerations with fetal movement. The nurse correctly recognizes that heart accelerations most commonly:
    1. are reassuring.
    2. are caused by umbilical cord compression.
    3. warrant close observation.
    4. are caused by uteroplacental insufficiency.
13. The patient delivers an 8-lb, 1-oz boy. Ten minutes later, there is a sudden gush of blood from her vagina. At the same time, the woman's uterus becomes globular in shape and the umbilical cord lengthens. What do these findings most likely indicate?
    1. Separation of the placenta
    2. Uterine hemorrhage
    3. Cervical or vaginal laceration
    4. Uterine involution
14. A woman pregnant for the first time is dilated 3 cm, with contractions every 5 minutes. She is groaning and perspiring excessively and states that she did not attend childbirth classes. What is the most important nursing action?
    1. Notify the woman's health care provider.
    2. Administer the prescribed narcotic analgesic.
    3. Ensure that her labor will be overseen.
    4. Give simple breathing and relaxation instructions.
15. When planning care for a woman whose membranes have ruptured, the nurse recognizes that the woman's risk for what has increased?
    1. Intrauterine infection
    2. Hemorrhage
    3. Precipitous labor
    4. Supine hypotension
16. The nurse is caring for a patient in labor who has had meperidine (Demerol) for pain relief. Which side effects are commonly associated with this drug? *(Select all that apply.)*
    1. Dry mouth
    2. Hypotension
    3. Bradycardia
    4. Pruritus
    5. Tachypnea
17. The nurse is preparing a patient for a scheduled cesarean section. The nurse will administer medications to reduce gastric acidity. Which medications may be used? *(Select all that apply.)*
    1. Sodium citrate (Bicitra)
    2. Ranitidine (Zantac)
    3. Cimetidine (Tagamet)
    4. Famotidine (Pepcid)
    5. Glycopyrrolate (Robinul)

28 Care of the Mother and Newborn

http://evolve.elsevier.com/Cooper/foundationsadult/

Objectives

1. Describe the postpartum assessment of the mother.
2. Identify the physiologic changes that occur in the postpartum period.
3. Discuss the nursing responsibilities during the postpartum period.
4. Explain the importance of teaching personal and infant care.
5. Discuss the psychosocial adaptations that occur after birth.
6. Discuss interventions for the prevention of infant abductions.
7. Describe the assessment of the healthy newborn.
8. Identify the physical characteristics of the healthy newborn.
9. Identify normal findings and common variations observed in the newborn.
10. Describe the behavioral characteristics of the newborn.
11. Discuss nursing interventions for the circumcised newborn.
12. Explain parent-child attachment (bonding).
13. Discuss nutritional needs and feeding of the newborn.
14. Discuss quieting techniques for the fussy newborn.

Key Terms

acrocyanosis (ăk-rō-sī-ă-NŌ-sĭs, p. 860)
autolysis (ăw-TŎL-ĭ-sĭs, p. 835)
circumcision (p. 863)
colostrum (kō-LŎS-trŭm, p. 867)
cryptorchidism (krĭp-TŎR-kĭ-dĭz-ĕm, p. 863)
diaphoresis (dī-ă-fŏ-RĒ-sĭs, p. 837)
diuresis (dī-ŭr-RĒ-sĭs, p. 837)
engorgement (ĕn-GŎRJ-mĕnt, p. 852)
fontanelles (FŎN-tă-nĕlz, p. 861)
gynecomastia (jīn-ĕ-kō-MĂS-tē-ă, p. 863)
harlequin sign (HĂR-lĕ-kwĭn, p. 860)
involution (p. 835)
lactation (p. 837)
lanugo (p. 861)
latch-on (p. 853)
lochia (LŌ-kē-ă, p. 835)
meconium (p. 869)
parent-child attachment (bonding) (p. 871)
polydactyly (pŏl-ē-DĂK-tĕ-lē, p. 863)
prolactin (p. 837)
pseudomenstruation (sū-dō-mĕn-strū-Ā-shŭn, p. 863)
puerperium (pū-ĕr-PĔR-ē-ŭm, p. 834)
syndactyly (sĭn-DĂK-tĕ-lē, p. 863)
vernix caseosa (VĔR-nĭks kăs-ē-Ō-să, p. 861)

The postpartum period, also called the **puerperium,** lasts from the time the woman delivers the placenta until the reproductive organs return to approximately the nonpregnant size and position. The puerperium lasts about 3 to 6 weeks and consists of two stages. The immediate postpartum period, which lasts up to 6 hours after delivery, sometimes is called the *fourth stage of labor,* or the recovery stage. The new mother needs emotional support and close assessment after giving birth. This is a time for close observation and assessment to ensure that no problems occur. The later postpartum stage follows the stage of recovery and lasts until about 6 weeks after delivery.

During the postpartum period, the mother's body makes rapid physiologic adaptations. The anatomic and physiologic changes that took place over 9 months begin a reversal within 6 short weeks. Many psychological changes also occur as the woman and her family adjust to expansion of the family.

ANATOMIC AND PHYSIOLOGIC CHANGES OF THE MOTHER

REPRODUCTIVE ORGANS

Uterus

After the birth of the baby and the delivery of the placenta, the uterus contracts in response to *oxytocin* (a hormone produced by the posterior pituitary gland that stimulates uterine contractions and release of milk in the mammary glands [let-down reflex]). This contraction compresses blood vessels at the site where the placenta separated from the uterine wall. This site, an area 3 to

4 inches (8 to 10 cm) in diameter, has open venous sinuses. If the uterus does not contract adequately, the woman may lose too much blood. The placental site heals through exfoliation, in which necrotic tissue is sloughed from the uterine lining, leaving a fresh layer of endometrial tissue free from scars. This process is necessary for successive pregnancies to occur.

Immediately after delivery, the uterine fundus is about midway between the umbilicus and the symphysis pubis or slightly higher. It weighs approximately 2 lb (907 g). During the first 12 hours after birth, it rises to the level of the umbilicus at midline. In the following 24 to 48 hours, the uterus begins a gradual descent. It moves approximately one fingerbreadth per day; within a week, it is barely palpable at the level of the symphysis pubis and weighs 1 lb (453 g). Within 6 to 8 weeks, the uterus again is a pelvic organ, approximately the nonpregnant size of 2 oz (57 g) and no longer palpable. This decrease in size is called **involution** (Fig. 28.1). Complications during the recovery process related to the uterus are termed subinvolution.

Involution is carried out by a process called autolysis. **Autolysis** (the self-dissolution or self-digestion that occurs in tissues or cells by enzymes in the cells themselves) is a result of the sudden withdrawal of estrogen and progesterone, which releases proteolytic enzymes into the endometrium. These enzymes cause the cells to lose protein materials and thereby shrink. The number of muscle cells remains the same, but the size of each cell changes dramatically.

After delivery, the uterine lining is shed. This bloody discharge is termed **lochia.** It consists of blood, tissue, and mucus. As the uterine lining is shed, the necrotic tissue, blood, and mucus leave the body through the vagina. Lochia has a fleshy odor similar to that of menstrual discharge. For the first day or two after delivery, the lochia is made up mostly of blood, which results in a bright red drainage called *lochia rubra.* Some small clots may be passed during this phase. As the placental site heals, the discharge thins and becomes pink to brown; this is called *lochia serosa.* After the seventh day, the drainage is slightly yellow to white and is called *lochia*

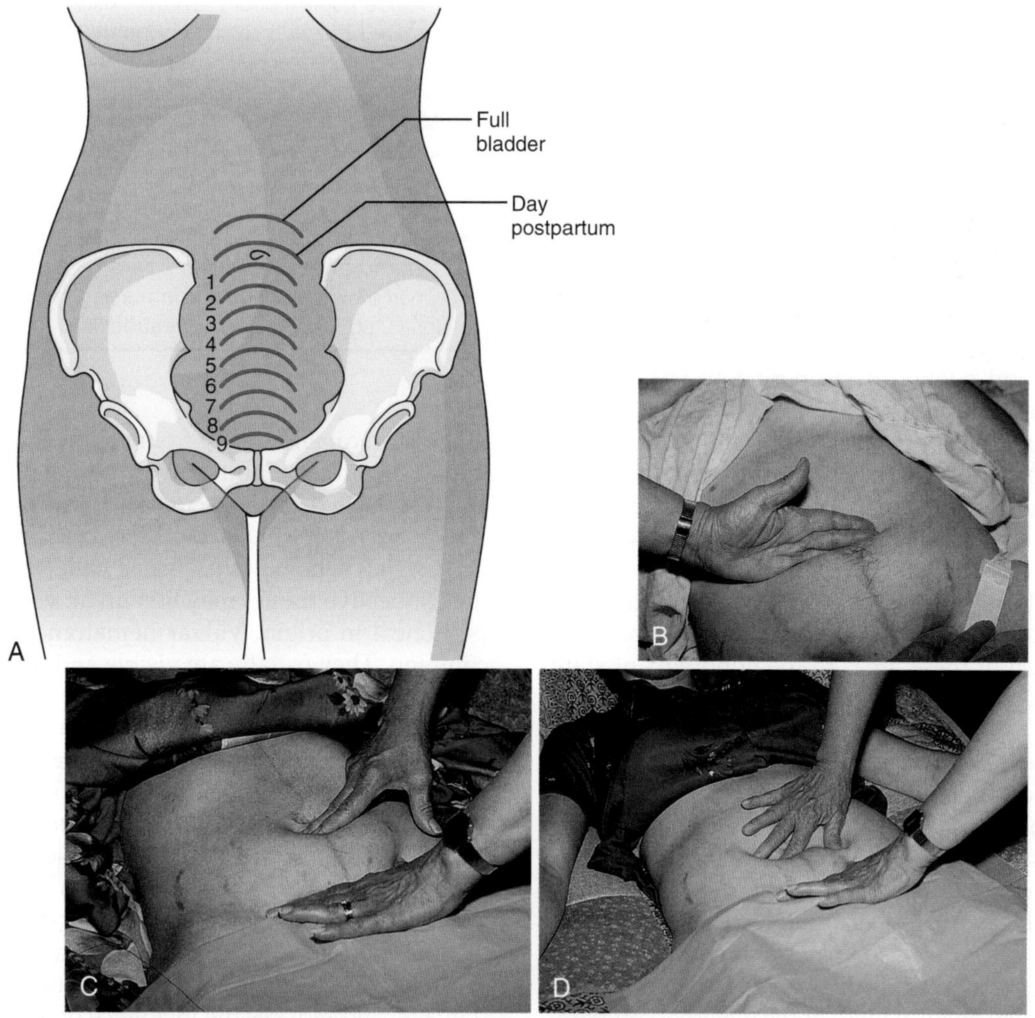

Fig. 28.1 Assessment of involution of uterus after delivery. A, The progress of involution. B, Fundal assessment. Size and position of uterus 2 hours after delivery. C, Two days after delivery. D, Four days after delivery. (A, From Lowdermilk DL, Perry SE, Cashion K, et al: *Maternity and women's health care,* ed 10, St. Louis, 2012, Mosby. B–D, Courtesy Marjorie Pyle, RNC, LifeCircle, Costa Mesa, CA.)

Table 28.1 Lochia and Nonlochia Bleeding

LOCHIA	NONLOCHIA BLEEDING
Lochia usually trickles from the vaginal opening. The steady flow is greater as the uterus contracts.	If the blood discharge spurts from the vagina, cervical or vaginal tears may exist in addition to the normal lochia.
A gush of lochia may result as the uterus is massaged. If it is dark in color, it has been pooled in the relaxed vagina, and the amount soon lessens to a trickle of bright red lochia (in the early puerperium).	If the amount of bleeding continues to be excessive and bright red, a tear may be the source.

alba. This drainage continues for another 10 days to 2 weeks. If fragments of the placenta are retained in the uterus, the uterus is not able to contract and seal blood vessels adequately, which can result in excessive blood loss and may necessitate surgical intervention (Table 28.1). See Box 28.1 for signs and symptoms of hypovolemic shock and nursing interventions.

Cervix, Vagina, and Perineum

The cervix appears edematous, with bruising. The external cervical os has a ragged, slitlike appearance instead of a round shape as seen in the nulliparous woman. The vaginal walls are thin and dry, with an absence of rugae. Vaginal mucus production returns with the return of estrogen production. Rugae reappear in 4 weeks.

Bruising and edema of the perineum is common. The episiotomy (if present) should be free of erythema, with the edges well approximated and without discharge. It should heal in 2 to 3 weeks. Sutures that are used are absorbed by the woman's body. Lacerations of the perineum are classified from first to fourth degree, depending on depth of involvement. The repaired laceration also should have well-approximated edges and no drainage. Healing time depends on laceration depth. Return of these areas to the nonpregnant state should be complete in 6 to 8 weeks.

Lacerations of the genital tract. Lacerations of the cervix, the vagina, and the perineum are also causes of postpartum hemorrhage. Hemorrhage related to lacerations should be suspected if bleeding continues despite a firm, contracted uterine fundus. This bleeding can be a slow trickle, an oozing, or frank hemorrhage.

Factors that can lead to obstetric lacerations of the lower genital tract include operative birth, precipitous birth, congenital abnormalities of the maternal soft parts (vulva perineum), and a contracted pelvis. Other causes include size, abnormal presentation, and position of the fetus; relative size of the presenting part to the size of the birth canal; scarring from prior vaginal infections, injury, or surgery; and vulvar, perineal, and vaginal varicosities. Extreme vascularity in the labia and periclitoral area often results in profuse bleeding if laceration occurs. Pelvic hematomas (i.e., a collection of blood in the connective tissue) may be vulvar, vaginal, or retroperitoneal in origin. Vulvar hematomas are the most common. They usually are visible and painful. Vaginal hematomas typically are associated with a forceps-assisted birth, episiotomy, or primigravidity. Retroperitoneal hematomas are the least common, but they are life threatening. They are caused by laceration of one of the vessels attached to the hypogastric artery, usually because of the rupture of a cesarean scar during labor.

Most acute injuries and lacerations of the perineum, the vagina, the uterus, and their support tissues occur during childbirth. Ideally, injuries are repaired at the time of delivery, which facilitates healing, limits residual damage, and reduces the incidence of infection. Future gynecologic problems, including pelvic relaxation, uterine prolapse, cystocele, and rectocele, may be attributed to childbirth.

Box 28.1 Hypovolemic Shock

SIGNS AND SYMPTOMS

- Woman has persistent significant bleeding (perineal pad soaked within 15 minutes); this bleeding may not be accompanied by a change in vital signs or maternal color or behavior.
- Woman states she feels weak, lightheaded, "funny," or "sick to my stomach" or she "sees stars."
- Woman begins to act anxious or exhibits air hunger.
- Skin turns ashen or grayish.
- Skin feels cool and clammy.
- Pulse rate increases.
- Blood pressure declines.

INTERVENTIONS

- Notify primary health care provider.
- If uterus is atonic, massage gently and expel clots to cause uterus to contract; compress uterus manually, as needed, with two hands. Add oxytocic agent to IV drip, as ordered.
- Give oxygen via face mask or nasal prongs at 8 to 10 L/min.
- Tilt the woman to her side or elevate the right hip; elevate her legs to at least a 30-degree angle.
- Provide additional or maintain existing IV infusion of lactated Ringer's solution or normal saline solution to restore circulatory volume.
- Administer blood or blood products, as ordered.
- Monitor vital signs.
- Insert an indwelling urinary catheter to monitor perfusion of kidneys.
- Administer emergency drugs, as ordered.
- Prepare for possible surgery or other emergency treatments or procedures.
- Chart incident, medical and nursing interventions instituted, and results of treatments.

The tendency to sustain lacerations varies with each woman; in some women, the soft tissue may be less distensible. Heredity may be a factor. For example, the tissue of light-skinned women, especially those with reddish hair, is not as readily distensible as that of darker-skinned women, and healing may be less efficient.

Perineal lacerations. Perineal lacerations are the most common of all injuries in the lower genital tract. They usually occur when the fetal head is being born. The extent of the laceration is defined in terms of its depth (Fig. 28.2):

- *First-degree:* Laceration extends through the skin and structures superficial to muscles.
- *Second-degree:* Laceration extends through muscles of perineal body.
- *Third-degree:* Laceration continues through the sphincter muscle.
- *Fourth-degree:* Laceration also involves the anterior rectal wall.

Perineal injury often is accompanied by small lacerations on the medial surfaces of the labia minora below the pubic rami and to the sides of the urethra and the clitoris. Lacerations in this vascular area often result in profuse bleeding and necessitate repair with absorbable sutures.

When caring for the woman with a third-degree or fourth-degree laceration, assess the bowel habits. Include assessment of fecal continence. The initial stool after delivery may be uncomfortable, and measures to promote soft stools should be implemented. Some health care providers may prescribe stool softeners. Additional measures include promoting fluid intake and encouraging increased dietary fiber and activity such as walking. Rectal treatments such as enemas or suppositories are contraindicated for women who have third-degree or fourth-degree lacerations. Antimicrobial therapy may be used in some cases.

Vaginal and urethral lacerations. Vaginal lacerations often occur in conjunction with perineal lacerations. Vaginal lacerations tend to extend up the lateral walls (sulci) and, if deep enough, involve the levator ani muscle. Additional injury may occur high in the vaginal vault near the level of the ischial spines. Vaginal vault lacerations may be circular and may result from forceps rotation, especially in cases of cephalopelvic disproportion, rapid fetal descent, and precipitous birth. Lacerations also can occur around the urethra (periurethral) and in the area of the clitoris.

Cervical injuries. Cervical injuries occur when the cervix retracts over the advancing fetal head. These cervical lacerations occur at the lateral angles of the external os; most are shallow, and bleeding is minimal. Larger lacerations may extend to the vaginal vault or beyond the vault into the lower uterine segment; serious bleeding may occur. Extensive lacerations may follow if the woman is allowed to push before full cervical dilation is achieved. Injuries to the cervix can affect pregnancies and childbirths.

Nursing interventions for episiotomy, lacerations, and hemorrhoids are listed in Box 28.2.

Breasts

Breast changes begin early in pregnancy. Increased amounts of estrogen stimulate enlargement of breast size by increasing adipose tissue and fluid retention. Estrogen also stimulates the growth of the milk ducts to prepare for **lactation** (function of secreting milk or period during which milk is secreted).

The first secretion produced by the breast is colostrum. This precursor to milk is thin, watery, and slightly yellow. It is rich in protein, calories, antibodies, and lymphocytes. Colostrum production begins in the second trimester. Expectant mothers begin to leak colostrum in the later weeks of the third trimester. Its production continues for about 2 days after delivery, when true milk production begins.

Lactation is a combination of hormonal, neurologic, and psychological responses. After delivery, estrogen and progesterone levels diminish rapidly. As they drop, the level of prolactin increases. **Prolactin,** a hormone secreted by the anterior pituitary gland, is responsible for stimulating milk production in the mammary alveolar cells. Stimulation of the nipples, particularly by the infant's sucking, causes the release of oxytocin from the posterior pituitary gland. Oxytocin stimulates contraction of the mammary ducts, and milk is ejected from the breast. This cycle is called the *let-down reflex.*

OTHER BODY SYSTEMS

Cardiovascular

Blood volume is reduced to nonpregnant levels by 2 to 4 weeks after delivery. **Diuresis** (the increased formation and secretion of urine) and **diaphoresis** (the secretion of sweat, especially when profuse) account for most of the fluid loss. Blood loss during delivery accounts for an additional 300 to 500 mL (600 to 800 mL with cesarean delivery). Cardiac output also declines rapidly. The patient is at risk for thrombus formation as a result of elevation of platelets in the early postpartum period.

Urinary

After childbirth, as a result of trauma, increased bladder capacity, and the effects of conduction anesthesia, women have a decreased urge to void. In addition, pelvic soreness and edema caused by forceps used during labor, vaginal lacerations, or the episiotomy reduce or alter the voiding reflex. Decreased voiding combined with postpartal diuresis may result in bladder distention. Immediately after giving birth, the woman may bleed excessively if the bladder becomes distended because it pushes the uterus up and to the side and prevents the uterus from firmly contracting. Later in the puerperium, overdistention can make the bladder more susceptible to infection and delay the return of normal voiding. With adequate emptying of the bladder, bladder

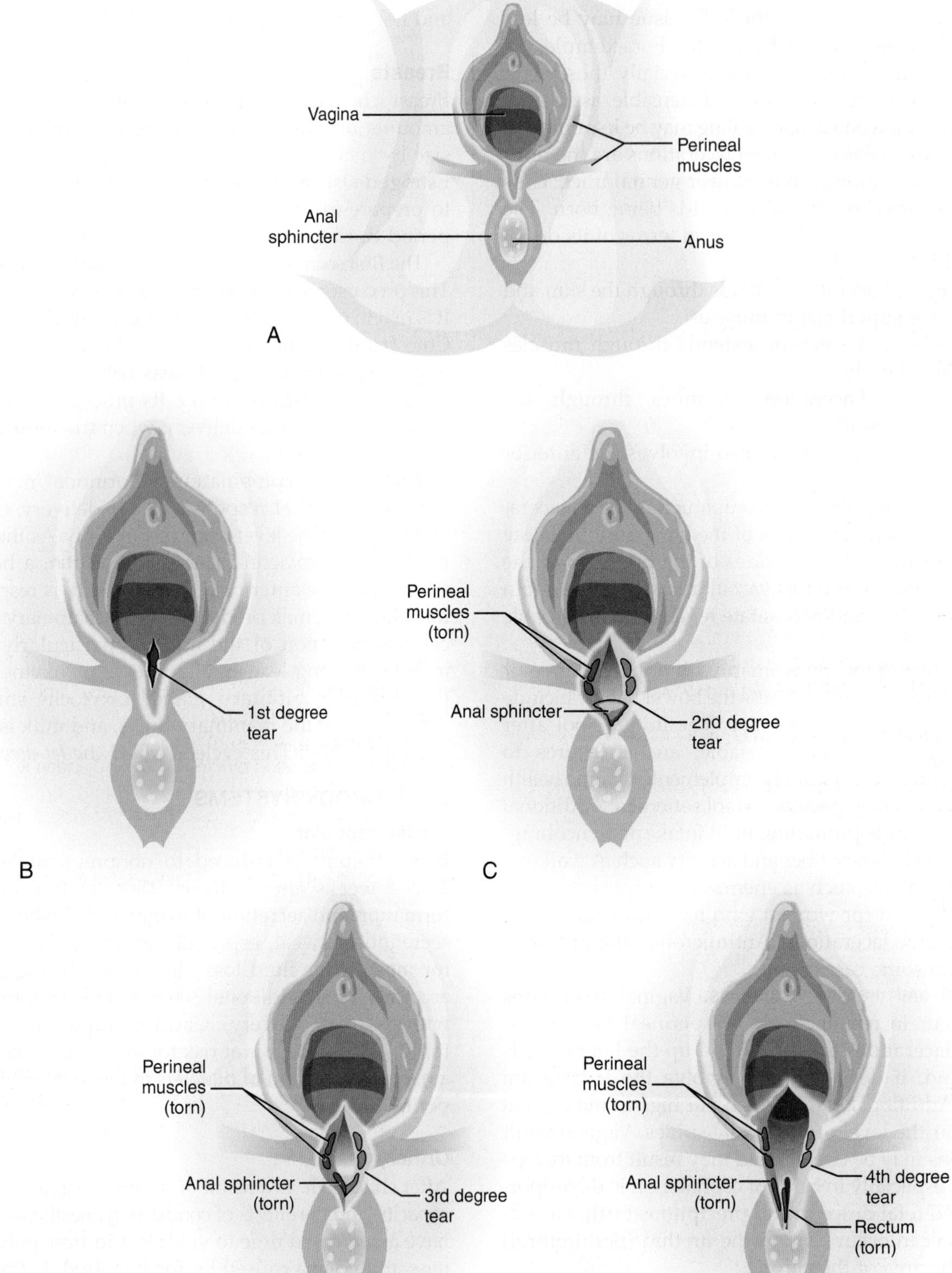

Fig. 28.2 Vaginal lacerations.

Box 28.2 Interventions for Episiotomy, Lacerations, and Hemorrhoids

CLEANSING
- Wash hands before and after cleaning perineum and changing pads.
- Explain procedure.
- Wash perineum with mild soap and warm water at least once daily.
- Cleanse from symphysis pubis to anal area.
- Apply peripad from front to back, protecting inner surface of pad from contamination.
- Wrap soiled pad and place in covered waste container.
- Change pad with each void or defecation or at least four times per day.
- Assess amount and character of lochia with each pad change.

ICE PACK
- Apply a covered ice pack to perineum from front to back:
  - During first 2 hours after the birth, to decrease edema formation and increase comfort
  - After the first 2 hours, to provide anesthetic effect

SQUEEZE BOTTLE
- Demonstrate for and assist woman; explain rationale.
- Fill bottle with tap water warmed to approximately 100.4°F (38°C; comfortably warm on the wrist).
- Instruct woman to position nozzle between her legs so that squirts of water reach perineum as she sits on toilet.
- Explain that it takes a whole bottle of water to cleanse perineum.
- Remind her to blot dry with toilet paper or clean wipes.
- Remind her to avoid contamination from anal area.
- Apply clean pad.

SITZ BATH
Built-in Type
- Prepare bath by thoroughly scrubbing with cleaning agent and rinsing. Pad with towel before filling.
- Explain procedure.
- Fill one-half to one-third with water of correct temperature (100.4° to 105°F [38° to 40.6°C]). Some women prefer cool sitz baths; add ice to lower the temperature to a comfortable level.
- Encourage woman to use at least twice a day for 20 minutes.
- Place call bell within easy reach.
- Teach woman to enter bath by tightening gluteal muscles and keeping them tightened and then relaxing them after she is in the bath.
- Place dry towels within reach.
- Ensure privacy.
- Check on woman in 15 minutes; assess pulse as needed.

Disposable Type
- Clamp tubing and fill bag with warm water.
- Raise toilet seat, place bath in bowl with overflow opening directed toward back of toilet.
- Place container above toilet bowl.
- Attach tube into groove at front of bath.
- Loosen tube clamp to regulate rate of flow; fill bath to half full; continue as previously described for built-in sitz bath.

DRY HEAT
- Inspect lamp for defects.
- Cover lamp with towels.
- Position lamp 50 cm from perineum; use three times a day for 20-minute periods.
- Provide draping over woman.
- If same lamp is used by several women, clean it carefully between uses.
- Teach woman regarding use of 40-watt bulb at home.

TOPICAL APPLICATIONS
- Apply anesthetic cream or spray; use sparingly three or four times a day.
- Offer witch hazel pads (Tucks) after voiding or defecating; woman pats perineum dry from front to back, then applies witch hazel pads. Explain rationale.

tone usually is restored 5 to 7 days after childbirth, with daily urinary output of up to 3 L common.

Neurologic

Neurologic changes during the puerperium result from a reversal of maternal adaptations to pregnancy or from trauma during labor and childbirth. Pregnancy-induced neurologic discomforts abate after birth. Through diuresis, edema is eliminated, which relieves carpal tunnel syndrome by easing compression of the medial nerve. The periodic numbness and tingling of fingers that affect 5% of pregnant women usually disappear after birth, unless lifting and carrying the baby aggravate the condition.

Headache requires careful assessment. Postpartum headaches may be caused by various conditions, including gestational hypertension, stress, and leakage of cerebrospinal fluid into the extradural space during placement of the needle for epidural or spinal anesthesia. Depending on the cause and the effectiveness of the treatment, the headaches can last from 1 to 3 days to several weeks.

Gastrointestinal

Appetite generally returns to normal immediately after delivery. However, gastric motility may continue to decline, leading to constipation. Normal bowel elimination should resume within 2 or 3 days after delivery. Decreased abdominal tone and tenderness from the episiotomy or hemorrhoids may make the patient reluctant to strain for a bowel movement.

Endocrine

Placental hormone levels rapidly fall after delivery and are soon undetectable or at their nonpregnant values. Estrogen and progesterone levels drop markedly after expulsion of the placenta and reach their lowest levels 1 week into the postpartum period. Decreased estrogen levels are associated with breast engorgement and with the diuresis of excess extracellular fluid that has accumulated during pregnancy. The estrogen levels in nonlactating women begin to rise by 2 weeks after birth and are higher by postpartum day 17 than in women who breast-feed. The anterior pituitary secretes prolactin, but only in response to nipple stimulation. Other endocrine glands (thyroid, adrenal, and pancreas) return to prepregnant size and function.

Musculoskeletal

Abdominal muscle tone returns and joint stabilization occurs over a 6- to 8-week period after delivery. The return of muscle tone depends on previous tone, proper exercise, and the amount of adipose tissue. Some pelvic joints may never return fully to their prepregnant position. Patients may feel discomfort in the joints immediately after delivery because of secretion of the hormone relaxin. However, even when all other joints return to their normal pregnant state, those of the parous woman's feet do not. The new mother may notice a permanent increase in shoe size.

Integumentary

Chloasma of pregnancy usually disappears at the end of pregnancy. Hyperpigmentation of the areola (the area encircling the nipple) and linea nigra (a dark line on the abdomen of a pregnant woman, usually extending from the symphysis pubis midline to the umbilicus) may not disappear completely after childbirth. Some women have permanent darker pigmentation of those areas. Striae gravidarum (stretch marks) on the breasts, the abdomen, and the thighs may fade but usually do not disappear.

Vascular abnormalities such as spider angiomas (nevi), palmar erythema, and epulis generally regress as estrogen rapidly declines after the end of pregnancy. For some women, spider nevi persist indefinitely.

The abundance of fine hair seen during pregnancy usually disappears after birth; however, any coarse or bristly hair that appears during pregnancy usually remains. Fingernails return to their prepregnancy consistency and strength.

Profuse diaphoresis in the immediate postpartum period is the most noticeable change in the integumentary system. This is common, especially at night, during the first week postpartum.

Immune

No significant changes in the maternal immune system occur during the postpartum period. Whether the mother needs a rubella vaccination or Rh_o(D) immune globulin (RhoGAM) for prevention of Rh isoimmunization should be determined. Pregnant women are screened routinely for immunity to rubella early in the prenatal period. Women who are not immune are immunized early in the postpartum period before discharge. Patients who are Rh negative are screened in pregnancy for isoimmunization. If they are not found to be sensitized and give birth to infants who are Rh positive, they must receive RhoGAM within 72 hours of delivery.

TRANSFER FROM THE RECOVERY AREA

After the initial recovery period of 1 to 2 hours, the woman may be transferred to a postpartum room in the same or another nursing unit. In labor, delivery, recovery, postpartum (LDRP) room settings, the nurse who provided care during the recovery period usually continues to care for the woman. In the labor, delivery, recovery (LDR) room or a traditional setting, the woman is transferred to a separate unit where the postpartum nursing staff provide her care. In some settings, the baby remains with the mother wherever she goes. In other facilities, the baby is taken to the nursery for several hours of observation during the mother's initial recovery period.

The move to another area of the maternity unit requires the nurse to prepare a transfer report. The information to be provided to the nurse accepting the patient must be accurate and concise. Sources of information include the admission record, the birth record, and the recovery record. The postpartum nurse should be advised about the name of the primary care provider; gravidity and parity; age; anesthetic used; medications given; duration of labor and time of rupture of membranes; oxytocin induction or augmentation; type of birth and repair; blood type and Rh status; rubella immunity status; syphilis and hepatitis serology test results; intravenous (IV) infusion of any fluids; physiologic status since birth; description of fundus, lochia, bladder, and perineum; infant's gender and weight; time of birth; pediatrician; chosen method of feeding; any abnormalities noted; and assessment of initial parent-infant interaction.

Most of this information also is documented for the nursing staff in the newborn nursery. In addition, specific information should be provided on the infant's Apgar scores, weight, voiding, and feeding since birth. Also nursing interventions that have been completed (e.g., prophylaxis, vitamin K injection) should be recorded.

NURSING ASSESSMENT OF AND INTERVENTIONS FOR THE MOTHER

HEALTH MANAGEMENT AND HEALTH PERCEPTION

In the early 1980s, the average length of stay after childbirth was 4 days for a vaginal delivery and 1 to 2 days longer for a cesarean birth. During the early 1990s, discharge time shrunk. The movement was largely the result of changes in insurance coverage. Resistance to the progressively shorter stays was swift and vocal. Many states began enacting legislation to restrict facilities,

Box 28.3 Postpartum Maternal Danger Signs

- Fever with or without chills
- Malodorous vaginal discharge
- Excessive amount of vaginal discharge
- Bright red vaginal bleeding after it has changed to pink or rust
- Edema; erythematous or painful area on the legs
- Pain or burning sensation with urination or an inability to void
- Breast changes, such as localized pain, heat, edema, or malodorous drainage
- Pain in the perineal or pelvic area

health care practitioners, and insurance companies from requiring women be discharged in less than 48 hours after a vaginal delivery or 96 hours after a cesarean. Of course, women still may voluntarily choose to be discharged sooner if their health and readiness allow. Early discharge is usually a patient's choice. Currently the majority of women (64%) who experience vaginal deliveries are hospitalized 2 to 3 days. Some women who have uneventful, uncomplicated deliveries may opt to stay 24 hours or less. The length of stay for a woman after a cesarean section ranges from 2 to 4 days (CDC, 2015). Regardless of the timing of the discharge, the woman's ability to meet her needs and those of her infant must be assessed. The assessment must include physiologic and psychological parameters.

Discuss the home situation. If any aspect of the home situation appears unsafe or questionable, confer with the health care provider and discuss a referral to social services before discharge. Self-care concerns, including postpartum danger signs (Box 28.3), the importance of medical follow-up, infant care, and family planning should be incorporated.

Parent-Newborn Relationships

The nursing assessment must include the mother's reaction to the sight of her newborn. Some new mothers may appear excited, laughing, talking, and even crying; some exhibit apparent apathy. A polite smile and nod may acknowledge the comments of nurses and primary care practitioners. Occasionally, the mother appears angry or indifferent, turns away from the baby, concentrates on her own pain, or makes hostile comments. These varying reactions can arise from pleasure, exhaustion, or deep disappointment. Whatever the reaction and cause may be, the mother needs continuing acceptance and support from all the staff. Consider the woman's age, placement within Erikson's stages of growth and development, and unique circumstances surrounding the pregnancy. For example, a teen mother may be more self-absorbed and less able to focus on the needs of her infant. A woman who has given birth to an unwanted pregnancy may have impaired bonding. Documentation in the nurse's notes concerning bonding behaviors noted is needed. Observations should include verbal and nonverbal behaviors of the parents (Box 28.4).

Box 28.4 Assessment of Attachment Behaviors

- When the infant is brought to the parents, do they reach out for the infant and call the infant by name? (Recognize that in some cultures parents may not name the infant in the early newborn period.)
- Do the parents speak about the infant in terms of identification, such as who the infant looks like, what appears special about their infant compared with other infants?
- When parents are holding the infant, what kind of body contact is there? Do parents feel at ease changing the infant's position? Do they use fingertips or whole hands? Are there parts of the body they avoid touching or parts of the body they investigate and scrutinize?
- When the infant is awake, what kinds of stimulation do the parents provide? Do they talk to the infant, to each other, or to no one? How do they look at the infant? With direct visual contact, avoidance of eye contact, or looking at other people or objects?
- How comfortable do the parents appear in terms of caring for the infant? Do they express any concern regarding their ability or disgust for certain activities, such as changing diapers?
- What type of affection do they demonstrate to the newborn, such as smiling, stroking, kissing, or rocking?
- If the infant is fussy, what kinds of comforting techniques do the parents use, such as rocking, swaddling, talking, or stroking?

Childbearing practices and rituals of other cultures may be different from standard practices associated with bonding in the Anglo-American culture. For example, Chinese families traditionally use extended family members to care for the newborn so that the mother can rest and recover, especially after a cesarean birth. In some cultures, women do not initiate breastfeeding until their breast milk comes in. In other cultures, families do not name their babies until after the confinement month. The amount of eye contact also varies among cultures.

Become knowledgeable about the childbearing beliefs and practices of diverse cultural and ethnic groups. Because individual cultural variations exist within groups, clarify with the patient and family members or friends what cultural norms the patient follows. Incorrect judgments may be made about mother-infant bonding if you do not practice culturally sensitive care.

Some warning signs of possible difficulties in parent-child relationships, apparent immediately after delivery, are listed in Box 28.5.

Maternal Self-Image

An important assessment concerns the woman's self-concept, body image, and sexuality. How a new mother

Box 28.5 Postpartum Danger Signs for Parent-Newborn Relationships

- Passive reaction, either verbal or nonverbal. (Parents do not touch, hold, or examine baby or talk in affectionate terms or tones about baby.)
- Hostile reaction, either verbal or nonverbal. (Parents make inappropriate verbalization, glances, or disparaging remarks about child's physical characteristics.)
- Disappointment over gender of baby.
- Lack of eye contact.
- Nonsupportive interaction between parents. (If interaction seems questionable, talk to nurse and physician involved with delivery for further information.)

feels about herself and her body during the puerperium may affect her behavior, adaptation to parenting, and sexuality.

Feelings related to sexual adjustment after childbirth often cause concern for new parents. Women who recently have given birth may be reluctant to resume sexual intercourse for fear of pain or damage to healing perineal tissue. Because many new parents are anxious for information but reluctant to bring up the subject, postpartum nurses should include the topic of postpartum sexuality in a matter-of-fact manner. This may be addressed during the routine physical assessment and reinforced during the discharge teaching period (Box 28.6). This approach assures the woman and her partner that resuming sexual activity is a legitimate concern for new parents and indicates the nurse's willingness to answer questions.

Promoting Parenting Skills

Parents are responsive to praise of their newborn. Many need reassurance that the baby's blue appearance after delivery is normal until respirations are well established. Review the reason for the molding of the baby's head. Repeat information about the hospital's routine for future parent-child contacts. Encourage siblings to get acquainted with the new family member (Fig. 28.3). The hospital staff, with their interest and their concern, can do much to make this experience satisfying for parents, family, and significant others.

New parents may feel anxious about their abilities to care for their child. They may demonstrate uncertainty when attempting to perform care. Educate new parents about the needs of the baby and reassure them. Parents first become acquainted with their new baby as the nurse performs a physical examination and describes any normal variations. Nurses act as role models by providing compassionate attentive care (Boxes 28.7 and 28.8). As one nurse described it:

> I found the mother crying and distraught as she wrapped and unwrapped her baby. She said, "I don't seem to be doing anything right." I took the baby from her and talked

Box 28.6 Resumption of Sexual Intercourse

- A woman can resume sexual intercourse safely when bleeding has stopped and the episiotomy has healed. The mother should be scheduled to see her primary care provider at 6 weeks postpartum. At that time, the woman's perineum and cervix are assessed for readiness for sexual intercourse. For the first 6 weeks to 6 months postpartum, the vagina does not lubricate well.
- The physiologic reactions to sexual stimulation for the first 3 months after birth are slower and less intense. The strength of the orgasm is reduced.
- A water-soluble gel, cocoa butter, or a contraceptive cream or jelly may be used for lubrication. If some vaginal tenderness is present, the partner can insert one or more clean lubricated fingers into the vagina and rotate them within the vagina to help relax it and to identify possible areas of discomfort. A position in which the woman has control of the depth of the insertion of the penis also is useful. The side-by-side or female-on-top position may be more comfortable.
- The presence of the baby influences postbirth lovemaking. Parents hear every sound made by the baby; conversely, they may be concerned that the baby hears every sound they make. In either case, any phase of the sexual response cycle may be interrupted by hearing the baby cry or move, leaving both partners frustrated and unsatisfied. In addition, the amount of psychological energy expended in child care activities may lead to fatigue.
- Some women report feeling sexual stimulation and orgasms when breast-feeding their babies.
- Instruct the woman to correctly perform Kegel exercises to strengthen the pubococcygeal muscle. This muscle is associated with bowel and bladder function and with vaginal feeling during intercourse.

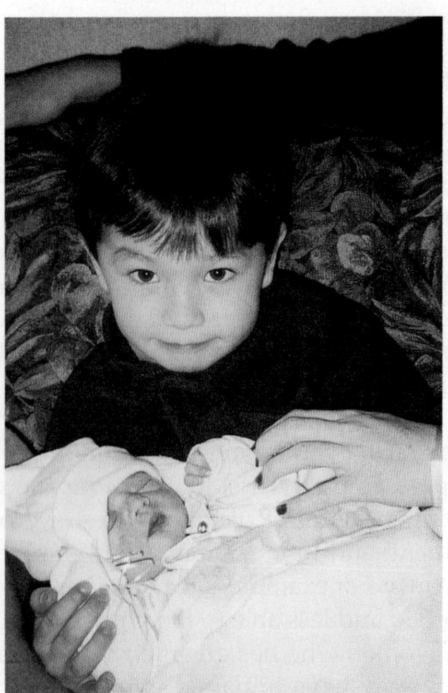

Fig. 28.3 Sibling involvement.

Box 28.7 Postpartum Maternal Teaching Summary

FUNDUS (HEIGHT, MASSAGE)
- Fundus height shrinks one fingerbreadth a day.
- It is back into pelvis in 10 days.
- It feels firm, like a softball.
- Report bogginess to primary care practitioner immediately.
- Cramping may occur with nursing.

LOCHIA (AMOUNT, CHANGES, WARNING SIGNS)
- For the first 3 days, lochia is dark red, like menstrual flow; 2 or 3 days after this, it is pinkish brown.
- Moderate flow consists of four to eight lightly saturated pads a day.
- Flow continues for 3 to 4 weeks.
- In the last couple of weeks, lochia is a yellowish color with a musty, stale odor.
- Report any foul-smelling or bright red discharge or large clots.
- Flow may increase with overactivity. Rest; if flow does not subside, notify primary care practitioner.

PERINEUM (EPISIOTOMY CARE, CLEANSING, HEALING, DOUCHING, TAMPONS)
- Take sitz baths two or three times daily with vaginal delivery.
- Cleanse from front to back.
- Use perineal spray water bottle after voiding.
- Change pad frequently—after each voiding and when soiled.
- Do not douche or use tampons until after first office visit when primary care practitioner says it is okay.
- Continue using witch hazel (Tucks pads) for discomfort and to aid in healing.
- Episiotomy heals in approximately 3 weeks (when the lochia has stopped).

BREASTS
- *Breast-feeding* (nipple care, engorgement, feeding techniques, breast pump)
  - Air dry; use proper technique to break infant's suction to the nipple; wear a good supportive bra.
  - Pregnancy can occur while nursing; use a contraceptive.
  - For engorgement, apply heat, warm shower; may pump to enable baby to latch on.
  - Feeding techniques: demonstrate proper use; advise where to purchase materials; demonstrate manual expression; expressed milk may be frozen in plastic bottles or bags for up to 2 weeks.
  - May take a mild analgesic 1 hour before nursing.
- *Dry breasts* (engorgement, fluid intake)
  - Wear supportive, well-fitting bra.
  - Avoid breast stimulation (warm showers).
  - Apply ice bags for 20 minutes four times a day.
  - Suppression of lactation takes about 5 days.
  - Do not drink excessive amounts of fluids (normal: six to eight 8-ounce glasses).

NUTRITION (NURSING, DIETING)
- Continue prenatal vitamins until gone.
- Nursing: need 500 kcal more than prepregnant diet; need increased protein, 400 mg calcium each day, 8 to 10 glasses of fluid each day; avoid onions, cabbage, chocolate, spices, and foods that may distress infant; no dieting during breast-feeding.

SEXUALITY (SEXUAL ACTIVITY)
(See Box 28.6)
- 45% of nonnursing mothers resume menses by sixth week.
- Breast-feeding does not protect against pregnancy.
- Avoid sexual activity until after first postbirth office visit and approval by primary care practitioner.
- If episiotomy is not healed and sexual activity is resumed, there is increased discomfort and chance of infection.

EXERCISE (WHEN, HOW MUCH)
- Increased lochia or pain means you need to reevaluate activity.
- Do not resume strenuous exercises until primary care practitioner approves.
- Gradually increase activity.

EMOTIONS (BONDING, "BABY BLUES")
- Parent-child attachment (bonding): schedule time to enjoy baby; use eye contact, cuddling, and caressing; enjoy infant feedings.
- Postpartum blues:
  - Mother may be tearful or anorexic and have difficulty sleeping.
  - Hormonal factors and fatigue are often responsible.
  - Notify primary care practitioner if prolonged, increased, or unmanageable.

CESAREAN BIRTH (INCISION, ACTIVITY)
- Notify primary care practitioner of any redness, drainage, separation of incision, temperature greater than 100.4°F (38°C).
- Do not lift anything heavier than baby, gradually increase activity.
- Take pain medications as ordered and needed.

REPORT TO PRIMARY CAREGIVER
- Temperature greater than 100.4°F (38°C)
- Chills
- Change in lochia: foul odor, return to bright red, excessive amount
- Calf pain, tenderness, or swelling
- Evidence of mastitis: breast tenderness, cracking, redness, or a feeling of discomfort or uneasiness
- Urinary urgency, burning, or frequency
- Severe or incapacitating depression

SAFETY (CAR SEAT SAFETY VIDEO, CAR SEAT DEMONSTRATION)
- Review infant safety from baby discharge sheet.
- Review car seat safety video if available.
- Volunteers have car seats to rent.
- Demonstrate proper use of car seat.

Box 28.8 Newborn Teaching Summary

SECURITY

- Know the caregiver. Check references.
- Ask others who are trusted to babysit.
- Do not leave baby alone on flat surface because the baby could roll over and fall off the surface.
- Do not lay baby on abdomen; place on the side or back to prevent sudden infant death syndrome (SIDS).
- Car seat safety and the law:
  - Use until age 4 years or 40 lb.
  - Infant in car seat should be secured in back seat, facing the rear of the car.
  - These are the laws in most states; if you are stopped, you could be fined.

BATH DEMONSTRATION AND NORMAL SKIN CONDITIONS

- Skin should be soft, pinkish, and dry.
- Clean perineum from front to back to prevent urinary tract infections.
- Use hypoallergenic soap. Most babies need bathing only every other day.
- Keep diaper area as clean as possible. (Use no talc.)
- Keep head clean, rinsing well after each shampoo to prevent cradle cap.

UMBILICAL CORD CARE

- Use alcohol on cord stump daily. (Be careful to prevent alcohol from dripping down to perineal area.)
- Keep area dry; fold diaper down with plastic side on outside to prevent moisture retention.
- Sponge bathe for 7 to 10 days until umbilical cord comes off. (Do not soak in bath water.)
- Report any redness, drainage, or foul odor coming from umbilical area.

CIRCUMCISION CARE

- If a Gomco or Mogen clamp was used, apply petroleum jelly–covered gauze to penis after every diaper change. Keep area clean to prevent infection; cleanse penis carefully with warm water at least every 4 hours.
- If a Plastibell is used, the plastic rim remains in place for about a week while healing takes place, after which the Plastibell falls off. Petroleum gauze is not necessary.
- Do not allow pressure on circumcised area. Loose diapering is necessary.
- Do not be alarmed when a yellowish crust forms; this is part of the normal healing process. Do not attempt to remove this crust; it lasts only 2 or 3 days. Fanfold the diaper so that it does not press on the area.

EYE CARE

- Wash with water from inner to outer corner with a different area of the washcloth for each eye.
- Note that a special treatment was administered to baby's eyes on delivery. This may cause some swelling and redness. Do not be alarmed; this is normal.

DIAPER AREA CARE

- Change diaper as soon as possible.
- Wash from front to back, especially on girls, to prevent urinary tract infection.
- Cleanse with warm water and mild soap; dry well.
- If rash persists, call the health care provider.
- Use no powder. Air out diaper area when possible.

FEEDING METHOD

Breast

- Position: Entire body of infant should face the breast.
- Feed baby before he or she gets frantic and very hungry.
- Lightly brush the infant's lips with the nipple to start the rooting reflex.
- Alternate breasts with each feeding.
- Direct the nipple into infant's mouth with as much of the areola tissue as possible in the baby's mouth and over the tongue.
- Gently hold breast away from baby's nostrils; babies are nose breathers.
- To break suction, place finger between the baby's lips and the breast; do not pull breast away from baby.
- Mothers who have cesarean births need to support infant so that he or she does not rest on the abdomen for long periods.
- Burping baby:
  - Burp between breasts, over the shoulder, sitting up supported by your hands, or lying across your lap.
- Length of time to nurse:
  - Feed for 10 to 15 minutes from each breast.
  - Emptying both breasts is important because an empty breast signals the woman's body to produce more milk.
- Supplement: You may pump your breasts while away from baby; keep breast milk cold during transport.
- Breast milk can be safely stored in a refrigerator for 24 to 48 hours.
- If breast milk will not be used within 48 hours, it should be frozen immediately after being expressed. Breast milk may be frozen for 2 weeks.
- To thaw, gently shake container under warm tap water or place breast milk in a container of warm water. Thawed breast milk should be used immediately. It should not be refrozen. Do not use a microwave to thaw or heat breast milk.
- After the milk supply is established, an occasional bottle does not affect lactation or breast-feeding.
- Stooling pattern: Stools of breast-fed babies are loose. Some infants have a stool with each feeding.

BOTTLE

- Positions:
  - Never prop the bottle.
  - Hold the bottle so that fluid fills the nipple and none of the air in the bottle is allowed to enter the nipple.
  - Avoid overfeeding; be alert to infant cues that enough formula has been taken (e.g., falls asleep, turns head to side, or ceases to suck).
- Burping baby:
  - Burp baby every 0.5 to 1 oz of milk.
  - Position baby over the shoulder, sitting up supported by your hands, or lying across your lap.
- Preparing bottles:
  - Purchase formula in ready-to-use powder or in liquid concentrate to be mixed with water.
  - Many helpful pamphlets on formula preparations are available.

Box 28.8 Newborn Teaching Summary—cont'd

- Prepare formulas with scrupulous cleanliness; if home conditions or the water supply is unsafe (such as from a private well), then water should be boiled for 15 minutes.
- Give formula at room temperature; test formula temperature on inner wrist or back of hand.
- Opened container of ready-to-feed or concentrated formula should be discarded after 24 hours; date the opened container.
- After feeding, position baby on right side to discourage regurgitation.

CLOTHING
- Dress infant for the season.
- Dress infant in soft, comfortable clothing.
- Dress infant as you are dressed.

VAGINAL AND BREAST SECRETIONS
- As the maternal hormones clear the infant's bloodstream, the infant may have a mucus-like, bloody vaginal discharge.
- Girl and boy babies may have a swelling of the breast tissue, and sometimes a thin discharge may be seen; this subsides as the mother's hormones are eliminated from infant's body.

BULB SYRINGE
- Squeeze out air to establish suction by compressing the bulb and holding it in.
- Gently insert tip of syringe into the side of infant's mouth and release; then suction the nares.
- Clean well after each use.

INFANT CARDIOPULMONARY RESUSCITATION
- Be sure to see video before dismissal if available.
- Teaching:
  - Give fingertip compressions (5 to 1).
  - Give puffs for breaths (1 to 5).
  - Cover baby's nose with cheek as you cover mouth.
  - Avoid stretching back too far in the head-tilt/chin-lift.

PHENYLKETONURIA, BIOTINIDASE, AND THYROID TESTING
- These tests should be performed on all newborns.
- Undetected abnormalities could lead to brain damage or death. With early detection and proper treatment, these are preventable.

AFTER DISCHARGE
- Keep, read, and refer to pamphlets if you have any questions.
- Use medication prescribed only by a physician. (Do not use nose drops because aspiration may result in lung complications.)

WHEN TO CALL PHYSICIAN
- If baby has sudden fever, rash, excessive vomiting, diarrhea, distended abdomen, or bleeding from circumcision, call the physician.
- Normal body temperature ranges from 97.6° to 99°F (36.4° to 37.2°C) when taken via the axillary route. This method is recommended until age 6 years.

to him, "What are you doing to your mother? You have her all upset!" The baby alerted to my voice and looked at me. Then, I said to the mother, "Now you talk to him." She said, "You're a big, lovely boy; don't cry so much." The baby, hearing her voice, promptly turned his head to look at her. I said, "You see, he knows his mother's voice and prefers it to mine." The mother was surprised and seemed very pleased and excited. We then reviewed how to wrap a baby snugly.

NUTRITIONAL AND METABOLIC ISSUES

Recovery Stage

After the time and exertion involved in labor and delivery, the mother is often hungry. Most women do not have dietary restrictions after vaginal childbirth. After a cesarean section, women often have restrictions that limit oral intake to ice or liquids for the first day with a gradual reintroduction to the diet. Fluids are important during the recovery phase to replace the fluids and blood lost during delivery; offer a variety of fluids such as water and juices. If the physician orders IV fluids, administer them promptly. When a general anesthetic has been used, such as during a cesarean delivery, verify the *presence of bowel sounds* before giving solid food.

If the woman used mouth-breathing techniques during labor, she may have dry mucous membranes, cracked lips, and noticeable breath odor. Good oral hygiene relieves these symptoms and reduces discomfort. A complete sponge bath or a shower with assistance enhances well-being and comfort by removing perspiration and other waste products from the skin.

Later Postpartum Stage

Diet remains an important concern postpartum. Many women are concerned about the weight gained during pregnancy and wish to lose the excess as soon as possible. Dieting must not deprive the woman of necessary nutrition. If the woman has not gained excessive weight during pregnancy, she usually returns to her prepregnant weight in 6 to 8 weeks without significant dietary restrictions. Most physicians do not recommend any weight-loss diets until after this time. Women who are not breast-feeding should continue to eat a well-balanced diet that follows MyPlate suggestions. Women who are breast-feeding generally continue the diet recommended during pregnancy because the body needs extra calories, vitamins, and minerals for lactation. The breast-feeding mother should maintain the increased caloric intake of 300 to 500 kcal/day as part of a well-balanced diet and should maintain a daily fluid intake of 2 to 3 L.

HYGIENE

During the postpartum stage, excessive perspiration is normal. The lochia has a characteristic musty odor. It should not have a foul or decaying smell. Encourage regular bathing (showers are preferred) to minimize odors and promote comfort. Most women are permitted to be up as tolerated within hours of giving birth, but they may experience vertigo as a result of vascular shifts related to the heat of the shower. If this occurs while the woman is standing in the shower, she may experience syncope and injure herself. The first time the newly delivered woman takes a shower, provide for safety by instructing her on use of the emergency call signal and the length of shower time recommended and by placing a chair in the shower room. Also, check the patient frequently during her first shower to verify she is safe. Tub baths are not recommended until after the postpartum examination at 6 weeks so that no water that has been contaminated with body wastes enters the vaginal canal or uterus until healing is completed.

Sitz baths may be used to provide cleansing, reduce discomfort, and promote healing of the perineum. Vasodilation from the warm water helps reduce edema and speed tissue repair. Instruct the patient about water temperature and length of time. Proper cleaning of equipment must take place between patients if community facilities are used. Most facilities use a personal, portable sitz bath that the patient can take home at discharge (Fig. 28.4).

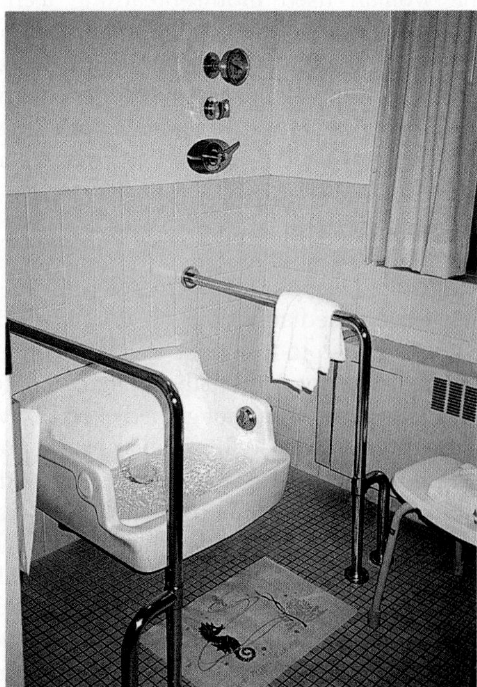

Fig. 28.4 Sitz bath for perineal care. (From Perry AG, Potter PA, Elkin MK: *Nursing interventions and clinical skills*, ed 4, St. Louis, 2008, Mosby.)

If the woman has delivered via cesarean section, she has an abdominal incision with sutures or staples. Assess this incision in the same manner as any other surgical incision. It should remain approximated with no erythema, little exudate, and no malodor (foul odor). Traditionally, the patient has a dressing covering the incision the day of surgery. This usually is removed the next day by the surgeon. The incision likely is left open to the air. Those patients with staples closing their wounds have them removed in approximately 3 days. Adhesive strips may be applied after their removal and remain on for the next 5 to 7 days. Care should be taken so that clothing does not irritate the incision. The patient may shower with the incision that contains sutures or staples. Wounds with adhesive strips must be protected from the direct flow of water during a shower.

ELIMINATION

Recovery Stage

Diuresis and diaphoresis are common immediately after delivery. If the woman received IV fluids, urinary output may be increased. Support the bladder above the symphysis pubis and palpate it to check for fullness. Encourage voiding because a full bladder may interfere with complete contraction of the uterus, potentially causing hemorrhage.

The initial voiding should occur within 4 to 6 hours after delivery. Tissue edema from the delivery may cause difficulty with voiding. In addition, some women may have reduced sensitivity and are unaware that the bladder is full. Some agencies have a policy to assess voiding three times in measurable amounts of 300 mL or more after delivery to determine urinary elimination. Try measures to stimulate voiding. If the patient is unsuccessful voiding a sufficient quantity, catheterization may be necessary. If repeated catheterization is needed, a Foley catheter may be inserted. An indwelling catheter is inserted routinely before cesarean delivery and may remain in place for 1 or 2 days after delivery.

Later Postpartum Stage

Women may not have a strong sense of urgency when the bladder is full. The perineum also may be sore, resulting in a reluctance to regularly void. Encourage the woman to void at regular intervals of 2 to 4 hours. Urinary retention should be considered if a woman is voiding small amounts (less than 100 mL) frequently. The assessment of voiding patterns should include inquiries about symptoms urgency and frequency or dysuria. Incomplete emptying of the bladder prevents the uterus from contracting normally and predisposes the patient to urinary tract infections.

Review proper cleansing technique after delivery. Instruct the woman to cleanse gently and pat dry from the anterior to posterior of the perineum. This method of cleansing prevents microorganisms from the rectal area being transported to the cleaner urinary or vaginal areas. A "peri bottle" (a plastic squeeze bottle) may be used after each urination or bowel movement. Water should be warm (100°F [37.7°C]). Cleansing with toilet tissue is discouraged until the episiotomy or laceration is healed.

The shortened length of hospitalization after childbirth may result in the woman being discharged before she has a bowel movement. Health care providers differ on requirements that the new mother have a bowel movement before discharge. Fear of discomfort from the episiotomy, lacerations, or hemorrhoids may result in the woman's resisting the urge to defecate. Bowel peristalsis may continue to be slow. Constipation may result when these factors are combined with a decrease in activity and loss of abdominal tone. Stool softeners may be prescribed. Promote good bowel habits by encouraging activity, fluid intake, and increased fiber in the diet. Occasionally, suppositories or fleet enemas are administered to promote bowel evacuation. Enemas and suppositories are contraindicated for women who have experienced third-degree or fourth-degree lacerations or extensions to their episiotomies. Sitz baths also can soothe the perineum and promote bowel elimination.

Patients with cesarean births, particularly those who received general anesthesia, are likely to develop problems with bowel function. The combination of general anesthesia and lost abdominal tone increases the risk of ileus, so pay close attention to bowel function and report any abnormal observations promptly. To promote bowel function, assist with and encourage the patient to ambulate periodically throughout the day.

Perineal pads, worn to absorb vaginal drainage, should be changed after each urination or defecation. Teach the woman the importance of correct application and changing of the pad. Pads should be applied and removed from anterior to posterior and secured so as not to move about. If they are not worn correctly, contaminated areas could touch cleaner areas of the perineum and increase the risk of infection. Stress correct and scrupulous handwashing before and after changing to prevent cross contamination.

MAINTENANCE OF SAFETY

ACTIVITY AND EXERCISE

Recovery Stage

Monitor vital signs every 15 minutes for the first hour and then hourly for the next 4 hours during the recovery stage (Table 28.2). Ensure the mother is settled comfortably in bed. A patient who has just given birth may need to remain in bed for a time to allow her body systems to adjust to fluid volume changes. Early ambulation is key in the prevention of complications. Consider the baseline blood pressure, amount of blood lost, type

Table 28.2 Vital Signs and Blood Pressure After Delivery

NORMAL FINDINGS	DEVIATIONS FROM NORMAL FINDINGS AND PROBABLE CAUSES
Temperature	
During first 24 h, temperature may rise to 100.4°F (38°C) as a result of dehydrating effects of labor. After 24 h, the woman should be afebrile.	A diagnosis of puerperal sepsis is suggested if a rise in maternal temperature to 100.4°F (38°C) is noted after the first 24 h after delivery and recurs or persists for 2 days. Other possibilities are mastitis, endometritis, urinary tract infection, and other systemic infections.
Pulse	
Bradycardia is common for the first 6 to 8 days after delivery. It is caused by increased cardiac output and stroke volume. The pulse returns to nonpregnant levels by 3 mo after delivery. A pulse rate between 50 and 70 beats/min is considered normal.	A rapid pulse rate or one that is increasing may indicate hypovolemia as a result of hemorrhage.
Respirations	
Respirations should fall to within the woman's normal predelivery range.	Hypoventilation may follow an unusually high subarachnoid (spinal) block.
Blood Pressure	
Blood pressure is altered slightly, if at all. Orthostatic hypotension, as indicated by feelings of vertigo or syncope immediately after standing up, can develop in the first 48 h as a result of the splanchnic engorgement (the excessive filling or pooling of blood within the visceral vasculature after removal of pressure from the abdomen) that may occur after delivery.	Low or falling blood pressure may reflect hypovolemia as a result of hemorrhage. However, it is a late sign, and other symptoms of hemorrhage usually alert the staff. An increased reading may result from excessive use of vasopressor or oxytocic medications. Because gestational hypertension can persist into or begin in the postpartum period, routinely evaluate blood pressure. If a woman reports headache, rule out hypertension as a cause before administering analgesics. If the blood pressure is elevated, confine the woman to bed and notify the physician.

and amount of analgesic or anesthetic medications administered during labor and birth, and level of pain when preparing to assist the woman to ambulate for the first time. The rapid decrease in intraabdominal pressure after birth results in a dilation of the blood vessels that supply the intestines (known as splanchnic engorgement), which causes blood to pool in the viscera. This contributes to orthostatic hypotension; when a woman who has recently given birth stands up, she may faint or feel lightheaded.

Instruct the patient to use her call bell to summon help before she attempts to get out of bed. Assess her color, pulse, and level of consciousness (LOC) in response to conversation and then assist her in ambulating to the bathroom. Once the woman has reached the bathroom, remain close with frequent inquiries as to her well-being. Have a wheelchair available in the room or just outside in case the woman is too weak to walk back to bed. Encourage her to rest after the ambulation so that she can regain her strength. Keep aromatic ammonia ampules on hand; these can be broken if necessary to revive the patient who is ambulating for the first time.

The patient who received conduction anesthesia (epidural block) is kept in bed until she can fully move, feels sensation in her legs, and has blood pressure and pulse within normal limits. Assess her ability to communicate, her LOC, and her vital signs for stability (within normal limits) before allowing her to get out of bed. The patient should wear slippers when ambulating to prevent slipping or sliding.

The patient who has received analgesics must be observed closely until she is recovered fully from the medication (i.e., vital signs are stable within her normal range and she is fully awake).

During the first 24 hours after giving birth, the woman's temperature may be elevated slightly if she is dehydrated. Elevations noted after the first 24 hours may signal the onset of an infection, and temperatures higher than 100.4°F (38°C) are significant and should be reported. Many women feel chilled after giving birth and appreciate an extra blanket or one that has been warmed. Sometimes a beverage such as hot tea or warm milk provides comfort. Tell the patient this chilling is a normal reaction to the stress of labor.

Slight bradycardia, 50 to 70 beats/min, sometimes is observed and is not considered abnormal if the other vital signs are within normal limits. Tachycardia also may occur in response to increased blood loss or physical exertion.

Blood pressure may be slightly elevated from exertion, from excitement, and possibly from the oxytocic medications. If the blood pressure is consistently elevated, or if the patient also reports headache or visual disturbances, complications related to gestational hypertension could be occurring. These often persist even after delivery. Notify the physician immediately. A decrease in blood pressure could be caused by altered intraabdominal pressure or hemorrhage. Watch changes closely and report them.

Later Postpartum Stage

Vital signs normally stabilize within the first 2 hours after delivery; report immediately any abnormality that persists longer than this. If vital signs have not stabilized within this time, continue to monitor them every 15 minutes to 1 hour and report significant changes.

A temperature of 100.4°F (38°C) or higher on 2 successive days during the first 10 days after delivery (not including the first 24 hours) is considered indicative of puerperal infection. Closely monitor any signs and symptoms of infection during the postpartum stage. Use good aseptic technique when caring for the postpartum patient. Review the signs and symptoms of infection with the new mother before discharge, and stress the importance of contacting the physician promptly if any of these occur (see Box 28.3).

Also assess pulse and blood pressure. Bradycardia may persist up to 10 days after delivery. Elevated blood pressure readings or a continued decrease in blood pressure may be significant and should be reported promptly.

Thrombophlebitis is a potential complication of the postpartum period. Early and frequent ambulation is the key to preventing this problem. Encourage new mothers to get out of bed and move about in the room. If the baby is kept in a nursery away from the mother's room, this is a good target for ambulation. If the perineum is uncomfortable, teach the woman to stand using the muscles of the legs while squeezing the buttocks together. This technique also helps when she attempts to sit. If she appears unsteady, accompany her when she ambulates. Ambulation is important for women who delivered via cesarean birth and may be initiated as early as the same day of surgery. Remember that inactivity predisposes patients to development of thrombophlebitis.

The flow of lochia may increase suddenly when the patient gets out of bed; secretions that pooled in the vagina drain out of the body when she stands. Once the lochia has changed to *serosa* or *alba,* excessive exercise or activity may result in the lochia changing back to *rubra.* This is a sign to slow down and increase activity gradually.

The physician indicates when postpartum exercises are suitable for the new mother, whether she delivered vaginally or via cesarean. The woman should begin gradually and avoid vigorous exercise until after the examination at 6 weeks, when the physician releases her to do so. Teach her isometric exercises that help toning without causing undue exertion.

REST AND SLEEP

Rest and sleep are important through the postpartum period. After the difficulties most women encounter at the end of pregnancy, it is a pleasure to sleep in any position desired. Many women report that the night after delivery, they get the best sleep they have experienced in weeks.

Hospital noises interrupt the sleep of many new mothers. Keeping environmental noise to a minimum to promote rest and sleep is helpful. Do not disturb the patient's sleep unless it is necessary to protect her well-being.

If she is breast-feeding, the new mother nurses her baby at 2- to 3-hour intervals during the night. This interrupted sleep pattern may persist for weeks until the infant is capable of sleeping for 5 or 6 hours without a feeding. Encourage the patient to take advantage of periods during the day when the baby is sleeping to rest and nap to compensate for lost sleep. If sleep deprivation is prolonged, it may interfere with milk production and the let-down reflex.

REPRODUCTIVE ISSUES

Recovery Stage

Check the fundus and lochia every 15 minutes for the first 1 or 2 hours after delivery. The fundus should remain contracted, firm, and midline. This is critical because severe bleeding may result if the uterus does not tightly constrict the placental site. A full bladder can displace the uterus and prevent its contraction. Encourage the patient to empty her bladder before checking the fundus. Palpate the uterus by placing one hand over the lower segment of the uterus near the pubic bone. Use the side of the other hand to feel the location and consistency of the uterus (see Fig. 28.1B).

If the fundus is not firm, it may be difficult to locate. An atonic uterus, one that has lost muscle tone, feels soft or boggy. Gently massage the fundus to increase contractility. Small clots frequently are expressed during this maneuver, and the uterus regains good contracted tone. If this does not result in contraction, the primary care provider should be notified. Oxytocic medications may be prescribed. Examples include oxytocin (Pitocin) and methylergonovine maleate (Methergine). These usually are administered intravenously to obtain prompt response. Methylergonovine also may be administered intramuscularly or orally. Monitor vital signs closely if these medications are given, because they may cause elevated blood pressure, bradycardia, nausea, headache, vertigo, and other side effects (Table 28.3).

While palpating the uterus, observe the amount of lochia. If the uterus is contracting well, small to moderate amounts of drainage are observed. If tone is poor, the amount of lochia is increased. Learn what amount is considered scant, light, moderate, and heavy. This usually is determined by the number of absorbent pads saturated in a period, such as pads per hour (Fig. 28.5). The time factor is important when assessing lochia. One pad saturated in 30 minutes is more serious than one pad saturated in 4 hours. Pay attention to the patient who has a small but steady trickle of lochia; the blood loss may be significantly greater than in those who seem to bleed larger amounts (see Table 28.1). Also, be sure to check under the buttocks of the patient who remains in the supine position; often gravity causes drainage to miss the pad and pool under the patient.

Later Postpartum Stage

Perform daily assessments of the breasts, the fundus, lochia, the perineum, the rectum, and the vascular condition of the legs.

As in the recovery stage, assess the location and consistency of the uterine fundus for the normal signs of involution. It normally is located at the level of the umbilicus on the day of delivery. The first day postpartum it may be one fingerbreadth above or at the level of the umbilicus; after that, it normally descends at the rate of one fingerbreadth per day (see Fig. 28.1A). When assessing the fundus of a woman who delivered via cesarean, carefully palpate the sides of the incision to determine uterine tone and position.

As during the early recovery stage, the fundus should remain firmly contracted. Manage any atony as described. If massage does not result in adequate contraction, notify the physician. Lochia may begin to change within the first 2 days from the rubra to the serosa form. Assess the amount of drainage. Frequently, less lochia is observed after cesarean deliveries, because the uterine cavity is suctioned as part of the surgical procedure. The odor of the lochia should remain fleshy. If a fetid odor is detected, infection may be present; report this promptly.

Inspect the perineum and the rectum by having the woman assume a lateral position with the upper leg drawn toward the chest. The perineum should be approximated. If an episiotomy was performed, the tissue may appear edematous. Erythema is common. Ecchymosis is also common, particularly after a difficult delivery. Many physicians order some form of topical anesthetic, such as witch hazel (Tucks pads), to soothe the perineum (see Table 28.3). This should be applied to the perineum with a clean, lint-free tissue, not the fingers.

If localized edema, discoloration, and intense pain are observed in the perineal area, a hematoma may be present. This hematoma is caused by excessive bleeding into the tissue. A hematoma is most common after deliveries in which forceps were used. Hematomas may be obvious or may be concealed in the vaginal canal. If the woman reports persistent perineal pain or fullness in the vagina, notify the physician. This problem necessitates medical attention and perhaps surgical intervention.

Although the rectum and legs are not part of the reproductive system, these areas typically are included in postpartum assessments. Hemorrhoids (varicosities of the rectum) usually disappear quickly after delivery if there is no longstanding history of this problem. Use

Table 28.3 Medications for the Mother and Newborn

GENERIC NAME (TRADE NAME)	ACTION	SIDE EFFECTS	NURSING IMPLICATIONS
benzocaine (Dermaplast spray or ointment)	Local anesthetic that inhibits conduction of nerve impulses from sensory nerves, temporarily reducing perception of local discomfort	Urticaria, edema, contact dermatitis	Cleanse area with clear, warm water after each trip to the toilet. Hold spray 6–12 inches from affected area and spray liberally. Use up to four times a day.
codeine (with acetaminophen; Tylenol #3) oxycodone terephthalate (with acetaminophen; Percocet)	Pain reliever, narcotic	Drowsiness, sedation, nausea, vomiting, constipation, respiratory depression, urinary retention, allergic reactions, rash, urticaria	Avoid concomitant use of alcohol or other central nervous system–depressant drugs; tell patient to avoid driving or other hazardous tasks while taking these medications; warn patient that extended use may result in dependency; avoid overdosing mother on acetaminophen.
dibucaine ointment (Nupercainal)	Topical anesthetic	Allergic reactions, burning, stinging	Instruct mother that it is for external use only (application to severely denuded tissue may result in systemic absorption).
erythromycin ophthalmic ointment or drops	Ophthalmic antibiotic agent	Irritation of eye that lasts 24 to 48 h Vision may be blurred temporarily	Apply to conjunctival sacs of baby. Wear gloves. Cleanse eye first, if necessary. Spread the ointment from the inner canthus to the outer canthus on lower lid. Do not touch the tube to the eye. After 1 min, wipe off excess ointment. Observe eyes for irritation.
ibuprofen (Advil, Motrin, Nuprin)	Nonsteroidal antiinflammatory with antipyretic and analgesic properties	Heartburn, nausea, pruritus, lightheadedness, gastrointestinal bleeding	Give 1 h before or 2 h after meals; with gastrointestinal intolerance, give with meals; instruct patient to avoid taking aspirin or acetaminophen concurrently; teach patient to avoid alcohol intake and to report gastrointestinal distress or bleeding.
methylergonovine maleate (Methergine)	Oxytocic agent, stimulates uterine contraction, used to control postpartum bleeding	Headache, dizziness, nausea, chest pain, tachycardia, hypertension	Contraindicated in patients sensitive to ergot derivatives.
oxytocin (Pitocin)	Oxytocic agent, stimulates uterine contractions	*Mother:* nausea, vomiting, uterine spasm or rupture, water intoxication, seizures, cardiac arrhythmias, hypotension *Fetus:* cardiac arrhythmias, central nervous system or brain damage	Carefully monitor intake and output; fetal heart tones; and length, duration, and force of uterine contractions.

Table 28.3 **Medications for the Mother and Newborn—cont'd**

GENERIC NAME (TRADE NAME)	ACTION	SIDE EFFECTS	NURSING IMPLICATIONS
purified lanolin cream	Retains the skin's natural moisture and protects the mother's nipple from further abrasions	None; does not need to be washed off for the next feeding	Applied to the mother's nipple. Mothers with a history of wool allergy should not use lanolin before a skin test can be done.
Rh_o(D) immune globulin (RhoGAM)	Gamma globulin solution containing immunoglobulins (IgG); provides passive immunity by suppressing antibody response and formation of anti-Rh(D) in Rh-negative individual exposed to Rh-positive blood	Injection site irritation; slight fever and lethargy	Check lot number, administer IM only to mother, using deltoid muscle within 72 h of pregnancy termination.
rubella vaccine	Live virus vaccine	Rash, joint pain, pain at site Does not harm breast-feeding mothers	Administer IM in deltoid muscle during postpartum period; warn patient to avoid pregnancy for at least 3 mo. Obtain informed consent.
simethicone (Mylicon)	Antiflatulent	None	Instruct patient to chew tablet thoroughly before swallowing; give after meals.
vitamin K (AquaMEPHYTON)	Antidote for inadequate absorption and synthesis of vitamin K in neonate	With a large dose: hyperbilirubinemia, hemolytic anemia, kernicterus	Administer 0.5–1 mg IM in the middle third of the infant's vastus lateralis muscle of thigh after delivery. Stabilize leg firmly.
vitamin, prenatal (Materna)	Vitamin supplement	Nausea, vomiting	Tell patient it is important that pregnant women take prenatal vitamins and not regular vitamin supplements and that prenatal vitamins contain extra folic acid, which is needed for normal fetal development.
witch hazel (Tucks pads, cream)	Astringent	Local irritation	Instruct mother that it is for external use only; use for relief of perineal discomfort.

NOTE: Hepatitis B vaccine is no longer given at birth while the patient is still in the hospital but in the physician's office, as determined by the health care provider.
IgG, Immunoglobulin G; *IM,* intramuscularly.

topical anesthetics to relieve pain if ordered by the physician. Sitz baths also provide relief and should be offered if the physician has ordered them. Suppositories may be ordered for hemorrhoid treatment.

Examine the patient's legs closely for warmth and redness. Question the patient about the sensation of pain in the legs. Early ambulation is the leading means of prevention of this potential complication.

The postpartum assessment can be organized as a head-to-toe assessment with the eight-letter mnemonic BUBBLE-HE (Box 28.9).

Lactation and breast-feeding. All new mothers should be encouraged to wear a bra regardless of breast size. The bra should be comfortable and fitted to provide support. Encourage breast-feeding mothers to use bras large enough to accommodate the growth that occurs with lactation. Nonnursing mothers need a bra that provides adequate compression to inhibit lactation without being uncomfortable.

With the bra removed, inspect and palpate the breasts. Observe for erythema, heat, edema, and engorgement. Visually assess the nipples for cracking and blisters.

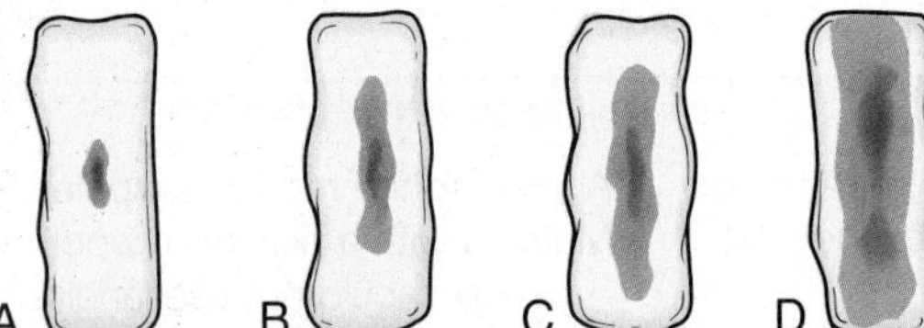

Fig. 28.5 Suggested guidelines for assessment of lochia volume. The pad may also be weighed and compared with the weight of a clean dry pad (1 g of weight equals 1 mL). A, Scant, less than 1 inch (2.5 cm). B, Light, less than 4 inches (10 cm). C, Moderate, less than 6 inches (15 cm). D, Heavy, pad saturated within 1 hour. (From Lowdermilk DL, Perry SE: *Maternity and women's health care,* ed 9, St. Louis, 2007, Mosby.)

Engorgement is an uncomfortable fullness of the breasts that occurs when the milk supply initially comes in. Three interrelated factors—congestion, increased vascularity, and the accumulation of breast milk—are the underlying causes. Filling of the breast with milk usually begins in the axillary region, so palpate the body and the tail of the breast. The condition may range from feelings of fullness to hard, painful breast tissues. In severe cases women may even experience numbness and tingling of the arms and hands. Engorgement usually is observed about the third day postpartum and resolves in about 48 hours but may continue up to a week. Because most patients are home by the time engorgement occurs, teach the new mother the symptoms of engorgement and methods of obtaining relief. If the patient is breast-feeding, interventions such as manual expression of milk and application of warm, moist heat are most useful. If the patient is not breast-feeding, compression of the breasts with a firm bra, wrapped ice packs, and analgesics are recommended most often. The use of cabbage leaves has been shown in some research studies to provide relief and reduction of engorgement (Gagandeep, 2013). Lactation experts recommend the placement of clean cabbage leaves inside the bra over the breasts. Some recommend the use of room temperature leaves and others suggest refrigerated, cooled leaves.

Inspect the nipples for inflammation, fissures, or tenderness. The nipples generally do not cause problems for nonlactating mothers; however, if the patient is breast-feeding, the nipples should be kept soft and supple. Most physicians recommend avoiding soap or other chemicals because they dry the skin and may be ingested by the infant. Plain water and air drying may prevent problems. Some physicians recommend allowing the nipples to dry after feeding without removing the milk residue. If additional moisturizer is needed, small amounts of unscented lanolin or a nipple cream may be used to soften and soothe dry, tender nipples. Modifications in the positioning of the baby may be needed if tender or cracked nipples continue to be a problem.

In addition to assessing the breasts, help the breast-feeding mother succeed in establishing lactation. To establish the lactation response, the breast must be

Box 28.9 Postpartum Assessment: BUBBLE-HE

Breast: For assessment of the breast, have the patient lie down and remove her bra. Palpate both breasts for engorgement or nodules. Inspect nipples for pressure, soreness, cracks, or fissures.

Uterus: The top of the uterus, the fundus, should remain very firm. If it becomes soft, the uterine muscles probably are not contracting properly or the uterus has retained placental fragments. Both conditions predispose the patient to hemorrhage. Gently massage the uterus to help the muscles contract and expel placental fragments.

Bladder: The new mother may urinate frequently the first few days after giving birth. Be alert for signs and symptoms of infection. Also note any dysuria or urinary retention.

Bowel: Because of early discharge from the hospital, many women leave without having had a bowel movement. Assess for bowel sounds, encourage activity with rest periods, and encourage adequate fluid intake.

Lochia: Lochia has a definite fleshy scent, but if it has a fetid odor, it may indicate infection. Assess carefully.

Episiotomy: Most new mothers have an episiotomy and, in some cases, a laceration. (NOTE: There is a move away from doing an episiotomy on the side—either left or right—and possibly even away from doing episiotomies at all, but midline is the site of choice. For a lateral episiotomy, use the following procedures.) Position the patient on her affected side. Instruct her to flex her top leg at the knee and draw it up toward her waist. Use a flashlight and wear gloves. Stand behind the patient and gently lift her top buttock to expose the perineum. Also assess for hemorrhoids.

Homans' sign: For patient assessment, position the legs flat on the bed while she reclines in the supine position. Dorsiflex her foot toward the ankle. Assess both extremities. If she reports calf pain, Homans' sign is positive; further assessment is needed because a blood clot in a vessel in the leg is indicated.

Emotional status: Consider the three phases most new mothers pass through:

1. The first is "taking in," the time immediately after birth. She sleeps, depends on others for nurturing and food, and relives the events surrounding the birth.
2. Over the next few days, she is "taking hold." She is preoccupied with the present and concerned about her health and her baby's condition. She cares for herself and wants to learn to care for her newborn.
3. The next phase, "letting go," comes later in the postpartum period. She reestablishes relationships with other people.

Monitor the patient's emotional status, noting how she interacts with her family, her level of independence, sleep and rest patterns, mood swings, irritability, or crying.

Modified from Ferguson H: Planning letter-perfect postpartum care. *Nursing* 1987;17(5):50.

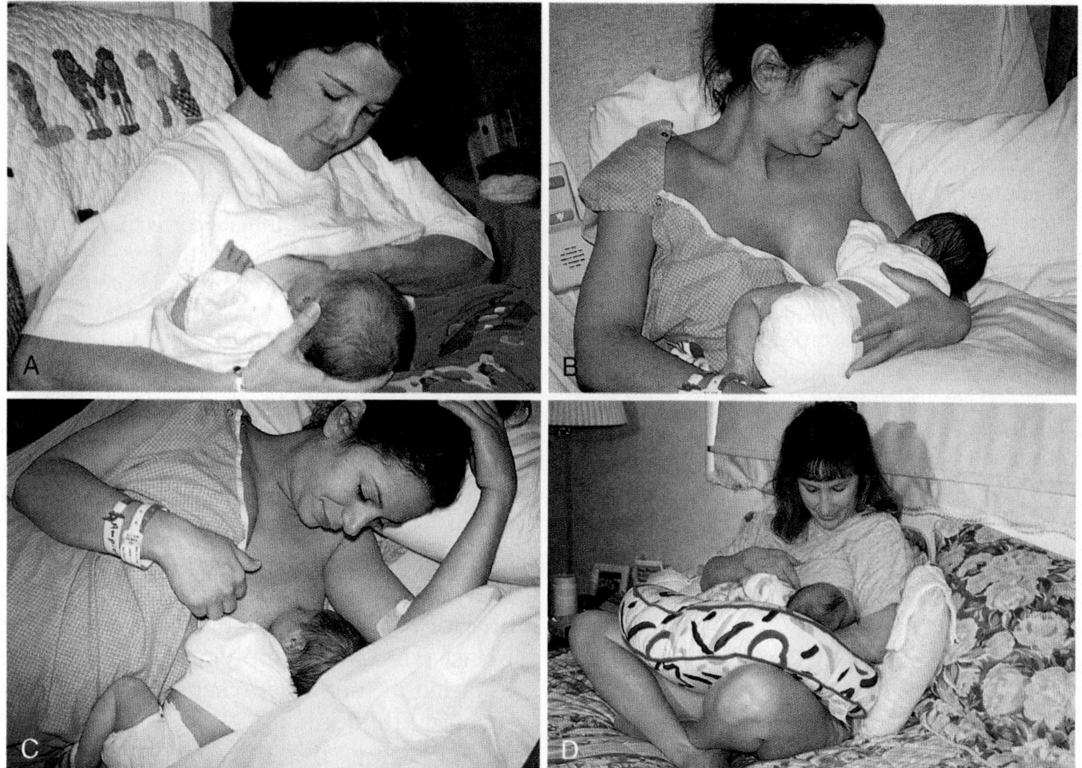

Fig. 28.6 Positioning the baby for breast-feeding. A, Football hold. B, Cradling. C, Lying down. D, Across the lap. (B–D, Courtesy Marjorie Pyle, RNC, LifeCircle, Costa Mesa, CA.)

stimulated adequately so that prolactin can be released by the anterior pituitary. Once the milk supply is established, prolactin production decreases, and oxytocin, released as the baby suckles, primarily maintains the supply of milk.

The mother may feel a tingling or prickling sensation, known as the *let-down reflex,* when feeding time approaches. If the mother nurses the baby at regular, frequent intervals and empties the breasts, the supply of milk increases in response to the baby's demands. If the breast is not stimulated adequately, the lactation response may not be established. This can happen when the baby has a weak suck or is not put to breast often enough. If the breast is not emptied adequately, the pressure of the milk in the alveoli also can suppress milk production. Incorrect placement at the breast also may lead to problems. If the baby's mouth grasps only the nipple and does not apply pressure on the lactiferous glands (mammary glands or Montgomery's glands, consisting of 20 to 24 glands in the areolae of the nipples), milk is not released and the needed stimulation does not occur. This also may lead to nipple trauma and soreness.

Become knowledgeable about correct breast-feeding techniques so that you can instruct the breast-feeding mother. These techniques include correct position and placement of the nipple and areola in the baby's mouth, stimulation of the infant to enable correct **latch-on** (attachment of the infant to the breast for feeding), frequency and length of nursing, and care of the breasts.

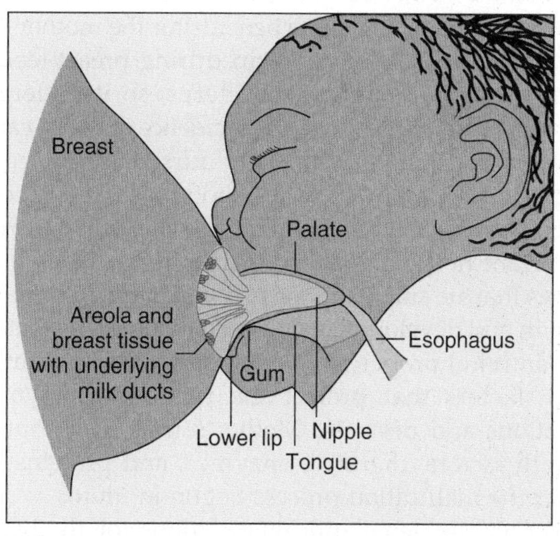

Fig. 28.7 Correct attachment (latch-on) of infant at breast. (From Lowdermilk DL, Perry SE: *Maternity and women's health care,* ed 9, St. Louis, 2007, Mosby.)

Also assist the mother's efforts by providing support and encouragement. Lactation consultants, teaching videos, and support groups such as La Leche League are excellent resources that supplement and reinforce teaching by the nurse (Figs. 28.6 and 28.7).

Manual pumping of the breasts may be necessary in some cases. The mother whose infant is unable to suckle at the breast at birth may pump to establish

Box 28.10 Advantages of Breast-Feeding

- *Antiinfective properties:* Immunoglobulins, lymphocytes, and other immune components that are present in breast milk protect the infant against infection. The bifidus factor in breast milk encourages growth of normal bacterial flora in the infant's gastrointestinal tract.
- *Nutrition:* Breast milk is specifically made for the human infant. Its protein, carbohydrate, and fat ratios are thought to be ideal for growth and development. It is well digested and readily absorbed.
- *Growth and development:* Breast-feeding promotes better tooth and jaw alignment. It may be less likely to produce obesity in the child, and it may favor optimal bonding between mother and infant.
- *Allergy:* Breast-feeding may reduce the incidence of allergies in infants at high risk for allergic conditions.
- *Maternal benefits:* Hormones produced in breast-feeding help contract and shrink the uterus. Breast-feeding requires no formula preparation or bottle sterilization and is more economical than formula feeding.

lactation and provide milk that can be fed to her baby by alternate means. The mother who must spend an extended time away from her infant, such as while at work, may pump to maintain lactation and provide breast milk for her baby during her absence.

Breast-feeding has many benefits for the mother (Box 28.10). The release of oxytocin during breast-feeding stimulates contraction of the uterus, so it undergoes more rapid involution. A lower incidence of breast cancer is found in women who have nursed for at least 3 months. Also, many women who breast-feed report a special closeness to their infants because they provide important nourishment. Human milk provides many factors that are suited uniquely to the infant and enhance growth and development. Human milk has antibacterial and antiviral properties, immunoglobulin, and antiallergy factors that protect the infant against many infections and diseases. Mother's milk also contains growth factors, digestive enzymes, and proteins that foster the maturation process begun in utero.

Patient problems and interventions for the breast-feeding patient include but are not limited to the following:

Patient Problem	Nursing Interventions
Insufficient Nutrition, related to nutritional demands during lactation	Review dietary choices Instruct patient to continue diet recommended during pregnancy Arrange consultation with a dietitian Inform patient of Women, Infants, and Children (WIC) supplemental food program
Anxiousness, related to initiating feedings as a result of inexperience	Evaluate patient's readiness to initiate feedings Initiate feedings as soon as possible Position mother and infant for comfort Initiate correct latch-on and position correctly Support and encourage mother in breast-feeding attempts

Bottle feeding is another choice for the new mother. If the mother chooses not to breast-feed, lactation must be suppressed. This can be accomplished by mechanical means, starting before milk production begins. The woman wears a supportive bra within 4 to 6 hours after delivery. Ice to the breasts also decreases the discomfort that may result from engorgement. She should avoid any form of breast stimulation, such as pumping the breasts, and avoid applying heat to the breasts, such as facing the hot water when showering. Do not restrict maternal fluid intake.

PSYCHOSOCIAL ASSESSMENT

COPING AND STRESS TOLERANCE

Many new mothers feel overwhelmed by the responsibility of motherhood. They may be intimidated by the nurses' capability and skill with the newborn. They often feel inept and may not wish to ask questions that may be viewed as unintelligent. Establishing rapport, listening, and anticipating fears and anxieties are important nursing measures. False reassurances are not helpful; thorough teaching and encouragement are far more beneficial.

Often women experience a period of depression after delivery that is triggered by rapid hormonal shifts. This so-called postpartum depression, or "baby blues," may be mild or severe. It often appears between 2 and 7 days postpartum. Prepare the woman for the possibility of this and plan a course of action if it occurs.

SIGNS OF POTENTIAL PROBLEMS

No assessment of psychosocial needs is complete without an assessment for signs of potential problems. Not all potential psychosocial problems are identified easily. However, some signs may indicate a need for further evaluation by a caregiver skilled in that area (Box 28.11). The presence of one or more of these signs does not prove that a problem exists but may indicate a need for further assessment (see Chapter 29).

ROLES AND RELATIONSHIPS

The addition of a new family member has a major effect on roles and relationships. These changes are most obvious when the first child is born, but adjustments take place whenever another child joins a family. Time,

Box 28.11 Signs of Potential Psychosocial Problems

- Inability or refusal to discuss labor and birth experience
- Refusal to interact with or care for baby (e.g., does not name baby, does not want to hold or feed baby)
- Refusal to attend infant care (including breast-feeding) classes
- Refusal to discuss contraception
- References to self as ugly and useless
- Excessive preoccupation with self (body image)
- Marked depression
- Lack of support system
- Partner or other family members reacting negatively to baby
- Expression of disappointment over baby's sex
- View of baby as messy or unattractive
- Baby reminding mother of family member or friend she does not like

Table 28.4 Transition to Fatherhood: A Three-Stage Process

STAGE	CHARACTERISTICS
Stage 1: Expectations	Father has preconceptions about what life will be like after baby comes home.
Stage 2: Reality	Father realizes that expectations are not always based on fact. Common feelings experienced are sadness, ambivalence, jealousy, and frustration. Father has overwhelming desire to be more involved. Some fathers are pleasantly surprised at ease and fun of parenting.
Stage 3: Transition to mastery	Father makes conscious decision to take control and become more actively involved with infant.

money, and environmental and emotional resources must be divided to include the new member.

In our society, the mother still fills the role of the child's primary caregiver and faces the greatest number of changes. The responsibility of this role, 24 hours a day, 7 days a week, is overwhelming to many women. Today, because many women are independent wage earners, the loss of freedom is a difficult adjustment. The transition to motherhood can lead to feelings of guilt and confusion. Be sensitive to the mother's concerns.

The responsibilities of fatherhood often become a reality when the father sees his child for the first time. The realization that a totally dependent individual needs him is frightening to many men. The financial concerns of feeding, clothing, and sheltering his family take on new significance. A formerly two-income family may have only one income, the father's wages, at least temporarily. Even if the mother returns to work, there are new expenses for child care. Both parents find that the child's needs take priority over their own needs or wishes. Freedom and spontaneity give way to a life circumscribed by feeding schedules, diaper bags, and babysitters.

Some men have little knowledge or experience in caring for infants; simple things, such as feeding, changing diapers, or even carrying a baby, may be intimidating. Help alleviate these fears by including the father in teaching whenever possible and by allowing him to verbalize his fears and concerns. Fathers go through a predictable three-stage process during the first 3 weeks of their transition to parenthood (Table 28.4).

Additional role adjustments relate to friends and the extended family. Friendships and socialization may take lower priority. Siblings assume a new position in the family order. Parents now become grandparents, and in-laws share grandchildren. These situations are all dynamic, and each family makes a variety of accommodations in incorporating their new roles.

SELF-PERCEPTION

The new mother commonly wishes to discuss her perception of the labor and delivery. The new mother may spend considerable time with friends or in telephone conversation relating her experiences of labor and delivery. Allow time for her to verbalize and work through her experiences. Reality may differ greatly from her expectations. She may need explanations to clarify things in her mind.

The new mother may be passive for the first day or two. This is called the taking-in stage (see Box 28.9). During this time, the mother needs supportive care. Her primary focus may be on herself and on personal needs such as sleep, food, and attention. She may defer to the nurses and let others care for the baby. This is followed by the taking-hold stage, when the woman is ready to assume greater authority and responsibility for herself and her baby.

Mood swings are common early in the postpartum period, related to recent stresses, fatigue, and rapid hormonal changes. Explain this to the new mother so that she does not become unduly concerned.

New mothers, particularly primiparas, commonly expect that they will regain their prepregnancy figures quickly after delivery. Many bring clothes that they hoped to wear home, only to be sadly disappointed. Be supportive and explain that it takes time for the body to regain the prepregnancy tone and shape.

COGNITIVE AND PERCEPTUAL ISSUES

Control of discomfort during the postpartum period is necessary for the woman to resume a normal activity level and get adequate rest. The most common discomforts experienced are perineal pain from the episiotomy and *afterbirth pains.* Afterbirth pains are cramping sensations that result from the contraction of the uterus. They are more common and may be more severe in multiparas and breast-feeding mothers.

Most physicians prescribe analgesics for these discomforts. Acetaminophen commonly is used, with or without codeine. Codeine is generally effective but is a controlled substance and also has side effects, such as constipation and vertigo, which may be undesirable in the postpartum patient (see Table 28.3). Salicylates, such as aspirin, usually are avoided because they may interfere with clotting mechanisms. Recently ibuprofen (Motrin) has been popular. Ibuprofen is an analgesic, an antiinflammatory, and a prostaglandin inhibitor. It is often effective in reducing the severity of the cramping without altering the contraction of the uterine muscle. CAUTION: Ibuprofen is to be used with caution in people with kidney or heart disease or those taking diuretics.

Another major challenge of the postpartum period for the mother involves learning how to care for herself and the newborn. This can be overwhelming for the first-time mother. The nurse has limited time to teach all the necessary information. Most hospitals have teaching lists and printed handouts or booklets that cover all the key areas (see Box 28.7). To prevent the woman from becoming overwhelmed, pace teaching throughout the hospital stay, rather than leaving it until discharge. Be sure to document teaching about newborn care (see Box 28.8).

❖ NURSING PROCESS FOR THE POSTPARTUM MOTHER

The role of the licensed practical nurse/licensed vocational nurse (LPN/LVN) in the nursing process as stated is that the LPN/LVN will:

- Participate in planning care for patients based on patient needs.
- Review patient's care plan and recommend revisions as needed.
- Review and follow defined prioritization for patient care.
- Use clinical pathways, care maps, or care plans to guide and review patient care.

◆ ASSESSMENT

Assessment begins with admission of the patient to the postpartum unit from the labor and delivery unit. Review the prenatal history for obstetric history, prenatal care, and health status during the pregnancy. Also review the events of labor, delivery, and recovery, including the onset of labor, the mother's physical and emotional status during labor, progress of labor, status of fetus, birth, and status of neonate. A physical and psychosocial assessment should follow. Areas assessed should include reproductive system, cardiovascular status, nutrition, elimination, activity and rest, maternal self-concept, knowledge level, parenting role, attachment, home environment, and support system. Physical and psychosocial assessments are ongoing during the postpartum stay.

◆ PATIENT PROBLEM

Nursing assessment helps identify the needs of the postpartum patient. Care then can be based on these needs. Possible patient problems for the postpartum patient include but are not limited to the following:

- *Alteration in family processes*
- *Alteration in Urinary Elimination*
- *Anxiousness*
- *Compromised Parenting Skills*
- *Compromised Tissue Integrity*
- *Impaired Self-Esteem due to Current Situation*
- *Ineffective Sleep Pattern*
- *Infrequent or Difficult Bowel Elimination*
- *Insufficient Knowledge*
- *Insufficient Nutrition*
- *Potential for Compromised Parenting Skills*
- *Potential for Inadequate Fluid Volume*
- *Potential for Infection*
- *Recent Onset of Pain*

◆ EXPECTED OUTCOMES AND PLANNING

The care plan focuses on the needs of the postpartum patient and the nurse's ability to meet those needs effectively (Nursing Care Plan 28.1). Each patient has differing needs; care must be individualized accordingly.

The care plan focuses on goals and outcomes specific to the patient problem. Examples include the following:

Goal 1: Patient will experience relief of pain at episiotomy site.

Outcome: Patient uses appropriate pain relief measures, such as a sitz bath, topical anesthetic spray, and medication, as necessary.

Goal 2: Patient will provide appropriate safe care to infant.

Outcome: Patient demonstrates competence in bathing, feeding, diapering, and comforting infant.

◆ IMPLEMENTATION

Nursing interventions during the postpartum period include the following:

- Assess progress of involution by monitoring vital signs, breasts, fundus, lochia, and episiotomy.
- Administer oxytocics, analgesics, and stool softeners as ordered.
- Use aseptic techniques, good handwashing, and standard precautions when caring for patient and baby.
- Teach or demonstrate the following (see Boxes 28.7 and 28.8):
    - Breast care measures
    - Signs and symptoms of infection and prevention measures
    - Nutritional and dietary requirements for healing and lactation

Nursing Care Plan 28.1 The Mother With a Newborn

Baby Caleb is a 39-week-gestation male neonate, 7 lb, 3 oz, and 21 inches long, born today to Philip and Anne P. Caleb was born via vaginal delivery after a 7-hour labor. Ms. P. had epidural anesthesia. Her pregnancy and medical history were unremarkable. Caleb is Philip and Anne's first child, and Ms. P. has begun breast-feeding. Caleb will be circumcised tomorrow. He has been nursing every 3 hours for approximately 20 minutes with a strong suck. At the initial assessment of Caleb 1 hour after birth, findings were all within normal limits. He was given 0.5 mL vitamin K (AquaMEPHYTON) in the left anterolateral thigh, and erythromycin (Ilotycin) was placed in both eyes. His temperature on admission to the nursery was 97.5°F (36.4°C) axillary. After he spent an hour under the radiant warmer, his temperature was 98.6°F (37°C) axillary, and he was given his initial bath. Caleb currently is rooming with his mother, who is asking numerous questions about his care.

INFANT PATIENT PROBLEM

Potential for Inability to Regulate Body Temperature, related to exposure to cool environment

Patient Goals and Expected Outcomes	Nursing Interventions	Evaluation
Stable infant temperature will be established and maintained	Dry infant immediately after birth. Wrap infant in warm blanket. Place infant under radiant warmer on admission to nursery. Place cap on infant's head. Keep infant away from drafts, exterior walls, and windows. Keep infant off cold surfaces. Monitor temperature q 30 min until normal, then q 4 hr. Delay bath until temperature is above 97.7°F (36.5°C) axillary.	Infant's temperature remains greater than 97.7°F (36.5°C) axillary. Infant is placed under radiant warmer on admission to nursery. Infant is properly dressed. Infant shows no signs of cold stress.

MATERNAL PATIENT PROBLEM

Insufficient Knowledge, Maternal, related to being a first-time parent

Patient Goals and Expected Outcomes	Nursing Interventions	Evaluation
Mother will verbalize understanding of infant care Mother will demonstrate infant bath and diaper change Mother will verbalize correct safety practices Mother will use correct breast-feeding techniques	Demonstrate and encourage return demonstration of infant bath, including umbilical cord care, circumcision care, and dressing. Demonstrate diaper change and cleaning of genital area. Teach correct positioning of infant. Teach techniques for breast-feeding. Teach methods to maintain infant's temperature.	Mother correctly bathes and diapers infant. Mother practices safe technique when handling infant. Mother successfully breast-feeds infant with correct techniques.

CRITICAL THINKING QUESTIONS

1. Even though Caleb is nursing well at each feeding, Ms. P. is anxious about her ability to successfully breast-feed. She asks how she will know whether Caleb is getting enough breast milk and whether she should supplement with formula, juice, or cereal. How should the nurse answer her?
2. A Gomco circumcision is performed on Caleb. After the procedure is completed, Caleb is returned to his mother's room. What should the nurse tell Ms. P. in response to her questions regarding diaper changes and care of the circumcision? How should the nurse describe the expected appearance of the circumcised penis?

    - Postpartum exercises
    - Infant care techniques
- Provide comfort and pain-relief measures.
- Encourage patient and family to express feelings.
- Make referrals to community agencies as appropriate.

Implementation of nursing care involves putting into practice specific activities that should result in the expected outcomes planned for each individual patient.

◆ EVALUATION

Continually evaluate the success of the interventions. As the postpartum period progresses, the goals and interventions may change. Refer to the goals and outcomes to determine whether the plan was successful and the outcomes met. Examples include the following:

Goal 1: Patient will experience relief of pain at episiotomy site.

Evaluative measures: Patient uses sitz bath twice a day, applies topical anesthetic spray with each peripad change, and requests analgesics for episiotomy pain.

Goal 2: Patient will provide appropriate safe care to infant.

Evaluative measures: Patient demonstrates appropriate infant bathing techniques, use of infant car seat, and feeding techniques.

VALUES AND BELIEFS

Cultural beliefs and practices are important determinants of parenting behaviors. They influence the interactions with the infant and the parent's or family's caregiving style. For example, Asian mothers may remain at home with the baby for at least 30 days after birth and are not supposed to engage in household chores, including care of the infant. Many times the grandmother takes over the baby's care immediately, even before discharge from the hospital. Similarly, a Jordanian mother may have a 40-day lying-in after birth, during which her mother or sisters care for the baby. Hispanics may practice a 40-day period after birth during which the mother is expected to recuperate and get acquainted with her infant. Traditionally this involves many restrictions concerning food (spicy or cold foods, fish, pork, and citrus are avoided; tortillas and chicken soup are encouraged); exercise; and activities, including sexual intercourse. Abdominal binding is a traditional practice, and many grown women avoid tub bathing and washing their hair. A traditional Hispanic husband does not expect to see his wife or infant until both have been cleaned and dressed after birth.

People in all cultures desire and value children. In Asian families, children are valued as a source of family strength and stability, are perceived as wealth, and are objects of parental love and affection. In the Yup'ik culture of the Alaskan Eskimos, where sharing traditionally has been necessary for survival, children are looked on as security. There is no concept of illegitimacy; every child is welcomed and loved. Adoption is common and is usually within the extended family.

Differing cultural values can influence parents' interactions with health care professionals. Because all members of a cultural group do not necessarily adhere to traditional practices, validate which cultural practices are important to individual parents. Knowledge of cultural beliefs can help with accurate assessments and diagnoses of observed parenting behaviors. For example, nurses may become concerned when they observe cultural practices that appear to reflect poor maternal-infant bonding.

Traditionally, Asians are taught to be humble and obedient. They are brought up to not question authority figures (such as a nurse) and to avoid confrontation and respect the yin-yang balance in nature. Because of these learned values, an Asian mother may not confront the nurse about the length of time before she receives the medication requested for her episiotomy pain. A mother may nod and say "Yes" in response to the nurse's directions for using an iced sitz bath but then not use the bath. The "Yes," in this case, is a courtesy, meaning "I'm listening," rather than an indication of agreement. The mother does not use the iced sitz bath because of her traditional avoidance of bathing and cold in the puerperium.

An Algerian mother may not unwrap and explore her infant as part of the acquaintance process, because in Algeria babies are wrapped tightly in swaddling clothes to protect them physically and psychologically. A Vietnamese woman may care for her infant but refuse to cuddle or further interact with her child. This apparent lack of interest in the newborn is this cultural group's attempt to ward off "evil spirits" and actually reflects an intense love and concern for the child. An Asian mother may be criticized for almost immediately relinquishing care of her infant to grandmothers and not even attempting to hold her baby when he or she is brought to the room. Family members show their support for a new mother's rest and recuperation by assisting with the care of the baby. Contrary to the guidance given to mothers in the United States about "nipple confusion," a mix of breast-feeding and bottle feeding is standard practice for Japanese mothers. This is out of concern for the mother's rest during the first 2 to 3 months and does not interfere with lactation; breast-feeding is widespread among Japanese women.

In helping new families adjust to parenthood, follow principles that facilitate nursing practice within transcultural situations (see the Cultural Considerations box).

PREVENTING INFANT ABDUCTION

An unfortunate but essential nursing role is protecting the infant from abduction (kidnapping). Precautions include teaching parents how to recognize the picture identification badge worn by birth facility personnel; providing parents with written and oral information, including a picture of staff identification badges, and cautioning parents to never give their infant to anyone who does not have proper identification.

Staff members who are working temporarily on the unit are assigned special identification badges that are monitored carefully so that they cannot be removed from the premises without alerting the staff. In some agencies, an electronic sensor is attached to each infant with a bracelet or tag. The sensor activates an alarm if it goes near an exit or if it is cut or removed from the infant. With some systems, all exits lock automatically if an alarm is activated.

Entrances to the maternity unit should be in areas where staff can watch people enter and leave. Unit doors may be locked at all times. Entrance requires knocking, pressing a call signal, or using a card key or a code on the lock. Visitors to maternity units may be required to check in with security guards or other staff members and wear special visitor identification tags. Remote exits are locked and often equipped with video cameras and alarms. Staff must respond quickly whenever a door alarm sounds.

Newborns usually are abducted by women who are familiar with the birth facility and its routines. They are of childbearing age, are often overweight, and may live near the birth facility. They usually visit several times to learn the routines so that they can impersonate

Cultural Considerations

Postpartum Period

- Many cultures emphasize certain postpartum rituals for mother and baby. In some cultures, including Chinese, Mexican, Korean, and Southeast Asian, these rituals may include bathing, activity, and dietary restrictions designed to restore the hot-cold (yin-yang) balance of the body:
  - The mother may observe a long period of seclusion and rest with avoidance of physical activity. Household responsibilities and infant care are provided by other female family members. The period of seclusion may last from 2 weeks to 40 days.
  - These cultures avoid cold and maintain increased body warmth; avoid bathing, hair washing, exercise, and exposure to wind for 7 to 30 days after childbirth; and add extra heat (cover with blankets).
  - The woman may avoid cold and raw foods and water. She may eat only warm foods and drink hot beverages to replace blood loss and to restore the balance of hot and cold in her body. Traditional foods of culture are encouraged.
- The woman may wear an abdominal binder. She may prefer not to give her baby colostrum.
- In other cultures, breast-feeding practices are not established until after milk comes in because of belief that colostrum is "bad" for the baby.
- A low-income mother may need to contend with stressors that distract her from developing a relationship with her baby. Inability to pay for infant supplies or child care, chaotic home situations, and worry over eligibility for social and health care services deplete the woman's mental and physical energy.
- An Arabic woman may eat special meals designed to restore her energy. She is expected to stay at home for 40 days after delivery to avoid illness from exposure to the outside air.
- A Haitian woman may request to take the placenta home to bury or burn.

birth facility staff to gain access to a newborn. They often know the layout of the facility and the locations of exits well. The woman may have had a previous pregnancy loss or be unable to get pregnant. She may want an infant to solidify her relationship with her husband or boyfriend. Although the woman plans the kidnapping scheme, she waits for an appropriate opportunity to take an infant (Box 28.12).

DISCHARGE: BEFORE 24 HOURS AND AFTER 48 HOURS

Early postpartum discharge, shortened hospital stays, and *1-day maternity stays* are all terms for the length of hospital stays of a mother and her baby after a low-risk birth. The trend of shortened hospital stays is based largely on efforts to reduce health care costs, coupled with consumer demands to have less medical intervention and more family-focused experiences.

Box 28.12 Precautions to Prevent Infant Abductions

- All personnel must wear appropriate identification that is easily visible at all times. No one without appropriate identification should handle or transport infants.
- Enlist parents' help in preventing kidnapping. Teach them to allow only hospital staff with proper identification to take their infant from them.
- Teach parents and staff to transport infants only in their cribs and never by carrying them. Question anyone walking in the hallway carrying an infant.
- Investigate anyone with a newborn near an exit or in an unusual part of the facility.
- Be suspicious of anyone who does not seem to be visiting a specific mother or who asks detailed questions about nursery or discharge routine.
- Be suspicious of unknown people carrying large bags or packages that could contain an infant.
- Respond immediately when an alarm sounds signaling that a remote exit has been opened or an infant has been taken to an unauthorized area.
- Never leave infants unattended at any time. Teach parents that their infant must be observed at all times. If no family members are present, the mother can take her infant into the bathroom with her or send the infant back to the nursery if she wishes to nap.
- Take infants to mothers one at a time. Never leave an infant in the hallway unsupervised.
- When an infant is left in a mother's room, place the crib away from the doorway.
- If entrances to the maternity unit or nurseries are equipped with locks that open to codes or card keys, protect them from others.
- When a parent or a family member comes to the nursery to take an infant, always match the infant and adult identification bracelet numbers. Never give an infant to anyone without the correct identification bracelet or other proper identification.
- Alert hospital security immediately of any suspicious activity.
- Suggest that parents not place announcements in the newspaper or signs in their yard that may alert an abductor that a new baby is in the home.

Laws Relating to Discharge

Health care providers have expressed concern with shortened stays, because some medical problems do not show up in the first 24 hours after birth. New mothers do not have sufficient time to learn how to care for their newborns and identify problems such as jaundice and dehydration related to breast-feeding difficulties.

The concern for the potential increase in adverse maternal-infant outcomes from hospital early discharge practices led the American College of Obstetricians and Gynecologists, the American Academy of Pediatrics, and other professional health care organizations to promote the enactment of federal and state maternity length-of-stay bills to ensure adequate care for the mother and the newborn. The Newborns' and Mothers' Health Protection Act of 1996 provides minimum federal standards for health plan coverage for mothers and their newborns. The act requires all health plans to allow the new mother and the newborn to remain in the hospital for a minimum of 48 hours after a normal vaginal birth and 96 hours after a cesarean birth, unless the attending provider, in consultation with the mother, decides on early discharge.

MATERNAL FOLLOW-UP CARE

After delivery, the woman is instructed to make a follow-up appointment with her health care provider in 6 weeks. Some birthing units require this appointment be made before discharge. If the nurse schedules the appointment, the patient needs prompt notification of the date and time of the appointment. Women with complications may be seen sooner.

WELL BABY FOLLOW-UP CARE

Healthy infants are seen by the physician at 2 weeks of age. Babies who are discharged before 48 hours of age traditionally are seen by the health care provider within 3 to 5 days after discharge. The purpose of this appointment is to review nutritional status, elimination, and the presence of jaundice. The schedule of appointments for a well baby is every 2 to 3 months until age 18 months. Milestone visits are planned for ages 2 and 3 years and then every 2 years. These visits focus on preventive care such as health education, nutritional assessments, review of growth and development, and routine immunizations (see Chapter 30).

ANATOMY AND PHYSIOLOGY OF THE HEALTHY NEWBORN

ASSESSMENT IMMEDIATELY AFTER DELIVERY

In addition to Apgar scoring (see Chapter 27), which is done immediately after delivery, other assessments are performed to establish the newborn's gestational age. Gestational age is the actual number of weeks since conception. This age is important because many problems observed in newborns are age related. Because many women are unsure of the exact date of conception, calendar-based gestational age is unreliable. Physical and neurologic assessments based on established criteria are more reliable. Evaluate physical characteristics within the first few hours of life. Neurologic assessment is done 24 hours later, after the nervous system has had the opportunity to stabilize from the trauma of delivery.

CHARACTERISTICS

Body Size and Shape

The newborn's head is disproportionately large for the body. The abdomen is prominent, with a smaller chest and narrow hips. The body usually is held in a moderately flexed position. A wide variation of size is seen in healthy newborns. The average newborn weighs 7 lb, 8 oz (3400 g) and is approximately 20 inches (50 cm) long. Charts are available for plotting height and weight. The head circumference averages 13 to 14 inches (33 to 35.5 cm) and is generally about 1 inch (2.5 cm) larger than the chest circumference, which averages 12 to 13 inches (30.5 to 33 cm).

Vital Signs

Respiratory rate averages from 30 to 60 breaths/min with brief periods of apnea. Breathing is diaphragmatic and should be effortless, without evidence of respiratory distress. Rate and rhythm vary with activity. Pulse rate averages 120 to 160 beats/min, with higher and lower variations depending on activity.

The heartbeat should have a regular rate and rhythm. Auscultate the apical beat between the fourth and fifth intercostal spaces. This is best done when the infant is asleep. Murmurs are common in the newborn. The physician determines whether they are significant. The blood pressure averages 60 to 80/40 to 50 mm Hg and should be approximately the same in all four extremities. A drop in systolic blood pressure (about 15 mm Hg) in the first hour after birth is common. Crying and moving usually cause increases in systolic blood pressure. The axillary temperature of the newborn should be between 97.6° and 98.6°F (36.4° and 37°C), with stabilization of temperature occurring within 8 to 10 hours after birth.

Skin

The infant's skin can exhibit a wide range of rashes and color changes (Box 28.13). Most are not significant and disappear within a few days. However, parents may be concerned until the changes are explained.

Color. The white newborn is usually pink to slightly reddish in appearance. The black newborn may appear pinkish or yellowish brown. Newborns of Spanish descent may have an olive tint or a slight yellow cast to the skin. Newborns of Asian descent may be a rosy or yellowish tan. The color of Native American newborns depends on the tribe and can vary from a light pink to a dark, reddish brown. By the second or third day, the skin turns to its more natural tone and is drier and flakier. The ruddiness results from normally elevated red blood cell concentration.

The hands and feet may appear slightly blue; this is called **acrocyanosis** and is caused by poor peripheral circulation. Acrocyanosis can last for 7 to 10 days. It is observed most commonly when the infant becomes cold. Mottling, a lacy pattern with dilated vessels on pale skin, is also common. Another normal variation is called the **harlequin sign;** half of the newborn's body appears deep red and the other half appears pale as a result of vasomotor disturbance, with some vessels constricting while others dilate. When the infant is placed on one side, the dependent half is noticeably pinker than the superior half. This may last for up to 20 minutes. Although disturbing to view, it is not harmful.

Box 28.13 Common Skin Observations in the Newborn

- *Milia* are small white spots usually seen on the nose and chin. They are a result of occluded sebaceous glands and disappear spontaneously within a few weeks.
- *Newborn rash,* or erythema toxicum neonatorum, is an elevated, hivelike rash that may result in small white vesicles. It is not contagious and, like milia, disappears without treatment.
- *Telangiectatic nevi,* "stork bites," are flat pink or red marks often seen on the eyelids, nose, or nape of the neck. These are dilated capillaries that become more vivid when the infant cries. They are not significant to the health of the infant and disappear at 1 to 2 years of age.
- *Mongolian spots* are areas of increased pigmentation. The lumbar dorsal area is the most common location. The area may appear bluish black. These are most often seen in darker-skinned people.
- *Nevus flammeus,* port-wine stain, is a reddish purple discoloration often seen on the face. This is a capillary angioma below the epidermis. Unfortunately, these do not disappear spontaneously. Medical techniques have been developed that reduce or remove port-wine birthmarks.
- *Strawberry birthmarks,* nevus vasculosus, are capillary hemangiomas. These may continue to increase in size for several months. They normally then begin to shrink spontaneously and usually disappear early in childhood.

The newborn's hemoglobin and hematocrit levels frequently are elevated; hemoglobin may range from 14 to 24 g/dL, and hematocrit from 44% to 64%. These elevated levels are needed by the fetus to assist with oxygen transport. After delivery, the neonate does not require these same levels. As the infant's body begins to manage this elevation and cells are broken down, jaundice results. *Jaundice,* a yellow discoloration caused by deposits of bile pigments and known as *icterus neonatorum,* is detected first over bony prominences on the face and the mucous membranes. Normally occurring jaundice results approximately 48 hours after birth and is termed physiologic jaundice. It gradually disappears by the 7th to 10th day. Jaundice that occurs sooner than 48 hours after birth is termed pathologic jaundice. This type of jaundice is not normal and may be the result of a maternal-fetal blood incompatibility. Further assessment of jaundice is necessary. The physician may order laboratory and diagnostic tests to determine the nature of the problem and begin treatment to prevent complications. Causes of jaundice are discussed further in Chapter 29.

Appearance. At birth, the skin is covered with a yellowish white, cream cheese–like substance called **vernix caseosa.** This substance protects the infant's skin from the amniotic fluid. When the vernix caseosa is removed, the skin may appear dry and may crack, flake, and peel. Another common finding is **lanugo** (downy, fine hair characteristic of the fetus between 20 weeks of gestation and birth). Lanugo is most noticeable over the shoulders, forehead, and cheeks, but it is found on nearly all parts of the body, except the palms, soles, and scalp.

Good turgor and tissue elasticity normally are observed. Desquamation of the skin of the term infant does not occur until a few days after birth. Its presence at birth is an indication of postmaturity.

Head

The **fontanelles** (broad area or soft spot that consists of a strong band of connective tissue contiguous with [touching] cranial bones and located at the junction of the bones) should be palpable. The *anterior fontanelle* is normally large and diamond shaped and closes at approximately 18 months of age. The *posterior fontanelle* is smaller and triangular and normally closes at 2 months of age. The sagittal suture may be felt by running the fingers between the two fontanelles (see Chapter 27, Fig. 27.2).

The newborn's head may manifest many variations. Most of these are a result of the birth process and disappear without treatment shortly after the delivery.

- *Molding* is overlapping of the bones of the skull. The head may appear elongated and misshapen; this condition is a result of compression during delivery and normally disappears within a day or two.
- *Caput succedaneum* commonly is seen with molding. It is the result of edema in the soft tissue of the scalp. The tissue feels spongy and may be felt over suture lines. This also disappears without treatment (Fig. 28.8A).
- *Cephalhematoma* is caused by bleeding within the periosteum of a cranial bone. It is confined to a particular bone and does not cross suture lines. This is usually a result of difficult labor. Cephalhematomas generally appear 1 or 2 days after birth. These normally absorb without treatment. Large hematomas may lead to anemia and jaundice, which necessitate medical intervention (Fig. 28.8B).

Face. The newborn's chin is receding, and the nose is relatively flat. Fat pads make the cheeks appear full and round. Movements of the face should be symmetric. The mouth should open freely, and the oral cavity should be intact with a closed palate. Small white nodules called *Epstein's pearls* may be observed on the hard palate. These are a result of epithelial cells and disappear spontaneously within a few weeks. Rarely, an infant is born with teeth; these teeth should be watched closely, because they may become loose and be aspirated. The oral cavity should be clean and free from lesions. A fungal infection may be acquired during passage through the birth canal if the mother is infected with *Candida albicans.* This results in thrush, a white, patchy coating

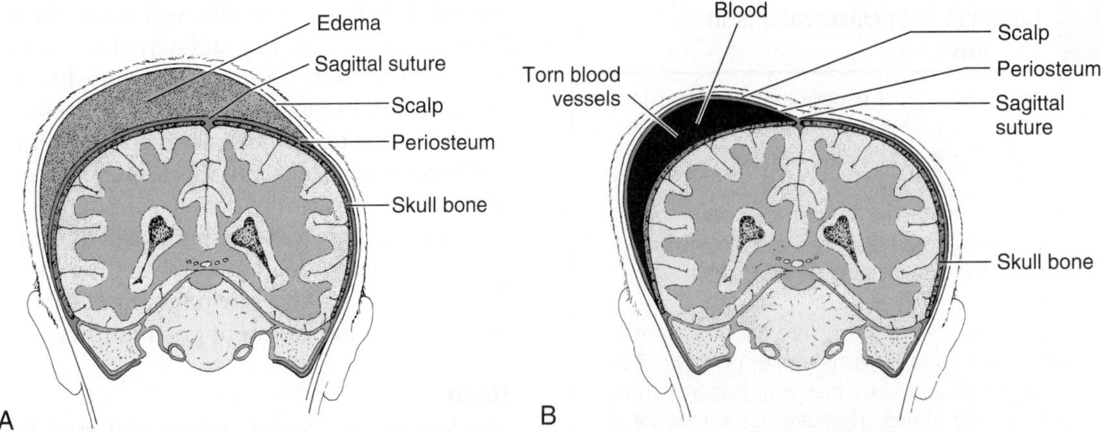

Fig. 28.8 Differences between caput succedaneum and cephalhematoma. A, Caput succedaneum: edema of scalp noted at birth; crosses suture line. B, Cephalhematoma: bleeding between periosteum and skull bone that appears within first 2 days; does not cross suture lines. (From Lowdermilk DL, Perry SE: *Maternity and women's health care,* ed 9, St. Louis, 2007, Mosby.)

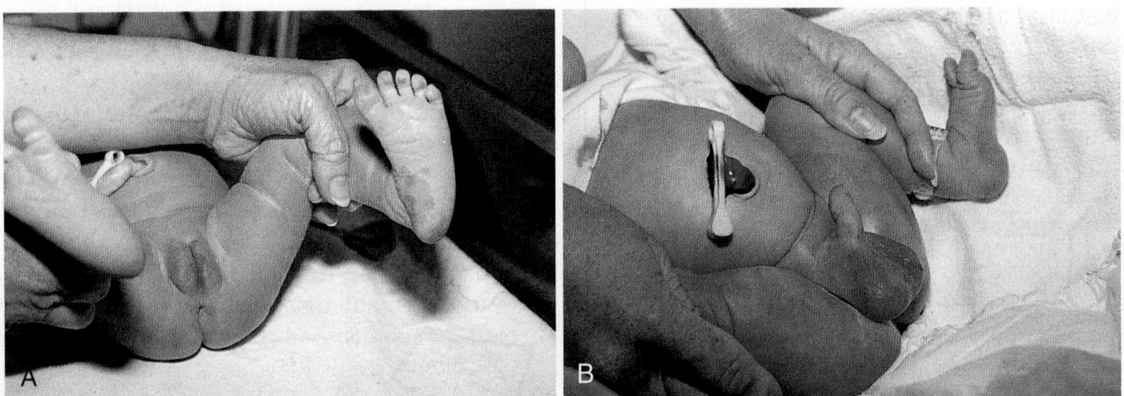

Fig. 28.9 External genitalia. A, Genitalia in female term infant. Note mucoid vaginal discharge. B, Genitalia in male infant. Uncircumcised penis. Rugae cover scrotum, indicating term gestation. Cord has been swabbed with ethylene blue to prevent infection. (Courtesy Marjorie Pyle, RNC, LifeCircle, Costa Mesa, CA, in Lowdermilk DL, Perry SE, Cashion K, et al: *Maternity and women's health care,* ed 10, St. Louis, 2012, Mosby.)

of the mucous membranes that cannot be wiped off. Treatment with antifungal medications such as nystatin or gentian violet is necessary.

Eyes. The eyelids may appear edematous because of prophylactic antibiotic medication that was applied to the eyes after birth to prevent *ophthalmia neonatorum* (infection in the neonate's eyes, usually resulting from gonorrheal or other infection contracted when the fetus passes through the birth canal [vagina]). The eyes appear wide set. *Strabismus* (crossed eyes) and *nystagmus* (abnormal motion of the eyes) are commonly seen as a result of the newborn's immature nervous system. Most white infants have slate-gray to blue irises at birth; in darker skinned infants, the irises may appear darker. The newborn does not produce tears because the lacrimal structures have not fully matured. Tears may not be present during crying for the first few months of life. Vision has been found to be more acute than previously believed. Newborns are nearsighted and can see objects best at 8 to 10 inches; most prefer simple patterns in black and white and human faces. Make certain the parents know this, because eye contact with the baby is an important part of bonding.

Ears. The ears normally are positioned with the upper insertion of the pinna located even with the outer canthus of the eye. Low-set ears may indicate a chromosomal disorder. Newborns are most attentive to high-pitched sounds and the mother's voice. The fetus becomes familiar with the mother's voice in utero.

Umbilical Cord

The umbilical cord is whitish blue-gray with three vessels (one vein and two arteries) and contains a gelatinous tissue called Wharton's jelly. Inspect the cord for the number of vessels, because a two-vessel cord may indicate congenital anomalies. In Fig. 28.9, note the cord

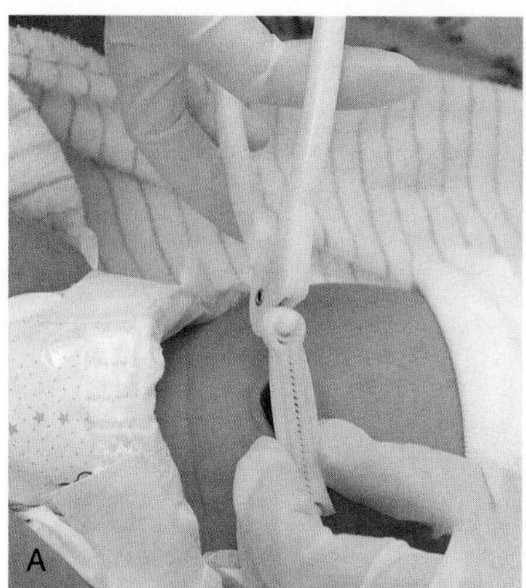

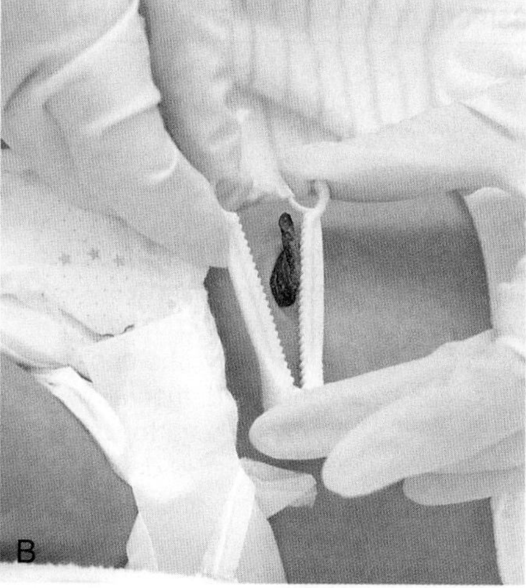

Fig. 28.10 The cord clamp is removed when the end of the cord is dry and crisp. The clamp is cut (A) and separated (B). NOTE: No triple dye was used; the diaper is folded down away from the cord area. (From McKinney ES, James SR, Murray SS, et al: *Maternal-child nursing*, ed 3, Philadelphia, 2009, Saunders.)

stump in *A* and the cord stump in *B* (triple dye gives it the purplish color).

Providing cord care. Check the cord for bleeding or oozing during the early hours after birth. The cord clamp must be fastened securely with no skin caught in it. Purulent drainage or redness or edema at the base indicates infection. The cord becomes brownish black within 2 or 3 days and falls off in about 10 to 14 days.

Care of the cord varies in different agencies. It may be treated with a bactericidal substance, such as triple-dye solution (see Fig. 28.9B), antibiotic ointment, or alcohol, three times a day or allowed to dry naturally. None of the treatments commonly used is better at keeping the cord clean and dry than the others. When soiled, the cord should be cleaned with water. This natural treatment of cords may shorten the time to cord separation and does not lead to increased infections. The diaper is folded below the cord to keep the cord dry and free from contamination with urine.

Remove the cord clamp about 24 hours after birth if the end of the cord is dry (Fig. 28.10). Although the base of the cord is still moist, it does not bleed if the end is dry and crisp.

Reflexes

Healthy newborns exhibit a wide variety of reflexes (Table 28.5). Some are protective reflexes, such as the rooting, sucking, gag, swallow, blink, burp, hiccup, and sneeze reflexes. Other reflexes, such as the Babinski's, Moro, tonic neck, and stepping reflexes, are related to the immature nervous system. Many are present for a limited time and then disappear.

Genitalia

The genitalia in female newborns may be edematous (see Fig. 28.9A). Discharge of blood-tinged mucus from the vagina, called **pseudomenstruation,** may occur in response to maternal hormones. Either gender may have enlarged breasts. This is called **gynecomastia** and is also a result of maternal hormones. The labia majora cover the minora in term infants (see Fig. 28.9A). The scrotum in the male may be enlarged and edematous, which indicates a hydrocele. The testicles normally are descended in term infants (see Fig. 28.9B); in preterm infants, they may not be descended **(cryptorchidism).** If the testicles are not descended, the condition is monitored until they do descend. In the event they have not by the age of 18 months to 2 years, surgical intervention is necessary. Inspect the penis for position of the urethral meatus. Abnormal placement may result in problems with voiding. **Circumcision** (the surgical removal of the foreskin) normally is not done if there is any malplacement, because the foreskin may be used as part of the surgical correction.

Spine

The spine should be straight without curves. The normal cervical and lumbar curves develop once the infant begins to stand. Also, examine the spine for dimples, tufts of hair, and masses that may indicate abnormalities of spinal column development.

Extremities

The arms and hands generally are flexed against the body. Both arms should move evenly. Trauma during delivery may result in fracture of the clavicle or in brachial palsy. Both hands should be free from webbing (**syndactyly,** malformation of digits, commonly seen as webbing or fusion of two or more digits to form one structure) or extra digits **(polydactyly).** A single crease in the palm of the hand, a simian line, may indicate chromosomal disorders such as *Down syndrome* (mongolism or trisomy 21, caused by an extra chromosome 21 in the G group) (see Chapter 31). Nails often extend beyond the fingertips. Legs should be equal in length.

Table 28.5 Assessment of Reflexes in the Healthy Newborn

EXPECTED BEHAVIORAL RESPONSE	COMMENTS	
Moro (Startle) Reflex		
Sudden jarring or change in equilibrium causes extension and abduction of extremities and fanning of fingers, with index finger and thumb forming a C shape, followed by flexion and adduction of extremities; legs may weakly flex; infant may cry.	Elicit reflex by holding the infant above the examining table in a supine position with one hand beneath the sacrum and the other supporting the upper back and head; then allow the infant's head to suddenly fall about 30 degrees. Disappears after 3 to 4 mo; usually strongest during first 2 mo.	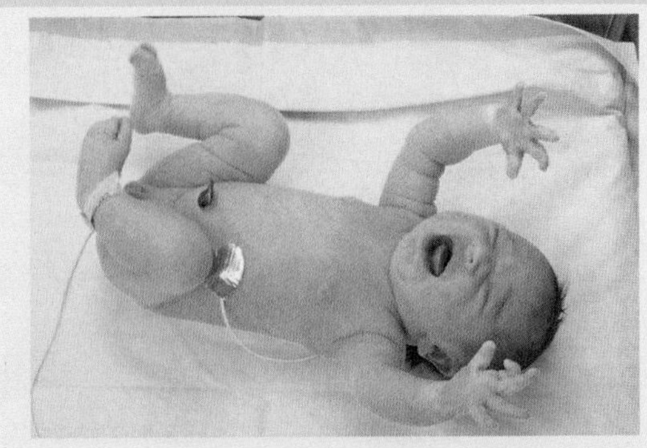
Tonic Neck Reflex		
When infant's head is quickly turned to one side, arm and leg extend on that side, and opposite arm and leg flex; posture resembles a fencing position.	Disappears by 3 to 4 mo of age, to be replaced by symmetric positioning of both sides of body.	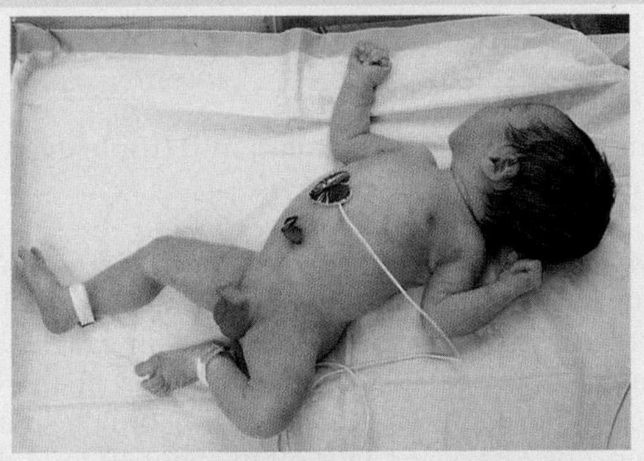
Dance or Stepping Reflex		
If infant is held so that sole of foot touches a hard surface, there is a reciprocal flexion and extension of the leg, simulating walking.	Disappears after 3 to 4 wk, to be replaced by deliberate movement.	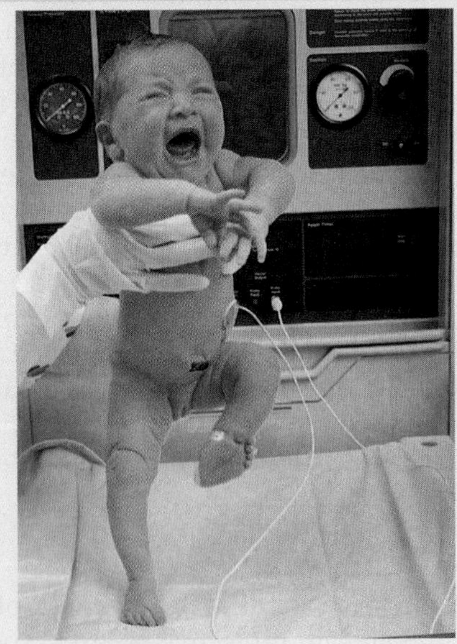

Table 28.5 Assessment of Reflexes in the Healthy Newborn—cont'd

EXPECTED BEHAVIORAL RESPONSE	COMMENTS	
Babinski's Reflex		
When the sole of the foot is stroked along side of sole beginning at heel and then moving across ball of foot to big toe, toes fan out with dorsiflexion of big toe.	Disappears by 1 yr. Absence laterally indicates central nervous system damage.	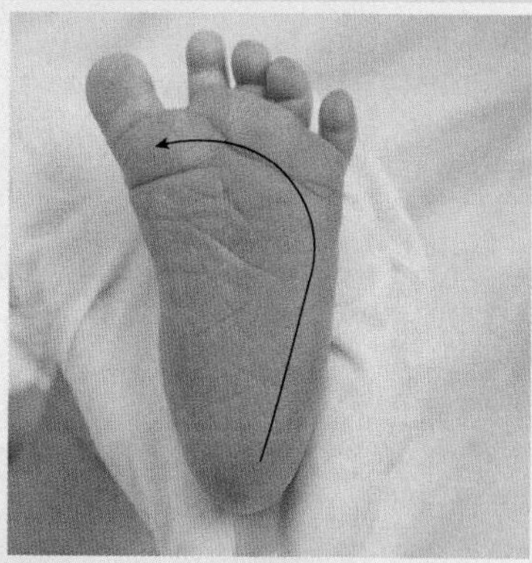
Grasp Reflex		
Palmar. Place finger in the palm of the hand. Infant's fingers curl around examiner's fingers.		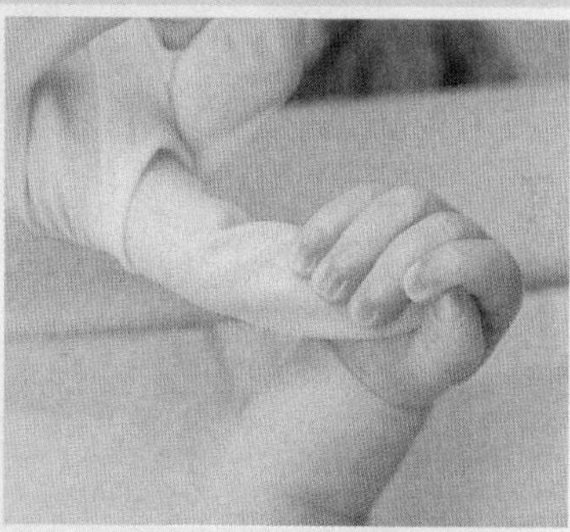
Plantar. Place fingers at the base of the toes. Toes curl downward.		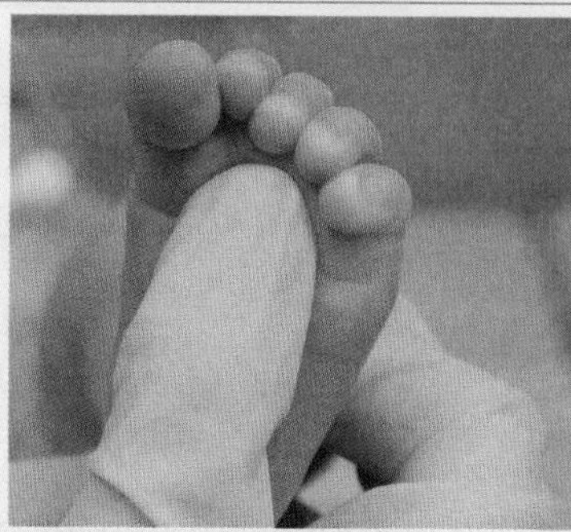
Pull to Sit (Traction) Reflex		
Pull infant up by the wrist from supine position with head in midline. Head lags until infant is in upright position, then head is held in the same place with chest and shoulder momentarily before falling forward; infant attempts to right head.		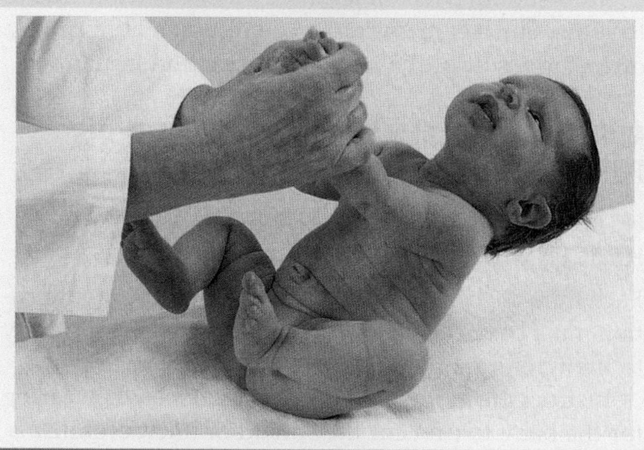

Moro, tonic neck, step, Babinski's, palmar, and plantar grasp reflex images from McKinney ES, James SR, Murray SS, et al: *Maternal-child nursing,* ed 4, St. Louis, 2013, Saunders. Pull to sit reflex image from Jarvis C: *Physical examination and health assessment,* ed 5, Philadelphia, 2008, Saunders.

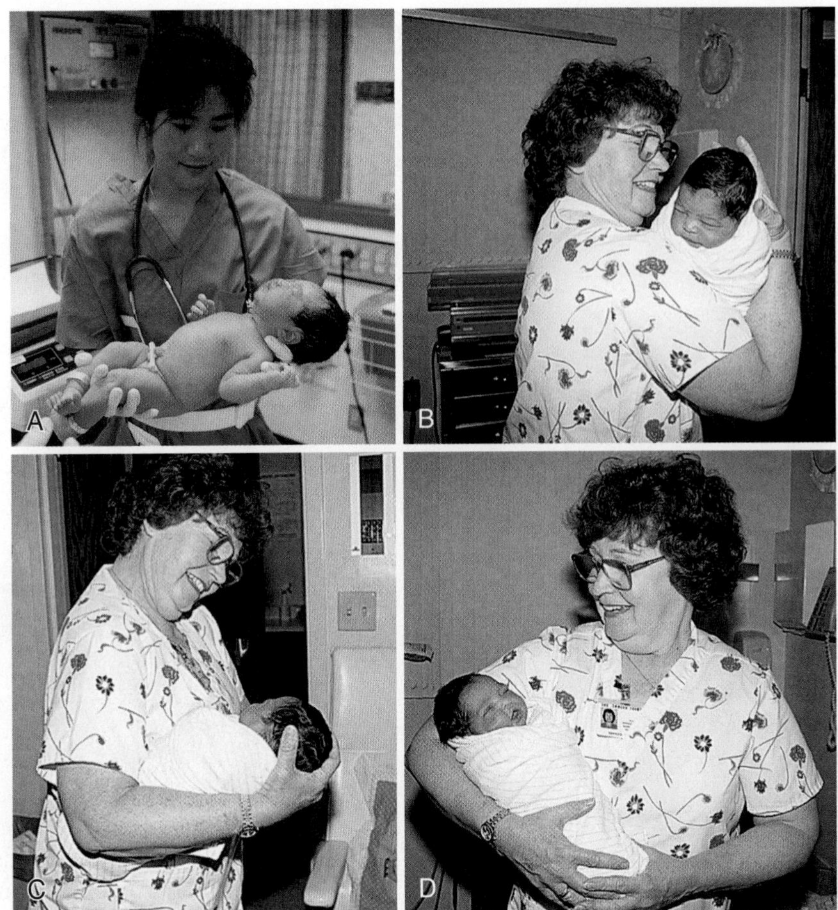

Fig. 28.11 Holding baby securely with support for head. A, Holding newborn while moving from one place to another. B, Holding newborn upright in burping position. C, Football hold. D, Cradle hold. (A, Courtesy Kim Malloy, Knoxville, IA. B–D, Courtesy Marjorie Pyle, RNC, LifeCircle, Costa Mesa, CA, in Lowdermilk DL, Perry SE, Cashion K, et al: *Maternity and women's health care,* ed 10, St. Louis, 2012, Mosby.)

If one leg appears longer or if the gluteal or popliteal folds are *asymmetric* (unequal in size or shape), congenital hip dysplasia may be suspected. The hips should move freely.

Also assess the feet for syndactyly or polydactyly. Creases should cover at least the anterior two-thirds of the sole. The feet may appear to be turned abnormally, often the result of the newborn's position in utero.

NURSING ASSESSMENT AND INTERVENTIONS FOR THE NEWBORN

HEALTH MANAGEMENT AND HEALTH PERCEPTION

Each time the baby is given to the mother, the identification must be checked to prevent giving the wrong baby to the wrong mother.

Instruct the mother about hand hygiene when caring for the baby to prevent the spread of microorganisms. Stress the importance of hand hygiene after performing personal care and before caring for the infant.

Instruct the new mother in safety practices to reduce the likelihood of injury to the infant. Education should include positions that provide head support to the infant during handling (Fig. 28.11). The mother must recognize the safety hazards of leaving the baby unattended in unsafe locations, such as the bed or changing table. To reduce the incidence of sudden infant death syndrome (SIDS), instruct parents to place babies on their back for sleeping. Include discussions concerning the risk to the infant from secondhand smoke. Babies exposed to smoke are more likely to die of SIDS. To prevent aspiration, the infant should not be placed immediately in the prone position after feeding (CDC, 2018). The environment should be kept free of hazards, such as pins or other sharp objects. Demonstrate bathing techniques and temperature taking. Bottles should never be propped for feeding, because this may lead to choking or aspiration. All 50 states have legislation mandating the use of car seats for infants (Governors Highway Safety Association, 2014).

NUTRITIONAL AND METABOLIC ISSUES

Each state has laws requiring that newborn screening testing be completed. The laws vary by state. These tests are done to detect conditions that result in serious complications, such as neurologic disorders and cognitive impairment. With early detection and proper

Table 28.6 **Standard Laboratory Results for a Full-Term Infant**[a]

PARAMETER	VALUE
Hematocrit	14–24 g/dL
Glucose	40–60 mg/dL
Bilirubin, direct	0–1 mg/dL
Hemoglobin	14–24 g/dL

[a]Heel-stick capillary blood.

treatment, many complications can be eliminated or reduced. Most of the diseases tested for involve inborn errors of metabolism in which the newborn is unable to metabolize various nutrients. Some of the more common tests are done to detect phenylketonuria, maple sugar urine disease, galactosemia, and hypothyroidism. These tests involve either blood or urine samples. For accurate results, the newborn must have consumed an adequate amount of nutrition (human milk or commercial infant formula preparation). This period is traditionally after 48 hours of age. Infants discharged before this period have an initial screening completed and are required to return for the remaining screening from 2 to 5 days of age. The parents must understand the importance of the tests and when the newborn is to be tested (Table 28.6).

Newborns have low prothrombin levels at birth and are at risk for hemorrhage. Because they are not able to synthesize vitamin K in the colon until they have adequate intestinal flora, a vitamin K injection (AquaMEPHYTON) is administered routinely. Injections are best administered in the vastus lateralis muscle, because it is more developed than the newborn's other muscles.

Monitor weight daily. A newborn normally loses up to 10% of body weight in the first week of life, from a combination of factors. More weight is lost through the passing of meconium and urine than is taken in by the newborn. This is particularly true in breast-fed babies. Most newborns regain their birth weight within the second week.

Nutritional Requirements

The healthy newborn needs approximately 120 kcal/kg of body weight each day. This includes proteins, carbohydrates, fats, vitamins, and minerals. Breast milk and prepared formulas are balanced to meet the newborn's needs. Because newborns cannot concentrate urine efficiently, fluid intake needs are high; 140 to 160 mL/kg/day is necessary (1 kg = 2.2 lb).

With the improved formulas available today, the infant's fluid and nutritional needs can be met with either breast-feeding or bottle feeding. The mother can choose the method she prefers. Provide support and teaching appropriate to the mother's chosen method.

Breast milk is produced in three stages. **Colostrum**, the first substance produced, is thin, watery, and slightly yellow. It is rich in protein and calories in addition to antibodies and lymphocytes. It also contains high levels of immunoglobulins, which transfer some immunity to the newborn. The mother begins producing colostrum in the last trimester of pregnancy and continues for 2 to 4 days after delivery; she then produces transitional milk for about 1 week. This milk may appear thinner and more watery but is high in fats, lactose, and water-soluble vitamins and contains more calories than colostrum. Mature milk generally is established by 2 weeks after delivery. This milk may appear very thin and watery. It provides 20 kcal/oz and contains lactose, proteins, minerals, and vitamins. If the mother is eating properly, only supplemental vitamin D may be needed. The primary care provider should be consulted.

Because human milk is designed uniquely to meet the needs of the human infant, it is used as the standard for all infant feedings. Infants who are not breast-fed should be given commercial formulas. Low-income families should be referred to WIC to determine their eligibility for services through the program, which provides iron-fortified infant formula.

Bovine milk (cow's milk) is the basis of most formulas. Infants with an allergic reaction to cow's milk formula may experience diarrhea, rash, colic, vomiting, and, in extreme cases, failure to thrive. Soy milk formula is acceptable for some of these infants, but others are allergic to soy protein. If hypersensitivity to cow's milk protein is suspected, a hydrolyzed casein formula may be effective; however, these special formulas are expensive.

Formulas are produced by modifying cow's milk to make it more similar to human milk. It appears thicker and richer but also contains 20 kcal/oz. Formulas are available in ready-to-feed, powdered, and concentrated forms. Instruct the mother in proper preparation and storage to prevent nutritional or digestive problems in her infant.

In bottle-fed infants, the first feeding is normally 15 to 30 mL of sterile water. This must be given with caution to verify that the infant is able to swallow normally and has no anomalies of the digestive tract. If the infant takes the water without difficulty, begin bottle feeding. Breast-fed newborns can be put to breast to nurse immediately after birth, without a sterile water feeding.

Regurgitation of mucus after the first few feedings is normal for infants. Food intake is necessary to prevent hypoglycemia, which is stressful to the newborn. Some facilities have a policy that requires a blood glucose determination test. Excessive maternal glucose results in fetal hyperglycemia and fetal hyperinsulinism. After birth, the neonate's high levels of insulin deplete the glucose stores, and hypoglycemia results. If the infant's blood glucose level is 40 mg/dL or less, sterile glucose water is given in the first hours after birth.

The frequency of feeding depends on the type of feeding. Breast-fed babies tend to do best on an "on demand" schedule, generally nursing at 2- to 3-hour intervals. Bottle-fed babies tend to eat less frequently, usually every 2 to 4 hours, because formula is digested more slowly. Each baby establishes a pattern over time. It is important not to overfeed, particularly with bottle-fed babies, because this can lead to regurgitation. Breast-fed infants are not normally given glucose water supplements, because doing so may interfere with the process of establishing lactation; the neonate may not be adequately hungry when put to breast. Exceptions may be made in cases in which the newborn's blood glucose is low.

Bottle-fed and breast-fed babies need to be burped at intervals. While sucking, the baby normally swallows air; if this air is not cleared from the stomach, the infant may feel satisfied and stop eating. When the air clears the stomach, the infant may again appear hungry.

Before starting, the mother should choose a feeding position that is comfortable and that facilitates the flow of milk into the infant's stomach. Many different positions are suitable for breast-feeding or bottle feeding (see Fig. 28.6).

Hypothermia

Maintenance of body temperature is a major concern in the care of newborns. Prolonged exposure to a cold environment can result in increased oxygen consumption and depleted glycogen reserves. Newborns have a relatively large surface area and a limited amount of protective adipose tissue. They lose heat through radiation, evaporation, conduction, and convection. Be aware of this and take precautions to reduce the losses (Table 28.7).

Monitor temperature with a skin sensor or thermometer. Verify that the anus is patent. The rectal method of temperature assessment is used rarely because of the chance of rectal irritation or perforation. Most facilities use the axillary route because it is considered safest. The normal axillary temperature is 97.6° to 98.6°F (36.4° to 37°C). Mercury thermometers are used rarely in health care settings today, although they may still be used in the home.

Table 28.7 Precautions to Minimize Heat Loss in Infants

TYPES OF HEAT LOSS	NURSING INTERVENTIONS TO PREVENT HEAT LOSS
Radiation: Loss that occurs when heat transfers from the body to cooler surfaces and objects not in contact with the body	Keep body well wrapped to prevent radiant loss. Work quickly to avoid excessive time with skin exposed. Use radiant warmer to minimize loss. Locate crib away from outside wall.
Evaporation: Loss when water is converted into a vapor	Dry infant thoroughly after delivery and promptly when bathing.
Conduction: Loss of heat to a cooler surface via direct skin contact	Pad surfaces under infant, including tables and scales. Warm other equipment, such as stethoscopes, before use.
Convection: Loss of heat to cooler air currents	Reduce drafts from open doors, windows, or air conditioning; wrap newborn to protect from cold.

Hygiene

Inspection and bathing of the neonate take place after the body temperature has stabilized. The frequency and type of baths depend on facility policies. Bathing serves a number of purposes: complete cleansing, observation of the infant's condition, comfort, and parent-child socialization.

Gather all bathing articles and the infant's change of clothing before bathing. The room temperature should be 75°F (24°C), and the bathing area should be free of drafts to prevent heat loss. The bath water should be approximately 100°F (38°C). Heat loss in the infant is greater than heat loss in the adult because of the relatively large ratio of the skin surface to body mass in the newborn. To conserve the infant's energy, control heat loss by bathing the infant quickly, padding cold surfaces, exposing only a portion of the body at a time, and thoroughly drying the infant. Until the initial bath is completed, wear gloves when handling the newborn.

The Centers for Disease Control and Prevention regulations related to standard precautions against human immunodeficiency virus and other bloodborne pathogens have increased the use of soap solutions for bathing newborn infants. Use a nonmedicated mild soap for the initial bath. Shampoo the hair and use a brush or a comb to remove dried blood and vernix caseosa. Use cotton balls, not gauze, to cleanse the nostrils and ears. Careful drying reduces the heat lost during bathing. The order of the bath is essentially the same as for an adult, beginning with the eyes, the face, and the head and ending with the anal region. Do not vigorously remove vernix caseosa (the white material that looks like cold cream), because it is attached to the upper, protective layer of the skin. Vernix caseosa may be left on for 48 hours; if it persists beyond that time, wash it off gently. Some nurses advocate massaging the vernix caseosa gently into the skin. No studies have confirmed the benefits or disadvantages of this technique.

Reassess the temperature 30 minutes after completion of the bath.

After the initial bath, washing with warm water is sufficient for the first week. Full submersion into a tub of water should not be done until the cord has fallen off. The infant's skin is thin and delicate. The infant's fragile skin can be injured by vigorous cleansing. Daily bathing is not needed; however, the perineal area should be washed carefully with nonmedicated mild soap and warm water and carefully dried with each diaper change. Parents may make personal decisions about the brand and type of cleaning agents used. Recommendations are that oils and scented products should be avoided.

After the bath, talc use should be limited because it may cause aspiration if too close to the nose and mouth.

Discuss the choice of cloth or disposable diapers with parents. Cloth diapers today are different from those used years ago with plastic or rubber pants. Exclusive use of disposable diapers is the most expensive and most popular method. Over 1 or 2 years, the cost can be considerable, particularly if more than one child is wearing diapers. However, some disposable diapers may help prevent diaper dermatitis.

Pay special attention to care of the umbilical area. At delivery, the cord is moist. Over the next few days, a drying process called *mummification* (producing a dry, hard mass) begins. Avoid getting the cord wet during bathing. Most facilities have a routine to promote drying with use of alcohol or other substances (triple dye) that inhibit microbial growth. Odor or exudate from the cord is abnormal and should be reported promptly. Delay tub bathing until the fully dried cord drops off at about 10 days of age.

Give the mother a demonstration of temperature taking and bathing the newborn. If possible, encourage her to bathe the infant while you observe. This helps her gain confidence and provides an opportunity to answer questions about care. It is also a good time to demonstrate safe methods of holding and positioning the infant.

Circumcision refers to the surgical removal of the foreskin. Many parents elect to have the procedure performed on their newborn infant. A review of the procedure's rates for 1997 to 2010 showed an overall decline. The national rate in 1997 was 64.5% and in 2010 it was 58.3%. There are regional differences across the country. Rates of circumcision are highest in the southern and midwestern states and lowest in the west. The reasons parents opt to have their sons circumcised are varied. Some parents choose circumcision to follow "family tradition," and others out of concern for their son's reproductive health. The Jewish faith promotes the circumcision of infant boys. Jewish families who follow the time-honored ritual of their faith opt to have the circumcision performed 7 days after birth. The procedure is performed in a religious ceremony by a religious figure. The American Academy of Pediatrics (AAP) reported in 1999 that acknowledged health benefits were associated with circumcision but that these benefits were not significant enough to warrant a recommendation to mandate this procedure for all male infants. In 2012 the AAP again reaffirmed this position (American Academy of Pediatrics, 2012). The AAP further states that analgesia should be used if a circumcision is performed; a consent form for both is required.

If circumcision is performed, keep the area clean and assess it for bleeding every hour for the first 12 hours after surgery. Apply gentle pressure to the bleeding area with a folded gauze pad. Sterile petroleum gauze usually is applied to the penis after a Gomco or Mogen circumcision and is left in place for 24 hours; it is replaced if it becomes dislodged prematurely. If a Plastibell circumcision is performed, the petroleum gauze is not needed, because the plastic bell that covers the glans does not stick to the diaper.

Wash the penis gently at diaper changes to remove urine and feces, and reapply fresh sterile petroleum gauze. Do not attempt to remove the dried yellow exudate that forms in 24 hours and persists for 2 to 3 days; this is part of the normal healing process. Some practitioners may recommend the use of cloth diapers during the first week to promote healing. Loose diapering is necessary. If bleeding is not controlled, continue application of intermittent pressure, notify the physician, and prepare for blood vessel ligation. If the infant has undergone this procedure without anesthesia, he should be comforted until he is quieted and then returned to his crib. These infants usually are fussy for about 2 to 3 hours and may refuse a feeding.

Teach the parents appropriate home care before discharge of the newborn. Teaching should include measures to promote hygiene and thus reduce the risks of infection. Educate the parents to report immediately any unusual signs and symptoms such as edema; purulent, malodorous discharge; elevated temperature; and delayed healing.

ELIMINATION

The newborn should void within 24 hours of delivery. If this does not occur, notify the physician. The average newborn voids small amounts of poorly concentrated urine; it is normally clear and odorless. Occasionally, a small pink or brownish discharge may be observed as a result of uric acid crystals that were formed in the bladder in utero. As fluid intake increases and kidney function improves, urination becomes more frequent and assumes the normal color.

Bowel elimination should occur within 24 hours of birth. The newborn's initial stools are odorless, black-green, and sticky. This is called **meconium** and is made up of vernix, strands of lanugo, mucus, and other substances from the amniotic fluid. Occasionally, the first stool is encased in mucus and called a *meconium plug*. If no stool is observed, notify the physician so that an examination can be performed to determine the problem. Once the infant begins to take nourishment, the stool changes. Transitional stools, which occur on about the second day, tend to be greenish and loose. These are seen until about the fourth day, when the milk stool is seen. Breast-fed babies tend to pass stool frequently, sometimes with every feeding. The stool is pale yellow and sweet smelling. Small curds may be observed. Babies who are bottle fed tend to have fewer stools, usually two or three per day after the first 2 weeks. These are bright yellow and pasty in consistency; the odor may be slightly stronger than that of breast-fed babies. This type of stool continues until solid food is introduced. Very watery stools, green stools (after the

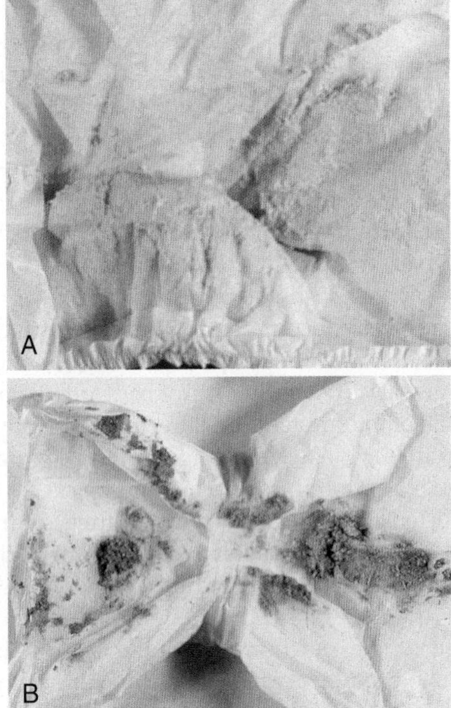

Fig. 28.12 Infant stool. A, Breast-fed. B, Formula fed. (From Zitelli BJ, McIntire SC, Nowalk AJ: *Zitelli and Davis' atlas of pediatric physical diagnosis*, ed 6, St. Louis, 2012, Saunders.)

transition), or stools expelled with force may indicate gastrointestinal irritation or infection and should be reported promptly (Fig. 28.12). Newborns can lose a great deal of fluid rapidly and become dehydrated (see Box 28.14 for stooling patterns of newborns). (Note that newborns normally give the impression of straining with a stool because their muscles are underdeveloped. This can cause parents undue concern if they are not advised about it. The straining subsides as growth and maturity continue.)

The skin of the perineum and buttocks can become irritated if waste products are left in contact for too long. Teach the parents to wash the skin, wiping from anterior to posterior, after each voiding or stool, and to change diapers promptly. Recommend minimal use of creams, which can irritate the skin. Disposable or cloth diapers may be chosen.

REST AND SLEEP

Most newborns spend 16 to 20 hours per day sleeping. They may be observed to startle and make sucking motions during sleep. Breathing may be regular and even or irregular, depending on the sleep state. The time awake is spent crying, eating, or in quiet alertness. Each infant establishes a unique pattern, which may be erratic but stabilizes over time as the nervous and digestive systems mature. Most infants do not exceed 5 continuous hours of sleep for some months, which can be disruptive to the sleep of others in the household.

Box 28.14 Change in Stooling of Newborns

MECONIUM

- Infant's first stool is composed of amniotic fluid and its constituents, intestinal secretions, shed mucosal cells, and possibly blood (ingested maternal blood or minor bleeding of alimentary tract vessels).
- Passage of meconium should occur within the first 24 to 48 hours, although it may be delayed up to 7 days in very low-birth-weight infants.
- Colostrum has a laxative effect that aids the infant to expel the meconium.

TRANSITIONAL STOOLS

- Transitional stools usually appear by the third day after initiation of feeding.
- They are greenish brown to yellowish brown, thin, and less sticky than meconium; they may contain some milk curds.

MILK STOOL

- Milk stools usually appear by the fourth day.
- In *breast-fed* infants, stools are yellow to golden, are pasty in consistency, and have an odor similar to that of sour milk.
- In *formula-fed* infants, stools are pale yellow to light brown, are firmer in consistency, and have a more offensive odor.

ACTIVITY AND EXERCISE

Maintenance of a clear airway is critical. Many infants need suctioning to remove mucus from the nose and mouth. Newborns are obligate (necessary or required) nose breathers; they must be able to breathe through the nose while suckling. Therefore the nasal passageway must be kept open and free from mucus. A small bulb syringe commonly is used. Compress it before insertion and then gently release it to suction secretions. Explain to parents the use of the bulb syringe before the first feeding. For the first few days, a bulb syringe always should be kept with the newborn, particularly during feeding.

Crying is the newborn's only means of communication. The cry can indicate hunger, pain, the need for attention, or fussiness. The newborn's cry should be strong, vigorous, and of medium pitch. As mother and infant become more adept at interpreting each other's behavior, some mothers can distinguish the reason for crying. The following report indicates that mother and baby are communicating effectively:

> I can tell when she's hungry. Crying starts in a plaintive [sorrowful, sad] way and then becomes more and more demanding. When she is hurt, she lets out a startled yell as though she couldn't believe it was happening to her. Sometimes when she is put down to sleep, she starts a kind of talking cry, jerky and demanding; it gets louder, and if nothing happens, fades away in little spurts. The fussy cry is the hardest to take—nothing seems to work; like a complaining that goes on and on.

A high-pitched cry may indicate neurologic problems and should be observed further and evaluated by a physician. See the Patient Teaching box for infant quieting techniques.

Patient Teaching

Infant Quieting Techniques

- Many newborns feel insecure in the center of a large crib. They prefer a small, warm, soft space that reminds them of intrauterine life. Try a smaller bed, such as a bassinet, portable crib, buggy, or cradle, or use a rolled-up blanket to turn a corner of the big crib into a smaller place.
- Carry baby in a front pack or backpack.
- Swaddle newborn snugly in a receiving blanket. Swaddling keeps the newborn's arms and legs close to his or her body, similar to the intrauterine position. It makes the newborn feel more secure. Swaddling never should be used when a baby is not placed on the back to sleep. Swaddling is viewed as safe for the first 2 months of life (Healthychildren.org, 2017).
- Prewarm the crib sheets with a hot water bottle or heating pad that is removed before putting the baby to bed. Some babies startle when placed on a cold sheet.
- Some newborns need extra sucking to soothe themselves to sleep. Breast-feeding mothers may prefer to let their infant suckle at the breast as a soothing technique. Other mothers choose to use a pacifier. Stroke the pacifier against the roof of the baby's mouth to encourage him or her to suck it during the first 2 weeks. Around age 3 months, infants can find and suck their thumbs as a way of self-consoling.
- A rhythmic, monotonous noise that simulates the intrauterine sounds of the maternal heartbeat and blood flow may help the infant settle down. Some parents have found it helpful to put a fussy baby in a portable crib beside the dishwasher or washing machine.
- Movement often helps quiet a baby. Take the baby for a ride in the car or an outing in a stroller or carriage. Rock the baby in a rocking chair or cradle.
- Place the baby on his or her stomach across the lap; pat and rub the back while gently bouncing legs or swaying them from left to right.
- Babies enjoy skin-to-skin contact. A combination of this and warm water often helps soothe a fussy baby. Fill the tub with warm water. Get in and let the baby lie on the chest so that the baby is immersed in the water up to his or her neck. Cuddle the baby.
- Let the baby see your face. Talk in a soothing voice.
- The baby may simply need more stimulation. Bring him or her into the room where the family is gathered. Change the baby's position; many babies like to be upright, such as being held up on the shoulder.

PARENT-CHILD ATTACHMENT

The human infant is born defenseless and could not survive without a caregiver. The parents are responsible for the infant's physical and psychological development.

Parenting is not instinctive; a new parent must bond with the baby first. **Parent-child attachment (bonding)** is defined as the initial phase in a relationship characterized by strong attraction and a desire to interact (Fig. 28.13). Without bonding, parents find the energy needed to meet the newborn's needs difficult to maintain. The nurse cannot make bonding occur but can facilitate its development.

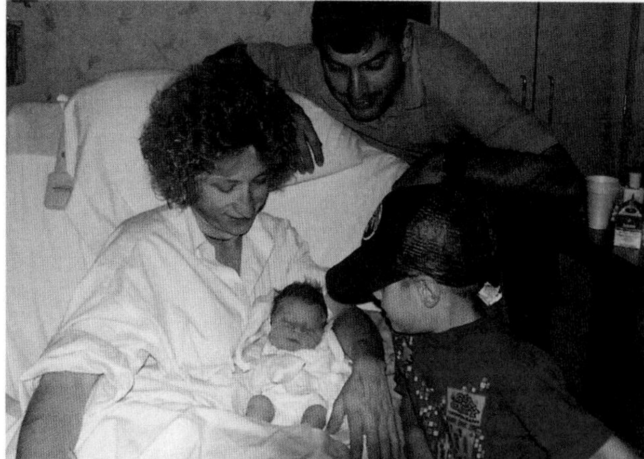

Fig. 28.13 Parents and sibling interacting with a newborn.

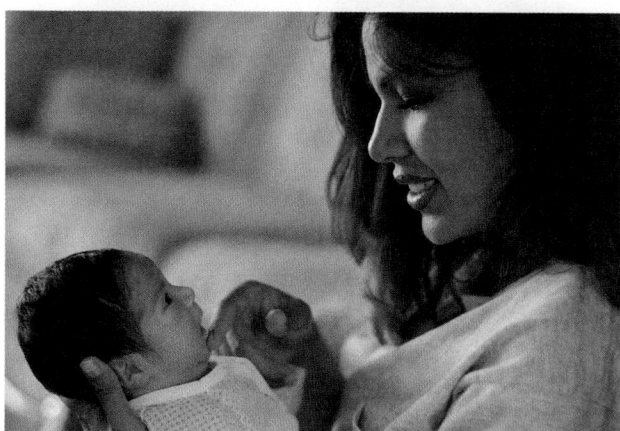

Fig. 28.14 The infant is quiet and alert during the initial sensitive period. The newborn gazes at the mother and responds to her voice and touch. (From McKinney ES, Murray SS: *Foundations of maternal-newborn nursing,* ed 5, Philadelphia, 2010, Saunders.)

Early contact with the infant is important to establish bonding. A new mother normally wishes to touch and explore her baby. Holding the infant close and looking eye to eye (the en face position) helps bonding occur (Fig. 28.14). It is normal for a new mother to talk in high-pitched tones to the baby. Encourage early and frequent interaction between the newborn and the parents (Fig. 28.15). Attachment increases when the infant begins to respond.

The newborn has amazing capabilities. The infant is a socially responsive human who can probably learn better on the first day of life than ever again. Immediately after birth, the baby stares intently at the parents' faces and sees them. In fact, the newborn prefers looking at the mother's face, especially the eyes, to looking at other objects. The newborn also can recognize an approaching

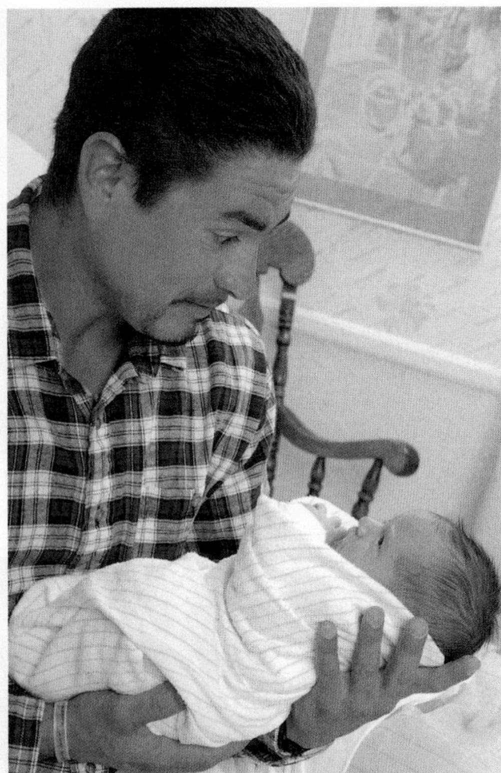

Fig. 28.15 The behavior of fathers at initial contact with their infant often corresponds to maternal behaviors. The intense fascination that fathers exhibit is called engrossment. Note eye-to-eye contact between father and infant. (From McKinney ES, Murray SS: *Foundations of maternal-newborn nursing*, ed 5, Philadelphia, 2010, Saunders.)

object as a threat and turns away to avoid it. He or she reaches for an object and usually comes close to touching it. The newborn imitates another person's facial expressions, such as sticking out the tongue, opening the mouth, and pursing the lips. Newborn babies are active stimulus seekers where repetition and the level of stimulation are important. The baby can shut out stimuli and may even turn his or her head at the sound of the mother's voice.

Indeed, babies are not passive and unresponsive creatures to be hurried off to the hospital nursery after birth. The affectionate bond between parents and child begins at the moment of birth (see Figs. 28.13 and 28.15). As long as the newborn is responding normally, immediate skin-to-skin contact with the parents is important in bonding. The newborn has difficulty opening the eyes under bright spotlights but looks around if the lights are dimmed. (If necessary, dim the main lights in the delivery area and keep a light focused over the perineum for episiotomy repair or other procedures.) Shielding the infant's face with a hand or a blanket also provides enough protection from the light to encourage the baby to open the eyes. Objects are in clearest range for the newborn at about 8 to 10 inches. Newborns prefer faces over other patterns. Refraining from using prophylactic eye drops and weighing and measuring the baby for 30 minutes to 1 hour after birth allows the parents time alone with their baby so that the attachment process can proceed without interruption. The mother may wish to breast-feed in the first hour after birth; the nurse or the father can assist her.

Periods of quiet alertness are best for interaction. Explain the different levels of alertness to the parents so that they can recognize them. Time care so that the mother is available to enjoy quiet moments with her newborn.

Patient problems for the newborn infant may include the following:

- *Inability to Maintain Adequate Breathing Pattern*
- *Inability to Regulate Body Temperature*
- *Potential for Infection*
- *Potential for Injury*
- *Potential or Inability to Clear Airway*
- *Recent Onset of Pain*

Get Ready for the NCLEX® Examination!

Key Points

- During the 6 weeks after delivery, the reproductive organs return to approximately the prepregnant size and location.
- The new mother should avoid dieting and excessive activity during the early postpartum period.
- Postpartum fatigue and depression are common as a result of hormonal and physiologic changes.
- Complications can occur during the postpartum period. Each woman must be assessed carefully.
- Before discharge, provide instruction concerning the danger signs of the postpartum period and verify that the woman knows when and how to contact her physician.
- Hormonal changes enable the woman to produce enough milk to meet the nutritional needs of the growing infant. Nutritional needs of the lactating woman are similar to those during pregnancy.
- Motherhood is a learned skill. The new mother needs extensive teaching and encouragement about parenting skills.
- Early discharge necessitates that the nurse provide essential teaching in a brief period. Be careful to document teaching.
- Supplement teaching with written materials so that the new mother has something to refer to when at home.
- Conduct assessment of the newborn in a head-to-toe format. Thoroughly review each body system.

- Newborns exhibit a wide range of normal variation. Verify any questionable observations with another nurse or physician.
- Hypothermia and infection are two major areas of concern in care of the newborn.
- Circumcision is an elective surgical procedure.
- The newborn has social and physical needs.
- Injuries to the cervix can have adverse effects on future pregnancies. Repair should be immediate.
- In preparing the transfer report, the recovery nurse uses information from the admission record, the birth record, and the recovery record.
- In helping new families adjust to parenthood, provide culturally sensitive care following principles that facilitate nursing practice within transcultural situations.
- Infant abduction from hospitals in the United States has been on the increase. Parents and nurses must work together to ensure the safety of newborns in the hospital environment.
- Provide demonstration and teaching to educate the mother about the newborn's hygiene needs.
- Whether or not this is the couple's first baby, parents appreciate anticipatory guidance in the care of their child.
- Parent-child attachment (bonding) is the process by which parent and child come to love and accept each other.

Additional Learning Resources

SG Go to your Study Guide for additional learning activities to help you master this chapter content.

evolve Be sure to visit the Evolve site at *http://evolve.elsevier.com/Cooper/foundationsadult/* for additional online resources.

Review Questions for the NCLEX® Examination

1. A primigravida has delivered a baby vaginally after 6 hours of labor. She had an uneventful pregnancy and is in good general health. She is transferred from the recovery room to the postpartum unit. What interventions are included in routine postpartum care? *(Select all that apply.)*
   1. Assessment of intake and output until the patient is voiding in sufficient quantities
   2. Insertion of a catheter to assess residual urine after the initial voiding
   3. Firm massage of the fundus every 15 minutes
   4. Assessment of the emotional status of the new mother
   5. Checking of breasts for engorgement and cracking of nipples
2. The nurse is performing a routine postpartum assessment. Which action is indicated before the fundal height is measured?
   1. Massage the uterus.
   2. Apply pressure to the fundus to check for clots.
   3. Elevate the head of the bed.
   4. Ask the patient to empty her bladder.
3. The nurse finds bright red bleeding on a patient's peripad. The stain is about 6 inches long. What is the correct description of the character and amount of lochia?
   1. Lochia rubra, moderate
   2. Lochia serosa, heavy
   3. Lochia rubra, heavy
   4. Lochia serosa, light
4. The nurse is teaching breast care for the lactating woman. What information should be included? *(Select all that apply.)*
   1. Expose the nipples to air for 20 to 30 minutes daily.
   2. Wear a supportive bra 24 hours a day for the first few weeks.
   3. Wash breasts and nipples with soap and water before each feeding.
   4. Use plastic liners in bras.
   5. Use ice packs every 4 hours as needed for discomfort associated with engorgement.
5. A woman asks the nurse how she will know her baby is getting enough milk. The nurse's response is based on understanding that which is the best determinant?
   1. The baby awakens every 4 to 6 hours to eat.
   2. The baby stops nursing when full.
   3. The baby has 6 to 10 wet diapers per day.
   4. The baby cries when hungry.
6. In evaluating maternal adjustment, which behavior leads the nurse to believe that the patient is still in the taking-in phase? *(Select all that apply.)*
   1. The mother states she is "starving" and can't wait to eat.
   2. The majority of the mother's time is spent talking about her delivery experience.
   3. The mother takes a shower and washes her hair.
   4. The mother asks the nurse to teach her how to give her baby a bath.
   5. The mother reports she feels as if she needs to get more rest.
7. A baby boy is 1 hour old when admitted to the newborn nursery. He weighs 7 lb, 3 oz; is 21 inches long; has irregular respirations of 42 breaths/min with adequate chest movement, a heart rate of 145 beats/min, and a temperature of 35.6°C, axillary; and is acrocyanotic. What is an appropriate goal for this baby within the next 2 hours, based on these findings?
   1. Color will remain unchanged.
   2. Respirations will slow.
   3. Temperature will stabilize at 36.5° to 37°C.
   4. Heart rate will decrease to 100 beats/min.
8. When teaching parents how to bathe their baby, which point should the nurse stress?
   1. Avoid immersing the baby in water until after the umbilical cord has fallen off.
   2. Use only mild medicated or scented soap.
   3. Apply baby powder after the bath to keep the skin dry.
   4. Apply baby oil after the bath to keep the skin soft and smooth.

9. When providing education to parents about care of the umbilical cord, what information should be included? *(Select all that apply.)*
   1. Cleaning the cord with an alcohol swab
   2. Keeping the diaper folded below the cord
   3. Applying triple dye to the cord
   4. Keeping the cord moist to promote healing
   5. Oiling the cord to facilitate it falling off
10. A baby has a Gomco circumcision. What instruction should the nurse give his parents for care of the circumcised penis?
    1. Soak the penis in warm water daily.
    2. Cover the glans with a petroleum gauze dressing.
    3. Clean the glans with alcohol to promote healing.
    4. Remove any yellowish exudate that forms within 24 hours.
11. On examining a woman who gave birth 5 hours previously, the nurse finds that the woman has saturated a perineal pad within 15 minutes. What action is the nurse's first priority?
    1. Increase the drip rate of an IV infusion of Ringer's lactate solution.
    2. Assess the patient's vital signs.
    3. Call the patient's primary health care provider.
    4. Palpate the woman's fundus.
12. A woman gave birth 48 hours ago to a healthy baby girl. She has decided to bottle feed. During the assessment, the nurse notices that both breasts are swollen, warm, and tender on palpation. The patient should be advised that this is best treated with which action?
    1. Running warm water over her breasts during a shower
    2. Applying ice to the breasts for comfort
    3. Expressing small amounts of milk from the breasts to relieve pressure
    4. Wearing a loose-fitting bra to prevent nipple irritation
    5. Wearing a snug bra
13. A first-time mother is to be discharged from the hospital tomorrow with her baby girl. Which maternal behavior indicates a need for further intervention by the nurse before she can be discharged?
    1. The mother leaves the baby on her bed while she takes a shower.
    2. The mother continues to hold and cuddle her baby after she has fed her.
    3. The mother reads a magazine while her baby sleeps.
    4. The mother changes her baby's diaper, then shows the nurse the contents of the diaper.
14. The nurse observes several interactions between a postpartum woman and her new son. Which behavior, if exhibited by this woman, does the nurse identify as maladaptive regarding parent-infant attachment?
    1. The mother talks and coos to her son.
    2. The mother seldom makes eye contact with her son.
    3. The mother cuddles her son close to her.
    4. The mother tells visitors how well her son is feeding.
15. The nurse can help a father in his transition to parenthood with what action?
    1. Pointing out that the infant turned to his voice
    2. Encouraging him to go home to get some sleep
    3. Taping the baby's diaper a different way
    4. Suggesting that he let the baby sleep in the bassinet
16. A breast-feeding mother reports to the nurse that her breasts are very firm and tender. What information should be included in the response by the nurse? *(Select all that apply.)*
    1. "Avoiding breast-feeding for several hours will be helpful."
    2. "Let's try to apply lettuce leaves to your breasts."
    3. "This is known as engorgement."
    4. "More frequent breast-feeding will be helpful in managing this condition."
    5. "Let's take off your bra for a few hours."
17. The nurse helps the breast-feeding woman change her newborn's diaper after the baby's first bowel movement. The mother expresses concern because of a large amount of sticky, dark green—almost black—stool. She asks the nurse if something is wrong. What information should be included in the nurse's response?
    1. Tell the woman not to worry because all breast-fed babies have this type of stool.
    2. Explain that this type of stool is called meconium and is expected for the first few bowel movements of all newborns.
    3. Ask the woman what she ate at her last meal before giving birth.
    4. Suggest that the mother ask her pediatrician to explain newborn stool patterns.

Care of the High-Risk Mother, Newborn, and Family With Special Needs

29

http://evolve.elsevier.com/Cooper/foundationsadult/

Objectives

1. List conditions that increase maternal and fetal risk.
2. Compare and contrast abruptio placentae and placenta previa, noting signs and symptoms, complications, and nursing and medical management.
3. Identify diagnostic tests used to determine high-risk situations.
4. Compare and contrast hypertensive disorders experienced during pregnancy.
5. Identify preexisting maternal health conditions that influence pregnancy.
6. List the infectious diseases most likely to cause serious complications.
7. Discuss the care of the pregnant adolescent.
8. Discuss the problems created by alcohol and drug abuse.
9. Identify concerns related to preterm infants.
10. Explain the hemolytic diseases of the newborn.
11. Discuss patient problems related to high-risk conditions of the mother and the newborn.
12. Identify nursing interventions for the pregnant woman with a cardiac disorder.
13. Explain the care of a pregnant woman with a pulmonary disorder.

Key Terms

anasarca (ăn-ă-SĂR-kă, p. 890)
atony (ĂT-ō-nē, p. 888)
brown fat (p. 909)
cerclage (sĕr-KLĂHZH, p. 883)
direct Coombs' test (p. 912)
dizygotic (dī-zī-GŎT-ĭk, p. 879)
eclampsia (ĕ-KLĂMP-sē-ă, p. 890)
erythroblastosis fetalis (ĕ-rĭth-rō-blăs-TŌ-sĭs fĕ-TĂL-ĭs, p. 911)
gestational diabetes mellitus (GDM) (jĕs-TĀ-shŭn-ăl dī-ă-BĒ-tēz MĔL-ĭ-tŭs, p. 897)
gestational hypertension (GH) (jĕs-TĀ-shŭn-ăl hī-pĕr-TĔN-shŭn, p. 890)
glycosylated hemoglobin (glī-KŌ-sĭ-lāt-ĕd HĒ-mō-glō-bĭn, p. 898)
high-risk pregnancy (p. 877)
hydramnios (hī-DRĂM-nē-ŏs, p. 888)
hyperbilirubinemia (hī-pĕr-bĭl-ĭ-rū-bĭ-NĒ-mē-ă, p. 912)
incompetent cervix (p. 883)
indirect Coombs' test (p. 912)
infant mortality (p. 875)
kernicterus (kĕr-NĬK-tĕr-ŭs, p. 912)
kick count (p. 892)
monozygotic (mŏn-ō-zī-GŎT-ĭk, p. 879)
morbidity (p. 877)
phototherapy (p. 912)
placental barrier (plă-SĔN-tăl, p. 911)
preeclampsia (prē-ĕ-KLĂMP-sē-ă, p. 890)
severe preeclampsia (p. 890)
TORCH (p. 895)

One of the indicators considered in the health of the nation is the rate of **infant mortality** (the number of infants who die within the first year of life, expressed as the number per thousand live births). The infant mortality rate is higher in the United States than in many other countries in the world. The last available ranking for this statistic placed the country 30th in line for this statistic (Centers for Disease Control [CDC], 2009). This number is troubling in a nation considered a super power. Approximately 4 million babies are born in the United States each year. The mortality rate is 5.6 per 1000 live births. Factors primarily associated with mortality rates are prematurity and low birth weight, birth defects, maternal complications, sudden infant death syndrome, and injuries (Statista, 2018). Nearly 10% of babies are born prematurely (CDC, 2017b). The rate of low–birth weight babies is 8.07% (CDC, 2017a). Prevention of morbidity and mortality among mothers and infants depends on identification of the risk, along with appropriate and timely intervention during the perinatal period.

With the changing demographics in the United States, more women and families are at risk for complications because of nonphysiologic factors. For example, increasing numbers of homeless, single, and uninsured pregnant women have no access to prenatal care during any stage of pregnancy. Behaviors and lifestyles that pose a risk to the health of the mother and fetus also contribute to the problem (Box 29.1).

Although most pregnancies proceed normally, complications and high-risk situations can occur at any stage of the childbearing process. Be aware of these so that you can take appropriate, timely action (see the Cultural Considerations box on high-risk pregnancies).

Box 29.1 Classification of High-Risk Factors of Pregnancy

BIOPHYSICAL

- *Genetic considerations:* Genetic factors may interfere with normal fetal or neonatal development, result in congenital anomalies, or create difficulties for the mother.
- *Nutritional status:* Adequate nutrition, without which fetal growth and development cannot proceed normally, is one of the most important determinants of pregnancy outcome.
- *Medical and obstetric disorders:* Complications of current and past pregnancies, obstetric-related illnesses, and pregnancy losses put the patient at risk.

PSYCHOSOCIAL

- *Smoking:* A strong, consistent, causal relationship has been established between maternal smoking and reduced birth weight.
- *Caffeine:* Birth defects in humans have not been related to caffeine consumption. High intake (three or more cups of coffee per day) has been related to a slight decrease in birth weight.
- *Alcohol:* Alcohol exerts adverse effects on the fetus, resulting in fetal alcohol syndrome, fetal alcohol effects, learning disabilities, and hyperactivity.
- *Drugs:* The developing fetus may be affected adversely by drugs through several mechanisms. Drugs can cause metabolic disturbances, produce chemical effects, or depress or alter central nervous system function. This category includes medications prescribed by a health care provider or bought over the counter, and commonly abused drugs such as heroin, cocaine, and marijuana.
- *Psychological status:* Childbearing triggers profound and complex physiologic, psychological, and social changes, with evidence to suggest a relationship between emotional distress and birth complications. This risk factor includes conditions such as specific intrapsychic disturbances and addictive lifestyles.

SOCIODEMOGRAPHIC

- *Low income:* Poverty underlies many other risk factors and leads to inadequate financial resources for food and prenatal care, poor general health, increased risk of medical complications of pregnancy, and greater prevalence of adverse environmental influences.
- *Lack of prenatal care:* Failure to diagnose and treat complications early is a major risk factor that arises from financial barriers or lack of access to care; cultural beliefs that do not support this need; and fear of the health care system and its providers.
- *Age:* Women at both ends of the childbearing age spectrum have a higher incidence of poor outcomes; however, age may not be a risk factor in all cases.
- *Adolescents:* More complications are seen in young mothers (less than 15 years old), who have a 60% higher mortality rate than those over age 20 years, and in pregnancies that occur less than 3 years after menarche. Complications include anemia, gestational hypertension (GH), prolonged labor, and contracted pelvis and cephalopelvic disproportion. Long-term social implications of early motherhood are lower educational status, lower income, increased dependence on government support programs, higher divorce rates, and higher parity.
- *Mature mothers:* The risks to mothers over 35 years old are not from age alone but from other considerations, such as number and spacing of previous pregnancies, genetic disposition of the parents, medical history, lifestyle, nutrition, and prenatal care. Medical conditions more likely to be experienced by mature women include hypertension and GH, diabetes, extended labor, cesarean birth, placenta previa, abruptio placentae, and death. Her fetus is at greater risk for low birth weight.
- *Parity:* The number of previous pregnancies is a risk factor that is associated with age and includes all first pregnancies, especially a first pregnancy at either end of the childbearing age spectrum. The incidence of GH and dystocia is higher with a first birth.
- *Marital status:* The increased mortality and morbidity rates for unmarried women, including a greater risk for GH, often are related to inadequate prenatal care and a younger childbearing age.
- *Residence:* The availability and quality of prenatal care varies widely with geographic residence. Women in metropolitan areas have more prenatal visits than those in rural areas, who have fewer opportunities for specialized care and consequently a higher incidence of maternal mortality.
- *Ethnicity:* Although ethnicity is not a major risk factor, race is an indicator of other sociodemographic risk factors. Nonwhite women are more than three times as likely as white women to die of pregnancy-related causes. Black babies have the highest rates of prematurity and low birth weight, with an infant mortality rate more than double that for whites.

ENVIRONMENTAL

- Various environmental substances can affect fertility and fetal development, the chance of a live birth, and the child's subsequent mental and physical development. Environmental influences include infections; radiation; chemicals such as pesticides, therapeutic drugs, illicit drugs, industrial pollutants, and cigarette smoke; stress; and diet.
- Paternal exposure to mutagenic agents in the workplace has been associated with an increased risk of spontaneous abortion.

Box 29.2 Factors That Place the Postpartum Patient and the Newborn at Risk

MOTHER
- Hemorrhage
- Traumatic labor or birth
- Infection
- Psychosocial factors
- Abnormal vital signs
- Previous medical conditions (e.g., diabetes, cardiovascular disease)

INFANT (FACTORS FOR ADMISSION TO NEONATAL INTENSIVE CARE UNIT)
High-Risk Category
- Continuing or developing signs of respiratory distress syndrome
- Asphyxiation (Apgar score, 6 at 5 minutes); resuscitation necessary at birth
- Preterm infants
- Cyanosis or suspected cardiovascular disease; persistent cyanosis
- Major congenital malformations that necessitate surgery; chromosomal anomalies
- Convulsions, sepsis, hemorrhagic diathesis (constitutional predisposition to certain disease conditions), or shock
- Meconium aspiration syndrome
- Central nervous system depression for longer than 24 hours
- Hypoglycemia
- Hypocalcemia
- Hyperbilirubinemia

Moderate-Risk Category
- Dysmaturity (premature weight between 2000 and 2500 g)
- Apgar score of less than 5 at 1 minute
- Feeding problems
- Multifetal birth
- Transient tachypnea
- Hypomagnesemia or hypermagnesemia
- Hypoparathyroidism
- Jitteriness or hyperactivity
- Cardiac anomalies that do not necessitate immediate catheterization
- Heart murmur
- Anemia
- Central nervous system depression for less than 24 hours

Provided care must offer concern and protection for the welfare of the mother and the child.

COMPLICATIONS OF PREGNANCY

All members of the obstetric team and other medical personnel collaborate closely to care for the patient at high risk. A **high-risk pregnancy** is one in which the life or health of the mother or the infant is jeopardized by a health concern. The condition may be preexisting, or it may be the result of pregnancy. For the mother, the high-risk status extends (based on medical judgment) through the puerperium (6 weeks after delivery). Postdelivery maternal complications usually are resolved within a month, but perinatal **morbidity** (state of having disease) may continue for months or years.

A better understanding of human reproduction has greatly reduced morbidity and mortality (quality or state of being subject to death). Knowledge about fetal and neonatal disorders has increased dramatically in the past 15 to 25 years. As a result, infant mortality rates have decreased, with a drop from 26 per 1000 live births in 1960 to the just less than 6 deaths per 1000 live births in 2014. However, less significant improvements have occurred in perinatal morbidity and mortality rates when only high-risk pregnancies are considered. Furthermore, the US mortality rate remains higher than that of many other industrialized countries. Infant mortality rates vary widely by racial and ethnic groups and geographically, with the highest rate among infants born to black mothers in the largest US cities (CDC, 2018). Understanding the high-risk patient allows individualized therapeutic nursing interventions. Nurses can be instrumental in educating the public about the importance of obtaining early and regular care during pregnancy. See Box 29.2 for factors that place the postpartum woman and neonate at high risk.

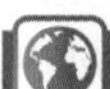 **Cultural Considerations**

High-Risk Pregnancies
- Providers must consider culturally based differences that could affect the treatment of diverse groups of women, and women must share practices and beliefs that could affect their nursing care or their willingness to comply. Health care providers are obligated to respect their patients' various sources of information and beliefs about sickness and health.
- Recognize that many women may be reluctant to disrobe and may avoid physical examination unless absolutely necessary.
- Consider who in the family traditionally makes the "major" decisions. In some families, the husband may be charged with these decisions, including those that affect the woman's health.
- Religious beliefs may dictate a care plan (e.g., with birth control measures or blood transfusions).
- Folk medicine, homeopathy, prayer, or a combination of these may be preferred to traditional Western medicine. Even the perceived effectiveness of medications may be affected by route of administration or color of pills.

HYPEREMESIS GRAVIDARUM

Etiology

Mild nausea and vomiting occurring during the first trimester of pregnancy are common and, to some extent, normal symptoms known as morning sickness. However, if the nausea and vomiting are severe and the symptoms last well beyond the first trimester, it may result in electrolyte, metabolic, and nutritional imbalances. This condition, termed hyperemesis gravidarum (also called pernicious vomiting), is a serious complication.

Hyperemesis is associated with weight loss, dehydration, acidosis from starvation, elevated blood and urine ketones, alkalosis from loss of hydrochloric acid in gastric juices and fluid, and hypokalemia. Short-term hepatic dysfunction with elevated liver enzymes may occur. Thiamine deficiency can cause encephalopathy.

The exact cause of this condition is not known. Elevated levels of human chorionic gonadotropin (HCG) are thought to be a factor. The disorder is more common with conditions that involve high levels of HCG, such as hydatidiform mole (gestational trophoblastic disease) or multifetal pregnancies. Women who have experienced the disorder in past pregnancies are at higher risk. Primigravidas also have a higher risk for developing the condition. Psychogenic factors also may play a role. Hyperemesis gravidarum is one of the most common nutrition-related discomforts of pregnancy.

Clinical Manifestations

The mother with hyperemesis gravidarum experiences vomiting and retching far worse than the usual morning sickness. The nausea and vomiting are not limited to the morning hours. Women may border on starvation and become severely dehydrated. Many serious complications that endanger the mother and the fetus can result. Acid-base imbalance related to the loss of excessive amounts of hydrochloric acid or intestinal juices may result in alkalosis or acidosis. Potassium may become depleted, leading to cardiac arrhythmias. Vitamin deficiencies can lead to jaundice and hemorrhage.

Assessment

Assess, record, and report the frequency, amount, and character of emesis. Carefully measure fluid intake and output (I&O). Obtaining the patient's daily weight for comparison purposes also is recommended. Assess the patient's skin turgor and mucous membranes. Psychosocial assessment includes asking the woman about anxiety, fears, and concerns related to her own health and the effects on her pregnancy. Assess family members' anxiety and their role in supporting the woman.

Assessment of the status of the fetus is also important. Monitor fetal heart rate (FHR) regularly and immediately report any significant changes (see Chapter 26).

Medical Management

Medical treatment is directed at meeting nutritional needs, thereby maintaining acid-base and electrolyte balance. An electrolyte profile should be obtained to determine the impact of the vomiting. Oral intake is restricted until the vomiting ceases. Once oral intake is resumed, it may be increased gradually, beginning with clear liquids and advancing the diet as tolerated. Intravenous fluid replacement is initiated. Fluids used in the replacement often include normal saline and lactated Ringer's solution (Khan, 2016). Additives in the fluids administered often include multivitamins, magnesium, potassium chloride, pyridoxine, and thiamine.

Complications may result if the woman is not hydrated adequately and electrolyte imbalances result. Observe the patient for any signs of complications, such as metabolic acidosis, jaundice, premature labor, and hemorrhage. Alert the physician if these occur.

Nursing Interventions and Patient Teaching

Ideally, the woman who experiences nausea and vomiting can maintain adequate hydration and nutritional intake. Consuming small, frequent meals is helpful. Avoidance of greasy or spicy foods is encouraged. High-protein snacks and intake of carbonated beverages may be beneficial. Ingesting dry crackers before getting out of bed is encouraged.

The patient is hospitalized and given parenteral fluids. Oral hygiene is essential because the mouth may be irritated by the vomitus. Weigh the woman daily during acute illness, and test the urine for ketones. Weight loss and ketones in the urine suggest that fat stores and protein are being metabolized to meet energy needs. A consultation with a dietitian is recommended (see Chapter 19 for further diet modification suggestions). Take steps to reduce the mother's emotional distress; commonly she fears for herself and her fetus. Provide emotional support and explanations. Include the family in the care plan whenever possible. Their participation may help alleviate some of the emotional stress associated with hospitalization. Complementary therapies may be included in the management of the condition. Acupuncture, Sea-Bands, and aromatherapy may be used.

More severe cases of hyperemesis may require pharmacologic intervention. Currently doxylamine-pyridoxine (Diclegis) is the only medication listed with FDA approval to treat vomiting in pregnancy. Other medications may be prescribed as deemed appropriate by the physician (see Table 29.3).

After several days of treatment in the hospital, most women return home, with nourishment by mouth. A few women continue to experience intractable nausea and vomiting throughout pregnancy. Rarely, a woman may need enteral, parenteral, or total parenteral nutrition to provide adequate nutrition for the mother and fetus.

Patient problems and interventions for the patient with hyperemesis gravidarum include but are not limited to the following:

Patient Problem	Nursing Interventions
Insufficient Nutrition, related to nausea and persistent vomiting secondary to pregnancy	Monitor food intake; caloric record may be desirable Offer dry crackers and bland food as tolerated Provide a pleasant atmosphere at mealtimes

Patient Problem	Nursing Interventions
	Administer antiemetics as prescribed Measure and record intake and output (I&O) Weigh daily Encourage oral fluids, slowly increasing amount as tolerated Maintain a calm, compassionate, and sympathetic manner Encourage patient to discuss concerns Encourage family participation
Fearfulness, related to concern for self and fetus	Convey acceptance of patient's perception of fear Help patient identify personal strengths and previous coping mechanisms Help patient identify sources of support Provide opportunities to verbalize fears Provide continuity of care; refer to social worker as indicated

Patient teaching includes: (1) arranging for dietary consultation; (2) educating patient regarding condition, including signs of improvement or deterioration, and treatment measures; (3) teaching patient how to assist with her own treatment (e.g., eating small, frequent meals with high carbohydrate content); and (4) providing referrals for follow-up treatment, such as psychological counseling, or for support from a social worker.

Prognosis

In most instances, hyperemesis gravidarum responds to therapy, and the prognosis is good. If untreated, hyperemesis gravidarum can result in maternal and fetal death.

MULTIFETAL PREGNANCY

Etiology

Pregnancy involving twins occurs in approximately 33.4 in 1000 live births in the United States. Triplets naturally occur in 101.4 to 100,000 live births (CDC, 2017c). Pregnancies that involve more than three fetuses are even rarer. Between 1998 and 2014 the occurrence of triplet and higher-order multiple births declined. Women who become pregnant with multiple fetuses most often are nonwhite, have a family history of multifetal pregnancies, or have taken fertility treatments.

Twins are classified as monozygotic (identical) or dizygotic (fraternal). **Monozygotic** twins begin with one fertilized ovum; the embryonic disk divides, causing identical twins. Because the genetic message is identical, the twins are of the same sex and carry an identical genetic code. They sometimes share a placenta or amniotic sac, but each has a separate umbilical cord.

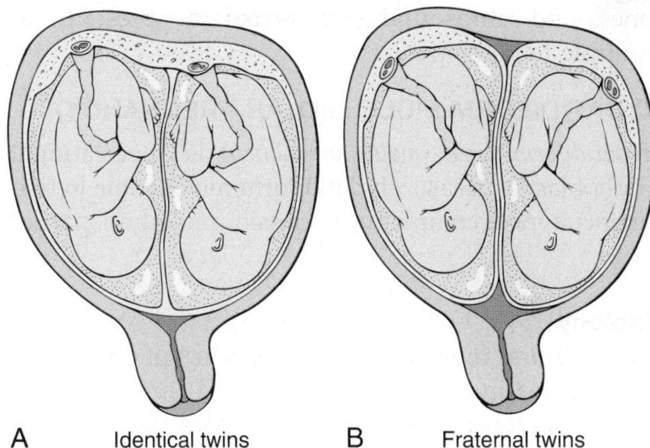

Fig. 29.1 Multiple pregnancies. A, Monozygotic (identical) twins develop from one ovum and one sperm. B, Dizygotic (fraternal) twins develop from two ova and two sperm. (From Frazier MS, Drzymkowski JW: *Essentials of human diseases and conditions,* ed 5, St. Louis, 2013, Saunders.)

Dizygotic twins are the result of two separate ova being fertilized at the same time. These twins almost always have separate placentas. The sexes can be different, and the genetic makeup varies; they are no more closely related than siblings born at different times (Fig. 29.1). Dizygotic twinning may be hereditary in some families, presumably because the woman inherited a tendency to release more than one ovum per cycle.

Pathophysiology

Maternal and fetal risks increase during a multiple pregnancy. Spontaneous abortions, maternal anemia, gestational hypertension (GH), hydramnios, and bleeding from placenta previa or abruptio placentae are more common in women with twins. The fetuses are more likely to have congenital anomalies, problems with entangled cords, and growth problems. An incomplete separation of the embryonic disk can result in conjoined twins.

Labor may be complicated by the loss of uterine tone that results from overstretching of the musculature, abnormal presentations, and preterm labor. Many twin pregnancies and almost all with more than two fetuses require a cesarean delivery.

Because of overdistention of the uterus, twins usually deliver before term and may have extended hospital stays. Twins may be a double joy, but they are also double the responsibility and expense of one baby. The parents need a great deal of support before and after the twins arrive. Breast-feeding of twins is possible. The mother may need additional help, because breast-feeding multiples consumes a lot of time and energy.

Clinical Manifestations

A multiple pregnancy is suspected when uterine enlargement exceeds the anticipated rate for growth, excess nausea and vomiting occurs, or levels of HCG are significantly elevated. Abdominal palpation with Leopold maneuvers, auscultation of two distinct heart tones, and ultrasound scan reveal the presence of multiple fetuses.

HYDATIDIFORM MOLE (MOLAR PREGNANCY)

Hydatidiform mole (molar pregnancy) is a gestational trophoblastic disease. Hydatidiform moles come in two distinct types: complete (or classic) mole and partial mole.

Etiology

Hydatidiform mole formation occurs in 1 of every 1200 pregnancies in the United States and Europe, but a higher incidence rate has been reported in women of Asian descent (Moore, 2016). The cause is unknown, although an ovular defect may occur. Women are at higher risk for hydatidiform mole formation if they have undergone ovulation stimulation with clomiphene (Clomid), are in their early teens, or are older than 40 years of age. The risk of a second mole is 1% to 2%.

Pathophysiology

The complete mole results from fertilization of an egg whose nucleus has been lost or inactivated. The nucleus of a sperm (23X) duplicates itself (resulting in the diploid number 46XX), because the ovum has no genetic material or the material is inactive. The developing cells resemble a cluster of grapes. The fluid-filled vesicles grow rapidly, causing the uterus to be larger than expected for the duration of the pregnancy. Usually the complete mole contains no fetus, placenta, amniotic membranes, or fluid. With no placenta to receive maternal blood, hemorrhage into the uterine cavity and vaginal bleeding occur. About 20% of cases of complete mole progress toward choriocarcinoma.

Clinical Manifestations

The signs and symptoms of a complete hydatidiform mole in the early stage cannot be distinguished from those of normal pregnancy. Early in pregnancy, the uterus in approximately half of affected women is significantly larger than expected based on the date of the last menstrual period. The percentage of women with an excessively enlarged uterus increases as the pregnancy advances. Approximately 25% of affected women have a uterus smaller than would be expected from menstrual dates.

Later, vaginal bleeding occurs in almost 95% of cases. The vaginal discharge may be dark brown (resembling prune juice) or bright red and either scant or profuse. It may continue for a few days or off and on for weeks.

Anemia from blood loss, excessive nausea and vomiting (hyperemesis gravidarum), and abdominal cramps caused by uterine distention are relatively common findings. Preeclampsia occurs in about 15% of cases, usually between 9 and 12 weeks of gestation, but any symptoms of GH before 20 weeks of gestation may suggest hydatidiform mole. Hyperthyroidism and pulmonary embolization of trophoblastic elements occur infrequently but are serious complications of hydatidiform mole. Partial moles cause few of these symptoms and may be mistaken for an incomplete or missed abortion.

Passages of vesicles (grapelike clusters) may occur around 16 weeks of gestation. There is no fetal movement, FHR, or palpable fetal parts. Some women have signs and symptoms of hyperthyroidism.

Diagnostic Measures

Diagnosis can be made with ultrasound scan, amniography, and measurement of HCG level in the blood. The ultrasound shows an enlarged uterus with no identifiable fetal parts. The uterine trophoblastic cells will be visualized. In most cases, the mole is discovered when abortion is threatened or in progress.

Medical Management

The molar pregnancy traditionally is managed with a suction curettage. After this is completed, the woman's medical management includes the assessment of HCG levels. The levels are assessed weekly until they are negative. Once the levels are negative, the monitoring is repeated monthly. A return to positive findings may signal the presence of carcinoma. Rho(D) immune globulin is administered to women who are Rh negative to prevent isoimmunization. Women who have experienced a molar pregnancy must avoid becoming pregnant for a year. Even with removal of the products of conception, cells may remain behind and develop into a malignancy.

Nursing Interventions and Patient Teaching

The woman and her family need information about the disease process, the necessity for a long course of follow-up, and the possible consequences of the disease. Help the woman understand and cope with pregnancy loss and recognize that the pregnancy was abnormal. Encourage the woman and her family to express their feelings, and provide information about support groups or counseling resources if needed. Explain the need to postpone a subsequent pregnancy the next year, and provide contraception counseling to emphasize the importance of consistent, reliable use of the method chosen.

ECTOPIC PREGNANCY

Etiology

In ectopic pregnancy, implantation occurs somewhere other than within the uterus, most commonly the fallopian tube (Fig. 29.2). An estimated 1% to 2% of reported pregnancies are ectopic. About 95% of all ectopic pregnancies occur in the fallopian tube. Other sites include the abdominal cavity, an ovary, ligaments, and the cervix (Fig. 29.3). Rarely the ectopic pregnancy is located in the abdomen (1% of ectopic pregnancies); in this case, the pregnancy may be salvageable. Tubal pregnancy occurs when, for some reason, the progress

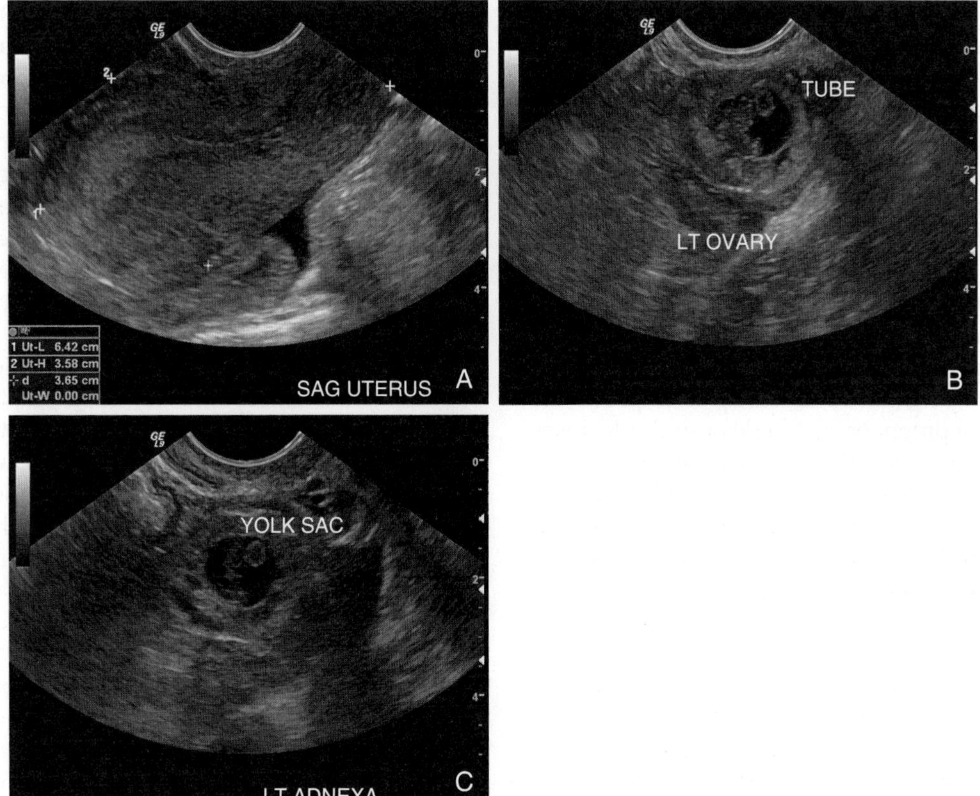

Fig. 29.2 Ectopic pregnancy, abdominal.

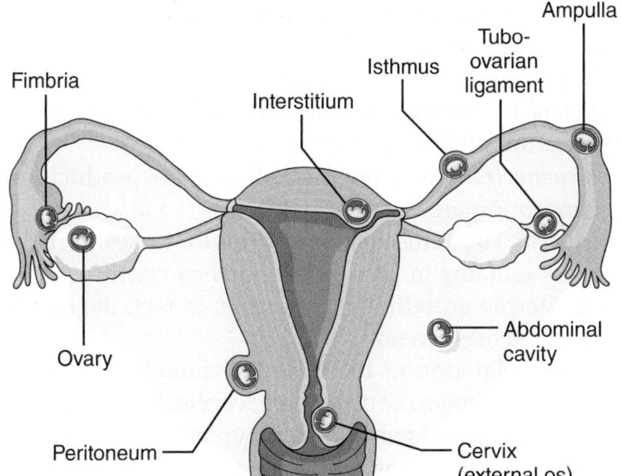

Fig. 29.3 Sites of implantation of ectopic pregnancies in order of frequency of occurrence: ampulla, isthmus, interstitium, fimbria, tuboovarian ligament, ovary, abdominal cavity, and cervix (external os).

of the fertilized ovum through the fallopian tube is slowed or obstructed. The incidence of ectopic pregnancy has increased dramatically throughout the world in the past 20 years. Ectopic pregnancy rates are higher in nonwhite and older women, particularly those over age 35 years. Risk factors for the development include history of pelvic inflammatory disease, tubal structural defects, endometriosis, history of surgery to the reproductive organs, smoking, the use of assistive reproductive techniques, and low progesterone levels.

Pathophysiology

Once the fertilized ovum implants, it begins to grow and develop. It becomes too large to be contained. This results in pain. If the pregnancy is not aborted, it ultimately results in rupture of the tube and bleeding into the abdominal cavity. At least three-fourths of ectopic pregnancies become symptomatic and are diagnosed during the first trimester. Ectopic pregnancy is a significant cause of maternal morbidity and mortality, even in developed countries.

Clinical Manifestations

The woman already may have had pregnancy confirmed with an HCG test. She may have experienced symptoms associated with pregnancy such as amenorrhea, nausea and vomiting, and breast tenderness. The woman often has lower abdominal pain. The pain may be diffuse or one sided. Uterine examination reveals enlargement in 25% of cases. Vaginal bleeding may be present. If the fallopian tube has ruptured, she may have vaginal bleeding, referred shoulder pain, and abdominal rigidity. The risk for hypovolemic shock is present.

Medical Management and Nursing Interventions

The initial management includes confirmation of the condition. HCG testing is performed and levels are traditionally lower than normal for the stage of gestation. Ultrasound scans are done to assess for the location of the pregnancy. A vaginal examination also is performed. Management of the ectopic pregnancy may be done surgically or pharmacologically. Surgical treatment, a laparotomy, requires removal of the pregnancy and related damaged tissue. It may necessitate removal of the fallopian tube (salpingectomy) or repair of the damaged tube (salpingostomy). If the fallopian tube is ruptured and significant bleeding occurs, blood transfusions may be necessary.

Pharmacologic therapy, when applicable, may allow for preservation of the tube and help to improve the chances of future pregnancies. Single or multiple doses of methotrexate may be prescribed for treatment of the unruptured ectopic pregnancy. Methotrexate is a folic acid antagonist that has been used for years to treat actively proliferating trophoblastic disease. It destroys the rapidly dividing cells. Not all women are candidates for the use of methotrexate. The fallopian tube must be unruptured and the size of the pregnancy less than 3.5 cm. The woman must be free of blood, liver, or kidney disorders. The medication may be administered once or twice if needed. Administration of Rho(D) immune globulin (RhoGAM) is indicated for those women who are Rh negative.

The woman and her family often need support to resolve emotions that may include anger, grief, guilt, and self-blame. The woman also may be anxious about her ability to become pregnant. Unfortunately, conditions that led to the ectopic pregnancy may exist in the other tube, placing the woman at increased risk for a repeated ectopic pregnancy. Be aware that these women may feel an acute sense of loss similar to that of women suffering miscarriage. Clarify the physician's explanation and use therapeutic communication techniques that help the woman deal with her anxiety and grief.

Prognosis

The prognosis varies. Maternal death from ectopic pregnancy occurs in about 1 in 800 cases in North America. The rates of maternal morbidity and secondary surgery are high, however, principally because of inaccurate or delayed diagnosis. The physician must rule out uterine abortion, ruptured corpus luteum cyst, appendicitis, salpingitis, ovarian cysts, torsion of the ovary, and urinary tract infection. The perinatal mortality rate in ectopic pregnancy is virtually 100%. Ectopic pregnancy recurs in approximately 10% of women, but more than 50% of women who have had an ectopic pregnancy achieve at least one normal pregnancy thereafter. The diagnosis and management of this condition are changing rapidly with technological advances.

SPONTANEOUS ABORTION

Etiology

Abortion is the termination of pregnancy before the age of viability—or 20 weeks of gestation in the United States. The two types of abortion are (1) spontaneous abortion, which results from natural causes, and (2) therapeutic abortion (including elective abortion), which is the interruption of the pregnancy for medical or personal reasons. Spontaneous abortion is referred to generally as a miscarriage. Most spontaneous abortions occur during the first trimester of pregnancy. Estimates are that as many as 10% to 15% of all pregnancies end in first-trimester spontaneous abortion. Many of these go unrecognized, with the woman merely thinking that her menstrual period was delayed.

More than half of all spontaneous abortions are caused by abnormal embryonic development, chromosomal defects, and inheritable disorders. Most other spontaneous abortions result from maternal causes, such as advancing maternal age and parity, chronic infections, chronic debilitating diseases, poor nutrition, and recreational drug use. The reasons for the remainder are open to speculation.

Pathophysiology

The pathophysiology depends on the specific cause.

Clinical Manifestations

The main presenting symptom is bleeding, which may or may not be accompanied by cramps or backache. Spontaneous abortions are classified as follows:

- *Threatened:* Unexplained bleeding and cramping occur. The fetus may or may not be alive. Membranes remain intact, and the cervical os remains closed.
- *Inevitable:* Bleeding increases, and the cervical os begins to dilate. Membranes may rupture.
- *Complete:* All products of conception are expelled from the uterus.
- *Incomplete:* Some, but not all, of the products of conception are expelled.
- *Missed:* The fetus dies and growth ceases, but the fetus remains in utero. Amenorrhea continues, but no uterine growth is measurable. In fact, the uterus may decrease in size.
- *Septic:* Malodorous bleeding, elevated temperature, and cramping may be present; cervical os is opened; and abdominal tenderness is typical.
- *Habitual:* This often is referred to as recurrent spontaneous abortion, when the woman has aborted spontaneously in three or more consecutive pregnancies; emotional trauma is increased, especially with subsequent pregnancies.

Medical Management

When a spontaneous abortion occurs, administer intravenous (IV) fluids and replace blood loss with transfusions, as ordered. A dilation and curettage (D&C) or dilation and evacuation (suction; D&E) may be indicated to remove retained placental tissue (Box 29.3). If significant blood loss occurred, iron supplementation may be ordered. Rh-negative women need the administration of RhoGAM.

Box 29.3 Types of Spontaneous Abortion and Therapeutic Management

- *Threatened:* Decreased activity, sedation, and avoidance of stress and orgasm are recommended. Further treatment depends on patient's course.
- *Inevitable, incomplete:* Prompt termination of pregnancy is accomplished, usually by dilation and evacuation (D&E).
- *Complete:* No further intervention may be needed if uterine contractions are adequate to prevent hemorrhage and if there is no infection.
- *Missed:* If spontaneous evacuation of the uterus does not occur, pregnancy is terminated with method appropriate to duration of pregnancy. Blood clotting factors are monitored until uterus is empty. Disseminated intravascular coagulation (DIC) and incoagulability of blood with uncontrolled hemorrhage may develop in cases of fetal death after 12th week if products of conception are retained for longer than 5 weeks (see discussion of DIC).
- *Septic:* Pregnancy is terminated immediately with method appropriate to duration of pregnancy. Cervical culture and sensitivity studies are done, and broad-spectrum antibiotic therapy (e.g., ampicillin) is started. Treatment for septic shock is initiated if necessary. If signs of uterine infection are seen, such as an elevated temperature, vaginal discharge with a foul odor, or abdominal pain, evacuation of the uterus is delayed until antibiotic therapy is initiated.

Patient Teaching

Patient teaching should include the need for rest (see the Patient Teaching box on spontaneous abortion).

 **Patient Teaching**

Spontaneous Abortion

- Refer patient to appropriate support groups, clergy, or professional counseling.
- Advise patient to report any heavy, profuse, or bright red bleeding to physician.
- Reassure patient that a scant, dark discharge may persist for 1 to 2 weeks.
- Instruct patient not to use tampons or douches until bleeding has stopped.
- Instruct patient to avoid sexual intercourse until bleeding has stopped.
- Acknowledge that patient has experienced a loss and that time is needed for recovery. She may experience mood swings and depression.
- Instruct patient to take antibiotics as prescribed.
- Advise patient that attempts to become pregnant are not recommended for at least 2 months or as recommended by the healthcare provider to allow the body to recover.

INCOMPETENT CERVIX

Late abortion and preterm delivery may be associated with **incompetent cervix.** This condition traditionally was defined as the passive and painless dilation of the cervix during the second trimester. A more recent idea is that cervical competence is variable and is determined in part by cervical length. Other related factors include composition of the cervical tissue and the individual circumstances associated with the pregnancy, such as maternal stress and lifestyle.

Etiology

Etiologic factors include a history of cervical lacerations during childbirth, excessive cervical dilation for curettage or biopsy, and the patient's mother's ingestion of diethylstilbestrol during pregnancy with the patient. Other instances may result from a congenitally short cervix or cervical or uterine anomalies. Reduced cervical competence is a clinical diagnosis, based on a history of short labors and recurring loss of the pregnancy at progressively earlier gestational ages. Ultrasound scan is used to diagnose this condition objectively. A short cervix (less than 20 mm long) is indicative of reduced cervical competence. Often, but not always, the short cervix is accompanied by effacement of the internal cervical os.

Medical Management

Women with a history of painless cervical dilation and effacement in a previous pregnancy or with a previous second-trimester loss in which short cervix and effacement were documented with ultrasound scan are candidates for prophylactic **cerclage,** a technique that uses suture material to constrict the internal os of the cervix (Fig. 29.4). Prophylactic cerclage is placed at 10 to 14 weeks of gestation. It is typically an outpatient procedure. After the placement of the cerclage, the woman is observed for approximately 1 to 2 hours. During the observation period, fetal heart tones and vital signs are assessed. Discharge teaching provided includes instructions to refrain from intercourse and to avoid prolonged standing and heavy lifting. The signs of premature labor and preterm rupture of membranes must be reviewed with the patient. She is instructed to contact her health care provider if she experiences cramping, bleeding, rupture of membranes, or elevated temperatures. She is monitored over the course of her pregnancy with ultrasound scans to assess for cervical shortening and effacement. The cerclage is removed electively (usually with an office or clinic procedure) when the woman reaches 37 weeks of gestation, or it may be left in place and a cesarean birth performed. Approximately 80% to 90% of pregnancies treated with cerclage result in live, viable births. If removed, the cerclage must be replaced with each successive pregnancy.

A woman whose reduced cervical competence is diagnosed during the current pregnancy may undergo emergency cerclage placement. Risks of the procedure include premature rupture of membranes, preterm labor, and *chorioamnionitis* (an inflammatory reaction in fetal membranes to bacteria or viruses in amniotic fluid).

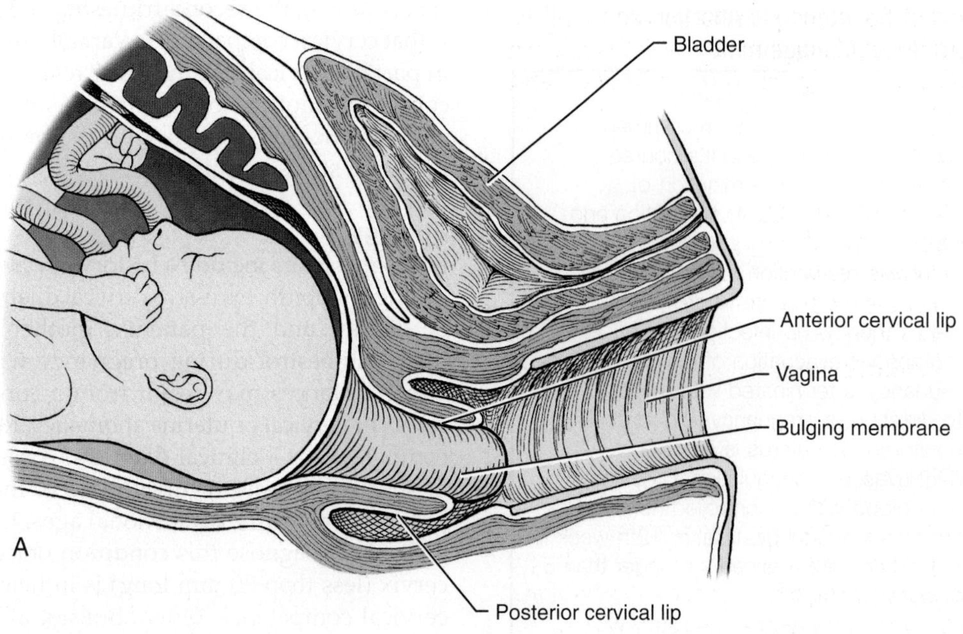

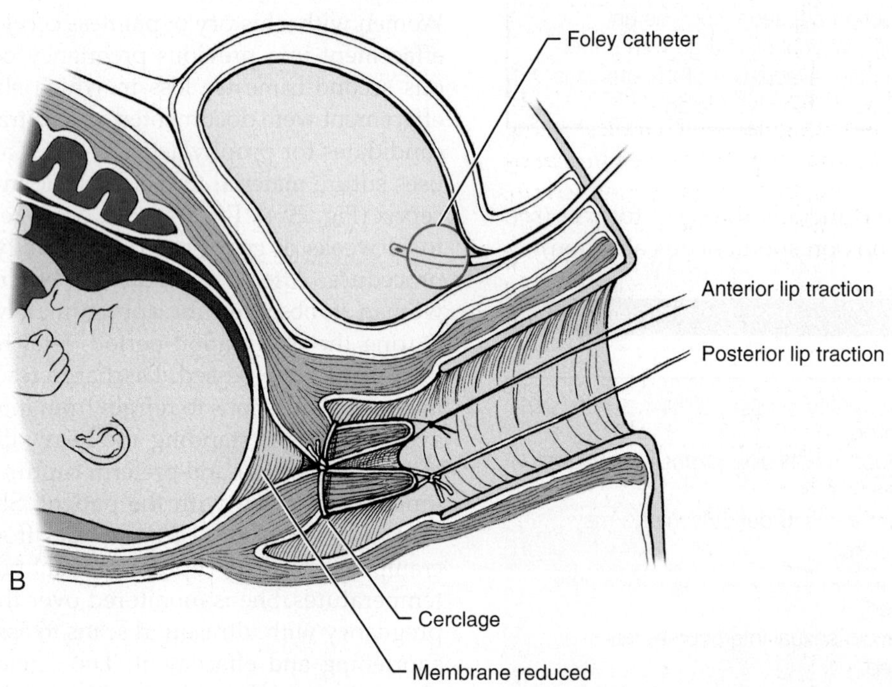

Fig. 29.4 A, Cerclage correction of recurrent premature dilation of cervix. B, Cross section of closed internal os. (From Shiland BJ: *Mastering healthcare terminology*, ed 6, St. Louis, 2019, Elsevier.)

Because of these risks and because bed rest and *tocolytic therapy* (drugs used to relax the uterus) can be used to prolong the pregnancy, cerclage rarely is performed after 26 weeks of gestation.

After a cervical cerclage is performed, monitor the woman for contractions, signs of rupture of membranes, and infection. Make referrals as appropriate for assistance once she is discharged to her home. Make certain she understands the rationale for the treatment and needed follow-up care. Because the diagnosis of reduced cervical competence usually is not made until the woman has lost one or two pregnancies, she may feel guilty or to blame for this impending loss; therefore assess the patient for previous reactions to stress and appropriateness of coping responses. She needs the support of her health care providers and her family. If management is unsuccessful and the fetus is born before viability, provide appropriate grief support. If the fetus is born prematurely, appropriate anticipatory guidance and support are necessary.

Prognosis

Prognosis for the fetus in the woman who has an incompetent cervix is based on early recognition and prompt medical management. The woman with the incompetent cervix likely will continue to face spontaneous abortions and premature labor if not managed with each pregnancy. Complications beyond pregnancy are very limited.

BLEEDING DISORDERS

Vaginal bleeding during pregnancy warrants investigation. Instruct the patient to contact her physician if any bleeding occurs. Depending on the stage of pregnancy, several different conditions may cause the bleeding.

PLACENTA PREVIA

Etiology

Placenta previa occurs when the placenta implants in the lower uterine segment. Placenta previa is described by the degree to which the placenta covers the internal cervical os: complete with total coverage; partial with incomplete coverage; and marginal, which indicates that only an edge of the placenta approaches the internal os (Fig. 29.5). The term *low implantation* is used when the placenta is situated in the lower uterine segment away from the internal os. In the second trimester, approximately 45% of all placentas are implanted in the lower uterine segment. As the lower uterine segment lengthens (stretches), the placenta seems to migrate upward.

Placenta previa occurs in 1 in 200 pregnancies. The cause is unknown. Risk factors include cesarean birth, possibly related to endometrial scarring; multiple gestation (because of the larger placental area); closely spaced pregnancies; and advanced maternal age (older than 35 years).

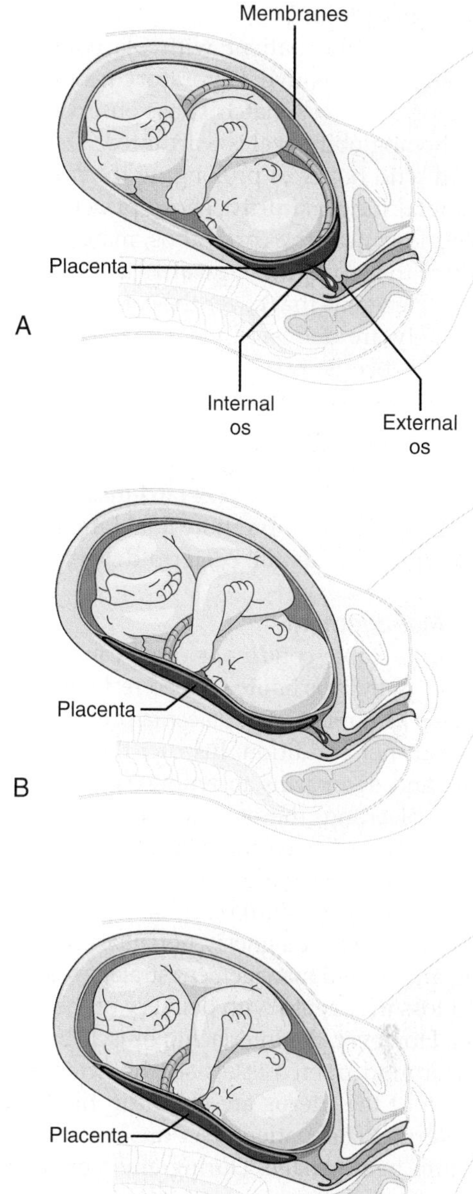

Fig. 29.5 Types of placenta previa after onset of labor. A, Incomplete, or partial. B, Complete, or total. C, Marginal, or low lying.

Pathophysiology

In the last trimester of pregnancy, uterine size increases and the cervix begins to dilate and efface. As the placenta separates from the uterus at the internal os of the cervix, sinuses at the site begin to bleed. The amount of bleeding depends on the amount of separation that occurs.

Clinical Manifestations

The main presenting symptom of placenta previa is painless, bright red, vaginal bleeding that occurs after 20 weeks of gestation. The bright red bleeding may be intermittent, may occur in gushes, or more rarely, may be continuous. It may start while the patient is resting or during any activity.

Abdominal examination usually reveals a soft (relaxed), nontender uterus of normal tone.

Diagnostic Testing

Obstetric ultrasound scan is the diagnostic method of choice. Vaginal examinations are restricted in the pregnant woman with undiagnosed vaginal bleeding. If done, the vaginal examination is performed by the primary care provider. The vaginal examination is performed in a care environment that allows for a *double setup*. This allows for the availability of a staffed operating room, with trained personnel and equipment available to manage an immediate vaginal or cesarean birth. Manipulation of the lower uterine segment or cervix may result in profound hemorrhage; preparation for immediate delivery is necessary.

Medical Management

Medical care of the patient with placenta previa is traditionally conservative. Laboratory testing includes blood typing and cross-match. Close observation of the patient's hemoglobin level is warranted. The patient is monitored with hopes of prolonging the pregnancy to promote fetal lung maturity. Those placentas that are implanted low, near the cervical os, may be delivered vaginally if they "migrate upward" as the pregnancy continues. Placentas that cover the cervical os partially or completely are delivered via cesarean section. The common practice is to schedule the cesarean birth at 36 weeks of gestation. If bleeding cannot be controlled or labor begins, delivery is indicated. Blood transfusions may be indicated to manage large volumes of blood loss or low hemoglobin levels. Betamethasone, a steroid, may be administered to promote fetal lung maturity in preparation for a potential preterm delivery.

Nursing Management

Patients with stable conditions often can be managed from home. Activity is limited to bed rest with bathroom privileges. The patient with placenta previa needs education about her condition. Instruct the patient about the signs and symptoms to report, such as increases in vaginal bleeding, the onset of labor, or rupture of membranes. The woman should be advised to count fetal movements daily. Sexual intercourse is not allowed in the patient diagnosed with placenta previa. Emotional support related to the diagnosis, potential compromise to the fetus, and related management strategies is indicated.

Blood loss may cease with delivery of the infant and placenta. However, the interlacing muscle bundles that contract around open vessels so characteristic of the upper part of the uterus are absent in the lower part of the uterus. The patient has an elevated risk for postpartum hemorrhage. During emergency preparations, constantly provide reassurance to reduce the woman's anxiety and that of her family.

Prognosis

Maternal mortality rate in placenta previa is low, about 0.6%. Fetal outcomes are related directly to the level of bleeding and the gestational age of the fetus at the time of delivery.

ABRUPTIO PLACENTAE

Etiology

Abruptio placentae is premature separation of the normally implanted placenta from the uterine wall. This generally occurs late in pregnancy, frequently during labor. Abruptio placentae occurs in about 1% of all pregnancies. The cause is unknown. Predisposing factors include trauma, chronic hypertension, and GH. Abruptio placentae is three times more likely to occur in women with gravidity of more than five. Women who use cocaine during pregnancy have a significant incidence of premature separation of the placenta. Blunt external abdominal trauma, usually the result of motor vehicle accidents or maternal battering, is an increasingly significant cause of placental abruption.

Table 29.1 Classification of Placental Abruption

TYPE	SEVERITY
Grade I (mild, 1)	The woman has vaginal bleeding perhaps with uterine tenderness and mild tetany (extremely prolonged uterine contraction), but neither mother nor baby is in distress. Approximately 10% to 20% of placental surface is detached.
Grade II (moderate, 2)	The woman has uterine tenderness and tetany, with or without external evidence of bleeding. The mother is not in shock, but there is fetal distress. Approximately 20% to 50% of the total surface is detached.
Grade III (severe, 3)	Uterine atony is severe, the woman is in shock (although the bleeding may not be obvious), and the fetus is dead. Often the woman has coagulopathy (defect in blood-clotting mechanisms). More than 50% of the placental surface area is detached.

Pathophysiology

When the placenta separates from the uterine wall, bleeding from uterine sinuses occurs, as in placenta previa. The most common classification of placental abruption is according to type and severity (Table 29.1).

Clinical Manifestations

The major symptoms of abruptio placentae are sudden, severe pain accompanied by uterine rigidity. The uterus also may increase in size because of the hemorrhage. The first sign during labor may be strong and constant contractions (tetany). Symptoms vary with the degree of separation. The presence of vaginal bleeding is determined by the location of the abruption.

Assessment

When any vaginal bleeding occurs during pregnancy, assess the following:

- *Duration, amount, color, and characteristics of the bleeding:* This includes assessment of: (1) the time since the onset of bleeding; (2) what, if any, activity preceded the bleeding episode; (3) the number of pads saturated per hour; and (4) the color of the bleeding (bright red, dark red, or brown). If a clot or tissue is passed, save it for examination by the health care provider.
- *Vital signs:* Depending on the origin and severity of the bleeding, signs of shock may be present. In addition to pulse and blood pressure, observe for pallor; diaphoresis; cool, clammy skin; and dyspnea. These

physical signs seem out of proportion to the amount of bleeding if the hemorrhage is concealed, as in central abruptio placentae.

- *Pain:* Note the location, nature, and duration of pain and whether bleeding is painless. This helps the physician determine the cause of the bleeding.
- *FHR:* Depending on the stage of pregnancy, measure FHR with a fetoscope or Doppler amplifier. If pregnancy is in the early stages, fetal heart sounds may not be heard. In labor, when there is uteroplacental insufficiency, the fetus, in its struggle to obtain more oxygen, may be restless and active. The FHR either accelerates greatly or slows.
- *Emotional response:* In addition to a physical assessment, address the emotional response of the expectant mother and her partner. They most likely are anxious, fearful, confused, and overwhelmed by the activity. They may have little knowledge of medical management and may not realize that the fetus must be delivered as quickly as possible and that a surgical procedure is necessary. Moreover, they may fear for the life of the woman and the fetus. Also, the fetus may be dead when the mother is admitted, adding shock and grief to their anxiety.

Diagnostic Tests

The most common laboratory tests include measurement of hemoglobin and hematocrit levels to determine the amount of blood lost. Blood typing and cross-matching are ordered in case blood replacement is necessary. Ultrasound scans may be done to determine placental location and fetal life. Vaginal examinations are avoided because they may increase the bleeding.

Medical Management

Abruptio placentae constitutes an obstetric emergency. The treatment often, but not always, includes delivery via cesarean birth and blood replacement.

A modified side-lying position with a wedge placed under the patient's right hip facilitates uterine-placental perfusion. Carefully monitor blood and fluid replacement therapy. Insert a retention catheter to monitor urinary output. The fetus is monitored and delivered when indicated. If signs of fetal compromise such as hypoxia are present or if the expectant mother exhibits signs of excessive bleeding, either obvious or concealed, the fetus is delivered immediately. Intensive monitoring of the woman and the fetus is essential because rapid deterioration in the condition of either can occur.

A woman undergoing immediate cesarean delivery may feel powerless as the health care team hurriedly prepares her for surgery. If possible, explain anticipated procedures to the woman and her family to reduce their fear and anxiety.

Nursing Interventions

Nursing measures are structured to support and promote optimal physical and psychological functioning.

Oxygen should be available. If blood loss is significant, oxygen-carrying capability is decreased; oxygen may be ordered to prevent maternal or fetal hypoxia.

IV or blood replacement therapy may be necessary, so be prepared for this. Possible loss of the pregnancy is a crisis. Be supportive of the patient's and family's emotional needs. Remain with the woman as much as possible, listen to her concerns, give clear explanations about medical treatment, and prepare her for the possible loss.

Patient problems and interventions for the patient with abruptio placentae include but are not limited to the following:

Patient Problem	Nursing Interventions
Insufficient Cardiac Output, related to excessive bleeding secondary to abruptio placentae	Monitor and record vital signs q 15 min until stable, then q hr as indicated Measure and record I&O Weigh daily Assess skin turgor and mucous membranes Help patient ambulate Monitor blood replacement therapy
Potential for Grief, related to possible loss of pregnancy	Allow time for patient to verbalize concerns about loss Assist with grieving processes Encourage contact with support system Encourage session with spiritual advisor if patient desires Foster active participation of significant other

Prognosis

Premature separation of the placenta is a serious disorder and accounts for about 15% of all perinatal deaths. Maternal mortality rate approaches 1% in abruptio placentae; this condition remains a leading cause of maternal death. The mother's prognosis depends on the extent of placental detachment, overall blood loss, degree of disseminated intravascular coagulation (DIC), and time between the placental separation and delivery.

Approximately one-third of infants of women with premature separation of the placenta die. More than 50% die as a result of preterm delivery, and many others die of intrauterine hypoxia.

DISSEMINATED INTRAVASCULAR COAGULATION

Etiology

Disseminated intravascular coagulation (DIC) is a potentially life-threatening disorder that results from alterations in the normal clotting mechanism. DIC is always a secondary diagnosis. It may be seen with abruptio placentae, incomplete abortion, hypertensive disease, or infectious process. It may occur with a postterm delivery.

Pathophysiology

In DIC, the body's attempts to prevent excessive blood loss put stress on the coagulation processes. The body produces excessive amounts of thrombin, stimulating the conversion of fibrinogen to fibrin. Elevated fibrin levels result in multiple small clots forming in small blood vessels, which may lead to obstruction of vessels, ischemia, and damage to vital organs. This clot formation also traps platelets and can result in generalized hemorrhage.

Clinical Manifestations

The onset of symptoms is sudden. The patient may report chest pain or dyspnea and become extremely restless and cyanotic, occasionally expectorating frothy, blood-tinged mucus. Profound circulatory shock from hemorrhage may occur rapidly. Fetal and maternal death may result.

Assessment

All women with complications that may result in DIC should be observed closely for signs of bleeding, such as epistaxis (nosebleeds), bleeding gums, or petechiae, particularly around the blood pressure cuff on the patient's arm. Excessive bleeding may occur from a site of slight trauma, such as venipuncture sites, intramuscular or subcutaneous injection sites, nicks from shaving of perineum or abdomen, and injury from insertion of urinary catheter. Continue to monitor the maternal and fetal conditions with assessment of vital signs, FHR, and I&O and with general careful assessment.

Diagnostic Tests

Blood testing includes determination of hemoglobin and hematocrit levels. Clotting factor studies, such as fibrinogen levels, platelet counts, prothrombin time (PT), and partial thromboplastin time (PTT), typically are ordered for the patient. Laboratory tests may reveal various degrees of anemia and decreased fibrinogen and platelet counts. Prolonged PT and PTT are also typical.

Medical Management

Emergency care for DIC includes IV administration of fibrinogen, blood, and other substances that help restore normal clotting mechanisms. Paradoxically, DIC therapy may include heparin via continuous infusion pump (although its use is controversial) and oxygen therapy with a tight-fitting mask at 10 to 12 L/min. If the fetus is not yet born, delivery should occur as soon as possible. Carefully monitor urinary output (it must be maintained at more than 30 mL/h), because renal failure is one consequence of DIC.

If the woman is still pregnant, position her in a side-lying tilt to maximize blood flow to the uterus.

Nursing Interventions

Nursing interventions are directed at supporting medical treatment. Report signs and symptoms promptly. Use caution when providing care to minimize the risk of additional trauma to tissue, which may lead to further bleeding. Recognize and support the emotional needs of the patient and the family.

Prognosis

DIC is a life-threatening disorder. The prognosis depends on the degree and extent of the underlying disorder and the response of the woman to prompt and proper treatment.

POSTPARTUM HEMORRHAGE

Etiology

Postpartum hemorrhage (PPH) is classified as early or late. Early PPH is blood loss greater than 500 mL after vaginal childbirth or 1000 mL after cesarean birth. Estimating blood loss is difficult, especially when bleeding is brisk or hemorrhage is concealed. Hemorrhage is one of the leading causes of maternal morbidity and mortality in the first 24 hours after delivery; late PPH occurs after the first 24 hours. At least 5% of women experience PPH. Studies have shown that women who have an extended second stage of labor, instrument-assisted delivery, large-for-gestational-age newborn, or induction or augmentation of labor or who are obese have an increased incidence of PPH.

The most common causes of early hemorrhage are uterine **atony,** *retained placental fragments,* and *perineal lacerations. Uterine atony* (lack of normal tone or strength) has several potential causes, including excessive distention of the uterus from multiple pregnancy, **hydramnios** (excessive amount of amniotic fluid), and a large infant. Atony is also more prevalent in grand multiparas or when labor is prolonged or traumatic. Pharmacologic therapies also may be linked to PPH. Magnesium sulfate and nifedipine are associated with PPH. Placental disorders, including implantation in the lower uterine segment and failure of the placenta to detach as in placenta accrete, are implicated as well. Infection is another contributing factor to PPH. The most common cause of late PPH is retained placental fragments.

Pathophysiology

Contraction of the uterus seals the uterine sinuses, aiding in the prevention of postpartum hemorrhage. Hemorrhage results when loss of tone or tissue remaining in the cavity prevents adequate uterine contraction. In addition, hemorrhage may result when there is unchecked bleeding from lacerations or tears. These tears may be uterine, perineal, or cervical.

Assessment

Nursing assessment of uterine contraction and lochia is part of routine postpartum assessment. If the uterus is boggy (soft, uncontracted) or the flow of lochia is heavy, suspect hemorrhage. Bleeding accompanied by a boggy uterus is consistent with atony. Bleeding that occurs in the presence of a firm, contracted uterus should be investigated, because potential causes include lacerations or tears. Vital sign changes such as tachycardia and hypotension are reflective of excessive blood loss. Compare findings with the patient's baseline values.

PPH can progress rapidly to shock. Symptoms consistent with advancing PPH include oliguria, restlessness, air hunger, and ultimately collapse. Review the history for factors that predispose to PPH.

For the first 24 hours after childbirth, the uterus should feel like a firmly contracted ball roughly the size of a large grapefruit. It should be located easily at about the level of the umbilicus. Lochia should be dark red and moderate in amount. Saturation of more than one peripad per hour is considered a large amount, and saturation of more than one peripad in 15 minutes is excessive. Realize that, although bleeding may be profuse and dramatic, a constant trickle or dribble is just as dangerous.

Assess the bleeding color, amount, and, if possible, source. Note the time of the last pad change. If the pad is loose, blood may pool under the patient, so assessment must include checking under the patient.

Vital signs may not be reliable indicators of shock in the immediate postpartum period because of physiologic adaptations of this stage. Data should include assessment for bladder distention, because a full bladder lifts and displaces the uterus and prevents effective contraction of the uterine muscles. Help the mother urinate or catheterize her as necessary.

Medical Management

Medical management begins with determination of the cause of bleeding. Diagnostic studies include complete blood count and type screen and cross-match. The presenting hemoglobin and hematocrit levels are compared with baseline studies. Intravenous fluid replacement is initiated. Transfusion with packed red blood cells may be performed. Treatment is based on the underlying case of the bleeding. Retained placental fragments are managed with a dilation and evacuation (D&E) to remove the tissue surgically. Lacerations are identified and repaired.

The management for uterine atony includes fundal massage, with the bladder kept empty. Fluid replacement is initiated with intravenous therapy. Oxytocic agents such as Methergine and Pitocin are administered. Failure to control bleeding may necessitate a hysterectomy.

Nursing Interventions

Nursing interventions are directed at the early identification of excess blood loss and the prevention of hemorrhage. If the uterus is boggy, massage is initiated. If the uterus remains atonic, the primary care provider may prescribe an oxytocic. If a D&E is necessary, preparation of the patient for surgery is completed by the nurse. Provide emotional support. Other surgical preparations include obtaining signed consent forms; verifying that laboratory data are on the chart, the patient has had nothing by mouth, and identification and allergy bands are in place; completing skin preparations as ordered; having the patient empty her bladder or inserting an indwelling catheter; removing jewelry, contact lenses, and dentures; obtaining vital signs; administering preoperative medication as scheduled; monitoring safety with side rails up; and documenting all preoperative care.

Trauma. If the fundus is firm but bleeding is excessive, the cause may be laceration of the cervix or birth canal. Inspect the perineum for a laceration in that area. Lacerations of the cervix or vagina are not visible, but bleeding when the uterus is contracted suggests a laceration. This sign warrants examination of the vaginal walls and the cervix by the health care provider (see Chapter 28 and Box 28.2).

If the mother reports deep, severe pelvic or rectal pain or if vital signs or skin changes suggest hemorrhage but excessive bleeding is not obvious, the cause may be concealed bleeding and the formation of a hematoma. Examine the vulva for a bulging mass or skin discoloration. A hematoma in the vagina or in the retroperitoneal area is not obvious. Notify the health care provider.

Keep the woman on bed rest to increase venous return and maintain cardiac output. The Trendelenburg position may interfere with cardiac function and is not advised. Continue assessments; call for assistance; and save all pads, linen savers, and linen so that blood loss can be estimated accurately. Assistance is necessary so that one nurse can continue to massage the uncontracted uterus and perform and record assessments while the other notifies the health care provider of the mother's condition.

The unusual activity of the hospital staff may make the mother and her family anxious. Keeping the family informed is one of the most effective ways of reducing anxiety.

Patient problems and interventions for the patient with PPH include but are not limited to the following:

Patient Problem	Nursing Interventions
Insufficient Knowledge, related to signs of hemorrhage	Select teaching strategies appropriate to patient's need and willingness to learn Demonstrate postpartum checks of fundus and lochia Observe patient performing self-check Review importance of contacting the health care provider if signs are abnormal or questionable
Inadequate Fluid Volume, related to hypovolemia secondary to excessive blood loss	Perform fundal massage until firm Monitor vital signs and I&O closely Assess blood loss by pad saturation Monitor fluid replacement therapy Monitor for signs and symptoms of infection Teach patient fundal massage Encourage fluids by mouth unless contraindicated

Patient Teaching

Because patients leave the hospital in a relatively short time, teach them how to perform the postpartum checks of the fundus and lochia. Late PPH, which typically occurs without warning 7 to 14 days after delivery, can be dangerous for the unsuspecting mother. Alert her to call the physician if bleeding is excessive or persists longer than expected.

Prognosis

Maternal mortality is estimated at 17.3 women per 100,000 live births in the United States (Smith, 2017). PPH is among the top three causes. Although all possible medical, surgical, and nursing interventions are attempted, maternal mortality may still occur.

HYPERTENSIVE CONDITIONS IN PREGNANCY

Etiology

During pregnancy, blood pressure levels normally are reduced during the first trimester. This results in response to the reduced vascular resistance caused by the hormone progesterone. The blood pressure levels gradually return to the prepregnancy baseline levels by 20 weeks' gestation, where they remain until delivery. Some women may experience blood pressure elevations in pregnancy. The conditions are categorized by the period of gestational onset.

Chronic hypertension: Present in women before pregnancy or occurs before 20 weeks' gestation. It may be caused by other conditions, such as renal disease. Patients with chronic hypertension have a 1:4 likelihood for development of preeclampsia during the pregnancy.

Gestational hypertension (GH): Formerly referred to as pregnancy-induced hypertension (PIH), GH is a disease encountered during pregnancy or early in the puerperium, characterized by increasing hypertension. The condition begins after 20 weeks' gestation. Unlike preeclampsia, it is not accompanied by proteinuria.

***Preeclampsia** and **eclampsia**:* Formerly referred to as toxemia, results in increasing blood pressure after 20 weeks' gestation. The hypertension is accompanied by albuminuria and generalized edema. The condition may be mild or severe. Additional symptoms of the condition include headache, visual disturbances, and epigastric pain. These symptoms may signal worsening of the condition.

Risk factors for the condition include first pregnancy, African American race, history of chronic or gestational hypertension, obesity, family history of preeclampsia, diabetes, and gestational trophoblastic disease. Age is also a factor, because women under age 18 years or over 35 years have increased occurrences.

Mild preeclampsia. Early preeclampsia has few clinical symptoms. Change in the blood pressure readings (an increase of 30 mm Hg systolic and 15 mm Hg diastolic, or a reading of 140/90 mm Hg in a woman whose blood pressure has been normal) indicates a problem. The blood pressure readings are reflective of hypertension when taken two times 6 hours apart. The reading should be taken with the woman seated and the appropriate cuff size. Generalized edema may be evident in the face, the hands, and the ankles. Periorbital edema may be a more ominous finding. Weight may increase as much as 3 pounds (1.4 kg) per month in the second trimester and 1 pound (0.5 kg) per week in the third trimester. Urine testing frequently shows 1+ to 2+ albumin readings. The urinary output is at least 500 mL/24 h.

Severe preeclampsia. The symptoms of **severe preeclampsia** may appear suddenly. Blood pressure readings increase; readings of 160/110 mm Hg or higher on two separate occasions 6 hours apart with the pregnant woman on bed rest are common. The presence and location of edema were once considered key criteria for the diagnosis of preeclampsia. Currently, the medical community promotes the monitoring of edema but does not use its occurrence as a determinant of the severity of the condition. Edema becomes increasingly obvious and may be observed in the face, the hands, the sacral area, the abdomen, and throughout the lower extremities. Weight increases dramatically. The woman may gain as much as 2 pounds (0.9 kg) in a matter of a few days or a week. Urine testing for albumin shows 3+ to 4+ readings. The urinary output is less than 500 mL/24 h. The patient often reports headache, blurred vision, and epigastric discomfort. The assessment reveals hyperreflexia. Clonus is noted with pending seizure activity.

Eclampsia. Eclampsia is the most severe form of preeclampsia. The most dramatic characteristic is seizure activity. The patient exhibits tonic (pertaining to or characterized by muscular tension) and clonic (spasmodic alteration of muscular contractions) phases. This generally is followed by a coma that lasts from minutes to hours. Other signs are elevated blood pressure, albuminuria, and oliguria. If untreated, this sequence of seizure-coma may repeat, and death may follow.

Assessment

Assess blood pressure routinely throughout pregnancy, labor, delivery, and the postpartum period. GH can occur any time after the 20th week and persist until 2 days after delivery. Record weight at each prenatal visit and compare it with norms. Excessive or rapid weight gain, particularly when accompanied by edema, should be reported promptly. Assess for edema at each visit (see Fig. 8.17 in *Adult Health Nursing*). Edema typically is described with a scale of 1+ to 4+:

1+ Minimal edema on pedal and pretibial area
2+ Obvious edema of lower extremities
3+ Edema of face, hands, sacrum, and abdomen
4+ Massive, generalized edema **(anasarca)**

Test urine for albumin with dipstick reagents at each visit and on admission for labor. (If the bag of waters is ruptured, these dipstick readings may be inaccurate.)

Certain symptoms, such as continuous headache, drowsiness, or mental confusion, indicate poor cerebral perfusion and may be precursors of convulsions. Visual disturbances, such as blurred or double vision or spots before the eyes, indicate arterial spasms and edema in the retina. Some symptoms such as epigastric pain or "upset stomach" are particularly ominous, because they indicate distention of the hepatic capsule and often warn that a convulsion is imminent. Decreased urinary output indicates poor perfusion of the kidneys and may precede acute renal failure.

If the patient is hospitalized for GH, monitor deep tendon reflexes (Table 29.2 and Fig. 29.6) and urinary output; also electronically monitor FHR.

Diagnostic Tests

Serum laboratory tests include hematocrit, blood urea nitrogen, complete blood cell count, clotting studies, liver enzymes, type and screen, and possible cross-match. Urine screenings, such as specific gravity and protein, and a 24-hour urine collection are obtained to measure creatinine and protein clearance. Electrolyte panels commonly are drawn. If symptoms indicate severe preeclampsia or eclampsia, liver function and platelet count evaluations also are done. If the health care provider is considering induction of labor before term, gestation tests to establish fetal maturity are indicated. These tests include amniocentesis and ultrasound scan. Nonstress tests, contraction stress tests, and biophysical profiles may be performed to assess fetal well-being.

Table 29.2 Assessment of Deep Tendon Reflexes

DEGREE	GRADING
Hyperactive response (brisk with intermittent or transient clonus)	4+
More than normal (brisk), slightly hyperactive	3+
Normal, active, expected response	2+
Sluggish or diminished	1+
No response	0

Medical Management

The woman may or may not need to be hospitalized, depending on the severity of symptoms. Mild preeclampsia may be managed at home. Activity at home is restricted, with rest strongly encouraged. Severe symptoms necessitate hospitalization. Bed rest typically is ordered, preferably in the left lateral recumbent position, to reduce pressure on the inferior vena cava and promote venous return. A well-balanced diet with adequate protein is important. Moderate sodium intake is allowed, but high-sodium foods should be avoided. Patients with gestational hypertension and preeclampsia do not face restricted-sodium diets. Balance is more the goal. Intravenous access is needed to provide a line if emergency medications are to be administered. The infant's status is monitored with vital signs and testing to ensure fetal well-being. In cases of severe preeclampsia or eclampsia, medication therapies including magnesium sulfate ($MgSO_4$) may be prescribed parenterally to prevent seizure activity. Antihypertensive medications are not used routinely for the patient with mild preeclampsia or gestational hypertension. Antihypertensive medications are prescribed for blood pressure readings that exceed 160/100 mm Hg. The administration of

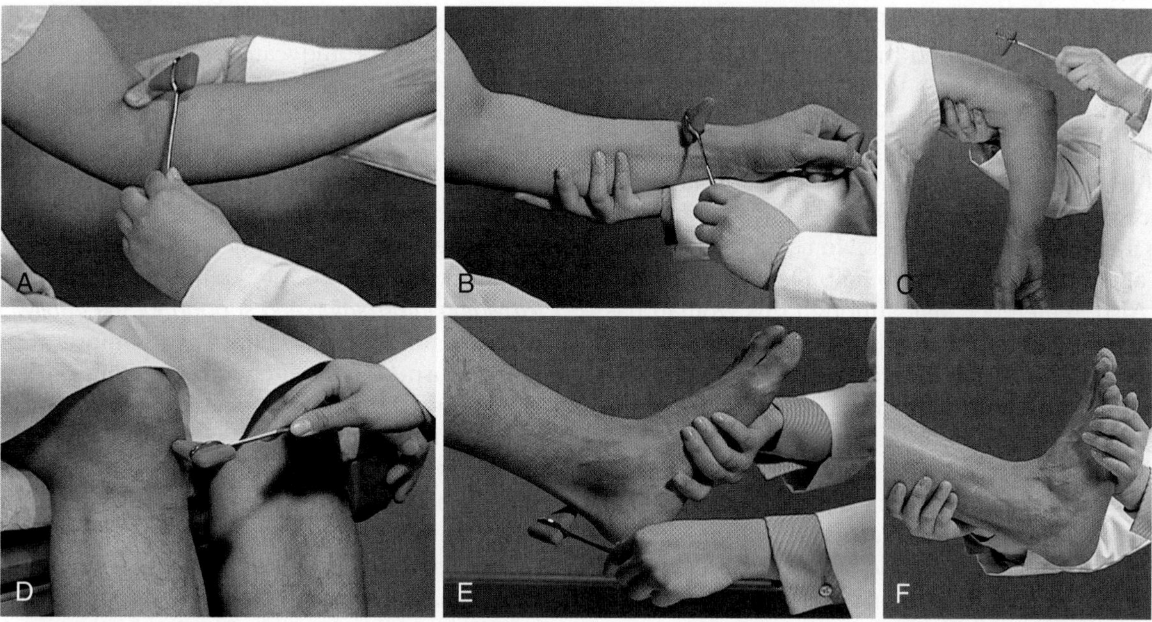

Fig. 29.6 Location of tendons for evaluation of deep tendon reflexes. A, Triceps. B, Biceps. C, Brachioradial. D, Patellar. E, Achilles. F, Evaluation of ankle tonus. (From Seidel HM, Ball, JW, Dains, JE, et al: *Mosby's guide to physical examination,* ed 7, St. Louis, 2011, Mosby.)

medications in less severe conditions may impair perfusion to the fetus.

Nursing Interventions

Nursing care for the woman with elevations of blood pressure during pregnancy focuses on assessment of the expectant woman, monitoring of the fetus, administration of prescribed medications, and emotional support. Subtle changes in blood pressure should be noted and reported. The assessment of the woman's mental status and any noteworthy changes necessitates consultation with the health care provider.

In mild cases, monitor routine I&O; in severe cases, it may be necessary to insert an indwelling catheter and record hourly urinary output. Monitor fetal condition carefully. In mild cases, routine auscultation of FHR is adequate. Severe cases necessitate continuous fetal monitoring. Record the patient's daily weight. Evaluate daily weight changes in conjunction with intake and output to determine levels of fluid retention.

Some practitioners request a **kick count,** a daily count of fetal movements felt in 1 hour while the mother is resting. Kick counts are recommended beginning at 28 weeks' gestation. Fetal activity of less than three kicks per hour is considered serious and must be reported. Fetal activity decreases in the presence of hypoxia.

Monitor blood pressure every 4 hours or more frequently if condition indicates. Encouraging compliance with treatment can help prevent the patient from convulsing. Because stress may exacerbate this condition, keep the environment quiet and nonstressful. Maintaining a stress-free environment is difficult, however, because enforced bed rest may last for several weeks. Enforced bed rest or hospitalization can be highly disruptive for the patient and her family; there are financial implications, and the woman's condition can affect family dynamics. Explain the necessity of treatment and the care and the treatment that will be given (Box 29.4).

Emotional and psychological support are essential in helping the woman and her family cope. Their perception of the disease process, the reasons for it, and the care received affects their compliance with and participation in therapy. The family needs to use coping mechanisms and support systems to help them through this crisis. Also, remember that, although this woman has a high-risk condition, she is first of all having a baby. A care plan designed for the woman with preeclampsia must be integrated with the nursing care all women need during labor and birth.

Protecting the woman and fetus during a convulsion. The nurse's primary responsibilities to protect the woman and the fetus during a convulsion include the following:

- Remain with the woman and press the emergency bell for assistance.
- If she is not on her side already, attempt to turn the woman onto her side when the tonic phase begins. The left side-lying position permits greater circulation through the placenta, and it may help prevent aspiration.
- Note the time and sequence of the convulsion.
- Insert an airway after the convulsion, and suction the woman's mouth and nose to clear secretions and prevent aspiration. Provide oxygen by mask at 8 to 10 L/min to increase oxygenation of the placenta and all maternal body organs.
- Observe fetal monitor patterns for nonreassuring signs, such as bradycardia, tachycardia, or decreased variability. These usually resolve within a few minutes as maternal oxygenation is restored.
- Notify, or have another nurse notify, the physician that a convulsion has occurred. Administer medications and prepare for additional medical interventions as directed by the physician.

Box 29.4 Eclamptic Seizure Precautions and Interventions

- Keep the environment quiet and nonstimulating, with subdued lighting.
- For seizure precautions, use padded side rails and have suction and oxygen administration equipment and airway ready to use.
- Keep the call button within easy reach.
- Emergency medication tray is immediately accessible.
- Hydralazine (antihypertensive vasodilator) and magnesium sulfate are in or adjacent to woman's room.
- Calcium gluconate is immediately available in a well-labeled syringe at the bedside as an antidote to magnesium sulfate toxicity.
- Emergency birth pack is accessible.
- Reduce noise when the door must be opened or closed.
- Keep noise to a minimum, including blocking incoming telephone calls or visitors.
- Group nursing assessments and care to allow the woman periods of undisturbed rest.
- Move carefully and calmly around the room and avoiding bumping into the bed or startling the woman.
- Collaborate with the woman and her family to restrict visitors.

Providing information and support for the family. Explain to the family what has happened without minimizing the seriousness of the situation. A convulsion is frightening for anyone who witnesses it, and the family often is reassured when the nurse explains that the convulsion lasts only a few minutes and that the woman probably will not be conscious for some time afterward. Acknowledge that the convulsion indicates worsening of the condition and that the physician needs to determine future management; this may include delivery of the infant as soon as possible. Vaginal birth is preferred if the maternal and fetal conditions permit because of abnormalities in coagulation and other body systems.

Patient problems and interventions for the patient with GH include but are not limited to the following:

Patient Problem	Nursing Interventions
Insufficient Diversional Activity, related to environmental lack of stimulation	Find out about hobbies or interests that the woman can perform while resting Involve patient in conversation while performing care Encourage family to visit and bring books or other recreational items Encourage relaxation techniques Encourage listening to music Gentle exercise such as range of motion, stretching, Kegel exercises, pelvic tilt (important in maintaining muscle tone, blood flow, regularity of bowel function, and a sense of well-being)
Potential for Injury, related to elevated blood pressure and central nervous system irritability	Determine prepregnant baseline vital sign values Monitor blood pressure q 4 hr (or more frequently as necessary) in supine and lateral recumbent positions Assess for headache and visual disturbances Weigh patient daily Monitor I&O Assess deep tendon reflexes and for the presence of clonus Monitor urine for protein Observe for pitting edema of upper extremities, periorbital area, and face. Monitor laboratory values Maintain bed rest as needed

Patient Teaching

Teach all pregnant women the danger signs of complications in pregnancy and the importance of regular medical supervision. Many of the symptoms of GH, particularly the mild, early symptoms, are detected only with regular physician contact. If GH is diagnosed, explain the consequences of failure to comply.

Encourage high-quality protein, vitamin, and mineral intake. Salt restriction below the normal dietary levels (4 to 6 g/24 h) usually is not recommended.

Be certain that the patient understands that bed rest is vital because it slows metabolism and relieves dependent edema.

Prognosis

Delivery of the baby is the only cure for preeclampsia and GH. The condition remains a cause for concern for 6 weeks during the postpartum period. Potential complications associated with the condition include bleeding problems, placental abruption, liver rupture, stroke, and death. Immediate and continuous care by the obstetric team is mandatory to prevent maternal and fetal morbidity and mortality.

HELLP SYNDROME

The *HELLP syndrome (H,* hemolysis; *EL,* elevated liver enzymes; *LP,* low platelet count) represents an extension of the pathology of severe preeclampsia and eclampsia. The initial symptoms of the HELLP syndrome usually appear early in the third trimester, although they may appear in the early postpartum period.

For a woman to be diagnosed with the HELLP syndrome, her platelet count must be less than 100,000/mm^3, her liver enzyme levels (aspartate aminotransferase and alanine aminotransferase) must be elevated, and some evidence for intravascular hemolysis must be present. The hemolysis accounts for the large drop in the hematocrit value, out of proportion to blood loss, that occurs in most new mothers with HELLP syndrome during the postpartum period. A unique form of coagulopathy (not DIC) occurs with the HELLP syndrome.

Recognition of the clinical and laboratory findings of the HELLP syndrome is essential to initiate early, aggressive therapy and prevent maternal and fetal mortality.

The prominent symptom of the HELLP syndrome is pain in the right upper quadrant, the lower chest, or the epigastric area. The woman may have tenderness from liver distention. Additional signs and symptoms include nausea, vomiting, and severe edema. Avoid traumatizing the liver with abdominal palpation, and use care in transporting the woman. A sudden increase in intraabdominal pressure, including a seizure, could lead to rupture of a subcapsular hematoma, resulting in internal bleeding and hypovolemic shock (see Chapter 28 and Box 28.1).

Women with HELLP syndrome should be managed in a setting with full intensive care facilities available. Their treatment is the same as for preeclampsia or eclampsia. After delivery, most women begin recovering within 72 hours.

Intrapartum nursing care of the woman with severe preeclampsia or HELLP syndrome involves continuous monitoring of maternal and fetal status as labor progresses. Continue the assessment and prevention of tissue hypoxia and hemorrhage, both of which can lead to permanent compromise of vital organs throughout the intrapartum and postpartum period.

An unfavorable (uneffaced and undilated) cervix and the aggressive nature of this disorder support the need for cesarean birth. Prolonged induction of labor could increase maternal morbidity. Fresh-frozen plasma may be needed if bleeding occurs and persists. The major laboratory manifestations of the disease, however, may not appear until the early postpartum period (48 to 72 hours). Delayed transfusion of packed red blood cells (RBCs) and platelets often is necessary because of the continued hemolysis. Attempt to lower the blood pressure if the diastolic pressure is consistently greater than 110 mm Hg. However, blood pressure may be normal or slightly elevated; thus it is not an adequate indicator of the severity of the disease. Hypoglycemia may be present in the woman with HELLP syndrome and, when the blood glucose is less than 40 mg/dL, is associated with a high maternal mortality rate.

COMPLICATIONS RELATED TO INFECTION

Mother and fetus must be considered in the assessment of maternal infection. In some diseases, such as tuberculosis, the fetus almost always is spared, even though the mother may be dying. With other infections, such as rubella, the fetus may be critically compromised, while the mother is only slightly ill.

Pregnancy generally is regarded as an immunosuppressed condition. Hormonal changes provide protection to the fetus by reducing the chance it will be expelled. Altered immune responses during pregnancy may decrease the maternal ability to fight infection. In addition, genital tract changes may affect susceptibility. As pregnancy advances, vaginal walls engorge, the cervix enlarges, and vaginal pH decreases, contributing to susceptibility.

Some consequences of maternal infection, such as infertility and sterility, last a lifetime. Psychosocial problems as a result of maternal infections may include altered interpersonal relationships and lowered self-esteem. Other conditions, such as a congenitally acquired infection, often affect the length and quality of a child's life.

Education and counseling are important in the prevention of maternal infections. Adolescent mothers are at risk because of earlier onset of intercourse and increased likelihood of multiple partners. The recent trend of exchanging sex for drugs is contributing to a rise in infection rates, especially among urban, poor, and minority women.

The prevention of disease and reduction of maternal and neonatal complications continue to be enormous challenges. Many microorganisms can increase maternal and fetal risk. Mortality and morbidity rates are increased when infection is present; thus it is important to prevent infection or at least to recognize and treat it promptly.

MASTITIS

Mastitis, an infection of the lactating breast, occurs most often during the second and third weeks after childbirth, although it may develop at any time. It usually affects only one breast.

Mastitis often is caused by *Staphylococcus aureus.* The bacteria typically are carried on the hands of the mother or agency staff or in the newborn's mouth. The organism may enter through an injured area of the nipple, such as a crack or blister, although there may be no sign of injury. Nipple soreness may result in insufficient emptying of the breast.

Engorgement and stasis of milk frequently precede mastitis, often when a feeding is skipped, when the infant begins sleeping through the night, or when breast-feeding is stopped suddenly. Constriction of the breasts from a tight bra may interfere with emptying all of the ducts and may lead to infection. The mother who is fatigued or stressed or who has other health problems that compromise her immune system is at increased risk for mastitis.

Initial symptoms may be flulike, with fatigue and aching muscles. Symptoms progress to include fever of 101.1°F (38.3°C) or higher, chills, malaise, and headache. Mastitis is characterized by a localized area of redness and inflammation.

Antibiotic therapy, antiinfective agents (antimicrobial agents), and continued emptying of the breast with breast-feeding or breast pump constitute the first line of treatment. With early antibiotic treatment, mastitis usually resolves in 24 to 48 hours. Approximately 5% of women with mastitis develop a breast abscess, which is treated with surgical drainage and antibiotics.

Supportive measures include application of heat or ice packs, breast support, and analgesics. The mother should continue to breast-feed from both breasts. If the affected breast is too sore, she can use a breast pump. Regular emptying of the breast helps prevent abscess formation. If an abscess forms and ruptures into the breast ducts, breast-feeding on that side should be discontinued and a breast pump used to empty the breast temporarily. Milk obtained should be discarded.

Nursing Interventions and Patient Teaching

Mastitis rarely occurs before discharge from the birth facility, so provide information for prevention and discuss symptoms to report to the health care provider. Measures to prevent mastitis include correctly positioning the infant and avoiding nipple trauma and milk stasis. The mother should breast-feed every 2 to 3 hours. She should avoid formula supplements and nipple shields, and she should change nursing pads when they are wet. She also should avoid continuous pressure on the breasts from tight bras or infant carriers.

Once mastitis occurs, nursing measures are aimed at increasing comfort and helping the mother maintain lactation. Moist heat promotes comfort and increases circulation. A shower or hot packs should be used before feeding or pumping the breasts. Cold packs can be used between feedings to reduce edema. The woman should complete the entire course of antibiotic therapy to prevent recurrence or a breast abscess.

The woman should empty the breast completely at each feeding to prevent stasis of milk, which can result in an abscess. If she is too sore to breast-feed on the affected side or if she is taking medications that are contraindicated during lactation, instruct her to express the milk or use a pump to empty the breasts. Breast-feeding or pumping every 1½ to 2 hours makes the mother more comfortable and prevents stasis. Starting the feeding on the unaffected side causes the milk-ejection reflex to occur in the painful breast and makes the process more efficient. Massage over the affected area before and during the feeding helps ensure complete emptying. Unless contraindicated, fluid intake should be 3000 mL/day. Analgesics may be needed to relieve discomfort.

The mother with mastitis is likely to be discouraged and may decide to stop breast-feeding because of the discomfort involved. Weaning during an episode of mastitis may increase engorgement and stasis, leading to abscess formation or recurrent infection. Therefore encourage the mother to continue breast-feeding.

TORCH INFECTIONS AND HUMAN IMMUNODEFICIENCY VIRUS

TORCH infections—or *T*oxoplasmosis, *O*ther infections such as hepatitis, *R*ubella virus, *C*ytomegalovirus, and *H*erpes simplex viruses—are a group of organisms capable of crossing the placenta and adversely affecting the development of the fetus (Box 29.5).

Transmission of human immunodeficiency virus (HIV), a retrovirus, occurs primarily through the exchange of body fluids. Severe depression of the cellular immune system characterizes acquired immunodeficiency syndrome (AIDS) (Box 29.6). Although the populations at high risk have been well documented, assess all women for the possibility of HIV exposure. HIV infection in women commonly is reported at a later stage in the disease; patients usually enter the hospital for initiation of treatment when the illness is more severe. The delay may be due in part to the fact that the symptoms are different from those in men. Chronic vaginitis and candidiasis are common presenting problems.

Obstetric risk in people with HIV infection is difficult to determine because so many other factors are often present. Many women who are HIV positive also have drug and alcohol addiction, poor nutrition, limited access to prenatal care, or concurrent sexually transmitted infections (STIs). Women who are HIV positive are probably at risk for preterm labor and birth, premature rupture of membranes, intrauterine growth restriction (IUGR), perinatal mortality, and postpartum endometritis (see Chapter 16 in *Adult Health Nursing*).

Etiology

Numerous infectious diseases may cause complications during pregnancy. Some are airborne or ingested, but most are spread via direct contact, usually through sexual transmission. Others are contracted with use of contaminated needles or blood transfusions.

Nursing Interventions

The presence of infection is not always evident. Because of the increased incidence of serious infectious diseases, the Centers for Disease Control and Prevention recommends use of standard precautions with all patients. These precautions are most important when dealing with blood and body fluids. Those caring for mothers and newborns frequently are exposed to blood and body fluids and must be particularly alert. Wear gloves, masks, gowns, and glasses during procedures that involve splashing of body fluids, such as amniotomy. Use gloves when cleaning or assessing the breasts or perineal area. Also use gloves when performing the initial newborn bath or changing diapers. Thorough handwashing, as always, is essential. Suction or resuscitate the infant with use of mechanical barriers or equipment such as mouth shields, suction devices, and ventilators. Take care when handling needles and syringes; dispose of these in special containers without breaking or recapping.

During the birthing process, every effort should be made to decrease the neonate's exposure to infected maternal blood and secretions. If feasible, the membranes should be left intact until the birth. Women who give birth within 4 hours after membrane rupture are less likely to transmit the virus to their neonates than women who experience a longer interval between rupture and birth. Avoid fetal scalp electrodes and scalp pH sampling, because these procedures may result in inoculation of the virus into the fetus. Likewise, avoid the use of forceps and a vacuum extractor when possible. Episiotomy and cesarean birth do not seem to influence the infection rate greatly.

The cleansed neonate can be with the HIV-infected mother after birth, but breast-feeding is discouraged because of possible HIV transmission in breast milk. (The World Health Organization has not discouraged breast-feeding in nonindustrialized nations because of the decreased availability of infant formula and hygiene risks in the preparation of formula but may be changing its recommendation.) After discharge, the woman and her infant are referred to physicians who are experienced in the treatment of AIDS and associated conditions.

Psychological support is important to the patient with an infectious disease. Because many of these diseases are life threatening to the mother, the fetus, or the newborn, fear and anxiety are common. If the infection results in fetal mortality or defects, the mother may express guilt. Nurses also must cope with their own feelings about these serious infectious diseases. Caring for mothers and newborns with AIDS and other such diseases can create judgmental feelings in nurses that they must resolve.

Patient Teaching

Education on prevention of infection should start long before pregnancy. Infections acquired by a woman before she becomes pregnant can seriously affect the outcome of pregnancy. Immunization for rubella before childbearing years is essential; stress to all new mothers the importance of having children routinely immunized. Review hygiene practices such as careful hand washing and proper storage and preparation of meats. Discuss safer sex practices, including use of condoms, with

Box 29.5 TORCH Infections

T: TOXOPLASMOSIS

- Toxoplasmosis is caused by a protozoan, *Toxoplasma gondii,* which can be contracted by eating raw contaminated meats or having contact with feces of infected cats.
- Toxoplasmosis is one of the common accompanying opportunistic infections of acquired immunodeficiency syndrome (AIDS). The mother may be free of symptoms or may have development of myalgia, enlarged posterior cervical lymph nodes, malaise, and rash that disappear in a matter of days. Acute infection in pregnancy produces flulike symptoms and lymphadenopathy.
- Diagnosis is confirmed with blood studies, and women in at-risk groups should have toxoplasmosis titer evaluated.
- The effects on the fetus can be profound: spontaneous abortion, stillbirth, neonatal death, blindness, retardation, and a wide range of congenital anomalies.
- Teach all pregnant women to avoid undercooked meats.
- If cats are present in the woman's environment, she should wear gloves whenever chance of contact with feces exists.

O: OTHER

- The primary infection in this category is hepatitis. Hepatitis A is a virus spread by droplets or hands and is associated with poor handwashing after defecation.
- Pregnancy effects include spontaneous abortion and flulike signs and symptoms: fever, malaise, and nausea. If the fetus is exposed in the first trimester and is untreated, possible effects include fetal anomalies, preterm birth, fetal or neonatal hepatitis, and intrauterine death. Gamma globulin vaccination is given to mothers and newborns for prophylaxis.
- Hepatitis B is a virus transmitted in a manner similar to that of human immunodeficiency virus (HIV). Routes of transmission include contaminated needles, syringes, or blood products; sexual intercourse; and body fluid exchange.
- During pregnancy, common signs and symptoms include fever, rash, anorexia, malaise, myalgias, and jaundice if the liver is affected acutely. Fetal and newborn effects are the same as those listed for hepatitis A. Vaccination during pregnancy is not thought to pose a risk to the fetus. Hepatitis B vaccine is recommended for all mothers and neonates.
- The "other" group includes other miscellaneous infections that may affect the mother or fetus (or both). Varicella zoster and mumps are included in this listing.
- Urinary tract and vaginal infections can cause fever, chills, dysuria, pain, malaise, and changes in vaginal drainage. Report any of these symptoms promptly to the physician. Culture and sensitivity tests usually reveal the specific organism. Treatment is based on the causative organism and the severity of the problem. Treatment must be done cautiously because of the possibility of teratogenic effects from the antibiotics.
- Sexually transmitted infections (STIs) are also a serious concern. Syphilis can cross the placental barrier and infect the fetus. Chlamydia may cause pneumonia or eye infections in the newborn. Gonorrhea can cause pelvic inflammatory disease in the mother and eye infections in the newborn.
- Human immunodeficiency virus (HIV) is an infection that has potentially lethal implications for both the mother and fetus. See Box 29.6.

R: RUBELLA, GERMAN MEASLES, OR 3-DAY MEASLES

- Rubella is a viral infection transmitted by droplets. Fever, rash, and mild lymphedema usually are seen in the affected mother. If contracted during the first trimester, rubella can cause a wide range of congenital defects, including congenital heart disease, mental retardation, deafness, and cataracts.
- Diagnosis is made with serologic tests for rubella titer.
- Immunization ideally should be given before a woman reaches childbearing age. If a pregnant woman does not have immunity, caution her to avoid risk of exposure to the disease.
- Because this immunization involves administration of an attenuated (diluted to reduce virulence of pathogenic microorganism) virus, it is given after delivery, frequently just before discharge. This is one time the physician can be certain that the woman is not pregnant.
- Further caution the woman to avoid becoming pregnant for 2 to 3 months after vaccination, because the attenuated virus used for immunization may still be present.

C: CYTOMEGALOVIRUS

- Cytomegalovirus (CMV) is a virus and belongs to the herpesvirus group.
- CMV is a common infection that can be spread by close contact, breast-feeding, sexual relations, and kissing.
- More than half of all adults have antibodies to the virus.
- This virus is capable of crossing the placental barrier and causing serious damage to the fetus, including cognitive impairment, hearing problems, and congenital anomalies. It is unusual in that the mother may be totally asymptomatic, and it does not always cause fetal complications.
- Pregnant health care providers should observe standard precautions to avoid exposure to droplets of infected secretions such as saliva, urine, and respiratory discharges.

H: HERPES GENITALIS

- Herpes genitalis also is called herpesvirus type 2. It causes painful lesions on the external genitalia and also can involve the cervix.
- Intrauterine infection of the fetus can occur if the membranes rupture or vaginal delivery takes place when active lesions are present. If the virus is not treated, the neonatal mortality rate is extremely high.
- Diagnosis is made on the basis of maternal symptoms and a culture of the lesions.
- Women with active herpes infection should deliver via cesarean birth.
- The pregnancy effects of primary genital herpes infection include spontaneous abortion, preterm labor, and intrauterine growth restriction.
- Health care providers with herpes simplex virus (HSV) infections should take precautions. Anyone with oral HSV lesions should wear a mask if in close contact with newborns, and anyone with skin lesions should not give direct care until lesions are dried and crusted. Scrupulous handwashing is essential.

Box 29.6 Acquired Immunodeficiency Syndrome

- Acquired immunodeficiency syndrome (AIDS) is a major health concern. It has had a significant effect on all areas of health care, including maternal nursing.
- The causative organism is the human immunodeficiency virus (HIV), which enters the body through blood, blood products, or sexual contact. It is capable of crossing the placental barrier and infecting the fetus in utero, causing congenital defects such as microcephaly (abnormal smallness of the head) and facial deformities.
- Because of the long incubation period, infants born to HIV-seropositive mothers may show no indication at birth but develop signs of the infection later. These signs include failure to thrive, recurrent infection, interstitial pneumonia, and neurologic abnormalities.
- Studies place the risk of perinatal transmission at 20% to 50%. Most children diagnosed with AIDS die within the first few years of life.
- All pregnant women diagnosed with HIV benefit from antiretroviral therapy. Most mother-to-fetus transmissions occur in the final weeks of pregnancy.
- Rapid HIV testing is available for women who come in for delivery without having had prenatal care. Results are rapidly available and allow for safer management of mother and baby.
- Vaginal birth is strongly discouraged, and cesarean delivery is advisable. Cesarean births have been shown to reduce contact with maternal virus.

Box 29.7 Comfort Measures for the Pregnant Woman With a Vaginal Infection

- Pour warm water over the urethra and vulva.
- Take warm sitz baths for 15 minutes three to five times daily.
- Avoid strong deodorant soaps, creams, and ointments.
- Dry the genital area with a blow dryer. (To prevent burning, beware of high temperatures.)
- Wear 100% cotton underwear.
- Do not wear tight-fitting jeans.
- Do not wear panties or pantyhose with nylon inserts.
- Obtain early and regular Papanicolaou (Pap) smears.
- Avoid any sexual contact during outbreaks.

individuals at risk, and stress the importance of regular medical care and treatment.

Counseling the pregnant woman with a vaginal infection also should include measures to deal with the discomfort (Box 29.7).

Prognosis

The success of the prevention measures depends on the conscientious effort of the health care worker in carrying out all recommended procedures carefully and the patient's willingness to comply with preventive measures or prescribed therapy.

COMPLICATIONS RELATED TO EXISTING MEDICAL CONDITIONS

DIABETES MELLITUS

Etiology

Diabetes mellitus is an endocrine disorder that affects metabolism and the utilization of glucose. This disease is not curable and is often difficult to control. In pregnancy, hormonal changes and stresses placed on all the maternal body systems result in even more complex medical and nursing management.

Pathophysiology

In diabetes mellitus, the pancreas does not produce adequate amounts of insulin to metabolize glucose normally. Because glucose does not enter the cells without adequate insulin, blood glucose levels remain high. The cells release stored fat and protein for energy, leading to ketosis and a negative nitrogen balance.

Diabetes is classified into various forms. Type 1 (formerly called insulin-dependent diabetes mellitus) requires regular administration of insulin for control. Type 2 (formerly called non–insulin-dependent diabetes mellitus) is controlled most often with diet or oral hypoglycemic medications. *Pregestational diabetes mellitus* is the label sometimes given to type 1 or type 2 diabetes that exists before pregnancy.

Gestational diabetes mellitus (GDM) is the inability to produce enough insulin to maintain normal glucose levels during pregnancy. Increased dietary glucose needs, along with insulin resistance from placental hormones, cortisol, and insulinase, result in hyperglycemia and GDM. The patient with GDM usually is diagnosed in the middle of the pregnancy and may have sustained hyperglycemia in the early months of the pregnancy. Thus she may be at greater risk for fetal complications than a woman with preexisting diabetes. Risk factors for the development of gestational diabetes includes older than age 25 years at the time of pregnancy, family history of diabetes, history of gestational diabetes, nonwhite race, obesity, and hypertension.

Improved control of this disease process has reduced the risk to mother and fetus; however, the incidence of complications is still significant. Maternal complications include infections (urinary tract and vaginal), difficult labor related to increased fetal size (which frequently results in cesarean birth), vascular complications (including retinopathy), azotemia, ketoacidosis, hypertensive disorders such as preeclampsia, and cesarean birth. Fetal complications include stillbirth, spontaneous abortion, hydramnios (excessive amniotic fluid), large placenta, alteration in size for gestational age (macrosomia), congenital anomalies, neonatal hypoglycemia, neonatal hyperbilirubinemia, respiratory distress syndrome, and fetal or neonatal death.

Clinical Manifestations

Alteration in blood glucose levels is the major manifestation of the disease. Blood glucose levels greater than

Box 29.8 Signs and Symptoms of Maternal Hypoglycemia and Hyperglycemia

HYPOGLYCEMIA
- Shakiness (tremors)
- Sweating
- Pallor; cold, clammy skin
- Disorientation, irritability
- Headache
- Hunger
- Blurred vision

HYPERGLYCEMIA
- Fatigue
- Flushed, hot skin
- Dry mouth, excessive thirst
- Frequent urination
- Rapid, deep respirations; odor of acetone on breath
- Drowsiness, headache
- Depressed reflexes

120 mg/dL significantly increase the risk of complications. When blood glucose levels are elevated, the classic symptoms of diabetes—polyuria, polydipsia, and polyphagia—may be observed (Box 29.8).

Assessment

Perform urine testing at all prenatal visits. If testing indicates the presence of glucose, additional testing is necessary. For the patient with known diabetes, assess diet, activity, and medication compliance. Assess the vascular system regularly for possible complications, and watch the patient closely for signs of infection. Also assess the condition of the fetus with serial ultrasound scans and other medical measures.

Diagnostic Tests

A 1-hour, 50-g diabetes screening test or glucose tolerance test is scheduled routinely between 24 and 28 weeks' gestation. Women with a history of gestational diabetes or who present with risk factors for development of the condition are tested earlier in the pregnancy. Results that indicate hyperglycemia in the fasting portion of the test (blood sugar [BS], >92 mg/dL) or the 1-hour reading (180 mg/dL) result in an order for the woman to undergo the 3-hour glucose tolerance test. The results from the 3-hour test are used to confirm the diagnosis. Any two results of displaying elevations establish the diagnosis (Davidson et al, 2012).

- Fasting, 95 mg/dL
- 1 hour, 180 mg/dL
- 2 hours, 155 mg/dL
- 3 hours, 140 mg/dL

Glycosylated hemoglobin (Hgb A_{1C}) is not a reliable test during pregnancy.

Diagnostic techniques for fetal surveillance often performed during pregnancy are complicated by diabetes mellitus. Tests to evaluate fetal well-being include nonstress test, contraction stress test, alpha-fetoprotein, biophysical profile (Table 29.3), and serum estriols (the major estrogen secreted by the placenta, measured to determine placental functioning). The patient who is diagnosed with gestational diabetes or who has been diagnosed with diabetes mellitus before pregnancy often has labor induced before the due date in an effort to avoid complications. Determination of the estimated due date (EDD) and assessments as the pregnancy progresses to determine fetal lung maturity are performed. Try to determine the estimated date of birth. A baseline ultrasound scan is done to assess the fetus's gestational age. Follow-up ultrasound examinations are performed as often as every 4 to 6 weeks to monitor fetal growth and development and to assess for congenital abnormalities. Biochemical analysis of amniotic fluid is performed to ascertain fetal lung maturity, typically in the third trimester.

Nursing Interventions

Nursing care is directed at maintaining the patient in a euglycemic (normal blood glucose) status. The patient's insulin requirements change significantly throughout pregnancy, labor, and delivery. Assess the patient carefully at each visit, complete all blood glucose level evaluations as ordered, and report any abnormalities to the health care provider promptly. Because of possible teratogenic effects, patients with type 2 diabetes mellitus have oral hypoglycemic medications discontinued and insulin prescribed. The initial plan of action for patients diagnosed with gestational diabetes is control of the condition with dietary interventions. In the event this is not successful, insulin therapy is prescribed. Regular and intermediate-acting insulin are most often administered. Blood glucose monitoring is recommended at fasting and then 1 to 2 hours after meals.

A patient problem and interventions for the patient with GDM include but are not limited to the following:

Patient Problem	Nursing Interventions
Impaired Health Maintenance, related to deficient knowledge of the effects of pregnancy on diabetes control	Review pathophysiology of the disease Assist the patient in formulating questions for the physician Clarify misconceptions Teach home monitoring of blood glucose levels Review effects of diabetes on the pregnant patient Explain in simple terms the advantages to the fetus of maintaining a normal maternal blood glucose level; advantages include an optimal pattern of growth, the increased likelihood that the baby will be born near term, and fewer complications associated with prematurity

Continued

Table 29.3 **Medications for the Mother and Newborn at Risk**

GENERIC NAME (TRADE NAME)	ACTION	SIDE EFFECTS	NURSING IMPLICATIONS
Metoclopramide	Antiemetic	Headache, weakness, fatigue	IV administration deliver dosage over 15 minutes.
doxylamine-pyridoxine (Diclegis)	Antiemetic	Drowsiness, headache, constipation	Take on an empty stomach with water. Do not crush or chew pill.
Methotrexate	Antimetabolite compound that interferes with DNA synthesis	Nausea, vomiting, skin redness	Administer intramuscularly. Review lab records to ensure patient is hemodynamically stable. Instruct patient of signs and symptoms to report.
valacyclovir (converts to acyclovir; Valtrex)	Antiviral	Topical: Stinging, burning, rash, pruritus Systemic: Headache, seizures, renal toxicity, phlebitis at intravenous site	Topical: Use glove to apply, cover lesion completely. Adequate hydration to prevent crystallization in kidneys; give IV dose for 1 h.
Hepatitis B immune globulin (HBIG)	Series provides immunity to hepatitis B	Pain, redness and itching at site of injection. Headache, fatigue and fever	Provide education on scheduling of subsequent injections in the series.
hydralazine	Arterial vasodilator	Headache, flushing, tachycardia	Assess for tachycardia, hypotension, urinary output; maintain bed rest.
Lung surfactant: colfosceril palmitate (Exosurf [synthetic]) beractant (Survanta [natural lung surfactant])	Replaces natural lung surfactant that maintains lung inflation and prevents lung collapse; used to treat and prevent respiratory distress syndrome in premature neonates	Synthetic: Apnea, pulmonary hemorrhage, pulmonary air leak Natural: Transient bradycardia, oxygen desaturation, hypotension, apnea	Administer endotracheally only; suction before administration (drug may reflux into endotracheal tube during administration); slow or stop administration until tube is clear.
Magnesium sulfate ($MgSO_4$)	See Chapter 26.		
oxytocin (Pitocin)	See Chapter 27.		
$Rh_o(D)$ immune globulin (RhoGAM)	See Chapter 27.		
ritodrine	See Chapter 26.		
Rubella vaccine	See Chapter 27.		
naloxone hydrochloride (Narcan)	Reverses central nervous system and respiratory depression caused by narcotics (opiates) Competes with narcotics at receptor sites	If given to an infant of a mother addicted to drugs, causes withdrawal and may cause seizures	Prepare the syringe before birth by drawing up more than is needed. After birth, remove excess from the syringe and give the amount according to the estimate of the infant's weight. Inject rapidly. Monitor for response and be prepared to give repeated doses if necessary. Use resuscitation measures as necessary.

Continued

Table 29.3 Medications for the Mother and Newborn at Risk—cont'd

GENERIC NAME (TRADE NAME)	ACTION	SIDE EFFECTS	NURSING IMPLICATIONS
terbutaline[a]	Stimulates beta-adrenergic receptors of the sympathetic nervous system Results primarily in bronchodilation and inhibition of uterine muscle activity Increases pulse rate and widens pulse pressure	Maternal and fetal tachycardia, palpitations, cardiac arrhythmias, chest pain, wide pulse pressure, dyspnea, tremors, weakness, dizziness, headache, hyperglycemia, nausea, vomiting, skin flushing, and diaphoresis	Explain common side effects, which usually are well tolerated. Assess FHR, usually with continuous fetal monitoring. Assess maternal pulse, respirations and blood pressure by the same schedule as for FHR. Maintain adequate hydration. Encourage patient to urinate q 2 hr. Report any significant or unacceptable side effects. Repeat continuing or recurrent uterine activity. Teach signs and symptoms of recurrent preterm labor and follow-up medical care after discharge.
nifedipine (Procardia)	Relaxes smooth muscles (tocolytic) Inhibits uterine contractions in preterm labor Not approved by the FDA for inhibiting uterine activity, although it is widely used for this purpose	Dizziness, headache, palpitations, weaknesses, shortness of breath, feelings of warmth, and tightness in chest	See nursing implications for terbutaline.
penicillin	Used for group B streptococcus Administered after culture and sensitivity is completed	Interferes with contraception usage	Assess for allergies; hypersensitivity reaction may be delayed. Assess respiratory system for abnormalities such as rate, status, character, any tightness in chest.

[a]Not approved by the FDA for inhibiting uterine activity, although it is widely used for this purpose; research has been mixed regarding the drug effects of terbutaline for this purpose, but its lower risk for adverse side effects, combined with some efficacy, has encouraged its use.
FDA, US Food and Drug Administration; *FHR*, fetal heart rate; *IV*, intravenous.

Patient Problem	Nursing Interventions
	Teach danger signs of diabetes and whom to notify (provide written as well as oral instructions) Stress importance of weekly prenatal visits during second half of pregnancy Refer patient to community diabetic support groups

Patient Teaching

The need for teaching differs with the classification of the disease and the patient's willingness to learn. A woman who has been diagnosed before pregnancy needs reinforcement of diet, medication, and health practices. Also explain the effects pregnancy has on diabetes throughout the course of pregnancy, labor, delivery, and the postpartum period.

The patient with newly diagnosed gestational diabetes needs a great deal of education. It is important to stress the necessity of good control of the disease. The training normally provided to a patient with newly diagnosed diabetes mellitus also may be helpful.

Be an active listener and allow time for the woman and her family to express concerns and feelings. Convey acceptance of expressed feelings whether they are negative or positive. Sharing emotions helps the woman cope with her anxiety and frustration and thus promotes her active participation in her care.

Prognosis

Maintenance of glycemic control is needed to promote improved outcomes. Potential complications for the mother include increased risk for operative birth and tissue trauma resulting from vaginal delivery of a large-for-gestational-age infant. Complications in the infant include risk for preterm delivery and macrosomia. Insulin does not cross the placental barrier (placental tissue limits passage of certain substances); consequently, control of the mother's diabetes is vital to the health of the fetus. Most women benefit from praise when diabetic control is well maintained. They feel competent and trusted by the health care team and motivated to continue.

CARDIAC DISEASE

Pregnancy increases the demands on the cardiovascular system. This is not a problem for the normal, healthy heart, which is able to adapt to the increased demands. However, women who have preexisting cardiac disease face increased risk when cardiac function is challenged by pregnancy. About 1% of pregnancies are complicated by heart disease. The degree of disability is often more important than the type of cardiovascular disease in the treatment and prognosis during pregnancy.

Etiology

The most common cardiac problems of maternity patients result from rheumatic heart disease, congenital heart defects, and mitral valve prolapse. Occasionally, a condition called peripartum *cardiomyopathy* (disease of the myocardium, especially as a result of primary diseases of the heart muscle) is observed in pregnant patients who have no history of cardiac problems. This may be seen in the last month of pregnancy or during the postpartum period. The symptoms are similar to those of congestive heart failure.

With successful treatment of congenital cardiac anomalies or mitral stenosis from rheumatic heart disease, many girls are now reaching childbearing age and bearing children. Rheumatic heart disease, a complication of streptococcal infection, is not common in the United States but may be found in recent immigrants. Hypertensive heart disease, often a secondary effect of obesity, can be expected to affect more childbearing women because of the growing incidence in the general population. Cardiomyopathy is a disorder of the muscle structure of the heart that may have any of several causes. Congestive heart failure may result from underlying heart disease or from treatment for other conditions.

Pathophysiology

During pregnancy, increased blood volume, heart rate, and cardiac output are normal. In the woman with existing cardiac problems, the muscle, the valves, or the vessels are overly stressed by these changes. Symptoms of the underlying pathologic condition are exacerbated, which results in cardiac decompensation, congestive failure, and other medical problems.

Clinical Manifestations

The symptoms depend on the underlying pathologic condition. Edema, cyanosis, tachycardia, palpitations, arrhythmias, chest pain, dyspnea, and fatigue may occur. Physical exertion may increase the severity of the symptoms. Clinical findings are those of heart failure (left ventricular failure). The patient has decreased cardiac output and pulmonary congestion, with fluid collecting in the lungs. Pulmonary edema and pleural effusion also occur, and pulmonary crackles, hemoptysis, and cough may be present.

Assessment

At each prenatal visit, measure the patient's vital signs and evaluate her ability to participate in activities. Unusual fatigue with activity may reveal problems. Monitor for edema, weight gain, murmurs, cough, dyspnea, and abnormal lung sounds. Compare these data with normal changes during pregnancy. The patient with preexisting heart disease also should be followed by her cardiologist during her pregnancy.

The pregnant woman with cardiac disease needs detailed assessment to determine the potential for optimal maternal health and a viable fetus throughout the peripartum period. If she chooses to continue the pregnancy, assess the condition of the woman with a high-risk pregnancy as often as weekly.

Diagnostic Tests

Chest x-ray evaluation, electrocardiograms, echocardiograms, and auscultation are used to determine the type and severity of the cardiac problem. Blood gas analysis may be performed if severe decompensation is observed. A woman's sudden inability to perform activities that she previously was comfortable doing may indicate cardiovascular decompensation.

Nursing Interventions

Nursing care is directed at helping the woman maintain normal physical and psychosocial function. During pregnancy, teach the importance of diet, medications, paced activity, and adequate rest. This includes education about the specific disease and its management. Iron intake must be adequate to prevent anemia, which further stresses the heart. Sodium may be restricted to control the fluid volume and decrease cardiac stress. Stool softeners may be prescribed to decrease use of the Valsalva maneuver (holding the breath while bearing down) when defecating. The activity level is dictated by the severity of the cardiac problem. Be aware of the medical recommendations and help the woman incorporate these into her daily life. Patients with more severe cardiac problems need the greatest adjustments. Be highly sensitive to personal and family needs.

If cardiopulmonary arrest occurs during pregnancy, cardiopulmonary resuscitation may be performed within certain guidelines.

During labor, the semi-Fowler's or side-lying position with the head elevated enhances respiratory effort and improves circulation. During every contraction, 300 to 500 mL of blood shifts from the uterus and placenta into the central circulation. This extra fluid causes a sharp rise in cardiac workload; therefore careful management of IV administration is essential to prevent fluid overload. The efforts of labor may necessitate oxygen administration to increase the blood oxygen saturation, which is monitored with pulse oximetry. Administer medications such as cardiotonics, diuretics, prophylactic antibiotics, sedatives, and analgesics as directed by the physician. Reduce discomfort to a minimum. Also try to eliminate unnecessary activity by the patient during labor. Resting between contractions and using shorter, open-glottis pushing are recommended to conserve energy. Closely monitor fetal condition for any signs of distress; use a fetal monitor for continuous assessment. Calmly explain everything to decrease anxiety.

A vaginal delivery is recommended for a woman with heart disease unless there are specific indications for a cesarean birth. Vacuum extraction or outlet forceps often are used to minimize the mother's use of the Valsalva maneuver when pushing during the second stage.

Postpartum care varies according to the severity of the cardiac problem. Explore methods of incorporating care of the infant into the mother's activities. Because extravascular fluid returns to the bloodstream after delivery, the mother is at risk for development of cardiac decompression during the 48 hours after the birth.

To promote normal parent-child attachment, establish contact as early as possible. Discuss breast-feeding with the physician because the physical effort may be excessive for the mother and the transfer of medications in the breast milk may be harmful to the infant. As in all other areas of nursing, continue to assess the patient's status and give explanations for all care.

Amnioinfusion. *Amnioinfusion,* an infusion of fluids directly into the amniotic sac, may be performed during pregnancy to treat patients with *oligohydramnios,* a deficit in the level of amniotic fluid. During labor, amnioinfusion may be performed with saline or lactated Ringer's solution to manage women with cord compression resulting in variable decelerations. Amniotic fluid provides buoyancy to the fetus, preventing cord compression and promoting musculoskeletal development.

Prognosis

In cardiac complications, the maternal mortality rate has been estimated in the range of 30% to 60%; the infant mortality rate is approximately 10%. The prognosis is good if cardiomegaly is not persistent after 6 months. The prognosis for women whose hearts remain enlarged is not as favorable. Future pregnancies usually result in some cardiac failure (50% to 88%). The mortality rate may be as high as 60%. Oral contraceptives are contraindicated because of the risk of thromboembolism.

COMPLICATIONS RELATED TO AGE

ADOLESCENTS

Adolescent patients present the nurse with a unique challenge. A significant number are sexually active and in need of contraceptive counseling; many become pregnant. The pregnant adolescent, her family, and her partner need sensitive, competent nursing interventions. The young woman may choose to terminate the pregnancy or carry it to term. She may place the infant up for adoption or elect to keep the baby. The nurse plays a vital role in helping the patient make informed decisions and in supporting her, physically and emotionally, in carrying out her chosen option. Never recommend a choice.

Growth and Development

The period of adolescence is divided into three stages: early, middle, and late. The higher the developmental level, the greater the readiness to accept responsibility for self and others.

Adolescent development is characterized by physical, cognitive, and behavioral development that approximates chronologic age. Adolescents are egocentric, concrete thinkers and have feelings of invincibility, which lead to risky behaviors, such as smoking, drug and alcohol abuse, and unprotected sex with multiple partners.

Before children can become mature adults, they must accomplish the developmental tasks of adolescence, including acceptance of body image, acceptance of sexual identity, development of a personal value system, preparation for making a living, independence from parents, development of decision-making skills, and development of an adult identity. These tasks vary from culture to culture and with individual adolescents and their goals.

Pregnancy interrupts the process of identifying formation and developmental tasks. Attempting to accomplish developmental tasks of pregnancy and of normal adolescence simultaneously may be overwhelming. The psychological burden may lead to depression and to postponement in attaining an adult identity. The pregnant adolescent faces further developmental tasks of parenthood. These tasks are as important to the new adolescent parents as they organize ways to behave in their environment as they are for the adult (see lifespan discussion in Chapter 24).

Although the number of adolescent pregnancies in the United States has not increased in the past 5 to 10 years, pregnancies have increased significantly among very young adolescents (ages 10 to 14 years). This trend is attributed to many sociologic factors, including breakdown of the traditional family and changes in social mores that result in earlier sexual activity. Teenagers account for an increasingly large percentage of births and abortions. Physiologic immaturity, incomplete education, and unresolved developmental tasks are complicating factors.

Several physiologic concerns are associated with the young pregnant adolescent. These include an increased risk for GH, cephalopelvic disproportion that results in cesarean birth, abruptio placentae, low birth weight, IUGR, anemia, infection, preterm delivery, and perinatal death. Pregnant teenagers also commonly fear or deny the pregnancy and go without medical attention until late in pregnancy. Lack of prenatal care increases the risk to the pregnant teenager and her infant.

Sociocultural concerns are seen in educational and economic arenas. The pregnancy frequently ends the adolescent's formal education, which leads to reduced job opportunities because of lack of training. This results in an increased poverty risk with potentially prolonged dependence on public assistance.

Assessment

Assessment of all health patterns for each adolescent is essential. When prenatal care is initiated early and consistently, and confounding variables (e.g., socioeconomic factors) are controlled, very young pregnant adolescents are at no greater risk (nor are their infants) for an adverse outcome than older pregnant women. The nurse's role in reducing the risks and consequences of adolescent pregnancy is twofold: to encourage early and continued prenatal care, and to refer the adolescent, if necessary, for appropriate social support services, which can help reverse the effects of a negative socioeconomic environment.

Nursing Interventions

When caring for the pregnant adolescent, be aware of the patient's unique nature and incorporate physical and psychological interventions into the care plan. An understanding of adolescent growth and development is necessary to successfully relate to and care for this patient.

Patient problems and interventions for the pregnant adolescent patient include but are not limited to the following:

Patient Problem	Nursing Interventions
Insufficient Knowledge, related to choices regarding pregnancy, childbirth experiences, and parenthood	Examine own views regarding sexuality to be able to maintain nonjudgmental approach Listen and give honest answers Create a safe and stable environment that engenders trust Evaluate which stage of development the adolescent is experiencing Teach the adolescent about pregnancy choices, childbirth, and parenthood Encourage questions and verbalization of fears and concerns Compliment teens on the questions asked and efforts made to learn about issues Encourage support personnel to attend and participate in prenatal care Refer to childbirth and parenthood class and community support and information groups
Imbalanced Nutrition, related to inadequate diet	Perform 24-h diet recall to establish dietary habits Assess height and weight and compare with norms for age Assess for frequent dieting, eating disorders, smoking, alcohol use, and substance abuse Assess fat content of diet Assess fluid intake for caffeine levels Explain fetal need for weight gain Refer to dietitian for nutrition counseling Provide sample menus, including increased vitamins, minerals, and calories Refer to the Women, Infants, and Children (WIC) program for dietary supplements

Labor and birth. The very young adolescent may be frightened of needles, pelvic examinations, noises from other women in labor or from equipment, and birth rooms. Provide a single, private room when possible. Ensure the patient has the support of a knowledgeable coach, whether husband, friend, parent, or nurse. Many teenagers come to labor lacking preparation; they are frightened and often alone. If they are admitted early in the first stage, teach about relaxation with contractions, ambulation, side-lying positions, and comfort measures. The adolescent is more concerned with how the baby will get out than with fetal well-being.

Pregnant young adolescents often are still growing, so there is an increased chance of cephalopelvic disproportion and cesarean birth. This provides an additional fear for the laboring adolescent. Be prepared to provide the necessary support and encouragement. Always provide anticipatory guidance and explain procedures. Many adolescents keep their infants and are responsive to staff members who share their delight. For these young parents, efforts to promote parent-child attachment are particularly important.

Postpartum care. Physically, the adolescent mother needs the same care as any woman who has given birth. Provide explicit directions for self-care and infant care. Most adolescents view the care of the infant as their primary area of concern. Continue to assess the new mother's parenting abilities during the postpartum period. In addition, continue to support the patient by involving grandparents or other family members, making home visits, and referring to group sessions for discussion of infant care and parenting problems. Outreach programs concerned with self-care, parent-child interactions, child injuries, and failure to thrive, and those that provide prompt and effective intervention prevent more serious problems.

Postpartum contraception is a high priority for almost every young adolescent. The risk of repeat pregnancy in adolescence is high, and all the accompanying risks of adolescent pregnancy increase with each subsequent pregnancy. Almost universally, postpartum adolescents say that they will never have sex again and therefore need no birth control. Nonetheless, adolescents need to leave the hospital with barrier methods (foam and condoms) and the knowledge of how and when to use them. Very young adolescents may be shy or embarrassed about touching their genitalia to use barrier methods. In addition, they are not likely to anticipate intercourse. For these reasons, some health care providers send adolescents home on a regimen of oral contraceptives. This practice is controversial because of the increased risk of thromboembolic disease in the immediate postpartum period (first 4 weeks). Thus the decision must be based on the adolescent and her life situation. Medroxyprogesterone (Depo-Provera) and levonorgestrel (Norplant) currently are encouraged strongly as contraceptives for adolescents. Cultural values and practices also should be considered.

Adolescent males must be considered and included in any interventions in sexuality education, family planning, and parent education.

The adolescent mother needs support if she is considering adoption for her child. Avoid use of phrases that give negative connotations to the adoption process. Phrases such as "put up for adoption" and "give up for adoption" imply the biologic parents are uncaring. Neither should the terms "real parents" or "natural parents" be used exclusively for genetic parents. The adoptive parents are the "real parents," because they care for the child. Neutral language, such as "arranging for an adoption," "biologic parent" or "birth mother," and "adoptive parent," is preferred. Give the mother the option of either remaining on the postpartum floor or transferring to another unit. Assure her that she will have as much access to the baby as she desires.

Grief results from actual or perceived loss. The adolescent may experience grief from thoughts about adoption, the birth of a preterm infant who may be in intensive care, or the infant's death. Help the patient move through the grieving process. The adolescent who gives birth to a preterm infant or one who is small for gestational age may find it difficult to reconcile this tiny, scrawny infant with her fantasized "Gerber baby." She may be afraid of caring for the child introduced to her in the intensive care unit. The confidence in her abilities gained during the prenatal period may be replaced by feelings of being overwhelmed and incompetent. Intensive teaching and continual support programs are essential to keep the young mother and her vulnerable infant from becoming estranged.

Many young mothers pattern their parenting on what they experienced. Therefore it is vital to determine the kind of support that those close to young mothers are able or prepared to give and the kinds of community aid that can supplement this support. The adolescent may have conflict with dependence versus independence issues as she performs her mothering role within the framework of her family of origin. The adolescent's family also may need help adapting to their new roles.

Adolescent father. The adolescent father also faces immediate developmental crises: completing the developmental tasks of adolescence and making a transition to parenthood and, sometimes, to marriage. These transitions can be stressful. Begin interacting with the adolescent father by asking his pregnant partner to bring him to the clinic with her so that he may participate in the birth. With the pregnant teen's agreement, the father also may be contacted directly.

To include the young father in all aspects of the care, assess four areas: (1) the couple's relationship; (2) levels of stress, concern, and coping; (3) educational and vocational goals; and (4) level of health care knowledge. Like all fathers, adolescent fathers need support to discuss their emotional responses to the pregnancy. The nurse's nonjudgmental attitude is essential for open communication. Recognize the father's feelings of guilt, powerlessness, or bravado and their negative consequences for parents and child. Counseling must be reality oriented. Discuss topics such as finances, child care, parenting skills, and the father's role in the birth experience. Teenage fathers also need knowledge of reproductive physiology and birth control options.

The adolescent mother's partner and family affect how she deals with her pregnancy, labor, birth, and subsequent parenthood. The adolescent father may continue to be involved with the young mother. In many instances, he plays an important role in the decisions she faces in pregnancy, including whether to continue the pregnancy, have an abortion, keep the child, or arrange for adoption.

Support the young father by helping him develop realistic perceptions of his role as "father of a child." Encourage his use of coping mechanisms that are not detrimental to his, his partner's, or his child's well-being. Enlist support systems, parents, and professional agencies on his behalf. Encourage mutual responsibility for birth control.

Patient Teaching

Education of the pregnant adolescent is essential. To work effectively with adolescents, be sensitive, nonjudgmental, and knowledgeable about the stages of adolescence. Because no two adolescents are alike, use a wide range of skills to reach each individual (see the Patient Teaching box on adolescent parents). Patient teaching may have to be directed toward the adolescent mother, who is often the primary caregiver. Efforts should be made to keep the adolescent in school. Many high schools have programs to assist adolescent parents in their educational endeavors.

Patient Teaching

Adolescent Parents

- Nutrition is a major area of concern for the teenager. The teen often is still growing, and her nutritional intake must meet her own needs and those of the fetus. Fad diets and food idiosyncrasies are common in teenagers; take this into account when teaching nutrition. Body image disturbance is a problem even for a mature woman. The teenager, particularly one who has not yet accepted the fact of pregnancy, may limit food intake to avoid gaining weight. This can be exceedingly dangerous to mother and infant.
- Preparation for labor and delivery is also essential. Many adolescents have little knowledge of human anatomy and have fears and misconceptions about the process of childbirth. They may have heard stories from friends that increase their anxiety. Be factual without being harsh when describing the birth process.
- Many adolescents plan to raise their infants; therefore instruction should include child care, growth, and development. Refer the women to community agencies that provide ongoing support.
- Do not ignore the adolescent father. Consider the effect of pregnancy on him, particularly if he remains meaningfully involved with the teenage mother. Counseling is important for both because the physical, financial, and emotional consequences of the pregnancy will affect both of them for the rest of their lives.

OLDER PREGNANT WOMAN

At the other end of the reproductive cycle are women who have their first child after they are 35 years of age. These women have a somewhat increased risk of maternal and fetal complications. Issues and concerns related to the over-35 age group have become increasingly prominent in the past decade. Some women have always borne children at a later age, either by choice or because of lack or failure of contraception during the perimenopausal years. Today this group also includes women who have postponed pregnancy because of careers or other reasons and women with infertility problems who become pregnant through technological advances that have expanded alternatives for couples desiring children.

Many women become aware of the so-called biologic clock as menopause approaches and wish to have a child while they are still able to do so. The potential for infertility increases with age. Although most women who wait until later in life are well educated and have decided to become pregnant, conception and pregnancy are not always easy. The incidence of ectopic pregnancy, placenta previa, and various medical conditions such as diabetes or hypertension increases with age. If the woman does become pregnant, each year after age 35 years increases the risk of conceiving a child with Down syndrome or other chromosomal anomalies. Amniocentesis and chorionic villus sampling are performed commonly to detect genetic problems (ACOG, 2017). Detection of genetic disorders can raise ethical dilemmas regarding aborting or raising a disabled child.

Older women who are without medical problems have a much lower risk for problems than previously thought. Those who do have some complications often can have a successful pregnancy with good medical and nursing care. As women maintain better overall health and fitness, increased age appears to be less of an impediment to a normal pregnancy. Most first-time mothers older than 35 years have waited and chosen this specific time for pregnancy; this choice is influenced by their awareness of the increasing possibility of infertility or of genetic defects in the infants of older women. Many women seek information about pregnancy from books and friends. They actively try to prevent fetal disorders and are careful in searching for the best possible maternity care. They identify sources of stress in their lives. They are concerned about having enough energy and stamina to meet the demands of parenting and their new roles and relationships.

Psychosocial adjustment to parenthood at this time of life depends greatly on the individual and her situation. Changes in income, lifestyle, and work routines can present challenges that are stressful, even if the pregnancy is desired.

Peer support may be less available for the mature primigravida. Many friends have teenage children and do not relate to the concerns of a new mother. Younger mothers have some of the same concerns, but they often do not share the perspective of older mothers. Family support may also be lacking. The woman's parents are usually in their 60s or 70s and may not be able to assist with child care to the extent that younger grandparents can.

Mature gravidas also worry about complications that may affect the fetus or their own health. They are aware that they may not have another opportunity for pregnancy because of their age. They may be concerned about their ability to balance their career with increased family responsibilities.

Emphasize measures to assist the mother in regaining strength and muscle tone (e.g., prenatal and postnatal exercises). Some older mothers may find that the care of the newborn infant exhausts their physical capabilities. Many women may benefit from referral to supportive resources in the community.

ADOPTION

Some women carry the pregnancy to term and then give up the newborn to the care of another family for adoption. The decision to place the infant for adoption is a painful one that can produce long-lasting feelings of ambivalence and sorrow. On one hand, the birth mother may be satisfied that the infant is going into a stable home where a child is wanted and will receive excellent care. On the other hand, the social pressures and personal feelings against giving up one's child are often intense.

The relationship between the birth mother and the adoptive parents varies greatly. The adoptive parents may be unknown to the birth mother, or she may have chosen them. Some adoptive mothers participate in the birth. The birth mother may never see the infant again or may keep in contact and participate in the child's life.

Nurses are sometimes unsure of how to communicate with the woman who is giving up her infant. First, the nursing staff who come into contact with the woman must be informed of her decision to place the infant for adoption. Information prevents inadvertent comments that could cause distress. Second, remember that adoption is an act of love, not one of abandonment, as the woman gives the newborn to a family who is better able to provide financial and emotional support.

Also be prepared to respect any special wishes that the mother may have about the birth. For instance, most birth mothers want to know all about the infant. They may want to see and hold the newborn and give the child a name. Many take photographs or save the crib card. Such actions provide memories of the infant and help the mother through the grieving process that may accompany adoption of the child.

Try to establish rapport and a trusting relationship with the mother. Acknowledgment of the situation at the initial contact with the woman is helpful: "Hello, my name is Claire, and I'll be your nurse today. I understand the adoptive family is coming this morning. What can I do to help you get ready?" This communication is more helpful than ignoring the event that is of primary concern to the mother. It also provides an opening for her to express feelings such as attachment to the infant, ambivalence about her decision, and profound sadness.

Nurses also teach adoptive families how to care for the newborn and what to expect in growth and development. Teaching requires adequate time and a private place. This family benefits from all the teaching provided to other new parents. They may be anxious, and demonstrations and return demonstrations are appropriate.

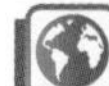 Cultural Considerations

Contraception

- Birth control as a government mandate for mainland China has been lifted. Previously, most Chinese women had an intrauterine device inserted after the birth of their first child. Some Chinese women do not want hormonal methods of contraception because they fear putting these medications in their bodies, but many now choose birth control because of the benefits of having only one child.
- Saudi Arabian and Hispanic women are likely to choose the rhythm method because of religious beliefs.
- (East) Indian men are encouraged to have voluntary sterilization via vasectomy.
- Muslim couples may practice contraception by mutual consent as long as its use is not harmful to the woman. Acceptable contraceptive methods include foam and condoms, the diaphragm, and natural family planning.
- Hmong women highly value and desire large families, which limits birth control practices.
- Arabic women value large families, and their sons are especially prized.

CONTRACEPTION

Contraception refers to actions taken to avoid becoming pregnant. Women and men actively engage in family planning and determine when to attempt to conceive a child or avoid pregnancy. A wide variety of birth control products are available. Selection of one involves a review of personal preferences and consideration of the woman's medical history and age. The assessment should include methods of interest and lifestyle concerns with a goal of paring the best option for the couple. Provide information about the use, effectiveness in preventing pregnancy, cost, potential protection from STIs, and pros and cons of the method selected. A visit with her primary care provider or health care professional also is advised. Also consider cultural values and practices (see the Cultural Considerations box on contraception).

POSTPARTUM THROMBOPHLEBITIS

Development of a blood clot in the interior of a blood vessel that results from inflammation or obstruction of a vessel is known as a *thrombosis.* The postpartum period may be affected by three types of thrombosis:

- *Superficial venous thrombosis:* Venous inflammation just below the skin's surface
- *Deep vein thrombosis:* A blood clot in a vein deep within the body, usually in the lower extremities
- *Pulmonary embolism:* Occlusion of the pulmonary artery by a blood clot traveling from elsewhere in the body

Incidence and Etiology

Thromboembolic disease is seen in less than 1% of postpartum women. Early ambulation after childbirth helps reduce the incidence. Risk factors for thromboembolic disease are increasing age, obesity, surgery, multiparity, and immobility.

Clinical Manifestations

Pain and tenderness in the lower extremities, along with warmth, redness, and hardening over the involved vessel, are common manifestations of superficial venous thrombosis.

During pregnancy, calf tenderness or leg pain and swelling may indicate deep vein thrombosis. The positive Homans' sign is not considered a definitive test, because it may be associated with other conditions. Be alert for the respiratory changes of dyspnea and tachycardia, which may signal pulmonary embolism.

Diagnosis is not based solely on the physical examination. Doppler ultrasound scan provides a noninvasive means to confirm the presence of thromboembolic disease. Compression ultrasound or magnetic resonance imaging also may be used.

Medical Management

A conservative approach is used to manage superficial venous thrombosis. Pharmacologic management includes the use of nonsteroidal antiinflammatory medications. Administer pain medications as needed, and limit activity. The goal is to rest the affected extremity in an elevated position. Heat applications and elastic stockings also are recommended.

The acute phase of treatment for deep venous thrombosis includes intravenous anticoagulant therapy, activity restriction, leg elevation, and pain management. Once the symptoms have eased, elastic stockings are applied, and the woman is able to ambulate. Begin administration of oral anticoagulant medications during this phase. Oral therapy can be anticipated for 3 months.

Management of a pulmonary embolism involves IV heparin therapy. Warfarin is contraindicated in pregnancy. After the acute phase of the illness, the patient takes subcutaneous heparin or oral anticoagulant therapies for 6 months. The use of aspirin is contraindicated in patients taking anticoagulant medications because of the increased risk for bleeding.

Nursing Interventions

To assess the woman with a thrombosis, observe and gently palpate the affected area, palpate peripheral pulses, measure the circumference of the leg for comparison, observe for signs of bleeding, and determine the presence of crackles or respiratory distress.

Evaluate the effectiveness of anticoagulant therapy in part with laboratory values. The PT or PTT is drawn and reviewed throughout the therapy. Report to the physician any laboratory values that fall outside the recommended therapeutic range.

During the acute phase of the illness the patient requires emotional support and education to ensure her compliance with the treatment regimen. Assistance with self-care may be needed. Provide instruction about positions to avoid in the bed such as crossing the legs. Encourage leg elevation. Instruct her to change positions frequently.

Nursing care of a woman experiencing a thrombosis involves patient and family education and ongoing assessment. Teach the patient about the diagnosis and treatment plans. Activity limitations may be difficult, so educate the patient about the risks associated with noncompliance. Massage of the thrombus is contraindicated because it may cause the clot to break free and travel to vital body organs.

Discharge teaching also should include information about the prescribed medication regimen and follow-up appointments with the laboratory and the physician. Medication education includes scheduling, dosages, potential side effects, and problems to report. Laboratory monitoring is needed throughout the therapy. The risk for injury is increased as a result of the anticoagulant therapy, so advise her to use a soft toothbrush and electric razor. Warfarin is associated with birth defects, so have a frank discussion about the need for contraception.

COMPLICATIONS RELATED TO THE NEWBORN

NEWBORNS AT RISK

Many maternal conditions can place the newborn in increased danger of illness or death. Identify any maternal risk factors as soon as possible to decrease the risk to the fetus or the newborn. Once these risks are identified, all medical and nursing measures possible should be undertaken to minimize the consequences to the mother and the newborn.

When risk factors are identified early, care providers can prepare to meet the needs of the newborn at risk. New equipment, such as fetal monitors and more sensitive diagnostic tests, has made problems during labor and delivery easier to recognize. Despite all progress, however, many infants still are born in need of special attention.

Assess the newborn at the time of delivery. The Apgar score gives important information about the newborn's status at 1 and 5 minutes after delivery (see Chapter 27). This is followed by a more detailed assessment of size related to gestational age. Distinguish between infants who are preterm and those who are small for gestational age. Although both groups are at risk, the problems they present are different.

GESTATIONAL AGE

Gestational age is a significant factor in neonatal mortality and morbidity (Figs. 29.7 and 29.8). Preterm and

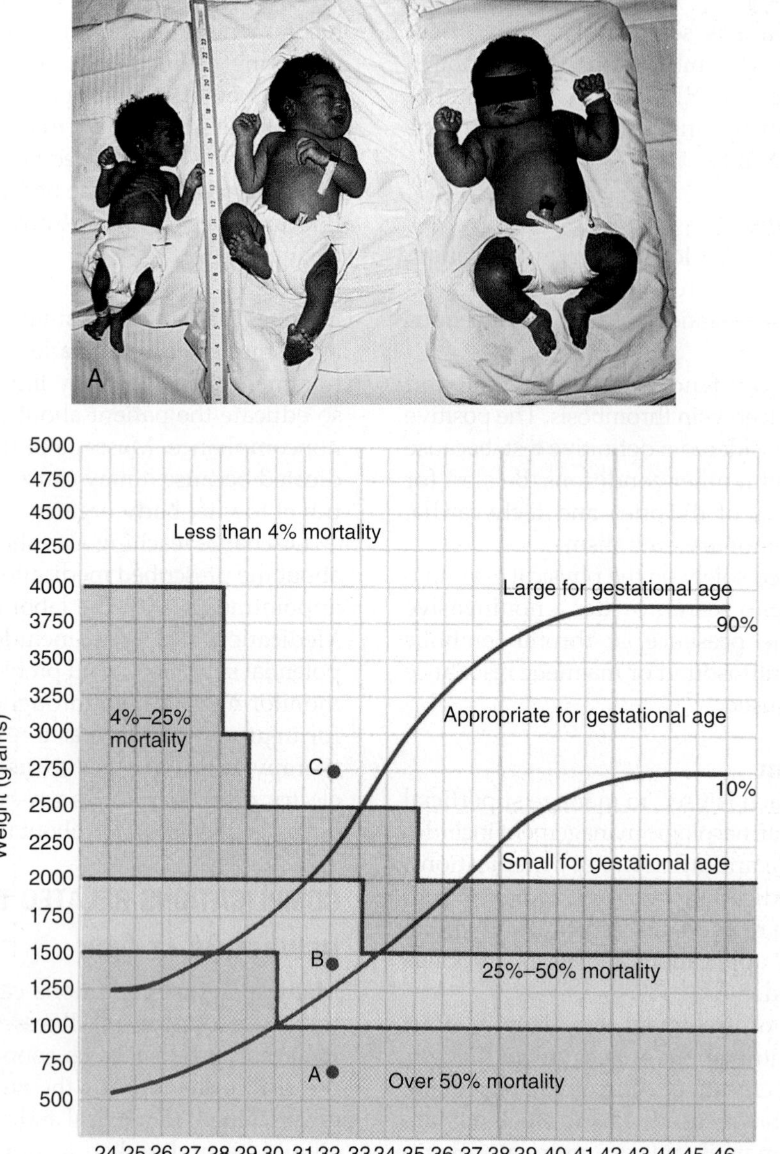

Fig. 29.7 A, Three babies of the same gestational age, with weights of 600, 1400, and 2750 g, respectively, from *left* to *right.* Their weights are plotted in B at points *A, B,* and *C.* B, Intrauterine growth status for gestational age and according to appropriateness of growth. (*A,* From *Perinatal assessment of maturation,* National Audiovisual Center, Washington, DC. *B,* Modified from Battaglia FC, Lubchenco LO: A practical classification of newborn infants by weight and gestational age. *J Pediatr* 1967;71[2]:59–63.)

postterm infants are at risk. Gestational age is classified as follows:

- *Preterm:* 20 to 37 completed weeks' gestation
- *Term:* 38 to 41 completed weeks' gestation
- *Postterm:* 42 weeks' gestation

Physical assessment procedures to determine gestational age are based on the method devised by Lilly and Victor Dubowitz, South African physicians. Their method is based on 21 strictly defined physical and neurologic signs and provides the correct gestational age ±2 weeks in 95% of infants. Most birthing facilities use this scale or one similar for determination of gestational age. Ideally the tests are performed between 2 and 8 hours of age. For the first hour, the infant is recovering from the stress of birth, and this is reflected in muscle movements; for example, the arm recoil is slower in a fatigued infant. After 48 hours, some responses change significantly. The plantar creases on the soles of the feet appear to increase in number and become visible as the skin loses fluid and dries. Fig. 29.8 shows newborn maturity ratings and classification.

NEUROMUSCULAR MATURITY

	−1	0	1	2	3	4	5
Posture							
Square Window (wrist)	> 90°	90°	60°	45°	30°	0°	
Arm Recoil		180°	140° - 180°	110° - 140°	90° - 110°	< 90°	
Popliteal Angle	180°	160°	140°	120°	100°	90°	< 90°
Scarf Sign							
Heel to Ear							

PHYSICAL MATURITY

	−1	0	1	2	3	4	5
Skin	sticky friable transparent	gelatinous red, translucent	smooth pink, visible veins	superficial peeling or rash, few veins	cracking pale areas rare veins	parchment deep cracking no vessels	leathery cracked wrinkled
Lanugo	none	sparse	abundant	thinning	bald areas	mostly bald	
Plantar Surface	heel-toe 40-50 mm: -1 <40 mm: -2	>50 mm no crease	faint red marks	anterior transverse crease only	creases ant. 2/3	creases over entire sole	
Breast	imperceptible	barely perceptible	flat areola no bud	stippled areola 1-2 mm bud	raised areola 3-4 mm bud	full areola 5-10 mm bud	
Eye/Ear	lids fused loosely: -1 tightly: -2	lids open pinna flat stays folded	sl. curved pinna; soft; slow recoil	well-curved pinna; soft but ready recoil	formed & firm instant recoil	thick cartilage ear stiff	
Genitals (male)	scrotum flat, smooth	scrotum empty faint rugae	testes in upper canal rare rugae	testes descending few rugae	testes down good rugae	testes pendulous deep rugae	
Genitals (female)	clitoris prominent labia flat	prominent clitoris small labia minora	prominent clitoris enlarging minora	majora & minora equally prominent	majora large minora small	majora cover clitoris & minora	

MATURITY RATING

score	weeks
-10	20
-5	22
0	24
5	26
10	28
15	30
20	32
25	34
30	36
35	38
40	40
45	42
50	44

Fig. 29.8 Estimation of gestational age. New Ballard scale for newborn maturity rating. Expanded scale includes extremely premature infants and has been refined to improve accuracy in more mature infants. (From Ballard JL, Khoury JC, Wedig K, et al: New Ballard score, expanded to include extremely premature infants. *J Pediatr* 1991;119[3]:417–423.)

PRETERM INFANT

Etiology and Pathophysiology

The exact causes of preterm labor are unknown. In some cases, it is related to maternal or placental problems, but in other cases, the cause cannot be determined. The end result is delivery of an infant at 37 weeks or less of gestation.

The preterm infant is developmentally immature. The lungs do not produce enough surfactant to allow adequate oxygenation. Circulation may not have adapted from fetal to neonatal, as it usually does in a term infant, which leads to oxygenation problems.

Problems with heat conservation stem from lack of subcutaneous fat, a large surface area relative to body weight, and poor reserves of glucose and **brown fat** (a source of heat unique to neonates that is capable of greater thermogenic [heat-producing] activity than ordinary fat; deposits are found around the adrenals, the kidneys, and the neck; between scapulae; and behind the sternum for several weeks after birth). The digestive system is formed, but problems with absorption of nutrients are common. The renal system is immature and ineffective. Fluid and acid-base imbalance frequently is observed. The infant is also neurologically immature; the gag, suck, and swallow reflexes may be weak or absent, and other normal reflexes may be absent or atypical.

The preterm infant is at risk because of immaturity of organ systems and lack of reserves. The morbidity and mortality rate for preterm infants is three to four times higher than that of older infants of comparable weight. The potential problems and care needs of the preterm infant of 2000 g differ from those of the term, postterm, or postmature infant of equal weight.

Preterm infants are at a disadvantage when they face the transition from intrauterine to extrauterine life. The degree of disadvantage depends primarily on their level of maturity. Physiologic disorders and anomalous malformations affect their response to treatment as well. In general, the closer they are to the normal term infant in gestational age and birth weight, the easier is their adjustment to the external environment.

Clinical Manifestations

The preterm newborn's posture is froglike or flaccid. The color is usually ruddy, and cyanosis may be present immediately after birth and for the first few hours of life. The head appears large in proportion to the body, and the bones of the skull are pliable with large, flat fontanelles. The skin is thin and translucent with obvious blood vessels and little subcutaneous fat. A layer of fine hair (lanugo) may coat large areas of the body. Cartilage in the ears is pliable, and the ears can be easily folded. The genitalia in boys are small, and frequently the testes are undescended. In girls, the labia majora are small and less prominent than the labia minora. The cry is weak, and reflexes are immature or absent.

Assessment

Assess all systems of the preterm newborn carefully and continually; changes occur rapidly and necessitate continuous monitoring. Preterm infants typically are placed in an intensive care nursery and receive care from nurses specially trained to meet their needs.

The preterm infant's greatest potential problem is respiratory distress syndrome, which results from an immature respiratory system (see Chapter 31). The first symptom of respiratory distress is usually grunting on expiration, followed by nasal flaring, circumoral cyanosis, substernal retractions, and tachypnea. It is treated with oxygen therapy and artificial surfactant. Providing periods of rest and maintaining body temperature are important components of treatment.

An accurate assessment of gestational age is a good indicator of the problems a preterm newborn is likely to experience. Follow a systematic approach in assessment. The preterm infant's response to extrauterine life is different from that of the term infant. Knowledge of the physiologic basis of these differences helps in assessment of these infants, understanding of their responses, and determination of which potential problems are most likely to occur.

Diagnostic Tests

A wide range of diagnostic tests may be performed, based on the newborn's specific needs.

Nursing Interventions

The specifics of care of the preterm newborn are beyond the scope of this text. The major goals include maintaining and stabilizing the conditions of preterm newborns until they mature adequately. Respiratory regulation, thermoregulation, fluid and electrolyte regulation, sensory stimulation, and promotion of bonding with the parents are major areas of concern for the nurse.

Patient problems and interventions for the preterm infant include but are not limited to the following:

Patient Problem	Nursing Interventions
Potential for Inability to Regulate Body Temperature, related to immature temperature regulation center, large body surface in relation to body weight, and minimal brown fat stores	Use skin probe to measure skin temperature and take steps to maintain it at 97° to 98°F (36.1° to 36.7°C) Monitor heart rate and rhythm Keep infant well covered and wrapped in blankets Pad cold surfaces Use radiant warmer if infant is uncovered for extended periods Keep skin dry Avoid drafts Keep crib, warmer, or Isolette away from windows and cold external walls Monitor for signs and symptoms of cold stress: decreased temperature, lethargy, and pallor (cold stress increases oxygen requirements) Avoid taking rectal temperature Obtain axillary temperatures and compare with registered skin probe temperature every 30 min for 2 h and until stable
Potential for Anxiousness (parental), related to preterm birth, separation, and breastfeeding	Encourage parents to stay with baby in the neonatal intensive care unit Encourage parents to actively participate in all aspects of care, if possible Encourage parents to hold baby and examine baby en face Encourage mother to breast-feed Explain the use of all equipment being used Discuss baby's behavioral cues and physical characteristics

Patient Problem	Nursing Interventions
	Encourage parents to express their feelings about the pregnancy, the labor, and the birth Discuss parents' feeding decisions Facilitate milk expression and storage by providing equipment or referral for lactation consultation

POSTTERM INFANT

The postterm infant may show signs of placental insufficiency, because the aging placenta was not fully functioning. Fetal malnutrition may occur as a result of deteriorating metabolic exchanges in the aging placenta. The infant also may be at increased risk for perinatal mortality from intrauterine hypoxia during labor and birth. This infant is at risk for asphyxia, respiratory distress, and hypoglycemia.

GESTATIONAL SIZE

Newborns are also classified according to their weight at any given gestational age. An infant may be as follows:

- *Small for gestational age (SGA):* Weight is less than the 10th percentile for age.
- *Appropriate for gestational age (AGA):* Weight is between the 10th and 90th percentiles.
- *Large for gestational age (LGA):* Weight is greater than the 90th percentile.
- *Low birth weight:* Weight is 2500 g or less at birth.

An SGA infant may be preterm, term, or postterm; an AGA infant may be preterm, term, or postterm; and an LGA infant may be preterm, term, or postterm.

The SGA infant may be small because of problems in the first trimester, such as infections or chromosomal abnormalities, or a later reduction in the fetal oxygen supply and fetal nutrition as a result of smoking, maternal hypertension, or malnutrition. Problems seen with SGA infants include asphyxia, meconium aspiration syndrome, hypoglycemia, and hypothermia. LGA infants often have hypoglycemia, respiratory distress, birth injuries, and asphyxia.

INFANT OF A MOTHER WITH DIABETES

The infant of a mother with diabetes, whether preterm, term, or postterm, is at risk. This infant frequently exhibits macrosomia (excessive size and stature), hypoglycemia, perinatal asphyxia, hypocalcemia, respiratory difficulties, and hyperbilirubinemia. The infant of the mother with gestational diabetes also may have congenital anomalies as a result of the uncontrolled maternal blood glucose levels in early pregnancy. The infant born to a woman with long-term and poorly controlled diabetes mellitus may be small for gestational age as a result of poor perfusion to the placenta and fetus.

HEMOLYTIC DISEASES

Etiology

Hemolysis may result from basic incompatibility of blood groups, such as ABO or Rh incompatibility, or from a transfer of antibodies through the placenta.

Pathophysiology

Understanding Rh incompatibility requires an understanding of basic genetics. Rh incompatibility occurs only when the mother is Rh negative and the fetus is Rh positive. For this to occur, the father of the fetus must be Rh positive (Fig. 29.9).

The term *Rh negative* indicates that the woman does not possess a specific blood antigen. If the woman is sensitized (i.e., exposed to the antigen), she produces antibodies. Exposure can occur through blood transfusion of incompatible blood or during pregnancy, when some fetal blood cells enter the maternal circulation. This transfer of antigen may occur in cases of abortion or abruption or at the time of delivery. Once the mother develops Rh antibodies, they remain in her blood, as do other antibodies.

When the woman becomes pregnant, maternal antibodies may cross the **placental barrier** (the boundary provided by placental tissue between the fetal and maternal circulations; small substances, excluding blood cells, may cross this barrier). If the fetal RBCs contain the Rh antigen, the maternal Rh antibodies cause hemolysis (destruction) of the fetal RBCs. The higher the level of maternal antibodies, the greater the destruction of fetal RBCs. This destruction of fetal RBCs results in pathologic jaundice, which occurs within the first 24 hours after birth.

Because sensitization most often occurs at delivery, the firstborn fetus generally has no signs of hemolysis; successive fetuses are most likely to be affected. Today, serious problems related to Rh incompatibility, such as **erythroblastosis fetalis** (a type of hemolytic anemia that occurs in newborns as a result of maternal-fetal blood group incompatibility, especially involving the Rh factor and ABO blood groups), usually are prevented (see Fig. 29.9).

ABO incompatibility is also an antigen-antibody process. Type O blood naturally contains anti-A and anti-B antibodies. These antibodies cross the placenta and cause hemolysis if the fetus has blood type A or B. Incompatibility is also possible if the mother is A and the infant is B or if the mother is B and the infant is A. No sensitization is necessary, and it may affect the first and all successive pregnancies.

Clinical Manifestations

The mother shows no clinical symptoms. Hemolysis may occur in utero, and detection must be made with diagnostic tests on amniotic fluid, suspected by changes in fetal condition, or maternal diagnostic tests. Jaundice present at birth or in the first 24 hours

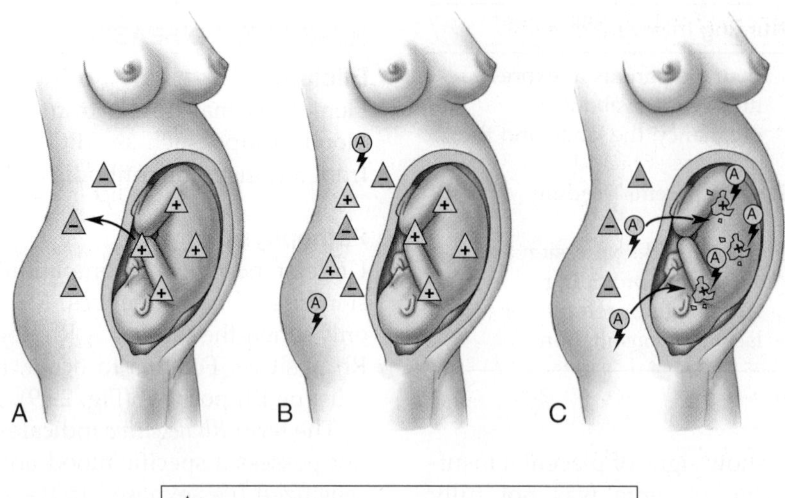

Fig. 29.9 Mechanisms of erythroblastosis fetalis, which is caused by Rh incompatibility. A, Rh-positive fetus is carried by Rh-negative mother. Rh protein crosses placental barrier and invades mother's bloodstream. B, Mother's system manufactures antibodies to destroy foreign Rh protein. C, Antibodies cross back over placenta and destroy fetus's blood cells, which are associated intimately with Rh protein. (From Herlihy B: *The human body in health and illness*, ed 4, St. Louis, 2011, Saunders.)

of life is considered an indicator of a pathologic condition. **Kernicterus** (an abnormal toxic accumulation of bilirubin in central nervous system tissues caused by **hyperbilirubinemia** [an excess of bilirubin in the blood of the newborn]) may result in neurologic damage or death. Anemia caused by RBC destruction is also possible.

Assessment

Determine the maternal blood type and Rh factor during pregnancy. If the mother is Rh negative, find out the father's blood type. If he is also Rh negative, no Rh-based problem will occur. If the father is Rh positive, problems are possible. Also assess the woman's history for any events that may have caused sensitization, such as previous pregnancy, birth, abortion, or amniocentesis and transfusion with Rh-positive blood, which causes immediate sensitization. Even premature separation of the placenta and trauma may cause sensitization.

Diagnostic Tests

Blood typing reveals situations that require follow-up. An **indirect Coombs' test** of maternal blood measures the number of maternal antibodies. Antibody titer tests determine the level of maternal antibodies. If the titer exceeds 1:16, amniocentesis may be performed to obtain fluid for further testing. Optical density studies, which measure bilirubin level, can be done on this fluid to assess fetal condition. (If the fetus is determined to be in grave danger, intrauterine transfusion may be necessary.) After delivery, a **direct Coombs' test** is done on infant blood to determine the presence of antibody-coated RBCs. Bilirubin levels of infant blood indicate the extent of RBC destruction.

Nursing Interventions

Maternal. If the results of an Rh-negative mother's indirect Coombs' test are negative, the mother is given an intramuscular injection of RhoGAM. This currently is recommended at 28 weeks of pregnancy and again within 72 hours of delivery. RhoGAM provides passive antibodies and prevents development of naturally occurring maternal antibodies. RhoGAM also should be given to an Rh-negative mother in cases of abortion, ectopic pregnancy, and amniocentesis. Give the mother an identification card with vital information, including date of last injection of RhoGAM. She should carry this card with her always.

Newborn. Carefully observe the newborn affected by a hemolytic process; jaundice and anemia may become severe and lead to other complications. Monitor the bilirubin, hemoglobin, and hematocrit levels and notify the physician of any abnormal results. The infant with severe jaundice may be treated with phototherapy or may need transfusion. Phototherapy usually is begun when the bilirubin levels reach 12 to 15 mg/dL.

Phototherapy requires several precautions. **Phototherapy** involves exposure of the skin to fluorescent lights, which converts the bilirubin to a water-soluble form that can be excreted in the urine. Maintain body temperature and protect the infant's eyes during this

Box 29.9 Home Phototherapy With a Biliblanket

Information for parents:

- As much of the infant's skin as possible should be in direct contact with the lighted section of the pad. The infant's back or chest should be placed directly on the pad, with the tip of the pad at the shoulder and the cable at the feet.
- Follow the equipment supplier's instructions regarding safety and use of the phototherapy unit.
- Phototherapy can be discontinued for brief periods without harming your baby.
- Temperature instability may occur when starting and stopping phototherapy and when collecting laboratory specimens.
- Effects of phototherapy may include changes in frequency and color of the infant's stools and rash from an increase in the number of loose stools.

Notify your child's health care provider if:

- A notable change is seen in activity level.
- The infant's temperature is not maintained at 97° or 100°F (33.3° to 37.7°C).
- The infant is feeding poorly.
- The infant is not voiding six times per day or does not void within a 6-hour period.
- Infant vomits two or more feedings.

Notify your home care agency if:

- Phototherapy is discontinued.
- An equipment malfunction occurs.

From University of California San Francisco Home Health Care: Guidelines for home therapy, San Francisco, 2001, University of California. In Lowdermilk DL, Perry SE, editors: Maternity and women's health care, ed 9, St. Louis, 2007, Mosby.

treatment. Phototherapy may be carried out at home with the use of a biliblanket (Box 29.9).

Eye patches should be removed and lights turned off during feedings and bathing to allow infant stimulation and face-to-face interaction with the mother or other caregiver. Stools may be loose and the urine contains excessive waste products, so it is important to maintain skin integrity with careful cleansing and frequent diaper changes. Because fluid loss is increased, adequate fluids are important to maintain necessary hydration.

Patient problems and interventions for the patient with hemolytic disease include but are not limited to the following:

Patient Problem	Nursing Interventions
Potential for Inadequate Fluid Volume, related to insensible weight loss and dehydration	Do not clothe infant; diapering is questionable Maintain thermoneutral phototherapy environment Maintain axillary temperature at 97.7°F (36.5°C) Assess axillary temperature at least q 2 hr and as needed Avoid exposure of skin temperature probe to phototherapy lights Weigh infant daily unclothed at the same time on the same scale before feeding Measure accurate I&O Check urine specific gravity every shift Test strength of bililight according to hospital's and manufacturer's policy
Potential for Compromised Parenting Skills, related to disruption of parent-infant interaction secondary to phototherapy	Explain need to provide adequate fluid intake, including water between feedings Discuss signs and symptoms to report to physician, such as recurrence of jaundice or persistent diarrhea Emphasize importance of having laboratory tests done as ordered Emphasize importance of follow-up care Encourage parent participation in infant care activities such as feeding, bathing, and cuddling Review care of infant with hyperbilirubinemia as necessary with parents Permit siblings to visit according to hospital policy When parents visit, turn off lights and remove eye shields for the time period ordered by physician Reinforce explanation of phototherapy, reasons for particular interventions, and care plan

Patient Teaching

Rh-negative women should be aware of the process involved in Rh sensitization. Answer all questions that the woman or her partner may have. Phototherapy is likely to be disturbing to the parents and can interfere with parent-child attachment. Explain the reasons for treatment and provide opportunities for maternal-infant interaction. Today many newborns are sent home receiving this form of therapy. Many insurance companies recognize the therapeutic value of phototherapy at home and include phototherapy in their policies. Teach the parents correct use of the equipment and the special care needed by the infant.

SUBSTANCE ABUSE

The use of legal substances, such as alcohol and tobacco, or illicit drugs, such as cocaine and marijuana, increases the risk for medical complications in the mother and poor birth outcomes in the infant. Approximately 1 in 10 infants is exposed to one or more mood-altering drugs during pregnancy. Although tobacco, alcohol, and marijuana are the most commonly abused drugs, the use of cocaine and heroin has had a major effect on health care for pregnant women and their offspring.

When the pregnant woman takes a substance, the fetus experiences the same systemic effects as the expectant mother but often more severely. For instance, cocaine raises the blood pressure of the woman and the fetus and puts both at risk for intracranial bleeding. A drug that causes intoxication in the woman causes it for prolonged periods in the fetus. The fetus cannot metabolize drugs efficiently and experiences the effects long after they have disappeared in the woman. Maternal, fetal, and neonatal effects of commonly abused substances are summarized in Table 29.4.

Nursing Interventions

Nursing care for the infant is directed at prevention of further injury, particularly during the withdrawal phase. Infants of known drug and alcohol users generally are placed in a neonatal intensive care unit. Physical care includes careful temperature regulation and monitoring of vital signs. Observe the newborn to detect increasing instability. Provide small feedings, and observe the infant for diarrhea, regurgitation, and vomiting. Positioning on the right side helps prevent aspiration. IV therapy may be necessary. Administer medications as ordered to prevent the most serious withdrawal symptoms. Reduce stimuli that may aggravate seizures. These infants are often inconsolable, which makes caring for them difficult and stressful.

Include the newborn's parents in care whenever possible. Depending on the severity of the problems encountered, the infant may remain in the hospital, be discharged to the parent, or be placed in the custody of social services. It is a major challenge to establish a therapeutic relationship with the chemically dependent

Table 29.4 Maternal and Fetal or Neonatal Effects of Commonly Abused Substances

SUBSTANCE	MATERNAL EFFECTS	FETAL OR NEONATAL EFFECTS
Caffeine (coffee, tea, cola, chocolate, cold remedies, analgesics)	Stimulation of CNS and cardiac function, vasoconstriction, mild diuresis; half-life triples during pregnancy	Crosses placental barrier and stimulates fetus; teratogenic effects are undocumented
Tobacco	Decreased placental perfusion, anemia, PROM, preterm labor, spontaneous abortion	Prematurity, LBW, fetal demise, developmental delays, increased incidence of SIDS, pneumonia
Alcohol (beer, wine, mixed drinks, after-dinner drinks)	Spontaneous abortion	Fetal demise, IUGR, FAS (facial and cranial anomalies, developmental delay, mental retardation, short attention span), fetal alcohol effects (milder form of FAS)
Cocaine ("crack")	Hyperarousal state, generalized vasoconstriction, hypertension, increased incidence of spontaneous abortion, abruptio placentae, preterm labor, cardiovascular complications (stroke, heart attack), seizures, increased STIs	Tachycardia; stillbirth; prematurity; LBW; tremors; IUGR; irritability; decreased ability to interact with environmental stimuli; poor feeding reflexes; nausea, vomiting, diarrhea; decreased intellectual development; distended, flabby, creased abdomen (prune-belly syndrome) caused by absence of abdominal muscles
Narcotics (heroin, methadone, morphine)	Spontaneous abortion, PROM, preterm labor, increased incidence of STIs, HIV exposure, hepatitis, malnutrition	IUGR, perinatal asphyxia, intellectual impairment, neonatal abstinence syndrome, neonatal infections, fetal or neonatal death (SIDS, child abuse, and neglect)
Sedatives (barbiturates, tranquilizers)	Lethargy, drowsiness, CNS depression	Neonatal abstinence syndrome, seizures, delayed lung maturity, possible teratogenic effect
Amphetamines ("speed," "crystal," or "ice" when processed in crystals to smoke)	Malnutrition, tachycardia, withdrawal symptoms (lethargy, depression)	Increased risk for IUGR, prematurity, cardiac anomalies, cleft palate, abruptio placentae, hypoglycemia, sweating, poor visual tracing, "glassy-eyed" look, lethargy, feeding problems
Marijuana ("pot" or "grass")	Often used with other drugs (alcohol, cocaine, tobacco), increased incidence of anemia and inadequate weight gain	Unclear, more study needed; believed related to prematurity, IUGR, tremors, sensitivity to light

CNS, Central nervous system; *FAS,* fetal alcohol syndrome; *HIV,* human immunodeficiency virus; *IUGR,* intrauterine growth restriction; *LBW,* low birth weight; *PROM,* premature rupture of membranes; *SIDS,* sudden infant death syndrome; *STIs,* sexually transmitted infections.
From McKinney ES, James SR, Murray SS, et al: *Maternal-child nursing,* ed 2, St. Louis, 2005, Saunders.

parent. Consult with social welfare or other departments that are best able to protect the newborn and help the parent obtain the treatment needed to overcome an addiction.

COMPLICATIONS RELATED TO POSTPARTUM MENTAL HEALTH DISORDERS

Mental health disorders have implications for the mother, the newborn, and the entire family. Such conditions can interfere with attachment to the newborn and family integration, and some may threaten the safety and well-being of the mother, the newborn, and other children. Because birth usually is thought to be a happy event, a new mother's emotional distress may confuse family and friends and leave them unable to act. At a time when she most needs the caring attention of loved ones, they may either criticize or withdraw because of their own anxiety.

MOOD DISORDERS

Mood disorders are the predominant mental health disorder in the postpartum period, typically occurring within 4 weeks of childbirth. Most women with mood disorders experience a mild depression, or "baby blues," after the birth of a child. Others can have more serious depression that eventually can incapacitate them to the point of being unable to care for themselves or their babies. Postpartum depression (PPD) leads to moderate to severe disturbances in the interaction of mothers and infants, which are predictive of poorer infant learning outcomes. In rare cases, a disturbed mother may kill her infant, herself, or other family members. Nurses are positioned strategically to offer anticipatory guidance, to assess the mental health of new mothers, to offer therapeutic interventions, and to provide referrals when necessary. Failure to do so may have tragic consequences.

Many women feel guilty about being depressed at a time when they believe they should be happy. They may be reluctant to discuss their symptoms or their negative feelings toward the child. A prominent feature of PPD is rejection of the infant, often caused by abnormal jealousy. The mother may be obsessed by the notion that the offspring will take her place in her partner's affections. Attitudes toward the infant may include disinterest, annoyance with care demands, and blaming because of her lack of maternal feeling. The woman may appear awkward in her responses to the baby. Obsessive thoughts about harming the child frighten her. Often she does not share these thoughts because of embarrassment, but when she does, other family members become frightened as well.

Medical Management

The natural course is one of gradual improvement over the 6 months after birth. Supportive treatment alone is not effective for major PPD; pharmacologic intervention is needed in most instances. Treatment options include antidepressants, anxiolytic agents (a sedative or minor tranquilizer), and electroconvulsive therapy. Psychotherapy focuses on the mother's fears and concerns regarding her new responsibilities and roles and monitoring for suicidal or homicidal thoughts. For some women, hospitalization is necessary.

❖ NURSING PROCESS FOR THE MOTHER AND NEWBORN AT RISK

The role of the licensed practical nurse/licensed vocational nurse (LPN/LVN) in the nursing process as stated is that the LPN/LVN will:

- Participate in planning care for patients based on patient needs.
- Review patient's care plan and recommend revisions as needed.
- Review and follow defined prioritization for patient care.
- Use clinical pathways, care maps, or care plans to guide and review patient care.

◆ ASSESSMENT

Nursing process for the patient at risk begins with assessment, which focuses on the history of the pregnancy and the patient's symptoms. Assessment includes physical and psychological arenas. Specific assessment items depend on the patient's disorder. Assessment also should include medical history, obstetric history, and social history.

◆ PATIENT PROBLEM

Nursing assessment helps identify the needs of the patient at high risk. Care then can be based on these needs. Patient problems depend on the high-risk condition and symptoms observed (see patient problem statements throughout the chapter).

◆ EXPECTED OUTCOMES AND PLANNING

The care plan focuses on the needs of the patient at high risk and the nurse's ability to meet those needs effectively. Each patient has different needs, and care is individualized accordingly. The care plan focuses on goals and outcomes specific to the patient problem. Examples include the following:

Goal 1: The patient with hyperemesis gravidarum will maintain caloric intake adequate to provide for fetal health and growth.

Outcome: Patient eats and retains 1800 kcal/day and drinks 2000 mL of fluid per day.

Goal 2: The preterm neonate will maintain skin temperature of 97.5° to 98.6°F (36.4° to 37°C) axillary while in an open crib.

Outcome: Neonate's temperature is 97.8° to 98.6°F (36.6° to 37°C) axillary on three successive occasions 4 hours apart.

◆ IMPLEMENTATION

Nursing interventions for the patient at high risk are determined by the patient problem and goals for the specific condition being treated.

◆ EVALUATION

Continually evaluate the success of the interventions. As the high-risk patient's situation changes, so too may the goals and interventions. Refer to the goals and outcomes to determine whether the plan was successful and the outcomes met. For example:

Goal 1: The patient with hyperemesis gravidarum will maintain caloric intake adequate to provide for fetal health and growth.

Evaluative measures: Patient ate six small meals totaling 1500 kcal with one emesis of 200 mL. Fluid intake of water and tea was 1200 mL.

Goal 2: The preterm neonate will maintain skin temperature of 97.5° to 98.6°F (36.4° to 37°C) axillary while in an open crib.

Evaluative measure: Neonate's temperature was 98.6°F (37°C) axillary at 0600, 98.2°F (36.8°C) axillary at 1000, and 98.9°F (37.2°C) axillary at 1400.

Get Ready for the NCLEX® Examination!

Key Points

- Complications can occur during any stage of the childbearing process.
- Continually assess pregnant women and newborns for any signs of complications.
- Educate all pregnant women about danger signs that indicate complications, stressing the importance of prompt medical attention.
- Hemorrhage is a danger sign during pregnancy and after delivery.
- Bleeding disorders of pregnancy are medical emergencies that demand expert teamwork from health care professionals.
- Premature separation, or placental abruption, is characterized by painful vaginal bleeding. A concealed bleed is possible depending on the location of the separation. Concealed bleeding is associated with abdominal rigidity.
- Placenta previa results from an abnormal location of implantation of the placenta, completely or partially covering the cervical os. This is associated with third trimester and painless vaginal bleeding.
- The type of spontaneous abortion determines the management.
- The cause of GH is unknown, and no known reliable tests are available for predicting women at risk for preeclampsia.
- Magnesium sulfate, the anticonvulsant agent of choice for prevention of eclampsia, necessitates careful monitoring of reflexes, respirations, and urinary output; its antidote, calcium gluconate, should be at the bedside.
- A wide range of infectious diseases present a threat to the mother and the newborn.
- The Rh-negative mother may need special interventions to prevent sensitization, which may affect future pregnancies.
- Preexisting health conditions, such as cardiac problems or diabetes mellitus, increase the risks of childbearing.
- Routine screening for GDM is performed for most women during the second trimester. Women with increased risk factors or those who are suspected of having diabetes-related issues may be tested earlier in gestation.
- The mother's age is significant in childbearing. The very young and the older mother are at increased risk.
- Adolescents can develop trusting relationships with helping professionals whom they respect.
- Drug and alcohol use have a serious impact on the developing fetus.
- Approximately 80% to 90% of pregnancies treated with cerclage result in live, viable births.
- The woman who is addicted to narcotics may have infections that compound the risk to the infant, including hepatitis; septicemia; and STIs, including AIDS.
- Newborns born to drug-abusing or alcohol-abusing mothers may manifest a variety of anatomic and neurologic defects.
- Infants born preterm or postterm and SGA or LGA are at greater risk for complications.
- Preterm infants are physiologically immature and at risk for respiratory distress syndrome, hypoglycemia, hyperbilirubinemia, and thermoregulation problems.

Additional Learning Resources

SG Go to your Study Guide for additional learning activities to help you master this chapter content.

evolve Be sure to visit the Evolve site at *http://evolve.elsevier.com/Cooper/foundationsadult/* for additional online resources.

Review Questions for the NCLEX® Examination

1. The nurse is reviewing the plan of care for a patient being treated for acute deep vein thrombosis. Which can be anticipated to be included in the plan of care at this time?
   1. Frequent ambulation
   2. Extremity elevation
   3. Intravenous anticoagulant therapies
   4. Oral anticoagulant therapies
   5. Activity restriction

2. A patient is admitted to the hospital with a diagnosis of suspected ectopic pregnancy. Which findings in the patient's history and assessment would be supportive of this diagnosis? *(Select all that apply.)*
   1. History of genital herpes simplex
   2. History of pelvic inflammatory disease
   3. Positive serum HCG test results
   4. Uterine enlargement
   5. Abdominal pain
3. A patient has been diagnosed with placenta previa. Which symptom is considered the classic diagnostic criterion for placenta previa?
   1. Painful vaginal bleeding
   2. Uterine irritability
   3. Elevation of temperature
   4. Painless vaginal bleeding
4. A patient is in labor and suddenly reports sharp fundal pain. She begins to have vaginal bleeding as well. What is the most likely cause of her symptoms?
   1. Preterm labor
   2. Abruptio placentae
   3. Pelvic inflammatory disease
   4. Placenta previa
5. A patient is diagnosed with an inevitable abortion. Which assessment finding distinguishes an inevitable abortion from a threatened abortion?
   1. Uterine cramping
   2. Vaginal bleeding
   3. Cervical dilation
   4. History of previous abortions
6. A patient is suspected of having gestational hypertension. Which assessments are likely to be included in the nursing assessment? *(Select all that apply.)*
   1. Deep tendon reflexes
   2. Determination of when she last ate
   3. Daily weight
   4. Intake and output
   5. Nitrazine testing
7. What is the most common cause of postpartum hemorrhage?
   1. Cervical lacerations
   2. Uterine atony
   3. Cesarean birth
   4. Disseminated intravascular coagulation
8. A baby boy was born at 38 weeks of gestation to a mother with type 1 diabetes. Into which category does this infant most likely fall?
   1. Premature
   2. Average for gestational age
   3. Intrauterine growth restriction
   4. Large for gestational age
9. A baby girl was born at 34 weeks of gestation. At 3 hours old, she is diagnosed with respiratory distress. What is an early symptom of respiratory distress?
   1. Nasal flaring
   2. Expiratory grunting
   3. Cyanosis
   4. Substernal retractions
10. A patient is Rh negative and delivers an infant with Rh-positive blood. RhoGAM is prescribed. What is the rationale for the use of this medication?
    1. To stimulate formation of maternal blood antigens
    2. To stimulate production of maternal blood antibodies
    3. To prevent production of maternal blood antibodies
    4. To prevent production of fetal blood antigens
11. After giving birth to a healthy baby boy, a primiparous woman, age 16 years, is admitted to the postpartum unit. An appropriate patient problem statement for her at this time is *Potential for Compromised Parenting Skills, related to deficient knowledge of newborn care*. In planning for the woman's discharge, the nurse should include what in the care plan?
    1. Tell the woman how to feed and bathe her baby.
    2. Give the woman written information on bathing her baby.
    3. Advise the woman that all mothers instinctively know how to care for their babies.
    4. Provide time for the woman to bathe her baby after she views a baby bath demonstration.
12. A newborn is jaundiced and receiving phototherapy. What is an appropriate nursing intervention when caring for an infant with hyperbilirubinemia who is receiving phototherapy? *(Select all that apply.)*
    1. Apply an oil-based lotion to the newborn's skin to prevent drying and cracking.
    2. Lay the baby down with the back directly on the biliblanket.
    3. Place eye shields over the newborn's eyes.
    4. Place the cord of the device near the head of the bed.
    5. Change the newborn's position every 3 to 4 hours.
13. A 26-year-old pregnant woman, gravida 2, para 1, is 28 weeks pregnant when she experiences bright red, painless vaginal bleeding. On her arrival at the hospital, what is an expected diagnostic procedure?
    1. Amniocentesis for fetal lung maturity
    2. Ultrasound scan for placental location
    3. Contraction stress test
    4. Internal fetal monitoring
14. In planning care of a 30-year-old woman with pregestational diabetes, what is the most important factor that affects pregnancy outcome?
    1. Mother's age
    2. Number of years since diabetes was diagnosed
    3. Amount of insulin required prenatally
    4. Degree of blood glucose control during pregnancy
15. When caring for a pregnant woman with cardiac problems, the nurse should be alert for what signs and symptoms that suggest cardiac decompensation? *(Select all that apply.)*
    1. Hypotension
    2. Hypertension
    3. Bradycardia
    4. Tachycardia
    5. Shortness of breath

30 Health Promotion for the Infant, Child, and Adolescent

http://evolve.elsevier.com/Cooper/foundationsadult/

Objectives

1. Identify the 12 leading health indicators cited in *Healthy People 2020.*
2. List three benefits of regular physical activity in children.
3. Identify barriers to health promotion and maintenance for the pediatric population.
4. State the American Academy of Pediatrics' recommendations for immunization administration in healthy infants and children.
5. State three strategies to promote dental health.
6. State the causes and prevention of accidental poisonings.
7. Describe four strategies to prevent aspiration of a foreign body.
8. Discuss the proper use of infant safety seats in motor vehicles.
9. List safety precautions important in educating parents to prevent environmental injuries to children.
10. Identify health risks for adolescents and interventions to reduce them.
11. Discuss the impact of social media on children.

Key Terms

anticipatory guidance (p. 918)
botulism (BŎT-ū-lĭzm, p. 927)
nursing bottle caries (p. 926)

The focus of health promotion is to assist individuals to realize their full potential. Active participation by patients and family is needed to develop and maintain a lifestyle that optimizes wellness. Traditionally, the primary care of children has fostered health promotion through health supervision and health maintenance visits, immunizations, screenings and surveillance, and **anticipatory guidance** (psychological preparation, based on developmental stage, of a person for an event expected to be stressful, as in preparing a child for surgery by explaining what will happen and what it will feel like; also used to prepare parents for normal growth and development of their children). Health promotion activities are essential in identifying risks and encouraging healthy behaviors in children and their families. Ideally these undertakings begin before the birth of the baby as the parents are prepared for the needs of their growing family. This lays a foundation for continued health promotion in subsequent years.

One of the major roles in nursing is promoting wellness and disease prevention. Pediatric nursing provides many unique opportunities to participate in this role. The pediatric population offers several challenges not found in the adult population. Pediatric nurses need to use a multidisciplinary approach to meet the demands related to the promotion of wellness and disease prevention concerning the pediatric population.

To assist a population in the achievement of optimal states of health and wellness it is necessary to understand the barriers standing in the way of these initiatives. Obstacles for care can be grouped as financial and nonfinancial. Financial barriers include available monetary resources to pay for the care or items that are not covered readily by any existing insurance. Families having insurance also may experience problems locating a desired provider who will accept their insurance. Aside from financial related barriers there are other identified areas of concern (Kullgren et al, 2011). Access to care may not be convenient to the family because of work conflicts, availability of reliable transportation, and location of provider in relation to the family. Psychosocial barriers also may play a role in the accessing of health services. Language and cultural beliefs may affect ability and willingness to use care resources. Finally, an understanding and belief in the importance of health promotion affect a family's willingness to participate in care services (Unite for Sight, n.d.). Nurses have a key role in the identification of real and perceived barriers. Once these have been highlighted, the nurse, in conjunction with the other members of the health care team, can initiate a plan to assist families in the achievement of health promotion and maintenance.

This chapter identifies health promotion and disease prevention factors unique to the pediatric population. The primary focus of this chapter is the indicators identified in *Healthy People 2020* (Office of Disease Prevention and Health Promotion [ODPHP], 2018), and dental health, poisoning, aspiration, and burn injuries related to children. Healthy People 2030 is being developed at the time of this publication.

HEALTHY PEOPLE 2020

Healthy People 2020 has identified 26 leading health indicators (LHI). These indicators are those topics of concerns to the health and well-being of Americans. The LHI have been organized within 12 topics. These topics are as follows:

1. Access to health services
2. Clinical preventive services
3. Environmental quality
4. Injury and violence
5. Maternal, infant, and child health
6. Mental health
7. Nutrition, physical activity, and obesity
8. Oral health
9. Reproductive and sexual health
10. Social determinants
11. Substance abuse
12. Tobacco

All the indicators have specific target goals related to children and adolescents. Environmental quality and access to health care do not have specific target goals that address the pediatric population; however, goals for the population in general are included (see the Health Promotion box). Additional information concerning the *Health People 2020* initiatives is available at *www.healthypeople.gov/2020/topicsobjectives2020/default.aspx.*

ACCESS TO HEALTH CARE

Health promotion and the care and treatment of disease is affected most by the access the family has to health care. The inability to engage in health care services can result in the absence or delay in receiving education about healthful practices. It can cause delays in the diagnosis and treatment of disease. Millions of American children do not have any type of health care insurance. There are racial divides regarding the coverage of children with health insurance. An estimated 10% of Hispanic children do not have insurance in comparison with 4% for white non-Hispanic and black non-Hispanic children. The rates for how the coverage is provided is also racially significant: the majority of white non-Hispanic children (68%) are privately insured; black non-Hispanic (34%) and Hispanic children (31%) are privately insured at a much-lower rate. This creates a somewhat impassable obstacle for people seeking health care services.

Other common barriers associated with access to health care, in addition to the financial one, include lack of primary care providers, cultural and spiritual differences, language barriers, discrimination, and concerns about confidentiality. All health care providers have a responsibility to improve health care access for all people.

NUTRITION, PHYSICAL ACTIVITY, AND OBESITY

Physical activity and a balanced diet are for the healthy growth and development of children and adolescents. Diet and exercise lay a foundation to maintain health throughout the lifetime. Diet and exercise aid in the prevention of diseases such as hypertension, cancer, and heart disease. Unfortunately, many American children do not follow the recommended dietary guidelines. Fewer than 1 in 3 children eat the recommended daily intake of vegetables. Exercise is also a concern, with more than 80% of adolescents not achieving the recommended level of physical activity.

Diet and exercise are intertwined with obesity in children. The number of overweight children in the United States is increasing and seems to be approaching epidemic status. In economically developed countries, the most common disease seen in childhood and adolescence is now obesity. An estimated 1 in 6 (16.67%) of American children are overweight. This number reflects a slight increase from 14.94% noted in 2010 (CDC, 2017). Children with a body mass index (BMI) between the 85th and 95th percentiles are considered overweight, and obesity is defined as a BMI greater than the 95th percentile. Children in the 99th percentile are considered extremely obese. Racial differences are noted: blacks (19.5%) and non-Hispanic blacks (21.9%) have higher rates of obesity than non-Hispanic whites. The rates of obesity climb with age. In children ages 2 to 5 years the rate of obesity is 8.9%. This rate soars in teens with rates of 7.5% in 6- to 11-year-olds and 20.5% in 12- to 19-year-olds (CDC, 2017).

Regular physical activity lowers death rates in adults and reduces the risk for development of heart disease, high blood pressure, diabetes mellitus, and colon cancer. In children, regular physical activity increases bone and muscle strength and helps decrease body fat. Psychological benefits of regular physical activity include improvement in self-esteem and reduction in stress and depression (Fig. 30.1). The establishment of health-seeking behaviors in childhood affects the long-range health status of those same individuals as they reach adulthood.

Nurses have the opportunity to promote physical activity in the pediatric population by educating parents, teachers, school administrators, and daycare providers. Physical activity in children is often reflective of the adults within their environment. Positive role modeling is another way to promote healthy living. Programs geared toward combining healthy eating and activity are most effective (Table 30.1).

Physical risks associated with excess weight include high blood pressure, high cholesterol, type 2 diabetes mellitus, fatty liver disease, heart disease, stroke, gallbladder disease, arthritis, sleep apnea, and problems breathing. Psychological risks associated with excess weight include discrimination, social stigmatization, lowered self-esteem, social isolation, and feelings of depression and rejection.

Many factors contribute to the excess weight carried by children. Some of the most common factors are lack of physical activity, increased fast food consumption, working mothers, and poverty. Although not all of these factors are possible to eliminate, many of them are amenable to significant improvement.

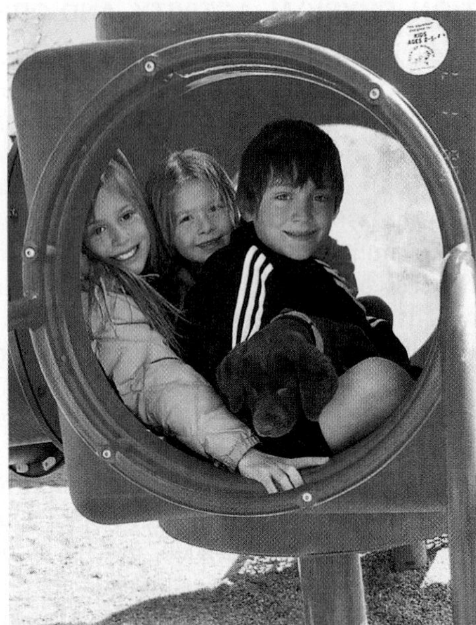

Fig. 30.1 Children engaging in physical activity.

Nutrition

Families today often are pressed for time. The convenience of fast food combined with the increase in families with two working parents has contributed to poor eating habits for many children. A review of the top three caloric sources for children ages 2 to 17 years reflects grain-based desserts, yeast breads, and pizza. The top choices reflect dietary selections with limited nutritional value. This is a definite cause for concern about the dietary intake of children. Children's diets contain an estimated 11% to 15% of calories from saturated fat instead of the American Heart Association's recommendation of a maximum of 7%. Children tend to consume high-calorie, poorer-quality diets that do not meet federal dietary recommendations for healthy growth and development. Childhood obesity results from a diet high in calories from saturated fat and lack of exercise (Mayo Clinic, 2012).

Table 30.1 National Resources for Childhood Physical Activity and Dietary Intake

RESOURCE	WEBSITE	MAJOR RECOMMENDATIONS
Physical Activity		
Physical Activity Guidelines for Americans	*https://health.gov/paguidelines/guidelines/children.aspx*	60 minutes or more of physical activity daily Most activity should be of moderate or vigorous intensity[a] Muscle-strengthening activity at least 3 days per week[b] Bone-strengthening activity at least 3 days per week[c]
Dietary		
Dietary Guidelines for Americans	*http://www.cnpp.usda.gov/dietaryguidelines.htm*	Build a healthy plate Cut back on foods high in solid fats, added sugars, and salt Eat the right number of calories for you Be physically active your way Use food labels to help you make better choices
Combined		
5-2-1-0 Let's Go!	*http://www.letsgo.org*	Five or more fruits and vegetables daily Two hours or less of screen time daily One hour or more of physical activity daily More water and low-fat milk, no sugary drinks
Let's Move!	*https://letsmove.obamawhitehouse.archives.gov*	Children: have fun being active and eating healthy Parents: get on track to eat well and stay fit Schools: add healthy living to the lesson plan Community leaders: empower families to make healthy decisions Health care professionals: educate and support patients in living healthier

[a]Examples of aerobic activity: running, biking, swimming, and dancing.
[b]Examples of muscle-strengthening activity: playing on playground equipment, climbing trees, and lifting weights.
[c]Examples of bone-strengthening activity: running, jumping rope, and basketball.
Modified from Health.gov: Children and Adolescents (https://health.gov/paguidelines/guidelines/children.aspx); United States Department of Agriculture: Dietary Guidelines (https://www.cnpp.usda.gov/dietary-guidelines); MaineHealth: Let's Go (https://mainehealth.org/lets-go); Let's Move! America's Move to Raise a Healthier Generation of Kids (https://letsmove.obamawhitehouse.archives.gov/).

 Health Promotion

Encouraging Healthy Behaviors in the Infant, Toddler and Child, and Adolescent

INFANT
- Encourage parental bonding.
- Monitor growth and development through well-baby clinic appointments.
- Encourage breast-feeding, if appropriate.
- Use prescribed baby formula to provide necessary nutrients and vitamins.
- Introduce baby foods as recommended. Begin with rice cereal and introduce one new food per week to monitor for allergic reactions.
- Monitor transitioning stools as the gastrointestinal system matures.
- Provide age-appropriate play to encourage physical and mental development.
- Transport infant in child carrier that faces the rear of the car (birth to 20 pounds).
- Maintain immunization schedule as recommended.

TODDLER AND CHILD
- Encourage a healthy diet to include high-nutrient foods such as fruits, vegetables, whole grains, and low-fat dairy and protein products (child and adolescent).
- Continue to provide health care, including immunizations and dental care.
- Encourage developmentally appropriate play.
- Remember that autonomy and initiative are paramount, and offer toddler and child choice of nutritionally dense foods.
- Teach parents and child appropriate methods for good hygiene, such as handwashing and covering mouth when coughing or sneezing.
- Mandate use of seatbelts while riding in vehicle:
  - Toddler, 20 to 40 pounds: Front-facing safety seat secured in rear seat
  - Child, more than 40 pounds: Secured in booster seat with lap and shoulder belt
- Children should wear protective helmets when riding tricycles and bicycles.
- Maintain immunization schedule as recommended.

ADOLESCENTS
- Instruct parents to monitor adolescent for use of drugs or alcohol by noting changes in behavior.
- Adolescents should wear protective helmets when riding bikes or motorcycles, or when skateboarding.
- Provide nutritionally dense foods and snacks to support this period of growth.
- Allow privacy in telephone use and interactions with friends.
- Allow the child to establish an identity even if it is different from that of the parents.
- Insist on mandatory use of seatbelts when in vehicle.
- Maintain immunization schedule as recommended.
- Encourage dental care.
- Encourage safe sun practices:
  - Teach that the long-term effects of sun exposure, such as tanning, include premature aging of the skin, increased risk of skin cancer, and, in susceptible individuals, phototoxic reactions.
  - Teach that the long-term effects of tanning machines are similar to those of the sun; dermatologists do not recommend suntanning by this means.
  - Provide education that the use of sunscreens, including hypoallergenic products, with a sun protective factor (SPF) of at least 15 and a nonalcohol base without lanolin or fragrance is important.

In contrast, the *Dietary Guidelines for Americans* (USDA, 2010), written jointly by the US Department of Health and Human Services and the US Department of Agriculture, recommends that children ages 2 years and older consume a diet of an assortment of foods that includes fruits, vegetables, grains (especially whole grains), fish, lean meats, poultry, and beans. Fat restriction is not appropriate for toddlers; 30% of their calories optimally come from fat. Children under the age of 2 years should drink whole milk or 2% milk. Children who are at risk for obesity or who have a family history of heart disease or high cholesterol may be moved to the lower-fat option after 12 months of age (Chapman, 2008). It is acceptable for the child and the adolescent to consume low-fat or fat-free milk products.

Promoting Lifestyle Changes

The nurse's most important role in relation to overweight and obese children is in education. Education of children and parents concerning dietary choices is essential. The *Dietary Guidelines for Americans* (USDA, 2016) recommends that children and adolescents ages 6 to 17 years get at least 60 minutes of physical activity per day. There are no specific recommendations for children who are under age 6 years. Teaching about the optimal types and amounts of physical activity is important. Many parents do not realize the magnitude of this problem; however, simply by acquiring an awareness of the need, many parents are motivated to make significant lifestyle changes for their children.

TOBACCO USE

Cigarette smoking continues to be the single most preventable cause of death and disease in the United States. A significant number of children and teenagers smoke. According to the Centers for Disease Control and Prevention (2013), in 2009, more than 19% of high school students reported smoking one or more cigarettes in the past month. Smokeless tobacco use was reported by more than 9%. Behaviors associated with teen smoking were use and approval of smoking by peers or siblings, smoking parents, accessibility of tobacco products, low self-esteem, and exposure to advertising for tobacco products. Many states have implemented laws that restrict the sale of tobacco products to minors. Cigarettes are considered to be a gateway drug, and teenagers who smoke are more likely to use illicit drugs.

Other forms of tobacco exposure that also arouse concern include smokeless tobacco, cigar smoking, and environmental tobacco smoke, commonly referred to as secondhand smoke. Adolescents rarely understand the risks involved in smokeless tobacco. These risks include lip, gum, throat, and stomach cancers. There is also a heightened risk for heart disease and hypertension. There is also an impact on pregnancy with stillbirths increasing with use of smokeless tobacco (ACS, 2015). Cigar smoking became more popular in the 1990s, especially among women. Nearly 4% of middle school students and 14.9% of high school students actively smoke cigars. Environmental tobacco smoke results in increased risk for heart and lung disease, particularly asthma and bronchitis in children. Parents often point out that they do not smoke in front of their child; however, the damaging smoke often is trapped in clothing, drapes, and household furnishings.

New pastimes related to smoking involve ENDS (electronic nicotine delivery systems). ENDS include hookahs, e-cigarettes, and vaping (Fig. 30.2). Initially ENDS were not under the purview of the FDA; however, in 2016 they became regulated by the FDA. Forty states have regulations prohibiting the sale of ENDS to minors. Hookah uses water and a special type of tobacco, which often is flavored. In a study 23 high school seniors had participated in hookah smoking in the past year. Some who enjoy hookah smoking activities feel it is a safer alternative. The practice still allows exposure to nicotine and other toxins of tobacco. Hookah smoking traditionally takes place in a hookah establishment, where numerous others are engaged in the practice. When the hookah is smoked, a repetitive puffing and inhalation pattern is used. This may increase the concentration of the toxin exposure. The Centers for Disease Control and Prevention report, "A typical 1-hour-long hookah smoking session involves 200 puffs, whereas an average cigarette is 20 puffs. The amount of smoke inhaled during a typical hookah session is about 90,000 milliliters, compared with 500 to 600 milliliters inhaled when smoking a cigarette" (CDC, 2016). Hookah smoking is associated with the same health risks as cigarettes (Box 30.1).

Box 30.1 Electronic Nicotine Delivery Systems (ENDS)

- More than 3 million middle and high school students were current users of e-cigarettes in 2015, up from an estimated 2.46 million in 2014.
- 16% of high school and 5.3% of middle school students were current users of e-cigarettes in 2015, making e-cigarettes the most commonly used tobacco product among youth for the second consecutive year.
- During 2011 to 2015, e-cigarette use rose from 1.5% to 16.0% among high school students and from 0.6% to 5.3% among middle school students.
- In 2013–2014, 81% of current youth e-cigarette users cited the availability of appealing flavors as the primary reason for use.

From FDA.gov *http://www.fda.gov/TobaccoProducts/Labeling/ProductsIngredientsComponents/ucm456610.htm.*

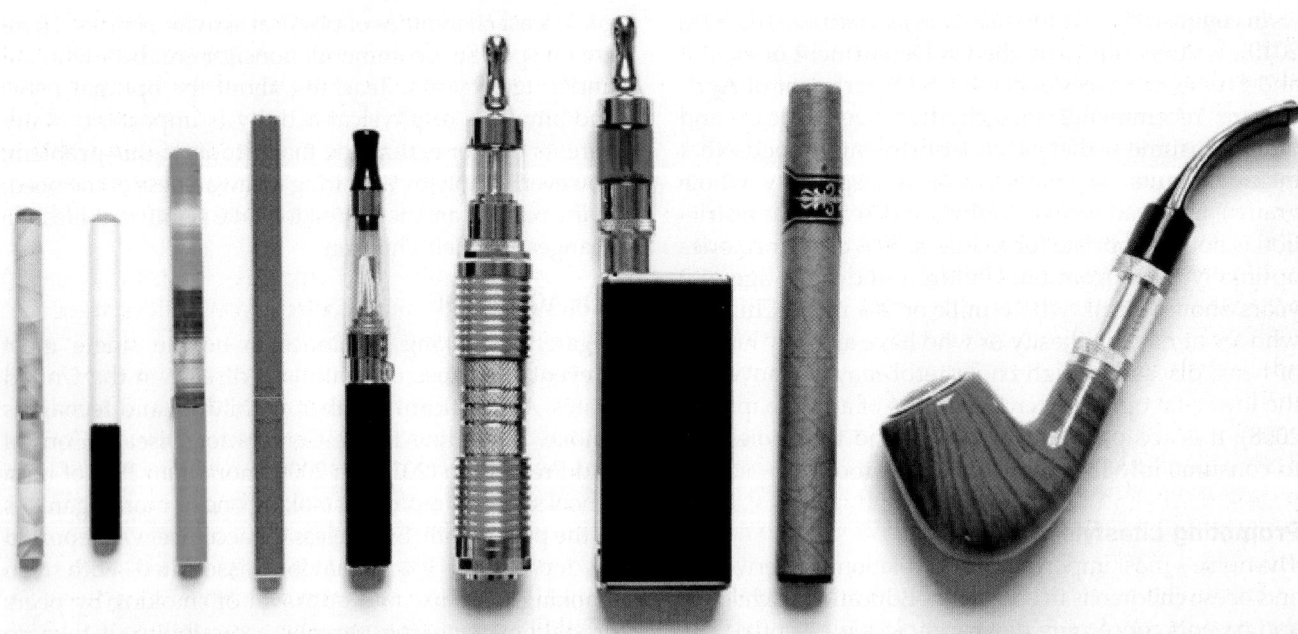

Fig. 30.2 Electronic nicotine delivery systems (ENDS). (From *http://www.fda.gov/TobaccoProducts/Labeling/ProductsIngredientsComponents/ucm456610.htm.*)

Electronic cigarettes and vaping are increasing in popularity. Many incorrectly feel they are not a danger and are much safer than traditional cigarettes. These provide an aerosolized nicotine to the user. There are concerns they carry the same risks as their paper and tobacco predecessor (CDC, 2014).

The American Cancer Society (ACS) and many other organizations offer excellent programs and resource materials aimed at educating children and adolescents concerning the dangers involved in tobacco use. These programs are available at no cost to schools, civic organizations, and health care professionals. Some teens volunteer with these programs to discourage tobacco use. Knowledge of available resources and the ability to promote their use are part of every pediatric nurse's toolbox and professional responsibility.

SUBSTANCE ABUSE

Statistics from 2013 demonstrate that drug use increases through the teen years. Children ages 12 to 13 reported a 2.5% rate of drug use within the previous 30-day period. These rates increase with age, showing a rapid climb of nearly 16% by the age of 17 years. Studies indicate that the early age onset for use of alcohol and drugs is a large determining factor in dependency on them later in life. *Healthy People 2020* seeks to reduce this statistic. Substance abuse is associated with many social problems found in the United States. These problems include domestic violence, sexually transmitted infections (STIs), teen pregnancy, school failure, motor vehicle accidents (MVAs), increased health care costs, decreased worker productivity, and increased homelessness. Teens who engage in alcohol and drug use are less likely to participate in healthy relationships with their peers and face more problems related to discipline and school truancy (Whitten, 2013). Adolescents experiment with marijuana, cocaine, crack, heroin, acid (LSD), inhalants, methamphetamines, ecstasy, and other street drugs and with misuse of prescription drugs. Recently, abuse of prescription and synthetic drugs has become a concern for professionals who work with children and adolescents. In addition, health professionals are concerned about the use of alcohol and volatile substances (such as gasoline, spray paint, antifreeze, and organic solvents) that are inhaled to achieve altered sensorium. The good news reported in *Healthy People 2020* is that substance abuse among adolescents remains below the all-time high reported in 1979. However, an increase has been seen in children ages 12 and 13 years who are experimenting with drugs. This is of particular concern because the younger a person is when drug use (abuse) becomes habitual, the stronger the addiction, and the more difficult the task of breaking it.

Encourage parents to talk with their children about the risks of substance abuse and to plan appropriate child care and supervision. Children who are left unattended are more likely to experiment with drugs. After-school programs are available in many areas. Also, help educate parents regarding the signs of potential drug use in their children.

TELEVISION, VIDEO GAMES, AND THE INTERNET

Parents and child development specialists are concerned about the influence that television, the Internet, and social media have on child development and behavior. Children in the United States spend more than 3 hours per day watching television (FCC, 2017). Many spend an equal number of additional hours using the computer. Time spent using these services reduces time available for other activities such as family, school, and friends. Electronic media time and television viewing are largely sedentary activities.

Children with televisions in their bedrooms spend on average 1½ hours more time watching television than those children do who do not have televisions in their bedrooms (University of Michigan, 2010). The average American home has three or more televisions. Teens who watched more television were more overweight than those who watch less (Herrick et al, 2014). Although television is capable of producing positive learning outcomes, the values and attitudes represented on television are often not realistic, and at times, they clash with the values that the child has been taught. Television seldom represents the actual daily experiences that a child faces. The American Psychiatric Association reports that by the time a child in the United States reaches the age of 18 they will have witnessed 200,000 acts of violence and 16,000 simulated murders on television alone. These numbers do not include video games or the Internet (Parents Television Council, 2018). Parental control of television viewing is beneficial to ensure the appropriateness of programming selected.

Sufficient evidence shows that exposure to violence on television is not conducive to the well-being of children. Research shows more aggressive behavior and increased fearfulness and decreased sensitivity in some children who watch violent television programs. Children who view violent television have been noted to be less likely to prevent or stop a fight. They also have nightmares, obsessive thoughts, and sleep disturbances (APA, 2004).

There are critics and supporters of children's and adolescents' exposure to video games. Critics argue that video games have detrimental effects, which include preventing children from completion of their homework, producing tension and violence, and causing sleeplessness. Critics also suggest video games have potentially negative physical and psychological results. Adverse physical effects possibly include triggering of epileptic seizures. However, video games possibly may have a positive influence on children. Supporters believe video games improve eye-hand coordination, inductive reasoning skills, and perception. They also suggest that video games are a positive substitute for the passivity involved in watching television (Gray, 2012).

Box 30.2 Social Media Use

Top Social Media Platforms for Teens % of all teens 13 to 17 who use:	
Facebook	71%
Instagram	52%
Snapchat	41%
Twitter	33%
Google+	33%
Vine	24%
Tumblr	14%
Different social media site	11%

Source: PEW Research Center's Teens Relationships Survey, Sept 25-Oct 9, 2014 and Feb 10-Mar 16, 2015 (n = 1,060 teens ages 13 to 17).

More than 70% of teens use a social media site (Lenhart, 2015). It is estimated that children spend on average 2 hours daily engaged in the pastime (AACAP, 2011). The increasing popularity of social media sites has brought some benefit but also challenges for children. As of 2018 an estimated 90% of teens ages 12 to 17 have a personal cellphone. Ready access to social media can promote socialization and communication (Box 30.2). There also is easily obtained health information online. Concerns related to social media use in children include cyberbullying and online harassment, privacy violations, sexting, and Facebook depression. Researchers have identified and defined this depression as "depression that develops when preteens and teens spend a great deal of time on social media sites, such as Facebook, and then begin to exhibit classic symptoms of depression" (News Medical Life Sciences, 2012). This condition leaves teens vulnerable, and studies show they are at increased risk for social isolation, use of risky Internet sites and blogs, unsafe, high-risk sexual behaviors, and drug use (Schurgin O'Keefe and Clarke-Pearson, 2011).

In the United States, 71% of families who have children ages 8 to 17 years have computers. Computers and the Internet provide valuable educational and recreational information, but just as in television programming, there are many dangers. Children sometimes are exposed to dangerous or illegal material and negative contact with others through e-mail or in chat rooms. Sharing of personal data or meeting with strangers puts the child and the family at financial and physical risk. Parents and children need to be educated about the potential risks involved in accessing the Internet, and the child always needs adult supervision.

Parents and teachers can provide safeguards by limiting the amount of time that children are allowed to watch television, play video games, or be online. Advise them to monitor content and to increase access to educational alternatives. The goal is balance with activities using electronic devices and media with time dedicated toward friends, family, and school.

RESPONSIBLE SEXUAL BEHAVIOR

Teens are waiting longer to engage in sexual activity than in they did in past decades. Statistics from 2016 show that the average age for the onset of sexual activity is 17 (Guttmacher Institute, 2017). Between 2006 and 2008, approximately 11% of females and 15% of males reported having sexual intercourse before age 15 years. In 1995 this number was 19% and 21%, respectively. Although this is a positive change, sexual activity in teens continues to be a concern. The major risks associated with irresponsible sexual behavior include unintended pregnancy, STIs, and human immunodeficiency virus and acquired immunodeficiency syndrome (HIV/AIDS). Approximately one half of all new HIV cases in the United States occur among people younger than 25 years of age.

Although abstinence is the only protection that is 100% effective, proper use of condoms helps prevent unintended pregnancies and transmission of STIs. This topic always has been a controversial issue with parents, school officials, and health care professionals. The rate of contraceptive use has increased to 79% from 2011 to 2013 from a frightening 48% in 1982 (Guttmacher Institute, 2017). The lack of either full compliance with the use of contraception or total abstinence indicates that education still is needed. It does not matter who provides the education. The bottom line is the necessity of teaching adolescents about responsible sexual behavior, because it is often a matter of life and death.

MENTAL HEALTH

Healthy People 2020 cites target areas related to adolescents and mental health. The initiatives have identified the following areas for improvement for children:

- Reduce suicide attempts by adolescents
- Reduce the proportion of adolescents who engage in disordered eating behaviors in an attempt to control their weight
- Reduce the proportion of adolescents age 12 to 17 years who experience major depressive episodes

The teenage years are among the most difficult times of a person's life. Teenagers want to fit in. They need to belong. They want to look and act like others their age. Parents often forget how difficult this time is for the adolescent.

Mental health issues often are considered less important than physical illnesses. Nurses who feel confident to help with physical symptoms all too commonly feel powerless when confronting matters concerning mental health.

Pediatric nurses are obliged to treat patients holistically, which means addressing physical and mental health. Nurses often underestimate the effect they can have on their patients' mental health. Keep these mental health issues in mind in the practice of pediatric nursing: depression, suicide, eating disorders, and substance abuse.

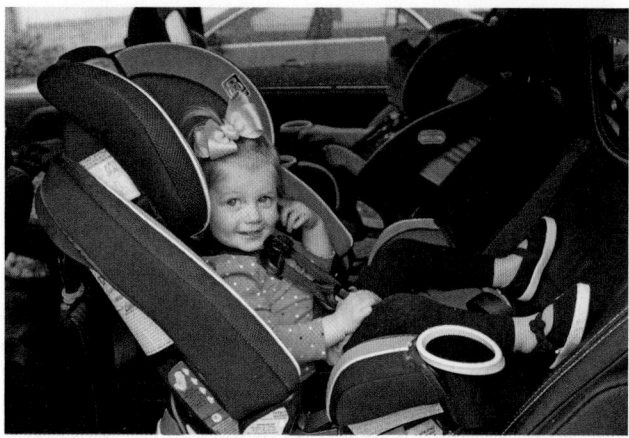

Fig. 30.3 Toddler in rear-facing safety seat, secured in the rear seat.

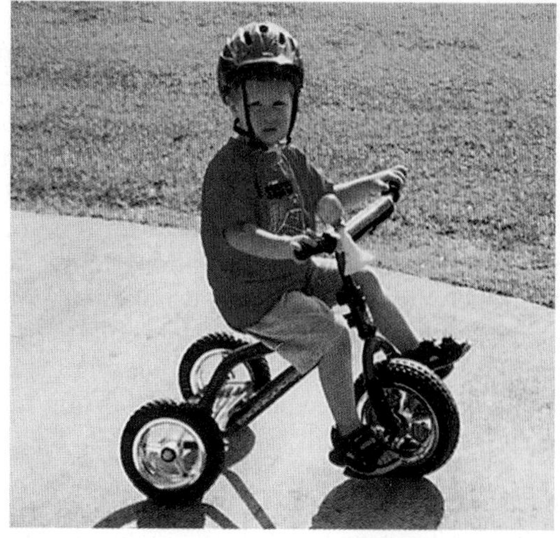

Fig. 30.4 Proper use of a safety helmet begins at an early age.

INJURY AND VIOLENCE

Injuries historically have been a problem in the pediatric population. Common injuries found in children and adolescents involve MVAs, accidental poisoning, suffocation, drowning, falls, aspiration of foreign bodies, and burns. Accidental firearm injuries continue to occur in the pediatric population. Premeditated intentional shootings also occur more frequently among today's adolescents.

The target goals related to injury and violence involving children and adolescents include a reduction in pediatric deaths caused by MVAs and homicides. The nurse contributes to these goals by encouraging proper use of child safety restraints and seatbelts. Advise parents of the following guidelines:

- Use infant car seats designed according to federal safety guidelines:
  - Birth to 20 pounds: Rear-facing safety seats secured in the rear seat (Fig. 30.3)
  - Toddlers 20 to 40 pounds: Front-facing safety seats secured in the rear seat
  - Children more than 40 pounds: Secured in booster seats with lap and shoulder belts. The properly fitted shoulder belt lies across the chest, and the lap belt sits below the hip bones to prevent internal injuries in the event of a vehicular accident.
- Teach the child pedestrian safety: "Stop, Look, Listen" at crosswalks; use sidewalks; wear light-colored clothing at night.
- Supervise children when playing outdoors—no playing at the curb or behind parked cars.
- Insist that the child wear an approved helmet when riding tricycles, bicycles, scooters, mopeds, and skateboards (Fig. 30.4). Protective wrist, elbow, and knee pads are necessary during play involving skateboards and while roller-skating or in-line skating.
- Reinforce the danger of using drugs or alcohol when driving, and insist that no child ride in a car with a person who has been drinking alcohol or using drugs.
- Emphasize rules for safe driving with the adolescent driver.

The role in pediatric nursing in the reduction of pediatric deaths by homicide includes assessment for potential violent behaviors and mental health disorders. Encourage parents to monitor their children's activities. Parents need to be aware of where their children are going and with whom. Encourage teachers, parents, and students to report strange behavior or threats made by other students.

Other significant injury prevention concepts call for awareness and concern. Poisoning, aspiration, and burn injuries in children are addressed subsequently in this chapter.

"Bullying is repeated verbal, physical, social or psychological aggressive behavior by a person or group directed towards a less powerful person or group that is intended to cause harm, distress or fear" (Victoria State Government, 2017). In the United States an estimated 28% of students in grades 6 to 12 report being the victim of a bully. The risk factors for being bullied include the following:

- Have a history of depression
- Are viewed by others as not "fitting in"
- Are overweight or have some other physical characteristic that makes them stand apart from the rest of the peer group

Bullies also have some characteristics placing them at risk for the behavior, including the following:

- Display aggression
- Have friends who bully others
- Have limited parental involvement
- Are experiencing problems at home
- Have difficulty following rules

The methods used vary and can be combined by the attacker (Stopbullying.gov, n.d.). Some assaults are by cyber methods. In this case the bullying may involve sending threatening messages, texts, or photographs.

Emotional attacks may include spreading rumors with the intent to harm the reputation of the victimized individual. Physical attacks may include hitting, tripping, or other types of violence. The verbal attack is just as powerful and may involve shaming, name calling, or rude comments. The impact of bullying can result in physical injuries and long- and short-term emotional harm. It can cause feelings of isolation, depression, or despair. When providing care for at-risk youth, include an assessment for bullying in the data collected. Make certain that the child is aware that bullying behaviors are not acceptable. Determine what reporting may be necessary.

ENVIRONMENTAL QUALITY

Environmental quality concerns specific to children and adolescents include exposure to environmental tobacco smoke (ETS), ozone (outdoor) standards, and (for infants and young children) exposure to lead-based paint. Make sure parents are aware of potential exposure to lead-based paint in older housing and possibly furniture, such as cribs. They need additional education regarding proper testing for lead levels in children, who are in some circumstances at risk for lead poisoning.

See the previous section on tobacco for a discussion of exposure to ETS and the potential problems related to it. Nursing responsibilities regarding ozone standards include awareness of any dangers in the area and of possible measures to take for prevention or avoidance and sharing of this information with others.

IMMUNIZATION

Immunizations are an excellent way to prevent the occurrence and spread of certain infectious diseases. Nearly 60% of all children in the United States have received a full schedule of recommended immunizations (ODPHP, 2014). *Healthy People*'s goal for immunizations is to vaccinate 80% of all children in the United States. Immunization standards offer a challenge for the pediatric nurse because these standards often change. With modern advances in medical research, new immunizations are being developed. The most recent recommended childhood immunization schedule for the United States, valid as of February 2018, was approved by the Advisory Committee on Immunization Practices (ACIP), the American Academy of Pediatrics (AAP), and the American Academy of Family Physicians (AAFP). It can be reviewed at *www.cdc.gov/vaccines/schedules/hcp/child-adolescent.html.* Children who are vaccinated according to the recommended immunization schedule are protected against 10 vaccine-preventable childhood diseases by age 2 years.

Gardasil and Cervarix are three-dose vaccines to prevent infection from human papillomavirus (HPV), the main cause of genital warts and cervical cancer (US Food and Drug Administration, 2009). Gardasil offers coverage against HPV types 6, 11, 16, and 18; Cervarix is effective against HPV types 16 and 18. The National Institute of Allergy and Infectious Diseases (NIAID, 2009) recommends that girls and young women up to age 26 years be vaccinated before becoming sexually active. These vaccines are not effective after exposure to HPV.

Barriers to proper immunization include lack of insurance and funding, lack of transportation, lack of education about the importance of immunizations, and personal and cultural beliefs. Vaccination assistance programs provide vaccinations to children whose parents are unable to pay. Know the current recommended immunization schedule and be able to answer parents' questions regarding immunizations.

DENTAL HEALTH

A multidisciplinary approach to all aspects of pediatric health promotion is fundamental to safeguarding the physical and emotional health of all children. Dental health promotion, an aspect of proper health care, is best to begin with the eruption of the primary teeth, usually at about 6 months of age; advise parents to begin it no later than when the child has reached 2½ years of age, the average age when deciduous dentition is complete. Although the incidence of dental caries has decreased considerably since the introduction of fluorides and increased dental health education and promotion, nursing bottle caries continues to be a significant concern for infants and toddlers. **Nursing bottle caries** is tooth decay that is the result of prolonged drinking from a bottle after the infant has been put to bed, when the milk, juice, or other fluid is allowed to bathe the teeth, thus providing sugar to oral bacteria for growth. During sleep, decreased salivary flow prevents clearance of the liquid from the mouth, and the liquid pools on the teeth (Fig. 30.5). The nurse is in a unique position to prevent these and other problems by promoting good dental health through counseling and education.

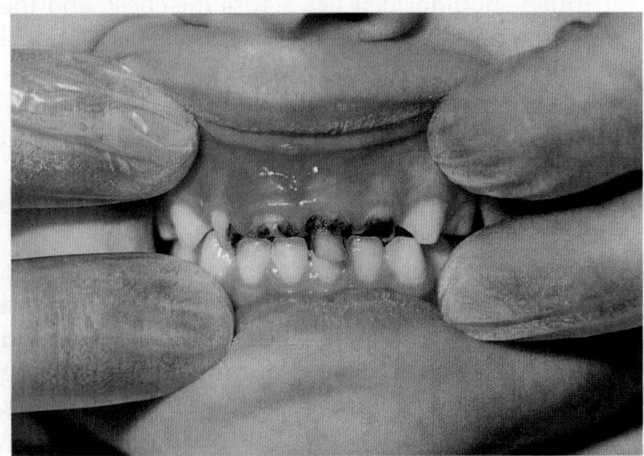

Fig. 30.5 Nursing bottle caries. (From Swartz MH: *Textbook of physical diagnosis: History and examination*, ed 4, Philadelphia, 2005, Saunders.)

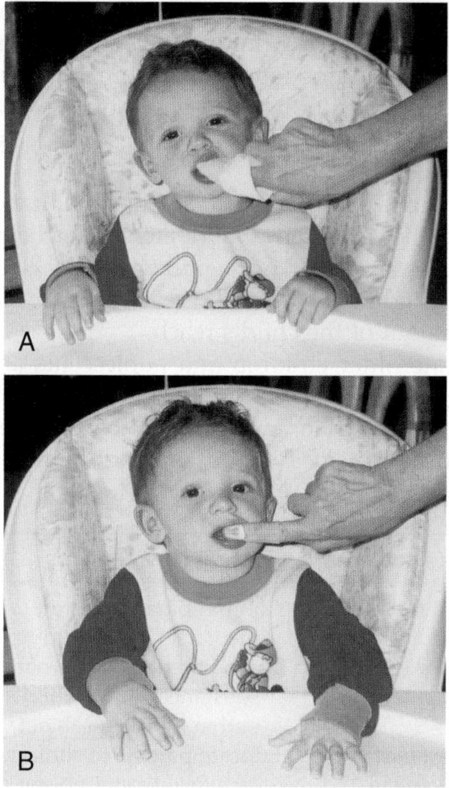

Fig. 30.6 For the infant, wipe the oral cavity and teeth with a damp washcloth. A, Cleansing with a damp washcloth. B, Cleansing with a finger cot toothbrush.

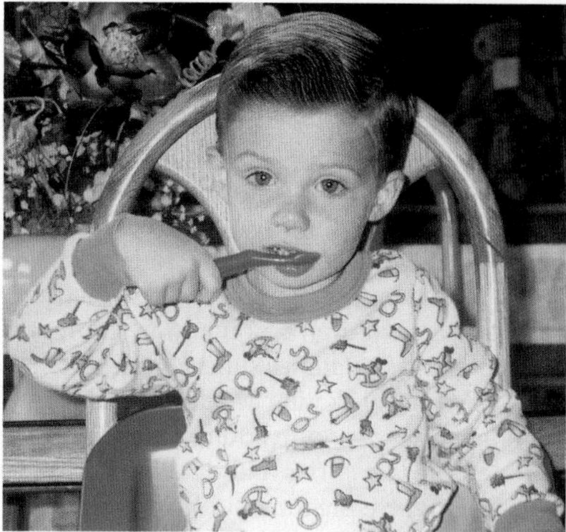

Fig. 30.7 Young children can participate in toothbrushing, but parents need to brush all the child's teeth thoroughly.

STRATEGIES TO PROMOTE DENTAL HEALTH

Make early institution of good dental hygiene and practices to prevent dental caries a part of the anticipatory guidance for all children and their parents. Help children and parents by teaching them to use the following strategies:

- Begin cleansing the oral cavity in infancy by wiping the teeth and gums with a damp washcloth (Fig. 30.6). A toothbrush usually is too harsh for an infant's tender gums. As an infant gets more teeth, use a small soft-bristled toothbrush with plain water to cleanse the teeth and gums. Avoid use of toothpaste during this age, especially if fluoridated, because swallowing by the infant leads to ingestion of excessive amounts of fluoride.
- Initiate fluoride supplementation at 6 months of age if the water in the infant's residential area is not fluoridated. Fluoride supplementation no longer is recommended for infants under 6 months of age.
- Encourage proper nutrition during infancy and childhood to promote good dental health. Avoid, or use sparingly, food with concentrated sugars. In addition, advise against use of honey during the first year of life because some cases of infant **botulism** (an often-fatal form of food poisoning caused by an endotoxin produced by the bacillus *Clostridium botulinum*) have been associated with it. Other foods associated with an increased incidence of dental caries include molasses, corn syrup, and dried fruits such as raisins.

Specific interventions are possible to prevent nursing bottle caries. Give the last bottle *before* bedtime, with proper cleansing of the teeth and gums *before* putting the child down to sleep. Use water in the bedtime bottle instead of juice or milk. Do not use sugar-coated or honey-coated pacifiers. Offer juice in cups, which the child drinks from and then sets down, rather than in bottles.

After infancy, dental hygiene and health care needs continue through the various stages of development.

- For preschool children, when the eruption of the deciduous teeth is complete, continued good dental hygiene is important. Parental assistance and supervision is necessary with brushing; also teach parents to perform flossing (Fig. 30.7). Promote continuation of professional dental care and fluoride supplementation. Encourage proper nutrition (see Chapter 19).
- Eruption of permanent teeth begins during the school-age years. Good dental hygiene and professional dental supervision are especially important during this period. Screening for malocclusion problems that result from abnormal eruption of permanent teeth is also important. Teach or reinforce correct brushing and flossing techniques. Have children brush teeth after meals and snacks and at bedtime. Encourage the child to decrease the ingestion of sugary food.
- Although the rate of caries formation slows during the adolescent years, continuing good dental practices is still important. Adolescence is often when orthodontic appliances are applied to correct malocclusions. Adolescents typically are concerned with body image and often must be reminded of the temporary nature of these devices and their proper use and care.

INJURY PREVENTION

Injuries in children are associated with age, developmental level, and the physical and cognitive skills of the child. The inexperience of infants with the environment and their immature motor skills make them vulnerable to falls and suffocation. Toddlers and preschoolers are at increased risk of injuries from water-related accidents, poisoning, and burns as they acquire new skills. School-age children become more competitive in their activities and sometimes suffer injuries from bicycle accidents, MVAs, and skating accidents. In their struggle to gain independence and freedom, adolescents become more vulnerable to injuries and death from MVAs and accidents that involve firearms, alcohol, and illegal drugs. *Anticipatory guidance* education has been the most widely used approach to educate parents in accident prevention. Use every opportunity to educate parents about injury prevention (see the Safety Alert box).

POISONING

The ingestion of harmful or poisonous substances is a common cause of morbidity and mortality in children younger than age 5 years. Children in the 1-year to 2-year age group are at increased risk because of their natural curiosity to explore their environment once they become mobile. The Poison Prevention Packaging Act of 1970, which requires childproof packaging of medications, has reduced greatly the incidence of poisoning; however, continued strategies and educational efforts are needed to reduce the morbidity and mortality of this preventable cause. Children are vulnerable to becoming poisoned from a variety of substances, including pharmaceuticals (especially acetaminophen, cough and cold preparations, iron, vitamins, and oral contraceptives) and nonpharmaceuticals (cleaning products, lead, plants, insecticides and pesticides, mouthwashes, and cosmetics).

Prevention

All parents must be educated to prevent accidental poisoning. Despite parents' best efforts, children are still at risk, especially when visiting the homes of relatives or friends. Parents must know the number of the poison control center (PCC) in their area. Advise parents to place the PCC telephone number close to each telephone in the home and program it into their cell phones. The PCC hotline number usually is found in the front of the telephone directory. The US Poison Control Center no longer recommends syrup of ipecac for routine treatment of poisoning. Help parents institute prevention strategies by instructing them to do the following:

- Never refer to medicines as candy; medicines are drugs. Store them with childproof caps, and keep them out of reach or in a locked cabinet.
- Place cleaning supplies and other toxic substances, including batteries, up high and out of reach of curious youngsters or in a locked cabinet.
- Do not keep large quantities of toxic agents (e.g., pesticides, cleaning fluids, drugs) in the home.
- Inspect the home for possible sources of lead contamination, including lead-based paint on windowsills, stair rails, and door moldings and peeling wall paint.
- Keep toxic plants out of reach of small hands.
- Remember that many grandparents take medications, and they, too, need to keep them in a locked cabinet or up high and out of the reach of children. Keep purses out of the child's reach.
- Educate older children and adolescents about the dangers of drugs and alcohol.

A patient problem and interventions for the patient with poisoning include but are not limited to the following:

Patient Problem	Nursing Interventions
Potential for Injury, related to lack of knowledge of safeguarding child's environment from harmful, poisonous substances	Counsel parents to store medicines with childproof caps Teach parents to store harmful substances out of child's reach and in a locked cabinet Educate parents to contact health care facility and poison control center immediately if suspected ingestion of harmful substance is noted

ASPIRATION OF A FOREIGN BODY

In children younger than 1 year of age, the leading cause of fatal injury is asphyxiation by aspiration of foreign materials into the respiratory tract. Although all children younger than age 3 years are at risk, the older infant 6 months to 1 year of age is at greatest risk because of the normal hand-to-mouth activities common in this age group. The severity of respiratory tract obstruction depends on the location and the type of material aspirated. Foods that pose the greatest danger include hot dogs, round candy, nuts, grapes, popcorn, peanuts, cookies or biscuits, other meats, carrots, apples, peanut butter, and beans. Common objects that are aspirated easily include buttons on clothing or toys, beads, coins, balloons, pins, and barrettes. Toys with small or loosely attached parts and pacifier nipples that become detached from the shield are also dangerous. More recently, the caps of medication syringes also have been implicated when caretakers forget to remove them before administering medication to a child.

Families need to be cognizant of choking hazards for small children. Counsel families about prevention strategies. Box 30.3 summarizes areas to discuss with parents during routine health supervision visits.

BURN INJURIES

Burns are the result of thermal damage to skin and tissues. Severity is related to the temperature and

Safety Alert

Infant, Toddler and Child, and Adolescent

INFANT
- Keep your hands on the infant at all times when crib rail is down.
- Use an infant car safety seat restraint that has been federally approved.
- Always place an infant who weighs less than 20 pounds (9 kg) or who is younger than 1 year of age in a rear-facing child safety seat in the back seat of the automobile. Never place an infant in the front seat of a vehicle.[a]
- Leave no gaps between crib side and mattress.
- Place infants on the back to sleep. The risk of sudden infant death syndrome (SIDS) is increased in infants placed in side-lying or prone position.
- Check all toys for small parts to reduce risk of choking or wounds.
- Support head, and shield head from injury.
- Do not prop bottle.
- Place infant in upright position when feeding solid foods.
- Use clean bowl and spoon to feed, and do not feed directly from jar; this prevents contamination of food.
- *Never* leave infant unattended in or near water.
- *Never,* under any circumstances, leave infant unsupervised in bathtub.
- Apply a sunscreen when infant is exposed to sunlight (year round).

TODDLER AND CHILD
- Use a toddler car safety seat restraint that has been federally approved; the safety seat restraint can be switched to forward facing once the child weighs more than 20 pounds and is older than 1 year.[a]
- Use car booster seats, also known as belt-positioning devices, for children less than 4 feet 9 inches tall and weighing more than 40 pounds, typically between 4 and 8 years.
- *Never* leave toddler unattended in vehicle or shopping cart.
- Protect from falls, burns, and collisions with objects that result from running and climbing.
- Use washable toys without small parts or sharp edges.
- Supervise closely when near any source of water.
- *Never* leave unsupervised in a bathtub.
- Cover electrical outlets with protective plastic caps.
- Do not allow toddler or child to play on curb or behind a parked car.
- Supervise tricycle and bicycle riding; have child wear helmet.
- Teach child to obey pedestrian safety rules.
- Never leave infant or toddler unattended in high chair.
- Supervise at playgrounds; select safe play areas.
- Apply a sunscreen when toddler or child is exposed to sunlight (year round).
- Stress danger of open flames.
- Always check bath water temperature; adjust water temperature to 120°F (48.9°C) or cooler (infants, toddlers, children).
- Place all potentially toxic agents out of reach or in a locked cabinet.
- Discard all unused refrigerators, ovens, and other appliances; if storing an old appliance, remove door.
- Keep venetian blind cords out of reach of a toddler or child.
- Teach child to never go with strangers.
- Teach child to tell parents if anyone makes child feel uncomfortable in any way.

ADOLESCENT
- Adolescents feel indestructible and tend to be more prone to deliberate (suicide) or nondeliberate accidents, such as in the use of guns, drugs, or motor vehicles.
- Emphasize and encourage safe pedestrian behavior.
- At night, walk with a friend.
- Do not walk in secluded area; take well-traveled walkways.
- Provide competent driver education; encourage judicious use of vehicle; discourage drag racing, "playing chicken"; maintain vehicle in proper condition (e.g., brakes, tires).
- Teach and promote safety and maintenance of two-wheeled vehicles.
- Promote use of seatbelts.
- Promote and encourage wearing of safety apparel, such as helmet or long pants, when skateboarding and bike riding.
- Reinforce the dangers of using drugs, including alcohol, when operating a motor vehicle.
- Teach nonswimmer to swim.
- Teach basic rules of water safety; stress the need to make sure water is of sufficient depth for diving.
- Reinforce proper behavior in areas that involve contact with burn hazards (gasoline, electrical wires, fires).
- Advise regarding excessive exposure to natural or artificial sunlight (ultraviolet burn); encourage use of sunscreen.
- Discourage use of all tobacco products.
- Educate in hazards of drug use, including alcohol.
- Promote acquisition of proper instruction in sports and use of sports equipment.
- Instruct in safe use of and respect for firearms and other devices with potential danger (e.g., power tools, fireworks).

[a]Data from Hockenberry MJ, Wilson D: Wong's nursing care of infants and children, ed 8, St. Louis, 2007, Mosby.

length of time the skin is exposed to the heat source. Burns occur as a result of flames, chemicals, hot objects, radiation, or electricity. Burns are the third leading cause of accidental death in children 1 to 4 years of age, the second in children 5 to 9 years of age, and the third in children 10 to 14 years of age. Up to 75% of all burn injuries occur in the home; children younger than age 2 years experience more scald burns, and children older than 5 years more frequently have flame burns.

Box 30.3 Foreign Body Aspiration Prevention Strategies

- Keep small objects and toys away from infants and young children, who are developmentally unable to obey restrictions. Small children may place small objects in the nose or the ear, causing obstruction.
- Inform parents of the dangers of round foods to children too young to chew these foods properly; they are acceptable to introduce when the child is older.
- When administering medications via syringe, stress to parents the need to remove the cap first.
- Encourage parents to choose one-piece pacifiers that do not come apart and cause aspiration. Have the parents check the pacifier frequently by pulling on the nipple. If it becomes separated from the shield, it is to be discarded.

Prevention

As infants and children acquire new motor skills, they are more vulnerable to accidental burns and other injuries. The nurse has a unique opportunity to educate parents to avoid risks and provide a safe environment for their children. Teach the following safety precautions:

- Keep the hot water heater set at no more than 120°F (49°C).
- Turn all pot handles on the stove toward the back of the stove.
- Keep hot objects, such as cigarettes, coffee pots, and hot liquids or foods, out of the reach of small hands.
- Remove hanging tablecloths and electrical cords, especially around children who crawl or walk.
- Teach older children safe cooking methods and emphasize that it is never acceptable to wear loose clothing near the stove or other heat source (e.g., fireplace, wood-burning stove).
- Use guardrails or guards around fireplaces, space heaters, and other heating sources.
- Use and maintain smoke detectors in the home.
- Keep electrical wires hidden and out of the reach of children.
- Use plastic caps to cover electrical outlets.
- Keep small, hot appliances such as curling irons and steam irons out of the reach of children.
- Keep a fire extinguisher in the home and know how to operate it.
- Use a cool mist rather than a hot mist vaporizer.
- Use a hat and sunscreen on children when outdoors, especially during peak sun hours.
- Teach older children the potential of burn hazards, such as gasoline, matches, barbecue grills, candles, and fireworks (e.g., Roman candles).
- Have parents map out an escape route in the home and practice fire drills with family members.
- Keep the telephone numbers of the fire and rescue squads near the telephone (911 in most areas). Teach small children "nine-one-one" (911), because how to dial nine-eleven is not necessarily a concept they are able to grasp.

Get Ready for the NCLEX® Examination!

Key Points

- Anticipatory guidance is education of parents to prepare them for normal growth and development of their children. It is also psychological preparation of a person for an event expected to be stressful, as in preparation of a child for surgery by explaining what will happen and what it will feel like.
- *Healthy People 2020* identified 12 leading health indicators for health promotion and disease prevention.
- Initiate fluoride supplementation at 6 months of age if the water in the infant's residential area is not fluoridated.
- The development of immunizations against communicable diseases has significantly reduced the morbidity and mortality associated with many diseases.
- Injuries in children are associated with age, developmental level, and the physical and cognitive skills of the child.
- Use infant safety seats designed according to federal safety guidelines: birth to 20 pounds, rear-facing safety seats secured in the rear seat; toddlers 20 to 40 pounds, front-facing safety seats secured in the rear seat; children over 40 pounds, secured in booster seats with lap and shoulder belts per federal safety protocol.
- The use of electronic media is a strong presence in the lives of children. The healthful balance of the media and other activities is needed.

Additional Learning Resources

SG Go to your Study Guide for additional learning activities to help you master this chapter content.

evolve Be sure to visit the Evolve site at *http://evolve.elsevier.com/Cooper/foundationsadult/* for additional online resources.

Review Questions for the NCLEX® Examination

1. When counseling the parents of a 6-month-old about dental health, the nurse includes which statement(s)? *(Select all that apply.)*
   1. "Begin cleansing the oral cavity by wiping teeth and gums with a damp washcloth."
   2. "Avoid toothpaste at this age, especially if it is fluoridated."
   3. "Initiate fluoride supplementation at 6 months of age if infant's home water supply is not fluoridated."
   4. "It is acceptable to prop a bottle with juice or milk for the infant if limited to nighttime periods."
   5. "Dilute fluids made with tap water if fluoridation is present."
2. The nurse is planning a program for parents and adolescents in the community related to obesity. What information is most appropriate for inclusion in the information that will be provided?
   1. Because more mothers work outside the home, children and adolescents eat only fast foods.
   2. Obese children always become obese adults.
   3. Being overweight or obese sometimes results in major physical and psychological health problems.
   4. It is best for families to have more meals at home.
3. Responsible sexual behavior among young people most importantly should include what characteristic?
   1. Having sexual activity only with someone you know
   2. Abstaining from sexual activity or properly using condoms
   3. Having sexual activity only once a month
   4. Requiring sexual partners to be tested for HIV
4. A 15-year-old male patient states that he does not smoke. Further assessment reveals he uses chewing tobacco. What information should the nurse provide to the patient about smokeless tobacco?
   1. The use of smokeless tobacco carries a similar risk for the development of lung cancer.
   2. Individuals using smokeless tobacco have an increased risk for the development of lip, gum, and throat cancer.
   3. People using smokeless tobacco are at an elevated risk for becoming a smoker later in life.
   4. The use of the tobacco must stop immediately.
   5. Heart disease risk is increased by the use of smokeless tobacco.
5. The parents of a 10-month-old are concerned about motor vehicle safety. What education should be provided from the nurse to the parents?
   1. Children who weigh more than 35 pounds must be secured with a lap and shoulder belt.
   2. Infants from birth to 20 pounds must be in a rear-facing safety seat.
   3. When using a lap and shoulder belt, have the lap belt rest above the hip bones.
   4. When using a lap and shoulder belt, have the shoulder belt fit across the upper abdomen.
6. Proper counseling of the parent of a 1-year-old regarding safety includes which instruction(s)? *(Select all that apply.)*
   1. Fence pools with a self-locking gate.
   2. Keep drapery cords out of children's reach.
   3. Place infant on back to sleep.
   4. Do not tie pacifiers on a string around the infant's neck.
   5. Limit bottle feeding to the periods before bedtime.
7. Human papillomavirus (HPV) vaccine is recommended for what population?
   1. Carriers of the disease
   2. Women with sexual partners who are carriers of the virus
   3. Girls from age 13 to 26 years who are not sexually active
   4. Girls who have been sexually active for less than 12 months
8. HPV infection is associated with what health complication?
   1. Infertility in women
   2. Menorrhagia
   3. Pelvic inflammatory disease
   4. Cervical cancer
9. The nurse is discussing dietary intake with the mother of an 18-month-old child. What statement(s) by the mother indicate(s) the need for further instruction? *(Select all that apply.)*
   1. "Whole milk is not a good option for my child."
   2. "I need to begin to decrease the amount of milk my child is allowed to drink."
   3. "2% milk is a good alternative to whole milk for my child."
   4. "Until my child is 3 years of age, whole milk is recommended."
   5. "I can continue to provide 2% milk for my child to drink."
10. The parents of a 13-year-old boy report their son spends several hours on the Internet and social media sites each day before and after school. What information should be provided by the nurse? *(Select all that apply.)*
    1. As long as the child's school grades are good, this is a safe practice.
    2. Excessive hours on social media can result in an imbalance between the rest of the social activities of the child.
    3. Social media use may result in mental health concerns.
    4. Social media has some benefits including improved communication with others.
    5. The Internet can provide educational benefits.

11. A 16-year-old teen reports he uses smokeless tobacco. Which statements by the teen indicate the need for further instruction?
    1. "Smokeless tobacco is safer for me than a cigarette."
    2. "As long as I brush my teeth after use I am going to be OK."
    3. "My breath may have a foul odor from smokeless tobacco."
    4. "I can become sterile from smokeless tobacco use."
    5. "I am at increased risk for heart disease from using this product."
12. When preparing snacks for an 18-month-old child, which would be appropriate? *(Select all that apply.)*
    1. Sliced apples
    2. Peanuts
    3. Grapes
    4. Orange segments
    5. Crackers
13. The nurse is discussing planned well child appointments with the mother of a toddler who frequently misses them. What actions should be taken by the nurse? *(Select all that apply.)*
    1. Assess the parent's beliefs on the importance of the health promotion activities.
    2. Determine if the family has transportation for the appointments.
    3. Seek family input on the dates and times for scheduling the appointments.
    4. Report the family to Child Protective Services.
    5. Review the family's ability to pay for health care.

Basic Pediatric Nursing Care

31

http://evolve.elsevier.com/Cooper/foundationsadult/

Objectives

1. Identify events that were significant to the health care of children in the United States in the 20th century.
2. Discuss the works of Abraham Jacobi and Lillian Wald.
3. Describe the purposes and outcomes of the White House Conferences on Children between 1909 and the 1980s.
4. Discuss the personal characteristics and professional skills of a successful pediatric nurse.
5. Identify key elements of family-centered care.
6. Describe areas in which the pediatric nurse uses principles of growth and development.
7. Discuss how to use the head-to-toe method for the physical assessment of a child.
8. Describe metabolism in the child and its relationship with nutrition.
9. List general strategies to consider when talking with children.
10. Describe the three categories of child abuse.
11. Outline several approaches for making the hospitalization of children a positive experience for them and their families.
12. Discuss pain management in infants and children.
13. Explain the needs of parents during their child's hospitalization.
14. Discuss common pediatric procedures.
15. Discuss administration of pediatric medications.
16. Discuss hazards and accident prevention in the pediatric population.

Key Terms

anterior fontanelle (fŏn-tă-NĔL, p. 959)
anticipatory guidance (p. 938)
birth defects (congenital anomalies) (kŏn-JĔN-ĭ-tăl ă-NŎM-ă-lēz, p. 935)
body surface area (BSA) (p. 966)
children with special needs (p. 936)
cognitive impairment (p. 937)
en face position (ăhn FĂS, p. 944)
family-centered care (p. 936)
morbidity (mŏr-BĬD-ĭ-tē, p. 969)
mortality (mŏr-TĂL-ĭ-tē, p. 933)
primary (deciduous) teeth (dĕ-SĬD-ū-ŭs, p. 945)
vastus lateralis muscle (VĂS-tŭs lăt-ŭr-Ă-lĭs, p. 967)
weaning (p. 947)

HISTORY OF CHILD CARE: THEN AND NOW

In today's society, children are recognized as individuals with unique medical needs that are different than those of adults. The care of children has not always been viewed as an important stage of life. For centuries, children were considered miniature adults.

In colonial America, children had to assume adult responsibilities as soon as they were capable. The value of children was related directly to the work they could perform. Infant and childhood **mortality** (or death) rates were high. Epidemic diseases were common, and there was no control over or treatment for such diseases as smallpox, diphtheria, measles, dysentery, mumps, chickenpox, yellow fever, cholera, or whooping cough. Farm accidents and burns from open fireplaces and gunpowder also contributed to high mortality rates.

Industrialization in America resulted in a population shift from rural to urban settings, where people lived in overcrowded and unsanitary conditions. Often unsanitary conditions were caused by lack of knowledge about how disease occurs. For instance, milk was not refrigerated and contained hundreds of millions of bacteria, which contributed to the development of diarrhea and tuberculosis. In addition to poor living conditions, children were treated as adults, working in factories for 12 to 14 hours a day. With no legal rights for children and no workplace laws, family life was sacrificed to focus on survival.

Children's health care needs were not considered different from those of adults until 1860, when Abraham Jacobi, a New York physician referred to as the "father of pediatrics," first lectured to medical students on the special diseases and health problems of children. With several other physicians, Dr. Jacobi pioneered the scientific and clinical investigation of childhood diseases. One outstanding achievement during Dr. Jacobi's era was the establishment of "milk stations " in 1893, in partnership with New York merchant Nathan Straus. At these free stations, infants were weighed and mothers were taught how to prepare milk before giving it to their babies. Mothers also had access to nurses who taught them the benefits of fresh air, clean water, and adequate clothing and how to satisfy the recreational needs of children. The crusade for pure milk resulted in improved sanitation, the advent of pasteurization of milk, and increased interest in infant care. Despite a remarkable decline in the infant mortality rate, 20% of children still died before their second birthday, and 50% died before age 21 (CDC, 1999).

During the late 1800s, increasing concern developed for the social welfare of children, especially those who were poor, homeless, immigrants, tenement residents, or employed as factory laborers. Reformer Lillian Wald (1867–1940) founded the Henry Street Settlement in New York City, which provided nursing services, social work, and an organized program of social, cultural, and educational activities. She is regarded as the founder of public health or community nursing. Wald believed that public health nurses should treat social and economic problems for the entire neighborhood. Her work had far-reaching effects on child health and nursing.

As medical and scientific advances revealed more causes of disease, emphasis was placed on isolation and asepsis. In the early 1900s children with contagious disease were isolated from adult patients. Parents were prohibited from visiting because of the possibility of transmitting disease to and from home. The works of Spitz (1945, 1946) and Robertson (1990) on institutionalized children helped health care professionals recognize how isolation and maternal deprivation affected children. The growing interest in the psychological health of children resulted in changes for hospitalized children, such as rooming in, prehospitalization, parent education, and hospital schooling.

Influenced by social reformers such as Lillian Wald, national leaders began to take action to improve children's living conditions. In 1909 President Theodore Roosevelt called the first White House Conference on Children. The conference focused on such issues as child labor, dependent children, and infant care. In 1912 the US Children's Bureau was established as a direct result of that conference. Its charge was to investigate all aspects of child care, including infant mortality, child labor laws, conditions of social agencies, and the country's birthrate.

The second White House Conference on Children convened in 1919, after World War I. This conference addressed the socioeconomic situation of mothers and children and resulted in the first federally supported health programs for mothers and children. The Great Depression of 1929 paralyzed the United States and resulted in devastating social and economic conditions. A White House Conference on Children was called in 1930 to study the economic effects of the Great Depression on the health and well-being of children. Thereafter a conference was held at the beginning of each decade until the 1980s. These conferences have been responsible over the years for many changes in child health and welfare, including funding for essential programs, legislation, and shifting the focus from treatment of diseases to preventive health care. Attendees were professionals who worked with children, representatives of federal and state agencies and volunteer organizations, and members of various citizen groups. Although the group did not have legislative powers, together its members raised the consciousness of public officials and private citizens regarding the status of children and families.

The United States did not recover from the Great Depression for many years. In the interim, the Children's Bureau was able to propose legislation to assist children. Some of the most remarkable pieces of legislation were those authorized by the Social Security Act of 1937, which was signed by President Franklin D. Roosevelt. The health care needs of children were incorporated into the provisions of Title V, Maternal and Child Health Services, which, among other accomplishments, recognized for the first time the needs of disabled children. Another important milestone was the Women, Infants, and Children (WIC) program, which opened its first distribution site in 1974. WIC offers assistance with food and nutrition counseling for low-income pregnant, breast-feeding, and non–breast-feeding postpartum women and infants and children under the age of 5 years.

Today the Office of Child Development, established in 1967, oversees children's programs. It houses the Children's Bureau and the Bureau of Child Development Services, which operates such programs as Head Start. The Secretary of Health and Human Services is the cabinet officer responsible for all their activities. In December 1987 the United States Congress and President Ronald Reagan created the National Commission on Children to serve as a forum on behalf of the children of the nation. In May 1991 after 2½ years of intensive investigation and deliberation, the 34-member commission concluded that the United States was failing many of its children. For example, the proportion of children who were not immunized adequately for preventable childhood diseases had increased dramatically since the early 1980s. Lack of immunization resulted in 26,500 cases of measles and 60 deaths from measles in 1990. The commission's final report listed numerous recommendations for addressing pressing children's issues, such as the need to ensure income security, improve health, increase educational achievement, prepare adolescents for adulthood, strengthen and support families, and protect vulnerable children and their families.

Children are the focus of many of our century's reform initiatives, and solutions are sure to emphasize collaboration between various disciplines. For example, violence, once considered solely a criminal justice problem, now is acknowledged as a preventable public health problem. The most effective solutions for this and other multifaceted problems require the expertise of health care professionals, and law enforcement and criminal justice officials, social workers, economists, and educators.

PEDIATRIC NURSING

The nursing of infants and children is consistent with the revised definition of nursing proposed by the Social Policy Task Force of the American Nurses Association (ANA) in 2003. The definition states that "nursing is the protection, promotion, and optimization of health and abilities; prevention of illness and injury; alleviation of suffering through the diagnosis and treatment of human response; and advocacy in the care of individuals, families, communities, and populations" (ANA, 2010, p. 10). This definition incorporates the four essential features of nursing practice:

1. *Human responses* of individuals to actual or potential health problems of concern to nurses, including any observable need, concern, condition, or fact of interest that may be the target of evidence-based nursing practice.
2. *Theory application* is built on understanding theories of nursing and other disciplines as a basis for evidence-based nursing actions.
3. *Nursing actions* are theoretically derived and evidence based and require well-developed intellectual competencies to prevent illness and injury, to alleviate suffering, and to advocate for all populations.
4. *Outcomes of nursing actions* produce beneficial results in relation to identified human responses. Evaluation of those actions determines whether they have been effective. Findings from nursing research provide rigorous scientific evidence of beneficial outcomes of specific nursing actions.

According to Hockenberry and Wilson (2015), "The major goal of pediatric nursing is to improve the quality of healthcare for children and their families." This can be attained by mechanisms such as improvements with immunization rates, nutrition counseling, teen pregnancy prevention, and improved oral health.

CHARACTERISTICS OF A PEDIATRIC NURSE

Pediatric nursing is different from other clinical specialties. First, the nurse must enjoy working with children of all ages and have enhanced growth and development knowledge. Second, when a child has a health problem, the child, family, and the disease become a nursing focus, and none of the three components can be separated from the other two during care consideration. Pediatric nursing is family-centered nursing in its truest sense. It is important for the family to be totally involved and have a feeling of control over the decision making concerning their child's health care. Provide care to the child while also identifying family stressors and providing care for other members of the family. Working with pediatric patients requires the nurse to have specialized skills, including excellent assessment skills; the ability to establish trust; teaching ability; and the ability to serve as a patient advocate.

By watching children play or perform certain tasks, a nurse should be able to assess their developmental ages. Not all **birth defects (congenital anomalies)** (any abnormality present at birth, particularly a structural one that is possible to inherit genetically, acquire during gestation, or acquire during the parturition [process of giving birth]) are diagnosed in the neonatal period. Sometimes nurses identify a problem as a result of the nursing assessment. When children are very ill, minor changes in their physical status sometimes result in a variety of complications; therefore any changes must be noted as early as possible.

Often the nurse is involved in supporting children through a difficult procedure or serious illness. Such an endeavor not only includes preparation for the event but also requires a level of trust that permits children to express their fear, apprehension, and anxiety. To establish a trusting relationship, convey respect to children, talk with them at a level they can understand, and, most importantly, be honest.

Teaching is ongoing in pediatrics and can be direct or indirect. Innumerable opportunities are available to help children and parents adapt to a chronic illness or disorder through direct teaching, but these require a nurse's knowledge of community resources or volunteer agencies. Be aware of the indirect teaching that occurs through example. A pediatric nurse serves as a role model for children by demonstrating appropriate health promotion and prevention behaviors, such as maintaining good nutrition, a healthy lifestyle, and personal hygiene, and for parents by exhibiting age-appropriate responses to children.

Another role the nurse fills is that of child and family advocate, whether the situation involves ethical decision making or the quality of care given. Sometimes this takes the form of coordinating the activities of a health team and collaborating with members of different disciplines to provide a child with the expert care that is necessary. The nurse often is the intermediary person between the child, family, and other health care providers, providing information, encouragement, clarification, and support.

To enjoy a career and continue working in pediatrics, the nurse needs the ability to recognize and appreciate the uniqueness that each child or adolescent brings to the nurse-patient relationship. It is that special quality—uniqueness—that anyone who provides care for children must understand, respect, and cherish.

CHILDREN WITH SPECIAL NEEDS

Medical advances over the past two decades have resulted in significant changes in the pediatric population. Fragile or premature infants and children with severe injuries or disabilities are now surviving, unlike in the past. With the aid of technology, babies born long before their due dates live into childhood and beyond, but they may face lifelong chronic or debilitating conditions. The term **children with special needs** refers to infants and children with congenital abnormalities; chronic physical conditions, such as malignant disease, gastrointestinal (GI) disease, or central nervous system (CNS) anomalies; and chronic developmental, behavioral, and emotional conditions. Many of these children need specialized care throughout childhood and into other developmental stages as they age.

Although children with special needs make up a large percentage of the hospitalized children, many forms of technology previously found only in hospital settings have been adapted for home use. With appropriate services and support, even children with severe disabilities can live at home with their family and attend school with their peers.

FAMILY-CENTERED CARE

Family-centered care is a philosophy of care that recognizes the family as the constant in the child's life and holds that systems and personnel are called on to support, respect, encourage, and enhance the strengths and competence of the family (Box 31.1). Nurses and others in the community support families in their natural caregiving and decision-making roles by building on existing unique strengths and acknowledging their expertise in caring for their children within and outside the hospital setting.

Two basic concepts in family-centered care are enabling and empowering. Professionals *enable* families by creating opportunities for all family members to make use of their abilities and competencies and to acquire new ones that are necessary to meet the needs of the child and the family. Professionals *empower* families to establish or confirm a sense of control over their lives. Empowerment frees families to foster their own strengths, abilities, and actions and thus enables them to make positive changes in their lives.

Box 31.1 Key Elements of Family-Centered Care

- Identify and mobilize internal and external strengths.
- Access appropriate resources in the extended family and community.
- Recognize and enhance positive communication patterns.
- Decide on a consistent discipline approach and access parenting programs if needed.
- Maintain comforting cultural and religious traditions and sources of healing.
- Engage in joint problem solving.
- Acquire new knowledge by providing information about a specific health problem or issue.
- Become empowered.
- Allocate sufficient privacy, space, and time for leisure activities.
- Promote health for all family members during times of crisis.

From James SR, Nelson KA, Ashwill JW: *Nursing care of children: Principles and practice*, ed 4, St. Louis, 2013, Saunders.

The *parent-professional partnership* is a powerful mechanism for enabling and empowering families. Parents serve as respected equals with professionals and have the right to decide what is important for themselves and their family. The professional supports and strengthens the family's ability to nurture and promote family development. In a parent-professional partnership, all persons involved in the care of the patient work together and share their talents and resources to provide the best care possible for the patient. The pediatric nurse should assist family members with identifying their strengths and needs and encourage family members to contribute to the plan of care. Last, all professionals involved in the care of the patient also must work together as a team to benefit the child(ren) and family.

Mutual respect is the foundation for effective partnerships with parents. Parents know their child better than anyone else and are able to provide the nurse with important information that cannot be obtained in any other way. Parents of a child with special needs also often become experts on their child's condition. The tradition of the authoritarian nurse has been replaced by a system in which nurses are consultants to the parents and share their unique knowledge and decision-making responsibility (Box 31.2).

Children are vulnerable to the major stressors inherent in hospitalization, such as separation from family and familiar environment, loss of control, bodily trauma, and pain. Many factors, including the child's age, available family support, coping skills, and diagnosis influence the child's response to the illness and hospitalization. Family-centered care is better understood with a comparison of the typical handling of child hospitalization or care needs in the past with today's family-centered approach to care. In the past, parents usually were denied access to their child's medical records or hospital chart. With a family-centered care approach, parents have the same access to information about their child as do all other members of the child's health care team. Other changes, such as hospitals welcoming parents 24 hours a day, reflect increased acknowledgment of the importance of family to the child and of family well-being to members of the family unit. A family-centered approach to care is an important concept in the nursing care of all children. However, it is crucial for optimum care of children with special needs, who are likely to experience repeated contact with the health care system throughout their life.

FUTURE CHALLENGES FOR THE PEDIATRIC NURSE

The present shift in focus from treatment of disease to promotion of health is likely to expand nurses' roles

Box 31.2 Implementation of Family-Centered Care

Although professionals readily accept the concept of family-centered care, they have been slow to implement practices that embody "the family as the patient." This lag has occurred in part because family-centered care requires a shift in orientation regarding the provision of services. The philosophy behind family-centered care requires stretching beyond clinical practices that have become traditional because of their convenience to the institution and personnel.

- Common examples of *system-based care* are exclusionary policies, such as not allowing family members to stay with their children during a procedure and restricting visiting hours and the number and the age of visitors.
- Family-centered care means putting families at the center of the caregiving process, with their input serving as the major determinant of the interventions provided. For example, exclusionary policies are replaced with *family-based care,* such as parental and child *choice* regarding separation during procedures, open visiting hours, and no limitations on the age or the number of visitors, except per family request. In fact, the question arises: Are we misusing the word *visitor* altogether? Family members certainly are not visitors to their child; nurses and other staff are.
- Even *child-based care* is not synonymous with family-based care. For example, often the hospital dietary service provides selections for children but fails to provide inexpensive meals for parents or consider family cultural and religious traditions. Primary nurses at times focus on the child's needs but place little emphasis on the family's concerns.
  - In your practice, what policies can be considered system-based, child-based, or family-based care? How can those that are not family-based be changed? What reasons do staff give for preferring system-based care?
- Compare your agency's policies with its mission statement and purpose. Fortunately, models of family-centered care do exist and have documented benefits:
  - Families experience greater feelings of confidence and competence and less stress in caring for their children.
  - The dependence of families on professional caregivers decreases.
  - Costs of care decrease.
  - Professionals experience greater job satisfaction.
  - Parents and providers are empowered to develop new skills and expertise.

further in ambulatory and outpatient care, with an emphasis on prevention and health teaching. Childhood diseases such as obesity and diabetes will continue to be a major challenge in the years ahead. The need for home care and community health services will make it imperative for nurses to become more independent and acquire skills well beyond those needed in traditional care settings.

Of the 73.9 million children in America, 65% live in a home with two married parents. Although the number of total children in America is on the decline, the number of minority children has increased slightly. Of the children ages 5 to 17 years, 22% speak a language other than English at home; 22% of children live in poverty; and an estimated 10% of children are without health care insurance (Forum on Child and Family Statistics, 2012). This results in limitations in access to affordable care. The provision of family-centered care to these children and their family is the challenge presented to the pediatric nurse.

NURSING IMPLICATIONS OF GROWTH AND DEVELOPMENT

The nurse must know the basic principles of normal growth and development to understand what can be expected from infants and children, what their needs are, and why they behave as they do. Although each child is unique, groups of children of the same age are more alike than they are different. For example, significant differences are found among the babies in a newborn nursery, but a number of general statements can be made about them. In knowing their similarities, the nurse is better able to perform assessments, develop interventions, identify problems, and promote healthy development (see the Health Promotion box).

Growth and development are complex processes that occur in stages as the body grows, the mind develops, and the personality unfolds. The newborn moves through infancy, toddlerhood, preschool, school age, and adolescence, and each stage consists of predictable, orderly events. Knowledge of the normal milestones of a 6-year-old, for example, makes for easier identification of a developmental delay in a 6-year-old who has not mastered the expected developmental milestones. Differences occur in the rate or the timing with which a child accomplishes a particular task. One infant may sit up at 5 months of age, perhaps, and another at 7 months. However, most infants do so by 6 months of age. Illness or a lack of stimulation interferes with normal development. Other variables that affect development include a baby's genetic makeup and a host of factors such as ethnic background, religion, family size, socioeconomic bracket, and education of the parents.

Growth and development is an important aspect of pediatric nursing. One of the nurse's primary responsibilities is to identify an infant or child who is demonstrating **cognitive impairment** (the preferred term for mental retardation). The earlier intervention takes place, the greater the likelihood of improvement or remediation. The pediatric nurse also has the opportunity to play a significant role in other types of interventions. For example, the nurse may caution expectant mothers on the hazards of consuming alcohol or smoking while pregnant, refer children with suspected delays to early interventionists, teach parents therapeutic activities and exercises to use with their children, and become

 Health Promotion

Characteristics of the Infant, Toddler, Child, and Adolescent: Encouraging Healthy Behaviors at Each Stage

INFANT

- Weight doubles by 6 months and triples by 1 year.
- Vision at birth is approximately 20/400; by 12 months, vision is 20/100.
- Play requires stimulation activities that involve motor skills, language, and social skills.
- Infants like toys that bang, shake, or can be pulled and enjoy playing "peek-a-boo."
- Infants like verbal praise and encouragement.

Guidance

- Encourage parents to not use baby talk but to instead pronounce words correctly.
- Sleep usually is established by the spacing of feedings. Encourage parents to give care during awake times either before or after feedings.

TODDLER AND CHILD

- Weight gain from 1 to 3 years is about 5 pounds per year. The weight is usually four times the birth weight by 3 years of age.
- This period consists of intense activity and exploration.
- The toddler or child takes 1 or 2 naps a day and sleeps up to 9 to 12 hours a night.
- Bowel and bladder control usually are achieved by 3 years of age.
- The toddler or child practices parallel play.
- Cognition regarding thinking and reasoning is based on magical or egocentric processes.
- The toddler or child experiences physiologic anorexia, which causes the child to either binge or be picky depending on individual growth spurts and plateaus.

Guidance

- Recommend milk as a drink of choice because of increased needs for calcium. Milk should be fat free or low fat to avoid a large number of "empty calories." Lactose-free milk and soymilk are available for those who are lactose intolerant.

ADOLESCENT

- Adolescents need to be more independent and vacillate between independent and dependent roles, which may be reflected in mood swings.
- Concern about body image, looks, and clothes increases.
- Interest in the opposite sex is heightened.
- Adolescents exhibit logical thought and reasoning and often question the values of parents.
- Adolescents prefer being with peers to establish identity, spending less time with parents and more time with friends.

knowledgeable about resources in the community that serve children and their families.

Knowledge of child development allows the nurse to use a developmental rather than a chronologic approach to pediatric nursing care. A developmental approach emphasizes the child's abilities and strengths rather than disabilities and weaknesses. It considers children's individuality and personalities and builds on what they *can* do rather than concentrating on what they *cannot* do.

Box 31.3 Children's Concepts of Illness

INFANTS
Perceive illness as generalized discomfort and pain.

PRESCHOOLERS
Conceive of illness as a punishment for bad thoughts or behavior; believe that adults have the power to magically cure the illness if they want.

SCHOOL-AGE CHILDREN
Sometimes perceive illness as a result of bad or indiscreet behavior; sometimes have an accurate awareness of the location of body parts and a beginning understanding of body processes and functions.

ADOLESCENTS
Focus on discrete symptoms rather than overall effect of illness; often intellectually question and deal with information about illness; at times use denial of illness or overcompensate in areas not affected.

An understanding of normal growth and development enables the nurse to select age-appropriate toys for the infant or young toddler and devise activities that appeal to the school-age child or adolescent. Children learn through every opportunity made available to them. For example, observe a 2-year-old playing with a large box, which demonstrates a child's curiosity and creativity.

Age and developmental level influence the ways in which children perceive and make sense of experiences such as illness or disability and therefore make an impact on their ability to cope. Knowledge of these levels prepares nurses to develop appropriate nursing plans of care. Some generalizations are possible to make regarding children's concept of illness at different stages of development (Box 31.3). Keep in mind that children, particularly very young ones, sometimes change very rapidly physically and developmentally. Therefore be sure to reassess and modify nursing care plans continually to reflect these changes.

Knowledge of growth and development is also the basis for anticipatory guidance with parents. **Anticipatory guidance** (psychological preparation) is preparation for what is likely to occur in the coming weeks and months so that it is possible to lay the groundwork now to protect and promote the child's well-being at that time. For example, parents learn that their 9-month-old or 10-month-old will begin to crawl from one place to another. It is normal, it is expected, and it must be allowed. However, parents have to remove any harmful objects from the child's reach.

Once a child becomes mobile, the environment should be made "childproof" so that it is safe for the curious crawler. Play is the work of childhood. It is best done in a safe environment, with toys that are safe. The nurse plays an important role in assisting parents to understand the physical and behavioral changes that occur rapidly in the developing infant or toddler. These principles also are useful in working with school-age children, who are exposed to many new experiences once they start school, and preadolescents, who need to be ready to manage the hormonal and growth changes they will experience. The parents of the adolescent are usually as confused and perplexed as the youngster is about changes and behavior at this stage of development. Nurses play an important role in supporting and guiding parent and adolescent through this trying time of life.

PHYSICAL ASSESSMENT OF THE PEDIATRIC PATIENT

Children's rate of growth, level of understanding, and means of communicating differ from adults'. Each stage of childhood is unique. The challenges that children present are constant, exciting, and satisfying. Different assessment skills must be used with children of different age groups.

As in the adult, the sequence of assessment of a child follows a head-to-toe direction. Sometimes you must alter the sequence to accommodate the child's developmental needs, but the findings are documented in the traditional way.

To prepare a child for a physical assessment, use developmental and chronologic age as the main criteria for the choice of method to assess each body system (Boxes 31.4 and 31.5).

GROWTH MEASUREMENTS

Measurement of physical growth is a key element in evaluation of the health status of children. The growth parameters include weight, height, and head

Box 31.4 Guidelines for Pediatric Physical Assessment

- Perform examination in appropriate, nonthreatening area:
  - Have room well lit and decorated with neutral colors.
  - Have room temperature comfortably warm.
  - Place all strange and potentially frightening equipment out of sight.
  - Have some toys, dolls, stuffed animals, and games available for child.
  - If possible, have rooms decorated and equipped for children of different ages.
- Provide privacy, especially for school-age children and adolescents.
- Provide time for play and becoming acquainted.
- Look for behaviors that signal child's readiness to cooperate:
  - Talking to nurse
  - Making eye contact
  - Accepting offered equipment
  - Allowing physical touching
  - Choosing to sit on examining table rather than parent's lap
- If you observe no signs of readiness, use the following techniques:
  - Talk to patient; gradually focus on a favorite object, such as a doll.
  - Make complimentary remarks about child, such as appearance, dress, or a favorite object.
  - Tell a funny story or play a simple magic trick.
  - Have a nonthreatening "friend" available, such as a hand puppet, to "talk" to child for the nurse.
- If child refuses to cooperate, use the following techniques:
  - Assess reason for uncooperative behavior; consider that a child who is unduly afraid has perhaps had a previous experience that was traumatic.
  - Try to involve child and parent in process.
  - Avoid prolonged explanations about examining procedure.
  - Use a firm, direct approach regarding expected behavior.
- Perform examination as quickly as possible.
- Have attendant gently restrain child.
- Minimize any disruptions or stimulations: limit number of people in room; use isolated room; use quiet, calm, confident voice.
- Begin examination in a nonthreatening manner for young children or children who are fearful:
  - Use approaches such as "Simon says" to encourage child to make a face, squeeze a hand, stand on one foot, and so on.
- Use "paper-doll" technique:
  1. Lay child supine on an examining table or floor that is covered with a large sheet of paper.
  2. Trace around child's body.
  3. Use body outline to demonstrate what will be examined, such as drawing a heart and listening with the stethoscope before performing the activity on child.
- Involve child in examination process:
  - Provide choices, such as sitting on the bed or the chair.
  - Allow child to handle or hold equipment.
  - Encourage child to use equipment on a doll, family member, or examiner.
  - Explain each step of the procedure in simple language.
  - Examine child in a comfortable and secure position: sitting in parent's lap; sitting upright if in respiratory distress.
- Proceed to examine the body in an organized sequence (usually head-to-toe) with the following exceptions: examine painful areas last; in emergency situation, examine vital functions (airway, breathing, and circulation) and injured area first.
- Reassure child throughout examination, especially about bodily concerns that arise during puberty.
- Discuss findings with family at end of examination.
- Praise child for cooperation during examination; give reward such as small toy, stickers, or sucker.

Box 31.5 Assessment of Body Systems

Use of developmental and chronologic age as the main criteria for the choice of method to assess each body system accomplishes several goals:

- It minimizes stress and anxiety associated with assessment of various body parts.
- It fosters a trusting nurse-child-parent relationship.
- It allows for maximum preparation of the child.
- It preserves the essential security of the parent-child relationship, especially with young children.
- It maximizes the accuracy and reliability of assessment findings.

Table 31.1 Expected Growth Rates at Various Ages

AGE	EXPECTED GROWTH RATE PER YEAR cm	inches
1 to 6 mo	18–22	7.2–8.8
6 to 12 mo	14–18	5.6–7.2
Second year	11	4.4
Third year	8	3.2
Fourth year	7	2.8
Fifth to tenth years	5–6	2–2.4

circumference and sometimes skinfold thickness and arm circumference. Plot the child's measurements with percentiles on growth charts and compare them with those of the general pediatric population to determine deviations from the norm. Evaluation of growth trends demonstrated by the child is imperative because growth is a continuous but uneven process, and therefore the most reliable evaluation lies in comparison of growth measurements of each child over a prolonged time (Table 31.1).

The most commonly used growth charts in the United States are from the National Center for Health Statistics (NCHS). The growth charts include 3rd and 97th smoothed percentiles for all charts, and the 85th percentile for the weight-for-stature and BMI-for-age charts.

Children whose growth necessitates further investigation include the following:

- Children whose height and weight percentiles are widely disparate (e.g., height in the 10th percentile and weight in the 90th percentile, especially with above-average skinfold thickness).
- Children who fail to show the expected growth rates in height and weight, especially during the rapid growth periods of infancy and adolescence.
- Children who show a sudden increase, except during puberty, or a decrease in a previously steady growth pattern.

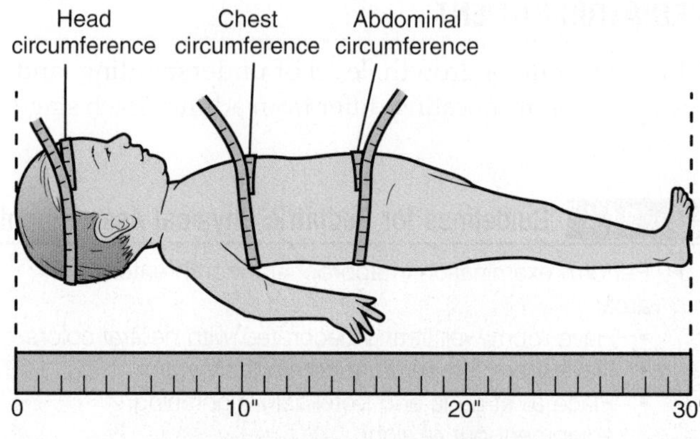

Fig. 31.1 Measurement of head, chest, and abdominal circumference and crown-to-heel measurement (recumbent length).

Common Measurements

Head circumference is measured in children up to 36 months. Head circumference usually is measured above the eyebrows and pinna of the ears and around the occipital prominence at the back of the skull (Fig. 31.1).

Length refers to measurements taken when children are supine. Until children are 2 years old, recumbent length is measured. Request assistance in holding the child's head in midline while you extend the child's legs to take a measurement.

Height refers to a measurement when a child stands upright.

Weight

A child's weight reflects fluid loss and inadequate calories, especially in the infant and the toddler. Because of the information that the child's weight conveys, consider the following:

- Use the same scale and weigh the child at the same time every day.
- Perform weight measurements in a warm room.
- What children wear and what is attached to them affects weight.
- If equipment has been added or removed, document this on the graphic sheet.
- Usually older children are weighed with underpants or a light gown (Fig. 31.2).
- Respect the privacy of all children.

Skinfold Thickness and Arm Circumference

Skinfold thickness is determined at one site, with at least two measurements taken for the greatest reliability (Box 31.6).

Arm circumference measures muscle mass. The same procedure is followed as for skinfold thickness, except the measurement is made with a tape measure rather than calipers.

VITAL SIGNS

Key elements in evaluation of physical status are vital signs: temperature, pulse, respiration, and blood pressure. (For best results taking vital signs of an infant,

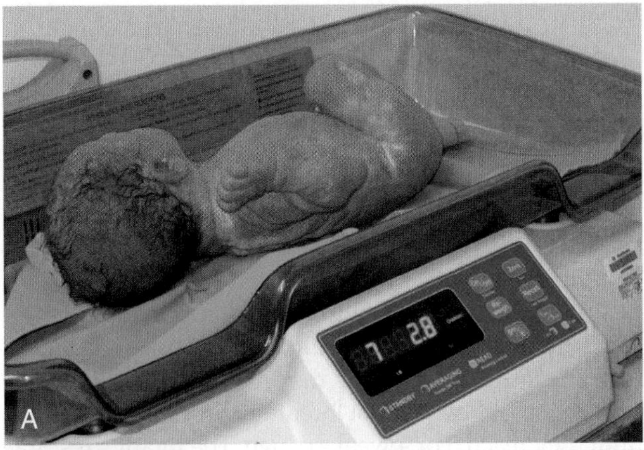

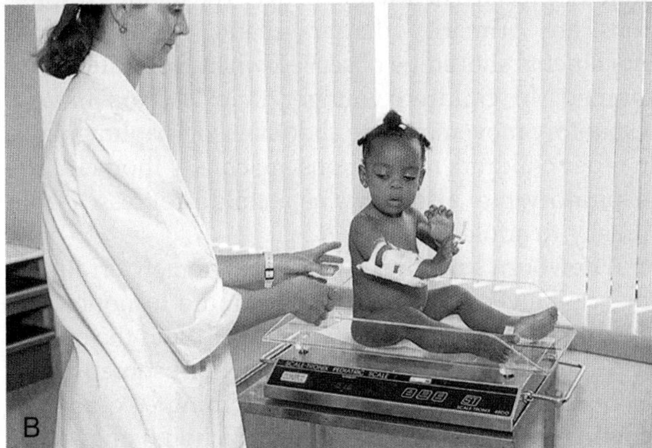

Fig. 31.2 A, Infant on scale. B, Toddler on scale. (B, From Hockenberry MJ, Wilson D: *Wong's essentials of pediatric nursing*, ed 8, St. Louis, 2009, Mosby.)

Box 31.6 Measurement of Triceps Skinfold Thickness

- With child's right arm flexed 90 degrees at elbow, mark midpoint between acromion and olecranon on posterior aspect of arm.
- With arm hanging freely, grasp a fold of skin between thumb and forefinger 1 cm above midpoint.
- Gently pull fold away from underlying muscle and continue to hold through the remaining steps until measurement is completed.
- Place caliper jaws over skinfold at midpoint mark; if a plastic catheter (e.g., Ross Adipometer) is used, apply pressure with thumb to align lines on caliper; follow directions for use of other calipers.
- Estimate reading to nearest millimeter, 2 or 3 seconds after applying pressure.
- Take measurements until you obtain two readings that agree within 1 mm.

count respirations first, before the infant is disturbed; take pulse second, and temperature last.)

Temperature

Body temperature, which also reflects metabolism, is fairly stable from infancy through adulthood. After the unstable regulatory ability in the neonatal period, heat production steadily declines as the infant grows into childhood. In an air-conditioned delivery room, the newborn's temperature sometimes drops to 97°F (36.1°C) or lower, which accounts for the use of radiant warmers for newborns after delivery. Newborns also tend to have difficulty dissipating heat in an overheated environment, which increases the risk of hyperthermia.

Table 31.2 Normal Temperature in Children

AGE	TEMPERATURE °F	TEMPERATURE °C
3 mo	99.4	37.5
6 mo	99.5	37.5
1 yr	99.7	37.7
3 yr	99.0	37.2
5 yr	98.6	37.0
7 yr	98.3	36.8
9 yr	98.1	36.7
11 yr	98.0	36.7
13 yr	97.8	36.6

Despite the ability to regulate their temperature, infants and toddlers are prone to wide variations, especially after crying for extended periods or after active play. Temperature elevations also occur rapidly in young children when infections are present.

Beginning at approximately 12 years of age, girls display a temperature that remains relatively stable, whereas the temperature in boys continues to fall for a few years longer. Females maintain a temperature slightly above that of males throughout life (for normal temperature in children, see Table 31.2).

The primary purpose of body temperature measurement is detection of abnormal values. In patients with febrile conditions, the chief concern is the temperature of the brain, because very high temperatures have the capacity to cause neural damage. Thus the best sites for measurement of temperature are those closest to the brain, which reflect central, or core, body heat. Other core sites are the esophagus and the bladder. However, these sites involve invasive thermometry and are impractical for routine temperature measurement.

The oral and axillary sites are used commonly in clinical practice. Other sites that also are used for temperature measurement are the tympanic membrane and temporal artery (temporal artery thermometry). Historically, the temperatures of infants and young children were taken rectally. Safety concerns and the availability of safer and more reliable methods have made this practice rare today. In infants and young children, tympanic or axillary temperatures often are preferred. Oral temperatures are acceptable when children are old enough to be cooperative and understand directions, typically around 5 or 6 years old.

Many facilities now use tympanic temperatures for all ages. The ear's proximity to the hypothalamus, the body's temperature-regulating center, makes it a desirable area for reflecting true core temperature. In comparisons with rectal, oral, or axillary temperature assessments in children, tympanic membrane measurements are fairly insensitive in detecting fevers and should be used with caution for children younger than 3 years of age. The size of the probe has the potential to influence the reading. Many ear probes are too large to be placed correctly in the pediatric ear canal. Use of correctly sized pediatric materials and supplies is important. Technique is another important factor. For the sensor to detect heat from the drum, instead of from the cooler canals, straighten the ear canal. When the ear is pulled back and down and the probe tip points at the midpoint between the eyebrow and the sideburn on the opposite side of the face, the most accurate temperature readings are obtained.

In considering all the findings for and against different sites of temperature measurement, think critically about why the temperature is needed, how clinically significant a small difference in temperature between routes really is, and how much the procedure upsets the child and the caregiver. Finally, in deciding which route to use, consider which method will be the least traumatic to the child. Children are less upset having their temperature measured via the ear route than via the rectal route. Parents also sometimes have objections to the rectal route.

Heart Rate or Pulse

Variations exist in the heart rates of children. Although an average apical beat of a newborn is around 120 per minute, the heart rate gradually slows to an average of 70 beats per minute by adolescence (Table 31.3). The presence of infection increases the heart rate, as does physical activity. During sleep, a child's pulse is at its slowest rate.

In assessment of the heart rate, note the rhythm and any irregularities. Count the pulse rate for 1 full minute.

Table 31.3 Vital Signs (Averages)

AGE	HEART RATE (beats/min)	RESPIRATIONS (breaths/min)	BLOOD PRESSURE (mm Hg)
Newborn	120	35	70/50
1–11 mo	120	30	90/60
2 yr	110	25	96/68
4 yr	100	23	100/70
6 yr	100	21	105/70
10 yr	90	20	108/70
12 yr	88	20	110/70
16 yr	70	20	120/70

An apical pulse measurement, heard at the apex of the heart (located at the fifth intercostal space on the left side), is more reliable if taken while the patient is asleep. For assessment for murmurs of the heart, listen at the second intercostal space. Whereas an apical pulse is taken in infants and young children, with children 5 years of age and older, a radial pulse often is taken.

Respiration

Respirations are counted in the pediatric patient in the same manner as in the adult. Newborns are obligate nasal breathers, meaning they breathe only through their noses; they do not breathe through the mouth until they reach 3 or 4 weeks of age. The infant's respirations are primarily diaphragmatic; the abdominal movements should be observed when respirations are counted. In children younger than 7 years of age, respiratory movements are abdominal or diaphragmatic. In older children, respirations are chiefly thoracic. The respiratory rate also slows as a child progresses from infancy to adolescence.

A newborn's respiratory rate is extremely erratic, so for accuracy, count it for 1 full minute to notice any irregularities. Assess the rate, the depth, and the quality of respirations. The rate in the newborn sometimes is as rapid as 40 to 50 breaths per minute, gradually slowing to 25 to 32 per minute by 36 hours of age (see Table 31.3 for normal respiratory rate in children).

Blood Pressure

Blood pressure typically is not measured until a child reaches 3 years of age (Box 31.7). Children with symptoms of hypertension, and those in intensive care, at high risk, and in emergency departments, need to have their blood pressure measured.

Blood pressure is low in a newborn. Gradually it rises, so by the end of adolescence it is about 120/78 mm Hg (see Table 31.3).

To ensure accuracy with a blood pressure reading, use the correct cuff size. Be sure the cuff covers two-thirds of the length of the upper arm or leg (Box 31.8).

See sites for measuring children's blood pressure in Fig. 31.3.

The technique for measuring blood pressure in children is the same as that for an adult. Because children are upset easily by unfamiliar procedures, an explanation

Box 31.7 Calculation of Normal Blood Pressure

Use the following quick formula to calculate normal systolic blood pressure:

- *1 to 7 years:* Age in years + 90 mm Hg
- *8 to 18 years:* (2 × Age in years) + 83 mm Hg

Use the following quick formula to calculate normal diastolic blood pressure:

- 1 to 5 years: 56 mm Hg
- 6 to 8 years: Age in years + 52 mm Hg

of each step is helpful. For preschool and early school-age children, explain how the cuff will feel, such as "tight feeling," "arm hug," or "I want to feel your muscle." Use an explanation such as, "I want to see how strong your muscle is."

Box 31.8 Correct Blood Pressure Cuff Size

- In choosing cuffs, use an appropriately sized one.
- A cuff of proper size covers two-thirds of the length of the upper arm or leg.
- If a cuff of the correct size is not available, use an oversized cuff rather than an undersized one, or use another site that more appropriately fits the cuff size.
- Do not choose a cuff based on the name of the cuff (e.g., an "infant" cuff is too small for some infants).

Because results are best when the child is quiet and relaxed during the procedure, measure blood pressure before performing any anxiety-producing procedures. Infants and small children are often quieter if the blood pressure is taken while they are sitting on the parent's lap. Never place the blood pressure cuff on any limb with an intravenous site.

HEAD-TO-TOE ASSESSMENT

Skin

Genetic factors influence assessment of skin color, as do physiologic factors. Edema decreases intensity of skin color, sometimes producing false pallor. Pallor is a sign of potential anemia, chronic disease, edema, or shock. Compare pallor or cyanosis (bluish tone) against the color change normally produced by blanching, with use of the nonpigmented nail: press down on the free

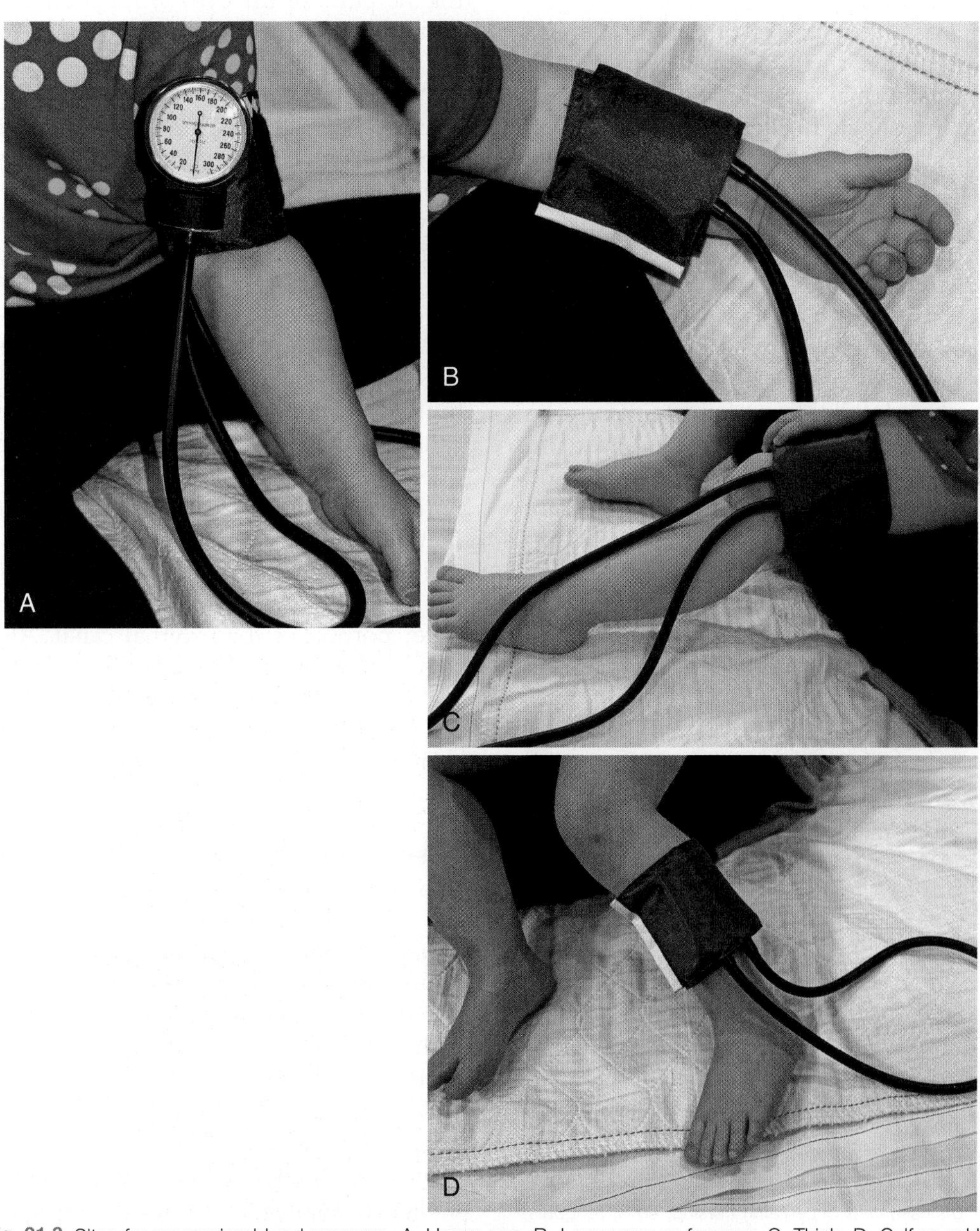

Fig. 31.3 Sites for measuring blood pressure. A, Upper arm. B, Lower arm or forearm. C, Thigh. D, Calf or ankle.

edge of the nail and observe return blood flow. Apply pressure to the lips or gums of dark-skinned individuals to observe color change. A yellow tint may indicate jaundice.

Erythema usually is the result of increased temperature, local inflammation, or infection. Normal skin texture in the young child is smooth, soft, and slightly dry to the touch.

Accessory Structures

Scalp hair is usually lustrous, silky, and elastic. Genetic factors influence the appearance of hair. Tufts of hair anywhere along the spine, especially the sacrum, are significant because they sometimes mark the site of spina bifida occulta.

Healthy nails are pink, convex, smooth, and hard but flexible, not brittle. Dark-skinned individuals sometimes have more deeply pigmented nail beds. Variation in color, such as blueness, suggests cyanosis.

Each person has a distinct set of handprints and footprints. The palm normally shows three flexion creases. If grossly abnormal lines or folds are observed, a specialist may investigate further. Note that the skin and accessory structures change with the aging process of an individual.

Eyes

The eyes of a newborn undergo many changes before vision is comparable with that of an adult. The baby achieves clear vision only at very close range. At birth, visual acuity is normally around 20/400, which makes it important for the adult holding a baby to assume an **en face position** (position in which the adult's face and the infant's face are approximately 8 inches apart and on the same plane, as when the mother holds the infant up in front of her face or when she nurses the infant) (Fig. 31.4). Teach parents to hold the baby comfortably so that they can make eye contact and the newborn can gaze on the face of the holder. Although tears are absent immediately after birth, by the second week of life, tear glands begin to function. Newborns develop the ability to follow bright, colorful objects by the second or third week of life.

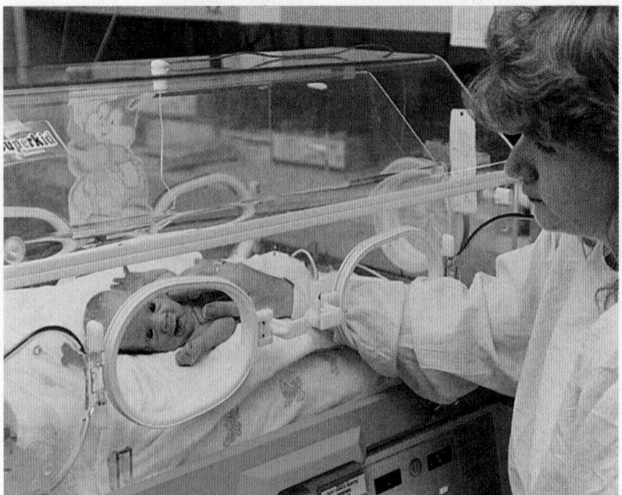

Fig. 31.4 Promoting bonding may require the mother overcome a physical barrier to achieve the en face position. (From Hockenberry MJ, Wilson D: *Wong's essentials of pediatric nursing*, ed 8, St. Louis, 2009, Mosby.)

Although visual acuity is typically 20/200 by the fourth or fifth month, depth perception does not develop before the ninth or tenth month. One-year-olds, who enjoy playing with large objects (blocks, toys, and boxes), often bump into obstacles because their vision is only about 20/100. Vision improves to 20/30 to 20/22 by age 2 to 3 years. When a child starts school, *accommodation* (changes in ciliary muscle and the lens in bringing light rays from various distances to focus on the retina) and *refraction* (the production by the normal eye of the proper image of the object on the retina) also are present. Almost 6 years of continual development are needed for the parts of the eyes to function as they do in an adult.

Ears

The tops of the ears, or pinnae, are generally on a horizontal line with outer canthus of eye. The pinna should be flexible with cartilage present. Low-set ears may be indicative of some congenital anomalies, and additional investigation may be necessary to determine the difference between signaling a significant anomaly or only as a familial trait (dad's ears). The ears should be inspected for general hygiene. If the ear canal appears free of *cerumen* (a waxy substance produced by the ceruminous gland in the outer portion of the canal), ask about ear-cleaning methods. It is best to question the parent and child about ear cleaning by remarking on how clean the ears are and asking how they remove wax. This approach is more likely to yield an honest answer. Advise parents and children to clean the ears with a washcloth and to gently wipe only the outer portion of the external canal. Also advise that they can soften any cerumen that is hard by instilling 2 or 3 drops of mineral oil into the ear for a few days and then rinsing the external canal with an ear syringe. Discourage the use of cotton swabs in the ear canal.

Nose, Mouth, and Throat

The nose normally lies from the center point between the eyes to the notch of the upper lip. No discharge usually is emitted from the nose. Inspect the lining of the mouth. Ask the child to open the mouth wide, to move the tongue in different directions, and to say "Ahh," which depresses the tongue for full view of the mouth.

Infants and toddlers, however, usually resist and do not open their mouth. Place the tongue blade along the side of the tongue, not the center where the gag reflex is elicited. Frequently, a protrusion of the tongue is seen in children with cognitive impairment.

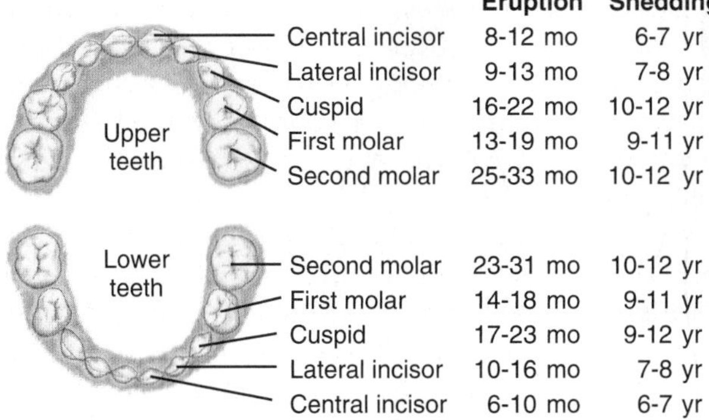

Eruption Shedding
Upper teeth
Central incisor 8-12 mo 6-7 yr
Lateral incisor 9-13 mo 7-8 yr
Cuspid 16-22 mo 10-12 yr
First molar 13-19 mo 9-11 yr
Second molar 25-33 mo 10-12 yr
Lower teeth
Second molar 23-31 mo 10-12 yr
First molar 14-18 mo 9-11 yr
Cuspid 17-23 mo 9-12 yr
Lateral incisor 10-16 mo 7-8 yr
Central incisor 6-10 mo 6-7 yr

Fig. 31.5 Sequence of eruption of primary teeth. (Modified from James SR, Nelson KA, Ashwill JW: *Nursing care of children: Principles and practice,* ed 4, St. Louis, 2013, Saunders.)

The number of teeth is also important to check. The **primary (deciduous) teeth** (the set of 20 teeth that normally appear during infancy) begin to descend between the sixth and ninth months of life. The central incisors are normally the first teeth to appear. By a child's third birthday, all 20 primary teeth are typically present. The exact mechanisms responsible for the eruption of teeth are not fully understood. The eruption of teeth is distressing to most babies, whose gums become erythematous and edematous. The fussiness demonstrated sometimes results in a refusal to eat. A cold teething ring and numbing (locally anesthetizing) agents provide some relief to painful gums. See Fig. 31.5 for the sequence of eruption of primary teeth.

Permanent teeth begin to appear at about 6 years, and most are present by 12 years.

Good dental hygiene should begin as soon as the primary teeth erupt. The first dental visit should be conducted by age 1 year. The promotion of dental health is important in the lives of children (American Academy of Pediatrics [AAP], n.d.). Dental caries are the leading chronic disease in children in the United States. Fluoride is a mineral that protects against tooth decay. Almost all water contains naturally occurring fluoride, but at levels that are not high enough to prevent tooth decay. Fluoride often is added to community drinking water and toothpaste to provide tooth protection benefits (Centers for Disease Control [CDC], 2016).

Lungs

Guidelines for effective auscultation of lung sounds in children are seen in Box 31.9 and Fig. 31.6.

Chest

During infancy, the chest appears circular. As the child grows, the chest size normally increases symmetrically. Asymmetry in the chest indicates the possibility of serious underlying problems such as cardiac enlargement (bulging on left side of ribcage) or pulmonary dysfunction. In an older child, a barrel-shaped chest sometimes indicates chronic obstructive pulmonary disease such as cystic fibrosis or asthma.

Box 31.9 Guidelines for Effective Auscultation of Lungs

- Be sure the child is relaxed and not crying, talking, or laughing. Record if the child is crying.
- Check that the room is comfortable and quiet.
- Warm the stethoscope before placing it against the skin.
- Apply firm pressure on the chest piece but not enough to prevent vibrations and transmission of sound.
- Avoid placing the stethoscope over hair or clothing, moving it against the skin, breathing on the tubing, or sliding fingers over the chest piece, all of which often cause sounds that falsely resemble pathologic findings.
- Use a symmetric and orderly approach to compare sounds.
- Ask the child to "blow out" the light on an otoscope or pocket flashlight; discreetly turn off the light on the last try so that the child feels successful (see Fig. 31.6).
- Place a cotton ball in the child's palm; ask the child to blow the ball into the air, and have the parent catch it.
- Place a small tissue on the top of a pencil and ask the child to blow off the tissue.
- Have child blow a pinwheel, a party horn, or bubbles.

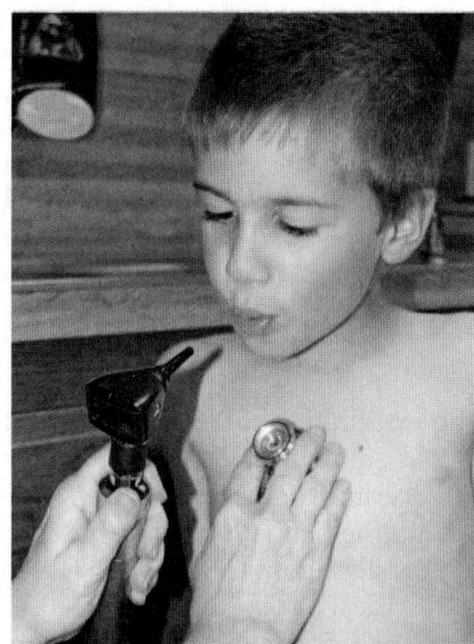

Fig. 31.6 Auscultation of lungs while child "blows out" otoscope light.

Back

The back of a newborn is C-shaped (Fig. 31.7A). As growth occurs, the typical S-shaped curve is seen in the older child and the adult. Marked curvature in posture is abnormal. Symmetry of the spine in the adolescent may be a sign of *scoliosis* (lateral curvature of the spine) (Fig. 31.7C). Scoliosis is an important childhood problem that is more common in females.

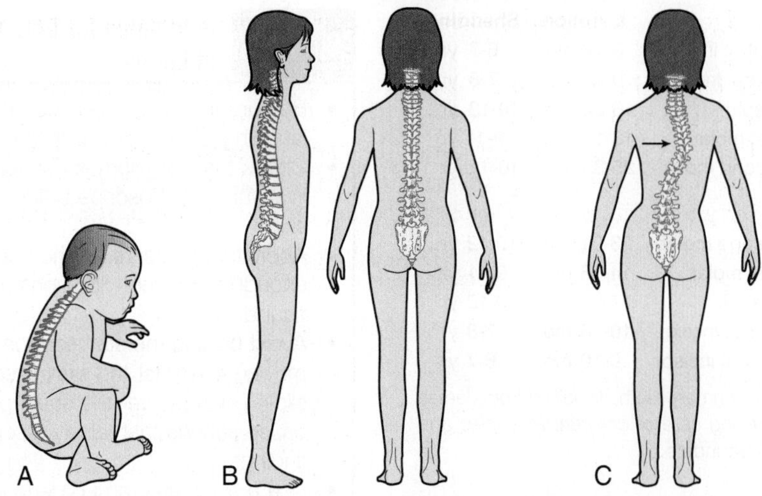

Fig. 31.7 A, Newborn showing normal "C" spinal curvature. B, Normal spine. C, Scoliosis.

Abdomen

Examination of the abdomen involves the following:

- *Inspection:* Done while the child is erect and supine. Normally in infants and young children, the abdomen appears slightly rounded. In the supine position, the abdomen appears flat.
- *Auscultation:* Heart or the lung sounds can be heard with a stethoscope placed gently on the skin, but the diaphragm of the stethoscope must be pressed firmly against the abdominal surface to hear bowel sounds.

The most important sound to listen for is peristalsis, which you may possibly hear every 10 to 30 seconds. Normal peristalsis sounds like metallic clicks and gurgles. Report the absence of bowel sounds or hyperperistalsis, because either usually denotes an abdominal disorder. The abdomen should be auscultated among all four quadrants for a full 3 minutes before absent bowel sounds are reported.

Extremities

Examine the extremities at birth for symmetry, range of motion, and signs of malformation. Count fingers and toes to be certain of normal numbers. As a toddler begins to walk, the legs are usually bowlegged until lower body and leg muscles develop. The infant and the toddler also must be observed for arch development and correct gait. By school age, the walking posture is more graceful and balanced. During puberty, adolescents sometimes experience awkward posture that results from rapid growth of extremities.

Renal Function

All structural components are present in the renal system of a newborn, but functional deficiency is found in the kidneys' abilities to concentrate urine and to cope with conditions of fluid and electrolyte fluctuation, such as dehydration or fluid overload. Infants are more prone to fluid volume fluctuations, because glomerular filtration and absorption are low as a result of the immature kidney function. The kidneys in children are not protected by padding and become susceptible to injury.

Urine output varies and depends on the size of the infant or child. Table 31.4 identifies average volumes excreted at given ages. The urine is colorless and odorless and has a specific gravity of approximately 1.020.

Table 31.4 Kidney Function and Urine Output

AGE	VOLUME OF URINE OUTPUT
Preterm newborn	1–3 mL/kg/h
Full-term newborn	3–4 mL/kg/h
6 mo	12 mL/h
1 yr	22 mL/h
5 yr	28 mL/h
12 yr	33–35 mL/h

Anus

Assess history of bowel movements for diarrhea, constipation, or rectal bleeding. Different stooling patterns are noted by feeding method and age. The stool of a baby who is breast-fed exclusively is typically light mustard color, grainy in texture, and runny in consistency. The stool of a formula-fed baby is usually tan, yellow, or light brown in color and firmer than that of the breast-fed baby. The presence of lesions or skin irritations near the anus necessitates further investigation. Reports of itching may signal parasitic infections.

Genitalia

Genitalia examination is usually uneventful for infants. It can be anxiety producing for toddlers, older preschoolers, school-age children, and adolescents.

The genital examination is an excellent time for eliciting questions concerning body functions or sexual activity. It provides an opportunity to increase or reinforce the child's knowledge of reproductive anatomy and explain its function.

During the male genital examination, assess the external appearance of the glans and the shaft of the penis, the prepuce, the urethral meatus, and the scrotum. Edema, skin lesions, inflammation, or other irregularities are possible signs of underlying disorders, especially sexually transmitted infections (STIs). The examination of the female genitalia usually is limited to the inspection and palpation of external structures.

FACTORS THAT INFLUENCE GROWTH AND DEVELOPMENT

NUTRITION

A holistic look at the child requires an assessment of current family nutrition. Nutrition is probably the single most important influence on growth. During infancy and childhood, the demand for calories is great because of rapid increase in height and weight. Growth is uneven during infancy and adolescence. A child's appetite fluctuates in response to growth spurts. Good nutrition begins before conception and is related closely to good health throughout life.

Infants begin life outside the womb nursing at the breast or ingesting formula or breast milk by bottle or tube. Human milk is the most desirable complete diet for the infant for the first 6 months of life. The American Academy of Pediatrics recommends breast-feeding exclusively until the infant reaches 6 months of age. Exclusive breast-feeding means that the infant receives only breast milk and no additional foods (except vitamin D) or fluids unless recommended by the primary health care provider (NICHD, n.d.). Whole cow's milk should be advised against until the child passes the 12-month mark because cow's milk contains high amounts of protein and minerals, which can stress an infant's immature kidneys. Skim or low-fat milk is not recommended because the essential fatty acids are inadequate and the solute concentration of protein and electrolytes, such as sodium, is too high. An allergy to protein in milk can cause the infant to be fussy and irritable.

Most infants are given solid foods at 4 to 6 months of age when they begin to need more iron in the diet and their teeth begin to erupt. Iron-fortified cereal is the first solid food most parents give to a baby. Rice cereal is digested easily and has low allergenic potential, so it is a common choice. However, oatmeal and barley are high-protein cereals and also make good options. After several months of breast milk or formula, the addition of solid foods to an infant's diet is a significant developmental step.

Although the order of introduction of foods other than cereal is arbitrary, the usual sequence is strained fruits, fruit juices, strained vegetables, and strained meats. As more teeth erupt, suggest offering finger food, such as zwieback (teething biscuit). This helps infants develop a hand-to-mouth cycle, which is basic to feeding themselves.

Each new food must be introduced at weekly intervals to allow recognition of any food allergies (an allergic response sometimes takes several days to appear). Development of a rash, wheezing, or diarrhea is a common sign that indicates the presence of an allergy to a food.

By 9 months, several teeth have erupted, and junior foods can be offered, which are of much coarser texture. These fruits, vegetables, and meats taste different, and their different texture encourages the infant to chew. Good choices of finger foods to give at this time include small pieces of fruit (excluding grapes, which could choke the infant) and cooked vegetables.

The cost of baby foods is significant; therefore, as the infant acquires more teeth and does not experience difficulty eating solids, encourage parents to prepare these foods at home. Canned foods, other than those prepared for infants, often contain excessive sodium or sugar. If sweetening is needed, refined sugar is acceptable to use, but advise against using honey and corn syrup because of the risk of infant botulism. Encourage cooking fresh or frozen foods and using a blender or food processor. By 12 to 15 months, toddlers usually are eating table food prepared for the family. Although use of a spoon is messy, typical toddlers become angry and frustrated when they are "ready" to feed themselves and parents continue to feed them.

Weaning (gradually eliminating breast-feeding or bottle feeding and instituting cup and table feedings) is a major accomplishment of toddlerhood. The earlier method of feeding has provided the child with a great deal of pleasure and satisfaction, and giving it up is sometimes difficult for child and parent. Breast-feeding should be continued until 12 months of age. After 12 months, the American Academy of Pediatrics states that the discontinuation of breast-feeding is a personal choice. The American Academy of Pediatrics (2010) recommends weaning bottle-fed infants by 15 months of age. Solid foods also are pleasing to the taste buds, but when toddlers feed themselves with a spoon, they may turn it upside down as they navigate the utensil toward their mouth, and they lose much of the food. The same occurs with a cup. A plastic cup with a spout decreases the amount of milk or juice that is spilled. Most 9-month-old or 10-month-old infants who can sit in a high chair begin to demonstrate a readiness to wean. They become much more active and squirm when they are held for feedings. In addition, they observe siblings and adults drinking from cups or glasses and desire to do the same. Gradually, parents replace bottle feedings or breast-feeding with the cup. Usually the bedtime feeding is the last one parents discontinue. A parent should never allow a child to take a bottle of milk or any sweetened liquids to bed and should never prop a bottle, because this is a major cause of dental caries in deciduous teeth.

If the child needs a bottle at bedtime, the parent should give water.

Ideally, concentrated sugars and high-carbohydrate snacks are absent from the young child's diet. The form of sugar in foods is important. Cariogenic (promoting or producing tooth decay) foods are those that are sticky and hard and remain in the mouth longer (e.g., lollipops). Help parents plan meals and snacks that include foods less damaging to teeth.

As children move through toddler and preschool stages, they often develop fads with strong preferences. Teach the school-age child and the parent the value of a diet balanced to promote growth. Adolescent problems include dietary imbalance and excesses. Excess intake of calories, sugar, fat, cholesterol, and sodium are common. Inadequate intake of certain vitamins is evident among teens. These dietary patterns can contribute to an increased risk of such chronic illnesses as heart disease and osteoporosis and some types of cancer later in life. The American Academy of Pediatrics recommends cholesterol testing for children whose parents or grandparents have total cholesterol levels of 240 mg/dL or higher and for children whose parents or grandparents have had heart attacks or have been diagnosed with blocked arteries at age 55 or earlier in men or age 65 or earlier in women. For children in these categories, the first cholesterol test should be after 2 years of age but no later than 10 years of age (Cleveland Clinic, 2016).

Each year, approximately 24.2 per 1000 women between the ages of 15 and 19 give birth (DHHS, 2016). The pregnant teen exhibits food preferences, eating behaviors, and lifestyle habits similar to nonpregnant peers. Frequent snacking on foods high in fat and sugar and low in essential nutrients (calcium, iron, zinc, folate, and vitamins B_6, A, and C) causes special concerns during pregnancy. Nurses play a central role in meeting the needs of pregnant teenagers. The nurse is frequently the one the young girl turns to for help and guidance in her dilemma and the one she relies on for support and reassurance. The nutritional assessment should focus on the dietary adequacy of iron, calcium, and multivitamins with folic acid.

METABOLISM

Metabolic needs vary among individuals. The rate of metabolism is highest in the newborn infant because the ratio of total body surface area to body weight is much greater in the infant than it is in the adult. This proportion decreases as the child grows and matures. The basal metabolic rate (BMR) is a measure of metabolism when the body is at rest; it changes dramatically as the body increases in size. Newborns double their birth weight by 5 to 6 months and triple it by about 1 year of age, which demonstrates the rapid rate at which metabolism occurs in very young children.

The body uses energy provided by foods. Whereas the energy requirements for an infant are highest during the first 6 months of life, they are fairly constant from 4 to 10 years and vary in adolescence, depending on the teen's physical development (Table 31.5).

Table 31.5 Daily Caloric Needs of Infants, Children, and Adolescents

AGE GROUP	CALORIC NEEDS
Infants	
Birth to 6 mo	108 kcal/kg
6–12 mo	94.4 kcal/kg
Children	
1–3 yr	100 kcal/kg
4–6 yr	90 kcal/kg
7–10 yr	71.4 kcal/kg
Adolescents	
Males	
11–14 yr	55.6 kcal/kg
15–18 yr	45.5 kcal/kg
Females	
11–14 yr	47.8 kcal/kg
15–18 yr	40 kcal/kg

Modified from *https://www.merckmanuals.com/professional/nutritional-disorders/nutrition-general-considerations/overview-of-nutrition#v881783*, 2016.

Because metabolism is so high in infants and children, their ability to recover from surgery or a fractured bone is swift compared with that of an adult. With the accelerated rate of all bodily functions, healing occurs quickly, provided all necessary nutritional components are in place. For example, a fractured femur at birth is united in 3 weeks, but an 8-year-old with the same type of fracture needs 8 weeks for union, and a 20-year-old takes 20 weeks to heal.

SLEEP AND REST

Children spend less total time sleeping as they mature. The newborn sleeps much of the time not occupied with feeding and other aspects of care. Most babies sleep through the night by the latter part of their first year and take one or two naps a day. Most 12- to 18-month-olds usually nap once a day. The 3-year-old child usually has given up all daytime naps.

The best way to prevent sleep problems with the infant and child is to establish bedtime rituals that do not foster problematic patterns. One of the most constructive ways is to place infants awake in their own crib or bed. Advise using the bed for sleeping only, not as a playpen.

SPEECH AND COMMUNICATION

Crying at birth is the earliest evidence of speech, wordless though it is. Infants use this method of communication when they are hungry or in pain or need to be changed. Crying is followed gradually by other sounds, such as cooing, laughing, or babbling. By 9 months, infants practice the noises they can make and painstakingly repeat them. Infants enjoy the sounds of their own voice. While they begin to express themselves, they also begin to imitate the vocal sounds of an adult. It is possible to have an actual conversation with the infant. Although no formal words are exchanged, it is a pleasant experience. The adult speaks, the infant responds, the adult answers, and so on. As the infant begins to enjoy experimenting with these sounds, encouragement of these vocalizations is important; it is positive reinforcement for oral communication.

A 1-year-old has a three-word or four-word vocabulary. It usually includes *mama* and *dada*. In toddlerhood, more words are understood than expressed. Children usually know 25 to 50 words by 18 months, but by 2 years, they often know more than 250 words. Speech develops rapidly at this stage, as children practice and learn new words and their meanings. Soon they are able to say a two-word or three-word sentence. Preschoolers have a fairly extensive vocabulary to convey their wants, needs, and desires.

Speech ability is determined by the child's stage of development, the amount of stimulation or encouragement received from adults, the child's health status, and many other factors. In addition, the development of language does not occur in isolation; it is related to the physiologic, neurologic, and psychosocial progress that is occurring simultaneously. Children learn the complex symbol system of language with astonishing speed.

It is important to know what typifies speech at each stage of childhood for identification of problems. For example, the lack of babbling or the inability of a 9-month-old to imitate sounds is a possible indication of deafness or hearing impairment. All babies make verbal sounds until 6 or 7 months of age, but then the child who is unable to hear decreases these verbalizations in favor of gesturing or some expression of body language (or nonverbal communication).

Verbal communication is used in a variety of ways in nursing practice. Talking softly to infants while cuddling them is an important part of establishing trust in a relationship with babies. Although the toddler is leery of strangers, if the nurse talks with a parent first, the 2-year-old senses the trusting attitude of the adult and begins to participate in the conversation. As a result of improving verbal skills, preschoolers and school-age children understand more and share their concerns more easily. Teaching 8- to 10-year-olds is particularly satisfying because they are eager to learn. On the other hand, adolescents who have refined their verbal abilities communicate a significant amount of information nonverbally through body language, gestures, and facial expressions. General strategies to consider when talking with children include the following:

- Use a calm, unhurried, and confident voice.
- Speak clearly, be specific, and use as few words as possible. As a general guide, use sentences whose sum of words is equal to the child's age in years plus one.
- State directions and suggestions in a positive way; for example, say, "You need to stay very still," rather than, "Don't move."
- Because children see things only in relation to themselves and from their viewpoint, focus communication on them.
- After greeting the child, continue to talk to the child and the parent while pursuing activities that do not involve the child directly.
- Use play as a strategy for getting to know the child. For example, if the child has a doll or a stuffed animal, begin by speaking to the toy. Then, initiate conversation with the child by asking simple questions about the toy.
- Listen to and observe the child at play. Often children express important information, such as complicated or difficult feelings, through this familiar medium.
- Look for opportunities to offer the child choices, but offer them only when they really exist. (Children are confused by choices being offered when there actually are none.) For example, when a child needs to change into a gown, a statement such as, "I need your dress off so that I can listen to your chest. Shall I help you take it off?" gives the child an explanation, a choice, and some control.
- Be honest with children. However, be careful about creating overly scary impressions. Instead of saying, "This will hurt" before a procedure, it is better to prepare the child with a statement such as, "Children tell me different things about how this feels. Some say it feels like a cat or dog scratching. Afterward, will you tell me what it felt like for you?"
- Use direct and concrete communication with young children because they are unable to work with abstractions or to separate fact from fantasy. For example, they attach literal meanings to such common phrases as "a frog in the throat" or "hold your horses."
- Avoid use of a phrase that is open to a young child's misinterpretation. For example, the statement, "Let's see how warm your body is," is preferred to "Let's take your temperature," because young children may wonder what you are going to do with their temperature once you have it and whether you are planning to give it back. Words such as "shot" are frightening if a child envisions a shot from a gun. Instead substitute "putting some medicine under the skin."
- Children between 5 and 8 years want concrete explanations and reasons for everything because they rely more on what they know than what they see when faced with new problems. Continue to use relatively simple explanations, remembering that their expanding vocabulary facilitates communication.

One of the most important points to remember is to speak with a child according to the child's stage of development. A conversation with a 2-year-old differs greatly from a conversation with a 12-year-old. To be successful in establishing relationships with children and to be effective in teaching or sharing information, be sure to communicate with them at the appropriate level.

Nonverbal Communication

Young children become very adept at understanding nonverbal communication. They sense anxiety or fear by the rise in pitch of the parent's voice. Nodding of the head, using direct eye contact, tapping finger or foot, avoiding eye contact, and using sign language are nonverbal symbols. Sometimes nonverbal behaviors are necessary to receive confirmation from the children in return. Children are very sensitive to nonverbal cues.

CHILD MALTREATMENT

The maltreatment of children is a complicated and prevalent problem in today's society. The problem of maltreatment is not confined to one specific race, religion, or socioeconomic level. Although certain groups have higher reported rates of abuse, this problem occurs in every level of society. *Child maltreatment* is a broad term used to describe physical and emotional neglect and physical, emotional, and sexual abuse of children. In recent years, the number of reported cases of child maltreatment has increased dramatically. The 2015 statistics from the US Department of Health and Human Services' (DHHS) Children's Bureau showed that nearly 683,000 children were abused or neglected. The leading age of the victims was from birth to age 1 year. The statistical difference in the rate of abuse in boys and girls is limited. Unfortunately, many cases of child maltreatment are insidious and go undetected and unreported.

CHILD NEGLECT

Neglect can be divided into two broad categories: physical neglect and emotional neglect. *Physical neglect* is the failure of a parent or caretaker to supply a child with adequate food, clothing, shelter, education, or health care despite being financially able to do so or offered financial or other means to do so. *Emotional neglect,* in contrast, is the failure by a parent or caretaker to meet a child's needs for emotional nurturance, affection, and attention.

CHILD ABUSE

Child abuse can be divided into three broad categories: physical, emotional, and sexual. *Physical abuse* is the intentional infliction of physical injury on a child, usually by the child's caregiver. *Emotional abuse* is the intentional attempt by a parent or caretaker to impair or destroy the mental or emotional state of a child. *Sexual abuse* is defined as commission of a sexual offense by a person responsible for the child's care, such as a parent, relative, acquaintance of the family, or babysitter, against a child who is dependent or developmentally immature, for the purpose of the perpetrator's own sexual stimulation or gratification.

Statistics show that in 2015, 75.3% of abused children were victims of neglect, and another 25.6% were victims of physical, sexual, or emotional forms of abuse (DHHS, 2015).

Etiology

Many factors contribute to the cause of child maltreatment, including parental, child, and situational factors. Parental factors include the parent's culture (see the Cultural Considerations box); socialization history and history of abuse as a child; the parent's age and developmental level; attitudes toward the child and child rearing; knowledge of normal child behavior and development; and the parent's psychological state. Characteristics of the child sometimes place the child at risk for maltreatment. Many factors—including temperament, age, exceptional physical needs, disabilities, and health or behavior problems—have the potential to increase the potential for maltreatment by a parent or caretaker. Situational factors include sources of stress and support within the family's environment. Other factors sometimes present include marital problems, financial difficulties, drug or alcohol abuse, lack of social support or the inability of the parent or caretaker to ask for support, poor social network, and poor relationships with extended families. These factors have the power to increase the potential for an abusive reaction by adding stress to an environment in which a parent or caretaker is already lacking resources.

 Cultural Considerations

Child Abuse

Uninformed health professionals run the risk of mistaking many cultural practices for evidence of child abuse. An understanding of these practices is important, yet the family should be informed that the practices are possibly harmful and may place them in jeopardy with child protective services. Examples of such practices include coining (repeatedly rubbing the edge of a coin on a child's skin, producing welts, to rid the body of a disease; practiced primarily by the Vietnamese) and moxibustion (a Southeast Asian practice of burning small areas of the skin to treat temper tantrums and enuresis).

Clinical Manifestations

Children who have been abused or neglected often manifest certain physical or behavioral indicators that suggest maltreatment. Table 31.6 summarizes these manifestations.

Nursing Interventions

The most important role for any health care provider, especially nurses, is the identification of a child who is being maltreated. Often the nurse is the first person to interact with the child and the parent. A thorough history

Table 31.6 Clinical Manifestations of Possible Child Maltreatment

BEHAVIORAL INDICATORS	PHYSICAL INDICATORS
Physical Neglect	
Begging or stealing food Extended stays at school Fatigue or listlessness at school Delinquency Alcohol or drug abuse	Failure to thrive (the abnormal retardation of growth and development of the infant resulting from conditions that interfere with normal metabolism, appetite, and activity) Lag in growth and development Consistent hunger Poor personal hygiene Inappropriate dress for season Unattended medical needs Abandonment
Physical Abuse	
Frequent injuries explained as accidents Conflicting stories about the "accident" or injury from the parents or others Wary of contacts with parents or other adults Apprehension when other children cry Fear of parents or going home Concealing clothing worn to hide injuries Low self-esteem Suicide attempts	Ecchymosis, welts, and bite marks Ecchymosis reflecting the shape of object used to inflict injury (electrical cord, belt buckle, iron, radiator, or a hand) Evidence of human bites Lacerations or abrasions Burns that are symmetric and have no "splash marks" Cigar or cigarette burns on soles, palms, back, or buttocks Fractures: • To skull, nose, or face • Multiple or spiral • Various stages of healing • Discovered during examination, not reported by caretaker
Sexual Abuse	
Nonspecific symptoms such as sleep disturbances or abdominal pain noted by provider Promiscuous behavior Unwillingness to change for gym Withdrawal, fantasy, or infantile behavior Age-inappropriate sexual knowledge Poor peer relationships Delinquency Prostitution Forcing of sexual acts on other children Fear of being touched Suicide attempts Low self-esteem Excessive or public masturbation Declining school performance	Difficulty in walking or sitting Torn, stained, or bloody underclothing Pain or pruritus in genital area Ecchymosis or bleeding in external genitalia, vaginal, or anal areas Ecchymosis to the hard or soft palate Sexually transmitted diseases in preteens Adolescent pregnancy Enuresis or encopresis Vaginal or penile discharge Foreign bodies in vagina or rectum Presence of semen Recurrent urinary tract infections
Emotional Neglect and Abuse	
Stranger anxiety Emotional withdrawal Inappropriate fearfulness Delinquency Lag in emotional and intellectual development Language difficulties Suicide attempts	Failure to thrive Feeding difficulties Enuresis or encopresis Sleep disturbances

and physical examination are the most effective diagnostic tools in recognizing a child who has been abused or neglected. A behavioral or physical indicator of maltreatment should be a cue to investigate further, because these indicators rarely appear as single factors. Carefully document any manifestations of abuse in the medical record, along with the caretaker's explanation for these findings. When documenting, use direct quotes, and report only objective findings. Pay special attention to injuries that are unexplained or inconsistent with the parent's or caretaker's explanation of how the injury was incurred.

If abuse is suspected, the child and the parent must be questioned separately. A child rarely betrays a parent and admits the abuse. Even the most battered of children remain loyal to the *perpetrators* (those guilty of committing the act). The use of drawings, play, diagrams, and anatomically correct dolls sometimes help a child to express what has happened.

All states have regulations for the mandatory reporting of child maltreatment when a health professional has reason to suspect that child abuse or neglect has occurred or is occurring. The professional does not need to be certain or prove that a child has been maltreated; it is enough for the reporter to distrust or doubt the caretaker's explanation of what has been observed in the child. Many states have a toll-free number where reports are taken by a state central registry and then referred to the social services office in the locality where the child resides. All health care providers are obliged to be alert to, assess, and report any abusive situations to proper authorities.

If the child needs hospitalization as a result of the abuse, a nonjudgmental attitude must be maintained toward the parents or caretakers. Establishing a rapport with the family promotes a trusting and open relationship between you and the parents. The hospitalization provides a unique opportunity to demonstrate positive caretaking activities and offer education through role modeling. Consistency in the caregivers assigned to the child is important. Explain all procedures and treatment to the child to prevent the child from misinterpreting invasive or painful events. If the child is to return to the parents' care, integrate their participation into the daily routine. In this situation, document interactions between the child and the parents in an objective and factual manner.

Prevention of child maltreatment is an area in which the nurse can play an active role. During the prenatal period, identify any families at risk for abuse and refer them for intervention. During the child's health care visits, identify families at risk when you observe behaviors indicating a lack of understanding of the child's care requirements or when the support systems available to the family in stress are assessed. Encourage parents to search for and make use of resources that provide supportive services. Reinforcement of positive caretaking behaviors is an effective way of affirming positive parenting practices.

HOSPITALIZATION OF A CHILD

Hospitalization is an anxiety-producing experience for children and their families, primarily because of a basic fear of not knowing what will occur. It creates an interruption in the child's normal development. Every member of the family is affected by the hospitalization because of the disruption it brings about in routines. Hospitalization is often the first crisis children face. How a child deals with this crisis is influenced by developmental age, previous illness experience, separation coping skills, seriousness of the illness, and support of parents and staff. An experience sometimes can be made less traumatic with *anticipatory guidance,* explanations and preparation to help relieve fear and anxiety. However, infants and toddlers are not able to understand; therefore separation is especially painful for them. Preparation for a scheduled admission is possible; however, emergencies arise, and unplanned hospitalizations occur. In those instances, always give explanations whenever possible and as soon as feasible to avoid aggravating an already traumatic situation.

Adequate preparation makes the transition from the security of a home to the unfamiliar atmosphere of a hospital less difficult. When it is best to begin preparation and how much information is right to give varies. The age of the child has a significant influence. A physician provides a family with details about a treatment plan, the length of stay, and expected results or outcomes. Parents then can reinforce the information by providing explanations to the child, using simple, age-appropriate terms. Usually time and opportunity are available before the actual admission for the child to talk about what will occur.

PREADMISSION PROGRAMS

Many hospitals have orientation programs for children who are to be admitted. In some hospitals, nurses conduct preadmission programs; other hospitals use *child life specialists* (health care professionals with extensive knowledge of child growth and development and the special emotional needs of children who are hospitalized).

The programs are based on the child's level of understanding and stage of development, with the purpose of familiarizing the child with hospital surroundings. These programs help to dismiss the child's fantasies and correct misconceptions. The programs include tours and audiovisual aids, such as movies, videos, and puppet shows. The child is given simple explanations of equipment used during surgery and hospitalization.

It is helpful for children to handle some of the items they will see while hospitalized, such as masks and gowns, stethoscopes, anesthesia masks, and syringes (without the needles attached). Be sure time is allowed for questions. Encourage children to talk about what they have seen or heard so that you can identify problem areas or areas of concern. Some hospitals distribute coloring books or storybooks that focus on the information covered in the orientation program. This material reinforces information and helps parents answer their child's questions. Many programs send the parents away with a brochure that describes hospital routines and lists items the hospital permits children to bring with them to the hospital. Keep written information simple, clear, and at an understandable level.

Timing of the orientation is important. Enough advance time must be allowed for the child to be able to assimilate the information after the program, but not

 Communication

Developmental Considerations: Communicating Effectively With Young Children

INFANTS

- Consider your body language, such as gestures and posture, and the pitch, intonation, and intensity of your voice.
- Nonverbal approaches work especially well for infants, with cuddling, patting, or some other form of gentle physical contact often quieting them.
- Maintain a calm voice and avoid sudden, loud noises. The actual words spoken are not as important as the way they are spoken.
- Because infants often begin fearing strangers at ages as young as 6 months, holding out the hands and asking the older infant to "come over" is seldom successful. If handling is necessary, the best approach is to pick up the infant firmly without using gestures.
- Infants are usually more at ease when upright and in visual contact with and proximity to their parents.

PRESCHOOL AND YOUNG SCHOOL-AGE CHILDREN

- Avoid quick approaches with preschool and young school-age children. Let them make the first move whenever possible.
- Broad smiles and other facial contortions sometimes have a threatening appearance.
- Avoid extended eye contact until after the child is comfortable.
- Position yourself at the child's eye level. You appear less threatening to the child, and you deemphasize the child's smallness.
- Children are often more responsive when they remain close to the parent, such as when they sit on the parent's lap.
- New or intimidating situations, such as hospitalization, are potentially stressful; thus children have even more difficulty grasping the new words they encounter in this environment, even simple words that express unfamiliar ideas. Avoid use of expressions with dual meanings, such as "put to sleep."
- Substitute words that have potentially threatening interpretations with words that are less emotionally charged, such as replacing "stick" with "gently slide," or "hurt" with "feel uncomfortable."

OLDER SCHOOL-AGE CHILDREN

- Give children an opportunity to express their thoughts, concerns, and feelings. Listen and respond to underlying messages rather than just verbal content. Be attentive, try not to interrupt, and avoid making comments that convey disapproval or surprise.
- Avoid prying, asking embarrassing questions, and lecturing when giving advice.

ADOLESCENTS

- Be prepared to deal with a wide range of emotions and behaviors with adolescents. Give concrete explanations that focus on the teenager's concerns, even though the adolescent's capacity to think in abstract terms increases with age.
- Fluency in teen jargon is not necessary, but ask for clarification when necessary.
- To enhance communication, exchange information without using questions that back the teenager into a corner. Initially confine discussions to less-threatening topics to allow time for trust to develop.
- Ask broad, open-ended questions before specific questions, such as "How's school?" before asking, "What is the best (or worst) thing about school?"

so much time that the child forgets the information. Generally, the younger the child, the shorter the period between when the child is told about pending hospitalization and the actual admission date. Usually, a toddler is told only days before. However, school-age children have a better understanding of time and the future; therefore they can be told that they are going to the hospital "in 2 weeks." Tell adolescents as far in advance as possible to allow them time to inform peers and solicit their support.

Children must be allowed to prepare for this new experience in their own way. This preparation involves telling friends and selecting pictures of family members, toys, or clothes they wish to take, if they are permitted. Packing a bag with these items reinforces the event's reality.

Parents also benefit from such orientation programs. They receive information that is helpful in answering a child's questions at home. Printed materials provide parents a reference guide for reviewing what the child has been told.

Emergency Admission

An emergency admission, in contrast to a well-planned and well-prepared-for admission, thrusts the child into an unknown environment with strange equipment, frightening sounds, and many unfamiliar adults. The incident that results in the hospitalization usually is sudden, serious, and possibly painful. The speed with which a health team responds to the emergency is critical, and little time is available for explanations. Whenever possible, explain to the child and family what is happening. This can prevent an escalating crisis situation. When the child is stable and awake, assess the child's perception of what happened, correct any misconceptions, and provide information not given initially.

ADMISSION

Confidentiality is important while interviewing the hospitalized pediatric patient and is particularly important with adolescents when they have concerns related to issues such as substance use or sexual behaviors.

Adolescents are more likely to participate in health care services when caring, respectful professionals are the ones providing them. Characteristics of good providers include compassion, warmth, understanding, an ability to communicate with the adolescent, a willingness to be straightforward and honest, and competency.

Pediatric units are usually bright, colorful, and cheery areas with cartoon figures on the walls (or ceilings of treatment rooms), many pictures, and large photographs of sports figures and popular singers. Often the unit or room is decorated to reflect the age group admitted there. For example, an infant and toddler unit usually has many age-appropriate toys, high chairs, playpens, and strollers. A typical adolescent area has a lounge with a television, video games, DVD player, CD player, and computers with age-appropriate software and Internet access. To decrease anxiety, most hospitals try to make the pediatric environment different from adult units and include many items that are found in the child's normal home or school environment.

First impressions are important and have the potential to color the child's entire hospital stay. Therefore be sure to greet children warmly and welcome them by name when they arrive on the unit. After they see their room and meet their roommate(s), give them a tour of the unit. Two important locations to point out are the area in which snacks or liquid refreshments are available and the playroom (or activity room when speaking to adolescents), where they will spend time when allowed out of bed. The play area is a safe, secure place for children. It contains an assortment of toys, games, and crafts for diversional activities. Newly admitted children also need explanations about when meals are served, how to operate the bed, and how to communicate with nurses by using a call bell or intercommunication system.

Sometimes anxiety levels about a hospital admission are high. Perhaps heart surgery is scheduled or a brain tumor is suspected. In those instances, a tour or an in-depth orientation may be postponed. The development of a therapeutic relationship with the family very possibly seems more important, because it has the potential to affect the entire course of a hospitalization. Inform parents that a tour and further orientation are available and that the timing of such events is the parent's choice.

After the child is admitted, obtain a nursing history. An identification bracelet, usually worn on the wrist, is important to verify identity when medications are given or procedures are done. Often these bands are placed on the ankles of infants and toddlers because they are curious about items on their wrists. When applying the band, allow enough space for one finger to fit between the band and the skin. Be sure the band is not constrictive, and check the skin underneath for its integrity.

Assess vital signs, including blood pressure. Measure and record the height (or length for infants) and weight. These are important baseline data. The height and weight are used in calculating a child's body surface area, especially when treating a child with burns or in calculating fluid and electrolyte requirements. Most medical centers use body weight in kilograms to compute drug dosages. An important nursing responsibility is identifying the scale used to weigh a child, if more than one is available, so that all staff use the same scale for subsequent weighings.

A laboratory technician draws routine blood samples on all newly admitted infants and children. Some hospitals make efforts to reduce the number of "sticks" a child receives by coordinating various physician requests whenever possible. A urine specimen also typically is collected. The laboratory values provide a physician with baseline information and are sometimes diagnostic. The physician orders additional x-ray examinations or procedures as appropriate to the child's specific health problem.

HOSPITAL POLICIES

Changes in hospitals' policies over recent years reflect their changed attitude toward parents. Most hospitals no longer consider parents "visitors" and welcome their presence throughout the child's hospitalization. Many hospitals have developed a system of family-centered care. This philosophy of care validates the integral role of the family in a child's life and acknowledges the family as an essential part of the child's care and illness experience. In this kind of system, the family becomes a partner in the care of the child.

Hospitalization is especially traumatic to very young children, and the presence of supportive parents increases their feelings of security. The typical fear and apprehension children experience when they are isolated from their parents and family is known as *separation anxiety* and causes major stress for the hospitalized child, especially between ages 15 to 30 months. Many hospitals have facilities that allow one parent to live in or room in, which means a parent can stay 24 hours a day. Make parents aware that beds, meals, and shower facilities are available for their use. Allowing parents or other family members to stay with the pediatric patient alleviates stress and is therapeutic for the patient.

Parents who are involved in care have a sense of contributing to the child's recovery, which is an important consideration. The presence of a parent increases the available teaching opportunities. It also enables the nurse to assess a family's strengths, needs, and potential problem areas. However, parents need time to relax and to get away from the child's bedside periodically. Rooming-in is sometimes an exhausting experience. Parents need breaks and relief to remain effective in supporting the child. Hospitals with a family-centered philosophy set aside a room or other specified area on the nursing unit for parents where they have the chance to socialize, support each other, and share their thoughts. Note that the presence of parents does not mean that nurses give up their responsibilities in caring for these children.

Some hospitals allow children to wear their own clothes, which is especially important for a hospitalized adolescent. However, if a child is scheduled for surgery or needs an IV line, hospital gowns usually are required.

DEVELOPMENTAL SUPPORT FOR THE CHILD

Hospitalization not only interrupts children's normal routines but also threatens their normal developmental process. Children often regress when hospitalized. For instance, some young school-age children resume the practice of thumb sucking. Often regression persists for several months after a child is discharged.

Some of the traumatic effects of hospitalization on a child's normal development can be alleviated or even eliminated in several ways. A child's developmental level influences his or her understanding and response to hospitalization. Strategies for supporting children are likely to be more effective when developmental concerns and needs are considered (Table 31.7).

Take particular care to meet the psychosocial needs of children with special needs who are hospitalized. Because of the nature of their conditions, these children are even more likely to experience invasive and traumatic procedures during frequent and lengthy hospital stays. These factors result in a group of children more vulnerable to the emotional and developmental consequences of hospitalization.

PAIN MANAGEMENT

Health care professionals, including nurses, tend to underestimate pain in children. Some people falsely believe that infants or young children are not able to feel pain. Another explanation for this tendency is a misconception of what playing or reading or any other activity means about a child's comfort level. Anything that is painful to adults should be assumed to be painful to infants and children. Children, like adults, engage in activities for distraction, as a method of coping with pain. These behaviors do not signal the absence of pain.

Pain is known commonly as the fifth vital sign, and it must be documented during each shift assessment. A critical component in management of pain is its assessment. However, pain assessment, especially for children who have limited cognitive and language skills,

Table 31.7 Age-Related Concerns and Needs of Children Who Are Hospitalized

CONCERNS	POSSIBLE RESPONSES	POSITIVE PARENT AND NURSE RESPONSES
Infancy		
Anxiety is common during this age because of separation from the parent(s).	Bonding is often an issue as well as distrust; skills may be delayed because of anxiety experienced by the infant.	Encourage rooming in of parent(s); teach parents procedures they are capable of being taught to perform; assign the same nurse when possible to maintain consistency.
Toddler/Preschool		
Separation from parents is a major issue because of stranger fear and separation anxiety. The toddler fears bodily injury and pain.	It is common for the hospitalized toddler to be uncooperative, throw temper tantrums, and show regression in behavior.	Praise for appropriate behavior (e.g., dressing or feeding self); set appropriate limits on negative behavior and encourage parents to do so; encourage home routines and rituals, such as bedtime stories.
School-Age		
The school-age child is concerned with bodily injury related to medical procedures. In addition to anxiety resulting from separation from parents, the school-age child also is anxious from separation from friends and school, and other family members.	The school-age child may show some level of regression. In addition, anger, acts of aggression, boredom, isolation, and withdraw from family may occur.	Encourage friends and family to visit and/or encourage talking to them on the phone if visits are not possible; ensure homework is obtained for child if condition permits; include the child in decision making.
Adolescence		
Adolescence is a time for establishment of identity. Inability to interact with peers is especially difficult during this time. Loss of control and fear of the unknown are paramount during this phase.	Rejection of the parents is a common reaction as well as being uncooperative and regression in regard to coping behaviors. Fear and anxiousness are typical reactions.	Always include the adolescent in decisions; encourage visits from peers or talking to them on the phone; in some situations the adolescent does not want the parent to be present as much as with previous ages.

Data modified from *http://www.austincc.edu/adnlev3/ol_hosp_child/care_plans_psychosocial_need.htm.*

MY PAIN RATING SCALE*

Please keep a record of how well your child's pain medicines are working. Rate your child's pain before and after pain medicine is given.

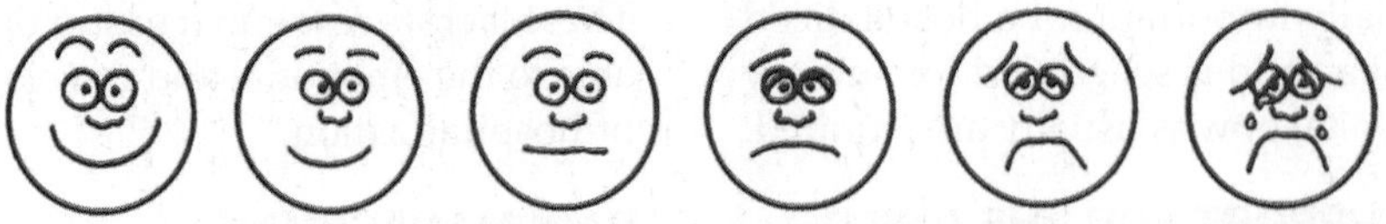

0	1	2	3	4	5
No Hurt	Hurts Little Bit	Hurts Little More	Hurts Even More	Hurts Whole Lot	Hurts Worst

Explain to your child that each face is for a person who has no hurt (pain) or some or a lot of hurt (pain). Point to each face and say the words under the face. Ask the child to pick the face that best describes how much hurt he (or she) has. Record the number of that face in the Pain Rating column. If your child's pain is above 2, or if you have other concerns with pain, let your nurse or physician know.

Date and time	Pain rating	Medicine I took	Side effects, such as drowsiness or upset stomach

Fig. 31.8 Wong-Baker FACES Pain Rating Scale. Explain to the patient that each face is for a person who feels happy because he has no pain (hurt) or sad because he has some or a lot of pain. Face 0 is very happy because he does not hurt at all. Face 1 hurts just a little bit. Face 2 hurts a little more. Face 3 hurts even more. Face 4 hurts a whole lot. Face 5 hurts as much as you can imagine, although you do not have to be crying to feel this bad. Ask the patient to choose the face that best describes now how he or she is feeling. Recommended for children ages 3 years or older. (From Hockenberry MJ, Wilson D: *Wong's essentials of pediatric nursing*, ed 8, St. Louis, 2009, Mosby.)

continues to be a challenge for health care providers. The pain that occurs in a child and the intensity of the pain are often difficult to ascertain. Infants are not able to verbalize that they are in pain or the pain's location. Rely on physiologic variables and behavioral variables, such as vocalization, facial expressions, and body movements. Pain assessment tools such as the Wong-Baker FACES Pain Rating Scale (Fig. 31.8) are helpful in the assessment of pain in children. Remember that some children are reluctant to let you know they are experiencing pain for fear of getting pain medication via injection. Advocate for IV analgesic administration, particularly when IV lines are already in place, and promote oral analgesic administration as soon as possible.

Reasons other than inaccurate pain assessment also lead to undertreatment of pain in children. Fear of respiratory depression or addiction sometimes means that a child does not receive an adequate amount of analgesic, does not receive it often enough, or is not considered a candidate for certain opioids. Although respiratory depression is a possible side effect with opioids in children older than 3 months of age (and possibly younger), opioids cause no greater respiratory depression than in adults. As for addiction, nothing indicates that children are at any increased risk of physiologic or psychological dependence from the use of opioids for pain management.

In addition to learning to assess pain accurately in children and advocating for and administering adequate analgesics, encourage parental presence and use sensitive care practices to lessen children's pain. Try integrating soothing talk or musical tapes into care practices. Infants often derive benefit from pacifiers, swaddling, rocking, or simply being held. Take care, whenever possible, to let the child's needs determine the timing of care routines, procedures, and tests. Also take appropriate action to reduce noise and other disturbing sensations to create a soothing and calming environment for the child in pain.

SURGERY

Undergoing a surgical procedure tends to be an especially stressful event for children and their families. Children who face surgery without information and preparation often develop misconceptions about the surgical event or any of the series of events that led up to or occur after surgery. Fantasies built on misconceptions typically lead to fears, which in turn often lead to negative reactions and long-term consequences, such as behavioral problems or an inability to trust others. Preparing a child for surgery entails providing information to parents and child about what will happen and what the child will experience. Addressing the events surrounding surgery that are most difficult for children

Table 31.8 **Age-Related Fears Associated With Surgery**

AGE	PRIMARY CONCERNS	INTERVENTION
Younger than 5 yr	What will happen when I wake up? Where will I be? Who will be with me?	Show recovery room, if possible. Tell when parents will visit after surgery. Encourage parents to be with child as soon as possible.
School-age	Anesthesia	Show mask.
Younger	That I might wake up during surgery	Explain "gas" or "medicine" and how it works.
Older	How doctor knows when, or if doctor knows how, to awaken me	Stress concept of "special sleep." Explain that it is a special person's job to control the sleep.
	Same as above plus the following: • Operation • Mutilation • Possible death	Same as above. Provide knowledge about procedure.
Adolescent	Same as above plus the following: • Special anxiety for change in body image • Loss of control while under anesthesia (in terms of behavior and for body integrity) • Peer reaction to scars • Effect on sexuality • Effect on adolescent mode of dress	Same as above. Reassure that only what is supposed to be done will be performed. Introduce to peer with similar surgery.

is a good place to begin. Six stress points are common for children undergoing surgery: (1) admission; (2) blood tests; (3) the afternoon of the day before surgery; (4) injection of preoperative medication; (5) the moments before and during transport to the operating room; and (6) return from the postanesthesia care unit (PACU). Think through each stress point from the child's perspective, and develop an individualized preparation plan. Explain the hospital system to the parents and inform them of the operation's progress.

Age influences the types of fears and concerns a child is likely to experience regarding surgery. Table 31.8 lists common age-related fears and effective interventions. Use of children's ages as a guide increases the likelihood that children are prepared adequately for surgery and all the surrounding events.

PARENT PARTICIPATION

An effective working relationship with parents must be established as soon as possible. Parents are the most significant individuals to a child. Also, they know their child better than anyone else and often play an important role in assessing the child's responses. Therefore take care to project a positive attitude toward parents: give them a warm greeting, smile, and establish eye contact. Gain the trust of the parents by: (1) reviewing and interpreting information from the physician as needed; (2) asking the parents whether they have any questions; (3) conveying concern for the parents' well-being; (4) listening and being available; and (5) respecting them as experts on their child and soliciting their input. These activities are time consuming, and yet for a nurse who works with families, they are some of the most satisfying.

When obtaining a nursing history, select a quiet place on the unit to listen to parents' responses and to provide them with opportunities to ask questions. Even if the physician sees the reason for hospitalization as minor, in some cases a parent perceives it as very serious. Parents experience fear and anxiety because of the seriousness of the illness, the procedures involved, or the pain the child will experience. Their apprehension then is transmitted to the child. Therefore convey interest and concern and try to decrease their anxieties.

Parents experience a series of reactions when a child is hospitalized. They too are in an unfamiliar environment, meeting different groups of people who ask many questions and give them much information. Perhaps the tests or procedures mentioned are unknown to them. They may become frustrated because they do not understand much of what is being told to them. Parents often do not know hospital rules and regulations and what is expected of them. They lose control in this setting and feel powerless. To this point, they alone have cared for their son or daughter. Now a nurse assumes control over the child's care. If an accident is the cause for hospitalization, parents sometimes blame themselves and feel guilty.

On admission, parents need specific information on routines, hospital policies that affect them, any limitations that exist, and what is expected of them. When parents receive information that they can apply immediately, their anxiety levels decrease and they feel more comfortable. When the emotional needs of a parent are met, that parent is better able to support the child (Box 31.10).

Later, be sure to explain to the parents any diagnostic tests, medications, or procedures that the physician

Box 31.10 Factors That Affect Parents' Reactions to Their Child's Illness

- Seriousness of the threat to the child
- Previous experience with illness or hospitalization
- Medical procedures involved in diagnosis and treatment
- Available support systems
- Personal ego strengths
- Previous coping abilities
- Additional stresses on the family system
- Cultural and religious beliefs
- Communication patterns among family members

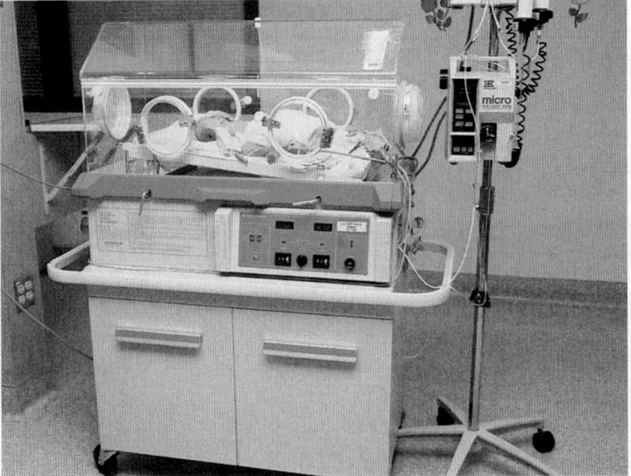

Fig. 31.9 A parent can easily feel overwhelmed by the equipment that surrounds an infant. (From Hockenberry MJ, Wilson D: *Wong's essentials of pediatric nursing*, ed 8, St. Louis, 2009, Mosby.)

plans. Keep in mind that anxiety and the sheer volume of information they have to absorb sometimes results in parents becoming confused or forgetting what they have heard. Any change in plans has the potential to generate anxiety and result in a parent being unable to process the information. Be sure to explain the tests and treatments thoroughly. Offer information several times to the parents, if necessary, to be certain they fully comprehend it.

As the parents' comfort increases, they become more involved in meeting their child's physical needs. Mothers tend to spend more time with their hospitalized children and participate early in providing care. Fathers are often more reluctant, so encourage them to become involved. When parents participate, they contribute to the child's recovery. Another strategy is to ask for parents' assistance in establishing goals or revising a care plan.

The equipment that surrounds a child is often overwhelming, with the strange-sounding alarms or with electrodes placed on different parts of the child's body (Fig. 31.9). When the function of a monitor or some other device is explained, it often becomes less threatening. However, use terms the parent can understand.

Initially parents watch the nurse perform a procedure for their child. When the nurse describes what is being done and why, parents become more interested. Information exchange, demonstrations, and teaching motivate parents to perform the procedure and improve their overall confidence in caregiving activities. Parents often become skillful in performing a variety of technical skills if taught in a patient, nonthreatening manner. Some activities in which parents become involved include gastrostomy tube feedings, tracheostomy suctioning, and subcutaneous injections.

Be sure parents are confident and knowledgeable in their ability to perform given tasks in their child's care, and encourage them to participate only in as many activities as they feel comfortable performing. Generally, the extent of parental involvement is a good measure of the nurse's effectiveness as a teacher.

The last phase of adaptation for parents of a child who is hospitalized relates to discharge. Do not postpone teaching until the time of discharge. Teaching begins at admission and is an ongoing process throughout the hospitalization. The child often has some activity restrictions, care requirements, or ongoing follow-up after discharge, but after you have instructed them and ascertained their competence, parents usually are able to provide any nursing interventions that are needed at home.

COMMON PEDIATRIC PROCEDURES

Some of the following procedures are for general care of children and procedures that healthy children experience in the home. Others take place primarily in health care settings. Many events that are common in health care settings are sometimes frightening for children. As is appropriate to the child's age, prepare children and their parents for all procedures, even those that you consider insignificant. Preparing children for procedures increases their cooperation, helps them cope, and promotes a sense of self-esteem and mastery.

A sensation-based approach is the most effective method of preparation. Provide information about what the child is likely to feel, see, smell, hear, or taste, along with emotions commonly experienced. For example, children scheduled for x-ray examinations or computed tomographic (CT) scans perhaps feel frightened, anxious, guilty ("Am I being punished for being bad?"), powerless, or curious. The sights they see probably include a "big machine" or "camera" over them and a lead shield or apron on themselves, the x-ray technician, and a parent if present. They hear noises of the machine "buzzing" and the sliding of x-ray plates. The room and the table most likely feel cold, and the lead shield heavy.

Timing is important in preparing the child. Young children are usually best to prepare close to the time of the procedure. Older children may be prepared further in advance. Preparation just before less-complicated procedures, such as injections, finger sticks, or vital sign assessments, is acceptable for children of all ages.

BATHING

Bathing the child provides the nurse with the opportunity to do a complete skin assessment. When giving a bath, protect the infant from drafts and chilling. Usually the best time to bathe the infant is before a feeding to avoid stimulating regurgitation or vomiting. Check the water temperature. If the umbilical cord is still attached, give a sponge bath. Clean the cord and the area around it with alcohol, which helps drying.

Use only water to clean areas around the eyes. Use a mild soap on the rest of the body; start with the face and move downward. Expose, wash, rinse, and dry one section of the body thoroughly before bathing another area. A baby's creases need special attention. Babies have very short necks; if they are not cleaned and dried thoroughly, skin impairment is possible.

If a sponge bath is given at the bedside, place the infant across the width of the bed facing you. This practice allows greater control of any movement by the baby and decreases the likelihood of the baby rolling out of the crib. Never use cotton-tipped applicators to clean the ear canal because injuries are possible; a washcloth is adequate. Give special care to the genitalia. In females, separate the labia and wash them in the anterior-to-posterior direction. Wash the penis and the scrotum of a circumcised male. In an uncircumcised male, daily external washing and rinsing are all that is necessary. It is best not to attempt to retract the foreskin because it is almost always attached to the glans. Forcing the foreskin back risks harm to the penis, causing pain, bleeding, and possibly adhesions. No ointments or powders usually are advised.

Infants enjoy being placed in basins or bathtub seats for baths. After washing the baby's face, lather the trunk and extremities. When placing the infant in the basin, use dry hands to pick up the infant more securely. The head needs the support of one hand; use the other hand to rinse the infant. Allow the baby to play and splash the water, which encourages development. After the infant is removed from the basin, wrap the infant in a towel and dry the infant thoroughly.

Hold the infant "football style" when washing the infant's head. In this position, the infant's hip rests on your hip. Your hand supports the baby's head, and the baby's back rests on your forearm. This position allows the infant to look at your face while the hair is washed. After the hair is lathered well, rinse the head over the basin at the bedside. Sometimes parents ask about the baby's soft spot (**anterior fontanelle**) (a space, roughly diamond-shaped, covered by tough membranes between the bones of an infant's cranium; the posterior fontanelle is triangular). Assure them that the area is not injured by shampooing.

Most toddlers love to be placed in a tub for their baths. Provide toys for the child to use in splashing, water play, and bathing. For most young children, 15 to 30 minutes is enough time to allow them to enjoy themselves in a tub. Remember that water is fascinating to a toddler because it has no shape or form. Safety is an issue: **never** leave a child in a tub without supervision.

The school-age child sometimes is reluctant to bathe, and many children are not accustomed to a daily bath. With encouragement, children who are feeling fairly well usually participate in their daily care. Use judgment of the child's physical and mental condition and advice from the child's parents to determine how much supervision a particular child needs.

Most adolescents become accustomed to bathing or showering as part of their daily routine. The need for an underarm deodorant usually becomes evident during puberty. Privacy when bathing and dressing is paramount during the teenage years.

FEEDINGS

Breast-Feeding

Breast milk is the preferred nutrition for the full-term infant, and a mother should be encouraged to continue breast-feeding her baby who is ill or hospitalized. Assist the mother by providing a quiet environment and a comfortable chair for her to sit in when nursing her baby. Some mothers are unable to be present for every feeding, or the baby is unable to take milk directly from the breast. Encourage the mother in this case to use a breast pump, and provide a private place for this activity. Bottles of breast milk may be frozen and given later by bottle or tube feeding.

Bottle Feeding

The correct position for feeding an infant is one that is comfortable for adult and infant. The caregiver holds the infant securely. Place a table or stand within arm's reach so that it is possible to set the bottle aside while *burping* (inducing belching or eructation) the baby. If a burp is not elicited by one position, try another.

Hold the bottle so that formula fills the nipple entirely to decrease the amount of air the baby swallows in the course of the feeding. Infants are not able to push the bottle voluntarily away when finished, so feed them only as much as they actively consume to prevent overfeeding. During the feeding, remove the bottle and burp the infant periodically. Newborns need burping more often than older babies.

Burping and Finishing a Feeding

There are three common methods of burping an infant. One way is to place the infant in a sitting position on the lap. With one hand over the infant's chin and chest supporting the body as the infant leans forward, use the other to gently pat or rub the infant's back from the waist to the shoulders. The infant also may be placed flat across the lap, face down, with one hand used to rub or pat the back and the other hand used to secure the body. The third position is with the baby upright against the body, looking backward over the shoulder. One arm holds the baby, and the other hand is free to rub the infant's back from the waist to the shoulders. Once the baby has released any trapped air, resume the feeding if the baby has not yet finished. Repeat this process until the infant has consumed the desired amount, ending with burping.

After feeding, position the infant on the right side to permit the feeding to flow toward the lower end of the stomach and allow any swallowed air to rise above the fluid and through the esophagus. Place infants only on their back to sleep; this measure helps prevent sudden infant death syndrome (SIDS). The Academy of Pediatrics (2017) has recommended the use of a pacifier at naptime and bedtime as a protective mechanism against the incidence of SIDS during the first year of life.

Solids

When the infant starts solid food, assist the parent to learn the proper feeding position. The parent feeds the infant in an infant seat. Always secure the safety strap. In an infant seat, the baby can focus the eyes on the adult, and both hands of an adult are free to introduce solids to the infant. Once an infant achieves control, caregivers can hold the baby in their arms. Older infants (8 or 9 months old) can sit in a high chair with a safety strap in place. Additional support is sometimes necessary. Try rolling up baby blankets and placing them on either side of the infant's trunk.

> It is important to wait to start solid foods until the baby is ready. Children do better with feeding if they have some control over the process, which is usually around 6 months of age. The semireclining baby has very little control over the spoon-feeding process. The sitting baby can look at the spoon, feel the food with his fingers, and get his fingers to his or her mouth. Babies who are sitting up can open their mouths and lean forward if they want to eat; they can close their mouths and turn their heads away if not interested. It is easy for a parent to pick up and understand feeding cues from a baby who is sitting up and eating solid food. It is much harder if the baby is really too little, lying back in an infant seat.
>
> Once a toddler has begun walking, placement in a high chair is a confinement that may be resisted vigorously. In climbing out of a high chair, a toddler may fall and sustain a significant injury, despite the fact that a safety strap was used. There are alternatives such as a booster seat, or pushing the high chair up to the table, or stools with backs/arm rests. Make sure the toddler's feet are supported—not dangling. Make sure toddlers are at a height where they do not have to reach "up" to get their food. Make sure they are close enough to the table to be somewhat confined so that their attention is on eating. Ideally the family eats at the same time as the toddler; therefore there is less risk for injury because parents can prevent the child from climbing. (Sometimes the ideal does not occur.) It is important to consider that the toddler appetite decreases at this age (physiologic anorexia), which is normal. Also, resistance to the high chair may be intense, and an injury can occur. It may be advantageous to try an alternative. Although they take in less solid food, toddlers continue to drink liquids freely.
>
> Parents should have three regular meals and planned snacks each day so that the child eats about every 2 to 3 hours.
>
> Also, children should sit down to eat. Choking is more likely if children eat on the run.
>
> —Modified from Kristen Maughan, RD; educator and mother of four.

Gavage

Some infants and children need gavage feedings. Gavage involves passing of a feeding tube through the nose or mouth, down the esophagus, and into the stomach. Although in many health care settings, nurses are required to have additional training before performing this function, the nurse usually assists with the tube placement and is permitted to perform the actual tube feedings.

To measure the tube before placing it, a qualified staff member uses one of the following procedures: (1) measure from the nose to the distal area of the earlobe and then to the end of the xiphoid process or (2) measure from the nose to the earlobe and then to a point midway between the xiphoid process and the umbilicus.

Some restraint of infant activity is likely to be necessary when passing the tube. Pulling up the bottom of the shirt over both arms is often all that is needed to restrain the newborn. Some infants may need to be wrapped in a mummy type of safety reminder device before proceeding. (See the description of the mummy safety reminder device in a later section.) In the unlikely event that a premature infant needs restraint, a small towel folded across the chest and secured beneath the shoulders is usually sufficient; take care not to compromise breathing.

Because infants are nose breathers, the mouth is the preferred route for tube insertion. The tube often is passed through the nose for older infants and children. Ask children who are able to understand to swallow while the tube is being inserted. A tube that will be indwelling is inserted almost always through the nose; to prevent irritation, use alternate nostrils for reinsertion. Once the tube is inserted, tape it in place. If the tube is inserted through a nostril, tape the tube to the cheek, not to the forehead, to prevent possible structural and cosmetic damage to the nostril.

Before feedings, check tube placement by (1) aspirating for stomach contents and (2) injecting a small amount of air (0.5 to 1 mL in premature or very small infants to 5 mL in larger children) through the syringe into the tube while simultaneously listening with a stethoscope over the stomach area for sounds of gurgling or growling. If any doubt exists about tube placement, do not proceed with feeding, and consult the practitioner. Sometimes radiographic data are necessary to confirm proper tube placement (see Chapters 15 and 19).

Whenever possible, hold the infant during the feeding. If this is impossible, position the infant or child on his or her back or toward the right side with the head and chest elevated. Give infants a pacifier during feedings to encourage sucking and help them associate sucking with satisfying hunger. Warm the formula to room temperature and, after a gentle push with the plunger, allow it to flow into the stomach via gravity. To prevent nausea and regurgitation, use rates of no more than 5 mL every 5 to 10 minutes in premature and very small infants and 10 mL per minute in older infants and children. At the completion of the feeding, flush the tube with sterile water (using from 1 or 2 mL for small tubes to 5 mL or more for large ones). Clamp or cap indwelling tubes after feeding. If the tube is to be removed, pinch it firmly to prevent escape of fluid and withdraw it quickly. Keep the child positioned on the right side for at least 1 hour to keep the possibility of regurgitation and aspiration to a minimum. Burp the infant if the medical condition permits. Record the type and the amount of feeding given and the child's response.

Gastrostomy

A gastrostomy tube (G tube) often is used in children in whom a nasogastric tube is contraindicated or in children who need tube feeding over an extended period. The physician places the tube during surgery when the child is under general anesthesia, or percutaneously with an endoscope with the child under local anesthesia. The practitioner inserts the tube through the abdominal wall into the stomach and secures it with a purse-string suture and anchors the stomach to the peritoneum at the operative site. Feeding is carried out in the same manner and rate as in gavage feeding. After feedings, place the child on the right side or in Fowler's position. The tube is left open and suspended or clamped between feedings, depending on the child's condition.

Total Parenteral Nutrition

When feeding by way of the GI tract is impossible, inadequate, or hazardous, total parenteral nutrition (TPN; also called IV alimentation or hyperalimentation) is an option. A highly concentrated solution of protein, glucose, and other nutrients is passed intravenously through conventional tubing with a special filter attached to remove particulate matter and microorganisms. Wide-diameter vessels, such as the subclavian vein, are the usual sites of infusion. In most health care settings, the nurse is required to have additional training before assisting with TPN. Nursing responsibilities include control of sepsis, monitoring of the infusion rate, and continuous observations. **Never** confuse this method of feeding with the use of "kangaroo" feedings, in which a mechanical pump is used to regulate the volume and rate of continuous gastric feedings per gastrostomy tube.

SAFETY REMINDER DEVICES

For safety reasons, children sometimes must be restrained after surgery or during a procedure or examination. Safety reminder devices (SRDs) are used only as a last resort. The SRD is used to ensure that safe care is given to the patient. The following clinical situations allow for the use of SRDs:

- Maintenance of oxygen therapy without interruption
- Protection from harm if child has an indwelling catheter, IV tubes, pacemaker wire, or sutures
- Patients who are confused, agitated, or unable to comprehend instructions (Hockenberry and Wilson, 2015)

Make sure to apply the SRD correctly, and closely monitor circulation and skin integrity. Remove the SRD every 2 hours to permit exercise of the body area. If you need to restrain the extremities, release them one at a time so that the child cannot pull out an IV or NG tube. Attach the ties of all SRDs to bed frames only, not to side rails.

Elbow Safety Reminder Devices

Elbow SRDs prevent flexion or bending of elbows. They allow an infant or toddler to move the upper extremities but prevent them from touching the head and neck area; thus, for example, they protect the newly repaired cleft lip or palate or scalp vein infusion site. Slip clean tongue blades into the parallel pockets of a wraparound SRD. Pull the shirt or pajama sleeve down to the wrist, and place the elbow in the center of this SRD. Wrap the SRD around the arm and tie it securely. Cuff the sleeve over the bottom of the SRD to protect the skin. Check the axilla and the wrist routinely for skin impairment.

Mummy Safety Reminder Device

A mummy SRD is used when it is necessary to immobilize head, neck, trunk, and upper and lower extremities. A jugular venipuncture or the insertion of an NG tube sometimes calls for this type of SRD. Place a square baby blanket on a crib, and fold over one corner. Place the infant on his or her back on the blanket so that the shoulders are at the level of the fold and arms are at the sides. Wrap one corner of the blanket over the right arm, and tuck it under the infant's left side. Place the opposite corner over the left arm, and place it securely under the right side of the body (Fig. 31.10). A commercially prepared mummy SRD is also available.

A modified version sometimes is needed so that it is possible to expose the chest. While you place one corner of the blanket around the right arm and tuck it under the baby's body, encircle the left arm with the opposite corner and secure it too. Bring the corner beneath the feet up to the abdomen and pin it, thereby leaving the chest exposed.

Clove-Hitch Safety Reminder Device

This type of four-point SRD is for use on all extremities of a child. Rolls of Kerlix, roller bandage, or strips of muslin can be used. Pad the wrists and ankles with gauze squares or other soft material. A clove hitch is

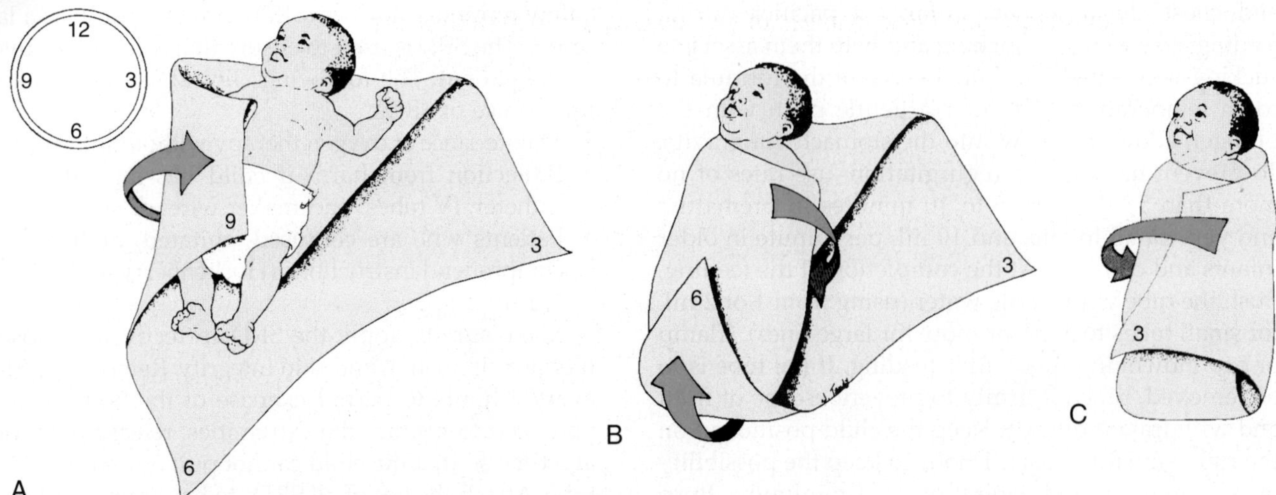

Fig. 31.10 Mummy restraint. A, Fold material over the right arm, and then tuck the corner under the left side. B, Fold the bottom up and the opposite corner over the infant's left arm. C, Tuck it under the right side to secure it. (From Lowdermilk DL, Perry SE: *Maternity and women's health care*, ed 9, St. Louis, 2007, Mosby.)

not a square knot. Make a figure-8 with the material, slip it over the padded wrist or ankle, and tighten it gently (see Chapter 10). Check each SRD frequently to be sure that circulation is not affected and pressure is not excessive. Use a slip knot to tie the ends of this SRD to the bed frame.

Jacket Safety Reminder Device

Sometimes a jacket SRD is needed to keep an extremely active older infant or toddler safely in bed or in a high chair. It resembles a vest and has ties in the back. Pull the child's arms through the jacket, and tie the jacket in the back. Attach the long ties to a bed frame or under the seat of a high chair. Although children are able to move all body parts, they cannot climb out of beds or high chairs.

OXYGEN THERAPY

Supplemental oxygen helps improve the child's respiratory status by increasing the amount of oxygen in the blood. It also is used in children who have cardiac or neurologic disorders. When administering oxygen to a newborn or infant, remember the harmful effects of oxygen on the developing pulmonary system. Oxygen is forced through sterile water to humidify it to counteract its drying effect. Check oxygen levels frequently (every 2 hours).

Monitor infants and children receiving oxygen with an oximeter, a flexible noninvasive photoelectric device with adhesive backing that is placed on the foot or the hand of an infant or the finger of an adolescent. The monitoring screen gives an instant reading of the oxygen saturation of blood. Correlation is high between this measurement and the arterial oxygenation. Table 31.9 presents advantages and disadvantages of various oxygen delivery systems.

Hood and Incubator

Oxygen often is delivered to small infants through a plastic hood that fits over the baby's head (Fig. 31.11). It is an efficient method of providing oxygen at well-controlled levels. More important, the body is accessible for starting an IV line or performing a procedure.

A less-efficient method of delivering oxygen to an infant is use of a closed incubator. Incubators have imperfectly fitted lids, uncovered vents, and portholes that must be opened to perform an activity on the infant, all of which contribute to fluctuations in oxygen levels. Maintenance of a constant temperature within the incubator is a problem as well. As an infant's metabolism increases in an effort to maintain body temperature, larger amounts of oxygen are needed.

Mist Tents

The purpose of a mist tent is to improve a child's respiratory status by liquefying pulmonary secretions. The child is observed easily through the plastic canopy. All of the device's working parts are outside of the tent, which is a distinct advantage when a toddler needs this form of therapy. Compressed air or oxygen runs through sterile water to form the therapeutic mist. A disadvantage is that the canopy must be opened for the treatments and procedures, which lowers the concentration of the mist.

Organize all activities and thus limit the number of times the tent is opened, to make maintenance of desired concentrations possible and to give the child longer rest periods. Tuck the tent under the mattress of a crib to maintain humidity levels. If the tent is functioning efficiently, dampness within it is significant, and frequent (every 3 to 4 hours) linen and clothing changes often are necessary.

Table 31.9 **Advantages and Disadvantages of Various Oxygen-Delivery Systems**

SYSTEM	ADVANTAGES	DISADVANTAGES
Oxygen mask	Delivers a more precise concentration of oxygen than the nasal cannula (most precise mask is the Venturi mask). Oxygen delivery is achieved even if child is a nose breather.	Patient unable to eat. Talking is muffled. Mask may be irritating to the face. Depending on the age of the child the mask may increase the chance of aspiration if patient vomits.
Nasal cannula	The child can eat and talk normally. Child is typically more compliant with nasal cannula than a mask because it is less intrusive.	Less precise concentration of oxygen delivered. Skin irritation is more likely along cheeks and over ears from tubing. May insert prongs in wrong direction, thus decreasing amount of oxygen received.
Oxygen tent	Child can eat and talk normally. Humidification easily achieved. Less intrusive than other devices.	Delivery of oxygen is interrupted when tent is open. May cause child to feel cold from moisture. Child may feel isolated in tent.
Oxygen hood, face tent	Less intrusive than a tent. Can administer higher concentration of oxygen than with a nasal cannula.	Child is unable to eat with hood or face tent. Excess moisture.

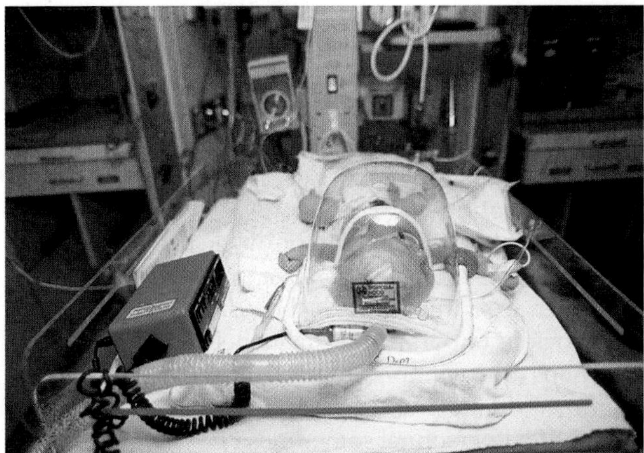

Fig. 31.11 Oxygen is administered to an infant by means of a plastic hood (Oxy-Hood). (From Wong DL, Perry SE, Hockenberry MJ, et al: *Maternal-child nursing care*, ed 3, St. Louis, 2006, Mosby.)

Nasal Cannula

Delivery of oxygen to newborns and all ages of children is possible by means of a nasal cannula. This mode of delivery is used commonly with infants with bronchopulmonary dysplasia (abnormal development of the bronchi and the lungs). Maintenance of the cannula's placement is often problematic in the infant, whose random head and hand movements disturb its position. Clear plastic tape placed around the oxygen tubing and over the nose and cheek helps prevent this. Adjusting the device at the back of an infant's head allows the tubing to be fitted to the child, and hooking it over the pinnae helps stabilize it. In older children, keep the nasal cannula in place by using the adjustable elastic straps on the child's head.

SUCTIONING

Patent airway maintenance sometimes necessitates suctioning. Air passages in children become occluded more commonly because of the small size of their respiratory tract structures. Signs that a child possibly needs suctioning include pallor; restlessness or anxiety; increased pulse, respiration, and temperature; dyspnea; bubbling (copious amounts of thin secretions); rattling (thick, tenacious secretions); drooling; mouth breathing; nasal flaring; grunting; gasping; retractions; cyanosis; and erythema (flushed face). Infants often have an anxious look in their eyes or fidget constantly. An older child perhaps constantly seeks attention with no explanation, tosses and turns in bed, or fingers the edge of a blanket.

Use suctioning when secretions are audible in the airway or when signs of airway obstruction or oxygen deficit are present. Various devices can be used to suction children, such as a bulb syringe or a straight suction catheter of the proper size for the child. In nonemergency situations, demonstrate how the suction machine operates by suctioning some water from a cup. Reassure the small child that the machine is only suctioning excess fluid from the mouth or nose, not body contents. Recommended pressures for airway suctioning with wall suction range from 50 to 95 mm Hg for infants to 95 to 110 mm Hg for children.

The use of artificial airways has become a routine life-sustaining measure in the pediatric and neonatal population. Depth, timing, and frequency are important considerations when suctioning a tracheostomy or endotracheal tube:

- *Depth:* Approximately ¼ to ½ inch beyond the tip of the artificial airway; determine placement by placing an appropriately sized suction catheter into an artificial airway of the same size, insert the catheter to the appropriate depth, mark with tape, and keep at the bedside as a reference.
- *Timing:* Limit suctioning to not more than 5 seconds.
- *Frequency:* Allow 30 seconds between suctioning attempts (two or three attempts at most).

INTAKE AND OUTPUT

Many health disorders necessitate accurate monitoring of the amount of solids and liquids taken in and the amount excreted. For example, measuring and recording intake and output (I&O) is extremely important in infants with diarrhea, toddlers with burns, or adolescents with renal disorders. Infants who are hospitalized because they fail to thrive or to grow as expected are placed on "calorie counts," which call for the careful recording of all food ingested and liquids given. This intake is recorded at the bedside, and a nutritionist calculates the calories the child actually consumes. It is helpful in determining whether the cause is organic or the result of an inadequate intake. These causes are ruled out before a maternal-infant problem is considered.

All fluids given to a child are documented on a record kept at the bedside. Adolescents are usually able to assume this responsibility after an explanation.

Many fluids are acceptable for encouraging fluid intake in the hospital and at home. They include diluted fruit juices, liquid or solid gelatin, sweetened tea, flavored ice pops, and sports electrolyte replacement drinks and infant solution (e.g., Pedialyte).

Persuading a reluctant child to drink fluids is often a nursing challenge. Offer fluids in small amounts at frequent intervals to prevent dehydration. Do not force them, and do not awaken the child from rest for this purpose.

When teaching parents about fluid management, determination of whether they understand the concept of clear liquids is always wise. Emphasize that milk is not a liquid because it forms curds when it comes in contact with the stomach lining. Caution parents about broths because most are high in sodium.

Encourage parents to relax any pressure on a child to eat during an acute illness. They need to understand that liquids can provide the necessary fluid and calories.

Infants and children who are unable or not permitted to take fluids by mouth face obligatory parenteral fluid therapy. Before an IV infusion is started, prepare the child and the family for this stressful procedure.

An understanding of the child's feeding habits often helps increase consumption after the child is able to step up the diet from fluids to solids. Once the child feels better, appetite begins to improve. Take advantage of any hungry period by serving high-quality foods and snacks. With the permission of the health care provider, encourage parents to bring in food items from home. This is especially important if the family's cultural eating habits differ from what hospital food services provide. The importance of recording all intake is key to preventing complications.

Measure all urine voided before discarding it. Remind older children to save all urine. Measuring urine output in the infant or toddler who is not toilet trained is sometimes a challenge. Most hospitals require routine weighing of diapers (before and after voiding) of all children who are not toilet trained. Subtract the weight of a dry disposable diaper from the weight of the wet diaper. The difference in the weight in grams equals the milliliters voided: 1 g equals 1 mL of urine.

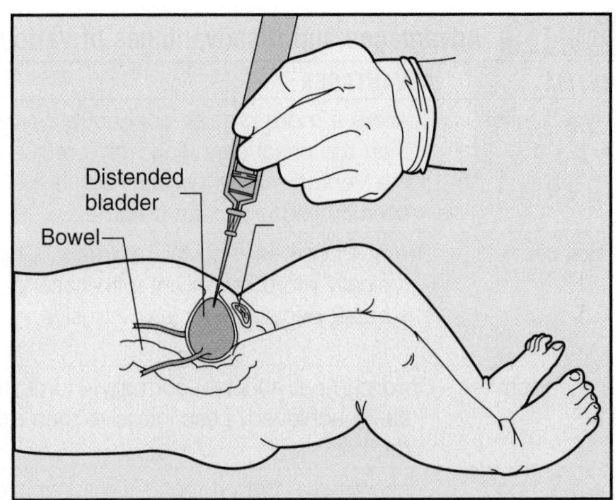

Fig. 31.12 Suprapubic bladder aspiration.

SPECIMEN COLLECTION

Urine Collection

Collection of a urine specimen when the child is not toilet trained is sometimes a major problem in pediatrics. It is often a routine part of the admission procedure and provides important information. In addition, kidney infections are common, so urine must be collected and examined often.

Qualified personnel sometimes perform suprapubic bladder aspiration on newborns and infants (Fig. 31.12). Contamination is a minimal concern with this method. Place an infant in a froglike position for the procedure, similar to the position described subsequently for femoral venipuncture. A qualified health care provider prepares the skin above the bladder and inserts a 20-gauge or 21-gauge needle into the bladder and removes several milliliters of urine. Gently prevent the legs from excessive movement, which has the potential to cause injury at the insertion site, by holding the infant's legs in a froglike position. Usually the best time for the procedure is 30 to 60 minutes after voiding.

Plastic urine collection bags sometimes are used for specimen collection. They must be applied correctly. Application of skin preparation to the area increases the adhesiveness of these bags (Fig. 31.13). In girls, give special attention to the narrow area between the vagina and the rectum. If the adhesive backing is not attached securely to this area, the anus is covered, and stool may contaminate the specimen.

When the bag is in place, cut a slit into the disposable diaper before it is placed on the child. This makes it possible to pull the urine bag through to the outside so that you can monitor it. As soon as the child voids,

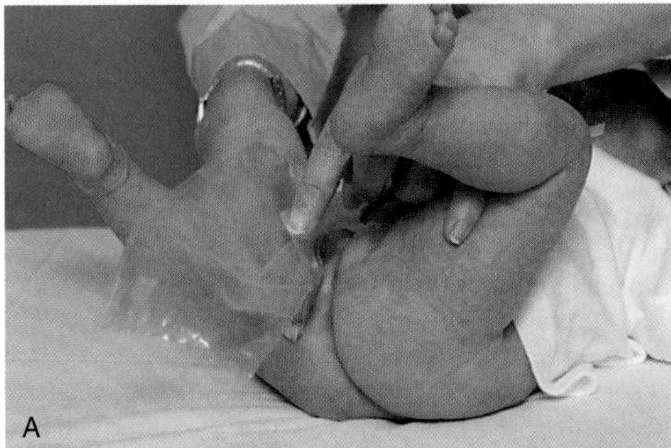

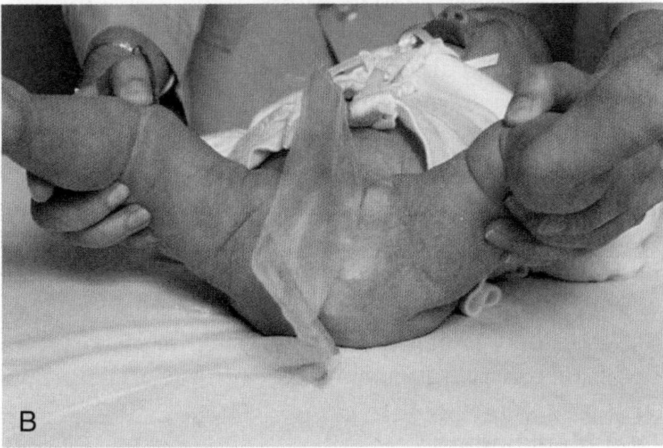

Fig. 31.13 Application of a urine collection bag. A, On female infant, apply adhesive portion to exposed and dried perineum first. B, Bag adheres firmly around perineal area to prevent urine leakage. (From Wong DL, Perry SE, Hockenberry MJ, et al: *Maternal-child nursing care,* ed 3, St. Louis, 2006, Mosby.)

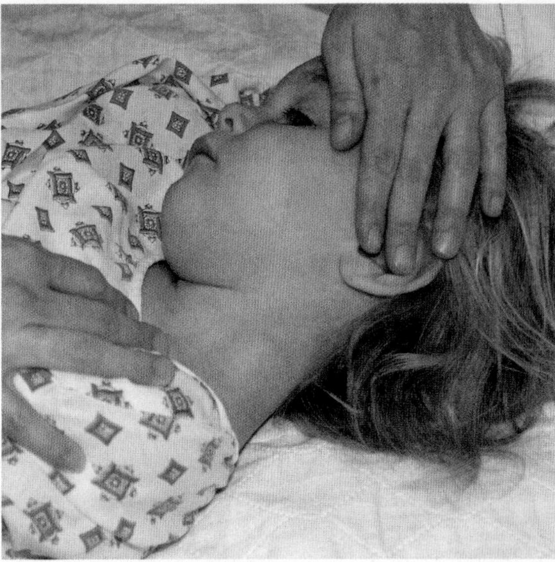

Fig. 31.14 Correct position for jugular venipuncture procedure.

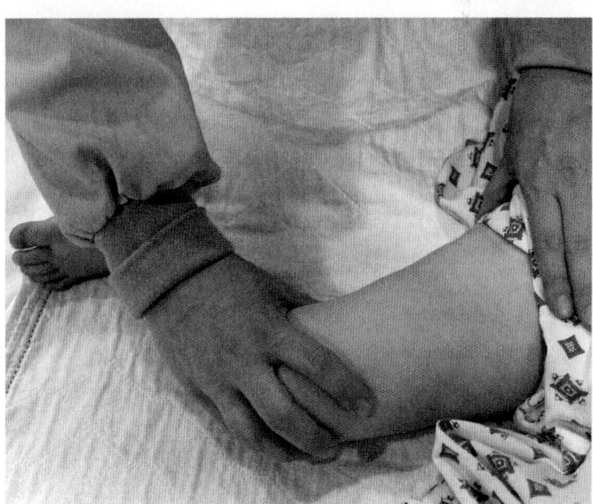

Fig. 31.15 Position for femoral venipuncture procedure.

remove the bag, so there is less chance of losing the urine specimen.

Catheterizations are done occasionally. Because of the high possibility of contamination, especially in regard to introducing organisms into the urinary system, practitioners use this procedure as little as possible.

Venipunctures to Obtain Blood Specimens

In infants and young children, the physician sometimes uses a jugular or femoral vein to obtain a blood specimen. The nurse prepares, positions, and restrains the child. Holding the head or lower extremities absolutely immobile is critical.

When a jugular vein is used, place the child in a mummy SRD beforehand. Place the child's body on the examining table so that the shoulders are at the edge of the table. Turning the infant's head 45 degrees provides the best angle for successful entry (Fig. 31.14). For a femoral venipuncture, place the infant on the back with both legs in a froglike position (Fig. 31.15).

Gentle pressure to both knees is necessary to restrict movement. Once the needle has been removed from the vein, apply pressure to the site to prevent the formation of a hematoma.

Sometimes the chosen site for venipuncture is one of the veins of the extremities, especially the arm and the hand. Older children, with appropriate explanation, preparation, and support, usually need only minimal, if any, restraint. One way of restraining younger children is to have the technician on one side of the child's bed and the nurse on the other. Lean across the child's upper body to prevent movement, and immobilize the venipuncture site with an arm.

Lumbar Puncture

Lumbar punctures are often frightening for children and parents. Explain the procedure to the parents and the child (if old enough to understand), and answer any questions they have. Application of EMLA (eutectic mixture of local anesthetics), a local anesthetic cream,

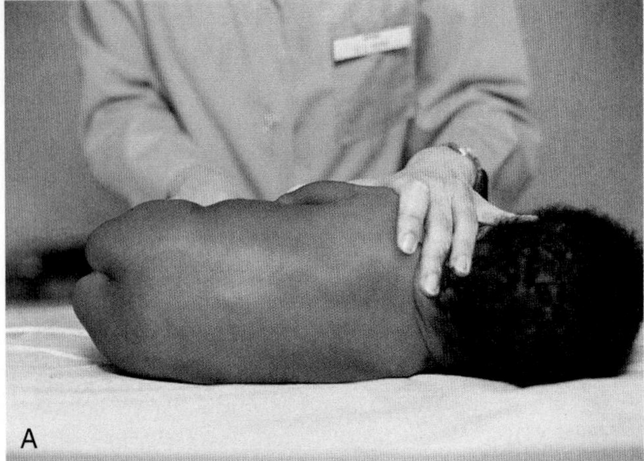

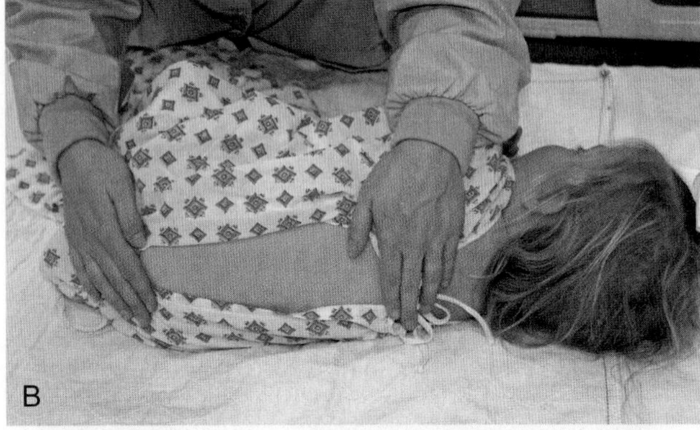

Fig. 31.16 A, Modified side-lying position for lumbar puncture. B, Older child in side-lying position. (A, From Wong DL, Perry SE, Hockenberry MJ, et al: *Maternal-child nursing care*, ed 3, St. Louis, 2006, Mosby.)

to the lumbar area usually is permitted. However, the EMLA cream should be applied at least 1 hour before the procedure.

This procedure requires positioning the child at the edge of the examining table or bed, on the side, facing you. Often the infant is placed in a sit ting position. Gently flex the neck and the legs, as shown in Fig. 31.16. This angle increases the spinal curvature and helps the physician gain entry into the subarachnoid space of the lumbar spinal canal. The child must be observed for any signs of difficulty. The toddler's legs may have to be wrapped in a blanket to decrease activity. Hold the child gently and securely in that position until the physician completes the spinal tap. Label the spinal fluid specimen immediately, and send it to the laboratory for analysis.

Normal spinal fluid pressure ranges from 60 to 180 mm Hg; the lower end of the range is typical in infants. Help adolescents avoid headache after a lumbar puncture by advising them to lie flat for several hours; young children usually do not have headaches, and quiet play after the procedure is generally appropriate.

MEDICATION ADMINISTRATION

A critical responsibility of a pediatric nurse is the administration of pediatric medications. For safety reasons, have a second nurse check all computed dosages. Do not forget the "six rights" of medication administration discussed in Chapter 17: Give the *right* medication and the *right* amount of the *right* medication to the *right* child at the *right* time and by the *right* route with the *right* documentation. Also remember to assess and document the child's response to the drug. Factors related to growth and maturation alter the child's capacity to metabolize and excrete drugs (see the Safety Alert box).

Immaturity or defects in all or part of the process of absorption, distribution, or excretion have the potential to alter the effect of a drug. Newborn and young children are more susceptible than adults to the toxic effects of certain medications because of their immature organ system's limited ability to detoxify or eliminate drugs. The side effects and toxic signs and symptoms are difficult to evaluate in a preverbal child.

Unit doses are not used in pediatrics because children are of various ages and weights. Methods of calculating dosages for children consider age, body weight, and **body surface area (BSA)** (total area exposed to the outside environment).

Also, see Chapter 21 for a detailed explanation of pediatric considerations in medication administration.

Oral Medications

When administering liquids, take care to prevent aspiration. With the infant held in a semireclining position, place the medicine in the mouth using a spoon, plastic cup, plastic dropper, or plastic syringe (without the needle). Place the dropper or syringe along the side of the infant's tongue and administer the liquid slowly, waiting for the infant to swallow between deposits. Another option is to use an empty nipple to deposit liquid medication. Remove the nipple as soon as the infant consumes all of the medication. Young children who refuse to cooperate or who resist despite explanation will need mild physical coercion at times. If this is necessary, carry it out quickly, kindly, and carefully. Remember the possibility that a crying child will aspirate medication when lying on his or her back.

To encourage the child's acceptance of oral medications:

- Give the child an ice pop or small ice cube to suck to numb the tongue before giving the drug.
- Mix the drug with a small amount (about 1 tsp) of a sweet-tasting substance, such as honey (except in infants because of the risk of botulism), flavored syrups, jam, fruit purées, or ice cream; avoid using essential food items because the child may later refuse to eat them.
- Give a "chaser" of water, juice, a soft drink, or an ice pop or frozen juice bar after the drug.
- If nausea is a problem, give a carbonated beverage poured over finely crushed ice before or immediately after the medication.

Safety Alert

Administering Medication to the Infant, Toddler and Child, and Adolescent

INFANT

- The health care provider is responsible for prescribing drugs in the correct dosage to achieve the desired effect without endangering the health of the child.
- The nurse must understand the safe dosage of medications being administered to children, and of the expected action, possible side effects, and signs of toxicity.
- Calculate dosage for all medications using the method desired by the facility. Any small differences in dosage have the potential to result in toxemia.
- A second nurse must check all computed dosages.
- When an ordered dose is outside the usual range or some question exists regarding the preparation or the route of administration, always check with the prescribing practitioner before proceeding with the administration of the drug. The nurse is legally liable for any drug administered.
- The vastus lateralis muscle is an acceptable injection site, because it is the most developed and not located close to any major circulatory or nerve structures.
- The ventrogluteal muscle is situated away from major nerves and blood vessels and is identified easily by a prominent bony landmark. It is the preferred injection site for children of all ages.
- Administer oral medications with a disposable plastic syringe (remove needle), releasing them slowly into buccal pouch; medication also can be placed in an empty nipple and the infant allowed to suck.

TODDLER AND CHILD

- Usually 1 mL is the maximal volume that is acceptable to administer parenterally (intramuscular [IM] or subcutaneous [SQ]) in a single site to small children.
- The ventrogluteal site is relatively free of major nerves and blood vessels, is a relatively large muscle, and is a safe injection site for young children.
- Allow toddler or child choices of drink to consume with oral medications.
- If possible, allow child to choose chewable or liquid medication if available.
- Never mix oral medications with essential foods, liquids, or honey (because of risk of botulism); use nonessential foods like applesauce or pudding.
- Use childproof tops on all medications for safety.
- Provide for sufficient help in restraining young child before giving IM or SQ injections; children are often unable to cooperate, and their behavior is usually unpredictable.
- Apply EMLA (eutectic mixture of local anesthetics, a topical anesthetic) over IM site if time permits (at least 60 minutes before giving injection). Applying LMX cream (lidocaine) is possible if time interval must be shorter.

ADOLESCENT

- The adolescent is capable of logical thought and reasoning and needs an explanation of hospital routine and purpose of treatments and medications.
- Older children and adolescents usually pose few problems in selecting a suitable site for IM injections.
- When administering medications to an adolescent, follow the same protocol as for an adult.
- The ventrogluteal site is the preferred site for IM injections for the adolescent.

- When medication has an unpleasant taste, have the child pinch the nose and drink the medicine through a straw. Much of what we taste is associated with smell.

Many pediatric medications are given via drops or dropper. A misunderstanding of these terms on parents' part creates a risk of overdose. In addition, many droppers that come with medications are marked in tenths of cubic centimeters. If parents use a syringe instead, which is marked in cubic centimeters, they run the risk of administering 4 cc instead of 0.4 cc. Parents also do not realize that cubic centimeters (cc) and milliliters (mL) are considered the same. If the prescription is written in cubic centimeters, parents often do not know what to do when droppers are in milliliters. Provide education to parents on correct methods for measuring and giving medication. Demonstrate the technique.

Intradermal, Subcutaneous, and Intramuscular Medications

Injections are a source of discomfort and fear for children, so drugs usually are given via injection only when other routes cannot be used. Table 31.10 lists recommendations for injection sites and needles. The primary site for IM injections are the vastus lateralis muscle (Fig. 31.17) and the ventrogluteal muscle (Fig. 31.18). The deltoid muscle is possible to use in children who are 18 months or older as a site for intramuscular injections and in infants who are receiving their hepatitis B vaccine (Hockenberry and Wilson, 2015) (Fig. 31.19). If time permits, apply EMLA, a local anesthetic cream, to the injection site at least 1 hour before the injection. Wearing gloves prevents anesthesia from affecting the nurse's fingers.

Injections administered with care seldom produce trauma to the child. Repeated use of a single site has been associated with fibrosis of the muscle and subsequent muscle contracture. Most children are unpredictable, and few cooperate totally when receiving an injection. It is advisable to have someone available to help gently restrain the child.

To estimate the needle length for IM injections, first grasp the **vastus lateralis muscle** (the largest of the four muscles of the quadriceps femoris, situated on the lateral

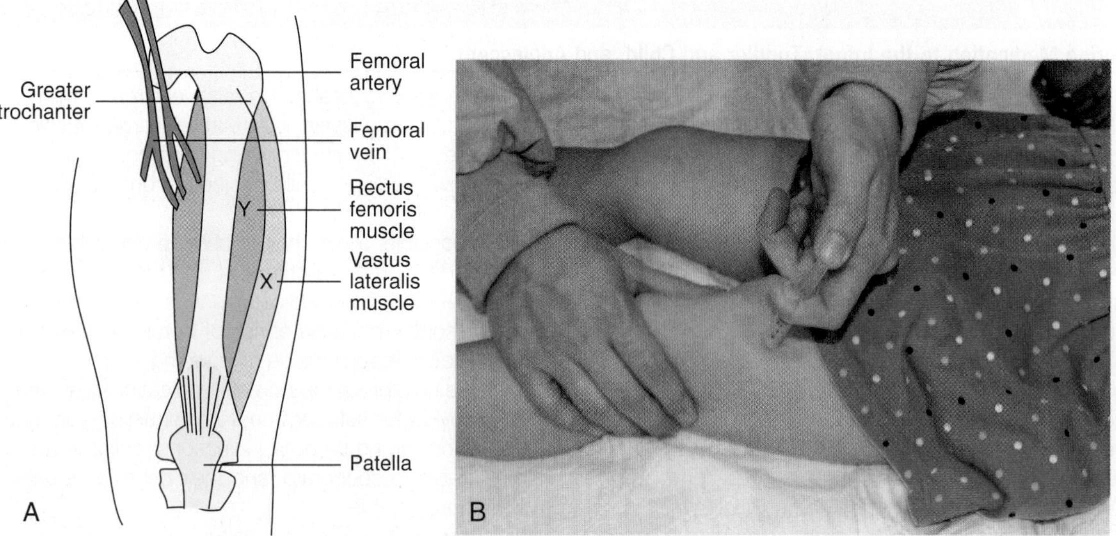

Fig. 31.17 Intramuscular injection sites. A, The middle third of the vastus lateralis muscle is the primary site for intramuscular injections in the thigh. B, Infant's leg is stabilized for intramuscular injection. The needle penetrates the midlateral thigh on a front-to-back course.

Table 31.10 Needle and Site Recommendations for Selected Injections

NEEDLE	SITE
Intradermal (ID)	
⅜-inch to ½-inch 25-gauge to 27-gauge	Primary: ventral forearm
Subcutaneous (SQ)	
⅜-inch to ⅝-inch 24-gauge to 26-gauge	Primary: upper outer aspect of arm; lower abdomen; anterior thigh
Intramuscular (IM)	
⅝-inch to 1-inch	Primary: 0–2 yr, vastus lateralis, ventrogluteal
20-gauge to 25-gauge	2–12 yr: vastus lateralis; ventrogluteal; deltoid

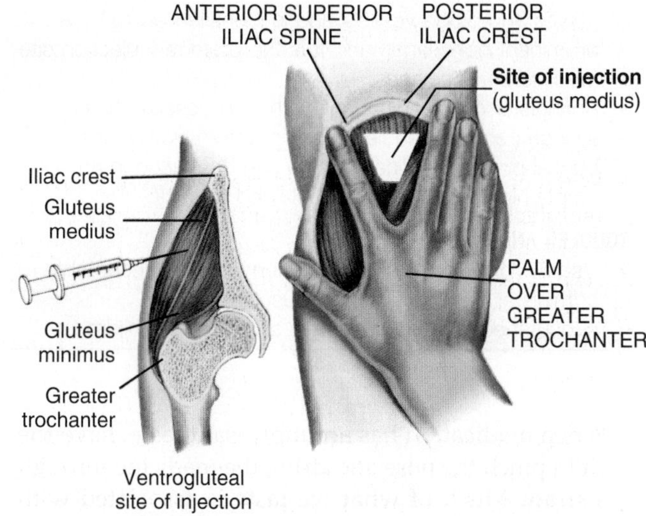

Fig. 31.18 Ventrogluteal site for intramuscular injection. (From Hockenberry MJ, Wilson D: *Wong's nursing care of infants and children*, ed 9, St. Louis, 2011, Mosby.)

side of the thigh; see Fig. 31.17A) or the deltoid muscle (see Fig. 31.19), and choose a needle length that is approximately half the distance between the thumb and index finger. With the ventrogluteal site, grasp only subcutaneous tissue, so choose a needle length that is slightly more than half the distance (see Fig. 31.18). Needle length should allow for a small portion of the needle to be exposed at the skin surface as a precaution if the needle breaks off from the hub.

Factors to consider when selecting a site for IM injection on an infant or child include the following (Box 31.11):

- The amount and character of the medication to be injected
- The amount and the general condition of the muscle mass
- The frequency or number of injections to be given during treatment
- The type of medication being given
- Factors that will possibly impede access to or cause contamination of the site
- The ability of the child to assume the required position safely

Intravenous Medications

The IV route of administering a medication often is selected for the following reasons:

- Medication is distributed almost immediately to tissues, and prompt physiologic action occurs.

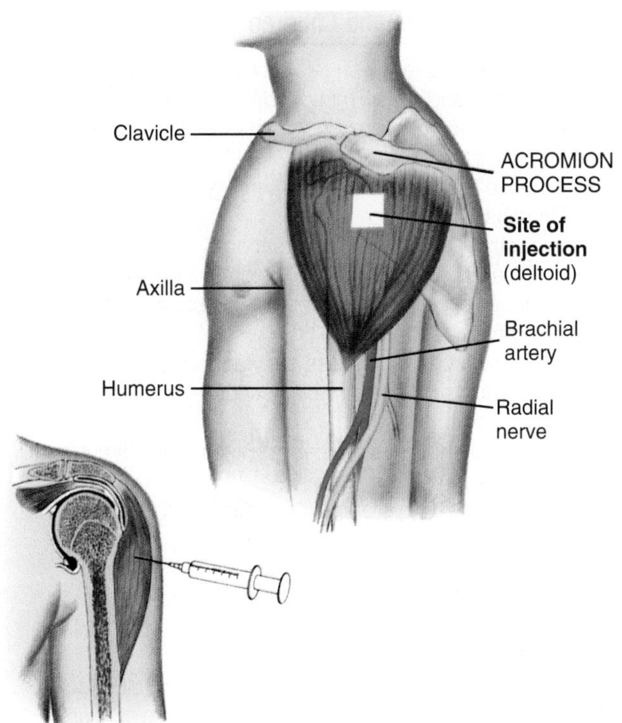

Fig. 31.19 Deltoid site for intramuscular injection. (From Hockenberry MJ, Wilson D: *Wong's nursing care of infants and children*, ed 9, St. Louis, 2011, Mosby.)

- With consecutive doses, predictable drug levels and maintenance of therapeutic effects are possible.
- After initial insertion, IV administration is more comfortable for the child than other types of parenteral injections.
- The IV sites in children differ from those of adults. A superficial scalp vein is used commonly in infants younger than 9 months of age, because these veins have no valves, so it is possible to insert a needle in either direction. In addition, the child can move the head from side to side without dislodging the needle. Any accessible vein is acceptable to use in older children. The use of peripheral lines in a child's lower extremities impedes ambulation.
- An infusion line may be converted to a saline lock when a child does not need additional IV fluids but still needs additional medications, such as antibiotics or pain medication. With a saline lock, a child can move about except for those brief periods when drugs are infused. Irrigate the tube regularly to keep the line open as per agency policy.

OCULAR, OTIC, AND NASAL ADMINISTRATION

A few differences are found in administering eye, ear, and nose medication to children or adults. Gaining children's cooperation is necessary for these procedures, and the child may need to be restrained.

Instilling eye drops in infants can be difficult, because infants often clench their lids together. One approach is to place drops in the nasal corner where the lids meet. When the child opens the lids, medication flows into the conjunctiva. For younger children, playing a game tends to be helpful. If eye ointment and eye drops are ordered, give drops first, wait 3 minutes, and then apply the ointment to allow each drug to work. When possible, administer eye ointments before bedtime or naptime because the child's vision will be blurred for a while.

Instill eardrops with the child restrained. For children 3 years of age and younger, straighten the external auditory canal by pulling the pinna downward and back. For children older than 3 years of age, pull the pinna upward and back. After instillation, have the child remain lying on the opposite side for a few minutes. Gentle massage of the area in front of the ear usually facilitates entry of the drops. Sterile cotton may be placed loosely in the ear to prevent infected material from being forced into the mastoid area.

For nasal administration, position the child with the head hyperextended to prevent the strangling sensations caused by medication trickling into the pharynx rather than up into the nasal passages.

RECTAL ADMINISTRATION

The rectal route is less reliable but sometimes is used when the oral route is difficult or contraindicated. Lubricate the suppository with water-soluble jelly or warm water, and insert it quickly and gently into the rectum beyond the rectal sphincters. Then hold the buttocks together firmly to relieve pressure on the anal sphincter until the urge to expel the suppository has passed (5 to 10 minutes).

Enema

The procedure for an enema for a child does not differ essentially from that for an adult (Table 31.11). Use an isotonic solution in children. Do not use plain water, because it is hypertonic and has the potential to cause rapid fluid shift and overload.

Proper insertion of the catheter tip, especially in infants, is essential to prevent rectal damage and perforation. If insertion of the enema tip causes discomfort, remove the tip and notify the physician.

SAFETY

Protecting a child from harm is paramount in pediatrics. Anticipatory guidance for parents of infants and toddlers and health teaching for school-age children and adolescents are two methods of preventing accidents. However, hazards and dangers are everywhere—in the home, at the playground, at school, and in the hospital.

Injuries cause more deaths and disabilities in children than all causes of disease combined. The risk-taking activities of adolescents also contribute to the **morbidity** (an illness or an abnormal condition or quality) and mortality of adolescence. Table 31.12 identifies common developmental characteristics, potential hazards, and

Box 31.11 Guidelines for Intramuscular Administration of Medication in Infants and Children

1. Use all usual safety precautions in administering medication (e.g., check child's identification). Apply EMLA cream (eutectic mixture of local anesthetics, a topical anesthetic) over site if time permits.
2. Prepare medication.
   - Select needle and syringe appropriate to the following:
     - Amount of fluid to be administered (syringe size)
     - Viscosity of fluid to be administered (needle gauge)
     - Amount of tissue to be penetrated (needle length)
     - Maximal volume to be administered in a single site is 1 mL for older infants and small children.
3. Determine the site of injection, and be certain muscle is large enough to accommodate volume and type of medication.
   - Older children: select site as with adult patient; allow child some choice of site, if feasible.
   - Vastus lateralis muscle and ventrogluteal muscle are acceptable sites for infants and small or debilitated children.
   - Dorsogluteal muscle is insufficiently developed to be a safe site for infants and small children. **The dorsogluteal muscle is not used for infants or children of any age.**
4. Administer medication.
   - Provide for sufficient help in restraining child; children are often uncooperative, and their behavior is usually unpredictable.
   - Explain briefly what is to be done and, if appropriate, what child can do to help.
   - Expose injection area for unobstructed view of landmarks.
   - Select a site where skin is free of irritation and danger of infection; palpate for and avoid sensitive or hardened areas. With multiple injections, rotate sites.
   - Place child in a lying or sitting position; child is not allowed to stand for the following reasons:
     - Landmarks are more difficult to assess.
     - Restraint is more difficult.
     - The child could faint and fall.
   - Use a new, sharp needle with smallest diameter that permits free flow of the medication.
   - Grasp muscle firmly between thumb and fingers to isolate and stabilize muscle for deposition of drug in its deepest part; in obese children, spread skin with thumb and index finger to displace subcutaneous tissue, and grasp muscle deeply on each side.
   - Allow skin preparation to dry completely before penetrating skin.
   - Have medication at room temperature.
5. Decrease perception of pain:
   - Distract child with conversation.
   - Give child something on which to concentrate (e.g., squeezing a hand or bed rail, pinching own nose, humming, counting).
   - Place a cold compress or wrapped ice cube on site about a minute before injection, or apply cold to contralateral site.
   - Say to child, "If you feel this, tell me to take it out, please."
   - Have child hold a small bandage and place it on puncture site after intramuscular (IM) injection is given.
6. Insert needle quickly, using a dartlike motion.
7. Avoid tracking any medication through superficial tissues:
   - If withdrawing medication from an ampule, use a needle equipped with a filter that removes glass particles; then use a new, nonfilter needle for injection.
   - Use the Z-track or air-bubble technique as indicated.
   - Do not depress the plunger at all during insertion of the needle.
8. Aspirate for blood.
9. If blood is found, remove syringe from site, change needle, and reinsert into new location.
10. If no blood is found, inject into a relaxed muscle.
11. Inject medication slowly (over 20 seconds).
12. Remove needle quickly; hold gauze sponge firmly against skin near needle when removing it to avoid pulling on tissue.
13. Apply firm pressure to site after injection; massage site to hasten absorption unless contraindicated, as with irritating drugs.
14. Place a small bandage on puncture site; with young children, decorate bandage by drawing a smiling face or other symbol of acceptance.
15. Hold and cuddle young child and encourage parents to comfort child; praise older child.
16. Allow expression of feelings.
17. Discard syringe and uncapped needle in puncture-resistant container located near site of use.
18. Record time of injection, drug, dose, and injection site.

preventive measures that help decrease the incidence of accidents and injuries.

Parents and children need to talk and listen to each other to prevent many accidents. Maintaining open communication between and among all members of a family is one method of prevention. The adult who is a role model, who thinks about safety, and who identifies potential dangers in the environment or a particular activity has immense power to influence a child.

Table 31.11 Guidelines for Administration of Enemas to Children

AGE	AMOUNT	INSERTION DISTANCE
Infant	120–240 mL	1 inch
2–4 yr	240–360 mL	2 inches
4–10 yr	360–480 mL	3 inches
11 yr	480–720 mL	4 inches

Table 31.12 Prevention of Accidents

BEHAVIOR OR AGE-RELATED FACTOR	ACCIDENT OR HAZARD	PREVENTION
Newborn		
Sleeping Poor head control Somewhat capable of moving body around	Suffocation	Do not tuck blankets in. Do not use pillows. Do not use plastic bags in crib. Avoid soft, moldable mattresses. Place healthy infants in supine or side-lying positions for sleep.
	Accidents	Use an approved car seat and follow manufacturer's instructions. Check crib slats; have them no more than 2⅜ inches apart.
	Burns	Test bath water temperature. Never smoke or drink hot liquids while holding baby.
	Falls	Never leave baby alone or unattended on bed, sofa, or counter. Always have one hand on baby. Carry newborn with two hands.
	Lead poisoning	Eliminate or reduce the child's exposure to any surfaces or substances that contain lead.[a]
1–6 Months		
Head control improving	Suffocation	Keep crib free of plastic bags. Do not use pillows.
Placing objects in mouth	Foreign body aspiration Injury from toys: loose parts or sharp edges	Inspect all toys; remove button eyes or detach small wheels. Do not offer foods that pose risk of choking, such as grapes, nuts, potato chips, and raisins. Remove open safety pins, needles, and nails from baby's reach.
Moving body from one place to another	Falls	Do not leave baby unattended on bed, sofa, or counter.
Beginning to pull self to sitting position	Burns	Test bath water; hold infant securely. Keep hot liquids in cups away from child's grasp.
7–12 Months		
Sitting up	Falls, drownings	Never leave infant unattended in high chair, on bed, or in tub.
Crawling	Accidents	Use gates at bottom and top of stairs. Place guards around fireplaces; never leave infant alone near space heater.
	Suffocation	Do not leave plastic bags or balloons in crib or playpen or within infant's reach.
Feeding self	Aspiration, ingestion	Do not offer foods on which child is likely to choke, such as popcorn; small, hard candies; gum; or hot dogs. Lock up all medications and poisonous household substances. Purchase medicines and household cleaners in childproof containers. Keep number of local poison control center by telephone. Childproof the entire house, including placing poisonous houseplants out of reach.
1–2 Years		
Holding on or walking	Falls, lacerations, abrasions	Keep furniture with sharp edges and glass tabletops out of child's way or protect with special corner protectors. Keep sharp kitchen utensils and garden equipment out of reach or locked up.
Exploring environment	Electrical injuries	Always know where the toddler is playing. Supervise all outdoor play activities.

Continued

Table 31.12 Prevention of Accidents—cont'd

BEHAVIOR OR AGE-RELATED FACTOR	ACCIDENT OR HAZARD	PREVENTION
Running		Do not allow child to run with objects in mouth. Begin teaching safety outdoors, including dangers of traffic, climbing, and walking in front of swings at playgrounds.
	Motor vehicle accidents	Always use an approved car seat and follow manufacturer's instructions. Keep toddler in fenced area. Install childproof locks on car doors. Teach child to cross street holding an adult's hand. Keep car doors locked in garage or driveway. Do not allow play in driver's seat without adult present.
	Ingestion, inhalation	Keep insecticides, medications, and all harmful cleaners locked up.
	Suffocation	Supervise play with balloons. Do not allow plastic bags in play. Remove doors of refrigerators or chain shut before discarding.
	Drowning	Keep bath water level low in tub. Never leave child alone in tub or wading pool; empty wading pool after use. Supervise child closely at beach. Never allow child near water without an adult. Fence around swimming pool. Enroll toddler in swimming class.
	Burns	Remove matches and lighters from reach. Teach fire safety. Keep handles of pots toward center of stove when cooking. Keep child away from stove while preparing meals. Keep child away from charcoal fires.
3–5 Years		
Climbing Running Exploring environment outside the home Improving motor skills	Falls, lacerations, and abrasions	Check yard, playground, and daycare center for potential hazards. Begin teaching: safety in using playground equipment; dangers of pushing and shoving playmates; and avoiding strangers. Supervise child using scissors, tricycles, and Big Wheels. Discourage approaching animals without an adult present. Teach child his or her own name, address, and telephone number.
	Drowning	Supervise action-related activities, such as swimming. Never leave child alone in bathtub or wading pool. Never allow child near water without an adult.
	Motor vehicle and pedestrian accidents	Use car seat or safety belts in car according to Department of Transportation (DOT) standards. Review acceptable behavior in a moving car. Review crossing street at corner, watching lights and flow of traffic.
	Assault, abuse	Teach child to keep parent informed of whereabouts. Confine play to yard; do not allow child to play in street.
	Burns	Practice fire drills in the home. Implement other practices similar to those for 1- to 2-yr-olds.
	Firearms	Never keep loaded guns or rifles in house or garage. Keep service guns locked. Instruct child never to touch gun or bullets.

Table 31.12 Prevention of Accidents—cont'd

BEHAVIOR OR AGE-RELATED FACTOR	ACCIDENT OR HAZARD	PREVENTION
6–11 Years		
Motor skills continuing to improve Enjoying large muscle activities Becoming increasingly independent Engaging in competitive sports, unsupervised activities	Motor vehicle and pedestrian accidents, injuries, fractures	Review traffic safety. Use safety belts. Teach skateboard safety: control speed; refrain from jumping; use helmet, knee, and elbow pads. Teach bicycle safety: rules of the road, use of reflectors, proper signaling, use of helmets. Review safety regarding use of lawn mowers, farm equipment, and tools. Teach child not to hide in or play near cars.
	Assault, abuse	Caution child about playing in vacant buildings, quarries, or sand pits. Teach proper use of protective gear in competitive sports. Teach child not to throw objects at people or moving vehicles. Teach child how to call fire department, police, and emergency medical assistance.
	Drownings	Review swimming and boating safety. Do not allow ice skating on pond unless its safety has been determined. Never allow the child to swim or skate alone.
	Inhalation, ingestions	Evaluate health education programs at school. Emphasize the hazards of glue sniffing and drug or alcohol use. Encourage family discussions about substance abuse.
12–18 Years		
Rapid growth spurt Demonstrating risk-taking behaviors Demonstrating increased independence Engaging in extracurricular activities Reacting to peer group influence Driving a car	Motor vehicle, motorcycle, and bicycle injuries and fractures	Evaluate the high school's safety and health education programs. Review bicycle and motorcycle safety, including use of helmets. Enroll child in driver education classes. Establish limits regarding care, use, and consequences of drinking alcohol and driving.
	Sporting injuries	Encourage group participation in outdoor activities, such as running or jogging. Supervise competitive sports activities. Encourage enrolling in first aid classes. Maintain a physical conditioning program.
	Drownings	Review water safety in seasonal activities. Discourage risk-taking behaviors at pool or beach. Discuss dangers of swimming and skating alone.
	Firearms	Keep guns empty and locked up. Teach proper care of firearms. Supervise target practice in isolated areas.

[a]Continued attention to this precaution is necessary throughout childhood.

Get Ready for the NCLEX® Examination!

Key Points

- Knowledge of basic principles of normal growth and development is important to understand what infants and children are like, what is possible to expect from them, what their needs are, and why they behave as they do.
- Knowledge of physical assessment with the systematic (head-to-toe) method is important for accurate documentation.
- Metabolism is highest in the newborn.
- Nutrition is probably the single most important influence on growth and is closely related to good health throughout life.
- By understanding that hospitalization is an anxiety-producing experience for the child and the family, the nurse is better able to address the needs of both.
- The goal of the pediatric nurse is to promote the highest state of health in each child.
- Family-centered care is a philosophy of care that recognizes the family as the constant in the child's life and holds that systems and personnel are called on to support, respect, encourage, and enhance the strengths and competence of the family.
- By understanding parents' responses to hospitalization of a child, the nurse is better able to address the parents' needs.
- Children in different age categories show varying concerns and needs while hospitalized.
- One way to decrease the traumatic effects of a child's hospitalization is to have the child and the parents attend a preadmission orientation program.
- Rooming-in facilities allow a parent to become as involved as desired and provide the child with the security of an adult who is known, trusted, and loved.
- Preparing children for pediatric procedures increases their cooperation, helps them cope, and promotes a sense of self-esteem and mastery.
- Always provide explanations to children at an age-appropriate level so that the child is able to understand them. Age and developmental level influence the ways in which children perceive and make sense of experiences such as illness or disability and therefore make an impact on their ability to cope.
- The administration of pediatric medications is a serious responsibility.
- The preparation of medication for a child requires precise computation of dosage.
- Accidents are a leading cause of death in children and adolescents, and identification and avoidance of potential hazards is necessary.

Additional Learning Resources

SG Go to your Study Guide for additional learning activities to help you master this chapter content.

evolve Be sure to visit the Evolve site at *http://evolve.elsevier.com/Cooper/foundationsadult/* for additional online resources.

Review Questions for the NCLEX® Examination

1. The nursing student is reviewing what he/she knows about the development of pediatrics as a discipline. The nursing student recognizes which of the following individuals as being credited with being the "father of pediatrics"?
   1. Hippocrates
   2. Abraham Jacobi
   3. James Mott
   4. R.E. Behrman

2. Lillian Ward, founder of the Henry Street Settlement in New York City, focused on which of the following? *(Select all that apply.)*
   1. Nursing services
   2. Social work
   3. Recreational sports
   4. Educational activities

3. The first White House Conference on Children focused on issues of child labor, dependent children, and infant care. As a result, what was established in 1987 on behalf of children?
   1. US Children's Bureau
   2. Office of Child Development
   3. National Commission on Children
   4. Women, Infants, and Children program

4. A 4-year-old child is to be hospitalized for the first time, and the parents voice anxiety about his condition and hospitalization. Which action by the nurse best addresses the concerns of the child's parents?
   1. Provide only necessary information.
   2. Provide an orientation to the child before hospitalization.
   3. Provide a tour of the entire hospital.
   4. Provide anticipatory guidance and explain all procedures.

5. Which method is the most effective when preparing a child for a pediatric procedure?
   1. Problem-solving approach
   2. Sensation-based approach
   3. Symbol-based approach
   4. Autonomy-based approach

6. A 16-month-old child is admitted to the pediatric floor after surgery to repair a cleft palate. The child's mother asks why her child is restrained. The nurse explains that the elbow SRD is being used to:
   1. monitor pressure to the suture line.
   2. prevent excessive movement in bed.
   3. help to prevent injury to the operative site.
   4. reduce the likelihood your baby will fall out of the bed.

7. Which statement by the new pediatric nurse indicates an understanding of medication administration to children? *(Select all that apply.)*
   1. "Children and adults are susceptible to toxic effects of medication at the same rate."
   2. "There are unit doses for children."
   3. "BSA is a reliable method of calculating children's medication dosage."
   4. "The route of choice is always the rectal route."
   5. The six rights of medication must be followed when administering medication.
8. A 7-year-old is about to have a finger-stick blood draw. Which statement by the nurse is most effective?
   1. "It will hurt, but you are a big girl, so you can just grin and bear it."
   2. "It will hurt a lot, and you can cry if you want to."
   3. "Some children say that they feel a little pinch."
   4. "Close your eyes, and don't look; it will be over in a minute."
9. An 18-month-old is hospitalized for surgery in the morning. Which intervention is most helpful in relieving the child's stress?
   1. Maintaining a normal routine
   2. Providing opportunities for play
   3. Encouraging parental presence and rooming-in
   4. Encouraging self-care activities
10. The mother of a 6-month-old is worried because the child's grandmother is concerned that the child is "slow" because she is not yet crawling. What action by the nurse is most appropriate?
    1. Assure the parent that grandmothers are often overly concerned when it comes to grandchildren.
    2. Ask the mother at what age her other children began crawling.
    3. Refer the mother for additional evaluation because most children do crawl by 6 months of age.
    4. Assure the mother that children develop at their own rate, but most children do not crawl at age 6 months.
11. An accurate apical heart rate measurement is assessed at the _______________ intercostal space.
12. A nurse is meeting a new 4-year-old patient for the first time. Which intervention is most effective when entering the patient's room for the first time?
    1. Speak only to the parents because the child will be very scared.
    2. Explain all procedures in detail because the child will want to know what is going on.
    3. Be careful not to use words that may be misinterpreted by the child, such as "take your temperature."
    4. Tell the parents they must leave the room until the physical assessment is complete.
13. The nurse is providing postoperative care instructions to parents of a 5-month-old who is recovering from surgery. Which statement indicates that the teaching was effective? *(Select all that apply.)*
    1. "The baby will perhaps be comforted by sucking on a pacifier, being swaddled, or being rocked."
    2. "Analgesics are best given only if the child will not stop crying."
    3. "At 5 months of age, the baby has immature pain receptors and therefore will not need analgesics."
    4. "The baby will have less pain if left alone in the bed for all activities."
    5. "I can continue to breast feed as soon as my child is able to eat."
14. What is true regarding the child's nutrition? *(Select all that apply.)*
    1. The toddler needs to eat twice as much as a 6-month-old infant.
    2. Infants can begin solid foods at 4 to 6 months of age.
    3. The toddler is too busy to eat, so give finger foods such as hot dogs, grapes, and nuts.
    4. The toddler has no risk of food allergies.
    5. Solid foods should be introduced one at a time and a new one each week.
15. What is the most accurate method to measure urine output in an infant?
    1. Weigh the diaper before and after the infant voids.
    2. Weigh the infant after each wet diaper.
    3. Have the parents try to catch the urine in a plastic cup.
    4. Insert a Foley catheter for all infants who are not potty trained.
16. What is true of intramuscular injections in children younger than 2 years old? *(Select all that apply.)*
    1. Not possible to give because of poor muscular development.
    2. Possible to give in the vastus lateralis muscle.
    3. Possible to give in the ventrogluteal muscle.
    4. Possible to give in the deltoid muscle.
    5. Apply EMLA cream 15 minutes before injection.
    6. Possible to give in the dorsogluteal muscle.
    7. Help should be obtained to restrain the child.
17. The most common asymmetry with lateral curvature of the spine in the adolescent is known as _______________.
18. What is the appropriate method to examine a 6-month-old's ear with an otoscope?
    1. Pull the ear up and back.
    2. Pull the ear down and forward.
    3. Pull the ear up and forward.
    4. Pull the ear down and back.

32 Care of the Child With a Physical and Mental or Cognitive Disorder

http://evolve.elsevier.com/Cooper/foundationsadult/

Objectives

1. Describe the etiology and pathophysiology, types, clinical manifestations, diagnostic tests, and medical management of and nursing interventions, patient teaching, and prognosis for children affected by the following:
   - Congenital heart defects
   - Iron-deficiency anemia, sickle cell anemia, and aplastic anemia
   - Hemophilia and idiopathic thrombocytopenia purpura
   - Leukemia
   - Acquired immunodeficiency syndrome (AIDS)
   - Juvenile rheumatoid arthritis
   - Disorders of the respiratory system, including respiratory distress syndrome, bronchopulmonary dysplasia, pneumonia, sudden infant death syndrome, upper respiratory tract infections, tonsillitis, croup, bronchitis, respiratory syncytial virus, pulmonary tuberculosis, cystic fibrosis, and bronchial asthma
   - Disorders of the gastrointestinal system, including cleft lip and cleft palate, dehydration, diarrhea, gastroenteritis, constipation, gastroesophageal reflux, hypertrophic pyloric stenosis, intussusception, and Hirschsprung's disease
   - Disorders of the genitourinary system, including nephrotic syndrome, acute glomerulonephritis, and Wilms tumor
   - Disorders of the endocrine system, including hypothyroidism, hyperthyroidism, and diabetes mellitus
   - Disorders of the musculoskeletal system, including hip dysplasia, Legg-Calvé-Perthes disease, osteomyelitis, talipes, Duchenne muscular dystrophy, and septic arthritis
   - Disorders of the nervous system, including meningitis, encephalitis, hydrocephalus, cerebral palsy, seizures, spina bifida, neonatal abstinence syndrome, and neuroblastoma
   - Lead poisoning
   - Disorders of the integumentary system, including contact dermatitis, diaper dermatitis, eczema, seborrheic dermatitis, acne vulgaris, herpes simplex virus type I, tinea infections, candidiasis, and parasitic infections
   - Disorders of the sensory system, including otitis media, refractive errors (myopia, hyperopia), strabismus, periorbital cellulitis, and allergic rhinitis
2. Discuss the parent teaching necessary to assist in prevention of urinary tract infection in infants and children.
3. Identify six possible causes of cognitive impairment.
4. Describe the clinical manifestations of Down syndrome.
5. Discuss the appropriate nursing interventions in caring for a child with autism.
6. Demonstrate an understanding of the medical management and nursing interventions for a child with a learning disability.
7. Describe four nursing interventions for a child with attention deficit/hyperactivity disorder.
8. Identify six clinical manifestations of depression in children.
9. Discuss three nursing interventions for the child who is suicidal.

Key Terms

acquired heart disorders (ŭ-KWĪRD HŎRT dĭs-ŌR-dŭrz, p. 977)
alpha-fetoprotein (ĂL-fŭ fē-tō-PRŌ-tēn, p. 1032)
amblyopia (ăm-blē-Ō-pē-ă, p. 1047)
attention deficit/hyperactivity disorder (ADHD) (ŭ-TĔN-shŭn DĔF-ĭ-sĭt hī-pŭr-ăk-TĬV-ĭ-tē dĭs-ŌR-dŭr, p. 1052)
autism (AW-tĭz-ŭm, p. 1050)
chelation therapy (kĕ-LĀ-shŭn THĔR-ŭ-pē, p. 1034)
cognitive impairment (KŎG-nĭ-tĭv ĭm-PĀR-mŭnt, p. 1048)
congenital heart disease (CHD) (kŏn-JĔN-ĭ-tŭl HŎRT dĭz-ĒZ, p. 977)
"currant jelly" stools (KŪR-ŭnt JĔL-ē STŪLZ, p. 1010)
Down syndrome (DOUN SĬN-drōm, p. 1049)
glomerulonephritis (glō-mĕr-ū-lō-nĕf-RĪ-tĭs, p. 1014)
Gowers sign (GOU-ŭrz SĪN, p. 1024)
intelligence quotient (IQ) (ĭn-TĔL-ĭ-jŭns KWŌ-shŭnt, p. 1048)
Legg-Calvé-Perthes disease (LĔG kăl-VĀ PĔR-tēz dĭz-ĒZ, p. 1020)
lichenification (lī-kĕn-ĭ-fĭ-KĀ-shŭn, p. 1036)
neural tube (NŪ-rŭl TŪB, p. 1031)
Nissen fundoplication (NĬS-ĕn fŭn-dō-plĭ-KĀ-shŭn, p. 1008)
nuchal rigidity (NŪ-kŭl rĭj-ĬD-ĭ-tē, p. 1026)
pica (PĪ-kŭ, p. 1034)
pneumothorax (nū-mō-THŌ-răks, p. 994)
priapism (prī-ŭ-PĬZ-ŭm, p. 985)
prodromal (prō-DRŌ-măl, p. 1042)

psychogenic (sī-kō-JĔN-ĭk, p. 1054)
school avoidance (SKŪL ŭ-VOYD-ŭns, p. 1051)
sickled cell (SĬK-ŭld sĕl, p. 985)
somatization disorders (sō-măt-ŭ-ZĀ-shŭn dĭs-ŌR-dŭrz, p. 1053)
subluxation (sŭb-lŭk-SĀ-shŭn, p. 1019)

Many of the health problems that affect children differ from those of adults, and management of these problems also can be different. Nurses must be aware of the unique way they provide care to children and their families. When providing nursing interventions to children, include parents as much as possible, delegating to them any interventions that are appropriate. It is also necessary to provide them with resources within their community so that they can provide for the continued health of their child after hospital discharge.

This chapter provides the reader with an understanding of the physical, mental, and cognitive (the process of knowing) disorders affecting children. Although it is dedicated to the understanding of the most prevalent health issues affecting children, it is beyond the scope of this chapter to address all disorders that may affect children.

PHYSICAL DISORDERS

DISORDERS OF CARDIOVASCULAR FUNCTION

Many cardiovascular disorders in children are the result of **congenital heart disease (CHD)**, an abnormality or anomaly of the heart that is present at birth. Consequences of many of these defects include heart failure, predisposition to infection, hypoxia, and alterations in growth. Another group of cardiovascular disorders, **acquired heart disorders**, comprises abnormalities occurring after birth that compromise the heart's function.

Any type of cardiovascular disorder tends to be frightening to the child and parents. It is important to educate and prepare them regarding the disorder and its management.

Congenital Heart Disease

It is estimated that 5% to 10% of full-term newborns have CHD. The rate is even higher among infants born prematurely.

Etiology and pathophysiology. The causes of many congenital heart defects are unknown, although genetics and maternal medication use may play a role. There are several probable environmental and genetic risk factors for the various types of defects. Environmental factors include intrauterine rubella exposure, maternal alcoholism, diabetes mellitus, advanced maternal age, and maternal drug ingestion (e.g., lithium, thalidomide, or phenytoin [Dilantin]). Genetic risk factors include the presence of a sibling or parent with a CHD, chromosomal anomalies (trisomy G [trisomy 21, Down syndrome]; trisomy D [trisomies 13, Patau syndrome; 14; and 15]; and monosomy X [Turner syndrome]), and the presence of other noncardiac congenital anomalies (Mayo Clinic, 2018a).

Principles of fetal and postnatal circulation. During fetal development, the placenta is the source of oxygen and nutrients. Oxygenated blood is brought to the fetus by the umbilical vein and enters the fetal heart via the inferior vena cava. The fetal lungs, which are collapsed and full of fluid, pose a strong resistance to the right side of the heart, increasing the pressures in the right atrium and the right ventricle. Because of the increased pressure in the right side of the heart, blood entering the heart from the inferior vena cava is directed across the right atrium through the foramen ovale to the left atrium. This blood is then ejected from the left ventricle into the aorta. Thus the blood richest in oxygen is pumped through the aorta to the coronary arteries, the brain, and the upper extremities. Venous blood returning from this region returns to the right atrium through the superior vena cava and is directed downward through the tricuspid valve into the right ventricle. From there it is pumped into the pulmonary artery, where the majority of the blood is shunted to the descending aorta through the ductus arteriosus and perfuses the lower body (Fig. 32.1). Only a small amount enters the fetal lungs for structure development, owing to high pulmonary resistance (Fig. 32.2A).

At delivery, with the first breath, the newborn's lungs expand, and the fluid within them is absorbed into the pulmonary circulation. As a result, pulmonary and right-sided heart pressures fall and, with the removal of the placenta, systemic pressures rise. The foramen ovale closes as the pressure in the left atrium exceeds the pressure in the right atrium. The ductus arteriosus closes with the increased oxygen content of the newborn's blood (see Fig. 32.2B).

Types of defects. In the past, diagnoses were based on a classification into two basic categories of CHD: disorders related to symptoms of color (cyanotic or acyanotic) and disorders related to the direction of blood flow (left-to-right shunt or right-to-left shunt). These categories sometimes have been difficult to understand because it was not possible to classify all disorders by these criteria.

A new classification system of CHD has emerged. The most current CHD categories are related to four physiologic characteristics: increased pulmonary blood flow, decreased pulmonary blood flow, obstruction to systemic blood flow, and mixed blood flow.

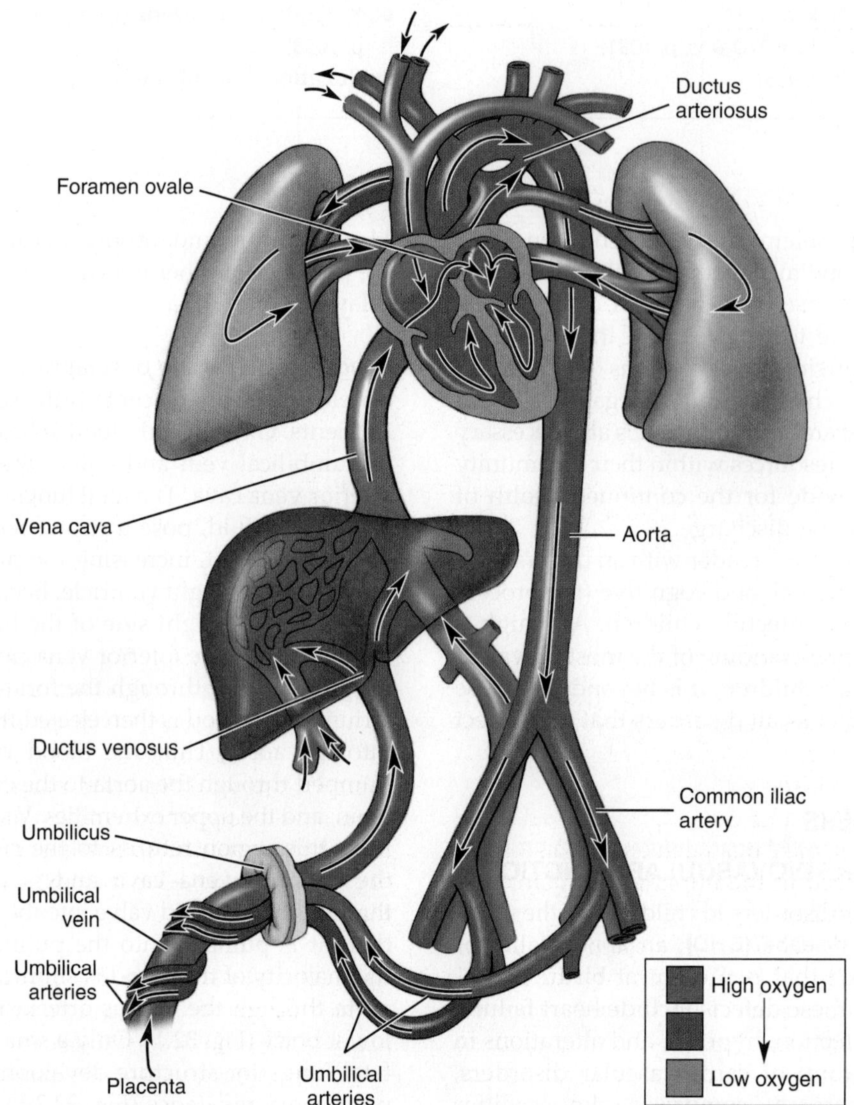

Fig. 32.1 Fetal circulation. (From Herlihy B: *The human body in health and illness*, ed 4, St. Louis, 2011, Saunders.)

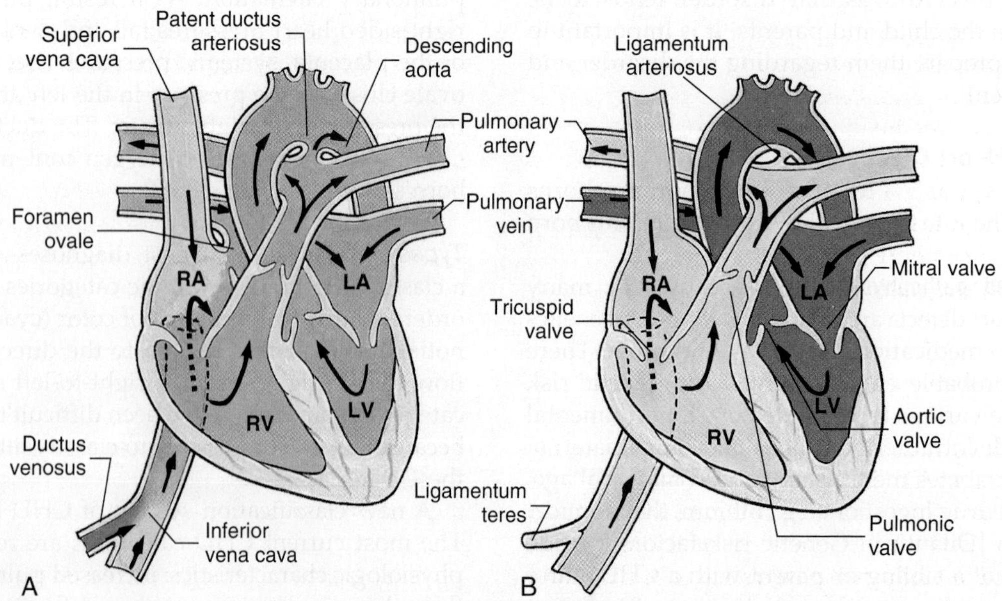

Fig. 32.2 Changes in circulation at birth. A, Prenatal circulation. B, Postnatal circulation. *Arrows* indicate direction of blood flow. *LA,* Left atrium; *LV,* left ventricle; *RA,* right atrium; *RV,* right ventricle. (From Hockenberry MJ, Wilson D: *Wong's essentials of pediatric nursing*, ed 9, St. Louis, 2013, Mosby.)

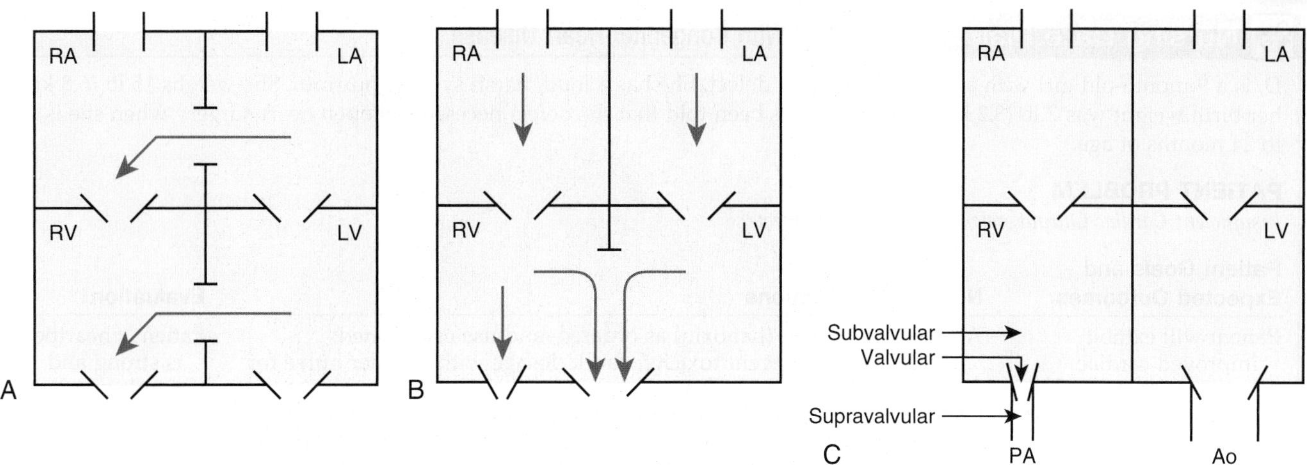

Fig. 32.3 Hemodynamics in congenital heart disease. A, Increased pulmonary blood flow. B, Decreased pulmonary blood flow. C, Obstruction to systemic blood flow. *Ao*, Aorta; *LA*, left atrium; *LV*, left ventricle; *RA*, right atrium; *RV*, right ventricle.

Fig. 32.3 illustrates hemodynamics related to the first three categories. The figure does not illustrate mixed blood flow, which includes many possible combinations of the mixing of oxygenated and unoxygenated blood in the heart or great vessels.

In this chapter, several of the major CHDs, clinical manifestations, and medical management are discussed. They also are described in the nursing care plans and critical thinking activities.

Clinical manifestations. Children with suspected cardiac dysfunction may exhibit cyanosis, pallor, cardiomegaly, pericardial rubs, murmurs, additional heart sounds (S_3 or S_4), discrepancies between apical and radial pulses, tachypnea, dyspnea, grunting, digital clubbing, hepatomegaly, splenomegaly, discrepancies between upper and lower extremity blood pressures, crackles, and wheezing. (See the discussions of specific clinical manifestations of common congenital heart defects throughout this chapter.)

Diagnostic tests. Many invasive and noninvasive tests are available to diagnose cardiovascular disorders. The choice of studies the health care provider orders will vary according to the nature of the suspected disorder. The more frequently conducted tests include urine culture, arterial blood gases (ABG), electrocardiography, echocardiography, fluoroscopy, angiography, cardiac catheterization, and cardiac magnetic resonance imaging (MRI).

Defects Involving Increased Pulmonary Blood Flow

Defects involving increased pulmonary blood flow are the most common CHDs. In this type of defect, there is a communication of some type between the right and the left sides of the heart. Because of the increased pressure of the left side of the heart, some of the blood is pushed back to the right side of the heart. The increased blood on the right side of the heart then is moved to the lungs. The size of the defect and the amount of increase in blood volume determine the severity of the symptoms of heart failure.

The most common defects involving increased pulmonary blood flow are patent ductus arteriosus, atrial septal defect, and ventricular septal defect (VSD). The clinical manifestations and medical management of each are discussed in the next sections (Nursing Care Plan 32.1).

Patent ductus arteriosus. The ductus arteriosus is a fetal artery that connects the pulmonary artery to the aorta (see Fig. 32.1). Failure of the ductus arteriosus to close within the first weeks of life allows oxygenated blood to shunt from the high-pressure aorta to the low-pressure pulmonary artery, which causes the blood to become deoxygenated (Fig. 32.4).

Clinical manifestations. Sometimes a small patent ductus arteriosus is asymptomatic. Children with larger defects often exhibit signs and symptoms of heart failure, including poor eating, poor growth patterns, and fatigue. Other possible clinical manifestations include a typical machine-like murmur audible at the upper left sternal border; widened pulse pressure; and bounding pulses.

Medical management. Administration of indomethacin (a prostaglandin inhibitor) often has been effective in closing the ductus arteriosus in full-term and premature newborns. Surgical correction involves ligating the ductus arteriosus through a thoracotomy incision (surgical opening into the thoracic cavity).

Surgeons are using a new technique in some cases. Three small incisions are made on the left side of the chest, and then a thoracoscope and instruments are used to place a clip on the ductus arteriosus.

Atrial septal defect. An atrial septal defect is an abnormal opening in the atrial septum that enables oxygenated blood to flow from the higher pressure left atrium to

Nursing Care Plan 32.1 A Child With Congenital Heart Disease

D. is a 9-month-old girl with a ventricular septal defect. She has a loud, harsh systolic murmur. She weighs 15 lb (6.8 kg); her birth weight was 7 lb (3.2 kg). The family has been told that the defect necessitates open heart surgery when she is 18 to 24 months of age.

PATIENT PROBLEM

Insufficient Cardiac Output, related to structural defect

Patient Goals and Expected Outcomes	Nursing Interventions	Evaluation
Patient will exhibit improved cardiac output; heartbeat will be strong, regular, and within normal limits for age	Administer digoxin (Lanoxin) as ordered, and use established precautions to prevent toxicity; check dosage with another nurse for safety. Count apical pulse for 1 full minute before administering drug. Withhold medication, and notify health care provider if pulse rate is less than 90–110 bpm (infants) or 75–85 bpm (older children), depending on previous pulse readings. Monitor serum potassium levels (decrease in levels enhances digoxin toxicity).	Patient's heartbeat is strong and regular.

PATIENT PROBLEM

Potential for Infection, related to debilitated physical status

Patient Goals and Expected Outcomes	Nursing Interventions	Evaluation
Patient will exhibit no evidence of infection	Use meticulous hand hygiene. Avoid contact with infected people. Monitor for signs of infection, including elevated temperature and elevated white blood cell count, which indicate possible infection. Provide frequent rest periods. Provide adequate nutrition; assess nutritional status, including daily weight. Be alert for signs of complications: • Heart failure • Digitalis toxicity • Increased respiratory effort • Hypoxemia • Cerebral thrombosis • Cardiovascular collapse	No evidence of infection is noted; temperature and white blood cell count remain within normal limits.

PATIENT PROBLEM

Potential for Inability to Tolerate Activity, related to imbalance between oxygen supply and demand

Patient Goals and Expected Outcomes	Nursing Interventions	Evaluation
Patient will maintain adequate energy levels	Allow for frequent rest periods. Encourage quiet, age-appropriate games and activities. Help child select activities appropriate to age, condition, and capabilities. Avoid extremes of environmental temperatures.	Patient is receiving adequate rest periods and is maintaining adequate energy levels.

PATIENT PROBLEM

Potential for Atypical Growth and Development, related to inadequate oxygen and nutrients to tissues

Patient Goals and Expected Outcomes	Nursing Interventions	Evaluation
Patient will achieve normal growth and development	Provide a diet high in nutrition. Provide pleasant environment for eating. Encourage patient to eat small, frequent meals. Provide snacks several times a day. Provide frequent rest periods between meals and activities. Encourage activities appropriate to the child's age and developmental level. Monitor for signs of heart failure and decreased cardiac output during activities. Arrange for continued family involvement during the child's hospitalization.	Patient is achieving normal growth and developmental milestones.

Nursing Care Plan 32.1 A Child With Congenital Heart Disease—cont'd

PATIENT PROBLEMS

Potential for Injury, related to cardiac condition and therapies
Insufficient Knowledge, related to the disorder and methods of treatment

Patient Goals and Expected Outcomes	Nursing Interventions	Evaluation
Family will demonstrate an understanding of the disorder and its treatments	Assess the family's understanding of the diagnosis. Reinforce the health care provider's explanation of the child's disorder and its treatments. Provide written instructions regarding medication schedules and treatment protocols. Encourage the family to verbalize questions, fears, and concerns. Allow the family to participate in the child's care when appropriate. Provide emotional support to the child and the family.	Family demonstrates understanding of child's cardiac condition as evidenced by verbal responses and therapeutic interventions.

CRITICAL THINKING QUESTIONS

1. You enter D.'s room and notice her mother sitting at her bedside crying. She states, "I don't know how I will deal with her having heart surgery." What would be an appropriate initial response to D.'s mother?
2. The mother states that D. has a very poor appetite. What two helpful suggestions may help educate the mother?
3. The mother mentions that she is concerned that D. will get an infection and become acutely ill. What are two therapeutic nursing interventions for patient teaching?

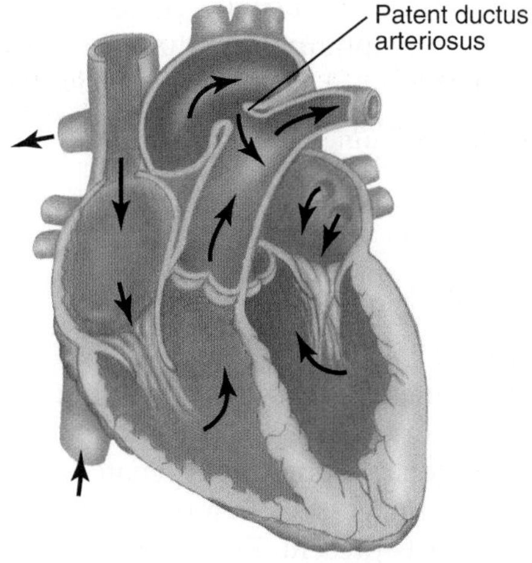

Fig. 32.4 Patent ductus arteriosus. (From James SR, Nelson KA, Ashwill JW: *Nursing care of children: Principles and practice,* ed 4, St. Louis, 2013, Saunders.)

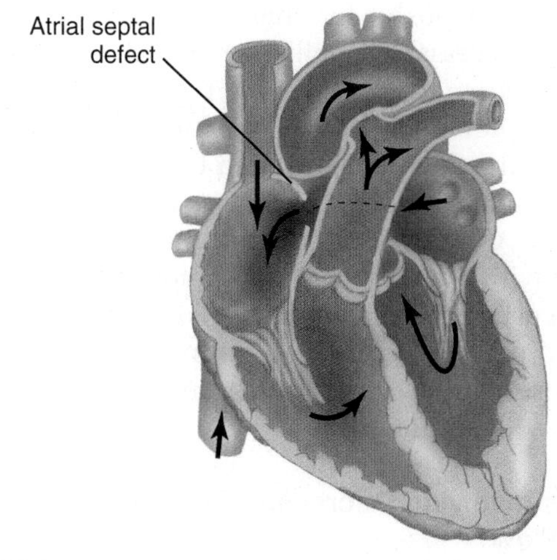

Fig. 32.5 Atrial septal defect. (From James SR, Nelson KA, Ashwill JW: *Nursing care of children: Principles and practice,* ed 4, St. Louis, 2013, Saunders.)

the lower pressure right atrium, which causes the blood to become deoxygenated (Fig. 32.5).

Clinical manifestations. Smaller defects (less than 5 mm in diameter) are often asymptomatic or do not produce symptoms until later in life. Larger defects produce manifestations consistent with heart failure. Additional manifestations include frequent respiratory infections and difficulty breathing. A characteristic harsh systolic murmur may be heard during auscultation over the third intercostal space ("Atrial septal defect [ASD]," 2015).

Medical management. Minor cases that are not producing symptoms often are not treated but are monitored for changes. Surgical correction consists of open heart surgery with cardiopulmonary bypass. The surgeon repairs small defects with purse-string sutures and moderate to large defects with a polyester fiber (Dacron) patch.

Ventricular septal defect. A ventricular septal defect (VSD) is an abnormal opening in the interventricular septum, resulting in the flow of oxygenated blood from the higher pressure left ventricle to the lower pressure right ventricle, which causes the blood to become deoxygenated. The possible scope of the defect ranges from a pinhole-sized opening to absence of the entire septum (single ventricle) (Fig. 32.6).

Clinical manifestations. Initially, such defects may be asymptomatic, but signs of heart failure eventually manifest. Other clinical manifestations include a loud, harsh systolic murmur and a palpable thrill.

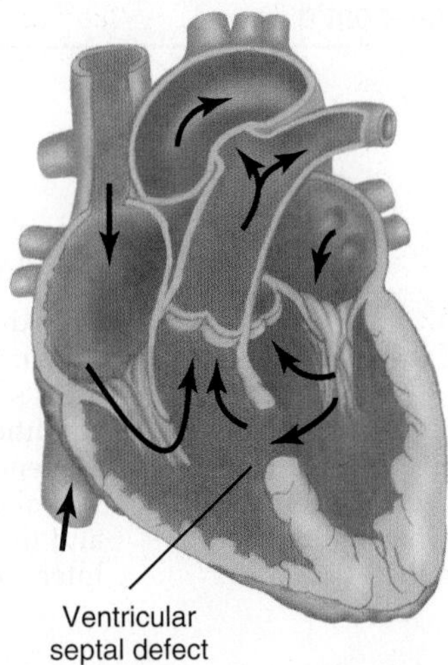

Fig. 32.6 Ventricular septal defect. (From James SR, Nelson KA, Ashwill JW: *Nursing care of children: Principles and practice*, ed 4, St. Louis, 2013, Saunders.)

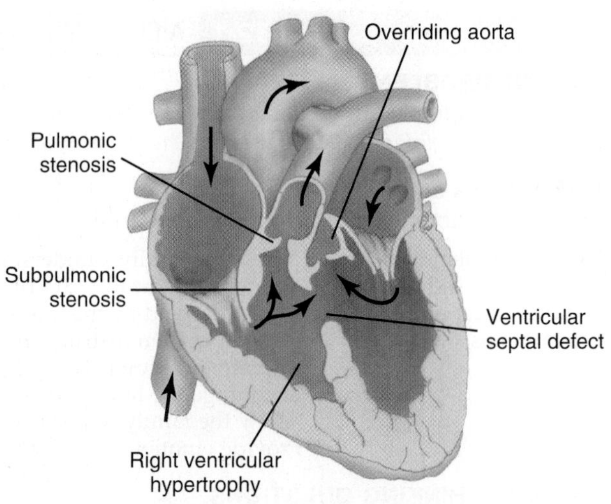

Fig. 32.7 Tetralogy of Fallot. (From James SR, Nelson KA, Ashwill JW: *Nursing care of children: Principles and practice*, ed 4, St. Louis, 2013, Saunders.)

Medical management. Approximately 50% of VSDs close spontaneously; for the remainder, open heart surgery is necessary. A palliative procedure, known as *pulmonary artery banding*, can be performed in infants with symptomatic VSDs. This procedure involves impeding the flow of blood from the right ventricle to the pulmonary circulation, thus reducing pulmonary congestion. Complete surgical repair involves open heart surgery with the use of cardiopulmonary bypass. The surgeon usually repairs the defect with a polyester fiber (Dacron) patch; smaller defects sometimes necessitate only observation or sometimes necessitate surgical closure with sutures.

Defects Involving Decreased Pulmonary Blood Flow

Defects involving decreased pulmonary blood flow result when there is some type of obstruction of blood flow to the lungs or if there is no connection between the right side of the heart and the lungs. Examples of defects involving decreased pulmonary blood flow include pulmonary stenosis, pulmonary atresia, and tetralogy of Fallot. The amount of obstruction or lack of connection determines the symptoms. The most common CHD resulting in decreased pulmonary blood flow is tetralogy of Fallot.

Tetralogy of Fallot. Tetralogy of Fallot involves a combination of four defects: (1) pulmonary stenosis, (2) VSD, (3) right ventricular hypertrophy, and (4) overriding aorta (Fig. 32.7).

Clinical manifestations. Affected infants tend to be profoundly cyanotic at birth and often experience acute episodes of severe cyanosis and hypoxia (blue spells). Older children with tetralogy of Fallot sometimes exhibit a systolic ejection murmur, clubbing of the nail beds, dyspnea, squatting, poor growth, mental slowness, syncope (fainting), and stroke.

Medical management. In infants with profound cyanosis and hypoxia, surgeons usually perform a palliative procedure. This temporary procedure, most commonly a Blalock-Taussig shunt, creates an artificial connection between the pulmonary artery and the aorta and thus redirects blood flow back to the lungs to allow for oxygenation. Complete surgical correction involves closure of the VSD, a pulmonic valvotomy, and repair of the overriding aorta.

Mixed Defects

Mixed defects include those that do not fit into one of the other categories. These defects often include the mixing of oxygenated and unoxygenated blood in the heart or the great vessels. Symptoms are specific to the type of defects present. Examples of mixed defects include transposition of the great vessels, truncus arteriosus, and hypoplastic left heart syndrome.

Transposition of the great vessels. In transposition of the great vessels, the pulmonary artery arises from the left ventricle and the aorta arises from the right ventricle. Therefore venous blood returning to the right side of the heart exits through the aorta without being oxygenated, and oxygenated blood returning from the pulmonary system is returned via the pulmonary artery to the lungs (Fig. 32.8). Some affected infants are born with associated defects that allow for communication between the two circulations.

Clinical manifestations. Infants born with minimal communication between the two circulations have profound cyanosis. Those who are born with an associated defect such as patent ductus arteriosus, atrial septal defect, or VSD sometimes have less cyanosis and experience manifestations of heart failure. Cardiomegaly is usually apparent on x-ray study.

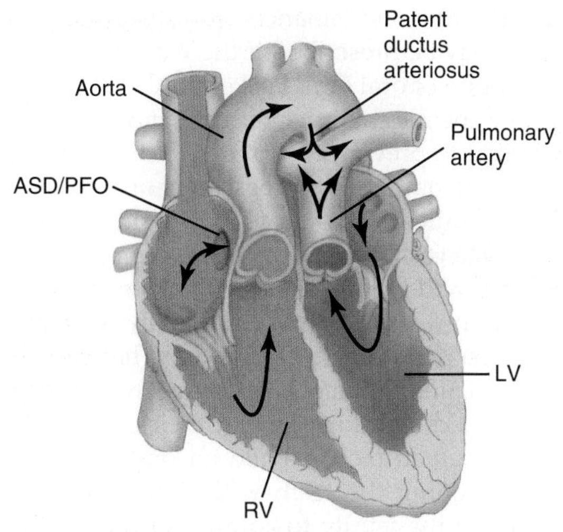

Fig. 32.8 Transposition of the great vessels. *ASD/PFO,* Atrial septal defect/patent foramen ovale; *LV,* left ventricle; *RV,* right ventricle. (From James SR, Nelson KA, Ashwill JW: *Nursing care of children: Principles and practice,* ed 4, St. Louis, 2013, Saunders.)

Medical management. Initially, the health care provider performs palliative procedures to provide mixing, either by enlarging an atrial septal defect that is already present or by creating one by pulling a balloon catheter through the atrial septum. Complete correction of transposition of the great vessels entails open heart surgery and involves switching the great vessels to their proper positions.

Defects Involving Obstruction to Systemic Blood Flow

Defects involving obstruction to systemic blood flow result in inability of the blood to reach the body from the heart. With this type of defect, symptoms include lack of oxygenation and decreased peripheral blood flow as a result of the obstruction, as well as symptoms of heart failure, because the blood backs up into the lungs. Defects resulting in obstruction to systemic blood flow include aortic stenosis, pulmonary stenosis, and coarctation of the aorta.

Coarctation of the aorta. Coarctation of the aorta is a narrowing of the lumen of the aorta (usually at the site of the ductus arteriosus), resulting in increased pressure proximal to the defect (head and upper extremities) and decreased pressure distal to the defect (body and lower extremities) (Fig. 32.9).

Clinical manifestations. The blood pressure in the arms is 20 mm Hg higher than that in the legs (reversal of normal pattern). Other manifestations include bounding pulses in the lower extremities, signs of heart failure, leg cramping on exertion in older affected children, and epistaxis.

Medical management. Surgical correction involves removal of the narrowed portion of the aorta with an end-to-end anastomosis (a connection between two vessels) or graft replacement if the narrowing is extensive.

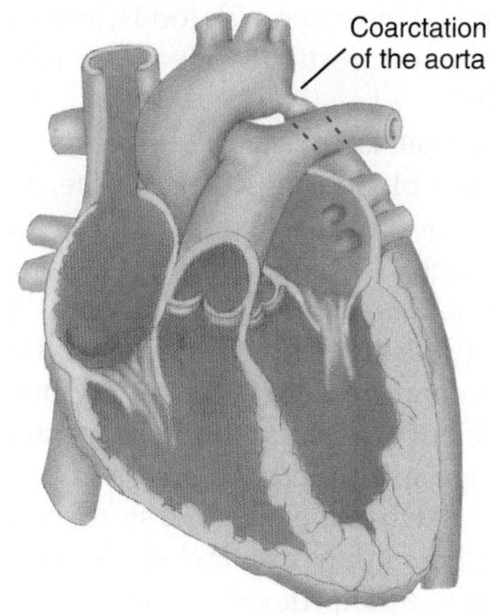

Fig. 32.9 Coarctation of the aorta. (From James SR, Nelson KA, Ashwill JW: *Nursing care of children: Principles and practice,* ed 4, St. Louis, 2013, Saunders.)

Acquired Heart Disease

Acquired heart disease refers to those disorders whose onset comes after birth. They result from a variety of reasons, including autoimmune processes, infection, familial tendencies, and environmental factors. One disease that has resurfaced and has caused concern to health care professionals is rheumatic fever.

DISORDERS OF HEMATOLOGIC FUNCTION

Childhood blood disorders encompass wide ranges of cause, severity, treatment, and prognosis. The majority of hematologic disorders occurring in infants and children stem from chronic systemic illness, nutritional deficits, and inherited blood disorders.

Anemias

Iron-deficiency anemia. Iron-deficiency anemia is the most prevalent blood disorder in infancy and early childhood; the incidence peaks between ages 6 and 24 months in children from lower-income backgrounds. The prevalence has decreased, probably in part because of families' participation in the Women, Infants, and Children (WIC) program, which provides iron-fortified formula for the first year of life.

Full-term, healthy infants have sufficient iron stores for the first 4 to 6 months of life. Breast-fed infants should receive adequate amounts of iron from the breast milk for the first 6 months of life. Infants who are not breast-fed should receive iron-fortified formulas for the first 9 to 12 months. Once introduction of foods begins, iron-fortified cereals and foods containing iron provide the necessary amount. The recommended daily allowance of iron for infants between the ages of 7 and 12 months is 11 mg of iron per day (NIH, 2018a). Toddlers require 7 mg/day of iron, and to meet this requirement, a diet of iron-rich foods, such as red meat, legumes, and iron-fortified cereals, is recommended (NIH, 2018).

Etiology and pathophysiology. *Anemia* is defined as a decrease in red blood cell (RBC) volume, a decrease in hemoglobin, or both. Anemia reduces the oxygen-carrying capacity of the blood and sometimes results in tissue hypoxia. Anemia is classified as either *hypoproliferative* (defective production of erythrocytes) or *hemolytic* (premature destruction of erythrocytes).

Iron-deficiency anemia develops at about 4 to 6 months of age in full-term infants and earlier in premature infants, when the maternal stores of iron become depleted and the infant becomes dependent on dietary sources of iron. Infants develop iron-deficiency anemia because milk is a poor source of iron and infants drink milk to the exclusion of solid foods. Infants who drink cow's milk have a 50% chance of increased fecal loss of blood. Anemic infants appear pale, may have poor muscle tone, and may be at increased risk for infection. Premature infants are at high risk because of a lower fetal iron supply.

Adolescents are also at risk for iron-deficiency anemia because of their rapid growth rate, combined with poor eating habits. The most common cause of anemia in adolescents is an inadequate intake of dietary iron, which is essential for hemoglobin synthesis. Other causes include acute or chronic blood loss and malabsorption of dietary iron secondary to chronic diarrhea or malabsorption syndromes.

Clinical manifestations. The clinical signs and symptoms of mild to moderate anemia (hemoglobin values: 6 to 10 g/dL) are often vague and nonspecific. They include irritability, weakness, decreased play activity, and fatigue. When the hemoglobin value falls below 5 g/dL, the child has anorexia, skin pallor, pale mucous membranes, glossitis, concave or "spoon" fingernails, inability to concentrate, tachycardia, and systolic murmurs. Children with chronic, long-term anemia often exhibit growth retardation and developmental delays.

Diagnostic tests. The diagnostic evaluation begins with an accurate history, including the information about the child's diet, appetite, activity, weight and rate of growth, and any recent blood loss. Initial laboratory tests include a complete blood cell count (CBC); reticulocyte count; and measurements of serum ferritin (a major iron-storage protein), serum iron concentration, and total iron-binding capacity. It is recommended that infants be screened for iron deficiency and iron deficiency anemia between the ages of 9 to 12 months of age (Mayo Clinic, 2016).

Medical management. Therapeutic management involves iron replacement therapy, nutritional counseling, and treatment of any underlying conditions (hemorrhage or malabsorption). Health care providers usually prescribe oral iron supplementation (ferrous sulfate) until the hemoglobin level returns to normal. Citrus fruits or juices with iron supplements may be advisable because ascorbic acid enhances iron absorption. Parenteral iron may be prescribed if there is a problem with the absorption of oral iron. Packed RBCs are given only to severely anemic children. Permanent dietary changes are essential to prevent recurrence. Mothers of infants should be encouraged to breast-feed or provide iron-fortified formulas and to provide iron-rich solid foods.

Nursing interventions. Dietary counseling is of primary importance, and the nurse's assistance to the family in choosing iron-rich foods is valuable. Advise giving oral preparations of iron three times daily between meals with citrus fruits or juices to enhance iron absorption. Parents should be informed that their child will have dark, tarry, green stools while on oral iron therapy. To avoid staining the teeth with liquid preparations of iron, teach the family to administer the medication with a syringe placed toward the back of the mouth for infants; older children can take the preparation through straws.

Patient teaching. A primary nursing objective is to educate the family in how to prevent nutritional anemia. For infants, discuss with parents the importance of using iron-fortified formula and the introduction of solid foods at the appropriate age. The best solid food source of iron is commercial infant cereals.

A difficulty encountered in discouraging the parents from feeding milk to the exclusion of other foods is dispelling the popular myth that milk is a perfect food. Many parents believe that milk is best for the infant and equate the weight gain with a healthy child and good parenting. They may not be concerned about providing other foods as long as the child continues to take milk. Stress that overweight is not synonymous with good health.

Diet education of teenagers is especially difficult, because teenage girls in particular are tempted to follow weight-reduction diets. Emphasizing the effects of anemia on appearance (pallor) and energy level (difficulty maintaining popular activities) is sometimes useful.

Prognosis. Serum iron levels usually return to normal within 2 months of treatment. Iron-deficiency anemia in infants and children may lead to difficulties in learning, a decrease in the attention span, and reduced alertness. In addition, iron deficiency can cause the body to absorb too much lead when exposed to the mineral.

Sickle cell anemia. Sickle cell anemia is one of a group of diseases collectively termed *hemoglobinopathies,* in which normal adult hemoglobin (hemoglobin A [HbA]) is replaced partially or completely by abnormal sickle hemoglobin (hemoglobin S [HbS]). Sickle cell anemia is a genetic disorder characterized by the abnormal form of hemoglobin within the erythrocyte. In the United States, the disease is most common in the African American population, with an incidence of 1 per 500 live births. Sickle cell anemia is classified as either sickle cell trait or active sickle cell disease. Sickle cell trait rarely results in clinical manifestations; however, children with sickle cell trait are carriers of sickle cell anemia. It is estimated that 1 per 13 African Americans have the sickle cell trait (Centers for Disease Control and Prevention [CDC], 2017). The rest of this discussion focuses on active sickle cell disease, which is the most severe and potentially fatal form of the disorder.

Etiology and pathophysiology. When oxygen is released into the tissues, the abnormal hemoglobin becomes more viscous and crystallizes, causing the erythrocyte to change from its characteristic round shape to an elongated, crescent shape (**sickled cell**). As sickled cells clump, circulation slows, resulting in obstructions with severe tissue hypoxia and necrosis. Sickling is an intermittent phenomenon; the usual precipitating factors are infection, fever, hypoxemia, dehydration, high altitudes, cold, or emotional stress.

Clinical manifestations. Children with sickle cell disease tend to first experience pallor, irritability, fatigue, and jaundice. Growth impairment becomes apparent as the child's height and weight fall below average. Cardiomegaly and heart failure develop in response to hypoxia and decreased cardiac output. In older affected children, the joints and surrounding tissue often become edematous and painful. If sickling causes cerebral occlusion, strokes can occur, which result in sensory deficits, paralysis, or death. Persistent penile erection (**priapism**) sometimes occurs in response to occluded penile veins. Severe sickling leads to recurrent sickle cell crisis, an acutely painful period that occurs intermittently throughout the life of a child with sickle cell disease (Fig. 32.10). A sickle cell crisis is classified as one of three types: vasoocclusive, sequestration, or aplastic (Box 32.1).

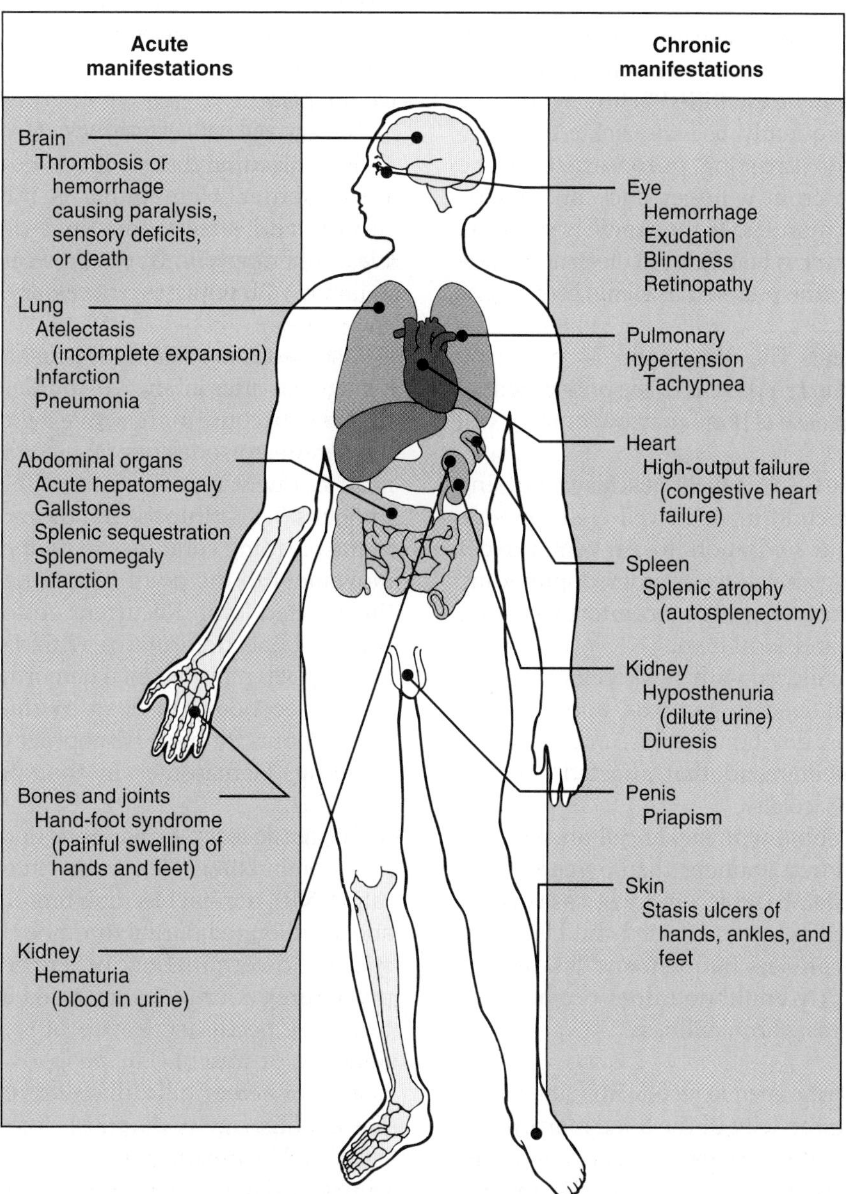

Fig. 32.10 Clinical manifestations of sickle cell disease. (From McCance KL, Huether SE: *Pathophysiology: The biologic basis for disease in adults and children*, ed 6, St. Louis, 2010, Mosby.)

Box 32.1 Types and Medical Management of Sickle Cell Crises

Vasoocclusive crisis: Obstruction of the small blood vessels of the hands and feet, resulting in edema, impaired range of motion, and pain
- Medical management: Palliative (analgesics, hydration, oxygen)

Sequestration crisis: Pooling of blood in the spleen and the liver, resulting in hepatosplenomegaly; sometimes progresses to cardiovascular collapse and death
- Medical management: Analgesics, volume expanders, transfusions; recurrent episodes treated by splenectomy

Aplastic crisis: Profound anemia, caused by premature destruction of erythrocytes
- Medical management: Transfusion of packed red blood cells

Diagnostic tests. Neonatal screening for sickle cell anemia is mandatory in most of the United States so that affected infants can be identified before symptoms occur. Institutions frequently use the sickle-turbidity test (SICKLEDEX) for screening purposes. It can be performed on blood from a finger stick and yields accurate results in 3 minutes. If the result is positive, the next step is to perform hemoglobin electrophoresis to determine whether the patient has sickle cell trait or sickle cell disease.

Medical management. The treatment is primarily palliative and is outlined in Box 32.1. The only potential cure for sickle cell disease is bone marrow or stem cell transplantation.

Nursing interventions and patient teaching. Nursing interventions for the child in sickle cell crisis include maintaining adequate hydration to prevent further sickling; administering analgesics as ordered; providing adequate oxygenation; and applying comfort measures such as warm baths and local heat.

Teach families of children with sickle cell anemia to avoid situations that lead to hypoxia and sickling: infection, dehydration, emotional stress, and strenuous physical activity. Recommend that affected children wear medical alert bracelets.

Prognosis. Most people with sickle cell anemia live into adulthood. Children younger than 5 years are at the highest risk for death, which in most cases is the result of severe infections. As an affected child becomes an adolescent, crises are less frequent and less severe; however, death in early adulthood does occur. Sickle cell anemia is a serious, chronic illness.

Aplastic anemia. Aplastic anemia results from the failure of the cell-generating capacity of the bone marrow. All formed elements of the blood are defective, underdeveloped, or absent, which results in severe anemia, leukopenia, and thrombocytopenia (pancytopenia). In some instances, aplastic anemia arises as a result of neoplastic disease of the bone marrow or, more commonly, from destruction of the bone marrow by exposure to toxic chemicals, ionizing radiation, or certain antibiotics or other medications. A failure of cell-producing capacity by aspirated bone marrow is diagnostic for aplastic anemia. In aplastic anemia, RBCs, white blood cells (WBCs), and platelets are deficient, and the red bone marrow becomes yellow and fatty. Treatment aims at restoring the function of the marrow through immunosuppressive treatment or at replacing the defective marrow through bone marrow transplantation. Survival rates at 5 years are about 70%. The rate of survival is highest in patients who received the transplant from close relatives (National Marrow Donor Program, n.d.).

Coagulation Disorders

Coagulation disorders in children characteristically involve abnormal bleeding into the skin or from internal organs, secondary to clotting factor defects, platelet dysfunction, or vascular compromise.

Hemophilia

Etiology and pathophysiology. Hemophilia is a serious, lifelong bleeding disease inherited as an X-linked recessive disorder. Hemophilia is transmitted by female carriers and affects boys in 1 per 5000 male births. Classic hemophilia (type A) is caused by a deficiency in factor VIII, which is a necessary component of blood coagulation.

Clinical manifestations. It is usually possible to make a diagnosis after infancy. In toddlerhood, when children typically become more active, hemophilic boys tend to have more episodes of oral bleeding and bruising. The most frequent types of internal bleeding occur within the joints (hemarthrosis) and the muscles. Pain intensifies as the bleeding continues to fill the joint cavity, limiting movement to the point where the child refuses to use the affected joint. Recurrent episodes of hemarthrosis lead to bone deformities with resulting contractures and crippling. Intracranial hemorrhage, either spontaneous or secondary to head trauma, is life threatening and accounts for more hemophilic deaths than any other bleeding. Hematomas in the spinal cord can cause paralysis.

Diagnostic tests. Laboratory findings include normal prothrombin time (PT), normal international normalized ratio (INR), normal bleeding time, normal platelet count, and a prolonged partial thromboplastin time (PTT). For specific determination of factor deficiencies, assay procedures normally performed in specialized laboratories are necessary. Levels of factors VIII and IX are deficient or absent. For people with a known family history of hemophilia, diagnosis can be made in utero. The average age of diagnosis for children is 9 months. Nearly 100% are diagnosed by the age of 2 years (Mayo Clinic, 2018b).

Medical management. For the most common type of hemophilia, small cuts and scrapes typically are treated with regular first aid (cleaning the cut, then applying pressure and a bandage). Deep cuts or internal bleeding may require that the missing clotting factor be administered so that a clot can form and the bleeding can be stopped (National Hemophilia Foundation, n.d.). Fibrin sealants also can be applied to wounds to promote direct clotting and healing of a wound. Antifibrolytics are clot-preserving medications that can help prevent clots from breaking down. Regular infusions of the hormone desmopressin (DDAVP) help in preventing bleeding from occurring (Mayo Clinic, 2018b).

Nursing interventions. Early recognition of the signs and symptoms of internal bleeding is very important, and the child should be treated aggressively with factor concentrate replacement therapy.

Nursing interventions focus on teaching the child and the family to avoid injury and control bleeding. The parents should be advised to give the child age-appropriate toys without rough or sharp edges, to remove throw rugs, and to place barriers at stairs. Playtime should be supervised to minimize hazards and injuries. Physical activity, such as swimming, softball, bicycling, hiking, bowling, golf, and running, should be recommended to promote muscle development and psychological well-being. The child should be advised against contact sports, such as football, hockey, or soccer, because of their potential for injury. Early dental visits with a dentist knowledgeable about hemophilia help minimize the risk of bleeding gums. Children with hemophilia should wear medical alert bracelets. The family also should be informed about the National Hemophilia Foundation, which is a good resource for financial, medical, and psychological assistance.

Patient teaching. Parents of children with hemophilia should be educated regarding the RICE method: *r*est, *i*ce, *c*ompression, and *e*levation. When external bleeding occurs, the affected area should be elevated while pressure and ice are applied. The child and family also should be instructed in safely administering factor products at home. Parents should seek emergency medical care if the child has signs of increased intracranial pressure, which sometimes indicates intracranial bleeding: severe headache, slurred speech, vomiting, disorientation, and loss of consciousness. The parents should be taught how to protect the child, but at the same time they should be encouraged not to be overprotective.

Prognosis. Medical advances have given children with hemophilia a normal life expectancy. Unfortunately, those who received blood transfusions before the use of the current purification techniques (before 1985) were at risk for exposure to the human immunodeficiency virus (HIV). People in whom hemophilia was diagnosed in the 1990s and have been treated with recombinant factor products are not at risk for developing HIV infections (Hockenberry and Wilson, 2015).

Gene therapy is a major focus of research. Some promising studies are being conducted in gene therapy that include infusion of the correct version of the gene that codes for clotting factor IX (Regalado, 2016).

Idiopathic thrombocytopenia purpura

Etiology and pathophysiology. Idiopathic (cause unknown) thrombocytopenia purpura (ITP) is characterized by a marked decrease in the number of circulating platelets with resultant bleeding beneath the skin. ITP is the most common thrombocytopenia of childhood, with onset most frequently among children aged 2 to 10 years. It occurs in either acute or chronic form. As its name implies, the cause of ITP is unknown; however, the condition is believed to be an autoimmune response to disease-related antigens. The acute form of ITP usually follows a viral infection (such as a respiratory infection, rubella, rubeola, mumps, or chickenpox; or after infection with parvovirus B19) and is self-limiting; the chronic form has periods of remission.

Clinical manifestations. Other than bleeding, the affected child appears healthy. The platelet count drops to below 20,000/mm^3, so clotting is impaired. Platelet counts lower than 10,000/mm^3 are potentially life threatening. Ecchymosis and a pinpoint petechial rash are usually the first signs of ITP, and the areas most commonly involved are over bony prominences. Other manifestations include bleeding gums, bleeding lips, and epistaxis (nosebleeds). The most serious complication of ITP is intracranial hemorrhage (bleeding into the subdural, subarachnoid, or intracerebellar space), and characteristic signs are hematuria (blood in urine), hemarthrosis, melena (black, tarry stools), hematemesis (blood in vomitus), and menorrhagia (abnormally heavy menstrual periods).

Diagnostic tests. Criteria indicating the possibility of this diagnosis are clinical manifestations. The platelet count is reduced to less than 20,000/mm^3. Microscopic examination reveals not only a decreased number of platelets but also platelets that are large. Bleeding time and clot reaction time are prolonged, and the tourniquet test for capillary fragility, in which a blood pressure cuff is inflated to 100 mm Hg and left in place for 5 minutes, yields a positive result: the appearance of more than 15 petechiae.

Medical management. ITP is a self-limiting illness in most cases, and about three-fourths of affected children recover without complications within 3 months. In most cases, health care providers allow ITP to run its course with supportive management. Some prescribe a short course of corticosteroids to suppress the immune attack on platelets, thereby reducing the severity of the disease. Transfusions of packed RBCs are sometimes necessary in treating severe, life-threatening hemorrhage. Use of intravenous gamma globulin (IVGG) and anti-D antibody therapy has achieved some success in treating chronic cases of ITP. Anti-D antibody therapy is a relatively new treatment that is much less expensive than IVGG. Children with symptomatic recurrent or chronic ITP that fails to respond to treatment for a year or longer usually undergo splenectomy, which eliminates the site of antiplatelet antibody production. Splenectomy removes the risk of hemorrhage, as well as the need for parents to closely monitor their child's activities. Before considering splenectomy, health care providers generally recommend waiting until the child is older than 5 years of age because of the increased risk of bacterial infection. In general, health care providers order pneumococcal and meningococcal vaccines before splenectomy. The child also receives penicillin prophylactically after splenectomy. The length of prophylactic therapy is controversial, but the usual recommendation is for a minimum of 3 years.

Nursing interventions and patient teaching. Nursing interventions are largely supportive. Preventing bruising and controlling bleeding are of primary importance in managing ITP. Offer education and emotional support.

The family must be taught to protect the child while the platelet count is lower than 100,000/mm^3, to restrict the child's activity, and to help the child avoid injury. It is best for children with ITP not to participate in any contact sports, bike riding, skateboarding, roller skating, gymnastics, climbing, or running. In addition, counsel the family never to depend on salicylate drugs (e.g., aspirin) for pain, because salicylates inhibit platelet function; salicylate substitutes such as acetaminophen (Tylenol) should be used instead. Instruct parents to notify their health care provider immediately if the child experiences acute head trauma and especially if the child exhibits symptoms of intracranial hemorrhage: headaches, visual disturbances, lethargy, vomiting, or disorientation.

Prognosis. For most children with ITP, the course is self-limited, with complete recovery within 6 months. For children who develop a chronic form of ITP, a splenectomy may be advised.

Neoplastic Disorders

Neoplastic disorders are the leading cause of death from disease in children past infancy. Although therapeutic advances in drug treatment (chemotherapy), radiation therapy, and surgical techniques have increased the potential for a normal lifespan, cancer remains a catastrophic, emotionally devastating diagnosis for the child and family.

Leukemia. *Leukemia* is the name given to a group of malignant diseases of the bone marrow and the lymphatic system. Leukemia is the most common malignancy of childhood and is more common in boys than in girls with an incidence peak between the ages of 2 and 6 years. It is, however, one of the forms of cancer for which survival rates have improved dramatically. Among children with acute lymphoid leukemia, the 5-year rate of survival is more than 85% (American Cancer Society, 2016a).

Etiology and pathophysiology. The type of leukemia that is most common in children is acute lymphoid leukemia (ALL), followed by acute nonlymphoid (myelogenous) leukemia. Although its cause is unknown, its pathologic characteristic is the uncontrollable proliferation of blast cells (immature WBCs), which accumulate in the marrow and cause crowding and depression of other healthy cells (mature WBCs, RBCs, and platelets).

Leukemia involves an overproduction of WBCs, although in the acute form of the disease, the WBC count is low. Bone marrow and peripheral blood smears show numerous, immature WBCs or blasts. Although the normal blood cells and vascular tissue are not destroyed directly by the leukemic cells, the leukemic cells infiltrate and crowd the normal cells, depriving them of the nutrients necessary for metabolism. Three problems and effects develop as a result: (1) the decrease in RBCs causes anemia, (2) neutropenia leads to infection, and (3) the decrease in platelets causes bleeding (Hockenberry and Wilson, 2015). As nonfunctional blast cells infiltrate the lymph nodes, liver, kidneys, and spleen, they cause organ enlargement, which produces the clinical manifestations of acute leukemia.

Clinical manifestations. Anemia, with pallor and fatigue, is often severe and often the first symptom of leukemia. Other signs are leukopenia, fever, infection, thrombocytopenia, bleeding, bruising, and petechiae. Blast cells also may invade bones, which results in bone and joint pain, limping, and edema. Bone fractures are the result of the weakening of the bone caused by the infiltration of the bone marrow by leukemic cells. Hepatosplenomegaly and enlargement of lymph nodes are often present at diagnosis. Involvement of the central nervous system (CNS) is secondary to leukemic infiltration, which sometimes causes increased intracranial pressure.

Diagnostic tests. Diagnosis is based on review of the patient's symptoms, medical history, and results of a complete physical examination. A CBC typically indicates pancytopenia (decreased amounts of RBCs, WBCs, and platelets). Diagnostic findings in bone marrow aspirate and peripheral blood smear are immature blastic leukocyte cells. Performing a lumbar puncture is an option to determine whether the CNS has been infiltrated.

Medical management. The health care provider institutes a highly individualized treatment protocol immediately after diagnosis. Many of the drugs used to bring about remission have the capacity to cause a serious depletion of blood elements. Therefore the period immediately after remission is characterized by vulnerability to serious infection and hemorrhage. Supportive therapy is critical until the bone marrow recovers.

Almost immediately after confirmation of the diagnosis, induction therapy begins and lasts for 4 to 6 weeks. The principal drugs that serve for induction in ALL are corticosteroids (especially prednisone), vincristine, and L-asparaginase, with or without doxorubicin. Drug therapy for ALL includes doxorubicin or daunorubicin (or daunomycin) and cytosine arabinoside.

To prevent the development of CNS leukemia, prophylactic treatment has become a standard protocol. However, the blood-brain barrier prohibits most systemic drugs from penetrating the CNS; therefore the intrathecal route (in which the health care provider injects the drugs directly into the cerebrospinal fluid via lumbar puncture) is the route of choice for CNS prophylaxis. Methotrexate, the drug of choice, is given intrathecally but also may be given intravenously, along with other chemotherapeutic agents, such as triple intrathecal agent (consisting of methotrexate, cytarabine, and hydrocortisone). Once remission has occurred, the health care provider initiates maintenance therapy in an effort to maintain remission and further reduce leukemic cells. The protocol includes daily doses of 6-mercaptopurine, weekly doses of methotrexate, and monthly doses of prednisone and vincristine for 2 to 3 years.

Nursing interventions. An important nursing intervention in dealing with children with any type of childhood cancer is to be available to the family, especially in the early phases of diagnosis and treatment.

Patient problems and interventions for a child with cancer include but are not limited to the following:

Patient Problem	Nursing Interventions
Potential for Infection, related to impaired immune system	Provide private room; use neutropenic precautions if necessary Restrict all visitors and health care providers with active infection Use strict hand hygiene technique Monitor the patient's temperature Use aseptic technique for all skin punctures Administer granulocyte colony–stimulating factor subcutaneously, as prescribed, to reduce the incidence and duration of infection in children receiving chemotherapy treatment for cancer In some research centers, special germ-free environments are available during complete myelosuppression from intensive chemotherapy or for bone marrow transplantation
Potential for Insufficient Nutrition, related to • Nausea • Vomiting • Anorexia	Encourage the patient to eat frequent, small meals of any food tolerated; plan to improve quality of food selections when appetite increases Take advantage of hungry period; serve small snacks Fortify foods with nutritious supplements, such as powdered milk or commercial supplements Allow child to be involved in food preparation and selection when appropriate
Anxiousness, related to unknown outcome	Instruct patient and family about treatments Promote atmosphere of open communication Encourage patient and family to ventilate feelings Recognize developmental fears associated with illness, procedures, and disturbance in self-esteem

Patient teaching. When working with families of children with cancer, the nurse has a significant supportive role in helping them understand the therapies; preventing or managing expected side effects or toxic effects; observing for late effects of treatment; and helping the child and family live as normal a life as possible and cope with the emotional aspects of the disease. Education is a constant feature of the nursing role, especially with regard to new treatments, clinical trials, and home care. Monitor the children closely after completion of treatment to evaluate for possible recurrence or to note any long-term complications as a result of the treatment.

Prognosis. Children younger than 1 year and older than 10 years when ALL is diagnosed are considered patients at high risk. Girls appear to have a slightly more favorable prognosis than do boys. African American and Hispanic children with ALL tend to have a slightly lower cure rate than do children of other races. Of children with acute nonlymphoid (myelogenous) leukemia, those younger than 2 years tend to respond better to treatment than do older children. With both types of leukemia, children who respond quickly to treatment are more likely to have a favorable outcome (American Cancer Society, 2016a).

Hodgkin's lymphoma. Childhood Hodgkin's lymphoma is a malignant lymphoma distinguished by painless, progressive enlargement of lymphoid tissue, fever, night sweats, and weight loss. Although the exact cause is unknown, it is believed to develop in one specific site and to spread to nearby lymph nodes through the lymphatic vessels. Infection with the Epstein-Barr virus is a risk factor for developing the disease. Classical Hodgkin's lymphoma and nodular lymphocyte-predominant Hodgkin's lymphoma are the two types of childhood Hodgkin's lymphoma. The most common sites for Hodgkin's lymphoma to develop are in the chest, the neck, and under the arms, and groin. Lymph node biopsy helps determine the presence of Reed-Sternberg cells, an abnormal type of B lymphocyte that is the main diagnostic feature of Hodgkin's lymphoma (NIH, National Cancer Institute, 2018).

Prognosis. If the diagnosis of childhood Hodgkin's lymphoma is detected early and treated promptly, the prognosis is favorable for curing the disease. Factors such as the stage of the cancer, features of the cancer cells, and how well the tumor responds to treatment determine the prognosis and curability (NIH, National Cancer Institute, 2018).

DISORDERS OF IMMUNE FUNCTION

Immunodeficiency disorders result from impairment of immune function with alteration of the immune (self-defense) response. Immunodeficiency disorders are classified as primary or secondary. Primary immunodeficiency disorders result from genetic or congenital abnormalities and include X-linked agammaglobulinemia (defect in B cell development), DiGeorge's syndrome (congenital absence of thymus and parathyroid glands), and severe combined immune deficiency (absence of B and T lymphocytes and of phagocytic cells). Secondary immunodeficiency disorders, the most common form of immunodeficiency, are disorders acquired in association with certain drug therapies such as corticosteroids, cancer chemotherapy, and antibiotics; radiation therapy; splenectomy; and viral infections. The common indicator in all immunodeficiency disorders is the development of unusual or recurrent, severe infections.

Human immunodeficiency virus (HIV) and acquired immunodeficiency syndrome (AIDS)

Etiology and pathophysiology. AIDS is a chronic and usually fatal disease caused by an acquired dysfunction of the immune system. AIDS is caused by HIV, which has been found in blood and in varying amounts in body fluids (semen, vaginal secretions, breast milk, tears, saliva, and urine). Children may become infected with HIV by their mother while in utero, during delivery, or through breast-feeding. Additional means of infection include sexual abuse by an infected offender and participation in high-risk behaviors such as intravenous (IV) drug use and unsafe sexual activity. Children living with HIV in the United States reflect a relatively small portion of the population of children infected worldwide (UNAIDS Fact Sheet, 2017).

HIV targets the cells that have the $CD4^+$ molecules on their surface, especially the T helper lymphocytes. These cells are targeted because they have more $CD4^+$ receptors on their surfaces than do any other cells. Immune dysfunction occurs as a result of the destruction of T helper cells by HIV. A normal $CD4^+$ lymphocyte count is 500/µL to 1600/µL of blood. The immune system remains healthy when $CD4^+$ counts exceed 500 cells/µL. Severe immune problems occur when the $CD4^+$ count falls below 200/µL, which heightens the risk for opportunistic diseases and death from AIDS (HIV.gov, 2017).

Transmission of HIV to the infant during pregnancy, labor, and delivery has decreased to less than to 10% since the 1990s. Interventions that have led to the decrease in the transmission rate include the use of antiretroviral drugs for prophylaxis, the avoidance of breast-feeding, and elective cesarean delivery (CDC, 2018a).

Clinical manifestations. Symptoms of HIV and AIDS infection in children range from no symptoms to severe, life-threatening illnesses. Signs and symptoms common to HIV and AIDS in children include failure to thrive; weight loss; meningitis; delayed physical and developmental growth; frequent and long lasting fevers and sweats; and frequent viral and bacterial infections (cytomegalovirus, herpes simplex virus, otitis media, sinusitis, enterocolitis, recurrent pneumonia, and septicemia).

The greatest threat to an HIV-infected infant younger than 1 year is *Pneumocystis jiroveci* (formerly *Pneumocystis carinii*) pneumonia, which is sometimes life threatening (Boston Children's Hospital, n.d.). Unique findings in the pediatric population with AIDS include lymphocytic interstitial pneumonia, oral and diaper-area candidiasis, and chronic ear infections. One of the most common causes of CNS mass lesions in HIV-infected children is malignant CNS lymphoma. In contrast to HIV-infected adults, infected children rarely contract Kaposi's sarcoma. Male and female infected adolescents demonstrate more adult-oriented symptoms; girls exhibit gynecologic manifestations similar to those seen in infected women. When caring for an HIV-infected adolescent, remember that the patient is still a child and still developing cognitively, physically, and emotionally.

Diagnostic tests. In children older than 18 months, health care providers establish the diagnosis of HIV infection by using the same serologic tests for the presence of serum HIV antibodies—enzyme-linked immunosorbent assay (ELISA) and Western blot—as in adults. The individual's blood is tested with ELISA or enzyme immunoassay (EIA), antibody tests that detect the presence of HIV antibodies. If the ELISA or EIA result is positive for HIV, then the same blood is tested a second time. If the result on the second test is positive, a more specific confirming test such as the Western blot is performed. Blood that is reactive or positive in all three steps is reported to be HIV positive. The diagnosis in a child younger than 18 months is complicated by the fact that in the seropositive mother, maternal HIV antibodies cross the placenta to the fetus. In most exposed infants up to 18 months of age, tests yield results positive for HIV antibodies, but it is unclear whose antibodies are being detected during this time.

A polymerase chain reaction (PCR) test, which tests for the presence of HIV, not for the antibody, is available to definitively diagnose HIV infection early in infants younger than 18 months. The benefits of this type of testing include early identification and treatment of the HIV-infected infant, as well as decreased anxiety and waiting time for HIV-negative parents with HIV-exposed infants.

Medical management. There is currently no cure for HIV. Treatment is aimed at slowing the progression of the virus, prevention and treatment of opportunistic

Box 32.2 Antiretroviral Drugs

NUCLEOSIDE REVERSE TRANSCRIPTASE INHIBITORS (NRTIs)
- lamivudine and zidovudine (Combivir)
- lamivudine, 3TC (Epivir)
- zidovudine, azidothymidine, AZT, ZDV (Retrovir)
- didanosine, ddI (Videx)
- abacavir sulfate, ABC (Ziagen)

NON-NUCLEOSIDE REVERSE TRANSCRIPTASE INHIBITORS (NNRTIs)
- rilpivirine (Edurant)
- efavirenz, EFV (Sustiva)
- nevirapine, NVP (Viramune XR)

PROTEASE INHIBITORS (PIs)
- tipranavir, TPV (Aptivus)
- saquinavir mesylate, SQV (Invirase)
- lopinavir and ritonavir, LPV/RTV (Kaletra)
- nelfinavir mesylate, NFV (Viracept)

HIV INTEGRASE STRAND TRANSFER INHIBITOR
- elvitegravir

infections, maintaining normal growth and development, and maintaining quality of life.

Combinations of antiretroviral drugs help prevent reproduction of new virus particles. Antiretroviral therapy does not cure the HIV-infected patient but does assist in preventing further destruction of the immune system. The antiretroviral drugs used in HIV therapy are listed and organized by category in Box 32.2. A combination of several antiretroviral drugs is prescribed to prevent resistance to the drugs from developing. Research continues in the development of treatment for HIV-positive patients. Therapy is lifelong, which makes adherence to the regimen difficult. Laboratory markers (CD4$^+$ lymphocyte count, viral load) assist in monitoring disease progression and response to therapy.

It is important that HIV-infected children keep current with all childhood immunizations. The weakened immune system may not produce antibodies to vaccines. Therefore, after exposure to childhood diseases such as varicella, measles, and rubella, prophylaxis treatment may be advised.

Nursing interventions. The nursing interventions are basically the same for the adult and pediatric populations. However, it is necessary to monitor HIV-infected children closely for signs of abnormal growth and development, which are common in this population. Complications of HIV-related infections often cause severe failure to thrive and numerous nutritional deficiencies. Because of anorexia, nausea, and diarrhea associated with recurrent illness, it is often difficult to maintain adequate nutrition. If the child exhibits weight loss and slowing of growth and development, the health care provider initiates intensive nutritional interventions (Hockenberry and Wilson, 2015). If the family is involved in the child's care, nursing interventions should be directed at emotionally supporting the family. Whenever possible, make arrangements for the intervention of social services and home health and nutritional services, such as the Women, Infants, and Children (WIC) program.

Patient problems and interventions for a child with HIV include but are not limited to the following:

Patient Problem	Nursing Interventions
Potential for Infection, related to • Impaired body defenses • Presence of infective organisms	Restrict contact with people who have infections, including family, other children, friends, and members of staff Practice thorough hand hygiene Place child in room with noninfectious children; restrict visitors with active illnesses Advise visitors (and hospital personnel) to practice thorough hand hygiene Promote body's remaining natural defenses (e.g., good nutrition)
Compromised Social Interaction, related to • Physical limitations • Hospitalizations • Social stigma surrounding AIDS	Administer medication as prescribed Assist child in identifying personal strengths Educate school personnel and classmates about AIDS Encourage child to participate in activities with other children
Potential for Complex Grief, related to having a child with a potentially fatal illness	Identify stage of grieving process that the family is experiencing Provide opportunities for the family to express emotions Help the parents deal with their feelings, which allows them more emotional reserve to meet the needs of their children Encourage the parents to share their moments of sorrow with their children Facilitate the family's assistance with the child's care

Patient teaching. The adolescent population is contracting HIV infection with increasing incidence. Changing moral standards, increased sexual freedom, increased IV drug use, and misinformation about the disease in this age group render adolescents at high risk for exposure to the disease. As a patient advocate, educate adolescents directly by counseling them on matters such as avoiding casual sex and using a condom during intercourse. Promote educational messages in the media, such as radio and social media, and in places that youths frequent.

Prognosis. Infants infected in the perinatal period generally have more rapid disease progression than do children infected at older ages or adults. It has been reported that the risk of dying is higher for children in whom AIDS is diagnosed early in life and in those who develop *P. jiroveci* pneumonia. Early recognition and improved medical treatments have changed the course of HIV infection in children from a rapidly fatal illness to a chronic but still terminal disease of childhood. The ultimate prognosis for children with perinatal HIV infection depends strongly on counseling pregnant women about HIV infection, voluntary testing, and the methods currently in practice for the prevention of perinatal transmission.

Juvenile idiopathic arthritis

Etiology and pathophysiology. *Juvenile idiopathic arthritis (JIA)*—also known as *juvenile rheumatoid arthritis*—is chronic arthritis occurring during childhood. JIA is the most common chronic form of joint inflammation in children, affecting girls twice as often as boys. The condition may manifest as early as 6 months of age. In most affected children, it is diagnosed by age 16 years.

JIA is characterized by chronic inflammation of the synovium with joint effusion. This inflammatory process leads to erosion, destruction, and fibrosis of the articular cartilage. The exact cause of the inflammatory process is unknown, but the supposition is that the tissue injury arises from a previous infectious process. There are several different types of JIA. The different types are classified partly on the basis of the areas of the body affected and the condition manifestations.

Clinical manifestations. JIA may affect a single joint or numerous joints. The affected joints may be stiff and warm to the touch. Systemic manifestations may include fever and rash. The physical examination may reveal swelling in the spleen, liver, and lymph nodes. Eye involvement, such as uveitis or iritis, also may be noted. Changes in vision may include red eyes and photosensitivity, although most children with eye involvement have no symptoms, so routine eye examinations are essential to detect early clinical manifestations.

Diagnostic tests. The diagnosis is made by the clinical presentation of the patient as well as diagnostic testing. Children who have the condition may exhibit normal findings on the traditional battery of tests performed to diagnose the disease. Initially, the history is reviewed, and other potential causes are ruled out. Laboratory tests include measurement of the erythrocyte sedimentation rate, which is elevated in the condition; CBC; measurement of C-reactive protein, to measure levels of inflammation; and search for antinuclear antibodies (ANA), which are present in the condition. Radiographic studies in early-onset JIA sometimes show the widening of joint spaces and, later, fusion and articular destruction. Regular eye examinations are indicated for a child with the condition.

Medical management. The goals of management include the prevention of joint contractures, preservation of joint function, and relief of signs and symptoms. There is no specific cure for JIA. Nonsteroidal antiinflammatory drugs (NSAIDs), which include naproxen (Naprosyn) and ibuprofen (Motrin), are the first line of drug treatment. Stronger prescription NSAIDs may be ordered by health care providers if over-the-counter NSAIDs are not effective. In addition, corticosteroids may be ordered to control exacerbations of inflammation. Health care providers usually add slower-acting antirheumatic drugs (SAARDs) to the drug therapy when one or two of the NSAIDs no longer effectively control signs and symptoms. The SAARDs include methotrexate, sulfasalazine (Azulfidine), and hydroxychloroquine (Plaquenil).

The class of medications known as disease-modifying antirheumatic drugs (DMARDs) is used when other treatment options become ineffective. DMARDs include methotrexate (Trexall) and sulfasalazine (Azulfidine) and can be used in combination with NSAIDs. The disadvantage of this class of medications is the increased chance of infection. Tumor necrosis factor (TNF)–blocking agents such as etanercept (Enbrel) and adalimumab (Humira) are the next step of treatment when SAARDs do not control symptoms. TNF blockers help in reducing pain, morning stiffness, and joint swelling. The disadvantage of TNF blockers is the increased the risk for infections, as well as the increased chance that lymphoma or another type of cancer will develop. Immune suppressants such as abatacept (Orencia) and rituximab (Rituxan) help slow the overactivity of the immune system in JIA. Symptom treatment for JIA includes physical therapy to improve joint mobility. Surgical intervention is sometimes necessary for children experiencing severe JIA that is unresponsive to therapy. Surgical procedures are performed to relieve pain or correct joint deformities. Joint replacement surgery also may be necessary.

Nursing interventions. A key role of the nurse in care of a child with JIA begins with a thorough collection of data. Assessment of difficulties and activity intolerance should be evaluated closely. Emotional support and teaching about planned diagnostic testing are indicated. The family and child should be encouraged to express fears and concerns. The patient and parents need instruction concerning the best means to conserve strength while attempting to participate in the normal activities of daily living. Rest, exercise, and pharmacologic therapies are the cornerstones of treatment. Independence, when possible, should be stressed. Suggested physical activity for the affected child includes walking, bicycling, and swimming. Disease management strategies, such as the use of heat and cold and range-of-motion exercises, are included in the topics of education. Suggest support groups for the child and the parents that provide the necessary education and resources to cope effectively with a chronic, debilitating illness. Referrals to the Arthritis Foundation *(www.arthritis.org)* and *www.kidsgetarthritistoo.org* can provide this assistance.

Patient problems and interventions for a child with JIA include but are not limited to the following:

Patient Problem	Nursing Interventions
Prolonged Pain, related to joint inflammation	Provide as much relief as possible with antiinflammatory medication and other therapies to help the child tolerate the pain and cope as effectively as possible (although complete pain relief is desirable, it is probably unattainable) Apply moist heat to relieve pain and stiffness (the most efficient and practical method is tub baths)
Compromised Physical Mobility, related to joint discomfort and stiffness	Promote activities of daily living to provide satisfactory exercise and increase mobility Encourage lying in the prone position to straighten hips and knees Instruct patient and family in the purpose and correct use of any splints and appliances Instruct in use of elevated toilet seat for independent toileting

Prognosis. The course of JIA is highly variable. Children who have systemic involvement may not achieve remission and may require long-term treatment into adulthood. These children may experience joint damage and disability. Early recognition and treatment of the disease may prevent permanent joint damage, and some children will experience complete remission.

DISORDERS OF RESPIRATORY FUNCTION

Acute respiratory infections are extremely common in infants and children. The possibilities range from minor to life-threatening illnesses. Most respiratory illnesses involve viral pathogens. Bacterial infections most commonly involve groups A- and β-hemolytic streptococci (GABHS), *Staphylococcus aureus,* and *Haemophilus influenzae.*

Disorders Involving the Entire Respiratory Tract

Respiratory distress syndrome

Etiology and pathophysiology. *Respiratory distress syndrome (RDS), idiopathic respiratory distress syndrome,* and *hyaline membrane disease* are synonymous terms for the severe lung disorder that is the major cause of morbidity and mortality in the neonatal period. RDS is caused by a deficiency of surfactant and occurs almost exclusively in preterm infants of low birth weight. RDS occurs more often in boys and in infants delivered by cesarean section. Other predisposing factors include maternal diabetes, asphyxia, maternal hemorrhage, and shock. Surfactant reduces the surface tension of fluids that line the alveoli, thereby enabling expansion of the lungs and alveolar inflation. Without sufficient production of surfactant, the infant is unable to keep the lungs inflated and the alveoli collapse at the end of expiration, resulting in hypoxia, atelectasis, and respiratory acidosis.

Clinical manifestations. Respiratory signs and symptoms become apparent immediately after birth. Signs and symptoms include nasal flaring; expiratory grunting; intercostal, subcostal, or substernal retractions; dusky color involving the skin, nail beds, and mucous membranes; tachypnea (up to 80 to 120 breaths/min) initially and dyspnea; and low body temperature. Manifestations as the disease progresses include apnea, flaccidity, absence of spontaneous movement, unresponsiveness, and mottling. In severe cases, infants sometimes die within hours of the onset of signs and symptoms; those who survive gradually show improvement by the fourth day.

Diagnostic tests. Criteria for the diagnosis of RDS consist of the clinical manifestations and the radiographic findings. Blood gas analysis indicates the degree of respiratory and metabolic acidosis.

Medical management. The treatment of RDS is entirely supportive and aims to correct imbalances. Supportive measures include maintaining a neutral thermal environment, providing adequate oxygenation either by increasing ambient (pertaining to the surrounding area) oxygen concentration or by ventilatory assistance, and correction of respiratory and metabolic acidosis. To prevent hypoxia and the toxic effects of high concentrations of oxygen, it is necessary to evaluate oxygen therapy continually by measuring arterial oxygen. Health care providers order nutritional support through parenteral therapy during the early acute stage to prevent aspiration. Nipple and gavage feeding are contraindicated in any situation that creates a marked increase in respiratory rate because of the greater hazards of aspiration.

In infants at high risk of developing or who have developed RDS, the administration of exogenous (originating outside the body) pulmonary surfactant has reduced greatly the rates of morbidity and mortality associated with the disorder. Exogenous surfactant is administered by an endotracheal tube directly into the infant's trachea and lungs shortly after birth. Additional doses sometimes are given. In some cases, the mother is given corticosteroids such as betamethasone before delivery to increase the production of surfactant in the preterm infant.

Nursing interventions and patient teaching. The primary nursing consideration in caring for an infant with RDS is to observe and assess the infant's response to therapy. Continuous monitoring and assessment are essential to adjust oxygen concentrations and ventilator settings in response to the infant's blood gas measurements and pulse oximetry readings. Perform frequent respiratory assessments, observe the infant's behavior, and observe for signs of respiratory complications and sepsis. Perform suctioning as needed, on the basis of assessment findings in the infant (auscultation, increased infant irritability, excessive moisture in the endotracheal tube). Suctioning must never be performed on a routine basis; frequent, vigorous suctioning increases the risk of bronchospasm, airway damage, infection, **pneumothorax** (a collection of air or gas in the pleural space that causes the lung to collapse), hypoxia, and increased intracranial pressure that can lead to intraventricular hemorrhage in the neonate. Help the infant maintain an open airway by positioning the infant on the side with the head supported in alignment. Assess the infant's skin frequently and protect the skin from impairment by frequent repositioning and the use of water mattresses or pillows and sheepskin. A water-soluble ointment is applied to reduce irritation to the nares or around the mouth, and frequent oral hygiene with water is performed to help relieve dryness caused by oxygen therapy.

Parents of such infants need emotional support. Encourage them to discuss their anxieties and concerns. Encourage parents to touch, hold, and talk to their infant and participate in the care whenever possible to promote bonding.

Prognosis. RDS is a self-limiting disease. Infants with RDS who survive the first 96 hours have a reasonable chance of recovery. Surfactant replacement therapy tends to improve the survival rate and reduce the severity of RDS.

Prevention. Prevention of premature delivery is the most effective preventive measure for RDS. Amniocentesis can determine fetal lung maturity before delivery.

Bronchopulmonary dysplasia

Etiology and pathophysiology. Bronchopulmonary dysplasia (BPD) is a chronic pulmonary disorder that develops in premature infants. BPD arises in association with meconium aspiration, RDS, high concentrations of oxygen, positive-pressure ventilation, and endotracheal intubation. Chronic lung changes include thickening and necrosis of alveolar walls with impairment of oxygen diffusion from the alveoli to the capillaries. Edema and inflammation of the capillary bed can cause some alveoli to collapse, some to hyperinflate, and others to rupture. Diffuse infiltrates, hyperinflation, and chronic pulmonary insufficiency characterize the disorder.

Clinical manifestations. The clinical signs and symptoms of BPD vary. Most affected infants show evidence of respiratory distress (wheezing, retracting, nasal flaring, irritability, abundant secretions, and cyanosis when stressed). These children are vulnerable to upper respiratory infections and frequently require hospitalization because of poor respiratory status.

Diagnostic tests. No specific signs, symptoms, or laboratory data confirm a diagnosis of BPD. Radiographic examination and ABG determinations are often helpful in making the diagnosis. Pulmonary function tests typically help determine the degree of lung dysfunction.

Medical management. Medical management involves taking precautions to prevent RDS and to reduce requirements for ventilation and oxygen. When ventilation and oxygen are necessary, meticulous management is necessary in using the lowest concentration of oxygen and ventilatory pressures to maintain adequate gas exchange to avoid further damage of lung tissue. During weaning, bronchodilators may be used to decrease airway resistance and increase lung compliance. Management includes nutritional support, provided initially by total parenteral nutrition and later by nasogastric, gavage, or breast-feeding or formula feeding.

Nursing interventions and patient teaching. Rest periods should be planned to decrease respiratory effort and conserve energy. When it is time to begin oral feedings, provide small, frequent feedings to prevent overdistention of the stomach, which can interfere with respiratory effort. You are instrumental in emotionally supporting parents and should encourage them to participate in their infant's care.

Parents also need counseling regarding ways to reduce the risk of respiratory infections. Instruct them to notify their health care provider at the first sign of a respiratory infection in their child. Teach parents cardiopulmonary resuscitation and how to manage any other possibly anticipated emergency.

Prognosis. Infants with BPD have a high mortality rate in the first year. Infants who survive are at risk for chronic lung disease. The use of exogenous surfactant in newborns with RDS has reduced the incidence of BPD greatly and its morbidity in at-risk infants.

Pneumonia

Etiology and pathophysiology. Pneumonia is an acute inflammation of the pulmonary parenchyma (tissue), small airways, and alveoli. Pneumonia is classified according to the causative agent: bacterial, viral, mycoplasmal, or foreign body aspiration. Pneumonia is common throughout childhood, occurs more frequently in infants and young children, and usually is associated with an upper respiratory infection. Pneumonias are most common in the winter months, from November through March. Viral pneumonias are more common than bacterial pneumonias. Respiratory syncytial virus (RSV) accounts for the largest percentage of infections in infants and young children. Bacterial pneumonias most common in infants and children are caused by streptococci, staphylococci, pneumococci, and *H. influenzae.*

Clinical manifestations. The clinical manifestations of viral and bacterial pneumonias are given in Box 32.3.

Diagnostic tests. Radiographic examination establishes the location and the extent of infection. Peripheral blood tests sometimes reveal an elevated WBC count, which is higher with bacterial infection than viral infection. Identification of the causative organism includes culture and Gram stain of respiratory secretions and the blood, as well as diagnostic thoracentesis if fluid is suspected in the pleural cavity. In the laboratory, nasal or

Box 32.3 Clinical Manifestations of Pneumonia in Children

- Abdominal pain
- Anorexia
- Chest pain
- Cough
- Fever
- Headache
- Irritability
- Lethargy
- Malaise
- Myalgia
- Nasal discharge
- Respiratory distress
- Wheeze or crackles

nasopharyngeal secretions are analyzed for RSV antigen detection. If no bacterial microorganism is identified, the pneumonia is considered viral.

Medical management. The goal of therapy in the management of pneumonia is to improve oxygenation and prevent dehydration. Treatment includes antibiotic therapy (for bacteria-based infections), oxygen therapy, chest physiotherapy, suctioning, fluid administration, and bronchodilators. Many health care providers order antipyretics to control fever.

Premature infants, infants with CHD, and infants with chronic lung disease are considered at high risk for RSV infection. A preventive therapy for RSV, palivizumab, is recommended for these infants. Palivizumab is a genetically engineered RSV monoclonal antibiotic. At-risk infants may receive the medication monthly for a prescribed length of time, depending on their identified risk factor, to aid in prevention of RSV (Munoz, et al, 2017).

Nursing interventions and patient teaching. Observation of respiratory status, including skin color and respiratory effort, and monitoring of cardiovascular status are two important nursing measures. Infection control measures should be followed according to hospital protocol. Supportive nursing management includes providing adequate rest periods to conserve energy, maintaining hydration by monitoring prescribed IV fluids, administering oxygen and antibiotics as prescribed, and gentle suctioning with a bulb syringe when necessary. Oral fluids, if allowed, should be given with caution to help prevent aspiration and to decrease the possibility of aggravating a fatiguing cough.

Encourage parents to participate in their child's care, guiding them in the proper methods to feed and hold their child while in the mist tent to prevent dislodgment of IV catheters.

Prognosis. The prognosis for children with pneumococcal and streptococcal pneumonias is generally good, with rapid resolution when detection and treatment occur early. Staphylococcal pneumonias typically run a longer course, but early detection and treatment are usually effective.

Sudden infant death syndrome. The sudden, unexpected, and unexplained death of an apparently healthy infant evokes a variety of familial responses ranging from hysteria and denial to stoicism (being impassive, indifferent to joy or pain). Nurses have an important role in assisting the family through the death and grieving process.

Etiology and pathophysiology. Sudden infant death syndrome (SIDS) is the sudden, unexpected death of an apparently healthy, normal infant younger than 1 year in which a postmortem examination, investigation of the death scene, and review of the case history fail to establish a cause of death. In the United States, the rate of mortality from SIDS has declined more than 50% since 1990. Health care providers attribute the dramatic decrease to the Safe to Sleep Campaign led by the National Institute of Child Health and Human Development. SIDS always occurs during sleep and is the leading cause of death among infants aged 1 to 12 months (NIH, 2017). The statistics show that 2 out of every 1000 infants die from SIDS, with most occurring between the ages of 1 to 4 months of age. Male infants have a higher incidence than female infants.

Native Americans and African Americans are most often affected, and it occurs more frequently among infants in lower socioeconomic classes. The cause of SIDS is unknown, but SIDS often is associated with premature birth and low birth weight, multiple births, and CNS and respiratory dysfunctions. There is also an association between SIDS and maternal smoking, drug addiction, and maternal age of less than 20 years. Smoking by the mother during the prenatal period and smoking in the home are linked to the incidence of SIDS. Breast-fed infants have a lower incidence of SIDS. Sleep position on the abdomen has been associated with SIDS, along with congenital abnormalities, sleep apnea, and depressed ventilator response to increased carbon dioxide or decreased oxygen blood levels. Sleeping in a prone position possibly predisposes the infant to oropharyngeal obstruction or affects ventilatory arousal. Soft, polystyrene-filled mattresses or pillows have the potential to cause suffocation in the infant sleeping in a prone position (see the Safety Alert box on preventing SIDS).

Clinical manifestations. Death occurs during sleep, and there is no audible cry or sign of distress.

Diagnostic tests. Confirmation of the diagnosis occurs at postmortem examination, which reveals pulmonary edema and intrathoracic hemorrhages.

Medical management. Therapeutic management consists of emotionally assisting the family who has just lost an infant to SIDS.

Nursing interventions. The death of an infant from SIDS propels the family into a crisis situation. The initial response is one of extreme shock and disbelief. As

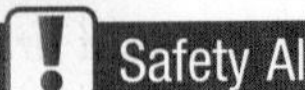

Safety Alert

Preventing Sudden Infant Death Syndrome

- Maternal smoking, prenatally and postnatally, is a possible cause of SIDS that some authorities have proposed, as are poor prenatal care and low maternal age.
- Bed sharing increases the risk of SIDS. Unlike a crib, whose design has to meet safety standards for infants, adult beds and sofas do not meet such specifications, and they carry a potential risk for accidental entrapment and suffocation.
- The infant should not be bundled too heavily. The infant should be dressed in lightweight clothing, and the room should be kept at a comfortable temperature.
- Infants always should be placed on their back for sleep until 1 year of age. Infants should be placed on a firm sleep surface. The crib or bassinet must meet current safety standards.
- Do not use soft bedding such as pillows or quilts under the infant for bedding.
- Remove items such as stuffed animals or towels from the crib while the infant is asleep to prevent possible asphyxia.
- Breast-feeding lowers the incidence of SIDS.

Information from National Institutes of Health (NIH): *Safe to sleep: Ways to reduce the risk of SIDS and other sleep-related causes of infant death*, 2017. Retrieved from *https://www.nichd.nih.gov/sts/about/risk/Pages/reduce.aspx*.

parents try to cope, they often experience feelings of guilt and blame.

The nurse becomes instrumental in assisting families with grief and mourning. Clean the infant, wrap the infant in a sheet or blanket, and tidy the room where the family will be able to spend time with the infant. For coming to terms with the death, ensure that the parents' last moments with their infant are quiet, peaceful, and as meaningful as possible. Offer to stay with the family or allow them private time if they wish.

Upper Respiratory Tract Infections

Acute pharyngitis (sore throat)

Etiology and pathophysiology. Acute pharyngitis is an inflammation of the pharynx. The majority of cases of acute pharyngitis are viral in origin, whereas less are diagnosed as bacterial (GABHS). Acute pharyngitis occurs frequently between the ages of 4 and 12 years, when children increasingly are exposed to infections outside the home. The infecting organism in children younger than 3 years with pharyngitis is usually *H. influenzae.* These children must be monitored for neurologic signs and symptoms that indicate possible meningitis. However, the use of the vaccine against *H. influenzae* type B (Hib vaccine) has begun to decrease the number of infections involving this organism. Acute cases of pharyngitis are more common in later winter and early spring.

Clinical manifestations. Viral pharyngitis causes low-grade fever, malaise, anorexia, pharyngeal erythema, and throat soreness. Many affected children also complain of headache, cough, hoarseness, rhinitis, and conjunctivitis. Streptococcal pharyngitis causes high fever, throat soreness, white exudates on the posterior pharynx and tonsillar region, vomiting, and abdominal pain.

Diagnostic tests. Although the majority of all cases of acute pharyngitis are of viral origin, a throat culture is performed to rule out GABHS.

Medical management. Viral pharyngitis is treated symptomatically with lozenges, gargles, and acetaminophen. Streptococcal pharyngitis must be treated with a 10-day course of antimicrobial therapy to prevent complications (acute rheumatic fever and acute glomerulonephritis). Penicillin derivatives are the drugs of choice for streptococcal pharyngitis. Other medications that also treat streptococcal pharyngitis include erythromycin, azithromycin, clarithromycin, cephalosporins, and amoxicillin.

Nursing interventions and patient teaching. To relieve throat discomfort in viral and bacterial infections, administer saline gargles, lozenges, warm compresses to the neck, and acetaminophen. Encourage the child to drink cool liquids (nonacid) until the throat feels better; then soft, bland foods may be introduced. Emphasize follow-up care after streptococcal pharyngitis to ensure eradication of the causative organism.

The family should be instructed in antimicrobial therapy, with emphasis on the need to finish the medication completely even though the child feels better. When a throat culture for streptococcal infection yields positive results, remind the child to discard his or her toothbrush and replace it with a new one after taking antibiotics for 24 hours.

Prognosis. The prognosis for children with acute pharyngitis is usually excellent. Inadequately treated streptococcal infections sometimes trigger a response in the heart (rheumatic fever) or kidneys (acute glomerulonephritis).

Tonsillitis

Etiology and pathophysiology. The tonsils are masses of lymphoid tissue located in the pharyngeal cavity. They are believed to protect the respiratory and alimentary tracts from invasion by pathogenic microorganisms. They probably also play a role in antibody formation. Tonsillitis usually occurs as a result of pharyngitis and has either viral or bacterial (streptococcal) causes.

Clinical manifestations. The signs and symptoms of viral and bacterial tonsillitis are similar and include sore throat, headache, edematous and tender cervical lymph glands, fever, hoarseness, and cough. In addition, many children with streptococcal tonsillitis exhibit vomiting, complain of muscle aches, and have difficulty swallowing or breathing.

Diagnostic tests. The WBC count sometimes is elevated significantly. A throat culture is performed to detect streptococcal tonsillitis.

Medical management. The treatment for bacterial and nonbacterial tonsillitis includes the comfort measures described in acute pharyngitis. In addition, treatment for bacterial tonsillitis comprises a 10-day course of penicillin (or erythromycin) to prevent complications.

Tonsillectomy is a surgical procedure that completely removes the tonsils. The primary care provider or ear, nose, and throat (ENT) specialist determines if the patient's condition warrants a tonsillectomy. Infrequent cases of pharyngitis typically do not warrant the need for a tonsillectomy. Repeated infections of the pharynx, especially streptococcal bacterial infections, may lead to a discussion regarding the pros and cons of a tonsillectomy.

Nursing interventions. The nursing interventions for tonsillitis are the same as those described for acute pharyngitis. Before any indicated surgery, prepare the child psychologically. Assess the child for signs of infection and loose teeth and check the child's laboratory data, including findings from bleeding and clotting studies. Postoperatively, the child should be kept in a semiprone position to facilitate drainage; also the child should be monitored frequently for excessive bleeding, which causes frequent swallowing even during sleep. Analgesics should be given as prescribed; and, after recovery from analgesia, fluids should be provided (with the exception of acidic, grape, red, or chocolate drinks so that you can distinguish fresh or old blood in emesis from ingested liquid). A soft diet follows. Postoperative hemorrhage is unusual but possible; therefore observe the child's throat directly for evidence of bleeding, with a good source of light and, if necessary, by carefully inserting a tongue depressor. Signs of hemorrhage include increased pulse (>120 bpm), pallor, frequent clearing of the throat or swallowing by a younger child, and vomiting of bright red blood. Restlessness, an indication of hemorrhage, is sometimes difficult to differentiate from general discomfort after surgery. Decreasing blood pressure is a late sign of shock.

Patient teaching. Appropriate discharge instructions include the following:

- Avoid foods that are irritating or highly seasoned.
- Avoid the use of gargles or vigorous brushing of the teeth.
- Try to avoid coughing or clearing the throat.
- Use mild analgesics or an ice collar for pain.
- Do not use aspirin.

Hemorrhaging is possible 5 to 10 days after surgery as a result of tissue sloughing from the healing process. If parents see any signs of bleeding, they must notify the health care provider immediately.

Prognosis. The prognosis is generally excellent. Improperly treated streptococcal infections potentially result in rheumatic fever or acute glomerulonephritis.

Croup: laryngotracheobronchitis and acute epiglottitis. Croup is an acute viral disease of childhood, marked by a resonant barking cough, suffocative and difficult breathing, and laryngeal spasm.

Etiology and pathophysiology. Laryngotracheobronchitis (LTB) is the most common form of croup. It affects children 3 months to 3 years of age and is usually viral in origin. LTB usually follows an upper respiratory infection that descends to the lower respiratory tract and has a gradual, progressive onset.

Acute epiglottitis is a severe, potentially life-threatening bacterial infection of the epiglottis in older children and usually is caused by *H. influenzae* type B. The inflamed epiglottis becomes cherry-red and edematous, which has the potential to lead to total airway obstruction. Since the advent of the Hib vaccine, the number of episodes of epiglottitis caused by *H. influenzae* type B has been decreasing.

Clinical manifestations. Children with LTB initially demonstrate hoarseness; inspiratory stridor; tachypnea; nasal flaring; suprasternal, substernal, and intercostal retractions; and characteristic barking cough. Body temperature is usually normal or mildly elevated. A child with epiglottitis is acutely ill with high fever, muffled voice, drooling, progressive respiratory distress, anxiety, and fear.

Diagnostic tests. Diagnostic criteria for LTB consist of a history of a preceding upper respiratory infection, CBC with differential, the clinical signs and symptoms, and physical examination.

Clinical signs and symptoms establish a tentative diagnosis of acute epiglottitis, which is considered a medical emergency. The child is taken to the operating or ambulatory surgery room, where emergency equipment is available for immediate intubation or tracheostomy in the event of further obstruction during examination of the pharynx. Health care providers sometimes obtain lateral neck radiographs in the operating room to observe for soft tissue edema and an area of obstruction. Skilled personnel with the equipment necessary to perform immediate intubation or tracheostomy never leave the child's side. The trend away from early intubation of children with LTB emphasizes the importance of nursing observation and the ability to recognize impending respiratory failure so that intubation is possible without delay. The child is put under anesthesia for visual examination of the pharynx and invasive procedures such as blood collection and insertion of IV lines. The laboratory performs culture and sensitivity testing on tracheal secretions collected at the time of intubation.

Medical management. Management of LTB and acute epiglottitis focuses on maintaining patency of the airway. A child with LTB receives high cool-mist humidity with low-concentration (approximately 30%) oxygen by mist tent. Administration of epinephrine by aerosol helps decrease airway edema by vasoconstriction and improve oxygenation by bronchodilation. The effects of epinephrine are short lived, however, and repeated doses are needed if and when the airway edema returns a few hours after epinephrine administration. Therefore it is necessary to monitor children receiving epinephrine very closely. During the acute phase, affected children receive nothing by mouth (NPO status), because the typically rapid respirations predispose to aspiration. IV administration of fluids provides adequate hydration. The use of sedatives is contraindicated, because they mask restlessness, which is a clinical indication of hypoxia and a deteriorating condition.

Immediate treatment of a child with acute epiglottitis includes establishing an artificial airway. Respiratory care includes humidification, gentle oral suctioning, and constant observation of respiratory status. Health care providers order oxygen for moderate respiratory distress and aerosolized epinephrine to decrease airway edema by local vasoconstriction. IV antibiotics and fluids are administered as ordered. Epiglottal edema usually decreases after 24 hours of antibiotic therapy. By the third day, the epiglottis is nearly normal in size, and it is safe to extubate the child.

Nursing interventions and patient teaching. LTB or acute epiglottitis tends to be a frightening experience for the child and the family. Never attempt to examine the mouth or throat in a child with LTB, because this results in epiglottal spasm and cessation of breathing. Respond quickly in a calm manner, emotionally supporting and reassuring parents that everything possible is being done for their child. Continually assess the child for signs of response to therapy or increasing obstruction. Nursing observations often provide the rationale for any treatment changes. The child is maintained in the Fowler's position, and respirations are monitored for rate, depth, retractions, and nasal flaring. Monitor the child's cardiac status because restlessness and tachycardia are signs of increasing hypoxia. Check vital signs frequently. Intubation and tracheostomy sets are kept at the child's bedside in case of respiratory failure. Nursing interventions must be planned carefully to include frequent rest periods for the patient to conserve energy. Keep parents informed of their child's progress and encourage them to participate in care.

Prognosis. In most affected children, LTB is relatively mild. Gradual improvement to recovery occurs in 3 to 7 days. The most serious complication, and the one responsible for most deaths from croup, is laryngeal obstruction.

Without prompt diagnosis and treatment, the rapid course of epiglottitis has the potential to cause death within a few hours.

Lower Respiratory Tract Infections

Bronchitis (tracheobronchitis)

Etiology and pathophysiology. Bronchitis (tracheobronchitis) is an inflammation of the large airways, the trachea, and the bronchi. It usually follows an upper respiratory infection and is almost always viral in origin. The most common cause is rhinovirus, although parainfluenza, adenovirus, and RSV are other known causes. *Mycoplasma pneumoniae* is a common cause of bronchitis in children older than 6 years. Bronchitis occurs mainly in the winter months, primarily in children younger than 4 years (although it has potential to affect any age group).

Clinical manifestations. The onset is gradual with signs and symptoms of an upper respiratory tract infection (cough, coryza, little or no fever). After 2 to 3 days, the nonproductive, hacking cough becomes productive and worsens at night.

Diagnostic tests. For a child with severe signs and symptoms, a radiographic examination of the chest is necessary. In the majority of affected children, chest radiographs appear normal.

Medical management. Treatment is basically palliative. If the cough interferes with resting or eating, then cough drops, lollipops, and pediatric cough preparations are usually effective. Cough suppressants are contraindicated in bronchitis unless the condition significantly affects sleep. Sometimes health care providers prescribe acetaminophen for fever. Antibiotics are not necessary in viral bronchitis. If the cough lasts beyond 10 days, a secondary bacterial infection is suspected.

Patient teaching. Suggest the use of a cool-mist humidifier to relieve the child's cough and help liquefy secretions. Encourage consumption of fluids to decrease viscosity of secretions and prevent dehydration.

Prognosis. Acute bronchitis is self-limiting.

Respiratory syncytial virus and bronchiolitis

Etiology and pathophysiology. Bronchiolitis is an acute viral inflammation of the smaller airway passages, the bronchioles; the bronchioles become inflamed, which causes edema. The accumulation of mucus and exudate has the potential to partially or completely obstruct the lumen. RSV is the organism responsible for most cases. Bronchiolitis occurs in children younger than 2 years. The incidence peaks at 6 months of age. Cases of bronchiolitis usually begin in the fall, and the incidence peaks in the winter. The virus is transmitted through respiratory secretions. RSV can survive for hours outside a host on such items as countertops and contaminated tissues.

Clinical manifestations. Signs and symptoms of an upper respiratory infection predominate during the first few days and worsen as respiratory distress develops. Affected infants exhibit retractions, tachypnea, nasal flaring, paroxysmal nonproductive coughing, and wheezing. Some affected infants have low-grade or very high fever; are irritable, fussy, and anxious; and have difficulty eating. Respiratory distress becomes progressively more severe during the first 72 hours. Severe disease is followed by a rise in arterial carbon dioxide tension (hypercapnia), which leads to respiratory acidosis and hypoxemia.

Diagnostic tests. The diagnosis is based on the age of the child and the clinical signs and symptoms. Radiographic examination of the chest shows areas of atelectasis and hyperinflation. Tests providing positive identification of RSV are either ELISA or rapid immunofluorescent antibody assays of specimens obtained from direct aspiration of nasal secretions or nasopharyngeal washings.

Medical management. There is no definitive antiviral medication suggested for use in most cases of bronchiolitis. Treatment is aimed at treating the symptoms. Hydration and oxygenation are the primary treatment modalities. High humidity, administered via mist tent, loosens secretions. If hypoxemia is present, the health care provider orders oxygen therapy with mist therapy. IV fluids are necessary if the infant is unable to tolerate oral feedings. Use of bronchodilators is sometimes an aspect of management in severe cases of bronchiolitis (Maraqa, 2018).

Nursing interventions and patient teaching. Follow respiratory isolation precautions. Practice and encourage thorough hand hygiene to prevent cross-contamination, along with the use of contact precautions (gloves, gowns, masks, and goggles). Another infection control measure includes making patient assignments so that nurses assigned to children with RSV do not take care of other patients at high risk for RSV infection. Acute nursing interventions focus on promoting adequate oxygenation, frequent monitoring of respiratory status, and maintaining hydration. As with any respiratory condition, parents need reassurance and emotional support during this stressful period.

Prognosis. The disease typically lasts 7 to 10 days. With prompt treatment the prognosis is very good. Overall, the mortality in children hospitalized for bronchiolitis in different series ranges from 0.2% to 7%, depending on such factors as the stage of the infection upon diagnosis and when treatment was started (Maraqa, 2018).

Pulmonary tuberculosis

Etiology and pathophysiology. Pulmonary tuberculosis (TB) is a chronic bacterial lung infection caused by the bacillus *Mycobacterium tuberculosis.* TB remains a leading cause of death in many underdeveloped countries. It continues to be a public health problem in the United States primarily because of immigration, infection with HIV, and multiresistant strains of *M. tuberculosis.* The most important risk factor in the progression from TB infection to active disease is an inadequate immune response, as a result of age or an impaired immune system, as in young infants, elderly people, or people infected with HIV. Immunocompromised children and children younger than 3 years are at greatest risk for TB, but the risk increases again during the postpubertal adolescent years. The primary source of *M. tuberculosis* infection in children is exposure to an infected adult, usually a family member, babysitter, or frequent visitor.

Clinical manifestations. When first infected, most children do not exhibit any clinical signs and symptoms. Signs and symptoms are extremely variable and develop so gradually that they often go unnoticed until the disease has progressed significantly.

Diagnostic tests. Although not diagnostic, the tuberculin skin test, formerly known as the *Mantoux test,* is the most important screening measure in identifying infected children at risk for disease. To confirm the diagnosis, bacteriologic sputum cultures for *M. tuberculosis* must yield positive results. Infected infants and young children do not cough and expectorate sputum. Instead, they usually swallow mucus from the respiratory tract. Therefore the best way to obtain sputum samples from infants and children is by gastric aspiration. Chest radiographs are also important in determining the presence and the extent of active lesions. The medical management and nursing interventions are basically the same as in adults with active TB.

Patient teaching. Because the success of therapy depends on compliance with the drug regimen, it is necessary to instruct parents regarding the importance of giving medications as often and for as long as ordered. The optimal duration of therapy is unknown, but the usual course of treatment is no less than 12 months for an initial infection or 18 to 24 months for more serious forms of the disease.

Prognosis. The prognosis relies greatly on the stage of the disease at the time of diagnosis. The rate of success in treating early-onset TB is high. Complications of pulmonary TB include pneumonia, pneumothorax, and stenosis of the airways. TB of the small intestine may result in obstruction, fistula formation, and malabsorption.

Cystic fibrosis

Etiology and pathophysiology. Cystic fibrosis (CF) is a genetic disorder that a child inherits from both parents. This is a disorder of the exocrine (mucus-producing) glands, with the characteristic presence of excessive thick mucus that obstructs the lungs and the gastrointestinal (GI) system. CF is a multiorgan disease, but death usually is caused by pulmonary failure. The incidence of CF is greater than 30,000 people in the United States with approximately 1000 new cases diagnosed every year. More than 75% of cases are diagnosed by the age of 2 years. Fifty percent of those living with CF are over the age of 18 (Cystic Fibrosis Foundation, n.d.).

The abnormally thick mucus that collects in the lung airways and organ ducts causes obstruction. Bronchiolar obstruction predisposes the lung to infection, bronchiectasis, and cystic dilations. Complications include bronchial and bronchiolar obstruction, pulmonary hypertension, and cor pulmonale. Obstruction of the pancreatic ducts leads to dilation and fibrosis and a decrease in levels of pancreatic enzymes (lipase, amylase, and trypsin), which results in malabsorption. The earliest manifestation of CF is meconium ileus in the newborn, in which the small intestine is occluded with tenacious putty-like, mucilaginous meconium. Obstruction in the hepatic system leads to biliary cirrhosis, portal hypertension, and splenomegaly. Sodium chloride concentrations in the sweat and the saliva are elevated as a result of the abnormal reabsorption of chloride by epithelial cells.

Clinical manifestations. Pancreatic insufficiency and malabsorption result in steatorrhea (bulky, foul-smelling, fatty stools), growth failure, protuberant abdomen, and thin, wasted extremities. Rectal prolapse is a common GI manifestation of CF. Appetite often is increased early in the illness in response to poor absorption. Malabsorption also has the potential to lead to a vitamin K deficiency, which results in bleeding disorders, esophageal varices, and ecchymosis. As a result of diminished subcutaneous fat, the skin appears sallow and transparent. Pulmonary complications constitute the most serious threat to life in children with CF. Many such children demonstrate respiratory symptoms before 1 year of age; others may not develop symptoms for weeks, months, or years. Pulmonary involvement is evident in chronic cough, wheezing, sputum production, and dyspnea, which results in hypoxia, clubbing of the fingers and toes, and cyanosis. Hyperinflation of the lungs sometimes causes the chest to become barrel shaped.

Diagnostic tests. All states in the United States screen newborns for CF using a genetic test or a blood test. Diagnostic criteria for CF consist of a family history of the disorder, absence of pancreatic enzymes, chronic pulmonary involvement, and a positive result of a chloride sweat test. Typically two sweat tests are performed to diagnose the disease. For this test, the doctor triggers sweating on a small patch of skin on an arm or leg. The provider rubs the skin with a sweat-producing chemical and then uses an electrode to provide a mild electrical current. Sweat is collected, then tested. A sweat chloride level higher than 60 mEq/L is diagnostic for CF. The normal level of sweat chloride is below 29 mmol/L in infants 6 months and younger; below 39 mmol/L for any age over 6 months (Johns Hopkins, 2018). Chest radiographs show patchy atelectasis and evidence of obstructive emphysema. Pulmonary function tests measure ventilation and diffusion of gas across the alveolar capillary membrane and reveal evidence of pulmonary problems.

Medical management. The goals of therapy include good nutrition, prevention and control of respiratory infections, and enabling as normal a lifestyle as possible for the child. Pulmonary therapy to ensure airway clearance is the single most important aspect of treatment. Chest physiotherapy and high-frequency chest wall oscillations have greatly improved the pulmonary status of the patient with CF. Breathing exercises are beneficial to improve aeration. Inhalation therapy with bronchodilators before chest physiotherapy facilitates secretion removal. Expectorants, mucolytic agents, and antibiotics help relieve obstruction and resolve infections. Chest physiotherapy is usually necessary twice daily (on rising and in the evening) and sometimes more frequently, especially during pulmonary infection. Positive expiratory pressure (PEP) therapy is another source of treatment. This therapy involves breathing through a device that provides resistance while exhaling. This pressure keeps the small airways of the lungs open to improve the mobility of the secretions. Digestive and nutritional therapies include pancreatic enzyme replacement, administration of fat-soluble vitamins (A, D, E, and K), and a diet high in calories, protein, and salt.

Nursing interventions. Nursing interventions for a child with CF are highly complex and can be challenging. Management focuses on improving pulmonary function and facilitating lung clearance, preventing or managing respiratory infections, promoting normal growth and development, optimizing nutritional status, educating the patient and family about the illness and its management, planning for home care and community support, referring for counseling when needed, providing long-term emotional support and follow-up, and encouraging compliance with the medication regimen.

Improving pulmonary function involves chest physiotherapy, breathing exercises, and inhalation treatment. Chest physiotherapy performed two or more times daily helps loosen secretions in the lung with high-frequency chest wall oscillations, and postural drainage facilitates the removal of these thick secretions. To encourage breathing exercises, suggest blowing bubbles or pinwheels to help prevent tracheobronchial obstruction. The nurse or the respiratory therapist sometimes performs nebulizer treatments. Assess the child's tolerance of therapy and monitor its effectiveness. Infection control measures are instituted to prevent cross-contamination, and the family is taught to protect the child from exposure to people with respiratory infections. Strongly recommend yearly influenza immunizations. Early in the course of the illness, some children exhibit excessive appetite; as the disease progresses, the appetite decreases, and children usually experience anorexia. Before meals and snacks, administer a mix of pancreatic enzymes, needed to digest proteins, fats, and carbohydrates, together with a carbohydrate.

Children with CF have frequent hospitalizations, which are likely to interfere with normal development and impair socialization; these issues must be addressed with psychological support and appropriate activities. One of the most critical aspects in providing care to children with CF and their families is assisting them with positive coping strategies and providing emotional support. Support groups are often a source of great comfort and assistance to children with newly diagnosed disease and to their families. The Cystic Fibrosis Foundation provides education and services to families and professionals.

Patient teaching. The family is instructed in improving the nutritional status of the child to ensure adequate growth and development. The nurse is responsible primarily for coordinating counseling, referrals to community support, and home care services, as well as for educating the child and the family in the disease process

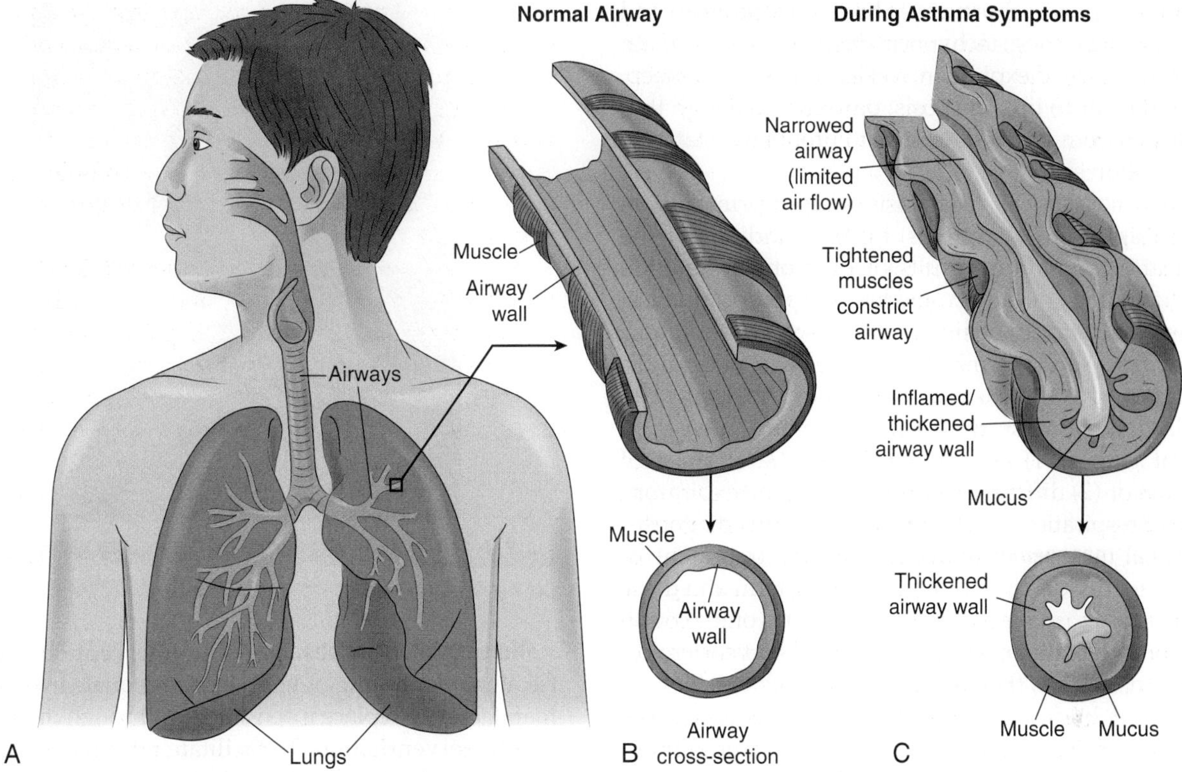

Fig. 32.11 Illustrations of lung anatomy. A, The location of the lungs and airways in the body. B, A cross section of a normal airway. C, A cross section of an airway during asthma symptoms. (Redrawn from the National Heart, Lung, and Blood Institute: *What is asthma?* 2012. Retrieved from *www.nhlbi.nih.gov/health/health-topics/topics/asthma.*)

and its management. The child should receive all childhood vaccinations as recommended.

Prognosis. CF is a chronic, incurable disease. According to the Cystic Fibrosis Foundation Patient Registry, treatment of the disease has improved substantially since the 1950s. In 1955 children with CF were not expected to live long enough to attend school. The median length of survival in 2009, in contrast, was in the mid-30s. Today, 45% of the population with CF are 18 years of age or older. Currently the life expectancy of a baby born in 2016 with CF is 47 years of age or older. Therapies and treatments for patients with CF are now individualized to provide the best possible outcomes, including mucus thinners, antibiotics, antiinflammatories, and bronchodilators (Marshall, 2017).

Bronchial asthma

Etiology and pathophysiology. Asthma is a chronic inflammatory disorder of the airways in which many cells (mast cells, eosinophils, and T lymphocytes) play a role. Bronchial asthma is a reversible obstructive respiratory disorder. Asthma accounts for the greatest number of school absences and visits to the emergency department by children. It is a leading cause of chronic disease in children with 6.2 million children affected (CDC, 2017b).

Bronchial asthma has a familial tendency and frequently occurs in association with allergic rhinitis and atopic dermatitis. A common cause of bronchial asthma is an allergic hypersensitivity to environmental factors. The common factors associated with bronchial asthma include bronchospasm, mucosal edema, and increased mucosal secretions. Bronchospasm of the bronchial smooth muscle causes bronchial edema with a decrease in the diameter of the bronchi and bronchioles; edematous mucous membranes produce thick, tenacious secretions, which cause a further narrowing of the air passages. Mucous plugs that occlude the smaller air passages cause obstruction and air trapping distal to the obstruction, which result in hypoxemia and increased respiratory effort (Fig. 32.11).

The National Heart, Lung, and Blood Institute's National Asthma Education and Prevention Program (2007) classified asthma based on symptoms that indicate the severity of the disease. The classifications are (1) mild intermittent, (2) mild persistent, (3) moderate persistent, and (4) severe persistent. These categories aid in the medical and environmental treatment of asthma.

Pulmonary function tests are useful in children after age 5 or 6 years. These tests help evaluate the presence and the degree of lung disease and responses to therapy. Health care providers often order skin testing for allergens in children with asthma to help identify and treat specific allergies.

Clinical manifestations. Initially, many children having an asthma attack complain of a sensation of tightness in the chest, and an audible expiratory wheeze may be detected. As the attack progresses, other signs and symptoms appear: shortness of breath; inspiratory and expiratory wheezing; tachypnea; dyspnea; coarse breath sounds; prolonged expiration; restlessness; anxiety; deep, dark red color to lips; cyanosis; paroxysmal cough that progresses from dry and hacking to productive; fatigue; and diaphoresis.

Diagnostic tests. The diagnosis is based primarily on clinical signs and symptoms; history; findings of the physical examination; results of pulmonary function tests, including spirometry and bronchoprovocation test (to assess sensitivity of airways); and serum laboratory tests such as ABG determinations and CBC. Radiographic examination of the chest and electrocardiography are standard imaging tests to rule out other disease. In general, either (1) chronic cough in the absence of infection or (2) diffuse wheezing during the expiratory phase of respiration is sufficient to establish a diagnosis.

Medical management. Medications for treatment of asthma are divided into those given long term and those administered to manage acute exacerbations of the condition. Long-term therapies include inhaled corticosteroids, cromolyn sodium, fluticasone (Flovent Diskus, Flovent HFA), and budesonide (Pulmicort Flexhaler). These medications are administered via a nebulizer and aid in the prevention of airway inflammation. Omalizumab (anti–immunoglobulin E), which is administered by injection once or twice per month, works to prevent the body from reacting to asthma triggers. Inhaled, long-acting beta-agonists may be administered to improve control of the condition. Leukotriene modifiers such as montelukast sodium (Singulair) and zafirlukast (Accolate) reduce inflammation and work to keep the airways relaxed. Long-term medications are not suitable for an acute exacerbation, because they do not work quickly enough to treat the condition.

Quick-relief (rescue) medications include short-acting $beta_2$-agonists such as albuterol (ProAir, Ventolin) and levalbuterol (Xopenex HFA). These medications act by dilating the bronchi within minutes after administration, and the effects of these medications may last for several hours. Oral and IV corticosteroids such as prednisone may be used to decrease bronchial inflammation in severe cases of asthma, but they are not used for long-term treatment because of their systemic effects on other organs. Metered-dose inhalers are used frequently to administer quick-relief and long-term medications. Health care providers typically administer nebulized medications to infants and young children who are not able to use a metered-dose inhaler. In young school-age children, the use of a spacer helps ensure that the child receives the full dose prescribed. The spacer provides a reservoir for the medication to allow the child time to inhale the full dose (Fig. 32.12). Chest physiotherapy is prescribed by some health care providers to help children with asthma strengthen their respiratory muscles and develop more efficient breathing patterns. Chest physiotherapy is not effective during an acute exacerbation of asthma.

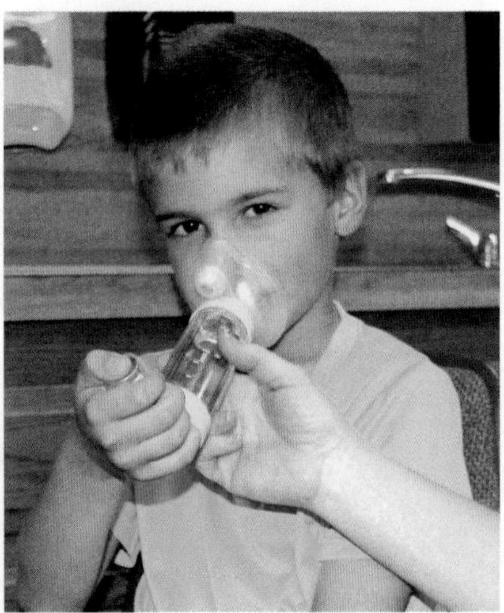

Fig. 32.12 Child using a metered-dose inhaler with spacer.

Nursing interventions. Nursing interventions include frequent monitoring of vital signs. Adequate hydration is maintained to replace insensible loss through diaphoresis and hyperventilation. To facilitate optimal ventilation, the child is kept in high Fowler's position, rest periods are provided, and breathing exercises are taught. It is extremely important to provide a calm atmosphere and reassurance for the anxious child and family. Parents and children need to understand the illness and how to allay or prevent attacks at home. Allergens can be identified through skin testing, and then measures can be instituted to eliminate or avoid them.

A patient problem and interventions for a child with bronchial asthma include but are not limited to the following:

Patient Problem	Nursing Interventions
Inability to Maintain Adequate Breathing Pattern, related to allergenic response in bronchial tree	Teach and supervise breathing exercises and controlled breathing Teach correct use of prescribed medications Assist patient and family in selecting activities appropriate for child's capabilities and preferences Encourage regular exercise Encourage good posture Encourage physical exercise involving stop-and-start activity that does not overtax the respiratory mechanism Discourage physical inactivity

Patient teaching. Parents need to understand the nature of the disease and, when the allergens are determined, know how to avoid or relieve asthma attacks. Teach parents and older children with asthma how to use the

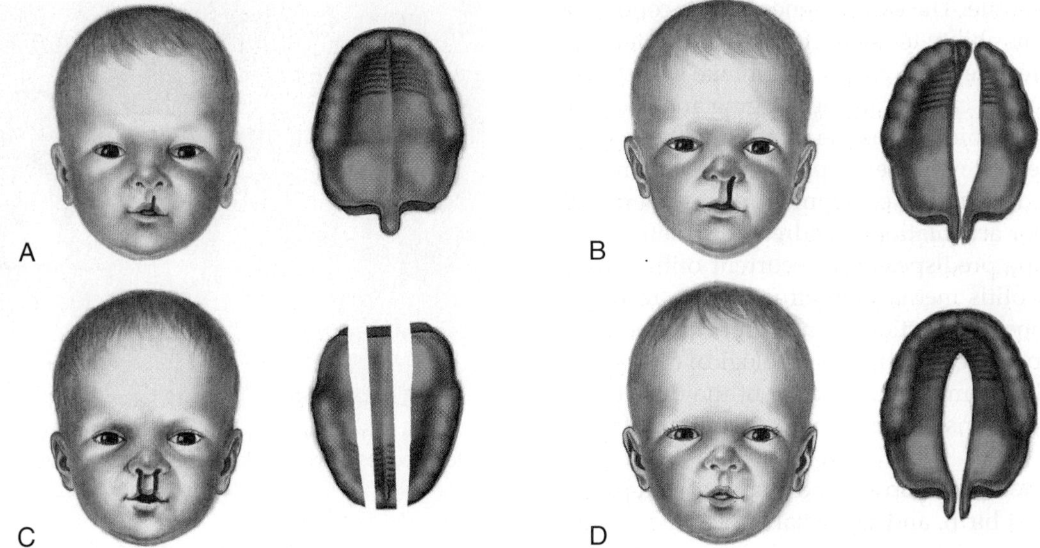

Fig. 32.13 Variations in clefts of lip and palate at birth. A, Notch in vermilion border, no cleft in palate. B, Unilateral cleft lip and palate. C, Bilateral cleft lip and palate. D, Cleft palate alone. (From Hockenberry MJ, Wilson D: *Nursing care of infants and children,* ed 9, St. Louis, 2011, Mosby.)

medications prescribed to relieve bronchospasms (see Fig. 32.12). Teach early signs and symptoms of an impending attack so that control is possible before symptoms become distressing. Older children who use a nebulizer or an aerosol device to deliver adrenergic drugs need instruction on how to use a metered-dose inhaler. The parents must be taught to avoid exposing the child to excessive cold, wind, or other extremes of weather and to smoke, sprays, or other irritants. Self-care is a hallmark of effective asthma management, and self-management programs are important in helping the child and the family cope with the disease.

Prognosis. The outlook for children with asthma varies widely. Many children lose the signs and symptoms at puberty, but no known factor predicts which children will "outgrow" their asthma. Although death from asthma is rare, the death rate has been rising steadily since 2000 despite improvements in treatment. It is important that children with asthma be assessed carefully and treated aggressively.

DISORDERS OF GASTROINTESTINAL FUNCTION

The primary function of the GI tract is the absorption and metabolism of nutrients necessary to support and promote optimal growth and development. Because the GI tract is responsible for processing nutrients for all parts of the body, an alteration in GI function has potential to affect other body systems. Failure to diagnose or treat a GI problem is likely to affect the overall health of the child. Conversely, any disease process has potential to result in manifestations of GI disturbance, even if it does not directly affect the GI tract.

Cleft lip and cleft palate. Clefts of the lip and the palate are facial malformations that occur during embryologic development. A combination of cleft lip and palate is more common than an isolated occurrence of either. Approximately 2650 babies are born with a cleft palate, and 4440 babies are born with a cleft lip with or without a cleft palate.

Etiology and pathophysiology. Cleft lip is caused by a failure of the medial nasal and maxillary processes to join (Fig. 32.13). Cleft of the palate is caused by a failure of the palatal shelves to fuse. Clefts in the palate sometimes involve only the soft palate and sometimes extend into the hard palate.

Cleft lip and palate has been linked to several environmental factors, including a folic acid deficiency in the maternal diet, maternal intake of alcohol during pregnancy, and smoking during pregnancy. Some folklore has mistakenly attempted to link the cause of cleft lip and palate to prenatal influences (see the Cultural Considerations box).

Cultural Considerations

Cleft Lip

Beliefs in folklore and superstitions have always surrounded pregnancy and birth. Some people believe that prenatal influences affect the outcome of an unborn child, specifically with regard to birth defects. Some people believe, for example, that if a pregnant woman encounters a rabbit or hare during her pregnancy, her child will be born with a "harelip" (cleft lip).

Clinical manifestations. Severity of cleft lip and palate may vary significantly. The cleft in the lip may be limited to a small open notch, or it may extend all the way to the base of the nose. The cleft in the palate may involve either one side or both sides of the roof of the mouth. The two clefts may combine and involve the lip and palate. Nasal shape irregularities should signal the need for further investigation. Manifestations that result from the condition may include feeding difficulties from the breast or the bottle. The extensiveness of the condition determines this ability to feed. Affected infants tend to have an ineffective suck. Saliva and intake sometimes leak into the nasal cavity, causing gagging and choking and leading to aspiration as the infant breathes.

Speech delays may develop. The most common speech-related issue is development of a hypernasal tone with poor articulation. Children with cleft palate also tend to be predisposed to recurrent otitis media or persistent otitis media with effusion as a result of eustachian tube dysfunction. Many older children with cleft lip and palate experience psychological difficulties because of the cosmetic appearance of the defect and because of problems with impaired speech and faulty dentition.

Diagnostic tests. Cleft lip and most cases of cleft palate are apparent at birth, and the facial appearance of the infant is of immediate concern to the parents. Digital examination of the mouth cavity is performed to assess the level of severity.

Medical management. Cleft lip usually is closed within the first few months of age. Cleft palate repair occurs within the first 18 months of age. Surgical repair during this period allows for palatal changes associated with normal growth. During the period before surgical repair, the infant may be fitted with a prosthetic device that mimics the palate to improve feeding abilities. For the most positive outcome after surgical repair, interventions involve a multidisciplinary health care team that includes a pediatric plastic surgeon, an orthodontist, an otolaryngologist, a speech and language pathologist, an audiologist, nurses, and social workers (CDC, 2017c).

Nursing interventions. Nursing interventions for a child with cleft lip and palate are focused initially on ensuring adequate nutritional support for the infant and helping the parents to deal with the diagnosis. Before surgical correction of cleft lip and palate, feeding is often a considerable problem. In addition to ensuring adequate food intake, a primary goal for nursing is to prevent aspiration. The best method for feeding is to support the infant's head in an upright position and to use care and patience during each feeding. Because infants with cleft lip and palate cannot generate the suction necessary to feed through a normal nipple or breast, the parents require assistance with learning to use special feeding devices. A variety of special "cleft-palate" nipples have had some success. However, large, soft nipples with large holes or long, soft lamb's nipples appear to offer the best means for nipple feeding (Fig. 32.14). Breast-feeding may be possible with the use of a breast shield with a specially designed nipple. The ESSR feeding technique works especially well for infants with cleft lip/palate before corrective surgery. ESSR stands for the following:

*E*nlarge the nipple.
*S*timulate the suck reflex.
*S*wallow fluid appropriately.
*R*est when infant signals with facial expression.

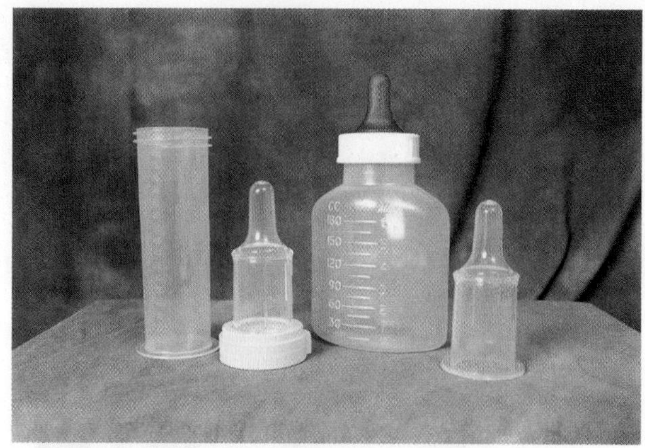

Fig. 32.14 Some devices used to feed an infant with a cleft lip and palate. (Courtesy Texas Children's Hospital, Houston.)

During feedings, these infants require frequent burping because they tend to swallow large amounts of air.

Another important goal is to assist the parents in dealing with the diagnosis of cleft lip and palate and to promote bonding between the parents and the infant. To accomplish this goal, try emphasizing positive aspects of the infant's appearance and behavior. Parents may benefit greatly from viewing photographs of children who have had cleft lip and palate repairs to illustrate the positive results of surgical intervention. Postoperative nursing interventions include protecting the integrity of the suture line, promoting optimal nutrition, and continuing emotional support of the child and parents. Such infants should be positioned only on their side or back; positioning on the abdomen allows them to rub the face on the sheets. Place safety reminder devices on the child's elbows to prevent touching or rubbing of the suture line. Periodically remove the safety reminder devices to enable movement of the arms, to provide an opportunity to observe the skin underneath for signs of impairment or pressure, and to cuddle the infant.

Immediately after surgery, the infant usually is kept on NPO status until the effects of the anesthesia have disappeared. Then the infant gradually is introduced to liquids, beginning with clear liquids (water and dextrose water) and gradually progressing to formula. A soft rubber-tipped feeder is generally preferred; slip the rubber tip of the feeder into the side of the infant's mouth carefully, avoiding contact with the suture line. Breast-feeding usually is contraindicated immediately after surgery. Help the mother if she wishes to pump her breasts to promote the continued production of milk until the infant is able to feed directly from the breast. After feedings, gently cleanse the suture line with a saline-soaked cotton-tipped swab. Then place the infant in an infant seat or on the right side to promote digestion and prevent aspiration of regurgitated formula. In addition, careful aspiration of the oral and nasopharyngeal cavities is sometimes necessary to remove collections of mucus, blood, and saliva and to prevent aspiration. Analgesics should be administered as ordered.

Postoperative care after surgical repair of cleft palate is similar to that after cleft lip repair. A child with cleft palate repair should lie on the abdomen, because this will facilitate drainage of mucus and serosanguineous exudate from the oral cavity. Administer analgesics as ordered. Liquid nourishments usually are provided by cup. Use of straws, pacifiers, and eating utensils is not advisable because they may injure the suture line. The child should advance gradually from a liquid diet to a blenderized diet, and parents are instructed to continue this diet after discharge until the surgeon instructs them otherwise.

Patient teaching. Assist the family by providing them with information on agencies that provide services, information, and emotional support to families with a child who has cleft lip and palate. These agencies include the Cleft Palate Foundation *(www.cleftline.org)* and the March of Dimes *(http://marchofdimes.com)*. Throughout the child's development, an important goal is the development of a healthy personality and self-esteem.

Prognosis. After surgery, speech impairments and middle ear infections continue to be a problem for most children with cleft lip or palate. Teach parents the signs and symptoms of upper respiratory and ear infections so that early treatment can be obtained. Early intervention is necessary in the development of normal speech patterns.

Dehydration. When the body loses more fluid than it absorbs, as in the presence of diarrhea, or when it absorbs less water than it excretes, as in the presence of vomiting, dehydration results. Dehydration occurs basically whenever the total fluid intake is less than the total fluid output. The most accurate method of assessing a child's degree of dehydration is by noting changes in the body weight. Mild, moderate, and severe dehydration correspond to fluid deficits of 5%, 10%, and 15%, respectively.

Etiology and pathophysiology. Dehydration is the result of many possible disease processes that cause abnormal fluid losses through the skin, respiratory, renal, and (most commonly) GI systems.

Clinical manifestations. The physical signs of dehydration are primarily the result of a deficiency in fluid volume. Because accurate record of weight before the episode of dehydration is not always available for comparison, it is easier to diagnose the degree of dehydration on the basis of its clinical manifestations (Table 32.1).

Diagnostic tests. Health care providers diagnose dehydration on the basis of observed clinical manifestations (see Table 32.1). Laboratory tests to support diagnosis and determine severity include measurements of serum sodium, serum glucose, serum bicarbonate, and blood urea nitrogen. In general, weighing the child daily also yields useful information about the degree and severity of dehydration.

Table 32.1 Clinical Manifestations of Dehydration

ASSESSMENT PARAMETER	SIGNS AND SYMPTOMS
Skin	Cold, dry, gray, loss of turgor
Mucous membranes	Dry
Eyes	Sunken
Fontanelle	Sunken
Behavior	Lethargic
Pulse	Rapid, weak
Blood pressure	Low
Respirations	Rapid

Medical management. Refer to the discussion of medical management of diarrhea (in the section "Diarrhea and Gastroenteritis").

Nursing interventions and patient teaching. Careful nursing assessment and intervention are important in the clinical detection and management of dehydration. An essential nursing function is to assess for any clinical manifestations of dehydration. This assessment begins with a general survey of the child and continues with specific observations.

Observation includes the measurement of intake and output (I&O). This measurement accounts for oral and parenteral intake and losses from sweat, wound drainage, urine, stools, vomiting, nasogastric drainage, and fistulas. For children who are not toilet trained, wet diapers should be weighed to assess the amount of output. By subtracting the weight (in grams) of a dry diaper from the weight of the wet diaper, calculate the actual fluid content of the diaper. The volume of fluid in milliliters is equal to the weight of the fluid measured in grams. Other data that assist in the assessment of dehydration include vital signs, body weight, skin color, temperature and turgor, capillary refill, presence or absence of edema, moisture and color of mucous membranes, sensation of thirst, and, in infants, assessment of the fontanelles.

Teach the parents that infants and young children have a greater need for water than do adults and are more vulnerable to alterations in fluid and electrolyte balance. In comparison with older children and adults, infants have a greater fluid I&O relative to size. Water and electrolyte disturbances occur more frequently and more rapidly, and infants and children adjust less promptly to these alterations.

Prognosis. Shock is common with severe depletion of extracellular fluid. When medical management and nursing interventions are effective, the prognosis is favorable.

Diarrhea and gastroenteritis. Diarrhea is one of the most common disorders affecting children; it has the capacity to quickly render the child vulnerable to fluid deficits and electrolyte imbalances. Diarrhea is a disturbance in intestinal motility, characterized by an increase in frequency, fluid content, and volume of stools. The diarrhea may be acute or chronic, and it may be either infectious or noninfectious. Diarrhea caused by an inflammatory process, such as infection, is called *gastroenteritis.*

Etiology and pathophysiology. Although diarrhea results from a variety of causes, the most common is bacterial or viral invasion of the intestinal mucosa. The most prevalent bacterial pathogens are *Salmonella, Shigella,* and *Rotavirus* organisms. Many factors can predispose a child to diarrhea. Infants have a greater susceptibility to diarrhea, and the results are more serious because infants have a small extracellular fluid reserve. When this reserve is depleted suddenly and quickly, dehydration rapidly ensues. Children who are malnourished, debilitated, or immunocompromised are more prone to diarrhea. Poor hygiene, contaminated food or water, warm weather, and crowded and substandard living conditions also predispose children to diarrhea. Other common causes of diarrhea are the ingestion of large quantities of fruit juices, such as apple juice; food sensitivities; antibiotics; and formula intolerance.

When a pathogen invades the intestinal mucosa, the resulting enterotoxins stimulate an inflammatory reaction. As a result, water and electrolytes are secreted, and the pathogen invades and destroys the epithelial cells of the GI mucosa. Serious disturbances, such as renal failure, dehydration, metabolic acidosis, shock, and circulatory collapse, may follow.

Clinical manifestations. In addition to the increased number of stools and the increased fluid content of stools, diarrhea has other clinical effects (Box 32.4). Assess for these, as well as for any signs of dehydration, which is a common complication of diarrhea (see Table 32.1).

Diagnostic tests. Document the history carefully, including information regarding recent travel, exposure to infected agents, personal contact, allergies, food or formula sensitivities, living conditions, and contact with contaminated water or food. Laboratory evaluation typically includes a stool culture, examination of the stool for ova and parasites, and CBC.

Box 32.4 Clinical Effects of Diarrhea

- Cool, pale skin
- Irritability progressing to lethargy
- Low blood pressure
- Malodorous stools
- Normal or elevated temperature
- Poor skin turgor
- Rapid pulse and respirations
- Sunken eyes
- Sunken fontanelles
- Vomiting
- Weight loss

Medical management. The goals of management are to restore the fluid and electrolyte balance and to treat the underlying cause. The American Academy of Pediatrics (since 2004) no longer recommends withholding food or fluids for 24 hours after the onset of diarrhea or administering the traditional diet of bananas, rice, applesauce, and toast or tea ("BRAT" diet). It is acceptable to offer a commercially available oral rehydration solution in small amounts for the first 4 to 6 hours after the onset of diarrhea. The infant who has been breast-feeding should continue doing so as a supplement to the oral rehydration solution. Administer oral maintenance doses of the solution for the remaining first 24 hours. An older child is permitted to take clear liquids. When the number and fluid content of stools have decreased, the infant is advanced gradually to full-strength formula. In an older child, solid foods should be offered when rehydration is complete. Initially, foods that are nonirritating to the bowel should be offered. The child may resume a regular diet gradually.

In cases of severe diarrhea, hospitalization and IV therapy are required. IV administration of a saline solution containing 5% dextrose enables rehydration. This solution provides the child with fluid, sodium, and calories. Once kidney function has been verified, it is acceptable to add potassium to the IV solution to correct any potassium depletion. IV rehydration must be continued until the diarrhea becomes less severe. Once rehydration has begun and the severe effects of the diarrhea and dehydration have abated, the focus of management shifts to determining and treating the underlying cause. This includes antimicrobial therapy as indicated.

Nursing interventions and patient teaching. Nursing interventions for the infant or child with diarrhea focus on assessment, including the careful recording of I&O; promotion of rehydration; correction of electrolyte imbalances; provision of age-appropriate nutrition; prevention of the spread of the diarrhea; prevention of complications; and emotional support of the child and family.

Patient problems and interventions for a child with diarrhea and gastroenteritis include but are not limited to the following:

Patient Problem	Nursing Interventions
Inadequate Fluid Volume, related to excessive GI losses in stool	Offer oral fluids as indicated and as tolerated Monitor IV fluids as prescribed Maintain strict record of I&O (urine and stool); monitor urine specific gravity Weigh patient daily Assess vital signs, skin turgor, mucous membranes, and mental status q 4 hr or as indicated

Patient Problem	Nursing Interventions
Compromised Skin Integrity, related to irritation caused by frequent, loose stools	Change diaper frequently Cleanse buttocks gently with bland, nonalkaline soap and water, or immerse patient in a bath for gentle cleansing Apply protective ointment (type of ointment often varies according to individual patient, and sometimes a trial period is necessary) Expose slightly erythematous intact skin to air whenever possible; apply protective ointment to very irritated or excoriated skin Observe buttocks and perineum for infection, such as *Candida*
Anxiousness, related to • Separation from parents • Unfamiliar environment • Distressing procedures	Provide mouth care and pacifier for infants who are on NPO status Encourage family visitation and appropriate participation in care Touch, hold, and talk to patient as much as possible Provide sensory stimulation and diversion appropriate for patient's developmental level

Parents should be instructed to avoid the use of antidiarrheals such as diphenoxylate (Lomotil) or kaolin and pectin (Kaopectate). Discuss hygiene practice and instruct the parents on hand washing after changing diapers to prevent the spread of infection. It is necessary to dispose of properly or thoroughly clean soiled diapers, bed linens, and clothes.

Prognosis. Mild or moderate diarrhea can be managed at home by simple methods. Severe diarrhea necessitates hospitalization with IV fluid therapy. When treatment is effective, the prognosis is usually excellent.

Constipation. *Constipation* is best defined as the passage of hardened stools, and it often occurs in association with failure to evacuate the colon completely with defecation. It is possible for constipation to manifest as a primary disorder or in association with a wide variety of GI tract or systemic disorders.

Etiology and pathophysiology. Constipation is possible in children of any age. Newborns normally pass a first meconium stool within 24 to 36 hours after birth. Failure to do this indicates possible intestinal atresia (congenital closure of a body part usually open; in this case, any part of the intestine) or stenosis (constriction or narrowing of a passage or orifice), Hirschsprung's disease, meconium ileus (ileus of the newborn caused by obstruction of the bowel with meconium), or a meconium plug. In formula-fed infants, constipation may result from a high fat or protein content or inadequate fluid in the formula. In children, constipation sometimes occurs in connection with environmental factors such as medications (e.g., iron supplements, anticonvulsant therapy, low-fiber diet, or antacids) or results from a learned repression of the urge to defecate. In children who have constipation, passage of hardened stools is painful. As a result, the child may repress the urge to defecate. Continuous repression results in dilation of the rectum, reduced sensation of the need to defecate, and decreased muscle tone in the lower rectum. This cycle results in chronic, incomplete evacuation of the colon, and the constipation becomes severe. Episodes of diarrhea or *encopresis* (leakage around the firm stool in the rectum) often lead to accidents or soiling.

Clinical manifestations. In infancy, constipation sometimes occurs in association with hard stools or evidence of fresh blood in the stools. Accompanying symptoms may include cramping abdominal pain, anal fissures, pain on defecation, loss of appetite, and irritability.

Diagnostic tests. Diagnosis of constipation rests largely on a thorough health history. The parents should be asked to describe the infant's or child's bowel patterns. A discussion of diet and medications is also indicated. The health care provider will perform a physical examination of the anus and rectum.

Medical management. In the newborn, simple measures often effectively alleviate constipation. Modifying the formula with addition of more fluid or carbohydrates sometimes corrects the situation. For infants older than 5 to 6 months, adding foods with bulk (fruits and vegetables) and increasing fluid intake sometimes correct the problem. If the constipation is the result of a tightened anal sphincter or anal stenosis, the health care provider may instruct parents to dilate the sphincter manually two or three times daily until sufficient dilation is attained. The management of simple constipation in children focuses on emptying the rectum completely of stool with the use of mild laxatives or enemas and instituting dietary modifications, such as increased fluid intake and addition of high-fiber foods, to prevent further constipation. The treatment of chronic constipation in children aims at complete evacuation of the rectum and bowel retraining therapy. It is usually possible to achieve complete evacuation of the rectum through the use of enemas, manual disimpaction, and stool softeners. After complete evacuation is attained, the health care provider institutes bowel retraining therapy to sustain evacuation. This generally consists of behavioral modification, with positive reinforcement for toilet sitting and defecation, and emotional support.

Nursing interventions and patient teaching. Nursing interventions begin with a careful history of bowel patterns, including stool characteristics (color, consistency, frequency, and associated pain), diet, and concomitant medications. If dietary modifications are to be instituted, educate the parents regarding these and ensure their understanding. Sometimes parents also need instruction about normal stool patterns and what constitutes constipation. Discussion of the parent's expectations and attitudes regarding toileting is helpful.

Providing emotional reassurance to the parents and child is beneficial.

Instruct parents to avoid the use of raw or unpasteurized honey and corn syrup products as a home remedy for constipation in young infants. Use of these products may be associated with the development of infant botulism.

Prognosis. Simple measures ordinarily correct constipation. The underlying cause and child's age will largely affect resolution. In the more complex situations, counseling and bowel retraining are often necessary.

Gastroesophageal reflux. Gastroesophageal reflux (GER) is the effortless regurgitation of the gastric contents into the esophagus. The passage of the gastric esophageal contents into the oropharynx is called *regurgitation.* Vomiting is the expulsion of refluxed gastric contents from the mouth. The health care provider diagnoses GER disease when gastric contents are regurgitated into the esophagus or oropharynx and produce symptoms. In affected infants, GER usually begins within 1 week of birth, and regurgitation occurs immediately after a feeding or when the infant is laid down after a feeding.

Etiology and pathophysiology. GER results primarily from an incompetent lower esophageal (or cardiac) sphincter. As a result, gastric contents can regurgitate into the esophagus.

Clinical manifestations. Vomiting or spitting up is the primary manifestation in the first week of life. Aspiration of the gastric contents has potential to lead to respiratory signs such as apnea, choking or gagging after feedings, and aspiration pneumonia. In affected young children, a chronic cough, wheezing, and recurrent pneumonia are common. Growth and weight gain are a problem with a majority of affected children. Continuous irritation of the esophageal lining with gastric acid can lead to esophageal ulceration and bleeding. This usually manifests as anemia, hematemesis, or blood in the stools.

Diagnostic tests. Diagnosis begins with an evaluation of the health history and of growth and weight patterns. More invasive studies such as barium esophagography, esophageal pH, and an upper endoscopy can be performed.

Medical management. Conservative management of GER includes feeding and positioning practices. Feeding small, frequent feedings that have been thickened with infant cereal may be implemented (Schwarz, 2017). If the infant is breast-feeding, the mother should express milk manually and mix it with cereal for feedings. The prone position improves gastric emptying and decreases GER; however, as previously discussed, to aid in preventing SIDS it is recommended to place infants to sleep on their backs. Prone positioning should be used only while the infant is awake, especially after feedings. The infant should be supervised carefully when placed in the prone position.

Pharmacologic therapies also may be prescribed. H_2-histamine receptor antagonists, such as cimetidine (Tagamet), ranitidine (Zantac), or famotidine (Pepcid), are effective in reducing the amount of acid present in gastric content and sometimes prevent esophagitis. It is also possible to give metoclopramide (Reglan) before meals and at bedtime to accelerate gastric emptying. Proton pump inhibitors such as omeprazole (Prilosec or Prevacid) and lansoprazole (Prevacid) reduce acid secretion.

Surgical management of GER sometimes is indicated in severe cases. A **Nissen fundoplication**, which involves wrapping the fundus of the stomach around the distal esophagus to prevent reflux of the stomach contents into the esophagus, is the most commonly performed surgical procedure.

Nursing interventions and patient teaching. The nurse is often the first health care provider to whom the condition is reported. A nursing priority is to collect supportive data. The problem is distressing for children and their parents, necessitating emotional support and reassurance that the condition is physiologic in nature and not caused by emotional problems or faulty feeding patterns. Teach the plan of treatment, prescribed medications, and signs and symptoms to report.

Prognosis. In the majority of affected infants, GER is mild and normal function is achieved by 6 to 7 weeks of age. Most cases improve by about 1 year of age. Medical therapy is required in more severe cases. If GER is severe and treatment remains unsuccessful, multiple complications such as esophageal strictures and recurrent respiratory distress with aspiration pneumonia can occur.

Hypertrophic pyloric stenosis. Hypertrophic pyloric stenosis (HPS) is an obstructive disorder in which the gastric outlet is obstructed mechanically by a congenitally hypertrophied pyloric muscle. It is also the most common reason for an abdominal operation during the first 6 months of life. Boys are affected more often than girls. HPS most often manifests within the first 3 months of life. Genes may play a role, because children of parents who had pyloric stenosis are more likely to have this condition.

HPS occurs most often in infants younger than 6 months. It is more common in boys than in girls.

Etiology and pathophysiology. The exact cause of HPS is not known. The incidence is higher in siblings and offspring of affected people. Other risk factors include certain antibiotics, too much acid in the first part of the small intestine (duodenum), and certain congenital diseases, such as diabetes. The circular muscle that surrounds the valve between the stomach and the duodenum becomes diffusely enlarged as the result of hypertrophy and hyperplasia (Fig. 32.15). As a result, the passage becomes narrower, and it is difficult for the stomach to empty. At approximately 4 to 6 weeks of age, infants with HPS begin to vomit almost immediately after feedings. As the condition progresses, the vomiting becomes more forceful and becomes projectile, the hallmark sign of HPS.

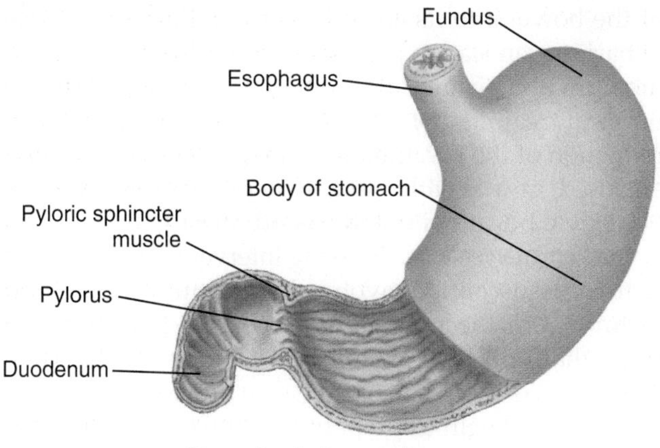

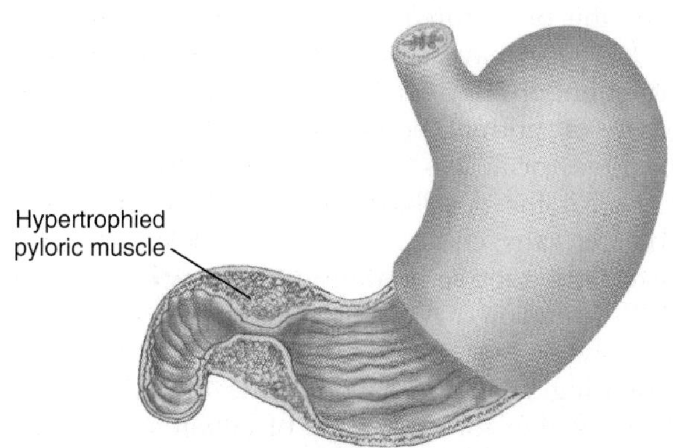

Fig. 32.15 Comparison of normal pyloric opening with evidence of pyloric stenosis. (From Ashwill JW, Droske SC: *Nursing care of children: Principles and practice*, ed 3, Philadelphia, 2007, Saunders.)

Clinical manifestations. Initially, the signs begin as regurgitation that progresses to projectile vomiting 30 to 60 minutes after feeding. As the condition progresses, the affected infant exhibits lethargy, weight loss, poor skin turgor, sunken fontanelles, and loss of subcutaneous tissue as dehydration ensues (Box 32.5).

Diagnostic tests. Examination of the abdomen is often a key assessment that assists in the diagnosis and reveals signs of HPS. Peristaltic waves that move from left to right across the epigastric region are sometimes visible, and palpation sometimes reveals an olive-shaped mass in this area to the right of the midline. If it is not possible to establish the diagnosis after history and physical examination, an ultrasonic examination usually is indicated. Ultrasonography demonstrates an elongated sausage-shaped mass with an elongated pyloric channel. If ultrasonography fails to demonstrate hypertrophy of the pylorus, health care providers order upper GI radiography to rule out other causes of vomiting.

Medical management. Surgical relief of the pyloric obstruction as soon as establishment of the diagnosis is the standard treatment of HPS. The surgical correction of HPS consists of a pyloromyotomy, in which the pylorus muscle is surgically split down to, but not including, the submucosa; this allows for enlarging of the lumen. This procedure has a high success rate when the infant receives careful preoperative preparation to correct fluid and electrolyte imbalances.

Box 32.5 Clinical Manifestations of Hypertrophic Pyloric Stenosis

- Projectile vomiting: vomitus is sometimes ejected 3 to 4 feet (0.9 to 1.2 m) from the child when child is in a side-lying position, 1 foot (0.3 m) or more when child is in a back-lying position:
  - Usually occurs shortly after feeding (may not occur for several hours)
  - May follow each feeding or appear intermittently
  - Nonbilious (no bile) vomitus; may be blood tinged
- Appetite: hungry, avid nurser; infant eagerly accepts a second feeding after vomiting episode
- No evidence of pain or discomfort except that of chronic hunger
- Weight loss
- Signs of dehydration
- Distended upper abdomen
- Readily palpable olive-shaped mass in the epigastrium just to the right of the umbilicus
- Gastric peristaltic waves that are visible and move from left to right across the epigastrium

Nursing interventions and patient teaching. Nursing interventions for an infant with HPS primarily involve assisting with the establishment of a diagnosis, providing adequate nutrition, managing preoperative and postoperative care, and emotionally supporting the family. A carefully documented history, with assessment for signs and symptoms of HPS, is essential for the prompt diagnosis. Correction of any metabolic disturbances and dehydration before surgery is essential. In general, this is possible through IV administration of fluid and electrolytes. It is necessary to keep the affected infant on NPO status to eliminate vomiting. Fluid replacement needs must be assessed and are determined largely by I&O. Postoperative nursing interventions are focused on preventing complications by monitoring I&O, observing physical signs, and instituting oral feedings. Feedings of glucose water usually begin 4 to 6 hours postoperatively; then, if feedings are retained for 24 hours, full feedings are started. Encourage parents to express their concerns, visit their infant frequently, and participate in the care when appropriate. Barring complications, affected infants usually are discharged within 1 to 2 days after surgery.

Prognosis. Most infants with HPS recover completely and rapidly after pyloromyotomy. Small feedings typically are initiated within a few hours postoperatively. Postoperative complications include persistent pyloric obstruction and wound dehiscence.

Intussusception. Intussusception is the most common cause of intestinal obstruction in children between 3 months and 6 years of age. It is twice as common in male children. In general, health care providers are unable to determine the cause of intussusception.

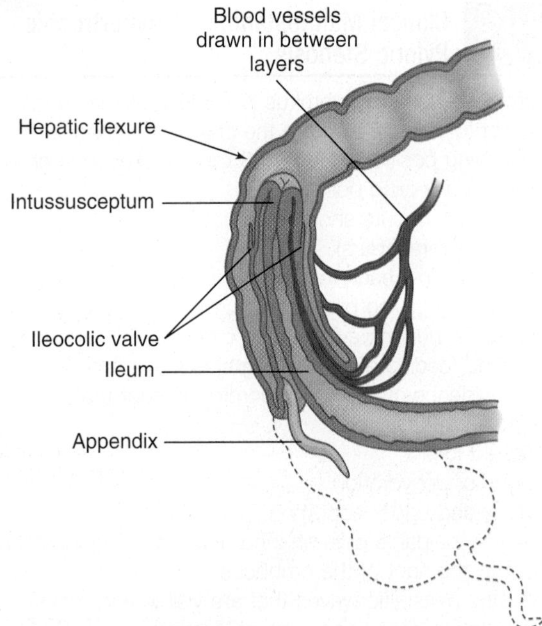

Fig. 32.16 Ileocolic intussusception. (From Hockenberry MJ, Wilson D: *Nursing care of infants and children*, ed 9, St. Louis, 2011, Mosby.)

Etiology and pathophysiology. Intussusception is the result of the telescoping of one portion of the intestine into another (Fig. 32.16). The site most commonly affected is the ileocecal valve, at the juncture of the distal ileum and the proximal colon. As the ileum telescopes into the colon, the passage of intestinal contents distal to the defect becomes obstructed. Subsequently, as the mucosa of the intestinal walls rub against each other, blood and mucus from the mucosa leak into the intestinal lumen and form **"currant jelly" stools** (feces mixed with blood and mucus from the intestinal mucosa), a hallmark sign of intussusception. Serious complications include peritonitis, intestinal ischemia, infarction, perforation, and shock. If the condition is not treated, the child may die within 2 to 5 days.

Clinical manifestations. In most cases, there is a sudden onset of severe abdominal pain in a previously well child. The child assumes a fetal position in an effort to guard the abdomen. Vomiting and lethargy usually occur. Within 12 hours of the onset of abdominal pain, the child usually passes the characteristic "currant jelly" stool.

Diagnostic tests. The signs and symptoms collected during the history and physical aid in the diagnosis of the disorder. Radiographic studies may show a perforation. Ultrasound and CT scans demonstrate intestinal obstruction caused by intussusception. Imaging of all three examinations may show a "bull's-eye," representing the intestine coiled within itself. An air or barium enema also may be used for diagnosis (Mayo Clinic, 2018c).

Medical management. In 90% of cases either of these diagnostic tests actually may correct the intussusception when the air or barium is instilled (Mayo Clinic, 2018c). The force exerted by the flowing barium from the enema sometimes successfully forces the telescoped portion of the bowel into its correct position. Because the use of barium can lead to peritonitis, water-soluble contrast medium and air pressure sometimes are used instead. Surgical treatment of intussusception involves manual reduction of the invagination (the process of becoming enclosed in a sheath) and, if necessary, resection of nonviable bowel with end-to-end anastomosis.

Nursing interventions. Nursing interventions for a child with intussusception involve documenting a thorough history from the parents and observing for physical signs that will help establish a prompt and accurate diagnosis. As soon as the health care provider establishes a diagnosis, begin to prepare the parents for the diagnostic barium enema study. Inform them that in many cases, this procedure is corrective, but if it is unsuccessful, surgery may be required. After the hydrostatic reduction, observe for the passage of barium and the return of normal bowel movements. The child is observed for at least 24 hours after the procedure to assess for the possibility of recurrence. If surgery is indicated, the child is kept on NPO status with a nasogastric tube set to intermittent low suction. Begin an IV infusion to supply adequate hydration and electrolytes. Postoperative care of the child involves measuring vital signs, monitoring the operative site, and assessing for the return of bowel sounds. When peristaltic function has returned, it is appropriate to gradually introduce oral feedings.

Prognosis. In many patients with intussusception, treatment with hydrostatic reduction is successful. Surgery is required for patients in whom the water-soluble contrast medium enema with air pressure was unsuccessful. If untreated, most patients suffer worsening or die of complications such as perforation, peritonitis, and sepsis. With early diagnosis and treatment, serious complications and death are rare.

Hirschsprung's disease. Hirschsprung's disease, also known as *megacolon* (congenital aganglionic megacolon), is a functional intestinal obstruction caused by the absence of parasympathetic ganglion cells in a portion of the colon. The incidence is 1 per 5400 to 7200 live births, with a predominance in boys. Hirschsprung's disease is more common in children with trisomy 21 (Down syndrome) (Wagner, 2017).

Etiology and pathophysiology. In Hirschsprung's disease, there is an absence of innervation to a segment of the bowel. In most cases, the lower portion of the sigmoid colon just above the anus is affected. As a result, there are no peristaltic waves in the affected portion of the colon to propel the fecal contents, which causes an intestinal obstruction and distention of the bowel proximal to the defect (Fig. 32.17).

Clinical manifestations. Clinical manifestations often vary according to age. Early observation of an affected newborn typically reveals a failure to pass meconium within 48 hours and signs of partial or complete intestinal obstruction, such as abdominal distention, vomiting,

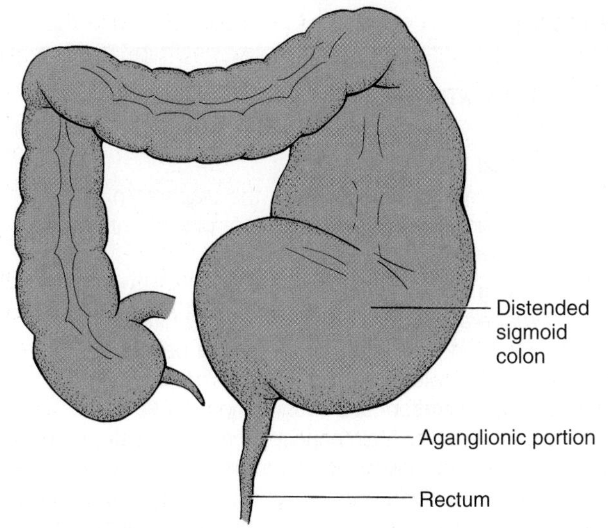

Fig. 32.17 Appearance of the affected portion of the bowel in Hirschsprung's disease. (From Hockenberry MJ, Wilson D: *Wong's essentials of pediatric nursing*, ed 9, St. Louis, 2013, Mosby.)

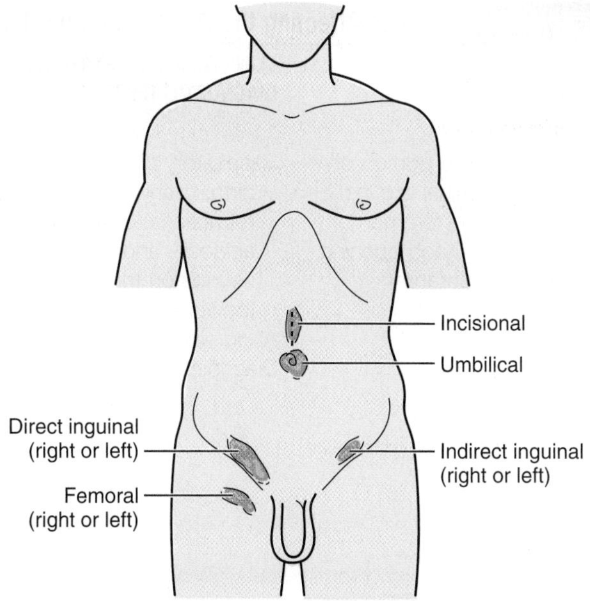

Fig. 32.18 Locations of hernias. (From Phillips N: *Berry and Kohn's operating room technique*, ed 12, St. Louis, 2013, Mosby.)

and poor feeding. Affected infants sometimes have a history of constipation or intermittent constipation and diarrhea. Dehydration, failure to thrive, abdominal distention, and fever are other possible manifestations. In affected older children, there is an association between Hirschsprung's disease and chronic constipation; abdominal distention; ribbon-like, foul-smelling stools; poor weight gain; malnourishment; anemia; palpable fecal mass; and visible peristalsis.

Diagnostic tests. A carefully obtained history, associated clinical manifestations, and a barium enema study assist in making a diagnosis of Hirschsprung's disease.

Medical management. Immediate treatment involves surgical removal of the affected portion of the bowel. The surgeon proceeds in two stages. The first stage involves placement of a temporary colostomy in the portion of normal, innervated colon just proximal to the defect. This allows for a period of rest, during which the normal bowel regains its tone. The second stage involves excising the affected segment and pulling the normal, innervated segment down through the anus, anastomosing it to the anal canal. This procedure, known as the *Soave endorectal pull-through,* usually is performed when the child reaches a weight of 20 pounds.

Nursing interventions and patient teaching. The nursing interventions for the infant or child with Hirschsprung's disease are focused on assisting the parents in adjusting to the diagnosis, promoting parent-infant bonding, preparing the parents for surgery, and educating them regarding colostomy care. Preoperatively, direct nursing interventions are focused on restoring the child's nutritional status with a low-fiber, high-protein, high-calorie diet or, in severe cases, total parenteral nutrition. Sometimes you must evacuate the patient's bowel with daily enemas and stool softeners. Oral antibiotics, if prescribed, are administered to decrease intestinal flora. Measure the patient's abdominal girth daily. Prepare the child, when developmentally appropriate, and the parents for the colostomy. Stress that this is a temporary procedure unless a large portion of the bowel is involved, which would necessitate a permanent ileostomy. Postoperative care includes assessing vital signs and bowel sounds, observing for the passage of flatus and stools, and monitoring the operative site. Surgeons generally place a nasogastric tube set to low intermittent suction during the surgery and order its removal as soon as peristalsis has returned, usually within 24 hours, and when a diet appropriate for age can be introduced.

Before discharge, parents need instruction regarding colostomy care; refer them as needed to a visiting nurse for assistance in caring for the colostomy.

Prognosis. After fluid and replacement therapy, the infant undergoes surgery, during which the surgeon creates a colostomy. One or more corrective surgeries will follow, after which time the colostomy can usually be reversed.

Hernias. A *hernia* is the protrusion of organs or portions of an organ through a structural defect or weakened muscle wall. A complication of herniation arises when the circulation to the protruding organ is impaired (known as a *strangulated hernia*) or when the pressure of protruding organs impairs the function of other organs. Incarceration of a hernia occurs when the hernia cannot be reduced manually. Fig. 32.18 and Table 32.2 illustrate and describe hernias affecting the diaphragm and the abdominal wall.

DISORDERS OF GENITOURINARY FUNCTION

Disorders of the genitourinary tract are common in children and arise from a variety of etiologic factors.

Table 32.2 Hernias Affecting the Diaphragm and the Abdominal Wall

HERNIAS TYPE	CLINICAL MANIFESTATIONS AND DIAGNOSTIC TESTS	INTERVENTIONS
Diaphragmatic		
Protrusion of a portion of the abdominal organs through the foramen of Bochdalek (and opening in the diaphragm)	Respiratory distress within hours of birth; cyanosis, tachypnea, retractions, dyspnea, respiratory acidosis, and absence of breath sounds on the affected side (bowel sounds may be present) Abdominal pain, vomiting Diagnosis made by radiography	**Medical** Immediate surgical repair of the diaphragm with replacement of the herniation; placement of chest tubes **Nursing** *Preoperative:* Support of respiratory function; comfort measures; placement of patient in semi-Fowler's position; suctioning, oxygen administration, and monitoring of IV fluids *Postoperative:* Maintenance of routine postoperative care and monitoring; placement of patient in semi-Fowler's position; physiotherapy and positive pressure ventilation; monitoring of oxygenation; comfort measures; emotional support of parents
Hiatal		
Intermittent protrusion of the stomach through the esophageal opening in the diaphragm	Vomiting, dysphasia, dyspnea, gastroesophageal reflux, respiratory distress, bleeding Diagnosis based on history and radiography	**Medical** Surgical repair of the esophageal opening **Nursing** Routine preoperative and postoperative care, as for diaphragmatic hernia
Inguinal		
Prolapse of a loop of intestine through the inguinal ring above the scrotal sac because of muscle weakness; can be either unilateral or bilateral	Usually asymptomatic and found only in the course of routine examination; can become strangulated or incarcerated (i.e., a portion of the intestine becomes tightly caught in the hernia sac, restricting blood supply) Sometimes accompanied by hydrocele or undescended testes	**Medical** Usually possible to reduce by gentle manipulation of the trapped intestine; after surgery (herniorrhaphy), overnight hospital stay not necessary **Nursing** Applying ice to the scrotum to reduce edema; comfort measures and quieting of the patient with an incarcerated (trapped) inguinal hernia so that the surgeon can reduce the incarceration; no diapers used postoperatively, even if the child is not toilet trained; instruction of parents not to give tub baths until healing is complete
Umbilical		
Protrusion of the intestine through a weakness in the abdominal wall around the umbilicus	Inspection and palpation of abdomen High incidence in African American infants Spontaneous closure at 1 to 2 years of age	**Medical** Spontaneous closure by age 2 yr with small defects (<2 cm); surgical closure if condition persists after age 2–5 yr or for defects larger than 2 cm **Nursing** Discouraging use of home remedies (i.e., coins, belly bands, abdominal taping); reassurance of parents

The genitourinary system is responsible for maintaining fluid and electrolyte balance within the body. Disorders of the genitourinary system alter the delicate balance of fluid and electrolytes within the body and sometimes become life threatening.

Urinary tract infection. Urinary tract infections (UTIs) affect the upper urinary tract (kidneys and ureters), the lower urinary tract (bladder and urethra), or both. They are more prevalent in girls, uncircumcised boys, and sexually active adolescents. UTIs are caused primarily by bacteria, most frequently gram-negative organisms. Because the female urethra is short (approximately 2 cm [0.8 in] in young girls and 4 cm [1.6 in] in mature women), it provides an efficient access route to the bladder for organisms that are common to the perineal and perianal regions. Another factor that sometimes leads to UTIs is urinary stasis. The urine is typically sterile, but the warm climate within the bladder provides an excellent growth medium for bacteria. Teaching parents correct perineal cleansing is imperative. In infant boys, it is necessary to retract and cleanse the foreskin with each diaper change. When older boys begin bathing themselves, it is necessary for parents to monitor this cleaning. For girls, cleansing the perineal area from front to back helps prevent UTIs from *Escherichia coli.* Some children also have a congenital anomaly such as urethral stenosis or vesicoureteral reflux (backward flow of urine from the bladder to the ureters) that can lead to urinary stasis and the development of a UTI. Signs and symptoms of UTIs are often subtle, and parents may not realize anything is wrong with the child. In affected infants, fever, weight loss, failure to thrive, feeding difficulties, vomiting, and diarrhea are common. In affected children, urinary frequency, pain during urination, foul-smelling urine, incontinence after successful toilet training, abdominal or flank pain, hematuria, and vomiting are common signs and symptoms.

Nephrotic syndrome (nephrosis). Nephrotic syndrome is a clinical state characterized by proteinuria, edema, hyperlipidemia, and hypoproteinemia. Nephrotic syndrome has three forms: (1) idiopathic, or primary; (2) secondary (occurring as a result of glomerular damage caused by a known cause); and (3) congenitally acquired. In children, the idiopathic form is most common.

Etiology and pathophysiology. For most children (90%), the cause of the syndrome is unknown. For the other 10% the most common cause is minimal change disease. Children with minimal change disease typically outgrow nephrotic syndrome by the time they reach their teen years. Minimal change disease has unknown cause, but it can be related to infections, tumors, allergic reactions, and overuse of over-the-counter medications such as ibuprofen and acetaminophen. The underlying pathologic abnormality is glomerular damage that renders the glomerulus permeable to protein (proteinuria). Loss of protein in the urine causes a decrease in the level of protein in the blood (hypoproteinemia), which causes a decrease in colloidal osmotic pressure in the capillaries. This results in hyperpermeability of the capillaries and causes fluid to leak into the interstitial spaces (edema). Children typically experience swelling around their eyes, abdomen, feet, and ankles (National Kidney Foundation, n.d.).

Clinical manifestations. The development of manifestations is subtle. Initially, children may develop periorbital edema, which is noticed primarily on awakening. Abdominal distention is sometimes apparent as fluid accumulates in the abdominal cavity (ascites). As the syndrome progresses, the edema becomes generalized and severe (anasarca) (Fig. 32.19). Vomiting, anorexia, diarrhea, and irritability are common. Increased body weight, decreased urine output, and marked edema are hallmark signs. Other signs include white nails, lusterless hair, and soft ear cartilage.

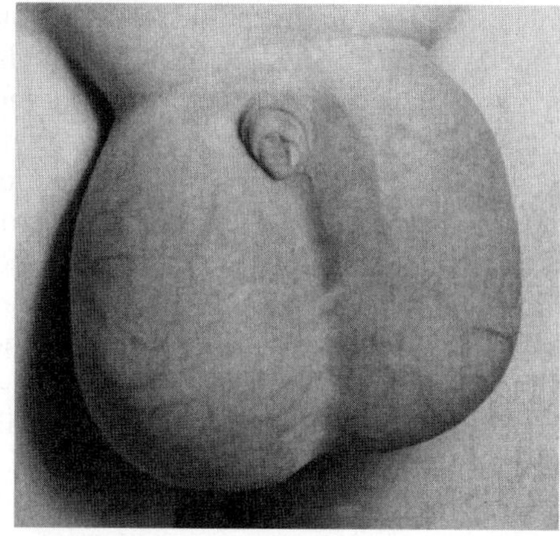

Fig. 32.19 Appearance of the genitals of a boy with nephrotic syndrome. (Courtesy Harry C. Shirkey, Fort Thomas, Kentucky.)

Diagnostic tests. A thorough physical examination and clinical manifestations such as weight gain, edema, and lab analyses are used in the diagnosis of nephritic syndrome. Analysis of the urine reveals marked proteinuria with a high specific gravity. The urine is frequently dark and frothy. RBCs, hyaline casts, and fat bodies also may be present. Serum protein levels are reduced, and serum lipid levels are elevated. A renal biopsy may help determine the extent of glomerular damage and evaluate the response to therapy.

Medical management. The principal goal of management of nephrotic syndrome is to reduce the edema. Steroid therapy is the primary means to accomplish this. Health care providers order adrenocortical steroids (prednisone) to reduce the proteinuria and subsequently the edema. This response usually occurs within 7 to 21 days of initiation of the therapy; administration of the steroids slowly tapers over a period of several weeks and discontinues when the child has no symptoms. Bed rest is encouraged in the acute phase of the illness, with progression to ambulation as the edema subsides. The child typically is placed on a low-sodium diet during the period of severe edema. A child with nephrotic syndrome may receive diuretic therapies to reduce edema. Treatment for relapses consists of a repeated course of high-dose steroid therapy (American Kidney Fund, n.d.).

Nursing interventions and patient teaching. Nursing interventions focus on clinical observation of the child in the acute phase and monitoring the effects of therapeutic interventions. Careful monitoring of I&O, body weight, and abdominal girth is essential in assessing the status of fluid retention or excretion. Provide meticulous skin care to prevent impairment of edematous skin and secondary infections. Frequent monitoring of vital signs is necessary to detect early signs of complications, such as infection or shock. Because children with nephrotic syndrome have a poor appetite, nutrition is likely to be a challenge. It is essential that the child have a good protein intake to offset the loss of protein through the urine. Preferred foods should be offered frequently in small amounts and served in an attractive manner. Dietary restrictions include low levels of salt and fluid restrictions. Because increased susceptibility to infection is a common side effect of steroid therapy, it is necessary to keep the child free of exposure to communicable diseases and sources of infection. As the edema decreases, it is appropriate to increase the child's activity. Provide continuous emotional support to the family during the acute phase of the illness and while the child recovers.

Teach parents about testing urine for albumin, administration of medications, diet restrictions (if any), and the common effects of steroid therapy. Instruct parents about preventing contact with infected playmates, although it is permissible for the child to attend school. Parents should learn how to assess for signs of relapse; ensure they understand to seek immediate medical attention if these signs occur.

Prognosis. The chance for ultimate recovery in most cases is good. The response is more likely to be satisfactory when detection of any relapses and institution of therapy occur promptly. Remissions are longer when the prescribed treatment regimen is followed. Most affected children actually outgrow the disease during their teens or by early adulthood. Even if a child has numerous attacks, most will not develop permanent kidney damage. The children who do not outgrow it or who do not respond to treatment may become candidates for kidney transplantation (National Kidney Foundation, n.d.).

Acute glomerulonephritis. **Glomerulonephritis** is inflammation of the glomeruli of the kidney. Most commonly, it occurs after a pneumococcal, streptococcal, or viral infection. *Acute poststreptococcal glomerulonephritis* (APSGN) is the most common form. APSGN affects primarily children of early school age, with onset peaking at ages 6 to 7 years, and the disease occurs twice as often in boys as in girls.

Etiology and pathophysiology. APSGN follows a streptococcal infection of the throat or skin. Immune complexes that develop as a result of infection with certain strains of group A β-hemolytic streptococci become fixed to the basement membrane of glomeruli. Most streptococcal infections do not cause APSGN. A latent period of 10 to 21 days occurs between onset of the streptococcal infection and the onset of clinical manifestations. The glomeruli become edematous and infiltrated with WBCs. As a result, the glomerular filtration rate decreases, which causes an accumulation of sodium and water in the blood, which in turn leads to circulatory congestion and edema. Inflammation and damage to the glomeruli result in increased permeability, allowing protein molecules to escape into the urine (proteinuria).

Clinical manifestations. Manifestations of APSGN usually appear 10 to 14 days after the streptococcal infection occurs. Initial characteristics are a sudden onset of hematuria, proteinuria, and oliguria. The child's urine sometimes appears cloudy, smoky brown, or what parents describe as tea or cola colored. Edema, abdominal pain, pallor, low-grade fever, anorexia, vomiting, and headache are sometimes present. Hypertension and heart failure are possible results of hypervolemia. Fluid retention does not explain completely the hypertension associated with acute glomerulonephritis. Overproduction of renin also sometimes occurs.

Diagnostic tests. Urinalysis reveals proteinuria, hematuria, and elevated specific gravity. Some patients have elevated levels of blood urea nitrogen and creatinine as a result of impaired glomerular filtration. Results of the urine culture are typically negative. Cultures of the throat or skin yield positive results for the streptococcal organism. The *antistreptolysin O titer* (antibodies formed against streptococci) is elevated, indicating that the patient has had a recent streptococcal infection. Renal ultrasonography, renal biopsy, electrocardiography, and chest radiography also commonly are performed to determine the extent of the disease.

Medical management. The acute phase of glomerulonephritis generally lasts 1 to 2 weeks. During this time, health care providers usually recommend bed rest, although many children set their own limits according to their tolerance of activity. Dietary fluid, sodium, potassium, and phosphate are restricted initially. Regular measurement of vital signs, body weight, and I&O is necessary to monitor the progression of the disease and detect any complications. It is necessary to anticipate acute hypertension and identify it early. Antihypertensive medications and diuretics help control hypertension. Antibiotic therapy is indicated only for children who have a persistent streptococcal infection.

Nursing interventions and patient teaching. Nursing interventions focus on promoting rest and adequate nutrition, preventing and detecting complications, and providing emotional support to the child and family. During the acute phase of the illness, some health care providers place the child on bed rest. Provide activities that require minimal energy expenditure and will keep the child's interest. Ensure that meals reflect the child's preferences and yet adhere to any dietary restrictions that have been ordered. Measurements of vital signs, body weight, and I&O provide information about the disease's progression and help detect the presence of complications.

Educate the parents about the disease and its therapy and allow them to express their feelings and concerns.

Prognosis. Most children with APSGN recover completely, with few or no complications. Specific immunity is conferred so that subsequent recurrences are uncommon. Dialysis is required if the disease is not controlled and causes acute or chronic renal failure. If acute renal failure occurs, kidney transplantation is considered.

Wilms tumor (nephroblastoma). Wilms tumor (or nephroblastoma) is the most common renal and intraabdominal malignant tumor of childhood, accounting for 5% of all cancers in children. About 500 new cases of Wilms tumor are diagnosed each year in the United States. The incidence of these tumors peaks at ages 3 to 4 years. It is uncommon in children older than 6 years of age (American Cancer Society, 2016b).

Etiology and pathophysiology. Wilms tumor most commonly affects the left kidney. Both kidneys are affected in 10% of cases. Wilms tumor has hereditary and nonhereditary origins. The most common sites for metastasis are the lungs, the lymph nodes, the liver, the brain, and bone.

Clinical manifestations. Most Wilms tumors manifest as enlarging, asymptomatic, and firm abdominal masses. Other manifestations of the tumor include abdominal pain, hematuria, fever, hypertension, weight loss, and fatigue. If Wilms tumor has metastasized, dyspnea, cough, and chest pain may be present.

Diagnostic tests. Parents may detect many tumors when they feel an enlarged abdominal mass while bathing, dressing, or carrying the child. In addition to a thorough history and physical examination, diagnostic studies include radiography, abdominal ultrasonography, abdominal and chest computed tomography, MRI, and hematologic and chemistry studies. The definitive (final) diagnosis is based on findings of surgical biopsy. Because the tumor is encapsulated, it is important not to palpate the child's abdomen more than is necessary for diagnosis. This decreases the possibility of rupture of the capsule and spillage of the malignant cells into the abdominal cavity.

Medical management. Treatment of Wilms tumor involves surgical resection as soon as possible after diagnosis, usually within 24 to 48 hours of admission. The surgeon performs an exploration of the abdomen to determine the extent of the disease and whether the tumor has metastasized. If one kidney is affected, the surgeon removes the tumor, the kidney, and the adrenal gland, with meticulous care during resection to avoid rupture of the capsule and spread of cancer cells throughout the abdomen. The other kidney is examined for evidence of disease. If both kidneys are involved, the surgeon removes part of the kidney on the less affected side and the entire kidney on the opposite side. Most children with Wilms tumor receive radiotherapy after surgery. Chemotherapy is indicated for all affected children. The usual course of treatment ranges from 6 to 15 months.

Nursing interventions and patient teaching. Preoperative nursing interventions involve preparing the child and family for surgery. This is a challenging responsibility for the nurse because most surgeries take place within 24 hours of diagnosis. Postoperative nursing interventions are similar to those provided to children undergoing abdominal surgery with an emphasis on monitoring renal function. Be sensitive to the parents' feelings about their child's diagnosis; it is common for parents to believe that they should have identified the mass earlier.

The overall objective in discharge planning is to return the child to a normal preoperative lifestyle. Emphasize the usual needs for discipline and moderate protection from infection. Help plan treatment schedules to allow uninterrupted school attendance. Because the child is left with one kidney, certain precautions, such as avoiding contact sports, should be recommended to prevent injuring the remaining organ. Prompt detection and treatment of any genitourinary signs or symptoms are mandatory.

Prognosis. Reinforce to parents that prognosis is excellent and survival rates have improved with the development of new treatment protocols. Children with a localized tumor (stages I and II) have a 90% chance of cure with appropriate therapy.

Structural defects of the genitourinary tract. Structural defects of the genitourinary tract have serious implications for the psychological well-being of the child. Prompt correction is necessary to avoid a negative psychological effect on the child, as well as to prevent physical complications. The major structural defects and their medical management are presented in Table 32.3 and hypospadias is depicted in Fig. 32.20.

Nursing interventions and patient teaching. Nursing interventions for a child with a defect of the genitourinary tract are focused on assisting with diagnosis and preparing the child and family for procedures and corrective surgeries. Provide the child and the parents with emotional support and opportunities to express their concerns, questions, and fears.

Prognosis. Surgical repair is successful for the more common disorders and takes place or begins as early as possible.

DISORDERS OF ENDOCRINE FUNCTION

The endocrine system is responsible for the production and secretion of the major chemical regulators of the body, namely, the hormones. Disorders are caused primarily by an undersecretion or oversecretion of these hormones. Endocrine system dysfunctions affect all aspects of body function, including appearance, growth, and physical and psychological well-being.

Hypothyroidism. Hypothyroidism results from deficient production of thyroid hormone by the thyroid gland. The main function of the thyroid gland is to regulate metabolism by the production of thyroxine (T_4), triiodothyronine (T_3), and calcitonin. Thyroid-stimulating hormone (TSH) from the anterior pituitary controls the secretion of these hormones.

Etiology and pathophysiology. Hypothyroidism has two forms: primary and acquired. Primary causes include (1) congenital defects and (2) defective synthesis resulting from an autoimmune process. Acquired causes of hypothyroidism include (1) insufficient stimulation of the gland by the pituitary gland or the hypothalamus and (2) systemic resistance to thyroid hormone.

Table 32.3 Defects of the External Genitourinary Tract

DEFECT	MEDICAL MANAGEMENT
Hypospadias	
Urethral opening located along the ventral (anterior) surface of the penile shaft (see Fig. 32.20)	Surgical correction involves extending the urethra to a normal position. After repair, the child is expected to have normal reproductive and urinary function.
Epispadias	
Urethral opening located along the dorsal (posterior) surface of the penile shaft	Surgical correction involves penile and urethral lengthening and possibly bladder neck reconstruction.
Phimosis	
Narrowing or stenosis of the opening of the foreskin	Mild cases are treated with manual retraction. Severe cases are treated with circumcision.
Hydrocele	
Fluid in scrotal sac	Surgical correction is indicated if spontaneous resolution has not occurred in 1 yr.
Cryptorchidism	
Failure of one or both of the testes to descend into the scrotum	Medical management involves administration of human chorionic gonadotropin. Surgical correction consists of orchiopexy, which is surgical fixation of a testis. Treatment is aimed at preventing testicular damage and malignancies.
Inguinal Hernia	
Protrusion of the abdominal organs through the inguinal canal and into the scrotal sac (see Fig. 32.18)	Surgical correction involves closure of the inguinal canal.

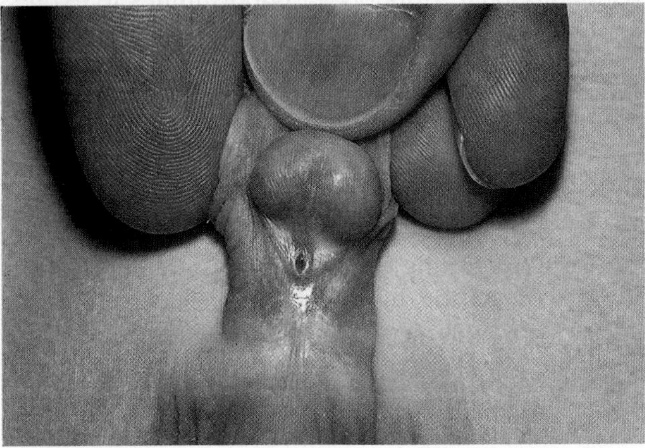

Fig. 32.20 Hypospadias. (Courtesy H. Gil Rushton, MD, Children's National Medical Center, Washington, D.C. From Hockenberry MJ, Wilson D: *Nursing care of infants and children*, ed 9, St. Louis, 2011, Mosby.)

Box 32.6 Clinical Manifestations of Hypothyroidism

CONGENITAL
- Cool, mottled skin
- Dyspnea
- Hypothermia
- Lethargy
- Poor appetite
- Poor sucking reflex
- Prolonged jaundice

ACQUIRED
- Constipation
- Dry skin
- Growth delay
- Lethargy
- Mental slowness
- Puffy eyes

Clinical manifestations. The clinical manifestations of hypothyroidism are described in Box 32.6.

Diagnostic tests. It is also possible to detect hypothyroidism when serum levels of thyroid hormone (T_4 and T_3) are decreased and serum TSH levels are increased (if the defect is in the thyroid) or decreased (if the defect is in the pituitary gland). A screening test for hypothyroidism is mandatory at birth. The screening is performed with a blood sample taken from the baby's heel.

Medical management. The treatment of choice for congenital and acquired hypothyroidism is oral thyroid hormone replacement therapy. Prompt treatment is especially critical in an infant with congenital hypothyroidism to avoid permanent cognitive impairment.

Nursing interventions and patient teaching. In addition to assisting in detection of the condition and implementation of thyroid hormone replacement therapy, nursing interventions focus on assisting the child and family in compliance with the medical regimen and periodic monitoring of its effects. As the child begins to mature, it is appropriate to place responsibility for treatment with the child.

Prognosis. If hypothyroidism is congenital, it is necessary to start treatment shortly after the patient's birth for normal physical and intellectual growth to occur. The most significant factor adversely affecting eventual intelligence appears to be inadequate treatment, which in some cases is related to noncompliance with the medical regimen.

Hyperthyroidism. Hyperthyroidism is rare in young children; it affects primarily young adolescents. The most common form of childhood hyperthyroidism is Graves' disease.

Etiology and pathophysiology. Although the exact causal mechanism is unknown, the most accepted theory is an autoimmune process that results in the production of immunoglobulins that have thyroid-stimulating properties.

Clinical manifestations. The clinical manifestations of hyperthyroidism are described in Box 32.7.

Diagnostic tests. In addition to clinical manifestations, the diagnosis of hyperthyroidism is based on increased serum levels of T_4, T_3, and radioactive iodine uptake. An ultrasound study of the neck also may assist in determining the presence of nodules or inflammation.

Medical management. The management of hyperthyroidism aims to decrease the rate of thyroid hormone secretion. To accomplish this, the child receives antithyroid medications, including propylthiouracil and methimazole (Tapazole); subtotal thyroidectomy; or administration of radioactive iodine (iodine-131).

Nursing interventions and patient teaching. Nursing interventions for a child with hyperthyroidism are focused on intervening with the physical manifestations of the disease. Sudden episodes of crying or elation exemplify the emotional lability typical of many affected children. Promote rest and provide a quiet, nonstimulating environment in the initial phase of treatment. To alleviate heat intolerance, the child should be dressed in lightweight clothing, the room temperature should be adjusted, and lightweight blankets should be offered for sleeping comfort. Dietary modifications include increased calories and daily vitamin supplementation. If surgery is recommended, inform the child and family of the nature of the surgery, where the incision will be located, and what to expect postoperatively. Postoperative care includes strict observation of bleeding and complications. The child's neck should be kept slightly flexed and supported to prevent strain on the suture line.

On discharge, make a referral to a public health nurse, school nurse, or home health care nurse to facilitate continuity of care and increase compliance with the medical regimen.

Prognosis. In general, after drug treatment, improvements are noted within the first 2 weeks. In many affected children, complete remission of the disorder follows an initial treatment course of 1 to 2 years. Those who experience relapse sometimes benefit from a second course of medication therapy, but some of them are also candidates for surgical intervention.

Box 32.7 Clinical Manifestations of Hyperthyroidism

- Accelerated growth
- Advanced bone age
- Excessive appetite
- Exophthalmos (protruding eyeballs)
- Heat intolerance
- Hyperactivity
- Hypertension
- Irritability
- Nervousness
- Palpable thyroid gland
- Tachycardia
- Tachypnea
- Thyroid storm: rapid onset with severe hyperthermia, vomiting, diarrhea, severe tachycardia; may advance to delirium, coma, death
- Tremors
- Warm skin
- Weight loss

Diabetes mellitus. Diabetes mellitus is a syndrome characterized by a deficiency of insulin that results in alterations in protein, carbohydrate, and fat metabolism. Type 1 diabetes mellitus is the endocrine disorder most frequently diagnosed in children.

The terms currently used for diabetes mellitus are *type 1* and *type 2*. Type 1 was classified previously as insulin-dependent diabetes mellitus and type 2 as non–insulin-dependent diabetes mellitus. These previous classifications could be confusing because the disease name could contradict the actual treatment (some people with type 2 diabetes required insulin).

Type 1 diabetes. Type 1 diabetes usually begins in childhood or early adulthood, but its onset can occur in adults. Each year, approximately 18,000 cases of type 1 diabetes are diagnosed in young people (American Diabetes Association, 2018). In type 1 diabetes, there is destruction of the pancreatic beta cells that produce insulin, which generally results in total insulin deficiency. In type 1 diabetes, a person with a genetic predisposition who is exposed to a precipitating event, such as a viral infection, experiences autoimmune destruction of the beta cells.

Type 2 diabetes. In the past, type 2 diabetes was most common in people who were older than 40 years, had a family history of diabetes, and were overweight. Type 2 diabetes results from insulin resistance and the body's improper use of insulin with relative—not absolute—insulin deficiency.

There has been a substantial increase in the number of cases of type 2 diabetes diagnosed in young children.

Contributing factors to the rise of type 2 diabetes in children include a low level of physical activity, exposure to diabetes in utero, and an obesity epidemic in the United States. Type 2 diabetes typically is diagnosed in children between the ages of 10 and 19 years, who are obese, who have a strong family history for diabetes, and who have insulin resistance. Nearly 6000 children are diagnosed with type 2 diabetes yearly (American Diabetes Association, 2017).

Etiology and pathophysiology. Hyperglycemia results when there is no insulin or not enough insulin is being secreted from the pancreas. This is due to the inability of glucose to enter the cells without the presence of sufficient amounts of insulin. Carbohydrates, fats, and proteins can only enter nerve cells and vascular tissue cells without the presence of insulin, resulting in damage to these tissues. When glucose levels rise above normal, the renal threshold is exceeded and glucose spills into the urine (glycosuria). When this occurs, glucose attracts water into the bladder, resulting in excessive urination (polyuria). Polyuria leads to dehydration and potential electrolyte imbalances. Dehydration causes excessive thirst (polydipsia).

When glucose does not enter the cells, the body breaks down protein to convert it to glucose in the liver (glucogenesis), again resulting in hyperglycemia. The body breaks down body fat and protein because it cannot use carbohydrates because of the insulin deficiency. The cells' lack of glucose causes excessive hunger (polyphagia). The three cardinal signs of type 1 diabetes are polyuria, polydipsia, and polyphagia.

Ketoacidosis. As discussed above, because glucose cannot be used for energy in diabetics the body breaks down fats for energy. Ketones are the product of fat metabolism and are formed by the fatty acids and glycerol that build up during this process. The ketone bodies are an alternative source of fuel; however, the rate of their use in the cells is limited. The body eliminates excess ketone bodies in the urine (ketonuria) or the lungs (acetone breath). The excessive ketone bodies in the blood (ketonemia) are toxic to the body and create strong acids (hence the term acidosis), thus resulting in ketoacidosis. As the serum pH decreases during acidosis hyperventilation, occurs to help the body eliminate carbon dioxide (acid) from the body. The characteristic Kussmaul respirations (abnormally deep and rapid respirations) are present during ketoacidosis.

Diabetic ketoacidosis is a life-threatening condition. The blood glucose level continues to rise during diabetic ketoacidosis and can reach levels that result in coma and death. The patient is treated in an acute care setting for this disorder.

Diagnostic tests. Diabetes mellitus is diagnosed on the basis of test results, including an 8-hour fasting glucose test, random blood glucose testing, and hemoglobin A_{1C}. The normal fasting glucose level for a child is less than 100 mg/dL. A fasting glucose level of 100 to 125 mg/dL is considered prediabetes. A fasting level higher than 125 mg/dL and a random blood glucose level higher than 200 mg/dL, accompanied by classic signs of diabetes, such as (1) glycosuria, polyuria, weight loss despite good appetite and (2) manifestations of metabolic acidosis with or without stupor or coma. The level of glycosylated hemoglobin (hemoglobin A_{1C}) is another important parameter. Nondiabetic hemoglobin A_{1C} levels are between 4% and 6.5%. A hemoglobin A_{1C} value of 6.5% or higher on two separate tests is indicative of diabetes in children. Ketoacidosis is diagnosed when blood glucose levels are greater than 200 mg/dL, ketones are highly present in the blood plasma, and ABG determinations demonstrate metabolic acidosis (pH less than 7.30), glycosuria, and ketonuria (Raghupathy, 2015).

Medical management. Medical management of diabetes mellitus in the child is a lifelong commitment to the prescribed regimen. A multidisciplinary approach must involve the family, the child (if appropriate), and a team of professionals that may include a pediatric endocrinologist, a diabetes nurse educator, a dietitian, and an exercise physiologist. Insulin therapy is necessary for the child. There are four types of therapeutic insulin: rapid, short acting, intermediate acting, and long acting. All insulins are prepared in strengths of 100 U/mL. The dosage of insulin for a child varies according to levels of glucose in the blood. Blood glucose monitoring is discussed in Chapter 23.

The appropriate daily insulin dosage depends on food intake, activity level, and exercise level. Management for children involves various types of insulin and must be determined through a consideration of the child's normal activities, eating schedule, and disease process. Possible insulin regimens may include a twice-daily insulin protocol combining rapid-acting insulin, such as lispro (Humalog), or short-acting insulin, such as regular insulin (e.g., Humulin R or Novolin R), with intermediate-acting insulins, such as Humulin N or Novolin N. The child receives the injections of insulin before breakfast and before dinner. Long-acting insulin therapy may be used alone or in combination with the other categories of insulin. Long-acting insulin is given once a day, usually before bedtime; formulations include glargine (Lantus) and detemir (Levemir). It is necessary to adjust the insulin dosage during growth spurts, periods of increased exercise, illnesses, infections, and surgery.

The insulin pump, which mimics the release of the insulin hormone from the islet cells of the pancreas, is also an option for children. The insulin pump delivers predetermined amounts of insulin continuously, or the dosage can be adjusted to meet the needs for dietary intake, glucose level, or activity. Blood glucose monitoring is necessary throughout the day to ensure that the correct dosage of insulin is being delivered. Education about the pump, as well as follow-up evaluation of the correct use of the pump, is important. The insulin pump comprises a small device that houses the insulin container and that is clipped to a belt or waist of clothing. Tubing attaches the insulin container to a very small needle that is embedded in the subcutaneous tissue and covered with a transparent dressing. The needle typically is changed every 48 hours, and the site of insertion is rotated. The insulin pump often affords better glucose control because repeated injections are not required, and it is not necessary to carry the equipment for injections.

Because the management of diabetes mellitus in children also centers on nutrition and exercise, a dietitian or nutritionist is an important resource person for the child and family. The diet is essentially the same healthy diet that is encouraged for all children, with an emphasis on avoiding foods high in sugars, carbohydrates, and fats. Choosemyplate.gov *(www.choosemyplate.gov)* is an excellent resource for meal planning. The amount of exercise also effects the food consumption needed and the amount of insulin required to maintain a normal glucose level. Exercise should be encouraged because it helps in lowering blood glucose levels.

Nursing interventions and patient teaching. Nursing interventions for a child with diabetes mellitus should focus on educating the child and the family about the disease and its treatment and possible complications, along with providing emotional support and reassurance. Because the treatment of diabetes mellitus relies on principles of self-management, it is essential that the child and the family understand the disease and its treatment. Encourage the parents and the child to express their questions, fears, and concerns about the disease and its management. Provide emotional support to the child and the family in their adjustment to the disease and provide them with concrete suggestions that will have a positive effect on their attitudes about diabetes mellitus and its management.

It is important that the child and family receive instruction about meal planning from a nutritionist and for the nurse to reinforce these instructions. The child and family need to be educated about the action of insulin, including the onset, peak, and duration of action, as well as about manifestations of hyperglycemia and hypoglycemia. They must also be aware of how to recognize manifestations of diabetic ketoacidosis. Instruct the child and the family in the proper techniques of insulin injections or use of the insulin pump. They should be taught to develop a rotation pattern if insulin injections are administered daily so that they do not give injections repeatedly in the same sites. Teach the parents and the child the principles and techniques of home glucose monitoring (see the Health Promotion box).

Prognosis. Advancements in diabetes treatment have improved the prognosis of patients living with diabetes and have decreased the risk of long-term complications. This improved outlook is highly dependent on the compliance of the patient with the prescribed long-term treatment plan. Diabetes mellitus affects the vasculature of all organs, especially those of the eyes, kidneys, and heart. Diabetic retinopathy, renal failure, and heart disease are complications of diabetes mellitus that may result but are less likely to have a major effect if diabetes is well controlled (National Institutes of Health, n.d.).

DISORDERS OF MUSCULOSKELETAL FUNCTION

Musculoskeletal problems in childhood are common and are a result of genetics, rapid growth, or the child's natural tendency to engage in active mobility. Many musculoskeletal conditions are temporary, and normal function ultimately returns.

Developmental dysplasia of the hip

Etiology and pathophysiology. Developmental dysplasia of the hip (DDH) is a developmental abnormality of the femoral head, the acetabulum, or both. The abnormality has familial tendencies and is more prominent in girls. DDH is associated with such conditions as first pregnancy, spina bifida, and breech presentation. The defining characteristic of subluxation of the hip is incorrect position, or partial dislocation, of the femoral head in the acetabulum. **Subluxation** is the degree of DDH most common in infants. In dislocation, the femoral head has no contact with the acetabulum.

Clinical manifestations. In affected infants, the femur on the affected side is shortened; thigh and gluteal folds are uneven (or increased on the affected side) when the infant is placed in the prone position, and abduction of the hip on the affected side is limited (Fig. 32.21). In children who are able to stand and walk, the affected leg is shorter than the other, and they demonstrate a waddling gait or limping.

Diagnostic tests. Early diagnosis of DDH in the newborn tends to enhance the success of treatment and minimize complications. Nursing assessment of the previously listed manifestations alerts the health care provider to the possibility of DDH. Physical assessment by the health care provider reveals an audible clunking sound when the hips are manually manipulated. In addition, radiographic examination is sometimes helpful in establishing the diagnosis.

Medical management. Once DDH is diagnosed, treatment begins immediately. Any delay in treatment is likely to result in worsening of the deformity and a poorer prognosis. Treatment depends on the severity of the dysplasia and the age of the infant. Treatment for infants younger than 6 months consists of positioning the head of the femur within the acetabulum and maintaining the hip in abduction for 4 to 6 months with the use of a Pavlik harness (Fig. 32.22). Once this therapy achieves abduction, a hip spica cast maintains positioning for several months until the hip is stable. Treatment for a child with DDH between the ages of 6 and 24 months may require manipulation of the head of the femur into the socket while the child is under anesthesia. Surgical open reduction is necessary in some cases if soft tissue obstructs the head of the femur from entering the acetabulum. Immobilization in a hip spica cast

Health Promotion

Child With Diabetes Mellitus

- Blood glucose self-monitoring has improved diabetes management and is used successfully by children from the onset of their diabetes. By testing their own blood, children and parents can adjust the insulin regimen to maintain the blood glucose level. The normal range in children is 70 to 99 mg/dL. Diabetes management depends to a great extent on self-monitoring.
- Essentially, the nutritional needs of children with diabetes are no different from those of unaffected children. Children with diabetes require no special foods or supplements. They need sufficient calories to balance daily expenditure for energy and to satisfy the requirement for growth and development. They also need consistent intake and timing of food.
- There is no one diet for diabetes. General guidelines exist, such as to eat less fat and saturated fat and to eat more whole grains, fruits, and vegetables. Sugars and sweets, or simple sugars, do not raise blood glucose any more quickly than do starches, or "complex carbohydrates." Healthy nutrition advice is to eat sugars and sweets in moderation. It is important to base diabetes meal plans on individual needs and develop them with expert assistance from a registered dietitian.
- Exercise should be encouraged and never restricted unless other health conditions indicate the need to do so. It is part of diabetes management, and planning it around the child's interests and capabilities is important. However, in most instances, children's activities are not rigidly scheduled. Parents should compensate for the inevitable decreases in the blood glucose level by providing extra snacks before (and, if prolonged, during) the activity. Besides providing a feeling of well-being, regular exercise aids in the body's use of food and often decreases insulin requirements.
- Even a child with well-controlled diabetes typically experiences occasional mild symptoms of hypoglycemia, but if the child and caretakers recognize the signs and symptoms early and relieve them promptly with appropriate therapy, it is not usually necessary to interrupt the child's activity for more than a few minutes.
- Families need to understand the treatment method and the insulin prescribed, including the effective duration, onset, and peak action. They also need to know the characteristics of the various types of insulin and the proper mixing of insulin. The amount of time that insulin is considered acceptable to use once opened is dependent on the type of insulin and whether it is stored at room temperature or refrigerated. The manufacturer's guidelines for each type of insulin should be followed.
- Insulin must never be stored at very cold (<36°F [2.2°C]) or very hot (>86°F [30°C]) temperatures. Extreme temperatures destroy insulin.
- The site selected for insulin injection may depend on who administers the insulin. The upper arms, the thighs, the hips, and the abdomen are usual injection sites for insulin. The child can reach the thighs, the abdomen, and part of the hip and arm easily, but sometimes help is needed to inject other sites. For example, a parent can pinch a loose fold of skin on the arm while the child injects the insulin.
- Some children are candidates for continuous subcutaneous insulin infusion with a portable insulin pump. The health care provider teaches the child and the parents to operate the device, including the mechanics of the pump, battery changes, and alarm systems. They learn how to load the syringe, insert the catheter, adjust the insulin flow for routine needs and for illnesses, and connect and disconnect the catheter. Nurses should become familiar with the operation of the specific device that their facility uses and the protocol of the regimen.
- Self-management techniques that the child and the family need to master are the testing of blood, administration of insulin, and adjustment of insulin and diet with alterations in day-to-day activities and unusual occurrences.

follows open reduction. The management of affected children older than 24 months is more extensive because adaptive changes have taken place. Open surgical reduction, osteotomy, and arthroplasty are sometimes necessary. A hip spica cast is necessary after these procedures.

Nursing interventions and patient teaching. Nurses play an important role in identifying signs of DDH and other congenital defects in newborns, and the earlier the defect is identified and treated, the better is the chance for a favorable outcome. The primary goals in caring for a child in a corrective device or cast are to maintain the position of the hip joint, prevent complications, and provide the stimulation necessary for the developing infant or child. As early as possible, involve parents in caring for their baby to build confidence in their ability to provide care at home. Box 32.8 provides general guidelines for the nursing interventions for a child in a corrective device or cast.

Parents and all other caregivers need to understand that children in corrective devices need involvement in all the activities of any child in the same age group. They must not confine the child or exclude the child from family activities.

Prognosis. With early treatment, the prognosis is more favorable for the restoration of normal body function. It is essential that parents make follow-up visits to ensure that treatment is effective. These visits are necessary until the child's growth is complete.

Legg-Calvé-Perthes disease (coxa plana)

Etiology and pathophysiology. **Legg-Calvé-Perthes disease** (coxa plana) is a disorder caused by decreased blood supply to the femoral head, which results in

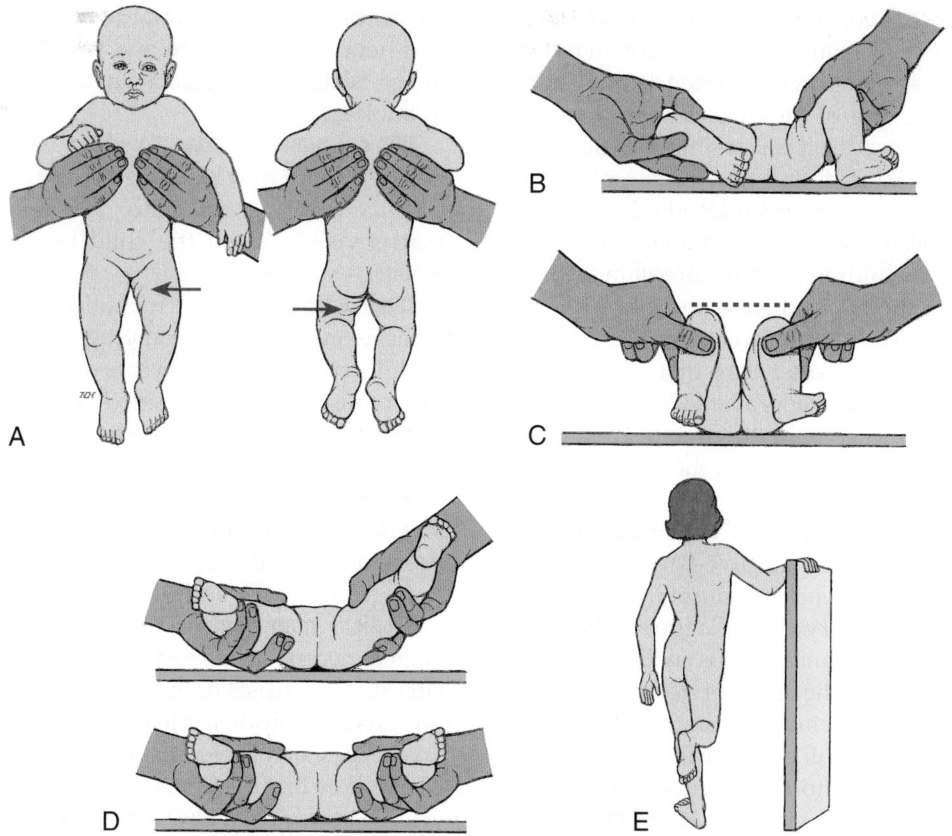

Fig. 32.21 Signs of congenital dislocation of the hip. A, Asymmetry of gluteal and thigh folds. B, Limited hip abduction, as seen in flexion. C, Apparent shortening of femur, as indicated by level of knees in flexion. D, Ortolani's click (if infant is younger than 4 weeks). E, Positive Trendelenburg sign or gait (if child is weight bearing). (From Hockenberry MJ, Wilson D: *Wong's essentials of pediatric nursing,* ed 9, St. Louis, 2013, Mosby.)

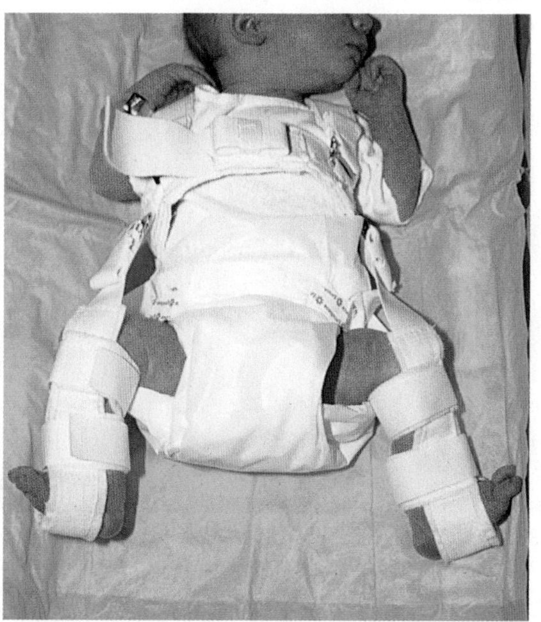

Fig. 32.22 Child in Pavlik harness. (From Ashwill JW, Droske SC: *Nursing care of children: Principles and practice,* ed 3, Philadelphia, 2007, Saunders.)

Box 32.8 Care of a Child in a Cast or Corrective Device

- Perform neurovascular assessment of the five *P*s (impairments to be reported immediately): *p*ain, *p*allor or cyanosis, *p*aresthesia (numbing or tingling, decrease in sensation), *p*ulselessness, and *p*uffiness.
- Monitor skin frequently for erythema or tenderness.
- Wash and dry skin at least daily.
- Smooth or pad a sharp cast or brace edges with gauze or adhesive tape.
- Teach the family cast or brace maintenance and cleaning.
- Assess circular dressings for excessive tightness.
- Stimulate circulation with gentle massage over pressure areas.

epiphyseal necrosis and degeneration of the femoral head, followed by regeneration or calcification. It occurs more often in boys and affects children from 4 to 10 years of age. The cause of the disorder is unknown, and the disease process itself is self-limited. The blood supply usually is restored, and new cells replace the necrotic bone. This entire process may take 2 to 3 years.

Clinical manifestations. Signs and symptoms are usually insidious. Affected children usually complain of pain, exhibit a limp on the affected side, and have limited range of motion (ROM). The disease in the affected hip causes the leg to be shorter than that on the unaffected side. The condition is aggravated by activity and improves with rest. Knee pain, thigh and groin pain, hip stiffness, and muscle atrophy in the thigh are also common.

Diagnostic tests. The presence of the common signs raises the suspicion of Legg-Calvé-Perthes disease. Radiographic examination helps confirm the diagnosis. MRI is sometimes necessary if the diagnosis cannot be determined from clinical manifestations and radiographs.

Medical management. The goal of treatment is to maintain the head of the femur within the acetabulum so that the femoral head will preserve its normal shape as it regenerates. If this effort is successful, full ROM can be maintained. Bracing may help keep the head of the femur contained within the acetabulum. Physical therapy and ROM exercises, along with antiinflammatory medications, help prevent joint stiffness and pain. Activities such as running may be limited, and nighttime traction may be used to prevent the head of the femur from becoming displaced. Bed rest is necessary only to treat bouts of severe pain. Surgical procedures are required only if all other treatments are ineffective.

Nursing interventions and patient teaching. While the child is in traction or in casts, braces, or harnesses, skin care and neurovascular assessment are essential. Box 32.8 details care of the child in a cast or corrective device. Appropriate education of the family and child includes purpose, function, application, and care of the corrective device. Correct use of the corrective device is vital for the long-term success of treatment. It is important that the child and parents understand how to use the device properly.

Prognosis. With patient compliance and early diagnosis, the prognosis is excellent. Legg-Calvé-Perthes disease is self-limiting, and early, efficient treatment and the age at onset are important factors in a positive outcome. If the diagnosis is made after the age of 6, the child is at higher risk for a hip deformity and osteoarthritis in later years.

Scoliosis

Etiology and pathophysiology. The most common skeletal deformity of adolescence is scoliosis. The condition is a lateral curvature of the spine that causes changes in the shapes of the spine, the chest, and the hips. Severe curvature has the potential to affect cardiopulmonary and neurologic function and result in a negative self-image. Scoliosis can occur at any age but is most common in adolescent girls.

Clinical manifestations. A child with idiopathic scoliosis has unequal hip heights and shoulder heights, scapular and rib prominence, and a posterior rib hump that is visible when the child bends forward at the waist.

Diagnostic tests. Early identification and treatment of scoliosis are vital for a good prognosis. Routine screening of children from 10 to 15 years of age involves posterior observation of the undressed child (bending forward at the waist with arms and head hanging downward) for curvature, asymmetry, and rib hump. Radiographs confirm the diagnosis. If the health care provider suspects an underlying cause for the scoliosis, such as a tumor, he or she orders additional tests, including MRI, computed tomography (CT), and bone scan.

Medical management. Curvatures of less than 20 degrees necessitate no treatment. Treatment for moderate curvatures consists of bracing, which potentially slows the progression of scoliosis until the spine is mature. Two types of braces are used to treat scoliosis: the Milwaukee brace and the thoracolumbosacral orthotic (TLSO) brace. The TLSO brace is used most commonly. It fits under the arm and is shaped to conform to the body (Fig. 32.23). The Milwaukee brace covers the entire torso and has a ring that encircles the neck with rests for the chin and the back of the head. This brace typically is used only if the TLSO brace is not effective. Surgical intervention is indicated in severe scoliosis or scoliosis that does not respond to bracing. Surgery consists of spinal fusion and the insertion of a stabilizing rod such as a Harrington rod or an L-rod.

Nursing interventions and patient teaching. Many adolescents who must wear casts or braces have difficulty

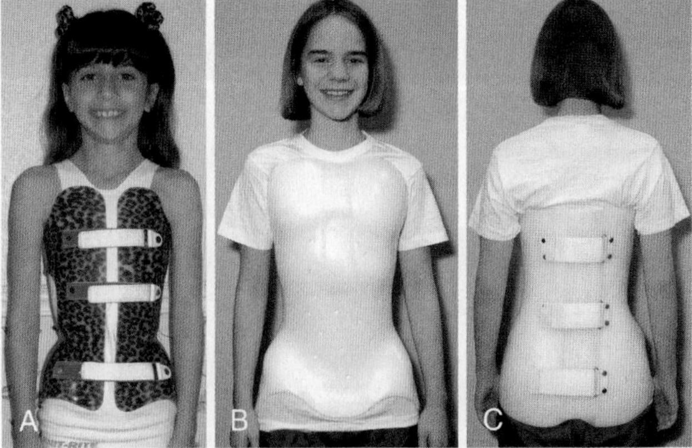

Fig. 32.23 Braces for idiopathic scoliosis. A, Standard thoracolumbosacral orthotic (TLSO) brace. Note the color and design incorporated into the brace to make it more acceptable to children and adolescents. B, Variation of a standard TLSO brace that fastens in the back (C) to provide needed support for the spine curvature. (From Hockenberry MJ, Wilson D: *Wong's essentials of pediatric nursing,* ed 9, St. Louis, 2013, Mosby.)

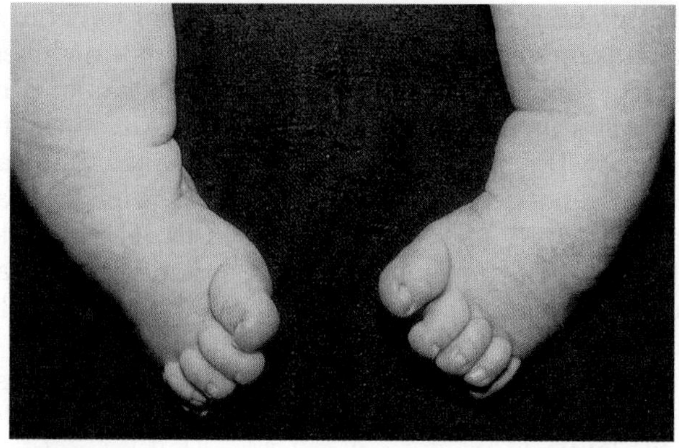

Fig. 32.24 Bilateral congenital talipes equinovarus (congenital clubfoot) in a 2-month-old infant. (From Zitelli BJ, McIntire SC, Davis HW: *Zitelli and Davis' atlas of pediatric physical diagnosis*, ed 6, St. Louis, 2012, Saunders.)

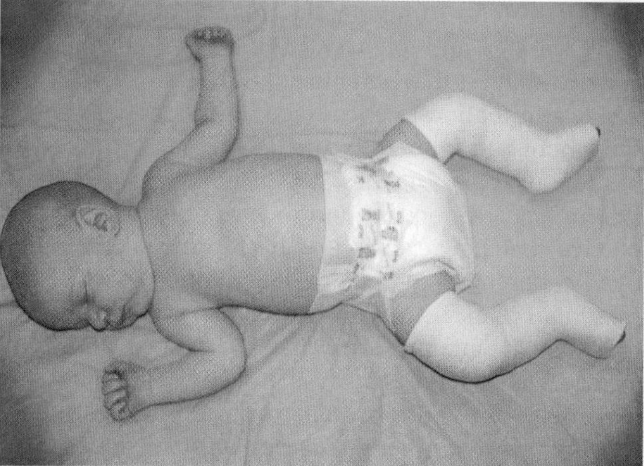

Fig. 32.25 Casting of feet for correction of bilateral congenital talipes equinovarus. (From Perry S, Hockenberry M, Lowdermilk D, et al: *Maternal-child nursing care*, ed 3, St. Louis, 2007, Mosby.)

complying with the treatment plan. Developmentally, adolescents are trying to fit in with peers by conforming to peer norms and need plenty of reassurance to feel attractive and worthwhile during treatment. Instruction on maintaining skin integrity is essential for adolescents in a brace or cast. Box 32.8 outlines care for the child in a corrective device or cast.

Provide proper instruction to the child and the parents regarding the appliance, the anticipated results, and the desired goal.

Prognosis. Treatment for scoliosis is a lengthy process, inasmuch as it occurs during a major growth period of the child. The prognosis depends on the severity of the condition and compliance with the prescribed treatment. Information and techniques for providing emotional support of the patient are available from the National Scoliosis Foundation (*www.scoliosis.org*).

Talipes equinovarus (clubfoot)

Etiology and pathophysiology. Talipes equinovarus is the most common congenital deformity of the foot and ankle. The incidence is 1 per 1000 live births and is twice as high among boys as among girls. The cause of talipes equinovarus is not known, but theories point to an inherited or environmental disorder. The incidence of talipes equinovarus is higher in families that already have a child with the defect (Patel, 2017).

Clinical manifestations. Talipes equinovarus varies in severity. It most commonly involves one foot but may involve both feet. In talipes equinovarus, the foot is pointed downward and inward (Fig. 32.24). The muscles of the affected calf and foot may be smaller and shorter than normal.

Diagnostic tests. Talipes equinovarus is evident at birth, and examination, manipulation, and radiographs are used to make the diagnosis.

Medical management. Treatment of talipes equinovarus consists of manipulation and the application of a series of short leg casts (Fig. 32.25). The earlier the treatment begins, the more favorable the outcome, and serial casting typically begins shortly after birth. The health care provider gently manipulates the foot into a more normal position and then applies a cast to maintain the correction. The health care provider changes the cast weekly to allow for further manipulation and to accommodate the rapidly growing infant. The manipulation and the application of casts continues until marked overcorrection is reached. After completion of the casting series and correction of the deformity, the foot (or feet) undergo a combination of passive stretching exercises and corrective splints or shoes to prevent the deformity from recurring. The child usually must wear a brace or corrective shoes, depending on the surgeon's preference, for several years.

In severe cases, casting may not successfully correct the deformity, and surgical intervention is required. A minor surgical procedure, called a *tenotomy,* is the surgical release of the Achilles tendon. The tenotomy, followed by additional serial casting, may be all the surgery that is required. More extensive surgery involves the repositioning of the anterior tibial tendon.

Nursing interventions and patient teaching. After the diagnosis of talipes equinovarus, parents need emotional support and education. Very often, parents need time to adjust to the distressing fact that their child has a deformity. Educate parents while encouraging them to express their feelings and concerns. Nursing care for an infant with casts is the same for any child in a cast (see Box 32.8). Many affected newborns receive the cast before discharge from the hospital. Keeping casts clean and dry is relatively easy with a small infant. The parents should be taught to inspect casts carefully for rough edges, which will irritate newborn skin. They should observe the toes frequently for coldness, pain, blueness, or edema, which, if present, must be reported to the health care provider immediately. Casts are cumbersome and heavy. Assist the parents to find comfortable positions for feeding, playing, and cuddling. Sponge baths are necessary until the infant no longer needs casting.

Casts also tend to hinder the infant's ability to kick, move the legs, and roll over. During this time of limited activity, suggest that parents provide audio, visual, and tactile stimulation to encourage normal development. Treatment and follow-up care usually take place on an outpatient basis.

Nursing responsibilities include the teaching of passive stretching exercises with a return demonstration by the parent, if parent participation is part of the treatment plan. Teach parents about cast care and how to handle the infant. Instruct them to perform stretching exercises several times a day; many parents find it easier to remember to perform the exercises if they do them together with another regular activity such as diaper changing or after feedings.

Prognosis. Some feet respond to treatment rapidly; some respond only to prolonged, vigorous, and sustained efforts; and the improvement in others remains disappointing even with maximal effort on the part of all concerned. Serial casting achieves the most reliable correction of talipes equinovarus. If surgical intervention is required, scar tissue can result in long-term pain and stiffness.

Duchenne muscular dystrophy

Etiology and pathophysiology. Duchenne muscular dystrophy (DMD) is a sex-linked inherited disorder whose defining characteristic is gradually progressive skeletal muscle wasting and weakness. The pattern of inheritance is such that primarily only girls are affected. Women, however, can be carriers of the gene. DMD is the most severe and most common form of all dystrophies. The onset of signs and symptoms typically occurs between ages 2 and 4 years.

Clinical manifestations. Initial signs and symptoms, which are mild and progress gradually, are easy to overlook. Parents tend to be the first to notice that the child is clumsy, frequently falls, has a waddling gait, and experiences difficulty running, climbing, and riding a bicycle. The muscles of the pelvic girdle are frequently involved, and the child shows evidence of this weakness by rising from the floor in a classic manner: The child lies on the side and flexes the knees (or gets on all fours), then extends the knees and uses the hands to "walk up" the thighs (**Gowers sign**). As the disorder progresses, there is severe muscle wasting, which results in contractures and deformities. By 12 years of age, ambulation may no longer be possible. Respiratory tract infection usually occurs in the final stages, when the diaphragm and the accessory muscles used in respiration become affected.

Diagnostic tests. The health care provider considers the possibility of DMD based on the clinical signs and symptoms and the family history. Electromyography, elevated levels of serum creatine kinase and aspartate aminotransferase, and muscle biopsy that reveals fibrous and fatty tissue confirm the diagnosis. Because of the frequent cardiac complications, the American Academy of Pediatrics recommends that the patient undergo a complete cardiac evaluation early in childhood and then undergo annual follow-up at the age of 10 years and on.

Medical management. There is no effective treatment to arrest DMD. Therefore the goals are to maintain ambulation and independence for as long as possible. Physical therapy serves to optimize ROM and to delay muscle atrophy; braces sometimes help provide additional support; and surgical intervention to release muscle contractures is another element of management.

Nursing interventions and patient teaching. The most important nursing consideration in the care of a child with DMD is to assist the child and the family in developing positive coping strategies to deal with the progressively debilitating aspects of the illness. The goal is to maintain independence for as long as possible. Because of the progressive nature of the illness, assess the child's capabilities frequently. The care of a child with DMD, or any child with a chronic, debilitating terminal illness, is extremely demanding and stressful for the family. Help the family lessen their anxiety and fears through teaching and active listening. The family also needs assistance with anticipatory grieving. A referral to the Muscular Dystrophy Association of America opens the door to many supplementary services to patients and their families.

Help the family plan an exercise program to encourage muscle strength and delay the onset of some of the physical disabilities. Counsel the family about good nutrition to prevent obesity, which sometimes causes affected children to become prematurely wheelchair bound.

Prognosis. As the condition progresses, cardiomyopathy, congestive heart failure, and scoliosis are noted with increasing frequency. Affected children rarely live past age 20; death results from respiratory or cardiac complications.

Septic arthritis (septic joint, suppurative arthritis)

Etiology and pathophysiology. Septic arthritis (septic joint, suppurative arthritis) is an infection of a joint, which possibly arises from bacteria in the blood or as a direct extension of an existing infection such as osteomyelitis. Potential causes include ear infections, bites (human, cat, dog, rat, or tick), infected wounds, and open fractures. The infection causes joint irritation and damage to the synovial membrane; synovial fluid increases and causes distention within the joint. As the infection progresses, pus accumulates and breaks down the articulating cartilage (which does not have the capacity to regenerate) and leads to permanent damage. In infancy, the incidence of septic arthritis is equal among boys and girls; in the adolescent age group, it occurs predominantly in boys. The joints most commonly affected are the hip, knee, shoulder, wrist, and ankle. Streptococci and staphylococcus are the most common bacteria. In rare cases, fungal and viral infections may be the culprits.

Clinical manifestations. The affected joint is erythematous, edematous, warm, and excruciatingly painful. The temperature of the joint also is elevated. ROM usually is limited. The child maintains the affected extremities in a flexed position. If the lower extremities are involved, the child often limps or refuses to walk. Except in infants, fever is usually present. The onset of septic arthritis is very rapid, and the condition is considered a medical emergency.

Diagnostic tests. Radiographic examination may reveal joint edema. The health care provider aspirates the synovial fluid and sends purulent matter for Gram stain examination and culture. A blood culture is necessary. Serologic testing reveals leukocytosis and elevated erythrocyte sedimentation rate in children; infants do not always demonstrate these findings.

Medical management. Joint aspiration and surgical irrigation are essential for managing the condition. Surgical drainage and irrigation ensure that the joint is decompressed, safeguard the vasculature, clear the joint of destructive purulent matter, eradicate the infection, and prevent secondary bloodborne spread of infection. The health care provider initiates broad-spectrum IV antibiotic therapy and switches it to more specific antibiotics once the laboratory has identified the organism. IV therapy continues for 10 to 14 days; once the IV response is good, the regimen can change to oral antibiotics. Oral therapy continues to complete a 4-week course. Additional pharmacologic interventions may include antipyretics and analgesics.

Nursing interventions. Because of the lengthy pharmacologic therapies, parents need education concerning the importance of compliance with the regimen. Discuss which signs and symptoms of medication side effects to report. Range-of-motion exercises to main joint strength and flexibility are included in the regimen.

Prognosis. The prompt management of this condition is paramount for a successful outcome. Left untreated, the condition may result in permanent damage and destruction of the joint and adjacent structures. Involvement of the hip joint—where avascular necrosis can develop and cause deformity—may result in long-term disability.

Fractures. Although any bone can be fractured, the most common fracture sites in children are the long bones of the extremities, the clavicles, the wrists, the fingers, and the skull. Fractures vary from complete (bone and periosteum separate completely) to incomplete or greenstick (the bone splits but does not completely break). Spiral fractures affect the length rather than the width of the bone and are frequently the result of child abuse.

Clinical manifestations. A bone fracture usually manifests with deformity, loss of normal function, and swelling. Pain and tenderness are also often present.

Diagnostic tests. Physical assessment of the affected area helps provide an initial diagnosis. The diagnosis ultimately is confirmed with radiographic studies. Fractures that protrude through the skin (open or compound) also are evaluated with serologic testing, including a CBC and probably subsequent culture and sensitivity testing to detect the possibility of infection.

Medical management. Upon confirmation of the fracture, the treatment includes realignment of the bones. This may be done in either a closed or open reduction. The closed reduction entails the external manipulation of the bones to return to a point of normal alignment, after which casting is performed to maintain this positioning. An open reduction requires surgical intervention to realign the bones. Pins, wires, plates, and screws are devices used to secure the bone fragments and maintain alignment to allow for healing. The open reduction may be followed by casting or traction. Pharmacologic therapies may include analgesic or antiinflammatory medications. Open fractures necessitate prophylactic antibiotic therapy.

Nursing interventions. Evaluating a possible traumatic injury involves assessment of the injury and soft tissue damage. The affected area is assessed for pain and point of tenderness, color, sensation, motion, and pulses distal to the injury. Limitations in function also should be noted. If the child is upset, it is necessary to calm and reassure the child and the parents.

Assist in care of the child as the health care provider realigns the extremity. If the injury necessitates casting, specific nursing measures are instituted. Assess pain and administer comfort measures and analgesics as prescribed. After alignment, nursing interventions include maintaining skin integrity and monitoring skeletal traction sites, as applicable, for infection. Observe for complications of immobility, especially circulatory compromise and muscle spasms. Patients undergoing surgical management for a fracture require routine postoperative care interventions.

Prognosis. Most fractures in children heal without incidence. Complications, although rare, include nonunion of the bones (bones do not heal together at the site of the fracture) and osteomyelitis (infection within the bone).

DISORDERS OF NEUROLOGIC FUNCTION

Disorders that affect neurologic function belong to three major categories: (1) increased intracranial pressure, (2) hypoxia, and (3) seizure activity. The residual effects of neurologic disorders often have profound effects on the child's function and future performance. It is essential to identify neurologic impairments at an early stage so that they can be diagnosed properly and interventions can be instituted.

Meningitis. Meningitis is a significant cause of illness in the pediatric age group. Meningitis is an infection of the meninges (protective covering of the brain). Most cases affect children younger than 5 years. Its importance lies primarily in the frequency with which it occurs in infancy and childhood and the unnecessarily high death rates and residual damage caused by undiagnosed and untreated or inadequately treated cases.

Etiology and pathophysiology. Although many bacterial, viral, and fungal organisms have the capacity to cause meningitis, bacterial meningitis is the most common. The advent of antimicrobial therapy has had a marked effect on the course and prognosis of bacterial meningitis, although the use of Hib vaccine, beginning in 1990, led to the most dramatic decrease in bacterial meningitis caused by *H. influenzae.* Bacterial meningitis caused by other organisms remains a serious illness in children. Organisms generally spread to the meninges after an upper respiratory infection, by lymphatic drainage, or by direct deposit through a lumbar puncture or skull fracture. After it invades the meninges, the organism enters the cerebrospinal fluid (CSF) and travels throughout the subarachnoid space, spreading the infection. As the meninges become infected, an inflammatory process ensues, causing a thick exudate and WBC accumulation. With continued inflammation, CSF flow becomes occluded, and the brain becomes hyperemic (increased blood to a part) and edematous.

Clinical manifestations. Meningitis manifests sometimes insidiously and sometimes suddenly, beginning with fever, vomiting, headache, irritability, photophobia, and **nuchal rigidity** (pain and stiffness in the neck when flexed) or opisthotonos (arched back); level of consciousness may decrease, and seizures may occur. Affected infants typically exhibit a bulging fontanelle and a characteristic high-pitched cry. Classic signs of meningeal irritation include a positive *Kernig's sign* (resistance to knee extension in the supine position with the hips and knees flexed against the torso) and a positive *Brudzinski's sign* (flexion of the knees and hips when the neck is flexed rapidly onto the chest). Meningococcal meningitis, the most readily transmissible type of meningitis, sometimes also produces petechiae and rapidly progresses to death if proper treatment is not initiated promptly.

Diagnostic tests. The diagnosis of meningitis is based on a carefully documented history, results of a physical examination, and analysis of CSF obtained by a lumbar puncture. CSF culture and sensitivity testing that shows an elevated WBC count, elevated protein level, and decreased glucose level indicates a bacterial infection. If signs of increased intracranial pressure (papilledema, neurologic deficits, and a bulging fontanelle) are present, a lumbar puncture is contraindicated because of the risk of brainstem herniation. CT or MRI also is used to assess the level of meningeal irritation.

Medical management. The management of bacterial meningitis involves immediate IV administration of appropriate antibiotic therapy. Therapy continues for at least 10 days or until the CSF culture result is negative. Intensive care often is employed until the antibiotic therapy has been under way for at least 24 hours.

If seizures occur, antiseizure medications are ordered. The choice of antibiotic is based on the known sensitivity of the pathogen. Appropriate hydration, antipyretics, and comfort measures are important aspects of management. Closely observe the child for complications of meningitis, including seizures, disseminated intravascular coagulation syndrome, and shock. After discharge, the health care provider monitors the child closely to assess for any sequelae of the disease, such as hearing impairments and cognitive, perceptual, language, and behavioral problems.

Nursing interventions and patient teaching. Initial nursing interventions focus on rapid identification of a child with meningitis and prompt institution of appropriate antibiotic therapy. Take all necessary isolation precautions to prevent the spread of the disease.

Promote rest for the child in the initial phase of the disease and minimize environmental stimuli (especially noise and bright lights). Institute safety measures because the child may develop seizures. The child is likely to be most comfortable without a pillow and with the head of the bed elevated. Observe vital signs, level of consciousness, I&O, and neurologic signs at frequent intervals. Provide emotional support to families throughout the course of the disease; they are usually unprepared for the sudden acuteness of the disease and may feel guilty for not recognizing it earlier.

Prevention. The spread of bacterial meningitis can be avoided in the exposed siblings by administration of prophylactic rifampin. Primary prevention strategies consist of vaccine administration.

Meningococcal polysaccharide (Menomune) and quadrivalent meningococcal conjugate (Menactra) are two available vaccines in the United States to immunize children against meningitis. The choice of vaccine is based on the patient's age. The mortality rate associated with bacterial meningitis is high, but early immunization can spare families from experiencing the tragic death or disability of a child from this disease. The nurse plays a significant role in educating families regarding preventive measures.

Prognosis. Although antimicrobial therapy often has a significant effect on the course of illness, meningitis remains a potentially life-threatening disease. The age of the child, the type of causative organism, the severity of the infection, the duration of the illness before the onset of therapy, and the sensitivity of the organism to antimicrobial drugs are important factors in the prognosis. Residual deficits are possible; these include communicating hydrocephalus and possible hearing loss, blindness, seizures, learning disorders, and attention-deficit disorder.

Encephalitis. Encephalitis is defined as an inflammation of the CNS: namely the brain tissue and the spinal cord. The course of the disease closely resembles that of meningitis and the care for each is similar.

Etiology and pathophysiology. Encephalitis is a rare condition and its cause is varied. A variety of organisms have the capacity to cause encephalitis, such as bacteria, spirochetes, fungi, protozoa, and viruses. Most cases of encephalitis occur as a result of direct invasion of the CNS by a virus or from postinfectious involvement after a viral illness, such as measles, mumps, or varicella. Other factors that may result in encephalitis include contact with infected respiratory secretions and insect bites (NIH, 2018b).

Clinical manifestations. An upper respiratory tract infection or GI infection may precede the onset of symptoms. The onset of encephalitis may be gradual or sudden, and manifestations may include malaise, fever, headache, dizziness, nuchal rigidity, nausea, vomiting, ataxia, tremors, seizures, and coma.

Diagnostic tests. The diagnosis of encephalitis is based on clinical manifestations associated with the disease and, if possible, identification of the virus. Laboratory detection of the virus is possible through serologic tests or CSF cultures. MRI and CT also are performed to assess inflammation.

Medical management. A child suspected of having encephalitis is hospitalized promptly for strict observation and supportive care. Treatment is primarily supportive, focusing on controlling fever, ensuring adequate hydration and nutrition, monitoring vital signs, and observing for complications. Pharmacologic therapies include organism-specific antibiotics or antiviral medications. Corticosteroids such as dexamethasone are prescribed to reduce brain inflammation. In addition, antiseizure and antipyretic agents may be prescribed. Analgesics are used with extreme caution because they may mask neurologic changes.

Nursing interventions and patient teaching. Nursing interventions for children with encephalitis are the same as those for children with meningitis. The major focus of care is on administering medication, controlling fever, monitoring neurologic status and vital signs, and providing emotional support to the child and the family.

Follow-up care with periodic reevaluation and rehabilitation is important for survivors with residual effects of the disease. Encourage the parents to keep appointments for follow-up examinations.

Prognosis. The prognosis depends on the child's age, the type of organism, and any residual neurologic damage. Children younger than 2 years of age sometimes exhibit increased neurologic disability, including learning disabilities and seizure disorders. In severe cases, encephalitis may lead to death.

Hydrocephalus. Hydrocephalus is a condition whose defining characteristic is an excess of fluid within the cranial vault, the subarachnoid space, or both. It is caused by an imbalance between the production and the absorption of CSF within the ventricular system. Hydrocephalus can develop during infancy (as a congenital lesion) and throughout life.

Etiology and pathophysiology. Hydrocephalus is caused by increased production of CSF, by obstruction within the ventricular system (noncommunicating hydrocephalus: no passage of fluid between the ventricles), or by defective reabsorption of the CSF (communicating hydrocephalus: passage of CSF between the ventricles). Overproduction of CSF results most commonly from a tumor in the choroid plexus. Obstruction within the ventricular system is caused most frequently by atresia (the absence of a normal body opening, duct, or canal), most commonly along the aqueduct of Sylvius (Fig. 32.26). Other causes of obstruction include a hemorrhage, a growing tumor, or an infection. Defects in the body's reabsorptive process are sometimes caused by an extensive hemorrhage within the subarachnoid space, which obscures the absorptive surface of the membrane.

As CSF accumulates within the cranium, the brain is compressed against the skull, and the ventricular vessels become dilated, which increases intracranial pressure (see Fig. 32.26). If hydrocephalus occurs before the fusion of the cranial sutures, the skull becomes markedly enlarged.

Clinical manifestations. In early infancy, manifestations of hydrocephalus include widening and bulging of the fontanelles, separation of the cranial sutures, dilation of scalp veins, thin and shiny scalp, and rapidly increasing head circumference. As CSF accumulation continues, frontal bossing (prominence of the forehead) becomes

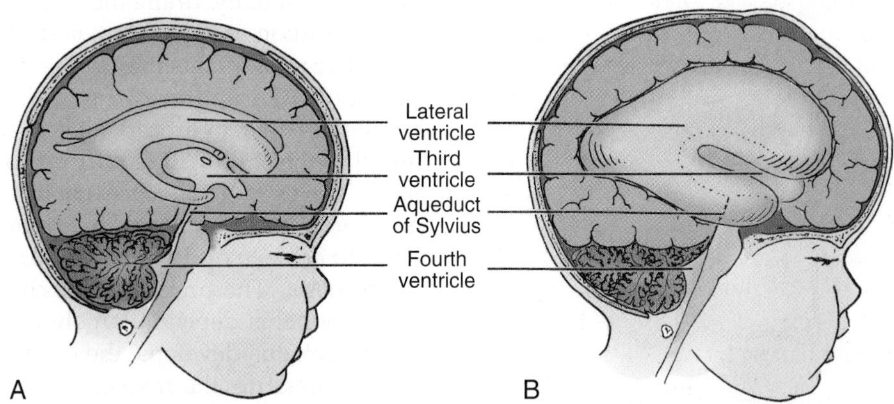

Fig. 32.26 Appearance of the brain with normal cerebrospinal fluid flow and in hydrocephalus. A, Normal: patent cerebrospinal fluid circulation. B, Hydrocephalus: enlargement of lateral and third ventricles, caused by obstruction of cerebral spinal fluid circulation at the aqueduct of Sylvius. (From Hockenberry MJ, Wilson D: *Nursing care of infants and children*, ed 9, St. Louis, 2011, Mosby.)

apparent. Other manifestations are depression of eyes with setting sun sign (sclera is seen above the iris), slow pupil response to light, irritability, high-pitched cry, difficulty in being consoled, lethargy, altered level of consciousness, and difficulty in sucking and feeding. In children, manifestations may include headache on awakening, hyperactive reflexes, strabismus, unsteady gait, irritability, papilledema (edema of the optic disk), lethargy, disorientation, and progression to stupor.

Diagnostic tests. In infants, measurement of the head circumference is the most important diagnostic technique. It is important to measure the head circumference routinely in all infants. Any measurement that crosses one or more grid lines on the growth chart within a 2- to 4-week period is suggestive of hydrocephalus. Other diagnostic assessments include observation of neurologic signs that indicate the possibility of increased intracranial pressure, CT, and MRI.

Medical management. Treatment of hydrocephalus is aimed at relieving the pressure on the ventricles and correcting the cause of the ventriculomegaly. Complications that occur as a result of the hydrocephalus must be identified and treated. If a tumor is the cause of hydrocephalus, the surgeon removes it. If the cause of the hydrocephalus is obstruction, the treatment involves surgical diversion of excess CSF from the ventricles to the peritoneum with a ventriculoperitoneal shunt (Fig. 32.27). Revisions in the ventriculoperitoneal shunt are needed when the shunt malfunctions, becomes infected, or becomes too short as the child grows.

Nursing interventions. Nursing interventions for a child with hydrocephalus involve assisting with prompt diagnosis, observing for complications of the disease and shunt placement, and providing emotional support and education to the family. Nutrition is likely to become an issue if intracranial pressure increases. The child should not be handled before, during, and after feedings because handling sometimes leads to vomiting. Small, frequent feedings are usually better tolerated, and it is best to place infants on their sides after feedings to avoid aspiration. After the child's surgery, observe the child for signs of increasing intracranial pressure, assess vital signs, and closely monitor I&O. Usually the child is placed on the nonoperative side to avoid putting pressure on the shunt site. Perform meticulous skin care, especially to the scalp, preoperatively and postoperatively. A sheepskin pad should be placed under the child's head, and the child's position should be changed every 2 hours. Provide emotional support to the family during the hospitalization and prepare them for discharge.

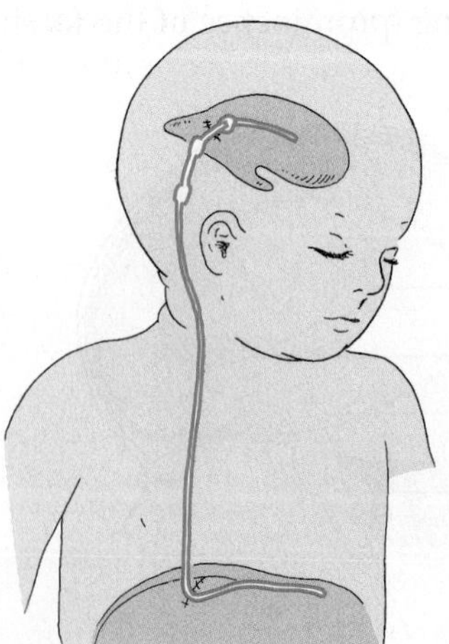

Fig. 32.27 Ventriculoperitoneal shunt placement. Catheter is threaded subcutaneously from small incisions at the sites of ventricular and peritoneal insertions. (From Hockenberry MJ, Wilson D: *Wong's essentials of pediatric nursing*, ed 9, St. Louis, 2013, Mosby.)

Patient problems and interventions for a child with hydrocephalus include but are not limited to the following:

Patient Problem	Nursing Interventions
Potential for Infection, related to presence of mechanical drainage system	Perform hand hygiene before contact with patient Limit visitors to reduce the number of organisms in patient's environment, and restrict visitation by individuals with any type of infection Encourage adequate diet to maintain optimal nutritional status Maintain asepsis for dressing changes and wound care
Impaired family processes, related to situational crisis (child with a physical defect)	Facilitate family's acceptance of infant: • Allow family's expression of feelings • Convey attitude of acceptance of infant and family Indicate by behavior that infant is a valuable human being

Patient teaching. To prepare for the child's discharge and home care, instruct the parents in how to recognize signs that indicate shunt malfunction or infection and how to manually drain the shunt if necessary. Safe transportation is an essential issue to discuss with parents. Small infants may be restrained in a reclining position in an approved car bed. It is important to emphasize that hydrocephalus is a lifelong problem and that the child will require evaluation on a regular basis. The overall aim is to establish realistic goals and an appropriate educational program that will assist the child to achieve optimal potential.

Prognosis. The prognosis for children with treated hydrocephalus depends largely on the rate at which hydrocephalus develops, the duration of raised intracranial pressure, the frequency of complications, and the cause of hydrocephalus. With prompt diagnosis and proper shunt functioning, the survival rate for children with hydrocephalus is 80%.

Cerebral palsy. Cerebral palsy is the most common permanent physical disability of childhood, with an average prevalence of 3.3 per 1000 live births in the United States. It occurs more often in boys than girls (CDC, 2017d). Cerebral palsy is a general term for a group of nonprogressive disorders of motoneuron impairment that result in motor dysfunction. In addition, affected children sometimes exhibit intellectual, visual, language, and neurologic impairments. The primary manifestations of cerebral palsy involve abnormal muscle tone and poor coordination.

Etiology and pathophysiology. Many antenatal, perinatal, and postnatal factors share some of the responsibility in the development of cerebral palsy. Antenatal factors include maternal infections, maternal drug ingestion, hypoxia in utero, and blood incompatibilities. Perinatal factors include cerebral trauma and anoxia during birth. Anoxia plays the most significant role in the pathologic process of brain damage. Anesthesia or analgesia during labor and delivery, prematurity, and metabolic or electrolyte disturbances are also factors. Postnatal factors include infection, head trauma, cerebrovascular accident, and poisoning.

Clinical manifestations. The clinical manifestations of cerebral palsy range from moderate to severe and are described in Box 32.9.

Diagnostic tests. The diagnosis of cerebral palsy is based on history and physical examination. A thorough antenatal and birth history must be documented. A thorough neurologic examination is an essential component of the physical examination process and often aids in establishing a diagnosis of cerebral palsy. Additional tests may include CT, cranial sonography, electroencephalography, MRI, and a serum metabolic screening.

Medical management. There is no cure for cerebral palsy. Common treatments include medicine, surgery, braces, and physical, occupational, and speech therapy. Treatment of the disorder should start as soon as the diagnosis is determined. The Individuals with Disabilities Education Act consists of two parts: A and B. This law ensures care for children during the first 36 months of age (part A) and supplies services to children from 3 to 21 years of age (part B). Braces, orthopedic devices, wheelchairs and walkers, and communication aids may be necessary in the treatment for the child with cerebral palsy (CDC, 2017d). These assistive devices often are used to aid in increasing patients' ability to manage the activities of daily living.

Botulinum toxin (Botox) is a drug used in the treatment of spasticity for cerebral palsy. Botox is injected into the muscle, where it acts to inhibit the release of acetylcholine into a specific muscle group, thereby preventing abnormal contractions. When administered early in the course of the disease, it often can prevent contractures, particularly in lower extremities, and eliminate the need for surgical procedures with possible adverse effects. The goal is to allow stretching of the muscle as it relaxes and permit ambulation with an ankle-foot orthosis. The major reported adverse effect of Botox injection is pain at the injection site.

Intrathecal or oral baclofen therapy is best suited for children with severe spasticity that interferes with activities of daily living and ambulation. The medication suppresses the release of excitatory neurotransmitters, thus reducing spasticity. If the medication is administered by the intrathecal route, a pump is implanted surgically. Benzodiazepines are used for seizure activity that may occur in the patient with cerebral palsy. Several other classes of drugs may be used as well to treat symptoms of cerebral palsy (Medscape, 2016).

Nursing interventions. Nursing interventions for a child with cerebral palsy focus on early recognition and prompt institution of interventions to enable optimal development. Adaptive eating utensils are used to facilitate eating. Encourage self-feeding and a high-calorie diet. It is important to encourage mobilization. Devices such as braces, wheeled scooters, and walkers are available to assist with mobility. Encourage use of protective headgear when these children are first learning to walk. Praise the children when goals are attained and encourage them to be as independent as possible within their limitations.

Patient problems and interventions for a child with cerebral palsy include but are not limited to the following:

Patient Problem	Nursing Interventions
Compromised Physical Mobility, related to neuromuscular impairment	Encourage sitting, crawling, and walking at appropriate ages Carry out therapies that strengthen and improve control Assist the child in using appropriate leg motions when the child is learning to walk Provide incentives to promote mobility Ensure that the child has rested before attempting locomotion activities

Continued

Box 32.9 Clinical Manifestations of Cerebral Palsy

- Arching of back
- Delayed gross motor development
- Developmental disabilities
- Difficulty swallowing and excessive drooling
- Exaggerated deep tendon reflexes
- Feeding difficulties
- Hypertonic muscles
- Involuntary movements
- Persistence of primitive reflexes
- Poor sucking
- Scissor-like gait with knees crossing
- Vision and hearing impairments

Patient Problem	Nursing Interventions
	Incorporate play that encourages desired behavior Employ aids that facilitate locomotion, such as parallel bars and crutches
Inability to Bathe, Dress of Feed Self, related to physical disability	Encourage the child to assist with care as age and capabilities permit Select toys and activities that allow maximal participation by the child and that improve motor function and sensory input Assist with jaw control during feeding Adapt utensils, foods, and clothing to facilitate self-help (e.g., large-bowled spoon with padded handle; finger foods and foods that adhere to, rather than slip from, utensil; and clothing that opens in front with self-adhering closings rather than buttons) Assist parents in toilet training the child

Patient teaching. Teach parents proper handling of their child and how to assist with activities of daily living. The family should learn to perform stretching and passive range-of-motion exercises and to select play activities that provide for maximal stimulation and participation. The parents also need education about the disorder and the resources available to them so that they can ensure optimal development for their child. Support groups are also beneficial to children and families. Information may be found at the MyChild website *(www.cerebralpalsy.org)*.

Prognosis. Cerebral palsy is a chronic neurologic disability. There is no cure, but promotion of an optimal developmental course is vital so that affected children can realize full potential within the limits of the brain dysfunction.

Seizure disorders

Etiology and pathophysiology. The term *seizure* refers to a sudden, excessive, disorderly discharge of abnormal electrical impulses by the brain's neurons, causing a temporary alteration in CNS function. Some seizures are the result of such conditions as tumors, trauma, hypoxia, infections, poisons, fever, and metabolic disturbances; however, most seizures have no identifiable cause. Children are most prone to seizures during the period between birth and 2 years. More than 750,000 children between the ages of 0 to 17 years in the United States have epilepsy or recurrent seizures (CDC, 2016). The current classification system divides seizures into two major categories: partial and generalized.

Diagnostic testing. Data collection and review of the health history provide invaluable tools in the evaluation and diagnosis of seizure disorders. The health care provider performs a detailed neurologic examination. Electroencephalography is the most useful tool for evaluating seizure disorders. Additional diagnostic tests include CT and MRI. Single-photon emission CT gives a three-dimensional view of the brain and its vasculature. It often is used to help pinpoint the specific location of seizure activity.

Medical management. The treatment of seizure disorders primarily involves drug therapy. Anticonvulsants that are most valuable in controlling partial or generalized seizures include carbamazepine (Tegretol), phenytoin (Dilantin), fosphenytoin (Cerebyx), and valproic acid (Depakote or Depakene). The drugs of choice for absence seizures, which belong to the class of partial seizures, are ethosuximide (Zarontin) and valproic acid. Reducing the number of drugs taken improves quality of life; therefore experts currently recommend single-drug therapy. Additional seizure management has been achieved with gabapentin (Neurontin), lamotrigine (Lamictal), and felbamate (Felbatol). The use of felbamate is controversial because of the side effects of aplastic anemia and hepatic failure. Anticonvulsant therapy continues for a prolonged period. The health care provider modifies the dosage as the child grows. In children with a normal electroencephalogram who have been seizure free for at least 2 years, it is possible to discontinue anticonvulsant medications without increasing the risk of seizure recurrence. Discontinuing the medication gradually over 1 to 2 weeks is best. Abrupt withdrawal of anticonvulsants has the potential to result in an increase in the number and severity of seizures and sometimes even precipitates an episode of status epilepticus (continuous seizure activity).

The initial treatment of status epilepticus focuses on supporting and maintaining vital functions, including securing a patent airway, administering oxygen, establishing venous access, providing hydration, and administering lorazepam (Ativan), diazepam (Valium), or phenobarbital, as ordered. After the continuous seizure is stopped, the child will possible receive a loading dose of phenytoin to ensure sustained control of seizures.

Nursing interventions. Nursing interventions for a child with a seizure disorder involve assisting with the diagnosis, providing acute care during a seizure, providing for long-term management of the seizure disorder, and emotionally supporting and assisting the child and the family. To assist with the diagnosis of a seizure disorder, observe the child during a seizure and carefully document events, including any precipitating factors, if known or suspected; behavior before the seizure; time when the seizure began and ended; clinical manifestations of the seizure; and postseizure behavior and signs and symptoms. Recognize precipitating factors and prevent or minimize the child's exposure to them. Protect the child from injury during a seizure. Measures to prevent injuries during a seizure include padding the bed side rails and keeping the side rails upright; easing the child to the floor from a sitting or standing position; moving furniture out of the way; loosening restrictive clothing; and turning the child's head to the side to prevent aspiration of secretions. It is important not to force an object (e.g., tongue blade, airway) between the child's teeth during a seizure because doing so sometimes causes oral trauma. Staying with the child during and after a seizure and providing reassurance, emotional support, and explanations help minimize the child's anxiety.

A significant nursing goal is to promote a positive self-image in the child through encouragement and identification of the child's strengths and assets. Providing emotional support to the family is also essential. Encourage parents to express their fears and concerns and assist them to understand their child's condition. The family needs education regarding the nature of the disorder and possible precipitating factors, seizure precaution measures, dosage and side effects of medications, and the importance of maintaining as normal a lifestyle as possible.

Patient teaching. The family must acknowledge the need to continue the medication regularly, without interruption, for as long as required. Help the parents plan the administration of the medication at convenient times to keep disruption of family routine to a minimum. Most neurologists prefer that patients take anticonvulsant medications in tablet or capsule form for more equal and accurate distribution of the medication. During periods of growth, medication dosage must be adjusted. Education concerning the prescribed dosages and common side effects also is needed. Teenage girls of childbearing age must be advised that selected antiseizure medications may reduce the effectiveness of hormone-based contraceptives. Individuals with seizure activity are advised to wear identification (e.g., bracelets) that highlights their seizure condition.

Prognosis. The incidence of seizures can be controlled or greatly reduced in the majority of affected children, and new studies hold the promise of progress in future treatment. Seizures do not shorten the life of the child, and the child is able to attend school, marry, and have children.

Spina bifida (myelomeningocele). *Spina bifida* is a term that describes a variety of congenital defects of closure of the **neural tube** (the tube formed from the fusion of the neural folds and from which the brain and spinal cord arise). When the neural tube fails to close during embryonic development, a defect arises that can involve anything from a small area of the neural tube to its entire length (Fig. 32.28). Many infants with spina bifida occulta have a tuft of hair, a cleft, or a small, fatty mass over the defect. Myelomeningocele is one form of spina bifida in which portions of the spinal cord, the meninges, spinal fluid, and nerves protrude through the neural tube defect (Fig. 32.29).

Etiology and pathophysiology. The cause of neural tube defects is generally unknown. Approximately 3000 children are born each year with a neural tubal defect. Poor nutrition and advanced maternal age have been implicated as contributing factors, as well as genetics, maternal antiseizure medications, and maternal obesity and diabetes. It is recommended that women of childbearing age consume 400 to 800 mcg of folic acid per

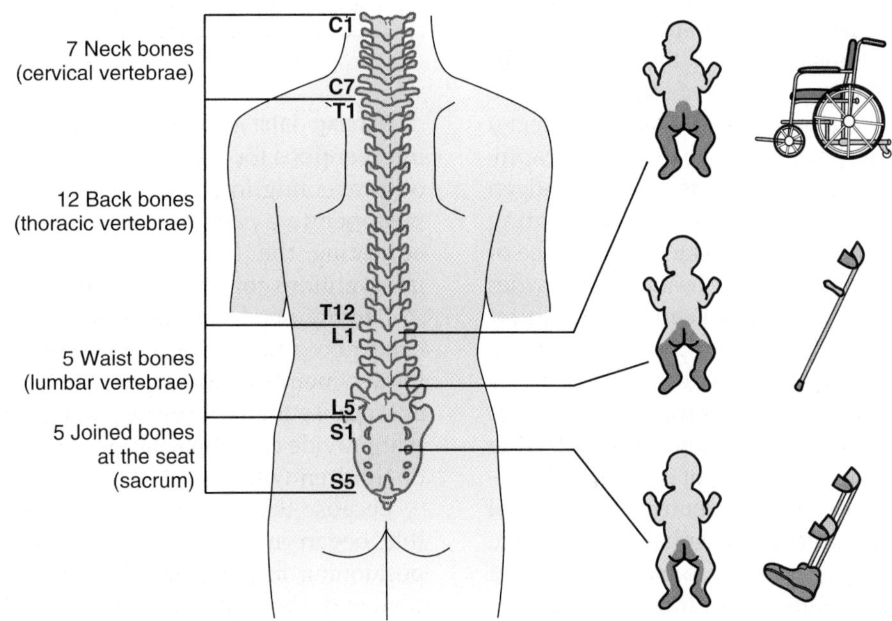

Fig. 32.28 Neural tube defect: effects at each level of the defect. (From Phillips N: *Berry and Kohn's operating room technique*, ed 12, St. Louis, 2013, Mosby.)

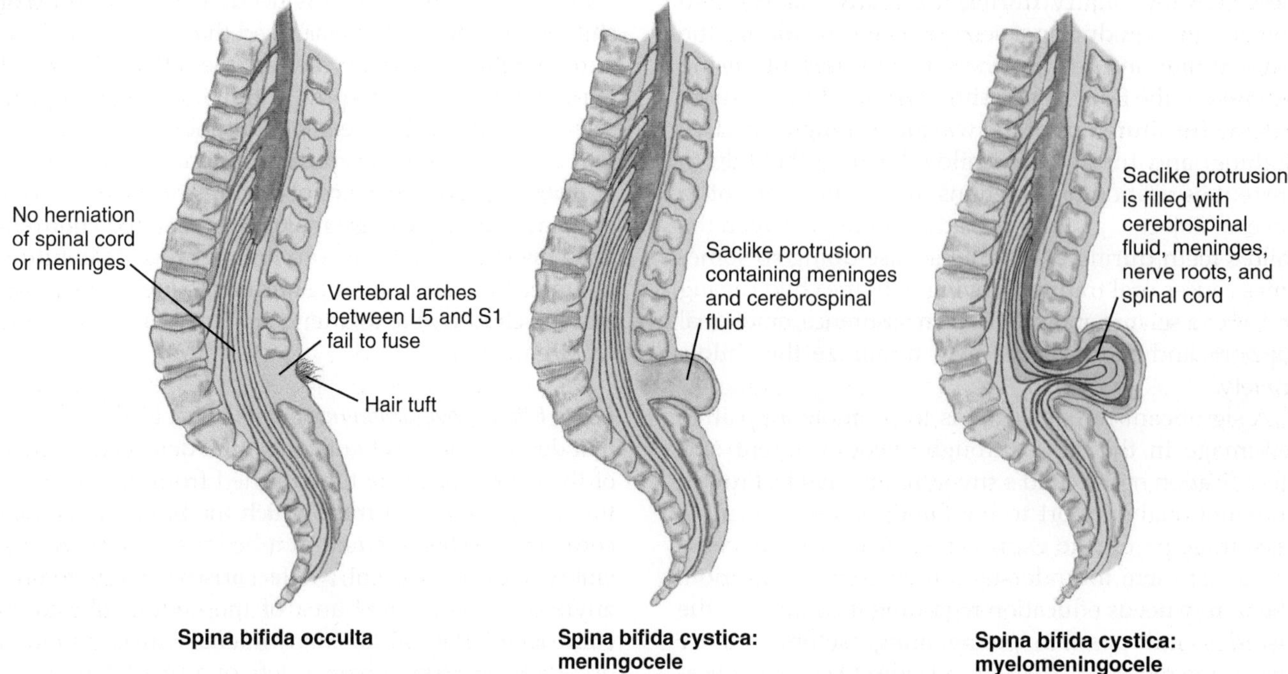

Fig. 32.29 Three forms of spina bifida. (From James SR, Nelson KA, Ashwill JW: *Nursing care of children: Principles and practice*, ed 4, St. Louis, 2013, Saunders.)

day to help prevent neural tube defects. Studies show that if all women of childbearing age met these dietary requirements, 70% or more of neural tube defects could be prevented (March of Dimes, 2016).

Clinical manifestations. In spina bifida, the spinal cord most commonly ends at the defect; therefore all motor and sensory function below the defect is absent. Most myelomeningoceles involve the lumbar and lumbosacral areas. Depending on the level of the defect, affected infants usually have flaccid paralysis and sensory deficits of the lower extremities, bowel and bladder incontinence, talipes equinovarus defects, and a subluxated hip (a partial or incomplete dislocation of the hip). Hydrocephalus is present in the majority of affected infants.

Diagnostic tests. It is sometimes possible to detect a neural tube defect prenatally. Uterine ultrasonography and elevated levels of maternal **alpha-fetoprotein** (antigen present in the human fetus that helps in evaluating fetal development) sometimes indicate the presence of a myelomeningocele. After birth, the health care provider makes the diagnosis on the basis of clinical manifestations. In some cases, the health care providers order a CT to assess for the presence of hydrocephalus.

Medical management. Treatment for myelomeningocele involves surgery to place the neural contents back within the sac to eliminate the possibility of infection. Sometimes it is necessary to insert a ventriculoperitoneal shunt to provide relief from hydrocephalus. Corrective surgeries are sometimes necessary to manage hip and lower extremity deformities. Additional measures include continuous neurologic assessments and assisting the family to deal with the diagnosis and surgery.

Box 32.10 Nursing Interventions for a Child With Myelomeningocele

PREOPERATIVE
- Position child on abdomen.
- Cover sac with sterile, saline-soaked gauze.
- Protect sac from contact with feces and urine.

POSTOPERATIVE
- Position child on abdomen for 10 to 14 days (until incision is healed).
- Monitor vital signs.
- Observe for signs of bleeding and infection.

Nursing interventions and patient teaching. Nursing interventions for a child with myelomeningocele focus on preventing infection and complications, providing postoperative care, and emotionally supporting and educating the family. Box 32.10 describes nursing interventions for children with myelomeningocele.

Parents need explanations regarding their child's condition and the surgery it necessitates. Encourage family members to express their fears and concerns and advise them of resources within their community that provide emotional support and services for families of children with spinal defects.

Because the parents will continue at home the care that began in the hospital, they need instruction on positioning, feeding, bowel training, bladder catheterization, and physical exercises.

Prognosis. The early prognosis for a child with myelomeningocele depends on the neurologic deficits present at birth, including motor ability, bladder and bowel innervation, and the presence of associated cerebral anomalies. Improved surgical techniques do not alter either the major physical disability and deformity or the chronic urinary tract and pulmonary infections and constipation that affect the quality of life for these children.

Neuroblastoma. Neuroblastoma is a malignant tumor composed principally of cells resembling neuroblasts that give rise to cells of the sympathetic nervous system. After brain tumors, neuroblastomas are the most common solid tumors in childhood, with approximately 700 new cases in children per year. The average age of diagnosis is 1 to 2 years of age with 90% diagnosed by age 5. Neuroblastoma has a high rate of dissemination, and approximately 67% of patients have metastatic disease at the time of diagnosis (ACS, 2018).

Etiology and pathophysiology. These tumors originate from embryonic neural crest cells that normally give rise to the adrenal medulla and the sympathetic ganglia. Consequently, most tumors develop in the adrenal gland or the retroperitoneal sympathetic chain. Other sites include the head, neck, chest, and pelvis. The most common sites for metastatic disease include the liver, skin, lymph nodes, bone, and bone marrow.

Clinical manifestations. The clinical manifestations of neuroblastoma depend on the location of the tumor. The most common location is the abdomen, and manifestations may include a palpable, firm, irregular mass that crosses the midline; anorexia; bowel and bladder alterations related to compression by the tumor; and spinal cord compression. If the tumor is located in the upper chest, manifestations include dyspnea, difficulty swallowing, and neck and facial edema. Many of the manifestations at the time of diagnosis are the result of metastatic disease. Manifestations of metastasis are hepatomegaly, splenomegaly, anemia, bone and joint pain, skin nodules (especially in infants), periorbital edema, weight loss, pallor, and weakness.

Diagnostic tests. Initial diagnostic studies focus on locating the primary tumor site and areas of metastasis. In addition to a complete history and physical examination, studies include skeletal survey, bone scan, CT, abdominal ultrasonography, MRI, bone marrow aspiration and biopsy, and urine collection for metabolites of catecholamines (biologically active amines, epinephrine, and norepinephrine; adrenal tumors stimulate the production of catecholamines). A biopsy of the tumor provides a definitive diagnosis and staging information.

Medical management. The management of neuroblastoma involves a combination of surgery, radiation therapy, and chemotherapy. If the tumor is localized, the surgeon removes the tumor, and radiation therapy follows. If disease is widely disseminated, the surgeon removes as much of the tumor as possible, and the child receives follow-up chemotherapy and radiation therapy.

Nursing interventions and patient teaching. Initial nursing interventions focus on preparing the child for diagnostic and operative procedures. Postoperative care is similar to that for any child undergoing abdominal surgery, including observation for any postoperative complications. Psychological support of the family is essential and involves helping them to prepare for the diagnostic and operative procedures and postoperative complications. Parents need an opportunity to express their fears and concerns. Because of the high incidence of metastasis at diagnosis, parents sometimes feel guilty that they did not seek medical attention sooner.

Parents also must be educated about any chemotherapy or radiation therapy that is needed.

Prognosis. Because this tumor is so frequently invasive, the prognosis for children with neuroblastoma is poor. In general, the younger the child is at diagnosis (especially younger than 1 year of age), the better the survival rate is. Neuroblastoma is one of the few tumors that may regress spontaneously, possibly as a result of maturity of the embryonic cell or the development of an active immune system.

Lead poisoning. Lead poisoning is one of the most common, preventable, serious health care problems affecting children in the United States. The CDC defines lead poisoning as a blood lead level higher than 10 mg/dL. Lead levels too low to produce symptoms nonetheless can cause neurologic deficits insidiously. Lead levels as low as 10 μg/dL may cause significant health concerns in children, including long-term cognitive and behavioral problems.

Etiology and pathophysiology. The leading cause of lead poisoning is ingestion or inhalation of environmental lead. Sources include lead-based paint, contaminated soil, and lead-contaminated pipes. The use of lead as an ingredient in household paint has been illegal in the United States since 1978. Older architectural structures still pose a threat to children's safety. Additional dangers for contamination may lurk in older painted toys and furniture. There are nearly 24 million housing units in which the children living in them are being exposed to lead because of deterioration of walls with lead paint (CDC, 2014).

Ingested lead is excreted slowly from the body through the GI and genitourinary tracts. Any lead that is retained is stored in the bone, where it remains inactive. When the level of lead exceeds the amount that bone can absorb, lead travels through the circulatory system and causes anemia. Lead poisoning occurs more rapidly in children with iron deficiencies. Lead poisoning can damage the CNS seriously and is particularly dangerous to younger children.

Clinical manifestations. Manifestations of lead poisoning include anemia, anorexia, abdominal pain, lethargy, aggression, impulsiveness, irritability, learning difficulties, delinquency, decreased attention span, decreased curiosity, hearing deficits, growth and developmental failure, and **pica** (craving to eat nonfood substances). Neurocognitive effects are possible results from lead poisoning and lead to long-term complications such as lowered IQ scores, developmental delays, speech and language problems, reading deficits, lower academic achievements, visual-spatial problems, and visual-motor problems.

Diagnostic testing. Direct measurement of blood levels remains the primary diagnostic technique in the assessment of lead poisoning. A complete history and physical examination and an environmental assessment provide valuable information that identifies exposed children and environments at highest risk. Lead paint screening begins with blood testing. Screening is mandated for children in some states. Although blood lead levels higher than 10 mg/dL are considered diagnostic, counseling and follow-up are needed for children whose blood levels of lead exceed 2 mg/dL. CBCs, coagulation studies, and iron levels also are evaluated. Radiographic studies of the abdomen and long bones also may be performed. Lead lines (areas of increased density) near the epiphyseal lines may be identified.

Medical management. The management of lead poisoning varies according to the blood level of lead. The primary objective of treatment is to remove lead from the body and prevent further exposure to lead. Pharmacologic treatment, such as **chelation therapy** (in toxicology, the use of a compound to bind to a toxic substance and render it nonactive and thus nontoxic), is a key intervention for children who have excessive lead levels. The precise course of therapy and the chelating agent depend on the preference of the health care provider and the severity of the child's condition. There is also an emphasis on ameliorating nutritional deficiencies and preventing infection.

Nursing interventions and patient teaching. The challenges of lead poisoning provide a unique opportunity for pediatric nurses. The main goal of prevention strategies is to identify and deal with lead sources for the population of children at risk and the communities in which they live. To reach this goal, a thorough environmental and health questionnaire is completed at each routine health examination. The questionnaire is used to assess the child's risk for lead exposure. Provide parents with referrals to help them access resources for help with this problem.

Parent guidelines for reducing lead in the child's environment are described in Box 32.11.

Prognosis. Although most of the pathophysiologic effects of lead are reversible, the most serious consequences of high- and low-level lead exposure are the effects on the CNS. In children with lead-induced encephalopathy, permanent brain damage results in cognitive impairment, behavior changes, possible paralysis, and seizures. Low-dose exposure also has the potential to cause permanent neurologic deficits. The neurologic deficits common with lead exposure include impulsivity, short attention span, distractibility, learning disabilities, and failure in school. With treatment, improvement may be seen in children with moderate lead poisoning.

Box 32.11 Parent Guidelines for Reducing Blood Lead Levels

- Make sure child does not have access to peeling paint or chewable surfaces painted with lead-based paint, especially window sills and wells.
- If house was built before 1960 and has hard-surfaced floors, wet mop them at least once a week with a high-phosphate solution such as trisodium phosphate (available in hardware stores). Wipe other hard surfaces (such as window sills and baseboards) with a similar solution. Do not vacuum hard-surfaced floors or window sills or wells because this spreads dust. Use vacuum cleaners with agitators to remove dust from rugs rather than vacuum cleaners with suction only.
- Wash child's hands and face before the child eats.
- Wash toys and pacifiers frequently.
- If soil around home is likely to be contaminated with lead (e.g., if home was built before 1960 or is near a major highway), plant grass or other ground cover; plant bushes around outside of house so that child is not able to play there.
- During remodeling of older homes, be sure to follow correct procedures. Be certain children and pregnant women are not in the home, day or night, until work is completed. After deleading, thoroughly clean house with wet mopping before inhabitants return.
- In areas where lead content of water exceeds the drinking water standard, run water for at least 2 minutes from cold-water tap for drinking, cooking, and making formula; use first-flush water for purposes other than consumption.
- Do not store food in open cans, particularly if cans are imported.
- For food storage or service, do not use pottery or ceramic ware that was inadequately fired or is meant for decorative use.
- Avoid folk remedies that contain lead.
- Make sure that parental occupations or hobbies are not causing exposure in the home. Household members who are employed in occupations such as lead smelting should shower and change into clean clothing before leaving work.
- Make sure child eats regular meals because more lead is absorbed on an empty stomach.
- Make sure child's diet contains plenty of iron, calcium, protein, and zinc.

Modified from Centers for Disease Control and Prevention: *Preventing lead poisoning in young children,* Atlanta, 2012, Author.

Neonatal abstinence syndrome. Because opioids readily cross the placental membrane, women who use drugs while they are pregnant cause a passive addiction in their unborn children. Opioids commonly abused by women during pregnancy include cocaine (including "crack"), heroin, and methadone. Shortly after birth, the affected infant exhibits signs and symptoms of drug withdrawal, including irritability, disturbed sleeping and feeding patterns, tremors, seizures, hyperreflexia (increased reflex reaction), clonus (abnormal neuromuscular activity characterized by rapidly alternating involuntary contraction and relaxation of skeletal muscles), high-pitched cry, hypertonic muscles, tachypnea, frantic sucking of hands, vomiting, diarrhea, and inability to maintain body temperature. Signs and symptoms of opioid withdrawal sometimes persist for 3 to 4 months. For infants suspected of having opioid abstinence syndrome, health care providers usually order urinalysis for metabolites of the drug. It is essential to obtain a urine sample from the infant immediately after birth because the by-products of the drugs are cleared quickly from the body.

Infants who are experiencing neonatal abstinence syndrome are most comfortable in a nonstimulating environment that is free from bright lights and loud noises. They often prefer to be tightly swaddled in a blanket, with a pacifier to satisfy their vigorous sucking needs. It is essential to monitor such infants' I&O and vital signs. Nursing interventions should be organized in a manner that reduces the amount of disturbance to the infant.

On discharge, affected infants need a referral to an early intervention program, because they are at risk for neurologic problems; parent-infant bonding difficulties; and developmental, behavioral, and learning disabilities. Their mothers need referral for parental education and drug treatment programs to enable an optimal outcome for the child and family.

DISORDERS OF INTEGUMENTARY FUNCTION

Skin function is affected by genetic factors, cleanliness, hydration, and nutrition. Dermatologic disorders in children are the reason for a significant proportion of children's visits to health care provider's offices and clinics. Many of these disorders are painful for the child and distressing for the family.

Noninfectious Disorders of the Skin

Contact dermatitis

Etiology and pathophysiology. Contact dermatitis is an inflammatory, delayed immune response of the skin resulting from contact with environmental antigens to which a person is hypersensitive. Contact dermatitis has the highest incidence in infants and toddlers, and many patients have a family history of allergy. The most commonly affected areas include face, neck, hands, feet, and legs. The allergens that are most commonly responsible in children include soaps, detergents, bubble baths, shoe components, metals, chemicals, cosmetics, and plants such as poison ivy, oak, and sumac.

Clinical manifestations. The contact area becomes erythematous, edematous, and pruritic. Papules (solid, red, raised areas less than 0.5 cm in diameter) and vesicles (circumscribed raised areas filled with serous fluid and less than 0.5 cm in diameter) form and can weep and ooze if broken.

Diagnostic tests. The health care provider makes the diagnosis by observing the pattern and the location of the rash and by documenting an accurate history to identify the causative agent. Skin testing is also helpful at times in the identification of suspected plants, foods, or animals.

Medical management. The hypersensitive reaction is usually self-limiting; therefore, in most cases, the health care provider directs treatment toward identifying and eliminating the cause and relieving signs and symptoms. Cool, wet dressings dipped in Burow's solution (solution of aluminum acetate, used as a drying agent for weeping skin lesions) or oatmeal baths help soothe the affected area. Calamine lotion may be recommended to manage pruritus without a prescription. It is acceptable to apply topical, over-the-counter steroid creams to mild contact dermatitis areas. In more severe cases, health care providers often prescribe systemic corticosteroids. Oral antihistamines such as diphenhydramine (Benadryl) are helpful in controlling pruritus.

Nursing interventions and patient teaching. Advise the family to keep the child's fingernails clipped short to prevent scratching, which can result in a secondary bacterial infection. Loose, lightweight clothing during the healing phase is also comfortable and decreases irritation.

Teach parents to keep an accurate history of possible causative agents. Once it is clear what the primary irritant is, teach them to avoid it. If the skin does come in contact with the causative agent, teach parents to wash the affected area with a mild soap and water and dry it thoroughly. It is best to avoid talcum powder, overheating, and hot baths. Teach the parents to apply topical medications only as directed by a health care provider.

Prognosis. The reaction is usually self-limiting and normally resolves within 2 weeks.

Diaper dermatitis

Etiology and pathophysiology. Diaper dermatitis is one of the most common skin disorders in infancy and the cause of great concern for many parents. Diaper dermatitis is a form of contact dermatitis and usually caused by an external irritant (Fig. 32.30). The most common irritating agents include prolonged exposure to urine or feces; inadequate cleaning of the diaper area; soaps, detergents, or fabric softeners; excessive use of powders or ointments; and the use of plastic pants. Fair-complexioned infants tend to have more sensitive skin and are more vulnerable to diaper rash than are infants with darker complexions. The occurrence peaks at 9 to 12 months of age, and the incidence is higher in formula-fed infants than in breast-fed infants.

Clinical manifestations. The rash appears as erythematous papular lesions (similar in appearance to a scald) on the areas that come into direct contact with the diaper:

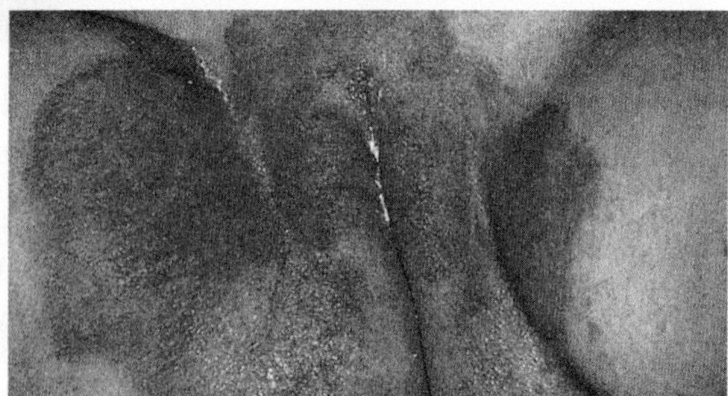

Fig. 32.30 Diaper dermatitis. (From Habif TP: *Clinical dermatology: A color guide to diagnosis and therapy*, ed 3, St. Louis, 1996, Mosby.)

the buttocks, the labia or the scrotum, the inner thighs, and the mons pubis. Skinfolds frequently are spared. In many cases, excoriation in the perianal area is caused by frequent diarrhea. The inflammation does not take on a specific configuration; rather, a variety of patterns are possible. The moist, warm, dark environment created by the diaper also tends to promote the growth of secondary bacterial or fungal infections. An infant with diaper dermatitis is usually uncomfortable and likely to be fussy, irritable, and restless.

Diagnostic tests. Clinical observation of the characteristics and the location of the rash and an assessment of possible irritants are diagnostic for diaper dermatitis. Bacterial or fungal cultures are sometimes necessary to investigate persistent secondary infections.

Medical management. Keeping the diaper area clean and dry is of primary importance. Measures to promote healing and prevent diaper dermatitis from recurring include changing diapers as soon as they become soiled, thoroughly cleansing the diaper area with a mild soap and water and then gently drying at each diaper change, exposing the affected area to the air several times a day, and avoiding occlusive plastic pants. For more severe cases, a topical glucocorticoid sometimes is required.

Nursing interventions and patient teaching. The prophylactic use of protective ointments such as Desitin, A+D ointment, or zinc oxide is often helpful. Keep the diaper area clean. An excessive amount of powder is contraindicated because in the presence of moisture, the powder will cake, hold the moisture, and excoriate the skin (Box 32.12).

Teach parents the basics of diaper and skin care as outlined previously. To prevent the infant's inhalation of powder dust, instruct parents to put a small amount in their hand and apply it to the infant's diaper area (see Box 32.12).

Prognosis. Quick recognition with prompt therapy leads to a good prognosis.

Atopic dermatitis (eczema)

Etiology and pathophysiology. Atopic dermatitis is a pruritic, allergic response common in infancy and childhood. *Atopy* refers to an allergy for which there is a genetic or inherited predisposition. The exact cause is unknown. Many affected children have a familial history of asthma, allergic rhinitis, or dry skin. The disease also occurs in association with hypersensitivity to histamine, as well as with food allergies and abnormal skin function. Infantile atopic dermatitis can occur between 2 and 5 months of age and sometimes continues to be problematic to age 2 or 3 years, when many children seem to "outgrow" the illness. Childhood atopic dermatitis usually occurs at age 2 or 3 years and persists to 5 years of age in some cases. Adolescent atopic dermatitis usually is seen at 12 years of age and in some cases lasts indefinitely.

Clinical manifestations. In infantile eczema, the primary lesions consist of erythema, vesicles, and papules, which typically ooze and form crusts. They appear most often on the cheeks, scalp, trunk, and extensor surfaces of the extremities. In childhood eczema, the lesions appear as erythematous, scaly patches on the trunk, elbows, knees, ankles, hands, and feet and behind the ears. The skin becomes thick and leather-like (**lichenification**). In adolescent eczema, the lesions are the same as in childhood, but the distribution involves mainly hands, feet, neck, and face. At any age, the unaffected skin is usually very dry, and the pruritus may be extremely intense. Affected children are often uncomfortable and restless. Affected infants unable to scratch often rub their faces on linens or clothing in an effort to relieve the itch. Scratching or rubbing also has the potential to lead to secondary infections, and many children

Box 32.12 Parent Guidelines for Controlling Diaper Rash

- Keep skin dry.
- Use superabsorbent disposable diapers to reduce skin wetness. If cloth diapers are used, use only overwraps that allow air to circulate; avoid using rubber pants.
- Change diapers as soon as they are soiled, especially with stool, whenever possible and preferably once during the night.
- Expose healthy or only slightly irritated skin to air, not heat, to dry completely.
- Apply ointment, such as zinc oxide or petrolatum, to protect skin, especially if skin is very erythematous or has moist, open areas.
- When the area is soiled, wipe off top layer of ointment and reapply.
- To completely remove ointment, especially zinc oxide, use mineral oil; do not wash vigorously.
- Avoid overwashing the skin, especially with perfumed soaps or commercial wipes that are potentially irritating. It is acceptable to use a moisturizer or nonsoap cleanser, such as cold cream or Cetaphil, to wipe urine from skin. Gently wipe stool from skin with water and mild soap, such as Dove.

with atopic dermatitis have an increased susceptibility to bacterial *(S. aureus)*, viral (herpes simplex), and fungal skin infections. The signs and symptoms are better in humid climates and worse in fall and winter, when homes are heated and environmental humidity is lower.

Diagnostic tests. The diagnosis is based on clinical observation of the type and distribution of the lesions, a positive family history of allergy, and severity of pruritus. In general, skin testing is important in severe cases to help determine specific allergens.

Medical management. The therapeutic management includes hydration of the skin, controlling pruritus, decreasing inflammation, and preventing secondary infections. Skin hydration can be accomplished in a variety of ways. Tepid baths followed by the administration of an unscented cream or lotion help trap moisture in the skin. The application of occlusive creams or ointments helps relieve dry skin. To decrease inflammation, the health care provider orders thin applications of topical steroid creams or lotions. The strength and the type of topical steroid vary according to the degree of inflammation and the age of the child. Oral antihistamines such as diphenhydramine (Benadryl) or hydroxyzine are useful in controlling pruritus. New therapies include topical immunomodulators, which are steroid-free medications that aid in the reduction of inflammation. Tacrolimus (Protopic) and pimecrolimus (Elidel) are examples of topical immunomodulators. Secondary bacterial infections are managed with systemic antibiotics (Nowicki, Trzeciak, et al, 2015).

Nursing interventions. The nurse's role in caring for a child with atopic dermatitis involves measures to control pruritus, promote skin integrity, and provide emotional support to the child and family. Compresses with Burow's solution (aluminum acetate) soothe itching and moisten skin. Hot baths and hot showers should be discouraged because of their drying effect on the skin. Suggest adding cornstarch to tepid bath water to provide some relief from itching, as well as to hydrate skin. Teach the child and the family to use only a mild, unscented soap such as Dove or Neutrogena, if they use any soap at all. To prevent new lesions or secondary infection, it is essential to minimize scratching. For the infant, covering the hands with mittens or socks helps reduce scratching. For the older child, gloves allow for more dexterity. At times, it may be necessary to use safety reminder devices to discourage scratching; however, it is important that the infant or child be free from these restrictions periodically.

Patient teaching. Overheating usually intensifies itching; therefore parents need to understand that dressing their child in lightweight, loose clothing made from cotton or cotton blends is preferable. They should wash and double-rinse clothing, linens, and blankets to ensure removal of all soap residue. It is important for parents to understand that they must apply lubricants frequently—especially after bathing, while the skin is still damp—to seal in moisture. Teach parents to keep the child's fingernails and toenails clipped short and clean to keep the risk of infection to a minimum. At any age, keeping the child's hands busy with play activities provides the distraction needed to discourage scratching. The appearance, discomfort, and irritability displayed by children with atopic dermatitis are often very upsetting for family members. Encourage parents to verbalize their feelings and provide reassurance. Teaching stress-reduction techniques is often helpful to the child and the parents because stress tends to aggravate the severity of the condition.

Prognosis. Atopic dermatitis can be controlled but not cured. Most young children with atopic dermatitis outgrow their condition before adolescence, but some continue to have symptoms throughout adulthood.

Seborrheic dermatitis

Etiology and pathophysiology. Seborrheic dermatitis, or cradle cap, is a chronic inflammatory reaction of the skin that is common in infancy. Although the cause of the condition is unknown, there appears to be a connection to sebaceous gland activity. Many affected infants have no family history of allergy.

Clinical manifestations. Seborrheic dermatitis most commonly affects the scalp and appears as thick, white or yellowish, crusty or scaly patches. Mild pruritus sometimes accompanies the disorder. Other commonly affected areas include the eyebrows or eyelids (blepharitis), the postauricular area (behind the ear), the external ear (otitis externa), the nasolabial (nose and lip) folds, and the inguinal region (seborrheic diaper dermatitis).

Diagnostic tests. Diagnosis is based on clinical observation of the characteristics and location of crusty patches. Skin biopsy of the affected area may be performed.

Medical management. Management of seborrheic dermatitis consists of treating the signs and symptoms and simple preventive measures. The nurse and the parents can remove crusty, scaly patches by applying mineral oil to soften the affected areas (except the eyelids) and help loosen crusts, followed by shampooing with a mild, tear-free shampoo and thoroughly rinsing. Then a soft baby brush or a soft toothbrush is used to brush the hair and remove flakes from the hair. A fine-tooth comb also works well. Preventive measures include daily shampooing with an antiseborrheic shampoo. Topical corticosteroids are rarely needed.

Nursing interventions and patient teaching. Soak crusts with warm water and cotton (or clean washcloth) compresses until the crusts are loosened. Then cleanse the eye area with clean cotton (or a clean washcloth) and warm water, starting at the inner canthus and continuing to the outer canthus. For each stroke, a clean piece of cotton (or clean area on the washcloth) should be used.

Patient Problems and Nursing Interventions for Children With a Disorder of Integumentary Function

Patient Problem	Nursing Interventions
Compromised Skin Integrity, related to irritation	Assess for signs of scratching Advise parents to keep the child's fingernails short or to cover the child's hands with mittens or socks Keep affected areas clean and dry Apply medications as directed
Potential for Infection, related to scratching and skin impairment	Assess for signs of infection Change diapers as soon as they are soiled Administer appropriate antibiotics as directed Implement standard precautions (see Chapter 7) Maintain careful hand hygiene Teach and reinforce positive habits of hygienic care
Distorted Body Image, related to perceptions of appearance	Encourage child to express feelings about personal appearance and perceived reactions of other people Hold child (remember that there is no substitute for the stimulation and comfort of human contact) Touch and caress unaffected area Teach self-care when appropriate Involve child in planning treatment schedules Emotionally support and encourage child in efforts to deal with multiple problems that sometimes occur in association with disorder, including discomfort, rejection, discouragement, and feelings of self-revulsion Encourage child to maintain usual activities

Often parents need reassurance that shampooing their infant's hair will not cause harm to the fontanelles. A demonstration on how to shampoo the hair is sometimes necessary. If cradle cap is extensive, inform parents that several treatments may be necessary to loosen and remove all crusts. If the eyelids are involved, teach the parents how to clean these areas safely.

Prognosis. The crusts may appear shortly after birth and until old age, with periods of remissions and exacerbations.

Acne vulgaris. Acne is an inflammatory process of the skin. It is slightly more common in boys and men. Acne most often occurs in teenagers, but it can occur at any age. Acne is a disease that involves the pilosebaceous follicles (the hair follicles and sebaceous gland complex) of the face, the neck, the shoulders, the back, and the upper chest.

Medical management. Treatment success depends on the commitment of the adolescent. Before treatment is prescribed, it is best to determine the adolescent's level of comfort and readiness to begin treatment.

Tretinoin (Retin-A) is the only drug that effectively interrupts the abnormal follicular keratinization that produces microcomedones, the invisible precursors of the visible comedones. Tretinoin alone is usually sufficient for management of comedonal acne. The medication should not be applied for at least 20 to 30 minutes after washing, to decrease the burning sensation. It is important to emphasize the need to avoid sun and use sunscreen daily, because sun exposure has potential to result in severe sunburn. Adolescents are advised to apply the medication at night and to use a sunscreen with a sun protection factor (SPF) of at least 15 in the daytime.

Topical benzoyl peroxide is an antibacterial agent that inhibits the growth of *Propionibacterium acnes* organisms. It is effective against inflammatory and noninflammatory acne and is an effective first-line agent. This medication is available over the counter and by prescription as a cream, lotion, gel, or wash.

When inflammatory lesions accompany the comedones, some health care providers prescribe a topical antibacterial agent. These agents prevent new lesions and treat preexisting acne. Clindamycin, erythromycin, metronidazole, azelaic acid, and the combination of benzoyl peroxide with either erythromycin (Benzamycin) or glycolic acid are options for topical antibacterial therapy. The combination of 5% benzoyl peroxide and 3% erythromycin is especially beneficial. Tretinoin improves the penetration of other topical agents, and combination therapy with tretinoin and an antibacterial is helpful.

Some health care providers turn to systemic antibiotic therapy when moderate to severe acne does not respond to topical treatments. Oral antibiotics are considered safe to use to treat acne. These antibiotics include tetracycline, erythromycin, minocycline, doxycycline, clindamycin, and trimethoprim-sulfamethoxazole.

Girls and women with mild to moderate acne sometimes respond well to topical treatment and the addition of an oral contraceptive pill. These pills reduce the endogenous androgen production, which may result in a decrease in acne.

Isotretinoin, or 13-*cis*-retinoic acid (Accutane), is a very potent and effective oral agent that is reserved for severe cystic acne that has not responded to other treatments. Isotretinoin is the only agent available that affects factors involved in the development of acne. However, it is essential for a dermatologist to manage any course of treatment with isotretinoin. Adolescents with multiple, active, deep dermal or subcutaneous cystic and nodular acne lesions receive treatment for 20 weeks. Multiple side effects are possible, including dry skin and mucous membranes, nasal irritation, dry eyes, decreased night vision, photosensitivity, arthralgia, headaches, mood changes, aggressive or violent behaviors, depression, and suicidal ideation. Adolescents who take this drug must be monitored for depression, depressive symptoms, and suicidal ideation. It is important to give this drug *only* at the recommended dosage for no longer than the recommended duration. The most significant side effects of this drug are teratogenic (cause developmental abnormalities in the fetus). Isotretinoin is *absolutely contraindicated* in pregnant women. Sexually active young women must use an effective contraceptive method during treatment and for 1 month after treatment. Patients receiving isotretinoin also must be monitored for elevated cholesterol and triglyceride levels. Significant elevation sometimes necessitates discontinuation of the medication.

Nursing interventions and patient teaching. An affected adolescent must be informed that benzoyl peroxide and retinoic acid are incompatible together, and thus the prescriber directs the adolescent to use them on alternate days or to use one in the morning and the other at night. The adolescent also must be informed of the side effects of topical medications, especially the erythematous skin that sometimes results from compliance with the regimen prescribed by the dermatologist. Assess the psychosocial effect of acne on the adolescent's self-image. Depression, anxiety, and low self-esteem sometimes occur during the adolescent task of developing identity. Adolescents with acne need a great deal of emotional support in dealing with feelings of self-consciousness and frustration, especially during periods of exacerbations. Teenagers should avoid oil-based cosmetics. Emphasize meticulous skin care, including removal of cosmetics at night. Involving the adolescent in developing the plan of care is sometimes the key to ensuring successful compliance with the treatment measures.

Although the disease is self-limited and not life-threatening, it is highly significant to adolescents, and it is a mistake to underestimate the effect it sometimes has on young people. See the patient problem box for patient problem statements with nursing interventions for a child with a disorder of integumentary function.

Prognosis. Acne resolves spontaneously over time, depending on the individual. Severe acne may result in scarring of the skin.

Psoriasis. Psoriasis is a chronic, proliferative skin disorder characterized by thick, scaly patches and inflammation. Psoriasis usually is not seen in children younger than 6 years of age. The disorder has characteristic remissions and exacerbations. Affected people are otherwise healthy. Humidifiers sometimes help in winter.

Traumatic Injuries

Animal, insect, and human bites in children account for a considerable number of visits to clinics and health care providers' offices. Most bites from dogs or cats are from pets belonging to the family or neighbors. Dog bites involve lacerations or tissue avulsion injuries, whereas cats inflict more puncture-like wounds. Animal bites most often occur on the child's face, scalp, and upper extremities because children tend to keep their heads close to the animal during play. Human bites occur in young children during rough or aggressive play or when they become frustrated; bites are also possible as the result of child abuse. The most common traumatic injuries in children and their manifestations, management, and nursing interventions are outlined in Table 32.4.

Infectious Disorders of the Skin

Bacterial infections. Impetigo, folliculitis, and cellulitis are common bacterial infections in childhood. The assessment of systemic signs and symptoms, areas involved, and appearance of lesions is helpful in establishing the type of infection. Table 32.5 lists the etiology, the clinical manifestations, the management, and the nursing interventions for these infections.

The prognosis for children with bacterial infections of the skin is favorable with proper treatment.

Herpes simplex virus type 1. Herpes simplex virus type 1 (HSV-1) is a common infection. HSV-1 is transmitted by direct contact of infected body fluids with nonintact skin or mucous membranes. The children most susceptible to HSV are immunosuppressed children (those receiving steroid therapy or chemotherapy, with leukemia, or who are HIV positive), children with burns, and infants with diaper rash or eczema.

The prognosis for children with viral infections of the skin is usually good; however, the infection is sometimes fatal in children with depressed immunity. Healing occurs without scarring unless secondary infection develops.

Tinea capitis, tinea corporis, tinea cruris, and tinea pedis (ringworm). Tinea infections are common fungal infections of the skin in children. The infections are classified according to the area of the body that is involved. Tinea capitis is a common infection of the scalp among school-age children. Tinea corporis occurs on the trunk and on the extremities in young children; tinea cruris ("jock itch") affects the inguinal area of pubescent boys; and tinea pedis ("athlete's foot") occurs between the toes.

The prognosis for children with fungal infections of the skin, with treatment, is good.

Candidiasis (thrush)

Etiology and pathophysiology. The fungus *Candida albicans* causes candidiasis, or thrush. The infection is a common disorder in infants younger than 6 months and is transmitted by contaminated hands, nipples, and pacifiers. In some newborns, candidal infection results from passage through the mother's infected vagina at birth. The candidal lesion begins as a pustule on an inflammatory base. As inflammatory cells accumulate,

Table 32.4 **Traumatic Injuries**

CLINICAL MANIFESTATION	MANAGEMENT	PREVENTION
Animal Bites (Dogs, Cats)		
Lacerations, punctures, tissue avulsion	Wound care	Supervise children during play with pets. Educate children in appropriate ways to handle pets. Teach understanding of animal behavior and respect for animals. Never leave infants alone with a pet.
Human Bites		
Lacerations	Wound care	Supervise young children at play.
Insect Bites (Fleas, Mosquitoes, Flies, Gnats)		
Hypersensitive reactions; papular urticaria; firm papules	Cool compresses, topical antihistamines, pramoxine (Caladryl) lotion	Use insect repellents (should not contain >10% *N,N*-diethyl-meta-toluamide [DEET]). Remove source by treating furniture, mattresses, carpets, and pets.
Insect Stings (Hornets, Wasps, Bees)		
Nonhypersensitive: local erythema, edema, tenderness, pruritus	Carefully scrape off stinger, if present; cleanse with soap and water; use cool compresses, antipruritic agents	Avoid insect breeding or nesting areas. Wear clothes that cover the extremities and feet.
Hypersensitive: systemic reactions and anaphylaxis	Intramuscular epinephrine and immediate medical attention; epinephrine kits available for home and school to prevent anaphylactic shock and death	
Sunburn		
Mild: erythema, tenderness, mild edema	Cool compresses, moisturizers	Use topical sunscreens containing para-aminobenzoic acid (PABA) and sun protection factor (SPF) 30. Limit time spent in sun during period of maximum exposure (11 a.m. to 3 p.m.); at higher elevations, limit time on fresh snow and water, especially when sun is directly overhead.
Severe: severe erythema, pain, edema, vesicular formation	Immediate medical attention	

whitish yellow or whitish gray curdlike patches appear over the infected area. The incidence of candidiasis is higher in immunocompromised children, infants of diabetic mothers, and children with oronasal malformations (cleft lip or palate).

Clinical manifestations. The white patches of *C. albicans* frequently appear on moist tissues because the organism cannot grow on dry skin. Common areas affected include the tongue, the buccal cavity, the GI tract, and the vagina. Parents often mistake thrush for a formula coating on the tongue. In general, the condition is asymptomatic and easily treated. Severe cases sometimes result in pain, which leads to refusal to eat or drink and thus causes risk for dehydration.

Diagnostic tests. Diagnosis is based on careful documentation of history and on clinical observation of the plaques. To distinguish thrush from formula, rinse the area with water or gently wipes the area with a wet washcloth. If the white coating remains, thrush is present. Scraping lesions is contraindicated because they bleed easily.

Medical management. Nystatin suspension is the most common antifungal agent used to treat oral *C. albicans* infections. Nystatin suspension is administered after feedings and applied directly onto the lesions and to each side of the mouth before the child swallows. Other drugs useful in the treatment of thrush include amphotericin B, clotrimazole, fluconazole, and miconazole. Treating infections early often prevents more serious complications, such as candidal infections of the upper airway and the GI tract. When a child has oral candidiasis, it is important to also inspect the diaper area for signs of infection. Nystatin cream is prescribed for diaper candidiasis.

Nursing interventions and patient teaching. Instruct parents to complete the full 7-day course of nystatin suspension, even though candidal lesions may no longer be present. Prevention of reinfection includes teaching

Table 32.5 Bacterial Infections of the Skin

ETIOLOGY	CLINICAL MANIFESTATIONS	MANAGEMENT
Impetigo		
Staphylococcus aureus, group A β-hemolytic streptococci, or both	Erythematous papules that progress to vesicles with exudative and honey-colored crusting stages; involves face, buttocks, and extremities; pruritus is common	Mupirocin; topical or systemic treatment with penicillin or erythromycin *Nursing interventions:* Teaching family the measures to control spread of infection; instruction in careful hand hygiene
Folliculitis		
S. aureus	Pustule with surrounding erythema of the hair follicle of the scalp or extremities; possible progression to a furuncle (a boil from the primary folliculitis), with extension into the surrounding dermis Systemic effects: malaise, if severe	Topical antibiotics and local, warm, moist compresses; in more severe cases, sometimes incision and drainage, followed by antibiotic therapy *Nursing interventions:* Teaching family the measures to control spread of infection and hygiene measures, such as careful hand hygiene
Cellulitis		
S. aureus, group A β-hemolytic streptococci, *Haemophilus influenzae* type b	Possible anywhere on the body; area is erythematous, edematous, warm, and painful; adjacent tender lymph node enlargement; sometimes progresses to abscess formation Systemic effects: fever, malaise	Antibiotic therapy, rest, and warm, moist compresses Neonates with herpes simplex virus type 1: hospitalization Children younger than 3 years of age with facial cellulitis: usually hospitalization *Nursing interventions:* Gently cleansing area with saline; observing for complications; administering antibiotics and analgesics as prescribed; instituting wound drainage precautions if drainage develops; teaching family the measures to control spread of infection, such as careful hand hygiene

parents to sterilize bottles, nipples, pacifiers, and teething objects. Emphasize proper hand hygiene. Instruct parents to report any oral discomfort that results in poor fluid intake. Review signs of dehydration with the family. If the mother is breast-feeding, advise her to wash her nipples with soap and water before and after feedings. Some health care providers also recommend the application of nystatin cream to the mother's nipples.

Prognosis. The prognosis for children with candidiasis (thrush) is good with prescribed therapy.

Parasitic Infections

Scabies and pediculosis. Scabies is an infectious parasitic disorder caused by a mite. Scabies is most common in school-age children. The scabies mite burrows under the skin, leaving behind debris, feces, and eggs. The condition causes a linear, papular rash and intense pruritus. Transmission occurs by direct contact with an infected person, infested bed linen, or infested clothing.

Pediculosis capitis (head lice) is a scalp infection that causes intense pruritus. It is common among preschool- and school-age children. The adult louse attaches to the skin and feeds by sucking blood. On the hair shaft, the mature female louse lays her eggs (nits), which hatch in 7 to 10 days. The louse does not jump or fly and is not carried or transmitted by pets. Infestations usually occur as a result of sharing contaminated combs, brushes, hats, or clothing that comes in contact with the head. Box 32.13 outlines medical management and nursing interventions for scabies and pediculosis.

Patient teaching is as follows:

- Remove dead lice and remaining nits with a fine-tooth comb. Tweezers are necessary to remove the nits if the comb is ineffective.
- Machine wash all washable clothing, towels, and bed linens on the hot water setting of the washer and dry in a hot setting of the dryer for at least 20 minutes. Dry clean nonwashable items.
- Thoroughly vacuum carpets, car seats, pillows, stuffed animals, rugs, mattresses, and upholstered furniture.
- Seal nonwashable items in plastic bags for 14 days if they cannot be dry cleaned or vacuumed.
- Soak combs, brushes, and hair accessories in lice-killing products for 1 hour or in boiling water for 10 minutes.

The prognosis is good with treatment.

Box 32.13 Medical Management and Nursing Interventions for Parasitic Infections

- Lindane (Kwell) 1% lotion, cream, or shampoo (contraindicated for children younger than 2 years because of neurotoxicity)
- Occlusive treatments such as petroleum jelly
- Simultaneous treatment of family members
- Hydroxyzine (Atarax) or diphenhydramine (Benadryl) for pruritus
- Cleansing of contaminated clothing and linens on hot water setting of washer
- Shampooing carpets and cleaning automobile interiors
- Discarding or treating stuffed animal or fabric toys
- Education of parents:
    - Carefully inspect the head (at the nape of the neck) of a child who scratches the head more than usual for bite marks, erythema, and nits.
    - Read directions carefully before beginning therapy.
    - Be aware of psychological effects, which can be highly stressful to children.

NOTE: Examiners should wear gloves when assessing for head lice.

COMMUNICABLE DISEASES AND IMMUNIZATIONS

The development and use of vaccines have reduced significantly the incidence of many communicable diseases and the serious complications associated with them. However, health care providers occasionally encounter children with a preventable communicable disease. You may be the first person to observe signs of illness, such as a rash, that may be related to a communicable disease. It is important to be able to identify potentially infectious cases to institute measures to prevent exposure and transmission to others. In assessing a child with suspect signs and symptoms, determine whether the child has had any recent exposure to a known case and whether the child is experiencing any **prodromal** symptoms (early signs of a developing condition or disease). The immunization status of the child and a history of the illness often help rule out certain communicable diseases. The goals of nursing interventions for a child with a communicable disease are to prevent transmission of disease to other people, prevent complications, and promote supportive management. Table 32.6 describes the communicable diseases common in childhood and their medical management, specific nursing interventions, and possible complications. With accurate diagnosis, prompt treatment, and prevention of complications, the prognosis is usually good.

DISORDERS OF SENSORY ORGAN FUNCTION

Sensory impairment in young children increases the risk for serious adverse outcomes in growth and development. Prevention, early detection, and management are essential for favorable outcomes.

Hearing

Otitis media

Etiology and pathophysiology. Otitis media, an infection of the middle ear, is a common infection in children aged 6 months to 2 years and often follows an upper respiratory infection. A significant cause of otitis media is the accumulation of bacteria in the nasopharynx. In young children, the eustachian tube, which connects the nasopharynx and the middle ear, is shorter, more horizontal, and wider, allowing passage and trapping of nasopharyngeal flora in the middle ear. Feeding practices also have been implicated in the incidence of otitis media. It is possible that formula-fed babies have a higher incidence of otitis media than do breast-fed babies because of the more supine position assumed during bottle feeding. Always evaluate toddlers and young children for foreign bodies (pieces of toys, beads, pebbles, vegetables, and so on) in the ear canal, which have the potential to lead to hearing loss and local infection.

Clinical manifestations. The infant or young child with acute otitis media is likely to experience otalgia (earache), fever, rhinitis, fussiness, irritability, and decreased appetite. In an affected infant, pulling, tugging, or rubbing the affected ear or rolling the head from side to side indicates possible acute otitis media. Affected older children usually complain of ear pain. On occasion, purulent discharge is present in the ear canal, which is indicative of a ruptured tympanic membrane. When this occurs, ear pain ceases suddenly.

Diagnostic tests. Visualization of the tympanic membrane by otoscopic examination, along with clinical signs and symptoms, usually confirms the diagnosis. If drainage is in the ear canal, the material may be cultured.

Medical management. The management of acute otitis media includes administration of antibiotics for 10 days and acetaminophen for fever and discomfort. On completion of antibiotic therapy, the health care provider examines the child to determine the effectiveness of treatment and observe for complications. An accumulation of fluid that remains in the middle ear space is often an indication for surgical insertion of tympanostomy tubes to drain the fluid and relieve the pressure. In children with chronic otitis media, some health care providers opt for tympanostomy tubes to prevent hearing loss. Tympanostomy tubes remain in the ear an average of 6 months before being ejected spontaneously.

Nursing interventions and patient teaching. Children usually begin to feel better after 48 to 72 hours of antibiotic therapy. The application of heat or cold (whichever provides the greatest comfort) over the affected ear with the child lying on the affected side often also helps alleviate pain. This position also facilitates drainage of the exudate if the eardrum has ruptured or after a myringotomy. If the ear is draining, clean the external canal with sterile cotton swabs or pledgets

Table 32.6 Childhood Communicable Diseases

DISEASE	CLINICAL MANIFESTATIONS	MEDICAL MANAGEMENT	NURSING INTERVENTIONS
Rubeola (Measles)			
Etiology: Paramyxovirus *Transmission:* Direct contact from respiratory tract secretions, blood, or urine of infected person *Incubation period:* 7–12 days *Communicable period:* 4 days before to 5 days after rash appears	*Prodrome:* Fever, malaise, cough, coryza, conjunctivitis; Koplik's spots (pinpoint red spots with central white speck in buccal cavity opposite lower molars) 3–4 days before rash *Acute phase:* Rash, appearing as irregular macular erythema, beginning on face and behind ears and spreading to feet, and lasting up to 7 days; possibly vomiting, diarrhea, anorexia, lymphadenopathy *Complications:* Otitis media, pneumonia, laryngotracheitis, encephalitis	*Supportive management:* Acetaminophen, fluids, and bed rest until fever subsides; dim lights or sunglasses if patient is photophobic	Institute seizure precautions (high fever is possible: 104°F [40°C]). Cleanse patient's eyes to remove crusting and decrease rubbing. Use a cool-mist humidifier for cough. Offer small, frequent meals of bland foods. Keep patient's skin clean and dry; administer tepid baths. Restrict to quiet activities until child feels better, usually by day 6 of rash. Use airborne precautions to prevent spread of infection. Teach and encourage good hand hygiene technique. Notify health care provider of ear pain, chest pain, difficulty breathing, headaches.
Rubella (German Measles)			
Etiology: Rubivirus *Transmission:* Direct contact with nasopharyngeal secretions of infected person; indirect contact with contaminated articles (fomites); transplacental transmission *Incubation period:* 14–21 days *Communicable period:* 7 days before to 5 days after rash appears	*Prodrome:* Young children—possible lymphadenopathy; adolescents and adults—low-grade fever, headache, sore throat, anorexia, clear nasal discharge, cough, lymphadenopathy for 1–5 days *Acute phase:* Pinkish red maculopapular rash beginning on face; spreads to trunk, then extremities within 3 days *Complications:* Usually none; rare complications include arthritis, encephalitis; birth defects as virus crosses placenta (teratogenic)	*Supportive management:* Acetaminophen for fever or discomfort	Provide airborne precautions to prevent spread of infection. Teach and encourage good hand hygiene technique. Institute comfort measures as needed. Isolate child from pregnant women. Reassure parents of benign nature of illness in affected child.
Roseola Infantum (Exanthema Subitum)			
Etiology: Human herpesvirus, type 6 *Transmission:* Unknown; occurs in children aged 6–24 mo *Incubation period:* Unknown *Communicable period:* Unknown	Sudden-onset, persistent high fever, lasting up to 4 days; child appears well otherwise; fever rapidly falls to normal, followed by rose-pink macular or maculopapular rash on trunk and spreads to rest of body; rash lasts 1–2 days and is nonpruritic *Complications:* Febrile seizures	*Supportive management:* Acetaminophen for fever; seizure precautions if child is prone to febrile seizures; encourage child to drink fluids	Teach parents how to lower fever safely. Reassure parents as to benign nature of illness. If child is prone to seizures, discuss appropriate precautions. Follow standard precautions.

Continued

Table 32.6 Childhood Communicable Diseases—cont'd

DISEASE	CLINICAL MANIFESTATIONS	MEDICAL MANAGEMENT	NURSING INTERVENTIONS
Varicella (Chickenpox)			
Etiology: Varicella zoster virus (herpesvirus) *Transmission:* Direct contact with respiratory tract secretions; indirect contact with contaminated articles; airborne droplets *Incubation period:* 10–21 days (usually 13–17 days) *Communicable period:* 1 day before eruption until all lesions crusted (1 wk after onset)	*Prodrome:* Low-grade fever, malaise, anorexia for 24 h *Acute phase:* Pruritic rash on trunk, face, proximal extremities, mucous membranes for 3–5 days, beginning as macules, progressing to papules and then vesicles on erythematous base; vesicles rupture, causing oozing and crusting; all three stages present in various intensities *Complications:* In children—possibly secondary bacterial skin infections; in adults—pneumonia, encephalitis, laryngeal edema, hemorrhagic varicella, thrombocytopenia	*Supportive management:* Acetaminophen for fever; systemic or topical antipruritics or systemic antihistamines; keeping skin clean and dry; antiviral treatment consisting of acyclovir (Zovirax); varicella zoster immune globulin within 3 days of exposure in children at high risk (those who are immunocompromised or have leukemia; newborns)	Keep patient's nails short and smooth; give daily baths without soap; dress patient in lightweight, loose clothing; administer antipruritics or antihistamines as ordered; teach child to apply pressure on itch rather than scratching; place mittens on hands of young children. Use airborne and contact precautions in hospital. If patient is at home, instruct parents to isolate ill patient from siblings, children at high risk, and adults until lesions dry. Teach and encourage good hand hygiene technique. Administer acetaminophen as ordered. Encourage patient to drink fluids.
Erythema Infectiosum (Fifth Disease)			
Etiology: Human parvovirus B19 *Transmission:* Respiratory tract secretions and blood *Incubation period:* 4–14 days but up to 20 days *Communicable period:* Unknown; probably before signs and symptoms develop; communicability unlikely once rash develops	*Prodrome:* In children with aplastic crisis—fever, malaise, myalgia; rash usually absent *Acute phase:* Rash appears in three stages: • First stage: red rash on face, "slapped cheek" appearance (fades in 1–4 days), circumoral pallor • Second stage: maculopapular, lacelike rash on upper extremities spreading to trunk and thighs; lasts 1 week or longer • Third stage: possible for rash to recur periodically for weeks in response to heat, sunlight, cold *Complications:* Arthralgia, arthritis (infrequent in children but common in adults); encephalitis, myocarditis (rare); maternal infection (low risk for fetal hydrops)	*Supportive management:* Acetaminophen for fever; analgesic or anti-inflammatory drugs	For hospitalized child, use droplet precautions for 7 days after onset: no isolation is necessary at home. Teach and encourage good hand hygiene technique. Institute comfort measures as necessary.

Table 32.6 Childhood Communicable Diseases—cont'd

DISEASE	CLINICAL MANIFESTATIONS	MEDICAL MANAGEMENT	NURSING INTERVENTIONS
Scarlet Fever			
Etiology: Group A β-hemolytic streptococci *Transmission:* Direct contact with respiratory tract secretions of infected person *Incubation period:* 2–5 days (average, 3 days) *Communicable period:* During incubation and acute illness phases	*Prodrome:* Sudden-onset high fever, vomiting, headache, chills, malaise *Acute phase:* Tonsillitis, pharyngitis, white strawberry tongue (tongue has white coating and papillae become red and edematous) by day 1 or 2; by day 4, white coating sloughs, leaving red strawberry tongue; sandpaper-like red rash appears about 12 h after prodrome and is intense in skinfolds; cheeks are flushed and circumoral pallor is present; desquamation begins by end of first week and continues for 3 wk or longer *Complications:* Otitis media, pneumonia, sinusitis, glomerulonephritis, carditis, peritonsillar abscess	*Antimicrobial treatment:* Full course of penicillin or, for patients allergic to penicillin, erythromycin *Supportive management:* Bed rest, analgesics, fluids	Institute respiratory precautions until completion of first 24 h of antimicrobial treatment. Teach and encourage good hand hygiene technique. Offer soft diet if child can chew; encourage drinking fluids. Restrict to quiet activities until child feels better. Offer lozenges, gargles, and cool-mist humidifier for throat. Maintain good oral hygiene. Advise parents to consult health care provider if fever persists after therapy begins. Discuss procedures for preventing spread of infection.
Diphtheria			
Etiology: Corynebacterium diphtheriae *Transmission:* Direct contact with nose, eye, throat discharges or skin lesions of infected person; in rare cases, fomite transmission or foodborne outbreaks *Incubation period:* 2–5 days *Communicable period:* Untreated person: 2 wk to several months	Clinical manifestations vary according to diphtheritic membrane affected: • Nasal: nasal discharge—serosanguineous and mucopurulent, possible progression to epistaxis • White membrane on nasal septum • Tonsillar or pharyngeal: pharyngitis; malaise; anorexia; fever (low grade) • Membrane over tonsils, pharynx; lymphadenitis; laryngeal: cough, fever, hoarseness *Complications:* Airway obstruction, thrombocytopenia, myocarditis, vocal cord paralysis	*Antimicrobial treatment:* Penicillin or erythromycin; antitoxin, usually IV, preceded by skin testing for horse serum sensitivity; possible tracheostomy for respiratory obstruction	Institute droplet precautions. Maintain bed rest. Offer liquid or soft diet. Perform gentle suctioning, as necessary. Observe for signs of respiratory distress or obstruction: dyspnea, apprehensiveness, cyanosis; report such findings to health care provider. Keep tracheostomy set at patient's bedside. Regulate humidity for optimal liquefaction of secretions.

Continued

Table 32.6 Childhood Communicable Diseases—cont'd

DISEASE	CLINICAL MANIFESTATIONS	MEDICAL MANAGEMENT	NURSING INTERVENTIONS
Mumps (Parotitis)			
Etiology: Paramyxovirus *Transmission:* Direct contact with respiratory tract secretions of infected person *Incubation period:* 16–18 days *Communicable period:* Up to 7 days before parotid edema to 5–9 days after onset of signs and symptoms	*Prodrome:* Fever, malaise, headache *Acute phase:* Unilateral or bilateral edema and tenderness of parotid glands by day 3; chewing aggravates "earlike" pain *Complications:* Meningoencephalitis, epididymoorchitis, arthritis, sensorineural deafness, myocarditis, sterility in male patients (rare)	*Supportive management:* Acetaminophen for fever, analgesics for pain; intravenous (IV) fluids sometimes necessary for a child who refuses to eat or drink	Institute droplet precautions for 9 days after onset of edema or until edema has subsided. Teach and encourage good hand hygiene technique. Offer soft, bland diet; encourage child to drink fluids. Use warm or cool compresses for edema. Dress boy in tightly fitting underpants or scrotal support for orchitis.
Pertussis (Whooping Cough)			
Etiology: Bordetella pertussis *Transmission:* Direct contact or droplet spread of respiratory tract secretions of infected person *Incubation period:* 7–20 days *Communicable period:* From prodromal stage through fourth week	*Prodrome:* Upper respiratory tract infection signs and symptoms for 1–2 wk; cough, sneezing, little or no fever, headache, anorexia *Acute phase:* Paroxysmal stage—dry, hacking cough followed by prolonged inspiration ("whoop" sound) most often at night; paroxysms usually followed by vomiting of thick, stringy mucus; lasts 4–6 weeks *Convalescent stage:* Decrease in coughing and whooping; lasts 1–2 wk *Complications:* Pneumonia, hypoxia, atelectasis, otitis media, seizures, dehydration, weight loss, prolapsed rectum, hernia, hemorrhage (epistaxis, subconjunctival), cerebral edema, and central nervous system (CNS) disturbances	*Antimicrobial treatment:* Erythromycin or trimethoprim-sulfamethoxazole (Bactrim, Septra) for 7–10 days *Antiseizure treatment:* For patients experiencing seizures; phenytoin; supportive management—hospitalization required for infants or children with underlying pulmonary or cardiac disease, dehydration, or severe signs and symptoms; gentle suctioning to prevent choking, high humidified oxygen therapy; IV fluids; intubation set at patient's bedside for emergency	Institute droplet precautions. Enforce strict hand hygiene. Maintain bed rest if child is febrile; offer quiet activities. Offer liquids: small amounts frequently; if child vomits, refeed. Monitor cardiac and respiratory status. Observe for signs of airway obstruction (dyspnea, restlessness, cyanosis) and report such findings to the health care provider. Provide high humidity and gentle, frequent suctioning to prevent choking. Reassure parents during paroxysms. Teach parents in the use of a cool-mist humidifier to avoid triggers of paroxysms (dust, smoke, chilling, sudden change in temperature, excitement). Teach parents how to recognize signs of respiratory distress, and arrange for a public health nurse to visit after discharge from hospital.

soaked in hydrogen peroxide. If ear wicks or lightly rolled sterile gauze packs are placed in the ear after surgical treatment, ensure that they are loose enough to allow accumulated drainage to flow out of the ear; otherwise the infection may migrate to the mastoid process. The wicks must be kept dry during shampoos or baths.

Emphasize the importance of taking the medication for the fully prescribed course to ensure eradication of the infection. To educate parents in the prevention of otitis media, teach them to hold their infant in an upright position when feeding. If the child has tympanostomy tubes, teach parents postoperative care. They must protect the ear during bathing, shampooing, and swimming, because bacteria from the water can be introduced into the ear.

Prognosis. The most common complication of otitis media is mild to moderate hearing loss as a result of chronic or recurrent effusion. The episodic (temporary) hearing loss that sometimes occurs during occasional bouts of otitis media is usually reversible; however, conductive hearing loss associated with chronic otitis media is in some cases permanent and has potential to interfere with language and cognitive development.

Vision

Refractive errors (myopia and hyperopia). Refractive errors occur when light rays entering the lens are bent and fall in front of or behind the retina, which prevents the image from falling on a single point on the retina as it normally does. Two of the most common refractive errors in childhood are myopia (nearsightedness) and hyperopia (farsightedness), which result in loss of visual acuity. Screening tests that measure visual acuity assist in identifying refractive errors. Treatment consists of corrective lenses and periodic reevaluation. The nurse plays a vital role in ensuring vision screening, especially in the preschool years.

Strabismus. In strabismus, a lack of coordination in the extraocular musculature results in a cross-eyed appearance. Strabismus is caused by muscle imbalance, results from paralysis, or in some cases is congenitally acquired. The condition affects sometimes one and sometimes both eyes and causes the brain to receive two images (instead of one). Common clinical manifestations include squinting, closing one eye, tilting the head (to block out one image), and difficulty focusing or picking up objects. Medical management varies according to the cause of the strabismus. There is no treatment that will align the eyes perfectly. The goal is to align them as close to normal as possible. The injection of botulinum toxin (Botox) into the extraocular muscle has been effective in relaxing the muscles in strabismic patients. Often the stronger eye is patched in an attempt to strengthen the muscles of the weakened eye. Surgical intervention may be required if other measures are not effective. Nursing intervention includes adequate explanation of the treatment plan, care of corrective lenses, instruction in eye exercises, and reinforcement of occlusive patches if they become loose.

Left untreated, strabismus increases the risk for **amblyopia** (lazy eye; reduction or dimness of vision, especially in which there is no apparent pathologic condition of the eye), in which visual acuity is lost. This complication can be prevented if the underlying problem is corrected before the child is 6 years of age.

Periorbital cellulitis

Etiology and pathophysiology. Periorbital cellulitis is a serious inflammation of the eyelid and periorbital area. The condition is usually unilateral and has the potential to affect the eye and the CNS. Conjunctivitis, impetigo, insect bites, and trauma are all possible causes of periorbital cellulitis. Common causative organisms include *H. influenzae, S. aureus,* and group A β-hemolytic streptococci.

Clinical manifestations. Children with periorbital cellulitis usually experience pain, tenderness, fever, erythema (of distinctive magenta color), and edema of the eyelids and periorbital area. Headache and purulent nasal discharge are also sometimes present.

Diagnostic tests. Cultures of the eye, the nose, and the blood help identify the causative agent. Ultrasonography and CT of the orbit are sometimes useful for ruling out abscess.

Medical management. Because of the emergency nature of the illness, the child is hospitalized for aggressive IV antibiotic administration. Analgesics and antipyretics commonly are administered for pain and fever. Warm compresses also help relieve discomfort.

Nursing interventions and patient teaching. As the edema decreases, the skin around the eye becomes dry and begins to peel. Preserving skin integrity involves the application of a thin layer of petrolatum to the area.

Reassure parents that eye discoloration sometimes persists for several days and that most children recover completely without complication.

Prognosis. The edema usually subsides within 36 hours of antibiotic therapy. With appropriate treatment, the prognosis is usually excellent.

Nasal Cavity

Allergic rhinitis

Etiology and pathophysiology. Allergic rhinitis occurs in about 40% of the pediatric population (Asthma and Allergy Foundation of America, n.d.). Allergic rhinitis is either seasonal or perennial, and affected children have a familial predisposition to allergy. Exposure to an inhaled allergen triggers the allergic response.

Clinical manifestations. The signs and symptoms common in the pediatric population include congestion, sniffling, mouth breathing, itchy nose, and postnasal drip. Often there is a line in the skin that is visible across the nose as a result of nasal rubbing ("allergic salute"). The medical management and nursing interventions for children with allergic rhinitis are the same as those for affected adults.

MENTAL AND COGNITIVE DISORDERS

DISORDERS OF COGNITIVE FUNCTION

A child's mental health is an integral part of the total well-being of the child. A variety of factors influence the personality and the developmental capabilities of a child, including genetic composition, environment, social support, and culture. It is appropriate to assess children for emotional as well as physical problems during all visits with a health care provider. Children in whom a cognitive impairment has been diagnosed require prompt intervention by specialists in the field of mental health, as do their families. The nurse is instrumental in providing appropriate referrals and offering emotional support to the child and the family (see the Health Promotion box).

Health Promotion

Encouraging Healthy Behaviors for Children With a Mental or Cognitive Disorder

DOWN SYNDROME

- Provide information to parents about expected delays in milestones.
- Encourage stimulating play.
- Provide nutritionally dense foods.
- Encourage physical activity and exercise.
- Praise child for accomplishments.
- Provide consistency in matters relating to discipline.
- Ensure patients have been evaluated for atlantoaxial instability before rigorous physical activity.

ATTENTION DEFICIT/HYPERACTIVITY DISORDER (ADHD)

- Provide a routine for daily activities.
- Maintain a nonstressful environment, but set limits and provide rewards.
- Encourage parents to seek training in behavioral therapy to learn effective ways of dealing with their child.
- Allow child time to explain events or interactions to aid in reducing stress.
- Encourage parents to continue therapeutic regimen and to monitor for medication side effects if medications are prescribed.

DEPRESSION

- Establish a trusting family relationship.
- Review treatment plan with parents as needed.
- To discourage social isolation, provide positive reinforcement when child participates in group activities.
- Identify support groups within the community for the child and for the parents.

SUICIDE

- Alert parents to signs that include depression, social isolation, social withdrawal, changes in grades, giving away important possessions, preoccupation with death, and changes in eating and sleeping habits.
- Encourage parents and child to stay in contact with school, peers, and relatives for emotional support at this time.

Cognitive Impairment

Cognitive impairment (formerly called *mental retardation*) is the most common developmental disability. It refers to significantly subaverage general intellectual functioning that exists concurrently with deficits in adaptive behavior and is manifested during the developmental period. Cognitive impairment is classified in four general categories, each corresponding to a range of the **intelligence quotient (IQ)** (an index of relative intelligence determined through the subject's answers to arbitrarily chosen questions): (1) *mild* (educable cognitive impaired), reflected by an IQ of 50 or 55 to approximately 70; (2) *moderate* (trainable cognitive impaired), reflected by an IQ of 35 or 40 to 50 or 55; (3) *severe*, reflected by an IQ of 20 or 25 to 35 or 40; and (4) *profound*, reflected by an IQ below 25.

Etiology and pathophysiology. The causes of cognitive impairment are varied and include biochemical, infectious, genetic, endocrine, and idiopathic factors. Specific causes include chromosomal abnormalities, such as Down syndrome; perinatal infections, such as cytomegalovirus, rubella, syphilis, and toxoplasmosis; perinatal anoxia; maternal drug or alcohol abuse; metabolic disorders, such as phenylketonuria; lead poisoning; hypothyroidism; and prematurity.

Clinical manifestations. Manifestations vary according to the child's age and degree of impairment. Affected children typically fail to achieve developmental milestones at appropriate ages. In general, they tend to manifest delays in motor, social, cognitive, or language skills, or some combination of these.

Diagnostic tests. In a child suspected of having cognitive impairment, it is important to begin assessment as soon as the parents or the health care provider realizes that the child is not developing normally. Diagnostic studies include neurologic examination, CT, serum metabolic screening, developmental screening tests (e.g., DENVER II), standardized intellectual tests (e.g., Stanford-Binet Intelligence Scale; Wechsler Intelligence Scale for Children, Revised), and chromosomal analysis and genetic screening.

Nursing interventions. Nursing interventions for a child with a cognitive impairment focus on promoting optimal development and providing the family with emotional support, education, and referrals. The family needs support at the time of initial diagnosis, as well as encouragement to verbalize their fears and concerns. Encourage parents to enroll the child in an early intervention program that will facilitate the child's self-care abilities and assist the family with future needs. When teaching, break up each task into small, specific steps because the child cannot always understand the task as a whole. The parents are encouraged to keep their focus on the normal needs of all children—including love, social interaction, and play—regardless of children's cognitive ability (see the Safety Alert box).

Patient and family teaching. Provide parents with information about normal developmental milestones, stimulation techniques, safety, normal speech development, sexual development, and the role of positive self-esteem in motivating children to accomplish goals within their limitations.

Prognosis. Cognitive impairment is a chronic condition. The philosophy of care toward people with cognitive impairment has undergone major changes since the 1960s. Children with cognitive impairment are no longer automatically admitted into institutional settings; many remain at home.

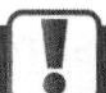

Safety Alert

Children With a Mental or Cognitive Disorder

DOWN SYNDROME

- It is not uncommon for children with Down syndrome to have the disorder atlantoaxial instability. Approximately 15% of Down syndrome children have the disorder but are asymptomatic, leading to the increased change for injury (Leas, 2017). This disorder is characterized by excessive movement at the junction between cervical vertebra 1 (C1) and cervical vertebra 2 (C2). Injury to the spinal cord can result, especially with physical activity. It is essential to ensure that parents are educated about this disorder and that children have been evaluated for atlantoaxial instability. Symptoms of the disorder include neck pain, weakness, and torticollis (abnormal, asymmetric head or neck position). Affected children are at risk for spinal cord compression, which places the child at risk of losing established motor skills and bladder or bowel control.
- Report immediately to a health care provider any child with the following signs of spinal cord compression:
  - Persistent neck pain
  - Loss of established motor skills and bladder or bowel control
  - Changes in sensation
- Monitor the child's airway clearance.
- Measures to decrease respiratory infections include clearing the child's nose with a bulb type of syringe, rinsing the mouth with water after feedings, increasing fluid intake, and using a cool-mist vaporizer to keep the mucous membranes moist and the secretions liquefied. Other helpful measures include changing the child's position frequently, performing postural drainage with percussion if necessary, practicing good hand hygiene, and properly disposing of soiled articles such as tissues.
- Monitor for adequate nutritional and fluid intake. The protruding tongue also interferes with feeding, especially of solid foods. Parents need to know that the tongue thrust is not an indication of refusal to feed but a physiologic response. Advise parents to use a small but long straight-handled spoon to push the food toward the back and side of the mouth. If the child thrusts the food out, the parent feeds it in again. Decreased muscle tone affects gastric motility, which predisposes the child to constipation. Dietary measures such as increased fiber and fluid intake promote evacuation. It is important to supervise dietary intake. It is sometimes necessary to scrutinize the child's eating habits to prevent obesity.

ATTENTION DEFICIT/HYPERACTIVITY DISORDER (ADHD)

- Keep in mind that children with ADHD often are distracted easily by extraneous stimuli and may have difficulty following directions.
- Also keep in mind that such children may have difficulty sequencing, storing, or retrieving data.
- Use pictures, demonstrations, or written lists for teaching and learning.

DEPRESSION

- Assess for diminished affect, fatigue with reduced motor activity, solitary play or lack of interest in play, tearfulness or crying, dependency and clinging behavior, and aggressive and disruptive behavior.
- Identification of the depressed child with suicidal tendencies and making appropriate referrals are important nursing functions.

SUICIDE

- Hospitalization is sometimes necessary for the child's self-protection.
- Provide constant monitoring to prevent self-injury.

Down syndrome. Varying degrees of cognitive impairment and multiple defects characterize **Down syndrome**, a congenital chromosomal abnormality. It is the most common chromosomal abnormality, affecting 1 per 800 live births (CDC, 2018b).

Etiology and pathophysiology. The incidence of Down syndrome in the United States is 1 per 800 live births. Although the risk of having a child with Down syndrome increases with maternal age, the majority of all infants with Down syndrome are born to mothers younger than 35 years old, because the majority of all babies are born to mothers in this younger age group (CDC, 2018b).

Clinical manifestations. Children with Down syndrome have a characteristic facial appearance (Fig. 32.31). Most frequently, manifestations in the infant include a small, rounded skull with a flat occiput; upward-slanting eyes with epicanthal folds; broad, flat nose; protruding tongue; short, thick neck; hypotonic extremities; mottled

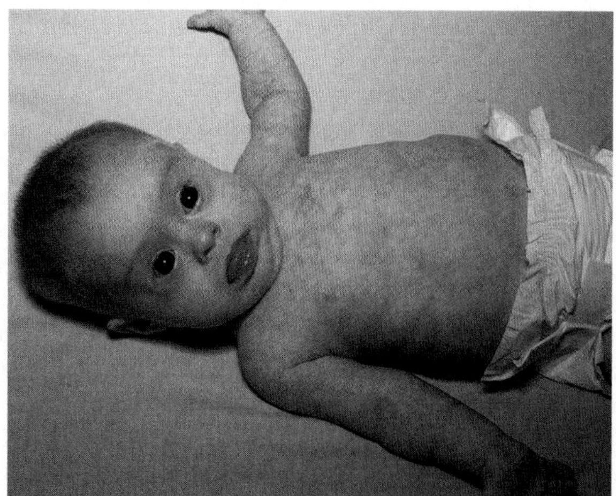

Fig. 32.31 Down syndrome in infant. Note small, square head; upward slant to the eyes; flat nasal bridge; protruding tongue; mottled skin; and hypotonia. (From Hockenberry MJ, Wilson D: *Wong's essentials of pediatric nursing*, ed 9, St. Louis, 2013, Mosby.)

skin; low-set ears; and a simian crease on the palmar side of the hand. All children with Down syndrome have some degree of intellectual impairment, ranging from low normal intelligence to severe cognitive impairment. Individual abilities vary greatly, but in general, children with Down syndrome typically display the following:

- Strengths in visual processing over auditory
- Weaknesses in grammar and language
- Delays in motor development

Children with Down syndrome are prone to upper respiratory infections and frequent otitis media, and many such children have congenital heart defects, which are the chief cause of death, particularly during the first year of life. Other associated health problems include increased incidence of leukemia, dysfunction of the immune system, and thyroid dysfunction, especially congenital hypothyroidism.

Diagnostic tests. As an adjunct to the characteristic manifestations indicating the diagnosis of Down syndrome, a chromosomal analysis helps confirm the chromosomal abnormality. Individuals with Down syndrome have a higher incidence of cardiac disorders. Cardiovascular system testing, including electrocardiography and radiographic studies, may be performed to assess function and potential abnormalities.

Medical management. In addition to routine medical care, corrective surgery is indicated in some cases for congenital heart defects. Auditory and vision screening are standard in assessing for any sensory impairments. Treatment of otitis media is necessary to prevent auditory loss, which can hamper cognitive function. Most experts also recommend thyroid function tests. If growth is delayed, it is important to carefully monitor and document nutrition, height, and weight. In an attempt to increase height, health care providers give growth hormones in some cases.

Nursing interventions. Care for children with Down syndrome is similar to that discussed earlier for children with a cognitive impairment. Primary nursing goals include emotionally supporting the family at the time of diagnosis and referring the child and family to agencies that provide support and services.

Patient and family teaching. The family needs education regarding their child's condition. Information regarding services available to children with Down syndrome should be conveyed to family members. The goal of treatment is to help the child reach their highest potential. Services available include speech, occupational, and physical therapy. In the United States virtually every state has early intervention programs for these children, so treatment can be initiated promptly.

Prognosis. The life expectancy for people with Down syndrome has improved over recent decades. Many people with Down syndrome live to the age of 50 and beyond (MCWL, 2018). Down syndrome is associated with earlier aging. As the prognosis continues to improve for these individuals, it is important to provide for their long-term health care and for their social and leisure needs.

Autism. **Autism** is a developmental disorder of brain functioning. Autism affects normal development of intelligence and behavior and results in impairments in social interactions and communications and in repetitive behaviors. *Autism spectrum disorder* refers to a broad group of developmental disabilities that vary in severity. Autism occurs include 1 in 68 children, with 1 in 42 boys and 1 in 189 girls. Autism typically is diagnosed between the ages of 2 and 3 years of age but can be diagnosed as early as 18 months of age in some cases (Autism Speaks, 2018).

Etiology and pathophysiology. The cause of autism remains unknown. The condition results in brain development that affects how a person perceives and socializes with others. Children and adults with autism spectrum disorder experience problems in social interaction and communication. Depending on the severity, functioning in society is often difficult.

There are several different genetic abnormalities that have been found to lead to autism spectrum disorder. Some genes are thought to affect brain development or the way that brain cells communicate. Other genetic disorders resulting in autism are related to fragile X syndrome, whereas some are related to inherited factors. Some research indicates that environmental factors also may play a role in the development of the disorder (Mayo Clinic, 2018d).

Thimerosal, a mercury-based preservative that previously was used in most childhood vaccines, was rumored to be a cause of autism. Thimerosal is no longer used in vaccinations (with the exception of some influenza vaccines). Multiple research studies have failed to demonstrate any relationship between vaccinations and autism (Mayo Clinic, 2018d).

Clinical manifestations and diagnostic tests. Children with autism may demonstrate alterations in social interactions, communication, and behavior. One hallmark characteristic is the inability to maintain eye contact with another person. Parents of autistic children have noted difficulties that their infants had at a very early age with eye contact and avoidance of body contact. Children with autism also display limited functional play and sometimes interact with toys in an unusual manner.

Children with autism may display stereotypical motor activities such as rhythmic rocking of their bodies, flapping of their hands, or spinning in circles. These are referred to as *self-stimulation behaviors.* One or all the body senses may be employed in the behaviors. Some autistic children have significant GI symptoms; constipation is a common one. Social development is affected; an autistic child may be unable to understand other people's feelings. Not all children with autism have the same manifestations. Some have mild forms that necessitate minimal supervision, and some have severe forms in which self-abusive behavior is common. The majority of children with autism have some degree of cognitive disability, with scores typically in the moderate to severe range. Very low intelligence scores are more common among affected girls than among affected boys. Despite their relatively moderate to severe disability, some children with autism excel in particular areas, such as art, music, memory, mathematics, or perceptual skills, such as puzzle building.

Speech and language delays are also common in autistic children. The American Academy of Pediatrics recommends that all children be screened for developmental delays at well-child visits at the ages of 9 months, 18 months, and 24 months. It is further recommended that all children be screened for autism at 18 and 24 months of age (CDC, 2015). Early recognition, referral, and intervention are important for improving outcomes for children with autism.

Nursing interventions. Therapeutic intervention for a child with autism is a specialized area involving professionals with advanced training. Although there is no cure for autism, numerous therapies can be attempted. The most promising results have been achieved through highly structured and intensive behavior modification programs. In general, the objective in these programs is to promote positive reinforcement, increase social awareness of other people, teach verbal communication skills, and decrease unacceptable behavior. Providing a structured routine for the child to follow is key in managing autism.

When these children are in the hospital, the parents must be included in planning care and ideally stay with the child as much as possible. Recognize that not all children with autism have the same problems and that each one requires individual assessment and treatment. Decreasing stimulation by using a private room, avoiding extraneous auditory and visual distractions, and encouraging the parents to bring in possessions that the child is attached to usually help lessen the disruptiveness of hospitalization. Because physical contact often upsets these children, minimal holding and eye contact are sometimes necessary to prevent behavioral outbursts. Take care when performing procedures on, administering medicine to, or feeding these children, because many are fussy eaters who at times willfully starve themselves or gag to avoid eating, and many are indiscriminate gorgers, swallowing any available edible or inedible items, such as a thermometer. Eating habits of autistic children tend to be particularly problematic for families and often involve food refusal, mouthing objects, eating inedible items, and smelling and throwing food.

Children with autism need to be introduced slowly to new situations. Visits with staff caregivers should be kept short whenever possible. Because these children have difficulty organizing their behavior and redirecting their energy, they need to be told directly what to do. Communication should be at the child's developmental level, brief, and concrete.

Prognosis. Autism encompasses a broad spectrum of behaviors and levels of severity. Some children with autism ultimately achieve independence, but others may require lifelong adult supervision. Aggravation of psychiatric symptoms occurs in about half of these children during adolescence; affected girls have a tendency for continued deterioration. The earlier the diagnosis and treatment are, the better is the chance for a more positive outcome. Family involvement is needed to promote the best possible outcome. Additional information may be found at the Autism Speaks website (*www.autismspeaks.org*).

SCHOOL AVOIDANCE (SCHOOL PHOBIA, SCHOOL REFUSAL)

School avoidance occurs when a physically healthy child repeatedly stays home from school or is sent home from school for physical symptoms of an emotional origin. School avoidance is the most common cause of vague physical symptoms in school-age children. It affects approximately 5% of elementary school–age children and 2% of middle school students. It is possible that the incidence of school avoidance is decreasing as more mothers are in the workplace. This trend requires young children to master the conflict of separation at an earlier age.

Etiology and pathophysiology. For some children, school avoidance is related to anxiety. Often they are worried about academic progress, peer conflicts, or marital discord in the home. Separation anxiety is also common among these children even after the normal age when this issue is mastered (3 to 4 years). These children tend to have an overprotective parent. Other children may not be anxious at all but receive secondary gains from their avoidance at school. These children stretch out an illness until they get extremely behind in their studies. Some parents of these children are too lenient, some place little value on education, and others are unconcerned about the ramifications of missing school.

Clinical manifestations. Children who are anxious tend to have physiologic symptoms of anxiety, including headache, recurrent abdominal pain, vomiting, diarrhea, insomnia, pallor, palpitations, and hyperventilation. The child who receives secondary gains typically exaggerates or fabricates symptoms such as sore throat, leg pain, coughing tics, chest pain, and fatigue. Upon physical examination and laboratory testing, no organic cause is found. The child usually sounds very sick but appears to be well. Symptoms usually appear in the morning and decrease once the child is told he or she is not going to school.

Diagnostic tests. Diagnostic tests are usually not indicated. Specific complaints help determine which laboratory tests, if any, may be indicated.

Medical management and nursing interventions. Once the health care provider establishes the diagnosis, the nurse's primary role is to assist in convincing parents that their child is physically healthy, explain the diagnosis of school avoidance to them, and assist in returning the child to regular school attendance. Parents need to be educated that school avoidance occurs in "normal" children and that it is stress related and not a psychiatric disorder. Once parents are convinced that their child is healthy, it is necessary that the child immediately return to school. Parents are told to be firm in the morning if the child is refusing to go to school. It is important to bring any somatic complaints to the attention of the primary care provider and, if the condition is minor or without an organic cause, to then send the child to school. Reassure the child that nothing is physically wrong with him or her and that he or she is in good health. Together with the parents explain to the child that attendance at school is not negotiable. They provide emotional support and reassurance to the child who is anxious about peer or academic issues.

LEARNING DISABILITIES

It is estimated that learning disabilities affect approximately 13%, or 6.6 million, of all school-age children in the United States (National Center for Education Statistics, 2018). Learning disabilities impair a child's ability to understand, assimilate, recall, or produce information. Children with learning disabilities usually score significantly poorly on tests of academic achievement in mathematics, reading, writing, or some combination. The factors that underlie learning problems typically exist before school entry but often do not become apparent until academic demands are placed on the child.

Etiology and pathophysiology. The cause of learning disabilities is multifactorial, and a specific cause often cannot be identified. Some affected children have a family history of learning disabilities. Learning problems are sometimes the result of various physiologic or environmental factors, or both, such as intrauterine exposure to alcohol, drugs, or infection; birth trauma; seizures; attention-deficit disorders; head trauma; malnutrition; and exposure to toxic substances, such as lead. Hearing or vision impairments sometimes lead to learning problems, and it is important to include the necessary screening procedures in the diagnostic assessment before the diagnosis is established. Genetic syndromes such as fragile X syndrome or Prader-Willi syndrome sometimes occur in association with learning disabilities.

Clinical manifestations. Children with learning disabilities sometimes manifest problems with speech, behavior, or motor coordination or a combination of these; failure to master basic, grade-appropriate academic skills in one or more subject areas; and a progressive decline in school performance. Other possible manifestations include delayed acquisition of language milestones, deficient social skills, avoidance behavior in response to challenging tasks, low frustration tolerance, disorganization, and somnolence.

Diagnostic tests. A thorough history and physical examination sometimes reveal specific indications to measure the lead level and perform electroencephalography, chromosomal studies, and hearing and vision screenings. General intelligence and achievement testing and neuropsychological testing help to identify cognitive strengths and weaknesses and in developing a comprehensive educational plan.

Medical management and nursing interventions. Learning disabilities are managed primarily through appropriate educational referrals. Parents need to be educated about the special education process. Federal law requires that all schools provide a comprehensive evaluation on written request from the parents to the school principal. Therapeutic manipulation of the educational setting may include special arrangements within a regular classroom, alternative classroom placement, tutoring, and remediation assistance. Reevaluation for special education is required at least every 3 years, more frequently in certain situations, depending on age, severity of disability, and academic progression. An important referral source for parents of a child with a learning disability is the National Center for Learning Disabilities (*www.ncld.org*).

Prognosis. With early identification, appropriate referrals, and proper educational interventions, the negative consequences of difficulty in school can be avoided, and children with a learning disability are usually able to function optimally within their limitations.

ATTENTION DEFICIT/HYPERACTIVITY DISORDER

Attention deficit/hyperactivity disorder (ADHD) is a group of behaviors—hyperactivity, inattentiveness, and impulsivity—that appear early in a child's life, persist throughout childhood and adolescence, and sometimes extend into adulthood. ADHD is being diagnosed at an increasing rate in America. Some studies indicate that 5% of children have ADHD, whereas other studies estimate the number of children affected to be 11%. ADHD is more prevalent in boys than girls (CDC, 2013).

Etiology and pathophysiology. The exact cause of ADHD is unknown. The disorder does appear to have a genetic basis. Several studies have revealed a genetic link within families. Studies of twins help support the familial link. Certain environmental factors have also been linked to the disorder, such as maternal cigarette smoking and alcohol use during pregnancy. Children who are exposed to high levels of lead at young ages have a higher risk of developing ADHD. Premature delivery and low birth weight are additional causes linked to ADHD (CDC, 2013).

Clinical manifestations. Children with ADHD sometimes exhibit decreased attention span, impulsivity, failure to follow instructions, hyperactivity, poor self-regulation, noncompliance, aggression, fidgeting, immaturity during play, failure to follow rules of play in games, lack of turn-taking during play, and easy distraction by extraneous stimuli. Associated problems include poor school performance; learning disabilities; antisocial behaviors such as lying, cheating, and stealing;

excessive anxiety; sleep disturbances; poor peer relationships; limited fine motor skills; and additional psychiatric diagnoses.

Diagnostic tests. No single test is available for ADHD, and the diagnosis requires a thorough evaluation of the child over an extended period of time. Information should be obtained from the child's parents, pediatrician, teachers, as well as specialists. Vision, hearing, and other medical testing should be performed to rule out a medical cause for the child's behavior.

Medical management. Behavioral counseling, educational intervention, and pharmacotherapy are essential components in the treatment of ADHD. Interventions aim at achieving optimal academic, emotional, social, and vocational outcomes and preserving good self-esteem. Behavior therapy is encouraged as the first line of treatment, especially with younger children.

Nursing interventions. A critical role for the nurse is parent counseling. It is most important to allay any inappropriate feelings of guilt or responsibility that the parents may have. Educate the parents about discipline, teach them how to set limits that are appropriate and provide rewards, and encourage them to establish a strict daily routine. The parents need information about the dangers of controversial therapies (e.g., megavitamin and herbal therapies). Stress the importance of accident prevention and safety. Explain the need for increased supervision and yet foster additional responsibilities and independence. Assist in the development of the educational plan as appropriate. If the child is taking medication, explain the reasons and minimal risks of such therapy to the child's teacher and school officials as needed. Parents also need to be informed of the importance of routine follow-up of children on medication. Children should be checked for medication side effects every 6 months, and the ongoing need for medication therapy should be assessed every year or more often.

Prognosis. With intervention, ADHD can be managed successfully throughout childhood and adolescence. Symptoms may persist into adulthood. Eating healthy diets, proper exercise, and adequate sleep help in managing the disorder.

OTHER DISORDERS

Anorexia nervosa and bulimia nervosa. Anorexia and bulimia are eating disorders with significant underlying psychological and emotional issues. Although these disorders affect primarily adolescents, younger children are sometimes affected. For a thorough discussion of anorexia and bulimia, refer to Chapter 35.

Substance abuse. Substance abuse is commonly a problem of adolescence; however, it sometimes occurs in elementary school–age children. In children, substance abuse usually points to significant problems for the child, the family, or both, and professional counseling is warranted. In adolescents, the incentives are usually experimental and recreational. Drug, alcohol, and tobacco use by the adolescent tends to be symbolic of maturity or serve purposes of peer group acceptance, stress reduction, or rebellion (see Chapter 30).

Depression. Depression is defined generally as a mood disturbance with overall feelings of sadness, despair, worthlessness, or hopelessness. The prevalence of depression among young children in the United States is approximately 2%, while the prevalence for teens is approximately 8% (Anxiety and Depression Association of America, n.d.). The rate of depression is higher in girls than in boys.

Etiology and pathophysiology. The causes of major depression have not been established. Possible risk factors are genetic or environmental. Many studies have shown that children of a parent suffering from a major affective disorder have a rate of depression three to six times higher than that in the general population. Cognitive theories attribute the development of depression to feelings of hopelessness and helplessness secondary to an actual or perceived loss. Psychosocial theories point to factors such as disturbance in family dynamics or in the parent-child relationship, a family move, the death of a loved one, divorce, or abuse or maltreatment.

Clinical manifestations. Depressive symptoms vary with age and developmental level of the child. In infancy, separation from the primary caretaker may lead to protest (crying, panic) followed by apathy, blank staring, and sad facial expressions. School-age children with depression often demonstrate sad facial expressions, irritability, crying easily, accident proneness, social withdrawal, and eating and sleeping disturbances. Some are also likely to manifest anxiety symptoms, physical aggression, and academic underachievement. Depressed adolescents typically show signs of impulsiveness, **somatization disorders** (characterized by recurrent, multiple physical complaints and symptoms with no organic cause), eating disorders, drug or alcohol use, antisocial behavior, withdrawal, fatigue, and suicidal ideation.

Diagnostic tests. Structured questionnaires or interviews (e.g., Children's Depression Inventory, Children's Depression Scale, Depression Self-Rating Scale) are useful for diagnosing depression in children and adolescents. No definitive biologic tests are specific for depression.

Medical management. Antidepressant medication, along with psychological therapies, is the mainstay of treatment of major depression. Tricyclic antidepressants or selective serotonin reuptake inhibitors such as fluoxetine (Prozac), trazodone, sertraline (Zoloft), bupropion (Wellbutrin), venlafaxine (Effexor XL), and paroxetine (Paxil) are helpful in alleviating symptoms. Parents must be aware of suicidal tendencies during the first and second weeks of therapy. In 2004 the US Food and Drug Administration ordered pharmaceutical companies to add a "black box" warning on all antidepressants to alert health care providers of an increased risk of suicidal thoughts or ideation in pediatric patients.

Psychological therapies include play therapy; art therapy; and various talk therapies, including family therapy.

Nursing interventions. Once the mental health care provider and the primary health care provider establish the treatment plan, establish a trusting relationship with the child. In addition, provide emotional support to the child's family, using open and honest communication. Stress the importance of meeting with therapists on a regular basis when warranted.

Patient and family teaching. Review the treatment plan with the family and ensure that the child and the family understand the importance of following the prescribed regimen.

Prognosis. For the child and family motivated to develop better social supports and relationship skills, the prognosis is often good. Depressive episodes may recur.

Patient problems and interventions for the patient with depression include but are not limited to the following:

Patient Problem	Nursing Interventions
Social Seclusion, related to feelings of hopelessness	Encourage a therapeutic, trusting relationship Provide supportive reassurance as needed Provide positive reinforcement when child participates in group activities or interacts with others
Insufficient Knowledge (of child, family, or both), related to lack of information about depression and its treatment	Assess child and family's understanding of depression and its treatment Instruct child, family, and significant others about depression and its treatment Identify support groups within their community

Suicide. *Suicide* is defined as the deliberate act of self-injury with the intent that the injury result in death. Suicide is the third leading cause of death among 5- to 14-year-olds in the United States (National Library of Medicine, n.d.). Few prepubertal children actually kill themselves, although many of them are knowledgeable about suicide. Although girls make more suicide attempts than do boys, boys more often complete the act of suicide. Girls tend to use more passive methods, such as medication ingestion or carbon monoxide poisoning, whereas boys traditionally use more violent methods, such as hanging, firearms, or wrist slashing. Drug overdose is the most common method of attempted suicide.

Etiology and pathophysiology. Suicide is not a result of a single factor; rather, suicide is the culmination of multiple factors. These include depression (which is a common preceding factor), loss of a loved one or relationship, and social isolation. The most important individual factor is the presence of an active psychiatric disorder (e.g., depression, bipolar disorder, psychosis, substance abuse, or conduct disorder). Comorbidity of an affective disorder and substance abuse also increase the risk of suicide. In addition, not having attained a sense of identity, a major task of adolescence, leads to self-doubt and low self-esteem.

Clinical manifestations. Many completed suicides are the result of previous attempts. Warning signs of impending suicide include depression, preoccupation with death, perceived or actual social isolation, withdrawal, poor school performance, drug or alcohol abuse (or both), appetite and sleep disorders, and loneliness. Symptoms are usually present for at least 1 month before the attempted or completed suicide.

Diagnostic tests. Diagnostic tests for depression (see earlier section "Depression") are useful when early recognition of depressive symptoms is part of a comprehensive effort to prevent suicidal ideation and attempts.

Medical management. Responsibility for a suicidal patient should be shared among as many people as possible. It indicates that other people care. Individual, family, and group therapy are all helpful for adolescents. Although ordinary health care providers may be able to manage an acute depressive reaction without difficulty, the child or adolescent who has made a serious attempt or has a specific plan for suicide must receive immediate attention and competent psychiatric care.

Nursing interventions. Mental health assessments of children and adolescents are a necessary part of every health visit. Children and adolescents are often surprisingly open in communicating their feelings with a trusted nurse in a confidential setting. If there are any concerns, ask directly whether the patient has thoughts of death or suicide, when the thoughts occurred, how long these thoughts lasted, and whether the patient has a plan. Any threat of suicide must be taken very seriously, particularly if the child has a plan, along with immediate evaluation by a mental health care provider. Help the child develop positive coping strategies in stressful situations (e.g., deep-breathing exercises, meditation, school or peer counseling) (Nursing Care Plan 32.2).

Prognosis. Prognoses vary. The children at greatest risk are those who verbalize suicidal thoughts and those who attempt suicide. It is possible for appropriate mental health care to help these children to alleviate depression and develop a more positive self-image.

Psychogenic abdominal pain (recurrent abdominal pain). Recurrent abdominal pain (RAP) is usually multifactorial, organic, dysfunctional, or **psychogenic** (originating from the mind). Psychogenic RAP is most common in school-age and adolescent children and is a diagnosis

Nursing Care Plan 32.2 A Child Who Attempts Suicide

S. is a 12-year-old girl who arrives at the hospital after taking 12 of her grandmother's anti-dysrhythmia pills in an attempt to end her life. She has been despondent since her mother died of breast cancer 6 months ago. Her school performance has been declining, and she has become increasingly isolated. She is admitted to the pediatric intensive care unit and then transferred to the adolescent psychiatric unit.

PATIENT PROBLEM

Potential for Injury, related to poisoning and cardiac dysfunction

Patient Goals and Expected Outcomes	Nursing Interventions	Evaluation
Patient will exhibit improved cardiac function	Maintain open airway and air exchange. Maintain cardiac function. Monitor patient for effects of the medications. Treat any dysrhythmias.	Telemetry reveals normal sinus rhythm; no dysrhythmias noted.

PATIENT PROBLEM

Impaired Coping, related to depression

Patient Goals and Expected Outcomes	Nursing Interventions	Evaluation
Patient will develop and use healthy coping skills	Develop a therapeutic relationship. Encourage patient to verbalize feelings and concerns. Maintain a safe environment: • Remove potentially harmful objects. • Provide direct observation monitoring as needed. • Use physical restraints as needed to prevent self-injurious behaviors. Report any changes in affect or behavior to the health care provider. Reassure child and family of the plan to protect child from suicidal attempts.	Patient is beginning to verbalize great sadness and emptiness over mother's death.

PATIENT PROBLEM

Impaired Self-Esteem due to Current Situation, related to feelings of worthlessness

Patient Goals and Expected Outcomes	Nursing Interventions	Evaluation
Patient will express feelings of positive self-worth	Encourage expression of feelings. Approach interactions with patient in a nonjudgmental manner. Provide positive feedback for all successes and reassurance after failures. Reinforce child's and family's strengths.	Patient is making a list of her positive strengths.

PATIENT PROBLEM

Insufficient Knowledge (of Child, Family, or Both), related to no previous experience with suicide

Patient Goals and Expected Outcomes	Nursing Interventions	Evaluation
Patient and family will verbalize understanding of signs of potential risk of suicide	Assess current level of understanding. Make appropriate referrals as needed to psychiatrist or psychologist; social worker; peer support group; hotlines. Provide information about early warning signs of ineffective coping that potentially lead to suicidal attempt or gesture: insomnia, change in weight, excessive fatigue, isolating behaviors, thoughts of death, giving away belongings, lack of interest in future, decreased social network. Encourage importance of follow-up; schedule appointments and provide phone numbers.	Patient verbalizes willingness to attend follow-up counseling sessions.

CRITICAL THINKING QUESTIONS

1. Upon entering S.'s room, the nurse notices that she is crying. She states, "I can't live without my mother; I want to be with her." What is an appropriate initial response?
2. S.'s father is concerned about taking her home after discharge. What are two therapeutic nursing interventions for patient and family teaching?
3. S. begins to express interest in others and in activities in her hospital unit. What nursing interventions would be appropriate to encourage her?

that warrants consideration in children with episodes of abdominal pain that recur monthly for at least 3 consecutive months once other causes have been ruled out.

Etiology and pathophysiology. Psychogenic RAP often is related to emotional factors in the child or family members, or both, such as poor self-esteem, anxiety, depression, school phobia, maternal depression, marital problems and divorce, or health problems in other family members. Organic causes—such as infections of the urinary tract, the GI tract, and the reproductive tract—should be assumed until proven otherwise.

Clinical manifestations. Children with RAP are usually afebrile and sometimes have occasional vomiting and constipation. The abdominal pain is usually nonspecific, or the child complains of episodic periumbilical or epigastric pain that is unrelated to eating, defecation, or exercise.

Diagnostic tests. For a child with RAP, it is necessary to rule out organic causes. Tests include a CBC, measurement of sedimentation rate, urinalysis and culture, serum albumin and amylase measurements, stool assessment for occult blood, and culture for bacteria and parasites. In the adolescent girl, a pregnancy test also should be considered.

Medical management. Once the health care provider has ruled out organic causes, it is necessary to identify and address stressors in the child's life. Consultation with a mental health care provider is often helpful. Children with psychogenic RAP sometimes must be seen as often as once every 2 or 4 weeks for pain evaluation and reassurance.

Nursing interventions. Once the family has been advised that there is no organic cause for the abdominal pain, encourage parents to maintain a normal schedule for their child with regard to school, play, and exercise. Overprotective parents need a great deal of emotional support in helping them deemphasize their child's complaints. Also give the family instructions to call if the child's symptoms worsen.

Prognosis. Once the stressors have been addressed, the prognosis is very good.

Get Ready for the NCLEX® Examination!

Key Points

- Common skin disorders of infancy and childhood include diaper dermatitis, atopic dermatitis, and seborrheic dermatitis.
- For children with many of the musculoskeletal disorders seen in infancy, treatment initiated immediately on diagnosis often results in a better prognosis.
- Cleft lip and palate, the most common facial malformations, usually involve nutritional, dental, and speech alterations and necessitate a multidisciplinary approach to treatment.
- Congenital heart defects are classified as either acyanotic or cyanotic.
- Nursing interventions in the care of a child with heart failure are to assist in improving cardiac function, decreasing cardiac demands, reducing respiratory distress, maintaining nutritional status, promoting fluid loss, and providing emotional support to the family.
- The most common form of neoplasm in childhood is acute lymphoblastic leukemia.
- Nursing interventions for a child with hemophilia involve preventing bleeding by decreasing the risk of injury, recognizing and managing bleeding with coagulation factor replacement, preventing the crippling effects of joint degeneration, and preparing and emotionally supporting the child and the family for home care.
- For a child with iron-deficiency anemia, it is best to give oral iron preparations between meals with citrus fruits or juices to enhance absorption.
- Croup is a group of signs and symptoms of varied origin. Characteristic manifestations are obstruction or edema in the region of the larynx, which produces inspiratory stridor, hoarseness, and a cough described as "barking."
- When first infected with *M. tuberculosis*, most children do not exhibit any clinical signs or symptoms; therefore routine skin screening is an important measure in diagnosis.
- Characteristic signs of hypertrophic pyloric stenosis are projectile vomiting, malnutrition, dehydration, and a palpable mass in the epigastrium.
- Diabetes mellitus is a syndrome whose primary characteristic is a deficiency of insulin, resulting in alterations in protein, carbohydrate, and fat metabolism.
- Hearing, vision, and speech deficits in infants and children can be recognized early through periodic screenings and assessments.
- Although meningitis has many causes, bacterial meningitis is the most common.
- Environmental exposure through inhalation or ingestion continues to be the most important contributing factor in lead poisoning.
- Acquired immunodeficiency syndrome is associated with certain drug therapies, radiation, splenectomy, and viral infections.
- Cognitive impairment (formerly called *mental retardation*) is significantly below-average general intellectual functioning that exists concurrently with deficits in adaptive behavior and manifested during the developmental period.
- The majority of cases of Down syndrome are attributable to an extra chromosome on the twenty-first pair, hence the term *trisomy 21*.
- Autism is a complex developmental disorder of brain function that occurs in the presence of a broad range and severity of intellectual and behavioral deficits.
- Learning disabilities are sometimes the result of various physiologic or environmental factors such as intrauterine exposure to alcohol, drugs, or infection;

birth trauma; seizures; attention deficit disorders; head trauma; malnutrition; and exposure to toxic substances, such as lead.

- Medications, especially CNS stimulants such as methylphenidate (Ritalin), are highly effective in improving the behaviors of children with ADHD. Positive results include increased attention span, normalization of activity level, and reduced impulsiveness.
- Suicide is the third leading cause of death among children aged 10 to 19 years in the United States.
- Psychogenic recurrent abdominal pain (RAP) often is related to emotional factors in the child or family member, such as poor self-esteem, anxiety, depression, school phobia, maternal depression, marital problems and divorce, or health problems in other family members.

Additional Learning Resources

SG Go to your Study Guide for additional learning activities to help you master this chapter content.

evolve Be sure to visit the Evolve site at *http://evolve.elsevier.com/Cooper/foundationsadult/* for additional online resources.

Review Questions for the NCLEX® Examination

1. The nurse is caring for a patient with nephrotic syndrome. What assessment finding does the nurse expect to find?
   1. Gross hematuria, albuminuria, temperature of 101°F (38.3°C) to 103°F (39.4°C)
   2. Elevated blood pressure, weight loss, hematuria
   3. Albuminuria, edema, puffiness of face
   4. Edema, albuminuria, hypotension

2. The student nurse is preparing a community presentation on urinary tract infections. What should the student include as risk factors? *(Select all that apply.)*
   1. A short urethra in young girls
   2. Frequent emptying of the bladder
   3. Increased fluid intake
   4. Ingestion of highly acidic juices
   5. Cleaning the perineal area from back to front

3. The nurse is answering questions from a parent whose child has acute glomerulonephritis. Which explanation of the disease is most accurate?
   1. It is a syndrome in which there is reabsorption of bicarbonate or in which excretion of hydrogen ions is impaired.
   2. It occurs after an antecedent streptococcal infection.
   3. It is a disorder manifested by gross bacteria.
   4. It is a disorder associated with a defect in the ability to concentrate urine.

4. A pediatric patient has received a diagnosis of Wilms tumor. Which statement regarding Wilms tumor is true?
   1. The tumor manifests as a firm, nontender, intraabdominal mass.
   2. The tumor is sometimes difficult to distinguish from the spleen.
   3. The tumor usually crosses the midline.
   4. If the surgeon successfully removes the tumor without a tear in its capsule, no chemotherapy is needed.

5. The LPN/LVN is assisting in preparing a care plan for a patient who has received a diagnosis of a seizure disorder. What is an important nursing intervention that should be included in caring for a child who is experiencing a seizure?
   1. Describe and record the seizure activity observed.
   2. Restrain the child when seizures occur to prevent bodily harm.
   3. Place a tongue blade between the teeth if they become clenched.
   4. Suction the child during a seizure to prevent aspiration.

6. In an assessment of a newborn, what findings are suggestive of hydrocephalus?
   1. Bulging fontanelle, dilated scalp veins
   2. Depressed fontanelle, decreased blood pressure
   3. Constant low-pitched cry, restlessness
   4. Closed fontanelle, high-pitched cry

7. A newborn was admitted to the nursery with a complete bilateral cleft lip and palate. The health care provider explained the plan of therapy and its expected good results; however, the mother refuses to see or hold her baby. What is the most therapeutic initial approach to the mother?
   1. Restate what the health care provider has told her about plastic surgery.
   2. Encourage her to express her feelings.
   3. Emphasize the normal characteristics of her baby and the baby's need for mothering.
   4. Keep the baby and mother apart until the lip has been repaired.

8. How is Hirschsprung's disease best described?
   1. Absence of parasympathetic ganglion cells in a segment of the colon
   2. Passage of excessive amounts of meconium by the newborn
   3. Results in excessive peristaltic movements within the GI tract
   4. Results in frequent evacuation of solids, liquids, and gas

9. The nurse is caring for a 4-month-old patient with severe infantile diarrhea. What condition is this patient most likely to experience as a result?
   1. Metabolic acidosis
   2. Metabolic alkalosis
   3. Respiratory acidosis
   4. Respiratory alkalosis

10. A 6-month-old patient is suspected of having cystic fibrosis. What diagnostic tests does the nurse expect to be ordered for this patient? *(Select all that apply.)*
    1. Bronchoscopy, with pulmonary washings
    2. Chest x-ray study
    3. Upper GI series
    4. Sweat test
    5. Pulmonary function tests
11. A 5-year-old patient is admitted to the pediatric unit in sickle cell crisis. Which nursing intervention will be included in the plan of care? *(Select all that apply.)*
    1. Strenuous exercise of the extremities to increase oxygen to the area
    2. Administration of IV fluids to improve circulation and hydration
    3. Administration of analgesics as ordered
    4. Administration of oxygen as ordered
    5. Applying ice packs to the affected areas
12. The nurse is caring for a child with nephrotic syndrome. The nurse is correct in questioning the health care provider's order of which class of medications? *(Select all that apply.)*
    1. Antibiotics
    2. Diuretics
    3. Vitamins
    4. Corticosteroids
    5. Antifungals
13. When interviewing parents of an infant with hypertrophic pyloric stenosis, the nurse expects the parents to report which symptom?
    1. Diarrhea
    2. Projectile vomiting
    3. Poor appetite
    4. Constipation
14. When caring for a patient who is 2½ years old and has Wilms tumor, what assessment is most likely to reveal clinical manifestations of the disease?
    1. Auscultation of lung sounds
    2. Palpation of the abdomen
    3. Assessment of skin turgor
    4. Palpation of femoral and dorsalis pedis pulses
15. The nurse is educating a new mother about infectious diseases. The mother demonstrates understanding of teaching by identifying which disorders as being contagious? *(Select all that apply.)*
    1. Impetigo
    2. *S. aureus* infection
    3. Infantile eczema (atopic dermatitis)
    4. Pediculosis
    5. Cystic fibrosis
16. In a discussion about an 11-month-old patient's diet, which statement by her mother indicates a possible cause for iron-deficiency anemia?
    1. "Formula is so expensive. We switched to regular milk early on."
    2. "She almost never drinks water."
    3. "She doesn't really like peaches or pears, so we stick to bananas for fruit."
    4. "I give her a piece of bread now and then. She likes to chew on it."
17. When caring for a 9-month-old patient who underwent surgery to repair a cleft palate, what is the priority intervention?
    1. Referral to a parent support group
    2. Maintaining adequate nutrition
    3. Keeping an IV line open
    4. Keeping the patient sedated
18. Which statement made by a 12-year-old patient with type 1 diabetes indicates a need for more teaching?
    1. "My pancreas is sick and needs insulin until it gets better."
    2. "I will need to take my insulin every day."
    3. "I need to keep a piece of candy in my pocket in case I start to feel shaky."
    4. "My mom has to give me insulin shots twice a day."
19. The nurse is discussing possible causes of a 4-year-old child's cognitive impairment with his mother. Which causes would the nurse be correct in including in the discussion?
    1. Metabolic disorders, perinatal anoxia, hyperthyroidism
    2. Perinatal infection, metabolic disorders, and postmaturity
    3. Lead poisoning, prematurity, perinatal anoxia
    4. Iron supplementation, toxoplasmosis, maternal drug use
20. A 2-month-old infant receives a diagnosis of Down syndrome. Which clinical manifestation supports this diagnosis?
    1. Pointed nose
    2. Small, rounded skull with flat occiput; simian crease
    3. Small tongue
    4. Downward-slanting eyes
21. When a child is beginning antidepressant medications, it is important for parents to be alert for signs of ______________ ______________ for the first 2 weeks of treatment.
22. The parents of a 12-year-old patient are concerned about the child's recent diagnosis of school avoidance. Which response by the nurse would be the most appropriate?
    1. Emphasize that the child is sick and needs to stay home from school.
    2. Discuss the importance of the child's returning to school.
    3. Ignore any somatic complaints the child may have.
    4. Instruct them that this is a psychiatric disorder.
23. A 14-year-old patient has a positive test result for human immunodeficiency virus (HIV) and expresses a desire to kill herself. What would be the most appropriate initial response of the nurse?
    1. Tell her that they are very close to discovering a cure for HIV.
    2. Encourage her to talk to her pastor.
    3. Arrange a visit with another adolescent who is HIV positive.
    4. Immediately report the threat to a mental health care provider.

24. A 7-year-old patient has a diagnosis of recurrent abdominal pain (RAP). What nursing interventions would be most appropriate to include in the plan of care? *(Select all that apply.)*
   1. Encourage the parents to maintain a normal schedule for their child with regard to school.
   2. Support the parents in deemphasizing their child's complaints.
   3. Educate the parents to contact the health care provider if symptoms worsen.
   4. Help the parents choose appropriate exercise for the child.
   5. Discourage the parent from allowing the child to play with other children until symptoms subside.

25. A 3-year-old patient has received a diagnosis of a cognitive impairment. Which intervention is most important in dealing with the patient and her family?
   1. Encourage the family to enroll the child in an early intervention program.
   2. Discourage play with "normal" children to prevent feelings of inadequacy.
   3. Instruct the family not to discuss their feelings in front of the child.
   4. Educate the family that they should treat the child in a special manner because she is "slow."

26. The mother of a child with Down syndrome expresses concerns about her child's physical health. Which response by the nurse would be the most appropriate?
   1. "Children with Down syndrome are prone to upper respiratory infections."
   2. "Congenital heart defects are uncommon in children with Down syndrome."
   3. "Your child will probably need to be institutionalized before the age of 18."
   4. "Most children with Down syndrome develop leukemia."

27. The health care provider has diagnosed depression in a 16-year-old patient. Which statement by the parents indicates that they have a proper understanding of the diagnosis?
   1. "My child will need to be placed in an inpatient mental health facility."
   2. "My child will have to take antidepressive medications for life."
   3. "The recovery process for my child is likely to be a slow, lengthy process."
   4. "Depression is nothing to worry about in a child of this age."

28. The nurse is assessing a newly admitted patient. What clinical manifestations would probably indicate that the child has autism? *(Select all that apply.)*
   1. Avoidance of body contact with other people
   2. Speech and language delays
   3. Deficits in social development
   4. Good eye contact with the nurse during the assessment
   5. Increased sensitivity to stimuli

33 Health Promotion and Care of the Older Adult

http://evolve.elsevier.com/Cooper/foundationsadult/

Objectives

1. Discuss health and wellness in the aging population of the United States in relation to the aims of *Healthy People 2020.*
2. Identify some of the common myths concerning the older adult.
3. Describe biologic and psychosocial theories of aging.
4. Discuss common psychosocial events that occur with the older adult.
5. Describe changes associated with aging for each of the body systems.
6. List methods of assessment used for each body system.
7. Identify patient problems appropriate to common health concerns of the older adult.
8. Describe appropriate nursing interventions for common health concerns of the older adult.
9. Discuss changes that occur with aging in intelligence, learning, and memory.
10. Discuss leading safety and security issues faced by older adults.
11. Identify ways to preserve dignity and to increase self-esteem of the older adult.
12. Discuss how finances and housing are major concerns for the older adult.
13. Compare how older adults differ from younger individuals in their response to illness, medications, and hospitalization.

Key Terms

ageism (Ā-jĭzm, p. 1063)
akinesia (ă-kĭ-NĒ-zhă, p. 1089)
aphasia (ă-FĀ-zhă, p. 1090)
ataxia (ă-TĂK-sē-ă, p. 1090)
Baby Boomers (p. 1062)
chronologic age (p. 1060)
claudication (klăw-dĭ-KĀ-shŭn, p. 1075)
dementia (dĕ-MĔN-shă, p. 1088)
dysarthria (dĭs-ĂHR-thrē-ă, p. 1090)
dysphagia (dĭs-FĀ-jă, p. 1071)
hemiplegia (hĕm-ĭ-PLĒ-jă, p. 1090)
kyphosis (kĭ-FŌ-sĭs, p. 1076)
nocturia (nŏk-TŪ-rē-ă, p. 1073)
orthostatic hypotension (ŏr-thō-STĂT-ĭk hī-pō-TĔN-shŭn, p. 1075)
presbycusis (prĕz-bē-KYŪ-sĭs, p. 1085)
presbyopia (prĕz-bē-Ō-pē-ă, p. 1084)
pruritus (prū-RĪ-tŭs, p. 1067)
respite care (p. 1065)
sandwich generation (p. 1065)
senility (p. 1087)
shearing forces (p. 1067)

HEALTH AND WELLNESS IN THE AGING ADULT

OLDER ADULTHOOD DEFINED

Older adulthood begins at about age 65 and continues until death, a possible span of 40 years or more. Older adulthood has been divided into four subgroups:

- Young-old: 65–74 years
- Middle-old: 75–84 years
- Old-old: 85–99 years
- Elite-old: 100 years and older

Other terms that may be used to refer to the aging population include *frail elderly,* which refers to those individuals older than 75 years of age with health concerns. *Centenarians* are those who are older than 100 years of age (Ignatavicius and Workman, 2016).

Although older adulthood is tied to **chronologic age** (age of an individual expressed as time elapsed since birth), chronologic age may not be an accurate predictor of health or behavior. Some individuals may be considered "old" in their 50s because of their appearance, behaviors, or health status. Today more people are living longer, active lives. Most consider maintaining activities and participating in healthy living behaviors as deflectors of typical aging perils (Fig. 33.1).

DEMOGRAPHICS

In the United States in 2015, 47.9 million people were 65 years of age and older, more than 14.9% of the population (US Census Bureau, 2014a).

In the past two decades, the population of older adults (ages 65 and older) has grown twice as quickly as the

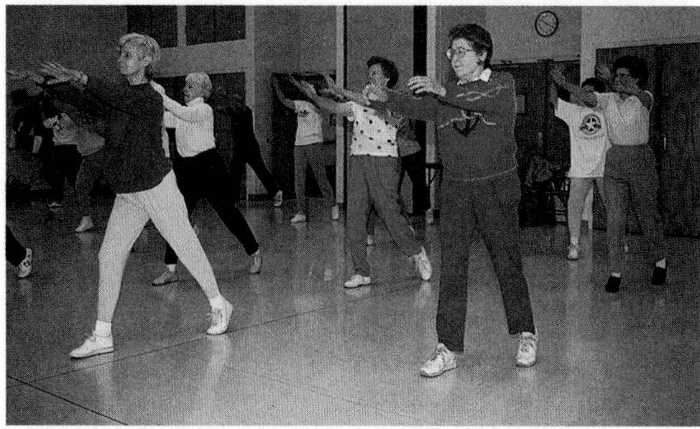

Fig. 33.1 Exercise and activity contribute to a healthier lifestyle for older adults. (From Sorrentino SA: *Mosby's textbook for nursing assistants*, ed 8, St. Louis, 2011, Mosby.)

rest of the population, and this increase is expected to continue. The US Census Bureau (2014b) estimates that by the year 2050 there will be 83.7 million people over the age of 65 living in the United States—more than double the number today, making them about 23.55% of the population. Approximately 54% of these will be women and 46% men. Estimates are that in 2060, most older adults will still be non-Hispanic white (56%). Hispanic older adults will make up 21.2% of the population. Non-Hispanic African Americans will make up 12.5%, with other races making up the final 10.3% (US Census Bureau, 2012). In 2015 the life expectancy in the United States was 79.3 years. This placed the United States at a ranking of 30th overall in the world (World Health Rankings, 2015). In the past 50 years, life expectancy for Americans has increased by almost 10 years.

Health care for older people has become more complex for several reasons:

- Scientific advances in treating life-threatening conditions of the past
- Substantially increased life expectancy
- Greater focus on ethical and legal issues related to life, disease, research, and dying

Older adults are a diverse group in terms of age, life experiences, the aging process, health habits, attitudes, and response to illnesses. To best meet the challenge of delivering age-appropriate care, know the differences between normal aging versus illness or disease-related changes and be able to assess effectively older adults with delirium, dementia, and depression. To promote the patient's return to health and increase the speed of recovery, be familiar with rehabilitation care services. Older adults often are concerned about losses of function, and they need their care providers to provide respectful care that allows them to maintain their dignity.

WELLNESS, HEALTH PROMOTION, AND DISEASE PREVENTION

Wellness is more than just the absence of disease. *Wellness* is the individual operating at the optimal level of function, and even during chronic illness and dying, some level of well-being is attainable. Wellness involves a balance among the individual's emotional, spiritual, social, cultural, and physical states. Box 33.1 lists the traits of a healthy person. The role of the nurse is to assist individuals to adapt to their life situation to achieve this balance.

Box 33.1 Traits of a Healthy Person

Self-responsibility: Is attuned to body messages and knowledgeable about health status and feels empowered to make healthy choices.

Nutritional awareness: Learns about healthy eating habits that reduce the risk for heart disease, high blood pressure, diabetes, osteoporosis, and cancer and that assist in achieving and maintaining a healthy body weight.

Physical fitness: Engages in regular physical activity, including aerobics, and activities that improve balance, muscle flexibility, and muscle strength.

Stress management: Identifies ways of coping with the stresses of life to be able to work productively and connect with others in the community.

Environmental sensitivity: Designs personal space to include a healthy physical and social environment with opportunities for time with friends, supportive network, giving and receiving affection, and reinforcing wellness behaviors.

From the US Department of Health and Human Services (US DHHS): National prevention strategy, 2012. Retrieved from *www.healthcare.gov/prevention/nphpphc/strategy/report.html*.

Health promotion takes a positive approach to health and emphasizes the strengths, resources, and abilities of an individual. Primary prevention stresses exercise to prevent cardiovascular disease, falls, and depression. Older people who quit smoking can reduce their risk of heart disease and improve lung function and circulation. A well-balanced diet without excessive sugar, fat, or alcohol is another important aspect of primary prevention. Primary prevention also includes recommended vaccinations. Immunizations recommended for older adults include an annual influenza vaccine, a tetanus/diphtheria (Td) booster every 10 years, a zoster (shingles) vaccine for those over the age of 60, and the pneumococcal vaccines (PCV13 and PPSV23) after 65 (Centers for Disease Control, 2018). Secondary prevention in older adults focuses on early detection and treatment of disease, including screening for heart disease and hypertension, cancer, infectious disease, polypharmacy (misuse of multiple medications), nutrition, oral health, osteoporosis, falls, and social isolation (Table 33.1).

HEALTHY AGING

Healthy People 2020 set forth the goals of the US Department of Health and Human Services (US DHHS) to prevent health risks, unnecessary disease, disability, and death. These recommendations are in the process of being updated in *Healthy People 2030* (USDHHS, 2018a). A summary of the current 2020 goals as they relate to older adults appears in Box 33.2. The focus of

Table 33.1 **Suggested Screening for Preventive Health for People 50 Years Old and Older**

EXAMINATION OR TEST	GROUP	FREQUENCY
Complete physical, including cholesterol	Men and women	Every 1–3 yr to age 75, then annually
Blood pressure	Men and women	Every 2 years for blood pressure measurements <120/80 mm Hg; every year if systolic blood pressure measurements of 120 to 139 mm Hg or diastolic blood pressure measurements of 80 to 89 mm Hg; otherwise as directed by the health care provider
Pelvic examination, Papanicolaou (Pap) test, and breast examination	Women	Every 3–5 yr
Mammogram	Women	Yearly for women ages 50 to 54; every 2 years for women 55 and older
Breast self-examination	Women	Monthly
Prostate examination	Men	Patients with average risk should begin discussing possible screening tests at age 50
Testicular self-examination	Men	Monthly
Stool for occult blood	Men and women	Yearly
Eye examination	Men and women	As recommended by the health care provider
Glaucoma test	Men and women	As recommended by the health care provider
Dental examination and cleaning	Men and women	Every 6 mo for those with own teeth; every 2 yr for denture wearers
Hearing test	Men and women	As recommended by the health care provider

Data from Johns Hopkins Medicine, *https://www.hopkinsmedicine.org/healthlibrary/prevention/women_age,50_64*; and Cancer Screening Guidelines by Age, *https://www.cancer.org/healthy/find-cancer-early/cancer-screening-guidelines/screening-recommendations-by-age.html.*

these goals is on improving functional independence and the quality of life.

A growing number of adults are living into their 90s and beyond. A significant number of this population maintain their health and remain active up until the time of their death. The age of 65 is no longer considered old. This reality changes the circumstances of life planning, social services, employment, and social policy and the focus of health care. Keeping this population healthy, active, and moving necessitates a high standard of assessment and health promotion.

Born between 1946 and 1964, more than 70 million people are **Baby Boomers**. They make up approximately 29% of the nation's population. The older Baby Boomers are entering and approaching young-old adulthood. More than 1.5 million of them will live to 100 years of age. This group is extremely diverse and better educated, more mobile, and more aware of how to achieve and maintain good health than any previous generation. They recognize the importance of nutrition, exercise, and a healthy environment. Many are concerned about the future in terms of available health care.

As more people take charge of their own health, many have found limitations in conventional medical approaches and have begun using alternative health strategies such as meditation, visualization, massage, magnets, aromas, and acupressure or acupuncture (see Chapter 20). Some of these therapies are effective; some are not. A method effective for one individual may not be for another. The patient must be cautioned to investigate the qualifications of the provider thoroughly, research the method under consideration, and use only one therapy at a time to allow sufficient time to identify reactions.

A holistic definition of health does not limit health to its physical and mental aspects but rather views health as a state of being, an attitude. It seems only natural to encourage people to make decisions that affect their own lives, but health care providers frequently fail to do so. Given sufficient information, most individuals make appropriate decisions.

Knowing the value others assign to us and being treated with respect build and sustain self-esteem (Fig. 33.2). Addressing an older individual as "Gramps" or "Grandma," "Honey," or any other similar term of familiarity is inappropriate unless the person is the caregiver's grandparent. Older adults should be called by name or by what they choose to be called; this indicates respect. Use of the person's first name is also inappropriate unless the person so specifies. Forcing changes that exceed the individual's ability to cope sometimes results in mental deterioration, physical illness, and even death. The role of the nurse includes affirmation, enhancement, and support of each person's movement through the aging process and encouragement of health and wellness.

MYTHS AND REALITIES

Some of the myths and stereotypes of aging and older adults are presented in Box 33.3. Most myths are generalizations that focus on the negative aspects of

Box 33.2 *Healthy People 2020*

GOAL FOR OLDER ADULTS

Improve the health, function, and quality of life.

The *Healthy People 2020* objectives for older adults are designed to promote healthy outcomes for this population. Many factors affect the health, function, and quality of life of older adults. Specifically the focus is on:

- Individual behaviors that promote health, such as participation in physical activity, self-management of chronic diseases, or use of preventive health services, and can improve health outcomes;
- Social environmental factors that promote health, such as housing and transportation services that affect the ability of older adults to access care; and
- Health and social services available to older adults and their caregivers to assist them in managing chronic conditions and long-term care needs effectively.

EXAMPLES OF OBJECTIVES FOR OLDER ADULTS, AND THEIR TARGETS AND BASELINE DATA

Prevention

OA–2.1: Increase the proportion of males age 65 and older who are up to date on a core set of clinical preventive services. Target: 50.9%. Baseline: 46.3% of males aged 65 years and older were up to date on a core set of clinical preventive services in 2008. Target setting method: 10% improvement.

OA–2.2: Increase the proportion of females age 65 years and older who are up to date on a core set of clinical preventive services. Target: 52.7%. Baseline: 47.9% of females aged 65 years and older were up to date on a core set of clinical preventive services in 2008. Target setting method: 10% improvement.

OA–3: (Developmental) Increase the proportion of older adults with one or more chronic health conditions who report confidence in managing their conditions.

OA–5: Reduce the proportion of older adults who have moderate to severe functional limitations. Target: 25.5%. Baseline: 28.3% of older adults had moderate to severe functional limitations. Target setting method: 10% improvement.

OA–6: Increase the proportion of older adults with reduced physical or cognitive function who engage in light, moderate, or vigorous leisure-time physical activities. Target: 37.1%. Baseline: 33.7% of older adults with reduced physical or cognitive function engaged in light, moderate, or vigorous leisure-time physical activities in 2008. Target setting method: 10% improvement.

OA–7.3: Increase the proportion of registered nurses with geriatric certification. Target: 1.5%. Baseline: 1.4% of registered nurses had geriatric certification in 2004. Target setting method: 10% improvement.

Long-Term Services and Supports

OA–10: Reduce the rate of pressure ulcer–related hospitalizations among older adults. Target: 887.3 pressure ulcer–related hospitalizations per 100,000 people aged 65 years and older. Baseline: 985.8 pressure ulcer–related hospitalizations per 100,000 people aged 65 years and older occurred in 2007. Target setting method: 10% improvement.

OA–11: Reduce the rate of emergency department (ED) visits due to falls among older adults. Target: 4711.6 ED visits per 100,000 due to falls among older adults. Baseline: 5235.1 ED visits per 100,000 due to falls occurred among older adults in 2007 (age adjusted to year 2000 standard population). Target setting method: 10% improvement.

OA–12.1: Increase the number of States and the District of Columbia that collect and make publicly available information on the characteristics of victims, perpetrators, and cases of elder abuse, neglect, and exploitation. Target: 4 States and the District of Columbia. Baseline: 3 States collected and made publicly available information on the characteristics of victims, perpetrators, and cases of elder abuse, neglect, and exploitation in 2004. Target setting method: 10% improvement.

From US Department of Health and Human Services: Older adults, 2012. Retrieved from *www.healthypeople.gov/2020/topicsobjectives2020/overview.aspx?topicId=31.*

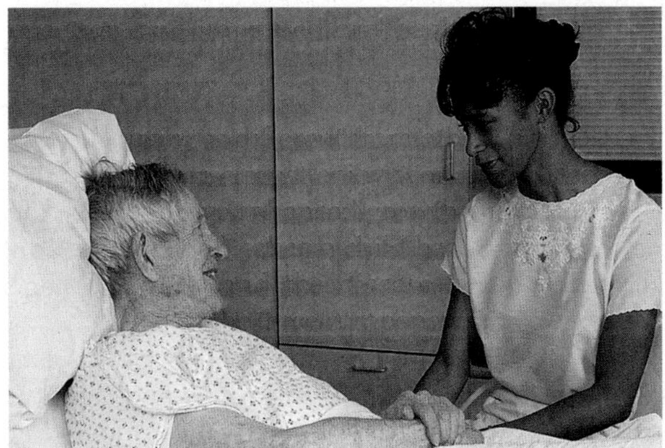

Fig. 33.2 Self-esteem is vital for successful aging. (From Perry AG, Potter PA, Elkin MK: *Nursing interventions and clinical skills,* ed 4, St. Louis, 2008, Mosby.)

aging. In many cases, research has proved such myths to be inaccurate.

THEORIES OF AGING

Our current knowledge about aging and the aging process is limited. In an attempt to explain aging and an individual's response to aging, experts have proposed a number of theories (Box 33.4). Biologic theories attempt to explain why the body ages; psychosocial theories try to give reasons for the responses and interactions older adults have with society during late adulthood (see Chapter 24).

AGEISM

Ageism is a term that describes prejudice against older adults. It reflects a negative response by younger

Box 33.3 Common Myths Associated With Aging

Myth: All people become senile when they become old.
Reality: Decline is not inevitable. Creativity and intelligence do not appear to change. Memory and learning ability sometimes show slight decline because they are functions of the nervous system, which does experience some age-related changes. Serious decline in mental capabilities is generally a result of disease process, not age. In people over the age of 65 only 6%–8% have dementia. In those over the age of 85 years only one-third are affected by dementia (Tan, 2011).

Myth: Becoming forgetful means that dementia will occur.
Reality: There are many causes of memory loss. Medications, stress, and depression are among possible culprits of forgetfulness.

Myth: Older adults are isolated and alone.
Reality: Most older adults have at least weekly contact with family. Many live within a 30-minute drive of at least one family member. Although it is assumed that the family is the main support and source of social activity, many older people have also developed a network of friends who provide support and relationships.

Myth: Most older adults are in nursing homes or care facilities.
Reality: About 80% of older adults own and live in their own homes.

Myth: Older adults do not have much energy and are always tired.
Reality: Energy is largely determined by lifestyle and attitude. Sedentary individuals do not have as much energy-geared initiative.

Myth: Older adults are ill and disabled.
Reality: Most older people have at least one chronic condition, but these conditions generally do not limit their ability to manage their household and activities of daily living. In a study of noninstitutionalized older adults, approximately 7 of 10 individuals reported their health as "good" or "excellent" as compared with that of others their own age.

Box 33.4 Common Theories of Aging

BIOLOGIC

Programmed Aging

Cells in the body can reproduce only 40 to 60 times. Aging takes place when more and more cells no longer have the capacity to regenerate themselves.

GENETIC FACTORS

People inherit a genetic program that determines their specific life expectancy.

IMMUNOLOGIC

The immune system becomes less effective or less able to distinguish between foreign and host cells, and aging is a result of the consequentially diminished protection from infection or disease, and the immune system destroying body cells that it misreads as defective or foreign.

FREE RADICAL

In the course of the metabolic activity of the body that produces energy, extra electrons are released that build up in the body and combine chemically, damaging cells and interfering with normal body function, resulting in aging.

WEAR AND TEAR

Cells of the body wear out from internal and external stress, including chemical damage, trauma, or dysfunction of body systems, and buildup of waste products.

PSYCHOSOCIAL

Erikson's Developmental Stages

In the last stage of life, the task is acceptance of life and one's own lifestyle, which potentially results in ego integrity. Inability to achieve a level of acceptance results in anger and despair.

Disengagement Theory

Aging is a process in which older adults and society gradually withdraw from each other to the mutual satisfaction of both.

Exchange Theory

Aging is reduced interaction between older adults and society as a result of the decreasing value that the interaction has for both.

Activity Theory

Older adults develop a positive concept of self as a result of maintaining ongoing social interactions. Well-being in later life is enhanced by substituting new roles in relation to family, recreation, and volunteer services for previous occupational roles.

Continuity Theory

Personality remains the same, and behavior becomes more predictable as people age.

people—a personal dread of growing old or becoming disabled, and a fear of powerlessness, uselessness, and death. Ageism systematically stereotypes and discriminates against people because they are old, just as racism and sexism stereotypes and discriminates against people on the basis of skin color and sex. To enhance the quality of life for older adults, support the patient's hope, pride, confidence, security, and integrity. All members of the health care team should work toward eliminating negative attitudes and discriminatory practices.

LEGISLATION THAT AFFECTS OLDER ADULTS

The first major legislation that attempted to provide financial security for older adults was the Social Security Act of 1935. At the time this law was passed, few people lived long enough to collect significant benefits. Over time, increasing numbers of politically active older adults sought and achieved legislation designed to benefit themselves (Table 33.2).

In 1965 the Older Americans Act (OAA) was established; it aimed to preserve the rights and dignity of the nation's older citizens. This act was updated and amended in 2006. The amendments retain provisions for low-income minorities and add emphasis on older individuals who reside in rural areas.

Table 33.2 Legislation That Has Helped Older Adults

YEAR	LEGISLATION
1935	Social Security Act
1965	Medicare and Medicaid established Administration on Aging established
1967	Age Discrimination Act passed
1972	Supplemental Security Income Program instituted Social Security indexed to reflect inflation, COLA (cost of living adjustments) Nutrition Act passed, which allows for provision of nutrition programs for older adults
1973	Council on Aging established
1978	Mandatory retirement age changed to age 70 yr
1986	Mandatory retirement age eliminated for most employees
1987	Omnibus Budget Reconciliation Act (OBRA)
1988	Catastrophic health insurance established as part of Medicare
1990	Self-Determination Act: Responsibilities of care providers. Advance directives for health care provide legal clarification of an individual's wishes for limiting treatment in the event of acute illness and in dying
2004	Prescription drug plans instituted
2010	Patient Protection and Affordable Care Act (ACA) • Free Medicare preventive services • Medicare drug discount for eligible seniors who are in the "donut hole" • The health care law cracks down on waste, fraud, and abuse while providing new protections for seniors
2016	The Older Americans Act Reauthorization Act • Improved protection for vulnerable elders • Improved nutrition services

The increasing number of older adults also raises the issue of the needs of their caregivers. The National Family Caregiver Support Program provided a means of addressing the growing needs of caregivers (USDHHS, 2017). In 2000 an additional program was added to support caregivers of American Indian elders (USDHHS, 2018b).

The Patient Protection and Affordable Care Act (ACA) was signed into law in 2010. The results of this legislation are still developing, but the law encourages payment for preventive services to Medicare recipients and provides a drug discount for eligible seniors in the "donut hole" (USDHHS, n.d.a). The "donut hole" is a coverage gap that exists in most Medicare D prescription plans. The plans pay a percentage of the cost of medications up to a certain amount. When that amount is reached, Medicare recipients must pay 100% of the cost of prescriptions up to a yearly maximum out-of-pocket limit. After the maximum limit is met, the coverage gap ends and the prescription plan pays a percentage of the cost of covered drugs again. Proponents of the ACA state that the law provides new protections for seniors and cuts down on waste, fraud, and abuse. Since its inception the ACA has been met with concern over costs to those it was developed to cover and by insurers. The nation's legislators continue to propose changes in the scope, cost, and implementation of the act.

PSYCHOSOCIAL CONCERNS OF THE OLDER ADULT

STRESSES OF CAREGIVING

Older people receiving care may feel they are being a burden, be angry or frustrated about giving up their independence, or become demanding in an attempt to regain control. Caregivers often feel overloaded, finding themselves pulled in many directions. There simply may not be enough time to meet all demands. Caregivers are at high risk for stress-related problems, including depression, anxiety, and increased vulnerability to physical health problems. The caregiver's coping style, how it affects caregiving, and the quality of the caregiver's support system are important to assess. Conflict is possible between family members who live near an older person and those who live at a distance because of different perspectives. It is often helpful to remind distant family members not to let apparent differences between what they see and what the local caregiver has said discredit the caregiver. Local caregivers often must compromise with the older person and accept imperfect solutions to problems.

One group of caregivers are known as the "**sandwich generation**." These are individuals who are faced with caring for their parents while also caring for their own children. There are an estimated 44 million caregivers to the elderly in the United States. The clear majority (75%) are employed. This places stress on the "sandwiched" person. The pull of the workplace, home, and the elder can result in loss of time at work. Such situations are estimated to cost US businesses $34 billion per year.

The nursing assessment should include the needs of the caregiver. Review the demeanor and responses of the caregiver and the patient that may indicate fatigue in relation to the provision of care for the loved one. Referrals to social services and available community resources may be indicated. **Respite care** refers to the provision of care by nonfamily members with a goal of allowing the primary caregivers the opportunity for relief from the stressors and strains imposed by caring for an ill or debilitated family member.

LOSS, GRIEF, AND DEPRESSION

Significant psychosocial changes experienced by older adults typically include personal, social, and economic losses resulting from role changes, retirement, and the loss of significant others—parents, siblings, children, spouses, and friends. Physical changes often result in loss of independence and space. For some older adults, losses may occur suddenly, concurrently, or within a short period, thus increasing their impact. The ability to cope with grief and the related losses depends on many factors. Successful coping strategies to deal with grief may include avoiding isolation and self-pity, helping others, joining groups, adopting a pet, setting goals, maintaining independence, and retaining a sense of humor (see Chapter 25 for additional information).

Short-term or long-term depression may result in response to the grief from real and perceived losses. Fatigue, sadness, insomnia, anorexia, helplessness, crying, agitation, and hypochondria are frequent symptoms of depression in older adults. These symptoms are misunderstood commonly as changes that normally occur with aging. Misunderstanding and misdiagnosis too often result in many older adults failing to receive the needed treatment for depression. Depression is more common in the older adult than any other age-related group. Older people who receive psychotherapy for depression show improvement.

Patient problems and interventions for older adults with loss, grief, or depression include but are not limited to the following:

Patient Problem	Nursing Interventions
Complex grief, related to losses (specify)	Encourage verbalization of feelings regarding losses Acknowledge reality of grief Plan care to promote consistency and reduce stress Encourage participation in activities to provide distraction Refer to spiritual counselor or other sources of support Spend time with isolated individual
Helplessness, related to personal, social, and economic losses	Allow older person to make choices whenever possible Encourage person to do as much for self as possible Adapt environment to support independence Explain reasons for changes in plan of care

END-OF-LIFE CARE

Nurses who work with older adults assist the entire health care team to meet the physical, spiritual, and psychosocial needs of dying patients or residents. Caring for the families is an important part of this care. Knowledge about a person's culture and religious beliefs helps the team provide compassionate care.

Nurses caring for patients at the end of life need to understand the 1991 Patient Self-Determination Act (PSDA) as it relates to advance directives, living wills, durable powers of attorney, and do-not-resuscitate (DNR) orders. The health care team works closely with the patient or resident and the family to ensure that the patient's wishes are respected (see Chapter 25).

AGING BODY

Physiologic changes affect a person's biologic, psychological, social, and environmental status. Physiologic changes in the aging process result in a decreased immune response, a decrease in compensatory reserve, and a loss of the body's ability to repair damaged tissue efficiently.

Numerous physiologic changes occur in all body systems during the natural aging process. There is strong evidence that inactivity is the most important contributor to declining physical mobility and function. Positive lifestyle modifications, including physical activity and proper nutrition, help optimize physical abilities and promote healthier aging. The degree and rate at which changes occur vary among individuals, systems, and organs, as does a person's ability to compensate.

In this chapter, common patient problems and nursing interventions related to each system are identified for selected age-related changes. Additional patient problem statements and nursing interventions may be appropriate to meet the individual needs of the older adult. See specific chapters for the discussion of nursing interventions that are appropriate regardless of age.

INTEGUMENTARY SYSTEM

Age-Related Changes

Aging skin is dry and thin and loses tone and elasticity. The loss of fat under the skin makes wrinkles increasingly apparent. Age spots called *lentigo* are tan or brown macules brought on by sun exposure and are more common in middle-aged and older people (Table 33.3). Hair grays and thins, and the distribution patterns often change, resulting in baldness. Nails grow slowly and often become thicker and more brittle, develop ridges, and turn yellow. Touch sensation often changes as a result of thinning skin, disease process, and responses to medication therapy. Susceptibility to infection, ecchymosis, and tearing increases with aging. Wounds tend to heal more slowly than those in a younger adult.

Assessment

- Observe skin hydration status. Pay close attention for signs of excessive dryness. Observe for skin tears or lesions. Note presence, location, and amount of exudate.
- Examine for lesions that have changed size, color, or shape. Lesions that are irregularly shaped, raised, crusted or pitting, or bleed easily should be examined by a dermatologist.
- Observe hair for excessive loss, dryness, or oiliness.
- Observe the nails for color, length, shape, symmetry, and cleanliness. Nursing interventions are indicated to manage cleanliness, excessive length, sharp edges, brittleness, increased thickening, and color changes.

Table 33.3 Integumentary Changes With Aging

PHYSIOLOGIC CHANGE	RESULTS
Decreased vascularity of dermis and decreased amount of melanin	Increased pallor in white skin
Decreased sebaceous gland function	Increased skin dryness
Decreased sweat gland function	Decreased perspiration
Decreased subcutaneous fat	Increased wrinkling
Decreased thickness of epidermis	Increased susceptibility to trauma
Increased localized pigmentation	Increased incidence of brown spots (senile lentigo)
Increased capillary fragility	Increased purple patches (senile purpura)
Decreased density of hair growth	Decreased amount and thickness of hair on head and body
Decreased melanin production in the hair bulb	Graying hair
Decreased hormone production	Decreased vaginal secretions and breast tissue mass and decreased speed of erection and the ability to maintain an erection Increased brittleness of nails
Decreased peripheral circulation	Increased thickening and yellowing of nails
Decreased rate of nail growth	Increased longitudinal ridges on nails
Increased androgen-to-estrogen ratio	Increased facial hair in women

Common Concerns and Nursing Interventions

Pruritus. Older people may report dryness and itching (**pruritus**) of the skin. This is more common in cold, dry weather because of reduced glandular secretions and moisture. Because soap tends to be drying, older adults should use soap sparingly and rinse the residue completely away. Antibacterial soap is very drying and usually is not a good option.

Skilled nursing facilities may have schedules for showering and shampooing. On nonshower days a partial bath is provided, which includes the washing of face, hands, axillary region, and perineal area.

In general, less frequent bathing is recommended for sedentary older adults because of a decrease in body oils and perspiration. Water-based or light oil-based lotions, rather than alcohol-based lotions, are best to use. Application of water-based lotions to dry areas, especially after bathing, usually increases most individuals' comfort and avoids the feeling of oil residue that some people find uncomfortable.

Moles. Most moles are benign. However, sun-related skin changes, including precancerous actinic keratosis, basal cell or squamous cell carcinoma, and malignant melanoma, sometimes develop on sun-exposed areas. Ask a dermatologist to examine any suspicious-looking lesions.

Nail abnormalities. Bilateral clubbing of fingers indicates possible pulmonary or cardiac disease. Yellowed nails indicate possible fungal infection. Splintered nails indicate possible malnutrition, and pitting sometimes signals peripheral vascular disease, psoriasis, diabetes mellitus, or syphilis. Brittle nails are often associated with fluctuations in hormones that occur during menopause.

Pressure injury. According to the National Pressure Ulcer Advisory Panel (NPUAP), more than 2.5 million US residents develop pressure injury every year (NPUAP, 2012). Pressure injury is a significant risk for older adults and patients with chronic disease. Thin skin and lack of subcutaneous fat predispose older adults to pressure injury development when their fragile skin is compressed between bony prominences of the body and other objects. Damage to the skin at these pressure points is best prevented by repositioning the patient at least every 2 hours. Many pressure-reducing pads and aids are available, but only those that do not restrict circulation or create pressure on surrounding areas should be used.

Fragile skin bruises and tears easily. Measures should be instituted to prevent pressure, friction, **shearing forces** (forces that can injure small blood vessels by sliding on a rough surface) (Fig. 33.3), and moisture (most commonly associated with incontinence).

Friction occurs when fragile skin rubs against the bed sheets. In addition to the normal safety precautions taken to prevent injury to any patient, gentle handling during turning and transfer is necessary. Additional assistance or equipment may be needed to lift and move a resident to avoid friction burns and tearing of the skin during repositioning in bed. The use of tape on the skin of older adults should be kept to a minimum, because fragile skin can easily tear in the process of removing tape. Urine, drainage, or fecal material left in contact with the skin even for a short time potentially causes the skin to become impaired. Urine and stool tend to accelerate the formation of pressure injury at

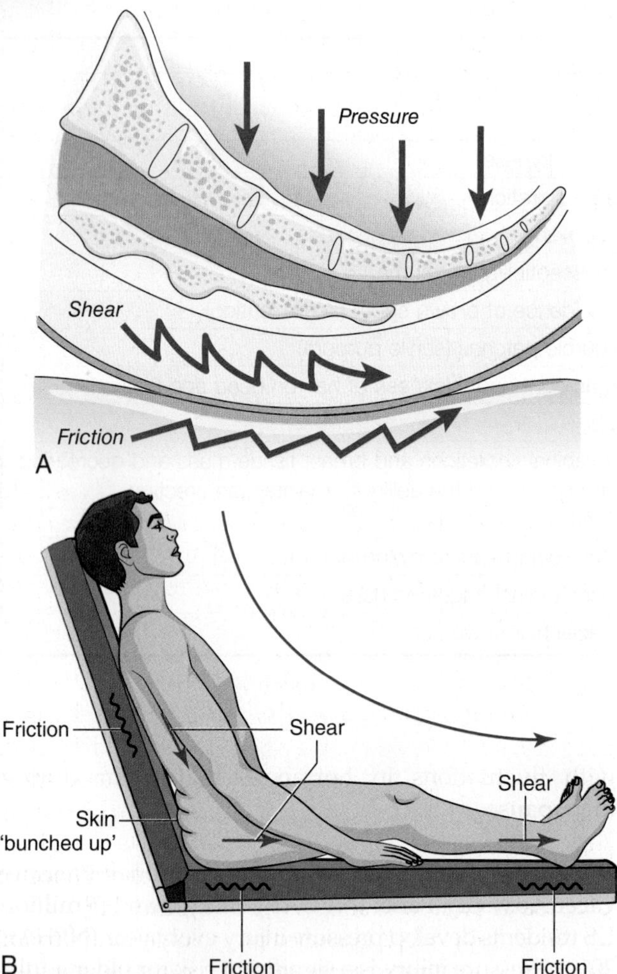

Fig. 33.3 Shearing forces that result from pressure against the skin impair circulation to underlying tissues.

pressure points such as the coccyx or hip. Urine, drainage, and fecal material must be removed, and the skin washed, rinsed with clear water, and patted dry.

Prevention and healing of any pressure ulcer depend on good nutritional status and adequate hydration. A well-balanced diet with attention to protein, vitamins, and minerals plays an important role in maintaining skin integrity in the older adult.

Patient problems and interventions for a resident with pressure injury include but are not limited to the following:

Patient Problem	Nursing Interventions
Potential for Compromised Skin Integrity, related to fragile skin associated with aging	Perform daily skin inspection Reduce frequency of bathing Use mild, nonirritating soaps, and rinse thoroughly Use emollients and lotions to maintain skin moisture Turn and reposition frequently Move and transfer carefully Reduce sources of pressure Keep linens clean, dry, and free from foreign objects
Compromised Skin Integrity, related to inadequate nutritional intake	Assess nutritional intake Explain importance of nutrition Provide adequate protein, vitamins, minerals, and fluids
Potential for Infection, related to impaired skin integrity	Assess wounds daily, including size, location, and depth Obtain wound cultures if appropriate Follow strict aseptic technique when performing wound care per the health care provider's orders Use photographs to document healing or changes in pressure injury

GASTROINTESTINAL SYSTEM

A balanced diet provides fuel for the body. Good nutrition is essential to health, function, and quality of life, regardless of age. An inadequate or imbalanced diet can be tied to numerous chronic conditions, including obesity, hypertension, diabetes, cancer, and cardiovascular disease. Older adults may experience a reduction in the sense of taste and smell. Medications may alter the taste of foods or result in a decrease in saliva production. Older adults living alone may report a lack of interest in preparing solo meals or may have limited financial resources to obtain nutritional foods. These occurrences contribute to undernutrition. Inactivity, boredom, and mental health concerns may result in excessive food consumption. This may result in overnutrition. Assess the patient's nutritional status. Interventions for nutritional issues can help the older adult attain higher self-esteem, improved physical well-being, and a better quality of life.

Age-Related Changes

Older adults have decreased secretion of saliva and a diminished gag response, which increases the chances of choking and aspiration. In addition, many medications taken by older adults may compound the problem by further reducing saliva production. The stomach of the older adult has decreased gastric motility as well as decreased production of bicarbonate and gastric mucus. Aging also can cause decreased production or lack of production of the intrinsic factor causing the body to become unable to use ingested vitamin B_{12}, leading to pernicious anemia.

Enzymes in the intestinal tract also are altered. The abdominal wall becomes less firm, and abdominal muscles weaken. Decreased tone of the intestine occurs, and it is common for peristalsis to become slower, leading to increased constipation (Table 33.4). The normal changes of aging often are intensified by medications commonly prescribed for other conditions, lack of fluids or dietary roughage or fiber, and lack of exercise or

Table 33.4 Gastrointestinal Changes With Aging

PHYSIOLOGIC CHANGE	RESULTS
Increased dental caries and tooth loss	Decreased ability to chew normally Decreased nutritional status
Decreased gag reflex	Increased incidence of choking and aspiration
Decreased muscle tone at sphincters	Increased incidence of pyrosis (heartburn); esophageal reflux
Decreased gastric secretions	Decreased digestion
Decreased peristalsis	Increased constipation and bowel impaction

activity. Liver function often decreases, making drug metabolism less efficient.

Assessment

- Assess oral cavity for presence of lesions; dental caries; loose, broken, or missing teeth; dentures that do not fit well; edematous gums; and halitosis.
- Assess ability to chew and swallow.
- Assess for reports of heartburn and nausea.
- Assess dietary intake, especially of high-fiber foods, fat, and sodium. Note amount and type of food and fluid intake. Assess appetite.
- Assess weight. Compare with norms, and monitor for significant changes.
- Assess frequency, amount, odor, and consistency of bowel elimination. Assess abdomen for tenderness, distention, and active or diminished bowel sounds. Ask about intestinal cramping.
- Assess individual's ability to control defecation.
- Assess bowel elimination routines and use of laxatives.
- An annual fecal occult blood test is recommended for adults more than 50 years of age for detection of colorectal cancer, the second leading cause of cancer deaths in the United States.
- A stool DNA test may be completed for detection of colorectal cancer.

Common Concerns and Nursing Interventions

Obesity. Defined as weighing at least 20% more than ideal body weight, obesity is common in older adults. Older adults should consume less food than they did in their earlier, more physically active years. Adults 75 to 90 years of age need approximately 30 calories per kilogram of body weight (14 calories/lb), compared with 40 calories per kilogram (18 calories/lb) for people 20 to 37 years of age. This normally represents a diet of 1800 to 2400 calories daily, depending on gender and ideal weight. Along with fewer calories, older adults need to consume quality foods, such as grains, vegetables, and fruits, which contain vitamins, minerals, roughage, and fiber, to meet their daily needs without large amounts of sugar and fat. They also need foods that provide protein and are good sources of calcium.

Some foods are not as well tolerated because of changes in the digestive tract or difficulty with chewing or swallowing. Individual food preferences should be respected. A well-balanced diet is generally accepted as adequate without vitamin supplements. Vitamins A, C, and E and niacin may help slow the aging process, counteract the effects of free radicals, and extend life.

Weight loss. Gradual weight loss over time is a normal response to loss of body mass. This typically occurs with changes in body composition of fat, muscle, and fluid. Decreased nutrient intake in aging because of decreased appetite, lower metabolic rate, and diminished energy output also produces weight loss. Rapid weight loss may indicate an illness and should be reported to the health care provider. Unexplained weight loss totaling more than 5% of weight in 6 months to 1 year necessitates a medical evaluation (Mayo Clinic, 2018).

Fluids and dehydration. Fluids are necessary for the body to function and to remove the waste products of metabolism. An older person needs a minimum of 1500 mL of fluids daily. Because of arthritis or other conditions, some older adults have difficulty pouring liquids and drinking from a cup. Older adults sometimes decrease their fluid intake to control incontinence or because of an illness such as heart failure (HF).

When fluid deficit is caused by the older adult trying to control incontinence, the most appropriate interventions are to make fluids readily available and toilet facilities more easily accessible. Arranging the room so that access to the bathroom is unobstructed often helps. Sometimes the older adult needs assistance to the bathroom on a schedule, usually every 2 hours during waking hours and every 4 hours at night. If needed, a commode or urinal should be placed where the person can easily use it. Older adults who have difficulty picking up a cup or bending the neck often find that an adapted cup with a double handle (Fig. 33.4) or a cutout for the nose is a good solution. Some older adults who are disoriented likely need to be prompted to drink. Those with severe impairments often must be assisted to drink fluids on a scheduled basis.

Oral hygiene. Loss of teeth often is assumed to be normal in old age, but this is a misconception. It is *not* part of the normal aging process. Many of today's older population matured before the introduction of many modern methods of dental prophylaxis, which affects their dental health in addition to individual oral hygiene habits and the possibility of untreated periodontal disease. In the future, with good oral hygiene practices throughout life, many people will maintain their natural teeth for life.

Missing teeth make chewing difficult and tiring. Loose-fitting dentures tend to make chewing difficult and often allow food to collect under the denture, resulting

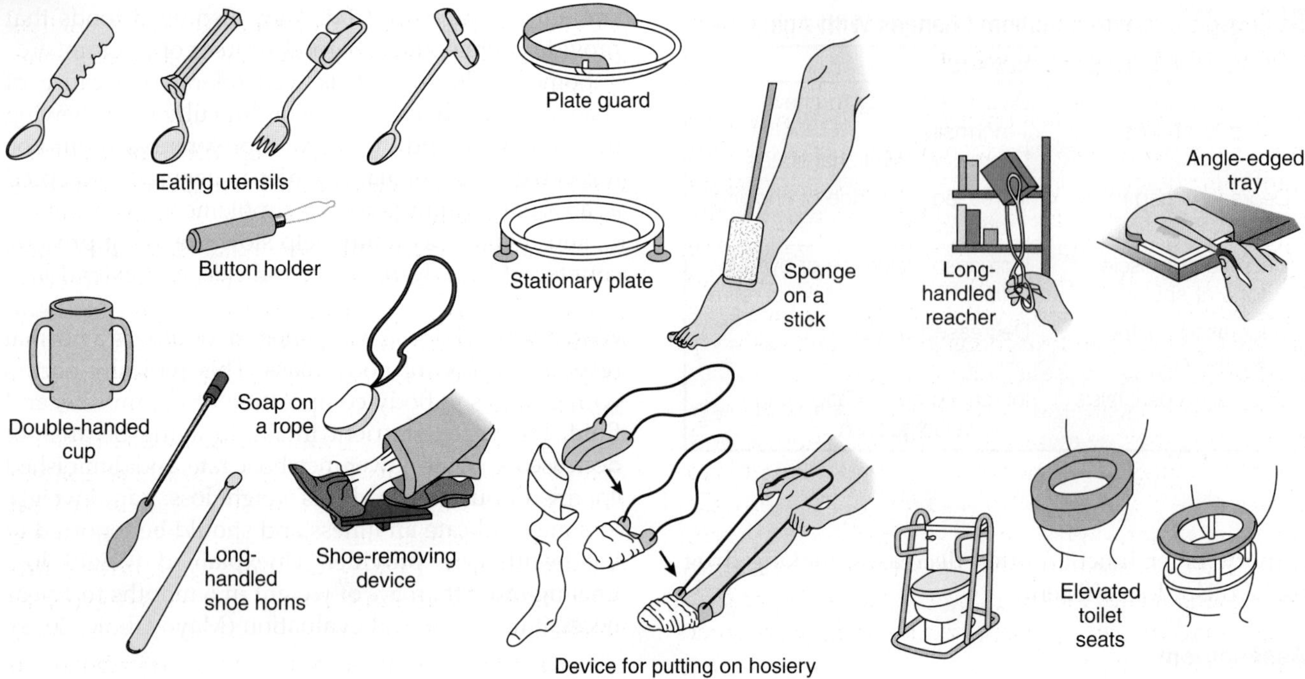

Fig. 33.4 Assistive devices for older adults.

in lesions. Both of these problems decrease a person's desire to eat. Oral hygiene is essential to eliminate debris that has the potential to interfere with taste or cause lesions. Recommended mouth care for older adults consists of a thorough cleansing of the entire mouth with a soft-bristled toothbrush or foam-stick applicator in the early morning and at bedtime. Mouth care is also important when an older adult has dentures. In addition to cleaning the dentures, brush the gums and the tongue, and rinse the mouth. If dentures are damaged, loose, or exert pressure on the oral mucous membranes, refer the person for dental services.

Loss of appetite. Older adults frequently experience a loss of appetite. Changes as a result of decreased saliva production and a decreased number of taste buds sometimes make food unappealing. Gastric motility slows because of the loss of smooth muscle in the stomach, which causes a delay in emptying time, distention, and early satiety. Anorexia and weight loss often result. In addition, many medications taken by older adults can produce side effects such as dyspepsia, nausea, vomiting, anorexia, diarrhea, and constipation, which affect the appetite.

Interventions to counteract the lack of taste buds or the lack of interest in eating may include preparing the food with color and garnishes, using attractive dishes and table settings with good lighting and bright colors, and providing foods that have more seasoning if there are no restrictions. Encourage the patient or caregiver to prepare homemade frozen dinners from extra portions of a favorite meal as an easy and effective way to provide a meal that will be enjoyed.

Individuals who have *impaired mobility* or *activity intolerance* that interferes with the ability to prepare food may benefit from community-based programs such as Meals on Wheels or home-delivered meals from a senior nutrition site. In addition, a wide variety of fresh, canned, and frozen foods in small or single servings is available in stores. Older adults should check the sodium content in canned or frozen to avoid consuming excessive amounts of sodium.

For most individuals, eating also is associated with a social setting. Dining alone may make eating less appealing. When an older individual has lost a spouse, or is unable to leave the house, *Despair, Grief,* and *Social Seclusion* are patient problem statements to be considered. Interventions that may assist the older adult in improving nutritional intake include community meal programs, church dinners, or senior citizen programs that provide transportation, meals, and opportunities to socialize.

Gastric reflux. Reflux occurs when the sphincter at the opening to the stomach becomes less efficient, which allows food and digestive enzymes to flow back into the esophagus. Symptoms include heartburn, sour stomach, and regurgitation of sour, bitter material. Reflux can be controlled by eating small meals, avoiding eating before bedtime, and elevating the head of the bed. Achieving and maintaining ideal body weight are also helpful.

Food intolerance. Lactose, primarily found in milk, is a common source of food intolerance. Dairy products are an important source of calcium, which is needed to prevent osteoporosis. Lactose-intolerant individuals may need to replace milk with cheese and yogurt, which is processed and easier to digest.

Dysphagia. Difficulty swallowing (**dysphagia**) may arise from many possible causes, including a stroke or other neurologic dysfunction, local trauma, and obstruction with a tumor. Assessment should focus on whether the dysphagia is with liquids, solids, or both and on the time frame for the progression of the symptoms. The older adult often has more difficulty swallowing fluids or foods that contain firm foods in liquid such as soup than swallowing semisolid or solid food.

Interventions for individuals who have difficulty swallowing include avoiding liquids, positioning, and verbal coaching. Thickeners can be added to liquids to improve the ability to control swallowing. The upright position, leaning slightly forward with the chin down, enlists the assistance of gravity to improve swallowing. Placing food on the unaffected side, reducing distractions in the room, and cueing the person to swallow are other ways to facilitate success.

Patient problems and interventions for the older adult with gastrointestinal system changes include but are not limited to the following:

Patient Problem	Nursing Interventions
Compromised Swallowing Ability, related to neurologic or vascular conditions	Refer to speech therapist for evaluation Assess individual's unique needs and problems Verify condition of teeth or fit of dentures Assist to sitting position with chin flexed toward chest Allow adequate time for meals Feed slowly Give frequent verbal cues to swallow Reduce distractions during meals. Keep suctioning equipment available in case of problems
Insufficient Nutrition, related to lack of interest in food	Assess reasons for loss of interest, such as depression or grief Monitor daily intake Weigh weekly Determine individual food preferences Provide oral hygiene before meals Serve meals in attractive manner; assist as needed Supplement meals with nutritious snacks if permitted Consult with dietitian Provide for social interaction during meals

Failure to thrive. Failure to thrive in older adults is characterized by refusal to eat, loss of weight and lean body mass, and subsequent malnutrition. This complex situation is associated with mental disorders, such as dementia and depression, and social and economic factors.

Specialized nutritional support. A patient's or resident's inability to ingest, digest, or absorb nutrients is in some cases an indication for enteral tube feedings. Feeding tubes can be placed into the stomach or the small intestine. A nasogastric or nasointestinal tube is inserted through the nose. A gastrostomy tube or percutaneous endoscopic gastrostomy (PEG) is inserted directly through the abdominal wall. Another option is a jejunostomy.

Standard enteral formulas contain whole proteins and complex carbohydrates. Other formulas contain modified protein (peptides) or amino acids. Enteral feedings sometimes are ordered short term after surgery, traumatic injury, or burns to improve nutritional intake. Transition to an oral diet occurs as soon as is feasible.

Long-term use of feeding tubes contributes to increased health risks and discomfort. The use of feeding tubes for cognitively impaired individuals is declining. The use of a tube feeding is not recommended for patients with advanced dementia. As a result, the use of feeding tubes has declined from 11.7% of patients with advanced dementia who had feeding tubes in 2000 to 5.7% in 2014 (Mitchell et al, 2016). Racial disparities have been noted with the use of feeding tubes. In 2000 8.6% of white patients with advanced dementia had feeding tubes compared with 37.5% of black patients. In 2014 the numbers had decreased to 3.1% and 17.5%, respectively (Mitchell et al, 2016). Many nursing home residents are provided with speech therapy to obtain recommendations for successful hand-feeding (Fig. 33.5).

Gastrointestinal cancer. Follow-up and diagnostic testing is indicated in the presence of the following:

- Change in bowel or bladder habits
- Persistent oral lesions
- Visible or occult blood
- Indigestion or difficulty swallowing
- Unexplained weight loss
- Constipation
- Persistent bloating

Constipation has been defined broadly as an abnormally infrequent or difficult passage of hard, dry feces. Failure to relieve constipation creates the risk of a fecal impaction. Constipation can be acute or chronic. Older adults are often very attentive to their bowel function. Problems often are reported when a deviation occurs from what is perceived as normal elimination, even with relatively minor physiologic changes. Assessment relating to constipation includes dietary intake of fiber and fluids; use of medications such as opioid analgesics, antacids, iron preparations, anticholinergics, or overuse of laxatives; mechanical obstruction from

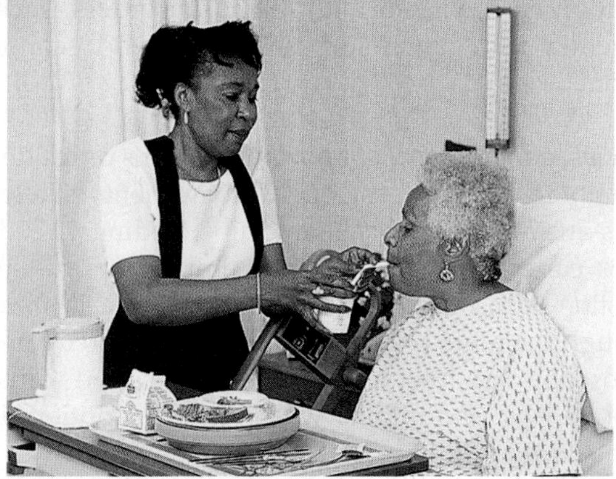

Fig. 33.5 Hand-feeding often averts the need for feeding tubes. (From Perry AG, Potter PA, Elkin MK: *Nursing interventions and clinical skills*, ed 4, St. Louis, 2008, Mosby.)

Table 33.5 Urinary Changes With Aging

PHYSIOLOGIC CHANGE	RESULTS
Decreased number of functional nephrons	Decreased filtration rate
Decreased blood supply	Decreased removal of body wastes Increased concentration of urine
Decreased muscle tone	Increased volume of residual urine, stress incontinence, nocturia
Decreased tissue elasticity	Decreased bladder capacity
Increased size of prostate	Increased risk of infection Decreased stream of urine Increased hesitancy, frequency, nocturia

fecal impaction, volvulus, adhesions, strangulated hernia, or cancer; activity and exercise patterns; and limitations such as inability to reach the toilet or a lack of privacy. Depression can be a contributing factor in some instances.

Nursing interventions include adequate fluids, exercise, and a diet that contains fiber. Bran is a good source of fiber for older adults who are unable to eat enough vegetables and fruits. Up to 10 g of bran per day may be included in the diet. This is achievable if the daily meals include two slices of whole-grain bread, two bran muffins or biscuits, and two spoonfuls of bran added to or sprinkled over other foods.

A patient problem and interventions for the older adult with constipation include but are not limited to the following:

Patient Problem	Nursing Interventions
Infrequent or Difficult Bowel Elimination, related to inadequate intake of fiber and fluids	Assess frequency and consistency of bowel movements Increase dietary fiber by encouraging cereals such as bran and fruits such as prunes Determine fluid preferences Keep fluids at bedside, and offer them at frequent intervals Administer stool softeners as ordered

Fecal incontinence. The most common cause of bowel incontinence in the older adult is fecal impaction associated with immobilization and inadequate fiber and fluid intake. A soft or liquid stool may ooze around the impaction, giving the appearance of diarrhea. Underlying diseases such as cancer, inflammatory bowel disease, colitis, and neurologic disease have the potential to cause fecal incontinence. A digital rectal examination by the primary health care provider may be needed to determine the nature of the problem.

Gastrointestinal bleeding. Older people have less protective mucus secretion, and therefore they are more susceptible to gastrointestinal (GI) bleeding. Assess for blood in the stools in the presence of dizziness, pallor, tachycardia, or hypotension. Rectal bleeding can be a sign of hemorrhoids, rectal fissures, or cancer. In older adults, consider a guaiac-positive stool an indication of pathologic disturbance until proven otherwise. Laxatives, iron supplements, cimetidine (Tagamet), anticoagulants, aspirin and nonsteroidal antiinflammatory drugs (NSAIDs), and foods such as red meat may yield a false-positive guaiac result.

GENITOURINARY SYSTEM

Age-Related Changes

Overall kidney function decreases with age (Table 33.5). Even with a decrease of 50%, the body has adequate reserve to support normal body functions unless kidney disease is present. Bladder capacity decreases approximately 50% with age. Some bladders in older adults only hold 150 mL.

Incontinence sometimes occurs because bladder capacity decreases, urine residual increases, and bladder contractions increase. A decrease of bladder tone causes urine to remain in the bladder on emptying, which results in the sensation of a full bladder (frequency) within a brief period. Urinary tract infections also may trigger incontinence. In the older adult confusion may by the first symptom of an infection.

Urinary incontinence (UI), which affects more than 17% of women and 11% of men older than age 65 years, is embarrassing and debilitating. It is not a normal part of aging, although many believe that it is and do not seek treatment.

Changes specific to women are related to perineal changes as estrogen levels decline. Intercourse may become painful as the vaginal opening constricts and the vagina shortens, loses tone, and dries. Abnormal postmenstrual bleeding may indicate endometrial cancer and must be investigated.

Changes specific to men include enlargement of the prostate gland, which results in the occlusion of the urethra, obstructing the flow of urine; also, the scrotum becomes more pendulous. Although a man's libido does not normally decrease, erections may develop more slowly and orgasms become less intense.

Assessment

- Assess frequency, amount, odor, color, and consistency of urine.
- Assess individual's ability to control urination.
- Assess satisfaction with sexuality and affectionate relationships.

Common Concerns and Nursing Interventions

Nocturia. At least 50% of older men and 70% of older women have to get up two or more times during the night to empty their bladders, a condition known as **nocturia** (urination at night). The decrease in bladder capacity may be associated with the increase in voiding at night. This condition should be evaluated. It may also be attributed to other factors. Although nocturia does not jeopardize an individual's physical health, it is inconvenient, interferes with sleep, and tends to contribute to fatigue. Nursing interventions to decrease nocturia include limiting fluids in the evening, giving diuretic medications in the morning, and preventing fall hazards when an individual has to get up to urinate. A history of nocturia or an increase in the number of episodes necessitates medical evaluation, because it may indicate an infection and the need for medical treatment.

Urinary incontinence. Another related problem for many older individuals is incontinence. Some older adults do not leave their home for fear they will have an accident in public. The several types of incontinence include stress, urge, overflow, and functional incontinence. These types may occur in combination, causing a mixed incontinence that is common in older adults.

Stress incontinence is involuntary loss of a small amount of urine with increased abdominal pressure, such as coughing or sneezing. It is common in older women who have had multiple vaginal births or loss of muscle tone.

Urge incontinence is associated with cystitis, urethritis, tumors, stones, and central nervous system (CNS) disorders such as stroke, dementia, and Parkinson's disease. Urge incontinence is characterized by involuntary urine loss after a sudden urge to void.

Overflow incontinence occurs when a chronically full bladder increases bladder pressure to a higher level than urethral resistance is able to counter, resulting in a loss of a small volume of urine. It is accompanied by a weak urine stream, difficulty starting to pass urine, interrupted voiding, or feeling of incomplete emptying. This may be the result of an atonic bladder from diabetic neuropathy, a side effect of anticholinergic medication, spinal cord injury, or mechanical obstruction (e.g., prostatic hypertrophy or a large cystocele).

Functional urinary incontinence occurs as a result of inability or unwillingness to get to the toilet because of physical limitations, depression, or confinement to bed or use of restraints. It may be related to dependence on a caregiver for assistance to the toilet.

Nursing interventions begin with an understanding that an older adult is *not* trying to get attention by requesting to go to the bathroom frequently and is not incontinent by choice. Never reprimand or humiliate an older adult for having to urinate or having accidents.

Careful evaluation of incontinence often helps identify *treatable* factors contributing to the incontinence. Treatment options include pharmacology, surgery, use of urethral inserts, and transvaginal or transrectal electrical nerve stimulation. Pharmacologic treatment possibilities include longer-acting versions of oxybutynin and tolterodine, which have fewer side effects. Behavioral therapies, such as pelvic floor–muscle training and bladder retraining, alone or in combination with medication, have the potential to improve UI without adverse effects. Bladder retraining encourages a gradual increase in the time between voidings by designating timed intervals between voidings, rather than responding to each urge to urinate. Pelvic floor–muscle training, also known as Kegel exercises, has been effective in some cases of stress incontinence among women who performed them daily. Biofeedback techniques can be used to teach the exercises to participants by providing observable information about the location and contraction of muscles of the pelvic floor. Many other therapies are also available to assist with stress incontinence, including vaginal cone therapy, electrical stimulation devices, and a urethral plug. Be certain that an older adult has frequent and easy access to a bathroom or a urinal or commode. When other treatments are unsuccessful, many ambulatory older adults are comfortable going out in public if fitted with external collection devices, panty liners, or absorbent briefs. Never refer to an absorbent brief as a diaper when using it for an older adult.

Patient problems and interventions for the older adult with urinary system changes include but are not limited to the following:

Patient Problem	Nursing Interventions
Inability to Control Urination	Collect baseline bladder diaries to assess bladder habits, including frequency of urination and frequency of urinary incontinence Assess circumstances that precipitate incontinence (i.e., coughing, sneezing, position changes, or urgency) Assess awareness of dribbling and ability to control urine elimination

Continued

Patient Problem	Nursing Interventions
	Assess general health, current medications, and past medical problems, current medications, and medical, surgical, and obstetric history Assess use of incontinence products or other responses to incontinence Assess for other urinary symptoms (i.e., burning, pain, blood in the urine, difficulty getting a stream, urgency, or difficulty emptying the bladder) Assess physical and mental factors that may cause the patient to be unable to get to the bathroom on time Assess caregiver's willingness to participate in a behavioral program to treat incontinence
Inability to Control Urination, due to physical stress	Encourage the patient to use the toilet at appropriate intervals Teach pelvic floor exercises Provide toileting assistance and incontinence supplies as needed
Inability to Control Urination, due to urgency	Implement bladder training to increase awareness of the need to toilet Encourage the patient to use the toilet at appropriate intervals Provide information on urge inhibition Teach pelvic floor exercises Restrict caffeine intake, allowing no caffeine in the evening
Inability to Control Urination/ Urgency Due to Overflow	Allow sufficient time for voiding Teach patients the Credé's method (manual expression of urine from the bladder) and encourage double voiding (urinate, relax, and repeat voiding attempt in 5 minutes) Notify the physician for an order for assessment of postvoid residual
Functional Inability to Control Urination	Teach caregiver to implement a prompted voiding program, increasing awareness of the need to toilet and prompting the use of the toilet at appropriate intervals Encourage fluid intake of 1500–2000 mL per day unless contraindicated Modify environment to maximize the patient's ability to get to the bathroom Obtain referral for physical or occupational therapy if indicated

CARDIOVASCULAR SYSTEM

Age-Related Changes

In general, cardiovascular changes with aging involve loss of structural elasticity (Table 33.6). Because the chambers are less elastic, the heart takes longer to contract and the chambers longer to fill. The heart valves become thicker and more rigid. A decrease in pacemaker cells occurs, and the electrical conduction is slowed or altered, which can lead to dysrhythmias. With aging, the resting heart rate tends to decrease, and the heart loses some of its capacity to increase the rate in response to exercise. Arteriosclerosis develops as the blood vessels become less elastic and are lined with deposits, resulting in increased blood pressure. In the past the definition of hypertension in the older adult was less than or equal to a systolic pressure of 140 mm Hg. Some studies identify hypertension in the elderly as a systolic of 150 mm Hg (Ferri et al, 2017). The patient's health care provider will determine the diagnosis of hypertension in the elderly based on individualized factors.

The leading cause of death in the United States is heart disease. Two classifications are used for risk factors: nonmodifiable and modifiable. Age, gender, and family history are nonmodifiable risk factors. Modifiable risk factors include smoking, high blood pressure, a high-fat diet, obesity, physical inactivity, and stress.

Disparities. Although stroke death rates have been decreasing in older adults, the condition remains a growing problem for the African American community. More than 45% of African American men and women have cardiovascular disease (AHA/ASA, 2018). The rate of stroke in this population is twice that of whites (National Stroke Association, n.d.). In addition, those African Americans affected are more likely to die.

Assessment

- Assess for difficulty breathing (dyspnea or orthopnea) aggravated by exertion.
- Assess cough onset and duration.
- Assess for signs of pallor, rubor, or cyanosis.

Table 33.6 Cardiovascular Changes With Aging

PHYSIOLOGIC CHANGE	RESULTS
Decreased cardiac output	Increased incidence of heart failure Decreased peripheral circulation
Decreased elasticity of heart muscle and blood vessels	Decreased venous return Increased dependent edema Increased incidence of orthostatic hypotension Increased varicosities and hemorrhoids
Increased atherosclerosis	Increased blood pressure Increased myocardial infarction

- Assess for chest pain, including onset, duration, relationship to activity, character (aching, burning, crushing), location, radiating, and severity, using a scale of 0 to 10.
- Assess apical and peripheral pulses. Compare both extremities when assessing characteristics of peripheral pulses.
- Assess capillary refill time.
- Assess for presence of vertigo, syncope, and fatigue.
- Assess blood pressure in lying, sitting, and standing positions. Note any significant change between positions (**orthostatic hypotension**).
- Assess for edema. Note location and severity.

Common Concerns and Nursing Interventions

Hypertension. Hypertension (HTN) contributes to coronary artery disease and stroke. It also contributes to the development of heart failure (HF), renal failure, and peripheral vascular disease. Pharmacologic treatment for hypertension in people older than age 60 has decreased the incidence rate of coronary events significantly.

Coronary artery disease. Elevated serum cholesterol level is a major risk factor for coronary artery disease (CAD). A total cholesterol level of 130 mg/dL raises the risk for cardiac disease. Decreasing saturated fat content in the diet assists in reducing cholesterol levels. No more than 7% of calories should come from saturated fat, and no more than 200 mg of cholesterol should be consumed per day (American Heart Association, 2017). The American Heart Association recommends 20 to 30 minutes of moderate intensity exercise three to five times a week. Advise older adults to begin an exercise program with a 10- to 15-minute warm-up to achieve 75% of their maximal heart rate safely. Walking is the best aerobic exercise for older adults. They can set their own pace and choose the location. Encourage older adults with CAD to participate in cardiac rehabilitation programs to restore their physical and mental health to the highest level of function. This often involves several phases, beginning in the hospital and continuing in an outpatient setting (see the Patient Teaching box). A maintenance phase of counseling, exercise, and socialization may continue indefinitely.

Dysrhythmias. Changes in the structure of the heart, the blood supply to the heart, and the pacemaker system sometimes make the heart more susceptible to irregular heart rhythms (dysrhythmias). Dysrhythmias cause the heart to be less effective in supplying blood to the body and have the potential to lead to heart failure. Nursing interventions for patients with dysrhythmias include checking vital signs frequently; noting the rate, regularity, and strength of the pulse; accurately monitoring fluid intake and output (I&O); and observing and reporting an older person's response to medications. Other nursing interventions include keeping stress on the heart to a minimum by monitoring the response to activity and providing appropriate rest periods before and after activity.

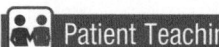

Patient Teaching

Coronary Artery Disease

- Assess the knowledge and understanding of the disease process.
- Discuss the diagnosis, symptoms, and potential complications.
- Explain the purpose, dosage, side effects, and special considerations of all prescribed medications.
- Assess for modifiable cardiac risk factors and instruct the patient on the reduction of risks including:
  - Diet (see Chapter 19)
    - Assess dietary intake.
    - Limit salt intake.
    - Limit intake of canned or processed foods.
  - Exercise
    - As allowed by the health care provider, implement an exercise program.
    - As allowed by the health care provider, implement an exercise program.
    - Seniors should attempt to engage in 150 minutes per week (Traywick, n.d.).
  - Obesity
    - Manage caloric intake to reduce BMI of 18.5–25.9 kg/m^2.
  - Smoking
    - Refrain from tobacco use.
    - Avoid exposure to secondhand smoke.
  - Diabetes mellitus
    - Monitor blood glucose levels daily or as recommended.
    - Maintain prescribed dietary regimens.
    - Exercise as directed.
- Avoid tobacco exposure.
- *Psychological state:* Identify sources of stress and changes that can be made to reduce these stressors.
- Implement positive sleep hygiene habits to ensure rest.

Peripheral vascular disease. Vascular changes affect the arteries or veins of the older adult. Spasms or atherosclerosis allow insufficient amounts of oxygenated blood to circulate to tissues in the legs and feet. Some older adults have inadequate circulation to the muscles, which results in cold feet, numbness, and intermittent **claudication** (cramping pain in the calves). Inadequate supply of arterial blood to the lower extremities results in a condition called peripheral vascular disease (PVD). Another common condition is varicose veins, which involves failure of the valves to close adequately because of distention and weakening of the venous walls.

Nursing interventions include techniques to promote circulation, including walking to stimulate venous return, avoiding standing in one place for long periods, and not crossing the legs. Compression stockings provide support for varicose veins.

When inadequate circulation results in skin ulcerations and altered sensation (numbness), nursing interventions may include compression stockings, pneumatic compression pumps, Unna boots, maintenance of the cleanliness of the feet and legs, adequate shoes that give protection, and education of the older adult to be aware of situations that may cause injury, because sensation for hot and cold is decreased.

A patient problem and interventions for the older adult with peripheral vascular disease include but are not limited to the following:

Patient Problem	Nursing Interventions
Compromised Blood Flow to Tissue, related to circulatory changes with aging	Assess peripheral tissue for color, temperature sensation, movement, and the presence of pain Assess rate, rhythm, and volume of peripheral pulses Assess for the presence of edema. Apply antiembolism stockings as ordered Teach patient to avoid constrictive clothing Establish a walking program to slowly and steadily increase walking distance without pain Administer vasodilating or cardiotonic medications as ordered Handle gently to avoid skin tears. Avoid temperature extremes Discourage smoking

RESPIRATORY SYSTEM

Age-Related Changes

The tissues of the lungs and bronchi become less elastic and more rigid with age. The ribs become less mobile, and osteoporosis and calcification of the cartilage lead to rigidity and stiffness of the thoracic cage. Oxygen-carrying capacity (hemoglobin) often is diminished in older adults. Muscles associated with respiration sometimes weaken so that lung expansion and vital capacity are decreased. Older adults also tend to have a decrease in the number and effectiveness of cilia in the tracheobronchial tree, which results in increased difficulty in clearing secretions and increased risk of respiratory infections. This, together with less elastic alveoli, decreases vital capacity and leads to shortness of breath with activity.

Kyphosis is an abnormal curve in the upper spine sometimes called "dowager's hump." The chest wall is less able to expand because of changes in the skeletal system (Table 33.7). Overall, the older person's air exchange is reduced, and secretions and residual air remain in the lungs.

Table 33.7 Respiratory Changes With Aging

PHYSIOLOGIC CHANGE	RESULTS
Decreased body fluids	Decreased ability to humidify air
Decreased number of cilia	Decreased ability to trap debris
Decreased tissue elasticity	Decreased gas exchange Increased pooling of secretions in lower lobes
Decreased number of capillaries	Decreased gas exchange
Increased calcification of cartilage	Increased rigidity of ribcage Decreased lung capacity
Possible development of kyphosis, an abnormal curve in the upper spine called "dowager's hump"	Chest wall less able to expand because of changes in the skeletal system

In addition, *lifestyle factors* affect lung function. Exercise has a positive effect on the respiratory and cardiovascular systems, whereas immobility has a negative effect. The lung damage that is caused by smoking and by prolonged exposure to secondhand smoke in the lungs of nonsmokers is well known. Obesity results in markedly reduced pulmonary function and increased breathlessness. Diminished cough and arousal reflexes increase the likelihood of aspiration during sleep. The increased sleep time of older adults increases the risk of aspiration and oxygen desaturation from diminished ventilatory drive and a loss of upper airway tone that predisposes to apnea or hypopnea.

Assessment

- Assess depth, rhythm, and rate of respiration at rest and with activity.
- Inspect the chest for shape and symmetry, body position, and use of accessory muscles for respiration.
- Assess breath sounds for adventitious sounds, including crackles and wheezing (inspiratory or expiratory).
- Assess the amount of activity the individual is able to tolerate. Note activities that result in increased respiratory effort.
- Ask the patient to evaluate breathlessness on a scale of 0 to 10.
- Assess for the presence of cough. Note whether cough is productive or nonproductive. Assess amount, frequency, and color of sputum production.

Common Concerns and Nursing Interventions

Chronic obstructive pulmonary disease. A common respiratory condition of older adults, chronic obstructive pulmonary disease (COPD) is not a single disease but commonly a combination of chronic bronchitis, chronic asthma, and emphysema in varying degrees as a result of progressive changes that are seen as individuals become older. A smoking history increases the risk of debilitating COPD. Assessment reveals diminished breath sounds, crackles, and wheezes and a "barrel chest" characterized by an increased anteroposterior diameter. By age 90, nearly everyone has some degree of COPD.

Nursing interventions for older adults with mild to moderate COPD include pulmonary hygiene, breathing retraining, chest physiotherapy, medications, smoking cessation, and exercise programs. Pulmonary hygiene includes encouraging the patient to drink plenty of fluids to liquefy secretions and teaching deep diaphragmatic breathing and a variety of coughing techniques to remove secretions and improve airway clearance. Techniques such as pursed-lip breathing help empty the lungs of used air, which in turn promotes inhalation of adequate oxygen. Chest physiotherapy (CPT) includes chest percussion, postural drainage, vibration, and rib shaking. Postural drainage consists of positioning the patient in a head-down position to facilitate drainage of pulmonary secretions. Medications may be given orally, via a metered-dose inhaler (MDI), or via nebulizer. Oxygen therapy also is considered a medication. The patient and the family need to learn correct oxygen liter flow, when it is to be used, and care and use of the equipment.

Patients must be taught how to adapt their lifestyles and activities of daily living (ADLs). Doing moderate intensity exercises for 20 to 30 minutes 3 to 5 days a week reduces cardiovascular disease risks, improves musculoskeletal function, helps promote weight loss, and helps prevent bone loss in older adults. In the presence of COPD, a program must be started in very small increments, such as walking for 3 to 5 minutes daily. Appropriate exercise intensity maintains a heart rate of at least 55% of the maximal rate for a patient's age, that is, a rate of 88 for a 60-year-old and 80 for a 75-year-old. Classes and exercise times usually allow for socialization with others, emotional support, and the opportunity to get out of the home.

Additional interventions include avoiding smoking and air pollution, preventing infections by avoiding crowds and people with upper respiratory infections, and receiving the flu vaccines annually. Older patients with COPD often find smoking cessation difficult, if not impossible. Success partly depends on the support of family and friends. Programs are available through the American Lung Association, the American Cancer Society, and many community hospitals.

Because respiratory function affects many other systems and the functional ability of the individual, other nursing diagnoses and interventions are likely to be appropriate for a patient with COPD.

Pneumonia. Age-related changes and decreased resistance to respiratory infections cause more older individuals to contract and die of pneumonia than younger people. Even with modern antibiotics and sophisticated medical treatment, pneumonia has the potential to be life threatening for the older adult. This is especially true if an older adult is hospitalized and has other chronic illnesses.

Older individuals do not always exhibit the usual signs and symptoms of pneumonia, such as high fever, cough, pain, and headache. In contrast, they often show signs and symptoms only of lethargy, disorientation, anorexia, and low or mild fever. Older adults who show such signs and symptoms should consult their health care provider for diagnosis and treatment.

Interventions focus on liquefying secretions through adequate intake of fluids, taking prescribed medications, assisting removal of secretions by teaching proper coughing technique to improve airway clearance, and turning and deep breathing to improve gas exchange and prevent stasis of secretions (see the Home Care Considerations box).

Home Care Considerations

Respiratory Disorders

- Encourage fluid intake of 8 to 10 glasses of water a day, if not contraindicated.
- Encourage the older adult to exercise within capacity to promote thoracic muscle conditioning.
- Monitor for smoking and exposure to secondhand smoke. Encourage family members to not smoke in the presence of the older adult.
- Encourage pursed-lip breathing to control breathlessness and improve oxygenation.
- Monitor pulse oximetry to assess oxygenation.
- Encourage frequent small meals to reduce breathlessness associated with eating.
- If home oxygen is used, assess the home environment for potential safety hazards, including the possibility of the older adult tripping over oxygen tubing.
- Assess for confusion, occipital headaches, and forgetfulness. These symptoms may be indicative of carbon dioxide retention. Teach family caregivers these signs as well.

Modified from Meiner SE: *Gerontologic nursing,* ed 4, St. Louis, 2011, Mosby.

Patient problems and interventions for the older adult with respiratory changes include but are not limited to the following:

Patient Problem	Nursing Interventions
Inability to Clear Airway, related to excessive tenacious secretions	Assess respiratory patterns, effort, and lung sounds Observe for signs of cyanosis Teach effective breathing and coughing Promote adequate hydration Suction secretions if necessary Administer supplemental oxygen and nebulizer treatments as ordered

Continued

Patient Problem	Nursing Interventions
	Encourage use of spirometry as ordered
Inefficient Oxygenation, related to elevated CO_2 (carbon dioxide)	Monitor oximetry readings for oxygen saturation Administer oxygen per protocol

Lung cancer. Lung cancer is the leading cause of cancer deaths. It is rare in people under the age of 40 but increases in incidence between ages 60 and 70. Risk factors for developing lung cancer include use of tobacco or marijuana; recurring inflammation; exposure to asbestos, talcum powder, or minerals or, less frequently, to radon; heredity; vitamin A deficiency; and air pollution. The most common form of lung cancer is small-cell lung carcinoma (SCLC), which sometimes metastasizes to the central nervous system, the bones, and the liver. Often no signs or symptoms are evident, or the signs are ignored or attributed to smoking or a preexisting lung disease. Nonspecific signs and symptoms may include cough, chest pain, and hemoptysis. The diagnosis of lung cancer is based on clinical history and chest x-ray studies or computed tomographic (CT) scan of the chest. Lung cancer staging provides the basis for treatment. Stage I is treatable with surgery. Treatment modalities for other stages include surgery, radiotherapy, and adjuvant chemotherapy. Stage IV treatment is palliative and includes radiotherapy, chemotherapy, and laser therapy. Nursing interventions include relief of pain, emotional support, counseling, and discussion of options and alternatives.

MUSCULOSKELETAL SYSTEM

Age-Related Changes

Some of the most obvious changes associated with aging occur in the musculoskeletal system. A gradual reduction is seen in the number and the size of active muscle fibers, and muscle tone, mass, and strength are decreased. The joints become less elastic and flexible with the loss and the calcification of cartilage. An alteration occurs in the equilibrium between bone deposition and resorption (Fig. 33.6). Falling estrogen levels in women increases bone resorption and decreases calcium deposition, resulting in bone loss and decreased bone density. The long bones and the vertebrae are especially vulnerable to the reduction of bone density. In the spine, narrowing of the intervertebral spaces results in a loss of 1½ to 3 inches of height. The lumbar curve of the lower back changes, which results in a shift in the center of gravity. Structural and postural changes may result in changes to the gait. The risk of fractures is increased in this population as a result of the interrelated factors (Table 33.8).

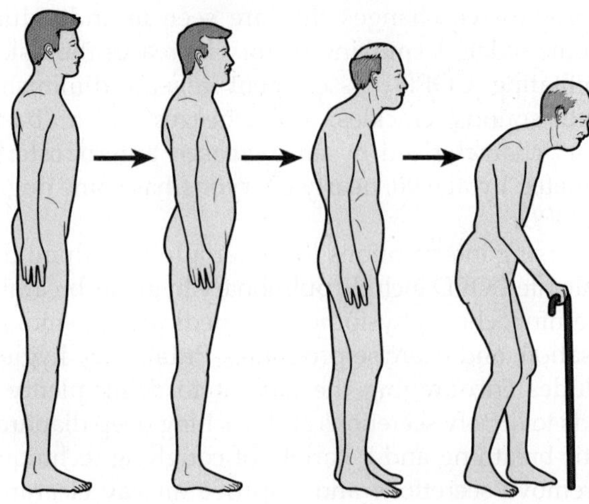

Fig. 33.6 Posture changes with aging.

Table 33.8 Musculoskeletal Changes With Aging

PHYSIOLOGIC CHANGE	RESULTS
Decreased bone calcium	Osteoporosis Increased curvature of the spine (kyphosis)
Decreased fluid in intervertebral disks	Decreased height
Decreased blood supply to muscles	Decreased muscle strength
Decreased joint mobility	Decreased mobility and flexibility
Decreased muscle mass	Decreased strength Increased risk of falls

Assessment

- Assess active and passive range of motion of each joint for stiffness and limitation of movement.
- Assess joints for edema, erythema, pain, and crepitus with particular motions.
- Assess ability to perform personal care (i.e., eating, bathing, dressing, grooming, and elimination) and other activities (i.e., housework, driving, climbing stairs, caring for pets).
- Assess standing and gait, including balance, posture, base of support, size of steps, and ability to turn.
- Assess for limping, numbness or tingling, deformity, and change in skeletal contour.
- Assess for muscle weakness, paralysis, tremors, spasms, clumsiness, muscle wasting, and muscle aches.
- Assess pain using a scale of 0 to 10, location, type, onset (sudden or gradual), aggravating or alleviating factors, and position of comfort.
- Assess history of falls, traumatic injury, surgeries on joint or bone, and back problems.

Common Concerns and Nursing Interventions

Arthritis. Two forms of arthritis may occur in the older adult. Rheumatoid arthritis, a systemic inflammatory

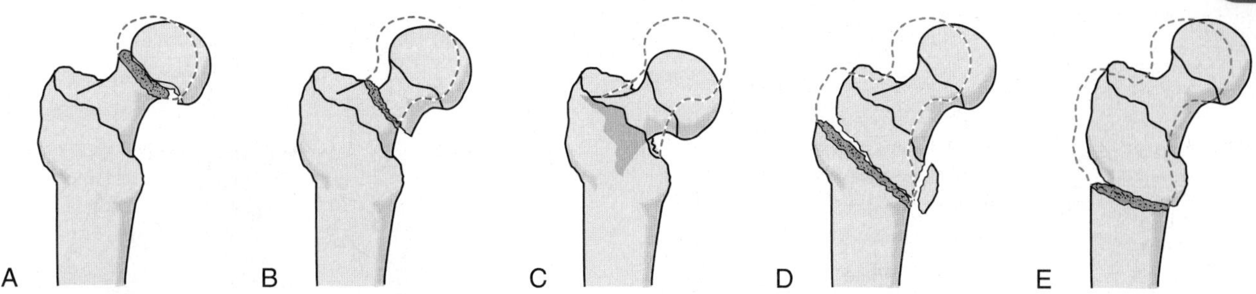

Fig. 33.7 Types of fractures of the hip. A, Subcapital fracture. B, Transcervical fracture. C, Impacted fracture of the base of the neck. D, Intertrochanteric fracture. E, Subtrochanteric fracture. (From Monahan FD, Sands J, Neighbors M, et al: *Phipps' medical-surgical nursing: Health and illness perspectives*, ed 8, St. Louis, 2007, Mosby.)

disease thought to be of immune factor origin, has the potential to affect people of any age. Osteoarthritis, or degenerative joint disease, is a noninflammatory disorder in which the cartilage in the joints deteriorates and new bone forms on the surface. This is the most common type of arthritis in older adults. Affected joints most commonly include the hands, fingers, and toes and the knees, hips, and spine.

Because the chronic nature of osteoarthritis affects an individual's functional ability and lifestyle, interventions for older individuals with arthritis involve joint protection and energy conservation through a balance between rest and exercise. Simple measures such as a warm bath or shower in the morning often reduce early morning stiffness. Recommend range-of-motion and other forms of mild exercise to maintain muscle strength and joint motion. Heat or cold therapy and gentle massage usually help to control pain and muscle spasms. Health care providers often prescribe NSAIDs and nonopioid analgesics. Injections of steroids into the joints two or three times yearly may help with chronic pain.

In more advanced situations, use of assistive devices is common (i.e., splints, walkers, adapted utensils, and clothes with Velcro fasteners). With increasing disability and severe pain, many people consider surgical options. Joint arthroplasty, a surgical replacement of the involved joint, is successful in treating arthritic pain in the shoulders, elbows, fingers, hips, and knees. Other surgical options include joint fusion, which increases function and decreases pain while eliminating some joint movement.

Hip fractures. According to the CDC (2016), one out of five falls result in serious injuries, such as broken bones or a head injury, and more than 800,000 patients are admitted each year because of head injuries or hip fractures resulting from a fall. The most frequently occurring fractures among older adults are hip, vertebral, and clavicular fractures. Fractures fall into two categories, open or closed, and vary according to location and type. The history of the patient with a fracture usually includes trauma followed by immediate local pain. Tenderness, edema, muscle spasm, deformity, bleeding, and loss of function are other manifestations common with fractures.

A fall may not be the precipitating factor in hip fractures. Commonly, weakening of the upper femur from osteoporosis causes the bone to break—and then the fall occurs (Ignatavicius and Workman, 2016). Hip fractures are the most disabling type of fracture in older adults. A significant percentage of patients with hip fracture die within 1 year after injury. Clinicians use the locations of hip fractures to classify them. Intracapsular or subcapital fractures occur within the hip capsule. Extracapsular fractures occur below the capsule and include intertrochanteric and subtrochanteric (Fig. 33.7).

When a hip fracture occurs, the affected extremity usually is rotated externally and shortened. Tenderness and severe pain at the fracture site are often present. Immobilization of the joint is necessary. Surgical repair is the preferred treatment when the patient's condition has stabilized. Surgery depends on the location and type of fracture and often includes open reduction and internal fixation (ORIF) with pins, plates, and screws for extracapsular fractures (Fig. 33.8A) or prosthetic replacement of the femoral head for intracapsular fractures (bipolar or hemiarthroplasty; Fig. 33.8B).

Nursing interventions after surgery require monitoring of vital signs and I&O. Frequent turning, deep breathing, coughing, and an incentive spirometer are used to prevent respiratory complications. Monitor the operative site for signs of infection and bleeding. Assess movement, circulation, and sensation of the extremity to detect impaired circulation. Monitor mental status. Postoperative delirium is possible from the anesthesia, the analgesic medications, pain, immobility, and loss of familiar surroundings. Opioid analgesics should be used cautiously. Practitioners often use lower doses of opioids to prevent changes in mental status, respiratory depression, and oversedation.

The affected extremity is kept in alignment to help keep pain to a minimum. Use pillows between the knees or an abduction splint to accomplish this. Patients who have hemiarthroplasty are at risk for dislocation, which is most likely to occur when the joint is adducted and internally rotated. Avoid movements such as crossing

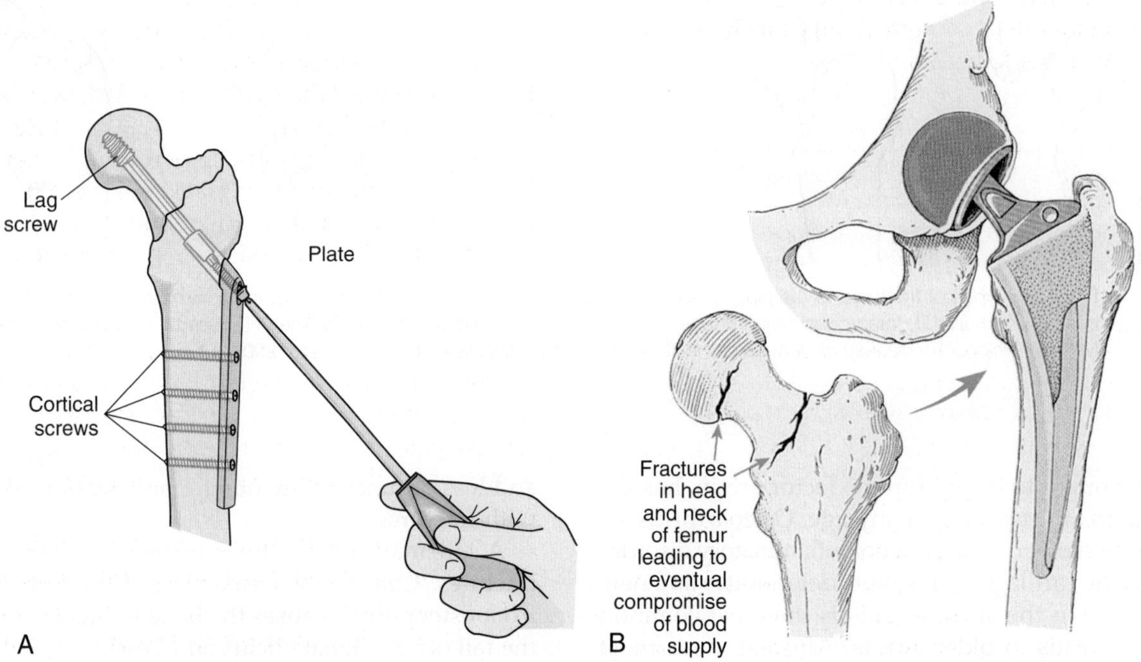

Fig. 33.8 A, Open reduction and internal fixation (ORIF) with nails, screws, or rods. B, Bipolar or hemiarthroplasty. (A, From Monahan FD, Sands J, Neighbors M, et al: *Phipps' medical-surgical nursing: Health and illness perspectives,* ed 8, St. Louis, 2007, Mosby.)

the legs and feet while the patient is seated and adducting the legs when the patient is lying on the unoperated side. Instruct patients to use a raised toilet seat and a shower chair, and avoid activities that have potential to cause dislocation of the hip for 6 weeks or more after surgery until the muscles that surround the joint are healed and the joint has stabilized.

Comprehensive multidisciplinary rehabilitation focuses on the goal of returning the patient to the previous level of function. Specific areas of treatment include gait and transfer training, muscle strengthening through active assistive exercises, and teaching the use of assistive devices such as walkers and canes. During recovery, it is important to prevent depression resulting from limited independence. Consistently point out the patient's strengths, give positive feedback, and reinforce progress.

Osteoporosis. Osteoporosis, a systemic skeletal disease, is one of the most common conditions in older women. The characteristic low bone mass and deterioration of bone tissue result in a significantly increased risk of fractures. Fractures are possible in the course of routine activities such as bending, lifting, coughing, and straining at stool. Osteoporosis of the spinal vertebrae may cause a loss of height of 1½ to 3 inches or kyphosis, the development of a C shape to the cervical vertebrae, which causes a stoop that is at times severe. The visible hump on the back is also called the dowager's hump. Although osteoporosis tends to be considered a disease of old age, it actually begins in younger women. Prevention begins with children and adolescents. A diet high in calcium and vitamin D and regular weight-bearing exercise lay the foundation for later life. Bone density testing helps identify older women at risk for fractures and points the way to instituting preventive measures. Advise all women to avoid smoking and excessive alcohol and limit caffeine consumption. Additional information for osteoporosis education is available through the National Osteoporosis Foundation at *www.nof.org*.

For some women, osteoporosis prevention includes reducing estrogen deficiency from perimenopause with hormone replacement therapy (HRT), but its use is controversial. Although HRT has a positive effect on calcium absorption, it possibly contributes to an increased incidence of endometrial cancer, an increased risk for breast cancer, and an increase in cardiovascular disease and stroke; therefore practitioners generally do not prescribe estrogen for osteoporosis except for limited periods.

Older women need 1200 to 2000 mg of calcium daily and 600 to 800 IU daily (Mayo Clinic, 2015). Sixty percent of patients with hip fractures have a deficiency of vitamin D. Bisphosphonates are the most common classification of medications prescribed to treat osteoporosis. These include alendronate (Fosamax), risedronate (Actonel), zoledronic acid (Reclast), and ibandronate (Boniva). These medications improve bone density and lessen the rate of bone loss.

Patient problems and interventions for the older adult with musculoskeletal system changes include but are not limited to the following:

Patient Problem	Nursing Interventions
Self-care deficit, related to weakness • Bathing/hygiene • Dressing/grooming • Feeding • Toileting	Assess ability to dress, feed, bathe, and toilet self Develop plan to enhance highest level of function Allow adequate time to perform activities Provide assistive devices as indicated Consult with physical and occupational therapy Modify environment to facilitate self-care
Potential for Falling, related to age-related changes	Assess balance, gait, strength, medications that cause vertigo or drowsiness, sensory problems, and impaired mobility Maintain a regular weight-bearing exercise routine that is enjoyable Provide good lighting and assistive devices (walkers or canes) to assist balance Eliminate environmental hazards, clutter, uneven walking surfaces, and scatter rugs Encourage moving slowly from lying to standing to keep orthostatic hypotension (a sudden drop in blood pressure when standing up quickly) to a minimum

ENDOCRINE SYSTEM

Age-Related Changes

The levels of hormones secreted and the response of body tissue to hormones change with age (Table 33.9). Thyroid disturbances, especially hypothyroidism and diabetes mellitus, are the common endocrine disorders in the older adult.

Assessment

- Assess laboratory results and report abnormal calcium, glucose, or thyroid hormone levels.

Common Concerns and Nursing Interventions

Type 2 diabetes mellitus. There are two general types of diabetes mellitus (DM): type 1 (formerly called insulin-dependent diabetes mellitus [IDDM] or juvenile diabetes), in which the body fails to produce insulin; and type 2 (formerly called non–insulin dependent [NIDDM] or adult-onset diabetes), which is characterized by the body's inability to produce and use insulin appropriately. Type 2 DM is more common than type 1 DM, and it affects 85% to 90% of adults with diabetes. Patients do not always exhibit the usual signs or symptoms of thirst, increased appetite, and large amounts of urine, as seen in type 1 diabetes mellitus. Repeated infections, slow healing, blurred vision, and weight gain or loss tend to be the initial signs and symptoms of diabetes mellitus that are more commonly seen in older adults.

The goal of interventions in type 2 diabetes mellitus is to achieve and maintain a stable metabolic state through diet management, weight control, and exercise. Diabetic education includes topics such as medication, the disease process, monitoring of blood glucose, signs and symptoms of hyperglycemia and hypoglycemia, sick-day management, foot care, eye care, and various other complications. Active involvement of the patient and family in the disease and plan of treatment promotes retention of information and compliance. Resources for patient educational handouts are available from the American Diabetes Association (ADA), and other sources.

When working with the older adult, assist in adapting a diet that meets the recommendations but also encompasses as many of the individual's personal dietary preferences as possible. This helps improve compliance. Goals should focus on achieving a BMI and weight within an acceptable range for the height and weight. A reduction in weight reduces the insulin resistance of the body's cells. Advise the person to balance intake with recommended amounts of protein, carbohydrates, fats, vitamins, and minerals. Encourage limiting refined sugar and choosing a high-fiber diet.

Older adults with DM are at a higher risk for foot problems because of changes in peripheral nerves and blood vessels. Inadequate blood flow to the feet and nerve damage contribute to the development of ulcers and infections. Hyperglycemia also plays a role because

Table 33.9 Endocrine Changes With Aging

PHYSIOLOGIC CHANGE	RESULTS
Decreased pituitary excretions of adrenocorticotropic hormone (ACTH) and steroids	Decreased muscle mass
Decreased production of thyroid-stimulating hormone	Decreased basal metabolic rate
Decreased production of parathyroid hormone (seen with osteoporosis)	Increased blood calcium levels
Decreased production and use of insulin	Increased blood glucose levels
Decreased release of testosterone, estrogen, and progesterone	Menopause in women and multiple system changes

a blood glucose level of 200 mg/100 mL or higher is associated with an altered immune system leukocyte response. Although the rate of limb amputations in patients with diabetes has declined over the past two decades to a rate of 4 per 1000 patients, the operative loss of a limb is life altering to the patient. *Peripheral neuropathy* is the presence of abnormal sensation, numbness, and burning sensations in the extremities. This condition increases with age, particularly in people who have DM. Decreased awareness of pain, temperature changes, and diminished circulation result in risk for injury. Undetected injuries become infected easily and, if untreated, in some cases necessitate eventual amputation. Activities that promote good circulation include avoiding smoking, avoiding constricting footwear, and keeping legs uncrossed.

To prevent foot injuries, recommend daily cleansing of the feet with nondrying agents and daily inspection of the feet for blisters, cuts, or infections with a mirror. Nails are best cut or filed straight across to prevent skin injury. Recommend regular visits to a podiatrist or a health care provider who inspects the feet. Counsel individuals with neuropathy of the feet, hyperglycemia, or a history of foot infections to seek care at the first sign of a foot injury or infection.

Hypothyroidism. Aging has an impact on the thyroid gland. Over time the thyroid's function may become impaired. Neoplasms and hypothyroidism and hyperthyroidism increase in likelihood with aging. The clinical manifestations of hypo- and hyperthyroidism are more subtle. Of people older than 65 years of age 20% have thyroid problems, the most frequent of which is hypothyroidism (Touhy and Jett, 2012). Decreased thyroid function often appears in a subclinical form, and the health care provider becomes aware of it through the results of routine serum testing. Almost all cases are inconspicuous and progress slowly toward thyroid failure. Signs frequently linked to hypothyroidism in older adults include unexplained elevation in triglycerides or plasma cholesterol, nonspecific cognitive impairment, slow metabolism, chest pain or atrial fibrillation, constipation, macrocytic anemia, vague arthritic reports, cold intolerance, and depression with underlying apathy and withdrawal. The goal for interventions is stabilization of thyroid levels with medication (levothyroxine). The practitioner monitors the response to therapy through thyroid-stimulating hormone (TSH) levels. Nursing interventions center on patient and family education related to disease signs and symptoms and medication therapy. Careful management of medication therapy is essential. With treatment, patients generally experience increased energy and weight loss.

REPRODUCTIVE SYSTEM

Age-Related Changes

The major changes in the reproductive system related to aging are diminished levels of estrogen and progesterone in women and diminished levels of androgen and testosterone in men. The process of aging diminishes sexual function but does not put a halt to it. The lack of the circulating hormone testosterone in men and estrogen, progesterone, and androgen in women results in changes with arousal, orgasm, post-orgasm, and genitalia. Although it takes longer for a man to be sexually aroused and achieve erection and ejaculation, men maintain the ability for sexual function into their 80s and 90s. For women, menopause is marked by a decrease in hormones, the inability to procreate, and tissue atrophy of ovaries, fallopian tubes, cervix, and vulva. A decrease is seen in the amount of vaginal secretions, and the pH becomes more alkaline. Although age-related changes occur, they do not diminish the older woman's capacity to achieve orgasm and enjoy sexual relations (Table 33.10).

The provision of holistic care requires the introduction of subjects that may be difficult. Sexuality and any related concerns should be included in the assessment. To begin the assessment, consider making a general statement about the continuing sexual needs of older adults. After this, open-ended questions regarding the patient's sexuality are likely to be useful. For example:

"Tell me how you express your sexuality."

"What concerns do you have about fulfilling your continuing sexual needs?"

"In what ways has your sexual relationship with your partner changed as you have aged?"

The PLISSIT model has been used to assess and manage adults' sexuality. The model includes obtaining

Table 33.10 Reproductive Changes With Aging

PHYSIOLOGIC CHANGE	RESULTS
Female	
Decreased estrogen levels	Vagina shortens, narrows, and loses some of its elasticity Decreased vaginal secretions Decreased pubic hair Increased vaginal tissue fragility and irritation Decreased size of uterus and vagina Increased pain with intercourse (dyspareunia) Decreased breast tissue mass
Increased vaginal alkalinity	Increased risk of infection
Male	
Decreased testosterone	Decreased amount of facial and pubic hair Lack of energy Erectile dysfunction Decrease in libido
Decreased circulation	Decreased rate of ejaculation Decreased force of ejaculation Decreased speed gaining erection

permission from individuals to initiate sexual discussion, providing the *l*imited *i*nformation they need to function sexually, giving *s*pecific *s*uggestions for individuals to proceed with sexual relations, and providing *i*ntensive *t*herapy regarding the issues of sexuality. The goal of assessment is to gather information that allows individuals to express sexuality safely and to feel uninhibited by normal or pathologic problems.

Nurses and nursing students commonly feel uncomfortable with assessing the sexual desires and functions of older patients. Regardless, a sexual assessment is a necessary part of the routine nursing assessment. Skill and comfort come with practice.

Assessment

- Assess past experiences or difficulties and sexually transmitted infections (STIs).
- Assess for signs of vaginal or penile ulceration, edema, or discharge.
- Assess for presence of lumps, dimpling, or drainage from the breast.

Common Concerns and Nursing Interventions

Sexual function. The misconceptions that older adults are impotent and asexual or that they are perverse if they are sexually active are common reasons for sexual dysfunction in older adults. If individuals continue to be sexually active on a regular basis, they retain the capability to respond sexually. If an older adult indicates that sexual intercourse is difficult or uncomfortable because of vaginal dryness, suggest use of estrogen creams or water-soluble lubricants to relieve the discomfort.

Research and information from a variety of sources indicate that aging individuals have the potential to be sexual, continue to have interest in sex, and are indeed sexual beings. For many older adults, the lack of a sexual partner is the main factor for decreased sexual activity.

Sexuality also encompasses sexual identity as a man or woman, intimacy (emotional closeness to others), and touch. Regardless of age, it is important to feel good about oneself as a male or female and to have close relationships with other people. Sexual intimacy is more than intercourse; it includes caressing, stroking, and kissing and being an emotional companion to the partner. A positive correlation exists between sexuality and physical health. This relationship makes the preservation of sexual activity and function a source of health promotion. To best assist patients and their significant others, examine your feelings about sexuality and aging and become informed about age-related changes in sexual function. The sexuality of older adults can also be supported by encouraging and helping them to look their best, complimenting them when they look nice, respecting and allowing them to have their privacy, allowing their expressions of affection for one another, and using touch to communicate acceptance. A pat on the arm or a hug is a potential way to communicate concern and caring to almost anyone.

A patient problem and interventions for the older adult with sexual dysfunction include but are not limited to the following:

Patient Problem	Nursing Interventions
Impaired Sexual Expression, related to lack of privacy	Allow verbalization of concerns regarding sexual needs Provide privacy for interaction between alert, consenting individuals Assist individual to maintain good physical hygiene and meet cosmetic needs Provide distraction and alternative activities for disoriented individuals who masturbate; if unsuccessful, provide privacy

SENSORY PERCEPTION

Age-Related Changes

The senses provide a link with the environment by receiving and interpreting various stimuli including but not limited to vision, hearing, taste, and smell (Table 33.11). Visual and hearing impairments interfere

Table 33.11 Sensory Changes With Aging

PHYSIOLOGIC CHANGE	RESULTS
Vision	
Decreased number of eyelashes	Increased risk of eye injury
Decreased tear production	Increased risk of eye irritation
Increased discoloration of lens	Decreased color perception
Decreased tissue elasticity	Increased blurring
Decreased muscle tone	Decreased diameter of pupil Increased refractive errors Decreased night vision Increased sensitivity to glare
Hearing	
Decreased tissue elasticity	Decreased ability to distinguish high-frequency sounds
Decreased joint mobility	Decreased ability to distinguish high-frequency sounds Decreased hearing ability
Decreased number of hair cells in inner ear	Increased problems with balance
Taste and Smell	
Decreased number of papillae on tongue	Decreased ability to taste
Decreased number of nasal sensory receptors	Decreased ability to detect smells

with communication, social interactions, and mobility, leading to social isolation. In the past, we recognized five senses: sight, hearing, taste, smell, and touch. Today we acknowledge additional senses and categorize all senses into two major groups: general and special. General senses include touch, pressure, pain, temperature, vibration, and proprioception. Special senses are produced by highly localized organs and sensory cells including sight, hearing, taste, smell, and balance. Sensation, or perception, is the conscious awareness and interpretation of sensory stimuli by sensory receptors.

Vision. Visual changes increase with aging. Significant changes are associated with ages over 65 years. The pupil is reduced in size. Acclimating to changes in light in the room becomes increasingly difficult. The muscles of the eyes become less effective causing changes in visual acuity. Discerning differing colors of similar hue becomes difficult. Tear production is also lessened (US National Library of Medicine, 2018). Visual impairments can lead to injury because of falls. The four leading causes of visual impairment are cataracts, glaucoma, macular degeneration, and diabetic retinopathy (Stibich, 2017). Undiagnosed visual disorders are increasing among older adults, especially in ethnic and cultural minorities.

Age-related changes in vision include **presbyopia** (farsightedness resulting from a loss of elasticity of the lens of the eye), or narrowing of the peripheral field of vision, decreased ability to focus on near objects, and a decrease in visual acuity as the pupil becomes smaller and less responsive to light. There is some clouding of the lens of the eye. Yellowing of the lens and changes in color perception cause older adults to have difficulty differentiating shades of some colors such as green, blue, and violet. Depth perception is distorted, and vision in dim light becomes difficult. General vision screening for individuals who wear glasses or contact lenses involves observation of reading print from a newspaper. Note the distance from the eyes the person holds the newspaper, and verify the person's ability to see print clearly (Fig. 33.9). Limited vision indicates the need for a more detailed eye examination. Although age-related changes decrease visual capability, blindness is not a normal result of aging.

Glaucoma. Glaucoma, the second leading cause of blindness in the United States, is caused by an occlusion in the drainage of the fluid in the anterior chamber of the eye, which produces an increase in intraocular pressure. Pressure transfers to the optic nerve, where damage or blindness is a possible result. Primary open-angle glaucoma, the most common type, makes up 90% of all cases of primary glaucoma. This type of glaucoma has the capacity to reduce vision so gradually and painlessly that a person is unaware of a problem until the optic nerve is badly damaged. Visual loss begins with deteriorating peripheral vision. Early diagnoses

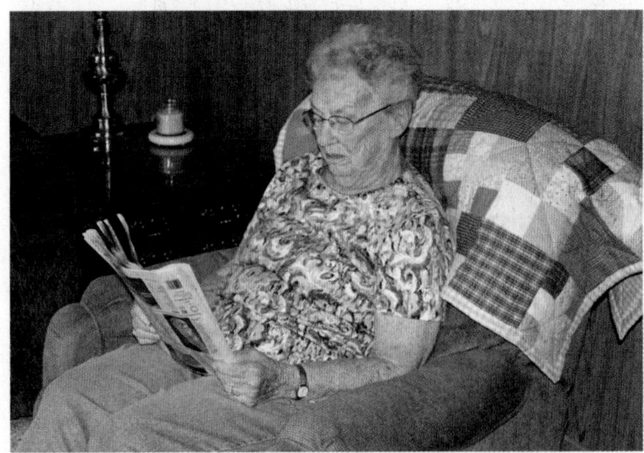

Fig. 33.9 Vision screening with use of a newspaper.

of primary open-angle glaucoma allows for control and prevention of serious visual impairment (National Eye Institute, 2015).

In contrast, acute angle-closure glaucoma occurs suddenly as a result of complete occlusion in the path of the aqueous humor. Signs and symptoms of acute angle-closure glaucoma include severe eye pain, erythema, clouded or blurred vision, nausea and vomiting, rainbow halo surrounding lights, pupil dilation, and a steamy appearance of the cornea. Severe problems develop in acute angle-closure glaucoma when intraocular pressure rises above 50 mm Hg (normal range is 10 to 22 mm Hg). In the absence of emergency medical attention, severe vision loss occurs; blindness results in 2 days. An iridectomy is a helpful option to reduce the intraocular pressure (Glaucoma Research Foundation, 2017).

Medical follow-up and eye medication are required for the rest of the person's life. Eye drops are necessary to continue even in the absence of symptoms. After administration of eye drops, pressure on the lacrimal duct for 1 minute prevents rapid systemic absorption. Use a medical-alert bracelet or card to identify glaucoma and the prescribed eye drop solution.

Cataracts. Cataracts are the most common disorder found in the aging eye. By the age of 80 an estimated 50% of people either have cataracts or have had surgery to correct them. A cataract is a clouding of the normally clear and transparent lens of the eye. Degenerative changes to the lens protein and fatty deposits (lipofuscin) in the lens are causative factors in the development of cataract. The lens focuses light on the retina to produce a sharp image. When a cataract forms, the lens sometimes becomes so opaque that the transmission of light to the retina becomes impossible. The size and the location of a cataract determine the amount of interference with sight. Cataract symptoms include dimmed, blurred, or misty vision; the need for brighter light to read; and sensitivity to glare and light.

Management and treatment of cataracts is conservative until visual impairments affect normal activities such as reading and driving. Several types of surgery exist, but the most recent technique involves the use of ultrasound to break the lens into small fragments, which allows removal from a tiny incision. A substitute lens is used to restore vision, which is a permanent, plastic intraocular lens. Cataract surgery is highly successful.

Hearing and balance. It is possible to consider the organs of hearing and balance in three parts: the external ear, the middle ear, and the inner ear. The inner ear is involved in hearing and balance. Hearing loss is not a normal part of aging and is necessary to evaluate.

The incidence of hearing impairments in older adults is frequent. Losses may be sudden in onset or occur over gradually. Between the ages of 65 and 74 years about one-third of people have a hearing impairment. For those over the age of 75 years this sharply increases to almost half of this population. Aging causes rigidity of the ossicles, which results in a loss of elasticity (National Institute on Deafness and Other Communication Disorders, 2017). Atrophic changes of the auditory nerve and end organs of the inner ear affect hearing. Because of exposure to a variety of loud noises throughout life and age-related changes, older individuals often have hearing losses of different tones, which cause some sounds to be distorted and others to be absent. Older adults often deny their hearing loss and need encouragement and support to explore various methods to improve hearing.

Cerumen impaction is a reversible, often overlooked cause of conductive hearing loss. Assess for itching and a feeling of ear fullness. Removal of the blockage sometimes restores hearing acuity and relieves symptoms associated with impaction. Removal includes instillation of a softening agent. The health care provider then irrigates the ear with a syringe device on its low setting, and finishes by draining excessive fluid from the ear.

Hearing impairment falls into three categories: conductive, sensorineural, and mixed. Conductive hearing loss results from interruption of the transmission of sound through the external auditory canal and middle ear and usually is related to cerumen impaction, otitis media, and fixation of the auditory ossicles.

Sensorineural hearing loss results when the inner ear, the auditory nerve, the brainstem, or the cortical auditory pathways do not function properly so that sound waves are not interpreted correctly. Mixed hearing loss is a conductive hearing loss superimposed on a sensorineural hearing loss.

Presbycusis is a sensorineural hearing loss and the most common form of loss in older adults. Typically, the loss is bilateral, resulting in difficulty hearing high-pitched tones and conversational speech. The sounds usually lost first are *f, s, th, ch,* and *sh.* As hearing loss progresses, the sounds of *b, t, p, k,* and *s* also become difficult to distinguish. The cause is unclear. Indications of hearing loss include behaviors such as increasing the volume on the television or the radio, tilting the head toward the person speaking, cupping a hand around one ear, trouble following conversation when more than one person is speaking, watching the speaker's lips, speaking loudly, and not responding when spoken to. Diagnosis involves audiometric evaluation. Treatment options include surgical placement with a cochlear implant, hearing devices, and auditory rehabilitation to facilitate communication.

Nursing interventions to improve communication with hearing loss include providing good visual contact to allow lip reading, avoiding situations in which there is glare or shadows on the person's field of vision, reducing or eliminating background noise, and speaking at a normal rate and volume. Do not overarticulate or shout. Use short sentences, and pause at the end of each sentence. Use facial expressions or gestures to give clues. Ask listeners what assists them to hear better, and be patient.

Touch. Touch involves tactile information involving pressure, vibration, and temperature. Age-related changes that affect the sense of touch and position include a decrease in the number of receptor cells throughout the skin and joints. Older adults have increasing difficulty sensing temperature and maintaining balance, which places them at risk for burns and falls. The most common disorders to affect tactile ability include stroke, PVD, and diabetic neuropathy. All these conditions involve decreased blood flow to various parts of the body. Nursing interventions should focus on prevention of accidental trauma and injury in the affected limbs.

Smell and taste. Olfactory receptors decline in number, which tends to reduce or alter a person's ability to smell. A decrease is also seen in the number of taste buds, which often influences appetite and causes the person to use more seasoning.

Assessment of the Sensory Organs

- Assess eyes for dryness, tearing, or signs of irritation.
- Assess ability of individual to see close up and at a distance. Ask about problems with or recent changes in vision.
- Assess hearing; note use of hearing aids and effectiveness.
- Assess for reported changes in taste or smell.

Common Concerns and Nursing Interventions

Decreased vision. With increasing age comes decreasing visual capability. Many interventions are possible to compensate for age-related changes in vision; be sure the patient's eyeglasses are clean and are available, increase the amount of light in the environment, reduce glare with use of shades on windows and lights, and use nightlights to avoid abrupt light-to-dark changes. The use of low-vision aids such as large print, strongly contrasting colors (black on a white background), and magnifying glasses helps compensate for the decrease in visual acuity.

Decreased hearing. The decreased ability to hear is frequently a frustration to the older adults who are affected and the individuals who are trying to talk to them. Hearing aids sometimes help in situations in which amplification has the potential to improve hearing, but hearing aids do not compensate for nerve damage or effectively screen out other distracting noises. To communicate with an individual with a hearing loss, face the individual and speak at a normal or slightly slower pace without exaggerating or shouting, lower the tone of voice (because hearing loss is frequently in the higher tones), and eliminate background noise whenever possible. Another effective communication technique is using nonverbal communication such as gestures, smiles, nodding the head with the verbal message, and written communication. When communication is difficult, carefully avoid expressing annoyance or impatience to the patient who has a hearing loss (Fig. 33.10).

A patient problem and interventions for the older adult with altered senses include but are not limited to the following:

Patient Problem	Nursing Interventions
Disturbed sensory perception (specify)	Assess for sensory changes Alert all caregivers to sensory problems of the individual Determine most effective methods of communicating with individual with sensory impairment Modify environment to remove hazards and reduce risks Verify that assistive devices such as hearing aids or glasses are clean and functional

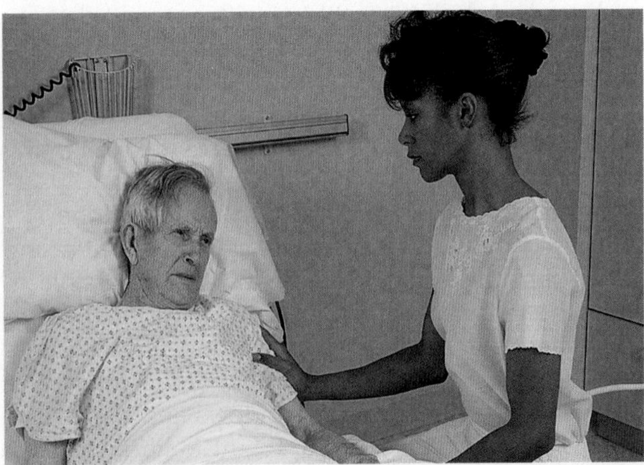

Fig. 33.10 The nurse listens to the frustrated older adult with patience and compassion.

NERVOUS SYSTEM

Age-Related Changes

Structural and functional changes of the nervous system are complex and depend on a number of variables, including the individual's genetic makeup and the specific brain regions affected. Changes associated with aging include a decline in the number of brain cells and peripheral nerve cells and fibers, and synaptic changes that affect transmission and the sensitivity of target cells to neurotransmitters. Physiologically, nerve impulse transmission in the nervous system slows, resulting in a longer reaction time for older adults. Until recently, neuron death was accepted widely as an inevitable result of normal aging. Age-related declines in neuron numbers are not a significant part of normal aging. Unless pathologic degeneration occurs, changes in neuron size and weight bring few if any negative behavioral effects. Autonomic nervous system changes include decreased efficiency in maintaining normal body temperature and in the pulse returning to normal after exercise or stress (Table 33.12).

Functional ability in older people does not consistently decline. Changes in sensorimotor and motor function, memory, cognition, sleep patterns, and proprioception occur at varying rates. Distinctive patterns of behavior, thoughts, and emotions, which constitute an individual's personality, generally remain consistent during normal aging.

Memory. Common memory concerns for older adults include forgetting names, misplacing items, and poor recall of recent events or conversations. Changes in short-term memory are common with aging. Long-term recall usually is maintained. Strategies for adapting, such as making lists or posting reminders, are useful to manage short-term memory loss.

Cognition. The process by which information is acquired, stored, shared, and used is termed cognitive function. The elements of this process include state of consciousness, general appearance and behavior, orientation, memory, language, intelligence, perception, insight and problem-solving ability, judgment, attention span, and mood and affect. Outcomes from cognitive function are thinking, remembering, perceiving, communicating,

Table 33.12 Neurologic Changes With Aging

PHYSIOLOGIC CHANGE	RESULTS
Decreased number of brain cells	Decreased reflexes
Decreased number of nerve fibers	Decreased coordination
Decreased number of neuroreceptors	Decreased perception of stimuli Decreased motor responses

and calculating. Many people think that cognitive abilities decline in old age. Only some older people experience some deficits, and the decline occurs at different times in their lives. Generalizations about cognitive decline in older adults are inappropriate. Intelligence and continued ability to learn is possible throughout the lifetime. Teaching strategies may need modification, and learning may require reinforcement because of the age-related changes in the senses and nervous system.

Sleep. Sleep disturbances are reported frequently by older adults. The causes for these complaints are varied. Difficulty sleeping may be related to an inability to go to sleep or interrupted sleep. Reports may include feelings that the sleep achieved is not of a good restful quality. Causes may be physiologic and relate to a disease such as Alzheimer's disease, changes to the body's natural clock, or secondary to pain from another illness. The roots of sleep disorders may be psychological and linked to depression or other mental health concerns. Medications including diuretics and corticosteroids may interrupt sleep. Alcohol and drugs can alter the pattern of sleep or totally interrupt it. The intake or use of stimulants such as nicotine or caffeine will limit sleep.

Proprioception. Proprioception, the ability to maintain an upright position without falling, depends on the ability to use balance, posture, and movement. This requires a great deal of sensory input, motor output, and central integration of balance and locomotion. Aging results in slower reflexes, diminished strength of muscles for posture, and increased postural sway. Conditions such as damage to the structures of the inner ear may affect peripheral and central control of mobility and thus affect balance. The ability to achieve proprioception declines with age.

Personality. Personality remains stable during normal aging. Consider any signs of impaired emotional control, diminished initiative, or withdrawal as indicators of other problems or an initial sign of brain dysfunction.

Assessment

- Assess level of consciousness including alertness, eye opening, verbal responses, and ability to follow simple commands.
- Assess appropriateness of behavior and responses.
- Assess mental status. Mental status examination tools vary depending on the setting. The Mental Status Questionnaire (MSQ) and Mini-Mental State Examination (MMSE) are examples. These assess orientation, immediate and recent memory, attention, calculation, and language and motor skills.
- Assess for the presence of pain. Note severity, location, quality, duration, and precipitating events.
- Assess sleep patterns. Note onset, duration, and quality of sleep and daytime napping.
- Assess laboratory results for electrolyte imbalance, anemia, liver function, thyroid function, drug levels, and vitamin B_{12}.
- Assess CT scan or magnetic resonance imaging (MRI) results if there is reason to suspect tumor, subdural hematoma, or stroke.

Common Concerns and Nursing Interventions

Insomnia. It is not unusual for older adults to report difficulty with sleep. It is commonly known that the sleep pattern changes with age. With aging, there are fewer periods of deep sleep and frequent periods of wakefulness, giving the impression of sleeplessness even though the total sleep time is the same or only slightly reduced from that of young adulthood.

Nursing interventions to help an older person sleep begin with encouraging a bedtime ritual and promoting an environment conducive to sleep. For most people, this typically includes brushing the teeth, reading a book or the paper, using a favorite pillow, and listening to the radio. Exercise and activity during the day increase the likelihood of falling asleep easily at night. Activities or dietary intake that promotes stimulation should be avoided before retiring.

To manage sleep disorders, older adults may resort to either over-the-counter preparations or mediations prescribed by their health care provider. Sleep aids can be habit forming, and their use must be monitored closely. In addition, sleep aids may cause safety concerns related to falls.

Delirium. **Senility** (the state of mental and physical deterioration associated with aging) is a fear and a myth associated with aging. Delirium is a reversible condition of rapid onset. It has a fluctuating and traditionally brief course. The symptoms of delirium may manifest as behavioral changes including restlessness, agitation, or appearing withdrawn. Emotional changes may be strong, such as personality changes or mood shifts or subtler changes including apathy or depression.

Delirium is not a disease of the nervous system; it is a syndrome that results from one or more causes, including the following:

- Fever or infection
- Dehydration or malnutrition
- Electrolyte imbalances (hyponatremia or hypocalcemia)
- Sleep deprivation
- Alcohol or drug use, abuse or withdrawal
- Pain
- Medications (analgesics, hypnotics, psychotropics)
- Physiological conditions resulting in inadequate oxygenation to the brain

When an older adult has sudden mental changes, it is important to look for a cause. Once the cause of the delirium is identified, treatment is possible. Research is focused on identifying risk factors and prevention strategies (Meiner, 2011). See Table 33.13 for a comparison

Table 33.13 **Comparison of Characteristics Associated With Delirium, Dementia, and Depression**

	DELIRIUM	DEMENTIA	DEPRESSION
Onset	Sudden	Insidious, relentless	Sudden or insidious
Duration	Hours to days	Persistent	For longer than 2 wk
Time of day	Increases and decreases during the day	Stable or no change	Throughout the greater part of the day
Cognitive impairment	Impairment of memory, attentiveness, consciousness, numerous errors in assessment tasks	Minimal cognitive impairment initially, progresses to impaired abstract thinking, judgment, memory, thought patterns, calculations, agnosia	Impaired concentration, reduced attention span, indecisiveness, slower thought processes, impaired short-term and long-term memory
Activity	Increased or decreased; may fluctuate	Unchanged from usual behavior	Insomnia or excessive sleeping, fatigue, restlessness, anxiety, increased or decreased appetite
Speech and language	Rambling and irrelevant conversation, illogical flow of ideas, incoherent	Disordered, rambling, or incoherent; struggles to find words	Slower speech
Mood and affect	Rapid mood swings; fearful and suspicious	Depressed, apathetic, uninterested	Sad, hopeless, feels worthless, loss of interest or pleasure
Delusions or hallucinations	Misperceptions, illusions, hallucinations, and delusions	Misperceptions usually absent, delusions, no hallucinations	No delusions or hallucinations
Reversibility	Potential	No; progressive	Can be treated

From Seidel HM, Ball JW, Dains JE, et al: *Mosby's guide to physical examination*, ed 7, St. Louis, 2011, Mosby.

of characteristics associated with delirium, dementia, and depression.

Nursing interventions to prevent delirium include education of nursing staff about the signs and symptoms of delirium, orientation and communication, mobilization, environmental modifications, education of caregivers, pain control, and management of elimination, medication management, and discharge planning.

Reality orientation. Reality orientation is a useful intervention for delirium. Guidelines for reality orientation include the following:

- Call patients by their correct names or by the name they wish to be called.
- Make eye contact.
- Converse about familiar subjects.
- Provide familiar objects in the older adult's environment.
- Explain events and procedures in concise, simple language.
- Be honest.
- Set a routine and be consistent.
- Engage the older adult in familiar and simple activities that have a purpose, such as washing the face or brushing the teeth.

Dementia and Alzheimer's disease. Experts define **dementia** as a progressive impairment of intellectual (cognitive) function. The reduction in mental performance affects interpersonal relationships and other activities. It is characterized by loss of memory and at least one other disturbance of intellectual function (e.g., orientation, attention, calculation, language, motor skills). Dementia affects short-term, intermediate, and long-term memory. The individual has difficulty with abstract thinking, and it is not uncommon for those experiencing dementia or Alzheimer's disease to have difficulty with identifying object or choosing words to use in conversation. Aphasia (inability to understand words), agnosia (inability to recognize familiar objects), apraxia (problems manipulating things), and agraphia (difficulty writing and drawing) are symptoms of dementia, as well as noticeable changes in the personality.

Alzheimer's disease is the most common cause of dementia. Dementia of the Alzheimer's type is a progressive disorder in which the brain atrophies. Research has focused on genetic, viral, environmental, immunologic, and other causes. It usually arises in individuals older than 60 years of age and includes loss of cortical neurons, enlarged ventricles, and senile plaques and neurofibrillary tangles that appear in the cortex of the brain. Experts divide the progression of Alzheimer's disease into three stages. The early stage consists of a gradual onset of memory loss and difficulty focusing attention. The middle stage involves difficulty with language, object recognition, and judgment. The terminal (final) stage is characterized by some urinary and fecal incontinence, inability to ambulate or provide self-care, and inability to communicate. There is little or no response to surroundings or recognition of family members. In late stages, the individual becomes mute and bedridden. The average duration of the illness is 8 years, but it can last as long as 20 years or more.

Multiinfarct dementia. Multiinfarct dementia (MID, vascular dementia) is the second most common cause of dementia in older adults. It results from the interruption of blood flow to the brain. As a result, multiple strokes occur. This condition is related to vascular disorders within the brain that possibly result from stroke and severe hypertension; characteristics of the condition are periods of remission (absence of symptoms), preservation of personality, and mood swings. Risk factors for development of MID include arteriosclerosis, blood dyscrasias, cardiac decompensation, hypertension, atrial fibrillation, cardiac valve replacements, systemic emboli arising from other causes, DM, peripheral vascular disease, obesity, smoking, and vasospasms in the brain called transient ischemic attacks (TIAs). The usual progression of MID follows a stair-step decline rather than the slow, steady decline of Alzheimer's disease. Symptoms depend on the location of the infarct. Abrupt-onset symptoms include confusion and problems with recent memory; wandering; getting lost in familiar places; moving with rapid shuffling steps; loss of bladder or bowel control; inappropriate display of emotions; and difficulty following instructions. Some intellectual impairment is common.

Other dementia-related diseases. Dementia may also occur in patients who have other diseases including Huntington's disease, Creutzfeldt-Jakob disease, and human immunodeficiency virus (HIV) (Table 33.14).

In management of dementia-related diseases, the goals are to maintain maximum self-care abilities and prevent injury. Activities of daily living (ADLs) such as dressing often must be broken down into small steps, and each step should be explained to the patient in specific and simple terms. The individual may need coaching about what to do when eating, and often it is better to give finger foods or only one item at a time. Keep the environment calm and eliminate distracting stimuli. Care of an older adult with dementia or Alzheimer's disease requires patience. Routine is very important, and changes should be introduced very slowly. Remember that the individual no longer thinks logically or understands the surroundings.

When understanding and communication become impaired, nonverbal communication becomes more important. Use a calm pleasant tone of voice and gestures that correspond to the verbal message, maintain contact through touch, and use listening skills. Music has a positive influence, including improved capacity to communicate, reminisce, and recall memories. Reminiscence therapy uses the exchange of information between the affected individual their caregivers, family, and friends. It employs the use of photographs, familiar smells and tastes, and objects that carry some autobiographical meeting for the individual. The processes may provide a link to things past, assist with conflict resolution, and provide closure in dealing with unresolved issues.

Alterations in cognition make the assessment of pain challenging. Unrelieved or chronic pain can lead to depression, social isolation, feelings of worthlessness, and a sense of a loss of personal power. Visual analog scales, word descriptor scales, and numeric scales have not been tested for accuracy of pain assessment in older adults, so using two types of assessments may yield a more accurate response.

Wandering is a behavior frequently associated with dementia. In some situations, it is an attempt to find the bathroom or familiar surroundings; for some individuals, it is their way of coping with anxiety. For individuals unable to locate the bathroom or their own rooms, easily read signs with universally accepted symbols and familiar objects are a means to help them find the way. Safety measures to prevent falls are essential.

Table 33.14 Other Dementia-Related Diseases

DISEASE	CHARACTERISTICS
Huntington's disease	Age range at diagnosis is 5–70 yr; not necessarily a disease of old age. Characterized by uncontrollable writhing movements and mental deterioration that terminates in severe dementia. Begins with disturbances of gait and slurred speech. Life expectancy after diagnosis is 16 yr.
Creutzfeldt-Jakob disease	Rare and rapidly progressive; associated with viral etiology, although isolation of a specific virus has not occurred. Average age of onset 50–60 yr. Terminal within 6–12 mo. No known treatment.
HIV-associated dementia	Characterized by forgetfulness, slowness, poor concentration, and difficulties in problem solving. Rapidly progressive.

Parkinson's disease. Parkinson's disease is the second most common disorder that affects the nervous system in the older adult. It is a progressive, degenerative disease whose defining characteristics are muscle rigidity, tremors, and **akinesia** (an abnormal state of motor and psychic hypoactivity). The individual has a masklike appearance, drooling, and shuffling gait and often experiences emotional instability. In most cases, stress and frustration increase signs and symptoms.

Medication therapy with levodopa, amantadine, and anticholinergics such as benztropine mesylate and trihexyphenidyl HCl sometimes helps to slow the process of the disease or in some cases temporarily improves a patient's condition, but side effects from the drugs also have potential to cause disorientation, blurred vision, delirium, and drowsiness.

Nursing interventions for an older adult with Parkinson's disease include observing the response to medication therapy and maintaining mobility through exercise and activity. Range-of-motion exercises and massages help relieve muscle spasms and maintain joint mobility. Interventions for a safe environment, such as removing throw rugs and furniture from walkways and providing handrails and good lighting, are important because the patient's lack of balance and general unsteadiness typically contribute to falls and injuries. Canes, walkers, and adaptive aids for ADLs sometimes prolong the independence of an individual with Parkinson's disease.

Intellectual function is not impaired, but the tremors and involuntary movements cause difficulty in communication and much frustration for the individual and others with whom he or she is trying to communicate. Give the individual time to respond, encourage efforts to communicate, and show acceptance of the individual through actions and nonverbal communication to help alleviate some of the feelings of frustration.

Transient ischemic attacks. The changes in the vascular system in older adults include thickening of the vessel walls and the presence to some degree of atherosclerosis and arteriosclerosis. Specific medical diagnoses related to arterial conditions common in the older adult are TIAs and cerebral vascular accident (CVA), or stroke.

TIAs are small spasms or occlusions in the cerebral vessels of the brain. Signs and symptoms of TIA vary, depending on the vessel's location in the brain. The most common signs and symptoms are changes in vision, headache, disorientation, **ataxia** (impaired ability to coordinate movement), and drop attacks (falling without losing consciousness). Symptoms sometimes last for as little as 20 minutes. One in three individuals who experience a TIA has a stroke within 5 years. The patient with a TIA must have a neurologic examination and screening to determine whether there are atherosclerotic plaque–like formations in the carotid arteries or other pathologic changes in the cerebral vasculature. The occurrence of strokes can be reduced greatly by identifying high-risk or stroke-prone older adults and providing the appropriate prophylactic interventions.

Stroke. Cerebrovascular accident (stroke) is the third leading cause of death in the United States and increases in likelihood after 55 years of age. Many of the risk factors for a stroke also are seen with increasing age. These include heart disease, diabetes mellitus, and physical inactivity. Possible symptoms of a stroke include **hemiplegia** (paralysis of one side of the body), **dysarthria** (difficult, poorly articulated speech, resulting from interference in the control over the muscles of speech), *dysphagia* (difficulty in swallowing), sensory changes such as *hemianopia* (defective vision or blindness in half of the visual field), **aphasia** (an abnormal neurologic condition in which language function is defective or absent because of an injury to certain areas of the cerebral cortex), and intellectual and emotional changes.

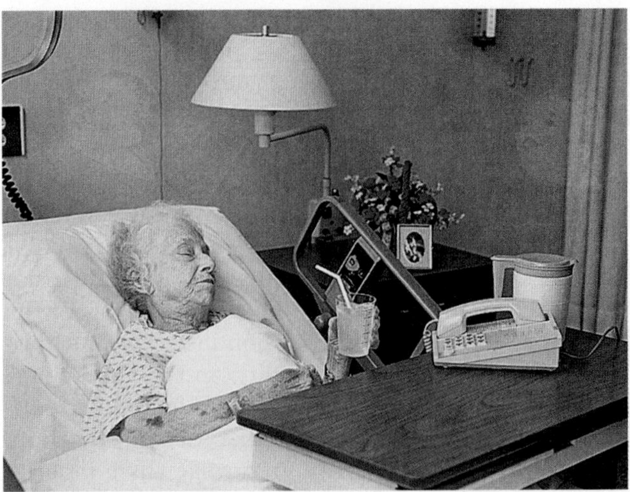

Fig. 33.11 Hemiplegia of dominant right side necessitates learning to use nondominant hand for activities of daily living (ADLs). (From Perry AG, Potter PA, Elkin MK: *Nursing interventions and clinical skills*, ed 4, St. Louis, 2011, Mosby.)

Nursing interventions immediately after the stroke involve support of life functions. Although some of the initial neurologic involvement is likely to disappear in 3 to 6 months, most individuals have some residual dysfunction. Interventions focus on rehabilitation to accomplish ADLs and to be as independent as possible. Older adults sometimes need to learn to use the nondominant hand because of hemiplegia (Fig. 33.11) and often require adaptive and assistive devices for ADLs, such as special utensils, reaching devices, and pull-on or easily secured clothing. Wheelchairs and canes are sometimes necessary for weakness, loss of balance, and loss of leg control. Encourage or assist the patient to do the exercises and activities the therapist prescribes.

Communication techniques for older adults with aphasia include listening carefully, turning down or decreasing competing stimuli such as the radio or the television, using pictures and appropriate gestures, speaking slowly, using short direct statements, and not interrupting. With all interventions, be sure not to rush the older adult, and give encouragement and praise for effort and success in performing tasks. In many settings, physical therapy and occupational therapy provide a valuable role in assessment and treatment of changes related to neurologic problems.

Patient problems and interventions for the older adult with neurologic problems include but are not limited to the following:

Patient Problem	Nursing Interventions
Compromised Verbal Communication, related to memory loss and difficulty focusing attention	Assess communication patterns. Provide calm environment with minimal distraction Use gestures to match simple verbal messages

Patient Problem	Nursing Interventions
	Use touch to increase attention Use familiar music to enhance recall
Excessive Demand on Primary Caregiver, related to difficulty coping with cognitive losses and progressive deterioration of self-care abilities	Assess family support network and available resources Establish opportunities for respite or timeout from caregiver role Access community support groups Provide stress management strategies Assess for signs of depression
Inability to Perceive or Use One Side of the Body, related to neurologic involvement	Position bed so that people approach and provide care from the unaffected side Ensure that affected body parts are safely positioned Provide range-of-motion exercises to affected side Adapt the environment to focus on the unaffected side (placement of personal items, television, or reading materials) Keep side rails up on affected side

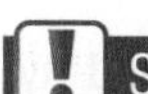
Safety Alert

General Fall Prevention Guidelines

GENERAL CARE
- Assess shoes for safety.
- Avoid wearing back-less shoes or flip flops.
- Wear leather or rubber-soled shoes.
- Illuminate darkened areas.
- Avoid storing items in overhead compartments.
- Assess assistive walking devices to ensure the tips and wheels are intact and functional.
- Use caution when standing from a sitting position. Allow time for the body to acclimate to positional changes.
- Avoid the use of alcohol.
- Do not use ladders or step stools unattended.

STEPS AND FLOOR SURFACES
- Avoid the use of throw rugs.
- Assess carpets for holes or frayed areas.
- To avoid missing a step count them to ensure placement.
- Install banisters in stairways.
- Keep walk areas clear.
- On landings, use carpeting that has color contrast.

BATHROOM
- Use assistive rales in the bath and shower area.
- Use a shower stool as needed.

SAFETY AND SECURITY ISSUES FOR OLDER ADULTS

FALLS

Falls are the leading cause of accidental death in individuals older than age 65. Approximately 25% of adults older than 65 years fall each year. Falls are considered an underreported occurrence between the older adult and the health care provider. The falls are caused by a combination of an environmental factor (e.g., a wet floor, stairs) and a physiologic problem (e.g., impaired vision or cognition, gait problems) or secondary to a disease or age-related change (see the Safety Alert box). Decreased circulation to the brain; diminished coordination, space, and position perception; decreased ability to balance; decreased muscle strength; changes in gait; and slowed nervous system responses are some of the major factors. Others include limited activity, side effects of medications, disorientation, and environmental hazards such as poor lighting and objects obstructing the pathway.

Prevention *begins* with exercise that increases strength, balance, endurance, and body awareness. Exercise must be weight bearing to maintain strength of muscles and bones and must be pleasurable to be continued in the long term.

For a reduced risk of falls, an environment that is free of hazards must be maintained. Some adaptations to prevent falls include providing assistive devices such as walkers and canes to aid balance, raised toilet seats, handrails on stairs, grab bars in the bathroom, nonskid shoes, and removal of small scatter rugs. Teach older adults to sit on the side of the bed when they arise and to stand for a minute or so before walking as a technique to cope with orthostatic *hypotension* (sudden low blood pressure that occurs when an individual assumes the standing posture) that sometimes arises from poor vascular perfusion or medications.

POLYPHARMACY

Polypharmacy refers to the use of five or more medications. Medications may be those prescribed by a health care provider or purchased over the counter. Although medications have therapeutic benefits, each has side effects and a risk for adverse effects. With each medication added, the risk intensifies. Between the ages of 65 and 69 the average number of medications taken is 14. After the age of 70 this number climbs to 18! Polypharmacy has been tied to 28% of hospital admissions. It also has been cited as the fifth leading cause of death in the United States (Health Research Funding, 2014). Among commonly used medications are laxatives, analgesics, cardiovascular medications, vitamins and supplements, and psychoactive medications (Table 33.15).

Medication therapies are implemented initially to manage a health concern. There are some individuals who are at a higher risk for an adverse effect of their medications. This includes those who are on increasing numbers of medications; borrow medications from friends or families; do not regularly check in with their

Table 33.15 Common Groups of Medications Used by the Older Adult

MEDICATION GROUP	NURSING INTERVENTIONS
Antacids	Observe for signs and symptoms of diarrhea, constipation. Teach older adult to check sodium and sugar content on the label. Encourage older adult to take antacid 1 hour after meals and not with other medications. Caution about use with a history of cardiac or renal conditions.
Antibiotics	Observe for disorientation, changes in hearing. Encourage fluid intake. Monitor weight, intake and output (I&O), specific gravity of urine. Observe for secondary yeast or fungal infections of mouth, vagina.
Antidepressants, antipsychotics	Observe for tremor, spasms. Teach techniques to use with vertigo when changing positions and methods to counteract dry mouth. Caution about use with glaucoma, prostate, or cardiac conditions. Observe for urinary retention.
Antihistamines	Observe for changes in blood pressure. Observe for anticholinergic effects—restlessness, delirium. Caution about use with glaucoma, prostate, or cardiac conditions.
Antihypertensives	Observe for depression, anxiety, disorientation. Monitor for bradycardia, angina, hypotension.
Antiinflammatory agents	Teach importance of taking with food. Explain need for avoidance with a history of peptic ulcer. Observe for nausea, vomiting, gastrointestinal (GI) bleeding. Observe for psychological disturbances and masking of infections.
Cardiovascular agents	Explain importance of keeping appointments for laboratory examinations. Observe for orthostatic hypotension. Monitor heart rate, rhythm, and blood pressure. Observe for adverse reactions—disorientation, depression, vertigo, lethargy.
Diuretics	Observe for orthostatic hypotension, delirium, changes in mental function. Explain reasons for taking in the morning. Observe for hypokalemia. Weigh daily. Record I&O.
Opioids	Observe for hypotension. Observe for adverse or idiosyncratic reactions—hallucinations, agitation, disorientation. Monitor respiratory function.
Oral anticoagulants	Monitor prothrombin time (PT) and international normalized ratio (INR). Observe for bleeding. Explain importance of keeping appointments for laboratory examinations. Explain the need to avoid aspirin-containing products. Institute safety measures to prevent injury.
Oral hypoglycemic agents	Observe for signs of hypoglycemia—weakness, headache, malaise. Monitor blood glucose levels.
Tranquilizers and sedatives	Observe for signs of oversedation—lethargy, disorientation, agitation. Explain the need to avoid other depressants and alcohol. Observe for adverse and idiosyncratic reactions—delirium, orthostatic hypotension, cardiac dysrhythmia.

health care provider when refilling medications; or combine prescribed medications with over-the-counter medications without consultation with their providers. A review of all medications, including over-the-counter medications, is essential in assessment. Ask patients when each was prescribed, its purpose, and how it affects them. Encourage use of one pharmacy for all medications so that the pharmacist can check for dangerous interactions.

Age-related changes in body function also contribute to some adverse reactions (Fig. 33.12). Research indicates that the body's ability to absorb, transport, and eliminate medications declines with age because of impaired circulation, changes in vessel walls, and a decrease in the number and efficiency of the glomeruli in the kidneys. Metabolism of medications also is reduced as a result of decreased blood flow in the liver, fewer functioning liver cells, and a decrease in the liver

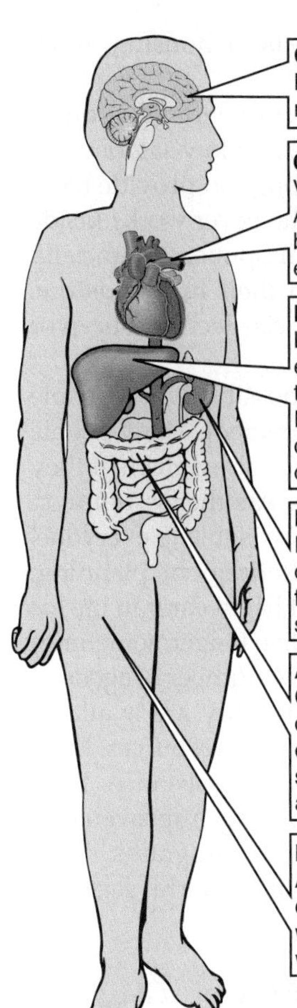

Central Nervous System
Brain receptors become more sensitive, making psychoactive drugs very potent.
Circulation
Vascular nerve controls grow less stable. Antihypertensives, for example, may drop blood pressure too low. Digoxin, for example, may slow the heart rate too much.
Metabolism
Liver mass shrinks. Hepatic blood flow and enzyme activity decline. Metabolism drops to 1/2 to 2/3 the rate of young adults. Enzymes lose ability to process some drugs that reduce irregular heart rhythms or breathing disorders.
Excretion
In kidneys, renal blood flow, and number of functional nephrons decline. Blood flow and waste removal slow and drugs stay in the body longer.
Absorption
Gastric enzymes and secretions decrease; gastric pH rises. Gastric emptying rate and gastrointestinal motility slow. Absorption capacity of cells and active transport mechanism declines.
Distribution
Adipose stores increase. Total body water declines, raising the concentration of water-soluble drugs, such as digoxin, which can cause heart dysfunction.

Fig. 33.12 Changes in the aging body alter medication effects. (From Lewis SL, Heitkemper MM, Dirksen SR, et al: *Medical-surgical nursing: Assessment and management of clinical problems,* ed 8, St. Louis, 2008, Mosby.)

enzymes that function to break down and transform medications. Because of all the changes, many medications remain in the body of an older adult longer than in a younger person. Dosages sometimes must be reduced to prevent toxicity because the normal adult dosage is typically for a 150-lb, 20-year-old individual. Many older adults also have conditions such as liver or kidney disease that further impair the body's ability to metabolize and excrete medications.

Nursing interventions begin with assessing the older person's ability to take medications properly. Most older adults are interested in learning about the medications they are taking and appreciate techniques that help them take the correct dose at the correct time, such as a chart or pill box with compartments labeled with the time and where the pills can be placed for each time they are to be taken. Also, be alert to the possibility of medication interactions and signs and symptoms of toxicities, which are easy to misinterpret as "signs of old age." Disorientation, fatigue, anorexia, falls, and vertigo are frequent indications of a medication reaction; these must be reported to the health care provider for evaluation. Nursing actions and patient teaching for homebound older adults promote safe medication practices in the home environment (see the Health Promotion box).

Health Promotion

Medication Practices for Homebound Older Adults

- During each home visit, assess the prescription and the nonprescription medications being taken by the homebound older adult.
- Document and notify the primary health care provider of the homebound older adult's medication regimen and of multiple health care provider sources for medications.
- Teach the possible complications and interactions of all over-the-counter medications to homebound older adults and their caregivers.
- Collaborate with social workers to identify community resources for financial assistance with pharmaceutical needs.
- Use laboratory parameters to monitor overuse and underuse of medications and interactive states of medications.
- Monitor urinary output status of older adults, because changes in renal excretion sometimes necessitate a decrease or increase in drug dosage.
- Teach the homebound older adult to set up a daily or weekly schedule of medications with a method or tool that fosters safe, independent administration.
- Reduce the chance of medication error by labeling or color coding medication bottles.
- Keep an accurate record of the homebound older adult's weight, because many medication dosages are calculated by body weight.
- Teach drug safety in the home environment by instructing older adults to do the following:
  - Keep drugs in original, labeled container.
  - Dispose of outdated medications appropriately; never dispose of them in the trash within reach of children.
  - Never "share" drugs with friends or family members.
  - Always finish a prescribed medication; do not save it for a future illness.
  - Read labels carefully and follow all instructions.
- Instruct older adults who have difficulty opening childproof containers to request their health care providers ask for non-childproof containers when writing prescriptions.

Modified from Meiner SE: *Gerontologic nursing,* ed 4, St. Louis, 2011, Mosby.

ELDER ABUSE AND NEGLECT

Abuse and neglect of the older adult refer to violence toward individuals older than age 65. Increasing concern has led the American Medical Association (AMA) to issue guidelines for the identification and treatment of abuse in five classifications: (1) physical or sexual abuse; (2) psychological abuse; (3) misuse of assets; (4) medical abuse (withholding necessary treatment or aids for ADLs); and (5) neglect. Common reasons for abuse and neglect include frustration and exhaustion of a caregiver; alcoholism; turbulent lifestyles; and

Box 33.5 Types of Elder Mistreatment*

Physical abuse: The use of physical force that has potential to result in bodily injury, physical pain, or impairment.
Sexual abuse: Nonconsensual sexual contact of any kind with an elderly person, including those individuals unable to give consent.
Emotional or psychological abuse: The infliction of anguish, pain, or distress through verbal or nonverbal acts, including intimidation or enforced social isolation.
Medical abuse: Subjecting a person to unwanted medical treatments or procedures; medical neglect occurs when a medically necessary and desired treatment is withheld.
Financial or material abuse or exploitation: The illegal or improper use of older adult's funds, property, or assets.
Neglect: The refusal or failure to fulfill any part of a person's previously agreed obligation or duties to an elder dependent on the person for care or assistance.
Abandonment: The desertion of an elder by an individual who had assumed the responsibility of providing care or assistance.

*Elder mistreatment implies that the recipient of the mistreatment is in a situation or condition in which the ability to protect oneself is limited in some way. Otherwise the actions are more accurately described as domestic violence, sexual assault, or fraud.
From Touhy T, Jett K: *Toward healthy aging: Human needs and nursing response,* ed 8, St. Louis, 2012, Mosby.

lack of financial, emotional, family, and community resources. The National Center on Elder Abuse identifies the two most important indicators of abuse as: (1) an older person's frequent unexplained crying; and (2) an older person's unexplained fear of or suspicion of a particular person(s) in the home. Older adults are often afraid to admit that they are being abused or neglected. Most states now have mandatory laws that require the reporting of older adult mistreatment. Be aware of the reporting policies within your area of practice (Box 33.5).

FINANCES

When asked what concerns them the most in their later years, older adults often answer "health" and "finances." The two are frequently related. For older people, health care often becomes a major expense and can devastate their financial security. Because of chronic health problems in addition to acute episodes, older adults spend a greater percentage of their income on health care than younger individuals do. Older adults may be assisted financially by Medicare, Medicaid, or both. Older adults who can afford to pay the premiums for Medicare supplemental insurance have a coinsurance, which pays the 20% of expenses that Medicare does not cover. Medicare Part D prescription drug plans are also available through insurance companies and private companies approved by Medicare. Some Medicare Advantage plans also have prescription plans. Many older adults are on a fixed income from Social Security or retirement pensions and have only limited savings to pay for the rising costs of housing, food, and health care.

For individuals in lower socioeconomic groups, pensions are not always available, and low salaries and seasonal work prevent saving enough to provide basic needs later in life. Some women who never work outside the home depend entirely on their spouses financially and become impoverished when their husbands die; others may be eligible to receive Social Security survivor benefits.

Financial problems are all too possible when people have not planned carefully for retirement. Many people assume that adequate pensions will be available if they have to retire or if their spouse dies. Another assumption is that Social Security benefits are available to everyone. Unfortunately, this is not true. Retirement planning, including financial planning, must begin early in life for men and women. Because people live longer, sometimes retirement lasts as long as 40 years. A number of agencies and senior programs in the community are available to help older adults who have limited resources. Such programs can include homemaking assistance, legal services, low-cost housing or housing improvement, heating assistance, multiservice senior programs, recreation programs, and information and referral services.

HOUSING

Housing represents a certain degree of self-concept and status. The insecurity that older adults feel when moving from one site to another in their later years is difficult for many to comprehend. In addition to the stress of relocation and the initial anxiety of adapting to a new setting, older adults typically move to more restrictive environments, sometimes against their wishes. Moving also may entail parting with possessions that have been acquired over a lifetime, making this transition more difficult. Housing is often the largest budgetary expenditure.

Relocation may be necessary as a result of physical or financial concerns. Ideally, the new setting should be as close to the old one as possible to reduce the stress of the move. Options may include downsizing to a smaller home or apartment. There are various arrangements for maintaining independent living, as long as people use some energy to develop the plan creatively. Renting may reduce the upkeep associated with home ownership. Older adults who are unable to live alone may decide to move in with their adult children.

Some older adults choose assisted living in a long-term care residence. Assisted-living facilities do not provide 24/7 skilled nursing care, but they do provide more assistance than an older adult receives in an independent-living environment. Assisted-living facilities are more expensive than completely independent settings; however, they are less costly than skilled nursing homes. Currently the average cost of an assisted living facility exceeds $3000 per month, compared to a skilled nursing long-term care facility, with an average monthly cost of $6500 to $7500 (AssistedLivingFacilities .org, n.d.).

CONTINUUM OF OLDER ADULT CARE

As the nation's population ages, nurses will care for increasing numbers of older adult patients. The increase in the aging population correlates to an increase in consumption of health care resources. An estimated 80% of older adults have a chronic illness, and half of those over the age of 65 have at least two chronic conditions.

HOSPITALIZATION, SURGERY, AND REHABILITATION

Age-related changes place the older adult at risk when faced with illness. Increased risks for the development of complications such as drug reactions, falls, infection, and delayed healing require knowledge of the specialized needs of the older adult. Although responses are individual, older adults have less reserve to cope physically and emotionally with the effects of hospitalization and surgery. They need longer postoperative recovery and convalescent periods. The normal effects of immobility on body systems, including stasis of secretions, orthostatic hypotension, and digestive and perceptual disorders, must be kept to a minimum. When adults in their 80s and 90s undergo surgery, their rehabilitation must begin as soon after surgery as their condition stabilizes.

Especially important are measures to prevent complications of immobility and techniques to support coping skills and independence. Turning, deep breathing, coughing, or other techniques for ventilation and removal of respiratory secretions are important with older adults because of the age-related changes in the respiratory tract that increase the risk of atelectasis and pneumonia. Depending on the type of surgery, older individuals are best ambulated within 8 to 24 hours to decrease the risks of stasis in the circulation, kidneys, bladder, and respiratory tract. Getting up, even to stand or take a few steps, usually helps to stimulate peristalsis, peripheral vascular circulation, and muscle activity; expand the lungs; and improve mental outlook (Fig. 33.13).

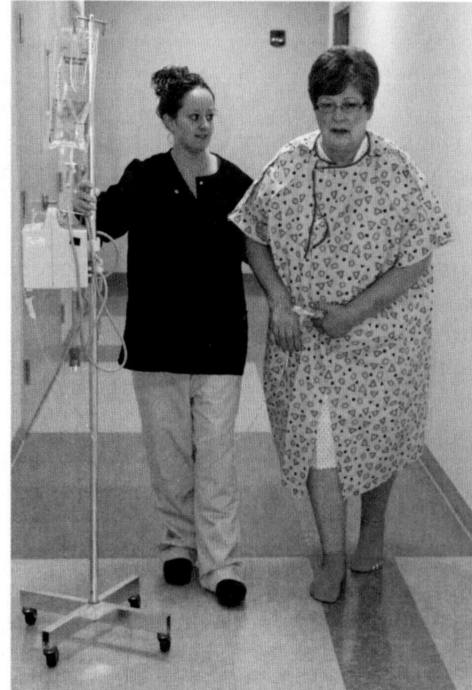

Fig. 33.13 Ambulation decreases the risks of stasis in the circulation, kidneys, bladder, and respiratory tract.

Encourage older individuals to perform self-care activities at their own level of tolerance and with rest periods. Remember that the hospitalization and the surgical intervention have the potential to increase signs and symptoms of other chronic conditions, such as arthritis, which sometimes is cause for reports of discomfort or difficulty in ADLs.

DISCHARGE PLANNING

Older adults need to have the necessary knowledge, skill, and resources to meet self-care needs at home before discharge from a health care facility. Planning begins with assessment of the biophysical, psychosocial, educational, self-care, and environmental needs. Strategies depend on physical and emotional readiness to learn, educational level, and family and community resources available. Written or visual guidelines that reinforce verbal instructions should be provided. Learning is enhanced when the older adult is actively engaged in the learning process (see the Patient Teaching box on discharge planning). Preserving as much of the older adult's autonomy as possible is a prime consideration. First consider the individual's physical strength and remaining functional abilities, not just the current disabilities, before making any modification to the home environment.

Patient Teaching

Discharge Planning for the Older Adult

- Teach when the older adult is alert and rested. Allow for several shorter sessions, watching for signs of fatigue.
- Involve the individual in discussion or activity.
- Focus on the person's strengths.
- Use approaches that adapt for the presence of pain and impaired range of joint motion, impaired reception of stimuli such as slower reaction time, muscular weakness, reduced pain and temperature perception, reduced depth perception and color discrimination, and reduced visual acuity.
- Consider need for adaptive devices, such as a syringe magnifier.
- As needed, enlist the help of the patient's significant other, or provide assistive personnel.

HOME CARE

Hospital lengths of stay are getting shorter for most illnesses. Early discharge for older adults may present unique challenges. Referrals to community-based services may be indicated to promote their independence and ability to return home.

To be eligible for the Medicare home health benefit, an individual must be homebound; have a condition that requires skilled, intermittent care; and have a referring health care provider who approves the plan of treatment in writing. The home health nurse assesses the physical, functional, emotional, socioeconomic, and environmental well-being of patients and works in collaboration with other members of the home health team, including the physical therapist, occupational therapist, speech therapist, social worker, and home health aide (HHA) or personal care attendant (PCA). Nurses initiate the plan of care and provide care that requires judgment and skill including health and self-care teaching; this teaching includes medications, medication administration, wound and decubitus care, urinary catheter care, ostomy care, postsurgical care, and care of the terminal patient. Some home health nurses provide intravenous therapy, enteral and parenteral nutrition, and chemotherapy. Once the registered nurse (RN) establishes the plan of care, licensed practical or vocational nurses (LPNs/LVNs) are permitted to provide skilled nursing and HHAs to provide personal care such as ADLs, hygiene, vital signs, and other tasks ordinarily done by the patient or family. Families often hire PCAs for cases in which only a sitter is required rather than personal or skilled care. They usually prepare meals, assist patients to the bathroom, assist with dressing and ambulation, and perform light housekeeping.

ASSISTED LIVING

Assisted living is one of the fastest growing industries in the United States. Placed between home health and the long-term care facility in the continuum of long-term care settings, assisted living offers meals, assistance with bathing and dressing, social and recreational programs, laundry and housekeeping services, transportation, emergency call system, health checks, and medication administration. Many services are purchased individually as needed by the resident.

Other options for living arrangements include retirement villages, senior housing apartments, single-family homes, group living, and sharing of a home.

LONG-TERM CARE FACILITIES

Emphasis on reducing costs in the hospital setting through earlier discharge has led to the shift of more acutely ill residents to skilled nursing facilities, traditionally referred to as nursing homes or long-term care facilities. Skilled nursing facilities may include care such as intravenous infusions, feeding tubes, ventilator care, wound vacuum-assisted closure devices, and peritoneal dialysis. Each skilled facility differs in the level of care provided and the type of patients they can accept based on the skill set of the nurses and the resources available.

Resident Characteristics

People who live in skilled or long-term care facilities are referred to as residents. The facility is their temporary or permanent home, and some residents need nursing care until death. Approximately 1.6 million individuals are currently living in these facilities in the United States. Estimates project a sharp increase in this number as the older population, particularly those over 85 years of age, grows exponentially over the next 30 years. The demographic of nursing facility residents is 67% female. The majority (69%) are over the age of 75 years.

Long-term care residents usually need 24-hour care, which is not possible to provide in the home environment because of the increased scope of needs and the family's inability to provide the necessary care. The facility usually provides medical, nursing, dietary, recreational, rehabilitative, social, and spiritual care.

Care Costs

The average cost of a long-term care facility is affected by location. The average cost for a semi-private room is $83,000 annually. Some Americans purchase long-term care insurance; however, individuals or state and federal Medicaid programs pay the majority of costs. Medicare covers the cost of only the first 20 days of skilled and rehabilitative care. Significant co-pay from Medicare supplemental insurance is needed for the cost of care for the next 80 days if the need for care continues. Medicaid provides coverage for all levels of care, if the resident qualifies. Presently government officials are trying to address concerns about the abilities of the state and federal governments to continue shouldering these costs. Future legislation undoubtedly will focus on this matter.

Quality of Care

Long-term care facilities are highly regulated. The Omnibus Budget Reconciliation Act (OBRA) of 1987 and subsequent revisions aimed to improve the quality of care and have had a positive outcome. OBRA requirements include comprehensive resident assessments, increased training requirements for unlicensed assistive personnel (UAP), a greater number of nursing staff, availability of social workers, standards for nursing home administrators, and quality assurance activities.

Legislation has been passed to protect the rights of residents of nursing homes, and it is mandatory to inform the residents of these rights. Staff are required to promote and protect these rights, which are posted in the long-term care facility so that the residents are readily able to see them (Box 33.6). The Long-Term

Box 33.6 Bill of Rights for Long-Term Care Residents

- The right to voice grievances and have them remedied.
- The right to information about health conditions and treatments and to participate in one's own care to the greatest extent possible.
- The right to choose one's own health care providers and to speak privately with one's health care providers.
- The right to consent to or refuse all aspects of care and treatments.
- The right to manage one's own finances if capable or choose one's own financial advisor.
- The right to be transferred or discharged only for appropriate reasons.
- The right to be free from all forms of abuse.
- The right to be free from all forms of restraint to the extent compatible with safety.
- The right to privacy and confidentiality concerning one's person, personal information, and medical information.
- The right to be treated with dignity, consideration, and respect in keeping with one's individuality.
- The right to immediate visitation and access at any time for family, health care providers, and legal advisors; the right to reasonable visitation and access for others.

NOTE: This list of rights is a sampling of federal and several states' lists of rights of residents or participants in long-term care. Nurses should check the rules of their own state for specific rights in law for that state.

From Touhy T, Jett K: *Toward healthy aging: Human needs and nursing response,* ed 8, St. Louis, 2012, Mosby.

Ombudsman Program is a national effort to support the rights of the residents and the facilities. Each long-term care facility is obliged to post the name and the contact information of the ombudsman assigned to each facility.

Residents' rights include the following: the right to autonomy and active participation and decision making in their care and life, including the right to self-administer medications; the right to informed consent for the use of side rails and chemical and physical restraints; and the right to withdrawal or withholding of life-sustaining treatments.

Interdisciplinary functional assessment of residents is the cornerstone of clinical practice in long-term care. The minimum data set (MDS) is a tool intended to develop a complete picture of each resident. It includes a comprehensive assessment of background information, cognition, communication, hearing, vision, physical function, mood, behavior, activity, bowel and bladder continence, disease diagnoses, nutrition and dental status, skin condition, medication use, and special treatments and procedures. This information is used to develop an individualized, comprehensive plan of care for each resident.

Get Ready for the NCLEX® Examination!

Key Points

- Although the efficiency of body systems declines with age, the body has reserves and compensatory mechanisms that normally, in the absence of disease, allow an individual to function well in late adulthood.
- Regardless of age, individuals have the same basic needs for physiologic function, safety, security, belonging, and self-esteem.
- Although older adulthood is tied to chronologic age, note that *chronologic age* may not be an accurate predictor of health or behavior.
- Wellness is based on a belief that each person has an optimal level of function and that even in chronic illness and dying some level of well-being is attainable.
- The role of a nurse includes affirmation, enhancement, and support of each person's movement through the aging process and encouragement of health and wellness.
- *Ageism* is a term that describes prejudice against older adults. All members of the health care team should work toward eliminating negative attitudes and discriminatory practices in the treatment of the elderly.
- Symptoms of depression are commonly misunderstood as changes that normally occur with aging. As a result, few older adults receive treatment for depression, although depression is common in this age group.
- Pressure injuries are a significant risk for older adults and patients with chronic disease. The best way to prevent damage to the skin is to reposition patients at least every 2 hours.
- Nutritional problems account for one-third to one-half of all health problems in older adults. Many independently living older adults have nutritional deficiencies.
- Urinary incontinence is not a normal part of aging, although many believe that it is and do not seek treatment.
- COPD is not a single disease but commonly a combination of chronic bronchitis, chronic asthma, and emphysema in varying degrees as a result of progressive changes as individuals age. By 90 years of age, nearly everyone has some degree of COPD.
- Repeated infections, slow healing, blurred vision, and weight gain or loss are often the initial signs and symptoms of diabetes mellitus in older adults.

- A common reason for sexual dysfunction in older adults is the misconception that older adults are impotent and asexual or that they are perverse if they are sexually active; however, if individuals continue to be sexually active on a regular basis, they retain the capability to respond sexually.
- About one-fifth of people older than age 70 years have visual impairments that limit activity and increase the risk of falls. Age-related changes in vision include presbyopia, a decrease in visual acuity, clouding of the lens of the eye, yellowing of the lens, and changes in color perception and depth perception.
- Cognitive decline is not a universal process of aging. Research indicates that most older people retain their intelligence and are capable of learning throughout their lives.
- Unless they are necessary for the treatment of medical symptoms, it is against the law for chemical or physical restraints to be used in long-term care facilities and skilled nursing facilities.
- Cerebrovascular attack (stroke) is the third leading cause of death in the United States and increases in likelihood after 55 years of age.
- Falls are the leading cause of accidental death in individuals older than the age of 65 years. Approximately one-third of people 70 years or older report falls in a single year.
- Forty percent or more of adults use alternative pharmacotherapy. Encourage older adults to avoid taking any herb, supplement, or other over-the-counter products without contacting the health care provider or a pharmacist who will review the complete drug profile.

Additional Learning Resources

SG Go to your Study Guide for additional learning activities to help you master this chapter content.

evolve Be sure to visit the Evolve site at *http://evolve.elsevier.com/Cooper/foundationsadult/* for additional online resources.

Review Questions for the NCLEX® Examination

1. Which statement best describes demographic changes in relation to the aging population in the United States?
   1. The older adult population is growing twice as fast as the rest of the population.
   2. Aging is a gradual process that has a predictable pattern based on gender and race.
   3. The term *old-old* refers to those more than 100 years of age.
   4. In the past 50 years, life expectancy for older Americans has increased by almost 10 years.
   5. Of the population older than age 65 years, approximately 60% are men and 40% are women.
2. The nursing student is discussing older adults. Which statements demonstrate an understanding of the population? *(Select all that apply.)*
   1. "Most people become senile when they become old."
   2. "Approximately 33% of older Americans have impaired hearing."
   3. "Most older adults have at least weekly contact with family."
   4. "Approximately 25% of the older adult population resides in a long-term care facility."
   5. "Most older people have at least one chronic condition and rate their health as 'good.'"
3. According to the "disengagement theory," people who are aging:
   1. inherit a genetic program that determines their specific life expectancy.
   2. gradually withdraw from society.
   3. have the inability to achieve a level of acceptance, which results in anger and despair.
   4. experience a change of personality and behaviors related to illness and loneliness.
4. Which assessment finding is associated with normal aging? *(Select all that apply.)*
   1. The integumentary system loses elasticity.
   2. There is loss of muscle tone, which increases the incidence of choking and aspiration.
   3. There is a gradual loss of weight because of loss of muscle tissue and fluid.
   4. There is increased resistance to infection from improved immune response.
   5. Personality changes are anticipated as the individual approaches age 70 years.
5. When caring for an older adult patient who is resistant to getting light exercise, the nurse should tell the patient that which of the following are benefits of this activity? *(Select all that apply.)*
   1. Improved circulation
   2. Decreased constipation
   3. Reduced incidence of osteoporosis
   4. Reduced incidence of gouty arthritis
   5. Enhanced hearing
6. Which change is suggestive of osteoporosis?
   1. Decreased muscle strength and joint mobility
   2. Increased curvature of the spine and decreased height
   3. Loss of balance and unsteady gait
   4. Nocturia and sleep pattern disturbances
7. What description for the term dementia is most appropriate?
   1. A sudden change in mental status that results from hypoxia, electrolyte imbalances, or some other treatable condition
   2. A state of physical and mental deterioration associated with normal aging
   3. Loss of awareness of person, place, and time
   4. A progressive impairment of intellectual function that interferes with normal activities

8. When administering medications to older adults, it is important that the nurse keep what concepts in mind? *(Select all that apply.)*
   1. Absorption, transport, and elimination of medications tend to decrease with age.
   2. Doses sometimes must be increased to achieve desired effects.
   3. Many older adults have conditions such as liver or kidney disease that impair the body's ability to metabolize and excrete medications.
   4. Up to 40% or more adults use alternative pharmacotherapy, such as herbal remedies, that have the potential to alter the effectiveness of certain prescribed medications.
   5. Older people use a high percentage of over-the-counter (OTC) medications, which enhance the excretion of other drugs.
9. The nurse is caring for an older adult patient who has been diagnosed with depression. The nurse correctly recognizes what characteristics about depression in the older adult as being correct?
   1. Depression is uncommon in older adults.
   2. Older people who receive psychotherapy for depression show improvement.
   3. Symptoms of depression are commonly misunderstood as normal changes of aging.
   4. Many older adults are treated for depression.
   5. Symptoms of depression in older adults may include crying, agitation, and hypochondria.
10. A patient has been experiencing visual changes from a loss of elasticity of the lens of the eye. What condition is associated with this phenomenon?
    1. Cataracts
    2. Presbyopia
    3. Glaucoma
    4. Macular degeneration
11. Older adults often have an *atypical response* to illness or infection. What is an *atypical response* in a previously active and alert older adult?
    1. Disorientation, weakness, or incontinence
    2. Fever, loss of appetite, pain
    3. Cough, shortness of breath, and fever
    4. Purulent drainage, redness, and warmth at the site of an injury
12. A patient with three school-age children cares for her mother who has Alzheimer's disease. Her mother can no longer safely stay at home alone and needs continual supervision. A nursing diagnosis of *caregiver role strain* is made. Which nursing intervention is most appropriate?
    1. Provide a calm environment with minimal distraction.
    2. Access community support to provide opportunity for the caregiver to do errands and spend time with her children.
    3. Assess communication patterns between the patient and her mother.
    4. Encourage the use of gestures and touch to enhance communication.
13. Which is an appropriate nursing diagnosis for an older adult male with neurologic problems? *(Select all that apply.)*
    1. Decreased cardiac output
    2. Impaired verbal communication
    3. Impaired urinary elimination
    4. Risk for disturbed sensory perception
    5. Risk for infection
14. In data collection from an older adult, the patient discusses intimacy concerns. When developing the plan of care, the nurse correctly recognizes which of the following as the primary reason for decreased sexual activity in many older adults?
    1. Painful sexual intercourse because of vaginal dryness or pain
    2. Loss of interest as a normal part of the aging process
    3. Treatment of other conditions with medications that induce impotence
    4. Lack of a sexual partner
15. Aging often causes a decreased production of intrinsic factor from the stomach, thus interfering with the body's ability to use vitamin B_{12}. What disease develops from this deficiency?
    1. Iron-deficiency anemia
    2. Aplastic anemia
    3. Pernicious anemia
    4. Sickle cell anemia
16. In a review of the patient's medical record, the intraocular pressure is noted within normal limits. What range confirms this finding?
    1. 2 to 8 mm Hg
    2. 10 to 22 mm Hg
    3. 25 to 32 mm Hg
    4. 50 to 60 mm Hg

34 Concepts of Mental Health

http://evolve.elsevier.com/Cooper/foundationsadult/

Objectives

1. Describe the mental health continuum.
2. Identify defining characteristics of people who are mentally healthy and those who are mentally ill.
3. Describe the parts of personality.
4. Describe the factors that influence an individual's response to change.
5. Identify factors that contribute to the development of emotional problems or mental illness.
6. Identify barriers to health adaptation.
7. Identify sources of stress.
8. Identify stages of illness behavior.
9. Identify major components of a nursing assessment that focuses on mental health status.
10. Identify basic nursing interventions for those experiencing illness or crisis.

Key Terms

adaptation (ăd-ăp-TĀ-shŭn, p. 1106)
anxiety (ăng-ZĪ-ŭ-tē, p. 1105)
behavior (bē-HĀV-yŭr, p. 1100)
conflict (p. 1106)
coping responses (KŌ-pĭng rē-SPŎNS-ŭz, p. 1106)
crisis (KRĪ-sĭs, p. 1108)
defense mechanisms (dē-FĔNS MĔK-ŭn-ĭz-ŭmz, p. 1106)
deinstitutionalization (dē-ĭn-stĭ-TŪ-shŭn-ŭl-ĭz-Ā-shŭn, p. 1102)
frustration (p. 1106)
humoral theory (HYŪ-mōr-ăl THĒR-ē, p. 1101)
illness (ĬL-nŭs, p. 1108)
mental health (MĔN-tŭl HĔLTH, p. 1100)
mental health continuum (MĔN-tŭl HĔLTH kŏn-TĬN-yū-ŭm, p. 1103)
mental illness (MĔN-tŭl ĬL-nŭs, p. 1101)
motivation (p. 1106)
Omnibus Budget Reconciliation Act (OBRA) (ŎM-nĭ-bŭs BŬD-jĭt rĕ-kŏn-sĭl-ē-Ā-shŭn ĂKT, p. 1103)
personality (pŭr-sŭn-ĂL-ŭ-tē, p. 1104)
self (SĔLF, p. 1104)
self-concept (SĔLF KŎN-sĕpt, p. 1105)
stress (STRĔS, p. 1105)
stressor (STRĔS-ŭr, p. 1105)

A licensed practical/vocational nurse (LPN/LVN) is likely to use mental health nursing principles in a variety of health care settings. Basic mental health concepts are useful in understanding a patient's behavioral responses to disease and dysfunction. **Behavior** can be defined as the manner in which a person performs any or all of the activities of daily life. Individuals respond differently to changes in daily activities, such as the changes created by illness and hospitalization. All individuals have unique personalities and resources that affect their behavior in dealing with changing situations and the changing environment. An individual's mental health sometimes varies in accordance with the situation and the available support systems.

Mental health can be defined as a person's ability to cope with and adjust to the recurrent stresses of everyday living. Mental health is dynamic and fluctuates along a continuum. Mentally healthy individuals are individuals who are able to enjoy life's activities, adapt successfully to changes, set realistic goals, solve problems, have satisfying working relationships, and maintain interpersonal relationships with family and friends (Fig. 34.1).

Factors affecting mental health include inherited characteristics, childhood nurturing, and life's circumstances. The influence of these factors on the individual's response to daily stressors in life is sometimes positive and sometimes negative. Possible positive influences include inherent adequate coping ability, mother-child bonding at birth, success in school, good physical health, and financial security. Possible negative influences include cognitive impairment, schizophrenia, extreme

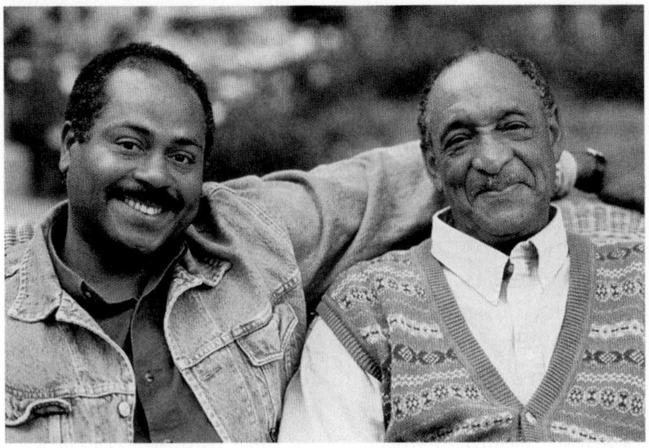

Fig. 34.1 Maintaining interpersonal relationships with family members provides a positive influence that affects mental health. (From Lewis SL, Heitkemper MM, Dirksen SR, et al: *Medical-surgical nursing: Assessment and management of clinical problems*, ed 7, St. Louis, 2007, Mosby.)

sibling rivalry, parental rejection, deprivation of maternal love, poor physical health, poverty, and dysfunctional relationships.

Evidence of **mental illness** often consists of a pattern of behaviors that are conspicuous, threatening, and disruptive of relationships or that deviate significantly from behaviors that are considered socially and culturally acceptable. Mental illness or disorder is a manifestation of dysfunction (behavioral, psychological, and biologic).

Changes in society and in the economy have altered the status and situation of many individuals. According to the National Institute of Mental Health (2017), 18.1% of adults in the United States received treatment for a mental health problem in 2014. This population includes all adults who received inpatient or outpatient care or used prescription medication for mental or emotional problems. Twice as many people actually have a mental health disorder. An astounding 50% of people in the United States will develop a mental health disorder in their lifetime. The discrepancy between individuals seeking treatment and those not treated for mental illness should serve as an alert to nurses who in their practice encounter patients and families who have mental health concerns (Centers for Disease Control and Prevention, 2011). The nurse may have daily contact with battered spouses, abused children, people who are homeless as a result of mental illness, substance abusers, or patients experiencing depression, anxiety, or other mental health alterations. Regardless of the practice setting, nurses frequently encounter patients who are in need of emotional support.

Nurses can help patients by providing nursing interventions in situations involving interpersonal exchanges. Patients express their feelings in a variety of ways. The nurse is responsible for assessing and intervening while maintaining a caring relationship of trust with the patient. The emphasis of the mental health aspect of nursing is to assist the patient and family to achieve satisfying and productive ways of dealing with the positive and the negative aspects of daily living and to cope with situations that necessitate a change in lifestyle.

HISTORICAL OVERVIEW

The history of mental health care began in ancient times. During early history, people thought that a physically or mentally ill person was possessed by evil spirits. For mental illness, the shamans or medicine men focused on removing evil spirits by magical treatments such as spells, potions, noises, or sacrifices and by physical treatments such as vomiting, bleeding, massage, and trephining (cutting holes in the skull to release evil spirits). If these tribal rites were unsuccessful, the community abandoned the affected individual to die by starvation or attack by wild animals.

Historical records show that there was an interest in mental health and illness and its treatment in the Greco-Roman era. The Greeks introduced the idea that it is possible to explain mental illness by observation of behavior. Hippocrates viewed mental illness as an imbalance of humors based on the fundamental elements of the world: air, fire, water, and earth. Each basic element corresponded to a particular fluid in the body: blood, yellow bile, phlegm, and black bile, respectively. This view of illness is called the **humoral theory** (pertaining to body fluids or substances contained in them). Roman physicians were interested in making their patients comfortable by providing physical care such as warm baths, massage, and music.

During medieval times, about AD 500 to 1400, society lost track of this concept of mental illness. The church became powerful and kept much knowledge locked away in the monasteries. Early Christians believed that mental illness was punishment for sins committed, evidence of possession by the devil, or an effect of witchcraft. Exorcisms, physical punishment and imprisonment, or banishment became the treatment for mental illness. Toward the end of the medieval period, Arabic influences in Europe reawakened awareness of the relation between emotions and disease and medical treatment for mental illness. The first English institution for the mentally ill was Bethlehem Royal Hospital, founded in the 16th century under Henry VI. The English word for a place of confusion and disorder, *bedlam,* originated from this hospital's nickname (Fig. 34.2). This term is still used today. To raise money to run the institution, it was common to shackle or cage the residents and display them for a price to people who were curious to see them. This practice continued for several hundred years.

During the Renaissance and the Reformation (15th and 16th centuries), little changed in the treatment of mental illness. The Reformation brought the closing of many Catholic institutions, which put the poor, the sick, and the insane back onto the streets.

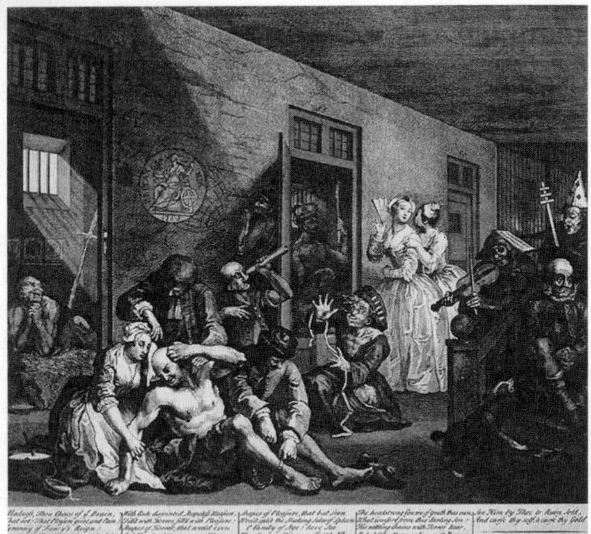

Fig. 34.2 Artist's representation of Bethlehem Royal Hospital, London, otherwise known as *Bedlam.* (From "The Rake in Bedlam," c. 1735. From the series titled *The Rake's Progress*, copyright The Trustees of the British Museum, London, England.)

The 17th and 18th centuries were a period of further growth of the sciences, literature, philosophy, and the arts, but conditions for the mentally ill were worse than ever. Common treatments included bleeding, starving, beating, purging, and confinement. During the last half of the 18th century, psychiatry became a separate branch of medicine.

Dr. Philippe Pinel, director of two Paris hospitals, changed the concept of care for the mentally ill. Pinel advocated humane care and maintenance of case history and conversation records. He classified illnesses by behaviors. In England about the same time, William Tukes, a Quaker, built an asylum similar to a Quaker household. His philosophy of care was to encourage acceptable behavior by providing a nurturing atmosphere. This concept of care became very popular.

In the United States, Dr. Benjamin Rush, a signer of the Declaration of Independence, established the Pennsylvania Hospital (1731) in Philadelphia for treatment of the mentally ill. Harsh treatment of the mentally ill still prevailed in the United States, as it did in Europe. Some newer therapies and devices (e.g., the tranquilizing chair) were used to encourage the rational mind to come forth. Dr. Rush used the newer, more humane therapies in his practice. He became known as the father of American psychiatry. The first public psychiatric hospital in the United States, Eastern Psychiatric Hospital, opened in 1773 in Williamsburg, Virginia.

The 19th century saw the flourishing of institutions and asylums. Overcrowding and bureaucracy brought the decline of care these institutions were able to provide. Dorothea Dix, a retired schoolteacher, was appalled by the care of the mentally ill and set out to change it. She surveyed jails, almshouses, and asylums throughout the United States, Canada, and Scotland and presented her findings to anyone who would listen: presidents, legislatures, civic groups, and concerned citizens. As a result of her efforts, millions of dollars were raised for the development of mental hospitals throughout the United States. In 1882 McLean Hospital in Waverly, Massachusetts, provided the first psychiatric training school for nurses.

The 20th century ushered in the reform of mental health care as the population became increasingly interested in social issues. Clifford Beers, a college student who had attempted suicide, spent 3 years as a patient in a mental hospital. Upon his release, he wrote *A Mind That Found Itself,* in which he described the beatings, isolation, and confinement that he experienced and witnessed while he was institutionalized. As a result of Beers's work, the Committee for Mental Hygiene formed in 1909. This committee focused on prevention of mental illness and removal of the stigma of mental illness. Around this same time, Sigmund Freud, a neurophysiologist now known as the father of psychiatry, was introducing his elaborate theories and treatment for mental illnesses.

During the 1930s, mental health practitioners developed electroconvulsive therapy and insulin shock therapy and used them to treat schizophrenia. Frontal lobotomy—a surgical procedure in which the frontal lobes are severed from the thalamus—was also used to eliminate violent behaviors. By 1939 about half of all nursing schools offered psychiatric courses in their curriculum.

In the 1940s the passage of the National Health Act and the establishment of the National Institute of Mental Health were among the most important developments in psychiatric medicine in the United States. The institute established research funding for the causes, the prevention, and the treatment of mental illnesses.

In the 1950s psychotherapeutic drugs were introduced. This allowed psychiatric patients to be treated in regular hospital settings. These drugs also allowed individuals to control their behavior and thus spend more time in the community, which was a primary goal of mental health care. At this time, the government started the movement of **deinstitutionalization,** the release of psychiatric patients from institutions to live and receive treatment in the community setting. During the 1960s and 1970s, legislatures brought about further changes in mental health treatment at the community level. A goal of community treatment is to return the individual to the home environment as soon as possible and to provide a support system within the community to facilitate treatment and bring about functioning as near to normal as possible.

President Jimmy Carter established the President's Commission on Mental Health in 1978. This commission assessed mental health care needs of the nation and made recommendations of action for the government to take. Martha Mitchell, a nurse educator and clinical specialist in psychiatric–mental health nursing, was among those appointed to this commission. This was the first time nursing had representation in a commission of this type. From this commission's recommendations, the most comprehensive mental health care bill in US history, the Mental Health Care Systems Act, was passed in 1980.

During President Ronald Reagan's administration, the **Omnibus Budget Reconciliation Act (OBRA)** of 1981 was passed; it drastically reduced funding for the mental health system and put remaining funds into block grants for use and disbursement at the community level. Rapid, if not indiscriminate, deinstitutionalization was one consequence of the severe fiscal cuts. Continued declines in federal and state budgets have resulted in the loss of services to vulnerable populations. Between 2009 and 2012, $1.6 billion was cut from state-based mental health programs. In 2013, 35 states increased funding for mental health services but in 2014 only 29 states increased funding. This overall reduction in funding has translated into reduced availability of housing, reduced access to care providers, and limited access to psychotropic medications, therapy, and crisis services (NAMI, 2014).

In the 21st century health care providers put mental health concepts and principles into practice in a variety of settings, including public health and home health care agencies, outpatient settings, and acute care hospitals. Psychiatric and mental health care centers are not the only settings in which mental health care is practiced. There are patients in need of emotional support in every health care setting. The community-based mental health movement and the holistic health movement have brought awareness to the public that all individuals, sick or well, have emotional needs to be met.

BASIC CONCEPTS RELATED TO MENTAL HEALTH

Nursing is a person-oriented profession. Every interaction that a nurse has with a patient affords an opportunity for assessment of the patient's emotional state. The nurse has the power and responsibility to create an environment that allows the patient to have as positive an experience as possible. Most people have an innate ability to heal themselves that is influenced by mental attitude. The nurse can help the patient use this inner healing capacity through nursing interventions.

MENTAL HEALTH CONTINUUM

Mental health and mental illness are the opposite ends of a **mental health continuum** (Fig. 34.3). Functioning is normal on the healthy end of the mental health continuum. This form of wellness includes an assertive communication style, acceptance of strengths and weaknesses, and available energy to deal with life's situations. The influences of daily stressors, although affecting the mentally healthy individual, do not normally disrupt mental health. Continued stressor exposure results in a deterioration of mental health and alterations in behaviors. The longer and the more intense the exposures are, the more likely behaviors are to become dysfunctional. Loss of contact with reality can result when an individual is at the illness end of the continuum. The midpoint on the continuum represents normal mental health. Although a person at this point probably displays some lack of insight, this midpoint level is characterized by adequate coping skills, problem-solving ability, and satisfactory responses or adjustments to life changes with some growth or possibly some mild regression. Although many individuals function in a relatively healthy manner, periods of crisis or biochemical imbalance have the potential to decrease functional capacity, moving one toward the illness end of the continuum (Box 34.1).

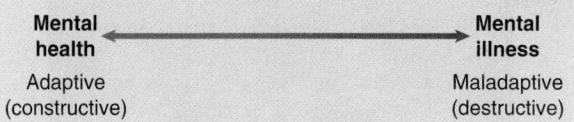

Fig. 34.3 Mental health continuum.

Box 34.1 Characteristics Identified in Mental Illness

- Poor self-concept
- Feelings of inadequacy
- Dependent behavior resulting from feelings of inadequacy
- Pessimism that is constant
- Poor judgment
- Inability to cope with daily events
- Irresponsibility
- Inability to accept responsibility for actions
- Avoidance of problems (no attempt to handle them)
- Inability to recognize own talents
- Inability to recognize limitations
- Inability to perceive reality
- Maladaptive behavior
- Demanding or seeking immediate gratification
- Inability to establish a meaningful relationship

To determine a patient's placement on the continuum, it is necessary to assess several components of mental health. These components include a positive self-concept, awareness of responsibility for one's own behavior and its consequences, maintenance of satisfying interpersonal relationships, adaptability to change, effective communication, awareness and acceptance of emotions and their expression, effective problem solving, and recognition and use of supportive systems (Fig. 34.4).

The point at which a person is deemed to be mentally ill is determined by the behavior the person exhibits, as well as the context in which the behavior occurs. Mental illness results from an inability to cope with a situation that an individual finds overwhelming. The maladaptive behavior is often part of a response to acute anxiety (see Box 34.1).

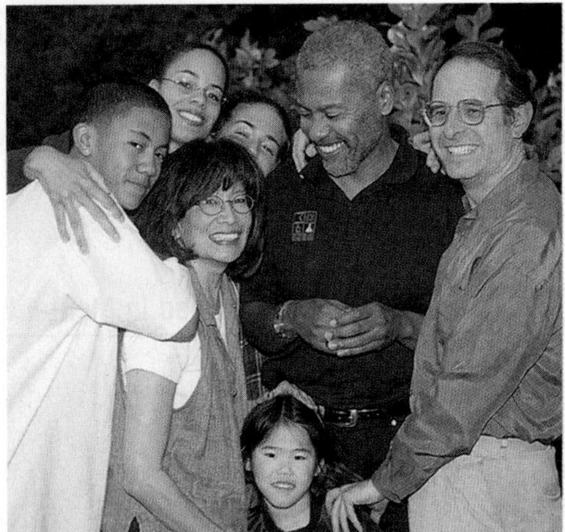

Fig. 34.4 Recognition and use of a support system of family and friends is one of the mental health components that determines placement on the mental health continuum. (From Varcarolis EM: *Foundations of psychiatric mental health nursing*, ed 5, Philadelphia, 2006, Saunders.)

PERSONALITY AND SELF-CONCEPT

Personality refers to the relatively consistent set of attitudes and behaviors particular to an individual. **Personality** consists of unique patterns of mental, emotional, and behavioral traits, woven together. Thoughts, feelings, values, and beliefs evolve into a consistent set of such traits that characterize an individual. Personality development comes under the influence of genetics and interactions with the environment. From infancy and throughout life, individuals have interactions that affect their personal security, values, personal identity, and relationships with others. Personality may be viewed as the total of internal and external patterns of adjustment to life. There are many theories about growth process and the development of personality. All are attempts to explain why people behave the way they do, as well as how each individual evolves emotionally and physically.

Erik Erikson provided a framework for understanding personality development in terms of task mastery (see Chapter 24). Erikson is one of the most widely read and influential theorists of development, and his concepts of identity and identity crisis have had major professional influence throughout the social sciences. According to Erikson's framework, if a person does not master a given task, then it is possible to predict a certain set of behaviors.

Sigmund Freud described personality development as having three parts: id, ego, and superego (Box 34.2). The id functions on a primitive level; its aims are primarily experiencing pleasure and avoiding pain. The ego functions to integrate and mediate between the self and the rest of the environment. It is the ego that experiences anxiety. The superego is the moralistic censoring force. It develops from the ego in response to reward or punishment from other people. When all three substructures function in harmony, the individual

Box 34.2 Parts of the Personality According to Freud

ID

- Basic innate drive for survival and pleasure
- Characterized by a demand for constant gratification
- Constitutes the individual's entire personality at birth
- Is not changed by experience because it is not in contact with the external world
- Its goals: to reduce tension, to increase pleasure, and to keep discomfort to a minimum

EGO

- "Reality factor"
- Helps the individual perceive conditions accurately
- Determines decisions about how to act and when to act
- Portion of the psyche that is in contact with external reality: enables reasoning and good sense (whereas the id stands for untamed passion)

SUPEREGO

- Parental or societal value system
- Characterized by striving for perfection and morality
- Develops from the ego
- Serves as a judge or censor over thoughts and activities of the ego; Freud described three functions of the superego: conscience, self-observation, and the formation of ideals

Modified from Thornton SP: Sigmund Freud (1856–1939). *Internet encyclopedia of philosophy.* Retrieved from *www.iep.utm.edu/freud/#H3.*

experiences emotional stability; that person is considered to have a healthy self-concept. A mature, well-adjusted personality is under the leadership of the ego.

Freud delineated levels of awareness: conscious, preconscious, and unconscious. At the conscious level, experiences are within a person's awareness; an individual is aware of and able to control thoughts (Thornton, n.d.). *Preconsciousness* refers to thoughts, feelings, drives, and ideas that are outside of awareness but that can be recalled easily to consciousness. The preconscious state helps screen certain thoughts and repress unpleasant thoughts and desires. The unconscious level holds memories, feelings, and thoughts that are not available to the conscious mind. This is the most significant level because of the effect it has on behavior.

Self is a complex concept comprising four distinct parts that influence behavior: personal identity, body image, role, and self-esteem. Personal identity is the organizing principle of the self; it is the "I." A person with a strong personal identity knows who he or she is and is not in regard to such things as beliefs, values, and goals in life. Body image comprises the mental picture of and the feelings toward one's body. Body image includes feelings about the way an individual looks, the way his or her body functions, the person's gender, body size, and whether one's body helps the person realize personal gains. Manifestations of body image include stance, posture, clothing, and jewelry.

Role performance is the expected behavior of an individual in a social position. Roles are ascribed or assumed. An ascribed role—for example, being female or male—involves no personal choice. An assumed role (e.g., occupation) is selected by the individual. In a lifetime, individuals fill many overlapping roles, and combining these roles to achieve an integrated pattern of functioning is necessary. Self-esteem is the assessment someone makes about personal worth. Self-esteem comprises the thoughts and feelings that an individual holds about himself or herself.

Self-concept is more than the total of the four parts of self. It is the frame of reference used for all that a person knows and experiences. Self-concept includes all perceptions and values held and all behaviors and interactions performed.

Through the process of growth and development, individuals accumulate and process information that helps form a basic perception of who they are, how they look, and how others react to them. How a person sees himself or herself determines behavior and interactions with others. Disturbances in self-concept commonly arise in people with mental illness or emotional problems.

STRESS

Individuals are exposed continually to a variety of situations that produce stress, and their mental health fluctuates along with their ability to adapt to and deal with life situations or events. Any event that requires change leads to stress. It is possible for the event to be either pleasant or unpleasant. **Stress** is the nonspecific response of the body to any demand made on it. An individual's response to a stressful situation or event is often a learned or conditioned behavior.

A **stressor** is a situation, activity, or event that produces stress. Stressors are physical, social, economic, chemical, spiritual, or developmental, or some combination of all of these. The meaning of the stress to an individual determines whether that individual feels distress. Stress is highly subjective, uniquely perceived by the person experiencing it. Stress in itself is neither good nor bad; however, it has positive and negative effects. Stress that facilitates individual growth and development and promotes change and adaptation brings positive results. Some stressors have the potential to be overwhelming, yielding the negative results characteristic of ineffective coping.

Mental health nursing focuses on behavior, particularly a person's response to stressors. Health factors affect this response. The stress of being ill greatly influences a person's emotional well-being and coping ability. How a person perceives stress determines whether the stress produces anxiety. A person's response to a stressful situation or event is often a result of learned or conditioned behavior and thus is, at least in theory, amenable to change. The nurse can serve as a resource in helping a patient develop adaptive patterns of behavior.

ANXIETY

Anxiety can be defined as a vague feeling of apprehension that results from a perceived threat to the self, although the source is often unknown. Anxiety is said to be a universal emotion and is a response to a stressful event. Anxiety is an internal process that a person experiences when there is a real or perceived threat to the physical body or self-concept. Anxiety is a major component of all mental health disturbances. In mild forms, anxiety readies the body for action and reaction to danger. Mild levels of anxiety enable the body to meet stressful demands by promoting problem solving and constructive action. Higher levels of anxiety immobilize coping skills and result in emotional chaos. In severe forms, anxiety interferes with daily activities.

Anxiety usually is described in terms of levels, and each level is associated with certain behaviors (Box 34.3). Signs of higher levels of anxiety include vocal changes; rapid speech; increased pulse, respirations, and blood pressure; tremors; restlessness; increased perspiration;

Box 34.3 Levels of Anxiety

An individual's response in a given situation depends on the level of anxiety.

MILD

- Slight increase in vital signs measurements and an awareness of danger
- Ability to think and make connections; heightened awareness
- Readiness for action
- Increased motivation

MODERATE

- Feeling of tension
- Decreased perception
- Continuing alertness, but only to specific information
- May display a proneness to arguing, teasing, or complaining
- Appearance (often) of physical signs and symptoms: headache, diarrhea, nausea, vomiting, low back pain, and stronger vital signs

SEVERE

- Feeling of impending danger
- Significant narrowing and distortion of perceptual field
- Possible distortion of communication and difficulty in making self understood
- Feeling of fatigue
- Changes in vital signs, potentially evident on assessment

PANIC

- Extreme terror
- Possible immobilization
- Distortion of reality
- Potential further disintegration of personality
- Potential to cause harm to self and others

nausea; decreased appetite; diarrhea; frequent urination; and occasionally, vomiting.

Anxiety arises as the result of inner conflict, and subsequent behavior stems from the anxiety. Maladaptive behavior is often a defense against anxiety. Individuals learn a variety of ways to respond to anxiety as they move through the various stages of growth and development. Behavior exhibited in response to stress and anxiety results from many factors. The degree of anxiety experienced is influenced by the following:

- How the individual views the stressor
- The number of stressors the individual is handling at one time
- Previous experience with similar situations
- The magnitude of change that the event represents for the individual
- The degree of physical and emotional health being experienced at the time of the stress

Events that have the potential to precipitate feelings of anxiety include the following:

- *Threats to physical integrity:* Decreased ability to perform activities of daily living; impending physiologic disability (surgery, diagnosis of a life-threatening disorder, pain, infection, trauma)
- *Threats to self-esteem and insults to the identity:* Loss of significant relationships, loss of spouse, difficulty at work, loss of job, change in jobs, relocation to a new home

Anxiety is relieved through various coping and mental mechanisms. These mechanisms are partly conscious and partly unconscious; they protect individuals from situations perceived as dangerous. Anxiety is an inevitable part of life. Part of the emotional growth process is to learn to deal with stress and anxiety in an adaptive or corrective manner.

MOTIVATION

Motivation is the gathering of personal resources or inner drive to complete a task or reach a goal. This inner drive is generated by anticipation of the reward or the punishment an individual expects when the needed task is performed. Motivation is an important aspect in treating emotional problems. The motivation to participate in care helps the patient through the stages of recovery quickly.

FRUSTRATION

Frustration is the emotional response to anything that interferes with goal-directed activity. This concept is important for understanding the individual's response to frustration. Some people are more flexible and adaptable than others. When adaptive behavior fails, anxiety increases.

CONFLICT

Conflict is a struggle, usually a mental one, either conscious or unconscious. Conflict results from the simultaneous presence of opposing or incompatible thoughts, ideas, goals, or emotional forces, such as impulses, denials, or drives. Some conflicts are resolved easily, whereas others are more complicated and lead to serious levels of anxiety. An example of conflict is the situation in which a person is ill and needs to see a physician but does not for fear of getting bad news.

ADAPTATION AND COPING

Adaptation refers to the ability to adjust to changing life situations by using various strategies. Any kind of change in routines or patterns of living causes stress in varying degrees. Illness, family problems, lack of money, and inadequate transportation may be viewed as stressful. An inability to meet basic needs or role expectations has the power to precipitate emotional upheaval. Feelings and emotions are part of a person's behavior. An individual who develops ways to deal with stress and resolve it has achieved adaptation. Adaptation, however, may be viewed as positive or negative. Growth or regression is a possible result of a stress experience.

Coping responses are the responses used to reduce anxiety brought on by stress. Common coping responses include overeating, drinking, drug use, smoking, withdrawal, seeking out someone to talk with, yelling, exercising or other physical activity, fighting, pacing, or listening to music. People often use coping responses consciously and unconsciously to adjust to stress without changing their actual goal.

Use of defense mechanisms—unconscious, intrapsychic reactions that offer protection to the self from a stressful situation—is another way of coping with anxiety. **Defense mechanisms** are behavioral patterns that protect individuals against a real or perceived threat; they are used to block conscious awareness of threatening feelings. This type of behavior develops when an unconscious conflict or a threat to self-concept is experienced (Table 34.1).

If defense mechanisms are used inappropriately or overused to help one cope, the behavior is termed *maladaptive.*

HOW ILLNESS AFFECTS MENTAL HEALTH

There is a misconception that mental health principles are applicable only in a mental health care facility or center. In reality, all nurses address the mental health needs of each patient. The stress of being ill greatly influences an individual's mental state and level of functioning.

Individuals like to feel in control of their lives. Illness reduces that control and sometimes creates instability of circumstances, causing anxiety. When a person is hospitalized, the familiarity of home and work is exchanged for the unfamiliar hospital setting. Upon entering the hospital setting, the patient exchanges his or her clothes for hospital wear, submits bodily fluids for testing and body parts for imaging, and endures

Table 34.1 **Commonly Used Defense Mechanisms**

MODE	DESCRIPTION	EXAMPLE
Compensation	Making up for a "deficiency" in one area by excelling in or emphasizing another area.	A boy who is small in stature places his emphasis on academics rather than attempting sports.
Conversion	Turning emotional conflicts into a physical symptom, which provides the individual with some sort of benefit (secondary gain).	An individual who witnesses a murder then experiences sudden blindness with no organic cause.
Denial	Disregard for reality.	A patient who had a severe myocardial infarction is told that he will have to severely restrict his physical activity. The evening nurse finds him on the floor of his room, doing sit-ups and push-ups.
Displacement	Expression of emotions toward someone or something other than the actual source of the emotion. Unconsciously, the individual does not feel safe expressing the feelings directly to the actual source.	A man has an argument with his employer and comes home and yells at his family.
Dissociation	Separation and detachment of emotional significance and affect from an idea or situation.	A person who has been traumatically victimized retells her situation, while smiling and joking about it.
Identification	Incorporation of a characteristic (thought or behavior) of another individual or group. The individual does not give up personal identity.	A teenager who dresses like a favorite rock singer.
Introjection	A quality or attribute of another person is internalized and becomes part of the individual's behavior.	A child follows her parents' instructions when the parents are not present (e.g., carefully crossing the street).
Projection	Attributing problems to other characteristics that the person does not want to admit possessing; blaming personal shortcomings on someone else.	A student who does poorly on an examination states, "That test was unfair. The teacher did not present the material correctly."
Rationalization	A process of constructing plausible reasons to explain and justify one's behavior. The person denies actual thoughts and justifies actions by giving untrue, but seemingly more acceptable, reasons for the behavior.	A young boy who was instructed to make up his bed and clean his room before leaving for school chooses to play instead. In the afternoon, when he and his mother arrive home and she becomes angry at his disregard of her instructions, he states, "But Mom, Dad was in a hurry this morning and told me that if I wanted a ride to school, I'd better get in the car."
Reaction formation	Conscious behavior that reflects an emotion opposite to the emotion actually felt.	A person is excessively polite to an individual whom the person dislikes.
Regression	Exhibition of behavior, thoughts, or feelings used at an earlier stage of development.	An 8-year-old reverts to bedwetting and thumbsucking while hospitalized.
Repression	The unconscious process of barring from conscious thought of painful, disagreeable thoughts, experiences, and or impulses. Energy is expended in this process, so the individual has less available energy.	A patient who was incontinent after surgery suppresses the embarrassment and totally represses the event.
Sublimation	The discharge of sexual or aggressive energy and impulses in a socially acceptable way.	A teenager engages in many competitive sports.
Suppression	An intentional (conscious) exclusion of painful thoughts, experiences, or impulses. (Some authorities do not consider this a defense mechanism.)	A student fails to keep an appointment for academic counseling.

Box 34.4 Patient Problem Statements for Psychiatric-Mental Health Nursing

Anxiousness
Compromised Social Interaction
Compromised Verbal Communication
Despair
Distorted Body Image
Fearfulness
Grief
Impaired Coping
Impaired Decision-Making Ability
Impaired family processes
Impaired Personal Sense of Identity
Impaired Role Functioning
Impaired Sexual Expression
Inability to Sleep
Obstructive Denial
Potential for Impaired Self-Esteem due to Current Situation
Potential for Impaired Spiritual Beliefs
Potential for Ineffective Belief System

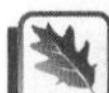

Lifespan Considerations

Older Adults

Aging and Mental Health

- Older people experiencing significant sensory changes in hearing or vision sometimes display behavioral changes that are easy to mistake for disorientation.
- Behavioral changes in elderly patients may be related to the many medications that they may be prescribed. The absorption, distribution, and clearance may be affected by aging and potentially by the interaction between medications.
- Social isolation of older adults is frequently a result of physical or financial limitations.
- The behavioral characteristics and personalities of older people are often an exaggeration of their behavior at a younger age.
- Many losses—including loss of loved ones, home, job, and independence—occur with aging. These losses result in varying amounts of grief. The number of losses and the rapidity with which they occur have the potential to affect the coping ability of the older person and result in anxiety, fear, and depression.
- Relocation from home to hospital or even from room to room has potential to cause stress in the older person, which manifests as behavioral change.
- Hopelessness, helplessness, and depression are common in older adults. These feelings sometimes lead older people to lose the will to live and even progress to committing suicide.
- Reminiscence and life review are effective techniques to help older adults cope with changing life circumstances.
- Alcoholism, often hidden or denied, is common among the older population. It is possible to use alcohol as an attempted means of coping with grief, depression, loneliness, or boredom. If unrecognized, alcoholism poses the risk of exacerbating medical conditions and leading to serious drug reactions.

the same questions again and again. Sometimes visitation with family and friends is limited. The patient must adapt to being one entry on someone else's scheduled daily duties: the nurse's.

Most people do not expect to become ill or have lifestyle alterations resulting from illness or accidents. Serious injury and illness have the capacity to alter dramatically a person's self-concept, body image, lifestyle, and role performance in family life, recreation, and work. Regardless of whether the situation is temporary or permanent, mental and emotional states undergo a disturbance. The nurse is able to provide effective nursing interventions only if the patient's emotional state is considered.

Meeting the psychosocial needs of the individual is a task for the health care team as a whole. Patients and their families remember the nurses who care for them, whether the nurse showed a little extra consideration or was short-tempered or judgmental. One of the steps to meeting these needs is effective patient education. It helps to build trust and encourages the patient to have faith in the care given. Patient support groups, family connections, and community involvement are important to maintain during an illness.

Box 34.4 lists psychiatric patient problem statements that nurses often use to address a patient's psychosocial needs (see the Lifespan Considerations for older adults box).

ILLNESS BEHAVIORS

Illness is a state of homeostatic imbalance. When an individual is ill or sick, he or she does not feel good. This is the body's way of saying, "Pay attention to my needs." The experience of being ill involves stages that are subjective and very personal. The illness experience starts with awareness of symptoms that are not healthy, and the individual takes on the sick role. The sick role allows the individual to be excused from everyday responsibilities, including social, to rest and heal. If an appropriate attempt at this stage does not cure the ailment, professional medical help is sought. The sick person receiving professional care assumes a dependent role—with the expectation of getting well. Keeping the patient informed and emotionally supported is a focus of professional care. Recovery and rehabilitation are the last stages of an illness event. The nurse assists the patient by setting attainable short-term goals to enable the patient to be aware of his or her recovery and rehabilitation.

CRISIS

A **crisis** can be defined as an unstable period in a person's life characterized by the inability to adapt to a change from a precipitating event. It most often results when a person is faced with a turning point in life, accumulating stressors, or illness. Successful management of a crisis period is needed to prevent disorganization within the individual or the family unit. Difficulty or inability to manage the crisis successfully results in physical illness or emotional breakdown. The manifestations associated with an inability to navigate a crisis situation may include denial, hostility, anger, vulgarity, noncompliance, aggression, manipulation, apathy, and depression.

The sick role often produces secondary gains as well as personal attention: for example, when a mother becomes very ill every time her daughter plans a trip out of town, or when a person obtains renewal of disability benefits because the injury flares up when reevaluation is scheduled. It is possible for the sick role to become a way of life. Secondary gains are sometimes a ploy used to manipulate and cope with various emotional conflicts. It is important for the nurse to recognize this to plan appropriate interventions to meet emotional and psychological needs of the patient who uses the sick role in a destructive manner (Box 34.5).

Behavior is learned through life experiences. Interactions between a patient and the health care system is influenced largely by the patient's past. A serious illness, the breakup of a relationship, a car accident, or the death of a loved one potentially can trigger a crisis response in an individual or family. Cultural and ethnic backgrounds affect the patient's and family's behavior during illness. For example, many men received the message as boys to be stoic or ignore feelings when hurt. As adults, these men are less likely to seek medical treatment in the early stages of disease. A family may provide home remedies that generations of their forebears used to treat colds and flu. The United States is teeming with cultural diversity; thus consider cultural influences on all patients' behavior (see Chapter 6). The nurse's responsibility is to note and to respond therapeutically to all behavior. By understanding the relationship of stressors, anxiety, and culture to behavior, nurses can facilitate healthy adaptation.

An *identity crisis* is a condition of instability that arises from an emotional or situational upheaval and results in extreme or decisive change. An identity crisis represents potential opportunity, as well as danger. From that period of vulnerability, personal growth and strength often are developed. Nurses deal with people in identity crises nearly every day.

Phases of crisis are similar to stages in grief and dying (see Chapter 25). The initial phase consists of confusion, disbelief, and high anxiety. This progresses to a denial phase, with grasping of the conviction that everything will be all right. Once the reality of the situation becomes evident, anger and remorse generally are expressed. Sadness and crying constitute a phase of grief seen during a crisis. In this phase, the individual acknowledges and expresses the loss of what was and never will be again. The final phase of reconciliation is reached with the person's acceptance that life will continue but will be different from how it had been, and adaptation occurs.

Help the individual or family to get through a crisis by providing accurate information that aids in realistic perception of the situation (see the Patient Teaching box).

Encourage expression of feelings and provide empathic gestures such as silent physical closeness, holding a hand, or giving a hug when appropriate (but not with an angry, hostile patient). These validate that individual's feelings of anger, denial, remorse, and grief as normal responses to crisis.

Identifying family supports and adequate coping mechanisms helps the nurse recognize family communication patterns. Dysfunction in relationships sometimes indicates a need to include other psychosocial professionals in the care of the individual or family in crisis. Active listening, restating the facts, and using other therapeutic communication techniques during family conferences are ways to help address the problem constructively. Offer as much flexibility in visiting hours as possible to reduce the frustration of separation in the individual and the family.

With or without crisis intervention, a crisis often tends to resolve over a 4- to 6-week period. The development of coping mechanisms and the redefinition of goals and roles in life often result from a crisis. The short-term active support the nurse provides in focusing on problem solving helps facilitate a positive resolution to the crisis (Box 34.6).

Box 34.5 Behaviors Common With Illness

DENIAL

A refusal to admit being ill. Short-term denial is often useful in mobilizing internal resources, but long-term denial usually results in maladaptive behavior patterns.

ANXIETY

Feelings of apprehension and uncertainty about the illness. Fear has the capacity to produce sympathetic nervous response (fight-or-flight response). The measurement of vital signs often helps in the assessment of level of anxiety.

SHOCK

An overwhelming emotion that paralyzes the individual's ability to process information. The individual is incapable of making decisions. The individual is unable to sort through information received.

ANGER

A response to feeling mistreated, injured, or insulted. Anger behaviors are directed inward, outward toward others, or both. Sometimes anger is an irrational response to minor events of the day and interrupts the person's social functioning.

WITHDRAWAL

Removal of self from interaction with others and the environment. Withdrawal is often a sign of depression. Family members sometimes withdraw from an ill person, or an ill person sometimes isolates herself or himself from the family.

Patient Teaching

Improving Mental Health

Teach the patient to do the following:

- Recognize constructive aspects of mild or moderate anxiety in learning, growth, and movement toward self-actualization.
- Recognize personal characteristics that indicate presence of anxiety.
- Describe current state of anxiety.
- Analyze current expectations, goals, beliefs, and values within the context of perceptions of what is actually happening.
- Recognize the healing power of positive thinking.
- Recognize sayings that support negative thinking, and change those sayings to reflect a positive feeling.
- Develop assertive communication skills.
- Develop problem-solving and decision-making skills.
- Use progressive muscle relaxation.
- Increase repertoire of strategies to reduce anxiety, including the following: talking or being with someone; simple, concrete tasks; walking; noncompetitive sports; professional assistance; listening to soothing music; meditating or prayer; deep-breathing exercises; and relaxation exercises.

Box 34.6 Crisis Intervention

GOALS

1. The victim's emotional stress will be decreased, and the nurse will protect the victim.
2. The nurse will assist the victim to organize and mobilize resources.
3. The victim will return to precrisis status or a higher functional level.

STEPS

1. Assess the situation and individual or individuals involved in the crisis.
2. Determine possible interventions with input from a spiritual care provider, other family members, significant others, or close friends, as well as health care providers.
3. Implement the intervention plan.

OUTCOME

The crisis resolves, and/or an anticipatory plan emerges from the solution to the problem.

Box 34.7 Assessment of Emotional Status

GENERAL APPEARANCE

Describe the patient's dress, makeup, and hygiene.

GENERAL BEHAVIOR

Describe the patient's general activity level, posture, gait, and response to examination.

SPEECH PATTERN

Describe the rate, tone, loudness, and quantity content of the patient's speech (descriptions include "response to questions too detailed"; "extreme distractibility"; "unable to complete an answer"; "uses rhyming").

CONTENT OF THOUGHT

Describe the patient's thinking: reality oriented, delusional, showing evidence of hallucinations, or showing evidence of ideas of reference or other non–reality-based thinking.

MOOD AND AFFECT

Describe the patient's overall feeling state and affect.

SENSORIAL FUNCTION

Describe the patient's orientation, memory, attention, and ability to think abstractly.

INSIGHT AND JUDGMENT

Assess whether the patient understands the current situation and what the individual is willing to do about it.

POTENTIAL FOR DANGER

Assess the patient's potential for violence or self-harm, degree of impulse control, and previous history of violence or aggression toward others.

APPLICATION OF THE NURSING PROCESS

In every setting, nurses use the nursing process to meet the many needs of patients. An LPN/LVN participates in the nursing process by observing patient behavior and assisting in establishing patient problem statements, as well as working with the registered nurse (RN) on outlining appropriate nursing interventions. The LPN/LVN and RN implement the plan by using therapeutic communication techniques and continue to observe and report behavior. Analysis of these observations makes it possible to adjust the plan of care appropriately.

Box 34.7 outlines basic nursing assessments of emotional status. Other possible assessments include observations for risk for violence, level of anxiety, use of defense mechanisms, and use of coping methods if the illness is severe or long lasting.

Get Ready for the NCLEX® Examination!

Key Points

- Historically, mental health care reflected fear and ignorance of mental illness that have directly influenced the attitude toward mental illness that prevails today.
- Individuals have unique personalities. According to Freudian theory, the personality consists of the id, the ego, and the superego.
- All behavior has meaning. An individual's behavior is the best that person is capable of within his or her current environment.

- Corrective emotional experiences assist the individual to change. The therapeutic relationship should be directed to facilitate this change.
- *Personality* refers to the relatively consistent set of attitudes and behaviors particular to an individual. Cultural and ethnic backgrounds influence personality development.
- Self is an important part of personality; self consists of identity, body image, role, and esteem.
- Anxiety is a universal response to a real or imagined threat to self.
- Defense mechanisms are automatic behaviors used to protect the personality in times of stress.
- Coping mechanisms are usually adaptive methods used to deal with uncomfortable feelings or stressors.
- Stress is the nonspecific response of the body to demands. Stressors are factors causing stress. High or chronic stress has the potential to hamper the immune response to illness.
- It is possible to view mental health and illness as existing on a continuum.
- Physical illness affects the mental health of an individual. Behavior incorporating the sick role and dependency until recovery occurs allows the individual to cope with body image changes and keep the self intact.
- The use of therapeutic communication is a dynamic method of interaction with patients for problem solving and growth.
- Observe and evaluate behavior to determine a patient's progress and the effectiveness of the care plan.

Additional Learning Resources

SG Go to your Study Guide for additional learning activities to help you master this chapter content.

evolve Be sure to visit the Evolve site at *http://evolve.elsevier.com/Cooper/foundationsadult/* for additional online resources.

Review Questions for the NCLEX® Examination

1. Who was the English Quaker who advocated humane care and built an asylum to reflect a household?
   1. Florence Nightingale
   2. William Tukes
   3. Sigmund Freud
   4. Benjamin Rush
2. Changes in the delivery of mental health care that resulted from the development of electroconvulsive therapy and psychotherapeutic drugs brought about which phenomenon in the 20th century?
   1. Behavioral therapy
   2. Personality disorganization
   3. Deinstitutionalization
   4. Brain surgery
3. What is the best description of personality?
   1. The level of mental health that a person attains in life
   2. The relatively consistent set of attitudes and behaviors particular to an individual
   3. The result of a positive self-concept and acceptable behavior
   4. The ability to manage stress
4. The nurse is reviewing the assessment findings for a patient hospitalized with a stress disorder. What findings support the diagnosis? *(Select all that apply.)*
   1. A vague feeling of depression
   2. An assumed role to protect the ego
   3. A main reason for all mental illnesses
   4. A distortion of reality in response to a stressor
   5. A response to any demand made upon the individual
5. The nurse is caring for a patient who is currently voicing feelings of anxiety. The nurse correctly recognizes what as the best description of the feelings that the patient is experiencing?
   1. A vague feeling of apprehension
   2. Feelings of paranoia
   3. Emotional stability
   4. Concerns about the impressions that others have of her
6. An assembly-line manager in a factory was told that he would be laid off if his line did not meet the hourly quota. He promptly went to his workers and threatened to fire anyone who was found taking even 1 minute extra on a break. What is the manager displaying?
   1. Denial
   2. Regression
   3. Displacement
   4. Identification
7. Punishment and abandonment were how mentally ill people were treated in medieval times. These practices continued until the 17th and 18th centuries. Which care practice that is still being used today did Dr. Philippe Pinel of France advocate?
   1. Electroshock therapy for melancholy
   2. Humane care with record keeping of behaviors
   3. Psychoanalysis
   4. Home care in the community
8. The student nurse is working on a presentation regarding OBRA. What was the result of this landmark legislation? *(Select all that apply.)*
   1. Deinstitutionalization
   2. Prohibition of electroshock therapy
   3. Limited access to psychotropic medications
   4. Approved surgical treatment for schizophrenia
   5. Increased construction of state facilities for residential mental health care
9. A 52-year-old patient experienced cardiac arrest from a myocardial infarction. During his acute care stay in the hospital, the patient flirts with all his female nurses. When he is asked to stop, he withdraws and later complains of chest heaviness. What is a possible explanation for the patient's behavior?
   1. Boredom from restricted activity
   2. Lack of motivation to recover
   3. Frustration from illness
   4. Threatened self-concept

10. A 14-year-old tells the school nurse that she is self-conscious about her recent breast development. She reports that the boys in her class are teasing her. What is the first step for the nurse to take?
 1. Call her parents.
 2. Ask her to describe what happened.
 3. Ask who her friends are.
 4. Provide her with a pamphlet outlining the changes associated with puberty.
11. The nurse is instructing a wife to give insulin injections to her husband. The wife is unable to sit still, frequently asks to repeat parts of the instruction for understanding, and sighs often with rapid respirations. What degree of anxiety is the wife experiencing?
 1. Mild
 2. Moderate
 3. Severe
 4. Panic
12. A 17-year-old patient was admitted to the orthopedic unit with pelvic fracture, wrist fracture, and multiple contusions and abrasions from an auto accident. She yells for the nurse every 5 minutes, refuses to use her call light, and breaks out in tears when she does not get her way. How would this behavior best be described?
 1. Regression
 2. Compensation
 3. Denial
 4. Displacement
13. A college student is brought to the emergency department by her roommate. The roommate states that when the patient returned from her date, she was crying and said she had been raped. The patient recounts the evening's events, cracking jokes about her date's trouble keeping an erection and asking if the nurse knows where she can get a replacement for her favorite outfit, which has been torn. How is this defense mechanism best described?
 1. Displacement
 2. Compensation
 3. Denial
 4. Dissociation
14. A teenager wrecks the family car by rear-ending a truck turning left. The teenager says, "It wasn't my fault. I came over the hill and that truck was just sitting there. It was his fault for turning left." What defense mechanism is the teenager using to deal with his situation?
 1. Compensation
 2. Conversion reaction
 3. Projection
 4. Rationalization
15. After a few days of hospitalization, a patient is participating in plans to be transferred to a rehabilitation facility to continue therapies to enhance his activities of daily living. Which statement indicates the patient is beginning to adjust to his new situation and future? *(Select all that apply.)*
 1. "I know that once I can walk without assistance, I can go back to my own home."
 2. "My wife will not be able to help take care of me until I get stronger."
 3. "I'm going to show everybody that I can make it on my own; just you wait!"
 4. "I don't know why everybody is making a big deal; I was by myself before I got sick."
 5. "I am ready to get started with therapy so I can hopefully go home soon."
16. What factor is most predictive of the onset of a crisis for an individual?
 1. The individual has no support system.
 2. The individual perceives a stressor to be threatening.
 3. The individual is exposed to a precipitating stressor.
 4. The individual experiences a stressor and responds with ineffective coping efforts.
17. During crisis intervention, what is the highest priority of nursing care?
 1. Managing anxiety
 2. Identifying situational supports
 3. Patient safety
 4. Teaching specific coping skills that the patient lacks
18. The leader of a self-help group is discussing the use of defense mechanisms. What information should be included about their use? *(Select all that apply.)*
 1. Once used, they are irreversible.
 2. Defense mechanisms are pathologic.
 3. They are a means of managing conflict.
 4. Defense mechanisms are predominantly unconscious.
 5. Defense mechanisms are primarily used to blame others.
19. What interventions can the nurse use to enhance the assessment of an older adult patient? *(Select all that apply.)*
 1. Identify and accommodate physical needs first.
 2. Pledge complete confidentiality on all topics to the patient.
 3. Interpret information with consideration of the patient's spiritual or cultural background.
 4. Adhere firmly to the sequence of questions on the standardized assessment tool.
 5. Determine whether there are any sensory changes in hearing or vision before beginning the assessment.
20. The nurse manager has completed an educational program with her staff regarding patient education and improving mental illness. Which statement by a participant would indicate a need for further education? *(Select all that apply.)*
 1. "I need to teach my patients ways to recognize and describe their levels of anxiety."
 2. "My patients will not need to worry about learning relaxation skills if they don't want to."
 3. "Patients who use passive communication skills have better mental health than those who use assertive communication skills."
 4. "Learning problem-solving skills can help improve a person's overall mental health."
 5. "The power of positive thinking patterns is a topic I need to discuss with my patients."

Care of the Patient With a Psychiatric Disorder

35

http://evolve.elsevier.com/Cooper/foundationsadult/

Objectives

1. Identify and describe the major mental disorders.
2. List five warning signs of suicide.
3. Identify basic interventions for patients experiencing various mental health problems.
4. Describe the general care and treatment methods for patients experiencing mental health problems.
5. Name two alternative therapies used for mental disorders.

Key Terms

anorexia nervosa (ăn-ō-RĔK-sē-ă nŭr-VŌ-să, p. 1128)
anxiety (ăng-ZĪ-ŭ-tē, p. 1122)
bulimia nervosa (bū-LĒ-mē-ă nŭr-VŌ-să, p. 1129)
compulsions (kŭm-PŬL-shŭnz, p. 1125)
cyclothymic disorder (sī-klō-THĪ-mĭk dĭs-ŌR-dŭr, p. 1122)
delirium (dĭ-LĬR-ē-ŭm, p. 1114)
delusion (dĭ-LŪ-zhŭn, p. 1114)
dementia (dĭ-MĔN-shŭ, p. 1114)
depression (dĭ-PRĔSH-ŭn, p. 1121)
hallucination (hă-lū-sĭ-NĀ-shŭn, p. 1120)
hypomanic episode (hī-pō-MĂN-ĭk ĔP-ĭ-sōd, p. 1121)
illusions (ĭl-LŪ-zhŭnz, p. 1126)
mania (MĀ-nē-ŭ, p. 1121)
multiaxial system (mŭl-tē-ĂK-sē-ăl SĬS-tŭm, p. 1113)
neurosis (nū-RŌ-sĭs, p. 1113)
obsessions (ŏb-SĔSH-ŭnz, p. 1125)
paraphilias (păr-ă-FĬL-ē-ŭz, p. 1127)
phobia (FŌ-bē-ŭ, p. 1125)
psychosis (sī-KŌ-sĭs, p. 1113)
schizophrenia (skĭt-sō-FRĒ-nē-ŭ, p. 1114)
serotonin syndrome (sĕr-ō-TŌ-nĭn SĬN-drōm, p. 1133)
somatic (sō-măt-ĭk, p. 1127)
sundowning syndrome (SŬN-DOUN-ĭng SĬN-drōm, p. 1114)

All nurses need to have a basic understanding of the classifications of human responses and methods of treatment for mental illness. Many patients on a medical unit have, in addition to a physiologic disorder, a history of psychiatric problems. An even more common situation is the ill patient's experience of emotional disturbance from the effects of the illness. It is important to be able to interact therapeutically with the physical and the emotional aspects of patient care.

A person's ability to handle a stressful event depends on that person's psychological state. **Neurosis** is a term describing ineffective coping with stress that causes mild interpersonal disorganization. People with a neurosis have insight that they have a psychiatric problem. A person with a neurosis remains oriented to reality but has some degree of distortion of reality manifested by a strong emotional response to the trigger event. The trigger event may be an everyday stressor, such as environmental stressors or family relationships. Various complaints of nervousness or emotional upset, compulsions, obsessiveness, and phobias are common with a neurosis. Many neurotic people exhibit poor self-esteem and have social relationships that are impaired by the various complaints noted. Treatment for patients with a neurosis usually is completed in an outpatient setting, if they seek treatment at all.

In contrast, a person with **psychosis** is out of touch with reality and has severe personality deterioration, impaired perception and judgment, hallucinations, and delusions. A psychotic person does not recognize the fact that he or she has a psychiatric illness. Treatment for psychosis often necessitates hospitalization with follow-up regularly through an outpatient setting. Some psychotic patients seek voluntary admission for treatment. Involuntary admission (commonly called *probating*) is also possible when a person is thought to be a danger to self or others. Although laws vary from state to state, a judge and either a clinical psychologist or a physician, or both, must be involved to complete an involuntary admission.

The *Diagnostic and Statistical Manual of Psychiatric Disorders*, Fifth Edition (DSM-V), published by the American Psychiatric Association (APA, 2013), includes signs and symptoms for all psychiatric illnesses. In previous editions, the *DSM* described a **multiaxial system** to document psychiatric illnesses. This system is not currently being used. Most hospitals and health care providers in the United States today use the *DSM-V* to facilitate medical diagnosis and as a guide to clinical practice.

Mental disorders discussed in this chapter include the following:

- Organic mental disorders (e.g., delirium and dementia)
- Thought process disorders (e.g., schizophrenia)
- Affective (mood) disorders
- Anxiety disorders
- Personality disorders
- Sexual disorders
- Psychophysiologic (somatoform) disorders
- Eating disorders

A basic description of some of the major disorders and a summary of treatment, prognosis, and related nursing diagnoses are included in Table 35.1.

TYPES OF PSYCHIATRIC DISORDERS

NEUROCOGNITIVE MENTAL DISORDERS

Neurocognitive disorders differ from other mental health disorders. An identifiable brain disease or dysfunction is the basis for the behavior. These disorders affect cognitive or intellectual abilities. The effects range from mild lapses in memory to severe memory loss and behavioral changes. A predominant characteristic of the type of disorder is disorientation.

Delirium

Delirium is a change in consciousness that occurs rapidly over a short time. Occurrence of this disorder is possible at any age. Delirium is associated with reduced awareness and attention to surroundings, disorganized thinking, sensory misinterpretation, and irrelevant speech. Sleep patterns often are disturbed. Possible causes of delirium include physical illnesses, such as fever, heart failure, pneumonia, azotemia, or malnutrition; drug intoxication; and anesthesia. Treatment for delirium involves determining the cause and correcting it. If the cause is a homeostatic imbalance such as hypoxemia, electrolyte imbalance, or malnutrition, treatment is focused on the problem causing the imbalance. If the cause is chemical agents, the chemicals or drugs should be withdrawn or the dosage reduced. A person with nocturnal delirium, or **sundowning syndrome,** displays increased disorientation and agitation only during the evening and nighttime.

Dementia

Dementia is a term describing an altered mental state secondary to cerebral disease. Dementia is usually a slow and progressive loss of intellectual function that is often irreversible. Symptoms are often severe enough to interfere with activities of daily living. Alzheimer's disease is the most common type of dementia in the United States, accounting for 60% to 80% of dementia cases. According to 2018 statistics from the Alzheimer's Association, 5.7 million people in the United States have Alzheimer's disease. It is projected that 14 million people will have Alzheimer's disease by the year 2050 (Alzheimer's Association, 2018). Using reality orientation techniques and providing a safe environment are two key aspects of nursing interventions in caring for patients with dementia (see Table 35.1).

SCHIZOPHRENIA

The main characteristic of thought process disorders is bizarre, non–reality-based thinking. **Schizophrenia** is one of a large group of psychotic disorders whose defining characteristics are gross distortion of reality; disturbance of language and communication; withdrawal from social interaction; and the disorganization and fragmentation of thought, perception, and emotional reaction. Schizophrenia is one of the most profoundly disabling mental illnesses that a nurse will ever encounter. The onset of schizophrenia typically occurs in young adulthood. It occurs in both sexes equally, and approximately 1% of the population will experience schizophrenia at some point in their lives. Schizophrenia is a chronic disorder with residual disability in functioning. The family of a patient with schizophrenia typically experiences emotional and financial devastation. Schizophrenia is prone to exacerbation from stresses in life.

Research findings have indicated a biologic basis for the disease, dispelling the early theory of poor mother-child relationship as the cause, and researchers have noted brain tissue changes. The ventricles of the brain are larger than normal, with the left ventricle larger than the right, and the cerebral cortex is smaller than normal. This is thought to account for the disorganized thinking, hallucinations, and delusions. The neurotransmitter dopamine is present in excess amounts in the brain with schizophrenia. Pupils of the eyes differ in size, and blinking rate is sometimes faster or slower than normal. Clumsiness and difficulty in distinguishing the right and left sides of the body sometimes occur and are attributable to the enlargement of the ventricles of the brain.

Behaviors that individuals with schizophrenia display fall into different categories: positive, or excessive, and negative, or absent. The prognosis for individuals who exhibit positive behavior patterns is good; such patients have fewer structural changes in the brain and respond better to drug therapy. Positive behavior patterns include delusions, hallucinations, and disordered thinking. Negative behavior patterns include apathy, social withdrawal, and flat affect.

Positive Behavior Patterns

A **delusion** is a false, fixed belief that cannot be corrected by feedback and that other people in the same cultural context do not accept as true. The affected individual believes that a false premise is true. The individual fits this false premise logically into his or her interpretation of reality. Because of the strong logic supporting the false premise, it is difficult for the individual to accept what is really true. There are several types of delusions (Table 35.2).

Text continued on p. 1120

Table 35.1 Psychiatric Disorders

CHARACTERISTICS	TREATMENT AND PROGNOSIS	ASSOCIATED PATIENT PROBLEMS	NURSING INTERVENTIONS
Neurocognitive Psychiatric Disorders			
Dementia			
Slow and progressive worsening of symptoms: impaired memory and judgment, personality changes, decreased cognitive function, impaired orientation	Treatment depends on the cause. Prognosis is poor; essential feature of this condition is the slow deteriorating rate of mental function.	*Impaired Cognitive Function* *Fearfulness* *Potential for Injury* *Anxiousness* *Inability to Bathe Self* *Excessive Demand on Primary Caregiver*	*Reality orientation techniques:* Place large clock and calendar in view; keep curtains opened and lights on during the day; and use calm, supportive approach. *Decrease sensory stimuli:* Do not expose patient to crowds; give instructions one step at a time, and keep in simple terms. *Provide for safety:* Place bed in lowest position; side rails useful to aid patient in turning. Ensure that hallway rails, chair, bed alarms, and call light are within reach; place personal articles within reach; and ensure sufficient night lighting. *Adequate nutrition:* Reduce dining distractions such as television; encourage snacks if patient is unable to eat a sufficient amount at one time; monitor weight monthly; and have family bring in patient's favorite foods. *Self-care support:* Assist as needed with ADLs and toileting; encourage mobility and other activities that use large muscle groups with activities such as "Simon says" or armchair aerobics; try to keep the daily routine the same times of each day; and, if possible, have same group of staff assist with ADLs.
Delirium			
Acute, rapid onset of symptoms: disorientation, incoherent thought content, impaired cognitive function, symptoms worsen at night, illusions, hallucinations	Treatment depends on the cause. Prognosis is guarded.	*Potential for Injury* *Potential for Harming Others* *Impaired Cognitive Function* *Inability to Bathe Self*	
Schizophrenia			
Inappropriate emotional responses, bizarre behaviors, impaired communications, delusions, illusions, hallucinations, inability to relate to other people, self-care deficit, symptoms present at least 6 mo, with positive behaviors for 1 mo or more	Treatment is milieu therapy (environment), psychotherapy, antipsychotic drug therapy, and long-term social support. Prognosis is variable and depends on the extent of the symptoms and responses to treatments. Many patients with paranoid type of schizophrenia are reluctant to seek treatment.	*Impaired Cognitive Function* *Disturbed Sensory Perception* *Anxiousness* *Inability to Bathe Self* *Inability to Dress Self* *Compromised Social Interaction* *Impaired Role Functioning* *Impaired Family Processes* *Ineffective Sleep Pattern* *Impaired Coping* *Impaired Personal Sense of Identity*	*Establish therapeutic relationship:* Be available and listen actively; use clear, simple statements in communications; ensure that your body language is in tune with the message; and avoid hand gesturing when talking, to prevent distraction from the message. *Reality orientation techniques:* Use verbal reminding; place large clock and calendar in view; reduce stimuli to help patient focus on reality; and establish and reinforce a daily routine. *Reduce anxiety:* Avoid having patient make choices; problem solve with patient on ways to reduce anxiety; encourage socialization by invitation, not assignment; decrease sensory stimuli; and accept and support patient's feelings (empathy reduces anxiety). *Manage positive behaviors:* Ask patient directly about his or her hallucinations; watch for cues that indicate that the patient is hallucinating; focus on reality; do not argue with the patient or enter into the patient's hallucination; if the patient is having delusions, be open and honest in interactions to reduce suspicion; respond calmly and matter-of-factly to suspicions; have the patient describe who "he" or "she" is, but do not argue the logic; and if the delusion is very strong, try to help the patient find a distraction from the delusion so as not to dwell upon it. Remember that hallucinations and delusions have the potential to provoke aggressive behavior. Watch for signs of growing agitation. Provide safety. *Manage negative behaviors:* Encourage self-care, assist only as indicated; help patient recognize own feelings of the event that just occurred; and encourage social participation, but do not force it onto the patient. *Medication management:* Be alert for early recognition of serious side effects; administer medications in liquid form if you suspect the patient of hoarding pills; encourage the patient to take medications routinely, to adjust to ideas of taking them for rest of life; and provide good nutrition.

Continued

Table 35.1 Psychiatric Disorders—cont'd

CHARACTERISTICS	TREATMENT AND PROGNOSIS	ASSOCIATED PATIENT PROBLEMS	NURSING INTERVENTIONS
Affective (Mood) Disorders			
Major Depression			
Prolonged, intense unhappiness Symptoms: apathy, pessimism, multiple physical complaints, guilt feelings, anxiety, isolation, suicidal thoughts, appetite disturbance, fatigue, sleep disturbance, constipation, limited attention span, short-term memory disturbance	Treatment possibilities include antidepressant drug therapy, individual family or group psychotherapy, and electroconvulsive therapy when drug therapy is ineffective or drugs are contraindicated. An estimated 50% of all individuals have at least one additional episode of depression.	*Potential for Violence Upon Self* *Despair* *Impaired Coping* *Inability to Bathe Self* *Inability to Dress Self* *Compromised Verbal Communication* *Ineffective Sleep Pattern* *Helplessness* *Potential for Insufficient Nutrition* *Impaired Belief System*	*Establish therapeutic relationship:* Use a kind but firm manner in addressing the individual; be honest and consistent; and show compassion, composure, and patience. Remember that depressed individuals have slower-than-normal physical responses. Manic individuals are not able to stay focused. *Communications: For depression:* Encourage expression of negative feeling; point out any specific improvement; reinforce assertive behavior; recognize and point out manifestations of self-destructive thoughts or behavior to the individual; and discuss and practice alternative ways to respond to stress. *For mania:* Keep directions specific and simple; use a calm approach; present reality without arguing; be consistent and keep to the rules; attempt to provide a focus in the conversation; interrupt to slow the individual down in conversation; and phrase questions that require a brief answer. *Planned activity:* Avoid competitive activities that require the individual to continually pay attention in order to participate (e.g., volleyball). Bowling and exercise such as yoga are better choices for group activities. When providing activities for the patient, do so in patient's room to reduce distractions. Small-group activities help build self-esteem. Allow for rest periods. *Nutritional risk:* Select well-balanced meals and snacks, and include high-fiber foods in the diet to reduce constipation. Handheld foods (e.g., individual sandwiches, fresh vegetables and fruits, crackers) work well for manic patients. Avoid junk food (snacks that are high in concentrated sugar and fats). Monitor for dehydration. Weigh weekly. *Do not remove salt* from the diet while a patient is taking lithium. (Reduced salt intake can contribute to lithium toxicity.) *Drug therapy:* Monitor lithium levels. Normal loading range is 1–1.5 mEq/L; common range for maintenance is 0.6–1.2 mEq/L. In charting, note presence or absence of adverse effects of lithium. Note changes in individual's behavior and thoughts individual expresses. Document all behaviors that can be considered a suicide threat or action. Remind patient that antidepressant medications take about 2 to 4 wk to produce any effects.
Bipolar Affective Disorder			
Mood swings with manic episodes, alternating with or without episodes of depression Symptoms of mania: grand or self-confident mood, overresponsiveness to stimuli, insomnia without fatigue, impaired judgment, irritability, psychomotor overactivity	Treatment possibilities include psychotherapy; antimanic drugs (lithium); and family and individual support, with education regarding drug use. Prognosis depends on response to medication and treatment.	*Potential for Injury* *Inability to Tolerate Activity* *Potential for Violence Upon Self or Others* *Impaired Cognitive Function* *Compromised Social Interaction* *Potential for Insufficient Nutrition*	

Anxiety Disorders			
Generalized Anxiety			
Characterized by a steady, pervasive level of anxiety; possible at any age but commonly occurs around ages 20–30; lasts 6 mo or longer Symptoms: apprehension, irritability, insomnia, poor concentration, fear of unknown, can be either preoccupied with or neglectful of self-care, autonomic hyperactivity; conversation dominated by physical complaints	Treatment possibilities include relaxation techniques, exercise, visual imagery, massage, biofeedback imagery, and antianxiety drug therapy. Prognosis is variable; condition sometimes lasts 6 mo or longer.	*Impaired Coping* *Anxiousness* *Insufficient Nutrition* *Fearfulness*	*Establish therapeutic relationship:* Encourage the patient to share thoughts and feelings. Be supportive and provide assistance. Encourage the patient to use more realistic thoughts, such as "Whatever happens, I can deal with it" or "I've been through this procedure before, and I handled it." Encourage self-care and simple decision making. Avoid reinforcing concerns over physical complaints, but do not ignore them without further assessment. *Reduce anxiety:* Decrease environmental stimuli to reduce agitation. It is sometimes a good idea to restrict visitors to decrease stimuli, but allow the patient that control. Instruct about staff routine. Teach the individual relaxation techniques such as the following: 1. Practice abdominal or deep breathing. 2. Imagery: In comfortable position, use deep breathing and focus on a pleasant image and all its details. 3. For painful procedures, have the patient imagine how a favorite hero or role model would tolerate the procedure. 4. Brisk walks, back rubs, hot showers or baths, or a heating pad also can help the patient relax. *Communications:* Include in therapeutic communications explanations of all procedures and treatments, and keep family informed about the hospital regulations (e.g., visiting hours) and the goals of the care provided (e.g., the need to reduce stimuli). Be punctual with treatments and medications. This builds trust. Anticipate needs.
Panic Disorders			
Severe anxiety, intense fear; exhibiting physical manifestations suddenly without apparent reason; onset frequently in late 20s Types of posttraumatic stress disorder: acute (occurs within 6 mo of event), chronic (lasts more than 6 mo), and delayed (starts 6 mo or more after event)	Use treatments for generalized anxiety disorders. Attacks last minutes to hours and possibly recur several times a week. Debriefing techniques (as used by the military) are often helpful.	*Anxiousness* *Fearfulness* *Impaired Coping* *Physical or Sexual Assault Trauma Condition* *Impaired Family Processes*	Panic attacks are a form of Generalized Anxiety Disorder. In addition to interventions for Generalized Anxiety Disorder the nurse can help the patient reduce anxiety during a panic attack by: 1. Remaining calm during the panic attack. 2. Giving the patient space during the attack so they do not feel smothered. 3. Encouraging distractions such as physical activity, which also reduces stress.

Continued

Table 35.1 Psychiatric Disorders—cont'd

CHARACTERISTICS	TREATMENT AND PROGNOSIS	ASSOCIATED PATIENT PROBLEMS	NURSING INTERVENTIONS
Phobias			
Characterized by persistent and irrational fear of a specific object, situation, or activity; leads to lifestyle of self-protective avoidance; social phobias are more common in women	With desensitization, patient learns to relax while reentering phobia-producing situation in imagination and then in real life. Anxiety and fear are kept to a minimum. Prognosis is variable and depends on response to treatment.	*Anxiousness* *Impaired Coping* *Fearfulness* *Impaired Family Processes*	Phobias are a form of Generalized Anxiety Disorder. In addition to interventions for generalized anxiety disorder the nurse can help the patient reduce anxiety experienced with a phobia by: 1. Reassuring the patient that they are safe. 2. Be accepting of the patient's fear. 3. Help the patient to identify stressors.
Obsessive-Compulsive Disorders (OCDs)			
Anxiety condition characterized by inability to stop persistent, irrational, and uncontrollable acts (compulsions) or thoughts (obsessions) contrary to person's standards or judgment; usually appears after adolescence, resulting from fear, guilt, and anticipation of punishment; person is usually orderly, meticulous, dependable, and scrupulous, although with tendency to be rigid and stubborn; mild forms are common; equally distributed between men and women; increases with stress	Treatment often consists of psychotherapy, to uncover the basic fears and to help the person distinguish objective dangers from imagined dangers. Drug therapy with clomipramine (Anafranil) has been of great value. Prognosis is more severe than with other anxiety disorders; complete recovery is rare. However, complete disability occurs only in a minority of cases.	*Impaired Coping* *Anxiousness* *Fearfulness* *Altered Thought Processes* *Ineffective Sleep Pattern* *Social Seclusion* *Impaired Role Functioning*	OCDs are a form of Generalized Anxiety Disorder. In addition to interventions for Generalized Anxiety Disorder the nurse can help the patient reduce anxiety experienced with OCD by: 1. Involving family with the treatment plan. 2. Helping the patient to recognize irrational thoughts and how best to address them. 3. Encouraging participation in support groups for those diagnosed with OCD.

Personality Disorders			
Range of behaviors, depending on the type of disorder present Common characteristics: poor impulse control (heavy drinking, overeating, substance abuse, assaultive behavior), self-destructive acts (such as self-mutilation), manipulation of or dependency on other people, inappropriate behavior for situation, disregard for rules; usually accompanied by denial of maladaptive behaviors	Treatment possibilities include psychotherapeutic drug therapy, group therapy, reality therapy, support groups, and family counseling. Prognosis is guarded; antisocial personality disorder is the more socially malignant of the disorders and appears to have the most severe consequences.	*Compromised Social Interaction* *Impaired Coping* *Impaired Family Processes* *Potential for Violence Upon Self or Others* *Compromised Parenting Skills* *Stress Response Condition*	*Establish therapeutic relationship:* Maintain a therapeutic environment. Be firm and consistent. *Set limits on behaviors:* Establish consequences for violating limits. Provide positive feedback for appropriate behavior; encourage ventilation of feelings. *Communications:* Encourage decision making and patient participation. Discuss incidents with patient. Approach in a calm, confident manner. *Safety and security:* Know where patient is at all times. Be alert for manipulating behaviors. Assist in ADLs as necessary.

Table 35.2 Types of Delusions

TYPE OF DELUSION	DEFINITION	EXAMPLE
Grandeur	Belief of being someone with great powers to control any situation	"I am God."
Ideas of reference	Belief that an event has special personal meaning	"The lady on TV is telling me to buy the soap."
Persecution	Belief that someone is out to harm him or her	"They put a transmitter in my tooth to monitor my every word."
Somatic delusions	False belief pertaining to body function or image	"I have diabetes." (in the absence of the disease)
Thought broadcasting	Belief that others know his or her ideas without action on his or her part to convey the thoughts	"You all know the thoughts I have been having today."
Thought insertion	Belief that ideas are put in his or her mind	"You put these thoughts in my head for your own pleasure."
Thought withdrawal	Belief that thoughts are being removed from his or her mind	"You have been stealing my thoughts."

A **hallucination** is a sensory experience without a stimulus trigger. Auditory hallucinations are the type that people experience most often. Visual, olfactory, and tactile hallucinations are also possible in the individual with schizophrenia.

Disordered thinking occurs when the individual is not able to interpret information being received in the brain. Loose association-making in speech sometimes makes this evident; conversation does not flow logically. *Concreteness* is sometimes a sign of disordered thinking. For example, when someone is taking a picture and the individual with schizophrenia hears "Watch the birdie!," the individual will look up into the tree for the bird instead of smiling for the camera.

Negative Behavior Patterns

Negative, or absent, behavior patterns also are associated with schizophrenia. They may manifest alone or together with positive behavior patterns. Negative behavior includes apathy (avolition), social withdrawal, alogia, blunted emotional responses, and anhedonia. *Apathy* is a lack of energy or interest. An unkempt appearance or lack of appropriate hygiene is often a reflection of apathy. *Social withdrawal* occurs in an attempt to reduce stimuli to the brain. Some individuals with schizophrenia are frightened or overwhelmed by the experience of trying to communicate with other people and find it easier to withdraw from the contact. *Alogia* is defined as reduced content of speech. Alogia sometimes occurs as part of the overload of information that occurs in conversation; the individual with schizophrenia needs time to sort out the message received. *Affect* is the outward display or expression of emotion that is felt. Flat affect and anhedonia are terms describing the lack of expressed feelings. *Flat affect* is the lack of nonverbal expression of emotions, such as by means of facial expression or tone of voice, and *anhedonia* is the inability to experience happiness or joy. Other behaviors sometimes exhibited by an individual with schizophrenia include bizarre posturing or behaviors such as laughing when receiving news about a death in the family. Adverse effects of drugs also have the potential to produce negative or absent behaviors. It is important to assess the situation surrounding the behavior.

Subtypes of Schizophrenia

Schizophrenia is a cluster of behaviors. There are five subtypes of this category of illness:

1. *Disorganized:* Flat or inappropriate affect, incoherence; prognosis is poor.
2. *Paranoid:* Delusions, auditory hallucinations; prognosis is good with treatment.
3. *Catatonic:* Stupor, negativism, rigidity, excitement, posturing; prognosis is fair.
4. *Undifferentiated:* Delusions, hallucinations, incoherence, gross disorganization (does not fit criteria of other types); prognosis is fair.
5. *Residual:* Typical signs and symptoms associated with schizophrenia without evidence of gross disorganization, incoherence, delusions, and hallucinations; prognosis is poor.

Stages of Schizophrenia

The course of schizophrenia involves four stages and features acute episodes of psychosis alternating with periods of relatively normal function. The *prodromal phase* often begins in adolescence and begins with lack of energy or motivation and withdrawal. Other symptoms common in this stage are as follows: affect becomes blunted; beliefs and ideas become odd; the person sometimes develops an excessive interest in philosophy or religion; self-care and personal hygiene decline; emotional lability is present; speech is difficult to follow; and the person often complains about multiple physical problems. Magical thinking, or believing that one's thoughts control events, is also a symptom.

Quiet, passive behavior is typical of the *prepsychotic phase.* The individual prefers to be alone. Hallucination and delusions sometimes occur in this stage. Odd, unusual, or eccentric behavior patterns are present. Family members report that they feel the individual has changed into a stranger.

During the *acute phase,* signs and symptoms sometimes vary widely, but disturbances in thought, perception, emotion, and behavior are very apparent. Often the individual loses contact with reality and is unable to function in the most basic ways.

The *residual phase* features a group of symptoms similar to that in the prodromal phase. The residual phase follows the acute phase. Following the residual phase is a remission period, in which the individual is able to experience some relief of symptoms and to manage some basic activities in life. Prognosis for recovery is fair to poor because of the complex aspects of this disorder.

Treatment for schizophrenia involves a number of psychotherapies to allow the individual self-expression, antipsychotic drug therapy to control symptoms, and a therapeutic relationship maintained over the years to provide continuity for the individual with a lifelong illness.

MAJOR MOOD DISORDERS

Mood disorders, also known as *affective disorders,* are any of a group of psychotic disorders whose defining characteristics are severe and inappropriate emotional responses, prolonged and persistent disturbances of mood and related thought distortions, and other symptoms associated with either depressed or manic states. *Mood,* as defined by the *DSM-V* (APA, 2013), is a prolonged emotion that affects a person's psyche. Extremes in mood range from depression to mania. Hereditary factors account for 60% to 80% of cases of mood disorders. The levels of the neurotransmitters norepinephrine and serotonin are deficient in depressed individuals, and the level of norepinephrine is excessive in manic individuals. Neurotransmitter imbalances are sometimes the result of heredity and sometimes are caused by environmental factors such as prolonged stress or brain trauma. Most people experience some type of depression and maintain their life; however, the individual with a mood disorder has these extreme moods for months or years without relief.

Depression

Depression is a mood disturbance characterized by exaggerated feelings of sadness, despair, lowered self-esteem, loss of interest in former activities, and pessimistic thoughts. Depression is more than a state of mind; in any given 2-week period, almost 8% of Americans report symptoms of moderate or severe depression (Centers for Disease Control and Prevention [CDC], 2018). Depression is found in all races, ethnic groups, age groups, and socioeconomic levels. Women are affected twice as often as men.

Depression can be so severe at times that an affected person contemplates, or actually succeeds at, committing suicide. Suicide falls in the top 10 leading causes of death in the United States; where the statistic falls in the top 10 depends on the age group (CDC, 2017). Many deaths supposedly caused by accidental overdoses, automobile accidents, and refusal of medical care may be viewed as hidden suicides even though they are not reported as such. Suicide attempts also are not included in the statistics. Although the highest rate of suicide is among the older population, suicide among teenagers is on the rise in this country. Children must be taught effective coping skills.

There is great controversy over the terminally ill patient's right to commit suicide. Some people believe that deliberately ending one's life is a rational decision in certain circumstances, such as terminal illness, and defend the right to commit suicide. There is growing support for right-to-die legislation, which removes the criminal stigma from suicide. Most people who commit suicide in the hospital setting have received the diagnosis of an incurable or painful illness. It is important to evaluate terminally ill individuals and treat them for depression, as well as for their physical disorders, to ease their pain and enhance their quality of life.

To help prevent suicide, recognize warning signs and learn the kinds of actions that often can avert suicide attempts (Box 35.1). Consider as warning signals verbal statements such as "I wish I were dead" or "You won't see me coming back here again" and questions about specific methods of suicide. Actions such as giving away possessions, refusing medications, or neglecting hygiene are also possible warning signals. Many people have anxiety because of a moral conflict within themselves. Many suicidal individuals manage to leave that anxiety behind by making the decision to commit suicide.

Major depression, or *persistent depressive disorder,* is defined as repeated, severe depressive episodes lasting more than 2 years (National Institute of Mental Health, 2018). Estimates are that up to 15% of people with major depressive disorder die from suicide. *Dysthymic disorder* is daily moderate depression that lasts more than 2 years. This disorder often ends up as a lifestyle in which the individual is able to function but not enjoy life.

Bipolar Disorders

Bipolar disorders, or *manic-depressive disorders,* feature shifts between emotional extremes from depression to mania. **Mania** is a mood disorder whose major characteristic is persistent, abnormal overactivity and a euphoric state. The early phase of a manic episode often is referred to as a **hypomanic episode** when symptoms are not severe. Often the manic person is engaging, outgoing, and charming, as well as achieving and successful; has excessive energy and optimism; and is possibly a very productive member of the community. Unfortunately, a manic episode has potential to accelerate.

As it intensifies, the episode of mania changes from cheerfulness into excessive feelings of euphoria, rapid

Box 35.1 Suicide Warnings and Precautions

WARNING SIGNS OF SUICIDE

- Withdrawing from family or friends
- Talking about death, the hereafter, or suicide
- Giving away prized possessions
- Drug or alcohol abuse
- Personality changes, such as unusual anger, boredom, or apathy
- Unusual neglect of appearance; difficulty concentrating on work or school; complaints of physical problems that have no organic cause; disturbed sleeping or eating patterns; loss of self-esteem; feelings of helplessness, hopelessness, extreme anxiety, or panic
- Previously failed attempts with verbalized regrets of failure

SUICIDE PRECAUTIONS IN THE HOSPITAL ENVIRONMENT

- Remove articles that can be used for suicide: belts, straps, shoelaces, sheets, breakable items for sharp edges, razor blades, curtain cords, bed coils, and personal care items.
- Remove any furniture that can be used for self-injury, as well as doors to closets. Make sure windows are shatterproof.
- Designate a room close to the front desk of the unit or a room with a closed TV monitor.
- Check the patient approximately every 15 minutes on an irregular schedule around the clock.
- Instruct visitors not to leave gifts in the room until the staff examines them for anything that can be used for self-injury.
- Make sure the patient swallows all medications administered. Administer liquid forms when available. Administer injectables if the patient refuses oral forms as ordered.
- Attend the patient during meals, and keep track of eating utensils and dinnerware. Make sure used trays are not sitting where the patient has the opportunity to walk by and remove tableware.
- Make frequent therapeutic verbal contact.

speech, flight of ideas, unrealistic beliefs in abilities, no sleep, poor judgment, denial that anything could possibly go wrong, increased sex drive, and obnoxious or provocative behavior such as robbing a store without the fear of being caught. If untreated, delirium may ensue, and death from exhaustion or accident is possible.

Cyclothymic disorder is a pattern that also involves repeated mood swings of hypomania and depression, although they are less intense. There are no periods of normal function with this condition. It is considered a muted version of bipolar disorder. Many individuals with cyclothymic disorder progress to bipolar disorder.

Other affective disorders are seasonal affective disorder (SAD) and postpartum depression. Both of these disorders are connected with hormonal imbalances and respond well to treatment. Practitioners treat SAD, also known as *winter depression,* with phototherapy. Postpartum depression often clears within days, but it is best to further investigate the problem if symptoms continue longer than 2 weeks.

Medical Treatment

Medical treatment for mood disorders includes antidepressants and lithium, electroconvulsive therapy (ECT), and psychotherapy. Antidepressants, such as fluoxetine (Prozac), trazodone, amitriptyline, and venlafaxine (Effexor XR), take 2 to 4 weeks to alleviate the depression. Some antidepressants such as amitriptyline work best when taken at bedtime because of a transient adverse effect of sedation; this regimen sometimes also helps normalize the sleeping pattern. Selective serotonin reuptake inhibitors (SSRIs), such as fluoxetine (Prozac) and paroxetine (Paxil), do not seem to produce as many of the anticholinergic and sedating side effects that sometimes cause patients to stop taking their medications. Some antidepressants, such as fluoxetine, work best when taken in the morning to prevent the adverse effect of insomnia. (See the later section on antidepressant medications for further discussion.)

Practitioners frequently use lithium to treat bipolar disorder. Lithium has a narrow therapeutic range, and patients who take it must be monitored closely for safety. Patients taking lithium also need to monitor the amount of sodium in their diet and fluid intake.

Other drugs in the pharmacologic toolbox to treat mental illness symptoms include duloxetine (Cymbalta), bupropion (Wellbutrin), and mirtazapine (Remeron). Bupropion is also a first-line medication for smoking cessation.

ECT is an option to consider when drug therapy is ineffective or is contraindicated (Box 35.2 and Nursing Care Plan 35.1).

ANXIETY DISORDERS

Anxiety is a normal response to stress or threat. **Anxiety** is a state or feeling of apprehension, uneasiness, agitation, uncertainty, and fear resulting from the anticipation of some threat or danger. Experts describe many types of anxiety. *Signal anxiety* is a learned response to an event such as test taking. *Free-floating anxiety* is associated with feelings of dread whose source cannot be identified. *Anxiety trait* is a learned aspect of personality. Individuals with anxiety trait have anxious reactions to relatively nonstressful events. Such individuals respond more quickly and more strongly to stress and are slower than normal to calm down. (See discussion of normal anxiety response in Chapter 34.)

Generalized anxiety disorders are characterized by a high degree of anxiety and/or avoidance behavior. An individual with generalized anxiety disorder tends to worry or fret over many things and finds it difficult to concentrate on the task at hand (Fig. 35.1).

Panic can be defined as an attack of acute, intense, and overwhelming anxiety accompanied by a degree of personality disorganization, such as inability to solve problems or think clearly. In a panic attack, symptoms

Box 35.2 Electroconvulsive Therapy

Electroconvulsive therapy (ECT) is administered on either an inpatient or an outpatient basis.

PATIENT PREPARATION

1. Purpose of ECT is relief from depression. Patient signs forms of consent for treatment.
2. Common side effects include headache, confusion upon awakening, and short-term amnesia. Patient should take acetaminophen (Tylenol) for persistent headache.
3. Patient needs to be on nothing-by-mouth (NPO) status for at least 8 hours before treatment.
4. Patient should wear loose-fitting clothes with access to the arm for intravenous line insertion.
5. Patient must arrange for someone to accompany him or her to and from the treatment. No treatment will take place if patient is unaccompanied.
6. Patient must avoid driving or operating machinery for at least 1 day after treatment.
7. Patient should avoid making any major decisions—about job, finances, relationships, and so forth—until the course of treatment is completed.
8. Patient should take any prescribed medications on time.

TREATMENT

1. Nurse measures baseline vital signs.
2. Nurse applies cardiac, blood pressure, and oximetry monitors to the patient.
3. Nurse establishes an intravenous line for administration of sedative and neuromuscular blockade.
4. Nurse applies electroencephalographic monitor to the patient.
5. After administration of intravenous drugs to patient, practitioner establishes an airway and delivers electrical shock for a few seconds.
6. A controlled seizure lasts 30 to 60 seconds. Neuromuscular blockade eliminates most body flexion, thereby reducing risk of spinal injury, bone fracture, or muscle tears.
7. Patient usually sleeps for about 1 hour after treatment.

POSTTREATMENT CARE

1. Nurse monitors vital signs and level of consciousness.
2. It is acceptable to discharge the patient with a responsible adult when patient is alert and walking. Confusion is sometimes present, and some patients do not remember coming to the hospital for treatment and leaving afterward.

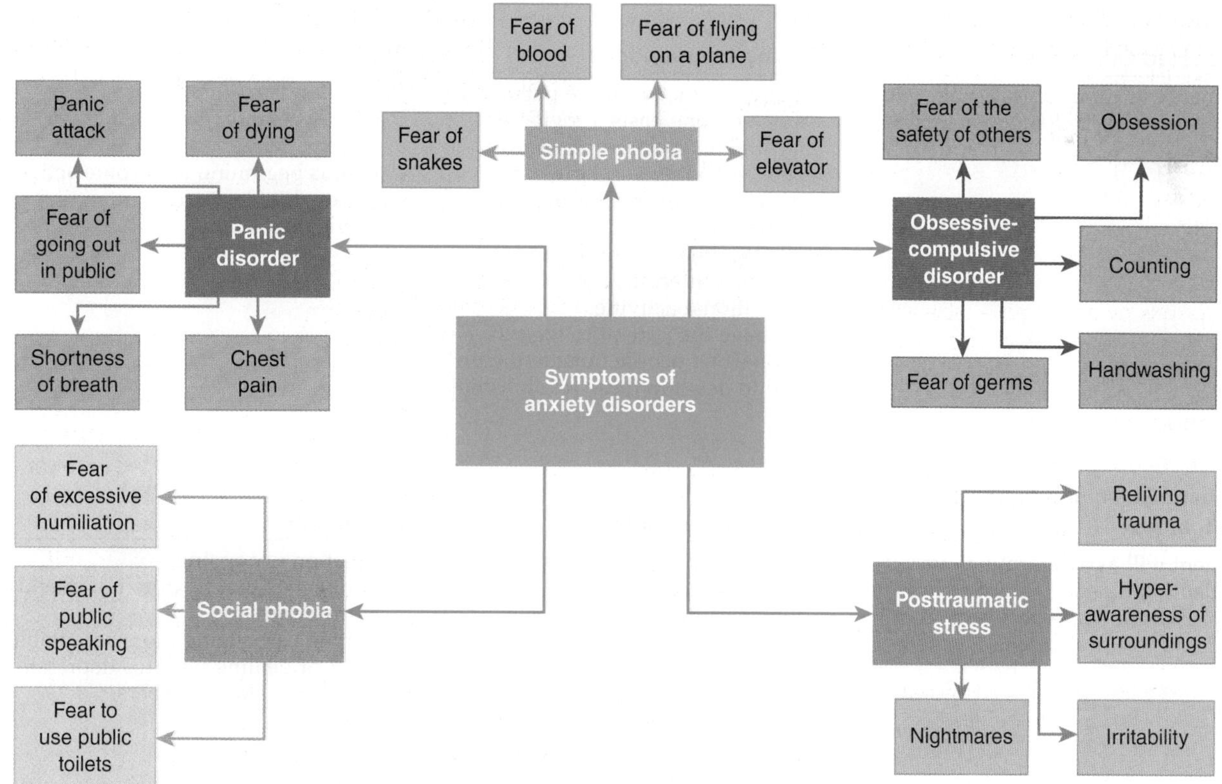

Fig. 35.1 Anxiety disorders. (Modified from Pathways Real Life Recovery, Sandy, Utah.)

occur abruptly and peak within 10 minutes. Panic attacks are characterized by at least four of the following: heart palpitations or accelerated heart rate; sweating, trembling, or shaking; feelings of dyspnea or choking; chest pain; nausea or abdominal distress; feeling dizzy or faint; fear of losing control or going crazy; fear of dying; paresthesias (a sensation experienced as numbness, tingling, or "pins and needles"); and chills or hot flashes. Panic disorders are more common in women than in men.

 Nursing Care Plan 35.1 **The Patient With Depression**

Mr. W. is a 69-year-old widower whose wife died from cancer 9 months ago. He entered the open psychiatric unit with the diagnosis of major depression. Mr. W.'s unmarried daughter lives out of state and is a partner in a law firm. Mr. W. has severe hypertension and early-stage chronic obstructive pulmonary disease (COPD). On admission, Mr. W. states, "I just can't go on all alone like this. … I have so little energy, and I can't sleep the way I used to." Mr. W. has lost 32 pounds in the past 6 months; he weighs 145 pounds and is 5 feet 11 inches tall. Mr. W. rarely leaves his house, although friends ask him out frequently. He is tearful at times, sighs often, and has poor eye contact during the admission interview. When asked, he admits to thoughts of killing himself. He states that he attempted to do so with an overdose of his hypertension medication, but he wanted to see his daughter one last time before he dies, so he came to the emergency department.

PATIENT PROBLEM

Impaired Coping

Patient Goals and Expected Outcomes	Nursing Interventions	Evaluation
Patient will engage in reality-based interactions Patient will express feelings directly and express anger or hostility outward in a safe manner	Establish a therapeutic relationship; keep staff assignment as consistent as possible. Use a firm, kind manner; tell patient that you can see that he is sad but that he still needs to complete his personal hygiene and activities of daily living. If the patient is ruminating, convey that you will talk about reality or his feelings, but limit the attention you give to repeated expressions of rumination.	Evaluation is ongoing. Weekly care meetings of staff to discuss the patient's progress. Good daily documentation reflecting the patient's progress. Patient is beginning to verbalize to staff his feelings of loss and grief resulting from his wife's death. Patient is expressing need to interact more with his daughter.

PATIENT PROBLEM

Compromised Social Interaction

Patient Goals and Expected Outcomes	Nursing Interventions	Evaluation
Patient will communicate with others Patient will participate in activities	Initially, interact with the patient on a one-on-one basis. Progress to facilitating social interactions between patient and other patients, from small groups to larger groups. Encourage the patient to pursue personal interests, hobbies, and recreational activities. Encourage the patient to identify supportive people outside the unit and to develop these relationships.	Evaluation is ongoing. Patient is beginning to interact with other patients. Patient is beginning to become active in personal interests (e.g., attending a movie or reading a book).

PATIENT PROBLEM

Potential for Violence Upon Self

Patient Goals and Expected Outcomes	Nursing Interventions	Evaluation
Patient will avoid harming himself Patient will identify alternative ways of dealing with stress and emotional problems	Determine appropriate level of suicide precautions, and institute the precautions immediately. Convey that you care about the patient and that you believe he is a worthwhile individual. Involve the patient as much as possible in planning his treatment. Plan with the patient how he will recognize and deal with feelings and situations that have precipitated suicidal feelings in the past.	Evaluation is ongoing. Patient states that he does not intend to harm himself. Patient is verbalizing more acceptable ways of dealing with his depression with other staff members.

Nursing Care Plan 35.1 The Patient With Depression—cont'd

PATIENT PROBLEM
Insufficient Nutrition

Patient Goals and Expected Outcomes	Nursing Interventions	Evaluation
Patient will maintain a regular, adequate eating pattern Patient will maintain normal body weight	Monitor patient's eating. Keep intake and output records. Encourage consumption of fluids (e.g., water, juices). Find out what foods the patient likes and dislikes. Try six small feedings per day. Discourage use of nonnutritional substances such as artificial sweeteners, coffee creamers, diet soda, tea, and coffee.	Evaluation is ongoing. Patient is eating 50% to 60% of each meal. Patient is beginning to demonstrate interest in sitting down and eating with a group.

PATIENT PROBLEM
Ineffective Sleep Pattern

Patient Goals and Expected Outcomes	Nursing Interventions	Evaluation
Patient will sleep 5 to 6 h per night before discharge Patient will verbalize ability to use relaxation techniques when awake at night	Plan for the patient to engage in physical activity while awake. Encourage only planned naps. Teach progressive relaxation exercises. Help the patient establish a consistent time to go to sleep.	Evaluation is ongoing. Patient is sleeping about 6 h per night. Patient is going to sleep at a scheduled time each night.

CRITICAL THINKING QUESTIONS

1. Mr. W. is admitted to the psychiatric unit and placed on suicide precautions. He sits stoically staring out the window and does not respond to the nurse's greeting. What safety interventions should the team incorporate into Mr. W.'s care to prevent his self-destruction?
2. Mr. W. sleeps poorly, approximately 2 to 3 hours a night. What therapeutic interventions should be used to correct his sleep pattern disturbance?
3. Mr. W. has lost 32 lb. What are some options for the staff to help him meet adequate nutritional requirements?

Agoraphobia is considered a type of panic disorder. Agoraphobia is extreme anxiety brought on by situations in which a panic attack is possible. People with agoraphobia avoid people, places, or events that have the potential to trigger an attack. Fear of not receiving any help or embarrassment when an attack occurs in a public place are characteristics of agoraphobia.

Treatment for panic disorders focuses on educating the individual about the nature of the disorder, assisting the individual to develop better coping mechanisms with anxiety, and blocking attacks pharmaceutically. Emotional support and reassurance are important nursing measures for individuals suffering with panic disorder.

Phobias

A phobia is different from normal fear. A **phobia** is irrational fear, in which the thoughts of the individual tend to dwell on the object of the phobia. The individual sometimes recognizes the irrationality of the fear but is still unable to control paralyzing anxiety. Characteristics of phobias vary with the culture. In some cultures, fear of hexes, magical spirits, snakes, and unseen forces have the power to trigger phobic fear reactions. Consider the patient's cultural background when assessing the phobic response.

Obsessive-Compulsive Disorder

Obsessive-compulsive disorder has two features. **Obsessions** are thoughts that are recurrent, intrusive, and senseless. These thoughts are anxiety producing and distressing in that they are uncontrollable. **Compulsions** are behaviors that are performed in response to an obsessive thought. The repetitive, ritualistic behaviors, such as checking the locks 10 times before going to bed, typically reduce the anxiety and tension produced by the obsession. Affected patients sometimes recognize the behavior as absurd but still are compelled to perform the ritual to relieve tension. Such patients tend to have difficulty expressing emotions and are often introspective. Stopping the repetitive act results in extreme anxiety. Depression is a feature that often occurs in association with this disorder. Individuals may isolate themselves or try to "make up" for actions as a way of trying to prevent anxiety. Interpersonal relationships and occupations suffer because of the time-consuming behaviors.

Experts believe that activity addictions such as compulsive gambling, sexual promiscuity, excessive Internet use, or overeating arise from obsessive-compulsive behavior disorders. See Chapter 36 for more information concerning addiction.

Posttraumatic Stress Disorder

Posttraumatic stress disorder (PTSD) describes a response to an intensely traumatic experience beyond the usual range of human experiences. These experiences—such as war, rape, a major auto accident, being tortured or observing someone being tortured, or witnessing a violent death—tend to evoke feelings of terror and helplessness. One such experience was witnessing the attack on New York City's World Trade Center on September 11, 2001. The people who escaped the World Trade Center towers before the collapse and emergency personnel who responded to the attack were the most likely to suffer from PTSD. Also at high risk are veterans returning from Iraq, Afghanistan, and other war-torn areas of the world. The experience often is relived repeatedly in dreams or flashbacks. Flashbacks often arise in response to a trigger, a stimulus that resembles the experience or perhaps the anniversary of the event. Flashbacks sometimes include **illusions** (false interpretation of extreme sensory stimuli, usually visual or auditory, such as a mirage in the desert or the sound of voices in the wind) and hallucinations. Avoidance behavior associated with this disorder sometimes includes emotional detachment, guilt about being a survivor, amnesia of the event, insomnia, irritability, difficulty concentrating, and wariness. Physical response to severe anxiety occurs with each relived episode. Depression and substance abuse often occur in association with PTSD.

There are three types of PTSD: acute, chronic, and delayed. In acute PTSD, symptoms occur within 6 months of the event and last about 6 months. Chronic PTSD is characterized by symptoms that last 6 months or longer. Delayed PTSD involves symptoms that start 6 months or more after the event.

Treatment for PTSD includes antidepressant or antiseizure medications; cognitive therapy, which focuses on breaking negative thought patterns; and behavioral therapy, which aims to break off a conditioned response that has become automatic. Debriefing people right after the event is one strategy that practitioners recommend to prevent PTSD.

PERSONALITY DISORDERS

Personality disorders are inflexible, maladaptive patterns of behavior or thinking that accompany significant impairment of functioning. The disorder usually surfaces during adolescence or earlier and continues through adulthood. The associated behaviors are generally more troublesome to other people than to the affected individual (Box 35.3). Personality disorders are characterized by the following:

- Lack of insight; concrete thinking; poor attention; inability to understand the consequences of behavior or learn from them
- Distorted self-perception; either hatred or idealization of self
- Impaired relationships; projecting own feelings onto others; poor impulse control; inability to maintain healthy interpersonal relationships
- Inflexible behavioral response patterns that do not allow the individual to handle change easily

The *DSM-V* (APA, 2013) has classified 10 distinct personality disorders. These disorders can be clustered into groups of similar behavior. Cluster A includes disorders with odd or eccentric behavior. Cluster B includes behaviors that are dramatic, emotional, or erratic. Cluster C disorders include behaviors that are anxious and fearful (see Box 35.3).

Box 35.3 Personality Disorders

CLUSTER A: ODD OR ECCENTRIC BEHAVIOR
- Schizoid personality disorder
- Paranoid personality disorder
- Schizotypal personality disorder

CLUSTER B: DRAMATIC, EMOTIONAL, OR ERRATIC BEHAVIOR
- Antisocial personality disorder
- Borderline personality disorder
- Narcissistic personality disorder

CLUSTER C: ANXIOUS FEARFUL BEHAVIOR
- Avoidant personality disorder
- Dependent personality disorder
- Obsessive-compulsive personality disorder

Data from Mayo Clinic: Personality disorders, 2016. Retrieved from *http://www.mayoclinic.org/diseases-conditions/personality-disorders/symptoms-causes/dxc-20247656*.

SEXUAL DISORDERS

Sex is ranked as a basic need in Maslow's hierarchy of human needs (Maslow, 1970). Human sexuality is the sum of physical and psychological attributes that express a person's gender identity and sexual behavior. Sexual disorders are of either physical or psychological origin, but often physical and psychological factors play a part in the perceived disorder.

Defining normal sexual behavior is difficult against the inescapable backdrop of cultural influences, religious institutions, and societal laws that affect an individual's beliefs regarding acceptable and unacceptable sexual behavior. Sexual behavior may be thought of on a continuum from adaptive sexual behavior to maladaptive sexual behavior. Adaptive sexual behaviors occur in private between two consenting adults, are satisfying, and are not forced on each other. Maladaptive sexual behaviors are harmful to self or others and possibly are performed publicly and sometimes without the consent of all those involved.

Sexual orientation is the preference or choice for a sex partner. *Heterosexual* is the term describing individuals who express their sexuality with members of the opposite sex. *Homosexual* is the term describing individuals who express their sexuality with members of the same sex. The *DSM-V* (APA, 2013) lists sexual and gender identity disorders in three main clusters: (1) sexual dysfunctions, (2) paraphilias, and (3) gender dysphoria. This list does not address sexual dysfunction caused by medical problems, such as impotence secondary to diabetic neuropathy.

Sexual dysfunction is a disturbance during sexual response. *Dyspareunia* (painful intercourse), hypoactive sexual desire, and premature ejaculation are examples of sexual dysfunction that have a possible psychological component, as well as a physical component. Some medications cause sexual dysfunction by altering sexual desire or the ability to perform. Medications are now available to treat men with erectile dysfunction, if the dysfunction has physical causes.

Paraphilias are a group of sexually gratifying activities that are not common in the general public and are illegal in some countries, including the United States. The suffix *-philia* means "attraction to." Adding a descriptive prefix, such as *pedo-*, rounds out the descriptions of what the sexual attraction is to. Thus *pedophilia* means fondling or pursuing other sexual activities with a prepubescent child by an adult.

Other paraphilic disorders include *exhibitionism* ("flashing"), which means exposing one's genitals to one or more unsuspecting people to achieve sexual arousal; *voyeurism,* which means obtaining sexual gratification by observing others during intercourse or viewing another's genitals; *frotteurism,* which is sexual arousal achieved by rubbing against or touching a nonconsenting individual; and *fetishism,* which is the use of an object, usually an article of clothing, to attain sexual arousal. Masturbation usually accompanies or follows an act of fetishism. *Transvestic fetishism* involves wearing clothing of the opposite sex (cross-dressing) to obtain sexual gratification.

Other paraphilic disorders are sexual sadism and masochism. *Sadism* refers to achieving sexual arousal from inflicting pain or humiliation on another person. Possible manifestations of sexual sadism vary from mild behavior, such as spanking, to more violent behavior, such as stabbing or strangulation. *Sexual masochism* refers to sexual arousal by receiving mental or physical abuse. A diagnosis of sexual masochism is appropriate if a person finds punishment necessary to achieve sexual gratification.

Gender identity is one of the first parts of personality development established. With gender dysphoria, biologic sex identity conflicts with gender perception. Many individuals with gender dysphoria truly believe that they were born with the wrong body. *Transsexualism* is a persistent desire to be the opposite sex and to have the body of the opposite sex. Transvestic fetishism is associated with this disorder. For a biologic sex change to take place, psychological counseling, hormone treatments, and major surgical procedures must occur over the course of several years. The surgical procedure is not reversible, which is one of the reasons for the lengthy counseling.

Therapeutic interventions depend on the type of disorder. Treatment for most individuals takes place on an outpatient basis. Some psychosexual problems are complex, and treatment requires the skill of specially educated health care providers, nurses, or sex therapists.

Many nurses encounter medical-surgical patients who also have a sexual disorder. Nurses must be aware of their own attitudes and values about sexual behaviors. A nurse's nonverbal messages of disapproval have the capacity to hinder development of a therapeutic relationship and affect the quality of nursing judgment.

SOMATIC SYMPTOM DISORDERS

Physical signs of emotional distress are sometimes very real. Just as eating too much at the Thanksgiving table can cause nausea, so can receiving a very distressing piece of news. The term **somatic** symptom disorder refers to a physical disorder arising as a result of a psychological trigger. This term developed a negative connotation because it acquired the implication that "it's all in your head." The more recent term somatic *illness* addresses the stress-related problems that have the potential to result in physical signs and symptoms. Somatic symptom disorders are thought to have an emotional basis, manifested as a physical illness.

The body responds to continual or repeated stress by overactivating its stress response mechanism; this tends to result in many physical signs and symptoms, such as diarrhea, heart palpitations, backaches, and headaches. The gastrointestinal tract appears to suffer the most from chronic stress.

Physical disorders thought to have psychological underpinnings include ulcerative colitis, irritable bowel syndrome, hypertension, cardiac disease, asthma, arthritis, some skin disorders, irregular menstruation, and migraine headache.

The typical characteristics of somatic symptom disorders are recurrent, multiple, physical complaints and symptoms for which there is no organic cause. It is a process by which an individual's feelings, needs, and conflicts are manifested physiologically. To establish the diagnosis of somatoform disorder, all possible physical causes of dysfunctions, all drug or other toxic substance reactions, and all mental health problems that are possibly related to the symptoms must be eliminated.

EATING DISORDERS

An eating disorder is an illness that disrupts the normal eating pattern. The three most common eating disorders are anorexia nervosa, bulimia nervosa, and binge eating. These are complex psychiatric disorders related to a number of factors, including individual mental and emotional processes, family relationships, cultural values, and genetic predisposition. Eating disorders are serious, potentially life-threatening conditions affecting emotional and physical health. Eating disorders frequently appear during the teen years or young adulthood; however, younger children and older adults also develop these disorders. Statistics show that eating disorders affect mostly girls and women, but increasing numbers of boys, older women, and men are affected (Fig. 35.2). Because of the secretiveness and shame associated with eating disorders, many cases may go unreported. Early detection and treatment of eating disorders increase the likelihood of recovery. Table 35.3 lists the diagnostic criteria used to identify eating disorders.

Recognizing and treating eating disorders early offers some hope of lessening their effects. Table 35.4 lists some danger signs of these disorders. In educating patients about eating disorders, place the greatest focus on prevention and concentrate on good health rather than on thinness. Encourage individuals to respect and value their uniqueness.

Anorexia Nervosa

Anorexia nervosa is an eating disorder characterized by self-imposed starvation. It typically develops in the early to middle stages of adolescence.

Common characteristics in individuals with this disorder include an intense drive for thinness, an intense fear of gaining weight or becoming fat, and a distorted body image such that individuals view themselves as "fat" even when their weight is much less than average for their height. Some affected patients exhibit obsessive-compulsive behaviors toward food, attempting to maintain strict control over intake by counting calories meticulously, practicing unusual food behaviors and rituals, making excuses to avoid eating, and hiding food that they claim to have eaten. Some affected patients enjoy food vicariously by cooking it, serving it, or being around it without eating it. Periods of starvation, compulsive exercising, and purging after meals are among the most common behaviors. Common purging behaviors are self-induced vomiting and the misuse of diuretics, laxatives, emetics, and enemas.

Weight loss and maintenance of weight at or below 85% of goal weight are apparent physical symptoms. Other physical symptoms include cessation of menstruation in women, loss of sexual drive, cold intolerance, the growth of fine hair on the body and the face (lanugo), hypotension, and heart irregularities. Bone density is compromised, which leads in some cases to compression of vertebrae and stress fractures. The gastrointestinal tract is affected, with delayed gastric emptying, slowed peristalsis, and severe constipation. The lining of the digestive tract often deteriorates so that when the patient does eat, he or she experiences malabsorption, flatulence, and diarrhea. This further compounds the negative perception of food. Brain activity is affected, leading to altered thinking patterns, disturbed sleep, and bad dreams. There is also evidence of structural brain abnormalities (tissue loss), some of which may be irreversible. Personality and emotional changes often are pronounced. Depression and apathy are possible.

A multidisciplinary approach to treatment is best and involves nutrition therapy and individual psychological counseling along with family counseling. Nutritional goals include increasing and improving dietary intake to reverse nutrient deficiencies, achieving a healthy weight for height, and reestablishing normal eating patterns.

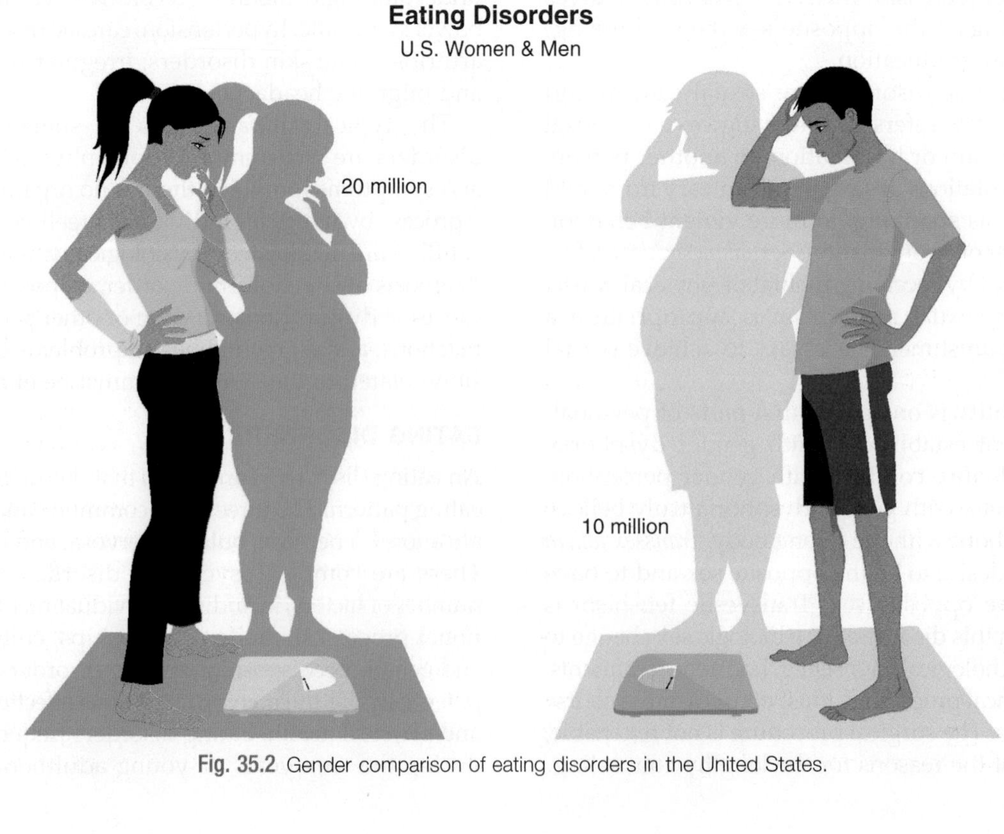

Fig. 35.2 Gender comparison of eating disorders in the United States.

Table 35.3 Comparison of Eating Disorder Diagnoses

CHARACTERISTIC	ANOREXIA NERVOSA	BULIMIA NERVOSA	BINGE-EATING DISORDER
Body weight and other physical indicators	Body weight at or below 85% of normal for age, sex, and height Amenorrhea (in women)	Possibly underweight, normal weight, or overweight	Usually obese
Eating behaviors	1. Restricting type: self-imposed starvation or semistarvation 2. Binge-eating or purging type: regular episodes of binge eating (eating an amount of food the patient considers to be excessive)	Recurrent episodes of binge eating: the compulsive eating of an excessive amount of food while feeling a lack of control over eating Binge eating or purging occurs at least twice per week for a period of 3 mo or more	Recurrent episodes of binge eating: the compulsive eating of an excessive amount of food while feeling a lack of control over eating Episodes occur at least twice per week for a period of 6 mo and are associated with at least three of the following: 1. Eating until uncomfortably full 2. Eating when not physically hungry 3. Eating rapidly 4. Eating alone because of embarrassment 5. Feeling guilt, disgust, or depression after overeating
Compensatory behaviors (purging)	1. Restricting type: may use excessive exercise 2. Binge-eating or purging type: regular episodes of self-induced vomiting or misuse of laxatives, diuretics, or enemas	1. Purging type: regular episodes of self-induced vomiting or the misuse of laxatives, emetics, diuretics, or enemas 2. Nonpurging type: use of fasting or excessive exercise	None
Psychological indicators	Distorted body image: patient perceives self as fat Intense fear of becoming fat Denial of the problem and its seriousness	Feelings of self-worth disproportionately based on body weight, shape, and size Usually awareness that there is a problem	Poor self-esteem, possible depression Awareness that there is a problem

Bulimia Nervosa

Bulimia nervosa is an eating disorder characterized by periods of binge eating followed by purging or other inappropriate compensatory behavior to prevent weight gain. Binge eating is the compulsive eating of an amount of food considered excessive in normal circumstances. Binge eating is followed by purging—self-induced vomiting and the misuse of diuretics, laxatives, emetics, and enemas—or by other compensatory behaviors such as severe caloric restriction, excessive exercising, or the use of diet pills.

People with bulimia are usually within a normal weight range and are aware that their eating patterns are abnormal. However, bulimic people may express a lack of control over the eating. They often experience fear of not being able to stop eating and experience depression, guilt, and remorse after a binge. In addition, bulimia tends to occur in combination with other psychiatric disorders such as depression, obsessive-compulsive disorder, substance abuse, and self-injurious behavior. Clinical symptoms of bulimia include possible tooth erosion, calloused knuckles, swollen parotid (salivary) glands, broken blood vessels in the eyes or face, stomach lacerations, and esophageal and sinus infections resulting from excessive vomiting. Electrolyte imbalances lead to muscle weakness and cramps, abnormal heart rhythms, cardiac complications, and, occasionally, sudden death. Proper treatment for bulimia, like that for anorexia nervosa, is multidisciplinary. Psychological counseling and therapy are necessary. Nutritional goals include improving dietary intake to correct nutritional deficiencies and electrolyte imbalances, and cessation of binge-purge behavior with reestablishment of normal eating patterns.

Table 35.4 Signs and Symptom of Eating Disorders

CATEGORY	SIGNS OR SYMPTOMS
Emotional	1. Change in attitude or performance 2. Inability to concentrate 3. Body image complaints or concerns: • Refers to self as fat, gross, ugly; overestimates body size; believes he or she is fat when of normal weight or thin • Unable to accept compliments • Constantly compares self to others; self-disparaging comments • Mood affected by thoughts about appearance; seeks outside reassurance about looks 4. Appears sad, depressed, anxious; expresses feelings of worthlessness 5. Obsessed with maintaining low weight to enhance performance in sports, dance, acting, modeling, and the like
Physical	1. Sudden weight loss, gain, or fluctuation in a short time 2. Abdominal pain; feeling full or "bloated"; bouts of constipation or diarrhea 3. Feeling fatigue or faint, "weak," or "dizzy" 4. Dry hair or skin, dehydration, poor circulation in hands and feet 5. Cold intolerance 6. Lanugo hair (fine hair on body and face) 7. Edematous glands in the neck or beneath the jaw 8. Erosion of tooth enamel, cavities, tooth pain, changes in tooth appearance 9. Amenorrhea in women of childbearing age 10. Insomnia
Behavioral	1. Caloric restriction and preoccupation with dieting 2. Chaotic food intake; skipping meals; exhibiting peculiar eating rituals 3. Extreme preoccupation with food; constantly talking about food 4. Secretive eating; binge eating 5. Carrying own food; eating small amounts or nothing in front of others 6. Wearing baggy clothes: • To hide a very thin body • To hide weight gain • To hide a normal-sized body because of distorted body image 7. Spending increasing amounts of time alone; withdrawal from family and friends 8. Displaying compulsive or obsessive behaviors 9. Spending frequent and increasing amounts of time in the bathroom 10. Abusing laxatives, diuretics, enemas, or diet pills 11. Excessive amounts of exercise

Modified from National Eating Disorders Association: Educator toolkit. Retrieved from *www.nationaleatingdisorders.org/sites/default/files/Toolkits/EducatorToolkit.pdf.*

Binge-Eating Disorder

Binge-eating disorder is a disorder sometimes referred to as *compulsive overeating*. Some authorities believe that this is the most common eating disorder, affecting millions of Americans. Binge-eating disorder is characterized by frequent, recurrent episodes of binge eating; that is, eating a larger amount of food than normal during a short period of time. People with a binge-eating disorder often report a feeling of lack of control over eating during the binge episode. Unlike bulimia nervosa, binge-eating disorder is not associated with purging or inappropriate compensatory behavior.

Many people with binge-eating disorder are obese. Encourage them to consider treatment that focuses on their binge-eating behavior before they attempt to lose weight. Treatment typically includes some combination of cognitive-behavioral therapy, interpersonal psychotherapy, antidepressants, and self-help groups.

TREATMENT METHODS

COMMUNICATION AND THE THERAPEUTIC RELATIONSHIP

Therapeutic communication is an important technique that practitioners use in treatment of psychiatric disorders. Psychiatric nursing is a science and an art. Each individual has unique value and potential for growth. Applying your own self-concept in the context of a therapeutic relationship requires self-knowledge.

The key component in psychiatric–mental health treatment is the development of a helping-trust relationship. The relationship maximizes the patient's strengths, maintains self-esteem, and assists the patient in developing and using coping skills. The helping-trust relationship is a therapeutic professional relationship; it is not social. In a therapeutic relationship, the nurse assists the patient in learning new ways of responding to people and situations.

Therapeutic communication is a dynamic process in which both participants (the nurse and the patient) share meaning and interact in the interests of problem solving and growth. To be therapeutic, communication must assist with the corrective experiences that help the patient in meeting predetermined goals. Therapeutic techniques for communication are described in Chapter 4. These techniques can be used in every nursing situation. The therapeutic dialogues in the Communication box demonstrate therapeutic nurse-patient interactions.

There are different types of relationships. Most are social; that is, the participants are involved equally in exchanging information and meeting individual needs. In a therapeutic relationship, both participants agree on goals and work toward them. The nurse assists the patient to learn new ways of interacting to function more effectively. The nurse attempts to establish rapport with the patient and obtain trust to facilitate positive interactions that will lead to corrective behavior. In day-to-day interactions with a patient, the patient is more responsive and amenable to instruction if the nurse has obtained the patient's trust and the patient sees the nurse as a competent professional.

Psychotherapy

In treating psychiatric problems, health care providers often use one or more of the following psychological techniques. *Behavior therapy* relieves anxiety through the conditioning and retraining of behavioral responses by repetition. It is often possible to resolve phobias with this technique. *Cognitive therapy* focuses on breaking

Communication

Starting the Conversation

Possibilities for starting a conversation with a patient include several approaches:

- "What circumstances brought you to the hospital?"
- "Tell me a little about what has been going on with you."
- "Ms. J., I am Linda, and I'll be your nurse today."
- "Tell me how you are feeling."

THERAPEUTIC DIALOGUE 1

Ms. J. underwent a hysterectomy 1 week ago for several fibroid tumors. She is 32 years of age and has a 3-year-old child. She has been married 5 years. The nurse who admitted her after surgery enters the room and finds her crying.

Nurse: (Walks over to Ms. J., touches her arm, and stands there quietly.)

Patient: (Continues to cry but looks up at the nurse and starts to quiet.)

Nurse: You look upset; please tell me what's upsetting you. (Pulls up a chair and sits at eye level.)

Patient: My whole life is ruined.

Nurse: Your life is ruined?

Patient: I wanted other children; we were going to have a large family.

Nurse: Tell me what a large family means to you.

Many patients experiencing loss need to cry. Crying begins to release emotion; the patient needs the nurse to accept it. The nurse's close physical presence and touch communicate acceptance. Acknowledgment of feelings encourages further expression, and then it is possible to explore the patient's sense of loss.

THERAPEUTIC DIALOGUE 2

Mr. H., 65 years of age, has received a diagnosis of cancer of the lung. The day nurse is making initial patient rounds and enters the room. The nurse notices that Mr. H. looks uncomfortable.

Nurse: (Walks over to the bed.) Good morning, Mr. H. You look uncomfortable.

Patient: I'm tired; I stayed awake all night.

Nurse: You had difficulty sleeping?

Patient: I have a lot on my mind. I couldn't sleep.

Nurse: (Sits down next to the patient and pats his hand.) Tell me what has been worrying you.

Encourage patients to talk (ventilate). Be observant for nonverbal communication and for underlying meanings in the stated words. Talking reveals emotions, at which point it is possible to identify and deal with them.

You and the patient bring your physiologic, psychological, developmental, and spiritual components into the therapeutic relationship. Other elements that you bring into the relationship are previous life experiences, needs, aspirations, and frustrations. You have an opportunity to help the patient explore a life event and the meaning that it has for the patient.

THERAPEUTIC DIALOGUE 3

Ms. K., who has been pacing the halls, is now staring out the window. She is toying with a ring on her finger. You notice that Ms. K. is vigorously tapping one foot on the floor.

Nurse: (Walks over to patient and sits beside her.) Ms. K., I have noticed that you seem a little restless. Is something troubling you?

Patient: No, not really. Well, maybe I am a little upset.

Nurse: Is there something in particular that is upsetting you?

Patient: I don't know. I'm just anxious.

Nurse: Tell me how you feel.

Patient: I feel jittery and nervous.

Nurse: Is there something specific that is worrying you right now?

Patient: My husband is going to lose his job in another month, and here I am in the hospital. I just don't know how we'll pay the bills. It scares me.

Nurse: Have you and your husband discussed this situation?

Patient: (Continues to share her feelings with the nurse.)

Anxiety is an unpleasant feeling of tension and apprehension. A person experiencing anxiety is sometimes unaware of the exact source of the tension. An array of physical and psychological symptoms usually accompanies anxiety. Resolution of the anxiety begins with awareness of the anxiety's source. A person seeks ways to resolve the tension (problem solving) to be rid of the tension.

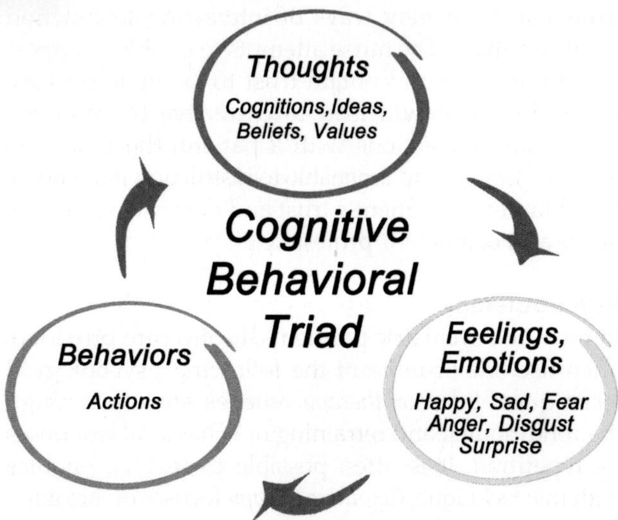

Fig. 35.3 Cognitive behavioral therapies. (Copyright © vaeenma/iStock/Thinkstock.)

negative thought patterns and developing positive feelings about memories or thoughts. These therapy types are interrelated and build upon each other. As individuals become aware of the negative actions and embrace the positive feelings, they are able to begin the process of demonstrating therapeutic behaviors (Fig. 35.3). *Group therapy* is often a useful modality in a hospital setting or day treatment programs. A group of patients with similar problems obtain insight through discussion and role playing. *Play therapy* often helps children express themselves by using toys such as puppets as their "spokesperson" of feelings.

Hypnosis helps a patient recover deeply repressed emotions and speed recovery. It also helps a patient change habits such as smoking.

Psychoanalysis was developed by Sigmund Freud. It is a long-term and intense form of therapy that enables the patient to bring unconscious thoughts to the surface. *Free association* (speaking thoughts without censorship) and dream interpretation are among the tools in psychoanalysis.

Adjunctive therapies include occupational therapy, recreational therapy, music therapy, magnetic therapy, art therapy, and hydrotherapy. These types of therapy allow expression of feelings, help increase self-esteem, and promote positive interaction and reality orientation. Such forms of adjunctive therapy can be used in a group setting or individually.

Limits of Confidentiality

Confidentiality is sometimes a dilemma when therapeutic effectiveness of care depends on the patient's willingness to talk about feelings and thoughts. It is important that the patient knows that each member of the health care team will share any information he or she receives with the others. No one member of the team keeps any secrets from the others. This practice also curtails patients' manipulating the staff or pitting one staff member or patient against another.

Just as the nurse has a duty to report child abuse, the nurse also has a duty to warn. Sometimes a patient expresses intent to kill someone when he or she is released, and the nurse is obligated to notify the appropriate authorities. Families of victims have filed—and won—lawsuits against health care workers for not warning the victim.

ELECTROCONVULSIVE THERAPY

In the late 1930s, two Italian physicians, Ugo Cerletti and Lucio Bini, introduced electroconvulsive therapy (ECT) to treat psychiatric disorders. Over the years, ECT has been refined. Muscle relaxants and anesthesia are now part of the therapy; these reduce the incidence of fracture, contusion, and sprains from the induced seizure.

ECT is a treatment for depression, mania, or schizoaffective disorders that do not respond to other treatment modalities. The course of ECT usually consists of approximately 10 treatments over several weeks. Only a very small amount of electrical current is required to trigger a tonic-clonic (grand mal) seizure; thus there is no risk of electrocution. Temporary memory loss after treatment is expected and lasts from a few hours up to a few days. Confusion right after a treatment usually dissipates in a few hours.

ECT usually is provided on an outpatient basis. There is a potential danger with the treatment, and it necessitates a great deal of care. When administered properly, for the right illness, ECT can help as much as or more than any other treatment.

Before a patient receives ECT, it is necessary to perform several tests. A thorough physical examination (which includes a blood chemistry survey, complete blood count, and urinalysis) detects any unsuspected conditions.

The practitioner completes a thorough mental examination. Electroencephalography is performed to rule out any existing electrical abnormalities. Chest and lumbosacral spine radiography rule out any skeletal abnormalities. Electrocardiography is also necessary because the treatment can put a strain on the heart.

In preparing the patient for ECT, treat the patient as a surgical candidate. In collecting data, make sure that all tests have been completed and that the health care provider has received the reports. Measure vital signs, height, and weight. If the patient has a knowledge deficit about the procedure, answer all of the patient's questions before the patient can sign a consent form. Describing the steps of the day, the room where the treatment is given, and where recovery takes place helps reduce anxiety.

Ensure that the patient is on nothing-by-mouth (NPO) status for at least 8 hours before the treatment. Just before the treatment, the patient is instructed to void.

The patient must remove all watches, jewelry, glasses or contact lenses, dentures, and hairpins. If the patient is an outpatient, it is acceptable to wear loose clothing such as a sweat suit or a hospital gown.

Administer ordered pre-ECT medications, usually including a sedative. An intravenous line is established for the anesthesiologist to use during the treatment.

Post-ECT care is similar to that for any postsurgical patient in the recovery room. Once the patient is fully awake and his or her gag reflex is present, the patient should be given a light meal or snack with acetaminophen. Assisting with mobility after the patient regains consciousness is sometimes also part of the care. Sometimes the patient is confused afterward and needs supervision and reassurance. Make sure family members understand the need to attend to the patient constantly because of the temporary confusion. Do not allow the patient to drive until the confusion is gone.

Continual reassurance, support, and attentiveness before and after each treatment help the patient deal with anxiety about ECT (see Box 35.2).

PSYCHOPHARMACOLOGY

Psychotropic (psychoactive) medications in conjunction with other therapies help modify a patient's behavior. Medication helps control symptoms. Monitoring for signs of effectiveness and evidence of side effects is a very important nursing responsibility. Understanding the medications used is clearly part of the nurse's role (Table 35.5).

Antidepressants

There are many antidepressant medications. In the newest class are the SSRIs and SNRIs, which include fluoxetine (Prozac), sertraline (Zoloft), venlafaxine (Effexor XR), citalopram (Celexa), and paroxetine (Paxil). As mentioned earlier, clinicians and patients tend to prefer these drugs over the other classes because they have fewer side effects. Other classes of antidepressants are tricyclic agents; monoamine oxidase inhibitors (MAOIs); and triazolopyridines, which are similar to tricyclic agents and include trazodone (Desyrel). Bupropion (Wellbutrin) is of the aminoketone subclass of MAOIs.

These medications work in different ways in the brain to alleviate signs and symptoms of depression, such as decreased appetite or sleep pattern disturbances, prolonged sadness, and lack of concentration. None of them take effect immediately; they generally take 2 to 4 weeks to effect any improvement. Patients often describe the change that drug therapy accomplishes in depression as a "fog lifting." Antidepressant therapy must be maintained for several months to a year to prevent symptom recurrence.

Serotonin syndrome. **Serotonin syndrome** is a potentially life-threatening condition that occurs usually as a result of an interaction between an SSRI and another serotonergic agent. It also can occur in older adult patients taking only an SSRI. Symptoms include altered mental status, autonomic dysfunction, and neuromuscular abnormalities.

Confusion, delirium, agitation, and mutism are some of the altered mental states that practitioners sometimes fail to recognize as side effects in chronically ill older adults living in long-term care facilities, a population in which the rate of depression is sometimes as high as 50%. Autonomic dysfunction can include blood pressure fluctuation, tachycardia, hyperthermia, marked pupil dilation (mydriasis), shivering, and diaphoresis. Possible neuromuscular symptoms include some that are similar to those produced by antipsychotic medications (see the later, more detailed, discussion of extrapyramidal symptoms): akathisia (a jittery feeling inside that causes restlessness), ataxia (incoordination), dystonia, dyskinesia, hyperreflexia, tremors, and seizures. Older adult patients are more likely to display neuromuscular side effects, which raises their risk of injury from falls. Serotonin syndrome worsens Parkinson's disease. Laboratory values indicative of serotonin syndrome include an elevated level of creatine phosphokinase as a result of muscle disintegration, elevated levels of white blood cells and transaminases, and a decreased level of serum bicarbonate.

Treatment for serotonin syndrome is to decrease the dosage of the drug slowly. Sudden discontinuation has potential to cause dizziness, nausea, vomiting, muscle pain, headaches, fatigue, anxiety, crying spells, and irritability. Instruct the patient about calling for assistance in ambulating until side effects have subsided. In the home setting especially, it is a good idea for the home health care nurse to encourage the patient to take an active role in managing medications by reporting even minor side effects or concerns. Review any over-the-counter medication that the patient takes. Emphasize the importance of informing the nurse and the prescribing health care provider when the patient uses an over-the-counter medication.

When assessing the patient for efficacy of antidepressants, be familiar with the actions of each drug, possible drug interactions, and serious side effects.

Antimanic Agents

Lithium carbonate is the primary drug that health care providers use to stabilize the mood and behavior of a patient with mania. A therapeutic blood level is required and sometimes takes 7 to 10 days to achieve. During the interim, practitioners frequently prescribe antipsychotic medications to control behavior. Toxicity is a problem with lithium usage. Poor fluid intake and salt restriction in the diet increase the risk of toxicity. Be aware of the signs of toxicity: nausea, vomiting, diarrhea, drowsiness, muscle weakness, and ataxia. If the patient does not stop taking the drug, toxicity potentially leads to seizures and death. Stopping the medication abruptly can also cause increased anxiety, nausea, and significant mood changes. Patient education is an important factor in lithium administration. The therapeutic level of

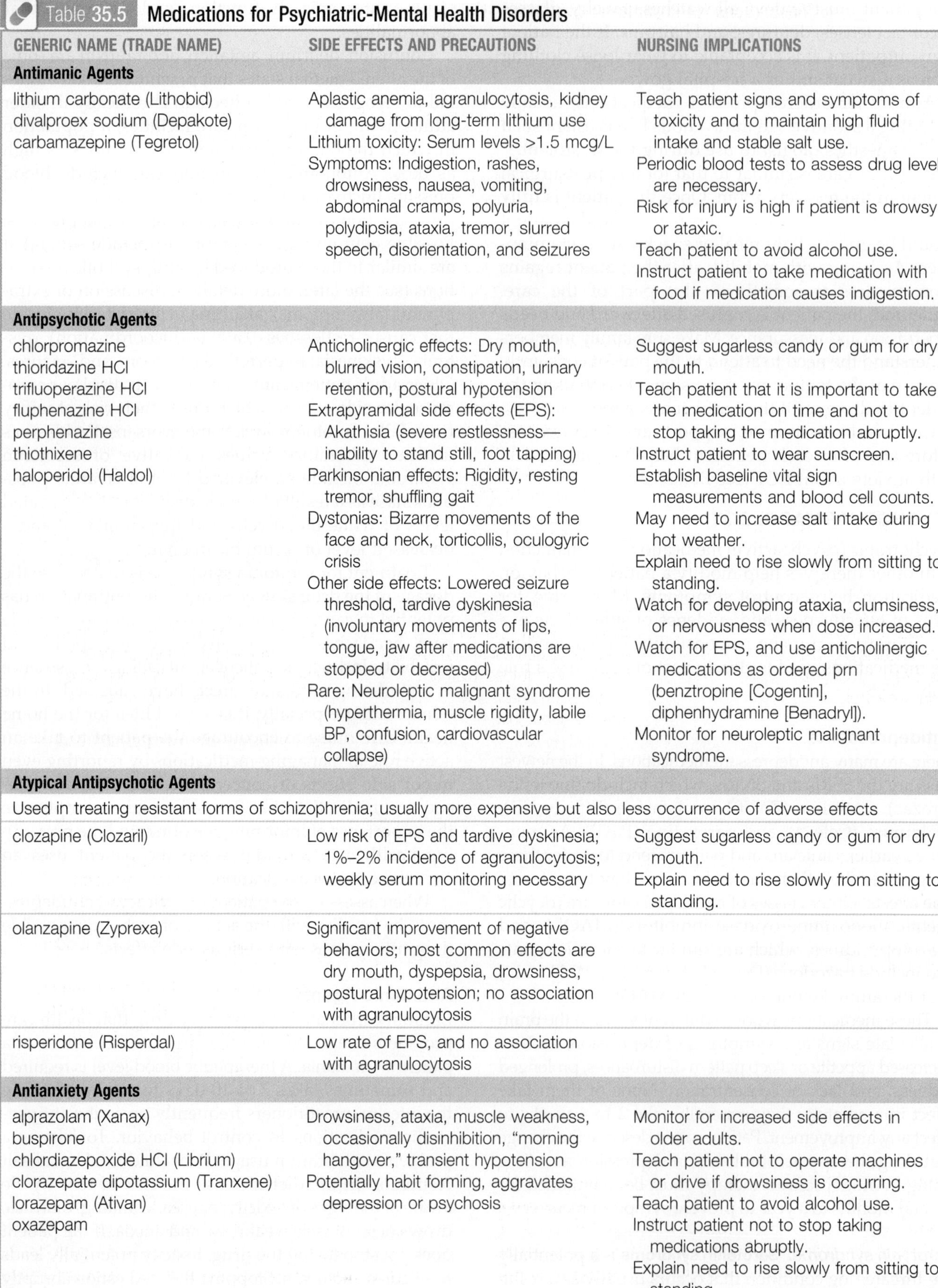

Table 35.5 Medications for Psychiatric-Mental Health Disorders

GENERIC NAME (TRADE NAME)	SIDE EFFECTS AND PRECAUTIONS	NURSING IMPLICATIONS
Antimanic Agents		
lithium carbonate (Lithobid) divalproex sodium (Depakote) carbamazepine (Tegretol)	Aplastic anemia, agranulocytosis, kidney damage from long-term lithium use Lithium toxicity: Serum levels >1.5 mcg/L Symptoms: Indigestion, rashes, drowsiness, nausea, vomiting, abdominal cramps, polyuria, polydipsia, ataxia, tremor, slurred speech, disorientation, and seizures	Teach patient signs and symptoms of toxicity and to maintain high fluid intake and stable salt use. Periodic blood tests to assess drug level are necessary. Risk for injury is high if patient is drowsy or ataxic. Teach patient to avoid alcohol use. Instruct patient to take medication with food if medication causes indigestion.
Antipsychotic Agents		
chlorpromazine thioridazine HCl trifluoperazine HCl fluphenazine HCl perphenazine thiothixene haloperidol (Haldol)	Anticholinergic effects: Dry mouth, blurred vision, constipation, urinary retention, postural hypotension Extrapyramidal side effects (EPS): Akathisia (severe restlessness—inability to stand still, foot tapping) Parkinsonian effects: Rigidity, resting tremor, shuffling gait Dystonias: Bizarre movements of the face and neck, torticollis, oculogyric crisis Other side effects: Lowered seizure threshold, tardive dyskinesia (involuntary movements of lips, tongue, jaw after medications are stopped or decreased) Rare: Neuroleptic malignant syndrome (hyperthermia, muscle rigidity, labile BP, confusion, cardiovascular collapse)	Suggest sugarless candy or gum for dry mouth. Teach patient that it is important to take the medication on time and not to stop taking the medication abruptly. Instruct patient to wear sunscreen. Establish baseline vital sign measurements and blood cell counts. May need to increase salt intake during hot weather. Explain need to rise slowly from sitting to standing. Watch for developing ataxia, clumsiness, or nervousness when dose increased. Watch for EPS, and use anticholinergic medications as ordered prn (benztropine [Cogentin], diphenhydramine [Benadryl]). Monitor for neuroleptic malignant syndrome.
Atypical Antipsychotic Agents		
Used in treating resistant forms of schizophrenia; usually more expensive but also less occurrence of adverse effects		
clozapine (Clozaril)	Low risk of EPS and tardive dyskinesia; 1%–2% incidence of agranulocytosis; weekly serum monitoring necessary	Suggest sugarless candy or gum for dry mouth. Explain need to rise slowly from sitting to standing.
olanzapine (Zyprexa)	Significant improvement of negative behaviors; most common effects are dry mouth, dyspepsia, drowsiness, postural hypotension; no association with agranulocytosis	
risperidone (Risperdal)	Low rate of EPS, and no association with agranulocytosis	
Antianxiety Agents		
alprazolam (Xanax) buspirone chlordiazepoxide HCl (Librium) clorazepate dipotassium (Tranxene) lorazepam (Ativan) oxazepam	Drowsiness, ataxia, muscle weakness, occasionally disinhibition, "morning hangover," transient hypotension Potentially habit forming, aggravates depression or psychosis	Monitor for increased side effects in older adults. Teach patient not to operate machines or drive if drowsiness is occurring. Teach patient to avoid alcohol use. Instruct patient not to stop taking medications abruptly. Explain need to rise slowly from sitting to standing.

Table 35.5 **Medications for Psychiatric-Mental Health Disorders—cont'd**

GENERIC NAME (TRADE NAME)	SIDE EFFECTS AND PRECAUTIONS	NURSING IMPLICATIONS
Antidepressants		
Tricyclic Agents amitriptyline amoxapine desipramine HCl (Norpramin) imipramine HCl (Tofranil) nortriptyline HCl (Pamelor)	Anticholinergic effects (see Antipsychotic Agents) Should not be administered to patients with severe liver disease or after myocardial infarction; should be administered with caution to patients with cardiac disease Sudden stoppage of medication sometimes causes sleep disturbance	Monitor BP for hypotension. Suggest sugarless candy or gum for dry mouth. Explain that appetite sometimes increases. Caution against strenuous exercise or high temperature because of reduced diaphoresis.
Monoamine Oxidase Inhibitors (MAOIs)		
phenelzine sulfate (Nardil) tranylcypromine sulfate (Parnate)	Orthostatic hypotension, headache, abnormal heart rate and rhythm, blurred vision, dry mouth, fatigue, nausea, vomiting, constipation, urinary hesitancy and retention Hypertensive crisis may result from eating foods containing tyramine (red wine, beer, aged cheese, chocolate, licorice, yogurt, caffeine-rich foods, liver, and broad beans)	Monitor BP; explain need to rise slowly from sitting to standing. Teach patient that tyramine-rich foods pose risk of life-threatening effects and their intake must be restricted. Teach patient to consult health care provider before taking over-the-counter cough or cold medicines. Teach patient drug interactions; consult resource when health care provider prescribes additional medications. Monitor intake and output.
Selective Serotonin Reuptake Inhibitors (SSRIs)		
fluoxetine (Prozac) fluvoxamine (Luvox) paroxetine HCl (Paxil) sertraline (Zoloft)	Anticholinergic effects (see Antipsychotic Agents), appetite loss, transient fatigue, weight loss, diarrhea or constipation, diaphoresis, anxiety, tremors, insomnia, tachycardia, sexual dysfunction	Because of insomnia, take medication in the morning and early afternoon. Avoid alcohol use. Call health care provider before taking other medications. Use cautiously in patients with renal or hepatic impairment. Monitor for symptoms of serotonin syndrome.
Other Antidepressants		
venlafaxine (Effexor) maprotiline nefazodone bupropion (Wellbutrin) trazodone mirtazapine (Remeron)	Same as for SSRIs	Same as for SSRIs. Instruct patient to take bupropion in three divided doses to minimize seizure risk. Suggest taking trazodone with food to decrease vertigo. Instruct patient not to take mirtazapine within 14 days of MAOI use: It has potential to cause hypertension, seizures, and death. Assess complete blood cell count and liver function periodically.

lithium is fairly narrow—0.4 to 1.3 mEq/L—and each patient must be evaluated individually and carefully monitored. The blood lithium level must be checked frequently to determine whether the therapeutic level has been obtained. Initially, daily level measurements may be ordered. Once a therapeutic level has been obtained, monthly measurements of the level typically are ordered.

Antipsychotic Agents

Antipsychotic medications or major tranquilizers are used for acute and chronic management of (1) schizophrenia, (2) organic mental disorders with psychosis, and (3) the manic phase of bipolar mood disorder. These drugs provide symptom control but are not a cure. Responses to these drugs are highly individualized. It is best to use the lowest effective dose.

A number of dose-related side effects occur in association with antipsychotic agents. Postural hypotension and sedation are common when patients first start taking these drugs. Consider implementing safety measures to prevent falls. Photosensitivity is another side effect; patients should wear sunscreen, hats, special clothing, and sunglasses to prevent sunburn. Autonomic reactions include urinary retention, dry mouth, constipation, edema, and weight gain. Increasing fluid intake not only relieves dry mouth but also actually triggers the body to release excess fluid from the tissues.

Various abnormal neuromuscular symptoms occur in association with these drugs. The extrapyramidal symptoms include pseudoparkinsonism (e.g., tremor with rigid posture); *akathisia,* or an inability to sit still, with continuous hand, mouth, or body movements (e.g., foot tapping); *dystonias,* or aberrant posturing (e.g., hand spasms); and *dyskinesia,* or involuntary movements (e.g., lip smacking or tongue protruding). *Tardive dyskinesia* is an extrapyramidal reaction that occurs in long-term use of neuroleptic agents and it is sometimes a permanent effect. Immediate action is necessary to combat extrapyramidal effects. Options to consider include stopping the drug or reducing the dosage, administering parenteral diphenhydramine (Benadryl), and follow-up use of antiparkinsonian drugs such as trihexyphenidyl or benztropine (Cogentin).

Antianxiety Agents

Antianxiety drugs (anxiolytics) or minor tranquilizers often help individuals experiencing moderate to severe anxiety. Practitioners prescribe benzodiazepine sedatives such as lorazepam (Ativan) to relieve the tension without sacrificing motivation. Abuse of drugs in this category is common.

Ongoing maintenance for severe persistent (chronic) mental illness is often very challenging for the patient and the family. Rehospitalization, when it occurs, reminds them that a cure for the disorder is not available and that close monitoring is still necessary, even when the patient is relatively free of symptoms. The special needs of long-term mentally ill individuals must be addressed by community mental health care and support, partial hospital programs, and assisted living environments.

ALTERNATIVE THERAPIES

Use of natural or herbal medications has become tremendously popular (see Chapter 20). However, their use has been integrated very little into the current system, which is based on prescription and over-the-counter drugs. The control and manufacture of these medications does not fall under the laws of the US Food and Drug Administration; as a result, the quality and the potency vary from manufacturer to manufacturer. Claims and clinical study results are not always consistent. Nonetheless, millions of people use herbal medicine on the basis of only advertising claims. When obtaining a drug history from the patient, inquire about the use of herbs.

St. John's wort *(Hypericum perforatum)* is one of the most common weeds in the world, and studies have shown its possible effectiveness in treating mild depression with few side effects when the patient takes therapeutic doses. St. John's wort potentially interacts with MAOIs and has the capacity to trigger hypertension if taken with allergy medication that contains monoamines or phenylalanine or with amino acid supplements containing tyrosine.

Kava *(Piper methysticum)* is an herb taken by some people to treat anxiety and insomnia because of its sedative effects. Scaly rash on the backs of the hands and forearms and on the soles of the feet is a common side effect. Alcohol potentiates the sedative effect and, if kava is taken with benzodiazepines, it produces toxicity and induces coma. Other side effects are neuromuscular abnormalities similar to the side effects of antipsychotics. Another herb useful in treating anxiety is gotu kola *(Centella asiatica)*, an herb that practitioners of ayurvedic medicine prescribe. The effectiveness of gotu kola is comparable to that of diazepam in reducing anxiety.

Ginkgo *(Ginkgo biloba)* and ginseng (various *Panax* spp.) are also popular herbs that some people believe improve memory and boost energy. Ginkgo provides moderate memory and cognitive improvement in treatment of early Alzheimer's disease by promoting cerebral blood flow, but it sometimes potentiates the action of anticoagulant drugs such as aspirin and warfarin (Coumadin), which poses the risk of fatal hemorrhage. Ginkgo has the capacity to affect insulin secretion, and ginseng sometimes lowers blood glucose in diabetic patients.

Many foods and beverages now contain herbs. Instruct the patient to read labels and avoid drug interactions with herbal additives. Encourage the patient to seek information about herbs from the pharmacist or health care provider before any herbs are used.

Aromatherapy has gained a foothold in the American way of life; however, its effects are limited. Its use is generally to enhance or potentiate another remedy. It is used in the forms of scented oils for massage, volatile oils to sniff or inhale, and scented candles or incense. Users believe that certain odors trigger chemical activity in the brain to relieve imbalance in the body.

Citrus essences, peppermint, cedarwood, rosemary, sandalwood, chamomile, and lavender are a few essential oils that many people believe help relieve stress and anxiety. It is possible to use such oils in a variety of ways—for example, chamomile tea, a sandalwood candle, or a hot bath with lavender oil. Aromatherapy focuses on the atmosphere of the moment and uses the body's senses to try to achieve mental balance. It has a definite place in holistic care.

APPLICATION OF THE NURSING PROCESS

In the psychiatric setting, as in every setting, the nurse uses the nursing process to meet the many needs of the patient, including assessment, formulation of patient problem statements, planning, intervention, and evaluation. The licensed practical nurse/licensed vocational nurse (LPN/LVN) participates in the nursing process as a member of the mental health care team that includes nurses, therapists, and health care providers. The LPN/LVN's observations of patient behavior and therapeutic communications with the patient assist the registered nurse (RN) in collecting data to form nursing diagnoses. The LPN/LVN's contributions in developing patient problem statements with the RN ensure appropriate interventions for the patient. The LPN/LVN and the RN work together to implement the plan of care for a therapeutic nurse-patient relationship.

Health promotion interventions are focused on preventing relapse and managing symptoms by practicing a healthy lifestyle. Patient teaching is most successful when it is simple, concrete, and clear. Patients need to realize that it is possible to manage their behaviors by recognizing when these behaviors are becoming problematic and by talking with their health care provider, therapist, or both.

Evaluation of the patient will be ongoing. At intervals or when the patient's response dictates, update the care plan. Examination of the documentation and personal observations are considerations when the plan of care is evaluated.

Clearly document all phases of the nursing process. Most of the documentation methods the nurse uses are ongoing and include the assessment criteria that the health care team uses. Ensure notes are accurate and descriptive. Terms such as "appears depressed" should be avoided; instead, specify behaviors, such as "no eye contact noted during conversation." Documentation of the patient's actual conversation is very valuable.

Working with patients who have a mental disorder is always a challenge. Honesty with a caring attitude goes a long way in helping such a patient deal effectively with his or her problem.

Get Ready for the NCLEX® Examination!

Key Points

- The nurse uses the nursing process in the psychiatric context; it includes assessment, formulation of patient problem statements, planning, intervention, and evaluation. The care plan documents this process.
- To help prevent suicide, it is necessary to recognize its warning signs and learn the kinds of actions that are possible to avert it.
- Therapeutic communication is a dynamic method of interacting with patients for problem solving and growth.
- In psychiatry, medications assist patients in dealing with feelings and behaviors.
- The nurse and the health care team observe and evaluate behavior to determine a patient's progress and the effectiveness of the care plan.

Additional Learning Resources

SG Go to your Study Guide for additional learning activities to help you master this chapter content.

evolve Be sure to visit the Evolve site at *http://evolve.elsevier.com/Cooper/foundationsadult/* for additional online resources.

Review Questions for the NCLEX® Examination

1. An 82-year-old man was admitted to the long-term care facility with moderate to severe heart failure and is unable to take care of himself at home. After dinner, the patient becomes agitated and confused. There are no significant changes in vital signs, and he has received the same medications he had been taking at home. What cause of acute confusion should the nurse consider?
   1. Alzheimer's disease
   2. Sundowning syndrome
   3. Electrolyte imbalance
   4. Acute renal failure
2. A patient with Alzheimer's disease continually wanders. Which snack will best meet the patient's nutritional needs? *(Select all that apply.)*
   1. Candy bars and ice cream sundaes
   2. Eggnog milk shakes and oatmeal-raisin cookies
   3. Protein bars and juice
   4. Root beer and potato chips
   5. Cheese and crackers and milk

3. The psychiatrist makes a diagnosis with the use of which system guide?
   1. *The Physicians' Desk Reference*
   2. *The Diagnostic and Statistical Manual*, Fifth Edition
   3. The hospital formulary
   4. Freud's *The Ego and the Id*
4. A delusional patient becomes agitated while watching television and states, "If I don't buy Crest toothpaste right now, I will have cavities." What is the nurse's best response?
   1. "The advertisement on the TV is saying its product will reduce tooth decay if you use their product regularly."
   2. "If you feel that it is absolutely necessary, we can go to the store now and purchase Crest toothpaste."
   3. "You can't believe everything you hear or see on TV."
   4. "Any toothpaste can be used to help prevent cavities; not just Crest toothpaste."
5. The nurse is assessing a patient with a diagnosis of schizophrenia for negative, or absent, behavior patterns. For which symptoms would the nurse assess? *(Select all that apply.)*
   1. Delusions
   2. Social withdrawal
   3. Hallucinations
   4. Disordered thinking
   5. Apathy
6. The nurse is assessing a patient admitted with depression. Which symptoms would the nurse expect the patient to exhibit? *(Select all that apply.)*
   1. Extreme fatigue
   2. Restlessness
   3. Flight of ideas
   4. Hallucinations
   5. Low self-esteem
7. What is the therapy of choice for bipolar, or manic-depressive, disorder?
   1. Chlorpromazine
   2. Lithium carbonate
   3. Electroconvulsive therapy
   4. Fluoxetine
8. A patient admitted to the emergency department is complaining of a panic attack. What manifestations are consistent with an anxiety attack? *(Select all that apply.)*
   1. Hypotension and bradycardia
   2. Lethargy and thready pulse
   3. Hyperventilation and tachycardia
   4. Hallucinations and apathy
   5. Inability to solve problems or think clearly
9. A 47-year-old patient is in the hospital for severe depression. She is unkempt and has lost 15 pounds in the past 2 months. Her family states that she always keeps a knife in her purse. The nurse will consider which intervention for this patient?
   1. Suicide precautions to prevent self-injury
   2. Occupational therapy to build self-esteem
   3. Art psychotherapy to help her express feelings
   4. Large-portioned meals to improve nutritional status
10. Antipsychotic medications have a number of side effects that discourage compliance by the patient. Which effect has the potential to lead to a serious permanent problem?
    1. Photosensitivity
    2. Postural hypotension
    3. Chronic constipation
    4. Tardive dyskinesia
11. A patient says the anchorwoman on the television news talks to him and told him that there was a car bombing in Israel today. What is the nurse's best response?
    1. "I don't think you understand how television projection works."
    2. "She is reporting the world news to everyone in the room. It only appears she is looking at you but she is looking in a TV camera that sends a picture to the TV."
    3. "If you look in the back of the TV console, you will see there is no person inside."
    4. "You are delusional. That is only a projected image of a person reading the news to a camera far away."
12. A 24-year-old woman was admitted for medication adjustment for bipolar disorder. The patient has not slept for 2 days and is unable to sit for more than a few minutes at a time. She has lost 11 pounds in the past week. Which factor will facilitate the best nutrition for the patient while she is in her manic phase?
    1. Have her take her meals in her room to reduce distracting stimuli.
    2. Have the kitchen double her meal portions, because she eats only half of the food served.
    3. Allow the patient to snack on candy bars between meals to gain back her lost weight.
    4. Keep sandwiches, granola bars, fruit, and noncaffeinated beverages available at the desk.
13. A patient who was sexually abused as a child recently married but finds sexual intercourse painful. She confides in her friend, who is a nurse. What is the appropriate response from her friend?
    1. "You should see your gynecologist right away in case you have torn tissues."
    2. "It is normal to have pain at first, but you will adjust to your husband over time."
    3. "You should seek counseling and make sure to get a good physical examination."
    4. "Did you report this abuse to the police?"
14. A patient is a broker on Wall Street who smokes half a pack of cigarettes a day. He avoids caffeine because he has trouble sleeping. He also often complains of an aching lower back. His physician was not able to find anything wrong physically. What is a possible cause of his back pain?
    1. Congenital anomaly
    2. Psychophysiologic origins
    3. Possible renal calculi forming
    4. Dependent personality disorder

15. A 17-year-old patient is worried about her weight. When she is out with friends, she eats junk food until she vomits and then exercises the next day for 4 hours. If she does not have a daily bowel movement, she takes a laxative. Her dentist has noticed her front teeth have signs of erosion. Her family has noticed her hair falling out, and now they have decided to take her to the family health care provider. What diagnosis do these symptoms support?
    1. Anorexia nervosa
    2. Laxative addiction
    3. Bulimia nervosa
    4. Gastroenteritis
16. A 37-year-old patient is not responding to drug therapy for depression. The health care provider has recommended ECT treatments for 1 week as an outpatient. The nurse will stress which point in the pretreatment teaching? *(Select all that apply.)*
    1. "You will need someone to take you to and from the clinic."
    2. "You may take acetaminophen after the treatment if you experience a headache."
    3. "Eat a good breakfast because you will sleep through lunch."
    4. "Scrub your forearms before coming to the clinic."
    5. "Take a laxative the night before so that you won't have an accident during the treatment."
17. The nurse is aware of the phases of schizophrenia. Arrange the following symptoms in the correct order according to the phases of schizophrenia.
    1. Odd or eccentric behavior
    2. Loss of contact with reality
    3. Lack of energy and motivation
    4. Some relief of symptoms
18. A 17-year-old boy tells his mother he is writing a paper for class on all the rock stars who have killed themselves. In the past few months, he has let his hair grow long, bathes only once a week, and stays in his room when he is at home. He is tired and irritable. His mother asks a friend who is a nurse if this is normal teenage behavior. What is the best response?
    1. "Yes; all teenagers go through a grunge stage."
    2. "Yes; he is just tired from the rapid growth spurt during adolescence."
    3. "No, and if he doesn't snap out of it, you might want to take him to a health care provider."
    4. "No; he should see a health care provider or counselor right away."
19. A 70-year-old patient is in the hospital for pneumonia and has been taking sertraline (Zoloft) for 1 year for depression. On the third day of her hospitalization, the patient has a pulse rate of 100 beats/min, demonstrates trembling in her hands, has an oral temperature of 103°F, and is diaphoretic. What is the nursing assessment?
    1. Anxiety, related to hospitalization
    2. Increased cranial pressure
    3. Impaired airway
    4. Serotonin syndrome
20. To effectively communicate with a patient demonstrating manic, elevated mood behaviors, the nurse will incorporate which technique into the plan of care?
    1. Provide detailed explanations to the patient.
    2. Joke and use puns with the patient.
    3. Be brief and concrete with the patient.
    4. Offer prn medications to the patient.
21. What is the priority nursing intervention when working with the patient with a personality disorder?
    1. Encouraging group activity participation
    2. Reassuring the patient that he or she is a "good person"
    3. Setting limits with the patient
    4. Supporting the patient's decisions consistently
22. When providing care for a depressed patient, what assessment data warrant immediate attention from the nurse?
    1. Anorexia and weight loss
    2. Lowered self-esteem
    3. Inability to care for self effectively
    4. Suicidal ideation
23. The nurse is assessing a patient diagnosed with schizophrenia and has noted several symptoms that correlate this diagnosis. Which symptoms would the nurse document as positive symptoms? *(Select all that apply.)*
    1. Auditory hallucinations
    2. Delusional belief that he is the president
    3. Avolition
    4. Apathy
    5. Tardive dyskinesia

36 Care of the Patient With an Addictive Personality

http://evolve.elsevier.com/Cooper/foundationsadult/

Objectives

1. Name two traits that characterize an addictive personality.
2. Describe the three stages of dependence.
3. Describe one legal effort that has decreased the incidence of substance abuse.
4. Describe three disorders associated with alcoholism.
5. Explain the two phases of recovery: detoxification and rehabilitation.
6. Identify six types of drugs of abuse.
7. Describe possible steps to help the chemically impaired nurse.

Key Terms

abuse (ŭ-BŪS, p. 1140)
addiction (ŭ-DĬK-shŭn, p. 1140)
addictive personality (ŭ-DĬK-tĭv pŭr-sŭn-ĂL-ĭ-tē, p. 1141)
Alcoholics Anonymous (AA) (ăl-kŭ-HŎL-ĭks ŭ-NŎN-ĭ-mŭs, p. 1146)
alcoholism (ĂL-kŭ-hŏl-ĭz-ĭm, p. 1140)
amotivational cannabis syndrome (ā-mō-tĭ-VĀ-shŭn-ăl KĂN-ă-bĭs SĬN-drōm, p. 1152)
cannabis (KĂN-ă-bĭs, p. 1152)
club drugs (KLŬB DRŬGZ, p. 1148)
delirium tremens (DTs) (dŭ-LĬR-ē-ŭm TRĔM-ĭnz [dē-TĒZ], p. 1143)
depressants (dĭ-PRĔS-ŭntz, p. 1148)
detoxification (dē-tŏk-sĭ-fĭ-KĀ-shŭn, p. 1145)
gateway drug (GĀT-wā DRŬG, p. 1143)
group therapy (GRŪP THĔR-ŭ-pē, p. 1146)
hallucinogens (hă-LŪ-sĭ-nō-jĕnz, p. 1151)
Healthcare Integrity and Protection Data Bank (HIPDB) (HĔLTH-căr ĭn-TĔG-rĭ-tē ĂND prō-TĔK-shŭn DĀ-tŭ BĂNGK, p. 1155)
huffing (HŬF-ĭng, p. 1153)
inhalants (ĭn-HĀ-lŭnts, p. 1153)
peer assistance programs (PĒR ŭ-SĬS-tŭns PRŌ-grămz, p. 1155)
psychoactive drugs (sī-kō-ĂK-tĭv DRŬGZ, p. 1141)
raves (RĀVZ, p. 1148)
street drugs (STRĒT DRŬGZ, p. 1148)
tolerance (TOL-ŭr-ŭns, p. 1142)

The treatment of patients with addictive behaviors is an important concern for nurses. Problems associated with the **abuse** or misuse of alcohol, tobacco, caffeine, nicotine, and other drugs consume a major proportion of current health care dollars. Many patients seeking care from acute care facilities and a variety of outpatient settings also suffer from some type of addictive behavior. Nurses often encounter problems of substance abuse and addiction in patients suffering from other medical conditions. It is not uncommon for patients to deny or hide their substance abuse problem. Substance abuse may not be addressed until withdrawal symptoms become apparent. Patients suffering with chronic pain have a high risk of developing tolerance of and addiction to opioids. Patients suffering from anxiety and depression sometimes self-medicate with alcohol, marijuana, or other substances. Investigate what the patient does to relieve stress or pain when you collect data about the patient. These data often help identify addictive behavior patterns that can impede the patient's recovery from acute illness.

ADDICTION

Addiction consists of four elements: (1) excessive use or abuse of a substance, (2) display of psychological disturbance, (3) decline of social and economic function, and (4) uncontrollable consumption of the substance, indicating dependence. **Alcoholism** is the addiction to alcohol. It is possible to suffer from more than one addiction at the same time. For example, an alcoholic person also may be a smoker and a compulsive gambler.

In the adult population (age 18 years and older), 87.4% report having consumed an alcoholic drink in the past 12 months. About 6% of these people have an alcohol use disorder (National Institute on Alcohol Abuse and Alcoholism, 2018). Age at the onset of drinking is strongly predictive of the development of alcohol dependence in the lifespan; of people who start drinking at the age of 14 or younger, 44% develop alcoholism. Alcohol and drug abuse are increasing in the older population. Older adults sometimes turn to alcohol, prescription and nonprescription drugs, caffeine, and nicotine to help cope with physiologic and sociologic changes associated with aging. Aging causes changes in absorption, distribution, metabolism, and excretion of drugs; thus the risk of misuse and abuse increases with age.

Alcohol is involved in 31% of all deaths caused by motor vehicle accidents. About 88,000 deaths each year are related to alcohol consumption. Approximately 70% of these deaths are among males. These statistics make alcohol consumption the fourth leading cause of preventable death in the United States (National Institute on Alcohol Abuse and Alcoholism, 2018).

The use of alcohol and drugs predates recorded history. In cultures from many parts of the world, alcohol and drugs have been used as medicine, in celebrations, and as a part of worship services. In the history of the United States, legal positions on the use of alcohol have varied. The temperance movement in the 1800s stressed moderation in or total avoidance of the use of alcohol. The Eighteenth Amendment to the US Constitution, known as *Prohibition,* which forbade the production, transport, and sale of alcoholic beverages, was passed in 1919 and later repealed in 1933. There has been a decrease in alcohol use over the years that experts attribute to education of the public and laws set forth to limit availability of alcohol to minors.

Although there has been a long-term decline in overall alcohol use, many people still use illicit drugs. In 2015, 10% of the United States population acknowledged that they had used illicit drugs in the previous month. Approximately 80% of these users admitted to using only marijuana (Centers for Disease Control and Prevention [CDC], 2017a). The goal of the Comprehensive Drug Abuse and Controlled Substance Act of 1970 (commonly referred to as the *Controlled Substance Act*) was to provide legal control over drugs that previous federal drug-related laws did not cover. The Bureau of Drug Abuse Control moved from the US Food and Drug Administration to the Department of Justice and later merged into the Drug Enforcement Agency, which today is the leading agency responsible for enforcing the 1970 act. All prescribing physicians and dispensing pharmacies register with the Drug Enforcement Agency. Smuggling and other illegal activities provide the public with illicit drugs.

Certain common traits have been identified in addicted people. These traits often have been grouped under the term **addictive personality** (exhibiting a pattern of compulsive and habitual use of a substance or practice to cope with psychic pain from conflict and anxiety). These personality traits include low tolerance for stress, dependency, negative self-image, feelings of insecurity, and depression. It is not clear whether these traits are present before the development of dependence or result from it.

STAGES OF DEPENDENCE

Psychoactive drugs, including alcohol, make the user feel good. Social use of drugs creates a relaxed atmosphere, encouraging people to socialize more openly. Movies, television commercials, and other media have suggested that individuals "need a drink" after a hard day at the office. Unfortunately, every psychoactive drug, including caffeine and nicotine, can be abused or become addicting. In the 1970s alcoholism and drug addiction acquired recognition as diseases. Experts published diagnostic criteria and established treatment centers for addiction in the United States—a psychoactive drug–oriented society. When does substance abuse become a disease and a problem? The indicator appears to be the loss of control. The disease of dependence is a chronic, incurable, progressive one with three characteristic stages of dependence: early, middle, and late (Box 36.1).

Box 36.1 Stages of Dependence

EARLY STAGE	MIDDLE STAGE	LATE STAGE
Increased drug tolerance	Moderate impairment	Severe impairment in all areas of function
Strong denial	Withdrawal signs with abstinence	Continuous use but inability to achieve "normal" feeling
Defending drug use in response to family concerns	Using drug to feel "normal"	Worsening medical problems; organ involvement
More socializing with users	Established pattern of use	Worsening malnutrition
Increased tardiness to or time off from work/school	Further alienation from family	Poor problem solving and judgment
Possible legal problems	Drug-related behavior such as lying, stealing, mood swings	Manipulativeness; denial of problems
Good prognosis for recovery, even without a treatment program	Decline in physical health	Unemployment
	Noticeable weight loss	Often homelessness
	Blackouts	No chance of improvement without treatment
	Financial/legal problems	
	Job loss or frequent job changes	
	Low chance of recovery without treatment	

EARLY STAGES

As a person uses an increasing amount of an addicting substance and uses it more frequently to achieve the same effect, **tolerance** develops. The user experiences the untoward effects of insomnia, anxiety, cramps, heart palpitations, changes in sexual libido, and accidental injury. Some users decrease or stop to prove that they have control of their substance use. Family and friends probably comment about their concern for the user's overinvolvement with drugs. The user may make light of the concern or become hostile and defensive. Some users avoid family and socialize only with other users. Users are prone to legal problems, such as charges of driving while intoxicated. Users sometimes miss work or show up late for work after a weekend of use. A pattern of absenteeism emerges. If a user is a student, truancy and falling grades with an uncaring attitude are common. Mood swings, decreased self-esteem, shame, guilt, remorse, resentment, and irritability are typical, with a tendency for these feelings to focus on drug use. Financial difficulties arise in connection with greater expenditures for drug use.

The prognosis with treatment is good in this early stage, and recovery without treatment is possible.

MIDDLE STAGE

In this stage, the dependent user is moderately impaired. With difficulty, the user makes efforts to decrease or stop, but these efforts are followed by heavier use. Abstinence brings on signs and symptoms of withdrawal. The user now uses the substance just to feel "normal." The user has a pattern of use in regard to time, place, and situation. Family relationships and friendships are weakened by drug-related behavior such as arguing, lying, stealing, incest, physical abuse, and child neglect. Physical health declines. Common problems that arise during this stage include weight changes; anorexia; malnutrition; gastrointestinal problems such as nausea, diarrhea, and gastritis; suicide attempts; blackouts of short-term memory; sexual problems; sexually transmitted infection; accidental injury; infections; and overdose. Job loss is common because of absenteeism, drug use on the job, and uncooperative attitudes. Employers sometimes ask users to seek treatment. Social isolation increases, and users continue to have legal and crime-related problems. Some dependent users stay in this stage a long time; with multidrug use, however, progression into the late stage is faster.

Very few people in this stage recover without treatment.

LATE STAGE

In this stage, the dependent user displays severe impairment in all areas of function. Drug use is nearly continual in an attempt to avoid emotional and physical pain, but the user is not able to achieve a feeling of normality. Medical problems worsen. Liver disease, pancreatitis, toxic psychosis, kidney failure, sexual impotence, and stroke are possible, along with malnutrition. Users in the late stage neglect personal hygiene. Intravenous drug users are at great risk for infection with human immunodeficiency virus (HIV) or hepatitis B or C virus and for developing septicemia, abscesses, or infective endocarditis. Some users become suicidal or homicidal. Users are manipulative, are in denial of their problems, and have poor problem-solving ability and judgment. Users in this stage are usually unemployed, associate only with dealers or other users, and may be homeless.

People in this stage cannot recover without treatment.

ALCOHOL ABUSE AND ALCOHOLISM

Alcoholism is a national health problem whose prevalence is surpassed only by those of heart disease and cancer. No one theory explains the cause of alcoholism. Several factors probably contribute to the development of alcoholism. Some authorities believe that people are more likely to develop alcoholism because of some biologic reason, such as an inner urge controlled by the nervous system or a dysfunction of the endocrine system. Alcoholism is determined, in part, genetically. The incidence of alcoholism in members of certain families is high: the sons of alcoholic men are four times more likely to develop alcoholism over their lifetime (National Council on Alcoholism and Drug Dependence, n.d.). Deficiencies in some hepatic enzymes necessary to metabolize alcohol contribute to the development of alcoholism in some people. Many Asians, Native Americans, and Inuits have deficiencies in these enzymes; alcoholism rates are higher in these ethnic groups than in the general public. Jews, Mormons, and Muslims have very low rates of alcoholism, whereas people of French descent and those of Irish descent have high rates.

Other theories rest on the belief that some part of the personality leads to the development of alcoholism. Some people still believe that alcoholism develops as a result of a moral fault. This theory provided the basis for much of the early treatment of alcoholic patients. Health care providers trained to provide treatment regimens that are based on this moral theory have difficulty assimilating newer biologic theories into their care.

Wide cultural differences concerning drug and alcohol use have been found in US society. Most young people in the United States have their first drink at an early age. In the past, girls were typically older than boys when they took their first drink of alcohol. Currently there are conflicting studies on what age girls and boys begin drinking. One study shows that the average age a girl has her first drink is 13 while for a boy, it's 11 (*Helpguide.org*, n.d.). From 2015–2016 approximately 13% of adolescents age 12 to 17 years reported using alcohol (Office of Disease Prevention and Health Promotion, n.d.). Alcohol sometimes serves as an informal rite of passage into adulthood. Drinking beer or other alcoholic beverages is the way many Americans celebrate certain holidays (e.g., St. Patrick's Day). Experts consider drinking to be the leading health problem in the African American community. Hispanic populations and many other ethnic groups celebrate life while drinking alcohol. Alcohol often serves as a **gateway drug.** Many multidrug users began by abusing alcohol and progressed to abusing other substances.

Etiology and Pathophysiology

Alcohol is a central nervous system (CNS) depressant. The so-called stimulating effect occurs because the first areas affected by alcohol are the higher centers of the brain, including the frontal cortex, which govern self-control. Judgment is blocked, but memory of pleasure is retained. As a person continues to ingest alcohol, it affects the nucleus accumbens in the limbic system (the most primitive part of the brain; it regulates hunger, thirst, and sexual desire). Repeated alcohol consumption affects the basal ganglia of the brain, where it unbalances compulsion controls, leading to obsessive-compulsive behavior. Rapid, large-quantity consumption can lead to unconsciousness, during which respiration is sometimes affected. Death from acute alcohol poisoning is possible.

The active ingredient of alcoholic beverages is ethyl alcohol or ethanol. There are similar amounts of alcohol in 12 ounces of beer, 4 ounces of wine, and 1½ ounces of hard liquor. Alcohol does not require digestion, and the body absorbs it readily in the stomach and the intestines. An empty stomach increases the rate of absorption. After ingestion, the body loses small amounts through breathing and in the urine, but 90% is metabolized by the liver.

Alcohol has a diuretic effect. The urine of a heavy drinker sometimes contains increased amounts of electrolytes, especially potassium, magnesium, and zinc. Prolonged use of alcohol has a toxic effect on the intestinal mucosa that results in decreased absorption of vitamin B_1 (thiamine), vitamin B_9 (folic acid), and vitamin B_{12} (cobalamin).

Alcohol does not undergo conversion to glycogen; it does provide the body with calories but no minerals or vitamins. One ounce of alcohol provides 200 kcal but no other nutritional value. Blood alcohol levels depend on the amount of alcohol ingested and the size of the individual. Most states designate blood alcohol serum levels of 80 mg/dL (0.08%) as the legal limit for driving a motor vehicle. Increasing blood alcohol serum levels have increasingly serious side effects (see Chapter 16, Table 16.1).

DISORDERS ASSOCIATED WITH ALCOHOLISM

Fetal Alcohol Syndrome

Fetal alcohol syndrome is a congenital anomaly resulting from maternal use of alcohol during pregnancy. Although the condition is more common in mothers who drank heavily during pregnancy, no specific amount of alcohol has been identified as the amount that results in the syndrome. As few as two drinks per day have the potential to cause adverse effects in an infant. Experts agree that during pregnancy, it is best to avoid alcohol ingestion completely. The damage seems to be greater when alcohol is consumed during the first trimester of pregnancy. Birth defects related to alcohol use include mental retardation; growth disorders; craniofacial abnormalities, including wide-set eyes and a flattened face; and malformed body parts. The effect on the pregnancy may include spontaneous abortion or stillbirth.

Alcohol Withdrawal Syndrome

Alcohol withdrawal syndrome occurs in a person who has developed physiologic dependence and quits drinking abruptly. The risk for having alcohol withdrawal syndrome is highest in older adults, people who have previously suffered delirium tremens, malnourished people, and people who have another acute illness. The range of possible signs and symptoms varies from mild tremor and flulike signs and symptoms to severe agitation and hallucinations. Signs and symptoms associated with the cessation of alcohol consumption include diaphoresis; tachycardia; hypertension; tremors; nausea or vomiting, or both; anorexia; restlessness; disorientation; hallucinations; and seizures.

The tremors from alcohol cessation occur 6 to 48 hours after the last drink and sometimes last for 3 to 5 days. Tremors usually occur in the hands but also may be present in the tongue, the chin, the trunk, and the feet. Seizures can occur 12 to 24 hours after alcohol cessation. Usually these are tonic-clonic (grand mal) seizures and often are not preceded by an aura.

Delirium Tremens

Delirium tremens (DTs) is a complication of alcohol withdrawal. This acute psychotic reaction is a result of excessive alcohol consumption over a long period. The risk of death from this complication is as high as 15%, even with treatment. Signs of DTs are tremors; increase in activity, sometimes to the point of extreme agitation; disorientation; fear with an appearance of panic; hallucinations; and elevated temperature (Burns, 2013). DTs most often occur 1 to 4 days after cessation of alcohol use and usually last from 2 days to a week.

Korsakoff Psychosis and Wernicke Encephalopathy

Korsakoff psychosis and Wernicke encephalopathy are two brain disorders that sometimes occur in people with chronic alcoholism. Characteristics of Korsakoff psychosis are short-term memory loss, disorientation, muttering, delirium, insomnia, hallucinations, polyneuritis, and painful extremities, with footdrop affecting the gait. Wernicke encephalopathy occurs in association with thiamine (vitamin B_1) deficiency, causing brain damage in the temporal lobes of the brain. It features memory loss, aphasia, involuntary eye movement and double vision, lack of muscle coordination, and disorientation with confabulation (i.e., the patient fills in memory gaps with inappropriate words).

Because alcohol affects all tissues in the body, chronic alcohol ingestion has the potential to cause damage to

Table 36.1 Disorders Associated With Alcoholism

SYSTEM	DISORDERS
Gastrointestinal (GI)	Gastritis; pancreatitis; cancer of mouth, esophagus, and stomach; esophageal varices; GI bleeding; malabsorption of nutrition; ascites
Hepatic	Hepatitis, cirrhosis, fatty liver, liver failure, hepatic encephalopathy
Cardiovascular and hematologic	Hypertension, enlarged heart, high cholesterol, heart failure, portal hypertension, low blood glucose level, anemia, poor clotting ability, increased susceptibility to infection
Respiratory	Decreased cough reflex, aspiration pneumonia
Urologic/ reproductive	Prostatitis, impotence, urinary flow problems
Musculoskeletal	Myopathies, bone fractures from falls, joint damage from injury
Neurologic	Neuritis, organic brain diseases such as Wernicke encephalopathy and Korsakoff psychosis, nerve palsies, gait changes, short-term memory loss

all parts of the body. Table 36.1 lists other disorders arising from chronic alcohol use.

❖ NURSING PROCESS

◆ Assessment

It is important to collect subjective and objective data about the patient who has a substance abuse or dependence problem. *Subjective data* include the person's normal using or drinking pattern, as well as the date and time of the last drink or use of a drug. The specific substance and the quantity the person uses are important. Other complaints such as nausea, indigestion, sleep disturbance, or pain sometimes indicate the simultaneous occurrence of another disease process, in addition to the side effects of substance abuse. Assessment of normal dietary patterns, the presence of any disease that necessitates treatment with prescribed medications, and regular use of any over-the-counter drugs help complete the picture of the patient's present state of wellness. Obtain this information in as much detail as possible by asking about drug allergies or unusual responses to anesthesia, sedatives, or preoperative medications. Maintaining a concerned, nonjudgmental attitude when asking for details helps reassure the patient, as does the promise of confidentiality about this private part of his or her life.

Assess for any history of tremors, hallucinations, delusions, seizures, or DTs. Note any past periods of abstinence. Ask about any problems with occupation, family, or legal matters. Document any family history

Box 36.2 CAGE Questions

Two or more affirmations to these questions indicate probable alcoholism:

1. Have you ever felt you ought to ***c***ut down on your drinking?
2. Have people ***a***nnoyed you by criticizing your drinking?
3. Have you ever felt bad or ***g***uilty about your drinking?
4. Have you ever had a drink first thing in the morning to steady your nerves or for your hangover (i.e., ***e***ye-opener)?

of substance dependency. Remember that denial is strong in people with untreated substance abuse or dependence, and information from such patients is often inaccurate. It is helpful to validate information with families or significant others if possible. Beneficial in affirming alcohol abuse is the CAGE questionnaire, whose title arises from an acronym formed from among the tool's four questions (Box 36.2).

Objective data include height, weight, vital sign measurements, and findings of physical assessment. The presence of tremor or skin conditions, especially on the forearms, should be noted. Needle tracks and small scabs on forearms, backs of hands, and insteps indicate intravenous use. Acne-like facial rash is possibly related to use of 3,4-methylenedioxymethamphetamine (MDMA, or Ecstasy). Excessive gum and tooth erosion and extreme vasoconstriction may indicate methamphetamine ("meth") use.

Frequent sniffling, stuffy nose, or harsh nonproductive cough is possibly related to drug use. Assess general behavior and cognitive abilities for impairment. The presence of tachycardia, hypertension, petechiae, and neuropathies is significant. A urine or blood sample positive for drugs or alcohol or the presence of ascites alerts the nurse to the need for further investigation of the patient's history.

◆ Diagnostic Tests

Blood and urine tests help screen for toxins. Certain foods sometimes cause a false-positive reading in a urine screen. If a person ate a poppy seed roll and later gave urine for a drug screen, the result may appear positive for heroin. Abnormalities in routine blood tests are sometimes directly related to alcoholism. Elevated levels of liver enzymes, hypoglycemia, and abnormal blood protein levels occur with alcoholism. Magnesium levels are decreased in some cases. Anemia and other evidence of poor nutrition are common in addicted patients. Some practitioners also order testing for hepatitis and HIV.

◆ Patient Problem

Patient problems and interventions for the patient with an addiction cover emotional needs and physical needs (Box 36.3).

Box 36.3 Possible Patient Problems for Addiction[a]

PHYSICAL CONDITIONS	EMOTIONAL CONDITIONS	EDUCATIONAL CONDITIONS
Acute confusion	Defensive coping	Deficient knowledge
Functional urinary incontinence	Disturbed personality identity	Ineffective family therapeutic regimen management
Impaired physical mobility	Dysfunctional family processes	Readiness for enhanced family processes
Insomnia	Impaired individual resilience	Readiness for enhanced self-concept
Risk for electrolyte imbalance	Ineffective impulse control	Risk-prone health behavior
Risk for imbalanced fluid volume	Risk for compromised human dignity	
Risk for impaired liver function	Social isolation	
Risk for poisoning	Spiritual distress	
Sleep deprivation	Stress overload	

[a]List is not all inclusive.
From Ralph S, Taylor C: *Nursing diagnosis reference manual*, ed 9, Philadelphia, 2014, Wolters-Lippincott.

Nursing Interventions

Care for the addicted patient starts with **detoxification,** the removal of the poisonous effects of a substance. A controlled setting in which the patient can be observed closely and treated for any complications is important during this acute phase of recovery.

Safety of the patient is a primary concern. If the patient is intoxicated, a patent airway must be maintained. The side-lying position and oral suctioning should be considered if oral secretions can be aspirated or if vomiting could occur. If swallowing is intact, the head of the bed should be elevated at least 30 degrees to encourage better air exchange. Intravenous (IV) fluids may be administered to correct the patient's fluid and electrolyte imbalance. The IV site must be monitored often, especially if the patient is restless. The facility's seizure precautions—such as padded side rails, floor pads, and moving patient to a room close to the nurse's station—should be instituted.

Practitioners usually treat tremors, nervousness, and restlessness with drugs such as chlordiazepoxide (Librium) or lorazepam (Ativan). Scheduled doses must be given on time. Environmental stimuli should be reduced. The patient should be allowed to ambulate or perform other benign activities that help ease nervousness, but the patient must refrain from overexertion. The patient should be attended while ambulating if he or she is unsteady from coordination disturbance or lack of conditioning. As weakness subsides, a regular exercise regimen should be included in the care plan (Nursing Care Plan 36.1).

Cardiorespiratory distress is a possible result of stimulant abuse. Health care providers sometimes prescribe beta-adrenergic agents such as propranolol (Inderal) and calcium channel blockers such as nifedipine (Procardia) and oxygen. Continuous cardiac monitoring and frequent checks on vital signs with respiratory assessment help the nurse detect any adverse changes early, before they have the chance to become life threatening.

Keep explanations to the patient simple. Speak in a calm voice, planning time for the patient's verbalizations. Therapeutic conversation techniques are used to assist the patient in understanding himself or herself (self-realization). Reinforce teaching about the disease concept of addiction. Denial is confronted in a nonjudgmental manner. The family is encouraged to participate in planning for sobriety. Counselors sometimes initiate individual therapy to assist the patient into the rehabilitation phase of recovery.

For patients who are extremely restless, health care providers sometimes order magnesium sulfate to raise the seizure threshold or another anticonvulsant medication such as phenytoin (Dilantin). High doses of chlordiazepoxide (Librium) have potential to cause urinary retention. Intake and output measurements are appropriate in some cases.

Disorientation is possible, especially at night. Nightlights in the room and frequent visits by nurses tend to help. If a patient is not able to sleep at night, he or she should sit up and have a snack; then give the patient a back rub and encourage him or her to rest. If the patient appears fearful or panicky and unable to reacquire orientation to reality, notify the supervising nurse. Check vital signs (including temperature) before the health care provider is notified. Physical restraints have the potential to escalate aggressive behavior but are sometimes necessary if the patient poses a risk for harm to self or others.

Many addicted patients are malnourished and suffer from loss of appetite. Incorporating nutritious foods and inquiring about food preferences help meet nutritional deficits. Providing between-meal snacks is also helpful. Administration of multivitamins and thiamine as ordered help the patient improve his or her nutritional state.

Rehabilitation

After detoxification, the acute phase of recovery, it is time to start rehabilitation. The object of rehabilitation is to help the patient abstain from substance abuse. Because there is no cure for addiction, abstinence is the practical equivalent to the control of the disease. Administration of disulfiram (Antabuse) is sometimes a way to encourage abstinence. It causes facial flushing, nausea, tachycardia, dyspnea, dizziness, and confusion when the patient consumes alcohol. The purpose is to

Nursing Care Plan 36.1 The Patient Who Abuses Alcohol

Mr. J., 56 years of age, was a corporate executive. His employer confronted him about his increasing tendency to call in sick, last-minute rescheduling of meetings, and excessive alcohol use during luncheon meetings. Later, after the confrontation, the police cited him for driving while intoxicated for the third time and jailed him. Sentencing included the requirement to complete a treatment program for alcoholism.

PATIENT PROBLEM

Obstructive denial, related to inability to admit being alcoholic

Patient Goals and Expected Outcomes	Nursing Interventions	Rationale
Patient will participate in program Patient will identify negative effects of drinking on other people Patient will abstain from alcohol use Patient will express acceptance of alcoholism as a disease Patient will express acceptance of responsibility for own behavior Patient will maintain abstinence after discharge	Confront the patient's denial by relating incidents and problems to its use. Reinforce teaching about the disease of alcoholism. Encourage the patient to identify behaviors that have caused problems in his or her life. Do not allow the patient to rationalize or to blame others.	It is necessary to address the problem of alcoholism first. Providing knowledge about the disease and having the patient identify the relationship between alcohol and his or her problems will help the patient overcome denial. Blaming others is an excuse to continue drinking behavior.

PATIENT PROBLEM

Impaired Coping, related to abnormal use of alcohol

Patient Goals and Expected Outcomes	Nursing Interventions	Rationale
Patient will express feelings directly and express anger or hostility outward in a safe manner Patient will practice using nonchemical alternatives to deal with stress or difficult situations Patient will verbalize increased self-esteem	Encourage the patient to explore alternative ways of dealing with a stressful situation. Involve the patient in a group to provide confrontation, positive feedback, and sharing of feelings. Avoid discussion of unanswerable questions, such as why he drinks.	Patient perhaps has minimal experience of dealing with stress without alcohol. Groups of peers are honest and supportive. Asking why when there is no answer is dwelling on the negative and in the past. Focus on positive and the future, for which change has the power to make a difference.

CRITICAL THINKING QUESTIONS

1. During Mr. J.'s assessment, the nurse notes that he has tremors, is agitated, and verbalizes visual hallucinations. What therapeutic interventions are appropriate to perform to prevent injury to the patient?
2. As Mr. J.'s physical condition improves, he discloses his hopelessness and lack of desire to continue living. What is an appropriate response by the nurse?
3. During group therapy, Mr. J. states, "Now that I am physically better, I know I will be able to stop drinking. I don't need any help. There really isn't anything wrong with me." What is the appropriate staff intervention at this time?

reduce alcohol consumption by aversion conditioning. Treatment programs often include family members in part of the treatment plan. Some of these programs are inpatient, and some are outpatient or day-treatment programs.

Group therapy. Group therapy is an effective treatment modality. **Group therapy** provides a caring, emotionally supportive atmosphere in which the patient is able to acknowledge the relationship of substance abuse with negative consequences in his or her life. The group tends to point out negative defense mechanisms such as denial or displacement and to offer possible solutions to its members. Families should be encouraged to attend support groups to help the patient and family to grow together, not apart. Group therapy sometimes continues after completion of an inpatient program. Group therapy is an important part of all recovery programs.

Alcoholics Anonymous. **Alcoholics Anonymous (AA)** is an international nonprofit organization that began in 1935 as a way for abstinent alcoholic people to help

Box 36.4 Twelve Steps of Alcoholics Anonymous

1. We admitted we were powerless over alcohol—that our lives had become unmanageable.
2. Came to believe that a Power greater than ourselves could restore us to sanity.
3. Made a decision to turn our will and our lives over to the care of God *as we understood Him.*
4. Made a searching and fearless moral inventory of ourselves.
5. Admitted to God, to ourselves, and to another human being the exact nature of our wrongs.
6. Were entirely ready to have God remove all these defects of character.
7. Humbly asked Him to remove our shortcomings.
8. Made a list of all people we had harmed, and became willing to make amends to them all.
9. Made direct amends to such people wherever possible, except when to do so would injure them or others.
10. Continued to take personal inventory and when we were wrong promptly admitted it.
11. Sought through prayer and meditation to improve our conscious contact with God *as we understood Him,* praying only for knowledge of His will for us and the power to carry that out.
12. Having had a spiritual awakening as a result of these Steps, we tried to carry this message to alcoholics, and to practice these principles in all our affairs.

From Alcoholics Anonymous: The twelve steps of Alcoholics Anonymous, 2016. Retrieved from *http://www.aa.org/assets/en_US/smf-121_en.pdf.*

other alcoholic people become and stay sober through group support, shared experiences, and faith in a power greater than themselves. There are regular meetings in most communities. Listings for local AA chapters may be found in the telephone book, in the newspaper, or on the Internet. The foundation of AA is a 12-step program that assists the dependent person in admitting powerlessness over alcohol (Box 36.4). Other groups have followed up on the success of AA, usually using similar models for rehabilitation; these groups include Overeaters Anonymous, Al-Anon (for friends and family of alcoholic people), and Narcotics Anonymous.

Treatment centers. Residential treatment centers provide the opportunity for detoxification. There is no direct medical intervention; instead, trained nurses provide close physical monitoring with the assistance of counselors and recovered peers. After detoxification, the patient enters a drug- and alcohol-free residence. A primary goal of this type of treatment is the rebuilding of social skills that do not involve drug use as the primary method of interaction. The length of the stay in a treatment center ranges from 1 to 6 months; most centers operate on an ability-to-pay basis, with some governmental funding.

Box 36.5 Addiction Issues to Consider

The medical community has overcome its fear of addiction and focuses on providing adequate pain management for acute and chronic pain conditions.

- Postoperative care with the use of opioids in patient-controlled administration devices has shown that opioid need and the severity of pain decrease. Many patients are using nonopioid medications for pain control by the third postoperative day. No development of tolerance or addiction occurs. However, the patient sometimes suffers undue fears of addiction when told that opioids will be used to control postoperative pain. Explanation of the pain management regimen usually helps allay the patient's fears of addiction. The patient's use of the self-medication before activities helps the patient heal more quickly.
- Chronic pain management involves more than just a pill to relieve pain. It is very important to use imagery, physical therapy, and other methods to help the patient relieve pain without chemical intervention. Side effects of high doses of NSAIDs are not tolerated by some patients; in such cases, it is possible to use narcotics to control pain. Although opioid addiction is always a possibility, health care providers sometimes consider opioids to be cheaper and more effective than treating the serious side effects of high-dose NSAID therapy. If the patient is dying, addiction to opioid agents is not an issue, but close monitoring is necessary to avoid acute overdose.
- Acute pain management for addicted patients presents a challenge to the health care team. Accidents and surgery are usually the cause of the acute pain. Circumstances of an injury sometimes trigger withdrawal symptoms within 24 hours of admission to an acute care facility. Most often, health care providers order medications to relieve pain and suppress withdrawal symptoms. Cross-tolerance and multidrug abuse necessitate careful consideration of minor changes in the patient's condition. In the plan of care, discuss referral for rehabilitation; the initial steps of rehabilitation will, in some cases, be part of the patient's acute phase of recovery.

Pain management. Pain management sometimes involves the use of addicting substances, which sometimes complicates pain management for an addicted person. The medical community has improved greatly the regimen options for effective pain management with combinations of nonopioid, opioid, and antianxiety agents, along with nonchemical interventions. Nursing interventions require not only careful assessment of pain but also observation for developing patterns of drug-seeking behavior that indicate the patient's tolerance or addiction to the drug. Encouraging the patient to practice and use nonchemical interventions to ease pain will reduce the risk of chemical dependency for relief (Box 36.5).

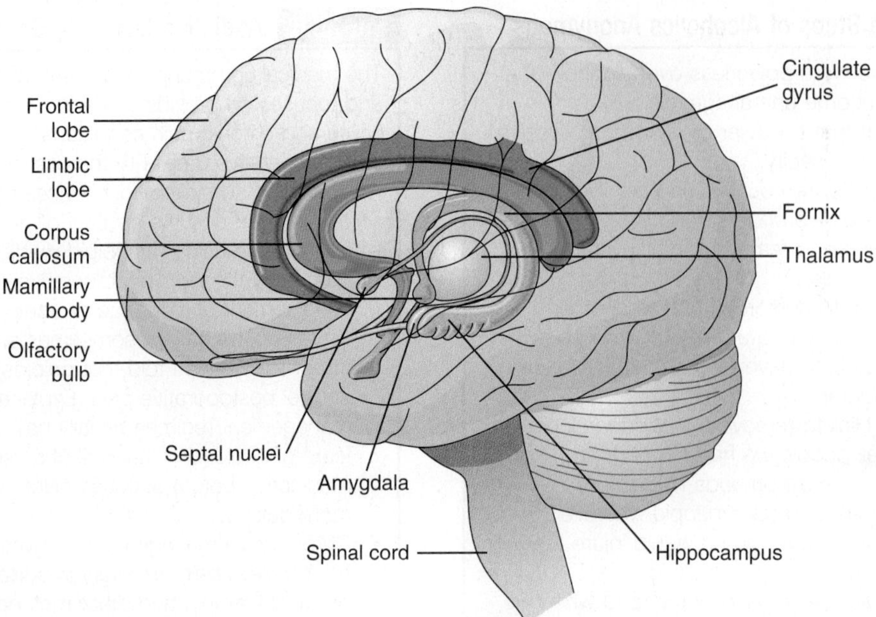

Fig. 36.1 Limbic system. The limbic system is considered to be the emotional center of the brain. An emotional response to an incoming stimulus is produced and then stored in memory. (From Copstead-Kirkhorn LE, Banasik J: *Pathophysiology*, ed 5, St. Louis, 2013, Mosby.)

DRUG ABUSE

Although alcohol abuse is present most frequently in patients fighting addiction or in patients who are being treated for other health problems, drug abuse is also a growing problem in the health care setting. Many people think only of illegal drugs when drug abuse is mentioned, but abuse of prescription and over-the-counter drugs is common. More than 46 people die every day because of a prescription drug overdose (CDC, 2017). Prescription drugs are sometimes traded or shared. Drug abusers may seek excessive prescriptions from their health care providers, purchase them on the streets, or divert them from the supplies of friends or family members. Rationalizations such as "If it worked for me, it will work for my friend" and "If one pill works, two pills will work better" often deny or justify misuse or abuse of many prescription and over-the-counter drugs.

When a person takes drugs for reasons other than medical issues or in a dose higher than recommended, the term *misuse* or *abuse* applies. **Club drugs** refer to substances that people frequently take for euphoric effect at parties, concerts, dance clubs, or all-night **raves** (also called trance parties: dance parties with extremely loud music). Club drugs are often street drugs. **Street drugs** are substances that users buy from illegal drug dealers. These drugs come from illegal manufacturers without strict controls, are illegally obtained prescription drugs, or are not approved for use in the United States. Chronic abuse has the potential to lead to psychological or physical dependence, or both. Many commonly abused drugs act on the limbic system of the brain and potentially cause permanent damage to that area (Fig. 36.1 and Box 36.6). Commonly abused drugs discussed in this chapter are depressants, opioids, stimulants, hallucinogens, cannabis, and inhalants (Box 36.7).

Box 36.6 Limbic System of the Brain

The structures of the limbic system, which are sometimes referred to as the *limbic lobe*, are involved in feeding, defense, reproduction, emotional responses, and the consolidation and retention of memory. The limbic lobe is not a separate structure; rather, it comprises border areas of the frontal, parietal, and temporal lobes with inner brain structures around the ventricles. Structures included are basal ganglia, amygdala, hippocampus, thalamus, hypothalamus, nucleus accumbens, cerebral cortex, olfactory cortex, and connecting nerve tracts.

DEPRESSANTS

CNS **depressants** include alcohol, sedative-hypnotic medications, and opioid analgesics. The sedative-hypnotic medications most often abused include barbiturates and benzodiazepines (minor tranquilizers). People usually take them orally in tablet or capsule form. Box 36.8 lists the effects of depressants.

Barbiturates entered into medical use in the beginning of the 20th century; they are useful in the clinical context for their sedative, hypnotic, anesthetic, and anticonvulsant effects. Problematic side effects include respiratory depression, rapid tolerance, and dependency; untoward effects (e.g., seizures or status epilepticus) accompany sudden withdrawal. In the 1960s benzodiazepines

Box 36.7 Commonly Abused Drugs and Their Street Names

Amphetamines: Speed, truck drivers, copilots, black beauties, crank, go
Barbiturates: Reds, blues, yellow jackets, rainbows, bluies
Benzodiazepines: Downers, chill pill, vitamin V
Chloral hydrate: Mickey Finn, mickey
Cocaine: Snow, crack, blow, coke, nose candy, toot, white dust, toot sweet
Gamma-hydroxybutyrate (GHB): Soap, easy lay, Georgia homeboy, liquid ecstasy
Heroin: H, smack, scag, junk, caca
Ketamine: Special K, vitamin K
Lysergic acid diethylamide (LSD): Acid, windowpane, gelcap, microdots, blotter, purple haze
Marijuana: Pot, reefer, grass, dope, weed, green, cannabis, Jamaican, Acapulco gold
Methamphetamine: Speed, crystal, ice
3,4-methylenedioxymethamphetamine (MDMA): Ecstasy, E, XTC, hug, love bug, beans, Adam, Molly
Nitrous oxide: Nitrous, whippets
Phencyclidine (PCP): Angel dust, rocket fuel, wack, ozone
Psilocybin: Shroom, magic mushroom
Rohypnol: Roofies, rough, rope, roach

Box 36.8 Signs and Symptoms Produced by Central Nervous System Depressants

- Ataxic gait (staggering)
- Decreased respirations
- Memory loss
- Nausea and vomiting
- Passiveness, listlessness
- Pinpoint pupils (opioid effect)
- Reduced hunger or thirst
- Reduced sexual drive
- Slurred speech
- Sense of heaviness in extremities

became popular as a safer alternative to barbiturates. Flurazepam (Dalmane) and chlordiazepoxide (Librium) were the first benzodiazepines, and diazepam (Valium) became available shortly after.

Valium soon became the most frequently prescribed antianxiety agent. The effects of addiction and overdose with benzodiazepines were not apparent at first, but by 1981 Valium dropped to the sixth most prescribed drug in the United States. In the 1990s alprazolam (Xanax) was the most frequently prescribed benzodiazepine for treatment of acute anxiety (American Society of Addiction Medicine, n.d.). Xanax is prescribed for anxiety and also is used as a drug of abuse.

Another benzodiazepine that gained notoriety in the 1990s was flunitrazepam (Rohypnol). Perpetrators of sexual assault frequently have administered this drug to victims, and people thus sometimes refer to it as a "date-rape drug." It is easy to mix it secretly into an alcoholic drink so that the victim consumes it unknowingly. Its effects include muscle relaxation and amnesia. Alcohol increases these effects; the two together are sometimes a lethal combination. Flunitrazepam is not legal for use in the United States. Klonopin (clonazepam) is a common benzodiazepine drug that is now prescribed for anxiety and recently has been seen as a drug of abuse.

Some people in the United States have abused gamma-hydroxybutyrate (GHB) for its euphoric, sedative, and body-building (anabolic) effects. Its abuse as a synthetic steroid is common at fitness centers and gyms. As with flunitrazepam, GHB has been associated with club drug use and sexual assault. Flunitrazepam and GHB are odorless, tasteless, and colorless. They are easy to mix with drinks and quickly cause unconsciousness. These drugs also rapidly cause relaxation of voluntary muscles and potentially cause the victim to have long-term amnesia for events occurring while the victim is under the influence of the drug.

OPIOID ANALGESICS

Opioid analgesics are drugs made from the opium poppy. Hippocrates praised the poppy's pain-relieving properties. During the 16th century, laudanum, an opium compound, was the most popular medication in Europe. Heroin is a widely abused drug in the United States. In 2016 about 948,000 Americans reported using heroin in the past year, with 626,000 of heroin users being dependent on the drug (National Institute on Drug Abuse, 2018). Heroin is a schedule I drug that has no medical use. People take heroin by snorting, smoking, or injecting it into a vein. Morphine and its synthetic derivatives are schedule II drugs. They can be taken orally or injected. Opioids replace natural endorphins in the CNS, which makes these drugs highly addictive. Besides being excellent pain suppressants, opioids act as cough suppressants, slow peristalsis in the gastrointestinal system, and mildly contract the bladder. Tolerance develops rapidly, but abstinence reverses tolerance. Cross-tolerance with other opioids is possible. Three general types of opioid abusers are (1) street abusers who get opioids illegally, (2) abusers of opioids from medical sources (prescription opioids), and (3) methadone abusers. Nurses often deal with people in the second group, who are predominantly middle-class older adults, health care professionals, women, and patients with chronic pain syndrome.

Symptoms of acute opioid overdose include severe respiratory depression, pinpoint pupils, and stupor or coma. Aspiration is possible. Treatment involves supporting ventilation and administering naloxone (Narcan) as prescribed. Health care providers sometimes prescribe clonidine (Catapres) to help reduce withdrawal symptoms. It is important to continue monitoring for recurrent symptoms of toxicity when naloxone is discontinued.

In addicted people who consume huge amounts of morphine and heroin, predictable withdrawal signs and symptoms typically begin approximately 6 hours after the last dose. Withdrawal symptoms include flulike signs and symptoms and body aches, watery eyes and runny nose, dilated pupils, vomiting, cramps and diarrhea, diaphoresis, tachycardia, hypertension, and chills and fever. The term "cold turkey" comes from the gooseflesh that is common during withdrawal. Intensity of signs and symptoms usually peaks in 2 to 3 days. Signs and symptoms subside within 5 to 10 days.

Methadone (Dolophine) is a synthetic opioid that helps suppress withdrawal symptoms in the morphine or heroin addict. Once the patient's condition stabilizes, the methadone dosage decreases daily until the addict is methadone free. Methadone is sometimes a drug of abuse for people formerly addicted to heroin. Success of any cessation program depends on the motivation of the user.

STIMULANTS

CNS stimulants include a wide variety of substances. The category ranges from caffeine (the most widely consumed substance in the world) to cocaine and amphetamines. Box 36.9 lists the effects of stimulants.

Caffeine

Caffeine is present in foods such as coffee, tea, chocolate, and soft drinks and in over-the-counter medications such as cold and sinus medications and appetite suppressants. It is chemically related to theophylline, which is useful in the treatment of chronic obstructive pulmonary disease. Stimulant effects of caffeine are usually mild and typically last 5 to 7 hours after consumption.

Box 36.9 Signs and Symptoms Produced by Central Nervous System Stimulants

- Anorexia
- Anxiety and paranoia
- Bronchodilation
- Bruxism (grinding of teeth)
- Delirium and hallucinations
- Diarrhea
- Dilated pupils
- Drug-induced psychosis
- Elation
- Euphoria
- Hostility and anger
- Hyperreflexia
- Hypertension
- Increased concentration
- Insomnia
- Mental alertness
- Nausea
- Peripheral vasoconstriction
- Tachycardia
- Twitching and tremors

Abrupt cessation of habitual use of five to seven cups of caffeinated beverages per day can cause withdrawal symptoms of headache, fatigue, and irritability. Caffeine potentially can aggravate anxiety disorders and schizophrenia, as well as heart conditions.

Nicotine

Nicotine is a drug present in tobacco. Tobacco use is a legally sanctioned form of substance abuse. The number of Americans who smoke is declining, but the number of female smokers and underage smokers is rising. The effects of nicotine include increased alertness and concentration, appetite suppression, and vasoconstriction. People who smoke heavily or persistently quickly develop tolerance and dependence. Smokers sometimes switch to smokeless, oral forms of tobacco (snuff or chew) to reduce hazards from smoke. People who smoke heavily and stop suddenly experience withdrawal symptoms that include craving, irritability, restlessness, impatience, hostility, anxiety, confusion, difficulty in concentration, disturbed sleep, increased appetite, and decreased heart rate. Treatment for nicotine dependence includes use of agents that deliver decreasing doses of nicotine. These agents include nicotine gum, transdermal patches, and nasal spray; agents that block the reinforcing effect of smoking; an antidepressant, bupropion (Zyban); and combinations thereof. Behavioral therapy is also often beneficial in remaining smoke free. As many as 70% of people who quit smoking experience relapse within 1 year.

Cocaine

Cocaine is a white powder that is used as a topical, local, and regional anesthetic and as a vasoconstrictor for some types of surgery of the eye, the ear, the nose, and the throat. Crack cocaine is an inexpensive form of cocaine mixed with baking soda. Freebasing is a method of smoking a drug, such as cocaine. To use powder cocaine, it is arranged into lines on a flat surface and snorted. Cocaine also can be taken intravenously. The rush occurs within 30 seconds, but the effect is very short lived. The "crash" that follows the rush consists of intense craving, agitation, and moderate to severe depression. Crack cocaine addiction occurs rapidly. The cravings have the potential to persist months into abstinence, which makes treatment difficult. The use of powder and crack cocaine became epidemic in the 1980s and 1990s.

Cocaine is a strong CNS stimulant. Chronic abuse by snorting erodes the nasal septum and often causes sinusitis and rhinitis. Smoking cocaine poses the risk of bodily injury from burns, and the caustic chemicals that people use to make it sometimes cause hemoptysis and pneumonitis. Overdose potentially produces cardiorespiratory distress and seizures. It is best to hospitalize the user to stabilize heart abnormalities and protect him or her from suicide if profound depression occurs. Health care providers have used dopaminergic drugs such as amantadine and bromocriptine (Parlodel), which assist treatment of Parkinson's disease, to reduce the craving. If psychotic symptoms do not resolve in 3 days, it is appropriate to start conventional treatment. Neonates of addicted mothers need close monitoring for complications. Swaddling or wrapping such babies snugly is often comforting; stimuli such as bright lights, loud noises, and excessive handling should be minimized.

Amphetamines

Amphetamines and their analogues (e.g., methylphenidate [Ritalin]) gained popularity as club drugs in the 1990s. Amphetamine is a powder that is snorted, smoked, or injected. People often mix it with other drugs such as heroin or marijuana. Methamphetamine is a potent, addictive amphetamine that causes powerful release of the neurotransmitter dopamine. Over time, dopamine depletion in the brain results in parkinsonian-like symptoms. Brain cell damage is sometimes permanent. CNS stimulation is so strong that hallucinations and paranoia are possible. Weight loss and malnutrition from the anorexia effect are sometimes severe. Overstimulation of the heart sometimes raises blood pressure, which potentially causes damage to blood vessels, leading to heart attack or stroke. Brain damage at the cellular level and sudden death have occurred with amphetamine use. Treatment for withdrawal corresponds to the severity of the symptoms. People who suffer from chronic abuse typically exhibit flat affect, forgetfulness, and difficulty in concentration as a result of irreversible brain damage after they complete detoxification.

HALLUCINOGENS

Hallucinogens, either natural or synthetic, affect several areas of the brain. These drugs alter perception and thinking, and some of their effects sometimes last 6 to 12 hours. Deaths have occurred as a result of altered perceptions that have the potential to trigger the fight-or-flight response, which then leads to possible cardiac arrest or dangerously altered thinking, such as the user's notion that he or she has the ability to fly.

Drugs in this group are phencyclidine (PCP); lysergic acid diethylamide (LSD); 3,4-methylenedioxy-methamphetamine (MDMA), known as Ecstasy, and its parent drug, methylenedioxyamphetamine (MDA); ketamine; mescaline; and psilocybin.

Phencyclidine

Phencyclidine (PCP) entered the street scene in the 1960s and quickly gained a reputation for causing adverse drug reactions. PCP is a powder that easily dissolves in water or alcohol; users often sprinkle it in other drugs such as marijuana. Some people take it without knowing, unaware that PCP is mixed into another street drug. Experts consider it addictive with regular use. In low to moderate doses, symptoms of generalized numbness and poor coordination occur. Flushing and sweating occur with a rise in blood pressure and pulse. Some users report feelings of increased strength and power. Overdosage of PCP sometimes becomes apparent through symptoms of schizophrenia-like psychosis with extreme violence or attempted suicide. Seizures and coma are possible. At high doses, a drop in respirations, pulse, and blood pressure accompanies loss of balance, blurred vision, nausea, and vomiting.

Lysergic Acid Diethylamide

Lysergic acid diethylamide (LSD) also entered the street scene in the 1960s. It is one of the most potent hallucinogenic drugs. Because its effects potentially last more than 12 hours, an LSD experience is referred to as a "trip." Dilation of pupils, sweating, loss of appetite, dry mouth, sleeplessness, and tremors occur. Crossover of sensory perception such as "hearing colors" and "seeing sounds" occurs. Altered perceptions such as melting walls and fear of insanity and death sometimes trigger panic attacks. Flashback of symptoms is possible, occurring suddenly within a few days or more than a year after LSD use. These flashbacks usually occur in chronic users. Risks of LSD use include flashbacks, bad "trips," lingering mental disorders such as severe depression and schizophrenia, and general impairment of mental function. LSD does not produce compulsive drug-seeking behavior, and experts consider it nonaddictive.

3,4-Methylenedioxymethamphetamine

3,4-Methylenedioxymethamphetamine (MDMA), also known as Ecstasy or Molly, has been a popular club drug since the 1980s. MDMA use is estimated to reach approximately 7% among high school seniors, and 12.9% among the 18- to 25-year-old age group in 2013 (National Institute on Drug Abuse, 2013b). It is considered a hallucinogenic stimulant that is neurotoxic, causing release of the neurotransmitter serotonin until it is depleted in the brain cells (Fig. 36.2). Because serotonin is involved with regulating mood, aggression, sex drive, sleep, and pain perception, there are many risks of lingering problems. Normal growth and development are altered in adolescents who use MDMA.

MDMA produces physical symptoms of muscle tension, bruxism (grinding of the teeth), nausea, blurred vision, chilling or sweating, and faintness. In high doses, it can trigger malignant hyperthermia, which leads to kidney and heart failure. MDMA gives the user a feeling of euphoria, like being in love. Many people with MDMA addiction use baby pacifiers to ease the teeth-grinding effect. Heat exhaustion results from physical exertion (movement eases muscle tension) and excess fluid loss. Drug effects potentially last 6 hours or longer. Users report drug craving and lasting psychological difficulties such as confusion, sleep disturbance, poor concentration, and anxiety.

MDMA's parent drug, MDA, has properties similar to those of MDMA and is related to the amphetamine

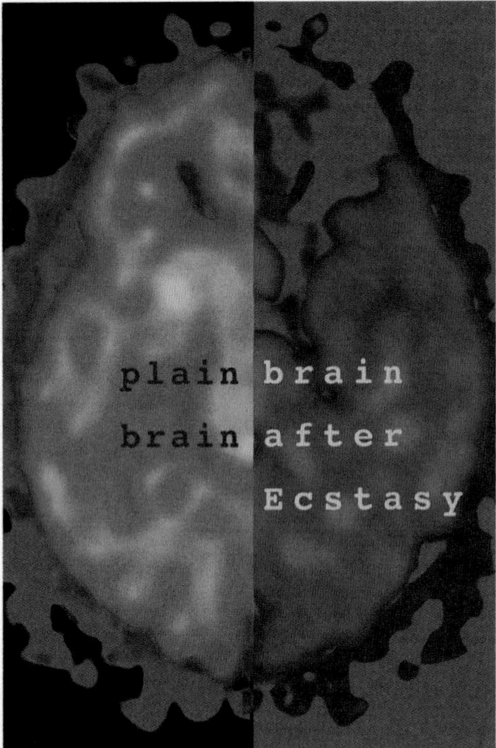

Fig. 36.2 Differences in human brain function with regard to drugs. *Left,* Scan of the brain of an individual who never used drugs; *right,* scan from an individual who had used the club drug 3,4-methylenedioxyamphetamine (MDMA or Ecstasy) many times but had not used any drugs for at least 3 weeks before having the scan. The left, bright-reddish half shows active serotonin sites in the brain. The dark sections in the right half represent serotonin sites that are not present even after 3 weeks without any drugs. In addition to these changes in serotonin sites, Ecstasy injures serotonin neurons. Although these have the capacity to regrow, they do not grow back normally, or sometimes they grow back but in the wrong location. (From National Institute on Drug Abuse, Bethesda, MD, 1999, National Institutes of Health.)

group. Lingering parkinsonian-like tremor has been reported with regular use of this drug.

Ketamine

Ketamine is an anesthetic drug that the US Food and Drug Administration has approved for human and veterinary use. Most ketamine that people sell legally in the United States is intended for veterinary use. Ketamine users either snort or inject it. It produces a dreamlike state with hallucinations. At higher doses, amnesia, impaired motor function, and delirium are possible. Sometimes it is used as a date-rape drug. Fatal respiratory problems have occurred. Emergency departments in the country's larger cities have reported increased use among youth since 2008 (American Society of Addiction Medicine, n.d.).

Mescaline and Psilocybin

Mescaline and psilocybin are naturally occurring hallucinogens. Mescaline is derived from peyote cactus. When dried, the round cactus looks like a button. Descendants of the Apache Native American tribe won the legal right to continue peyote use in their religious ceremonies. Psilocybin comes from a mushroom. Both produce the same types of hallucinations and side effects of LSD, but their effects are not as long lasting as those of LSD. Because of the general lack of availability, the abuse potentials of these drugs are low.

CANNABIS

People have used **cannabis** or marijuana for thousands of years. Its first descriptions are in Chinese writings of 2700 BC. No other drug has evoked so much controversy over the appropriateness of legalization and use for medical purposes. Marijuana remains a schedule I drug because of its high abuse and addiction potential in the absence of proven medical use. Evaluation of its therapeutic use as an analgesic, an antiemetic for chemotherapy, a tranquilizer, glaucoma medication, and an antispasmodic for multiple sclerosis has shown only fair results. Medicinal use of marijuana is legal in some states.

Marijuana and hemp are common names for the herb *Cannabis sativa.* Hashish is the concentrated resin from the plant. Delta-9-tetrahydrocannabinol (THC) is the main active ingredient present in marijuana. Users usually smoke marijuana in a cigarette (or "joint" or "nail") or in a pipe (or "bong"). Marijuana eaten in foods such as brownies produces a longer lasting effect. Physical effects are short lived, but THC potentially does accumulate in the body because of its fat solubility. THC sometimes remains in the body up to a month or longer after last use; thus tests for this illegal drug may yield positive results for a long time.

Effects of marijuana include distorted perception; difficulty in problem solving, memory, and learning; euphoria; uncontrolled laughter; increased appetite; dreamy or sleepy affect (being "stoned"); anxiety and panic attacks; dry mouth and dry eyes; increased sexual interest; loss of coordination; and increased heart rate.

Chronic abuse sometimes has long-lasting effects. Some physical effects include stuffy nose, bronchitis and asthma, lung cancer, abnormal sleeping and eating patterns, decreased testosterone and sperm count, and decreased immune function. Accidents occur because of altered perception and judgment. Some observers report craving and drug-seeking behavior. Psychological effects include panic reactions, hallucinations, and delusions from acute toxicity; organic brain syndrome; and amotivational cannabis syndrome.

Characteristics of **amotivational cannabis syndrome** are decreased goal-directed activities, abrupt mood swings, abnormal irritability and hostility, apathy, and decline of personal grooming. Depression, paranoia, and suicidal thoughts or attempts are possible. Abstinence reverses this syndrome.

Research on marijuana use among people 18 years of age and younger has shown a trend of lower achievement than in nonusers, more acceptance of deviant and delinquent behavior, poorer relationships with parents, and greater rebelliousness. Marijuana use among 12th graders has been unchanged at approximately 6% over the last 5 years. Many of those teenagers that use marijuana as seniors continue to use marijuana into adulthood. It remains the most commonly used illicit drug in the United States.

Some experts consider marijuana a gateway drug similar to alcohol. Many people who abuse other drugs have reported starting with marijuana. Each year, more people enter treatment centers for their primary addiction to marijuana. Some people report withdrawal symptoms, which suggests that physical dependence as well as psychological dependence is possible.

INHALANTS

Inhalants are volatile chemicals that have the capacity to alter thinking and emotions when people inhale them. This group includes solvents, glues, aerosols, refrigerants, and anesthetic gases. Use of inhalants during religious rites and healing ceremonies dates back to ancient Egypt. Today, inhalants are favorite drugs of abuse among young people between the ages of 14 and 17. Inhalants serve, in some cases, as gateway drugs to more dangerous drug abuse.

In the 1960s the number of reports about abuse of model airplane glue, lighter fluid, and cleaning fluids grew rapidly. The federal government banned the use of carbon tetrachloride after reports attributed a number of deaths to it and benzene. Rates of use are higher among people from minority groups, such as Mexican Americans and Native Americans. Men are more likely to abuse inhalants than are women. Users in a group setting sometimes put solvents onto a cloth or into a paper or plastic bag and pass it around; inhaling in this way is sometimes called **huffing.** Effects are short lived and include a euphoric or intoxicated feeling, auditory hallucinations, feeling weightless or floating on air, ataxia, slurred speech, wheezing, cough, photophobia, irregular heartbeat, anorexia, and nausea. High doses pose the risk of respiratory arrest and irreversible damage to the brain, kidneys, or other organs. Most fatalities have occurred with butane, adhesive solvents, and cleaning fluid solvents containing toluene and other halogenated hydrocarbons.

Some people used anesthetic gases, chloroform, and ether as anesthetics and parlor entertainment until less flammable gases gained notoriety. Nitrous oxide (laughing gas), which dentists use today, is available as a street drug and in balloons at outdoor festival activities. After inhalation, its effects last only a few minutes. "Whippets" are nitrous oxide cartridges for commercial use. Amyl nitrate and butyl nitrate ("poppers"), whose proper use is to treat heart disease, are cloth-covered ampules that a user has to break and inhale.

Most inhalants are not detected in a routine drug screen, but people who use them chronically sometimes develop organic brain disorders, general myalgia and neuritis, mood disorders, and cognitive impairment. Liver and kidney failure are possible results of chronic exposure to inhalants (Table 36.2).

CHEMICALLY IMPAIRED NURSES

An estimated 10% of nurses in the United States have a drug dependency problem. The high-stress work environment, potential for work-related injuries, and accessibility to drugs are believed to be contributing factors. In 1982 the American Nurses Association adopted a policy that recommends offering treatment to chemically impaired nurses before taking disciplinary action. Today, according to the National Council of State Boards of Nursing, 41 states have programs that offer chemically impaired nurses the option to receive treatment and rehabilitation in order to keep their license (American Nurses Association, n.d.).

Nurses are as vulnerable as the general public to substance abuse and addiction. Denial by the abuser as well as by colleagues may be intense. Many of the same indicators of substance abuse that are evident in patients appear in addicted nurses. Family history, a chronic medical condition necessitating opioid analgesics, physical signs and symptoms of use, memory loss, mood swings, and changes in work performance and work relationships sometimes point to substance abuse.

Some nurses who abuse drugs request to work night shift or assignments that facilitate access to drugs. Behaviors indicating possible use on the job include frequent trips to the bathroom, with behavioral changes noted afterward, and sudden absence from the unit. Impaired nurses become illogical and careless in performing documentation responsibilities and duties. Discrepancies in narcotics counts, patients who feel less pain relief when a particular nurse is on duty, and unusual variation in the quantity of medications dispensed to the patients on the unit are indications of drug diversion by an impaired nurse.

As addiction progresses, an impaired nurse sometimes signs out medications and reports spillage. Some impaired nurses steal drugs from patients' bedsides after supply count for the shift is done. Some nurses have stolen entire deliveries with the sign-out sheets and then claimed that it was an accounting error (Box 36.10).

Impaired nurses put their patients at risk for injury, medication error, and slower recovery. It is important for nursing colleagues to report suspect behavior. It is the duty of every nurse to uphold the standards of the profession. Most state boards of nursing accept anonymous tips. Although it is easy to ignore or cover up the problem, reporting suspicious behavior anonymously or to the supervisor will begin the healing process for an impaired nurse. Other nurses

Table 36.2 Acute Intoxication and Withdrawal of Psychoactive Substances

SIGNS AND SYMPTOMS	TREATMENT	WITHDRAWAL SYMPTOMS
Alcohol		
Behavior dependent on blood serum levels: slurred speech; ataxia; blurred vision; decreased level of consciousness; possible nausea, vomiting, and diarrhea; loss of consciousness and respiratory depression with high blood level	Maintain ventilation. Position unconscious patient lying on the side. Monitor vital signs every 30–60 min until they are stable. Check emesis and stool for occult blood. Offer fluids and small amounts of bland foods when swallowing ability is intact. Allow patient to get up as tolerated, but prevent overexertion. Give thiamine as ordered; possible to give IM or IV initially, then PO daily. Give sedative as ordered for tremor and restlessness; watch for urine retention with high dosage of chlordiazepoxide (Librium); some health care providers order naltrexone or lorazepam (Ativan). Seizure medications such as phenytoin (Dilantin) or magnesium sulfate may be given if indicated. Provide teaching of health risks. Encourage patient to seek a recovery program such as AA.	Mild to severe tremors of the hands, jaw, torso Restlessness, pacing Illogical thinking Demanding, drug craving Manipulating Diaphoresis Chain smoking Visual and auditory hallucinations Confusion If patient is unable to reorient, appears panicked, and temperature is elevated, suspect DTs.
CNS Depressants (Including Barbiturates, Benzodiazepines, Narcotics)		
Range of relaxation to sleepiness to coma; depressed vital signs; pinpoint pupils; respiratory depression	Lavage if ingestion was recent. Maintain ventilation. Position unconscious patient lying on the side. Monitor vital signs every 15–30 min until stable. Administer drugs as ordered for cardiac dysrhythmias. Barbiturate dosages must be tapered down to reduce risk of status epilepticus. Maintenance therapy can start with methadone or LAAM. Clonidine may be given for opioid withdrawal, as may naltrexone (ReVia). Provide teaching concerning health risks. Encourage patient to seek a recovery program.	Opioids: restlessness, yawning, lacrimation, diaphoresis, rhinorrhea, anorexia, abdominal cramping, body ache, tremors, gooseflesh, insomnia, drug craving, possible seizures with barbiturates, symptoms such as DTs
CNS Stimulants (Including Cocaine, Amphetamines, MDMA)		
Elevated vital sign values, cardiac dysrhythmias, flushing or pallor, agitation, paranoia, fever, convulsions, cardiac arrest	Monitor vital signs. Provide a quiet environment. Reorient patient to reality. Encourage consumption of fluids and nutrition. Give cardiac drugs as ordered; beta blockers (Inderal) and calcium channel blockers (Procardia) can be administered for dysrhythmias. Amantadine (Symmetrel) and other antiparkinsonian drugs may be given to reduce cocaine craving. Provide teaching concerning health risks. Encourage patient to seek a recovery program.	Mild withdrawal: apathy, somnolence, fatigue, irritability, depression Severe withdrawal: drug craving, "crashing," depression, paranoia, suicidal ideation, tachycardia, heart failure, malnutrition
Hallucinogens (Including LSD, PCP, Ketamine, MDMA)		
Strong psychological effects; emotional lability (laughing or crying); acute panic attacks; acute psychosis from a bad "trip"; flashback episodes	Provide a quiet supportive environment. Remind patient that experience from drug will subside when the drug is out of the body. Monitor vital signs routinely. Some health care providers order an antianxiety drug for severe anxiety or agitation. Encourage consumption of fluids. Provide teaching concerning the health risks and possible permanent damage.	No evidence of withdrawal symptoms

Table 36.2 Acute Intoxication and Withdrawal of Psychoactive Substances—cont'd

SIGNS AND SYMPTOMS	TREATMENT	WITHDRAWAL SYMPTOMS
Cannabis		
Mild anxiety to panic attacks, emotional lability, increased appetite, dilated pupils, dry mouth, dry eyes, drowsiness	Provide supportive environment. Give antianxiety medication as ordered for agitation. Provide teaching concerning health risks and amotivational cannabis syndrome.	Mild withdrawal symptoms: drug craving, irritability, anorexia, insomnia
Inhalants		
Usually short-acting effects: euphoria, intoxication	Usually chronic use impairs cardiopulmonary function and causes hepatic and renal failure. Provide teaching concerning health risks (e.g., plastic bags lead to possible suffocation death).	No withdrawal symptoms; drug craving by chronic users noted

AA, Alcoholics Anonymous; *CNS,* central nervous system; *DTs,* delirium tremens; *IM,* intramuscular (route); *IV,* intravenous (route); *LAAM,* levo-alpha-acetylmethadol; *LSD,* lysergic acid diethylamide; *MDMA,* 3,4-methylenedioxymethamphetamine; *PCP,* phencyclidine.

Box 36.10 Warning Signs of Nurse Impairment

The Texas Peer Assistance Program for Nurses lists the following behavior patterns as warning signs that a nurse is possibly impaired by chemical dependence or a mental health disorder.

ALCOHOLISM

- Blackouts (periods of temporary amnesia)
- Elaborate excuses for behavior; unkempt appearance
- Impaired motor coordination, slurred speech, flushed face, bloodshot eyes
- Increased social isolation from other people
- Irritability, mood swings
- Numerous injuries, burns, bruises, and so on, with vague explanations for same
- Smell of alcohol on breath, or excessive use of mouthwash, mints, and so forth

DRUG ADDICTION

- Consistently signing out more or larger amounts of controlled drugs than anyone else; excessive "wasting" of drugs
- Excessive discrepancies in signing and documenting procedures of controlled substances
- Frequent absence from unit; frequent use of restroom
- Increased social isolation from other people
- Increased somatic complaints that necessitate prescriptions of pain medications
- Often volunteering to medicate other nurses' patients; wearing long sleeves all the time
- Possibly working a lot of overtime; usually arriving early and staying late
- Rapid changes in mood, performance, or both
- Reports from patients that pain medication is not effective or that they did not receive medication

MENTAL HEALTH DISORDER

- Depression, lethargy, inability to focus or concentrate, apathy
- Erratic behavior or mood swings
- Inappropriate or bizarre behavior or speech
- Making many mistakes at work
- Sometimes exhibiting some of the same or similar characteristics as chemically dependent patients

From Texas Peer Assistance Program for Nurses—Texas Nurses Association. Retrieved from *www.texasnurses.org/displaycommon.cfm?an=1&subarticle nbr=103.*

should report observations objectively and keep a diary in case it becomes necessary to recall an event. When action is necessary, the supervisor or the state board of nursing contacts the peer assistance program. Sometimes investigation reveals that mental illness, rather than drug abuse, is responsible for the behavioral manifestations. Either way, people in authority will approach the nurse and ask him or her to seek treatment.

Peer assistance programs (called *diversion programs* in some states) are usually under the jurisdiction of the state board of nursing. These programs administer contract agreements requiring that the nurse undergo treatment and monitoring for a period of several years to keep his or her license in good standing. Many programs have requirements of continued attendance at Alcoholics Anonymous or Narcotics Anonymous, with random drug screening as part of the monitoring during return to work. Some job modification is necessary in some cases to reduce stress and decrease opportunity for relapse. These programs maintain confidentiality as much as possible, but it is necessary for a nurse to notify employers if he or she is in the program. It is not permitted in most states to subpoena any records the program keeps.

In 1999 the US Department of Health and Human Services established a national data bank, **Healthcare Integrity and Protection Data Bank (HIPDB).** It requires federal and state government agencies (including nursing boards and health agencies) to report all final adverse actions taken against a health care provider, supplier, or practitioner since August 1996. This provides incentive for impaired nurses to enter treatment and avoid any final action that must be reported to the HIPDB.

Finally, nurses who are suffering from addiction or another health problem that affects performance on the job must be truthful and seek help. Being proactive results in benefits to his or her own personal life and career, to the welfare of patients, and to the overall functioning of the health care setting.

Get Ready for the NCLEX® Examination!

Key Points

- Many patients who enter acute care facilities with other diagnoses also have problems of drug and alcohol abuse.
- *Substance abuse* and *drug dependency* are terms often used interchangeably in reference to addiction.
- Alcoholism is a chronic, incurable, progressive disease.
- Common traits of an addictive personality include low tolerance for stress; dependency; negative self-image; depression; and feelings of insecurity.
- The three distinct stages of dependence disease are early, middle, and late.
- Morality-based theories about alcoholism are falling from favor because of biologic findings. Changes in brain activity, hepatic enzyme deficiencies, and genetic links prove the existence of a disease process.
- Alcohol and drug use weaves its way into the multicultural society of the United States through family traditions, peer pressure, and mass media advertising.
- Chronic alcohol abuse is toxic to multiple organs and results in development of physical disorders.
- Denial and delusions are coping mechanisms common among untreated substance abusers.
- Maintaining a professional, nonjudgmental attitude when communicating about use sometimes allows the user to be honest about use.
- The goal of detoxification is to keep the patient free from complications while ridding the body of the substance.
- Safety is of primary concern during detoxification.
- Malnourishment occurs in many people who chronically abuse alcohol or drugs.
- Like illegal drugs, over-the-counter drugs and prescription drugs are abused.
- Street drugs pose a risk of severe side effects and sometimes permanent damage because there are no controls in the manufacturing of these drugs.
- Peer assistance programs are available for helping impaired nurses into recovery without taking away the privilege to practice nursing.

Additional Learning Resources

SG Go to your Study Guide for additional learning activities to help you master this chapter content.

evolve Be sure to visit the Evolve site at *http://evolve.elsevier.com/Cooper/foundationsadult/* for additional online resources.

Review Questions for the NCLEX® Examination

1. An early age at the onset of drinking alcohol is a strong risk factor for developing which disorder?
   1. Alzheimer's disease
   2. Alcohol or substance abuse
   3. Resistance to chemical dependency
   4. Immunity to alcohol

2. In all deaths related to motor vehicles and fatal intentional injuries, alcohol is involved in what percentage of them?
   1. 7%
   2. 10%
   3. 17%
   4. 38%

3. Two days after surgery, a patient is agitated and asking to be discharged home because he cannot get any rest in the hospital. Slight tremors in his hands are noted. The admission records indicate that the patient states he does not use alcohol or drugs. Which coping mechanism is this patient probably using?
   1. Denial
   2. Regression
   3. Guilt
   4. Hostility

4. A patient was found unconscious in his apartment with four empty bottles of whiskey and was brought to the hospital by his family. Upon admission, he moans out loud and is having dry heaves and diarrhea. What is the best way to maintain his airway?
   1. Elevate the head of the bed to ease breathing, and place an emesis basin on the patient's lap.
   2. Place the patient in the side-lying position until the swallowing reflex is intact.
   3. Adjust the bed to the reverse Trendelenburg position until the patient regains consciousness.
   4. Tape an oral suction catheter in place to avoid aspiration.

5. What area of the brain is affected most often by psychoactive substances and has the potential to sustain permanent damage?
   1. Brainstem
   2. Limbic system
   3. Cerebellum
   4. Corpus callosum

6. A patient with a history of alcoholism nervousness has escalated, and this evening he keeps looking over his shoulder. He shouts out, "There's a fire!" Upon entering his room, the nurse finds the patient huddled in a corner, diaphoretic and with a fearful expression. The nurse reassures him that there is no fire and assesses him, finding the following: blood pressure of 160/95, pulse rate of 132, respiration rate of 30, and temperature of 100°F. Which of these manifestations is consistent with delirium tremens? *(Select all that apply.)*
   1. Fever
   2. Abdominal cramping
   3. Nervousness
   4. Fear
   5. Disorientation

7. A 25-year-old patient entered the hospital with diagnoses of septicemia and infective endocarditis. He admits to using IV heroin regularly. For what withdrawal symptoms should the nurse monitor?
   1. Red rash similar to that of chickenpox
   2. Head cold and flulike signs and symptoms
   3. Intractable singultus
   4. Severe joint pain and back pain
8. The nurse is caring for a patient who is in the emergency department after a suspected "date rape." What benzodiazepine drug is most likely to be suspect?
   1. Diazepam (Valium)
   2. Flunitrazepam (Rohypnol)
   3. PCP
   4. LSD
9. The nurse is caring for a patient who has been using MDMA (Ecstasy). Why is this substance considered to be neurotoxic?
   1. Serotonin is depleted in the brain, which damages brain cells.
   2. Dehydration causes neurologic damage.
   3. Heart damage results from malignant hyperthermia.
   4. Inner ear damage leads to deafness.
10. Amotivational cannabis syndrome is suspected in a patient. What findings would support this diagnosis? *(Select all that apply.)*
    1. Periods of euphoria
    2. Obsession with personal hygiene
    3. Apathy
    4. Sharp increases in appetite, commonly referred to as the "munchies"
    5. Irritability
11. A nurse with a history of drug-related charges has action taken against her practitioner's license. Where is this reported?
    1. National Health and Welfare Records Department
    2. Healthcare Management Organization of the United States
    3. Federal Drug Enforcement Agency
    4. Healthcare Integrity and Protection Data Bank
12. A patient is scheduled for abdominal surgery. He tells the nurse that his uncle became addicted to narcotics after his surgery; fearing that he too could become addicted, he does not want to receive any narcotics. What is the nurse's most appropriate response?
    1. "Don't worry. You can refuse to take them."
    2. "Usually narcotics are given in the first few days after surgery; then you will be given a milder pain reliever for your pain. You will not be given narcotics long enough to become addicted."
    3. "Your fear of addiction is unfounded, but I will tell your health care provider about your concern."
    4. "I've never heard of anyone getting hooked on narcotics after surgery."
13. The nurse is ready to give the end-of-shift report to the nurse in charge of the unit for the next shift. When the oncoming nurse arrives 15 minutes late, she does not make eye contact, she smells of mints, her hands are trembling, her uniform is disheveled, and her shoes are untied. She asks no questions regarding any patients, and leaves the room when the report is completed. What should the first nurse do?
    1. Go home because the shift is completed.
    2. Call the supervisor and report observations.
    3. Stay on the unit until she is sure the oncoming nurse has no questions regarding the patients.
    4. Call the state board of nursing and report the oncoming nurse's behavior.
14. A patient has begun a substance abuse outpatient treatment program and is allowed to return to work with supervision. Which statement by the patient indicates that she is recovering from her substance abuse problem?
    1. "I wish I knew who turned me in to administration; I would like to give that nosy witch a piece of my mind!"
    2. "Just because I had a glass of wine with a meal before I came to work once or twice, I'm going to be watched like a hawk. What a pain!"
    3. "I realize that I'm going to have to regain the trust of my coworkers and administrators, but I can do that, one day at a time."
    4. "If other people took their jobs as seriously as I take mine, they wouldn't have time to rat on other people."
15. The nurse is performing a physical assessment on a patient who has a history of long-term cocaine use. Which finding is indicative of long-term cocaine use?
    1. Constricted pupils
    2. Red, irritated nostrils
    3. Conjunctival redness
    4. Muscle aches
16. A person addicted to heroin is likely to exhibit which symptoms of withdrawal? *(Select all that apply.)*
    1. Nausea and vomiting, diarrhea, and diaphoresis
    2. Tremors, insomnia, and hypotension
    3. Incoordination and unsteady gait
    4. Decreased heart rate and flushing
    5. Chills and fever
17. A patient has begun attending AA meetings. Which statement reflects the patient's understanding of the purpose of this organization?
    1. "I will attend meetings and have a support person to help me stay sober. I must not drink any alcohol again."
    2. "I'll dry out in AA, and then I can have a social drink once in a while."
    3. "AA is only for people who have reached the bottom."
    4. "If I lose my job, AA will help me find another."

18. The nurse is caring for a patient who is in the acute care unit for elective surgery. What findings during the patient's hospitalization would be consistent with alcohol withdrawal? *(Select all that apply.)*
1. Euphoria and hyperactivity
2. Depression and hypersomnia
3. Diaphoresis and nausea
4. Below normal temperature and bradycardia
5. Vomiting and tremors

19. The nurse has completed an educational program on impaired nurses. Which statements by a participant indicated the teaching was successful? *(Select all that apply.)*
1. "Impaired nurses tend to work day shift so their patients are awake and will request more pain medication."
2. "Frequent bathroom breaks with varied behavior may be an indication of an impaired nurse."
3. "Impaired nurses commit all medication errors."
4. "Patients being cared for by impaired nurses may complain of inadequate pain control."
5. "Nurses who are impaired cannot work as a nurse until they complete a recovery program."

20. The nurse is reviewing a patient's chart admitted with substance abuse. The nurse notes that the previous nurse charted that the patient has developed tolerance. Which statement by the patient would support this?
1. "When I wake up in the morning, my hands shake until I take my first drink."
2. "I used to drink 4 to 5 drinks every night but now I drink 10 to 12 drinks to feel the same way."
3. "My wife won't quit nagging me to quit drinking. I work hard and deserve the chance to relax."
4. "I think I've hit rock bottom. I need help to quit drinking."

Home Health Nursing

37

http://evolve.elsevier.com/Cooper/foundationsadult/

Objectives

1. List at least three types of home health agencies.
2. Summarize governmental financing possibilities for home health nursing.
3. Discuss new developments that are occurring in home health care, including remote electronic monitoring.
4. Relate seven steps to breaking through cultural barriers to communication.
5. List at least four services possible to provide with home health care.
6. Define skilled nursing services.
7. Describe the role of the licensed practical/vocational nurse (LPN/LVN) in the delivery of skilled nursing care.
8. Relate the nursing process to home health care practice.
9. List two sources of reimbursement for home care services.

Key Terms

accreditation (ă-crĕd-ĭ-TĀ-shŭn, p. 1161)
certification (sŭr-tĭ-fĭ-KĀ-shŭn, p. 1161)
diagnosis-related groups (DRGs) (p. 1160)
home health care (p. 1159)
Medicaid (p. 1169)
Medicare (p. 1169)
telehealth services (p. 1161)

Recently, a shift to community-based care has led to an increased number of acutely ill home care patients, which changes demands on health care providers. **Home health care** services enable individuals of all ages to remain in the comfort and security of their home while receiving health care. Family support, familiar surroundings, and participation in the care process contribute to feelings of worth and dignity. Possible services include skilled nursing, physical therapy, psychiatric therapy, pain education and management, speech and language therapy, occupational therapy, social services, intravenous therapy, nutritional support, respiratory therapy, acquisition of medical supplies and equipment, home health aide, homemaker, pet care assistance, and companion care.

Patients most often receive referrals for home health services on discharge from the hospital. However, the patient, the family, or the health care provider can request home health care at other times.

For qualified coverage by Medicare, a health maintenance organization (HMO), or various types of insurance, the patient must be "homebound," meaning unable to leave the home or needing a great deal of effort to travel for appointments to see the health care provider. The patient also has to be in need of intermittent skilled services, nursing, or therapy (Medicare.gov, n.d.).

Patients older than 65 years account for more than 82% of all home health patients, with 26% 85 years and older. Patients of all ages with various diagnoses account for the rest (Jones, et al, 2012). On discharge from a hospital or a rehabilitation center, patients who have had a stroke, chronic obstructive pulmonary disease, fractured hips with or without surgical interventions, and joint replacement procedures often are referred to home health agencies. Home health care includes wound care, ostomy assistance, setting up of oral medications, prefilling of insulin syringes, administration of injections, intravenous (IV) administration, postoperative assistance for patients who have undergone total hip and total knee replacements, and monitoring of patients with heart failure, diabetes, and hypertension (National Association for Homecare and Hospice, 2014). The frequency and length of home health visits vary depending on the services needed. The visits occur sometimes as often as twice daily and as seldom as monthly.

Health care providers are referring patients to home care more today than ever before. Advancing technology has enabled more care to be delivered in the home. Americans are living longer and thus have more health concerns that necessitate care. The length of hospital stays continues to shrink, resulting in an increasing number of patients who need nursing care on discharge from the facility.

The best approach to patient care is one of teamwork and blending of disciplines. The licensed practical/vocational nurse (LPN/LVN) is a valuable member of this important health care team. Registered nurses (RNs) are involved primarily in case management, the administration and management of agencies, and the supervision of nursing interventions. Although home care traditionally has been a part of public and community health services, its focus is now much narrower.

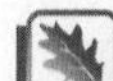
Lifespan Considerations

Older Adults

Home Care Services

- The growing number of older adults has resulted in increased need for home health care services.
- Early discharge policies have resulted in very ill older adults leaving the hospital. This increases the importance of patient teaching, early discharge planning, and appropriate referral to home health agencies by hospital staff nurses.
- Many older adults do not need total care but do need a limited amount of assistance. Home care reduces disruption of lifestyle and is more cost effective than institutional placement.
- Transfer to a hospital or nursing home even on a temporary basis increases the stress level of older people. Stress is decreased if they receive care in a familiar environment.
- Caregivers must learn the importance of preserving the older adult's autonomy and make any modifications to the home environment with consideration of the older adult's physical strengths and remaining functional abilities, not just the patient's disabilities.
- Many agencies assist older adults in their communities. The services offered by some of these agencies include Meals on Wheels, home health aides, homemakers, and home-based physical therapy services. Be familiar with home health services available in your area of service.

HOME HEALTH CARE DEFINED

Home health care preserves individual independence and integrity and keeps families together. The following are definitions of home health care as viewed from four different perspectives:

- *Official:* A component of comprehensive health care in which individuals and their families receive services in their place of residence for the purpose of promoting, maintaining, or restoring health, or of minimizing the effects of illness and disability.
- *Patient:* Skilled and compassionate care provided on a one-to-one basis in the comforting and familiar surroundings of the home. Providers base care on individual needs and personalized schedules and do so over a given period to enable adjustment, change, and learning to take place effectively.
- *Family:* A means to keep the family together as a functioning, integrated unit. The goals are learning to adapt to change, preventing dysfunctional patterns from setting in, and attaining family wellness within the scope of an individual member's illness or disability. It provides needed emotional support and linkage with the larger community support systems.
- *Provider:* Challenges all disciplines involved to provide excellent care in often less-than-excellent conditions and surroundings. Independence, creativity, communication, and excellent clinical skills are integral aspects of daily practice. It is an opportunity for nurses to demonstrate the best of their profession and themselves in cooperation with the health care team to patients and families with physical and psychological needs.

HISTORICAL OVERVIEW

A series of legislative events have facilitated the growth and expansion of home health care. In 1965 Title XVIII (known as Medicare) and Title XIX (known as Medicaid) amendments to the Social Security Act were passed, which directly affected home health care. Medicare provided direct federal funds for the health care of all citizens 65 years and older (or disabled), regardless of socioeconomic status. The companion Medicaid bill covered the care needs of the poor and indigent of all ages. When Medicare became effective in 1966, it revolutionized home care by (1) changing it to a medical rather than nursing model of practice; (2) defining and limiting the services it reimbursed; and (3) changing the payment source and even changing the reason for providing home care (see the Lifespan Considerations for older adults box).

The next major influence on home care occurred in 1983. Congress enacted the prospective payment system (PPS) as a part of the Tax Equity and Fiscal Responsibility Act for hospitals receiving Medicare reimbursement. This system, based on major diagnostic categories and **diagnosis-related groups (DRGs),** pays a set rate (according to diagnosis) for the hospitalized patient's care rather than the "cost," or charges an institution traditionally bills according to its own schedule of fees. The net effect of the change was a major shift of patients out of hospitals and into their homes, extended-care facilities, or skilled nursing facilities. Discharge for such patients occurred earlier in their convalescence; thus the patient needed more nursing care. This created a challenge to home care in terms of volume of patients seen, the need to provide more skilled nursing care over more intensive periods, and the evolution of highly technical procedures in the home. Existing agencies expanded, and new ones developed to meet the demand.

In an effort to control home health expenditures, Congress imposed new limits on home health payments through a provision of the Balanced Budget Act of 1997 (BBA) called the interim payment system (IPS). Until BBA, there were no limits on payment for covered home health services provided to qualifying patients as long as visit costs were within "reasonable" cost limits. To reduce the growth in home health, the IPS imposed lower per-visit limits and imposed a new agency-specific, aggregate per-beneficiary limit based on agencies' federal fiscal year spending in 1994 (CMS, 2018a).

The effects of IPS were more far reaching than either Congress or the Health Care Financing Administration (HCFA) intended, producing a reduction in beneficiaries served and a reduction in overall expenditures, leading to a reduction to use of home health care services in some instances. The effect on individual agencies that were unable to maintain costs within per-visit and per-beneficiary limits was devastating. Once the current prospective payment system was put into place in the year 2000, home health care use saw a rise again. According to 2016 statistics over 12,181 Medicare certified home health agencies were in operation throughout the United States. The number of beneficiaries receiving home health care services was 3,507,659, and 110,277,728 home visits were made (CMS, 2018b).

BBA provided the authority for development of a prospective payment system (PPS) for home health (HH), which went into effect in 2000. With HH PPS, Medicare pays providers of home health services at fixed predetermined rates for services and supplies to cover an episode of care during a specific 60-day period. The goal of PPS is to produce incentives for the home health provider to be more efficient in the delivery of home health services and still remain financially viable. The goal is for home health care agencies to be more cognizant of limiting excess expenditures, thus saving money paid out by Medicare. This is especially important given the concerns that have arisen the last several years about the amount of funds available through Medicare.

Home care visits and Medicare expenditures for home care quadrupled between 1980 and 1991. This was attributed directly to shorter hospitalizations, more seriously ill patients being discharged to home, and increased acceptance of the delivery of higher technological care in the home. Home health care grew five times faster than the average of other health care industries between 1990 and 1997 and accounted for more than 6% of health service jobs. The annual growth rate for home health care had been 1.7% in 2010, a 20% increase from 2002 with a slight decrease in costs. Cuts in home health care are expected over the next several years (Morse, 2017).

TYPES OF HOME CARE AGENCIES

In the broadest terms, delivery of home care services is possible by any individual, service group, organization, or agency with the desire to provide services to the older adult, disabled, or ill of any age. The type and qualifications of personnel used, the quality of services delivered, and the standards of care can vary widely, and these often depend on funding sources. The agency typically has to comply with federal, state, and local laws and regulations via the following:

- *Licensure by the state.* This gives legal permission to operate within that state only. Regulations vary widely. Not all states have such laws.
- *Certification by the state certifying body that the federal government designates.* The federal government sets the rules that govern **certification** (a process in which the government evaluates and recognizes an individual, institution, or educational program as meeting certain predetermined standards). Only certified agencies are permitted to receive Medicare payments. Many states piggyback Medicaid reimbursement to certification, as do some insurers.
- *Certificate of need:* Some states grant this according to rules and formulas that state regulators devise. Cost of starting and running the agency, availability of personnel, and need for their services generally are considered in this process.
- *Accreditation by an outside agency that evaluates and judges how well the agency meets certain standards that the accrediting organization sets.* An agency sometimes obtains this **accreditation** (a process whereby a professional association or nongovernmental agency grants recognition to a school or institution for demonstrated ability in a special area of practice or training) from organizations such as the National League for Nursing Community Health Accreditation Program, The Joint Commission, or the Community Health Accreditation Partner (CHAP). Other groups sometimes grant accreditation to special programs or specialized agencies. Some of these national accrediting agencies are seeking "deemed status" from federal regulators, which allows their accreditation also to serve as the required certification. This eliminates the need for separate surveys for some agencies.

Before Medicare, the provision of home health care was primarily the task of visiting nurse associations, nursing divisions of state or local health departments, and hospitals. Now agencies are classified according to (1) *tax status,* for profit or not for profit; (2) *location,* freestanding or institution-based; and (3) *governance,* private or public. Table 37.1 summarizes the six generally accepted types of home health agencies. The structure of some of these agencies is subject to change and variation. For example, some visiting nurse associations have reorganized and placed their home health agencies into private, nonprofit structures to ensure reimbursement that covers the cost of providing services.

Growth in number of agencies has mirrored the growth of home care. Although the late 1980s saw a decrease in agencies, the numbers rebounded, largely because of increases in hospital-based agencies and specialized agencies that provide highly technical types of care, including intravenous therapies, peripherally inserted central catheter (PICC) line care, and ventilator-dependent care services. A newer method of care delivery is **telehealth services.** This innovative approach to the provision of care allows for patient and care provider interaction and monitoring through the use of telephones, computers, televisions, and two-way

Table 37.1 Home Health Agencies

STATUS	GOVERNANCE	SOURCE OF SUPPORT	SERVICES OFFERED	NATURE OF STAFF	TIME OF SERVICE	EXAMPLE
Voluntary						
Public; nonprofit; freestanding	Community-based board of directors	Tax-deductible contributions; grants; fees from all sources	Community health; public health; home health	RN; LPN/LVN; aide; homemaker; social worker; therapists	Generally 30 min to 8 h	Visiting nurse association
Official						
Public; nonprofit; freestanding	State, county, city, or other local unit of government and volunteer board representatives of the area	State, local, or county revenues; grants; fees from limited sources; charitable contributions	Community health; public health; home health	RN; LPN/LVN; aide; homemaker; social worker; therapists	Generally 30 min to 4 h	State health departments; county health departments; city health departments
Combination						
Public; nonprofit; freestanding	Jointly operated by the two types of agencies previously mentioned under a combined board of directors	State, local, or county revenues; grants; fees from limited sources; charitable contributions	Community health; public health; home health	RN; LPN/LVN; aide; homemaker; social worker; therapists	Generally 30 min to 4 h	County-based visiting nurse association
Hospital						
Private; nonprofit or for profit; institution-based; hospital	Hospital board of directors	Fees from all sources	Home health; community health (limited)	RN; LPN/LVN; aide; social worker; therapists	Generally 30 min to 4 h	XYZ hospital home health agency
Proprietary						
Private; for profit; freestanding	Governed and owned by individual, corporation, or other organization; many paid boards of directors appointed by owner	Fees from most sources; some do and some do not participate in Medicare-Medicaid	Some offer limited home health; private duty; homemaker	RN; LPN/LVN; aide	1 to 24 h	Home health care of XYZ
Private Not for Profit						
Private; not for profit; freestanding	Governed and owned by individual, corporation, or other organizational structure; board appointed by owner	Fees from most sources; some do and some do not participate in Medicare-Medicaid	Some offer limited home health services; private duty; homemaker	RN; LPN/LVN; aide	30 min to 24 h	ABC home health agency
Other						
Private; for profit or nonprofit; institution-based	Based within formalized institution; governed by that board or designated board	Fees from all sources	Home health services; limited homemaker	RN; LPN/LVN; aide; therapists; may have homemaker; social worker	30 min to 8 h	ABC nursing home—home health agency; ABC rehabilitation facility; home care

LPN/LVN, Licensed practical/vocational nurse; *RN,* registered nurse.

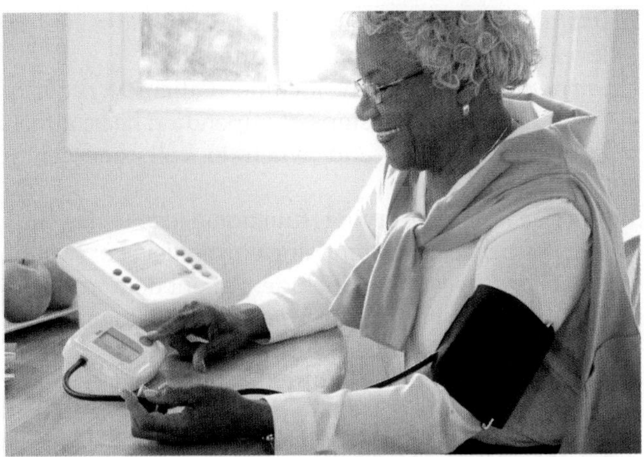

Fig. 37.1 Telehealth care. (Courtesy Philips Healthcare. Used with permission.)

monitors. The use of technology allows patient care to take place outside of the traditional inpatient setting. A computerized system can call a patient on the telephone at home and ask recorded questions such as, "What is your blood pressure?" The patient is able to respond by using the phone's keypad. In this way the nurse is able to review the patient's progress efficiently without making a home visit. Over the past several years, advances in technology and forward-thinking home health agencies have helped spur a jump in the adoption of telemonitoring for home health patients. Advantages include a return of the patient to the family unit, conservation of financial resources, family participation in care delivery, and increased care delivery options in rural settings or settings at a distance from the health care provider (Nelson and Staggers, 2014) (Fig. 37.1). For example, a patient with recently diagnosed diabetes can receive telehealth monitoring with the use of a glucometer to read blood sugar, which may be transmitted electronically to a health care provider, who then may evaluate the results for the need of additional intervention without having to visit the patient.

CHANGES IN HOME HEALTH CARE

Some recent changes have occurred in home health care, including the establishment of ethics committees to handle ethical issues that arise in the home. Another includes Medicare reimbursing psychiatric nurse clinicians for home visits. Psychiatric patients are required to be under the care of a psychiatrist and have a psychiatric diagnosis. The psychiatric nurse clinician provides therapy and education and counsels family members.

Social workers have been taking a more active role in home health care. Social workers provide assistance with a patient's emotional, financial, and household problems, thus allowing the nurse more time to perform nursing interventions.

More home health agencies are employing nurse pain specialists to assess and manage pain control in the home. They can provide education to patients and staff and provide greater benefits in relief of pain and reduce the cost of ineffective pain management.

Most agencies are obtaining a separate Medicare certification to provide hospice care. Medicare-certified hospices receive per diem payments rather than a fee for visit. This method of payment is more economical for insurers and taxpayers.

Pet care programs are a new inclusion in some areas to reduce stress for home health patients who are too ill to care for their pets. A "durable power of attorney for pet care" allows patients to make arrangements for pet care if they become hospitalized or die. Some home health agencies provide special pet services, such as transportation of pets to veterinarian appointments or in-home pet care.

One of the most rapidly growing segments in home health is home infusion therapy; an increasing number of home health agencies are offering home infusion services in an effort to compete for patient referrals. Health care facilities are eager to have home health agencies provide this service because home IV therapy complements their cost-cutting strategies. Until the 1980s patients needing infusion therapies were managed by admission to hospitals or long-term care facilities, resulting in elevated costs to patients and insurers. Antibiotics, hydration, and total parenteral nutrition (TPN) are three of the most common forms of home IV therapy, and the practitioner may order them for patients at home without prior hospital admission. The list of medications for home intravenous therapies has grown and includes analgesics, chemotherapeutic agents, hormones, and antiemetic agents.

SERVICE COMPONENTS

Most home health agencies follow the basic Medicare model of services they offer. State licensing boards and professional organizations dictate functions and scopes of practice. Primary services include the following:

- Skilled nursing
- Physical therapy
- Speech-language therapy
- Occupational therapy
- Medical social services
- Homemaker–home health aide

Other therapy services (e.g., respiratory) or professional services (e.g., nutritional counseling, pharmacy, podiatry, dentistry, and psychiatric or mental health) are sometimes offered. Provision of support services (e.g., homemaker, companion, and respite) is common but not directly reimbursable by Medicare. The service mix depends on patient diagnosis, patient and family needs, and availability of resources. The agency commonly provides medical supplies, including durable medical equipment (DME). Home medical equipment ranging from the traditional hospital bed to highly sophisticated items such as respirators and apnea monitors is possible to buy or lease from companies that specialize in equipment provision (see the Health Promotion box).

Health Promotion

Home Care

- The most common diagnoses for home care patients are diabetes mellitus, hypertension, heart and circulatory diseases, osteoarthritis, stroke, acute and chronic wounds, chronic obstructive pulmonary disease, cancer, and endocrine disorders (National Association for Homecare and Hospice, 2014).
- Commonly performed treatments in the home include administration of infusion therapy (i.e., antibiotic administration), patient-controlled analgesia for pain management, enteral feedings, parenteral nutrition, chemotherapy, hydration therapy, and psychiatric counseling and education.
- The nurse and a rehabilitation team member sometimes also provide medical equipment in the home to facilitate medical treatment and safety, such as electrical beds, wheelchairs, commodes, walkers, and other assistive devices.

Medicare and Medicaid home care services are based on the medical model of treatment and depend on the physician for entry into the formalized system. Medicare requires a plan of treatment signed by the physician that outlines all disciplines, treatment, frequency, and duration. The physician or a designated medical provider (nurse practitioner or physician assistant), working in conjunction with the physician, must provide a face-to-face visit with the patient. If the patient is to receive home care benefits beyond the original 60-day period, a recertification must be completed for each subsequent 60-day period. This recertification requires a face-to-face encounter and the medical provider and each of the primary disciplines involved to sign the plan of treatment (CMS, 2011). Third-party payers sometimes do and sometimes do not have similar requirements. This chapter explains only the primary services.

SKILLED NURSING

Currently licensed RNs provide and direct skilled nursing services. Some agencies require that nurses have a bachelor's degree in nursing, whereas others employ nurses from differing educational levels (e.g., LPN) of all types of RN programs and teach them agency policies and specific procedures. Not all nurses have the ability to be effective home health nurses. The LPN/LVN provides nursing care under the direction of the RN whose responsibility is development of the plan of care.

Service Goals

Skilled nursing services revolve around four major goals:

1. *Restorative:* Returning to a previous level of functioning as appropriate and realistic.
   Restorative goals may include: Patient able to feed self without signs of choking.
2. *Improvement:* Achieving better health and a higher level of functioning than at admission.
   Improvement goals may include: Patient verbalizes understanding of signs of impending heart attack or brain attack and when to call emergency assistance.
3. *Maintenance:* Preserving functional capacities and independence by maintaining current level of health.
   Maintenance goals may include: Patient demonstrates compliance with daily exercise routine to maintain strength and prevent further decline.
4. *Promotion:* Teaching healthy lifestyles that keep the effect of illness or disability to a minimum and prevent the recurrence of illness.
   EXAMPLE: The patient who just had a stroke
   Promotion goals may include: Patient demonstrates compliance in low-fat, low-cholesterol, low-sodium diet.

Provider Attributes

Nurses who practice in the home setting are caregivers, teachers, counselors, case managers, and advocates. Attributes of an effective home health nurse are technical proficiency and self-motivation, good organizational skills, innovation, independence in decision making, and response to problems promptly. The home care patient must be able to depend on the honesty and reliability of the assigned nurse. Positive communication skills and rapport with the patient are essential. Ongoing assessment and reinforcement of the teaching plan are crucial in caring for patients in their homes. When services are provided in the patient's home, the nurse needs to feel comfortable with the unknown and accept differences in ethnic cultures and value systems. Nurses who prefer the structure of the institutional setting and benefit from immediate direction and frequent peer support find the independence of home care practice difficult.

Those working in the home care setting must remember that they are walking into the home of the patient and family. In doing so, remember, as a guest in this home, to respect the cultural values and beliefs. At times, this may include the use of alternative or complementary medicine. Always remember to include the use of herbal remedies and alternative treatments in the assessment and to incorporate these in the plan of care if not contraindicated and if approved by the medical provider signing the plan of care.

Strong communication skills are essential for teaching, counseling, interviewing, and listening. A high energy level, cheerfulness, and a positive attitude are valuable attributes because nurses often are called on to work with patients and families who are under stress. Respect for the patient's dignity, privacy, and need for autonomy is an integral part of providing effective nursing services. Commitment to professional standards of practice, ongoing continuing education, and skills updates are important.

ROLE OF THE LPN/LVN

RNs have been the primary providers of skilled service by tradition and regulation. However, skilled service has become a growing field of practice for the LPN/LVN as agencies cope with increased staffing needs, nursing shortages, and recognition of the many contributions the LPN/LVN makes to home care.

An RN has to supervise LPN/LVNs. Although LPN/LVNs are not empowered to make detailed patient assessments or clinical judgments, their observations, reporting, documentation, teaching, and technical care capabilities are important to home care.

Provider Attributes

Personal and professional attributes described for RNs also apply to the LPN/LVN. Independent practice is not allowed, but self-direction, motivation, creativity, clinical proficiency, flexibility, compassion, empathy, and patience are essential attributes. Good communication skills—written and spoken—are necessary. The ability to work alone, follow directions, recognize important changes in condition, and assist in patient teaching is needed. Evaluation of care interventions and recommendations for alteration of the plan of care constitute a part of the role. It is important to understand and practice the concept of teamwork.

Functions

Depending on the agency, agency policies, and state practice acts, the LPN/LVN may provide the following services in the home as directed by the plan of care established:

- Bowel and bladder training
- Catheter care and teaching
- Emotional support
- Enemas for special conditions
- Finger sticks for blood glucose readings
- Injection administration
- Insertion of urinary catheter, irrigation, and observation for infections
- Monitoring of physical status (such as lung sounds, bowel sounds, pulses, edema, and weight)
- Nutrition; assessment of nutrition and hydration status; teaching about prescribed diet; administration of nasogastric, gastrostomy, and jejunostomy tube feedings, and teaching families about tube feedings
- Ostomy care and teaching
- Pain management
- Patient and family teaching (Fig. 37.2)
- Prefilling of insulin syringes
- Preventive health measures
- Respiratory care, management of oxygen therapy, mechanical ventilation, and physiotherapy
- Specimen collection
- Teaching, monitoring, or setting up medications
- Therapeutic diet teaching or reinforcement
- Tracheostomy care, including suctioning

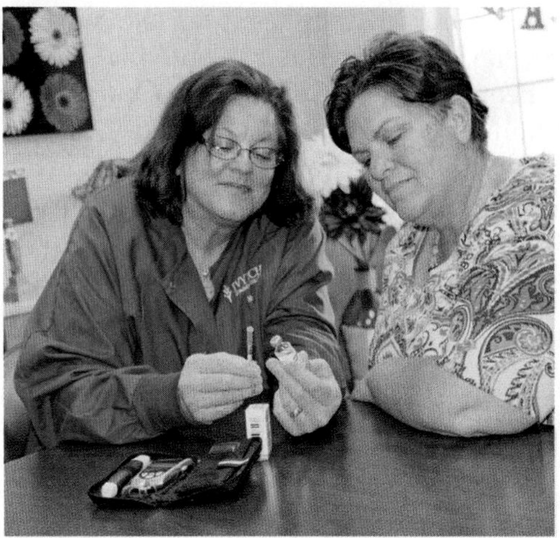

Fig. 37.2 Educating the patient in the home setting.

- Vital signs
- Wound care and sterile dressing changes

Safety Alert

Home Oxygen Use

MASK OR CANNULA

- Ensure that the straps are not too tight.
- Remove the straps two or three times a day to wash, dry, and stimulate skin.
- Pad any pressure points.
- Observe the tops of the ears for skin impairment from pressure points.

ORAL AND NASAL MUCOUS MEMBRANES

- Assess oral and nasal mucous membranes two or three times a day.
- Use water-based gel on lips and nasal mucosa.
- Provide frequent oral hygiene.
- Provide humidification via humidifier or nebulizing device.

DECREASING RISK FOR INFECTION

- Remove mask or collar and cleanse with water two or three times a day.
- Cleanse skin carefully at this time and observe for cuts, scratches, and ecchymosis.
- Change disposable equipment frequently.
- Remove secretions that are expectorated.

DECREASING RISK OF FIRE INJURIES

- Post "No Smoking" warning signs in home where they are clearly visible.
- Do not allow open flames, wool blankets, or mineral oils in the area where oxygen is in use.
- Do not allow smoking in the home.

Assistance with highly technical procedures, such as IV therapies, home dialysis, and respirator management, is occurring in home health care.

Home health care offers a new and challenging area of practice for the LPN/LVN who enjoys practicing nursing in a less restrictive environment. LPN/LVNs employed in home health agencies cite satisfaction in terms of flexibility, pay, and one-on-one relationships with patients. The need for this level of nursing practice will continue to grow. Commitment to quality of care is a common thread through skilled nursing services; the LPN/LVN has the responsibility also to pursue frequent in-service updates and continuing education to ensure current practice.

PHYSICAL THERAPY

A qualified and licensed physical therapist is required to provide services. A physical therapy assistant under the supervision of the licensed therapist is permitted to deliver limited services. The goals of treatment have to be restorative for Medicare reimbursement but in some cases are for maintenance or prevention for other payer sources. The therapist completes a detailed assessment of the patient and then determines treatment, education, and assistive devices needed for rehabilitation. These are included as a part of the physician-approved plan of treatment. Treatments range from muscle strengthening to transcutaneous nerve stimulation and ultrasound treatments, which also may aid in pain management. Patients who have orthopedic conditions, such as repair of a fractured hip or a total hip or total knee replacement, frequently receive physical therapy services in the home care setting. Other common reasons for home health physical therapy include wound care, heart failure complications, and diabetes medication teaching. The therapist actively teaches the patient and the family the rehabilitation plan to promote self-care and independence. Communication with the physician and the RN is mandatory and promotes continuity of care.

SPEECH-LANGUAGE THERAPY

For Medicare reimbursement, a master's-prepared clinician who has been certified by the American Speech and Hearing Association is required to provide speech services. Other insurers sometimes accept a practitioner prepared at the bachelor's level. Therapy goals include reducing to a minimum communication disorders and their physical, emotional, and social impact. Independent functioning and maximum rehabilitation of speech and language abilities are primary treatment goals. Often the provision of services occurs after stroke or surgery. Possible therapies range from language relearning to working with eating or swallowing disorders or teaching lip-reading to those with hearing disorders. Pathologists work closely with the patient and family for rehabilitation or adjustment to a new disability.

OCCUPATIONAL THERAPY

Occupational therapy services deal with life's practical tasks. Therapists have the opportunity to earn the occupational therapist, registered (OTR) designation if they meet the registration requirements of the National Occupational Therapy Association. The certified occupational therapy assistant is permitted to provide some services under the supervision of the OTR. On the basis of a complete evaluation of functional level, the therapist chooses and teaches therapeutic activities designed to restore functional levels. Services include the following:

1. Techniques to increase independence
2. Analysis of activities as they relate to patients' skin, their environment, their families, and their routines
3. Expanding the disease management approach into a lifestyle management approach
4. Design, fabrication, and fitting of orthotic or self-help devices
5. Assessment for vocational training

Occupational therapists assist patients to improve in their performance of activities of daily living (ADLs), and their sensory-motor, cognitive, and neuromuscular functioning. Patient-centered education is an integral part of attaining independence in self-care (Bureau of Labor Statistics, 2015).

MEDICAL SOCIAL SERVICES

Social workers prepared at the master's level provide medical social services. Workers with bachelor's degrees are permitted to provide services under the supervision of a social worker with a master's degree (Master of Social Work, MSW). Their focus is on the emotional and social aspects of illness. The patient, the family, or other support systems undergo evaluation for social, emotional, and environmental factors. The care plan includes education, counseling, payment source identification, and referrals. Coping with stress and crisis intervention are also part of social worker services. Social services in home health are generally short term.

HOMEMAKER–HOME HEALTH AIDE

Medicare refers to the homemaker–home health aide (HM-HHA) as a home health aide (HHA). These workers are an integral part of the home health care team. They provide the basic support services that sometimes enable an elderly individual, disabled adult, or dependent child to remain at home. Medicare requires that a primary skilled or therapy service (speech or physical) be provided before HHA services are arranged. Medicaid and some insurers have less stringent requirements. Many insurers do not reimburse this care. Family members and individuals are often willing to pay privately to prevent institutionalization.

Most aide services fall into one of three categories: (1) *personal care,* or assistance with bathing, oral hygiene, eating, dressing, and toileting (see the Coordinated Care box); (2) *physical assistance* with transfers, medications, and ambulation; or (3) *household chores,* or cooking, light housekeeping, shopping, and laundry. Medicare does not cover visits made solely for the third reason.

Although training of aides has long been required by Medicare, rules governing type, length, and content of preparation have been nonexistent; hence skills and standards were not uniform. Part of the Omnibus Budget Reconciliation Act of 1987 involved the formulation of

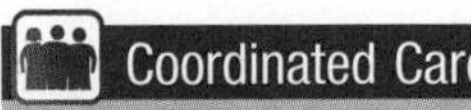

Coordinated Care

Delegation

Patient Bathing

Skills of bathing are often acceptable to delegate to unlicensed assistive personnel (UAP); however, skin and range-of-motion (ROM) assessments require the critical thinking and knowledge application unique to the nurse. As a nurse, do the following:

- Instruct the care provider as to which type of bath (complete, partial assist, tub, shower) is appropriate to the patient's diagnosis, needs, and ability.
- Remind the care provider to notify you of any skin integrity problems so that you can be sure to inspect areas of impairment or potential impairment.
- Remind the care provider to use an organized approach and reassuring tone of voice so that the patient feels safe and comfortable during bathing.
- Instruct the care provider to encourage the patient to report any concerns or discomfort during the bath.
- Instruct the care provider to encourage as much independence in the patient's self-care skills as appropriate and to provide positive feedback.

new standards for training and competency evaluation that are now in effect.

Medicare and Medicaid require on-site supervision of the aide every 2 weeks, principally by the RN. Supervision by a licensed physical therapist is acceptable if skilled nursing is not involved (US Government Publishing Office, 2011). Private payers, however, often do not have such requirements. Aide services sometimes are provided in blocks of time ranging from 1 to 2 hours for Medicare to 8 to 24 hours for private or other payment sources.

TYPICAL HOME HEALTH PROCESS

REFERRAL

The entry point to the home health care system is by referral. This comes from the patient, the family, a social service agency, the hospital, the physician, or another agency. Agencies have a variety of methods of intake for referrals, ranging from a formalized hospital discharge planning process with a central agency intake coordinator to a direct call from the patient's physician to the agency staff.

ADMISSION

The RN makes the initial evaluation and admission visit within 24 to 48 hours of the referral. In some instances, if nursing is not necessary at the start of care, the physical therapist may be the one completing this admission process. The physician often gives general orders before this visit, but agencies sometimes make an evaluation visit without orders if agency policy permits. The evaluation and admission process generally includes at least the following:

1. Complete patient evaluation, including physical and psychosocial factors
2. Environmental assessment relating specifically to safety and ability to provide services effectively in the home
3. Identification of primary functional impairments
4. Identification of the impact of the disease or disability on the patient and the family
5. Assessment of the support system of the family or the significant other
6. Determination of knowledge and adherence to treatments and medications
7. Determination of desire for care and services
8. Involvement of the patient and the family in the development of the plan of care and goals
9. Notification of the patient of rights as a patient, along with information on costs, payment sources, and billing practices
10. Explanation of the patient's right to self-determination, including information and implementation policies for advanced directives
11. Provision of initial nursing interventions (obtain an initial set of orders from the health care provider and proceed with providing the specific interventions ordered)

The admission process typically takes a minimum of 1 hour. It takes longer if the patient is disoriented or in need of nursing interventions. Some hospital-based agencies initiate an abbreviated evaluation visit while the patient is still in the hospital.

CARE PLAN

If the agency is to admit the patient, the physician must be contacted for specific orders before delivery of care. Agency staff drafts a treatment plan cooperatively with the physician. This plan describes the current physical status of the patient, medications, treatments, the disciplines needed to provide care, the frequency and the duration of services, the goals and outcomes, and the time frame for implementation. The physician is required to sign the plan of treatment, which serves as the traditional physician orders. The treatment plan is possible to alter at any time (based on patient needs) through additional written, signed orders, and it is obligatory to review and renew it on a regular schedule for Medicare and Medicaid patients. Separate care plans that are discipline specific, such as nursing and physical therapy, are possible. A separate, detailed home health aide care plan always is required.

VISITS

Skilled visits for interventions by the disciplines are conducted according to the orders in the plan of treatment and serve to meet the patient-centered goals and make progress toward identified outcomes. Skilled nursing interventions typically take 30 to 45 minutes, but duration potentially increases to several hours for complex procedures. Therapy visits range from 30 minutes to 1 hour. With increasing federal pressure to decrease home care and hospice costs, and with the current Medicare PPS, clinical efficiency is critically necessary within the industry. The current method of developing individual care plans, that is, having a home care nurse visit a patient for a predetermined number of visits per week during each episode of care, is no longer tenable. Patients who use telemonitoring are "seen" daily, thereby allowing agencies to plan home visits, not for regular patient assessment (such as vital signs), but to provide hands-on intervention or face-to-face teaching when necessary. The purpose of telehealth is not to replace nurses but to generate data that professional caregivers need to make critically important clinical decisions, which allows them to use their time and talents more effectively and efficiently (HealthIT, 2017). Aide visits average 1 to 2 hours but sometimes are longer, depending on needs and payment source. Patients receive visits as infrequently as once a month for diabetic monitoring to several times a day over a short period to provide complex care. Some patients receive only skilled nursing services, and others receive assistance from all disciplines. Greater and more frequent use of LPN/LVNs is occurring when clinically appropriate. Patients sometimes remain on the caseload for a week or years, depending on the needs of the patients.

DOCUMENTATION

Throughout the care process, concise and complete documentation is essential. This documentation may be handwritten. With increasing frequency, agencies are moving toward computerization. These systems are beneficial on many fronts. They provide the following benefits (HealthIT, 2018):

- Provide extended periods of health information
- Allow medical documentation to be accessible by varying members of the health care team
- Monitor patient compliance and care needs
- Promote quality of care

Many agencies are beginning to use various problem classification schemes linked with patient problems (Box 37.1), specific interventions, and defined patient outcomes. Documentation that follows the nursing process model provides an accurate picture of the type and the quality of care. It reflects the effectiveness of the plan of care and progress toward goals and outcomes, or it reflects the nature of and the reasons for lack of progress or deterioration and includes alternative interventions. Communications with the home care team and referral sources are also necessary to document.

Other factors also influence documentation. Staff members must recognize the record as a legal document subject to close scrutiny at any time. Professional standards, accountability, and quality of care are linked closely to legal implications and to internal evaluation purposes. Reimbursement sources have a major influence on documentation requirements by setting forth specific forms and formats that are necessary to follow. Medicare requires extensive paperwork. Private insurer requirements are generally less cumbersome.

Box 37.1 Selected Patient Problems for Home Health Care

Inability to Bathe Self, related to:
- *Decreased endurance*
- *Musculoskeletal impairment*
- *Neurologic impairment*
- *Pain*

Excessive Demand on Primary Caregiver, related to:
- *Inability to manage the care needs of the family member*
- *Inability to participate in activities away from the home*

Insufficient Knowledge, related to:
- *Cognition limitation*
- *Lack of experience*

Insufficient Nutrition, related to:
- *Economic deprivation*
- *Inability to absorb nutrients*
- *Inability to ingest or digest food*

Compromised Skin Integrity, related to:
- *Impaired circulation (pressure)*
- *Inadequate nutrition*
- *Physical immobility*
- *Radiation*

Impaired Family Processes, related to:
- *Changes in family resources*
- *Illness-necessitated role changes*

Discomfort, related to:
- *Chronic illness (e.g., rheumatoid arthritis)*
- *Terminal cancer*

Potential for Infection, related to:
- *Inadequate acquired immunity*
- *Inadequate primary or secondary defenses*
- *Malnutrition*

Social Seclusion, related to:
- *Feelings of being homebound with ill family member*
- *Limited contact with family and friends*

DISCHARGE PLANNING

Discharge planning for home care, as in hospitals, begins with admission. When patient goals or other specific criteria are met, the discharge occurs. Agencies encourage patient and family participation in discharge planning. The agency consults the physician regarding the discharge, and the physician issues the final order. Many agencies follow up on a postdischarge basis to track patient progress and elicit patient satisfaction information. The purpose of discharge planning is to promote continuity of care in the patient's home.

QUALITY ASSURANCE, ASSESSMENT, AND IMPROVEMENT

Quality assessment programs provide documentation for outside organizations and for internal measures for improvements and refinements of policies and procedures. Assessment of quality involves evaluation of all aspects of the agency operation. Quality management is the guidelines and techniques used to meet the needs of the home care clients and continuously improve (continuous quality improvement) the quality of care provided. Three major elements are included:

1. *Structural criteria:* The agency's overall organization, philosophy, policies, procedures, bylaws, personnel practices, supervision, orientation, contracts, and physical facilities.
2. *Process criteria:* Evaluation of care delivery. Authorities scrutinize the activities of the health professionals and paraprofessionals and support in the management of patient care, documentation, and patient care conferences.
3. *Outcome criteria:* Measurement of change in patient behavior, the results of patient care in terms of changes, health indicators, and satisfaction. Care standards and expected outcomes are integral parts of this area.

Those responsible for quality assessment develop specific criteria and measures in each area and evaluate them for compliance and effectiveness. Evaluation is possible to accomplish in some areas by management, and in others by a multidisciplinary committee or by groups of outside professionals and consumers.

In the past, measures of quality of the agency, the care delivered, and the staff were subjective, with little standardization and agreement. Quality assessment plans now reflect standards, objectives, and measurable outcomes and include plans for remediation or improvement as an integral part of the process. There is a move by a national accreditation body (The Joint Commission) and many businesses to redefine quality assessment activities in terms of quality improvement. The following major principles are involved:

- Quality of patient care and desired outcomes are possible to improve by assessing and improving governance, management, and clinical and support processes that affect patient outcomes.
- Processes are carried out by individuals (managers, clinicians, support) and jointly by these groups.
- Coordination and integration of processes are necessary.
- Employees of an organization are motivated and competent to carry out processes. It is appropriate to give them opportunities to improve continuously through continuing education and certification.

This move will have a direct effect on all staff members and provide a different emphasis on how many agencies will operate.

REIMBURSEMENT SOURCES

Reimbursement for home health services comes from a variety of sources, and covered services and disciplines vary. Medicare and Medicaid are primary sources of income for the majority of agencies, but reliance on these sources for reimbursement has decreased in recent years.

MEDICARE

Medicare is a federal program that requires agencies to be certified as meeting the federal conditions of participation, which set forth specific requirements for organization, staffing, training, types of services covered, and agency evaluation. Regulations further mandate eligibility requirements. Beneficiaries of services are required to be 65 years or older or disabled or have end-stage renal disease. In addition, they have to be under the care of a licensed physician. In 2011 it was mandated through the Affordable Care Act that beneficiaries of services must be seen in a face-to-face visit with a physician or nurse practitioner up to 90 days before or 30 days after the beginning of home health care for payment to occur. This face-to-face visit may be an office visit or telehealth visit (Center for Medicare Advocacy, 2016). Home care recipients also must be homebound and in need of skilled nursing or therapy services on an intermittent basis. Types of services covered and length of coverage are delineated further in guidelines developed by the Health Care Financing Administration (HCFA). Ten regional fiscal intermediaries, who act on behalf of the HCFA, receive claims for payment, process reimbursement, and determine coverage.

MEDICAID

The **Medicaid** program pays for home care services to indigent and low-income people of all ages. The state administers it, but state and federal funding subsidize it. Many states require Medicare certification for participation in the Medicaid program. Services covered vary from state to state, but most include the basic services covered by Medicare plus expansion of aide and personal care services.

THIRD PARTY

Third-party insurers pay for limited home care services. Coverage, requirements, and payment rates vary. Reimbursement often is tied to posthospitalization recoveries. A few progressive companies are paying for nursing and aide services for new mothers who return home within 24 hours of delivery.

There is wide practice of case management by or on behalf of insurance companies and worker compensation plans. A case manager (commonly a nurse or social worker) determines and arranges for a mix of home care, therapy services, counseling, supplies, and equipment for a patient. The availability of these combined, paid-for services often allows earlier discharges and provides a planned approach to rehabilitation.

A similar approach to case management for the older adult is commonly the goal of area Agencies on Aging, social service departments, community or public health agencies, independent case managers, or contracts with groups or companies that provide such services. Costs sometimes are fully paid, depending on how the service is provided.

PRIVATE PAY

Individuals sometimes also pay directly for home health services. Possible charges range from the standard full charge to scaled-down rates based on the ability of the patient to pay.

OTHER SOURCES

Health maintenance organizations (HMOs) and preferred provider organizations (PPOs) have negotiated contracts with home health agencies to provide services to their patients. Both organizations are prepaid health plans operated independently or through employer groups. Again, requirements and coverage differ.

CULTURAL CONSIDERATIONS

Nurses encounter great diversity in a variety of cultural interactions. This factor must be considered when providing nursing interventions in the hospital, the nursing home, or the community. Culture is present in the lives of patients, families, and health care providers and is especially apparent in the home environment. Frustration occurs when values conflict, thus increasing the complexity involved in nursing interventions. As a nurse, you need to anticipate potential cultural problems and identify your own and other's values. Cultural health practices are acceptable to incorporate with traditional medical care in the home environment provided it does not conflict with the prescribed treatment.

Apply all of the strategies you use to communicate with patients in general and to patients from different cultures. In addition, several other steps should be taken to ensure clear and effective communication with patients from other cultures (see the Cultural Considerations box; see Chapter 6).

 Cultural Considerations

Breaking Through Cultural Barriers to Communication

STEP 1: ASSESS YOUR ATTITUDES ABOUT PEOPLE FROM OTHER CULTURES
- Review your personal beliefs and past experiences.
- Set aside any attitudes, values, and biases that are judgmental.

STEP 2: ASSESS COMMUNICATIONS VARIABLES FROM A CULTURAL PERSPECTIVE
- Learn as much as possible about the patient's cultural customs and beliefs.
- Encourage the patient to reveal cultural interpretation of health, illness, and health care.
- Be sensitive to the uniqueness of the patient.
- Identify sources of discrepancy between the patient's and your own conceptions of health and illness.
- Communicate at the patient's level of functioning.
- Assess cultural factors that have the potential to affect your relationship with the patient and respond appropriately.

STEP 3: MODIFY COMMUNICATION TO MEET CULTURAL NEEDS
- Be attentive to signs of fear, anxiety, and confusion in the patient. Be alert for feedback that the patient does not understand the communication taking place.
- Respond in a reassuring manner in keeping with the patient's cultural orientation.
- Be alert to words the patient seems to understand and use them frequently.
- Keep messages simple and repeat them frequently.
- Avoid using medical terms and abbreviations that the patient perhaps does not understand.
- Be aware that in some cultural groups discussion with others concerning the patient possibly will cause offense and impede nursing practices.
- Use an appropriate language dictionary or chart.
- Use appropriate language translation service according to agency policy.

STEP 4: RESPECT PATIENTS AND THEIR COMMUNICATED NEEDS
- Use a kind and attentive approach to convey respect.
- Learn how people signal that they are listening in the patient's culture; then use appropriate active listening techniques.
- Adopt an attitude of flexibility, respect, and interest to help bridge barriers imposed by culture.
- Be considerate of reluctance to talk when the subject involves sexual matters; be aware that in some cultures, people do not discuss sexual matters freely with members of the opposite sex.

STEP 5: COMMUNICATE IN A NONTHREATENING MANNER
- Use a caring tone of voice and facial expression to help alleviate the patient's fears.
- Speak slowly and distinctly but not loudly.
- Conduct the interview in an unhurried manner.
- Follow acceptable social and cultural amenities.
- Ask general questions during the information-gathering stage.
- Be patient when the respondent gives information that seems unrelated to the patient's health problem.
- Develop a trusting relationship by listening carefully, allowing time, and giving the patient your full attention.
- Use gestures and pictures to help the patient understand.
- Repeat the message in different ways if necessary.

STEP 6: USE INTERPRETERS TO IMPROVE COMMUNICATION
- Ask the interpreter to translate the message, not just the individual words.
- Obtain feedback to confirm understanding.
- Use an interpreter who is culturally sensitive.
- Speak to the patient not to the interpreter.

Modified from Giger JN, Davidhizar RE: *Transcultural nursing: Assessment and intervention*, ed 5, St. Louis, 2007, Mosby.

NURSING PROCESS FOR HOME HEALTH CARE

The role of the licensed practical/vocational nurse (LPN/LVN) in the nursing process as stated is that the LPN/LVN will:

- Participate in planning care for patients based on patient needs
- Review patient's plan of care and recommend revisions as needed
- Review and follow defined prioritization for patient care
- Use clinical pathways, care maps, or care plans to guide and review patient care

Home health nursing uses the basic nursing process to assess the needs, establish a patient-centered plan of care, implement nursing actions, evaluate the effectiveness of actions, and plan for modification or resolution of identified problems. Possible interventions range from wound care to intravenous chemotherapy. Teaching sometimes involves diabetes mellitus instruction or perhaps the management of complex support equipment in the home. Teaching is always patient centered, with the primary goals being self-care and independent functioning within the confines of the illness or disability (Fig. 37.3). In the counseling role, the nurse sometimes provides emotional support to the dying patient and the family or provides skilled psychiatric interventions (if properly qualified). Case management possibly includes only supervision of the home health aide or involves the coordination of complex care plans with services, supplies, and equipment provided by many different disciplines.

ASSESSMENT

Begin assessment by considering the patient and the family members and the patient's attitude toward the family. Also assess functions of the patient and the family. These include the ability of the family to provide emotional support for the patient, the ability to cope with the current health problem or situation, ways that goals are set, and progress everyone makes toward the achievement of goals. Work within the structure of the family when providing care.

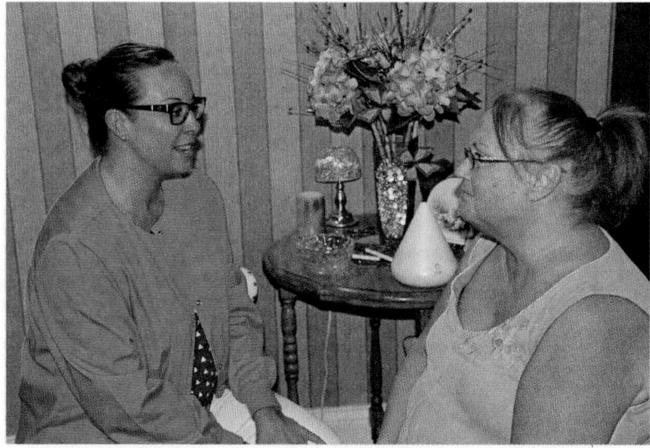

Fig. 37.3 In the home, the nurse encourages the patient to use imagery to relax and relieve pain.

PATIENT PROBLEM

The patient problem often focuses on the family's ability to cope with the illness of the family member. During times of acute illness, the family in some cases becomes extremely distressed and possibly focuses solely on the patient, neglecting the needs of other members. While caring for a patient, sometimes you will learn of such difficulties and have the opportunity to help or refer the family to other resources. Maintain a family nursing perspective. Possible patient problems related to the home health patient and family are included in Box 37.1.

EXPECTED OUTCOMES AND PLANNING

When planning nursing interventions for the patient, work with the patient and the family in setting goals. The patient and the family must understand and agree on the goals as you set them together. Also consider ways that the older adult affects family structure. The following is an example of a family-oriented goal and outcome:

Goal: The patient and family voice understanding and demonstrate effective coping with the health problems of its member.

Outcome: The patient and family are able to meet the needs of all members.

IMPLEMENTATION

After goal setting has taken place, assist the patient and family to learn health promotion practices. Providing accurate health information about the diagnosis and the prognosis helps the patient and the family members to understand the patient's experience and the best ways to be effective caregivers.

EVALUATION

Be prepared to revise a plan of care depending on the findings of the evaluation. Determine whether expected outcomes have been met. An example of a goal and evaluative measure related to the family follows:

Goal: The family voices understanding and demonstrates effective coping with the health problems of its members.

Evaluative measure: The family members are able to perform care measures correctly.

CONCLUSION

Current trends support the growth of home care as an economic, compassionate, preferred health delivery system for many types of care. Advances in medical knowledge, coupled with high-technology health care, have increased the number of individuals surviving birth traumas, prematurity, infectious diseases, acute illnesses, accidents, and other maladies that were formerly fatal.

Medical management and control rather than cure are the standard of care for many illnesses. This has increased the number of potentially debilitating chronic illnesses. Dependency and disability are more prevalent in all age groups. Home care provides the assessment and evaluation of chronic illnesses necessary to prevent acute episodes. Aides and homemakers have the capacity to provide necessary support in ADLs to enable the patient to remain in the home.

The birth rate has declined, resulting in an aging population. In the 1900s only 2% of the US population was 65 years or older. That figure was 13% (40 million people) in 2010 and is projected to reach 20% by 2030. Nearly 20% of this group falls into the categories of the poor or the near-poor. Some 80% of this group is estimated to have at least one chronic disability. The age group of older than 85 years is the fastest growing group today, with a projection of growing from 5.5 million in 2010 to possibly 19 million by 2050. About 40% of those 85 years and older need help with physical activities (Federal Interagency Forum on Aging-Related Statistics, 2012). Assistance in daily living is essential to this group. Skilled nursing and therapy offer rehabilitation and prevention of deterioration, and methods to cope with physical changes.

Federal and private insurers are trying to cap the rapidly rising cost of health care by shortening hospital stays and controlling admissions. Home care agencies are filling the gap for patients who are released early but still need complex care or rehabilitation. In many cases, home care services offer the means to prevent hospitalization by providing enteral, parenteral, intravenous, and blood transfusion services.

The movement toward deinstitutionalization of technology-dependent children and adults now is becoming feasible as Medicaid and third-party payers change reimbursement criteria. Home care support makes "family life" a reality for people who once thought of hospital personnel as parents because of their dependency on various machines for sustaining life.

Home health providers support an emphasis on healthy living and illness prevention as part of the plan of care. This one-on-one education teaches specific techniques to prevent recurrences of illness or deterioration of condition. Individuals want to be at home as long as possible. Care provided by home health agencies and support from social service agencies and others are now making this possible throughout the lifespan.

Get Ready for the NCLEX® Examination!

Key Points

- Home health care allows individuals to maintain personal control and to participate in the direction of their own care.
- Families are an important part of the success of home care services as health care workers provide care, supervision, assistance, and support in attaining the care plan goals.
- Home health care is not a new concept; however, legislative, regulatory, and current health care trends have changed the way it is provided.
- A number of different professional and paraprofessional disciplines provide home care services based on a coordinated plan of care approved by a physician. Teamwork is an essential component of the concept.
- Home health agencies are organized groups that employ or contract with professionals and paraprofessionals to provide services. Different types of agencies usually are subject to varying federal, state, and local laws and regulations.
- Skilled nursing care is the most frequently provided service. RNs and LPN/LVNs under the supervision of RNs provide direct care of different levels of complexity.
- Providers of care in the home must possess special qualities to practice effectively in this nontraditional environment.
- Home health care agencies strive to provide the highest quality of services economically. Success is evaluated through quality assurance plans.
- Home health services are reimbursed by federal, state, local, group, and private sources.
- Congress imposed new limits on home health payments through a provision of the Balanced Budget Act of 1997 (BBA) called the Interim Payment System (IPS), which later became the prospective payment system (PPS).
- Quality assessment of safe and effective care in the home is significant.
- Although some aspects of nursing interventions in the home are the same as those practiced in other health care settings, home health care nurses pay particular attention to interaction and cooperation among family members, the patient, and other members of the health care team.
- The acuity levels of patients who need care in their homes continue to rise, and the technological aspects of care, including use of mechanical equipment and invasive procedures such as intravenous therapies, are increasing in home care. These factors, when combined with shorter hospital stays, require extensive discharge planning to prepare patients and family for home health care.

Additional Learning Resources

SG Go to your Study Guide for additional learning activities to help you master this chapter content.

evolve Be sure to visit the Evolve site at *http://evolve.elsevier.com/Cooper/foundationsadult/* for additional online resources.

Review Questions for the NCLEX® Examination

1. A 79-year-old patient recently fractured her hip and had a hemiarthroplasty (bipolar) hip repair. Her daughter works during the day but provides care in the evening. Which service agency is most appropriate to provide for this patient's daily care?
   1. Private duty agency
   2. Home health care agency
   3. Nursing home facility
   4. Outpatient rehabilitation agency
2. A student nurse asks her nurse educator why there is an increased demand for home health care. Which response is the most accurate for the nurse educator?
   1. More family members want to care for their ill members at home.
   2. There is a shortage of nurses who want to work in acute hospital care settings.
   3. There is an increase in the number of older patients with chronic illnesses.
   4. There is increased technology in hospitals, which provokes anxiety in many patients.
3. The nurse is assigned to home health care for an 83-year-old patient with a stroke who has right-sided hemiplegia, difficulty swallowing, and speech impairment. He is receiving care in his home from his wife and daughter. Which should the home care nurse provide?
   1. Strict regimen and care plan
   2. Holistic, nonjudgmental philosophy
   3. Teaching plan for all family members
   4. Means of transporting the patient to his physician
4. Which is an example of an evolving future health care trend?
   1. Increased reimbursement for home health care services
   2. Keeping patients in the hospital longer because of the severity of their illnesses
   3. Increased use of telehealth
   4. Slowed growth in number of agencies involved in home care
5. A 68-year-old patient is recovering from an abdominoperineal resection with a permanent colostomy. Her physician has ordered home health care nursing on her discharge. What is the primary patient goal?
   1. The patient will be able to return to previous lifestyle.
   2. The patient will avoid dependency on medication therapy.
   3. The patient will establish self-care and independence.
   4. The patient will maintain a friendly relationship with family members.
6. The home health nurse has been assigned to provide care for a patient with cultural values that differ from the nurse's. What is the best action for the nurse to take? *(Select all that apply.)*
   1. Ask for an assignment change to allow a colleague who has cultural values more in line with those of the patient to be assigned.
   2. Accept the assignment and provide the patient with information on the values of the nurse to facilitate communication.
   3. Take time to consider the differences between the values held and those of the assigned patient.
   4. Research the culture of the assigned patient.
   5. Review past experiences with cultural dilemmas.
7. When arranging home care for a patient, from whom should the home health care nurse collect data? *(Select all that apply.)*
   1. Home care agency
   2. Patient
   3. Primary care provider
   4. Community volunteer agencies
   5. Family members as per patient wishes
8. The nurse is reviewing a patient's eligibility for home services reimbursed by Medicare. What criteria are needed to be eligible? *(Select all that apply.)*
   1. Age 60 years or older
   2. Under the care of a nurse practitioner
   3. Homebound
   4. In need of intermittent skilled nursing services
   5. In acute renal failure
9. A group of nursing students is preparing a presentation on the major diagnostic categories and diagnosis-related groups. What is the correct name for this system?
   1. Prospective payment system (PPS)
   2. Medicaid
   3. Medicare
   4. Older American Act
10. Which 1997 congressional act imposed new limits on home health payments?
    1. Social Security Administration
    2. National Institutes of Health (NIH)
    3. Balanced Budget Act (BBA)
    4. Human and Health Services (HHS)
11. What was instituted by the Health Care Financing Administration (HCFA) in 2000?
    1. A new payment system for home health agencies
    2. Medicare-certified agencies
    3. The Joint Commission
    4. Rules governing certification of home health agencies
12. What are the major nursing considerations crucial for patients in their homes and in structured facilities? *(Select all that apply.)*
    1. Immediate medical direction
    2. Nursing assessment
    3. Frequent peer support
    4. Reinforced patient teaching
    5. Individualized care

13. A patient is discussing the need for home health care services with the primary care provider. Which statement by the patient indicates the need for reinforced teaching? *(Select all that apply.)*

1. "My Medicaid will pay for a nurse to stay at my house for up to 60 days."
2. "Having home health care will let my doctor make house calls."
3. "My home health nurse can help set up my daily medications."
4. "I will be able to receive my IV medications at home instead of coming in to the hospital."
5. "The federal government pays for all of the Medicaid bills."

14. Over the past several years, technology advances have helped increase the adoption of __________ to monitor the patient's vital signs, oxygen saturation, and weight in the home by the home health agency.

15. The nurse is beginning orientation for a position in a medical practice that employs telehealth. What statement by the nurse indicates an understanding of telehealth?

1. "The patient must have a computer in the home to utilize the services."
2. "Blood glucose monitoring may be performed with telehealth services."
3. "Telehealth is more expensive than traditional health care services."
4. "Insurance rarely covers telehealth-related expenses."

Long-Term Care

38

http://evolve.elsevier.com/Cooper/foundationsadult/

Objectives

1. Describe settings of long-term care services.
2. Identify patients of long-term care services.
3. Discuss federal and state regulations related to long-term care.
4. Identify the sources of reimbursement for long-term care services.
5. Define chronic and acute health services.
6. Describe goals of long-term care health services.
7. Describe long-term care nursing services.
8. Describe services available from each type of agency: home health agency, hospice agency, adult daycare, assisted living facility, continuing care community, and long-term care facility.
9. Identify 2017 Nursing Care Center Safety Goals and strategies to meet these goals.

Key Terms

activities of daily living (ADLs) (p. 1177)
adult daycare (p. 1178)
assisted living (p. 1179)
continuing care retirement community (CCRC) (p. 1180)
functional assessment (p. 1183)
hospice (HŎS-pĭs, p. 1178)
instrumental activities of daily living (IADLs) (p. 1179)
long-term care (p. 1175)
Medicaid (p. 1182)
Medicare (p. 1182)
minimum data set (MDS) (p. 1183)
Omnibus Budget Reconciliation Act (OBRA) (p. 1182)
palliative care (p. 1178)
quality of life (p. 1175)
resident assessment instrument (RAI) (p. 1183)
residential care (p. 1179)
restorative nursing care (p. 1182)
skilled nursing care (p. 1180)
subacute unit (p. 1180)

Long-term care is defined by the US Centers for Medicare and Medicaid Services as an array of services an individual may find necessary to help in meeting various personal care needs (Medicare.gov, n.d.). Rather than medical care, most long-term care residents only require assistance with meeting their activities of daily needs. The goal of all long-term care is to keep people as independent as possible. The need for long-term care arises when an individual is not capable of meeting daily needs independently, perhaps because of physical or psychological impairment. The term *long-term care* often makes people think of older adults in a nursing home setting, but patients of all age groups may need long-term care at any given time, in various types of facilities. Long-term care encompasses a range of services, including health maintenance and care, rehabilitation, treatment of disease processes, and assistance with activities of daily living (ADLs). The need for these services may follow an acute illness such as a traumatic injury or may be for the effects of a chronic illness such as diabetes or schizophrenia.

There are various settings for and a broad spectrum of long-term care services. The types of setting and services necessary depend on the individual and unique needs of each patient. Care is aimed at providing patient-centered care and maintaining quality of life. The term **quality of life** is an individualized concept, but it generally refers to an individual's overall well-being and feeling of physical, social, and spiritual happiness. Quality of life is important in maintaining self-esteem and a sense of well-being and in experiencing the pleasures of life (Fig. 38.1). *Healthy People 2020* includes the initiative health-related quality of life (HRQoL; Healthypeople.gov, 2010). HRQoL addresses the need for physical, mental, emotional, and social well-being and the impact a person's health status has on quality of life.

Culture is a system of values, beliefs, and practices that guides a person's behavior. Culture plays a large role in shaping patients' beliefs about health and illness and therefore greatly influences health behaviors. Religion is one of the universal components of culture (see the Cultural Considerations box on religion among older adult populations). Ethnicity is a person's identification with a certain ethnic group based on shared traditions, national origin, physical characteristics, and other markers such as language, religion, food, and dress. The composition of the older adult population is changing—racial and ethnic diversity is increasing

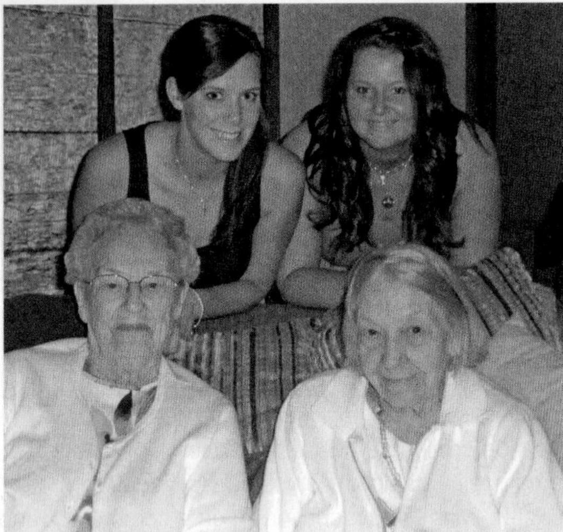

Fig. 38.1 Family is important in helping to maintain quality of life for the older adult.

(see the Cultural Considerations box on diversity in the long-term care setting). For example, as of 2017, there were 48.2 million Americans aged 65 and over and 6.4 million aged 85 and over living in the United States. Hispanics totaled approximately 8% of this older population (US Census Bureau, 2017). The 65 and older total populations is expected to double by the year 2060 with 22% being of Hispanic decent. (Administration for Community Living [ACL], 2015). Knowledge of cultural and ethnic groups is important to the ability to provide comprehensive nursing interventions.

Cultural Considerations

Religion Among Older Adult Populations

- In the long-term care facility, one goal of the interdisciplinary team is to provide opportunities for residents to participate in worship services that support their religious beliefs. Worship services to meet spiritual needs are important; visitation and support from clergy of any denomination also are encouraged.
- Nursing, social services, and the dietary department provide support through an interdisciplinary team approach.
- Dietary services take into consideration any food preferences or foods to avoid, based on the resident's culture and religion.
- The long-term care facility consistently provides opportunities to practice one's religious faith.

Historically, providers of long-term care have managed these services based on a medical model that includes expert nursing services and medical management. Patient safety in any setting has been and always will be a priority. As the patient population changes, health care in the long-term care industry will evolve to meet the needs of older adults with functional impairments related to normal changes of aging, in addition to any health disorders they experience.

Cultural Considerations

Diversity in Long-Term Care Facilities

Although residents of long-term care facilities are currently predominantly white women, residents are becoming older and ethnically more diverse. The population in the United States is expected to grow from 310 million in 2010 to 439 million in the year 2050. By 2042 the ethnicity that now makes up the minority of the population is expected to become the majority. By 2030 1 in 5 residents in the United States will be 65 years of age and older. By 2050, 42% of the population will be of older age. Between 2010 and 2050 the white elderly population is projected to decrease from 87% to 77%. The Asian elderly population will increase from 3% to 9% by 2050, and the African American elderly population will increase from 9% to 12%. By 2050 the elderly population of the American Indian and Alaskan Native will increase from 235,000 to 918,000 and the Hawaiian and other Pacific Islander elderly population will grow from 39,000 to 219,000. The largest growth of cultural diversity in this age group will be in those who are of two or more races, with an increase from 278,000 in 2010 to 1.3 million in 2050.

Data from the US Census Bureau: The older population in the United States: 2010 to 2050, 2010. Retrieved from *www.aoa.gov/Aging_Statistics/future_growth/DOCS/p25-1138.pdf.*

SETTINGS FOR LONG-TERM CARE

As the population of older adults continues to grow, so will the need for long-term care. Many changes are occurring in the long-term care system in regard to types of settings, criteria for admission, services offered, and reimbursement. Approximately 9 million Americans over the age of 65 years needed long-term care in the year 2012. By 2020 that number is estimated to increase to 12 million. Most of these individuals will be cared for in the home setting, which leaves approximately 40% who need admission to a nursing home facility. Of those admitted to the nursing home, about 10% will remain in the facility for 5 years or longer (Medicare.gov, n.d.a). Long-term care will continue to evolve over the coming years. At present, there are numerous settings for long-term care, including the home, community, and specialized facilities (Fig. 38.2).

HOME

Most older adults live in a home setting, with only a small percentage of those age 65 and older residing in an institutional setting. In 2014 only 1.4 million of the elderly population over the age of 65 in the United States lived in a long-term care setting (CDC, 2017). Ethnicity and race play a factor in which population of the elderly live at home. From 2011-2015 single-person households were comprised of mostly white American women, followed by Hispanic, African-American, Asian, and other race/ethnicity respectively (Johnson and Appold, 2017). Women being the majority of elderly living at home is not surprising since the age expectancy of women is higher than for men.

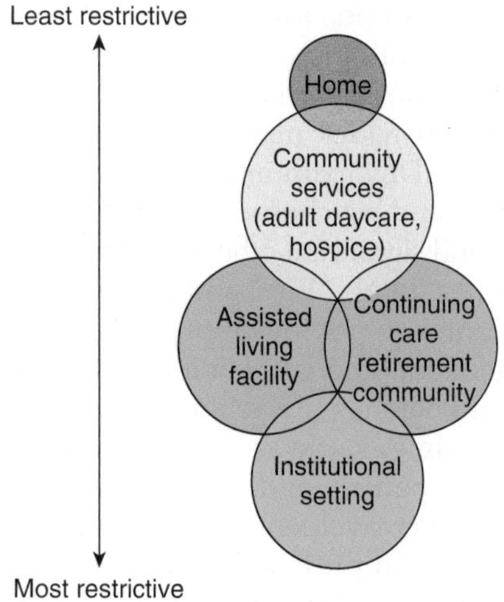

Fig. 38.2 Available settings that provide long-term care services.

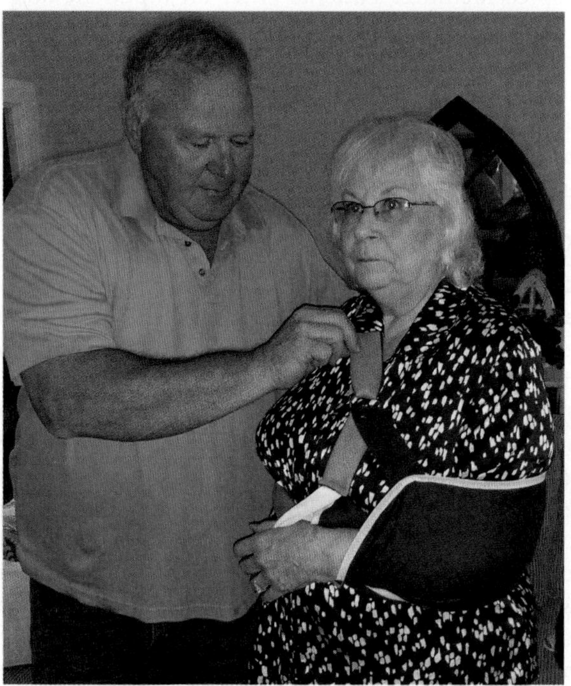

Fig. 38.3 Caring for aging parents is one of the tasks of middle adulthood. Women who care for aging parents often find their own needs and the needs of others difficult to balance.

Care of the older adult at home sometimes involves a great deal of participation from loved ones. Caregivers also may be caring for a spouse, children, grandchildren, and even great-grandchildren in a multigenerational household (Fig. 38.3). Without the support of families, there undoubtedly would be even more admissions to long-term care facilities. The cost savings to society cannot be ignored. Care for an older adult at home costs approximately half as much as care in a long-term care facility, unless the older adult has a great degree of physical impairment. Many of those who care for older adults at home rely on valuable community services to assist them (Box 38.1).

One of these services, the home health agency, strives to fulfill the needs of homebound patients for as long as possible (see Chapter 37). The increased rate of growth of the over-65 population and the increased cost of institutional long-term care continue to be driving forces in the continued progression of home health care. The needs of the home health care patient range from complex skills such as central line intravenous care or mechanical ventilation to more simple needs such as help with **activities of daily living (ADLs).** ADLs are daily routines of hygiene, dressing and grooming, toileting, eating, and ambulating each person carries out independently throughout life.

Box 38.1 Services to Support Home Care Providers for Older Adults

- *Respite care:* Scheduled stays for the older adult who needs care at a long-term care facility to give the caregiver a break from the responsibility of providing care.
- *Daycare:* A setting that provides structured age-appropriate activities during the day; frequently used by family members and caregivers who work during the day.
- *Home health care:* Includes homemakers, shoppers, respite care workers, personal care attendants, home health aides, and nursing care staff.
- *Nutrition programs:* Community programs, such as senior centers, or home delivery of one hot meal per day (Meals on Wheels); some programs are funded by the community, and others charge a small fee for services.
- *Senior centers:* Government or community-funded centers that provide recreational activities, lunch, health screening, exercise classes, educational classes, and transportation to and from the site if needed.
- *Transportation services:* Community or government funded service to grocery shopping or medical appointments. Some of these services may charge a fee.

Data from the National Institute on Aging: Long-term care: Facility-based services, n.d. Retrieved from *http://nihseniorhealth.gov/longtermcare/communitybasedservices/01.html.*

Home health agencies provide services that focus on rehabilitation with physical therapy, occupational therapy, speech therapy, respiratory therapy, access to social services, nutritional support by a registered dietitian, the rental or purchase of durable medical equipment, and nursing services. Home health agencies offer nursing services from shoppers, respite care workers, personal care attendants, certified nursing assistants (CNAs), home health aides (HHAs), licensed practical/vocational nurses (LPN/LVNs), as well as registered nurses (RNs) to provide the more complex care and education.

Medicare and Medicaid offer a program called Program of All-Inclusive Care for the Elderly (PACE), which helps people remain in their homes while still receiving necessary care. Services are offered by an interdisciplinary team in the home, community, and

PACE centers. To qualify for PACE a person must be 55 years or older, live in a service area that has a PACE organization, qualify for nursing home–level care, and be deemed safe to live at home with the help of PACE services. Payment is dependent on the patient's financial state. Some of the services include dentistry, home care, meals, adult day care, physical therapy, and medications (Medicare.gov, n.d.b).

Role of the Licensed Practical Nurse/Licensed Vocational Nurse and the Registered Nurse in the Home Care Setting

Often the role of the LPN/LVN in the home health care setting involves private duty or shift work. Responsibilities sometimes include home visits to gather data to evaluate care provided by the personal care attendants, CNAs, and HHAs. The LPN/LVN also provides a valuable human resource as staffing coordinator, intake coordinator, or medical chart auditor or reviewer. The staffing coordinator receives information from the intake coordinator describing the requested home care for the patient. The staffing coordinator, on the basis of established protocols, schedules the appropriate care provider to meet the needs of the patient and verifies financial coverage for the care. A medical chart auditor or reviewer uses knowledge of health care to fulfill the quality assurance documentation guidelines (see the Coordinated Care box).

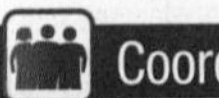
Coordinated Care

Delegation

Licensed Practical/Vocational Nurse as Staff Coordinator

An important example of delegation of care by the LPN/LVN is the role of staffing coordinator. As with any delegation, the LPN/LVN must consider the scope of practice and the individual abilities of the caregiver when scheduling and assigning care. In some states, LPN/LVNs are not authorized to delegate; only RNs have the power to delegate, by regulation.

In home health care, the RN provides intermittent visits for holistic care, supervisory home visits, comprehensive assessments, referrals, nursing interventions, health care education, health maintenance, and home management. Within the home health care agency, the RN also functions as a manager and administrator.

HOSPICE

Hospice agencies provide services to patients and families as the end of life approaches. These services are available to any age group, not just older adults. Medical certification is required for terminal care. Hospices care for terminally ill cancer patients and a growing number of patients with other chronic, life-threatening illnesses, such as end-stage heart and lung disease, and amyotrophic lateral sclerosis (ALS) (see Chapter 40).

The philosophy of the overriding value of maintaining comfort as death approaches is central to hospice care. **Palliative care** extends the principles of hospice care to a broader population that has the possibility to benefit from comfort care earlier in an illness or disease process. This agency provides nursing interventions to meet basic needs, ADLs, pain and symptom management, and spiritual and psychosocial support for the patient, the family, and significant others. Care providers include CNAs, HHAs, LPN/LVNs, and RNs for case management. Volunteers provide respite relief for caregivers and socialization and companionship for the patient. If the patient belongs to a religious community, parish nurses sometimes serve as an adjunct to hospice care to assist the patient and family with psychosocial concerns and bereavement issues. Hospice or terminal care is possible to provide in the home setting; in an inpatient hospice unit located in an institutional setting, such as a long-term care facility; and in a stand-alone hospice facilities. Patients enter an inpatient hospice unit generally for one of the following reasons: pain or symptom management, respite for the family, or terminal care. If hospice care is given in the home setting, family members or loved ones are the primary caregivers with hospice staff making regular visits while available 24 hours a day (see Chapter 40).

COMMUNITY RESOURCES

Adult Daycare

Adult daycare services are community-based programs designed to meet the needs of functionally or cognitively impaired adults through supervised health care and social and recreational activities. These structured, comprehensive programs provide a variety of services, including physical care, mental stimulation, socialization, assistance with health maintenance, and health referrals, during any part of the day, but for less than 24 hours a day (Box 38.2). These centers generally operate during regular business hours, with the patient returning home to family or caregivers at night, although some offer services during evening and weekend hours.

Adult daycare centers are designed to serve adults who need supervision, social opportunities, or assistance because of physical or cognitive impairment. The typical

Box 38.2 Typical Services Offered by Adult Daycare Centers

- Transportation
- Social services
- Meals
- Limited nursing care
- Personal care
- Counseling
- Therapeutic activities
- Rehabilitation therapies
- Crafts
- Recreational activities

Data from the National Institute on Aging: Long-term care: Facility-based services, n.d. Retrieved from *http://nihseniorhealth.gov/longtermcare/communitybasedservices/01.html.*

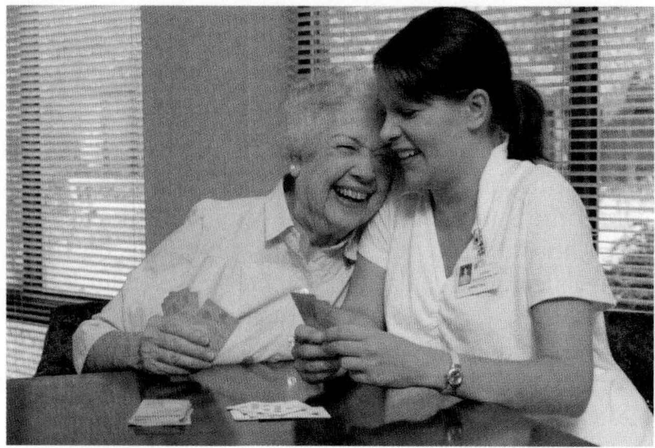

Fig. 38.4 Social interaction and acceptance are important aspects of care for the older adult.

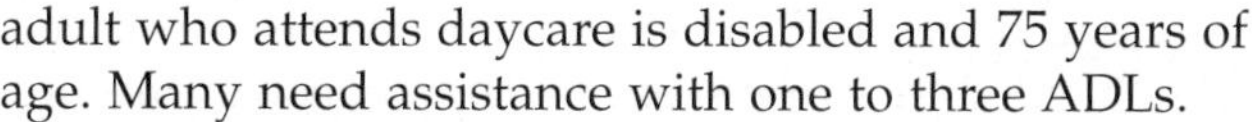

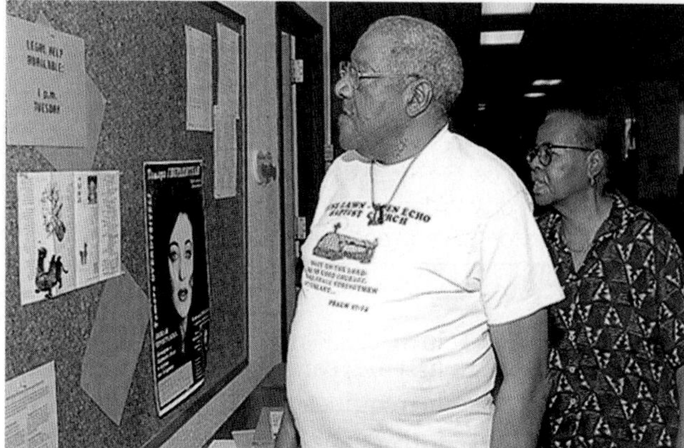

Fig. 38.5 A bulletin board at a senior center shows times when legal help is available.

adult who attends daycare is disabled and 75 years of age. Many need assistance with one to three ADLs.

Adult mental health centers and senior centers are additional places where families are able to turn for adult daycare services. These centers sometimes are located in churches or public-use areas within the community. Their staff includes a director, an activities coordinator, and a personal care attendant. The director of an adult daycare center is usually either a social worker or an RN. The activities coordinator typically has specialized training and education in activities to promote maintenance of functional abilities and independence in the environment (Fig. 38.4). The personal care attendant assists with ADLs. The CNA or personal care attendant has to meet state requirements of training in assistance with ADLs and basic observation skills.

Transportation Services

Transportation services are offered in many communities to older or disabled people. These services may be funded by the community or may be operated privately and charge a fee. Transportation is provided to and from health care–related appointments, shopping centers, grocery stores, and other community agencies.

Respite Care

Respite care is care provided to give family members or caregivers a "break" from the responsibility of care to patients who are unable to care for themselves. Respite care is available for as little as 1 hour to as much as days. The service is available in various settings, including the person's home, long-term care facilities, and respite care facilities. Respite care is reimbursed by some private and some government-sponsored insurance.

RESIDENTIAL CARE SETTINGS

Residential care settings serve the older adult population and the mentally or physically disabled person and offer a wide variety of services. Among the most popular types of residential care facilities are assisted living facilities, congregate care facilities, and continuing care retirement communities. In the following section, two of the more popular types of settings, assisted living and continuing care retirement communities, are discussed.

Assisted Living

Assisted living is a type of residential care setting in which the adult patient rents a small one-bedroom or studio-type apartment and has the option of receiving several personal care services such as bathing, dressing, and administration of medications. Assisted living services are possible to provide in freestanding residences, near or integrated with skilled nursing homes or hospitals, as components of continuing care retirement communities, or at independent housing complexes. Virtually unheard of before 1990, in 2014 there were 30,200 residential care communities in the United States according to the CDC (Caffrey, Harris-Kojetin, and Sengupta, 2015). These communities provide the availability of 1 million beds nationwide. Of the beds available, there are over 835,000 living in these facilities, with the majority being over the age of 85. (National Center for Assisted Living [NCAL], n.d.a). Approximately 60% of these residents will live in these facilities for an average of 22 months before moving to a skilled nursing facility (NCAL, n.d.b.).

Personal care services included in assisted living environments include housekeeping and laundry. The patient receives encouragement to partake in communal dining and various social activities. Some facilities offer transportation for organized recreational activity or personal business (Fig. 38.5). Nursing care varies from minimal care for patients with impairments in ADLs or **instrumental activities of daily living (IADLs)** to more complex daily tasks such as shopping and using the telephone and assistance with medications, to more complex care such as tube feeding and oxygen therapy. Some facilities even contract for outside hospice care. Key features of assisted living are listed in Box 38.3.

Staffing requirements for caregivers in assisted living facilities vary from state to state, as do regulations for the facilities. Many states have age and skill requirements

Box 38.3 Key Features of Assisted Living

- Services and supervision available 24 hours per day
- Services to meet scheduled and unscheduled needs
- Care and services provided or arranged to promote independence
- Emphasis on resident's dignity, autonomy, and choice
- Emphasis on privacy and a homelike environment

for caregivers (e.g., first aid, cardiopulmonary resuscitation [CPR]), and some require special credentialing such as CNA or HHA. Administrators are sometimes RNs or LPN/LVNs, and others are licensed long-term care administrators.

Continuing Care Retirement Communities

A **continuing care retirement community (CCRC)** offers a complete range of housing and health care accommodations, from independent living to 24-hour skilled nursing care. Usually, older adults enter a CCRC when they are in relatively good health and capable of living independently or with little assistance. In most cases, signing a contract to enter a CCRC is a lifetime commitment. CCRCs offer residents this complete range of housing and care for the rest of their lives, enabling older adults the opportunity to experience a gradual transition from independent living to continuous skilled nursing care (if needed) while remaining at the same location. For an older couple, the knowledge that they will be able to stay together is comforting, even though one of them may come to need long-term care (AARP, n.d.).

CCRCs offer apartments, townhomes, or detached dwellings, or a combination of these; they sometimes accommodate several hundred residents, although they sometimes also provide much smaller settings. Facilities range from luxurious settings with tennis courts, swimming pools, and hotel-style dining rooms to more modest facilities with similar but less plush amenities. Many CCRCs have long waiting lists for admission.

Nursing interventions for a resident in a CCRC depend on the functional abilities of the older adult. With more independent residents, a personal care attendant, CNA, or HHA can provide assistance with ADLs or IADLs. Nursing interventions are possible for residents who need skilled nursing interventions by LPN/LVNs or RNs. Some CCRCs contract with outside agencies to provide needed services, such as hospice care. Some CCRCs contract with nursing registries to provide personnel for long-term care in a resident's apartment. The reward of nursing in this setting is, again, the opportunity to care for a patient over a longer time frame.

INSTITUTIONAL SETTINGS

Subacute Unit

The **subacute unit** is a type of institutional setting that has become extremely popular since the late 1980s, when the advantage became clear of a less expensive alternative to acute care for patients with high-acuity medical and nursing intervention needs. The subacute unit is possible to view as a bridge between acute care and long-term care. Most subacute units are located in long-term care facilities, which provide **skilled nursing care;** others are former hospital units that have been reclassified to provide subacute care. Subacute units have a stronger rehabilitative focus and shorter length of stay than a long-term care facility. The level of care that subacute units provide is at nearly the same acuity as in the hospital. In fact, the typical older adult in a subacute unit today corresponds to some medical-surgical patients.

Subacute care has become necessary because of our increased lifespan as well as changes in hospital reimbursement. Modern medicine now saves lives that, before technological advances, were unable to be saved. This has led to a ripple effect. The intensive care unit (ICU) cares for patients whose condition is so critical that they formerly would not have survived. Patients whose condition is so serious that they formerly would have been cared for in the ICU are now on the medical-surgical unit. Patients who would have been on the medical-surgical units are now discharged out of the hospital, but often their conditions are too complicated for home care, hence the evolution of the subacute unit.

In the acute care setting, strict rules about length of stay and limitations in cost reimbursement limit the amount of time an adult can be hospitalized. The reimbursement rules for acute care are different from those that apply to subacute care provided in a skilled nursing facility setting. Therefore, cost savings are an important reason for the growth of subacute care.

Patients with numerous disorders make up much of the population in a subacute facility. Patients are able to receive numerous therapies, including intravenous medication administration via peripheral or central venous catheters, complex dressing changes, peritoneal dialysis, and even mechanical ventilation. Some of the most common patient care needs in subacute care are physical rehabilitation, stroke rehabilitation, wound care, and recovery from hip fracture. The nurse employed in a subacute unit needs to have a variety of assessment, rehabilitative, medical-surgical, and leadership skills. The assessment and technical skills of a medical-surgical nurse are required, along with the knowledge about reimbursement and interdisciplinary team skills of a long-term care nurse.

Long-Term Care Facility

Commonly known as a nursing home or extended-care facility, this institutional setting mostly provides services to adults, primarily older adults (older than age 65), although a person of any age can be cared for in a long-term care setting. Long-term care facilities provide 24-hour care to individuals who do not need expensive inpatient hospital services but who do not have options for care at home or by other community agencies or services. Because the long-term care facility becomes a home for the adult, on either a long-term or a short-term basis, the adult is referred to as a resident rather than a patient. As of 2015 approximately 43 million people age 65 and older live in the United States (Statista, 2018). In 2014 the number of residents of the age of 65 and older in long-term care was 1.4 million (CDC, 2017). With the projected increase in the elderly population, these numbers are expected to grow.

Most residents of long-term care facilities have more than one health disorder when they are admitted. The most common disorders on admission include cardiovascular disease, hypertension, depression, dementia, and type 2 diabetes.

It is a common misconception that most older adults live in long-term care facilities. As noted in the previously mentioned statistics the vast number of the population over the age of 65 do not live in long-term care facilities.

Although cardiovascular disorders are the most common diagnoses on admission, they are not necessarily the main reasons why an older adult enters into long-term care. Cognitive impairment, incontinence, inability to perform ADLs, and the state of being single or widowed and unable to care for oneself are also important factors that determine placement into a long-term care facility. Patients with cognitive disorders, such as Alzheimer's disease, pose a challenge to manage at home or in other less restrictive care environments because of the patient's short-term memory loss, confusion, disorientation, restlessness, wandering, and hallucinations. A major safety event, such as forgetting to turn off the stove, is often the precipitating event in long-term care facility placement. As patients with Alzheimer's disease advance in age, their ability to participate in their ADLs declines and eventually they become totally dependent on others for care. In the final stages of the disorder, they often have impaired mobility.

Two categories of residents generally are found in a long-term care facility. The first category is the short-term resident, sometimes called the short-stay resident. Typically, these residents have been transferred from an acute care facility to which they had been admitted for an acute illness or the worsening of a chronic illness. The residents are admitted principally for rehabilitation and are expected to be discharged within 6 months. These residents and the residents of a subacute unit have many similarities. The second category is the traditional type of resident who lives in the facility on a long-term basis. Such residents usually stay in the facility until they die or are transferred to an acute care facility. These residents have numerous nursing intervention needs and are sometimes cognitively impaired. Most residents in the typical long-term care facility are of the traditional category, although the trend is toward admitting more short-term residents. As a result, the

Box 38.4 Selection of a Nursing Home

CONSIDERATIONS WHEN CHOOSING A NURSING HOME

- Five-star quality rating based on health inspections, staffing, and quality measures
- Health inspections from regulatory agencies. Evaluation includes management of medications, protection of residents from physical or mental abuse, general care of the residents, environment of the facility, and storage and preparation of food
- Staffing ratios of licensed and nonlicensed personnel to residents
- Fire safety standards
- Medicare published quality measures, which include whether residents are receiving flu vaccines, weight loss statistics, and pain control measures

Data from *https://www.medicare.gov/what-medicare-covers/part-a/choose-nursing-home-step-2.html.*

overall nursing interventions of long-term care residents have become increasingly complex.

The long-term care facility industry is large and will continue to grow as the population ages, although it is changing. Fewer, but larger, long-term care facilities are found today. The greatest population growth is occurring in the older adult group, the oldest-old or frail elderly, those older than age 85. The philosophy in a long-term care facility is to maintain and restore health and functional abilities to the resident's highest level and to provide a homelike atmosphere, promoting dignity, independence, restoration, maintenance, and assistance in ADLs, and skilled nursing interventions (Box 38.4).

Long-term interdisciplinary care team. The long-term care facility is an interdisciplinary setting. In this setting, health care professionals work together as an interdisciplinary team to meet the needs of the resident. Members of the team possibly include the resident, nursing personnel (gerontologic clinical nurse specialists, RNs, LPN/LVNs, CNAs), the primary or facility health care provider, social worker, pharmacist, dietitian, activities director, and rehabilitation specialists (from the areas of physical therapy, occupational therapy, and speech therapy), and a podiatrist, psychiatrist, audiologist, and dentist. As mentioned, the long-term care industry is now challenged to provide a homelike environment and an individualized approach to residents with more complex care needs than this setting used to accommodate. The interdisciplinary care planning meetings (often called ICPs) are mandated by the Omnibus Budget Reconciliation Act (OBRA) to occur on a regular basis. The team meets regularly to review a resident's care plan, with each team member offering a unique perspective.

The goal is to have a plan of care that accurately reflects the resident's needs and goals and, as much as possible, retains life as it was at home. The care plan sometimes has many components and properly includes input from the direct care providers, CNAs, and nurses. In some states, the resident's family members or significant others, or health care power of attorney, are required to receive an invitation to attend these interdisciplinary team meetings. If CNAs are not part of the official meeting, it is up to the LPN/LVN to communicate closely with them. LPN/LVNs must make sure their viewpoints are represented, because they are usually the ones who work most closely with the older adults, performing the majority of physical care in the long-term care setting. Involvement of all categories is crucial to successful implementation of the interventions developed at the meeting.

The long-term care facility is managed by an administrator and a director of nursing (DON). The facility has nursing services, social services, dietary services, activities or recreation, rehabilitation or physical therapy, building maintenance, and housekeeping departments. These departments and the provision of care are highly regulated by state and federal agencies to ensure quality services are supplied to a potentially vulnerable population, the frail older adult.

Nursing services is the largest department, as it is in most health care facilities. The DON is an RN. Depending on the size of the facility or the number of beds, the facility sometimes has an assistant director of nursing (ADON), a staffing coordinator, and RNs as managers of nursing units and shift charge nurses. In many facilities, LPN/LVNs function in these management roles and provide direct nursing care. LPN/LVNs are sometimes facility supervisors, medical record technicians, staff development assistants, and admission coordinators because of their nursing assessment and data collection abilities. Within the nursing department, CNAs provide the largest percentage of nursing care. The CNA receives educational preparation to encourage the patient's independence within the environment, offer restorative nursing interventions, and assist with ADLs. This group of nursing care providers also learns basic observation, reporting, and recording skills to support nursing care.

A unique member of the caregiving team in the long-term care facility setting in some states is the certified medication aide or certified medication technician (CMA/CMT). This caregiver is first required to be a CNA and then has the option to complete an educational course in administration of medications. In the long-term care facility, medication administration is permitted by the RN, the LPN/LVN, and the CMA/CMT. The CMA/CMT works under the guidance of the licensed nurse and is prohibited from administering certain type of medications. In regard to medication administration, the difference between long-term care and acute care is the vast number of patients to whom the medication administration person sometimes administers medications. In some states, this ratio is as high as one medication administration person to 60 residents; in long-term care, there is a 2-hour window for legal administration of medications (1 hour before the scheduled time to 1 hour after), although the individual facility's policy is important to check. Restorative nursing assistants are CNAs who have completed an educational program that focuses on **restorative nursing care,** or basic concepts of physical therapy for maintenance of functional mobility and physical activity.

Legal, Ethical, and Financial Issues

Legal and ethical issues among long-term care agencies are similar, but subtle differences exist depending on the provider setting. Most providers are subject to regulation by federal and state guidelines or use them as minimal standards for health care services, reimbursement, or quality indicators. The **Omnibus Budget Reconciliation Act (OBRA)** of 1987, also known as the nursing home reform legislation, was a landmark law that affected long-term care facilities. OBRA defines requirements for the quality of care given to residents and covers many aspects of institutional life, including nutrition, staffing, qualifications required of personnel, and many others.

Some of the positive outcomes of OBRA include empowerment of residents, focus on residents' rights, reduction or elimination of physical restraint use, and improved staffing, although many nurses believe that staffing continues to need greater improvement in many facilities. The enactment of OBRA led to the requirement for long-term care facilities to use greater numbers of licensed nursing staff, which led to greater opportunities for employment for the LPN/LVN. Other aspects of the OBRA law helped expand the role of the LPN/LVN to include areas such as intravenous therapy and team leading.

The Health Care Financing Administration (HCFA) administers and monitors the OBRA guidelines through institutional surveys. Surveyors are required by law to visit the long-term care facility unannounced (on an annual basis and as needed) to assess the quality of life for the residents by assessing each department and its services, the physical layout of the facility, and records. The HCFA makes available the information it obtains about quality of long-term care facilities to beneficiaries, providers, researchers, and state surveyors. The Patient Protection and Affordable Care Act is the newest legislation implemented for the protection of the elderly population. It was passed in 2013 (Box 38.5).

The long-term care facility is able to receive **Medicare** (a federally funded national health insurance program in the United States for people older than age 65) funding by adhering to the HCFA guidelines for reimbursement. **Medicaid** (a federally funded, state-operated program of medical assistance to people with low incomes), financial assistance provided to anyone who qualifies, is a large source of revenue for the long-term care facility. More recently, individuals have invested in long-term

Box 38.5 Patient Protection and Affordable Care Act

The Patient Protection and Affordable Care Act (PPACA) is the first comprehensive law in a generation to improve the care and safety of the elderly and people with disabilities in nursing homes and other long-term care settings. When they were fully implemented in 2013, its Nursing Home Transparency and Elder Justice provisions in the law provided:

- Information to guide families in one of the most difficult decisions they ever make: the choice of a nursing home to care for a loved one. The PPACA expands information about the quality of individual nursing homes on the Medicare website, Nursing Home Compare; helps consumers avoid homes that provide poor care; and creates incentives for Medicare and Medicaid providers to improve staffing, services, and safety in their facilities.
- Public disclosure of nursing home owners and operators that allows government regulators, and consumers, to identify who is responsible for care in facilities.
- More accountability in individual facilities and better oversight of corporations that operate nursing homes in multiple states.
- A stronger consumer complaint system.
- Disincentives for nursing homes to delay compliance by filing meritless appeals.
- Adequate notification and appropriate relocation of residents when facilities decide to close.
- Training of nursing assistants in the care of people with dementia and in prevention of abuse.
- Better training for long-term care ombudsmen and state inspectors.
- A program to support national criminal background checks on people who work with vulnerable adults who receive long-term care in institutions or in their own homes.
- Mandatory reporting of the abuse, neglect, or exploitation of anyone in a long-term care facility that receives federal funds.
- Better coordination among agencies that prevent, investigate, and prosecute neglect, exploitation, and abuse of the elderly.

care insurance in anticipation of the possibly of needing these services as they age. Private pay is another method of payment for care in a long-term care facility. Unfortunately, private pay often results in older adults spending all of their assets in a short time. The resident sometimes then qualifies for Medicaid to cover the continued costs of living in a long-term care facility.

Long-term care facilities, like all other health care providers, come under the regulation of the Occupational Safety and Health Administration (OSHA). The inclusion of long-term care facilities in the OSHA guidelines significantly increases the cost of care in this setting but ensures a safe environment for the personnel, which is mandatory today.

Box 38.6 Other Ethical Issues Related to Long-Term Care

- Adherence to a patient's bill of rights
- Advance directives
- Do-not-resuscitate (DNR) orders
- Guardianship
- Power of attorney
- Responsible party designation

Resident rights are a universal priority in all long-term care settings (Box 38.6). Residents and staff of each agency receive communications about setting-specific interpretations as a part of orientation for the personnel and orientation to the services for the recipient of health care services. Advance directives are imperative and valuable in the long-term care facility. Do-not-resuscitate (DNR) orders from the physician are always the result of discussion with the resident, family, and significant others, and documentation by the physician is required. These directions help promote dignity in the last stages of life.

Power of attorney, guardianship, and responsible party designation are all varying degrees of decision-making mechanisms for the resident. The legal system is the route to establish power of attorney and guardianship, and documentation (legal papers) in the resident's chart is necessary. A responsible party is a person the patient designates, not necessarily with legal formality, to take care of financial and business affairs.

Functional assessment and documentation. Several different types of nursing are present in the long-term care setting: team nursing, functional nursing, total resident care, or a combination of these. The goal remains the same—that is, to provide nursing interventions to a special population over a long period, based on individual assessment and fulfillment of the resident's wishes and needs at this time in life.

The interdisciplinary **functional assessment** of the resident is the cornerstone of clinical practice in this setting. OBRA prescribed the method of resident assessment and care plan development in an instrument known as the **resident assessment instrument (RAI).** The LPN/LVN is permitted to complete this assessment tool under the direction of the RN, but it must be signed by the RN. The RAI consists of three parts: the **minimum data set (MDS),** the resident assessment protocols (RAPs), and the utilization guidelines. The MDS provides a system for assessment of each resident's functional, medical, mental, and psychosocial status on admission to a facility and at regular intervals thereafter. It is an assessment instrument that consists of more than 400 items that usually help identify a resident's problems, strengths, needs, and preferences so that a resident's function can be maintained or enhanced.

After the nurse completes the MDS on a resident, responses to specific items trigger further assessment with the RAPs. RAPs are assessment guides that address common clinical problems, such as delirium, falls, and urinary incontinence. RAPs have accompanying utilization guidelines, the third component. These contain a wealth of clinical information to assist in assessment and care planning. The functional status of the resident is the ability to perform normal, expected, or required activities. In reference to the older adult, it is the capacity to perform self-care activities (ADLs), and the more complex personal, household, and social activities (IADLs) necessary for independent living. The MDS incorporates many of the same assessment factors as a functional assessment tool and requires input from nursing and social services within a specified time frame. The comprehensive assessment provided by the RAI is intended to lead to improved care planning and provision of care for long-term care facility residents.

In this setting, documentation of the resident's condition is different from that in the acute care setting. A summary, including vital signs and weights, is required only monthly. The exception to this charting is a condition change, acute illness, or incident reporting, which is necessary to document at or soon after the time of occurrence.

SAFETY ISSUES IN THE LONG-TERM CARE SETTING

To aid in meeting the safety needs of residents in the long-term care setting, The Joint Commission has established national patient safety goals (TJC, 2017). In addition, The Joint Commission has also provided suggestions on strategies to meet these goals. The five major patient safety goals are:

- Identify residents correctly
- Use medicine safely
- Prevent infection
- Prevent residents from falling
- Prevent pressure injuries

Strategies to meet each of these goals can be found in Box 38.7. Chapter 10 addresses all other safety concerns of patients and residents in health care facilities, including the long-term care setting.

Box 38.7 2017 TJC Nursing Care Center National Patient Safety Goals

SAFETY GOAL	STRATEGY TO MEET GOAL
Identify residents correctly	Use a minimum of two identifiers for patients or residents. Suggestions are name and date of birth.
Use medicines safely	Use caution with patients or residents on anticoagulants. Upon admission ensure a current medication list is obtained. Follow policy to confirm correct medications are administered.
Prevent infection	Use good hand hygiene at all times to prevent the spread of infection among patients or residents. Follow policy to prevent infection in the blood during care of central lines. Care for catheters and provide urinary system hygiene care according to facility policy.
Prevent residents from falling	Determine which patients or residents are at risk for falls. Institute fall protocol for these patients or residents according to facility policy.
Prevent bed sores	Perform skin assessments to identify patients or residents at risk for impaired skin integrity. Institute measures to prevent skin breakdown in these patients or residents according to facility policy.

Data from The Joint Commission: 2017 Nursing Care Center National Patient Safety Goals, 2016. Retrieved from *https://www.jointcommission.org/ncc_2017_npsgs/*.

NURSING PROCESS

The role of the licensed practical nurse/licensed vocational nurse (LPN/LVN) in the nursing process as stated is that the LPN/LVN will:

- Participate in planning care for patients based on patient needs
- Review patient's plan of care and recommend revisions as needed
- Review and follow defined prioritization for patient care
- Use clinical pathways, care maps, or care plans to guide and review patient care

The nursing process is used in long-term care on admission to the facility and is an ongoing process.

ASSESSMENT

The assessment of a long-term care resident occurs on admission and is an ongoing process for collection of data and information to meet a resident's needs. Communication with the resident, significant other, or family member is essential for complete data collection. The nursing assessment includes a health history, medication history (including herbal products and nutritional supplements) and current medication usage, a functional assessment related to ADLs, personal preferences (e.g., routines, likes and dislikes, hobbies), a physical assessment to document baseline information, and a mental status assessment. The MDS and nursing admission forms document a great deal of this information. In long-term care, the interdisciplinary team reviews the resident's plan of care every 90 days for resolution of problems or revision of goals and interventions.

Safety Alert

Herbal Products and Nutritional Supplements

When eliciting a medication history and current medication usage patterns, ask about the use of herbs and nutritional supplements. These products, which are marketed as "safe" and "natural," are unregulated by the US Food and Drug Administration (FDA) and potentially have actions and side effects similar to medications. They also have the potential to interact with medications the health care provider prescribes for the resident and in some cases affect medical conditions (either beneficially or detrimentally). Take a complete history of vitamin and mineral usage (and look at the label on the bottle if available); some multivitamin and multimineral products actually contain multiple herbs as well. Residents sometimes are unaware that they are consuming herbal products.

◆ PATIENT PROBLEM

The nurse and the team identify patient problems from the assessment. Prioritize risk patient problems for the long-term care resident according to that individual's needs. Possible selections are available in the following list of patient problems (which is not all inclusive):

- *Anxiousness, related to financial difficulties*
- *Complex Grief, related to multiple losses*
- *Compromised Physical Mobility, related to abnormal gait*
- *Functional Ability to Control Urination, related to decreased bladder capacity*
- *Impaired Cognitive Thinking, related to cognitive impairment*
- *Inability to Bathe Self, related to musculoskeletal weakness*
- *Inability to Clear Airway, related to chronic respiratory conditions and musculoskeletal weakness*
- *Inefficient Oxygenation, related to chronic respiratory conditions*
- *Insufficient Cardiac Output, related to cardiovascular disease*
- *Insufficient Nutrition, related to decreased appetite and cognitive impairment*
- *Potential for Aspiration Into Airway, related to impaired swallowing, ill-fitting dentures, musculoskeletal weakness, and medical conditions such as stroke*
- *Potential for Compromised Skin Integrity, related to malnutrition*
- *Potential for Inadequate Fluid Volume, related to altered thirst mechanism*
- *Potential for Injury, related to forgetfulness, impaired balance*
- *Prolonged Confusion, related to cognitive impairment*
- *Prolonged Low Self-Esteem, related to physical impairment*
- *Social Seclusion, related to homebound status*

◆ EXPECTED OUTCOMES AND PLANNING

The planning process must be patient centered and individualized to meet the needs of the patient. Priorities begin with consideration of meeting basic physiologic needs (airway, breathing, and circulation) and go on to consider the patient's multiple conditions or needs. Emotional and psychosocial needs of the patient are also necessary to consider and include in the plan of care.

Properly formulated, the expected outcomes reflect the input of the patient, significant others, and the interdisciplinary team. Expected outcomes have to be measurable, be specific to the patient problem, and include a time element. Examples are as follows:

Expected outcome 1: Patient will have respirations of 16 to 20 breaths per minute during the next 90 days.

Expected outcome 2: Patient will have pulse rate between 60 and 100 beats per minute during the next 90 days.

Expected outcome 3: Patient will verbalize two positive attributes about his or her appearance within 2 days.

◆ IMPLEMENTATION

Nursing interventions basic to long-term care include making rounds and monitoring for resident safety *every* 2 hours. The interpretation of this includes seeing the resident, changing the resident's position, assessing for incontinence, providing skin care, and offering fluids. For example, the LPN/LVN or RN has the responsibility of assessing and intervening to support progress toward the first patient-centered expected outcome in the previous section with the following interventions. Assess the resident for the following:

- Respiratory rate, noisy respirations, signs of suprasternal or intercostal retractions, or nasal flaring
- Color of skin, lips, mucous membranes, and nail beds; cyanosis
- Adventitious lung sounds: describe character and phase of the respiratory cycle (inspiration or expiration) when they occur
- Oxygen administration: note the method of oxygen delivery (nasal cannula versus mask); verify flow rate with physician order; post a "No Smoking" sign on room door; secure the tank for safety; assess tubing or mask for proper fit on resident's face; assess skin for impairment; maintain tubing off the floor
- Offer a sip of water cautiously to assess resident's ability to swallow fluids
- Assess for cough, sputum characteristics, and ability to expectorate
- Elevate the head of the bed to 30 degrees or greater
- Offer periods of rest between activities
- Alternate foods and fluid when assessing with meals

◆ EVALUATION

Although the RN is officially responsible for the evaluation and modification of the plan of care for the patient, the LPN/LVN's contribution is crucial. The data gathered, along with observation of changes in the patient, make the difference in whether the plan of care is successful.

Nursing evaluation must be aimed directly at the patient outcomes. The outcomes identified earlier in the chapter are straightforward and objective, and they require nursing assessment and data gathering to evaluate progress. Evaluation of other outcomes possibly requires additional investigation, such as consulting various sources of information (including reading the progress notes, discussing the plan with the resident, speaking with family and significant others, listening to the nursing report, and investigating laboratory data). In addition, the nursing evaluation also has to take into consideration individual interventions used and which ones were effective and which ones were less useful. This written evaluation is helpful for all nurses implementing the care plan.

The evaluation of care is based on questions such as the following: Was the expected outcome reached for and with the resident? Is the outcome what the resident wishes to accomplish? Are significant others and family members supportive of the outcomes developed by the interdisciplinary team with the resident? After consideration and analysis of the evaluative measures, with use of the nurse's knowledge base, the team makes a decision to continue the current regimen or to implement a change in the nursing interventions to better achieve the patient-centered expected outcome and offer a better quality of life the resident desires. For example:

Expected outcome 1: Patient will have respirations of 16 to 20 breaths per minute.

Evaluative measure: Is the resident experiencing shortness of breath during activity or rest? Is there a color change of lips during activity? What is the resident's respiratory rate before, during, and after activity?

The nursing services in long-term care center on functional assessment. Nursing interventions also must be provided based on the following prioritized list of nursing needs: airway, breathing, circulation, nutrition, fluids, elimination, sexuality, safety and security, belonging, self-esteem, and self-actualization.

Get Ready for the NCLEX® Examination!

Key Points

- The need for long-term care services arises after the acute stage of an illness has resolved, when the patient continues to need services to maintain the current and changing physical and psychosocial status and functional abilities.
- Settings that provide long-term care include the home, residential care settings, and institutional settings.
- Services that assist those caring for older adults in the home include adult daycare, hospice, home health agencies, and other community agencies and services.
- Residential care settings offer a wide variety of services to the older adult; two of the more popular types are assisted living facilities and continuing care retirement communities.
- Institutional facilities include subacute units and long-term care facilities.
- Most long-term health care providers are under regulation by federal and state guidelines or use them as minimal standards for health care services, reimbursement, and quality indicators.
- Ethical issues related to long-term care services include adherence to a patient's bill of rights, advance directives, DNR orders, power of attorney, guardianship, and responsible party designation.
- In the long-term care facility, the resident's plan of care is reviewed every 90 days for resolution of problems or revision of expected outcomes and interventions by the team.
- Identification of safety concerns, goals, and ways to meet safety goals are an important aspect of care in the long-term care setting.

Additional Learning Resources

SG Go to your Study Guide for additional learning activities to help you master this chapter content.

evolve Be sure to visit the Evolve site at *http://evolve.elsevier.com/Cooper/foundationsadult/* for additional online resources.

Review Questions for the NCLEX® Examination

1. The student nurse is researching long-term care. What does the student identify as being the overall goal for residents in long-term care?
   1. The resident will remain free of disease.
   2. The resident will return home as soon as possible.
   3. The resident will enjoy their long-term care experience.
   4. The resident will remain as independent as possible in the long-term care setting.
2. Which person would benefit most from long-term care services?
   1. A 98-year-old widow who lives at home independently and can perform ADLs but needs a ride to church every Sunday
   2. A 65-year-old widower who is recovering from a stroke and is unable to move his left side
   3. A 75-year-old woman who lives with her husband and has arthritis and osteoporosis with reports of mild to moderate stiffness every morning
   4. A 70-year-old man who lives alone and has a history of coronary artery disease and hypertension

3. The nurse identifies which patient as having the highest priority need for hospice care?
   1. A 65-year-old woman who has metastatic lung cancer and receives home health services
   2. A 77-year-old man who has end-stage prostate cancer and lives in a long-term care facility
   3. A 44-year-old woman who has AIDS and lives in a continuing care retirement community
   4. A 70-year-old woman who recently was diagnosed with ovarian cancer
4. A patient is receiving hospice care for his end-stage cardiac disease. Which statement by his wife alerts the nurse for the need for further education regarding hospice care? *(Select all that apply.)*
   1. "What are the side effects of my husband's pain medication?"
   2. "Are there support groups to help with the grieving process?"
   3. "My husband finally slept for more than 2 hours last night."
   4. "How will I know when it is time to call 9-1-1?"
   5. "We will only need hospice care until my husband gets better."
5. What institutional setting is a bridge between acute care and long-term care?
   1. Subacute care
   2. Nursing home care
   3. Residential care
   4. Adult daycare
6. Which scenario best illustrates the effect OBRA has had on the professional practice of LPN/LVNs in the long-term care setting? *(Select all that apply.)*
   1. The LPN/LVN may be responsible for administering intravenous therapy.
   2. The LPN/LVN provides direct bedside resident care.
   3. The LPN/LVN performs dressing changes.
   4. The LPN/LVN functions as medication nurse.
   5. The LPN/LVN has the responsibility of being a team leader.
7. Which is the best example of an interdisciplinary team?
   1. Director of nurses, charge nurse, staff nurse, CNA, resident
   2. Resident, nurses, physician, social worker, pharmacist, dietitian, activities director, rehabilitation specialists, podiatrist, psychiatrist, audiologist, dentist
   3. Attending physician, resident physician, intern, medical student, CNA, CMA/CMT, physical therapist
   4. Gerontologic clinical nurse specialist, physician, pharmacist, social worker, clergy, resident
8. The new nurse has questions about palliative care. Which response by the nurse best describes this type of care?
   1. "Palliative care is usually provided in acute care facilities."
   2. "Palliative care is typically recommended for individuals with less than 6 months' life expectancy."
   3. "Palliative care is usually affiliated with a church and provided by parish nurses."
   4. "Palliative care extends the principles of hospice care to a broader population that has the possibility to benefit from comfort care earlier in the disease process."
9. Which statement by the student nurse is most accurate in regard to the elderly population?
   1. Most live in a long-term care facility.
   2. Most attend an adult daycare facility.
   3. Most live in a home setting.
   4. Most live in an assisted living setting.
10. The nurse working in an outpatient clinic refers which patient to PACE based on the nurse's assessment?
    1. A 52-year-old who is being treated for hypertension and lives alone
    2. A 70-year-old who has no support system and has chronic venous ulcers requiring treatment at the local wound center
    3. A 90-year-old who has type 2 diabetes controlled by oral diabetic agents and lives with family
    4. A 49-year-old who is disabled because of a chronic debilitating neuromuscular disease and requires physical therapy services three times per week
11. In accordance with National Patient Safety Goals for Nursing Care Centers, which action by the nurse demonstrates and understanding of these goals? *(Select all that apply.)*
    1. The nurse asks the patient to state his or her name and hospital ID number before administering them their medication.
    2. The nurse provides indwelling catheter care to a patient by following facility policy and procedures.
    3. The nurse performs a thorough skin assessment of a new resident upon admission to the health care facility.
    4. The nurse performs a sterile dressing change to the central line of a resident as directed by facility policy.
    5. The nurse asks the resident's family to bring in all home medications to ensure the list given by the patient upon admission to the facility is accurate.

39 Rehabilitation Nursing

http://evolve.elsevier.com/Cooper/foundationsadult/

Objectives

1. Define the philosophy of rehabilitation nursing.
2. Identify patients who would benefit from rehabilitation services.
3. Discuss the goals of rehabilitation therapies.
4. Describe the interdisciplinary rehabilitation team concept and the function of each team member.
5. Discuss the role of the nurse in the specialized practice of rehabilitation.
6. Recognize the importance and significance of family-centered care in rehabilitation.
7. Discuss two major disabling conditions.
8. Recognize polytrauma as a difficult challenge for rehabilitation.
9. Recognize how important it is for the nurse on the rehabilitation team to be knowledgeable about posttraumatic stress disorder (PTSD) and assess for its presence.
10. Describe the goals of pediatric and gerontologic rehabilitation nursing.

Key Terms

chronic illness (KRŎN-ĭk ĬL-nĭs, p. 1189)
Commission on Accreditation of Rehabilitation Facilities (kŭ-MĬSH-ŭn ŎN ŭ-krĕd-ĭ-TĀ-shŭn ŬV rē-ŭ-bĭl-ĭ-TĀ-shŭn fŭ-SĬL-ŭ-tēz, p. 1190)
comprehensive rehabilitation plan (kŏm-prē-HĔN-sĭv rē-ŭ-bĭl-ĭ-TĀ-shŭn PLĂN, p. 1190)
disability (dĭs-ŭ-BĬL-ŭ-tē, p. 1189)
exacerbation (p. 1189)
family-centered care (FĂM-ŭ-lē SĔN-tŭrd KĀR, p. 1193)
functional limitation (FŬNG-shŭn-ŭl lĭm-ĭ-TĀ-shŭn, p. 1189)
gerontologic rehabilitation nursing (jĕr-ŏn-tŭ-LŎJ-ĭk rē-ŭ-bĭl-ĭ-TĀ-shŭn NŬR-sĭng, p. 1200)
impairment (ĭm-PĀR-mĭnt, p. 1189)
interdisciplinary rehabilitation team (ĭn-tŭr-DĬS-ŭ-plĭn-ăr-ē rē-ŭ-bĭl-ĭ-TĀ-shŭn TĒM, p. 1191)
multidisciplinary rehabilitation team (mŭl-tē-DĬS-ŭ-plĭn-ăr-ē rē-ŭ-bĭl-ĭ-TĀ-shŭn TĒM, p. 1191)
pediatric rehabilitation nursing (pē-dē-ĂT-rĭk rē-ŭ-bĭl-ĭ-TĀ-shŭn NŬR-sĭng, p. 1200)
physiatrist (fĭz-ē-ĂT-rĭst, p. 1190)
posttraumatic stress disorder (PTSD) (pōst-trăw-MĂT-ĭk STRĔS dĭs-ŌR-dŭr, p. 1195)
spinal cord injury (SCI) (SPĪ-nŭl CŌRD ĬN-jŭr-ē, p. 1196)
transdisciplinary rehabilitation team (trănz-DĬS-ŭ-plĭn-ăr-ē rē-ŭ-bĭl-ĭ-TĀ-shŭn TĒM, p. 1191)
traumatic brain injury (TBI) (trăw-MĂT-ĭk BRĀN ĬN-jŭr-ē, p. 1199)

The focus of rehabilitation nursing is to support patients in the restoration of a health state or in the adaptation of changes that have resulted from chronic illness, disability, or injury. Rehabilitation nursing is holistic. The patient's physical, mental, emotional, and social needs are assessed and incorporated into the plan of care. The participation of the family is encouraged. In rehabilitation nursing, these concepts are used throughout the continuum of care and across the lifespan of the patient.

Rehabilitation is possible to define in a variety of ways. This chapter will focus on rehabilitation from a medical aspect. Mental health focused rehabilitation is addressed in Chapters 34 through 36. Rehabilitation is a process of outcome-focused patient care delivered by an interdisciplinary team (such as nurses, physical and occupational therapists, speech therapists, and mental health professionals) with the goal of restoring the patient to the fullest physical, mental, social, vocational, and economic capacity of which he or she is capable. Rehabilitation helps an individual regain function or adjust to a new set of needs by finding new ways to do the things previously done. The underlying philosophy of rehabilitation is to focus on abilities rather than disabilities, to continually make the most of the abilities that remain intact. The individual, the family, and the support system are the focus of all rehabilitation efforts. Quality rehabilitation results in the person continually striving to reach his or her highest potential. The setting for rehabilitative activities may be inpatient or outpatient.

NEED FOR REHABILITATION

Rehabilitation is required and valuable in a variety of circumstances. What precipitates the need for rehabilitation may include one or more of the following:

- **Impairment:** Any loss or abnormality of psychological, physical, or anatomic structure or function.
- **Disability:** The loss of ability to participate in one or more major life activities as a result of mental, emotional, or physical impairments. This includes activities such as school, employment, home, community, or social events (ADA National Network, n.d.). The impairment may limit participation in a manner within a range of ability that is considered normal.
- **Functional limitation:** Any loss of ability to perform tasks or activities of daily living.
- **Chronic illness:** A chronic illness generally refers to a condition or state that lasts for 3 months or longer. A chronic illness can have periods of remission and **exacerbation**.

It is important to recognize the differences between these terms and the uniqueness of each term. In rehabilitation nursing, the individual is recognized to have a disability, and the focus is on the individual rather than on the disability. Thus rehabilitation nurses work with people who have disabilities, rather than "the disabled."

CHRONIC ILLNESS AND DISABILITY

Although managing chronic illness and disability is one of the biggest health care problems facing developed countries, the US health care system is not yet positioned to provide optimal care for the individuals who need it. The emphasis on acute care persists, even though the largest group of health care consumers consists of people with chronic illnesses: 113 million Americans have a chronic illness. This accounts for 40% of the population. The risk of chronic illness intensifies with age: an estimated 80% of individuals aged 65 and older are living with a chronic disease (National Rehabilitation Information Center, 2016). Children are not exempt from this plight. In the population aged 5 to 17 years, 8% experience loss of functionality related to a chronic condition. Medical costs for chronic conditions represent about 86% of these health care expenditures (Centers for Disease Control and Prevention, National Center for Chronic Disease Prevention and Health Promotion, 2018). The US Department of Health and Human Services (DHHS) developed a systematic approach for managing chronic illness and improving the quality of life for people with disabilities, titled *Healthy People 2020* (US DHHS, 2013). The set of objectives outlines health goals, starting with identifying people with disabilities and reducing the difficulty in accessing needed care (Box 39.1). A concerned public, as well as committed and knowledgeable professionals, are necessary to accomplish these goals.

Box 39.1 *Healthy People 2020* Focus Areas Related to Chronic Illness and Disability

- Access to health services
- Arthritis, osteoporosis, and chronic back conditions
- Cancer
- Chronic kidney disease
- Dementias, including Alzheimer's disease
- Diabetes
- Disability and health
- Hearing and other sensory or communication disorders
- Heart disease and stroke
- Human immunodeficiency virus (HIV) infection
- Mental health and mental disorders
- Respiratory diseases
- Vision

Health care providers must learn to recognize the special needs of the person with a chronic illness or disability and to organize, plan, and provide care to meet these needs. To appreciate the need for a specific, unique approach to planning and providing care for individuals with chronic illnesses and disabling conditions, providers first need to understand the concepts of chronicity and disability.

CHRONICITY

Unlike acute illnesses, which are usually abrupt in onset and self-limiting (the illness is either resolved or death ensues), chronic illnesses have the potential to be either abrupt or insidious in onset and, by definition, persist for an extended and indefinite period. Affected patients are still able to function but often with some limitation because of the chronic illness.

SCOPE OF INDIVIDUALS REQUIRING REHABILITATION

Rehabilitation is a bridge for the patient, spanning the gap between uselessness and usefulness, between hopelessness and hopefulness, between despair and happiness. The scope of conditions that necessitate rehabilitation is broad and spans the life continuum. Living longer in the United States presents an interesting paradox between retiring and enjoying the so-called golden years and a strong probability of acquiring one or more chronic, disabling conditions. Chronic illness and physiologic changes of aging increase the likelihood of physical limitations and disability disproportionately for older people in comparison with younger adults. Although many families continue to care for older people with disabling conditions in their homes, many also live in nursing homes. Whether an older patient is in the acute stage of an illness or injury or in the community, rehabilitation services are built around maintaining functional abilities, ensuring safety, promoting effective coping, preventing complications, and modifying the environment for maximal independence.

A disability has a number of potential effects on the patient and the family, including behavioral and emotional changes and changes in roles, body image, self-concept, and family dynamics.

GOALS OF REHABILITATION

Rehabilitation is a goal-oriented (outcome-oriented) process. These goals are personal, and the rehabilitation team individualizes them to meet the holistic needs of each patient served. To determine goals, a collaborative goal-setting process includes the members of the rehabilitation team, with the patient and the family at the center of the process.

It is appropriate to include the following criteria in all rehabilitation goals:

- The goals maximize the quality of life of the patient.
- The goals address the patient's specific needs.
- The goals assist the patient with adjusting to an altered lifestyle.
- The goals are directed toward promoting wellness and minimizing complications.
- The goals assist the patient in attaining the highest degree of function and self-sufficiency possible.
- The goals assist the patient with home and community reentry.

All rehabilitation efforts must be outcome focused and comprehensive and must constitute an educational process.

CORNERSTONES OF REHABILITATION

Rehabilitation involves several important aspects of care in helping the patient meet agreed-upon goals. The following are important factors to keep in mind in helping the patient to reach these goals:

- *Focus on the individual:* All efforts of rehabilitation are centered on the patient's goals and objectives. When the patient sets or holds goals that are not realistic, the team works with the patient in reshaping expectations.
- *Community reentry:* Rehabilitation is considered successful if the patient is able to reenter the community through participation in social, vocational, and recreational activities.
- *Independence:* The goals of rehabilitation focus on promoting and maintaining the patient's physical and emotional independence.
- *Functional ability:* Progress in rehabilitation is measured in terms of functional outcomes.
- *Team approach:* Rehabilitation goals are achieved through the work of the rehabilitation team members, including the patient and the family.
- *Quality of life:* Goals focus on improving the quality of life, rather than increasing the quantity of life.
- *Prevention and wellness:* Because many problems that necessitate rehabilitation are long standing, rehabilitation goals focus on preventing complications and maximizing function.
- *Change process:* Patients who experience a disabling condition or chronic illness experience the change process, as do their families. The rehabilitation team is responsible for directing the change in as positive a manner as possible.
- *Adaptation:* Although patients with disabilities do not always accept their disability, learning to adapt to the circumstances created by the limits of their abilities is a positive method of coping.
- *Patient and family education:* Knowledge and skills are essential components of the rehabilitation program. Patients with substantial disability have the potential to obtain a degree of independence through patient education, which enables them to direct their own care.

COMPREHENSIVE REHABILITATION PLAN

The more comprehensive the rehabilitation program is, the better are the chances for higher functional outcomes of the people served. According to the **Commission on Accreditation of Rehabilitation Facilities** (a nonprofit, private, international standard-setting and accreditation body whose mission is to promote and advocate the delivery of quality rehabilitation), it is necessary to initiate an overall individualized **comprehensive rehabilitation plan** of care within 24 hours of the patient's hospital admission and have it ready for review and revision by the rehabilitation team within 3 days of the admission. The results of the interdisciplinary admission assessment provide the basis for developing the plan. Underlying it are individual goals incorporating the unique strengths, needs, abilities, and preferences of the patient. This plan reflects the environment where the patient will go upon hospital discharge. The goals must be measurable, must be described in functional or behavioral terms, and must have associated time frames for achievement, and the responsible team member or members must be listed.

All clinicians treating the patient use this comprehensive plan of care. Evaluation conferences and family conferences take place on a regular basis. The active participation of the patient and family is an integral part of planning and implementing the discharge process.

REHABILITATION TEAM

Because a single discipline does not offer the knowledge and expertise necessary to provide all the components of the rehabilitation program, the rehabilitation team is composed of people from multiple disciplines. The patient's specific illness and needs ultimately determine the team's composition. Members of the interdisciplinary team may include a physician, a nurse practitioner, a **physiatrist** (physicians specializing in physical medicine or rehabilitation; American Association of Physiatrists, 2013), a physical/occupational/speech therapist, a recreational therapist, a nutritionist, a psychologist, a spiritual adviser, and a social worker; and it always

Table 39.1 Rehabilitation Team

MEMBER	ROLE	ACTIONS
Patient	Key member	Participates in goal setting Takes control of own life
Physiatrist	Rehabilitation physician	Is team leader and coordinator of program
Rehabilitation RN	Coordinator, educator	Provides support Educates patient and family concerning rehabilitation process Promotes independence
Rehabilitation LPN/LVN	Care provider; patient's advocate	Provides support Reinforces education to the patient and family concerning the rehabilitation process Assists in treatment plan and implementation
Physical therapist	Designing exercise program	Provides therapy Assesses patient's needs Provides training
Occupational therapist	Assessing independent living needs	Recommends equipment modifications Adapts equipment
Speech-language pathologist	Performing assessment of communication and swallowing abilities Designing rehabilitation communication program	Helps patient regain communication skills Teaches patient
Therapeutic recreation therapist	Recreation planner	Plans leisure activities Promotes patient's interest in activities
Clinical psychologist	Emotional evaluator	Assesses patient's position on the mental health continuum Promotes patient's independence by maximizing active participation Assists patient in developing realistic positive attitudes
Chaplain	Spiritual consultant	Provides spiritual support and guidance
Vocational rehabilitation counselor	Vocational planner	Helps patient obtain training for new or current employment

LPN/LVN, Licensed practical nurse or licensed vocational nurse; *RN*, registered nurse.

includes the patient. The team coordinates the comprehensive rehabilitation program for each patient in an individualized manner (Table 39.1 and Fig. 39.1).

MODELS OF TEAM FUNCTIONING

There are three primary models of rehabilitation team functioning. One model, primarily of service in the past, is the **multidisciplinary rehabilitation team.** Characteristic of this model are discipline-specific goals, clear boundaries between disciplines, and outcomes that are the sum of each discipline's efforts. Effective communication is the key to success for this type of team.

The type of team most commonly used today in rehabilitation hospitals is the **interdisciplinary rehabilitation team.** This type of team collaborates to identify individual's goals and features a combination of expanded problem solving beyond the boundaries of the individual disciplines, together with discipline-specific work toward goal attainment.

A third type of team is the **transdisciplinary rehabilitation team.** What characterizes this model is the blurring of boundaries between disciplines, as well as cross-training and flexibility to minimize any duplication of effort toward individual goal attainment.

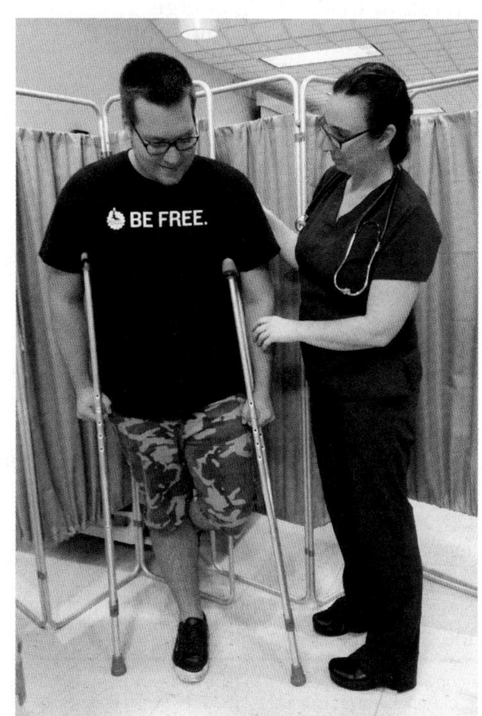

Fig. 39.1 Members of the rehabilitation team helping a patient with ambulation.

Major strengths of the team methods of care delivery are that they are well established, promote good communication and collaboration among disciplines, address comprehensive aspects of care, energize staff, and view the patient holistically. These models provide a structure for rehabilitation. It is still necessary to integrate services to ensure a comprehensive, appropriate experience.

REHABILITATION NURSE

The rehabilitation nurse with diverse expertise, roles, and work settings plays a vital, unique role on this team. Rehabilitation nurses are with the patient on a 24-hour basis. Because of this constant exposure, nurses can notice small, often imperceptible changes. It is necessary for rehabilitation nurses to have broad knowledge of the pathophysiology of a wide range of medical-surgical conditions and highly specialized knowledge and skills regarding rehabilitation (Box 39.2).

In addition to a set of specialized knowledge and skills, rehabilitation nursing is an attitude. In rehabilitation, the work is predicated on the belief that individuals with functional disabilities or chronic illnesses have an intrinsic worth that transcends the disability or illness. William Barclay put it this way:

> One of the highest of human duties is the duty of encouragement…It is easy to laugh at men's ideals; it is easy to pour cold water on their enthusiasm; it is easy to discourage others. The world is full of discouragers…We have a duty to encourage one another. Many a time a word of praise or thanks has kept a man on his feet. Blessed is the man who speaks such a word.

Rehabilitation nurses are obliged to offer encouragement on a regular basis. The role of a rehabilitation nurse is to put the individual in charge of his or her own care rather than taking charge.

Box 39.2 Roles of the Rehabilitation Nurse

- Educator
  - Reinforces the teaching delivered by other members of the health care team
  - Discusses wellness and health promotion activities
  - Provides information about the disease process and the plan of care
- Provider of care
  - Performs holistic patient assessments
  - Provides or oversees physical care of the patient
  - Plans nursing care
- Collaborator
  - Work to streamline the interactions of the health care team
  - Develops realistic, patient focused goals
- Patient advocate
  - Actively listens to the needs and wishes of the patient
  - Seeks to incorporate the requests of the patient in the plan of care

The Association of Rehabilitation Nurses (2016) gives the following definition:

> Rehabilitation nursing is a specialty practice area within the scope of professional nursing. It involves the diagnosis and treatment of human responses of individuals and groups to actual or potential health problems resulting from altered functional ability and altered lifestyle.
>
> The goal of rehabilitation nursing is to assist individuals with disabilities and chronic illness in the restoration, maintenance, and promotion of optimal health. The rehabilitation nurse is skilled at treating alterations in functional ability and lifestyle resulting from injury, disability, and chronic illness.
>
> Rehabilitation nurses provide comfort, therapy, and education; promote health-conducive adjustments; support adaptive capabilities; and promote achievable independence. Rehabilitation nurses provide holistic, comprehensive, and compassionate end-of-life care, including promotion of comfort and relief of pain.

Specialized training is necessary to become an effective team member. Although each team member contributes to the rehabilitation process, it is the rehabilitation nurse who reinforces teaching and training completed by the other disciplines on a 24-hours-a-day, 7-days-a-week basis. Efficacious rehabilitation nursing is essential for a successful rehabilitation outcome.

Rehabilitation nursing is practiced in a variety of settings across the continuum of care: primary care clinics, home health agencies, outpatient services, hospitals and rehabilitation facilities, skilled nursing facilities, subacute or transitional care facilities, residential facilities, daycare agencies, insurance companies, and private companies. The rehabilitation nurse is a vital member of the interdisciplinary rehabilitation team and is responsible for taking on many roles: educator, caregiver, counselor, care coordinator, case manager, patient advocate, consultant, researcher, administrator or manager, and expert witness.

The focus in rehabilitation is on enabling the patient to move from a totally dependent state to a level of independence. In the optimal scenario, each patient receives individual treatment from specific nurses and therapists so that bonds of trust and friendship can develop through the difficult rehabilitation process. Extensive family and patient education, modern adaptive equipment, numerous community integration activities, specialized programs, and professional, effective team therapies combine to help patients learn to make the most of their lives.

Basic rehabilitation can be used whether the patient is suffering from arthritis, multiple sclerosis, mental illness, brain attack or stroke, spinal cord injury, burn, or traumatic brain injury. The nurse's responsibility is to apply appropriate concepts and techniques throughout the continuum of care. All basic nursing measures are essential; these include position changes and maintaining body alignment, which prevent skeletal and muscular deformities (contractures) and pressure ulcers.

Rehabilitation nursing is a challenge that requires knowledge, teamwork, coordination, planning, and patience. To care for people with disabilities, it is important for rehabilitation professionals to learn and stay abreast of current knowledge and techniques.

The phenomenon of change as it relates to the human experience is a central concept in nursing. This is especially true for rehabilitation nurses, who regularly interact with people experiencing great change. The focus of this chapter is on the individual patient, who is the central member of the rehabilitation team. Understanding and promoting the change process is therefore an integral part of the role of a rehabilitation nurse.

Nursing Assessment

The nurse begins to develop a plan of care for the patient by assessing the ability of the patient to perform activities of daily living in a safe manner; this assessment helps the nurse determine the patient's level of independence. This assessment is performed best through observation of the patient completing different basic tasks, such as ambulation and bathing. Observation of the abilities or disabilities of the patient provides information on which to base the plan of care. Additional areas to observe include ability of the patient to dress himself or herself, including fastening clothing, and self-feeding ability, including holding utensils and chewing and swallowing food and liquids.

Patient Problem

The major patient problem for a patient receiving rehabilitation services is related to performing activities of daily living (ADLs). Based on assessment findings, any of the following patient problem statements could be used in relation to inability to perform ADLs:

- *Inability to Bathe Self*
- *Inability to Dress Self*
- *Inability to Feed Self*
- *Inability to Toilet Self*

Additional patient problems for consideration in the rehabilitation setting include the following:

- *Compromised Maintenance of Health*
- *Excessive Demand on Primary Caregiver*
- *Helplessness*
- *Insufficient Knowledge*
- *Interrupted Family Processes*
- *Potential for Inability to Tolerate Activity*

NURSING INTERVENTIONS

Nursing interventions are geared to support and reinforce activities included in the interdisciplinary plan of care. Additional nursing interventions may include the following:

- Assisting the patient with repetition and practice of exercises
- Minimizing distractions that would prevent patient participation in therapy
- Providing cues and reminders as needed

The following five-step approach is an option to guide this process:

1. Assess the patient's and the family's needs, abilities, and concerns.
2. Plan interventions on the basis of these needs, abilities, and concerns.
3. Implement the educational plan.
4. Document the educational process.
5. Evaluate and revise the educational plan.

FAMILY AND FAMILY-CENTERED CARE

Family-centered care is a philosophy that recognizes the pivotal role of the family in the lives of children with disabilities or other chronic conditions. It is a philosophy by which health care providers strive to support families in their natural caregiving roles by building on the parents' unique strengths as individuals. This perspective promotes normal patterns of living at home and in the community, and families and professionals are viewed as equals in a partnership committed to excellence at all levels of health care. The ability and willingness of nurses and health care providers to share knowledge and control of health resources with families, empowering them to act as advocates for themselves and their children, is an integral part of family-centered care.

The key elements of family-centered care are as follows:

- Incorporating into policy and practice the recognition that the family is the constant in a child's life, whereas the service systems and support personnel within those systems are transitional
- Facilitating family-professional collaboration at all levels of hospital, home, and community care
- Exchanging complete and unbiased information between families and professionals in a supportive manner at all times
- Encouraging and facilitating family-to-family support and networking
- Appreciating the unique characteristics of families and children with a recognition of the wide range of strengths, concerns, emotions, and aspirations beyond their need for specialized health and developmental services and support (Bamm and Rosenbaum, 2008)

Collaboration between family and professional is essential for providing appropriate and optimal care.

Family-centered care is an evolving concept. It is a process that differs according to variations in situations, families, cultures, health care settings, and providers. Family-centered care requires learning new ways of relating to and working with families, in rehabilitation and throughout the continuum of care.

CROSS-CULTURAL REHABILITATION

Society is in a state of transformation. Many countries are experiencing considerable demographic shifts along with an increasingly wide range of ethnic identification, religions, material reality, beliefs, and behaviors, all leading to rich diversity and cultural complexity. At the same time, health professionals, including rehabilitation teams, are becoming much more aware of the need to become culturally knowledgeable to be effective in their interaction with patients.

Rehabilitation team members must engage in genuine collaboration with patients and colleagues, including community-level workers and those trained in other disciplines, to obtain the best possible functional outcome for the patient. Disability exists in all societies, but the definition and significance of disability in an individual culture depends on that culture's values. Attitudes also vary toward individuals with a disability; toward concepts of rehabilitation; toward the sociocultural, biologic, and economic implications of disability; and toward policy affecting individuals with a disability. (See Chapter 6 for a detailed discussion of culture and ethnic considerations.)

Cultural competence requires the acknowledgment and awareness of one's own cultural norms. Then it involves the awareness and acceptance of those cultural values and behaviors of another. The incorporation of cultural competence into the assessment, planning, and delivery of care enables the patient to receive holistic care.

The following describes a culturally competent practitioner:

- Has the capacity for cultural self-assessment
- Provides health care that is sensitive to the culture and values of the patient and is linguistically appropriate
- Is conscious of the dynamics of difference
- Disseminates cultural knowledge
- Adapts to diversity in race, color, ethnicity, national origin, immigration status, religion, age, gender, sexual orientation, political beliefs, social and economic status, education, occupation, spirituality, and any other differences (Cultural Competency Advisory Group, 2009)

In summary, what characterizes cultural competence is acceptance and respect for difference, continuing self-assessment regarding culture, vigilance toward the dynamics of difference, ongoing expansion of cultural knowledge and resources, and adaptability of services.

People develop *cultural proficiency* when they hold culture in high regard. The culturally proficient professional recognizes the need to conduct research, disseminates the results, and develops new approaches that promise to increase culturally competent practice. Rehabilitation professionals have an ethical responsibility to strive for cultural competence and cultural proficiency.

ISSUES IN REHABILITATION

In rehabilitation, several forces drive the rendering of care. The issues involved include but are not limited to the following:

- *Quality of life versus quantity of life:* Rehabilitation focuses on continually improving the quality of the person's life, not merely maintaining life itself.
- *Care versus cure:* Because of the suddenness and catastrophic effect of many conditions that necessitate rehabilitation, it is necessary to consider the care of the individual in relation to the cure of the condition. Many conditions are irreversible; therefore the focus of care is on adapting and accepting an altered life rather than resolving an illness.
- *High cost of interdisciplinary care versus long-term care:* Rehabilitation is expensive, mainly because the care is delivered by a team of highly trained professionals. Studies of resource allocation have shown that starting rehabilitation early saves thousands of dollars and increases the chance that the patient will be able to live independently and return to the workforce, thereby eliminating the expense of a caregiver or residential long-term care (American Physical Therapy Association, 2014; Lipshutz et al, 2012). In some cases, the success of rehabilitation is viewed as a person's return to productive employment; in other cases, a disability means that two people become unemployed: the individual with the disability and the caregiver. Rehabilitation in this scenario can be successful, and the savings still considerable, if the individual with the disability becomes independent enough to not require a caregiver even though he or she remains unable to return to work.

CHRONIC CONDITIONS NECESSITATING REHABILITATION THERAPY

CARDIAC REHABILITATION

An insult to the cardiovascular system, such as a myocardial infarction or cardiac surgery, may require the patient to participate in rehabilitation to improve function and return to normal activities. A cardiac rehabilitation program is designed to meet the needs of the patient through exercise, education about heart healthy living, and counseling in stress reduction in an effort to reduce modifiable risk factors associated with cardiac disease and to prevent future hospitalizations (National Heart, Lung, and Blood Institute, 2013). The rehabilitation team evaluates baseline levels of physical fitness and develops an individualized program. The focus is also on improving the patient's emotional adaptation to the cardiac condition and related limitations.

PULMONARY REHABILITATION

Patients with chronic breathing problems, such as chronic obstructive pulmonary disease, and those who require or have just recently undergone lung surgery may benefit from pulmonary rehabilitation. This type of rehabilitation includes an exercise program; counseling regarding diet and nutrition; education regarding the lung disease process; and management, energy conservation techniques, and breathing strategies (American Lung

Association, 2018). The program may be located in the hospital or offered on an outpatient basis in the community. Home-based services are common. Health care team members involved in pulmonary rehabilitation include primary care providers, nurses, respiratory therapists, physical and occupational therapists, dietitians, and nutritionists. Social services also may be represented.

POLYTRAUMA AND REHABILITATION NURSING

Soldiers wounded in conflicts, including those in Iraq, Afghanistan, and Syria, brought about challenges to today's health care system. These soldiers experience multiple traumas with variable patterns, a phenomenon known as polytrauma–blast-related injury (PT/BRI), as a result of explosions (Pennardt, 2016). Rehabilitative nurses in the military and in the Veterans Administration have responded to these challenges (Fig. 39.2).

Blast-related injuries are categorized as primary, secondary, tertiary, or quaternary (miscellaneous) (Medscape, 2016). Air-filled cavities in the body (ears, lungs, and gastrointestinal tract) and organs enveloped by fluid (brain and spinal cord) are most susceptible to compression damage from high explosive blasts. These injuries are considered primary blast-related injuries. Injuries from airborne debris, bomb fragments, and shrapnel embedded in any body part are considered secondary blast-related injuries. Any injury sustained from being thrown as the result of an explosive shock wave or dynamic overpressure is a tertiary blast-related injury; examples include broken bones and traumatic head and spinal cord injuries. Inhalation of and exposure to toxic chemicals, traumatic amputations of limbs, and burns are examples of quaternary injuries (Stevenson, 2009).

In an effort to deal more effectively with PT/BRI, medical treatment of these soldiers is focusing on postacute care with the goal of reducing disabilities associated with these injuries (Rosenfeld and Ford, 2013). The rehabilitation teams for soldiers who have experienced PT/BRI gear their care toward discovering and treating additional injuries that were not detected during the postacute phase, as well as treating those originally identified injuries (Rosenfeld and Ford, 2013). The earlier the injuries are identified, the more successful treatment outcomes are and the lower the costs incurred during treatment are (Rosenfeld and Ford, 2013).

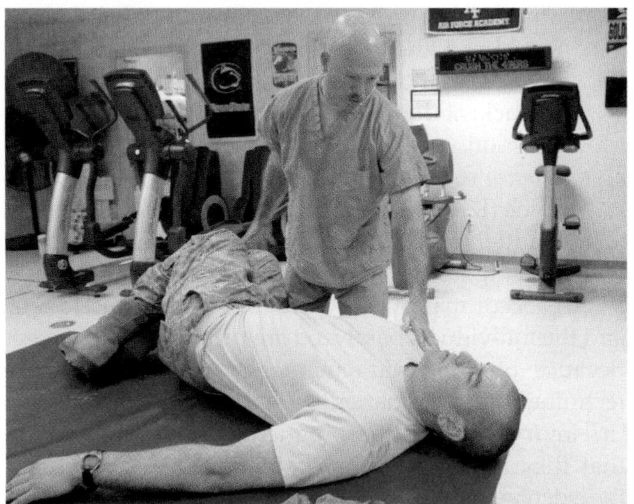

Fig. 39.2 Wounded army veteran receiving rehabilitative nursing care. (US Army photo by Spc. Cody Barber/Released.)

It is important to understand, identify, and treat PT/BRIs to avoid focusing care solely on the more visible injuries. Identification of this newly identified group of injuries allows successful treatment of a variety of conditions, ranging from concussions that cause cognitive and vestibular deficits to posttraumatic stress disorder (Rosenfeld and Ford, 2013).

POSTTRAUMATIC STRESS DISORDER

Posttraumatic stress disorder (PTSD) is defined as a mental health condition related to the experiencing of or witnessing of a traumatic event outside the normal range of human experience (Mayo Clinic, 2018). Instead of getting better over time, the symptoms get worse. It is repeatedly experiencing the traumatic event through flashbacks or nightmares, causing difficulty in sleeping and concentrating. A person experiencing PTSD tries to avoid people, places, and activities that serve to remind of the traumatic event (Anxiety & Depression Association of America, 2017).

The American Psychiatric Association first identified PTSD in 1980. Before 1980 the field described soldiers who experienced the symptoms now known as PTSD as suffering from "shell shock" or "war neurosis" (Glass, 1969), and many people believed that affected soldiers were making up the symptoms to avoid being involved in further combat (Clark, 1997). After the Vietnam War, PTSD received acceptance as a psychiatric diagnosis, and other forms of trauma, such as rape and natural disasters, also were identified as causes of PTSD (American Psychiatric Association, 1980).

Events such as the September 11, 2001, terrorist attacks in the United States, Operation Iraqi Freedom, and Hurricane Katrina have again brought attention to PTSD in survivors. However, the veracity of the disorder still raises doubt among some family members and health care providers. PTSD diagnosis is considered if the symptoms do not improve or even worsen after at least 1 month and are dependent on the identification of a traumatic event, either personally experienced or witnessed, and/or the re-living of the traumatic events either through dreams or reoccurring vivid memories or flashbacks, interfering with normal life functions (Mayo Clinic, 2016).

Without proper identification and treatment, PTSD has been known to lead to other mental health problems such as depression, anxiety, alcohol or drug use, and even suicidal thoughts or actions. Effective treatments for PTSD have included psychotherapy and pharmacotherapy. Studies have shown that a combination of cognitive and prolonged-exposure therapy is the most effective in treating the disorder, sometimes with the aid of medications such as selective serotonin reuptake inhibitors (National Center for PTSD, 2013).

For the nurse on the rehabilitation team, it is important to be aware that other psychological conditions often accompany PTSD. The nurse plays a critical supportive role during rehabilitation in assisting the patient to adapt or regain control over the symptoms of PTSD (Rehabilitation Institute of Chicago, 2013). Through early assessment of PTSD symptoms and the use of therapeutic communication, nurses are able to assist patients in achieving the goal of treatment. Therapeutic communication techniques include listening, reframing, normalizing responses, and working to develop trust in the nurse-patient relationship. Nurses also need to be aware of their own reactions, emotions, and communication skills when caring for trauma victims. Nurses who are feeling overwhelmed sometimes need to consult with a mental health care provider.

DISABILITY

The Americans with Disabilities Act became law in 1990. This landmark legislation provides protection against discrimination for people with disabilities. Universally accepted, the Americans with Disabilities Act defines an individual as disabled if he or she has a physical or mental impairment that substantially limits one or more major life activities, has a record of such an impairment, or is regarded as having such an impairment.

As is the case with chronic illness, it is important to recognize that having a disability is just one of many variants of the normal human experience. One way to look at it is to assert that all individuals are only temporarily able-bodied and that at some point in life, everyone experiences some form of disability. It is essential to develop this level of awareness to avoid labeling groups of people in ways that risk disenfranchising them.

People with disabilities are not defined by their illness or their disability. They are complex individuals with unique combinations of skills, and identifying them as such is obligatory. The basis for planning care that promotes health and positively affects the quality of life is a holistic, person-first approach in which the shared experience of being human, along with the uniqueness of the individual, is honored and the strengths, as well as impairments, are recognized.

Furthermore, providers are called on to offer interventions that address the need of people with chronic illnesses or disabilities to develop personally within the context of that illness or disability.

The following sections concern two of the major conditions for which dedicated rehabilitation efforts are necessary.

SPINAL CORD INJURIES

A **spinal cord injury (SCI)** is any injury in which the spinal cord undergoes compression by fracture or displacement of vertebrae, by bleeding, or by edema. Injury at each level has its unique characteristics, but in general, the higher the injury point is, the greater is the loss of function. The body parts and the functions located above the injury point continue to operate as they should. Injury to the spinal cord is irreversible in that the cord is unable to repair itself. Spinal function is sometimes present below the level of the lesion. In general, however, the effects of an injured spinal cord include paralysis, loss of normal bowel and bladder function, and loss of sensation (Fig. 39.3). Terminology associated with SCI includes but is not limited to the following:

- *Complete injury:* No motor or sensory function below the level of injury
- *Incomplete injury:* Some or all motor or sensory function below the level of injury
- *Quadriplegia:* Damage to the cervical spine or the neck that involves weakness or paralysis in all four extremities
- *Paraplegia:* Damage below the cervical area that involves weakness or paralysis in the trunk and lower extremities
- *Paresis:* A slight paralysis, incomplete loss of muscular power, or weakness of a limb
- SCIs are categorized as follows:
  - *Cervical cord injury:* Level of injury is at the cervical spine (C2 to C7) and involves paralysis of all extremities and trunk, respiratory failure, bladder and bowel disturbance, bradycardia, perspiration, elevated temperature, and headache.
  - *Thoracic cord injury:* Level of injury is at the thoracic spine (T1 to T12) and involves paralysis of lower extremities. Initially after the injury, muscles are flaccid (weak, soft, flabby, lacking normal muscle tone) and later become spastic (having spasms or other uncontrolled contractions of the skeletal muscles). Other potential symptoms are paralysis of bladder, bowel, and sphincters; pain in chest or back; abdominal distention; and loss of sexual function.
  - *Lumbar cord injury:* Level of injury is at the lumbar spine (L1 to L2) with paralysis of lower extremities, bladder, and rectum and loss of sexual function (see Fig. 39.3).

SCIs occur mainly as a result of traumatic accidents, and the individuals paralyzed are primarily young men. Because of improved emergency and medical care techniques, typical patients are more likely to survive the injury. Most of these patients are young enough that they have vocational potential. Injury level and the extent of damage to the spinal cord largely determine functional disabilities. Functional limitations occur in nearly every aspect of an individual's life after an SCI.

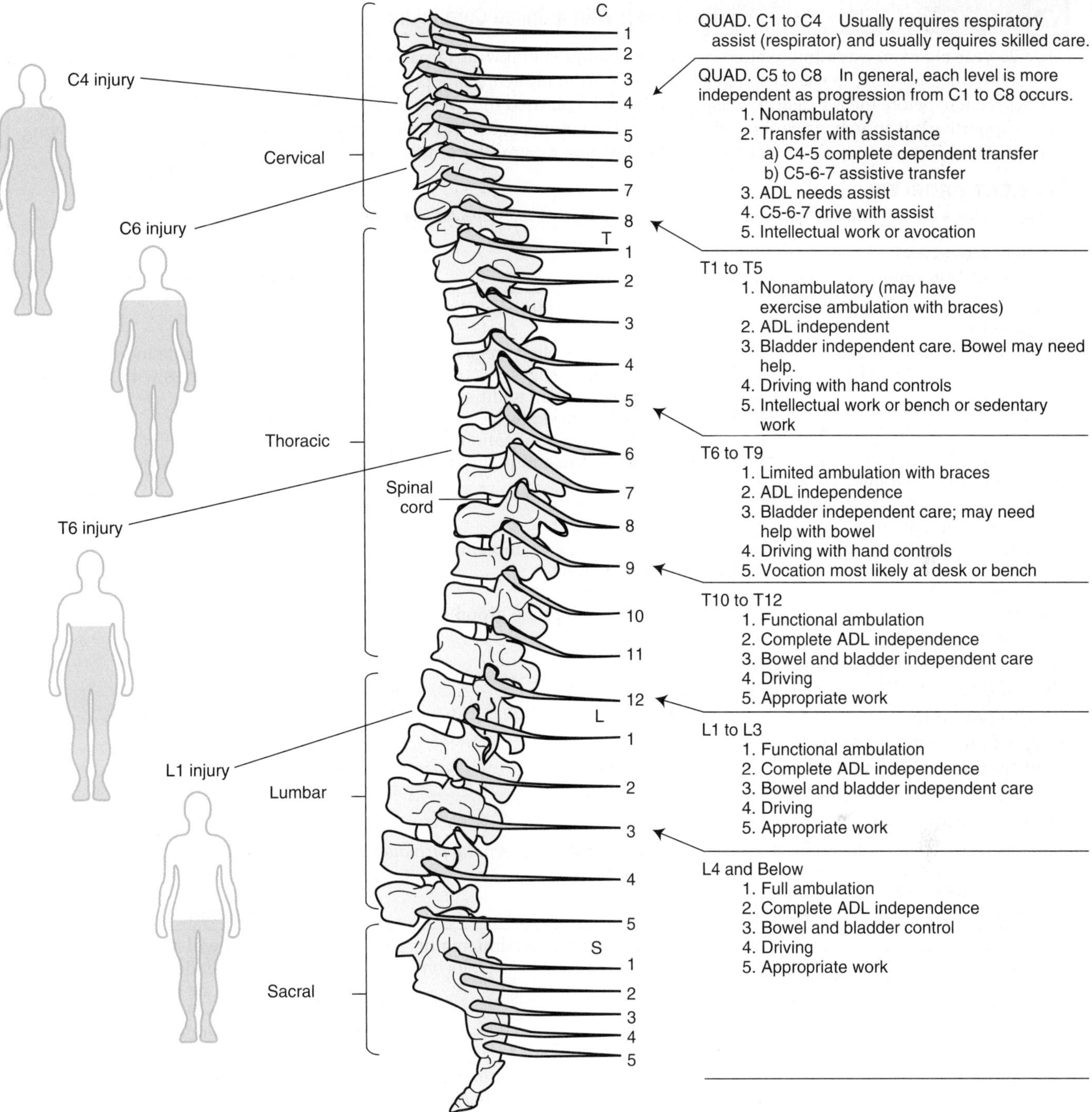

C4 injury
C6 injury
T6 injury
L1 injury
Cervical
Thoracic
Lumbar
Sacral
Spinal cord
C
T
L
S
QUAD. C1 to C4 Usually requires respiratory assist (respirator) and usually requires skilled care.
QUAD. C5 to C8 In general, each level is more independent as progression from C1 to C8 occurs.
1. Nonambulatory
2. Transfer with assistance
a) C4-5 complete dependent transfer
b) C5-6-7 assistive transfer
3. ADL needs assist
4. C5-6-7 drive with assist
5. Intellectual work or avocation
T1 to T5
1. Nonambulatory (may have exercise ambulation with braces)
2. ADL independent
3. Bladder independent care. Bowel may need help.
4. Driving with hand controls
5. Intellectual work or bench or sedentary work
T6 to T9
1. Limited ambulation with braces
2. ADL independence
3. Bladder independent care; may need help with bowel
4. Driving with hand controls
5. Vocation most likely at desk or bench
T10 to T12
1. Functional ambulation
2. Complete ADL independence
3. Bowel and bladder independent care
4. Driving
5. Appropriate work
L1 to L3
1. Functional ambulation
2. Complete ADL independence
3. Bowel and bladder independent care
4. Driving
5. Appropriate work
L4 and Below
1. Full ambulation
2. Complete ADL independence
3. Bowel and bladder control
4. Driving
5. Appropriate work

Fig. 39.3 Levels and loss of function by location of spinal cord injury. *ADL*, Activities of daily living.

The effect of SCI on the individual remains one of the most compelling challenges in the field of rehabilitation. Patients with SCI often require considerable motivation and reeducation to regain a satisfying quality of life and to ensure community reintegration. Crucial for rehabilitation is the communal effort of an interdisciplinary team whose members work together to meet the specific needs of the patient and the family.

Common medical complications experienced by patients with SCI include but are not limited to postural hypotension, autonomic dysreflexia, heterotopic ossification, and deep vein thrombosis. Patient problems for a patient with SCI include but are not limited to those listed in Nursing Care Plan 39.1.

Postural Hypotension

Some patients with spinal cord injuries have a marked drop in blood pressure while sitting in a wheelchair. It is common for many quadriplegic patients to have a blood pressure of 90/60 mm Hg (or lower) when sitting as a result of the pooling of the blood in the lower extremities and in the abdominal area. Returning the patient to the horizontal position usually stops dizziness. To lessen hypotension, raise the head of the bed 15 to

Nursing Care Plan 39.1 The Patient With a Spinal Cord Injury

T., a 26-year-old man, was admitted to the acute rehabilitation unit with T1 paraplegia secondary to a motor vehicle accident 10 days earlier. Initially he was in spinal shock, and during his acute care phase he had periods of despondency and signs of depression. Before the accident, T. was scheduled to be married in 2 weeks. His future wife and his family were attentive and supportive but apprehensive about their future. The young couple was in the process of purchasing a house and moving out of state, where T. was scheduled to begin employment as a mechanical engineer.

PATIENT PROBLEM

Grief, related to loss of function, perceived decreased ability to meet role expectations, and changes in family processes

Patient Goals and Expected Outcomes	Nursing Interventions	Evaluation
Patient will acknowledge disability	Offer guidance and support through early stage of grieving.	
Patient will verbalize sense of loss from enforced changes	Encourage expression of feelings regarding disability and enforced lifestyle changes.	Patient is able to verbalize his distress with his altered lifestyle.
	Assist patient in using current abilities in the performance of self-care skills, leisure activities, and family and community socialization.	
Patient and family will reorganize life on the basis of patient's current strengths and abilities	Guide realistic goal setting and planning to meet goals.	Patient and fiancée set alternative wedding date.
Patient will refocus energies to promote positive changes	Reinforce active planning and implementation of future vocational options.	Patient is exploring alternative employment options.
Patient will participate in social interaction	Provide contacts for appropriate group support.	
Patient will participate in leisure activities or verbalize plan to incorporate leisure activities		
Patient will identify value in altered lifestyle		

PATIENT PROBLEM

Compromised Bed Mobility, related to inability to move the body purposefully, including bed mobility, transfer, and ambulation

Patient Goals and Expected Outcomes	Nursing Interventions	Evaluation
Patient will be able to perform independent bed mobility skills, transfers, and wheelchair mobility	Instruct and assist the patient in maximizing his ability to move around in the environment (e.g., locomotion by wheelchair).	Patient will achieve optimal independence in transfers from one surface to another. Patient will achieve independence in wheelchair mobility.
Patient will demonstrate the ability to direct others to assist him to achieve optimal mobility	Instruct and assist the patient in maximizing his ability to transfer from one surface to another (e.g., bed to chair). Instruct and assist the patient in the use of adaptive or assistive equipment. Instruct and assist the patient in methods that help increase mobility in bed. Instruct and assist the patient in methods that help maximize energy and maintain safety during movement.	Patient will learn to use adaptive equipment to achieve his optimal level of independence in performing activities of daily living.
	Instruct and assist the patient in maintaining optimal body alignment to promote skin integrity and prevent contracture.	Patient will maintain intact skin integrity. Patient will be free of contractures.

CRITICAL THINKING QUESTIONS

1. Describe the stimuli or precipitating factors associated with bowel functioning or management that have potential to cause autonomic dysreflexia. What are the appropriate interventions if it does occur?
2. The patient has T1 quadriplegia. How is it possible to lessen the patient's potential for developing orthostatic hypotension?
3. When explaining orthostatic hypotension to a new nursing assistant, what commonly occurring signs and symptoms should the nurse describe, and what instructions should be given to the nursing assistant?

20 minutes before moving the patient to the wheelchair. Elastic stockings (thromboembolic disease [TED] hose) and abdominal binders may also be used.

Autonomic Dysreflexia

Patients with spinal cord lesions above T5 sometimes experience sudden and extreme elevations in blood pressure, caused by a reflex action of the autonomic nervous system. It is the result of some stimulation of the body below the level of the injury, usually bladder distention from a blocked catheter. Any stimulation has potential to produce the syndrome, including constipation, diarrhea, sexual activity, pressure ulcers, position changes (from lying to sitting), and even wrinkles in clothing or bed sheets. In addition to high blood pressure, possible symptoms include diaphoresis, shivering or goose bumps, flushing of the skin, and a severe, pounding headache.

Treatment for autonomic dysreflexia is to find and remove the source of irritation. Once the irritation is gone, the blood pressure returns to normal within a few minutes. The patient should be raised into a sitting position immediately. This helps reduce the elevated blood pressure before damage occurs.

Heterotopic Ossification

Heterotopic ossification is the abnormal formation of bone cells in joints. It commonly arises in people with SCIs and occurs below the level of the lesion. The formation of extra bone in these joints usually results in limited range of motion. The most commonly affected joints are the hips and sometimes the knees. It occurs most frequently 1 to 4 months after the injury and rarely occurs more than 1 year afterward. Symptoms include localized edema around the area; after several days, a firm mass can be palpated in underlying tissue. After several weeks, range of motion is diminished. Treatment options involve aggressive range-of-motion exercises, medications, and occasionally surgery.

Deep Vein Thrombosis

Patients with spinal injuries have the potential to develop deep vein thrombosis in the lower extremities. Deep vein thrombosis is a clotting of blood within vessels of the legs caused by slowing of the circulation or an alteration in the blood vessel walls. Clinical signs include localized swelling, redness, and heat in the involved area. If these signs are present, aggressive movement to that leg is unwise because it has the potential to detach the blood clot, which in turn has the potential to lodge in the lung (as an embolus). Anticoagulants (blood thinners) prevent deep vein thrombosis. Passive and active range-of-motion exercises are other possible preventive measures.

TRAUMATIC BRAIN INJURIES

Every year an estimated 2 million Americans suffer from **traumatic brain injury (TBI)**, ranging from mild concussion to the more devastating kind that renders injured people comatose for the remainder of their lives. Although some people are fortunate enough to return to their previous functioning level shortly after receiving their injury, statistics related to TBI are depressing. Of the 75,000 to 100,000 people who die each year from TBI, many are children and young adults. Of the individuals who do survive, 500,000 receive injuries severe enough to necessitate hospitalization, and 90,000 of the injuries result in severe and permanent disability. Most brain-related disabilities, including physical, cognitive, and psychosocial difficulties, necessitate at least 5 to 10 years of difficult and painful rehabilitation; many affected patients require lifelong treatment and attention. When these statistics expand to include families of individuals with brain injuries, the number of people whose lives are forever altered by TBI rises to staggering proportions.

The primary goal of the rehabilitation professional treating the survivor of brain injury is to restore the patient to the highest possible level of independent functioning.

Head injuries are classified as either penetrating or closed-head injuries. In penetrating injuries, an object lacerates the scalp, fractures the skull, and injures the soft tissue in its path, thus destroying nerve cells. In a closed-head injury, some application of force causes the brain to collide with an inner surface of the skull. There is often violent twisting action, which causes the upper section of the brain to rotate while the lower end remains securely anchored in a stationary position. This results in widespread damage called *shearing* (when the brain mass is rotated in the cranial vault). Brain injuries are also possible as a result of other traumas (e.g., electrocution, drug overdose).

Brain injuries are classified as *mild, moderate, severe,* or *catastrophic.* Brief or no loss of consciousness characterizes mild brain injury, which is the majority of head injuries. Neurologic examination findings are often normal. Postconcussive syndrome sometimes persists for months, years, or indefinitely. Signs and symptoms include fatigue, headache, vertigo, lethargy, irritability, personality changes, cognitive deficits, decreased information processing speed, and difficulties with memory, understanding, learning, and perception. These symptoms can lead to feelings of incompetence, guilt, and frustration. Family members also may become impatient and frustrated at times.

Moderate brain injuries are characterized by a period of unconsciousness ranging from 1 to 24 hours. Cognitive skills—including planning, sequencing, judgment, reasoning, and computation skills—are usually impaired. In general, some psychosocial problems also occur, such as self-centeredness, denial, mood swings, agitation, depression, lethargy, sexual dysfunction, emotional lability, low tolerance for frustration, poor judgment, and behavioral outbursts.

Patients with severe brain injuries experience unconsciousness or posttrauma amnesia for longer than 8 days. Cognitive, psychosocial, and behavioral disabilities result.

In catastrophic brain injury, a defining characteristic is a coma lasting several months or longer. Affected individuals sometimes appear to be awake. However, they generally never regain significant, meaningful communication with their environment.

The nurse performing a rehabilitative assessment of the patient with TBI commonly observes inconsistent performance, anger, and frustration. However, ineffective problem-solving strategies can be modified (unless the injury is neurogenic). Cognitive barriers to rehabilitative recovery include problems in thinking and reasoning (impaired memory), impaired concentration and attention, and impaired informational processing speed. Psychosocially, the patient appears to lack initiative; however, this is a normal consequence of a head injury. Egocentric (self-centered) behavior often is noted in brain-injured individuals, as is depression. In general, the more the memory improves, the more the patient becomes depressed. Abstinence from alcohol is a primary injunction for any patient with a brain injury, because alcohol increases the chance of abnormal electrical impulses and seizure activity.

Continuous and honest involvement of the family, as a victim of the injury and an equal participant in the rehabilitation process, is crucial for successfully rehabilitating a patient with TBI. Rehabilitation professionals must be available and honest when reporting to families. Equal communication with all family members is important, as is encouraging the family to become involved in counseling and education. Family members should be reminded to be aware of each other's needs and interests. Help them become involved in a support group and inform them of available community resources.

Regardless of personality types, any disability, particularly a TBI, is a crisis that threatens many aspects of the patient's and family's life: job income, pleasures, family, community ties, health, and life. The fears are valid.

Patient problems for a patient with TBI include but are not limited to those in Nursing Care Plan 39.2.

PEDIATRIC REHABILITATION NURSING

Pediatric rehabilitation nursing is a specialty practice area that also continues to expand within the field of rehabilitation. The field of pediatric rehabilitation has undergone marked development since the early 1900s. The number of children with chronic disabling conditions has increased as a result of improved rates of survival from illnesses and injuries that once were fatal.

Since the 1990s the field has evolved from a mere combination of pediatrics and rehabilitation into a true specialty committed to the care of children with disabilities or other chronic conditions and their families. Nurses in this field, in a collaborative relationship with the interdisciplinary team, provide a continuum of care so that affected children can become contributing members of society and function at their maximal potential. Infants, children, and adolescents with a variety of disabling conditions receive specialized care from hospital to home, from clinic to school. Physical, emotional, social, cultural, educational, developmental, and spiritual dimensions are subjects of consideration in a holistic approach to care. The goal is to cherish and foster the unique qualities of each child.

The primary difference between rehabilitation of children and rehabilitation of adults is the developmental potential of each child. Children and adolescents can receive an injury resulting in disability at any age, with very different consequences for the patient's future, depending on the age and developmental level at which the trauma occurred. Children who are born with genetic disorders, who are premature, or whose fetal development is affected by maternal disease, injury, or substance abuse require services focused on habilitation rather than rehabilitation. Whereas *rehabilitation* refers to the relearning of skills or behaviors lost as a result of disease or injury, *habilitation* refers to the process of acquiring skills and behaviors by an individual whose development has been affected by disease or other disabling conditions since birth or very early childhood.

In summary, as leader, advocate, and educator, the pediatric rehabilitation nurse has the power to have a very positive influence on the lives of children with disabilities and chronic conditions, as well as on their families. By facilitating transition from hospital to home and community and by offering counseling and support to families, the nurse provides assistance in meeting identified needs. By designing an individualized plan of care that incorporates the values and beliefs supported in rehabilitation, the nurse has the opportunity to affect the quality of the child's life for the better and to facilitate the child's interactions with family and friends within the community.

GERONTOLOGIC REHABILITATION NURSING

Gerontologic rehabilitation nursing is a specialty practice that focuses on the unique requirements of older adult rehabilitation patients. Because the needs of older adults differ from those of the rest of the population, the knowledge and skill needed to provide quality patient care warrants special attention. Gerontologic rehabilitation nurses are knowledgeable about techniques of caring for the aged and rehabilitation concepts and principles. This unique type of nursing combines knowledge of the aging process and rehabilitation practice in the specialized task of caring for older adults with a disability or long-term health problem.

A primary goal in gerontologic rehabilitation nursing is the assistance of older adult patients in achieving

Nursing Care Plan 39.2 The Patient With Traumatic Brain Injury

J. is a 33-year-old man employed as a chemist for a large pharmaceutical company. He lives alone in a second-floor apartment. After not reporting to work for 2 days, he was found unconscious on the floor of his bathroom. He was taken to the hospital, where he remained in a deep coma for 5 days as a result of electrocution that caused anoxic encephalopathy. After 4 weeks, J. was transferred to an acute rehabilitation unit.

PATIENT PROBLEM

Impaired Neurovascular Function, related to increased intracranial pressures as demonstrated by the following:

- Disturbance in orientation
- Disturbance in memory
- Disturbance in attention and concentration
- Disturbance in judgment
- Disturbance in reasoning and problem solving

Patient Goals and Expected Outcomes	Nursing Interventions	Evaluation
Patient will provide accurate responses to orientation testing	Provide reality orientation and testing.	Patient is able to consistently respond accurately when reality testing is done.
Patient will have increased attention span	Implement memory training program. Implement visual and auditory cues. Control environmental stimuli when working with patient.	Patient is able to follow a three-step command consistently. Patient is able to recall names and activities completed during the previous 3 days. Patient is able to complete a task once it is begun.
Patient will demonstrate appropriate behavior that is based on reality	Provide appropriate level of interactions with a gradual increase in socially appropriate interactions.	Patient is able to demonstrate good judgment in abstract problem-solving situations given to him.
Patient will demonstrate improved accuracy in problem solving	Cue patient on the focus of task before he starts, and reorient him as required. Implement sensory stimulation program.	Patient is able to use information to reach appropriate conclusions.

PATIENT PROBLEM

Potential for Injury, related to neurologic deficit resulting in the following:

- Impaired judgment
- Impaired mobility
- Impaired coordination
- History of injuries
- Decreased sensation
- Omission of safety measures (e.g., locking of wheelchair, positioning feet)

Patient Goals and Expected Outcomes	Nursing Interventions	Evaluation
Patient will demonstrate an awareness of potential safety hazards Patient will demonstrate safety in activities of daily living (ADLs) and mobility activities Patient will demonstrate knowledge and use of safety devices Patient will obtain assistance for activities appropriately to ensure safety Patient will remain injury free	Initiate appropriate safety precautions to protect patient from injury. Establish behavior modification program for isolated safety activities. Use verbal cueing to prevent injury in all activities. Reinforce use of appropriate measures to compensate for the patient's physical or cognitive deficits. Explain side effects of medications that have potential to affect the patient's safety. Anticipate the patient's needs (e.g., toileting, eating, and drinking) to minimize impulsive movement. Use calm, controlled, and consistent manner. Use short-term, goal-directed techniques. Assume nothing: review, review, review.	Periodically evaluate and document patient's progress toward prevention of injury. Consult with other health care professionals on methods to prevent patient from sustaining injury.

CRITICAL THINKING QUESTIONS

1. Deficits with socialization, motivation, and sexual behaviors that occur after brain injury result from damage to which portion of the brain? Discuss appropriate nursing interventions for a patient with this type of injury.
2. A patient recovering from a traumatic brain injury has problems telling the difference between objects that have a similar shape. What is this type of deficit, and what nursing interventions are appropriate for a patient with this deficit?
3. What interventions are most appropriate to begin establishing communication with a patient who is just emerging from coma after a brain injury?

From CDC: The Primer, n.d. Retrieved from *https://www.cdc.gov/masstrauma/preparedness/primer.pdf.*

their personal optimal level of health and well-being through holistic care in a therapeutic environment. This aim is similar to that of general rehabilitation nursing but with a special focus on the geriatric population, considering their special needs, roles, and social relationships, and the potential physical limitations that are possible as a result of the aging process.

Gerontologic rehabilitation nurses strive not only to provide rehabilitative care but also to teach prevention. Thus gerontologic rehabilitation nurses have an opportunity to function within primary, secondary, and tertiary levels of care, with the universal goal of helping older adult patients to achieve optimal wellness and self-care.

CONCLUSION

Rehabilitation nursing is a career with several key requirements and rewards. This type of responsibility should be taken seriously because it can significantly affect the future of patients with disabilities. Rehabilitation nurses facilitate the change from resistance to openness, turning inertia into action. The focus must be maintained on the assets and the successes of people who have disabilities.

Ralph Waldo Emerson (1803–1882) summed it up succinctly when he wrote, "It is one of the most beautiful compensations of this life that no man can sincerely try to help another without helping himself."

Get Ready for the NCLEX® Examination!

Key Points

- Rehabilitation is the process of maximizing an individual's capabilities or resources to foster optimal independent functioning.
- The patient is the most important team member and must be involved in planning the programs and learning in detail about the disabilities, the ways of accomplishing the goals, and the options available.
- Rehabilitation nursing aims toward preventing complications of disease or trauma and toward maintaining or restoring function.
- Basic rehabilitation is possible regardless of the cause of disability. The rehabilitation team individualizes care by developing a goal-directed, comprehensive care plan for each patient.
- A disability has a number of potential effects on both the patient and the family, including behavioral and emotional changes and changes in roles, body image, self-concept, and family dynamics.
- Holistic nursing interventions are used to assist the patient in attaining an optimal level of functioning and well-being.
- A comprehensive rehabilitation plan is multifaceted and properly involves a functional assessment, an evaluation conference, and a family conference.
- The focus of all rehabilitation is on the patient's abilities, not on his or her disabilities.

Additional Learning Resources

SG Go to your Study Guide for additional learning activities to help you master this chapter content.

evolve Be sure to visit the Evolve site at *http://evolve.elsevier.com/Cooper/foundationsadult/* for additional online resources.

Review Questions for the NCLEX® Examination

1. When setting goals for an elderly patient, the nurse should consider what primary goal of rehabilitation?
   1. Enabling patient's return to work
   2. Teaching safe mobility
   3. Improving quality of life
   4. Reducing cellular destruction

2. A 19-year-old patient is seen in the emergency department after a diving accident. She is noted as having a spinal cord injury at the cervical level (C3). Which patient problem is likely?
   1. *Inability to Maintain Adequate Breathing Pattern, related to neurogenic injury*
   2. *Inadequate Fluid Volume, related to osmotic diuresis*
   3. *Prolonged Pain, related to disease process*
   4. *Insufficient Knowledge, related to disease process*

3. An 11-year-old boy had a head injury from being struck in the skull by a baseball bat. When he awakens in the hospital 3 weeks later, how would his head injury be classified?
   1. Mild brain injury
   2. Moderate brain injury
   3. Severe brain injury
   4. Catastrophic brain injury

4. A patient has been in the intensive care unit for several days after a head injury. His condition is stable, but today he has shown no signs of improvement. Over the past shift, the patient's father has seemed increasingly upset over small concerns. Toward the end of the shift, he yells at the nurse when the intravenous (IV) alarm goes off. What would be the most appropriate response by the nurse?
   1. "You sound upset."
   2. "I am going to get my supervisor for you."
   3. "You need a break."
   4. "Maybe you had better speak to the physician."

5. What term is the student nurse referring to that describes a disadvantage for a person that results from an impairment or a disability and limits that person's fulfillment of his or her normal roles?
   1. Disability
   2. Impairment
   3. Handicap
   4. Inconvenience
6. The nurse is considering a position on a rehabilitation care unit that uses the concept of a transdisciplinary rehabilitation team. The nurse must be aware that this type of care will require what characteristics? *(Select all that apply.)*
   1. The ability to work with all members of the rehabilitation team
   2. Organized approaches to care
   3. Skills in all therapies that are provided
   4. Willingness to cross-train with other disciplines
   5. Developing expertise in a limited number of skills
7. Which are barriers to cultural competence? *(Select all that apply.)*
   1. Respect for the beliefs of others
   2. Knowing all members of a cultural group are not necessarily alike
   3. Believing that one's own culture is better than others
   4. Treating one group better than another on the basis of culture or race
   5. Performing self-assessment of awareness of various cultural beliefs
8. As part of the rehabilitation treatment team, why is the nurse often the first professional to detect symptoms of posttraumatic stress disorder (PTSD)?
   1. Nurses are more intuitive than other members of the team.
   2. The rehabilitation team has no need to address this issue.
   3. Nurses are the only members of the team knowledgeable about PTSD.
   4. Nurses are in the unique position of having extended time to talk with patients and hear their concerns, feelings, and needs.
9. The nurse is caring for a veteran who has shrapnel embedded in his eye as a result of a polytrauma–blast-related injury (PT/BRI). How should the nurse classify this injury?
   1. Primary
   2. Secondary
   3. Tertiary
   4. Quaternary
10. When caring for a patient with PTSD, what should the nurse's initial action with the patient be?
    1. The nurse should first communicate the planned routine for the rehabilitation unit.
    2. The nurse should first work with the patient to establish goals for the plan of care.
    3. The nurse should first determine the family's level of involvement with care.
    4. The nurse should establish a therapeutic nurse-patient relationship.
11. Which nurse is demonstrating a desired quality of a rehabilitation nurse? *(Select all that apply.)*
    1. The nurse is focusing on helping the patient work toward a cure for his condition.
    2. The nurse includes the patient's family in the plan of care.
    3. The nurse helps the patient achieve the goal of reentry into the home or community.
    4. The nurse uses therapeutic communication skills with the patient and family.
    5. The nurse encourages the patient to delay rehabilitation until his strength increases.
12. When dealing with the patient, what must the rehab nurse remember?
    1. The nurse is frequently interacting with people experiencing change.
    2. The nurse must ensure change is occurring with each patient.
    3. The nurse is always changing.
    4. The nurse is the center of change.
13. Family centered care recognizes that when caring for a child with disabilities, which of the following is true?
    1. The family needs assistance.
    2. The family and professional are equals in a partnership.
    3. The family is in charge.
    4. The family must understand they must change.
14. Reasons a patient may be admitted for rehabilitation include which of the following? *(Select all that apply.)*
    1. Post coronary bypass
    2. Cardiopulmonary disease
    3. Diabetic ketoacidosis
    4. Urinary tract infection
    5. Cardiovascular accident
15. A 10-year-old patient keeps crying and saying "No, no," moving as if uncomfortable, then returns to sleep every few hours throughout the night. Her mother is not sure why this is happening. What should the nurse suspect?
    1. The patient is not comfortable in her bed and should be awakened to assess comfort level.
    2. The patient may have experienced a traumatic event, which may need further investigation.
    3. The mother is upsetting the patient by staying in the room.
    4. The patient is acting out because of staying in a strange place.

40 Hospice Care

http://evolve.elsevier.com/Cooper/foundationsadult/

Objectives

1. Discuss the philosophy of hospice care.
2. Differentiate between palliative care and curative care.
3. Discuss four criteria for admission to hospice care.
4. Name the members of the interdisciplinary team, and explain their roles.
5. Develop a care plan with patient goals related to the common symptoms of terminal illness.
6. Discuss the usefulness of pain assessments and when it is best to complete them.
7. Discuss the role of hospice in families' bereavement period.
8. Discuss two ethical issues in hospice care.

Key Terms

adjuvant (ĂJ-ŭ-vănt, p. 1212)
bereavement (bĭ-RĒV-mĭnt, p. 1210)
cachexia (kă-KĔK-sē-ŭ, p. 1215)
curative treatment (KYŪR-ŭ-tĭv TRĒT-mĭnt, p. 1206)
holistic (hō-LĬS-tĭk, p. 1207)
hospices (HŎS-pĭs-ĕz, p. 1205)
interdisciplinary team (ĭn-tŭr-DĬS-ŭ-plĭn-ăr-ē TĒM, p. 1207)
pain assessment (PĀN ŭs-SĔS-mĭnt, p. 1211)
palliative care (PĂL-ē-ă-tĭv KĂR, p. 1205)
primary caregiver (PRĪ-măr-ē KĂR-gĭv-ŭr, p. 1207)
psychosocial (sī-kō-SŌ-shŭl, p. 1209)
respite care (RĔS-pĭt KĂR, p. 1209)
terminal illness (TŬR-mĭn-ŭl ĬL-nŭs, p. 1204)
titrated (TĪ-trāt-ĭd, p. 1212)

The philosophy of hospice is to provide care and support to patients with a **terminal illness** (a disease in an advanced stage with no known cure and poor prognosis) and their families. An interdisciplinary team promotes comfort, care, and support through compassion, interest, and genuine concern (Box 40.1) to promote quality of life as the end approaches. With hospice support, the patient and the family recognize that dying is a natural part of life. The goals are to maximize the quality of life and keep the patient as comfortable as possible in the home or setting that he or she chooses. Studies have shown that patients cared for in a hospice setting have a higher quality of pain management accompanied by pain-related assessments than those patients not in a hospice setting (Goldstein and Glaser, 2011).

HISTORICAL OVERVIEW

"Hospice" is from the Latin word *hospitium,* meaning "hospitality" and "lodging." The concept originated in Europe, where hospices were resting places for travelers. Monks and nuns believed that service to one's neighbor was a sign of love and dedication to God. Typical medieval hospices run by monks and nuns were a combination guesthouse and infirmary. They were places of refuge for the poor, the sick, and travelers on religious journeys. They provided food, shelter, and care to ill guests until the guests were strong enough to continue their journey or died. As centuries passed and hospices developed into hospitals, the emphasis on physical care increased, and spiritual care became less important.

The idea of hospice was renewed in the 1960s in London, when Dame Cicely Saunders, a nurse and physician, realized that terminally ill patients needed a different kind of care. She had a patient who was dying of a terminal illness, and she found that quality of life was not the main emphasis of his care. She then devoted her life to improving pain management and symptom control for people who were dying. She believed it is important for each patient to know his or her own contribution to life and that his or her life had meaning. She began her work at St. Joseph's Hospice, operated by the Irish Sisters of Charity. In 1968 St. Christopher's Hospice of London was opened, and this hospice continues to serve as a national and international education, training, and research center for professionals involved in the hospice approach to care of terminally ill patients.

The philosophy of hospice migrated to the United States in the early 1970s; the first hospice program opened in Connecticut in 1971. Since then, health care providers, nurses, clergy, social workers, and many nonprofessional volunteers have worked together to

Box 40.1 Hospice Nurse's Perspective

Frequently I am asked whether it is depressing to work with terminally ill patients and death every day. Frankly, I cannot think of doing anything else. Death is as much a part of life as is birth, and through hospice, I am challenged to find very individualized and innovative ways to give back the control that dying patients have lost while being treated for various kinds of terminal illnesses.

As a hospice nurse, I am guided by a dedicated interdisciplinary team to achieve symptom control so that quality of life can again be realized. Many hopes and dreams can become reality once a patient is comfortable. Frequently comfort enables our patients to take one more family trip, attend a great family reunion, and go to a special wedding, graduation, or anniversary. What could be more rewarding than playing a part in that and seeing the joy it brings? Together we rejoice in the celebration of life, see families reunited, see peace made with God, review each triumph, and weep over each disappointment and loss. Families are enabled to say all the things they could not find words for before: "Thank you"; "I'm sorry"; "Forgive me"; "I love you"; and finally the good-byes.

Of course there is sadness, but there are also reconciliation, peace, and beauty, for this is a part of life and these are the important things in life. Daily, I feel so personally grateful for every person I have known and loved and lost, for I know that I have learned far more about living from them than I could ever teach them about dying. Through it all, I have become closer to God, more compassionate, more open to people, and more sensitive to the needs of others. Hospice nursing has given me direction and hope.

Kathleen Carsten, CRNH
Hospice Nurse

develop more than 4000 hospice programs serving between 1.6 and 1.7 million patients throughout the United States. Despite the rates of hospice use there are some consistent myths. These include the following (Morrow, 2018a):

- Myth 1: Hospice means giving up hope.
- Myth 2: Hospice means I must sign a DNR order.
- Myth 3: Hospice is only for cancer patients.
- Myth 4: Hospice is only for patients actively dying or close to death.

Hospices serve patients with various primary disease processes, the most common being cancer, which accounts for 27.2% of the patient population. Dementia-related disease processes account for 18% of the client population, and cardiac and lung diseases account for almost 18.7% of the primary diagnoses of the patients served by hospice (National Hospice and Palliative Care Organization, 2018).

Hospices vary in structure and organization. Inpatient facilities and residences may be hospital based or freestanding. The freestanding hospices have an atmosphere that is more like that of a friendly dormitory than that of a hospital. The patients usually wear their own clothes, move about the hospice as they choose, and socialize with each other and with the staff. The kitchen is always open for individually prepared food, as well as for conversation. Some hospices are operated by a home health agency or community-based organization in which care usually is provided in the patient's home, wherever that home may be. Hospice care also may be given in a long-term care setting. On occasion, a hospice patient goes into the hospital and receives hospice services for control of acute pain or for 5-day respite care for the family or care provider on an occasional basis. Hospice care can be delivered intermittently or continuously. Skilled team members, including health care providers, nurses, hospice aides, social workers, spiritual leaders, bereavement coordinators, and volunteers, make visits to the home or wherever the patient most often resides. The team provides comfort measures, as well as medications and therapy. The team members also educate the patient and the caregiver with regard to disease processes, medication administration, and how to provide daily care. Expert help and support is available to the patient and the caregiver 24 hours a day, either by phone or in person.

The Medicare Hospice Benefit came into effect in 1983, and today hospice services are reimbursable through Medicare, Medicaid, and most private insurance companies. Medicare certification or state licensure ensures quality hospice services (see the Lifespan Considerations for older adults box).

Lifespan Considerations

Older Adults

Hospice Care

- The Hospice Medicare Benefit covers all expenses for palliative care related to the terminal illness, including professional staff visits, medication, equipment, occasional short periods of respite for caregivers, and acute care when needed for the control of symptoms.
- Hospice often provides dying older adults with a higher level of control and dignity than do other types of health care.
- The primary caregiver is often a member of the immediate family, such as the spouse or adult child.
- The Hospice Medicare Benefit provides for bereavement follow-up care for up to 1 year after the patient's death.

From Centers for Medicare & Medicaid Services: Coverage of hospice services under hospital insurance. Medicare benefit policy manual (Publication No. 100-02), 2015. Retrieved from *www.cms.gov/Regulations-and-Guidance/Guidance/Manuals/downloads/bp102c09.pdf.*

PALLIATIVE VERSUS CURATIVE CARE

Palliative care, as defined by the World Health Organization (2017), is an approach that improves the quality of life of patients and their families facing the problem associated with life-threatening illness, through the prevention and relief of suffering by means of early identification and impeccable assessment and treatment of pain and other problems, physical, psychosocial, and

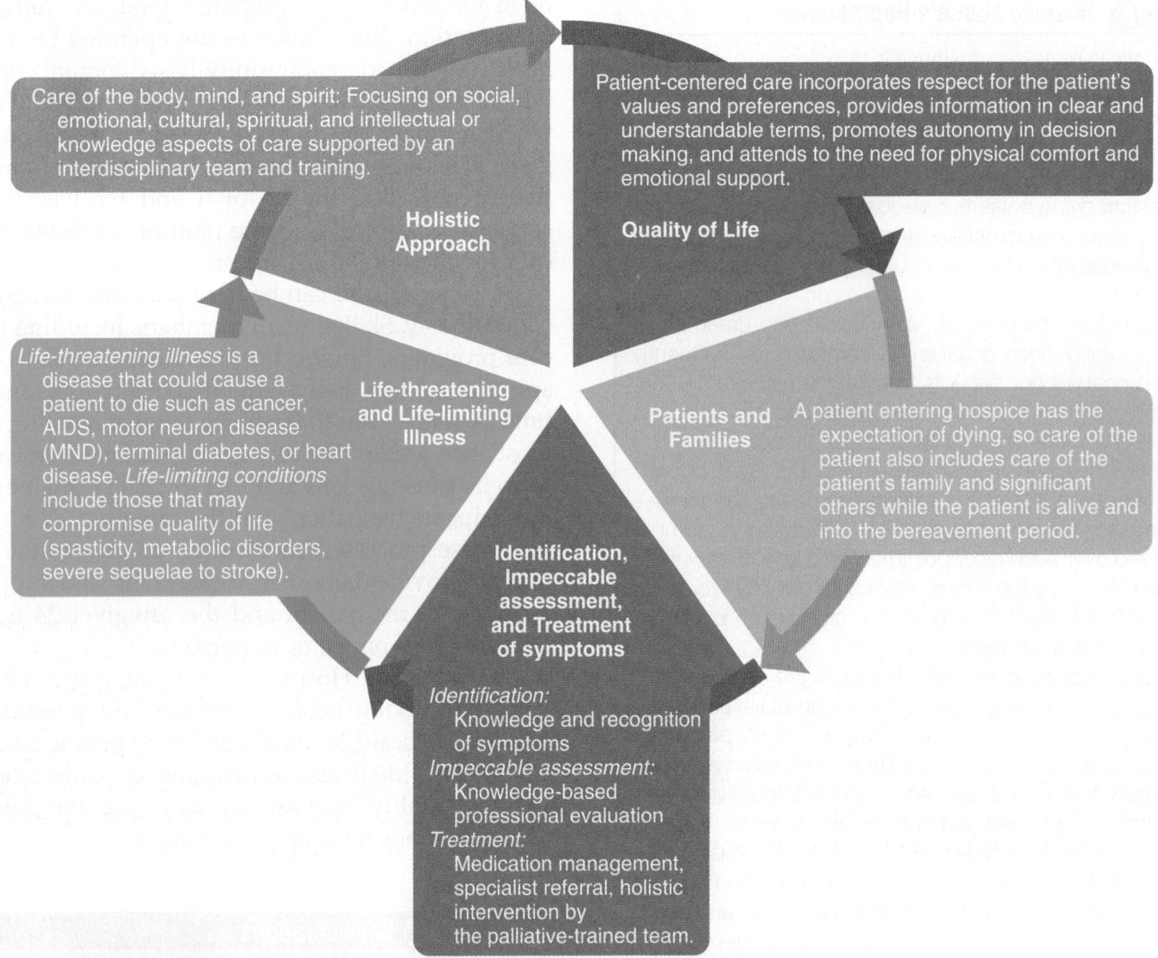

Care of the body, mind, and spirit: Focusing on social, emotional, cultural, spiritual, and intellectual or knowledge aspects of care supported by an interdisciplinary team and training.
Patient-centered care incorporates respect for the patient's values and preferences, provides information in clear and understandable terms, promotes autonomy in decision making, and attends to the need for physical comfort and emotional support.
Holistic Approach
Quality of Life
Life-threatening illness is a disease that could cause a patient to die such as cancer, AIDS, motor neuron disease (MND), terminal diabetes, or heart disease. Life-limiting conditions include those that may compromise quality of life (spasticity, metabolic disorders, severe sequelae to stroke).
Life-threatening and Life-limiting Illness
Patients and Families
A patient entering hospice has the expectation of dying, so care of the patient also includes care of the patient's family and significant others while the patient is alive and into the bereavement period.
Identification, Impeccable assessment, and Treatment of symptoms
Identification: Knowledge and recognition of symptoms
Impeccable assessment: Knowledge-based professional evaluation
Treatment: Medication management, specialist referral, holistic intervention by the palliative-trained team.

Fig. 40.1 Components of palliative care. (From Abernethy AP, Wheeler JL, Bull J: Development of a health information technology–based data system in community-based hospice and palliative care. *Am J Preventive Med* 2011;40[5 Suppl 2]:S217–S224.)

spiritual (Fig. 40.1). **Curative treatment** is aggressive care in which the goal and intent are curing the disease and prolonging life at all cost. When a patient with a life-threatening illness has undergone all reasonable treatment and the disease has not been arrested or cured, it is necessary for the patient to decide whether continued active therapy is feasible or beneficial. By that time, the patient already may have experienced many debilitating physical and emotional symptoms as a result of the treatments or the progression of the disease. This situation leads the patient and family to decide whether to continue with curative treatments or to transition to palliative measures. Palliative care is not curative but aims to relieve pain and distress and to control symptoms of disease. It is important to give the patient and caregiver honest and accurate information so that they are able to make appropriate decisions.

CRITERIA FOR ADMISSION TO HOSPICE

The patient is required to meet certain criteria to be admitted into hospice:

- The health care provider must certify that the patient's illness is terminal and that the patient has a prognosis of 6 months or less to live. The health care provider must have a doctorate of medicine or osteopathy to make the prognosis determination.
- For the patient to qualify for Medicare or Medicaid assistance, two health care providers are required to verify that the patient is dying and has less than 6 months to live. This must be documented by the medical provider in a narrative that supports the reason for the limited life expectancy. The hospice patient who continues to live beyond the estimated time period still qualifies for Medicare if hospice criteria are still met (Medicare.gov, n.d.).
- It is mandatory that the patient desires the services. The patient and caregiver must understand that all treatment will be palliative and that no further curative treatment will be rendered.
- The patient and caregiver are required to understand and agree that hospice staff will plan the care according to comfort and that they will not necessarily perform life-support measures.
- The patient and caregiver—or, if the patient is unable to participate, the caregiver—are required to understand the prognosis and be willing to participate in the planning of care.

Many hospices in the United States request that the patient have a **primary caregiver** (a person who assumes ongoing responsibility for health maintenance and therapy for the illness). The caregiver is sometimes an immediate family member and sometimes a significant other, a friend, or a hired caregiver. Caregivers' services become vital when patients are no longer able to care for themselves safely. If a patient resides in a freestanding hospice residence, a long-term care facility, or a residential home, the nursing staff is designated as the primary caregiver.

Once the criteria are met and a patient is admitted to hospice, the staff performs complete physical, psychosocial, and spiritual assessments, and those involved discuss the care openly. The patient and caregiver receive a complete explanation of the hospice program and the philosophy of hospice, along with the interdisciplinary team concept.

GOALS OF HOSPICE

To provide effective hospice care, an understanding of the philosophy and its relationship with the patient's responses and points of view is beneficial. The basic goals of hospice address the following:

- Controlling or alleviating the patient's symptoms
- Allowing the patient and caregiver to be involved in the decisions regarding the plan of care
- Encouraging the patient and caregiver to live life to the fullest
- Providing continuous support to maintain patient and family confidence
- Educating and supporting the primary caregiver in the home setting that the patient chooses

INTERDISCIPLINARY TEAM

In this approach of hospice, defined as **holistic** (pertaining to the total patient care in which the physical, emotional, social, economic, and spiritual needs of the patient are considered), an interdisciplinary team manages the problems (Fig. 40.2). The **interdisciplinary team** (a multiprofessional health team whose members work together in caring for a terminally ill patient) develops and supervises the plan of care in conjunction with all those involved with the care. The core interdisciplinary team members are the medical director, the nurse coordinator, the social worker, and the spiritual coordinator. To provide support to the dying patient and the caregiver, the interdisciplinary team considers all aspects of the family unit. They include the family in all decisions and care planning because families also experience the stresses of the terminal illness and death of the patient (Fig. 40.3). These stresses also extend into the bereavement period after the patient dies.

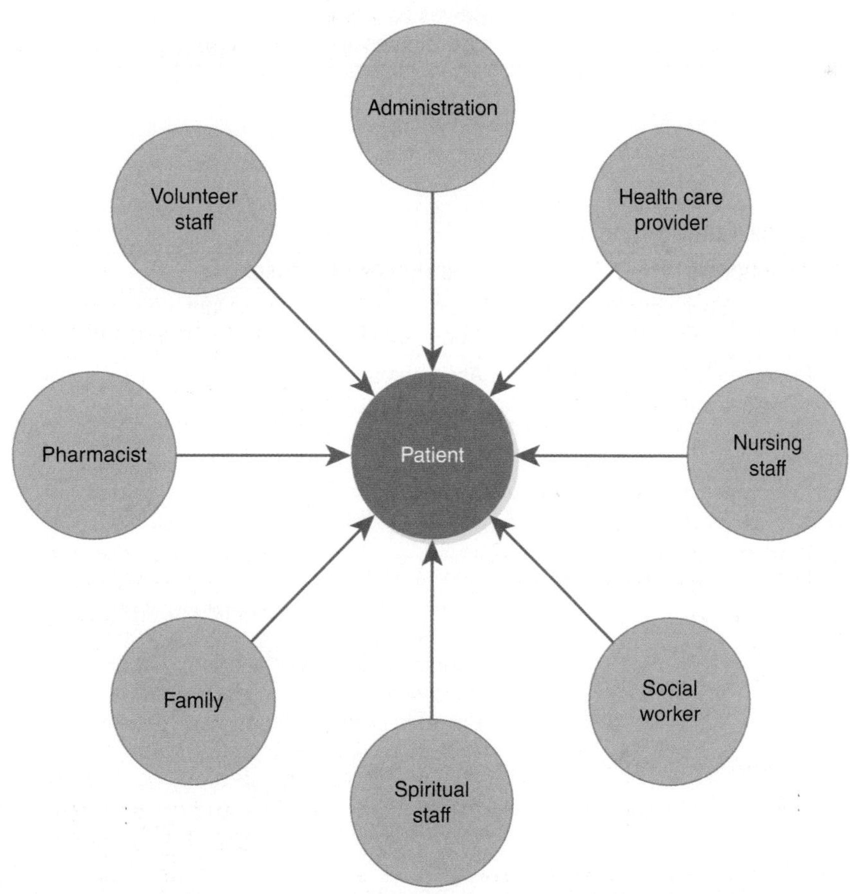

Fig. 40.2 The relationship between the hospice team members and the patient.

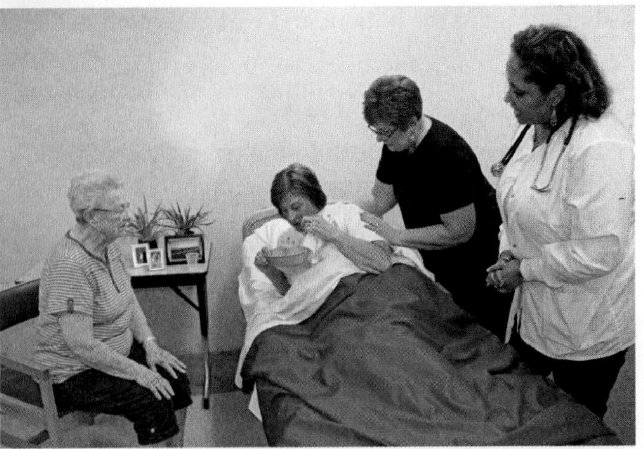

Fig. 40.3 Family member participation with the hospice care team.

Each hospice patient is assigned a primary team that consists of the patient's own health care provider, the primary hospice nurse, the social worker, a primary hospice aide, a primary volunteer, and a spiritual leader. This group of professionals, along with the interdisciplinary team, develops and is responsible for carrying out the plan of care. Regular and frequent team meetings are held to discuss the patient's physical, mental, and spiritual conditions; the plan of care is revised as needed. The effectiveness of the plan of care is also discussed. The team meeting is the forum for bringing together all members' observations and thoughts respectfully, and the team strives to function as a cohesive unit to use all expertise and resources in the interest of providing quality patient care (Tables 40.1 and 40.2).

Table 40.1 Core Interdisciplinary Hospice Team

TEAM MEMBER	BACKGROUND	FUNCTION OR RESPONSIBILITY
Medical director	Licensed physician	Mediates between the hospice team and attending medical provider Provides consultation relative to the medical aspect of care
Nurse coordinator	Licensed registered nurse	Manages the patient's care Explains the service, admits the patients, assigns the primary team
Social worker	Bachelor's degree in social work	Evaluates the patient's psychosocial needs Serves as resource for potential community services Assists with counseling in grief issues
Spiritual coordinator	Seminary degree	Serves as liaison between the patient and the spiritual community Coordinates spiritual support

Table 40.2 Primary Hospice Team

TEAM MEMBER	BACKGROUND	FUNCTION OR RESPONSIBILITY
Volunteer coordinator	Experience in volunteer work	Recruits and trains the volunteers Coordinates assignments of volunteers
Bereavement coordinator	Professional with grief experience	Assesses and supports the bereaved survivor Facilitates support groups
Hospice pharmacist	Licensed registered pharmacist	Provides drug consultation
Primary health care provider	Licensed physician	Responsible for the medical aspect of symptom control for patient
Primary nurse	Licensed registered nurse	Serves as liaison between (1) patient and (2) caregiver, health care provider, and interdisciplinary team Evaluates patient's response to treatment Educates the patient and family in disease process and care Assesses symptom management Provides emotional support to patient and caregiver
Primary spiritual leader	As required by religious group	Supports patient and caregiver in coping with fears and uncertainty about spiritual issues
Hospice volunteer	Completion of volunteer training	Provides companionship for patient and caregiver Available for short periods of respite care
Hospice aide	Certified as a home health aide	Administers personal care and assistance with bathing

MEDICAL DIRECTOR

The medical director has a doctorate of medicine or osteopathy and assumes overall responsibility for the medical component of the hospice patient's care program. The medical director does not take the place of the patient's health care provider but acts as a consultant for the health care provider. The medical director, with consultation from the interdisciplinary team, medically certifies the patient's eligibility for hospice care. The medical director is a mediator between the interdisciplinary team and the health care provider. He or she oversees the plan of care, ensuring that the care being provided and ordered is palliative in nature.

NURSE COORDINATOR AND HOSPICE NURSES

The nurse coordinator is a registered nurse who coordinates the implementation of the plan of care for each patient. The nurse coordinator often performs the initial assessment, admits the patient to the hospice program, and develops the plan of care along with the interdisciplinary team. The nurse coordinator also ensures that the plan of care is being followed, coordinates assignments of the hospice nurses and aides, facilitates meetings, and determines methods of payment.

Hospice nurses coordinate services of the hospice team, which includes hospice health care providers, pharmacists, dietitians, physical therapists, social workers, clergy, certified nursing assistants, and hospice volunteers. Hospice nurses must possess compassion, excellent teaching skills, and the ability to adapt therapeutically to the hospice patients' many needs. It is also necessary for a hospice nurse to be especially adept in pain and symptom control.

SOCIAL WORKER

The social worker evaluates and assesses the **psychosocial** (a combination of psychological and social factors) needs of the patient. The social worker assists with accessing community resources and filing insurance papers, supports the patient and caregiver with emotional and grief issues, and, in some cases when communication difficulties are present, also assists with counseling. The social worker provides these services under the direction of the health care provider and in accordance with the plan of care.

SPIRITUAL COORDINATOR

The spiritual coordinator, who may be affiliated with any religion, is the liaison between the spiritual community and the interdisciplinary team. The spiritual coordinator assists with the spiritual assessment of the patient and, in keeping with patients' and families' beliefs, develops the plan of care with regard to spiritual matters. If the patient desires spiritual assistance and does not have a spiritual home, the spiritual coordinator assists in finding the spiritual support desired. The spiritual coordinator is vital in assisting the patient and caregiver to cope with fears and uncertainty. Possible support includes dealing with unfinished business and regrets and providing opportunities for reconciliation, prayer, and spiritual healing. Funeral planning and performing funeral services also are included in this role, as is continued support for the family throughout the bereavement period. In addition, the spiritual coordinator is one resource to assist with cultural differences (see the Cultural Considerations box).

Cultural Considerations

Death and Dying

- The United States is becoming increasingly multicultural, and hospice care is challenged to meet the needs of people from other cultures.
- Compassionate and empathic care bridges cultures, but it is necessary to learn as much as possible about a patient's culture to provide appropriate assistance. Each person has a different reaction and tradition regarding death and dying, but all people experience grief.
- A cultural assessment of the patient and the family must include factors such as the following:
  - Religious beliefs
  - Primary decision-making person and process
  - Dietary preferences
  - Preferred language and the need for translation services as needed, as well as written information provided in the language of preference for the patient and the family
  - Support measure preferences such as alternative medicine, as well as who is allowed to support the patient
  - The patient's perspective of death, dying, and burial
  - The family's grief processes, burial practices, and perspective of death
- The team may need to be prepared for a change in expectations regarding the death of the patient because of differences in belief systems between the patient and the surviving family members.
- Changes regarding the plan of care must not be made without discussing them with all family members.

The following sections describe additional members of the team whose services are needed to provide adequate care for the patient.

VOLUNTEER COORDINATOR

The volunteer coordinator must have experience in volunteer work. The volunteer coordinator assesses the needs of the patient and caregiver for volunteer services. When families are responsible for the total care of the patient in the home, caregiver "burnout" becomes a concern. This is when the services of volunteers become vital. They provide companionship, caregiver relief through **respite care** (a period of relief from responsibilities of caring for a patient), and emotional support. Appropriate services for the volunteer to provide are what are considered typical of a good neighbor: perhaps grocery shopping, yard work, reading to the patient, or keeping the patient company while the caregiver leaves the home for short periods. The volunteer coordinator ensures that the volunteer is adequately trained and prepared for working with the dying patient. Responsibilities also include assigning the proper volunteer to the appropriate patient. Hospice volunteers are an instrumental part of the hospice experience. To retain funding, agencies that receive Medicare and Medicaid funding are required to demonstrate that at least 5% of the work being completed is done by volunteers. Training is needed to ensure the volunteers have an understanding of the role and clear expectations relating to what they will encounter as a hospice volunteer. Training program vary and normally last about 30 hours (Morrow, 2018b).

BEREAVEMENT COORDINATOR

Bereavement is a period of mourning or an expression of grief in reaction to the death of someone close. The bereavement coordinator is a professional who has experience in dealing with grief issues. The bereavement coordinator assesses the patient and the caregiver at admission to the hospice program and identifies potential risk factors that may arise after the death of the patient. The bereavement coordinator follows the plan of care for the bereaved caregiver for at least a year after the death. The bereavement coordinator facilitates support groups and assigns bereavement volunteers to visit the caregiver.

The bereavement coordinator sometimes also provides counseling but has the option to refer the family to other counseling if the issues are too extensive. The goals of bereavement counseling for loved ones during the patient's illness and after the death are (1) to provide support and (2) to assist survivors in the transition to a life without the deceased person. It is appropriate to incorporate grief support into the plan of care.

HOSPICE PHARMACIST

The hospice pharmacist must be a licensed pharmacist and available for consultation about the drugs the hospice patient may be taking. The pharmacist evaluates for drug-drug or drug-food interactions, appropriate drug doses, and correct administration times and routes. The pharmacist typically gives information and advice about common drugs used, administration time, and doses (Table 40.3).

NUTRITION CONSULTANT

Licensed medical nutritional therapists (LMNTs) or licensed dietitians are available for hospice consultations and for diet counseling. The hospice nurse performs the nutritional assessment at the patient's admission. If the nurse notes nutritional problems, a referral may be made to the LMNT or dietitian for assistance with diet counseling and meal planning. The LMNT or dietitian also assists with educating the caregiver about nutritional issues in end-stage diseases.

HOSPICE AIDE

The hospice aide is a certified nurse's aide who works under the supervision of the hospice nurse. The hospice aide follows the plan of care that the interdisciplinary team develops and assists the patient with bathing and hygiene, including hair, nail, oral, and skin care. The hospice aide sometimes also assists the patient or the caregiver with light housekeeping services. The patient and the hospice aide often develop a close relationship,

Table 40.3 Medications Commonly Used in Hospice Care

GENERIC NAME (BRAND NAME)	INDICATIONS	SIDE EFFECTS	NURSING INTERVENTIONS
morphine sulfate: immediate-release	Acute and severe pain	Constipation, nausea and vomiting, sedation	Assess pain control by using pain assessment; instruct about administration routinely.
morphine sulfate: controlled-release (MS Contin)	Moderate and severe pain	Constipation, nausea and vomiting, sedation	Assess pain control and medication effectiveness.
fentanyl transdermal system (Duragesic patch; an opioid)	Moderate and severe pain	Confusion, hypoventilation, nausea and vomiting, constipation	Instruct caregiver to clean patient's skin with water only and dry before application.
droperidol (Inapsine)	Emesis	Hypotension and tachycardia, drowsiness, dizziness	Ensure that caregiver is administering the antiemetic appropriately and routinely.
prochlorperazine	Emesis	Extrapyramidal symptoms, dry mouth, depression	Assess control of nausea, and ensure that caregiver is administering the antiemetic appropriately and routinely.
senna (Senokot)	Constipation	Nausea and vomiting, diarrhea, abdominal cramping	Encourage patient to drink fluids; assess gastrointestinal status, and administer the laxative routinely if patient is taking pain medication.
lorazepam (Ativan)	Anxiety	Dizziness, drowsiness, orthostatic hypotension, tachycardia	Administer routinely; instruct patient in safety issues regarding rising slowly and not driving.

and in some cases, the patient shares feelings with the aide more easily than with any other member of the team.

OTHER SERVICES

Other services, if needed, are available from a physical therapist, a speech-language pathologist, and an occupational therapist. These services are available not for rehabilitative purposes but to assist with improving the quality of life and care for the patient and the caregiver. The physical therapist assists with teaching the caregiver transferring skills, exercises that are sometimes useful to relieve muscle cramps, and wheelchair fittings. The speech-language pathologist helps with difficulties in communication or swallowing. The occupational therapist helps with positioning for comfort, providing adaptive equipment for the patient, or other assistance for comfort and for activities of daily living.

PALLIATIVE CARE/HOSPICE

The goal and emphasis of hospice is symptom management and palliative care. The team of caregivers routinely assesses, reassesses, and documents the severity, the treatment, and the control of symptoms of the illness.

When the patient's is admitted and with each subsequent visit, the nurse and the team must assess the comfort level of the patient. One assessment tool that often is used is the Edmonton Symptom Assessment System. This tool addresses the areas of pain, tiredness (lack of energy), drowsiness, nausea, appetite, shortness of breath, depression (feeling sad), anxiety or nervousness, and overall feeling of well-being. The patient is asked to rate each of these areas on a scale of 0 to 10. Having the patient participate in this way allows the patient to say where he or she has the most discomfort or area of greatest concern (National Palliative Care Research Center, 2013).

PAIN

Of all the symptoms that a dying patient experiences, pain is the most dreaded and feared; therefore pain management is a priority in hospice. Pain disrupts activities as well as the quality and enjoyment of life. To a healthy person, pain is usually temporary and tolerable, but to a terminally ill patient, it can be excruciating, constant, and terrifying. Pain takes many forms, such as physical, psychosocial, and spiritual, and addressing and alleviating it is correct and proper. It is all too easy for the caregiver caring for people experiencing pain to become frustrated and feel helpless as he or she tries to control the discomfort, which leads to feelings of guilt and inadequacy.

Initially, the health care provider may order diagnostic tests to determine the exact cause of the pain. Findings may reveal the pain to be related to tumor invasion, compression of organs or nerves, erosion of tissue, or other pathologic factors. Removing the cause is not always possible in some cases; therefore controlling the symptoms becomes central to the successful management of pain for terminally ill patients. Initial and routine assessments are vital for managing pain, and the patient is the primary source of information. The patient's self-report of intensity, quality, and management of pain provides the most significant data. The **pain assessment** (evaluation of the factors that alleviate or exacerbate a patient's pain) should include information about the severity and the history of the pain and what brings relief to the patient. Pain assessment begins with the patient's self-report, and the patient rates the pain on a scale of 0 (no pain at all) to 10 (the worst imaginable pain). Any pain the patient rates at 5 or higher on the pain scale has a great effect on the quality of life.

Clinicians use many different pain assessments, such as OLD CARTS, which stands for *o*nset, *l*ocation, *d*uration, *c*haracter of pain, *a*ggravating factors, *r*elieving factors, *t*reatments, and *s*everity. Use the pain assessment tool available at your practicing institution. Assessment of pain is ongoing; any change in the intensity or type of pain necessitates changes to the plan of care (Box 40.2).

The answers to the questions in Box 40.2 help the hospice team determine the appropriate mode of therapy

Box 40.2 Pain Assessment Questionnaire

1. Throughout our lives, most of us have had pain from time to time such as minor headaches, sprains, and toothaches. Have you had pain other than everyday kinds of pain today?
2. Where is the pain? (The use of a body chart often helps the patient to identify the location.)
3. Using the scale of 0 to 10, with 0 being no pain and 10 being the worst pain imaginable, rate the pain at its worst in the past 24 hours.
4. Using the same scale of 0 to 10, rate the pain at its lowest point in the past 24 hours.
5. Using the same scale of 0 to 10, rate the pain on the average.
6. Describe your pain. (The words the patient uses to describe the pain help you to understand the type of pain for treatment purposes.)
7. What treatments or medications are you using to control the pain?
8. Using the scale of 0 to 10, with 0 being no relief and 10 being complete relief, rate the amount of relief received from the treatment.
9. What causes or increases the pain?
10. Does the pain interfere with any of the following?
    - General activity
    - Mood
    - Walking ability
    - Normal work
    - Relations with other people
    - Sleep
    - Appetite
    - Enjoyment of life

Box 40.3 Pain Control

- It is never right for a patient to suffer pain.
- Ask the question "Are you experiencing any pain?" If the answer is yes, ask the patient to describe the pain using the pain assessment questionnaire.
- Pain is treated with medications such as morphine singularly or in combination with other medications to provide maximal relief while at the same time avoiding maximal side effects.
- Proper pain relief is provided on a regular around-the-clock basis.
- Medications should be available to manage episodes of breakthrough pain.
- Nonpharmacologic interventions should be included in the plan of care.
- The need for palliative care worldwide is enormous and will continue to increase. Symptom management and adequate pain control must be the prime objectives for the hospice nurse; at the same time, the nurse must always strive to maintain the patient's dignity and capacity to contribute to society as a full human being (Gordon, 2001).

that will be effective in managing the patient's pain. The goal of therapy is to prescribe a dose of effective drug sufficient to alleviate pain and allow the patient to remain alert enough to participate in activities of daily living (Box 40.3).

To effectively treat pain, it is important to determine which of the three main types of pain the patient is experiencing. *Somatic pain* arises from the musculoskeletal system and is described as aching, stabbing, or throbbing. Nonsteroidal antiinflammatory drugs, nonopioid drugs, and opioid drugs are often effective in treating somatic pain.

Pain that originates from the internal organs is called *visceral pain.* The words people commonly use to describe this are "cramping," "pressure," "dull pain," or "squeezing pain." Health care providers typically prescribe an anticholinergic medication alone or as an **adjuvant** (additional drug or treatment that is added to assist in the action of the primary pain treatment) to nonopioids or opioids.

Neuropathic pain arises from the nerves and the nervous system. Tingling, burning, or shooting pains often have neuropathic causes. Health care providers sometimes order anticonvulsants to be administered as an adjuvant to assist with pain control.

Lifestyle considerations are important in determining the route and the type of medication to administer for pain control. Oral medications may be preferable because they help the patient and the caregiver manage the scheduling and administration more easily. After the severity of pain and the type of medication to be used are determined, the dosage of the medication must be **titrated** (slowly increased to the level at which the drug is therapeutic). Mild to moderate pain sometimes can be managed with nonsteroidal antiinflammatory drugs; as the pain increases in severity with progression of the patient's condition, the health care provider often switches the analgesic regimen to an opioid drug, with or without adjuvant drugs. Nonsteroidal drugs can be administered along with the opioid to enhance the medication's effectiveness. Oral administration of analgesics is not always feasible because of nausea and vomiting, obstruction, or inability to swallow, and other routes (sublingual, subcutaneous, parenteral, rectal, or topical) may be considered. Morphine derivatives are often the drugs of choice in caring for hospice patients, because they can be delivered by all routes and the dosage can be titrated to control the pain. Breakthrough pain management is a primary need of hospice patients. Analgesics should be administered as needed.

Long-acting medications such as morphine sulfate (MS Contin), oxycodone (OxyContin), or fentanyl (Duragesic) patches often provide better pain control and are more convenient for the patient and the caregiver. As the pain increases, it is important to monitor the amount and frequency of medications administered. Increases in dosages may be needed to manage breakthrough pain.

As the patient's condition deteriorates and pain increases, the expert knowledge and skill of the hospice personnel in titrating and managing the pain are invaluable.

Ineffective pain management usually is associated with undermedication as a result of common myths and fears. The myths and fears are addiction, tolerance, and respiratory depression. With careful and expert monitoring by the hospice team, along with reassurance and support, these fears can be relieved.

An individualized approach is needed to manage pain successfully. Various alternative pharmacologic and nonpharmacologic options are available. Radiation therapy, nerve blocks, and psychological or physical methods can be tried in appropriate circumstances. Hot or cold packs at the site of discomfort, repositioning the patient, music therapy, relaxation techniques, acupuncture, and even transcutaneous electric nerve stimulation (TENS) are sometimes good alternatives.

Nursing Interventions and Patient Teaching

The nurse's role is to focus on the effectiveness of the care plan: that is, to ensure that the plan achieves good control of the symptoms (Nursing Care Plan 40.1). It is necessary to assess and reassess constantly the pain and the symptoms to ensure that their management is adequate. The patient and the caregiver must be educated in the appropriate administration, scheduling, and effects of the medication to help them become aware of signs and symptoms of increasing pain. The patient and the caregiver must understand that it is possible to control pain and that using large doses of opioids is common and necessary to achieve that control. Assist

Nursing Care Plan 40.1 The Hospice Patient With Metastatic Prostate Cancer

Mr. B. is a 74-year-old who has prostate cancer with bone metastasis. He complains of severe pain in his right leg and in his ribs, which he rates as a 7 to 8 on a scale of 0 to 10. Mr. B. also has shortness of breath. He is on a regimen of morphine sulfate: MS Contin, 20 mg every 12 hours, and Roxanol, 20 mg every 4 hours.

PATIENT PROBLEM

Pain, related to the cancer that has metastasized to the bone, manifested by complaints of pain, rating 7 to 8 on a scale of 0 to 10

Patient Goals and Expected Outcomes	Nursing Interventions	Evaluation
Pain will be controlled at a rating of 2 or less on a scale of 0 to 10	Assess pain control and pain level by using the pain assessment scale of 0 to 10 every visit. Assess patient's and caregiver's understanding of medication administration. Assess for compliance with medication schedule. Assess for side effects of the medications, and educate patient and caregiver accordingly. Notify the interdisciplinary team of any uncontrolled pain. Educate patient and caregiver of other pain control methods such as transcutaneous electric nerve stimulation (TENS), repositioning methods, and heat and cold treatments. Have the patient and caregiver keep a pain diary.	Patient rates pain at 7 or 8 on the pain scale of 0 to 10.

PATIENT PROBLEM

Inability to Maintain Adequate Breathing Pattern, related to disease process manifested by shortness of breath

Patient Goals and Expected Outcomes	Nursing Interventions	Evaluation
Patient will not complain of shortness of breath	Assess respiratory status and effort at every visit. Ask patient to rate respiratory effort on the scale of 0 to 10 at every visit. Assess need for oxygen use by measuring oximetry level as ordered. Administer oxygen per nasal cannula as needed. Notify the interdisciplinary team of any complaints of respiratory distress. Educate patient and caregiver about methods that ease respiratory distress (e.g., relaxation techniques, diaphragmatic breathing, medication usage, positioning). Provide emotional support to patient and caregiver at each visit.	Patient rates respiratory distress at 6 on a scale of 0 to 10. Oxygen is administered at 3 L/min by nasal cannula.

CRITICAL THINKING QUESTIONS

1. Mr. B.'s wife complains to the hospice nurse that her husband has not had a bowel movement in 3 days. What will be included in an appropriate nursing intervention that would provide relief for Mr. B.?
2. The nurse notes that Mr. B. is restless and demonstrates dyspnea. She performs an oximetry check on Mr. B. and notes that oxygen saturation is 83%. List three nursing interventions to improve his respiratory distress.

the caregiver in setting a schedule for administering the medications and then monitoring the patient's response to and compliance with the established plan. This should be documented by the caregiver and monitored by the nurse at each visit to ensure compliance and to help in determining when a change in the plan of care is necessary. Encourage the use of alternative treatment such as music therapy and relaxation methods to aid in pain control. It is important to give encouragement and positive reinforcement to the patient and the family in their efforts at following the plan.

NAUSEA AND VOMITING

Nausea and vomiting tend to be very upsetting to the patient and the caregiver. Many patients consider nausea to be worse than vomiting, because sometimes it is noticeable only to the patient and therefore is overlooked by caregivers and health care professionals. It is important to assess for the cause of nausea and vomiting, and to remove the cause if at all possible. Nausea is a possible side effect of chemotherapy and can result from obstruction, tumor, uncontrolled pain, constipation, and even food smells. At times, the treatment of the nausea is as simple as bringing in food already prepared so that the cooking smells do not bother the patient. Sometimes the drugs used for pain control cause nausea; antiemetics may be administered with the opioid analgesic. Nausea is a common side effect with the initiation of opioid treatment. This side effect usually subsides after a time, and the best response is to use an antiemetic rather than discontinue the opioid. Anxiety also has been known to cause nausea, which then leads to vomiting. Patients who vomit are typically anxious about why they are vomiting, which often worsens the symptoms.

Nursing Interventions and Patient Teaching

Educate the patient and the caregiver regarding the cause or the prevention of nausea and vomiting. Managing nausea and vomiting will include close monitoring of labs to ensure electrolyte imbalances are corrected, re-hydration and the administration of anti-emetic medications. In the acute phases of the nausea and vomiting, intravenous administration is needed. Then, oral medications can be used. Determining an effective pharmacologic regimen may be challenging. No single medication will work for each patient. Combinations of medications may be needed. Serotonin (5-HT3) angatonist medications such as ondansetron (Zofran) and dolasetron (Anzemet) and phenothiazine medications such as prochlorperazine and promethazine are frequently prescribed.

Eating slowly and in a pleasant atmosphere, with relaxation and rest periods after eating, is a good way to control the nausea. If vomiting occurs, discourage eating for a short time until peristalsis stabilizes. When the nausea and vomiting have subsided, the patient may begin drinking liquids to avoid dehydration or start eating soft, bland foods. Small, light, bland meals should be served, and sweet, greasy, spicy, or strong-smelling foods should be avoided. If anxiety and fear are causing nausea and vomiting, verbalizing the fears is often helpful. Under no circumstances is it ever acceptable to force the patient to eat food or drink fluids if he or she has no desire to eat because this also has potential to compromise dignity and be detrimental to the patient's well-being.

Patients may achieve relief from dehydration with the use of hypodermoclysis. Hypodermoclysis involves the administration of fluids subcutaneously through a butterfly needle; 0.9% sodium chloride is administered by gravity infusion. The individual state nurse practice act may allow this intervention to be performed by the LPN/LVN (Vidal et al, 2016).

CONSTIPATION

One of the most common problems of terminally ill patients is constipation. Constipation has many possible causes, and assessment as to the cause is fundamental for treating it adequately. Sometimes this problem causes more anxiety and discomfort than pain itself. Because constipation has the capacity to cause other symptoms, such as abdominal pain, nausea, or vomiting, prevention of the problem is important. Factors that contribute to constipation are poor dietary intake, poor fluid intake, hypercalcemia, hyponatremia, tumor compression of the bowel, use of opioids for pain control, and decrease in physical activity. Opioid administration can be followed by administration of a stool softener and a stimulant as well. Some opioids are more likely to cause constipation than are others; in such cases, a different opioid may be helpful. Changing the rate of administration sometimes also provides some relief. As with other drugs, if inability to swallow or nausea and vomiting are also a problem, other routes, such as suppositories or enemas, should be considered. A rectal examination may be necessary to check for an impaction, along with manual removal of stool. A small volume enema helps soften and dissolve a hard impaction whose removal is otherwise a painful procedure. Premedicating the patient with an anxiolytic and an analgesic before the removal of an impaction may help the patient better tolerate the procedure.

Nursing Interventions and Patient Teaching

Supporting and educating the patient and the caregiver are the nurse's primary concerns. The following points should be covered with the patient and the caregiver:

- A decrease in oral intake will also decrease the amount of stool expelled.
- Even though a patient does not have oral intake, bowel movements can still occur in some cases.
- Opioids pose a risk of constipation, so patients who receive opioids should also take laxatives.
- Comfort is the all-important factor. If the patient has not had a bowel movement, discomfort, bowel sounds, and firmness of abdomen must be assessed before any active treatment.

ANOREXIA AND MALNUTRITION

Anorexia and malnutrition are major anxiety-producing symptoms of terminal illness. Poor appetite potentially arises from nausea, vomiting, constipation, dysphagia, stomatitis, tumor invasion, general deterioration of the body, depression, or infections. These complications lead to difficulty in eating, which in turn causes loss of appetite. Odors of food cooking, inability to tolerate sweet foods, or a bitter taste in the mouth also contribute to the problem. This makes food less enjoyable, so the patient does not eat.

Disease processes change the body's metabolism and appetite; these changes sometimes lead to **cachexia** (malnutrition marked by weakness and emaciation), usually in association with a serious disease such as cancer and resulting in muscle weakness and weight loss. If poor oral intake of either food or fluids is affecting the quality of life, it is necessary to make adjustments to the plan of care.

Nursing Interventions and Patient Teaching

Complete nutritional assessments routinely and apply the findings to the hospice plan of care as appropriate. Assess and treat causes of manifestations such as nausea, vomiting, and constipation. For depression or infection, treatment options should be discussed with the medical provider and interdisciplinary team. If anorexia is related to stomatitis or infections, good oral hygiene is important. A technique to alleviate discomfort of the mouth is to use sponge-tipped oral swabs soaked in mouthwash. Patients who have oral ulcerations may experience discomfort with mouthwash; therefore water-soaked swabs may be a better option. Small frequent drinks, crushed ice, or artificial saliva are often useful in relieving a dry mouth. If the odor of food causes anorexia, the patient should not be in the kitchen during meal preparation, or family, friends, or volunteers may bring in meals. The meals should be made as attractive as possible, consisting of foods the patient chooses. High-protein supplements are helpful when eating is difficult. Avoid weighing the patient because sometimes the patient becomes depressed and discouraged by attention to weight loss.

Often the caregiver needs additional support when a patient is not eating; many caregivers think that a reduced diet will hasten death, and therefore, if they manage to get the patient to eat, the food will prolong life. Nurses often must reassure the patient and the caregiver that anorexia is part of the end-of-dying process and that forcing the patient to eat may be harmful. If the cause of the anorexia is untreatable, as in the case of tumor invasion, the patient and the caregiver may need additional emotional support. Rarely do artificial hydration, total parental nutrition, and tube feedings come into consideration. These may slow the overall cachexic effect, but they have the potential to do more harm than good, and the long-term result and quality of life will not change.

DYSPNEA AND AIR HUNGER

Dyspnea is a symptom that arises from a variety of possible conditions, such as heart failure, dysrhythmias, infection, ascites, or tumor growth. Breathing effectively is difficult for many patients, especially during the final stage of the illness. Air hunger is sometimes caused by tumor pressure, fluid and electrolyte imbalance, or anemia. Anxiety resulting from fear or panic may accompany this problem. Some respiratory distress is relieved by oxygen, morphine, or bronchodilators. Oxygen may not actually relieve the dyspnea, but it often eases the anxiety of the patient and the caregiver. Sublingual morphine helps relax the patient's respiratory effort, thus enabling greater respiratory efficiency. Bronchodilators sometimes ease respiratory obstructions and ease the respiratory distress. In many cases, 24 to 48 hours before death, the patient exhibits the "death rattle," which is the result of an accumulation of mucus and fluids in the posterior area of the pharynx. The sound that air makes as it passes through the mucus is coarse and loud and can upset the caregiver. Anticholinergic drugs, such as transdermal scopolamine or atropine given sublingually, are sometimes helpful in preventing excess secretions.

Nursing Interventions and Patient Teaching

The main nursing focus is in relieving the anxiety and supporting the patient and caregiver. Education on positioning, use of a fan to circulate air, use of morphine to decrease the work of respiration, use of anxiolytics to ease anxiety, and maintaining good oral hygiene help the patient and ease the caregiver's anxiety. Suctioning should be minimized, because it actually increases mucus production and is very uncomfortable for the patient. Suctioning should be performed only if the patient is choking and unable to recover.

PSYCHOSOCIAL AND SPIRITUAL ISSUES

Spiritual unrest and issues are often interrelated with psychosocial problems and have the potential to surface, especially when symptoms are uncontrolled. It is always necessary to respect any religious or spiritual concerns and meet the patient's wishes if at all possible. Spiritual assessments are meant to gather information regarding the patient's feelings and needs. When confronted with a terminal illness, some patients question their faiths and beliefs, and some search for the spiritual support that they have never had. Many symptoms such as depression, the need to suffer, bitterness, anger, hallucinations, or dreams of fire are, in some cases, indicative of unmet spiritual needs.

Nursing Interventions and Patient Teaching

Spiritual issues should be referred to the spiritual coordinator and not used as an opening to share personal feelings and beliefs unless the patient specifically asks for that perspective. The hospice organization determines whether the nurse or the spiritual coordinator performs the spiritual assessment. It is essential for the assessor to be nonjudgmental and accepting of the patient's and the caregiver's spiritual beliefs. The social worker also may assist with the relationship between the patient and the caregiver and provide counseling to resolve conflict. The social worker does not "fix" the conflicts but assists in problem solving. The development of trust between the patient and the interdisciplinary team is critical and is invaluable in dealing with these issues.

OTHER COMMON SIGNS AND SYMPTOMS

Weight loss and dehydration sometimes lead to a decrease in soft tissue, especially on the bony areas of knees, hips, elbows, and buttocks, which can lead to skin impairment.

Increased weakness is also notable in the last stages of a terminal illness; it often leads to activity intolerance and causes the patient to spend most of the time reclining. This leads to a risk for skin impairment and the formation of pressure ulcers. Poor nutrition, decreased circulation, and decreased mobility contribute to an increased risk for skin impairment. Education provided frequently to the family and the patient is necessary to promote integrity of the skin. The caregiver should observe the patient's skin and report any erythema or impairment. Instruct the caregiver to reposition the patient for comfort, use alternating air or egg-crate mattresses, and to perform good hygiene to prevent skin impairment.

Weakness is accompanied by safety issues of instability and falling. Patients often exhibit signs of depression and may make comments regarding suicide. Comments regarding suicide do not always come from the actual desire to kill oneself but are, in some cases, rather a statement of a desire for independence. Sleeplessness and insomnia sometimes occur as a result of an accumulation of signs and symptoms, and exhaustion has the potential to cause an exacerbation of all other signs and symptoms.

Nursing Interventions and Patient Teaching

It is important at this time to teach the patient and the caregiver the basics of good skin care. Cleanliness promoted by bathing is often refreshing, as well as therapeutic in promoting comfort and the feeling of self-worth. The skin should be inspected frequently and kept as dry and clean as possible. Stress the need to avoid harsh soaps, strong detergents, and irritation by buttons, snaps, or food crumbs. An egg-crate mattress, sheepskin, or an air-flotation mattress, as well as heel and elbow protectors, help cushion the bony areas. The hospice aide is often very helpful to the patient in assisting with personal care, hygiene, and bathing. If pressure ulcers occur, cleaning with normal saline, drying well, and applying a skin protector are helpful measures. Caregivers must be able to prevent falls and injuries; provide information regarding home safety. Listening and providing emotional support are important nursing interventions for the patient with depression and suicidal thoughts. The social worker is influential in these situations.

The hospice interdisciplinary team realizes that a terminal illness is potentially the most difficult time in a person's life. The team takes as honest and straightforward an approach as possible in all matters affecting the patient and caregiver. It is thought that the fear of the unknown is always greater than the fear of the known. Because of this, education is an important part of the care that the team provides to the patient. Educating the caregiver about symptom management, hands-on care of the patient, caring for body functions, and the signs and symptoms of approaching death are important to help relieve fears (Table 40.4).

PATIENT AND CAREGIVER TEACHING

BEREAVEMENT PERIOD

Hospice care does not conclude once the patient dies. Loss and grief are individualized emotions. The need for support is provided by the hospice for an extended period after the death. The family, especially the primary caregiver, continues to need support after the patient dies. Even though the family feels they have prepared for the death, facing the future without the person who died is difficult. Many people believe that four full seasons must pass before bereaved persons are able to think of the deceased without feeling intense emotional pain, but this period is different for everyone. The death of a loved one is a devastating agony that takes time to heal and subside. Depending on the size of the program, special bereavement teams with counselors may be available for the caregiver and family. Some teams facilitate a bereavement support group that meets on a regular basis, providing these families the opportunities to communicate and share their feelings. Volunteers and pastors keep in touch by visits, phone calls, cards, and remembering the bereaved person on holidays and anniversaries.

The hospice staff also goes through a grieving period for each patient who dies. It is a good idea to encourage the team members to attend funeral services, attend memorials, or visit the caregivers as appropriate after the death to help ease their grief. Each hospice provides support to its staff with support meetings and time to vent their feelings and to heal.

ETHICAL ISSUES IN HOSPICE CARE

Ethical issues that sometimes arise when dealing with hospice patients include withholding or withdrawing nutritional support, the right to refuse treatment, allowing a natural death, and do-not-resuscitate (DNR) orders. Families find it difficult to discontinue nourishment, even when death is clearly approaching. If the patient is unconscious, decision making regarding these issues sometimes falls on one family member, which has

Table 40.4 Signs and Symptoms of Approaching Death

SIGNS AND SYMPTOMS	NURSING INTERVENTIONS
The arms and legs of the body sometimes become cool to the touch, and the underside of the body sometimes becomes darker.	Keep warm blankets on the patient to prevent feeling of coldness.
The patient may spend more and more time sleeping during the day and at times is difficult to arouse.	Assist caregiver in planning time to be with the patient when the patient is most alert.
The patient may become increasingly confused about time, place, and identity of close and familiar people.	Reorient the patient as appropriate to the time of day and who is present. Do not upset the patient.
Incontinence of urine and bowel movements often happens when death is imminent. Sometimes there is a significant decrease in urine output.	Educate the caregiver in keeping the patient clean and dry. Provide pads or adult diapers as needed.
Oral secretions sometimes become more profuse and collect in the back of the throat. This produces the sound often referred to as the "death rattle."	Provide a cool-mist humidifier to increase the humidity in the room when oral secretions build up. Elevate the head of the bed with pillows or obtain a hospital bed to make breathing easier.
Clarity of hearing and vision decrease slightly.	Keep lights on in the room when vision decreases, and never assume that the patient is not able to hear you.
Restlessness, pulling at the bed linen, and having visions of people or things that do not exist sometimes occur.	Talk calmly and assuredly with the confused patient so as not to startle or frighten him or her further.
The patient's need for food and drink decreases.	Inform the caregiver that the patient will not starve to death or die of dehydration. Much reassurance is needed in this area.
Breathing patterns change to an irregular pace; there are sometimes 10- to 30-second periods of no breathing (apnea).	Elevating the head of the bed often relieves the patient who has irregular breathing patterns. Oxygen sometimes is and sometimes is not beneficial.
Changes in vital signs occur, with decreased blood pressure and elevated pulse.	Inform the family that these changes are normal and expected and are not uncomfortable for the patient.

potential to create guilt feelings if other family members disagree. There are no simple answers to any of these concerns. It is helpful when the patient makes his or her wishes known in advance, as in a living will or an advance directive, or assigns a durable power of attorney.

An advance directive is a document prepared while an individual is alive and competent. It provides guidance to the family and the health care team in the event that the individual is no longer capable of making decisions. The directive states the individual's preferences concerning life-support measures and organ donations and sometimes gives authority to another person to make decisions for the individual, who at that point may be in a coma.

Physician Orders for Life-Sustaining Treatment (POLST) is a form completed by the medical provider and the patient to inform health care providers of the patient's wishes. This form may be referred to by other names in different states. It is a shorter form than the advance directive with a few simple questions that can be filled out in a few minutes. This may be used in addition to or instead of the advance directive; it has proven to be more effective in preventing medical errors that arise from not following patients' wishes. Completion of this form is encouraged for all nursing home patients and for patients entering a hospital or hospice; 23 states are endorsing the POLST and 25 states are still in the process of disseminating this form (National POLST Paradigm, n.d.).

Nurses must be aware of their organization's ethics policies and procedures so that they and their colleagues are able to address any questions and concerns appropriately and correctly. No discrimination is ever tolerable for patients in hospice, regardless of sex, race, age, religion, and diagnosis. It is never acceptable for hospices to exclude or refuse patients who need high-cost care; their mandate is to serve everyone regardless of ability to pay. Services are to be available 7 days a week, 24 hours a day.

A hospice patient may have suffered many losses throughout the illness: health, job, independence, self-esteem, family, and financial security. Hospice attempts to assist the patient in maintaining dignity and control. Hospice places the emphasis on living and not dying. It is important for the hospice team to be sensitive to the patient's and the caregiver's needs and to maintain honesty at all times. The team must make sure to include the patient and the caregiver in all aspects of care and decision making. Provide opportunities for expressing concerns and fears, because this will make the process less fearful and threatening. Allowing the patient and the caregiver to live fully, comfortably, and with dignity until death occurs naturally is the main goal of hospice care.

FUTURE OF HOSPICE CARE

Trends indicate that as more patients and families are educated about its many benefits, hospice is increasingly attractive as an alternative to facing death in a clinical setting. Nevertheless, only a fraction of people who have the option of hospice care choose to participate in it. Health care providers, patients, and family members may be unwilling to begin hospice care for several reasons. The patient or family sometimes believe that availing themselves of the services of hospice denotes giving up hope, and some health care providers are hesitant to prescribe hospice care if they perceive the patient's worsening condition a personal failure on their part. The average length of service is 17.4 days. Clearly the process of death and dying for the chronically ill often exceeds this timeframe. This statistic highlights the need for increased attention and education to the benefits of hospice to patients, families, and members of the health care team (NHPCO, 2013).

Get Ready for the NCLEX® Examination!

Key Points

- Hospice is a philosophy of care about providing support to patients with a terminal illness and to their families.
- "Hospice" is from the Latin word *hospitium*, meaning "hospitality" and "lodging."
- Hospice care is appropriate when active treatment is no longer effective and supportive measures are necessary to assist a terminally ill patient through the dying process.
- The Hospice Medicare Benefit covers all expenses for palliative care related to the terminal illness, including professional staff visits, medication, equipment, respite care, and acute care.
- Hospice care emphasizes quality, not quantity, of life.
- Palliative care is appropriate when a cure is not possible but care is still necessary.
- The goal of palliative care is to control pain and other symptoms for the prevention of distress.
- Palliative care is the treatment used to relieve or reduce discomfort of disease processes and may be used at any point during treatment, but is used most often when curative therapy has failed.
- Entering a hospice program is the decision of a patient and family.
- An important criterion for the patient to be admitted into hospice is certification by the attending health care provider and a second health care provider that the patient has a prognosis of 6 months or less to live.
- Hospice care consists of a blending of professionals and nonprofessionals to meet the total needs of the patient and family.
- Hospice care is delivered by an interdisciplinary team because no individual or individual profession is able to meet all the needs of terminally ill patients and families all the time.
- Hospice care accounts for all aspects of the lives of patients and their families. Stresses and concerns have the potential to arise in many ways when families are faced with a terminal illness.
- In a hospice care program, the patient and family are considered together as the unit of care because families experience much stress and pain during the terminal illness of one of their members.
- Family participation in caregiving is an important part of palliative care.
- Hospice care is available 24 hours a day, 7 days a week, because needs may arise at any time.
- Hospice care entails respect for all patient and family belief systems, wherein resources to meet the physical, psychosocial, and spiritual needs of the family unit are sought.
- Hospice care for the family continues into the bereavement period. Needs of the family continue after the patient dies.

Additional Learning Resources

SG Go to your Study Guide for additional learning activities to help you master this chapter content.

evolve Be sure to visit the Evolve site at *http://evolve.elsevier.com/Cooper/foundationsadult/* for additional online resources.

Review Questions for the NCLEX® Examination

1. The health care provider is explaining to a 74-year-old patient that his prostate cancer is progressing and that curative treatment is no longer feasible. The health care provider has recommended hospice to the patient and his wife. What information may be included with a recommendation to hospice?
   1. "We can provide support and control your symptoms and discomfort so that you have good quality days."
   2. "With hospice, we would continue with aggressive curative care."
   3. "There is no hope left for you, and you should just go home and wait to die."
   4. "We can no longer guarantee controlled symptoms or a dignified life, but we can still provide sympathy."

2. The patient's wife calls the hospice nurse and reports that her husband is complaining of pain in his leg and is not able to get comfortable. What action by the hospice nurse may be implemented?
   1. Explain to the wife that pain will increase because of the progression of the disease and there is nothing to be done.
   2. Ask the wife how the patient rates his pain and whether he has taken any medication for breakthrough pain.
   3. Advise the wife that her husband must be a complainer.
   4. Advise the wife to wait until morning and call the health care provider.
3. When the nurse makes a home visit, the patient is experiencing shortness of breath and has increased anxiety. Place the hospice nurse's interventions in order.
   1. Assess the respiratory status.
   2. Increase morphine dosage to the higher end of the prescribed scale.
   3. Check pulse oximetry.
   4. Contact the primary care provider for a possible order for oxygen.
4. The patient is experiencing a decreased appetite and voices concerns about his weight loss. What action by the hospice nurse is most appropriate?
   1. Encourage the patient's wife to cook all of his favorite foods, and maybe he will eat.
   2. Tell the patient to force himself to eat.
   3. Explain to the patient that decreased appetite is normal.
   4. Contact the primary care provider for an order for an appetite stimulant.
5. The patient's wife is exhausted and expresses a need to get away for a short time. How can the volunteer coordinator help in this situation?
   1. Advise the wife that a volunteer will not help the situation at all.
   2. Instruct the wife that it is best for her to just stay with her husband because he might die while she is away.
   3. Assign a volunteer to sit with the patient for a couple of hours two or three times a week so that the wife is able to either take a nap or to leave for a short time to do errands.
   4. Assign a volunteer to do errands so that the patient's wife does not have to leave.
6. As a part of the hospice program, the patient has a core interdisciplinary team that manages his care. What members make up the core interdisciplinary team? *(Select all that apply.)*
   1. Spiritual coordinator
   2. Physical therapist
   3. Nurse coordinator
   4. Social worker
   5. Medical director
7. The patient's wife tells the hospice aide that she is having problems meeting their financial obligations. What action by the hospice aide is most appropriate?
   1. Tell no one because this is confidential information.
   2. Ask her for permission to report this to the interdisciplinary team, and have the social worker make a visit to see whether it is possible to provide assistance.
   3. Report this to the patient's church to see whether there is some financial assistance available.
   4. Encourage the patient's wife to consider government assistance during this difficult time.
8. The patient is complaining of constipation. He has had very little food intake the past 4 days. What action by the nurse is most appropriate?
   1. Advise his wife to stop all food and water.
   2. Assess for bowel sounds, abdominal distention, and possible impaction.
   3. Explain that reduced intake will result in reduced stool output.
   4. Instruct him to bear down to assist in elimination of his stool.
9. The patient is complaining of pain at a 5 on a pain scale of 0 to 10. What action by the nurse is indicated?
   1. Assume that because the pain is rated a 5, no further treatment is necessary or no changes are appropriate.
   2. Ask the patient what he wants his pain goal to be; if it is below 5, then you will have to notify the health care provider.
   3. Explain that the patient needs to try to tolerate a pain rating 5 or less.
   4. Automatically give the patient an additional analgesic.
10. The _______ is the mediator between the hospice team and the attending health care provider.
11. The nurse is discussing hospice with the spouse of a patient who has been diagnosed with dementia. During the session, which statement by the patient's spouse indicates the need for further discussion?
   1. "My wife will be happier that we can keep her at home during her hospice care."
   2. "My wife does not meet the criteria for using hospice."
   3. "The hospice care team is available around the clock."
   4. "I am glad to know that my family does not have to sign any documents allowing her to be without resuscitation should the time come."

12. The patient is nearing death. His wife, who is the primary caregiver, asks the nurse if it is still appropriate to turn the patient every 2 hours even as it creates discomfort and causes him to become restless. What would be the nurse's best response?
  1. "You should always reposition the patient every 2 hours no matter what."
  2. "Yes, you do not want the patient to develop pressure ulcers."
  3. "Position changes at this stage can be limited and performed only when he appears to be uncomfortable."
  4. "Position changes should be avoided from this point on."

13. The patient has never attended church and on hospice admission requested no spiritual support. Now he is within days of death and voiced some spiritual concerns to the nurse. What action by the nurse is indicated?
  1. Share personal spiritual beliefs with him.
  2. Advise him that it is too late and no church would accept him.
  3. Contact the interdisciplinary team to ask that the spiritual coordinator make a home visit.
  4. Communicate this information to the social worker.

14. The patient died peacefully and with dignity, but his wife is still having problems dealing with the death. What services by the hospice team can be anticipated?
  1. Continued bereavement support for her for the next year.
  2. Dismiss the wife from all hospice services.
  3. Encourage her to begin to explore activities outside of the home.
  4. Have the hospice aide continue with her visits to the home.

15. For the patient to qualify for assistance from Medicare or Medicaid for hospice care, which criteria are necessary? *(Select all that apply.)*
  1. The health care provider's statement that the patient has less than 6 months to live
  2. The fact that the patient is receiving chemotherapy or radiation
  3. Two health care providers' verification that the patient is dying
  4. The patient's prognosis of less than 1 year to live
  5. The patient or caregiver's understanding of the plan of care

16. The bereavement coordinator on the hospice team follows a plan of care for the bereaved caregiver for what length of time after the death of the patient?
  1. 3 to 4 months
  2. 9 to 10 months
  3. Up to 13 months
  4. Up to 3 years

17. What elements are included in the definition of palliative care according to the World Health Organization? *(Select all that apply.)*
  1. Focusing on controlling pain and other symptoms, as well as reducing psychological, social, and spiritual distress for the patient and the family
  2. The active total care of patients whose disease is not responsive to curative treatment
  3. The framework for hospice care
  4. The active total care of patients by providing treatments to assist in improving patient prognosis
  5. The care in this setting initiated at the final stages of the dying process

Introduction to Anatomy and Physiology

41

http://evolve.elsevier.com/Cooper/foundationsadult/

Objectives

1. Identify the difference between anatomy and physiology.
2. Define the term anatomical position.
3. List and define the principal directional terms and sections (planes) used in describing the body and the relationship of body parts to one another.
4. Use each word from a given list of anatomical terms in a sentence.
5. List the nine abdominopelvic regions and the abdominopelvic quadrants.
6. List and discuss in order of increasing complexity the levels of organization of the body.
7. Differentiate among tissues, organs, and systems.
8. Identify and define three major components of the cell.
9. Discuss the stages of mitosis and explain the importance of cellular reproduction.
10. Differentiate between active and passive transport processes that move substances through cell membranes, and give two examples of each.
11. Describe the four types of body tissues.
12. Discuss the two types of epithelial membranes.
13. List the 11 major organ systems of the body and briefly describe the major functions of each.

Key Terms

active transport (p. 1227)
anatomy (p. 1221)
cell (p. 1224)
cytoplasm (SĪ-tō-plăzm, p. 1225)
diffusion (dĭ-FŪ-zhŭn, p. 1228)
dorsal (p. 1223)
filtration (p. 1228)
homeostasis (hō-mē-ō-STĀ-sĭs, p. 1224)
membrane (p. 1225)
mitosis (mĭ-TŌ-sĭs, p. 1226)
nucleus (p. 1225)
organ (p. 1224)
osmosis (ŏz-MŌ-sĭs, p. 1228)
passive transport (p. 1227)
phagocytosis (făg-ō-sī-TŌ-sĭs, p. 1227)
physiology (fĭz-ē-ŎL-ō-jē, p. 1221)
pinocytosis (pī-nō-sī-TŌ-sĭs, p. 1227)
quarks (p. 1224)
system (p. 1224)
tissue (p. 1224)
ventral (p. 1222)

Caring for a person who is sick or injured requires understanding how the human body normally functions, so nurses must be familiar with basic human anatomy and physiology principles. **Anatomy** is the study, classification, and description of structures and organs of the body. **Physiology** explains the processes and functions of the various structures and how they interrelate. The normal, healthy human body is like a finely tuned machine; each part performs a special function. Like a machine, when the body malfunctions, the repairer must understand how to make the necessary repairs to return the body to homeostasis; otherwise, illness, disease, or death may result.

ANATOMICAL TERMINOLOGY

Study of the human body first requires mastery of terms that aid in locating specific structures. To understand the following terms, consider the body in a normal anatomical position, that is, standing erect with the face and palms facing forward (Fig. 41.1):

- *Anterior (or ventral):* To face forward; the front of the body. The chest is located anterior to the spine.
- *Posterior (or dorsal):* Toward the back. The kidneys are posterior to the peritoneum.
- *Cranial:* Toward the head. The brain is located in the cranial portion of the body.

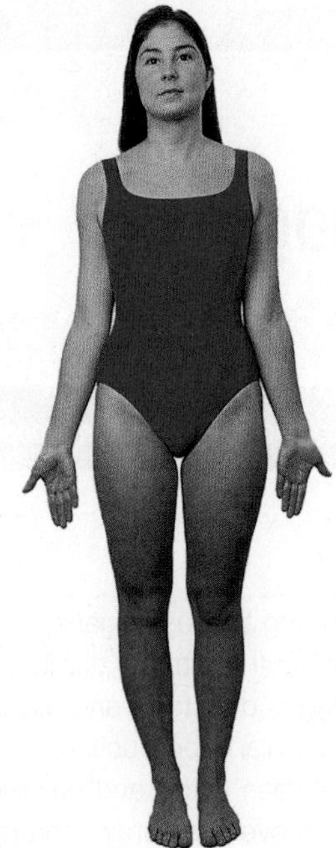

Fig. 41.1 Anatomical position. The body is in an erect or standing posture with the arms at the sides and palms forward. The head and feet also point forward. The right and left sides of the body are mirror images of each other. (From Frank ED, Long BW, Smith BJ: *Merrill's atlas of radiographic positioning and procedures*, ed 1, St. Louis, 2012, Mosby.)

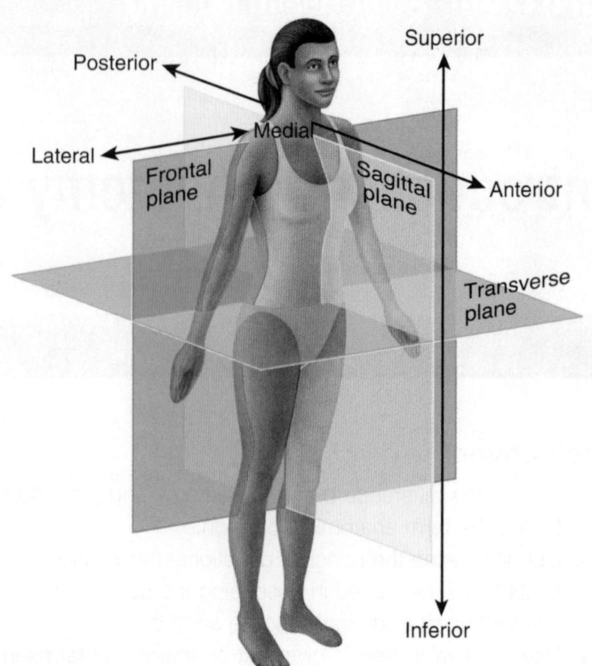

Fig. 41.2 Directions and planes of the body. (From Harkreader H, Hogan MA, Thobaben M: *Fundamentals of nursing: Caring and clinical judgment*, ed 3, St. Louis, 2007, Saunders.)

- *Caudal:* Toward the distal end of the body (trunk). A caudal anesthetic may be given.
- *Superior:* Toward the head, or above. The neck is superior to the shoulders.
- *Inferior:* Lower, toward the feet, or below another. The foot is inferior to the ankle.
- *Medial:* Toward the midline. The sternum (breastbone) is located in the medial portion of the chest.
- *Lateral:* Toward the side. The outer area of the leg, the area located on the side, is called lateral.
- *Proximal:* Nearest the origin of the structure; nearest the trunk. The elbow is proximal to the forearm.
- *Distal:* Farthest from the origin of the structure; farthest from the trunk. The fingers are distal to the palm of the hand.
- *Superficial:* Nearer the surface. The skin of the arm is superficial to the muscles below it.
- *Deep:* Farther away from the body surface. The bone of the upper arm is deep to the muscles that surround and cover it.

BODY PLANES

To make it easier to study individual organs or the body as a whole, divide the body into three imaginary planes: the sagittal, the coronal (frontal), and the transverse (Fig. 41.2):

1. The sagittal plane runs lengthwise from the front to the back. A sagittal cut gives a right and a left portion of the body. A midsagittal cut gives two equal halves.
2. The coronal (frontal) plane divides the body into a ventral (front) section and a dorsal (back) section.
3. The transverse plane cuts the body horizontal to the sagittal and frontal planes, dividing the body into caudal and cranial portions.

BODY CAVITIES

Although the body appears to be a solid structure, it is not. It is made up of open spaces, or cavities, that contain compact, well-ordered arrangements of internal organs. The body has two major cavities that are subdivided and contain compact, well-ordered arrangements of internal organs. The two major cavities are the ventral and the dorsal body cavities (Fig. 41.3 and Table 41.1).

Ventral Cavity

The **ventral** cavity consists of the thoracic (or chest) cavity and the abdominopelvic cavity (see Fig. 41.3), which are separated by the diaphragm (a muscle directly beneath the lungs).

The thoracic cavity contains the heart and the lungs. Its mid-portion is a subdivision of the thoracic cavity, the mediastinum, which contains the trachea, the heart, and the blood vessels. Its other subdivisions are the right and left pleural cavities, which contain the lungs.

The abdominal cavity contains the stomach, the liver, the gallbladder, the spleen, the pancreas, the small intestine, and parts of the large intestine. The pelvic cavity is a subdivision of the abdominal cavity and contains the lower portion of the large intestine (lower sigmoid colon, rectum), the urinary bladder, and the internal structures of the reproductive system. Because the abdominal and pelvic cavities are not separated by any structure, they are referred to collectively as the abdominopelvic cavity (see Table 41.1).

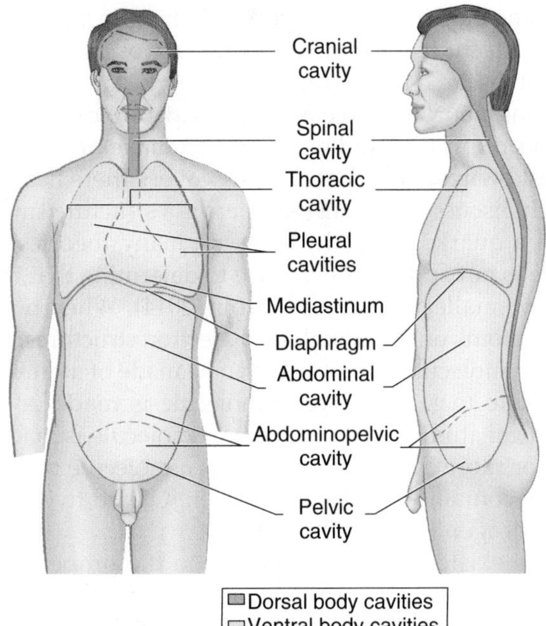

Fig. 41.3 Location and subdivisions of the dorsal and ventral body cavities as viewed from the front (anterior) and the side (lateral). (From Thibodeau GA, Patton KT: *Structure and function of the body,* ed 14, St. Louis, 2012, Mosby.)

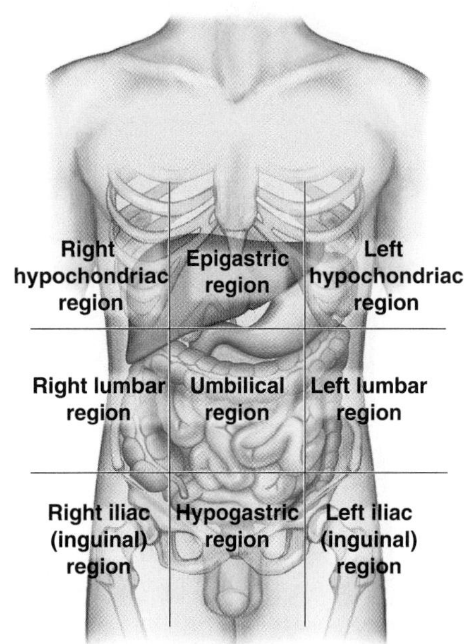

Fig. 41.4 The nine regions of the abdominopelvic cavity. The most superficial organs are shown. Can you identify the deeper structures in each region? (From Patton KT, Thibodeau GA: *The human body in health and disease,* ed 7, St. Louis, 2018, Elsevier.)

Table 41.1 Body Cavities

BODY CAVITY	ORGAN(S)
Ventral Body Cavity	
Thoracic Cavity	
Mediastinum	Trachea, heart, blood vessels
Pleural cavities	Lungs
Abdominopelvic Cavity	
Abdominal cavity	Liver, gallbladder, stomach, spleen, pancreas, small intestine, parts of large intestine
Pelvic cavity	Lower (sigmoid) colon, rectum, urinary bladder, reproductive organs
Dorsal Body Cavity	
Cranial cavity	Brain
Spinal cavity	Spinal cord

Dorsal Cavity

The **dorsal** cavity is composed of the cranial and spinal body cavities. The cranial body cavity houses the brain, whereas the spinal cavity contains the spinal cord. The dorsal body cavity is smaller than the ventral cavity (see Table 41.1).

ABDOMINAL REGIONS

For convenience in locating abdominal organs, anatomists divide the abdomen into nine imaginary regions. The nine regions are identified from right to left and from top to bottom (Fig. 41.4).

The most superficial organs located in each of the nine abdominal regions are shown in Fig. 41.4. The visible organs in each region are as follows: (1) right hypochondriac region, the right lobe of the liver and the gallbladder; (2) epigastric region, parts of the right and left lobes of the liver and a large portion of the stomach; (3) left hypochondriac region, a small portion of the stomach and large intestine; (4) right lumbar region, parts of the large and small intestine; (5) umbilical region, a portion of the transverse colon and loops of the small intestine; (6) left lumbar region, additional loops of the small intestine and a part of the colon; (7) right iliac region, the cecum and parts of the small intestine; (8) hypogastric region, loops of the small intestine, the urinary bladder, and the appendix; and (9) left iliac region, portions of the colon and the small intestine (Patton, 2019).

ABDOMINOPELVIC QUADRANTS

Health professionals frequently divide the abdomen into four quadrants to describe the site of abdominopelvic pain or to locate an internal pathologic condition such as a tumor or abscess (Fig. 41.5). Horizontal and vertical lines passing through the umbilicus (navel) divide the abdomen into right and left upper quadrants and right and left lower quadrants.

STRUCTURAL LEVELS OF ORGANIZATION

Before studying the structure and function of the human body and its many parts, think about how those parts are organized and how they may fit together into a functioning whole. Fig. 41.6 illustrates the different levels of organization that influence body structure and

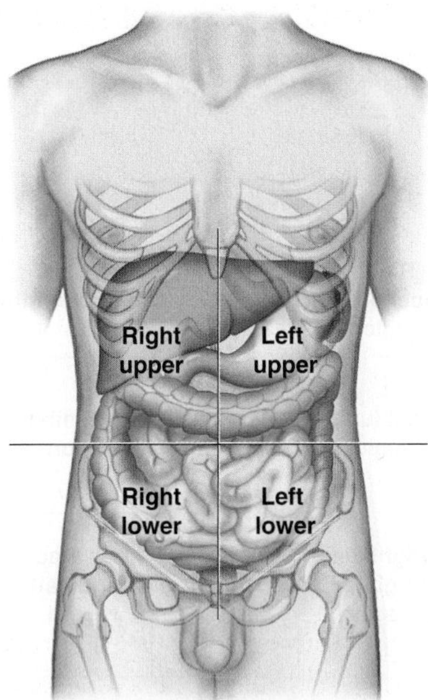

Fig. 41.5 Horizontal and vertical line passing through the umbilicus (navel) divides the abdomen into right and left upper quadrants and right and left lower quadrants. (From Patton KT, Thibodeau GA: *The human body in health and disease,* ed 7, St. Louis, 2018, Elsevier.)

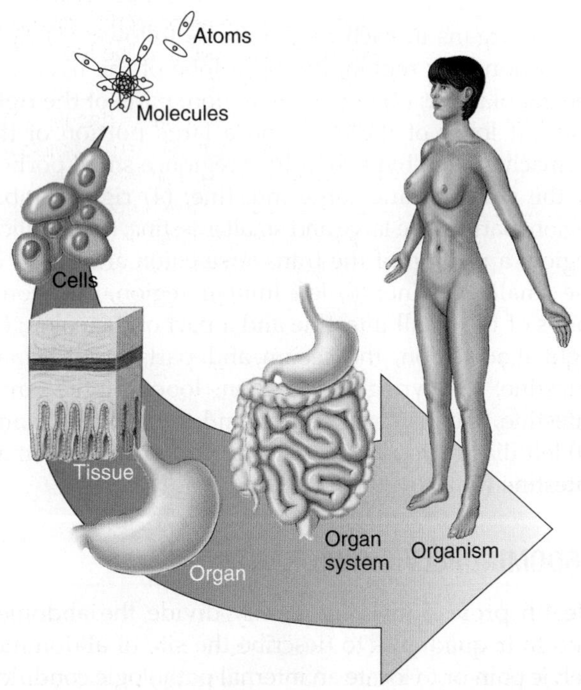

Fig. 41.6 Structural levels of organization in the body. (From Herlihy B: *The human body in health and illness,* ed 5, St. Louis, 2014, Saunders.)

function. The levels of organization progress from the least complex (chemical level) to the most complex (body as a whole). The structural levels of organization in the body are cells, tissues, organs, and systems.

Although the body is a single structure, it is made up of billions of smaller structures. Atoms and molecules often are referred to as the chemical level of organization (see Fig. 41.6). Atoms are small particles that form the building blocks of matter, once thought to be the smallest complete units of which all matter was made. More recent research has identified the quark. Atoms contain protons, neurons, and electrons; **quarks** are the building blocks of protons and neutrons that make up the atom (Moskowitz, 2012). Since this discovery there has been much discussion of whether there is a structure smaller than a quark. Presently, there are many theories, but there is not sufficient evidence to determine that there is any smaller structure (Lincoln, 2014). When two or more atoms unite through their electron structures, they form a molecule. A molecule can be made of atoms that are alike (e.g., the oxygen molecule is made of two identical atoms), but more often a molecule is made of two or more different atoms (e.g., a molecule of water [H_2O] contains one atom of oxygen [O] and two atoms of hydrogen [H]) (see Fig. 41.6).

The existence of life depends on the proper levels and proportions of many chemical substances in the cytoplasm of cells. The cell is considered the smallest living unit of structure and function in our bodies. Although cells are considered the simplest units of living matter, they are extremely complex units.

Tissues are even more complex than cells. A **tissue** is an organization of many similar cells that act together to perform a common function. Cells are held together and are surrounded by varying amounts and types of gluelike, nonliving intercellular substances.

Organs are more complex than tissues. An **organ** is a group of several different kinds of tissues arranged to perform a special function. The stomach and intestines shown in Fig. 41.6 are an example of organization at the organ level.

Systems are the most complex units that make up the body. A **system** is an organization of varying numbers and kinds of organs arranged to perform complex functions for the body. The organs of the gastrointestinal system, shown in Fig. 41.6, permit digestion of ingested food and excretion of waste products. Major organs of the digestive tract include the mouth, esophagus, stomach, and the small and large intestines.

CELLS

In the mid-1660s scientist Robert Hooke discovered the first cell while examining plant fragments under the microscope. The structures reminded him of the cells in a monastery, so he coined the term **cell** (the fundamental unit of all living tissue) (Fig. 41.7; famousscientists .org, 2014). Many living things are so simple that they consist of just one cell. Conversely, the human body is so complex that it has trillions of cells.

All cells are microscopic but differ greatly in size and shape. Despite their differences, all cells exhibit five unique characteristics of life: growth, metabolism, responsiveness, reproduction, and homeostasis. **Homeostasis** is achieved when the body's internal environment is relatively constant; this state is maintained naturally by adaptive responses that promote healthy survival.

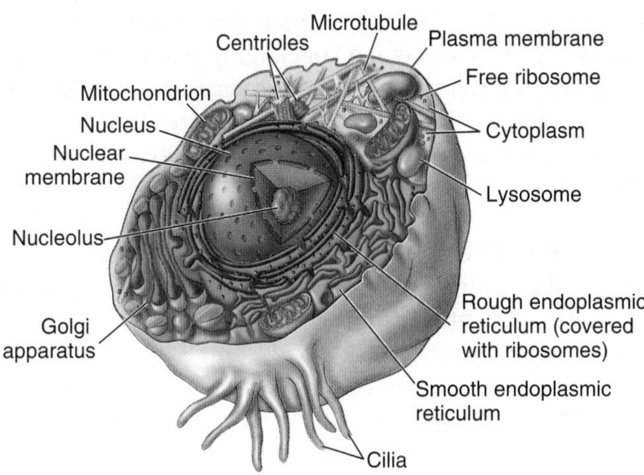

Fig. 41.7 A typical cell. (From Herlihy B: *The human body in health and illness*, ed 6, St. Louis, 2018, Elsevier.)

Structural Parts of Cells

The three main parts of a cell are the plasma membrane, the cytoplasm, and the nucleus (see Fig. 41.7).

Plasma membrane. The plasma membrane encloses the cytoplasm and forms the outer boundary of the cell. The plasma membrane is a thin and an extremely delicate structure. Despite its size and delicacy, it has a precise, orderly structure.

Even though it seems fragile, the plasma membrane is strong enough to keep the cell whole and intact. It also performs other life-preserving functions for the cell, serving as a gateway between the fluid inside the cell and the fluid around it. The plasma membrane is selectively permeable. This means the **membrane** permits certain substances to enter and leave while not allowing other substances to cross. This membrane separates the cell contents from the dilute saltwater solution called interstitial fluid, or tissue fluid, which surrounds every cell in the body. The plasma membrane also has distinct surface proteins that identify a cell as coming from one individual. This fact is the basis of tissue typing, a procedure performed to determine compatibility before an organ transplantation can occur. Carbohydrate chains attached to the surface of cells often help identify cell types.

Cytoplasm. **Cytoplasm,** found only within cells, is the internal living material of cells. Also known as protoplasm, it is a sticky, gel-like substance that contains approximately 70% water, as well as food, minerals, enzymes, and other specialized materials. Lying between the plasma membrane and the nucleus of the cell, cytoplasm contains numerous organelles (tiny functioning structures) that help with the processes of the cell. Because organelles are so small, they were not discovered until the development of the powerful electron microscope. (Table 41.2 lists major cell structures and their functions.)

Table 41.2 Some Major Cells and Their Functions

CELL STRUCTURE	FUNCTION(S)
Plasma membrane	Serves as the cell's boundary; protein and carbohydrate molecules on outer surface of plasma membrane perform various functions (e.g., serve as markers that identify cells of each individual or as receptor molecules for certain hormones)
Endoplasmic reticulum (ER)	Ribosomes attach to rough ER to synthesize proteins; smooth ER synthesizes lipids and certain carbohydrates
Ribosomes	Synthesize proteins; the cell's "protein factories"
Mitochondria	Synthesize adenosine triphosphate (ATP); the cell's "powerhouses"
Lysosomes	Serve as cell's "digestive system"
Golgi apparatus	Synthesizes carbohydrate, combines it with protein, and packages the product as globules of glycoprotein
Centrioles	Function in cell reproduction
Cilia	Short, hairlike extensions on the free surfaces of some cells capable of movement; often have specialized functions such as propelling mucus upward over cells that line the respiratory tract
Flagella	Single projections of cell surfaces, much larger than cilia; an example in humans is the "tail" of a sperm cell; propulsive movement makes it possible for sperm to "swim" or move toward the ovum once they are deposited in the female reproductive tract
Nucleus	Dictates protein synthesis, thereby playing an essential role in other cell activities, namely, active transport, metabolism, growth, and heredity
Nucleoli	Play an essential role in the formation of ribosomes

Nucleus. The **nucleus** is the largest organelle within the cell. It is responsible for cell reproduction and control of the other organelles. The nucleus is surrounded by the nuclear membrane. It contains nucleoplasm, a refined form of cytoplasm, and the nucleolus, the largest structure in the nucleus. The nucleolus is critical in the formation of ribonucleic acid (RNA).

Endoplasmic reticulum. Throughout the cytoplasm lies a system of membranes, or canals, called the endoplasmic reticulum (ER). ER functions as a miniature circulating system for the cell by carrying substances from one part of the cell to another. There are two types of ER: (1) smooth, which is found in cells that deal with fatty substances, and (2) rough, which is found in cells that manufacture proteins (Patton and Thibodeau, 2015).

Ribosomes. Ribosomes are tiny structures floating free in the cytoplasm or attached to the rough ER. They are called protein factories because they produce enzymes and other proteins.

Mitochondria. The mitochondria are the powerhouses of the cells. They are bean shaped with a folded interior membrane. They take food and convert it to a complex energy form, adenosine triphosphate (ATP), for use by the cell. ATP supplies the energy for all activities.

Lysosomes. Lysosomes are small saclike structures containing enzymes that digest food compounds and microbes that have invaded the cell.

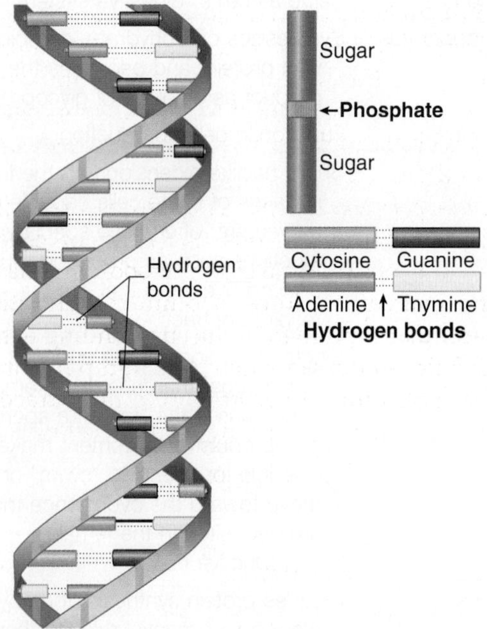

Fig. 41.8 Deoxyribonucleic acid (DNA) molecule. Note that each side of the DNA molecule consists of alternating sugar and phosphate groups. Each sugar group is united to the sugar group opposite it by a pair of nitrogenous bases (adenine-thymine or cytosine-guanine). The sequence of these pairs constitutes a genetic code that determines the structure and function of a cell. (From Patton KT, Thibodeau GA: *Anatomy & physiology*, ed 10, St. Louis, 2019, Elsevier.)

Golgi apparatus. The Golgi apparatus usually is located near the nucleus. It is the "packaging plant" of the cell. It packages certain carbohydrate and protein compounds into globules. Then it moves outward through the cell membrane, where it breaks open and releases its contents.

Centrioles. The centrioles are paired, rod-shaped organelles. During cell division (mitosis) they aid in the formation of the spindle, a structure necessary for cell reproduction.

Protein Synthesis

Protein is a vital component of every cell in the body. Protein production relies on nucleic acids in the cell's cytoplasm and nucleus. Two important nucleic acids are (1) DNA (Fig. 41.8), which is located only in the nucleus, and (2) ribonucleic acid (RNA), which is located in the nucleus and cytoplasm. The DNA encodes a message for protein synthesis as RNA and sends the RNA to ribosomes in the cytoplasm, where the protein is produced. For this reason, DNA is called the chemical blueprint, and RNA is called the chemical messenger.

Cell Division

All cells in the body, except sex cells, reproduce by **mitosis**, which is a type of somatic (pertaining to nonreproductive cells) cell division in which the original cell divides to form two daughter cells. Each daughter cell has the same characteristics (including the nucleus and cytoplasm) as the original cell. Each daughter cell contains the same number of chromosomes as the parent cell. Each chromosome in the daughter cells contains the complete genetic information of the original chromosome because of duplication of the DNA molecule during interphase (Fig. 41.9).

The chromosomes (spindle-shaped rods) in the cell's nucleus carry the genes that are responsible for the organism's traits, including such hereditary factors as hair and eye color. These chromosomes are composed of DNA. Each body cell in humans contains 46 chromosomes, which exist in pairs. At the time of fertilization, one member of each pair is received from the father and one is received from the mother to form a total of

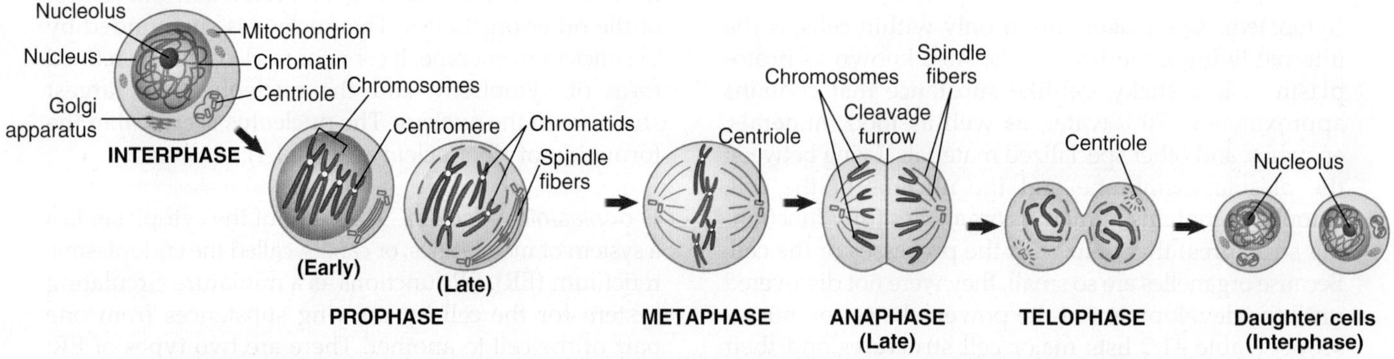

Fig. 41.9 Mitosis. (From Thibodeau GA, Patton KT: *Structure and function of the body*, ed 14, St. Louis, 2012, Mosby.)

23 pairs of chromosomes. These paired chromosomes, except for the pair that determines sex, are alike in size and appearance and carry genes for the same traits.

During mitosis the cell goes through four phases: prophase, metaphase, anaphase, and telophase:

1. *Prophase:* In the nucleus the chromosomes form two strands called chromatids. In the cytoplasm the centrioles form a network of spindle fibers.
2. *Metaphase:* The nuclear membrane and nucleolus disappear, and the chromosomes are aligned across the center of the cell. The centrioles are at the opposite ends of the cell, and spindle fibers are attached to each chromatid.
3. *Anaphase:* The chromosomes are pulled to the opposite ends of the cell, and cell division begins.
4. *Telophase:* During this final phase of cell division, the two nuclei appear and the chromosomes disperse. At the end of the phase, two new daughter cells appear.

Movement of Materials Across Cell Membranes

For a cell to survive, it must receive food and oxygen and secrete its waste products. A number of processes allow for mass movement of substances into and out of the cells. These transport processes are classified under two general headings: passive transport and active transport.

The difference between active and passive transport is based on whether energy is required. **Active transport** involves chemical activity that allows the cell to admit larger molecules than would otherwise be possible. Active processes require the cell to expend energy. **Passive transport** processes, on the other hand, do not require energy expenditure. The cell obtains energy for active transport from an important chemical substance called ATP. ATP is produced in the cell from nutrients and releases energy so that the cell can work.

Active transport processes. Active transport is an extremely important process. It allows cells to move certain ions or other water-soluble particles to specific areas. Certain enzymes play a role in active transport, providing a chemical "pump" that helps move substances through the cell membrane. For example, insulin binds with glucose and transports the glucose into the cell. Other active transport processes (Table 41.3) include the following:

- **Phagocytosis** (Greek for "cell-eating"): The process that permits a cell to engulf (or surround) any foreign material and to digest it. The white blood cells in the human body often perform this function.
- **Pinocytosis** (Greek for "cell-drinking"): The process by which extracellular fluid is taken into the cell. The cell membrane develops a saclike indentation filled with extracellular fluid and then closes around it and digests it.
- *Sodium-potassium pump:* The process of actively transporting sodium ions (Na^+) out of cells and potassium ions (K^+) into cells. The sodium-potassium pump maintains a lower sodium concentration in intracellular fluid than in the surrounding extracellular fluid. At the same time, this pump maintains a higher potassium concentration in the intracellular fluid than in the surrounding extracellular fluid.

Table 41.3 Active Transport Processes[a]

DESCRIPTION		EXAMPLE(S)
Ion Pump		
Movement of solute particles from an area of low concentration to an area of high concentration (up the concentration gradient) by means of a carrier protein structure	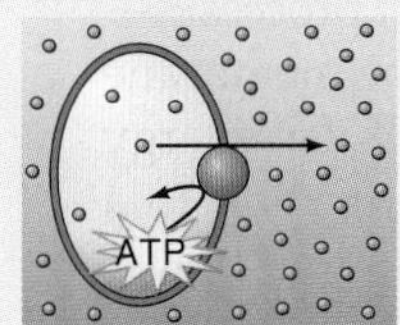	In muscle cells, pumping of nearly all calcium ions to special compartments or out of the cell
Phagocytosis		
Process that permits a cell to engulf or to surround any foreign material and to digest it	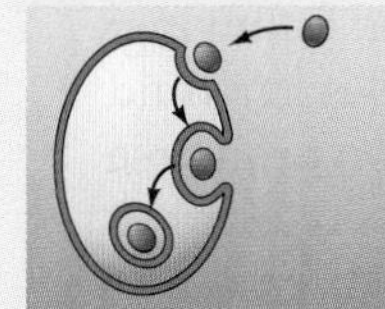	Trapping of bacterial cells by phagocytic white blood cells
Pinocytosis		
Movement of fluid and dissolved molecules into a cell by trapping them in a section of plasma membrane that pinches off to form an intracellular vesicle; type of endocytosis	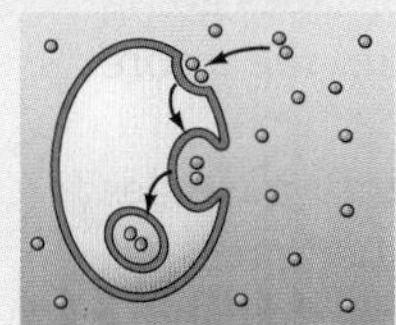	Trapping of large protein molecules by some body cells

[a]The energy required for active transport processes is obtained from ATP (adenosine triphosphate). ATP is involved in all active transport processes.
From Patton KT, Thibodeau GA: *The human body in health and disease*, ed 7, St. Louis, 2018, Elsevier.

Table 41.4 Passive Transport Processes

DESCRIPTION		EXAMPLE(S)
Diffusion		
Movement of solute particles through a membrane from an area of high concentration to an area of low concentration (down the concentration gradient)	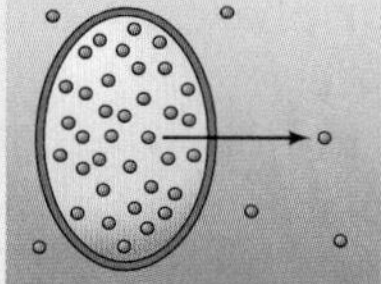	Movement of carbon dioxide out of all cells; movement of sodium ions into nerve cells as they conduct an impulse
Osmosis		
Diffusion of water through a selectively permeable membrane in the presence of at least one impermeable solute	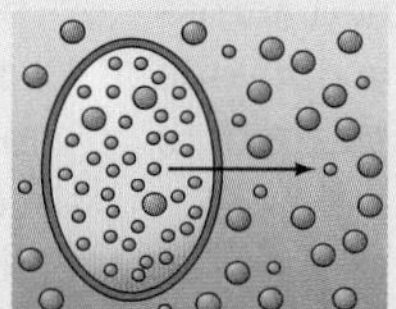	Diffusion of water molecules into and out of cells to correct imbalances in water concentration
Filtration		
Movement of water and small solute particles, but not larger particles, through a filtration membrane; movement occurs from an area of high pressure to an area of low pressure	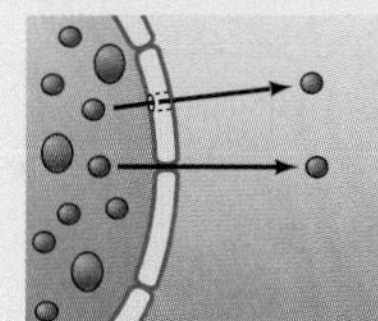	In the kidney, movement of water and small solutes from blood vessels but lack of movement by blood proteins and blood cells; begins the formation of urine

From Patton KT, Thibodeau GA: *The human body in health and disease*, ed 7, St. Louis, 2018, Elsevier.

This active transport pump operates in the plasma membrane of all human cells and is essential for healthy cell survival.

- *Calcium pump:* Active calcium carriers in the membranes of muscle cells (for example) that allow the cells to force nearly all the intracellular calcium ions (Ca^{2+}) into special compartments or out of the cell entirely. This is important because a muscle cell cannot operate properly unless the intracellular Ca^{2+} concentration is kept low during rest.

Active transport processes require cellular energy to move substances from a low concentration to a high concentration. In contrast, passive transport processes—the movement of small molecules across the membrane of a cell by diffusion—do not require cellular energy and move substances from a high concentration to a lower concentration.

Passive transport processes. The primary passive transport processes (Table 41.4) include the following:

- **Diffusion:** A process in which solid particles in a fluid move from an area of higher concentration to an area of lower concentration, resulting in an even distribution of the particles in the fluid (Fig. 41.10).
- **Osmosis:** The passage of water across a selectively permeable membrane, with the water molecules going from the less concentrated solution to the more concentrated solution (Fig. 41.11).
- **Filtration:** The movement of water and particles through a membrane by force from either pressure or gravity. This membrane contains spaces that allow liquid to pass but are too small to be permeated by solid particles. Movement is from areas of greater pressure to areas of lesser pressure.

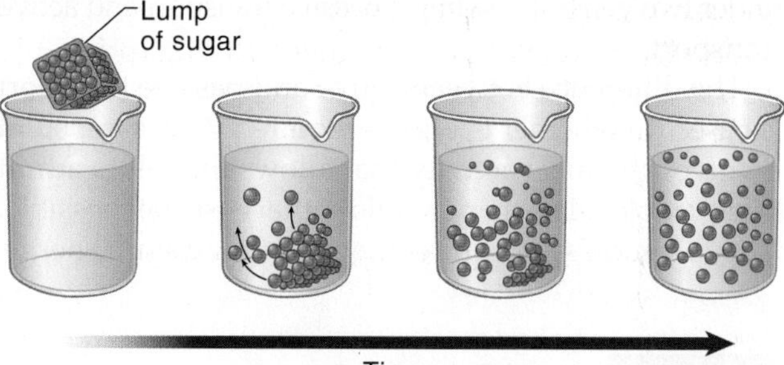

Fig. 41.10 Diffusion. The molecules of a lump of sugar are very densely packed when they enter the water. As sugar molecules collide frequently in the area of high concentration, they gradually move away from each other toward the area of lower concentration. Eventually the sugar molecules are distributed evenly. (From Patton KT, Thibodeau GA: *The human body in health and disease*, ed 7, St. Louis, 2018, Elsevier.)

TISSUES

Tissues are groups of similar cells that work together to perform a specific function. The body and its organs are composed of the following four main types of tissues: epithelial, connective, muscle, and nervous (Table 41.5).

Epithelial Tissue

Epithelial cells are packed closely together and contain no blood vessels. Epithelial tissue covers the outside of the body and some of the internal structures. The four types of epithelial tissue are (1) simple squamous, (2) stratified squamous, (3) simple columnar, and (4) stratified transitional (see Table 41.5).

Epithelial tissue serves several important functions in the body, including the following:

- *Protection:* By covering the body and many of its organs, epithelial tissue is a protective barrier against invasion.

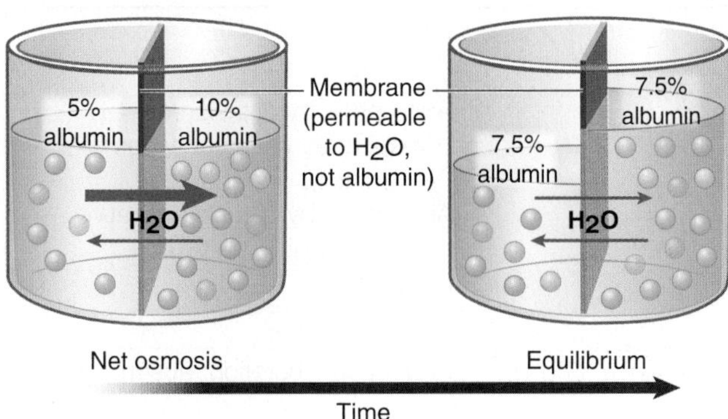

Fig. 41.11 Osmosis. Osmosis is the diffusion of water through a selectively permeable membrane. The membrane shown in this diagram is permeable to water but not to albumin. Because there are relatively more water molecules in 5% albumin than in 10% albumin, more water molecules osmose from the more dilute into the more concentrated solution (as indicated by the *large arrow* in the diagram on the left) than osmose in the opposite direction. The overall direction of osmosis, in other words, is toward the more concentrated solution. Movement across the membrane continues until the concentrations of the solutions equalize. (From Patton KT, Thibodeau GA: *The human body in health and disease*, ed 7, St. Louis, 2018, Elsevier.)

- *Absorption:* Certain specialized epithelial cells can absorb material in the body (e.g., the lining of the small intestine can absorb digested nutrients).
- *Secretion:* Mucus is secreted in areas such as the respiratory and digestive tracts.

Connective Tissue

As the name suggests, connective tissue "connects," or joins, tissues or structures of the body, and it supports and protects them. Connective tissue is the most abundant and widely distributed tissue in the body. It exists in various forms: thin and delicate, tough and cordlike, or liquid (blood). Mast cells, plasma cells, and white blood cells are found in connective tissue; red blood cells are not unless blood vessels have been injured. Unlike the closely packed epithelial tissue, the connective tissue cells are spaced out and surrounded by intercellular fluid, which is composed of protein complexes and tissue fluid.

Some of the most important forms of connective tissue are loose fibrous (areolar) connective tissue, adipose (fat) tissue, fibrous connective tissue, bone, cartilage, blood, and hematopoietic tissue (see Table 41.5).

Muscle Tissue

Muscle tissue is composed of cells that contract in response to a message from the brain or the spinal cord. The three types of muscle cells are (1) skeletal (striated, voluntary), (2) cardiac (striated, involuntary), and (3) visceral (smooth, involuntary) (Fig. 41.12).

Skeletal muscle cells are striated (have a striped appearance) and attach to bones to produce voluntary movement. Skeletal muscle is also known as voluntary muscle because a person has voluntary control over skeletal muscle contractions (see Fig. 41.12A).

Cardiac muscle cells are striated with fibers that branch to form many networks, or webs. These networks are found only in the walls of the heart, and the regular contractions of cardiac muscle produce the heartbeat. In general, cardiac muscle cells are involuntary; that is, a person cannot contract them at will (see Fig. 41.12B).

Smooth (visceral) muscle cells are nonstriated and appear in the viscera, or internal organs, such as the stomach and the intestines as well as in the walls of blood vessels and the uterus. Contractions of smooth muscle propel food and fluid through the digestive tract and help regulate the diameter of blood vessels. Contraction of smooth muscle in the tubes of the respiratory system, such as the bronchioles in the lungs, can impair breathing and result in asthma attacks and labored respiration. In general, smooth muscles are involuntary, but some control can be exerted with biofeedback techniques (see Fig. 41.12C).

Nervous Tissue

Nervous tissue allows rapid communication between the brain or spinal cord and body structures and allows control of body functions. Nervous tissue is composed of two types of cells: neurons and glial cells. The neurons are the nerve cells and transmit impulses or messages. They are the system's functional or conducting units. The glial cells are connecting and supporting cells; they support and nourish the neurons.

Each neuron has three parts: (1) dendrites, which carry impulses toward the cell body; (2) a cell body; and (3) an axon, which carries impulses away from the cell body (see Chapter 54, Fig. 54.1).

MEMBRANES

Membranes are thin sheets of tissue that serve many functions in the body. They cover body surfaces, line and lubricate hollow organs, and protect and anchor organs and bones. The two major types of membranes are epithelial and connective tissue membranes.

Epithelial Membranes

Epithelial membranes usually are composed of a thin layer of epithelial cells with an underlying layer of connective tissue for strength. Epithelial membranes are divided into two subgroups: mucous membranes and serous membranes.

Mucous membranes. Mucous membranes secrete mucus (a thick, slippery material), which keeps the membranes moist and soft and protects against bacterial invasion. Mucous membranes line the body surfaces that open to the outside environment. Examples include the nose; the mouth; and urinary, respiratory, gastrointestinal, and reproductive tracts. The type of epithelium in the mucous membrane varies, depending on its location and function. The esophagus, for example, contains a tough, abrasion-resistant, stratified squamous epithelium. A thin layer of simple columnar epithelium covers the walls of the lower segments of the digestive tract.

Table 41.5 Tissues

TISSUE	LOCATION	FUNCTION
Epithelial		
Simple squamous	Alveoli of lungs	Absorption by diffusion of respiratory gases between alveolar air and blood
	Lining of blood and lymphatic vessels	Absorption by diffusion, filtration, and osmosis
Stratified squamous	Surface of lining of mouth and esophagus	Protection
	Surface of skin (epidermis)	Protection
Simple columnar	Surface layer of lining of stomach, intestines, and parts of respiratory tract	Protection; secretion; absorption
Stratified transitional	Urinary bladder	Protection
Connective[a]		
Areolar	Between other tissues and organs	Connection
Adipose (fat)	Under skin	Protection
	Padding at various points	Insulation; support; reserve food
Dense fibrous	Tendons; ligaments	Flexible but strong connection
Bone	Skeleton	Support; protection
Cartilage	Part of nasal septum; covering articular surfaces of bones; larynx; rings in trachea and bronchi	Firm but flexible support
	Disks between vertebrae	
	External ear	
Blood	Blood vessels	Transportation
Hematopoietic	Liquid matrix with dense arrangement of blood cell–producing cells located in red bone marrow	Blood cell formation
Muscle		
Skeletal (striated voluntary); see Fig. 41.12A	Muscles that attach to bones	Maintenance of posture, movement of bones
	Eyeball muscles	Eye movements
	Upper third of esophagus	First part of swallowing
Cardiac (striated involuntary); see Fig. 41.12B	Wall of heart	Contraction of heart
Smooth (nonstriated involuntary or visceral); see Fig. 41.12C	In walls of tubular viscera of digestive, respiratory, and genitourinary tracts	Movement of substances along respective tracts
	In walls of blood vessels and large lymphatic vessels	Changing diameter of blood vessels
	In ducts of glands	Movement of substances along ducts
	Intrinsic eye muscles (iris and ciliary body)	Changing diameter of pupils and shape of lens
	Arrector muscles of hair follicles	Erection of hairs (gooseflesh)
Nervous	Brain; spinal cord; nerves	Irritability; conduction

[a]Connective tissues are the most widely distributed of all tissues.

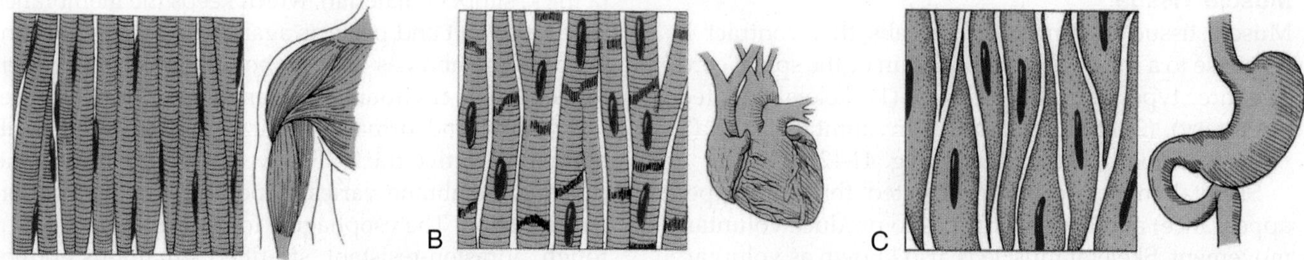

Fig. 41.12 Types of muscle. A, Skeletal muscle. B, Cardiac muscle. C, Smooth muscle.

In addition to protection, the mucus produced by mucous membranes also serves other purposes. For example, mucus in the digestive tract lubricates food as it moves through the digestive tract, and mucus secreted in the respiratory tract acts as a defense mechanism by trapping microorganisms and preventing their invasion into the respiratory system.

Serous membranes. Serous membranes secrete a thin, watery fluid that prevents friction when organs rub against one another. These membranes line the body surfaces that do not open to the outside environment. Examples include the lungs (pleura), the intestines (peritoneum), and the heart (pericardium). Like epithelial membranes, serous membranes are composed of two distinct layers of tissue: (1) the epithelial sheet, a thin layer of simple squamous epithelium, and (2) the connective tissue layer, a very thin sheet that holds and supports the epithelial cells.

The serous membrane that lines body cavities and covers the surfaces of organs in those cavities is a single, continuous sheet covering two different surfaces. The parietal membrane lines the wall of the cavity, whereas the visceral membrane covers the surface of the viscera (organs within the cavity).

Connective Tissue Membranes (Synovial Membranes)

Connective tissue (or synovial) membranes are smooth and slick and secrete synovial fluid (a thick, colorless lubricating fluid). Synovial membranes line the joint spaces and prevent friction between the ends of the bones, allowing free movement of the joints. Synovial membranes also line small, cushion-like sacs called bursae, which are found between some moving body parts. Unlike serous and mucous membranes, connective tissue membranes do not contain epithelial components.

ORGANS AND SYSTEMS

When several kinds of tissues are united to perform a more complex function than any tissue alone, they are called organs. Examples are the heart, stomach, and kidneys. These organs working together for the same general purpose make up organ systems, which maintain the whole body. Systems perform a more complex function than any one organ can perform alone (Table 41.6).

Table 41.6 Organ Systems and Their Functions

STRUCTURE	FUNCTION
Integumentary System	
Hair Nails Oil glands Sense receptors Skin Sweat glands	• Protection • Regulation of body temperature • Sense organ • Synthesis of chemicals
Skeletal System	
Bones Joints	• Blood cell formation • Movement (with joints and muscles) • Storage of minerals • Support
Muscular System	
Involuntary or smooth muscles Voluntary or striated muscles	• Maintenance of body posture • Movement • Production of heat
Nervous System	
Brain Nerves Sense organs Spinal cord	• Communication • Contains body's control center • Control • Control is fast acting and of short duration • Integration • Recognition of sensory stimuli • Responsible for all the coordination of body's activities • System functions by production of nerve impulses caused by stimuli of various types
Endocrine System	
Adrenal glands Hypothalamus Ovaries (female) Pancreas Parathyroid glands Pineal gland Pituitary gland Testes (male) Thymus gland Thyroid gland	• Control is slow and of long duration • Examples of hormone regulation: growth, metabolism, reproduction, and fluid and electrolyte balance • Same as nervous system—communication, integration, control • Secretion of special substances (hormones) directly into the blood (e.g., insulin from the pancreas)
Cardiovascular (Circulatory) System	
Blood vessels Heart	• Immunity (body defense) • Regulation of body temperature • Transportation for nutrition, water, oxygen, and wastes
Lymphatic System	
Lymph nodes Lymphatic vessels Spleen Thymus Tonsils	• Maintains body's internal fluid environment by producing, filtering, and conveying lymph • Production of various blood cells • Protection • Transportation
Respiratory System	
Nose Larynx Pharynx Trachea Lungs Bronchi	• Area of gas exchange in the lungs called alveoli • Exchange of waste gas (carbon dioxide) for oxygen in the lungs • Filtration of irritants from inspired air • Regulation of acid-base balance

Continued

Table 41.6 Organ Systems and Their Functions—cont'd

STRUCTURE	FUNCTION	STRUCTURE	FUNCTION
Digestive System		**Reproductive System**	
Primary Organs		**Male**	
Mouth Pharynx Esophagus Stomach Small intestine (duodenum, jejunum, ileum) Large intestine (ascending, transverse, descending, sigmoid) Rectum Anal canal	• Absorption of nutrients • Mechanical and chemical breakdown (digestion) of food • Undigested waste product that is eliminated is called feces	Gonads (testes) Genital ducts (epididymis, vas deferens, ejaculatory duct, urethra) Accessory glands (prostate, seminal vesicles, Cowper's glands) Supporting structures (penis, scrotum)	• Fertilization of female sex cells • Production of sex cells (sperm) • Production of sex hormones • Survival of species • Transfer of sperm to female sex cells
Accessory Organs		**Female**	
Teeth Salivary glands Tongue Liver Gallbladder Pancreas Appendix	• Appendix is a structural but not a functional part of the digestive system • Function of other structures can be found in the digestive system chapters (see Chapters 45 and 46)	Gonads (ovaries) Accessory organs (uterus, fallopian tubes [oviducts], vagina) External genitalia (vulva) • Mons pubis • Labia majora • Labia minora • Clitoris Accessory glands (Skene's glands, Bartholin's glands) Mammary glands (breasts)	• Development and birth of offspring • Nourishment of offspring • Production of sex cells (ova) • Production of sex hormones • Survival of species
Urinary System			
Kidneys Ureters Urinary bladder Urethra	• Acid-base balance • Clearing or cleaning blood of waste products; waste product excreted from the body is called urine • Electrolyte balance • Urethra has urinary and reproductive functions (in male) • Water balance		

Get Ready for the NCLEX® Examination!

Key Points

- Anatomy is the study, classification, and description of structures and organs of the body. Physiology explains the function of the various structures and how they interrelate.
- The normal anatomical position of the body is standing erect with the face and the palms of the hands forward.
- For the purposes of study, the body is divided into three imaginary planes: sagittal, coronal (frontal), and transverse.
- The body is divided into two large cavities: the dorsal and the ventral. The dorsal cavity contains the cranial and spinal cavities. The ventral cavity contains the thoracic, abdominal, and pelvic cavities.
- For the purposes of study, the abdominal region is divided into nine regions: right hypochondriac region, epigastric region, left hypochondriac region, right lumbar region, umbilical region, left lumbar region, right inguinal region, hypogastric region, and left inguinal region.
- The cell's major structures are the cytoplasm, nucleus, endoplasmic reticulum, ribosomes, mitochondria, lysosomes, Golgi apparatus, and centrioles.
- Organization is a fundamental characteristic of body structure.
- Cells are considered the smallest living units of structure and function in the body. Although long recognized as the simplest units of living matter, cells are extremely complex.
- Tissues are groups of similar cells that work together to perform a specific function.
- Organs are structures made up of two or more kinds of tissues organized so that they can perform a more complex function than they could alone.
- Systems are groups of organs arranged so that they can perform a more complex function than they could alone.

- To receive nutrition and oxygen and to rid itself of wastes, the cell performs passive transport (diffusion, osmosis, filtration) and active transport (phagocytosis and pinocytosis, as well as the sodium-potassium pump and the calcium pump).
- The body is composed of four main types of tissues: epithelial, connective, muscle, and nervous tissues.
- The major systems of the body are integumentary, skeletal, muscular, nervous, endocrine, cardiovascular (circulatory), lymphatic, respiratory, digestive, urinary, and reproductive.

Additional Learning Resources

SG Go to your Study Guide for additional learning activities to help you master this chapter content.

evolve Be sure to visit the Evolve site at *http://evolve.elsevier.com/Cooper/foundationsadult/* for additional online resources.

Review Questions for the NCLEX-PN® Examination

1. The nurse is caring for a patient who is experiencing back pain located in the lower portion of the spine. The nurse is correct in documenting this as what area?
 1. Medial
 2. Caudal
 3. Proximal
 4. Dorsal

2. The nurse correctly identifies which organs as being found in the abdominopelvic cavity? *(Select all that apply.)*
 1. Spleen
 2. Urinary bladder
 3. Pancreas
 4. Gallbladder
 5. Rectum

3. The student nurse correctly identifies __________ as when a person's body is maintaining a balanced state within its internal environment.
 1. Homeostasis
 2. Mitosis
 3. Lysosomes
 4. Protein synthesis

4. What process has occurred when the patient inhales oxygen and it passes through the lungs and into the bloodstream (area of higher concentration to an area of lower concentration)?
 1. Phagocytosis
 2. Pinocytosis
 3. Osmosis
 4. Diffusion

5. The nurse correctly identifies which mechanism as the movement of materials across the membrane of a cell by means of chemical activity requiring the expenditure of energy by the cell?
 1. Passive transport
 2. Active transport
 3. Telophase
 4. Transcription

6. What type of tissue is composed of cells that contract in response to a message from the brain or spinal cord?
 1. Epithelial
 2. Connective
 3. Membrane
 4. Muscle

7. The student nurse demonstrates knowledge of basic human anatomy and physiology with which statement?
 1. "Mucous membranes line many organs, open to the outside environment, and are part of the body's defense mechanism against invasion of microorganisms."
 2. "Serous membranes line many organs, open to the outside environment, and are part of the body's defense mechanism against invasion of microorganisms."
 3. "Striated smooth muscle lines many organs, open to the outside environment, and are part of the body's defense mechanism against invasion of microorganisms."
 4. "Visceral, involuntary smooth muscle lines many organs, open to the outside environment, and are part of the body's defense mechanism against invasion of microorganisms."

8. When the body recognizes a foreign body invasion and responds by engulfing or surrounding the foreign material and digesting it, the nurse is accurate in identifying this process as what?
 1. Mitosis
 2. Pinocytosis
 3. Phagocytosis
 4. Filtration

9. A type of cell division of somatic cells in which each daughter cell contains the same number of chromosomes as the parent cell is called what?
 1. Flagella
 2. Mitosis
 3. ER synthesis
 4. Mitochondria

10. When a group of several different kinds of tissues is arranged to perform a special function, the nurse correctly uses which term to describe it?
 1. Cell
 2. Organ
 3. Tissue
 4. System

11. The hypogastric region of the abdominopelvic cavity is located where? *(Select all that apply.)*
 1. Inferior to the umbilical region
 2. Lateral to the left iliac region
 3. Medial to the right iliac region
 4. Lateral to the epigastric region
 5. Superior to the right lumbar region

12. A patient is being admitted to the intensive care unit following a motor vehicle accident that resulted in serious injury to organs in the dorsal cavity. Which organs does the nurse suspect are involved?

1. Right kidney
2. Spinal cord
3. Liver
4. Gallbladder
5. Brain

13. The patient had a gunshot wound that damaged the structure that divides the thoracic cavity from the abdominal cavity. The nurse is aware that what structure has been affected?

1. Mediastinum
2. Diaphragm
3. Lungs
4. Stomach

14. The nurse is caring for a patient with a disease of the endocrine system. Which organs does the nurse identify as possibly not functioning correctly based on this patient's disease? *(Select all that apply.)*

1. Pituitary gland
2. Pancreas
3. Thyroid gland
4. Spleen
5. Adrenal glands

Matching

Match each directional term in Column B with its opposite term in Column A.

COLUMN A	COLUMN B
15. _____ Superior	a. Posterior
16. _____ Distal	b. Superficial
17. _____ Anterior	c. Medial
18. _____ Lateral	d. Proximal
19. _____ Deep	e. Inferior

Match the function in Column B with the correct system in Column A.

COLUMN A	COLUMN B
20. _____ Integumentary	a. Provides movement, body posture, and heat
21. _____ Skeletal	b. Uses hormones to regulate body functions
22. _____ Muscular	c. Transports fatty nutrients from the digestive system to the blood
23. _____ Nervous	d. Makes physical and chemical change in nutrients and absorbs nutrients
24. _____ Endocrine	e. Cleans the blood of metabolic wastes and regulates electrolyte balance
25. _____ Cardiovascular	f. Protects underlying structures, provides for sensory reception, and regulates body temperature
26. _____ Lymphatic	g. Transports substances from one part of the body to another
27. _____ Respiratory	h. Ensures the survival of the species rather than the individual
28. _____ Digestive	i. Uses electrochemical signals to integrate and control body functions
29. _____ Urinary	j. Exchanges oxygen and carbon dioxide and regulates acid-base balance
30. _____ Reproductive	k. Provides a rigid framework for the body and stores minerals

Care of the Surgical Patient

42

http://evolve.elsevier.com/Cooper/foundationsadult/

Objectives

1. Identify the purposes of surgery.
2. Distinguish among elective, urgent, and emergency surgery.
3. Explain the concept of perioperative nursing.
4. Discuss the factors that influence an individual's ability to tolerate surgery.
5. Discuss considerations for the older adult surgical patient.
6. Describe the preoperative checklist.
7. Explain the importance of informed consent for surgery.
8. Explain the procedure for turning, deep breathing, coughing, and leg exercises for postoperative patients.
9. Differentiate among general, regional, and local anesthesia.
10. Explain conscious (moderate) sedation.
11. Describe the roles of the circulating nurse and the scrub nurse during surgery.
12. Discuss the initial nursing assessment and management immediately after transfer from the postanesthesia care unit.
13. Identify the rationale for nursing interventions designed to prevent postoperative complications.
14. List the assessment data for the surgical patient.
15. Identify the information needed for the postoperative patient in preparation for discharge.
16. Discuss the nursing process as it pertains to the surgical patient.

Key Terms

ablative (ăb-LĀ-tĭv, p. 1236)
anesthesia (ăn-ĕs-THĒ-zē-ă, p. 1254)
atelectasis (ă-tē-LĔK-tā-sĭs, p. 1246)
cachexia (kă-KĔK-sē-ă, p. 1265)
catabolism (kă-TĂB-ō-lĭsm, p. 1270)
conscious (moderate) sedation (sĕ-DĀ-shŭn, p. 1258)
dehiscence (dē-HĬS-ĕns, p. 1265)
drainage (p. 1263)
embolus (ĔM-bō-lŭs, p. 1248)
evisceration (ĕ-vĭs-ĕr-Ā-shŭn, p. 1265)
extubate (ĕks-TŪ-bāt, Table 42.7, p. 1264)
exudate (ĔKS-yū-dāt, p. 1263)
incentive spirometer (ĭn-SĔN-tĭv spĭ-RŎM-ĕ-tĕr, p. 1245)
incisions (ĭn-SĬZH-ŭnz, p. 1253)
infarct (ĬN-făhrkt, p. 1248)
informed consent (p. 1243)
intraoperative (ĭn-tră-ŎP-ĕr-ă-tĭv, p. 1237)
palliative (PĂL-ē-ă-tĭv, p. 1236)
paralytic ileus (păr-ă-LĬT-ĭk ĬL-ē-ŭs, p. 1270)
perioperative (pĕr-ē-ŎP-ĕr-ă-tĭv, p. 1237)
postoperative (pōst-ŎP-ĕr-ă-tĭv, p. 1237)
preoperative (prē-ŎP-ĕr-ă-tĭv, p. 1237)
prosthesis (prŏs-THĒ-sĭs, p. 1259)
singultus (SĬNG-gŭl-tŭs, p. 1270)
surgery (p. 1235)
surgical asepsis (ā-SĔP-sĭs, p. 1262)
thrombus (THRŎM-bŭs, p. 1248)

Surgery is the area of medicine that addresses diseases, conditions, and traumatic injuries that are difficult or impossible to treat only with medicine. Since the discovery of anesthesia in the 1840s and the development of antiseptic and aseptic practices, surgical procedures have become much safer and more refined. However, patients are frequently fearful of surgery. Nurses can help alleviate much of this fear by providing support and educating patients about their procedures.

Surgery is classified as elective, urgent, or emergent. Elective surgery is not necessary to preserve life and may be performed at a time the patient chooses. Urgent surgery is required to keep additional health problems from occurring. Emergent surgery is performed immediately to save the individual's life or to preserve the function of a body part or system. Surgical procedures also may be categorized as either major or minor, although all surgeries have an element of risk.

Surgery is performed for various purposes, including diagnostic, ablative, palliative, reconstructive, curative, preventive, transplant, constructive, and cosmetic (Table 42.1). Table 42.2 presents frequently used surgical terminology.

Traditionally, surgical procedures were performed in hospitals. With the discovery of new technologies and the current emphasis on decreasing health care

Table 42.1 **Classification of Surgical Procedures**

TYPE	DESCRIPTION AND EXAMPLES
Admission Status	
Ambulatory (outpatient)	Patient enters setting, has surgical procedure, and is discharged on the same day (e.g., breast biopsy, cataract extraction, hemorrhoidectomy, scar revision).
Same-day admit	Patient enters hospital, undergoes surgery on the same day, and remains for convalescence (e.g., carotid endarterectomy, cholecystectomy, mastectomy, vaginal hysterectomy).
Inpatient	Patient is admitted to hospital, undergoes surgery (surgery may occur on a day other than the day of admission), and remains in hospital for convalescence (e.g., amputation, heart transplant, laryngectomy, resection of aortic aneurysm).
Seriousness	
Major	Involves extensive reconstruction or alteration in body parts; poses great risks to well-being (e.g., coronary artery bypass, colon resection, gastric resection).
Minor	Involves minimal alteration in body parts; often designed to correct deformities; involves minimal risks compared with those of major procedures (e.g., cataract extraction, skin graft, tooth extraction).
Urgency	
Elective	Performed on basis of patient's choice (e.g., bunionectomy, plastic surgery).
Urgent	Necessary for patient's health (e.g., excision of cancerous tumor, removal of gallbladder for stones, vascular repair for obstructed artery [e.g., coronary artery bypass]).
Emergency or Emergent	Must be done immediately to save life or preserve function of body part (e.g., removal of perforated appendix, repair of traumatic amputation, control of internal hemorrhaging).
Purpose	
Diagnostic	Surgical exploration that allows physician to confirm diagnosis; may involve removal of tissue for further diagnostic testing (e.g., exploratory laparotomy [incision into peritoneal cavity to inspect abdominal organs], breast mass biopsy).
Ablative	Excision or removal of diseased body part (e.g., amputation, removal of appendix, cholecystectomy).
Palliative	Surgery for relief or reduction of intensity of disease symptoms; will not produce cure (e.g., colostomy, debridement of necrotic tissue).
Reconstructive	Restoration of function or appearance to traumatized or malfunctioning tissue (e.g., internal fixation of fractures, scar revision, breast reconstruction).
Curative	Surgery that cures the problem or condition.
Preventative	Surgical procedure that prevents any problems or damage from occurring.
Transplant	Replacement of malfunctioning organs (e.g., cornea, heart, joints, kidney).
Constructive	Restoration of function lost or reduced as result of congenital anomalies (e.g., repair of cleft palate, closure of atrial-septal defect in heart).
Cosmetic	Alteration of personal appearance (e.g., rhinoplasty to reshape nose).

Table 42.2 **Surgical Terminology**

TERM/SUFFIX	INTERPRETATION WITH EXAMPLE
Anastomosis	Surgical joining of two ducts or blood vessels to allow flow from one to another; to bypass an area (e.g., Billroth I, joins stomach and duodenum).
-ectomy	Surgical removal of (e.g., cholecystectomy, removal of the gallbladder).
Lysis	Destruction or dissolution of (e.g., lysis of adhesions, removal of adhesions).
-orrhaphy	Surgical repair of (e.g., herniorrhaphy, repair of a hernia).
-oscopy	Direct visualization with a scope (e.g., cystoscopy, direct visualization of the bladder and urethra by means of a cystoscope).
-ostomy	Opening made to allow the passage of drainage (e.g., ileostomy, formation of an opening of the ileum onto the surface of the abdomen for passage of feces).
-otomy	Opening into (e.g., thoracotomy, surgical opening into the thoracic cavity).
-pexy	Fixation of (e.g., cecopexy, fixation or suspension of the cecum to correct its excessive mobility).
-plasty	Plastic surgery (e.g., mammoplasty, reshaping of the breasts to reduce, lift, reconstruct).

Box 42.1 Common Surgical Settings

Inpatient: Patient hospitalized for surgery.
One-day (same-day surgery): Patient is admitted the day surgery is scheduled and discharged the same day.
Outpatient: Patient (not hospitalized) is admitted either to a short-stay unit or directly to the surgical suite (sometimes referred to as ambulatory surgery).
Short-stay surgical center: Independently owned agency; surgery is performed when overnight hospitalization is not required (also called an ambulatory surgical center or 1-day surgery center).
Short-stay unit: Department or floor where a patient's stay does not exceed 24 hours (sometimes referred to as an outpatient/observation unit).
Mobile surgery unit: A unit that moves from place to place; it moves to the patient instead of the patient traveling to the unit.

costs, the surgical suite may now be in a variety of settings. Although facilities use different terms for surgical settings and processes, some common variations are listed in Box 42.1.

PERIOPERATIVE NURSING

The **perioperative** period encompasses the **preoperative** phase (before surgery), **intraoperative** phase (during surgery), and **postoperative** phase (after surgery). Perioperative nursing stresses the importance of providing continuity of care for the surgical patient by using the nursing process. In many hospitals, perioperative nurses assess a patient's health status preoperatively, identify specific patient needs, teach and counsel, attend to the patient's needs in the operating room (OR), and then monitor the patient's recovery. In other facilities, different nurses care for the patient during each phase. Nurses also may delegate certain aspects of perioperative care to appropriate personnel (Box 42.2). It is the nurse's responsibility to ensure that safe, consistent, and effective nursing care is provided during each phase of surgery.

Box 42.2 Delegation Considerations in Perioperative Nursing

- The skills of assessment that are part of preparing a patient for surgery require the critical thinking ability and knowledge application unique to a nurse. For these skills, delegation is inappropriate. However, unlicensed assistive personnel (UAP) may obtain vital signs and weight and height measurements. Instruct UAP on proper precautions for these delegated procedures as needed.
- The skills of preoperative teaching require the critical thinking and knowledge application unique to a nurse. For these skills, delegation is inappropriate. However, UAP may reinforce and assist patients in performing postoperative exercises.
- Review with UAP any precautions for a particular patient (e.g., turning method).
- Be certain staff members know when to inform the nurse if the patient is unable to perform the exercises correctly.
- Coordinating the patient's preparation for surgery requires the critical thinking and knowledge application unique to a nurse. However, UAP may administer an enema or douche; obtain vital signs; apply antiembolic stockings; and assist patient in removing clothing, jewelry, and prostheses.
- Instruct UAP in proper precautions when preparing a patient for surgery.
- Instruct UAP in proper observations and precautions if the patient has an intravenous (IV) catheter in place.
- The skills of sterile gowning and gloving can be delegated to a surgical technologist or a nurse who has acquired the proper skills.
- The skill of initiating and managing postoperative care of a patient requires the critical thinking and knowledge application unique to a nurse. However, UAP may obtain vital signs, remove and replace a nasal cannula or oxygen mask during transfers, and provide basic comfort and hygiene measures.

INFLUENCING FACTORS

Every surgical procedure is stressful for the patient. Observing the patient's nonverbal communication and listening to questions help identify the patient's feelings and concerns. By helping the patient to express the concerns, the nurse can offer support, reassurance, and information to address fear of the unknown. Numerous factors (1) affect the individual's ability to tolerate surgery and (2) influence the development of intraoperative and postoperative complications.

Age

Young and old patients do not tolerate major surgical procedures as well as patients in other age groups. Because of their metabolism, patients in these extreme age groups may have a slower response to physiologic changes such as temperature variations, cardiovascular shifts, respiratory needs, and renal function. Therefore nursing assessments and appropriate interventions must be ongoing (see the Lifespan Considerations box).

Physical Condition

Patients in good overall general health have smoother and faster recovery periods than patients with coexisting health problems. The nurse should assess each body system to identify actual and potential problems and determine measures to prevent postoperative complications (Box 42.3).

Nutritional Factors

The body uses carbohydrates, proteins, and fats to supply energy-producing glucose to its cells. Carbohydrates and fats are the primary energy producers, and

Lifespan Considerations

Older Adults

Undergoing Surgery

- Older adults undergoing surgery have higher morbidity and mortality rates than younger people.
- Surgery places a greater stress on older people than on younger people. The patient's physiologic status and coexisting conditions, such as diabetes mellitus or cardiac disease, should be evaluated carefully. The individual's current health status is a more important factor than age when considering the benefits and risks of surgery. Consequently, increasing numbers of older patients are undergoing surgery, and nurses need to know the age-related factors that affect their response to surgical procedures.
- Older patients tend to recover from surgery more slowly than younger patients. Recovery is affected by the level of mental functioning, individual coping ability, and the availability of support systems.
- Older adults have an increased risk of aspiration, atelectasis (collapsed lung), pneumonia, thrombus formation, infection, and altered tissue perfusion because of age-related changes to various body systems.
- Older adults are more likely to experience disorientation or toxic reactions after the administration of anesthetics, sedatives, or analgesics. These reactions result from age-related changes in the hepatic and renal systems and may persist for days after receiving the medication. The health care staff should, however, be cautioned to avoid undermedicating an older adult solely based on age, remembering that many elders are in very good physiologic health.
- Preoperative and postoperative teaching may require extra time. The nurse should allow time for the patient to process any information presented. Repeating and reinforcing directions is sometimes necessary.
- When communicating with older adult patients, the nurse should be aware of any auditory, visual, or cognitive impairments.

protein is essential to build and repair body tissue. Under stressful conditions such as recovering from surgery, the body's need for energy and repair increases. Nutritional needs are affected by a patient's age and physical requirements; patients who maintain a sound nutritional diet tend to recover more quickly.

A complete diet history identifies the patient's usual eating habits, nutritional patterns, and food preferences. Dietary practices are influenced by a patient's ethnic, cultural, religious, and socioeconomic background. Consider this information when offering the patient appropriate foods that are high in energy-producing nutrients. Surgery may decrease a patient's appetite and alter metabolic functions, so observe the patient for signs of malnutrition. If malnutrition is identified promptly, tube feedings, intravenous (IV) therapy, or total parenteral nutrition can be initiated (see Chapters 15 and 18 in *Foundations of Nursing*).

Box 42.3 ABCDEF Mnemonic Device to Ascertain Serious Illness or Trauma in the Preoperative Patient

A *Allergy* to medications, chemicals, and other environmental products such as latex. All allergies are reported to anesthesia and surgical personnel before the beginning of surgery. Place an allergy band on the patient's arm immediately.

B *Bleeding* tendencies or the use of medications that deter clotting, such as aspirin or products containing aspirin, heparin, or warfarin sodium. Herbal medications also may increase bleeding times or mask potential blood-related problems.

C *Cortisone* or steroid use.

D *Diabetes mellitus,* a condition that not only requires strict control of blood glucose levels but also is known to delay wound healing. Patients with diabetes also may have elevated blood glucose levels even after being placed on NPO (nothing by mouth) status because of the body's stress response.

E *Emboli.* Previous embolic events (such as lower leg blood clots) may recur because of prolonged immobility.

F *Fighting ability.* Patients whose immune systems are suppressed are at a much higher risk for development of postoperative infection and are less capable of fighting that infection.

PSYCHOSOCIAL NEEDS

As the patient and family plan for surgery, they frequently express concern and fears about possible outcomes (Box 42.4). Preoperative fear has been linked to intraoperative and postoperative behavior. The preoperative anxiety level influences the amount of anesthesia required, the amount of postoperative pain medication needed, and the speed of recovery from surgery. Each patient's perceptions, emotions, behavior, and support systems should be evaluated to identify factors that may influence the individual's progress through the perioperative period. Patiently and actively listening to the patient, the family, and significant others allows the nurse to address fears and help reduce anxiety (Fig. 42.1).

While the patient prepares for the upcoming surgery, family members and support people are also trying to cope. Families may have additional burdens, such as financial obligations, living changes, and added personal responsibilities. In addition to nursing and medical personnel, social workers, clergy, or patient advocates can provide support for patients and families during this stressful time (see the Patient Teaching box on preoperative care).

SOCIOECONOMIC AND CULTURAL NEEDS

The United States is a nation of diverse individuals of various social, economic, religious, ethnic, and cultural origins. Even regional factors affect the way a patient

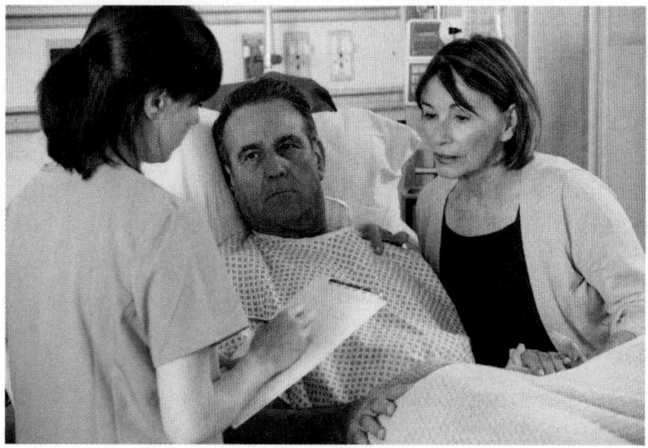

Fig. 42.1 Knowledge deficits often occur when a patient is undergoing his or her first surgical experience.

Box 42.4 Common Fears Associated With Surgery

- Fear of loss of control is associated primarily with anesthesia. The patient becomes almost totally dependent on the health care team during the surgical experience—even for basic needs such as breathing and life support—while under the influence of anesthesia.
- Fear of the unknown may result from uncertainty about the surgical outcome or a lack of knowledge regarding the surgical experience.
- Fear of anesthesia may include fears of unpleasant induction of or emergence from anesthesia. The patient may fear waking up during the operation and feeling pain while under anesthesia. This fear often is related to loss of control and fear of the unknown.
- Fear of pain or inadequate postoperative analgesia is common. Reassure the patient and significant others that the pain will be controlled.
- Fear of death is a legitimate fear. Even with the great strides in surgery and anesthesia, no anesthetic or operation is perfectly safe for all patients.
- Fear of separation from the usual support group may arise because the patient is separated from spouse, family, or significant others, as well as other support groups, and is cared for by strangers during this highly stressful period.
- Fear of disruption of life patterns relates to surgery and recovery interfering in varying degrees with activities of daily living, social activities, work, and professional activities.
- Fear of change in body image and mutilation is not unusual. Surgery disrupts body integrity and threatens body image.
- Fear of detection of cancer produces a high anxiety level.

responds to surgery. Therefore it is important to allow patients and families to express themselves openly.

A multicultural perspective (see Chapter 6 in *Foundations of Nursing*) helps nurses approach patients with respect and individually tailor care to promote recovery (see the Cultural Considerations box).

Patient Teaching

Preoperative Care

The nurse may assist preoperative patients and their families by providing information about the following:

- Preoperative tests: Reason, preparation
- Preoperative routines: Sequence of events
- Special equipment needed, especially if the patient is undergoing same-day surgery and being discharged home. Items that may be necessary include crutches, orthopedic boots or splints, wheelchair, walker, bedside commode, and shower chair
- Transfer to operating room: Time, checking procedures
- Medications that may be prescribed at discharge: Addressing how the patient will obtain prescribed medication is especially important for the patient who does not have insurance
- Recovery room or postanesthesia care unit
- Place where the patient will awaken
- Frequent monitoring of vital signs
- Return to room when vital signs are stable
- Probable postoperative therapies
- Need for increased mobility as soon as possible
- Need to keep respiratory passages clear
- Anticipated treatments such as an intravenous line, dressing changes, and incentive spirometry
- Pain medication routines (timing sequence, "as needed" [prn] status), other modalities of management such as patient-controlled analgesia and patient-controlled epidural analgesia

MEDICATIONS

Review of the patient's current medication regimen is essential. Polypharmacy (concurrent use of multiple medications) occurs in all age groups but is more common with older adults. The National Council on Patient Information and Education (NCPIE) reported that approximately 34% of prescription drugs and 30% of over-the-counter medications were taken by elderly people. Two out of five Medicare recipients report taking an average of five or more prescription drugs (NCPIE, 2018). The use of multiple medications can lead to adverse drug reactions and interactions with other medications in the perioperative setting.

During the perioperative period, health care providers use medications and agents from several pharmacologic categories, including anesthetics, antimicrobials, anticoagulants, hemostatic agents, steroids, diagnostic imaging dyes, diuretics, central nervous system agents, and emergency protocol medications. An acutely ill patient may receive several drugs at one time. The larger the number of medications, the greater the chance of an adverse interaction.

People also frequently use herbal remedies as alternative or complementary therapy. It is essential to ask the patient about the use of herbal preparations, either as dietary supplements or as medicines, because most patients do not think of them as medications. Even

Cultural Considerations

The Surgical Patient

- Use of the patient's language helps put an anxious patient at ease. Use an interpreter when possible. Learn some key phrases in foreign languages. Use references such as medical dictionaries, which usually have key phrases listed in an appendix.
- Because some older Asians, older Native Americans, and those from Middle Eastern cultures may avoid eye contact and consider it disrespectful, consider limiting eye contact when dealing with these patients.
- Chinese Americans may not ask for pain medication and may need teaching to help understand how comfort and relief from pain promote healing and a quicker recovery.
- Native Americans are often stoic when ill. Complaints of pain to the nurse may be in general terms such as, "I am uncomfortable." Undertreatment of pain is common.
- Among Arab Americans, verbal consent often has more meaning than written consent because it is based on trust. Fully explain the need for written consent. The patient may be expressive regarding pain. Pain may cause intense fear. Prepare the patient for painful procedures, and develop a care plan to prevent pain. Assistance with toileting or other intimate care also may be an area of concern in which the nurse must consider male/female roles.
- For Vietnamese patients, having an interpreter is important, depending on the sensitivity of the subject under discussion, because of modesty. A female family member is expected to be at the bedside to provide care and comfort. Men are the decision makers and support the family; therefore speaking with the male head of the family may be necessary. Eye contact and touch should be avoided in many instances.

Data from Centers for Disease Control and Prevention (CDC), 2010.

though herbs are natural products, they act like drugs and may interact with or potentiate other medications or interfere with surgical procedures (Table 42.3). Vitamin use also must be addressed because of vitamins' physiologic actions (e.g., vitamin E may prolong bleeding times).

Some medications may be stopped before the patient goes to surgery. The nurse needs to know the purposes and actions of drugs because they may be critical for a patient with coexisting conditions. For example, if a patient with diabetes has the insulin dose withheld before surgery, the nurse must monitor the patient's blood glucose level pre- and postoperatively. The anesthesiologist, in collaboration with the patient's health care provider and surgeon, determines whether such medications should be taken the day of surgery and postoperatively. Common medications that are not stopped and are given with a sip of water the morning of surgery include antiseizure and cardiac drugs.

Assess the patient for allergies to drugs that may be given during any phase of the perioperative period. If the patient is allergic to a drug, ask him or her to describe specifically the type of reaction. Determine nondrug allergies, including allergies to foods, chemicals, pollen, antiseptics used to prepare the skin for surgery, and latex products. A patient with a history of allergic responsiveness is more likely to have a hypersensitivity reaction to anesthesia agents. Many facilities require such patients to wear an allergy identification band during surgery. Follow facility policy for posting allergy alerts in the patient's medical record.

EDUCATION AND EXPERIENCE

When teaching patients, consider the patient's age, educational level, and communication abilities. Communicate at a level that patients understand. The care plan should include provisions to ensure the patient has understood any new information presented. For example, ask the patient to summarize the information given or to perform a return demonstration.

PREOPERATIVE PHASE

Before surgery, patients require a thorough health assessment. Acute or chronic diseases hinder the body's ability to repair or to adjust to surgical treatment. Disorders of the systems identified in Table 42.4 present high-risk conditions for surgery. Each system is affected further by the patient's age, health, nutritional status, and mental state. Assessment questions regarding the patient's use of chemicals, alcohol, and recreational substances help the health team select medications. When possible, postoperative care also is adjusted to prevent potential complications. For example, a patient who smokes cigarettes may have impaired alveoli and reduced lung capacity. Mucus and anesthesia by-products may become trapped in the lungs, causing atelectasis and pneumonia. After surgery, breathing exercises and treatments for smokers aid in lung expansion and decrease the risk of respiratory complications.

Additional preoperative questions identify allergies, past surgeries, and infection and disease history. The patient should be asked for a complete list of prescription drugs, over-the-counter medications, as well as vitamins, minerals, and herbal products taken, including home remedies. The patient's vital signs, height, and weight should be measured before surgery to have a baseline for postoperative comparison.

PREOPERATIVE TEACHING

Patient teaching before surgery helps reduce (1) the patient's anxiety associated with fear of the unknown, (2) the amount of anesthesia needed, (3) postsurgical pain, and (4) corticosteroid production. Decreasing postsurgical complications through preoperative teaching speeds wound healing.

Include the patient and family when providing preoperative teaching, and remember that basic terminology and information are easier for them to understand than complex explanations. Frequently verify the patient's

Table 42.3 Preoperative Considerations for Commonly Ingested Herbs

HERB	COMMON USES	PREOPERATIVE CONSIDERATIONS
Echinacea	Treat cold symptoms	Possible negative impact on the liver. Subsequent interference with hepatic metabolism of certain anesthesia medications.
Ephedra sinica	Decongestant Weight loss	Increased risk of cardiac dysrhythmias. May reduce effectiveness of medications used to treat hypotension.
Feverfew	Migraine prevention	Has anticoagulation factors; potential for increased bleeding. Preoperative assessment should include clotting studies. Discontinue before surgery.
Garlic	Improved immunity High blood pressure and cholesterol	Potential for increased bleeding.
Ginger	Motion sickness Cough Menstrual cramps Intestinal gas	Risk of prolonged clotting times. Preoperative assessment should include clotting studies. Discontinue before surgery.
Ginkgo biloba	Brain function and alertness Tension Erectile dysfunction	Potential for increased bleeding.
Ginseng	Overall well-being Diabetes	May increase anesthetic agent requirements. Potential for hypoglycemia in patients taking insulin or oral diabetes agents.
Guarana	Mental alertness Fatigue	May reduce the efficacy of warfarin. May potentiate sympathetic nervous system stimulants, leading to cardiac complications. May decrease cerebral blood flow.
Kava	Sleep aid Anxiety, tension	May potentiate muscle relaxants. May increase effects of certain antiemetics. Potential for serious liver damage and subsequent decreased hepatic metabolism of certain anesthetic agents.
Licorice	Asthma, eczema, rheumatoid arthritis Expectorant Gastritis	May cause hypertension. Potential for hypokalemia and associated cardiac dysrhythmias.
St. John's wort	Antidepressant Antiviral properties Antiinflammatory action	Should not be used with other psychoactive drugs, monoamine oxidase inhibitors, or serotonin reuptake inhibitors. Discontinue before surgery because of possible drug interactions.
Valerian root	Sedative or tranquilizer effect Sleep aid	Should not be used with sedatives or anxiolytics. May increase effects of central nervous system depressants.

understanding of information, ask questions, and encourage responses. Avoid asking questions that can be answered "yes" or "no." Instead of saying, "Do you have any questions?" try asking, "What questions do you have?" If using printed material for preoperative teaching, make sure that the patient is able to read and that the printed material is within the patient's reading level. Printed or video material used in preoperative teaching sessions should be documented. Older adults may have difficulty reading small print or hearing audio material. If the patient does not understand English, an interpreter should explain the information presented. Also, patients should understand that a nurse will be with them throughout the entire surgical experience.

For surgical procedures that have potential long-term effects, support groups can offer assistance preoperatively. Cancer organizations, amputation support groups, and enterostomal associations are examples of large national organizations that offer peer support.

Ideally the patient is seen in the surgeon's office and preoperative teaching is provided when the surgery is scheduled, when anxiety is not as high. The surgeon provides information regarding the actual surgical procedure, as well as the risks, benefits, and possible outcomes. The surgeon's nursing staff typically provides teaching regarding preoperative instructions, such as any gastrointestinal cleansing preparation, or the need for assistive devices to be obtained for use immediately after surgery (e.g., crutches or orthopedic boots). The

Table 42.4 Surgical Effects on Body Systems

DISEASE OR DISORDER	SURGICAL EFFECTS
Cardiovascular (See Chapter 48)	
Recent myocardial infarction, dysrhythmias, and heart failure Hypertension	Hypotension and cardiac dysrhythmias are the most common cardiovascular complications of the surgical patient. Early recognition and management before these complications become serious enough to diminish cardiac output depend on frequent assessment of the patient's vital signs.
Endocrine (See Chapter 51)	
Type 1 and type 2 diabetes	Diabetes increases susceptibility to infection and may impair wound healing because of altered glucose metabolism and associated circulatory impairment. Fluctuating blood glucose levels may cause central nervous system malfunction during anesthesia.
Gastrointestinal (See Chapter 45)	
Hiatal hernia	
Ulcers	Preoperative and postoperative medication may be necessary to control gastric acidity.
Esophageal varices	Risk of hemorrhage may increase because of intubation.
Liver disease	Liver disease alters metabolism and elimination of drugs administered during surgery and impairs wound healing because of alterations in protein metabolism.
Immune (See Chapter 55)	
Acquired immunodeficiency syndrome; allergies; immunodeficiency	Disease slows the body's ability to fight infection. Immunologic disorders increase risk of infection and delay wound healing after surgery. Hypothermia during surgery decreases immune function.
Musculoskeletal (See Chapter 44)	
	Osteoporosis and increased risk for fractures in the older adult place patient at increased risk for injury during surgery.
Neurologic (See Chapter 54)	
Seizures	Ensure anti-seizure medications are at therapeutic levels to prevent postoperative seizures.
Myasthenia gravis	Muscle relaxants may need to be excluded because of patient's decreased ability to reverse their effects.
Cerebrovascular accident	Impaired verbal communication, defective perception of the body, paralysis, and visual disturbances place patient at high risk for injury.
Peripheral vascular disease	Patient has a decreased threshold for peripheral pain.
Respiratory (See Chapter 49)	
Tumors Chronic obstructive pulmonary disease Emphysema Asthma	Lung capacity is decreased and gas exchange slowed. Anesthetic agents reduce respiratory function, increasing risk for severe hypoventilation.
Urinary (See Chapter 50)	
Renal failure	Impaired kidney function decreases excretion of anesthesia and alters acid-base balance.
Tumors	Prostate enlargement may increase risk of urinary tract infection.

nurse clarifies what the physician has explained to the patient, reviews the time of the surgery, and witnesses the patient signing the informed consent. If the patient is already in the hospital and a surgery is scheduled, the nurse on the unit provides similar information that the office staff provides, as well as information about the recovery area (e.g., previously assigned units, intensive care, specialty units, or outpatient area). Facilities often have an established teaching program, which includes a systematic preoperative teaching plan and checklist. If a transfer is planned after surgery, it is helpful to take the patient and family on a tour of the new unit. The nurse also should explain that vital signs, dressings, and tubes are assessed every 15 to 30 minutes until the patient is awake and stable.

PREOPERATIVE PREPARATION

Preparation for surgery depends on the patient's age and physical and nutritional status, the type of surgery, and the surgeon's preference. For surgery in a short-stay or ambulatory setting, the workup normally occurs a few days in advance. If the patient is admitted to the hospital, testing may be conducted to assess for potential problems. Preparation frequently includes in-facility testing and evaluation of test results that were completed before admission.

Laboratory Tests and Diagnostic Imaging

Testing before surgery depends on the institution's policies, the health care provider's directives, and the patient's condition. Laboratory tests commonly reviewed before surgery include a urinalysis; a complete blood count; and a blood chemistry profile to assess endocrine, hepatic, renal, and cardiovascular functions. Serum electrolytes are evaluated if extensive surgery is planned or if the patient has associated problems. One essential electrolyte assessed is potassium; abnormal serum potassium levels can lead to dysrhythmias during and after surgery, and the patient's recovery may be delayed by general muscle weakness. A chest x-ray evaluation and electrocardiogram are used to identify disease processes or existing respiratory or cardiac damage. Additional tests are conducted to assess the organ involved in surgery. A blood chemistry profile tests several blood levels, including lipids, blood urea nitrogen (BUN), and creatinine (kidney function), proteins and electrolytes, as well as liver function.

Informed Consent

The Patient's Bill of Rights affirms that patients must give **informed consent** (i.e., permission to perform a specific test or procedure) before any procedure is begun. In signing the consent form, the patient must be competent and agree to have the procedure that is stated on the form. The surgeon must explain the risks involved, identify expected benefits, and describe consequences or alternatives for the presenting problem. The nurse frequently is a witness when a patient signs the consent form. A witness only verifies that this is the person who signed the consent and that it was a voluntary consent; the witness cannot verify that the patient understood the procedure. Ideally, the surgeon discusses the surgical procedure with the patient in advance. In some institutions, the surgical consent is completed in the physician's office or in the admissions department before the patient is admitted to the unit. Informed consent should not be obtained if the patient is disoriented, unconscious, mentally incompetent, or, in some agencies, under the influence of sedatives. The nurse must follow agency policy (see Chapter 2, Fig. 2.1 in *Foundations of Nursing*).

If the patient has vision or hearing impairment, additional time may be necessary to explain and obtain the patient's signature on the consent form. For patients who do not understand English, an interpreter may be necessary. A patient should never be coerced into signing a consent that he or she does not understand or that contains information different from that originally given. If necessary, inform the physician that the patient does not understand the procedure. (Refer to Chapter 2 in *Foundations of Nursing* for discussion of informed consent.)

In an emergency, the patient may not be able to give consent for surgery. Every effort is made to locate family members to assume this responsibility. In many cases consent will be provided by the spouse. In the absence of a spouse, this role may be passed to another legally identified individual (e.g., advance directive). On occasion, telephone permission may be obtained. Hospitals have standard guidelines for obtaining verbal consent. If the patient's life is in danger and family members cannot be located, the surgeon may legally perform surgery. If the patient is deemed incompetent to provide consent, there is a legal process for identifying a legal guardian eligible to provide the consent. If family members object to surgery that the physician believes is essential, a court order may be obtained for the procedure. This practice is used only in extreme circumstances (e.g., when a child's life is in danger). The nurse must follow agency policy in any of these circumstances.

Gastrointestinal Preparation

In the past, the standard gastrointestinal preparation included placing the patient on nothing by mouth (NPO) status at midnight the night before surgery to decrease the risk of intra- and postoperative vomiting and aspiration. Several studies have shown that being NPO for extended periods of time before surgery does not significantly decrease the risk for aspiration and actually increases the patient's risk for dehydration, insulin resistance, and muscle wasting and places a strain on the immune system. In addition, prolonged NPO status increases the patient's anxiety level, thirst, dizziness, and hunger. Newer recommendations suggest allowing the patient to have clear liquids up to 2 hours before surgery unless the patient has a condition that delays gastric emptying. Regardless of studies, many health care providers continue to place patients on NPO status at midnight before surgery. The nurse must follow any preoperative orders issued by the health care provider (Blanchard, 2012).

The patient can have oral care while NPO but should be cautioned not to swallow any fluids used. A wet cloth on the lips helps relieve dryness. If the patient needs to be hydrated or requires special IV medications, the health care provider may order parenteral fluids or medication. Depending on the procedure, many patients resume eating and drinking on the same day following the surgery.

Because anesthesia relaxes the bowel, a bowel cleanser may be ordered to evacuate fecal material and lessen postoperative gastrointestinal (GI) problems (nausea and vomiting). A cleansing enema or a general laxative may be used. If a bowel preparation is given, chart the type of preparation used, the patient's tolerance to the procedure, and the results. Some studies indicate that there is no benefit to mechanical bowel preparation before surgery (Harris et al, 2009; Scabini et al, 2012). Follow the order of the health care provider. Before bowel surgery, medication (neomycin, sulfonamides, erythromycin) may be given over a period of days to detoxify and sterilize the GI tract. This lessens the chance of infection if fecal contamination occurs during surgery.

Skin Preparation

Before surgery the surgeon may order hair removal at the surgical site. Typically, hair removal is ordered only if it may interfere with exposure, closure, or dressing of the surgical site. During hair removal, the operative site must be treated carefully to remove the hair without injuring the skin (Skill 42.1).

Studies indicate no significant difference in surgical site infection (SSI) rates when comparing the results of no hair removal with hair removal by shaving, clipping, and depilatory cream (Kowalski et al, 2016). Shaving the hair before surgery can create microscopic cuts that increase the risk of SSI. The Centers for Disease Control and Prevention strongly recommend not removing hair unless it would interfere with the surgery (CDC, 2012). Debate also continues regarding when to perform hair removal if it is indicated. Some surgeons prefer patient hair removal close to the time of the surgical procedure to decrease the time for growth of bacteria and lower

Skill 42.1 Performing a Surgical Skin Preparation

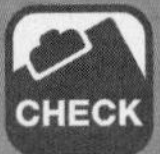

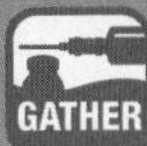

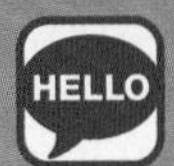

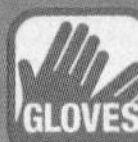

NURSING ACTION *(RATIONALE)*

1. Refer to medical record, care plan, or Kardex for special interventions. *(Provides basis for care.)*
2. Obtain equipment. *(Organizes procedure.)*
   a. Appropriate light
   b. Operating room prep kit:
      Basin
      Razor
      Sponge with soap
      Waterproof pad
      Cotton-tipped applicators
   c. Clean gloves
3. Introduce self. *(Decreases patient's anxiety.)*
4. Identify patient. *(Identifies correct patient for procedure.)*
5. Explain procedure to patient. *(Improves cooperation and decreases anxiety.)*
6. Perform hand hygiene and, if appropriate, don clean gloves. Know agency policy and guidelines from the Centers for Disease Control and Prevention (CDC) and the Occupational Safety and Health Administration (OSHA). *(Reduces spread of microorganisms.)*
7. Prepare patient for intervention:
   a. Close door to room or pull curtain. *(Provides privacy.)*
   b. Drape for procedure if necessary and position patient. *(Promotes proper body mechanics.)*
8. Raise bed to comfortable working level. *(Promotes proper body mechanics.)*
9. Place towel or waterproof pad under area to be shaved. *(Protects bed and linen from soiling.)*
10. Fill basin with warm water. *(Allows nurse to lather soap and rinse skin.)*
11. Place bath blanket over patient. *(Exposes only area to be shaved.)*
12. Adjust lighting. *(Allows thorough assessment of skin and helps decrease chance of skin impairment.)*
13. Lather skin with antiseptic soap and warm water. *(Cleanses skin, softens hair, and reduces friction from razor.)*
14. If using a razor, hold razor at a 30- to 45-degree angle to skin. *(Minimizes chances of cutting or nicking skin.)*
    a. Shave small areas while holding skin taut.
    b. Use short, smooth strokes. *(Prevents pulling skin.)*
    c. Shave hair in same direction it grows. *(Removes hair close to skin surface.)*
15. Rinse razor frequently. *(Removes accumulation of hair from razor and prevents contamination from dirty water.)*
16. After entire area is shaved, cleanse it with a washcloth and clean, warm water. Dry skin. *(Removes excess shaved hair, body oils, and soil on skin. Reduces number of microorganisms. Promotes patient comfort.)*
17. Reassess skin for cuts, nicks, or hair. *(Prevents growth of microorganisms and possible infections from skin impairment.)*
18. Return patient to appropriate position. *(Provides patient comfort and safety.)*
19. Clean and dispose of equipment. *(Reduces spread of microorganisms.)*
20. Remove and dispose of soiled gloves and wash hands. *(Reduces spread of microorganisms.)*
21. Document. *(Verifies procedure.)*

Special concerns for patients undergoing a surgical skin preparation are as follows:

- Small children may be easily frightened by this procedure, and it may have to be done in the operating room (OR).
- Older adults need a detailed explanation to relieve their anxiety.
- Older adults have less subcutaneous tissue, less skin elasticity, and more delicate skin tissue. Take extreme care when shaving the older adult.
- Older adults are usually more susceptible to infections.

the potential for infection. Some surgical departments prepare the patient either in a surgical holding room or in the operating room (OR). Each facility should have policies and protocols regarding the timing, the method, and the staff responsible for the preoperative skin preparation of surgical patients.

Facility policy or specific surgeon order dictates preoperative skin preparation. The nurse reviews agency policy and the patient chart to determine the area to be prepared. Before the skin preparation, the surgical site is assessed carefully for the presence of any skin impairment (e.g., infection, irritation, bruises, lesions). The patient also is assessed for any skin allergies. Any abnormal assessment findings must be recorded and reported to the surgeon. Some surgeons require patients shower with an antimicrobial solution the night before or the day of surgery, or both.

Once the patient is in the OR, an antiseptic solution to kill adherent and deeper-residing bacteria is used. Common surgical antiseptic solutions include povidone-iodine (Betadine) and chlorhexidine. The surgeon may place a transparent sterile drape directly over the skin before making an incision.

Latex Allergy Considerations

A focused assessment helps identify patients who may be at risk for latex allergy response. Assessing the patient's experience helps identify those at risk for a systemic reaction (e.g., the patient may relate stories of complicated anesthesia events, hives from blowing up a balloon, or severe swelling of the labia with a urinary catheterization).

With the advent of universal precautions (now called standard precautions) in the late 1980s, the use of latex gloves dramatically increased, and latex allergies were detected much more often. Gloves are worn by all staff members providing health care to patients. Most gloves are powdered to make them easier to put on. The powder absorbs protein allergens from the latex and deposits them on skin and into surgical wounds; it also aerosolizes the protein allergens. Aerosolized latex allergens are carried in ventilation systems, requiring further preventive measures.

Latex allergy occurs in three ways: (1) as irritant contact dermatitis, (2) as type IV allergic reactions, and (3) as type I allergic reactions. The irritant reaction, which is seen most commonly, is actually a nonallergic reaction and results in itchy, dry, and irritated hands. The type IV allergic reaction to latex is a cell-mediated response to the chemical irritants found in latex products. The true latex allergy is the type I allergic reaction, and it occurs shortly after exposure to the proteins in latex rubber. The type I reaction is an immunoglobulin E–mediated systemic reaction that occurs when latex proteins are touched, inhaled, or ingested (Asthma and Allergy Foundation of America, n.d.).

Factors influencing the risk for latex allergy response are the individual's susceptibility and the route, duration, and frequency of latex exposure. Risk factors (Mayo Clinic Staff, n.d.) include the following:

- A job with daily exposure to latex (health care, food handlers, rubber industry workers)
- Children with spina bifida (about 50% with disorder) due to early and repeated exposure to latex products through necessary health care provided frequently, beginning at birth
- Food allergies (specifically kiwi, bananas, avocados, chestnuts)
- History of allergies and asthma
- History of reactions to latex (balloons, condoms, gloves)
- Multiple surgical procedures (especially from infancy)

To provide a latex-safe environment for susceptible patients, all surgical patients should be screened for the risk for latex allergy response before admission. Identification of patients at risk is the first step in preventing a reaction.

When a patient with a suspected or known latex allergy is scheduled for surgery, all latex use is avoided, and the patient is admitted directly to the OR as the first case of the day, if possible. Many facilities have converted isolation rooms into latex-safe environments for patients with latex allergy. Nurses must ensure that everyone on the health care team is aware that a patient is, or may be, allergic to latex. A medical alert or allergy band must be placed around the patient's wrist and clearly flagged on the patient's medical record. All natural rubber latex products are removed from the area, and latex-free measures are used for medication preparation. The crash cart must be stocked with latex-free equipment, supplies, and drugs for treating anaphylaxis. Some surgeons order preoperative prophylactic treatment with glucocorticoid steroids and antihistamines. Box 42.5 lists interventions based on NIC (Nursing Interventions Classifications) for the perioperative care of the patient at risk for a latex allergy response (Nursing Interventions and Rationales, 2013).

Respiratory Preparation

If a general anesthetic is administered, it is essential to ventilate the lungs postoperatively to prevent or treat atelectasis, improve lung expansion, improve oxygenation, and prevent postoperative pneumonia. Because the lungs do not expand fully during surgery, mucus and gases remain in the lungs until expelled. Pulmonary exercises can help to expand the lungs and remove these by-products. Preoperative introduction to incentive spirometry has proven helpful.

The nurse usually instructs the patient about the **incentive spirometer** (IS). The patient should use the IS at the bedside at regular intervals to promote deep breathing (Skill 42.2 and the Patient Teaching box on incentive spirometry). A chart included inside the IS package helps predict IS capacity based on gender, height, and age. The initial postoperative goal is one third of the predicted value. The amount of air inspired

Box 42.5 Responding to a Patient's Risk for Latex Allergy

LATEX ALERT PATIENT (HIGH RISK FOR ALLERGIC RESPONSE)

- Recognize the problem.
- Avoid exposing the patient to latex.
- Notify surgeons and operating room nurses and staff.
- Be prepared to treat anaphylaxis should it occur.
- Be alert to signs and symptoms of a reaction postoperatively.

LATEX ALLERGY PATIENT (SUSPECTED OR KNOWN ALLERGIC RESPONSE)

- Administer prophylactic treatment with steroids and antihistamines preoperatively.
- Prepare a latex-safe environment, include latex-safe supply cart and crash cart.
- Apply cloth barrier to patient's arm under a blood pressure cuff.
- Use medications from glass ampules.
- Do not puncture rubber stoppers with needles.
- Wear synthetic gloves.
- Use latex-free syringes.
- Use latex-safe (polyvinyl chloride) intravenous (IV) tubing.
- Do not use latex equipment (i.e., tubing and spikes on tubing) on IV bags.

is measured, and the patient is encouraged to attain the established goal. When the patient is able to reach that goal on a regular basis, the goal should be increased. A respiratory therapist may provide preoperative teaching of IS use if the patient is considered at high risk for **atelectasis** (an abnormal condition characterized by the collapse of lung tissue). Conditions such as chronic respiratory disease and thoracic or abdominal surgery increase the risk for atelectasis.

Patient Teaching

Incentive Spirometry

- After performing incentive spirometry exercises, the patient should practice controlled coughing techniques.
- Teach the patient to examine his or her sputum for consistency, amount, and color changes.
- Before discharge, ask the patient to demonstrate the correct procedure for use of incentive spirometer.
- Administer breathing treatments before the patient's meals to prevent nausea and vomiting.
- To encourage patient use, place the spirometer close by, on the bedside stand. The usual rate of use is 10 breaths hourly during waking hours.

Skill 42.2 Incentive Spirometry or Positive Expiratory Pressure Therapy and "Huff" Coughing

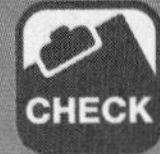

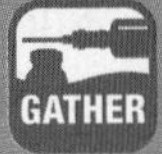

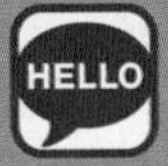

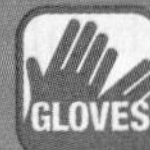

NURSING ACTION *(RATIONALE)*

1. Refer to physician's orders, care plan, or Kardex. *(Health care facilities frequently require a medical order for incentive spirometry.)*
2. Assess patient's respiratory status and lung sounds. Indications for spirometry are (a) asymmetric chest wall movement, (b) increased respiratory rate, (c) increased production of sputum, and (d) diminished lung expansion postoperatively. *(Alerts health care personnel to those patients at risk for respiratory complications during illness or after surgery.)*
3. Explain procedure, and instruct patient in the correct use of the spirometer. Frequently the respiratory therapist will do this. However, it may be the nurse's responsibility to follow up and promote proper technique. *(Understanding improves compliance with use.)*
4. Obtain supplies and equipment. *(Organizes procedure.)*
   a. Incentive spirometer or positive expiratory pressure (PEP) therapy device
   b. Emesis basin
   c. Tissues
   d. Bedside trash bag
   e. Clean gloves (if soiling is likely)
5. Wash hands and don gloves (if soiling is likely). Know agency policy and guidelines from the Centers for Disease Control and Prevention and the Occupational Safety and Health Administration. *(Reduces spread of microorganisms.)*
6. Place prescribed incentive spirometer at the bedside. *(Prepares equipment for procedure.)*
7. Place patient in semi-Fowler's or high Fowler's position. *(Promotes optimal lung expansion.)*

Skill 42.2 Incentive Spirometry or Positive Expiratory Pressure Therapy and "Huff" Coughing—cont'd

8. Place tissues, emesis basin, and bedside trash bag within easy reach. *(Enables sanitary disposal of respiratory secretions expectorated during procedure.)*

9. Incentive spirometry

a. Instruct patient to completely cover mouthpiece with lips (use a nose clip if patient is unable to breathe through the mouthpiece) and to (a) inhale slowly until maximum inspiration is reached, (b) hold breath 2 to 3 s, and (c) slowly exhale (see Fig. 42.2). *(Promotes maximum inspiration.)*

b. Instruct patient to relax and breathe normally for a short time. *(Prevents patient from hyperventilating and prevents fatigue.)*

c. Instruct and encourage patient to gradually increase depth of inspiration. *(Promotes maximum lung expansion.)*

d. Offer oral hygiene after spirometry is completed. *(Patients often find this refreshing.)*

e. Store spirometer in an appropriate place, such as the bedside table, until next scheduled time. *(Provides a convenient place for repeated use.)*

10. PEP therapy and "huff" coughing

a. Wash hands. *(Reduces transmission of microorganisms.)*

b. Set PEP device for setting ordered. *(The higher the setting, the more effort required.)*

c. Instruct patient to assume a semi-Fowler's or high Fowler's position, and place nose clip on patient's nose. *(Promotes optimum lung expansion and expectoration of mucus.)*

d. Instruct patient to place lips around mouthpiece and (1) take a full breath and exhale two or three times longer than inhalation and (2) repeat this pattern for 10 to 20 breaths. *(Ensures that all breathing is done through the mouth and that the device is used properly.)*

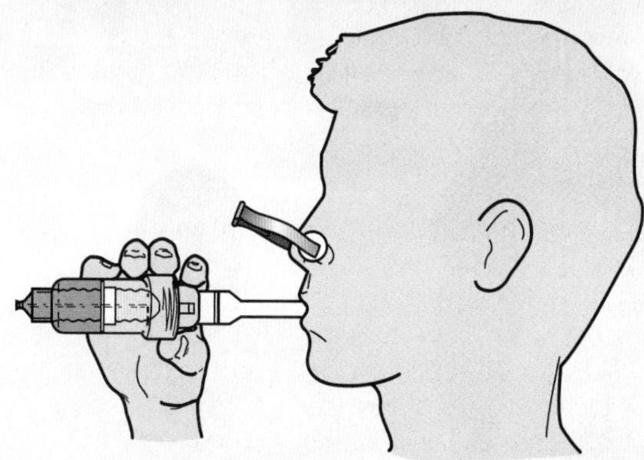

e. Remove device from mouth, and have patient take a slow, deep breath and hold for 3 s. *(Promotes lung expansion before coughing.)*

f. Instruct patient to exhale in quick, short, forced "huffs." *("Huff" coughing, or forced expiratory technique, promotes bronchial hygiene by increasing expectoration of secretions.)*

11. Position patient as desired or as ordered. *(Helps maintain patient comfort and promotes maximum chest expansion.)*

12. Place call light within easy reach. *(Maintains patient safety.)*

13. Remove and dispose of soiled gloves and wash hands. *(Reduces spread of microorganisms.)*

14. Assess respiratory status and evaluate patient's response to spirometry. *(Provides a basis for repeated use.)*

15. Document in nurse's notes patient's respiratory status before and after incentive spirometry, type of spirometry, and any adverse effects from the procedure. *(Verifies patient care. Some agencies require such documentation for third-party reimbursements.)*

16. Carry out patient teaching (see the Patient Teaching box on incentive spirometry).

Figure from Potter PA, Perry AG, Stockert PA, et al: *Fundamentals of nursing,* ed 9, St. Louis, 2017, Elsevier.

There are two general types of incentive spirometer:

1. *Flow-oriented inspiratory spirometer:* This type of incentive spirometer is inexpensive and measures inspiration. It contains one or more clear plastic cylinder chambers that contain freely movable, colored, lightweight plastic balls or a disk. Instruct the patient to place the mouthpiece in the mouth and inhale slowly and deeply; this raises the balls or disk in the cylinders. Encourage the patient to keep the colored balls or disk floating or raised for at least 2 to 3 seconds. The degree of elevation is marked on the cylinders so that this, plus the length of time the patient maintains elevation, can be recorded (Fig. 42.2).
2. *Volume-oriented spirometer:* This form of incentive spirometer maintains a known volume of inspiration. Encourage the patient to breathe with normal inspired capacity.

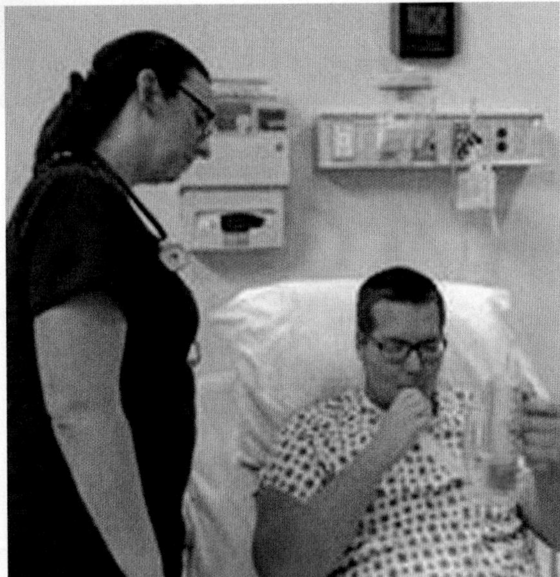

Fig. 42.2 Flow-oriented spirometer.

Before surgery, help the patient practice coughing (Skill 42.3 and the Patient Teaching box on controlled coughing technique), turning, and deep breathing (Skill 42.4). Because coughing increases intracranial pressure, it usually is contraindicated in cranial and spine-related surgeries. Coughing also is contraindicated after most types of eye surgery (Box 42.6). Patients frequently ambulate within a few hours of surgery or sooner to return cardiovascular and respiratory functions to normal more quickly.

Cardiovascular Considerations

Accompanying the need to turn, cough, and deep-breathe is the need to practice leg exercises (see Skill 42.4). Because blood stasis occurs when the body lies flat, encourage the patient to do leg exercises to assist venous blood flow. Slow venous blood flow can lead to the formation of a **thrombus** (an accumulation of platelets, fibrin, and cellular elements of the blood attached to the interior wall of a vessel, sometimes occluding the lumen). If a thrombus is dislodged, it can travel as an **embolus** (a traveling or mobilized clot) to the lungs, heart, or brain, where the vessel can be occluded. Without an adequate blood supply, an **infarct** (localized area of necrosis) can occur. Antiembolism stockings (thromboembolic deterrent stockings) and/or sequential compression devices (SCDs) with an intermittent external pneumonic compression system may be ordered to provide support and to prevent venous thrombus in the lower extremities. Newer models of SCDs are battery operated so that the patient does not have to be tethered to a motor, allowing for use at any time (Skill 42.5 and the Patient Teaching box on use of thromboembolic deterrent stockings and sequential compression devices).

 Patient Teaching

Controlled Coughing Technique

- For the patient entering the hospital for same-day surgery, controlled coughing can be taught in the physician's office, in the preoperative area, or postoperatively.
- The home health nurse may need to reinforce the importance of coughing once or twice an hour during waking hours for the patient receiving home care services.
- Young children or older adults may not understand fully the importance of controlled coughing, and continual reinforcement of teaching and assistance may be needed.
- Teach family members of a young child the procedure so that they may assist the child.
- After brain, spinal, head, neck, or eye surgery, coughing often is contraindicated because of a potential increase in intracranial pressure.
- Instruct the patient to cough instead of just clearing the throat.
- Teach the patient how to splint the incision with a small pillow or blanket, that controlled coughing will not injure the incision, and that there will be less discomfort with splinting.
- Teach the patient to examine the sputum for odor, consistency, amount, and color changes.

Box 42.6 Surgeries for Which Coughing Is Contraindicated or Modified

Intracranial: Coughing increases intracranial pressure (ICP), leading to cerebrospinal fluid leakage.
Eye: Coughing increases ICP, which then increases intraocular pressure, causing pressure on suture line.
Ear: If patient must cough, mouth must be kept open to prevent pressure backup through eustachian tube to middle ear, causing pressure on suture line.
Nose: If patient must cough, mouth must be kept open to prevent dislodgment of a clot with subsequent bleeding.
Throat: Vigorous coughing may dislodge a clot with subsequent bleeding.
Spinal: Coughing increases spinal canal pressure.

Consider the following points when applying antiembolism stockings:

- The postoperative patient with abdominal or thoracic incisions will not be able to bend and pull on his or her own stockings.
- Measurements should be taken according to the manufacturer's guidelines to ensure proper size and fit.
- Stockings may be difficult to apply for some patients; the nurse or family members will need to assist.

Skill 42.3 Teaching Controlled Coughing

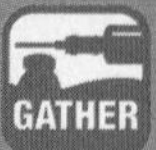

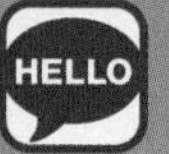

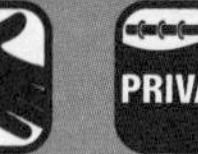

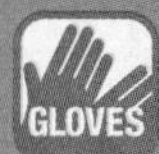

GLOVES

NURSING ACTION *(RATIONALE)*

1. Refer to medical record, care plan, or Kardex for special interventions. *(Provides basis for care.)*
2. Obtain equipment. *(Organizes procedure.)*
   a. Pillow or bath blanket
   b. Gloves
   c. Emesis basin
   d. Facial tissues
   e. Chair or bed
3. Introduce self. *(Decreases patient's anxiety.)*
4. Identify patient. *(Ensures correct patient for procedure.)*
5. Explain procedure. *(Improves cooperation and decreases anxiety.)*
6. Wash hands and don clean gloves according to agency policy and guidelines from the Centers for Disease Control and Prevention and the Occupational Safety and Health Administration. *(Reduces spread of microorganisms.)*
7. Assist patient to upright position. Place pillow between bed or chair and patient. *(Facilitates deep breathing and optimum chest expansion.)*
8. Demonstrate coughing exercise for patient (see illustration). *(Allows patient to observe nurse and to ask questions.)*
   a. Take several deep breaths. *(Deep breaths expand lungs fully so that air moves behind mucus and facilitates effect of coughing.)*

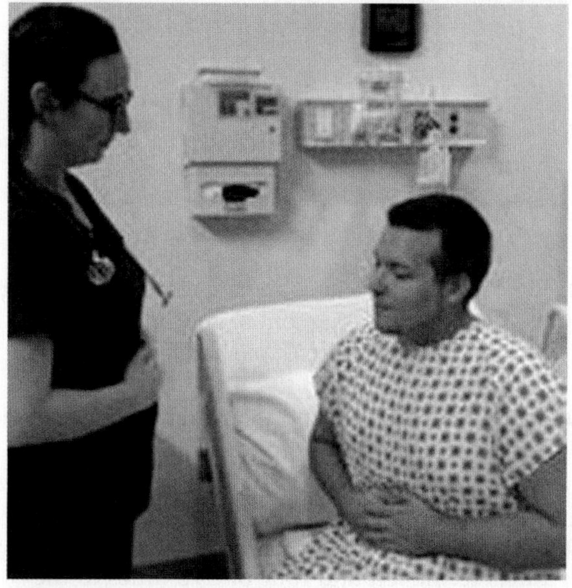

   b. Inhale through nose.
   c. Exhale through mouth with pursed lips.
   d. Inhale deeply again and hold breath for count of three.
   e. Cough two or three consecutive times without inhaling between coughs. *(Consecutive coughs remove mucus more effectively and completely than one forceful cough.)*
9. Caution patient against just clearing the throat instead of coughing. *(Clearing the throat does not remove mucus from deep in airways.)*
10. Before the patient coughs, abdominal or thoracic incision can be splinted with hands, pillow, towel, or rolled bath blanket (see illustration). *(Surgical incision cuts through muscles, tissues, and nerve endings. Deep breathing and coughing place additional stress on suture line and cause discomfort. Splinting incision provides firm support and reduces incisional pulling.)*

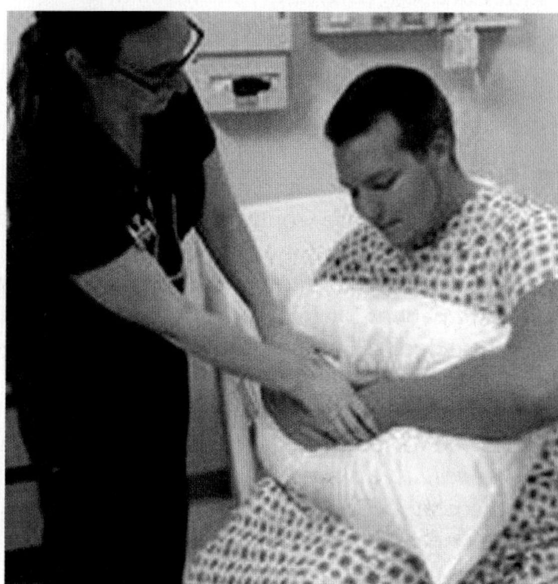

11. Encourage patient to practice coughing once or twice an hour during waking hours, while splinting incisional area. Assist patient as indicated. *(Helps effectively expectorate mucus with minimal discomfort.)*
12. Remind patient to use tissues and emesis basin for any mucus expectorated. *(Reduces spread of microorganisms.)*
13. Teach patient to examine sputum for consistency, amount, and color changes. *(Changes could indicate respiratory complications such as pneumonia.)*
14. Provide wash cloth and warm water for washing hands and face, provide for oral hygiene, and return patient to comfortable position. *(Provides for patient comfort.)*
15. Remove and dispose of soiled gloves and wash hands. *(Reduces spread of microorganisms.)*
16. Document exercises performed and patient's ability to perform them independently. *(Verifies care given and patient teaching.)*
17. Carry out patient teaching (see the Patient Teaching box on controlled coughing technique).

Skill 42.4 Teaching Postoperative Breathing Techniques, Leg Exercises, and Turning Exercises

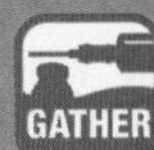

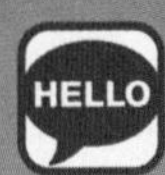

PRIVACY

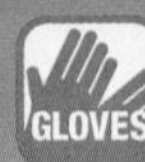

NURSING ACTION *(RATIONALE)*

1. Refer to medical record, care plan, or Kardex for special interventions. *(Provides basis for care.)*
2. Obtain equipment. *(Helps organize procedure.)*
   a. Support pillow, towel, or folded bath blanket
   b. Gloves
   c. Emesis basin
   d. Facial tissues
3. Introduce self. *(Decreases patient's anxiety.)*
4. Identify patient. *(Verifies correct patient for procedure.)*
5. Explain procedure to patient. *(Improves cooperation and decreases anxiety.)*
6. Perform hand hygiene and don clean gloves. Know agency policy and guidelines from the Centers for Disease Control and Prevention and the Occupational Safety and Health Administration. *(Reduces spread of microorganisms.)*
7. Prepare patient for intervention.
   a. Close door to room or pull curtain. *(Provides privacy.)*
   b. Drape for procedure if necessary.
8. Raise bed to comfortable working level. *(Promotes proper body mechanics.)*
9. Premedicate with pain medication, if indicated. *(Elicits patient compliance.)*

POSTOPERATIVE BREATHING TECHNIQUES

10. Place pillow between patient and bed or chair. *(Allows for fuller chest expansion [bed or chair is too firm to provide expansion].)*
11. Sit or stand, facing patient. *(Allows patient to observe nurse.)*
12. Demonstrate taking slow, deep breaths. Avoid moving shoulders and chest while inhaling. Inhale through nose. *(Prevents panting and hyperventilation. Moistens, filters, and warms inhaled air.)*
13. Hold breath for a count of three, and slowly exhale through pursed lips. *(Allows for gradual expulsion of air.)*
14. Repeat exercise three to five times. Have patient practice exercise. *(Allows patient to observe appropriate technique. Allows nurse to assess patient's technique and correct errors.)*
15. Instruct patient to take 10 slow, deep breaths q 2 hr until ambulatory. *(Helps prevent postoperative complications.)*
16. If there is an abdominal or chest incision, instruct patient to splint incisional area, using pillow or bath blanket, if desired, during breathing exercises. *(Provides support and additional security for patient.)*

LEG EXERCISES

17. Lifting one leg at a time and supporting joints, gently flex and extend leg 5 to 10 times. *(Stimulates circulation and helps prevent thrombus formation.)*

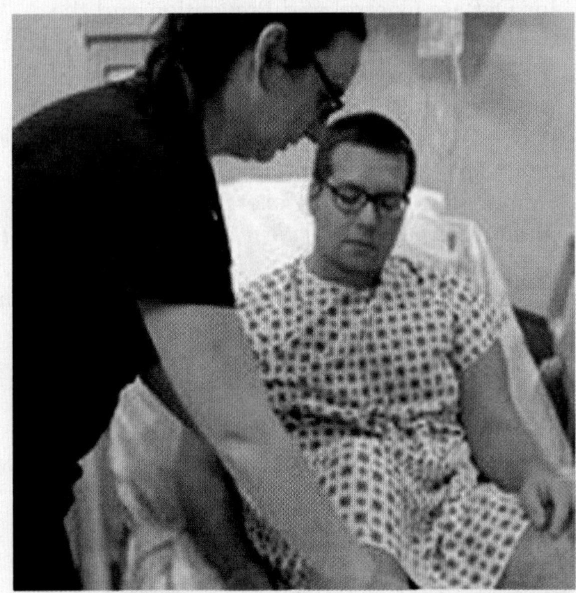

18. Repeat exercise with opposite extremity. Lifting leg while supporting joints, gently flex leg 5 to 10 times. *(Stimulates circulation and helps prevent thrombus formation.)*
19. Flex ankle with toes pointed toward head, then extend ankle with toes pointed toward foot of bed. *(Uses additional muscle flexion and contraction to stimulate circulation.)*
20. Make circle with ankles of both feet four or five times to the left and four or five times to the right. *(Further stimulates circulation through muscle contraction and flexion.)*
21. Assess pulse, respiration, and blood pressure. *(Aids in determining complications from exercise.)*

Skill 42.4 Teaching Postoperative Breathing Techniques, Leg Exercises, and Turning Exercises—cont'd

TURNING EXERCISES

22. Instruct patient to assume supine position on right side of bed. Have side rails on both sides of bed in up position. *(Positioning begins on right side of bed so that turning to left side will not cause patient to roll toward bed's edge. Side rails in the raised position promote patient safety.)*

23. Instruct patient to place left hand over incisional area to splint it. *(Supports and minimizes pulling on suture line during turning.)*

24. Instruct patient to keep left leg straight and to flex right knee up and over left leg. *(Straight leg stabilizes patient's position. Flexed right leg shifts weight for easier turning.)*

25. Instruct patient to turn q 2 hr while awake. *(Reduces risk of vascular and pulmonary complications.)*

26. Remove and dispose of soiled gloves and wash hands. *(Reduces spread of microorganisms.)*

27. Document. *(Records patient education and verifies procedure.)*

Skill 42.5 Applying Thromboembolic Deterrent Stockings and Sequential Compression Devices

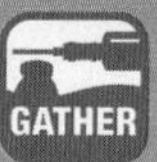

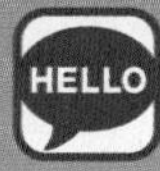

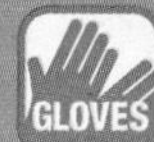

NURSING ACTION *(RATIONALE)*

1. Refer to medical record, care plan, or Kardex for special interventions. *(Provides basis for care.)*
2. Obtain equipment. *(Organizes procedure.)*
   a. Thromboembolic deterrent stockings (TEDs) or sequential compression devices (SCDs)
   b. Clean gloves (when appropriate)
   c. Tape measure
3. Introduce self. *(Decreases patient's anxiety.)*
4. Identify patient. *(Identifies correct patient for procedure.)*
5. Explain procedure. *(Improves cooperation and decreases anxiety.)*
6. Perform hand hygiene and, if appropriate, don clean gloves. Know agency policy and guidelines from the Centers for Disease Control and Prevention and the Occupational Safety and Health Administration. *(Reduces spread of microorganisms.)*
7. Prepare patient.
   a. Close door to room, pull curtain, and drape for procedure, if necessary. *(Provides privacy.)*
8. Raise bed to comfortable working level. *(Promotes proper body mechanics.)*
9. Examine legs and assess risk for conditions. *(Helps nurse determine presence of pigmentation around ankles, pitting edema, or peripheral cyanosis, which may indicate inadequate circulation.)*
10. Assess patient for calf pain, redness, tenderness, warmth, and/or swelling. *(May indicate presence of thrombophlebitis.)*
11. Measure legs for stockings according to agency policy, and order stockings. *(Promotes the correct size to accomplish purpose of stockings.)*

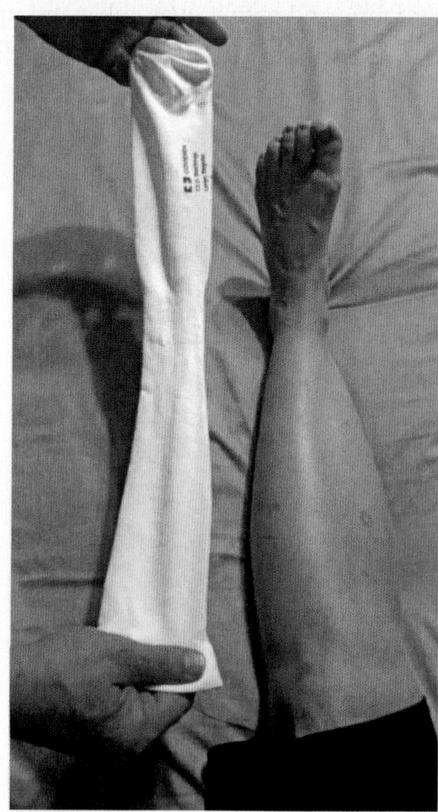

Continued

Skill 42.5 Applying Thromboembolic Deterrent Stockings and Sequential Compression Devices—cont'd

THROMBOEMBOLIC DETERRENT STOCKINGS

12. Assist patient to supine position to apply stockings before patient rises. Patient should be recumbent for at least 30 min before application. *(Prevents veins from becoming distended or edema from occurring.)*

13. Turn stockings inside out as far as heel. Place thumbs inside foot part, and slip stocking on until heel is correctly aligned. *(Positions stocking for appropriate application.)*

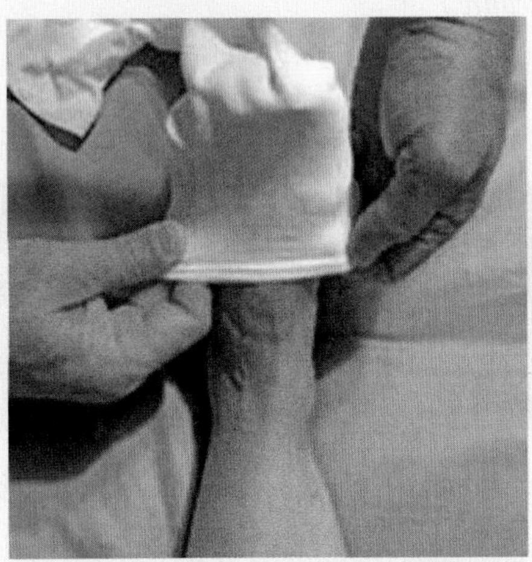

14. Gather fabric and ease it over ankle and up the leg. *(Prevents bunching of stocking, which can cause local pooling of blood.)*

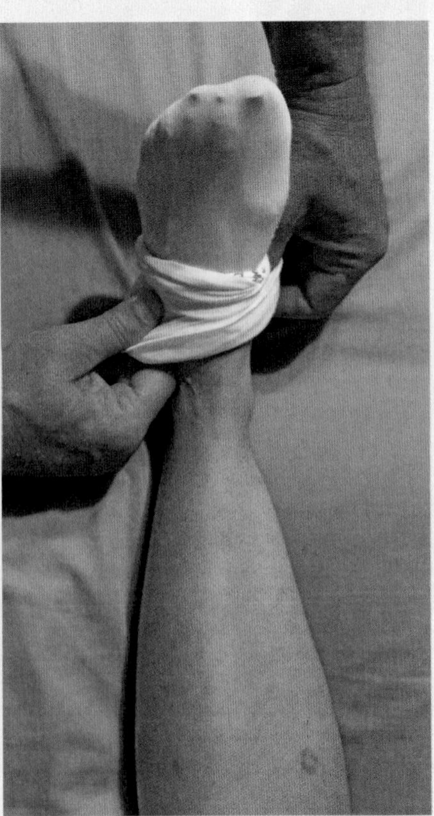

15. Pull leg portion of stocking over foot and up as far as it will go, making certain that gusset lies over femoral artery. Adjust stocking to fit evenly and smoothly with no wrinkles. *(Allows appropriate fit and application, which are vital for maintaining even pressure. Prevents irritation and impediments to circulation.)*

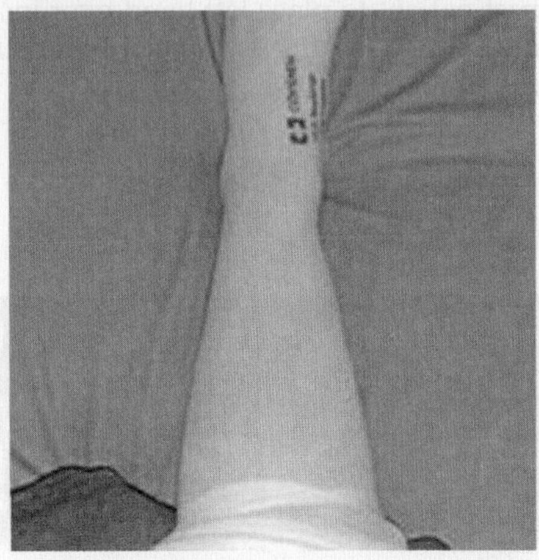

16. Repeat steps 12 to 15 for opposite extremity. *(Ensures appropriate application.)*

SEQUENTIAL COMPRESSION DEVICES

17. Place sleeve under patient's leg, with fuller portion at top of thigh. *(Ensures correct fit.)*

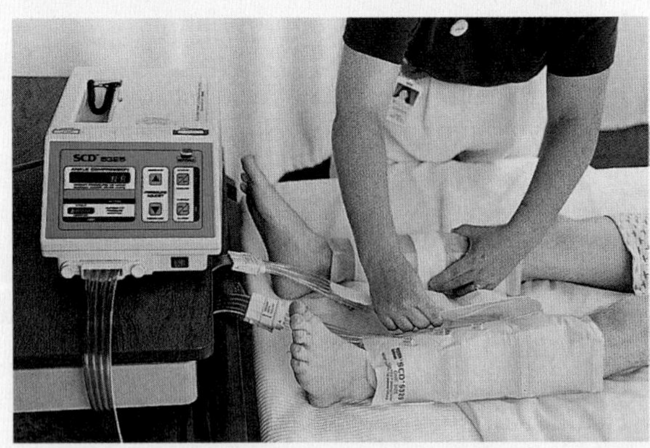

Skill 42.5 Applying Thromboembolic Deterrent Stockings and Sequential Compression Devices—cont'd

18. Apply sleeve with opening at front of knee and closed portion behind knee. *(Ensures appropriate placement and desired effect.)*
19. When the SCD is in place, make sure there are no wrinkles or creases in stockings. Fold Velcro strips over to secure stockings. *(Allows proper functioning of stockings and prevents irritation.)*
20. Attach tubing to SCD after both sleeves are applied. Align arrows for correct connection and appropriate effect. Plug in unit. *(Allows air to inflate stockings in sequential order.)*
21. Assess patient periodically. *(Determines presence of edema or cyanosis.)*
22. Assess stocking at regular intervals. *(Ensures that top has not rolled down or loosened and that no wrinkles are present.)*
23. Remove and dispose of soiled gloves and wash hands. *(Reduces spread of microorganisms.)*
24. Document. *(Verifies patient care.)*
25. Carry out patient teaching (see the Patient Teaching box on use of thromboembolic deterrent stockings and sequential compression devices).

Step 17 from Elkin MK, Perry AG, Potter PA: *Nursing interventions and clinical skills*, ed 4, St. Louis, 2007, Mosby.

 Patient Teaching

Use of Thromboembolic Deterrent Stockings and Sequential Compression Devices

- Teach the patient how to correctly apply antiembolism stockings.
- Teach the patient appropriate care of the stockings. (Hand wash in warm water and mild soap, do not wring dry, and lay over flat surface to dry.)
- Instruct the patient not to massage legs because of the risk of dislodging a thrombus.
- Teach the patient the signs of possible complications. (If stockings or devices are too restrictive, edema and pain could result.)

Vital Signs

Vital signs mirror the body's response to anesthesia and surgery. Explain to the patient before surgery that it is normal for blood pressure, temperature, pulse, and respiration to be monitored before and after surgery, until the patient stabilizes. The schedule for monitoring vital signs depends on the facility's protocol and the patient. Preoperative vital signs provide a baseline for determining postoperative stability or identifying related problems. Postoperative vital signs are discussed later in this chapter.

Genitourinary Considerations

After general anesthesia, the urinary bladder's tone is decreased, leading to urinary retention. Assess the patient's normal bladder habits preoperatively and identify when the bladder is full and distended postoperatively. If the patient does not urinate within 8 hours after surgery, assess the patient by palpating above the symphysis pubis to determine if the bladder is distended (Fig. 42.3). Once the patient is awake and tolerating fluids, encourage an adequate fluid intake. Occasionally a urinary catheter is inserted to monitor urinary output. This procedure normally is reserved for a patient undergoing urinary surgery or who may have difficulty voiding or needs the output closely monitored postoperatively. The catheter is removed as soon as possible, based on the patient's condition, either at the conclusion of the surgery or 1 or 2 days postoperatively, to reduce the chance of bladder infection. Once it is removed, encourage the patient to drink 8 ounces of fluids per hour while awake unless contraindicated. Also, monitor intake and output (I&O) values until the patient's normal voiding pattern returns. Urinary retention is a common postoperative complication.

Surgical Wounds

Incisions (cuts produced surgically by a sharp instrument to create an opening into an organ or body space) are closed in a variety of ways: with sutures, staples, Steri-Strips, transparent strips, or tissue adhesives. Knowing the type of closure enables the nurse to explain its appearance to the patient. Some surgeries require the removal of exudate, often with a drain. The purpose of the drain should be explained to the patient and monitored and cared for appropriately. Wound care, dressing changes, and drainage systems are described in more detail in Chapter 22 of *Foundations of Nursing*.

Pain

Many individuals undergoing surgical procedures fear the prospect of postoperative pain. Discussion of various pain relief measures should be included in the preoperative teaching. If the patient is considering nonpharmacologic analgesia (e.g., imagery, biofeedback, relaxation techniques), these techniques should be reviewed with the patient, and practice time should be planned. Most patients choose traditional analgesia. Some patients fear

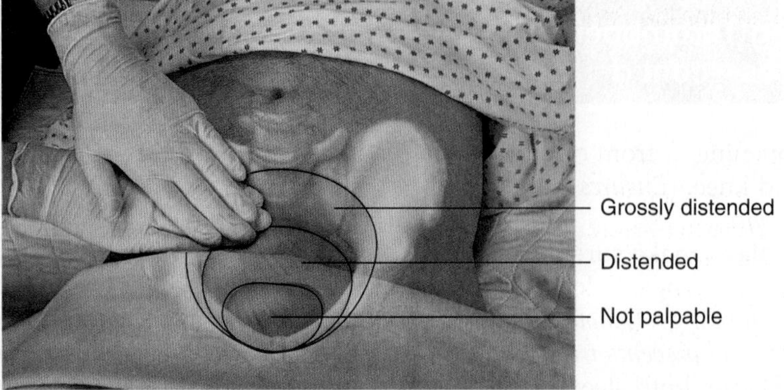

Fig. 42.3 Assess the bladder by palpating the lower abdomen for distention. (From Harkreader H, Hogan MA: *Fundamentals of nursing: Caring and clinical judgment*, ed 3, Philadelphia, 2007, Saunders.)

that addiction to pain medications may occur, so it is important to reassure patients that addiction to analgesics rarely occurs in the time frame needed for comfort. For the patient who is apprehensive about intermittent injections, patient-controlled analgesia (PCA) and opioids injected into the epidural space (patient-controlled epidural) offer safe and effective relief for postoperative pain. When the patient can resume oral intake, oral analgesics coupled with nontraditional methods are often effective (see Chapter 21 in *Foundations of Nursing*). Nurses must listen to patient complaints of postoperative pain.

Tubes

Depending on the surgery, patient teaching includes information about nasogastric (NG) tubes, wound drainage units, and IV and oxygen therapy. Allowing patients to view related equipment and understand their purpose lessens the fear associated with them. (See Chapters 14 and 15 in *Foundations of Nursing* for more detailed discussion of the tubes and drains used in the postoperative patient.)

Preoperative Medication

Preoperative medication reduces the patient's anxiety, decreases the amount of anesthetic needed, and reduces respiratory tract secretions. The patient should be told what to expect from preoperative medications. Barbiturates and tranquilizers (e.g., phenobarbital and diazepam [Valium]) sometimes are given for sedation to reduce the amount of anesthetic required. Opioid analgesics (meperidine and morphine) may be administered by intermittent injection or PCA if the patient has pain before surgery; this also reduces the amount of anesthetic required. An introduction to PCA preoperatively helps the patient understand the concept and how the equipment works. Anticholinergics such as atropine reduce spasms of smooth muscles and decrease gastric, bronchial, and salivary secretions (Table 42.5).

The patient frequently becomes drowsy, notices a dry mouth, and experiences vertigo after receiving a preoperative medication. If the preoperative medication is given on the nursing unit, the patient should be encouraged to void before receiving the medication and must remain in bed after administration of the medication to prevent falls. Safety measures should be instituted, such as placing the bed in a low position and raising side rails and monitoring the patient every 15 to 30 minutes until the patient leaves for surgery. Reassurance and support should be given to the patient as well as providing a quiet environment on the nursing unit while waiting for transport to the surgical suite. In many institutions, the preoperative medication is given by the anesthesiologist or anesthesia provider, such as a certified registered nurse anesthetist (CRNA), in the preoperative holding area.

For the patient scheduled for surgery, all medications ordered before surgery usually are stopped preoperatively except for those prescribed for long-term conditions, such as phenytoin (Dilantin) for seizure control (Table 42.6). After surgery, the surgeon prescribes or re-orders the necessary medication, as does the primary health care provider.

Anesthesia

Anesthesia means the absence of all sensation, including pain (*an*, meaning "without," plus *esthesia*, meaning "awareness of feeling"). Anesthesia is divided into four categories: general, regional, local, and conscious (moderate) sedation.

General anesthesia. General anesthesia produces amnesia, analgesia, muscle paralysis, and sedation. The patient is in a state of unconsciousness that is reversible. General anesthesia is used for major surgery requiring extensive tissue manipulation. Modern anesthetics are much easier to reverse, and they allow the patient to recover with fewer unwanted effects than in the past.

Table 42.5 **Medications for the Perioperative Period**

GENERIC NAME (TRADE NAME)	DOSAGE AND ROUTE	ACTION	NURSING IMPLICATIONS
Benzodiazepines			
midazolam	Dosage depends on the amount of sedation necessary for surgery	• Decrease anxiety and produce sedation • Induce amnesia	Monitor for respiratory depression, hypotension, drowsiness, and lack of coordination.
diazepam (Valium)	5–20 mg PO		
lorazepam (Ativan)	44 mcg/kg to 2 mg IV		
Opioid Analgesics			
morphine	5–15 mg IM or IV	• Decrease anxiety • Allow decreased anesthetics	Monitor for respiratory depression, nausea, vomiting, orthostatic hypotension, and pruritus.
fentanyl citrate (Sublimaze)	50–100 mcg/mL IM or slow IV		
H_2 Receptor Antagonists			
famotidine (Pepcid)	20 mg IV	• Reduce gastric acid volume and concentration	Monitor for confusion and dizziness in older adults.
ranitidine (Zantac)	50 mg IV		
Antiemetics			
metoclopramide (Reglan)	10 mg IV or IM	• Enhance gastric emptying • Tranquilizing effect • Prevent postoperative nausea and vomiting	Monitor for sedation and extrapyramidal reaction (involuntary movement, muscle tone changes, and abnormal posture). Instruct patient to report any difficulty in breathing.
droperidol (Inapsine)	2.5–10 mg		
ondansetron HCl (5-HT3 receptor antagonist) (Zofran)	4 mg IV		
Anticholinergics			
atropine sulfate	0.4–0.6 mg IM or IV	• Reduce oral and respiratory secretions to decrease risk of aspiration • Decrease vomiting and laryngospasm	Monitor for confusion, restlessness, and tachycardia. Prepare patient to expect dry mouth.
glycopyrrolate (Robinul)	0.1–0.3 mg IM or IV		
Antibiotics			
cefazolin sodium (Ancef)	1–2 g q 6 hr Maximum, 12 g/day	• Bactericidal • Minimizes risk of wound infection	If large doses are given, therapy is prolonged, or patient is at high risk, monitor for signs and symptoms of superinfection, including abdominal pain, moderate to severe diarrhea, severe anal or genital pruritus, and severe mouth soreness. Determine patient's history of allergies. If dosing continues, space drug evenly around the clock. Advise patient to complete therapy.
cefotaxime sodium (Claforan)	1 g IM or IV 30–90 min before surgery	• Bactericidal • Used for perioperative prophylaxis	
ceftriaxone	1 g IM or IV 0.5–2 hr before surgery	• Bactericidal • Used for perioperative prophylaxis	
Adrenocortical Steroid			
methylprednisolone (Depo-Medrol, Solu-Medrol)	Adults: 10–250 mg (succinate) IV q 4–6 hr Oral, 2–60 mg in four divided doses IM, 10–80 mg (acetate)	• Decreases inflammation	Determine whether patient has hypersensitivity to drug. Determine whether patient has diabetes mellitus, and anticipate an increase in antidiabetic drug regimen because of raised blood glucose level.
Nonsteroidal Antiinflammatory Drug (NSAID)			
ketorolac	50 mg/mL IM; 30 mg/mL IV push over at least 15 s	• Reduces intensity of pain • Reduces inflammation	Assess the duration, location, onset, and type of pain the patient is having. Evaluate patient for therapeutic response.

Continued

Table 42.5 Medications for the Perioperative Period—cont'd

GENERIC NAME (TRADE NAME)	DOSAGE AND ROUTE	ACTION	NURSING IMPLICATIONS
Anticoagulants			
enoxaparin sodium (Lovenox)	30 mg/0.3 mL to 150 mg/mL subQ in prefilled syringes	• Produces anticoagulation • Prevents new clot formation or secondary embolic complications	Do not give IM, but give subQ. Tell the patient not to take aspirin or similar over-the-counter drugs.
heparin sodium (Heparin)	10 units/mL to 15,000 units/500 mL subQ Heparin sodium flush syringes: 10 units/mL, 100 units/mL Vials (most use saline for flush): 10 units/mL, 100 units/mL		Cross-check heparin dose with another nurse before administering. Use constant rate IV infusion pump. Monitor the patient's partial thromboplastin time diligently. Assess patient's gums for erythema and gingival bleeding; skin for bruises or petechiae; and urine for hematuria.
warfarin sodium (Coumadin)	5-mg vials, IM; 1–10 mg PO tablets or IV		Observe patient for evidence of hemorrhage such as abdominal or back pain, decreased blood pressure, increased pulse rate, and severe headache. Urge patient not to ingest alcohol or make drastic dietary changes. If administration continues, urge patient to notify the physician if he or she experiences black stools; bleeding; brown, dark, or red urine; coffee-ground vomitus; or red-speckled mucus from a cough.

IM, Intramuscular; *IV,* intravenous; *mcg,* microgram; *PO,* per os (by mouth); *q 4–6 hr,* every 4 to 6 hours; *subQ,* subcutaneously.
Data from *Mosby's 2017 Nursing Drug Reference,* St. Louis, 2017, Elsevier.

Table 42.6 Medications With Special Implications for the Surgical Patient

DRUG CLASS	IMPLICATIONS FOR THE SURGICAL PATIENT
Anticoagulants	Anticoagulants such as warfarin and aspirin are stopped several days before surgery. Anticoagulants prolong clotting times, which may lead to hemorrhage.
Antihypertensives	Antihypertensives may cause hypotension when combined with anesthetic agents and narcotics used for pain control.
Antiseizure drugs	Long-term use of certain antiseizure drugs (e.g., phenytoin [Dilantin], phenobarbital) can interact with anesthetic agents.
Corticosteroids	If used for an extended period, corticosteroids may prolong bleeding and hamper the body's ability to heal. These drugs also may decrease the body's ability to deal with the stress of surgery as a result of suppression of the adrenal glands.
Diuretics	Because of fluid loss during surgery, diuretics may cause hypotension after surgery and decreased serum potassium level.
Herbal therapies	Several herbal therapies can affect clotting times. Ginseng may increase hypoglycemia with insulin therapy (see Chapter 20 in *Foundations of Nursing,* Complementary and Alternative Therapies boxes for potential complications that may occur when herbal therapies are combined with traditional medications).
Insulin	Blood glucose levels fluctuate, so insulin levels may require adjustment. A patient with diabetes may have reduced need for insulin after surgery because nutritional intake is decreased; conversely, stress response and intravenous administration of glucose solutions can increase dosage requirements after surgery.
Nonsteroidal antiinflammatory drugs (NSAIDs)	NSAIDs inhibit platelet function and may prolong bleeding, leading to possible hemorrhage.

An anesthesiologist or a CRNA administers general anesthetics through the four stages of anesthesia. Common anesthetic agents include propofol (a nonbarbiturate intravenous anesthetic), nitrous oxide gas, and desflurane and sevoflurane vapors; muscle relaxants also may be used as an adjunct.

In the induction phase, the patient is awake and the anesthetic often is given intravenously. This phase is complete when the patient loses consciousness. Intubation with an endotracheal tube or use of a laryngeal mask airway (Fig. 42.4) is done at this time to establish an airway.

During the maintenance phase, the patient is kept anesthetized at appropriate levels throughout the surgical procedure. Anesthesia may be maintained using a combination of inhalation of gases and vapors and IV medications. The patient also receives a continuous supply of oxygen and adjunct medications such as opioid analgesics and muscle relaxants. A combination of small amounts of several medications can mean a significant reduction in dose compared with using a single drug.

The duration of anesthesia depends on the length of surgery. Surgical risks influence the duration of surgery. The greatest risks from general anesthesia are the adverse effects of anesthetic agents, including cardiovascular depression or irritability, respiratory depression, and liver and kidney damage.

Patients emerge from anesthesia when procedures are complete and reversal agents are given. Because of the short half-life of the anesthetic agents currently used, emergence often occurs in the OR. The oropharynx is suctioned to decrease the risk of aspiration and laryngeal spasm after extubation. Extubation or removal of the laryngeal airway mask may occur before transfer to the postanesthesia care unit (PACU), depending on the patient's ability to maintain a patent airway. If the patient is having difficulty maintaining a patent airway after extubation, an oral airway may be used to maintain an open airway until the patient is fully conscious (Fig. 42.5).

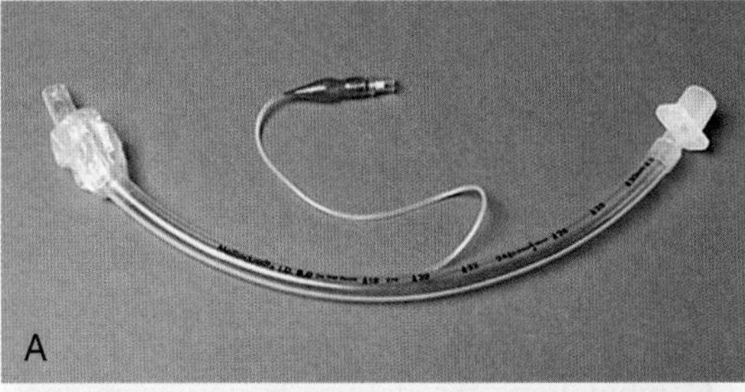

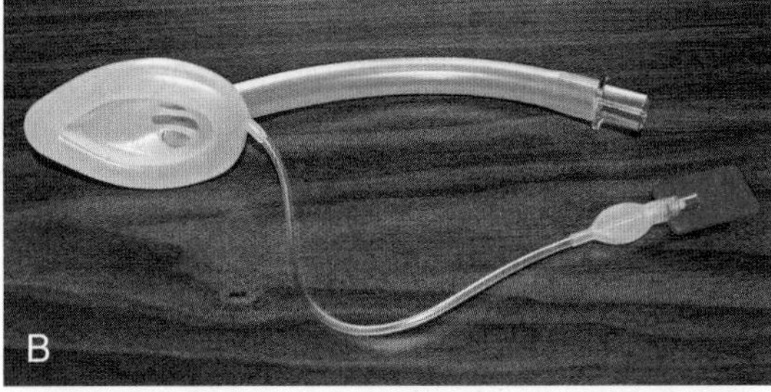

Fig. 42.4 A, Endotracheal tube. B, Laryngeal mask airway. (From Monahan FD, Neighbors M, Sands JK, et al: *Phipps' medical-surgical nursing: Health and illness perspectives,* ed 8, St. Louis, 2007, Mosby.)

Regional anesthesia. Regional anesthesia causes loss of sensation in an area of the body and is used for some surgical procedures and pain management. The patient does not lose consciousness with regional anesthesia but usually is sedated. The anesthesiologist or CRNA administers regional anesthetics by infiltration and local application. Fig. 42.6 shows common sites where spinal or epidural anesthetics are administered to achieve a regional block. The sensory pathway that is anesthetized depends on the method of induction.

Infiltration of anesthetic agents may involve one of the following induction methods:

- *Epidural anesthesia:* This procedure is safer than spinal anesthesia because the anesthetic agent is injected into the epidural space outside the dura mater and the depth of anesthesia is lighter. Epidural anesthesia blocks sensation in the vaginal and perineal areas and thus often is used for obstetric procedures. The epidural catheter may be left in so that the patient can receive medication via continuous epidural infusion after surgery.
- *Nerve block:* Local anesthetic is injected into a nerve (e.g., brachial plexus in the arm), blocking the nerve supply to the operative site. This type of anesthesia is used commonly for orthopedic surgery involving extremities.
- *Spinal anesthesia:* The anesthesiologist or CRNA performs a lumbar puncture and introduces local anesthetic into the cerebrospinal fluid in the subarachnoid space. Anesthetic effects can extend from the tip of the xiphoid process down to the feet. The position of the patient influences the movement of the anesthetic agent up or down the spinal cord. Spinal anesthesia often is used for lower abdominal, pelvic, and lower extremity procedures; urologic procedures; and surgical obstetrics.

Infiltrative anesthesia involves risks, particularly with spinal anesthesia, because the anesthetic agent may move upward in the spinal cord and affect breathing. This migration of anesthetic depends on the drug type and amount and on patient position. The patient's blood pressure may drop suddenly because of extensive vasodilation caused by the anesthetic block to sympathetic vasomotor nerves and pain and motor nerve fibers. If the level of anesthesia rises, respiratory paralysis may develop, requiring resuscitation by the anesthesiologist. Elevation of the upper body prevents respiratory paralysis. The patient must be monitored carefully during and immediately after surgery.

The patient under regional anesthesia is awake throughout the procedure unless the physician orders a tranquilizer that promotes sleep and/or amnesia.

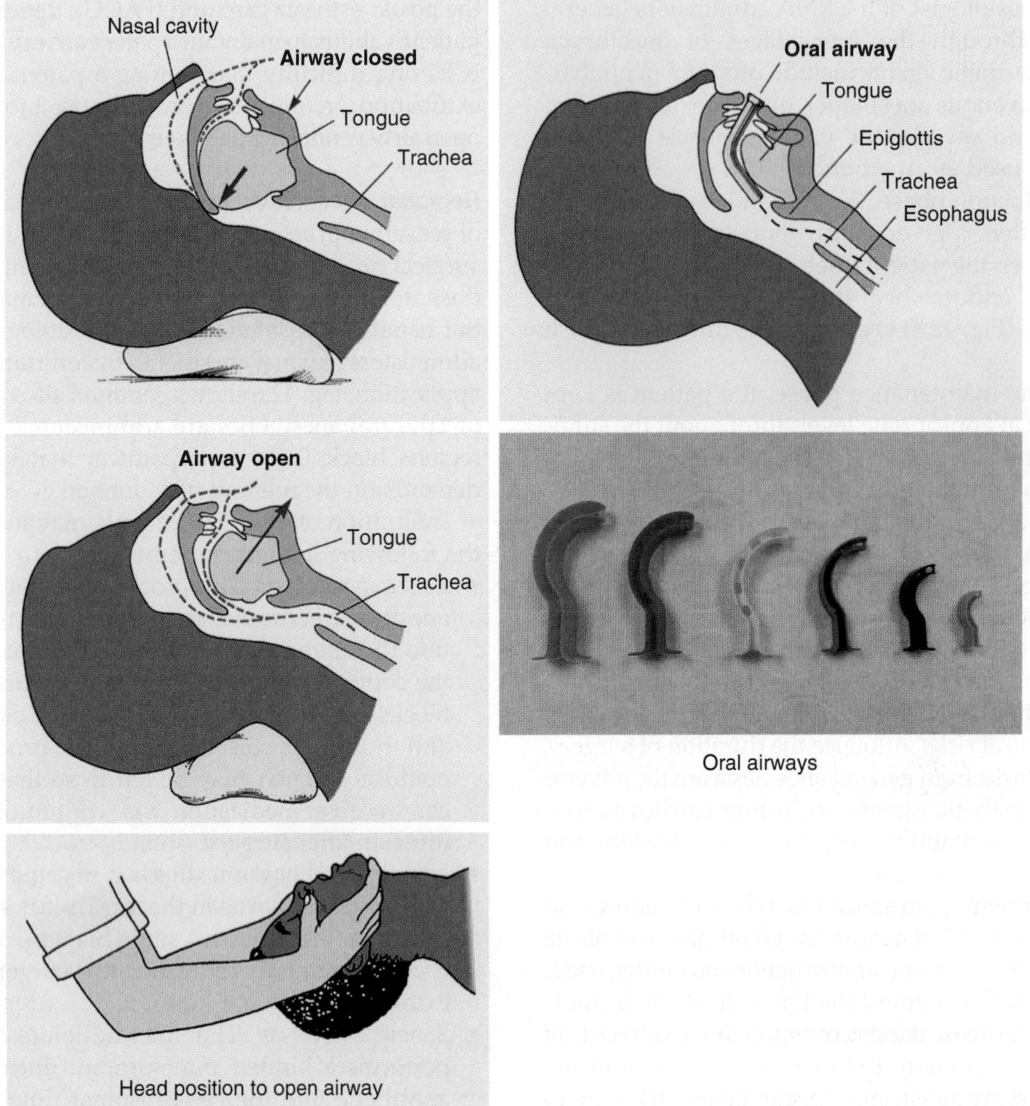

Fig. 42.5 Oral airways that may be used during the postoperative period. (Line drawings from Elkin MK, Perry AG, & Potter PA: *Nursing interventions and clinical skills*, ed 4, St. Louis, 2007, Mosby.)

Because the patient is responsive and capable of breathing voluntarily, the anesthesiologist or CRNA does not need to insert an endotracheal tube.

Local anesthesia. Local anesthesia involves loss of sensation at the desired site (e.g., a growth on the skin or the cornea of the eye). The anesthetic agent (e.g., lidocaine) inhibits nerve conduction until the drug is diffused into the circulation. Local anesthetics usually are injected or applied topically. The patient loses sensation of pain and touch, and control over motor and autonomic activities (e.g., bladder emptying). Local anesthesia is used commonly for minor surgical procedures, such as a biopsy of a tumor or removal of a growth. Physicians also may infiltrate the operative area with a local anesthetic to promote postoperative pain relief.

Conscious sedation (moderate sedation). In **conscious sedation,** more recently referred to as *moderate sedation,* the patient is given drugs that depress the central nervous system or provide analgesia to relieve anxiety or provide amnesia during surgical diagnostic procedures. Combinations of sedatives, tranquilizers, anesthetics, or anesthetic gases commonly are used for conscious (moderate) sedation. It is used routinely for procedures that do not require complete anesthesia but rather a depressed level of consciousness. A patient under conscious (moderate) sedation must retain independently a patent airway and airway reflexes and be able to respond appropriately to physical and verbal stimuli.

Advantages of conscious (moderate) sedation include adequate sedation and reduced fear and anxiety as well as minimal risk, amnesia, relief of pain and noxious stimuli, mood alteration, elevation of pain threshold,

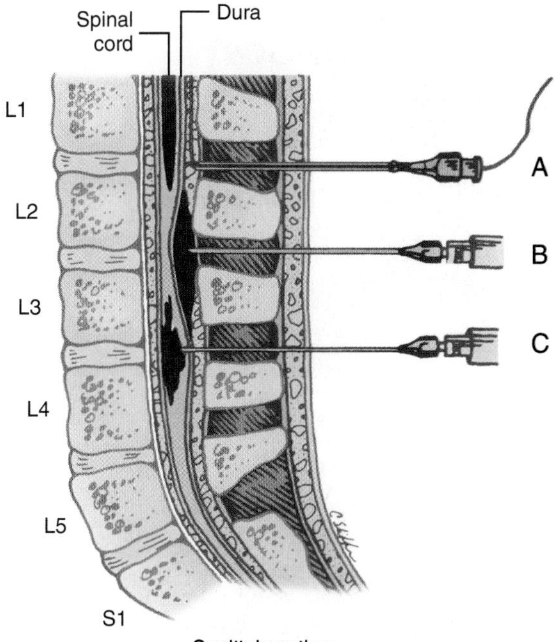

Fig. 42.6 Spinal column—side view with spinal and epidural anesthesia needle placement. A, Epidural catheter. B, Single injection epidural. C, Spinal anesthesia. (Interspaces most commonly used are L4-L5, L3-L4, and L2-L3.) (From Rothrock JC: *Alexander's care of the patient in surgery*, ed 16, St. Louis, 2019, Elsevier.)

enhanced patient cooperation, stable vital signs, and rapid recovery. Conscious (moderate) sedation is appropriate for a variety of diagnostic and therapeutic procedures, such as burn dressing changes, endoscopic procedures, certain biopsy procedures, and dental surgeries.

Nurses assisting with the administration of conscious (moderate) sedation must be knowledgeable about anatomy, physiology, cardiac dysrhythmias, procedural complications, and pharmacologic principles related to the particular sedation agents. Nurses also must be able to assess, diagnose, and intervene if an adverse reaction occurs and provide airway management and oxygen delivery. Resuscitation equipment must be readily available.

Positioning the patient for surgery. During general anesthesia the nursing personnel and surgeon often wait to position the patient until he or she is relaxed completely. The choice of position usually is determined by the surgical approach (Fig. 42.7). Ideally the patient's position provides good access to the operative site and sustains adequate circulatory and respiratory function, but it should not impair neuromuscular structures. The surgical team must consider the patient's comfort and safety, including such issues as age, weight, height, nutritional status, physical limitations, and preexisting conditions. These then are documented for staff members who care for the patient postoperatively. Nurses in postoperative divisions must recognize the discomfort a patient may feel after surgery (e.g., discomfort of the left arm or side of a patient whose right kidney was removed).

An alert person maintains normal range of joint motion by pain and pressure receptors. If a joint is extended too far, pain reminds the person that the muscle joint strain is too great. In a patient who is anesthetized, however, normal defense mechanisms cannot guard against joint damage, muscle stretch, and strain. The muscles are so relaxed that it is relatively easy to place the patient in a position he or she could not assume while awake. The patient often remains in a given position for several hours. Although it may be necessary to place a patient in an unusual position, it is important that the surgical team attempt to maintain correct alignment and protect the patient from pressure, abrasion, and other injuries (e.g., corneal abrasion). Attachments to the OR table allow protection and padding of extremities and bony prominences. Positioning should not interfere with normal movement of the diaphragm or circulation to body parts. If restraints are necessary, the surgical team should pad the area to be restrained to prevent skin trauma (see Chapter 10 in *Foundations of Nursing*).

Preoperative Checklist

A preoperative checklist often is used by facilities to ensure that all required care has been performed and that the patient is prepared properly for surgery. This form is completed before the patient leaves the nursing unit (Fig. 42.8). Signing the preoperative checklist means that the nurse assumes responsibility for all areas of care included on the list. If the preoperative medication is to be given on the nursing unit, the preoperative checklist must be completed before the medication is administered. Any **prosthesis** (an artificial replacement for a missing part of the body), contact lenses, dentures, and jewelry and other valuables are removed and either given to family members or placed in a secure area. Some facilities allow patients to wear dentures while in surgery and remove them later. If the patient wears rings and does not want them removed, they should be secured with tape and noted in the chart. The patient should void before the preoperative medication is administered, or 1 hour before surgery is scheduled. Although most patients become drowsy after administration of a preoperative medication, a few either become hyperactive or demonstrate no side effects. The nurse should remind the patient to remain in bed, and side rails should be raised and the call light within reach to ensure patient safety.

Eliminating Wrong Site and Wrong Procedure Surgery

The Joint Commission (TJC) established Universal Protocol guidelines to prevent surgeons from performing surgery at the wrong site or performing the wrong procedure. If an invasive surgical procedure is planned,

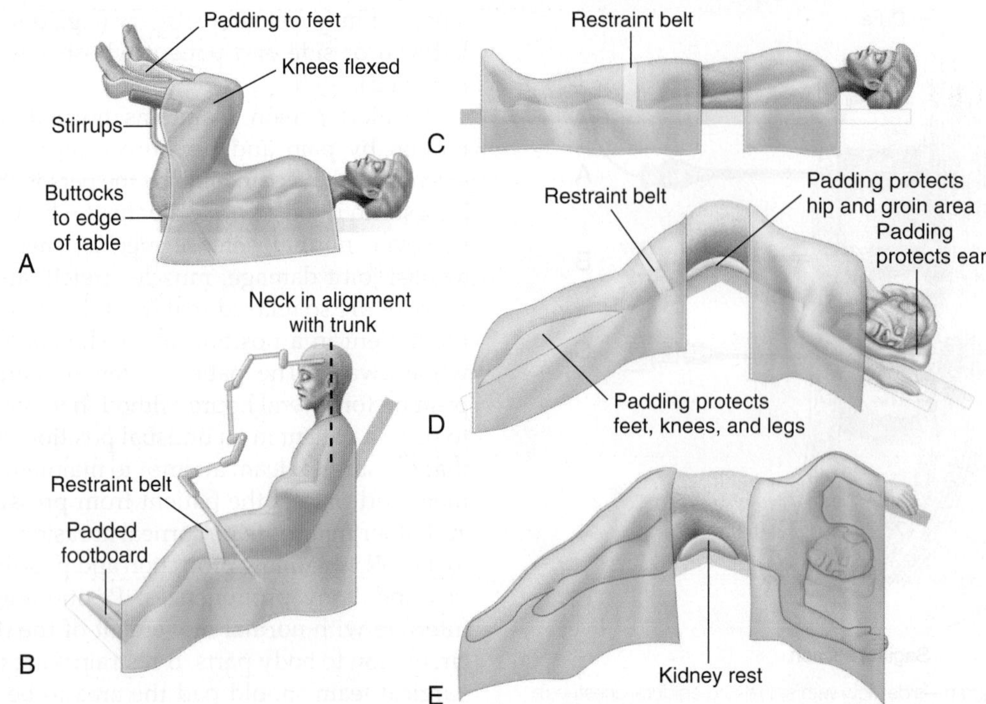

Fig. 42.7 Common perioperative positions and the padding provided to relieve pressure in each position. A, Lithotomy position, used for vaginal and perineal procedures. B, Sitting position, used for neurologic procedures. C, Supine position (the most common position). Potential pressure points are the occiput, scapula, olecranon, thoracic vertebrae, sacrum, coccyx, and calcaneus. D, Jackknife position, used for gluteal and anorectal surgeries. E, Lateral kidney position, used for procedures requiring a retroperitoneal approach. (From Harkreader H, Hogan MA: *Fundamentals of nursing: Caring and clinical judgment,* ed 3, Philadelphia, 2007, Saunders.)

this protocol must be implemented regardless of location (ambulatory surgery centers, hospital, or health care provider's office). The protocol consists of three main steps:

1. Conduct a preoperative verification process that guarantees all relevant documents and test results are available and that they meet the patient's expectations.
2. Mark the operative site with indelible ink, including marking left or right, multiple structures (e.g., toes), and vertebral level(s) of the spine.
3. Just before the start of the procedure, all members of the surgical and procedure team have a timeout to verify they have the correct patient, procedure, site, and any implants.

A legally designated representative or an active patient must be included in all the protocol steps. If the representative or patient refuses to allow marking of the operative site, this must be noted on the procedure checklist (TJC, 2013).

Transport to the Operating Room

Personnel in the OR notify the nursing unit when it is time for surgery. The transporter checks the patient's identification bracelet against the patient's medical record to be sure the correct person is going to surgery. For transportation on a gurney, the nurses and transporter help the patient safely transfer from bed to gurney. The ambulatory surgery patient may walk to the OR, allowing more control over the event. The trip to surgery should be as smooth as possible so that the sedated patient does not experience nausea or dizziness.

Family should be allowed to visit before the patient is transported to the OR and then directed to the appropriate waiting area. If family members plan on leaving the facility during the procedure, the nurse should ensure there is a way to contact them.

Preparing for the Postoperative Patient

If the patient was hospitalized before surgery and will return to the same nursing unit, the bed and room should be prepared for the patient's return. The bed is placed in the high position with the bed rails down on the receiving side and up on the other side. A postoperative bedside unit should include the following items:

- Bed pads to protect bed linen from drainage
- Clean gown
- Emesis basin
- Extra pillows for positioning
- IV pole and pump
- Oxygen equipment
- PCA pump, if ordered
- Sphygmomanometer, stethoscope, and thermometer
- Suction equipment
- Wash cloth, towel, and facial tissues

Kell-Russell Memorial Hospital

Patient name:
Date of Birth (DOB):
Medical ID number:

Check the appropriate box and initial	Surgery/Procedure Checklist			
Items Assessed	**Check for yes and initial**	**Non-applicable (N/A) and initial**	**Comments**	**Date**
1. Informed consent witnessed and signed				
2. ID band on				
3. Blood transfusion consent signed and ID band on				
4. Allergies identified and allergy band on				
5. Allergies, list				
6. Surgical site identified and marked				
7. Height and weight documented in chart				
8. Prosthetic devices removed (eyeglasses, contacts, dentures-full or partial, artificial eye, etc.)				
9. Nail polish, artificial nails, makeup, jewelry, hairpins removed				
10. Skin prep, list				
11. Hospital gown				
12. Anti-embolism stockings				
13. Time of NPO				
14. Lab results in chart				
15. ECG, scans, x-rays, etc. in chart				
16. History and physical in chart				
17. Pre-op vital signs				
18. Voided or catheterized				
19. Pre-op medications administered				
20. Mode of transfer to OR				
Signature of Nurse: *Kate Nicoli, LPN*	Initials of Nurse: *KN*	Signature of Nurse:	Initials of Nurse:	

Fig. 42.8 Preoperative assessment form. *BP,* Blood pressure; *CBC,* complete blood count; *DNR,* do not resuscitate order; *IV,* intravenous; *P,* pulse rate; *R,* respiratory rate; *T,* temperature; *TED,* thromboembolic deterrent stockings.

INTRAOPERATIVE PHASE

Intraoperative (within the surgical suite) care focuses on care and protection of the patient. When the patient enters the OR (Fig. 42.9), the patient is identified verbally and by the identification band and medical records. Nursing interventions include warm, personal contact with the patient to humanize the OR's cold, aseptic, and highly technical environment. During surgery and particularly while anesthetized, patients cannot protect themselves from sources of possible harm. Essential elements for monitoring and promoting patient safety include being aware of the potential for harm, recognizing body areas most susceptible to injury, strictly adhering to principles of positioning and asepsis, and monitoring sites for impairment or early signs of injury. The nurse must ensure that small or potentially dangerous objects such as needles and syringes are not placed near the patient. Side rails and safety straps are used, even for the fully conscious patient, to protect the patient from injury. Safety reminder devices may be necessary to protect the delirious, semicomatose, or disoriented patient from injury.

HOLDING AREA

In many facilities the patient enters a surgical care unit called a preanesthesia care unit (or holding area) outside the OR, where the nurse completes the preoperative preparations. Nurses in this unit are usually part of the OR staff and wear surgical scrub suits.

The nurse, anesthesiologist, or CRNA inserts an IV catheter into the patient's vein to establish a route for fluid replacement and IV medications. A large-bore IV catheter is used for optimal infusion of all fluids and possible blood products.

The temperature in the OR is usually cool to aid in hindering the growth of bacteria, so the patient should be offered an extra blanket for warmth and relaxation. This blanket often is placed in a warmer before covering the patient with it. The patient's stay in the holding area is generally brief.

NURSE'S ROLE

In the intraoperative phase, the nurse assumes one of two roles during the surgical procedure: scrub nurse or circulating nurse (Box 42.7). Everyone (nurses, physicians, anesthesia providers) in the OR must practice **surgical asepsis** (using sterile technique to protect against infection before, during, or after surgery) to prevent microbial contamination of the operative site. The patient is at risk for introduction of infecting organisms through catheters, drains, and the surgical wound. Standards and guidelines for surgical scrubs and skin preparation should be followed strictly. The operation's success and ease greatly depend on group dynamics as professionals work to achieve common goals (Fig. 42.10).

POSTOPERATIVE PHASE

IMMEDIATE POSTOPERATIVE PHASE

During the postoperative phase the OR nurse assists in transferring the patient to the PACU (Fig. 42.11), the recovery room, or the intensive care area. The staff reviews information about the patient's status, including IV fluids, medications, and blood products administered; the surgical dressing; any complications in the OR; and unusual risks for hemorrhage or cardiac irregularities. The OR nurse is an important resource in planning the patient's postoperative care.

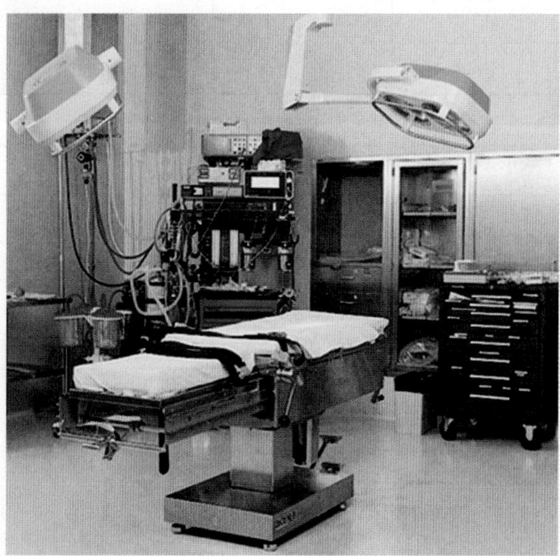

Fig. 42.9 Traditional operating room. (From Lewis SL, Heitkemper MM, Dirksen SR, et al: *Medical-surgical nursing: Assessment and management of clinical problems*, ed 10, St. Louis, 2017, Elsevier.)

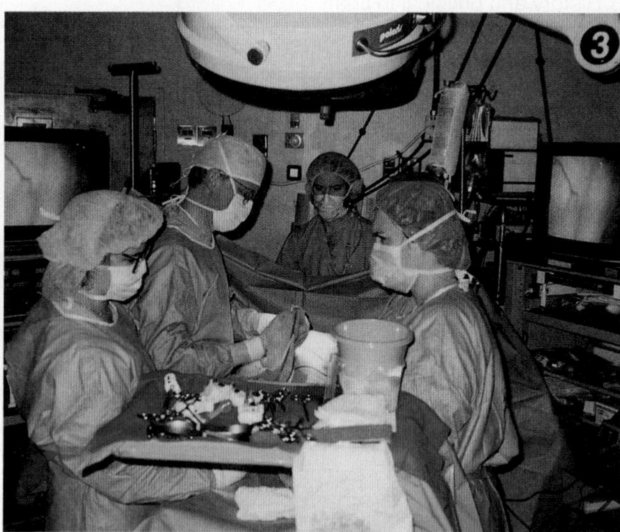

Fig. 42.10 Safe, effective intraoperative care requires team effort. (From Harkreader H, Hogan MA: *Fundamentals of nursing: Caring and clinical judgment*, ed 3, Philadelphia, 2007, Saunders.)

Box 42.7 Responsibilities of the Circulating Nurse and the Scrub Nurse

RESPONSIBILITIES OF THE CIRCULATING NURSE

- Prepares operating room with necessary equipment and supplies and ensures that equipment is functional.
- Arranges sterile and unsterile supplies; opens sterile supplies for scrub nurse.
- Sends for patient at proper time.
- Visits with patient preoperatively; explains role, identifies patient, verifies operative permit, and answers any questions.
- Performs patient assessment.
- Confirms patient assessment.
- Checks medical record for completeness.
- Assists in safe transfer of patient to operating room table.
- Positions patient on operating room table in accordance with type of procedure and surgeon's preference.
- Places conductive pad on patient if electrocautery is to be used.
- Counts sponges, needles, and instruments with scrub nurse before surgery.
- Assists scrub nurse and surgeons by tying gowns.
- May prepare patient's skin.
- Assists scrub nurse in arranging tables to create sterile field.
- Maintains continuous astute observations during surgery to anticipate needs of patient, scrub nurse, surgeons, and anesthesiologist.
- Provides supplies to scrub nurse as needed.
- Observes sterile field closely for any breaks in aseptic technique and reports accordingly.
- Cares for surgical specimens according to institutional policy.
- Documents operative record and nurse's notes.
- Counts sponges, needles, and instruments when closure of wound begins.
- Transfers patient to gurney for transport to recovery area.
- Accompanies patient to the recovery room and provides a report.

RESPONSIBILITIES OF THE SCRUB NURSE

- Performs surgical hand scrub.
- Dons sterile gown and gloves aseptically.
- Arranges sterile supplies and instruments in manner prescribed for procedure.
- Checks instruments for proper functioning.
- Counts sponges, needles, and instruments with circulating nurse.
- Gowns and gloves surgeons as they enter operating room.
- Assists with surgical draping of patient.
- Maintains neat and orderly sterile field.
- Corrects breaks in aseptic technique.
- Observes progress of surgical procedure.
- Hands surgeon instruments, sponges, and necessary supplies during procedure.
- Identifies and handles surgical specimens correctly.
- Maintains count of sponges, needles, and instruments so that none will be misplaced or lost in wounds.

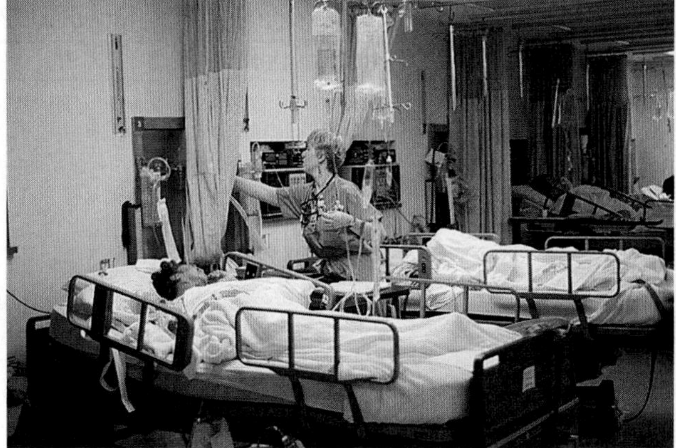

Fig. 42.11 Nurse in a postanesthesia care unit. (From Potter PA, Perry AG: *Fundamentals of nursing,* ed 7, St. Louis, 2009, Mosby.)

Immediate postoperative observation and interventions are focused on maintaining and monitoring the patient's airway, breathing, consciousness, circulation, and system review (Table 42.7). Vital signs are assessed every 15 minutes during the recovery period, and respiratory and GI functions are monitored. The wound is evaluated for any **drainage** or **exudate** (fluids from a body cavity, wound, or other source of discharge that slowly seeps from cells, tissue, or blood vessels through small pores or breaks in cell membranes). Once the patient has a patent airway and stable vital signs, is conscious, and responds to stimuli, the anesthesia provider or surgeon approves transfer to the nursing unit. As the patient regains consciousness, relief from pain is often the first need expressed. Frequently, medication is given in the recovery area. Staff members on the nursing unit review documentation from the surgical suite and recovery room to assess how well the patient tolerated the surgery.

The patient's body temperature must be monitored closely. Hypothermia—a rectal temperature of less than 96°F (35.6°C) or an oral temperature of less than 95°F (35°C)—frequently occurs because of body exposure in a cold OR, the effects of cold solutions, or as a possible consequence of some anesthetics. The heat loss in the OR can continue in the PACU, so warmed blankets may be used to increase the patient's body temperature. Another therapy may be used to provide warmth to the patient, convective warming. This therapy uses a disposable cover inflated with warm air from a heating unit placed over the patient; warm air passes out through the underside, so the warm air is moving constantly. In the PACU, the patient's temperature and vital signs are monitored every 15 minutes until vital signs are stable, or more frequently if they are unstable. The frequency and duration of monitoring are dictated by facility PACU policy. Patients are monitored until they are discharged from the PACU, usually at least 1 hour. Before discharge from the PACU, the patient must meet minimum criteria as established by the facility. This often is scored using a system based on assessment of

Table 42.7 Interventions Associated With Immediate Postoperative Recovery Phase

ASSESSMENT MODE	INTERVENTION
A: Airway	• Maintain patency: keep head tilted up and back; may position on side with the face down and the neck slightly extended. • Note presence or absence of gag or swallowing reflex; stay at bedside until gag reflex returns. • Suction until awake and alert. • Provide oxygen if necessary.
B: Breathing	• Evaluate depth, rate, sounds, rhythm, and chest movement. • Assess color of mucous membranes. • Place hand above patient's nose to detect respirations if shallow. • Initiate coughing and deep breathing exercises as soon as patient is able to respond. • Chart time oxygen is discontinued. • Monitor oxygen saturation levels (SaO_2) by pulse oximetry checks.
C: Consciousness	• **Extubate** patient (remove endotracheal tube from airway). • Confirm that patient responds to commands. • Confirm that patient verbalizes responses. • Confirm that patient reacts to stimuli.
C: Circulation	• Monitor temperature, pulse, respirations, and blood pressure q 10–15 min; take axillary, tympanic, or rectal temperature if warranted. • Assess rate, rhythm, and quality of pulse. • Evaluate color and warmth of skin and color of nail beds. • Check peripheral pulses as indicated. • Assess incision and dressing (monitor wound drainage output). • Monitor intravenous lines: solution, rate, site. • Cardiac monitors are usually in place for patients who had general anesthesia.
S: System review	• Assess neurologic functions, muscle strength, and response. • Monitor drains, tubes, and color and amount of output. • Check for pressure, type, and condition of dressings. • Evaluate pain response; may need to give analgesic and monitor patient response. • Observe for allergic reactions. • Assess urinary output if Foley catheter is in place.

the patient. Assessment variables that determine when the patient may be discharged include the patient's pain level, the presence of nausea or vomiting, ability to urinate, vital signs, cognitive level, and the amount bleeding from the surgical site.

The PACU nurse must be aware that malignant hyperthermia also can occur in the PACU and repeatedly assess the patient for signs of this condition. Malignant hyperthermia is a rare genetic disorder characterized by uncontrolled skeletal muscle contractions leading to cardiac dysrhythmia and potentially fatal hyperthermia. It occurs when patients predisposed to the disorder are given a combination of certain anesthetic agents. Unless the triggering event is stopped and the body is cooled, death results.

LATER POSTOPERATIVE PHASE

Immediate Assessments

When the patient returns to the nursing unit, the nurse performs a thorough postsurgical assessment. Common initial assessment criteria include a review of vital signs, the IV and incisional sites, any tubes, and postoperative orders. A review of each body system identifies when body functions return and provides a guideline for further assessments. Unless otherwise indicated, it is standard practice in most facilities to monitor vital signs and make general assessments using the "times 4" factor—every 15 minutes times 4 (for 4 times); every 30 minutes times 4; every hour times 4; then every 4 hours, or until assessments are within expected ranges. Table 42.8 details body temperature responses to surgery. A postoperative flow sheet (Fig. 42.12) is used frequently to document the patient's progress. This is often a computerized form. Significant observations are critical for the patient after surgery.

Although the patient may respond, the level of consciousness is altered; therefore it is important to keep the side rails up and the call light within reach for safety. Until the patient is fully conscious, a pillow should not be placed under the patient's head because this may cause the tongue to obstruct the airway. The patient should be positioned on the side, depending on the type of surgery, or the head of the bed should be raised to a 45-degree angle. Positioning the head higher than the chest reduces the chance of the patient aspirating vomitus. Because nausea and vomiting are normal in the first 12 to 24 hours, an emesis basin should be kept at the bedside. If the patient vomits, the amount should be measured and carefully described in the documentation. Any red or coffee-ground emesis must

Table 42.8 Temperature Assessment and Intervention

CAUSE	ASSESSMENT AND INTERVENTION
Hypothermia	
Within First 12 Hours	
Response to surgery, anesthesia, and body exposure	• Monitor temperature readings. • Assess for warmth. • Provide warm blankets. • Do not expose for long periods. • Assess orientation.
Hyperthermia	
24–48 Hours	
Dehydration Decreased lung activity Inflammatory response to surgery	• Monitor temperature readings. • Monitor intravenous rate. • Encourage fluids. • Assess intake and output (I&O). • Have patient turn, cough, and breathe deeply. • Provide incentive spirometer. • Assess lung sounds. • Observe incision.
After Day 2	
Infection: Respiratory, wound, urinary, or circulatory	• Monitor temperature readings. • Assess lung sounds and expectoration of sputum. • Evaluate incision and drainage. • Monitor I&O. • Encourage fluids (6–8 oz/h) unless contraindicated. • Note urine color, odor, amount, and consistency, and patient's complaints of burning on micturition. • Perform leg exercises q 2 hr, and ambulate q 4 hr.

be reported immediately, because this is an indication of GI bleeding. Frequently the patient remains on NPO status for the first few hours after surgery; fluids are introduced gradually. The surgeon may order ice chips followed by clear or full liquids.

Postoperative complications can occur suddenly, making ongoing assessments critical. Vital signs, coupled with the patient's behavior, are an early indication of postoperative complications. A pulse that increases and becomes thready, a declining blood pressure, cool and clammy skin, reduced urinary output, narrowing pulse pressure, and restlessness are usually indicative of hypovolemic shock. Hypovolemic shock in the postoperative period can be a life-threatening emergency and frequently is caused by internal hemorrhage or excessive loss of blood or fluids during surgery (Box 42.8). A drop in blood pressure slightly below a patient's preoperative baseline reading is common after surgery. However, a significant drop in blood pressure, accompanied by an increased heart rate, may indicate hemorrhage, circulatory failure, or fluid shifts. Impending hypovolemic shock cannot be based on one low blood

Box 42.8 Possible Causes of Postoperative Shock

- Cardiac dysrhythmias
- Cardiac failure
- Inadequate ventilation
- Loss of blood and other body fluids
- Movement of patient from operating table to gurney
- Pain
- Patient (gurney) being jarred during transport
- Reactions to drugs and anesthesia

pressure reading. If the patient's blood pressure is showing a trend of dropping, measurements of the pressure should be taken every 5 minutes for 15 minutes to determine the variability. Fluctuations in blood pressure also can mean that the anesthetic is wearing off or that the patient is experiencing severe pain.

In addition to hypotension, manifestations of shock include tachycardia (rapid heartbeat), restlessness, apprehension, and cold, moist, pale, or cyanotic skin. When a patient appears to be going into shock, standard protocol in most facilities includes the following steps: (1) administer oxygen per facility protocol or increase its rate of delivery, unless contraindicated by a respiratory disease or disorder such as chronic obstructive pulmonary disease (COPD); (2) raise the patient's legs above the level of the heart; (3) increase the rate of IV fluid administration as per facility protocol, unless contraindicated because of fluid excretion problems or other existing conditions; (4) notify the anesthesia provider and the surgeon; (5) provide medications as ordered; and (6) continue to assess the patient and the patient's response to interventions.

Incision

The incisional dressing must be monitored to assess for bleeding or excessive drainage (e.g., dressings saturated with bright red drainage, or bright red drainage occurring 24 to 48 hours after surgery warrants notifying the surgeon). Normally dressings are not changed but are reinforced during the first 24 hours. To accurately measure the amount of drainage, circle the shadowed drainage markings on the dressing and write the time and date; this technique makes evident any increased bleeding or drainage over time. **Dehiscence** (the separation of a surgical incision or rupture of a wound closure) may occur 3 days to more than 2 weeks postoperatively. Wound separation in the first 3 days usually is related to technical factors, such as the sutures. Separation within 3 to 14 days postoperatively usually is associated with postoperative complications such as distention, vomiting, excessive coughing, dehydration, or infection. Wound separation after 2 weeks usually is associated with metabolic factors, such as **cachexia** (ill health, malnutrition, and wasting as a result of chronic disease), hypoproteinemia, increased age, malignancy, radiation therapy, and obesity. Wound **evisceration** (protrusion of an internal organ through a wound or surgical

Kell-Russell Memorial Hospital	Post-operative Assessment			Patient name:
				Date of Birth (DOB):
				Medical ID number:
Surgeon:	**Operative Procedure:**	**Date and Time patient received:**	**Anesthetic Type:**	**Allergies:**
Time	B/P, P, R, T	Pain Level (0-10 scale)	O_2 Saturation	Assessment
1300	90/60, 100, 32, 98.4	1	95% on O_2 @2L N/C	Pt. received from PACU via stretcher. Drowsy but able to answer questions. Surgical dressing clean, dry, and intact. See flow sheet for remainder of assessment.
1315	96/62, 98, 28, 98.2	1	96% on O_2 @2L N/C	Remains drowsy but continues to answer questions. Dressing remains clean, dry, and intact.
1330	98/62, 94, 26, 98.3	2	93% on O_2 @2L N/C	Drowsy. Encouraged to take deep breaths. Pinpoint shadowed area of sanguineous drainage on dressing. Area marked with time.
1345	110/70, 94, 28, 98.7	4	96% on O_2 @2L N/C	Less drowsy, reports incisional pain at a 4/10. Encouraged to press PCA for bolus. Patient complied. No increase in drainage on dressing.
Signature of Nurse: Kate Nicoli, LPN	Initials of Nurse: KN		Signature of Nurse:	Initials of Nurse:

Fig. 42.12 Postoperative assessment form. *BP-P-R*, Blood pressure–pulse rate–respiratory rate; *PACU*, postanesthesia care unit; *PCA*, patient-controlled analgesia; *ROM*, range of motion; *O_2 saturation*, arterial oxygen saturation.

incision, especially in the abdominal wall) also may occur. Wound dehiscence and evisceration require prompt attention (Fig. 42.13). If the patient feels a sudden "give," sutures or staples may have broken. Cover the wound immediately with a sterile dressing moistened with sterile normal saline and notify the surgeon. Tension on the abdomen may be decreased by placing the patient in a Fowler's or semi-Fowler's position with the knees slightly flexed. Reassure the patient regarding the situation and inform him or her that surgery will be required. Begin preparing the patient for surgery by placing him or her on NPO status as well as following other facility protocol. Sterile technique procedures—including dressing change and care of the surgical incision with phases of wound healing—are discussed in Chapter 22 in *Foundations of Nursing*.

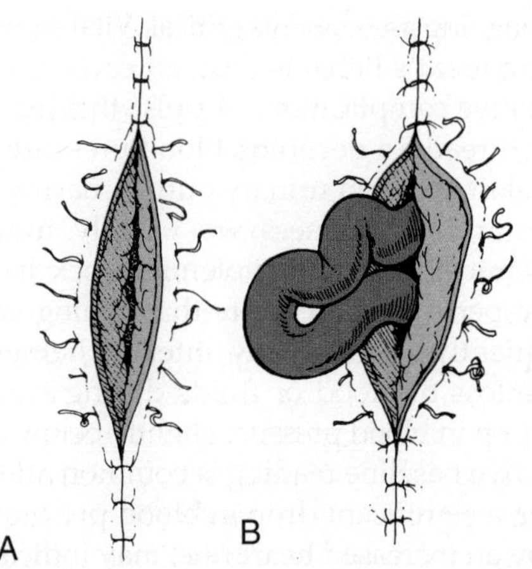

Fig. 42.13 A, Wound dehiscence. B, Evisceration.

Ventilation

Immediate postoperative hypoventilation can result from drugs (anesthetics, narcotics, tranquilizers, sedatives), incisional pain, obesity, chronic lung disease, or pressure on the diaphragm. Inadequate ventilation leads to hypoxemia. Arterial oxygen saturation (SaO_2) is monitored either by arterial blood gas measurements or by pulse oximetry.

Because lung ventilation is vital, the patient should be helped to turn, cough, and breathe deeply every 1 to 2 hours until the chest is clear. Having practiced this combination preoperatively, the patient is usually able to remove adequately trapped mucus and surgical gases. To ease the pressure on the incision, help the patient support the surgical site with a pillow or rolled bath blanket. The hand can be used to splint the incision, but it is not the ideal method. Administration of analgesics, as prescribed, to control pain before coughing and deep-breathing exercises will increase the effectiveness of these activities. Early mobility and frequent position changes facilitate secretion clearance and improve the ventilation and perfusion in the lungs. Respiratory infections frequently are caused by shallow breathing and poor coughing. The LPN/LVN (licensed practical nurse/licensed vocational nurse) should auscultate (i.e., listen to) the lungs at least every 2 hours to determine the presence of any adventitious (i.e., unusual or abnormal) breath sounds as an early indication of postoperative complications.

If the patient feels chest pain or has a fever, productive cough, or dyspnea (difficulty breathing), atelectasis or pneumonia may be developing. Sudden chest pain along with dyspnea, tachycardia, cyanosis (i.e., a slightly bluish, gray, or dark purple discoloration of the skin), diaphoresis (excessive sweating), and hypotension is a sign of a pulmonary embolism. Raise the head of the bed immediately to decrease dyspnea and immediately report signs and symptoms to the health care provider, because this is a medical emergency. Frequently oxygen therapy is instituted to assist with breathing.

Whenever air exchange is reduced, postoperative recovery slows. Medication, suctioning, and oxygen therapy may be needed to assist the patient in respiratory distress. Mechanical devices, such as incentive spirometers, are used to stimulate deep breathing (see Skill 42.2). Patients are encouraged to take 10 deep breaths every hour while awake.

If respiratory complications develop, the health care provider may order nebulizer treatments to deliver bronchodilators and/or steroids or antiinflammatory medications, or intermittent positive-pressure breathing (IPPB) treatments to deliver a mixture of air and oxygen; medication can be added to enhance respirations. IPPB treatments use positive pressure to expand the lungs for better distribution of medication. Chest percussion and postural drainage constitute a form of chest physiotherapy that combines positioning and percussion movements to lung areas to help dislodge and move secretions; this also may be ordered by the health care provider. This treatment, as well as IPPB, usually is delivered by a respiratory therapist.

Pain

Because postoperative pain is to be expected, it is important for the nurse to monitor and assess the patient for pain postoperatively. Effective pain management allows for early ambulation, promotion of adequate rest, and fewer postoperative complications. Depending on the type of surgery, acute pain usually begins to subside within 24 to 48 hours, and pain medication is adjusted as necessary. In the early stages of recovery, comfort interventions may help ease pain. After the acute phase, comfort measures may be the only interventions required (Box 42.9).

A patient's level of pain can be difficult to evaluate. If the patient is able to communicate verbally, ask the patient to rate the pain on a scale of 0 to 10 or 0 to 5, depending on facility policy. There are standard pain indexes (restlessness, moaning, grimacing, diaphoresis), but some patients may not exhibit signs outwardly.

Box 42.9 Postoperative Comfort Measures for Pain

DECREASE EXTERNAL STIMULI

- Darken room; close drapes.
- Keep TV and radio off or low.
- Monitor hall traffic and noise.
- Assess staff interruptions.
- Check room for noise—dripping water, buzzing lights, constant intercom messages.

REDUCE INTERRUPTIONS

- Plan care to allow rest.
- Post "Do Not Disturb" sign.
- Unplug telephone, if acceptable to patient.
- Restrict visitors.
- Pull curtains around bed.

ELIMINATE ODORS

- Discuss offending odors and assess elimination.
- Remove from room all dressings that are soiled with exudate.
- Remove food trays immediately after meals.

NURSING INTERVENTIONS

- Ask patient about normal relaxation patterns and practices.
- Have patient practice deep-breathing and relaxation techniques.
- Plan rest periods.
- Provide back rub.
- Engage patient in conversation; ask about concerns and fears.
- Encourage diversional activities.
- Reposition and support with pillows, bed rolls.
- Check tube placement.
- Offer warm fluids if indicated.
- Reduce room clutter.
- Provide restful environment.

Objective pain factors are signs that the body is responding to "pain"; these include vital sign changes (blood pressure lowers in the immediate postoperative period and elevates in response to pain after about 12 hours, and pulse increases), restlessness, diaphoresis, and pallor. The patient's description of discomfort represents subjective pain factors. Pain behaviors are influenced by the patient's culture and past experiences. Behaviors include moaning, grimacing, and favoring a body area.

The effectiveness of analgesic measures differs with each person; if relief is not obtained, changing the medication or administration schedule may provide effective pain control. Many patients wait to request or accept analgesics until pain is at its worst. Explain that pain medication is more effective if taken at the onset of pain. Remember that each patient interprets pain differently and has a personal pain tolerance level; pain is whatever the patient says it is.

The success of pain management depends on the surgery, the patient's emotional state, and postoperative complications. Patients experiencing chronic pain may have more difficulty obtaining relief than individuals with acute episodes. Commonly used analgesic measures are nurse-administered narcotics, patient-controlled IV medications (see Chapter 21 in *Foundations of Nursing*), and pain control via a transcutaneous electrical nerve stimulation (TENS) unit (Fig. 42.14). When attached to the skin, the TENS unit applies electrical impulses to the nerve endings and blocks transmission of pain signals to the brain. The PCA system is a pump that is programmed to dispense only a given amount of medication. The patient can self-administer an analgesic by pressing a control button. The PCA system must be monitored by the nurse at least every 3 to 4 hours, or as directed by facility policy. Nonpharmacologic pain control measures such as repositioning and diversional activities may be effective in treating pain. (Refer to Chapter 21 in *Foundations of Nursing* for pain management.)

Urinary Function

Anesthesia depresses urinary function, so it is important for the nurse to assess the bladder area for distention and changes in renal function. It routinely takes 6 to 8 hours for voiding to occur after surgery. If patients do not void within 8 hours, catheterization may be necessary, but it should be used only if necessary. Before use of catheterization to treat urinary retention, try noninvasive measures such as having the patient listen to running water, placing the hands in warm water, or ambulating to the bathroom or bedside commode, if able, to facilitate voiding. Helping male patients stand often encourages voiding. Usually I&O is measured while a Foley catheter is in place, while the patient is receiving IV therapy, and immediately after a Foley catheter has been removed. The urine measurement should continue until the patient is voiding without difficulty. Determination of serum blood urea nitrogen may be ordered by the health care provider daily until the patient has recovered.

Fluid deficit may result from inadequate replacement of body fluids lost during surgery or from continued fluid losses. Fluid excess may occur from large amounts of IV fluids when kidney function is inadequate. A urinary output of 30 mL/h is considered acceptable postoperatively. Unless the patient has had urinary tract surgery, urine should be clear and yellow and smell like ammonia.

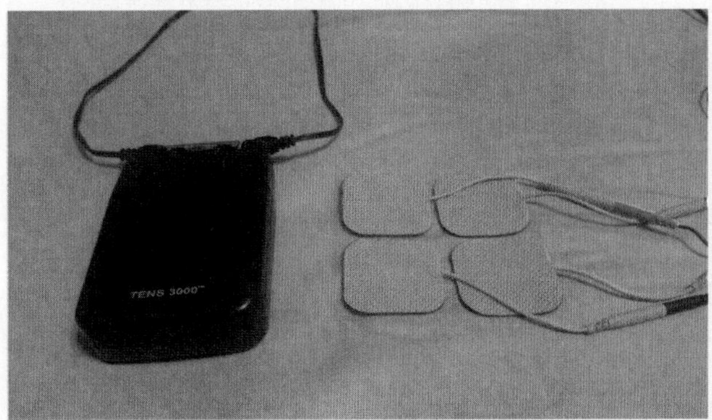

Fig. 42.14 Transcutaneous electrical nerve stimulation (TENS) unit.

Venous Stasis

Venous stasis (a disorder in which the normal flow of fluid through a vessel of the body is slowed or halted) is the underlying cause of thrombus formation. Performing leg exercises every 2 hours and using intermittent pneumatic compression devices and compression stockings aid the circulatory system and help prevent deep-vein thrombosis. Assessment of the feet and legs includes palpating for pedal pulse (i.e., pulse on upper surface of foot) and noting the skin's color and temperature. If edema, aching or cramping, sensitivity, redness, inflammation, warmth, or pain occurs in the calf or leg, thrombophlebitis should be suspected. The patient is to remain in bed until the health care provider can perform an evaluation. The patient should be instructed not to cross the legs when in bed and be encouraged to be out of bed as much as possible (if not contraindicated) to prevent venous stasis. If the bed has a knee gatch (i.e., a bed jointed to allow knee flexion), it should not be used with the postoperative patient because this promotes venous stasis in the lower legs.

Surgical patients are at increased risk of developing life-threatening deep vein thrombosis and pulmonary embolism. Not only does surgery injure blood vessels, but anesthesia and inactivity also cause venous stasis. Surgery, however, is not the only risk factor. Others include pregnancy, myocardial infarction, heart failure, stroke (cerebrovascular accident or brain attack), cancer, sepsis, and immobility. Effective methods to prevent deep vein thrombosis include early and frequent ambulation and leg exercises. Antiembolism stockings and pneumatic compression devices are also useful preventive measures.

The external sequential compression device (SCD) (see Skill 42.5) is used on many postoperative patients, especially those patients who are at increased risk of developing deep vein thrombosis and pulmonary embolism. Many surgeons require that the device be placed on the patient preoperatively so that therapy can be initiated during surgery or in the immediate postoperative period without delay. This device includes an air pressure pump and cuffs, one for each entire leg, calf, or foot. Continuous inflation and deflation of the cuffs decrease pooling of venous blood in the legs and improves venous return to the heart. The pressure cuffs automatically inflate to the prescribed setting and deflate in cycles, with inflation lasting about 12 seconds and deflation lasting about 48 seconds. This system is contraindicated for any patient with acute thrombophlebitis or deep vein thrombosis.

When ambulating the patient, turn the pump off and remove the cuffs. The SCD should not be disconnected for more than 30 minutes. If the patient is scheduled for diagnostic examinations that require leaving the nursing unit for longer than 30 minutes, the compression pump, the cuffs or sleeves, and the instructions on operation should travel with the patient if traditional SCDs are used. If battery-operated SCDs are used, ensure that the batteries are charged fully.

The treatment usually continues for 72 hours postoperatively or until the patient is ambulating well. The cuffs should be removed daily to assess skin integrity and to provide skin care. Documentation of the use of the intermittent external pneumatic compression system and any abnormal reaction, such as numbness or tingling, should be included in the patient's record.

Activity

Early ambulation is a significant factor in hastening postoperative recovery and preventing postoperative complications. The exercise of getting in and out of bed and walking during the early postoperative period has numerous benefits (Box 42.10). Ambulation usually is contraindicated for patients with severe infection or thrombophlebitis.

Assessment. Before helping the patient ambulate for the first few times after major surgery, assess the following:

1. Level of alertness: Ask the patient simple questions or to follow simple commands
2. Cardiovascular status (orthostatic hypotension, i.e., a drop of 25 mm Hg in systolic pressure and a drop of 10 mm Hg in diastolic pressure when moving from a lying to sitting position)
   a. Assess pulse and respiratory rate and depth while patient is supine, and then after sitting.
   b. Observe skin color for pallor while patient is sitting.
   c. Note complaints of vertigo while patient is sitting.
3. Motor status
   a. Assess muscle strength of patient's legs.
   b. Assess sitting ability.

Box 42.10 Effects of Early Postoperative Ambulation

- Increased circulation
- Increased kidney function
- Increased mental alertness from increased oxygenation to brain
- Increased metabolism
- Increased micturition (urinary elimination)
- Increased peristalsis
- Increased rate and depth of breathing
- Nutrients required for healing are more available to wound
- Prevention of abdominal distention and gas pain
- Prevention of atelectasis and hypostatic pneumonia
- Prevention of constipation
- Prevention of loss of muscle tone
- Prevention of paralytic ileus
- Prevention of thrombophlebitis
- Prevention of urinary retention
- Promotion of expulsion of flatus
- Restoration of nitrogen balance

It is also important to consider any preoperative limitations to ambulation. The patient with arthritis or arteriosclerosis may take longer to move and to adjust to standing and walking. The patient who used a walker preoperatively needs assistance for a longer time before using the walker again. Family members are important in assisting patients with any physical limitation and in providing emotional support during postoperative recovery.

Nursing interventions. Nursing interventions are as follows:

1. Encourage muscle-strengthening exercises before ambulation.
   a. Have patient bend knees, lower knees, press back of knees hard against bed.
   b. Have patient alternately contract and relax calf and thigh muscles 10 times, using the following cycle: contract, relax, rest.
2. Obtain vital signs, and if within normal limits, have patient sit on side of bed (legs dangling) to adapt to the upright position before ambulating for the first time. Be certain that the pulse has stabilized (returned to baseline) before patient attempts ambulation.
3. If the patient has a nasogastric (NG) tube, clamp it while the patient ambulates and then reconnect it.
4. Keep urinary tube connected to drainage bag, and keep the drainage receptacle below the level of bladder to prevent reflux of urine.
5. Attach IV bag to a movable pole.
6. Make sure two people assist in ambulating an unsteady patient receiving IV fluids.
7. Encourage the patient to walk farther at each ambulation.

The word *ambulate* means to move from place to place or to walk. Sitting in a chair is not ambulation. After ambulating, the patient may sit in a chair but should be advised to stand and walk at intervals and to elevate the legs while sitting to prevent venous pooling in the extremities. The patient should avoid sitting in a chair for long periods (see Chapter 8 in *Foundations of Nursing*).

GASTROINTESTINAL STATUS

Abdominal distention frequently occurs after surgery. Because anesthesia, surgical manipulation, administration of narcotics, and introduction of carbon dioxide into the abdominal cavity during surgery slow peristalsis (i.e., the normal propulsion of food through the digestive tract), it may take 3 or 4 days for bowel activity to return. Auscultate for bowel sounds in the abdomen to assess the return of peristalsis. Normal peristalsis is indicated by hearing 5 to 30 gurgles per minute. Bowel sounds are auscultated in all four quadrants. If bowel sounds are absent (each quadrant must be assessed for 3 to 5 minutes to determine absence of bowel sounds), **paralytic ileus** (a significant decrease in or absence of intestinal peristalsis that may occur after abdominal surgery, peritoneal trauma, severe metabolic disease, and other conditions) may have developed. This finding can develop into a medical emergency within 24 to 48 hours. If inactivity continues, the physician usually orders placement of an NG or nasointestinal tube to help remove any gas that has formed in the stomach and small intestine, as well as fluid that has accumulated. When listening for bowel sounds in patients who have an NG or nasointestinal tube, turn off the suction machine during the assessment and then turn it back on.

If the patient has developed abdominal distention, it should be assessed by measuring the patient's abdominal girth. To ensure the measurement is accurate, mark the placement for the tape measure at the level of the umbilicus. Assess and chart the expelling of flatus, bowel sounds, and abdominal girth. On occasion, analgesics (meperidine) and other medications may slow peristalsis; charting the patient's GI habits helps identify causative factors.

Encouraging movement (turning every 2 hours, early ambulation) helps restore GI activity. The health care provider may order a rectal tube to be inserted to relieve pain from intestinal gas (see Chapter 15 in *Foundations of Nursing*). For the patient who has difficulty with flatus, limiting iced beverages and offering warm liquids may help resolve the discomfort. The patient may have fluids and food withheld until flatus is expelled. As the patient returns to previous eating habits, bowel function slowly resumes its preoperative state. Constipation is also a frequent problem after surgery. The same aids for abdominal distention assist in alleviating constipation. If the patient does not pass feces within 2 or 3 days after resuming solid foods, a suppository, stool softener, or a small-volume enema may be ordered.

Singultus (hiccup) is an involuntary contraction of the diaphragm followed by rapid closure of the glottis. Singultus results from irritation of the phrenic nerve. Sedatives may be necessary in extreme cases. Abdominal distention is sometimes the cause, so this is another important reason for thorough assessment of the patient's abdomen for proper GI function. Abdominal distention usually is caused by gas in the intestinal tract but may be related to internal bleeding. Proper assessment can help determine the cause of abdominal distention.

FLUIDS AND ELECTROLYTES

Fluid is lost during surgery through blood loss and increased insensible fluid loss through the lungs and skin. For at least the first 24 to 48 hours after surgery, the body attempts to retain fluids as part of the stress response to trauma and the effect of anesthesia.

Sodium and potassium depletion can occur after surgery as a result of the loss of blood or body fluids during surgery or the loss of GI secretion because of vomiting and NG tubes. Potassium is also lost during **catabolism** (tissue breakdown), especially after severe trauma or crush injuries. Loss of gastric secretions can result in chloride loss, producing metabolic alkalosis. Electrolytes often are added to the IV solution in the form of potassium chloride (KCl).

The nurse is responsible for closely monitoring fluid tolerance and electrolyte values during the postoperative period. When the patient returns from the recovery room, IV therapy will be in progress. Until the patient is past the nausea and vomiting period and can tolerate oral fluids, parenteral therapy most likely will be maintained. The IV line must be assessed for patency and ordered fluid rate; the IV site also should be monitored for erythema, edema, heat, and pain. The IV solution may become infiltrated because of movement or inadvertent dislodgment of the needle when the patient ambulates; infiltration is indicated by the presence of swelling that is cool to the touch at the IV site, sluggish or absent flowing of the fluid, and/or absence of a blood return. The assessment for rate of infusion is extremely important for older patients or patients with cardiac and pulmonary disorders, who may quickly experience fluid overload and pulmonary edema.

Muscles and nerves require ongoing nourishment to function adequately, and parenteral fluids contain the necessary glucose and electrolytes. Depending on the type of surgery and the patient's nutritional needs, IV therapy lasts from a few hours to a few days. As long as the patient is receiving parenteral fluids, I&O status should be measured. If the patient's overall nutritional state is in question, daily weights should be obtained (see Chapter 19 in *Foundations of Nursing*).

As oral fluids are introduced, the patient should be encouraged to drink small amounts frequently (6 to 8 oz/h). A review of the diet history reveals fluids normally enjoyed by the patient. Unless otherwise ordered, patients usually begin by ingesting clear liquids (clear soda, water, tea, broth, gelatin) and progress as the GI system returns to normal functioning. Unless the patient has other problems (e.g., decreased renal excretion because of renal failure or advanced age), encourage the patient to drink 2000 to 2400 mL in 24 hours. Because iced and carbonated beverages cause GI disturbances in some individuals, patients should avoid these fluids until active peristalsis is noted. If nausea and vomiting persist, an antiemetic such as promethazine (Phenergan), benzquinamide (Emete-Con), ondansetron (Zofran), or prochlorperazine (Compazine) may be ordered to be administered intravenously or rectally.

NURSING PROCESS FOR THE SURGICAL PATIENT

The role of the LPN/LVN in the nursing process is that the LPN/LVN will:

- Participate in planning care for patients based on patient needs
- Review patients' care plans and recommend revisions as needed
- Review and follow defined prioritization for patient care
- Use clinical pathways, care maps, or care plans to guide and review patient care

ASSESSMENT

General assessment of the preoperative patient includes obtaining a nursing history. This consists of any prior surgery, allergies, current medications, use of other drugs or alcohol, and smoking status. The patient's physical condition and at-risk data, emotional status of the patient and family members, and patient's preoperative diagnostic data also are assessed. It is important for the patient and family to understand the surgical procedure and the expected outcomes. In the intraoperative stage, any procedures such as skin preparation or catheterization are completed. During surgery and recovery, the patient's condition is assessed continually. Postoperative care should be tailored to prevent and detect postoperative complications and return the patient to wellness.

PATIENT PROBLEMS

Determining patient problems establishes the direction for the care to be provided during one or all surgical phases (Boxes 42.11 and 42.12). Identification of the patient problems may focus on preoperative, intraoperative, and postoperative risks. Preventive care is essential for effective management of the surgical patient.

EXPECTED OUTCOMES, GOALS, AND PLANNING

The care plan begins before surgery and follows through the postoperative period to provide the best nursing interventions possible. It is important to include the patient in health care planning. A patient informed about the surgical experience is less likely to be fearful and is better able to prepare for expected outcomes.

Goals and expected outcomes for the surgical patient may include the following:

Goal: Patient achieves physical comfort by demonstrating effective coughing and deep-breathing technique.

Outcome: Patient verbalizes relief of pain (optimally, 3 or below on a 10-point scale during the immediate postoperative phase), based on pain scale assessment.

IMPLEMENTATION

Nursing interventions before surgery physically and psychologically prepare the patient for the surgical procedure. The nurse should act as an advocate for the patient during and after surgery to ensure that the patient's dignity and rights are protected at all times (Nursing Care Plan 42.1).

EVALUATION

Evaluation of the effectiveness of the care plan is essential, and revision of the plan should be addressed

Box 42.11 Preoperative Patient Problem Statements

- *Inability to Clear Airway*
- *Anxiousness*
- *Insufficient Knowledge*
- *Impaired Family Coping*
- *Impaired Role Functioning*
- *Fearfulness*
- *Insufficient Nutrition*
- *Potential for Compromised Skin Integrity*

Box 42.12 Postoperative Patient Problem Statements

- *Compromised Oral Mucous Membrane, related to nothing by mouth (NPO) status, irritation of endotracheal tube or NG tube*
- *Compromised Physical Mobility, related to pain, postoperative activity restrictions*
- *Compromised Verbal Communication, related to endotracheal tube placement*
- *Fluid Volume Overload, related to excess IV fluid replacement, decreased circulation*
- *Grief, related to patient's critical condition*
- *Impaired Coping, related to constraints imposed by surgery, postoperative condition*
- *Inability to Bathe Self, Dress Self, Feed Self, Toilet Self*
- *Inability to Clear Airway, related to diminished cough, prolonged sedation, retained secretions*
- *Inability to Maintain Adequate Breathing Pattern, related to incisional pain, effects of anesthetic, narcotic pain medications*
- *Potential for Compromised Skin Integrity, related to wound exudate, immobility, insufficient nutritional intake*
- *Potential for Inability to Regulate Body Temperature*
- *Potential for Inadequate Fluid Volume, related to wound drainage, decreased fluid intake*
- *Potential for Infection, related to surgical incision, indwelling catheter, wound drainage tubes*
- *Recent Onset of Pain*

Nursing Care Plan 42.1 The Postoperative Patient

Mr. S. is a 40-year-old, obese patient weighing 280 lb who was admitted with bowel obstruction and a scheduled right hemicolectomy. Mr. S. has hypertension and a history of poor wound healing.

PATIENT PROBLEM

Inability to Clear Airway, related to incisional pain

Patient Goals and Expected Outcomes	Nursing Interventions	Evaluation and Rationale
Patient will cough deeply in 24 hours. Patient's lung sounds will clear after coughing.	Medicate with analgesia to control pain. Raise head of bed to full Fowler's position during exercises. Splint incision with rolled bath blanket. Have patient turn, cough, and deep-breathe q hr while awake. Use incentive spirometer hourly. Take vital signs q 4 hr and note evidence of dyspnea or restlessness. Monitor intravenous fluids. Offer sips of fluid q hr if permissible.	Providing pain relief enables patient to cough and breathe deeply without discomfort. In Fowler's position the diaphragm falls, which permits lung expansion. Splinting incision provides abdominal support during coughing. Turning, coughing, and deep breathing aid in mobilizing secretions. Adequate lung expansion can prevent atelectasis. Increased fluid intake helps prevent thickening of mucus.

PATIENT PROBLEM

Inability to Maintain Adequate Breathing Pattern, related to poor body mechanics

Patient Goals and Expected Outcomes	Nursing Interventions	Evaluation and Rationale
Patient will effectively use incentive spirometer.	Encourage deep breathing q 1–2 hr while awake. Reposition q 2 hr; support joints and incision. Continue oxygen at 2 L per cannula; cleanse nares q 4 hr; post "No Smoking" sign. Encourage use of incentive spirometer, 10 breaths q hr.	Adequate lung expansion helps prevent atelectasis. Turning promotes lung expansion. Additional oxygen ensures adequate tissue oxygenation. "No Smoking" sign promotes safety. Adequate lung expansion helps prevent atelectasis.
Patient's respirations will be even and unlabored.	Record respirations q 4 hr, noting depth, rate, and quality. Assess skin and nail beds q 4 hr; report slow blanching color and condition. Darken room; decrease stimuli, monitor pain, and offer analgesic prn (as needed).	Regular assessments help detect early signs and symptoms of respiratory complications. A change in color of skin and nail beds signals poor oxygenation. Comfort measures promote rest and relaxation and decrease pain level.

PATIENT PROBLEM

Potential for Infection, related to open surgical incision and draining wound

Patient Goals and Expected Outcomes	Nursing Interventions	Evaluation and Rationale
Patient's wound will not be erythematous or produce purulent exudate. Patient's vital signs will remain within normal range.	Perform hand hygiene appropriately. Monitor wound q 4 hr, noting amount and color of drainage; assess skin for warmth, color, and sensation. Mark drainage on dressing q 4 hr; reinforce prn. Use surgical asepsis when changing dressing. Monitor vital signs q 4 hr. Monitor white blood cell (WBC) level as ordered.	Hand washing helps prevent transmission of microorganisms. Regular assessments reveal early signs and symptoms of wound infection. Containing wound drainage within dressing provides comfort to the patient and enables the nurse to correctly determine the type of drainage. Surgical asepsis prevents the transmission of microorganisms. Elevation of WBCs indicates an infectious process and its severity.

CRITICAL THINKING QUESTIONS

1. On the second postoperative day, Mr. S. is taking shallow breaths and having difficulty complying with coughing and deep breathing. His temperature is 101.8°F (38.8°C), and he has adventitious breath sounds bilaterally in the bases. List several nursing interventions to assist Mr. S.
2. In his third postoperative day Mr. S. has an erythematous incision with moderate amounts of purulent exudate from the Penrose drain site. List the correct nursing interventions.
3. What signs and symptoms would the nurse note when assessing Mr. S. for dehydration secondary to elevated temperature and decreased fluid intake?

as needed. An example of a goal and an evaluative measure is as follows:

Goal: Patient achieves physical comfort.

Evaluative measure: Observe patient for nonverbal signs of discomfort, such as guarding the painful area and grimacing. Also check that patient verbalizes decrease or elimination of pain based on pain scale assessment.

DISCHARGE: PROVIDING GENERAL INFORMATION

Preparation for the patient's discharge is an ongoing process throughout the surgical experience, beginning during the preoperative period. The informed patient therefore is prepared as events unfold and gradually assumes greater responsibility for self-care during the postoperative period. As discharge approaches, it is important that the patient be given certain vital information (Box 42.13). If the health care provider has not provided information about diet or activity restrictions, the nurse verifies this information with the health care provider before instructing the patient. Being careful to provide complete discharge instructions may prevent needless distress for the patient and prevent complications at home. Written instructions are important for reinforcing verbal information. The nurse must document specifically in the record the discharge instructions provided to the patient and family as well as any return demonstrations by the patient or caregivers that occur after discharge teaching. Documentation of information related to the patient's mental status (ability to understand importance of teaching for patient and family members) is necessary. For the patient, the postoperative phase of care continues into the recuperative period. Assessment and evaluation of the patient after discharge may involve a follow-up call or a visit from a home health nurse.

AMBULATORY SURGERY DISCHARGE

The patient leaving an ambulatory surgery setting must be able to provide a degree of self-care and must be mobile and alert. Postoperative pain and nausea and vomiting must be controlled. Overall, the patient must be stable and near the same level of functioning as before surgery. At discharge, the patient and family or responsible party are given specific and general instructions—verbally and reinforced with written directions. The patient may not drive and must be accompanied by a responsible adult at the time of discharge. Health care personnel often phone the patient to schedule a follow-up evaluation and to address any specific questions and concerns the day after discharge.

Box 42.13 Vital Information for the Patient Being Discharged

- Action and possible side effects of any medications; when and how to take them
- Activities allowed and prohibited; when various physical activities can be resumed safely (e.g., driving a car, returning to work, sexual intercourse, leisure activities)
- Answers to any individual questions or concerns (allow time for questions)
- Care of wound site and any dressings
- Dietary restrictions or modifications
- Symptoms to be reported (e.g., development of incisional tenderness or increased drainage, discomfort in other parts of the body)
- Where and when to return for follow-up care

Get Ready for the NCLEX® Examination!

Key Points

- The time before, during, and after surgery is the perioperative period. It is divided into preoperative, intraoperative, and postoperative phases.
- Perioperative nursing interventions take place before, during, and after surgery.
- The ability to tolerate surgery is influenced by nursing interventions, previous illness, and past surgeries.
- Older adult patients are at surgical risk from their declining physiologic status.
- All medications taken before surgery are discontinued automatically after surgery unless a physician reorders the medications, except for medications for long-term conditions such as phenytoin for seizure control.
- Family members are important in assisting patients with physical limitations and in providing emotional support during the postoperative recovery.
- Preoperative assessment of vital signs and physical findings provides an important baseline for comparing perioperative and postoperative assessment data.
- A patient's feelings about surgery can have a significant effect on relationships with nursing staff and the patient's ability to participate in care.
- Clinical problems of the surgical patient may require interventions during one or all phases of surgery.
- Informed consent should not be obtained if a patient is confused, unconscious, mentally incompetent, or under the influence of sedatives. Know agency policy.
- Structured preoperative teaching positively influences postoperative recovery.
- A routine preoperative checklist is a guide for final preparation of the patient before surgery.
- Nurses in the OR focus on protecting the patient from potential harm.

- Assessment of the postoperative patient centers on the body systems most likely to be affected by anesthesia, immobilization, and surgical trauma.
- Because a surgical patient's condition may change rapidly during immediate postoperative recovery, monitor the patient's status at least every 15 minutes.
- The PACU nurse reports to the nurse on the postoperative unit information pertaining to the patient's current physical status and risk for postoperative complications.
- From the time of admission, plan for the surgical patient's discharge.
- Discharge planning identifies home care measures to promote recovery that involve patient and family.
- Evaluation of all perioperative care is sometimes difficult, because the patient may be discharged from the nurse's care before the outcome is certain.

Additional Learning Resources

SG Go to your Study Guide for additional learning activities to help you master this chapter content.

evolve Be sure to visit the Evolve site at *http://evolve.elsevier.com/Cooper/foundationsadult/* for additional online resources.

Review Questions for the NCLEX® Examination

1. A patient is being discharged and the nurse is teaching the patient how to do daily dressing changes at home. What is the most important point to include in the teaching plan?
   1. Discussion of surgical asepsis
   2. Discussion of hand hygiene
   3. Instruction in sterilization
   4. Demonstration of gloving
2. To assist a patient in the prevention of postoperative pulmonary complications, what interventions will be most helpful preoperatively? *(Select all that apply.)*
   1. Ask the surgeon to prescribe IPPB treatment.
   2. Teach the patient to do leg exercises.
   3. Teach the patient how to properly use an incentive spirometer.
   4. Tell the patient that lack of an effective cough may result in the need for suctioning.
   5. Ask the patient to perform a return demonstration of controlled coughing.
3. A patient underwent surgery for lysis of adhesions. He is transferred from the PACU to his room on the surgical floor. During the immediate postoperative period on the surgical floor, how often should the nurse measure blood pressure, pulse, and respirations?
   1. Every 15 minutes
   2. Every 5 minutes
   3. Every 20 minutes
   4. Every 30 minutes
4. The nurse is assessing the bowel sounds of a patient who had a suprapubic prostatectomy 2 days ago. To confirm that no bowel sounds are present, the nurse would need to auscultate each quadrant for how long?
   1. 1 minute
   2. 3 minutes
   3. 10 minutes
   4. 15 minutes
5. A patient is recovering from a right lobectomy. The nurse is going to assist in splinting the patient's incision so that the patient can cough and breathe deeply. When should an intramuscular analgesic be administered to achieve the most therapeutic effect?
   1. After the procedure so the patient can rest
   2. 15 minutes before the procedure
   3. 1 hour before the procedure
   4. 30 minutes before the procedure
6. A patient reports being allergic to penicillin. Which question would elicit the most useful information?
   1. "When did the reaction occur?"
   2. "What infection did you have that required penicillin?"
   3. "What type of allergic reaction did you have?"
   4. "Did you notify your physician of the allergy?"
7. Which patient is at greatest risk for surgical and anesthetic complications?
   1. A 3-year-old patient scheduled for hernia repair
   2. An 80-year-old patient scheduled for exploratory laparotomy
   3. An 18-year-old patient scheduled for an appendectomy
   4. A 42-year-old patient scheduled for breast biopsy
8. An alert 75-year-old patient is to undergo elective surgery. Who must sign the operative permit?
   1. The patient
   2. The patient and the patient's spouse
   3. Either the patient or the patient's spouse
   4. The patient and the surgeon
9. What is the best nursing intervention to help a patient cope with fear of pain associated with surgery?
   1. Describe the degree of pain expected.
   2. Explain the availability of pain medication.
   3. Inform the patient of the frequency of pain medication.
   4. Divert the patient when talking about pain.
10. A patient tells the nurse that "using this tube thing [incentive spirometer] is a waste of time." Which statement by the nurse best explains the purpose of the incentive spirometer?
    1. "It helps by directly removing excess secretions from the lungs."
    2. "It increases pulmonary circulation."
    3. "It helps promote lung expansion and prevent pulmonary complications."
    4. "It helps stimulate the cough reflex and keeps your lungs working."

11. When a patient is prepared for surgery, which interventions are appropriate during the preoperative period? *(Select all that apply.)*
    1. Provide sips of water for a dry mouth.
    2. Remove the patient's makeup and nail polish.
    3. Remove the patient's gown before transport to the OR.
    4. Leave on all of the patient's jewelry.
    5. Teach the patient postoperative breathing and coughing exercises.
12. Which statement is accurate regarding a patient who receives general or regional anesthesia in an ambulatory surgery center?
    1. The patient will remain in the unit longer than a hospitalized patient.
    2. The patient is allowed to ambulate as soon as he or she is admitted to the recovery area.
    3. The patient's level of consciousness must be near the level of preoperative functioning before dismissal.
    4. The patient is immediately given liberal amounts of fluid to promote excretion of the anesthesia.
13. After abdominal surgery, a patient is suspected of having internal bleeding. Which finding is most indicative of this complication? *(Select all that apply.)*
    1. Increased blood pressure
    2. Incisional pain
    3. Increased abdominal distention
    4. Increased urinary output
    5. Increased respirations
14. An obese patient is at risk for poor wound healing postoperatively for what reasons? *(Select all that apply.)*
    1. Ventilation capacity is reduced.
    2. Fatty tissue has a poor blood supply.
    3. The risk for dehiscence is increased.
    4. Clotting factors are delayed.
    5. Thrombophlebitis risk is increased.
15. A patient asks the nurse why the nurse asked for the name and dosage of all prescription and over-the-counter medications (including herbal remedies) taken before surgery. Which response by the nurse is most accurate?
    1. "These medications may cause allergies to develop."
    2. "These medications are automatically ordered postoperatively."
    3. "These medications should be taken the morning of surgery with sips of water."
    4. "These medications may create a greater risk for complications or interact with anesthetic agents."
16. The nurse is correct when identifying a patient who smokes two packs of cigarettes per day as being at most risk for which postoperative complication?
    1. Infection
    2. Pneumonia
    3. Hypotension
    4. Cardiac dysrhythmias
17. A postoperative abdominal surgery patient complains that he "felt something give way" in his incision. On assessing the wound, the nurse notes a large amount of serosanguineous drainage and that wound edges are not approximated. Intestines are protruding from the wound. What nursing action is appropriate?
    1. Encourage the patient to turn, cough, and deep-breathe while splinting the opening.
    2. Cover the protruding internal organs with sterile gauze moistened with normal saline.
    3. Paint the open wound with an antimicrobial solution to prevent infection.
    4. Reinsert the organs and apply a pressure dressing to prevent further organ protrusion.
18. On admission of a patient to the PACU from surgery, on what should the nurse place the highest priority for assessment?
    1. Patient's level of consciousness
    2. Condition of the surgical site
    3. Adequacy of airway and breathing
    4. Fluid and electrolyte balance
19. The nurse is admitting a patient into the room on the surgical unit after abdominal surgery. There is a 1.5-cm–diameter spot of serosanguineous drainage on the dressing. What should the nurse do at this time?
    1. Notify the physician of bleeding from the wound.
    2. Note the amount of drainage and continue to monitor.
    3. Remove the dressing to check for bleeding from the suture line.
    4. Apply gentle pressure to the site for 5 minutes.

43 Care of the Patient With an Integumentary Disorder

http://evolve.elsevier.com/Cooper/foundationsadult/

Objectives

Anatomy and Physiology

1. Discuss the primary functions of the integumentary system.
2. Describe the differences between the epidermis and dermis.
3. Discuss the functions of the three major glands located in the skin.

Medical-Surgical

4. Discuss the general assessment of the skin.
5. Discuss the viral disorders of the skin.
6. Discuss the bacterial, fungal, and inflammatory disorders of the skin.
7. Identify common parasitic disorders of the skin.
8. Describe the common tumors of the skin.
9. Identify the disorders associated with the appendages of the skin.
10. State the pathophysiology involved in a burn injury.
11. Identify the methods used to classify the extent of a burn injury.
12. Discuss the stages of burn care with appropriate nursing interventions.
13. Discuss how to use the nursing process in caring for patients with skin disorders.
14. Identify general nursing interventions for the patient with a skin disorder.

Key Terms

alopecia (ăl-ō-PĒ-shē-ă, p. 1312)
autograft (ĂW-tō-grăft, p. 1319)
contractures (kŏn-TRĂK-chŭrz, p. 1317)
Curling's ulcer (KŬR-lĭngz ŬL-sĕr, p. 1317)
débridement (dă-BRĒD-mĕnt, p. 1318)
eschar (ĔS-kăr, p. 1318)
excoriation (ĕks-kŏr-ē-Ā-shŭn, p. 1291)
exudate (ĔKS-ū-dāt, p. 1286)
heterograft (xenograft) (HĔT-ĕr-ō-grăft; ZĒ-nō-grăft, p. 1319)
homograft (allograft) (HŌ-mō-grăft; ĂL-ō-grăft, p. 1319)
keloids (KĒ-loydz, p. 1309)
macules (MĂK-ūlz, p. 1294)
nevi (NĒ-vī, p. 1310)
papules (PĂP-ūlz, p. 1298)
pediculosis (pĕ-dĭk-ū-LŌ-sĭs, p. 1306)
pruritus (prū-RĪ-tŭs, p. 1279)
pustulant vesicles (PŬS-tū-lănt VĔS-ĭ-kŭlz, p. 1294)
rule of nines (p. 1314)
suppuration (sūp-ū-RĀ-shŭn, p. 1296)
urticaria (ŭr-tĭ-KĂ-rē-ă, p. 1300)
verruca (vĕ-RŪ-kă, p. 1310)
vesicle (VĔS-ĭ-kl, p. 1286)
wheals (wēlz, p. 1300)

The skin, or *integument,* is a major organ and the outer covering of the body making it essential to life. Together with its appendages—hair, nails, and special glands—it makes up the integumentary system. People spend a great deal of time and money on grooming hair, cleansing skin, applying cosmetics, and manicuring nails. However, beyond its value in appearance, the integument is the body's protector, its first line of defense against infection and injury.

ANATOMY AND PHYSIOLOGY OF THE SKIN

FUNCTIONS OF THE SKIN

By covering the body, the skin protects the internal organs. It works to maintain homeostasis by monitoring and adapting to changes in temperature and environmental conditions. The skin is subjected continuously to temperature variances, humidity, environmental changes, and risk for exposure to pathogens, trauma, ecchymosis (bruising), and daily wear and tear. The skin carries out numerous functions to protect and maintain the body (Box 43.1).

Protection

Sensory receptors within the skin receive information about the environment. Messages about heat, cold, pressure, and touch are received and relayed to the central nervous system for interpretation. Healthy skin protects the body from absorbing many chemicals and foreign substances. In addition, as long as it remains intact, skin provides a barrier to many microorganisms in the environment. Internal organs are cushioned and protected by a subcutaneous layer of fat (adipose tissue). The skin aids in elimination of waste products, prevents dehydration, and serves as a reservoir for food and water. Keratin, a fibrous water-repellent protein found in skin, is tough and protects the skin from excessive fluid loss. It also helps the skin resist injury and prevents the entry of harmful substances. Melanin, another skin protein, forms a protective shield that guards the keratinocytes and nerve endings from ultraviolet light.

Temperature Regulation

Skin helps the body maintain a constant temperature under varying internal and external conditions. It allows blood vessels near the surface to constrict when the environment is cold to preserve heat and allows them to dilate when it is hot to release excess body heat. Sweat glands release moisture, which cools the body as it evaporates. A layer of adipose tissue insulates by retaining heat.

Box 43.1 Functions of the Skin

- Aids in excretion of waste products
- Has nerve endings that provide the brain with sensory information related to pain, heat and cold, touch, pressure, and vibration
- Insulates body and protects from trauma through subcutaneous layer of fat
- Prevents excessive water loss (dehydration)
- Protects from pathogenic organisms and foreign substances; provides a natural barrier against infection
- Regulates temperature
- Synthesizes vitamin D

Vitamin D Synthesis

Cholesterol compounds in the skin are converted to vitamin D when bare skin is exposed to the sun's ultraviolet rays. Vitamin D is necessary for healthy bone development. Although exposure to the sun is important for vitamin D synthesis, prolonged exposure to the sun's rays, which include ultraviolet radiation, should be avoided because of the increased risk of developing skin cancer. Synthesis occurs with very limited periods of exposure. There is no universally established period of time recommended for exposure. Many factors, such as skin color, determine how much sunlight is needed. In addition to sunlight, our bodies rely on food sources for vitamin D.

STRUCTURE OF THE SKIN

Skin consists of two primary layers: the outermost layer, called the epidermis; and the innermost layer, called the dermis or corium. Beneath these layers of skin lies the subcutaneous layer, or superficial fascia (Fig. 43.1).

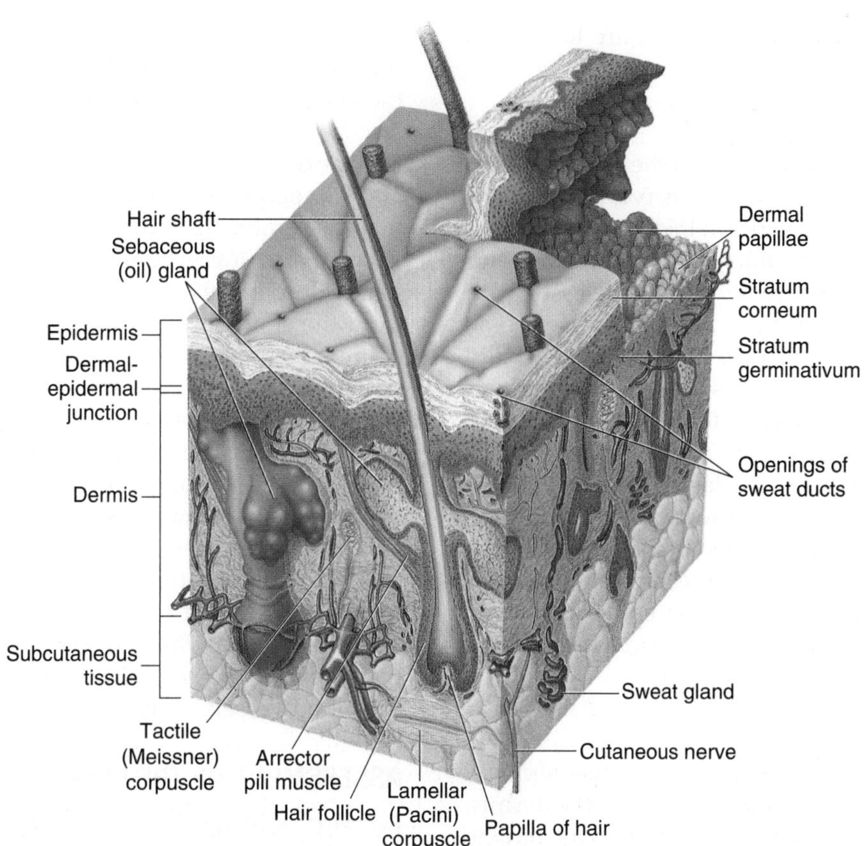

Fig. 43.1 Structures of the skin. (From Patton KT, Thibodeau GA: *The human body in health and disease,* ed 7, St. Louis, 2018, Elsevier.)

Epidermis

The *epidermis,* the outermost layer of the skin, is composed of stratified squamous (from the Latin *squama,* meaning "scale") epithelium. The cells of the epidermis are packed tightly and have no distinct blood supply (i.e., avascular). The epidermis is divided into layers, or strata: an outer, dead, cornified portion and a deep, living, cellular portion. The inner layer is called the *stratum germinativum;* it is the only layer of the epidermis able to undergo cell division and reproduce. It receives its blood supply and nutrition from the underlying dermis through a process called *diffusion.* The stratum germinativum provides a constant new supply of cells for the upper layer and enables the skin to repair itself after injury. As these cells push their way to the surface, their internal structures are destroyed and the cells die. By the time they reach the outermost epidermal layer, called the *stratum corneum,* they are flat and the cell structure is filled with a protein called *keratin.* The keratin makes the cells dry, tough, and somewhat waterproof.

Another layer in the epidermis contains highly specialized cells called *melanocytes.* These cells give rise to the pigment *melanin,* a black or dark brown pigment occurring naturally in the hair, the skin, and the iris and choroid of the eye. Melanin is responsible for the skin's color. Higher concentrations of melanin result in darker skin tones. Sometimes irregular patches with greater concentrations of melanin occur, producing freckles. Melanin levels are determined genetically. Although skin color is inherited, exposure to the sun and other factors can influence skin color.

Dermis

The *dermis,* or *corium,* often is called the true skin. It is well supplied with blood vessels and nerves and contains glands and hair follicles. It varies in thickness throughout the body but tends to be thickest on the palms and soles. The dermis is composed of connective tissue with cells scattered among collagen and elastic fibers. The dermis receives strength from the collagen and flexibility from the elastic connective fibers. The cells throughout this layer are bathed in tissue fluid, called interstitial fluid. The skin wrinkles with the normal aging process, as the dermis loses some of its elastic connective fibers and the subcutaneous tissue directly beneath it loses some of its adipose tissue. Located in the upper portion of the dermis are small finger-like projections called *papillae* that project into the lower epidermal layer. Without the dermal papillae, the epidermal layer would be unable to survive.

Subcutaneous Layer

The subcutaneous layer, sometimes called the *superficial fascia,* is the layer of tissue directly beneath the dermis. The subcutaneous layer connects the skin to the muscle surface. This layer is composed of adipose tissue and loose connective tissue. It serves several important functions, including (1) storing water and fat, (2) insulating the body, (3) protecting the organs lying beneath it, and (4) providing a pathway for nerves and blood vessels. The distribution of subcutaneous tissue throughout the body provides shape and contour. A woman's body usually contains more subcutaneous tissue than a man's; thus her body is softer and appears more rounded.

APPENDAGES OF THE SKIN

Sudoriferous Glands

The *sudoriferous* (sweat) *glands* are coiled, tubelike structures located in the dermal and subcutaneous layers. The tubes open into pores on the skin surface. Approximately 3 million sweat glands are located throughout the integumentary system. These glands excrete sweat, which cools the body's surface. Sweat is composed of water, salts, urea, uric acid, ammonia, sugar, lactic acid, and ascorbic acid.

Ceruminous Glands

Ceruminous glands are modified sudoriferous glands. They secrete a waxlike substance called *cerumen* and are located in the external ear canal. Cerumen is thought to protect the canal from foreign body invasion. However, too much cerumen, causing impaction in the ear canal, can cause difficulty with hearing and can make the ear canal a breeding ground for infection.

Sebaceous Glands

The *sebaceous* (oil) *glands* secrete *sebum* (an oily secretion) through the hair follicles distributed on the body. Their function is to lubricate the skin and hair that covers the body. Sebum also inhibits bacterial growth.

Hair and Nails

Hair is composed of modified dead epidermal tissue, mainly keratin. It is distributed all over the body in varying amounts. The root of the hair is enclosed in a follicle deep in the dermis. The shaft of the hair protrudes from the skin. Surrounding the hair follicle is a band of muscle tissue called *arrector pili* (see Fig. 43.1). A sensation of cold or fear causes these muscles to contract, making the hair stand upright and dimpling the skin surrounding it. The effect is called piloerection, "gooseflesh," or "goosebumps."

Nails also are composed mainly of keratin, but the keratin is more compressed. The base of the nail, the root, is made up of living cells and is covered mostly by the cuticle. Part of the root, the lunula, is exposed and looks like a white crescent. The remainder of the nail is called the *nail body.* It appears pink because of the blood vessels lying immediately beneath it.

ASSESSMENT OF THE SKIN

INSPECTION AND PALPATION

A thorough assessment of the skin helps identify many diseases. Skin assessment provides information about conditions taking place in other body systems.

Begin the assessment by obtaining a careful health history from the patient. Ask the patient about (1) recent skin lesions or rashes, (2) where the lesions first appeared, and (3) how long the lesions have been present. Also ask questions about personal and family history. Inquire about conditions such as asthma, seasonal rhinitis, or allergies. Explore all complaints of pain, **pruritus** (the symptom of itching), tingling, or burning. Ask the patient about personal skin care and about (1) any recent skin color changes; (2) exposure to the sun, with or without sunscreen; and (3) family history of skin cancer.

Assess the skin under natural lighting, and use the senses of sight, touch, and smell while inspecting and palpating the skin. Expose the area to be assessed while maintaining privacy. Remember to wear gloves when inspecting the skin, mucous membranes, and any other involved area. In the hospital, the morning bath provides an excellent opportunity to assess the patient's skin without exposure or embarrassment.

Observe the color of the skin. The color depends on many physiologic factors, including the following:

- Amount of hemoglobin in the blood
- Amount of melanin in the epidermis
- Amount of substances such as bilirubin, urea, or other chemicals in the blood
- Oxygen saturation of the blood
- Quality and quantity of blood circulating in the superficial blood vessels

Skin lesion assessment includes a description of the appearance (size, shape, color), degree of moisture present, drainage, and location. Details assist the health care provider in determining the diagnosis and help the nurse to provide care. Disorders of the integument are characterized by the type of lesion involved. Most disorders have only one or two types of lesion. Some of the typical clinical manifestations of skin disorders are shown in Table 43.1.

Text continued on p. 1284

Table 43.1 Primary Skin Lesions

DESCRIPTION	EXAMPLES		
Macule			
Flat, circumscribed area that is changed in color; <1 cm in diameter	Freckles, flat moles (nevi), petechiae, measles, scarlet fever		Measles[a]
Papule			
Elevated, firm, circumscribed area; <1 cm in diameter	Warts (verrucae), elevated moles, lichen planus		Lichen planus[b]
Patch			
Flat, nonpalpable, irregularly shaped macule; >1 cm in diameter	Vitiligo, port-wine stains, mongolian spots, café-au-lait spots		Vitiligo[b]

Continued

Table 43.1 Primary Skin Lesions—cont'd

DESCRIPTION	EXAMPLES		
Plaque			
Elevated, firm, rough lesion with flat-topped surface; >1 cm in diameter	Psoriasis, seborrheic keratosis, actinic keratosis	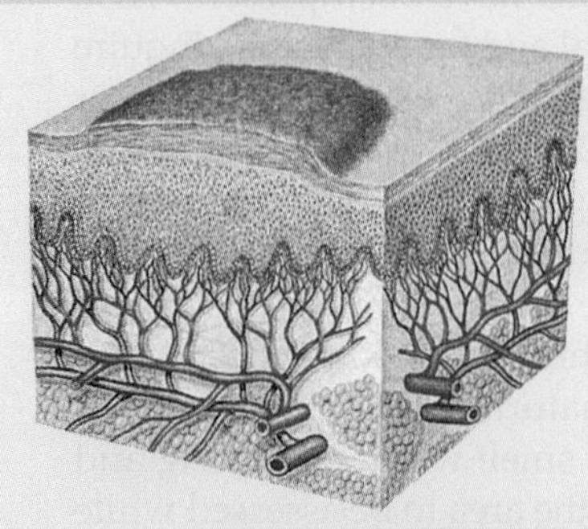	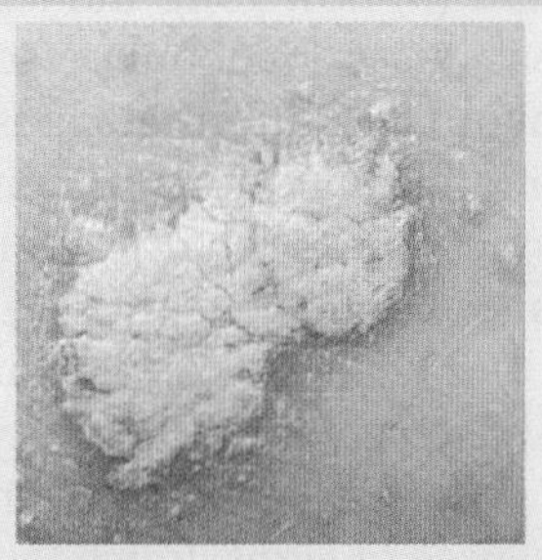 Plaque[a]
Wheal			
Elevated, irregularly shaped area of cutaneous edema; solid, transient; variable diameter	Insect bites, urticaria, allergic reaction	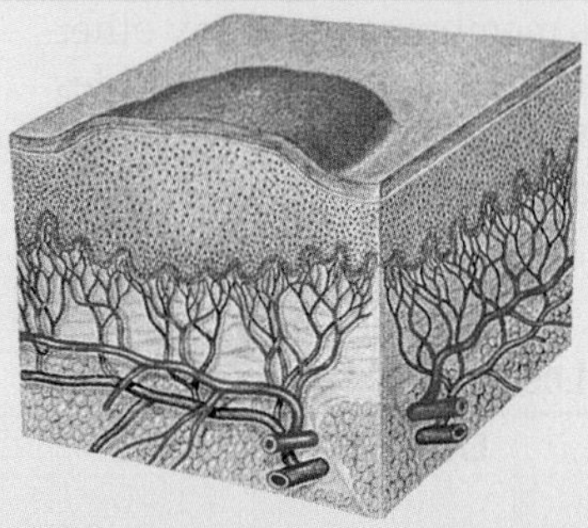	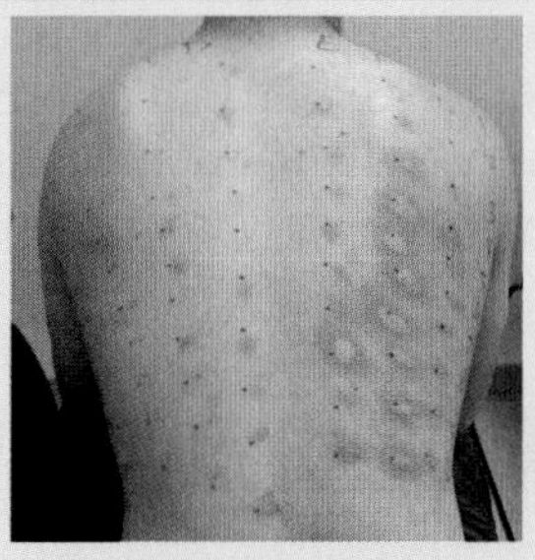 Wheal
Nodule			
Elevated, firm, circumscribed lesion; deeper in dermis than a papule; 1–2 cm in diameter	Erythema nodosum, lipomas	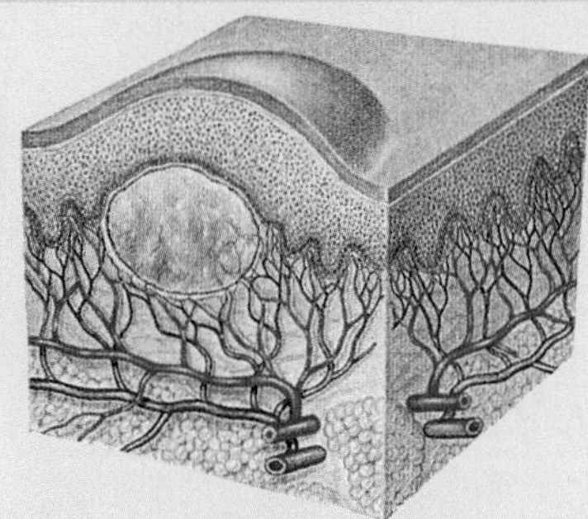	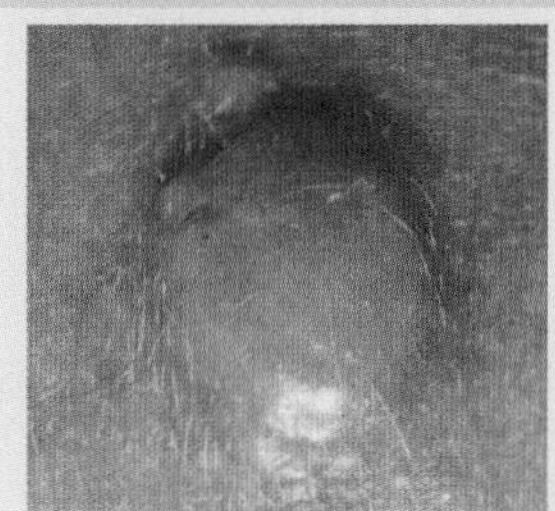 Hypertrophic nodule[a]
Tumor			
Elevated and solid lesion; may or may not be clearly demarcated; deeper in dermis; >2 cm in diameter	Neoplasms, benign tumor, lipoma, hemangioma	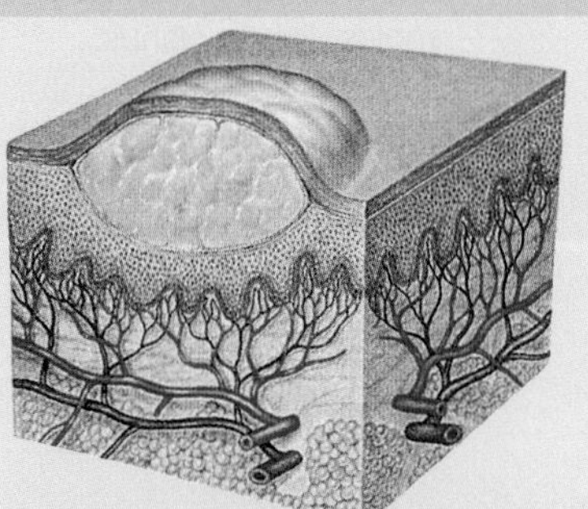	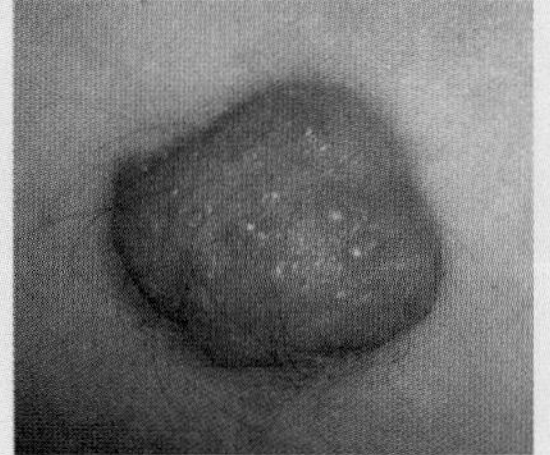 Hemangioma[b]
Vesicle			
Elevated, circumscribed, superficial, not into dermis; filled with serous fluid; <1 cm in diameter	Varicella (chickenpox), herpes zoster (shingles)	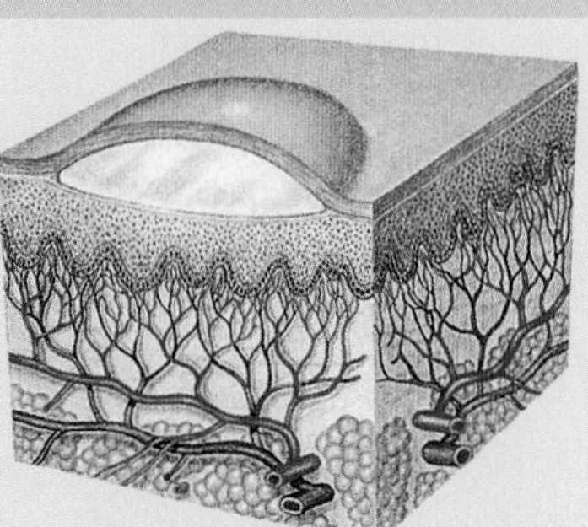	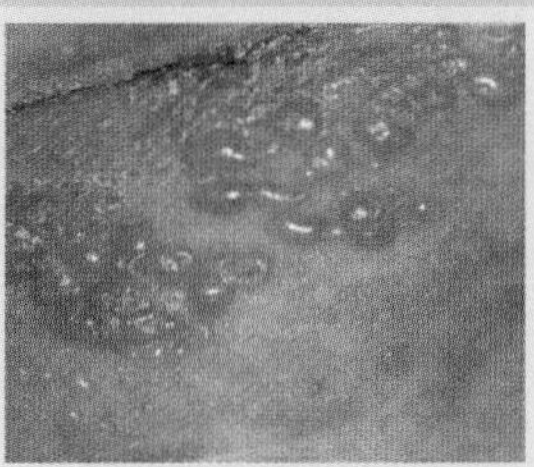 Vesicles caused by varicella[b]

Table 43.1 Primary Skin Lesions—cont'd

DESCRIPTION	EXAMPLES	
Bulla		
Vesicle >1 cm in diameter	Blister, pemphigus vulgaris	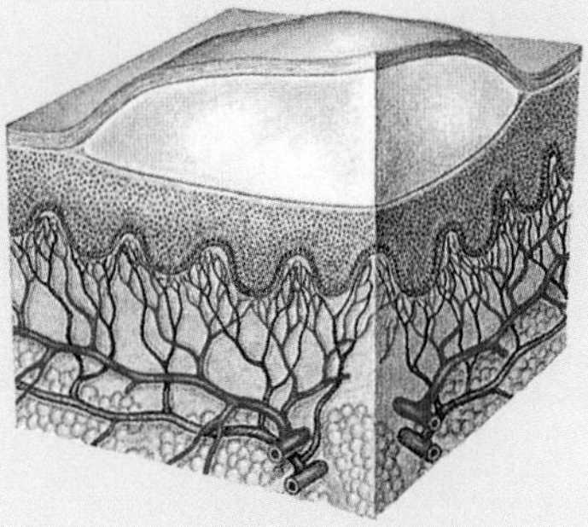 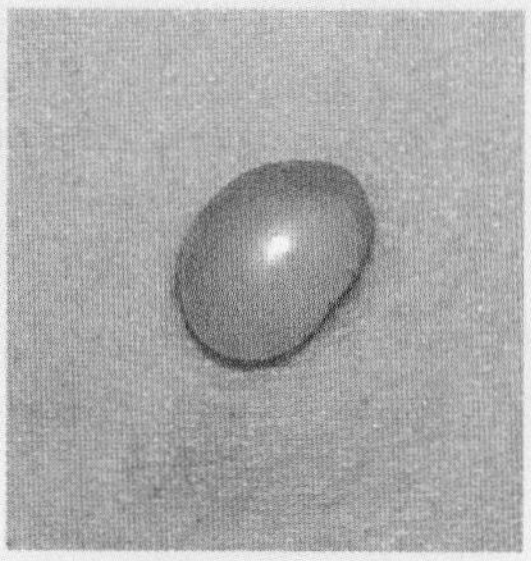 Blister[d]
Pustule		
Elevated, superficial lesion; similar to a vesicle but filled with purulent fluid	Impetigo, acne	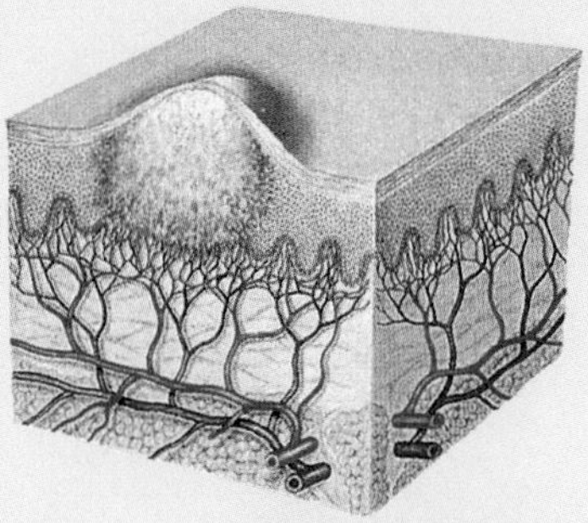 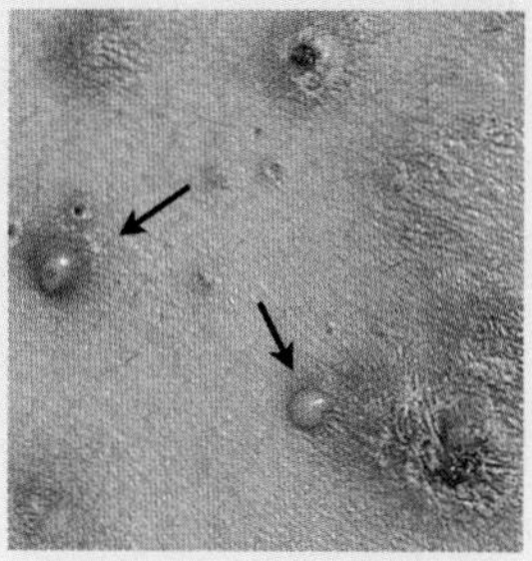 Acne[b]
Cyst		
Elevated, circumscribed, encapsulated lesion; in dermis or subcutaneous layer; filled with liquid or semisolid material	Sebaceous cyst, cystic acne	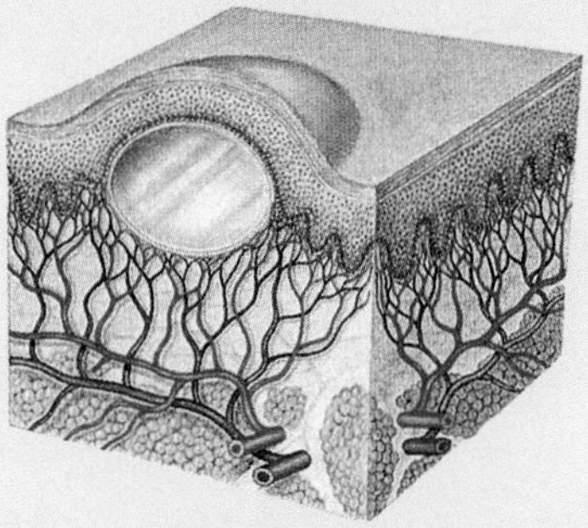 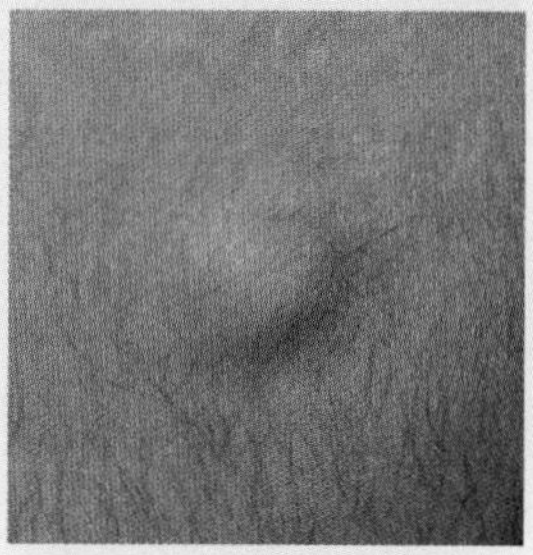 Sebaceous cyst[b]
Telangiectasia		
Fine, irregular red lines produced by capillary dilation	Telangiectasia in rosacea	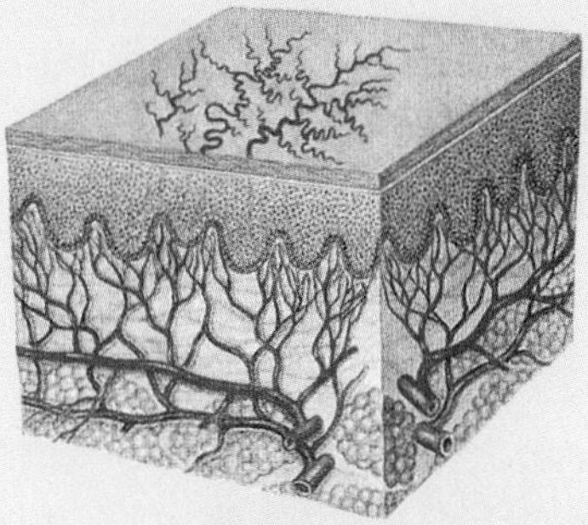 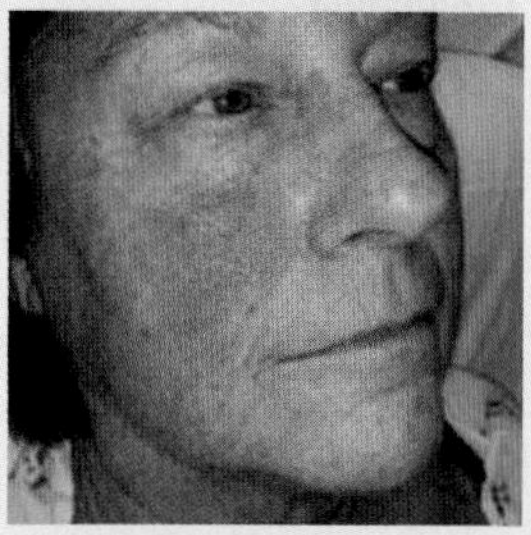 Rosacea
Scale		
Heaped-up keratinized cells; flaky skin; irregular; thick or thin; dry or oily; variation in size	Flaking of skin with seborrheic dermatitis after scarlet fever, or flaking of skin after a drug reaction; dry skin	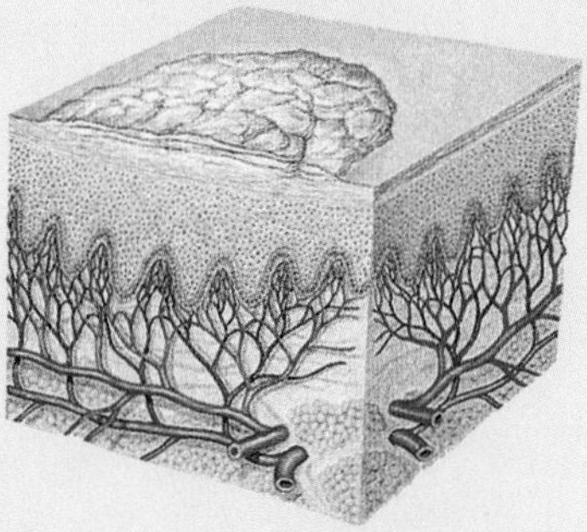 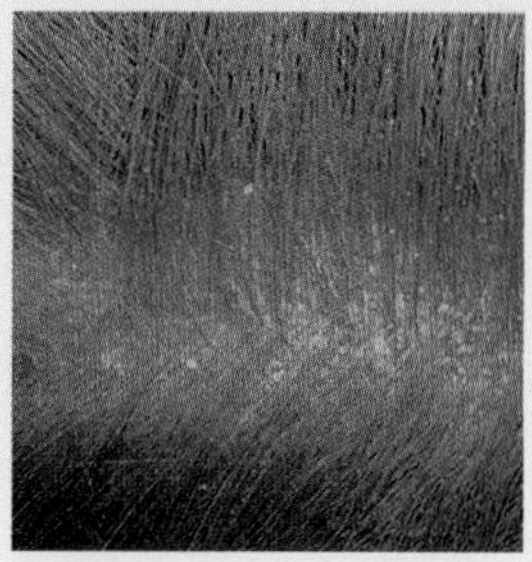 Fine scaling[c]

Continued

Table 43.1 Primary Skin Lesions—cont'd

DESCRIPTION	EXAMPLES		
Lichenification			
Rough, thickened epidermis secondary to persistent rubbing, itching, or skin irritation; often involves flexor surface of extremity	Chronic dermatitis	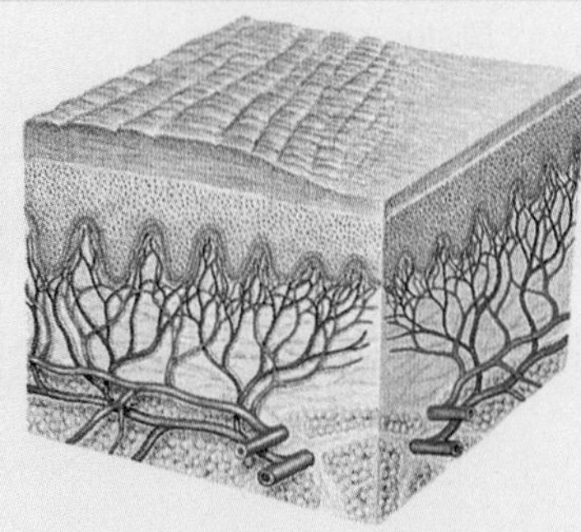	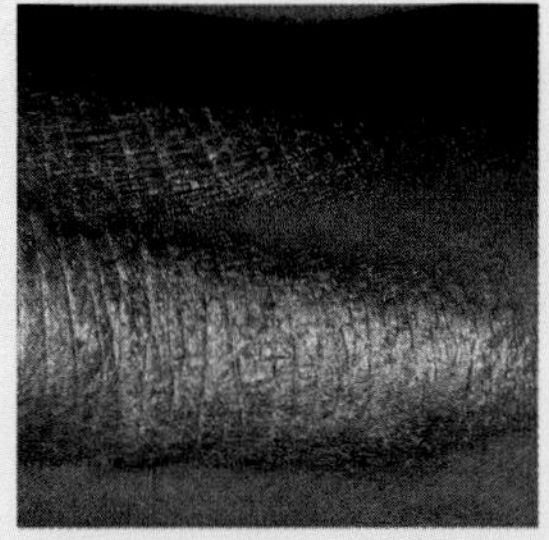 Stasis dermatitis in an early stage[b]
Keloid			
Irregularly shaped, elevated, progressively enlarging scar; grows beyond the boundaries of the wound; caused by excessive collagen formation during healing	Keloid formation after surgery	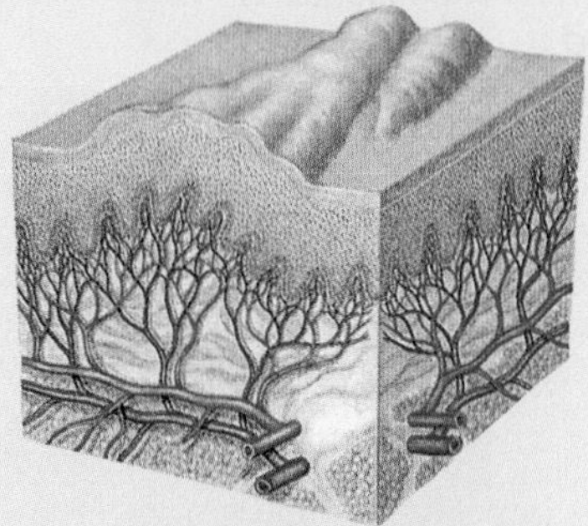	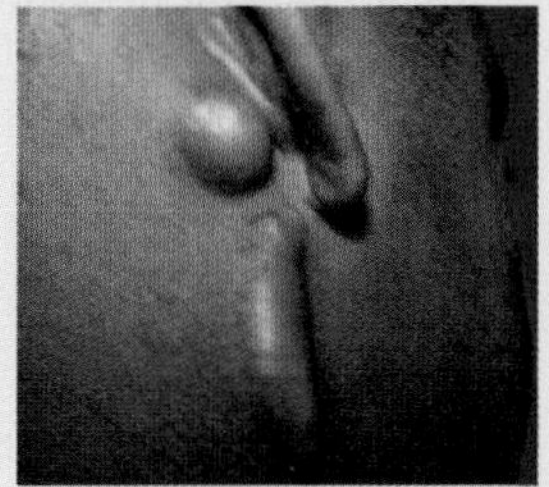 Keloid[b]
Scar			
Thin to thick fibrous tissue that replaces normal skin after injury or laceration to the dermis	Healed wound or surgical incision	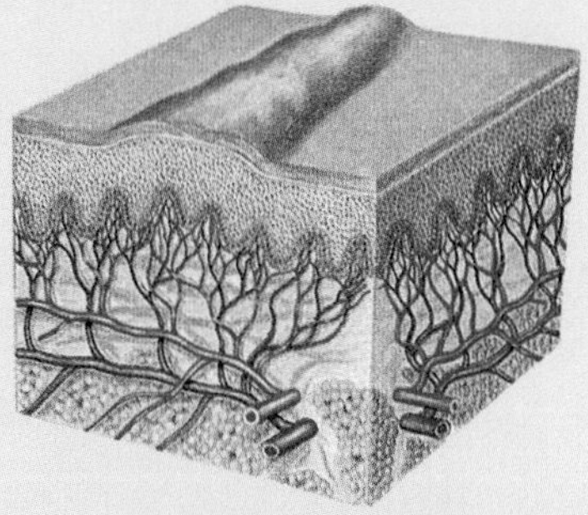	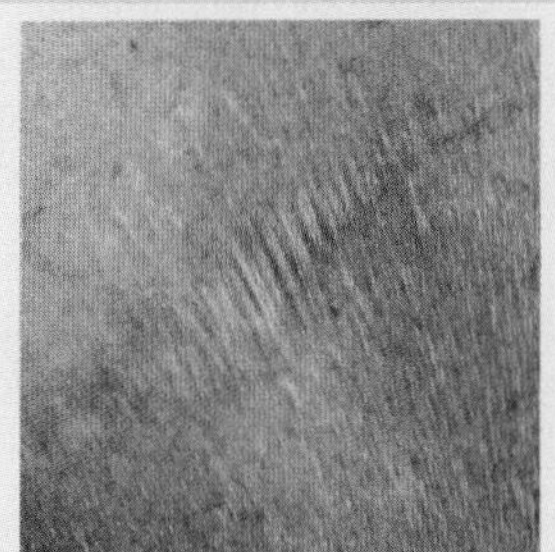 Incisional scar
Excoriation			
Loss of the epidermis; linear hollowed-out crusted area	Abrasion or scratch, scabies	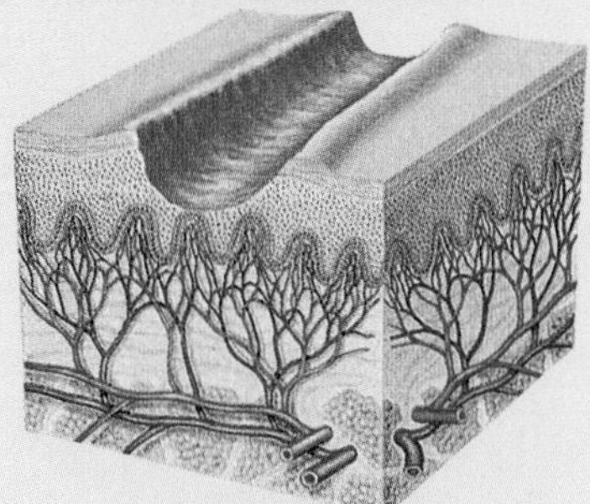	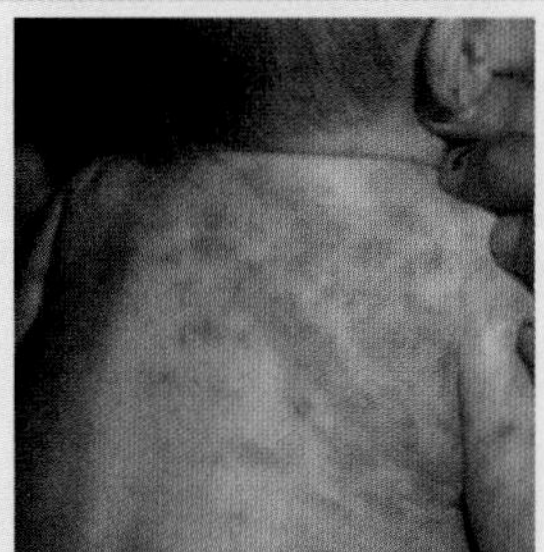 Scabies[b]
Fissure			
Linear crack or break from the epidermis to the dermis; may be moist or dry	Athlete's foot, cracks at the corner of the mouth	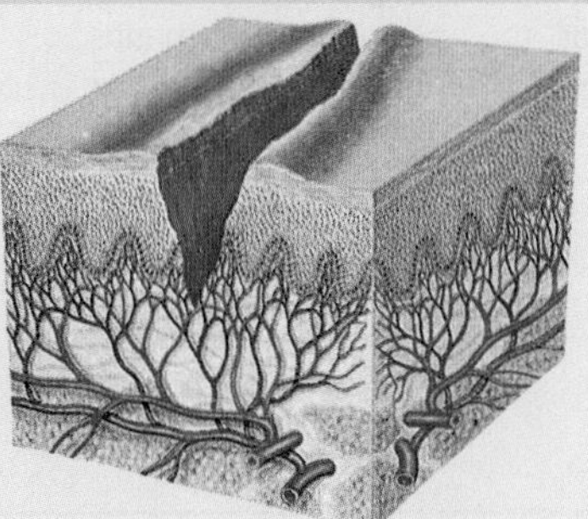	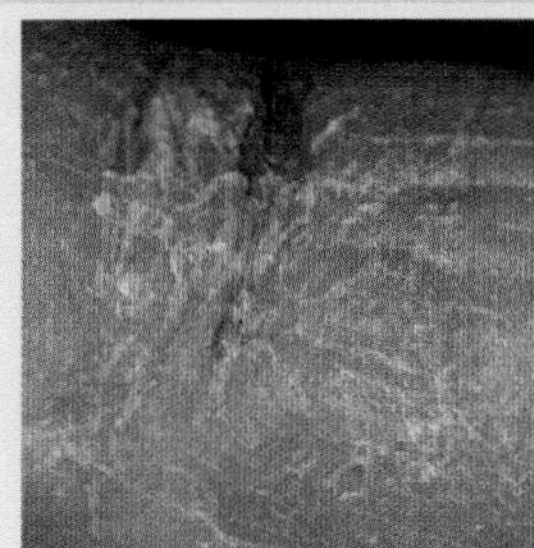 Fissures[b]

Table 43.1 Primary Skin Lesions—cont'd

DESCRIPTION	EXAMPLES
Erosion	
Loss of part of the epidermis; depressed, moist, glistening; follows rupture of a vesicle or bulla	Varicella, variola after rupture
	Erosion[d]
Ulcer	
Loss of epidermis and dermis; concave; varies in size	Pressure sores, stasis ulcers
	Stasis ulcer
Crust	
Dried serum, blood, or purulent exudate; slightly elevated; size varies: brown, red, black, or tan	Scab on abrasion, eczema
	Scab[b]
Atrophy	
Thinning of skin surface and loss of skin markings; skin translucent and paper-like	Striae; aged skin
	Aged skin

[a]Zitelli BJ, McIntire SC, Nowalk AJ: *Zitelli and Davis' atlas of pediatric physical diagnosis,* ed 6, St. Louis, 2012, Saunders.
[b]Weston WL, Lane AT, Morelli JG: *Color textbook of pediatric dermatology,* ed 4, St. Louis, 2007, Mosby.
[c]Baran R, Dawber RPR, Levene GM: *Color atlas of the hair, scalp, and nails,* St. Louis, 1991, Mosby.
[d]Potter PA, Perry AG: *Fundamentals of nursing,* ed 7, St. Louis, 2009, Mosby.
[e]Cohen BA: *Pediatric dermatology,* London, 1993, Wolfe.
Modified from Thompson J, Wilson S: *Health assessment for nursing practice,* St. Louis, 1995, Mosby.

Assessment also includes noting the presence of rashes, scars, lesions, or ecchymoses and the distribution of hair. Assess temperature and texture by touch, using the palms of the hands to compare opposite body areas. For example, feel both legs before concluding that the left leg is cold. Use a cotton-tipped applicator to touch the sole of the foot and assess sensation. Inspect the nails for normal development, color, shape, and thickness. Clubbing (broadening) of the fingertips indicates decreased oxygenation (hypoxemia) and should be reported. Inspect the hair for thickness, dryness, or dullness. Assessment also includes inspecting the mucous membranes for pallor or cyanosis (blue discoloration). Document profuse sweating or any sign of impaired skin integrity. Examine the ceruminous and sebaceous glands for activity. Ask the patient to describe any occasions on which perspiration has been excessive or troubling as well as whether earwax has ever been removed by the health care provider.

A growing segment of the population has begun to embrace body art, such as piercing, tattoos, and carving/branding (used to facilitate the development of a keloid-type scar). Note the presence of any body art and its location. Allergic reactions to tattoo ink may occur years after application of the art.

The incidence of self-harm or self-injury (formerly known as self-mutilating) activities such as cutting, carving, or burning is increasing. The arms, legs, and anterior torso are the body areas most commonly affected. Persons who self-harm are most often female teens or young adults. Depression, personality disorders, or anxiety disorders may underlie such behavior. The presence of any injuries suspected as being self-inflicted must be documented (Mayo Clinic, 2017b).

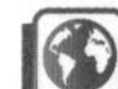 Cultural Considerations

Skin Care

- The darker a person's skin, the more difficult it is to assess for changes in color. Establish a baseline in natural lighting if possible or with (at least) a 60-watt light bulb.
- Assess baseline skin color in areas with the least pigmentation, such as palms of the hands, soles of the feet, underside of forearms, abdomen, and buttocks.
- All skin colors have an underlying red tone. Pallor in black-skinned individuals is seen as ashen or gray. Pallor in brown-skinned individuals appears as yellowish. Assess pallor in mucous membranes, lips, nailbeds, and conjunctivae (i.e., the inner surface of the lower eyelids).
- To assess rashes and skin inflammation in dark-skinned individuals, rely on palpation for warmth and induration (i.e., an abnormally hard spot) rather than observation.
- Some folk remedies may be misdiagnosed as injuries. Three folk practices of Southeast Asia can leave marks on the body that can be mistaken for signs of abuse or violence. *Cao gio* is the rubbing of the skin with a coin to produce dark blood or ecchymotic strips; it is done to treat a thrombus or symptoms of the flu. *Bat gio* is skin pinching on the temples to treat headaches or on the neck for a sore throat. The treatment is considered a success if petechiae or ecchymoses appear. *Moxibustion* refers to the burning of the skin with a stick containing dried herbs. It is believed the burning will cause the noxious element that causes the pain to leave the body.*

Assessment of Dark Skin

Skin color, which is determined genetically, depends on how much light is reflected when it strikes melanin, the underlying skin pigment. Melanin is produced by melanocytes deep in the epidermis. Melanocytes with increased activity, producing large amounts of melanin, account for darker skin colors. This increased melanin forms a natural sun shield, accounting for the lower incidence of skin cancer in people with dark skin.

The structures of dark skin are no different from those of lighter skin, but they are more difficult to assess due to their darker pigmentation. Practice is necessary. Assessment is easier in areas where the epidermis is thin, such as the lips and mucous membranes. Rashes are often difficult to observe and may have to be palpated.

Dark skin is predisposed to certain skin conditions, including pseudofolliculitis, keloids, and mongolian spots. Color cannot be used as an indicator of systemic conditions in darker-skinned individuals (e.g., flushed skin with fever) (see the Cultural Considerations box).

CHIEF COMPLAINT

When skin lesions accompanying a skin disorder are found, document the exact location, length, width, general appearance, and type. A helpful mnemonic for assessing the chief complaint is to remember *PQRST:*

P **P**rovocative and **P**alliative factors (factors that cause the condition)
Q **Q**uality and **Q**uantity (characteristics and size) of the skin problem
R **R**egion of the body
S **S**everity of the signs and symptoms
T **T**ime (length of time the patient has had the disorder)

An important objective in skin assessment is to identify possible malignancies. The three most common are melanoma, basal cell carcinoma, and squamous cell carcinoma. When assessing growths or changes in a mole, ask the following questions, using the mnemonic device *ABCDE:*

A Is the mole **A**symmetric?
B Are the **B**orders irregular?
C Is the **C**olor uneven or irregular?
D Has the **D**iameter of the growth changed recently?
E Has the surface area become **E**levated?

Promptly report a positive finding of any of these characteristics to a health care provider. After completing the assessment, document the findings. Proper assessment and identification serve as a baseline for evaluating nursing care and determining whether changes are needed.

PSYCHOSOCIAL ASSESSMENT

Integumentary disorders may be acute or chronic. Recovery may be lengthy with little visible outward improvement. A person's body image and self-esteem may be affected. Society's reaction to a skin condition has a significant effect on the patient. Personal appearance is a primary concern to many individuals. Others may think the condition is infectious and may isolate the patient socially. An integumentary disorder can have a negative effect on a patient's self-concept because of the value society places on a person's physical characteristics.

Assess the patient's coping abilities by using open-ended questions to encourage him or her to talk and ventilate feelings. Also assess the patient's interaction with family and others. Nonverbal behavior such as covering the involved area and avoiding eye contact may indicate a self-image problem. Validate or correct a patient's knowledge base. Be skilled and knowledgeable about skin care. Rarely are skin diseases fatal, and few are contagious. Work through your feelings about a patient's skin appearance before you can be a source of encouragement. Your attitude and interventions should be nonjudgmental, warm, and accepting.

A patient with a skin disorder may have a problem with anxiety. Decrease the patient's anxiety by implementing the following interventions:

- Provide the patient with consistent information related to his or her care plan.
- Include the family in the treatment plan. The family may be able to help the patient follow the instructions, which helps to decrease anxiety.
- Provide positive feedback concerning the patient's efforts and progress, no matter how large or small.
- Refer the patient to a support group as soon as possible (if appropriate).

PRESSURE INJURIES

The National Pressure Ulcer Advisory Panel (NPUAP) has announced that the term *pressure injury* will be used to replace the term *pressure ulcer* in the staging system. The NPUAP has determined that the term pressure injury more accurately describes injuries to intact and ulcerated skin, especially because previously stage 1 was referred to as a pressure injury and the remaining stages were referred to as ulcers. The numbering system also was changed at this time to Arabic numerals (NPUAP, 2016).

Skin breakdown can result from a variety of causes. Pressure injuries are responsible for many hospitalizations and health care–related expenses, in addition to the pain and suffering of patients. If a pressure injury is discovered, immediate action is required to ensure that the wound receives proper care and does not increase in size and develop additional complications.

The following sections summarize the revised stages of pressure injury development according to the NPUAP (2016). Additional information regarding pressure injuries can be found at *www.npuap.org*.

STAGE 1

A stage 1 pressure injury is a localized area of skin, typically over a bony prominence, that is intact with nonblanchable redness. Skin with darker tones may not have visible blanching, but its color is likely to differ from the surrounding area. The wound characteristics vary: areas may be painful, firm, soft, warm, or cool compared with adjacent tissue. This stage is typically difficult to detect in patients with dark skin tones.

STAGE 2

A stage 2 pressure injury involves partial-thickness loss of dermis. It appears as a shallow open injury, usually shiny or dry, with a red-pink wound bed without slough or bruising. (Bruising raises the suspicion of deep tissue injury.) Some stage 2 injuries manifest as intact or open (ruptured) serum-filled blisters. Do not use the term stage 2 to describe skin tears, tape burns, perineal dermatitis, maceration, or excoriation.

STAGE 3

A stage 3 pressure injury involves full-thickness tissue loss, in which subcutaneous fat is sometimes visible, but bone, tendon, and muscle are not exposed. If slough is present, it does not obscure the depth of tissue loss. Possible features are undermining and tunneling. The depth of a stage 3 pressure injury varies depending on its anatomic location. On the bridge of the nose, the ear, the occiput, and the malleolus, which lack subcutaneous tissue, these injuries are shallow. Extremely deep stage 3 pressure injuries develop in areas with significant layers of deep adipose tissue.

STAGE 4

A stage 4 pressure injury involves full-thickness tissue loss with exposed bone, tendon, cartilage, or muscle. Sometimes slough or eschar is present on some parts of the wound bed. The injury often includes undermining or tunneling. As with stage 3 pressure injuries, stage 4 pressure injuries vary in depth depending on their location. Because these injuries extend into muscle and supporting structures, the patient is at risk for osteomyelitis.

UNSTAGEABLE/UNCLASSIFIED

An unstageable pressure injury involves full-thickness tissue loss, a wound base covered by slough (yellow, tan, gray, green, or brown), and eschar in the wound bed that usually is tan, brown, or black. The true depth and stage of the injury cannot be determined until the base of the wound has been exposed. Stable eschar on the heels provides a natural biologic cover: do not remove it.

SUSPECTED DEEP TISSUE PRESSURE INJURY

During this stage, the wound appears as a localized purple or maroon area of discolored intact skin or a blood-filled blister. This is caused by underlying soft tissue damage from pressure or shear. Characteristics of the area range from painful, firm, mushy, boggy, or warm to cool compared with adjacent tissue. In patients with dark skin tones, deep tissue injury is sometimes difficult to detect but often starts with a thin blister over a dark wound bed. The wound sometimes becomes covered with thin eschar. Even with prompt treatment, some wounds evolve rapidly, exposing additional layers of tissue.

NURSING INTERVENTIONS

Nursing interventions for patients with pressure injuries include ongoing assessment and evaluation of improvement. Assessment data include the size and the depth of the injury, the amount and color of any exudate, the presence of pain or odor, and the color of the exposed tissue. Healing is a long-term process; therefore make sure the plan of care is consistent over time and evaluate it for effectiveness.

WOUND CARE

The skin serves as the body's first defense. Impairments in the integument provide a portal for infection. Management of wounds and the prevention of their development are essential for health maintenance. During wound care, the type and size of the wound primarily will determine the dressing and treatment plans (Table 43.2).

VIRAL DISORDERS OF THE SKIN

HERPES SIMPLEX

Etiology and Pathophysiology

Herpes simplex virus (HSV) causes cold sores and genital herpes. It is one of the most common skin infections. Genital herpes affects an estimated one in six adults between the ages of 14 and 49 years. Two types of the virus are known:

- Type 1 (HSV-1) is the most common. It causes cold sores, often referred to as *fever blisters,* and usually is associated with febrile conditions. The infection is generally self-limiting, that is, it usually clears up by itself, requiring no treatment.
- Type 2 (HSV-2) causes lesions in the genital area known as genital herpes (Centers for Disease Control and Prevention [CDC], 2018a). HSV-2 is also a member of the herpesvirus family, as is HSV-1, and is discussed in Chapter 52.

Both types of viruses may be transmitted by direct contact with any open lesion. The primary mode of transmission for type 2 is through sexual contact. Lesions appear 2 days to 2 weeks after exposure. The lesions are usually present for 2 to 3 weeks and are most painful during the first week. Complications may be severe if the disease spreads to other body areas. HSV-1 herpes simplex is associated with oral lesions, but it may manifest anywhere on the body, including the perineal and genital regions. Most commonly found in the genital region, HSV-2 may present in facial or other areas of the body. Herpes simplex may have severe consequences in pregnancy. Miscarriage and premature delivery have been linked to herpes simplex. Herpesvirus may be fatal to the newborn when transmitted during childbirth. Studies indicate that the transmission rate of herpesvirus from an infected mother to a newborn is high, approximately 30% to 50% among women who acquire genital herpes near the time of delivery. The transmission rate is much lower (<1%) in mothers who previously knew they were infected or those who were aware they contracted the infection during the first half of a pregnancy (CDC, 2015). Women who have active herpes lesions at the time of childbirth give birth by cesarean section.

Clinical Manifestations

HSV-1 is characterized by a **vesicle** (circumscribed elevation of skin filled with serous fluid; smaller than 0.5 cm) at the corner of the mouth, on the lips, or on the nose. It is commonly known as a *cold sore* (Fig. 43.2). At first the involved area is usually erythematous and edematous (i.e., red and swollen). The vesicle then appears, ulcerates, and encrusts. When the vesicle ruptures, it produces a burning pain. The patient experiences general malaise and fatigue. Cold sores typically occur after an acute illness or infection.

Type 2, genital herpes, produces various types of vesicles that rupture and encrust, causing ulcerations. The cervix is the most common site in women, and the penis is the most common area in men. Flulike symptoms occur 3 or 4 days after the vesicles erupt. Headache, fatigue, myalgia, fever, and anorexia are common. Patients experiencing severe outbreaks in the genital region may experience difficulty voiding. In general, the initial outbreak is the most severe.

Assessment

Assessment involves primarily inspection of the skin. Obtain a complete health history to support assessment data. *Subjective data* (symptoms described by the patient, but that cannot be measured) include complaints of fatigue along with pruritus and burning pain in the mouth for HSV-1 and in the genital area for HSV-2. Patients experiencing a genital herpes outbreak may report pain with urination.

Objective data for HSV-1 include an edematous, erythematous area on the face. The most common location is the lips, but it may spread to the eyes. In HSV-2, the labia, vulva, or penis appears edematous and erythematous. The vesicular lesions may rupture, developing a dried **exudate** (fluid, cells, or other substances that have been slowly exuded, or discharged, from cells or blood vessels through small pores or breaks in cell membranes). Lymph nodes may be tender and enlarged.

Table 43.2 Characteristics and Uses of Wound-Dressing Materials

CATEGORY	EXAMPLES	DESCRIPTION	APPLICATIONS
Alginate	AlgiSite, Comfeel, Curasorb, Kaltogel, Kaltostat, Sorbsan, Tegagel	Alginate dressings are made of seaweed extract containing guluronic and mannuronic acids, which provide tensile strength; and calcium and sodium alginates, which confer an absorptive capacity. Some can leave fibers in the wound if they are not thoroughly irrigated. These dressings are secured with secondary coverage.	These dressings are highly absorbent and useful for wounds with copious exudate. Alginate rope is particularly useful to pack exudative wound cavities or sinus tracts.
Debriding agents	Hypergel (hypertonic saline gel), Santyl (collagenase), Accuzyme (papain urea)	These products provide some chemical or enzymatic débridement.	Débriding agents are useful for necrotic wounds as an adjunct to surgical débridement.
Foam	Lyofoam, Spyrosorb, Allevyn	Polyurethane foam has absorptive capacity.	These dressings are useful for cleaning granulating wounds with minimal exudate.
Hydrocolloid	CombiDERM, Comfeel, DuoDerm CGF Extra Thin, Granuflex, Tegasorb	Hydrocolloid dressings are made of a microgranular suspension of natural or synthetic polymers, such as gelatin or pectin, in an adhesive matrix. The granules change from a semihydrated state to a gel as the wound exudate is absorbed.	Hydrocolloid dressings are useful for dry necrotic wounds, wounds with minimal exudate, and for clean granulating wounds.
Hydrofiber	AQUACEL, AQUACEL-Ag, Versiva	An absorptive textile fiber pad, hydrofiber is also available as a ribbon for packing of deep wounds. This material is covered with a secondary dressing. The hydrofiber combines with wound exudate to produce a hydrophilic gel. Aquacel-Ag contains 1.2% ionic silver that has strong antimicrobial properties against many organisms, including methicillin-resistant *Staphylococcus aureus* and vancomycin-resistant enterococci.	Hydrofiber dressings are absorbent and used for exudative wounds.
Hydrogel	Aquasorb, DuoDerm, IntraSite gel, GranuGEL, Normlgel, Nu-Gel, Purilon gel, K-Y jelly	Hydrogel dressings are water-based or glycerin-based semipermeable hydrophilic polymers; cooling properties may decrease wound pain. These gels can lose or absorb water depending on the state of hydration of the wound. They are secured with secondary covering.	These dressings are useful for dry, sloughy, necrotic wounds (eschar).
Low-adherence dressing	Mepore, Skintact, Release	Low-adherence dressings are made of various materials designed for easy removal without damaging the underlying skin.	These dressings are useful for acute minor wounds, such as skin tears, or as a final dressing for chronic wounds that have nearly healed.
Transparent film	OpSite, Skintact, Release, Tegaderm, Bioclusive	Transparent films are highly conformable acrylic adhesive films with no absorptive capacity and little hydrating ability. They may be vapor permeable or perforated.	These dressings are useful for clean, dry wounds with minimal exudate. They also are used to secure an underlying absorptive material, to protect high-friction areas and areas that are difficult to bandage (e.g., heels), and to secure intravenous catheters.

From Daley BJ: Drugs, diseases, & procedures: Wound care treatment and management. Retrieved from *http://emedicine.medscape.com/article/194018-treatment.*

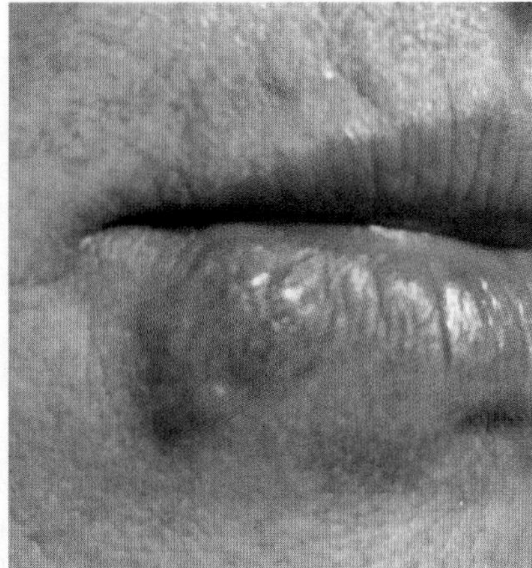

Fig. 43.2 Herpes simplex.

Diagnostic Tests

Diagnosis of herpesvirus is made by laboratory assessment of cultures from the lesion. Inspection and health history support the diagnosis. Patients also should be assessed for human immunodeficiency virus (HIV).

Medical Management

Herpesvirus infection has no cure. Lesions spontaneously resolve if there are no complications. Treatment focuses on symptom relief. For HSV-1 outbreaks, over-the-counter topical treatments often are effective if used within the first 1 to 2 days of the outbreak. Antiviral drugs such as acyclovir (Zovirax) administered orally, topically, or intravenously can shorten the outbreak and lessen its severity (Table 43.3). The initial outbreak often is treated for 7 to 10 days, and subsequent outbreaks are managed with a 5-day course of therapy. Oral acyclovir therapy can be continued safely and effectively for up to 5 years, but therapy should be interrupted after 1 year to assess the patient's rate of recurrent episodes. Adverse reactions to acyclovir are usually mild and include headache, occasional nausea and vomiting, and diarrhea. The safety of systemic acyclovir during pregnancy has not been established. Acyclovir ointment appears to be of no clinical benefit in treating recurrent lesions, either in speed of healing or in resolution of pain. Intravenous (IV) acyclovir is reserved for severe or life-threatening infections in which the patient is hospitalized for the treatment of CNS infections (meningitis) or pneumonitis. High-dose IV use can produce nephrotoxicity.

A patient with frequent outbreaks may be prescribed a daily suppressive therapy such as valacyclovir (Valtrex) (CDC, 2015). Patients who are immunosuppressed are not candidates for suppressive therapies. Acetaminophen (Tylenol) may be given for relief of discomfort. Pain may require a local anesthetic such as lidocaine (Xylocaine) or systemic analgesics such as codeine and aspirin. Nonsteroidal antiinflammatory drugs such as ibuprofen may be used to manage inflammation.

Nursing Interventions and Patient Teaching

Nursing interventions focus primarily on treating symptoms and preventing spread of the disease. Lesions should be kept clean and dry. Loose, absorbent underclothing is usually more comfortable than tight-fitting clothing. Sitz baths decrease lesion discomfort and enhance urinary and bowel elimination. The patient can use warm compresses to relieve pain and severe pruritus. The specific patient problems related to herpes infection are based on the assessment data gathered. Type 2 herpesvirus (HSV-2; genital herpes) may be transmitted by viral shedding even during periods of remission. Frank discussions concerning safe sexual practices, including condoms, are indicated. Infection control and hand washing should be discussed. Management of recurrent outbreaks should be reviewed.

Problem identification and interventions for the patient with herpes include but are not limited to the following:

Patient Problem	Nursing Interventions
Recent Onset of Pain, related to pruritus	Assess factors that precipitate pruritus Apply local anesthetic Apply drying agent to lesions Apply warm compresses Have patient wear loose-fitting, cotton clothing that does not constrict movement or occlude circulation
Compromised Skin Integrity, related to open lesions	Inspect lesions for drainage, color, and location Wash hands before and after contact Keep area dry Administer antiviral agents as ordered In genital herpes, a hair dryer can be used to dry the lesions and promote patient comfort
Potential for Infection, related to skin excoriation	Use standard precautions Teach patient proper skin care Wash hands before and after care Keep area dry Administer antiviral drugs as prescribed

Preventing infection is the priority when caring for a patient with an open skin lesion. Patient teaching focuses on the principles of medical asepsis and includes specific measures to prevent spread of the disease. Using good hygiene in all areas of care is critical to prevent secondary infections. Include the complications and precipitating factors in patient teaching and discharge planning.

Prognosis

Herpes simplex has no cure. The healing time for an HSV-1 infection is 10 to 14 days without treatment. HSV-2 lesions are usually present for 7 to 14 days. After outbreaks the virus goes dormant. Unfortunately, 75% of all patients have at least one recurrence, and two thirds have one to five recurrences annually. However,

Table 43.3 Medications for the Integumentary System

GENERIC NAME (TRADE NAME)	ACTION	SIDE EFFECTS	NURSING IMPLICATIONS
acyclovir (Zovirax)	Antiviral	*Topical:* Burning, rash, pruritus, stinging *Systemic:* Headache, seizures, renal toxicity, phlebitis at IV site	*Topical:* Use gloves to apply; cover lesion completely. *Systemic:* Ensure adequate hydration to prevent crystallization in kidneys; administer IV dose for at least 1 h.
Alpha Keri	Emollient	Local irritation, allergic reactions	For external use only; exercise caution when using in tub to avoid slipping.
Aluminum acetate solution (Burow's solution)	Astringent	Local irritation, allergic reactions	For external use only; do not use with occlusive dressings.
Antihistamines, including: diphenhydramine (Benadryl) hydroxyzine (Vistaril)	Blocks histamine at H_1 receptor site, inhibiting many allergic reactions	Drowsiness, dizziness, confusion, dry mouth, urinary retention	If drowsiness occurs, avoid activities that require concentration; avoid using with alcohol or other CNS depressants.
Benzoyl peroxide	Antiacne agent	Excessive drying of skin, allergic reactions	Discontinue use if excessive drying or peeling occurs; avoid contact with hair or fabric.
Calamine lotion	Astringent	Local irritation	For external use only.
chlorhexidine gluconate (Hibiclens)	Antimicrobial skin cleanser	Irritation, dermatitis, allergic reactions	For external use only; do not use on broken skin unless directed by a health care provider.
Coal tar (Estar gel, PsoriGel, others)	Treatment of pruritic dermatoses, including eczema and psoriasis	Photosensitivity, dermatitis, allergic reactions	Avoid exposure to sunlight for 72 h after use; may stain clothes and bathtub; for external use only.
Corticosteroids (topical), including: fluocinonide (Lidex) triamcinolone (Kenalog) betamethasone	Antiinflammatory agent	Local irritation, maceration, superinfection, atrophy, itching, and drying of skin (more severe local reactions and systemic effects possible with higher doses and potency or when used with occlusive dressings)	Do not use occlusive dressings unless directed by a health care provider; washing or soaking area before application increases drug penetration.
crotamiton (Eurax)	Scabicidal and antipruritic	Local irritation, allergic reactions	For external use only; do not apply to severely irritated skin.
Curel, Eucerin, Lubriderm	Emollient	Local irritation, allergic reactions	For external use only.
fluconazole (Diflucan)	Antifungal	Headache, nausea, vomiting, diarrhea	May elevate liver function test results; monitor BUN, creatinine.
griseofulvin	Antifungal agent	Hypersensitivity reactions, photosensitivity, nausea, fatigue, mental confusion	Avoid exposure to sunlight; drug absorption increased when given with meals; clinical response may appear only after full course of therapy.
isotretinoin	Antiacne agent	Severe dryness of skin, mouth, eyes, mucous membranes, nose, and nails; skin fragility; epistaxis; joint and muscle pain; nausea; abdominal pain	Absolutely contraindicated in pregnant women or women contemplating pregnancy; women of childbearing age must practice contraception during therapy and 1 mo before and after therapy; give drug with meals; do not give vitamin supplements containing vitamin A; avoid exposure to sunlight.

Continued

Table 43.3 Medications for the Integumentary System—cont'd

GENERIC NAME (TRADE NAME)	ACTION	SIDE EFFECTS	NURSING IMPLICATIONS
itraconazole (Sporanox)	Antifungal agent	Hypertension, headache, nausea, anorexia	Give with food; check hepatic function; can increase PT.
lindane	Scabicide, ovicide	Local irritation, dizziness, seizures (rare)	For external use only; avoid applying to open skin lesions.
Lubriderm	Emollient	Local irritation, allergic reactions	For external use only; exercise caution when using in tub to avoid slipping.
methoxsalen (Oxsoralen-Ultra)	Skin-pigmenting agent	Severe photosensitivity, nausea, nervousness, insomnia, headache, hypopigmentation	Avoid all exposure to sunlight for 8 h after oral ingestion and for several days after topical application; wear UVA-absorbing sunglasses for 24 h after oral ingestion; use sunscreen to prevent exposure to sunlight; give agent with food or milk or in divided doses; clinical response may not appear for several months.
povidone-iodine (Betadine)	Topical antimicrobial agent	Local irritation	For external use only; may stain skin and clothing.
pyrethrin (RID, others)	Pediculicide	Local irritation	For external use only; do not use for infestations of eyebrows or eyelashes.
Salicylic acid	Keratolytic agent	Local irritation, erythema, scaling	For external use only; may damage clothing, plastic, wood, and other materials on contact.
terbinafine (Lamisil)	Antifungal agent	Pruritus, local burning, erythema	For external use only; do not use occlusive dressings unless directed by a health care provider.
tetracycline	Antibacterial agent	*Topical:* Stinging, burning, slight yellowing of skin may occur *Systemic:* Nausea, diarrhea, photosensitivity	*Topical:* Avoid contact with sunlight *Systemic:* Give on empty stomach; avoid concomitant administration of dairy products, laxatives, antacids, and products containing iron; avoid contact with sunlight; may cause permanent tooth discoloration when used in children.
tolnaftate (Tinactin, Aftate, others)	Antifungal agent	Local irritation	For external use only.

BUN, Blood urea nitrogen; *CNS,* central nervous system; *IV,* intravenous; *PT,* prothrombin time; *UVA,* ultraviolet A.

the recurrences are sometimes milder and of shorter duration than the primary infection. Certain triggers can reactivate the virus, causing the patient to experience lesions. Triggers to an outbreak include fatigue, illness, emotional stress, and for HSV-2 lesions, genital irritation. Subsequent outbreaks are typically of shorter duration and less painful (NLM, 2012b).

HERPES ZOSTER (SHINGLES)

Etiology and Pathophysiology

Herpes zoster, commonly known as *shingles,* and chickenpox (varicella) are caused by the same virus: varicella-zoster virus (sometimes called human herpesvirus type 3). A person with shingles has a history of chickenpox infection. An estimated one in three people who have had chickenpox will also get shingles (CDC, 2018a). The varicella virus lies dormant until the person's resistance to infections becomes lowered. Risk factors for shingles include suppressed immunity, aging, infection, and stress. The virus causes an inflammation of the spinal ganglia and produces skin lesions of small vesicles along the peripheral nerve fibers of the spinal ganglia (Fig. 43.3). Sometimes the virus may affect a single nerve, such as the trigeminal nerve.

Clinical Manifestations

Eruption of the vesicles is preceded by pain. The rash generally occurs in the thoracic region but also may affect the lumbar, cervical, and cranial areas. Vesicles erupt in a line along the involved nerve. The vesicles rupture and form a crust, and the serous fluid in the

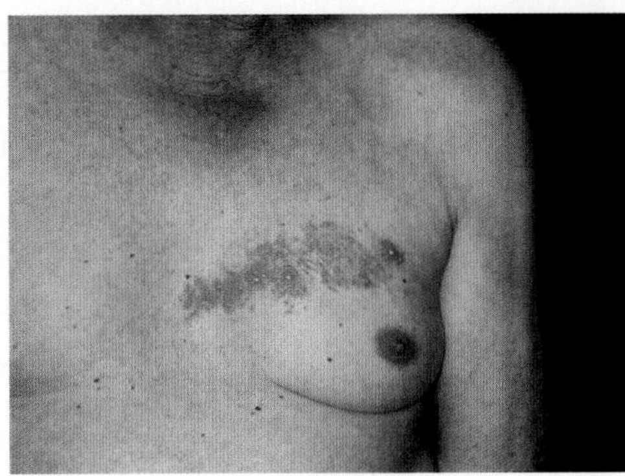

Fig. 43.3 Herpes zoster. (Courtesy Department of Dermatology, School of Medicine, University of Utah, Salt Lake City, Utah.)

vesicles may become purulent. This painful condition lasts 7 to 28 days.

The pain associated with herpes zoster is severe; most patients describe it as burning and knifelike. Extreme tenderness and pruritus occur in the affected area. The patient with herpes zoster needs frequent analgesic therapy during the acute episode.

Herpes zoster is usually not permanently disabling to a healthy adult. The greatest risk is for a patient with a lowered resistance to infection, such as one receiving chemotherapy or large doses of prednisone. In a patient with a compromised immune system, the disease can be fatal.

Assessment

Assessment of the patient should include obtaining a thorough health history and performing a careful inspection to gather relevant data.

Subjective data include (1) sharp, burning pain, usually on one side; (2) severe pruritus of the lesions; (3) general malaise; and (4) a history of chickenpox (varicella).

Objective data include (1) evidence of skin **excoriation** (injury to the surface layer of skin caused by scratching or abrasion) related to scratching, (2) patches of vesicles on erythematous skin following a peripheral nerve pathway, and (3) demonstration of tenderness to touch in the involved area. Other objective signs may include frequent requests for analgesics.

Diagnostic Tests

The diagnostic test for herpes zoster is a culture that isolates the virus. Other diagnostic measures are physical examinations and a thorough health history obtained on admission to the health care facility.

Medical Management

Medical interventions are directed at controlling the pain and preventing secondary complications. Early diagnosis and initiation of treatment are key in the resolution of the outbreak. Oral and intravenous acyclovir, when administered early, ideally within 72 hours of onset of the development of symptoms, reduces the pain and duration of the virus. Analgesics, often opioids, are given for the pain. Steroids may be given to decrease inflammation and edema. Lotions (Kenalog, Lidex) may be used to relieve pruritus, and corticosteroids may be used to relieve pruritus and inflammation. Recovery generally occurs in 2 to 3 weeks. Approximately 20% of patients experience some form of neuralgia after the episode. A vaccine to prevent herpes zoster, called Zostavax, is now available. It is recommended for adults over 60 years of age and who have had varicella (chickenpox) (CDC, 2016).

Nursing Interventions and Patient Teaching

Nursing interventions are directed at education about the disease and plan of treatment, relieving pain and pruritus, and preventing secondary complications. Tranquilizers such as lorazepam (Ativan) are prescribed to decrease the anxiety associated with severe pain. Analgesics are given to control pain. The nurse must understand and be able to apply the principles of pain management to provide nursing interventions. Medicated baths and warm compresses may be ordered to soothe the skin. Use aseptic technique when caring for open lesions (Nursing Care Plan 43.1).

Problem identification and interventions for the patient with herpes zoster include but are not limited to the following:

Patient Problem	Nursing Interventions
Recent Onset of Pain, related to inflammation of the involved nerve pathways	Assess pain and pruritus for necessary relief measures Administer medications for pain and pruritus Teach stress relaxation techniques, and offer diversional activities
Potential for Infection, related to tissue destruction	Assess factors that contribute to infection, such as an immunocompromised patient (one who has decreased white blood cell count) Monitor for signs of infection, such as pyrexia and leukocytosis Stress aseptic hand hygiene technique Maintain aseptic technique when providing care Limit visitors

Begin patient teaching by assessing the patient's knowledge and readiness, including the following: (1) methods for controlling pain, (2) application of medication and wet dressings, (3) methods for inhibiting the spread of disease, (4) techniques to prevent secondary infections, and (5) proper diet with vitamin C to promote healing.

Health care staff who have received two doses of the varicella vaccine should be assessed for symptoms 8 to 21 days after exposure to a patient with shingles. Any staff member who develops symptoms consistent

Nursing Care Plan 43.1 The Patient With Herpes Zoster

Ms. L., a 28-year-old teacher, is admitted with herpes zoster located around her left eye. She has several vesicles that have crusted and several vesicles that are still intact. She is complaining of pruritus and pain. She keeps asking the nurse if the lesions will leave a scar.

PATIENT PROBLEM

Compromised Skin Integrity, related to open lesions around the left eye

Patient Goals and Expected Outcomes	Nursing Interventions	Evaluation and Rationale
Patient's skin integrity will improve as shown by:		
• No signs of infection such as erythema, purulent drainage, and elevated white blood cell count during hospitalization	Assess skin, especially eye area, for changes in color, texture, turgor, and increase in lesion size. Assess lesions for signs of infection. Monitor albumin and white blood cell levels as ordered.	The patient showed no signs of erythema or purulent drainage. The patient showed improvement of vesicles.
• Remaining skin showing no signs of impairment during hospitalization	Use principles of aseptic technique.	No skin impairment noted in remaining skin.
• Decrease in the number of lesions within 72 h	Monitor status of lesions q 12 h.	The number of lesions increased during the first day of hospitalization but decreased during the next 48 h.
• Patient stating pain level has decreased from a "9" to a "4" within 24 h	Administer or apply medications as ordered to decrease pain or pruritus Teach patient importance of using medical asepsis in care of lesions.	Patient stated that pain was a "3" within 24 h of medication administration.

PATIENT PROBLEM

Distorted Body Image, related to location of lesions as manifested by continual remarks to the nurse, "Will these sores leave a scar?"

Patient Goals and Expected Outcomes	Nursing Interventions	Evaluation and Rationale
The patient will verbalize and demonstrate acceptance of appearance as manifested by:		
• Verbalizing positive feelings about body image	Assess patient's feelings about personal appearance by encouraging patient to express her feelings.	The goal was met: The patient stated she believed the lesions would not be permanent.
• Participating in normal activities	Encourage patient to ask questions about her health problem. Provide reliable information, and reinforce the information already given. Clarify any misconceptions about the care the patient is receiving. Provide privacy, and avoid criticism. Teach patient about the disease and the course of the disease.	The goal was met: The patient returned to work after dismissal from the hospital before the lesions had completely healed.

CRITICAL THINKING QUESTIONS

1. Ms. L. turns on her call light. She is crying and states she is in severe pain. She describes the pain as a burning, stabbing pain over her left forehead and eye. She rates her pain as a 7 on a pain scale of 0 to 10. She also complains of pruritus. What would be the most appropriate nursing interventions to provide comfort and pain control for Ms. L.?
2. Ms. L. tells the nurse that a friend told her she could not visit because she has not had chickenpox. Her friend is afraid she might "catch chickenpox" from Ms. L.'s shingles. Describe the accurate patient teaching to give in response to Ms. L.'s statements.

with herpes zoster should be removed from active duty. Health care staff who have not received the two doses of varicella vaccine may be contagious for 8 to 21 days and should be moved to another duty location, away from patient care (CDC, 2017). Implementation of proper transmission-based precautions as directed by the infection control department prevent the transmission of the virus in the health care setting. The CDC suggests that immunocompromised patients should be placed in airborne and contact transmission-based precautions for disseminated herpes zoster until the infection is determined to be localized; if the infection is localized, standard precautions with the lesions covered are followed. For patients who are immunocompetent, the CDC suggests using standard precautions with the lesions covered if the infection is localized; for disseminated herpes zoster, airborne and contact precautions. Once the lesions are dry and crusted, the patient is no longer considered communicable (CDC, 2017).

Prognosis

The prognosis is generally good; however, older adults are more susceptible to complications such as postherpetic neuralgia (PHN), which may persist for several months or even years after the skin lesions have cleared. PHN is most common in adults older than age 60 years. Herpes zoster also can result in eye complications that can lead to blindness, deafness, brain inflammation, and death. Evidence indicates that the varicella-zoster virus remains latent in the body of a person once infected. A person lacking varicella (chickenpox) immunity or who is immunocompromised can acquire chickenpox from someone who has shingles (CDC, 2017).

PITYRIASIS ROSEA

Pityriasis rosea is a skin rash that may affect people of any age but is noted most often in young adults. It is not known what causes the rash, but it is thought to be linked to a viral infection. It is not considered contagious.

Etiology and Pathophysiology

Pityriasis rosea is caused by a virus, but it is not clear which virus. Some studies indicate it may be linked to certain strains of the herpesvirus, but not the type 1 herpesvirus. The rash generally disappears without treatment within 4 to 8 weeks (Mayo Clinic, 2015).

Clinical Manifestations

Pityriasis rosea begins as a single lesion referred to as a herald patch, a scaly area up to 4 inches in diameter (10 cm) with a raised border and a pink center that resembles ringworm (a fungal infection). Within 7 to 14 days after the initial eruption, smaller matching spots become widespread on both sides of the body. The rash consists of pink, oval-shaped spots that are ¼ to ½ inch across. The rash appears mainly on the chest, abdomen, back, groin, and armpits (axillae).

Assessment

Assessment involves inspecting the skin and gathering a detailed health history. Ask questions related to gathering subjective data.

Diagnostic Tests

Diagnosis of pityriasis rosea is based on inspection and subjective data provided by the patient. No specific laboratory tests support a definitive diagnosis.

Medical Management

Pityriasis rosea usually requires no treatment, but preventive interventions can control secondary infections related to pruritus. If the skin becomes dry, moisturizing cream may help. For pruritus, the patient should use 1% hydrocortisone cream two or three times a day. Ultraviolet light, such as sunbathing for 30 minutes, shortens the course of pityriasis rosea.

Nursing Interventions

The nursing interventions for pityriasis rosea include symptomatic relief of the symptoms such as pruritus. Analgesics and oatmeal baths may be ordered to help decrease the pain and pruritus. Antihistamines and topical steroids may be used to control the pruritus. Sun exposure aids in the resolution of the lesions.

Prognosis

The disease is self-limiting and resolves in a few weeks.

BACTERIAL DISORDERS OF THE SKIN

CELLULITIS

Etiology and Pathophysiology

Cellulitis, a potentially serious infection, involves the underlying tissues of the skin. Although it is not contagious, the bacteria that cause cellulitis can be spread by direct contact with an open area on a person who has an infection. The most common causes in adults are group A streptococci and *Staphylococcus aureus; Haemophilus influenzae* type B is more common in children. The risk is increased by venous insufficiency or stasis; diabetes mellitus; lymphedema; surgery; malnutrition; substance abuse; the presence of another infection; compromised immune function resulting from HIV; treatment with steroids or cancer chemotherapy; or autoimmune diseases, such as lupus erythematosus.

Cellulitis develops as an edematous, erythematous area of skin that feels hot and tender (Fig. 43.4). It occurs when bacteria enter the body through a break in the skin, such as a cut, scratch, or insect bite that is not cleansed with soap and water. The infection usually affects skin on the lower extremities or face, although cellulitis can occur on any part of the skin. The infection is usually superficial, but cellulitis may spread and

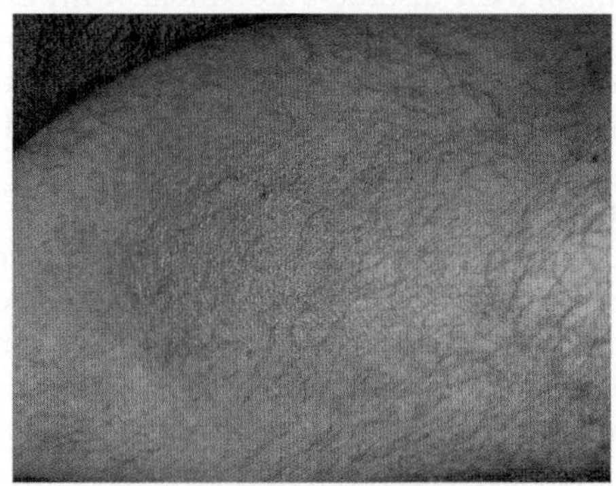

Fig. 43.4 Cellulitis.

become life threatening as the infection invades the deeper tissues, lymph nodes, and bloodstream.

Clinical Manifestations

Cellulitis is an infection of the skin and underlying subcutaneous tissues. The affected areas become erythematous, edematous, tender, and warm to the touch. Often a fever accompanies the other symptoms. The first signs and symptoms generally are erythema, pain, and tenderness over an area of skin. These signs and symptoms are caused by the bacteria and by the body's attempts to halt the infection. The infected skin may look slightly pitted, like an orange peel. Over time, the area of erythema spreads and small red spots may appear. Vesicles may form and burst, or large bullae may appear on the infected skin. As the infection spreads, nearby lymph nodes may become enlarged and tender (lymphadenitis). *Erysipelas* is one form of streptococcal cellulitis in which the skin is bright red and noticeably edematous, and the edges of the infected area are raised. Edema occurs because the infection occludes the lymphatic vessels in the skin. Most patients with cellulitis feel only mildly ill, but some have fever, chills, tachycardia, headache, hypotension, and confusion.

Assessment

Assessment involves primarily inspection of the skin. Collect a health history to support assessment data. Subjective data include complaints of fatigue, tenderness, pain, limited movement of the involved extremity, and general malaise. Objective data include edema, erythema, and areas that are warm to touch. Vesicles may be present. An elevated temperature accompanied by tachycardia and leukocytosis (elevated white blood cell count) often occurs.

Diagnostic Tests

Cellulitis is diagnosed by its appearance as well as the signs and symptoms. Cultures may be needed from blood, purulent exudate, or tissue specimens for laboratory identification of the bacteria. A complete blood count (CBC) reveals leukocytosis. A Gram stain can determine the appropriate antibiotic therapy. Sometimes tests are performed to differentiate cellulitis from deep vein thrombosis of the lower extremity because the signs and symptoms of these disorders are similar. X-ray examination, ultrasound, computed tomography, or magnetic resonance imaging may be used to determine the extent of inflammation and to identify abscess formation.

Medical Management

Prompt treatment with antibiotics can prevent cellulitis from spreading rapidly and reaching the blood and organs. Commonly used antibiotics include penicillin, cephalexin, and erythromycin. Most cases are treated with antibiotic therapy that is effective against streptococci and staphylococci (NLM, 2018). A patient with mild cellulitis may take oral antibiotics. If the patient has rapidly spreading cellulitis, high fever, or other evidence of a serious infection, the health care provider will order IV antibiotics.

Nursing Interventions and Patient Teaching

Nursing interventions involve treating the signs and symptoms and preventing the spread of the disease. Administer the antibiotic, monitor the patient's progress, assess pain, administer an analgesic, change dressings, and monitor the patient's nutrition and hydration status. The affected body part, when possible, should be immobilized and is elevated to help reduce edema. Warm, moist dressings applied to the infected area may relieve discomfort.

Signs and symptoms of cellulitis usually disappear after a few days of antibiotic therapy. However, they may worsen before they improve because, as the bacteria die, they release substances that damage tissue. When this occurs, the body continues to react even though the bacteria are dead. Antibiotics are continued for a minimum of 10 days. Teach the patient that it is important to take the entire prescription of antibiotics and to monitor for signs and symptoms of secondary diseases such as yeast infections. The specific patient problems related to cellulitis depend on the assessment data gathered and the extent of the infection. Analgesics such as acetaminophen or oxycodone-acetaminophen (Percocet) help control the pain and fever associated with cellulitis. Patients who develop blistering, increasing temperatures, or red streaks in the affected extremity should be advised to contact the primary care provider.

Prognosis

Cure is possible with 7 to 10 days of treatment. Cellulitis may be more severe in people with chronic diseases and those who are susceptible to infection, such as those with immunosuppression. Complications from cellulitis include sepsis, meningitis, and lymphangitis.

IMPETIGO CONTAGIOSA

Etiology and Pathophysiology

Impetigo is caused by *S. aureus,* streptococci, or a mixed bacterial invasion of the skin. It is a highly contagious inflammatory disorder, seen at all ages but particularly common in children. The lesions start as **macules** (small, flat blemishes flush with the skin surface), develop into **pustulant vesicles** (small, circumscribed elevations of the skin that contain pus), and then rupture and form a dried exudate. The crust is honey-colored and easily removed. Under the dried exudate is smooth, red skin (Fig. 43.5).

Clinical Manifestations

The exposed areas of the body most often affected are the face, hands, arms, and legs. The pustulant lesions are distributed randomly over the involved area. The honey-colored dried exudate ranges from pinpoint to the size of a nickel or larger. Impetigo is highly contagious

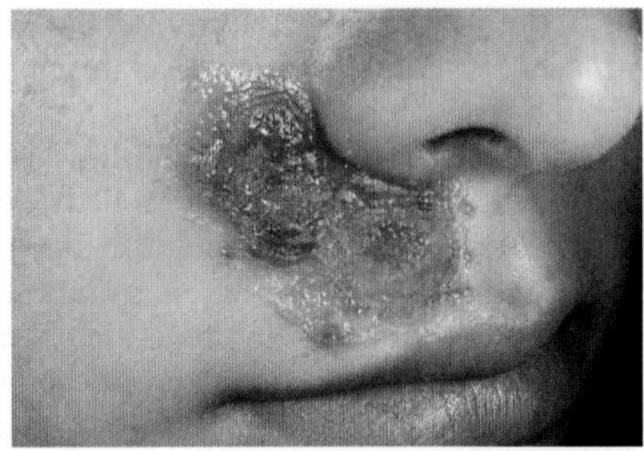

Fig. 43.5 Impetigo and herpes simplex. (Courtesy Department of Dermatology, School of Medicine, University of Utah, Salt Lake City, Utah.)

to a person who directly contacts the exudate of a lesion. The disease may be spread by touching personal articles, linens, and clothing of the infected person.

Assessment

Subjective data include symptoms of (1) pruritus, (2) pain, (3) malaise, (4) spread of the disease to other parts of the body, and (5) the presence of other diseases.

Objective data include all or some of the following: (1) erythema; (2) pruritic areas; (3) honey-colored crust over dried lesions; (4) smooth, red skin under the crust; (5) low-grade fever; (6) leukocytosis; (7) positive culture for *Streptococcus* or *S. aureus;* and (8) purulent exudate.

Diagnostic Tests

The diagnosis is made by taking a culture of the exudate and identifying the specific bacterium. Inspection and symptoms are the standard means of identifying the condition.

Medical Management

The health care provider prescribes systemic antibiotics (such as erythromycin, dicloxacillin, or a cephalosporin) based on the culture and sensitivity test. Topical antibiotics such as mupirocin (Bactroban) have proven effective when started early in the treatment, but most health care providers include a systemic antibiotic as well. Retapamulin (Altabax) was approved by the US Food and Drug Administration (FDA) for topical treatment of impetigo for adults and children over 9 months old for methicillin-susceptible *Staphylococcus aureus* and *Streptococcus pyogenes* (American Family Physician, 2007 and NLM, 2016). Medical treatment emphasizes the use of antiseptic soaps to remove crusted exudate and cleansing agents to clean the involved area thoroughly before applying an antibiotic cream, ointment, or lotion. A primary goal is to prevent glomerulonephritis (inflammation of the glomerulus of the kidney), which may occur after streptococcal infections.

Nursing Interventions and Patient Teaching

Interventions are aimed at disrupting the course of the disease and preventing the spread of infection. Antibiotics are used to arrest the disease process. Systemic parenteral penicillin is one of the most commonly used antibiotics. Cephalosporins or beta-lactam/beta-lactamase inhibitor combination are also used in a first line defense (Lewis and Steele, 2017). Don gloves and wash the lesions with an antibacterial agent.

The lesions usually are soaked with an antiseptic solution, and the dried exudate is removed with special instruments. Topical antibiotics are applied several times a day using sterile technique.

Problem identification and interventions for the patient with impetigo include but are not limited to the following:

Patient Problem	Nursing Interventions
Compromised Skin Integrity, related to S. aureus, *streptococci, or a mixed bacterial invasion as evidenced by crusted, open lesions*	Inspect lesions every day for drainage, size, and extent of body area covered Keep area clean and dry
Insufficient Knowledge, concerning the cause and spread of the disease	Assess patient's knowledge level and readiness to learn Demonstrate appropriate care and application of topical medications Stress importance of individual personal items, such as linens and towels Involve family in patient teaching

Assess the patient's level of knowledge, and instruct the patient and family members in the principles of hygiene. When demonstrating home care techniques, reinforce correct information and stress the importance of preventing the spread of the disease by contact.

Prognosis

With proper treatment the prognosis is good. Emphasize that the patient should complete the prescribed medication therapies.

FOLLICULITIS, FURUNCLES, CARBUNCLES, AND FELONS

Etiology and Pathophysiology

Folliculitis is an infection of a hair follicle, generally by *S. aureus* bacteria. The infection may involve one or several follicles. It often occurs after men or women shave. A stye resulting from an infected eyelash is an example of folliculitis.

A *furuncle* (boil) is an inflammation that begins deep in the hair follicles and spreads to the surrounding skin. Irritation is a common predisposing factor. Common locations are the posterior area of the neck, the forearm, buttocks, and the axillae (Fig. 43.6).

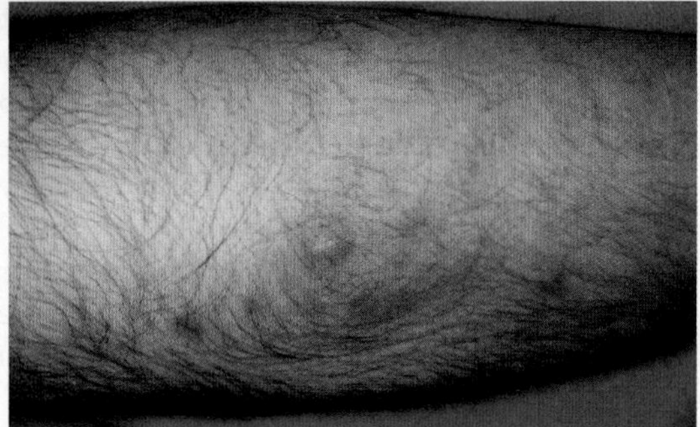

Fig. 43.6 Furuncle of the forearm. (Courtesy Department of Dermatology, School of Medicine, University of Utah, Salt Lake City, Utah.)

A *carbuncle* is a cluster of furuncles. It is an infection of several hair follicles that spreads to surrounding tissue. Obesity, poor nutrition, untreated diabetes mellitus, and poor hygiene contribute to the formation of carbuncles.

A *felon* is an infection of the soft tissue under and around an area such as the fingernail. The involved finger becomes erythematous, edematous, and tender to touch.

Clinical Manifestations

The involved area is usually edematous, erythematous, painful, and pruritic. After several days, the infected area becomes localized. The exact area may become shiny. The lesion may begin to present with a pointed head and point up; in a furuncle or carbuncle, the center turns yellow. Carbuncles can have four or five cores with spontaneous rupture of the core. The pain stops immediately on rupture. A surgical incision and drainage can be performed if the core does not rupture.

Assessment

Subjective data include the patient's general symptoms, such as tenderness and pain with movement. Ask about a family history of diabetes mellitus or the wearing of improperly fitting clothing. Objective data include noting erythema and edema in the involved area. The patient is often overweight and may have poor body hygiene.

Diagnostic Tests

Diagnosis is based primarily on a thorough physical examination, health history, and inspection of the area. The drainage may be cultured.

Medical Management

Medical treatment is aimed at preventing the spread of infection. Patients in the hospital are isolated, using wound and secretion precautions. Surgical treatment may include draining the lesion and applying topical antibiotics.

Nursing Interventions and Patient Teaching

Warm soaks, two or three times a day, can speed the process of **suppuration** (production of purulent material). When the lesion ruptures, discontinue the soaks to prevent damage of the surrounding skin and spread of the infection. Use good medical asepsis while caring for these patients. In the hospital, follow isolation procedures for drainage and secretion. If the lesion is incised and drained, use sterile technique to apply topical antibiotics. The affected part must be immobilized to prevent pain and elevated to decrease the edema.

Problem identification and interventions for the patient with bacterial disorders include but are not limited to the following:

Patient Problem	Nursing Interventions
Compromised Skin Integrity, related to infection of a hair follicle, as evidenced by exudates from wound	Assess wound daily for exudates and excoriation Apply skin protectant to opening
Recent Onset of Pain, related to infection of a hair follicle	Assess area for edema and tenderness Elevate involved body part above the level of the heart Apply hot soaks and immobilize affected part

Teach patients not to touch the exudate. Meticulous hand hygiene is a must before and after contact with the lesions. Demonstrate good hygiene practices and ask for return demonstrations by the patient and the family. Each family member needs his or her own toilet items and bath linens, which are not to be shared. They should be encouraged to use bacteriostatic soap and shampoo. Demonstrate proper disposal and cleaning of contaminated articles.

Prognosis

Patients make a full recovery when they follow the treatment plan. A follow-up examination with a health care provider may be needed to identify any underlying disease process, such as diabetes mellitus.

FUNGAL INFECTIONS OF THE SKIN

Fungal infections, which are known as *dermatophytoses,* are superficial infections of the skin. The most common types are tinea capitis, tinea corporis, tinea cruris, and tinea pedis.

Etiology and Pathophysiology

Tinea capitis is known commonly as ringworm of the scalp. *Microsporum audouinii* is the major fungal pathogen. The fungus is spread by contact with infected articles. Trauma or irritation breaks the skin and facilitates spread of the infection (Fig. 43.7).

Tinea corporis is known as ringworm of the body. It occurs on parts of the body with little or no hair.

Tinea cruris is known as jock itch. It is found in the groin area.

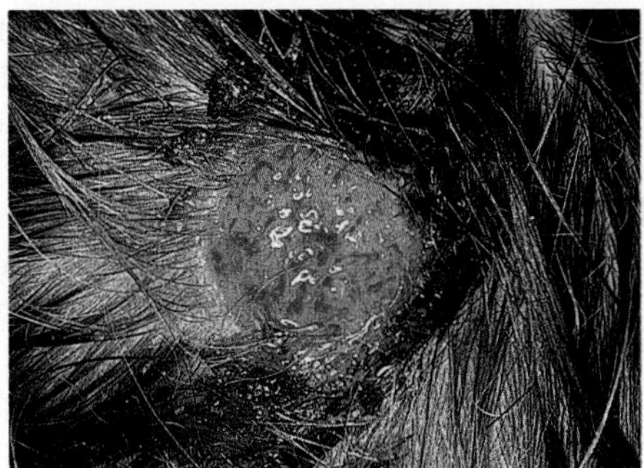

Fig. 43.7 Tinea capitis. (From Habif TP, Campbell JL Jr, Chapman MS, et al: *Skin disease: Diagnosis and treatment,* ed 3, St. Louis, 2011, Saunders.)

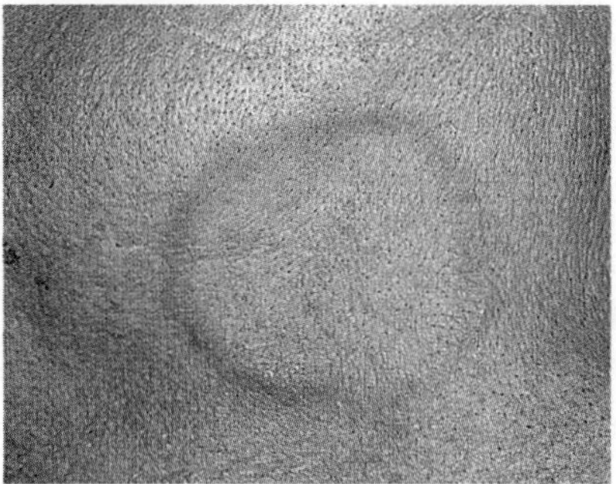

Fig. 43.8 Tinea corporis. (From Habif TP, Campbell JL Jr, Chapman MS, et al: *Skin disease: Diagnosis and treatment,* ed 3, St. Louis, 2011, Saunders.)

Tinea pedis is the most common of all fungal infections. Commonly known as athlete's foot, it occurs between the toes of people whose feet perspire heavily. The fungus also can be spread from contaminated public bathroom facilities and swimming pools.

Clinical Manifestations

Tinea capitis is usually an erythematous, round lesion with pustules around the edges (see Fig. 43.7). Temporary alopecia occurs at the site, and infected hairs turn blue-green under a Wood's lamp (an ultraviolet light).

Tinea corporis produces flat lesions that are clear in the center with erythematous borders. Scaliness also occurs, and pruritus is severe (Fig. 43.8).

Tinea cruris has brownish red lesions that migrate out from the groin area. Pruritus and skin excoriation from scratching are found.

Tinea pedis produces more skin maceration than the others. Commonly seen are fissures and vesicles around and below the toes, with occasional discoloration of the infected area.

Assessment

Subjective data include any symptoms of extreme pruritus and tenderness from excoriation of the area. Collection of objective data for tinea capitis includes an inspection and location of a round, scaled lesion that has pustules around the edges of the scalp. The involved area is erythematous and has no hair. In tinea corporis, the lesions are flat with clear centers and erythematous borders on nonhairy body parts. In tinea cruris, the groin area reveals brown to red lesions that radiate outward, with skin excoriation from intense scratching. In tinea pedis, fissures between the toes and soft skin are accompanied by vesicular lesions and thick toenails.

Diagnostic Tests

The diagnosis is primarily by visual inspection and, for tinea capitis, use of a Wood's lamp. The light causes hairs infected by the fungus to become brilliantly fluorescent. No other tests are performed, but a thorough health history supports the diagnosis of all fungal infections of the skin.

Medical Management

Medical treatment involves the use of topical or oral antifungal drugs. Griseofulvin (Fulvicin, Grifulvin) is the most common oral drug given; topical drugs do not penetrate the hair bulb. Antifungal soaps and shampoos are recommended. Antifungal agents such as tolnaftate 1% (Tinactin), miconazole (Lotrimin AF), (Monistat-Derm, Desenex), and butenafine (Mentax) can be applied directly. Treatment may last from 2 to 6 weeks. See Table 43.3 for a list of drugs commonly used for fungal and other integumentary infections.

Nursing Interventions and Patient Teaching

Nursing interventions for fungal infections involve two primary principles: (1) protect the involved area from trauma and irritation by keeping it clean and dry and (2) alleviate the fungus through proper application of medications and warm compresses.

Tinea pedis should be treated with warm soaks, using Burow's solution (5% aluminum subacetate), and topical antifungal agents. Burow's solution has antiseptic properties, relieves itching, and aids in the reduction of bacterial and fungal growth. It is available without prescription. Excellent foot care is stressed. The feet should be cleaned and dried thoroughly, paying special attention to the toes. Wearing sandals or going barefoot helps decrease foot moisture. Footwear, such as stockings, must be made of an absorbent material.

Problem identification and interventions for the patient with fungal infections include but are not limited to the following:

Patient Problem	Nursing Interventions
Compromised Skin Integrity, related to fungal infection, as evidenced by: • Increased moisture • Pruritus	Keep involved area clean and dry Have patient wear loose-fitting clothing and shoes Apply medications as directed

Patient education involves teaching proper skin care and comfort measures to relieve pruritus. Review the medications to be taken and the procedures for the patient to do at home, emphasizing that fungal skin disorders may take months to cure. Stress general information about athlete's foot and clarify the many misconceptions.

Prognosis

Prognosis for recovery is good. Few complications result when treatment is followed.

INFLAMMATORY DISORDERS OF THE SKIN

Superficial infection of the skin is known as *dermatitis.* It can be caused by numerous agents, such as drugs, plants, chemicals, metals, and food. Regardless of the precipitating factor, the lesions associated with dermatitis develop along the same pattern. The nurse first observes erythema and edema, followed by the eruption of vesicles that rupture and encrust. Pruritus is always present, which promotes further skin excoriation.

CONTACT DERMATITIS

Etiology and Pathophysiology

Contact dermatitis is caused by direct contact with agents in the environment to which the individual is hypersensitive. The epidermis becomes inflamed and damaged by repeated contact with the physical and chemical irritants. Common causes of dermatitis are detergents, soaps, industrial chemicals, and plants such as poison ivy.

Clinical Manifestations

Lesions appear first at the point of contact with the irritant. Usually the patient feels burning, pain, pruritus, and edema. The involved area is soon erythematous, with **papules** (small, raised, solid skin lesions less than 1 cm in diameter) and vesicles appearing most often on the dorsal surfaces.

Assessment

Thoroughly research the patient's activities. If necessary, ask the patient to write a log of activities for the 48 hours before development of symptoms.

Subjective data usually reveal that the patient has (1) tried a new soap, (2) been traveling and using different personal items, or (3) been working with plants or flowers. The patient may have severe pruritus and difficulty moving the involved area.

Objective data should reveal (1) erythema, (2) papules and vesicles that generally ooze and weep a clear fluid, (3) scratch marks resulting from intense pruritus, and (4) edema of the area.

Diagnostic Tests

The primary diagnostic test is an accurate health history to identify the agent and inspection of the skin. Intradermal skin testing may identify plants and environmental agents, and elimination diets are used to identify food allergies. Elevated serum immunoglobulin E (IgE) levels and eosinophilia support the diagnosis. Both tests are thought to be related to abnormalities of T cell function.

Medical Management

Medical intervention involves identifying the cause of the hypersensitive reaction. Symptomatic treatment for the inflammation, edema, and pruritus may include topical application of corticosteroids and the oral administration of antihistamines such as diphenhydramine (Benadryl). If the patient has a history of asthma (reactive airway disease), he or she may experience an acute asthmatic episode. Hydroxyzine (Atarax) and inhalation treatments provide prophylactic treatment for asthma.

Nursing Interventions and Patient Teaching

The primary goal is to identify the offensive agent to protect the skin from further damage. Identify the cause by first describing the pattern of the reaction.

Wet dressings using Burow's solution help promote the healing process. To prevent infection, use aseptic technique when applying corticosteroids to the open lesions.

Pruritus is responsible for most of the discomfort. A cool environment with increased humidity decreases the pruritus. Cold compresses may be applied to reduce circulation to the area (vasoconstriction). The patient should take daily baths with an application of oil to cleanse the skin. Fingernails should be cut at the level of the fingertips to decrease excoriation from scratching. Clothing should be lightweight and loose to decrease trauma of the involved area.

Problem identification and interventions for the patient with inflammation of the skin include but are not limited to the following:

Patient Problem	Nursing Interventions
Compromised Skin Integrity, related to direct contact with agents in the environment as evidenced by scratching and the appearance of papules	Assess for signs of scratching Have patient keep fingernails short and wear mittens Apply medications as directed
Recent Onset of Pain, related to pruritus	Assess degree of pruritus and discomfort every shift Keep environment cool Apply cold compresses Apply antipruritic medications as prescribed

Teach the patient to keep an accurate history of possible predisposing offensive agents. As soon as the primary irritant has been identified, the patient should avoid it. Irritants may include certain soaps or excessive heat and friction at the site and should be avoided. Any time the skin is exposed to the primary irritant, the affected area should be washed thoroughly. Topical creams may be applied only as directed by a health care provider.

Prognosis

Removal of the offensive agent results in full recovery. Desensitizing the individual may be necessary if recurrences are frequent.

DERMATITIS VENENATA, EXFOLIATIVE DERMATITIS, AND DERMATITIS MEDICAMENTOSA

Etiology and Pathophysiology

Dermatitis venenata results from contact with certain plants, commonly *poison ivy* and *poison oak.* The signs and symptoms include mild to severe erythema with pruritus. Initial exposure causes the body to form sensitizing antigens, resulting in an immunologic change in certain lymphocytes. Subsequent exposure to the antigen causes the lymphocytes to release irritating chemicals, leading to inflammation, edema, and vesiculation. The lesions are found mainly on the body part exposed to the sensitizing agent.

Exfoliative dermatitis can be caused by the ingestion of certain heavy metals, such as arsenic or mercury, or by antibiotics, aspirin, codeine, gold, or iodine. The skin sloughs off, and the area becomes edematous and erythematous. If severe pruritus with fever occurs, the patient may require hospitalization. Treatment is individualized. If the cause can be determined, the source should be removed or treated appropriately. Careful monitoring is essential to prevent secondary infection, avoid further irritation, and maintain fluid balance.

Dermatitis medicamentosa occurs when people are given a medication to which they are hypersensitive. An individual may present with a skin reaction to a medication that was taken in the past without incident. Any drug can cause a reaction, but the common agents are penicillin, codeine, and cephalosporins (WebMD, 2017).

Clinical Manifestations

Clinical manifestations range from mild to severe erythema with vesicular eruptions. In severe reactions, respiratory distress may occur. Any type of lesion may be found.

Assessment

Subjective data for dermatitis include complaints of pruritus and a burning pain in the involved area.

Objective data include observation of lesions that are white in the center and red on the periphery. Vesicles are common in dermatitis venenata. Patients with dermatitis medicamentosa may have severe dyspnea caused by respiratory distress.

Diagnostic Tests

A careful patient history is paramount in the diagnosis of dermatitis venenata, exfoliative dermatitis, and dermatitis medicamentosa. A laboratory examination for serum IgE and eosinophilia is ordered.

Medical Management

The medical treatment for dermatitis ranges from therapeutic baths to administration of corticosteroids. The medical treatment is directed at the cause.

Nursing Interventions and Patient Teaching

Pruritus is the primary symptom in all types of dermatitis. Calamine lotion, a common over-the-counter medication, is used to reduce itching. Therapeutic baths using colloid solution, lotions, and ointments also help relieve the pruritus. Emotional support is necessary. The patient's physical appearance is difficult for the patient and family members to accept.

In dermatitis venenata, instruct the patient to wash the affected part immediately after contact with the offending allergen. After the lesions appear, only cool, open, wet dressings should be used.

In dermatitis medicamentosa, identifying the drug and discontinuing its use are paramount. If the offending allergen cannot be pinpointed, no drugs should be given. Notify the health care provider, who will determine which medication is responsible. The lesions will disappear after the medication is discontinued. More specific nursing intervention is directed by individual patient symptoms.

Problem identification and interventions for the patient with dermatitis include but are not limited to the following:

Patient Problem	Nursing Interventions
Compromised Skin Integrity, related to exposure to the antigen as evidenced by encrusted, open lesions	Inspect lesions every day for exudate, size, and specific body area involved Keep area clean and dry
Potential for infection, related to break in skin	Assess skin for signs of infection Identify interventions to prevent or reduce the risk of infection Monitor vital signs; assess for elevated temperature Stress medical aseptic hand hygiene technique Keep involved areas dry
Insufficient Knowledge, related to the cause and spread of the disease	Assess patient's knowledge level and readiness to learn Demonstrate appropriate care and application of topical medications Stress importance of individual personal items, such as linens and towels Involve family in patient teaching

Advise the patient to wear a medical alert bracelet or necklace showing the name of the allergen and to notify all health care personnel of the medication allergy.

Prognosis

Full recovery occurs when the offending agent is removed.

URTICARIA

Etiology and Pathophysiology

Urticaria is the presence of wheals or hives in an allergic reaction, commonly caused by drugs, food, insect bites, inhalants, emotional stress, or exposure to heat or cold. The **wheals** (round elevation of the skin; white in the center with a pale red periphery) (see Table 43.1) of urticaria appear suddenly. Urticaria, or hives, is caused by the release of histamine in an antigen-antibody reaction.

Clinical Manifestations

In addition to wheals, the increased histamine causes the capillaries to dilate, resulting in increased permeability. Respiratory involvement may occur.

Assessment

Subjective data include patient complaints of pruritus, edema, a burning pain, and sometimes dyspnea.

Collection of objective data identifies transient wheals of varying shapes and sizes with well-defined erythematous margins and pale centers. Intense scratching may be seen, and in some cases respiration may be compromised. Assessment of respiratory status provides a baseline for future assessments.

Diagnostic Tests

A detailed health history is the primary tool to identify the cause of hives. An allergy skin test may be performed, using minute quantities of antigen, to identify the allergenic substances. A serum examination for IgE elevation may be ordered.

Medical Management

Administering an antihistamine and sometimes epinephrine provides relief from urticaria. Identification of the cause of the urticaria is important to prevent recurrence.

Nursing Interventions and Patient Teaching

Nursing interventions include helping the patient identify the cause and decreasing the discomfort from the pruritus. Teach the patient about possible causes and prevention methods. Explain medications thoroughly, and describe the procedure for therapeutic baths. Review the signs and symptoms of an anaphylactic reaction, including shortness of breath, wheezing, and cyanosis.

Prognosis

Patients recover fully when the offending agent is determined and avoided. Compliance with the therapeutic regimen influences the outcome.

ANGIOEDEMA

Etiology and Pathophysiology

Angioedema is a form of urticaria and is caused by the same offenders. It occurs in the subcutaneous tissue, whereas urticaria is a lesion of the skin and mucous membranes. Angioedema is characterized by local edema of an entire area, such as an eyelid, hands, feet, tongue, larynx, gastrointestinal (GI) tract, genitalia, or lips. Only a single edematous area usually appears at one time.

Assessment

Subjective data include symptoms of burning, pruritus, acute pain if in the GI tract, or respiratory distress if in the larynx.

The collection of objective data reveals edema (swelling); overlying skin appears normal.

Diagnostic Tests

A careful patient history is essential in the diagnosis of angioedema. Patients with a history of allergies are more likely to have angioedema.

Medical Management

Treatment to relieve angioedema may include antihistamine drugs such as diphenhydramine. Epinephrine injections and infusions of corticosteroids such as methylprednisolone (Solu-Medrol) also may be prescribed.

Nursing Interventions

A cold pack or cold compress may be used. Continual respiratory assessment is essential to detect respiratory distress. Instruct patients to wear a medical alert bracelet. Education is the key to prevent recurrent episodes.

Prognosis

With treatment, the prognosis is excellent.

ECZEMA (ATOPIC DERMATITIS)

Etiology and Pathophysiology

Eczema is a chronic inflammatory disorder of the integument. It usually is diagnosed in children, but exacerbations often continue into adulthood. There are associations with allergies to chocolate, wheat, eggs, and orange juice. The allergen causes histamine to be released, and an antigen-antibody reaction occurs.

Clinical Manifestations

Papular and vesicular lesions appear and are surrounded by erythema. The vesicles generally rupture, discharging a yellow, tenacious exudate that dries and encrusts. If the lesions become infected, the skin loses its pigment and becomes shiny with dry scales.

Assessment

Subjective data include complaints of pruritus and scratching. Children are generally fussy and irritable, and anorexia is common. The skin is sensitive to touch. A family history of allergies and asthma supports the findings in many cases.

Objective data include vesicles and papules found on the scalp, the forehead, the cheeks, the neck, and the surfaces of the extremities. The involved area is erythematous and dry. Tiny cracks in the epithelium allow fluid to escape and further promote dryness. The primary signs result from the scratching in response to pruritus. Scales accompanied by dryness in the involved area are a distinguishing characteristic of eczema.

Diagnostic Tests

The diagnosis generally is made during a thorough health history. Heredity is a prominent factor in the disease. An elimination diet and skin testing may be used to identify the specific substance to which the patient is hypersensitive. IgE serum tests provide data related to allergic response.

Medical Management

Medical treatment involves reducing the amount of allergen exposure. The eruptions and pruritus can be relieved if the aggravating factor is identified and controlled. The primary goal is to break the inflammation cycle.

Hydration of the skin is the key to treatment. The skin is dry because of tiny cracks that allow body fluids to escape. The skin may be hydrated by soaking the affected area in warm water for 15 to 20 minutes and then applying an occlusive ointment to retain the water. Examples of occlusive preparations are petrolatum and corticosteroid ointments. The skin should be patted dry after the bath and the occlusive preparation applied immediately to the damp skin.

Nursing Interventions and Patient Teaching

Nursing interventions are directed toward treatment of symptoms for the eczematous patient. Administer the therapeutic bath and occlusive preparations as directed. Use wet dressings to maximize hydration of the skin. Apply topical steroids to relieve discomfort.

When the lesions begin to heal, moisturizing lotions should be applied three or four times a day to add moisture to the skin. Wet wraps and occlusive preparations only hold water already present.

The emotional impact of having eczema ranges from anger to depression. The nurse provides an emotional outlet for these patients. Encourage the patient to share emotions by using effective listening skills and open-ended questions. This provides a means to establish a therapeutic rapport with the patient.

Before the development of steroids, coal tar products were used to reduce the skin inflammation. Coal tar products do not decrease inflammation as quickly as steroids, but they last longer and have fewer side effects, making them more suitable to treat chronic eczema. Preparations such as Estar gel and PsoriGel are applied once a day at bedtime with a moisturizer.

Problem identification and interventions for the patient with eczema include but are not limited to the following:

Patient Problem	Nursing Interventions
Compromised Skin Integrity, related to chronic inflammatory disorder as evidenced by open lesions	Assess skin for signs of secondary infection Monitor CBC for elevated white blood cell count Apply ordered medications, using medical aseptic technique
Potential for Impaired Self-Esteem due to Current Situation, related to change in body image	Assess patient's mental status Be an active listener Encourage verbalization of concerns the patient may be experiencing Observe interaction with family and staff members and assist in establishing a therapeutic rapport
Potential for Infection, related to open lesion	Report at once the signs of wound infection such as erythema, especially beyond the wound margins Increasing edema, purulent exudates, change in the description of the pain or increased pain, and increased warmth in the involved area are signs and symptoms of infection

ACNE VULGARIS

Etiology and Pathophysiology

Acne is an inflammatory papulopustular skin eruption that involves the sebaceous glands; it occurs primarily in adolescents. The exact cause is unknown. Factors that may contribute to the condition include stress, hormone fluctuations, medications, diet, oil production, dead skin cells, clogged pores, and bacteria (Mayo Clinic, 2017a).

Acne develops when the oil glands become occluded. At puberty androgens are secreted, increasing the size of the oil glands and causing the sebum to combine more readily with epithelial cells and bacteria. Sebum then may occlude a hair follicle, forming a comedo (plural, *comedones*). A comedo is a blackhead. It is dark because of the effect of oxygen on sebum, not because of the presence of dirt.

Clinical Manifestations

Acne is found most often on the face, neck, upper chest, shoulder, and back (Fig. 43.9). The first symptom is usually tenderness and edema in the area, followed by the comedo. The skin is oily and shiny, and the lesions last up to 10 days. Scarring results from large lesions that are traumatized when the person tries to rupture the comedo.

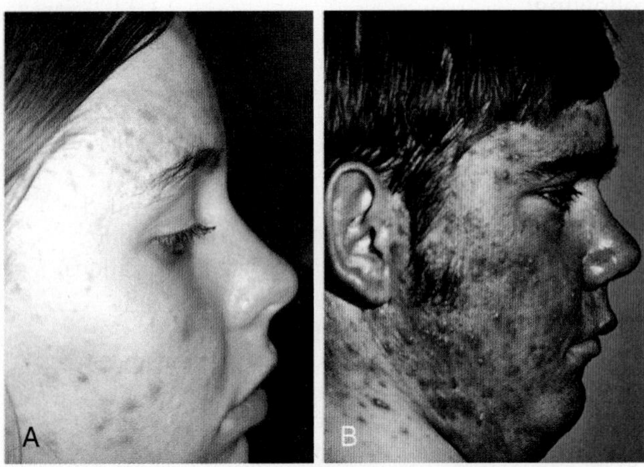

Fig. 43.9 Acne vulgaris. A, Comedones with a few inflammatory pustules. B, Papulopustular acne. (From Weston WL, Lane AT, Morelli JG: *Color textbook of pediatric dermatology,* ed 4, St. Louis, 2007, Mosby.)

Assessment

Acne can have psychological consequences that require treatment, so the collection of subjective data includes asking the adolescent how acne affects his or her lifestyle: Does it affect your participation in activities or group communication? Most patients acknowledge that acne affects their self-image. Common locations for acne lesions are the face and chin, which are highly visible areas. The number of lesions increases with emotional upsets and stress.

Collection of objective data includes noting the presence of edema in the involved area. Comedones (blackheads) are found on the skin of the face, back, or chest.

Diagnostic Tests

The medical diagnosis is made primarily by inspection of the lesions and a health history that supports the diagnosis.

Medical Management

Medical management can involve topical, systemic, or intralesional medications. The medications prescribed will cleanse, dry, reduce inflammation, reduce bacterial count, or reduce sebum production (Table 43.4). Women of childbearing age should receive counseling about

Table 43.4 Treatments for Acne Vulgaris

TREATMENT	APPLICATION	EFFECT	ADVERSE EFFECTS	COMMENTS
Retinoid therapies (tretinoin, adapalene, tazarotene)	Primarily topical for entire affected area	Reduces inflammation	Redness, burning, and sensitivity to sunlight Do not combine with OTC washes and medications	
isotretinoin (Accutane)	Oral	Reduces sebum production and abnormal keratinization of gland ducts	Destructive effect on fetal development Depression	Assess for: • Changes in behavior • Hepatotoxicity
benzoyl peroxide	Washes and soaps	Antimicrobial Reduces inflammation		
Antibiotic therapies (erythromycin, clindamycin, and tetracycline)	Oral	Reduce bacterial counts	Reduce effectiveness of oral contraceptives	Tetracycline may not be used for children under the age of 9 yr or for those who are pregnant or breastfeeding
Salicylic acid	Ointment	Reduces inflammation		
Hormone therapy (combination contraceptives containing estrogen and progestin)[a]	Oral	Reduces sebum production		
benzoyl peroxide medications	Topical, spot treatment	Dry skin lesions		

[a]Used only in females.
OTC, Over the counter.
Based on data from WebMD, 2017. Retrieved from *http://www.webmd.com/skin-problems-and-treatments/acne/acne-vulgaris-treatment-overview;* and Skidmore-Roth L: *Mosby's 2017 nursing reference,* ed. 30, St. Louis, 2016, Elsevier.

the need for reliable methods of contraception with some medications. Some of the therapies may be teratogenic to fetal development.

Nursing Interventions and Patient Teaching

When planning nursing interventions, consider the compliance of adolescents. Assess and consider what acne means to them. The actual extent of the condition is not as important as the adolescent's feelings. Appearance and acceptance by peers are important to the adolescent. Self-esteem may be hindered with acne.

In addition to psychological concerns, focus on preventive nursing interventions. The important areas are skin care, compliance, and emotional support. Prevention stresses identification of factors that directly exacerbate acne. Although poor hygiene may not be a cause, cleanliness decreases infection rate and promotes healing. The patient should keep the hands and hair away from the face, wear clothes that do not restrict affected areas, wash the hair daily, and wash the skin two or three times a day with medicated soap. Cosmetics must be water based. Improvement with the condition may take several weeks, making compliance difficult. Often 3 weeks of treatment are required before the patient, the family, or friends notice improvement (see the Health Promotion box).

Problem identification and interventions for the patient with acne vulgaris include but are not limited to the following:

Patient Problem	Nursing Interventions
Compromised Skin Integrity, related to occluded oil glands	Assess extent of occluded oil glands by inspecting lesions for size, color, and location Monitor for signs of infection Wash involved areas two or three times a day Apply medications to decrease occlusion of oil glands
Impaired Self-Esteem due to Current Situation, related to change in body image	Assess primary cause of low self-esteem and depth of feelings Assess family support Encourage verbalization of feelings about cosmetic appearance and ways to deal with the situation Observe nonverbal communication to discover patient's perception of the illness Stress the importance of not comparing oneself with others Have patient list current successes and strengths Give positive reinforcement

Health Promotion

Healthy Skin

- Adequate nutrition (fluids; protein; vitamins A, B complex, and C; iron; adequate calories; and unsaturated fatty acids) promotes healthy skin.
- Refrain from smoking to improve skin color and to prevent circulation difficulties.
- Drink eight glasses of water per day to help rid the skin of waste products.
- Exercise increases circulation and dilates blood vessels. Its psychological effects can improve one's appearance and mental outlook. Use caution to protect against overexposure to heat, cold, and sun during outdoor exercise.
- Wash the skin and hair often enough to remove excess oil and excretions and to prevent odor.
- The use of neutral soaps and avoidance of hot water and vigorous rubbing can noticeably decrease local irritation and inflammation.
- Older adults should avoid using harsh soaps and shampoos because of the increased dryness of their skin.
- Use moisturizers after bath or shower, while the skin is still damp, to seal in this moisture.
- Obesity has an adverse effect on the skin. Increased subcutaneous fat can lead to stretching and overheating. Overheating causes an increase in perspiring, which can impair normal or inflamed skin.

Teaching should center on the patient's physical and emotional needs. Address diet, hygiene, stress reduction, makeup, and medications. Coping skills may have to be retaught and counseling referrals made. The extensive treatment time should be covered in minute detail because this disease is chronic and exacerbations will occur. Helping the adolescent communicate about feelings will decrease any long-term effects that acne may have on his or her personality. The patient taking isotretinoin will develop dry skin; teach the patient measures to prevent it.

Prognosis

The prognosis for acne is good. However, lasting psychological effects can occur from the scarring that may result. In extreme cases eczema may develop from taking medications such as isotretinoin for acne.

PSORIASIS

Etiology and Pathophysiology

Psoriasis is a noninfectious skin disorder. It is a hereditary, chronic, proliferative disease involving the epidermis and can occur at any age. No specific predisposing factors are known. In psoriasis the skin cells divide much more rapidly than normal. The normal time for the entire skin to be replaced through sloughing and generation of new cells is 28 days; in psoriasis the time may decrease to 7 days. Severe scaling results from the rapid cell division.

Clinical Manifestations

The lesions appear as raised, erythematous, circumscribed, silvery scaling plaques. The primary lesion is papular. The papules become plaques, which are located on the scalp, the elbows, the chin, and the trunk (see Plaques in Table 43.1). The condition may be classified as mild, moderate, or severe.

Assessment

Subjective data initially include symptoms of mild pruritus. Patients sometimes express feelings of depression, frustration, and loneliness. They report that others stare and avoid contact with them, thus increasing their self-consciousness about their appearance.

Objective data include the observation of dull, erythematous, sharply outlined plaques covered with silvery scales on the elbows, the knees, and the scalp. Fingernails can be affected and show pitting with yellowish discoloration.

Diagnostic Tests

No specific diagnostic tests exist for psoriasis. Primary diagnosis is made by observing the patient and the signs displayed.

Medical Management

Medical management is aimed at slowing the proliferation of epithelial layers of the skin. Topical steroids and keratolytic agents are used in occlusive wet dressings to decrease inflammation. Keratolytic agents such as tar preparations and salicylic acid decrease shedding of the outer layer of the skin. Topical steroids used are hydrocortisone and betamethasone valerate (Valisone).

Another treatment, photochemotherapy, involves the use of a drug enhanced by exposure to light. This therapy combines methoxsalen (Oxsoralen), which is given orally, and the concurrent use of ultraviolet light A (UVA).

Methotrexate and vitamin D reduce epidermal proliferation in some cases. There are several systemic medications approved by the FDA to treat psoriasis, including methotrexate (an antimetabolite), cyclosporine (an immunosuppressant), and acitretin (a retinoid). Infliximab (Remicade) is an example of a biologic classification drug used to control the severe plaque form of the disease (National Psoriasis Foundation, 2016).

Nursing Interventions and Patient Teaching

Nursing interventions include proper administration of the therapeutic modality. Additional rest and measures to promote psychological well-being, such as counseling, are necessary. The patient's emotional needs are as important as the physical needs. Because this disease is chronic, encourage the patient to focus on positive attributes.

Problem identification and interventions for the patient with psoriasis include but are not limited to the following:

Patient Problem	Nursing Interventions
Compromised Skin Integrity, related to proliferation of epithelial cells	Assess extent of the scale Administer treatment method correctly Use medical aseptic technique
Impaired Self-Esteem due to Current Situation, related to change in body image	Assess patient's concept of body Help patient focus on positive aspects Discuss with patient ways to conceal obvious lesions
Social Seclusion, related to decreased self-esteem	Assess activity pattern and social outlets Demonstrate ways to conceal lesions with clothes Involve patient in a support group

The primary points in patient teaching include the nature of the disease, correct application of the therapeutic modality, and compliance with medical care. The patient should be taught about factors associated with exacerbation of the condition.

Prognosis

Psoriasis is a chronic disease. The clinical course is variable, but fewer than half of the patients have a prolonged remission. Severity ranges from a minimal cosmetic problem to a life-threatening emergency.

SYSTEMIC LUPUS ERYTHEMATOSUS

The Latin word for wolf, *"lupus,"* is used to describe the skin changes that resemble the erythema of a red wolf (Fig. 43.10). Discoid lupus is an inflammatory condition with skin manifestations that can lead to the autoimmune disease, systemic lupus erythematosus (SLE) (Lupus Foundation of America, 2017).

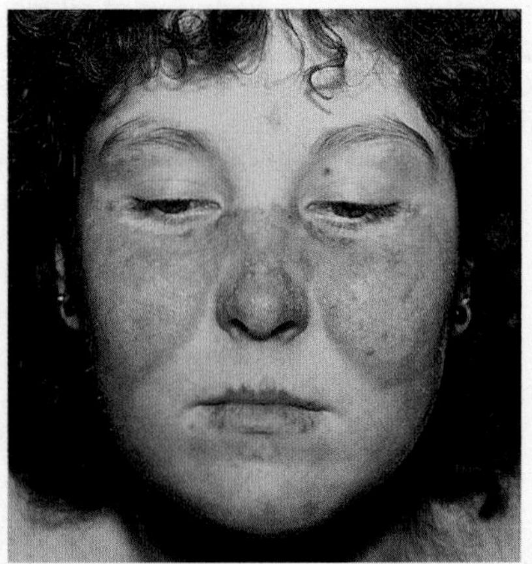

Fig. 43.10 Systemic lupus erythematosus flare. The classic butterfly rash occurs over the nose and cheek area in 10% to 50% of patients with acute cutaneous lupus erythematosus. (From Habif TP, Campbell JL Jr, Chapman MS, et al: *Skin disease: Diagnosis and treatment,* ed 3, St. Louis, 2011, Saunders.)

Etiology and Pathophysiology

SLE is an autoimmune disorder characterized by inflammation of almost any body part. It is a chronic, multisystem inflammatory disorder that occurs when the body produces antibodies against its own cells. The resulting antigen-antibody complexes damage connective tissues. SLE is a disease of exacerbations and remissions. It is distinguished by an inflammatory lesion that affects several organ systems: the skin, joints, kidneys, and serous membranes.

SLE is chronic and incurable, and it has multiple causes. Although the disease's origin remains unknown, increasing evidence suggests that immunologic, hormonal, genetic, and possibly viral factors may contribute to its onset. Genetic predisposition seems to play a role in most cases, coupled with a precipitating agent or factor. The person with SLE has a decreased number of T-suppressor cells, and the remaining T-suppressor cells have a limited function in antibodies developed against antigens.

SLE usually is found in women of childbearing age; only about 10% of cases are men. African Americans are three times more likely than whites to be affected. Survival rates have increased to more than 15 years from diagnosis. Despite advances in treatment, SLE remains a serious illness.

Clinical Manifestations

Clinical manifestations include oral ulcers, arthralgias or arthritis, vasculitis, rash, nephritis, pericarditis, synovitis, organic brain syndromes, peripheral neuropathies, anemia, leukopenia, thrombocytopenia, coagulopathies, immunosuppression, and dermatitis. Anemia tends to be the most common complication (Box 43.2).

Box 43.2 Pathogenic Conditions and Clinical Manifestations in Body Systems of People With Systemic Lupus Erythematosus

MUSCULOSKELETAL

Inflammation of vessels, tendons, and muscle tissue occurs because of deposits of fibrin. Polyarthralgia and polyarteritis occur in approximately 90% to 95% of patients.

GASTROINTESTINAL

Ulceration occurs on mucosal membranes because of degeneration of collagen tissue, with gastrointestinal manifestations of hemorrhage, abdominal pain, pancreatitis, cholecystitis, and bowel infarction.

RENAL

Glomerular sclerosis and glomerulonephritis occur with persistent proteinuria or cellular casts in urine.

HEMATOLOGIC

Cells are destroyed, and interference with coagulation occurs because of circulating antibodies. Anemia, leukopenia, lymphopenia, thrombocytopenia, and elevated erythrocyte sedimentation rate result.

CARDIOVASCULAR

Pericarditis is the most common cardiac manifestation. It often is the first clinical problem the patient manifests. Pericardial rub, commonly associated with pericarditis, can lead to dysrhythmias. Vasculitis in the small vessels may occur.

PULMONARY

Pleurisy and pleural effusions resulting from inflammation of the pleura are relatively common.

INTEGUMENTARY

Classic characteristics include the erythematous butterfly rash over the bridge of the nose and on the cheeks and linear erythema along the eyelids (see Fig. 43.10). Other features may include bullae, patchy areas of purpura, urticaria, and subcutaneous nodules.

NEUROLOGIC

Mental and neurologic signs and symptoms occur in 35% to 40% of patients with systemic lupus erythematosus. Signs and symptoms relate to the central nervous system, not to the peripheral nerves. Mental and behavioral changes may occur, as well as seizures, headaches, and strokes.

Diagnostic Tests

Diagnosis of SLE may require extensive evaluations over months or years. A detailed history, physical examination, and results of laboratory findings are required to confirm the diagnosis. Diagnostic tests for SLE (Box 43.3) often have positive results in the presence of inflammatory disease (Lupus Foundation of America, 2013; Mayo Clinic, 2014). No single test is considered conclusive for diagnostic purposes. However, positive results for one or more diagnostic tests along with at least three other criteria lead to the diagnosis of SLE. Criteria for diagnosis include the following:

- Alopecia (hair loss), with frontal alopecia seen more frequently in women
- Erythematous butterfly rash (see Fig. 43.10) over the nose and cheeks and along the eyelids
- Hematologic disorders, such as hemolytic anemia, leukopenia, lymphopenia, or thrombocytopenia without other diagnostic reasons
- Immunologic disorder identified with positive lupus erythematosus prep, antinuclear antibody (ANA), or double-stranded DNA
- Neurologic signs, such as seizures of unknown cause
- Oral ulcers
- Other skin features, including bullae, patchy areas of purpura, thickening of epidermis
- Photosensitivity
- Pleuritic pain, pleural effusion, pericarditis, and vasculitis
- Polyarthralgias and polyarthritis
- Positive ANA in the absence of patient use of drugs known to cause drug-induced lupus erythematosus
- Renal disorders as evidenced by protein or cellular casts in the urine

Box 43.3 Diagnostic Tests for Systemic Lupus Erythematosus

- Antinuclear antibody (ANA)
- Anti-Sm antibody
- Chest radiographic study
- Coagulation profile
- Complement
- Complete blood count (CBC)
- Coombs' test
- C-reactive protein (CRP)
- DNA antibody
- Erythrocyte sedimentation rate (ESR; not diagnostic, but used to monitor disease activity and effectiveness of therapy)
- Lupus erythematosus cell preparation (LE cell prep)
- Rapid plasma reagin (RPR)
- Rheumatoid factor (RF)
- Skin and renal biopsy
- Urinalysis

Medical Management

SLE treatment goals include relief of symptoms, remission of the disease, early alleviation of exacerbations, and prevention of untoward complications. Additional outcomes include therapeutic management of the signs and symptoms and suppression of inflammation.

Drug therapy includes nonsteroidal antiinflammatory agents such as acetylsalicylic acid (ASA; aspirin) and ibuprofen (Motrin), antimalarial drugs (hydroxychloroquine [Plaquenil] or chloroquine), and corticosteroids (such as prednisone) in low doses given several times a day. Methylprednisolone may be used intravenously in cases of exacerbation. Peak amounts of steroids help achieve remission. The steroid dosage is decreased slowly (tapered) until a maintenance dosage is reached. Topical corticosteroid creams are used to treat the distinctive SLE rash. Antineoplastic drugs such as azathioprine (Imuran) or chlorambucil (Leukeran) may be used to achieve remission or to control signs and symptoms.

Antimalarial drugs (e.g., hydroxychloroquine) are used to control discoid and other skin lesions and rheumatic manifestations. Because retinal toxicity may occur at high doses, patients should receive pretreatment and annual ophthalmic examinations.

Antiinfective agents are used to treat and to prevent infections in the patient with SLE. The specific antibiotic depends on the infection site. Urinary tract infections respond well to ciprofloxacin (Cipro).

Peritoneal dialysis or hemodialysis may be indicated in patients who have moderate to severe renal involvement. Laboratory tests assessing blood urea nitrogen (BUN) and serum creatinine provide information regarding kidney function. Analgesics and diuretics may be used to treat symptoms often found in patients with SLE. Supportive therapy such as a balanced diet, a balance between rest and activity, and reduced exposure to the sun also may be indicated.

Nursing Interventions and Patient Teaching

Because SLE is a multisymptom disease, a thorough assessment is indicated. Tailor the care plan to include (1) skin care, including teaching avoidance of direct sunlight and use of protective clothing and sunscreen; (2) a balance between rest and activity; (3) recognition of signs of exacerbation (i.e., fever, rash, cough, or increasing muscle and joint pain); (4) early recognition of signs and symptoms of infection; (5) stress reduction and management; and (6) balanced nutrition and reduced sodium intake. Because the disease is one of exacerbation and remission, each exacerbation will intensify the patient's stress and decrease his or her ability to cope. Provide psychosocial, emotional, and spiritual support for the patient.

The patient with an impaired immune system function must endure the consequences of chronic or incurable disease. A caring, gentle, and understanding approach to patient care will help reduce the burden and stress of SLE (Nursing Care Plan 43.2). The nurse's responsibilities in patient education are related to the information needed to help the patient live a normal life. Focus on activity level, prevention of infection, and potential complications.

Prognosis

SLE has no known cure. Management of the disease depends on the nature and severity of the manifestations and the organs affected. Early treatment of SLE contributes to a better prognosis.

PARASITIC DISEASES OF THE SKIN

PEDICULOSIS

Etiology and Pathophysiology

Pediculosis (lice infestation) is a parasitic disorder of the skin. Although the condition is commonly associated with poor living conditions and poor personal hygiene, these are not prerequisites; it can occur anywhere. Lice are transmitted by close contact with either infected individuals or their personal items such as hats, clothing, and grooming items. Once lice find a host, they seek blood. Lice can live only 1 to 2 days without a blood source. They leave their eggs (nits) on the skin surface, attached to hair shafts (Figs. 43.11 and 43.12; CDC, 2013).

Humans have three types of lice:

1. The head louse, causing pediculosis capitis
2. The body louse, causing pediculosis corporis
3. The pubic louse, causing pediculosis pubis

In pediculosis capitis, the head louse attaches itself to the hair shafts. The adult has a relatively short lifespan of 30 days. The adult female may lay up to 10 eggs per day. The eggs are visible at the back of the neck as gray, shiny, oval bodies.

In pediculosis corporis, the body louse is found around the neck, waist, and thighs. The louse generally is found in the seams of clothing and causes severe pruritus and pinpoint hemorrhages.

 Nursing Care Plan 43.2 **The Patient With Systemic Lupus Erythematosus**

Ms. T., age 34, is experiencing an acute exacerbation of systemic lupus erythematosus. She is admitted to the medical unit with severe joint pain, butterfly rash, generalized edema, and Sjögren's syndrome.

PATIENT PROBLEM

Compromised Skin Integrity, related to skin rash (butterfly across face), hair loss, skin atrophy, discoid lesions involving other parts of the body

Patient Goals and Expected Outcomes	Nursing Interventions	Evaluation and Rationale
Patient will verbalize understanding of skin care regimen and positioning schedule	Develop positioning schedule. Use appropriate devices such as air mattress, egg-crate mattress, sheepskin, or foam padding, where indicated.	Patient verbalizes understanding of the purpose of changing positions q 2 hr to prevent skin impairment.
Patient will demonstrate behaviors to promote skin healing	Assess and monitor skin and mucous membranes and describe lesions' size, characteristics, and changes noted. Assess nutritional status and areas at risk for pressure. Measure intake and output. Provide optimum nutrition.	Patient states she understands skin care regimen to promote skin healing.
Patient will experience improved wound and lesion healing	Monitor for signs of infection. Encourage patient to minimize sun exposure by wearing long-sleeved blouses or shirts and wide-brimmed hats and by using sunscreens with a sun protection factor of at least 15. Teach skin care maintenance.	Patient's skin lesions are beginning to show signs of healing.

PATIENT PROBLEM

Distorted Body Image, related to baldness and pathologic skin pattern conditions

Patient Goals and Expected Outcomes	Nursing Interventions	Evaluation and Rationale
Patient will verbalize understanding of altered body image	Assess patient's perception of body image; investigate what aspects are not pleasing and how she perceives changes as deviating from social norms.	Patient states she understands that skin changes and hair loss are part of the disease process of systemic lupus erythematosus.
Patient will have a positive, accepting, and realistic body image Patient will perform self-care activities within level of own ability	Teach patient ways to improve body image (e.g., improving personal hygiene, wearing makeup, changing type of clothes, protecting self from sun).	
Patient will identify personal community resources that can provide assistance	Encourage family members and significant others to maintain open communication with patient. Assess and document emotional status. Set limits on maladaptive behavior.	Patient talks about importance of open communication with her family and significant other concerning her feelings of body image disturbance.

CRITICAL THINKING QUESTIONS

1. Ms. T. has painful, edematous joints that greatly decrease her mobility. She has 4+ pitting edema to the lower extremities secondary to the loss of protein through her kidneys. What are the most appropriate nursing interventions to decrease Ms. T.'s pain level and to increase her mobility?
2. On entering the room, the nurse notes Ms. T. crying. She says that her lifestyle is severely altered because she is unable to be in the sun to work in her beloved garden. What nursing interventions would be most beneficial?
3. Ms. T. confides that she fears that this severe increase in her symptoms will lead to an early death. What initial response to this statement would be of greatest assistance?

The pubic louse, the parasite involved in pediculosis pubis, does not resemble the head or body louse. It looks like a crab with sharp pincers that attach to the pubic hair. Transmission can be through sexual contact or contact with infested bed linens or bath towels.

Clinical Manifestations

Nits or lice can be seen on the body. Pinpoint, raised red macules, pinpoint hemorrhages, and severe pruritus confirm the diagnosis. Excoriation is common because of the intense pruritus.

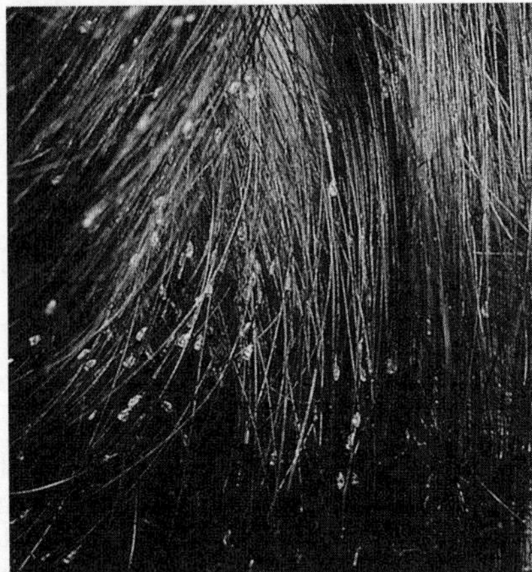

Fig. 43.11 Eggs of *Pediculus* (head lice) attached to shafts of hair. (From Baran R, Dawber RPR, Levene GM: *Color atlas of the hair, scalp, and nails*, St. Louis, 1991, Mosby.)

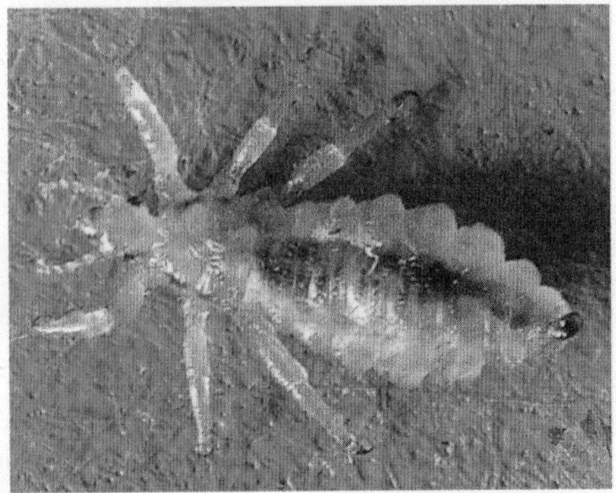

Fig. 43.12 Lice have six legs and are wingless. (From Habif TP: *Clinical dermatology*, ed 4r, St. Louis, 2004, Mosby.)

Assessment

Subjective data include complaints of pruritus in the area involved. Tenderness and difficulty wearing clothes also are noted.

Objective data include erythema, petechiae, and skin excoriation in the affected area.

Diagnostic Tests

The diagnostic test is a physical examination of the involved area. A health history supports the diagnosis. Removal of the parasite confirms the diagnosis.

Medical Management

Management may include over the counter (OTC) or prescription medications. Initial treatments traditionally begin with OTC preparations. Permethrin or pyrethrin with additives may be used. In the event the infestation is stubborn and repeated treatments are required prescription strength medications will be employed. Prescription medications include benzyl alcohol, malathion, and lindane. A topical pediculicide such as lindane or pyrethrin (RID) is applied to any contaminated area. The specific technique for applying these products varies and should be followed closely to eliminate lice. Once the lice-killing shampoos and rinses are used, the lice and nits will not simply fall off. They must be picked off, using a nit comb. The agents used to treat the conditions are pesticides. They cannot be used for children under the age of 2 years or for pregnant women. Occlusive (i.e., air- and water-tight) agents such as petroleum jelly are used to treat an infestation in these groups.

Nursing Interventions and Patient Teaching

The primary nursing intervention involves applying the medication to rid the patient of lice. Identify involved people and appropriate health teaching. Stress the nature and transmission of the disease. Assess each family member for nits, and teach measures to reduce pruritus, such as cool compresses and corticosteroid ointments. Furniture, carpeting, and car interiors also must be cleaned to prevent reinfection. Bed linens should be washed in hot water and dried in a dryer. Children's stuffed animals may be placed in a hot dryer for a full cycle. Items that cannot be washed may be isolated and bagged in plastic trash bags for a period of time, allowing the lice to die. Assessment of the patient's emotional needs is also important.

Prognosis

The prognosis is good; proper treatment results in full recovery.

SCABIES

Etiology and Pathophysiology

Scabies is caused by the human itch mite *(Sarcoptes scabiei)*. The mite penetrates the skin and makes a burrow. Once under the skin, the mite lays eggs that mature and rise to the skin surface. Scabies is transmitted most often by prolonged contact with an infected individual or contact with infected items such as clothing and bedding. Overcrowded living conditions, poverty, changing sexual behaviors, and world travel have increased the incidence of scabies. Scabies occurs in all age groups and socioeconomic classes.

Clinical Manifestations

Scabies causes wavy, brown, threadlike lines on the body, especially the hands, arms, body folds, and genitalia (see Table 43.1). Pruritus is severe, and secondary infections are common from the excoriation caused by scratching. The itching is more severe during the nighttime hours.

Assessment

Subjective data include the severe pruritus associated with scabies and the skin excoriation resulting from scratching.

Objective data include finding the wavy brown lines on the body and severe erythema from the scratching. The most common areas for the rash include the webbing between the fingers, wrists, elbows, arm pits, and waistline.

Diagnostic Tests

The condition is diagnosed most often by the presenting symptoms. Confirmation may involve a skin scraping, which may yield the mite.

Medical Management

Medical treatment attempts to eliminate the mite and prevent complications. Crotamiton (Eurax) and a 4% to 8% solution of sulfur in petrolatum may be prescribed to manage the condition. Treatment will also be extended to include sexual and other close contacts of the infected person. Treatment of pets is not necessary.

Nursing Interventions and Patient Teaching

Nursing interventions to restore skin integrity involve using medical aseptic techniques to improve hygiene and to apply medications. Proper application of medication is essential to destroy the parasite. The patient's emotional well-being is another focus of nursing care. Using open-ended questions and listening skills helps provide support.

A primary concern is to educate family members about the transmission of scabies. Each family member needs to treat the whole body with a scabicide. Clothing, bed linens, and bath articles should be washed in hot water and dried using the dryer's hot cycle. If clothes are line dried, they should be ironed. Stress the importance of compliance with the treatment. Parasitic infestations are often embarrassing and result in stress for the family. Conveying a nonjudgmental attitude is important.

Prognosis

The prognosis is good; with adequate treatment, full recovery results.

TUMORS OF THE SKIN

Overgrowth of the skin cells can develop from any layer or its appendages. Most skin tumors are benign. Outgrowths or tumors can be predisposing factors for skin cancer.

Etiology, Pathophysiology, and Clinical Manifestations

The specific signs and symptoms of skin tumors relate to the type of tumor. Keloids, which originate in scars, are hard and shiny. Angiomas resemble birthmarks. Warts (verrucae) are located on the arms and hands. Nevi are thought to predispose a person to cancer, and patients become anxious when they notice a color change. Skin cancers may be life threatening and occur wherever a patient's exposure to the sun was greatest.

Report any changes in a skin lesion to a health care provider, including changes in size, color, border, surface, or elevation. Also report the development of pain, bleeding, or pruritus.

Assessment

Subjective data should include a good health history. First assess the patient's risk factors, such as lifestyle, occupation, family history, and geographic location.

Objective data include observation of the lesion in detail. The size, the location, and any pain are significant factors in determining the type of skin tumor. The lesion's appearance can take several forms.

Diagnostic Tests

The diagnostic test for skin tumors is biopsy of the lesion. A health history and visual inspection support the diagnosis.

Medical Management

The primary medical intervention for skin tumors is surgical removal. Other treatment modalities are radiation therapy to reduce the size of the tumor and application of topical medications such as corticosteroids to decrease tumor size and inflammation.

Nursing Interventions and Patient Teaching

Patients are understandably concerned about the potential threat of malignancy. Careful explanations of treatments, medications, and tests help decrease anxiety. Nursing interventions center on preparing the patient for the treatment needed. Skin tumors may be a threat to the patient's self-image. Emotional care is important; encourage the patient to verbalize feelings of fear or anxiety.

Problem identification and interventions for malignant melanoma, discussed in an earlier section (see "Assessment of the Skin: Chief Complaint"), are applicable to most skin cancers. Although the tumors previously mentioned are not all malignant, the problems posed are the same until a definitive diagnosis is made.

Discharge instructions include skin care, dressing changes, and follow-up care. Involve the family in teaching so that they can support the patient. Discuss the signs and symptoms of infection with the patient who had a tumor surgically removed.

KELOIDS

Keloids (an overgrowth of collagenous scar tissue at the site of a skin wound) are seen more often in individuals of African descent than in whites. Collagen tissue becomes raised, hard, and shiny. The keloid may be red, pink, or flesh-colored. Keloids usually originate from a scar and can be located anywhere on the body (see Table 43.1). Individuals who are susceptible may develop keloid scarring with ear piercing, surgical intervention, or other injuries to the integument. Management options for the scarring may include corticosteroid injections, cryotherapy, laser surgery, radiation, or surgical removal. The keloid may recur at the same site. Enlargement with return is also a possibility.

ANGIOMAS

An angioma develops when a group of blood vessels dilate and form a tumor-like mass. A common angioma is a birthmark, such as the port-wine birthmark. This discoloration is not elevated and may be found on one side of the face or any part of the body. Treatment involves electrolysis or radiation.

A spider angioma, or telangiectasia, is associated with liver disease. A group of venous capillaries dilate and branch out like a spider. Spider angiomas usually resolve as the disease improves.

VERRUCA (WART)

A **verruca** is a benign, viral, warty skin lesion with a rough, papillomatous (nipple-like) growth pattern. Warts occur in many forms: they may occur singly or in groups and are thought to be contagious. Common locations are the hands, arms, and fingers, but warts can occur anywhere on the body. The plantar wart develops on the sole of the foot and is extremely painful. Treatment of warts depends on the type, location, and number. Cauterization, solid carbon dioxide (i.e., dry ice), liquid nitrogen, and preparations of salicylic acid are used to remove warts.

NEVI (MOLES)

Nevi (singular, *nevus*), or moles, are pigmented, congenital skin blemishes that are usually benign but may become cancerous. They are nonvascular tumors and also are called *birthmarks.* There are many types of nevi, and several may become malignant, especially if traumatized. The raised, black nevus is considered one of the most threatening, and removal is recommended to prevent it from becoming malignant. Any change in color, size, or texture or any bleeding or pruritus deserves investigation.

BASAL CELL CARCINOMA

Basal cell carcinoma is one type of skin cancer. Factors related to the development of skin cancer include frequent contact with certain chemicals, overexposure to the sun, and radiation treatment. Fair-skinned people are more likely to develop skin cancer, possibly because they have less melanin on the skin surface.

Basal cell carcinomas arise in the basal cell layer of the epidermis. They often are found on the face and upper trunk and may not be noticed by the patient. Metastasis is rare, but underlying tissue destruction can progress to include vital structures. Basal cell carcinoma is usually scaly in appearance. It may be a pearly papule with a central crater and waxy, pearly border.

With early detection and complete removal, the outcome is favorable; however, this type of cancer recurs in 40% to 50% of patients treated (Fig. 43.13).

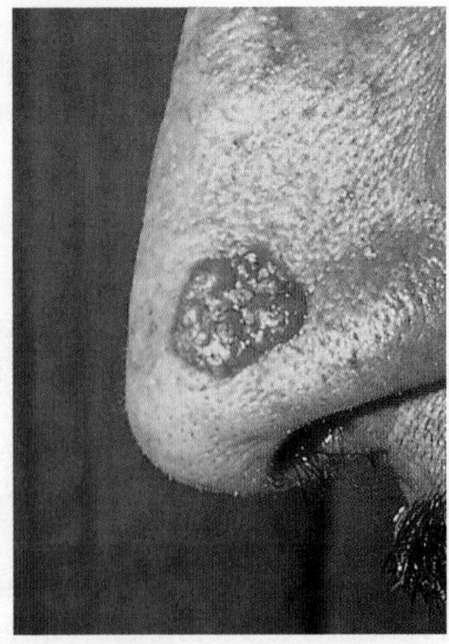

Fig. 43.13 Basal cell carcinoma. (From Belcher AE: *Cancer nursing,* St. Louis, 1992, Mosby.)

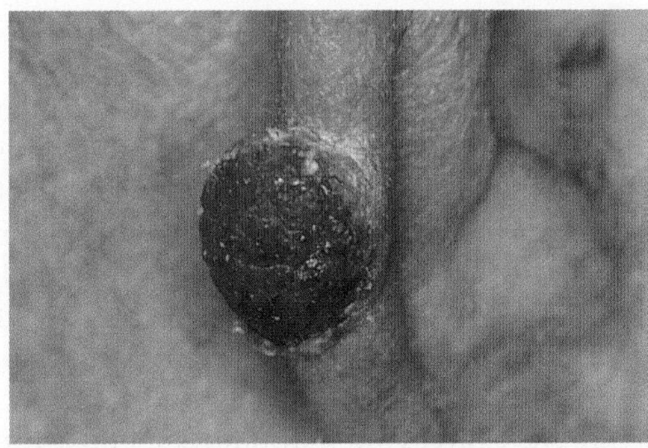

Fig. 43.14 Squamous cell carcinoma. (Courtesy Department of Dermatology, School of Medicine, University of Utah, Salt Lake City, Utah.)

SQUAMOUS CELL CARCINOMA

Squamous cell carcinoma arises in the epidermis. This cancerous neoplasm is a firm, nodular lesion topped with a crust or a central area of ulceration and indurated margins (Fig. 43.14). Ten percent of patients have rapid invasion with metastasis by way of the lymphatic system, so early detection and treatment are important. Larger tumors are more prone to metastasis.

Sun-exposed areas, especially the head, neck, and lower lip, are common places of occurrence. The cancer also occurs on sites of chronic irritation or injury (scars, irradiated skin, burns, and leg ulcers).

MALIGNANT MELANOMA

Etiology and Pathophysiology

A malignant melanoma is a cancerous neoplasm in which pigment cells (melanocytes) invade the epidermis, dermis, and sometimes the subcutaneous tissue. Several types of melanoma occur, and they are categorized by location and description. Most melanomas arise from melanocytes in the epidermis, but some may appear in preexisting moles. A melanoma can metastasize to any organ, including the brain and heart.

Melanoma is the most deadly skin cancer, and its incidence has doubled in the past two decades, a faster rate of growth compared with any other cancer (Fig. 43.15). The increased occurrence is associated with recreational exposure to the sun (see the Evidence-Based Practice box). Heredity is also a factor, and any person who has a large number of moles with a variety of sizes and colors should be monitored. The person with a history of skin cancer is at greater risk.

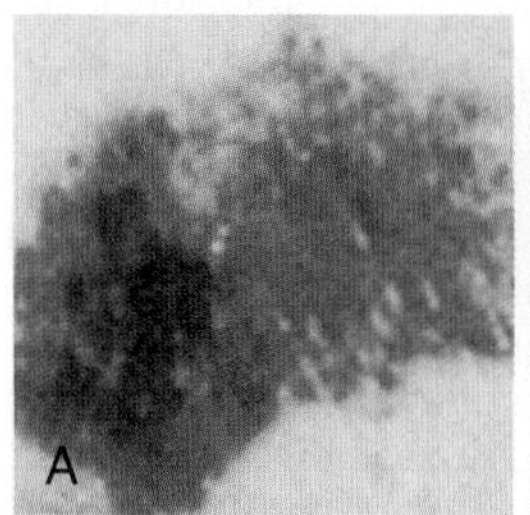

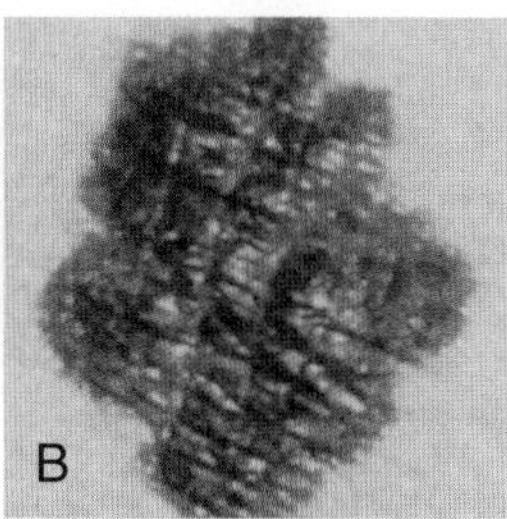

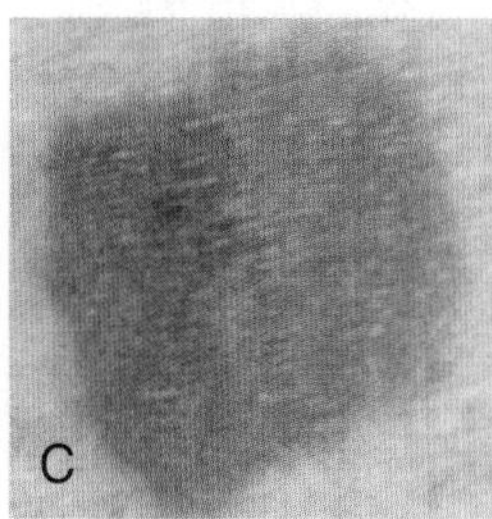

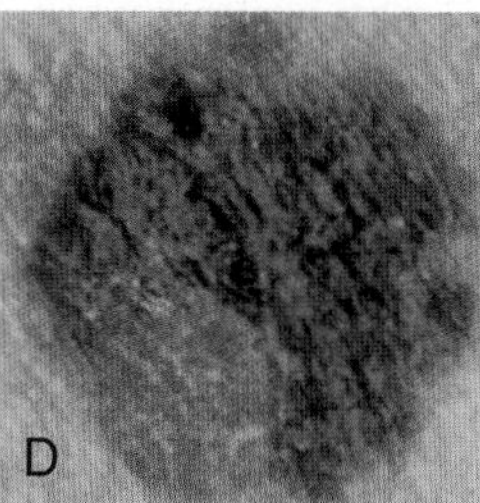

Fig. 43.15 The ABCDs of melanoma. A, Asymmetry (one half unlike the other). B, Border (irregularly scalloped or poorly circumscribed border). C, Color varied from one area to another; shades of tan and brown, black, and sometimes white, red, or blue; change in shape, size, or color of mole. D, Diameter larger than 6 mm as a rule (diameter of a pencil eraser). (From Habit TP: *Clinical dermatology,* ed 4, St. Louis, 2004, Mosby.)

Evidence-Based Practice

Skin Cancer Prevention

RESEARCH SUMMARY

What is cancer? More specifically, what is skin cancer? Cancer is an uncontrolled growth and spread of abnormal cells. Therefore skin cancer is characterized by abnormal skin cells, which can spread and invade other tissues. More importantly, what can we do about skin cancer? As nurses, it becomes our responsibility to assess for and educate our patients about all types of skin cancer, especially for the most serious form called melanoma. There are several risk factors for melanoma. The greatest risk is exposure to ultraviolet (UV) light. Additional factors include a family history of melanoma, a prior melanoma, and multiple or unusual moles. Other factors include a fair complexion/skin that is sensitive to the sun, and the use of tanning beds or booths.

Research has indicated that skin cancer, when detected early and treated properly, is highly curable. Overall survival rates for melanoma are 97% at 5 years and 95% at 10 years, so early intervention is of the utmost importance.

APPLICATION TO NURSING PRACTICE

The results of research studies have made it a nursing responsibility to screen patients and intervene when it is in their best interest. It is necessary that we promote self-screening for all patients and their family members. We also must educate the general public.

- Instruct patients to conduct a complete monthly self-examination of the skin and scalp, noting moles, blemishes, and birthmarks.
- Perform the examination after a bath or shower, including a head-to-toe check.
- Use a well-lit room and mirrors to examine all skin surfaces. If necessary, have the patient ask a family member/significant other to aid in the investigation.
- The American Cancer Society outlines the warning signs of skin cancer, using the ABCDE mnemonic: *A* is for Asymmetry—look for uneven shape; *B* is for Border irregularity—look for edges that are blurred, notched, or ragged; *C* is for Color—pigmentation is not uniform (blue, black, brown variegated and areas of pink, white, gray, blue, or red are abnormal); *D* is for Diameter—greater than the size of a typical pencil eraser; and *E* is for Evolving—in size, shape, or color.
- Teach your patients to contact their health care provider if a skin lesion or mole starts to bleed or ooze or feels different (swollen, hard, lumpy, itchy, or tender to the touch). Especially instruct older adults, who tend to have delayed wound healing.
- Inform your patients of ways to prevent skin cancer by avoiding overexposure to the sun:
  - Wear wide-brimmed hats and long sleeves.
  - Apply broad-spectrum sunscreens with a sun protection factor (SPF) of 15 or greater to protect against ultraviolet B (UVB) and ultraviolet A (UVA) rays approximately 15 minutes before going into the sun and after swimming or perspiring. Reapply every 2 hours.
  - Avoid tanning under the direct sun at midday (10 a.m. to 4 p.m.).
  - Do not use indoor sunlamps, tanning parlors, or tanning pills.
  - Inform patients who are on medications that make the skin more sensitive to the sun (e.g., oral contraceptives, antibiotics, antiinflammatories, antihypertensives, immunosuppressives) to take extra precautions when spending time in the sun.
  - Advise patients to protect their children from the sun. Severe sunburns in childhood greatly increase melanoma risk later in life.

These interventions will provide the patient with self-screening measures to detect, prevent, and seek early treatment for skin cancer.

Modified from Potter PA, Perry AG: *Fundamentals of nursing: Concepts, process, and practice,* ed 7, St. Louis, 2009, Mosby; American Cancer Society: *Cancer facts and figures 2006,* Atlanta, 2006, American Cancer Society; Hayes JL: Are you assessing for melanoma? *RN,* 66:36, 2003; Skin Cancer Foundation: Teacher resources, 2016. Retrieved from *https://www.skincancer.org.*

Clinical Manifestations

Malignant melanomas are divided into four primary types: (1) superficial spreading melanomas, (2) lentigo malignant melanomas, (3) nodular melanomas, and (4) acral lentiginous melanomas.

Superficial spreading melanomas are the most common and may occur anywhere on the body. These melanomas are slightly elevated, irregularly shaped lesions in varying hues; common colors are tan, brown, black, blue, gray, and pink. Lentigo malignant melanomas usually are found on the heads and necks of older adults. Characteristically these appear as tan, flat lesions that change in shape and size. Nodular melanomas appear as a blueberry-type growth, varying from blue-black to pink. The patient often describes the lesion as a blood blister that fails to resolve. Nodular melanomas grow and metastasize faster than the other types. Acral lentiginous melanomas occur in areas not exposed to sunlight and where no hair follicles are present. Common locations are the hands, the soles, and the mucous membranes of dark-skinned people.

Assessment

Subjective data should include a thorough health history related to skin cancer. Patients at greatest risk have fair complexions, blue eyes, red or blond hair, and freckles.

Objective data include the location, color, and appearance of the lesions.

Diagnostic Tests

Diagnosis depends primarily on the results of the tissue biopsy. The patient also is examined thoroughly for suspicious lesions. Monitor any lesion that is variegated in color, has an irregular border, or has an irregular surface. The tumor thickness at the time of diagnosis is a key factor in the prognosis of malignant melanoma.

Medical Management

Medical management depends on the site, level of invasion, thickness of the melanoma, and the patient's age and general health.

A wide surgical excision of the primary lesion with a margin of normal skin is the treatment of choice. Skin grafts sometimes are needed. Subsequent treatment modalities such as chemotherapy, nonspecific immunotherapy, chemoimmunotherapy, and radiation may be planned, depending on the stage of the disease.

Nursing Interventions and Patient Teaching

The major goals of nursing care include pain relief, reduction of anxiety, and palliative treatment of the disease. Fear of the unknown is a major concern for the patient with a melanoma. Explaining procedures and diagnostic tests in terms that the patient can understand may help decrease anxiety.

Problem identification and interventions for the patient with melanomas include but are not limited to the following:

Patient Problem	Nursing Interventions
Recent Onset of Pain, related to lesion	Use the mnemonic PQRST to assess the chief complaint[a] Provide nursing comfort measures, such as back rubs, to decrease pain Administer pain medication as needed Teach relaxation techniques
Anxiousness, related to cancer, its treatment, and prognosis	Listen to and accept expression of anger, sadness, and helplessness

[a]See "Assessment of the Skin: Chief Complaint" earlier in this chapter.

Discharge instructions include wound care, medication, cleansing, and follow-up care. Assess the family's knowledge about the seriousness and treatment of the disease. Explain to the patient the need for regular physical examinations and regular skin self-assessment. Encourage the patient to protect skin from the sun by using sunscreens and protective clothing and by limiting exposure. Stress the use of medical aseptic techniques to prevent a secondary infection.

Prognosis

The key prognostic factor in malignant melanoma is the thickness of the lesion. Individuals with lesions less than 1 mm thick have a survival rate of almost 100%, whereas those with lesions 3 mm thick or thicker have survival rates of less than 50%. If the cancer spreads to regional lymph nodes, the patient has a 50% 5-year survival rate. The tumor may metastasize by vascular or lymphatic spread, with rapid movement of melanoma cells to other parts of the body. If metastasis occurs, treatment is largely palliative (American Cancer Society, 2016; Melanoma Research Foundation, 2017).

DISORDERS OF THE APPENDAGES

ALOPECIA

Alopecia is the loss of hair. The cause can be aging, drugs such as antineoplastics, anxiety, or disease processes. Unless it is related to aging, alopecia is usually not permanent; the hair usually grows back but can take several months. Any time a patient loses hair, body image and self-esteem are threatened.

HYPERTRICHOSIS (HIRSUTISM)

Hypertrichosis is an excessive growth of hair in a masculine distribution. It can be hereditary or acquired as a result of hormone dysfunction and medications. Treatment is removal by dermabrasion, electrolysis, chemical depilation, shaving, tweezing, or rubbing with pumice. Treatment of the cause usually stops growth of additional hair.

HYPOTRICHOSIS

Hypotrichosis is the absence of hair or a decrease in hair growth. Skin disease, endocrine problems, and malnutrition are associated factors. Treatment involves identifying and treating the cause.

PARONYCHIA

Paronychia is a disorder of the nails. The nails get soft or brittle, and the shape can change as they grow into the soft tissue (ingrown nails). In paronychia, an infection of the nail develops and spreads around the nail, thus giving it the nickname "runaround." The nails are painful as they loosen and separate from the tissue. Wet dressings or topical antibiotics may be used. Sometimes a surgical incision and drainage of the infected area are performed.

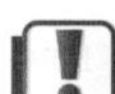

Safety Alert

Prevention of Burns

- The major cause of fires in the home is carelessness with cigarettes. Preventive education is imperative.
- Other causes of burns include hot water from water heaters set higher than 140°F (60°C), cooking accidents, space heaters, combustibles such as gasoline and charcoal lighter fluid, steam from radiators, and chemicals.
- Most burns can be prevented. The nurse is in a good position to conduct home safety assessments and to educate people about burn injuries before accidents occur. Home safety measures include using smoke alarms and fire extinguishers. Families should have fire drills, and each family member should know where to go and what to do in case of a fire.
- Local fire departments can inform the public of regional fire codes and perform home safety checks.
- Knowledge of potential sources of burn injury allows problem solving for burn prevention.

BURNS

Etiology and Pathophysiology

In 2016 approximately 486,000 people in the United States sought medical attention for burns. About 40,000 of them required hospitalization. The number of deaths from burn injuries or smoke inhalation was 3275 (American Burn Association, 2016). The survival rate for individuals admitted to burn facilities was 96.8% from 2005 to 2014 (American Burn Association, 2016). The high survival rate for burn patients stems from the creation of regional burn centers, as well as a national focus on fire safety, the use of smoke detectors, and occupational safety mandates.

Burns may result from thermal or nonthermal causes. Thermal burns are caused by flames, scalds, and thermal energy (heat) and are the most common type of burn injury. Nonthermal burns result from electricity, chemicals, and radiation. Skin destruction depends on the burning agent, the temperature of the burning agent, the condition of the skin before the injury, and the duration of the person's contact with the agent.

Teaching people the proper use of appliances (e.g., space heaters, electrical cords, wiring, outlets, outdoor grills, and water heaters) can prevent burn injury.

Burns cause dramatic changes in most physiologic functions of the body, beginning in the first few minutes to the first 12 to 24 hours after the burn injury. The burn's effect depends on two factors: the extent of the body surface burned and the depth of the burn injury. The extent of burn is measured in terms of the total body surface area (TBSA) injured. Burns exceeding 20% TBSA result in massive evaporative water losses and fluid loss into the interstitial spaces. Depth depends on the layers of the skin involved.

With any burn injury, a pathophysiologic process ensues. In the damaged area, the capillaries dilate, resulting in capillary hyperpermeability that lasts for about 24 hours. The increased cell permeability causes the fluid to shift from the capillaries into the surrounding tissues (interstitial spaces), resulting in edema and vesiculation (blistering). A larger burned area results in a more rapid shift of fluid from the intravascular area into the interstitial area (sometimes known as third spacing). This shift poses the greatest threat to life because the cells become dehydrated. As a result, the body experiences hypovolemic shock and hyperviscosity. Blood pressure and blood flow to the kidneys decrease, symptoms of hypovolemic shock develop, and acute renal failure may result.

The pathophysiology and care of burns may be divided into three stages:

Stage 1, the emergent phase, is from the onset of the injury until the patient stabilizes. Hypovolemic shock is the major concern for up to 48 hours after a major burn.

Stage 2, the intermediate or acute (or diuretic) phase, begins 48 to 72 hours after the burn injury. In this stage the greatest concern is circulatory overload. Circulatory overload may result from the fluid shift back from the interstitial spaces into the capillaries. The acute phase begins when the kidneys excrete large volumes of urine (hence the name diuretic stage).

Stage 3, the long-term rehabilitation phase, begins at the same time as burn wound treatment. In the third stage, the patient care outcome involves returning the patient to as normal a state as possible. A second outcome is freedom from wound infection.

In a burn injury, usually the greatest fluid loss occurs within the first 12 hours. The proteins, plasma, and electrolytes shift from the vascular compartment to the interstitial compartment. Red blood cells tend to remain in the vascular system, causing increased viscosity of the blood and a falsely elevated hematocrit level. Acute dehydration is present, and renal perfusion is seriously compromised. This fluid shift and the loss of intravascular fluids may lead to the development of burn shock. The rapid loss of fluid places a strain on the heart because the blood volume diminishes and the heart can no longer supply enough blood to perfuse the vital organs. The body responds by increasing the peripheral resistance. Burn shock is characterized by hypotension; decreased urinary output; increased pulse (tachycardia); rapid, shallow respirations (tachypnea); and restlessness. Most deaths from burns result directly from burn shock.

Fluids begin to shift back to the vascular compartment in approximately 48 to 72 hours. Fluid return denotes the end of the hypovolemic stage and the beginning of the diuretic stage. Reabsorption of the interstitial fluid back into the intravascular area causes an increase in blood volume. As the blood volume increases, the cardiac output increases, resulting in increased renal perfusion. The result includes diuresis. Rapid movement of fluid back into the intravascular space puts the patient at risk for fluid overload. Monitor the patient's vital signs, urinary output, and level of consciousness. Patients with preexisting cardiac problems, as well as the very young and very old, run the greatest risk for circulatory overload.

A burn victim may experience smoke inhalation damage from breathing the chemicals produced by the burn. The fumes damage the cilia and the mucosa of the respiratory tract. Alveolar surfactant decreases, and atelectasis can occur. Breathing difficulties may take several hours to appear. While assessing a patient who has sustained any burn to the upper chest, the neck, and the face, consider the patient at high risk for respiratory distress. Signs of respiratory difficulty include a hoarse voice or a productive cough. Other physical findings suggesting an inhalation injury include the following:

- Singed nasal hairs
- Agitation, tachypnea, flaring nostrils, or intercostal retractions
- Brassy cough, grunting, or guttural respiratory sounds
- Erythema or edema of the oropharynx or nasopharynx
- Sooty sputum

Clinical Manifestations

Traditionally, burns were classified as first, second, or third degree (Table 43.5). However, using only the visual characteristics of the burn wound results in an inaccurate description. A more accurate classification is superficial thickness injuries, partial-thickness injuries, and full-thickness injuries; these terms graphically describe the burn and indicate the depth and severity of the tissue injury (Figs. 43.16 to 43.18).

Assessment

The nursing assessment includes (1) depth of the burn, (2) causative agent, (3) temperature and duration of contact, and (4) skin thickness. The patient's age and other disease processes affect the outcome of the burn. The **rule of nines** determines the TBSA burned (Fig. 43.19). The rule of nines divides the body into multiples of nine. The entire head is 9%; the anterior and posterior aspects of the arms are a total of 9% each; the legs are 9% anterior and 9% posterior; the chest and back are 18% each; and the perineum is 1%.

NOTE: The rule of nines does not take into account the different levels of growth and is not accurate for children.

Subjective data include the causative agent, other diseases present, the temperature and duration of

Table 43.5 Causes and Factors Determining Depth of Burn Injury

DEPTH	CAUSE	APPEARANCE	COLOR	SENSATION
Superficial (first degree)	Flash flame, ultraviolet light (sunburn)	Dry, no vesicles Minimal or no edema Blanches with fingertip pressure, and refills when pressure is removed	Increased erythema	Painful
Partial thickness (second degree)	Contact with hot liquids or solids Flash flame to clothing Direct flame Chemicals Ultraviolet light	Large, moist vesicles that increase in size Blanches with fingertip pressure and refills when pressure is removed	Mottled with dull, white, tan, pink, or cherry red areas	Very painful
Full thickness (third degree)	Contact with hot liquids or solids Flame Chemicals Electrical contact	Dry with leathery eschar Charred vessels visible under eschar Vesicles rare, but thin-walled vesicles that do not increase in size may be present No blanching with pressure	White, charred, dark tan Black Red	Little or no pain Hair easily pulls out

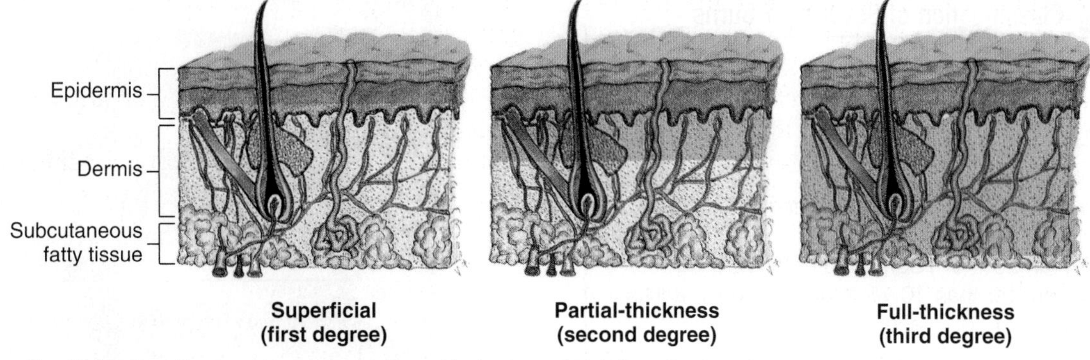

Fig. 43.16 Classification of burn depth. (From Hockenberry MJ, Wilson D: *Wong's nursing care of infants and children*, ed 8, St. Louis, 2007, Mosby.)

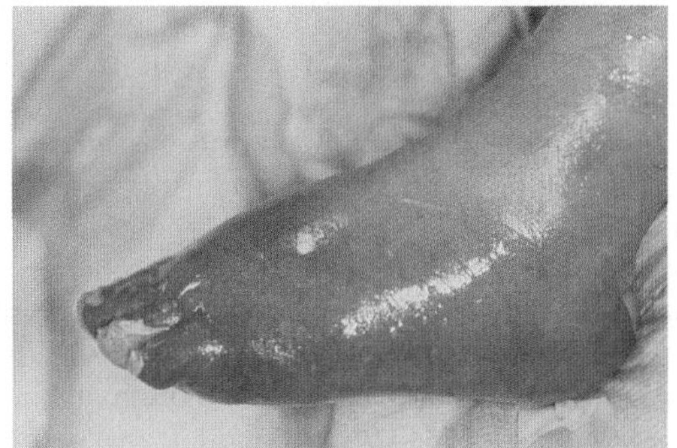

Fig. 43.17 Superficial partial-thickness injury. (Courtesy Intermountain Burn Center, University of Utah, Salt Lake City, Utah.)

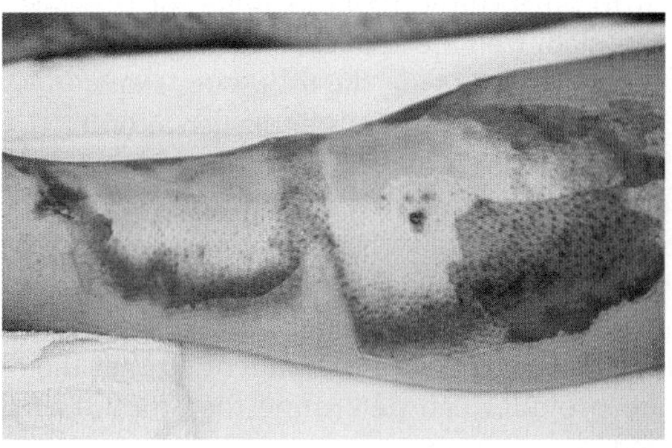

Fig. 43.18 Full-thickness thermal injury. (Courtesy Intermountain Burn Center, University of Utah, Salt Lake City, Utah.)

contact, and the patient's age. If the patient is able to communicate, ask him or her to rate the pain on a scale from 0 to 10.

Objective data include the depth of the burn, the skin thickness involved, the percentage of TBSA burned, the specific location, and any other injuries sustained. Any time a patient has a burn that involves the face, neck, or chest, observe for respiratory difficulty. Determine whether the victim has had a tetanus booster in the past 5 years.

The severity of the burn depends on several factors. Major burns require the most skilled nursing interventions. Moderate and minor burns require fewer nursing interventions. Factors determining a major, moderate, or minor burn are the (1) percentage of the TBSA burned,

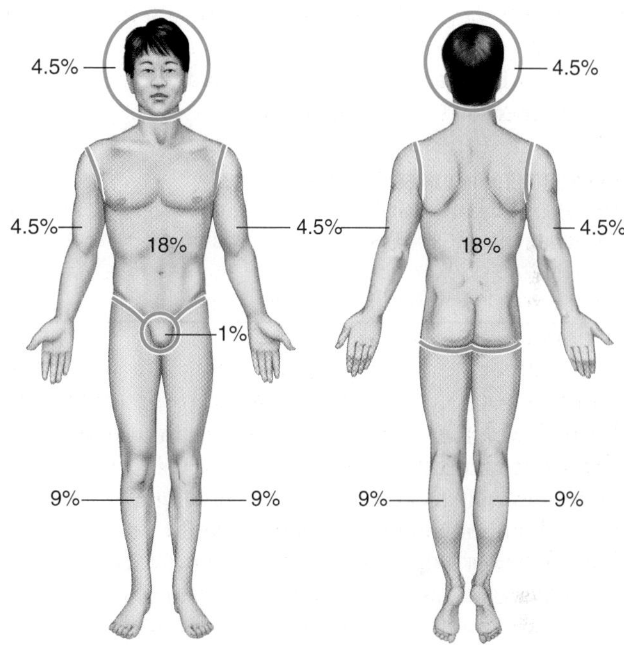

Fig. 43.19 Rule of nines. (From Patton KT, Thibodeau GA: *The human body in health and disease*, ed 7, St. Louis, 2018, Elsevier.)

(2) victim's age, (3) specific location of the burn, (4) cause of the burn, (5) other diseases present, (6) depth of the burn, and (7) injuries sustained during the burn (Box 43.4).

Diagnostic Tests

The primary diagnostic test is a physical examination to determine the amount of burned area. Blood assessments—such as those for electrolytes, CBC, serum chemistries, and arterial blood gases—may help establish the severity of dehydration. In inhalation burns, the carboxyhemoglobin level is evaluated. Most fatalities occur among survivors with severe asphyxiation or carbon monoxide intoxication. Carbon monoxide (CO) binds to hemoglobin with greater affinity than does oxygen, resulting in tissue hypoxia.

Medical Management

The medical treatment of burns is divided into three phases with differing priorities. Remember that these phases are not always clearly defined and may overlap.

Box 43.4 Classification of Severity of Burns

MAJOR BURN INJURIES

- Burns complicated by inhalation injury or major trauma
- Burns in patients with preexisting disease (diabetes, heart failure, or chronic renal failure)
- Electrical burns
- Greater than 10% of total body surface area (TBSA), full thickness
- Greater than 25% of TBSA (greater than 20% in children younger than 10 years of age, and in adults older than 40 years of age)
- Involvement of face, eyes, ears, hands, feet, perineum

MODERATE BURN INJURIES

- 15% to 25% TBSA in adults, partial thickness (10% to 20% TBSA in children younger 10 years of age and adults older than 40 years of age)
- Burns in patients with no preexisting disease
- Burns with no concurrent injury
- Less than 10% TBSA, full thickness

MINOR BURN INJURIES

- Burns in patients with no preexisting disease
- Less than 15% TBSA in adults (less than 10% in children or older adults)
- Less than 2% TBSA, full thickness

Emergent phase. The primary concern in the emergent phase is to stop the burning process, using the "stop, drop, and roll" technique. Also, removing clothing and shoes from the victim may eliminate the source of the burn to arrest skin damage. Do not apply ice to burns because it can cause rapid vasoconstriction, which may cause more trauma to the tissues by increasing the depth of the burn.

The second step is to provide an open airway; the third is to control bleeding. Fourth, remove all nonadherent clothing and jewelry (rings, watches). Fifth, cover the victim with a clean sheet or cloth. Sixth, transport the victim to the hospital. In the case of a chemical burn, it is important to rinse the skin generously with water to remove all chemicals. Electrical burns have an entry point and an exit point that must be identified. Most electrical burns result in cardiac arrest, and the patient requires cardiopulmonary resuscitation or astute cardiac monitoring.

During the primary survey assessment, quickly assess the ABCs (airway, breathing, and circulation) and look for life-threatening injuries, such as blunt chest trauma. Assessment of the patient's airway becomes and remains the priority of nursing care. Suspect an inhalation injury, especially if the burn occurred in a closed or confined area. Signs and symptoms of inhalation injury include singed facial hair, black-tinged sputum, soot in the throat, hoarseness, and neck or face burns. Stridor is a life-threatening sign.

Carbon monoxide (CO) poisoning is likely if the patient was in an enclosed area. CO displaces oxygen from hemoglobin. Do not rely on pulse oximetry to rule out CO poisoning. Oximeters cannot distinguish between oxyhemoglobin and carboxyhemoglobin. The carboxyhemoglobin level should be measured, when feasible, by means of a blood sample. Early signs of CO poisoning include headache, nausea, vomiting, and unsteady gait. Treatment includes administering 100% oxygen.

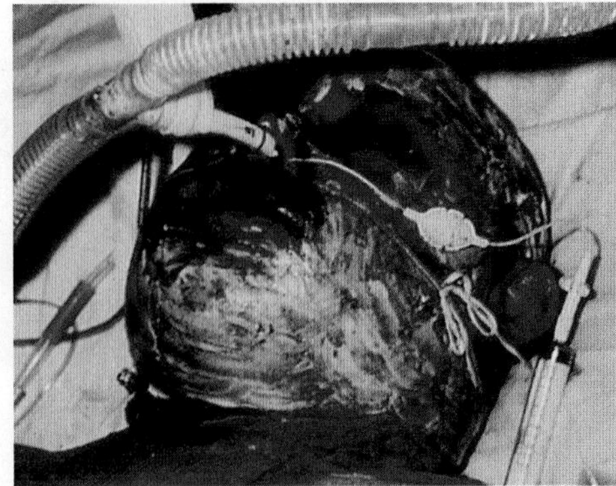

Fig. 43.20 Endotracheal intubation for patient with severe edema 5 hours after a burn injury. (Courtesy Burn Center, Cleveland Metropolitan General Hospital, Cleveland, Ohio.)

Once the patient is in the hospital, the severity of the burn dictates the care given. Perform a thorough assessment every 30 minutes to 1 hour in the emergent phase. Patients with major burns generally are transferred to burn care centers or units for treatment but must be stabilized first. Patients with moderate to severe burns are treated using the following steps:

1. Establish airway. Administer oxygen as ordered. Often the health care provider inserts an endotracheal tube to ensure a patent airway (Fig. 43.20).
2. Initiate fluid therapy. Begin intravenous fluid therapy with Ringer's lactate solution immediately. The amount of fluid given is related to the percentage of TBSA burned. Weigh the patient so that the health care provider can determine the amount of fluids needed.
3. Insert a Foley catheter to determine hourly urinary output. An hourly output of 30 to 50 mL is recommended. Intravenous fluids are given to maintain renal perfusion (Box 43.5).
4. Insert a nasogastric tube to prevent aspiration. Patients with severe burns often develop a paralytic ileus as a result of trauma.
5. Administer analgesics intravenously in small, frequent doses for pain control. Morphine may be used. Any degree of hypovolemia can increase the effects of medications. Carefully assess the patient's respiratory status when administering morphine.
6. Maintain airway and fluid status, and monitor vital signs.
7. Give tetanus immunization prophylaxis as needed. (Patients who have been immunized against tetanus do not need a tetanus toxoid booster unless the last injection was more than 5 years ago. If the patient

Box 43.5 Indications for Fluid Resuscitation

- Burns greater than 10% of total body surface area (TBSA) in children
- Burns greater than 20% of TBSA in adults
- Electrical burns
- Patient older than 55 or younger than 4 years of age
- Patient with preexisting disease that would reduce normal compensatory responses to minor hypovolemia (cardiac or pulmonary disease, diabetes)

has never had a tetanus immunization, administer tetanus serum and active immunization in the emergency department.)

The first 72 hours require diligent medical care. The primary goals in the emergent phase are to maintain respiratory integrity and to prevent hypovolemic shock, which may result in death (Box 43.6).

Acute phase. The acute phase begins when fluids shift back to the intravascular compartment, usually 72 hours after the burn. During the acute phase, the patient's metabolism increases. Urinary output also increases as the fluid shifts back into the blood circulation. As the urinary output increases, the edema in the tissues begins to decrease. The acute phase may last from 10 days to months. The two primary treatment goals are treatment of the burn wound and prevention and management of complications. Infection is the most common complication and cause of death after the first 72 hours. Other complications include heart failure, renal failure, **contractures** (shortening or tension of muscles that affects extension), paralytic ileus causing gastric dilation, and **Curling's ulcer** (a duodenal ulcer that develops 8 to 14 days after severe burns on the surface of the body; the first sign is usually vomiting of bright red blood).

Nursing interventions. Prioritizing nursing care, using the ABCs, remains the most important nursing intervention. After completing the ABCs, gather data in a head-to-toe assessment concerning (1) respiratory pattern, (2) vital signs, (3) circulation, (4) intake and output, (5) ambulation, (6) bowel sounds, (7) inspection of the wound itself, and (8) mental status.

Fluid-reshifting complications also may develop during the acute phase if renal damage has occurred. Monitor the patient for signs of acute renal failure such as elevated serum creatinine and BUN. Electrolyte levels also must be monitored closely. Serum potassium levels may rise sharply in the first 72 hours. Heart failure may develop as a result of the rapid increase in blood volume from the return of fluid from the interstitial spaces into the intravascular vessels. The primary goals in the acute phase include proper care of the burn wound to promote healing and prevent infection and the prevention and treatment of complications. Assessment for infection of the burn wound includes observing the wound for increasing erythema, odor, or a green or yellow exudate.

Box 43.6 Patient Problems Seen in the Emergent Phase of Burns

- *Compromised Skin Integrity, related to damage by the burns*
- *Compromised Swallowing Ability, related to mucosal edema*
- *Compromised Verbal Communication, related to breathing difficulties*
- *Inability to Clear Airway, related to edema of the respiratory passages*
- *Inadequate Fluid Volume (dehydration), related to shift of body fluids*
- *Inadequate Fluid Volume, related to capillary hyperpermeability with fluid moving out of the cells into the interstitial area*
- *Ineffective Sleep Pattern, related to hospital environment*
- *Insufficent Cardiac Output, related to hypovolemia*
- *Potential for Aspiration into Airway, related to decreased peristalsis*
- *Potential for Infection, related to impairment of skin integrity*
- *Recent Onset of Anxiousness, related to injury*
- *Recent Onset of Pain, related to loss of skin*

Local and systemic infections complicate recovery and increase recovery time. Wound cultures and sensitivities help pinpoint the type of organism present and the most effective antibiotic for treatment. Report any signs of an infection.

Once the patient's vital signs and urinary output stabilize and the acute phase begins, complete a nutritional assessment. Provision for adequate nutrition remains a cornerstone of burn care during the acute phase. Increased amounts of protein, calories, and vitamins help repair the damaged tissue; encourage oral intake of nutrients as soon as possible. The nutritional challenge includes providing enough nutrients to meet the body's increased metabolic requirement. Monitor nutritional status through daily measurement of weight, serum electrolytes, and serum albumin and through urinalysis. Adequate nutrition decreases healing time, whereas weight loss increases healing time. Skin grafts will not be successful unless nutrition is adequate.

Nursing interventions include measures to control pain and to support the patient's psychological well-being. Intravenous opioids in small, frequent doses provide relief from pain, but care must be taken to avoid jeopardizing respiratory integrity. Specific interventions include verbal support, unhurried care, truthful explanations, and effective listening. Excellent communication skills are essential.

Protective isolation is necessary when the skin is damaged. Wear a gown, mask, cap, and gloves during each contact with a patient with major burns. Follow strict surgical aseptic technique during dressing changes. Use of proper equipment and cleaning procedures is imperative. Hydrotherapy (e.g., whirlpool) can be a source of infection.

The standard treatment for partial-thickness burns includes débriding the wound, applying topical antibiotics, and changing dressings twice a day. A new treatment for burns includes temporary skin substitutes. Made from a variety of materials, skin substitutes promote faster healing for burn wounds and can eliminate painful dressing changes and minimize scarring. In 1997 TransCyte, a temporary bioengineered skin substitute, became the first such product to be approved by the FDA for burn treatment. TransCyte is designed as an alternative to silver sulfadiazine (Silvadene) for patients with partial-thickness burns and to cadaver skin for full-thickness burns and deep partial-thickness burns requiring surgical débridement. It is made from neonatal human fibroblast cells. The fibroblasts secrete human derma, collagen, matrix proteins, and growth factors. All these factors promote wound healing. TransCyte typically is applied only once, thus avoiding the frequent, painful dressing changes. TransCyte provides a temporary covering that helps protect against fluid loss and reduces the risk of infection.

A new and highly successful skin replacement therapy, based on the Integra Dermal Regeneration Template, is being used in the treatment of life-threatening, full-thickness, or deep partial-thickness burn wounds. Within the first few days of admission, the patient goes to surgery, the wound is débrided, and the Integra artificial skin is applied. The wound then is wrapped with dressings. The artificial skin stimulates regeneration of new dermis by the body. During a second surgical procedure, the artificial skin is removed and replaced by the patient's own autografts (US Food and Drug Administration, n.d.).

Traditional wound care involves the removal of the eschar that forms. **Eschar** is a black, leathery crust (i.e., a slough) that the body forms over burned tissue; eschar can harbor microorganisms and cause infection. It also may compromise circulatory status. An escharotomy often is done to relieve circulatory constriction (Fig. 43.21). Daily **débridement** (removal of damaged tissue and cellular debris from a wound or burn to prevent infection and to promote healing) and special cleansing support regeneration of the tissues. Hydrotherapy softens the eschar to make removal less painful. It also promotes range of motion to decrease contractures.

The specific wound care method depends on the severity of the burn. The open or exposure method may be used for burns of the face, neck, ears, and perineum. The area is cleaned and exposed to air. A hard crust forms, and regeneration of tissue follows.

Proper positioning and range-of-motion exercises (facilitated by the nurse and physical therapist) are vital for the burn patient's well-being. Special bed equipment is needed to prevent the burn from touching the linens. A bed cradle, a CircOlectric bed, or a Clinitron bed is recommended. Chilling may be controlled by keeping the room temperature at 85°F (29.4°C) and providing lights or heat lamps for additional warmth. Humidity should be between 40% and 50%.

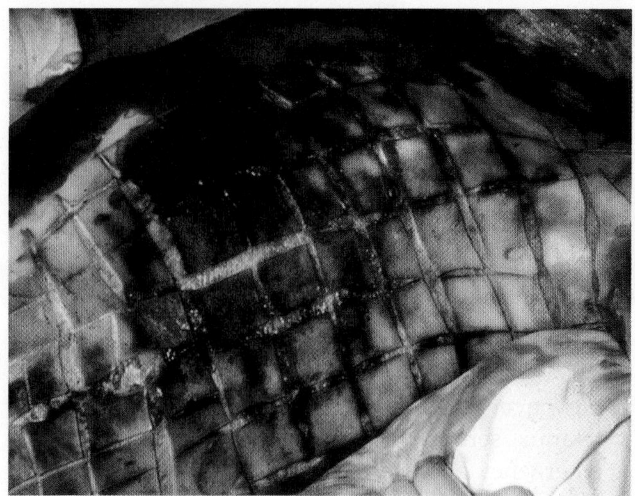

Fig. 43.21 Grid escharotomy used to alleviate circulatory and pulmonary constriction. (Courtesy Burn Center, Cleveland Metropolitan General Hospital, Cleveland, Ohio.)

Advantages to the open method are that (1) the wound can be observed more easily; (2) movement in bed is less restricted; (3) circulation of the body part is not restricted; and (4) exercises can be done more easily to prevent contractures. Disadvantages are (1) pain; (2) chilling; (3) contamination of wound by the health care provider; (4) unattractive appearance, which causes emotional distress; and (5) the need for protective isolation precautions for the immunocompromised patient.

Control the pain with intravenously administered opioids in the early days of the acute phase. Diazepam (Valium) has been found to be effective, but morphine commonly is used.

The closed (or occlusive) method involves cleaning the burn, applying the prescribed medication, and dressing the wound as ordered. Advantages of the closed method are that (1) it protects the burn area from injury and (2) it prevents contamination of the area by the health care provider. Circulation checks are important with pressure dressings to assess for adequate arterial perfusion to the involved areas.

The topical medications used to hasten healing and prevent infection vary. Topical administration is preferred because the capillaries are coagulated by the burn. Mafenide (Sulfamylon), silver sulfadiazine, and silver nitrate are drugs commonly used in burn care. Each drug has specific advantages and disadvantages (Table 43.6).

Burn care essentials include a lightweight dressing. A single layer of gauze covered with medication and a single wrap of Kerlix provide adequate coverage. When applying gauze to the burn area, place gauze between skin areas that touch to prevent skin-to-skin contact.

Table 43.6 Topical Medications for Burn Therapy Skin Grafts

GENERIC NAME (TRADE NAME)	ADVANTAGES	DISADVANTAGES
mafenide (Sulfamylon)	Bacteriostatic against gram-negative and gram-positive organisms Penetrates thick eschar	Metabolic acidosis Pain on application Allergic rash
silver sulfadiazine (Silvadene)	Broad antimicrobial activity against gram-negative, gram-positive, and *Candida* organisms No electrolyte imbalances Painless and somewhat soothing Not nephrotoxic	With repeated application, skin may develop slimy, grayish appearance, simulating an infection despite negative cultures Prolonged use may cause skin rash and depress granulocyte formation
silver nitrate	Bacteriostatic effect Lessens pain and eliminates odor Reduces evaporative water loss from burns	Electrolyte imbalances Stains everything it comes into contact with Does not penetrate eschar Pain on application
gentamicin sulfate	Broad antimicrobial activity Painless	Ototoxicity Nephrotoxicity Development of resistant bacterial strains
neomycin	Broad antimicrobial activity Causes miscoding in the messenger RNA of bacterial cells	Serious toxic effects Ototoxicity Nephrotoxicity
Xeroform	Nonantiseptic Débrides and protects donor site Protects graft	Removal may be painful because it sometimes adheres to wound Neither antiseptic nor antimicrobial
sodium hypochlorite (Dakin's solution)	Chlorine-based solution that is bactericidal Aids in debriding wounds Aids cleaning of copious drainage	Dissolves blood clots May inhibit clotting May irritate the skin
Sutilains ointment (Travase)	Topical enzymatic agent Dissolves necrotic tissue by proteolytic action Facilitates removal of eschar and purulent drainage	Mild, transient pain on application Paresthesia, bleeding, dermatitis Dressing must be kept moist at all times

RNA, Ribonucleic acid.
Based on data from WebMD, 2017. Retrieved from *http://www.webmd.com/skin-problems-and-treatments/acne/acne-vulgaris-treatment-overview;* and Skidmore-Roth L: *Mosby's 2017 nursing reference*, ed. 30, St. Louis, 2016, Elsevier.

Changing burn dressings is painful; therefore 30 minutes before the procedure, administer an analgesic, either 5 to 10 mg of intravenous morphine sulfate or a sedative. Most dressings are changed after hydrotherapy. Remove all old medication and eschar before applying any new medication. Failure to débride promotes infection, delays healing, and increases scarring.

Skin grafts are used as soon as possible to cover full-thickness burns. Grafting promotes healing and prevents infection. Grafting generally occurs during the first 3 weeks of care. Four types of grafts may be used:

1. An **autograft:** Surgical transplantation of any tissue from one part of the body to another location in the same patient
2. A **homograft (allograft):** The transfer of tissue between two genetically dissimilar individuals of the same species, such as a skin transplant from another person who is not an identical twin (often a cadaver)
3. A **heterograft (xenograft):** Tissue from another species, such as a pig or a cow, used as a temporary graft
4. A **synthetic graft substitute:** The autograft is permanent, whereas the other types are temporary

Grafts are applied by either the pedicle method (the tissue is left partially attached to the donor site and the other portion of the tissue is attached to the burn site) or the freestanding method (the tissue is removed completely from the donor site and is attached to the burn site) (Chrysopoulo, 2017).

Graft sites are a nursing challenge. Any movement that results in pulling the graft area can dislodge the graft. Do not change dressings until ordered. The donor site resembles a partial-thickness burn after the graft. Donor site care is as important as care of the burn site. Inspect the donor site for signs of infection, such as erythema and malodor (see the Patient Teaching box). Pain is a primary complaint after the graft and should be treated.

The nutritional aspect of burn care is another nursing challenge. Destroyed body proteins and fluid loss present problems as the body increases metabolism to meet the

Patient Teaching

Skin Grafts

- Do not remove dressing unless ordered.
- Keep surface of healed graft moistened daily with skin lotion for 6 to 12 months. (Grafted skin does not perspire; it dries and cracks easily.)
- Protect grafted skin from direct sunlight with a sunscreen lotion for at least 6 months.
- Report changes in the graft (hematoma, fluid collection) to health care provider.
- Wear a strong elastic stocking for 4 to 6 months for grafts on lower extremities.

extra demands for healing. Therefore the body requires enough energy to maintain homeostasis while meeting the increased need for repairing the injury.

Burn patients should eat by mouth as soon as their condition permits. Protein requirements are increased. Normal protein intake is usually 0.8 g/kg of body weight, whereas the burned patient requires 1.5 to 2.0 g/kg[5] of body weight. Thus a normal 150-lb person needs 55 g of protein per day; if burned, the same person needs 102 to 158 g of protein, depending on the extent of the burn. Daily caloric requirements range from 2000 to more than 6000 calories, depending on the burn. Meeting these enormous requirements requires diligent nursing interventions. Concentrated, high-calorie foods must be offered frequently. The body also requires additional amounts of vitamins A, B, and C to promote digestion, absorption, and repair of tissue. Increased amounts of calcium, zinc, magnesium, and iron are needed. Vitamin C and zinc aid in wound healing, and supplemental B complex vitamins help metabolize the extra protein and carbohydrate intake. Adding oral supplements such as Ensure and Sustacal can increase vitamin, mineral, and protein intake. Total parenteral nutrition provides an alternative to oral intake of proteins if the patient is unable to take in adequate nutrients by mouth (NutritionMD, n.d.).

Most burn victims have poor appetites and getting the patient to eat is difficult. Small, frequent feedings of high-calorie, high-protein, low-volume foods are the best way to meet the patient's nutritional needs. Some patients develop Curling's ulcer 8 to 14 days after the burn injury because of increased gastric acidity. The first sign is vomiting of bright red blood. The prophylactic treatment involves intravenous or oral administration of cimetidine (Tagamet), ranitidine (Zantac), omeprazole (Prilosec), or famotidine (Pepcid). Box 43.7 lists patient problems commonly seen during the acute phase of burns.

Rehabilitation phase. Rehabilitation of the burn patient begins at admission. However, the third phase of burn care begins when 20% or less of the TBSA remains burned. The goal becomes to promote independence so that the patient may have a productive life. The rehabilitation process addresses social and physical skills and may take years.

Mobility limitations constitute the major concerns. The patient requires a comprehensive physical therapy program for positioning, skin care, exercise, ambulation, and activities of daily living (ADLs). Contractures remain a concern in the care of a burn patient. Although physical therapists provide most of the rehabilitative care, the nurse helps to provide continuity of care. When planning the care, set realistic, short-term goals to motivate patients to try to achieve more.

Maintaining or restoring the patient's independence remains the primary rehabilitative goal. Given the possibility of a changed body image, encourage the patient to talk about fears and concerns. Working with others such as social workers and counselors, develop a holistic care plan to provide the comprehensive care needed. During visiting hours, assess family interactions. Helping the family cope with the changes in their loved one is a major nursing intervention.

Patient problems commonly seen with burn victims, as listed in Box 43.8, encompass family, patient, and social roles.

Box 43.7 Patient Problems Seen in the Acute Phase of Burns

- *Compromised Physical Mobility, related to burns*
- *Distorted Body Image, related to disfigurement from burns*
- *Fearfulness, related to chronic illness*
- *Helplessness, related to prolonged recovery and loss of income*
- *Impaired Coping, related to seriousness of injury*
- *Impaired Family Processes, related to long-term hospitalization*
- *Impaired Role Functioning*
- *Impaired Self-Care (in ADLs), related to area of burn involved*
- *Insufficient Diversional Activity, related to confinement during care*
- *Insufficient Knowledge in all areas, related to expected care*
- *Insufficient Nutrition: less than body requirements, related to increased metabolic demands*
- *Potential for Infection, related to open skin wounds*
- *Prolonged Pain, related to procedures performed*
- *Recent Onset of Anxiousness, related to change in body image*
- *Social Seclusion, related to perceived change in body image*

ADLs, Activities of daily living.

Patient Teaching

Before discharge, the burn patient and family need education. Provide written instructions that are complete, comprehensive, easy to understand, and realistic. Return demonstrations are the best way to determine that

Box 43.8 Patient Problems Seen in the Rehabilitation Phase of Burns

- *Anxiousness, related to role change*
- *Compromised Physical Mobility, related to splinting and dressings*
- *Distorted Body Image, related to scarring*
- *Excessive Demand on Primary Caregiver, related to prolonged recovery period*
- *Fearfulness, related to impending surgery*
- *Grief, related to loss of wellness*
- *Impaired Coping*
- *Impaired Coping, related to long-term rehabilitation*
- *Impaired Personal Identity, related to inability to return to previous lifestyle for prolonged period*
- *Impaired Self-Care* (in ADLs)
    - *Recent Onset of Pain*
    - *Lethargy or Malaise*
- *Inability to Clear Airway, related to edema of the respiratory passages*
- *Inability to Tolerate Activity, related to prolonged bed rest*
- *Insufficient Knowledge, related to impaired home maintenance management*
- *Post-Event Emotional Crisis, related to the cause of the burn*
- *Potential for Contractures or Muscle Atrophy, related to noncompliance*
- *Recent Onset of Pain*

ADLs, Activities of daily living.

learning has taken place. The major topics to cover are (1) wound care, (2) signs and symptoms of complications, (3) dressings, (4) exercises, (5) clothing, (6) ADLs, and (7) social skills (see the Home Care Considerations box).

Evaluation

Evaluation depends on meeting the stated goals. In evaluating the burn patient, ask the following questions:

- Can the patient take care of self?
- Can the patient ambulate without difficulty?
- Can the patient and family cope?
- Does the patient have contractures?
- Does the patient understand the treatment process?

Burn care is extensive, and the exact nursing interventions for each patient are individualized. Many times the patient must change vocation, and family relationships change. The degree of scarring—emotionally and physically—cannot be predicted; nor can the patient's acceptance by society.

Prognosis

The outcome for the patient with burns depends on the size of the burn; depth of the burn; the victim's age; the body part involved; the burning agent; and history of cardiac, pulmonary, endocrine, renal, or hepatic disease and other injuries sustained at the time of the burn.

Home Care Considerations

Burns

- Bathe twice a day with mild soap.
- Test the water temperature before getting into the shower because your skin is sensitive to extremes of hot and cold.
- Be certain to clean the tub well before each bath.
- If itching becomes severe, take a lukewarm bath with Alpha Keri lotion added to the bath water.
- Do not use lotions that contain lanolin or alcohol because they will cause blisters.
- Avoid direct sunlight. Wear light clothing to cover areas that have been burned because these areas burn easily.
- Discoloration and scarring are normal during healing. The color of the scar may remain red because of the healing process. Usually within 6 months to a year the scar loses its red color and becomes softer. Normal color to the area may take several months to return.
- Report to the health care provider:
    - Any signs of infection
    - Fever greater than 101°F (38.3°C)
    - Feeling of inability to cope

NURSING PROCESS FOR THE PATIENT WITH AN INTEGUMENTARY DISORDER

ASSESSMENT

Assessment of the skin is an important aspect of patient care. Skin changes can reflect specific skin disorders, but they also may alert the nurse to a systemic disorder. Skin assessment allows the identification of obvious and subtle changes in the patient's state of health. Effective skin assessment takes a critical eye and knowledge of the expected normal findings.

Because the skin usually is assessed at the same time as other body systems, nurses tend to underestimate the valuable information that can be obtained. Assessing the skin provides a baseline knowledge of the patient's hygiene measures, nutritional status, circulatory status, and sensory perception. The skin is the first line of defense against infection. Therefore ongoing assessment of the skin is important in the maintenance of health and the prevention of infection.

Assessment of the older adult can be challenging for the health care professional. Safe, effective patient care requires that the nurse understand the normal changes that occur with aging. The older patient population is growing, as are the opportunities for the student to assess the older patient (see the Lifespan Considerations box).

PATIENT PROBLEM

Assessment provides data to identify the patient's problems, strengths, potential complications, and learning needs. After defining the clinical problems, start formulating a care plan that meets the patient's needs,

Lifespan Considerations

Older Adults

Effects of Aging on the Integumentary System

- Physiologic changes make the skin of the older adult more fragile and susceptible to impairment.
- Aging changes include decreases in tissue fluid, subcutaneous fat, and sebaceous secretions, resulting in dryness, flaking, pruritus, loss of elasticity, altered turgor, and a wrinkled appearance.
- Hyperkeratotic changes are typically seen in the nails, which make them thick and difficult to care for. Podiatric care is recommended for older adults, particularly those with circulatory impairments and diabetes mellitus.
- Circulatory changes and decreased mobility increase the risk of senile purpura and decubitus ulcers.
- Significant hair and scalp changes can occur with aging:
  - Loss of pigmentation leading to graying
  - Decreased hair thickness or balding
  - Increased incidence of seborrheic dermatitis of the scalp requiring special care
  - Growth of facial hair on women, which can damage self-image
  - Localized clustering of melanocytes surrounded by areas of decreased pigmentation results in "age spots."
  - The incidence of basal and squamous cell carcinoma increases with age, particularly in individuals who have had excessive sun exposure. Inspect aging skin closely for changes in the appearance of moles or warts.

prioritizing problems from most to least important. Being able to prioritize nursing interventions contributes to a more predictable recovery for the patient. Possible clinical problems that should be considered for the patient with a skin disorder are as follows:

Patient Problem	Nursing Interventions
Anxiousness, related to altered appearance	Assess anxiety level every shift Observe verbal and nonverbal behavior Encourage the patient to share feelings Teach relaxation techniques
Recent Onset of Pain, related to loss of superficial skin layers	Assess patient for pain Initiate nursing measures to minimize or relieve pain
Insufficient Knowledge, related to cause of skin disorder	Assess patient for learning needs daily Involve patient in setting goals Use audiovisuals as teaching aids Evaluate patient's success
Potential for Infection, related to impaired skin integrity	Assess patient daily for risk factors such as abrasions, elevated white blood cell count, and temperature Implement nursing measures, such as using good hand hygiene and keeping patient's nails trimmed, to decrease risk factors
Insufficient Knowledge, related to treatment of pruritus	Assess factors contributing to pruritus Promote hydration of the skin by having patient avoid hot showers and apply emollients after bathing Encourage adequate fluid intake Implement nursing measures to decrease skin irritation, such as avoiding clothes made of rough weave Encourage patient to stop scratching by rubbing or applying pressure to the area Administer prescribed medications for pruritus such as corticosteroids and antihistamines
Potential for Trauma, related to excessive scratching	Assess onset and contributing factors of episodes of pruritus Encourage patient to stop scratching by rubbing or by applying pressure to the involved area
Social Seclusion, related to anticipated or actual response of others to disfiguring skin disorders	Encourage patient to discuss feelings of loneliness Identify available support systems to patient
Impaired Self-Esteem due to Current Situation, related to change in body image	Assess patient's feelings of self-worth by having patient describe feelings about self Implement nursing measures to assist patient in dealing with body image Accept feelings of anger or hostility from patient Suggest clothing to conceal changes in skin integrity

◆ EXPECTED OUTCOMES AND PLANNING

When planning patient care, look at the nursing diagnoses and establish the cause of the nursing problem. Determining the cause enables you to develop a care plan that includes nursing interventions to eliminate the cause if possible. Include the patient in this planning. Ascertain the patient's preferences and capabilities. Including the patient is one way to promote compliance. Most skin problems are chronic, and progress is often slow. Furthermore, many patients are older and require more time for healing.

Planning includes the development of realistic goals and outcomes that stem from the identified patient problems. Establish short- and long-term goals. Examples of measurable goals include the following:

Goal 1: Patient shows no signs of infection in abdominal wound as evidenced by the wound remaining free of erythema, purulent drainage, odor, and localized tenderness.

Goal 2: Patient is able to change dressing correctly as evidenced by the patient following the written guidelines during demonstration.

Goals should have a date when they will be evaluated. Failure to attain a goal means the nurse should reevaluate the chosen interventions and determine why the goals have not been met.

◆ IMPLEMENTATION

When providing nursing interventions related to the skin, (1) include ways to prevent skin problems, (2) provide education in home care management, and (3) provide safety tips for the patient. Patients with skin diseases usually are managed at home and need to be aware of the potential for infection because the skin is not intact (see Box 43.1 and the Home Care Considerations box).

Home Care Considerations

Home Care Guidelines for Baths and Soaks

- The water temperature should be comfortable, usually 90° to 100°F (32° to 38°C).
- Dissolve medication completely while tub is filling.
- The soak should last 20 to 30 minutes.
- When oils are added, assist the patient out of the water to prevent slipping.
- Pat the skin dry, rather than rubbing, to avoid skin irritation.
- Apply creams or ointments immediately after the bath to retain moisture.
- Drain water from the tub before the patient gets out.
- The door should not be locked, and a helper should be within hearing distance.
- Use a bath mat to prevent slipping.
- Hand rails may be needed in the shower or tub.
- A seat may be needed in the shower or tub.
- After a medicated bath, pour 1 cup of bleach into used tub water; let stand 5 minutes; wipe sides and bottom of tub; drain tub, and clean as usual.

Nursing measures for the skin include a variety of simple or complex interventions, including applying medications, dressings, and heat or cold application, and teaching the patient how to perform these measures at home. The principles of surgical and medical asepsis are important when providing nursing interventions. Incorporate nutritional guidelines for the patient to follow. Patients need extra nutrients, such as protein, for the building and repair of tissues.

Consider the patient's cultural beliefs, personal values, and economic resources when selecting the appropriate care. More people are using forms of treatment for integumentary disorders other than traditional medical therapy (see the Complementary and Alternative Therapies box). To promote compliance with planned treatment, consider the patient's independence, dignity, privacy, and physical strengths and limitations.

Complementary and Alternative Therapies

Integumentary Disorders

- The management of integumentary disorders is often difficult. Nutritional and herbal approaches to the treatment of skin problems have been shown to be effective for some disorders, often with fewer side effects than with conventional methods.
- Chinese herbs have long been used in Asian countries for the treatment of skin diseases. A landmark study in England showed the effectiveness of Chinese herbs in treating atopic dermatitis. This study was undertaken after dermatologists were impressed by the results in their patients who were also under the care of a Chinese herbalist. Participants in the study who received the active herbal formula reported decreases in the number of lesions and itching, as well as improved sleep.
- A traditional Australian plant remedy, tea tree oil (from *Melaleuca alternifolia*), has been effective in the treatment of acne.
- A topical mixture of the essential plant oils of thyme, rosemary, lavender, and cedarwood, in a carrier of jojoba and grapeseed oils, has been found to have significant effect in the treatment of alopecia areata.
- A published report from Taiwan states that acupuncture has been effective in the treatment of urticaria (hives).

From Sheehan MP, Rustin MH, Atherton DJ, et al: Efficacy of traditional Chinese herbal therapy in adult atopic dermatitis, *Lancet* 340:13–17, 1992.

◆ EVALUATION

During and after the planned nursing interventions, determine the outcomes. This is an ongoing process of continually trying to establish the most effective care plan.

Economic and home care implications are important. Patients are being discharged from the health care facility more quickly than in the past, and insurance companies are more selective in how they pay for the care and supplies the patient needs. Creativity and critical thinking are important skills to meet the needs of today's patient.

Evaluation involves determining whether the established goals have been met. The nurse and patient evaluate the goals to see whether the criteria for measurement have been met. For example, the goal is that the patient's wound would not become infected, as demonstrated by a lack of erythema, purulent drainage, and odor. If, at the end of the designated time frame, the wound shows no signs of infection, the goal has been met.

Get Ready for the NCLEX® Examination!

Key Points

- The skin, including nails, hair, and glands, makes up the integumentary system.
- The main functions of the integumentary system are protection, temperature regulation, and vitamin D synthesis.
- The two layers of true skin are the epidermis and dermis.
- The layer of tissue directly beneath the skin is the subcutaneous layer; it is composed of adipose tissue and loose connective tissue.
- The sudoriferous (sweat) glands release perspiration through the skin.
- The sebaceous (oil) glands secrete sebum, which lubricates the skin and prevents invasion of bacteria through the skin.
- Any injury to the skin poses a threat to a person's self-concept.
- It is important to establish a therapeutic relationship to meet the patient's psychological needs.
- Most skin disorders are not contagious and are rarely fatal. They are often chronic.
- Sterile technique and isolation techniques are required with any open, draining lesion.
- Wet dressings must be checked frequently. Constant moisture softens the skin and contributes to skin maceration.
- Medicines must be applied to clean skin.
- The nursing interventions for a skin disorder depend on the cause; however, common problems are decreased skin integrity, risk for infection, lack of knowledge concerning the disease, and ineffective coping.
- A primary nursing intervention is to teach the patient about the mode of transmission of the particular disease.
- The assessment of patients with skin disorders includes collection of subjective and objective data.
- Wet dressings and baths may be done to soothe, vasoconstrict, débride, or decrease pruritus.
- Before initiating heat and cold therapy, understand normal body responses to local temperature variations, assess the integrity of the body part, determine the patient's ability to sense temperature, and ensure proper operation of equipment.
- Prevent malignant skin diseases by educating the public about causes.
- Burns can be classified by depth and TBSA involved.
- The pathophysiology and care of burns involve three stages: the hypovolemic, or emergent, phase; the acute, or diuretic, phase; and the long-term, or rehabilitation, phase.
- The three phases of burn care overlap, with different goals and nursing interventions in each.
- A primary nursing intervention for the burn patient in the emergent phase is to establish and maintain an open airway.
- The treatment method for a burn patient depends on age, body surface area involved, location, depth, and other diseases present.
- The primary causes of death in burn victims are hypovolemic shock in the first 72 hours and infection during the acute phase.
- Suspect inhalation injury if the burn injury occurred in a closed or confined area.
- A treatment for burns is use of temporary skin substitutes derived from human fibroblast cells.

Additional Learning Resources

SG Go to your Study Guide for additional learning activities to help you master this chapter content.

evolve Be sure to visit the Evolve site at *http://evolve.elsevier.com/Cooper/foundationsadult/* for additional online resources.

Review Questions for the NCLEX® Examination

1. The health care provider has ordered oral griseofulvin for tinea capitis. The patient's mother asks the nurse why an oral medication is used rather than a cream. What information should be provided by the nurse?
   1. Topical creams do not reach the root of the hair to kill the fungus.
   2. Oral medications are more economical.
   3. Topical medications cause more pain when applied.
   4. It is more convenient to take the medication once a day rather than applying the cream once a day.
2. The nurse is caring for a patient with an open skin lesion. Which patient goal is the highest priority?
   1. The patient understands the treatment regimen.
   2. The patient does not develop an infection of the lesion.
   3. The patient voices concern regarding the appearance of the lesion.
   4. The patient seeks assistance for care of the lesion upon discharge.
3. Which of the following assessments should the nurse report to the health care provider immediately for an adult patient with partial-thickness burns over 25% of his body?
   1. Complaints of pain every 4 to 6 hours
   2. Decreasing appetite over the past 2 days
   3. Hourly urinary output of 10 to 15 mL
   4. Edema at the intravenous (IV) site
4. A patient has a rash on her back that began about 10 days ago with a raised, scaly border and a pink center. Now she has similar eruptions on both sides of her back. With what condition are these manifestations most consistent?
   1. Impetigo contagiosa
   2. Pityriasis rosea
   3. Contact dermatitis
   4. Infantile eczema

5. A patient complains of a burning pain on his lower thoracic area. On inspection, the area is found to be erythematous and edematous with a cluster of vesicles. What condition is most likely to be diagnosed?
   1. Herpes zoster
   2. Herpes simplex
   3. Varicella
   4. Impetigo
6. A patient states that he has basal cell carcinoma and is going to die. When planning the best response to make, the nurse should include what knowledge?
   1. Basal cell carcinoma is rarely terminal.
   2. Without proper medication it can result in melanoma.
   3. It is a hereditary disorder caused by decreased melanin.
   4. Treatment involves strong chemotherapeutic agents.
7. It is important to teach a patient the warning signs of skin cancer. Which characteristic(s) of a nevus is a warning sign of skin cancer? *(Select all that apply.)*
   1. Border irregularity
   2. Smooth surface
   3. Decreasing diameter
   4. Mole symmetry
   5. Delayed or prolonged lesional healing
8. A patient has an inhalation burn injury. Which is a medical emergency?
   1. Singed facial hair
   2. Neck or face burns
   3. Pallor
   4. Respiratory stridor
9. Which method of assessing burn size applies only to adults?
   1. Lund-Browder
   2. Rule of nines
   3. Parkland method
   4. Primary survey
10. The nurse just finished an assessment for a patient with systemic lupus erythematosus (SLE). Which clinical manifestation would the nurse expect to find? *(Select all that apply.)*
    1. Oral ulcers
    2. Urticaria
    3. Jaundice
    4. Diarrhea
    5. Erythematous rash over the nose and cheeks
11. The health care provider has scheduled a débridement for a patient who has partial-thickness burns on his chest and right upper leg. Which nursing intervention is most important?
    1. Ambulate the patient to increase the blood flow to the area.
    2. Administer an opioid analgesic intravenously before the débridement.
    3. Teach the patient to remove the old dressings, using clean technique.
    4. Explain to the patient that the procedure will be painful.
12. A patient is admitted with partial- and full-thickness burns on his right lower extremity. What is likely to be included in the plan of care initially?
    1. Closed dressing change every 3 hours
    2. Open dressing
    3. Temporary skin cover
    4. Incision and drainage of the wound
13. A patient is admitted with partial-thickness burns on his upper chest and face. What is the most important thing for the nurse to monitor in the patient on admission?
    1. Respiratory problems
    2. Burn shock
    3. Infection of the wound
    4. Cellulitis of the affected area
14. What should be included in the assessment of a patient with an electrical burn?
    1. Infection
    2. Cardiac irregularities
    3. Burn depth
    4. Hypovolemic shock
15. A patient is admitted with herpes zoster. The health care provider orders an antiviral medication to slow the progression of the virus. Which medication will the nurse administer?
    1. acyclovir (Zovirax)
    2. cefaclor
    3. acetaminophen (Tylenol)
    4. cimetidine (Tagamet)
16. A patient has been diagnosed with scabies. What does the nurse anticipate to assess with this patient? *(Select all that apply.)*
    1. Wavy brown lines on the skin
    2. Nocturnal pruritus
    3. Localized pain
    4. Skin paresthesia
    5. Hives
17. An adolescent patient is seen in the clinic with a mild case of acne. What does the nurse expect to assess?
    1. The patient reports a plan for suicide.
    2. The patient reports a sense of low self-esteem.
    3. The patient reports an increased intake of fatty foods.
    4. The patient reports a drastic change in weight.
18. A patient with thermal burns over 30% of his body has maintained a urinary output of 250 mL for the past 8 hours. What can the nurse infer from this information?
    1. Patient is not improving as expected
    2. Stage of hypovolemic burn shock is resolving
    3. Pain is decreasing
    4. Nutritional status is improving

19. A patient tells the nurse she has not gone out of the house for weeks because she could not cover the lesions on her face with makeup. What would be an appropriate patient problem?
    1. *Distorted Body Image, related to change in personal appearance*
    2. *Self-Protective Coping, related to lack of social contact*
    3. *Anxiousness, related to the fear of permanent disfigurement*
    4. *Inability to Tolerate Activity, related to lack of exercise*
20. When teaching a patient to care for herpes zoster lesions at home, which is the most important instruction for the nurse to provide?
    1. Clean the lesions with sterile saline daily.
    2. Wash hands before and after applying medication.
    3. Report to the health care provider when the lesions are crusted.
    4. Launder all clothes in vinegar.
21. The nurse is reviewing the history for a patient who has been admitted with cellulitis. Which condition(s) would predispose the patient to cellulitis? (*Select all that apply.)*
    1. Malnutrition
    2. Treatment with chemotherapy
    3. Venous insufficiency of the lower legs
    4. Idiopathic hypertension
    5. Diabetes mellitus
22. A parent tells the dermatologist that her daughter seems to be losing interest in school. Which medication could have caused the patient's change in behavior?
    1. isotretinoin
    2. minocycline (Minocin)
    3. tazarotene (Tazorac)
    4. penicillin
23. An African American patient is seen with impending shock after an accident. How would the nurse expect the skin to appear during the assessment of the patient?
    1. Ruddy blue
    2. Generalized pallor
    3. Ashen, gray, or dull
    4. Whitish, blue, or bright
24. The nurse planning the care for a patient who has impetigo expects to administer which topical drug to the patient?
    1. Acetaminophen
    2. Retapamulin
    3. Nystatin
    4. Corticosteroids
25. When teaching home care to a patient with recurrent genital herpes infection, it is important to include which information? *(Select all that apply.)*
    1. The infection is contagious only when lesions are visible.
    2. Antiviral agents are curative in the majority of cases.
    3. The patient will need to take antiviral agents daily for life.
    4. The patient will need to use protection even when no lesions are evident.
    5. Precautions for delivery must be made in the event of becoming pregnant.

Care of the Patient With a Musculoskeletal Disorder

44

http://evolve.elsevier.com/Cooper/foundationsadult/

Objectives

Anatomy and Physiology

1. List the five basic functions of the skeletal system.
2. List the two divisions of the skeleton.
3. Describe the location of major bones and muscles of the body.
4. List the types of body movements.
5. Describe three vital functions muscles perform when they contract.

Medical-Surgical

6. List diagnostic examinations for musculoskeletal function.
7. Compare medical and nursing care for patients suffering from gouty arthritis, rheumatoid arthritis, and osteoarthritis.
8. List at least four healthy lifestyle measures people can practice to reduce the risk of developing osteoporosis.
9. Describe the medical and nursing care for the patient undergoing a total hip or knee replacement.
10. Discuss nursing interventions for a patient with a fractured hip after open reduction with internal fixation and bipolar hip prosthesis (hemiarthroplasty).
11. Discuss the physiology of fracture healing (hematoma, granulation tissue, and callus formation).
12. Describe the signs and symptoms of compartment syndrome.
13. List nursing interventions for a fat embolism.
14. List at least two types of skin and skeletal traction.
15. Compare methods for assessing circulation, nerve damage, and infection in a patient who has a traumatic insult to the musculoskeletal system.
16. List four nursing interventions for bone cancer.
17. Describe the phenomenon of phantom pain.
18. Define lordosis, scoliosis, and kyphosis.

Key Terms

ankylosis (ăng-kĭ-LŌ-sĭs, p. 1342)
arthrocentesis (ăr-thrō-sĕn-TĒ-sĭs, p. 1334)
arthrodesis (ăr-thrō-DĒ-sĭs, p. 1352)
arthroplasty (ĂR-thrō-plăs-tē, p. 1352)
bipolar hip replacement (hemiarthroplasty) (hĕ-mē-ĂR-thrō-plăs-tē, p. 1358)
blanching test (p. 1387)
callus (p. 1362)
Colles' fracture (KŎL-ēz FRĂK-shŭr, p. 1361)
compartment syndrome (p. 1366)
crepitus (KRĔP-ĭ-tŭs, p. 1363)
fibromyalgia (fī-brō-mĭ-ĂL-jă, p. 1350)
kyphosis (kĭ-FŌ-sĭs, p. 1386)
lordosis (lŏr-DŌ-sĭs, p. 1386)
open reduction with internal fixation (ORIF) (p. 1363)
paresthesia (păr-ĕs-THĒ-zē-ă, p. 1378)
scoliosis (skō-lē-Ō-sĭs, p. 1386)
sequestrum (sĕ-KWĔS-trŭm, p. 1350)
subluxations (sŭb-lŭk-SĀ-shŭnz, p. 1379)
tophi (TŌ-fī, p. 1346)
Volkmann's contracture (VŎLK-mănz kŏn-TRĂK-shŭr, p. 1367)

ANATOMY AND PHYSIOLOGY OF THE MUSCULOSKELETAL SYSTEM

Bones and joints form the framework of the body, and muscles contract and relax to allow movement. All movement of the body is orchestrated by the functioning of the bones, the joints, and the muscles attached to the bones. This chapter discusses the structure and the function of bones and muscles and how they serve the body.

FUNCTIONS OF THE SKELETAL SYSTEM

The human skeletal system is composed of 206 bones and has five basic functions.

1. *Support:* The skeleton is the body framework that supports internal tissues and organs.
2. *Protection:* The skeleton forms a firm, cagelike structure that protects many internal structures. The cranium (skull) protects the brain, the vertebrae protect the

spinal cord, the ribs and the sternum (breastbone) protect the lungs and the heart, and the pelvis protects the digestive and reproductive organs.

3. *Movement:* Skeletal muscles are attached to the bones, which enables the bones to provide leverage for movement. As a muscle contracts, it pulls on the bone and movement occurs.
4. *Mineral storage:* The bones serve as a storage area for various minerals, particularly calcium and phosphorus. When the body's intake of these minerals is inadequate, the bones release the minerals.
5. *Hematopoiesis:* Hematopoiesis (blood cell formation) takes place in the red bone marrow. The red bone marrow is spongy bone found in the ends of the long bones. A child's bones contain a proportionately larger amount of red bone marrow than an adult's. As a person ages, much of the red bone marrow converts to yellow bone marrow, which is composed of fat cells.

STRUCTURE OF BONES

Bones are classified into four groups, based on their form and shape: long, short, flat, and irregular. Long bones are found in the extremities, short bones are found in the hands and feet, flat bones are found in the skull and sternum, and irregular bones make up the vertebrae (backbone).

ARTICULATIONS (JOINTS)

Bones cannot bend without damage. To allow movement, individual bones articulate (join) at joint sites (Fig. 44.1). Bones are held together by flexible connective tissue. The joint is the point of contact between the individual bones. The structure of the individual bones depends on the function of the area. Every bone in the body (except the hyoid bone, which anchors the tongue) connects, or articulates, with at least one other bone.

Joints perform two important functions: they hold the bones together to form the skeleton, and they allow movement and flexibility of the skeleton.

The most common way to classify joints is according to the degree of movement they permit. There are three types of joints:

1. *Synarthrosis:* No movement
2. *Amphiarthrosis:* Slight movement
3. *Diarthrosis:* Free movement

A goniometer measures the angle of a joint. It is used to determine the degree of joint mobility.

DIVISIONS OF THE SKELETON

The skeleton is divided into the axial and the appendicular skeletons (Box 44.1). The axial skeleton is composed of the skull, hyoid bone in the neck, vertebral column, and thorax (chest). The appendicular skeleton is composed of the upper extremities, lower extremities, shoulder girdle, and pelvic girdle (excluding the sacrum) (Fig. 44.2).

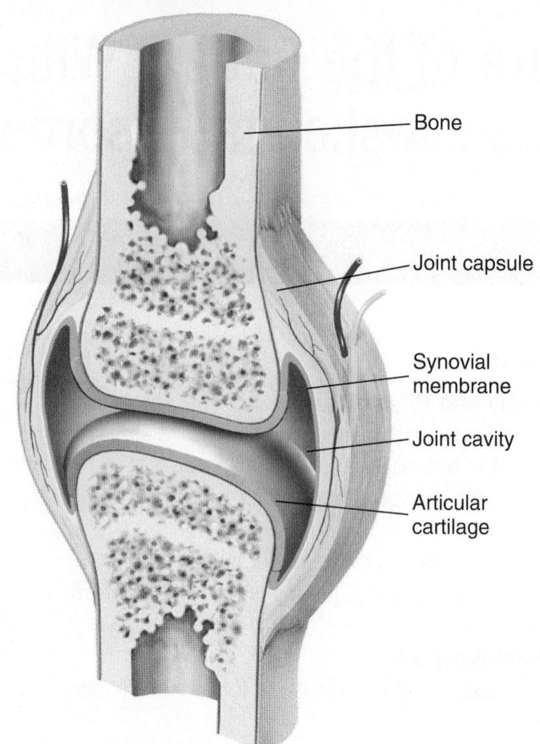

Fig. 44.1 Structure of a freely movable (diarthrotic) joint. Note these typical features: joint capsule, joint cavity lined with synovial membrane, and articular (hyaline) cartilage covering the end surfaces of the bones within the joint capsule. (From Patton KT, Thibodeau GA: *The human body in health and disease*, ed 7, St. Louis, 2018, Elsevier.)

Box 44.1 Main Parts of the Skeleton

AXIAL SKELETON	APPENDICULAR SKELETON
Skull	Upper extremities
• Cranium	• Shoulder (pectoral) girdle
• Ear bones	• Arms
• Face	• Wrists
Spine	• Hands
• Vertebrae	Lower extremities
Thorax	• Hip (pelvic girdle)
• Ribs	• Legs
• Sternum	• Ankles
	• Feet

FUNCTIONS OF THE MUSCULAR SYSTEM

The bones and joints provide the framework of the body, but the muscles are necessary for movement. This motion results from contraction and relaxation of the individual muscles. The body has more than 600 muscles, making up approximately 40% to 50% of the total body weight. They usually act in groups to execute a body movement (Table 44.1).

As muscles contract, they perform three vital functions: motion, maintenance of posture, and production of heat. Contraction also assists in return of venous blood and lymph to the right side of the heart.

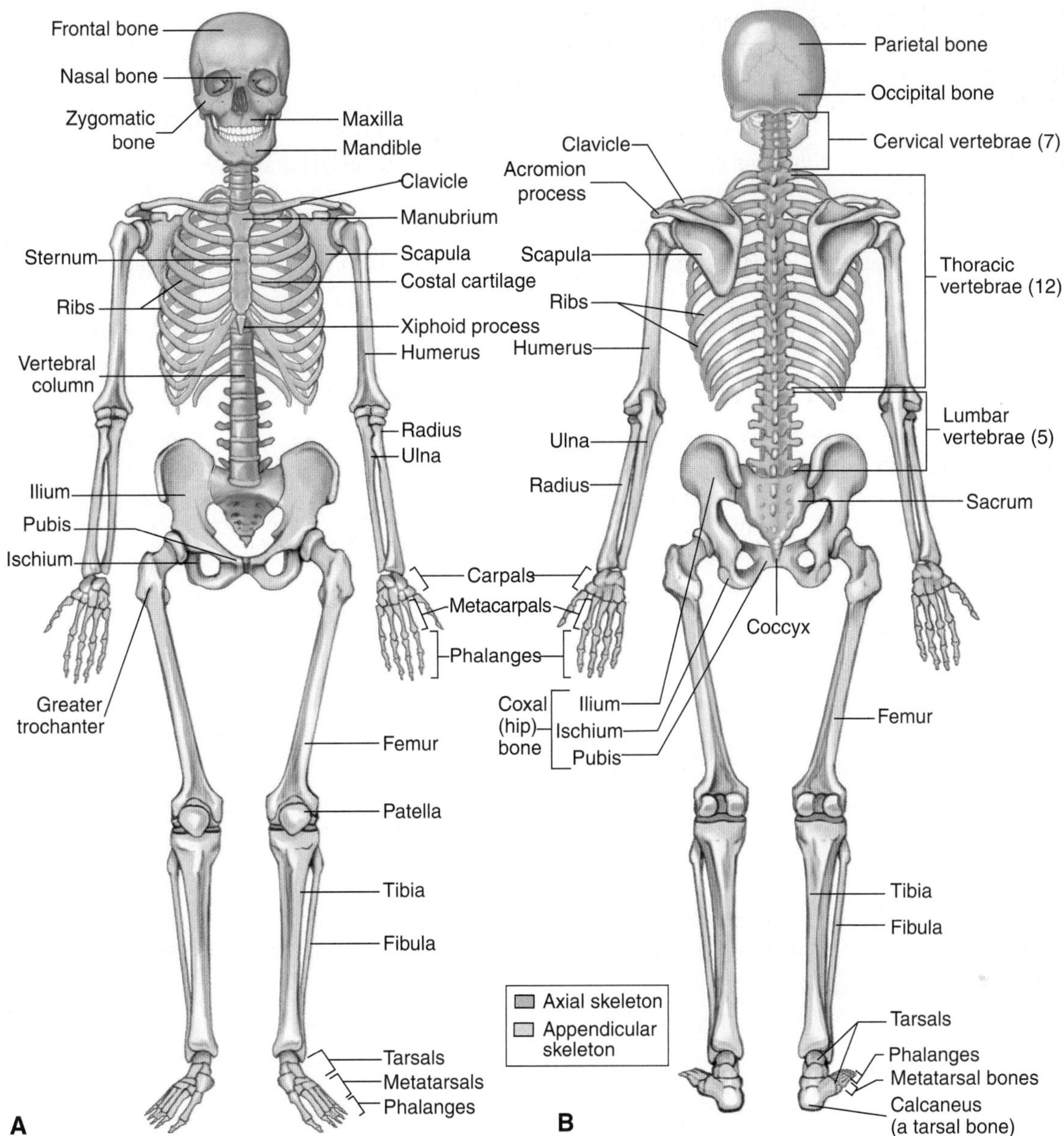

Fig. 44.2 Skeleton. Axial skeleton is shown in blue. Appendicular skeleton is bone colored. A, Anterior view. B, Posterior view. (From Patton KT, Thibodeau GA: *The human body in health and disease*, ed 7, St. Louis, 2018, Elsevier.)

All body movements rely on the integrated functioning of the bones, joints, and muscles. Muscle tissue is under voluntary or involuntary control. Voluntary muscle is under conscious control, whereas involuntary muscle tissue responds to internal commands without any conscious control of it. Involuntary motions include activities conducted by the internal organs, such as the heart beating, the gallbladder releasing bile, and the stomach churning food.

The contraction of certain skeletal muscles gives the body proper posture. These muscles pull on various bones, allowing the body to sit or stand.

As skeletal muscles contract, they produce body heat. Approximately 85% of all body heat is generated by the contraction of the skeletal muscles.

Skeletal Muscle Structure

A skeletal muscle is composed of hundreds of muscle fibers (cells). Each skeletal muscle is surrounded by a covering of connective tissue called the *epimysium.* The epimysium joins with two other inner coverings, the perimysium and the endomysium, and extends beyond the muscle to form a tough cord of connective tissue known as a *tendon.* Tendons anchor muscles to bones. As a muscle contracts, it pulls the corresponding tendon and bone toward it. This is how movement occurs. Tendons in the ankle and wrist are enclosed in *tendon sheaths,* which are sleeves or tubelike structures of connective tissue. Tendon sheaths contain synovial fluid and permit the tendons to slide easily; the sheaths also keep the tendons in place. All of the body's tendons,

Table 44.1 Principal Muscles of the Body

MUSCLE	FUNCTION	INSERTION	ORIGIN
Muscles of the Head and Neck			
Frontal	Raises eyebrow	Skin of eyebrow	Occipital bone
Orbicularis oculi	Closes eye	Maxilla and frontal bone	Maxilla and frontal bone (encircles eye)
Orbicularis oris	Draws lips together	Encircles lips	Encircles lips
Zygomaticus	Elevates corners of mouth and lips	Angle of mouth and upper lip	Zygomatic bone
Masseter	Closes jaw	Mandible	Zygomatic arch
Temporal	Closes jaw	Mandible	Temporal region of the skull
Sternocleidomastoid	Rotates and extends head	Mastoid process	Sternum and clavicle
Trapezius	Extends head and neck	Scapula	Skull and upper vertebrae
Muscles That Move the Upper Extremities			
Pectoralis major	Flexes and helps adduct upper arm	Humerus	Sternum, clavicle, and upper rib cartilages
Latissimus dorsi	Extends and helps adduct upper arm	Humerus	Vertebrae and ilium
Deltoid	Abducts upper arm	Humerus	Clavicle and scapula
Biceps brachii	Flexes lower arm	Radius	Ulna
Triceps brachii	Extends lower arm (called "boxer's muscle"—straightens the elbow when a blow is delivered)	Ulna	Scapula and humerus
Muscles of the Trunk			
External oblique	Compresses abdomen	Midline of abdomen	Lower thoracic cage
Internal oblique	Compresses abdomen	Midline of abdomen	Pelvis
Transversus abdominis	Compresses abdomen	Midline of abdomen	Ribs, vertebrae, and pelvis
Rectus abdominis	Flexes trunk	Lower ribcage	Pubis
Muscles That Move the Lower Extremities			
Iliopsoas	Flexes thigh or trunk	Ilium and vertebrae	Femur
Sartorius	Flexes thigh and rotates lower leg	Tibia	Ilium
Gluteus maximus	Extends thigh	Femur	Ilium, sacrum, and coccyx
Gluteus medius	Abducts thigh	Femur	Ilium
Adductor group			
• Adductor longus	Adducts thigh	Femur	Pubis
• Gracilis	Adducts thigh	Tibia	Pubis
• Pectineus	Adducts thigh	Femur	Pubis
Hamstring group			
• Semimembranosus	Flexes lower leg	Tibia	Ischium
• Semitendinosus	Flexes lower leg	Tibia	Ischium
• Biceps femoris	Flexes lower leg	Fibula	Ischium and femur
Quadriceps group			
• Rectus femoris	Extends lower leg	Tibia	Ischium
• Vastus lateralis, intermedius, and medialis	Extends lower leg	Tibia	Femur
Tibialis anterior	Dorsiflexes foot	Metatarsals (foot)	Tibia
Gastrocnemius	Plantar flexes foot	Calcaneus (heel)	Femur
Soleus	Plantar flexes foot	Calcaneus (heel)	Tibia and fibula
Peroneus group			
• Peroneus longus and brevis	Plantar flexes foot	Tarsals and metatarsals (ankle and foot)	Tibia and fibula

Table 44.2 Muscles Grouped According to Function

PART MOVED	FLEXORS	EXTENSORS	ABDUCTORS	ADDUCTORS
Upper arm	Pectoralis major	Latissimus dorsi	Deltoid and latissimus dorsi contracting together	Pectoralis major
Lower arm	Biceps brachii	Triceps brachii	None	None
Thigh	Iliopsoas and sartorius	Gluteus maximus	Gluteus medius	Adductor group
Lower leg	Hamstrings	Quadriceps group	None	None
Foot	Tibialis anterior	Gastrocnemius and soleus	Peroneus longus	Tibialis anterior

ligaments (which are like tendons, but anchoring bone to bone), and aponeuroses (very broad, flat, tendons) are composed of connective tissue in various sizes, shapes, and densities. These are known collectively as *fasciae.*

Nerve and Blood Supply

Because of the physical demands placed on the skeletal muscles, they need a constant supply of oxygen and nutrition. They are well supplied with blood vessels that carry oxygen and nutrition to the area and remove the waste products of metabolism.

The skeletal muscles are voluntary, so they need a constant source of information. Nerve cells or fibers continuously send impulses that stimulate the muscle cells. These impulses enter at the neuromuscular junction, the point of contact between the nerve ending and the muscle fiber. As a nerve impulse passes through this junction, chemicals are released that cause the muscle to contract.

Usually one artery, two veins, and one nerve penetrate a particular muscle. Each muscle cell comes in contact with several capillaries and a portion of a nerve cell. The muscle cells, in union with the nerve cell that controls them, are called a *motor unit.*

The impulse from the nerve cell must travel across a small gap because the nerve cell and the muscle cell do not directly touch each other. This small gap is called a *synaptic cleft* and is filled with tissue fluid. A special chemical *(neurotransmitter)* travels through the fluid to stimulate the muscle fiber. Acetylcholine is the neurotransmitter for skeletal muscle tissue. An enzyme called *cholinesterase* breaks down the acetylcholine once it has transferred the message. This allows the muscle cell to relax between impulses.

Muscle Contraction

Muscle stimulus. Muscle cells are governed by the "all or none" law; that is, when a muscle cell is stimulated or shocked adequately, it will contract completely. Because each skeletal muscle is composed of thousands of muscle cells that react to many different nerve cells, the muscle as a whole contracts according to the principle of graded response. The strength of the muscle contraction therefore depends on the number of individual muscle cells responding. These muscle responses allow us to tenderly brush a baby's cheek or swat an irritating mosquito.

Muscle tone. The skeletal muscles are in a constant state of readiness for action. At any given time, several muscle cells within a certain muscle are contracted and the remainder are relaxed. Muscle tone is necessary for good posture but does not provide movement. To understand the importance of muscle tone, observe an extremity that has become paralyzed; the muscles are flaccid, limp, or atrophied (wasted) and incapable of producing movement because the cells no longer receive stimuli from the nerve fibers.

Types of body movements. Some muscles can move some body parts in only two directions, whereas others can move certain body parts in several directions. The body's more common movements include flexion, extension, abduction, adduction, rotation, supination, pronation, dorsiflexion, and plantar flexion (Table 44.2, Box 44.2, and Fig. 44.3).

Skeletal Muscle Groups

Skeletal muscles usually are classified into two broad categories: axial and appendicular. The axial muscle groups are located on the head, face, neck, and trunk. The appendicular muscle groups are in the extremities. Fig. 44.4 shows the location of the muscles of the body.

LABORATORY AND DIAGNOSTIC EXAMINATIONS

RADIOGRAPHIC STUDIES

The diagnostic study frequently used for determining musculoskeletal system integrity is the radiographic, roentgenographic, or (as it is more commonly known) x-ray examination or diagnostic imaging.

A radiographic examination of a joint reveals fluid, irregularity of the joint with spur formation, or changes in the size of the joint contour. Radiographic examination is used to determine the presence of a skeletal fracture. To avoid potential damage to a growing fetus it is vital to ask women of childbearing age if there is any possibility that they are pregnant before performing x-ray examinations.

Laminography or *planography* (also called *body section roentgenography*) is useful in locating small cavities, foreign bodies, and lesions that are overshadowed by opaque structures.

Scanography, a method of producing a radiograph of internal body organs by means of a series of parallel beams that eliminate size distortion, allows accurate measurement of bone length.

Box 44.2 Types of Body Movement

- *Abduction:* A movement of an extremity away from the midline of the body.
- *Adduction:* A movement of an extremity toward the axis of the body.
- *Extension* (see Fig. 44.3): A movement allowed by certain joints of the skeleton that increases the angle between two adjoining bones. For example, extending the leg increases the angle between the femur and the tibia. If the extension angle is more than 180 degrees, the extremity is *hyperextended.*
- *Flexion:* A movement allowed by certain joints of the skeleton that decreases the angle between two adjoining bones. For example, bending the arm at the elbow decreases the angle between the humerus and the ulna.
- *Rotation:* A movement of a bone around its longitudinal axis (e.g., a pivot motion, such as shaking the head "no").
- *Supination:* A movement of the hand and forearm that causes the palm to face upward or forward.
- *Pronation:* A movement of the hand and forearm that causes the palm to face downward or backward.
- *Dorsiflexion:* A movement that causes the top of the foot to elevate or tilt upward.
- *Plantar flexion:* A movement that causes the bottom of the foot to be directed downward.

Myelogram

Myelographic examination involves injection of a radiopaque dye into the subarachnoid space at the lumbar spine to x-ray the spinal cord and the vertebral column. It is used to detect structural disorders such as a herniated disk, tumors, or the presence of infection. The test involves the same procedure as a lumbar puncture (spinal tap), which is discussed in Chapter 54. Contrast medium may be used. Assess for a history of allergies to iodine or seafood. Allergies of this nature cause reactions to the contrast medium. Notify the health care provider if any allergies exist. The examination can be performed without the use of contrast medium.

This examination may involve the entire spine or just the cervical or lumbar area. After the myelogram has been obtained, the dye, if oil-based, is removed through the spinal needle to prevent meningeal irritation. Water-soluble dye is used most often and does not have to be removed; the body absorbs it and excretes it in the urine. Inform the patient that the test is performed with the patient on a tilting table that is moved during the test to allow contrast medium to flow up to the cervical area.

The most common discomfort after a myelogram is headache. If water-soluble dye is used, the patient should lie quietly in a semi-Fowler's position for approximately 8 hours. Patient positioning is important to keep the dye in the lower spine. During this time, encouraging fluid consumption helps the body absorb the dye from the spinal column. If oil-based dye is used, the patient rests in a flat position for up to 12 hours. Tell the patient to inform the nurse if he or she has a headache, stiff neck, leg weakness, or difficulty voiding. Rare complications include seizure, infection, drowsiness, severe headache, numbness, and paralysis.

Patients needing a myelogram may express concern that the needle insertion may damage the spinal cord. Provide instructions to the patient explaining that the

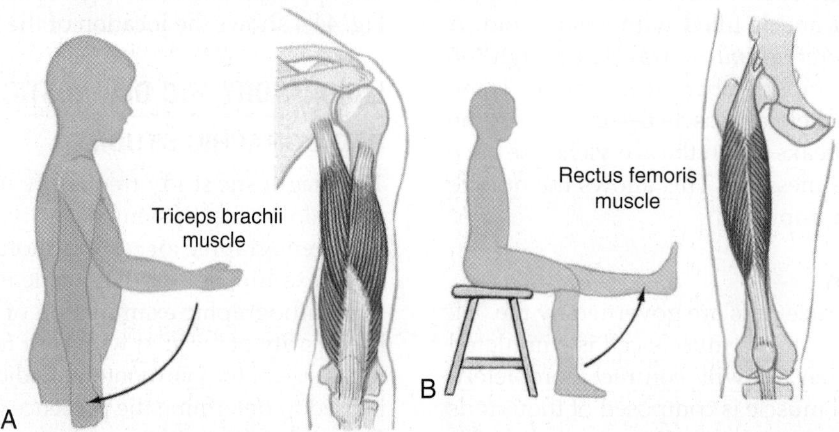

Fig. 44.3 Extension of the lower arm and lower leg. A, When the triceps brachii muscle *(right)* contracts, it extends the lower arm at the elbow joint *(left).* B, When the rectus femoris muscle (part of the quadriceps femoris muscle group) *(right)* contracts, it extends the lower leg at the knee joint *(left).* (From Thibodeau GA, Patton KT: *Structure and function of the body*, ed 13, St. Louis, 2008, Mosby.)

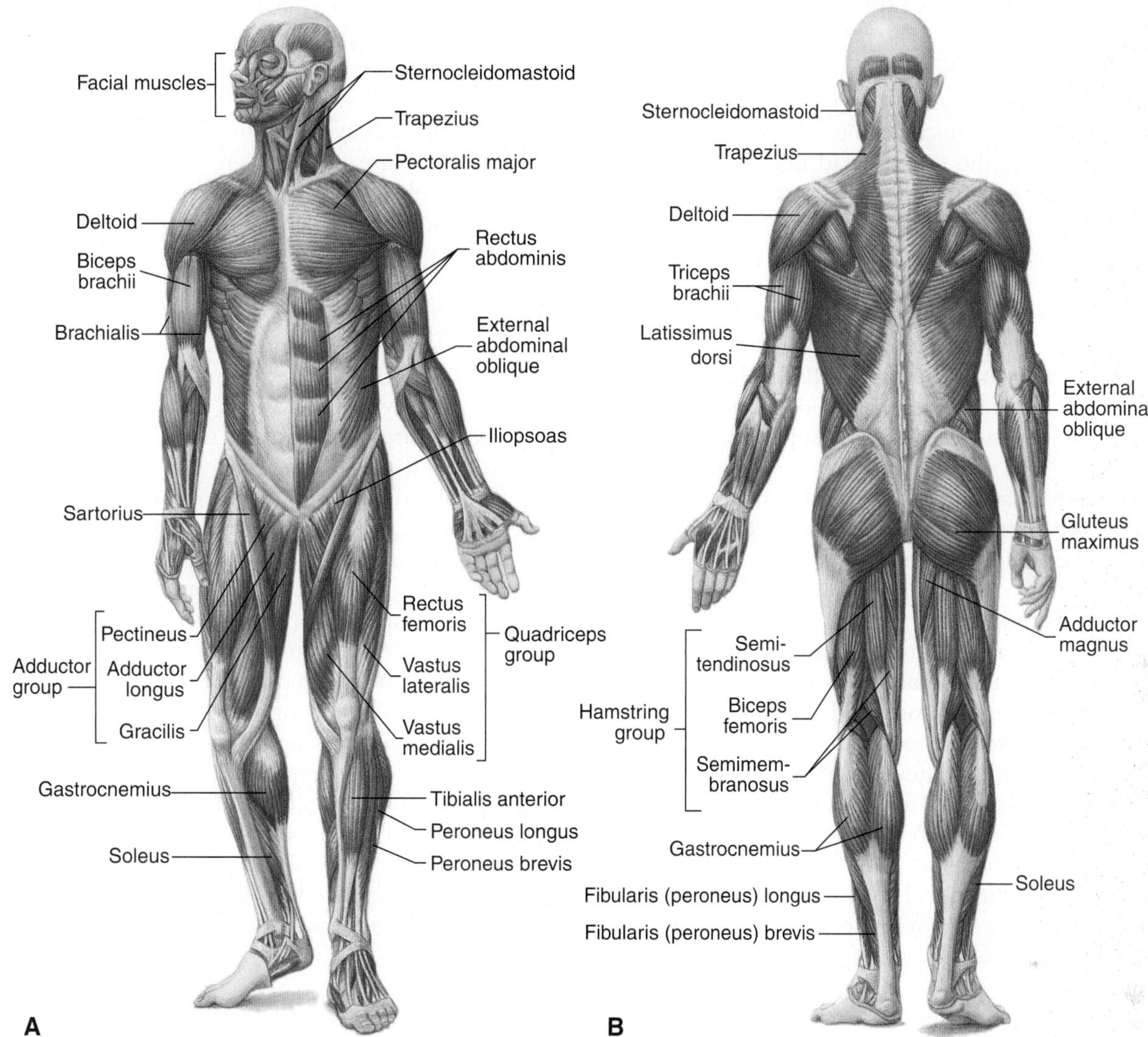

Fig. 44.4 A, Anterior view of the body. B, Posterior view of the body. (From Patton KT, Thibodeau GA: *The human body in health and disease*, ed 6, St. Louis, 2014, Mosby.)

needle is inserted below the level of the spinal cord at the fourth or fifth lumbar space (L4-L5).

Nuclear Scanning

Nuclear scanning tests are done in the nuclear medicine department, which has scanners or camera detectors that record images on radiographic film. Diagnostic tests use low doses of radioactive isotopes; precautionary measures that are required for radium therapy are not necessary.

Nursing interventions required when patients are scheduled for nuclear scanning procedures include (1) obtaining written consent from the patient, (2) informing the patient that the radioactive isotopes will not affect family or visitors, and (3) following the nuclear medicine department's instructions for special preparations for specific scans.

Magnetic Resonance Imaging

Musculoskeletal magnetic resonance imaging (MRI) assists in diagnosing abnormalities of bones and joints and surrounding soft tissue structures, including cartilage, synovium, ligaments, and tendons. The test uses magnetism and radio waves to make images of cross sections of the body. MRI can give much more detailed pictures of fluid-filled soft tissue and blood vessels than any other test.

In preparation, ask the patient to remove any metal, such as jewelry, clothing with metal fasteners, glasses, and hair clips. Patients with metal prostheses such as heart valves, orthopedic screws, or cardiac pacemakers may not be allowed to undergo MRI, depending on the type of metal used. Certain metals, such as titanium, are typically safe during an MRI. Persons who have been involved in an explosion, such as military personnel, may be excluded from an MRI due to metal shrapnel embedded in the body.

The standard machine looks like a narrow tunnel, which completely encloses the patient. Patients are required to lie still in this machine for 45 to 60 minutes. The patient enters the tunnel head first and may feel some anxiety or claustrophobia. The procedure is painless; however, if the patient is extremely anxious, a sedative is given. Encourage patients to use relaxation techniques, such as imagery, during the test. Newer machines called open MRIs are designed to be less confining and more comfortable than the traditional machine. Because the procedure requires the patient to be motionless, relaxation techniques that require flexing and relaxing the muscles are not appropriate during the test.

After the test, take routine vital sign measurements and allow the patient to resume pretest activities. There are no adverse effects.

Computed Tomography

Body sections can be examined from many different angles with a computed tomography (CT) scanner, which uses a narrow x-ray beam and produces a three-dimensional picture of the structure being studied. The CT scanner is approximately 100 times more sensitive than the radiograph machine and should not be used unnecessarily because of radiation exposure. Iodine contrast dye sometimes is used. A CT scan can be used for any part of the head and body. It is useful in locating injuries to the ligaments or tendons, tumors of the soft tissue, and fractures in areas difficult to define by other means.

Patient preparation includes (1) having the patient sign a consent form authorizing the examination if not included on the initial hospital consent form, (2) questioning the patient regarding allergies (e.g., iodine and seafood), (3) keeping the patient on NPO (nothing by mouth) status 3 to 4 hours before the test (in case contrast dye is used, because the dye can cause nausea and vomiting), (4) measuring vital signs to be used as a baseline, (5) having the patient void before the test, (6) removing metal articles such as jewelry and hairpins, and (7) telling the patient that he or she must lie still during the test and may feel warm and slightly nauseated for a few minutes when dye is injected.

After the test, observe the patient for delayed allergic reactions (if contrast dye was used). Encourage fluids unless contraindicated. Pretest diet and activity usually can be resumed.

Bone Scan

The bone scan test is especially valuable in detecting metastatic and inflammatory bone disease (osteomyelitis). This test involves the intravenous (IV) administration of nuclides (atomic material) approximately 2 to 3 hours before the test is scheduled. There are no food or fluid restrictions, and patients are encouraged to drink water over the next 1 to 3 hours to aid renal clearance of any radioisotope not picked up by the bone. After the patient has voided, a scanning camera reveals the degree of radionuclide uptake; areas of concentrated nuclide uptake may represent a tumor or other abnormality. These areas of concentration can be detected days or weeks before an ordinary radiograph reveals a metastatic lesion. The test takes approximately 30 to 60 minutes and requires the patient to lie still.

Aspiration

An aspiration procedure is done to obtain a specimen of body fluid. The health care provider inserts a needle into a cavity with the patient under local anesthesia. This procedure is performed using sterile technique. Commonly the health care provider takes a biopsy of tissue while doing the aspiration procedure. Nursing interventions are similar for all aspiration tests, with special emphasis on (1) having the consent form signed; (2) reinforcing the health care provider's explanation of the procedure; (3) encouraging the patient to remain immobile during the procedure; (4) having the patient void before the procedure; (5) maintaining sterile technique; (6) supporting the patient emotionally; (7) applying a sterile pressure dressing to the puncture site and maintaining the dressing until bleeding has stopped; (8) assisting with collecting, labeling, and transporting a specimen to the laboratory immediately; and (9) observing for emotional and physical distress after the procedure. Postprocedure care involves resting and elevation of the affected area. Ice may be used to prevent inflammation.

SYNOVIAL FLUID ASPIRATION

Arthrocentesis is the puncture of a patient's joint with a needle and the withdrawal of synovial fluid for diagnostic purposes. It is helpful in diagnosing trauma, systemic lupus erythematosus, gout, osteoarthritis, and rheumatoid arthritis (RA). It also may be used to instill medications for the patient with septic arthritis or to remove fluid from joints to relieve pain. Normally a patient's synovial fluid is straw colored, clear, or slightly cloudy. If trauma or a disease is present, the synovial fluid appears cloudy, milky, sanguineous (i.e., containing blood), yellow, green, or gray.

After the procedure, provide proper support to the affected extremity. Placing it on a pillow and maintaining joint rest for approximately 12 hours may be indicated. Apply ice to the affected joint for 24 to 48 hours unless otherwise ordered. An antiinfective or corticosteroid may be prescribed. Assess the patient for signs of infection. After the pressure dressing is removed from the site, an adhesive bandage can be used.

ENDOSCOPIC EXAMINATION

For endoscopy, a lighted tube is used to visualize inside a body cavity. Although some procedures require general anesthesia, most require only local anesthesia. Emotional support and complete explanations help relieve the patient's anxiety. Preparation for an endoscopic examination is similar to that for surgical preparation: (1) have the patient sign a consent form; (2) complete a preoperative checklist with special attention to removing jewelry, dentures, and contact lenses; (3) initiate NPO status 6 to 12 hours before the examination; (4) administer prescribed premedications, such as atropine and a sedative; (5) encourage the patient to void; (6) record vital signs; and (7) maintain bed rest with side rails up after giving the premedication.

Arthroscopy

Arthroscopy is an endoscopic examination that enables direct visualization of a joint. The procedure is used to (1) explore the joint to determine the presence of a disease process, (2) drain fluid from the joint cavity, and (3) remove damaged tissue or foreign bodies.

This examination is performed most commonly on the knee joint, with the synovium, articular surfaces, and meniscus (a curved, fibrous cartilage structure in the knee) visualized through the scope. The procedure involves insertion of a large-bore needle into the suprapatellar pouch and saline instillation into the joint. Arthroscopy also can be done on the hip or shoulder. The patient may be given a general or local anesthetic agent. After the arthroscopic examination, advise the patient to limit activities for several days.

Endoscopic Spinal Microsurgery

Surgeons can perform spinal surgery with less damage to surrounding tissues by passing endoscopic equipment through small incisions. Special scopes enable surgeons to successfully treat spinal column disorders (e.g., herniated disk, spinal stenosis) and spinal deformities (e.g., scoliosis, kyphosis). Spinal microsurgery can be performed with the patient under local anesthesia; discharge occurs after a brief stay. Candidates for microsurgery procedures are evaluated on the basis of information obtained from x-ray examinations, MRI scans, CT scans, and bone scans.

ELECTROGRAPHIC PROCEDURE

Electrographic procedures use electrodes to measure electrical activity in specific areas of the body.

Electromyogram

An electromyogram involves insertion of needle electrodes into the skeletal muscles so that electrical activity can be heard, seen on an oscilloscope (an instrument that displays a graphic representation of electron beams), and recorded on paper at the same time. Muscles do not produce an electrical charge at rest, but with neuromuscular disorders unusual patterns can be observed. Nerves can be observed for neuropathy and muscles for myopathy. Electromyography can be used to detect chronic low back pain based on muscle fatigue patterns.

LABORATORY TESTS

Specific laboratory tests are ordered when musculoskeletal disorders are suspected (Table 44.3).

EFFECTS OF BED REST ON MINERAL CONTENT IN BONE

Bone requires exercise to remain healthy much like the rest of the human body. Weight-bearing exercises help maintain bone density. Immobility causes the body to lose calcium. Every day of bed rest leads to further loss of total bone density. Loss of activity will result in bone resorption, causing a loss of density. If immobilization is limited to 1 to 2 months, it is possible for the bone loss to be reversed totally once weight-bearing activities are resumed. Studies conducted on astronauts experiencing loss of gravity support these findings regarding bone loss. Patients who are immobile and thus experiencing lost bone density face an increased risk for pathologic fractures (National Institutes of Health, 2016).

DISORDERS OF THE MUSCULOSKELETAL SYSTEM

INFLAMMATORY DISORDERS

Arthritis is a disease involving inflammation of the joints. An estimated 50 million Americans are affected by arthritis, and 4 million of these are dependent and unable to work, attend school, or participate in social functions. There are many types of arthritis, but the most common are rheumatoid arthritis (RA), rheumatoid spondylitis, osteoarthritis (degenerative joint disease [DJD]), and gout (gouty arthritis). Table 44.4 compares RA and osteoarthritis.

RHEUMATOID ARTHRITIS

Etiology and Pathophysiology

Rheumatoid arthritis (RA), the most serious form of arthritis, can lead to severe joint deformity. It is a chronic, systemic inflammatory autoimmune disease that affects approximately 1.3 million people (Rheumatoid Arthritis Support Network, 2016). RA is more common in women, affecting nearly three times as many women as men. Although it can affect women of any age, women 30 to 60 years of age are affected most often. There is also a noted genetic link. Smoking significantly increases the risk of RA in men and women who are predisposed genetically to the disease. Additional risk factors include bacterial and viral diseases.

RA is a systemic disorder and can affect many organ systems (lungs, heart, blood vessels, muscles, eyes, skin). RA is characterized by a chronic inflammation of the synovial membrane (synovitis) of the diarthrodial joints (also called synovial joints: the freely movable joints in which continuous bony surfaces are covered by cartilage and connected by ligaments lined with synovial membrane).

Table 44.3 Laboratory Tests for Musculoskeletal Disorders

NORMAL VALUE	POSSIBLE CAUSE FOR INCREASE OR DECREASE
Calcium: 9.0–10.5 mg/dL	Increased in metastatic tumor in the bone, Addison's disease, Paget's disease of the bone, acromegaly, acute osteoporosis, hyperparathyroidism, vitamin D deficiency, renal failure, malabsorption, and rickets.
Phosphorus: 2.5–4.5 mg/dL	Increased in acromegaly, bone metastases, excessive levels of vitamin D, hypocalcemia, renal failure. Decreased in acute gout, hypercalcemia, vitamin D deficiency.
Vitamin D, 25–dihydroxy: 6–52 ng/mL	Increased in vitamin D intoxication. Decreased in bowel resection, malabsorption, rickets.
Vitamin D_1, 25–dihydroxy: 15–60 pg/mL	Increased in liver disease; bone disease; healing fractures; metastatic tumor in bone; osteogenic sarcoma; osteoporosis; cancer of breast, colon, lung, or pancreas. Decreased in severe anemia, folic acid deficiency, pernicious anemia.
Alkaline phosphatase: 30–120 units/L	Increased in skeletal muscle injury or myocardial infarction.
Myoglobin: 5–70 mcg/dL	Decreased in rheumatoid arthritis.
Erythrocyte sedimentation rate (ESR): • *Males:* Up to 15 mm/hr • *Females:* Up to 20 mm/hr	A nonspecific test used to detect inflammatory, neoplastic, infectious, and necrotic processes. Indicates the presence of inflammation as seen in rheumatoid arthritis and rheumatic fever. One of the most objective measurements of rheumatoid arthritis severity. Increased as the disease worsens. Increased in multiple myeloma, acute myocardial infarctions, toxemia, bacterial infections, and gout. Decreased in congestive heart failure, sickle cell anemia, polycythemia vera, infectious mononucleosis, degenerative arthritis, and angina pectoris.
Rheumatoid factor (RF): 40–60 units/mL	An immunoglobulin found in approximately 80% of adults with rheumatoid arthritis; other diseases such as systemic lupus erythematosus may cause a positive RF result.
Uric acid (blood): • *Males:* 2.1–8.5 mg/dL • *Females:* 2.0–6.6 mg/dL	Increased in patients with gout, kidney failure, alcoholism, leukemia, metastatic cancer, multiple myeloma, or dehydration.

Data from Pagana KD, Pagana TJ: *Mosby's manual of diagnostic and laboratory tests*, ed 5, St. Louis, 2014, Mosby.

Clinical Manifestations

RA is believed to involve an immune reaction caused when the body's immune system chooses to attack one of its own proteins. The immune response causes an inflammatory response. The repeated inflammation of the joints and surrounding tissue may lead to gross deformity and loss of function (Fig. 44.5).

RA is characterized by periods of remission and exacerbation. Arthritic flare-ups may be attributed to a precipitating stressful event such as infection, work stress, physical exertion, childbirth, surgery, or emotional upset. During remission the inflammation, pain, stiffness, and edema subside, and progression of tissue damage is halted or reduced.

Assessment

Collection of *subjective data* is important in helping diagnose RA. According to the Arthritis Foundation (2017) the symptoms of RA include the following:

- Joint pain, tenderness, swelling or stiffness for 6 weeks or longer
- More than one joint is affected
- Morning stiffness for 30 minutes or longer
- Small joints (wrists, certain joints of the hands and feet) are affected
- The same joints on both sides of the body are affected

Other symptoms include fatigue and low-grade fever. The patient with RA has periods of remission and exacerbation. The common terminology used for an exacerbation of RA is a "flare." RA flares can last for days up to months. If prolonged inflammation goes untreated or has frequent recurrences, RA can affect the patient systemically. Organs that are affected commonly include the eyes (dryness and light sensitivity), oral cavity (irritation and ulcerations), skin (RA nodules), lungs and blood vessels (inflammation), and bone marrow (anemia) (Arthritis Foundation, 2017).

Collection of *objective data* includes observing the joints for edema, tenderness, subcutaneous nodules, limitation in range of motion (ROM), symmetric joint involvement, and fever.

Diagnostic Tests

No single test is definitive for RA. Diagnosis is based primarily on patient history and physical examination. The four classic symptoms most frequently reported

Table 44.4 Comparison of Rheumatoid Arthritis and Osteoarthritis

	RHEUMATOID ARTHRITIS (RA)	OSTEOARTHRITIS (OA)
Pathophysiology	Inflammation of synovial membrane; destruction of cartilage, joint capsule, bones, ligaments, and tendons	Degeneration of cartilage from wear and tear; bone spur formation
Joints most commonly affected	Symmetric joint involvement noted in wrists, knees, and knuckles	Often only one side of body affected with changes noted in hands, spine, knees, and hips
Clinical signs and symptoms	Edema, erythema, heat, pain, tenderness, nodule formation, fatigue, stiffness, muscle aches, and fever Systemic manifestations occur Vasculitis (inflammation of blood vessels) may be responsible for a variety of systemic complications, including peripheral neuropathy, myopathy, cardiopulmonary involvement, and ischemic ulcerations of the skin Potential complications include infection, osteoporosis, and Sjögren's syndrome. Dry mouth and decreased tearing occur in Sjögren's syndrome	Localized pain, stiffness, bony knobs of end joints of fingers (Heberden's nodes), edema (not as pronounced as in RA) No systemic involvement is present Constitutional symptoms such as fatigue or fever are not present Other organ involvement is absent as well, which is an important differentiation between OA and RA
Age at onset	Children nearing adolescence; adults between 20 and 50 yr	Ages 45–90 yr. Most people have some features with increasing age
Sex	Females affected more often than males, at a ratio of 3:1	Males and females affected equally
Heredity	Familial tendency	The form with knobby fingers can be hereditary
Diagnostic tests	Rheumatoid factor (RF) found in serum of about 85% of patients with RA. Erythrocyte sedimentation rate, C-reactive protein, complete blood count, x-rays, examination of joint fluid RF positive in 80% of patients	X-rays; no specific laboratory abnormalities are useful in diagnosing OA. RF negative
Treatment	Control inflammation and pain with medications Balance exercise with rest Provide joint protection; encourage weight control and stress reduction Surgically replace joints	Maintain activity level Control pain with medication Encourage exercise, joint protection, weight control, stress reduction Surgical joint replacement may be necessary

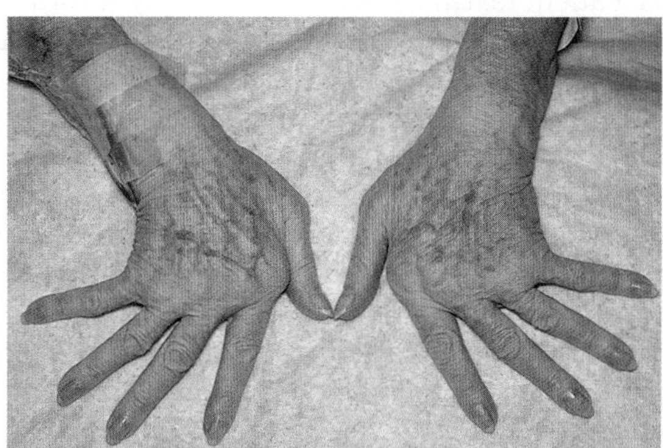

Fig. 44.5 Rheumatoid arthritis of the hands. (From Swartz MH: *Textbook of physical diagnosis,* ed 5, Philadelphia, 2006, Saunders.)

are morning stiffness, joint pain, muscle weakness, and fatigue. Swelling of joints is not uncommon. Radiographic studies reveal loss of articular cartilage and change in subchondral bone. The following laboratory tests are used often in supporting the diagnosis and in ruling out other diseases:

- *Anti-CCP (cyclic citrullinated peptide) antibody test:* Anti-CCP antibodies are found frequently in the blood of patients with RA. This test can identify RA before symptoms develop and identify the likelihood of patients developing severe RA.
- *Anti-nuclear antibody (ANA) titers and elevated C-reactive protein (CRP):* These are seen in some patients with RA.
- *C-reactive protein (CRP):* Indicates the presence of inflammation in the body.
- *Erythrocyte sedimentation rate (ESR):* An increase indicates the presence of an inflammatory reaction somewhere in the body.
- *Latex agglutination test:* This test detects the presence of the immunoglobulin M version of RF, which combines with antigen-coated latex particles to form a precipitate.
- *Red blood cell count:* This detects anemia, which is often present during chronic infection.
- *Rheumatoid factor (RF):* An elevation indicates an abnormal serum concentration of this protein.

Positive RF occurs in approximately 80% of patients with RA.

- *Synovial fluid aspiration:* Normal fluid is usually clear and highly viscous; however, when inflammation is present, the fluid is cloudy, yellow, less viscous, and contains increased protein.
- *Synovial fluid biopsy:* The biopsy shows changes in the synovial tissue.
- *X-rays:* To determine the presence of any joint damage.

Medical Management

The patient with RA benefits from aggressive treatment early in the course of the disease. The medical management of RA is directed toward (1) controlling the disease activity by administering disease-modifying and antiinflammatory drugs (Table 44.5); (2) providing pain relief; (3) reducing clinical symptoms in days to weeks with the rapid antiinflammatory effect of methotrexate (Rheumatrex); (4) prolonging joint function (often with physical therapy, traction, and splints); and (5) slowing the progression of joint damage by promoting activities of daily living (ADLs), an exercise program, and weight management.

Advances in cell and molecular biology have influenced the treatment of RA. Current medications actually target the pathophysiology of the disease. Disease-modifying antirheumatoid drugs (DMARDs) offer wider treatment options. These medications target a protein known as tumor necrosis factor (TNF). TNF is produced by the synovial cells and other cells of the body and is a proinflammatory substance—that is, it has the ability to produce signs and symptoms of inflammation (see Table 44.5). Complementary therapies to decrease inflammation include nonsteroidal antiinflammatory drugs (NSAIDs); capsaicin (Capzasin), a nonopioid topical analgesic; fish oil; and antioxidants (vitamins C and E and beta-carotene). Musculoskeletal surgery in the form of joint replacement is another option.

Nursing Interventions and Patient Teaching

Patient education is essential to help the patient and family understand what is happening and what to expect as the disease progresses. Fatigue can be a major concern. Achieving restful sleep is important. Additional sleeping periods and naps are indicated only during disease exacerbation. Exercise helps prevent the joints from "freezing" and the muscles from weakening. An initial exercise program calls for two or three 10- to 15-minute daily sessions of "quiet" exercise that gently put joints through ROM. Heat is used often to relax and soothe muscles. Strength training, aerobic exercise, and yoga also may be included. Some patients achieve comfort from warm packs and heat lamps, and applications of hot paraffin wax may be helpful. Rehabilitation is aimed at helping the patient adapt to physical limitations and promoting normal daily activities.

Problem statements and interventions for the patient with RA include but are not limited to the following:

Patient Problem	Nursing Interventions
Prolonged Pain, related to joint inflammation	Administer prescribed salicylate or nonsteroidal antiinflammatory drugs (NSAIDs) Assist patient with an exercise program prescribed by the health care provider Physical therapy referral as indicated to discuss proper body mechanics and use of a walker or cane During acute stages of disease, encourage patient to rest inflamed joints and maintain proper body alignment Application of heat (may include heating pads, warm compresses, heat patches, warm baths, or wax) Application of cold therapy (may include ice or cold packs) Assist and teach patient to extend joints as possible and to avoid external rotation of extremities; use sandbags or trochanter rolls Avoid use of pillow under knees and/or support joints
Prolonged Low Self-Esteem, related to negative self-evaluation about self or capabilities	Encourage patient to express feelings about health problems, progress, and prognosis concerning diagnosis Encourage patient to explore ways to remain active while experiencing limited mobility (e.g., doing tasks while sitting as opposed to standing or walking)

As with any chronic illness, patient teaching is perhaps the most important aspect of nursing interventions. Patient teaching includes providing information about joint protection and energy conservation techniques, proper balance of rest and activity, proper use of medications (i.e., names of drugs, dosages, precautions in administration, and side effects or toxic effects), plans for implementation of the exercise program prescribed by the health care provider or physical therapist, proper application of heat or cold packs, proper use of walking aids, safety measures to prevent injury, basics of good nutrition and the importance of avoiding weight gain, and the danger of following programs that promise a "cure."

Prognosis

The course of RA is variable but is marked by remissions and exacerbations. The prognosis is based on a variety of clinical and laboratory findings. Stage I represents early effects. Stage IV, the terminal category, includes marked joint deformity, extensive muscle atrophy, soft tissue lesions, bone and cartilage destruction, and fibrous or bony ankylosis.

Table 44.5 Medications for Rheumatoid Arthritis

GENERIC NAME (TRADE NAME)	ACTION	SIDE EFFECTS/TOXIC EFFECTS	NURSING IMPLICATIONS
Salicylates			
aspirin, salsalate choline salicylate choline magnesium	Antiinflammatory, analgesic, antipyretic; act by inhibiting synthesis of prostaglandins	GI irritation (dyspepsia, nausea, ulcer, hemorrhage) Prolonged bleeding time Exacerbation of asthma (aspirin-sensitive asthma) Tinnitus, dizziness with repeated large doses	Administer drug with food, milk, antacids as prescribed, or full glass of water; may use enteric-coated aspirin. Report signs of bleeding (e.g., tarry stools, bruising, petechiae, nosebleeds).
Nonsteroidal Antiinflammatory Drugs (NSAIDs)			
indomethacin (Indocin)	Analgesic, antiinflammatory	Headache, vertigo, insomnia; confusion, GI irritation; can decrease effect of ACE inhibitors	Give with food, milk, or antacid. Discontinue if CNS symptoms develop and notify health care provider. Monitor BP. Report signs of bleeding.
ibuprofen (Motrin, Advil)	Analgesic, antiinflammatory	Same as indomethacin but believed less irritating to GI tract Fluid retention Can cause hypertension	Know that delayed absorption occurs if taken with food. Monitor BP.
tolmetin sodium (Tolectin)	Analgesic, antiinflammatory	Same as ibuprofen	Give with food or milk.
naproxen (Naprosyn)	Analgesic, antiinflammatory	Same as ibuprofen Causes drowsiness	Give with food, milk, or antacid. Tell patient to avoid driving until dosage effect is established.
meloxicam (Mobic)	Antiinflammatory, analgesic, antipyretic	Dizziness, headache, insomnia, seizures, dysrhythmias, heart failure, hemorrhage, diarrhea, indigestion, nausea, pancreatitis, renal failure, leukopenia, thrombocytopenia, asthma, bronchospasm, angioedema Drug is contraindicated in women who are pregnant or plan to become pregnant	Monitor BP. Instruct patient to avoid using aspirin or products containing aspirin. Assess patient for history of allergic reactions to aspirin or other NSAIDs before starting drug. Tell patient the drug can be taken without regard to meals. Advise patient to report signs and symptoms of GI ulcers and bleeding. Advise patient to report any skin rash, weight gain, or edema. Alert patient with history of asthma that asthma may recur while taking the drug. Advise patient to avoid alcohol and tobacco products while taking the drug. NSAIDs can cause fluid retention; closely monitor patients with hypertension, edema, or heart failure. Inform patient that consistent pain relief may take several days of drug administration.
nabumetone (Relafen)	Analgesic, antiinflammatory	Dizziness, anxiety, depression, gastric irritation, edema, prolonged bleeding, rash	Give with meals or antacids. Advise patient to avoid alcohol, aspirin, or aspirin products or acetaminophen without health care provider's consent. Arthritic relief noted in 1–2 wk.
meclofenamate	Analgesic, antiinflammatory	Gastric irritation, headache, dizziness, edema	Advise patients to avoid aspirin and aspirin products. Give 30 min before or 2 hr after eating.

Continued

Table 44.5 Medications for Rheumatoid Arthritis—cont'd

GENERIC NAME (TRADE NAME)	ACTION	SIDE EFFECTS/TOXIC EFFECTS	NURSING IMPLICATIONS
COX-2 Inhibitor			
celecoxib (Celebrex)	Analgesic, antiinflammatory	Mild to moderate indigestion, risk of GI bleeding, diarrhea, abdominal pain Has been linked to an increased risk of cardiovascular events, such as MI or stroke	Give medication orally. It can be taken with or without food. Celebrex is indicated for relief of the signs and symptoms of osteoarthritis and RA. Do not administer to patients who have asthma, urticaria, or allergic reactions to aspirin or other NSAIDs. Do not give to patients who are allergic to sulfonamide. Use cautiously with ACE inhibitors, warfarin, lithium, and furosemide. Monitor patients for signs of GI bleeding.
Potent Antiinflammatory Agents			
Adrenocorticosteroids (e.g., prednisone)	Interfere with body's normal inflammatory responses	Fluid retention, sodium retention, potassium depletion, hypertension, decreased healing potential, increased susceptibility to infection, GI irritation, hirsutism, osteoporosis, fat deposits, diabetes mellitus, myopathy Adrenal insufficiency or adrenal crisis if abruptly withdrawn	Give with food, milk, or antacid. Do not increase or decrease dosage without health care provider supervision. Give in morning if given once a day.
Corticosteroids, intraarticular injections (e.g., methylprednisolone [Depo-Medrol])	Suppression of inflammation and modification of the normal immune response	Decreased wound healing and increased susceptibility to infection	Check injection site for signs of infection. Inform patient joint improvement can last weeks to months. Advise patient to avoid overuse of joint.
Slow-Acting Antiinflammatory Agents			
Antimalarials hydroxychloroquine (Plaquenil)	Antiinflammatory (mechanism unknown); effect not expected to be noted for 6–12 mo after beginning therapy	GI disturbances Retinal edema that may result in blindness	Instruct patient to obtain eye examination before beginning therapy and every 6 mo thereafter. Monitor CBC.
Gold Salts (IM) Gold sodium thiomalate	Antiinflammatory; effect not noted for 3–6 mo after beginning therapy	Renal and hepatic damage, corneal deposits, dermatitis, ulcerations in mouth, hematologic changes	Monitor urinalysis and CBC before each injection. Report dermatitis, metallic taste in mouth, or lesions in mouth to health care provider.
Oral gold salts (auranofin [Ridaura])	Antirheumatic	Stomatitis (lesions in mouth); thrombocytopenia and leukopenia	Minimize exposure to sunlight and provide meticulous oral hygiene.
Antineoplastic methotrexate (Rheumatrex, Trexall)	Alters the way the body uses folic acid, which is necessary for cell growth; decreases inflammation	Upset stomach, nausea, vomiting, anorexia, diarrhea, or sore mouth; headache, blurred vision, dizziness	Drug is taken orally or by injection. Monitor vital signs, WBC, platelets, I&O, appetite. Advise patient to avoid pregnancy while taking this drug and not to get vaccinations without health care provider's consent. Keep patient well hydrated.

Table 44.5 **Medications for Rheumatoid Arthritis—cont'd**

GENERIC NAME (TRADE NAME)	ACTION	SIDE EFFECTS/TOXIC EFFECTS	NURSING IMPLICATIONS
Disease-Modifying Antirheumatoid Drugs (DMARDs)			
etanercept (Enbrel)	Blocks the normal and inflammatory immune responses seen in RA; binds tumor necrosis factor (TNF), which is involved in immune and inflammatory reactions	Pain at injection site, upper respiratory tract infections and sinusitis; in severe cases, tuberculosis possible	Give twice weekly subcutaneously in the thigh, abdomen, or upper arm Refrigerate, but never freeze medication Use with caution in patients with chronic infections May cause or aggravate systemic lupus erythematosus.
leflunomide (Arava)	Reduces signs and symptoms of RA and retards structural bone damage	Diarrhea, elevated liver enzymes, alopecia, rash	Medication is taken orally. Monitor urinary output. Do not use with patients with hepatic impairment or positive for hepatitis B or C.
infliximab (Remicade)	An antibody that binds specifically to proinflammatory enzymes produced by the synovial cells	Upper respiratory tract infections, headache, nausea, sinusitis, rash, cough	Administer intravenously at 2 and 6 wk initially, then every 8 wk thereafter. Do not give to patients with a clinically active infection.
adalimumab (Humira)	Reduces infiltration of inflammatory cells	Increased risk of infection, headaches and rash; neutropenia; injection site reaction	Assess for signs of infection before injection. Do not give to patients with active infections. Monitor new infections closely.
sulfasalazine (Azulfidine, Salazopyrin)	Sulfonamide; antiinflammatory; blocks prostaglandin synthesis	GI effects (anorexia, nausea, vomiting); bleeding, bruising, jaundice; headache; rash, urticaria, pruritus	Advise patient that drug may cause orange-yellow discoloration of urine or skin. Space doses evenly around the clock, taking drug after food with 8 oz of water. Treatment may be continued even after symptoms are relieved. Monitor CBC.
penicillamine (Cuprimine, Depen)	Antiinflammatory; exact mechanism of action in RA unknown but may suppress cell-mediated immune response	GI irritation (nausea, vomiting, anorexia, diarrhea); reduced or altered taste; rash; proteinuria, hematuria; iron deficiency (especially in menstruating women)	Monitor WBC count, platelets, urinalysis. Advise patient to take medication 1 h before or 2 h after meals or at least 1 h away from any other drug, food, or milk.
anakinra (Kineret)	Blocks the action of interleukin-1, thus decreasing the inflammatory response	Injection site reaction, leukopenia, headache, abdominal pain, rash	Evaluate for relief of pain, swelling, stiffness; increase in joint mobility. Advise patient that injection site reaction generally occurs in first month of treatment and decreases with continued therapy. Evaluate renal function. Monitor for infection. Do not give drug with other TNF inhibitors.
abatacept (Orencia)	Modulates T cell activation; suppresses immune response	Headache, upper respiratory tract infection, nausea, sore throat, injection site reaction	Not recommended for concomitant use with TNF inhibitors. Evaluate for relief of pain, swelling, stiffness and increase in joint mobility.
rituximab (Rituxan)	Monoclonal antibody that targets B cells	Dizziness, palpitations, fever, itching, difficulty breathing, sore throat	Give in combination with methotrexate. Monitor for infection and bleeding. Advise patient not to receive virus vaccines with treatment. Monitor for low BP if also taking BP medication.

Continued

Table 44.5 Medications for Rheumatoid Arthritis—cont'd

GENERIC NAME (TRADE NAME)	ACTION	SIDE EFFECTS/TOXIC EFFECTS	NURSING IMPLICATIONS
Immunosuppressant			
azathioprine (Imuran) cyclophosphamide	Inhibits DNA, RNA, protein synthesis	GI irritation (nausea, vomiting, anorexia with large doses), rash	Evaluate for relief of pain, swelling, stiffness; increase in joint mobility. Advise patient to immediately report unusual bleeding or bruising. Advise patient that therapeutic response may take up to 12 wk. Advise women of childbearing age to avoid pregnancy.
Topical Analgesics			
capsaicin cream (Zostrix, Capzasin) 5% lidocaine	Depletes substance P from nerve endings, interrupting pain signals to the brain (substance P may participate directly or indirectly in the transmission process of certain neurons)	Rash, urticaria, localized burning sensation, erythema	Must be used regularly over time for maximal effect. Aloe vera cream may moderate burning sensation. Advise patient not to use cream with external heat source (heating pad) because of risk of burns. Available in OTC and prescription strengths. Advise patient to wear gloves when applying cream to other joints and to wash hands; avoid touching damaged or irritated skin, eyes, nose, and mouth.

ACE, Angiotensin-converting enzyme; *BP,* blood pressure; *CBC,* complete blood count; *CNS,* central nervous system; *DNA,* deoxyribonucleic acid; *GI,* gastrointestinal; *I&O,* intake and output; *IM,* intramuscular; *MI,* myocardial infarction; *OTC,* over the counter; *RA,* rheumatoid arthritis; *RNA,* ribonucleic acid; *TNF,* tumor necrosis factor; *WBC,* white blood cell count.

Data from Lewis SL, Heitkemper MM, Dirksen SR, et al: *Medical-surgical nursing: Assessment and management of clinical problems,* ed 10, St. Louis, 2016, Mosby, and Skidmore-Roth L: *Mosby's 2017 nursing drug reference,* ed 30, St. Louis, 2016, Elsevier.

ANKYLOSING SPONDYLITIS

Etiology and Pathophysiology

Ankylosing spondylitis (AS) is one of the types of arthritis that comprise the group of rheumatic disorders known as *spondyloarthritis,* or *SpA.* It is a chronic, progressive rheumatic disorder that affects primarily the spine. When other joints are involved, the disease commonly includes the sacroiliac and hip joints and the adjacent soft tissues. Another common type of arthritis that is part of the SpA group is psoriatic arthritis. This type of arthritis differs in that it largely effects the fingers and toes (causing swelling), back pain and stiffness, changes to the finger and toe nails (indentations or discoloration), and psoriatic lesions (Spondylitis Association of America, 2017). The exact cause of the disease is unknown. Genetic links are the strongest suspicion. A leading theory is that a trigger or stimulus from the environment or illness can trigger the disorder. Risk factors include testing positive for the HLA-B27 marker, a family history of the disease, and frequent gastrointestinal infections. It can affect both sexes but is seen more often in young men. The presence of human leukocyte antigen A and B27 (HLA-B27) in the serum of 90% of whites and 50% of African Americans with AS suggests a hereditary factor. The most common time for onset of AS is between 15 and 35 years of age. Women develop a milder form of AS than men, and fusion of the spine rarely is seen. It is sometimes referred to as *rheumatoid spondylitis* (Mayo Clinic, 2017).

Clinical Manifestations

The characteristic spinal inflammation of AS results in the bones of the spine fusing (growing together). The accompanying fixation of the joint is referred to as **ankylosis.** This fixation is often in an abnormal position.

The inflammation typically is located where the ligaments and tendons attach to the bone. AS can affect joints such as the neck, jaw, shoulders, knees, and hips. Progression of the disease causes the ligaments to become ossified (hardened). The cardiovascular system can be involved, and heart enlargement and pericarditis can occur. If the costovertebral joints (i.e., where the ribs connect with the spine) are affected, kyphosis can occur, leading to a forward curvature of the upper back and altered respirations. The patient may have difficulty expanding the ribcage while breathing. Many patients with the disease also have inflammatory bowel disease. Vision loss occurs with chronic AS, and blindness may result from glaucoma and pupil damage. The condition is characterized by periods of remission and exacerbations or "flares."

Assessment

Subjective data include complaints of low backache, stiffness, and alternating or bilateral "sciatica pain" that lasts for a few days and then subsides. Pain is more pronounced when the patient is in an erect position. Inactivity exacerbates the pain, and exercise gives relief. Complaints of weight loss, abdominal distention, visual problems, and fatigue are common. AS is present in 3% to 10% of patients with inflammatory bowel disease.

Collection of objective data includes assessment for tenderness over the spine and sacroiliac region. Peripheral joint edema and decreased ROM may be seen. Assessment of vital signs may indicate elevated temperature, tachycardia, and hyperpnea. Respiratory difficulties arise if there is limited expansion of the chest, as often is seen in kyphosis.

Diagnostic Tests

Patients with AS often have the following laboratory test results: (1) low hemoglobin and hematocrit, indicative of anemia; (2) elevated ESR and CRP, which are common in chronic inflammatory disease; (3) elevated serum alkaline phosphatase levels in patients who are immobilized or have bone resorption; and (4) presence of the HLA-B27 antigen. Radiographic examination often reveals sacroiliac joint and intervertebral disk inflammation with bony erosion and joint space fusion.

Medical Management

The health care provider usually prescribes oral analgesics and NSAIDs. Corticosteroid therapy with prednisone may be prescribed. TNF inhibitors are biologic response modifiers. They target the immune cells. Examples include etanercept (Enbrel), infliximab (Remicade), and adalimumab (Humira). Regular exercise is recommended. Exercise will help to prevent demineralization of bone and promote flexibility and improved posture. Swimming and walking are low-impact activities that may be considered for the regimen. Patients are encouraged to work toward exercising two or three times each week for 30 to 40 minutes. Patients who have been relatively sedentary will need to gradually build to this level of activity.

Surgery may be necessary to replace fused joints (commonly the hip or the knee). Cervical or lumbar osteotomy can be done for severe kyphosis.

Endoscopic microsurgery can be performed on select candidates. In microsurgery, the bone or tissue that is putting pressure on the spinal nerves is removed by using endoscopic equipment placed through small incisions. Most patients leave the hospital within 24 hours and start physical therapy within a few days.

Nursing Interventions and Patient Teaching

Nursing interventions are aimed at maintaining alignment of the spine. Providing a firm mattress, bed board, and back brace helps provide support. Encouraging the patient to lie on the abdomen for at least 15 to 30 minutes four times daily helps extend the spine. Turning and positioning every 2 hours helps prevent pressure sores. Postural and breathing exercises help compensate for the possibility of impaired gas exchange caused by the changes in posture and chest cavity size. Heat and cold also may be included in the plan of care. Heat will reduce pain and stiffness. Cold applications will aid in the reduction of inflammation and swelling.

Teach the patient the appropriate use of prescribed medications, postural exercises, and methods of applying heat to back and hips. Promote correct posture and prevent complications by encouraging the patient to use a firm mattress, sleep without a pillow, and do respiratory exercises.

Prognosis

AS is a chronic disease occurring in persons younger than age 30 years that generally "burns itself out" after a course of 20 years, leaving permanent, irreversible systemic involvement if not treated (Mayo Clinic, 2017).

OSTEOARTHRITIS (DEGENERATIVE JOINT DISEASE)

Etiology and Pathophysiology

Osteoarthritis (OA) sometimes is referred to as degenerative joint disease because it results from wear and tear on the joints. Osteoarthritis is a nonsystemic, noninflammatory disorder that begins with degeneration of the cartilage of joints, thus causing damage to bones. Degenerative joint changes traditionally are noticed beginning in middle age. By the age of 70 most adults have hypertrophic joint changes. Before age 55, osteoarthritis occurs with similar frequency in men and women. Women begin to outpace men with incidence after that point (Box 44.3). The disease is a consequence of aging and is a major cause of severe chronic disability. Osteoarthritis takes two forms: primary (cause is unknown) and secondary (caused by trauma, infections, previous fractures, RA, stress on weight-bearing joints from obesity, occupations placing abnormal stressors on joints such as professional athletics, and occupations requiring excessive stooping and bending such as plumbers). A comparison of RA and osteoarthritis is found in Table 44.4.

Clinical Manifestations

This disorder most commonly affects the joints of the hand, knee, hip, and cervical and lumbar vertebrae (Fig. 44.6) (National Institute of Arthritis and Musculoskeletal and Skin Diseases [NIAMS], 2016). Symptoms include pain and stiffness in the joints. The joints are stiffest in the morning hours upon awakening. With activity the stiffness reduces. Grating or cracking sounds may be noted with joint movement. The disease affects the hands in women more often, whereas in men the hips are affected.

Box 44.3 Osteoarthritis

- Osteoarthritis is the most common form of arthritis and the leading cause of disability in people older than age 65 years. Under age 55, men and women are affected equally. In older individuals, osteoarthritis of the hip is more common in men and osteoarthritis of the interphalangeal joints and the thumb is more common in women. Osteoarthritis occurs more frequently in people who are obese or who experience repetitive stress to the joints.
- More than 70% of total hip and knee replacements are for osteoarthritis.
- Overweight people have a higher risk of knee and hip osteoarthritis.
- Weight loss programs for overweight older adults lessen symptoms in those with the disease.
- Acetaminophen is recommended by the American College of Rheumatology for osteoarthritis pain because of fewer gastrointestinal and renal side effects compared with other drugs.
- Bicycling and swimming are considered good exercises for people with osteoarthritis of the knee; walking should be done on level ground.
- People with osteoarthritis of the knee or hip should avoid climbing stairs, bending, stooping, or squatting.

Assessment

Collection of subjective data includes questioning the patient about pain and stiffness (rest usually relieves pain in the early stages). Past illnesses, surgical procedures, or trauma may be relevant, and information about excessive weight gain and occupation may be significant. Complaints regarding reduced grip strength are common.

Collection of objective data includes assessment for joint edema, tenderness, instability, and deformity. *Heberden's nodes* appear on the sides of the distal joints of fingers (Fig. 44.7), and *Bouchard's nodes* appear on the proximal joints of fingers; these nodes are hard, bony, and cartilaginous enlargements. The patient's gait reveals a limp, especially if the hips or legs are affected.

Diagnostic Tests

There is no specific test to diagnose osteoarthritis. However, radiographic studies, MRI, arthroscopy, synovial fluid examination, and bone scans are used to provide supportive information.

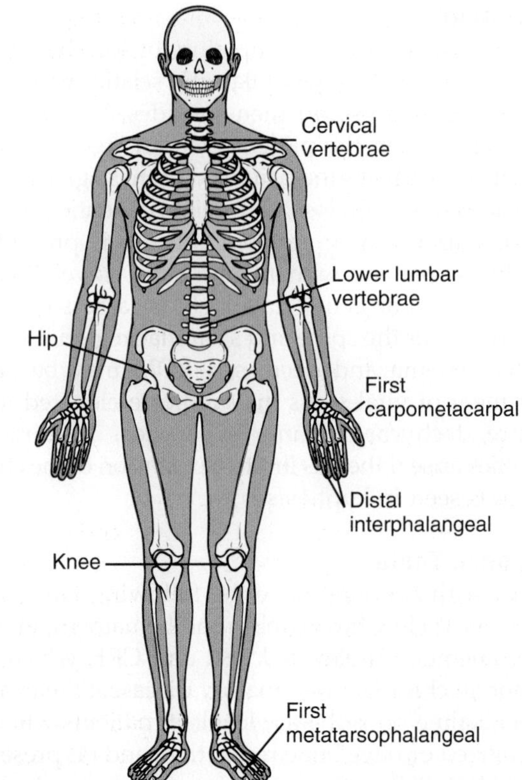

Fig. 44.6 Joints most frequently involved in osteoarthritis. (From Kamal A, Brocklehurst JC: *Color atlas of geriatric medicine*, ed 2, St. Louis, 1991, Mosby.)

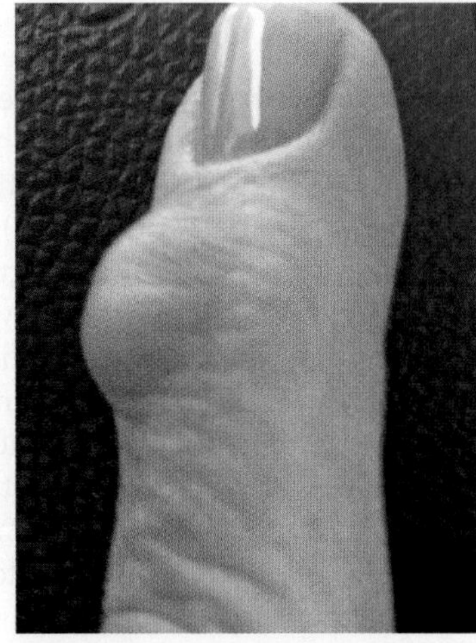

Fig. 44.7 Heberden's nodes.

Medical Management

The primary care provider prescribes an exercise plan that is balanced with rest periods. Physical therapy using heat application helps reduce stiffness, pain, and muscle spasms. Gait enhancers—such as canes, walkers, and shoe inserts—help relieve discomfort while using weight-bearing joints. Pharmacologic therapies begin with lower doses of over-the-counter medications such as acetaminophen (Tylenol) and progress to NSAID therapies, including salicylates (aspirin) and ibuprofen (Motrin) (NIAMS, 2016). Dosages are increased as tolerance and/or the condition progresses. A corticosteroid (cortisone) sometimes is used in low doses or injected into joints to produce immediate pain relief and temporarily halt the destructive process. Patients with hypertension must be screened carefully while taking NSAIDs because certain NSAIDs elevate blood pressure. Patients need to inform their health care provider if they have been prescribed hypertensive medication by another health care provider so that a safe and effective combination of drugs can be chosen. Indomethacin (Indocin) can decrease the effect of enalapril (Vasotec) (an angiotensin-converting enzyme inhibitor used for hypertension), and the combination of ibuprofen and lisinopril (Prinivil, Zestril) can trigger a hypertensive response. Acetaminophen is used commonly as an analgesic and does not affect the blood pressure. Tramadol hydrochloride (Ultram) is a synthetic analgesic used for moderate to severe pain and can be used for patients taking antihypertensives.

Alternatives to NSAIDs. The discomfort associated with acute or chronic RA, osteoarthritis, gouty arthritis, and AS also may be decreased through the use of nonpharmacologic measures. Measures such as relaxation techniques, massage therapy, imagery, and therapeutic touch have been proven effective in reducing discomfort and decreasing the need for NSAIDs.

Glucosamine is found in the body and acts as a lubricant and shock absorber necessary for repairing and maintaining healthy joint function. The aging process has been linked to the loss of glucosamine and other substances in the cartilage. Taking supplements of natural glucosamine enables the body to manufacture collagen and proteoglycans and resupply lubricant found in the synovial fluid necessary for restoring healthy cartilage (see the Complementary and Alternative Therapies box). Glucosamine supplements have been linked with reductions in articular pain, joint tenderness, and restricted joint movement in people suffering from arthritis. People with chronic medical problems, or women who are pregnant or lactating should not take supplemental glucosamine without conferring with a health care provider. Although glucosamine often is obtained from the shells of shrimp, crab, and lobster, there are no reports of allergic reactions by persons who are allergic to shellfish after using glucosamine (National Library of Medicine [NLM], 2016).

Surgical intervention, such as osteotomy, may help correct malalignment. Joint replacement may be necessary to replace all or part of the joint's articulating surface. Arthroplasty of the hip and knee is the most common surgical intervention.

Complementary and Alternative Therapies

Musculoskeletal Disorders

- Alternative therapies being considered in the treatment of osteoarthritis include compounds such as glucosamine and chondroitin. These substances appear to provide pain relief, perhaps even slowing the disease process. Glucosamine apparently stimulates cartilage cells to manufacture proteoglycans, whereas chondroitin inhibits enzymes that break down cartilage. Few adverse effects have been seen with glucosamine used up to 3 years.
- Chiropractic adjustment has been effective in patients with some types of back pain. Many insurance companies allow for this form of therapy.
- Other manual healing methods—therapy that includes touch and manipulation of soft tissues or realignment of body parts to correct a dysfunction that affects other body parts—include the following:
  - Acupuncture
  - Massage and other physical healing methods
  - Reflexology (a system of treating certain disorders by massaging the soles of the feet or the palms of the hands)
  - Rolfing (a technique of deep massage intended to realign the body by altering the length and tone of myofascial tissues)

Nursing Interventions and Patient Teaching

Nursing interventions include encouraging the patient to maintain ADLs and adapt to limitations of the disease. Alternating sitting, walking, and standing with periods of rest can help reduce joint discomfort and deterioration. Older patients may be physically capable of turning and moving in bed but may forget to do so because of alteration in their level of orientation. Assist the patient with a weight reduction plan if obesity is a problem. If splints are used to support a painful joint, assess for neurovascular impairment above and below the site of application. Also check gait enhancers for safety considerations, such as rubber tips on ends, proper size, and patient knowledge about use. If the patient has been taking aspirin over a period of time, gastrointestinal (GI) bleeding may occur. It may be necessary to perform a guaiac test on stool and emesis to determine the presence of occult blood.

As with RA, teaching the person with osteoarthritis about the disease process and the steps to control that process is the most important aspect of nursing interventions. Patient teaching should include the same information as for RA.

Prognosis

Osteoarthritis is a chronic disease that ultimately causes permanent destruction of affected cartilage and underlying bone with variable pain and disability. Bones rub against other bones because of the destruction of the cartilage between them; arthroscopic surgery to remove resultant bone spurs may help ease pain. Joint replacement is necessary for improved mobility and reduction in pain when severe OA is present.

GOUT (GOUTY ARTHRITIS)

Etiology and Pathophysiology

Gout is a metabolic disease resulting from an accumulation of uric acid in the blood. It is an acute inflammatory condition associated with ineffective metabolism of purines. Gout can be primary (linked with hereditary factors), secondary (resulting from use of certain medications or complication of another disease), or idiopathic (of unknown origin). It affects men approximately eight times more frequently than women and usually occurs in middle life. Women who experience gout traditionally are affected after menopause. Of all people with gout, 85% have a genetic tendency to develop the disease.

Tophi (calculi containing sodium urate deposits that develop in periarticular fibrous tissue, typically in patients with gout) result in inflammation of the joint; it is unclear why this occurs. More than 75% of people with gout experience big toe involvement. Other joints such as the foot, fingers, and wrists are affected with lesser frequency.

Clinical Manifestations

Onset occurs at night, with excruciating pain, edema, and inflammation in the affected joint. The pain may last a short time but return at intervals, or it may be severe and continuous for 5 to 10 days. The patient may have repeated attacks or only one attack in a lifetime. Tophi are seen around the rim of the ear and can cause disfigurement. Surgical removal may be necessary.

Assessment

Collection of subjective data includes noting a complaint of pain occurring at night involving the great toe or other joints. Take a dietary history, with specific questions on consumption of alcohol and foods high in purines, such as organ meats (brain, kidney, liver, heart), anchovies, yeast, herring, mackerel, and scallops.

Collection of objective data includes assessment of joints (especially the great toe) for signs of edema, heat, discoloration (may appear erythematous or purple), and limited movement. Vital sign data may reveal an elevated temperature and hypertension, tachycardia, and tachypnea. Carefully assess urinary output because tophi can form in the kidneys and alter kidney function. Assess the patient for tophi (typically seen on the earlobes, fingers, hands, and toes).

Diagnostic Tests

Laboratory tests used to diagnose gout include serum (see Table 44.3) and urinary uric acid levels (elevation is significant), complete blood count (CBC) (leukocytosis and anemia may be present), and elevated ESR. Radiographic studies reveal cysts and toe bone pockets. Synovial fluid contains urate crystals.

Medical Management

Several drugs are used to treat gout. For acute attacks, colchicine is administered orally or intravenously. The oral dosage is 0.5 mg hourly for 12 doses. The drug is discontinued if GI symptoms develop or pain is not relieved. Indomethacin suspension and injectable is an effective antiinflammatory drug in treating gout. Corticosteroids can be administered orally, intravenously, or intraarticularly and will relieve signs and symptoms within 12 hours. The health care provider may order allopurinol (Zyloprim) to decrease the production of uric acid. The medication probenecid (Probalan) is prescribed to inhibit renal tubular resorption of uric acid, which increases secretion of uric acid by the kidneys. The drug febuxostat (Uloric) has been prescribed to lower serum uric acid levels, but the US Food and Drug Administration (FDA) has warned that it has an increased risk for causing heart-related deaths and deaths from all causes (US FDA, 2017a). Aspirin inactivates the effect of uricosurics (e.g., probenecid), resulting in urate retention, and should be avoided while patients are taking uricosuric drugs.

Nursing Interventions and Patient Teaching

Nursing intervention is aimed at giving medications prescribed by the health care provider for relief of pain and inflammation. When giving colchicine, observe for side effects, such as diarrhea, nausea, and vomiting. Increasing the patient's fluid intake to at least 2000 mL daily helps eliminate the excess urinary urates. Approximately 10% to 20% of patients with gouty arthritis have uric acid kidney stones. Carefully document intake and output (I&O). Advise the patient to avoid excessive use of alcohol and consumption of foods high in purines, which include sardines, herring, anchovies, alcohol, and beer. Maintain bed rest and joint immobilization while the patient is symptomatic. Bed cradles prevent pressure from bed linens on the affected joints.

Problem statements and interventions for the patient with gout include but are not limited to the following:

Patient Problem	Nursing Interventions
Prolonged Pain, related to disease process	Maintain patient in a position of comfort with foot supported and in alignment; place bed cradle over foot; no weight-bearing Apply cold packs as ordered, keeping pressure off joint Administer analgesics and antigout and antiinflammatory agents as ordered; observe for side effects
Insufficient Knowledge, related to lack of information concerning medications and home care management	Provide medication schedule, including name, dosage, purpose, and side effects Discuss importance of diet, exercise, and rest program Encourage follow-up visits with health care provider

Patient teaching is aimed at giving information about the disease and stressing the importance of keeping the serum uric acid levels within the normal range by taking the prescribed medications; following the prescribed diet; and avoiding infections, lack of sleep, and stress. The patient may need to take colchicine, probenecid, and allopurinol as a maintenance dose even when signs and symptoms are not present.

Prognosis

The signs and symptoms are recurrent; episodes become longer each year. The disorder is disabling and, if untreated, can progress to the development of tophi and destructive joint changes.

OTHER MUSCULOSKELETAL DISORDERS

OSTEOPOROSIS

Etiology and Pathophysiology

Osteoporosis is a disorder that results in a loss in bone density. This reduction is sufficient to interfere with the mechanical support function of the bone. Nearly 25% of women over the age of 65 and 5.1% of men in the United States have osteoporosis (CDC, 2016). Women between the ages of 55 and 65 years are identified as a high-risk group for postmenopausal osteoporosis, and many researchers believe that this is related to the loss of the female hormone estrogen. An increase in type 1 (postmenopausal) osteoporosis suggests estrogen deficiency is connected with increased bone resorption and sensitivity to parathyroid hormone (a substance that weakens bone by increasing calcium movement from bone into the extracellular fluid). Type 2 (senile) osteoporosis is seen in people between ages 70 and 85 years and affects twice as many women as men. Each year, 700,000 people with osteoporosis experience compression fractures of the spine, and 2 million people overall experience some type of fracture related to the disease (American Academy of Orthopaedic Surgeons, 2016). Genetic and environmental factors, such as small bone structure and lack of exercise, can contribute to the rate of bone loss. Osteoporosis affects the vertebrae, neck of the femur, pelvis, hands, and wrists. Individuals most at risk for developing osteoporosis are small-framed, white (northern European descent) or Asian women. Smoking and alcoholism are also risk factors. Medical conditions associated with increased development of the disease include hyperthyroidism, chronic lung disease, cancer, inflammatory bowel disease, alcoholism, and vitamin D deficiency. Medications linked to the development of osteoporosis include steroids, anticonvulsants, immunosuppressant therapies, and heparin. Diets low in calcium or high in caffeine and protein also are implicated (see the Cultural Considerations box) (Mayo Clinic, 2016b).

Clinical Manifestations

Most patients with osteoporosis have no symptoms in the early stages of the disease. A fracture, usually of the vertebrae, is often the first symptom. Loss of height over time or a stooped posture may be an indication of the disease before a diagnosis is made.

Assessment

Collection of subjective data includes questioning the patient about lifestyle practices and complaints of pain (low thoracic and lumbar) that worsens with sitting, standing, coughing, sneezing, and straining.

Collection of objective data includes assessing the patient for dowager's hump (spinal deformity and height loss that result from repeated spinal vertebral fractures) and increased lordosis, scoliosis, and kyphosis (Fig. 44.8). Also assess gait impairment associated with inability to maintain erect posture.

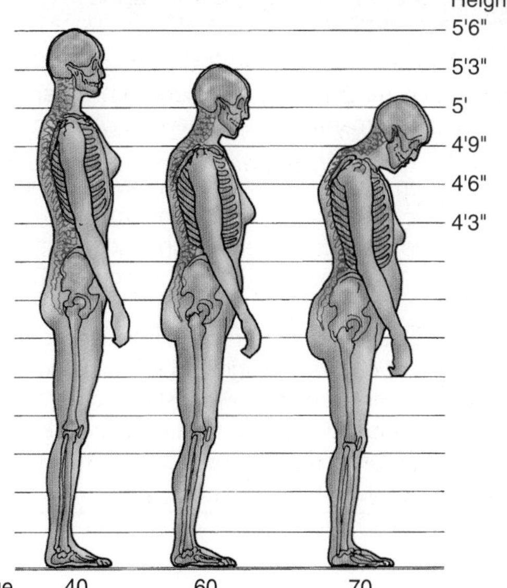

Fig. 44.8 A normal spine at age 40 years and osteoporotic changes at ages 60 and 70 years. These changes can cause a loss of as much as 6 inches in height and can result in the so-called dowager's hump *(far right)* in the upper thoracic vertebrae. (From Ignatavicius DD, Workman ML, Blair M, et al: *Medical-surgical nursing: Patient-centered collaborative care*, ed 8, St. Louis, 2016, Elsevier.)

Diagnostic Tests

The health care provider orders a CBC; serum calcium, phosphorus, and alkaline phosphatase; blood urea nitrogen (BUN); creatinine level; urinalysis; and liver and thyroid function tests. A bone mineral density (BMD) measurement is recommended for women around the time of menopause. BMD is determined by dual-energy x-ray absorptiometry (DEXA). The BMD test assesses the mass of bone per unit volume, or how tightly the bone is packed. Usually the hip and the spine are measured. The test takes about 10 minutes and involves low amounts of radiation. The World Health Organization has defined criteria for adult women as follows:

- Normal bones have a BMD within 1 standard deviation of the young female adult average.
- Low bone mass (osteopenia) is between 1 and 2.5 standard deviations below the young female adult average.
- Osteoporosis is 2.5 standard deviations or more below the young female adult average *of negative 1 or above* (International Osteoporosis Foundation, 2015).

Medical Management

The health care provider orders a treatment regimen aimed at increasing bone density and retarding bone loss. Calcium supplements that bring the total calcium intake per day to 1200 mg for men and postmenopausal women are recommended, with 2000 mg being the maximum amount (as well as vitamin D, 800 international

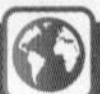

Cultural Considerations

Osteoporosis

- White women have a higher incidence of osteoporosis than Asian women, followed by African American women (Cauley, 2011).
- Like women, white and Asian men have a higher incidence of osteoporosis than other men; however, the rate of osteoporosis in men is significantly less than in women, 5.1% in men and 24.5% in women (CDC, 2016).
- Postmenopausal women are at the highest risk regardless of cultural background or ethnic group.
- Hispanic women are at a lower risk of osteoporosis than white and Asian women. The rate of osteoporosis for African American and Hispanic women is similar (NIAMS, 2015).

units daily). Alcohol intake should be limited because excessive intake interferes with absorption of calcium and vitamin D. Weight-bearing exercise programs to improve muscle tone, such as walking, help prevent further bone loss and stimulate new bone formation (Bethel, 2017b).

Alendronate (Fosamax), zoledronic acid (Reclast), and ibandronate (Boniva) are bone resorption inhibitors that assist in increasing bone density (Table 44.6). These drugs absorb calcium phosphate crystal in bone and are given orally to treat symptoms of osteoporosis. Administer these drugs first thing in the morning with 6 to 8 ounces of water at least 30 minutes before other medications, beverages, or food. Caution the patient to remain upright for 30 minutes after a dose to facilitate passage to the stomach and to minimize risk of esophageal irritation.

Risedronate (Actonel) is another bone resorption inhibitor. The drug adsorbs (i.e., binds) calcium phosphate crystal in bone and inhibits bone resorption without inhibiting bone formation or mineralization. It is given orally. The patient should sit upright for 30 minutes after a dose to prevent esophageal irritation. Another type of drug used in treating osteoporosis is selective estrogen receptor modulators, such as raloxifene (Evista). These drugs mimic the effect of estrogen on bone by reducing bone resorption.

Teriparatide (Forteo) is a form of parathyroid hormone approved for postmenopausal women who are at increased risk for osteoporosis fractures or who cannot use other treatments. The drug prevents sloughing of osteoblasts (bone cells that form new bone) in porous or spongy bones and increases bone mass in the spine and hip. Teriparatide treatment requires a daily subcutaneous injection of the drug and is limited to a 24-month period. The drug must be kept refrigerated. The most common side effects are nausea, dizziness, leg cramps, hypercalcemia, and orthostatic hypotension. The drug is not recommended for patients with an increased risk of osteosarcoma (Bethel, 2017a).

Surgical interventions for osteoporosis. Women with severe osteoporosis who are unresponsive to an analgesic may be candidates for a surgical procedure to relieve the pain. Vertebroplasty and kyphoplasty may be successful in relieving pain from compression fractures of the spine. Vertebroplasty (plastic surgery on a vertebra) involves high-pressure injection of poly(methyl methacrylate) cement into the spine, which pushes the vertebrae apart. The procedure is performed with the patient under a general or local anesthetic. Major complications involve damage to the posterior vertebral walls from the high pressure used to inject the cement and movement of the cement out of vertebral spaces into the spinal canal.

Kyphoplasty (plastic surgery on dowager's hump) involves inserting a balloon into the center of the collapsed vertebrae, which restores the position of the vertebrae and creates a space for injection of poly(methyl methacrylate) cement. Porous bone is packed around the outside edge. This procedure is less risky than vertebroplasty because the balloon removes the need to use high pressure for the cement placement (Bethel, 2017c).

Nursing considerations. Patients are admitted to the hospital and required to stay up to 24 hours after the procedure. Flat bed rest is ordered for the first 4 hours postoperatively, then patients are allowed to ambulate as able. A small dressing covers the operative site, and antibiotics and steroids typically are ordered for three doses after the procedure.

Nursing Interventions and Patient Teaching

Nursing interventions are aimed at preventing further bone loss and fractures. A diet rich in milk and dairy products provides most of the calcium in the diet (see the Patient Teaching box). Food and beverages that contain caffeine also contain phosphorus, which contributes to bone loss. Teach patients relaxation techniques

Patient Teaching

Dietary Needs in Osteoporosis

- Calcium is a mineral that can slow bone loss and may decrease fractures.
- A total of 1200 to 2000 mg of calcium is needed daily in the diet or through supplements.
- Food sources of calcium include milk products, many green vegetables, calcium-fortified orange juice, and soy milk.
- Vitamin D helps calcium absorption and stimulates bone formation.
- A diet low in sodium, animal protein, and caffeine is recommended.
- Foods that are high in calcium include whole and skim milk, yogurt, turnip greens, cottage cheese, ice cream, sardines with bones, and spinach.

Table 44.6 **Medications for Osteoporosis**

GENERIC NAME (TRADE NAME)	ACTION	SIDE EFFECTS/TOXIC EFFECTS	NURSING IMPLICATIONS
Bisphosphonates: alendronate (Fosamax), risedronate (Actonel), etidronate, pamidronate (Aredia), ibandronate (Boniva)	Slow bone loss and increase bone density	Difficulty in swallowing, chest pain, severe or recurring heartburn	Administer first thing in the morning with 6–8 oz plain water, 30 min before other medications, beverages, or food.
calcitonin-salmon injection (Miacalcin) or calcitonin-salmon nasal spray	Increases bone mass, particularly in the spine	Injection site reaction, nasal irritation	Monitor for injection site reaction. Advise patient to take medication exactly as directed.
Estrogen receptor modulator: raloxifene (Evista)	Prevents bone loss and spinal fractures	May increase tendency for deep vein thrombosis, myocardial infarcts, uterine bleeding, and breast abnormalities	Administer without regard to meals.
Parathyroid hormone: teriparatide (Forteo)	Prevents bone loss; promotes bone growth	Increased heart rate or dizziness	Administer subcutaneously into thigh or abdominal wall once daily.

Data from Skidmore-Roth L: *Mosby's 2017 nursing drug reference*, St. Louis, 2016, Mosby.

and encourage them to stop smoking. Safety measures, such as side rails, hand rails, bedside commodes with seat elevators, and rubber mats in showers, can help prevent falls in older adults. Efforts are made to keep patients with osteoporosis ambulatory to prevent further loss of bone substance as a result of immobility. Encourage weight-bearing exercise to increase bone density.

A patient problem statement and interventions for the patient with osteoporosis include but are not limited to the following:

Patient Problem	Nursing Interventions
Insufficient Knowledge, related to issues of home care	Stress importance of activity and rest; provide aerobic exercise schedule; caution patient to avoid jogging Advise patient to take recommended medications Instruct patient in how to maintain a healthy diet

To prevent osteoporosis, advise women to maintain an adequate daily intake of calcium and vitamin D; to avoid smoking; to decrease caffeine intake; to decrease excess protein in the diet; and to engage in moderate activity such as walking, bike riding, or swimming at least 3 days a week.

After menopause, the usual recommended daily allowance is 1000 mg of calcium in postmenopausal women taking estrogen and 1500 mg in postmenopausal women who are not taking estrogen. Vitamin D, which increases calcium absorption, may be added to the daily regimen of postmenopausal women according to the health care provider's orders. Encourage the patient to make follow-up visits to the health care provider for guidance on medication, diet, and exercise regimen.

Prognosis

Osteoporosis is a chronic disorder, but vitamin D and calcium, as well as pharmacologic therapy, may help stop the rate of bone loss. In postmenopausal women, therapy with estrogen decreases the rate of bone resorption but does not increase bone formation. Prevention of osteoporosis should begin before bone loss has occurred.

OSTEOMYELITIS

Etiology and Pathophysiology

Osteomyelitis (local or generalized infection of bone and bone marrow) can occur from bacteria introduced through trauma, such as a compound fracture or surgery. Bacteria also may travel by the bloodstream from another site in the body to a bone, causing an infection. Staphylococci are the most common causative agents. Other invading organisms include *Streptococcus viridans, Escherichia coli, Mycobacterium tuberculosis, Neisseria gonorrhoeae, Pseudomonas organisms,* salmonellae, and fungi.

Bacteria invade the bone, and bone tissue degenerates. If osteomyelitis becomes chronic, the bone tissue often is weak and predisposed to spontaneous fractures. Osteomyelitis can become chronic as a result of inadequate acute treatment. It is either a continuous persistent problem or a process of exacerbations and remissions. Over time, granulation tissue turns to scar tissue. This avascular scar tissue provides an ideal site for continued microorganism growth and is impenetrable to antibiotics.

Clinical Manifestations

The patient with osteomyelitis is subject to contractures in the affected extremity if positioned incorrectly. A new focus of infection can develop months and sometimes years after the initial infection is diagnosed.

Assessment

Collection of subjective data includes a complete history of injuries, surgical procedures, and diseases. Assess the patient's complaints of persistent, severe, and increasing bone pain and tenderness, as well as regional muscle spasm. Also inquire about any allergies, especially to medications, because antibiotics are given long term.

Collection of objective data includes careful inspection of any wounds. Assess the drainage for color, amount, and odor. Monitor vital signs for signs of infection (temperature elevation, tachycardia, and tachypnea). Note any edema, especially in joints with limited mobility.

Diagnostic Tests

Take a complete history, along with a physical examination. Radiologic tests may include radiographic studies, MRI, and CT scans. Laboratory studies may include a complete blood count (leukocytosis may be present), ESR, C-reactive protein (CRP), needle aspiration, and cultures of blood and drainage, if present (Cleveland Clinic, 2014).

Medical Management

Medical care for the patient with osteomyelitis includes wound management and antibiotic therapy. Necrotic tissue requires débridement. For some patients, surgery may be performed to remove a fragment of necrotic bone that is partially or entirely detached from the surrounding or adjacent healthy bone **(sequestrum)**. Hyperbaric oxygen therapy may be initiated. The administration of high levels of oxygen stimulates tissue growth and repair.

Vigorous and prolonged intravenous antibiotic therapy will be used. These antibiotics may include penicillin, nafcillin, neomycin, cephalexin (Keflex), cefoxitin (Mefoxin), and gentamicin (Garamycin). Parenteral antibiotics are usually necessary for several weeks but may be prescribed for as long as 3 to 6 months. Bed rest usually is prescribed (Kishner, 2016).

Nursing Interventions and Patient Teaching

Nursing interventions include gentleness in moving and manipulating the diseased extremity, because pain is severe in the early phase of infection. The affected part may need absolute rest, with careful positioning using pillows and sandbags for good alignment. Often wounds are irrigated with normal saline or with antiseptic or antibiotic solution and then covered with a sterile dressing, using strict surgical asepsis. Patients are placed on drainage and secretion precautions. Dietary planning includes a diet high in calories, protein, and vitamins. Monitor the patient for worsening infection. Assess vital signs. Review laboratory results.

Teaching includes information about the signs of infection, such as elevated temperature. Because chronic osteomyelitis may last a lifetime, warn the patient of the recurrence of signs and symptoms. Patients must avoid trauma to the affected bone because pathologic fractures are common.

Prognosis

Acute osteomyelitis may respond to treatment after several weeks. Abscess formation, deformity, sepsis, and loss of mobility, and fractures are potential complications. Chronic osteomyelitis may persist for years with exacerbations and remissions. A recurrence of the infection is not uncommon (Kishner, 2016).

FIBROMYALGIA SYNDROME

Etiology and Pathophysiology

Fibromyalgia is a chronic syndrome of unknown origin that causes pain in the muscles, bones, or joints. It is associated with soft tissue tenderness at multiple characteristic sites. It contributes to poor sleep, headaches, altered thought processes, and stiffness or muscle aches. Fibromyalgia affects approximately 5 million people; 80% to 90% of those diagnosed are women. The disorder is more common in people between ages 20 and 50 years. Fibromyalgia has been referred to as *fibrositis, fibromyositis, myofascial pain syndrome,* and *psychogenic rheumatism.* Clinical symptoms of fibromyalgia syndrome (FMS) can overlap those of chronic fatigue syndrome. It is not considered life threatening and does not cause permanent damage. It often is seen in patients who also have rheumatic conditions such as rheumatoid arthritis and lupus. The stress response appears hyperactive in patients with FMS (CDC, 2015).

Clinical Manifestations

Patients with FMS frequently complain of a generalized achiness in axial locations, such as the neck and lower back, accompanied by stiffness that is worse in the morning. Factors that aggravate the condition include cold or humid weather, physical or mental fatigue, excessive physical activity, and anxiety or stress. Difficulty sleeping is common, as well as headaches, tingling or numbness in the hands and feet, and painful menstrual periods. Mental health concerns reported by fibromyalgia sufferers include cognitive difficulties, anxiety, and depression (CDC, 2015).

Assessment

Collection of subjective data includes questioning the patient about muscle pain, often described as muscle ache; tension or migraine headaches; premenstrual tension; jaw pain; excessive fatigue; anxiety; and depression. Include questions about sensations of numbness, tingling, and perception of insects crawling on or under the skin. Complaints of being forgetful and unable to recall recent information—such as appointments, location of parked car, or how to get to familiar places—are significant.

Collection of objective data includes noting periodic limb movement, especially at night, or a persistent need to move the lower extremities day and night. Ask about sleep deprivation and the patient's ability to complete self-care activities.

Diagnostic Tests

No specific laboratory and radiographic tests diagnose FMS. Diagnosis confirmation for patients with fibromyalgia may take months to years. The process is one that eliminates other potential conditions. Blood chemistry screening, a CBC, rheumatoid factor, and ESR are normal in patients with FMS. A sleep study may be ordered in patients with a history suggestive of particular types of sleep disturbances; however, sleep study findings are typically normal in patients with FMS. Research is focusing on the relationships between neurotransmitter levels and fibromyalgia syndrome.

Medical Management

There is no cure for fibromyalgia. The primary treatment approach includes patient education and reassurance. Inform the patient with FMS that this is not a psychiatric disturbance and that symptoms are not uncommon in the general population. Although FMS has no single treatment, combining pharmacologic agents has been helpful. Tricyclic antidepressants are used in the treatment of uncontrollable pain disorders. Benefits of these agents include (1) antidepressant results, (2) antiinflammatory features, (3) central skeletal muscle relaxation, and (4) pain inhibition through suppression of serotonergic and noradrenergic pathways (Table 44.7).

Nursing Interventions and Patient Teaching

Nursing interventions are individualized, holistic, and goal oriented. Management of FMS focuses on functional goals that enable the patient to live as normal a life as possible. Treatment programs include education, exercise, and relaxation techniques. Patients are taught the basic principles of good sleep hygiene (see the Patient Teaching box). Exercise programs consist of gentle, progressive stretching, beginning with a muscle warm-up through either gentle exercise or warm baths. Stretching helps release tight muscles. Nonimpact exercise such as swimming, walking, or stationary cycling is helpful. Yoga benefits individuals in a variety of ways including promotion of relaxation, stress reduction, and increased flexibility.

Prognosis

Fibromyalgia is a challenging disorder to treat. Patients may have difficulty achieving remission of symptoms. Many patients report that the condition impairs their ability to successfully complete their activities of daily living. The emotional stressors of the condition affect their ability to maintain employment and remain active in family processes (University of Maryland Medical Center, 2016).

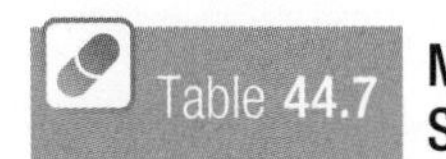

Medications for Fibromyalgia Syndrome

GENERIC NAME (TRADE NAME)	ACTION
amitriptyline (Endep)	Diminishes local pain and stiffness; improves sleep pattern
cyclobenzaprine	Diminishes local pain, improves sleep pattern, and decreases number of tender points
clonazepam (Klonopin)	Decreases symptoms of constant leg movement, especially at night
acetaminophen and tramadol	Used together or given alone for management of moderate to severe pain. Bind opioid receptors, inhibit reuptake of norepinephrine and serotonin
pregabalin (Lyrica)	An anticonvulsant that decreases pain severity and improves fatigue, sleep, and physical functioning
tizanidine (Zanaflex)	Eases pain by lowering substance P, which participates in the transmission process of certain neurons; improves sleep and physical functioning
sodium oxybate (Xyrem)	Improves deep sleep and growth hormone levels and helps reduce pain and fatigue
duloxetine hydrochloride (Cymbalta)	Reduces pain in patients with fibromyalgia with or without having symptoms of major depression

Patient Teaching

Sleep Hygiene

- Control environmental factors by avoiding large meals 2 to 3 hours before bedtime and keeping the sleep environment dark, quiet, and comfortable.
- Exercise regularly each day.
- Keep a diary recording sleep patterns.
- Maintain regular sleep patterns by going to bed and awaking the same time each day; avoiding long naps, and taking a hot bath within 2 hours of bedtime.
- Recognize how drugs such as nicotine, alcohol, and caffeine affect sleep.

SURGICAL INTERVENTIONS FOR TOTAL KNEE OR TOTAL HIP REPLACEMENT

Surgical procedures can prevent progressive deformities; relieve pain; improve function; and correct deformities resulting from RA, osteoarthritis, or other disorders. Tendon transplants can replace damaged muscles.

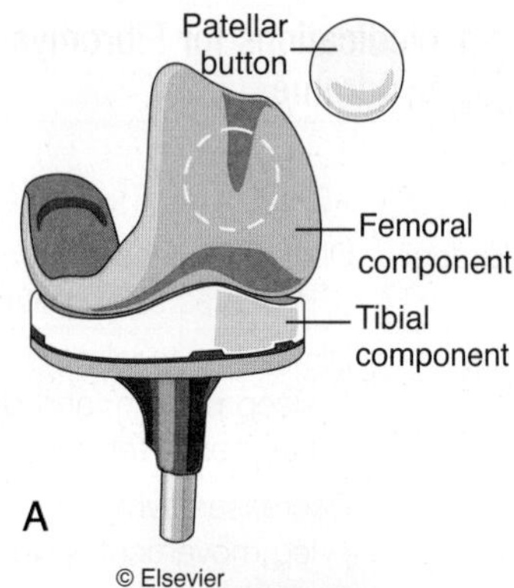

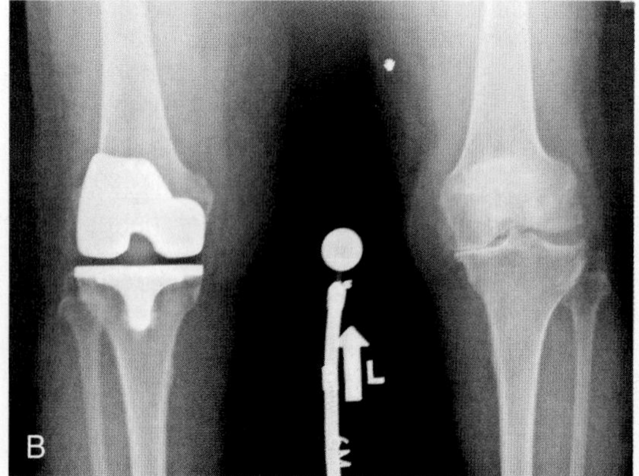

Fig. 44.9 A, Tibial and femoral components of total knee prosthesis. Patellar button, made of polyethylene, protects the posterior surface of the patella from friction against the femoral component when the knee is moved through flexion and extension. B, *(left)* Total knee prosthesis in place; *(right)* arthritic knee.

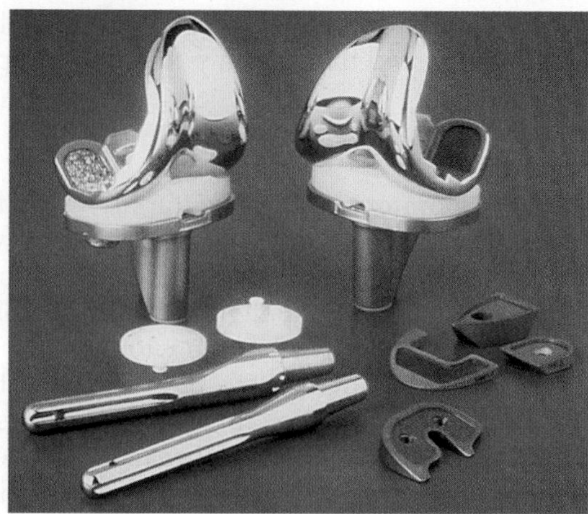

Fig. 44.10 Total joint replacements: knee.

Patients with RA may need a synovectomy (excision of synovial membrane) to maintain joint function. An osteotomy (cutting into bone to correct bone or joint deformities) can improve function and relieve pain. **Arthrodesis** (surgical fusion of a joint) can be performed when severe joint destruction has occurred. Total joint replacement **arthroplasty** (repair or refashioning of one or both sides, parts, or specific tissue within a joint) often is required on the elbow, hip, knee, or shoulder joint to restore or increase mobility.

KNEE ARTHROPLASTY (TOTAL KNEE REPLACEMENT)

The knee joint may be replaced to restore motion, relieve pain, or correct deformity. Figs. 44.9 and 44.10 show the tibial and femoral components of a knee prosthesis. Nursing interventions for the patient undergoing total knee replacement are shown in Box 44.4.

UNICOMPARTMENTAL KNEE ARTHROPLASTY

Unicompartmental knee replacement also is referred to as partial knee replacement. This modified surgical procedure is performed when only one of the compartments of the knee is affected by arthritic changes. If both sides of the bones in the knee, including the underside of the patella, are damaged, a total knee replacement is necessary (see Fig. 44.10).

The knee has three compartments: (1) the medial, or inside, compartment; (2) the lateral, or outside, compartment; and (3) the patellofemoral compartment, which is where the kneecap rests. Minimally invasive knee surgery removes only the most damaged areas of cartilage; a small plastic disk replaces the worn cartilage, providing a new cushion between the bones.

Partial knee surgery involves making a small incision over the knee and exposing the worn-out cartilage. The rough edges of the distal area of the femur and superior area of the tibia are cut flat and cleaned, and the unicompartmental device is put into place. Some of the devices are cemented in place.

Total knee arthroplasty (TKA) is performed on patients of all ages, from teenagers to patients in their nineties. The decision to perform TKA is based on the patient's overall health and expected outcome of the surgery. The patient must be able to withstand intensive physical therapy for several weeks to months after the replacement.

Assessment

Subjective data include a medical history of home medications, allergies, past surgeries, and significant medical problems. Assess the patient for complaints of pain on one or both sides of the knee with weight-bearing. Also gather information on the effectiveness of conservative treatments such as medications, cortisone injections, strengthening exercises, weight loss, and use of assistive devices such as gait enhancers.

Objective data include vital signs and weight. Patients who are obese or have significant inflammation are not candidates for the surgery. Blood tests, electrocardiogram (ECG), and chest x-ray examination are done to evaluate the patient's state of health. Also assess the patient's understanding of the surgical procedure.

Diagnostic Tests

An x-ray examination of the knee shows damage to the joint.

Box 44.4 Nursing Interventions for the Patient Undergoing Total Knee Replacement

PREOPERATIVE INTERVENTIONS

Same as for any major surgery (see Chapter 42).

POSTOPERATIVE INTERVENTIONS

1. Positioning
   a. Elevate the operative leg on pillows to enhance venous return for the first 24 hours only. Place pillows with caution to avoid flexing the knee.
   b. The patient may be turned from side to back to side.
2. Wound care
   a. Care of drains (usually Hemovac) as for total hip replacement.
   b. Assess patient for systemic evidence of loss of blood (hypotension, tachycardia) if bulky compression dressing is used because it may hold large quantities of drainage before drainage is visible.
   c. Remove bulky dressings before the patient begins continuous passive motion (CPM) flexion greater than 20 degrees.
3. Activity
   a. Passive flexion in a CPM machine within prescribed flexion-extension limits may be started in the postanesthesia care unit (see Fig. 44.11). Patient's leg should remain in machine as much as tolerated (up to 22 hours per day) to facilitate even healing of tissue. The physical therapist increases extension on CPM as patient tolerates. (Once the large bulky dressing is replaced with a smaller dressing, flexion degree is increased.) Many surgeons are opting to not use CPM but rely on active patient flexion and extension exercises. When CPM is not occurring, patient's leg is extended with no pillow under leg.
   b. Encourage patient to perform active dorsiflexion of the ankles; quadriceps setting; and, after the drain is removed, straight leg–raising exercises.
   c. Patient begins active flexion exercises three or four times a day about the fifth postoperative day.
   d. Light weight-bearing with an assistive device may be started as early as upon arrival to the hospital room after surgery and increased as the patient tolerates.
   e. Sitting in a chair with the leg elevated may be started on the first postoperative day.
   f. Encourage patient to wear a resting knee extension splint (immobilizer) on the operated leg until able to demonstrate quadriceps control (independent straight leg–raising).
4. Pain control
   a. For initial control of pain, use opioids (usually with a patient-controlled epidural or patient-controlled analgesia) and positioning; gradually decrease medication to nonopioid analgesics as patient tolerates.
   b. Encourage patient to use cool applications at 40°F (4.4°C) continuously on knee.
5. Discharge instructions
   a. Patient must observe partial weight-bearing restriction and use ambulatory aid for approximately 2 months after discharge.
   b. Patient should continue active flexion and straight leg–raising exercises at home.

Nursing Interventions and Patient Teaching

Nursing interventions are aimed at promoting healing and facilitating mobility. The typical postoperative stay for patients having TKA is one or two nights. Monitor pain and administer analgesics as needed. Help the patient deep breathe and cough every 2 hours. Also encourage use of an incentive spirometer. Begin clear liquids and advance to regular diet as tolerated. Monitor IV fluids and antibiotics. Change the dressing as needed.

Patients may resume weight-bearing postoperatively as soon as allowed by the surgeon, with some as soon as returning to their hospital room. Assess their ability to use an assistive device such as crutches or a walker. The day of surgery the physical therapist begins teaching basic postoperative exercises. Physical therapy continues either in a rehabilitation facility or at home upon discharge and then continues for several weeks or months. Also instruct the patient that prophylactic antibiotics are recommended before routine dental cleaning or any dental procedure up to 2 years after the surgery.

HIP ARTHROPLASTY (TOTAL HIP REPLACEMENT)

Hip arthroplasty, or total hip replacement, is performed commonly when arthritis involves the head of the femur and acetabulum. Additional indications for hip replacement include fractures, tumors, and injuries. The decision to have hip replacement surgery traditionally follows periods of lengthy pain and discomfort. The choice to have the surgery will in most cases result in reduced pain, improved mobility, and increased enjoyment of life.

Prosthetic devices may be cemented or uncemented. The cemented device is secured to the patient's healthy bone tissue with a gluelike adhesive (Fig. 44.11). Uncemented prosthetic devices are inserted and then the patient's body tissue grows into them for attachment. Several variations of hip replacement surgery are practiced, but each uses similar equipment. The Bechtol total hip system involves a white plastic cup cemented in place to replace the damaged acetabulum. A stainless steel or Vitallium ball on a stem replaces the head of the femur, which is removed surgically. The stem is cemented into the femoral canal, and the new head fits precisely into the plastic acetabulum, providing friction-free movement in the joint (US FDA, 2017b).

Assessment

Collection of subjective data includes assessing the patient's level of orientation, because older adults can become disoriented from a change in the environment

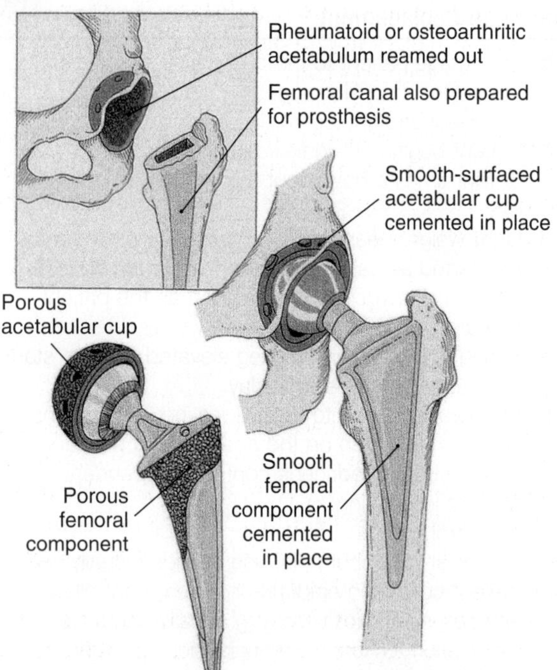

Fig. 44.11 Hip arthroplasty (total hip replacement).

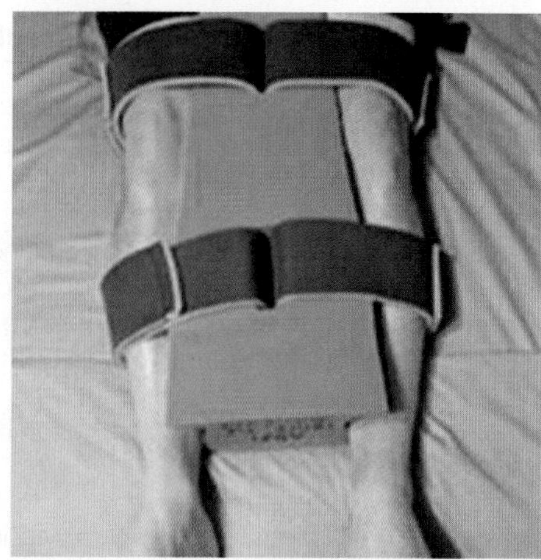

Fig. 44.12 Maintaining postoperative abduction after total hip replacement.

(home to hospital setting) and the effects of anesthesia and other prescribed medications. Complaints of unrelieved pain and numbness, tingling, or paresthesia indicate neurovascular impairment.

Collection of objective data includes assessment of the patient's compliance with nursing interventions to promote circulation; prevent impairment of skin integrity; and prevent hypostatic pneumonia by such means as coughing, turning (to the unaffected side; additional pillows are used to keep the affected leg abducted), deep breathing every 2 hours, and using an incentive spirometer. Assess vital signs for evidence of excessive bleeding, including hypotension, tachycardia, and tachypnea. Decreased urinary output is indicative of hypovolemia. Carefully assess drainage of the surgical wound at least every 4 hours. Hemovacs or other suction devices are placed in the wound during surgery to provide closed-wound suction. Assess approximation of the incision line and signs of inflammation (erythema, edema, fever, and pain). Also assess traction (if used) for the correct amount of weight, the proper alignment, and maintenance of the affected leg in an abducted position. Look for any reaction to the cement, signs of phlebitis (edema, erythema, and pain), and urinary retention (indwelling catheters may be used for the first 24 to 48 hours).

Nursing Interventions and Patient Teaching

Nursing interventions are aimed at the assessment of potential complications, the promotion of healing, and facilitating mobility. Take vital signs at least every 4 hours. Document intake and output. Measure oral intake and urinary output as well as intravenous fluids and fluids from drainage devices such as the Hemovac. Thigh-high antiembolism stockings are used before and after surgery. Early in the postoperative period the surgeon orders a plan of weight-bearing and physical therapy. Nursing education should focus on reinforcing this plan to the patient and family.

Encourage coughing and deep-breathing exercises at least every 2 hours. Give oxygen at 1 to 2 L per nasal cannula as needed. Instruct the patient in the use of the incentive spirometer every 2 to 4 hours.

Perform neurovascular checks every hour for 24 hours, then every 2 hours for the next 24 hours, and then every 4 hours. Check vital signs every 4 hours. Also carefully assess the patient for pain control. This includes monitoring patient-controlled epidural (PCE), patient-controlled analgesia (PCA), or oral medications, whichever is prescribed.

The surgical dressing will remain in place until removal is ordered by the surgeon; most surgeons prefer to remove the surgical dressing. Reinforce the dressing as needed. Report excessive drainage. Maintain the position of the operative area with a splint, an abduction pillow (Fig. 44.12), an immobilizer, or a brace; turn the patient to the nonoperative side.

Begin clear liquids, and advance diet as tolerated. Encourage fluid intake and high-fiber foods (if tolerated) to prevent constipation.

Bed rest is maintained for approximately 24 hours postoperatively. Teach the patient to do isometric exercises on the quadriceps and gluteal muscles of the affected extremity by keeping the toes pointed up, flexing the ankles, and flexing and extending the knee of the unaffected extremity. Physical therapy exercises begin on the first or second postoperative day. The exercises are either active or passive to all joints, excluding the operated joint, and include quadriceps setting, straight leg–raising, flexion and extension, or other individually prescribed exercises. The patient should be up with walker or crutches four times daily; increase ambulation as the patient is able with up to 25 pounds of weight-bearing on the operative limb, gradually increasing to full weight-bearing with crutches or a walker. The patient should be up but not bearing weight on the operative limb after the bed rest order expires. Some health care providers may permit touch-down weight-bearing. Protection of the integrity of the new joint requires the avoidance of hyperflexion of the hip. Chair sitting initially is limited to 10 to 15 minutes two or three times daily for the first week, and then for 20 to 30 minutes four times daily. Use of a toilet-seat riser prevents hyperflexion of the hip after total replacement. Patient problem and interventions for the patient with a total hip replacement include but are not limited to the following:

Patient Problem	Nursing Interventions
Prolonged Pain, related to: • Preoperative arthritic pain necessitating surgery • Incisional pain • Soft tissue trauma of surgery	Explain analgesic therapy, including medication, dose, and schedule If patient is a candidate for PCA or PCE, explain the concept and routine Respond quickly to pain complaints Obtain pain rating from patient Instruct patient to request analgesic before pain is severe Administer analgesics as ordered and per hospital policy or procedure Encourage use of analgesics 30 to 45 min before therapy; unrelieved pain hinders rehabilitation progress Change position (within hip precautions) q 2 hr Document all responses to analgesics
Compromised Physical Mobility, related to surgical procedure and discomfort	Allow patient to dangle feet at bedside several minutes before getting out of bed Reinforce physical therapist's instructions for exercises and ambulation techniques and devices; consistent instructions from interdisciplinary team members promote safe, secure rehabilitation environment Maintain weight-bearing status on affected extremity as prescribed Keep abduction pillow between legs while turning in bed (see Fig. 44.13) Do not have the patient lie on the operative side Maintain the leg in abduction when the patient is lying supine or on the nonoperative side Encourage the patient to use trapeze in bed to assist in mobility

Discharge instructions include teaching the patient to use an ambulatory aid, avoid adduction, and limit hip flexion to 90 degrees for approximately 2 to 3 months. A raised toilet seat should be obtained and used at home until flexion restrictions are removed. The patient should avoid leaning forward and use assistive devices to avoid bending. The patient may need a long-handled shoehorn and reacher to facilitate ADLs within flexion restriction.

FRACTURES

FRACTURE OF THE HIP

Etiology and Pathophysiology

Hip fractures are the leading type of fracture requiring treatment in a hospital facility (see the Lifespan Considerations and Health Promotion boxes). Women are at greater risk for hip fracture because of their increased likelihood to develop osteoporosis and longer life expectancy compared with men.

Fractures of the hip include intracapsular fractures, in which the femur is broken inside the joint (subcapital) or in the femoral head or neck (transcervical and basal) (Figs. 44.13A to C). Intracapsular fractures may disrupt the blood supply to the head of the femur, which subsequently develops avascular necrosis (Figs. 44.14 and 44.15). Therefore fractures of the head or proximal femoral neck may be treated with insertion of a femoral prosthesis (Fig. 44.16). The more common type of hip fracture is an extracapsular fracture, one that occurs outside the hip joint capsule. These are referred to as intertrochanteric or subtrochanteric fractures (see Fig. 44.13D). These fractures heal well, without vascular necrosis, with the use of compression screws or nails because the blood supply to the fracture site comes from the surrounding vessels outside the capsule (see Figs. 44.14 and 44.15). Side plates attached to the nails help maintain a stable reduction while healing progresses (Fig. 44.17A). An intertrochanteric fracture occurs below the lesser trochanter and frequently is seen in younger patients suffering from hip trauma (see Fig. 44.13D).

Clinical Manifestations

Signs and symptoms of hip fracture are severe pain and tenderness in the region of the fracture site or inability to move the leg voluntarily, and shortening or external rotation of the leg.

Assessment

Subjective data include an accurate history of the events before the injury. Assess the patient's level of orientation. Disorientation can occur, especially in older adults when they are in pain, are anxious, or are in an unfamiliar environment. The patient's medical and surgical history is significant, as is any family history of bone disease. Patients with gastroesophageal reflux disease who are taking antacids or using proton pump inhibitors are at increased risk of hip fractures, because these drugs cause malabsorption of calcium.

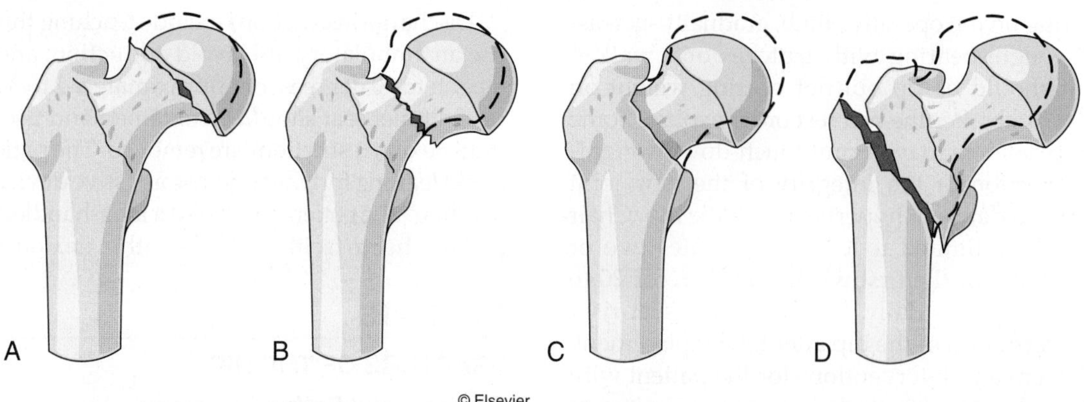

Fig. 44.13 Fractures of the hip. A, Subcapital fracture. B, Transcervical fracture. C, Impacted fracture of the base of the neck. D, Intertrochanteric fracture.

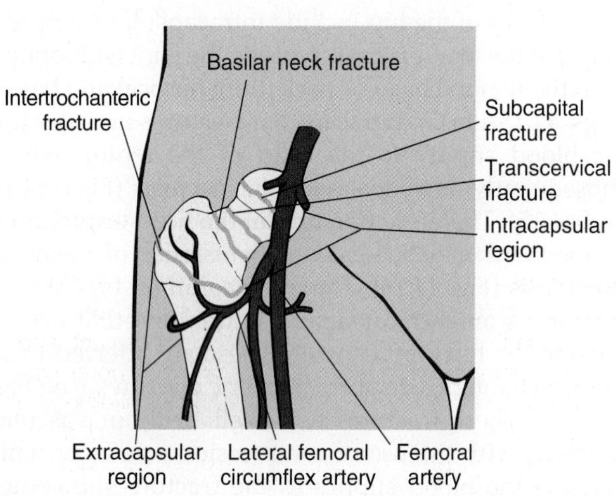

Fig. 44.14 Femur with location of various types of fractures. (From Lewis SL, Heitkemper MM, Dirksen SR, et al: *Medical-surgical nursing: Assessment and management of clinical problems,* ed 7, St. Louis, 2007, Mosby.)

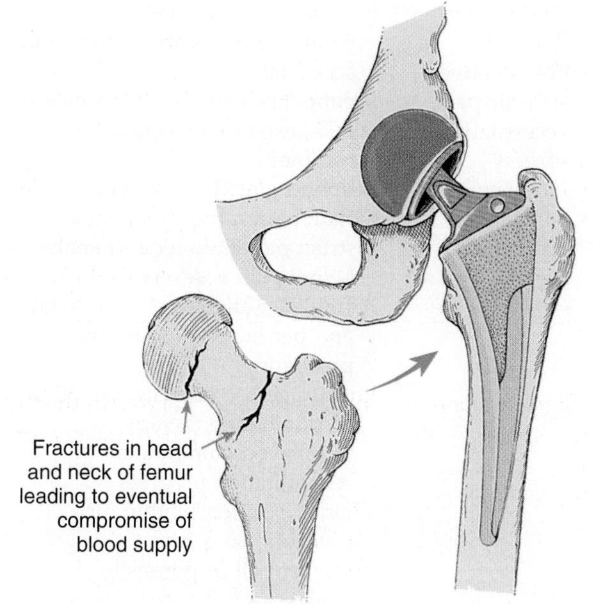

Fig. 44.16 Bipolar hip replacement (hemiarthroplasty).

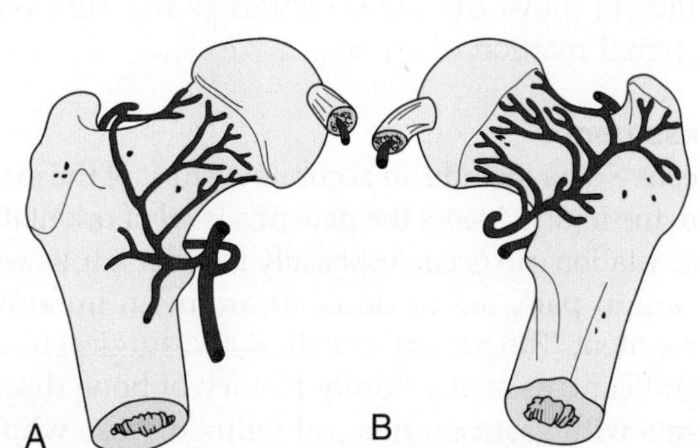

Fig. 44.15 A, Anterior arterial blood supply to hip joint. B, Posterior arterial blood supply to hip joint. (Modified from Mourad L: *Orthopedic disorders,* St. Louis, 1991, Mosby.)

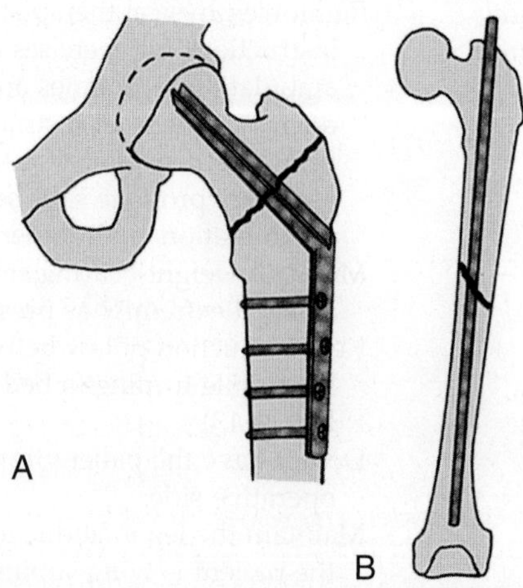

Fig. 44.17 A, Neufeld nail and screws in repair of intertrochanteric fracture. B, Küntscher nail (intramedullary rod) used in repair of midshaft femoral fracture. (From Monahan FD, Sands JK, Neighbors M, et al: *Phipps' medical-surgical nursing: Health and illness perspectives,* ed 8, St. Louis, 2007, Mosby.)

Lifespan Considerations

Older Adults

Musculoskeletal Disorder

- Physiologic changes of aging result in decreased joint flexibility and muscular strength.
- Changes in bone mass with aging increase the risk of fractures. Hip fractures and compression fractures of the spine are noted most frequently.
- Degenerative joint disease related to "wear and tear" on joints is associated with aging. Joint replacement is no longer considered a last resort for older adults and provides an opportunity for improvement in the quality of life.
- Changes in the foot can occur with aging, poorly fitted shoes, or heredity. Bunions and hammertoe are seen with increasing frequency in older adults, causing pain and possibly decreased mobility. Encourage older adults to wear properly fitted shoes to reduce discomfort. If discomfort is severe, surgical correction may be necessary.
- Check the homes of older adults for safety hazards such as rugs that could cause falls.
- Older adults should avoid climbing unsteady or uneven surfaces because coordination and balance change with age and falls may result.
- Instruct older adults in the correct use of assistive devices such as canes or walkers. Encourage them to use these regularly to prevent injury.

Signs and symptoms of a fracture vary with the type and location of the break. Usually the patient has some degree of discomfort that may be more pronounced with slight movement of the affected part. Most patients complain of pain in the affected leg after sustaining a fractured hip, although patients suffering from an impacted intracapsular fracture have little pain, if any, immediately after the fracture. Impaired sensation may indicate nerve damage from the bone fragments "pinching" or severing the nerve. Assess for edema, tenderness, muscle spasms, deformity, and loss of function. Patients may say they heard a "snap" or "pop" at the time the bone was injured. The patient may report simply sitting down and feeling or hearing the pop of the fracture.

Collection of objective data includes assessment for soft tissue injury, with erythema or ecchymoses noted. Look for differences between the injured limb and the uninjured limb. A change in the curvature or length of bone may indicate fracture. The affected leg is shorter, usually externally rotated approximately 90 degrees, and slightly flexed after an extracapsular hip fracture. With an intracapsular fracture, the upper thigh is more edematous than the area below it, and the affected leg is shortened with external rotation. Subtrochanteric fractures cause excessive bleeding into the soft tissue, and the affected leg is shortened and rotated anteriorly. Crepitus may be felt or heard as the broken bone ends rub together. Assess neurovascular status of the extremity (Box 44.5).

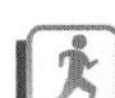

Health Promotion

Hip Fracture

- Factors that contribute to the incidence of hip fracture in older adults include an increased risk for falls, inability to correct a postural imbalance, inadequacy of local tissue to absorb shock (e.g., fat, muscle bulk), and underlying skeletal weakness.
- Factors that increase the risk of older adults falling include gait and balance problems, decreased vision and hearing, diminished reflexes, orthostatic hypotension, and medication use.
- Leading hazards that increase the risk of falls are loose rugs and slippery or uneven surfaces.
- Many falls are associated with getting in or out of a chair or bed.
- Falls to the side, the most common type in the frail elderly, are more likely to result in a hip fracture than forward falls.
- Two important factors influencing the amount of force imposed on the hip are the presence of energy-absorbing soft tissue over the greater trochanter and the state of leg muscle contraction at the time of the fall.
- Many older adults have poor muscle tone, an important factor in the severity of a fall.
- Older women often have osteoporosis and accompanying low bone density, which increases the risk of hip fracture.
- Targeted interventions to reduce hip fractures in older adults include a variety of strategies. Calcium and vitamin D supplementation, estrogen replacement, and drug therapy have been shown to decrease bone loss or increase bone density and decrease the likelihood of fracture. Be vigilant in planning interventions that are known to reduce the incidence of hip fracture in the older adult.

Keep the injured part still because movement of a fractured bone can cause additional damage and may turn a closed fracture into an open fracture. Also assess the patient's nutritional status. Thin and obese patients are at risk for impaired skin integrity if bed rest is ordered. After the fracture is reduced, regularly inspect skin areas in contact with cast edges or traction apparatus for signs of neurovascular compromise. Patients suffering from any trauma are at risk for shock. Treating the shock takes precedence over treating the fracture.

Diagnostic Tests

Diagnosis is confirmed by radiographic examination of the injured part. Blood tests, such as hemoglobin values, often show decreased laboratory values because of bleeding at the fracture site; the blood glucose level may be elevated because of the stress of the trauma.

Medical Management

Surgical repair is the preferred method of managing intracapsular and extracapsular hip fractures. Surgical treatment enables the patient to get out of bed sooner

Box 44.5 Circulation Check (Neurovascular Assessment)

- A circulation check is also known as a neurovascular assessment. The mnemonic CMS indicates the need to check circulation, motion, and sensation. The assessment is made on patients after musculoskeletal trauma; postoperatively if damage to nerves and blood vessels is suspected; and after casting, splinting, or bandaging.
- Assess the patient every 15 to 30 minutes for several hours and every 3 to 4 hours thereafter, with proper documentation of the findings.
- Subjective data include complaints of numbness or tingling not relieved by flexing the fingers and toes and repositioning the extremity. Objective data include cool, pale, or cyanotic skin above or below the altered site; edema; a capillary refill time greater than 2 seconds; and absent or diminished pulses.
- Remember the seven *P*s when completing the assessment:
  1. Pulselessness
  2. Paresthesia (numbness or tingling sensation)
  3. Paralysis or paresis
  4. Polar temperature
  5. Pallor
  6. Puffiness (edema)
  7. Pain
- Complaints of numbness or tingling may result from general decreased mobility and may be relieved by flexing the fingers and toes and repositioning the extremity. However, if the numbness and tingling are not relieved by these measures and the extremity feels cool to the touch, is slow in capillary refill, has diminished or absent pulses, and appears pale or cyanotic, these are significant symptoms of neurovascular impairment and the findings must be reported immediately.

and decreases the major complications associated with immobility.

The affected extremity may be immobilized temporarily by either Buck's or Russell's traction until the patient's physical condition is stabilized and surgery can be scheduled. The choice of fixation device depends on the fracture location and the potential for avascular necrosis of the femoral head and neck. The use of these devices is called internal fixation. Prosthetic implants, such as the **bipolar hip replacement (hemiarthroplasty)** (see Fig. 44.16), are used to replace the femoral head and neck in fractures when the vascular supply to the femoral head may be compromised. A Neufeld nail and screws are used in the repair of intertrochanteric fractures (see Fig. 44.17A). A Küntscher nail (intramedullary rod) is used to repair midshaft femoral fractures (see Fig. 44.17B). Sliding nails are used in repair of intertrochanteric fractures. Sliding nails usually permit the patient to bear weight to some degree because they "give" slightly without shifting their placement or penetrating the femur. Bone grafts, either autograft (patient's bone) or allograft (cadaver bone), may be used with internal fixation devices when excessive bone is lost at the fracture site. If a stable reduction cannot be achieved, the health care provider may do an arthroplasty (surgical reconstruction of a joint). Immobilization devices, such as casts or splints, also may be used with open reduction.

Nursing Interventions and Patient Teaching

Nursing interventions for a fractured hip are concerned with preventing shock and further complications. A primary concern is to maintain proper alignment through traction and abduction of the hip when turning a patient with a fractured hip from side to side. Some health care providers do not want patients turned onto their sides for several days after surgery; others may order the patient to be turned only on the nonoperative side. It is important to know the orders and to educate patients about activity restrictions. Patients who have had internal fixation for a fractured hip should avoid elevating the affected extremity when sitting. Elevate the head of the bed a maximum of 45 degrees to avoid acute flexion of the hip and strain on the fixation device. Instruct the patient *not* to cross the legs because this can adduct the affected extremity and dislocate the hip. Limit weight-bearing on the hip by providing walking assists such as a walker or crutches.

Postoperative interventions for a patient with hip fracture repair include wound assessment with special attention to color, amount, and odor of exudate. Assess vital signs, as well as the suture line for approximation of skin edges and intact sutures or staples, at least every 8 hours. Jackson-Pratt or Hemovac drains often are used during the initial postoperative days and must be assessed for amount and color of wound drainage at least every 4 hours. Document intake and output. Encourage the use of incentive spirometers to aid in adequate respiratory ventilation and prevent pneumonia. Turn and move the patient on schedule to maintain skin integrity and promote circulation.

Leg manipulation during surgery and immobility afterward place the patient at risk for deep vein thrombosis and pulmonary embolism. Antiembolism stockings, elastic wraps, or pneumatic compression stockings and foot and leg exercises increase venous flow to the heart. Remove the stockings once each shift to assess for compression points and skin integrity. Anticoagulation therapy with enoxaparin (Lovenox), aspirin, or warfarin (Coumadin) often is prescribed.

Special postoperative instructions regarding proper positioning, sitting, and turning are required for patients who have had a prosthetic implant or bipolar hip replacement (Fig. 44.18; and the Patient Teaching box on postoperative care of the patient who had a fractured hip). Isometric exercises are done on the quadriceps and gluteal muscles to strengthen the muscles used for walking (see the Patient Teaching box on quadriceps setting exercises).

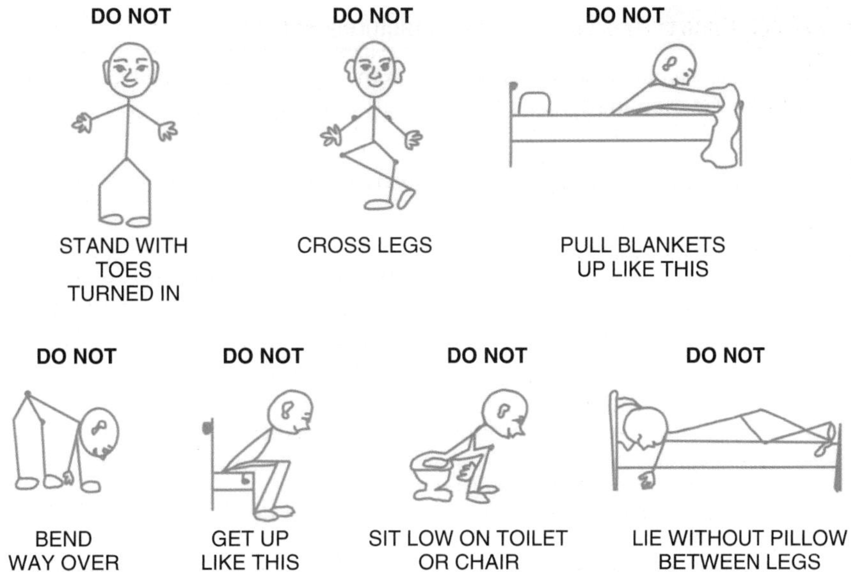

Fig. 44.18 Instruction sheet for the patient with a bipolar hip replacement (hip prosthetic implant).

Patient Teaching

Quadriceps Setting Exercises

Quadriceps and gluteal muscles must be strong for ambulation. The quadriceps muscles stabilize the knee joint. Teach the patient to do the following exercises 10 to 15 times hourly:

- To strengthen quadriceps muscles, push the knee down against the mattress while raising the heel of the foot off the bed; maintain the contraction for a count of five and relax for a count of five.
- For gluteal setting exercises, contract, or "pinch," the buttocks together for a count of five, then relax for a count of five.
- Strengthen the unaffected leg by pushing down against the footboard, holding for a count of five, releasing for a count of five, and repeating.

Nursing interventions also involve use of an abduction splint (a wedge-shaped foam bolster or pillow) for 7 to 10 days to ensure postoperative maintenance of leg abduction and to prevent dislocation of the prosthesis. Place the abduction splint between the patient's legs when in a supine position. Turn the patient with the extremities maintained in proper alignment by using the logrolling procedure with the assistance of at least two nurses. Most health care providers order the patient to be turned toward the unoperated side; check each order by the health care provider. Transfer the patient from bed to chair on the unoperated side by pivoting on the unaffected leg. The injured leg is kept extended forward to avoid extreme hip flexion and possible dislocation of the prosthesis. Provide a chair with a firm, nonreclining seat and arms; elevate the sitting surfaces as necessary with pillows or foam cushions to keep the angle of the hip within the prescribed limits when the patient is sitting. In general, patients who have had *any* kind of internal fixation for a fractured hip should avoid elevation of the operated leg when sitting in a chair, because this puts excessive strain on the fixation device (Nursing Care Plan 44.1).

Prognosis

Complications of hip fractures are the most common cause of death after age 75. Hip fractures in older adults often are complicated by other medical conditions such as diabetes mellitus, cardiac problems (e.g., heart failure), and neurologic disorders (e.g., stroke). A large bone such as the hip heals slowly in older patients, and this predisposes them to various complications. They are at high risk for pneumonia, deep vein thrombosis, fat embolus, pulmonary embolus, impaired skin integrity, urinary retention, constipation, mental disorientation, and depression.

OTHER FRACTURES

Etiology and Pathophysiology

A fracture is a traumatic injury to a bone in which the continuity of the tissue of the bone is broken. Most fractures result from an insult to the bone, such as a forceful blow (twisting or crushing), which places more stress on the bone than it can absorb. Fractures that occur without trauma are referred to as pathologic or spontaneous fractures and can be caused by a weakening of the bone by osteoporosis, metastatic cancer and tumors of the bone, Cushing's syndrome, malnutrition, and complications of long-term steroid therapy.

Fractures may result from (1) direct force, which causes a fracture at the site of the trauma; (2) torsion, as in a twisting injury in which the fracture occurs at a point remote from the trauma (e.g., forceful twisting of the wrist may fracture the arm); or (3) violent contractions involving highly developed muscles (e.g., severe muscle spasms may cause a fracture in a paraplegic patient).

Nursing Care Plan 44.1 The Patient With a Fractured Hip

A female, age 72, fell in her kitchen while removing cookies from the oven. She sustained a subcapital fracture of the right hip. The patient is scheduled in the morning for a bipolar (hemiarthroplasty) prosthesis.

PATIENT PROBLEM

Compromised Tissue Perfusion, related to vascular injury or interruption of arterial and venous flow secondary to edema

Patient Goals and Expected Outcomes	Nursing Interventions	Evaluation and Rationale
Patient's circulation will be maintained to fulfill body requirements	Palpate site for warmth. Observe site for color. Apply moderate pressure to nailbed, and subsequently observe speed of capillary refill. Assess pedal pulse bilaterally q 4 hr. Question patient regarding pain and paresthesia in injured part. Apply antiembolism stockings as ordered.	Distal pulses palpable; toes symmetric, warm, dry, and pink; sensation and mobility intact.
	Help and teach patient to cough q 2 hr and deep breathe q hr. Monitor vital signs q 2–4 hr.	Able to cough and deep breathe with assistance; oxygen saturation 92%, lungs clear.

PATIENT PROBLEM

Insufficient Knowledge, related to home care management

Patient Goals and Expected Outcomes	Nursing Interventions	Evaluation and Rationale
Patient and/or significant other will demonstrate understanding of home care and follow-up instructions through interactive discussion and return demonstration	Stress importance of prescribed rehabilitation plan of activity, rest, and exercise.	Patient demonstrates ambulation with walker, exercises, transfers, and precautions, verbalizes understanding of discharge instructions and home care.
	Provide diet instructions on type and amount of food to eat, and advise patient to avoid weight gain if applicable.	Discusses correct foods to eat for therapeutic results.
	Discuss medications: name, purpose, schedule, dosage, and side effects.	Verbalizes knowledge of medications for purpose, dosage, side effects, and correct schedule to prevent any drug errors.
	Discuss signs and symptoms to report to health care provider: severe pain; changes in temperature, color, or sensation in extremity; malodorous drainage from wound.	Verbalizes knowledge of need to report abnormalities to the health care provider including severe pain, abnormal temperature, color, or tingling in affected extremity as well as abnormal wound drainage.
	Stress home safety factors such as elimination of throw rugs, use of safety bars on the bathtub, elevated toilet seats.	Discusses home preparations for safety to include removal of throw rugs, placement of safety bars on bathtub, and availability of toilet riser. Safety knowledge will prevent accidents.
	Encourage follow-up visits with health care provider.	Notes the importance of postoperative follow-up visits with health care provider. Promotes postoperative recovery.

CRITICAL THINKING QUESTIONS

1. The first postoperative evening, the patient is restless and disoriented. What nursing interventions are needed to prevent dislocation of her bipolar hip prosthesis?
2. On the third postoperative day the nurse notes an erythematous area on the patient's coccyx. What therapeutic measures can prevent skin impairment?
3. On the third postoperative day the patient complains of pain in the right calf when the nurse performs dorsiflexion. What is the most appropriate immediate action by the nurse?

The more than 150 types of fractures can be classified in various ways. First, they are described as either closed (simple) or open (compound) (Fig. 44.19). In a closed fracture, the bone has not protruded through the skin; in an open fracture, it has. A closed fracture does not involve a break in the skin. These fractures sometimes can be realigned by external manipulation rather than invasive surgery. Open fractures are more serious because they involve more soft tissue damage, require surgical treatment to repair, and significantly increase the risk for infection.

Fractures can also be described in terms of appearance (Fig. 44.20).

- *Complete fracture:* Fracture line extends entirely through the bone, with the periosteum disrupted on both sides of the bone.
- *Comminuted fracture:* Bone is splintered into three or more fragments at the site of the break. There is more than one fracture line.
- *Transverse fracture:* Break runs directly across the bone at a right angle to the bone's axis.
- *Oblique fracture:* Break runs diagonally across the bone at approximately a 45-degree angle to the shaft of the bone.
- *Spiral fracture:* Break coils around the bone. This is sometimes called a torsion fracture and results from a twisting force.
- *Impacted fracture:* Sometimes called a *telescoped* fracture because one bone fragment is wedged forcibly into another bone fragment. In long bones, this can shorten the extremity.
- *Greenstick fracture:* Incomplete fracture in which the fracture line extends only partially through the bone. The bone is broken and bent but still secured at one side. This fracture is common in children because their bones are softer and more flexible than those of adults.

Fractures are described according to their location on the bone—for example, proximal, midshaft, or distal. Fractures also can be classified according to the force that caused the break. An example of this is the marching fracture, which can occur in the metatarsals as a result of a long march.

Fractures sometimes are named after the first health care provider to describe them. For example:

- **Colles' fracture:** Fracture of the distal portion of the radius within 1 inch of the wrist joint; commonly occurs when a person attempts to break a fall by putting the hands down.
- *Pott's fracture:* Occurs at the distal end of the fibula and is characterized by chipping off of a piece of the medial malleolus with a displacement of the foot outward.

Fractures sometimes are referred to as joint fractures if they involve or are close to a joint. An articulation fracture involves the surface of a joint. An extracapsular fracture involves a fracture near the joint but one that has not entered the joint capsule. An intracapsular fracture is a fracture within the joint capsule.

Fractures also can be described by their displacement. Figs. 44.19 and 44.20 show that fragments may be displaced sideways, can override the opposite fractured

Patient Teaching

Postoperative Care for the Patient Who Had a Fractured Hip

OPEN REDUCTION WITH INTERNAL FIXATION

Teaching for patients who had a fractured hip and received an internal fixation with nails or pins (see Fig. 44.18) would include the following:

- Assess patient's ability to understand instructions and limitations.
- Assist patient to dangle feet at bedside on first postoperative day and then to pivot to chair with no weight on operative leg, or touch-down weight if allowed.
- Stress that the operative foot should be placed on floor, but weight should be borne on the unoperative leg (refer to limb as either left or right leg so that the patient understands) to maintain safety in care.
- Turn patient every 2 hours; prop with pillows between legs or under the back to maintain position.
- Assist with range-of-motion exercises to maintain muscle strength.
- Help physical therapist walk patient with walker and with limited weight placed on operative limb (if assistance is needed) for comfort and safety.
- Encourage patient and family members to walk together for patient's safety. Instruct family about weight-bearing techniques for clarity and safety.
- If a stable plate and screw fixation is used to repair the fractured hip, the patient should not bear weight for 6 weeks to 3 months to protect the fracture site.
- A telescoping nail fixation allows minimal to partial weight-bearing during the first 6 weeks to 3 months.

HIP PROSTHETIC IMPLANT

Teaching for patients who had a fractured hip and received a hip prosthetic implant (hemiarthroplasty) (see Fig. 44.17) includes the following:

- Avoid hip flexion beyond 60 degrees for approximately 10 days.
- Avoid hip flexion beyond 90 degrees for 2 to 3 months.
- Avoid adduction of the affected leg beyond midline for 2 to 3 months.
- Maintain partial weight-bearing status for approximately 2 to 3 months.
- Avoid positioning on the operative side in bed.
- Maintain abduction of the hip by using a wedge-shaped foam bolster or pillows arranged in a wedge; this will require nursing assistance.

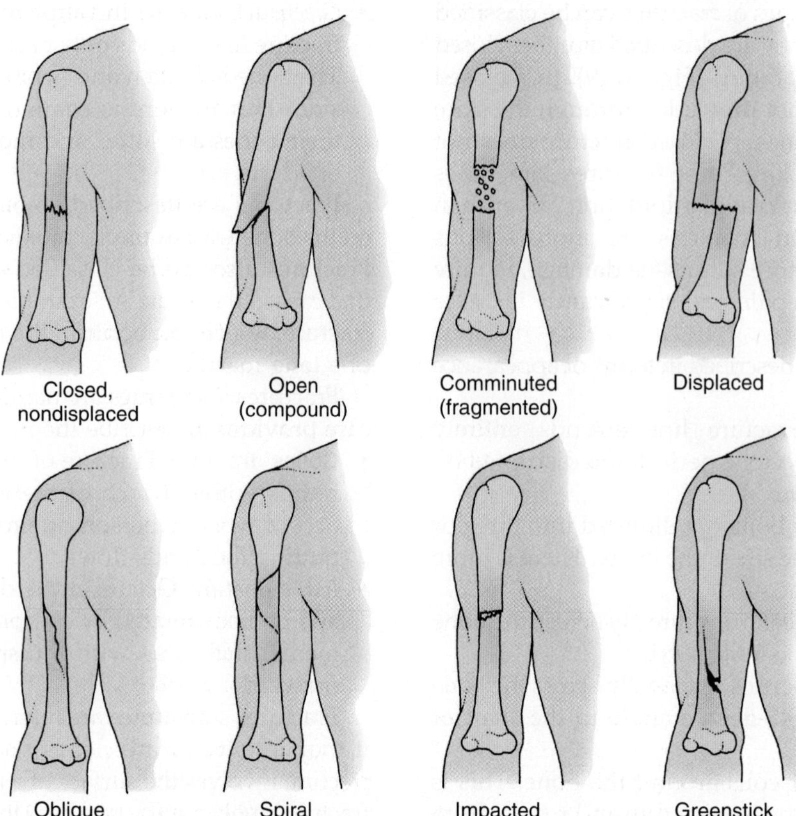

Fig. 44.19 Common types of fractures. (From Ignatavicius DD, Workman ML: *Medical-surgical nursing: Patient-centered collaborative care,* ed 8, St. Louis, 2016, Elsevier.)

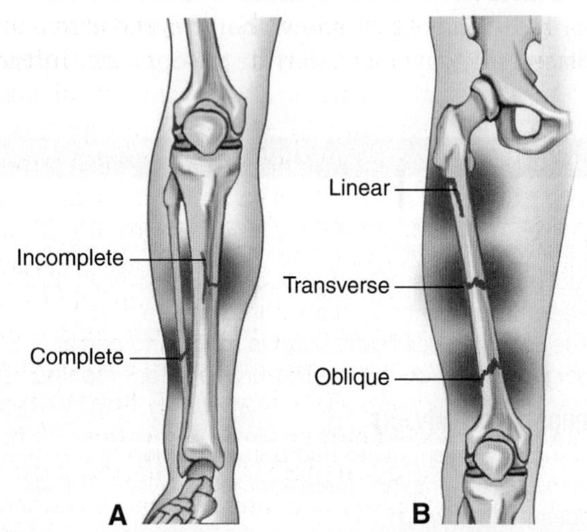

Fig. 44.20 Bone fractures. A, Incomplete and complete. B, Linear, transverse, and oblique. (From Patton KT, Thibodeau GA: *The human body in health and disease*, ed 7, St. Louis, 2018, Elsevier.)

surface, may angulate or create a bend in the bone, and may rotate away from the fracture site. When a bone is displaced, the bone fragments can cause soft tissue damage. The patient has severe pain, edema, and muscle spasms in the early stages of healing.

Bone is vascular; therefore, when a fracture occurs, bleeding occurs at the site of the fracture and in the surrounding tissue. A clot forms at the ends of the fractured bone. The next phase of healing occurs when the hematoma becomes organized as fibroblasts invade the area and a fibrin meshwork is formed. Inflammation is localized as the white blood cells wall off the area. Osteoblasts enter the fibrous area to help hold the union firm. Blood vessels develop, and collagen strands start to incorporate calcium deposits. **Callus** (bony deposits formed between and around the broken ends of a fractured bone during healing) forms when the osteoblasts continue to lay the network for bone buildup and osteoclasts destroy dead bone. The collagen strengthens and continues to incorporate calcium deposits. Remodeling is the final step and occurs when the excess callus is resorbed and trabecular bone is laid down along the lines of stress.

Clinical Manifestations

The signs and symptoms of fractures vary according to the location and function of the involved bone, the strength of its muscle attachment, the type of fracture sustained, and the amount of related damage. Pain, warmth over the injured area, and ecchymosis of the skin surrounding the injured area may not be present for several days. Some fractures may result in an obvious deformity and loss of normal function. The injured part may be incapable of voluntary movements; have a change in the curvature or length of bone (for a fractured hip, the affected leg will be shorter and externally rotated); and have a loss of sensation or paralysis distal to injury, which is indicative of nerve constricture.

Crepitus, or a grating sound, may be heard if the limb is moved gently (do not attempt to verify this sign when fracture is suspected because it may cause further damage and increase pain). The patient also may demonstrate signs of shock related to tissue injury, blood loss, and severe pain.

Assessment

Rapid orthopedic and peripheral vascular assessment. Perform the *seven* Ps *of orthopedic assessment* to establish a baseline and monitor changes in the patient's muscular function, bone integrity, distal circulation, and sensation:

1. Pain: Does it seem out of proportion to the patient's injury? Does the pain increase on active or passive motion?
2. Pallor
3. Paresthesia, or numbness
4. Paralysis
5. Polar temperature: Is the extremity cold compared with the opposite extremity?
6. Puffiness from edema or a hematoma
7. Pulselessness: A Doppler ultrasound device may be useful to determine the presence or absence of blood flow if unable to palpate distal pulses

Subjective data include pain at the site of the injury, loss of sensation or movement of the affected part, and cause of injury.

Objective data include warmth, edema, and ecchymosis; obvious deformity; loss of normal function in the injured part; signs of systemic shock; and signs of any circulatory, motor, or sensory impairment.

Diagnostic Tests

An accurate diagnosis of the fracture is made by radiographic examination or fluoroscopy.

Medical Management

Immediate management includes splinting and elevation to prevent edema of the affected part. Preservation of body alignment is also critical. Apply cold packs (during the first 24 hours) to reduce hemorrhage, edema, and pain. Administer analgesics as ordered. Observe the injured part for change in color, sensation, or temperature. Also observe the patient for signs of shock.

Secondary management for a closed fracture begins with optimal reduction: replacing bone fragments in their correct anatomic position. This can be accomplished through (1) closed reduction, which involves manual manipulations—moving bony fragments into position by applying traction and pressure to distal fragments; (2) traction; (3) **open reduction with internal fixation (ORIF),** a surgical procedure allowing fracture alignment under direct visualization while using various internal fixation devices applied to the bone; or (4) immobilization. Immobilization can be achieved through one or a combination of the following: (1) external fixation with a cast or splint; (2) traction; or (3) internal fixation devices such as pins, plates, screws, wires, and prostheses (see Fig. 44.18).

For an open fracture, additional measures are taken. The wound undergoes surgical débridement to remove dirt, foreign materials, devitalized tissue, and necrotic bone. The date of the last tetanus toxoid administration is needed. Patients having expired status must have the tetanus toxoid administered. A wound culture is indicated. Prophylactic antibiotic therapy is initiated. Observe the wound for signs of osteomyelitis, tetanus, or gangrene. Closure of the wound occurs when there is no sign of infection. Reduction and immobilization of the fracture then take place. Finally, observe for and treat any complications.

Nursing Interventions and Patient Teaching

The nursing interventions for patients with fractures are essentially the same as for any surgical patient. The care of the patient in traction and in a cast is discussed later in this chapter. Each healing phase after a fracture is enhanced by a balanced diet. Proteins, calcium, and vitamins are essential. The patient should be instructed on good food sources for each. Protein-rich foods include lean meats, eggs, nuts, and beans. Dark leafy green vegetables, low-fat dairy products, and soy are good sources for calcium. Vitamin D is found in many of the calcium-rich foods in addition to tofu, some seafood, and fortified cereals. Fluids should be encouraged as with any well-balanced diet. Exercise of the unaffected joints, muscle-setting exercises, skin care, and elimination are important considerations in patient care. Internal fixation has simplified nursing intervention for many patients with fractures and shortened the period of hospitalization, but many patients require longer periods of hospitalization. If activity is restricted, anticipate and prevent the complications that result from immobility.

Patient teaching includes (1) how to move comfortably in bed; (2) how to transfer safely in and out of bed; (3) weight-bearing restrictions and activity limitations, including how long these must be observed; (4) proper use of ambulatory assistive devices; (5) how to avoid edema in the affected part by proper elevation; (6) how to control pain or discomfort in the affected part; (7) exercises to perform to maintain strength and enhance circulation; and (8) proper method of cleansing pins, using surgical asepsis per the health care provider's protocol.

Prognosis

Bone production and fracture healing depend on the patient's age and general health. The presence of other systemic diseases complicates the healing process. Nutrition is a major factor as well in the bone healing process.

FRACTURE OF THE VERTEBRAE

Etiology and Pathophysiology

Injuries such as diving accidents or blows to the head or body can result in fractures of the vertebrae. Patients with osteoporosis and metastatic cancer are at risk for vertebral fractures. Motorcycle and car accidents (especially head-on collisions) occur more frequently with young men (ages 16 to 30 years).

Fractures of the vertebrae may involve the vertebral body, lamina, and articulating processes and may occur with or without displacement. If the fracture has displaced the vertebral structures, pressure may be placed on spinal nerves. The sharp bone fragments also may sever the spinal cord nerves, causing permanent paralysis from the point of injury downward.

Clinical Manifestations

Signs and symptoms of vertebral fracture include pain at the site of the injury; partial or complete loss of mobility or sensation below the level of the injury; and evidence of fracture or fracture dislocation on routine radiographic examination, myelography, or CT scans.

Assessment

Collection of subjective data includes assessment for pain (if the fracture has injured the spinal cord, pain may not be present), numbness, tingling, and inability to move extremities from below the level of the trauma site.

Collection of objective data includes careful assessment of neurologic function, such as pupillary reaction to light, hand grip, ability to move extremities, level of orientation, vital signs, and reaction to painful stimuli (see Chapter 54). Observe for fecal and urinary retention and for signs of hemorrhage such as hypotension, tachycardia, tachypnea, and decreased renal functioning.

Diagnostic Tests

Radiographic studies are done to determine whether the vertebral bodies are compressed. A spinal cord injury may result from a fracture or dislocation of a vertebra; if this is suspected, the health care provider performs a spinal tap to evaluate the spinal fluid. Spinal fluid is normally clear, and the presence of blood indicates trauma (see Chapter 54).

Medical Management

Stable injuries to the vertebrae that are not a threat to spinal cord integrity are treated with pain medication and muscle relaxants. Anticoagulant therapy may be ordered as a prophylaxis for thromboembolic complications. Maintaining erect posture can be enhanced by the use of a back support, corset brace, or a cast. The patient may be allowed to ambulate with assistance (gait enhancers) once discomfort subsides.

Unstable fractures that involve displacement are more serious. Treatment is aimed at fracture reduction through postural positioning and traction. Cranial skeletal traction is used with cervical spine fractures (see Chapter 54). A halo brace (Fig. 44.21), an external immobilization device in which a plaster or plastic brace that incorporates metal struts attached to pins is inserted into bone, is used to allow the patient to be mobile. Pelvic traction is used for lumbar spinal fractures. An open reduction may be necessary with internal fixation using a Harrington rod. After this surgical procedure, the patient is placed in a body cast.

Nursing Interventions and Patient Teaching

Nursing interventions are aimed at maintaining the stability of the fracture fixation by (1) logrolling the patient for position changes; (2) after the correct procedure for turning a patient in a special bed, such as a Stryker frame or Foster bed; (3) elevating the head of the bed no more than 30 degrees; (4) using stabilization devices for the head and back. Assess the continuity of traction (e.g., weights hanging free and ropes not twisted) and

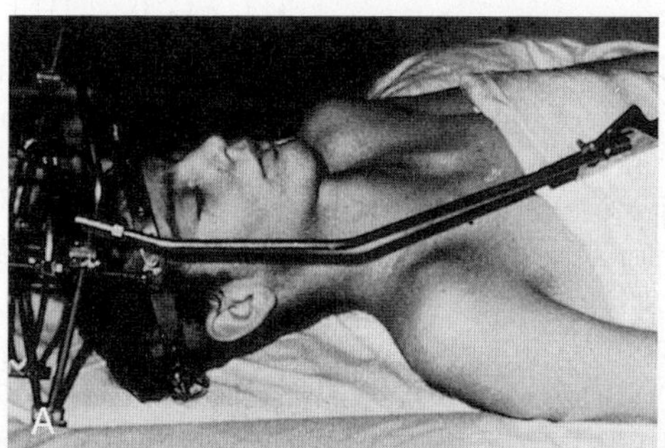

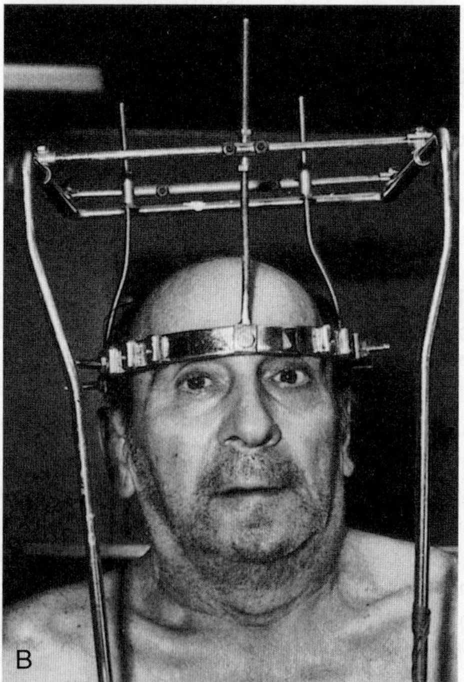

Fig. 44.21 A, Halo attached to body cast. Metal strut will be anchored firmly into body cast with additional plaster. B, Metal ring, or halo, that attaches to skull. (From Lewis SL, Heitkemper MM, Dirksen SR, et al: *Medical-surgical nursing: Assessment and management of clinical problems*, ed 7, St. Louis, 2007, Mosby.)

skin integrity (e.g., erythema, tenderness, and edema), as well as surrounding traction equipment.

Patient problem statements and interventions for the patient with a vertebral fracture include but are not limited to the following:

Patient Problem	Nursing Interventions
Potential for Infection, related to immobility and/or surgical intervention	Monitor patient for signs and symptoms of infection (elevated temperature, increased pulse rate, malodorous exudates, erythema, cloudy urine, diminished breath sounds, and crackles and wheezes) Monitor laboratory values (such as CBC) and blood and wound cultures Protect patient from cross-contamination by practicing good hand-washing techniques, maintaining surgical asepsis when changing dressings, and using strict surgical asepsis with catheter care Encourage coughing, deep breathing, and leg exercises Encourage use of incentive spirometer Prevent people with infectious processes from coming in contact with patient
Compromised Physical Mobility, related to: • Discomfort • Neuromuscular skeletal impairment • Pain	Maintain bed rest in correct body alignment; avoid lifting or twisting body Place patient in immobilization device, such as cervical head halter, skeletal traction, Stryker frame, or CircOlectric bed, as ordered; maintain cervical spine in extension Assess neurovascular status q 2 hr; monitor pulse, color, temperature, sensation, and mobility of all extremities Perform passive ROM or assist with and teach active ROM exercises for all extremities q 2 hr As fracture heals, traction is replaced with cast Assist patient with ambulation when ordered; monitor for vertigo and weakness; progress slowly

Patient teaching includes how to support the back by (1) using a firm mattress; (2) sitting in straight, firm chairs (for no longer than 20 to 30 minutes), when allowed; (3) using proper lifting techniques (using the leg muscles, not the back); and (4) doing back exercises to strengthen spinal extensor muscles.

Prognosis

Stable injuries to the vertebrae that are not a threat to spinal cord integrity have an excellent prognosis with full recovery. Unstable fractures are more serious, and the prognosis is guarded when spinal cord injury is involved.

FRACTURE OF THE PELVIS

Etiology and Pathophysiology

Most pelvic fractures result from trauma involving great force, such as falls from extreme heights, automobile accidents, or crushing accidents. When the trauma is severe enough to fracture the pelvis, vital abdominal organs, such as the bladder, vagina, uterus, liver, spleen, intestines, or kidneys, also may be damaged. Because the pelvis has a rich blood supply, a fracture can result in extensive blood loss (as much as 1 to 4 L).

Clinical Manifestations

The patient with a fractured pelvis is unable to bear weight without discomfort. Local tenderness and edema are common at the trauma site. Hematuria (blood in the urine) may result from trauma to the bladder. Hemorrhage is by far the most life-threatening complication to a patient with a pelvic fracture.

Assessment

Subjective data include complaints of pelvic pain or tenderness and backache. Complaints of restlessness, anxiety, and progressive disorientation may be signs of shock.

Collection of objective data includes assessment of muscle spasms in the pelvic region; ecchymoses over the pelvis, perineum, groin, or suprapubic area; inability to raise the legs when supine; and external foot rotation on the affected side with noticeable shortening of one leg. Vital sign assessment may indicate shock (hypotension, tachycardia, tachypnea, oliguria, and diaphoresis). Careful observation for fat embolism syndrome is especially pertinent for patients with pelvic fractures. Assess bowel sounds in all four quadrants and document the findings; large bowel and rectal lacerations are possible in patients with pelvic fractures. Assess color and amount of urinary output because of the possibility of laceration of the bladder.

Diagnostic Tests

Abdominal radiographic studies are done with the patient in the supine and lateral positions. CT provides an evaluation of the bony pelvis and intraabdominal contents. Intravenous pyelogram is performed to determine kidney damage. Interpretation of laboratory values for hemoglobin and hematocrit, urinalysis, and stool for occult blood helps determine whether the patient is bleeding and anemic.

Medical Management

The patient often remains on bed rest for 3 weeks and then walks with crutches for approximately 6 weeks. If the patient has a symphysis pubis fracture and an iliac fracture on the same side, the health care provider performs surgery. After surgery, skeletal traction is applied for approximately 6 weeks to maintain the leg position. When traction is released, the patient may ambulate without bearing weight for approximately 3 months. For a bilateral fracture of the pelvis, the health care provider may order a pelvic sling to support the fracture. To treat severe fractures that totally disrupt the pelvic ring and dislocate the sacroiliac joints, the health care provider may apply an external skeletal fixation device. He or she also may apply a spica or body cast to support the fracture.

Nursing Interventions and Patient Teaching

Nursing interventions involve monitoring the patient for signs of progressive shock (hypotension, tachycardia, tachypnea, and decreased urinary output). Measure the abdominal girth at least every 8 hours for signs of increased abdominal pressure that could result from internal hemorrhaging. Monitor I&O for signs of hypovolemia, laceration of the bladder, and potential kidney trauma. Insert a Foley catheter to monitor urinary output and color. Implement nursing interventions appropriate for impaired mobility, impaired skin integrity, fluid volume deficit, and pain management.

A patient problem statement and interventions for the patient with a pelvic fracture include but are not limited to the following:

Patient Problem	Nursing Interventions
Compromised Tissue Perfusion, related to: • Hemorrhage • Hypovolemia • Shock	Assess for ecchymosis over pelvis and perineum Monitor vital signs q 15 min for evidence of shock until stable Insert a Foley catheter per health care provider's order to monitor color and amount of urinary output Monitor parenteral fluids per health care provider's order Provide quiet, therapeutic environment Administer oxygen per health care provider's order Maintain bed rest per health care provider's order Monitor bowel sounds and measure abdominal girth to ascertain possible lacerated bowel

Reinforce the reasons for immobility and not bearing full weight; the patient may be too anxious to hear or understand initial explanations. Also explain measures for dealing with acute pain and changes in medications as pain decreases. In addition, explain turning and moving techniques to prevent skin impairment.

Prognosis

Hemorrhage is by far the most life-threatening complication. The long-term prognosis depends on the severity of the fracture, the patient's age, and the presence of other systemic disorders.

COMPLICATIONS OF FRACTURES

COMPARTMENT SYNDROME

Compartment syndrome is a pathologic condition caused by the progressive development of arterial vessel compression and reduced blood supply to one of the body's compartments, typically in an extremity. Muscle fascia lines the muscles, nerves, and blood vessels. It is a very fibrous, tough, and nonelastic structure. With an injury such as a fracture, inflammation leading to swelling often occurs. Expansion or inflammation of a compartment's contents can result in compression of the blood vessels, resulting in compartment syndrome. Compression of blood vessels may result from swelling or from a tight cast or dressing, resulting in muscle ischemia (decreased blood supply to the muscles) because of the inability of the compartment to expand. Irreversible muscle ischemia can occur within 6 hours as a result of compression of the arteries, nerves, and tendons entering the compartment. Paralysis and sensory loss follow, with contracture and permanent disability of the extremity seen within 24 to 48 hours.

Assessment

Collection of subjective data includes pain assessment. Usually the patient complains of sharp pain that increases with passive movement of the hand or foot. The patient experiences deep, unrelenting, progressive, and poorly localized pain unrelieved by analgesics or elevation of the extremity. Numbness or tingling in the affected extremity is common.

Collection of objective data includes assessment of the patient's inability to flex the fingers or toes, coolness of the extremity, and absence of pulsation in the affected extremity. Assess skin color for signs of pallor or cyanosis. Gentle palpation of the extremity reveals slowing of the capillary refill time (blanching). Close monitoring and proper documentation of vital signs are essential (especially temperature to detect signs of tissue necrosis) (see Box 44.5).

Medical Management

Prompt management of compartment syndrome is indicated to avoid permanent neurovascular damage. Surgical intervention, a fasciotomy (incision into the fascia) to relieve pressure and allow return of normal blood flow to the area, is indicated. The incision is often left open to heal by granulation (healing by second intention) (Fig. 44.22).

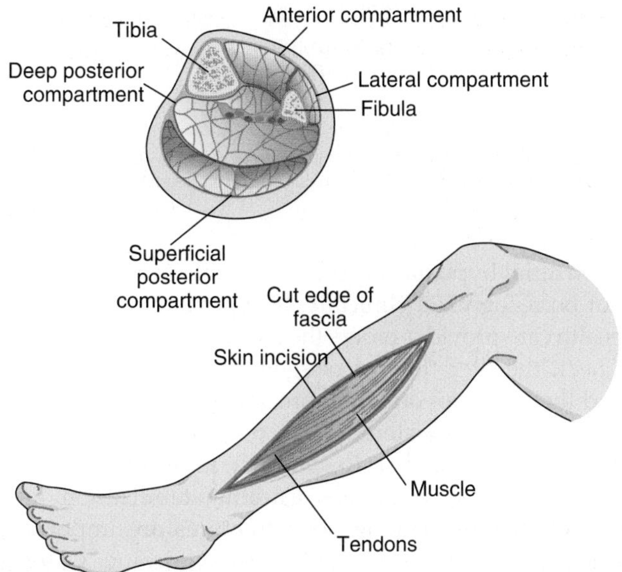

Fig. 44.22 Compartment syndrome. Often more than one compartment is involved, and the anterior compartment of the lower leg is especially vulnerable. Causes include trauma, severe burn, or excessive exercise. A single incision may open more than one compartment. (Courtesy Dr. Henry Bohlman, Cleveland, Ohio.)

Nursing Interventions

Nursing interventions include administration of analgesics with careful documentation of relief obtained. To slow further circulatory compromise, elevate the affected limb, no higher than heart level, to maintain arterial pressure. Apply cold packs and remove any constricting material, such as an elastic bandage. The most common complication when decompression is delayed is infection as a result of tissue necrosis. Purulent drainage from the dressing is a sign of infection and must be reported immediately. If drainage and secretion isolation are required, provide careful instructions to the patient, who may feel isolated. Encourage patients to express their fears and emotional needs. **Volkmann's contracture** is a permanent contracture (with clawhand, flexion of wrist and fingers, and atrophy of the forearm) that can occur as a result of compartment syndrome. Proper positioning and alignment can reduce the risk of this complication.

Prognosis

Compartment syndrome can result in a variety of complications if not treated promptly. A permanent contracture deformity of the hand or foot, muscle necrosis, or infection may result.

SHOCK

Bone is vascular. Shock can occur as a result of blood loss from a fractured bone or from severed blood vessels, seen especially in open fractures. Pain and fear also can cause shock.

Assessment

Collection of subjective data includes monitoring the patient's level of consciousness. Restlessness or complaints of anxiety may suggest a decrease in cerebral perfusion, resulting in brain hypoxia. Complaints of weakness and lethargy are common.

Collection of objective data includes monitoring vital signs. Typical signs of shock include hypotension, tachycardia, diaphoresis, and tachypnea. As shock progresses, hypothermia occurs. The patient may have pale, cool, moist skin. Oliguria (diminished urinary output) is present with shock.

Medical Management

The health care provider's priority concern is to restore blood volume to ensure a rapid return of oxygen to the tissues. Blood volume can be expanded with rapid intravenous fluid administration. Lactated Ringer's solution and 5% dextrose in normal saline are common selections. Whole blood, plasma, or plasma substitutes also may be given. Respiratory assistance may be given by administering oxygen. A central venous catheter may be inserted for accurate monitoring of vital signs to prevent pulmonary edema. Shock trousers may be applied. These are pneumatic trousers designed to counteract hypotension associated with internal or external bleeding and hypovolemia.

Nursing Interventions

Nursing interventions for IV fluid administration include monitoring the intravenous insertion site for signs that infusion solution is seeping into the tissue surrounding the vein; this is called *infiltration*. Signs of infiltration include edema, pain, and induration (hardening of tissue) at the IV site. Monitor the patient's vital signs every 15 minutes until stable. Monitor urinary output every hour. Decreased renal perfusion is indicated by output less than 30 mL/h. The patient should remain flat in bed. If there are no head injuries, raise the lower extremities to improve venous return to the major body organs. Trendelenburg's position presses the abdominal organs against the diaphragm, reducing the effectiveness of heart and lung functions, and should be avoided. Keep the patient warm, but avoid external heat. Give nothing by mouth. Sedatives, tranquilizers, and narcotics may reduce the level of consciousness and mask neurologic changes and therefore should be avoided. Be aware that the patient's family will be anxious and provide them with brief explanations of the patient's condition.

Prognosis

Shock can lead to a loss of consciousness or coma. Shock can be fatal within a few hours of injury; therefore immediate attention is required.

FAT EMBOLISM

Pulmonary fat embolism involves the embolization of tissue fat with platelets and circulating free fatty acids within the pulmonary capillaries. Fat embolism is rare but can be life threatening, because the fat droplets can occlude capillaries of the pulmonary circulation, causing brain hypoxia and tissue death. Risk factors include long bone and pelvic fractures, crush injuries, and hip replacement surgery. It can occur within 48 hours of the injuries. Pulmonary fat embolism syndrome is the most serious complication of long bone fractures.

Assessment

Collection of subjective data includes assessment of mental disturbances, such as irritability, restlessness, disorientation, stupor, and coma. These symptoms can result from effects of severe hypoxemia. The patient may complain of chest pain, especially on inspiration, and of localized muscle weakness, spasticity, and rigidity.

Collection of objective data includes assessing for tachypnea, dyspnea, hypoxemia, and auditory crackles and wheezes in the lung field. As the lung filters and traps embolic material, ventilation is disturbed. Assess the apical pulse to detect dysrhythmias. Patients are placed on cardiac monitoring for observation of dysrhythmias and cardiovascular collapse. Assess the patient for petechiae (a rash of red, pinpoint dots, especially in the buccal membranes, conjunctival sacs, hard palate, chest, and anterior axillary folds) caused by occlusion of capillaries. The appearance of petechiae on the conjunctiva of the eye, the neck, chest, or axillary region is a typical sign of a fat embolism (Kirkland, 2013).

Diagnostic Tests

The diagnosis is based on clinical signs and symptoms, which appear within 24 to 48 hours of injury. Blood gases indicate hypoxemia. Hemoglobin and hematocrit laboratory values are decreased. Fat is present in the blood and urine. The sedimentation rate is increased, and the platelet count is decreased.

Medical Management

Treatment for fat embolism is directed at prevention. Careful immobilization of a long bone fracture is probably the most important factor in the prevention of fat embolism. The health care provider orders the administration of IV fluids to prevent shock and dilute free fatty acids. Use of corticosteroids to prevent or treat fat embolism is controversial. Digoxin often is ordered to increase the patient's cardiac output. Oxygen is administered if the arterial oxygen pressure (PaO_2) is less than 70 mm Hg. Intubation or intermittent positive-pressure ventilation may be considered if a satisfactory PaO_2 cannot be obtained with supplemental oxygen alone. Incentive spirometry is ordered to improve lung expansion and oxygenation.

Nursing Interventions

Nursing interventions include close monitoring of the patient's arterial blood gases. Normal values include the following:

pH	7.35 to 7.45
$PaCO_2$	35 to 45 mm Hg
PaO_2	80 to 100 mm Hg
HCO_3	21 to 28 mEq/L
SaO_2	95% to 100%

HCO_3, Bicarbonate; *$PaCO_2$*, arterial carbon dioxide pressure; *PaO_2*, arterial oxygen pressure; *SaO_2*, oxygen saturation of arterial hemoglobin.

Arterial hypoxia is present with fat emboli and may not be recognized clinically. If hypoxia is present, the health care provider orders the administration of oxygen. Check the liter flow of oxygen and educate patients and their families on safety precautions necessary when oxygen is administered (e.g., no smoking or use of electrical equipment). Respiratory failure is the most common cause of death. Careful stabilization and immobilization of long bone fractures are important steps in preventing fat embolism syndrome. Careful support when turning and positioning the patient can prevent the manipulation of the fracture and reduce the risk of fat embolism syndrome. Reposition the patient as little as possible before fracture immobilization because of the danger of dislodging more fat droplets into the general circulation. An accurate record of I&O and daily weights is essential to monitor fluid balance.

Prognosis

Fat embolism can be life threatening.

GAS GANGRENE

Gas gangrene is a severe infection of the skeletal muscle caused by gram-positive clostridial bacteria, particularly *Clostridium perfringens,* which may occur in the presence of open fractures and lacerated wounds. Clostridial bacteria in these injuries can produce exotoxins that destroy tissue. The onset is usually sudden, generally 1 to 14 days after injury. These organisms are anaerobic (i.e., they grow and function without oxygen) and are spore formers. They normally are found in soil and the intestinal tracts of humans. As the clostridial bacteria invade devitalized tissue (especially where blood supply is diminished), they multiply and produce toxins that cause (1) hemolysis (breakdown of red blood cells and release of hemoglobin); (2) vessel thrombosis; and (3) damage to the myocardium, liver, kidneys, and brain.

Assessment

Collection of subjective data includes observation of pain, which is usually sudden and severe at the site of the injury. A characteristic finding is toxic delirium.

Collection of objective data includes careful inspection of the skin for gas bubbles at the site of the wound. The various *Clostridium* species produce a characteristic cellulitis in which gas is present under the skin. This causes crepitation (a crackling sensation when the skin is touched). Observe for signs of infection, including elevated temperature, tachycardia, tachypnea, and edema around the wound. The skin around the wound becomes necrotic and ruptures, revealing necrotic muscle. The wound discharge is thin, watery, and foul smelling. Carefully document the patient's response to antibiotic therapy (e.g., decline in temperature and decrease in amount of wound drainage).

Medical Management

Treatment of gas gangrene involves establishing a larger wound opening to admit air and promote drainage. Antibiotics, such as penicillin G or cephalothin, are ordered intravenously and must be administered as scheduled. Observe the patient for adverse reactions.

Nursing Interventions

Nursing interventions include wound care, using strict medical asepsis. Spore-forming bacteria are not destroyed by ordinary disinfecting methods. Therefore all contaminated equipment and linens must be autoclaved. Follow drainage and secretion isolation procedures to prevent the spread of the infection to other patients.

Prognosis

If left untreated, gas gangrene is rapidly fatal. Prompt treatment, including excision of gangrenous tissue and administration of penicillin G intravenously, saves 80% of patients. If massive gangrene develops, amputation is necessary.

THROMBOEMBOLUS

Etiology and Pathophysiology

Thromboembolus is a condition in which a blood vessel is occluded by an embolus carried in the bloodstream from the site of formation of the clot. It is associated with reduced skeletal muscle contractions and bed rest. The person with pelvic and hip fractures is at high risk for this complication.

Clinical Manifestations

The area supplied by an obstructed artery may tingle and become cold, numb, and cyanotic. An embolus in the lungs causes sudden, sharp thoracic or upper abdominal pain, dyspnea, cough, fever, and hemoptysis.

Assessment

Collection of subjective data includes careful investigation of complaints of pain in the lower extremities (especially the calf). A complaint of tenderness over the area is common. The patient may complain of a sharp pain in the thoracic area when an embolus is in the lung.

Collection of objective data includes assessing signs consistent with thromboembolus. The affected area may be erythematous, warm to the touch, and edematous. Assess for differences in leg size (circumference) bilaterally from thigh to ankle. (In the past, Homans' sign commonly was assessed and considered a positive finding for the condition. This involved the flexion of the foot. The presence of pain was consistent with a possible thromboembolus. This is not done in many facilities now because of fears of potentially dislodging the clot.) Also observe the patient for dyspnea and blood in the sputum if pulmonary embolus is present. When anticoagulant therapy is ordered, assess for signs of bleeding, such as petechiae, epistaxis, hematuria, hematemesis, and occult or gross blood in the stool.

Diagnostic Tests

A complete history is taken and a physical examination is performed. Laboratory studies, including a prothrombin time (PT), international normalized ratio (INR), D-dimer concentration, and CBC, may be performed. Diagnostic tests for deep vein thrombosis may include Doppler ultrasonography or duplex scanning. A spiral CT scan of the lung, a ventilation/perfusion scan, or a pulmonary arteriogram may be ordered to rule out pulmonary embolism.

Medical Management

Treatment includes administration of anticoagulants, such as heparin, enoxaparin, or warfarin. A surgical procedure known as a thrombectomy (removal of a thrombus from a blood vessel) may be done.

Nursing Interventions

Nursing interventions involve caring for the patient whose physical activity has been restricted. Often this involves bed rest with the foot of the bed elevated to aid venous return. Teach the patient to engage in active exercise, such as dorsiflexion (pointing backward) and plantar flexion (pointing forward) of the toes, several times each hour. This exercise stimulates circulation to the legs. Continuous hot, moist compresses usually are ordered. Antiembolism stockings and intermittent pneumatic compression devices are ordered while the patient is on bed rest and are maintained even after the patient is ambulatory. Assess lung sounds every 4 hours and adhere to the activity ordered. If the patient is receiving anticoagulants, closely monitor PT, INR, and partial thromboplastin times.

Prognosis

Obstruction of the pulmonary artery or one of its branches may be fatal (see the Safety Alert box). A thrombus in an extremity usually resolves with treatment, and a favorable prognosis is noted.

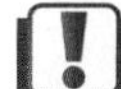

Safety Alert

Thromboembolus

Never massage a patient's lower extremities. Thromboembolus can be present without clinical signs and symptoms.

DELAYED FRACTURE HEALING

A *delayed union* is a fracture that fails to heal within the usual time. The healing is impaired but has not stopped completely and eventually will repair itself. *Nonunion* is when the ends of the fractured bone fail to unite and produce a stable union after 6 to 9 months. Potential causes of delayed union and nonunion include infection and poor perfusion. The calcification of cartilage and bone formation do not occur. Bone grafting, prosthetic implant, internal fixation, external fixation, or a combination of these methods can be used to correct the problem of delayed union or nonunion of bone fractures. Health care providers are using electrical stimulation as a new method of promoting healing of nonunion fractures. The use of electrical probes on bone stimulates bone production.

Prognosis

Bone production and fracture healing depend on the patient's age and general health. The presence of other systemic diseases complicates the healing process.

SKELETAL FIXATION DEVICES

EXTERNAL FIXATION DEVICES

External fixation devices are used to hold bone fragments in normal position. Casts, skeletal and skin traction, braces, and metal pins are examples of these devices.

Skeletal Pin External Fixation

One external fixation technique immobilizes fractures with pins inserted through the bone and attached to a rigid external metal frame (Fig. 44.23). This technique is becoming more popular because it provides rigid support of comminuted open fractures, infected nonunions, and infected unstable joints. The patient can use the muscles and joints above and below the fixation. Leaving the fracture open to air has the advantage of visibility of the area and accessibility for wound care.

This procedure is performed with the patient under general anesthesia. Reassure the patient that the pain after the insertion of the pins is minimal. Immediately after the procedure, the extremity is placed in balanced suspension traction to help relieve the edema. Assess the pins that are inserted through the bone at least every 4 hours. The position of each pin and surrounding skin should be documented in the assessment. Signs of infection, including drainage or odor, should be included. Remove dried exudate from around the pins as ordered, with the prescribed cleaning agent and surgical asepsis. Patients are permitted to ambulate on crutches when soft tissue edema is relieved. They are permitted to shower when the wounds have healed but must avoid salt or chlorinated water to prevent fixator corrosion.

NONSURGICAL INTERVENTIONS FOR MUSCULOSKELETAL DISORDERS

CASTS

Casts are immobilization devices. The materials most commonly used for casting are plaster and fiberglass. Material selection largely depends on the location of the fracture and the time needed for healing to take place. Body casts and long bones requiring more stabilization traditionally are casted with plaster, which is heavier and more durable. Fiberglass casts are relatively lightweight and are used commonly on arm fractures. Once the affected body part has been aligned, the casting material is applied. Alignment may be performed externally or internally through a surgical intervention. The process is relatively pain free. The patient experiences discomfort with the manipulation of the body part during the process. First a cotton or synthetic stockinette is applied to cover the length of

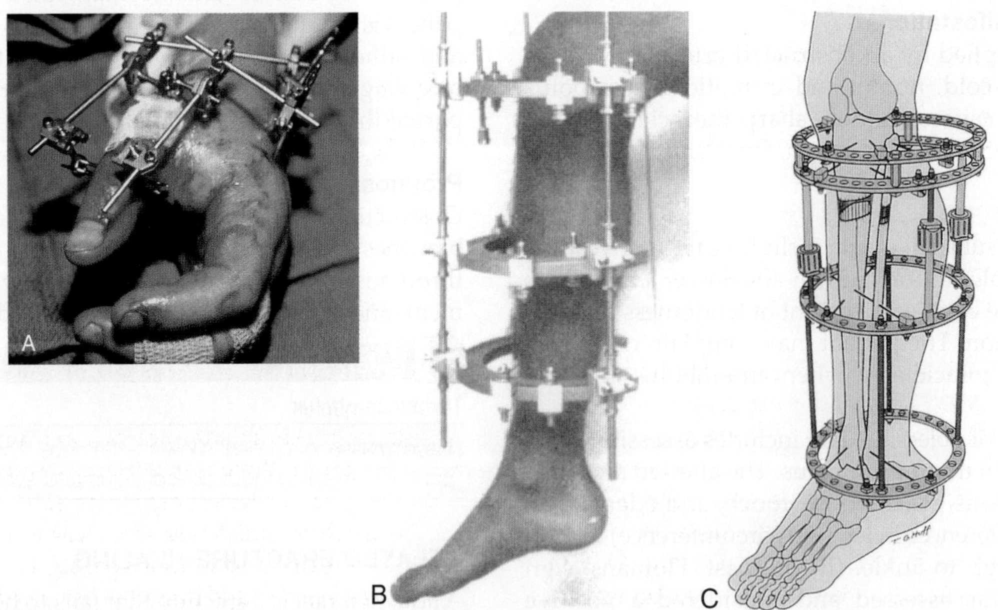

Fig. 44.23 External fixation apparatuses. A, Hoffmann. B, Monticelli-Spinelli circular fixator. C, Ilizarov apparatus with corticotomies for lengthening lower leg. (From Beare PG, Myers JL: *Adult health nursing*, ed 3, St. Louis, 1998, Mosby.)

the extremity. Cotton sheeting or wadding is applied next, followed by the casting material. Most health care providers bring the stockinette up and over the distal and proximal edges of the cast. Inspect these edges for rough pieces of casting that may irritate the skin. Superficial burns can occur as the cast begins to set up, especially if the patient is not appropriately padded or too much fiberglass material is used.

The application is similar to that for an elastic bandage. The type of cast used is indicative of the part of the body immobilized. Examples include (1) short arm cast, which extends from below the elbow to the proximal palmar crease; (2) long leg cast, which extends from the upper thigh to the base of the toes; and (3) spica cast or body cast, which covers the trunk and one or both extremities (Fig. 44.24). A cast may be bivalved to relieve pressure. This involves splitting the cast down both sides and securing the pieces so that the extremity is supported (Skill 44.1, Step 8a).

Cast Brace

The cast brace is an alternative appliance to the traditional leg cast. It provides the support and stability of the plaster cast, with additional support and mobility provided by a hinged brace. The appliance is most effective for fractures of the shaft of the femur and permits early ambulation and weight-bearing. It is used approximately 2 to 6 weeks after fracture reduction.

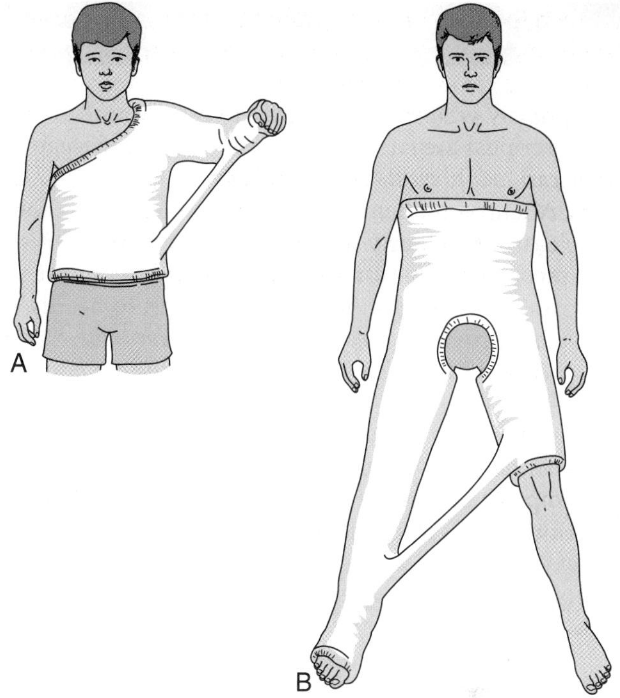

Fig. 44.24 Spica casts. A, Shoulder spica. B, One and one-half leg-hip spica. (From Thompson JM, Hirsch JE, Tucker SM, et al: *Mosby's clinical nursing,* ed 5, St. Louis, 2002, Mosby.)

Skill 44.1 Care of the Patient in a Cast

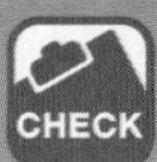

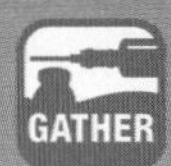

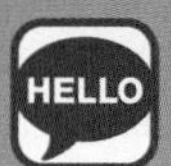

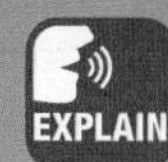

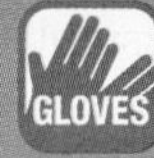

NURSING ACTION *(RATIONALE)*

1. Patient teaching. *(Ensures patient cooperation; reduces patient anxiety.)*
   a. Explain why the cast is being applied and how it will be applied. *(Sudden movement during procedure could cause injury.)*
   b. Advise the patient that the plaster cast will feel warm as it dries.
   c. Explain the extent of immobilization.
   d. Explain care of the cast and expectations after discharge.
   e. Instruct patient not to insert sharp objects (coat hangers or pencils) under the cast. *(These may abrade the skin and lead to infection.)*
2. Handling the new cast. *(A fiberglass cast dries immediately after application; a plaster extremity cast dries in approximately 24 to 48 hours; a plaster spica or body cast dries in 48 to 72 hours* [see Fig. 44.25].*)*
   a. Support wet cast with the flat of the hands or on pillows. *(Avoids indentations that will cause pressure on underlying skin.)*
   b. Place cotton blankets or other absorbent material under the cast. *(Aids drying of cast.)*
   c. Expose the cast to air as much as possible. *(Aids drying of cast.)*
   d. Turn the patient frequently. *(Aids drying of cast.)*
   e. Use a cast dryer or hair dryer on a warm (not hot) setting. *(Circulates air over the cast.)*
   f. Do not apply paint, varnish, or shellac to the cast. *(Plaster is a porous material that allows air to circulate to the skin.)*
3. Skin care. *(Decreases the chance of skin irritation or tissue injury.)*
   a. Inspect skin at edges of cast and underlying cast for erythema or skin impairment.
   b. Remove plaster crumbs from skin with a washcloth moistened with warm water.
   c. Use creams and lotions sparingly. *(They may soften the skin and cause the cast to stick to the skin.)*

Continued

Skill 44.1 Care of the Patient in a Cast—cont'd

d. Apply waterproof material to cast around perineal area. *(Prevents soiling of and damage to cast and prevents skin impairment.)*

e. Attend to patient's complaint of pain under the cast, particularly over bony prominences. *(This may indicate pressure on the skin.)* If discomfort is not relieved by repositioning, report to health care provider. *(Cast pressure may have to be relieved by windowing or bivalving [cutting into halves].)*

4. Turning: Turning to any position generally is permitted as long as the integrity of the cast is not compromised and the patient is comfortable; do not turn by grasping the abductor bar. *(It is not safe transport.)*
5. Toileting for a long leg or hip spica cast.
   a. Use a fracture pan with blanket roll or padding. *(Provides support under the small of the back.)*
   b. Elevate the head of the bed, if permitted, or place the bed in reverse Trendelenburg's position. *(Eases procedure.)*
6. Abdominal discomfort: Cast may be "windowed" (an opening cut into it). *(Provides relief of abdominal distention or a port for checking bladder distention.)*
7. Mobilization.
   a. The health care provider decides whether and how much weight-bearing is allowed.
   b. A cast shoe or a walking heel is incorporated into a lower extremity cast (see Fig. 44.26). *(Permits weight-bearing without damaging the cast.)*
8. Prevention of neurovascular problems: Establish baseline measurements and assess neurovascular status before cast application; palpate distal pulses; assess color, temperature, and capillary refill of the appropriate fingers or toes; assess neurologic function, including sensation and motion in the affected and unaffected extremity. *(Changes in neurovascular status may occur after casting, possibly further compromising already injured tissues. Note the baseline neurovascular status so that those changes, if they occur, can be assessed readily.)*
   a. Perform neurovascular checks every hour for at least 24 hours after cast application to detect difficulty from edema or pressure of cast on nerves or vessels; notify health care provider of color changes, alterations in sensation, or unrelieved discomfort; cast may need to be bivalved to relieve pressure.

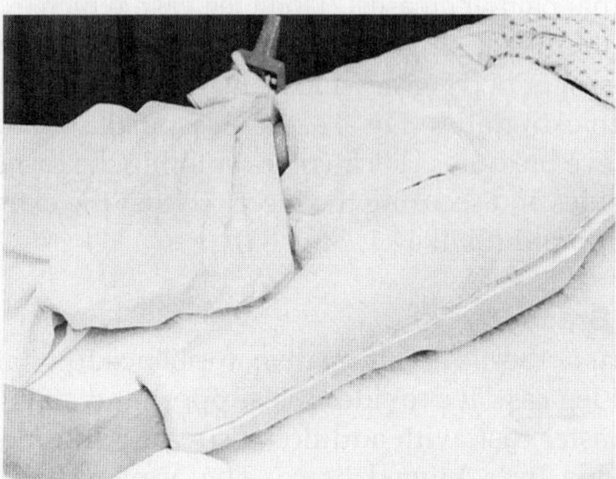

(Figure from Monahan FD, Sands JK, Neighbors M, et al: *Phipps' medical-surgical nursing: Health and illness perspectives*, ed 8, St. Louis, 2007, Mosby.)

   b. Elevate affected extremity on pillows. *(Danger of edema is usually 24 to 48 hours.)*
   c. After mobilization of patient with lower extremity or upper extremity cast, avoid keeping extremity in dependent position for prolonged periods. *(Prevents edema.)*
   d. After lower extremity cast is removed, encourage patient to wear elastic stocking and elevate affected leg while at rest until full mobility is regained. *(After immobilization, the involved joints and muscles will be weak, and range of motion may be limited. Activity must be resumed slowly. Elastic stockings enhance deep vein circulation.)*

Cast bracing is based on the concept that limited weight-bearing helps promote the formation of bone. A problem encountered frequently with cast bracing is edema around the knee. Instruct patients to elevate the leg when sitting to promote venous return. A cast shoe or walking heel incorporated into a lower extremity cast permits weight-bearing without damaging the cast (Fig. 44.25).

Assessment

Nursing assessment is similar regardless of what kind of casting material is used. Perform a neurovascular assessment, including capillary refill, every 15 to 30 minutes for several hours after casting and every 4 hours the first few days (see Box 44.5). Capillary filling time is a way to assess arterial flow to the extremities; squeeze the patient's nailbeds to produce blanching and observe for the return of color. With normal arterial capillary perfusion, the color returns to normal within 2 seconds (Fig. 44.26). Observe the skin at the cast edges for erythema and irritation. Compare the temperature and skin appearance on the casted side and noncasted side for comparison purposes. Assess the ability of the patient to move the fingers or toes on the affected side. Complaints of pain or discomfort should be evaluated closely. Determine the specific location and assess the effectiveness of any analgesics administered.

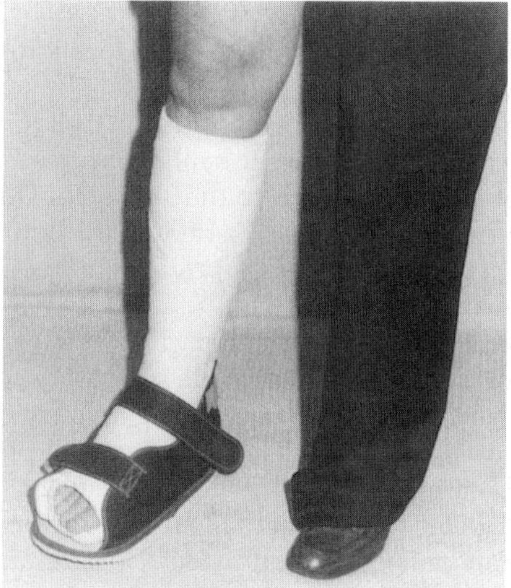

Fig. 44.25 Short-leg walking cast with cast shoe. (Courtesy Dr. Henry Bohlman, Cleveland, Ohio.)

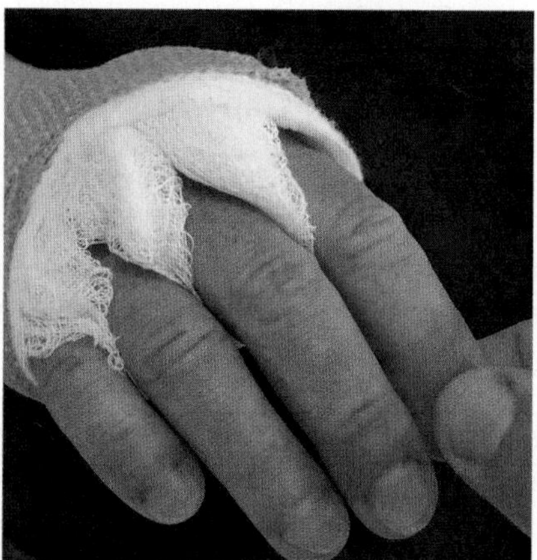

Fig. 44.26 Capillary refill assessment.

Nursing Interventions and Patient Teaching

Nursing interventions for the patient in a cast (see Skill 44.1) include patient education on preventing infection, irritation, neurovascular pressure, and misalignment of bone ends. Handle a wet cast gently and support it with the flat of the hand or on pillows to avoid indentations that cause pressure on the skin and lead to skin impairment. Never use the bar in a spica cast as support when turning the patient. Turning the patient frequently aids the drying process. If a cast dryer is used, set it on warm, never hot (drying a plaster of Paris cast too quickly from the outside may weaken the cast). Elevating the casted extremity reduces edema (usually elevation is recommended for 24 to 48 hours). Instruct patients using crutches to support their weight on their hands; weight borne on the axillae can damage the brachial plexus nerves (crutch paralysis).

Cast syndrome (superior mesentery artery syndrome) can occur after the application of a spica (body) cast (see Fig. 44.24) and involves acute obstruction of the duodenum. If nausea occurs, place the patient prone to relieve pressure symptoms and alert the charge nurse. Gastric decompression may be necessary, and if conventional measures fail, surgical intervention (duodenojejunostomy—making an opening into the small intestine) may be necessary.

Patient teaching includes information about cleaning around the cast site with a mild soap and rinsing away excessive soap so that it does not accumulate around the cast and impair the skin. A synthetic (fiberglass) cast can be flushed with water if it becomes soiled. It must be dried afterward to prevent skin impairment and maceration (softening). A synthetic (fiberglass) cast can be dried by blotting it with a towel and then using a blow dryer on the cool or warm setting in a sweeping motion across the cast. Proper drying may take as long as 1 hour.

Patients often complain of pruritus (itching) of the skin that is covered by a cast (especially after having the cast for a few weeks). Recommend diversion activities when the pruritus begins. Also advise the patient to gently rub the area below and above the cast to decrease the desire to scratch. Warn patients not to stick sharp objects underneath the cast to relieve the pruritus. This may impair the skin and result in serious complications.

Cast Removal

Casts are removed with an electric vibrating saw rather than a cutting saw. Reassure patients that there is little risk of the saw injuring the skin beneath the cast, even though it is noisy and looks like a cutting saw. Prepare the patient for the sight of the skin beneath the cast. Patients may be distressed by the appearance of their extremity after the cast is removed. Health care providers removing the cast should opt to wear masks to avoid respiratory irritation from the powder released when the cast is cut. If this powder is inhaled over a period of time, the plaster deposits can build up in the lungs' small air sacs and cause respiratory distress.

After removal of a cast, eliminate the buildup of secretions and dead skin on the affected extremity by gently washing and applying lotion or cream to the area. This may take several days, but caution the patient against trying to remove the devitalized material rapidly to avoid causing skin impairment. Muscle atrophy is common. Reassure the patient that the muscle will increase in strength and size with proper exercise through either physical therapy or home exercise programs.

TRACTION

Traction is the process of putting an extremity, bone, or group of muscles under tension by means of weights and pulleys. Traction may be used to (1) align and stabilize a fracture site by reducing the fractured part, (2) relieve pressure on nerves as in the case of herniated disk syndrome, (3) maintain correct positioning, (4) prevent deformities, and (5) relieve muscle spasms. The two general types of traction are skeletal and skin. Traction may be continuous or intermittent. To stabilize a fracture, continuous traction is applied; it must not be disconnected unless ordered by the health care provider. Cervical and pelvic traction sometimes is ordered as intermittent traction.

Skeletal Traction

Skeletal traction (Fig. 44.27) is applied directly to a bone. It normally is used for longer periods and employs heavier weights than skin traction. A surgeon inserts wires and pins through the bone distal to the fracture site while the patient is under local or general anesthesia. The pin protrudes through the skin on both sides of the extremity, and traction is applied with weights attached to a rope that is tied to a spreader bar. Skeletal traction can be used for fractures of the femur (see Fig. 44.27A), tibia (see Fig. 44.27B), humerus, and cervical spine (see Chapter 54).

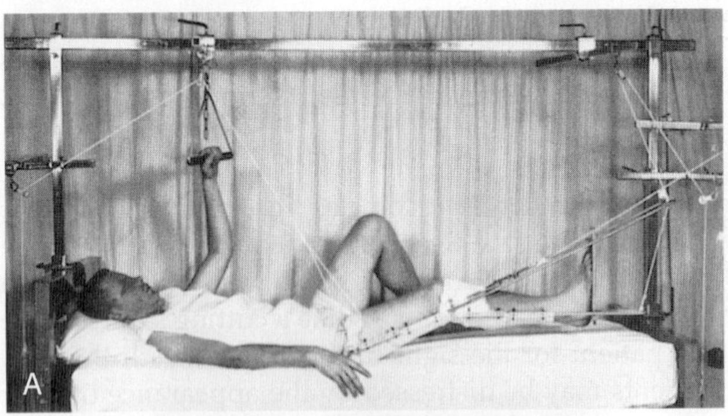

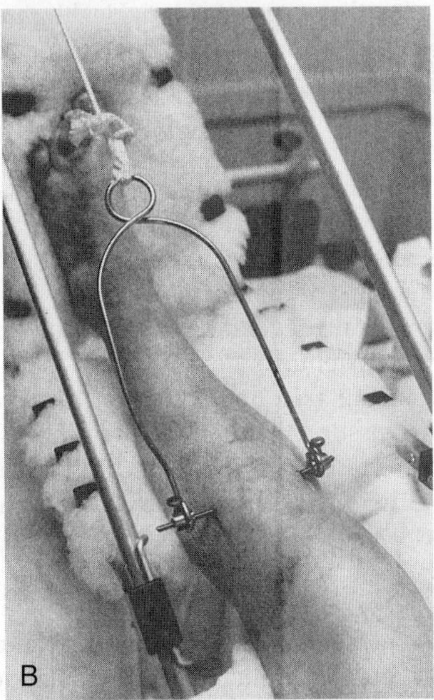

Fig. 44.27 A, Balanced suspension skeletal traction to the femur. B, Tibial pin traction with Steinmann pin used in treatment of distal femoral fracture. The bow attached to the pin provides a place of attachment for the rope that holds the traction weights. The pull exerted by the weight keeps the fracture fragments aligned. Pin sites must be inspected at least daily to detect signs of pin reaction or infection. (A, Modified from Mourad L: *Orthopedic disorders*, St. Louis, 1991, Mosby. B, From Monahan FD, Sands JK, Neighbors M, et al: *Phipps' medical-surgical nursing: Health and illness perspectives*, ed 8, St. Louis, 2007, Mosby.)

Skin Traction

Skin traction traditionally is intended for short-term use and uses lighter weights. The device is applied directly to the skin. Skin traction uses weight that pulls on sponge rubber, moleskin, and elastic bandage with adherent or plastic materials attached to the skin below the site of the fracture, with the pull exerted on the limb. Buck's, Russell's, and Bryant's are types of skin traction.

Buck's traction. Buck's traction (Fig. 44.28) is used as a temporary measure to provide support and comfort to a fractured extremity while waiting for more definitive treatment. Traction (pull) is in a horizontal plane with the affected extremity. This traction frequently is used to maintain the reduction of a hip fracture before surgery. It also can be used to treat muscle spasms and minor fractures of the lower spine.

Russell's traction. Russell's traction (see Fig. 44.28B) is set up similarly to Buck's traction. However, a knee sling supports the affected leg. It allows more movement in bed and permits flexion of the knee joint. Russell's traction is used commonly to treat hip and knee fractures.

Nursing Interventions

Nursing interventions for patients in traction include measures to maintain the body in proper alignment and careful assessment of traction equipment. The pulleys must remain off the floor to ensure correct alignment. Care of a patient in skeletal traction involves assessment of the pin sites. Pin site care includes cleansing with a prescribed agent, using a sterile cotton-tipped applicator. Antibiotic ointment may be prescribed for the pin insertion sites. Traction care is summarized in Box 44.6.

ORTHOPEDIC DEVICES

Frames can be used for orthopedic patients to assist with turning and positioning while maintaining proper alignment.

- The *Balkan frame* is a wooden or steel attachment to the hospital bed. It has adjustable pulleys and a trapeze bar attached to an overhead bar.
- The *Bradford frame* is made of rectangular steel with two pieces of canvas stretched tightly and laced to the frame. A space is left in the buttocks area for toileting and hygiene.
- The *CircOlectric bed* is a vertical turning bed that can be operated electrically by one person and placed in a variety of positions. Side-to-side movement can be accomplished while maintaining proper positioning if traction is ordered.
- The *microAIR alternating lateral rotation bed* regulates air with a series of valves that open and close. The bed has customizable turn times ranging from 10 to 60 minutes.
- The *RotoRest bed* can rock a patient as much as 62 degrees, 17 times per hour. The electric-powered bed can help heal pressure ulcers, prevent venous thrombosis, and reduce kidney stone formation.

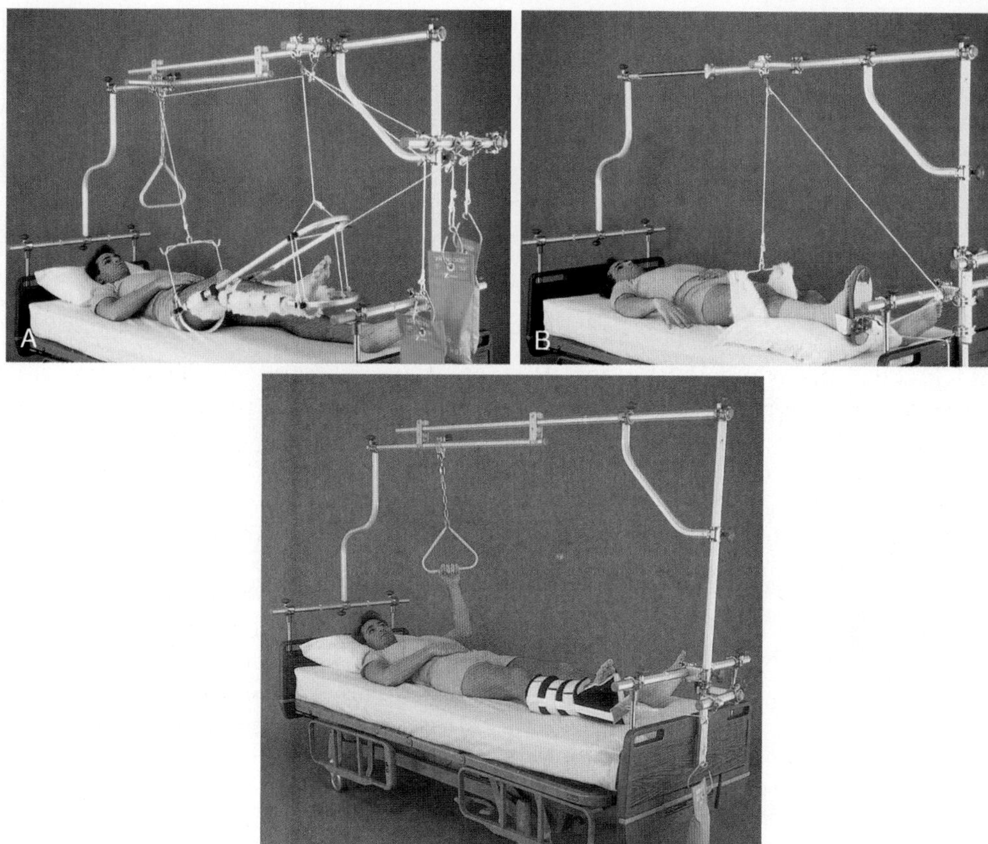

Fig. 44.28 A, Balanced traction with a Thomas ring and a Pearson attachment. B, Russell's traction. C, Buck's traction. (Courtesy Zimmer, Inc., Warsaw, Indiana).

- The *Stryker wedge turning frame* and *Foster bed* are similar and assist in changing the patient's position from supine to prone. Patients may become apprehensive when turned on a frame for fear of falling, so thorough explanations and reassurances are helpful.

Safety Alert

Crutch Safety

Crutch safety involves:

- Proper measurement (with weight on hands, not axillae, to avoid nerve and blood vessel damage in the axillary region); leave a 2-inch width between the axillary fold and the arm piece on the crutches
- Rubber tips on the ends of the crutches to prevent slippage
- Adequate muscle strength in the upper extremities to support the patient's weight

Splints, crutches, and *braces* are used to immobilize and assist with ambulation. There are numerous types of splints and braces, and nurses must understand the procedure for the proper application for each kind.

Safety is the first concern when ambulatory devices such as crutches are used (see Safety Alert box on crutch safety). Encourage the patient to do push-ups by pressing the hands against the mattress and lifting the upper body to gain muscle strength. Types of *crutch walking* depend on the number of points making contact with the floor (Fig. 44.29). For example, a three-point gait involves two crutch points plus one leg making contact with the floor (patient must have strong arms to support body weight). Instead of a three-point gait, patients may use the four-point gait (slower, but stable) or two-point gait (faster; requires balance). Another type of crutch walking is the swing-to or swing-through gait, in which the patient swings the body up to or beyond the two points of the crutch tips. Most crutch walking is taught by a physical therapist (Fig. 44.30). However, the nurse monitors the patient's progress.

Older patients are likely to use *cane walking* for balance and support. Instruct the patient to hold the cane in the opposite hand of the affected extremity and advance the cane at the same time the affected leg moves forward. An effective rubber tip on the point will help prevent slippage. Older adults also use walkers to maintain balance. Safety concerns are the same as those for the cane.

The Roll-A-Bout walker is a gait enhancer designed for patients who have an injury below the knee such as a fractured tibia, fibula, ankle, or foot. The Roll-A-Bout allows the patient to distribute weight evenly by placing the knee of the injured leg on the knee pad and propelling the Roll-A-Bout with the unaffected leg (Fig. 44.31).

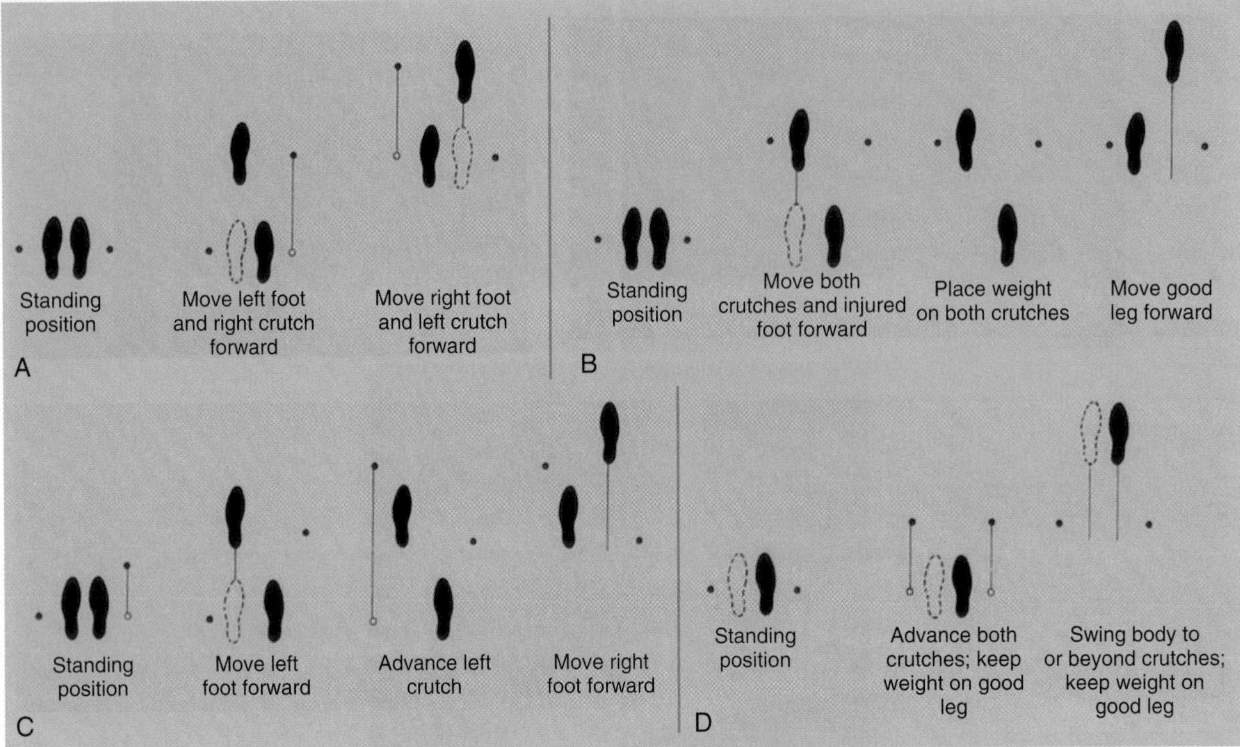
Standing position
Move left foot and right crutch forward
Move right foot and left crutch forward
A
Standing position
Move both crutches and injured foot forward
Place weight on both crutches
Move good leg forward
B
Standing position
Move left foot forward
Advance left crutch
Move right foot forward
C
Standing position
Advance both crutches; keep weight on good leg
Swing body to or beyond crutches; keep weight on good leg
D

Fig. 44.29 Crutch walking. A, Two-point gait. B, Three-point gait. C, Four-point gait. D, Swing-through gait. (From Harkness GA, Dincher JR: *Medical-surgical nursing: Total patient care*, ed 10, St. Louis, 1999, Mosby.)

Box 44.6 Nursing Interventions for the Patient in Traction

- Maintain the patient's body in proper alignment. The force or pull on the extremities should be in alignment with the long axis of the bone.
- Ensure that weights hang freely from the bed and are never removed without a health care provider's order.
- Question patients as to their understanding of the purpose of the traction, and assess their ability to use a trapeze bar for self-movement. Elevate the foot of the bed to help prevent the patient from sliding down toward the foot of the bed (countertraction).
- Observe the condition of the traction cords, making sure they are not weakened or frayed. All knots used on the rope or cord are to be square knots.
- Center the ropes on the traction pulley.
- Assess, document, and report neurovascular impairment.
- Ensure that the weight used is the correct weight as ordered by the health care provider.
- Carefully observe the skin for signs of impairment. Use sheepskin heel protectors and bed pads to reduce impairment.
- If skeletal traction is used, assess the pin site for signs of infection. Cleanse the pin site every 8 hours with hydrogen peroxide or normal saline, as ordered.
- Assess the distal pulses bilaterally for circulatory integrity of the extremities.
- Inspect for loss of sensation in the dorsal area of the foot with weakness and inversion of the foot (inside surface turned outward).

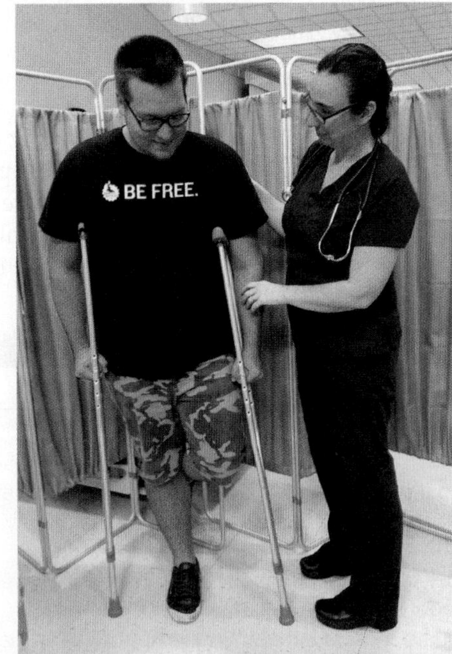
BE FREE.

Fig. 44.30 Assisting the patient with crutch walking. Note how the therapist guards the patient and how the patient's elbows are at no more than 30 degrees of flexion.

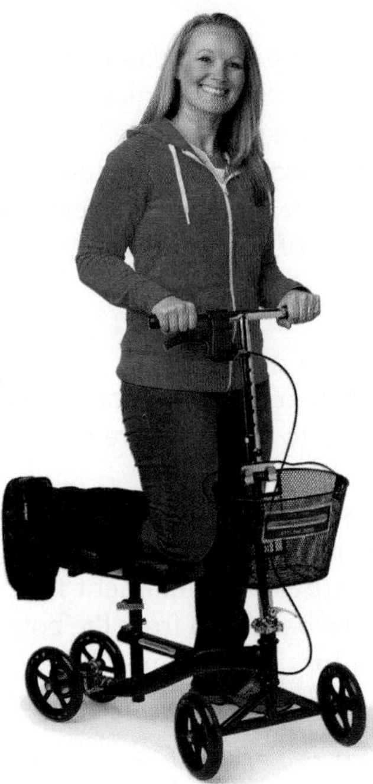

Fig. 44.31 The Roll-A-Bout walker. (Copyright 2013 Goodbye Crutches. Used with permission from Surgical Specialties Medical Devices, LLC.)

Safety Alert

Preventing Musculoskeletal Trauma

- Teach patients and community members to take appropriate safety precautions to prevent injuries while at home, at work, when driving, or when participating in sports.
- Be a vocal advocate for personal actions known to reduce injuries such as regularly using seatbelts, driving within posted speed limits, stretching before exercise, using protective athletic equipment (helmets and knee, wrist, and elbow pads), and not combining drinking and driving.
- Encourage older adults to participate in moderate exercise to aid in the maintenance of muscle strength and balance.
- To reduce falls, examine older adults' living environment to rule out the use of scatter rugs, to ensure adequate footwear and lighting, and to clear paths to bathrooms for nighttime use.
- Stress the importance of adequate calcium and vitamin D intake.

TRAUMATIC INJURIES

Traumatic injuries to the musculoskeletal system can occur in all age groups. However, older adults may have disorders that predispose them to musculoskeletal injuries (see the Safety Alert box on preventing musculoskeletal trauma). The more serious injuries involving fractures are treated in a hospital, whereas the less serious—such as contusions, sprains, or strains—may be treated in an outpatient facility.

CONTUSIONS

Etiology and Pathophysiology

Contusions are the most common soft tissue injury. An injury from a blow or blunt force causes local bleeding under the skin and possibly a hematoma (sac filled with blood). The severity of a contusion depends on the part of the body affected. A contusion of the brain is very serious, whereas a contusion of the arm is less serious. Large areas affected by soft tissue bleeding with slow absorption of the blood have a higher potential of developing into cellulitis (an infection of the subcutaneous tissue).

Medical Management

Most contusions are treated by applying ice bags or cold compresses for 15- to 20-minute periods over 12 to 36 hours for the vasoconstrictive effects of cold. The involved extremity is elevated to reduce edema and suppress pain.

Prognosis

The prognosis is excellent.

SPRAINS

Etiology and Pathophysiology

Sprains can result from a wrenching or hyperextension of a joint, tearing the capsule and ligaments. A sprain can involve bleeding into a joint (hemarthrosis). Common sites include the knee, ankle, and cervical spine (whiplash). Sprains are often the result of a sudden, twisting injury. Medical management is similar to that for contusions. Treatment usually consists of rest, ice, compression, and elevation (RICE) of the affected area.

Prognosis

The prognosis is excellent.

WHIPLASH

Etiology, Pathophysiology, and Clinical Manifestations

Injury at the cervical spine, or whiplash, is classified as a type of cervical disk syndrome. This means that there is compression or irritation of one or more cervical nerves. Whiplash is caused by an injury that involves hyperextension and flexion, which results in compression of the anatomic structures. This type of injury usually occurs as a result of sudden acceleration and deceleration, such as rear-end car collisions that cause violent back-and-forth movements of the head and neck. Symptoms of a whiplash (primarily pain) may not be obvious for a few days or even a week after the injury. Cervical fractures can accompany a whiplash injury.

Assessment

Collection of subjective data includes the patient's complaint of pain (the most common symptom), which usually begins in the cervical area but may radiate down the arm to the fingers and increase with cervical motion. The pain may increase sharply with coughing, sneezing, or any radical movement. Other signs and symptoms may be **paresthesia** (numbness or tingling), headache, blurred vision, decreased skeletal function, and weakened hand grip.

Objective data include edema in the cervical spine region with tightening of the muscles. Vital signs are usually within normal ranges. However, if the assessment findings indicate hypertension with widened pulse pressure and bradycardia, suspect increased intracranial pressure (ICP); report and document the findings immediately. Perform a neurologic assessment every 15 to 30 minutes to rule out increased ICP.

Diagnostic Tests

Physical examination and radiographic studies confirm the health care provider's diagnosis.

Medical Management

Symptoms commonly recur. A medical approach is used most often for the treatment of whiplash. Analgesics and muscle relaxants are prescribed, along with intermittent cervical traction. Surgery may be necessary if cervical fracture with displacement occurs (see "Herniation of Intervertebral Disk [Herniated Nucleus Pulposus]" later in this chapter).

Other treatments include special exercises, heat therapy, and administration of mild analgesics as ordered by the health care provider to control the pain. A soft foam rubber neck brace collar may be used for whiplash injuries to limit head movement.

Nursing Interventions

Nursing interventions include care of the patient with restricted activity to immobilize the cervical vertebrae, decrease irritation, and provide rest for the traumatized area. This is accomplished with cervical traction. If a neck brace is used, carefully inspect the skin around the neck and chin for signs of excoriation.

Prognosis

The prognosis depends on the extent of neurologic involvement. The prognosis is excellent with minor trauma, but because the spinal canal is full of neural tissue in the cervical area, more extensive injury can produce profound disability.

ANKLE SPRAINS

Etiology and Pathophysiology

An ankle sprain often is referred to as a twisted ankle and is caused by a wrenching or twisting of the foot and ankle (see Safety Alert box on strains and sprains).

Clinical Manifestations

The ankle area becomes edematous quickly, with spasms of the muscles and pain on passive movement of the joint.

Assessment

Collection of subjective data includes assessment of pain and tenderness in the affected ankle that intensifies with movement of the foot or ankle.

Collection of objective data includes assessment of the traumatized ankle for signs of edema, limited movement and function of the joint, and ecchymosis of the soft tissue around the ankle.

Diagnostic Tests

A radiographic examination of the injured area is the only accurate way to ensure there is no bone injury.

Medical Management

Surgery may be indicated for severe sprains. The health care provider sutures torn ligament fibers together. If the ligaments have been torn from the bone, the surgeon reattaches them by drilling small holes in the medial malleolus (rounded bony protrusion on the medial area of the ankle).

Nursing Interventions

The injured area must be elevated and kept at rest. Application of ice for 15 to 20 minutes intermittently for 12 to 36 hours—followed after 24 hours by the application of mild heat for 15 to 30 minutes, four times daily—will promote absorption of blood and fluid from the area. Use compressive dressings and splinting to help support the injured area. A neurovascular assessment is necessary to detect impaired tissue perfusion.

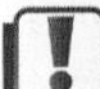
Safety Alert

Strains and Sprains

A strain and a sprain are not the same. Strains are produced by minute muscle tears and overstretching of tendons, whereas sprains are caused by a twisting of the joint.

Prognosis

With proper treatment, sprains and strains can be effectively treated. The prognosis is generally excellent.

STRAINS

Etiology and Pathophysiology

Strains are characterized by microscopic muscle tears as a result of overstretching muscles and tendons. An acute strain results when the muscles and tendons are overstretched in a forceful movement, such as unaccustomed vigorous exercise.

Assessment

Collection of subjective data includes noting the patient's complaint of sudden and severe pain away from the joint, which increases with activity. Chronic muscle strain can occur from repeated muscle overuse, and the pain may not appear for several hours. The patient typically complains of soreness, stiffness, and tenderness in the area.

Collection of objective data includes observation of stiffness, ecchymosis, and slight edema over the injury site. The most common sites are calf muscles, hamstrings, quadriceps, and the lumbosacral area. Edema can occur rapidly in the muscle and tendon area.

Diagnostic Tests

A radiographic study is necessary to rule out bone trauma.

Medical Management

Surgical repair is necessary if the muscle is ruptured completely. The health care provider orders analgesics and muscle relaxants. An exercise program almost always is prescribed if the strain is in the lumbosacral region. The exercises are aimed at strengthening the lower abdominal muscles.

Nursing Interventions

Nursing interventions for a strain are similar to those for a sprain. Ice application helps relieve pain, but some health care providers prefer heat application rather than ice. Back strains are among the most common strains. If the symptoms worsen, advise the patient to avoid strenuous activities, use a firm chair with rigid back support, avoid wearing high heels, use a firm mattress for sleep, and never sleep on the abdomen. Encourage the patient to do leg exercises to prevent development of thrombosis.

Prognosis

The prognosis is usually favorable.

DISLOCATIONS

Etiology and Pathophysiology

Dislocations usually involve tearing of the joint capsule; **subluxations** (partial or incomplete dislocations) involve stretching of the joint capsule. Both are temporary displacements of bones from their normal position within joints. A dislocation may be (1) congenital (e.g., congenital hip displacement), (2) caused by a disease process, or (3) caused by trauma. A dislocation or subluxation also may be accompanied by stretching and tearing of ligaments and tendons and by fractures. The displaced bone may rupture blood vessels. When subluxation occurs, the joint's articulating (movable) surfaces are partially separated.

Clinical Manifestations

Dislocation may or may not be visible. Sometimes a dislocation changes the length of an affected extremity. Pain and loss of function may be similar to those occurring with a fracture. However, dislocation partially immobilizes a joint, whereas a fracture site typically has abnormal free movement. Common dislocation sites include the shoulder, hip, and knee.

Assessment

Subjective data include the patient's description of the injury and pain. For shoulder dislocation, the patient complains of sensation loss and paresthesia.

Collection of objective data includes the assessment of any erythema, discoloration, edema, pain, tenderness, limitation of movement, and deformity or shortening of the extremity. Compare both sides for validation. Neurovascular assessment is important to determine whether vascular or nerve injury is present in the affected area. For shoulder dislocation, assess for an absent radial pulse, hypothermia of the hand, and wrist drop.

Diagnostic Tests

The diagnosis is based on complaints of discomfort, physical examination, and diagnostic radiographic examination of the injured site.

Medical Management

The health care provider may perform a closed reduction, which corrects the deformity through manipulation of the extremity. Surgical intervention to restore joint articulation sometimes is required.

Nursing Interventions and Patient Teaching

Nursing interventions include (1) reduction of edema and discomfort, (2) immobilization of the injured part to promote healing, and (3) patient education. Ice application is recommended for the first 24 hours after trauma. After 24 hours, heat may be used if there are no indications of bleeding. Elevation of the injured extremity on pillows and the application of elastic bandages help relieve edema. Immobilization of joints may involve application of a splint, sling, or elastic bandage. The air cast or air splint brace is an immobilization device. It is inflatable, lightweight, and conforms to the extremity's size and shape. When immobilization devices are used, perform a neurovascular assessment frequently (see Box 44.5 and the patient problem statements below). Administer analgesics as prescribed by the health care provider. Asking the patient to rate the pain on a scale from 0 to 10 is helpful in determining pain severity. For control of extreme pain, the health care provider may order an opioid, such as morphine. For mild to moderate pain, ibuprofen or acetaminophen (Tylenol) may be prescribed. Positioning and repositioning the injured part can help reduce discomfort.

Patient problem statements and interventions for the patient with impaired neurovascular integrity include but are not limited to the following:

Patient Problem	Nursing Interventions
Compromised Peripheral Tissue Perfusion, related to: • Injury • Treatment	Position extremities in alignment; elevate affected extremity Carefully monitor distal pulses, capillary refill, and temperature of involved area

Patient Problem	Nursing Interventions
Potential for Harm or Damage to the Body, related to neurovascular impairment	Compare affected extremity with unaffected extremity, using same hand for palpation Test capillary refill (blanching test) Check each digit for sensation and motion Document location and characteristics of pain Palpate pedal, tibial, or radial pulses, and compare with unaffected extremity Assess for edema with pallor, cyanosis, and coldness Ask patient to describe sensations Document all findings

Promoting an accident-free environment is essential. Areas of preventive medicine to explore with patients include the following:

- Grab bars mounted in the bathroom near the toilet or tub and rubber mats or slip guards in the tub and shower help prevent falls.
- Removing throw rugs and obstacles from the floor can prevent falls.
- A gait enhancer, such as a cane, crutches, or a walker, must be used correctly and with attention to safety precautions, such as using rubber tips on the points that make contact with the floor to prevent slippage.
- Patients in the hospital are at risk of falling out of bed if their disease, condition, or medication results in disorientation. Carefully assess their level of orientation, keep side rails up, and provide safety reminder devices to prevent self-injury.
- Using a safe ladder when climbing can help prevent a fall.
- Wearing protective clothing while engaging in dangerous work or contact sports is recommended.

Appropriate health teaching should be targeted for people at risk for musculoskeletal diseases, such as osteoporosis, which can predispose them to pathologic or nontraumatic fractures.

Prognosis

The prognosis is generally excellent.

AIRBAG INJURIES

Airbag deployment injuries include chemical burns, ocular trauma, cervical injury, soft tissue injury, and upper extremity and chest trauma. Orthopedic injuries tend to involve the upper extremities, especially the wrist, hand, and elbow. Injuries from airbag deployment can be life threatening in the very young. People at increased risk include older adults and small children. Airbag-induced injuries are associated with a rapid, forceful inflation, lasting less than 1 second from inflation to deflation. Management for these injuries will be based on the type and degree of injury. Treatments may include wound assessment and cleaning, application of ice to inflamed areas, and analgesic therapies.

MUSCULOSKELETAL DISORDER AND SURGICAL INTERVENTIONS

CARPAL TUNNEL SYNDROME

Etiology and Pathophysiology

Carpal tunnel syndrome is a painful disorder of the wrist and hand. It is caused by inflammation and edema of the synovial lining of the tendon sheaths in the carpal tunnel of the wrist. As a result, the tunnel space is narrowed, resulting in compression of the median nerve between the inelastic carpal ligament and other structures in the carpal tunnel (Fig. 44.32). The symptoms of *paresthesia* (any subjective sensation such as pricks of pins and needles) and *hypoesthesia* (a decrease in sensation in response to stimulation of the sensory nerves) of the thumb, index, and middle fingers may develop spontaneously or occur as a result of disease or injury.

This condition has a higher incidence in obese, middle-aged women and individuals employed in occupations involving repetitious motions of the fingers and hands (e.g., computing, hairdressing, manufacturing, basket weaving, meat carving, and typing). Carpal tunnel syndrome has become one of the three most common industrial or work-related conditions and is related to increased computer usage. Research also supports genetic links for the development of the condition. Edema of the tendon sheaths caused by RA can predispose a patient to carpal tunnel syndrome. Pregnant women also develop the syndrome during their last trimester of pregnancy. Fluid retention and edema experienced during pregnancy are thought to be the likely cause by compressing the nerves.

Clinical Manifestations

The clinical manifestations include gradual to increased numbness and tingling in the thumb, index, and middle

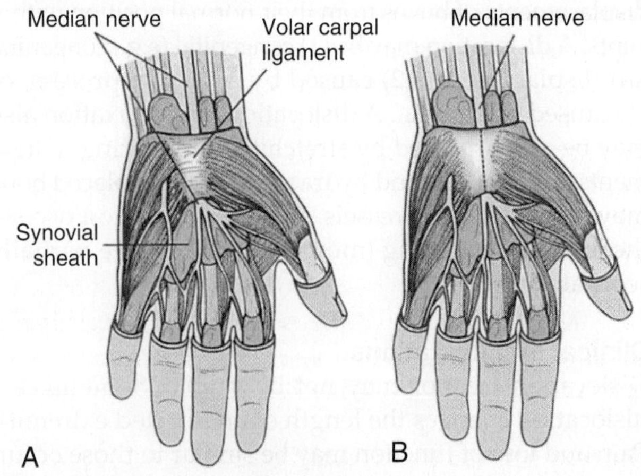

Fig. 44.32 A, Wrist structures involved in carpal tunnel syndrome. B, Decompression of median nerve. (From Thompson JM, Hirsch JE, Tucker SM, et al: *Mosby's clinical nursing,* ed 5, St. Louis, 2002, Mosby.)

fingers. These symptoms initially may appear then disappear but then become increasingly persistent as the nerve becomes consistently compressed or becomes damaged. The affected hand has altered ability to grasp or hold small objects. Atrophy of the thenar eminence (the padded area of the palm below the base of the thumb) is noted as the disease progresses.

Assessment

Subjective data include the patient's description of discomfort, such as burning pain or tingling in the hands, relieved by vigorously shaking or exercising the hands. Pain may be intermittent or constant and is often more intense at night. The patient also may complain of numbness (hypoesthesia) of the thumb, index, and ring fingers, especially after prolonged flexion of the wrist; and inability to grasp or hold small objects.

Collection of objective data includes assessment of the hand, wrist, or fingers for edema; muscle atrophy; or a depressed appearance of the soft tissue at the base of the thumb on the palmar surface.

Diagnostic Tests

Physical examination reveals deficits in sensory mapping along median nerve innervation pathways; positive Tinel's sign; increased tingling with a gentle tap over the tendon sheath on the ventral surface of the central wrist; edema of the fingers; and thenar surfaces of the palm thinner than normal (wasting). Having the patient hold the wrists against each other in forced palmar flexion for 1 minute can elicit sensory changes of numbness and tingling, which is a positive Phalen's maneuver test (one indication of carpal tunnel syndrome).

An electromyogram shows a weakened muscle response to stimulation. MRI shows compression and flattening of the median nerve, increased signal intensity within the median nerve, and abrupt changes in diameter of the median nerve. A handheld electroneurometer predicts motor latency of the median nerve, which is diagnostic of carpal tunnel syndrome.

Medical Management

If the symptoms are mild and surgery is not a desirable option, an immobilizer such as a splint can be used. Physical therapy and yoga have demonstrated improved strength and reduced discomfort. Hydrocortisone acetate suspension injected into the carpal tunnel can relieve mild symptoms. Surgery is indicated for severe symptoms with muscle atrophy. The standard surgical treatment is decompression of the median nerve by sectioning of the transverse carpal ligament. This can be accomplished by either an endoscopic technique or open surgery (Mayo Clinic, 2016a).

Nursing Interventions and Patient Teaching

Education concerning the need for frequent position changes and stretching of the hands and fingers is helpful in preventing discomfort. There are specialized tools for the office and desk to prevent median nerve compression.

If surgery is not required, the nurse is involved in the application of an immobilizer to promote comfort. General nursing interventions are use of a wrist cock-up splint to relieve pressure and to lessen wrist flexion, elevation to relieve edema, ROM exercises to lessen sense of clumsiness, and restriction of twisting and turning activities of the wrist.

If surgery is required, postoperative interventions include (1) elevating the hand and arm for 24 hours; (2) implementing and evaluating active thumb and finger motion within limits imposed by the dressing; (3) administering prescribed analgesics as needed; (4) monitoring vital signs (temperature elevation could indicate infection); and (5) checking fingers for circulation, sensation, and movement every 1 to 2 hours for 24 hours.

Encourage patients to use the affected hand in normal activities as soon as 2 to 3 days after surgery.

Prognosis

Mild symptoms of carpal tunnel syndrome are relieved by nonsurgical treatment; severe symptoms require surgical intervention with excellent prognosis. If the patient is pregnant, symptoms usually are relieved after delivery.

HERNIATION OF INTERVERTEBRAL DISK (HERNIATED NUCLEUS PULPOSUS)

Etiology and Pathophysiology

Herniated nucleus pulposus is a rupture of the fibrocartilage surrounding an intervertebral disk, releasing the nucleus pulposus that cushions the vertebrae above and below. This displacement puts pressure on nerve roots. Lumbar and cervical herniations are most common (Fig. 44.33). Herniated nucleus pulposus can occur suddenly (from lifting, twisting, or trauma) or gradually (from degenerative changes, as seen with DJD, osteoporosis, aging, and chronic diseases affecting bones). Herniations of the lumbar spine usually affect people 20 to 45 years old; cervical herniations are seen most in people 45 years and older. Men are more prone to this disorder than are women.

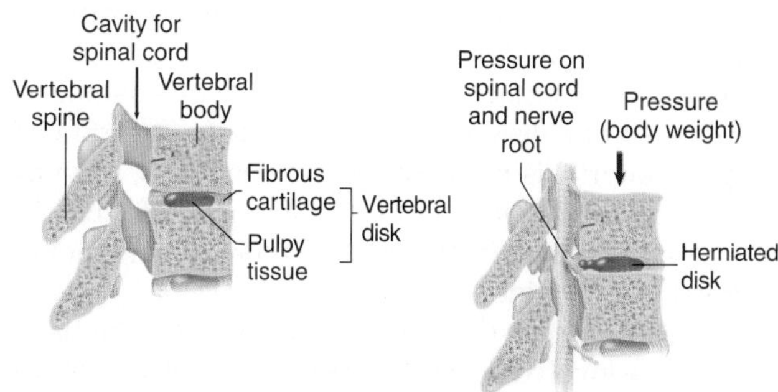

Fig. 44.33 Sagittal section of vertebrae showing normal *(left)* and herniated disks *(right)*. (From Patton KT, Thibodeau GA: *The human body in health and disease*, ed 7, St. Louis, 2018, Elsevier.)

Clinical Manifestations

Low back pain that occurs with the slightest movement is the most common symptom of lumbar herniation. The pain radiates over the buttock and down the leg, following the sciatic nerve pathway *(radicular pain)*, causing numbness and tingling in the affected leg. Complaints of pain in the back radiating down the leg (sciatica) are common. Complaints about activity intolerance and alteration in bowel and bladder elimination (constipation and urinary retention) are significant.

A patient with cervical herniation may experience neck pain, headache, and neck rigidity. Pain, numbness, and tingling are not uncommon to radiate down one or both arms. Loss of strength in the arm or arms may occur as well.

Assessment

Collection of subjective data includes assessing pain and asking patient about measures used for relief and other possible symptoms, such as activity intolerance and altered bowel and bladder function. Pain often gets worse with activity.

Collection of objective data includes observing for signs of limited spinal flexibility (limited forward bending) and gait alteration (patient may support weight on one extremity). An ineffective breathing pattern may result from pain and decreased mobility. Assessment includes determination of bowel and bladder elimination and maintenance of traction equipment.

Diagnostic Tests

Obtain a complete history and physical examination. The health care provider orders radiographic studies, MRI, CT, myelography, and electromyelography to determine nerve involvement.

Medical Management

The patient may follow a conservative approach initially, which includes physical therapy; local heat or ice; ultrasound and massage; and transcutaneous electrical nerve stimulation (TENS). The patient typically is treated with NSAIDs and muscle relaxants. Epidural corticosteroid injections by a pain specialist are used commonly if other conservative approaches are not successful. If the patient demonstrates neurologic deterioration or continued pain, a surgical procedure may be required, such as one of the following:

- *Artificial disk replacement:* Replacement of a damaged intervertebral disk with an artificial disk. The artificial disk material is made of various materials, such as medical-grade metal or plastic. The goal of artificial disk replacement is the return of more natural movement of the spine.
- *Chemonucleolysis:* Can be done on patients who have no nerve involvement. The procedure involves administering a local anesthetic agent and then guiding a needle into the nucleus pulposus to inject chymopapain (a drug that dissolves the nucleus pulposus).
- *Diskectomy:* Removal of the extruded disk material, often with a microscope. Percutaneous lateral diskectomy—cutting a window around the anulus fibrosus—is performed with the patient under local anesthesia.
- *Endoscopic spinal microsurgery:* Can be performed with the patient under local anesthesia. Special scopes enable the surgeon to remove herniated disks successfully with minimal damage to surrounding tissues.
- *Laminectomy:* Surgical removal of the bony arches or one or more vertebrae performed to relieve compression of the spinal cord caused by bone displacement from an injury or degeneration of a disk, or to remove a displaced vertebral disk.
- *Spinal fusion* (arthrodesis; the surgical immobilization of a joint; artificial ankylosis): Removal of the lamina and several herniated nuclei pulposi. A portion of bone taken from the patient's iliac crest or from a bone bank is used as a bone graft in the vertebral spaces.

Postoperative laminectomy care includes assessing the incision site for signs of infection such as drainage, edema, odor, and temperature elevation. Use of surgical asepsis when changing dressings and handling drainage decreases the chance of infection. After chemonucleolysis, carefully assess for signs of allergic reactions to chymopapain, such as urticaria and respiratory difficulties.

Nursing Interventions and Patient Teaching

Nursing interventions are aimed at providing nursing care appropriate for the following patient problems:

- *Anxiousness, related to discomfort, fear of the unknown, and lifestyle changes*
- *Recent Onset of Pain (back), related to muscle spasms and painful diagnostic tests*
- *Prolonged Infrequent or Difficult With Bowel Elimination and Retaining Urine or Inability to Urinate, related to pain, analgesics, immobility, and neurologic involvement*

Give the patient and family information about procedures and hospital protocol to help reduce their anxiety. Administer the medications prescribed on schedule, and document the effectiveness of the medication. Distraction, heat or ice application (if ordered), and moving (by logrolling) and positioning the patient every 2 hours (if not contraindicated because of need to maintain traction) can promote patient comfort. Dietary monitoring is important to ensure that the patient maintains a high-protein, iron- and vitamin-enriched diet.

Observe dressing for bleeding or cerebrospinal fluid leakage. Apply antiembolism stockings if ordered. Careful documentation of I&O provides information about bowel and bladder function. Ensure that the patient has voided in the first 8 hours, and use nursing measures to promote voiding before resorting to catheterization. Encourage the patient to sit in a straight, firm chair for no longer than 30 minutes at one time.

Monitor the patient for evidence of respiratory distress and paralytic ileus, complications that may occur in laminectomy patients.

Patient problem statements and interventions for the patient with a herniated disk include but are not limited to the following:

Patient Problem	Nursing Interventions
Insufficient Knowledge, related to home care management	Stress importance of rehabilitation plan of activity, rest, and exercise Provide diet instructions related to type and amount of food and weight maintenance (no gain) if applicable Discuss medications: name, purpose, schedule, dosage, and side effects Discuss signs and symptoms to report to health care provider: severe pain; changes in temperature, color, or sensation in extremity; and malodorous drainage from wound Encourage follow-up visits with health care provider
Helplessness, related to: • Decreased mobility • Pain	Use active listening and permit verbalization of anger and weakness Assist patient in identifying coping mechanisms that will reduce feeling of powerlessness; use those that have been successful in the past Offer positive recognition for increased activity level Assist patient in identifying areas that can be controlled Involve patient in decision-making process for own care

The patient may begin activity out of bed as early as 1 day after a simple laminectomy or 2 to 4 days after a laminectomy and fusion. Transfer the patient out of bed with as little time spent in the sitting position as possible. The patient may be permitted to walk as much as tolerated, with assistance if necessary. Braces or corsets, if prescribed, are applied before the patient gets out of bed. Encourage the patient to participate in ADLs within prescribed limits of mobility.

Instruct the patient not to lift or carry anything heavier than 5-10 lb (about 2.25 kg) for at least 8 weeks, not to drive a car until permitted by the surgeon, and to avoid twisting motions of the trunk. Reinforce the importance of follow-up visits to the health care provider.

Prognosis

With conservative treatment, some patients receive relief of symptoms; if a neurologic pathologic condition develops, surgical intervention is needed. The prognosis is usually favorable.

TUMORS OF THE BONE

Etiology and Pathophysiology

Tumors of the bone may be primary or secondary and may be benign or malignant. As with other types of tumors, the cause of bone tumors is not always known. Carcinoma of the prostate, lung, breast, thyroid, and kidney may metastasize to the bones. *Osteogenic* tumors are primary malignant bone tumors that occur most often in young people.

Osteogenic sarcoma is a fast-growing and aggressive tumor that affects the long bones of the body, particularly the distal femur, the proximal tibia, and the proximal humerus. Osteogenic sarcoma can metastasize to the lungs and to the rest of the body via the bloodstream. It affects males between the ages of 10 and 25 more often than females.

Osteochondroma is the most common benign osteogenic tumor. The incidence is highest in males between 10 and 30 years of age. Osteochondromas can occur as a single tumor or as multiple tumors. They usually affect the humerus, tibia, and femur.

Clinical Manifestations

When healthy bone cells are replaced by cancer cells, the bone's strength is altered and spontaneous fractures can occur. Anemia occurs when cancer invades the long bones and interrupts the manufacture of red blood cells in the bone marrow. Cancerous bone tumors metastasize and invade other bones and lung tissue.

Benign bone tumors can grow large enough to put pressure on blood vessels and nerves. Benign tumors do not spread. However, they may undergo cancerous changes and become malignant.

Assessment

Malignant and benign bone tumors cause pain in the affected bone site. Subjective data include complaints of pain, especially with weight-bearing. Pain may result from a spontaneous fracture. The patient also may complain of tenderness at the affected site.

Collection of objective data includes assessment of the painful part, which may reveal edema and discoloration of the skin.

Diagnostic Tests

Diagnosis is confirmed with radiographic studies, bone scan, bone biopsy, and laboratory studies, such as a CBC (which reveals bone marrow involvement), serum protein levels (elevated in multiple myeloma), and serum alkaline phosphatase level (elevated in osteogenic sarcoma).

Medical Management

The health care provider evaluates the tumor type, size, and location and plans the treatment accordingly. Larger, symptomatic benign tumors and malignant tumors require surgical intervention. The surgical procedure depends on the tumor size, location, and extent of tissue involvement. The surgery may involve (1) wide excision or resection, (2) bone curettage, or (3) leg or arm amputation.

Treatment is aimed at destroying or removing the malignant lesion. Amputation of the affected extremity may be necessary. Radiation and chemotherapy may be used before surgery to decrease tumor size or tissue involvement. Limb-salvage surgical procedures in combination with radiation and chemotherapy are being used more frequently for treatment of malignant bone tumors.

Chemotherapy is aimed at destroying cancer cells at primary and metastatic sites. Patients usually receive chemotherapy in 3- or 4-week cycles. Radiation therapy may be given internally and externally. The nurse must know the safety precautions and side effects of chemotherapy and radiation therapy. (See Chapter 57 for a discussion of care of the patient with cancer.)

Nursing Interventions and Patient Teaching

Preoperatively the patient and family need complete and concise information about procedures and postoperative expectations. Postoperative nursing interventions include (1) performing a neurovascular assessment (see Box 44.5); (2) monitoring vital signs; (3) administering analgesics and evaluating the effectiveness; (4) providing cast care or dressing changes with careful documentation of drainage, odors, and signs of circulation impairment; (5) cooperating with physical and occupational therapists to promote mobility and ADLs; and (6) educating the patient and family about home health care and early detection of tumor recurrence.

A patient problem statement and interventions for the patient with a bone tumor include but are not limited to the following:

Patient Problem	Nursing Interventions
Anxiousness, related to: • Fear of cancer • Body image • Lifestyle change • Possibility of death	Establish therapeutic relationship: acknowledge fear, encourage patient to acknowledge and express feelings Give accurate information about condition and therapies Refer patient to other resources when necessary (e.g., social worker, religious counselor)

Prognosis

The prognosis for bone tumors has improved in recent years with the combination of local surgery, chemotherapy, and radiation. Disease-free survival rates for patients whose osteogenic sarcoma is treated with surgery, chemotherapy, and radiation appear to be greater than 50% at 5 years.

AMPUTATION

The amputation of a portion of or an entire extremity may be necessary because of malignant tumors, injuries, impaired circulation (caused by diabetes mellitus or arteriosclerosis), congenital deformities, and infections. Most amputations are elective surgery unless they are related to trauma. Advances in microsurgical techniques enable surgeons to reattach severed extremities. Therefore traumatic amputations sometimes can be reversed by replantation if the severed limb is located, kept cooled, and presented to the emergency medical team.

Amputation of long bones can result in postoperative anemia. A traumatic or surgical amputation of an extremity can cause serious blood loss. Malignant bone tumors can metastasize via the bloodstream to other body systems.

Preoperative Assessment

Collection of subjective data includes questioning the patient about his or her understanding of the injury or disease process. Assess and document complaints of pain and symptoms of neurovascular impairment. Assess the patient's level of orientation, because many amputations occur in the older adult population as a result of impaired circulation.

Collection of objective data includes assessment of vital signs (temperature elevation, tachycardia, and tachypnea indicate infection). Assess arterial blood flow by palpation of bilateral pedal pulses and Doppler pressure measurements. Assess wound drainage for color, amount, and presence of odor. Evaluate upper body muscle strength and nutritional status.

Diagnostic Tests

A CBC is done to determine blood dyscrasias (i.e., an imbalance in the blood's cellular profile), such as anemia and bleeding tendencies, which could increase postoperative complications (such as hemorrhage, delayed wound healing, and disorientation). The health care provider orders laboratory studies such as BUN, potassium levels, and routine urinalysis. An ECG is performed to detect cardiac dysrhythmias, which are often present in older adult patients.

Medical Management

When the amputation results from traumatic injury to an extremity, the health care provider's interventions include measures to restore circulating blood volume, control pain, prevent infection in the wound, perform plastic surgical repair at the amputation site to facilitate the use of a prosthesis, and maintain adequate urinary output.

For elective amputations, the health care provider assesses the patient's physiologic, psychological, and emotional status. If infection is present in the body (gangrene may occur if circulation is impaired), treatment includes administration of antibiotics, and every attempt is made to control the infection before surgery. The health care provider discusses the possibility of the patient using a prosthesis. Much of the preoperative preparation focuses on the patient attaining a physical and emotional status conducive to wearing a prosthesis or achieving mobility through the use of a wheelchair or a gait enhancer such as crutches or a walker.

Postoperative Assessment, Nursing Interventions, and Patient Teaching

Collection of subjective data includes careful assessment of pain. *Phantom pain* (pain felt in the area of the missing extremity as if it were still present) may occur and be frightening to the patient. Phantom pain occurs because the nerve tracts that register pain in the amputated area continue to send a message to the brain; this is normal.

Collection of objective data includes observing for signs of hemorrhage, such as hypotension, tachycardia, tachypnea, pallor, decreased urinary output, restlessness, and progressive loss of consciousness. Monitor and document suction drainage, and assess and protect the remaining extremity. Observe for neurovascular impairment (done hourly in the immediate postoperative period) from tightly applied elastic wraps, dressings, or casts (see Box 44.5).

Nursing intervention is aimed at effective pain management and prevention of deformities (contractures, especially in the joint above the amputation, and abduction deformities are common). Flexion hip contractures can be prevented postoperatively by raising the foot of the bed slightly to elevate the residual extremity (with care taken not to flex the patient's hips by elevating the stump on a pillow), encouraging movement from side to side, and placing the patient in a prone position at least twice a day. This will stretch the flexor muscles. Teach the patient how to strengthen the remaining muscles to facilitate mobility and prevent muscle atrophy (push-ups from a prone position and sit-ups from a seated position). Apply elastic wraps to shrink and reshape the residual extremity into a cone and facilitate the proper fit and use of a prosthesis (Fig. 44.34). A prosthesis may be fitted as early as 2 or 3 weeks postoperatively. Because many amputations are performed in people between 60 and 70 years of age, observe the patient carefully for pulmonary complications (such as pulmonary embolus) and cardiovascular collapse. Keep suction equipment and oxygen at the bedside.

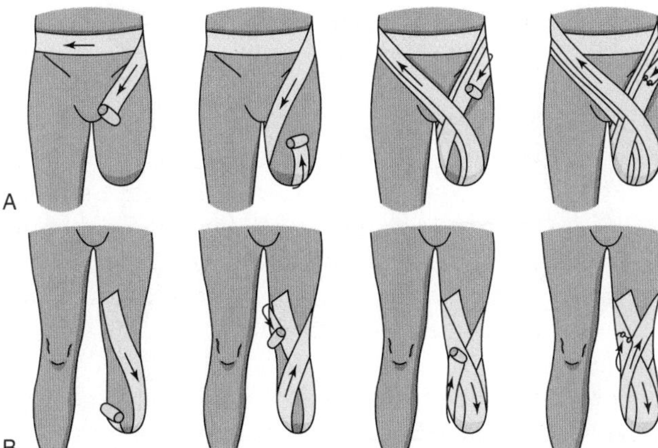

Fig. 44.34 Correct method of bandaging amputation stump. A, Anchor bandage around patient's waist. B, Method of bandaging midcalf stump, where bandage need not be anchored around waist. (From Beare PG, Myers JL: *Adult health nursing*, ed 3, St. Louis, 1998, Mosby.)

Patient education concerning phantom limb sensation, and the fact that it is a normal physiologic response, can help relieve patient fears. The patient may feel pain or other sensations, such as burning, tingling, throbbing, or pruritus in the area of the amputated extremity. These sensations can last for months or decades on a consistent or intermittent basis. Recommend that patients gently rub the residual extremity or take analgesics for relief.

For persistent, severe phantom pain, the following measures may be employed:

- Stump revision with reamputation at a higher level
- Local infiltration of the stump with procaine
- Mechanical percussion by striking the sensitive digital stump against a solid object—believed to shrink neuromas (small tumors that form in the scar tissue of the stump)
- Sympathetic nerve block

Encourage the patient to share his or her feelings over the loss of the extremity. Discuss the importance of allowing the grieving process to occur.

Patient problem statements and interventions for the patient undergoing an amputation include but are not limited to the following:

Patient Problem	Nursing Interventions
Distorted Body Image, related to loss of limb	Assess effects of amputation on body image Encourage patient to express feelings of mutilation, grief, anger, and loss to aid adaptation processes Encourage patient to help with dressing changes and wrapping of stump as able Teach family member wrapping techniques if necessary to increase competence and independence Use prescribed pain management techniques Encourage family members to walk with patient to maintain strength and social contacts Encourage grooming and wearing of personal clothing to maintain individuality and personality Encourage activities for self-care and ambulation to maintain positive outlook and maximum strength Encourage or arrange for social services consultation for economic and employment aid Arrange for follow-up care referral to aid rehabilitation

Continued

Patient Problem	Nursing Interventions
Compromised Physical Mobility, related to loss of limb	Assess ability to use remaining limbs Turn and position on side, back, and abdomen (after 24 hours) to maintain muscle and joint ROM Teach adduction and extension exercises and help patient perform them q 4 hr to prevent abduction and flexion contractures Assist with sitting in chair and ambulation with aid as able, to maintain muscle strength Prepare patient for physical therapy, transportation for exercises, and stump wrapping, if appropriate Encourage family members to walk with patient during initial ambulation periods, accompanied by health professionals, to increase independence Teach purposes of prone and extension positions to prevent contractures Assist prosthetist with prosthesis measurements and fitting as needed to aid rehabilitation

Before discharge, teach the patient and family proper positions, exercises, and ambulation techniques. Also demonstrate stump-wrapping techniques to the patient and family (see Fig. 44.34). Explain to them that prolonged phantom pain experiences are unusual and should receive medical attention. Discuss skin care with the patient and family so that they can take steps to prevent stump irritation or impairment. Also discuss the signs of a wound infection, and instruct them when it is necessary to call the health care provider.

Prognosis

The prognosis for successful adaptation to an amputation depends on the patient's age, the condition that resulted in amputation, other systemic disorders, emotional health, and support system.

NURSING PROCESS FOR THE PATIENT WITH A MUSCULOSKELETAL DISORDER

The role of the licensed practical nurse/licensed vocational nurse (LPN/LVN) in the nursing process as stated is that the LPN/LVN will:

- Participate in planning care for patients based on patient needs
- Review patient's care plan and recommend revisions as needed
- Review and follow defined prioritization for patient care
- Use clinical pathways, care maps, or care plans to guide and review patient care

ASSESSMENT

The musculoskeletal system provides protection, support, and movement for the body. Proper function of the musculoskeletal system is associated closely with proper function of the nervous and circulatory systems. Orthopedics is the branch of medicine that deals with the prevention or correction of disorders involving locomotor structures of the body. Permanent disability and crippling result if patients with musculoskeletal dysfunction do not receive prompt treatment.

Assess orthopedic function for all patients, especially those who are (1) having difficulty with gait; (2) experiencing muscle weakness; (3) suffering from trauma of soft tissue and bone; (4) unable to move and participate in activities for personal, economic, and social fulfillment; (5) experiencing diseases of the musculoskeletal system; or (6) chronically ill.

Assessment of a patient's mobility includes bone integrity, posture, joint function, muscle strength, gait, pain, and neurovascular disturbances related to pressure. Compare body symmetry. For example, assess both legs for same length and diameter and for comparable muscle strength. Observe the patient's gait for unsteadiness or irregular movements. Difficult ambulation associated with shortness of breath can indicate cardiovascular or respiratory system difficulties.

Assessment of posture and gait simply involves observing the patient walking. Common posture deformities include lateral (or S) curvature of the spine, known as **scoliosis;** a rounding of the thoracic spine (hump-backed appearance), known as **kyphosis;** and an increase in the curve at the lumbar space region that throws the shoulders back, resulting in a sway-backed gait, referred to as **lordosis** (Fig. 44.35). Rigidity of the spine can result from ankylosis, in which the vertebrae

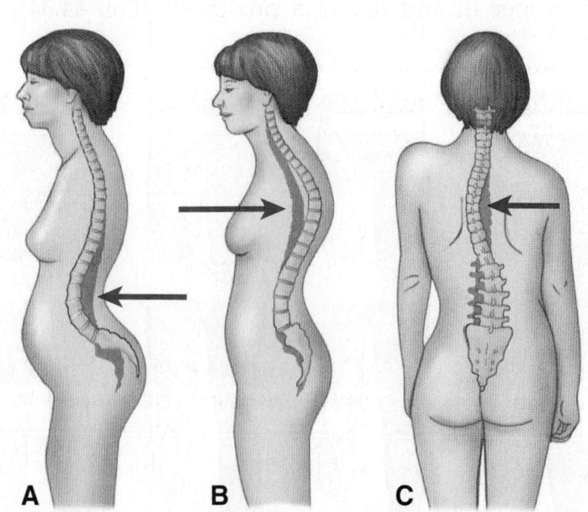

Fig. 44.35 Abnormal spinal curvatures. A, Lordosis. B, Kyphosis. C, Scoliosis. (From Patton KT, Thibodeau GA: *The human body in health and disease*, ed 7, St. Louis, 2018, Elsevier.)

are fused with loss of mobility, producing a rigid gait or "poker spine" appearance.

Assessment of neurologic and circulatory function is important if the patient has experienced a traumatic injury; damaged blood vessels and nerves can cause permanent disabilities.

Assess the skin for signs of coolness, pallor, sensation, or cyanosis to help determine the patient's circulatory status. A faint or absent pulse in an extremity indicates impaired circulation. Palpating the femoral, popliteal, and dorsalis pedis pulses on both extremities provides pertinent data about the lower extremities. If the pulse is not palpated readily with a light touch of the finger, a Doppler instrument can be used to magnify the sound of the pulsation. The absence of a pulse is serious and must be reported to the charge nurse immediately. Assess the brachial and radial pulses to determine circulation in the upper extremities. Palpating a pulse may be difficult if the patient has a cast or bandage. Reach under the cast or bandage if possible. Assess the pulse in the unaffected extremity for comparison.

The **blanching test** (meaning to whiten or pale) is a test of the rate of capillary refill, which signals circulation status. This is also referred to as a *capillary nail refill test.* Compress each fingernail or toenail of the affected extremity (noting the white color as pressure is applied), release the pressure, and note how quickly the pink color returns to the nailbed. The nailbed color should return to normal within 2 or 3 seconds. If the color is slow to return, circulation is impaired and requires prompt attention (see Box 44.5).

Neurovascular assessments are made on patients with musculoskeletal trauma or damage to nerves and blood vessels resulting from surgery, tight bandages, splints, or casts. Impaired circulation resulting in alteration of nerve function can cause loss of the use of an extremity; this impairment generally is seen in the extremities. See Box 44.5 for information concerning neurovascular (circulation) assessment.

◆ PATIENT PROBLEMS

Nursing assessment establishes the patient's needs regarding mobility. Care of the patient is based on the following problem statements:

- *Compromised Physical Mobility, related to musculoskeletal impairment*
- *Compromised Bed Mobility*
- *Inability to Tolerate Activity, related to musculoskeletal impairment*
- *Impaired Coping*
- *Anxiousness, related to changes in body integrity*
- *Prolonged Pain, related to musculoskeletal disorder*
- *Insufficient Knowledge, regarding therapeutic regimen*
- *Potential for Contractures or Muscle Atrophy*

◆ EXPECTED OUTCOMES AND PLANNING

The plan for facilitating mobility must center on improving and restoring performance and preventing deterioration. Nursing interventions help the patient adapt, reduce, or eliminate activities that cause pain.

Consider the amount of assistance needed for ambulation. Assessment of ROM and muscle strength helps decide whether the patient can ambulate safely. Ambulation after surgery often requires physical assistance in addition to the use of mobility aids such as walkers, canes, and crutches.

The care plan focuses on accomplishing individual goals and outcomes that relate to the identified patient problems. Examples of these include the following:

Goal 1: Patient will demonstrate the use of adaptive devices to increase mobility.

Outcome: Patient demonstrates more independence in mobility by meeting self-care needs.

Goal 2: Patient will demonstrate ambulation and state safety precautions before discharge from health care facility.

Outcome: Patient demonstrates ambulation skills and states correct safety precautions before discharge.

◆ IMPLEMENTATION

Improving the patient's mobility requires awareness of the health care provider's orders specific to ambulation. Check mobility aids for the correct size. Educate patients on safety measures, such as rubber tips in good condition on canes. Shoes that are easy to put on, have nonslip soles, and provide foot and ankle support are safer than bedroom slippers or stockings.

Activities must be alternated with rest periods. Administer analgesics at least 30 minutes before ambulation for patients experiencing pain. Encourage patients to pace themselves. Patient assistance may be necessary to complete ADLs such as ambulating to the bathroom or to a bedside commode.

Specific principles are involved with mobility:

- Bone loss occurs when patients are confined to bed rest.
- The activities of the human body depend on effective interaction between normal joints and the neuromuscular parts that pilot them.
- Muscles, tendons, ligaments, cartilage, and bones do their share to ensure smooth function.

Nurses working with patient mobility needs must support physical therapy department activities and goals. Assess a patient's perceptions to help determine his or her motivation for mobility independence. For example, when older adults think they are too fragile to walk, they may be afraid of trying. Use a safety belt when a patient's stability is questionable. The belt encircles the patient's waist; grasp the belt in the middle of the back to help the patient stand, gain balance, and ambulate.

Patients may have difficulty coping with mobility aids and perceive them as a visible sign of weakness. Point out that devices to help mobility are not unlike glasses to help eyesight. Mobility aids increase proficiency of activities and promote joint rest and protection.

◆ EVALUATION

Evaluate the success of interventions by noting a patient's progress during and after ambulation, based on stated goals and outcomes. For example, if the patient is not able to walk to the bathroom, a shorter distance may be more practical. The patient may increase mobility by using a bedside commode. When patients are unable to meet expected outcomes, be ready to revise the care plan to promote success. Examples of goals and their corresponding outcomes include the following:

Goal 1: Patient will demonstrate the use of adaptive devices to increase mobility.
Evaluative measure: Patient ambulates within physical environment.
Goal 2: Patient will understand safety precautions concerning use of mobility aids.
Evaluative measures: Patient checks rubber tips on mobility aid and uses equipment correctly.

Get Ready for the NCLEX® Examination!

Key Points

- The skeletal system has five basic functions: support of the body, protection of internal organs, movement of the body, storage of minerals, and blood cell formation.
- The skeleton is divided into the axial and the appendicular skeletons. The axial skeleton is composed of the skull, vertebral column, and thorax. The appendicular skeleton is composed of the upper extremities, lower extremities, shoulder girdle, and pelvic girdle.
- The three types of joints and their movement are (1) synarthrosis: no movement; (2) amphiarthrosis: slight movement; and (3) diarthrosis: free movement.
- Joints hold the bones together and allow movement and flexibility. Differences in the structure determine the amount of flexibility.
- Some of the more common movements that the body produces are flexion, extension, abduction, adduction, rotation, supination, pronation, dorsiflexion, and plantar flexion.
- The bones and joints provide the framework of the body, but the muscles are necessary for movement. Movement results from contraction and relaxation of the individual muscles.
- An erythrocyte sedimentation rate is the most objective laboratory test for determining the severity of rheumatoid arthritis (RA).
- RA affects a young population (ages 30 to 55 years) with crippling changes in the synovial membrane of the joints.
- Salicylates and NSAIDs are used to treat RA and osteoarthritis.
- Osteoarthritis is a degenerative joint disease that affects the population older than 40 years of age and causes articular cartilage degeneration.
- Porous and brittle bones caused by a lack of calcium are one of the physiologic changes noted in osteoporosis.
- Osteoporosis-related fractures occur in one in two women, compared with one in eight men, over the course of a lifetime.
- Vertebroplasty and kyphoplasty are surgical procedures used to relieve pain in women with osteoporosis who do not respond to other pain management programs.
- Arthroplasty procedures (such as hip and knee arthroplasty) commonly are performed on patients suffering from severe arthritis.
- Unicompartmental knee arthroplasty, also referred to as partial knee replacement, is performed on patients who have only one of the compartments of the knee affected by arthritis.
- Nursing intervention specific to the care of a patient suffering from a fractured hip involves maintaining abduction of the affected leg.
- Fractured hip fixation devices—such as hip prosthetic implant, plate and screw fixation, and telescoping nail fixation—require some degree of non–weight-bearing for 6 weeks to 3 months.
- The use of antacids and proton pump inhibitors increases a patient's risk of hip fractures.
- A significant postoperative nursing intervention for a patient with an amputation is proper care of the stump to facilitate the use of a prosthetic device.
- Herniated nucleus pulposus is seen most often in the cervical and lumbar spinal regions and can be treated surgically (laminectomy and spinal fusion) or medically (medication, traction, and physical therapy).
- Osteogenic sarcoma is a common primary malignant tumor seen in young people; it can metastasize to the lungs.
- Compartment syndrome, shock, fat embolism, gas gangrene, thromboembolus, and osteomyelitis are complications resulting from a fractured bone.
- Petechiae on the conjunctiva of the eye, the neck, the chest, or the axillary region is a typical sign of a fat embolism.
- External fixation devices such as casts, braces, metal pins, and skeletal and skin traction are used to hold bone fragments in normal position.
- Whether the casting material is plaster of Paris or a synthetic material, proper drying, cleansing, handling, and assessing are required to prevent patient complications.
- The nurse caring for a patient in traction is responsible for knowing (1) the purpose of the traction (traction applied for fractures must be continuous), (2) the equipment needed and appropriate safety measures, (3) the amount of weight ordered, and (4) the patient's understanding of the traction.

- Crutches, canes, walkers, and the Roll-A-Bout are used as gait enhancers for patients with altered mobility.
- Crutch walking involving the three-point gait is used most commonly for patients wearing leg casts.

Additional Learning Resources

SG Go to your Study Guide for additional learning activities to help you master this chapter content.

evolve Be sure to visit the Evolve site at *http://evolve.elsevier.com/Cooper/foundationsadult/* for additional online resources.

Review Questions for the NCLEX® Examination

1. Where does hematopoiesis take place?
   1. The lymph nodes
   2. The spleen
   3. The yellow bone marrow
   4. The red bone marrow
2. The nurse is repositioning a patient. During the movement the extremity is placed in a position away from the midline of the body. To document this position, what term is most appropriate?
   1. Adduction
   2. Pronation
   3. Flexion
   4. Abduction
3. A patient is suspected of having rheumatoid arthritis (RA). What diagnostic tests may be used to support the diagnosis? *(Select all that apply.)*
   1. Complete blood count
   2. Erythrocyte sedimentation rate
   3. Prothrombin time
   4. Urinary uric acid level
   5. C-reactive protein
4. The nurse is reviewing the assessment findings and medical history of a patient suspected of having gouty arthritis. What findings support the diagnosis?
   1. Heberden's nodes
   2. Pathologic fractures
   3. Tophi
   4. Homans' sign
5. A 55-year-old patient mentions that she is postmenopausal and is not taking estrogen supplements. A review of her normal dietary intake indicates a high consumption of caffeine and limited dietary ingestion of calcium. Based on her history, she faces an increased risk for what condition?
   1. Osteomyelitis
   2. Osteoarthritis
   3. Osteogenic sarcoma
   4. Osteoporosis
6. What is an appropriate nursing intervention for a patient suffering from a fractured hip with bipolar hip repair? *(Select all that apply.)*
   1. Release traction weight every 4 to 6 hours.
   2. Maintain abduction of the affected extremity.
   3. Maintain adduction of the affected extremity.
   4. Encourage active range of motion in the affected extremity.
   5. Ensure the head of the bed is not elevated more than 45 degrees.
7. A patient is being discharged after a prosthetic hip implant. She asks when she can begin to bear weight on the affected leg. What is a correct response by the nurse?
   1. "You will not be able to bear weight on the affected leg for 6 to 12 months."
   2. "Most patients bear weight in 5 days. I will check your orders."
   3. "You will use a gait enhancer and keep the majority of weight off the unaffected leg."
   4. "You will most likely require some degree of non–weight-bearing for 6 weeks to 3 months."
8. A patient has been seeing the health care provider for complaints of osteoarthritis. Today the patient is discussing concerns about their condition and asks what has caused the osteoarthritis. Which response by the nurse is most correct?
   1. "We don't really know what causes osteoarthritis."
   2. "Everyone your age has arthritis; you are fortunate you are still able to walk."
   3. "Wear and tear over the years have most likely caused the joints to begin to degenerate."
   4. "You probably did not exercise as much as you should have, and you should start vigorous exercising now to prevent further complications."
9. When providing care to a patient in skeletal traction what action would be included in the nurse's plan of care?
   1. Provide cast care.
   2. Cleanse pin sites and observe for signs of infection.
   3. Place patient on drainage and secretion precautions.
   4. Encourage patient to sit in a straight, firm chair for no longer than 20 minutes each time.
10. After a fracture of the forearm or tibia, complaints of sharp, deep, unrelenting pain in the hand or foot unrelieved by analgesics or elevation of the extremity indicate which complication?
    1. Fat embolism
    2. Compartment syndrome
    3. Gas gangrene
    4. Cast syndrome

11. A patient suffered a knee injury while playing football. The patient is scheduled for an arthroscopic examination and asks the nurse to explain the procedure. What information should be included in the nurse's response?
    1. "Your health care provider will insert a small scope into your knee joint to visualize the joint for damaged tissue."
    2. "The test involves the use of magnetism and radio waves to make images of cross sections of the body."
    3. "The radiographic technician will inject your knee joint with an atomic material and take a radiograph of your affected knee."
    4. "The health care provider will insert needle electrodes into the knee muscle to document electrical activity of the knee."
12. A patient with RA asks if there is a cure. What response by the nurse is most appropriate?
    1. "Yes, new drugs offer a cure."
    2. "No, but new drugs can interfere with the body's reaction to inflammation and better control the disease process."
    3. "Yes, but the patient must take medication for at least 10 years."
    4. "No, most patients with RA also develop osteoarthritis."
13. A patient is scheduled for endoscopic spinal microsurgery to correct a herniated disk. Select the most accurate statement concerning this type of surgery.
    1. "Endoscopic spinal microsurgery requires a general anesthetic."
    2. "Special scopes are placed through small incisions, causing minimal damage to surrounding tissue."
    3. "Patients older than 80 years of age are always candidates for endoscopic spinal microsurgery."
    4. "Endoscopic spinal microsurgery is limited to the repair of herniated disks."
14. A patient has osteoarthritis of the knee and is seeking information about glucosamine supplements. What would be an appropriate response by the nurse?
    1. "Glucosamine is a natural substance in the body, and it is not necessary to take a supplement."
    2. "Glucosamine supplements are relatively safe in people younger than 40 years of age."
    3. "Studies suggest that glucosamine supplements may be helpful in maintaining healthy joint function."
    4. "A healthy lifestyle with high-impact exercise is more important than taking a supplement."
15. Select the most appropriate nursing assessment for the patient problem of ineffective tissue perfusion, secondary to fractured hip.
    1. Assess for ecchymosis over pelvis and perineum.
    2. Protect patient from cross-contamination.
    3. Assess for adventitious lung sounds.
    4. Assess distal pulses.
16. A patient has just undergone total hip replacement. The patient asks why she cannot cross her legs when sitting but must do straight leg–raising exercises. What is the most correct response?
    1. "The exercises help strengthen the leg muscles; crossing your legs puts pressure on the joints and could damage the hip prosthesis."
    2. "The exercises keep you from getting too tired while you sit; when you want to cross your legs, it is time to rest."
    3. "The exercises strengthen the muscles in your upper legs to help you walk."
    4. "The health care provider ordered these exercises but did not order you to cross your legs."
17. Which objective signs will the nurse find during the assessment of a patient with compartment syndrome in the lower leg? *(Select all that apply.)*
    1. Hypotension
    2. Gas bubbles under the skin
    3. Positive Homans' sign
    4. Absence of pulsation in the affected extremity
    5. Pain that is unreleased by medication or elevation of the extremity
18. A patient had a compound fracture of his right femur 2 years before the present admission. His health care provider suspects osteomyelitis and has informed the patient that tests are needed to confirm the diagnosis. The patient wants to know what tests can be ordered to determine osteomyelitis. An appropriate response would include which test for osteomyelitis? *(Select all that apply.)*
    1. Goniometer
    2. BMX
    3. Bone scan
    4. Bone biopsy
    5. Erythrocyte sedimentation rate
19. A construction worker suffered a fracture of the femur 48 hours ago. The nurse notices that he has petechiae on the conjunctiva, chest, neck, and axillae. Petechiae in these locations are consistent with which condition?
    1. Compartment syndrome
    2. Deep vein thrombosis
    3. Gas gangrene
    4. Fat embolism

Care of the Patient With a Gastrointestinal Disorder

45

http://evolve.elsevier.com/Cooper/foundationsadult/

Objectives

Anatomy and Physiology

1. List in sequence each of the parts or segments of the alimentary canal and identify the accessory organs of digestion.
2. Discuss the function of each digestive and accessory organ.

Medical-Surgical

3. Discuss the laboratory and diagnostic examinations associated with the gastrointestinal system.
4. Identify nursing interventions associated with disorders of the gastrointestinal tract.
5. Explain the etiology and pathophysiology, clinical manifestations, assessments, diagnostic tests, medical-surgical management, and nursing interventions for the patient with disorders of the mouth, esophagus, stomach, and intestines.
6. Identify nursing interventions for preoperative and postoperative care of the patient who requires gastric surgery.
7. Compare and contrast the inflammatory bowel diseases of ulcerative colitis and Crohn's disease.
8. Identify nursing interventions for the patient with a stoma for fecal diversion.
9. Discuss the etiology and pathophysiology, clinical manifestations, assessment, diagnostic tests, medical management, and nursing interventions for the patient with acute abdominal inflammations (appendicitis, diverticulitis, and peritonitis), for the patient with hernias, and for the patient with colorectal cancer.
10. Differentiate between mechanical and nonmechanical intestinal obstruction, including causes, medical management, and nursing interventions.
11. Explain the causes, medical management, and nursing interventions for the patient with fecal incontinence.

Key Terms

achalasia (ăk-ăh-LĀ-zhē-ă, p. 1406)
achlorhydria (ă-khlŏr-HĪ-drē-ă, p. 1396)
anastomosis (ă-năs-tō-MŌ-sĭs, p. 1405)
cachexia (kă-KĔK-sē-ă, p. 1436)
carcinoembryonic antigen (CEA) (kăr-sĭn-ō-ĕm-brē-ĂN-ĭk ĂN-tĭ-jĕn, p. 1415)
dehiscence (dĕ-HĬS-ĕntz, p. 1416)
dumping syndrome (DŬMP-ĭng SĬN-drōm, p. 1416)
dyspepsia (dĭs-PĔP-sē-ă, p. 1408)
dysphagia (dĭs-FĀ-jhē-ă, p. 1401)
evisceration (ĕ-vĭs-ĕr-Ā-shŭn, p. 1416)
exacerbations (ĕg-zăs-ĕr-BĀ-shŭnz, p. 1421)
gluten (GLŪ-tĕn, p. 1419)
hematemesis (hĕ-mă-TĔM-ĕ-sĭs, p. 1407)
intussusception (ĭn-tŭs-sŭs-SĔP-shŭn, p. 1398)
leukoplakia (lū-kō-PLĀ-kē-ă, p. 1401)
lumen (LŪ-mĕn [adjectival, LŪ-mĕn-ăl], p. 1398)
melena (MĔL-ĕh-nă, p. 1397)
occult blood (ŏ-KŬLT, p. 1398)
paralytic (adynamic) ileus (pă-ră-LĬ-tĭk ā-dī-NĂM-ĭk Ĕ-lē-ŭs, p. 1434)
pathognomonic (păth-ŏg-nō-MŎN-ĭk, p. 1399)
remissions (rĕ-MĬSH-ŭnz, p. 1421)
steatorrhea (stĕ-ă-tō-RĒ-ă, p. 1426)
stoma (STŌ-mă, p. 1425)
tenesmus (tĕ-NĔZ-mŭs, p. 1418)
volvulus (VŎL-vū-lŭs, p. 1434)

ANATOMY AND PHYSIOLOGY OF THE GASTROINTESTINAL SYSTEM

DIGESTIVE SYSTEM

The digestive tract, or alimentary canal, is a muscular tube containing a mucous membrane lining that extends from the mouth to the anus (Fig. 45.1) and is approximately 9 m (30 ft) long. It consists of the mouth, pharynx, esophagus, stomach, small intestine, large intestine, and anus. *Peristalsis* is the coordinated, rhythmic, sequential contraction of smooth muscle that pushes food through the digestive tract, as well as bile through the bile duct.

Accessory organs aid in the digestive process but are not considered part of the digestive tract. They release

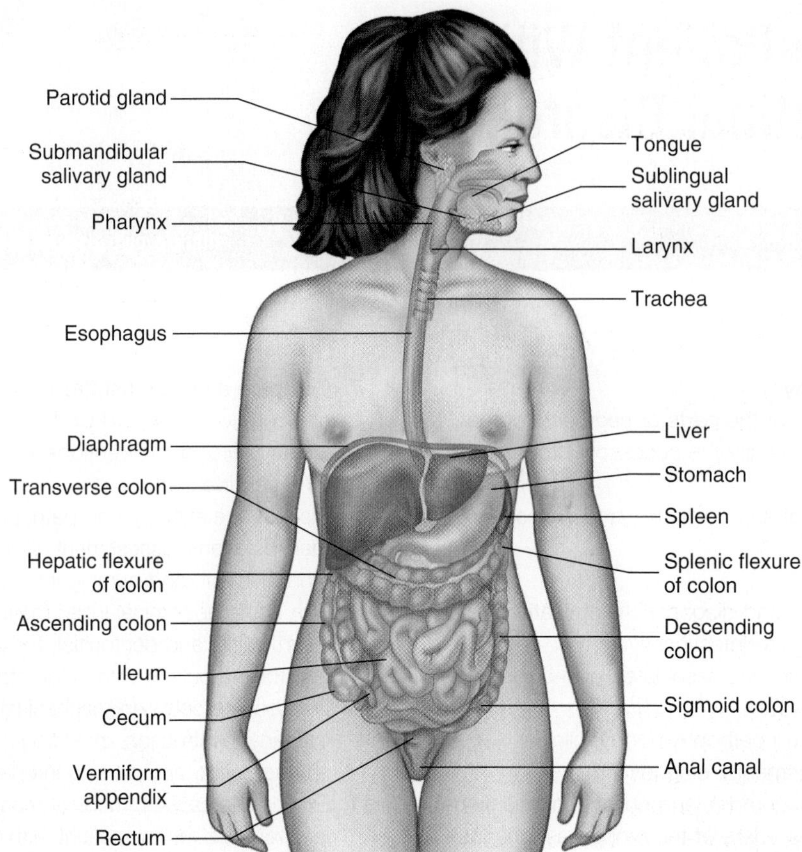

Fig. 45.1 Location of digestive organs. (From Patton KT, Thibodeau GA: *Anatomy & physiology*, ed 10, St. Louis, 2019, Elsevier.)

chemicals into the system through a series of ducts. The teeth, tongue, salivary glands, liver, gallbladder, pancreas, and appendix are considered accessory organs.

Organs of the Digestive System and Their Functions

Box 45.1 lists various organs of the digestive system and the accessory organs involved in digestion.

Mouth. The mouth marks the entrance to the digestive system. The floor of the mouth contains a muscular appendage, the tongue. The tongue is involved in chewing, swallowing, and the formation of speech. Tiny elevations, called *papillae,* contain the taste buds. They differentiate among bitter, sweet, sour, and salty sensations.

Digestion begins in the mouth. Here the teeth mechanically shred and grind food and enzymes begin the chemical breakdown of carbohydrates.

Teeth. Each tooth is designed to carry out a specific task. At the front of the mouth are the incisors, which are structured for biting and cutting. Posterior to the incisors are the canines, pointed teeth used for tearing and shredding food. The molars are to the rear of the jaw. These teeth have four cusps (points) and are used for mastication (the crushing and grinding of food).

Box 45.1 Organs of the Digestive System

ORGANS OF THE ALIMENTARY CANAL

- Mouth
- Pharynx (throat)
- Esophagus (food pipe)
- Stomach
- Small intestine
- Duodenum
- Jejunum
- Ileum
- Large intestine (colon)
- Cecum
- Ascending colon
- Transverse colon
- Descending colon
- Sigmoid colon
- Rectum
- Anal canal

ACCESSORY ORGANS

- Teeth and gums
- Salivary glands
- Parotid
- Submandibular
- Sublingual
- Tongue
- Liver
- Gallbladder
- Pancreas
- Vermiform appendix

Salivary glands. The three pairs of salivary glands are the parotid, submandibular, and sublingual glands (see Fig. 45.1). They secrete fluid called *saliva,* which is approximately 99% water with enzymes and mucus.

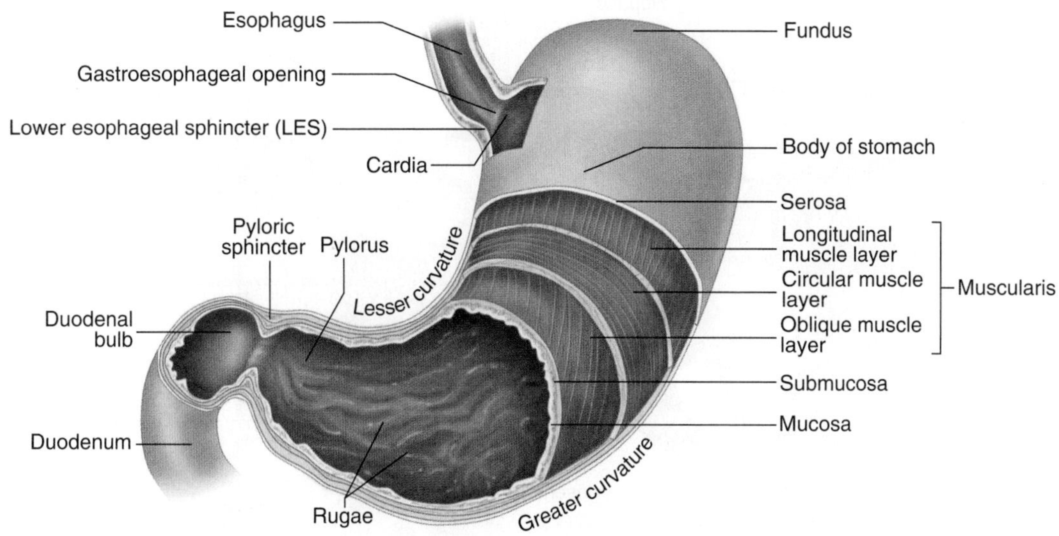

Fig. 45.2 Stomach. Cut-away sections show muscle layers and interior mucosa thrown into folds called *rugae*. (From Patton KT, Thibodeau GA: *The human body in health and disease*, ed 7, St. Louis, 2018, Elsevier.)

Normally these glands secrete enough saliva to keep the mucous membranes of the mouth moist. Once food enters the mouth, the secretion increases to lubricate and dissolve the food and to begin the chemical process of digestion. The salivary glands secrete about 1000 to 1500 mL of saliva daily. The major enzyme is salivary amylase (ptyalin), which initiates carbohydrate metabolism. Another enzyme, lysozyme, destroys bacteria and thus protects the mucous membrane from infections and the teeth from decay. After food has been ingested, the salivary glands continue to secrete saliva, which cleanses the mouth.

Esophagus. The esophagus is a muscular, collapsible tube that is approximately 25 cm (10 in) long, extending from the mouth through the thoracic cavity and the esophageal hiatus (a hole in the diaphragm) to the stomach. Digestion does not take place in the esophagus. Peristalsis moves the bolus (food broken down and mixed with saliva, ready to pass to the stomach) through the pharynx, to the esophagus, and then to the stomach in 5 or 6 seconds.

Stomach. The stomach is in the left upper quadrant of the abdomen, directly inferior to the diaphragm (Fig. 45.2). A filled stomach is the size of a football and can hold a volume of approximately 1 to 1.5 L. The stomach entrance is at the cardiac sphincter (so named because it is close to the heart); the exit is at the pyloric sphincter. As food leaves the esophagus, it enters the stomach through the relaxed cardiac sphincter. The sphincter then contracts, preventing reflux (splashing or return flow), which can be irritating to the esophagus.

Once the bolus has entered the stomach, the muscular layers of the stomach churn and contract to mix and compress the contents with the gastric juices and water.

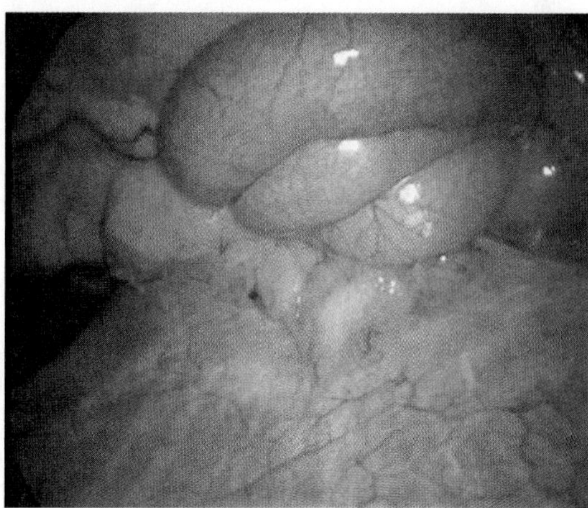

Fig. 45.3 Laparoscopic view of the small intestine. (From Abrahams P, Marks S, Hutchings R: *McMinn's color atlas of human anatomy*, ed 7, Philadelphia, 2013, Saunders.)

The gastric juices are secretions released by the gastric glands. Digestion of protein begins in the stomach. Hydrochloric acid softens the connective tissue of meats, kills bacteria, and activates pepsin (the chief enzyme of gastric juices that converts proteins into proteoses and peptones). Mucin is released to protect the stomach lining. Intrinsic factor (a substance secreted by the gastric mucosa) is produced to allow absorption of vitamin B_{12}. The stomach breaks the food down into a viscous, semiliquid substance called *chyme*. The chyme passes through the pyloric sphincter into the duodenum for the next phase of digestion.

Small intestine. The small intestine (Fig. 45.3) is a tube that is 6 m (20 ft) long and 2.5 cm (1 in) in diameter. It begins at the pyloric sphincter, ends at the ileocecal

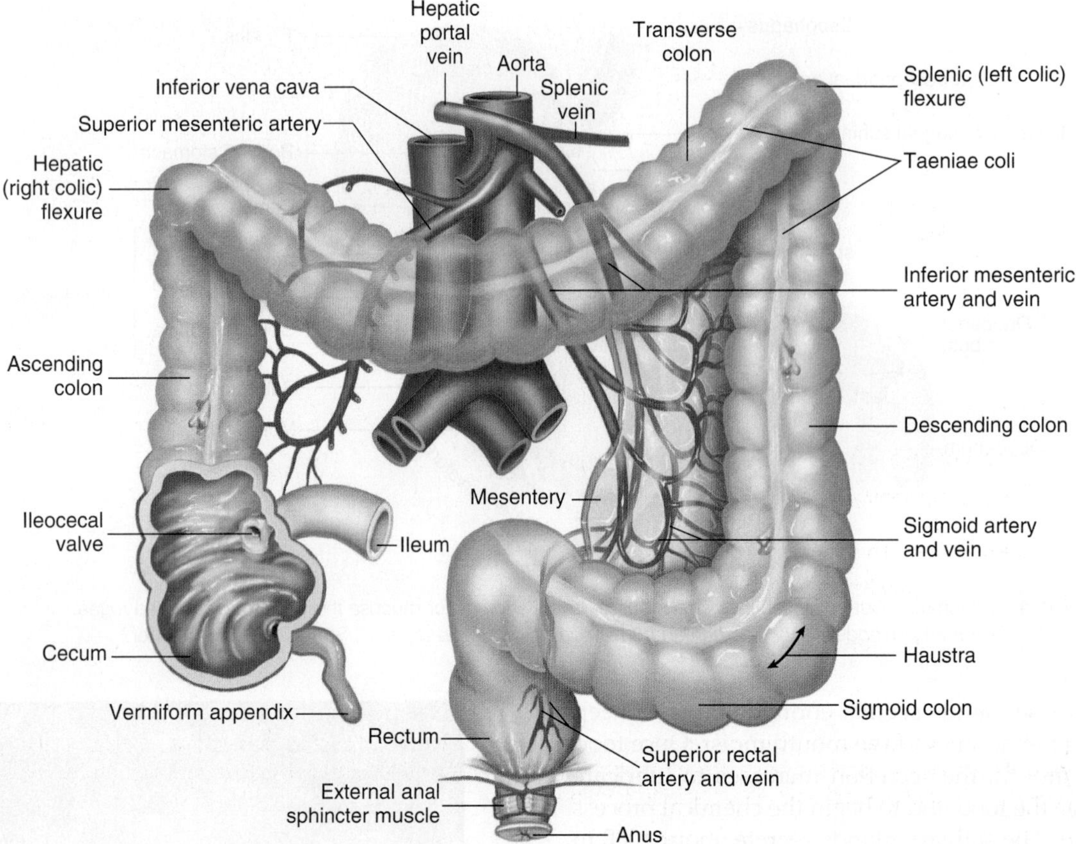

Fig. 45.4 Divisions of the large intestine. (From Patton KT, Thibodeau GA: *The human body in health and disease*, ed 7, St. Louis, 2018, Elsevier.)

valve, and is divided into three major sections: *duodenum, jejunum,* and *ileum.* Up to 90% of digestion takes place in the small intestine. The intestinal juices finish the metabolism of carbohydrates and proteins. Bile and pancreatic juices enter the duodenum. Bile from the liver breaks molecules into smaller droplets, which enables the digestive juices to complete their process. Pancreatic juices contain water, protein, inorganic salts, and enzymes. Pancreatic juices are essential in breaking down proteins into their amino acid components, in reducing dietary fats to glycerol and fatty acids, and in converting starch to simple sugars.

The inner surface of the small intestine contains millions of tiny finger-like projections called *villi,* which are clustered over the entire mucous membrane surface. The villi aid in the digestive process by absorbing the products of digestion into the bloodstream. They increase the absorption area of the small intestine by about 600 times. Inside each villus is a rich capillary bed, along with modified lymph capillaries called *lacteals.* The primary function of the lacteals is to absorb metabolized fats.

Large intestine. Once the small intestine has completed its tasks of digestion, the ileocecal valve opens and releases the contents of digestion into the large intestine. The large intestine is a tube that is larger in diameter (6 cm, or 2 in), but shorter at 1.5 to 1.8 m (5 to 6 ft), than the small intestine. The large intestine consists of the cecum; appendix; ascending colon, hepatic flexure, transverse colon, splenic flexure, descending colon, and sigmoid colon; rectum; and anus (Fig. 45.4). This is the terminal portion of the digestive tract, where the process of digestion is completed. The large intestine has four major functions: (1) completion of absorption of water, (2) manufacture of certain vitamins (such as vitamins K and B_7), (3) formation of feces, and (4) expulsion of feces.

Just inferior to the ileocecal valve is the cecum, a blind pouch approximately 2 to 3 in long. The vermiform appendix, a small, wormlike, tubular structure, dangles from the cecum. Research has revealed that the appendix functions as an area where nonpathologic bacteria live safely until they are needed for digestion. In addition, the appendix houses immune system cells and tissue (Rahman and Parash, 2013). The open end of the cecum connects to the ascending colon, which continues upward on the right side of the abdomen to the inferior area of the liver. The ascending colon then becomes the transverse colon. It crosses to the left side of the abdomen, where it becomes the descending colon. When the descending colon reaches the level of the iliac crest, the sigmoid colon begins and continues toward the midline to the level of the third sacral vertebra.

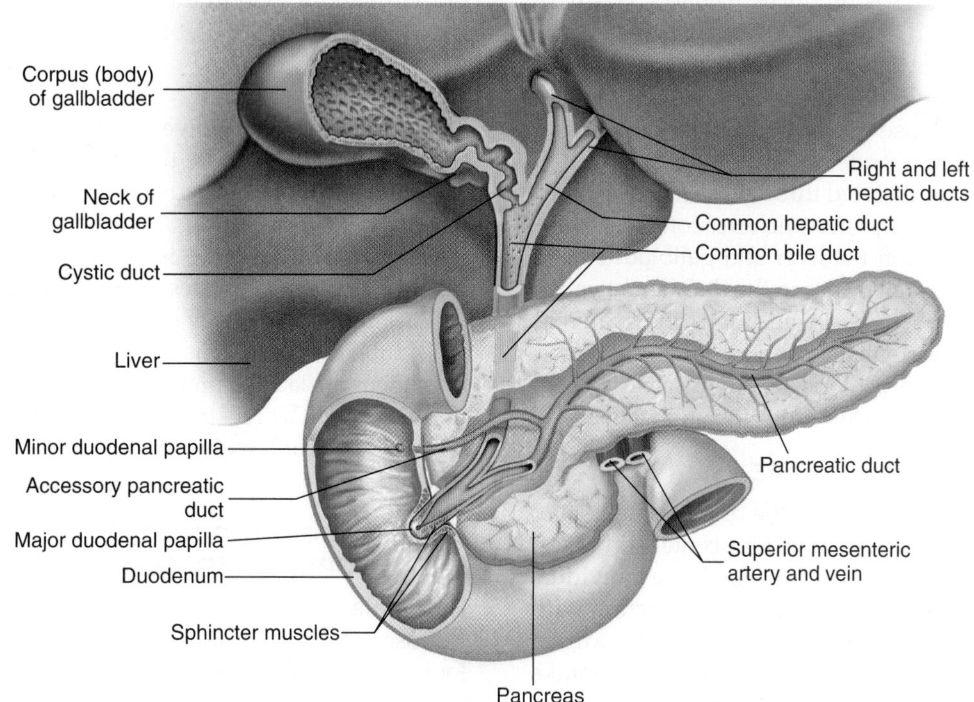

Fig. 45.5 Gallbladder and bile ducts. Obstruction of the hepatic or common bile duct by stone or spasm occludes the exit of the bile and prevents matter from being ejected into the duodenum. (From Patton KT, Thibodeau GA: *The human body in health and disease*, ed 7, St. Louis, 2018, Elsevier.)

Bacteria in the large intestine change the chyme into fecal material by releasing the remaining nutrients. The bacteria are also responsible for the synthesis of vitamin K, which is needed for normal blood clotting, and the production of some of the B-complex vitamins. As the fecal material continues its journey, the remaining water and vitamins are absorbed into the bloodstream by osmosis.

Rectum. The rectum is the last 20 cm (8 in) of the intestine, where fecal material is expelled. The anus is the opening to the outside of the body, where feces are passed.

ACCESSORY ORGANS OF DIGESTION

Liver

The liver is the largest glandular organ in the body, weighing approximately 1.5 kg (3 to 4 lb) in the adult, and is one of the more complex organs in the body. It is located just inferior to the diaphragm, covering most of the upper right quadrant and extending into the left epigastrium, and it is divided into two lobes. The lobes are further divided into several lobules (smaller lobes) containing small blood vessels. Approximately 1500 mL of blood is delivered to the liver every minute by the portal vein and the hepatic portal artery. The cells of the liver produce a product called *bile,* a yellow-brown or green-brown liquid; bile is necessary for the emulsification of fats. The liver releases approximately 500 to 1000 mL of bile per day, which then travels to the gallbladder through hepatic ducts. The gallbladder is a sac about 8 to 9 cm (3 to 4 in) long, located on the right inferior surface of the liver. Bile is stored in the gallbladder until it is needed for fat digestion (Fig. 45.5).

In addition to producing bile, the liver's functions include managing blood coagulation; metabolizing proteins, fats, and carbohydrates; manufacturing cholesterol; manufacturing albumin to maintain normal blood volume; filtering out old red blood cells (RBCs) and bacteria; detoxifying poisons (alcohol, nicotine, drugs); converting ammonia to urea; providing the main source of body heat at rest; storing glycogen for later use; activating vitamin D; and breaking down nitrogenous waste (from protein metabolism) to urea, which the kidneys can excrete as waste from the body.

Gallbladder

The gallbladder is a pear-shaped organ measuring approximately 7 to 10 cm (3 to 4 in) long. Areolar connective tissue connects it to the underside of the liver. The gallbladder can store 30 to 50 mL of bile, and its primary function is to store and eject bile into the duodenum for digestion of fats.

Pancreas

The pancreas is an elongated gland, approximately 12 to 15 cm (6 to 9 in) long, which lies posterior to the stomach (see Fig. 45.4). It is involved in endocrine and exocrine duties. In this chapter, discussion of the pancreas is limited to its exocrine activities.

Each day the pancreas produces 1000 to 1500 mL of pancreatic juice to aid in digestion. This pancreatic juice contains the digestive enzymes protease (trypsin), lipase (steapsin), and amylase (amylopsin). These enzymes are important because they digest the three major components of chyme: proteins, fats, and carbohydrates. The enzymes are transported through an excretory duct to the duodenum. This pancreatic duct connects to the common bile duct from the liver and gallbladder and empties through a small orifice in the duodenum called the *major duodenal papilla*. In addition, the pancreas contains an alkaline substance, sodium bicarbonate, which neutralizes hydrochloric acid in the gastric juices that enter the small intestine from the stomach.

REGULATION OF FOOD INTAKE

The hypothalamus, a portion of the brain, contains two appetite centers that affect eating. One center stimulates the individual to eat, and the other signals the individual to stop eating. These centers work in conjunction with the rest of the brain to balance eating habits. In addition to the hypothalamus, factors that also affect food intake include lifestyle, culture, eating habits, emotions, and genetics.

LABORATORY AND DIAGNOSTIC EXAMINATIONS

UPPER GASTROINTESTINAL STUDY (UPPER GI SERIES, UGI)

Rationale

The upper gastrointestinal (UGI) study consists of a series of radiographs of the lower esophagus, stomach, and duodenum, using barium sulfate as the contrast medium. A UGI series detects any abnormal conditions of the UGI tract, any tumors, or other ulcerative lesions.

Nursing Interventions

The patient should take nothing by mouth (NPO) and avoid smoking after midnight the night before the study. Explain the importance of rectally expelling all the barium after the examination. Feces (stools) are light in color until all the barium is expelled (up to 72 hours after the test). Eventual absorption of fecal water may cause a hardened barium impaction. Patients should be instructed to increase their fluid intake to help expel the barium, thus preventing constipation or blockage. The health care provider may order a laxative to be given in addition to increasing fluid intake.

TUBE GASTRIC ANALYSIS

Rationale

The stomach contents are aspirated to determine the amount of acid produced by the parietal cells in the stomach. The analysis helps determine the completeness of a vagotomy, confirm hypersecretion or **achlorhydria** (an abnormal condition characterized by the absence of hydrochloric acid in the gastric juice), estimate acid secretory capacity, or test for intrinsic factor.

Nursing Interventions

The patient should receive no anticholinergic medications for 24 hours before the test and should maintain NPO status after midnight to avoid altering the rate of gastric acid secretion. The patient also should be instructed that smoking is prohibited before the test because nicotine stimulates the flow of gastric secretions.

The nurse or radiology personnel inserts a nasogastric (NG) tube into the stomach to aspirate gastric content. Specimens are labeled properly and sent to the laboratory immediately. The NG tube is removed, and the patient may eat and drink without restrictions unless otherwise ordered.

ESOPHAGOGASTRODUODENOSCOPY (EGD, UGI ENDOSCOPY, GASTROSCOPY)

Rationale

Endoscopy (from *endo,* within, inward; and *scope,* to look) enables direct visualization of a particular hollow organ or cavity by means of a long, flexible fiberoptic scope (Fig. 45.6). An EGD visualizes the esophagus, stomach, and duodenum for routine screening as well as for examination of tumors, varices (abnormally enlarged veins), mucosal inflammation, hiatal hernias, polyps (small tissue growths projecting from a mucous membrane), ulcers, *Helicobacter pylori,* strictures (narrowings), and obstructions. The endoscopist also can remove polyps, coagulate sources of active GI bleeding, and perform sclerotherapy (injection of a solution into the vein causing it to shrink and eventually disappear) of

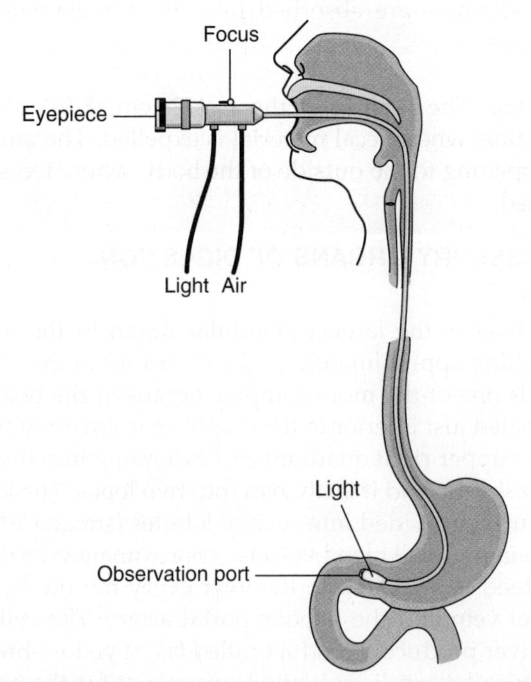

Fig. 45.6 Fiberoptic endoscopy of the stomach. (From Monahan FD, Neighbors M, Sands JK, Marek JF, Green CJ: *Phipps' medical-surgical nursing: Health and Illness perspectives*, ed 8, St. Louis, 2007, Mosby.)

esophageal varices. Areas of narrowing can be dilated by the endoscope or by passing a dilator through the scope. Camera equipment can be attached to the viewing lens to photograph a pathologic condition. The endoscope also can obtain tissue specimens for biopsy or culture to determine the presence of *H. pylori.*

Endoscopy enables evaluation of the esophagus, stomach, and duodenum. A longer fiberoptic scope allows evaluation of the upper small intestine. This is referred to as *enteroscopy.*

Nursing Interventions

The patient should maintain NPO status after midnight before the test, and an informed consent form must be signed. The patient usually is given a preprocedure intravenous (IV) sedative such as midazolam, and the patient's pharynx is anesthetized by spraying it with lidocaine hydrochloride (Xylocaine). After the procedure the patient will not be allowed to eat or drink until the gag reflex returns, which is usually soon after the procedure and can be assessed by placing a tongue blade to the back of the pharynx. Monitor the patient's vital signs and oxygen saturation after the procedure and assess for any signs and symptoms of perforation, including abdominal pain and tenderness, guarding, oral bleeding, **melena** (tarlike, fetid-smelling stool containing undigested blood), and hypovolemic shock.

CAPSULE ENDOSCOPY

Rationale

For capsule endoscopy, the patient swallows a capsule (approximately the size of a large vitamin) containing a camera that provides endoscopic evaluation of the GI tract. It commonly is used to visualize the small intestine and diagnose diseases such as Crohn's disease, celiac disease, and malabsorption syndrome. It also helps identify sources of possible GI bleeding in areas not accessible by upper endoscopy or colonoscopy. The camera takes tens of thousands of images during an 8-hour examination. The capsule relays images to a data recorder that the patient wears on a belt. After the examination, images are viewed on a monitor (Mayo Clinic, 2015a).

Nursing Interventions

The patient is NPO for approximately 12 hours before the test and should not smoke for 24 hours before the test. The patient may need to stop taking some medications before the procedure. The health care provider determines which, if any, medications must be halted before the patient ingests the capsule. The patient swallows the video capsule and usually is kept NPO for 2 hours and usually can eat a light meal 4 hours after swallowing the capsule. The procedure is comfortable for most patients. Peristalsis causes passage of the disposable capsule with a bowel movement, usually within 2 to 3 days or sooner, depending on the patient's rate of peristalsis. The pill camera does not have to be retrieved (Mayo Clinic, 2015a).

BARIUM SWALLOW AND GASTROGRAFIN STUDIES

Rationale

A barium swallow study allows a clearer view of the esophagus than that provided by most UGI examinations; this is because the esophageal movements do not show up well on x-rays. When the patient swallows barium, however, the outline of the esophagus is clear. As in most barium contrast studies, defects in luminal filling and narrowing of the barium column indicate tumor, scarred stricture, or esophageal varices. A barium swallow allows easy recognition of swallowing difficulties resulting from conditions such as cerebrovascular accidents (stroke or brain attack), and of anatomic abnormalities, such as hiatal hernia. Cancers of the esophagus, gastroesophageal reflux disease (GERD) and ulcers, and muscle disorders are other reasons for performing a barium swallow study (Johns Hopkins University, n.d.a).

Gastrografin (diatrizoate meglumine and diatrizoate sodium) is a product used in place of barium for patients who are susceptible to bleeding from the GI tract and who are being considered for surgery. Gastrografin is water soluble and rapidly absorbed, so it is preferable when a perforation is suspected. Gastrografin facilitates imaging through radiographs, but if the product escapes from the GI tract, it is absorbed by the surrounding tissue. In contrast, if barium leaks from the GI tract, it is not absorbed and can lead to complications (Drugs.com, 2018).

Nursing Interventions

The patient is NPO after midnight. Food and fluid in the stomach prevent barium from accurately outlining the GI tract, and the radiographic results may be misleading. Explain the importance of rectally expelling all barium. Stools will be light in color until this occurs. Eventual absorption of fecal water may cause a hardened barium impaction. The patient should be instructed to increase his or her fluid intake to help in expelling the barium, thus preventing constipation or blockage. The health care provider may order a laxative to be given in addition to increasing fluid intake.

ESOPHAGEAL FUNCTION STUDIES (BERNSTEIN TEST)

Rationale

The Bernstein test, an acid perfusion test, is an attempt to reproduce the symptoms of gastroesophageal reflux. It helps differentiate esophageal pain caused by esophageal reflux from that caused by angina pectoris. If the patient suffers pain with the instillation of hydrochloric acid into the esophagus, the test is positive and indicates reflux esophagitis (National Library of Medicine [NLM], 2014).

Nursing Interventions

The patient is NPO for 8 hours before the examination, and any medications that may interfere with the production of acid, such as antacids and analgesics, are withheld. An NG tube is inserted, and mild hydrochloric acid is instilled followed by saline. The patient should be asked if any pain or discomfort is felt during instillation of the hydrochloric acid.

EXAMINATION OF STOOL FOR OCCULT BLOOD

Rationale

Tumors of the large intestine grow into the **lumen** (the cavity or channel within a tube or tubular organ) and are subject to repeated trauma by the fecal stream. Eventually the tumor ulcerates and bleeding occurs. Sometimes the bleeding is so slight that gross blood is not seen in the stool. If this **occult blood** (blood that is obscure or hidden from view) is detected in the stool, a benign or malignant GI tumor is suspected. Tests for occult blood include the stool guaiac test, Hemoccult test, and Hematest.

Occult blood in the stool also may occur in ulceration and inflammation of the upper or lower GI system, as well as with internal hemorrhoids that are bleeding. Other causes include swallowing blood of oral or nasopharyngeal origin. For specimen collection the patient usually is asked to collect stool in an appropriate container.

Nursing Interventions

The patient is instructed to keep the stool specimen free of urine or toilet paper, because either can alter the test results. The nurse or patient should don gloves and use tongue blades or an appropriate specimen collection device for stool to transfer the stool to the proper receptacle. The patient should not eat any organ meat for 24 to 48 hours before a guaiac test. Use a specimen slide and developer to test the stool for occult blood. The health care provider sometimes orders that three consecutive stools be tested for occult blood.

SIGMOIDOSCOPY (LOWER GI ENDOSCOPY)

Rationale

Endoscopy of the lower GI tract allows visualization of the inner lining of the sigmoid colon and, if indicated, access to obtain biopsy specimens of tumors, polyps, or ulcerations of the anus, rectum, and sigmoid colon. The lower GI tract is difficult to visualize radiographically, but sigmoidoscopy allows direct visualization. Microscopic review of tissue specimens obtained using this procedure leads to diagnoses of many lower bowel disorders.

Nursing Interventions

The patient should maintain NPO status after midnight before the test, and an informed consent form must be signed. The specific bowel preparation is determined by the health care provider performing the procedure, usually a gastroenterologist, and usually consists of laxatives, enemas, or a combination of both. After the examination, observe the patient for evidence of bowel perforation (abdominal pain, tenderness, distention, and bleeding) and instruct the patient to watch for these symptoms at home.

BARIUM ENEMA STUDY (LOWER GI SERIES)

Rationale

The barium enema (BE) study consists of a series of x-rays of the colon used to detect the presence and location of abnormalities such as polyps, tumors, and diverticula. Barium sulfate also assists in visualization of mucosal detail. Therapeutically, a BE may be used to reduce (treat) a nonstrangulated ileocolic **intussusception** (infolding of one segment of the intestine into the lumen of another segment) in children (Punnoose, 2012). The contrast agent causes the infolded portion to move back into its normal position.

Nursing Interventions

The evening before the BE, cathartics such as magnesium citrate, or other cathartics designated by facility policy, are administered. A cleansing enema the evening before or the morning of the BE is administered if directed by the health care provider's order or facility policy. Fluids should be encouraged, and a laxative may be ordered after the BE to stimulate evacuation of the barium.

After the BE study, assess the patient for complete evacuation of the barium, or instruct the patient to monitor stools at home. Patients typically expel most of the barium before leaving the radiology department. Retained barium may cause constipation or a hardened impaction. Stool will be light in color until all the barium has been expelled.

COLONOSCOPY

Rationale

The development of the fiberoptic colonoscope has enabled examination of the entire colon, from the anus to the cecum, in most patients. Colonoscopy visualizes the mucosa of the colon and can detect lesions in the proximal colon, which would not be found by sigmoidoscopy. Benign and malignant neoplasms, mucosal inflammation or ulceration, and sites of active hemorrhage also can be visualized. Biopsy specimens can be obtained and small tumors removed through the scope. Actively bleeding vessels can be coagulated.

A less invasive test than a standard colonoscopy is called virtual colonoscopy. This test uses computed tomography (CT) scanning or magnetic resonance imaging (MRI) with computer software to produce images of the colon and rectum. For both procedures a small tube is inserted through the anus and into the rectum. With the CT procedure the colon is expanded by instillation of carbon dioxide gas to aid in visualization.

For the MRI method a contrast medium is given to expand the colon. The colon preparation is similar to that for a regular colonoscopic examination. Sedatives are not required and no scope is needed. One disadvantage of this procedure is that it does not allow for biopsies, removal of polyps, or coagulation of vessels (NIH, 2016). Patients who have had cancer of the colon are at high risk for developing a subsequent colon cancer; patients who have a family history of colon cancer are also at high risk. For these patients, colonoscopy allows early detection of any primary or secondary tumors.

Nursing Interventions

Informed consent is necessary for a colonoscopy to be performed. Dietary restrictions include a clear liquid diet for 1 to 3 days before the procedure to decrease the residue in the bowel, and then NPO status is maintained for 8 hours before the procedure. Laxatives and/or enemas, and premedication, such as a stool softener, are ordered to cleanse the bowel. The bowel preparation will depend on the health care provider's preference and the patient's condition.

After the colonoscopy, monitor the patient for evidence of bowel perforation (abdominal pain, guarding, distention, tenderness, excessive rectal bleeding, or blood clots). The stools should be examined for gross blood. Monitor the patient for hypovolemic shock.

STOOL CULTURE

Rationale

The feces (stool) can be examined for the presence of bacteria, ova, and parasites (a plant or animal that lives on or within another living organism and obtains some advantage at its host's expense). The health care provider may order a stool for culture of bacteria or of ova and parasites (O&P). Many bacteria (such as *Escherichia coli*) are indigenous in the bowel. Bacterial cultures usually are done to detect enteropathogens (such as *Staphylococcus aureus, Salmonella* or *Shigella* organisms, *E. coli* O157:H7, or *Clostridium difficile*) (Centers for Disease Control and Prevention [CDC], 2013a, 2013b).

When a patient is suspected of having a parasitic infection, the stool is examined for O&P. Usually at least three stool specimens are collected on consecutive days. Because culture results are not available for several days, they do not influence initial treatment, but they do guide subsequent treatment if bacterial infection is present.

Nursing Interventions

If an enema must be administered to collect specimens, only normal saline or tap water is used. Soapsuds or any other substance could affect the viability of the organisms collected.

Stool samples for O&P are obtained before barium examinations. Be sure that urine is not mixed with feces in the sample. Wear gloves for sample collection. The specimen is taken to the laboratory within 30 minutes of collection in a specified container.

OBSTRUCTION SERIES (FLAT PLATE OF THE ABDOMEN)

Rationale

The obstruction series is a group of radiographic studies performed on the abdomen of patients who have suspected bowel obstruction, paralytic ileus, perforated viscus (a *viscus* is any large interior organ in any of the great body cavities), or abdominal abscess. The series usually consists of at least two radiographic studies. The first is an erect abdominal radiographic study that allows visualization of the diaphragm. Radiographs are examined for evidence of free air under the diaphragm, which is **pathognomonic** (signs or symptoms specific to a disease condition) of a perforated viscus (hollow organ). This radiographic study also is used to detect air-fluid levels within the intestine (NLM, 2013).

Nursing Interventions

For adequate visualization, ensure that this study is scheduled before any barium studies.

DISORDERS OF THE MOUTH

Common disorders of the mouth and esophagus that interfere with adequate nutrition include poor dental hygiene, infections, inflammation, and cancer.

DENTAL PLAQUE AND CARIES

Etiology and Pathophysiology

Dental decay is an erosive process that results from the action of bacteria on carbohydrates in the mouth, which in turn produce acids that dissolve tooth enamel. Many Americans experience tooth decay at some time in their life. Dental decay can be caused by several factors:

- Dental plaque, a thin film on the teeth made of mucin and colloidal material found in saliva and often secondarily invaded by bacteria
- The strength of acids and the inability of the saliva to neutralize them
- The length of time the acids are in contact with the teeth
- Susceptibility of the teeth to decay

Medical Management

Dental caries are treated by removal of affected areas of the tooth and replacement with some form of dental material. Treatment of periodontal disease focuses on removal of plaque from the teeth. If the disease is advanced, surgical interventions on the gingivae and alveolar bone may be necessary.

Nursing Interventions and Patient Teaching

Proper technique for brushing and flossing the teeth at least twice a day is the primary focus for teaching patients. Plaque forms continuously and must be removed periodically through regular visits to the dentist. Stress the importance of prevention through continual care. Because carbohydrates create an environment in which caries develop and plaque accumulates more easily, include proper nutrition in patient teaching. When the patient is ill, the mouth's normal cleansing action is impaired. Illnesses, drugs, and irradiation interfere with the normal action of saliva. If the patient is unable to manage oral hygiene, assume this responsibility.

Patient problems and interventions for the patient with dental plaque and caries include but are not limited to the following:

Patient Problem	Nursing Interventions
Insufficient Knowledge, *related to:* • Inability to prevent dental caries • Periodontal disease	Assess and observe the oral cavity for moisture, color, and cleanliness Stress importance of meticulous oral hygiene Explain the need to see a dentist at least yearly for an examination

Modified from Ackley BJ, Ladwig GB: *Nursing diagnosis handbook: An evidence-based guide to planning care,* ed 11, St. Louis, 2017, Mosby.

The prevention and elimination of dental plaque and caries are related directly to oral hygiene, dental care, nutrition, and heredity. All but heredity are controllable factors. The prognosis is more favorable for people who brush, floss, regularly visit the dentist for removal of affected areas, eat low-carbohydrate foods, and drink fluoridated water.

CANDIDIASIS

Etiology and Pathophysiology

Candidiasis is any infection caused by a species of *Candida,* usually *C. albicans. Candida* is a fungal organism normally present in the mucous membranes of the mouth, intestinal tract, and vagina; it also is found on the skin of healthy people. This infection also is referred to as *thrush* or *moniliasis.*

This disease appears more commonly in the newborn infant, who becomes infected while passing through the birth canal. In the older individual, candidiasis may be found in patients with leukemia, diabetes mellitus, or alcoholism, and in patients who are taking antibiotics (chlortetracycline or tetracycline), are undergoing corticosteroid inhalant treatment, or are immunosuppressed (e.g., patients with acquired immunodeficiency syndrome [AIDS] or those receiving chemotherapy or radiation therapy).

Clinical Manifestations

Candidiasis appears as pearly, bluish white "milk-curd" membranous lesions on the mucous membranes of the mouth, tongue, and larynx. One or more lesions may be on the mucosa, depending on the duration of the infection (see Chapter 56, Fig. 56.5 for illustration). If the patch or plaque is removed, painful bleeding can occur.

Assessment

Assessment of the patient with oral candidiasis may reveal subjective complaints of soreness, and difficulty swallowing. Angular cheilitis (cracks at the corners of the mouth) is an objective sign of oral candidiasis. Failure to eat is an objective common sign of candidiasis of the GI tract that is seen in infants and adults.

Medical Management

Nystatin or amphotericin B (an oral suspension) or buccal tablets of anidulafungin (Eraxis) or fluconazole (Diflucan), one-third–strength hydrogen peroxide, and saline mouth rinses may provide some relief. In addition, eating unsweetened yogurt or taking acidophilus capsules or liquid can restore normal bacterial flora (Hidalgo and Bronze, 2017).

Nursing Interventions

Meticulous hand hygiene should be used to prevent spread of the infection. For infants, hand hygiene, care of feeding equipment, and cleanliness of the mother's nipples are important to prevent spread. The infant's mouth should be assessed regularly.

For adults, encourage the patient to use a soft-bristled toothbrush and to avoid hot, cold, spicy, fried, or citrus foods. Many patients find that a topical anesthetic such as a lidocaine or benzocaine oral solution eases the discomfort of eating and drinking if taken approximately an hour prior.

Prognosis

If the host has a strong defense system and medical treatment is initiated early in the course of the disease, the prognosis is good.

CARCINOMA OF THE ORAL CAVITY

Etiology and Pathophysiology

Oral (or oropharyngeal) cancer may occur on the lips, the oral cavity, the tongue, and the pharynx. The tonsils occasionally are involved. Most of these tumors are squamous cell epitheliomas that grow rapidly and metastasize to adjacent structures more quickly than do most malignant tumors of the skin. An estimated 49,670 new cases and 9700 deaths from oral cavity and pharynx cancer are expected to occur in 2017. The number of new cases has been consistent in the male population but has risen with women. The rise in the incidents of oral cancer in women is linked to infection with the human papilloma virus (HPV). Death rates have been decreasing over the past 30 years (American Cancer Society [ACS], 2017b).

Tumors of the salivary glands occur primarily in the parotid gland and are usually benign. Tumors of the submaxillary gland have a high incidence of malignancy.

These malignant tumors grow rapidly and may be accompanied by pain and impaired facial function.

Kaposi's sarcoma is a malignant skin tumor that occurs primarily on the skin or on mucosal surfaces such as in the mouth. It is seen at a rate of 6 cases per million people infected with AIDS, and at a rate of 1 in 200 for patients receiving immunosuppressive therapy after organ transplantation. The lesions are purple and nonulcerated. Irradiation is the treatment of choice (ACS, 2014b).

The types of cancers of the lip that usually are seen are basal cell carcinoma and squamous cell carcinoma. Cancer of the lip occurs most frequently as a chronic ulcer of the lower lip in men over the age of 50. The cure rate for cancer of the lip is high because the lesion is apparent to the patient and to others, so patients often seek early treatment. If early detection and treatment do not occur, metastasis to regional lymph nodes may occur. In some instances a lesion may spread rapidly and involve the mandible and the floor of the mouth by direct extension. On occasion, the tumor may be a basal cell lesion that starts in the skin and spreads to the lip (Skin Cancer Foundation, 2016).

Cancer of the anterior tongue and floor of the mouth may seem to occur together because their spread to adjacent tissues is so rapid. Because of the tongue's abundant vascular and lymphatic drainage, metastasis to the neck may occur. There is a higher incidence of cancers of the mouth and throat among people who are heavy drinkers and who have a history of tobacco use (e.g., cigar, cigarette, pipe, chewing tobacco) and exposure to human papillomavirus (HPV) (National Cancer Institute, n.d.a). Also, data show that men are twice as likely to be diagnosed with cancer of the tongue (ACS, 2014b).

Clinical Manifestations

Leukoplakia (a white, firmly attached patch on the mouth or tongue mucosa) may appear on the lips and buccal mucosa. These nonsloughing lesions cannot be rubbed off by simple mechanical force. They can be benign or malignant. A small percentage develop into squamous cell carcinomas, and biopsy is recommended if the lesions persist for longer than 2 weeks.

Assessment

Collection of subjective data includes understanding that malignant lesions of the mouth may be asymptomatic. The patient may feel only a roughened area with the tongue. As the disease progresses, the first complaints may be (1) difficulty in chewing, swallowing, or speaking; (2) edema, numbness, or loss of feeling in any part of the mouth; and (3) earache, facial pain, and toothache, which may become constant. Cancer of the lip is associated with discomfort and irritation caused by a nonhealing lesion, which may be raised or ulcerated. Malignancy at the base of the tongue produces less obvious symptoms: slight **dysphagia** (difficulty in swallowing), sore throat, and salivation. Most oral cancers occur in males over the age of 60, but do not overlook symptoms based on age and gender.

Diagnostic Tests

Direct and indirect laryngoscopy are important diagnostic tests for examination of the soft tissue. This procedure allows direct visualization of the oral cavity, and both can be performed in the health care provider's office. If necessary, panendoscopy—a more invasive form of laryngoscopy—may be performed with an endoscope. Radiographic evaluation of the mandibular structures is another essential part of the head and neck examination to rule out cancer. Excisional biopsy is the most accurate method for making a definitive diagnosis. Oral exfoliative cytology, in which a scraping of a lesion provides cells for cytologic examination, is used to screen intraoral lesions (ACS, 2016b).

Medical Management

Treatment depends on the location and staging of the malignant tumor. Stage I oral cancers are treated by surgery or radiation. Stage II and III cancers require surgery and radiation. Chemotherapy also may be used when surgery and radiation therapy fail or as the initial therapy for smaller tumors. Treatment for stage IV cancer may include all three treatment modalities, or treatment may be palliative if metastasis is extensive. The 5-year survival rate for patients with oral cancers that have metastasized depends on the degree of metastasis. For lip cancer the 5-year survival rate is 48% for regional metastasis and 53% for distal metastasis. The 5-year survival rate for cancer of the tongue is 63% for regional metastasis and 36% for distal metastasis. If the cancer is in the floor of the mouth, the 5-year survival rate is 38% for regional metastasis and 20% for distal metastasis (ACS, 2014a).

Small, accessible tumors can be excised surgically. Surgical options include a glossectomy, removal of the tongue; hemiglossectomy, removal of part of the tongue; mandibulectomy, removal of the mandible; and total or supraglottic laryngectomy, removal of the entire larynx or the portion above the true vocal cords.

Large tumors usually require more extensive and traumatic surgery. In a functional neck dissection of neck cancer with no growth in the lymph nodes, the surgeon removes the lymph nodes but preserves the jugular vein, the sternocleidomastoid muscle, and the spinal accessory nerve. In radical neck dissection, all these structures are removed, and reconstructive surgery is necessary after tissue resection. Patients may have drains in the incision sites that are connected to suction to aid healing and reduce hematomas. A tracheostomy also may be performed, depending on the degree of tumor invasion.

Because of the location of the surgery, complications can occur. These include airway obstruction, hemorrhage, tracheal aspiration, facial edema, formation of fistulas (abnormal passages connecting internal organs, or to the surface of the body), and necrosis of the skin flaps. If the patient has difficulty swallowing, a percutaneous endoscopic gastrostomy (PEG) tube may be inserted to allow for adequate nutritional intake. Neurologic complications can occur because of nerves being severed and manipulated during surgery.

Radiation therapy may involve (1) external radiation beam radiation therapy or (2) internal radiation by means of needles or seeds. The purpose of radiation therapy is to shrink the tumor. It can be given preoperatively or postoperatively, depending on the health care provider's preference and the patient's disease process. In more advanced cases, chemotherapy may be combined with radiation postoperatively to make the patient more comfortable. Other treatment options include laser excision.

Nursing Interventions and Patient Teaching

A holistic approach to patient care includes awareness of the patient's level of knowledge regarding the disease, emotional response and coping abilities, and spiritual needs. Nursing interventions must be individualized to the patient—beginning with the preoperative stage, continuing through the postoperative stage, and ending after the patient's rehabilitation in the home environment. Family members, hospice workers, close friends, social workers, and pastoral care staff may provide information and support during this potentially fatal disease.

Patient problems and interventions for the patient with oral cancer include but are not limited to the following:

Patient Problem	Nursing Interventions
Distorted Body Image and Impaired Personal Sense of Identity, related to: • Disfiguring appearance of an oral lesion • Reconstructive surgery	Provide alternative methods for communication if radiation therapy results in dysarthria (difficult, poorly articulated speech, resulting from interference in the control over muscles of speech) Provide information to the patient and family to help with difficult decisions related to surgery, radiation, or chemotherapy Provide support to the patient and family

Modified From Ackley BJ, Ladwig GB: *Nursing diagnosis handbook: An evidence-based guide to planning care*, ed 11, St. Louis, 2017, Mosby.

Prevention is the key to successful treatment or cure for cancer of the oral cavity and should include education on avoiding excess exposure to sun and wind on the lips, eliminating smoking or chewing tobacco, eliminating plaque and caries through good oral and dental care, and decreasing the intake of excessive amounts of alcohol. Individuals infected with HPV also should be monitored for the development of oral cavity cancer. Early detection of oral cancer can increase the patient's chance of survival. Any person with a mouth lesion that does not heal within 2 to 3 weeks is urged to seek medical care.

Provide instruction regarding preoperative and postoperative care, with full explanations regarding potential speech loss and alternative methods of nutritional intake if warranted by the extent of cancer or anticipated surgical procedure. Explanation of tracheostomy care and other tubes the patient may have on discharge helps reduce anxiety and increases the patient's sense of control over the situation.

Prognosis

Staging and biologic characterization of the neoplasm provide prognostic information. The prognosis of carcinoma in the oral cavity is related directly to the size of the primary tumor, the involvement of regional lymph nodes, and the presence or absence of metastasis. The patient's immunologic response and general condition also influence the prognosis and the choice of therapy.

Carcinomas of the lip generally can be detected early by the patient, the health care provider, or the dentist during examination, and the prognosis for cure is good. If the carcinoma is difficult to detect, as on the anterior tongue and the floor of the mouth, it is often in a more advanced stage when detected, making the prognosis poor.

DISORDERS OF THE ESOPHAGUS

GASTROESOPHAGEAL REFLUX DISEASE

Etiology and Pathophysiology

Gastroesophageal reflux disease (GERD) is a backward flow of stomach acid up into the esophagus. Symptoms typically include burning and pressure behind the sternum, often described by patients as heartburn. Most cases are thought to be caused by the inappropriate relaxation of the lower esophageal sphincter (LES) in response to an unknown stimulus. Symptoms of GERD develop when the LES is weak or experiences prolonged or frequent transient relaxation, conditions that allow gastric acids and enzymes to flow into the esophagus. Reflux is much more common in the postprandial state (after meals), because this position allows more reflux of gastric juices when the LES is relaxed. GERD occurs in all age groups and is estimated to affect approximately 20% of the population experience GERD on a weekly basis and 7% on a daily basis, making GERD one of the most common upper GI problem seen in adults (Noar, 2015).

Clinical Manifestations

The clinical manifestations of GERD are consistent but vary substantially in severity. The irritation of chronic reflux produces the primary symptom, which is heartburn *(pyrosis).* Heartburn often is described as a substernal or retrosternal burning sensation that tends to radiate upward and may involve the neck, the jaw, or the back. Heartburn usually is experienced after eating. An atypical pain pattern that closely mimics angina also may occur and must be differentiated carefully from true cardiac disease. The second major symptom of GERD is regurgitation. The individual experiences a feeling of warm fluid moving up the throat and may experience a sour taste in the mouth. Symptoms also may include a dry cough, a feeling of a lump in the throat, dysphagia, and hoarseness or a sore throat (Mayo Clinic, 2014b).

GERD can produce symptoms such as dysphagia or odynophagia (painful swallowing), dry cough, hoarseness, and a sore throat. Eructation (belching) and a feeling of flatulence are other common complaints. The frequency and severity of reflux episodes usually determine the severity of the symptoms.

Assessment

Subjective data include heartburn, a substernal or retrosternal burning sensation that may radiate to the back or jaw (in some cases the pain may mimic angina), and regurgitation, which causes a sour or bitter taste in the pharynx. Frequent eructation, flatulence, and dysphagia or odynophagia usually occurs only in severe cases.

Objective data include nocturnal cough, wheezing, and hoarseness.

Diagnostic Tests

When a mild case of GERD is suspected, treatment is initiated on the basis of the presumptive diagnosis. More involved cases may require other screening tools, such as an esophageal pH test. In this test the patient is fitted with a small nasogastric tube that remains in place and is connected to a small computer that may be worn on the belt or on a shoulder strap. The probe, in the esophagus, monitors acid levels for 24 to 48 hours. An esophageal motility test and Bernstein test can be performed in conjunction with pH monitoring to evaluate LES competence and the response of the esophagus to acid infusion. The barium swallow with fluoroscopy is used widely to document the presence of hiatal hernia. Endoscopy is performed routinely to evaluate for LES competence, potential scarring and strictures, and the presence and severity of esophagitis, and to rule out malignancy (Kahrilas, 2012).

Medical Management

In its simplest form, GERD produces mild symptoms that occur infrequently (twice a week or less). In these cases, encouraging the patient to avoid problem foods or beverages, stopping smoking, elevating the head of the bed, or losing weight may solve the problem. Medication therapy for GERD focuses on improving LES function, increasing esophageal clearance, decreasing volume and acidity of reflux, and protecting the esophageal mucosa. Treatment with antacids or acid-blocking medications called H_2 receptor antagonists—such as cimetidine (Tagamet), ranitidine (Zantac), famotidine (Pepcid), or nizatidine (Axid)—also may be used. More severe and frequent episodes of GERD can trigger asthma attacks, cause severe chest pain, result in bleeding, or promote a narrowing (stricture) or chronic irritation of the esophagus. In these cases, more powerful inhibitors of stomach acid production called proton pump inhibitors (PPIs), such as omeprazole (Prilosec), esomeprazole (Nexium), pantoprazole (Protonix), rabeprazole (Aciphex), and lansoprazole (Prevacid), may be added to the treatment prescribed. Sucralfate (Carafate) is an antiulcer drug that may be used in patients with GERD for its protective properties by forming a complex that adheres to an ulcer. Metoclopramide (Reglan) is used in moderate to severe cases of GERD. It is in a class of drugs called *promotility agents,* which increase peristalsis and therefore promote gastric emptying and reduce the risk of gastric acid reflux.

If conventional treatments fail, the health care provider may suggest a surgical procedure to treat the condition. *Nissen fundoplication* is a surgical procedure that can be performed to strengthen the sphincter. The procedure involves wrapping a layer of the upper stomach wall (fundus) around the sphincter and terminal esophagus to lessen the possibility of acid reflux (see Fig. 45.14). Surgery also may be performed to create a barrier that will prevent the backup of gastric acid. A device called an *EsophyX* folds the tissue at the base of the stomach, acting as a sphincter valve. Another surgical approach is the *Stretta procedure.* This procedure uses electrodes to heat the tissue in the esophagus to create scar tissue that strengthens the esophagus. The *LINX* is another surgical device that is used to treat GERD; it consists of a band of titanium beads with magnetic cores that, when implanted around the LES, strengthens it by closing the sphincter when necessary. If GERD is left untreated, serious pathologic (precancerous) changes in the esophageal lining may develop—a condition called *Barrett's esophagus* (esophageal metaplasia). In Barrett's esophagus the normal squamous epithelium of the esophagus is replaced by columnar epithelium. Because patients with Barrett's esophagus are at higher risk for esophageal cancer, they may need to be monitored regularly (every 1 to 3 years) by endoscopy and biopsy (Mayo Clinic, 2014b).

Nursing Interventions and Patient Teaching

Nursing interventions involve educating the patient about diet and lifestyle modifications that may alleviate symptoms of GERD.

Dietary instructions include the following: (1) eat four to six small meals daily; (2) follow a low-fat, adequate-protein diet; (3) reduce intake of chocolate, tea, and other foods and beverages that contain caffeine; (4) limit or eliminate alcohol intake; (5) eat slowly, and chew food thoroughly; (6) avoid evening snacking, and do not eat for 2 to 3 hours before bedtime; (7) remain upright for 1 to 2 hours after meals when possible, and never eat in bed; (8) avoid any food that directly produces heartburn; and (9) reduce overall body weight if needed.

Numerous lifestyle changes also are indicated in the treatment of GERD. Patients who smoke should be encouraged to stop. Cigarette smoking has been associated with decreased acid clearance from the lower esophagus. Advise patients to avoid constrictive clothing over the abdomen and avoid activities that involve straining, heavy lifting, or working in a bent-over position. Also, patients should be instructed never to sleep flat in bed. They should elevate the head of the bed at least 6 to 8 inches for sleep, using wooden blocks or a thick foam wedge.

Prognosis

If GERD is not controlled successfully, it can progress to serious and even life-threatening problems. Esophageal ulceration and hemorrhage may result from severe erosion, and chronic nighttime reflux is accompanied by a significant risk of aspiration. Adenocarcinoma can develop from the premalignant tissue (termed *Barrett's esophagus*). Gradual or repeated scarring can permanently damage esophageal tissue and produce strictures (NLM, 2018b).

CARCINOMA OF THE ESOPHAGUS

Etiology and Pathophysiology

Carcinoma of the esophagus is a malignant epithelial neoplasm that has invaded the esophagus and has been diagnosed as a squamous cell carcinoma or an adenocarcinoma. In 2017 16,940 new esophageal cancer cases were diagnosed, 13,360 in men and 3580 in women. Recent statistics reveal that about 15,690 deaths from esophageal cancer occur with 12,720 in men and 2970 in women. Risk factors for esophageal cancer include alcohol and tobacco use, acid reflux, and obesity. Environmental carcinogens, nutritional deficiencies, chronic irritation, and mucosal damage also have been considered as causes of esophageal cancer. Another risk factor is Barrett's esophagus. The longer a person has Barrett's esophagus, the greater the chance that it will progress to esophageal adenocarcinoma (ACS, 2017d) (see Health Promotion box on prevention or early detection of esophageal cancer).

Unfortunately, early esophageal cancer typically has no symptoms, making early diagnosis difficult. The stage of esophageal cancer greatly affects the 5-year survival rate. The overall 5-year survival rate for a person with cancer of the esophagus that is localized is approximately 40%; regional metastasis is approximately 20%; and distant metastasis is 4%. Less than 15% of all cases of esophageal cancer occur before the age of 55, and it is more prevalent in men (ACS, 2017d).

> **Health Promotion**
>
> **Prevention or Early Detection of Esophageal Cancer**
>
> - Patients with diagnosed gastroesophageal reflux disease and hiatal hernia need counseling regarding regular follow-up evaluation.
> - Health teaching should focus on elimination of smoking and excessive alcohol intake.
> - Maintenance of good oral hygiene and dietary habits (intake of fresh fruits and vegetables) may be helpful.
> - Patients diagnosed with Barrett's esophagus must be monitored, because this is considered a premalignant condition. Regular endoscopic screening with biopsy is required.
> - Encourage patients to seek medical attention for any esophageal problems, especially dysphagia.

Clinical Manifestations

The most common clinical symptom is progressive dysphagia over a 6-month period. The patient may have a substernal feeling, as though food is not passing through the esophagus.

Assessment

Collection of subjective data includes noting that initially the patient may have difficulty swallowing when eating bulky foods such as meat; later the difficulty occurs with soft foods and finally with liquids and even saliva. Another symptom is odynophagia (painful swallowing). Pain is a late symptom and indicates local extension of the malignancy. Additional subjective symptoms include chest pain, pressure, or burning; indigestion; heartburn; and fatigue.

Collection of objective data includes observing the patient for regurgitation (backward flowing or casting up of undigested food), vomiting, hoarseness, chronic cough, choking, and iron deficiency anemia. Weight loss may be related directly to the cancer or to the difficulty in swallowing. Hemorrhage may occur if the cancer erodes through the esophagus. Esophageal perforation may result in the formation of a tracheoesophageal fistula (an abnormal passage between two internal organs), causing the patient to cough when swallowing anything, including saliva. Esophageal tumors may enlarge enough to cause esophageal obstruction, causing increased dysphagia. The cancer spreads via the lymph system; the liver and lung are common sites of metastasis.

Diagnostic Tests

A barium swallow examination with fluoroscopy and endoscopy is used to detect esophageal cancer. An endoscopy with biopsy and cytologic examination provides a highly accurate diagnosis. Endoscopic ultrasonography is an important tool used to stage esophageal cancer. Computed tomography (CT), positron emission tomography (PET), and magnetic resonance imaging (MRI) also are used to assess the extent of the disease.

Medical Management

The treatment of esophageal cancer depends on the tumor's location and whether invasion or metastasis has occurred. Tumor staging must be determined to guide patient management. For esophageal cancer that has not metastasized, a wide excision removing the tumor and enough surrounding tissue to leave cancer-free margins may be effective. For more advanced cases an esophagectomy may be necessary. If the cancer has spread from the esophagus to the stomach, an esophagogastrectomy is performed. A description of these surgeries is described below (Mayo Clinic, 2018a).

Radiation therapy may be curative or palliative. Problems associated with radiation therapy include the development of a tracheoesophageal fistula and burning. The burning that occurs may result in sunburned-like skin when external radiation is used, or damage to nearby organs such as the lungs and heart if internal radiation therapy is used. Aspiration from the fistula and edema from the radiation are common as well. Chemotherapeutic agents such as cisplatin, paclitaxel (Taxol), and fluorouracil (5-FU) are used currently, as well as other chemotherapy agents, in combination with radiation before and/or after surgery (ACS, 2017e). Because of the extreme toxicity of these drugs, expect the patient to experience side effects of respiratory and liver dysfunction, nausea and vomiting, leukopenia, and sepsis. If the tumor is in the upper third of the esophagus, radiation is indicated. A tumor in the lower third usually is resected surgically.

The following four types of surgical procedures can be performed:

1. *Esophagogastrectomy:* Resection of a lower esophageal section with a proximal portion of the stomach, followed by **anastomosis** (surgical joining of two ducts, blood vessels, or bowel segments to allow flow from one to the other) of the remaining portions of the esophagus and stomach. Surrounding lymph nodes also are removed.
2. *Esophagogastrostomy* or *esophagectomy:* Resection of a portion of the esophagus with anastomosis to the stomach. Surrounding lymph nodes also are removed.
3. *Esophagoenterostomy:* Resection of the esophagus and anastomosis to a portion of the small intestine. Surrounding lymph nodes also are removed.
4. *Gastrostomy:* Insertion of a catheter into the stomach and suture to the abdominal wall; performed when the patient cannot take food orally because inoperable cancer of the esophagus interferes with swallowing

Nursing Interventions and Patient Teaching

Patient problems and nursing interventions for the patient with esophageal carcinoma include but are not limited to the following:

Patient Problem	Nursing Interventions
Inability to Maintain Adequate Breathing Pattern, related to: • Incisional pain • Proximity of incision to diaphragm	Monitor respirations carefully because of proximity of incision to diaphragm and patient's difficulty in carrying out breathing exercises
Insufficient Nutrition, related to: • Dysphagia • Decreased stomach capacity • Anorexia	Monitor intake and output (I&O) and daily weights to determine adequate nutritional intake Assess which foods patient can and cannot swallow to select and prepare edible foods Administer tube feedings through gastrostomy, if present

Discuss with the patient and family all aspects of care, including surgery, radiation, and chemotherapy. Psychological adjustment of the patient who cannot ingest food orally, whether temporary or permanent, is difficult. Thorough explanations of all diagnostic tests, medications, procedures, and the treatment plan help relieve the patient's anxiety. Give support to the patient with this serious diagnosis by allowing time for questions.

Prognosis

In carcinoma of the esophagus, the disease is often well advanced by the time symptoms appear. The delay between the onset of early symptoms and when the patient seeks medical advice may be extensive. High mortality rates among these patients are affected by the following issues: (1) the patient is generally older; (2) the tumor usually has invaded surrounding structures by the time diagnosis is made; (3) the malignancy tends to spread to nearby lymph nodes; and (4) the esophagus is close to the heart and lungs, making these organs accessible to tumor extension.

The esophagus has an extensive lymphatic network, which facilitates the rapid spread of malignant cells to various local and distant sites. As discussed earlier in this section, the stage of the disease when diagnosed directly affects the survival rate.

Collection of objective data includes observing for premalignant lesions, including leukoplakia. Unusual bleeding in the mouth, some blood-tinged sputum, lumps or edema in the neck, and hoarseness may be observed.

ACHALASIA

Etiology and Pathophysiology

Achalasia, also called *cardiospasm,* is an abnormal condition characterized by the inability of a muscle to relax, particularly the cardiac sphincter of the stomach. Although the cause is unknown, nerve degeneration, esophageal dilation, and hypertrophy are thought to contribute to the disruption of the esophagus's normal neuromuscular activity. This results in decreased motility and dilation of the lower portion of the esophagus, along with an absence of peristalsis. Thus little or no food can enter the stomach, and in extreme cases the dilated portion of the esophagus holds as much as a liter or more of fluid. This disease may occur in people of any age, but is more prevalent in middle-aged to older adults (NLM, 2018a).

Clinical Manifestations

The primary symptom of achalasia is dysphagia. The patient has a sensation of food sticking in the lower portion of the esophagus. As the condition progresses, the patient complains of regurgitation of food, which relieves prolonged distention of the esophagus. The patient also may have substernal chest pain.

Assessment

Observe for loss of weight, poor skin turgor, and weakness.

Diagnostic Tests

Radiologic studies show esophageal dilation above the narrowing at the cardioesophageal junction. The diagnosis is confirmed by manometry, which shows the absence of primary peristalsis. Esophagoscopy also is used to confirm the diagnosis.

Medical Management

Conservative treatment of achalasia includes drug therapy and forceful dilation of the narrowed area of the esophagus. Anticholinergics, nitrates, and calcium channel blockers reduce pressure in the lower esophageal sphincter.

Dilation is done by first emptying the esophagus. Then a dilator with a deflated balloon is passed down to the sphincter. The balloon is inflated and remains so for 1 minute; it may have to be reinflated once or twice.

The preferred surgical approach is a cardiomyotomy. The muscular layer is incised longitudinally down to but not through the mucosa. Two-thirds of the incision is in the esophagus, and the remaining one-third is in the stomach; this permits the mucosa to expand so that food can pass easily into the stomach.

Nursing Interventions and Patient Teaching

Nursing interventions for esophageal surgery are presented in Box 45.2.

Box 45.2 Nursing Interventions for the Patient Experiencing Esophageal Surgery

PREOPERATIVE NURSING INTERVENTIONS

1. Encourage improved nutritional status.
   a. Offer a high-protein, high-calorie diet if oral diet is possible.
   b. Total parenteral nutrition may be necessary for severe dysphagia or obstruction.
   c. Gastroscopy tube feedings may be indicated.
2. Give meticulous oral hygiene; breath may be malodorous.
3. Give preoperative preparation appropriate for thoracic surgery.
4. Give prescribed antibiotics before esophageal resection or bypass, as ordered.

POSTOPERATIVE NURSING INTERVENTIONS

1. Promote good pulmonary ventilation.
2. Maintain chest drainage system as prescribed.
3. Maintain gastric drainage system.
   a. Small amounts of blood may drain from nasogastric tube for 6 to 12 hours after surgery.
   b. Do not disturb nasogastric tube (to prevent traction on suture line).
4. Maintain nutrition.
   a. Start clear fluids at frequent intervals when oral intake is permitted.
   b. Introduce soft foods gradually, increasing to several small meals of bland foods.
   c. Have patient maintain semi-Fowler's position for 2 hours after eating and while sleeping if heartburn (pyrosis) occurs.

A patient problem and interventions for the patient with achalasia include but are not limited to the following:

Patient Problem	Nursing Interventions
Insufficient Nutrition, related to difficulty swallowing both liquids and solids	Encourage fluids with meals to increase lower esophageal sphincter pressure and to push food into stomach. Monitor liquid diet for 24 hr after dilation procedure

Discuss home care and follow-up care in preparation for dismissal. Include a family member or support person if possible, and involve the patient as an active participant in the planning. Explain the need to eat high-calorie, high-protein foods, and provide printed material in support of such a diet. Explain the need to sleep with the head elevated and to avoid bending over and stooping. Discuss medications if prescribed (including name, dose, time of administration, purpose, and side effects). Discuss ways to avoid constipation by eating high-fiber foods (if tolerated) and natural laxatives. Explain the importance of follow-up care with the health care provider. Finally, discuss symptoms of recurrence or progression of disease and the need to report these to the health care provider.

Prognosis

Surgical separation, in addition to bag dilation, permits the return of normal peristalsis in approximately 10% of patients with achalasia.

DISORDERS OF THE STOMACH

GASTRITIS (ACUTE)

Etiology and Pathophysiology

Gastritis is an inflammation of the lining of the stomach. Acute gastritis is a temporary inflammation associated with alcoholism, smoking, and stressful physical problems, such as burns; major surgery; food allergens; viral, bacterial, or chemical toxins; chemotherapy; or radiation therapy. Changes in the mucosal lining from gastritis damages the cells that secrete acid and pepsin. Acute gastritis is often a single incident that resolves when the offending agent is removed.

Clinical Manifestations

If the condition is acute, the patient may experience fever, epigastric pain, nausea, vomiting, headache, coating of the tongue, and loss of appetite. If the condition results from ingestion of contaminated food, the intestines are usually affected, and diarrhea may occur. Some patients with gastritis have no symptoms.

Assessment

Collection of subjective data includes observing for anorexia, nausea, discomfort after eating, and pain.

Collection of objective data includes observing for vomiting, **hematemesis** (vomiting blood), and melena caused by gastric bleeding.

Diagnostic Tests

Diagnosis is based on testing the stools for occult blood, noting white blood cell (WBC) differential increases related to certain bacteria, evaluating serum electrolytes, and observing for elevated hematocrit related to dehydration.

Medical Management

If medical treatment is required, an antiemetic—such as prochlorperazine, promethazine, or trimethobenzamide (Tigan)—may be prescribed. Antacids and cimetidine (Tagamet) or ranitidine (Zantac) may be given in combination. Antibiotics are given if the cause is a bacterial agent. IV fluids are used to correct fluid and electrolyte imbalances. Patients who experience GI bleeding from hemorrhagic gastritis require fluid and blood replacement and NG lavage.

Nursing Interventions and Patient Teaching

Monitor and record the patient's I&O. Withhold oral foods and fluids as prescribed until signs and symptoms of gastritis subside. Monitor tolerance to oral feedings and administer IV feedings as prescribed. Clear liquids are increased to a diet as tolerated when the patient's symptoms improve.

A patient problem and interventions for the patient with gastritis include but are not limited to the following:

Patient Problem	Nursing Interventions
Inadequate Fluid Volume, related to vomiting, diarrhea, and blood loss	Keep patient NPO or on restricted food and fluids as ordered, and advance as tolerated Monitor laboratory data for fluid and electrolyte imbalance (potassium, magnesium, sodium, and chloride) Maintain IV feedings Record I&O

Patient education includes explanations of (1) the effects of stress on the mucosal lining of the stomach; (2) how salicylates, nonsteroidal antiinflammatory drugs (NSAIDs), and particular foods may be irritating; and (3) how lifestyles that include alcohol and tobacco may be harmful. Assist the patient in locating self-help groups in the community to deal with these behaviors.

Prognosis

Because of the many classifications and causes of gastritis, prognosis is variable. In general, the prognosis is good for individuals who are willing to change their lifestyles and follow a medical regimen.

PEPTIC ULCER DISEASE

Etiology and Pathophysiology

Peptic ulcers are ulcerations of the mucous membrane or deeper structures of the GI tract. They most commonly occur in the stomach *(gastric ulcer)* and duodenum *(duodenal ulcer)*. The term *peptic ulcer* refers to acid in the digestive tract eroding the mucosal lining of the stomach, esophagus, or duodenum.

The stomach normally is protected from autodigestion by the gastric mucosal barrier. The GI tract has a high cell turnover rate, and the stomach's surface mucosa is renewed about every 3 days. As a result, the mucosa continuously repairs itself except in extreme instances when cell breakdown surpasses the cell renewal rate. In such cases, peptic ulcers can occur. The most common causes of peptic ulcer disease include the presence of *Helicobacter pylori (H. pylori)* bacteria in the stomach, regularly taking NSAIDs, smoking or chewing tobacco, and excessive alcohol intake.

Understanding of the factors that contribute to ulcer formation is developing rapidly. The discovery of the bacterium *H. pylori* provided new insight into ulcer formation. Approximately two-thirds of the people in the world have the bacteria in their stomachs (NLM, 2016). *H. pylori* has been identified in more than 80% of patients with gastric ulcers and 90% of those with duodenal ulcers. In Western cultures, half of all people over age 50 harbor *H. pylori,* yet most do not develop peptic ulcer disease. Scientists must still determine what triggers ulcers in those with *H. pylori* (Johns Hopkins University, n.d.b).

Stress ulcers develop as the result of physiologic trauma to the body. Examples of patients who develop stress ulcers include patients with burns, sepsis, or those who have prolonged stays in the hospital or intensive care units. A stress ulcer is a form of erosive gastritis. It is believed that the gastric mucosa of the stomach undergoes a period of transient ischemia in association with hypotension, severe injury, extensive burns, and complicated surgery. The ischemia is due to decreased capillary blood flow as blood is shunted away from the GI tract, so blood flow bypasses the gastric mucosa. This occurs as a compensatory mechanism in hypotension or shock. The decrease in blood flow produces an imbalance between the destructive properties of hydrochloric acid and pepsin and protective factors of the stomach's mucosal barrier, especially in the fundus portion. Multiple superficial erosions result, and these may bleed. Because of the possibility of development of physiologic stress ulcers and high morbidity, patients at risk receive prophylaxis with antisecretory agents, including H_2 receptor blockers and proton pump inhibitors.

Clinical Manifestations

Gastric and duodenal ulcers may have similar symptoms but may differ in timing, degree, or factors that worsen or alleviate the symptoms. Pain is the characteristic symptom and is described as dull, burning, or gnawing; it is located in the epigastric region.

Assessment

Collection of subjective data requires awareness that in patients with gastric ulcers, the pain is associated closely with food intake and usually does not awaken the patient at night. With duodenal ulcers the patient often complains of pain 1 to 2 hours after eating. Nausea, weight loss, eructation (belching), and distention are also common complaints made by patients with PUD. Upset stomach and other vague GI complaints are referred to as **dyspepsia.**

Collection of objective data includes observing for signs of complications of PUD. Hemorrhage is a potential complication.

- *Hematemesis and melena:* When GI bleeding occurs, one sign is the vomiting of blood (hematemesis) that is either bright red or has a "coffee grounds" appearance resulting from the action of the gastric acid on hemoglobin. The patient may produce melena (stool that is black and tarry with undigested blood), which occurs when the blood passes through the digestive tract. Salicylates and alcohol aggravate bleeding in patients with a history of peptic ulcers.
- *Hemorrhage:* Bleeding from a gastric ulcer can worsen quickly into an emergency situation if erosion is extensive. Hemorrhage, with accompanying symptoms of shock, occurs when the ulcer erodes into a blood vessel. Surgical intervention is indicated if the patient remains unstable after receiving blood over several hours.
- *Perforation:* Perforation occurs when the ulcer crater penetrates the entire thickness of the wall of the stomach or duodenum. The release of air, gastric acid, pancreatic enzymes, or bile into the peritoneal cavity causes pain, emesis, fever, hypotension, and hematemesis. Perforation is considered the most lethal complication of peptic ulcer. Bacterial peritonitis may occur within hours. The severity of the peritonitis is proportional to the amount and duration of the spillage through the perforation.
- *Gastric outlet obstruction:* Gastric outlet obstruction is a complication of benign peptic ulcer disease. It is a blockage, located close to the pylorus (the part of the stomach that connects to the duodenum) and is caused by acute inflammation or edema. The most common symptom is vomiting undigested food. Symptoms may be relieved by constant NG aspiration of stomach contents due to the inability for digestion to occur. This also helps relieve edema and inflammation of the pylorus. Medications to treat inflammation of the pylorus may be administered intravenously. If conservative treatment is not successful, surgery may be warranted to address the stenosis.

Diagnostic Tests

Fiberoptic endoscopy can detect gastric and duodenal ulcers. This is called *esophagogastroduodenoscopy (EGD).* Fiberoptic endoscopy is more reliable than barium contrast studies because of the maneuverability of fiberoptic scopes and direct visualization of the entire esophagus and gastric and duodenal mucosa. This procedure also can be used to determine the degree of ulcer healing after treatment. During endoscopy, specimens can be obtained for identification of *H. pylori* or tissue specimens for biopsy. The patient is sedated but remains conscious throughout the endoscopy procedure. Local anesthetics in the throat are used to decrease the gag reflex and minimize pain during the procedure. No liquids or food are allowed after the procedure until the patient's gag reflex returns.

A noninvasive test used for diagnostic purposes is a breath test to detect *H. pylori.* The test calls for the patient to drink a solution containing carbon-13–enriched urea, a natural, nonradioactive substance. If *H. pylori* infection is present, it breaks down the compound and releases carbon-13 dioxide ($^{13}CO_2$). Thirty minutes after drinking the solution, the patient exhales into a collection bag, which is sent to the manufacturer for analysis. A finding of $^{13}CO_2$ confirms *H. pylori* infection. The test may prove especially useful in determining whether antibiotic therapy eradicated an *H. pylori* infection. A fecal assay antigen test for *H. pylori* is another test that is especially useful to determine eradication of the bacteria after antibiotic treatment. An additional noninvasive way to confirm *H. pylori* infection is a serum or whole blood antibody test, in particular, immunoglobulin G. This test is approximately 90% to 95% sensitive for *H. pylori* infection but cannot distinguish active from recently treated disease (Johns Hopkins, n.d.b).

Barium contrast studies (UGI) are not as accurate as endoscopy, especially for small lesions, but still are used occasionally. Testing of feces for occult blood in the intestinal tract also is used for diagnosis.

Medical Management

The health care provider may order insertion of an NG tube to remove gastric contents and blood. Surgery usually is indicated for complications of perforation, penetration, or obstruction, or for PUD that is no longer responding to medical management.

Scar tissue builds up with repeat episodes of ulceration and healing, causing obstruction, particularly at the pylorus. The patient may experience gastric dilation, vomiting, and distention. When fluid and electrolyte balance is achieved, surgical intervention is possible.

The primary treatment for peptic ulcers is to reduce signs and symptoms by decreasing or neutralizing normal gastric acidity with drug therapy. The types of drugs most commonly used include the following (Table 45.1):

- *Antacids:* Neutralize or reduce the acidity of stomach contents (e.g., Maalox, Gaviscon, Rolaids, Tums, Mylanta, and Riopan).
- *Antisecretory and cytoprotective agent:* Inhibits gastric acid secretion and protects gastric mucosa (misoprostol [Cytotec]). Cytotec is approved in the United States for the prevention of gastric ulcers induced by NSAIDs and aspirin (Medscape, 2010).
- *Histamine receptor blockers:* Decrease acid secretions by blocking histamine (H_2) receptors (e.g., cimetidine, ranitidine, famotidine, and nizatidine). Do not give within 2 hours of antacids.
- *Mucosal healing agent:* Heals ulcers without antisecretory properties. Sucralfate is a cytoprotective drug. It accelerates ulcer healing, presumably because of the formation of an ulcer-adherent complex that covers the ulcer and protects it from erosion by pepsin, acid, and bile salts.
- *Proton pump inhibitors:* Antisecretory agents that inhibit secretion of gastrin by the parietal cells of the stomach (e.g., omeprazole, lansoprazole, pantoprazole, rabeprazole, and esomeprazole).

Antibiotic therapy eradicates *H. pylori*. The drugs used include metronidazole (Flagyl), tetracycline, amoxicillin, and clarithromycin (Biaxin). Treatment typically is combined in a therapeutic regimen with other medications, such as bismuth or omeprazole. Another weapon that has entered the battle against *H. pylori* is a combination of bismuth, metronidazole, and tetracycline. Marketed under the brand name Helidac, the medication kit contains a 14-day supply of the three drugs, with each daily dose packaged on a blister card to improve patient compliance.

Among patients whose *H. pylori* is treated with antibiotics, the peptic ulcer recurrence may be as low as 10%. Patients who do not receive antibiotics have a relapse rate of 75% to 90%.

Dietary modification may be necessary to avoid foods and beverages that irritate the ulcer. There is considerable controversy over the therapeutic benefits of a bland diet, because the rationale is not supported by scientific evidence. Therefore it is recommended that the patient eat smaller meals more frequently throughout the day to decrease the degree of gastric motor activity.

Smoking has an irritating effect on the mucosa, increases gastric motility, and delays mucosal healing. Smoking should be eliminated completely or severely reduced. The combination of adequate rest and cessation of smoking accelerates ulcer healing. Because caffeinated and decaffeinated coffee, tobacco, alcohol, and aspirin aggravate the mucosal lining of the stomach and duodenum, educate patients with ulcers about the need for lifestyle change.

Surgical intervention has decreased drastically with more effective diagnosis and medical treatment with antisecretory agents and antibiotics. Approximately 20% of patients with ulcers require surgical intervention. These are patients who are unresponsive to medical management, raising concerns about gastric cancer; patients whose ulcers are drug induced but who cannot be withdrawn from the drugs (e.g., patients with rheumatoid arthritis); or patients who develop complications. Surgical procedures that may be performed are the same as those listed for cancer of the stomach.

Nursing Interventions and Patient Teaching

NG or intestinal tube insertion, irrigation, and intermittent suctioning often are performed while the patient is feeling ill and uncomfortable from PUD. In addition to being skilled and knowledgeable in performing these procedures, the nurse is responsible for easing the patient's fears and anxieties. Patient cooperation not only makes the procedures easier but also reduces patient discomfort.

Helping patients through the experience of GI intubation requires understanding of the following points:

- For most patients, NG or intestinal tube placement is a new and frightening experience. Explain the rationale for this therapy to the anxious patient and family. Help the patient and family understand that the advantages far outweigh the discomfort.
- Inability to chew, taste, and swallow food and liquids may contribute to patient anxiety during GI intubation.
- A patient with an NG or intestinal tube is usually on NPO status. On occasion, ice chips are allowed.
- An NG or intestinal tube is connected to either continuous or intermittent suctioning, usually at 100 to 125 mm Hg for decompression.
- An NG or intestinal tube is a constant irritant to the nasopharynx and nares, requiring frequent care to the mouth and nose.

Table 45.1 Medications for Gastrointestinal Disorders

GENERIC NAME (TRADE NAME)	ACTION	SIDE EFFECTS	NURSING IMPLICATIONS
Antacids, e.g., aluminum, calcium, magnesium salts, and sodium bicarbonate (Maalox, Mylanta, Titralac, Alternagel, and others)	Neutralizes gastric acid; aluminum and calcium antacids also bind phosphates in patients with renal failure	Aluminum: Constipation, hypophosphatemia Calcium: Constipation, rebound hyperacidity, hypercalcemia Magnesium: Diarrhea, hypermagnesemia Sodium bicarbonate: Sodium and water retention, alkalosis, rebound hyperacidity	Monitor serum electrolytes with long-term use; do not give antacid simultaneously with other medications because absorption of the other medication may be affected; best to separate administration by 2 hr; magnesium salts are contraindicated in patients with renal disease
Antispasmodics, including atropine, scopolamine, hyoscyamine, dicyclomine, clidinium (Donnatal, Bentyl, and others)	Anticholinergic agents that decrease GI motility by relaxing GI smooth muscle	Dry mouth and skin, constipation, paralytic ileus, urinary retention, tachycardia, drowsiness, dizziness, confusion, altered vision	Avoid using other CNS depressants or alcohol at the same time; avoid driving or other potentially hazardous tasks until accustomed to sedating effects
bismuth subsalicylate (Pepto-Bismol)	Antidiarrheal agent; also used in peptic ulcer disease caused by *Helicobacter pylori*	Fecal impaction, tinnitus	May turn stools dark gray to black; avoid use with aspirin; consult health care provider if diarrhea is accompanied by high fever or lasts more than 2 days
cimetidine (Tagamet)	H_2 receptor antagonist; inhibits gastric acid secretion	Confusion, headache, gynecomastia, bone marrow suppression (rare)	Increases serum levels and clinical effects of oral anticoagulants, theophylline, phenytoin, some benzodiazepines, and propranolol (these medications may require dosage reduction)
dimenhydrinate (Dramamine, others)	Antiemetic agent; blocks central vomiting center	Drowsiness, dry mouth, constipation	Avoid use with other CNS depressants and alcohol; avoid driving or other hazardous activities until accustomed to sedating effects
diphenoxylate with atropine (Lomotil)	Antidiarrheal agent (diphenoxylate: narcotic; atropine: anticholinergic)	Drowsiness, sedation, constipation, dry mouth, urinary retention	Avoid use with other CNS depressants and alcohol; avoid driving or other hazardous activities until accustomed to sedating effects; do not use in infectious diarrhea
famotidine (Pepcid)	H_2 receptor antagonist; inhibits gastric acid secretion	Headache, dizziness, constipation, thrombocytopenia (rare)	Unlike cimetidine, does not affect serum levels of hepatically metabolized drugs (warfarin, phenytoin, theophylline)
kaolin-pectin (Kaopectate)	Antidiarrheal agent	Constipation	Shake well before using
ketoconazole (Nizoral)	Antifungal agent	Gynecomastia, impotence, hepatotoxicity, abdominal pain	Requires acid environment for absorption; do not use with antacids, H_2 receptor blockers, or omeprazole; do not use with loratadine (has caused dysrhythmias and death); monitor liver function tests often; monitor serum levels and clinical effects of warfarin, cyclosporine, and theophylline

Table 45.1 Medications for Gastrointestinal Disorders—cont'd

GENERIC NAME (TRADE NAME)	ACTION	SIDE EFFECTS	NURSING IMPLICATIONS
lansoprazole (Prevacid)	Binds to an enzyme in the presence of acid gastric pH, preventing the final transport of hydrogen ions into the gastric lumen	Drowsiness, abdominal pain, diarrhea, nausea	Sucralfate (Carafate) decreases absorption of lansoprazole (take 30 min before sucralfate); administer before meals. Assess patient routinely for epigastric or abdominal pain. May cause abnormal liver function test results
loperamide (Imodium)	Antidiarrheal agent	Drowsiness, dry mouth, constipation	Monitor for dehydration; do not use in infectious diarrhea
mesalamine (Rowasa, Asacol)	GI antiinflammatory agent	Abdominal cramps and gas, rash, headache, dizziness	Swallow tablets whole; give enema at bedtime, retain 10–15 min
misoprostol (Cytotec)	Prostaglandin analog that acts as gastric mucosal protectant against NSAID-induced ulcers	Diarrhea, nausea, vomiting, flatulence, uterine cramping	Absolutely contraindicated in pregnant women; women of childbearing age must use reliable contraception
nizatidine (Axid)	H_2 receptor antagonist, inhibits gastric acid secretion	Drowsiness, headache, dizziness, sweating, thrombocytopenia (rare)	Does not affect serum levels of hepatically metabolized drugs (warfarin, phenytoin, theophylline)
nystatin (Mycostatin, Nilstat, others)	Antifungal agent, available as oral suspension and topical product	*Oral:* Nausea, vomiting, diarrhea *Topical:* Local irritation	Long-term therapy may be needed to clear infection; use for entire course
olsalazine (Dipentum)	GI antiinflammatory agent	Diarrhea, abdominal pain and cramps, nausea, allergic reactions, arthralgia, rash, anaphylaxis	Take with food; notify health care provider if severe diarrhea occurs
omeprazole (Prilosec)	Proton pump inhibitor; totally eradicates gastric acid production	Headache, dizziness, abdominal pain, nausea, vomiting, rare bone marrow suppression	Inhibits hepatic metabolism of warfarin, phenytoin, benzodiazepines, and other drugs metabolized by liver; do not crush or chew capsule contents
ranitidine (Zantac)	H_2 receptor antagonist; inhibits gastric acid secretion	Headache, abdominal discomfort; granulocytopenia and thrombocytopenia (both rare)	Minimal effect on serum levels of hepatically metabolized drugs (phenytoin, warfarin, theophylline)
sucralfate (Carafate)	Gastric mucosal protectant agent; adheres to site of ulcer	Constipation, hypophosphatemia	Do not give with other drugs; coating action may interfere with the absorption of other drugs—separate by 2 hr
sulfasalazine (Azulfidine)	GI antiinflammatory agent	Nausea, vomiting, abdominal pain, photosensitivity, rash, Stevens-Johnson syndrome (rare), renal failure, bone marrow suppression (rare), allergic reactions, anaphylaxis	Ensure adequate hydration to prevent crystallization in kidneys; avoid exposure to sunlight; women taking oral contraceptives need to use alternative methods because of decreased effectiveness of oral contraceptives; monitor CBC and renal function; take with meals

CBC, Complete blood count; *CNS,* central nervous system; *GI,* gastrointestinal; *NSAID,* nonsteroidal antiinflammatory drug.
Data from Skidmore-Roth L: *Mosby's 2017 nursing drug reference*, ed 30, St. Louis, 2017, Elsevier.

Table 45.2 Purposes of Nasogastric Intubation

PURPOSE	DESCRIPTION	TYPE OF TUBE
Decompression	Removal of secretions and gaseous substances from GI tract; prevention or relief of abdominal distention	Salem sump, Miller-Abbott
Feeding (gavage)	Instillation of liquid nutritional supplements or feedings into stomach for patients unable to swallow fluid	Duo, Dobhoff
Compression	Internal application of pressure by means of inflated balloon to prevent internal GI hemorrhage	Sengstaken-Blakemore
Lavage	Irrigation of stomach in cases of active bleeding, poisoning, gastric dilation, or intestinal obstruction	Ewald, Salem sump

GI, Gastrointestinal.

- A patient with a GI tube may be afraid that moving will dislodge the tube. Implement frequent position changes to enhance tube functioning and prevent complications of immobility.

An NG tube is inserted through the nose, pharynx, and esophagus into the stomach. Various tubes are available, depending on the purpose (Table 45.2).

Nursing interventions depend on the stage of the ulcer disease. The emphasis in patient care always should be on prevention and early detection of pain in the epigastric region, hematemesis, melena, or tenderness and rigidity of the abdomen (see the Communication box on gastrointestinal bleeding and Nursing Care Plan 45.1).

Patient problems and interventions for the specific stages of ulcer care include but are not limited to the following:

Patient Problem	Nursing Interventions
Insufficient Knowledge, related to: • Medications • Diet • Signs and symptoms of bleeding, perforation, or gastric outlet obstruction	Provide verbal and written instructions on exact dosage and time intervals for medications and whether medication is taken with or without food Have dietitian provide instructions on therapeutic diet Explain that repeat episodes are not uncommon; listen carefully for aggravating factors
Nonconformity, related to: • Risk behaviors (use of tobacco or alcohol) • Dietary patterns	Assess patient's level of knowledge regarding food and other irritants to mucosal lining Teach preventive measures, such as quitting smoking Explain need for small and frequent meals Caution patient to avoid high-fiber foods, sugar, salt, caffeine, alcohol, and milk Remind patient to take fluids between meals, not with meals Explain the need to eat slowly and chew food well Discuss importance of adequate rest and exercise
Insufficient Nutrition, related to preoperative food and fluid restrictions	Maintain NPO status Connect NG tube to intermittent suction apparatus Note color and amount of gastric output q 4 hr Do not reposition tube Maintain patency of tube by irrigation with measured amounts of saline *only if ordered* NOTE: After gastrectomy, output is minimal Monitor parenteral fluids with electrolyte additives as ordered Measure I&O When bowel sounds return and flatus is expelled, administer clear liquids as ordered Progress to small, frequent meals of soft food as ordered. Avoid milk because it may cause dumping syndrome

It is necessary to form a trusting relationship with the patient with an ulcer because of the severity of the condition and the need for long-term treatment. Include the family in patient education sessions to increase understanding and support, and involve the patient in goal setting to increase compliance (see the Home Care Considerations box).

Instruct the patient to seek medical attention immediately if severe and sudden pain occurs. Assist the patient in describing signs and symptoms of weakness, anorexia, nausea, diarrhea, constipation, anxiety, or restlessness. When medications are prescribed, the patient must understand fully (1) the purpose of taking antibiotic therapy to eradicate *H. pylori;* (2) the importance of taking all medications such as H_2 receptor antagonists, antiulcer drugs, prostaglandin E analog, and proton pump inhibitors as prescribed; (3) why the antacids are taken in specific dosages and at the specific times ordered; and (4) the known side effects (diarrhea and constipation). Preventive teaching includes identifying high-risk behaviors, such as the use of tobacco,

 Nursing Care Plan 45.1 **The Patient With Gastrointestinal Bleeding**

Mr. D., 33 years of age, is admitted with pain in the epigastric region and copious hematemesis. He appears anxious; his skin is pale, cool, and clammy; and he is breathing rapidly. This patient has a history of recurrent episodes of vomiting blood that has a coffee grounds appearance. He denies passing blood rectally but admits his stools have changed in consistency.

PATIENT PROBLEM

Potential for Inadequate Fluid Volume, related to hemorrhage, vomiting, and diarrhea

Patient Goals and Expected Outcomes	Nursing Interventions	Evaluation
Patient will have normal fluid balance as evidenced by balanced intake and output (I&O) within 24 h, including stable weight Blood pressure, pulse, and respiratory rate will be within normal limits Patient will have normal tissue turgor within 24 h	Monitor IV and blood transfusion therapy as ordered. Accurately record I&O q hr until stable: emesis, urine, and stool. Document fluid losses for possible imbalance; urinary output less than 30 mL/h may indicate hypovolemia. Monitor for signs and symptoms of dehydration and fluid and electrolyte imbalance (dry mucous membranes, poor skin turgor, thirst, decreased urinary output, and changes in behavior) q 15 min until stable, then q 2 hr. Document characteristics of output. Test all emesis and fecal output for presence of blood as ordered. Prepare to assist with inserting a nasogastric (NG) tube and connecting it to wall suction. Irrigate NG tube with saline as ordered to promote clotting; irrigation removes old blood from the stomach.	Patient has urinary output of 1500 mL for prior 24-hour period. Patient's blood pressure, pulse, and respiratory rate are within patient's pre-gastrointestinal bleeding baseline levels. Patient's tissue turgor is normal.

PATIENT PROBLEM

Anxiousness, related to hospitalization and illness

Patient Goals and Expected Outcomes	Nursing Interventions	Evaluation
Patient will demonstrate decrease in anxiety as evidenced by ability to sleep or rest at frequent intervals, verbalization of feelings, and blood pressure and pulse within normal limits	Assess physiologic components of anxiety (restlessness, increased pulse and respirations, diaphoresis, and elevated blood pressure) at least q 8 hr. Provide concise explanations for all procedures; prepare patient for surgery if indicated. Develop rapport with patient and family members with each contact.	Patient is sleeping 5 to 6 h during the night and resting at intervals during the day. Patient verbalizes a feeling of less stress and anxiety. Therapeutic rapport with nurse, patient, and family members is noted.

CRITICAL THINKING QUESTIONS

1. Mr. D. has an NG tube connected to wall suction that is draining sanguineous fluid. He complains of severe fatigue and epigastric pain. He is pale and drawn, with a hemoglobin level of 5.1 g/dL. Mr. D. puts his call light on and requests the nurse to assist him to the bathroom for a bowel movement. What appropriate interventions will ensure Mr. D.'s safety?
2. During assessment of Mr. D., what signs and symptoms would indicate inadequate fluid volume?
3. Mr. D. says to the nurse that he fears he may die. He appears anxious and tremulous. What is the most therapeutic approach to help decrease his fears?

caffeine, and alcohol. Emphasize that the patient should eat six smaller meals daily and avoid any foods that cause noticeable stomach discomfort.

If surgery is required, explain the procedures thoroughly, including the reasons for them. Explain immediate postoperative care, including deep breathing; coughing; position changes; frequent monitoring of vital signs; IV tubing, NG tubing, catheters, and other drainage tubes; and the use of patient-controlled analgesia (PCA) or other medications for pain relief. The patient's ability to eat normally after healing depends on the type of surgery and when peristalsis returns. Help the patient realize that symptoms often recur and that he or she should seek medical care if they do.

Prognosis for Peptic Ulcers

Recurrence of an ulcer may happen within 2 years in about one-third of all patients. Among patients whose

 Communication

Patient With Gastrointestinal Bleeding

Nurse: You look like you are resting better, Mrs. S. How have you been feeling? *(Reaffirming a relationship that was begun yesterday.)*

Patient: My stomach pain is much better. The medicine helped.

Nurse: If you are comfortable, perhaps you and your husband have some questions about why you are here. *(Trying to determine whether the patient is receptive to patient teaching. A knowledge deficit was suspected on admission.)*

Patient: I was scared when I started to vomit blood. It has happened before but not this much. Where does the blood come from?

Nurse: You have a diagnosis of GI bleeding with questionable duodenal ulcer. This means that the bleeding is coming from somewhere in your digestive tract or from an ulcer that has formed in the first part of your small intestine. The ulcer is an erosion of the lining of your stomach or small intestine. Do you understand what I have said so far? *(The nurse begins with the admitting diagnosis and explains one thing at a time, making sure the patient verbalizes understanding before continuing. It is beneficial for the nurse to show the patient a diagram of the GI system.)*

Patient: Well, I understand where the bleeding is coming from, but why am I bleeding there?

Nurse: We are not sure yet, Mrs. S., but you are scheduled for a procedure that will allow the health care provider actually to look at the surface of the stomach and a portion of the intestine. It is called an endoscopy, and it will be done tomorrow morning. Did someone explain this to you? *(The nurse answers the patient's question openly and honestly and uses her answer to lead into further patient education.)*

 Home Care Considerations

Peptic Ulcer Disease

- The patient who has recurrent ulcer disease after initial healing must learn to live with a chronic disease.
- The patient may be angry and frustrated, especially if he or she has faithfully followed the prescribed therapy but failed to prevent the recurrence or extension of the disease process.
- Unfortunately, many patients do not comply with the care plan and experience repeated exacerbations.
- Changes in lifestyle are difficult for most people and may be resisted.
- The patient who is instructed to stop smoking or avoid alcohol may resist.
- The goal should be to adhere to the prescribed therapeutic regimen, including nutritional management, cessation of smoking, and decreased use of alcohol and caffeine.
- A patient with chronic ulcers needs to be aware of the complications that may result from the disease, the clinical manifestations indicating their presence, and what to do until the health care provider can be seen.
- Teach the patient to take all medications as prescribed. This includes antisecretory and antibiotic drugs. Failure to take prescribed medications can result in relapse.

H. pylori is treated with antibiotics, the peptic ulcer recurrence drops to 20%. Patients who do not receive antibiotics have a relapse rate of 85% to 90%. The likelihood of recurrence is lessened by eliminating foods that aggravate the condition and following prescribed therapies such as taking proton pump inhibitors and avoiding NSAIDs. If symptoms recur, the prognosis is better in patients who seek immediate medical treatment and comply with the prescribed regimen (Anand, 2017).

CANCER OF THE STOMACH

Etiology and Pathophysiology

Stomach, or gastric, cancer saw its peak in the 1930s, when it was the leading cause of death. Although those numbers have decreased significantly over the years, the American Cancer Society estimates that 2017 will see 28,000 new cases of stomach cancer in the United States and nearly 11,000 people will die from the disease. Of the new cases diagnosed 17,750 will be in men and 10,250 in women. The incidence and mortality rate are much higher outside of the United States, especially in less developed areas. Rates are highest in Japan, China, Southern and Eastern Europe, and South and Central America. Gastric cancer affects mostly the elderly population: nearly two-thirds of those diagnosed are over the age of 65, and the average age is 69 (ACS, 2017c). The most common neoplasm or malignant growth in the stomach is adenocarcinoma. The primary location is the pyloric area, but the incidence of proximal tumors seems to be rising. Because of its location, the tumor may metastasize to lymph nodes, liver, spleen, pancreas, or esophagus.

Many factors have been implicated in the development of stomach cancer, yet no single causative agent has been identified. Stomach carcinogenesis probably begins with a nonspecific mucosal injury as a result of aging; autoimmune disease; or repeated exposure to irritants such as bile, antiinflammatory agents, or smoking. Other factors include history of polyps, pernicious anemia, hypochlorhydria (deficiency of hydrochloride in the stomach's gastric juice), chronic atrophic gastritis, and gastric ulcer. Because the stomach has prolonged contact with food, cancer in this part of the body is associated with diets that are high in salt, smoked and preserved foods (which contain nitrites and nitrates), and carbohydrates, and low in fresh fruits and vegetables. Whole grains and fresh fruits and vegetables are associated with reduced rates of stomach cancer. Infection with *H. pylori,* especially at an early age, is considered a definite risk factor for gastric cancer.

Clinical Manifestations

The patient may be asymptomatic in early stages of the disease. Stomach cancer often spreads to adjacent organs before any distressing symptoms occur. With more advanced disease, the patient may appear pale and lethargic if anemia is present. With a poor appetite and significant weight loss, the patient may appear cachectic (weak and emaciated).

Assessment

Subjective data include complaints of vague epigastric discomfort or indigestion, early satiety, and postprandial (after meal) fullness. Some patients complain of an ulcer-like pain that does not respond to therapy. Anorexia and weakness are also common.

Objective data include weight loss, blood in the stools, hematemesis, and vomiting after drinking or eating. Anemia is common. It is caused by chronic blood loss as the lesion erodes through the mucosa or as a direct result of pernicious anemia, which develops when intrinsic factor is lost. The presence of ascites is a poor prognostic sign.

Diagnostic Tests

Endoscopic or gastroscopic examinations with biopsy remain the best diagnostic tool. The stomach can be distended with air during the procedure to stretch mucosal folds. Tissue samples for the growth-promoting protein, HER2/neu, can be obtained during endoscopic examination. Findings of increased levels are seen in gastric adenocarcinoma. Endoscopic ultrasound and CT and PET scans can be used to stage the disease. Stool examination provides evidence of occult or gross bleeding. **Carcinoembryonic antigen (CEA)** and carbohydrate antigen 19-9 tumor markers usually are elevated in advanced gastric cancer. Serum tumor markers correlate with the degree of invasion, liver metastasis, and cure rate. Laboratory studies of RBCs, hemoglobin, hematocrit, and serum B_{12} assist in the detection of anemia and determination of severity (ACS, 2016d).

Medical Management

Treatment depends on the staging of the disease. Often a combination of treatments, including surgery, chemotherapy, radiation therapy, and targeted drug therapy, is beneficial. Surgery may be done as an exploratory celiotomy to determine involvement. The surgical interventions used in treating gastric cancer are typically the same procedures used for peptic ulcer disease. A partial or total gastric resection is the treatment of choice for an extensive lesion. Surgery for advanced gastric cancer carries high morbidity and mortality rates (Mayo Clinic, 2018b). Types of surgical procedures include the following:

- *Antrectomy:* Removal of the entire antrum, the gastric-producing portion of the lower stomach, to eliminate the main stimulus to acid production.
- *Gastroduodenostomy (Billroth I)* (Fig. 45.7A): Direct anastomosis of the fundus of the stomach to the duodenum; used to remove ulcers or cancer located in the antrum of the stomach.

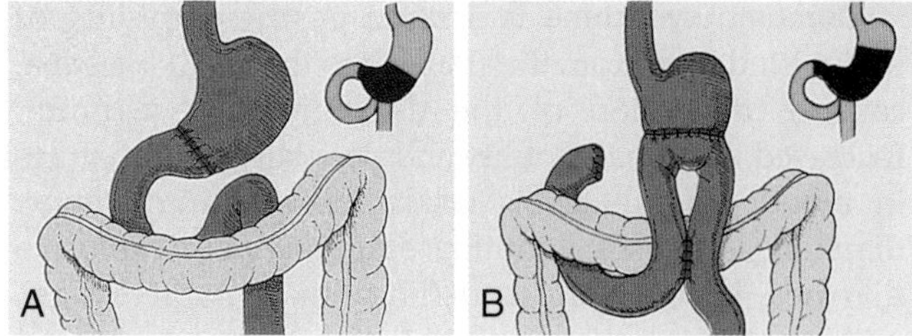

Fig. 45.7 Types of gastric resections with anastomoses. A, Billroth I. B, Billroth II.

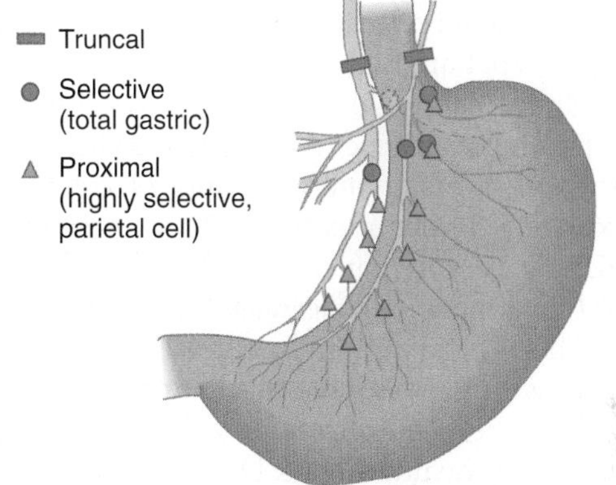

Fig. 45.8 Types of vagotomies: truncal, selective, and proximal or parietal cell. (From Black JM, Hawks JH: *Medical-surgical nursing: Clinical management for positive outcomes*, ed 8, St. Louis, 2009, Saunders.)

- *Gastrojejunostomy (Billroth II)* (Fig. 45.7B): Closure of the duodenum, and anastomosis of the fundus of the stomach into the jejunum; used to remove ulcers or cancer located in the body of the fundus.
- *Pyloroplasty:* Surgical enlargement of the pyloric sphincter to facilitate passage of contents from the stomach; commonly done after vagotomy or to enlarge an opening that has been constricted from scar tissue. A vagotomy decreases gastric motility and subsequently gastric emptying. A pyloroplasty accompanying vagotomy increases gastric emptying (Johns Hopkins, n.d.c).
- *Total gastrectomy:* Removal of the entire stomach; rarely used for patients with gastric cancer.
- *Vagotomy:* Removal of the vagal innervation to the fundus, decreasing acid produced by the parietal cells of the stomach (Fig. 45.8); usually done with a Billroth I or II procedure or with a pyloroplasty.

The choice of which procedure to use is difficult and depends on the surgeon's preference and results of diagnostic testing. Regardless of the procedure selected, postoperative complications are possible. Bleeding may occur up to 7 days after gastric surgery. Abdominal rigidity, abdominal pain, restlessness, elevated temperature, increased pulse, decreased blood pressure, and leukocytosis are possible indications of postoperative bleeding. Note the amount and type of drainage from the incision. Surgical intervention may be necessary to correct the bleeding.

Dumping syndrome is a rapid gastric emptying of undigested food from the stomach to the small intestine, causing distention of the duodenum or jejunum. Increased intestinal motility and peristalsis and changes in blood glucose levels occur. Patients may report diaphoresis, nausea, vomiting, epigastric pain, explosive diarrhea, borborygmi (rumbling noises made by gas passing through the liquid of the small intestine), and dyspepsia. Dumping syndrome is the direct result of surgical removal of a large portion of the stomach and the pyloric sphincter. Approximately one-third to one-half of patients experience dumping syndrome after peptic ulcer surgery. Treatment includes eating six small meals daily that are high in protein and fat and low in carbohydrates, eating slowly, and avoiding fluids during meals. Treatment also includes (1) anticholinergic agents to decrease stomach motility, and (2) reclining for approximately 1 hour after meals. To increase long-term compliance, reassure patients that following the recommended treatment will decrease symptoms within a few months. The symptoms are self-limiting and often disappear within several months to a year after surgery.

Several other complications after gastric surgery present serious health threats. Diarrhea is common and usually responds to conservative treatment of controlled diet and antidiarrheal agents. Diphenoxylate with atropine (Lomotil), loperamide (Imodium), paregoric, or codeine is often used. Reflux esophagitis and nutritional deficits—leading to weight loss, malabsorption, anemia, and vitamin deficiency—can also be life threatening.

Pernicious anemia is a serious potential complication for any patient who has had a total gastrectomy or extensive resections. This is caused by a deficiency of intrinsic factor, produced exclusively by the stomach, which aids intestinal absorption of vitamin B_{12}. Recommend that all patients with a partial gastrectomy have a blood serum vitamin B_{12} level measured every 1 to 2 years so that replacement therapy of vitamin B_{12} via a monthly injection, or weekly via the nasal route, can be instituted before anemia appears.

Wound healing may be disrupted by **dehiscence** (a partial or complete separation of the wound edges) or by **evisceration** (protrusion of viscera through the disrupted wound). Dehiscence and evisceration may be caused by problems in suturing the wound or by poor tissue integrity. Excessive coughing, straining, malnutrition, obesity, and infection also may increase the chances of dehiscence. Nursing interventions for dehiscence include instructing the patient to remain quiet, to cover the wound with a dry sterile dressing, and to avoid coughing or straining. Keep the patient in a dorsal recumbent position (on the back with the knees flexed) to remove stress on the wound and notify the surgeon. If evisceration occurs, keep the patient on bed rest and loosely cover the protruding viscera with a warm sterile saline dressing. Notify the surgeon immediately because treatment consists of reapproximating (i.e., drawing together) the wound edges.

Chemotherapy yields greater response and longer survival rates than radiation. Because the radiosensitivity of stomach cancer is low, radiation therapy is of little value. Radiation therapy may be used as a palliative measure to decrease tumor mass and temporarily relieve obstruction. The combination of chemotherapy and radiation therapy sometimes is used for patients who are at high risk for disease recurrence after surgery. These treatment modalities often are used in conjunction with surgery (Mayo Clinic, 2018b).

Nursing Interventions and Patient Teaching

Provide the patient and family with further clarification about the disease and the surgical intervention. Preoperative preparation includes improving the patient's nutritional status by monitoring total parenteral nutrition (TPN; complete nutrition provided intravenously) and providing supplemental feedings. Postoperative teaching is necessary to relieve anxiety and promote understanding of drainage tubes, feeding tubes, dressing changes, weakness, medications, and other routine care. Close monitoring of intake and output, maintenance of TPN, and being alert to weight loss are important in the postoperative period for surgeries involving the stomach.

Patient problems and interventions for the patient with cancer of the stomach include but are not limited to the following:

Patient Problem	Nursing Interventions
Potential for Harm or Damage to the Body, related to: • Aspiration • Infection • Hemorrhage • Anemia or vitamin deficiency	Monitor closely for elevated temperature, bleeding from incision, pallor, dyspnea, cyanosis, tachycardia, increased respirations, and chest pain Monitor laboratory results and activity tolerance because of possible anemia Change dressings, using sterile technique

Because care encompasses so many areas, instruction should be (1) planned according to the patient's needs and level of understanding, (2) given when the patient is free of pain, and (3) communicated verbally and in print. Address areas such as surgery, chemotherapy, radiation therapy, continued nutritional needs, pain relief, and support groups for psychosocial needs.

Weight loss indicates the need for additional caloric intake and can be measured by monitoring weight and comparing it with the patient's normal weight before illness. If a gastrostomy tube (G-tube) is necessary, prevention of skin excoriation around the G-tube site should be ensured. Hypermotility or diarrhea that follows radiation therapy can be treated with dietary therapy and/or medication. The debilitated patient and family may require referral for hospice care.

Prognosis

The prognosis for patients with gastric cancer depends on the stage at which the cancer was detected. If found and treated in the early stages, the 5-year survival rate is approximately 65%. For gastric cancer that has metastasized to nearby tissue or lymph nodes the 5-year survival rate is approximately 30%. Distant metastasis has a 5% survival rate in 5 years. The overall average 5-year survival rate is about 30% (URMC, 2017).

DISORDERS OF THE INTESTINES

INFECTIONS

Etiology and Pathophysiology

Intestinal infections are the invasion of the alimentary canal (both the small and large intestine) by pathogenic microorganisms that reproduce and multiply. The infectious agent can enter the body by several routes. The most common way is through the mouth in contaminated food or water. Some intestinal infections occur as a result of person-to-person contact. Fecal–oral transmission occurs through poor hand hygiene after elimination.

Bacterial flora grow naturally in the intestinal tract and help the immune system combat infection. Long-term antibiotic therapy can destroy the normal flora, resulting in pathogenic microorganisms entering the intestines. The impaired immune response in some individuals delays the body's attempt to destroy invading pathogens.

Infectious diarrhea causes secretion of fluid into the intestinal lumen. *Clostridium, Salmonella, Shigella,* and *Campylobacter* bacteria are associated with intestinal infections. These bacteria produce toxic substances, and the mucosal cells respond by secreting water and electrolytes, causing an imbalance. The amount of fluid secreted exceeds the ability of the large intestine to reabsorb the fluid into the vascular system (Guandalini, 2016).

One strain of *E. coli*—serotype O157:H7—often has a virulent course. Unlike other strains, *E. coli* O157:H7 is not part of the normal flora of the human intestine. Found in the intestines of approximately 1% of food cattle, in turkeys, and rarely in pigs, this strain can, even in small amounts, contaminate a large amount of meat, especially ground beef (Mayo Clinic, 2014a). It is transmitted in contaminated, undercooked meats such as hamburger, roast beef, ham, and turkey; in produce that has been rinsed with water contaminated by animal or human feces; or by a person who has been handling contaminated food. The bacterium also has been cultured in unpasteurized milk, cheese, and apple juice and can be found in lakes and pools that have been contaminated by fecal matter. Hemorrhagic colitis (which results in bloody diarrhea and severe cramping accompanied by diffuse abdominal tenderness) develops between the second and fourth days. Antidiarrheals should not be given because these medications prevent the intestines from getting rid of the *E. coli* pathogen. Antimotility drugs such as diphenoxylate with atropine or antibiotic therapy are not recommended because they increase the likelihood of developing hemolytic-uremic syndrome, a pathologic condition of the kidney. Poisoning with *E. coli* O157:H7 can be life threatening, particularly in the very young and in older adults. Usually little or no fever is present, and the illness resolves in 5 to 10 days. In approximately 2% to 7% of infections, particularly in young children, hemolytic-uremic syndrome occurs and the kidneys fail.

Sigmoidoscopic or colonoscopic examination and stool specimens are used to diagnose a type of inflammation or colitis called *antibiotic-associated pseudomembranous colitis* (AAPMC). Immunosuppressed patients and older adults are particularly susceptible. *C. difficile* is a facility-acquired infection, because hospitalized patients are often immunosuppressed, antibiotic therapy is common, and the spores can survive for up to 70 days on inanimate objects. *C. difficile* spores have been found on commodes, telephones, thermometers, bedside tables, floors, and other objects in rooms, as well as on the hands of health care workers. Health care workers who do not adhere to infection control precautions can transmit *C. difficile* from patient to patient. Washing hands with soap and water is necessary because antiseptic hand rub does not destroy *C. difficile.* This type of colitis is a complication of treatment with a wide variety of antibiotics, including lincomycin, clindamycin, ampicillin, erythromycin, tetracycline, cephalosporins, and aminoglycosides. A *C. difficile* test is ordered on stool specimens to aid in the diagnosis of AAPMC in inpatients and outpatients. Characteristic lesions of AAPMC are identified on tissues obtained through endoscopic examination.

Treatment with antibiotics (especially clindamycin, ampicillin, amoxicillin, and the cephalosporins) inhibits normal bacterial growth in the intestine. This inhibition of normal flora can lead to the overgrowth of other bacteria such as *C. difficile.* Under the right conditions, *C. difficile* produces two toxins, A and B. Toxins A and B are produced by *C. difficile* at the same time, and these toxins cause the tissue damage seen in AAPMC. The incidence of *C. difficile* toxin found in the stool ranges from 1% to 2% in a normal population to 10% in hospital inpatients and up to 85% to 90% in patients with proven AAPMC. The *C. difficile* test alone is not conclusive but does aid in the diagnosis of AAPMC.

Because the level of *C. difficile* antigens associated with the disease state may vary, a negative *C. difficile* test result alone may not rule out the possibility of *C. difficile*–associated colitis. Signs and symptoms of the disease such as the duration and severity of diarrhea should be monitored. These observations, along with the duration of antibiotic treatment and the presence of colitis or pseudomembranes, are factors the health care provider must consider when diagnosing AAPMC disease.

The health care provider treats a mild case of antibiotic-related *C. difficile*–associated diarrhea by simply discontinuing the antibiotic and providing fluid and electrolyte replacement. For mild to moderate cases of the infection, oral metronidazole (Flagyl) is recommended as initial treatment. In more severe cases the health care provider discontinues the antibiotic and starts antimicrobial therapy; the drug of choice is metronidazole or, if that is ineffective, vancomycin (Vancocin) (Aberra, 2016).

A treatment that is being used in some cases is fecal microbial transplantation. In this procedure a patient is prepped for a colonoscopy, a sample of feces is obtained from a donor (who has been screened for any infection) and is sent to the laboratory for processing, and the sample then is placed into the sigmoid colon of the recipient. The goal of this therapy is to promote growth of normal flora in the intestine that has been lost (Aroniadis and Brandt, 2013).

Clinical Manifestations

Diarrhea is the most common manifestation of an intestinal infection. The fecal output has increased water content, and if the intestinal mucosa is directly invaded, the feces may contain blood and mucus.

Assessment

Collection of subjective data includes noting complaints of diarrhea, rectal urgency, **tenesmus** (ineffective and painful straining with defecation), nausea, and abdominal cramping.

Objective data include a fever and vomiting. History taking provides useful information regarding number and consistency of bowel movements, recent use of antibiotics, recent travel, food intake, and exposure to noninfectious causes of diarrhea. Noninfectious diarrhea may be caused by heavy metal poisoning, shellfish allergy, and ingestion of toxins from mushrooms or fish. Diarrhea from noninfectious causes usually is characterized by a short incubation period (minutes to hours after exposure).

Diagnostic Tests

The key laboratory test for patients with intestinal infections is a stool culture. Stools are examined for blood, mucus, and WBCs. A blood chemistry study to monitor changes in the patient's fluid and electrolyte status may be included.

Medical Management

Usually the treatment of intestinal infections is conservative, letting the body limit the infection. Antibiotics rarely are used to treat acute diarrhea but may be given in cases of prolonged or severe diarrhea with a stool positive for leukocytes. If fluid and electrolyte replacement is necessary to offset the losses from diarrhea, the oral route is usually sufficient. The IV route is indicated if the patient cannot take sufficient fluids orally.

The use of antidiarrheals and antispasmodic agents actually may increase the severity of the infection by prolonging the contact time of the infectious organism with the intestinal wall. The health care provider determines when and if such medications should be prescribed.

Nursing Interventions and Patient Teaching

Perform a thorough assessment to aid the health care provider in determining the seriousness of the intestinal infection. Determining the onset of the disease and the number of people exposed is important, because the majority of GI infections are communicable and represent a community health problem. Also, assessment for fluid imbalance is important, including measurement of postural changes in blood pressure, skin turgor, mucous membrane hydration, and urinary output.

Patient problems and interventions for the patient with intestinal infections include but are not limited to the following:

Patient Problem	Nursing Interventions
Inadequate Fluid Volume, related to excessive losses from diarrhea and vomiting	If oral intake is tolerated, offer apple juice, clear carbonated beverages, clear broth, plain gelatin, and water If IV feedings are required to maintain intravascular volume, these fluids should have electrolytes added Maintain accurate I&O

Instruct the patient to report the number, color, and consistency of bowel movements; abdominal cramping; and pain. Ensure that the patient and family understand the importance of hand hygiene after bowel movements to interrupt the fecal–oral route of transmission. Information should be given to family members responsible for food preparation about the importance of proper methods of food preparation and storage to reduce the growth of infecting organisms. The patient at home may benefit from drinking water and rehydration solutions such as Gatorade (adults) or Pedialyte (infants and children).

Prognosis

Intestinal infections. The body may be able to defend itself successfully against the infection without medical intervention. In severe cases, medications and fluid replacement may be necessary. Prognosis is favorable unless the patient is severely debilitated by other conditions.

Antibiotic-associated pseudomembranous colitis. The prognosis for AAPMC is better when the disease is diagnosed early and the antibiotics are changed. This allows the normal growth of bacteria in the intestine to resume. The prognosis depends on the patient's overall condition.

CELIAC DISEASE (CELIAC SPRUE)

Etiology and Pathophysiology

Celiac disease is a genetic disorder that most commonly affects the small intestine but can affect any part of the GI system. It is considered an autoimmune disease that disrupts the absorption of nutrients from foods in response to the ingestion of **gluten** (a protein primarily found in wheat, rye, and barley). When these proteins are ingested, the immune system begins damaging the inner lining of the small intestine and destroying the villi (finger-like protrusions lining the intestine). Celiac disease affects approximately 1 in 100 people in the world. Among first-degree relatives of patients with celiac disease, the incidence increases to 1 in 10 people (Celiac Disease Foundation, 2017).

Clinical Manifestations

The patient with celiac disease experiences very individualized clinical manifestations. Commonly, abdominal pain and diarrhea after ingesting foods containing gluten is experienced. Malabsorption occurs because the damage to the lining of the small intestine prevents digestion from occurring. This manifestation may result in weight loss and vitamin deficiencies. Vitamin deficiencies may be so severe that the brain, peripheral nervous system, bones, liver, and other vital organs are affected.

Assessment

Subjective data include complaints of abdominal pain and bloating, irritability and depression, joint pain, muscle cramps, neuropathic complaints such as tingling in the legs and feet, and general weakness and fatigue.

Objective data include chronic intermittent diarrhea, weight loss, osteoporosis, mouth sores, dental problems, unexplained iron deficiency anemia, and pale, foul-smelling stools that contain a large amount of fat.

Diagnostic Tests

Blood tests for the presence of specific autoantibodies (anti–tissue transglutaminase antibodies [TGAs] or anti-endomysial antibodies [EMAs]) are performed while the patient still is ingesting gluten. False negatives may occur if gluten already has been eliminated from the diet. Intestinal biopsy via an endoscopy is performed if blood tests are positive for the disease (Celiac Disease Foundation, 2017).

Medical Management

There is no medical treatment for celiac disease other than following a gluten-free diet. Referral to a dietitian is most beneficial for a patient newly diagnosed with the disease. Vitamins and supplements may be ordered by the health care provider for severe deficiencies. Steroids also may be prescribed to treat extensive inflammation of the intestinal lining.

Nursing Interventions and Patient Teaching

The patient diagnosed with celiac disease must understand how to incorporate a gluten-free diet into his or her life. Foods containing wheat, rye, and barley are prohibited. Foods that commonly contain these ingredients are made with wheat flour, which includes most grains, cereal, pasta, and many processed foods. Replacing these foods with potato, rice, soy, amaranth, quinoa, buckwheat, and bean flour prevent the autoimmune response of celiac disease. In 2006 the Food Allergen Labeling and Consumer Protection Act (FALCPA) required that food labels identify wheat and other common food allergens in the list of ingredients. Many food labels clearly identify gluten-free products. Plain meat and fish, fruits, vegetables, and rice can be included into the diet because they do not contain gluten.

Prognosis

Patients who follow a strict gluten-free diet typically notice improvement in symptoms within a few days of changing their diet, and the damage to the intestine often is resolved within 3 to 6 months. Small amounts of gluten can damage the intestine even if symptoms are not apparent.

IRRITABLE BOWEL SYNDROME

Etiology and Pathophysiology

Irritable bowel syndrome (IBS) is considered a functional disorder characterized by episodes of altered bowel function and intermittent and recurrent abdominal discomfort and pain. Patients with IBS experience diarrhea, constipation, or a combination of both that occurs for months or years, and the cause of the disorder is not known.

IBS affects about 10% to 15% of the American population. More women than men are affected by IBS (two of three individuals with the disorder), and most people with IBS are under the age of 50. Approximately 20% to 40% of people who visit a gastroenterologist are seeking diagnosis or treatment for IBS symptoms (International Foundation for Functional Gastrointestinal Disorders [IFFGD], 2016).

The actual cause of IBS is unknown, but there are several commonalities among those diagnosed with the disorder and theories regarding the cause. One theory is that the brain, intestine, and nervous system interact in a way that causes greater than normal discomfort when stool passes through the colon. Another theory is that peristalsis contractions last longer and are stronger than normal, causing more discomfort, bloating, and frequency of stools. The opposite problem of slowed peristalsis, leading to hardened feces and causing discomfort, may be attributed to episodes of constipation. Psychological factors also are considered a possible cause for IBS. Anxiety disorders, depression, and forms of abuse, including physical, social, and sexual abuse, are considered possible causes of IBS (IFFGD, 2016).

Clinical Manifestations

Alterations of bowel function include abdominal pain relieved after a bowel movement; more frequent bowel movements with pain onset; a sense of incomplete evacuation; flatulence; and constipation, diarrhea, or both. Stress is not considered a cause of IBS but can exacerbate symptoms of diarrhea; usually weight loss does not occur. The physical examination is generally normal, and nocturnal symptoms are rarely present. The symptoms of IBS are deceptive and are frustrating for the patient to manage.

Assessment

Subjective data include complaints of abdominal distress, pain at onset of bowel movements, abdominal pain relieved by defecation, and feelings of incomplete emptying after defecation.

Objective data include the presence of mucus in stools, visible abdominal distention, and frequent or unformed stools.

Diagnostic Tests

The key to accurate diagnosis of IBS is a thorough history and physical examination. Emphasize symptoms, health history (including psychosocial aspects such as physical or sexual abuse), family history, and drug and dietary history.

Diagnosis of IBS occurs by exclusion. Patients who see the health care provider with symptoms of intermittent or chronic abdominal pain and altered bowel motility are screened for pathologic conditions such as Crohn's disease, ulcerative colitis, colorectal cancer, diverticulitis, and infections such as *Salmonella.* When no pathologic or structural abnormality is detected, IBS is a probable diagnosis. Symptom-based criteria for IBS have been standardized and are referred to as the *Rome criteria.* Rome III criteria include abdominal discomfort that occurs at least 3 days per month within the past 3 months and that has at least two of the following characteristics: (1) relieved with defecation, (2) onset associated with a change in stool frequency, and (3) onset associated with a change in stool appearance.

Medical Management

Stress management and behavioral therapy. Although stress does not cause IBS, it can make the symptoms worse. Stress management techniques, biofeedback, relaxation therapy, and hypnosis are some of the cognitive therapies used to manage IBS. Keeping a diary also may help with identifying lifestyle and diet issues that may worsen symptoms, thus allowing modifications of these issues.

Diet and bulking agents. Increasing dietary fiber may help to increase stool bulk and frequency of passage and to reduce bloating. Adequate fiber may be provided more reliably with over-the-counter bulking agents than with diet alone. The bulking agents seem to be most effective in treating constipation-predominant IBS, although they may alleviate mild diarrhea. If the patient's symptoms are exacerbated consistently after eating certain foods, those foods should be avoided. Advise the patient whose primary symptoms are abdominal distention and increased flatulence to eliminate common gas-producing foods (e.g., broccoli, cabbage) from the diet and to substitute yogurt for milk products to help determine whether he or she is lactose intolerant.

Medication. Anticholinergic drugs may help relieve abdominal cramps caused by spasm of the colon, and antidiarrheal medications may be necessary for bouts of diarrhea. Antianxiety drugs may help patients suffering from panic attacks associated with IBS. Antidepressants may be used sparingly for diarrhea-predominant IBS in patients with severe discomfort who have not responded to other measures, or for those experiencing depression from living with IBS. New drug therapies are in development. Drugs that affect serotonin receptors hold promise in the treatment of IBS. Newer medications that have been approved for the treatment of select patients with IBS include alosetron (Lotronex) and lubiprostone (Amitiza). Alosetron (Lotronex) is a nerve receptor antagonist that helps in relaxing the colon and slowing the movement of stool through the colon, and lubiprostone (Amitiza) is a chloride channel activator that works for those suffering from constipation by increasing fluid secretion in the small intestine to help with the passage of stool.

Some patients have reported benefits from the use of complementary therapies such as acupuncture, herbal therapy, chiropractic techniques, and yoga (see the Complementary and Alternative Therapies box). Although some studies have examined the use of such therapies in the treatment of IBS, clinical trial data are inadequate to determine their efficacy or to recommend any one as the sole therapy in the treatment of the syndrome.

Nursing Interventions and Patient Teaching

Many patients with IBS learn to cope with their symptoms enough to live in reasonable comfort. It is the nurse's role to assist in identifying those patients with IBS who need management. The nurse's skill in history taking, listening, nutrition planning, and understanding psychological effects on the body can assist the patient in setting goals to manage the disease. Emphasize the importance of keeping a daily log showing diet; number and type of stools; presence, severity, and duration of pain; side effects of medication; and life stressors that aggravate the disorder. This information assists in the diagnosis and treatment of IBS.

Complementary and Alternative Therapies

Irritable Bowel Syndrome

- Peppermint oil, an herbal extract, has been studied for its use in irritable bowel syndrome. It acts by relaxing smooth muscle in the colon. Peppermint may cause heartburn, so the patient should be advised to take enteric-coated tablets.
- Biofeedback is a relaxation training method that gives individuals a greater degree of awareness and control of physiologic function. Computer-based biofeedback equipment gives immediate feedback to the patient on changes in certain parameters, such as muscle electrical activity and skin temperature.
- Similar interventions have used various psychotherapy, stress management, and relaxation exercises, often in combination.
- Herbs that patients should avoid because they can cause GI upset include milk thistle *(Silybum marianum)*, goldenseal *(Hydrastis canadensis)*, ginger *(Zingiber officinale)*, kelp *(Fucus vesiculosus)*, comfrey *(Symphytum officinale)*, chaparral *(Larrea divaricata)*, cayenne *(Capsicum)*, and alfalfa *(Medicago sativa)*.
- Some people find that acupuncture or acupressure provides relief from nausea and vomiting and relaxation of muscle spasms in the colon.
- Some people experience improved blood flow to digestive organs and improved digestion after chiropractic adjustment.
- Probiotics are "good" bacteria that are found in the intestinal tract. One theory is that people with IBS have an insufficient amount of good intestinal bacteria. Therefore foods that are high in probiotics, such as yogurt, or dietary supplements sometimes are added to the diet as a complementary treatment method.
- Regular exercise, massage, yoga, and meditation may help in managing stress.

Patient problems and interventions for the patient with an irritable bowel include but are not limited to the following:

Patient Problem	Nursing Interventions
Discomfort, related to diet consumed and bowel evacuation	Have patient log the type of food consumed in terms of fiber content, consistency of stool, and degree of pain
Insufficient Knowledge, related to the effect of fiber content on spastic bowel	Educate patient regarding the relationship of fiber to constipation and diarrhea Teach patient about the use of bulking agents

IBS involves many personal feelings that the patient must recognize and be comfortable with before a care plan can be established. It is important to establish a strong relationship with the patient before patient teaching begins. Patient teaching includes diet management and ways to control anxiety in daily living. The goal of patient teaching is to empower the patient to control the disorder. Provide community resources for counseling if psychological problems seem related to increased or decreased elimination accompanied by pain and discomfort.

Prognosis

IBS does not damage the bowel. It is a functional problem that, if managed well, can interfere minimally with a person's daily life.

INFLAMMATORY BOWEL DISEASE

Ulcerative colitis and Crohn's disease are chronic, episodic, inflammatory bowel diseases. These are immunologically related disorders that commonly affect young adults, usually between the ages of 15 and 30 years. These diseases are distributed evenly between males and females; ulcerative colitis is slightly more prevalent in females, whereas Crohn's is slightly more prevalent in males. Individuals of Ashkenazi Jewish descent have a higher rate of inflammatory bowel disease (IBD), and there also seems to be a familial tendency for both disorders (CDC, 2014).

The causes of ulcerative colitis and Crohn's disease are unknown. Theories involve genetic and environmental factors, including bacterial infection, immunologic factors, and psychosomatic disorders. The fact that people with ulcerative colitis commonly have a relative with Crohn's disease and vice versa supports the existence of a common gene. Inflammatory bowel diseases are characterized by **exacerbations** (increases in severity of the disease or any of its symptoms) and **remissions** (decreases in severity of the disease or any of its symptoms).

The two diseases require similar nursing interventions but different surgical interventions and medical treatment. Certain criteria are used to differentiate ulcerative colitis from Crohn's disease (Table 45.3), but the diseases have much in common and cannot be differentiated in some cases. Patients have been known to have features of both diseases, making a definite diagnosis difficult.

ULCERATIVE COLITIS

Etiology and Pathophysiology

Because of difficulty in diagnosing and misclassification of the diseases, the data may not be completely accurate, but the incidence of ulcerative colitis appears to be higher than that of Crohn's disease. The causes of IBD may be attributed to the immune system and/or genetics. Regarding the immune system, it is believed that either a virus or bacterium invades the immune system, resulting in inflammation from the immune response; or an autoimmune reaction occurs, causing inflammation, with no pathogen provoking this response. Genetics are suspected because the disease is seen frequently among first-degree relatives.

Ulcerative colitis is confined to the mucosa and submucosa of the colon. The disease can affect segments

Table 45.3 Comparison of Ulcerative Colitis and Crohn's Disease

FACTOR	ULCERATIVE COLITIS	CROHN'S DISEASE
Cause of disorder	Unknown; autoimmune; genetic factors and environment play a role; various bacteria have been proposed	Unknown; possible cause is an altered immune state; autoimmune; various bacteria have been proposed Genetic and environmental factors play a role
Usual age at onset	Teenage years and early adulthood; second peak in sixth decade	Early adolescence; second peak in sixth decade
Area of involvement	Confined to mucosa or submucosa of the colon	Can occur anywhere along the gastrointestinal tract from the mouth to the anus Most common site is terminal ileum and proximal cecum
Area of inflammation	Mucosa and submucosa	Transmural (pertaining to the entire thickness of the wall of an organ)
Characteristics of inflammation	Tends to be continuous, starting at the rectum and extending proximally; limited to the mucosal lining	May be continuous or interspersed between areas of normal tissue; may extend through all layers of the bowel
Character of stools	Blood present No fat 15–20 liquid stools daily	No blood present Steatorrhea (fat in stool) 3 or 4 semisoft stools daily
Major complication	Toxic megacolon, fistulas, and abscesses (rare)	Malabsorption, bowel obstruction, fistulas, tissue abscesses
Major complaints	Rectal bleeding, abdominal cramping	Right lower abdominal pain with mass present
Reason for surgery	Poor response to medical therapy	Indicated to remove diseased areas that do not respond to aggressive medical therapy. Surgery does not cure the disease
Response to surgery	Removal of the colon cures the intestinal disease, but not extraintestinal symptoms, such as inflammation of joints and liver disease	Alleviation of symptoms caused from diseased portion of intestine
Cancer potential	Increased risk after 10 yr of disease	Small intestine incidence increased; colon incidence increased, but not as much as in ulcerative colitis
Biopsy findings	Architectural changes consistent with chronic inflammation	Architectural changes consistent with chronic inflammation; may show granulomas
Weight loss	May develop weight loss depending on severity	Cobblestoning of mucosa is common; may be severe
Malabsorption and nutritional deficiencies	Minimal incidence	Common; may be severe; frequent

Data from International Foundation for Functional Gastrointestinal Disorders (IFFGD): Statistics, 2016. Retrieved from *http://www.aboutibs.org/facts-about-ibs/statistics.html*; and Centers for Disease Control and Prevention (CDC): 2014. Irritable bowel disease. Retrieved from *https://www.cdc.gov/ibd/index.htm*.

of the entire colon, depending on the staging (phases or periods in the course of the disease). This disease usually starts in the rectum and moves in a continuous pattern toward the cecum. Although sometimes mild inflammation of the terminal ileum occurs, ulcerative colitis is a disease of the colon and rectum. The inflammation and ulcerations occur in the mucosal layer of the bowel wall. Because it does not extend through all bowel wall layers, fistulas and abscesses are rare. Capillaries become friable and bleed, causing the characteristic diarrhea containing pus and blood. Pseudopolyps (tissue that resembles polyps because of the cratering effect of surrounding ulcerations) are common in chronic ulcerative disease and may become cancerous. With healing and the natural formation of scar tissue, the colon may lose elasticity and absorptive capability.

Clinical Manifestations

The person diagnosed with ulcerative colitis often has periods of exacerbation and remission, and the degree of the illness can vary from mild to severe. Patients with severe ulcerative colitis may have as many as 15 to 20 liquid stools per day, containing blood, mucus, and pus. With severe diarrhea, losses of sodium, potassium, bicarbonate, and calcium ions may occur. Abdominal cramps may occur before the bowel movement. The urge to defecate lessens as scarring within the bowel progresses. This results in involuntary leakage of stool. In mild to moderate ulcerative colitis, diarrhea may consist of two to five stools per day with some blood present.

Complications are seen less in ulcerative colitis than with Crohn's disease. Complications of ulcerative colitis include bleeding from ulcerations of the colon, rupture of the bowel, and severe abdominal bloating. A less common complication is toxic megacolon (toxic dilation of the large bowel). The bowel becomes distended and so thin that it could be perforated at any time. Clinical manifestations of toxic megacolon include fever, abdominal pain and tenderness, severe abdominal distention, and shock. The patient with ulcerative colitis is at increased risk for colon cancer. Surgical interventions for treatment of this complication are usually necessary.

Assessment

Subjective data include complaints of rectal bleeding and abdominal cramping. Lethargy, a sense of frustration, and loss of control result from painful abdominal cramping and unpredictable bowel movements.

Objective data include weight loss, abdominal distention, fever, tachycardia, leukocytosis, and observation of frequency and characteristics of stools.

Diagnostic Tests

Double-contrast barium enema studies of the intestine, sigmoidoscopy and colonoscopy with biopsy, and stool testing for melena aid the health care provider in diagnosis. Additional studies include radiologic examination of the abdomen, serum electrolytes and albumin levels, liver function studies, and other hematologic studies.

Medical Management

The medical interventions chosen depend on the phase of the disease and the individual response to therapy. Common treatment modalities include medication, diet intervention, and stress reduction.

Drug therapy. The four major categories of drugs used are (1) those that affect the inflammatory response, (2) antibacterial drugs, (3) drugs that affect the immune system, and (4) antidiarrheal preparations.

Sulfasalazine (Azulfidine) is a common medication used for mild chronic ulcerative colitis. Sulfasalazine is broken down by bacteria in the colon into sulfapyridine and 5-aminosalicylic acid (5-ASA). It affects the inflammatory response and provides some antibacterial activity. It is effective in maintaining clinical remission and in treating mild to moderately severe attacks. Newer preparations have been developed to deliver 5-ASA to the terminal ileum and colon (e.g., olsalazine [Dipentum], mesalamine [Pentasa], and balsalazide [Colazal]). These drugs are as effective as sulfasalazine and are better tolerated when administered orally. Immune system suppressants such as cyclosporine (Gengraf), infliximab (Remicade), methotrexate, and ustekinumab (Stelara) commonly are prescribed.

Non-sulfa drugs such as mesalamine (Rowasa) can be given by retention enema.

Corticosteroids are antiinflammatory drugs effective in relieving symptoms of moderate and severe colitis; they can be given orally or intravenously if inflammation is severe.

Antidiarrheal agents are recommended over anticholinergic agents because anticholinergic drugs can mask obstruction or contribute to toxic colonic dilation. Loperamide may be used to treat cramping and diarrhea of chronic ulcerative colitis. Azathioprine (Imuran) is also beneficial (Mayo Clinic, 2015b).

Nutrition therapy. Diet is an important component in the treatment of inflammatory bowel disease, and a dietitian should be consulted. The goals of diet management are to provide adequate nutrition without making symptoms worse, to correct and prevent malnutrition, to replace fluid and electrolyte losses, and to prevent weight loss. Patients with inflammatory bowel disease must eat a balanced, healthy diet with sufficient calories, protein, and nutrients. Patients can use MyPlate guidelines to ensure that they get adequate portions from all the food groups. The diet for each patient is individualized.

Patients with diarrhea often decrease their oral intake to reduce the diarrhea. The anorexia that accompanies inflammation also results in decreases in food intake. Blood loss leads to iron deficiency anemia.

Inflammatory bowel disease has no universal food triggers, but patients may find that certain foods initiate diarrhea. A food diary helps them identify problem foods to avoid. Many patients are lactose intolerant and improve when they avoid milk products. High-fat foods also tend to trigger diarrhea. Cold foods and high-fiber foods (cereal with bran, nuts, raw fruit) may increase GI transit. Smoking stimulates the GI tract (increases motility and secretion) and should be avoided. Patients with significant fluid and electrolyte losses or malabsorption may need parenteral nutrition or enteral feedings, such as elemental diets. Elemental diets are high in calories and nutrients, lactose free, and absorbed in the proximal small intestine, which allows the more distal bowel to rest.

Stress control. Ulcerative colitis is aggravated by stress. Identifying the factors that cause stress is the first step in controlling the disease. Working with the patient to find healthful coping mechanisms is part of the holistic approach in nursing interventions.

Surgical intervention. If an acute episode does not respond to treatment, if complications occur, or if the risk of cancer becomes greater because of chronic ulcerative colitis, surgical intervention is indicated (Box 45.3). Approximately 25% to 40% of patients with ulcerative colitis need surgery at some time during their illness. Most surgeons prefer a conservative approach, removing only the diseased portion of the colon. The operations

Box 45.3 Surgical Interventions for Ulcerative Colitis

- *Colon resection:* Removal of a portion of the large intestine and anastomosis of the remaining segment
- *Ileoanal anastomosis:* Removal of the colon and rectum but leaving the anus intact, along with the anal sphincter; anastomosis formed between the lower end of the small intestine and the anus
- *Ileostomy:* Surgical formation of an opening of the ileum onto the surface of the abdomen, through which fecal matter is emptied
- *Kock pouch (Kock continent ileostomy):* Surgical removal of the rectum and colon (proctocolectomy) with formation of a reservoir by suturing loops of adjacent ileum together to form a pouchlike structure, nipple valve, and stoma
- *Proctocolectomy:* Removal of anus, rectum, and colon; ileostomy established for the removal of digestive tract wastes

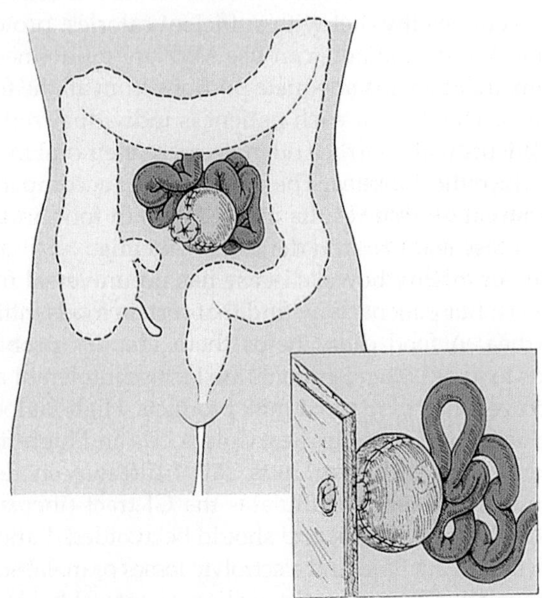

Fig. 45.9 Kock pouch (Kock continent ileostomy).

of choice may be a single-stage total proctocolectomy with construction of an internal reservoir and valve (Kock pouch, or Kock continent ileostomy) (Fig. 45.9); total proctocolectomy with ileoanal anastomosis with or without construction of an internal reservoir; and temporary ileostomy. In the case of a high-risk patient, a subtotal colectomy may be performed with ileostomy. After the patient's recovery (approximately 2 to 4 months), removal of the rectum or construction of an internal reservoir is possible.

Nursing Interventions

Nursing interventions include a thorough assessment of the patient's bowel elimination, support systems, coping abilities, nutritional status, pain, and understanding of the disease process and treatment required. Patients need a complete understanding of the care plan so that they can make informed choices. Prevention of future episodes is a goal for the patient with ulcerative colitis.

Preoperative care for these patients includes (1) selecting a stoma site, (2) performing additional diagnostic tests if cancer is suspected, (3) helping the patient accept that previous treatments were unsuccessful in curing the disease, and (4) preparing the bowel for surgery. The bowel is prepared 2 or 3 days preoperatively. A bland to clear liquid diet is ordered, along with a bowel prep of laxatives. Antibiotics, such an erythromycin and neomycin, frequently are given to decrease the number of bacteria in the bowel.

Postoperative nursing interventions depend on the type of procedure performed and the individual's response. Areas of concern are bowel and urinary elimination; fluid and electrolyte balance; tissue perfusion; comfort and pain; nutrition; gas exchange; infection; and, in the case of ostomy construction, assessment of the ileostomy and peristomal skin integrity.

A patient problem and interventions for the patient with chronic inflammatory bowel disease include but are not limited to the following:

Patient Problem	Nursing Interventions
Helplessness, related to loss of control of body function	Assist weakened patient with activities of daily living (bathing, oral hygiene, shaving, and other grooming needs) Offer choices to patient, when possible, to provide a sense of control

Patient problems for the surgical patient include *Potential for Impaired Coping, Impaired Self-Esteem due to Current Situation,* and *Distorted Body Image.* Nursing interventions include reinforcing the health care provider's explanation of the surgical procedure and expected outcomes. Providing reading material and demonstrating the care of an ostomy pouch when the patient seems ready reduces anxiety. A visitor from the United Ostomy Associations of America can provide hope, as a recovered and productive role model. Surgical intervention and the subsequent stoma are often difficult for the patient to cope with initially. Be supportive and encourage the patient to share fears. Box 45.4 lists postoperative nursing interventions.

Peristomal area integrity. Assess the peristomal skin for impaired integrity. Four primary factors contributing to loss of peristomal skin integrity are allergies, mechanical trauma, chemical reactions, and infection:

- Allergies to pouches, adhesives, skin barriers, powders, and paste are rare but are evident at areas of contact. The skin may appear erythematous, eroded, weeping, and bleeding. Changing the type of pouch, tape, or adhesive may resolve the problem.

Box 45.4 Postoperative Nursing Interventions for Ulcerative Colitis

1. Monitor nasogastric (NG) suction for patency until bowel function is resumed. Maintain correct wall suctioning. Accurately record color and amount of output. Irrigate NG tube as needed. Apply water-soluble lubricant to nares. Assess bowel sounds, being certain to turn off NG suction during auscultation.
2. Initiate ostomy care and teaching when bowel activity begins. Be sensitive to patient's pain level and readiness for teaching of ostomy care.
3. Observe **stoma** (an artificial opening of an internal organ on the body's surface) for color and size (should be pink/red and slightly edematous). Document assessment (e.g., "stoma pink and viable").
4. Select appropriate pouching system that has skin-protective barrier, accordion flange to ease pressure applied to new incisional site, adhesive backing, and pouch opening no more than 1/16 inch larger than the stoma. Stomas change in size over time and should be measured before new supplies are ordered.
5. Empty pouch when it is approximately one-third to one-half full to prevent breaking the seal, resulting in pouch leakage.
6. Explain that initial dark green liquid will change to yellow-brown as patient is allowed to eat.
7. Teach patient to care for the stoma; this includes having patient look at stoma and gradually assist with emptying, cleaning, and changing pouch. Teach patient that normal grieving occurs after loss of rectal function. Be supportive of patient's concerns.
8. Promote independence and self-care to decrease state of denial.
9. Instruct on follow-up home care, including changing skin barrier (a piece of pectin-based or Karaya wafer with measurable thickness and hydrocolloid adhesive properties) every 5 to 7 days. Using antacids, skin protective paste, and liquid skin barrier may be appropriate if skin excoriation is observed.
10. Patient may shower or bathe with or without pouch on.
11. Patient should avoid lifting objects heavier than 10 lb until health care provider says it is allowed.
12. A special diet is not necessary, but patients should drink 8 to 10 glasses of water a day, chew food well, and limit or avoid certain gas-forming foods.
13. Sexual relationships can be resumed when health care provider feels it is not harmful to the surgical area. Counseling may be appropriate if patient has fear of resuming this activity.

- Mechanical trauma caused by pressure, friction, or stripping of adhesives and skin barriers can be avoided by changing the pouch less frequently, using adhesive tape sparingly, and using skin preparation solutions. The skin must be protected when the pouch is removed.
- The most common chemical irritant is the stool from the stoma. Protect the skin from these digestive enzymes by using skin barriers before applying the pouch. Skin barriers include adhesives (Stomahesive), powders (Stomahesive powder), liquid skin barriers (Skin Prep), and caulking paste (Stomahesive paste).
- A common cause of infection of the peristomal skin is *Candida albicans.* People who have been taking antibiotics for 5 or more days may be prone to this problem. Treatment is the application of nystatin powder or cream, by health care provider order. A skin barrier should be applied over the medicated area to ensure that the adhesive sticks.

Patient Teaching

The patient and/or significant other must be taught the appropriate care of the ileostomy or colostomy to foster independence. This includes pouch change, cleansing, irrigation, and skin care. Providing a list of foods known to cause constipation, diarrhea, blockage, odors, and flatus is helpful. Before discharge the patient should be given a list of resource people; phone numbers; and supplies, including where to obtain them.

Prognosis

The prognosis for patients with chronic ulcerative colitis is related directly to the number of years they have had the disease and the severity. The incidence of carcinoma increases when the colon is extensively involved over time. The disease carries a higher mortality rate among patients who have had the disease for an extended period of time.

CROHN'S DISEASE

Etiology and Pathophysiology

Crohn's disease, although not as prevalent as ulcerative colitis, is increasing in incidence. Crohn's disease is characterized by inflammation of segments of the GI tract. The cause of the disease is not known, but there seems to be a strong association between Crohn's disease and altered immune mechanisms. Genetic and environmental factors seem to play a role. It most commonly occurs during adolescence and early adulthood but is also seen developing in patients between 50 and 60 years of age. Crohn's disease can occur anywhere in the GI tract from the mouth to the anus but occurs most commonly in the terminal ileum and proximal colon. The inflammation involves all layers of the bowel wall. It may involve only one segment of the bowel, or segments of diseased tissue may alternate with healthy tissue. In the early stages of the disease, tiny ulcers form on various parts of the intestinal wall. Over time, horizontal rows of these ulcers fuse with vertical rows, giving the mucosa a cobblestone appearance. Inflammation, fibrosis, and scarring often involving the entire thickness of the intestine are characteristics of Crohn's disease. Patients with Crohn's disease are likely to have a bowel obstruction, fistulas, fissures, and abscesses. In some patients the disease may involve the colon without any changes in the small intestine.

Malabsorption is the major problem when the small intestine is involved, and this contributes to nutritional problems. Pernicious anemia may result from decreased absorption of vitamin B_{12} in the small intestine. Fluid and electrolyte disturbances with acid-base imbalances can occur, particularly with depletion of sodium or potassium associated with diarrhea or with excessive small intestine drainage through fistulas associated with the pathologic process.

Clinical Manifestations

The manifestations depend largely on the anatomic site of involvement, extent of the disease process, and presence of complications. The onset of Crohn's disease is usually insidious, with nonspecific complaints such as diarrhea, fatigue, abdominal pain, weight loss, and fever. As the disease progresses, the patient experiences weight loss, malnutrition, dehydration, electrolyte imbalance, anemia, and increased peristalsis.

Assessment

Collection of subjective data for the patient with Crohn's disease includes noting the patient's list of complaints, including weakness, loss of appetite, abdominal pain and cramps, intermittent low-grade fever, sleeplessness caused by diarrhea, and stress. Right-lower-quadrant abdominal pain is characteristic of the disease and may be accompanied by a tender mass of thickened intestines in the same area.

Objective data include complaints of diarrhea—three or four semisolid stools daily, containing mucus and pus, but usually no blood. **Steatorrhea** (excess fat in the feces) also may be present if the ulceration extends high in the small intestine. With small intestine involvement, weight loss occurs from malabsorption. Scar tissue from the inflammation narrows the lumen of the intestine and may cause strictures and obstruction, a frequent complication. Intestinal fistulas are a cardinal feature and may develop between segments of bowel. Cutaneous fistulas, common in the perianal area, and rectovaginal fistulas may occur. Fistulas communicating with the urinary tract may cause urinary tract infections. Poor absorption of bile salts by the ileum may lead to watery stools. Fever and unexplained anemia also may occur.

Diagnostic Tests

The most definitive test to differentiate Crohn's disease from ulcerative colitis is colonoscopy with multiple biopsies of the colon and terminal ileum. The appearance of the mucosa in Crohn's disease can range from normal to severely inflamed, and areas of inflammation may be continuous or interspersed with areas that appear normal. The small bowel mucosa may show abnormalities such as a cobblestone appearance, as well as fistulas and strictures of the ileum. Blood tests for anemia also may be ordered. Because viewing the entire small intestine may be limited with traditional endoscopy, capsule endoscopy may be beneficial in the diagnostic process (Crohn's and Colitis Foundation of America [CCFA], n.d.).

Medical Management

Medications. Treatment is individualized depending on the patient's age, the location and severity of the disease, and any complications present. Once Crohn's disease has been diagnosed, the patient is started on drug therapy to try to get the disease in remission. Those with mild to moderate disease usually take antiinflammatory agents such as sulfasalazine, mesalamine, olsalazine, or balsalazide. When inflammation is severe, corticosteroids such as prednisone may be prescribed. Patients are weaned off steroids as soon as possible to prevent dependency and long-term complications. Multivitamins and B_{12} injections often are recommended to correct deficiencies. If first-line therapy fails, treatment with second-line drugs becomes necessary. These include immunosuppressive agents such as azathioprine; cyclosporine (Neoral, Sandimmune); methotrexate; and IV immunoglobulin. Biologic response modifiers such as infliximab (Remicade), adalimumab (Humira), and certolizumab pegol (Cimzia) may be used to treat Crohn's disease.

Diet intervention, stress reduction, and surgery also are used to manage Crohn's disease.

Diet. Bowel symptoms and diarrhea may be minimized by excluding from the diet (1) lactose-containing foods in patients suspected of having lactose intolerance; (2) certain gas-causing vegetables (e.g., cauliflower, broccoli, asparagus, cabbage, Brussels sprouts); (3) caffeine, beer, monosodium glutamate, and sugarless (sorbitol-containing) gum and mints; and (4) highly seasoned foods, concentrated fruit juices, carbonated beverages, and fatty foods.

Diets high in protein (100 g/day) are recommended for patients with hypoproteinemia caused by mucosal loss, malabsorption, maldigestion, or malnutrition. Some patients find small frequent meals to be beneficial to limiting symptoms. Liquids, especially water, should be increased to replace fluid lost. Placing the patient on NPO status and starting total parenteral nutrition may be necessary when the patient with Crohn's disease is having severe symptoms so that the colon can be allowed to rest.

Complications of inflammation with fibrous scarring, obstruction, fistula formation in the small intestine, abscesses, and perforation are indications for surgical excision and anastomosis. Resection is the preferred surgery because the bypass procedure has a greater failure rate.

Surgical treatment. About 75% of patients with Crohn's disease eventually require surgery. Although surgery produces remission, recurrence rates are high. Surgical removal of large segments of the small intestine can lead to short-bowel syndrome, a condition in which the absorption surface is inadequate to maintain life and parenteral nutrition is used. Surgery is reserved for emergency situations (excessive bleeding, obstruction, peritonitis) or when medical treatment has failed. One surgical technique for Crohn's disease is strictureplasty to widen areas of narrowed bowel. It is sometimes necessary to resect the diseased bowel and anastomose the ends. Unfortunately, the disease commonly recurs at the area of anastomosis. Emergency surgery is necessary when perforation allows bowel contents to drain into the abdominal cavity. Surgery to cleanse the peritoneal cavity and create a temporary ostomy frequently is performed.

Nursing Interventions

In caring for the patient with Crohn's disease, consider nutrition, fluid balance, elimination, medications, psychological aspects, and sexuality. Total parenteral nutrition may be ordered in cases of severe disease and marked weight loss. Tube feedings that allow rapid absorption in the upper GI tract are begun, and then oral intake of a low-residue, high-protein, high-calorie diet is introduced gradually. Vitamin supplements are frequently necessary, and vitamin B_{12} is given when there is a marked loss of ileum. When anemia is present, iron dextran (Dexferrum) is given by Z-track injection (because of irritation to the tissues) because oral intake of iron is ineffective because of intestinal ulceration.

Oral diets of 2500 mL/day to replace fluids and electrolytes lost from diarrhea are not uncommon. Monitor the patient for weight loss or gain. Monitor daily skin condition and I&O. A urinary output of at least 1500 mL/day is desired.

When a patient is hospitalized, a bedside commode or a bedpan must be accessible at all times because of the urgency and frequency of stools. Emptying the bedpan immediately and deodorizing the room maintain an aesthetic environment. The anal region may become excoriated from frequent stools. Assess the anal area regularly and keep it clean, using medicated wipes and sitz baths. These nursing interventions promote comfort and hygiene for the patient.

Most patients with Crohn's disease require emotional support from all health care personnel. The onset of the disease often occurs at a young age, before the person has the emotional development and maturity to cope. The support groups sponsored by the CCFA can play a major role in helping patients. Antidepressants and psychology or psychiatry services may be required when managing the disease. Current evidence suggests that Crohn's disease is not caused by psychological stress but that psychiatric disturbances are the result of the disease's symptoms and chronicity.

Patient problems and interventions for patients with Crohn's disease include but are not limited to the following:

Patient Problem	Nursing Interventions
Helplessness, related to exacerbations and remissions	Explore with patient factors that aggravate the disease Assist patient in listing factors that can be controlled: diet, stressors, medication compliance, self-monitoring of symptoms
Insufficient Nutrition, related to: • Bowel hypermotility • Decreased absorption	Emphasize the importance of weighing daily, following special diets, and assessing energy levels

Nursing Interventions and Patient Teaching

The patient must understand how diarrhea and rapid emptying of the small intestine affect the body's nutritional needs. This leads to acceptance of special diets and the ability to retain some personal control of the disease. The patient must also understand the relationship of emotional feelings to Crohn's disease. Identifying resources for emotional support in the family and community and among health professionals promotes coping skills and mental hygiene.

Prognosis

Crohn's disease is a chronic disorder; it has a high rate of recurrence, especially in patients younger than 25 years of age. Prognosis depends on the extent of involvement, duration of illness, and success of medical interventions. No known therapy keeps a patient with Crohn's disease in remission.

ACUTE ABDOMINAL INFLAMMATION

APPENDICITIS

Etiology and Pathophysiology

Appendicitis is the inflammation of the vermiform appendix, usually acute. If undiagnosed, it leads rapidly to perforation and peritonitis. Appendicitis is most likely to occur in persons between the ages of 10 and 30 years.

The vermiform appendix is a small tube in the right lower quadrant of the abdomen. The lumen of the proximal end is shared with that of the cecum, whereas the distal end is closed. The appendix fills and empties regularly in the same way as the cecum. However, the lumen is tiny and easily obstructed. The most common causes of appendicitis are obstruction of the lumen by a fecalith (accumulated feces), foreign bodies, and tumor of the cecum or appendix. If it becomes obstructed and inflamed, pathogenic bacteria *(E. coli)* begin to multiply in the appendix and cause an infection with the formation of pus. If distention and infection are severe enough, the appendix may rupture, releasing its contents into the abdomen. The infection may be contained within an appendiceal abscess or may spread to the abdominal cavity, causing generalized peritonitis.

Clinical Manifestations

Light palpation of the abdomen elicits rebound tenderness in the right lower quadrant (increased pain felt when using the fingertips to press on the abdomen on the opposite side of the suspected problem, then quickly releasing pressure). This is also referred to as Rovsing's sign. The abdominal musculature overlying the right lower quadrant may feel tense as a result of voluntary rigidity. The patient often lies on the back or side with knees flexed in an attempt to decrease muscular strain on the abdominal wall.

Assessment

Subjective data include the most common complaint of constant pain in the right lower quadrant of the abdomen, around McBurney's point (halfway between the umbilicus and the crest of the right ileum). The pain may be accompanied by nausea and anorexia.

Objective data include vomiting, fever, an elevated WBC count, rebound tenderness, a rigid abdomen, and decreased or absent bowel sounds.

Diagnostic Tests

The health care provider orders a WBC count with differential. Most patients have a WBC level above 10,000/mm^3 (the normal range is 4500 to 11,000/mm^3). An abdominal CT scan and abdominal ultrasound are excellent diagnostic tools. Urinalysis also may be performed to rule out a urinary tract infection as the source of pain.

Medical Management

Emergency surgical intervention is the preferred treatment for acute appendicitis, or surgery may be performed when a patient is having another abdominal surgical procedure. Because mortality correlates with perforation and peritonitis, and perforation correlates with duration of symptoms, early diagnosis and appendectomy are essential. Antibiotic therapy is given when perforation is likely. Complications include infection, intraabdominal abscess, and mechanical small bowel obstruction (see the Safety Alert box).

Nursing Interventions and Patient Teaching

Nursing interventions include following general preoperative procedure. Explain diagnostic tests and possible surgical procedures to relieve anxiety. Maintain bed rest and NPO status, provide comfort measures for pain relief so that symptoms are not masked by medication, and replace fluids and electrolytes. The patient's vital signs are monitored and documented every hour because of the threat of perforation with peritonitis.

Administer prescribed opioids after the health care provider has assessed the patient. Opioids can mask symptoms of acute appendicitis. In some cases an ice bag to relieve pain is given; no heat is applied because this increases circulation to the appendix and could lead to rupture. A cleansing enema is not ordered because of the danger of rupture. General postoperative care is performed.

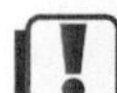

Safety Alert

Appendicitis

- Encourage the patient with abdominal pain to see a health care provider and to avoid self-treatment, particularly the use of laxatives and enemas.
- The increased peristalsis of laxatives and enemas may cause perforation of the appendix.
- Until the patient is seen by a health care provider, he or she should remain NPO to ensure the stomach is empty in case surgery is needed.
- An ice bag may be applied to the right lower quadrant to decrease the flow of blood to the area and impede the inflammatory process.
- *Heat is never used* because it could cause the appendix to rupture.
- Surgery usually is performed as soon as a diagnosis is made.

Patient problems and interventions for the patient with appendicitis include but are not limited to the following:

Patient Problem	Nursing Interventions
Recent Onset of Pain, related to inflammation	Support the patient and the family by listening and by explaining tests and procedures Administer opioids as soon as indicated after the health care provider assesses the patient Monitor for increases in pain, rebound tenderness (Rovsing's sign), and abdominal rigidity Take vital signs frequently (q hr)

Patient teaching may include the reason for IV fluids with gradual advancement of the diet from clear liquids to regular diet as peristalsis returns. If antibiotics or oral medications are continued postoperatively, ensure the patient understands the name, purpose, and side effects of each medication. If complications occur, necessitating an NG tube or drainage tubes, explain the reason for these interventions to the patient.

Prognosis

The rate of cure through surgical intervention is high in patients with appendicitis. The patient's prognosis is altered if peritonitis complicates this diagnosis.

DIVERTICULOSIS AND DIVERTICULITIS

Etiology and Pathophysiology

Diverticular disease has two clinical forms: *diverticulosis* and *diverticulitis.* Diverticulosis is the presence of pouch-like herniations through the circular smooth muscle of the colon, particularly the sigmoid colon (Fig. 45.10).

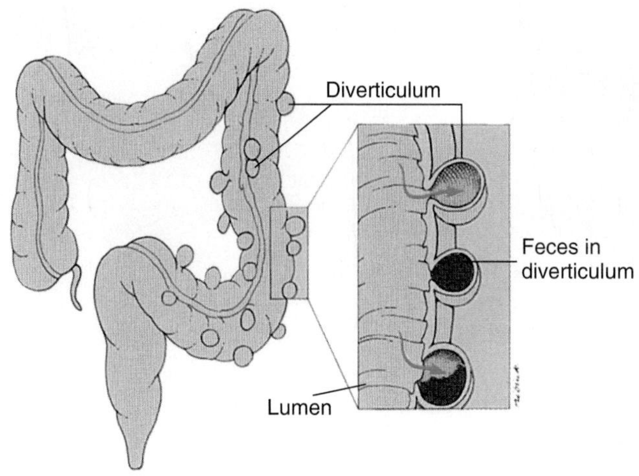

Fig. 45.10 Diverticulosis.

Diverticulitis is the inflammation of one or more of the diverticular sacs.

The incidence of diverticulosis is increased after the age of 40. Several factors are linked to the incidence of the diseases. Aging may lead to decreased strength and elasticity of the colon, resulting in the outward pouching. Lack of fiber in the diet and an increase in refined carbohydrates is also thought to be a contributing factor, causing high pressure in the lumen of the colon. Other contributing factors include lack of exercise, obesity, and smoking. Penetration of fecal matter through the thin-walled diverticula causes inflammation and abscess formation in the tissues surrounding the colon. With repeated inflammation, the lumen of the colon narrows and may become obstructed. When one or more diverticula become inflamed, diverticulitis results, which is a complication of diverticulosis. This inflammation can lead to perforation, abscess, peritonitis, obstruction, and hemorrhage. Diverticulitis is the most common cause of lower GI hemorrhage.

Clinical Manifestations

When diverticula perforate and diverticulitis develops, the patient complains of mild to severe pain in the left lower quadrant of the abdomen, has a fever, and has an elevated WBC count and erythrocyte sedimentation rate. If the condition goes untreated, septicemia and septic shock can develop. This patient is generally hypotensive and is tachycardic. Intestinal obstruction can occur, causing abdominal distention, nausea, and vomiting.

Assessment

Collection of subjective data includes an awareness that the patient with diverticulosis may not display any problematic symptoms. Complaints of constipation and diarrhea accompanied by pain in the left lower quadrant are common. Other common symptoms include increased flatus and chronic constipation alternating with diarrhea, anorexia, and nausea.

Objective data include abdominal distention, low-grade fever, leukocytosis, vomiting, blood in the stool, abdominal tenderness on palpation, and sometimes a palpable abdominal mass.

Diagnostic Tests

Ultrasound and CT scan with oral contrast are used to confirm the diagnosis and evaluate the severity of the disease. A CBC, urinalysis, and fecal occult blood test should be performed. A barium enema occasionally is used to determine narrowing or obstruction of the colonic lumen. Colonoscopy may help rule out polyps or a malignancy. A patient with acute diverticulitis should not have a barium enema or colonoscopy because of the possibility of perforation and peritonitis.

Medical Management

A diet high in fiber, mainly from fresh fruits and vegetables, and decreased intake of fat and red meat are recommended for preventing diverticular disease. High levels of physical activity also seem to decrease the risk.

Weight reduction is important for the obese person. Patients should avoid increased intraabdominal pressure, which may precipitate an attack. Factors that increase intraabdominal pressure are straining at stool; vomiting; bending; lifting; and wearing tight, restrictive clothing.

In acute diverticulitis, the goal of treatment is to allow the colon to rest and the inflammation to subside. Observe the patient for signs of possible peritonitis. Administer broad-spectrum antibiotics as ordered. Monitor the WBC count. Frequently, diverticulitis can be managed in an outpatient setting, and hospitalization is reserved for older adults or those with severe symptoms.

When the acute attack subsides, oral fluids are given initially, progressing to semisolids. The patient should be observed for a recurrent exacerbation. If the patient has a bowel resection or colostomy, the nursing care is the same as previously discussed.

Although diverticular disease is common, complications are rare. Bowel rest and antibiotic therapy are usually adequate. Surgical treatment is advised if long-term problems do not respond to medical management and is likely if complications (e.g., hemorrhage, obstruction, abscesses, or perforation) occur. In elective surgery a thorough bowel preparation is most important. Laxatives, enemas, or intestinal lavage are given to cleanse the bowel, depending on the surgeon's preference. Antibiotics are given orally and parenterally.

In cases of perforation, abscess, peritonitis, or fistula, resection of the bowel with a temporary colostomy is needed. Either the one-stage procedure (resection of the affected bowel with anastomosis and no diverting colostomy) or the two-stage procedure (resection of the diseased bowel with diverting colostomy) is performed.

The bowel diversion can be accomplished by Hartmann's procedure (Fig. 45.11A), in which the descending colon is resected, the proximal end is brought to the

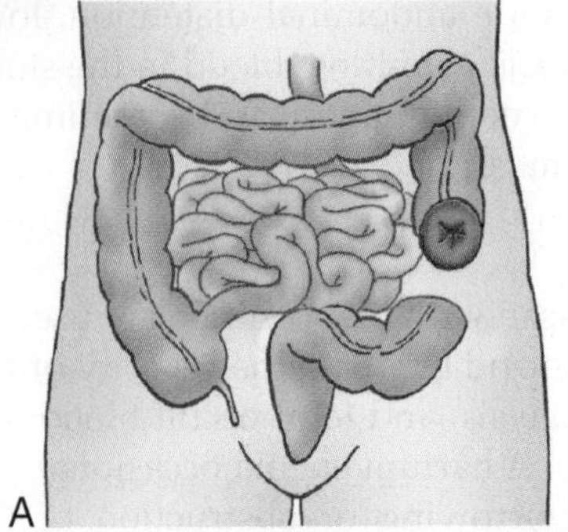

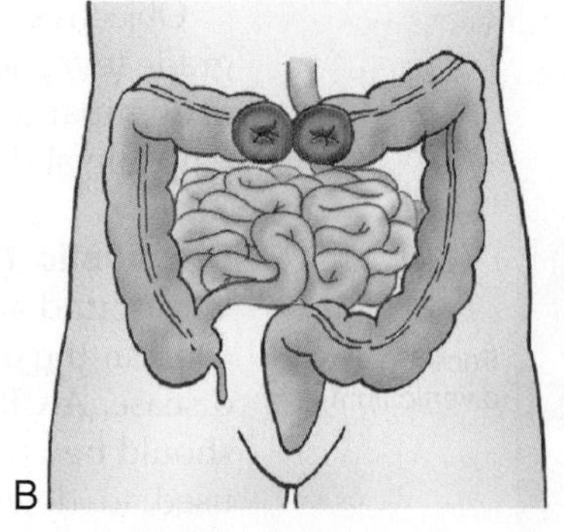

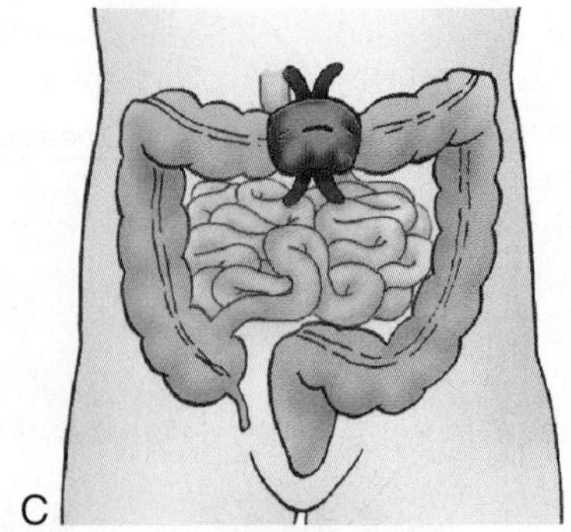

Fig. 45.11 A, Hartmann's pouch. B, Double-barrel transverse colostomy. C, Transverse loop colostomy with rod or butterfly. (Modified from Black JM, Hawks JH: *Medical-surgical nursing clinical management for positive outcomes*, ed 8, St. Louis, 2009, Saunders.)

abdominal wall surface, and the distal bowel is sealed off for later anastomosis. Other procedures are the double-barrel colostomy, in which the bowel is brought up through the abdominal surface (Fig. 45.11B), and transverse loop colostomy, in which a loop is formed and the bowel is held in place with a plastic butterfly bridge between the bowel and the abdomen (Fig. 45.11C). The bowel can be opened at the time of surgery or postoperatively. Removal of the affected bowel segment and reanastomosis of the bowel are included in the initial procedure.

Closure of the temporary colostomy is the desired goal in the case of diverticular disease. Usually this takes place 6 weeks to 3 months after the initial surgical procedure. Again, the bowel must be prepared for closure by a liquid diet; laxatives; antibiotics; intestinal lavage as mentioned; and a cleansing colostomy irrigation of the proximal and, in the case of the loop or double-barrel colostomy, distal end of the stoma.

Nursing Interventions and Patient Teaching

The return of bowel activity after closure may take several days. The patient will have IV fluids and an NG tube for the first few days postoperatively.

Nursing interventions include teaching the patient about the disease process and surgery, if planned. Assess the patient's nutritional status and reinforce the prescribed diet. Assess the patient's pain so that comfort measures or medication can be administered. Include the patient and family in setting goals for the teaching plan.

Patient problems and interventions for the patient with diverticular disease include but are not limited to the following:

Patient Problem	Nursing Interventions
Insufficient Knowledge, related to disease process and treatment	Instruct patient and family in disease process and signs and symptoms of acute diverticulitis attack
Insufficient Nutrition, related to decreased oral intake	Instruct patient about dietary fiber (for prevention) or bland, low-residue diet (for inflammatory phase) Assess daily weights, calorie counts, and I&O Monitor serum protein and albumin

When a colostomy is performed, ask the patient or family member to verbalize and demonstrate understanding of ostomy care. The teaching of colostomy care must not be rushed; the patient should be free of pain and receptive to learning. A family member may be taught to help until the patient is able to assume self-care, keeping in mind that the goal is patient independence. A home care referral may be needed so that the teaching process may continue after discharge.

Prognosis

With diverticulosis, the prognosis is good. Most patients have few symptoms except for occasional bleeding from the rectum. Diverticulitis has a good prognosis; some patients need bowel resection of the affected part in acute cases to reduce mortality and morbidity.

PERITONITIS

Etiology and Pathophysiology

Peritonitis is an inflammation of the abdominal peritoneum. This condition occurs after fecal matter seeps from a rupture site, causing bacterial contamination of the peritoneal cavity. Some examples are diverticular abscess and rupture, acute appendicitis with rupture, and strangulated hernia. Peritonitis also can be caused by chemical irritants, such as blood, bile, necrotic tissue, pancreatic enzymes (pancreatitis), and foreign bodies. Ascites that occurs with cirrhosis of the liver provides an excellent liquid environment for bacteria to flourish. Patients who use continuous ambulatory peritoneal dialysis are also at high risk. No matter what the cause, the resulting inflammatory response leads to massive fluid shifts (peritoneal edema and adhesions as the body attempts to wall off the infection). Sepsis can occur if peritonitis is not treated early enough or if it is not treated successfully.

Clinical Manifestations

Generalized peritonitis is an extremely serious condition characterized by severe abdominal pain. The patient usually lies on the back with the knees flexed to relax the abdominal muscles; any movement is painful. Rebound tenderness, muscular rigidity, and spasm are major symptoms of irritation of the peritoneum. The abdomen is usually tympanic and extremely tender to the touch.

Assessment

Collection of subjective data includes observing for severe abdominal pain. Nausea and vomiting occur, and as peristalsis ceases, constipation occurs with no passage of flatus. Chills, weakness, and abdominal tenderness (local and diffuse, often rebound) are other symptoms.

Collection of objective data includes noting a weak and rapid pulse, fever, and lowered blood pressure. Leukocytosis and marked dehydration occur, and the patient can collapse and die.

Diagnostic Tests

An abdominal x-ray is ordered to find out whether free air is present under the diaphragm as a result of visceral perforation. A CBC with differential is ordered to determine the degree of leukocytosis. A blood chemistry profile helps determine renal perfusion and electrolyte balance. Peritoneal aspiration may be performed and the fluid analyzed for blood, bile, pus, bacteria, or fungus. Ultrasound and CT scans may help identify ascites and abscesses.

Medical Management

Aggressive therapy includes correction of the contamination or removal of the chemical irritant by surgery and parenteral antibiotics. NG intubation is ordered to prevent GI distention. IV fluids and electrolytes are administered to prevent or correct imbalances. Analgesics are provided intravenously via PCA pump. The patient may be placed on total parenteral nutrition because of increased nutritional requirements. Early treatment to prevent severe shock from the loss of fluid into the peritoneal space is essential.

Nursing Interventions and Patient Teaching

Nursing interventions for the patient with peritonitis include the following:

- Place patient on bed rest in semi-Fowler's position to help localize purulent exudate in lower abdomen or pelvis.
- Give oral hygiene to prevent drying of mucous membranes and cracking of lips from dehydration.
- Monitor fluid and electrolyte replacement.
- Encourage deep-breathing exercises; patient tends to have shallow respirations as a result of abdominal pain or distention.
- Use measures to reduce anxiety.
- Use meticulous surgical asepsis for wound care.

Instruct the patient about the importance of ambulation, coughing, deep breathing, use of an incentive spirometer, and leg exercises. If the patient has a draining wound at discharge, teach surgical asepsis for dressing changes. Encourage a nutritious diet. Instruct the patient not to lift more than 10 lb until the health care provider approves it. Stress the importance of keeping health care provider follow-up appointments.

Prognosis

The mortality rate among patients with generalized peritonitis depends on how quickly the infection is diagnosed, as well as age, cause of the peritonitis, and overall condition of the patient. Early recognition and treatment yield a 5% mortality rate, whereas later treatment yields a mortality rate of greater than 30%. Up to 70% of patients who have bacterial peritonitis experience a recurrent episode within 1 year. Delayed treatment often leads to gastrointestinal bleeding, renal dysfunction, and liver failure (Daley, 2017).

HERNIAS

EXTERNAL HERNIAS

Etiology and Pathophysiology

A hernia is the protrusion of a viscus through an abnormal opening or a weakened area in the wall of the cavity in which it normally is contained. Most hernias result from congenital or acquired weakness of the abdominal wall or a postoperative defect, coupled with increased intraabdominal pressure from coughing, straining, or an enlarging lesion within the abdomen.

The various types of hernias include ventral hernia, femoral hernia, inguinal hernia, and umbilical hernia. A ventral, or incisional, hernia is due to weakness of the abdominal wall at the site of a previous incision. It is found most commonly in patients who are obese, who have had multiple surgical procedures in the same area, and who have inadequate wound healing because of poor nutrition or infection. An inguinal hernia is caused by a weakness in the lower abdominal wall opening, through which the spermatic cord emerges in men and the round ligament of the uterus emerges in women. A femoral hernia also is caused by a weakness in the lower abdominal wall, resulting in a bulging of tissue in the patient's groin.

A hernia may be reducible (able to be returned to its original position by manipulation) or irreducible (or incarcerated; unable to be returned to its body cavity). When the hernia is irreducible, it may obstruct intestinal flow. The hernia is strangulated when it occludes blood supply and intestinal flow. To prevent anaerobic infection in the area, immediate surgical intervention is performed when a hernia strangulates.

Factors such as age, wound infection, malnutrition, obesity, increased intraabdominal pressure, or abdominal distention can affect whether a hernia forms after surgical incisions. Fewer hernias occur with transverse incisions than with longitudinal incisions. Also, upper abdominal incisions are associated with fewer hernias than lower abdominal incisions.

Assessment

Collection of objective data includes palpation of the hernia area, revealing the contents of the sac as soft and nodular (omentum; the layer of tissue that surrounds the abdominal organs) or smooth and fluctuant (bowel). Never attempt to push a hernia back into place, because this can lead to complications such as rupture of the strangulated contents.

Subjective and objective signs and symptoms depend on where the hernia occurs. With an inguinal hernia, the patient may complain of pain, urgency, and a mass in the groin region.

Objective data include a visible protruding mass or bulge around the umbilicus, in the inguinal area, or near an incision; this is the most common objective sign. If complications such as incarceration or strangulation follow, the patient may have bowel obstruction, vomiting, and abdominal distention.

Diagnostic Tests

The diagnosis is aided by palpation of the weakened wall. Radiographs of the suspected area may be ordered.

Medical Management

Hernias that cause no discomfort can be left unrepaired unless strangulation or obstruction follows. Teach the patient to seek medical advice promptly if abdominal pain, distention, changing bowel habits, temperature elevation, nausea, or vomiting occurs. If the hernia can be reduced manually, an abdominal binder keeps the hernia from protruding and holds the abdominal contents in place.

Elective surgery for hernia repair may be done because of inconvenience to the patient or constant risk of strangulation. A procedure to close the hernial defect by approximating and suturing the edges of adjacent muscles or using a synthetic mesh is done on either an inpatient or outpatient basis.

Nursing Interventions and Patient Teaching

Nursing interventions for external hernia require observation of the hernia's location and size and tissue perfusion to the area. The patient may be limited in activity and the type of clothing worn.

Herniorrhaphy (surgical hernia repair) usually is performed by a laparoscopic procedure on an outpatient basis. Open abdominal surgery may be necessary for the patient with a strangulated hernia. The patient should be prepared for a longer hospitalization, which may include NG suctioning, IV antibiotics, fluid and electrolyte replacement, and parenteral analgesics until peristalsis returns.

Postoperatively, the patient is monitored for urinary retention; wound infection at the incision site; and, with inguinal hernia repair, scrotal edema. If scrotal edema is present, the scrotum is elevated on a rolled pad with an ice pack applied, and a supportive garment (scrotal support, jockstrap, or briefs) provided. The patient should deep breathe every 2 hours, but many surgeons discourage coughing. Teach the patient how to support the incision by splinting the area with a pillow or pad. This support, along with analgesics, helps relieve pain.

Patient problems and interventions for the patient with a hernia include but are not limited to the following:

Patient Problem	Nursing Interventions
Insufficient Knowledge, related to disease process	Instruct patient to observe and report hernias that become irreducible or edematous Instruct patient to report increased pain, abdominal distention, or change in bowel habits Explain reason to avoid prolonged standing, lifting, or straining Instruct patient to support weakened area by use of truss or manually as needed (as when coughing)
Compromised Blood Flow to Tissue, related to strangulation or incarceration of hernia	Monitor patient for increased pain, distention, changing bowel habits, abnormal bowel sounds, temperature elevation, nausea, and vomiting Report changes in appearance and signs and symptoms to health care provider

Follow-up care includes teaching the patient to limit activities and avoid lifting heavy objects or straining with bowel movements for 5 to 6 weeks. Also, the patient should report to the health care provider immediately any erythema or edema of the surgical area or increased pain or drainage.

HIATAL HERNIA

A hiatal hernia (esophageal hernia or diaphragmatic hernia) results from a weakness of the diaphragm. Hiatal hernia is a protrusion of the stomach and other abdominal viscera through an opening, or hiatus, in the diaphragm (Fig. 45.12). A hiatal hernia is a problem of the diaphragm that affects the alimentary tract. It is an

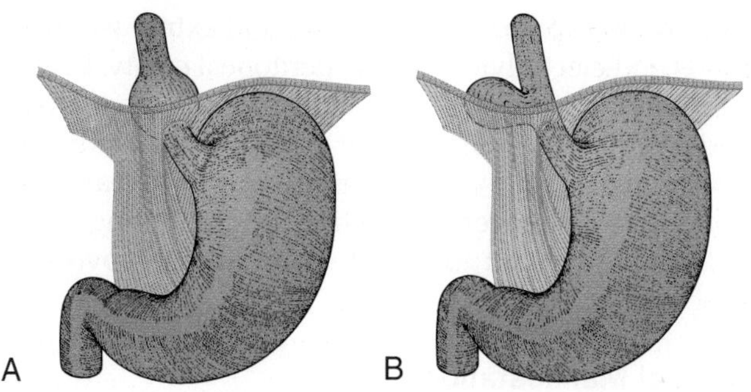

Fig. 45.12 Hiatal hernia. A, Sliding hernia. B, Rolling hernia.

anatomic condition, not a disease. This condition occurs predominantly in individuals over the age of 50 (MedlinePlus, 2018). The major difficulty in symptomatic patients is gastroesophageal reflux, manifested as pyrosis (heartburn) after overeating. Complications of strangulation, infarction, or ulceration of the herniated stomach are serious and require surgical intervention. Factors contributing to the development of these hernias include obesity, trauma, and a general weakening of the supporting structures as a result of aging (see the Lifespan Considerations box).

Lifespan Considerations

Older Adults

Gastrointestinal Disorders

- Loss of teeth and resultant use of dentures can interfere with chewing and lead to digestive complaints.
- Dysphagia commonly is seen in the older adult population and may be caused by changes in the esophageal musculature or by neurologic conditions.
- Hiatal hernias and esophageal diverticula are increased significantly with aging because of changes in musculature of the diaphragm and esophagus.
- Older adults have decreased secretion of hydrochloric acid (hypochlorhydria and achlorhydria) from the parietal cells of the stomach. This results in an increased incidence of pernicious anemia and gastritis in the older adult population.
- Peptic ulcers are common, but often the symptoms are vague and go unrecognized until there is a bleeding episode. Medications such as aspirin, nonsteroidal antiinflammatory drugs, and steroids that are taken for the chronic degenerative joint conditions common with aging should be used with caution because they can contribute to ulcer formation.
- Frequency of diverticulosis and diverticulitis increases dramatically with aging and can contribute to malabsorption of nutrients.
- Constipation is a problem for many older adults. Inactivity, changes in diet and fluid intake, and medications can contribute to this problem. Monitor bowel elimination and establish a bowel regimen to prevent impaction.

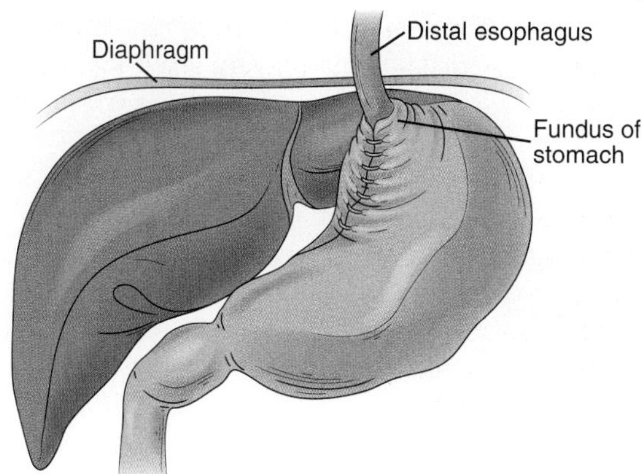

Fig. 45.13 Nissen fundoplication for hiatal hernia, showing fundus of stomach wrapped around distal esophagus and sutured to itself.

Medical Management

The health care provider may perform (1) a posterior gastropexy, in which the stomach is returned to the abdomen and sutured in place; or (2) a laparoscopically performed Nissen fundoplication, in which the fundus of the stomach is wrapped around the lower part of the esophagus and sutured in place (Fig. 45.13). The use of laparoscopic techniques has reduced the overall morbidity, complications, and cost of hospitalization associated with a thoracic or open abdominal approach. However, a thoracic or open abdominal approach may be used in selected cases.

Nursing Interventions

Nursing care of the patient after surgery is similar to that after gastric surgery or thoracic surgery, depending on the procedure performed.

Prognosis

The prognosis for hernias is good because surgical intervention is usually successful. The result can be altered if the patient is a poor surgical risk or has other complications.

DISORDERS OF THE SMALL AND LARGE INTESTINES

INTESTINAL OBSTRUCTION

Etiology and Pathophysiology

Intestinal obstruction occurs when intestinal contents cannot pass through the GI tract. Intestinal obstructions are considered mechanical (e.g., a tumor blocking the intestinal lumen) or nonmechanical (e.g., paralytic ileus after surgery). No matter the cause, an intestinal obstruction can become a life-threatening condition. Prompt assessment of symptoms by the nurse is vital. An obstruction may be partial or complete.

Mechanical obstruction. Mechanical obstruction may be caused by an occlusion of the lumen of the intestinal tract. Most obstructions occur in the ileum, which is the

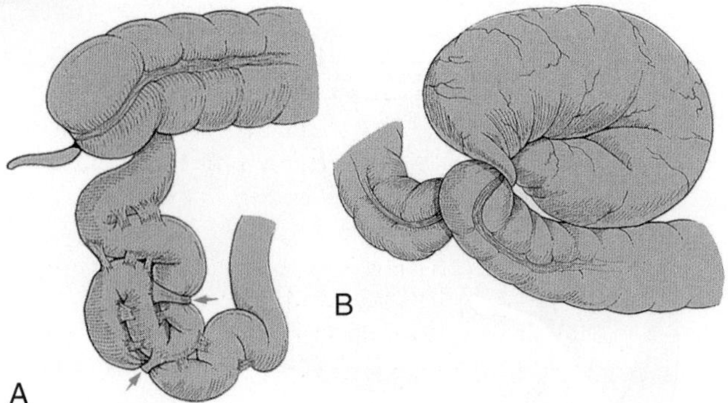

Fig. 45.14 Intestinal obstructions. A, Adhesions. B, Volvulus.

narrowest segment of the small intestine. Adhesions (Fig. 45.14A) from previous abdominal surgeries account for approximately 60% of all intestinal obstructions. Other mechanical obstructions include incarcerated hernias. Additional causes include impacted feces, diverticular disease, tumor of the bowel, intussusceptions, **volvulus** (Fig. 45.14B) (a twisting of bowel onto itself), or the strictures of inflammatory bowel disease. Residues from foods high in fiber, such as raw coconut or fruit pulp, also can obstruct the small bowel.

Nonmechanical obstruction. Nonmechanical obstruction may result from a neuromuscular or vascular disorder, or it may be the result of a general anesthetic during surgery. The cause is something that decreases the muscle action of the bowel and affects the ability of fecal matter and fluid to move through the intestines. **Paralytic (adynamic) ileus** (lack of intestinal peristalsis and bowel sounds) is the most common form of nonmechanical obstruction. It occurs to some degree after any abdominal surgery. Other causes include inflammatory responses (e.g., acute pancreatitis, acute appendicitis), electrolyte abnormalities (especially hypokalemia), and thoracic or lumbar spinal trauma from either fractures or surgical intervention. Vascular obstructions are rare and are due to an interference with the blood supply to a portion of the intestines. The most common causes are emboli and atherosclerosis of the mesenteric arteries. The celiac, inferior, and superior mesenteric arteries supply blood to the bowel. Emboli may originate from thrombi in patients with chronic atrial fibrillation, diseased heart valves, and prosthetic valves.

When the small intestine becomes obstructed, it interrupts the normal process of secretion and reabsorption of 6 to 8 L of electrolyte-rich fluid. Large amounts of fluid, bacteria, and swallowed air build up in the bowel proximal to the obstruction. Water and salts shift from the circulatory system to the intestinal lumen, causing distention and further interfering with absorption. As the fluid increases, so does the pressure in the lumen of the bowel. The increased pressure leads to an increase in capillary permeability and extravasation of fluids and electrolytes into the peritoneal cavity. Edema, congestion, and necrosis from impaired blood supply and possible rupture of the bowel may occur. The retention of fluid in the intestine and peritoneal cavity can lead to a severe reduction in circulating blood volume and result in hypotension and hypovolemic shock.

Clinical Manifestations

The signs and symptoms of intestinal obstruction vary with the site and degree of obstruction. During partial or early phases of mechanical obstruction, auscultation of the abdomen reveals loud, frequent, high-pitched sounds. However, when smooth muscle atony (weak, or lack of normal tone) occurs, bowel sounds are absent.

Assessment

Subjective data include the pattern of the patient's pain, including onset, frequency, and characteristics. Nausea and the inability to pass flatus are common symptoms. Early complaints of obstruction of the small intestine include spasms of cramping abdominal pain as peristaltic activity increases proximal to the obstruction. As the obstruction progresses, the intestine becomes fatigued, with periods of decreased or absent bowel sounds and increased abdominal pain. Note any history of previous bowel disorders or abdominal surgeries and changes in bowel elimination.

Collection of objective data begins with assessing the abdominal surface for evidence of distention, hernias, scars indicating previous surgeries, or visible peristaltic waves. Bowel sounds may be high pitched when assessed in early obstruction, progressing to hypoactive or absent bowel sounds later. Other objective data include vomiting; signs of dehydration caused by the fluid shift; abdominal distention, tenderness, and muscle guarding; and decreased blood pressure.

Obstruction of the colon causes less severe pain than obstruction of the small intestine, marked abdominal distention, and constipation. The patient may continue to have bowel movements, because the colon distal to the obstruction continues to empty.

Diagnostic Tests

Abdominal x-rays are the most useful diagnostic aids. Flat, upright, and lateral x-rays show gas and fluid in the intestines. Intraperitoneal air (sometimes referred to as *free air under the diaphragm*) indicates perforation. Radiographic examination reveals the level of obstruction and its cause. Sigmoidoscopy or colonoscopy may provide direct visualization of an obstruction in the colon. CT scans also may be used in diagnosis. The fluid and electrolyte balance are evaluated through laboratory test results. Elevated blood urea nitrogen and decreased serum sodium, chloride, potassium, and magnesium are common. The patient's hemoglobin and hematocrit levels may increase because of hemoconcentration associated with the fluid volume deficit.

Medical Management

Treatment is directed toward decompression of the intestine by removal of gas and fluid, correction and maintenance of fluid and electrolyte balance, and relief or removal of the obstruction. Treatment may include the evacuation of intestinal contents by means of an intestinal tube. An NG or nasojejunal tube is inserted and connected to wall suction to decompress the intestine. A long intestinal tube (10 ft [300 cm]; e.g., Miller-Abbott) may be used instead of an NG tube to decompress the bowel; however, its use is controversial and limited because it is more difficult and time consuming to insert and may not be more effective than an NG tube. Surgical repair is necessary to relieve mechanical obstructions caused by adhesions, volvulus, and strangulated hernias or if obstruction does not resolve within 48 hours after less invasive therapies have been initiated. Restore fluid and electrolyte balance by carefully monitoring IV infusion. Nonopioid analgesics usually are prescribed to avoid the decrease in intestinal motility that often accompanies the administration of opioid analgesics.

Nursing Interventions and Patient Teaching

Unless surgery is indicated, nursing interventions include carefully monitoring fluids and electrolytes, measuring the patient's urinary output, observing the function of tubes used to decompress and relieve distention, and administering analgesics.

For the patient with intestinal obstruction undergoing surgery, preoperative preparation includes explaining the procedure at a level the patient can understand. Provide emotional support for the patient because he or she is experiencing the stressors of pain and vomiting plus the added stressor of emergency surgery.

Postoperative nursing interventions are similar to those for any patient who has had abdominal surgery. Place the patient in a Fowler's position for greater diaphragm expansion. Encourage the patient to breathe through the nose and not swallow air, which would increase distention and discomfort. Encourage deep breathing and coughing. Continue nasointestinal suctioning until bowel activity returns. Assess for bowel sounds and abdominal girth and expulsion of flatus and stool to help determine the return of peristalsis. When the patient is ready to eat, usually within 24 to 48 hours after surgery or at the first sounds of peristalsis, provide a progressive diet as tolerated. Some patients require temporary bowel diversion via a double-barrel or loop colostomy to manage the obstruction.

To manage pain, administer all medications as prescribed. Medications may include opioids or opioid derivatives.

Patient problems and interventions for the patient with an intestinal obstruction include but are not limited to the following:

Patient Problem	Nursing Interventions
Recent Onset of Pain, related to increased peristalsis	Reposition patient frequently to help intestinal tube advance Irrigate suction tubing with 30 mL of sterile saline to keep tube patent Explain purpose of all procedures Provide comfort measures Administer analgesics as ordered

Follow-up teaching focuses on prevention, including diet and prevention of constipation, as well as early symptoms of recurrence and the need to seek prompt medical care. For the patient with a temporary ostomy, follow-up care is necessary as plans are made for closure of the stoma.

Prognosis

The prognosis depends on early detection of the obstruction and the type and cause of the obstruction, as well as the success of medical interventions. The prognosis is poorer for patients who develop complications such as hypovolemic shock.

CANCER OF THE COLON AND RECTUM (COLORECTAL CANCER)

Etiology and Pathophysiology

Malignant neoplasms that invade the epithelium and surrounding tissue of the colon and rectum are the third most prevalent internal cancers in the United States and the second leading cause of cancer deaths. The American Cancer Society estimates 95,520 new cases of colon cancer and 39,910 new cases of rectal cancer will be diagnosed in 2017. An estimated 50,260 deaths will result from these cancers (ACS, 2017a).

Most growths are seen in the sigmoid and rectal areas of the colon. Cancer occurs with the same frequency in men and women; 9 of 10 colorectal cancer cases occur in people 50 years of age and older.

The cause of colorectal cancer remains unknown, but certain conditions appear to make patients more susceptible to malignant changes. These conditions are termed *predisposing* or *risk factors.* Fortunately, about 85% of colorectal cancers arise from adenomatous polyps, which can be detected and removed from the rectum and sigmoid colon by sigmoidoscopy or colonoscopy. Some diseases, including ulcerative colitis and diverticulosis, increase the risk of colorectal cancer over time. Recent research has isolated a gene that causes colon cancer in certain families. Hereditary diseases (e.g., familial adenomatous polyposis) account for about 5% to 10% of colorectal cancer cases. Hereditary nonpolyposis colorectal cancer syndrome, also called Lynch syndrome, is the most common inherited form of hereditary colorectal cancer. History-taking and regular checkups are important preventive measures.

Other factors implicated in colorectal cancer include lack of bulk in the diet, high fat intake, and high bacterial counts in the colon. It is theorized that carcinogens are formed from degraded bile salts, and the stool that remains in the large bowel for a longer period as a result of too little fiber to stimulate its passage may overexpose the bowel to these carcinogens. Another theory is that the increased transit time for low-fiber foods to pass through the intestine is related to malignancy. These factors support certain dietary changes: decreased animal fat, reduced red meat, and increased high dietary fiber found in fruits, vegetables, and bran may have a protective effect and act as a primary preventive measure. Smoking, excessive intake of alcohol, obesity, and diabetes also have been identified as risk factors.

Clinical Manifestations

Signs and symptoms of cancer of the colon vary with the location of the growth. During the early stages, most patients are asymptomatic. Clinical manifestations are usually nonspecific or do not appear until the disease is advanced.

Assessment

Subjective data include changes in bowel habits alternating between constipation and diarrhea, excessive flatus, and cramps. Constipation is more likely with descending colon cancer, whereas ascending colon cancer may produce no change in bowel habits. Another complaint may be rectal bleeding (the most common sign of colorectal cancer), with the color varying from dark to bright red, depending on the location of the neoplasm. Later stages of colon cancer may involve subjective symptoms of abdominal pain, nausea, and **cachexia** (weakness and emaciation associated with general ill health and malnutrition).

Collection of objective data includes observing for vomiting, weight loss, abdominal distention or ascites, and test results that are compatible with the diagnosis. The most common clinical manifestations are chronic blood loss and anemia.

Diagnostic Tests

Early diagnosis of the tumor, including identification of the cell type involved, is the most important factor in treating the disease. Fecal occult blood tests are an early screening test used to assist in colon cancer detection. Because half of all cases are found in areas of the colon that are inaccessible by sigmoidoscopy, colonoscopy is considered the gold standard for colorectal cancer screening and the detection and removal of precancerous polyps. Other procedures include endorectal ultrasonography and CT scan of the abdomen and pelvis to localize the lesion or determine its size.

A baseline colonoscopy before age 50 should be performed on those who have a family history of colon cancer. Individuals with known gene mutations need to be monitored by colonoscopy every year.

Routine physical examinations should include a digital rectal examination, because rectal polyps and cancer can be reached with a finger, but this method should not be used for fecal occult blood testing. The American Cancer Society has established guidelines for colorectal cancer screening (see the Health Promotion box). In addition to these recommendations other laboratory and diagnostic studies include a UGI series, radiologic abdominal series, and barium enema. Hemoglobin, hematocrit, and electrolyte levels are examined and, if cancer and metastasis are suspected, a blood test is done to detect antibodies to carcinoembryonic antigen (CEA) (an oncofetal glycoprotein, found in colonic adenocarcinoma and other cancers and in nonmalignant conditions; *oncofetal* means occurring in both cancerous tissue and fetal tissue). Because the CEA level can be elevated in benign and malignant diseases, it is not considered a specific test for colorectal cancer. Its use is limited to determining the prognosis and monitoring the patient's response to antineoplastic therapy. Newer diagnostic studies used in colorectal cancer screenings and diagnostics include stool DNA testing. Cologuard DNA testing method was approved by the US Food and Drug Administration (FDA) in 2014 (Nelson, 2014). It detects minute amounts of blood in the stool. It also detects nine DNA biomarkers and three genes that have been found in colorectal cancers.

Health Promotion

Screening for Colorectal Cancer

Current recommendations from the American Cancer Society for colorectal cancer screening are as follows:

- Starting at the age of 50 years, fecal testing for occult blood every year
- Flexible sigmoidoscopy every 5 years (colonoscopy if test results are positive)
- Colonoscopy every 10 years
- Double-contrast barium enema every 5 years
- CT colonography (virtual colonoscopy) every 5 years
- Tests that are done mainly to find cancer:
  - Fecal occult blood test (FOBT) every year
  - Fecal immunochemical test (FIT) every year
  - Stool DNA (sDNA) test
  - Screening for high-risk patients beginning before age 50, usually by colonoscopy

Data from American Cancer Society (ACS): Colorectal cancer screening tests, 2017. Retrieved from *https://www.cancer.org/cancer/colon-rectal-cancer/early-detection/screening-tests-used.html.*

Medical Management

Medical treatment includes radiation, chemotherapy, and surgery. Radiation therapy often is used before surgery to decrease the chance of cancer cell implantation at the time of resection. Radiation can reduce the size of the tumor and decrease the rate of lymphatic involvement. Radiation before surgery has few side effects but some potential complications.

Postoperatively, those patients at high risk for recurrence or people whose disease has progressed may receive radiation administered over 4 to 6 weeks.

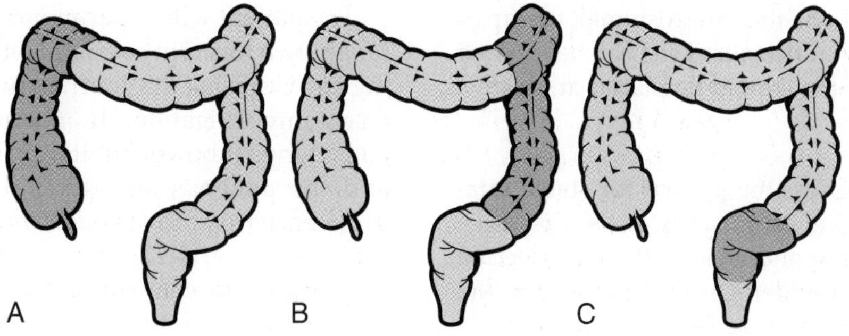

Fig. 45.15 Bowel resection. A, Right hemicolectomy. B, Left hemicolectomy. C, Anterior rectosigmoid resection.

Chemotherapy is given (1) to patients with systemic disease that is incurable by surgery or radiation alone; (2) to patients in whom metastasis is suspected (e.g., when a patient has positive lymph node involvement at the time of surgery); or (3) for palliative therapy to reduce tumor size or relieve symptoms of the disease, such as obstruction or pain. Health care provider opinion and individual patient response vary regarding use of chemotherapy for colorectal cancer.

Surgical interventions depend on the tumor's location, presence of obstruction or perforation of the bowel, possible metastasis, the patient's health status, and the surgeon's preferences. When obstruction has not occurred, a portion of the bowel on either side of the tumor is removed and an end-to-end anastomosis (EEA) is done between the divided ends. When obstruction of the bowel occurs, the commonly used procedures are as follows:

- One-stage resection with anastomosis
- Two-stage resection with (1) the ends of the bowel brought to the surface and creation of a temporary colostomy and mucus fistula or Hartmann's pouch (see Fig. 45.11A); (2) a double-barrel colostomy (see Fig. 45.11B); or (3) a temporary loop colostomy (see Fig. 45.11C), for closure later
- Surgical procedures for colorectal cancer include the following:
  - *Right hemicolectomy:* Resection of ascending colon and hepatic flexure (Fig. 45.15A); ileum anastomosed to transverse colon
  - *Left hemicolectomy:* Resection of splenic flexure, descending colon, and sigmoid colon (Fig. 45.15B); transverse colon anastomosed to rectum
  - *Anterior rectosigmoid resection:* Resection of part of descending colon, the sigmoid colon, and upper rectum (Fig. 45.15C); descending colon anastomosed to remaining rectum

In carcinoma of the rectum, the surgeon makes every effort to preserve the sphincter, often with an EEA. The use of EEA staplers allows lower and more secure anastomosis. The stapler is passed through the anus, where the colon is stapled to the rectum. This technique makes it possible to resect lesions as low as 5 cm from the anus. If the surgeon is unable to perform an anastomosis, an abdominoperineal resection may be done.

In the abdominoperineal resection, an abdominal incision is made and the proximal sigmoid is brought through the abdominal wall in a permanent colostomy. The distal sigmoid, rectum, and anus are removed through a perineal incision (Fig. 45.16). The perineal wound may be closed around a drain or left open with packing to allow healing by granulation. Possible complications are delayed wound healing, hemorrhage, persistent perineal sinus tracts, infections, and urinary tract and sexual dysfunction.

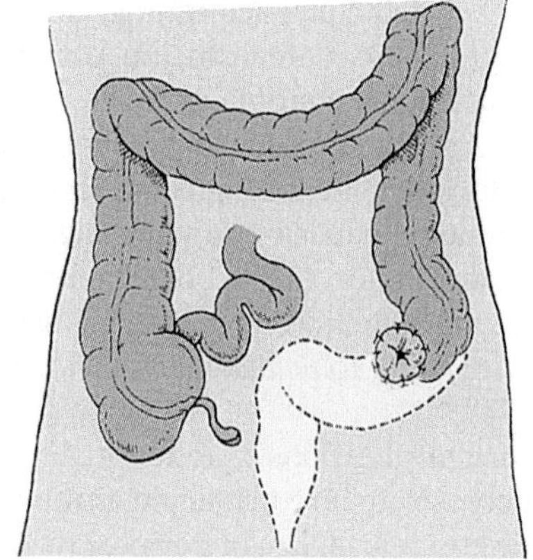
Fig. 45.16 Descending or sigmoid colostomy.

Nutritional status is important because of the threat of infection and a compromised postoperative healing process as a result of constipation, diarrhea, nausea, vomiting, and possible obstruction.

Nursing Interventions and Patient Teaching

Nursing interventions include assessment of bowel and urinary elimination, fluid and electrolyte balance, tissue perfusion, nutrition, pain, gas exchange, infection, and peristomal skin integrity, as discussed previously.

Preoperative care. The patient has some type of bowel preparation, which usually includes 2 or 3 days of liquid diets; a combination of laxatives, or enemas; and oral antibiotics to sterilize the bowel. The antibiotic of choice may be neomycin, kanamycin, or erythromycin; each suppresses anaerobic and aerobic organisms in the colon.

Before surgery, provide instruction in turning, coughing, and deep breathing; use of an incentive spirometer; wound splinting; and leg exercises. Inform the patient that he or she will have IV lines, a Foley catheter, possibly an NG tube, a Davol drain, and abdominal dressings after surgery.

If a stoma is planned, the enterostomal therapist should be notified so that the stoma site can be marked before surgery. The stoma should be placed at the best site for the patient.

Postoperative care. Assess the patient for stable vital signs and return of bowel sounds. Check the dressings for drainage or bleeding and change them as needed as per the health care provider's order. Monitor the NG tube, any wound drains, and the Foley catheter for rate of flow and color of output. Keep accurate I&O records to maintain the fluid and electrolyte balance. Other postoperative care includes coughing, deep breathing, early ambulation, adequate nutrition, pain control, and meticulous wound and stoma care.

Paralytic ileus, a common complication of abdominal surgery, produces the classic signs of increased abdominal girth, distention, nausea, and vomiting. Interventions include decompression of the bowel with an NG tube connected to wall suction, NPO status, and increased patient activity (refer to *Foundations of Nursing,* Chapter 15, Skill 15.7).

Long-term complications of abdominal resection with permanent colostomy are urinary retention or incontinence, pelvic abscess, failure of perineal wound healing, wound infection, and sexual dysfunction.

In addition to monitoring the stoma for color, size, location, and the condition of the peristomal skin, watch for possible complications, including necrosis and abscess. Necrosis results from compromised blood flow to the stoma; the stoma appears pale and dusky to black. Abscess caused by stoma placement too close to the wound, retention sutures, and drains must be assessed promptly. Report all complications promptly to the surgeon and document them in the medical record.

Patient problems and interventions for the patient with cancer of the colon include but are not limited to the following:

Patient Problem	Nursing Interventions
Distorted Body Image, related to loss of normal body function (colostomy)	Allow time for grieving Assist patient and family in accepting ostomy Encourage verbalization. Observe for signs of denial, grief, or anger Answer all questions, and explain treatment and procedure Provide care in positive manner; always avoid facial expressions connoting distaste Provide privacy and a safe environment. Encourage self-care and independence when patient demonstrates readiness Facilitate contact with individuals with similar changes in body image to provide realistic experiences of having ostomy

The patient with a permanent end colostomy can be taught two forms of colostomy management: (1) emptying and cleansing the pouch as needed and (2) managing colostomy irrigation. In planning patient teaching, consider past bowel habits; location of the colostomy; and the patient's age, general health, and personal preference (refer to *Foundations of Nursing,* Chapter 15, Skill 15.11 and 15.12).

Nerves that control the bladder may be damaged when a large amount of tissue is removed in an abdominoperineal resection or if radiation therapy has occurred. When the Foley catheter is removed after surgery, the patient may be unable to void or empty the bladder completely. If the problem does not resolve, the patient may need a Foley catheter and a urology consultation.

When a large amount of tissue is removed, as in an abdominoperineal resection, the cavity left is a sanctuary for bacteria, increasing the risk of infection. Monitor the drain site for increased pain, erythema, and purulent drainage, and monitor for elevated body temperature. The perineal wound may be closed using various techniques. The wound may be closed with a drain to suction. The semiclosed wound usually has either a Davol or Penrose drain left in place, with the drain shortened over time by the health care provider or nurse. The open wound (in which packing is used and later removed) may need irrigation and sitz baths to facilitate healing. Any changes in exudate color and odor and temperature elevation are reported to the surgeon.

Sexual dysfunction for men and women is related to removal of the rectum. Contributing factors may be partial to complete disruption of the nerve supply to the genital organs, psychological factors, or decreased activity associated with age. When the nurse and the patient have a comfortable relationship, it is easier to introduce the topic of sex. Exploring the patient's and the partner's fears and providing information on penile prosthesis surgery and simple suggestions to both partners help decrease anxiety concerning intercourse. Counseling may be necessary if the patient's and the partner's perceptions of body image have been altered. Support groups are available to the cancer patient in most communities. Above all, the nurse's silent communication of touch and eye contact can give the patient a message that he or she is accepted and valued.

Prognosis

The 5-year survival rate for stage I colon cancer is approximately 92%. For stage IIA of the disease, the 5-year relative survival rate is about 87%; for stage IIB cancer, the survival rate is about 63%. Stage III colon cancers range from 89% for stage IIIA to 53% for stage IIIC. Metastatic stage IV colon cancer has a survival rate of 11% (ACS, 2016b). For more information on the staging of colorectal cancer visit *www.cancer.org.*

HEMORRHOIDS

Etiology and Pathophysiology

Hemorrhoids are varicosities (dilated veins) that may occur outside the anal sphincter as external hemorrhoids or inside the sphincter as internal hemorrhoids. This is one of the most common health problems, with the greatest incidence from ages 20 to 50 years. Etiologic factors include straining at stool with increased intra-abdominal and hemorrhoidal venous pressures. With repeated increased pressure and obstructed blood flow, permanent dilation occurs. Hemorrhoids may be caused by constipation, diarrhea, pregnancy, congestive heart failure, portal hypertension, and prolonged sitting and standing.

Clinical Manifestations

The most common symptoms associated with enlarged, abnormal hemorrhoids are prolapse (protrusion outside the anal sphincter) and bleeding. The bright red bleeding and prolapse usually occur at time of defecation.

Assessment

Subjective data include complaints of constipation, pruritus, severe pain when dilated veins become thrombosed, and bleeding from the rectum that is not mixed with feces.

Collection of objective data includes observing external hemorrhoids and palpating internal hemorrhoids. Because bleeding and constipation are signs of cancer of the rectum, all patients with these symptoms should have a thorough examination to rule out cancer.

Diagnostic Tests

Internal hemorrhoids are diagnosed by digital examination, anoscopy, and sigmoidoscopy. External hemorrhoids can be diagnosed by visual inspection and digital examination.

Medical Management

Therapy is directed toward the causes and the patient's symptoms. A high-fiber diet and increased fluid intake prevent constipation and reduce straining, which allows engorgement of the veins to subside. Conservative interventions include the use of bulk stool softeners, as well as bran, and natural food fibers to relieve straining. Topical creams with hydrocortisone relieve pruritus and inflammation, and analgesic ointments relieve pain. Sitz baths usually are given to relieve pain and edema and promote healing.

Rubber band ligation is a popular and easy method of treatment (Fig. 45.17). Tight bands are applied with a special instrument in the health care provider's office, causing constriction and necrosis. The destroyed tissue sloughs off in about 1 week, and discomfort is minimal. Sclerotherapy (with a sclerosing agent injected at the apex of the hemorrhoid column), cryotherapy (tissue destruction by freezing), infrared photocoagulation (destruction of tissue by creation of a small burn), laser excision, and operative hemorrhoidectomy are additional interventions.

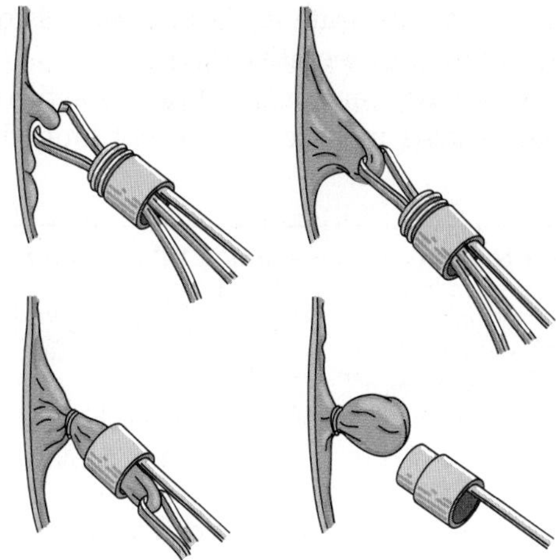

Fig. 45.17 Rubber band ligation of an internal hemorrhoid. (From Monahan FD, Sands JK, Neighbors M, et al: *Phipps' medical-surgical nursing: Health and illness perspectives*, ed 8, St. Louis, 2007, Mosby.)

Hemorrhoidectomy, the surgical removal of hemorrhoids, can be performed if other interventions fail to relieve the distressing signs and symptoms. Surgery is indicated for patients with prolapse, excessive pain or bleeding, or large hemorrhoids. In general, hemorrhoidectomy is reserved for patients with severe symptoms related to multiple thrombosed hemorrhoids or marked protrusion. Surgical removal may be done by cautery, clamp, or excision. After removal of the hemorrhoid, wounds can be left open or closed, although closed wounds are reported to heal faster. Hemorrhoidectomy is not considered a major procedure, but the pain may be acute, requiring opioids and analgesic ointments. Complications include hemorrhage, local infection, pain, urinary retention, and abscess.

Nursing Interventions and Patient Teaching

Rectal conditions can be embarrassing to the patient, and the nurse's direct but concerned attitude can decrease this embarrassment. Assess the knowledge level by asking patients about their condition, what they have been told about treatment, and what treatments have been done before surgery and why.

Observe the patient with a prolapsed hemorrhoid for edema, thrombosis, and ischemia. Ischemic tissue is dark red to necrotic (black). Explain that a low-bulk diet can produce chronic constipation (see the Evidence-Based Practice box on managing chronic constipation in older adults).

For the surgical patient, take vital signs frequently for the first 24 hours to rule out internal bleeding. Sitz baths are given several times daily. Early ambulation and a soft diet facilitate bowel elimination. The patient may have a great deal of anxiety concerning the first defecation; discuss this and provide an analgesic before the bowel movement to reduce discomfort. A stool softener such as docusate (Colace) usually is ordered for the first few postoperative days.

Patient problems and interventions for the patient with hemorrhoids include but are not limited to the following:

Patient Problem	Nursing Interventions
Recent Onset of Pain, related to edema, prolapse, and surgical interventions	Instruct patient to wash anal area after defecation and pat dry Sitz baths or local heat applied to site may be soothing Use of local anesthetics (dibucaine ointment or Tucks pads) may give relief Apply ice packs to hemorrhoids if thrombosed to prevent edema and pain Use cushion for sitting postoperatively
Anxiousness, related to: • Previous experiences • Fear of first bowel movement postoperatively • Lack of knowledge regarding diet	Establish a supportive relationship with patient Explain need for high-residue diet Administer laxatives and oil-retention enema as ordered Give analgesics before first bowel movement and a sitz bath for pain relief

Advise the patient to include bulk-forming foods in the diet, such as fresh fruits, vegetables, and bran cereals, as well as 8 to 10 glasses of fluid a day unless contraindicated. If the patient is anemic, discuss foods high in iron, such as red meats, liver, and dark green leafy vegetables. Sitz baths are recommended for 1 to 2 weeks postoperatively. Emphasize the need for moderate exercise and a routine time for a daily bowel movement. Also instruct the patient to report any signs of infection or delayed healing.

Prognosis

There are several preferred methods of treatment for hemorrhoids. Conservative modes of treatment and surgical intervention for hemorrhoids have good prognostic rates.

ANAL FISSURE AND FISTULA

An anal fissure is a linear ulceration or laceration of the skin of the anus. Usually it is the result of trauma caused by hard stool that overstretches the anal lining. The fissure is aggravated by defecation, which initiates spasm of the anal sphincter; pain; and, at times, slight bleeding. If the lesion does not heal spontaneously, the tract is excised surgically.

An anal fistula is an abnormal opening on the cutaneous surface near the anus. Usually this is from a local crypt abscess; it is also common in Crohn's disease. A perianal fistula may or may not communicate with the rectum. It results from rupture or drainage of an anal abscess. This chronic condition is treated by a fistulectomy (removal) or fistulotomy (opening of the fistula tract).

The postoperative care required for repair of an anal fissure or fistula is similar to that for the patient who has had a hemorrhoidectomy.

Prognosis

The prognosis for anal fissures and fistulas is good, whether the patient is treated with conservative measures or with surgical intervention.

Evidence-Based Practice

Management of Chronic Constipation in Older Adults

EVIDENCE SUMMARY

For adults over the age of 60, chronic constipation is a common occurrence. Primary, or functional, constipation refers to the passage of hard stools with normal frequency, infrequent defecation, or infrequent defecation along with bloating and discomfort. Secondary constipation refers to constipation that is related to disease conditions, medications, or psychosocial concerns. Approximately 50% of nursing home residents experience constipation. The study indicates that if a patient has constipation, there are two pathways to address the problem. If the assessment of the patient indicates a disorder may be present, the patient must be referred to a gastroenterologist. If there is no indication of a disorder, then the suggested line of treatment is (1) behavioral changes (increase fiber and fluids, schedule toileting after meals), if no improvement; (2) administer polyethylene glycol (Miralax), if no improvement; and (3) stool softeners and stimulant laxatives.

APPLICATION TO NURSING PRACTICE

- Note the subjective and objective assessment findings and communicate these findings to the health care provider.
- If the health care provider determines that there is no disorder present, first implement nursing measures to address the constipation.
- Ensure the patient receives a fiber intake of 20 to 35 g per day along with an adequate fluid intake, depending on the patient's condition.
- Ensure a toileting schedule is followed, including toileting after meals when the defecation impulse is generally high.
- Initiate health care provider orders if constipation continues, including polyethylene glycol (osmotic agent that causes water to be retained with the stool), and stool softeners and stimulant laxatives as needed.

REFERENCE

Mounsey A, Raleigh M, Wilson A: Management of constipation in older adults, *Am Fam Physician* 92(6):500–504, 2015.

FECAL INCONTINENCE

Etiology and Pathophysiology

Fecal incontinence is a complex problem that has a variety of causes. The external anal sphincter may be relaxed, the voluntary control of defecation may be interrupted in the central nervous system, or messages may not be transmitted to the brain because of a lesion within or external pressure on the spinal cord. The disorders that cause breakdown of conscious control of defecation include lesions of the cerebral cortex, spinal cord lesions or trauma, and trauma to the anal sphincter (e.g., from fistula, abscess, or surgery). Perineal relaxation and actual damage to the anal sphincter often are caused by injury from perineal surgery, childbirth, or anal intercourse. Relaxation of the sphincter usually occurs with the general loss of muscle tone in aging. The normal changes that occur with aging are usually not significant enough to cause incontinence, however, unless concurrent health problems predispose the patient to the disorder.

Normally the contents of the bowel are moved by mass peristaltic movements toward the rectum. The rectum then stores the stool until defecation occurs. Distention of the rectum initiates nerve signals that are transmitted to the spinal cord and then back to the descending colon, initiating peristaltic waves that force more feces into the rectum. The internal anal sphincter relaxes, and if the external sphincter is also relaxed, defecation results. Defecation is a reflex response to the distention of the rectal musculature, but this reflex can be inhibited voluntarily. Voluntary inhibition of defecation is learned in early childhood, and control typically lasts throughout life. The rectum is emptied when the external anal sphincter (under cortical control) relaxes, and the abdominal and pelvic muscles contract.

Reflex defecation continues to occur even in the presence of most upper or lower motor neuron lesions, because the musculature of the bowel contains its own nerve centers that respond to distention through peristalsis. Therefore, even when the patient has motor paralysis, reflex defecation often persists or can be stimulated. Defecation occurs primarily in response to mass peristaltic movements that follow meals or distention of the rectum. Any physical, mental, or social problem that disrupts any aspect of this complex learned behavior can result in incontinence.

Medical Management and Nursing Interventions

Biofeedback training is the cornerstone of therapy for patients who have motility disorders or sphincter damage that causes fecal incontinence. The patient learns to tighten the external sphincter in response to rectal distention. This technique has been proven effective with alert, motivated patients.

Bowel training is the major approach used with patients who have cognitive and neurologic problems resulting from stroke or other chronic diseases. If a person can sit on a toilet, he or she may be able to defecate automatically given a pattern of consistent timing, familiar surroundings, and controlled diet and fluid intake. This approach allows many patients to defecate predictably and remain continent throughout the day. Surgical correction is possible for a small group of patients whose incontinence is related to structural problems of the rectum and anus.

Patient Teaching

Bowel training requires significant amounts of time and effort on the part of the nursing staff, family, and patient. Incontinence is a major issue in home care and frequently is cited as the most common reason for older adults to be admitted to nursing homes.

To plan the most effective approach, gather specific information concerning the person's general physical and cognitive condition, ability to contract the abdominal and perineal muscles on command, and awareness of the need or urge to defecate. Also, collect data about the nature and frequency of the incontinence problem, particularly its relationship to meals or other regular activities.

Teach the family about the training program and how they can assist and support the effort. This includes the importance of providing a high-fiber diet and ensuring that the patient has a sufficient fluid intake. Evaluate the need for a regular stool softener or bulk former. When an optimal time for defecation has been established, usually after breakfast, a glycerin suppository may be inserted to stimulate defecation.

Despite efforts by family members, staff, and patient, fecal incontinence may remain uncontrolled. Efforts then shift to odor control, prevention of skin impairment, and support for the patient's psychological integrity. Commercially available protective briefs are expensive, but they can reduce the burden of care for the family substantially and provide the patient with a sense of security and dignity.

❖ NURSING PROCESS FOR THE PATIENT WITH A GASTROINTESTINAL DISORDER

◆ ASSESSMENT

To care for the patient admitted with a GI disorder, a thorough, immediate, and accurate nursing assessment is an essential first step. The assessment includes the patient's level of consciousness; vital signs; skin color; edema; appetite; weight loss; nausea; vomiting; and bowel habits, including color and consistency of stools. Assess the abdomen for distention, guarding, and peristalsis. Also obtain a past history of smoking or alcohol use, medications, epigastric or abdominal pain, and acute or chronic stressors and coping/stress tolerance.

◆ PATIENT PROBLEMS

Assessment provides the data for identifying the patient's problems, strengths, potential complications, and learning needs. Once the patient problem statements are defined, assist in formulating a care plan that meets the patient's needs and prioritizing nursing interventions. Possible patient problem statements that should be considered for the patient with a GI disorder include but are not limited to the following:

- *Anxiousness*
- *Compromised Maintenance of Health*
- *Compromised Tissue Perfusion*
- *Discomfort*
- *Distorted Body Image*
- *Fearfulness*
- *Frequent, Loose Stools*
- *Impaired Coping*
- *Inability to Tolerate Activity*
- *Inefficient Sleep Pattern*
- *Infrequent or Difficult Bowel Elimination*
- *Insufficient Nutrition: Less Than Body Requirements*
- *Potential for Compromised Skin Integrity*
- *Potential for Inadequate Fluid Volume*
- *Social Seclusion*

◆ EXPECTED OUTCOMES (GOALS) AND PLANNING

Care planning for the patient with a GI disorder involves looking at the patient problems and establishing nursing interventions to assist in eliminating the problems. Include the patient in planning to promote compliance with the nursing interventions.

The care plan may be based on one or both of the following goals:

Goal 1: Patient will have no evidence of excoriation around stomal area.

Goal 2: Patient will begin to adjust to disturbed body image.

◆ IMPLEMENTATION

Nursing interventions for the patient with a GI disorder may be simple or complex. Interventions include assessment, monitoring nutritional status, administering medications, promoting health, relieving pain, maintaining skin integrity, managing fluid and electrolyte imbalance, promoting normal bowel elimination patterns, preventing wound infection, health counseling to focus on elimination of smoking and excessive alcohol intake, and patient teaching for enterostomal therapy.

◆ EVALUATION

Determining the outcomes of the nursing interventions is an ongoing process that helps the nurse establish the most effective care plan. The nurse and the patient evaluate the goals to see whether the criteria for assessment have been met. Examples of goals and the corresponding evaluative measures are as follows:

Goal 1: Patient will have no evidence of excoriation around stomal area.

Evaluative measure: There is no impairment of skin integrity around stoma.

Goal 2: Patient will begin to adjust to disturbed body image.

Evaluative measures: Patient demonstrates adjustment to disturbed body image by expressing feelings about stoma and is beginning to assume some stoma and pouch care. Goal met.

Get Ready for the NCLEX® Examination!

Key Points

- The digestive tract begins with the mouth, extends through the thoracic and abdominal cavities, and ends with the anus.
- The major processes of digestion and absorption take place in the small intestine.
- The large intestine is responsible for the preparation and evacuation of feces.
- Diet therapy has an important role in the treatment of GI disorders.
- Treatment of esophageal disorders often involves providing the patient with a means of eating in addition to treating the disorder.
- Common causes of gastric disorders are alcohol, tobacco, aspirin, and antiinflammatory agents.
- Duodenal ulcers are the most common type of peptic ulcer disease.
- A relatively new diagnostic examination is capsule endoscopy, in which the patient swallows a capsule equipped with a camera to visualize the small intestine and diagnose diseases such as Crohn's disease.
- Surgical procedures are available as alternatives to the traditional ileostomy and colostomy.
- A nursing goal for the patient with an ileostomy or a colostomy is to foster patient independence in daily care when the patient demonstrates readiness.
- Keeping the surgical area free of contamination is paramount after rectal surgery.
- The approximate location of GI bleeding may be determined by the characteristics of the emesis or the fecal material.
- Explain the purpose of any diagnostic procedure, how the procedure is performed, and the preparation necessary for the procedure, and help the patient understand the results.
- *Helicobacter pylori* has been identified in more than 70% of patients with gastric ulcers and 95% of those with duodenal ulcers.

- Individuals with inflammatory bowel disease have a greater risk of developing cancer of the bowel.
- Early detection of cancer in the GI system facilitates early treatment and a better prognosis.
- An NG tube is inserted to keep the stomach empty until peristalsis resumes after a general anesthetic or any condition that interferes with peristalsis.
- Effective postoperative care begins with patient teaching during the preoperative period.

Additional Learning Resources

SG Go to your Study Guide for additional learning activities to help you master this chapter content.

evolve Be sure to visit the Evolve site at *http://evolve.elsevier.com/Cooper/foundationsadult/* for additional online resources.

Review Questions for the NCLEX® Examination

1. The nurse is caring for a patient who has had a partial gastrectomy. Which vitamin will the nurse anticipate educating the patient about?
   1. A
   2. B_{12}
   3. C
   4. K
2. The nurse is caring for several patients on a medical-surgical unit. Which patient is the nurse most concerned may develop a paralytic (adynamic) ileus?
   1. The patient with impacted feces, tumor of the colon, or pancreatitis
   2. The patient with an electrolyte imbalance, or acute inflammatory reactions
   3. The patient with adhesions or a strangulated hernia
   4. The patient with volvulus, intussusceptions, or electrolyte imbalances
3. The nurse is caring for a patient scheduled for an esophagogastroduodenoscopy. Which intervention should the nurse include in the patient's plan of care? *(Select all that apply.)*
   1. Allow the patient to drink fluids up to 4 hours before the examination.
   2. Withhold any anticholinergic medications before the procedure.
   3. Encourage the patient to not smoke before the examination.
   4. Maintain NPO status until the gag reflex returns postprocedure.
   5. Instruct the patient to contact the health care provider if intense abdominal pain occurs postprocedure.
4. A patient has been admitted with a diagnosis of peptic ulcers. Which drugs would the nurse expect this patient to be prescribed to decrease gastric acid secretion? *(Select all that apply.)*
   1. sodium polystyrene sulfonate
   2. ranitidine (Zantac)
   3. erythromycin (Ery-tab)
   4. sucralfate (Carafate)
   5. famotidine (Pepcid)
5. A patient is scheduled for a hemicolectomy for removal of a cancerous tumor of the ascending colon. The patient asks the nurse why he is taking intestinal antibiotics preoperatively. Which response by the nurse is correct?
   1. To decrease the bulk of colon contents
   2. To reduce the bacteria content of the colon
   3. To prevent pneumonia
   4. To eliminate the risk of postoperative wound infection
6. A patient was admitted during the evening shift with a tentative diagnosis of cancer of the esophagus. What complaint does the nurse anticipate finding in the initial assessment of the patient?
   1. Dysphagia
   2. Malnutrition
   3. Pain
   4. Regurgitation of food
7. When caring for a patient admitted with a bleeding peptic ulcer, the nurse will include what intervention in the patient's acute plan of care?
   1. Measuring the blood pressure and pulse rates each shift
   2. Frequently monitoring arterial blood levels
   3. Observing vomitus for color, consistency, and volume
   4. Checking the patient's stools for occult blood
8. A patient has undergone numerous diagnostic tests to determine whether a gastric malignancy is present. The patient asks the nurse what test will be most definitive for diagnosis. Which response by the nurse is correct?
   1. Radiographic GI series
   2. Breath test for *H. pylori*
   3. Serum test for *H. pylori* antibodies
   4. Endoscopy with biopsy
9. A patient has been prescribed infliximab (Remicade) for the treatment of Crohn's disease. What information should the nurse include in patient teaching regarding this medication?
   1. "This medication is given to suppress your immune system's overactive response."
   2. "This medication has been prescribed to treat the infection in your colon."
   3. "This medication is given to cure your Crohn's disease."
   4. "This medication will decrease the inflammation in your intestine."
10. During assessment of a patient with esophageal achalasia, what does the nurse expect the patient to report when the health history is obtained?
    1. A history of alcohol use
    2. A sore throat and hoarseness
    3. Dysphagia, especially with liquids
    4. Relief of pyrosis with the use of antacids

11. What nursing intervention is most appropriate to decrease postoperative edema and pain in a male patient after an inguinal herniorrhaphy?
    1. Applying a truss to the hernial site
    2. Allowing the patient to stand to void
    3. Supporting the incision during routine coughing and deep breathing
    4. Elevating the scrotum with a support or small pillow
12. The nurse is preparing a presentation on the differences between ulcerative colitis and Crohn's disease. What should the nurse include in the presentation? *(Select all that apply.)*
    1. Ulcerative colitis causes more nutritional deficiencies than Crohn's disease.
    2. Ulcerative colitis is confined to the mucosa and the submucosa of the colon.
    3. The intestinal disease of ulcerative colitis is curable with a colectomy, whereas Crohn's disease often recurs after surgery.
    4. Blood is often present in the stools with ulcerative colitis; fat is usually present in the stools with Crohn's disease.
    5. Patients with ulcerative colitis may have 3 or 4 semisoft stools per day; 15 to 20 liquid stools per day are common with Crohn's disease.
13. Which type of medication order should the nurse question when caring for a patient with *E. coli* O157:H7?
    1. Antiemetics
    2. Antimotility drugs
    3. Antilipidemic agents
    4. Beta blockers
14. The nurse is discharging a patient after a hemorrhoidectomy. Which teaching point should the nurse include in the discharge instructions?
    1. Do not use the Valsalva maneuver.
    2. Eat a low-fiber diet to rest the colon.
    3. Administer an oil-retention enema to empty the colon.
    4. Use a prescribed analgesic before a bowel movement.
15. The student nurse is teaching a patient about his Crohn's disease. The student is correct in identifying what complication as being the result of granulomatous cobblestone lesions of the small intestine?
    1. Malabsorption of nutrients
    2. Severe diarrhea of 15 to 20 stools per day
    3. A high probability of developing intestinal cancer
    4. An inability of the body to absorb water
16. After a transverse loop colostomy, the nurse inspects the patient's stoma. The stoma appears pale pink with some dusky discoloration at the lower border. What is the most appropriate action by the nurse?
    1. Clean the area around the stoma and record the observation in the nurses' notes.
    2. Carefully place a clean pouch over the stoma to prevent any tissue damage.
    3. Cover the stoma with petroleum gauze to prevent any further irritation to the stoma.
    4. Clean the area around the stoma, apply a clean pouch, and notify the health care provider about the discoloration.
17. The nurse is teaching a postgastrectomy patient about dumping syndrome. Which statement indicates that the patient needs further instruction?
    1. "I will lie down after eating a meal."
    2. "I will eat smaller portions of food, more frequently."
    3. "I will not drink liquids when I eat."
    4. "I will avoid fats and increase carbohydrates."
18. A patient has recently been diagnosed with celiac disease. What patient statement indicates the need for further teaching regarding the disease? *(Select all that apply.)*
    1. "I should add pasta and bread back into my diet gradually."
    2. "There is no cure for my disease, but I can manage it well with my diet."
    3. "I will likely need to have surgery to repair the damage to my intestine."
    4. "My children are at a higher risk for developing celiac disease because I have it."
    5. "I will need to eliminate foods containing wheat flour from my diet."
19. While obtaining the patient's health history and reviewing the medical records, which information will alert the nurse that the patient has an increased risk of developing peptic ulcer disease? *(Select all that apply.)*
    1. Excess of gastric acid or a decrease in the natural ability of the GI mucosa to protect itself from acid and pepsin
    2. Invasion of the stomach and/or duodenum by *Helicobacter pylori*
    3. Viral infection, allergies to certain foods, immunologic factors, and psychosomatic factors
    4. Taking certain drugs, including corticosteroids and antiinflammatory medications
    5. Having allergies to foods containing gluten in their ingredients

Care of the Patient With a Gallbladder, Liver, Biliary Tract, or Exocrine Pancreatic Disorder

46

http://evolve.elsevier.com/Cooper/foundationsadult/

Objectives

1. Discuss nursing interventions for the diagnostic examinations of patients with disorders of the gallbladder, liver, biliary tract, and exocrine pancreas.
2. Explain the etiology, pathophysiology, clinical manifestations, assessment, diagnostic tests, medical management, and nursing interventions for the patient with cirrhosis of the liver, carcinoma of the liver, hepatitis, liver abscesses, cholecystitis, cholelithiasis, pancreatitis, and cancer of the pancreas.
3. Discuss specific complications and teaching content for the patient with cirrhosis of the liver.
4. Define jaundice and describe signs and symptoms that may occur with jaundice.
5. State the six types of viral hepatitis, including their modes of transmission.
6. List the subjective and objective data for the patient with viral hepatitis.
7. Discuss the indicators for liver transplantation and the immunosuppressant drugs to reduce rejection.
8. Discuss the two methods of surgical treatment for cholecystitis and cholelithiasis.

Key Terms

ascites (ă-SĪ-tēz, p. 1452)
asterixis (ăs-tĕr-ĬK-sĭs, p. 1455)
biliary atresia (BĬL-ē-ăr-ē ă-TRĒZ-yă, p. 1450)
esophageal varices (ē-sŏf-ă-JĒL VĂR-ĭ-sēz, p. 1453)
flatulence (FLĂT-ū-lĕns, p. 1464)
hepatic encephalopathy (hĕ-PĂT-ĭk ĕn-sĕf-ă-LŎP-ă-thē, p. 1455)
hepatitis (hĕp-ă-TĪ-tĭs, p. 1448)
jaundice (JĂWN-dĭs, p. 1452)
occlusion (ŏ-KLŪ-zhĕn, p. 1468)
paracentesis (pă-ră-sĕn-TĒ-sĭs, p. 1452)
parenchyma (pă-RĔN-kĭ-mă, p. 1450)
sclerotherapy (SKLĔR-ō-THĔR-ă-pē, p. 1454)
spider telangiectases (SPĪ-dĕr tĕl-ĂN-jē-ĕk-TĀ-sēz, p. 1452)
steatorrhea (stē-ăt-ŏ-RĒ-ă, p. 1464)

Chapter 45 discussed the anatomy and function of the organs of the gastrointestinal system, as well as care of the patient with disorders involving the gastrointestinal system. This chapter discusses the care of the patient with disorders involving the accessory organs of the digestive system; specifically, the liver, the gallbladder, and the exocrine pancreas. These organs assist in digestion in various ways.

LABORATORY AND DIAGNOSTIC EXAMINATIONS IN THE ASSESSMENT OF THE HEPATOBILIARY AND PANCREATIC SYSTEMS

SERUM BILIRUBIN TEST

Bilirubin is the pigment that gives bile its yellow-orange color. It is formed when old or damaged red blood cells disintegrate and release their hemoglobin, which is broken down into its component parts, including heme. The heme in turn is converted into bilirubin. Unconjugated (water-insoluble; also called *indirect*) bilirubin passes through the bloodstream to the liver, where it is converted into conjugated (water-soluble; also called *direct*) bilirubin. From here the bilirubin is expelled into the bile. Normal values are as follows:

Direct bilirubin: 0.1 to 0.4 mg/dL
Indirect bilirubin: 0.2 to 0.8 mg/dL
Total bilirubin: 0.3 to 1.2 mg/dL

Rationale

Total serum bilirubin determination measures direct and indirect bilirubin. The total serum bilirubin level is the sum of the direct and indirect bilirubin levels. Testing for bilirubin in the blood provides valuable information for the diagnosis and evaluation of liver disease, biliary obstruction, and hemolytic anemia. Jaundice, the discoloration of body tissues caused by abnormally high blood levels of bilirubin, is visible when the total serum bilirubin exceeds 2.5 mg/dL.

Nursing Interventions

Keep the patient on NPO (nothing by mouth) status until after the blood specimen is drawn. Inform the patient about blood draws and what test is being performed. Monitor the venipuncture site for bleeding.

LIVER ENZYME TESTS

The normal values for liver enzyme test results are as follows:

- *Alkaline phosphatase:* Adult: 30 to 120 units/L. The alkaline phosphatase level is elevated in obstructive disorders of the biliary tract, hepatic tumors, cirrhosis, hepatitis, primary and metastatic tumors, hyperparathyroidism, metastatic tumor in bones, and healing fractures.
- *ALT* (alanine aminotransferase; formerly serum glutamic-pyruvic transaminase [SGPT]): Adult or child: 4 to 36 units/L. The ALT level is elevated in hepatitis, cirrhosis, hepatic necrosis, and hepatic tumors and by hepatotoxic drugs.
- *AST* (aspartate aminotransferase; formerly serum glutamic oxaloacetic transaminase [SGOT]): Adult: 0 to 35 units/L. The AST level is elevated in myocardial infarction, hepatitis, cirrhosis, hepatic necrosis, hepatic tumor, acute pancreatitis, and acute hemolytic anemia.
- *GGT* (gamma-glutamyl transpeptidase): Males and females older than age 45 years: 8 to 38 units/L; females younger than age 45 years: 5 to 27 units/L. Levels are elevated in liver cell dysfunction such as hepatitis and cirrhosis; in hepatic tumors; with the use of hepatotoxic drugs; in jaundice; and in myocardial infarction (4 to 10 days after), heart failure, alcohol ingestion, pancreatitis, and cancer of the pancreas.
- *LDH* (lactic acid dehydrogenase): Adult: 100 to 190 units/L. Values are increased in myocardial infarction, pulmonary infarction, hepatic disease (e.g., hepatitis, active cirrhosis, neoplasm), pancreatitis, and skeletal muscle disease.

Rationale

The liver is a storehouse of many enzymes. Injury or diseases affecting the liver cause release of these intracellular enzymes into the bloodstream, and their levels become elevated. Some of these enzymes also are produced in other organs, and injury or disease affecting these organs raises the serum level. Therefore, although elevation of these serum enzymes is found in pathologic liver conditions, the test is not specific for liver diseases alone.

Nursing Interventions

Provide information to the patient regarding blood draws and what test is being performed. Monitor the venipuncture site for bleeding.

SERUM PROTEIN TEST

The normal values for serum protein test results are as follows:

Total protein: 6.4 to 8.3 g/dL
Albumin: 3.5 to 5 g/dL
Globulin: 2.3 to 3.4 g/dL
Albumin/globulin (A/G ratio): 1.2 to 2.2 g/dL

Rationale

One way to assess the liver's functional status is to measure the products it synthesizes. One of these products is protein, especially albumin. When a disorder or disease affects liver cells (i.e., hepatocytes), they lose their ability to synthesize albumin and the serum albumin level falls markedly. A low serum albumin level also may result from excessive loss of albumin into urine (as in nephrotic syndrome) or into third-space volumes (as in ascites), as well as in liver disease, increased capillary permeability, or protein-calorie malnutrition.

Nursing Interventions

Provide information to the patient regarding blood draws and what tests are being performed. Monitor the venipuncture site for bleeding.

CHOLECYSTOGRAPHY

Rationale

The oral cholecystogram (OCG) provides roentgenographic visualization of the gallbladder after the oral ingestion of a radiopaque, iodinated dye. Adequate visualization requires concentration of the dye within the gallbladder. This test is used much less frequently than in the past. More often, the test is performed via a T-tube with contrast agents such as Hypaque or Renografin. Other options include using a CT scan using the iodine based dye Biliscopin intravenously to evaluate the biliary tree.

Nursing Interventions

To prevent an allergic reaction, determine whether the patient is allergic to iodine, because the dyes typically used for these tests are iodine based. The patient is put on NPO status from midnight. The patient may be given a high-fat meal or beverage to stimulate emptying of the gallbladder after the test has begun. No other food or fluids are allowed until after the examination.

INTRAVENOUS CHOLANGIOGRAPHY

Rationale

In intravenous cholangiography, intravenously administered radiographic dye is concentrated by the liver and secreted into the bile duct. The intravenous cholangiogram (IVC) allows visualization of the hepatic and common bile ducts and the gallbladder if the cystic duct is patent. An IVC is used to demonstrate stones, strictures, or tumors of the hepatic duct, common bile duct, and gallbladder. Intravenous cholangiography is a less commonly used method of visualizing the biliary tree. It should not be used in the jaundiced patient unless it is determined that there are no blocked ducts.

OPERATIVE CHOLANGIOGRAPHY

In operative cholangiography the common bile duct is injected directly with radiopaque dye. Stones appear as radiolucent shadows, and the presence of tumors causes partial or total obstruction of the flow of dye into the duodenum. Visualization of the biliary duct structures provides the surgeon with a "road map" of a difficult anatomic area. This reduces the possibility of inadvertently injuring the common duct.

If common duct stones are suspected, a cholecystectomy and a common duct exploration (CDE) are necessary. When intraoperative cholangiography is used routinely, CDE is performed only on those with positive cholangiograms.

T-TUBE CHOLANGIOGRAPHY

Rationale

T-tube cholangiography (postoperative cholangiography) is performed to diagnose retained ductal stones postoperatively in the patient who has undergone a cholecystectomy and a common bile duct (CBD) exploration to demonstrate good flow of contrast into the duodenum. The test is performed through a T-shaped rubber tube that the surgeon places in the bile duct during the operation. The end of the T tube exits through the abdominal wall, where dye is injected and radiographic films are taken.

Nursing Interventions

During the preoperative phase ensure the patient is not allergic to iodine. Preparation of the patient also includes maintaining NPO status after midnight and until the examination is completed. Administer a cleansing enema on the morning of the examination, if ordered.

Postoperatively, the patient is protected from sepsis by connecting the T tube (if left in place) to a sterile closed-drainage system. If the T tube is removed, cover the T tube tract site with a sterile dressing to prevent bacteria from entering the ductal system.

ULTRASONOGRAPHY OF THE LIVER, THE GALLBLADDER, AND THE BILIARY SYSTEM

Rationale

Ultrasonography (ultrasound, echogram) is an imaging technique that visualizes deep structures of the body by recording the reflections (echoes) of ultrasonic waves directed into the tissues. This diagnostic test is not effective in examining all tissue, because ultrasound waves do not pass through structures that contain air, such as the lungs, the colon, or the stomach. Although fasting is preferred, it is not necessary for ultrasonography. Because ultrasound requires no contrast material and has no associated radiation, it is especially useful for patients who are allergic to contrast media or are pregnant. Ultrasound is used to corroborate data already obtained by "questionable positive" cholangiograms, liver scans, and OCGs. Gallstones are detected easily with ultrasound.

Nursing Interventions

The patient is on NPO status from midnight before the test. If the patient has had recent barium contrast studies, request an order for laxatives because ultrasound cannot penetrate barium, and the study will not be adequate.

GALLBLADDER SCANNING

Rationale

The biliary tract can be evaluated safely, accurately, and noninvasively by intravenous (IV) injection of technetium (^{99}Tc; technetium-99m), and positioning the patient under a camera to record distribution of the tracer in the liver, biliary tree, gallbladder, and proximal small bowel. The primary use of this study is in the diagnosis of acute cholecystitis. This procedure is superior to oral cholecystography, ultrasonography, and computed tomography (CT) scanning of the abdomen for the detection of acute cholecystitis. Hepatobiliary iminodiacetic acid (HIDA) scanning is also useful for identifying diffuse hepatic disease (such as cirrhosis or neoplasm) and a nonfunctioning gallbladder.

Nursing Interventions

Reassure the patient that exposure to radioactivity is minimal, because only a trace dose of the radioisotope is used. The patient is on NPO status from midnight until the examination is complete.

NEEDLE LIVER BIOPSY

Rationale

Needle liver biopsy is a safe, simple, and valuable method of diagnosing pathologic liver conditions. A specially designed needle is inserted through the skin (making it a *percutaneous* procedure), between the sixth and seventh or eighth and ninth intercostal space, and into the liver. The patient lies supine with the right arm over the head. The patient is instructed to exhale fully and not breathe while the needle is inserted. This procedure often is done using ultrasound or CT guidance. A piece of hepatic tissue is removed for microscopic examination. The tissue sample is placed into a labeled specimen bottle containing formalin and sent to the pathology department. Percutaneous liver biopsy is used in the diagnosis of various liver disorders, such as cirrhosis, hepatitis, drug-related reactions, granuloma, and tumor.

Nursing Interventions

After the health care provider has explained the procedure to the patient, verify the patient has signed the consent form. Ensure that measurements of platelets, clotting or bleeding time, prothrombin time, and international normalized ratio (INR) have been ordered; report any abnormal values to the health care provider. After the procedure observe the patient for symptoms of bleeding. Monitor the patient's vital signs every 15 minutes (two times), then every 30 minutes (four times), and then every hour (four times). Keep the patient lying on the right side with a rolled towel against the puncture site for at least 2 hours to splint the puncture site. In this position, the liver capsule (a connective tissue layer covering the liver) is compressed against the chest wall, decreasing the risk of hemorrhage or bile leak.

Some pain is common. When leakage involves a large quantity of blood or bile, the peritoneal reaction is great and the resulting pain severe. Assess the patient for pneumothorax (collapsed lung) caused by improper placement of the biopsy needle into the adjacent chest cavity or for bile peritonitis. Immediately report to the health care provider signs and symptoms of pneumothorax such as shortness of breath, change in respiratory and cardiac rate, or decreased breath sounds on the affected side.

RADIOISOTOPE LIVER SCANNING

Rationale

A radioisotope liver scan is a procedure used to outline and detect structural changes of the liver. A radioisotope (also called a *radionuclide*) is given intravenously. Later, a gamma ray–detecting device (Geiger counter) is passed over the patient's abdomen. This records the distribution of the radioactive particles in the liver. The spleen also can be visualized by the detector when technetium-99m sulfur is used.

Nursing Interventions

The patient is on NPO status from midnight before the test. Assure patients that they will not be exposed to a large amount of radioactivity, because only trace doses of isotopes are used.

SERUM AMMONIA TEST

The normal serum ammonia test value is 10 to 80 mcg/dL.

Rationale

Ammonia is a by-product of protein metabolism. Most of the ammonia is made by bacteria acting on proteins in the intestine. By way of the portal vein, ammonia goes to the liver, where it normally is converted into urea and then excreted by the kidneys. When the patient has severe liver dysfunction or altered blood flow to the liver, ammonia cannot be catabolized, the serum ammonia level rises, and the blood urea nitrogen level decreases. The serum ammonia level is used primarily as an aid in diagnosing hepatic encephalopathy and hepatic coma. Elevated serum ammonia levels suggest liver dysfunction as the cause of these signs and symptoms.

Nursing Interventions

Notify the laboratory of any antibiotics the patient is currently taking. Certain broad-spectrum antibiotics such as neomycin can cause a decreased ammonia level, thus giving inaccurate test results.

HEPATITIS VIRUS STUDIES

A normal laboratory test result is negative for hepatitis-associated antigen.

Rationale

Hepatitis is an inflammation of the liver caused by viruses, bacteria, and noninfectious causes such as alcohol ingestion and drugs. Five viruses, designated A through E, can cause this disease. Hepatitis A, B, and C viruses are the most common hepatitis viruses. Hepatitis D virus is carried by the hepatitis B virus (HBV). Hepatitis D and E viruses are seen less frequently in the United States than are the hepatitis A, B, or C viruses. The various types of hepatitis virus can be detected by their antigen and antibody levels, and their different incubation periods must be considered.

Nursing Interventions

Use standard precautions and handle the serum specimen as if it were capable of transmitting viral hepatitis. Don gloves when handling any blood or body fluids, and wash hands carefully after handling equipment.

SERUM AMYLASE TEST

The normal serum amylase test value is 60 to 120 Somogyi units/dL, or 30 to 220 units/L (SI units).

Rationale

The serum amylase test can aid in quickly diagnosing pancreatitis in its early stages. Damage to pancreatic cells (as in pancreatitis) or obstruction to the pancreatic ductal flow (as in pancreatic carcinoma) causes an outpouring of this enzyme into the intrapancreatic lymph system and the free peritoneum. Blood vessels draining the free peritoneum and absorbing the lymph pick up this excess amylase. An abnormal rise in the serum level of amylase occurs within 2 hours of the onset of pancreatic disease. Because amylase is cleared rapidly by the kidney, serum levels may return to normal within 36 hours. Persistent pancreatitis, duct obstruction, or pancreatic duct leak (e.g., pseudocysts) cause persistent elevated serum amylase levels.

Nursing Interventions

Note on the laboratory order whether the patient is receiving intravenous dextrose or any medications, because these can cause a false-negative result.

URINE AMYLASE TEST

The normal urine amylase test value is up to 5000 Somogyi units/24 h, or 6.5 to 48.1 units/h.

Rationale

Levels of amylase in the urine remain elevated for 7 to 10 days after the onset of pancreatitis. Urine amylase is particularly useful in detecting pancreatitis late in the disease course. This fact is important for diagnosing pancreatitis in patients who have had symptoms for 3 days or longer.

Nursing Interventions

Record the exact time at the beginning and end of the collection period. A 2-hour spot urine or 6-hour, 12-hour, or 24-hour collection can be performed, depending on the health care provider's order. The collection begins after the patient empties the bladder and discards that specimen. All subsequent urine is collected, including the voiding at the end of the collection period. Keep the specimen on ice or refrigerated until it is sent to the laboratory.

SERUM LIPASE TEST

The normal value for serum lipase test results is 10 to 140 units/L.

Rationale

Like serum amylase, serum lipase is elevated in acute pancreatitis and is a helpful complementary test because other disorders (e.g., mumps, cerebral trauma, and renal transplantation) also may cause an increase in serum amylase. Lipase appears in the bloodstream after damage to the pancreas. The lipase levels rise a little later than amylase levels (4 to 48 hours after the onset of pancreatitis), peak around 24 hours, and remain elevated for at least 14 days. Because lipase peaks later and remains elevated longer than amylase, it is more useful in the diagnosis of acute pancreatitis later in the course of the disease.

Nursing Interventions

Instruct the patient to remain on NPO status from midnight, except for water.

ULTRASONOGRAPHY OF THE PANCREAS

Rationale

With the use of reflected sound waves, ultrasonography of the pancreas provides diagnostic information about this inaccessible abdominal organ. Ultrasound examination of the pancreas is used mainly to diagnose carcinoma, pseudocyst, pancreatitis, and pancreatic abscess. Because abnormalities seen on ultrasound persist from several days to weeks, it can support the diagnosis of pancreatitis even after the serum amylase and lipase levels have returned to normal. Furthermore, a follow-up ultrasound study is used to monitor the resolution of pancreatic inflammation and a tumor's response to therapy. A newer procedure using ultrasound is endoscopic ultrasound of the pancreas. In this procedure an ultrasound probe is passed through the patient's mouth and into the small intestine. The sound waves emitted by the probe allow examination of the structures surrounding the pancreas and for fine needle biopsy of the pancreas (the needle is passed through the stomach wall to the pancreas) or lesions of the pancreas to differentiate benign lesions from malignancies. The procedure is an esophagogastroduodenoscopy (EGD) (see Chapter 45) with a camera. In the event that a lesion is cancerous, this procedure also provides staging of the cancer by visualization via ultrasound of the surrounding structures.

Nursing Interventions

Fluids and food are withheld for 8 hours before the examination. If an endoscopic ultrasound is being performed, implement the same interventions as for an EGD (see Chapter 45). If the patient's abdomen is distended with gas or if the patient has had a recent barium examination, the study should be postponed, because gas and barium interfere with sound wave transmission.

COMPUTED TOMOGRAPHY OF THE ABDOMEN

Rationale

A CT scan of the abdomen is a noninvasive, accurate radiographic procedure used to diagnose pathologic pancreatic conditions such as inflammation, tumors, pseudocyst formation, ascites, aneurysms, cirrhosis, abscesses, trauma, cysts, and anatomical abnormalities. The recognizable cross-sectional image produced by a CT scan is especially important for studying the pancreas, because this organ is well hidden by the overlying peritoneal organs.

Nursing Interventions

Fluids and food are withheld from midnight until the examination is complete; however, this test can be performed on an emergency basis on patients who have eaten recently. If possible, show the patient a picture of the machine and encourage the patient to verbalize fears, because some patients suffer claustrophobia when enclosed in the machine.

ENDOSCOPIC RETROGRADE CHOLANGIOPANCREATOGRAPHY OF THE PANCREATIC DUCT

Rationale

Endoscopic retrograde cholangiopancreatography (ERCP) enables visualization not only of the biliary system but also of the pancreatic duct. The test involves inserting a fiberoptic duodenoscope through the oral pharynx, through the esophagus and the stomach, and into the duodenum (Fig. 46.1). Dye is injected for radiographic visualization of the common bile duct and pancreatic duct. ERCP of the pancreas is a sensitive and reliable procedure for detecting clinically significant degrees of pancreatic dysfunction. It also can be used to evaluate obstructive jaundice, remove common bile duct stones, and place biliary and pancreatic duct stents to bypass obstruction. Localized pancreatic duct narrowing indicates the presence of a tumor. Chronic

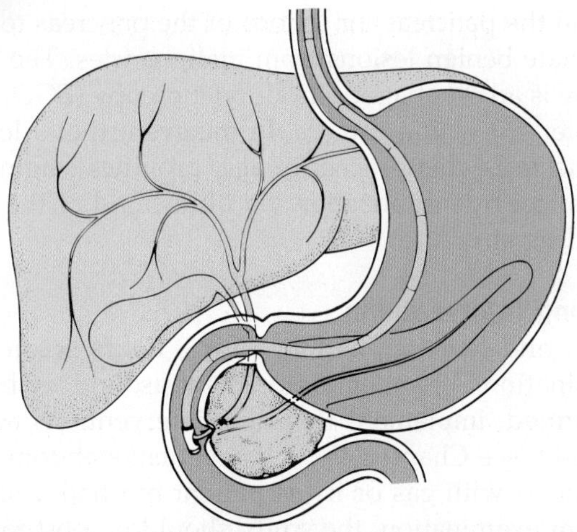

Fig. 46.1 Endoscopic retrograde cholangiopancreatography (ERCP). (From Pagana KD, Pagana TJ: *Mosby's diagnostic and laboratory test reference*, ed 12, St. Louis, 2015, Elsevier.)

pancreatitis is demonstrated by multiple areas of ductal narrowing, which can be visualized by ERCP.

Nursing Interventions

Withhold food and fluids for 8 hours before the examination, and obtain the patient's signature on a consent form. Assess prothrombin time and INR before the procedure. Tell patients that the test takes approximately 1 to 2 hours, during which time they must lie completely motionless on a hard x-ray table, which may be uncomfortable. After the procedure, keep the patient on NPO status until the gag reflex returns; assess for abdominal pain, tenderness, and guarding, which could be signs of perforation. Assess for signs and symptoms of pancreatitis (the most common ERCP complication), including increasingly intense abdominal pain, nausea, fever, chills, vomiting, and diminished or absent bowel sounds. Assess for signs of hypovolemic shock, including decreased blood pressure, increased pulse and respirations, shortness of breath, cool and clammy skin, and decreased urine output.

DISORDERS OF THE LIVER, BILIARY TRACT, GALLBLADDER, AND EXOCRINE PANCREAS

The liver, gallbladder, and exocrine pancreas are organs that assist with digestion. Review the anatomy and physiology of the accessory organs of digestion (see Chapter 45) and the hepatic portal circulation. Refer to Table 46.1 for medications used for disorders of the accessory organs of digestion.

CIRRHOSIS

Etiology and Pathophysiology

Cirrhosis is a chronic, degenerative disease of the liver in which the lobes become covered with fibrous (scar) tissue, the **parenchyma** (i.e., the functional tissue of an organ, as opposed to supporting or connective tissue) degenerates, and the lobules are infiltrated with scar tissue or fat. The liver normally can regenerate itself, but not when cirrhosis is present. In the early stages of the disease the liver can function, but as the disease progresses, the liver fails to perform its normal functions. The overgrowth of new and fibrous tissue restricts the flow of blood to the organ, which contributes to its destruction. Hepatomegaly (enlargement of the liver) and liver contraction (occurs later in the disease) cause loss of the organ's function (NIH, 2014).

Cirrhosis is ranked as the twelfth leading cause of death in the United States. Approximately 38,000 people die each year from the disease. Slightly more men are diagnosed with cirrhosis than women; more than 100,000 people have the disease (Centers for Disease Control and Prevention [CDC], 2016a).

There are several forms of cirrhosis, caused by different factors. *Alcohol-related liver disease* may occur with heavy alcohol consumption. The amount of alcohol that causes damage to the liver differs among individuals. The chances for developing alcohol-related cirrhosis increase for women when they ingest more than two or three alcoholic drinks per day, and for men when they drink three or four drinks per day. *Postnecrotic cirrhosis,* which occurs worldwide, is caused by viral hepatitis (especially hepatitis C, but also hepatitis B and D), exposure to hepatotoxins (e.g., industrial chemicals, drugs, medications), or infection. *Biliary cirrhosis* results from destruction of the bile ducts as a result of inflammation. The resulting damage to the ducts leads to bile backing up into the liver. Conditions such as chronic biliary tree obstruction from gallstones, chronic pancreatitis, a tumor, cystic fibrosis, or **biliary atresia** (the absence of or underdevelopment of biliary structures that is congenital in nature) in children lead to biliary cirrhosis. *Cardiac cirrhosis* results from longstanding, severe right-sided heart failure in patients with cor pulmonale, constrictive pericarditis, and tricuspid insufficiency. *Nonalcoholic fatty liver disease (NAFLD)* results from fat building up in the liver. The incidence of NAFLD is increasing as a result of the growing obesity population. NAFLD also is associated with diabetes, coronary artery disease, and use of corticosteroids.

The cause of cirrhosis is not always known. Alcoholism is by far the greatest factor leading to cirrhosis. It is believed to result from the combination of alcohol's hepatotoxic effect on the liver coupled with the common problem of protein malnutrition seen in alcoholics. Cirrhosis of the liver from severe malnutrition without alcoholism also has occurred.

With repeated insults, the liver progresses through the following stages: destruction, inflammation, fibrotic regeneration, and hepatic insufficiency. Although liver cells have great potential for regeneration, repeated scarring decreases their ability to replace themselves. As the blood supply continues to diminish and scar tissue increases, the organ atrophies.

Table 46.1 Medications for Disorders of the Gallbladder, Liver, Biliary Tract, and Exocrine Pancreas

GENERIC NAME (TRADE NAME)	ACTION	SIDE EFFECTS	NURSING IMPLICATIONS
cholestyramine	Binds bile acids in the GI tract, forming an insoluble complex; relief of pruritus associated with elevated levels of bile acids	Nausea, constipation, abdominal discomfort	Assess severity of pruritus and skin integrity
gemcitabine hydrochloride (Gemzar)	Exhibits antitumor activity; indicated as first-line treatment of locally advanced or metastatic adenocarcinoma of the pancreas	Myelosuppression; nausea and vomiting; macular papular pruritic rash	Monitor CBC. Provide antiemetic to control nausea and vomiting. Provide relief measures to control pruritus
lactulose	Acidifies colonic contents, thus decreasing absorption of ammonia from gut; also has cathartic laxative properties; primarily used in hepatic encephalopathy	Nausea, vomiting, diarrhea	Titrate dose to three or four loose stools per day; monitor for dehydration; monitor for serum ammonia levels and improved mental status
meperidine (Demerol)	Binds to opiate receptors in CNS; alters perception of and response to painful stimuli, while producing generalized CNS depression; used for biliary pain because morphine may cause spasms of the sphincter of Oddi	Sedation, confusion, respiratory depression, hypotension, bradycardia, nausea, vomiting, urinary retention	Assess type, location, intensity of pain before and 1 h after administration. If respiratory rate is <10 breaths/min, assess level of sedation
neomycin	Inhibits protein synthesis in bacteria at the level of the 30S ribosome subunit; decreases the number of ammonia-producing bacteria in the gut as part of management of hepatic encephalopathy	Ototoxicity; local stinging, burning; nephrotoxicity	Monitor neurologic status and renal function
pancrelipase (Pancrease)	Increased digestion of fats, carbohydrate, and proteins in the GI tract; treatment of pancreatic insufficiency associated with chronic pancreatitis, pancreatectomy	Diarrhea, nausea, stomach cramps, abdominal pain	Assess patient's nutritional status; monitor stools for high fat content; assess patient for allergy to pork; administer immediately before meals or with meals
propantheline	Antisecretory and antispasmodic agent; slows GI motility through anticholinergic activity; decreases pancreatic activity	Drowsiness, confusion, dry mouth, constipation, urinary retention, tachycardia, blurred vision	Avoid use with other CNS depressants or alcohol; avoid driving or other activities until accustomed to effects; may cause hypotension when given intravenously; do not use in patients with Parkinson's disease
spironolactone (Aldactone)	Competes with aldosterone at receptor sites in distal tubule, resulting in excretion of sodium chloride and water and retention of potassium and phosphate; used in cirrhosis of the liver with ascites	Headache, confusion, diarrhea, bleeding, dysrhythmias, impotence, hypokalemia	Assess electrolytes, sodium, chloride, potassium, BUN, serum creatinine. Weigh daily; monitor I&O. Administer in the morning to avoid interference with sleep
vasopressin	Synthetic pituitary agent; antidiuretic effects on kidney; a potent vasoconstrictor; used to treat bleeding esophageal varices	Hypertension; ischemia to heart, mesenteric organs, and kidneys; angina; myocardial infarction; water retention; hyponatremia	Use with caution in older adults and in patients with known coronary artery disease or known CHF; discontinue if chest pain develops; monitor urinary output and serum sodium

BUN, Blood urea nitrogen; *CBC,* complete blood count; *CHF,* congestive heart failure; *CNS,* central nervous system; *GI,* gastrointestinal; *I&O,* intake and output.
From Skidmore-Roth L: *Mosby's 2017 nursing drug reference*, ed 30, St. Louis, 2016, Mosby.

Functions of the liver are altered in several ways. The liver's ability to synthesize albumin is reduced as a result of liver cell damage. Obstruction of the portal vein as it enters the liver results in portal hypertension—increased venous pressure in the portal circulation caused by compression or occlusion of the portal or hepatic vascular system. In most instances, portal hypertension that is caused by cirrhosis is irreversible.

This increased pressure causes **ascites** (an accumulation of fluid and albumin in the peritoneal cavity). The damaged liver cannot metabolize protein in the usual manner; therefore protein intake may result in an elevation of blood ammonia levels. Reduced synthesis of protein and the leaking of existing protein result in hypoalbuminemia (reduced protein or albumin level in the blood), which reduces the blood's ability to regain fluids through osmosis. Protein must be present in adequate amounts to create colloidal osmotic pressure and "attract" the fluid to pass back into the blood vessels after it escapes in the capillaries. As fluid leaves the blood and the circulating volume decreases, the receptors in the brain signal the adrenal cortex to increase secretion of aldosterone to stimulate the kidneys to retain sodium and water. The normal liver inactivates the hormone aldosterone, but the damaged liver allows its effect to continue (hyperaldosteronism). Retention of fluid and sodium results in increased pressure in blood vessels and lymphatic channels, resulting in portal hypertension. Ascites is thus a result of portal hypertension, hypoalbuminemia, and hyperaldosteronism.

Hepatic insufficiency gradually causes distention of veins in the upper part of the body, including the esophageal vein. Esophageal varices develop and may rupture, causing severe hemorrhage.

Clinical Manifestations

Clinical manifestations of cirrhosis of the liver differ, depending on the stage of the disease. In the early stages the liver is firm and therefore easier to palpate, and abdominal pain may be present because rapid enlargement produces tension on the organ's fibrous covering. Later stages of the disease are characterized by dyspepsia, changes in bowel habits, gradual weight loss, ascites, enlarged spleen, malaise, nausea, jaundice, ecchymoses, and **spider telangiectases** (small, dilated blood vessels with a bright red center point and spider-like branches). Spider telangiectases occur on the nose, cheeks, upper trunk, neck, and shoulders. These later manifestations are the result of scarring of liver tissue that produces chronic failure of liver function and fibrotic changes that cause obstruction of the portal circulation.

When enough cells of the liver become involved to interfere with its function and obstruct its circulation, the GI organs and the spleen become congested and cannot function properly. Anemia occurs because of the body's decreased ability to produce red blood cells (RBCs). The cirrhotic liver cannot absorb vitamin K or produce the clotting factors VII, IX, and X. These factors cause the patient with cirrhosis to develop bleeding tendencies.

Assessment

Subjective data in the early stages include the patient's description of flulike symptoms (loss of appetite, nausea and vomiting, general weakness, and fatigue), indigestion, abnormal bowel function (either constipation or diarrhea), flatulence, and abdominal discomfort. The anatomic area most commonly affected is in the epigastric region or the right upper quadrant of the abdomen.

Subjective data in the later stages typically include the same early stage symptoms, but now more intense in the later stages. The patient may complain of dyspnea, pruritus, and severe fatigue that interfere with the ability to carry out routine activities. Pruritus results from an accumulation of bile salts under the skin, the result of jaundice.

Collection of objective data in the early stages includes observing low hemoglobin, fever, weight loss, and **jaundice** (yellow discoloration of the skin, mucous membranes, and sclera of the eyes [scleral icterus], caused by greater than normal amounts of bilirubin in the serum). Collection of objective data in the later stages includes noting epistaxis, purpura, hematuria, spider angiomas (telangiectases), and bleeding gums. Late symptoms include ascites, hematologic disorders, splenic enlargement, and hemorrhage from esophageal varices or other distended GI veins. The patient also may appear mentally disoriented and display abnormal behaviors and speech patterns because of increased ammonia levels in the brain. Any prolonged interference with gas exchange leads to hypoxia, coma, and ultimately death.

Diagnostic Tests

Many diagnostic tests aid in the diagnosis of cirrhosis. Poor liver function may be manifest as abnormal electrolyte values; elevated serum bilirubin, AST, ALT, LDH, and GTT; decreased total protein and serum albumin; elevated ammonia; low blood glucose (hypoglycemia) from impaired gluconeogenesis; prolonged prothrombin time; increased INR; and decreased cholesterol levels. Visualization through ERCP (to detect common bile duct obstruction), esophagoscopy with barium esophagography to visualize esophageal varices, scans and biopsy of the liver, and ultrasonography are used to diagnose cirrhosis. **Paracentesis** (a procedure in which fluid is withdrawn from the abdominal cavity) relieves ascites and also provides fluid for laboratory examination.

Medical Management

When possible causes have been identified, the initial treatment is to eliminate those causes, decrease the buildup of fluids in the body, prevent further damage to the liver, and provide individual supportive care. Eliminating alcohol, hepatotoxins (e.g., acetaminophen [Tylenol]), or environmental exposure to harmful chemicals is essential to prevent further damage to the liver. Diet therapy is aimed at correcting malnutrition, promoting the regeneration of functional liver tissue, and compensating for the liver's inability to store vitamins, while avoiding fluid retention and hepatic encephalopathy. A diet that is well balanced, high in calories (2500 to 3000 calories/day), moderately high in protein (75 g of high-quality protein per day), low in fat, low in sodium (1000 to 2000 mg/day), and with additional vitamins and folic acid usually meets the needs of the patient with cirrhosis and improves deficiencies. A protein-restricted diet may be prescribed for a patient recovering from an acute episode of hepatic encephalopathy.

Antiemetics may be prescribed to control nausea or vomiting. Monitor the patient closely for toxicity, which develops quickly when the poorly functioning liver cannot clear these drugs from the system. Diphenhydramine (Benadryl) or dimenhydrinate (Dramamine) may be given, whereas prochlorperazine maleate, hydroxyzine pamoate (Vistaril), ondansetron hydrochloride (Zofran), and hydroxyzine hydrochloride are contraindicated in severe liver dysfunction.

Later manifestations may be severe and result from liver failure and portal hypertension. Jaundice, peripheral edema, esophageal varices, hepatic encephalopathy, and ascites develop gradually (Fig. 46.2).

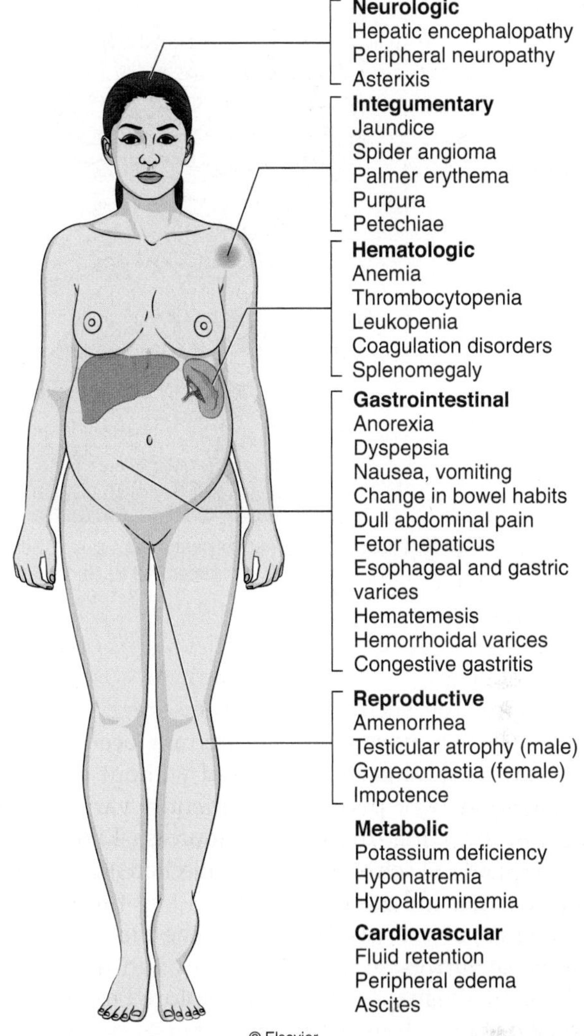

Fig. 46.2 Systemic clinical manifestations of liver cirrhosis.

Complications and treatment. The severity of fluid retention from ascites and edema determines the treatment. Initially the patient is placed on bed rest with accurate monitoring of intake and output (I&O). Restrictions are placed on the amount of fluid (500 to 1000 mL/day) and sodium (1000 to 2000 mg/day) consumed. Diuretic therapy may be added if the diet does not control the ascites and edema. Spironolactone (Aldactone) at 100 to 400 mg/day may be used to obtain the desired diuresis. Other diuretics may be added, including furosemide (Lasix) or hydrochlorothiazide. Vitamin supplements include vitamin K, vitamin C, and folic acid. Salt-poor albumin may be administered in an attempt to restore plasma volume if the intravascular volume is decreased significantly. Complications of diuretic therapy include plasma volume deficit, decreased renal function, and electrolyte imbalance.

Another method of treatment for ascites and edema is the LeVeen continuous peritoneal jugular shunt (Fig. 46.3). This procedure allows the continuous shunting of ascitic fluid from the abdominal cavity through a one-way, pressure-sensitive valve into a silicone tube that empties into the superior vena cava. Patients with this shunt are monitored for complications, which include congestive heart failure, leakage of ascitic fluid, infection at the insertion sites, peritonitis, septicemia, and shunt thrombosis.

Paracentesis (see *Foundations of Nursing*, Chapter 23), in which fluid is removed from the abdominal cavity by either gravity or vacuum, provides temporary relief from ascites. It is imperative that patients urinate immediately before the procedure to prevent puncture of the bladder. The patient should sit on the side of the bed or be placed in a high Fowler's position. An incision is made in the skin, and a hollow trocar, cannula, or catheter is passed through the incision and into the cavity. The fluid is removed over a period of 30 to 90 minutes to prevent sudden changes in blood pressure, which could lead to syncope. Monitor the patient closely for signs of hypovolemia and electrolyte imbalances. Apply a dressing over the insertion site, and observe for bleeding and drainage.

Esophageal varices (a complex of longitudinal, tortuous veins at the lower end of the esophagus) enlarge and become edematous as the result of portal hypertension. They are susceptible to ulceration and hemorrhage; avoiding this is a main goal of treatment. For patients who have not bled from esophageal varices, prophylactic treatment with nonselective beta blockers (e.g., propranolol [Inderal]) has been shown to reduce the risk of bleeding and bleeding-related deaths. Varices can rupture as a result of anything that increases abdominal

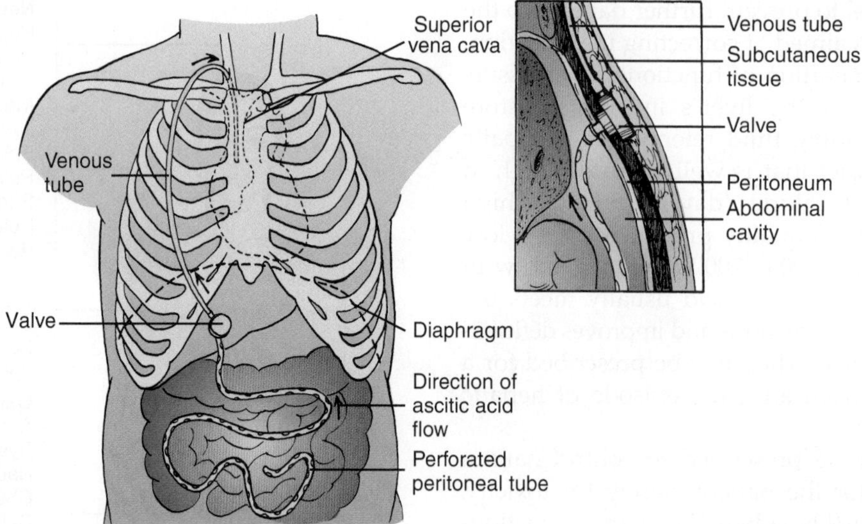

Fig. 46.3 LeVeen continuous peritoneal jugular shunt. (From Black JM, Hawks JH: *Medical-surgical nursing: Clinical management for positive outcomes*, ed 8, St. Louis, 2009, Mosby.)

venous pressure, such as coughing, sneezing, vomiting, or the Valsalva maneuver. Rupture may occur slowly over several days or suddenly and without pain. An endoscopy may be performed to identify varices or to rule out bleeding from other sources. Endoscopic therapies include **sclerotherapy** (the injection of chemicals used to cause inflammation, followed by fibrosis and destruction of the vessels causing the bleeding) and ligation of varices.

Therapeutic management of a ruptured esophageal varix is a medical emergency. The patient's airway must be maintained, the bleeding varix controlled, and IV lines established for fluids and blood replacement as needed. The hormone vasopressin (VP), administered intravenously or directly into the superior vena cava, is used to decrease or stop the hemorrhaging. VP produces vasoconstriction of the vessels, decreases portal blood flow, and decreases portal hypertension. Current drug therapy in some institutions is a combination of VP and nitroglycerin (NTG). NTG reduces the detrimental effects of VP, which include decreased coronary blood flow and increased blood pressure. VP should be avoided or used cautiously in the older adult because of the risk of cardiac ischemia (i.e., a restriction in blood supply to the heart). If the VP drip does not stop or control bleeding, a Sengstaken-Blakemore tube with openings at the tip may be inserted. This triple-lumen tube has a lumen for inflating the esophageal balloon, one for inflating the gastric balloon, and one for gastric lavage (Fig. 46.4). The tube is passed through the nose, and the balloon in the stomach, the one in the esophagus, or both are inflated to press against the bleeding vessels and control the hemorrhage. The gastric aspiration is attached to low, intermittent suction. When either balloon is inflated, a Levin tube is passed into the esophagus through the mouth and attached to low suction to drain the saliva that cannot drain into the stomach. The balloon must be deflated periodically to prevent necrosis. Give the patient nothing by mouth and elevate the head of the bed 30 to 45 degrees to help prevent aspiration of stomach contents and help the patient breathe.

Gastric lavage is performed to remove any swallowed blood from the stomach. Some facilities use iced isotonic saline solutions for the lavage to facilitate vasoconstriction. Endoscopic sclerotherapy also may be used to control the bleeding.

Other methods used to treat bleeding esophageal varices include band ligation. In this procedure an endoscope is passed into the esophagus and elastic bands are placed to tie off bleeding vessels. This procedure also is performed to prevent esophageal varices from bleeding. Band ligation has a small risk of causing scarring of the esophagus. The medication octreotide (Sandostatin) sometimes is used in combination with band ligation when treating bleeding varices. Octreotide (Sandostatin) slows the flow of blood from internal organs to the portal vein. This helps to reduce pressure in the portal vein and is administered for 5 days after an esophageal hemorrhage (Mayo Clinic, 2016a).

Patients suffering from portal hypertension and esophageal varices may benefit from surgical shunting procedures that divert blood from the portal system to the venous system. The portacaval shunt diverts blood from the portal vein to the inferior vena cava. The splenorenal shunt requires the removal of the spleen, and the splenic vein is anastomosed to the left renal vein. The mesocaval shunt involves anastomosis of the superior mesenteric vein to the inferior vena cava. These procedures are associated with a high mortality rate. They may be performed in an emergency to control acute esophageal varix bleeding or in a therapeutic situation when a patient already has

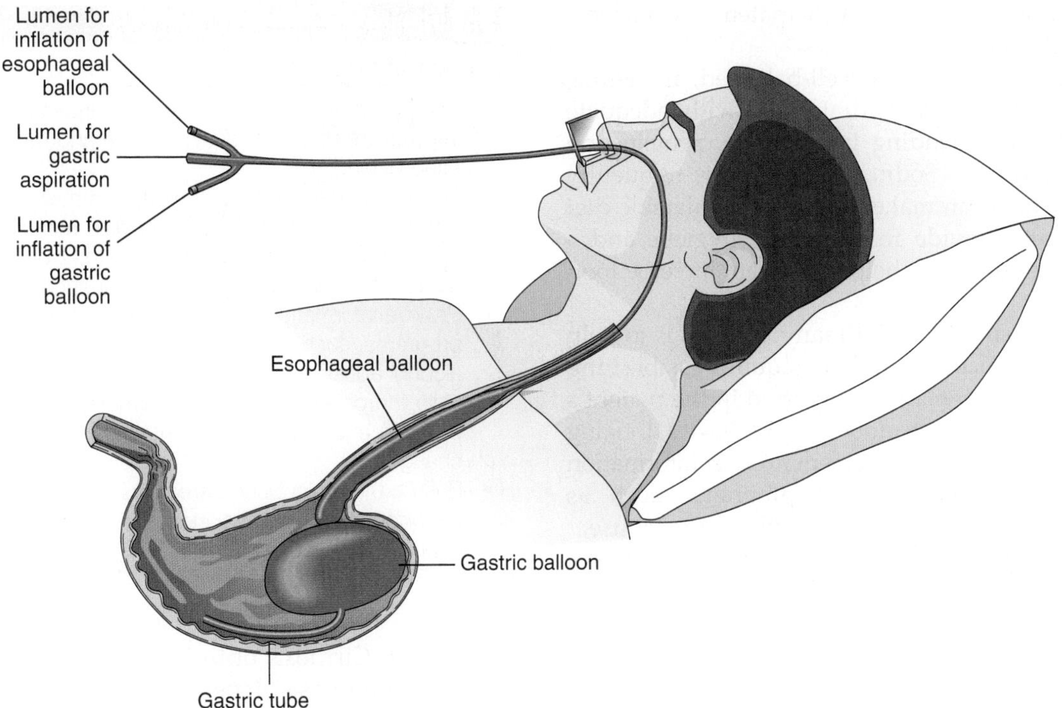

Fig. 46.4 Esophageal tamponade accomplished with a Sengstaken-Blakemore tube. (From Copstead-Kirkhorn LE, Banasik J: *Pathophysiology*, ed 5, St. Louis, 2013, Mosby.)

bled. Complications of surgical shunting procedures are hepatic encephalopathy, GI bleeding, ascites, and liver failure.

Care of the patient who has hemorrhaged from an esophageal varix includes maintenance of oxygen content levels within the blood and administration of fresh frozen plasma and packed RBCs, vitamin K (AquaMEPHYTON), histamine (H_2) receptor blockers such as cimetidine (Tagamet), and electrolyte replacements as needed without fluid overload. Ammonia buildup is avoided with the use of cathartics (e.g., lactulose) and neomycin. Preventing ammonia buildup prevents hepatic encephalopathy.

Hepatic encephalopathy is a type of brain damage caused by liver disease and consequent ammonia intoxication. It is thought to result from a damaged liver being unable to metabolize substances that can be toxic to the brain, such as ammonia. The patient's signs and symptoms progress from inappropriate behavior, disorientation, asterixis, and twitching of the extremities to stupor and coma. **Asterixis** is a hand-flapping tremor in which the patient stretches out an arm and hyperextends the wrist with the fingers separated, relaxed, and extended. A rapid, irregular flexion and extension (flapping) of the wrist occurs in the patient who is acutely ill. Treatment of the patient with hepatic encephalopathy consists of supportive care to prevent further damage to the liver.

In the past, a low-protein diet often was prescribed for patients with cirrhosis of the liver. Restricting protein intake was thought to decrease the amount of ammonia produced in the intestine, thus preventing hepatic encephalopathy. The current belief is that protein should not be restricted, because these patients often have existing malnutrition. On occasion, protein is decreased in the diet of a patient with an exacerbation of hepatic encephalopathy. In addition, carbohydrates are necessary for the patient with cirrhosis (US Department of Veteran Affairs, 2016). If the patient is unable to consume enough nutrients with food, liquid dietary supplements may be added to the diet. The content of supplements varies, so the health care provider should be consulted when choosing the proper supplement.

Teach the patient to avoid potentially hepatotoxic over-the-counter drugs such as acetaminophen and to abstain from alcohol. Medications may be given to cleanse the bowel and help decrease the serum ammonia level. Lactulose decreases the bowel's pH from 7 to 5, thus decreasing the production of ammonia by bacteria within the bowel. Lactulose may be administered orally, as a retention enema, or via nasogastric (NG) tube. It also functions as a cathartic. The lactulose traps ammonia in the gut, and the drug's laxative effect expels the ammonia from the colon. Antibiotics such as neomycin, which are poorly absorbed from the GI tract, are given orally or rectally. They reduce the bacterial flora of the colon. Bacterial action on protein in feces results in ammonia production. Because neomycin may cause renal toxicity and hearing impairment, lactulose frequently is preferred.

Nursing Interventions and Patient Teaching

Check vital signs every 4 hours or more often if evidence of hemorrhage is present. Observe the patient for GI hemorrhage as evidenced by hematemesis, melena, anxiety, and restlessness.

Most patients require a well-balanced, moderate, high-protein, high-carbohydrate diet with adequate vitamins. With impending liver failure, protein and fluids are restricted. Sodium restriction is frequently necessary, which can make providing a palatable diet more difficult. Provide frequent oral hygiene and a pleasant environment to help the patient increase food intake.

A major nursing focus for many patients is to help them deal with alcoholism. This requires establishing trust that the health team is interested in the patient's well-being. Patients must admit that they have a drinking problem before they can be helped. Provide information regarding community support programs, such as Alcoholics Anonymous, for help with alcohol abuse.

Because of pruritus, malnutrition, and edema, the patient with cirrhosis is prone to skin lesions and pressure sores. Initiate preventive nursing interventions to avoid impairment of skin integrity, such as an alternating pressure air mattress, frequent turning, and back rubs. Apply soothing lotion to relieve pruritus.

Observe the patient's mental status and report changes such as disorientation, headache, or lethargy. Assist in activities of daily living (ADLs) as needed to promote good hygiene while allowing the patient to conserve energy. Observe for edema by measuring ankles daily, and observe for ascites by measuring abdominal girth. Record accurate I&O and daily weight. Nursing intervention with concern and warmth regardless of physical changes is essential in helping the patient maintain self-esteem.

Refer to Nursing Care Plan 46.1 for a sample nursing care plan for the patient with cirrhosis of the liver. The patient with cirrhosis must understand the need for getting adequate rest and avoiding infections. Plan activity around complete bed rest until strength is regained. Turning the patient at least every 2 hours and providing range-of-motion exercises help avoid infection and prevent thrombophlebitis. Instruct the patient to use a soft-bristled toothbrush, use an electric razor, blow the nose cautiously, and avoid straining at stools to prevent bleeding as a result of a lack of vitamin K and certain clotting factors. Avoid soap, perfumed lotion, and rubbing alcohol, because they dry the skin. For pruritus caused by dry skin, administer diphenhydramine (Benadryl). Explain the relationship of the therapeutic diet to the diagnosis and the liver's ability to function.

Help the patient and family identify community resources for home health care and alcohol rehabilitation to assist them in dealing with problems that arise after discharge. Because of the seriousness of the disease, the patient and the family need understanding and support throughout the treatment (see the Home Care Considerations box).

 **Home Care Considerations**

Cirrhosis of the Liver

- The patient and the family need to understand the importance of continual health care and medical supervision.
- Encourage measures to achieve and maintain remission. These include proper diet, rest, avoidance of potentially hepatotoxic over-the-counter drugs (e.g., acetaminophen [Tylenol]), and abstinence from alcohol.
- Provide information regarding community support programs, such as Alcoholics Anonymous, for help with alcohol abuse.
- Help the patient maintain the highest level of wellness possible and initiate and maintain necessary lifestyle changes.
- Ensure the patient and caregivers understand the importance of a well-balanced diet. Provide sample diets for reference.

Prognosis. Cirrhosis of the liver cannot be cured; the patient's prognosis depends on many factors. If the cause of the liver damage can be treated or eliminated, the prognosis improves. Discontinuing drinking alcohol and treating the hepatitis help to slow and even stop the progression of cirrhosis. The patient's adherence to prescribed treatment also is a determining factor in the prognosis. Liver transplantation is an option for some patients, but this depends on many factors, including the cause of the cirrhosis and the patient's overall health status.

LIVER CANCER

Etiology and Pathophysiology

The American Cancer Society (ACS) estimates that *primary liver cancer* will be diagnosed in more than 40,000 people in the year 2017 (more than 29,000 men and more than 11,000 women). Of these newly diagnosed cases it is estimated that almost 30,000 will die of the disease. The type of primary liver cancer seen most frequently is hepatocellular carcinoma; the other primary tumors are cholangiomas or biliary duct carcinomas. Cirrhosis of the liver and infection with hepatitis C or hepatitis B are high-risk factors for primary liver cancer. Since 1980 the incidence of liver cancer has more than tripled. The increase in cases of primary liver cancer stems from the increased incidence of hepatitis B. More than 4 million people in the United States are infected with hepatitis B or C (CDC, 2018). Increasing age, obesity, type 2 diabetes, male gender, cirrhosis, and hepatotoxins are some of the risk factors tied to liver cancer.

Metastatic carcinoma of the liver, or *secondary liver cancer*, occurs more often than primary liver cancer (ACS, 2016a). The high rate of blood flow through the portal vein and its massive capillary structure make the metastasis of cancer cells to the liver more likely than to other organs. The pancreas, colon, stomach, breast,

 Nursing Care Plan 46.1 **The Patient With Cirrhosis of the Liver**

Mr. K., 49 years of age, is admitted with loss of appetite, generalized edema, pruritus, flappy tremors of the hands, ascites, and lethargy. He appears disoriented. His skin has areas of excoriation caused by scratching and a sallow appearance. His wife states that he has been unable to concentrate, appears confused and listless, and has been eating poorly. Mr. K. has been an alcoholic for the past 18 years. His total bilirubin is 4.5 mg/dL, GGT is 65 units/L, total protein is 4.8 g/dL, albumin is 2.8 g/dL, and blood ammonia is 160 mcg/dL. He is demonstrating signs and symptoms of hepatic encephalopathy.

PATIENT PROBLEM

Insufficient Nutrition, related to anorexia, nausea, and impaired utilization and storage of nutrients, as demonstrated by lack of interest in food, aversion to eating, inadequate food intake

Patient Goals and Expected Outcomes	Nursing Interventions	Evaluation/Rationale
Patient will eat 50% of meal Patient will maintain baseline body weight	Monitor weight to determine whether weight loss occurs Provide oral care before meals to remove foul taste and improve taste of food Administer antiemetics as ordered to relieve nausea and vomiting Provide small, frequent meals at times the patient can best tolerate them to prevent feeling of fullness and to maintain nutritional status Determine food preferences and allow these whenever possible to increase appeal of food for patient	Patient is eating 50% to 75% of his meals Patient has no weight loss, indicating maintaining satisfactory nutritional balance

PATIENT PROBLEM

Recent Onset of Confusion, related to increased formation of ammonia as demonstrated by inability to concentrate, lethargy, disorientation, and asterixis (hand flapping tremors)

Patient Goals and Expected Outcomes	Nursing Interventions	Evaluation
Patient will be oriented to person, place, time, and purpose	Monitor for hepatic encephalopathy by assessing patient's general behavior, orientation to time and place, speech, and ammonia levels, because liver is unable to convert accumulating ammonia to urea for renal excretion Encourage fluids (if not restricted), and give laxatives and enemas as ordered to decrease ammonia production Provide prescribed protein-restricted diet until acute clinical signs and symptoms of hepatic encephalopathy are decreased Administer lactulose or neomycin as prescribed Limit physical activity because exercise produces ammonia as a by-product of metabolism. Control factors known to precipitate hepatic coma	Patient responds appropriately to assessment of person, place, time, and purpose

CRITICAL THINKING QUESTIONS

1. Mr. K. is thrashing about in his bed and has attempted to climb over the side rails. He is disoriented to time and place. What appropriate nursing interventions will ensure Mr. K.'s safety?
2. Mrs. K. notes that her husband has a low-protein diet. She confides to the nurse that she thinks he needs more meat, eggs, and cottage cheese to improve his nutrition. What is the most appropriate response?

and lung are common primary sites of cancer that metastasizes to the liver.

Clinical Manifestations and Diagnostic Tests

Diagnosing carcinoma of the liver is difficult. In its early stages many of the clinical manifestations (e.g., hepatomegaly, weight loss, peripheral edema, ascites, portal hypertension) are similar to those of cirrhosis of the liver. Other common manifestations include dull abdominal pain in the epigastric or right upper quadrant region, jaundice, anorexia, nausea and vomiting, and extreme weakness. Palpation may reveal an enlarged, nodular liver. Patients frequently have pulmonary emboli. Tests to assist in the diagnosis are a liver scan, ultrasound, CT scan, magnetic resonance imaging, hepatic arteriography, ERCP, and needle liver biopsy. Serum liver function tests can be an early indication that the liver is not functioning properly, but this is not always a routine lab test. The test for alpha-fetoprotein (AFP) may be positive in hepatocellular carcinoma. AFP helps distinguish primary cancer from metastatic cancer (ACS, 2016b).

Medical Management and Nursing Interventions

Treatment of cancer of the liver is largely palliative. Surgical excision (lobectomy) sometimes is performed if the tumor is localized to one portion of the liver. Only a small percentage of patients have surgically resectable disease; usually the cancer is too advanced for surgery when it is detected. Surgical excision or transplantation offers the only chance for cure. Medical management is similar to that for cirrhosis of the liver. Chemotherapy may be used, but the response is usually poor. Portal vein or hepatic artery perfusion with chemotherapy agents such as 5-fluorouracil (5-FU) may be attempted.

Nursing interventions for the patient with liver carcinoma focus on keeping the patient as comfortable as possible. Because the problems are the same as with advanced liver disease, the nursing interventions discussed for cirrhosis of the liver apply.

Prognosis

The 5-year survival rate for liver cancer depends on the extent of the cancer when it is diagnosed. Localized liver cancer (cancer has not spread past the liver) 5-year survival rate is approximately 31%. Regional stage liver cancer (involves the liver and nearby lymph nodes and organs) 5-year survival rate is 11%. Unfortunately, the 5-year survival rate for distant liver cancer (metastases to distant organs or tissues) is 3%. If liver cancer is detected early and the patient has a liver transplant, the 5-year survival rate is 60% to 70% (ACS, 2016c).

HEPATITIS

Etiology and Pathophysiology

Hepatitis is an inflammation of the liver resulting from several types of viral agents or exposure to toxic substances. Rarely, hepatitis is caused by bacteria, such as streptococci, salmonellae, or *Escherichia coli*.

The five major types of viral hepatitis are caused by distinct but similar viruses that produce almost identical signs and symptoms in some of the strains but vary in their incubation period, mode of transmission, and prognosis. Hepatitis A (formerly called infectious hepatitis) is the most common form today and is a short-incubation virus (10 to 40 days). Hepatitis B (formerly called serum hepatitis) is a long-incubation virus (28 to 160 days). Hepatitis C has an incubation period of 2 weeks to 6 months (commonly 6 to 9 weeks). Hepatitis D (also called delta virus) only occurs in people infected with hepatitis B and may progress to cirrhosis and chronic hepatitis. The incubation period is 2 to 10 weeks. Hepatitis E (also called enteric non-A–non-B hepatitis) is transmitted through fecal contamination of water, primarily in developing countries. It is rare in the United States. The incubation period is 15 to 64 days. Hepatitis G virus is a little known strain that infects only 2% to 5% of the population. It frequently coexists with other hepatitis viruses, such as hepatitis C.

Health officials are required by law to report all cases of viral hepatitis to the Centers for Disease Control and Prevention (CDC) in Atlanta, Georgia. Modes of transmission for the various types of hepatitis are listed in Box 46.1.

The basic pathologic findings in the six forms of viral hepatitis are identical. A diffuse inflammatory reaction occurs, liver cells begin to degenerate and die, and the liver's normal functions slow down. The outcome may be affected by the virulence of the virus, the liver's preexisting condition, the health care given when the disease is diagnosed, and patient compliance with treatment.

Box 46.1 Modes of Transmission of the Six Types of Viral Hepatitis

- Hepatitis A spreads by direct contact through the oral-fecal route, usually by food or water contaminated with feces. The incidence of the infection in the United States has decreased significantly because of the availability of the hepatitis A vaccine. People traveling outside the United States should avoid untreated water sources and uncooked food.
- Hepatitis B is transmitted by contaminated serum via blood transfusion, contaminated needles and instruments, needlesticks, illicit intravenous (IV) drug use, and by direct contact with body fluids from infected people, such as breast milk and sexual contact. An ever-increasing risk comes from improper disposal of used needles and syringes. Sharing toothbrushes, razor blades, or personal items with an infected person also may lead to exposure.
- Hepatitis C (HCV) is transmitted through needlesticks, blood transfusions, illicit IV drug use, and unidentified means. HCV also can be transmitted by sharing contaminated straws used for snorting cocaine. In the past, hepatitis C could not be detected in banked blood, so it was transmitted more easily through transfusion. The advent of routine blood screening in 1992 greatly reduced the number of cases of transfusion-related hepatitis C.
- Hepatitis D is transmitted in the same way as hepatitis B; it appears as a coinfection with hepatitis B.
- Hepatitis E is transmitted by the oral-fecal route; it spreads through the fecal contamination of water.
- Hepatitis G is seen frequently as a coinfection with hepatitis C; it spreads through bloodborne exposure. Hepatitis G has been found in some blood donors and can be transmitted by transfusion. Transmission occurs through contaminated injectable drugs; contaminated blood, organs, or tissues; or unsafe methods of tattooing or body piercing.

From World Health Organization: What is hepatitis? 2016. Retrieved from *http://www.who.int/features/qa/76/en/*.

 Safety Alert

Prevention of Acute Viral Hepatitis

HEPATITIS A

- Hand washing is imperative. Hepatitis A virus (HAV) is transmitted when people eat food that is contaminated with fecal material (called "fecal–oral transmission"). Teach patients the importance of good hand hygiene after using the bathroom or changing a diaper, as well as proper food preparation, to prevent the spread of HAV. There are several documented cases of HAV being linked to food preparation and handling in restaurants.
- The best protection against HAV transmission is the two-dose HAV vaccine.

HEPATITIS B

- Wash hands.
- One of the best preventive measures against hepatitis B virus (HBV) is the HBV vaccine.
- Hepatitis B is transmitted via blood and body fluids.
- Children younger than 18 years of age are vaccinated routinely.
- People who are at risk for the virus, such as health care workers, should be vaccinated.
- People who play or work in inner-city parks and playgrounds are at risk for exposure to HBV from garbage containers and used needles and syringes. They should be vaccinated, as should men who have sex with men, individuals who use illicit IV drugs, and those who travel to areas with a high infection rate. Individuals who are traveling internationally should be vaccinated.
- People who are positive for HBV should not donate blood, organs, or tissue, and should not breastfeed.
- Ensure proper disposal of needles.
- Use standard precautions when handling blood products.
- Use needleless IV access devices if available.

HEPATITIS C

- Wash hands.
- Hepatitis C virus is transmitted by needle sharing among illicit IV drug users.
- Other significant risk factors include receipt of clotting factor made before 1987, hemodialysis, receipt of blood or solid organs donated before 1992, maternal-fetal transmission, and multiple or infected sex partners.
- Ensure proper disposal of needles.
- Use standard precautions when handling blood products.
- Use needleless IV access devices if available.

HEPATITIS D

- Modes of hepatitis D virus (HDV) transmission are similar to those of HBV. Sexual transmission of HDV is less efficient than for HBV. Educate patients regarding risky behavior.

HEPATITIS E

- Educate patients to avoid drinking water or beverages with ice in areas with uncertain water quality. They should refrain from eating raw shellfish and avoid raw produce unless it is prepared with purified water.
- Hepatitis E is seen most often in Southeast and Central Asia, the Middle East, Africa, and Mexico.

HEPATITIS G

- Hepatitis G has been detected in blood samples in Europe, Asia, and Australia.
- Transmission of hepatitis G virus occurs when tainted injectable drugs are used; tainted blood, organs, or tissues are received; or unsafe methods are used for tattooing or body piercing.

Clinical Manifestations

The clinical manifestations for viral hepatitis vary greatly; some patients are asymptomatic, whereas others develop hepatic failure or hepatic encephalopathy.

Assessment

Subjective data include patients' reports of general malaise, aching muscles, photophobia, lassitude, headaches, and chills. Abdominal pain, dyspepsia, nausea, diarrhea, and constipation are reported also. The patient may complain of pruritus from the buildup of bile salts in the skin. The patient complains of tenderness in the liver and remains fatigued for several weeks.

Collection of objective data includes observing hepatomegaly, enlarged lymph nodes, and weight loss. Jaundice appears because of the damaged liver's inability to metabolize bilirubin; the resultant signs are yellowish skin; discoloration of the sclera (scleral icterus) and mucous membranes; dark, tea-colored urine; and clay-colored stools. Relapses are common in the convalescent stage.

Diagnostic Tests

Changes in the liver caused by viral hepatitis result in elevated direct bilirubin, GGT, AST, ALT, LDH, and alkaline phosphatase levels; a prolonged prothrombin time and increased INR; and, in severe hepatitis, decreased serum albumin. Leukopenia (low white blood cell count) is common in these patients, followed by lymphocytosis (high white blood cell count). Hypoglycemia is present in approximately 50% of patients with hepatitis. Serum is examined for the presence of antigens associated with hepatitis A, B, C, D, or G. A CT scan of the abdomen reveals hepatomegaly.

Medical Management

Providing supportive therapy for existing signs and symptoms and preventing transmission of the disease are important aspects of treatment of the patient with viral hepatitis. Hospitalization is an option for patients whose bilirubin concentrations in the blood are more than 10 mg/dL and for those with a prolonged prothrombin time and increased INR, but usually patients are cared for at home. Bed rest for several weeks commonly is prescribed.

Drug therapy for chronic hepatitis B focuses on decreasing the viral load, decreasing the rate of disease progression, and monitoring for detection of drug-resistant HBV. Drugs that are considered first line treatment for chronic HBV include pegylated interferon alfa (PEG-IFN-a), entecavir (ETV), and tenofovir disoproxil fumarate (TDF). These are antiviral medications used to stop or reverse the progression of HBV. A serious side effect that is associated with these medications is lactic acidosis that is caused by the buildup of lactic acid in the bloodstream. Common symptoms of lactic acidosis include nausea, abdominal pain, elevated heart rate, muscle ache and weakness, and unintentional weight loss. Liver failure can result from this condition.

In chronic hepatitis C, drug therapy also is directed at reducing the viral load, decreasing progression of the disease, and promoting seroconversion. Treatment options for HCV are interferon alfa-2b (Intron A), ribavirin (Rebetol), and pegylated interferon alfa-2a (Pegasys). This combination therapy eradicates the virus more effectively than monotherapy. Another treatment option is liver transplantation. In fact, half of all liver recipients are HCV positive. Most transplanted livers eventually become infected with HCV, but recipients can increase quantity and quality of life by avoiding risky behaviors (US Food and Drug Administration, 2017).

The patient is not allowed alcohol for at least 1 year and may need supportive care from the community to comply. Most patients tolerate small, frequent meals of a low-fat, high-carbohydrate diet. If the patient is dehydrated, IV fluids are given with addition of vitamin C for healing, vitamin B complex to assist the damaged liver's inability to absorb fat-soluble vitamins, and vitamin K to combat prolonged coagulation time. Avoid all unnecessary medications, particularly sedatives.

Give gamma globulin or immune serum globulin as soon as possible to people who have been in direct contact with a person with hepatitis A during the infectious period (2 weeks before and 1 week after onset of symptoms). A dose of 0.1 to 0.2 mL/kg of body weight, given intramuscularly, is effective in preventing hepatitis A in 80% to 90% of cases. At present, three vaccines are used to prevent hepatitis A: Havrix and Vaqta.

Primary immunization consists of a single dose administered intramuscularly in the deltoid muscle. A booster is recommended between 6 and 12 months after the primary dose to ensure adequate antibody titers and long-term protection. However, primary immunization provides immunity within 30 days after a single dose (Mayo Clinic, 2014).

Until routine vaccination of children is feasible, people who are at risk for infection should be vaccinated for hepatitis A. This includes people traveling to countries where hepatitis A is endemic; sexually active homosexual and bisexual men; patients with chronic liver disease; injecting drug users; and people at risk for occupational infection, such as those who work with hepatitis A in research laboratory settings.

Individuals who have been exposed to HBV via a needle puncture or sexual contact should be protected with hepatitis B immune globulin. A dose is administered intramuscularly as quickly after exposure as possible. This dose is repeated 1 month later. People identified as being at high risk for developing hepatitis B should be vaccinated if they are not already immune. These people include the following:

- All health care personnel (especially emergency department, operating room, intensive care unit [ICU], and dialysis personnel; phlebotomists; and laboratory technicians)
- People with high-risk lifestyles (drug users, tattoo recipients, homosexual men, and prostitutes)
- Infants born to mothers who test positive for hepatitis B surface antigen
- Hemodialysis patients
- Individuals sharing a household with an infected person

The CDC (2016) recommends making hepatitis B vaccine a part of routine vaccination schedules for all newborns and adolescents. The protection program consists of three vaccinations: an initial vaccination, a vaccination 1 month later, and a third vaccination 6 months after the first injection. The hepatitis B vaccine has been shown to provide protection for 3 to 5 years in approximately 90% of the people treated. It is hoped that universal vaccination will lead to eventual prevention and control of hepatitis B (CDC, 2016b).

Hepatitis B, C, D, and G are spread through blood transfusions. The blood used should be screened for elevated ALT and anti–hepatitis B core, and for anti–hepatitis C, anti–hepatitis D, and anti–hepatitis G antigens.

Liver transplantation. Liver transplantation has become a practical therapeutic option for many people with end-stage liver disease, generally improving their quality of life. Indications for liver transplantation include congenital biliary abnormalities, inborn errors of metabolism, hepatic malignancy (confined to the liver), sclerosing cholangitis, and chronic end-stage liver disease. Liver disease related to chronic viral hepatitis is the leading indication for liver transplantation. Liver transplants are not recommended for patients with widespread malignant disease. There are approximately 16,000 people waiting for liver transplants. At present, only approximately 6000 transplants are performed annually (American Liver Foundation, 2016).

The major postoperative complications are rejection and infection. Liver transplant candidates must go through a rigorous presurgery screening. However, the liver seems to be less susceptible to rejection than the kidney.

The source of a liver used for transplantation may be a deceased donor or a live donor. The live donor donates only a portion of his or her liver to the recipient.

Within weeks the recipient and the donor's liver will grow to the size the body needs. The donor faces potential risks, such as liver and biliary problems, postoperative infection, and other common postoperative complications (see Chapter 42).

The most common complications for the recipient of a liver transplant include rejection of the new liver tissue and infection. The use of cyclosporine, an effective immunosuppressant drug, has been a major factor in improving the success rate of liver transplantation. It does not cause bone marrow suppression and does not impede wound healing. Other immunosuppressants used include azathioprine (Imuran), corticosteroids, tacrolimus (Prograf), and mycophenolate mofetil (CellCept). The interleukin-2 receptor antagonists basiliximab (Simulect) and daclizumab (Zinbryta), are being used in combination with other immunosuppressive agents to reduce rejection. Other factors in the improved success rate are advances in surgical techniques, better selection of potential recipients, and improved management of the underlying liver disease before surgery.

Patients who have liver disease secondary to viral hepatitis often experience reinfection of the transplanted liver with hepatitis B or C. HCV recurrence as evidenced by histologic damage is almost universal after transplantation. Approximately 20% to 30% of patients develop cirrhosis of the transplanted liver by the fifth year posttransplantation. Antiviral therapy for HCV initiated posttransplantation, even before the development of histologic evidence of recurrence, has failed to alter this recurrence pattern. Approximately 75% of patients survive more than 5 years after transplantation (American Liver Foundation, 2016).

NURSING INTERVENTIONS AND PATIENT TEACHING

The patient who has a liver transplant requires competent and highly skilled nursing interventions, in either an ICU or another specialized unit. Postoperative nursing care includes assessing neurologic status; monitoring for signs of hemorrhage; preventing pulmonary complications; monitoring drainage, electrolyte levels, and urinary output; and monitoring for signs and symptoms of infection and rejection. Common respiratory problems include pneumonia, atelectasis (collapsed lung), and pleural effusions. Have the patient use measures such as coughing, deep breathing, incentive spirometry, and repositioning to prevent these complications. Measure and record drainage from the Jackson-Pratt drain, NG tube suctioning, and T tube, and note the color and consistency of drainage. A critical aspect of nursing interventions after liver transplantation is monitoring for infection. The first 2 months after the surgery are critical. Infection can be viral, fungal, or bacterial. Fever may be the only sign of infection. Emotional support and teaching the patient and family are essential.

The care of the patient with viral hepatitis includes ensuring rest, maintaining adequate nutrition, providing adequate fluids, and caring for the skin. The care of the patient with hepatitis continues over time, and support and patient education are necessary throughout the entire illness.

Preventing transmission of the disease is paramount in caring for the patient with viral hepatitis. The patient, family, and health care providers must be knowledgeable about routes of transmission of the virus and take steps to avoid such transmission. Proper personal hygiene and good sanitation, as well as hepatitis A vaccination, help prevent the spread of hepatitis A. Thoroughly explain to patients the reasons for the precautions, and instruct them in the proper handling of their own secretions and body wastes and in thorough methods of hand hygiene. Wear gown and gloves when handling excreta, giving enemas, taking rectal temperatures, handling food waste, handling needles, disposing of urine, or carrying out any other procedure or hygiene measure that involves direct contact with the patient's body fluids.

Not all patients know they are infected with hepatitis, so following standard precautions with all patients prevents the spread of all bloodborne pathogenic diseases. Health care personnel always should take the utmost care in handling syringes, needles, and other instruments that are contaminated with the patient's serum. Maintaining standard precautions while exposed to blood and body fluids such as saliva, semen, and vaginal secretions is essential to prevent the transmission of hepatitis B. Follow appropriate transmission-based precautions as designated by facility policy. Use enteric precautions for 7 days after the onset of hepatitis A. Use standard precautions for all patients.

Patient problems and interventions for the patient with hepatitis include but are not limited to the following:

Patient Problem	Nursing Interventions
Potential for Harm or Damage to the Body, related to: • Poor nutrition • Prolonged clotting times	Pad side rails if necessary Assist weakened patient with activities Encourage use of electric razor and soft toothbrush
Insufficient Nutrition, related to: • Anorexia • Nausea • Vomiting • Altered metabolism of nutrients by the liver	Provide diet high in carbohydrates and low in fats, and encourage total fluid intake of 2500 to 3000 mL daily Monitor I&O Monitor daily weight Note color and consistency of stool and color and amount of urine Administer antiemetics as ordered Offer support and understanding Promote adequate rest

For the patient with viral hepatitis being cared for at home, teach the family necessary precautions. Patients should avoid sexual activity during the acute stage of hepatitis B, C, and D. Sexual precautions should be taken, and needles and razors should not be shared. Patients with hepatitis A must wash their hands thoroughly after toileting, must disinfect feces-soiled articles (boil for 1 minute), and must not prepare foods for others while symptomatic. If possible, the patient should use separate bathroom facilities. Personal care items and drinking glasses should not be shared. The patient's clothes should be laundered separately in hot water. Contaminated items should be disposed of properly. Sexual intercourse should be avoided while in the acute stage of hepatitis A.

Inform the patient and family about signs and symptoms associated with hepatitis, including light-colored stools, dark-colored urine, jaundice, fever, GI disturbances, unusual bleeding that may be indicative of a prolonged prothrombin time and increased INR, and tenderness or pain in the abdomen. The danger of alcohol use and its effect on the liver should be clearly understood.

Prognosis

The prognosis for the patient with hepatitis differs, depending on the causative agent. Recovery from hepatitis A is high, because the virus does not remain in the body after the infection has resolved. Within 3 months after diagnosis most people recover and nearly all recover within 6 months. For this reason, the mortality rate for hepatitis A is very low. The acute stage of the illness typically lasts up to 3 weeks, and it is usually 4 to 6 months before the liver returns to normal function. A small percentage of patients develop chronic hepatitis and cirrhosis as a result of hepatitis B infection. Patients who do develop chronic hepatitis are at a higher risk for liver cancer. Hepatitis B has a higher mortality rate than hepatitis A, but not as high as hepatitis C. Hepatitis C often progresses to chronic hepatitis, and the majority develop chronic infection. Cirrhosis and liver cancer are not uncommon with hepatitis C. The prognosis for patients with chronic hepatitis C infection has increased the demand greatly for liver transplants. The acute phase of hepatitis D typically improves within 2 to 3 weeks, and liver enzymes return to normal within 16 weeks. Almost all patients with hepatitis E recover completely. Hepatitis G infections frequently coexist with other hepatitis infections, such as hepatitis C. However, most hepatitis G infections are not associated with chronic hepatitis; thus the association of hepatitis G virus with liver disease is, at this time, uncertain.

Recovery from acute toxic hepatitis is rapid if the hepatotoxin is identified early and removed or if exposure to the agent has been limited. However, the prognosis is poor if the period between exposure and the onset of signs and symptoms is prolonged, because there are no effective antidotes.

LIVER ABSCESSES

If an infection develops anywhere along the GI tract, there is a chance of the infecting organisms reaching the liver through the biliary system, portal venous system, or hepatic arterial or lymphatic systems, and creating an abscess (a collection of pus). If an abscess is allowed to progress, it can become life threatening. The past mortality rate among patients with liver abscesses was 100% because of the vague clinical symptoms, inadequate diagnostic tools, and inadequate surgical drainage. Today medical management is more successful (Peralta, 2016).

Etiology and Pathophysiology

If the body does not successfully destroy the bacteria, the bacterial toxins attack neighboring liver cells, and the necrotic tissue produced is a protective wall for the organism. Meanwhile, leukocytes migrate into the infected area. The result is an abscess: a cavity full of a liquid containing living and dead leukocytes and bacteria. Pyogenic (pus-producing) abscesses of this type may be single or multiple. Common sources of liver abscess include abdominal infections such as appendicitis, diverticulitis, and perforated colon. Other causes include any infection in the blood or bile ducts, and trauma to the liver.

Clinical Manifestations

Patients with liver abscess often have vague signs and symptoms. Fever accompanied by chills, abdominal pain, and tenderness in the right upper quadrant of the abdomen are common complaints. Unintentional weight loss, jaundice, and weakness are additional symptoms (Peralta, 2016).

Assessment

Subjective data are related to the infection and to the inability of the liver to function normally. Symptoms include chills, complaints of dull abdominal pain, abdominal tenderness, and discomfort.

Objective data also are related to the infection and impaired function of the liver. Signs of liver abscess include fever, hepatomegaly, jaundice, and anemia. Clay-colored stools and dark urine also are commonly present because of the decreased amount of bile being excreted.

Diagnostic Tests

The diagnosis is established by demonstrating a space-occupying lesion in the liver radiographically (radiograph, ultrasound, CT, and liver scan). Liver biopsy may be performed to determine the presence of an abscess, and a culture may be initiated to determine the infective agent. Common laboratory testing that helps establish the diagnosis includes bilirubin levels, liver enzymes, blood cultures for bacteria, and a complete blood count (CBC). Amebic liver abscess (caused by a microscopic, single-celled parasite) also may be confirmed by serologic examination (in which ameba-specific antibodies are detected in the patient's serum) (Peralta, 2016).

Medical Management

Usually liver abscesses are managed by medical therapy. Treatment includes IV antibiotic therapy specific to the organism identified. Antibiotic therapy often is continued for 4 to 6 weeks.

Percutaneous (performed through the skin) drainage of a liver abscess is reserved for patients who do not respond to medical therapy or are at high risk for rupture. Open surgical drainage has been the standard in patients whose liver abscesses have ruptured into the peritoneal space, but some of these patients now are managed with percutaneous drainage. All patients require a full course of antibiotic therapy.

Nursing Interventions and Patient Teaching

Continuous monitoring and supportive care are indicated because of the seriousness of the patient's condition. Monitoring objective and subjective symptoms is important. Notify the health care provider if signs and symptoms increase in severity.

The patient's response to drug therapy is determined by a decrease in fever, tenderness and rigidity of the abdomen, chills, and discomfort. If percutaneous or open surgical drainage is instituted, observe the drainage for amount, color, and consistency.

A patient problem and interventions for the patient with a liver abscess include but are not limited to the following:

Patient Problem	Nursing Interventions
Potential for Inability to Regulate Body Temperature, related to infectious state	Check temperature as ordered by health care provider or as indicated by the patient's worsening condition, and report findings to health care provider Encourage fluids to prevent dehydration. Monitor IV fluids Explain how fever and drainage can deplete fluids in the body Record I&O Monitor oral mucous membranes and skin turgor

In addition to the relationship of infection and nutrition, teach preoperative and postoperative procedures if the patient requires percutaneous or open surgical drainage. A thorough explanation and assessment for the patient's understanding are necessary. The seriously ill patient becomes less anxious as the knowledge base increases and the patient feels more in control of the situation.

Prognosis

The prognosis for patients with liver abscesses was very poor in the past, with an extremely high mortality rate. Sepsis was commonly the cause of death. The prognosis today is much improved because of advanced diagnostic tests, including CT and liver scans, and aggressive medical and nursing interventions.

CHOLECYSTITIS AND CHOLELITHIASIS

Etiology and Pathophysiology

Disorders of the biliary system are common in the United States and are responsible for the hospitalization of hundreds of thousands of people each year. The two most common conditions are cholecystitis (inflammation of the gallbladder) and cholelithiasis (presence of gallstones in the gallbladder). These two diseases are seen more commonly in women than men; in Native Americans, white Americans, and African Americans; and in obese people, pregnant women, multiparous women (i.e., women who have given birth to two or more babies), women who use birth control pills, and people with diabetes.

Cholecystitis can be caused by an obstruction, a gallstone, a nonfunctioning gallbladder, or a tumor. The exact cause of stone formation in the gallbladder and the common bile duct is not known. However, altered lipid metabolism and female sex hormones play a role in the disease. The stones usually occur in multiples but can occur singly (Fig. 46.5).

When an obstruction is caused by gallstones or a tumor prevents bile from leaving the gallbladder, the

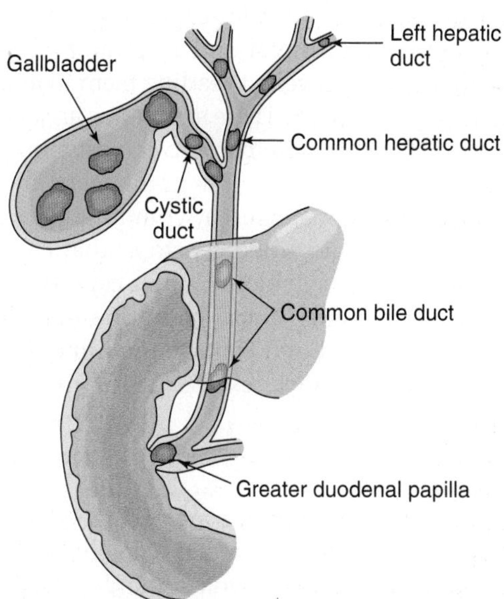

Fig. 46.5 Common sites of gallstones. (From Monahan FD, Sands JK, Neighbors M, et al: *Phipps' medical-surgical nursing: Health and illness perspectives*, ed 8, St. Louis, 2007, Mosby.)

trapped bile acts as an irritant, causing inflammatory cells to infiltrate the gallbladder wall after 3 to 4 days. A typical inflammatory response occurs, and the gallbladder becomes enlarged and edematous. The vascular occlusion along with bile stasis causes the mucosal lining of the gallbladder to become necrotic. At first, the bile in the gallbladder is sterile. Within a few days bacteria infiltrate and begin to grow. When the disease is severe enough, the gallbladder may become gangrenous, rupture, and spread infection to the hepatic duct and liver.

Clinical Manifestations

The condition may be acute, with a sudden onset of indigestion; nausea and vomiting; and severe, colicky pain in the right upper quadrant of the abdomen. The pain may be referred to the right shoulder and scapula. Pain resulting from cholecystitis or cholelithiasis sometimes is mistaken for a cardiac problem because of the pain that is felt in the epigastric region and radiating to the back. If the condition is chronic, the patient usually has had several milder attacks of pain and a history of fat intolerance. When gallstones move through the biliary ducts, the patient often complains of pain being intensified.

Assessment

Subjective data include complaints of indigestion after eating foods high in fat. The pain of acute cholecystitis is abrupt in onset, reaches peak intensity quickly, and remains at that level for 2 to 4 hours. It localizes in the right upper quadrant epigastric region. The pain radiates around the mid-torso to the right scapular area. Anorexia, nausea, vomiting, and **flatulence** (excess formation of gases in the stomach or intestine) also are noted. This pain is caused by the gallbladder contracting in an attempt to secrete bile for fat digestion. Patients may experience increased heart and respiratory rates and become diaphoretic (sweaty), leading them to think they are having a heart attack. These symptoms are decreased or absent in patients with chronic cholecystitis.

Objective data include a low-grade fever, increased pulse and respirations, nausea, vomiting, an elevated leukocyte count, mild jaundice, stools that contain fat **(steatorrhea)**, and clay-colored stools caused by a lack of bile in the intestinal tract. The urine may be dark amber to tea colored and contain urobilinogen as the kidneys try to remove excess bilirubin from the bloodstream.

Diagnostic Tests

A number of diagnostic studies are performed to confirm a diagnosis of cholecystitis and cholelithiasis. Fecal studies, serum bilirubin tests, ultrasound of the gallbladder and biliary system, a HIDA scan, and an OCG may be done. Ultrasound of the gallbladder is extremely accurate in diagnosing cholelithiasis. HIDA scanning is helpful in assessing the patency of the cystic and common bile ducts as well as the ability of the gallbladder to function efficiently. Operative cholangiography is a procedure in which the common bile duct is injected directly with radiopaque dye. This frequently is done at the time of gallbladder surgery.

Medical Management

If the attack of cholelithiasis is mild, the patient is treated conservatively. Bed rest is prescribed, an NG tube is inserted and connected to low suction, and the patient is placed on NPO status. This allows the GI tract, including the gallbladder, to rest. IV fluids are given to rehydrate the patient and to replace drainage from the NG tube.

Antispasmodic and analgesic drugs may be given to decrease pain. Meperidine (Demerol) and ketorolac are used commonly for pain management. An antispasmodic such as dicyclomine (Bentyl) may be used to decrease the incidence of spasms of the sphincter of Oddi (which controls the flow of pancreatic juices and bile into the duodenum). Morphine generally is not used for pain management because it often increases the tone of the sphincter of Oddi. Antibiotics may be given (1) prophylactically to prevent infection; (2) to treat an existing infection; and (3) after perforation, should it occur. A diet that is low in fat and cholesterol may be prescribed (see the Complementary and Alternative Therapies box).

Complementary and Alternative Therapies

Gallbladder, Biliary, and Pancreatic Disorders

- Fresh black root is used as an emetic. The dried root has a gentler action and is used to treat constipation and liver and gallbladder disease and to increase bile flow. Caution patients with gallstones or bile duct obstruction to avoid using it because it may worsen these diseases.
- Blessed thistle is used orally to treat digestive problems such as liver and gallbladder diseases.
- Dandelion traditionally is used as a bile stimulator to treat gallbladder ailments.
- Onion is used as a gallbladder stimulant. It increases the risk of hypoglycemia, so monitor patients with diabetes closely.
- Autumn crocus (active ingredient: colchicine) has been used to treat hepatic cirrhosis and primary biliary cirrhosis. Because of the plant's toxicity, internal use is not recommended.
- Papaya (pawpaw) is used to treat gastrointestinal tract disorders such as pancreatic insufficiency.
- Royal jelly (bee pollen complex) is used in treating liver disease and pancreatitis. Do not confuse royal jelly with bee pollen and honeybee venom. (Royal jelly should be used with extreme caution by patients with asthma, because allergic reactions to royal jelly have led to asthma attacks, anaphylaxis, and death.)

Lithotripsy. Extracorporeal shock wave lithotripsy is used to treat a patient who has mild or moderate

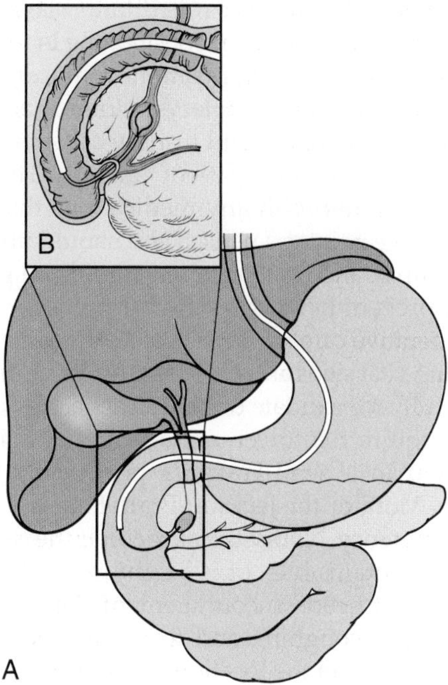

Fig. 46.6 A, During endoscopic sphincterotomy, a flexible endoscope is advanced through the mouth and the stomach until its tip sits in the duodenum opposite the common bile duct. B, After widening the duct mouth by incising the sphincter muscle, the health care provider advances a basket attachment into the duct and retrieves the stone. (From Lewis SL, Dirksen SR, Heitkemper MM, et al: *Medical-surgical nursing: Assessment and management of clinical problems,* ed 10, St. Louis, 2017, Elsevier.)

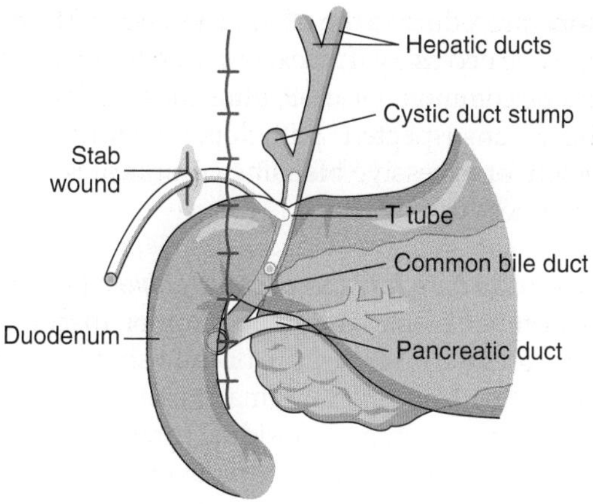

Fig. 46.7 T tube in common bile duct. (From Beare PG, Myers JL: *Adult health nursing,* ed 3, St. Louis, 1998, Mosby.)

symptoms caused by a few stones. The machine discharges a series of shock waves through water or a cushion that breaks the stones into fragments. The natural flow of bile carries the stone fragments out of the gallbladder and into the intestine for eventual excretion. Nursing intervention after the procedure is similar to that for patients undergoing liver biopsy.

Surgical intervention. The treatment of choice is cholecystectomy (removal of the gallbladder) with ligation of the cystic duct, vein, and artery. A laparoscopic cholecystectomy and open abdominal cholecystectomy are the two surgical procedures (see Fig. 46.6 for stone retrieval). A Jackson-Pratt, Penrose, or Davol drain (which promotes drainage and prevents pressure and fluid accumulation under the diaphragm) may be inserted if an open cholecystectomy is performed. If the stones are in the common bile duct and edema is present, a biliary drainage tube, or T tube, is inserted to keep the duct open and allow drainage of the bile until the edema resolves. The short end of the tube is placed in the common bile duct, and the longer end is brought to the surface through a stab wound (Fig. 46.7). The long end is attached to a closed drainage system (bile bag) that is placed below the level of the common bile duct.

The T tube also provides a route for postoperative cholangiography if desired (T-tube cholangiogram) to assess the patency of the common bile duct. The T tube is removed 24 hours after the cholangiogram if the edema is resolved and the common bile duct appears normal. The T tube is removed by cutting the anchoring stitches and pulling the tube out. The small opening is covered with an adhesive bandage or gauze dressing and heals on its own within a few days. The 24-hour period allows the dye to drain out of the common bile duct. If the edema does not resolve in this time, the patient may be discharged with the T tube in place.

The most common treatment for cholecystitis and cholelithiasis is with an endoscopic technique called *laparoscopic cholecystectomy,* in which a laser or cautery is used to remove the gallbladder. This procedure replaces the open surgical procedure 80% to 85% of the time. It involves removing the gallbladder through one of four small punctures in the abdomen (a comparatively minor procedure). During surgery, the abdominal cavity is inflated with 3 to 4 L of carbon dioxide to improve visibility. A laparoscope, which has a camera attached, is inserted into the abdomen. The surgeon removes the deflated gallbladder through the laparoscope. If the organ contains so much bile or gallstones that it cannot be collapsed, its contents will be aspirated first. Laparoscopic cholecystectomy offers several advantages over the common open abdominal cholecystectomy, including the following:

- It is less invasive (and thus there is less chance of wound infection or respiratory impairment) and has a shorter healing time and a shorter recuperative time.
- There is no unsightly scar.
- There is less pain and thus more rapid return to normal activities.

When a medical history, physical examination, and blood studies are complete, an ultrasound is done to locate gallstones and detect any dilation of the hepatic bile ducts. If *choledocholithiasis* (stones in the common bile duct) is confirmed, a sphincterotomy and stone extraction (see Fig. 46.6) are performed before laparoscopic surgery.

It is important to obtain informed consent for endoscopic and open cholecystectomy in case converting from one procedure to the other is necessary. The conversion may be necessary if an extensive adhesion, gallstones within the common bile duct, unusual vascular or ductal anatomy, unsuspected pathologic condition of the abdomen, or excessive bleeding complicates the endoscopic procedure.

Postoperative care for laparoscopic cholecystectomy. A small number of patients report minor discomfort at the laparoscopic insertion site or mild shoulder or neck pain resulting from diaphragmatic irritation secondary to abdominal stretching or residual carbon dioxide. Oral analgesics or antiinflammatory agents relieve these symptoms.

Oral liquids and a light meal are given the first night after surgery. The patient has four bandages at the puncture sites on the abdomen. Assess vital signs routinely. The patient should be ambulatory by the first postoperative night.

One of six patients is discharged the day of surgery. Most patients are discharged the next day. Patients are usually able to resume moderate activity within 48 to 72 hours.

Patient teaching. Before discharge, patients should be able to eat without difficulty and walk and should have no abdominal distention, evidence of bleeding, or bile leakage. Instruct them to immediately report to the health care provider any severe pain, tenderness in the right upper quadrant, increase in abdominal girth, leakage of bile-colored drainage from the puncture site, increase in pulse, or symptoms of low blood pressure. Patients are usually able to return to work in 3 days and resume full activity after 1 week.

Although there are contraindications for endoscopic cholecystectomies, most patients are treated with this less painful, less expensive procedure.

Nursing Interventions and Patient Teaching

Nursing interventions begin with careful assessment of the characteristics of pain (if it is present) and any signs of jaundice of the skin, sclera, and mucous membranes. Observe the patient's urine and stool for alterations in the presence of bilirubin.

When the patient is treated conservatively, nursing interventions center on keeping the patient comfortable by carefully administering the medications prescribed and monitoring the patient's response to the medications. The patient is kept on NPO status or on clear liquids. Administer antiemetics if nausea is present. Observe IV infusions for patency, correct rates, and entry sites that are free from erythema and edema. Measure I&O and describe carefully.

Preoperative care includes teaching the patient to turn, cough, and deep breathe and to use an incentive spirometer to facilitate air movement in and out of the lungs to prevent pneumonia and atelectasis. To enable the patient to follow postoperative instructions more easily, teach him or her how to splint the abdomen with the hands, small pillow, or rolled bath blanket before attempting a cough; practice repositioning in the hospital bed; and assume a sitting position from a standing or lying position. If an open cholecystectomy is anticipated, explaining the IV tubing and urinary catheter and their functions helps relieve patient anxiety. The patient should be familiar with any medications that may be used to relieve pain and nausea and should understand that vitamin K and antibiotics may be given preoperatively to prevent hemorrhage and infection.

Postoperative care for open cholecystectomy includes monitoring vital signs and observing dressings frequently and carefully for exudate or hemorrhage. The dressings usually require reinforcement at the drain site. Place the patient in a semi-Fowler's position to facilitate drainage. Monitor the Jackson-Pratt, Penrose, or Davol drain for patency. Notify the surgeon if the drainage is excessive, contains bile, or is bright red.

The patient needs encouragement to perform deep breathing and coughing and to use an incentive spirometer, because of the location of the incision. Provide analgesics frequently in the early postoperative period to facilitate movement and deep breathing. Help the patient to dangle (i.e., sit up with the legs hanging over the side of the bed) the night of surgery and ambulate the first postoperative day. Monitor the patient's neurologic status by checking ability to be aroused easily, orientation to the environment and family, and ability to move extremities equally on command.

Maintain fluid balance with IV therapy; potassium usually is added to compensate for loss from surgery. Check the health care provider's order before giving ice or clear liquids to the patient, and allow the patient to rinse the mouth frequently.

The nurse is responsible for the care of the T tube if one is placed. The drainage bag for the T tube is placed below the level of the common bile duct to prevent the reflux of bile. Position the bag so that the tube is not kinked and bile can drain from the liver. Frequently check the position of the bag and tube and the color and amount of exudate during the first 24 hours and record the results. Place a gauze roll under the tube, anchoring it to the patient's abdomen and preventing tension and pull on the tube from the weight of the bag. The T tube drains as much as 500 mL during the first 24 hours. The amount should decrease as the edema resolves and bile begins flowing through the common bile duct. Be careful not to dislodge the T tube when changing the patient's dressings, as prescribed by the health care provider.

After oral intake is resumed, the health care provider may order the T tube clamped for 1 to 2 hours before meals and unclamped 1 to 2 hours after the patient eats, to aid in the digestion of fat. While the T tube is clamped, the patient may show signs of distress, including abdominal pain, nausea, vomiting, light brown urine, and clay-colored stools. If distress occurs, unclamp the tube immediately. Increase the time that the T tube remains clamped as the patient tolerates the procedure.

The tube may be left in place for as long as 10 days. The health care provider removes the tube when the common bile duct is patent for drainage of bile.

Check bowel sounds every 8 hours for the return of peristalsis by auscultating the abdomen. Ask the patient if he or she is passing flatus. A clear liquid diet usually is ordered immediately or within the first 24 hours postoperatively and increased as tolerated. When the patient begins eating solid food, usually low-fat foods are best. Flatulence or nausea after eating certain foods may persist after surgery; instruct the patient to experiment with different foods.

The patient who undergoes a cholecystectomy must be observed for complications. These include jaundice (from an occluded common duct) and hemorrhage (indicated by decreased blood pressure, increased pulse, and increased exudate at the dressing site). An elevated temperature could indicate peritonitis or wound infection. Pancreatitis may occur after cholecystectomy.

Patients at high risk of not surviving a cholecystectomy may need a cholecystostomy (forming an opening into the gallbladder through the abdominal wall). This can be done using a local anesthetic. The opening provides a means of removing purulent exudate and possibly the stone. It also allows drainage of bile.

Patient problems and interventions for the patient with open cholecystectomy or cholecystostomy include but are not limited to the following:

Patient Problem	Nursing Interventions
Potential for Compromised Skin Integrity, related to: • Wound drainage • Accidental obstruction of bile drainage	Maintain patency and prevent tension on T tube; promote drainage of T tube by placing patient in low Fowler's to semi-Fowler's position Observe, describe, and record amount and character of drainage from T tube at least q 8 hr Empty bile bag when half full Clamp T tube as ordered by health care provider 3 to 4 days postoperatively Reinforce primary dressing and observe exudates; change and apply sterile, dry dressing as ordered; use Montgomery straps to secure if drainage is profuse Cleanse skin thoroughly at insertion site before applying sterile dressing Apply skin barriers as needed for added protection

Dietary teaching is necessary for the patient who is treated conservatively for cholecystitis, as well as for the patient who undergoes surgery. The patient who is treated conservatively must continue to avoid fatty foods, including fried foods, cream, whole milk, butter, margarine, peanut butter, nuts, chocolate, pastries, and gravies. For the postsurgical patient, provide instructions to try small amounts of foods that previously caused discomfort and gradually eliminate those that continue to do so. The patient usually can resume a normal diet without difficulty.

The patient should understand that stones may recur elsewhere in the biliary system. Teach the patient to identify the signs of complications that should be reported. These include jaundice caused by occlusion or stricture of a duct, hemorrhage or leakage of bile, elevated temperature, pain, and dietary intolerance associated with another attack. The patient also should be able to demonstrate care of the T tube, if present on discharge; identify activity restrictions; and identify a date for a return visit to the health care provider.

Prognosis

To prevent complications from cholecystitis or cholelithiasis, assess the patient for signs and symptoms of infection within the gallbladder, which can lead to death of the gallbladder from gangrene infection if the initial infection is not treated or does not respond to therapy. Other complications include abscess formation, and rupture of the gallbladder (which can lead to peritonitis). Stones may also lodge in various biliary ducts, including the common bile duct, leading to pancreatitis or obstructive jaundice.

With prompt treatment of cholecystitis and cholelithiasis, the prognosis is excellent. Laparoscopic surgery also has decreased the number of complications. The prognosis is not as favorable in patients who develop pancreatitis (see the Lifespan Considerations box).

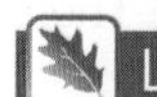

Lifespan Considerations

Older Adults

Gallbladder, Liver, Biliary Tract, or Exocrine Pancreatic Disorder

- The incidence of cholelithiasis increases with aging. Closely observe older adults with histories of this disease for changes in the color of urine and stool or other signs and symptoms of gallbladder problems.
- As the body ages, the number and size of hepatic cells decrease, which results in an overall reduced size and weight of the liver. The liver also has decreased ability to regenerate after injury or from hepatotoxic injury. Detoxification of substances is delayed.
- Older adults have a decrease in protein synthesis in the liver and possible changes in the production of enzymes that assist in the metabolism of drugs, particularly anticonvulsants, psychotropics, and oral anticoagulants.
- Be alert to the signs and symptoms of drug toxicity, even when the drugs are administered in normal doses, because the decreased metabolism in the liver can cause an accumulation of the drugs.
- The pancreas exhibits ductal hyperplasia and fibrosis with aging, but these changes are not necessarily associated with altered functioning. The output of pancreatic secretions steadily declines after age 40, but related problems with absorption cannot be documented.

PANCREATITIS

Etiology and Pathophysiology

Pancreatitis is an inflammatory condition of the pancreas that may be acute or chronic. The degree of inflammation varies from mild edema to severe hemorrhagic necrosis. Although the exact cause of pancreatitis remains unknown, many predisposing factors have been identified. Acute or chronic pancreatitis is generally the result of damage to the biliary tract (most common in women), alcohol consumption (most common in men), trauma, infectious disease, or certain drugs. Alcoholism and biliary tract disease are the two factors most commonly associated with pancreatitis. Pancreatitis can develop as a postoperative complication in patients who have had surgery of the pancreas, stomach, duodenum, or biliary tract. Pancreatitis also can occur after undergoing ERCP (see Fig. 46.1).

In the pathophysiologic process of pancreatitis, the enzymes cannot flow out of the pancreas because of **occlusion** (an obstruction or closing off) of the pancreatic duct (duct of Wirsung) by edema, stones, or scar tissue. The pancreatic enzymes build up and increase pressure within the duct. The duct ruptures, releasing enzymes that begin digesting the pancreas (autodigestion). In chronic pancreatitis, the enzyme-producing acinar tissue atrophies and is replaced with fibrotic tissue, resulting in the pancreas becoming necrotic.

The development of pseudocysts or abscesses in pancreatic tissue is a serious complication. After autodigestion occurs, the pancreas and occasionally the surrounding organs form walls around cystic fluid, including pancreatic enzymes, and necrotic debris. These pseudocysts can develop into an abscess.

Clinical Manifestations

Manifestations include severe abdominal pain radiating to the back. The pain usually is located in the left upper quadrant. The pain is sometimes relieved by leaning forward, taking the stomach weight off the pancreas. Jaundice may be noted if the common bile duct is obstructed.

Assessment

Pain is the most common subjective data associated with pancreatitis. Pain may be gradual or have a sudden onset and is often severe. The pain is caused by the enlargement of the pancreatic capsule, an obstruction, or chemical irritation from enzymes. The pain usually is decreased by flexing the trunk, leaning forward from a sitting position, or by assuming the fetal position. It is increased by eating or lying down. Other complaints include nausea, anorexia, malaise, and restlessness.

Collection of objective data includes noting the presence of low-grade fever, leukocytosis, hypotension, and vomiting. Jaundice often is seen if the common bile duct is obstructed. The abdomen usually appears swollen. Bowel sounds may be decreased or absent, leading to an ileus (paralysis of the bowel). The patient appears acutely ill (Mayo Clinic, 2016b).

Diagnostic Tests

Acute and chronic pancreatitis are diagnosed by radiologic studies (abdominal CT scan and ultrasound of the pancreas), endoscopy, and laboratory analysis of the pancreatic enzymes in the serum and urine. Laboratory tests reveal an increased level of serum amylase and lipase during the first few days and increased urine amylase thereafter. Amylase and lipase levels that are three times above normal are considered most definitive for pancreatitis. The amylase level is not a specific indicator for pancreatitis; abnormal levels also can be seen in cases of perforated peptic ulcer, perforated bowel, and diabetic ketoacidosis. Elevation of the pancreatic amylase level is a better indicator of pancreatitis. The level of lipase is more specific for diagnosing acute pancreatitis. The lipase level typically remains elevated for 12 days with pancreatitis. In chronic pancreatitis the serum lipase levels often remain elevated, and the serum amylase remains normal. Leukocytosis, an elevated hematocrit level, hypocalcemia, hypoalbuminemia, and hyperglycemia also may be present. Pancreatic insulin production may be diminished if the islets of Langerhans become infected, and some patients develop diabetes mellitus.

Medical Management

Treatment is medical unless the precipitating cause is biliary tract disease; then surgery may be indicated. Food and fluids are withheld to avoid stimulating pancreatic activity, and IV fluids are administered. The patient is on NPO status, and an NG tube is inserted to decrease pancreatic stimulation, to treat or prevent nausea and vomiting, and to decrease abdominal distention. Analgesics prescribed by the health care provider should be administered as needed to control the pain associated with pancreatitis. Analgesics may be combined with an antispasmodic to achieve optimum pain control.

Parenteral anticholinergic medication, such as atropine or propantheline, helps decrease pancreatic activity. This medication is contraindicated in paralytic ileus. Antacids or antihistamine H_2 receptor antagonists, such as cimetidine, may be given to prevent stress ulcers caused by decreased gastric pH. Some health care providers prescribe antibiotics to treat secondary infections.

Enteral feeding (i.e., tube feeding) is begun 24 to 48 hours after the onset of acute pancreatitis and is administered via the jejunum to prevent the release of pancreatic enzymes. Enteral feeding is preferred to the IV route because it is more nutritionally sound, is less costly, and has fewer complications. However, if enteral feeding is not tolerated in 5 to 7 days, the patient may need to be switched to total parenteral nutrition (TPN, intravenous feeding).

A clear liquid diet with gradual progression may be started once the patient's pain is under control for at least 24 hours. The diet should be low in fat and protein. The diet also should be free of caffeinated beverages because caffeine acts as a gastric stimulant. If the patient experiences increased pain from oral nutrition, hold all food and fluids and contact the health care provider. Oral hypoglycemic agents or insulin may be needed if there is destruction of the islets of Langerhans.

Nursing Interventions and Patient Teaching

Determine the presence and location of pain, as well as what aggravates or relieves the pain. Keep the patient as comfortable as possible through proper administration of analgesic and antispasmodic medications. The patient is usually on bed rest with bathroom privileges to decrease the flow of pancreatic enzymes. Nutritional needs are met by enteral feeding via the jejunum as long as necessary. If enteral feedings fail, the patient may need parenteral feedings. The patient who is addicted to alcohol may go through withdrawal while in the hospital. Be prepared to protect the patient from injury and provide supportive care to the patient and the family. Carefully monitor all replacement fluids and medications for proper administration.

Patient problems and interventions for the patient with pancreatitis include but are not limited to the following:

Patient Problem	Nursing Interventions
Recent Onset of Pain, related to stimulation of nerve endings caused by enlargement of pancreatic capsule, obstruction, or chemical irritation from enzymes	Administer medications as prescribed and monitor the response Restrict diet as necessary to prevent aggravation of pain (eliminate fats, alcohol, caffeine) Use alternative comfort measures: Repositioning, positive imagery, and time for listening Monitor NG tube hook-up to wall suction for functioning to prevent abdominal distention
Insufficient Nutrition, related to: • Anorexia • Nausea • Vomiting • Loss of enzymes necessary for the digestive process	Administer enteral feeding via jejunum as ordered Weigh patient daily at same time and using same scale Record I&O, including NG tube suctioning output Administer antacids and antiemetics as prescribed Instruct patient to follow a diet that is low in fat and high in protein and carbohydrates when tolerated

The patient remains on a low-fat, high-calorie, high-carbohydrate diet after discharge. Alcohol and beverages or foods containing caffeine are not allowed if full recovery is desired. Ensure that the patient understands the disease process and the severity of the disease and related complications.

Prognosis

The prognosis of pancreatitis depends on the course of the disease and complications, including pseudocysts and abscesses. In most patients, acute pancreatitis is mild, requiring less than 1 week of hospitalization. However, 5% to 25% of patients have a more complicated course. The severity of the disease varies according to the extent of pancreatic destruction. Some patients recover completely; others have recurring attacks. The overall mortality rate for acute pancreatitis is 10% to 15%. The mortality rate for patients with severe disease resulting in organ failure is approximately 30%. Complications can occur with mild, acute, chronic, or severe pancreatitis. Mortality rates for acute necrotizing pancreatitis are 20% and higher, depending on other organs that become involved (Mathew, 2017).

CANCER OF THE PANCREAS

Although once considered relatively rare, pancreatic cancer is now the fourth leading cause of cancer death in the United States and Canada. According to the American Cancer Society, it is estimated that more than 54,000 Americans will be diagnosed with pancreatic cancer during 2017 and that more than 43,000 Americans will die of the disease (ACS, 2017). A major factor in the high death rate from pancreatic cancer is the difficulty in diagnosing it at an early, curable stage. The disease usually occurs after middle age. The risk increases with age, with peak incidence occurring between 65 and 80 years of age.

Etiology and Pathophysiology

The most common environmental risk factor for pancreatic cancer is cigarette smoking. Smoking is seen in 30% of patients diagnosed with the disease. Other risk factors include exposure to chemical carcinogens, diabetes mellitus, cirrhosis, and chronic pancreatitis. Diets high in red meat and pork (especially processed meat such as bacon), fat, and coffee also are linked to pancreatic cancer. Obesity, genetics, and being an African American male increase the risk of developing pancreatic cancer.

The cancer may originate in the pancreas or be the result of metastasis from cancer of the lung, the stomach, the duodenum, or the common bile duct. Most often the head of the pancreas is involved and causes jaundice by compressing and obstructing the common bile duct. As the cancer spreads, it may invade the posterior wall of the stomach, the duodenal wall, the colon, and the common bile duct. Biliary obstruction and gallbladder dilation are subsequent complications. It is not uncommon for the tumor to grow rapidly and invade the vascular and lymphatic systems. Many patients live only 4 to 6 months after diagnosis because of the common late diagnosis.

Clinical Manifestations

The insidious onset of the disease with initially vague symptoms generally accounts for delays in diagnosis. Complaints of anorexia, malaise, nausea, and fatigue are common. Abdominal pain in the mid-epigastric region or back occurs in many of the patients. About half the patients develop diabetes mellitus if islet cells are involved.

Assessment

A psychosocial history taken during patient assessment may reveal that the patient belongs to one of the at-risk populations such cigarette smokers, coal- and gas-plant employees, chemists, and workers exposed to beta-naphthol and benzidine. Subjective data include anorexia; fatigue; nausea; flatulence; a change in stools; and steady, dull, and aching pain in the epigastrium or referred to the back. The pain is usually worse at night.

Objective data include weight loss, often gradual and progressive, which is one of the earliest signs. Jaundice usually is progressive and may occur late. Pruritus accompanies the jaundice. Many patients have recent onset of diabetes mellitus.

Diagnostic Tests

Diagnosis of pancreatic cancer is based on the patient's history, signs and symptoms, and diagnostic studies. Diagnostic studies include transabdominal ultrasound and CT, endoscopic ultrasound (EUS) with fine needle biopsy to obtain specimens for cytologic examination, ERCP, and pancreatic scans. ERCP allows for visualization of the pancreatic duct and biliary system. With ERCP, pancreatic secretions and tissues can be collected for analysis of various tumor markers (see Fig. 46.1).

The level of one tumor marker, cancer-associated antigen CA 19-9, is elevated in patients with pancreatic cancer. It is the most commonly used tumor marker to diagnose pancreatic adenocarcinoma and to monitor the patient's response to treatment. However, CA 19-9 can be elevated in other diseases such as cancer of the gallbladder and acute pancreatitis. Also, it is less sensitive in the early stages of the disease. CA 19-9 has proven to be more helpful for staging purposes and monitoring the patient posttreatment.

Medical Management

Often malignant tumors of the pancreas are inoperable by the time they are diagnosed. Treatment of pancreatic cancer is primarily surgical and has been associated with a high mortality rate. Cancer of the head of the pancreas usually is treated by pancreatoduodenectomy; the Whipple procedure involves resection of the antrum of the stomach, the gallbladder, the duodenum, and varying amounts of the pancreas. Anastomoses are constructed between the stomach, the common bile duct and the pancreatic ducts, and the jejunum (Fig. 46.8). In most cases, this procedure is performed by surgeons who are specially trained and experienced.

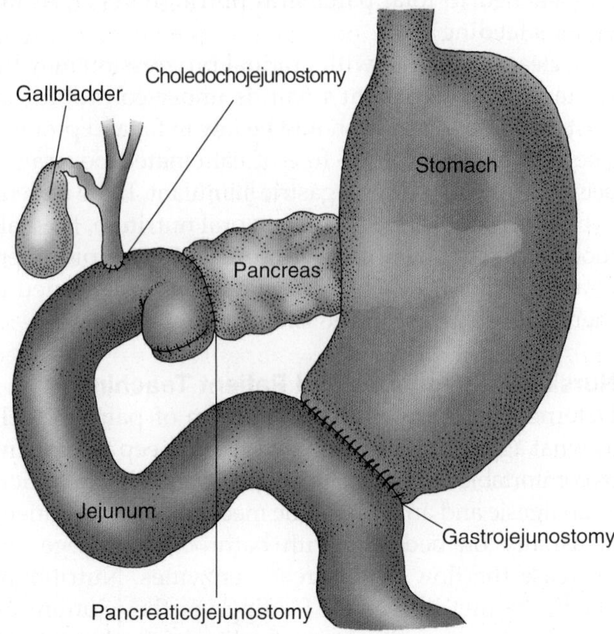

Fig. 46.8 The Whipple procedure, or radical pancreaticoduodenectomy. This surgical procedure involves resection of the proximal pancreas, adjoining duodenum, distal portion of the stomach, and distal portion of the common bile duct. The pancreatic duct, common bile ducts, and stomach are anastomosed to the jejunum. (From Ignatavicius DD, Workman ML: *Medical-surgical nursing: Patient-centered collaborative care*, ed 8, St. Louis, 2016, Elsevier.)

Another procedure is total pancreatectomy with resection of parts of the GI tract. Subtotal pancreatic resection has complications of postoperative pancreatic fistulas and is not recommended.

Combinations of drugs such as fluorouracil and gemcitabine (Gemzar) may produce a better response than a single chemotherapeutic agent. Gemcitabine is a main treatment for pancreatic cancer that has metastasized. The current role of chemotherapy in pancreatic cancer is limited. Adjuvant therapy—using surgical resection, radiation, and chemotherapy—is believed by some to be the most effective way to manage the almost always fatal cancer of the pancreas.

Nursing Interventions and Patient Teaching

Pancreatic surgery is radical and requires critical care nursing. Postoperative care focuses on maintaining fluid and electrolyte balance, preventing hemorrhage, preventing respiratory complications, and monitoring endocrine and exocrine functions of the pancreas.

Palliative care is crucial for the patient who is not a candidate or elects not to have treatment or surgery for pancreatic cancer. The patient may receive long-acting narcotic analgesics for chronic pain, supplemented by quick-acting opioids for breakthrough pain. Tricyclic antidepressants as well as antiemetics often are administered with the narcotic analgesic to potentiate (enhance) their effects. Nerve blocks or lysis of nerves of the celiac ganglia can be performed if pain control cannot be achieved with medications. Radiation therapy also is used to treat the pain associated with pancreatic cancer.

The health care provider caring for the patient with pancreatic cancer must offer compassionate physical and emotional assistance. Refer the patient and the family to social services and support groups. Hospice care is very beneficial to the family and patient.

A patient problem and interventions for patients with cancer of the pancreas include but are not limited to the following:

Patient Problem	Nursing Interventions
Potential for Compromised Skin Integrity, related to drainage from wound	Monitor for excoriation and infection; use skin barriers and disposable postoperative pouches and appliances to prevent enzymatic contact with the skin and to aid in the accurate collection and measurement of pancreatic drainage

The patient is facing a life-threatening illness, and family members and close friends are important for the patient's well-being. If the patient has an inadequate support system, it is important to use the resources that are available. Health care personnel, support groups, and hospice care are essential resources for supportive care.

Prognosis

The prognosis for patients with cancer of the pancreas is very poor because of the often late diagnosis. Median survival after diagnosis is only 5 to 12 months. Exocrine pancreatic cancer has a low 5-year survival rate. The 5-year survival rate for stage IA exocrine pancreatic cancer is approximately 14%. The 5-year survival rates decrease through the stages to 1% for stage IV. The 5-year survival rates for neuroendocrine pancreatic cancer is higher: 61% for stage I and 16% for stage IV. Prognosis is related to the tumor's location and the stage at which the disease is diagnosed (ACS, 2016d).

❖ NURSING PROCESS FOR THE PATIENT WITH A GALLBLADDER, LIVER, BILIARY TRACT, OR EXOCRINE PANCREATIC DISORDER

◆ ASSESSMENT

Nursing assessment of the patient with a gallbladder, liver, biliary tract, or exocrine pancreatic disorder must be performed accurately. Perform a head-to-toe assessment. Also assess the patient's knowledge of the disease process, nutritional status, pain, discomfort, current health problems, and signs and symptoms. Note changes in appetite and weight. Measure vital signs, noting any alterations from normal, such as hyperthermia, hypotension, hypertension, tachycardia, or tachypnea. Observe the skin, the sclerae, the mucous membranes, the urine, and the stool for alterations in the presence of bilirubin. Inspect, auscultate, and palpate the abdomen. Document any abdominal tenderness, pain, or abnormal bowel sounds.

◆ PATIENT PROBLEMS

Assessment provides data for identifying the patient's problems, strengths, potential complications, and learning needs. Patient problems for patients with disorders of the liver, biliary tract, or exocrine pancreas include but are not limited to the following:

- *Compromised Maintenance of Health*
- *Compromised Skin Integrity*
- *Helplessness*
- *Inability to Maintain Adequate Breathing Pattern*
- *Inability to Tolerate Activity*
- *Inadequate Fluid Volume*
- *Insufficient Knowledge*
- *Insufficient Nutrition*
- *Noncooperation or Nonconformity*
- *Potential for Harm or Damage to the Body*
- *Prolonged Pain*
- *Recent Onset of Confusion*
- *Recent Onset of Pain*

◆ EXPECTED OUTCOMES AND PLANNING

When planning care, look at the identified patient problem(s) and establish interventions. The overall goals for patients with disorders of the gallbladder, liver, biliary tract, and exocrine pancreas include (1) relief of pain and discomfort; (2) stabilization of fluid and electrolyte balance; (3) minimal to no complications; (4) ability to resume normal activities; (5) a return, if possible, to normal pancreatic and liver function without complications; and (6) a return to as normal a lifestyle as possible.

Planning includes the development of realistic goals and outcomes from the identified patient problems. Establish short- and long-term measurable goals. Examples of measurable goals are the following:

- Patient will feel rested enough to assist in ADLs.
- Patient will have increased activity tolerance by walking 100 ft.
- Patient will report that pain is less than a 4 on a scale of 0 to 10.

◆ IMPLEMENTATION

Maintaining the patient's optimal level of health is important in reducing biliary and pancreatic symptoms. Nursing interventions may include nutritional management, pharmacologic management, and health promotion and maintenance to prevent complications. Encourage the early diagnosis and treatment of liver, biliary tract, and pancreatic disease. Nursing interventions involve supportive care with special attention to nutrition, hydration, skin care, and pain relief.

◆ EVALUATION

During and after the planned nursing interventions, determine the outcomes of the interventions. This is an ongoing process of continually trying to establish the most effective care plan.

Evaluation involves determining whether the established goals have been met. Involve the patient in evaluating the goals to see whether the criteria for measurement have been met. Goals and evaluative measures for disorders of the liver, biliary tract, and exocrine pancreas may include the following:

Goal 1: Patient voices and demonstrates improved activity tolerance.

Evaluative measure: Observe patient exercise.

Goal 2: Patient remains free of bodily injury.

Evaluative measure: Ask patient to list factors that increase the risk of injury.

See the Cultural Considerations box.

Cultural Considerations

Gallbladder, Liver, Biliary Tract, or Exocrine Pancreatic Disorder

- Mortality from cirrhosis occurs more frequently among African Americans than among other ethnic groups.
- Primary hepatic cancer has a higher incidence among African Americans, Asian Americans, and Inuit (Eskimos) than among white Americans.
- Pancreatic cancer occurs more frequently among African Americans and Asian Americans than among white Americans.
- White Americans and Native Americans have a higher incidence of gallbladder disease than African Americans and Asian Americans.

Get Ready for the NCLEX® Examination!

Key Points

- Planned nursing interventions must be individualized according to each patient's and family's unique needs.
- The most common cause of cirrhosis of the liver is alcohol ingestion.
- Clinical manifestations of cirrhosis of the liver differ, depending on whether the patient is in the early or later stages of the disease.
- An important aspect of nursing interventions in patients with hepatitis and cirrhosis of the liver is the relief of pruritus.
- Prevention of the spread of viral hepatitis is a primary concern of health care professionals.
- Vaccines are available to prevent the development of hepatitis A and hepatitis B.
- If an infection develops anywhere along the GI tract, there is danger that the infecting organism may reach the liver through the biliary system, portal venous system, or hepatic arterial or lymphatic system and result in a liver abscess.
- Cholecystectomy (removal of the gallbladder by means of a laparoscopic or open abdominal procedure) is one of the most commonly performed surgical procedures.
- Pancreatic disorders may cause diabetes mellitus because of interference with insulin production.
- Clinical manifestations of acute pancreatitis include severe abdominal pain radiating to the back; the pain is sometimes relieved when the patient leans forward, taking the weight of the stomach off the pancreas.
- Tumor markers are used to establish the diagnosis of pancreatic adenocarcinoma and to monitor the response to treatment of cancer; CA 19-9 is elevated in pancreatic cancer and is the most commonly used tumor marker.

Additional Learning Resources

SG Go to your Study Guide for additional learning activities to help you master this chapter content.

evolve Be sure to visit the Evolve site at *http://evolve.elsevier.com/Cooper/foundationsadult/* for additional online resources.

Review Questions for the NCLEX® Examination

1. A patient is admitted with common bile duct obstruction related to cancer of the pancreas. Which clinical manifestations would the nurse expect to find? *(Select all that apply.)*
   1. Brown feces
   2. Scleral icterus
   3. Dark, tea-colored urine
   4. Jaundice
   5. Mid-epigastric pain
2. The nurse is caring for a postoperative cholecystectomy patient. The nurse includes coughing and deep breathing in the patient's care plan based on what criteria?
   1. The patient is often obese.
   2. The patient usually smokes.
   3. The patient is on bed rest for a prolonged period.
   4. The patient tends to take shallow breaths due to the location of the incision.

3. The nurse is caring for a patient with hepatic encephalopathy. While assessing the patient, the nurse notes rapid, irregular flexion and extension (flapping) of the wrist when the nurse requests that the patient stretch out the arm and hyperextend the wrist with fingers separated. How should the nurse document this finding?
   1. "Patient demonstrates the presence of varices."
   2. "Patient demonstrates the presence of asterixis."
   3. "Patient demonstrates the presence of pruritus."
   4. "Patient demonstrates the presence of bacterial toxins."
4. A patient has advanced cirrhosis of the liver with an acute exacerbation of hepatic encephalopathy. What type of food may be limited in his diet?
   1. Fruits
   2. Vegetables
   3. Meats
   4. Carbohydrates
5. The nurse is assessing a newly admitted patient. Which findings are most indicative of a liver abscess?
   1. Asterixis, ascites, and esophageal varices
   2. Fever accompanied by chills, abdominal pain, and tenderness in the right upper quadrant
   3. Enlarged spleen and spider telangiectases
   4. Constipation; left quadrant abdominal cramping; and loud, high-pitched abdominal sounds on auscultation
6. While discharging a patient after a laparoscopic cholecystectomy, the nurse hears the patient report mild shoulder pain. The nurse is aware that the pain is likely caused by which factor?
   1. Paralytic ileus with mesenteric irritation
   2. Incision along the rectus abdominis muscle
   3. Diaphragmatic irritation secondary to residual carbon dioxide
   4. Spasm of the duct of Wirsung
7. A patient has been admitted with right upper quadrant pain and has been placed on a low-fat diet. Which tray would be acceptable for the patient?
   1. Whole milk, veal, rice, and pastry
   2. Liver, fried potatoes, gelatin, and avocado
   3. Skim milk, lean fish, steamed carrots, and fruit
   4. Ham, mashed potatoes, creamed peas, and gelatin
8. The nurse is preparing a presentation on hepatitis types B and C. What should the nurse include in the presentation regarding the most common methods of becoming infected with the disease? *(Select all that apply.)*
   1. Recent blood transfusions
   2. Contaminated needles and instruments
   3. Direct contact with body fluids from infected people, such as through sexual contact
   4. Eating food prepared by someone with unclean hands
   5. Drinking contaminated water
9. A patient is scheduled for surgery for a common bile duct exploration. The nurse would expect the patient to return from surgery with which device in place?
   1. An underwater-seal drainage
   2. A T tube connected to gravity drainage
   3. A Penrose drain
   4. A nephrostomy tube
10. The nurse is caring for a patient with cholecystitis associated with cholelithiasis. Which statement by the nurse is most accurate when answering patient questions?
    1. "The disorder can be successfully treated with oral bile salts that dissolve gallstones."
    2. "Analgesics are usually not necessary to relieve the pain of bile duct spasms during an acute attack."
    3. "A heavy meal with a high fat content may precipitate the signs and symptoms of the disease."
    4. "A low-cholesterol diet is indicated to reduce the availability of cholesterol for gallstone formation."
11. Discharge teaching in relation to home management after a laparoscopic cholecystectomy should include which instructions?
    1. Keeping the bandages on the puncture sites for 48 hours
    2. Reporting any bile-colored drainage or pus from any incision
    3. Using over-the-counter antiemetics if nausea and vomiting occur
    4. Emptying and measuring the contents of the bile bag from the T tube every day
12. The student nurse asks the nurse why a patient with advanced cirrhosis has an abdomen that is so swollen. Which response by the nurse is correct?
    1. "A lack of clotting factors promotes the collection of blood in the abdominal cavity."
    2. "Portal hypertension and hypoalbuminemia cause a fluid shift into the peritoneal space."
    3. "Decreased peristalsis in the GI tract contributes to gas formation and bowel distention."
    4. "Bile salts in the blood irritate the peritoneal membranes, causing edema and pocketing of fluid."
13. When caring for a patient with acute exacerbation of hepatic encephalopathy, the nurse may give a lactulose enema, provide a low-protein diet, and limit physical activity. The nurse explains to the patient that these measures are taken for what reason?
    1. To promote fluid loss
    2. To eliminate potassium ions
    3. To decrease portal pressure
    4. To decrease ammonia production

14. If a patient is scheduled for an ultrasound of the pancreas, which situation would cause the examination to be postponed? *(Select all that apply.)*
    1. Low serum albumin
    2. MRI of abdomen
    3. ERCP examination
    4. Recent barium enema examination
15. The surgical procedure for cancer of the pancreas involves resection of the antrum of the stomach, the gallbladder, the duodenum, and varying amounts of the pancreas. Anastomoses are constructed between the stomach, the common bile and pancreatic ducts, and the jejunum. The nurse correctly identifies this procedure with which name?
    1. Whipple procedure
    2. Pancreatectomy
    3. Billroth I
    4. Billroth II
16. A patient's brother asks the nurse why the patient's pancreatic cancer is at stage IV so early after hearing the diagnosis. The nurse correctly identifies the late diagnosis and high mortality rates as being attributed to what factors? *(Select all that apply.)*
    1. It is difficult to diagnose pancreatic cancer at an early, curable stage.
    2. Patients with pancreatic cancer are often in denial.
    3. The majority of cancers have metastasized at the time of diagnosis.
    4. Early tumors often remain asymptomatic, or "silent," until their growth is advanced.
    5. Patients often attribute the vague early symptoms of pancreatic cancer to problems that do not warrant seeking medical attention.
17. While caring for a patient with hepatitis A, the nurse expects the stools of the patient to appear what color?
    1. Dark brown
    2. Black
    3. Clay-colored
    4. Green

Care of the Patient With a Blood or Lymphatic Disorder

47

http://evolve.elsevier.com/Cooper/foundationsadult/

Objectives

Anatomy and Physiology

1. Describe the components of blood.
2. Discuss factors necessary for the formation of erythrocytes.
3. Differentiate between the functions of erythrocytes, leukocytes, and thrombocytes.
4. Define the white blood cell differential.
5. Describe the blood-clotting process.
6. List the basic blood groups.
7. Describe the generalized functions of the lymphatic system and list the primary lymphatic structures.

Medical-Surgical

8. List common diagnostic tests for evaluation of blood and lymph disorders, and discuss the significance of the results.
9. Compare and contrast the various types of anemia in terms of etiology and pathophysiology, clinical manifestations, assessment, diagnostic tests, medical management, nursing interventions, patient teaching, and prognosis.
10. List six signs and symptoms associated with hypovolemic shock.
11. Discuss important issues to cover in patient teaching and home care planning for the patient with pernicious anemia.
12. Discuss the etiology and pathophysiology, clinical manifestations, assessment, diagnostic tests, medical management, nursing interventions, patient teaching, and prognosis for patients with acute and chronic leukemia.
13. Compare and contrast the disorders of coagulation (thrombocytopenia, hemophilia, disseminated intravascular coagulation) in terms of etiology and pathophysiology, clinical manifestations, assessment, diagnostic tests, medical management, nursing interventions, and prognosis.
14. Discuss the primary goal of nursing interventions for the patient with lymphedema.
15. Discuss the etiology and pathophysiology, clinical manifestations, assessment, diagnostic tests, medical management, nursing interventions, patient teaching, and prognosis for the patient with multiple myeloma, malignant lymphoma, and Hodgkin's lymphoma.
16. Apply the nursing process to the care of the patient with disorders of the hematologic and lymphatic systems.

Key Terms

anemia (ă-NĒ-mē-ă, p. 1483)
disseminated intravascular coagulation (DIC) (dĭ-SĔM-ĭ-nāt-ĕd, p. 1503)
erythrocytosis (ĕ-rĭth-rō-sī-TŌ-sĭs, p. 1493)
erythropoiesis (ĕ-rĭth-rō-pō-Ē-sĭs, p. 1476)
hemarthrosis (hē-măr-THRŌ-sĭs, p. 1501)
hemophilia A (hē-mō-FĒL-ē-ă, p. 1501)
heterozygous (hĕt-ĕr-ō-ZĪ-gŭs, p. 1490)
homozygous (hō-mō-ZĪ-gŭs, p. 1490)
idiopathic (ĭd-ē-ō-PĂTH-ĭk, p. 1499)
leukemia (lū-KĒ-mē-ă, p. 1495)
leukopenia (lū-kō-PĒ-nē-ă, p. 1494)
lymphangitis (lĭm-făn-GĪ-tĭs, p. 1506)
lymphedema (lĭm-fĕ-DĒ-mă, p. 1507)
multiple myeloma (MŬL-tĭ-pŭl mī-ĕ-LŌ-mă, p. 1505)
pancytopenic (păn-sī-tō-PĒN-ĭk, p. 1487)
pernicious (pĕr-NĬSH-ŭs, p. 1485)
recombinant (p. 1501)
Reed-Sternberg cells (rēd–STĔRN-bĕrg, p. 1508)
thrombocytopenia (thrŏm-bō-sīt-ō-PĒ-nē-ă, p. 1482)

ANATOMY AND PHYSIOLOGY OF THE HEMATOLOGIC AND LYMPHATIC SYSTEMS

The hematologic and lymphatic systems are vital for keeping the body in a state of homeostasis. Diseases and disorders that affect these two systems can cause serious and widespread problems in other body systems. Blood transports oxygen to cells, removes waste products from cells, and delivers nutrients throughout the body. The lymphatic system filters harmful substances out of the fluid that surrounds body tissues and maintains fluid balance.

CHARACTERISTICS OF BLOOD

Blood is a viscous (thick), red fluid that contains red blood cells (RBCs, or erythrocytes), white blood cells

(WBCs, or leukocytes), and platelets (thrombocytes). Plasma is the light yellow fluid of the blood and constitutes 55% of the blood's volume; the remaining 45% is composed of the blood cells and platelets. Blood is slightly alkaline, with a pH range of 7.35 to 7.45. It has a sodium chloride concentration of 0.9%. The average adult's blood volume is 5 to 6 L.

The blood performs three critical functions. First, it transports oxygen and nutrition to the cells and waste products away from the cells, and it transports hormones from endocrine glands to tissues and cells. Second, it regulates the acid-base balance (pH) with buffers, helps regulate body temperature because of its water content, and controls the water content of its cells as a result of dissolved sodium ions. Third, it protects the body against infection by transporting leukocytes and antibodies to the site of infection and prevents blood loss using special clotting mechanisms.

COMPONENTS OF BLOOD

Red Blood Cells

An RBC is the major cellular element of the circulating blood. A mature RBC, or *erythrocyte,* is a biconcave disk with no nucleus; it contains cytoplasm and hemoglobin, which give blood its rich red color. Hemoglobin (Hgb) is a substance in the blood that carries oxygen from the lungs to the cells and carbon dioxide away from the cells to the lungs. Hgb content is measured in grams per deciliter of blood. RBCs may be normochromic (normal amount of Hgb in a RBC giving it a normal color) or hypochromic (decreased amount of Hgb causing pallor of RBC). RBC size usually is described as macrocytic, microcytic, or normocytic. Men usually have approximately 5.5 million RBCs per cubic millimeter (mm^3) of blood; women usually have approximately 4.8 million RBCs per mm^3 (Table 47.1). The normal Hgb level is 14 to 18 g/dL for men and 12 to 16 g/dL for women. The average lifespan of an RBC is 120 days. Erythrocytes are produced continuously in the red bone marrow, principally in the vertebrae, ribs, sternum, and proximal ends of the humerus, pelvic girdle, and femur.

When the amount of oxygen delivered to the tissues by RBCs decreases, it triggers the kidneys to release a hormone, renal erythropoietic factor, or *erythropoietin.* Erythropoietin is carried to the bone marrow, where it initiates the development of mature RBCs. The increased number of RBCs allows more oxygen to be delivered to the tissues and thereby shuts off the signal to increase RBC production.

Erythropoiesis (the process of RBC production) depends on several factors, including healthy bone marrow and kidney function, and the presence of dietary substances such as iron, copper, and essential amino acids as well as certain vitamins, especially vitamin B_{12}, folic acid, riboflavin (vitamin B_2), and pyridoxine (vitamin B_6).

A common laboratory test, called the *hematocrit* (Hct), measures the volume percentage of red blood cells in whole blood. Hematocrit is expressed as a percentage of the total blood volume. RBCs usually make up about 42% to 52% of the blood volume in men and 37% to 47% in women, depending on the lab testing method.

Table 47.1 Diagnostic Blood Studies

BLOOD TEST	NORMAL VALUES	DESCRIPTION	CLINICAL SIGNIFICANCE
Red blood cells (RBCs)	Males: 4.7–6.1 million/mm^3 Females: 4.2–5.4 million/mm^3		Increased in dehydration, with polycythemia, at high altitudes, and with hypoxia; decreased in anemia, leukemia, and after hemorrhage.
Hemoglobin	Males: 14–18 g/dL Females: 12–16 g/dL	Measure of total amount of Hgb (Hb) in peripheral blood	Increased in polycythemia, dehydration, chronic obstructive lung disease; decreased in anemia and after hemorrhage.
Hematocrit	Males: 42%–52% Females: 37%–47%	Measure of the percentage of the total blood volume that is made up by the RBCs	Increased with severe burns, shock, severe dehydration, and polycythemia; decreased with severe blood loss, leukemia, and anemia.
Erythrocyte sedimentation rate (ESR)	Male: 0–15 mm/h Female: 0–20 mm/h	Rate at which RBCs settle out of a tube of unclotted blood in 1 h	Increased in tissue destruction; indicates infection when results are compared with elevation in WBC count; a fairly reliable indicator of the course of disease and therefore used to monitor disease therapy, especially for inflammatory autoimmune diseases.
Reticulocyte count	0.5%–2%	Number of reticulocytes in whole blood	Increased in bone marrow hyperactivity and hemorrhage; decreased in hemolytic disease.

Table 47.1 **Diagnostic Blood Studies—cont'd**

BLOOD TEST	NORMAL VALUES	DESCRIPTION	CLINICAL SIGNIFICANCE
Platelet count	150,000–400,000/mm^3	Actual cell count	Increased in granulocytic leukemia; decreased in thrombocytopenia or aplastic anemia.
Prothrombin time (PT)	11–12.5 s	Rapidity of blood clotting	Detects plasma clotting defects, screens for coagulation, and monitors warfarin (Coumadin) therapy; possible critical values >20 s.
International normalized ratio (INR)	0.7–1.8	World Health Organization has recommended that PT results now include the INR value; many hospitals report PT results in both absolute numbers and INR	Therapeutic INR usually considered to be 2–3.5.
Partial thromboplastin time (PTT)	60–70 s	Fibrin clot formation	Detects coagulation defects of the intrinsic system and deficiency of plasma clotting; used to monitor the appropriate dose of heparin.
Bleeding time	1–9 min (Ivy method)	Amount of time for a small stab wound to stop bleeding	Prolonged in hemorrhagic disease or with coagulation factor defect.
Clotting time	3–9 min	Amount of time for blood in a tube to clot	Prolonged with deficiency in coagulation factors or vitamin K; used to monitor anticoagulant therapy.
White Blood Cell (WBC) Count With Differential			
WBC	5000–10,000/mm^3	Actual cell count	Increased neutrophils with a number of bacterial infections, inflammatory but noninfectious diseases (collagen disorder, rheumatic fever, and pancreatitis); increased with infectious diseases (usually of bacterial origin) and with trauma or leukemia; decreased by chemotherapy, radiation, aplastic anemia, and agranulocytosis.
Neutrophils	60%–70%[a] 3000–7000/mm^3		Increased with burns, crushing injuries, diabetic acidosis, and infections; decreased in bone marrow failure after antineoplastic chemotherapy or radiation therapy or in agranulocytosis, dietary deficiencies, and autoimmune diseases.
Eosinophils	1%–4%[a] 50–400/mm^3		Increased with allergic and parasitic disorders.
Basophils	0.5%–1%[a] 25–100/mm^3		Increases uncommon; found with some forms of acute leukemia.
Lymphocytes	20%–40%[a] 1000–4000/mm^3		Increased in infectious mononucleosis, measles, certain viruses, infectious hepatitis, and lymphocytic leukemia; decreased in AIDS, lupus erythematosus, and Hodgkin's lymphoma.
Monocytes	2%–6%[a] 100–600/mm^3		Increased in the recovery phase of bacterial infections and chronic inflammatory conditions.

[a]Relative values: expressed as percentage of total WBCs.
AIDS, Acquired immunodeficiency syndrome.

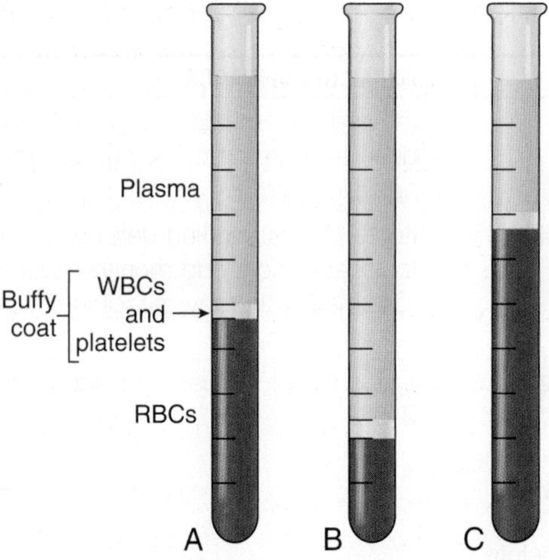

Fig. 47.1 Hematocrit (Hct) tubes showing normal blood, anemia, and polycythemia. Note the buffy coat located between the packed red blood cells (RBCs) and the plasma. A, A normal percentage of RBCs. B, Anemia (a low percentage of RBCs). C, Polycythemia (a high percentage of RBCs). *WBCs*, White blood cells. (From Patton KT, Thibodeau GA: *The human body in health and disease*, ed 7, St. Louis, 2018, Elsevier.)

The Hgb level and the Hct are based on whole blood and are affected by plasma volume. The Hgb and the Hct often test high if the patient is suffering from dehydration. Conversely, the Hgb level and Hct appear low with lab testing if the patient is in fluid overload (Fig. 47.1).

If Hgb falls below the normal level, as it does in anemia, an unhealthy chain reaction begins: less Hgb means less oxygen transported to cells, a slower breakdown and use of nutrients by cells, less energy produced by cells, and decreased cellular function. Understanding the relationship between Hgb and energy makes it clear why an anemic person complains of feeling "tired all the time."

White Blood Cells

Unlike erythrocytes, *leukocytes* (WBCs) have nuclei, are colorless, and have a lifespan ranging from a few days to several years. Body defense, such as the destruction of bacteria and viruses, is their primary function. Normal WBC levels are 5000 to 10,000/mm^3 of blood. Some WBCs leave the bloodstream and move through tissue spaces to fight foreign invaders such as bacteria. WBCs have two broad categories: granular and agranular WBCs, which are produced in the red bone marrow. The three types of granular WBCs are neutrophils, eosinophils, and basophils. The agranular WBCs include lymphocytes and monocytes. A *differential white blood cell count* measures the five types of WBCs and reports them as percentages of the total examined. They also may be reported as absolute counts (i.e., actual numbers).

Leukocytes respond predictably to symptoms of infection and recovery, so they are a reliable gauge of the state of the body's defenses. This is why the differential WBC count is such a common blood test. The differential WBC aid in diagnosing a disease, assist in discriminating between bacterial and viral infections, help in revealing activity that points to occult (hidden) infection, or may signal the intensity of chemotherapy.

Granulocytes develop from the red bone marrow and contain granules in their cytoplasm. The granules are demonstrated when the cells are stained with Wright's stain (a chemical solution). *Neutrophils* (granular circulating leukocytes essential for *phagocytosis*—the process by which bacteria, cellular debris, and solid particles are destroyed and removed) ingest bacteria and dispose of dead tissue. Neutrophils are the primary phagocytic cells involved in the acute inflammatory response. A mature neutrophil is called a segmental neutrophil, or "seg," because the nucleus is segmented into two to five lobes connected by strands. They also release lysozyme, an enzyme that destroys certain bacteria. The normal differential value for neutrophils is 60% to 70%.

Mature neutrophils have a short lifespan (approximately 7 hours), after which they die, along with the bacteria and debris they have engulfed. Bone marrow thus must manufacture neutrophils constantly; normally it stores approximately a 6-day supply. Because neutrophils respond in proportion to the severity of the infection, an overwhelming infection may deplete marrow reserves. When this happens, the marrow releases polymorphonuclear leukocytes ("polys") that are in the final stages of development. These immature neutrophils are called *bands*. When the band count exceeds 8% of the total number of polys, the marrow has used up its reserve. In the differential WBC count, an increase in the number of band neutrophils is called *bandemia*. Bandemia is seen in patients with serious bacterial infections. The presence of excess bands in the peripheral blood traditionally was called "a shift to the left." This term originated when cells were counted by hand using a manual counting machine, with the immature neutrophils recorded on the left side of the paper.

Eosinophils are WBCs that play a role in allergic reactions and are effective against certain parasitic worms. Normal values of eosinophils are 1% to 4%.

Basophils are WBCs that are essential to the nonspecific immune response to inflammation because they release histamine (vasodilator) during tissue damage or invasion. They have cytoplasmic granules that contain heparin, serotonin, and histamine. If a basophil is stimulated by an antigen or by tissue injury, it releases these substances from within the granules. This is part of the response seen in allergic and inflammatory reactions. Normal values of basophils are 0.5% to 1%.

Monocytes are WBCs that function like neutrophils: they circulate in the bloodstream and move into tissue, where they engulf foreign antigens and cell debris. Monocytes are the second type of WBC to arrive at the scene of an injury. They are useful in removing dead bacteria and cells in the recovery stage of acute bacterial infections. Normal values of monocytes are 2% to 6%.

Lymphocytes are WBCs that may be divided into two groups: T cells and B cells. T cells and B cells arise in the red bone marrow. T cells then migrate to the thymus, where the thymic hormones bring them to maturity (William and Hopper, 2015). T cells and B cells set up the antigen-antibody process, which protects the body. The B cells search out, identify, and bind with specific antigens. T cells, when exposed to an antigen, divide rapidly and produce large numbers of new T cells that are sensitized to that antigen. B cells produce antibody, a special protein that combats foreign invaders, or antigens. T cells work together with the B cells to destroy the foreign antigen. Normal values of lymphocytes are 20% to 40%.

Thrombocytes (Platelets)

Thrombocytes, or platelets, are the smallest cells in the blood. They are circular cell fragments that do not contain nuclei. They have a lifespan of 5 to 9 days and number 150,000 to 400,000/mm^3 of blood. They are produced in the red bone marrow and have a role in the process of hemostasis (the prevention of blood loss). They assist in forming clots, which seal off a break in the continuity of the walls of the blood vessels (Fig. 47.2).

Hemostasis

Hemostasis is a body process that arrests the flow of blood and prevents hemorrhage. Three actions take place: (1) vessel spasm, (2) platelet plug formation, and (3) clot formation. When a vessel has a tear or rupture, the smooth muscle in the walls of the vessel causes it to contract. Platelets rush in and attempt to seal the area, which is effective in small vessel tears. The third process, clot formation, is more detailed and occurs in larger injuries. This process can be summarized as follows (see Fig. 47.2):

1. Injury occurs, and a blood vessel is damaged.
2. Hemorrhage begins.
3. Platelets are activated and clump at the site of damage.
4. Thromboplastin, released from platelets, reacts with calcium ions.
5. In the presence of thromboplastin and calcium, prothrombin is converted to thrombin.
6. Thrombin links with fibrinogen.
7. Fibrinogen forms fibrin.
8. Fibrin traps RBCs and platelets, forming a blood clot.
9. The blood clot seals the damaged blood vessel.

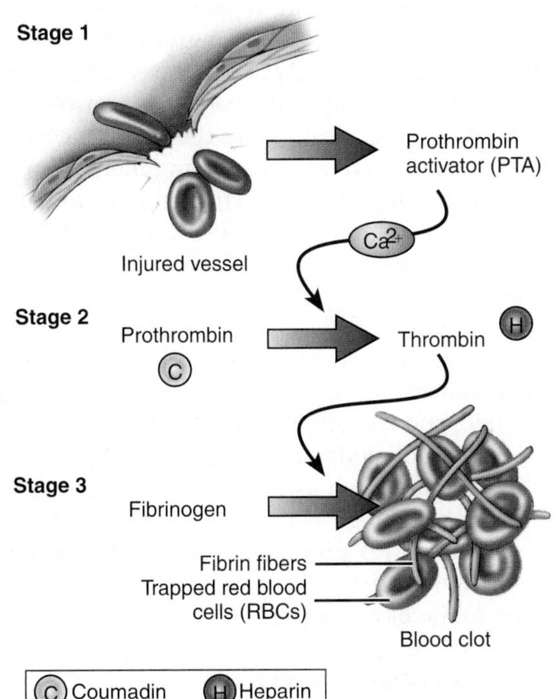

Fig. 47.2 Blood clotting. The extremely complex clotting mechanism can be distilled into three basic stages: *stage 1*, release of clotting factors from injured tissue cells and sticky platelets at the injury site; *stage 2*, formation of thrombin; and *stage 3*, formation of fibrin and trapping of red blood cells to form a clot. (From Herlihy B: *The human body in health and illness*, ed 6, St. Louis, 2018, Elsevier.)

Blood Types (Groups)

Genetics determines blood group or type; it is inherited from the parents. Blood types are determined by the presence or absence of specific antigens on the outer surface of the RBCs. In certain types of blood, the antigens on the RBCs are accompanied by antibodies found in the blood plasma. This is referred to as the ABO blood group system. According to this system, each person's blood type is one of the following: *A, B, AB,* or *O.* In ABO typing, red blood cells are isolated from the blood sample and mixed with antiserum (serum containing antibodies that are specific for one or more antigens) with a known antibody type. Cells marked with antigen A clump when mixed with antibody A, cells with B antigen clump when exposed to antibody B, AB antigens clump with either, and O clumps with neither. The type of positive clumping reaction determines blood type. Rh type (Rh factor is described in the next section) is determined in the same manner, with Rh-positive blood exhibiting a clumping reaction with Rh antibodies.

Harmful effects or death can result from a blood transfusion if antibodies in the recipient's plasma react to the donor's blood and the RBCs clump together (become agglutinated). If the donor's blood is type O, and therefore its RBCs do not contain any A or B antigen, the blood cannot be clumped by anti-A or anti-B antibodies. For this reason type O blood is known as *universal donor* blood; it can be used in an emergency as donor blood no matter what the recipient's blood type. Blood type AB has been called the *universal recipient* blood because it contains neither anti-A nor anti-B antibodies in its plasma. Therefore it does not clump any donor's RBCs containing A or B antigens. In acute clinical settings, however, all blood for transfusion is typed and cross-matched carefully to the blood of the recipient for a variety of factors. Fig. 47.3 shows the results of combinations of donor and recipient blood.

Recipient's blood		Reactions with donor's blood			
RBC antigens	Plasma antibodies	Donor type O	Donor type A	Donor type B	Donor type AB
None (Type O)	Anti-A Anti-B				
A (Type A)	Anti-B				
B (Type B)	Anti-A				
AB (Type AB)	(None)				

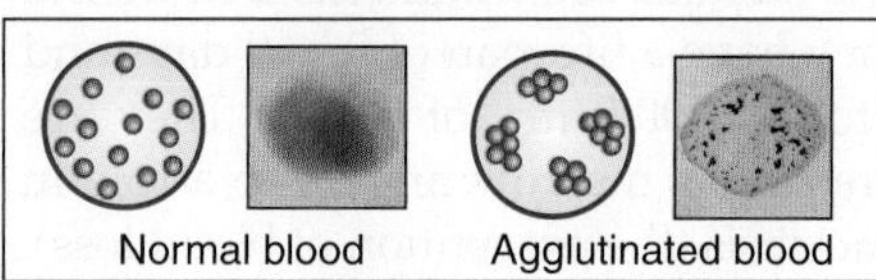

Fig. 47.3 Results of various combinations of donor and recipient blood. The *left columns* show the recipient's blood characteristics, and the *top row* shows the donor's blood type. (From Patton KT, Thibodeau GA: *The human body in health and disease,* ed 7, St. Louis, 2018, Elsevier.)

Two types of reaction can occur: agglutination and hemolysis. In agglutination the donor cells clump together because of the antibodies; this occludes arteries and can result in death. In hemolysis the antibodies cause the RBCs of the recipient to rupture and release their cell contents; this also can lead to death.

Rh Factor

Rh factor is located on the surface of the RBCs. People who have Rh factor are said to be Rh positive; people who do not have Rh factor are said to be Rh negative: 85% of humans have Rh factor; 15% do not. Normally human plasma does not contain Rh antibodies; these develop in response to an individual's receiving the wrong type of blood (i.e., if an Rh-negative person receives Rh-positive blood). Within approximately 2 weeks, Rh antibodies are produced and remain in the blood. If the Rh-negative person then receives more Rh-positive blood, a severe reaction occurs because the anti-Rh antibodies react with the donor blood. The antibodies hemolyze the donor RBCs, causing them to rupture and lose their contents. Unlike in the ABO system, antibodies to Rh antigens do not develop naturally. They develop only as an immune response after a transfusion or during pregnancy.

Rh incompatibility is seen most commonly in pregnancy. Fortunately, this incompatibility can be prevented. The first step in preventing hemolytic disease of the newborn (HDN) is to find out the Rh types of the expectant parents. If the mother is Rh negative and the father is Rh positive, the baby is at risk for developing HDN. The next step is to test the mother's serum to make sure she does not already have anti-Rh (also called anti-D) antibodies from a previous pregnancy or transfusion. This procedure is similar to blood typing. Finally, the Rh-negative mother is given an injection of Rh immune globulin (RhIg) at 27 to 28 weeks of gestation and again after delivery, if the baby is Rh positive. The RhIg attaches to any Rh-positive cells from the baby in the mother's bloodstream, preventing them from triggering anti-D antibody production in the mother. An Rh-negative woman also should receive RhIg after a miscarriage, abortion, or ectopic pregnancy.

LYMPHATIC SYSTEM

The lymphatic system is a subdivision of the cardiovascular system. It consists of lymphatic vessels, the lymph fluid, and the lymph tissue. In addition to lymph vessels and lymph nodes, the lymphatic system includes lymphatic organs such as the thymus and the spleen. The system has three basic functions: (1) maintenance of fluid balance, (2) production of lymphocytes, and (3) absorption and transportation of lipids from the intestine to the bloodstream.

Lymph and Lymph Vessels

The constancy of the fluid around each body cell can be maintained only if numerous homeostatic mechanisms function together in a controlled and integrated response to changing conditions. The circulatory system plays a key role in bringing many needed substances to cells and then removing the waste products that accumulate as a result of metabolism. This exchange of substances between blood and tissue fluid occurs in capillary beds of the circulatory system. Many other substances that cannot enter or return through the capillary walls, including excess fluid and protein molecules, are returned to the vascular system as lymph, transported by lymph capillaries and vessels. Lymph capillaries and vessels have one-way valves, as do veins of the circulatory system, but they are more numerous in the lymphatics (Williams and Hopper, 2015).

The lymphatic system consists of lymph vessels and lymph nodes found throughout the body. The lymph vessels collect lymphatic fluid, which consists of protein, water, fats, and wastes from cells. The lymph vessels transport the fluid to the lymph nodes, where waste and foreign materials are filtered out from the fluid. The fluid then is returned to the circulatory system. When lymphatic vessels are damaged or missing, the lymph fluid cannot move freely throughout the system and therefore accumulates. This results in abnormal swelling of the arm(s) or leg(s), and occasionally swelling in other parts of the body.

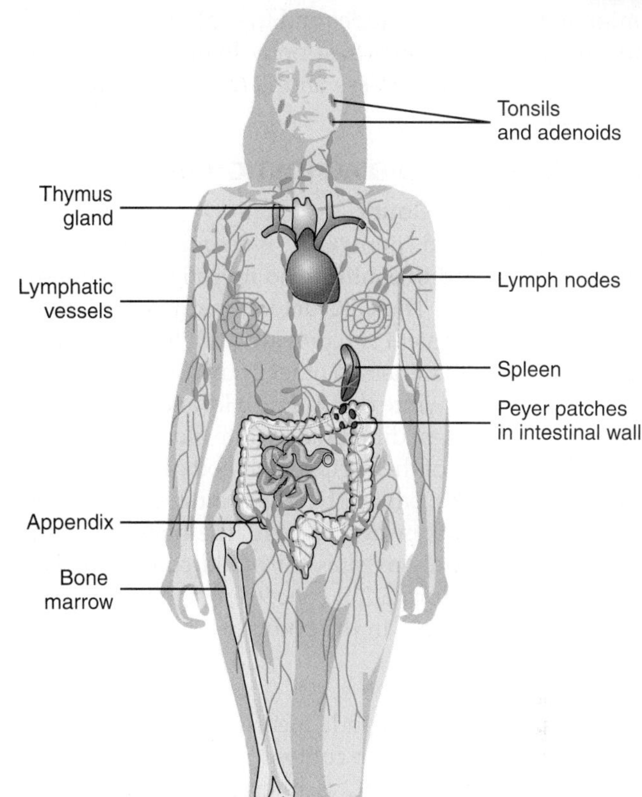

Fig. 47.4 Principal organs of the lymphatic system. (From Copstead-Kirkhorn LE, Banasik J: *Pathophysiology*, ed 5, St. Louis, 2013, Mosby.)

Lymphatic Tissue

Lymph nodes. Lymph nodes help fight infection by filtering foreign material, such as bacteria and cancer cells, from the lymphatic fluid, and fight infection by releasing stored lymphocytes (WBCs). The body contains 500 to 600 lymph nodes, found along the pathways of the lymph vessels, and lymph flows through these nodes on its way to the subclavian arteries. Lymph nodes are small, soft, round bean-shaped structures, usually appearing in groups. They range from 0.04 to 1 inch (1 to 25 mm) in length. Lymph nodes are found in the axilla (armpits), the abdomen, the thorax (chest), and the cervical (neck) and inguinal (groin) regions (see Fig. 47.4). As lymph passes through a lymph node, bacteria and other foreign material are destroyed by macrophages (phagocytic monocyte) through the process of phagocytosis. The collection of the foreign matter, such as bacteria, is the reason why lymph nodes become swollen during an infection. In addition, B cell lymphocytes exposed to pathogens in the lymphatic system produce antibodies that help the body fight infection (Vorvik and Zieve, 2016).

Tonsils. The tonsils are lymphatic tissue found in the mucous membrane of the pharynx. The tonsils contain lymphocytes and macrophages to protect the body and lungs against microorganisms. Like other lymph nodes in the body, the tonsils become enlarged when the filtering function becomes overwhelmed with a virus or bacteria. Tonsillitis often results when pathogens enter these tissues.

Spleen. The spleen is a soft, roughly ovoid, highly vascularized organ located in the left upper quadrant of the abdominal cavity, just below the diaphragm (see Fig. 47.4). The spleen is 5 to 6 in (12.7 to 15.2 cm) long and 2 to 3 in (5 to 7.6 cm) wide. It contains lymphatic nodules.

The spleen stores approximately 500 mL or 1 pint of blood, which can be released during emergencies, such as hemorrhage, in less than 60 seconds. This large amount of blood gives the spleen its deep purple color. One of the major functions of the spleen is hemolysis (destroying) of old or imperfect red blood cells. Other functions of the spleen are as follows: (1) it serves as a reservoir for blood; (2) it stores lymphocytes, monocytes, and plasma cells; (3) the white blood cells in the lining of the hollow cavities within the spleen engulf and destroy foreign materials, as well as damaged red blood cells, that pass through the spleen; and (4) it produces RBCs before birth (the spleen is believed to produce RBCs after birth only in cases of extreme hemolytic anemia).

Thymus. The thymus is located in the mediastinum (upper thorax posterior to the sternum and between the lungs) (i.e., the tissue and organs between the lungs) (see Fig. 47.4). The thymus functions in utero (before birth) and for a few months after birth to help develop the immune system. In particular, the thymus is responsible for the development of T lymphocytes, which take part in the cell-mediated immune response before they migrate to the lymph nodes and the spleen. At puberty the thymus gland begins to atrophy. In the mature adult, it is relatively functionless and is replaced by fat and connective tissue.

LABORATORY AND DIAGNOSTIC TESTS

Complete Blood Count

The complete blood count (CBC) is an important screening tool. It is used to confirm and investigate for many disease processes. The CBC detects many disorders of the hematologic system and provides data for diagnosing and evaluating disorders in other body systems. A CBC includes red and white cell counts, Hct and Hgb levels, erythrocyte indexes, differential white blood cell count, and examination of the peripheral blood cells (see Table 47.1). Prepare the patient by explaining that a blood sample will be taken from a vein. The hand and arm are used commonly as sites for blood collection. The CBC provides information concerning the presence of infection and anemia in the body.

Erythrocyte Indexes

Erythrocyte indexes include measurements of the size of RBCs and of their Hgb content. The average size, or volume, of a single RBC is referred to as the mean corpuscular volume (MCV). Mean corpuscular hemoglobin (MCH) is a measure of the average amount (weight) of Hgb within an RBC. Mean corpuscular hemoglobin concentration (MCHC) is a measure of the average concentration or the percentage of Hgb within an RBC.

Peripheral Blood Smear

A peripheral blood smear, along with the differential WBC count, allows examination of the size, shape, and structure of individual blood cells and platelets. This information is useful in differentiating various forms of anemias and dyscrasias (any abnormal physiologic condition, especially of the blood). All three hematologic cell lines (RBCs, WBCs, and platelets) can be examined. When adequately prepared and examined microscopically by an experienced technologist, a peripheral blood smear is the most informative of all hematologic tests.

Schilling Test and Megaloblastic Anemia Profile

The Schilling test is used to diagnose pernicious anemia (anemia caused by impaired intestinal absorption of vitamin B_{12}, which is needed to make RBCs). In the Schilling test, radioactive vitamin B_{12} is administered and measured before and after parenteral injection of *intrinsic factor* (a glycoprotein normally secreted by the stomach that is necessary for intestinal absorption of cyanocobalamin [vitamin B_{12}]), by examination of the urinary excretion of vitamin B_{12}. Normal findings are excretion of 8% to 40% of radioactive vitamin B_{12} within 24 hours. The Schilling test for pernicious anemia is being replaced by a serum test called a *megaloblastic anemia profile,* which measures levels of vitamin B_{12}, methylmalonic acid (produced when proteins in the body break down), and homocysteine (an amino acid).

Gastric Analysis

The Schilling test is performed rarely; gastric analysis is obligatory to determine intrinsic factor output. Gastric analysis is an older test for determining pernicious anemia. In pernicious anemia the gastric secretions are minimal, and the pH remains elevated, even after injection of histamine (a compound known to stimulate the stomach to secrete acid). Pernicious anemia is a consequence of intrinsic factor loss and neutralizing intrinsic factor antibody that impairs cobalamin absorption. Laboratory diagnosis rests on parietal cell antibody with or without intrinsic factor antibody, cobalamin-deficient megaloblastic anemia, and elevated serum gastrin from loss of acid secretion. This study is also important to eliminate the possibility that a patient has simple atrophic gastritis, a disease much more frequent than pernicious anemia (Cattan, 2011).

Radiologic Studies

Radiologic studies of the hematologic system involve primarily the use of computed tomography (CT) or magnetic resonance imaging (MRI) for evaluating the spleen, liver, and lymph nodes. In the past, lymphangiography (i.e., x-ray analysis of lymphatic vessels and nodes) with contrast dye was a common procedure for evaluating lymph nodes deep inside the body.

Bone Marrow Aspiration or Biopsy

Bone marrow aspiration and biopsy can help establish a diagnosis when there is a suspected hematologic issue. The most common site for this procedure is the posterior iliac crest. This site frequently is used because there are not vital organs, blood vessels, or nerves near this area. The tibia also can be used for bone marrow aspiration or biopsy, but this is not a preferred site.

The sternum also may be used, but generally only for aspiration. Normal bone marrow is soft and semifluid and can be removed by aspiration through a specialized needle device. Bone marrow aspiration is performed most commonly in people with marked anemia, neutropenia (decreased number of certain WBCs), acute leukemia, and **thrombocytopenia** (decreased number of platelets). The aspirate is examined for cell types, numbers, and degree of maturation. Although complications of bone marrow aspiration are minimal, there is a possibility of penetrating the underlying structures. This complication is greatest in an aspiration procedure involving the sternum.

DISORDERS OF THE HEMATOLOGIC SYSTEM

The hematologic and lymphatic systems include the blood and the organs of blood production, the bone marrow, and lymphatic tissue. Disorders of blood production, bone marrow, or lymphatic tissues affect all body systems. Disturbances in this delicate balance can produce life-threatening signs and symptoms, severe pain, and incapacitation.

DISORDERS ASSOCIATED WITH ERYTHROCYTES

ANEMIA

Anemia is a condition in which there is a below-normal amount of RBCs, causing a decrease in Hgb and Hct. Oxygen supply to tissues and cells is decreased because of the lack of oxygen carrying Hgb. Symptoms of anemia include fatigue, shortness of breath, and weakness.

Etiology and Pathophysiology

Anemia can be caused by many things, including excessive blood loss of short- and long-term duration such as hemorrhage, prolonged menstrual periods, and gastrointestinal bleeding. Additional conditions leading to anemia include impaired production of RBCs (bone marrow depression), increased destruction of RBCs (hemolysis), and nutritional deficiencies (long-term iron deficiency), acting alone or in combination. Hemorrhage, or blood loss, accounts for temporary anemia, whereas nutritional deficit can cause long-term iron deficiency anemia. Marrow failure may result from a disease process, toxic exposure, tumor, or unknown causes. Decreased RBC production or increased RBC destruction results in fewer circulating RBCs. In either case bone marrow hematopoietic function is unable to produce the needed quantity of RBCs.

Loss of Hgb, the oxygen-carrying element in the blood, results in a supply/demand imbalance in vital organs. The peripheral circulation compensates by shunting blood to vital organs, thus causing hypoxia in other areas of the body. Rapid hematopoietic effort may lead to blood cell irregularities (e.g., the presence of immature RBCs in the blood) and an inability to produce RBCs, with a resultant decrease in the RBC count.

Clinical Manifestations

The clinical manifestations of anemia depend on the individual's ability to compensate for the loss in oxygen-carrying capacity. If the onset of anemia is sudden, the symptoms are more dramatic. For example, a sudden loss of more than one-third of a patient's blood volume typically results in hypotension, respiratory distress, and acute mental status change, even in a young, previously healthy patient. Most of the symptoms can be contributed to the body trying to overcome decreased oxygenation. In cases of acute blood loss or when Hgb falls below 5 g/dL, patients may experience shock, severe hypotension, myocardial infarction, stroke, and confusion, and sometimes death.

On the other hand, chronic mild anemia may show no symptoms and is detected as an incidental finding on a routine laboratory test. With the more typical chronic development of anemia, the clinical changes are more subtle and depend on the patient's age and comorbid conditions. Common symptoms in this situation include general malaise, heart palpitations, shortness of breath on exertion, dizziness, and lightheadedness.

Assessment

Subjective data commonly include complaints of weakness, dyspnea, fatigue, and vertigo. Anorexia and dyspepsia may accompany headache and insomnia, but the patient generally does not link these complaints to the condition unless questioned. In older adult patients with impaired cardiopulmonary reserves, be alert to complaints of chest pain, dyspnea on exertion, palpitations, and dizziness.

Collection of objective data includes observing signs of bleeding or shock (hypovolemic anemia). Laboratory values show a low RBC count and Hct and low Hgb levels. Skin and mucous membranes are pale, and cardiac symptoms are related to anemia.

Diagnostic Tests

The CBC of a patient with anemia typically shows a low RBC count and below-normal Hgb and Hct levels. Serum iron, total iron-binding capacity, and serum ferritin levels also may be below normal. Serum folate (also called *folic acid*) may be measured if certain types of anemia are suspected. The reticulocyte (i.e., immature RBC) count may be increased because of the presence of high numbers of immature RBCs. A bone marrow study shows a deviation from normal findings. Peripheral blood smears enable identification of abnormalities in the shape and color of blood cells. A megaloblastic anemia profile reveals decreased levels of vitamin B_{12}.

Medical Management

Intervention depends on the cause. Correction of the disease process may correct or lessen the anemic condition. Transfusion is appropriate for blood loss; iron and vitamin B_{12} are replaced if these are deficient. Treatment is often specific to the particular anemia (see the Cultural Considerations box).

Nursing Interventions and Patient Teaching

Patient problems and interventions for the patient with anemia include but are not limited to the following:

Patient Problem	Nursing Interventions
Compromised Blood Flow to Tissue (cardiovascular), related to reduction of cellular components necessary for delivery of oxygen to the cells	Monitor changes in vital signs and change in LOC Monitor for cardiac rhythms Monitor Hgb, Hct, and RBCs Assess baseline arterial blood gases and electrolytes Note presence and degree of dyspnea, cyanosis

Continued

Patient Problem	Nursing Interventions
Insufficient Oxygenation, related to deficient: • RBCs • Hgb • Hct	Evaluate ability to manage activities of daily living (ADLs), related to oxygen decrease Assess activity tolerance, dyspnea, heart rate, oxygen saturation, nail beds for cyanosis Observe for cyanosis, hypoxia, and hypercapnia Maintain bed rest as necessary and provide range-of-motion (ROM) exercise Monitor oxygen saturations frequently by pulse oximetry Administer oxygen as ordered Explain activity–oxygen deficit relationship
Inability to Tolerate Activity, related to: • Tissue hypoxia • Dyspnea	Plan care to conserve energy after periods of activity Encourage the patient to limit visitors, phone calls, and unnecessary interruptions to conserve energy Assist the patient with self-care activities as needed Place articles within easy reach of the patient to reduce physiologic demands on the body Administer oxygen as ordered to relieve dyspnea Monitor Hgb and Hct levels

Tailor patient education to the individual's condition and needs.

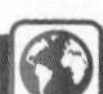 Cultural Considerations

Jehovah's Witness Opposition to Blood Transfusion

The nurse providing culturally appropriate nursing interventions to a Jehovah's Witness has many factors to consider. Jehovah's Witnesses are opposed to homologous blood transfusion (blood obtained from a blood bank or through donations). They believe that receiving blood products from another person carries eternal consequences. However, many (but not all) Jehovah's Witnesses may agree to certain types of autologous blood transfusions (sometimes called *autotransfusions*). One type of autologous transfusion that may be acceptable is blood retrieved through induced hemodilution at the start of surgery. This blood conservation technique involves removing blood from a patient—either immediately before or shortly after induction of anesthesia—while simultaneously replacing the blood with an equivalent volume of a blood volume expander (e.g., crystalloid [sodium chloride] and/or colloid). The withdrawn blood is anticoagulated and maintained at room temperature in the operating room for up to 8 hours. It is reinfused into the patient as needed during or after the surgical procedure (Chand, 2014; Lindstrom and Johnstone, 2010).

The consensus of the US Supreme Court has been that an adult—that is, a person who has reached the age of majority—has the right to refuse treatment but does not have the right to withhold a potentially life-saving treatment from a minor child.

Some Jehovah's Witnesses allow the use of certain blood volume expanders (colloids). Many Jehovah's Witnesses carry a card with the types of blood volume expanders permitted. Ask the patient for this card or, if the patient is unconscious, examine the patient's personal belongings to find this extremely important card (Chand, Subramanya, and Rao, 2014).

Data from Lindstrom E, Johnstone R: Acute normovolemic hemodilution in a Jehovah's Witness patient: A case report. *AANA J* 78(4):326-330, 2010; and Chand NK, Subramanya HB, Rao GV: Management of patients who refuse blood transfusion, *Indian J Anaesth* 58(5):658-664, 2014.

Hypovolemic Anemia (Blood Loss Anemia)

Etiology and pathophysiology. Secondary anemia occurs when deficiencies in RBCs and other components are caused by an abnormally low circulating blood volume resulting from acute or chronic blood loss. Loss of blood decreases the amount of circulating fluid and Hgb and thus decreases the amount of oxygen carried to the body tissues. The tissues must have oxygen to survive. The average adult has an approximate total blood volume of 6000 mL (6 L [12 pints]) and can tolerate a loss of up to 500 mL. Blood loss of 1000 mL or more in an adult can have severe consequences. This level of reduction in total blood volume can lead to hypovolemic shock. Such a loss usually is related to internal or external hemorrhage caused by a surgical procedure, gastrointestinal (GI) bleeding, menorrhagia (abnormally prolonged menstrual bleeding), trauma, or severe burns. The rapidity of blood loss is related to the severity and number of signs and symptoms.

Clinical manifestations. Signs and symptoms include restlessness; a subtle rise in respiratory rate; weakness; stupor; irritability; a pale, cool, moist skin; and a rapid, thready pulse (Box 47.1). Excessive blood loss results in shock. Shock occurs when there is a deprivation of oxygen and nutrients to organs. Hemorrhagic blood loss results in a decrease in blood volume. In shock, vasoconstriction occurs in blood vessels to noncritical organs such as skin, muscles, and intestines. This decreases the blood flow to these organs and shunts blood to the vital organs such as the heart and the brain.

The greater the amount of blood loss, the more the heart rate and blood pressure are affected. The body is able to compensate for blood loss less than 15% or 750 mL. The initial symptom may be only tachycardia, although there can be an initial rise in systolic blood pressure, then a fall to below 80 mm Hg. At 20% to

Box 47.1 Signs of Hypovolemia

- Anxiety or agitation
- Confusion
- Cool, clammy skin
- Decreased or no urine output
- Diaphoresis
- General weakness
- Hypotension
- Low body temperature
- Pale skin color (pallor)
- Pulse weak and thready
- Rapid breathing
- Tachycardia
- Unconsciousness

25% blood loss, tachycardia and mild to moderate hypotension are present. With a loss of 40% or greater (2000 mL) all clinical signs and symptoms of shock are present.

Hypovolemic anemia in a child often results in differing signs and symptoms initially than in adults. The child may be alert and have normal blood pressure, pulse, and perfusion initially. Signs and symptoms may progress to cool and clammy skin, hypotension, tachycardia, tachypnea, and reduced urine output. Treatment is similar to adults. IV fluid administration is the first treatment. If fluid administration is not effective, blood administration may be necessary.

The patient's clinical signs and symptoms of hypovolemic anemia are equally as important as the laboratory values. Be alert to the patient's expression of pain. Internal hemorrhage may cause pain because of tissue distention, organ displacement, and nerve compression. Pain may be localized or referred (*referred pain* is felt at a place other than where the damage actually is). Decreased RBC, Hgb, and Hct levels may not be evident until several days after severe blood loss has occurred. The severity of the patient's signs and symptoms correlates with the severity of the blood loss.

Assessment. Subjective data commonly include complaints of thirst, weakness, irritability, and restlessness.

Objective data include decreased blood pressure; rapid, weak, thready pulse; and rapid respirations. Cold, clammy skin with pallor is noted. Oliguria (urine output less than 400 mL in 24 hours) is often evident. Mental disorientation and physical collapse with prostration can occur.

Diagnostic tests. When blood loss is sudden and plasma volume has not yet had a chance to increase, the loss of RBCs is not reflected in laboratory data, and values may seem normal or high for 2 to 3 days. However, once the plasma is replaced, the RBC mass is less concentrated. RBC, Hgb, and Hct levels are severely decreased, often to half the normal values.

Medical management. In the case of massive hemorrhage, measures are taken to stop the blood loss and treat for shock and lost volume. Severe hemorrhaging often results in the need for mechanical ventilation. Oxygen therapy restores oxygen that is less available because of decreased Hgb in the blood. To replace fluid volume, intravenous (IV) saline is administered. In severe fluid volume depletion, a bolus of 2 L of normal saline (i.e., a 0.9% NaCl solution) is given. Current guidelines from the American Society of Hematology recommend transfusing packed RBCs when the Hgb falls below 7 g/dL for the patient in an acute care setting or in the intensive care setting (ICU), and when the Hgb falls below 8 g/dL for the patient who is symptomatic for anemia, for the postoperative cardiac and orthopedic patient, and the patient with cardiovascular disease. Often platelets, fresh frozen plasma (FFP), or cryoprecipitate is included in the treatment to control hemorrhage (Szczepiorkowski, 2013).

Monitor the Hgb level to note the effectiveness of the treatment. One unit of packed RBCs should increase the Hgb level by 1 g/dL or raise the Hct by 3%. The patient also may need supplemental iron because the availability of iron affects the marrow production of erythrocytes. Oral or parenteral iron preparations often are administered.

Nursing interventions and patient teaching. Monitor blood and fluid restoration and identify blood loss sites to control the bleeding. Keep the patient flat and warm. Take vital signs at frequent intervals (every 15 minutes or more frequently) until the systolic blood pressure is above 90 mm Hg. Take precautions to prevent injury to a restless or disoriented patient. Sedatives may be ordered if the patient is restless (Williams and Hopper, 2015). Measure intake and output (I&O), with careful monitoring of urinary output for oliguria caused by decreased renal perfusion. The decrease in urinary output correlates to the amount of blood lost. If a patient has a blood loss of 750 to 1500 mL, the urinary output is 20 to 30 mL/h; with a blood loss of 1500 to 2000 mL, the urinary output is less than 5 to 15 mL/h; and a blood loss of 2000 mL or more would result in a negligible (very low) urinary output (Wade, 2013).

If hemorrhage is caused by a chronic problem, teach the patient to monitor bleeding amounts and associated factors and to report to the health care provider immediately for treatment.

Prognosis. Without treatment, death results. With aggressive treatment, the prognosis is favorable.

Pernicious Anemia

Etiology and pathophysiology. **Pernicious** anemia is a disease that results from the body's inability to absorb vitamin B_{12} (cyanocobalamin). Vitamin B_{12} is necessary for the production of red blood cells. It is absorbed when the lower portion of the stomach's gastric mucosa secretes the glycoprotein called the intrinsic factor. When the intrinsic factor is not secreted, vitamin B_{12} is not absorbed in the small intestine. Intrinsic factor secretion fails because of gastric mucosal atrophy or a partial or total gastrectomy (surgical removal of part or all of the stomach). Pernicious anemia also may result from a progressive, megaloblastic, macrocytic anemia (i.e., characterized by abnormally large, immature [nucleated] RBCs), primarily affecting older adults.

In pernicious anemia intrinsic factor is not available to combine with vitamin B_{12}, preventing transport of this necessary vitamin to the ileum (vitamin B_{12} normally is absorbed in the distal ileum). Deficiency of vitamin B_{12} affects the growth and maturity of all body cells, including RBCs in the marrow. In the case of RBCs, the erythrocyte membrane becomes fragile and ruptures easily. Vitamin B_{12} also affects nerve myelination; its absence leads to progressive demyelination and degeneration of nerves and white matter.

Clinical manifestations. Pernicious anemia results in the same symptoms as anemia, which were discussed previously. In addition to these symptoms, the patient with pernicious anemia often has a smooth, thick, red tongue. Other symptoms include numbness and tingling in the hands and feet, various gastrointestinal complaints, and neurologic problems such as confusion and memory loss.

Assessment. Subjective data include the patient's complaints of palpitations, nausea, flatulence, constipation, diarrhea, and indigestion. The patient may complain that the tongue is tender and burning. Weakness and difficulty in swallowing (dysphagia) may occur. Neurologic symptoms include tingling of the hands and feet and loss of the sense of body position (impaired proprioception).

Collection of objective data includes observation of a smooth and erythematous tongue, with infection about the teeth and gums. Cerebral signs include mental disorientation, personality changes, and behavior problems. Severe neurologic impairments can result, including partial or total paralysis from destruction of the nerve fibers of the spinal cord.

Diagnostic tests. In addition to the patient's signs and symptoms, several laboratory tests are used to diagnose pernicious anemia. The complete blood count (CBC) is the most common test and helps in the preliminary diagnosis with the result of low Hgb and Hct levels. Further testing is required for an accurate diagnosis. These tests include reticulocyte count, which measures the number of red blood cells in the blood, indicating if the bone marrow is producing RBCs; serum folate, iron, and iron-binding capacity indicate if anemia is from vitamin B_{12} deficiency; mean corpuscular volume, which measures the size of the red blood cells (red blood cells are typically larger than normal in pernicious anemia); serum megaloblastic anemia profile, which reveals decreased serum levels of vitamin B_{12}, serum methylmalonic acid, and homocysteine; and bone marrow aspiration and biopsy if other tests are not conclusive of B_{12} deficiency. Bone marrow aspiration reveals abnormal RBC development. The erythrocytes appear large (macrocytic) and have abnormal shapes, probably the result of reduced serum cobalamin (B_{12}) levels. A gastric analysis may be done to determine the cause of the vitamin B_{12} deficiency. Gastric analysis is performed in the endoscopy suite. A nasogastric tube is inserted, and stomach contents are aspirated. The total absence of intrinsic factor is diagnostic of pernicious anemia; because the same stomach cells produce hydrochloric acid, achlorhydria (an absence of hydrochloric acid) is diagnostic as well (National Institutes of Health Clinical Center, 2016).

Medical management. Oral vitamin B_{12} replacement is ineffective if there is an absence of intrinsic factor in the stomach or a malabsorption problem in the ileum. Cyanocobalamin (B_{12}) injections, folic acid supplement, and iron replacement are ordered. If the anemia is severe, the patient may be transfused with packed RBCs. The standard treatment includes initiating vitamin B_{12} replacement therapy; without it, these individuals die within 1 to 3 years. Treatment is 1000 units of vitamin B_{12} administered intramuscularly daily for 2 weeks, and then weekly until the Hct is normal, and finally monthly for life. In addition, an intranasal form of cyanocobalamin (Nascobal) can be self-administered once weekly. Iron supplements may be prescribed to treat iron deficiency anemia. The most common side effect of iron supplements is stomach upset, including discomfort, nausea, diarrhea, constipation, and heartburn. Taking iron supplements often darkens stool color. Iron can interfere with the absorption of many other medications. Iron taken with birth control pills can increase serum iron levels. Cholesterol medication, antacids, and dairy products can reduce iron absorption. For this reason, it is best to take iron supplements at least 2 hours before or 2 hours after eating (University of Maryland Medical Center, 2013). The patient's blood values should return to normal within 2 months of B_{12} therapy. A CBC is necessary every 3 to 6 months to monitor the long-term success of treatment.

Nursing interventions and patient teaching. The nursing interventions depend to some extent on the stage of the disease. A symptomatic approach is appropriate. When the patient is confined to the hospital, the nurse checks vital signs every 4 hours and performs special mouth care several times daily. The diet should be high in protein, vitamins, and minerals. Anemic patients are especially sensitive to cold, so additional lightweight, warm blankets may be needed. Interventions should conserve energy and prevent injury. The room temperature may have to be increased for the patient's comfort.

Patient problems and interventions for the patient with pernicious anemia include but are not limited to the following:

Patient Problem	Nursing Interventions
Insufficient Nutrition, related to: • Sore mouth and tongue • Diarrhea • Constipation	Administer vitamin B_{12} and other medications prescribed to promote production of erythrocytes Instruct patient on balanced diet high in protein, vitamins, and iron, such as red meat, dairy products, and eggs, to increase intake of vitamin B_{12} Provide meticulous and frequent oral hygiene to promote improved appetite and prevent infection Provide six to eight small meals daily to conserve energy and decrease GI distress Monitor patient's bowel movements, noting color consistency and amount

To control the disease, the patient must understand the disease process and the importance of lifetime therapy with vitamin B_{12}. Discuss the importance of a diet high in vitamin B_{12}. Adjusting activities when signs and symptoms are present may lessen the patient's stress. The need for assistance with ADLs and for frequent rest periods should be impressed on the patient and significant people involved in the patient's care.

Prognosis. This condition, if untreated, can be considered terminal in 1 to 3 years. With treatment the patient may be asymptomatic. Because the potential for gastric carcinoma is increased in pernicious anemia, the patient should be monitored closely.

Aplastic Anemia

Etiology and pathophysiology. Aplastic anemia is a rare disorder but is serious when it occurs. The bone marrow does not produce enough RBCs for the body to function properly. There are numerous possible causes of aplastic anemia, including (Medline Plus, 2018):

- Autoimmune disorders
- Certain inherited conditions
- Certain medicines
- Infections such as hepatitis, Epstein-Barr virus, or HIV
- Pregnancy
- Radiation therapy and chemotherapy for cancer
- Toxic substances, such as pesticides, arsenic, and benzene
- Unknown causes

Depression of erythrocyte production results in lowered Hgb and RBCs. Leukopenia and thrombocytopenia may develop. Patients with aplastic anemia are usually **pancytopenic;** that is, all three major blood elements (red cells, white cells, and platelets) from the bone marrow are reduced or absent. The incidence of aplastic anemia is low, affecting approximately 4 of every 1 million people.

Clinical manifestations. The signs and symptoms of aplastic anemia may have an acute onset or develop slowly over several weeks to months. Lower-than-normal numbers of red blood cells, white blood cells, and platelets cause most of the signs and symptoms of aplastic anemia. With suppression of all three major blood elements, the patient may have signs and symptoms related to each. The most common symptoms of a low red blood cell count are fatigue, shortness of breath, dizziness, especially when standing up; headaches; coldness in your hands or feet; pale skin; and chest pain. Signs and symptoms of a low white blood cell count include fevers, frequent infections that can be severe, and flulike illnesses that linger. Common types of bleeding associated with a low platelet count include epistaxis, bleeding gums, petechiae, and blood in the stool. Women also may have heavy menstrual bleeding.

Assessment. Subjective data include a history of exposure to chemicals such as insecticides and drugs in addition to a family history of aplastic anemia. Ask the patient about the ability to carry out ADLs without fatigue.

Collection of objective data includes monitoring the patient for pallor, signs of infection, and bleeding tendencies. Also, dyspnea and tachycardia may be noted.

Diagnostic tests. The diagnosis of aplastic anemia begins with a CBC, in which all the values will be low. A reticulocyte count also results in below normal levels. Bone marrow aspiration and biopsy are common in the diagnosis of aplastic anemia and results in below-normal numbers of all three types of blood cells.

Medical management. The cause of aplastic anemia must be identified promptly and removed or discontinued. Bone marrow suppression is expected with certain antineoplastic medications or radiation therapy, and laboratory values should be monitored frequently to maintain control.

Avoid blood transfusions, if possible, to prevent iron overloading and the development of antibodies to tissue antigens. Platelet transfusions that are human lymphocyte antigen (HLA) matched are used to treat serious bleeding in a thrombocytopenic patient. Blood transfusions are used cautiously to minimize the risk of rejection for a bone marrow transplant candidate.

A splenectomy may be required in patients with hypersplenism that is destroying normal platelets. Steroids and androgens sometimes are used to stimulate the bone marrow. Immunosuppressive therapy with anti-thymocyte globulin and cyclosporine or high-dose cyclophosphamide has become important for patients who are not candidates for bone marrow transplantation or hematopoietic stem cell transplantation (SCT). Bone marrow transplantation or hematopoietic SCT is the treatment of choice for patients younger than 45 years and who have a compatible donor. Granulocyte-macrophage colony-stimulating factor (GM-CSF) is used as a biologic response modifier treatment for aplastic anemia.

Bone marrow transplantation. A bone marrow transplant is indicated for certain patients, such as those who are immunodeficient or who have cancer, leukemia, or recurrent aplastic anemia. It is essential, to avoid rejection or complications, that the patient have a matched donor. Specimens from twins, siblings, or the patient (autologous) while in remission are preferred.

After the patient has been emotionally and physically prepared, blood studies are performed to set baselines and assess the patient's status. Establish a pathogen-free environment, with the immunocompromised patient placed in neutropenic precautions (i.e., kept in an environment that protects the patient from being contaminated/infected by other people or objects). Monitor for fever or infection. The medication therapy used in this preparation may include immunosuppressants, antibiotics, and antianxiety agents.

Bone marrow transplants are used increasingly in hematologic malignancies after large doses of chemotherapy or radiation therapy have been administered. Ordinarily only a limited amount of chemotherapy or radiation can be administered because of its toxicity to the bone marrow; when bone marrow is transplanted, much larger therapeutic doses are possible.

Bone marrow is obtained by multiple marrow aspirations under general or spinal anesthesia, usually yielding 500 to 800 mL of marrow. The marrow is cryopreserved (frozen) until it is used. Shortly after chemotherapy (with or without radiation therapy) is completed, the patient receives the donated marrow through an IV catheter. This infusion of marrow is called the *rescue process.* The donated marrow travels through the bloodstream to the bone marrow, where it begins to manufacture new leukocytes, erythrocytes, and thrombocytes. The infused marrow repopulates the patient's marrow after several weeks. The patient runs a great risk of toxicity, including infections, marrow rejection, and graft-versus-host disease. Medications supporting graft acceptance include cyclosporine (immunosuppressant) and chemotherapy (to prevent graft-versus-host complications).

Splenectomy. In addition to aplastic anemia, there are several reasons why a spleen may have to be removed. The most common reason is to treat a condition called idiopathic thrombocytopenia purpura (ITP). Patients with ITP tend to bleed easily because their immune system attacks and destroys platelets (blood cells that aid in blood clotting). Hemolytic anemia (in which red blood cells are broken down at an abnormally high rate) requires spleen removal to prevent or decrease the need for transfusion. Hereditary (genetic) conditions that affect the shape of red blood cells, such as sickle cell disease and thalassemia, may require splenectomy. Patients with cancers of the cells that fight infection, for example, lymphoma or certain types of leukemia, often require spleen removal. When the spleen becomes enlarged, it sometimes removes too many platelets from the blood and must be removed. The spleen may be removed to diagnose or treat a tumor. Splenectomy also may be warranted when the blood supply to the spleen becomes infarcted (blocked) or the artery abnormally expands (aneurysm).

Preoperative assessment includes cardiovascular observation, respiratory function determination, and GI evaluation. Drugs such as aspirin, blood thinners, antiinflammatory medications (arthritis medications), and vitamin E must be stopped temporarily for several days to a week before surgery. Postoperatively, compare these observations with the patient's baseline evaluations, and observe the patient for infection or inflammation. Potential complications include infection, hemorrhage, shock, and paralytic ileus. Maintain parenteral therapy. Nasogastric (NG) suction may be ordered if a paralytic ileus develops. Address the patient's postoperative pain. Also maintain movement and use positioning to prevent infection or postoperative pneumonia.

Nursing Interventions and Patient Teaching

Proper observation and care after bone marrow study are essential. Patients with aplastic anemia are highly susceptible to infection; thus nursing interventions should be directed toward prevention. Adhere to strict aseptic techniques for dressing changes and IV site care. To prevent impaired skin and mucous membranes, avoid intramuscular injections, administration of rectal medications, and measurement of rectal temperatures. An air mattress can help protect the patient's skin. In the presence of thrombocytopenia, observe carefully for any signs of bleeding and prevent any risk for injury. Monitor the patient's urine and stool for occult or gross blood.

Patient problems and interventions for the patient with aplastic anemia include, but are not limited to, *Inability to Tolerate Activity, related to inadequate tissue oxygenation* and *Potential for Infection, related to increased susceptibility.*

Patients with aplastic anemia need to know how to protect themselves from excessive bleeding. Help the patient maintain a balance between rest and activity. Discuss with the patient how to avoid infection, especially of the respiratory or urinary tract (see the Safety Alert box).

Prognosis. The prognosis for the patient with untreated aplastic anemia is poor (fatal for approximately 75% of

Safety Alert

Aplastic Anemia

- Avoid contact with those who have infection.
- Avoid enemas or other rectal insertions.
- Avoid excessive workload or heavy lifting, and ask for assistance with strenuous activity.
- Avoid intramuscular injections.
- Avoid picking or blowing the nose forcefully.
- Avoid sharing eating utensils and bath linens.
- Avoid trauma, falls, bumps, and cuts; avoid contact sports.
- Avoid use of aspirin or over-the-counter (OTC) aspirin preparations (anticoagulant effect).
- Bathe or shower every day (or every other day if skin is dry); keep perineal area clean.
- Decrease activity if shortness of breath, dizziness, or sensation of heaviness in extremities occurs.
- Eliminate intake of raw meats, fruits, or vegetables.
- Immediately report signs of infection to health care provider.
- Increase time necessary for routine care.
- Keep mouth clean and free of debris.
- Observe for signs such as blood in urine or stool and petechiae, and report these to health care provider.
- Prevent fatigue.
- Prevent hemorrhage.
- Prevent infection.
- Report signs of increased fatigue.
- Take frequent rest periods between activities of daily living (ADLs).
- Use a soft toothbrush or swab for mouth care.
- Use adequate lubrication and gentleness during sexual intercourse.
- Use an electric razor.
- Use good hand hygiene technique.
- Use good oral hygiene.

patients). Advances in medical management have improved outcomes significantly in aggressively treated patients. The objective of care is to produce remission and prolong survival.

Iron Deficiency Anemia

Etiology and pathophysiology. Iron deficiency anemia is a condition in which the RBCs contain less Hgb than normal. Common causes of iron deficiency anemia are excessive iron loss, a diet low in iron sources, bleeding from gastric or duodenal ulcers, esophageal varices, hiatal hernias, colonic diverticula, and tumors, or nonabsorption of vitamin B_{12}. The major sources of chronic blood loss are from the GI and genitourinary systems (Box 47.2).

GI bleeding is often not apparent and may exist for a considerable time before being identified. Loss of 50 to 75 mL of blood from the upper GI tract is required for stools to appear black, or *melenic*. The color results from the iron in the RBCs. Blood losses related to menstruation or pregnancy are common causes of iron deficiency anemia in young women. Rarely, excessive losses occur through microhemorrhages into lung tissue or from intestinal parasites. Even without excessive blood loss, iron deficiency anemia can result when the body's demand for iron exceeds its absorption, which commonly occurs in infants, young adolescents, and pregnant women. Iron deficiency anemia also may result from malabsorption of iron caused by diseases such as celiac disease and sprue. Subtotal gastrectomy may lead to iron deficiency caused by *achlorhydria* (loss of hydrochloric acid), occult bleeding, and decreased iron in postgastrectomy diets. Deficiency caused by poor dietary intake is rare in middle-aged adults.

Box 47.2 Causes of Iron Deficiency Anemia

- Blood loss is a major cause of iron deficiency in adults. The major sources of chronic blood loss are from the GI and genitourinary systems. Common causes of GI blood loss are peptic ulcers, gastritis, esophagitis, diverticulitis, hemorrhoids, and neoplasms. The average monthly menstrual blood loss is about 45 mL and causes the loss of 22 mg of iron.
- Daily iron intake from food and dietary supplements is adequate to meet the needs of men and older women, but it may be inadequate for those with higher iron needs (e.g., menstruating or pregnant women).
- Iron deficiency may develop from inadequate dietary intake, malabsorption, blood loss, or hemolysis (breakdown of red blood cells).
- Malabsorption of iron may occur after certain types of gastrointestinal (GI) surgery and in malabsorption syndromes. Iron absorption occurs in the duodenum. Malabsorption of iron may involve disease of the duodenum, in which the absorption surface is altered or destroyed.

Approximately 1 mg of every 10 to 20 mg (5% to 10%) of iron ingested is absorbed in the duodenum. For example, the average daily iron requirement for infants (older than 6 months), children, adolescents, and adults is between approximately 7 mg and 11 mg. This amount of dietary iron meets the needs of men and older women, but it may be inadequate for people who have higher iron needs (e.g., ill children, pregnant and lactating women).

Clinical manifestations. The most common symptoms of iron deficiency anemia are pallor and glossitis (red, smooth tongue). Fatigue, weakness, and shortness of breath also often occur. Signs and symptoms typical of anemia, previously discussed, occur.

Assessment. In addition to typical signs and symptoms of anemia, assessment often reveals various GI symptoms such as glossitis and *pagophagia* (the desire to eat ice, clay, or starches). Weakness, cold extremities, and complaints of chest pain may be assessed.

Collection of objective data includes noting the signs, including pallor and tachycardia. Fingernails may be fragile and shaped like the head of a spoon with a central depression and raised borders. Mucous membranes of the mouth may be inflamed (stomatitis), and lips may be erythemic with cracking at the angles.

Diagnostic tests. The peripheral blood counts show that RBCs, Hgb levels, and Hct are decreased; serum iron levels are low.

Medical management. Administration of iron salts such as ferrous sulfate often is required. In 3 weeks the Hct level should rise 5% to 15%, and the Hgb level should rise by 2 to 5 g/dL. For the body to incorporate 100 mg of iron per day, 900 mg/day is administered. Iron is administered orally or by injection. Ascorbic acid (vitamin C) has been shown to enhance iron absorption. Food sources of iron include meat, fish, poultry, eggs, green leafy vegetables, whole grains, and dried beans (Box 47.3).

When the patient cannot tolerate oral preparations of iron, parenteral iron therapy is used. The Z-track method of giving iron dextran (Dexferrum) intramuscularly is preferable to prevent skin staining. Iron sucrose (Venofer) is an IV drug frequently used to treat iron deficiency anemia.

Nursing interventions and patient teaching. Because treatment is directed toward diagnosis and alleviation of the cause, the patient interview is important. Medication therapy for iron replacement is initiated as ordered. Plan for rest periods when fatigue is present. Education about nutritional needs relative to the condition may prevent this anemia (see Box 47.3).

Explanation of the side effects of iron therapy is essential to alleviate distress and to extend the therapy for the necessary time (see the Health Promotion box). The patient must know which signs and symptoms are significant and must be reported to the health care provider. Diarrhea or nausea is significant, but black, tarry stools are not (these are expected with iron therapy).

Prognosis. The prognosis is usually good with correction of the underlying cause and compliance with the medical treatment.

Box 47.3 Food Sources of Nutrients Needed for Erythropoiesis

IRON
- Dark green vegetables: spinach, Swiss chard, kale, greens (dandelion, beet, and turnip)
- Dried fruits: apricots, dates, figs, prunes, and raisins
- Eggs
- Iron-enriched or iron-fortified breads and cereals
- Legumes and nuts
- Muscle meats, especially dark meat from poultry
- Organ meats: liver, kidney, heart, and tongue
- Shellfish
- Whole-grain breads and cereals

FOLIC ACID
- Asparagus, broccoli
- Enriched and fortified breads and cereals
- Fish
- Green, leafy vegetables
- Legumes
- Meat
- Organ meats: Liver
- Whole-grain breads and cereals

VITAMIN B_{12}
- Eggs
- Milk and cheese
- Muscle meats
- Organ meats: liver and kidney

AMINO ACIDS
- Eggs
- Fish
- Legumes
- Meat
- Milk and milk products (cheese, ice cream)
- Nuts
- Poultry

VITAMIN C
- Cantaloupe
- Citrus fruits
- Leafy, green vegetables
- Strawberries

Sickle Cell Anemia

Etiology and pathophysiology. Sickle cell anemia is the most common genetic disorder in the United States, predominantly affecting those of African or Eastern Mediterranean heritage. A sickle cell is an abnormal, crescent-shaped RBC containing Hgb S (Hb-S), a defective Hgb molecule. This anemia is a severe, chronic, incurable condition that occurs in people **homozygous** (having two identical genes inherited from each parent for a given hereditary characteristic) for Hb-S. Sickle cell crisis is an episode of acute "sickling" of RBCs, which causes occlusion and ischemia in distal blood vessels. Sickling leads to clumping, or aggregation, of these misshapen RBCs, which lodge in small vessels. Sickle cell trait is the **heterozygous** (having two different genes) form of sickle cell anemia, whereby the individual has Hb-S and Hgb A (Hb-A) in the RBCs. Patients with sickle cell trait do not have signs or symptoms but risk passing the disorder on to their children.

Approximately 8.3% of African Americans have the sickle cell trait (about 2 million in the United States), and approximately 1 of every 600 (about 80,000 individuals in the United States) has sickle cell anemia (Lewis et al, 2007). It is estimated that sickle cell disease affects approximately 100,000 Americans: it occurs in 1 out of every 365 black or African American births and 1 out of every 16,300 Hispanic American births. About 1 in 13 black or African American babies is born with sickle cell trait (CDC, 2016).

Sickle cell trait (also known as being a carrier) occurs when a person has one gene for sickle Hgb and one gene for normal Hgb. People who are carriers generally do not have any medical problems and lead normal lives. A carrier cannot develop sickle cell disease.

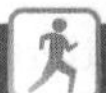 Health Promotion

Iron Administration

- Check for constipation or diarrhea. Record color (iron turns stools green to black) and amount of stool.
- Dilute liquid iron preparations in juice or water, and administer with a straw to avoid staining teeth. Provide oral hygiene after taking.
- Do not administer with antacids, because they reduce the absorption of iron.
- Dosages are determined by the elemental iron content of the preparation.
- If a dose is missed, continue with the schedule; do not double a dose.
- If side effects develop, the dose and type of iron supplement may be adjusted. Some people cannot tolerate ferrous sulfate because of the effects of the sulfate base. Ferrous gluconate may be an acceptable substitute.
- Iron is absorbed best from the duodenum and proximal jejunum. Therefore enteric-coated or sustained-release capsules, which release iron farther down in the GI tract, are counterproductive; they are also more expensive.
- Iron is best absorbed in an acidic environment. To avoid binding the iron with food, iron should be taken about an hour before meals, when the duodenal mucosa is most acidic. Taking iron with vitamin C (ascorbic acid) or orange juice, which contains ascorbic acid, also enhances iron absorption. Gastric side effects, however, may necessitate ingesting iron with meals.
- Iron is toxic, and caution must be taken to store iron preparations out of a child's reach.
- Iron may interfere with absorption of oral tetracycline antibiotics (quinolones [Cipro, Levaquin]). Do not take within 2 hours of each other.
- Iron preparations supplement the body's natural iron stores.
- Iron supplements may be contraindicated in peptic ulcer disease.
- Side effects include gastrointestinal (GI) upset (nausea, vomiting), constipation or diarrhea, and green to black stools. Elixir may stain teeth.

Tissue hypoxia and ischemia occur, causing pain and edema as a result of inflammation. Compared with a normal lifespan of about 120 days, an RBC affected by sickle cell disease has a lifespan of only 10 to 20 days (CDC, 2016; Lewis et al, 2017). Destruction of fragile RBCs thus inhibits the oxygen-carrying function.

Clinical manifestations. Usually the newborn with sickle cell anemia is asymptomatic for the first 10 to 12 weeks of age, until most of the fetal Hgb (Hb-F) has been replaced by Hb-S. However, periods of crisis then occur, accelerating the signs and symptoms. Many people with sickle cell anemia are in reasonably good health most of the time. The typical patient is anemic but asymptomatic except during painful episodes. Physical and emotional factors (stress) precipitate a painful episode. Physical factors include events that cause dehydration or change the oxygen tension in the body, such as infection, overexertion, weather changes (cold), ingestion of alcohol, and smoking.

Infections, such as those causing pneumonia, meningitis, influenza, and hepatitis, are a major complication of sickle cell anemia. Loss of appetite and irritability with weakness follow minor infections. Abdominal enlargement with pooling of blood in the liver, spleen, and other organs may accompany jaundice. Joint and back pain is noted, as is edema of the extremities. Complications include multisystem failure, infarctions, hemorrhage, and retinal damage leading to blindness.

Assessment. Collection of subjective data begins with assessing the patient's knowledge and feelings about the disease and factors that appear to precipitate crisis or exacerbate signs and symptoms. Fatigue may be reported when anemia is severe. The primary symptom associated with sickling is pain in the joints, especially those of the hands and feet. Abdominal pain is common with swelling of the spleen and engorgement of vital organs. Hypoxia occurs as fever and pain increase, causing the patient to breathe rapidly. A male patient may have a continuous painful erection (priapism) from impaired blood flow out of the erect penis. The pain associated with these attacks often is described as deep, gnawing, and throbbing. Acute chest syndrome is a serious complication of sickle cell disease that results from sickling in blood vessels of the lungs. This prevents oxygen from entering the lungs. The complication typically starts a few days after a painful crisis begins. Assess for signs and symptoms of chest pain, fever, shortness of breath, increased respirations, and a cough. Infection in the lungs also may develop (National Heart, Lung, and Brain Institute [NHLBI], 2017).

Further collection of objective data includes observing for abdominal enlargement and jaundice, edema of the extremities, and signs of hemorrhage. As a result of the accelerated RBC breakdown, the patient has a characteristic clinical finding of hemolysis (jaundice, elevated serum bilirubin levels).

Diagnostic tests. Electrophoresis of Hgb from a patient with sickle cell anemia is specific for detecting sickle cell crisis or anemia. More than 80% of sickle cell Hgb as shown by electrophoresis is Hb-S, not Hb-A. A stained blood smear detects anemia only. The Hct and Hgb levels are below normal values. WBCs are increased with infection. Skeletal x-rays demonstrate bone and joint deformities and flattening. MRI may be used to diagnose a stroke caused by occluded cerebral vessels from sickled cells.

Medical management. Sickle cell anemia has no specific treatment. Treatment is symptomatic, alleviating the symptoms that result from complications. Treatment should include adequate hydration, antibiotics for infections, and nonsteroidal antiinflammatory (NSAIDs) medications for pain. *Haemophilus influenzae*, pneumococcal conjugate, meningococcal, and hepatitis immunizations should be administered to prevent infections. A bone marrow transplant, which infuses healthy stem cells into the bone marrow, may be performed in select patients to treat severe cases of the disease. The challenge is finding a match for transplantation (Maakaron, 2017).

Sickle cell crisis may require hospitalization. Oxygen may be administered to alter hypoxia and control sickling. Encourage rest and administer fluids and electrolytes intravenously to reduce blood viscosity and maintain renal function. Use analgesics to treat pain. Sickle cell crisis pain often is undertreated. The nurse needs a clear understanding of the disease process and of current approaches to pain management.

Opioid pain management is often necessary when NSAIDs are no longer effective. Patient-controlled analgesia may be used during an acute crisis. After discharge, patients may continue taking oral opioid analgesics for a period of time. Blood transfusion of packed RBCs may be necessary to treat severe anemia. However, frequent transfusions can cause high levels of iron to build up in the body. *Chelation* therapy, a medicine to reduce the amount of iron in the body and the problems that iron overload causes, may be prescribed (NHLBI, 2017). These patients have an increased need for folic acid, so it is important that they take daily supplements. Iron therapy generally is not suggested.

Another medication, hydroxyurea, currently is being prescribed as maintenance therapy to help prevent anemia and to prevent acute episodes of pain. This medication boosts the levels of fetal Hgb (Hb-F). This lowers the concentration of Hb-S within a cell, resulting in less polymerization of the abnormal Hgb (NHLBI, 2017).

Sickle cell disease is associated with considerable morbidity and premature mortality. Hematopoietic stem cell transplantation (HSCT) is the only available therapy with curative intent. HSCT from matched sibling donors in pediatric patients has shown positive results. However, the availability of matched sibling donors and concerns regarding regimen-related toxicity have made this treatment problematic (Maakaron, 2017).

Nursing interventions and patient teaching. Supportive treatment depends on the signs and symptoms: hydration and analgesia during crises, and dilution of blood with increased fluid intake to reverse sickling. Monitoring the transfusion therapy for evidence of transfusion reaction is vital. Attention to fever and infection is important. Genetic counseling is indicated.

A patient problem and interventions for the patient with sickle cell anemia include but are not limited to the following:

Patient Problem	Nursing Interventions
Recent Onset of Pain, related to thrombotic crisis	Place patient in proper anatomic alignment, and protect joints Position patient by slow, gentle handling Apply warmth with soaks or compresses to relieve discomfort Give analgesics on a fixed time schedule to maintain a steady serum drug level, which improves pain control, minimizes complications, and decreases anxiety Medications may be administered by the nurse or a patient-controlled analgesic infusion pump provides a constant, low-dose infusion of an opioid for excellent pain control

Alert the patient to the need for family testing to determine the presence of Hb-S; genetic counseling is available for carriers. Explain how to avoid sickle cell crises: avoid high altitudes, flying in unpressurized planes, dehydration, extreme temperatures, iced liquids, alcohol, and vigorous exercise; use stress reduction methods. Patients should not smoke and should protect extremities from injury because of impaired circulation. Patients with sickle cell disease have frequent problems with infections. It is important for the patient to remain current with vaccinations and take prophylactic antibiotics to protect against these infections. Explain that young pregnant women with sickle cell anemia have a high risk for developing pulmonary and/or renal complications. Alert the patient to the signs and symptoms of increased intracranial pressure and to the need to blow the nose gently, avoid coughing, and avoid straining on elimination.

Practice ROM exercises with the patient and encourage regular physical activity to prevent bone demineralization. Instruct the patient in the need for a balance between rest (physical and mental) and activity, such as ROM and isometric exercises. Also discuss the principles of good nutrition, such as the importance of protein, calcium, vitamins, and adequate fluids. Provide patient education on how to monitor oral intake, urinary output, and urine protein.

Prognosis. In the past, people with sickle cell disease often died between ages 20 and 40. Earlier detection, improved treatments, and greater use of immunizations help patients with sickle cell disease live longer, more productive lives. People with sickle cell disease now can live to the age of 50 and beyond (National Library of Medicine [NLM], 2013). Still, the prognosis is guarded. In addition to hemolytic anemia, painful crises with multiple infarctions of most organ systems can occur. With repeated episodes of sickling, there is gradual involvement of all body systems, especially the spleen, lungs, kidneys, and brain. Bone marrow grafts from HLA-identical siblings are providing hope for patients with sickle cell anemia.

POLYCYTHEMIA (ERYTHROCYTOSIS)

Etiology and Pathophysiology

The two types of polycythemia are *primary polycythemia (polycythemia vera)* and *secondary polycythemia.* Their causes and pathophysiology differ, although their complications and clinical manifestations are similar.

Polycythemia vera is a blood disorder characterized by hyperplasia (overgrowth) of bone marrow; it manifests with an overproduction of circulating erythrocytes (**erythrocytosis**), granulocytes, basophils, and platelets. This results in increased blood viscosity and volume. Polycythemia vera develops gradually and is a chronic disease; patients are diagnosed at an average age of 60 years. It occurs slightly more frequently in men. Secondary polycythemia is caused by hypoxia rather than by a defect in the development of blood cells. Hypoxia stimulates the production of erythropoietin in the kidneys, which in turn stimulates erythrocyte production in the bone marrow. The need for increased oxygen may result from high altitude, pulmonary disease, cardiovascular disease, or tissue hypoxia. Secondary polycythemia is not a pathologic response, but a physiologic response in which the body tries to compensate for a hypoxic problem. In polycythemia vera the pathologic response is a malignancy of the blood cells.

Hyperplastic bone marrow elements can affect multiple organs. Because of the increased erythrocyte mass, chronic hypervolemia (increased volume) and hyperviscosity (increased "stickiness") of the blood result in congestion of tissues and organs. The sluggish circulatory process results in hypercoagulopathy (excessive clotting) that predisposes patients to infarctions of vital organs.

Clinical Manifestations

Polycythemia vera involves an increased number of red blood cells within the bloodstream. Affected individuals also may have excess white blood cells and platelets. These extra cells cause the blood to be thicker than normal, and abnormal blood clots are more likely to form and block the flow of blood through arteries and veins. Individuals with polycythemia vera have an increased risk of blood clots in the deep veins of the arms or legs (deep vein thrombosis [DVT]), the lungs (*pulmonary embolism* [PE]), the heart (causing a heart attack), and the brain (causing a stroke) (NIH, 2017a). Venous distention and platelet dysfunction cause esophageal varices, epistaxis, GI bleeding, and petechiae. Hepatomegaly and splenomegaly, the result of organ engorgement, may contribute to patient complaints of satiety and fullness.

Assessment

Subjective data include patient complaints of sensitivity to hot and cold. Generalized pruritus (often exacerbated by a hot bath) may be a striking symptom and is related to histamine release from an increased number of basophils. Headaches, vertigo, tinnitus, blurred vision, and painful burning of the hands and feet are often present.

Objective data include eczema and dermatologic changes. The skin may develop an erythemic appearance. Elevated blood pressure accompanies left ventricular hypertrophy and angina.

Diagnostic Tests

Plasma and RBC volume are increased. Elevations are seen in Hgb and Hct levels, reticulocyte and erythrocyte counts, platelets (thrombocytes), and WBC count with increased basophils. Elevated alkaline phosphatase, uric acid, and histamine levels are noted. Bone marrow examination in polycythemia vera shows hypercellularity of RBCs, WBCs, and platelets. The basal metabolic rate (BMR) is increased without thyroid function alteration. Splenomegaly is found in more than 75% of patients with primary polycythemia but does not accompany secondary polycythemia (Merck Manual, 2012).

Medical Management

Blood viscosity is decreased by repeated phlebotomy—removal of 500 to 2000 mL of blood until the Hct level is maintained at 45% to 48%. The procedure is repeated if the Hct rises to more than 50%. Once the diagnosis of polycythemia vera is made, treatment is directed toward reducing blood volume and viscosity and bone marrow activity. Myelosuppressive agents such as busulfan (Myleran), hydroxyurea (Hydrea), melphalan (Alkeran), and radioactive phosphorus often are given to inhibit bone marrow activity (Merck Manual, 2012). Allopurinol may reduce the number of acute gouty attacks.

Nursing Interventions and Patient Teaching

Polycythemia vera is not preventable. However, because secondary polycythemia is generated by any source of hypoxia, problems may be prevented by maintaining adequate oxygenation. Therefore controlling chronic pulmonary disease, smoking cessation, and avoiding high altitudes are vital.

When acute exacerbations of polycythemia vera develop, the nurse has several responsibilities. Judiciously evaluate fluid I&O during hydration therapy to avoid fluid overload (which further complicates the circulatory congestion) and dehydration (which can cause the blood to become even more viscous). If myelosuppressive agents are used, administer the drugs as ordered, observe the patient, and teach the patient about medication side effects.

Assess the patient's nutritional status with the dietitian if necessary to offset the inadequate food intake that can result from GI symptoms of fullness, pain, and dyspepsia. Institute activities, such as active or passive leg exercises and ambulation, to decrease the risk of thrombus formation.

Because of its chronic nature, polycythemia vera requires ongoing evaluation. Phlebotomy may be needed every 2 to 3 months, reducing the blood volume by about 500 mL each time. Evaluate the patient for the development of complications.

Patient problems and interventions for the patient with polycythemia vera include but are not limited to the following:

Patient Problem	Nursing Interventions
Compromised Blood Flow to Tissue (cardiopulmonary, cerebral, GI, and peripheral), related to: • Hyperviscosity of fluid • Potential bleeding	Keep patient in a comfortable position, turning frequently to relieve pressure Elevate head of bed, keeping legs in a nondependent position Use ROM exercises to stimulate circulation Assess peripheral pulses and color and temperature of extremities every 4 to 6 hours Assess for blood in urine and stools Assess for thrombus formation Monitor laboratory studies If patient has a bleeding tendency, avoid invasive procedures when possible Avoid trauma; provide education related to ADLs

Educate the patient about this condition. Emphasize the importance of compliance with the medical and nutritional regimen. Dietary teaching should emphasize avoiding foods that contain iron while increasing the intake of calories and protein (because of BMR increase).

Emphasize that certain signs and symptoms (such as pain, edema, or erythema associated with thrombosis) require medical supervision. Because this is a chronic illness, emotional support is imperative.

Prognosis

Polycythemia vera is a chronic, life-shortening disorder. Although the incidence is small, leukemia and lymphomas develop in some patients with polycythemia vera. This may occur as a result of the chemotherapeutic drugs used to treat the disease or may be secondary to a disorder in the stem cells that progresses to leukemia. The major cause of morbidity and mortality from polycythemia vera is thrombosis.

DISORDERS ASSOCIATED WITH LEUKOCYTES

AGRANULOCYTOSIS

Etiology and Pathophysiology

Agranulocytosis is a potentially fatal condition of the blood characterized by a severe reduction in the number of granulocytes (basophils, eosinophils, and neutrophils). The WBC count is extremely low **(leukopenia),** as is the differential neutrophil count (less than 200/mm^3 [neutropenia]). The normal neutrophil value is 3000 to 7000/mm^3.

Adverse medication reaction or toxicity is the primary cause of agranulocytosis. However, neoplastic disease, chemotherapy, and radiation therapy often are cited as causative. Viral and bacterial infections are possible causes of the condition. Heredity also is considered.

Suppression of the bone marrow by the causative agent reduces the number and production of WBCs. Leukocytes, formed in the bone marrow, protect the body against microorganisms. This protection is ineffective when bone marrow suppression has occurred.

Clinical Manifestations

Fever, chills, headache, and fatigue are symptoms associated with infection and the inflammatory process. Ulcerations of mucous membranes—mouth, nose, pharynx, vagina, and rectum—also are found. Bronchial pneumonia and urinary tract infections are complications that occur in the later stages.

Assessment

Subjective data include common complaints of fever, extreme fatigue, and prostration. All medications taken, whether prescription or over-the-counter, are considered as possible causes of the condition.

Objective data include fever over 100.6°F (38.1°C). Erythema and pain from ulcerations may occur. Ulcerations are cultured for microorganisms. Lung and bronchial auscultation reveals crackles and rhonchi (course rattling sounds) because of trapped exudates.

Agranulocytosis may be caused by autoimmune disorders; bone marrow diseases such as myelodysplasia or large granular lymphocyte leukemia; chemotherapy and bone marrow transplantation; and medications such as rituximab, penicillin, captopril, ranitidine, cimetidine, methimazole, and propylthiouracil.

Diagnostic Tests

The levels of leukocytes with neutrophils differential are below normal. A bone marrow study shows depression of activity.

Medical Management

The main objective of treatment is to alleviate the factors responsible for bone marrow depression and to prevent or treat infection. Blood cultures may be performed when fever is elevated, and cultures may be ordered if ulceration occurs. Transfusions of packed RBCs often are ordered. Granulocyte colony-stimulating factor (G-CSF) (filgrastim [Neupogen]), pegfilgrastim (Neulasta), and granulocyte-macrophage colony-stimulating factor (GM-CSF) (sargramostim [Leukine]) given subcutaneously or intravenously can be used to treat a neutropenic patient. Precautions to prevent infection in the neutropenic (immunocompromised) patient also may be instituted.

Nursing Interventions and Patient Teaching

A patient with a compromised WBC system is highly susceptible to life-threatening infections. Nursing interventions are directed toward protecting the patient from potential sources of infection. Monitor the patient conscientiously to detect the earliest signs of infection so that therapy may be initiated promptly. Restrict visitors and prevent personnel with colds from caring for the patient. Meticulous hand hygiene and universal precautions by medical and nursing personnel and strict asepsis are mandatory.

A patient problem and interventions for the patient with agranulocytosis include but are not limited to the following:

Patient Problem	Nursing Interventions
Potential for Infection, related to depressed WBC (leukocyte) production	Institute neutropenic precautions Restrict visitors or medical personnel with bacterial or viral infections Provide instruction on handwashing to patient and visitors Monitor for signs and symptoms of infection Maintain standard precautions Use strict asepsis for procedures Avoid fresh flowers and plants Provide high-protein, high-vitamin, high-calorie soft diet to maintain nutritional status Avoid raw foods, such as sushi, Caesar salad dressing (may have raw eggs), blue cheese, and fruits that cannot be peeled or vegetables that cannot be well cleaned Encourage increased fluid intake to prevent dehydration Monitor vital signs to assess for signs of infection Observe the patient for extreme fatigue, sore throat or mouth, and fever as signs of infection Monitor laboratory values Relieve fever with tepid bath or cooling blanket Administer antibiotics as prescribed Provide hygiene with adequate rest periods

In patient teaching, discuss the use of frequent and meticulous oral hygiene to treat or prevent mouth and pharyngeal infection. Explain the need to avoid crowds, people with infectious diseases, and cold or hot environments; also teach signs and symptoms of infection and appropriate interventions. Explain the need for a soft, bland diet (if mouth ulcers are present) high in protein, vitamins, and calories. Encourage a balance between rest and activity to prevent fatigue and generalized weakness.

Prognosis

Agranulocytosis is a potentially fatal condition because of the possibility of a life-threatening bacterial infection.

LEUKEMIA

Etiology and Pathophysiology

Leukemia is a malignant disorder of the hematopoietic system in which excessive numbers of abnormal leukocytes accumulate in the bone marrow and lymph nodes. Risk factors include genetics, viral infection, previous treatment with or exposure to radiation, chemotherapeutic agents, smoking, family history, and exposure to certain chemicals such as benzene (Mayo Clinic, 2018).

In leukemia, normal white blood cells in the bone marrow are replaced with abnormal numbers and forms of rapidly dividing cells, which then spread to the circulation and infiltrate the lymph nodes, spleen, and other organs, including those of the central nervous system. Leukemic infiltration leads to problems such as hepatomegaly, splenomegaly, lymphadenopathy, bone pain, meningeal irritation, and oral lesions. Hematopoietic function is disrupted by incompetent bone marrow. Increased susceptibility to infection results.

Classification

Leukemia comes in multiple forms and is classified by identifying whether it is acute or chronic and what type of blood cell is involved. There are four common types of leukemia (ACS, 2018):

- *Acute lymphocytic (lymphoblastic) leukemia (ALL):* ALL affects lymphoid cells and grows quickly. Nearly 6000 new cases will be diagnosed annually. The majority of cases are in children under the age of 5 years and in males. After children the next age group impacted are over the age of 50 years.
- *Acute myeloid leukemia (AML):* AML affects myeloid cells and grows quickly. More than 19,000 new cases will be diagnosed annually. While it occurs in both adults and children the majority of cases will be in adults.
- *Chronic lymphocytic leukemia (CLL):* CLL affects *lymphoid cells* (cells that become lymphocytes, often B cells) and usually grows slowly. Approximately 21,000 Americans will be diagnosed each year. The incidence is rare in children and young adults.

Diagnosis is most commonly made in the 7th decade of life.

- *Chronic myeloid leukemia (CML):* CML affects *myeloid cells* (cells that become any type of blood cell other than lymphocytes) and usually grows slowly at first. Approximately 8500 cases are diagnosed each year. Most cases involve older adults.

Clinical Manifestations

The clinical manifestations of leukemia vary. They relate to problems caused by bone marrow failure and the formation of leukemic infiltrates. Bone marrow failure results from (1) bone marrow overcrowding by abnormal cells and (2) inadequate production of normal marrow elements. The patient is predisposed to anemia and thrombocytopenia.

As leukemia progresses, fewer normal blood cells are produced. The abnormal WBCs continue to accumulate. The leukemic cells infiltrate the patient's organs, leading to problems such as splenomegaly, hepatomegaly, lymphadenopathy, bone pain, meningeal irritation, and oral lesions. Enlarged lymph nodes and painless splenomegaly may be the first signs of the disease in some patients.

Diagnostic Tests

A complete blood count is a test to check the number of white blood cells, red blood cells, and platelets. Leukemia also may cause low levels of platelets and Hgb, which is found inside red blood cells. It can cause the WBC count to be low, elevated, or excessively elevated. Anemia and thrombocytopenia are noted. Bone marrow biopsy shows immature leukocytes. Chest radiographic examination may show mediastinal lymph node and lung involvement and bone changes. Lymph node biopsy reveals excessive blasts (immature cells). Peripheral blood evaluation and bone marrow examination are the primary methods of diagnosing and classifying the type of leukemia. Further studies such as lumbar puncture and CT scan can be performed to determine the presence of leukemic cells outside of the blood and bone marrow.

Assessment

Subjective data include patient history and physical assessment. Patients often have pain in bones or joints, fatigue, malaise, decreased activity tolerance, and irritability.

Objective data include those signs listed in clinical manifestations. Data include laboratory studies of WBCs with differential. Cultures of throat, urine, stool, and blood are obtained to determine which organisms are present. Abnormalities of skin (petechiae, ecchymoses) and mucous membranes (bleeding) may be present.

Medical Management

The goal of treatment is to achieve remission or to control the symptoms. Treatment is aimed at eradicating the leukemia with chemotherapy or bone marrow transplant. Combination chemotherapy is the mainstay for treating leukemia. Multiple drugs are used to (1) decrease drug resistance, (2) minimize the drug toxicity by using multiple drugs with varying toxicities (with lower dosages of each), and (3) interrupt cell growth at multiple points in the cell cycle. Observation for drug toxicity is imperative (Table 47.2).

Tremendous progress in the treatment of leukemia has been made in recent years with the use of a complex combination of chemotherapeutic drugs and radiation therapy. Bone marrow transplantation and HSCT may be the treatment of choice in patients with suitable donors and initial remission of the acute leukemia (see Chapter 57). Before transplantation, the patient's bone marrow cells and leukemic cells must be killed by massive chemotherapy and total body irradiation. The patient may succumb to infection, hemorrhage, or graft-versus-host disease.

In chronic leukemia, which occurs almost exclusively in adults and develops slowly, the desired objectives of treatment depend on the kind of cells involved. Medications commonly used include chlorambucil (Leukeran), hydroxyurea, corticosteroids, and cyclophosphamide. Lymph nodes often are irradiated, and a blood transfusion may be given if anemia is severe. Although medications are not curative in chronic leukemia, they help to prolong life (see Table 47.2).

Nursing Interventions and Patient Teaching

Prevent infection by teaching the patient and family the appropriate precautions for the neutropenic patient and the avoidance of infectious agents. Leukopenia (an abnormal decrease in the number of WBCs to less than 5000 cells/mm^3) can be fatal. The usual inflammatory process to control infection is decreased; thus frequent observation for signs and symptoms of infection is necessary. Thrombocytopenia-induced hemorrhage may be life threatening; prevent this condition through safe, gentle care. Control pain through pharmacologic and nonpharmacologic measures. Coping mechanisms may be strained because of pain, complexities of treatment, side effects and toxicities, change in body image, or fear of death. Support the patient and family by developing a positive nurse-patient-family relationship and referring them to community support groups.

Palliative care of the dying child should allow the child and family to experience the best quality of life possible. The child's illness and palliative care affect the whole family. Therefore the pediatric nurse needs to establish and develop effective communication with the family and between the dying child, parents, and siblings to help allay unnecessary fears and distress about imminent death and to support anticipatory grieving. Varied communication methods should be used to enable the nurse to understand the dying child and siblings' thoughts and feelings. Drawings can communicate perceptions and emotions about death and dying. These can relate to anger, fear, loss, hope,

Table 47.2 Medications for Blood and Lymphatic Disorders

GENERIC NAME (TRADE NAME)	ACTION	SIDE EFFECTS	NURSING IMPLICATIONS
cyanocobalamin, vitamin B_{12} (Cobal 1000)	Needed for adequate nerve functioning, protein and carbohydrate metabolism, normal growth, RBC development, and cell reproduction	Flushing, diarrhea, itching, rash, hypokalemia	Assess GI functions and potassium levels at beginning of treatment; stress need for patients with pernicious anemia to return for monthly injections; give intramuscularly only
desmopressin acetate (DDAVP)	Promotes reabsorption of water by kidneys and increase in plasma factor VIII levels, which increases platelet aggregation, resulting in vasopressor effect	Nasal irritation, congestion, drowsiness, headache, flushing, nausea, abdominal cramps, heartburn, vulval pain, hypertension	Avoid overhydration; assess pulse and blood pressure when giving drug subcutaneously; monitor factor VIII antigen levels and aPTT
ferrous sulfate (Feosol, Fer-In-Sol)	Replaces iron stores needed for RBC development	Nausea, constipation, epigastric pain, black and red tarry stools, vomiting, diarrhea, discolored urine, staining of teeth	Between-meal dosing is preferable but can be given with some foods, although absorption may be decreased; give tablets with orange juice to promote iron absorption; to avoid staining teeth, give elixir iron preparations through straw; oral iron may turn stools black
filgrastim, G-CSF (Neupogen)	Stimulates proliferation and differentiation of neutrophils	Fever, alopecia, skeletal pain, nausea, vomiting, diarrhea, mucositis, anorexia	Monitor CBC and platelet count before treatment and twice weekly; refrigerate but do not freeze; avoid shaking; store at room temperature for at least 6 h; discard any vial that has been at room temperature for more than 6 h
folic acid, B complex vitamin	Needed for erythropoiesis; increases RBC, WBC, and platelet formation in megaloblastic anemias	Pruritus, rash, general malaise, bronchospasm, slight flushing	Drug may be administered by deep intramuscular, subcutaneous, or intravenous route; do not mix with other medications in same syringe for intramuscular injections
iron dextran (Dexferrum)	Released into the plasma and carried by transferrin to the bone marrow, where it is incorporated into Hgb	Stained skin at site of injection, fever, chills, headache, sweating, discolored urine, diarrhea	Administer 0.5-mL test dose by preferred route before therapy; wait at least 1 h before giving remaining portion

aPTT, Activated partial thromboplastin time; *CBC,* complete blood count; *G-CSF,* granulocyte colony-stimulating factor; *GI,* gastrointestinal; *RBC,* red blood cell; *WBC,* white blood cell.

and acceptance of dying and can assist the nurse in providing holistic care for the child and family. Facilitating creative activity satisfies a basic need and gives the dying child the chance to do something while respecting individual autonomy, choice, and control (National Cancer Institute, 2013a).

Palliative care supports the patient and family's goals for the future (including their hopes for cure or life prolongation) as well as their hopes for peace and dignity throughout the course of illness, the dying process, and death. The aims of palliative care include guiding the patient and family in making decisions that enable them to work toward their goals during their remaining time. Nurses facilitate shared decision making between health care professionals and patient/family, management of pain and symptoms, recognition and support of grief, and appropriate hospice referrals.

From a physical care perspective, it is challenging to make astute assessments and plan care to help the patient survive the severe side effects of chemotherapy. The life-threatening results of bone marrow suppression (anemia, thrombocytopenia, neutropenia) require aggressive nursing interventions. Additional complications of chemotherapy may affect the patient's GI tract, nutritional status, skin and mucosa, cardiopulmonary status, liver, kidneys, and neurologic system.

Understand all drugs being administered, including the mechanism of action, purpose, routes of administration, usual doses, potential side effects, safe handling considerations, and toxic effects. In addition, recognize laboratory data reflecting the effects of the drugs. Patient survival and comfort during aggressive chemotherapy are affected significantly by the quality of nursing intervention.

Include the patient and family by discussing procedures, meaning of treatments, and care plans. Be certain to cover the nature of the disease and previous information given the patient. Community resources for support and information are invaluable for educating the patient and the family. Examine expectations of physical abilities, remission, and future plans. Encourage continuation of the medical regimen and avoidance of situations in which infection can be transmitted. Most patients should receive the pneumococcal vaccine (Pneumovax) at diagnosis and every 5 years and an annual influenza vaccine (CDC, 2013). Encourage six to eight small meals a day that consist of a diet high in calories, protein, and vitamins; as well as soft, bland food to reduce irritation to the mouth. Inform patient about the common side effects of their antileukemic therapy and the importance of taking these and other medications on schedule (Williams and Hopper, 2015).

Prognosis

The prognosis for patients with acute myeloid leukemia (AML) is dependent on the age of the onset of the disease. The 5-year survival rate for adults is approximately 25%, and 65% for children and adolescents younger than 15 years of age (Nursing Care Plan 47.1). The prognosis for patients with acute lymphocytic leukemia (ALL) is about a 92% chance of experiencing remission in children, whereas adults have about a 69% 5-year survival rate. Adult patients with CLL generally have a 5-year survival rate of 83%. For adult patients with CML, the prognosis depends on the age of the patient, the stage of the disease, and the treatments used. The overall 5-year survival rate is approximately 59% (Leukemia and Lymphoma Society, 2013).

DISORDERS ASSOCIATED WITH COAGULATION

Etiology and Pathophysiology

Release of blood from the vascular system results from trauma or vessel damage, vessel inadequacy, disturbance of the function of platelets or clotting factors, or liver disease. When this happens, the body attempts to stop the flow of blood by clotting. Blood clotting, or coagulation, is one of the main ways the body maintains hemostasis.

Cells and proteins are involved in normal blood coagulation: some may sound familiar (platelets, prothrombin, thrombin, fibrinogen, and fibrin) and others less familiar (tissue factor, factors I through XIII, as well as other factors); all act in three separate chain reactions that together form the coagulation cascade.

The first step in the clotting mechanism is the production of a hemostatic plug, followed by blood clotting. Vasoconstriction inhibits capillary leakage; hematoma compression provides pressure. The body reacts by lowering arterial blood pressure. Any manifestation that alters this process predisposes the body to hemorrhage. The affected mechanism may be vascular, platelet dysfunction, or an alteration in plasma coagulation factor. The disorder may be congenital or acquired, possibly secondary to another disease or to medication toxicity.

Clinical Manifestations

Skin and mucous membrane manifestations include petechiae and ecchymoses. Epistaxis and gingival bleeding are common. Circulatory hypovolemia is noted through hypotension; pallor; cool, clammy skin; and tachycardia. GI tract bleeding is common, with abdominal flank pain caused by internal bleeding. CNS involvement ranges from altered response and malaise to loss of consciousness or affected speech.

Assessment

Subjective data include a history of bleeding after surgical or dental procedures. Exposure to toxic or hazardous agents or to radiation may be revealed. Complaint of headache, extremity pain, and numbness is noted. Medications taken (e.g., aspirin) may lead to suspicion of toxicity.

Collection of objective data involves observation of pain on pressure to the abdomen, revealing liver and spleen tenderness and perhaps enlargement. Skin and mucous membranes may have petechiae, ecchymoses, and occasionally hematoma. Emesis and stool may show signs of bleeding. Joint examination reveals motion pain.

Diagnostic Tests

The platelet count is low. The RBC count is low with a decreased Hgb level. Coagulation time is altered. Bone marrow studies show abnormal cells.

Medical Management

The underlying cause is assessed and corrected, and replacement transfusions may be ordered. Heparin therapy or other anticoagulant (blood-thinning) medications such as warfarin (Coumadin) and enoxaparin (Lovenox) are considered as a possible cause. The health care provider decreases or discontinues these medications as necessary. Infections and complications are prevented or treated.

Nursing Interventions

Medical intervention often depends on accurate reporting of signs and symptoms and nursing observations. In coagulation disorders, monitor vital signs to note any signs of hypovolemic shock. Move the patient gently to prevent trauma to the tissues. Monitor IV infusions and transfusions as ordered. Tapering of anticoagulant

 Nursing Care Plan 47.1 **The Patient With Leukemia**

Ms. M. is a 26-year-old patient diagnosed with acute lymphocytic leukemia. She is married and the mother of a 3-year-old daughter. Ms. M. has been receiving chemotherapy and is immunocompromised, with a differential white blood cell (WBC) count revealing a neutrophil count of 22%. Her Hgb is 8.8 g/dL, and her platelets are 55,000/mm^3. Her mouth appears edematous, and she complains of oral tenderness.

PATIENT PROBLEM

Potential for Infection, related to leukopenia

Patient Goals and Expected Outcomes	Nursing Interventions	Evaluation
Patient or caregiver will identify measures to prevent or control infection	Inspect all body sites for infection at least daily; note and report fever, sore throat, purulent exudate, chills, cough, burning with urination, erythema, edema, tenderness, and pain.	Patient will remain free of infection.
Patient or caregiver will verbalize and report signs and symptoms of infection	Monitor vital signs. Obtain cultures as ordered. Monitor WBC counts and culture reports. Administer antibiotics on time as ordered. Promote and maintain hygiene integrity of skin and mucous membranes. Use aseptic technique in treatments. Teach the patient and family: • Necessity of avoiding crowds or people with infections while WBC count is decreased. • Personal hygiene measures. • Signs and symptoms of infection.	Patient demonstrates no signs or symptoms of infection; temperature and WBC count are within normal range.

PATIENT PROBLEM

Impaired Coping, related to diagnosis and disease process

Patient Goals and Expected Outcomes	Nursing Intervention	Evaluation
Patient and family will demonstrate measures to effectively cope by verbalizing role of family, significant others, and support groups in therapeutic coping	Assess coping capabilities of patient and significant others. Discuss disease process and expectations. Alleviate knowledge deficit. Encourage questions and self-expression; listen actively, demonstrate compassion, reassure with touch and personal contact. Assess fear of threat of death; allow time for personal expression and provide one-on-one discussion opportunity.	Patient and family express factors that are causing anxiety and powerlessness.

CRITICAL THINKING QUESTIONS

1. What should the nurse do if a visitor with an obvious upper respiratory tract infection is seen approaching Ms. M.'s room?
2. What nursing interventions would be most appropriate in providing therapeutic oral hygiene for Ms. M.?
3. What personal hygiene and activities of daily living would be most beneficial for Ms. M.?

therapy must be followed as directed by the health care provider.

DISORDERS ASSOCIATED WITH PLATELETS

THROMBOCYTOPENIA

Etiology and Pathophysiology

A deficiency in the number of circulating platelets or change in the function of platelets alters the process of coagulation. *Thrombocytopenia* is an abnormal hematologic condition in which the number of platelets is reduced to fewer than 150,000/mm^3. Decreased production occurs in aplastic anemia, leukemia, tumors, and chemotherapy. Decreased platelet survival occurs when there is destruction by antibodies (i.e., an autoimmune process), infection, or viral invasion. Increased platelet destruction is caused by disseminated intravascular coagulation (DIC; discussed later). Splenomegaly, which can result from various disorders, entraps blood, including platelets, leading to thrombocytopenia.

The most common cause of increased destruction of platelets is *thrombocytopenic purpura,* which may be drug-induced or immune-mediated. Immune (originally called **idiopathic**) thrombocytopenic purpura, or ITP, is an autoimmune disease. In ITP, platelets become coated with antibodies. Although these platelets function normally, when they reach the spleen, the antibody-coated platelets are recognized as foreign and are

Box 47.4 Medications With Thrombocytopenic Effects

- Aspirin
- Digitalis derivatives
- Furosemide
- Nonsteroidal antiinflammatory agents (azathioprine, D-penicillamine, ibuprofen, indomethacin)
- Oral hypoglycemics
- Penicillins
- Quinidine
- Rifampicin
- Sulfonamides
- Thiazides

destroyed by macrophages in the spleen. Normal platelets survive 8 to 10 days, but with ITP, platelet survival is, on average, 1 to 3 days. If thrombocytopenia is medication induced (Box 47.4), the patient's platelet count usually returns to normal 1 to 2 weeks after the medication is withdrawn. The acute form of ITP is found mostly in children; the chronic form is found in patients of all ages but is more common in 20- to 40-year-old women. It is an autoimmune process caused by the production of an autoantibody (immunoglobulin G) directed against a platelet antigen.

Clinical Manifestations

The major signs of thrombocytopenia that are observable by physical examination are petechiae and ecchymoses on the skin. The severity of signs and symptoms correlates with the platelet count. As the level drops to less than 100,000/mm^3, the risk for bleeding from mucous membranes and in cutaneous sites and internal organs increases. Significant risk for serious bleeding occurs once the count is less than 20,000/mm^3. When the platelet count is less than 5000/mm^3, spontaneous, potentially fatal CNS or GI hemorrhage can occur.

Assessment

Collection of subjective data includes questioning the patient about recent viral infections (which may produce a transient thrombocytopenia), medications in current use, and the extent of alcohol ingestion.

Collection of objective data includes observing the patient's skin for petechiae and ecchymoses, or possibly hematoma. Epistaxis and gingival bleeding are common. Signs of increased intracranial pressure caused by cerebral hemorrhage may be detected. If bleeding occurs in the GI tract, the patient may vomit blood (hematemesis) or may pass blood in the stool, resulting in bright red blood in the stools from bleeding in the lower GI tract, or dark, tarry stools (melena) from bleeding higher in the GI tract.

Diagnostic Tests

To ascertain the characteristics of all blood cells, laboratory studies include platelet count, peripheral blood smear, and bleeding time. In addition, a bone marrow analysis is performed to determine the presence of immature platelets. Examination also reveals the presence or absence of primary bone marrow abnormalities, such as neoplastic invasion or aplastic anemia.

Medical Management

By treating the underlying cause of the thrombocytopenia, the patient's signs and symptoms may improve. Corticosteroids may help if the disorder is related to an autoimmune problem. Packed RBC or platelet transfusions are sometimes necessary. Other medical treatments for ITP include IV immunoglobulin (IVIG) and IV Rho immunoglobulin (RhIG) (Kessler and Sandler, 2013). Splenectomy is a last effort for treatment if all other methods of treatment are not successful (Mayo Clinic, 2015).

Nursing Interventions and Patient Teaching

Support the medical treatment regimen, using specific interventions for specific disease causes. If medication toxicity is the cause, the medication is discontinued. Prevent infections by meticulous asepsis, universal precautions, and gentle handling of the patient. Closely monitor plasma and platelet infusion and whole blood transfusions for reaction and effects on the patient's condition.

A patient problem and interventions for the patient with thrombocytopenia include but are not limited to the following:

Patient Problem	Nursing Interventions
Compromised Blood Flow to Tissues (cerebral, cardiopulmonary, renal, GI, peripheral), related to bleeding	Monitor vital signs and neurologic status Monitor platelet count and abnormal bleeding times Check for bleeding in urine, stool, and emesis Monitor invasive diagnostic procedure sites for bleeding Maintain comfort measures and bed rest Avoid trauma and infection Monitor intake and output for untoward signs Monitor potential sites of hemorrhage

The patient must understand the disease process and causative agents to provide self-care and to prevent trauma or infection. Provide instructions on signs, symptoms, and preventive measures: avoid trauma, use stool softeners, maintain a high-fiber diet to prevent constipation, check for the presence of blood, use a soft toothbrush, and blow the nose gently. Stress the importance of notifying the health care provider of signs and symptoms of bleeding.

Prognosis

The prognosis is variable, depending on the underlying cause. In ITP, treatment may be necessary for 3 to 4 weeks before a complete response is seen. More than 80% of children with immune ITP require no treatment and have a spontaneous recovery from the disorder within weeks after diagnosis. In chronic ITP, transient remissions occur. Approximately 75% of patients benefit from splenectomy, resulting in a complete or partial remission (Kessler and Sandler, 2013).

DISORDERS ASSOCIATED WITH CLOTTING FACTOR DEFECTS

HEMOPHILIA

Etiology and Pathophysiology

Hemophilia, a hereditary coagulation disorder, is characterized by the absence of certain blood-clotting factors. In **hemophilia A,** the more common type (representing 80% of the total incidence), the blood-clotting factor VIII is absent. In hemophilia B (Christmas disease), a much rarer type, factor IX is absent. Because these factors are absent or deficient, patients with hemophilia experience prolonged bleeding that ultimately may be fatal.

The genes causing hemophilia A and B are inherited according to a recessive, X chromosome–linked pattern. Hemophilia therefore affects mainly males; females are typically carriers.

In the past, patients with hemophilia frequently were treated with pooled plasma transfusions containing concentrated factor VIII or IX, and were therefore at risk for being infected with human immunodeficiency virus (HIV) and later developing acquired immunodeficiency syndrome (AIDS). Approximately 50% of patients with hemophilia who received blood products between the late 1970s to the mid-1980s became infected with HIV and subsequently developed AIDS. Viral detection processes and viral inactivation of blood products have restored safety to transfusing blood products. The management of people with hemophilia A has improved enormously over the past 50 years. There has been progressive improvement of virus-inactivation methods in plasma products. The introduction of methods used to screen for the presence of viruses in blood donations and plasma pools has led to an impressive increase in the safety of plasma-derived factor concentrates. Indeed, there have been no new cases of product-transmitted hepatitis viruses or HIV infection in the past 20 years. There has been no transmission of HIV to anyone receiving factor VIII or IX since 1987 (National Hemophilia Foundation, 2017).

The use of **recombinant** blood factors (the result of gene cloning) also is improving long-term survival rates. The development of recombinant (recombinant refers to artificial DNA) clotting factor VIII for hemophilia A and factor IX for hemophilia B has been a major step forward in the treatment of hemophilia. In the past, the life expectancy for a male with hemophilia was approximately 20 years because of uncontrolled spontaneous bleeding or bleeding after an injury. Recombinant factor VIII and IX replacement therapy has changed the prognosis drastically for the patient with hemophilia. Patients with hemophilia can expect a normal life without serious bleeding episodes. Potential improvements for recombinant factor VIII and IX include advances that would prevent spontaneous bleeding with fewer intravenous infusions (US FDA, 2014). Septic arthritis (infection in a joint, usually caused by bacteria) is a complication commonly occurring in the patient with hemophilia resulting from repeated bleeding into the joints (Hemophilia Federation of America, 2017). Advances with treatment would be expected to reduce the incidence of septic arthritis in hemophilia.

Clinical Manifestations

Clinical manifestations of hemophilia include severe bleeding episodes from minor injuries. Hemorrhage occurs with extensive, deep bruising (ecchymosis) of muscle tissue, which may show deformity; hemorrhage also occurs into joints, which eventually become ankylosed (i.e., fused or obliterated). **Hemarthrosis,** or bleeding into a joint space, is a hallmark of severe disease and usually occurs in the knees, ankles, elbows, shoulders, and hips. Pain, edema, erythema, and fever accompany hemarthrosis. Small cuts can prove fatal; blood loss from simple dental procedures may be significant.

Assessment

Subjective data include reports by patient and family of incidents of ecchymosis and hemorrhage from even the slightest trauma. Pain is associated with joint motion.

Collection of objective data includes noting blood in subcutaneous tissues, urine, or stool and noting edematous or immobile joints.

Diagnostic Tests

Factors VIII and IX are absent or deficient. Coagulation profiles reveal a normal platelet count and therefore bleeding time test result (the bleeding time test measures platelet response to injury; the platelets of patients with hemophilia are normal). The prothrombin time and international normalized ratio are also normal; it is the partial thromboplastin time that is prolonged. Notify laboratory personnel of the patient's disorder to alleviate further incidents of trauma as a result of diagnostic procedures (e.g., venipuncture).

Medical Management

Care focuses on preventing and treating bleeding and relieving pain. Transfusions and administration of factor VIII or IX concentrate may be prophylactic or used to stop the hemorrhage. Two different clotting factor concentrates made from human plasma can be used. One, cryoprecipitate, is a clotting factor concentrate rich in factor VIII. This treatment is used less because of the risk, although small, of viral disease transmission. In addition, home administration of cryoprecipitate is difficult because it must be stored at low temperatures. The second human-derived product, factor VIII concentrate, is used more often. A wide variety of these products are available; all are freeze-dried concentrates of factor VIII and factor IX and are prepared from pooled plasma from thousands of donors. These products are treated specially to inactivate any viral contamination (such as HIV or hepatitis viruses). A newer treatment is a synthetic hormone that stimulates the release of stored factor VIII. This therapy is used only for mild forms of hemophilia A (NHLBI, 2013).

Because human plasma products still carry a slight risk of infection transmission and require human donors, scientists have used genetic engineering to manufacture factor VIII. This product, recombinant factor VIII, is advantageous because of viral safety, unlimited supply, and lower cost. Recombinant replacement factor VIII is now commercially available for widespread use.

Nursing Interventions and Patient Teaching

Assess the patient's level of understanding of the clinical course of the disease and prevention of complications. Educate the patient and the entire family because many people may be involved in the patient care. Control hemorrhages in emergency situations by applying pressure and cold to the site. Support and reassurance are imperative. Monitor transfusions of factor VIII concentrate. Supportive care measures include pain management and genetic counseling. Do not give hemophilia patients aspirin or aspirin products, because they can further complicate the bleeding tendency.

Patient problems and interventions for the patient with hemophilia include but are not limited to the following:

Patient Problem	Nursing Interventions
Impaired Coping, related to long-term illness	
Inadequate Fluid Volume, related to bleeding	Assess for extent of hemorrhage Prevent further hemorrhage or extension
Compromised Blood Flow to Tissue, related to blood loss from coagulation deficit	Monitor vital signs and laboratory reports Apply cold compresses to bleeding areas Assess for anxiety, shock, disorientation Assess for decreased urinary output Teach safety precautions to prevent trauma Administer analgesia as ordered Move patient gently and slowly, supporting joints Prevent deformity through support, splints, and physical therapy

Discuss with the patient ways to avoid injury and control bleeding. Also discuss physical activity within limits. Encourage the patient to wear a medical-alert tag. Emergency care teaching includes immobilizing the affected part, applying ice, and notifying the health care provider. Discuss diet to prevent obesity, which puts excess pressure on joints. Regular dental care and preventive dental and medical measures are important aspects. Overprotection is sometimes a factor to discuss. Neither aspirin nor any other medication, including over-the-counter medications, should be taken except with the health care provider's knowledge (see the Home Care Considerations box).

Home Care Considerations

Hemophilia

- Home management is a primary consideration for a patient with hemophilia because the disease follows a chronic, progressive course.
- The quantity and length of life may be affected significantly by the patient's knowledge of the illness and understanding of how to live with it.
- Refer the patient and family to the local chapter of the National Hemophilia Foundation to encourage association with other individuals who are dealing with the problems associated with hemophilia.
- Teach the patient with hemophilia to recognize disease-related problems and to learn which problems can be resolved at home and which require hospitalization.
- Immediate medical attention is required for severe pain or edema of a muscle or joint that restricts movement or inhibits sleep and for a head injury, edema in the neck or mouth, abdominal pain, hematuria, melena, and skin wounds in need of suturing.
- Oral hygiene must be performed gently, without trauma.
- Aspirin and aspirin products should not be taken, because they decrease platelet aggregation.
- Understanding how to prevent injuries is an important consideration. The patient can learn to participate in noncontact sports (e.g., golf) and wear gloves when doing household chores to prevent cuts or abrasions from knives, hammers, and other tools.
- The patient should wear a medical-alert tag to ensure that health care providers know about the hemophilia in case of an accident.
- A person with hemophilia who is mature enough, or a family member, can be taught to administer some of the factor replacement therapies at home.

Prognosis

The use of recombinant blood factors (the result of gene cloning) is improving long-term survival rates. The development of recombinant factor VIII has been a major step forward in the treatment of hemophilia A. In the past, the life expectancy for a male with hemophilia was approximately 20 years because of uncontrolled spontaneous bleeding or bleeding after an injury. Recombinant factor VIII replacement therapy has changed drastically the prognosis for the patient with hemophilia. Most patients with hemophilia live to a normal life expectancy.

VON WILLEBRAND'S DISEASE

Etiology and Pathophysiology

von Willebrand's disease (vWD) is an inherited genetic bleeding disorder characterized by abnormally slow coagulation of blood and spontaneous episodes of GI bleeding, epistaxis, and gingival bleeding. The disease is caused by a deficiency of von Willebrand's factor (vWF), which is a protein that is critical for platelet adhesion (one of the earliest steps in blood coagulation). Because vWF is bound to factor VIII, protecting it from rapid breakdown in the blood, a patient with vWD also has low factor VIII levels. vWD is more common and generally less serious than hemophilia.

Researchers have identified many variations of vWD, but most fall into the following classifications (Pollak, 2017):

- *Type 1:* Partial quantitative vWF. Levels of vWF are lower than normal, and levels of factor VIII also may be reduced. Twenty-five percent of people with vWD have type 1.
- *Type 2:* Qualitative vWF deficiency. In people with type 2 vWD, the vWF has an abnormality. Depending on the abnormality, patients may be classified as having type 2a or type 2b, type 2M, and 2N. The classification of type 2 varies depending on specific molecular mutations that have varying treatment modalities. Approximately 66% of people with vWD have some form of type 2 vWD.
- *Type 3:* Total vWF deficiency. This is severe vWD. These people may have a total absence of vWF, and factor VIII levels are often less than 10%.

Desmopressin (DDAVP) has become the treatment of choice for patients who have the mild form of vWD. This drug is a synthetic form of the human antidiuretic hormone, vasopressin. It causes an increase in vWF release from storage sites in the body and of factor VIII. Desmopressin often is administered prophylactically to patients with mild vWD who require surgery or dental extractions. For patients with more severe forms of vWD, desmopressin is ineffective, and treatment involves administration of plasma concentrates containing vWF and factor VIII.

Observation and nursing interventions for hemophilia A and B can be adapted easily to vWD.

Prognosis

The prognosis is usually good for patients with early diagnosis and effective treatment. Most people who have type 1 vWD are able to live normal lives with only mild bleeding issues. Individuals with type 2 are at an increased risk of experiencing mild to moderate bleeding and complications. During times of infection, surgery, or pregnancy the patient often has increased bleeding. Type 3 poses an increased risk for severe bleeding, externally and internally. These patients have a normal life expectancy (Pollak, 2017).

DISSEMINATED INTRAVASCULAR COAGULATION

Etiology and Pathophysiology

Disseminated intravascular coagulation (DIC) is a grave coagulopathy resulting from the overstimulation of clotting and anticlotting processes in response to disease or injury, including septicemia, obstetric complications, malignancies, tissue trauma, transfusion reaction, burns, shock, and snake bites (Box 47.5). In DIC, widespread clotting (thrombosis) within small vessels occurs, with subsequent damage to multiple organs. In addition, the body-wide blood coagulation leads to the depletion of clotting factors in the plasma. This in turn leads to abnormal bleeding, sometimes happening simultaneously with the thrombosis.

Abruptio placentae (placental abruption, the premature separation of the placenta from the uterus) generally is considered one of the more common causes of the development of DIC. In addition, a mother whose fetus dies in utero, whether as a result of placental abruption or not, is at especially high risk for the development of DIC, especially when the delivery of the deceased fetus is delayed. For this reason, the death of one fetus in a multifetal pregnancy (i.e., twins, triplets, or other) presents a grave risk for the development of DIC.

Box 47.5 Disorders Usually Associated With Disseminated Intravascular Coagulation (DIC)

ACUTE DIC

- Acute liver failure
- Gram negative
- Gram positive
- Organ destruction
- Organ destruction (e.g., pancreatitis)
  - Severe tissue damage (burns, crushing)
  - Head trauma
  - Obstetric complications (e.g., abruptio placenta, low platelets [HELLP] syndrome), amniotic embolism, abruptio placenta, eclampsia
  - Abortion
  - Intravascular hemolysis
  - Severe blood transfusion reaction
- Sepsis (most common)
- Toxins
- Trauma

CHRONIC DIC

- Autoimmune disorders (transplant rejection)
- Cardiovascular diseases (e.g., valve stents, myocardial infarction, aneurysms)
- Hematologic disorders
- Inflammatory disorders
- Malignancy (especially solid tumors)
- Renal vascular disorders
- Retained fetal syndrome

Patients with preeclampsia or HELLP syndrome have a higher risk for the development of DIC. HELLP stands for the characteristics of the syndrome: H for hemolysis, the breaking down of red blood cells; EL for elevated liver enzymes; and LP for low platelet count. HELLP syndrome is a life-threatening pregnancy complication usually considered to be a variant of preeclampsia. About 4% to 12% of women with diagnosed preeclampsia develop HELLP syndrome. Both conditions usually occur during the later stages of pregnancy, or within 48 hours to 7 days after childbirth (American Pregnancy Association, 2015).

Clinical Manifestations

Bleeding is noted in mucous membranes, venipuncture or surgical sites, GI and urinary tracts, and generally from all orifices. Bleeding ranges from occult to profuse. Dyspnea; hemoptysis (blood-tinged sputum); and diaphoresis with cold, mottled digits are observed.

Assessment

Subjective data include patient complaints of bone and joint pain. Changes in vision occur.

Collection of objective data includes observing for occult or obvious bleeding. Purpura on the chest and abdomen, reflecting fibrin deposits in capillaries, is a common first sign of DIC. Note the color of skin and mucosa and the presence of petechiae. Abdominal tenderness may be present. GI bleeding, hematuria, pulmonary edema, pulmonary embolism, hypotension, tachycardia, absence of peripheral pulses, decreased blood pressure, restlessness, confusion, seizures, or coma may be present.

Diagnostic Tests

The coagulation profile shows prolonged prothrombin and activated partial thromboplastin times, as well as prolonged bleeding time. The platelet count is low, showing marked thrombocytopenia. Other tests show fibrinogen deficiency (hypofibrinogenemia; reflecting the consumption of fibrinogen in DIC) and deficits of factors V, VII, VIII, X, and XII.

D-dimer test results are elevated. D-dimer reveals the breakdown of fibrin and is a specific marker for the degree of fibrinolysis in the serum.

Medical Management

The underlying cause of DIC must be addressed and corrected. Administration of platelet transfusion and factor replacement therapy is initiated when extensive bleeding occurs. Heparin therapy may be ordered if the patient has widespread fibrin deposition without significant bleeding. Heparin blocks the formation of microemboli by inhibiting thrombin activity. It has no effect, however, on existing clots. The goal of administering heparin is to stop the rapid overproduction of microemboli and thus allow for reperfusion of vital organs and replenishment of clotting factors. Packed RBC transfusion may be initiated to reestablish normal hemostatic potential if the thrombosis is blocked by heparin. FFP (fresh frozen plasma) can be administered to replace other coagulation factors (Marcel and Schmaier, 2012).

Nursing Interventions and Patient Teaching

Protection from bleeding and trauma and application of pressure to sites of hemorrhage are essential nursing measures. Support and reassurance of the patient may aid in relieving high stress levels. Monitor the patient in a quiet, nonstressful environment. Make sure the patient's bed has padded side rails, and use foam or cotton swabs for mouth care. Monitor vital signs and administer heparin, blood and FFP transfusions, and factor replacement therapy as ordered. Use the blood pressure cuff infrequently to avoid subcutaneous bleeding.

Patient problems and interventions for the patient with DIC include but are not limited to the following:

Patient Problem	Nursing Interventions
Potential for Injury, Bleeding, and Fluid Deficit, related to: • Depleted coagulation factors • Adverse effect of heparin (excess heparin, insufficient heparin)	Monitor Hct and Hgb Assess skin surface for signs of bleeding; note petechiae; purpura; hematomas; oozing of blood from IV sites, drains, and wounds; and bleeding from mucous membranes Observe for signs of bleeding from GI and genitourinary tracts Note any hemoptysis or blood obtained during suctioning Monitor level of consciousness (LOC); institute neurologic checklist (mental status changes may occur with the decreased fluid volume or with decreasing Hgb) Monitor vital signs for signs of hemorrhage Observe for signs of orthostatic hypotension (drop of >15 mm Hg when changing from supine to sitting position indicates reduced circulating fluids) Avoid intramuscular injections; any needlestick is a potential bleeding site Apply pressure to bleeding site Prevent trauma to catheter and tubes by proper taping, minimum pulling

Discuss with the patient and family the signs and symptoms of DIC and have them repeat this information to the nurse or health care provider. Teach the patient to self-administer heparin therapy subcutaneously if prescribed. Instruct the patient and family to avoid mechanical trauma, such as from a hard toothbrush, blade razor, rough nose blowing, or contact sports.

Prognosis

Mortality rates from DIC vary, depending on severity. Death is usually a result of either uncontrolled hemorrhage, irreversible end-organ damage, or both.

DISORDERS ASSOCIATED WITH PLASMA CELLS

MULTIPLE MYELOMA

Etiology and Pathophysiology

Multiple myeloma, or plasma cell myeloma, is a malignant neoplastic disease of the bone marrow. Neoplastic plasma cells build up in the bone marrow and produce one or more tumors. The tumors destroy bone (osseous) tissue, especially in flat bones, causing pain, fractures, and skeletal deformities.

The specific immunoglobulin produced by the myeloma cells is present in the blood and/or urine and is referred to as *monoclonal protein, M protein,* or *paraprotein.* This protein is a helpful marker to monitor the extent of the disease and the patient's response to treatment. It is measured by serum or urine protein electrophoresis.

The older adult patient whose chief complaint is back pain and who has elevated total serum protein should be evaluated for possible multiple myeloma. It most frequently occurs in patients older than age 40 years, with a peak incidence around 65 years of age, and affects more men than women. Onset is gradual and insidious; the disease often goes unrecognized for years while the individual experiences frequent, recurrent bacterial infections (the result of immune dysfunction: there is too much of a particular nonfunctional immunoglobulin and not enough normal immunoglobulin). Early detection can decrease the amount of pain and disability resulting from bone destruction and pathologic fractures (National Cancer Institute, 2013b). The annual incidence of multiple myeloma in the United States is estimated to be more than 30,280 new cases (17,490 in men and 12,790 in women) with nearly 12,590 deaths (ACS, 2016a).

Clinical Manifestations

The disease process shows a proliferation of malignant plasma cells and development of single or multiple bone marrow tumors. This is followed by bone destruction with dissemination into lymph nodes, liver, spleen, and kidneys.

The skeletal system symptoms typically involve the ribs, spine, and pelvis. Osteolytic lesions are seen in the skull, vertebrae, and ribs. Vertebral destruction can lead to collapse of vertebrae with ensuing compression of the spinal cord. Patients complain of bone pain that increases with movement. About 30% develop pathologic fractures accompanied by severe pain.

In an individual with multiple myeloma, production of erythrocytes, platelets, and leukocytes is disrupted because the marrow is crowded by the abnormal proliferation of plasma cells. This leads to infection, anemia, and increased potential for bleeding. Calcium and phosphorus drain from bones, leading to hypercalcemia and renal problems. In addition, cell destruction contributes to the development of hyperuricemia (high uric acid in the blood), which, along with the high protein levels caused by the myeloma protein, can result in renal failure.

Assessment

Collection of subjective data includes assessment of the patient's complaints of pain, especially skeletal pain in the back, pelvis, the spine, and the ribs.

Collection of objective data includes assessing the patient's facial expression for signs of increased pain with movement, the ability to perform ADLs, increased body temperature, increased potential for bleeding, changes in urine characteristics, and effectiveness of medication administration.

Diagnostic Tests

Diagnosis of multiple myeloma is made with radiographic skeletal studies, bone marrow biopsy, and laboratory examination of blood and urine. A monoclonal antibody (M protein) may be present, as evidenced in serum or urine electrophoresis. Bony degeneration also causes loss of calcium in the bones, eventually causing hypercalcemia. Pancytopenia, hypercalcemia, hyperuricemia, and elevated creatinine may be found. In addition, an abnormal globulin known as Bence Jones protein is found in the urine and can result in renal failure.

Radiographic skeletal examinations reveal widespread demineralization, lytic lesions, and osteoporosis. Lytic lesions (destruction of an area of bone due to a disease process) may be seen on bone roentgenograms but are not well visualized on bone scans. Bone marrow studies reveal large numbers of immature plasma cells, which normally account for only 5% of marrow population.

Medical Management

Traditional chemotherapy may be used to treat multiple myeloma. A combination of drugs such as vincristine, doxorubicin, and bendamustine (Treanda) are more effective than a single drug. Corticosteroids are used commonly along with traditional chemotherapeutic drugs to help reduce nausea and vomiting. Immunomodulating drugs (see Chapter 57) often are prescribed. Other medications used to treat multiple myeloma include proteasome inhibitors (stop enzyme complexes, proteasomes, in cells from breaking down proteins important for keeping cell division under control); histone deacetylase (HDAC) inhibitors (affect which genes are active inside cells by interacting with proteins in chromosomes, referred to as histones); and interferon (similar to a hormone released by the WBCs that slows the growth of myeloma cells) (ACS, 2016a).

Hypercalcemia (resulting from bone destruction) and pain also should be addressed. Analgesics, orthopedic supports, and localized radiation help reduce the skeletal pain. Hospitalization to administer chemotherapy, corticosteroids, and fluids may be required.

Nursing Interventions and Patient Teaching

Care of the patient with multiple myeloma focuses on relieving pain, preventing infection and bone injury, administering chemotherapy and radiation, and maintaining hydration (Box 47.6). Encourage ambulation and adequate hydration to treat hypercalcemia, dehydration, and potential renal damage. Fluid intake of 3 to 4 L/day is encouraged to prevent dehydration and maintain a urinary output of 1.5 to 2 L/day. Patients with multiple myeloma with high tumor burdens (the total mass of tumor tissue carried by a patient with a malignancy) who receive chemotherapy have increased cell lysis and release of uric acid, resulting in hyperuricemia. Weight-bearing helps the bones reabsorb some calcium, and fluids dilute calcium and prevent protein precipitates from causing renal tubular obstruction.

Because of the potential for pathologic fractures, be careful when moving and ambulating the patient. A slight twist or strain on the bones may be sufficient to cause a fracture. Attention to the psychosocial, emotional, and spiritual needs is also extremely important.

Patient problems and interventions for the patient with multiple myeloma include but are not limited to the following:

Patient Problem	Nursing Interventions
Potential for Injury, related to: • Osteoporosis • Lytic lesions	Protect from bone injury; use logroll, turning sheet Use pillows to support bony prominences
Recent Onset of Pain, related to disease process	Administer analgesics as ordered (such as nonsteroidal antiinflammatory drugs, acetaminophen, or an acetaminophen-opioid combination). Combination drugs may be more effective than opioids alone in diminishing bone pain Provide comfort measures Assess contributing factors

Teach the patient how to avoid traumatic bone injury and infection. Discuss the importance of adequate hydration and review the pain control modalities available. It is also important to identify spiritual resources.

Box 47.6 Chemotherapy Side Effects

- Alopecia (hair loss)
- Appetite changes
- Bleeding problems
- Constipation/diarrhea
- Fatigue
- Infection
- Mouth and throat changes
- Nausea and vomiting
- Nerve changes
- Pain
- Sexual and fertility changes in women
- Skin and nail changes
- Swelling (fluid retention)
- Urination changes

Address the patient's understanding of the disease, verbalization of discouragement and hopelessness, and desires for emotional and spiritual support.

Prognosis

The prognosis for multiple myeloma is dependent on several factors, including stage when diagnosed, effectiveness of medical treatment, and comorbidities. According to the American Cancer Society (ACS, 2016a), if the disease is diagnosed and treatment is started, the life expectancy for stage I is 62 months, stage II is 44 months, and stage III is 29 months. Improvements with treatment should lend to an increase in life expectancy. If there is a relapse of the disease, life expectancy drops to 9 months.

DISORDERS OF THE LYMPHATIC SYSTEM

LYMPHANGITIS

Etiology and Pathophysiology

Lymphangitis is an inflammation of one or more lymphatic vessels or channels that usually results from an acute streptococcal or staphylococcal infection in an extremity.

Clinical Manifestations

Lymphangitis is characterized by fine red streaks from the affected area in the groin or axilla. The infection usually is not localized, and edema is diffuse. Chills, fever, and local pain accompany headache and myalgia (muscle pain). Septicemia may occur; lymph nodes enlarge.

Medical Management

Administration of antimicrobial drugs by oral or intravenous route controls the infection. Antiinflammatory medications may be ordered to reduce inflammation. Hot, moist heat (soaks or packs) brings comfort. Surgery may be required if any abscesses have formed (Phillips, 2012).

Nursing Interventions

The affected area should be kept clean to promote healing. Rest and extremity elevation may relieve the pressure and reduce any swelling that may have occurred.

Prognosis

With treatment, the prognosis is usually good.

LYMPHEDEMA

Etiology and Pathophysiology

Lymphedema is a primary or secondary disorder characterized by the accumulation of lymph in soft tissue and edema. The accumulation of lymph in soft tissue is caused by obstruction, an increase in the amount of lymph, or removal of the lymph channels and nodes. The condition also may be hereditary. If the lymphatic drainage function is disturbed, an inflammatory process may result.

Clinical Manifestations

Massive edema and tightness cause pressure and pain in the affected extremities. It progresses toward the trunk and is aggravated by standing; pressure; obesity; and warm, humid environments.

Assessment and Diagnostic Test

Subjective data include complaints of pain and pressure. Medical history of varicosities, pregnancy, or modified radical mastectomy is important.

Collection of objective data includes observation of the extremities for edema and palpation of peripheral pulses. Lymphoscintigraphy commonly is used to diagnose the disorder. This test involves injection of a radioactive substance under the skin between the first and second fingers or toes. Blockages then can be detected by scanning the flow of the dye through the lymph system (National Cancer Institute, 2013c).

Medical Management

Mechanical management includes special massage techniques referred to as manual lymph drainage. These techniques should be performed only by specially trained individuals (Mayo Clinic, 2016). Additional therapy includes compression bandaging, compression pumps, and elastic sleeves or stockings on the affected limb. Light exercise can help by increasing circulation, thus improving lymph drainage. Diet restrictions include limiting sodium intake.

Nursing Interventions and Patient Teaching

The primary goal of care is to increase lymphatic drainage and avoid trauma. Elevation of the extremities while asleep and periodically during the day facilitates drainage. Massage techniques previously discussed help improve lymph drainage. If the patient tolerates light exercise, it should be encouraged. Advise patients to avoid constrictive clothing, shoes, or stockings (except elastic stockings). Patients with lymphedema are at risk for infection in the affected extremity. Good skin care, avoiding injury, inspecting the skin daily for cuts or cracks in the skin, is important. Lotions can be applied to prevent dryness of the skin.

Emotional support for the patient is also important. Address body image disturbance related to the appearance of the lymphedematous extremity. Emphasize that lymphedema need not prevent the individual from engaging in routine activity.

A patient problem and interventions for lymphedema include but are not limited to the following:

Patient Problem	Nursing Interventions
Compromised Skin Integrity, related to altered lymphatic drainage	Protect engorged tissues Consider physical therapy or ROM exercises (aids lymphatic flow) Examine skin for impaired skin integrity Gently handle affected parts Apply skin-protecting moisturizers or emollients Teach application of supportive stockings or elastic sleeves

From Vaqas B, Ryan TJ: Lymphoedema: Pathophysiology and management in resource-poor settings: Relevance for lymphatic filariasis control programmes. Filaria J 2:4, 2003.

Make certain the patient is aware of the condition's progression and cause. If the disorder is long term and ongoing, discuss how to cope with its effects. Explain the rationale behind nursing interventions to enhance the ongoing medical regimen. Encourage the patient to maintain interests and socialize to enhance feelings of well-being.

Prognosis

Lymphedema has no cure, but signs and symptoms of the condition can be controlled by compliance with treatment. The goal of care is to prevent lymphedema when possible and to initiate prompt treatment when it does occur. Compliance with suggested treatment modalities can prevent complications of the disorder.

HODGKIN'S LYMPHOMA

Etiology and Pathophysiology

Hodgkin's lymphoma, also called Hodgkin's disease, is a malignant disorder characterized by painless, progressive enlargement of lymphoid tissue. It affects males twice as frequently as females, and the age incidence curve is bimodal (two separate populations), with a peak early in life at 15 to 35 years, and a peak later in life at 50 years. The two peaks in incidence may represent separate diseases. The first incident peak suggests a viral cause. Beginning as an inflammatory or infectious process, the condition develops into a neoplasm. The exact cause is unknown, but Hodgkin's lymphoma is thought to be an immune disorder (T cell disease).

Hodgkin's lymphoma has no major risk factors, but the disease occurs more frequently in people who have had mononucleosis (an infection caused by Epstein-Barr virus), have acquired or congenital immunodeficiency syndromes, are taking immunosuppressive drugs after organ transplantation, have been exposed to occupational toxins, or have a genetic predisposition. The presence of HIV increases the incidence of Hodgkin's lymphoma.

Lymphoid tissue enlargement usually is noticed first in the cervical nodes and is characterized by abnormal or atypical cells. **Reed-Sternberg cells** are atypical histiocytes consisting of large, abnormal, multinucleated cells in the lymph nodes found in Hodgkin's lymphoma. These cells increase in number, replacing normal cells. The main diagnostic feature of Hodgkin's lymphoma is the presence of Reed-Sternberg cells in lymph node biopsy specimens.

The disease is believed to arise in a single location (the lymph nodes in most patients) and then spread along adjacent lymphatics. It eventually infiltrates other organs, especially the lungs, spleen, and liver. In the majority of patients, the cervical lymph nodes are affected first. Unless they exert pressure on adjacent nerves, the enlarged nodes are not painful. When the disease begins above the diaphragm, it remains confined to lymph nodes for a variable period. Disease originating below the diaphragm frequently spreads to extralymphoid sites such as the liver.

Box 47.7 Cotswold-Modified Ann Arbor Staging System for Hodgkin Lymphoma

Stage I: Disease affecting a single lymph node region or lymphoid structure (e.g., spleen, thymus, Waldeyer ring).

Stage II: Disease affecting two or more discrete lymph node regions confined to the same side of the diaphragm.

Stage III: Disease affecting two or more discrete lymph node regions or lymphoid structures on both sides of the diaphragm.

Stage IV: Disease that has spread to one or more extranodal sites (that does not meet the criteria for E) or an extralymphatic structure including involvement of the bone marrow, liver, or lungs.

DESIGNATIONS

A: Absence of B symptoms[a]

B: Presence of B symptoms[a]

S: Involvement of the spleen

E: Single extranodal site or involvement of an extranodal site that is contiguous to an involved nodal region.

X: Bulky disease as defined as >1/3 mediastinum at its widest part or a nodal mass >10 cm at its greatest diameter.

[a]B symptoms: constitutional symptoms including night sweats, fevers, or weight loss (>10% over 6 months).

From Hoffman R, Anastasi J, Weitz J, et al: *Hematology: Basic principles and practice*, ed 7, St. Louis, 2018, Elsevier.

Clinical Manifestations

Painless enlargement of the cervical, axillary, or inguinal lymph nodes is most often the initial development. Anorexia, unexplained rapid weight loss, fever, night sweats, fatigue, and pruritus are complaints associated with this condition. One other unusual symptom is pain in the lymph nodes after ingesting alcohol (Mayo Clinic, 2017). Night sweats, weight loss, and fever, which are referred to as "B" symptoms, are associated with a worse prognosis (Box 47.7). Low-grade fever may occur. Anemia and leukocytosis follow, with development of respiratory tract infections.

Assessment

Subjective data include the common complaints of fatigue and appetite loss. Pruritus is often severe. After the ingestion of even small amounts of alcohol, individuals with Hodgkin's lymphoma may complain of a rapid onset of pain at the site of the disease. The cause for the alcohol-induced pain is unknown. Bone pain occurs later in the disease's course.

Collection of objective data includes palpating enlarged cervical and supraclavicular lymph nodes. Splenomegaly, hepatomegaly, and abdominal tenderness are found. Excoriation of skin and evidence of scratching from pruritus are noted. Clinical signs and symptoms vary depending on where the enlarged lymph nodes are located. If Hodgkin's lymphoma affects lymph nodes inside the chest, the swelling of these nodes may press on the trachea, stimulating a cough reflex or dyspnea. Some patients may complain of pain behind the sternum and difficulty swallowing (ACS, 2017a).

Diagnostic Tests

Peripheral blood studies show anemia (normocytic, normochromic), WBC increase, and an abnormal erythrocyte sedimentation rate. Other blood studies may show hypoferremia (low iron level in the blood) caused by excessive iron intake by the liver and the spleen, elevated leukocyte alkaline phosphatase from liver and bone involvement, hypercalcemia from bone involvement, and hypoalbuminemia from liver involvement. Chest radiographic examination may reveal a mediastinal mass. CT or MRI can detect retroperitoneal node involvement. Lymph node biopsy that includes laparoscopy for retroperitoneal nodes is performed. Bone marrow biopsy is an important aspect of staging. A CT scan and an ultrasound examination can indicate an enlarged spleen or liver. The presence of Reed-Sternberg cells remains a hallmark of Hodgkin's lymphoma.

Positron emission tomography (PET), CT scans, bone scans, and bone marrow biopsy aid in the staging of the disease by determining the extent of any metastasis (ACS, 2017a). The liver, lungs, and bone are common areas of metastasis.

Medical Management

Treatment depends on the staging process (see Box 47.7). The stage of Hodgkin's lymphoma must be established before selecting an appropriate treatment plan.

Combination chemotherapy is used in some early stages in patients believed to have resistant disease or to be at high risk for relapse. Chemotherapy and radiation therapy are used against the generalized forms (stages III and IV). Advances in treatment now enable some stage IIIB and stage IV diseases to be cured with high-dose chemotherapy and bone marrow or peripheral stem cell transplantation (SCT). The site of the disease and the amount of resistant disease after chemotherapy determine the role of radiation in supplementing chemotherapy.

Treatment of early-stage Hodgkin's lymphoma consists of two to four cycles of ABVD (doxorubicin, bleomycin, vinblastine, and dacarbazine) chemotherapy.

For advanced-stage Hodgkin's lymphoma some people have ABVD for up to eight cycles. Other possible combinations include Stanford V (mechlorethamine, doxorubicin, vinblastine, vincristine, bleomycin, etoposide, and prednisone), and BEACOPP (bleomycin, etoposide, doxorubicin, cyclophosphamide, Oncovin [vincristine], procarbazine, and prednisone (ACS, 2017a). If chemotherapy does not work well or the lymphoma comes back, some people have high-dose chemotherapy with stem cell transplantation (ACS, 2017a).

Nursing Interventions and Patient Teaching

Plan care according to the staging level. Awareness of side effects of radiation therapy or chemotherapy is important in preparing the patient to deal effectively with the treatment. Because the survival of patients with Hodgkin's lymphoma depends on their response to treatment, helping the patient deal with the consequences of treatment is extremely important. Comfort measures focus on skin integrity. Soothing baths with an antipruritic medication (as prescribed) can be effective. Control fever and moisture with medication (with attention to increased fluid intake) and linen changes as necessary to prevent further skin problems. Explain extensive tests to the patient to aid in reduction of anxiety and difficulty coping.

Patient problems include *Anxiousness* and *Fearfulness*, related to unknown outcome, and *Potential for Infection*, related to compromised immune system. An additional patient problem and interventions for the patient with Hodgkin's lymphoma include but are not limited to the following:

Patient Problem	Nursing Interventions
Compromised Skin Integrity, related to: • Pruritus • Jaundice • Diaphoresis	Assess skin and level of discomfort Administer skin care by baths and keep patient clean and dry Apply calamine lotion, cornstarch, sodium bicarbonate, and medicated powders to relieve pruritus Maintain adequate humidity and a cool room to decrease pruritus Monitor vital signs for fever; assess for perspiration and change linen, keeping it wrinkle free

Understanding the disease through education and teaching is important for the patient to perform self-care and retain independence. Fertility issues may be of particular concern because this disease frequently is seen in adolescents and young adults. Help ensure that these issues are addressed soon after diagnosis. The effect on the patient's life, as well as on significant others, is a prime consideration in patient attitude and adjustment. Realistic approaches to the illness and therapies are imperative. Referrals for patients seeking counseling for stress management can be helpful. Discuss special nutritional considerations concerning excess weight loss or an undernourished condition.

Prognosis

The staging of the disease is important in the prognosis. The disease is classified as stage I if the cancer is found in only one lymph node area or lymphoid organ, such as the thymus, or the cancer is found only in one area of a single organ outside the lymph system. Stage II is characterized by cancer being found in two or more lymph node areas on the same side of the diaphragm, or the cancer extends locally from one lymph node area into a nearby organ. Stage III is determined by the presence of cancer in lymph node areas on both sides of the diaphragm, or the cancer is in lymph nodes above the diaphragm and in the spleen. Cancer that has spread widely into at least one organ outside of the lymph system, such as the liver, bone marrow, or lungs is classified as stage IV Hodgkin's lymphoma (ACS, 2017a). In general, the earlier the stage of the cancer, the higher the survival rate and chance for a cure. The 5-year survival rate for those with stage I or II who have received proper treatment is approximately 90%. Those with stage III disease have a 5-year survival rate of 80% with proper treatment, and stage IV survival rate is approximately 65% (ACS, 2017a).

NON-HODGKIN'S LYMPHOMA

Etiology and Pathophysiology

Non-Hodgkin's lymphomas (NHLs) are a group of malignant neoplasms of primarily B or T cell origin, affecting people of all ages. B cell lymphomas constitute about 85% of NHLs. A third type is natural killer (NK) cells, which attack virus-infected cells or tumor cell. Previous infection with human T cell leukemia/ lymphoma virus and the Epstein-Barr virus have been found to be linked to the disease. The neoplasms are classified according to different cellular and lymph node characteristics. Patients with a compromised immune system and those who take immunosuppressive agents have a greater chance of developing NHL. In the United States NHL is more common in the white population and in men older than 60 years of age. Persons in farming communities have a higher incidence, which is believed to be due to exposure to pesticides and herbicides (Leukemia and Lymphoma Society, n.d.).

Common symptoms of NHL include enlarged lymph nodes, fever, sweating and chills, weight loss, and fatigue. Abdominal distension may result if lymph nodes of the abdomen, liver, or spleen are enlarged as a result of the disease process. If NHL is in the chest, the patient may experience pain in the chest, pressure, a cough, and shortness of breath (ACS, 2016c). There is no hallmark pathologic feature in NHL that parallels the Reed-Sternberg cell of Hodgkin's lymphoma. However, all NHLs involve lymphocytes arrested in various stages of development.

It is estimated that approximately 72,240 new cases of NHL will be diagnosed in 2017, and approximately 20,140 deaths will occur. NHL is estimated in 2017 to be seventh in new cases of cancer and will rank sixth in cancer deaths (National Cancer Institute, n.d.).

NHL is rare in children. When it does occur, it is more common in older children than in younger ones. It is also more common in boys than in girls and in white children than in black children. Most children with NHL do not have any known modifiable risk factors for this disease. Some of the factors that may put a child at increased risk are as follows:

- Congenital (present at birth) immune deficiency syndrome
- Epstein-Barr virus infection
- HIV/AIDS
- Organ transplantation: Children with transplanted organs (kidney, heart, liver) are treated with drugs that weaken their immune system
- Radiation exposure
- Weakened immune system

Risk factors in adults for non-Hodgkin's lymphoma include the following:

- Age (65 to 74 years old is most common range)
- Specific infections such as HIV, Epstein-Barr virus, *Helicobacter pylori*, hepatitis C virus
- Weakened immune system

(National Cancer Institute, n.d.).

Clinical Manifestations

The method of spread can be unpredictable when NHLs originate outside the lymph nodes. At the time of diagnosis, most patients have widely scattered disease. Painless, enlarged lymph nodes and fever, weight loss, night sweats, anemia, pruritus, fatigue, and susceptibility to infection may develop. Pressure-related symptoms in the involved areas are noted. Pleural effusion, bone fractures, and paralysis are complications. Because the disease usually is disseminated by the time it is diagnosed, other symptoms are present, depending on where the disease has spread (e.g., hepatomegaly with liver involvement).

Assessment

Subjective data include frequent patient complaints of fatigue, malaise, and anorexia.

Collection of objective data includes examination of the abdomen for splenomegaly. Enlarged lymph nodes are also evident. Fever, night sweats, and weight loss are usually present.

Diagnostic Tests

Biopsies of lymph nodes, liver, and bone marrow are performed to establish the cell type and pattern. A bone scan may reveal fractures, lesions, and tumor infiltration. PET scans, CT, MRI, and chest x-ray are common tests for diagnosing NHL. Common serum lab tests include the CBC, immunohistochemistry (detects specific antibodies), flow cytometry (identifies specific types of cells), and DNA/genetic testing. Diagnostic studies used for NHL resemble those used for Hodgkin's lymphoma (ACS, 2016c).

Staging, as described for Hodgkin's lymphoma, is used to guide therapy. The four-stage system used with Hodgkin's lymphoma is the same system used for NHL.

Medical Management

Once the diagnosis is made, the extent of the disease (staging) is determined. Accurate staging is crucial to determine the treatment regimen. The therapeutic regimen for NHLs includes chemotherapy and radiation. Indolent (slow-growing) lymphomas have a naturally long course but are difficult to treat effectively. In contrast, more aggressive lymphomas are more likely to be cured, because they are more responsive to treatment. Some chemotherapy agents used are cyclophosphamide, vincristine, prednisone, doxorubicin, bleomycin, and methotrexate. The monoclonal antibody rituximab (Rituxan) was approved for the treatment of follicular lymphoma. Ibritumomab (Zevalin) is another monoclonal antibody that can be used in patients who are refractory to rituximab, or in conjunction with it. Conventional chemotherapy used to treat patients with relapsed, aggressive NHL, who are still responding to salvage chemotherapy, is not as effective as high-dose chemotherapy with autologous (tissue derived from the same individual) hematopoietic stem cell transplantation (HSCT) (ACS, 2017b).

Patients with lymphoma commonly receive radiation to the chest wall, mediastinum, axillae, and neck—the region known as the "mantle field." Some patients also need radiation to the abdomen; paraaortic area; spleen; and, less commonly, the pelvis.

Chemotherapy remains the traditional method of treatment of NHLs that are not localized. High-dose chemotherapy with peripheral blood stem cell or bone marrow transplantation may be indicated. Interferon is being used to help in boosting the immune system. Monoclonal antibodies are being designed to attack a specific target, such as a substance on the surface of lymphocytes, and destroy cancer cells. Targeted cancer therapies such as the use of monoclonal antibodies promise to be more selective for cancer cells than normal cells, thus harming fewer normal cells, reducing side effects, and improving quality of life (ACS, 2016b).

Nursing Interventions and Patient Teaching

Supportive care of the patient during radiation and chemotherapy is primary in nursing management. Observation for complications follows. Further intervention is similar to that for Hodgkin's lymphoma.

Explanations of the extensive diagnostic workup and its importance for staging the disease and determining the treatment plan are an important focus of patient teaching during the diagnostic period.

Prognosis

The prognosis is influenced by the staging classification. The overall 5-year survival rate for NHL is 70%, whereas the 10-year survival rate is approximately 60% with early diagnosis and proper treatment. As with most cancers, a relapse within the first 2 years significantly worsens the prognosis (ACS, 2016b).

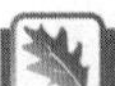

Lifespan Considerations

Older Adults

Blood or Lymphatic Disorder

- The subjective symptoms of hematologic disorders (e.g., fatigue, weakness, dizziness, and dyspnea) may be mistaken for normal changes of aging or attributed to other disease processes commonly seen in older adults.
- The most common blood disorders are forms of anemia.
- Decreased production of intrinsic factor in an aging gastric mucosa results in increased incidence of pernicious anemia.
- Many older adults suffer from conditions such as colonic diverticula, hiatal hernia, or ulcerations that can cause occult bleeding. Older adults with these conditions should be observed for iron deficiency anemia.
- Age-related problems such as altered dentition, limited financial resources, difficulty in food preparation, and poor appetite resulting from emotional upset or depression can cause an increased incidence of iron deficiency anemia.
- Severe or persistent anemia can place additional stress on the aging or diseased heart.
- Administer blood products with caution because older adults are at increased risk of developing congestive heart failure. Careful assessment of cardiopulmonary function and intake and output is essential.
- Oral administration of iron preparations increases the risk of gastrointestinal (GI) irritation and constipation in older adults.
- Ingestion of large amounts of aspirin and other antiinflammatory medications commonly taken by older adults increases the risk of GI bleeding and can lead to alteration in clotting.
- Chronic lymphocytic leukemia is the most common form seen among older patients. This form of leukemia usually progresses slowly in older adults and rarely is treated.

NURSING PROCESS FOR THE PATIENT WITH A BLOOD OR LYMPHATIC DISORDER

ASSESSMENT

Collect data from diverse sources: patient and family observation, physical examination, and diagnostic evaluation results (see Table 47.1).

The subjective data collected at the onset of the disease process are generally vague and nonspecific: malaise, fatigue, and weakness. The patient may relate a history of illness, easy bruising, bleeding tendencies with petechiae, and ecchymoses. Integumentary changes (including pruritus, nonhealing cuts and bruises, draining lesions, jaundice, and palpable subcutaneous nodules) may be reported. Edema and tenderness in lymph node regions may be accompanied by pain, sometimes severe. GI complaints are noted, as well as cardiovascular and respiratory changes. Neurologic complaints include headache, numbness, tingling, paresthesias, and behavioral alteration (see the Lifespan Considerations box).

Collection of objective data follows a system-by-system approach to confirm patient complaints. Manipulation of joints can reveal stiffness and hematoma and may produce pain. Examination of the oral cavity can reveal lesions, ulcers, signs of bleeding, or gingivitis. Cardiovascular and respiratory assessments include breath and heart sound variations. Note any patient anxiety, and observe for diminished comprehension. Listening and an unhurried interview may reveal many symptoms not previously mentioned.

PATIENT PROBLEM

Patient problems are determined from the assessment, which provides data for identifying the patient's problems, strengths, potential complications, and learning needs. Patient problems for the patient with a blood or lymphatic disorder include but are not limited to the following:

- *Compromised Blood Flow to Tissue*
- *Compromised Skin Integrity*
- *Impaired Coping*
- *Inability to Tolerate Activity*
- *Insufficient Knowledge of Condition and Disease Management*
- *Insufficient Oxygenation*
- *Lethargy or Malaise*
- *Potential for Harm or Damage to the Body, Potential for (Bleeding, Falls)*
- *Potential for Infection*
- *Prolonged Pain*
- *Recent Onset of Pain*

◆ EXPECTED OUTCOMES AND PLANNING

Most patients have more than one patient problem. Therefore the planning step in the nursing process involves determining the priority for nursing interventions from the list of patient problems. Use Maslow's hierarchy of needs to prioritize needs. Life-threatening needs such as *Insufficient Oxygenation* would have a higher priority than *Ineffective Coping*.

Planning includes developing realistic goals and outcomes that stem from the identified nursing diagnosis. Examples of expected patient outcomes for the patient with a blood or lymphatic disorder may include but are not limited to the following:

Goal 1: Patient is free of signs and symptoms of an infection.

Goal 2: Patient has no evidence of bleeding (any bleeding is quickly controlled).

◆ IMPLEMENTATION

The implementation of the nursing process is the actual initiation of the nursing care plan. Patient outcomes and goals are achieved by performance of the nursing interventions. Nursing interventions for the patient with a blood or lymphatic disorder may include the following:

- Place patient in private room; avoid contact with visitors or staff members who have an infection (for the immunocompromised patient).
- Stress careful hand hygiene to patient, significant others, and all caregivers.
- Assist in planning daily activities to include rest periods to decrease fatigue and weakness.
- Provide oxygen for dyspnea or excessive fatigue with exertion.
- Explain the disease process, and stress the importance of continued medical follow-up. Most important is the patient's ability to identify the body's signals that blood abnormalities are present. Petechiae, ecchymoses, and gingival bleeding are the warning signs to seek medical attention promptly.

◆ EVALUATION

To evaluate the effectiveness of nursing interventions, compare the patient's behaviors with those stated in the expected patient outcomes. Successful achievement of patient outcomes for the patient with a blood or lymphatic disorder is indicated by the following evaluative measures:

- Patient shows no sign of infection; temperature and WBC count are within normal limits.
- Patient has not fallen.
- Patient shows no signs of bleeding (e.g., petechiae, hemorrhage); any bleeding is controlled quickly.
- Patient is able to bathe self in 30 minutes without becoming fatigued.
- Patient is able to correctly explain measures to prevent infection by good hand hygiene techniques and avoidance of people with infectious conditions.
- Patient is able to explain measures to prevent hemorrhage by avoiding traumatic injury and intramuscular injections.
- Patient reports no shortness of breath with activity.

Get Ready for the NCLEX® Examination!

Key Points

- Blood is a thick, red fluid composed of plasma, a light yellow fluid; albumin, the most abundant protein in human blood plasma; RBCs; WBCs; platelets; and electrolytes, which regulate our nerve and muscle function, our body's hydration, blood pH, blood pressure, and the rebuilding of damaged tissue.
- The blood performs several critical functions: It transports oxygen and nutrients to the cells and waste products away from the cells; it regulates acid-base balance (pH) with buffers; and it protects the body against infection and prevents blood loss with special clotting mechanisms.
- Every person's blood is one of the following blood types in the ABO system of typing: A, B, AB, or O.
- The lymphatic system is a vast, complex network of capillaries, thin vessels, valves, ducts, nodes, and organs that helps to protect and maintain the internal fluid environment of the entire body by producing, filtering, and conveying lymph and by storing and releasing various immune cells.

- The tonsils are composed of lymphoid tissue and are responsible for filtering bacteria.
- The thymus gland is composed of lymphoid tissue in utero (before birth) and the early years of life. It aids in the development of the immune system.
- The spleen also is composed of lymphoid tissue and has many functions, such as filtering out old RBCs, storing a pint of blood, producing antibodies, and phagocytosing bacteria.
- Anemia may be caused by blood loss, impaired RBC production, increased RBC destruction, or nutritional deficiency.
- Shock occurs when organs are deprived of oxygen and nutrients. Shock is characterized by inadequate circulatory provision of oxygen, which causes vital organs and tissues to shut down. Blood pressure falls to a life-threatening low, either from reduced cardiac output or from reduced effective circulating blood volume.
- Hypotension, defined as a systolic blood pressure of less than 90 mm Hg and tachycardia of more than 120 bpm, occurs with blood loss of 1500 to 2000 mL. By the time blood pressure reaches this point, about 30% to 40% of the blood volume may have been lost, and end-organ damage may be irreversible.
- Weakness and fatigue are major symptoms of anemia. They result from decreased oxygenation from decreased levels of Hgb and increased energy needs required by increased RBC production.
- Ingestion of iron compounds or intramuscular Z-track administration of iron dextran is part of the therapy for iron deficiency anemia.
- Sickle cell anemia is a hemolytic anemia with a genetic basis; a sickle cell crisis occurs when the RBCs become deoxygenated and sickle shaped, thus causing stasis and obstruction of the microvasculature, leading to organ infarction and necrosis.
- Polycythemia vera is characterized by excessive bone marrow production that manifests with an increase in circulating erythrocytes, granulocytes, and platelets. Secondary polycythemia is caused by hypoxia rather than a defect in the development of the blood cells.
- Thrombocytopenia is a decrease in the number of circulating platelets and leads to bleeding; people with thrombocytopenia need to learn how to prevent injury and hemorrhage.
- Hemophilia is a hereditary coagulation disorder; hemophilia A is a lack of coagulation factor VIII, and hemophilia B is a lack of factor IX. Maintenance therapy consists of blood factor replacement therapy and prevention of injury.
- DIC is a coagulation disorder characterized initially by clotting and secondarily by hemorrhage. It results from an alteration in the balance between clotting factors and fibrinolytic factors; the person is usually critically ill.
- People with alterations of WBCs are at high risk of infection because leukocytes are a major factor in the body's defense against invading microorganisms.
- The leukemias are malignant disorders characterized by uncontrolled proliferation of WBCs and their precursors; the cause is unknown, but several theories have been proposed.
- Leukemias may be lymphocytic, or myelogenous, and acute or chronic. Acute leukemias have a rapid onset and a short course, if untreated; chronic leukemias have a more insidious onset and longer course. The major therapies for leukemias are chemotherapy and bone marrow transplantation.
- Multiple myeloma is a malignant neoplastic immunodeficiency disease of the bone marrow that affects the plasma cells. The specific immunoglobulin produced by the myeloma cells is present in the blood and urine and is referred to as the monoclonal protein.
- Lymphomas are malignant disorders of the lymphatic system. People with Hodgkin's lymphoma have defective cellular immunity and are therefore at high risk for infection. NHL is a group of lymphoid malignancies. Chemotherapy and radiation are the primary medical treatment for lymphomas.

Additional Learning Resources

SG Go to your Study Guide for additional learning activities to help you master this chapter content.

evolve Be sure to visit the Evolve site at *http://evolve.elsevier.com/Cooper/foundationsadult/* for additional online resources.

Review Questions for the NCLEX® Examination

1. What compound in the blood carries oxygen to the cells from the lungs and carbon dioxide away from the cells to the lungs?
   1. Leukocyte
   2. Thrombocyte
   3. Hemoglobin
   4. Erythrocyte
2. A universal donor has which blood type?
   1. Type A
   2. Type B
   3. Type AB
   4. Type O
3. The spleen is located in which quadrant of the abdominal cavity?
   1. Upper right
   2. Upper left
   3. Lower left
   4. Lower right
4. A patient's platelet count is 18,000/mm^3. What is the most appropriate nursing intervention?
   1. Provide oral hygiene four times per day.
   2. Institute bleeding precautions.
   3. Order a high-protein diet.
   4. Request an order for oxygen per nasal cannula.

5. A patient's spouse tells the nurse that her husband, who has been admitted to the hospital with advanced leukemia, is talking about dying and expresses fears of death. She asks for suggestions for helping her husband. Which response is best?
   1. "Your husband will probably die of another disease before he dies of leukemia."
   2. "Your husband is expressing a readiness to be admitted to a hospice."
   3. "Talk of death is natural at this time but will diminish as he feels better."
   4. "It's normal to want to talk about death; what we can do is be supportive by listening."
6. A 28-year-old man is admitted with fatigue; discomfort; enlarged, painless cervical lymph nodes; and pruritus. A lymph node biopsy leads to the diagnosis of Hodgkin's lymphoma. What are the abnormal cells noted by the pathologist in Hodgkin's lymphoma called?
   1. Rodem-Lee cells
   2. Bullus-Frendelenburg cells
   3. Reed-Sternberg cells
   4. Stevens-Jorgens cells
7. An adult patient is seen by the nurse at a health maintenance organization for signs of fatigue. The patient has a history of iron deficiency anemia. What data from the nursing history indicate that the anemia is not currently managed effectively?
   1. Pallor
   2. Poor skin turgor
   3. Heart rate of 68 bpm, weak pulse
   4. Respiration at 18 breaths/minute and regular
8. What is an important teaching point for a patient who has iron deficiency anemia?
   1. Use birth control to avoid pregnancy.
   2. Increase fluids to stimulate erythropoiesis.
   3. Decrease fluids to prevent sickling of RBCs.
   4. Alternate periods of rest and activity to balance oxygen supply and demand.
9. The nurse instructs a patient about foods rich in iron. Which foods should be included in the diet?
   1. Fresh fruit and milk
   2. Cheeses and processed lunch meats
   3. Dark green, leafy vegetables and organ meats
   4. Fruit juices and cornmeal bread
10. Which statement by the patient with pernicious anemia would indicate that she understood the teaching?
    1. "I'll be glad when I can stop the injections and take only oral medicine."
    2. "I'll have to take B_{12} shots for the rest of my life."
    3. "After a while I'll no longer need to take shots, just the pills."
    4. "I was glad to hear that pills are available to treat me."
11. A patient is admitted with polycythemia vera. The patient's Hgb value is 20 g/dL. Which treatment will be ordered?
    1. Whole blood transfusion
    2. Platelet transfusion
    3. Phlebotomy with removal of 800 mL of blood
    4. Vitamin B_{12} injection
12. Which laboratory finding is a strong indicator of disseminated intravascular coagulation (DIC)?
    1. An elevated platelet count
    2. An elevated D-dimer test result
    3. A normal prothrombin time
    4. An elevated fibrinogen level
13. The nurse is teaching the patient with pernicious anemia about the disease. The nurse explains that pernicious anemia results from the lack of:
    1. folic acid.
    2. intrinsic factor.
    3. extrinsic factor.
    4. an RBC enzyme.
14. A patient with sickle cell anemia asks the nurse why the sickling crisis does not stop when oxygen therapy is started. Which statement by the nurse is the most accurate answer?
    1. "Sickling occurs in response to decreased blood viscosity, which is not affected by oxygen therapy."
    2. "When red cells sickle, they occlude small vessels, which cause more local hypoxia and more sickling."
    3. "The primary problem during a sickle cell crisis is destruction of the abnormal cells, resulting in fewer RBCs to carry oxygen."
    4. "Oxygen therapy does not alter the shape of the abnormal erythrocytes but only allows for increased oxygen concentration in Hgb."
15. What nursing interventions are indicated for a patient during a sickle cell crisis? (*Select all that apply.*)
    1. Frequent ambulation
    2. Apply antiembolism hose
    3. Restrict sodium intake
    4. Increase the oral fluid intake
    5. Administer therapeutic doses of continuous opioid analgesics
16. Hodgkin's lymphoma occurs more frequently in individuals with which risk factor?
    1. A history of cancer treated with radiation
    2. Exposure to nuclear explosions
    3. Infection with the Epstein-Barr virus
    4. Infection with *Helicobacter pylori*
17. Which statement concerning Hodgkin's lymphoma is correct?
    1. The 10-year survival rate for stage I or II Hodgkin's lymphoma is more than 90%.
    2. Hodgkin's lymphoma commonly occurs between the ages of 15 and 35 years.
    3. Hodgkin's lymphoma is not a curable disease.
    4. The incidence of Hodgkin's lymphoma in the female population has increased.
18. What is an appropriate nursing intervention for a patient with hemophilia who is hospitalized with acute knee pain and edema?
    1. Wrapping the knee with an elastic bandage
    2. Placing the patient on bed rest and applying ice to the joint
    3. Gently performing ROM exercises to the knee to prevent adhesions
    4. Administering nonsteroidal antiinflammatory drugs as needed for pain

19. During a physical assessment of a patient with thrombocytopenia, the nurse would expect to find:
1. petechiae and purpura.
2. jaundiced sclera and skin.
3. tender, enlarged lymph nodes.
4. splenomegaly.

20. Which nursing interventions are necessary when caring for a patient who has a WBC count of 1800/mm^3? *(Select all that apply.)*
1. Prevent patient contact with people who have respiratory tract infections or influenza.
2. Perform hand hygiene before and after patient contact.
3. Report temperature elevation.
4. Monitor Hgb.
5. Assess for signs of bleeding.

21. Which are necessary for the maturation of a red blood cell? *(Select all that apply.)*
1. Vitamin B_{12}
2. Folic acid
3. Renal erythropoietic factor
4. Capric acid
5. Iron

22. Which represents the correct medical management for the patient with DIC? *(Select all that apply.)*
1. Addressing and correcting underlying cause
2. Transfusion replacement
3. Cryoprecipitate
4. Administering colony-stimulating factor (filgrastim [Neupogen])
5. Heparin therapy

48 Care of the Patient With a Cardiovascular or a Peripheral Vascular Disorder

http://evolve.elsevier.com/Cooper/foundationsadult/

Objectives

Anatomy and Physiology

1. Discuss the location, size, and position of the heart.
2. Identify the chambers and valves of the heart and their functions.
3. Discuss the electrical conduction system that causes the cardiac muscle fibers to contract.
4. Explain what produces the two main heart sounds.
5. Trace the path of blood through the coronary circulation.

Medical-Surgical

6. List diagnostic tests used to evaluate cardiovascular function.
7. For coronary artery disease, compare nonmodifiable risk factors with factors that are modifiable in lifestyle and health management.
8. Describe five cardiac dysrhythmias.
9. Compare the etiology and pathophysiology, clinical manifestations, assessment, diagnostic tests, medical management, nursing interventions, and prognosis for patients with angina pectoris, myocardial infarction, or heart failure.
10. Specify patient teaching for patients with cardiac dysrhythmias, angina pectoris, myocardial infarction, heart failure, and valvular heart disease.
11. Discuss the purposes of cardiac rehabilitation.
12. Discuss the etiology and pathophysiology, clinical manifestations, assessment, diagnostic tests, medical management, nursing interventions, and prognosis for the patient with pulmonary edema.
13. Compare and contrast the etiology and pathophysiology, clinical manifestations, assessment, diagnostic tests, medical management, nursing interventions, and prognosis for the patient with rheumatic heart disease, pericarditis, and endocarditis.
14. Identify 10 conditions that may result in the development of secondary cardiomyopathy.
15. Discuss the indications and contraindications for cardiac transplant.
16. Identify risk factors and the effects of aging associated with peripheral vascular disorders.
17. Compare and contrast signs and symptoms and discuss nursing interventions associated with arterial and venous disorders.
18. Compare essential (primary) hypertension, secondary hypertension, and malignant hypertension.
19. Discuss the etiology and pathophysiology, clinical manifestations, assessment, diagnostic tests, medical management, and nursing interventions and the importance of patient education for the patient with hypertension.
20. Compare and contrast the etiology and pathophysiology, clinical manifestations, assessment, diagnostic tests, medical management, nursing interventions, and prognosis for patients with arterial aneurysm, Buerger's disease, and Raynaud's disease.
21. Discuss the etiology and pathophysiology, clinical manifestations, assessment, diagnostic tests, medical management, nursing interventions, and prognosis and appropriate patient education for patients with thrombophlebitis, varicose veins, and stasis ulcer.

Key Terms

aneurysm (ĂN-ŭr-ĭ-zĭm, p. 1573)
angina pectoris (ăn-JĪ-nă PĔK-tŏr-ĭs, p. 1535)
arteriosclerosis (ăr-tē-rē-ō-sklĕ-RŌ-sĭs, p. 1570)
atherosclerosis (ăth-ĕr-ō-sklĕ-RŌ-sĭs, p. 1535)
B-type natriuretic peptide (BNP) (nā-trē-yū-RĔT-ĭk, p. 1525)
bradycardia (brăd-ĕ-KĂR-dē-ă, p. 1529)
cardioversion (kăr-dē-ō-VĔR-zhŭn, p. 1524)
coronary artery disease (CAD) (p. 1535)
coronary occlusion (ō-KLŪ-zhŭn, p. 1541)
defibrillation (dē-fĭb-rĭ-LĀ-shŭn, p. 1532)
dysrhythmia (dĭs-RĬTH-mē-ă, p. 1528)
embolus (ĔM-bō-lŭs, p. 1540)
endarterectomy (ĕnd-ăr-tĕr-ĔK-tō-mē, p. 1573)
heart failure (HF) (p. 1546)
hypoxemia (hī-pŏk-SĒ-mē-ă, p. 1524)
intermittent claudication (klăw-dĕ-KĀ-shŭn, p. 1564)
ischemia (ĭs-KĒ-mē-ă, p. 1536)
multigated acquisition (MUGA) scan (p. 1524)
myocardial infarction (MI) (mī-ō-KĂR-dē-ăl ĭn-FĂRK-shŭn, p. 1540)
orthopnea (ŏr-THŎP-nē-ă, p. 1549)
peripheral (pĕ-RĬF-ĕr-ăl, p. 1563)
pleural effusion (PLŪR-ăl ĕ-FŪ-zhŭn, p. 1521)
polycythemia (pŏl-ē-sī-THĒ-mē-ă, p. 1524)
pulmonary edema (PŪL-mō-nă-rē ĕ-DĒ-mă, p. 1552)
rubor (p. 1570)
tachycardia (tăk-ĕ-KĂR-dē-ă, p. 1528)

ANATOMY AND PHYSIOLOGY OF THE CARDIOVASCULAR SYSTEM

The cardiovascular (circulatory) system is the transportation system of the body. It delivers oxygen and nutrients to the cells to support their individual activities and transports the cells' waste products to the appropriate organs for disposal. This chapter discusses the structure and function of the blood vessels and the heart.

HEART

The heart is a remarkable organ, not much bigger than a fist (Fig. 48.1). It pumps 1000 gallons of blood every day through the closed circuit of blood vessels. It beats 100,000 times a day and transports the blood 60,000 miles through a network of blood vessels. The heart is a hollow organ composed mainly of muscle tissue with a series of one-way valves.

The heart is located in the chest cavity between the lungs in a region called the *mediastinum* (the organs and tissues separating the lungs; in addition to the heart and its greater vessels, the mediastinum contains the trachea and the esophagus). Two-thirds of the heart lies left of the midline. The wider *base* of the heart lies superior to and beneath the second rib. The *apex,* or narrow part, of the heart lies inferiorly, slightly to the left between the fifth and sixth ribs near the diaphragm.

Heart Wall

The heart wall is composed of three layers: pericardium, myocardium, and endocardium. The *pericardium* is a two-layered, serous membrane that covers the entire structure. Between the two thin membranes is a serous fluid that allows friction-free movement of the heart as it contracts and relaxes. The pericardium is the outermost layer of the heart. The *myocardium* forms the bulk of the heart wall and is the thickest and strongest layer of the heart. It is composed of cardiac muscle tissue. Contraction of this tissue is responsible for pumping blood. The *endocardium* (innermost layer) is composed of a thin layer of connective tissue. This structure lines the interior of the heart, the valves, and the larger vessels of the heart.

Heart Chambers

The heart is divided into right and left halves by a muscular partition called the *septum* (Fig. 48.2). The heart has the following four chambers:

1. The *right atrium* is the upper right chamber. It receives deoxygenated blood from the entire body. The superior vena cava returns blood from the head, the neck, and the arms. The inferior vena cava returns blood from the lower body. The coronary vein returns it from the heart muscle to the coronary sinus.
2. The *right ventricle* is the lower right chamber. It receives deoxygenated blood from the right atrium. The right ventricle pumps blood to the lungs via the *pulmonary artery* to release carbon dioxide and receive oxygen.
3. The *left atrium* is the upper left chamber. It receives oxygenated blood from the lungs via the *pulmonary veins.*

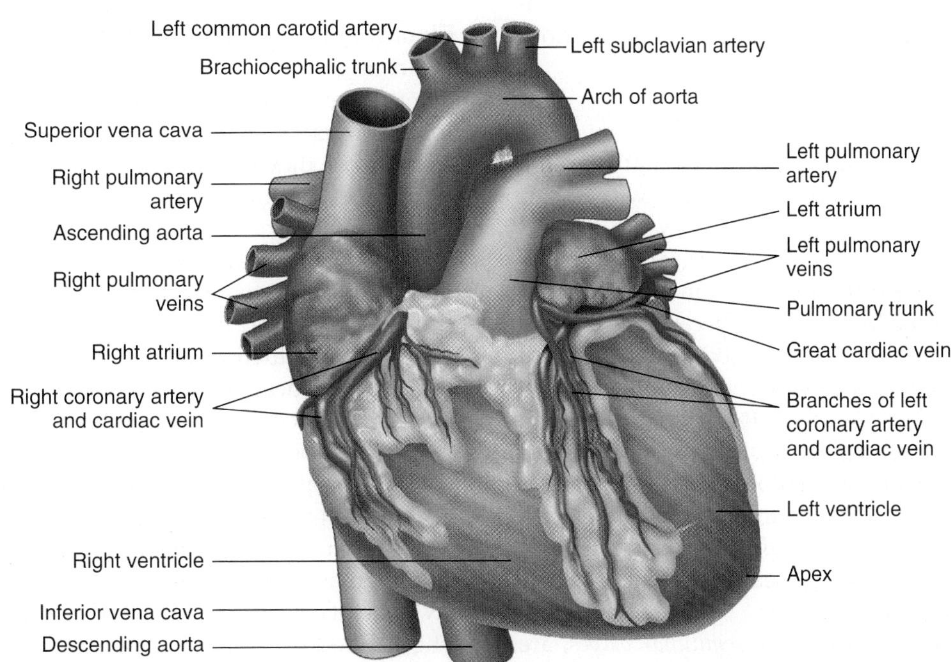

Fig. 48.1 Heart and major blood vessels viewed from the front (anterior). (From Patton KT, Thibodeau GA, Douglas MM: *Essentials of anatomy and physiology,* St. Louis, 2012, Mosby.)

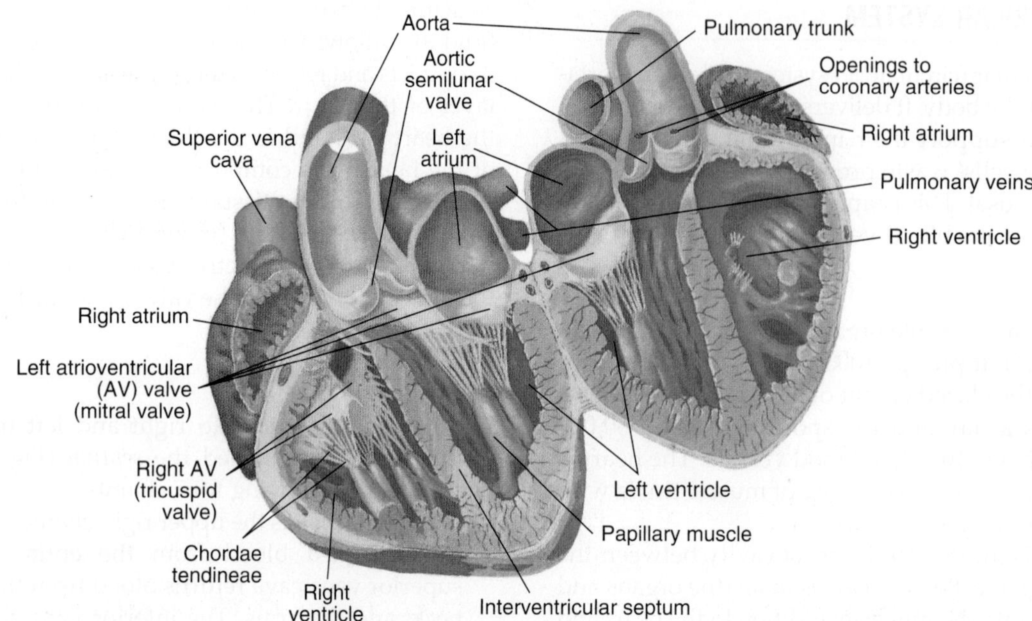

Fig. 48.2 Interior of the heart. This illustration shows the heart as it would appear if it were cut along a frontal plane and opened like a book. The front portion of the heart lies to the reader's right; the back portion of the heart lies to the reader's left. The four chambers of the heart—two atria and two ventricles—are easily seen. (From Patton KT, Thibodeau GA, Douglas MM: *Essentials of anatomy and physiology*, St. Louis, 2012, Mosby.)

4. The *left ventricle* is the lower left chamber. It receives oxygenated blood from the left atrium. It is the thickest, most muscular section of the heart and pumps the oxygenated blood out through the aorta to all parts of the body.

The heart functions as two separate pumps: (1) the right side receives deoxygenated blood and pumps it to the lungs, and (2) the left side receives oxygenated blood from the lungs and pumps it throughout the body.

Heart Valves

Located within the heart are four valves that keep the blood moving forward and prevent backflow. The heart has two *atrioventricular (AV) valves.* They are located between the atrium and the ventricles. The right AV valve, located between the right atrium and the right ventricle, is called the *tricuspid valve* because it contains three flaps, or cusps. The left AV valve is composed of two cusps (bicuspid) and commonly is called the *mitral valve.* It is located between the left atrium and the left ventricle. Both of these valves rapidly close to prevent backflow of blood. Small cordlike structures, *chordae tendineae,* connect the AV valves to the walls of the heart and work with the *papillary muscles* located in the walls of the ventricles to make a tight seal to prevent backflow when the ventricles contract.

The two remaining valves, the *semilunar valves,* are located at the points where the blood exits the ventricles. The *pulmonary semilunar valve* is located between the right ventricle and the pulmonary artery. Blood is pushed out of the right ventricle and travels to the lungs via the pulmonary artery. The *aortic semilunar valve* is located between the left ventricle and the aorta. When the left ventricle contracts, the blood is forced into the aorta and the aortic semilunar valve closes. Both of the semilunar valves have three cusps in the shape of a half moon, hence the name *semilunar* (see Fig. 48.2).

Electrical Conduction System

Heart muscle tissue has an inherent ability to contract in a rhythmic pattern. This ability is called *automaticity.* If heart muscle cells are removed and placed under a microscope, they continue to beat. In addition, they can respond to a stimulus in the same way that nerve cells do. This unique property is called *irritability.* Automaticity and irritability are two characteristics that affect the functions of the conduction system. Hormones, ion concentration, and changes in body temperature also affect the conduction of messages around the heart, initiation of heartbeat, and coordination of beating patterns between the atria and the ventricles.

The heartbeat is initiated in the *sinoatrial (SA) node,* which is located in the upper part of the right atrium, just beneath the opening of the superior vena cava (Fig. 48.3). Because it regulates the heartbeat, the SA node is known as the *pacemaker.* Impulses are passed to the AV node, which is located in the base of the right atrium. The AV node slows the impulses to allow the atrium to complete contraction and to allow the ventricles to fill. The impulses then pass to a group of conduction fibers called the *bundle of His,* which divides into right

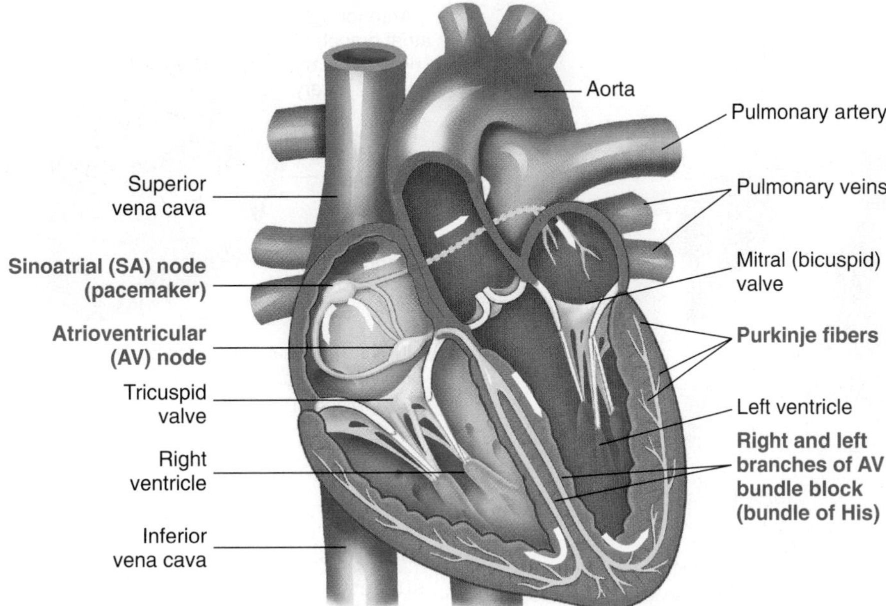

Fig. 48.3 Conduction system of the heart. Specialized cardiac muscle cells in the wall of the heart rapidly initiate or conduct an electrical impulse throughout the myocardium. The signal is initiated by the sinoatrial (SA) node (pacemaker) and spreads to the rest of the right atrial myocardium directly, to the left atrial myocardium by way of a bundle of interatrial conducting fibers, and to the atrioventricular (AV) node by way of three internodal bundles. The AV node then initiates a signal that is conducted through conduction fibers called the *bundle of His,* which breaks into right and left bundle branches to travel to smaller branches called the *Purkinje fibers,* which surround the ventricles. (From Thibodeau GA, Patton KT: *Structure and function of the body,* ed 14, St. Louis, 2012, Mosby.)

and left bundle branches to travel to smaller branches called the *Purkinje fibers,* which surround the ventricles. The message travels rapidly through the ventricles and causes contractions, which empty the ventricles.

The impulse pathway is as follows:

SA node → AV node → Bundle of His
Right and left bundle branches → Purkinje fibers

Cardiac Cycle

The cardiac cycle refers to a complete heartbeat. The two atria contract while the two ventricles relax. When the ventricles contract, the two atria relax. The phase of contraction is called *systole* (Fig. 48.4), and the phase of relaxation is called *diastole* (the period between contraction of the atria or the ventricles during which blood enters the relaxed chambers from the systemic circulation and the lungs [Fig. 48.5]). Complete diastole and systole of both atria and ventricles constitute a cardiac cycle; this takes an average of 0.8 second.

The heart sounds, *lub* and *dub,* are produced by closure of the valves. The first sound, *lub* (long duration and low pitch), is heard when the AV valves close. The second sound, *dub* (short duration, sharp sound), is heard when the semilunar valves close. On occasion, a murmur (swishing sound) can be heard. This can be a normal functional phenomenon produced by rapid filling of the ventricles, or it can be an abnormal condition produced by ineffective closure of the valves.

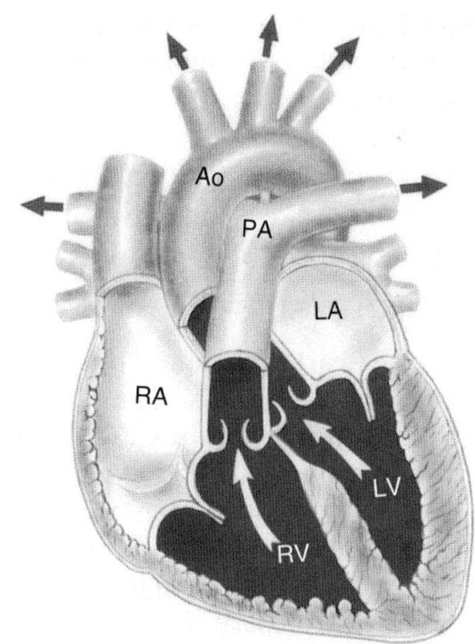

Fig. 48.4 Blood flow during systole. *Ao,* Aorta; *LA,* left atrium; *LV,* left ventricle; *PA,* pulmonary artery; *RA,* right atrium; *RV,* right ventricle. (From Canobbio M: *Mosby's clinical nursing series: Cardiovascular disorders,* St. Louis, 1990, Mosby.)

BLOOD VESSELS

Three main types of blood vessels are organized to carry blood to and from the heart: arteries, veins, and capillaries. The heart delivers the blood to large vessels called *arteries,* which carry blood away from the heart. The arteries branch into smaller vessels called *arterioles,*

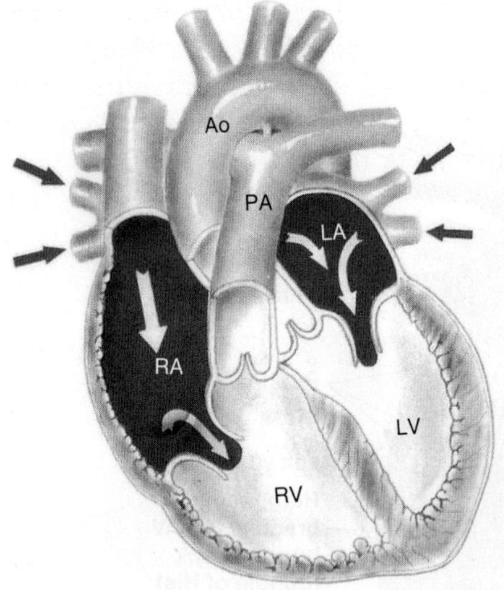

Fig. 48.5 Blood flow during diastole. *Ao,* Aorta; *LA,* left atrium; *LV,* left ventricle; *PA,* pulmonary artery; *RA,* right atrium; *RV,* right ventricle. (From Canobbio M: *Mosby's clinical nursing series: Cardiovascular disorders,* St. Louis, 1990, Mosby.)

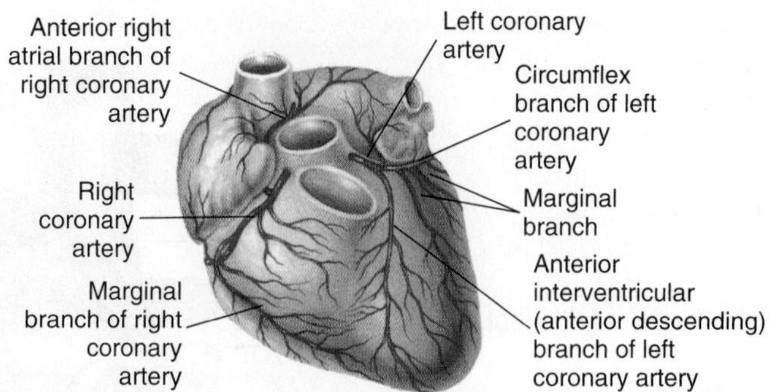

Fig. 48.6 Arterial coronary circulation (anterior). (From Canobbio M: *Mosby's clinical nursing series: Cardiovascular disorders,* St. Louis, 1990, Mosby.)

which deliver the blood to the tissues. Within the tissues, the arterioles divide into microscopic vessels called *capillaries,* which form an extensive (50,000-mile) network that allows exchange of products and by-products between the tissues and blood. The capillaries then join to form tiny veins, or *venules,* that link with larger *veins,* which carry the blood toward the heart. The pattern is as follows:

Artery → Arteriole → Capillary → Venule → Vein

CIRCULATION

CORONARY BLOOD SUPPLY

To sustain life, the heart must pump blood throughout the body on a continuous basis. As a result, the heart muscle (or myocardium) requires a constant supply of blood containing nutrients and oxygen to function effectively. The delivery of oxygen and nutrient-rich arterial blood to cardiac muscle tissue and the return of oxygen-poor blood from this active tissue to the venous system are called the *coronary circulation* (Fig. 48.6).

Blood flows into the heart muscle by way of two small vessels, the right and left coronary arteries. The coronary arteries wrap around the myocardium (see Figs. 48.1 and 48.6). The openings into these vessels lie behind the flaps of the aortic semilunar valves (see Fig. 48.6). The coronary arteries bring oxygen and nutrition to the myocardium. Once the circulation is completed and the carbon dioxide and waste products have been collected, the blood flows into a large coronary vein and finally into the coronary sinus, which empties into the right atrium. These two main arteries have many tiny branches that serve the heart muscle. If an artery becomes occluded (blocked or obstructed), these branches provide collateral circulation (alternate routes) to nourish the heart muscle. If the occlusion is severe, surgery and other procedures may be needed. These interventions are discussed later in this chapter.

SYSTEMIC CIRCULATION

Systemic circulation occurs when blood is pumped from the left ventricle of the heart through all parts of the body and returns to the right atrium. When the oxygenated blood leaves the left ventricle, it enters the largest artery (1 inch [2.5 cm] in diameter) of the body, the *aorta.* This is the main trunk of the systemic arterial circulation and is composed of four parts: the ascending aorta, the arch, the thoracic portion of the descending aorta, and the abdominal portion of the descending aorta. As the blood flows through the artery branches, the branches become smaller in diameter (arterioles). The blood continues to flow into the capillaries. The capillaries surround the cells and exchange oxygen and nutrients for carbon dioxide and other waste products. The blood flows to the tiny venules, then to the larger veins, and finally returns to the right atrium via the largest vein, the *vena cava* (one of two large veins returning blood from the peripheral circulation to the right atrium of the heart).

The blood is now deoxygenated and must be replenished with oxygen. In addition, the blood is carrying a high concentration of carbon dioxide. Note that the upper portion of the vena cava (superior vena cava) returns deoxygenated blood from the head, neck, chest, and upper extremities. The inferior vena cava returns deoxygenated blood from parts of the body below the diaphragm.

PULMONARY CIRCULATION

The deoxygenated blood now passes through the pulmonary circulation to pick up the needed oxygen. Blood is pumped from the right atrium to the right ventricle, where it leaves the heart to travel via the pulmonary artery to the lungs. Once the blood reaches the lungs, it travels through arterioles to microscopic capillaries surrounding the *alveoli* (air sacs), where oxygen diffuses into the bloodstream and carbon dioxide diffuses out. The capillaries then connect with the venules and finally with the four pulmonary veins, which return the oxygenated blood to the left atrium of the heart. It then is pumped to the left ventricle and to the aorta, and the systemic circulation then is repeated. The blood circulation pattern is as follows:

Superior or inferior vena cava → Right atrium
Tricuspid valve → Right ventricle
Pulmonary semilunar valve → Pulmonary artery
Capillaries in the lungs → Pulmonary veins
Left atrium → Bicuspid valve → Left ventricle
Aortic semilunar valve → Aorta

LABORATORY AND DIAGNOSTIC EXAMINATIONS

Many diagnostic tests are used to evaluate cardiovascular function. The nursing responsibilities are to prepare the patient physically for diagnostic procedures and to explain the examination to the patient.

DIAGNOSTIC IMAGING

Radiographic examination (i.e., an x-ray) of the chest provides a film record of heart size, shape, and position and outline of shadows. Lung congestion is also shown, indicating heart failure (HF), perhaps in the earliest stages. **Pleural effusion** (an abnormal accumulation of fluid in the thoracic cavity between the visceral and parietal pleurae) may be noted in left-sided HF. The nurse's role in preparation for this procedure is to explain the reasons for examination and what the examination shows.

Fluoroscopy allows observation of movement and is invaluable in pacemaker or intracardial catheter placement. Using a fluoroscope, the motion of internal structures such as the heart is examined with a device that emits x-rays that pass through the patient and fluoresce on a special screen, producing a sort of x-ray–based motion picture.

An *angiogram* is a series of radiographs taken after a contrast medium (dye) is injected into an artery or vein. Picturing the circulatory process aids in diagnosis of vessel occlusion, pooling in various heart chambers, and congenital anomalies. Angiography allows x-ray visualization of the heart, aorta, inferior vena cava, pulmonary artery and vein, and coronary arteries.

In an *aortogram,* the abdominal aorta and the major leg arteries are examined by x-ray visualization after a contrast medium is injected via a catheter (a thin, flexible tube) passed through the femoral artery and into the aorta. Aneurysms (abnormal bulges in the wall of a blood vessel) and many other abnormalities can be diagnosed. Contrast media also may be used to visualize the aortic arch and branches.

The nurse's role in preparing the patient for the examination is to explain the procedure. Because dye is involved, it is very important to make sure the patient does not have an allergy to ingredients in the dye. This type of procedure requires the patient's informed consent. After the procedure, check the site of catheter insertion (usually the groin area) for excess bleeding, ensure that a compression device is in place, and alert the health care provider if excess bleeding is noted. Check for circulation in the periphery below the site, monitor vital signs, and ensure that the patient remains supine (lying face up) for the recommended amount of time.

CARDIAC CATHETERIZATION AND ANGIOGRAPHY

Cardiac catheterization is an invasive procedure used to visualize the heart's chambers, valves, great vessels, and coronary arteries. This procedure aids in diagnosis, prevention of progression of cardiac conditions, and accurate evaluation and treatment of the critically ill patient.

In cardiac catheterization, a catheter is passed through a peripheral vessel and into the vessels or chambers of the heart. It can reveal heart abnormalities, such as valvular defects, arterial occlusion, and congenital anomalies. Cardiac catheterization allows (1) measurement of blood pressure within the heart and (2) assessment of the blood in the heart. Blood samples also may be obtained. Contrast dye may be injected to allow better heart and vessel visualization (angiography). Cardiac catheterization is performed under sterile surgical conditions. Its invasive nature requires a prior signed consent from the patient. Because the contrast medium contains iodine, it is important to determine whether the patient is sensitive to iodine before injection to avoid an allergic reaction. After the procedure, assess the circulation to the extremity used for catheter insertion. Check peripheral pulses, color, and sensation of the extremity every 15 minutes for 1 hour and then with decreasing frequency. Observe the puncture site for hematoma and bleeding. Monitor the vital signs and checks for abnormal heart rate, dysrhythmias, and signs of pulmonary emboli (indicated by respiratory difficulty). The patient lies supine for a designated period with a compression device over the pressure dressing at the insertion site to prevent hemorrhage.

ELECTROCARDIOGRAPHY

The electrocardiogram (ECG or EKG) is a graphic study of the electrical activities of the myocardium to determine transmission of cardiac impulses through the muscles and conduction tissue. Each ECG has three distinct waves, or deflections: the *P wave,* the *QRS complex,* and the *T wave. Depolarization* refers to the electrical activity when the heart contracts. *Repolarization* is the relaxation phase. The P wave represents the depolarization of the atria. The QRS complex represents the depolarization of the ventricles. The T wave represents the repolarization of the ventricles. Atrial repolarization is not represented but does occur; it is covered by the large QRS complex and cannot be seen on the ECG tracing.

A standard ECG has 12 electrodes attached to the skin surface to measure the total electrical activity of the heart. Each lead records the electrical potential between the limbs or between the heart and limbs. A conductive gel enhances the contact and transmission. The patient typically is placed in the supine position; ambulatory ECGs and exercise stress test ECGs require position variation. The machine, an electrocardiograph or galvanometer, records the energy wave of each heartbeat through a vibrating needle on graph paper, which feeds through the machine at a standard rate. Each ECG waveform represents a single electrical impulse as it travels through the heart (Fig. 48.7).

The ECG tracing is read or interpreted by a cardiac specialist (cardiologist) or by internal medicine specialists, family practitioners, pediatricians, and emergency department practitioners. The reading also may be displayed on the fluorescent screen (oscilloscope) of a cardiac monitor. A graphic tracing may be printed out by the monitor.

Ambulatory ECGs can be used to monitor heart rhythm over prolonged periods—12, 24, or 48 hours—and compared with various activities or symptoms recorded in a diary kept by the patient. A Holter monitor (small portable recorder) is attached to the patient by leads, with a 2-pound tape recorder carried on a belt or shoulder strap. The monitor operates continuously to record the patterns and rhythms of the patient's heartbeat. In conjunction with the diary, the health care provider can note various events, times, and medication

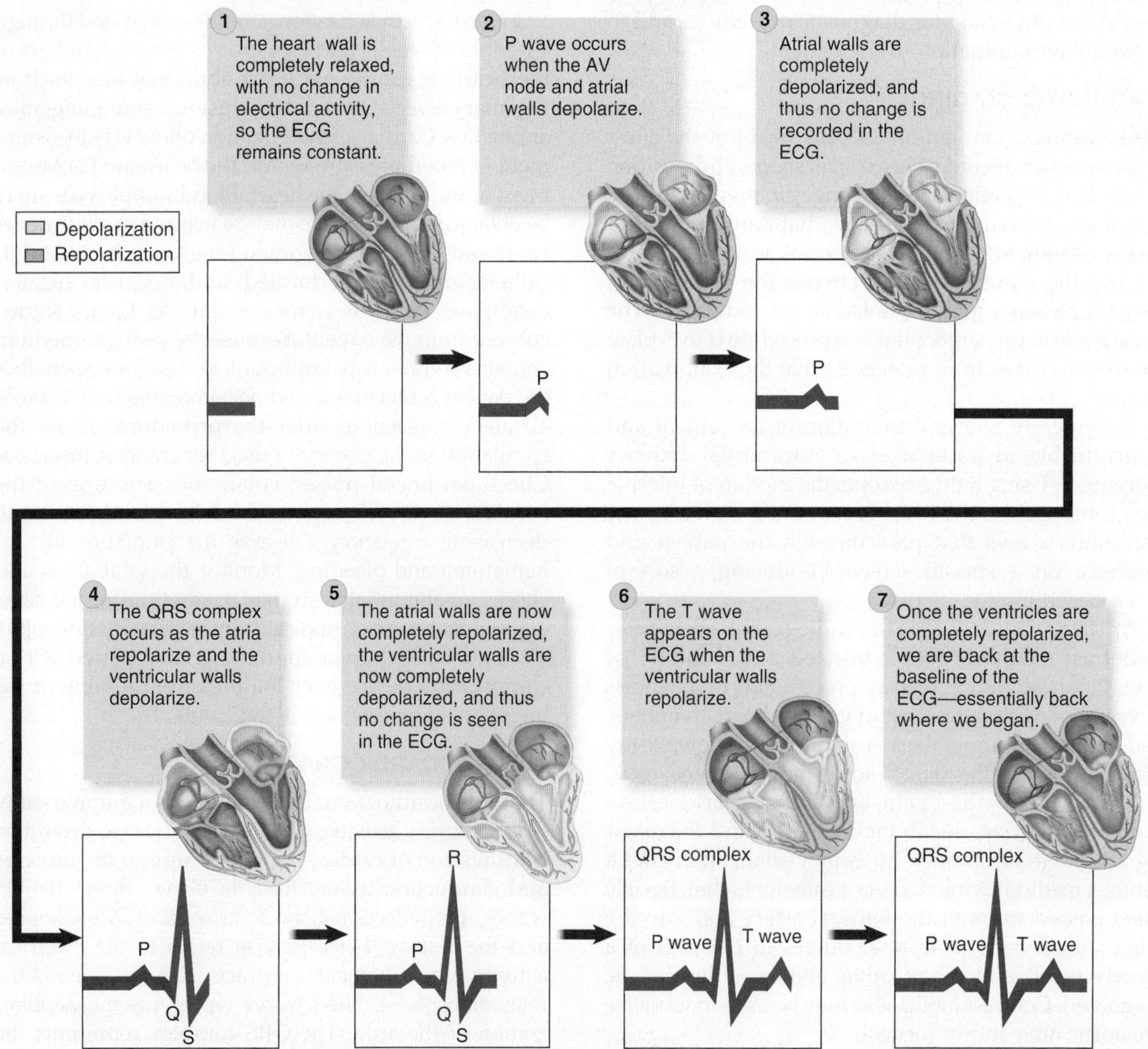

Fig. 48.7 Normal electrocardiographic (ECG) waves, or deflections. (From Thibodeau GA, Patton KT: *Structure and function of the body*, ed 14, St. Louis, 2012, Mosby.)

peaks that affect or precipitate dysrhythmias. An ambulatory ECG is particularly useful for patients whose clinical symptoms indicate heart disorders but who may have normal ECG tracings on a resting test. Thorough explanation by the health care provider is essential to ensure proper recordings by the patient, because this is an outpatient procedure.

CARDIAC MONITORS

It is common practice to assess continuously the cardiac electrical activity of patients who are known or suspected to have dysrhythmias or who are prone to develop dysrhythmias or acute cardiovascular symptoms. A cardiac monitor displays information on the electrical activity of the heart transferred via conductive electrodes placed on the chest.

Most monitors provide a visual display of cardiac electrical activity and the patient's heart rate. Preset alarms warn of heart rates that exceed or drop below limits considered acceptable for each patient and also warn of dysrhythmias.

Ambulatory patients (i.e., patients who are able to walk) are monitored more often by battery-powered ECG transmitters that do not connect the patient directly to an oscilloscope. This monitoring is called *telemetry,* which is the electronic transmission of data to a distant location. The electrodes placed on the patient's chest are attached to a transmitter the patient carries in a pocket or pouch. The transmitter sends a radio signal to a receiver, usually located at the nurses' station or a remote location within a hospital.

Patients need telemetry monitoring for various reasons, including a history of cardiac disease, angina pectoris, suspected dysrhythmias, a change in medications, an electrolyte abnormality, or unexplained syncope. Many of these patients are monitored in a centralized area such as an intermediate care or step-down unit (with monitors at the nurses' station). By remote telemetry, a patient on a medical-surgical unit may be monitored at a separate location, called the *home unit,* which is usually on a critical care unit. Remote telemetry patients are usually stable; but a stable patient's condition can change rapidly, and telemetry allows continuous heart monitoring to detect abnormalities.

Attachment to a cardiac monitor does not change a patient's need for nursing interventions. The monitoring electrodes are placed on the anterior thorax (chest) rather than the extremities, enabling the patient to be relatively free to carry on usual activities. Pay special attention to the electrode site to ensure a constant tight seal between the electrode and the skin and to note the development of any skin impairment. The conduction gel dries out, even if the pad is sealed; changing electrodes regularly is recommended. Check the telemetry pack for integrity of the lead wires and test the monitoring device's battery with a battery tester. Inform the monitoring area whenever the patient is moved off the unit for a diagnostic test, because the patient may go outside the monitor's range. Another important safety measure is *never* to remove the telemetry device and allow the patient to shower unless the health care provider has written the order to allow a shower. The patient could be subject to severe dysrhythmia, which would not be detected with the telemetry device removed.

Exercise-stress ECG is another form of monitoring the heart's capability, this time in a laboratory setting while the patient performs a prescribed exercise. Tasks include use of treadmills, stair climbing, and aerobic exercise. While being monitored carefully, the patient is coaxed to a limit of exertion to evaluate myocardial ischemia (reduced oxygen in the heart resulting from insufficient blood flow), dysrhythmia, and cardiac capability under extreme circumstances. The test sets the limit of exercise tolerance in cardiac disease. If the patient is unable to tolerate activity, a stress test can be done by administering dipyridamole (Persantine) or adenosine (Adenocard), which makes the patient's heart respond as if it were under stress or activity.

THALLIUM SCANNING

Thallium-201 is a radioactive isotope (radioisotope) that is transported actively into normal cells. If the cells are ischemic or infarcted, the thallium will not be picked up. Thallium concentrates in tissue with normal blood flow; tissue with inadequate perfusion appears as dark areas on scanning—a "cold spot." The radioisotope is injected intravenously while the patient exercises on a treadmill. (Note: Breast tissue in the female can produce artifact, leading to a false-positive result. Technetium-99m sestamibi may be used instead of thallium to minimize artifact and thus improve accuracy.) In a patient who cannot tolerate physical exercise, dipyridamole is given before the thallium to simulate physiologically exercise-induced stress. After the procedure is over, caution the patient to avoid driving for the next 4 hours and to stand slowly from a sitting or lying position to avoid orthostatic hypotension during that time.

ECHOCARDIOGRAPHY

Echocardiography uses high-frequency ultrasound directed at the heart. The echo, or reflected sound, is recorded graphically as a *sonogram,* outlining the size, shape, and position of cardiac structures. This test is used to detect pericardial effusion (collection of blood or other fluid in the pericardial sac), ventricular function, cardiac chamber size and contents, ventricular muscle and septal motion and thickness, cardiac output (ejection fraction), cardiac tumors, valvular function, and congenital heart disorder.

The ventricular ejection fraction (EF) on an echocardiogram can be gauged as follows:

- *Normal:* 55% to 70%
- *Moderate HF:* 40% to 55% (indicates damage, perhaps from a previous heart attack but not necessarily heart failure)
- *Moderate to severe HF:* Less than 40%

POSITRON EMISSION TOMOGRAPHY

Positron emission tomography (PET) is a computerized radiographic technique that uses radioactive substances to examine the metabolic activity of various body structures. In PET studies the patient either inhales or is injected with a radioactive biochemical substance. A computer interprets the data, depicting the various levels of metabolic activity as color-coded images. Used to study dementia, stroke, epilepsy, and tumors, PET is also useful in the diagnosis and treatment of cardiac disease. The ability of PET to distinguish between viable and nonviable myocardial tissue allows health care providers to identify the most appropriate candidates for bypass surgery or angioplasty. PET is also able to detect accurately coronary artery disease (CAD) noninvasively in an asymptomatic patient, prompting early intervention that can salvage a potentially ischemic myocardium.

MULTIGATED ACQUISITION (MUGA) SCAN

A **multigated acquisition (MUGA) scan** uses a radioactive tracer and a special camera. The camera takes pictures of the heart as it pumps. The test may be done while the patient is resting, exercising, or both. This test is considered a noninvasive procedure, although a radioisotope is injected to assess the ejection fraction of the left ventricle.

Before the procedure begins, ensure that the patient has had no food or drink for at least 6 hours before the test and has avoided caffeine and tobacco use as well.

After the scan is done, encourage the patient to drink plenty of fluids to flush out the radioactive dye. The patient should be able to resume normal activities after the procedure.

LABORATORY TESTS

The history, physical examination, and blood studies help the health care provider diagnose and monitor the cardiovascular disease process. The nurse's responsibility is to prepare the patient by explaining what the tests are for and the preparation required for each test.

Blood cultures to detect growth of bacteria in the blood are crucial to the diagnosis of infective endocarditis.

A *complete blood count (CBC)* is a determination of the number of red blood cells (erythrocytes) and white blood cells (WBCs; leukocytes) per cubic millimeter, as well as the proportions of the various kinds of white blood cells (the WBC differential), platelets, hemoglobin, and hematocrit (the volume percentage of red blood cells in whole blood). Lower hemoglobin levels reduce the ability of the blood to carry oxygen to the cells, resulting in anemia. An elevated WBC count indicates infection or inflammation. An elevated red blood cell count indicates that the body is compensating for chronic **hypoxemia** (an abnormal deficiency of oxygen in the arterial blood) by stimulating red blood cell production by the bone marrow, leading to secondary **polycythemia** (an abnormal increase in the number of red blood cells in the blood). Chronic hypoxemia often is found in heart failure.

Coagulation studies include prothrombin time (PT), international normalized ratio (INR), and partial thromboplastin time (PTT). These studies are used to monitor the patient receiving anticoagulant drug therapy, which is prescribed for patients after a myocardial infarction (MI) to dissolve the thrombus. Coagulation studies also are used in patients with chronic atrial fibrillation or those with atrial fibrillation who are undergoing electrical **cardioversion** (restoring the heart's normal sinus rhythm by delivering a synchronized electric shock through two metal paddles placed on the patient's chest).

The *erythrocyte sedimentation rate (ESR)* is determined to monitor or rule out inflammatory/infective conditions. The ESR is elevated with MI and infective endocarditis and decreases when healing begins. The ESR also indicates the extent of inflammation and infection in rheumatic fever.

Serum electrolyte tests focus on the body's balance of sodium, potassium, calcium, and magnesium, which are necessary for myocardial muscle function. Sodium (Na^+) helps maintain fluid balance. Potassium (K^+) is required for relaxation of cardiac muscle, and calcium (Ca^{2+}) is necessary for contraction of cardiac muscle. Magnesium (Mg^{2+}) helps maintain the correct level of electric excitability in the nerves and the muscles, including the myocardium and the cardiac conduction system. The health care provider compares serum electrolyte levels with ECG changes.

Serum lipids are associated with vascular disease, particularly CAD. Cholesterol and triglycerides bound to plasma proteins are found in the blood as lipoproteins. Density levels vary according to the protein-to-fat ratio. An elevated level of high-density lipoprotein (HDL) is desired, but an elevated level of low-density lipoprotein (LDL) or very-low–density lipoprotein (VLDL) increases the risk for cardiovascular disease (Box 48.1).

Arterial blood gases are measured to monitor oxygenation (PaO_2, the partial pressure of oxygen in the blood; and $PaCO_2$, the partial pressure of carbon dioxide in the blood) and acid-base balance (pH). These tests are used to monitor blood oxygenation in patients with unstable cardiac conditions and to evaluate patients in cardiac failure.

Serum cardiac markers are certain proteins released into the circulation as a result of damage to the cardiac cells. These markers, specifically serum cardiac enzymes and troponin I, are important screening diagnostic criteria for an acute MI. The increase in serum cardiac enzymes that occurs after cell death can show whether cardiac damage is present and the approximate extent of the damage. The levels of cardiac enzyme creatine kinase (CK) and its isoenzyme, creatine phosphokinase (CK-MB), start to rise within 2 to 3 hours after the beginning of an MI, peak in 24 hours, and return to normal within 24 to 40 hours. CK and CK-MB have

Box 48.1 Cholesterol Numbers: What Do They Mean?

YOUR TOTAL CHOLESTEROL NUMBER A total cholesterol level less than 200 mg/dL is considered desirable.	**TOTAL CHOLESTEROL LEVEL** *Desirable:* Less than 200 mg/dL *Borderline:* 200 mg/dL to 239 mg/dL *High:* 240 mg/dL or greater
HDL CHOLESTEROL NUMBER The higher the HDL cholesterol level, the better, because this means that there are more good lipoproteins to decrease the buildup of cholesterol from the arteries.	**HDL CHOLESTEROL LEVEL** *Low:* Less than 40 mg/dL in men and less than 50 mg/dL in women *High:* Greater than 60 mg/dL
LDL CHOLESTEROL NUMBER The higher the number of bad lipoproteins, or LDLs, in the blood, the risk of heart disease goes up.	**LDL CHOLESTEROL LEVEL** *Optimal:* Less than 100 mg/dL *Near to above optimal:* 100–129 mg/dL *Borderline high:* 130–159 mg/dL *High:* 160–189 mg/dL *Very high:* Greater than 190 mg/dL
TRIGLYCERIDES Fat build up in the arteries leading to narrowing of the vessel.	**LDL CHOLESTEROL LEVEL** Less than 150 mg/dL: normal 150–199 mg/dL: borderline to high 200–499 mg/dL: high Above 500 mg/dL: very high
LDL CHOLESTEROL NUMBER The higher the number of bad lipoproteins, or LDLs, in the blood, the risk of heart disease goes up.	**TRIGLYCERIDE LEVEL** Less than 150 mg/dL: normal 150–199 mg/dL: borderline to high 200–499 mg/dL: high Above 500 mg/dL: very high

HDL, High-density lipoprotein; *LDL*, low-density lipoprotein.
Data from Wedro B: *Cholesterol charts (what the numbers mean)*, n.d. Retrieved from *http://www.emedicinehealth.com/understanding_your_cholesterol_level/page2_em.htm.*

been the gold standard for years, but they have been replaced with troponins I and T. CK-MB also is found in skeletal muscle, and its blood level can be elevated by surgery, muscle trauma, and muscle diseases, making the differential diagnosis more difficult, so it is not a specific indicator for MI.

Troponins are myocardial muscle proteins released into the circulation after a myocardial injury. In the heart there are two subtypes: cardiac-specific troponin T and troponin I. These sensitive markers can indicate a very small amount of myocardial damage. Troponin T appears in the blood 3 to 5 hours after an MI, and its level may remain elevated for up to 21 days. Like CK-MB, the level of troponin T is affected by skeletal muscle injury and renal disease. Troponin I is a sensitive and specific cardiac marker, not influenced by skeletal muscle trauma or renal failure. The troponin I level rises 3 hours after MI, peaks at 14 to 18 hours, and may remain elevated for 1 to 2 weeks after MI. Troponin I is most useful in diagnosing an MI because it is cardiac muscle specific. The ability to measure the myocardial contractile proteins (troponins) in serum, which are often present in very small amounts, is a major advance in the diagnosis of acute MI and acute myocardial damage.

Myoglobin is released into circulation within a few hours after an MI. Although it is one of the first serum cardiac markers that increase after an MI, myoglobin is also present in skeletal muscle, so an increase can be associated with noncardiac causes. In addition, it is excreted rapidly in urine, and blood levels return to normal range within 24 hours after an MI.

B-type natriuretic peptide (BNP) is a hormone secreted by the heart in response to ventricular expansion and pressure overload. A BNP level above 100 pg/mL indicates HF. The higher the BNP level, the more severe the HF.

Homocysteine is an amino acid produced during protein digestion. Normal values range from 4 to 14 μmol/L. Elevated blood levels of homocysteine may be an independent risk factor for ischemic heart disease, cerebrovascular disease, peripheral arterial disease (PAD), and venous thrombosis. Homocysteine appears to promote the progression of atherosclerosis by causing endothelial damage, promoting LDL deposits, and stimulating vascular smooth muscle growth. Homocysteine plays an important role in blood clotting. An elevated level results in increased platelet aggregation. Screening for elevated homocysteine levels (greater than 14 μmol/L) should be considered in patients with progressive and unexplained atherosclerosis despite normal levels of lipoproteins and those who have no other risk factors. It also is recommended in patients with an unusual family history of atherosclerosis, especially at a young age.

Dietary deficiency of vitamins B_6 (pyridoxine), B_{12} (cobalamin), or folate is the most common cause of elevated homocysteine. Some researchers believe that an elevated level of homocysteine can be treated by giving vitamins B_6, B_{12}, and folate. Whether this treatment will reduce the incidence of MI remains to be proven (Spinler, 2014).

The liver produces *C-reactive protein (CRP)* during periods of acute inflammation. The presence of CRP is a predictor of cardiac events and is emerging as an independent risk factor for CAD. People with diabetes mellitus are already at high risk for developing cardiovascular disease. If a patient has both an elevated level of CRP and diabetes, the risk for a cardiovascular disorder becomes even greater (Shrivastava et al, 2015).

DISORDERS OF THE CARDIOVASCULAR SYSTEM

Cardiovascular disorders are a major health care problem in the United States. Public awareness, modifications in lifestyle, and improvements in medical treatment have contributed to a decline in overall deaths. The nurse's role in caring for patients with cardiovascular disorders includes being aware of the prevalence of cardiac disease, risk factors, and the disease process; implementing nursing interventions; and patient teaching.

EFFECTS OF NORMAL AGING ON THE CARDIOVASCULAR SYSTEM

By the time an individual reaches the age of 65 years, physiologic changes have reduced the heart's efficiency as a pump. However, the heart still is capable of functioning adequately unless there is underlying cardiac disease (see the Lifespan Considerations box). According to the American Heart Association (2017a), all adults over the age of 20 should have their cholesterol levels checked once every 4 to 6 years. Older adults with high cholesterol should take steps to lower their cholesterol levels, including taking cholesterol-lowering medications, stopping smoking, increasing their activity levels, continuing their blood pressure medications, decreasing their weight, and, if they have diabetes, continuing to control their blood glucose level (CDC, 2018).

RISK FACTORS

Risk factors indicate predispositions for developing cardiovascular disease. The presence of more than one risk factor is associated with an increased risk for developing cardiovascular disease. Risk factors are classified as *nonmodifiable* and *modifiable.*

Nonmodifiable Factors

An important aspect of caring for the patient with a cardiovascular disorder is understanding the risk factors for cardiovascular disease and incorporating them into patient teaching. The nonmodifiable risk factors (risk factors that cannot be changed) associated with cardiovascular disorders include age, genetics, and heredity.

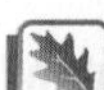

Lifespan Considerations

Older Adults

Cardiac Disease

- Changes in the cardiac musculature lead to reduced efficiency and strength, resulting in decreased cardiac output.
- Disorientation, syncope, and decreased tissue perfusion to organs and other body tissues can occur as a result of decreased cardiac output.
- Aging causes sclerotic changes in blood vessels and leads to decreased elasticity and narrowing of the lumen. Arterial disease resulting from the aging process causes hypertension because of the increased cardiac effort needed to pump blood through the circulatory system.
- Progressive coronary artery changes can lead to the development of collateral coronary circulation. This can modify the severity of signs and symptoms seen in MI. Angina symptoms may be less pronounced, and dyspnea may replace angina as a key symptom of acute infarction.
- Heart failure can result from rapid intravenous infusion.
- Edema secondary to heart failure may cause tissue impairment in the immobile older adult. Immobility leads to venous stasis (i.e., a slowing or stoppage of venous blood flow), venous ulcer, and poor wound healing. It also increases the risk of venous thrombosis and embolus formation.
- Older adults with cardiac disease often receive several medications, which often are prescribed at lower doses than for younger adults. Even with lower doses of medications, observe the older adult closely for signs of toxicity, because the rate of drug metabolism and excretion decreases with age.
- Independent older adults with cardiac conditions should receive adequate teaching regarding medication, diet, and warning signs of complications. Encourage them to maintain regular contact with the health care provider and to seek care at the first sign of problems.

Family history. A family member such as a parent or sibling who has had a cardiovascular problem before 50 years of age puts the patient at greater risk for developing cardiovascular disease.

Age. Normal physiologic changes that occur with aging and past lifestyle habits increase the patient's risk for developing cardiovascular disease with advancing age. CAD and MI occur most frequently among white, middle-aged men.

Gender. Middle-aged men are at greater risk of developing cardiovascular disease than middle-aged women. Although the incidence in men and women equalizes after age 65, cardiovascular disease is a more common cause of death in women than in men. Women develop CAD about 10 years later than men, because natural estrogen may have a cardioprotective effect before menopause. Despite this, the incidence of cardiovascular disease in women 50 years of age and older is increasing. Factors possibly responsible are increased social and economic pressures on women and changes in lifestyle. Ten times more women die from heart disease than die from breast cancer. The mortality rate for women with CAD has remained relatively constant even though cardiovascular disease remains the leading cause of death. Despite this statistic, only 15% of women consider CAD their greatest health risk. Recent research on CAD has shown that women often do not have the same signs and symptoms of an acute coronary event as those that are commonly seen in men (American Heart Association, 2017b).

Cultural and ethnic considerations. African Americans have a higher incidence of MI and stroke than other Americans, with more than 1.5 million of these disease cases combined. Almost 44% of African American men and 48% of African American women have some type of cardiovascular disease (CDC, 2014). The rate of cardiovascular disease in the Hispanic population is 33.4% of men and 30.7% of women (American Heart Association, 2013d).

Modifiable Factors

Smoking. Individuals who smoke cigarettes have a two to three times greater risk of developing cardiovascular disease than nonsmokers. The degree of risk is proportional to the number of cigarettes smoked. Individuals who quit smoking decrease their risk. Tobacco smoke contains nicotine, which causes the release of catecholamine (i.e., epinephrine, norepinephrine). Catecholamine causes tachycardia, hypertension, and vasoconstriction of the peripheral arteries. This increases the workload of the heart, thus reducing the amount of available oxygen to the heart muscle. The other chemicals in cigarettes, including tar and carbon monoxide, also contribute to heart disease. These chemicals cause atherosclerosis because of the buildup of fatty plaque in the vessels. Fibrinogen levels also rise as the result of these chemicals, leading to clot formation, which can cause MI or stroke (Texas Heart Institute, n.d.).

With the increased use of marijuana because of legalization in some states, studies are being conducted regarding the potential harm to various organs. A recent study from the American College of Cardiology (Kattoor and Mehta, 2016) showed that the active use of marijuana may double the risk of stress cardiomyopathy.

Hyperlipidemia. Hyperlipidemia is elevated concentrations of any or all lipids in the plasma. The ratio of HDL to LDL is the best predictor for the development of cardiovascular disease. Density levels vary according to the protein-to-fat ratio:

- VLDL contains more fat than protein (primarily triglycerides); triglycerides are the main storage form of lipids and constitute approximately 95% of fatty tissue.
- LDL contains an equal amount of fat and protein (approximately 50%) with moderate amounts of phospholipid cholesterol (see Box 48.1).
- HDL contains more protein than fat (which serves a protective function, removing cholesterol from tissues). It is suspected that HDL also removes cholesterol from the peripheral tissues and transports it to the liver for excretion. HDL may have a protective effect by preventing cellular uptake of cholesterol and lipids. Low levels (less than 40 mg/dL) are believed to increase a person's risk for CAD, whereas high levels (more than 60 mg/dL) are considered protective (see Box 48.1).

A diet high in saturated fat, cholesterol, and calories contributes to hyperlipidemia. Therefore dietary control is an important aspect in modifying this risk factor. An overall serum cholesterol level of less than 200 mg/dL is desirable, 200 to 239 mg/dL is borderline high, and more than 239 mg/dL is high.

Change in diet is probably the most important method of lowering the cholesterol level. Weight reduction in overweight patients with abnormal lipid profiles is an essential element of dietary intervention. In addition to lowering LDL levels, weight reduction leads to decreases in triglyceride level and blood pressure. A combination of weight reduction and physical exercise improves the lipid profile, with a decrease in LDL level, an increase in HDL level, and a decrease in triglyceride levels. Low HDL levels are often familial and only somewhat modifiable.

Cholesterol-lowering drugs often are included in treatment of hyperlipidemia. Cholesterol-lowering drugs are divided into six classes: (1) bile acid sequestrants; (2) nicotinic acid (niacin); (3) statins such as atorvastatin (Lipitor), simvastatin (Zocor), pravastatin (Pravachol), and rosuvastatin (Crestor); (4) fibric acid derivatives such as gemfibrozil (Lopid) and probucol; (5) the cholesterol absorption inhibitor ezetimibe (Zetia); and (6) combination drugs such as ezetimibe and simvastatin (Vytorin). Pravastatin reduces the risk of a first MI by about one-third in hypercholesterolemic patients with no history of coronary disease. Simvastatin now is allowed by the US Food and Drug Administration (FDA) to add a label statement that the drug can reduce deaths by lowering cholesterol.

Hypertension. Hypertension is called the "silent killer" because a patient with elevated blood pressure does not display signs and symptoms of heart disease until damage has begun to develop. This damage increases the risks of heart disease, stroke, heart failure, or cardiovascular death. Prehypertension is defined as blood pressure of 120 to 139/80 to 89 mm Hg, which requires monitoring yearly to decrease a patient's risk of developing cardiac disease.

Hypertension is blood pressure higher than 140/90 mm Hg, taken on two separate occasions. Adhering to diet, exercise, and the prescribed pharmacologic therapies to control elevated blood pressure helps modify the individual's risk.

Diabetes mellitus. Cardiac disease has been found to be more prevalent in individuals with diabetes mellitus. Diabetes poses a greater risk than other factors, possibly because an elevated blood glucose level damages the arterial intima (the innermost layer of an artery) and contributes to atherosclerosis. Patients with diabetes also have alterations in lipid metabolism and tend to have high cholesterol and triglyceride levels. Keeping the blood glucose level under control helps modify the individual's risk. The CDC estimates that 70% of individuals over age 65 who have diabetes will die of heart disease. More than 16% will die from a stroke (CDC, 2016a). Adults with diabetes and heart disease are two to four times more likely than adults without diabetes to die from cardiac-related complications. Blood pressure control decreases these risks by 33% to 50%. In general, every 10-mm Hg drop in systolic blood pressure decreases the risk by 12%. Patients with diabetes who decrease their diastolic blood pressure by 10 mm Hg decrease their chance of a cardiovascular event by 50%.

Obesity. Excess body weight increases the workload of the heart. It also contributes to the severity of other risk factors. The CDC estimates that 35.7% of Americans are obese. This correlates to 97 million Americans with a body mass index (BMI) of 30 or above. As the BMI increases, so do the risk factors for developing diabetes, cardiovascular events, and stroke. A weight reduction program and maintaining an ideal body weight help modify the individual's risk.

Sedentary lifestyle. Lack of regular exercise has been correlated with an increased risk of developing cardiovascular disease. Regular aerobic exercise can improve the heart's efficiency and help lower the blood glucose level, improve the ratio of HDLs to LDLs, reduce weight, lower blood pressure, reduce stress, and improve overall feelings of well-being. Individuals with sedentary lifestyles should work with their health care provider to plan an exercise program that fits their lifestyle. Some health care providers define regular physical exercise as exercising at least three to five times a week for at least 30 minutes, causing perspiration and an increase in heart rate by 30 to 50 beats per minute (bpm). Yoga has been receiving increasing research as a form of exercise that increases musculoskeletal strengthening, flexibility, and relaxation. Yoga movements also have therapeutic cognitive effects of distraction and mindfulness, thereby reducing stress on the body. Another form of exercise receiving national attention is walking. Walking is one of the best forms of exercise, because it is the simplest and easiest way to exercise. Walking can strengthen bones, tune up the cardiovascular system, and clear a cluttered mind. Walking is a remedy for stress as well.

Stress. The body's stress response releases catecholamines that increase the heart rate. Catecholamines are hormones produced by the adrenal glands and released during times of physical and emotional stress. Catecholamines also affect myocardial cells and may cause cellular damage. The vasoconstriction that occurs may contribute to the development of cardiovascular disease. Stress reduction measures may help modify an individual's risk.

Psychosocial factors. In the early 1970s, health care providers used the term "type A personality" to describe a person who is always in a hurry, impatient, and irritable, or always angry or hostile. Recent studies have found that the term *type A* does not always fit the person with cardiovascular risks. More recent studies have found that the type D personality is more likely to suffer from increased cardiovascular symptoms. The person with a type D personality has chronic negative emotions, is pessimistic, and socially inhibited. Type D personalities tend to have increased levels of anxiety, irritation, and depressed mood across most situations and times. Type D people do not share their feelings because they fear disapproval, thereby increasing their chance of a cardiovascular event.

CARDIAC DYSRHYTHMIAS

A cardiac **dysrhythmia** (or arrhythmia) is any cardiac rhythm that deviates from normal sinus rhythm. Normal sinus rhythm originates in the SA node and is characterized by the following:

- *Rate:* 60 to 100 bpm
- *P waves:* Precede each QRS complex (atrial depolarization)
- *P-R interval:* Interval between atrial and ventricular repolarization
- *QRS complex:* Ventricular depolarization
- *T wave:* Ventricular repolarization
- *Rhythm:* Regular

A dysrhythmia is the result of an alteration in the formation of impulses through the SA node to the rest of the myocardium. It also results from irritation of the myocardial cells that generate impulses, independent of the conduction system. Signs and symptoms of dysrhythmia vary, as do treatment options, depending on the type and severity of the dysrhythmia. A short overview of each dysrhythmia follows.

Types of Cardiac Dysrhythmias

Sinus tachycardia. Sinus **tachycardia** is a rapid, regular rhythm originating in the SA node. It is characterized by a heartbeat of 100 to 150 bpm or more.

Causes of sinus tachycardia include exercise, anxiety, fever, shock, medications, HF, excessive caffeine, recreational drugs, and tobacco use. Tachycardia increases the amount of oxygen delivered to the cells by increasing the amount of blood circulated through the vessels.

Clinical manifestations include occasional palpitations. Many patients are asymptomatic. Other signs and symptoms may include hypotension and angina, if cardiovascular disease is also present.

Medical management is directed at the primary cause. This is a normal rhythm and is not usually caused by a cardiac problem.

Sinus bradycardia. Sinus **bradycardia** is a slow rhythm originating in the SA node. It is characterized by a pulse rate of less than 60 bpm. Bradycardia can be life threatening if the cause is not found. Bradycardia caused by an SA node dysfunction or other undetermined causes may be managed by the insertion of a pacemaker. Causes of sinus bradycardia include obstructive sleep apnea, vomiting, intracranial tumors, MI, medications (especially overuse of digitalis, beta-adrenergic blockers, or calcium channel blockers), carotid sinus massage, vagal stimulation, endocrine disturbances, increased intracranial pressure, and hypothermia. When found in association with MI, it is a beneficial rhythm because it reduces myocardial oxygen demand. An athlete's resting heart rhythm may normally be slow, because of the training the athlete undergoes.

Clinical manifestations of bradycardia may not be manifested in some patients until the heart rate drops below 60 beats per minute and may include fatigue, lightheadedness, and syncope. Some patients are asymptomatic.

Medical management is directed toward the primary cause of the problem and maintaining cardiac output. If the cause is determined to be vagal stimulation, such as when bearing down with a bowel movement or vomiting, a stool softener is given or medication to stop the vomiting, and the patient is taught how to stop vagal stimulation. Atropine may be prescribed to increase the heart rate. A temporary or permanent, implantable pacemaker is sometimes necessary (Figs. 48.8 and 48.9). If the cause is suspected to be drug related, blood is drawn and the drug concentration is determined; if necessary, the drug is withheld.

Supraventricular tachycardia. Supraventricular tachycardia (SVT) is the sudden onset of a rapid heartbeat. It originates in the atria. It is characterized by a pulse rate of 150 to 250 bpm.

Causes of SVT include medications, alcohol, mitral valve prolapse, emotional stress, smoking, and hormone imbalance such as decreases in estrogen in postmenopausal women. The cause typically is not

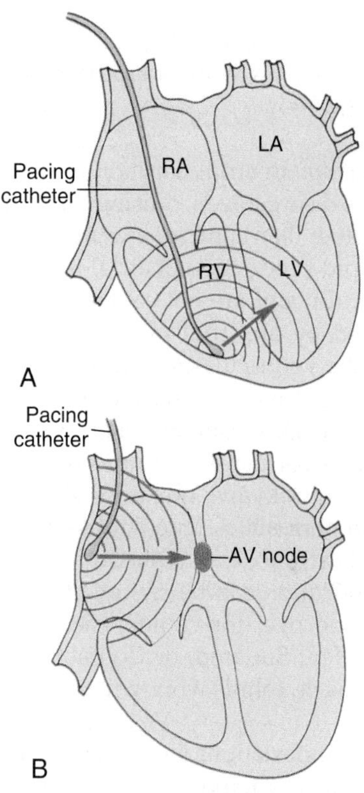

Fig. 48.8 A, Ventricular pacing. Impulses are initiated in the right ventricle. B, Atrial pacing. Impulses are initiated in the right atrium and travel to the ventricles via the normal conduction system through the atrioventricular (AV) node. *LA*, Left atrium; *LV*, left ventricle; *RA*, right atrium; *RV*, right ventricle.

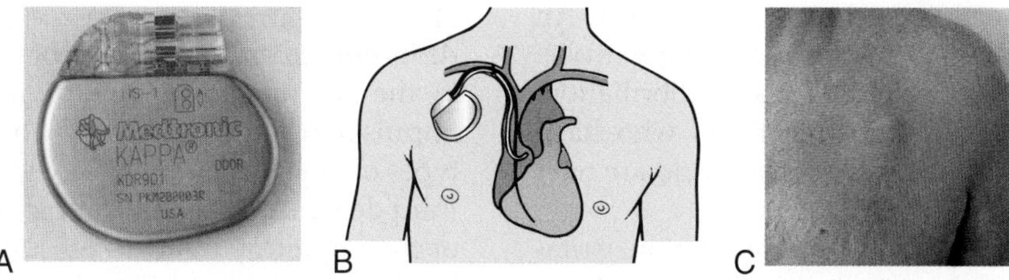

Fig. 48.9 A, A dual-chamber, rate-responsive pacemaker from Medtronic, Inc., is designed to detect body movement and automatically increase or decrease paced heart rates based on the level of physical activity. B, Cardiac leads, in the atrium and the ventricle, enable a dual-chamber pacemaker to sense and pace in both heart chambers. C, Pacemaker in subcutaneous tissue.

associated with heart disease. Clinical manifestations include palpitations, lightheadedness, dyspnea, and anginal pain.

Medical management first looks at how well the patient tolerates the dysrhythmia and at the overall clinical picture. The focus is aimed at decreasing the heart rate and eliminating the underlying cause. Specific treatments may include carotid sinus pressure, adenosine, digoxin (Lanoxin), calcium channel blockers (e.g., diltiazem [Cardizem]), beta-adrenergic blockers, propranolol (Inderal), antidysrhythmics, amiodarone, and cardioversion. Persistent, recurring SVT caused by the presence of an accessory pathway (i.e., a second, abnormal electrical conduction pathway; see the section "Electrical Conduction System" earlier in the chapter) ultimately may be treated by radiofrequency catheter ablation (i.e., cutting away or eradication) of the accessory pathway.

Atrial fibrillation. In atrial fibrillation, electrical activity in the atria is disorganized, causing the atria to fibrillate, or quiver, rather than contract as a unit. Atrial fibrillation is a very rapid production of atrial impulses. The atria beat chaotically and are not contracting properly. It is characterized by an atrial rate of 350 to 600 bpm. If untreated, the ventricular response rate may be 100 to 180 bpm.

Causes of atrial fibrillation include cardiac surgery, longstanding hypertension, pulmonary embolism, atherosclerosis, mitral valve disease, HF, cardiomyopathy, congenital abnormalities, chronic obstructive pulmonary disease, and thyrotoxicosis. Other not-so-obvious causes of atrial fibrillation can be energy drinks, high ingestion of caffeine, over-the-counter medications for colds such as Actifed, Sudafed, or Contact, and even some herbs, such as St. John's wort, which can interfere with clotting.

Clinical manifestations include pulse deficit, palpitations, dyspnea, angina, lightheadedness, syncope, fatigue, change in level of consciousness, and pulmonary edema. Because of ventricular rhythm irregularity and ineffective atrial contractions, decreased cardiac output may be noted, resulting in HF, angina, and shock. Thrombi (blood clots) may form in the atria as a result of ineffective atrial contraction and cause emboli (i.e., thrombi that have moved from one point in the body to another), thus affecting the lungs or periphery. An embolized clot may pass to the brain, causing a stroke. Risk of stroke increases fivefold with atrial fibrillation. Risk of stroke is even higher in patients who have structural heart disease and hypertension and are over 65 years of age.

Medical management focuses on treating the irritability of the atria, slowing the ventricular response to atrial stimulation, and correcting the primary cause. The goal of therapy is to prevent atrial thrombi from developing and embolizing, such as in the lungs or periphery. Specific pharmacologic treatments to achieve cardioversion may include (1) digitalis; (2) calcium channel blockers such as intravenous (IV) diltiazem (Cardizem) and verapamil (Calan); (3) antidysrhythmics such as procainamide, amiodarone, dofetilide (Tikosyn), flecainide (Tambocor), and propafenone (Rythmol) (St. Luke's Health System, n.d.); and anticoagulants such as heparin and warfarin (Coumadin). Outpatients typically take oral warfarin to maintain anticoagulation. The goal of anticoagulation is to maintain an INR between 2 and 3. If pharmacologic cardioversion fails, the patient may need electrical cardioversion. Transesophageal echocardiography (TEE) is used to detect a thrombus in the atria before proceeding with electrical cardioversion (American Heart Association, 2016a). The Joint Commission (2014) recommends that patients with atrial fibrillation be prescribed warfarin and long-term antidysrhythmic medication therapy at discharge.

There are several new anticoagulants on the market that are also being prescribed to treat deep vein thrombosis (DVT) and atrial fibrillation. Pradaxa (dabigatran etexilate mesylate) and Xarelto (rivaroxaban) are two of the newest that have been approved for this use. Unlike warfarin (Coumadin), these drugs do not require continuing modification of the dosages. Although these drugs do not require modification of dosages and long-term determination of PT, PT/INR blood levels, there are still issues with the drugs. Please see the Safety Alert box for drugs that interact unfavorably with Xarelto.

For patients who do not respond to medication therapy or electrical conversion, catheter ablation (cutting or removal) with radiofrequency energy is used to destroy the areas in the atria that trigger abnormal electrical signals. The catheter is inserted into the femoral vein and threaded via fluoroscopy to the heart. The special ablation catheter is placed in strategic areas, and bursts of radiofrequency energy destroy the irritable area (American Heart Association, 2017c).

Catheter ablation to treat atrial fibrillation usually is performed on younger patients because of a better response rate and fewer complications than in the older adult. After the catheter ablation procedure, perform neurovascular assessment checks at the peripheral sites distal to the catheter insertion site (American Heart Association, 2017c).

Atrioventricular block. AV block occurs when a defect in the AV junction slows or impairs conduction of impulses from the SA node to the ventricles. Three types of blocks are seen: first degree, second degree, and third degree. A third-degree block indicates worsening of the impairment at the AV junction and a complete heart block.

Common causes of AV block include atherosclerotic heart disease (ASHD), MI, and HF. Other causes may be digitalis toxicity, congenital abnormality, drugs, and hypokalemia (low potassium in the blood).

Safety Alert

Drugs That Interact Unfavorably With Xarelto (Rivaroxaban)

ANTIBIOTICS
- azithromycin (Zithromax)
- clarithromycin (Biaxin)
- erythromycin (Erythrocin)

BARBITURATES
- pentobarbital
- phenobarbital (Solfoton)
- secobarbital (Seconal)

CALCIUM CHANNEL BLOCKERS
- verapamil (Calan)

HEART AND BLOOD PRESSURE MEDICATIONS
- cardizem (diltiazem)
- cordarone (amiodarone)
- dronedarone (Multaq)
- felodipine

HERBALS
- St. John's wort

NONSTEROIDAL ANTIINFLAMMATORY DRUGS (NSAIDS)
- celecoxib (Celebrex)
- diclofenac (Voltaren, Flector patch)
- ibuprofen (Advil, Motrin)
- indomethacin (Indocin)
- meloxicam (Mobic)
- naproxen (Aleve)

QUININE
- quinidine

SALICYLATES
- aspirin (ASA)
- Pepto-Bismol

SEIZURE MEDICATIONS
- carbamazepine (Tegretol)
- phenytoin (Dilantin)
- primidone (Mysoline)

First-degree heart block is often asymptomatic. Vertigo, weakness, and irregular pulse are seen with second-degree block. Disease that is progressing, as with third-degree block, will be accompanied by hypotension, angina, and bradycardia. The heart rate is often low, often between 30 and 40 bpm.

Medical management involves evaluating the patient's response and determining the cause of the dysrhythmia. Atropine and isoproterenol may be prescribed. A pacemaker frequently is needed with third-degree block (see Fig. 48.8).

Premature ventricular contractions. Premature ventricular contractions (PVCs) are abnormal heartbeats that arise from the right or left ventricle. PVCs are early ventricular beats that occur in conjunction with the underlying rhythm, which is unchanged except for the PVC itself.

PVCs may originate from more than one location in the ventricles and be caused by irritability of the ventricular musculature, exercise, stress, electrolyte imbalance, digitalis toxicity, hypoxia, and MI.

Clinical manifestations depend on the frequency of PVCs and their effect on the heart's ability to pump blood effectively. Some patients are asymptomatic; others may experience palpitations, weakness, and lightheadedness. Other symptoms are associated with decreased cardiac output.

Medical management focuses on treating the underlying heart condition. Symptomatic PVCs can be treated with beta-adrenergic blockers such as carvedilol (Coreg), antianginals, propranolol (Inderal), and antidysrhythmics such as procainamide, amiodarone, or lidocaine (Xylocaine).

A PVC may be a single event or may occur several times in a minute or in pairs or strings. PVCs that last long enough to cause ventricular tachycardia may lead to death.

Ventricular tachycardia. Ventricular tachycardia (VT) occurs when three or more successive PVCs occur. In VT the ventricular rate is greater than 100 bpm (usually 140 to 240 bpm). The rhythm is regular or slightly irregular. Conditions that can cause its occurrence include hypoxemia, drug toxicity such as with digitalis or quinidine, electrolyte imbalance (e.g., potassium, magnesium), and bradycardia. Repeated and prolonged episodes of VT in the second week after MI may be a warning of ventricular fibrillation and require aggressive evaluation and treatment.

Medical management focuses on intravenously administered procainamide or amiodarone. These drugs depress excitability of cardiac muscle to electrical stimulation and slow conduction in the atria, bundle of His, and ventricles. Lidocaine is used only if acute myocardial ischemia or MI is considered to be the cause of VT. If pharmacologic measures are unsuccessful, the alternative is cardioversion. Catheter ablation can be helpful. Ongoing VT suppression is obtained with oral beta-adrenergic blockers or calcium channel blockers.

Ventricular fibrillation. Ventricular fibrillation occurs when the ventricular musculature of the heart is quivering. This medical emergency is characterized by rapid and disorganized ventricle pulsation.

The cause is usually myocardial ischemia or infarction. Other causes are untreated VT, electrolyte imbalances, digitalis or quinidine toxicity, and hypothermia. It also may occur with coronary reperfusion after thrombolytic therapy.

Clinical manifestations are the result of no cardiac output and include loss of consciousness, lack of a pulse, decreases in blood pressure and respirations, possible seizures, and sudden death if untreated.

Medical management focuses on providing emergency treatment, including cardiopulmonary resuscitation

(CPR), **defibrillation** (the termination of ventricular fibrillation by delivering a direct electrical countershock to the patient's precordium, i.e., that part of the patient's body surface covering the heart and stomach), and medications such as lidocaine or procainamide. Defibrillation is the most effective method of ending ventricular fibrillation and ideally should be performed within 15 to 20 seconds of onset to avoid brain damage from the lack of blood flow.

Assessment

Subjective data for the patient with a cardiac dysrhythmia include the patient's report of symptoms associated with the specific dysrhythmia. Symptoms may include palpitations, skipped beats, nausea, lightheadedness, vertigo, anxiety, dyspnea, fatigue, and chest discomfort.

Collection of objective data includes immediate visual observation of the patient when ECG monitoring indicates a dysrhythmia. Signs may include syncope, irregular pulse, tachycardia, and tachypnea. Noting the patient's response to the dysrhythmia is important to plan and implement appropriate nursing interventions. Monitor vital signs and observe for signs of decreased cardiac output.

Diagnostic Tests

Before treating a patient with a dysrhythmia, the health care provider needs to know if this is an abnormal or normal conduction occurrence of the heart. To find the cause or abnormality diagnostic tests are scheduled. Some of these can be performed without hospitalization.

ECG monitoring, telemetry, and Holter monitoring are used commonly to confirm the diagnosis of cardiac dysrhythmias and can be done without hospitalization. Laboratory work is also done to detect a medication toxicity. Treatment is aimed at the findings of the diagnostic tests.

Medical Management

Treatment varies according to the type of cardiac dysrhythmia (Table 48.1).

Nursing Interventions and Patient Teaching

Nursing interventions focus on symptomatic relief, promotion of comfort, relief of anxiety, emergency action as needed, and patient teaching.

Assess the patient's apical pulse to obtain an accurate pulse rate when dysrhythmias are present. Because the rhythm is irregular, take the apical pulse for 1 minute. Assess the patient's anxiety and degree of understanding, noting verbal and nonverbal expressions regarding diagnosis, procedures, and treatments.

Explain the diagnostic and monitoring devices in use. Monitor heart rate and rhythm. Administer antidysrhythmic agents as ordered and monitor response. Maintain a quiet environment; administer sedation or analgesic medication as ordered. Administer oxygen per protocol.

Table 48.1 Medications for Cardiac Dysrhythmias

GENERIC NAME (TRADE NAME)	ACTION	NURSING INTERVENTIONS
Cardiac Glycoside		
digoxin (Lanoxin)	Used to control rapid ventricular rate in atrial fibrillation and to convert paroxysmal supraventricular tachycardia to normal sinus rhythm Increases cardiac force and efficiency, slows heart rate, increases cardiac output	Monitor apical pulse to ensure rate is above 60 bpm (call health care provider if digoxin withheld) Monitor for digitalis toxicity (nausea, vomiting, anorexia, dysrhythmias, bradycardia, tachycardia, headache, fatigue, visual disturbance)
Antidysrhythmic Agents		
procainamide	IV solutions given for severe ventricular dysrhythmias Depresses excitability of cardiac muscle to electrical stimulation and slows conduction in atrium, bundle of His, and ventricle, thus increasing refractory period	Observe for new dysrhythmias, dry mouth, blurred vision, bradycardia, hypotension, nausea, anorexia, dizziness, visual disturbances
lidocaine (IV)	Suppresses the impulse that triggers dysrhythmias	Monitor heart rate and BP closely
disopyramide (Norpace CR)	Provides long-term treatment of premature ventricular contractions, ventricular tachycardia, and atrial fibrillation	Monitor BP and apical pulse

Table 48.1 **Medications for Cardiac Dysrhythmias—cont'd**

GENERIC NAME (TRADE NAME)	ACTION	NURSING INTERVENTIONS
adenosine (Adenocard)	Slows conduction through AV node, can interrupt reentry pathways through AV node, and can restore normal sinus rhythm in patients with paroxysmal supraventricular tachycardia (PSVT)	Monitor BP, pulse rate, and respirations Assess patient for headache, dizziness, gastrointestinal complaints, new dysrhythmias Do not give caffeine within 4–6 h of adenosine because caffeine inhibits the effect of the drug
amiodarone (Pacerone)	Prolongs duration of action potential and effective refractory period; provides noncompetitive alpha- and beta-adrenergic inhibition; increases P-R and Q-T intervals; decreases sinus rate; decreases peripheral vascular resistance. Used for severe ventricular tachycardia, supraventricular tachycardia, atrial fibrillation, ventricular fibrillation not controlled by first-line agents, cardiac arrest	Observe for headache, dizziness, hypotension, bradycardia, sinus arrest, heart failure, dysrhythmia Assess BP continuously for hypotension or hypertension Report dysrhythmia or bradycardia Monitor for dyspnea, chest pain
mexiletine propafenone (Rythmol)	Decrease excitability of cardiac muscle	Monitor pulse, BP Monitor for diarrhea, visual disturbances, respiratory distress
tocainide	Suppresses automaticity of conduction tissue	Notify health care provider if cough, wheezing, or shortness of breath occurs
Beta-Adrenergic Blockers		
propranolol (Inderal) sotalol (Betapace) acebutolol (Sectral) esmolol (Brevibloc) metoprolol (Lopressor) carvedilol (Coreg)	Used to treat supraventricular and ventricular dysrhythmias, persistent sinus tachycardia Decrease myocardial oxygen demand, decrease workload of the heart, decrease heart rate	Monitor heart rate and BP carefully. Use caution with patient with bronchospastic disease Monitor for bradycardia, hypotension, new dysrhythmias, dizziness, headache, nausea, diarrhea, sleep disturbances
Calcium Channel Blockers		
verapamil (Calan) diltiazem (Cardizem)	Treat supraventricular tachycardia and control rapid rates in atrial tachycardia Produce relaxation of coronary vascular smooth muscle, dilate coronary arteries	Use caution in patients with CHF Monitor apical pulse and BP Watch for fatigue, headache, dizziness, peripheral edema, nausea, tachycardia Verapamil and diltiazem increase the toxicity of digoxin
Inotropic Agent		
dobutamine (IV) dopamine (IV)	Used in severe CHF with pulmonary edema Increase myocardial contractility Increase cardiac output, increase BP, and improve renal blood flow	Monitor BP, heart rate, and urinary output continuously during the administration Palpate peripheral pulses; notify health care provider if extremities become cold or mottled
Anticoagulant		
warfarin (Coumadin)	Used in treatment of atrial fibrillation with embolization to prevent complication of stroke	Assess patient for signs of bleeding and hemorrhage Monitor prothrombin time and international normalized ratio (PT/INR) frequently during therapy Review foods high in vitamin K. Patient should have consistently limited intake of these foods because these foods will cause levels to fluctuate

AV, Atrioventricular; *BP,* blood pressure; *bpm,* beats per minute; *CHF,* congestive heart failure; *HCl,* hydrochloride; *IV,* intravenous.

Patient problems and interventions for the patient with a cardiac dysrhythmia include but are not limited to the following:

Patient Problem	Nursing Interventions
Discomfort, related to ischemia	Administer medications as ordered Teach relaxation techniques Institute position change and support Administer prescribed oxygen
Insufficient Cardiac Output, related to cardiovascular disease	Monitor heart rate and rhythm Reduce cardiac workload by encouraging bed rest Elevate head of bed 30 to 45 degrees for comfort Restrict activities as ordered; plan care to avoid fatigue Administer antidysrhythmic agents as ordered Monitor for signs of drug toxicity
Impaired Coping, related to fear of and uncertainty about disease process	Assist patient in identifying strengths and coping skills Supply emotional support Teach relaxation techniques Assess coping ability and level of family support Explain purpose of care as related to specific dysrhythmia

Teach the patient the importance of lifestyle changes such as avoiding or stopping smoking or use of nicotine products. Teach the patient about medication therapy and its purposes, desired effects, and dosage and the side effects to report to the health care provider. Explain the reason for and method of taking pulse rate and rhythm. Explain the need to avoid exercising beyond the tolerance level, to avoid strenuous or isometric activity, and to check with the health care provider regarding limitations and allowances. Instruct the patient regarding conserving energy for activities of daily living (ADLs): taking regular rest periods between activities and for 1 hour after meals; when possible, sitting rather than standing while performing a task; and stopping an activity or task if symptoms such as fatigue, dyspnea, or palpitations begin. Stress management is important to promote healing and prevent further cardiac events.

CARDIAC ARREST

The sudden cessation of cardiac output and circulatory process is termed *cardiac arrest*. Conditions leading to cardiac arrest are severe ventricular tachycardia, ventricular fibrillation, and ventricular asystole. The absence of oxygen–carbon dioxide exchange leads to symptoms of anaerobic tissue cell metabolism and respiratory and metabolic acidosis. Thus immediate CPR is necessary to prevent major organ damage. Signs and symptoms of cardiac arrest include abrupt loss of consciousness with no response to stimuli, gasping respirations followed by apnea, absence of pulse (radial, carotid, femoral, and apical), absence of blood pressure, pupil dilation, and pallor and cyanosis.

CPR is initiated by the first person to discover the condition. The aim is to reestablish circulation and ventilation. Prevention of severe damage to the brain, heart, liver, and kidneys as a result of anoxia (lack of oxygen) is of primary concern. Remember the CAB of CPR: *C*, circulation; *A*, restore airway; and *B*, restore breathing. Resuscitation measures are divided into two components: basic cardiac life support in the form of CPR and advanced cardiac life support (ACLS).

ACLS is a systematic approach to provide early treatment of cardiac emergencies. ACLS includes (1) basic life support, (2) the use of adjunctive equipment and special techniques for establishing and maintaining effective ventilation and circulation, (3) ECG monitoring and dysrhythmia recognition, (4) therapies for emergency treatment of patient with cardiac or respiratory arrest, and (5) treatment of patient with suspected acute MI.

Artificial Cardiac Pacemakers

A pacemaker is made of titanium with computer circuits that control the pacing system; one or more leads are placed into the heart and a lithium battery is used (American Heart Association, 2016b). It initiates and controls the heart rate by delivering an electrical impulse via an electrode to the myocardium. These catheter-like electrodes are placed within the area to be paced: right atrium, right ventricle, or both (see Figs. 48.8 and 48.9). A permanent pacemaker power source is placed subcutaneously, usually over the pectoral muscle on the patient's nondominant side. Most are demand pacemakers, which send electrical stimuli to pace the heart when the heartbeat decreases below a preset rate. Some pacemakers have a single-chamber device with one lead that paces the right atrium or right ventricle; other pacemakers are dual-chamber with separate leads that connect to both the right atrium and the right ventricle.

Another pacemaker, the biventricular pacemaker, has three leads, one lead for each ventricle and one lead for the right atrium. This device restores normal simultaneous contraction of the ventricles. A biventricular pacemaker significantly improves left ventricular ejection fraction and exercise tolerance. It improves the quality of life for patients with worsening HF (American Heart Association, 2016b).

A pacemaker maintains a regular cardiac rhythm by electrically stimulating the heart muscle. It is used when patients experience adverse symptoms because of dysrhythmias that cannot be managed by medications alone. These include second- and third-degree AV block, *bradydysrhythmia* (slow and/or irregular heartbeat), and *tachydysrhythmia* (rapid heartbeat that can be regular or irregular).

An external pacemaker is used in emergency situations on a short-term basis. Temporary pacemakers are used for cardiac support after some MIs or open-heart surgery. A permanent pacemaker is placed when other measures have failed to convert the dysrhythmia or conduction problem. The batteries used in permanent pacemakers today are small, weighing less than 1 ounce, and can last 15 years or more.

Nursing Interventions and Patient Teaching

After placement of a pacemaker, closely monitor heart rate and rhythm by apical pulse and by ECG patterns. Check vital signs and level of consciousness frequently until stable. Observe the insertion site for erythema, edema, and tenderness, which could indicate infection. The patient may be on bed rest with the arm on the pacemaker side immobilized for the first few hours. Discharge teaching includes instructions not to lift the arm on the surgical side over the head for 6 to 8 weeks. The patient needs to refrain from swimming, golfing, and weight lifting until given permission by the health care provider (American Heart Association, 2016b).

Inform the patient of the necessity to continue medical management, and advise that he or she wear medical-alert identification and carry pacemaker information. Emphasize the importance of reporting signs and symptoms of pacemaker failure: weakness, vertigo, chest pain, and pulse changes.

Teach the patient to avoid potentially hazardous situations. Each pacemaker manufacturer can provide a list of devices that patients with pacemakers should avoid getting close to. In the past patients had to avoid objects such as high-output electrical generators or large magnets such as a MRI scanner because these objects could cause interference resulting in the pacemaker going into a fixed mode. Because of the grade of titanium metals used, patients who have pacemakers placed in the past several years can have MRI testing without difficulty. The patient always should report the use of a pacemaker before having an MRI.

The pacemaker's pulse generator is set to produce a heart rate appropriate to the patient's clinical condition and the desired therapeutic goal. With rare exceptions, the rate is set between 70 and 80 bpm. If the heart rate falls below the preset level, notify the health care provider.

Teach the patient how and when to take a radial pulse. The pulse should be taken at the same time each day and when symptoms of vertigo or weakness occur. During patient education, remember to (1) list symptoms to expect and to report to the health care provider, (2) promote understanding of medication administration, (3) explain treatment outcomes, (4) explain the importance of maintaining prescribed diet and fluid amounts, and (5) explain the importance of not smoking. Teach the patient that shortness of breath occurring with exercise or exertion can be significant, because of the heart's inability to provide enough oxygen to the cells.

Prognosis

The patient can expect to lead a reasonably normal life with full resumption of most activities as prescribed by the health care provider.

DISORDERS OF THE HEART

CORONARY ATHEROSCLEROTIC HEART DISEASE

The coronary arteries arise from the base of the aorta just below the semilunar valves (see Fig. 48.6). These arteries curve and branch to adequately supply the heart muscle with oxygen and nutrients. The shapes, contours, and arrangements of the vessels allow for easy entrapment of substances that interfere with blood flow.

Coronary artery disease (CAD) is the term used to describe a variety of conditions that obstruct blood flow in the coronary arteries. **Atherosclerosis** (a common arterial disorder characterized by yellowish plaques of cholesterol, lipids, and cellular debris in the inner layers of the walls of large and medium-sized arteries) is the primary cause of ASHD. The *lumen* (a cavity or channel within any organ of the body) of the vessel narrows as the disease progresses. Blood flow to the heart is obstructed when this process occurs in the coronary arteries.

Atherosclerosis, the basic underlying disease affecting coronary lumen size, is characterized by changes in the intimal lining (the innermost layer) of the arteries. The severity of the disease is measured by the degree of obstruction within each artery and by the number of vessels involved. Obstructions exceeding 75% of the lumen of one or more of the three coronary arteries increase the risk of death.

The basic physiologic changes of the atherosclerotic process result in problems with myocardial oxygen supply and demand. When the myocardial oxygen demand exceeds the supply delivered by the coronary arteries, ischemia results (Fig. 48.10). The artery walls also become less elastic and less responsive to blood flow (see the Cultural Considerations box).

ANGINA PECTORIS

Etiology and Pathophysiology

Angina means a spasmodic, cramplike, choking feeling. *Pectoris* refers to the breast or chest area. **Angina pectoris** refers to the paroxysmal (severe, usually episodic) thoracic pain and choking feeling caused by decreased oxygen flow to or lack of oxygen (anoxia) of the myocardium.

Angina pectoris occurs when the cardiac muscle is deprived of oxygen. Atherosclerosis of the coronary arteries is the most common cause. The narrowed lumina

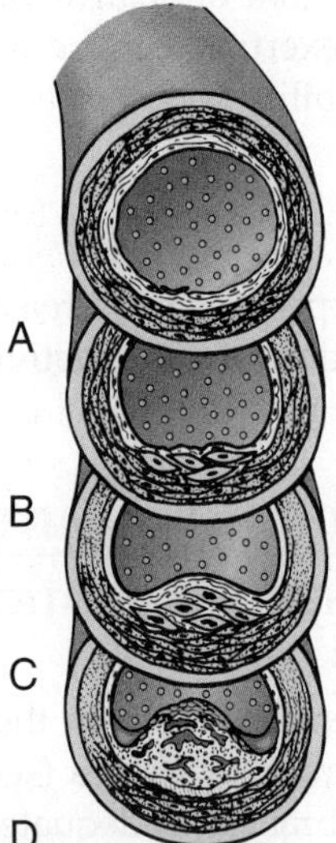

Fig. 48.10 Progressive development of coronary atherosclerosis. A, Injury to intimal wall. B, Lipoprotein invasion of smooth muscle cells. C, Development of fatty streak and fibrous plaque. D, Development of complicated lesion. (From Black JM, Hawks JH: *Medical-surgical nursing: Clinical management for positive outcomes*, ed 8, St. Louis, 2009, Mosby.)

of the coronary arteries are unable to deliver enough oxygen-rich blood to the myocardium. When the myocardial oxygen demand exceeds the supply, **ischemia** (decreased blood supply to a body organ or part, often marked by pain and organ dysfunction) of the heart muscle occurs, resulting in chest pain or angina. Typically angina occurs with an increased cardiac workload brought on by exposure to intense cold, exercise, unusually heavy meals, emotional stress, or any other strenuous activity.

CAD is the number one killer in the United States. Many people who die from the disease, however, experience several episodes of unstable angina first. If unstable angina were diagnosed accurately and promptly managed, many deaths and much of the disability associated with CAD could be avoided.

Cultural Considerations

Cardiovascular Disorder

- White, middle-aged men have the highest incidence of coronary artery disease (CAD).
- African Americans and Hispanics have a higher incidence of hypertension than do white Americans.
- African Americans have an early age of onset of CAD.
- African American women have a higher incidence of CAD than do white American women.
- Native Americans younger than 35 years of age have a heart disease mortality rate twice as high as that of other Americans.
- Hispanics have a lower death rate from heart disease than do non-Hispanics.
- Major modifiable cardiovascular risk factors for Native Americans are obesity and diabetes mellitus.

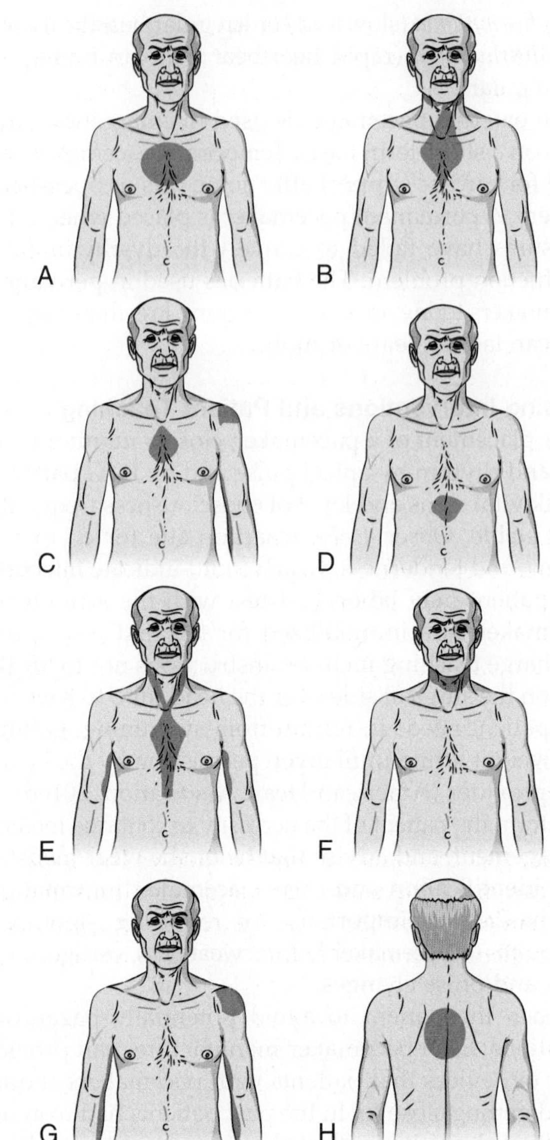

Fig. 48.11 Sites to which ischemic myocardial pain may be referred. A, Upper chest. B, Beneath sternum, radiating to neck and jaw. C, Beneath sternum, radiating down left arm. D, Epigastric. E, Epigastric, radiating to neck, jaw, and arms. F, Neck and jaw. G, Left shoulder and inner aspect of both arms. H, Intrascapular.

Unstable angina is defined as an unpredictable and transient episode of severe and prolonged discomfort that appears at rest, has never been experienced before, or is considerably worse than previous episodes. It mimics an MI in that the discomfort it causes often is described as tightness or a crushing sensation in the chest, arms, back, neck, or jaw. For some patients, unstable angina is a red flag that an MI will occur.

Clinical Manifestations

Pain is the outstanding characteristic of angina pectoris (Fig. 48.11). The patient usually describes the pain as a heaviness or tightness of the chest. At times it is thought to be indigestion. The pain is often substernal (below the sternum) or retrosternal (behind the sternum). Pain may radiate to other sites, or it may occur in only one site. The pain often radiates down the left inner arm to the little finger and also upward to the shoulder and jaw. Patients may also describe it as a pressure or a squeezing sensation, but usually not as a sharp pain. Sometimes a patient experiences posterior thoracic or jaw pain only. The chest pain may be accompanied by other signs and symptoms such as dyspnea, anxiety, apprehension, diaphoresis, and nausea. Symptoms of CAD in women vary and may be more subtle or generalized than in men. Women often report heaviness, squeezing, or pain in the left side of the chest, or pain in the abdomen, arm, mid-back, or scapular region. Women may also complain of palpitations and chest discomfort during rest, during sleep, or with exertion (American Heart Association, 2015).

The signs and symptoms of angina are often similar to those of MI. Anginal pain is believed to be caused by a temporary lack of oxygen and blood supply to the heart. It is often relieved by rest or medication such as nitroglycerin, which dilates the coronary arteries and increases the flow of oxygenated blood to the myocardium. Nitroglycerin administered sublingually usually relieves angina symptoms but does not relieve the pain from an MI. This is often used as a preliminary diagnostic tool to quickly differentiate angina from an MI.

Diabetes can cause damage to nerves (neuropathy) that can make the usual signs and symptoms of chest pain harder to detect because of the decrease in sensation. The patient with neuropathy may have no pain with an MI. Patients with diabetes may experience chest discomfort, sweating, shortness of breath, or nausea and/or vomiting during an MI. These symptoms should be treated as a medical emergency.

Assessment

Subjective data include the patient's statements regarding the location, intensity, radiation, and duration of pain. The patient may express a feeling of impending death. Assess precipitating factors that led to the development of symptoms. Determine what relief measures have been used. Identify whether the symptoms have changed in frequency or severity, indicating a worsening of the ischemia.

Collection of objective data includes noting the patient's behavior, such as rubbing the left arm or pressing a fist against the sternum. Monitor vital signs and note changes or abnormalities. Increases in pulse rate, blood pressure, and respiratory rate may be noted. Identify the presence of diaphoresis or anxiety.

Diagnostic Tests

The diagnosis of angina pectoris frequently is based on the patient's history. The ECG may reveal ischemia and rhythm changes. Holter monitoring correlates activity with precipitating factors. The exercise stress test determines ischemic changes in a controlled environment. Thallium-201 scanning and PET are used to diagnose ischemic heart disease. Coronary angiography may be done to determine the extent of CAD.

Medical Management

The focus of medical management is to control symptoms by reducing cardiac ischemia. Cardiovascular risk factors are identified and corrected if possible. Precipitating factors—such as exposure to intense cold, strenuous exercise, smoking, heavy meals, and emotional stress—are identified and avoided. Anti–platelet aggregation therapy is a first-line treatment of angina. Aspirin (acetylsalicylic acid, ASA) is the drug of choice. Taking low-dose aspirin is reasonable for adults, who are at increased risk of cardiovascular disease. The American Heart Association recommends that men older than age 50 and women older than age 60 who have more than one cardiovascular risk factor take low-dose aspirin (American Heart Association, 2018a). Risk calculations are aimed at people who have greater risk factors and are more likely to develop heart disease. For example, people who have a cholesterol level of 300 and smoke are at an increased risk of developing heart disease compared with someone who has a cholesterol level of 240 and does not smoke. Low-dose aspirin is indicated for people who have a calculated 10-year CAD risk of more than 10% (Lin, 2016). Aspirin, even at low doses (81 mg), is effective in inhibiting platelet aggregation. Medications such as ticlopidine or clopidogrel (Plavix) may be given as antiplatelet therapy. Medication therapy to dilate coronary arteries and decrease the workload of the heart consists of vasodilators (nitrates, especially nitroglycerin); beta-adrenergic blocking agents such as propranolol, metoprolol (Lopressor), nadolol (Corgard), atenolol (Tenormin), and timolol; and calcium channel blockers such as nifedipine (Procardia), verapamil, diltiazem, and nicardipine (Cardene). Give nitroglycerin sublingually for angina. Repeat the dose in 5 minutes if pain does not subside. Repeat two or three times at 5-minute intervals. Call the health care provider if pain has not subsided after a third nitroglycerin tablet. High-risk patients with unstable angina should be given supplemental oxygen.

Surgical interventions. *Coronary artery bypass graft:* Surgical management of the patient with ASHD or CAD may consist of performing a coronary artery bypass graft (CABG) after diagnosis by cardiac catheterization. Any number of grafts can be done, depending on the areas of occlusion in the coronary arteries. Blood flows to the myocardium through the grafts, which bypass the occluded coronary arteries. The grafts usually are taken from sections of the saphenous veins in the legs, or the internal mammary (breast) artery is used.

When the saphenous vein is used for the graft, one end is sutured to the aorta and the other end is sutured to the coronary artery distal to the occlusion. When an internal mammary artery is used, the distal end of this vessel is freed from the anterior chest wall and sutured

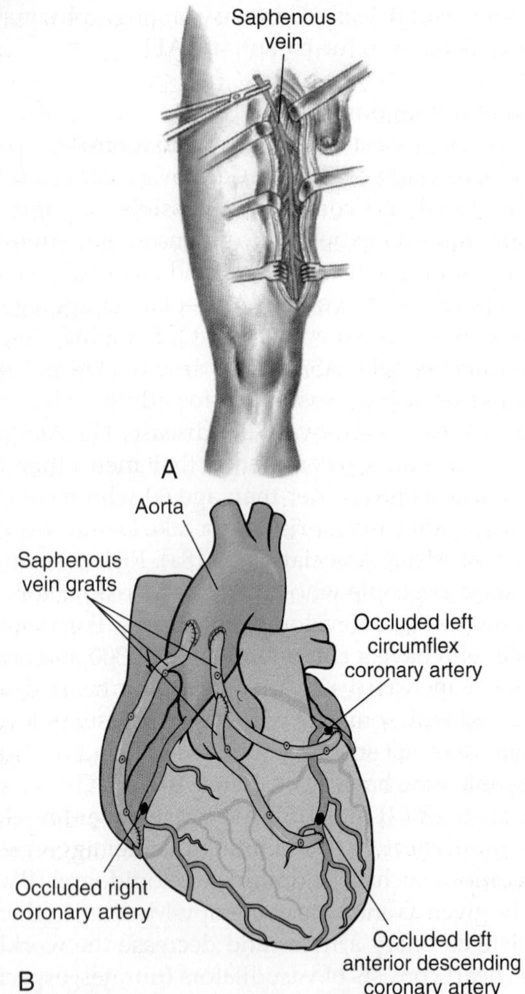

Fig. 48.12 A, Saphenous vein. B, Saphenous vein aortocoronary bypass or revascularization involves taking a piece of saphenous vein from the leg and creating a conduit for blood from the aorta to the area below the blockage in the coronary artery. A triple bypass is illustrated. (A, From Urden LD, Stacy KM, Lough ME: *Thelan's critical care nursing: Diagnosis and management,* ed 5, St. Louis, 2006, Mosby. B, From Lewis SL, Heitkemper MM, Dirksen SR, et al: *Medical-surgical nursing: Assessment and management of clinical problems,* ed 7, St. Louis, 2007, Mosby.)

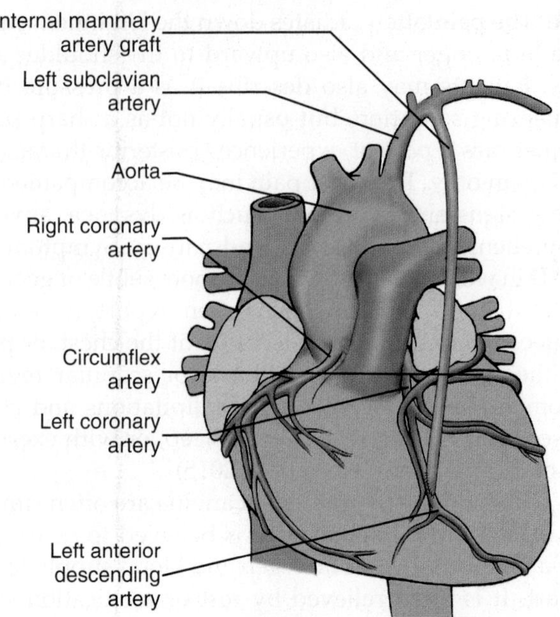

Fig. 48.13 Coronary artery bypass graft. Internal mammary artery is used; the distal end of this vessel is freed from the anterior chest wall and sutured in place distal to the occlusion in the coronary artery. (From Monahan FD, Sands JK, Neighbors M, et al: *Phipps' medical-surgical nursing: Health and illness perspectives,* ed 8, St. Louis, 2007, Mosby.)

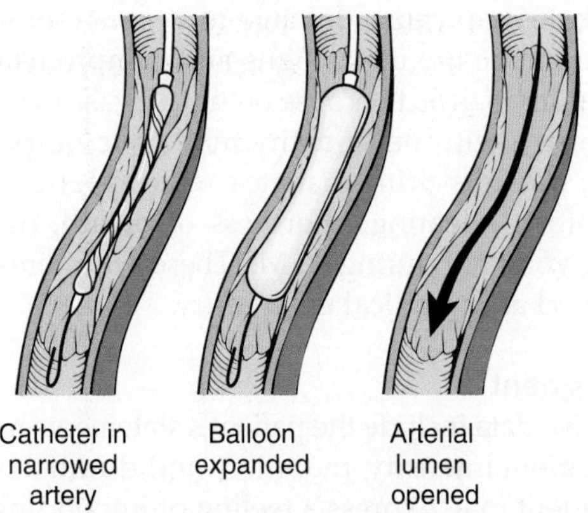

Fig. 48.14 Percutaneous transluminal coronary angioplasty (PTCA). (From Frazier MS, Drzymkowski JW: *Essentials of human diseases and conditions,* ed 5, St. Louis, 2013, Saunders.)

in place distal to the occlusion in the coronary artery. Internal mammary arteries are the preferred blood vessels for bypass surgery. A typical procedure involves one or two mammary arteries and saphenous vein grafts. Internal mammary arteries usually last more than 15 years, whereas saphenous vein grafts last an average of 5 to 10 years. Researchers continue to search for alternative blood vessels for CABG surgery (Figs. 48.12 and 48.13).

Percutaneous transluminal coronary angioplasty. Percutaneous transluminal coronary angioplasty (PTCA) is a surgical procedure for management of the patient with CAD. PTCA is an invasive procedure performed in the cardiac catheterization laboratory. In an *angioplasty,* the narrowing in a coronary artery is widened without open-heart surgery. *Percutaneous* indicates that the procedure is performed through the skin; *transluminal* means that it is done within the lumen of the artery. Patients undergoing PTCA are required to sign an informed consent form allowing CABG surgery, because of the possibility of complications developing during the procedure that would require immediate surgical intervention. Fluoroscopy is used to guide a catheter from the femoral or brachial artery to the coronary arteries to be treated. A balloon catheter is inflated once it is positioned (Fig. 48.14). The outward push of the balloon against the narrowed wall of the coronary artery reduces the constriction until it no longer interferes with blood flow to the heart muscle. Vessel patency (i.e., the state of being open, rather than blocked) is reestablished by angioplasty. This procedure may take 1 to 2 hours, with the patient usually awake but mildly sedated.

Postprocedure nursing interventions are to monitor the patient continually, as with any surgical recovery. Observe the area of catheter insertion for hemorrhage potential. Monitor the patient in the cardiac care unit, usually for 1 day before dismissal to the medical-surgical unit. The total hospitalization stay is 1 to 3 days compared with the 4- to 6-day stay after open heart surgery with a CABG; thus PTCA reduces hospital costs. Patients return to work rapidly (approximately 5 to 7 days after PTCA) rather than requiring the 2- to 8-week convalescence common after CABG.

Stent placement. Stents are used to treat abrupt or threatened vessel closure after PTCA. Stents are expandable, meshlike structures designed to maintain vessel patency by compressing plaque against the arterial walls and resisting vasoconstriction. Stents are placed carefully at the angioplasty site to hold the vessel open. Stents are thrombogenic and require the patient to take anticoagulants for at least 3 months. The primary complications from stent placement are hemorrhage and vascular injury. Less common complications are stent thrombosis, acute MI, emergency CABG, and coronary spasms. The possibility of dysrhythmias is always present.

Nursing Interventions and Patient Teaching

Nursing interventions are based on the patient's individual needs. They focus on achievement of five major patient outcomes.

1. *Ensure comfort.* Reduce or remove any known factors that are contributing to increased pain. Assess for causes of decreased pain tolerance, such as anxiety, fatigue, or lack of knowledge. Fatigue from increased oxygen demands with a decreased oxygen supply increases pain perception. Promote measures to reduce fatigue, such as providing rest periods. Provide a calm environment to decrease stress and anxiety. Administer sublingual vasodilators, such as nitroglycerin, as ordered. Administer oxygen for high-risk patients with unstable angina and those with cyanosis or respiratory distress.
2. *Promote tissue perfusion.* Instruct the patient to avoid becoming overly fatigued and to stop activity immediately in the presence of chest pain, dyspnea, syncope, or vertigo, which indicate low tissue perfusion.
3. *Encourage activity and rest.* Increase the patient's activity tolerance by encouraging slower activity or shorter periods of activity with more rest periods. Most people with angina pectoris are able to tolerate mild exercise such as walking or playing golf, but exertion such as running or climbing stairs rapidly causes pain. Nitroglycerin may be used prophylactically to prevent pain from strenuous activities. Isosorbide mononitrate and isosorbide dinitrate (Isordil) are nitrates used for acute treatment of angina attacks (sublingual only) or orally for prophylactic management of angina pectoris. Anginal pain occurs more easily in cold weather. The key is to avoid overexertion.
4. *Reduce anxiety and promote feelings of well-being.* Help the patient reduce the level of anxiety. The patient should minimize emotional outbursts, worry, and tension. People with angina may need continuing help in accepting situations. Supportive family members, a spiritual adviser, business associates, and friends can sometimes be of assistance. Relaxation techniques and music therapy may be beneficial. Peer support groups and behavioral change programs are available. An optimistic outlook helps to relieve the work of the heart. Many people who learn to live within their limitations live out their expected lifespan despite the disease.
5. *Provide education to the patient and the family.* Delay teaching until the patient is ready (see the Communication box). The patient needs to be relatively free of pain and anxiety to learn. Promote a positive attitude and active participation of patient and family to encourage compliance. The teaching plan should include information on medications, ways to minimize the events that trigger angina pectoris, effects of exercise on reduction of myocardial oxygen needs, the need to stop smoking because of the vasoconstriction of nicotine, and the need for regular medical follow-up (see the Patient Teaching box).

Patient problems and interventions for the patient with angina pectoris include but are not limited to the following:

Patient Problem	Nursing Interventions
Discomfort, related to myocardial ischemia	Administer oxygen as ordered Administer prescribed nitroglycerin. Repeat q 5 min, three times. If pain is unrelieved, notify health care provider Monitor blood pressure and pulse before and after administration of nitroglycerin Promote rest Maintain diet as ordered; if chest pain occurs while eating or immediately after, advise small meals rather than two or three large meals Balance rest with activity Instruct patient to stop activity at the first sign of chest pain or other symptoms of cardiac ischemia
Compromised Blood Flow to Cardiac Tissue, related to narrowing of coronary arteries	Administer prescribed oxygen Instruct patient that nitroglycerin may need to be taken before exercise and sexual activity to prevent cardiac ischemia Encourage less strenuous or shorter periods of activity interspersed with rest Avoid exercise in cold weather Take prescribed nitroglycerin before activities that will increase the workload of the heart

 Communication

Methods to Decrease Angina Pectoris Attacks

Mrs. M., a patient with angina, has been admitted for further care, diagnosis, and treatment. After the initial nursing assessment, the nurse interviews the patient about the course of her anginal episodes. With the data gathered, the nurse participates in the development of a program to educate Mrs. M. how to minimize or control the attacks.

Nurse: I would like to ask you some questions about the anginal pain you are experiencing.

Patient: I already told the doctor about those attacks when I visited his office. Her nurse has all those records.

Nurse: Your health care provider asked us to help you plan a program for preventing or minimizing these attacks. With the information we gather, we can set goals for your care. We can also identify how angina relates to some of your activities.

Patient: OK, I would like to understand it better. Perhaps I would be less frightened when it happens. My friend told me about her aunt who had angina—she died. That really worries me.

Nurse: We hope to decrease some of your fears by helping you understand. First, when do your attacks usually occur?

Patient: Oh, mostly after a really busy day, you know—shopping or gardening or housecleaning. But a few times I had problems after my sister-in-law visited. She and my husband always seem to get into upsetting discussions. They never got along well. She upsets us both—she criticizes everything!

Nurse: Have you noticed if a big meal is related to the pain?

Patient: No, not really … well, only when my sister-in-law is there. We hardly ever eat big meals anymore, except when she comes. She expects to be fed well. My husband and I have cut down a lot. Big meals upset our systems—and then her, that harping on old problems, and how she thinks we should run our lives! She upsets me so!

Nurse: Mrs. M., I think we should talk about how to handle stressful situations like visits from your sister-in-law. But first, could you describe the pain for me? Does it come on suddenly? How long does it last? What does it feel like?

Patient: Oh, no, not all of a sudden. It is just dull at times, like an upset stomach. But then, it travels up in my chest and gets really heavy, like pressure. Sometimes it makes my face and teeth hurt … and my arm, too—this one [left]—all the way down to my little finger. If it's a really bad attack, I sometimes feel like I am going to vomit.

Nurse: On a scale of 0 to 10, how would you rate most of your angina attacks?

Patient: Probably 5 to 6 would be the average, but sometimes it's a 10.

Nurse: Does your heart beat faster?

Patient: Oh, yes, and I just have to sit down and be quiet or I can't catch my breath. That's when I take the nitroglycerin. I carry it with me all the time now, in this special little container.

Nurse: I see. And how long does it take for the pain to stop after you take the medicine?

Patient: I used to think it took forever, but my husband—he times it for me—says it lasts about 15 to 20 minutes. I relax a little, and it passes.

Nurse: What about the weather? Have you noticed that it affects your attacks in any way?

Patient: I don't know if it is all those clothes or the weather, but I get more pains if I get out in the cold.

Nurse: Do you or your husband smoke?

Patient: Not anymore. I gave up cigarettes when this angina started on me. I noticed the difference, too. Now I can't even stay in a room if people are smoking. I also cut down on coffee when I retired. My doctor said that too much caffeine isn't good for my heart. All the good things, they have to go when you get old!

Nurse: Maybe with some understanding of how certain activities and other factors affect your condition, you can find new "good things" that you'll enjoy just as much. We'll talk again soon. There are some effective coping methods we can explore to decrease your stress when your sister-in-law visits.

Prognosis

The prognosis for the patient with angina pectoris may be grave. Attacks may be intermittent. The patient with diabetes who also has coronary artery disease may have the highest risk of all. A patient with diabetes may have nerve damage, making the normal warning signs of an MI more difficult to detect. Early management of the patient with diabetes includes teaching lifestyle changes as well as how to recognize the signs and symptoms of an MI. The mortality rate can be reduced with early and aggressive management of angina.

MYOCARDIAL INFARCTION

Etiology and Pathophysiology

A **myocardial infarction (MI),** or *heart attack,* is the necrosis (death) of heart muscle. It is caused by obstruction of a major coronary artery or one of its branches, either by an atherosclerotic plaque or by an **embolus** (a foreign object, a quantity of air or gas, a bit of tissue, or a piece of a thrombus that circulates in the bloodstream until it becomes lodged in a vessel). The obstruction leads to tissue ischemia (oxygen deprivation) because of the lack of blood supply. An occlusion can occur anywhere

Patient Teaching

Angina Pectoris

USING NITRATE MEDICATIONS

- Use nitroglycerin prophylactically to avoid pain known to occur with certain activities.
- A burning sensation on the tongue indicates nitroglycerin is activated.
- A throbbing sensation in the head and flushing may occur.
- When changing to a sitting or standing position, do it slowly after taking nitroglycerin. Postural hypotension is a side effect of nitroglycerin.
- Place a nitroglycerin tablet under the tongue at the onset of anginal pain; a second tablet can be taken after 5 minutes and a third tablet after another 5 minutes if pain is unrelieved.
- Call the health care provider if pain does not subside after the third nitroglycerin tablet; go to the nearest emergency department; do not drive yourself.
- Always carry nitroglycerin on your person.
- Store nitroglycerin in a dark bottle and keep it in a dry place.
- Replenish nitroglycerin supply every 6 months or before the expiration date.
- Remove all old nitrate ointment before application of new cream.
- Place nitroglycerin patches on skin in the morning and remove at bedtime. This prevents development of tolerance and maintains effectiveness.

MINIMIZING PRECIPITATING EVENTS

- Use caution when taking medications for erectile dysfunction. Nitrate medications may result in severe hypotension.
- Avoid overexertion. Take nitroglycerin before exercise.
- Try to reduce stress and anxiety, which cause blood vessels to constrict.
- Avoid overeating because it places an increased workload on the heart.
- Avoid cold weather (constricts coronary vessels to conserve body heat; hence anginal pain can develop more easily).
- Dress warmly in cold weather.
- Avoid hot, humid conditions (increases workload on the heart).
- Avoid walking uphill, in the cold, or against strong wind, because these activities increase the workload on the heart.
- Discontinue smoking. Nicotine causes vasoconstriction of the arteries.

EXERCISING TO REDUCE MYOCARDIAL OXYGEN NEEDS

- Engage in a regular exercise program, such as a walking program or yoga, to improve collateral circulation.
- Exercise conditions the heart muscle and can decrease oxygen demand during exertion.
- Space exercise period with rest periods.
- Take nitroglycerin before exertion.

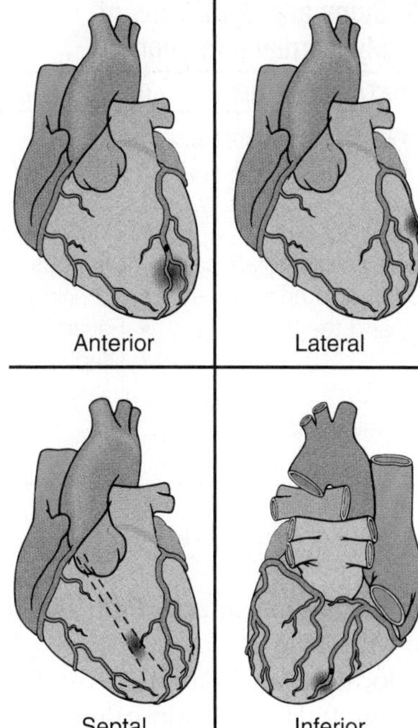

Fig. 48.15 Four common locations where myocardial infarctions occur. (From Lewis SL, Heitkemper MM, Dirksen SR, et al: *Medical-surgical nursing: Assessment and management of clinical problems,* ed 7, St. Louis, 2007, Mosby.)

in the body; **coronary occlusion** refers specifically to the obstruction or closing off of a coronary artery. Eighty to 90% of all acute MIs are the result of thrombus formation (USDDHS, n.d.), also called *coronary thrombosis.* Myocardial ischemia lasting more than 35 to 45 minutes produces cellular damage and necrosis. These conditions impair the ability of the cardiac muscle to contract and pump blood. The extent of damage to the surrounding tissues depends on the ability of the heart to develop collateral circulation. *Collateral circulation* is the development of new vessels in the heart that compensate for the loss of circulation from the occluded artery. The location of the occlusion and the extent of tissue damage affect the patient's response to the injury (Fig. 48.15).

The body's response to cell injury is inflammation. Within 24 hours leukocytes infiltrate the area in response to chemicals released by the injured cardiac cells. (Note: Dying cardiac cells also release enzymes that are important diagnostic indicators; see the sections "Laboratory Tests" [earlier] and "Diagnostic Tests" [later] for a discussion on serum cardiac markers.) Phagocytes (neutrophils and monocytes)—a kind of leukocyte—clear the necrotic debris from the injured area, and by 6 weeks after an MI, scar tissue has replaced the necrotic tissue.

Clinical Manifestations

Sometimes an asymptomatic MI or *silent MI* may occur. Many symptoms of MI are associated with irreversible ischemia, but they are similar to those of angina pectoris. In an MI, the symptoms are more severe and last longer

Table 48.2 Signs and Symptoms of Myocardial Infarction

SUBJECTIVE DATA (SYMPTOMS)	OBJECTIVE DATA (SIGNS)
• Heavy pressure or squeezing in center of chest behind sternum • Pain, retrosternal and in heart region, often radiating down the left arm and to the neck, jaw, and teeth • Anxiety • Dyspnea • Weakness, faintness • Nausea	• Pallor • Erratic behavior • Hypotension, shock • Cardiac rhythm changes • Vomiting • Fever • Diaphoresis

than during an angina attack. Pain is the foremost symptom of MI (Table 48.2).

The pain location and radiation to other sites are depicted in Fig. 48.11. The pain often is described as crushing or viselike, an oppressive sensation as though a heavy object is sitting on the chest. The pain is retrosternal (behind the sternum) and in the heart region. In men, it often radiates down the left arm and to the neck, jaws, teeth, and epigastric area. It may occur suddenly, or it may build up over a few minutes. It may occur in conjunction with intense emotion, during exertion, or at rest. The pain is prolonged and more intense than anginal pain. It lasts 30 minutes to several hours or longer. It is not relieved by changes in body position, nitroglycerin, or rest. Health care providers often tell patients who call complaining of chest pain to take an aspirin (chewable if they have it) and report to the hospital emergency department. Other signs and symptoms that may occur with the pain include nausea, dyspnea, dizziness, weakness, diaphoresis, pallor, ashen color, and a sense of impending doom. Early signs and symptoms of an acute MI in women are unusual fatigue, sleep disturbances, shortness of breath, weakness, indigestion, and anxiety. Often, acute chest pain is not present in women, causing health care providers to fail to identify an MI. The health care provider may begin testing for other disorders such as gallbladder disease or anxiety. Table 48.3 provides a comparison of signs and symptoms and the medical management of angina pectoris and MI.

Table 48.3 Coronary Artery Disorders

SIGNS AND SYMPTOMS	MEDICAL MANAGEMENT
Angina Pectoris	
Chest pain (substernal, retrosternal), may radiate to neck, jaw, left arm, and shoulder; great anxiety, fear of approaching death; face pale, ashen; pulse variable, usually tense and quick; blood pressure elevated during an attack; usually brought on by exertion, emotional upsets; relieved by rest, nitroglycerin	• Avoidance of precipitating factors • Reduction of modifiable risk factors • Medications: Nitrates, beta blockers, calcium channel blockers • Oxygen therapy • ECG monitoring • Aspirin for unstable angina
Myocardial Infarction	
Severe, crushing chest pain; prolonged heavy pressure or squeezing pain in center of chest; may spread to shoulder, neck, arm, fourth and fifth fingers on left hand, teeth, and jaw; may radiate as with angina; not relieved with rest or nitroglycerin; may be associated with dyspnea, diaphoresis, apprehension, nausea, and vomiting; signs and symptoms of cardiogenic shock may develop; the pain is prolonged and more intense than anginal pain In women, these classic symptoms are far less common; most frequent early warning symptoms are unusual fatigue, sleep disturbances, shortness of breath, weakness, indigestion, and anxiety; in one study, only 30% of women reported chest pain, and acute chest pain was absent in 43%	• Relief of pain (oxygen), morphine, and other analgesics • ECG monitoring • Thrombolytic therapy to dissolve clot • Reduction of oxygen demand (rest) • Prevention of complications (through use of stool softeners, anticoagulants) • Treatment of complications (dysrhythmias, HF) • Anticoagulants to prevent further clotting

ECG, Electrocardiogram; *HF*, heart failure.

Assessment

Subjective data include the onset, location, quality, duration, and radiation of pain. The patient may complain of shortness of breath, dizziness, weakness, anxiety, fear, or unusual fatigue. Identify precipitating factors. Inquire about measures the patient has tried to relieve the pain.

Collection of objective data includes observation of the patient's behavior to detect apprehension and anxiety. Typical vital signs reveal hypotension, pulse abnormalities such as tachycardia or a barely perceptible pulse, and early temperature elevation. Note the presence of diaphoresis; vomiting; ashen color; cool, clammy skin; labored respirations; and cardiac dysrhythmias. If possible, find out about risk factors. A respiratory assessment also is necessary.

Diagnostic Tests

Diagnostic tests are used to confirm the diagnosis of MI. Serum tests are obtained initially. Serum cardiac markers (e.g., CK-MB, myoglobin) are released into the vascular system when infarcted myocardial muscle cells die. A sensitive cardiac marker present in serum, called *troponin I*, has proven useful in detecting ischemic myocardial injury. Troponin I is cardiac specific and therefore a highly specific indicator of an MI. (See the section "Laboratory Tests," earlier, for a discussion on serum cardiac markers.) An elevated white blood cell count of 12,000 to 15,000/mm^3 is associated with severe infarcts. The increase begins a few hours after the onset of pain and lasts for 3 to 7 days. The ESR rises during the first week and may remain elevated for several weeks.

Twelve-lead ECG findings that support the diagnosis of MI include ST-segment elevation and the development of Q waves. An acute MI caused by complete interruption of blood flow that causes ST elevation, is referred to as a STEMI. The elevation is shown on the ECG and the management is different from that of a non–ST-elevation MI. STEMI MI causes more deaths. In time the ST segment returns to normal and the T wave inverts. These ECG changes are important in confirming the diagnosis of MI. ECG findings are significantly different for men and women. A woman experiencing an MI is far less likely than a man to have concurrent ST-segment elevation, resulting in misdiagnosis and failure to receive the correct treatment. A chest x-ray is performed to note size and configuration of the heart. More complex tests occasionally are done, including cardiac fluoroscopy, myocardial imaging (thallium scan), echocardiogram, PET, and multigated acquisition (MUGA) scanning. These tests may be done in conjunction with other tests to diagnose MI and determine the severity of CAD.

Medical Management

Medical management focuses on preventing further tissue injury and limiting the size of the infarction. It is extremely important that a patient with a suspected MI be diagnosed rapidly and treated to preserve cardiac muscle. Intervention is designed to restore cardiac tissue perfusion and reduce the workload of the heart. Promoting tissue oxygenation, relieving pain, preventing complications, improving tissue perfusion, and preventing further tissue damage are important medical considerations.

Medications such as morphine and diazepam (Valium) are used to alleviate pain and anxiety. A continuous IV infusion of amiodarone may be given to the patient who has frequent PVCs, which may precede ventricular fibrillation. Prophylactic lidocaine is not recommended by the American College of Cardiology practice guidelines for the treatment of acute MI. Lidocaine may be a treatment option for the patient who has sustained VT or ventricular fibrillation. The use of beta-adrenergic blockers such as atenolol, metoprolol, propranolol, nadolol, and carvedilol (Coreg) early in the acute phase of an MI and during a 1-year follow-up regimen can decrease morbidity and mortality. Angiotensin-converting enzyme (ACE) inhibitors may be used after MIs. Their use can help to prevent or slow the progression of HF (Table 48.4). Calcium channel blockers or longer-acting nitrates can be added if the patient is already on adequate doses of beta-adrenergic blockers or cannot tolerate beta-adrenergic blockers. Examples of calcium channel blockers are amlodipine (Norvasc), diltiazem, nifedipine, and verapamil. An example of a long-acting nitrate is isosorbide dinitrate. Oxygen is prescribed to facilitate cardiac tissue perfusion. Attention is given to respiratory difficulties, fluid overload, and cardiac dysrhythmias.

Medical therapy also is directed toward limiting the size and extent of injury by attempting to reperfuse (reinstitute blood flow to) the occluded coronary artery. Fibrinolytic agents such as streptokinase (Streptase), anistreplase, and a tissue plasminogen activator (tPA) such as alteplase currently are used to attempt reperfusion. Thrombolytic therapy is the standard practice in the treatment of acute MI. Thrombolytics salvage heart muscle by minimizing infarct size and maximizing heart function. They lyse (decompose or dissolve) the clot in the occluded coronary artery, reopening the vessel and allowing perfusion of the heart muscle.

The adage "Time is muscle" highlights the need for fast action and prompt treatment to restore myocardial blood flow, limit infarct size, preserve heart tissue, and improve the patient's chance of survival and recovery. To be effective, reperfusion must occur 3 to 5 hours after the onset of symptoms. Myocardial cells do not die instantly. In most patients, it takes approximately 4 to 6 hours for the entire thickness of the muscle to become necrosed. Mortality and infarction size can be reduced significantly if thrombolytic therapy starts within 30 to 60 minutes of symptom onset. Before a thrombolytic is administered, obtain a thorough history. Thrombolytics are not used for patients with active internal bleeding, suspected aortic dissecting aneurysm, recent head trauma, history of hemorrhagic stroke within the past year, or surgery within the past 10 days.

PTCA may be used instead of thrombolytic therapy as a primary treatment in some cases. This involves advancing a balloon-tipped catheter into the lumen of the obstructed coronary artery. The balloon is inflated intermittently to dilate the artery and improve blood flow (see Fig. 48.14). Along with balloon compression, stents may be used to prevent acute closure and restenosis (i.e., repeat narrowing of the blood vessel).

CABG surgery may be considered for patients with multiple vessel disease and when less invasive interventions, such as thrombolysis and PTCA, have failed (see Figs. 48.12 and 48.13).

Complications commonly associated with MI include ventricular fibrillation, cardiogenic shock (Box 48.2), HF, and dysrhythmias. Cardiogenic shock, often referred to as pump failure, is characterized by low cardiac output and peripheral vascular system collapse. Left ventricular function is severely decreased, resulting in an inadequate

Table 48.4 Medications for Myocardial Infarction

CLASSIFICATION	GENERIC NAME (TRADE NAME)	ACTION
Vasopressor	dopamine	Raises systemic arterial pressure and cardiac output
Anticoagulants	heparin warfarin (Coumadin)	Reduce incidence of clotting
Platelet aggregation inhibitor	ticlopidine aspirin (acetylsalicylic acid; ASA)	Decreases platelet release of thromboxane, so that vasoconstriction and platelet aggregation are decreased Decreases platelet aggregation
Analgesic	morphine	Controls pain; reduces myocardial oxygen demand
Tranquilizer	diazepam (Valium)	Decreases anxiety and restlessness
Thrombolytic agent	streptokinase (Streptase)	Thrombolytic (pertaining to dissolution of blood clots) agent used when acute MI symptoms have been present less than 6 h, preferably from 30 min to 1 h; restores blood flow and therefore limits infarct size in certain patients
Tissue plasminogen activator	alteplase (Activase, recombinant)	Dissolves blood clots and reduces blood viscosity
Nitrates	nitroglycerin isosorbide atenolol (Tenormin)	Dilate blood vessels by reducing coronary artery spasm, increase coronary artery blood supply, and decrease oxygen demands
Beta-adrenergic blockers	propranolol (Inderal) nadolol (Corgard) metoprolol (Lopressor) carvedilol (Coreg)	Block beta-adrenergic stimulation and decrease myocardial oxygen demands, thus decreasing myocardial damage; decrease mortality rate
Calcium channel blockers	nifedipine (Procardia) diltiazem (Cardizem) verapamil (Calan) amlodipine (Norvasc)	Dilate blood vessels, increase coronary artery blood supply, and decrease myocardial oxygen demands
Angiotensin-converting enzyme (ACE) inhibitors	captopril enalapril (Vasotec)	Can help prevent ventricular remodeling and prevent or slow the progression of HF Prevent conversion of angiotensin I to angiotensin II Decrease endothelial dysfunction
Salicylates	aspirin	Decrease platelet adhesion and thus decrease thrombosis formation
Antidysrhythmics	lidocaine (Xylocaine) IV	Treat ventricular dysrhythmias (rarely used except for ventricular tachycardia)
Stool softeners	docusate calcium (Surfak) docusate sodium (Colace)	Reduce straining at stool; prevent constipation produced by decreased mobility and use of constipating narcotics
Diuretics	furosemide (Lasix)	Control edema
Electrolyte replacement	potassium chloride (Slow-K)	May be necessary when diuretics are used
Inotropic agents	digoxin (Lanoxin) amrinone IV dobutamine	Increase the heart's pumping action (contractility) Indicated when left ventricle failure is present

HF, Heart failure; *IV*, intravenous; *MI*, myocardial infarction.

blood supply to the vital organs. Immediate detection and treatment are necessary to prevent irreversible shock and death. Cardiogenic shock proves fatal in 50% to 80% of cases. Other possible complications include ventricular aneurysm, pericarditis, and embolism.

Nursing Interventions and Patient Teaching

Administer oxygen per protocol or at 2 L/min for 24 to 48 hours or longer if pain, hypotension, dyspnea, or dysrhythmias persist. Administer medications as prescribed (see Table 48.4).

- Administer lipid-lowering agents such as simvastatin, atorvastatin (Lipitor), or rosuvastatin to prevent elevated cholesterol levels.
- Stool softener may be prescribed to prevent rectal straining. The Valsalva maneuver may cause severe changes in blood pressure and heart rate, which may trigger ischemia, dysrhythmias, or cardiac arrest.

Box 48.2 Cardiogenic Shock

CLINICAL MANIFESTATIONS	SIGNS AND SYMPTOMS	MEDICAL MANAGEMENT	NURSING INTERVENTIONS
Decreased cardiac output Myocardial ischemia Cerebral hypoxia Impaired tissue perfusion Decreased renal circulation Anaerobic metabolism with lactic acidosis Peripheral vascular system collapse Shock	Dysrhythmias, chest pain Anxiety, agitation, restlessness, disorientation Urinary output diminished or absent Lactic acid accumulation in blood Tachycardia, thready pulse, tachypnea Decreased blood pressure Narrowed pulse pressure[a] Cyanosis; cold, moist, pale, clammy skin Decreased peripheral pulses Capillary refill time decreased Hypoactive bowel sounds	Recognition and control of life-threatening signs and symptoms Oxygenation to promote tissue perfusion Parenteral fluid as a volume expander Drug therapy: • Vasopressors: Raise arterial blood pressure • Cardiac glycoside: Digoxin (Lanoxin) increases cardiac contraction (inotropic) and strengthens and corrects dysrhythmias • Adrenergic drugs: Dopamine at therapeutic levels increases cardiac output and blood pressure • Sodium bicarbonate: Combats lactic acidosis (given sparingly because it causes fluid retention)	Monitor vital signs q 5 min during acute stage and q 1 hr when stabilized Administer oxygen as ordered Maintain bed rest to reduce myocardial workload and increase oxygenation Monitor acid-base balance Monitor urinary output hourly to determine adequate kidney perfusion Allow nothing by mouth Initiate bed rest to minimize energy expenditure Administer medications as ordered Provide comfort measures

[a]Pulse pressure is based on blood pressure: It is the numeric difference between the systolic and diastolic blood pressure. For example, if the blood pressure is 100/70 mm Hg, the pulse pressure is 30.

To help the patient recovering from an MI minimize straining, offer the use of a bedside commode or nearby bathroom whenever possible. The patient may use the Valsalva maneuver when straining to pass stool. Teach mouth breathing to help decrease the severity of straining, which is contraindicated for the patient after an MI.

Instruct the patient to avoid excessive fatigue and to stop activity immediately when chest pain, dyspnea, or faintness occur. Plan nursing interventions to promote rest and minimize disturbances. Monitor the vital signs; document the rate and rhythm of the pulse.

The patient usually is placed on bed rest with commode privileges for 24 to 48 hours. Assist the patient with ADLs. During this period, sedation with diazepam or an equivalent may be prescribed to relieve anxiety and restlessness and to promote sleep. After the first 24 to 48 hours, encourage the patient to increase activity gradually, depending on the severity of the infarction. Continually monitor the patient for signs of dysrhythmias, cardiac pain, and changes in vital signs.

Food usually is withheld until the patient's condition becomes stable because the patient may need to undergo cardiac catheterization, PTCA, or a CABG procedure. A liquid diet progresses as tolerated to a regular diet with modifications. A low-fat, low-sodium, easily digested diet is desirable.

To prevent complications, antiembolic stockings are used. Continue to assess and report cardiac status, dyspneic condition, and pulse change (rate, rhythm, and volume).

During hospitalization, many patients experience denial, depression, and anxiety. Anxiety varies in intensity, depending on the severity of the perceived threat and the patient's success in coping.

Patient problems and interventions for the patient with an MI include but are not limited to the following:

Patient Problem	Nursing Interventions
Recent Onset of Chest Pain, related to myocardial ischemia	Assess original pain and location, duration, radiation, and onset of new symptoms Administer prescribed analgesics (usually morphine sulfate, which relieves pain, reduces anxiety, causes vasodilation of vascular smooth muscle, and reduces myocardial workload) Maintain bed rest and reduced patient activity Administer oxygen as prescribed Record patient's response to pain relief measures Employ alternative methods of pain relief Provide calm, restful environment

Continued

Patient Problem	Nursing Interventions
Insufficient Cardiac Output, related to conduction defects (dysrhythmias) and decreased myocardial pumping action	Assess and monitor vital signs q 4 hr Maintain bed rest with head of bed elevated 30 degrees for first 24–48 h to reduce myocardial oxygen demand Monitor IV feedings; infuse according to health care provider's order Administer prescribed medications such as antidysrhythmics, nitrates, and beta blockers Auscultate breath sounds and heart rate q 4 hr; increase activity level as prescribed Palpate for pedal pulses, assess capillary refill, auscultate bowel sounds, assess for pedal or dependent edema q 4 hr, and strictly monitor intake and output (I&O)

 Home Care Considerations

Exercise Program After Myocardial Infarction

- After discharge from the hospital, many patients are encouraged to begin a 2- to 12-week walking program. This is a structured program designed to have the patient walking 2 miles in less than 60 minutes by the end of 12 weeks.
- Encourage patients to work through this program at their own rate until they achieve a pace below a slow jog and their heart rate is below the prescribed rate set by the cardiologist.
- Not all patients are physiologically capable of participating in a rigorous exercise program after an MI.
- Eventually, most patients are encouraged to participate in a maintenance (lifetime), unsupervised, home-based exercise program designed specifically for them.
- Almost everyone can benefit from some type of cardiac rehabilitation.

Patients and their family members need to be reassured of recovery. More than 85% of patients with an uncomplicated MI return to work. Provide information on resuming sexual activities. The patient with an uncomplicated MI who is able to climb two flights of stairs without difficulty is usually able to resume sexual activities. Approximately 80% of all postcoronary patients resume sexual activity without serious risks. The other 20% need not abstain totally but should limit their sexual activity according to their cardiac capacity.

Cardiac rehabilitation. The health care provider may prescribe cardiac rehabilitation after an MI. Before discharge from the hospital, discuss how participation in a monitored exercise program and continuing education as part of outpatient cardiac rehabilitation help the patient recover faster and return to a full and productive life. Cardiac rehabilitation has two major parts:

1. Exercise training to teach the patient how to exercise safely, strengthen muscles, and improve stamina. The exercise plan is based on the individual's ability, needs, and interests.
2. Education, counseling, and training to help the patient understand his or her heart condition and find ways to reduce the risk of future heart problems. The cardiac rehabilitation team assists the patient in adjusting to a new lifestyle and dealing with fears about the future. Cardiac rehabilitation may last 6 weeks, 6 months, or longer. Cardiac rehabilitation has lifelong favorable effects (see the Home Care Considerations box and Health Promotion box).

Prognosis

Medical care must be instituted without delay. Many patients with an MI who are not treated before reaching the hospital die. The prognosis also depends on the area and extent of the damage and the presence or absence of complications.

HEART FAILURE

Etiology and Pathophysiology

When the heart cannot pump enough blood to sustain the body's metabolic needs, it is called heart failure or cardiac insufficiency. **Heart failure (HF)** traditionally is defined as circulatory congestion caused by the heart's inability to pump effectively. Many patients also have pulmonary or systemic congestion with HF, and the syndrome commonly was called *congestive heart failure (CHF)*. However, this term excludes patients who do not have congestion. HF is currently understood to be a neurohormonal problem that progresses because of the chronic release of substances such as catecholamines (epinephrine and norepinephrine). Epinephrine and norepinephrine are hormones of the sympathetic nervous system and they can produce harmful effects on the failing heart and circulatory system.

Circulatory congestion and compensatory mechanisms may occur. HF may develop after an MI, in response to prolonged hypertension or diabetes mellitus, or in relation to valvular or inflammatory heart disease. Other factors associated with HF include infection, stress, hyperthyroidism, anemia, and fluid replacement therapy. HF is the most common diagnosis for the hospitalized patient over 65 years of age. It affects about 5.7 million Americans and accounts for more than 200,000 deaths annually (CDC, 2016b). The increasing prevalence and incidence of HF result from people (1) living longer and (2) being more likely to survive cardiovascular disease.

According to the American Heart Association the most commonly used classification system for HF is

 Health Promotion

Myocardial Infarction

Teach the patient the following:

- The effects of MI, the healing process, and the treatment regimen.
- The effects of medications used to treat MI.
- The association between risk factors and coronary artery disease (CAD).
- How to identify nonmodifiable risk factors.
- How to identify modifiable risk factors (particularly cigarette smoking and stress). The patient should stop smoking and encourage family and significant others to stop.
- The effect of dietary restrictions on atherosclerotic heart disease or CAD. Recommended daily intake is 2 g of sodium, 1500 calories, low cholesterol, and fluid restrictions.
- To limit total fat intake to 25% to 35% of total calories each day. Limit intake of saturated fats to less than 7% of total fat intake. Saturated fats (e.g., shortening, lard, or butter) are solid at room temperature; better sources of fat include vegetable, olive, and fish oils.
- To avoid foods high in sodium, saturated fats, and triglycerides. Review alternative ways of seasoning foods to avoid cooking with salt. Explain the need to limit intake of eggs, cream, butter, and foods high in animal fat. Teach the patient and family how to read labels on foods.
- To eat 20 to 30 g of soluble fiber every day. Foods such as bran, beans, and peas help lower bad cholesterol (low-density lipoprotein).
- The effect of activity on the heart and the need to participate in a progressive activity plan.
- Refer the patient to social support groups as indicated.
- Stress the importance of participating in cardiac rehabilitation services.
- Explain cardiac warning symptoms. Patients and their partners are often unsure which symptoms should be reported. If nitroglycerin has been prescribed, advise the patient to take it when experiencing chest pain and to notify the health care provider if the pain is not relieved within 15 minutes. Other signs to report include shortness of breath, rapid heart rate, dizziness, insomnia, a persistent increase in heart rate or blood pressure, and extreme fatigue after sexual activity.
- Most patients have concerns about resuming sexual activity after an MI but may not express them to the nurse. Initiate the conversation and include the topic of sexual activity when discussing other physical activities. Explain what is safe and when. The joint guidelines of the American College of Cardiology and the American Heart Association recommend that after an "uncomplicated MI" (i.e., the patient's condition was stable with no complications), sexual intercourse can be resumed in 7 to 10 days. However, many patients tend to resume sexual activity more gradually than this. A "complicated MI" means that the patient required CPR or had hypotension, serious dysrhythmia, or heart failure while hospitalized. Patients with complicated MIs should resume sexual activity more slowly, depending on their tolerance for exercise and activity. Encourage patients to talk to their health care providers about resuming sexual activity; the type and extent of damage from the MI may influence recommendations.
- Explain the importance of taking prescribed medications such as beta blockers. Patients who take beta-adrenergic blockers for 1 year after an MI have a reduced chance of reinfarction and increased survival. The patient should also continue to take lipid-lowering agents such as simvastatin (Zocor), atorvastatin (Lipitor), lovastatin, pravastatin (Pravachol), or rosuvastatin (Crestor).

the New York Heart Association (NYHA) Functional Classification system (American Heart Association, 2017d). (See Box 48.3.)

Because the left ventricle is most often affected by coronary atherosclerosis and hypertension, HF usually begins there. If untreated, the condition progresses to right-sided failure. Right ventricular failure can occur separately from left ventricular failure, but its appearance is usually a consequence of left-sided failure. The signs and symptoms of HF result from decreased cardiac output, because of impaired cardiac pumping power, and congestion that involves the pulmonary and/or venous systems.

Left ventricular failure. When the left ventricle is unable to pump enough blood to meet the body's demands, major consequences occur. The first consequences are the signs and symptoms of decreased cardiac output. The second is pulmonary congestion. Increased pressure in the left side of the heart backs up into the pulmonary system, and the lungs become congested with fluid. Fluid leaks through the engorged capillaries and permeates air spaces in the lungs. If during each heartbeat the right ventricle pumps out just one more drop of blood than the left, then within only 3 hours the pulmonary blood volume will have expanded by 500 mL. Pulmonary edema and pleural effusion occur. Signs and symptoms of this condition include dyspnea; orthopnea; pulmonary crackles; wheezing; pink, frothy sputum; and cough.

Right ventricular failure. Right ventricular failure occurs when the right ventricle is unable to pump effectively against increased pressure in the pulmonary

Box 48.3 Classifying and Staging Heart Failure

NEW YORK HEART ASSOCIATION HEART FAILURE CLASSIFICATION

The New York Heart Association classification is a universal gauge of heart failure severity based on physical limitations.

CLASS I: MINIMAL
- No limitations.
- Ordinary physical activity does not cause undue fatigue, dyspnea, palpitations, or angina.

CLASS II: MILD
- Slightly limited physical activity.
- Comfortable at rest.
- Ordinary physical activity results in fatigue, palpitations, dyspnea, or angina.

CLASS III: MODERATE
- Markedly limited physical activity.
- Comfortable at rest.
- Less than ordinary activity causes fatigue, palpitations, dyspnea, or anginal pain.

CLASS IV: SEVERE
- Patient unable to perform any physical activity without discomfort.
- Angina or symptoms of cardiac inefficiency may develop at rest. Physical activity increases discomfort.

AMERICAN COLLEGE OF CARDIOLOGY AND AMERICAN HEART ASSOCIATION (ACC/AHA) HEART FAILURE STAGES

Stage A: Patient is at high risk for developing heart failure but has no structural disorder of the heart. The patient has a primary condition that is strongly associated with heart failure (such as diabetes mellitus, hypertension, substance abuse, or history of rheumatic fever) but no signs or symptoms of heart failure.

Stage B: Patient has a structural disorder of the heart, such as left ventricular remodeling, left ventricular hypertrophy, valvular heart disease, or previous myocardial infarction, but has never developed symptoms of heart failure.

Stage C: Patient has past or current symptoms of heart failure associated with underlying structural disease. The patient may display signs of dyspnea or fatigue but is responding to therapy.

Stage D: Patient has end-stage disease and requires specialized treatment strategies that may include mechanical circulatory support, continuous inotropic infusions, heart transplant, or hospice care. These patients are frequently hospitalized and cannot be discharged without symptom recurrence.

Data from American Heart Association: *Classes of heart failure,* 2017d. Retrieved from *http://www.heart.org/HEARTORG/Conditions/HeartFailure/AboutHeartFailure/Classes-of-Heart-Failure_UCM_306328_Article.jsp#.WajCAdEpD7M; and* Graham KE: Heart Failure ACC/AHA Staging System for Patients, n.d. Retrieved from http://heartfailurecenter.com/HF-ACCAHA.htm.

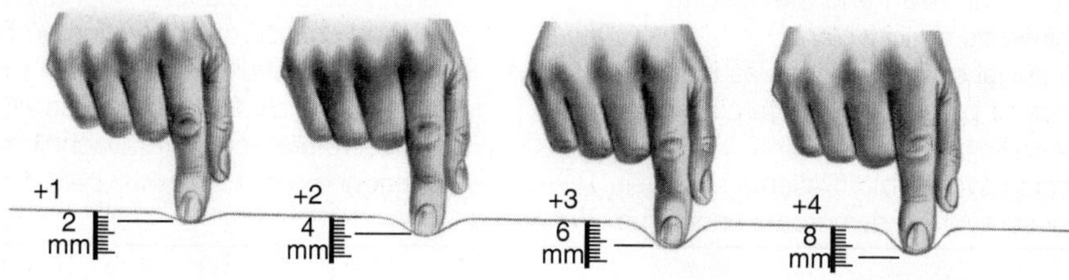

Fig. 48.16 Scale for pitting edema depth. (From Canobbio M: *Mosby's clinical nursing series: Cardiovascular disorders,* St. Louis, 1990, Mosby.)

circulation. The increased pressure usually is caused by blood backing up from a failing left ventricle, but right ventricular failure can also result from chronic pulmonary disease (cor pulmonale) and pulmonary hypertension. The right ventricle's inability to pump blood forward into the lungs results in peripheral congestion and an inability to accommodate all the venous blood that normally is returned to the right side of the heart. Venous blood is forced backward into the systemic circulation. Increased venous volume and pressure force fluid out of the vasculature into interstitial tissue (peripheral edema). Edema appears in dependent areas of the body such as the sacrum when the patient is supine and the feet and ankles while in an upright position. As right ventricular failure continues, edema may progress to pitting edema and move up the legs into the thighs, external genitalia, and lower trunk. To check for edema, press down on the tissue for several seconds and lift the finger. If the depression does not fill almost immediately, pitting edema is present (Fig. 48.16 and Table 48.5).

Table 48.5 Pitting Edema Scale

SCALE	DEGREE	RESPONSE
+1: Trace	2 mm (0–1/16 inch)	Rapid
+2: Mild	4 mm (0–1/4 inch)	10–15 sec
+3: Moderate	6 mm (1/4–1/2 inch)	1–2 min
+4: Severe	8 mm (1/2 inch)	2–5 min

One liter of fluid equals 1 kg (2.2 lb); therefore a weight gain of 2.2 lb signifies a gain of 1 L of body fluid. The liver may become congested, and fluid can accumulate in the abdomen (ascites). Distended neck veins may be observed when the patient is sitting.

Clinical Manifestations

Manifestations of HF are those associated with decreased cardiac output, left ventricular failure, and right ventricular failure (Box 48.4).

Assessment

Subjective data include complaints of dyspnea, **orthopnea** (an abnormal condition in which a person must sit or stand to breathe deeply or comfortably), paroxysmal nocturnal dyspnea (sudden awakening from sleep because of shortness of breath), and cough. The patient may report fatigue, anxiety, weight gain from fluid retention, and edema. Physical symptoms and impaired physical function cause psychosocial stress. Patients with New York Heart Association (NYHA) class III or IV HF are at high risk for major depression (American Heart Association, 2017d). Document any pain (anginal or abdominal) and the patient's stated ability to perform ADLs.

Box 48.4 Signs and Symptoms of Heart Failure

DECREASED CARDIAC OUTPUT
- Fatigue
- Anginal pain
- Anxiety
- Oliguria
- Decreased gastrointestinal motility
- Pale, cool skin
- Weight gain
- Restlessness

LEFT VENTRICULAR FAILURE
- Dyspnea
- Paroxysmal nocturnal dyspnea
- Cough
- Frothy, blood-tinged sputum
- Orthopnea
- Pulmonary crackles (moist popping and cracking sounds heard most often at the end of inspiration)
- Radiographic evidence of pulmonary vascular congestion with pleural effusion

RIGHT VENTRICULAR FAILURE
- Distended jugular veins
- Anorexia, nausea, and abdominal distention
- Liver enlargement with right upper quadrant pain
- Ascites
- Edema in feet, ankles, sacrum; may progress up the legs into thighs, external genitalia, and lower trunk

Collection of objective data includes noting the presence of respiratory distress, the number of pillows required to breathe comfortably while attempting to rest (orthopnea), edema (site, degree of pitting), abdominal distention secondary to ascites, weight gain, adventitious breath sounds, abnormal heart sounds (gallop and murmurs), activity intolerance, and jugular vein distention. Blood flow to the kidneys is diminished, resulting in reduction in the glomerular filtration rate and ultimately oliguria. Oxygen deficit in tissues results in cyanosis and general debilitation.

Diagnostic Tests

Diagnosis is based on presenting signs and symptoms of HF and is confirmed by various diagnostic tests. A chest radiograph reveals pulmonary vascular congestion, pleural effusion, and cardiomegaly (cardiac enlargement). ECG shows cardiac dysrhythmias. The most noninvasive diagnostic test for evaluating a patient with HF is an echocardiogram. Echocardiography helps to assess the valves and chambers of the heart. It can be used to identify valvular heart disease and detect the presence of pericardial fluid. Pulmonary artery catheterization is done to assess right and left ventricular function.

Exercise stress testing is performed to determine activity tolerance and the severity of underlying ischemic cardiovascular disease. *Cardiac catheterization* may be done to detect cardiac abnormalities and underlying cardiovascular disease. MUGA scanning is used to evaluate cardiac function, ejection fraction, and wall motion abnormalities.

Laboratory studies include electrolytes, sodium, calcium, magnesium, and potassium levels. Blood chemistry reveals elevated blood urea nitrogen (BUN) and creatinine resulting from decreased glomerular filtration; liver function values (alanine aminotransferase, aspartate transaminase, gamma-glutamyltransferase, alkaline phosphatase) are mildly elevated. BNP is a hormone secreted by the heart in response to ventricular expansion and pressure overload. A higher level of BNP correlates with an increase in the patient's signs and symptoms of HF:

- Less than 100 pg/mL (normal): The patient does not have HF
- Greater than 100 pg/mL: Suggestive of HF
- Greater than 700 pg/mL: Indicates decompensated HF (i.e., HF that is worsening)
- Arterial blood gases may show hypoxemia and acid-base imbalance.

Medical Management

Medical management of HF includes increasing cardiac efficiency with digoxin and vasodilators (nitroglycerin, isosorbide) for expanded output. Digoxin was once the cornerstone of HF treatment but is now used less often and at lower doses. Angiotensin-converting enzyme

(ACE) inhibitors such as captopril, enalapril (Vasotec), ramipril (Altace), benazepril (Lotensin), lisinopril (Prinivil, Zestril), quinapril (Accupril), and fosinopril decrease peripheral vascular resistance and improve cardiac output. These drugs improve the quality of life for the patient diagnosed with HF. Remodeling occurs when the left ventricle dilates, hypertrophies, and develops a more spheric shape. The shape change puts extra stress on the ventricle walls, increases the amount of blood regurgitated through the mitral valve, and decreases the ventricle's ability to work. Two beta blockers approved by the FDA to treat HF are carvedilol (an alpha blocker and nonselective beta blocker) and metoprolol. Beta blockers inhibit chronic activation of the sympathetic nervous system. Beta blockers are so effective at reducing symptoms, improving clinical status, and decreasing mortality and hospitalizations, that they have become the most significant drugs for HF management. Angiotensin II receptor blockers such as irbesartan (Avapro), losartan (Cozaar), and valsartan (Diovan) selectively and competitively block the vasoconstrictive and aldosterone-secreting effects of angiotensin, leading to vasodilation. Research for their use in HF continues. Angiotensin II receptor blockers are not a substitute for ACE inhibitors unless an ACE inhibitor is clearly not tolerated. Nesiritide (Natrecor) is used intravenously in patients with acutely decompensated HF who have shortness of breath (i.e., dyspnea) at rest or with minimal activity. Nesiritide is the first of the drug class called human BNPs. It reduces pulmonary capillary pressure, helps improve breathing, and causes vasodilation with increase in stroke volume and cardiac output.

Therapeutic management also includes lowering the oxygen requirements of body systems. This is done by elevating the head of the bed to 45 degrees or by having the patient sit on the edge of the bed with arms resting on the overbed table to reduce myocardial oxygen demand and decrease circulating volume returning to the heart. Oxygen therapy provides oxygen to the tissues if the patient is hypoxic.

Edema and pulmonary congestion are treated with diuretics, a sodium-restricted diet, and restricted fluid intake. Weigh the patient daily to monitor fluid retention.

The health care provider commonly initiates medication therapy with digoxin, ACE inhibitors, thiazide, and loop diuretics (Table 48.6). Once the workload of the heart is decreased and the tissue and organ engorgement has abated, the patient's activity level will increase.

A biventricular pacemaker can improve symptoms and function, improve quality of life, and decrease hospitalization for patients with HF who also have conduction system disorder. An implantable cardioverter-defibrillator can decrease the risk of sudden cardiac death for patients with a family history of sudden cardiac death, life-threatening dysrhythmias, or mild to moderate HF who have an ejection fraction of less than 30% (American Heart Association, 2016b) (see section on "Echocardiography").

Oxygen administration and pharmacologic therapies are the primary concerns in the management of acute HF. Decreasing oxygen requirements through rest slows the heart rate and increases cardiac and respiratory reserves. Anxiety produced by the signs and symptoms and the fear of a life-threatening situation can be allayed by reassurance and explanation. Accurate interventions, observation, and reporting reduce the threat of complications such as embolus, thrombophlebitis, MI, and pulmonary edema.

Nursing Interventions

Nursing interventions include measures to prevent disease progression and complications. Monitor vital signs for changes. Note any signs of respiratory distress or pulmonary edema. Carefully monitor signs and symptoms of left-sided versus right-sided HF. Urinary output is typically low, and edema is soft and pitting; legs are elevated to decrease edema.

Also note an increase in abdominal girth and total body weight as indicators of fluid retention, which is common in HF. Auscultate the lung fields to detect the presence of crackles and wheezes; also note coughing and complaints of dyspnea. Restful sleep may be possible only in the sitting position or with the aid of extra pillows. Activity intolerance is accompanied by extreme fatigue and anxiety. Assess patients for depression. Explain to patients with HF and depression that the depression is readily treatable and that several approaches can be used separately or in combination, including pharmacologic therapy, psychosocial and psychotherapeutic interventions, and cardiac rehabilitation.

Key components of care. The Institute for Healthcare Improvement recommends these components of care for all patients with HF (unless the patient cannot tolerate them or unless contraindicated):

- Assess left ventricular systolic function.
- At discharge from hospital (when left ventricular ejection fraction is less than 40%, indicating systolic dysfunction), administer ACE inhibitor or angiotensin.
- At discharge, administer an anticoagulant if the patient has chronic or recurrent atrial fibrillation.
- Encourage smoking cessation.
- Instruct the patient at discharge regarding activity, diet, medication, follow-up appointment, weight monitoring, and what to do if symptoms worsen.
- Provide influenza and pneumococcal immunization.
- At discharge, institute optional beta blocker therapy for stabilized patients with left ventricular systolic dysfunction who have no contraindications.

The new guidelines also recommend a discussion of end-of-life decisions with the patient and the family. Patients should talk with their health care providers

Table 48.6 **Medications for Heart Failure**

GENERIC NAME (TRADE NAME)	ACTION	NURSING INTERVENTIONS
Cardiac Glycosides		
Digitalis preparations, such as digoxin (Lanoxin)	Strengthen cardiac force and efficiency Slow heart rate Increase circulation, effecting diuresis	Monitor apical pulse to ensure rate greater than 60 bpm; monitor for toxicity (nausea, vomiting, anorexia, dysrhythmia, bradycardia, tachycardia, headache, fatigue, and blurred or colored vision)
Diuretics		
Thiazides, such as chlorothiazide (Diuril), hydrochlorothiazide	Increase renal secretion of sodium Are safe for long-term use Block sodium and water reabsorption in kidney tubules	Monitor electrolyte depletion; weigh daily to ascertain fluid loss
Sulfonamides (loop diuretic), such as furosemide (Lasix), bumetanide (Bumex)	Act rapidly for less responsive edema	Administer in the morning to prevent nocturia Monitor for electrolyte depletion Consider sulfa allergy (furosemide)
Aldosterone antagonist (potassium-sparing), such as spironolactone (Aldactone)	Relieves edema and ascites that do not respond to usual diuretics Blocks sodium-retaining and potassium-excreting properties of aldosterone	Monitor for gastrointestinal irritation and hyperkalemia
Potassium Supplements		
potassium (K-Lyte)	Restores electrolyte loss	Monitor blood potassium levels
Sedatives and Analgesics		
temazepam (Restoril)	Promotes rest and comfort	Monitor rest and sleep benefits
morphine	Relieves chest and abdominal pain, reduces anxiety, and decreases myocardial oxygen demands Lessens dyspnea	
Nitrates		
nitroglycerin	Dilates arteries, improves blood flow Reduces blood pressure	Monitor blood pressure for hypotension Monitor for headache and flushing
Angiotensin-Converting Enzyme (ACE) Inhibitors		
captopril enalapril (Vasotec) ramipril (Altace) benazepril (Lotensin) lisinopril (Prinivil; Zestril) quinapril (Accupril) fosinopril moexipril perindopril trandolapril (Mavik)	Act as antihypertensives, reduce peripheral arterial resistance, and improve cardiac output	Observe patient closely for a precipitous drop in blood pressure within 3 h of initial dose; monitor blood pressure closely Monitor blood potassium levels
Beta-Adrenergic Blockers		
carvedilol (Coreg)	Directly blocks the sympathetic nervous system's negative effects on the failing heart	Start at a low dose, increasing the dose slowly every 2 wk as tolerated by the patient Monitor blood pressure and notify health care provider of significant change Monitor pulse: If <50 bpm, withhold drug and call health care provider
metoprolol (Toprol-XL)	Blocks beta$_2$-adrenergic receptors in bronchial and vascular smooth muscle. Lowers blood pressure by beta-blocking effects; reduces elevated renin plasma levels	Monitor I&O, weigh daily Monitor apical or radial pulse before administration Notify health care provider of any significant changes, or if pulse <50 bpm

Continued

Table 48.6 Medications for Heart Failure—cont'd

GENERIC NAME (TRADE NAME)	ACTION	NURSING INTERVENTIONS
Inotropic Agents		
dobutamine dopamine	Low-dose dobutamine and low-dose dopamine are relatively safe on medical-surgical units; at low doses they dilate renal blood vessels, stimulating renal blood flow and glomerular filtration rate; this in turn promotes sodium excretion, often helping patients with CHF improve	Make certain patient is not taking monoamine oxidase (MAO) inhibitors, tricyclic antidepressants, phenytoin (Dilantin), or haloperidol (Haldol). Record accurate I&O; assess for dizziness, nausea, vomiting, headache. Assess vital signs carefully every 15 min for first 2 h, then every 2 h for the next 4 h, and finally once a shift. Observe carefully for extravasation, tachycardia, bradycardia, angina, palpitations, hypotension, hypertension, azotemia, and anxiety
Human B-Type Natriuretic Peptides		
nesiritide (Natrecor)	New class of synthetic HF drugs; causes arterial and venous dilation, thereby decreasing systemic vascular resistance and pulmonary arterial pressures; decreases blood pressure, promotes better left ventricle ejection, and increases cardiac output; may also promote diuresis; an IV treatment for patients with acutely decompensated CHF	Observe carefully for hypotension. Natrecor should not be used for patients with cardiogenic shock or with a systolic blood pressure <90 mm Hg

ACE, Angiotensin-converting enzyme; *bpm*, beats per minute; *CHF*, congestive heart failure; *HF*, heart failure; *I&O*, intake and output.

about treatment preferences, advance directives, living wills, power of attorney for health care, and life support issues. HF is progressive, and patients should make decisions concerning health care wishes and plans while they are capable of expressing choices. Hospice services, originally developed to assist patients with cancer, are appropriate for the patient with end-stage HF (see the Patient Teaching box, Nursing Care Plan 48.1, and Box 48.5).

Prognosis

Approximately 10% of patients diagnosed with HF die in the first year, and 50% within 5 years. HF is a chronic condition. With treatment advances, many people now live for years with damaged hearts. With the advent of ACE inhibitors and new research on the benefits of prescribed exercise, improvement in the quality of life for patients with HF is being seen.

PULMONARY EDEMA

Etiology and Pathophysiology

Pulmonary edema (the accumulation of extravascular fluid in lung tissues and alveoli, most often caused by HF) is an acute and extensive, life-threatening complication of HF caused by severe left ventricular dysfunction. Fluid from the left side of the heart backs up into the pulmonary vasculature and results in extravascular fluid accumulation in the interstitial space and alveoli. This causes the patient to "drown" in the secretions.

Clinical Manifestations

The patient exhibits signs of severe respiratory distress when pulmonary edema occurs. Frothy sputum is produced from air mixing with the fluid in the alveoli; the sputum is blood-tinged from blood cells that have exuded into the alveoli.

Assessment

See Box 48.6 for signs and symptoms of pulmonary edema.

Diagnostic Tests

Diagnosis is made by observing signs and symptoms and is supported by chest radiograph and arterial blood gas studies. PaO_2 and $PaCO_2$ (the partial pressures of oxygen and carbon dioxide, respectively, in the arterial blood) may reveal respiratory alkalosis or acidosis.

Medical Management

Medical management involves simultaneous interventions to promote oxygenation, improve cardiac output, and reduce pulmonary congestion. Respiratory failure

 Nursing Care Plan 48.1 **The Patient With Heart Failure**

Mr. D. is a 61-year-old clinical administrator. He was admitted to the hospital with the diagnosis of heart failure. He has a history of hypertension and coronary artery disease. Six months ago he had a myocardial infarction. He has felt tired for the past 3 wk and has been experiencing increased dyspnea. He has noticed some edema in his ankles and is concerned about gaining 5 lb in the past week and having an increasing intolerance to exertion. The nursing admission history revealed:

- Mr. D. has not been taking his antihypertensive medication regularly. He did not like the side effects and stopped taking the medication, but he was too embarrassed to call his health care provider.
- Vital signs revealed an elevated blood pressure.
- He has shortness of breath during activities and when lying down.
- Pitting edema is seen on both ankles.
- Crackles are heard bilaterally in the lungs.

PATIENT PROBLEM

Insufficient Cardiac Output, related to cardiovascular disease

Patient Goals and Expected Outcomes	Nursing Intervention	Evaluation
Patient will have decreased adventitious lung sounds when lying in bed within 24 h Patient will have oxygen saturations at 91% with prescribed oxygen within 24 h Patient will have vital signs within acceptable levels within 72 h Patient will have decreased edema and weight loss of 5 lb within 72 h	Maintain initial bed rest with stress-free environment. Maintain semi-Fowler's to high Fowler's position. Explain and encourage gradual increases in activity to prevent a sudden increase in cardiac workload. Monitor respirations, lung sounds, heart sounds, and vital signs q 4 hr. Palpate pedal pulses, and assess capillary refill q 8 hr. Administer digitalis, diuretics, angiotensin-converting enzyme inhibitors, vasodilators, beta blockers, and antihypertensive medication as prescribed. Monitor intake and output and weigh daily. Monitor oxygen saturation with pulse oximetry q 4 hr. Administer prescribed oxygen.	Patient has decreased crackles in lung fields within 24 h of admission. Patient has an oximetry reading of 91% oxygen saturation with oxygen prescribed within 24 h of admission. Patient has a heart rate of 80 bpm, respiratory rate of 22 breaths/min, and blood pressure of 148/86 mm Hg within 72 h of admission. Patient has a weight loss of 5 lb within 72 h of admission. Patient has pedal pitting edema decreased to 1+ within 2 days of admission.

PATIENT PROBLEM

Anxiousness, related to change in health status, lifestyle changes, fear of death, or threats to self-concept

Patient Goals and Expected Outcomes	Nursing Intervention	Evaluation
Patient will verbalize anxieties within 48 h of admission Patient will demonstrate reduction of anxiety by enjoying periods of rest and sleep undisturbed for 6 h within 48 h of admission	Identify coping techniques. Provide information to decrease fears. Identify support systems. Provide calm, relaxing environment. Administer antianxiety medications per health care provider's orders as needed. Help patient cope with lifestyle changes. He may feel anxious because of changes in body image, family and social roles, and finances. Focus on progress patient is making in managing his condition. Encourage patient to participate in health care decisions, and allow him to release anger and frustration. Allow patient to sleep undisturbed for 6 h when vital signs are stable.	Patient is verbalizing anger and frustration over current medical conditions within 48 h of admission. Patient is sleeping 5–6 h per night within 48 h of admission.

CRITICAL THINKING QUESTIONS

1. Mr. D. is experiencing severe dyspnea, with the presence of crackles bilaterally in all lung fields. His pulse is 108 bpm, and respirations are 33 breaths/min. When performing his morning ADLs, the nurse could perform which beneficial nursing interventions?
2. On assessing Mr. D.'s skin, the nurse notes 4+ pitting edema in his lower extremities. A weight gain of 6 lb in the past 24 hours also is noted. For therapeutic diuresis to occur, what would the medical management likely include?
3. Mr. D. puts his call light on to request assistance to ambulate. The nurse notes subclavicular retractions and cyanosis of his nailbeds. What would be the most appropriate nursing actions?

Box 48.5 Guidelines for Nursing Interventions for the Patient With Heart Failure

- Provide oxygenation.
- Administer oxygen by nasal cannula per protocol as prescribed for dyspnea.
- Patient should be well supported in semi-Fowler's or high Fowler's position.
- Reinforce importance of conservation of energy and planning for activities that avoid fatigue.
- Encourage activity within prescribed restrictions; monitor for intolerance to activity (dyspnea, fatigue, increased pulse rate that does not stabilize).
- Assist with activities of daily living as necessary; encourage independence within patient's limitations.
- Provide diversionary activity that will assist in conservation of energy.
- Monitor for signs of fluid and potassium imbalance; record daily weights, intake and output.
- Provide skin care, particularly over edematous areas; use prophylactic measures to prevent skin impairment.
- Assist in maintaining an adequate nutritional intake while observing prescribed dietary modifications (sodium restrictions).
- Monitor for constipation; give prescribed stool softeners.
- Give prescribed medications:
  - Digitalis (take apical pulse before administration)
  - Diuretics (assess for hypokalemia)
  - Vasodilators, angiotensin-converting enzyme inhibitors, beta blockers
  - Medications to reduce anxiety and promote sleep
- Provide the patient and the family opportunities to discuss their concerns.
- Teach the patient about the disorder and self-care.

Box 48.6 Signs and Symptoms of Pulmonary Edema

- Restlessness
- Vague uneasiness
- Agitation
- Disorientation
- Diaphoresis
- Severe dyspnea
- Tachypnea
- Tachycardia
- Pallor or cyanosis
- Cough; production of large quantities of blood-tinged, frothy sputum
- Audible wheezing, crackles
- Cold extremities

 **Patient Teaching**

Heart Failure

- Monitor for signs and symptoms of recurring heart failure and report them to the health care provider or clinic. The following signs and symptoms indicate worsening heart failure:
  - Weight gain of 2 to 3 lb (1 to 1.5 kg) over a short period (about 2 days)
  - Shortness of breath
  - Orthopnea
  - Swelling of ankles, feet, or abdomen
  - Persistent cough
  - Frequent nighttime urination
- Avoid fatigue and plan activity to allow for rest periods.
- Plan and eat meals within prescribed sodium restrictions. Avoid salty foods.
- Avoid drugs with high sodium content (e.g., some laxatives and antacids, Alka-Seltzer); read the product labels. Ideally, limit sodium intake to 2 g/day.
- Maintain low-fat diet, with fat intake less than 30% of total calories.
- Eat several small meals rather than three large meals per day.
- Take medications as prescribed.
- If several medications are prescribed, develop a method to facilitate accurate administration.
- When taking digoxin, check own pulse rate daily; report a rate of less than 60 bpm to the health care provider. Do not take digoxin if pulse is less than 60 bpm.
- Take diuretics as prescribed.
- Weigh self daily at same time and in similar clothes.
- Eat foods high in potassium and low in sodium (such as oranges and bananas) if the patient is not taking a potassium-sparing diuretic.
- Take all prescribed medications.
- Report signs of hypotension (lightheadedness, rapid pulse, syncope) to the health care provider.
- Avoid alcohol when taking vasodilators.
- Reinforce the importance of regular exercise once heart failure is stabilized. A thorough treatment regimen may allow the patient to increase activity level over time. The health care provider may ultimately recommend 30 to 45 minutes of aerobic exercise three or four times a week to improve patient's well-being.
- Report to the health care provider for follow-up as directed.

may occur without prompt emergency treatment (Table 48.7).

Nursing Interventions

Interventions include administering oxygen. The patient should sit upright with legs in a dependent position to decrease venous return to the heart, relieving pulmonary congestion and dyspnea. Monitor arterial blood gases and administer drugs as ordered. Auscultate lung sounds often. Provide emotional support; remain with the patient. Explain all procedures. Monitor vital signs, fluid I&O, and serum electrolytes.

Patient problems and interventions for the patient with pulmonary edema include but are not limited to the following:

Table 48.7 Medical Management for Acute Pulmonary Edema

INTERVENTION	RATIONALE
Patient in high Fowler's position or over side of bed with arms supported on bedside table	Promotes expansion of lungs; legs in dependent position causes venous pooling and reduction in venous return (preload)
Morphine sulfate, 10–15 mg IV; titrated	Decreases patient anxiety; relieves pain; slows respirations; reduces venous return; decreases oxygen demand; dilates the pulmonary and systemic blood vessels
Oxygen at 40%–100%; nonrebreather face mask; intubation as needed	Promotes oxygenation; increased tidal volume also promotes removal of secretions from alveoli
Administer sublingual nitroglycerin	Increases myocardial blood flow
Diuretics: furosemide (Lasix), bumetanide (Bumex) (IV)	Reduce pulmonary edema by decreasing the fluid in the lungs and increasing excretion through the kidneys
Insert Foley catheter	Allows patient to rest and conserve energy; monitors urinary output after IV furosemide has been administered
Inotropic agents: dobutamine, amrinone	Increase myocardial contractility without increasing oxygen consumption; increase peripheral vasodilation; increase cardiac output
Nitroprusside (Nitropress)	A potent vasodilator; improves myocardial contraction and reduces pulmonary congestion

IV, Intravenous.

Patient Problem	Nursing Interventions
Fluid Volume Overload, related to fluid accumulation in pulmonary vessels	Administer medications as ordered Carefully monitor I&O Weigh patient at same time each day Assess for edema
Inefficient Oxygenation, related to fluid in lungs	Assess for signs of hypoxia, such as restlessness, disorientation, and irritability Monitor arterial blood gases per health care provider's order Administer oxygen per health care provider's order Position patient in high Fowler's position with legs in dependent position, or sitting and leaning forward on overbed table to facilitate breathing

Prognosis

Pulmonary edema is a grave, life-threatening condition that is usually responsive to aggressive interventions.

VALVULAR HEART DISEASE

Etiology and Pathophysiology

Normal heart valves maintain the direction of blood flow through the right atrium, right ventricle, lungs, left atrium, and left ventricle and to the rest of the body. Heart valves passively open and close in response to pressure changes in the heart. The tricuspid valve is located between the right atrium and the right ventricle. The pulmonary semilunar valve allows blood to flow from the right ventricle, through the pulmonary artery and into the lungs. The mitral (bicuspid) valve is located between the left atrium and the left ventricle. The aortic semilunar valve allows blood to flow from the left ventricle into the aorta. Valvular disease occurs when the valves are damaged and do not open and close properly. Two valvular problems are *stenosis,* which is a thickening of the valve tissue, causing the valve to narrow; and *insufficiency,* which occurs when the valve is unable to close completely. Valvular heart disorders include mitral stenosis, mitral insufficiency, aortic insufficiency, aortic stenosis, tricuspid insufficiency, tricuspid stenosis, pulmonary insufficiency, and pulmonary stenosis.

Valvular disorders occur in children, adolescents, and adults, primarily from congenital conditions. A prominent factor in the development of valvular disease is a history of rheumatic fever. Clinical symptoms of valvular heart disease tend to occur 10 to 40 years after an episode of rheumatic fever. Rheumatic fever is caused by an untreated or undertreated streptococcal infection. The streptococcal infection in children may lie dormant for years in either the mitral or aortic valves. Valvular disorders are found when the patient becomes symptomatic, such as with shortness of breath on exertion or when the patient complains of "extra heartbeats felt." The greater blood volume and workload of the heart on the left side results in the increased impact on the mitral and aortic valves.

Clinical Manifestations

Signs and symptoms seen in valvular disorders are related to decreased cardiac output (Table 48.8).

Assessment

Subjective data include the patient's statement of a history of rheumatic fever and of an inability to perform activities and ADLs without fatigue or weakness. Ask the patient about chest pain, including its quality, duration, onset, precipitating factors, and measures that provide relief. The patient may complain of heart palpitations, lightheadedness, dizziness, or fainting. The history may include a patient statement of weight gain. Dyspnea, exertional dyspnea, nocturnal (nighttime) dyspnea, and orthopnea often are reported, depending on the degree of HF.

Collection of objective data includes observing for a heart murmur and noting the presence and character of any adventitious breath sounds (crackles, wheezes) and edema (pitting or nonpitting).

Table 48.8 Manifestations of Valvular Heart Disease

DIAGNOSIS	MANIFESTATIONS
Mitral valve stenosis	Dyspnea on exertion, hemoptysis; fatigue; atrial fibrillation on ECG, palpitations, stroke; loud, accentuated S_1; low-pitched, rumbling diastolic murmur
Mitral valve regurgitation	*Acute:* Generally poorly tolerated; new systolic murmur with pulmonary edema and cardiogenic shock developing rapidly *Chronic:* Weakness, fatigue, exertional dyspnea, palpitations; an S_3 gallop, holosystolic murmur
Mitral valve prolapse	Palpitations, dyspnea, chest pain, activity intolerance, syncope; holosystolic murmur
Aortic valve stenosis	Angina, syncope, dyspnea on exertion, heart failure; normal or soft S_1, diminished or absent S_2, systolic murmur, prominent S_4
Aortic valve regurgitation	*Acute:* Abrupt onset of profound dyspnea, chest pain, left ventricular failure, and cardiogenic shock *Chronic:* Fatigue, exertional dyspnea, orthopnea, paroxysmal nocturnal dyspnea; water-hammer pulse; heaving precordial impulse; diminished or absent S_1, S_3, or S_4; soft, high-pitched diastolic murmur, Austin Flint murmur
Tricuspid and pulmonic stenosis	*Tricuspid:* Peripheral edema, ascites, hepatomegaly; diastolic low-pitched murmur with increased intensity during inspiration *Pulmonic:* Fatigue, loud midsystolic murmur

ECG, Electrocardiogram; *S_1*, first heart sound (*lub*), produced by atrioventricular valve closure; *S_2*, second heart sound (*dub*), produced by semilunar valve closure; *S_3* and *S_4*, gallop rhythms.
Modified from Lewis SL, Dirksen SR, Heitkemper MM, et al: *Medical-surgical nursing: Assessment and management of clinical problems*, ed 9, St. Louis, 2014, Mosby.

Diagnostic Tests

The diagnostic tests used to confirm valvular heart disease are chest radiograph, ECG, echocardiogram, and cardiac catheterization.

Medical Management

Medical management includes activity limitations, sodium-restricted diet, diuretics, digoxin, and antidysrhythmics.

When medical therapy no longer alleviates clinical symptoms or when diagnostic evidence exists of progressive myocardial failure, surgery often is performed. The surgery may include the following:

- *Open mitral commissurotomy:* A surgical splitting of the fused mitral valve leaflet for treating stenosis of the mitral valve.
- *Valve replacement:* Replacement of the stenosed or incompetent valve with a bioprosthetic or mechanical valve. Commonly used valves include tilting disks, porcine (pig) heterografts (tissue taken from one species and grafted onto another), homografts (a graft of human tissue), and ball-in-cage valves.

Nursing Interventions and Patient Teaching

Nursing interventions focus on assisting with ADLs, relieving specific symptoms associated with decreased cardiac output, and promoting comfort. Administer the prescribed medications (diuretics, digoxin, and antidysrhythmics). Assess and review vital signs, breath sounds, and heart sounds for changes from the baseline assessment. Pulse oximetry is reviewed and evaluated at regular intervals. Maintain oxygen therapy as prescribed. Monitor fluid balance by assessing and recording the presence of edema, daily weight, and intake and output. Check for capillary perfusion and pedal pulses. Have the patient consume a sodium-restricted diet for control of edema. Discuss with the patient a plan for rest periods, and identify those ADLs that produce fatigue and require assistance.

Patient problems and interventions for the patient with valvular heart disease include but are not limited to the following:

Patient Problem	Nursing Interventions
Inability to Tolerate Activity, related to: • Weakness • Fatigue • Dyspnea	Balance activities with rest periods Identify fatiguing activities and obtain assistance as needed Use oxygen as prescribed by health care provider

Patient Problem	Nursing Interventions
Fluid Volume Overload, related to decreased cardiac output	Administer prescribed oxygen, digoxin, diuretics, and antidysrhythmics Monitor I&O Weigh patient daily at same time Perform respiratory assessment Perform cardiovascular assessment Inspect for presence of edema Obtain vital signs routinely Maintain sodium-restricted diet

Patient teaching focuses on medications, dietary management, activity limitations, diagnostic tests, surgical interventions, and postoperative care as appropriate. Describe the disease process and associated symptoms to report to the health care provider. Explain antibiotic prophylaxis to prevent infective endocarditis. Explain the importance of notifying the dentist, urologist, and gynecologist of valvular heart disease. The patient must remain on higher dosages of warfarin after valve replacement surgery. Carefully monitor the PT and INR. Explain the need to maintain good oral hygiene and make regular visits to the dentist.

Prognosis

The prognosis for the patient with valvular heart disease varies, depending on the specific disease. The prognosis after surgery for the affected valve is fair to good with improvement of signs and symptoms but often without resolution of all abnormalities.

INFLAMMATORY HEART DISORDERS

All cardiac tissues are susceptible to inflammation, and HF can be a serious and rapid result of the inflammatory process.

RHEUMATIC HEART DISEASE

Etiology and Pathophysiology

Rheumatic heart disease is the result of rheumatic fever and the clinical manifestation of carditis resulting from an inadequately treated childhood pharyngeal or upper respiratory tract infection (group A beta-hemolytic streptococci). By the 1980s rheumatic fever had almost disappeared in developed countries such as the United States. However, it has remained common and severe in most developing countries. Antibiotics, especially penicillin, are responsible for the decline in rheumatic fever.

Ineffective treatment of infection results in delayed reaction and inflammation of the cardiac tissues and the central nervous system, joints, skin, and subcutaneous tissues. Ninety percent of patients who get rheumatic fever are between 5 and 15 years of age. The onset of rheumatic fever is usually sudden, often occurring within 1 to 5 symptom-free weeks after recovery from pharyngitis (sore throat) or from scarlet fever. In some patients the rheumatic fever may progress without symptoms and go undiagnosed and untreated. Years later the patient may develop clinical manifestations of valvular heart disease.

Rheumatic heart disease can affect the pericardium, myocardium, or endocardium. The affected tissue develops small areas of necrosis, which heal, leaving scar tissue. The heart valves are typically the most affected by Aschoff's nodules (vegetative growth; in this context a "vegetative growth" refers to a growth of pathologic tissue), and they become fibrous and incompetent. With healing, the valves become thickened and deformed. These changes result in valvular stenosis and insufficiency, varying in extent and severity.

Clinical Manifestations

Fever, increased pulse, epistaxis, anemia, joint involvement, and nodules on joints and subcutaneous tissue may be noted. Carditis (inflammation of heart tissues) can develop. When valvular involvement occurs, signs and symptoms are specific to each condition.

Assessment

Collection of subjective data may reveal joint pain (polyarthritis) and chest pain. Lethargy and fatigue are also present.

Objective data include skin manifestations of small erythematous circles and wavy lines on the trunk and abdomen that appear and disappear rapidly (erythema marginatum). The nurse may observe involuntary, purposeless movement of the muscles if Sydenham's chorea (St. Vitus' dance), a disorder of the central nervous system, is present. Heart murmur may be auscultated if the patient has carditis with valve involvement. Rheumatic heart disease is characterized by heart murmurs resulting from stenosis or insufficiency of the valves.

Diagnostic Tests

Diagnosis is made through signs and symptoms and supported by laboratory study results. An echocardiogram is done to determine the extent of damage to the valves and myocardium. An ECG shows cardiac dysrhythmia. Cardiac murmurs or friction rub can be heard. No specific diagnostic test exists for rheumatic fever. The erythrocyte sedimentation rate and leukocyte count are elevated. The development of serum antibodies against streptococci (measured by antistreptolysin-O titer) may occur. CRP, elevated in a specimen of blood, is abnormally high.

Medical Management

Preventive measures are the most effective interventions. Rapid treatment for pharyngeal infection, usually with prolonged antibiotic therapy, is desired. Penicillin is the preferred antibiotic. Prolonged periods of bed rest were recommended, but now the patient without carditis may be ambulatory as soon as acute symptoms have subsided. When carditis is present, ambulation is postponed until HF is controlled. Symptomatic treatment and care are given. Nonsteroidal antiinflammatory drugs (NSAIDs) for joint pain and inflammation are accompanied by application of gentle heat. A well-balanced diet, following the personalized daily food choices and number of servings recommended by the US Department of Agriculture's My Plate food planning tool, is supplemented by vitamins B and C and high-volume fluid intake. In some patients, surgical commissurotomy or valve replacement is necessary.

Nursing Interventions and Patient Teaching

Signs and symptoms largely determine the type of nursing interventions. Bed rest during the acute phase is recommended when carditis is present. If the patient has polyarthritis, minimize joint pain by proper positioning. After the acute stage, the child or the adult is treated at home. Review a schedule of daily events with the patient and the parents.

Perform nursing interventions quickly and skillfully to minimize discomfort and avoid tiring the patient. Throughout the course of the disease, the patient and the family benefit from emotional support and appropriate diversions. Teaching focuses on increasing understanding of the disease process, signs and symptoms, and gradually increasing activity levels. Emphasize the importance of eating a nutritional diet and keeping appointments for medical checkups. Patients with a history of rheumatic fever or evidence of rheumatic heart disease should receive daily prophylactic penicillin by mouth or monthly intramuscular injections of penicillin to prevent streptococcal infection, at least during childhood and adolescence. Patients with evidence of deformed heart valves should be given prophylactic antibiotics before surgery and all dental procedures.

Prognosis

Prognosis depends on involvement of the heart; carditis can result in a serious heart disease, including valvular disease.

PERICARDITIS

Etiology and Pathophysiology

Pericarditis is inflammation of the membranous sac surrounding the heart. It may be an acute or a chronic condition. Bacterial, viral, or fungal infection is associated with acute pericarditis. It may occur as a complication of noninfectious conditions such as azotemia (too much urea and other nitrogenous compounds in the blood); acute MI; neoplasms such as lung cancer, breast cancer, leukemia, Hodgkin's disease, and lymphoma; scleroderma; trauma after thoracic surgery; systemic lupus erythematosus; radiation; and drug reactions (e.g., from procainamide and hydralazine). Fibrosis of the pericardial sac develops in the chronic form of pericarditis.

Fibrous constriction and thickening of the pericardium occur gradually, causing compression severe enough to prevent normal filling during diastole. Surgical removal of the pericardium may be necessary to restore normal cardiac output.

Clinical Manifestations

Pericarditis differs clinically from other inflammatory conditions of the heart in that patients often have debilitating pain, much like that of an MI. The pain is aggravated by lying supine, deep breathing, coughing, swallowing, and moving the trunk and is alleviated by sitting up and leaning forward. Dyspnea, fever, chills, diaphoresis, and leukocytosis are observed. The hallmark finding in acute pericarditis is pericardial friction rub; grating, scratching, and leathery sounds are detected, although this appears in only about half of cases.

Decreased heart function to the level of cardiac failure can occur when the heart is compressed by excess fluid in the pericardial sac. Normally 15 to 50 mL of fluid are found in the pericardial sac, but with pericarditis 150 to 200 mL or more may develop.

Assessment

Subjective data include the patient's description of muscle aches, fatigue, and dyspnea. Excruciating chest pain is said to originate precordially and radiate to the neck and shoulders with severe and sudden onset.

Collection of objective data includes noting expressed substernal chest pain that radiates to the shoulder and neck; such pain is evidenced by orthopneic positioning (i.e., sitting propped up in a bed or chair) and facial grimace on inspiration. Elevated temperature accompanies chills and may be followed by diaphoresis. A nonproductive cough is often present. Patients commonly verbalize anxiety, anticipation of danger, or uneasiness. Vital sign changes include a rapid and forcible pulse and rapid, shallow breathing. Pericardial friction rub heart sounds become muffled, and the health care provider may note a dysrhythmia.

Diagnostic Tests

ECG changes (dysrhythmia) are noted. Echocardiography shows pericardial effusion or cardiac tamponade (compression of the heart). Laboratory studies show leukocytosis (10,000 to 20,000/mm^3), and the erythrocyte sedimentation rate is elevated. Blood cultures may be ordered to identify the specific pathogen present. To rule out an MI, cardiac enzyme levels are determined. A C-reactive protein (CRP) blood level commonly is ordered to aid in diagnosis. Elevated CRP levels indicate inflammation, which occurs with an infectious process.

Chest radiographic findings are generally normal or nonspecific in acute pericarditis unless the patient has a large pericardial effusion.

Medical Management

Analgesia for comfort and relief of pain reassures the anxious patient. Oxygen and parenteral fluids usually are given. Antibiotics are used to treat bacterial pericarditis. The health care provider prescribes salicylates for increased temperature and antiinflammatory agents (e.g., indomethacin) and corticosteroids for a persistent inflammatory process. These medicines require nursing knowledge of troublesome effects and nursing implications for control of this condition. When pericardial effusion restricts heart movement *(cardiac tamponade)*, a pericardial tap *(pericardiocentesis)* may be performed to remove excess fluid and restore normal heart function. Surgical intervention—pericardial fenestration (pericardial window) or pericardiocentesis (pericardial tap)—may be performed to provide continuous drainage of pericardial fluid and restore normal heart function. Complications include atelectasis and introduction of infectious agents.

Nursing Interventions

Carefully evaluate vital signs and auscultate lung and heart sounds. Provide supportive measures and observe for complications. Maintain bed rest to promote healing and decrease the cardiac workload. Elevate the head of the bed to 45 degrees to decrease dyspnea. Hypothermia treatment may be necessary to reduce elevated temperature. Remain with the patient if he or she is anxious. Explain all procedures thoroughly.

Patient problems and interventions for the patient with inflammatory heart conditions include but are not limited to the following:

Patient Problem	Nursing Interventions
Insufficient Cardiac Output, related to inflammatory process	Maintain bed rest with head of bed elevated to 45 degrees Assess vital signs q 2–4 hr as indicated by patient's condition Administer medications as ordered Monitor I&O Provide planned rest periods
Discomfort, related to inflammatory process	Assess and record pain type and quality Administer analgesics according to need, as ordered. (Pain is what the patient says it is) Maintain the patient on bed rest with the head of the bed elevated to 45 degrees and provide a padded overbed table on which the patient may rest his or her arms Use comfort measures to provide physical and emotional support
Fluid Volume Overload, related to ineffective myocardial pumping action	Restrict sodium in diet as prescribed; monitor I&O Weigh daily; compare values Administer diuretic therapy as ordered; monitor electrolyte values Observe respiration and pulse quality Assess for dyspnea and peripheral edema

Prognosis

The prognosis is fair in early stages but extremely grave if purulent and fibrinous stages develop.

ENDOCARDITIS

Etiology and Pathophysiology

Endocarditis is an infection or inflammation of the inner membranous lining of the heart, particularly the heart valves. Classified on the basis of cause, it may result from invasion of an organism *(infective endocarditis)* or from injury to the lining. The term *bacterial endocarditis* has been replaced by *infective endocarditis* because causative organisms include fungi, chlamydiae, rickettsiae, viruses, and bacteria. The causative organisms—most commonly *Streptococcus viridans, S. pyogenes, Staphylococcus aureus, S. epidermidis,* and enterococci—are deposited on the heart lining or valves. As the organism embeds into the tissue, a vegetative growth perforates the chambers or valve leaflets. Fibrin and calciferous growths of the vegetation may ulcerate and scar the valves; or the growths may break away, causing emboli, infection, or abscess in organs where they lodge. The loss of portions of vegetative lesions into the circulation results in embolization. Systemic embolization occurs from left-sided heart vegetation, progressing to infarction of an organ (particularly the brain, kidneys, and spleen). Right-sided heart lesions embolize to the lungs. Endocarditis may develop after cardiac surgery, which is traumatic.

People at risk include patients with rheumatic, congestive, or degenerative heart disease. With the increasing use of valve replacement, the incidence of prosthetic valve endocarditis continues to rise. In some cases endocarditis occurs as a result of unhealthy teeth and gums (allows bacteria to enter the body), after invasive dental procedures, minor surgery, gynecologic examinations, needles used for tattooing or body piercing, or insertion of indwelling urinary catheters that cause urosepsis. People at high risk include those who use illegal IV drugs, which can cause bacteremia from contaminated needles and syringes. Conditions predisposing people to infective endocarditis have changed because of the decreasing incidence of rheumatic heart disease and increased recognition and treatment of mitral valve prolapse. Patients with heart valve replacement need to tell their dentists before dental procedures, because bacteria harboring inside the mouth and gums could be dislodged and cause an infection.

Clinical Manifestations

Endocarditis occurs in acute or subacute forms. Signs and symptoms progress rapidly during the acute phase or gradually in the subacute phase. Damage occurs over a long period of time.

Assessment

Subjective data include patient complaints of influenza-like symptoms with recurrent fever, undue fatigue, chest pain, headaches, joint pain, and chills.

Collection of objective data may reveal the significant signs of petechiae in the conjunctiva, oral mucosa, neck, anterior chest, abdomen, and legs. Splinter hemorrhages (black longitudinal streaks) may occur in the nailbeds. Other signs are nontender macular lesions (in this case, flat reddish spots) on the palms and soles, plus tender erythematous, elevated nodules on the pads of the fingers and toes. Microemboli, vasculitis, and embolism are responsible for the development of these signs. They also have the potential to cause serious complications such as stroke and renal or splenic damage (Mayo Clinic, 2017a). Weight loss may occur. Pulse is rapid. Infective endocarditis may cause a murmur, with the aortic and mitral valves most commonly affected.

Diagnostic Tests

ECG changes and chest radiographic examination reveal evidence of HF and cardiomegaly. TEE and digital imaging using two-dimensional transthoracic echograms can detect vegetation or thrombi and abscesses on valves. Laboratory findings indicate leukocytosis, increased ESR, anemia, and hyperglobulinemia. Blood cultures determine the causative organism, and sensitivity tests indicate the antibiotic needed for medical management.

Medical Management

The medical management of the patient with endocarditis includes support of cardiac function, destruction of the pathogen, and prevention of complications.

Embolization, a serious and common complication, can occur. An embolus may go to the brain, the lungs, the coronary arteries, the spleen, the bowel, and the extremities, with catastrophic results. The most frequent embolic events usually occur during the first 2 weeks of acute infective endocarditis. Anticoagulation is not recommended because of the risk of an intracerebral hemorrhage. A patient who was receiving anticoagulation therapy before developing endocarditis may continue therapy as long as neurologic function is monitored carefully (Mayo Clinic, 2017a).

Management relies on rest to decrease the heart's workload. Complete bed rest usually is not indicated unless the temperature remains elevated and there are signs of HF. After the blood cultures, massive doses of antibiotics are administered, usually parenterally, to combat the organism. Antibiotic therapy continues often as long as 1 to 2 months. Traditionally this has required a prolonged hospitalization for most patients, but with newer, more versatile antibiotics (and growing economic concerns), outpatient treatment of patients with infective endocarditis is more common.

Prophylactic antibiotic treatment is recommended for individuals who are considered at high risk for developing infective endocarditis. Patients at risk include those with previous valve surgery, preexisting valvular heart disease, or congenital abnormalities. Infective endocarditis precautions involve antibiotic therapy as prescribed by the health care provider before any invasive procedure such as dental work or minor surgery.

Surgical repair of diseased valves or prosthetic valve replacement may be necessary if the patient's condition is severe. Valve replacement has become an important adjunct procedure in the management of endocarditis (Mayo Clinic, 2017a).

Nursing Interventions and Patient Teaching

The nursing interventions are based primarily on the signs and symptoms. Observe for petechiae, location of pain, vomiting, and fever, and report these signs and symptoms if observed.

During the acute phase, maintain the patient on decreased activity and provide a calm, quiet environment. Take vital signs, including apical pulse, every 4 hours. When increased activity or ambulation begins, assess pulse before and after to determine the effects on the heart muscle.

Ensuring adequate nutrition is important. Frequently patients have a decreased appetite because of the disease process. Provide attractive meals with supplemental between-meal nourishment. Promote rest and comfort and prevent further inflammation and infection during hospitalization.

Patient teaching focuses on identifying causes, infective endocarditis precautions, dietary requirements, and gradually increasing activity levels. Advise the patient on the need for prophylactic antibiotics before any invasive procedure if the patient has preexisting valvular heart disease. Instruct the patient about signs and symptoms that may indicate recurrent infections such as fever, fatigue, malaise, and chills and the need to report any of these signs and symptoms to the health care provider.

Prognosis

Before the advent of antibiotics, patients with infective endocarditis had a poor prognosis with a high mortality rate. Prompt treatment with intensive antibiotic therapy now cures a majority of the patients with this condition.

MYOCARDITIS

Acute myocarditis is relatively rare. Inflammation of the myocardium may originate from rheumatic heart disease; viral, bacterial, or fungal infection; or endocarditis or pericarditis. In the United States, most significant cases of acute myocarditis are caused by coxsackie virus type B (Muller, 2017). However, sometimes the cause may be unknown.

Signs and symptoms vary. The patient may have upper respiratory tract symptoms such as fever, chills, and sore throat; abdominal pain and nausea; vomiting; diarrhea; and myalgia. These generally occur up to 6 weeks before the patient has signs and symptoms of myocarditis, such as chest pain and overt HF with dyspnea (Mayo Clinic, 2017b). Cardiac enlargement, murmur, gallop, and tachycardia typically are seen in myocarditis. Cardiomyopathy may develop as a complication. Enlargement of the myocardium may result in dysrhythmias.

Early detection can help in treating myocarditis before complications develop. Useful tests to help diagnose myocarditis are chest x-ray, ECG, echocardiography, MRI, and cardiac catheterization with endomyocardial biopsy (Mayo Clinic, 2017c).

Therapy is symptomatic and primarily follows the same approach as that of endocarditis: bed rest, oxygen, antibiotics, antiinflammatory agents, careful assessments, and correction of dysrhythmias.

The goals of treatment are to preserve myocardial function and to prevent HF and other serious complications such as dilated cardiomyopathy. Patients may recover but may later develop cardiomyopathy. As a result, the disease may have a long, benign course, or it may result in sudden death during exercise.

CARDIOMYOPATHY

Etiology and Pathophysiology

Cardiomyopathy is a term used to describe a group of heart muscle diseases that primarily affect the structural or functional ability of the myocardium. This primary dysfunction is not associated with CAD, hypertension, vascular disease, or pulmonary disease.

When cardiomyopathies are classified by cause, two forms are recognized: primary and secondary. Primary cardiomyopathy consists of heart muscle disease of unknown cause and is classified as dilated, hypertrophic, or restrictive:

- *Dilated cardiomyopathy:* Characterized by ventricular dilation, dilated cardiomyopathy is the most common type of primary cardiomyopathy.
- *Hypertrophic cardiomyopathy:* Hypertrophic cardiomyopathy results in increased size and mass of the heart because of increased muscle thickness (especially of the septal wall) and decreased ventricular size.
- *Restrictive cardiomyopathy:* In restrictive cardiomyopathy the ventricular walls are rigid, thus limiting the ventricles' ability to expand and resulting in impaired diastolic filling (American Heart Association, 2016c).

Secondary cardiomyopathy has a number of types: (1) infective (viral, bacterial, fungal, or protozoal myocarditis); (2) metabolic; (3) severe nutritional deprivation such as in anorexia nervosa, a mental disorder in which people see themselves as severely overweight and starve themselves; (4) alcohol (large quantities consumed over many years leading to dilated cardiomyopathy); (5) peripartum (unexplained cause; may develop in the last month of pregnancy or within the first few months after delivery); (6) drugs (doxorubicin or other medications); (7) radiation therapy; (8) systemic lupus erythematosus; (9) rheumatoid arthritis; and (10) "crack" heart, caused by cocaine abuse.

Cardiomyopathy caused by cocaine abuse causes intense vasoconstriction of the coronary arteries and peripheral vasoconstriction, resulting in hypertension. This can result in increased myocardial oxygen needs and decreased oxygen supply to the myocardium and can lead to acute MI or ischemic cardiomyopathy. Cocaine also causes high circulating levels of catecholamines, which may damage further myocardial cells, leading to ischemic or dilated cardiomyopathy. The cardiomyopathy produced is difficult to treat. Interventions deal mainly with the HF that ensues. The prognosis is poor.

Clinical Manifestations

Angina, syncope, fatigue, and dyspnea on exertion are common signs and symptoms. The most common symptom is severe exercise intolerance. The patient may have signs and symptoms of left-sided and right-sided HF, including dyspnea, peripheral edema, ascites, and hepatic dysfunction.

Diagnostic Tests

Diagnosis of cardiomyopathy is made by the patient's clinical manifestations and noninvasive and invasive cardiac procedures to rule out other causes of dysfunction. Diagnostic studies include ECG, chest radiograph, echocardiogram, CT scan, nuclear imaging studies, MUGA scanning, cardiac catheterization, and endomyocardial biopsy.

Medical Management

Medical management consists of treatment of the underlying cause and HF management to slow the progression of the disease and symptoms. Medications may include diuretics, ACE inhibitors, antidysrhythmics, and beta-adrenergic blockers. An automatic internal defibrillator occasionally is implanted. In patients with advanced disease that is not responding to medical treatment, cardiac transplantation should be considered. Advise the patient to avoid strenuous exercise because of the risk of sudden death.

Cardiac transplantation. The first heart transplant was performed in 1967 and has since become the treatment of choice for patients with end-stage heart disease who are unlikely to survive more than 12 months. Patients with cardiomyopathy are more than 50% of cardiac transplant recipients. Dilated cardiomyopathy is the most common type of cardiomyopathy requiring transplantation. Inoperable CAD is the second most common indication for transplantation, accounting for 40% of candidates (Box 48.7; Botta, 2016).

Once a patient meets the criteria for cardiac transplantation, the goal of the evaluation process is to identify patients who would most benefit from a new heart. In addition to the physical examination, psychological assessment of candidates is valuable. A complete history of coping abilities, family support system, and motivation to follow through with the transplant and the rigorous transplantation regimen is essential. The complexity of the transplant process may be overwhelming to a patient with inadequate support systems and a poor understanding of the lifestyle changes required after transplant.

Once potential recipients are placed on the transplant list, they may wait at home and receive ongoing medical care if their medical condition is stable. If their condition is not stable, they may require hospitalization for more intensive therapy. Unfortunately, the overall waiting period for a transplant is long, and many patients die while waiting for a transplant. A patient awaiting a heart transplant may use an external heart pump.

Box 48.7 Indications and Contraindications for Cardiac Transplantation

INDICATIONS
- Suitable physiologic and chronologic age
- End-stage heart disease that is not responding to medical therapy
- Dilated cardiomyopathy
- Inoperable coronary artery disease
- Vigorous and healthy individual (except for end-stage cardiac disease) who would benefit from procedure
- Compliance with medical regimens
- Demonstrated emotional stability and social support system
- Financial resources available

CONTRAINDICATIONS
- Systemic disease with poor prognosis
- Active infection
- Active or recent malignancy
- Type 1 diabetes mellitus with end-organ damage
- Recent or unresolved pulmonary infarction
- Severe pulmonary hypertension unrelieved with medication
- Severe cerebrovascular or peripheral vascular disease
- Irreversible renal or hepatic dysfunction
- Active peptic ulcer disease
- Severe osteoporosis
- Severe obesity
- History of drug or alcohol abuse or mental illness

Donor and recipient matching is based on body and heart size and ABO blood type. Tissue cross-matching between donor and recipient generally is not done because of difficulty in obtaining good matches and lack of correlation between match and outcome.

Most donor hearts are obtained at locations distant from the institution performing the transplant. The maximum acceptable ischemic time for cardiac transplant is 4 to 6 hours.

The recipient is prepared for surgery, and cardiopulmonary bypass is used. The usual surgical procedure involves removing the recipient's heart, except for the posterior right and left atrial walls and their venous connections. The recipient's heart is then replaced with the donor heart, which has been trimmed to match. Care is taken to preserve the integrity of the donor SA node so that a sinus rhythm can be achieved postoperatively.

Immunosuppressive therapy usually begins in the operating room. Regimens vary but usually include azathioprine (Imuran), corticosteroids, and cyclosporine. Cyclosporine is used with corticosteroids for maintenance immunosuppression. Its use reduces rejection and slows the rejection process so that early treatment can be instituted.

The postoperative care is similar to that of other open-heart surgeries. Endomyocardial biopsies via the right internal jugular vein are performed periodically to detect rejection. In addition, peripheral blood T-lymphocyte monitoring is done to assess the recipient's immune status.

Because the patient is immunosuppressed, nursing interventions involve prevention of infection, which is the leading cause of death in this population. Many deaths from infection occur during augmented immunosuppressive therapy for acute rejection episodes. Provide a great deal of emotional support and teaching for the patient and the family, because transplantation is a last resort. In addition, the patient is often far from home and significant others.

Advances in surgical technique and postoperative care have improved early survival rates after cardiac transplantation. Attention is directed toward improvements in immunosuppression and management of long-term complications. Nursing management focuses on promoting patient adaptation to the transplant process, monitoring, managing lifestyle changes, and educating the patient and the family. Ongoing data collection and research continue in regard to quality of life, functional level, and rehabilitation of the cardiac transplant recipient (American Heart Association, n.d.).

Nursing Interventions and Patient Teaching

Nursing interventions focus on relieving symptoms, observing for and preventing complications, and providing emotional and psychological support. Monitor the response to medications and monitor for dysrhythmias.

Teach patients to adjust their lifestyle to avoid strenuous activity and dehydration. Advise patients to space activities and allow for rest periods.

Prognosis

Most patients have a severe, progressively deteriorating course, and the majority (particularly those older than 55 years of age) die within 2 years of the onset of signs and symptoms. However, improvement or stabilization occurs in a minority of patients. Death is due to either HF or ventricular dysrhythmia. Sudden death resulting from dysrhythmia is a constant threat. The survival rate with cardiac transplantation is approximately 81.8% for 1-year posttransplantation, and a 5-year survival rate of 69.8%. A growing number of recipients survive more than 10 years after the procedure.

DISORDERS OF THE PERIPHERAL VASCULAR SYSTEM

Peripheral vascular disease is any abnormal condition that affects the blood vessels outside the heart and the lymphatic vessels. The word **peripheral** means pertaining to those areas away from the center (in this context, the heart). The peripheral vascular system consists of arteries, capillaries, and veins. This system supplies oxygen-rich blood to the upper and lower extremities of the body, and returns blood and carbon dioxide from those areas to the heart and lungs. Disorders of the peripheral vascular system occur when circulation to the upper and lower extremities is compromised.

EFFECTS OF NORMAL AGING ON THE PERIPHERAL VASCULAR SYSTEM

Degenerative changes occur in the vascular system as part of the normal aging process. These changes affect the walls of the blood vessels and lead to problems in the transport of blood and nutrients to the tissues. The inner walls of the blood vessels (tunica interna) become thick and less flexible. The middle walls of the blood vessels (tunica media) become less elastic. With marked decreases in the elasticity and flexibility of the vessels, peripheral vascular resistance increases, causing a rise in blood pressure and increasing a person's susceptibility to peripheral vascular disease (see the Lifespan Considerations box in the section "Effects of Normal Aging on the Cardiovascular System").

RISK FACTORS

Risk factors for peripheral vascular disorders are similar to those for cardiovascular disorders. An important aspect of caring for the patient with a peripheral vascular disorder is understanding the risk factors and incorporating them into patient teaching.

Nonmodifiable Factors

- *Age:* As a person ages, arteriosclerotic changes in the peripheral vascular system lead to increased peripheral vascular resistance and decreased blood flow to the tissues.
- *Gender:* Men are more susceptible than women to arteriosclerotic changes. This gender difference decreases after menopause, when the protective effects of estrogen are no longer present in women.
- *Family history:* A family history of atherosclerosis increases an individual's risk.

Modifiable Factors

- *Smoking:* Smoking is one of the major contributing factors in the development of peripheral vascular problems. The nicotine in cigarettes causes vasoconstriction and spasms of the arteries, elevates blood pressure, and reduces circulation to the extremities. The carbon monoxide inhaled in cigarette smoke reduces oxygen transport to the tissues.
- *Hypertension:* Increased blood pressure causes wear and damage to the inner arterial walls, resulting in a buildup of fibrous tissue. This in turn leads to further narrowing of the vessel and increased resistance to blood flow.
- *Hyperlipidemia:* An elevation in serum cholesterol and triglycerides contributes to the buildup of plaque inside the blood vessels. The patient should maintain a diet with decreased saturated fat and cholesterol. If serum cholesterol remains elevated, drug therapy must be considered.
- *Obesity:* Excessive body weight and body fat contribute to the severity of other risk factors. Extra weight in relation to bone structure and height places an increased workload on the heart and blood vessels and may contribute to congestion in the venous system. The body mass index (BMI) is an indictor of whether the patient is overweight or obese. Use the following formula for calculation: 703 × Patient's weight in pounds ÷ Patient's height in inches squared. The CDC defines obesity as a BMI of 30 or above (CDC, 2016c).
- *Lack of exercise:* Decreased activity may compromise the peripheral vascular system because of a lack of muscle tone. The contraction and relaxation of muscles facilitate the return of blood in the veins to the heart and the lungs. A sedentary person does not realize the benefits of regular physical activity, such as weight and stress reduction and improved vascular tone.
- *Emotional stress:* Stress contributes to increased blood pressure, increased production of cholesterol, and increased vasoconstriction of the blood vessels. Emotional stress is different with each patient. Some patients deal with stress with appropriate coping mechanisms, whereas other patients have difficulty coping with stress. Family and financial concerns impose the most stress on individuals.
- *Diabetes mellitus:* Uncontrolled elevated serum glucose levels contribute to the atherosclerotic process, although the exact mechanism by which diabetes mellitus leads to peripheral vascular disorders is

unknown. Elevated serum glucose levels result in circulatory disorders.

ASSESSMENT

Arterial Assessment

The first symptom of decreased arterial circulation is pain from arterial insufficiency and ischemia. Arterial insufficiency occurs when not enough blood is available or able to flow through the arteries to body tissues. Ischemia occurs when the tissue does not receive enough oxygen-rich blood to function normally. Ischemic pain in the lower extremities is usually a dull ache in the calf muscles. It is often accompanied by leg fatigue and cramping. The pain is brought on by exercise and relieved by rest. It is referred to as **intermittent claudication** (a weakness of the legs accompanied by cramplike pains in the calves caused by poor circulation of the arterial blood to the leg muscles). Pain also may be felt in the thighs and buttocks. As arterial disease progresses and becomes chronic, pain occurs even at rest. Burning, tingling, and numbness of the legs may occur at night while the patient is lying down.

Other nursing assessments include palpating and comparing pulses in the extremities. Pulses may be weak, thready, or absent in the affected extremity because of decreased blood flow. Several scales are used to measure pulses. To ensure that the patient's pulses are graded the same way each time, all nurses should use the same scale, such as the following:

0 Absent
+1 Barely palpable, intermittent
+2 Weak, possibly thready, but constantly palpable and with consistent quality
+3 Normal strength and quality
+4 Bounding, easily palpable, may be visible

A Doppler ultrasound device may be needed to check the patient's pulses if pulmonary vascular disease (PVD), low blood pressure, edema, or large amounts of subcutaneous tissue impede the assessment. If a Doppler device is used, record pulsation as *present* or *absent* rather than using the numeric scale. Many nurses will mark the area with a skin marker where the pulse was found with the Doppler to allow for better accuracy and less time for assessing the pulse later. Assess the affected extremity and compare it with the unaffected extremity for color, temperature, skin characteristics, and capillary refill time (Box 48.8).

For a uniform assessment and documentation technique for *veins* and *arteries*, the following mnemonic device, PATCHES, is helpful:

P for *pulses:* Assess the patient's affected extremity first. Then assess the apical pulse and bilateral temporal, carotid, brachial, radial, femoral, popliteal, posterior tibial, and dorsalis pedis pulses. Absence of pulses is generally a medical emergency that requires immediate treatment, but in some cases it may be normal. Compare the findings with previous ones or correlate them with the patient's signs and symptoms. The use of a Doppler ultrasound probe to assess pulses must be documented. This allows all nursing staff assessing peripheral pulses to assess in the same way for continuity of assessments and care.

A for *appearance:* Note whether the extremity is pale, mottled, cyanotic, or discolored red, black, or brown. Document areas of necrosis or bleeding and the size, depth, and location of ulcers. When assessing ulcers, note whether the edges are jagged or smooth and whether the area is painful to touch. Shiny skin often indicates the presence of edema or presence or absence of hair; a dull appearance may signal inadequate arterial blood supply. Look for superficial veins, erythema, or inflammation anywhere on the affected extremity. Standing allows the saphenous veins to fill, so varicosities in the saphenous system are evaluated best with the patient standing. If a line of color change is present, mark it with a skin marker and monitor for changes in location.

T for *temperature:* If the patient has an arterial problem, the affected extremity feels cool; if the problem is venous, the extremity feels normal or abnormally warm. However, problems in arteries and veins are not the only reasons for temperature changes in an extremity; aortoiliac disease, HF, hypovolemia, pulmonary embolism, and other conditions can also affect skin temperature by interfering with peripheral blood flow.

C for *capillary refill:* Capillary refill is normally less than 2 seconds, but it may be extended when the patient has PVD. Press on a nail until the nailbed blanches, and then release and count how many seconds it takes for normal color to return. Other sites to check capillary refill are the pads of the toes and fingers, the heel, and the muscles at the base of the thumb. Although abnormal capillary refill is not diagnostic, it adds valuable data to the assessment (see Box 48.8).

H for *hardness:* Palpate the extremity to determine whether the tissues are supple or hard and inelastic. Hardness may indicate longstanding PVD, chronic venous insufficiency, lymphedema, or chronic edema. Hardened subcutaneous skin also increases the risk of stasis ulcers.

E for *edema:* Pitting edema frequently indicates an acute process, and nonpitting edema may be seen with chronic conditions, such as venous insufficiency.

Box 48.8 Capillary Refill Time

1. Apply pressure to a toenail or fingernail for several seconds until it blanches (the area loses its color).
2. Relieve the pressure.
3. Note the amount of time it takes for the color to return.
   - The color should return almost instantly—in less than 2 seconds.
   - With an arterial disorder, it will take more than 2 seconds for the color to return.

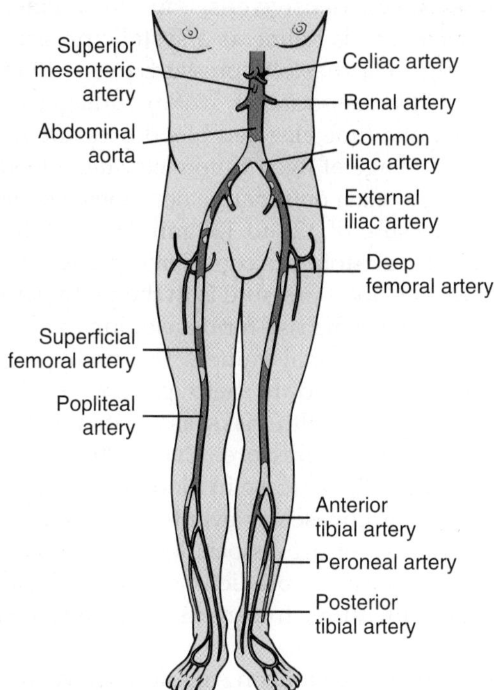

Fig. 48.17 Common anatomic locations of atherosclerotic lesions *(shown in yellow)* of the abdominal aorta and lower extremities. (From Lewis S, Dirksen SR, Heitkemper MM, et al: *Medical-surgical nursing: Assessment and management of clinical problems,* ed 8, St. Louis, 2011, Mosby.)

Table 48.9 Comparison of Signs and Symptoms Associated With Arterial and Venous Disorders

SIGNS AND SYMPTOMS	ARTERIAL DISORDER	VENOUS DISORDER
Pain	Aching to sharp cramping; brought on by exercise; relieved by rest	Aching to cramping pain; relieved by activity or elevating extremity
Pulses	Diminished or absent	Usually present
Edema	Usually absent	Usually present; increases at the end of the day and when extremity is in a dependent position
Skin changes	Cool or cold Dry, shiny Hairless Pallor develops with elevation; becomes erythematous with dangling	Warm, thick, and toughened Darkened pigmentation Stasis ulcers

Assess both extremities for edema and compare and document the findings. To assess for pitting edema, gently press the skin on the affected extremity for at least 5 seconds. Release and grade pitting as follows: +1, 2-mm indentation; +2, 4-mm indentation; +3, 6-mm indentation; and +4, 8-mm indentation (Fig. 48.17). The most accurate way to determine the degree of nonpitting edema is to measure the circumference of the extremity and compare measurements with the other extremity and subsequent measurements. Measure at the point of edema, and then mark the point with a skin marker so that everyone assesses the same area. Accuracy is greatest if the measurements are taken at the same time every day, preferably in the morning before the patient ambulates.

S for *sensation:* Vascular discomfort can originate in arteries, in veins, or in the microcirculation if the patient has diabetes mellitus. In addition to asking the patient about pain, ask if he or she has other abnormal sensations, such as numbness or tingling. Tingling or tenderness can result from peripheral tissue ischemia, and the patient may say the extremity feels abnormally hot or cold.

Venous Assessment

Decreased venous circulation leads to edema. When the venous system does not return sufficient blood from the tissues to the heart and the lungs (venous insufficiency), excess fluid is left in the tissues of the affected extremity (edema). Assess for edema in the affected extremity and compare it with the unaffected extremity.

Venous insufficiency may lead to changes in skin pigmentation. Assess the skin for darker pigmentation, dryness, and scaling in the affected extremity. Chronic edema and stasis of blood from venous insufficiency may lead to ulceration of the tissues. These ulcers are referred to as *stasis ulcers*. Peripheral pulses are usually present with venous insufficiency. Pain, aching, and cramping associated with venous disorders usually are relieved by activity and/or elevating the extremity. Refer to Table 48.9 for a comparison of signs and symptoms associated with arterial and venous disorders.

Diagnostic Tests

Diagnostic tests for peripheral vascular disorders include noninvasive procedures and invasive procedures.

Noninvasive procedures include the following:

- *Treadmill test:* This exercise test is used to determine blood flow in the extremities after exercising. It identifies pain associated with exercise such as claudication.
- *Plethysmography:* Plethysmography is used to assess changes in blood volume in the veins of the calf or other body extremities. The test can be done in either a health care provider's office or on an outpatient basis in the hospital. The patient is asked to recline in a semi-Fowler's position with the legs dangling. A blood pressure cuff in placed on the arm and leg of the affected side. The health care provider inflates the cuffs and a plethysmograph measures the pulses from each cuff.

- *Digital subtraction angiography:* Initially an IV contrast solution is administered. This allows blood vessels in the extremities to be visualized by radiography, using an image intensifier video system and a television monitor.
- *Doppler ultrasound:* A Doppler ultrasound flowmeter measures blood flow in arteries or veins to assess intermittent claudication, obstruction of deep veins, and other disorders of peripheral veins and arteries.

Invasive procedures include the following:

- *Venography:* A contrast medium is administered through a catheter placed in a foot vein. X-ray films are taken to detect filling defects. Venography is the gold standard by which to assess the condition of the deep leg veins and to diagnose DVT. Venography is invasive and costly, can be unpleasant, and may cause phlebitis. Before undergoing venography, the patient must sign an informed consent form, because the procedure involves the injection of a contrast medium. Because the contrast medium contains iodine, determine whether the patient is allergic to iodine or shellfish (the latter being an indication of sensitivity to iodine). Care after the procedure is similar to post-angiography care, including monitoring the pulse, assessing for edema, and monitoring sensation in the extremity.
- *Angiography:* This is done by injection of a contrast medium intravascularly and then visualizing the arteries by radiography.
- *D-dimer:* A serum venous blood test. D-dimer is a product of fibrin degradation (change to a less complex form). When a thrombus is present, plasma D-dimer concentrations are usually greater than 1591 ng/mL. The normal range for D-dimer is 68 to 494 ng/mL.
- *Duplex scanning:* This is a combination of ultrasound imaging techniques and Doppler capabilities to determine the location and extent of thrombi within veins (most widely used test to diagnose DVT).

HYPERTENSION

Hypertension is considered with peripheral vascular disorders, because it is a risk factor in atherosclerosis, which leads to peripheral vascular disease.

Etiology and Pathophysiology

Normal blood pressure is a reading of less than 120 mm Hg systolic and 80 mm Hg diastolic. Hypertension (or high blood pressure) occurs when a sustained elevated systolic blood pressure is greater than 140 mm Hg and/or a sustained elevated diastolic blood pressure is greater than 90 mm Hg. Stage 1 hypertension is defined as a systolic blood pressure of 140 to 159 mm Hg or a diastolic blood pressure of 90 to 99 mm Hg. Stage 2 and stage 3 hypertension have been combined into a single category, called stage 2, that is defined as a systolic blood pressure of 160 mm Hg or higher or a diastolic blood pressure of 100 mm Hg or higher. A hypertensive crisis, in which emergency care is necessary, is define as a systolic pressure over 180 mm Hg or a diastolic pressure over 110 mm Hg (American Heart Association, 2018b). A diagnosis is not based on a one-time elevated blood pressure reading, but on an average of two or more elevated blood pressure readings taken on separate occasions. People with a blood pressure of 120 to 139 mm Hg systolic or 80 to 89 mm Hg diastolic are considered prehypertensive. People whose blood pressure is in the prehypertensive range are at twice the risk for developing hypertension as people with normal values. The prehypertensive category was created to help patients understand the considerable health risks associated with small increases in blood pressure. Every 20 (systolic)/10 (diastolic)–mm Hg increase in blood pressure doubles the risk for cardiovascular events for people ages 40 to 70 (American Heart Association, 2018b). Although there is no way of predicting who will develop high blood pressure, hypertension can be detected easily.

Approximately 85 million Americans have hypertension, and an additional 25 million have prehypertension (American Heart Association, 2018b). It has been estimated that up to 30% of the adult population in the United States have undiagnosed hypertension. It is difficult to determine exact numbers, because most people are symptom free.

Arterial blood pressure is the pressure exerted by the blood on the walls of arteries. Systolic blood pressure is the greatest force caused by the contraction of the left ventricle of the heart. Diastolic blood pressure occurs during the relaxation phase between heartbeats. Blood flow is determined by the amount of blood the heart pumps with each contraction and how fast the heart beats. Peripheral vascular resistance is affected by the diameter of the blood vessels and the viscosity of the blood. Blood flow and peripheral vascular resistance play an important role in regulating blood pressure. Increased peripheral vascular resistance resulting from *vasoconstriction,* or narrowing of peripheral blood vessels, is a common factor in hypertension.

Vasoconstriction and vasodilation are controlled by the sympathetic nervous system and the renin-angiotensin system of the kidney. Stimulation of the sympathetic nervous system and the release of epinephrine and/or norepinephrine cause blood vessel constriction and increased peripheral vascular resistance. The activation of the renin-angiotensin system occurs with decreased blood flow to the kidney. Renin leads to the formation of angiotensin, which is a potent vasoconstrictor. Angiotensin stimulates the secretion of aldosterone, leading to the retention of sodium and water. The result is an increase in blood pressure.

The two main types of hypertension are *essential (primary)* hypertension and *secondary* hypertension. The incidence of hypertension increases with age and other risk factors.

Essential (Primary) Hypertension

Essential (primary) hypertension makes up the majority of all diagnosed cases. Although there is no general agreement on the cause of essential hypertension, theories to explain the mechanisms involved include arteriolar changes, sympathetic nervous system activation, hormonal influence (renin-angiotensin-aldosterone system stimulation), genetic factors, greater-than-ideal body weight, sedentary lifestyle, increased sodium intake, and excessive alcohol intake. For a long time many experts believed that an increase in systolic blood pressure was a normal part of aging. In fact, some believed that "100 mm Hg plus the patient's age" was a tolerable systolic blood pressure in the older adult. Treatment for hypertension was based primarily on the diastolic reading, and isolated systolic hypertension (ISH) often was not treated.

Clinical trials have reemphasized that ISH is believed to raise the risk of cardiovascular disease and stroke (Mayo Clinic, 2018). ISH is actually a better overall predictor of cardiovascular morbidity and mortality than diastolic pressure. (Diastolic pressure remains the better predictor of CAD in people younger than 45 years.) ISH is defined as an elevated systolic blood pressure of 140 mm Hg or more with a diastolic blood pressure below 90 mm Hg. The value of treating ISH in older patients has been established only recently, but now those findings are widely circulated. The recommendations are now aimed at keeping systolic blood pressure at 140 mm Hg or less, with a diastolic blood pressure not less than 70 mm Hg.

Prognosis. With prolonged untreated essential hypertension, the elastic tissue in the arterioles is replaced by fibrous tissue. This process leads to decreased tissue perfusion and deterioration, especially in the target organs—the heart, kidney, and brain. CAD and cerebrovascular accident (stroke), the major causes of death and disability, are much more frequent in those who have elevated blood pressure than in those who are normotensive. With treatment, the prognosis is usually good. Risk factors that contribute to the development of essential hypertension are listed in Box 48.9.

Box 48.9 Risk Factors for Essential Hypertension

NONMODIFIABLE RISK FACTORS

- *Age:* Risk increased as age advances past 30 years old
- *Gender:* Men more at risk than women
- *Race:* Risk twice as high in African Americans as in white Americans
- *Family history:* Risk increased with a family history of hypertension

MODIFIABLE RISK FACTORS

- *Smoking:* Nicotine constricts blood vessels
- *Obesity:* Associated with increased blood volume
- *High-sodium diet:* Increases water retention, which increases blood volume
- *Elevated serum cholesterol:* Leads to atherosclerosis and narrowing of blood vessels
- *Oral contraceptives or estrogen therapy:* May contribute to elevated blood pressure
- *Alcohol:* Increases plasma catecholamines (biologically active amines, epinephrine, and norepinephrine), which leads to blood vessel constriction
- *Emotional stress:* Stimulates the sympathetic nervous system, which leads to blood vessel constriction
- *Sedentary lifestyle:* Regular exercise helps lower blood pressure over time

Secondary Hypertension

Secondary hypertension is attributed to an identifiable medical diagnosis. Conditions associated with secondary hypertension are given in Table 48.10.

Prognosis. In most instances, secondary hypertension subsides when the primary disease process is treated or corrected. Because of the varied conditions causing secondary hypertension, problems can be anywhere in the body. The results of untreated secondary hypertension can lead to atherosclerosis; aneurysms; heart failure; weakened or narrowed vessels in the kidneys; thickened, narrowed, or torn vessels in the eyes; metabolic syndrome; as well as trouble with memory or understanding.

Malignant Hypertension

Malignant hypertension is a severe, rapidly progressive elevation in blood pressure (diastolic pressure greater than 120 mm Hg) that causes damage to the small arterioles in major organs (heart, kidneys, brain, eyes). A primary distinguishing finding is inflammation of arterioles (arteriolitis) in the eyes. This type of hypertension is most common in African American men younger than 40 years of age.

Prognosis. Unless medical treatment is successful, the course is rapidly fatal. The most common causes of death are MI, HF, stroke, and renal failure.

Clinical Manifestations

Hypertension is essentially a disease without symptoms until vascular changes occur in the heart, brain, eyes, or kidneys. Longstanding, untreated hypertension can cause target organ damage. Advanced target organ damage may account for left ventricular hypertrophy, angina pectoris, MI, HF, stroke or transient ischemic attack, nephropathy, peripheral arterial disease, or retinopathy. Signs and symptoms usually occur as a result of advanced hypertension. These signs and symptoms may include awakening with a headache, blurred vision, and spontaneous epistaxis (nosebleed).

Table 48.10 Causes of Secondary Hypertension

CONDITION OR DISORDER	MECHANISM
Renal vascular disease	Kidney disease (glomerulonephritis, renal failure, renal artery stenosis, physiologic changes related to type of disease) affects renin and sodium and results in hypertension
Diseases of the adrenal cortex • Primary aldosteronism • Cushing's syndrome • Pheochromocytoma	Atherosclerotic changes in renal arteries cause increase in peripheral vascular resistance Increase in aldosterone causes sodium and water retention and increases blood volume Increase in blood volume Excess secretion of catecholamines increases peripheral vascular resistance
Coarctation of the aorta (narrowing of the aorta)	Causes marked elevated blood pressure in upper extremities with decreased perfusion in lower extremities
Head trauma or cranial tumor	Increased intracranial pressure reduces cerebral blood flow and stimulates medulla oblongata to raise blood pressure
Pregnancy-induced hypertension	Cause unknown; generalized vasospasm may be a contributing factor

Assessment

Collection of subjective data includes assessing for morning headache in the occipital area and blurred vision. Assess the patient for risk factors (see Box 48.9). Determine the patient's understanding of hypertension, including the definition, meaning of systolic and diastolic readings, complications of hypertension, and possible concerns regarding treatment.

Collection of objective data includes measuring the blood pressure in both arms with the patient in supine and sitting positions. Compare the reading with previous blood pressure results. Take two or more blood pressure measurements on two separate occasions. Also measure and record height and weight. Assess and record heart sounds, and palpate and record peripheral pulses.

Diagnostic Tests

Diagnostic tests associated with hypertension evaluate the functions of the brain, heart, and kidneys. The results indicate the effects of hypertension on these organs and provide baseline information for future reference. These tests include CBC; serum levels of sodium, potassium, calcium, and magnesium; lipid profile; fasting blood glucose level; creatinine, BUN, urinalysis, and IV pyelography (i.e., radiography of the kidneys and ureters); renal arteriography (the gold standard for confirming renal artery stenosis); and chest radiography, ECG, and possible echocardiography (to determine any effect on the heart).

Medical Management

Medical management is directed at controlling hypertension and preventing complications. The goal in older adults is to keep the blood pressure at less than 140/90 mm Hg. The general goal for younger adults with mild hypertension is to achieve blood pressure of less than 130/80 mm Hg. Treatment is based on the severity of the hypertension, associated risk factors, and damage to major organs. Antihypertensive medications and nonpharmacologic measures are used to lower blood pressure.

Drug therapy. For stage 1 or 2 hypertension, drug therapy may include the following (American Heart Association, 2017e):

- Diuretics (thiazides, loop diuretics, potassium-sparing drugs)
- Beta-adrenergic blockers such as metoprolol, nadolol, propranolol, acebutolol (Sectral), atenolol, bisoprolol, timolol
- ACE inhibitors such as captopril, enalapril, lisinopril
- Angiotensin II receptor blockers such as valsartan, losartan, irbesartan, candesartan (Atacand), telmisartan (Micardis)
- Calcium channel blockers such as diltiazem, amlodipine, nifedipine, felodipine, verapamil
- Alpha-agonists such as clonidine
- Drug combinations such as Caduet, which contain Norvasc and Lipitor; Lotensin HCT, which contains benazepril and hydrochlorothiazide; and others, in an attempt to lower the number of pills taken so that patients will be more compliant in taking blood pressure–lowering medications
- Aliskiren hemifumarate (Tekturna), the first antihypertensive drug that is a direct renin inhibitor, decreases plasma renin activity and inhibits the conversion of angiotensinogen to angiotensin I (NIH, 2016)

Special considerations include using ACE inhibitors for diabetes mellitus; using ACE inhibitors and diuretics for HF; using beta blockers and ACE inhibitors for MI; using calcium channel blockers and diuretics for African Americans; and using diuretics and long-acting calcium channel blockers for older adults with ISH.

Nonpharmacologic therapy. Nonpharmacologic therapy for hypertension includes the following:

- *Lose excess weight:* Being overweight is associated with increased blood pressure, abnormally high blood lipid levels, diabetes mellitus, and CAD. Limiting calorie intake and increasing physical exercise are the keys to losing weight.

- *Exercise regularly:* Thirty to 45 minutes of aerobic exercise, three or four times a week, helps decrease the risk of hypertension and cardiovascular disease.
- *Reduce saturated fat:* A patient with high blood lipid levels may require dietary modification or drug therapy to normalize them. A cardinal rule is to limit fat intake to less than 30% of total calories. According to the Dietary Approaches to Stop Hypertension (DASH) study, a low-fat diet rich in fruits and vegetables is recommended.
- *Consume enough potassium, calcium, and magnesium:* Plenty of potassium in the diet helps decrease blood pressure, so eating potassium-rich fruits and vegetables may improve blood pressure control. Administering potassium supplements to a patient who is hypokalemic as a result of diuretic therapy also combats hypertension. A word of caution: Anyone receiving ACE inhibitors or potassium-sparing diuretics should receive potassium supplements only with extreme caution and close monitoring for hyperkalemia. Low dietary calcium and magnesium may contribute to hypertension (www.dashdiet.org); the National Heart, Lung, and Blood Institute suggests consuming adequate amounts of calcium and magnesium but does not recommend supplementation to combat hypertension.
- *Limit alcohol intake:* Excessive alcohol consumption may contribute to hypertension. A man of normal weight should not drink more than 1 ounce of ethanol per day (the equivalent of 24 ounces of beer, 10 ounces of wine, or 2 ounces of 100-proof whiskey). Women and lightweight men should restrict their intake to half this amount.
- *Reduce sodium intake:* High sodium intake can increase blood pressure, especially in African Americans, older adult patients with existing hypertension, and patients with diabetes mellitus. It is recommended that sodium intake be limited to 2.4 g/day. Encourage your patient to eat unsalted, unprocessed foods and to read labels when shopping.
- *Stop smoking:* Cigarette smoking is one of the leading risk factors for hypertension and heart disease. Smoking also inhibits the effect of antihypertensive medication, so techniques for stopping are an integral part of patient education. Counseling, support groups, and aids to stop smoking are effective. Individuals who discontinue smoking may gain weight. Provide information about weight management and exercise programs.
- *Use relaxation techniques and stress management:* Stress management and relaxation techniques have also been shown to offset hypertension and its symptoms.

Nursing Interventions and Patient Teaching

The main focus of nursing interventions is to maintain blood pressure management through patient teaching about hypertension, risk factors, and drug therapy. Patient compliance is improved with education about side effects of medications, dietary instruction, exercise, and stress-reduction techniques (Box 48.10).

Box 48.10 Measures to Increase Compliance With Antihypertensive Therapy

- Be certain that patient understands that absence of symptoms does not indicate control of blood pressure; remind patient that symptoms do not occur until advanced stages of the disease.
- Advise patient against abrupt withdrawal of medication; rebound hypertension can occur.
- Encourage patient to discuss unpleasant side effects of medication with a health care professional.
- If remembering to take medications is a problem, discuss alternative ways to remember, such as taking them with certain meals or placing medication in separate containers labeled with times of day.
- Suggest patient participate in an exercise program with a friend or pay for the program (more likely to participate "to get money's worth").
- Include family and significant others in the teaching process to provide support and promote adherence to regimen.
- Explain reason for regular health care follow-up (high blood pressure is a chronic disorder).
- Contact patients who consistently cancel follow-up appointments.

Patient problems and interventions for the patient with hypertension include but are not limited to the following:

Patient Problem	Nursing Interventions
Insufficient Knowledge, related to: • Disease process • Therapeutic management	Assess level of understanding Implement teaching plan for hypertension: • Disease process, risk factors • Prescribed medications and side effects; proper dosage and administration; necessity of taking medication, even when blood pressure readings are normal • Dietary restrictions • Exercise program • Relaxation techniques • Sexual dysfunction as a potential side effect of adrenergic inhibitors • Compliance with therapy and follow-up appointments Encourage the patient to promptly report any problems to health care professionals for counseling

ARTERIAL DISORDERS

ARTERIOSCLEROSIS AND ATHEROSCLEROSIS

Arteriosclerosis (a common arterial disorder characterized by thickening, loss of elasticity, and calcification of arterial walls, resulting in a decreased blood supply) is the underlying problem associated with peripheral vascular disorders. *Arteriosclerosis* and *atherosclerosis* frequently are used interchangeably.

Atherosclerosis is characterized by yellowish plaques of cholesterol, lipids, and cellular debris in the inner layers of the walls of large and medium-sized arteries. The result is narrowing of the artery and reduced nutrients and oxygen reaching the tissue, resulting in tissue ischemia. The arterial wall also loses its elasticity and becomes less responsive to changes in blood volume and pressure. Once plaque is formed in the arteries, it is thought to be irreversible. Lesions in the arteries formed from plaque may occlude an artery completely. Atherosclerosis can progress to obstruction, thrombosis, aneurysm, and rupture.

When the need for oxygen in the tissues exceeds the supply, ischemia occurs and may result in cell death and tissue necrosis. The degree of reduction in blood flow and oxygen determines the amount of ischemia and necrosis that occurs. Specific peripheral vascular disorders that stem from arteriosclerosis and atherosclerosis are discussed individually in this chapter.

PERIPHERAL ARTERIAL DISEASE OF THE LOWER EXTREMITIES

Etiology and Pathophysiology

Peripheral arterial disease (PAD) of the lower extremities is accompanied by narrowing or occlusion of the intimal and medial layers of the blood vessel walls. Plaque, as a result of the arteriosclerotic process, forms on the internal wall of the blood vessel, causing partial or complete occlusion. The result is little or no blood flow to the affected extremity. The artery is unable to supply blood and oxygen to the tissues whether the patient is exercising or at rest. Thus signs and symptoms associated with tissue ischemia appear.

Patients with PAD have atherosclerosis of the coronary and carotid arteries. The most common arteries affected in PAD of the lower extremities are the iliac, common femoral arteries, and superficial femoral arteries. Patients with diabetes mellitus are especially prone to develop PAD below the knees commonly in the anterior distal popliteal artery.

Clinical Manifestations

The severity of the signs and symptoms of PAD depends on the location and the extent of the atherosclerosis and on the amount of collateral circulation.

Pain is the first symptom that occurs from tissue ischemia. The pain generally occurs in the affected extremity in conjunction with sustained activity (see Table 48.9). This is because the oxygen demand of the tissue exceeds the available blood supply. The process of activity → ischemia → pain in an affected extremity is referred to as *claudication*. The pain of claudication subsides with rest; therefore it frequently is referred to as intermittent claudication (a weakness of the legs accompanied by cramping pains in the calves caused by poor circulation of the blood to the muscles). A burning pain at rest or at night occurs when the disease process is severe. Symptoms of coldness, numbness, and tingling may be associated with the pain. The signs and symptoms to watch for include the classic five *P*s of arterial occlusion: *pain, pulselessness, pallor, paresthesia,* and *paralysis*.

Assessment

Collection of subjective data focuses on pain associated with intermittent claudication. Does the pain occur with activity, and is it relieved by rest? Does pain occur at rest?

Collection of objective data includes assessment of pulses in the affected extremity, which may be weak or absent; comparison with pulses in the unaffected extremity; and assessment of capillary refill (more than 3 seconds indicates PAD) and ankle-brachial index (ABI; it is the ratio of the systolic blood pressure at the ankle to the systolic blood pressure in the arm). An ABI less than 0.70 indicates PAD. Other assessment findings may include pallor and hairless, shiny skin that is dry and cool to touch. Patients with chronic PAD may have **rubor** (discoloration or erythema [redness] caused by inflammation) or cyanosis, arterial ulcers, cellulitis, or gangrenous changes in the affected extremity.

Diagnostic Tests

A variety of tests are useful to diagnose PAD of the lower extremities. Treadmill testing, digital subtraction angiography, Doppler ultrasound, duplex imaging, MRI, and angiography are likely choices.

The ABI is a quick and noninvasive way to check for risk of peripheral artery disease. People who have a decreased ABI are at increased risk of developing a heart attack, stroke, poor circulation in the legs, and leg pain. The ABI is determined with the patient lying face up on a table while a technician measures the patient's blood pressure in both arms. Then the technician measures the patient's blood pressure in the two arteries in the left ankle, using an inflatable cuff and a hand-held Doppler ultrasound probe. The Doppler uses sound waves to produce images and lets the health care provider hear pulses in the ankle arteries after the blood pressure cuff is deflated. The test takes a few minutes, and no special precautions are necessary before or after the procedure. According to the American Heart Association and the American College of Cardiology, a borderline ABI of 0.91 to 0.99 puts the patient at minimal risk. An abnormal reading (anything below 0.9) puts the patient at higher risk of developing peripheral artery disease.

Medical Management

A patient with PAD is also at increased risk for developing ischemic stroke, MI, or other cardiovascular problems. Treatment should be aimed at preventing complications such as development of further cardiovascular disease and ischemic stroke. Smoking causes increased vasoconstriction, so smoking cessation is essential to decrease lower extremity ischemia in PAD and reduce the risk of MI and stroke.

Common oral antiplatelet treatment for patients with PAD is aspirin (160 to 325 mg/day) or clopidogrel (Plavix). These medications help prevent the development of thrombi or thrombophlebitis.

ACE inhibitors (e.g., ramipril) are prescribed for patients with PAD regardless of whether they have hypertension or left ventricular dysfunction (American Heart Association, 2016d). The use of ACE inhibitors decreases cardiovascular risks, improves arterial blood flow to the lower extremities, and improves walking stamina (American Heart Association, 2016d).

Two drugs commonly used to treat intermittent claudication are pentoxifylline and cilostazol. These drugs improve the distance the patient can walk without pain by increasing blood flow through the lower extremities (Mayo Clinic, 2015).

Fibrinolytics or thrombolytics are useful in dissolving existing thrombi. Urokinase (Abbokinase) is used in most patients with peripheral arterial occlusive disease. Unlike lytic therapy in MI or pulmonary embolism, in peripheral arterial occlusion the drug is administered directly into the thrombus through a central line that contains proximal and distal infusion wires (see the Complementary and Alternative Therapies box).

Surgical intervention for advanced disease includes embolectomy (removal of embolism) or endarterectomy (surgical removal of the lining of an artery, usually performed on any diseased or occluded major artery, such as the carotid, femoral, or popliteal), arterial bypass (Fig. 48.18), percutaneous transluminal angioplasty (PCTA), or amputation. If gangrene is extensive or all major arteries in the extremity are occluded, amputation, although the least desirable end-stage surgical option, may be required.

Nursing Interventions and Patient Teaching

Nursing interventions are based on assessment findings and nursing diagnoses. Patient problems and nursing interventions for the patient with PAD of the lower extremities include but are not limited to the following:

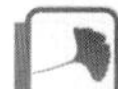

Complementary and Alternative Therapies

Cardiovascular and Peripheral Vascular Disorders

Herbs have been studied for their circulatory effects:

- *Ginkgo biloba* has been found to be minimally effective for treating intermittent claudication and decreased cerebral circulation leading to reduced function. Manifestations of decreased cerebral circulation include decreased memory, vertigo, tinnitus, and mood swings with anxiety. Gingko biloba cannot be taken with warfarin (Coumadin) as this increases the anticoagulant effect.
- Horse chestnut seed extract (HCSE, *Aesculus hippocastanum*) may be equivalent to use of compression stocking therapy to treat chronic venous insufficiency. German health authorities have approved HCSE to treat chronic venous insufficiency, pain and heaviness in the legs, and varicose veins. Gastrointestinal side effects may occur but are uncommon.
- Garlic has been studied for its effects on arteriosclerosis and lipids, but it has varying results. The amount of fresh garlic a person would need to eat for a therapeutic dose is large and likely to cause gastric upset. Garlic preparations vary widely in terms of their active constituents.
- Red yeast rice contains monacolins, which inhibit cholesterol synthesis. One of these, monacolin K, is known as mevinolin and as lovastatin. Lovastatin is a statin, that is, a cholesterol-lowering agent; some patients who cannot tolerate statins may not be able to use this herbal alternative.
- According to some studies, fish oil does not show the same promise of lowering cardiovascular risks as it once did, primarily because of the rise in methylmercury in fish oil.
- Flaxseed oil was once touted as an adjunct therapy to lower the risk of developing cardiovascular disease. New research has found that flaxseed oil does not lower serum lipids, but instead it suppresses oxygen radical production by white blood cells and prolongs bleeding times.
- Patients taking anticoagulants should be cautious regarding the use of herbs, including garlic, ginkgo, angelica, anise, bilberry, devil's claw, goldenseal, licorice root, parsley, and red clover. Although natural, these substances can have potent actions, possibly because of their anticoagulant effects, which may enhance the action of anticoagulant medications. Ask patients whether they are using such substances and monitor any interactions. Not enough controlled research is available to make definite predictions.
- Herbal remedies used to self-treat peripheral vascular disorders include those for hypertension, varicose veins, atherosclerosis, and vascular spasm. Herbs with antihypertensive action include garlic *(Allium sativum)*, hawthorn *(Crataegus oxyacantha)*, kudzu *(Pueraria lobata)*, nettle *(Urtica dioica)*, onion *(Allium cepa)*, purslane *(Portulaca oleracea)*, reishi mushroom *(Ganoderma lucidum)*, and valerian *(Valeriana officinalis)*, which is used as an antispasmodic. Antihypertensive spices include basil, black pepper, fennel, and tarragon.

Data from Rabito and Kaye, 2013.

Patient Problem	Nursing Interventions
Inability to Tolerate Activity, related to: • Ischemic pain • Immobility	Prevent hazards of immobility by turning, positioning, deep breathing, and performing isometric and range-of-motion exercises Encourage program of balanced exercise and rest to promote circulation Instruct the patient to use pain or intermittent claudication as a guide to limiting activity during exercise
Compromised Blood Flow to Tissue, peripheral, related to decreased arterial blood flow	Place patient's legs in a dependent position relative to the heart to improve peripheral blood flow Avoid raising feet above heart Promote vasodilation by providing warmth to extremities and keeping room warm Teach the patient to avoid vasoconstriction from nicotine, caffeine, stress, or chilling Teach the patient to avoid constrictive clothing such as garters, tight stockings, or belts Administer prescribed medications Teach the patient to avoid crossing the legs

Prognosis

In advanced disease, ischemia may lead to necrosis, ulceration, and gangrene (particularly of the toes and distal foot) because of the decreased circulation.

ARTERIAL EMBOLISM

Etiology and Pathophysiology

Arterial emboli are blood clots in the arterial bloodstream. They may originate in the heart from an atrial dysrhythmia, MI, valvular heart disease, or HF. Other foreign substances such as a detached arteriosclerotic plaque or tissue may result in arterial emboli. An embolus becomes dangerous when it lodges within and occludes a blood vessel. Blood flow to the area distal to the lodged embolus is impaired, and ischemia occurs. Signs and symptoms depend on the size of the embolus and the amount of circulation that is compromised.

Clinical Manifestations

Sudden loss of blood flow to tissues causes severe pain. Distal pulses are absent, and the affected extremity may become pale, cool, and numb. Necrotic changes may occur. Shock may result if the embolus occludes a large artery.

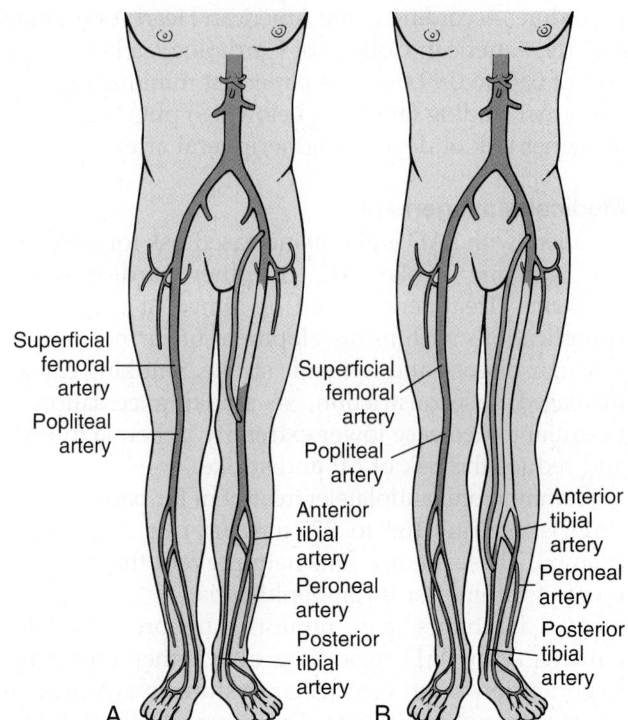

Fig. 48.18 A, Femoral-popliteal bypass graft around an occluded superficial femoral artery. B, Femoral posterior tibial bypass graft around occluded superficial femoral, popliteal, and proximal tibial arteries. (From Lewis S, Dirksen SR, Heitkemper MM, et al: *Medical-surgical nursing: Assessment and management of clinical problems*, ed 8, St. Louis, 2011, Mosby.)

Assessment

Collection of subjective data includes determining the onset of pain and numbness and the location, quality, and duration of these symptoms.

Collection of objective data includes assessing pulses in the affected extremity. Compare both extremities to determine skin temperature and color, in addition to pulse volume.

Diagnostic Tests

Doppler ultrasonography (see previously described studies on Doppler ultrasound) and angiography are indicated to obtain a diagnosis. An abnormal result may mean a blockage of an artery by a blood clot, fat embolism, or air embolism.

Medical Management

Medications used to treat obstructed arteries include anticoagulants and fibrinolytics or thrombolytics. Anticoagulants prevent further clot formation and inhibit extension of a clot. Thrombolytics and fibrinolytics dissolve an existing clot. See Table 48.6 for more information on anticoagulants and fibrinolytics.

Endarterectomy (the surgical removal of the intimal lining of an artery) may be the treatment of choice. This involves stripping arteriosclerotic plaque from the intima or inner media of arteries affected by atherosclerosis. Balloon catheters and other instruments are used to accomplish this. Removal of plaque and thrombi increases blood flow and lessens the danger of complications from further emboli or occlusion of an artery.

Embolectomy is another treatment used when larger arteries are obstructed. It is the surgical removal of a blood clot. Surgery must be done within 6 to 10 hours of the event to prevent necrosis and loss of the extremity. Endarterectomy and embolectomy may be done together to deal with the existing emboli and to prevent recurrence.

Nursing Interventions and Patient Teaching

Nursing interventions are similar to those for PAD in terms of preventing further arterial problems. During the acute phase monitor the patient for changes in skin color and temperature of the extremity distal to the embolus. Increasing pallor, cyanosis, and coolness of the skin indicate worsening or occlusion of arterial circulation to the extremity. Keep the extremity warm, but do not apply direct heat.

Patient problems and postoperative nursing interventions for the patient requiring an embolectomy and/or endarterectomy include but are not limited to the following:

Patient Problem	Nursing Interventions
Compromised Blood Flow to Tissue, related to decreased arterial blood flow	Monitor skin color and temperature of affected extremity every hour Assess sensation and movement in the distal extremity Assess peripheral pulses and capillary refill in the involved extremity: • Sudden absence of pulse may indicate thrombosis • Mark location of peripheral pulse with a skin pen to facilitate frequent assessment • Use a Doppler probe to monitor whether pulses of involved extremity are nonpalpable and compare with pulses of noninvolved extremity Monitor extremity for edema Check incision for erythema, edema, and exudates Monitor and immediately report signs of complications, such as increasing pain, fever, changes in drainage, absent or weakening pulse, changes in skin color, limitation of movement, or paresthesia Promote circulation: • Reposition patient q 2 hr • Tell patient not to cross legs • Use a footboard and overbed cradle to keep linens off extremity • Encourage progressive activity when permitted • Avoid sharp flexion in area of graft • Monitor for signs of bleeding secondary to anticoagulation therapy
Insufficient Knowledge, related to anticoagulant therapy	Teach patient general action and side effects of prescribed drug; instruct patient to avoid taking anticoagulant medications with aspirin, which also has anticoagulant effect Instruct patient to take anticoagulant at same time every day and to not stop taking it until advised by health care provider Have patient check for signs of bleeding (gums, epistaxis [nosebleed], ecchymosis [bruising], cuts that do not stop bleeding with direct pressure, blood in urine or stool); report promptly to health care professional Encourage patient to wear a medical-alert bracelet or to carry an identification card containing the drug name, drug dosage, and health care provider's name in case of emergency Have patient report for prescribed blood tests (PTT, PT, INR) used to adjust drug dosage Tell patient not to add dark green and yellow vegetables to diet (these contain vitamin K, which counteracts the anticoagulant drug effect) Instruct patient to restrict alcohol intake (increases anticoagulant effect)

Patient teaching is the same as for PAD, with an emphasis on anticoagulant therapy.

Prognosis

Prognosis depends on the size of the embolus, the presence of collateral circulation, and the proximity to a major organ.

ARTERIAL ANEURYSM

Etiology and Pathophysiology

An **aneurysm** occurs when the wall of an artery weakens, resulting in bulging of the artery when it fills with blood.

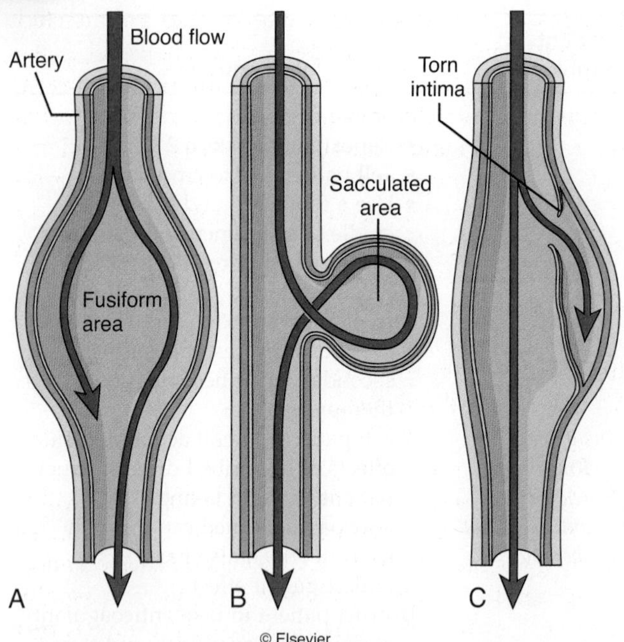

Fig. 48.19 Types of aneurysms. A, Fusiform. B, Saccular. C, Dissecting.

Aneurysms may be the result of arteriosclerosis, trauma, or a congenital defect. The force of blood pushing against walls of the artery combined with damage or injury to the artery's walls have caused the aneurysm. Aneurysms of the lower extremities commonly affect the popliteal artery. Other areas predominantly affected are the thoracic and abdominal aorta and the coronary and cerebral arteries. The aorta is especially prone to aneurysm and rupture, because it is continuously exposed to high pressures. Aortic aneurysms are most common in men in their 60s and 70s, especially if they have ever smoked. Other risk factors are hypertension, atherosclerosis, family history of aortic aneurysm, infarction, and trauma (National Heart, Lung, and Blood Institute, 2011). Dissections (separations and tears) and ruptures are more likely in the thoracic portion of the aorta than in the abdominal portion. An aneurysm starts with a weakened arterial wall that becomes dilated from blood flow and pressure in the area. The pathologic effect of this condition is differentiated according to shape and site of presentation (Fig. 48.19).

Clinical Manifestations

A large pulsating mass may be the only identifiable factor. Clinical signs and symptoms of a thoracic aortic aneurysm depend on its location. If it compresses adjacent structures, it can cause chest pain, shortness of breath, cough, hoarseness, or dysphagia. If it compresses the superior vena cava, the patient may have edema of the face, the neck, and the arms. In the early stages an abdominal aneurysm is unlikely to cause symptoms. As it expands, however, it may cause pain in the chest, the lower back, or, in men, the scrotum. A pulsatile, nontender upper abdominal mass may be palpated.

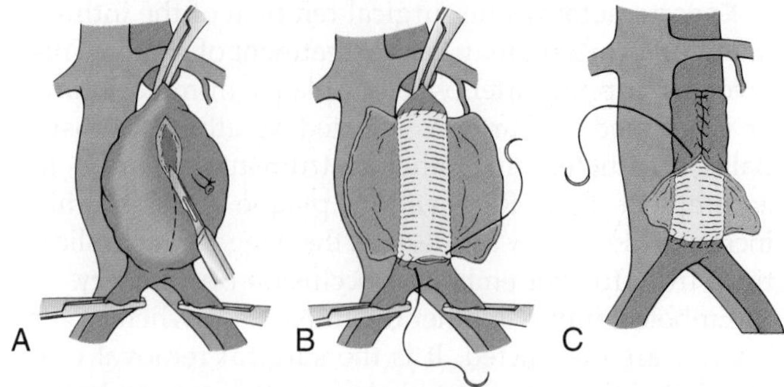

Fig. 48.20 Surgical repair of an abdominal aortic aneurysm. A, Incising the aneurysmal sac. B, Insertion of synthetic graft. C, Suturing native aortic wall over synthetic graft. (From Lewis S, Dirksen SR, Heitkemper MM, et al: *Medical-surgical nursing: Assessment and management of clinical problems*, ed 8, St. Louis, 2011, Mosby.)

Assessment

Collection of subjective data may reveal no subjective symptoms unless the aneurysm is large and impinges on other structures, causing pain and inequality of pulses. A thoracic aortic aneurysm can result in chest pain, shortness of breath, or dysphagia.

Collection of objective data includes palpation of a large, nontender, pulsating mass at the site of the aneurysm.

Diagnostic Tests

Fluoroscopy, chest radiographic studies, CT scan, ultrasound, contrast aortography, arteriography, MRI, and TEE are used to diagnose an aneurysm. It is recommended that all men who have ever smoked have an abdominal aneurysm screening (National Heart, Lung, and Blood Institute, 2011).

Medical Management

Aneurysms are monitored for complications such as dissection, rupture, formation of thrombi, and ischemia. Control of hypertension is the priority of care. An oral beta blocker reduces blood pressure, heart rate, and myocardial contractility. Surgical intervention may be necessary. The blood vessel may be ligated or grafts used to replace the section of the artery that contains the aneurysm or to bypass the aneurysm.

A fusiform or circumferential aneurysm (in which all the walls of the blood vessel dilate more or less equally, creating a tubular swelling) can be removed and repaired with a graft of synthetic fiber, such as Dacron or Teflon, or with a vessel taken from another region of the patient's body. Saccular aneurysms (an aneurysm, usually caused by trauma, that consists of a weak area on only one side of the vessel, causing an outpouching of the vessel wall that is attached to the artery by a narrow neck) can be removed and the vessel then sutured, or a patch graft can be used to replace the deformity (Figs. 48.20 and 48.21).

In repair of a popliteal aneurysm, popliteal blood flow is enhanced when a homograft (or *allograft*, tissue

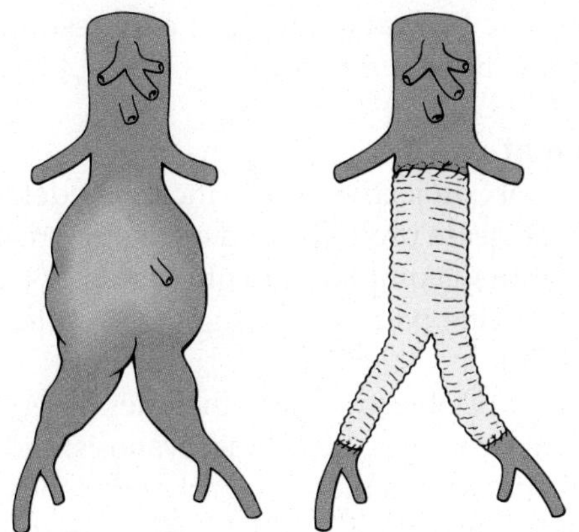

Fig. 48.21 Replacement of aortoiliac aneurysm with a bifurcated synthetic graft.

transferred between two genetically dissimilar individuals of the same species, such as two humans who are not identical twins) is used.

Nursing Interventions and Patient Teaching

Initial nursing interventions include monitoring the status of an existing aneurysm. Monitor the patient for signs of rupture of the aneurysm, such as paleness, weakness, tachycardia, hypotension, sudden onset of abdominal or chest pain, back pain, or groin pain and a pulsating mass in the abdomen.

Postoperative patient problems and interventions for the patient with arterial aneurysm include but are not limited to the following:

Patient Problem	Nursing Interventions
Compromised Blood Flow to Tissue, related to decreased arterial blood flow	Assess circulation (especially in extremities) by pedal pulse checks and capillary refill assessments Be alert for complications

Because aneurysm formation is associated most commonly with atherosclerosis, patient teaching focuses on managing risk factors, including control of hypertension, promotion of tissue perfusion, maintenance of skin integrity, and prevention of infection and injury.

Prognosis

An aneurysm may rupture and cause hemorrhage, resulting in death, unless emergency surgical intervention occurs. With surgical intervention, the prognosis is often good.

THROMBOANGIITIS OBLITERANS (BUERGER'S DISEASE)

Etiology and Pathophysiology

Thromboangiitis obliterans (Buerger's disease) is an occlusive vascular condition in which the small and medium-sized arteries become inflamed and thrombotic. The cause is not understood fully, but men between the ages of 25 and 40 years who smoke are affected most commonly by the disorder. Women, however, make up as much as 40% of patients with Buerger's disease. The disorder develops in the small arteries and veins of the feet and hands. Buerger's disease causes inflammation and damage to the arterial walls and is a type of arteritis (Mayo Clinic, 2017d). The wrists and lower legs also may be involved. Occlusion of the arteries leads to ischemia; pain; and, in later stages, infection and ulceration. There is a strong relationship between Buerger's disease and tobacco use. It is thought that the disease occurs only in smokers, and when smoking is stopped, the disease improves.

Clinical Manifestations

The main characteristic is inflammation of vessel walls. The most common symptom is pain with exercise affecting the arch of the foot, also called *instep claudication.* When the hands are involved, the pain is usually bilaterally symmetric (equal). Pain may occur at rest and be frequent and persistent, particularly when the patient also has atherosclerosis. The skin on the affected extremity may be cold and pale, and ulcers and gangrene may be present. Sensitivity to cold is an outstanding clinical manifestation. An early sign of Buerger's disease may be superficial thrombophlebitis.

Assessment

Subjective data include information about pain, claudication, and sensitivity to cold in affected extremities and risk factor assessment.

Objective data include presence of pulses, skin color, and temperature in the affected extremities.

Diagnostic Tests

No diagnostic tests are specific to Buerger's disease. Diagnosis is based on age of onset; history of tobacco use; clinical symptoms; involvement of distal vessels; presence of ischemic ulcerations; and exclusion of diabetes mellitus, autoimmune disease, and proximal source of emboli. Patients with Buerger's disease have a higher hematocrit level and more pronounced red blood cell rigidity, leading to greater blood viscosity, than do patients with peripheral arterial disease (Mayo Clinic, 2017d).

Medical Management

Medical management is directed at preventing disease progression. Modifying risk factors and smoking cessation are the major focus. Smoking causes vasoconstriction and decreases blood supply to the extremities. Treatment includes complete cessation of tobacco use in any form (including secondhand smoke and nicotine-replacement products). Continued smoking can lead to complete lack of blood flow to extremities. Trauma to the extremities must be avoided. Exercise to develop collateral circulation is encouraged. Surgical intervention, such as amputation of gangrenous fingers and toes, may be indicated. A sympathectomy (a surgical interruption of part of the sympathetic nerve pathways) to alleviate pain and vasospasm also may be performed.

Nursing Interventions and Patient Teaching

Nursing interventions focus on managing risk factors, promoting tissue perfusion, providing comfort measures, and patient teaching. Care of the extremities to prevent necrosis and gangrene includes hydration and cleanliness. Well-fitting shoes and socks alleviate pressure.

The hazards of cigarette smoking and its relationship to Buerger's disease are the primary focus of patient teaching. None of the palliative treatments are effective if the patient does not stop smoking. Nowhere are the consequences of smoking so dramatically seen as with Buerger's disease.

Prognosis

Buerger's disease is a chronic condition. Amputation may be necessary if the condition progresses to gangrene with chronic infection and extensive tissue destruction. The prognosis improves if the patient stops smoking. When patients are compliant with therapy, 94% of patients avoid amputation. The 8-year amputation rate for patients who continue to smoke is 43% (Nassiri, 2017).

RAYNAUD'S DISEASE

Etiology and Pathophysiology

Raynaud's disease is caused by intermittent arterial spasms. Intermittent attacks of ischemia, especially of the fingers, toes, ears, and nose, are caused by exposure to cold or by emotional stimuli. Raynaud's disease is either primary or secondary. The cause of primary Raynaud's is unknown, and the condition is usually mild. When symptoms occur in association with autoimmune diseases, a diagnosis of secondary Raynaud's disease is made. Primary Raynaud's disease usually occurs before 30 years of age, whereas secondary Raynaud's disease usually occurs after age 30. Secondary Raynaud's disease is associated with other conditions such as scleroderma (a relatively rare autoimmune disease affecting blood vessels and connective tissue), rheumatoid arthritis, systemic lupus erythematosus, drug intoxication, and occupational trauma. It usually affects women and is more prevalent during the winter months. The exact cause is unknown, but emotional stress, alterations in the nervous system and immunologic system, and hypersensitivity to cold may play a role in the development of signs and symptoms. Few arterial changes occur initially, but as the disease progresses, the intimal wall thickens and the medial wall hypertrophies.

Clinical Manifestations

The patient typically complains of chronically cold hands and feet. During arterial spasms, pallor, coldness, numbness, cutaneous cyanosis, and burning, throbbing pain occur. Chronic Raynaud's disease may result in ulcerations on the fingers and toes.

Assessment

Collection of subjective data includes determining underlying disease processes and evaluating risk factors. The patient may complain of cold hands or feet and a throbbing, aching pain with a tingling sensation (Mayo Clinic, 2017e).

Collection of objective data includes assessment of pallor; edema; coldness; blanching; cyanosis; and reactive hyperemia (increased blood in part of the body, caused by increased blood flow), which instigates rubor, after an arterial spasm. Inspect the fingers and toes for ulceration because of circulatory inadequacy and residual waste products.

Diagnostic Tests

A cold stimulation test is used to diagnose Raynaud's disease. Skin temperature changes are recorded by a thermistor attached to each finger. Submerge the patient's hand in an ice water bath for 20 seconds and record ongoing temperatures. A comparison is made for baseline data.

Medical Management

Medical therapy is aimed at prevention. Drug therapy may be prescribed to reduce pain and promote circulation. At present, first-line drug therapy involves calcium channel blockers, such as nifedipine and diltiazem, to relax smooth muscles of the arterioles. Nifedipine is preferred over diltiazem, because it has a stronger vasodilating effect and less effect on the calcium channels in the conduction system in the heart (Mayo Clinic, 2017e). Biofeedback techniques have been used to increase skin temperature and thereby prevent spasms. Relaxation training and stress management are effective for some patients. Temperature extremes should be avoided. The patient should stop using all tobacco products and avoid caffeine and other drugs with vasoconstrictive effects such as amphetamines and cocaine. Possible surgical interventions include sympathectomy for symptomatic relief. If the disease is advanced, with ulcerations and gangrene, the involved area may have to be amputated.

Nursing Interventions and Patient Teaching

Nursing interventions are similar to those for other arterial disorders: promoting tissue perfusion, maintaining comfort, and preventing injury and infection. Risk factor management includes stress reduction techniques and smoking cessation as well as decreasing the amount of alcohol consumption. Patients should be cautioned to avoid drastic temperature changes. Exercise is encouraged to increase blood flow. Stress reduction techniques help in preventing triggers for attacks. Patients should be educated on what to do if an attack occurs. Gentle warming of extremities is stressed. If patients are outdoors, they should get indoors or to a warmer environment. Moving the fingers, hands, and arms can increase circulation as well as placing the hands under the axilla and massaging hands and feet (Mayo Clinic, 2017e).

Patient problem statements and interventions stress patient teaching for the patient with Raynaud's disease, including but not limited to the following:

Patient Problem	Nursing Interventions
Insufficient Knowledge, related to: • Effects of cigarette smoking • Stress reduction • Avoidance of exposure to cold	Develop teaching plan to include the following: • Effects of smoking on vasoconstriction and arterial blood flow • Techniques for smoking cessation: Stop-smoking programs, biofeedback, hypnosis • Techniques for stress reduction: Massage, imagery, music, exercise, lifestyle changes • Ways to avoid exposure to cold: Layer clothing, wear mittens and warm socks during winter, use caution when cleaning the refrigerator and freezer, wear gloves when handling frozen food, and avoid occupations requiring constant exposure to cold

Prognosis

Raynaud's disease persists but may be controlled by protecting the body and extremities from the cold and using mild sedatives and vasodilators. No serious disability develops, but this condition sometimes is associated with rheumatoid arthritis or scleroderma.

VENOUS DISORDERS

Venous disorders occur when the blood flow is interrupted in returning from the tissues to the heart. Changes in smooth muscle and connective tissue make the veins less distensible. The valves in the veins may malfunction, causing backflow of blood. The major venous disorders are thrombophlebitis and varicose veins (Table 48.11).

THROMBOPHLEBITIS

Etiology and Pathophysiology

Thrombophlebitis is the inflammation of a vein in conjunction with the formation of a thrombus. It occurs more frequently in women and affects people of all races. The incidence increases with aging. Other factors associated with thrombophlebitis include venous stasis, hypercoagulability (excessive clotting) of the blood, and trauma to the blood vessel wall. Immobilized patients who have had surgical procedures involving pelvic blood vessel manipulation, such as total hip replacement or pelvic surgery, or patients with MI are prone to thrombophlebitis. Thrombophlebitis develops in deep veins (DVT) (Fig. 48.22) or in superficial veins

Table 48.11 Venous Disorders

SIGNS AND SYMPTOMS	MEDICAL MANAGEMENT AND NURSING INTERVENTIONS
Thrombophlebitis	
Entire extremity may be pale, cold, and edematous Area along vein may be erythematous and warm to touch Patient may have Homans sign: Pain in calf on dorsiflexion Superficial veins feel indurated (hard) and thready or cordlike and are sensitive to pressure Extremities have difference in circumference	Maintain bed rest during acute phase Apply warm, moist heat to reduce discomfort and pain per health care provider's orders Elevate extremity, but do not use pillows under the knees, and never bend the knees Assess circulation of the affected extremity, and skin condition and pulses in all extremities Measure calf circumference daily and record Use antiembolism stocking on unaffected extremity Administer heparin or enoxaparin (Lovenox) and warfarin (Coumadin) per health care provider's orders Administer fibrinolytics (streptokinase) to resolve the thrombus per health care provider's orders Begin exercise program after acute phase per health care provider's orders
Varicose Veins	
Veins appear as darkened, tortuous, raised blood vessels; more pronounced on prolonged standing Legs feel heavy Patient has fatigue Patient has pain and muscle cramps Legs are edematous Ulcers are seen on skin	Conservative treatment: • Elevate legs 10–15 min at least q 2–3 hr. • Wear elastic stockings. • Unna's paste boot is recommended for the older or debilitated person with cutaneous ulcers. • Avoid standing for long periods. • Avoid anything that impedes venous flow, such as garters, tight girdles, crossing the legs, and prolonged sitting. • Reduce weight if obese. • Inject sclerosing solutions for small varicosities. Surgery: • Venous ligation and stripping

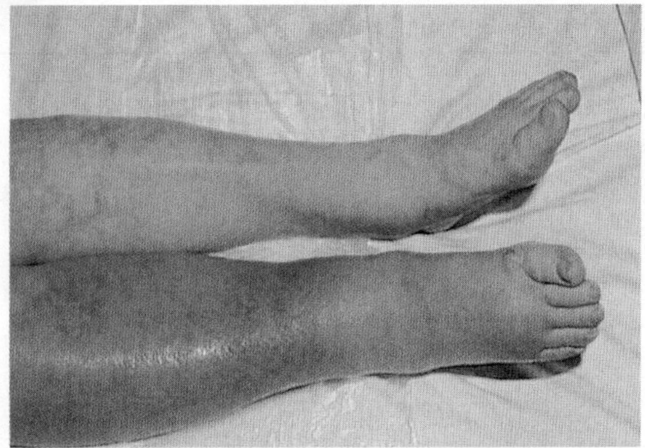

Fig. 48.22 Deep vein thrombosis. (From Lewis SL, Heitkemper MM, Dirksen SR, et al: *Medical-surgical nursing: Assessment and management of clinical problems*, ed 7, St. Louis, 2007, Mosby.)

(superficial thrombophlebitis). Thrombophlebitis usually occurs in an extremity, most frequently a leg. Superficial thrombophlebitis is often minor and is treated with elevation, antiinflammatory agents, and warm compresses. DVT is a condition involving a thrombus in a deep vein such as the iliac or femoral veins. It is of greater significance and the thrombus can prevent blood flow to an area or it can become dislodged, carried to the lungs via the bloodstream, and cause a pulmonary embolus. Pulmonary embolism is a life-threatening complication. The CDC (2017) estimates that 900,000 people could be affected by DVT (1 to 2 per 1000) each year in the United States, and 60,000 to 100,000 Americans die of DVT/PE (pulmonary embolism). The CDC also estimates that 10% to 30% of people will die within 1 month of diagnosis, and sudden death is the first symptom in about one-fourth (25%) of people who have a PE.

Clinical Manifestations

Pain and edema commonly occur when the vein is obstructed; however, some patients do not experience pain. The circumference of the calf or thigh may increase. In the past it was believed that active dorsiflexion of the foot may result in calf pain when thrombophlebitis is present. This is referred to as a positive Homans sign. *Homans sign* has been found to be an unreliable sign, because it is not specific for DVT and appears in only 10% of patients with DVT. Superficial thrombophlebitis may show signs of inflammation such as erythema, warmth, and tenderness along the course of the vein.

Assessment

Subjective data include characteristics of pain in the affected extremity, noting onset and duration and any history of venous disorders.

Collection of objective data includes inspecting the extremity and determining color and temperature (pale and cold if vein is occluded; erythematous and warm if a superficial vein is inflamed). Measure both legs for circumference and comparison and to detect edema. Signs of decreased circulation may occur distal to the area of the clot. The degree of blockage determines the severity of the symptoms.

Diagnostic Tests

Diagnostic tests for DVT include venous Doppler, duplex scanning (the most widely used test), and venography (phlebography). The results of a serum D-dimer test are elevated in DVT. D-dimer is a fibrin degradation fragment, the result of fibrinolysis. When a thrombus is undergoing lysis (destruction), it results in increased D-dimer fragments.

Medical Management

Anticoagulant therapy is used for DVT prevention and treatment. For an existing DVT, anticoagulant therapy prevents extension of the clot, development of a new clot, or embolization (embolus traveling through the bloodstream). Anticoagulants do not dissolve a clot, but they help the clot from growing in size. Heparin (warfarin) can be given subcutaneously or intravenously. Other common anticoagulants that are administered subcutaneously include enoxaparin (Lovenox), dalteparin (Fragmin), or fondaparinux (Arixtra). Lysis (destruction) of the clot begins immediately by the body's own fibrinolytic system, but for more serious thrombi, thrombolytics such as streptokinase and tissue-type plasminogen activator (tPA) may be administered intravenously or via a catheter placed with a cardiac catheterization. Venous filters may be necessary to prevent PE by blocking a moving clot if clots are large or if the patient cannot tolerate medications (Mayo Clinic, 2017f).

Low-molecular-weight heparin (LMWH) is effective for the prevention of venous thrombosis and any extension or recurrence. Enoxaparin and dalteparin are two types of LMWH. LMWH is administered subcutaneously in fixed doses, once or twice daily. LMWH has the practical advantage that it does not require anticoagulant monitoring and dose adjustment. LMWH has greater bioavailability, a more predictable dose response, and a longer half-life than heparin with less risk of bleeding complications.

The affected extremity is elevated periodically above heart level to prevent venous stasis and to reduce edema. Specific orders depend on the health care provider's preference. When the patient ambulates, elastic stockings (antiembolism stockings) are used to compress the superficial veins, increase blood flow through the deep veins, and prevent venous stasis. Warm compresses may be ordered if the thrombus is superficial.

Surgery is indicated only when conservative measures have been unsuccessful. A thrombectomy (removal of a clot from a blood vessel) or the transvenous placement of a grid or umbrella in the vena cava may be done to prevent the flow of emboli into the lungs. The inferior vena caval interruption device can be inserted percutaneously through the superficial femoral or internal jugular vein. When the filter device is opened, the spokes penetrate the vessel walls. The device creates

 Safety Alert

Patient on Anticoagulant Therapy

1. Teach patient receiving oral warfarin about the requirements for frequent follow-up with blood tests (PT, INR) to assess blood clotting and whether a change in drug dosage is required.
2. Teach patient side effects and adverse effects of anticoagulant therapy requiring medical attention.
   - Any bleeding that does not stop after a reasonable time (usually 10 to 15 minutes)
   - Blood in urine or stool or black, tarry stools
   - Unusual bleeding from gums, throat, skin, or nose, or heavy menstrual bleeding
   - Severe headaches or stomach pains
   - Weakness, dizziness, mental status changes
   - Vomiting blood
   - Cold, blue, or painful feet
3. Avoid any trauma or injury that may cause bleeding (e.g., vigorous brushing of teeth, contact sports, inline roller skating).
4. Do not take aspirin-containing drugs or NSAIDs because of the blood-thinning effects these drugs contribute.
5. Limit alcohol intake to small amounts. Alcohol interferes with metabolism of the drug.
6. Wear a medical-alert bracelet or necklace indicating what anticoagulant is being taken.
7. Avoid marked changes in eating habits, such as dramatically increasing foods high in vitamin K (e.g., broccoli, spinach, kale, greens). Do not take supplemental vitamin K.
8. Inform all health care providers, including dentist, of anticoagulant therapy.
9. Correct dosing is essential, and supervision may be required (e.g., for patients experiencing confusion).
10. Do not use herbal products that may alter coagulation (see the Complementary and Alternative Therapies box).

a "sieve-type" obstruction, filtrating clots without interrupting blood flow.

Nursing Interventions and Patient Teaching

Early mobilization is the easiest and most cost-effective method to decrease the risk of DVT. Patients on bed rest must be instructed to change position, dorsiflex their feet, and rotate their ankles every 2 to 4 hours. Ambulatory patients should ambulate at least three times per day. Elastic compression stockings (e.g., thromboembolic disease hose) and/or an intermittent compression device are used for hospitalized patients at risk for DVT. The major emphasis for the patient with thrombophlebitis is to prevent complications, promote comfort, and teach about the disease and how to prevent a recurrence. Patients should avoid extended periods of inactivity. When traveling, the patient must wear antiembolism stockings and take frequent breaks to ambulate.

Patient problems and interventions for the patient with thrombophlebitis include but are not limited to the following:

Nursing Diagnosis	Nursing Interventions
Compromised Blood Flow to Tissue, related to decreased venous blood flow	Confine patient to bed in acute phase Elevate affected extremity according to health care provider's orders Check circulation frequently (monitor pedal pulses, capillary refill) Administer prescribed anticoagulants, and fibrinolytics Measure calf or thigh circumference daily Assess site for signs of inflammation and edema Have patient wear elastic stockings when ambulatory Implement graded exercise program as ordered
Insufficient Knowledge, related to disease process and risk factors	Develop a teaching plan to prevent venous stasis, including the following: • Avoid prolonged sitting or standing; begin weight reduction if obese • Avoid crossing the legs at the knee and wearing tight stockings or garters • Elevate legs when sitting • Do flexion-extension exercises of feet and legs when sitting or lying down to promote circulation and venous return • Do not massage extremities because of danger of embolization of clots (thrombus breaking off and becoming an embolus) • Take prescribed medication

Prognosis

A major risk during the acute phase of DVT is dislodgment of the thrombus, which can migrate to the lungs, causing a pulmonary embolus. Postphlebetic syndrome also may develop after a DVT. Inflammation of the vein at the site of the thrombus may be temporary or may be a long-term complication. Postphlebetic syndrome results in swelling of the extremity. Elevation and antiembolism stockings generally are prescribed.

VARICOSE VEINS

Etiology and Pathophysiology

A varicose vein is a tortuous, dilated vein with incompetent valves. The highest incidence of varicose veins occurs in women ages 40 to 60 years. Approximately

15% of the adult population is affected. Causes of varicose veins include congenitally defective valves, an absent valve, or a valve that becomes incompetent. External pressure on the legs from pregnancy or obesity can place a strain on the vessels, and they become elongated and dilated. Poor posture, prolonged standing, and constrictive clothing also may contribute to this problem. The great and small saphenous veins of the legs are affected most often. The vessel wall weakens and dilates, stretching the valves and leaving the vessel unable to support a column of blood. Pooling of blood in the veins or varicosities is the result. Chronic blood pooling in the veins is referred to as *venous stasis.* Hemorrhage can occur if a varicose vein suffers trauma.

Clinical Manifestations

Varicose veins may be primary or secondary. Primary varicosities have a gradual onset and occur in superficial veins. Secondary varicosities affect the deep veins and result from chronic venous insufficiency or venous thrombosis. Often the only symptom is the appearance of darkened veins on the patient's legs. Symptoms include fatigue, dull aches, cramping of muscles, and a feeling of heaviness or pressure arising from decreased blood flow to the tissues. Signs and symptoms such as edema, pain, changes in skin color, and ulceration may occur as a result of venous stasis.

Assessment

Collection of subjective data includes gathering information about predisposing factors: a family history of varicose veins, pregnancy, or other conditions that could cause pressure on the veins. Also include symptoms the patient is experiencing such as aches, fatigue, cramping, heaviness, and pain.

Collection of objective data includes inspecting the legs for varicosities, edema, color, and temperature of the skin and observing for ulceration.

Diagnostic Tests

Trendelenburg's test is done to diagnose the ability of the venous valves to support a column of blood by measuring venous filling time. The patient lies down with the affected leg raised to allow for venous emptying. A tourniquet is applied above the knee, and the patient stands. The direction and filling time of the veins are recorded before and after the tourniquet is removed. When the veins fill rapidly from a backward blood flow, the veins are determined to be incompetent.

Medical Management

Mild signs and symptoms may be controlled with elastic stockings, rest periods, and leg elevation. Sclerotherapy consists of injection of a sclerosing solution at the sites of the varicosities. It is done as an outpatient procedure and produces permanent obliteration (complete occlusion of a part) of collapsed veins and good cosmetic results. Elastic bandages are applied for continuous pressure for 1 to 2 weeks. Surgical intervention is indicated for pain, progression of varicosities, edema, and stasis ulcers, and for cosmetic reasons. Surgery consists of vein ligation and stripping. The great saphenous vein is ligated (tied) close to the femoral junction. The great and small saphenous veins are stripped out through small incisions made in the inguinal area, above and below the knee and the ankle. The incisions are covered with sterile dressings, and an elastic bandage is applied and worn for at least 1 week. Newer, laser treatments are available for smaller varicosities.

Nursing Interventions and Patient Teaching

Nursing interventions focus on care of the patient after a surgical procedure, including maintaining comfort, maintaining peripheral circulation and venous return, and teaching the patient about varicose vein prevention and maintenance.

Patient problems and interventions for the patient with varicose veins include but are not limited to the following:

Patient Problem	Nursing Interventions
Compromised Blood Flow to Tissue, related to impaired venous blood return	Monitor for signs and symptoms of bleeding postoperatively. If bleeding occurs, apply pressure to the wound, elevate the leg, and notify the health care provider Keep elastic bandage snug and wrinkle free; do not remove bandage for daily dressing change Encourage deep breathing exercises and early ambulation to facilitate venous return Encourage dorsiflexion exercises while in bed or sitting to facilitate venous return
Insufficient Knowledge, related to disease process and measures to avoid venous stasis and promote venous return	Develop teaching plan to include the following: • Avoid anything that can increase pressure above the knees (crossing the legs, sitting in chairs that are too high, wearing garters and knee-high stockings) • Begin regular exercise to promote venous return by contraction of leg muscles • Avoid prolonged sitting or standing • Elevate legs when sitting • Maintain ideal weight • Wear elastic stockings for support for activities that require prolonged standing or when pregnant. These measures are aimed at those people who are at greater risk, to decrease occurrences

Prognosis

Varicosities are chronic conditions if not treated surgically; the affected person must know how to prevent venous stasis and encourage venous return. Prevention is the key to preventing complications. Patients should avoid prolonged sitting with regular exercise and weight reduction. Noncompliance can result in chronic swelling, pain, decreased circulation, and possibly ulcerations.

VENOUS STASIS ULCERS

Etiology and Pathophysiology

Venous stasis ulcers or leg ulcers occur from chronic deep vein insufficiency and stasis of blood in the venous system of the legs. Other causes include severe varicose veins, burns, trauma, sickle cell anemia, diabetes mellitus, neurogenic disorders, and hereditary factors. A leg ulcer is an open, necrotic lesion that results when an inadequate supply of oxygen-rich blood and nutrients reaches the tissue (Fig. 48.23). The results are cell death, tissue sloughing, and skin impairment. Decreased circulation to the area contributes to the development of infection and prolonged healing.

Clinical Manifestations

Patients may report varying degrees of pain, from mild discomfort to a dull, aching pain relieved by elevation of the extremity. The skin is visibly ulcerated and has a leathery appearance and dark pigmentation. Edema may be present. Ulcerations often occur around the medial aspect of the ankle. Pedal pulses are present.

Assessment

Subjective data include onset and duration of pain and successful relief measures. Predisposing factors such as thrombophlebitis, venous insufficiency, and diabetes mellitus are noted.

Collection of objective data includes inspection of ulcerated areas: size, location, and condition of skin; color; and temperature. Palpate pedal pulses and observe for edema.

Diagnostic Tests

Venography and Doppler ultrasonography are used to confirm venous insufficiency and stasis. See the section "Diagnostic Tests" under "Venous Assessment" for a description of what is included in these tests. They show slow progression of blood to the extremities.

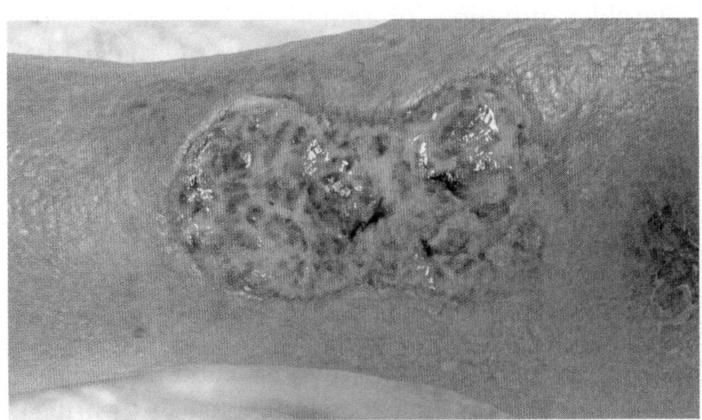

Fig. 48.23 Venous leg ulcer.

Medical Management

Management focuses on promoting wound healing and preventing infection. Diet is important to ensure adequate protein intake, because large amounts of protein in the form of albumin are lost through the ulcers. Also, vitamins A and C and the mineral zinc are administered to promote tissue healing. Débridement of necrotic tissue, antibiotic therapy, and protection of the ulcerated area are usual treatments. Débridement can be mechanical with a débriding instrument. Débridement also may be chemical; enzyme ointments such as fibrinolysin with DNase (deoxyribonuclease, Elase) are placed over the ulcer to break down necrotic tissue. Medihoney is currently a common treatment. It is a medical-grade honey product that promotes healing by providing a low pH-balanced moisture environment. Therapy for a venous stasis ulcer also may consist of saline irrigation with ultrasound therapy called MIST therapy. Surgical débridement using a scalpel is done when other measures are not successful.

Applying compression to the affected area is essential to promote venous ulcer healing and to prevent ulcer recurrence. Compression options include elastic wraps, custom-fitted compression stockings, and intermittent compression devices. Coban can be used to apply compression. Compression therapy usually is maintained for an average of 3 days; therefore circulation must be assessed to prevent decreased circulation from the extremity swelling or from the compression being applied too tightly. If copious amounts of drainage occur, compression therapy may be challenging. An Unna's paste boot can be used to protect the ulcer and provide constant and even support to the area (Fig. 48.24). Moist, impregnated gauze is wrapped around the patient's foot and leg. It hardens into a "boot" that may be left on for 1 to 2 weeks, although it may be changed more often if there is copious drainage. This treatment is not used as commonly today. Balanced nutrition to promote healing is important with an emphasis on increasing protein.

Nursing Interventions and Patient Teaching

Nursing interventions focus on promoting wound healing, promoting comfort, maintaining peripheral tissue perfusion, preventing infection, and patient teaching.

Patient problems and interventions for the patient with venous stasis ulcers include but are not limited to the following:

Patient Problem	Nursing Interventions
Compromised Skin Integrity, related to venous insufficiency as evidenced by open ulceration	Perform dressing changes per health care provider's order, using gauze, moistened with saline, topical drug treatments, and Unna's boot therapy Assess wound for signs and symptoms of infection

Continued

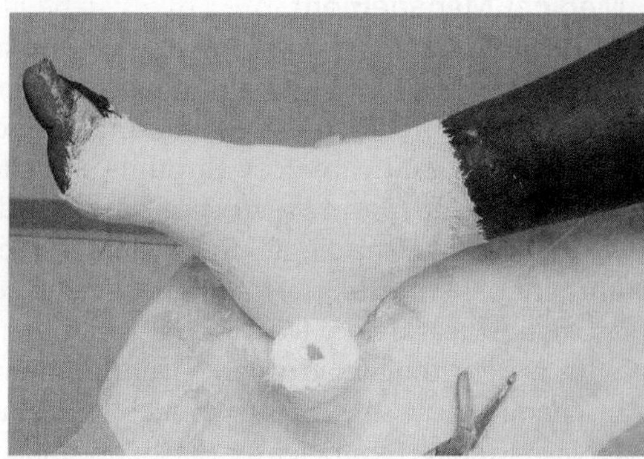
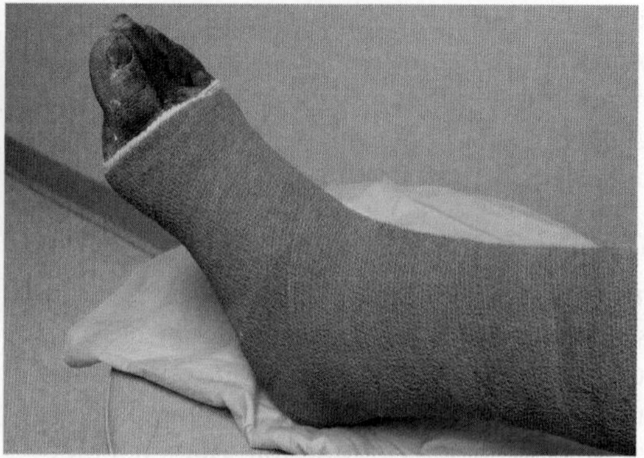

Fig. 48.24 The stages of application of the Unna's paste boot, using specially impregnated gauze. Most ulcers are on the inferior aspect of the patient's foot. (Cameron MH, Monroe LG: *Physical rehabilitation for physical therapist assistant*. St. Louis, 2011, Saunders.)

Patient Problem	Nursing Interventions
Compromised Blood Flow to Tissue, related to insufficient venous circulation	Provide antibiotic therapy as prescribed Encourage nutritional intake to promote wound healing Elevate extremities when sitting or lying down to promote venous return and decrease risk of edema and venous stasis Use overbed cradle to protect extremities from pressure of bed linens Use cotton between toes to prevent pressure on a toe ulcer Assess level of discomfort

Patient teaching focuses on preventing infection, maintaining peripheral tissue circulation, avoiding venous stasis, and providing proper wound care and dressing changes. See previous nursing diagnoses and interventions.

Prognosis

Venous stasis ulcers are a chronic condition caused by chronic venous insufficiency and delayed healing. Most venous ulcers heal with therapy.

NURSING PROCESS FOR THE PATIENT WITH A CARDIOVASCULAR DISORDER

The role of the licensed practical nurse/licensed vocational nurse (LPN/LVN) in the nursing process as stated is that the LPN/LVN will:

- Participate in planning care for patients based on patient needs
- Review patient's care plan and recommend revisions as needed
- Review and follow defined prioritization for patient care
- Use clinical pathways, care maps, or care plans to guide and review patient care

Systemic cardiac assessment provides baseline data useful for identifying the patient's physiologic and psychosocial needs.

ASSESSMENT

Begin assessment of the patient with a cardiovascular disorder by performing a complete health history and physical assessment. The physical assessment includes level of consciousness, vital signs, lung sounds (crackles, wheezes), bowel sounds, apical heart sounds (strength, regularity of rhythm), pedal pulses, capillary refill, skin color (pallor, cyanosis), turgor, temperature and moisture, and presence of edema. The history includes a description of symptoms, when they occurred, their course and duration, location, precipitating factors, and relief measures. Specific signs and symptoms to be aware of include the following:

- *Pain:* Note the character, quality, radiation, and associated symptoms. Ask the patient to rate pain on a scale of 0 to 10. Determine what, if anything, relieved the pain, such as rest or medication (e.g., nitroglycerin sublingually). Chest pain is the primary complaint when patients have symptoms of heart disease. Some patients with ischemia have pain in the jaw and left shoulder. The patient may describe the pain as dull, sharp, pressure, squeezing, crushing, viselike, grinding, or radiating. Note any factors precipitating the onset. Pain originating from cardiac muscle ischemia (decreased blood supply to a body organ or part) produces anxiety. It may lead to other signs and symptoms such as nausea, vertigo, or diaphoresis. Chest pain is significant in indicating cardiac ischemia or damage.
- *Palpitations:* Characterized by rapid, irregular, or pounding heartbeat, palpitations may be associated with cardiac dysrhythmias (any disturbance or abnormality in a normal rhythmic pattern) or cardiac ischemia. Patients may begin to notice the heartbeat

and describe it as "pounding" or "racing." This can be frightening for the patient.

- *Cyanosis:* A bluish discoloration of the skin and mucous membranes caused by an excess of deoxygenated hemoglobin in the blood. Cyanosis results from decreased cardiac output and poor peripheral perfusion.
- *Dyspnea:* Dyspnea is characterized by difficulty in breathing or shortness of breath. Observe for dyspnea with activity, referred to as *exertional dyspnea,* which commonly is associated with decreased cardiac function.
- *Orthopnea:* Orthopnea is an abnormal condition in which a person must sit or stand to breathe deeply or comfortably.
- *Cough:* The cough may be dry or productive and results from a fluid accumulation in the lungs. The patient may describe it as irritating or spasmodic. Dyspnea may be associated with it. The production of sputum should be observed for frothiness or hemoptysis (see the section "Pulmonary Edema").
- *Fatigue:* Exhaustion and activity intolerance are associated with decreased cardiac output. The patient may be unable to perform ADLs. Depression may accompany this or be a result of it.
- *Syncope:* Syncope or fainting is a brief lapse of consciousness caused by transient cerebral hypoxia. It usually is preceded by a sensation of lightheadedness. It can result from a sudden decrease in cardiac output to the brain as a result of dysrhythmia (bradycardia or tachycardia) or decreased pumping action of the heart.
- *Diaphoresis:* Sweating, especially profuse sweating, is associated with clamminess. Diaphoresis is a result of decreased cardiac output and poor peripheral perfusion.
- *Edema:* Weight gain of more than 3 pounds in 24 hours may be indicative of HF. The mechanism leading to edema in HF is the inability of the heart to pump efficiently or accept venous return, causing retrograde blood flow and an excessive amount of circulating blood volume. This increased blood volume results in increased hydrostatic pressure and an increase in fluid in the interstitial spaces.

◆ PATIENT PROBLEM

Assess the patient's cardiovascular system and identify characteristics that reveal a patient problem. Patient problems for cardiovascular problems may include the following:

- *Anxiousness*
- *Compromised Blood Flow to Cardiac Tissue*
- *Discomfort*
- *Fluid Volume Overload*
- *Inability to Tolerate Activity*
- *Inefficient Oxygenation*
- *Insufficient Cardiac Output*
- *Insufficient Knowledge (specify)*

◆ EXPECTED OUTCOMES AND PLANNING

Plan appropriate interventions to meet the needs of patients with cardiovascular problems. The nurse is uniquely qualified for ongoing patient monitoring and is able to participate in the development of nursing diagnoses, help select appropriate interventions, and document the care plan. Teaching throughout the hospital stay and when preparing for discharge is important. Reinforcement of good health habits improves the likelihood for compliance with the care plan.

◆ IMPLEMENTATION

Nursing interventions for the patient with a cardiovascular disorder include enhancing cardiac output, promoting tissue perfusion, promoting adequate gas exchange, improving activity tolerance, and promoting comfort. Patient teaching emphasizes adherence to diet and exercise and medication protocols and strategies for balancing activity, getting rest, and reducing stress.

◆ EVALUATION

Evaluate the expected outcomes as the final step of the nursing process and determine their effectiveness. Participate in the revision of the plan and nursing interventions when necessary.

Get Ready for the NCLEX® Examination!

Key Points

- The cardiovascular system is composed of the heart, blood vessels, and lymphatic structures.
- The functions of the cardiovascular system are to deliver oxygen and nutrients to the cells and to remove carbon dioxide and waste products from the cells.
- The heart is a large pump (the size of a human fist) that propels blood through the circulatory system.
- The heart is composed of four chambers: two atria and two ventricles.
- There are two coronary arteries; they supply the heart with nutrition and oxygen.
- The electrical impulse pathway starts at the SA node, which is the pacemaker of the heart; it initiates the heartbeat. The impulse travels to the AV node. From here the impulse travels to a bundle of fibers called the bundle of His, which divides into right and left bundle branches and finally to the Purkinje fibers.
- Three kinds of blood vessels are organized for carrying blood to and from the heart: the arteries, the veins, and the capillaries.

- Risk factors for developing CAD are classified as nonmodifiable and modifiable.
- Nonmodifiable risk factors for CAD include advancing age, male gender, black race, and a positive family history of CAD.
- Major modifiable risk factors for CAD include cigarette smoking, hyperlipidemia, stress, obesity, sedentary lifestyle, and hypertension. A diet high in cholesterol and saturated fats contributes to risk.
- An important aspect of caring for the patient with a cardiovascular disorder is understanding the risk factors and incorporating them into patient teaching.
- Major diagnostic tests to evaluate cardiovascular function include chest radiograph, arteriography, cardiac catheterization, ECG, echocardiogram, telemetry, stress test, PET, and thallium scanning.
- Common laboratory examinations to evaluate cardiovascular function are blood cultures, CBC, PT, INR, PTT, ESR, serum electrolytes, lipids (VLDL, LDL, HDL), triglycerides, arterial blood gases, BNP, and serum cardiac markers. Troponin I is a myocardial muscle protein released into the circulation after myocardial injury and is useful in diagnosing an MI.
- CAD includes a variety of conditions that obstruct blood flow in the coronary arteries.
- When the myocardial oxygen demand exceeds the myocardial oxygen supply, ischemia of the heart muscle occurs, resulting in chest pain or angina.
- Patient teaching to minimize the pain of angina pectoris includes taking nitroglycerin before exertion, eating small amounts more frequently rather than two or three larger meals in a day, balancing exercise periods with rest, stopping activity at the first sign of chest pain, avoiding exposure to extreme weather conditions, quitting smoking, and seeking a calm environment.
- Subjective data for the patient with MI may include heavy pressure or squeezing pressure in the chest, retrosternal pain radiating to left arm and jaw, anxiety, nausea, and dyspnea.
- Objective data for the patient with MI include pallor, hypertension, cardiac rhythm changes, vomiting, fever, and diaphoresis.
- Possible nursing diagnoses for the patient with MI include pain (acute), tissue perfusion (ineffective), activity intolerance, decreased cardiac output, anxiety, and constipation.
- Cardiac rehabilitation services are designed to help patients with heart disease recover faster and return to full and productive lives. Cardiac rehabilitation improves patient compliance.
- HF leads to the congested state of the heart, lungs, and systemic circulation as a result of the heart's inability to act as an effective pump. The most recent definition is that HF should be viewed as a neurohormonal problem that progresses as a result of chronic release in the body of substances such as catecholamines (epinephrine and norepinephrine). These substances may have toxic effects on the heart.
- It is important to realize that 1 L of fluid equals 1 kg (2.2 lb); so, a weight gain of 2.2 lb signifies a gain of 1 L of body fluid.
- Signs and symptoms of HF with left ventricular failure include dyspnea; cough; frothy, blood-tinged sputum; pulmonary crackles; and evidence of pulmonary vascular congestion with pleural effusion.
- Signs and symptoms of HF with right ventricular failure include edema in feet, ankles, and sacrum, which may progress into the thigh and external genitalia; liver congestion; ascites; and distended jugular veins.
- Medical management of HF includes increasing cardiac efficiency with digitalis, vasodilators, and ACE inhibitors; administering a beta blocker (carvedilol) for mild to moderate HF; lowering oxygen requirements through bed rest; providing oxygen to the tissues through oxygen therapy if the patient is hypoxic; treating edema and pulmonary congestion with a diuretic and a sodium-restricted diet; and weighing daily to monitor fluid retention.
- Nursing interventions for the patient with valvular heart disease include administering the prescribed medications (diuretics, digoxin, and antidysrhythmics); monitoring I&O and daily weight; auscultating breath sounds and heart sounds; taking blood pressure; and assessing capillary perfusion, pedal pulses, and presence of edema.
- Teaching for the patient with valvular heart disease includes dietary management, activity limitations, and the importance of antibiotic prophylaxis before invasive procedures.
- Most patients with cardiomyopathy have a severe, progressively deteriorating course, and the majority older than age 55 years die within 2 years of the onset of signs and symptoms.
- PVD is any abnormal condition that affects the blood vessels outside the heart and the lymphatic vessels.
- Arteriosclerosis is the underlying problem associated with PVD.
- Hypertension occurs when there is a sustained elevated systolic blood pressure greater than 140 mm Hg and/or sustained elevated diastolic blood pressure of greater than 90 mm Hg on two or more readings.
- Nursing interventions for hypertension primarily focus on blood pressure management through patient teaching, risk factor recognition, drug therapy, dietary management, exercise, and stress-reduction techniques.
- An aneurysm is an enlarged, dilated portion of an artery and may be the result of arteriosclerosis, trauma, or a congenital defect.
- The hazards of cigarette smoking and its relationship to thromboangiitis obliterans (Buerger's disease) are the primary focuses of teaching the patient with Buerger's disease.
- The two major venous disorders are thrombophlebitis and varicose veins.
- Thrombophlebitis may result in calf pain on dorsiflexion of the foot, which is referred to as a positive Homans sign. However, a positive Homans sign appears in only 10% of patients with DVT.
- The patient with thrombophlebitis should be taught to avoid prolonged sitting or standing, avoid dehydration, reduce weight if obese, perform dorsiflexion-extension exercises of the feet and legs, not cross the legs at the knees, and to elevate legs when sitting.

Additional Learning Resources

SG Go to your Study Guide for additional learning activities to help you master this chapter content.

evolve Be sure to visit the Evolve site at *http://evolve.elsevier.com/Cooper/foundationsadult/* for additional online resources.

Review Questions for the NCLEX® Examination

1. A patient is admitted to the hospital with a diagnosis of heart failure. Recently the patient's symptoms have been getting worse as a result of arteriosclerosis. In establishing a patient care plan, what is the primary goal of treatment?
   1. Reduce the workload of the heart.
   2. Promote rest for the heart.
   3. Reduce fluid retention.
   4. Reduce circulating blood volume.
2. What is the best nursing action that will lessen the severity of a patient's orthostatic hypotension?
   1. Turn him from side to side every 2 hours.
   2. Limit times he will have to get in and out of the bed.
   3. Change his position routinely, especially from horizontal to vertical.
   4. Encourage him to move very slowly.
3. When caring for a patient whose health care provider has ordered furosemide (Lasix), what will the nurse recognize when the medication is having the desired effect? *(Select all that apply.)*
   1. The patient becomes very thirsty.
   2. The patient's resting heart rate slows.
   3. The patient's blood pressure is reduced.
   4. Production of urine is increased.
   5. The patient's weight decreases
4. A patient receives a diagnosis of angina pectoris, with no subsequent cardiac involvement. The health care provider prescribes nitroglycerin. What explanation would the nurse give to this patient about why this medication is given sublingually?
   1. Superficial blood vessels promote rapid absorption of the medication.
   2. Stomach acids destroy the medication.
   3. Saliva helps break down the medication for absorption.
   4. The medication is too rapidly absorbed in the stomach.
5. Before administering a dose of digoxin to an assigned patient, the nurse observes that the patient's pulse rate is 52. What is the most appropriate nursing action?
   1. Notify the charge nurse.
   2. Recognize that these are signs of digoxin toxicity and withhold the dose.
   3. Administer the medication.
   4. Hold the medication and notify the health care provider.
6. The nurse is assessing a patient and suspects the patient is experiencing thrombophlebitis in the lower leg. What symptoms would the nurse assess? *(Select all that apply.)*
   1. Numbness along a vein
   2. Severe cramping
   3. Edema of the extremity
   4. Calf is warm to the touch
   5. Pain in the effected extremity
7. When a patient is receiving heparin therapy, what would be the nurse's most appropriate action?
   1. Observe him for cyanosis.
   2. Assess degree of edema in all extremities.
   3. Give the injection intramuscularly.
   4. Observe emesis, urine, and stools for blood.
8. A patient is admitted to the medical floor with a diagnosis of HF. Which assessment findings are consistent with the medical diagnosis? *(Select all that apply.)*
   1. Increase in abdominal girth
   2. Weight loss of 6 pounds in the past 2 weeks
   3. Pitting edema
   4. Nervous tremors
   5. Night sweats
9. A 10-year-old patient is diagnosed with rheumatic fever. Of all the manifestations seen in rheumatic fever, which is most likely to lead to permanent complications?
   1. Sydenham's chorea
   2. Erythema marginatum
   3. Subcutaneous nodules
   4. Carditis
10. A patient has a diagnosis of hypertension. When providing discharge teaching what should the nurse include? *(Select all that apply.)*
    1. Instruction in consuming a bland diet
    2. Instruction to limit sodium intake to 2 g/day
    3. Encouragement to begin a vigorous exercise program
    4. Monitoring and keeping a record of blood pressure measurements at home
    5. Education on continuing to take antihypertensive medications as prescribed
11. An 86-year-old patient is receiving an intravenous infusion at 83 mL/hour via an electronic infusion pump. Why is it so vital that the IV lines of older adult patients be monitored carefully?
    1. These patients do not become dehydrated very easily.
    2. These patients are at an increased risk for developing fluid overload of the circulatory system.
    3. These patients are at an increased risk for developing a venous infection.
    4. Aging patients present an increased risk for developing thrombophlebitis in the peripheral system.

12. A patient with a history of IV drug use is diagnosed with acute infective endocarditis. Which nursing intervention for this patient is most appropriate?
1. Early ambulation
2. Restricted activity for several weeks
3. Low-calorie diet
4. Dilution of blood by increased fluid intake

13. A patient has a history of angina pectoris. To decrease the pain from angina pectoris, what should the patient do?
1. Take a cardiac glycoside at the first symptom of cardiac pain.
2. Avoid taking more than three or four nitroglycerin pills daily.
3. Take nitroglycerin sublingually three times daily.
4. Take nitroglycerin sublingually prophylactically before strenuous exercise.

14. A 75-year-old patient is diagnosed with heart failure. The nursing diagnosis of *Activity Intolerance, related to dyspnea and fatigue,* would be appropriate. What nursing intervention would be most appropriate for this diagnosis?
1. Plan frequent rest periods.
2. Allow the patient to shower.
3. Encourage the patient to perform all ADLs.
4. Encourage fluid intake of 3000 mL/day.

15. A patient presents with dependent edema of the extremities, enlargement of the liver, oliguria, jugular vein distention, and abdominal distention. What does the nurse suspect the patient is experiencing?
1. Right-sided heart failure
2. Left-sided heart failure
3. Cardiac dysrhythmias
4. Valvular heart disease

16. What is the primary goal of patient teaching after a myocardial infarction?
1. Explaining the disease process
2. Assisting the patient in developing a healthy lifestyle
3. Describing the precipitating causes and onset of pain
4. Educating the patient on causative factors that initiate cardiac vasoconstriction

17. A patient experienced intense chest pain, anxiety, and nausea. The admitting diagnosis is suspected myocardial infarction. When providing care for the patient in the emergency department, the nurse must understand what about a myocardial infarction?
1. It involves a critical reduction in blood supply to the myocardium.
2. There is a marked increase in cardiac output.
3. A sudden irregularity of cardiac contraction occurs.
4. There is a marked decrease in cardiac output.

18. When providing patient teaching regarding coronary artery disease, the nurse can include which of the following when advising the patient about modifiable risk factors? *(Select all that apply.)*
1. Family history
2. Smoking
3. Cholesterol level
4. Obesity
5. Ethnicity

19. When a patient returns to the unit following cardiac catheterization, which nursing activity should follow immediately after taking of vital signs?
1. Placing the patient in a warm bed and encouraging sleep
2. Providing the patient with fluids
3. Assessing the patient's peripheral pulses
4. Reapplying the patient's dressing where the dye was injected

20. What is the most useful noninvasive diagnostic tool for evaluating the patient with heart failure?
1. Coronary angiography
2. Echocardiogram
3. Electrocardiogram
4. Thallium scanning

21. What actions would the nurse expect to be used to treat heart failure? *(Select all that apply.)*
1. Cardiotonic drugs (digitalis)
2. Diuretic agents
3. Generous fluid intake
4. ACE inhibitors, beta-adrenergic blockers (carvedilol), nitrates
5. Oxygen therapy

22. The nurse is aware that the patient will benefit from the administration of streptokinase and tissue plasminogen activators when administered how long after admission for acute MI signs and symptoms?
1. In the first 24 hours
2. In the first 30 minutes to 1 hour
3. In the first 72 hours
4. In the second 6 hours after an MI

23. A patient is admitted with a diagnosis of possible aortic abdominal aneurysm. What is the most important factor to monitor as a possible complication?
1. Body temperature
2. Skin turgor
3. Respiratory rate
4. Blood pressure

24. A patient has Buerger's disease. What is the most important aspect of patient compliance to decrease signs and symptoms of Buerger's disease?
1. Low-fat diet
2. Weight loss
3. Cessation of tobacco use
4. Keeping extremities warm

25. The nurse is providing patient teaching for a patient with Raynaud's disease. Which information should be included? *(Select all that apply.)*
1. Avoid cold.
2. Warm hands and feet with heating pad.
3. Practice stress reduction techniques.
4. Comply with smoking cessation.
5. Limit caffeine intake.

Care of the Patient With a Respiratory Disorder

49

http://evolve.elsevier.com/Cooper/foundationsadult/

Objectives

Anatomy and Physiology

1. Differentiate between external and internal respiration.
2. Describe the purpose of the respiratory system and discuss the parts of the upper and lower respiratory tracts.
3. List the ways in which oxygen and carbon dioxide are transported in the blood.
4. Discuss the mechanisms that regulate respirations.

Medical-Surgical

5. Identify signs and symptoms that indicate a patient is experiencing hypoxia.
6. Differentiate among sonorous wheezes, sibilant wheezes, crackles, and pleural friction rub.
7. Describe the purpose, significance of results, and nursing interventions related to diagnostic examinations of the respiratory system.
8. Describe the significance of arterial blood gas values and differentiate between arterial oxygen tension (PaO_2) and arterial oxygen saturation (SaO_2).
9. Discuss the etiology and pathophysiology, clinical manifestations, assessment, diagnostic tests, medical management, nursing interventions, and prognosis of the patient with disorders of the upper airway.
10. Discuss nursing interventions for the patient with a laryngectomy.
11. Discuss the etiology and pathophysiology, clinical manifestations, assessment, diagnostic tests, medical management, nursing interventions, and prognosis of the patient with disorders of the lower airway.
12. Differentiate between tuberculosis infection and tuberculosis disease.
13. List nursing assessments and interventions pertaining to the care of the patient with closed-chest drainage.
14. Compare and contrast the etiology and pathophysiology, clinical manifestations, assessment, diagnostic tests, medical management, nursing interventions, and prognosis for the patient with chronic obstructive pulmonary disease, including emphysema, chronic bronchitis, asthma, and bronchiectasis.
15. State three possible nursing diagnoses for the patient with altered respiratory function.

Key Terms

adventitious (ăd-vĕn-TĪ-shŭs, p. 1593)
atelectasis (ă-tĕ-LĔK-tă-sĭs, p. 1625)
bronchoscopy (brŏn-KŎS-kō-pē, p. 1595)
cor pulmonale (kŏr pŭl-mō-NĂ-lē, p. 1636)
coryza (kō-RĪ-ză, p. 1605)
crackles (KRĂK-ŭlz, p. 1593)
cyanosis (sī-ă-NŌ-sĭs, p. 1603)
dyspnea (DĬSP-nē-ă, p. 1592)
embolism (ĔM-bō-lĭz-ŭm, p. 1631)
empyema (ĕm-pī-Ē-mă, p. 1621)
epistaxis (ĕp-ĭ-STĂK-sĭs, p. 1598)
exacerbation (ĕg-zăs-ĕr-BĀ-shŭn, p. 1638)
extrinsic (ĕk-STRĬN-zĭk, p. 1640)
hypercapnia (hī-pĕr-KĂP-nē-ă, p. 1638)
hypoventilation (hī-pō-vĕn-tĭ-LĀ-shŭn, p. 1625)
hypoxia (hī-PŎK-sē-ă, p. 1593)
intrinsic (ĭn-TRĬN-zĭk, p. 1640)
orthopnea (ŏr-THŎP-nē-ă, p. 1593)
pleural friction rubs (PLŪ-răl FRĬK-shŭn rŭbz, p. 1593)
pneumothorax (nū-mō-THŌ-răks, p. 1626)
sibilant wheezes (SĬB-ĭ-lănt wēz-ĕz, p. 1593)
sonorous wheezes (sŏ-NŎR-ŭs wēz-ĕz, p. 1593)
stertorous (STĔR-tĕr-ŭs, p. 1600)
tachypnea (tăk-ĬP-nē-ă, p. 1625)
thoracentesis (thŏ-ră-sĕn-TĒ-sĭs, p. 1592)
virulent (VĬR-ū-lĕnt, p. 1613)

ANATOMY AND PHYSIOLOGY OF THE RESPIRATORY SYSTEM

All cells require a continuous supply of oxygen to carry out their specialized activities. *External respiration,* or breathing, is the exchange of oxygen and carbon dioxide between the lungs and the environment. The respiratory system works with the cardiovascular system to deliver oxygen to the cells, where it provides energy to carry out metabolism. *Internal respiration* is the exchange of oxygen and carbon dioxide at the cellular level. Oxygen enters the cells while carbon dioxide leaves them. The gases diffuse across the cell membrane into the bloodstream, which plays the role of transporter. Failure of

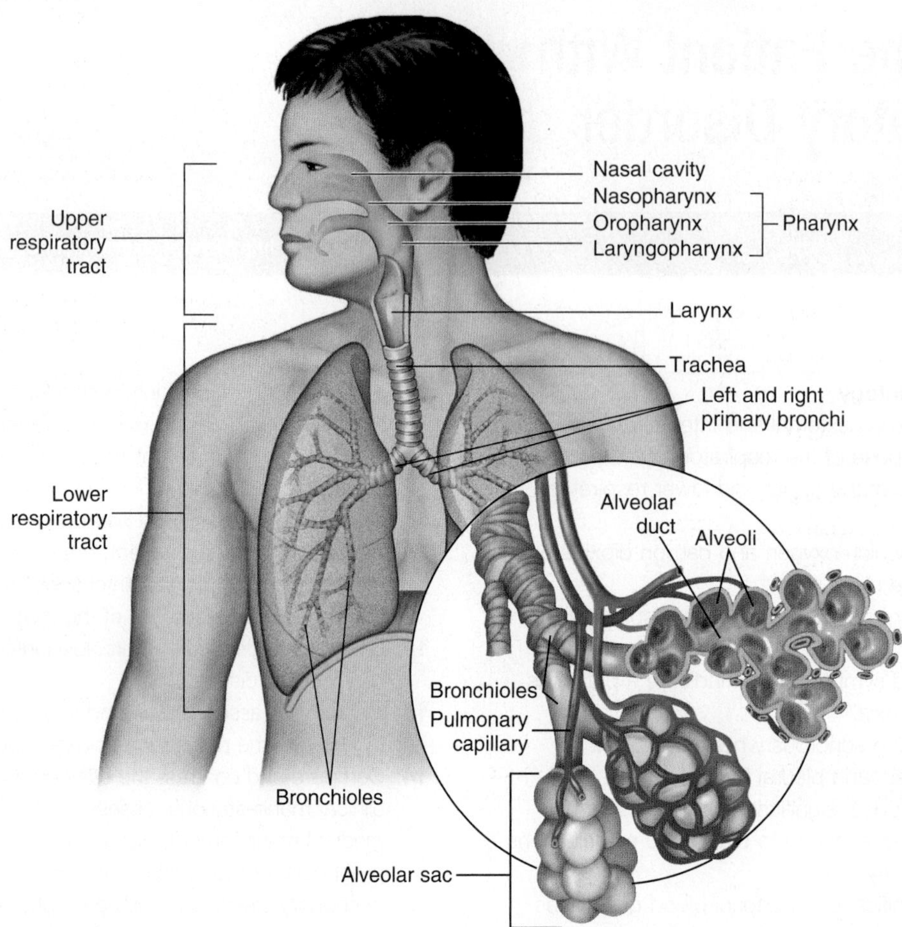

Fig. 49.1 Structural plan of the respiratory organs, showing the pharynx, trachea, bronchi, and lungs. The *inset* shows the grapelike alveolar sacs where the interchange of oxygen and carbon dioxide takes place through the thin walls of the alveoli. Capillaries surround the alveoli. (From Patton KT, Thibodeau GA: *Anatomy and physiology*, ed 8, St. Louis, 2013, Mosby.)

the respiratory system or cardiovascular system has the same result: rapid cell death from oxygen starvation. Fig. 49.1 shows the structure of the respiratory organs.

UPPER RESPIRATORY TRACT

Nose

Air enters the respiratory tract through the nose. The air is filtered, moistened, and warmed as it enters the two nasal openings (nares) and travels to the nasal cavity. The nasal septum separates the nares. This entire area is lined with mucous membrane, which is vascular. The mucous membrane provides warmth and moisture and secretes 1 L of moisture every day.

Lateral to the nasal cavities are three scroll-like bones called *turbinates* or *conchae* (Fig. 49.2), which cause the air to move over a larger surface area. This increase in surface area provides more time for warming and moisturizing the air. Lining the nasal cavities are tiny hairs, which trap dust and other foreign particles and prevent them from entering the lower respiratory tract.

Communicating with the nasal structures are paranasal sinuses (Fig. 49.3). They are called the *frontal, maxillary, sphenoid,* and *ethmoid cavities.* These are hollow areas that make the skull lighter and are believed to give resonance to the voice. They are lined with mucous membranes that are continuous with the nasal cavity. Because of this, nasal infections can cause sinusitis.

The receptors for the sense of smell are located in the mucosa of the nasal cavities. They are the nerve endings of the olfactory nerve, the first cranial nerve. The nasolacrimal ducts, or tear ducts, communicate with the upper nasal chamber. Therefore crying is accompanied by copious nasal secretions.

Pharynx

The *pharynx,* or throat (a tubular structure about 5 inches [13 cm] long extending from the base of the skull to the esophagus and situated just in front of the vertebrae), is the passageway for air and food. At the distal end of the pharynx are three subdivisions: (1) the *nasopharynx* (superior portion), (2) the *oropharynx* (posterior to the mouth), and (3) the *laryngopharynx* (directly superior to the larynx) (see Fig. 49.2).

The eustachian tubes enter on either side of the nasopharynx, connecting it to the middle ear. Because

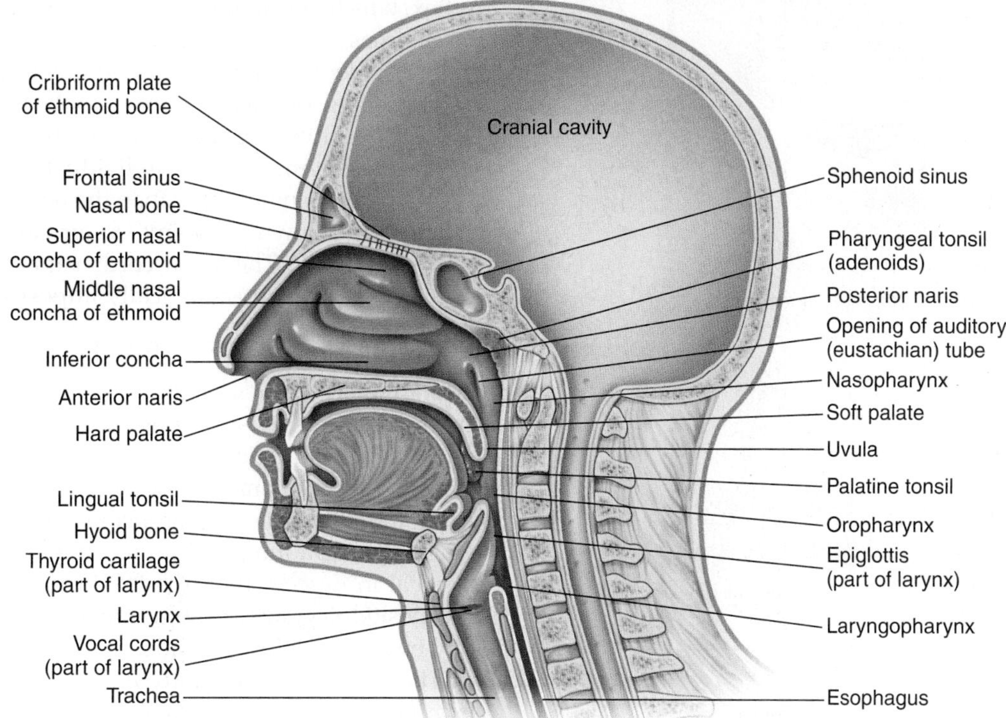

Fig. 49.2 Sagittal section through the face and the neck. (From Patton KT, Thibodeau GA: *The human body in health and disease,* ed 6, St. Louis, 2014, Mosby.)

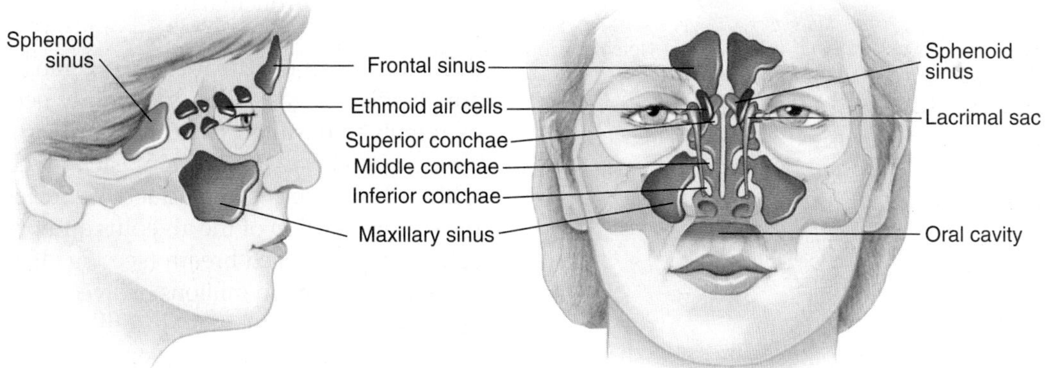

Fig. 49.3 Projections of paranasal sinuses and oral nasal cavities of the skull and the face. Note the connection between the sinuses and the nasal cavity. (From Patton KT, Thibodeau GA: *Anthonys textbook of anatomy and physiology,* ed 20, St. Louis, 2013, Mosby.)

the inner linings of the pharynx and the eustachian tube are continuous, an infection of the pharynx can spread easily to the ear. This is common in children. The adenoids (pharyngeal tonsils) are in the nasopharynx, whereas the palatine tonsils are in the oropharynx.

Larynx

The *larynx* (Fig. 49.4A), or the voice box, is supported by nine areas of cartilage and connects the pharynx with the trachea. The largest area of cartilage is composed of two fused plates and is called the *thyroid cartilage,* or *Adam's apple.* It is the same size in girls and boys until puberty, when it enlarges in boys and produces a projection in the neck. The *epiglottis,* a large leaf-shaped area of cartilage, protects the larynx when swallowing. It covers the larynx tightly to prevent food from entering the trachea and directs the food to the esophagus (see Fig. 49.4B).

The larynx contains the vocal cords. During expiration, air rushes over the vocal cords, causing them to vibrate. This enables speech to occur. The opening between the vocal cords is the glottis.

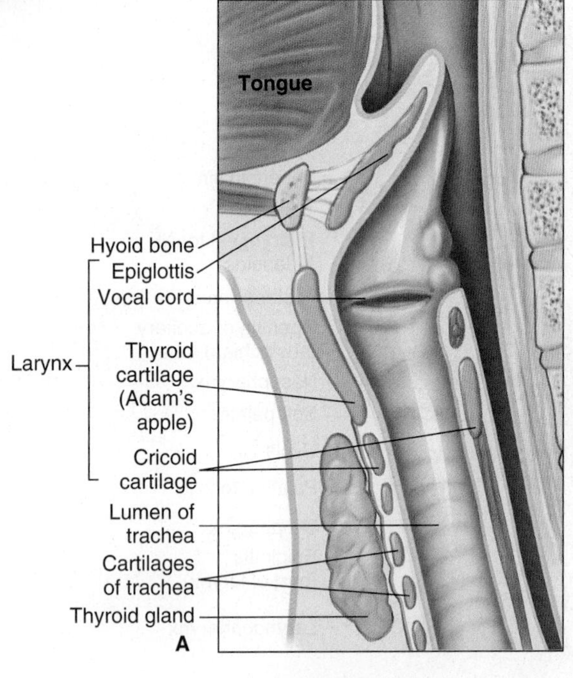

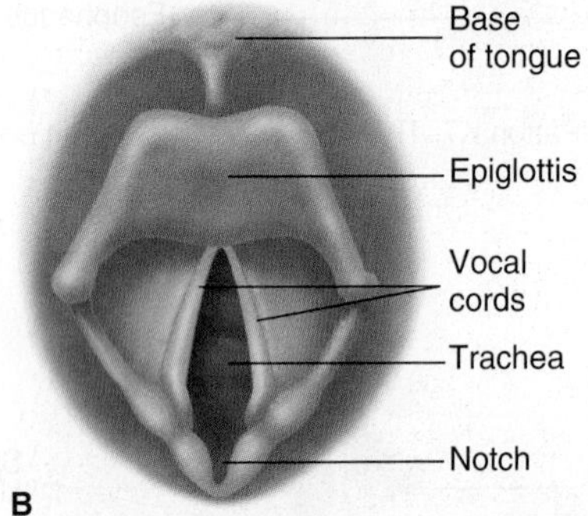

Fig. 49.4 A, Sagittal section through the larynx. B, Larynx and vocal cords as viewed from above, with a laryngeal mirror. (From Thibodeau GA, Patton KT: *Structure and function of the body*, ed 14, St. Louis, 2012, Mosby.)

Trachea

The *trachea* (Fig. 49.5), or windpipe, is a tubelike structure that extends approximately 4⅓ inches (11 cm) to the mid-chest, where it divides into the right and left bronchi. It lies anterior to the esophagus and connects the larynx with the bronchi. The ventral (anterior) surface of the tube is covered in the neck by the isthmus (narrow connection) of the thyroid gland. It contains C-shaped cartilaginous rings that keep it from collapsing. The open part of the C-shaped rings lies posterior to the column anterior to the esophagus, which allows the esophagus to expand during swallowing while maintaining patency of the trachea. This is necessary for uninterrupted breathing.

The entire structure is lined with mucous membranes and tiny *cilia* (small, hairlike processes on the outer surfaces of small cells, which produce motion or current in a fluid) that sweep dust or debris upward toward the nasal cavity. Any large particles initiate the cough reflex, which aids in the evacuation of foreign material. Sometimes, because of an airway obstruction, a health care provider performs a tracheotomy (i.e., creates a surgical opening, or tracheostomy, into the trachea through which an indwelling tube may be inserted). Once this procedure is completed, the individual breathes through the tracheal opening rather than the nose or mouth. The opening is below the larynx, so air cannot pass over the vocal cords. The vocal cords cannot vibrate, and speech becomes physiologically impossible.

LOWER RESPIRATORY TRACT

Bronchial Tree

As the trachea enters the lungs, it divides into the right and left bronchi. The left bronchus enters the left lung. It is smaller in diameter and slightly more horizontal in position than the right bronchus. The right bronchus enters the right lung. It is larger in diameter and more vertical in descent than the left bronchus. Because of this positioning, foreign objects that are aspirated generally enter the right bronchus.

The bronchi divide into smaller structures called *bronchioles*. These structures divide into smaller, tubelike structures called *terminal bronchioles* or *alveolar ducts*. All these structures are lined with ciliated mucous membrane, as is the trachea. The end structures of the bronchial tree are called *alveoli*. These saclike structures resemble a bunch of grapes. A single grapelike structure is called an *alveolus* (Fig. 49.6; see Fig. 49.1). In this terminal structure of the bronchial tree, gas exchange takes place. Each alveolus is surrounded by a blood capillary, where diffusion of carbon dioxide and oxygen occurs. Alveoli are effective in gas exchange, mainly because they are extremely thin walled; each alveolus lies in contact with a blood capillary. In addition, each alveolus is coated with a thin covering of surfactant. Surfactant reduces the surface tension of the alveolus and prevents it from collapsing after each breath (see Fig. 49.6).

The lungs contain millions of alveoli; these give shape and form to the lungs and are filled with air. Alveoli, which are tiny, grapelike structures, are the most important feature of the respiratory system. In the alveoli, oxygen diffuses into the cardiovascular system.

MECHANICS OF BREATHING

Thoracic Cavity

The thoracic cavity is enclosed by the sternum, ribs, and thoracic vertebrae. The space within the cavity is occupied primarily by the lungs. The centermost area is referred to as the mediastinum or interpleural space and contains the heart and great vessels.

Lungs. The lungs are large, paired, spongy, cone-shaped organs (see Fig. 49.5). The right lung weighs approximately 625 g; the left lung weighs approximately 570 g. The right lung has three lobes; the left lung has two lobes. Located approximately 1 inch (2.5 cm) above the

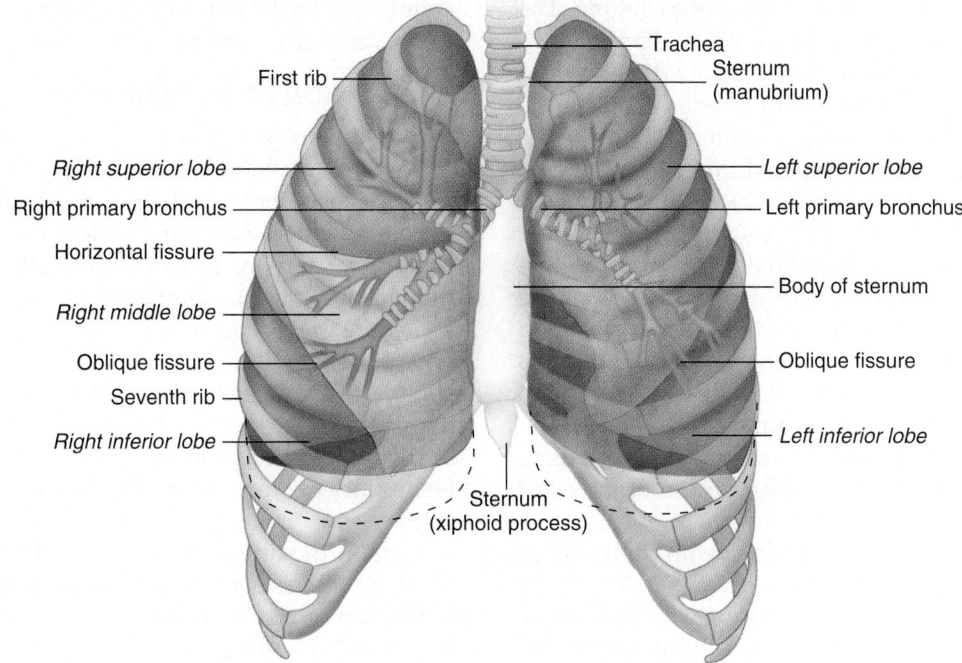

Fig. 49.5 Projection of the lungs and trachea in relation to ribcage and clavicles. *Dotted line* shows location of dome-shaped diaphragm at the end of expiration and before inspiration. Note that the apex of each lung projects above the clavicle. Ribs 11 and 12 are not visible in this view. (From Patton KT, Thibodeau GA: *Anatomy and physiology,* ed 8, St. Louis, 2013, Mosby.)

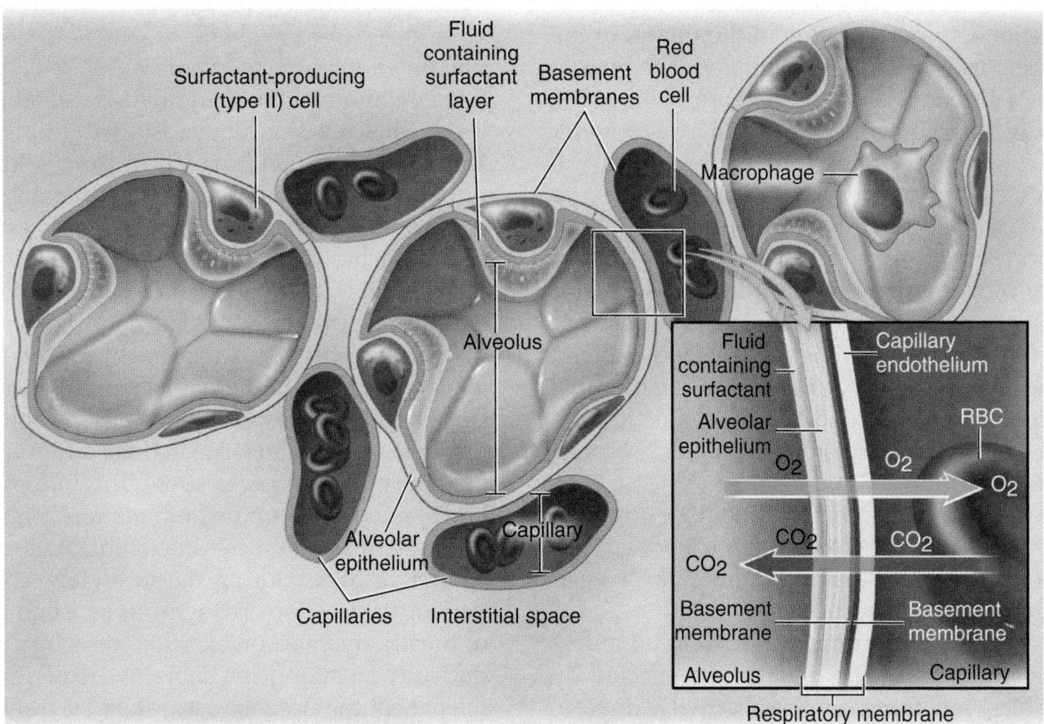

Fig. 49.6 Each alveolus is ventilated continuously with fresh air. *Inset* shows a magnified view of the respiratory membrane composed of the alveolar wall (surfactant, epithelial cells, and basement membrane), interstitial fluid, and the wall of a pulmonary capillary (basement membrane and endothelial cells). Carbon dioxide and oxygen diffuse across the respiratory membrane. (From Patton KT, Thibodeau GA: *The human body in health and disease,* ed 6, St. Louis, 2014, Mosby.)

first rib is the narrow part (the apex) of each lung. The broad, inferior part (the base) lies in the diaphragm.

The lungs receive their blood supply directly from the heart through the pulmonary arteries. Blood in the lung capillaries has little oxygen content. The air in the alveoli is rich in oxygen. Oxygen diffuses from the area of high concentration (alveolar air) to the area of low concentration (the lung capillaries). Blood in the lung capillaries is high in carbon dioxide, a waste product from the cells. Carbon dioxide also diffuses from the blood in the lung capillaries into the alveoli. After carbon dioxide has diffused into the alveoli and oxygen has diffused into the blood, carbon dioxide leaves the body by expiration of air from the lungs. The blood, now rich in oxygen and cleansed of its carbon dioxide, returns by the pulmonary veins to the left atrium of the heart for circulation to the rest of the body.

The surface of each lung is covered with a thin, moist, serous membrane called the *visceral pleura.* The walls of the thoracic cavity are covered with the same type of membrane, called the *parietal pleura.* The pleural cavity around the lungs is an airtight vacuum that contains negative pressure. The air in the lungs is at atmospheric pressure—higher than in the pleural cavity. The negative pressure assists in keeping the lungs inflated. The visceral and parietal pleura produce a serous secretion, which allows the lungs to slide over the walls of the thorax while breathing. Usually the body produces the exact amount of serous secretion needed. If too much serous secretion is produced, fluid accumulates in the pleural space; this is called *pleural effusion.* The pleural space becomes distended and puts pressure on the lungs, making it difficult to breathe. The health care provider may decide to remove the fluid by performing a **thoracentesis**—inserting a needlelike instrument into the pleural space and removing the fluid.

Respiratory Movements and Ranges

The rhythmic movements of the chest walls, ribs, and associated muscles when air is inhaled and exhaled make up the respiratory movements. The combination of one inspiration and one expiration equals one respiration. At rest the normal inspiration lasts about 2 seconds and expiration about 3 seconds.

Room air, when inhaled, contains about 21% oxygen; exhaled air contains 16% oxygen and 3.5% carbon dioxide. This represents the actual amount of oxygen used in a single breath.

The normal range of respiration for an adult at rest is 14 to 20 breaths/min. This rate can be affected by many variables, including age, sex, activity, disease, and body temperature. The respiratory rate is 40 to 60 breaths/min for a newborn, 22 to 24 breaths/min for an early school-age child, and 20 to 22 breaths/min for a teenager. The normal range for women is higher than that for men.

Members of the health care team should assess all factors influencing the patient's respirations and should count the respirations without the patient's awareness to prevent alterations in the breathing pattern.

REGULATION OF RESPIRATION

Nervous Control

The medulla oblongata and pons of the brain are responsible for the basic rhythm and depth of respiration. The body's demands can modify the rhythm. Other parts of the nervous system help coordinate the transfer from inspiration to expiration. Chemoreceptors clustered in areas of the carotid artery and aorta, called the carotid and aortic bodies, are specialized receptors. When stimulated by increasing levels of blood carbon dioxide, decreasing levels of blood oxygen, or increasing blood acidity, these receptors send nerve impulses to the respiratory centers, which in turn modify respiratory rates.

Carbon dioxide, which is present in the blood as carbonic acid, is considered the chemical stimulant for regulation of respiration. The normal pH of the blood is 7.35 to 7.45—a narrow range. If the blood pH goes outside this range, the patient develops either *acidosis* (too much acid, such as carbon dioxide, in the blood) or *alkalosis* (not enough carbon dioxide, or too much base, in the blood). After exhalation the blood becomes more alkaline.

ASSESSMENT OF THE RESPIRATORY SYSTEM

The function of the respiratory system is gas exchange (oxygen and carbon dioxide) at the alveolus-capillary level. This function depends on the lungs' ability to contract and expand, which in turn is influenced by musculoskeletal and neurologic functions.

Physical assessment of the patient's general health always includes the respiratory system. More extensive assessments are required for patients with acute or chronic respiratory or cardiac conditions, those with a history of respiratory impairment related to trauma or allergic reactions, or those who recently have undergone surgery or anesthesia. Because physical and emotional responses often are correlated, also inquire about any accompanying anxiety or stress. This information should be obtained in an unhurried, matter-of-fact manner.

The respiratory assessment includes collection of subjective data. During the interview, encourage the patient to describe any symptoms, such as shortness of breath, dyspnea on exertion, or cough. **Dyspnea,** or difficulty breathing, is a subjective experience that only the patient can describe accurately. Data should include onset; duration; precipitating factors; and relief measures, such as position and use of over-the-counter or prescribed medications. If the patient reports a cough, ask for a description of the cough: productive or nonproductive; harsh, dry, or hacking; and color and amount of mucus expectorated. Record this information as direct quotes from the patient when possible.

Table 49.1 Adventitious Breath Sounds

TYPE	CHARACTERISTICS	COMMENTS
Crackles (rales)	Brief, not continuous; more common in inspiration; interrupted crackling or bubbling sounds, similar to those produced by hairs being rolled between the fingers close to the ear	Caused by fluid, mucus, or pus in the small airways and alveoli
Fine crackles	As described above; high-pitched, sibilant crackling at end of inspiration	Found in diseases affecting bronchioles and alveoli
Medium crackles	As described above; medium pitch, more sonorous, moisture sound during mid-inspiration	Associated with diseases of small bronchi
Coarse crackles	As described above; loud, bubbly sound in early inspiration	Associated with diseases of small bronchi
Sonorous wheezes (rhonchi)	Deep, running sound that may be continuous; loud, low, coarse sound (like a snore) heard at any point of inspiration or expiration	Caused by air moving through narrowed tracheobronchial passages (caused by secretions, tumor, spasm); cough may alter sound if caused by mucus in trachea or large bronchi
Sibilant wheezes (wheezes)	High-pitched, musical, whistle-like sound during inspiration or expiration; sound may be several notes or one, and may vary from one minute to the next	Caused by narrowed bronchioles; bilateral wheeze is often the result of bronchospasm; unilateral, sharply localized wheeze may result from foreign matter or tumor compression
Pleural friction rub	Dry, creaking, grating, low-pitched sound with a machinelike quality during both inspiration and expiration; loudest over anterior chest	Sound originates outside respiratory tree, usually caused by inflammation; over the lung fields it suggests pleurisy; over the pericardium it suggests pericarditis with a pericardial friction rub. To distinguish the two, ask the patient to hold the breath briefly. If the rubbing sound persists, it is a pericardial friction rub because the inflamed pericardial layers continue rubbing together with each heartbeat; a pleural rub would stop when breathing stops

Next, gather objective data. Begin the assessment with observation. Assess respiratory rate and oxygen saturation. The patient's expression, chest movement, and respirations provide valuable visual clues. At times the patient cannot verbalize distress but has a wide-eyed, anxious look that reflects the fear of suffocating. Flaring nostrils indicate the patient is struggling to breathe, which is usually a late sign of respiratory distress. Initial observation yields information on the patient's skin color and turgor. Note any obvious respiratory distress, wheezes, or **orthopnea** (an abnormal condition in which a person must sit or stand to breathe deeply or comfortably).

To continue the assessment, auscultate all lung fields, anteriorly and posteriorly, comparing bilaterally. Note the presence of **adventitious** sounds (abnormal sounds superimposed on breath sounds, including sibilant wheezes [formerly called *wheezes*], sonorous wheezes [formerly called *rhonchi*], crackles [formerly called *rales*], and pleural friction rubs) (Table 49.1). **Sibilant wheezes** are musical, high-pitched, squeaking or whistling sounds caused by the rapid movement of air through narrowed bronchioles. **Sonorous wheezes** are low-pitched, loud, coarse, snoring sounds. They often are heard on expiration. **Crackles** are short, discrete, interrupted crackling or bubbling sounds that are heard most commonly during inspiration. Crackles sound like hairs being rolled between the fingers close to the ear. They are thought to occur when air is forced through respiratory passages narrowed by fluid, mucus, or pus. They are associated with inflammation or infection of the small bronchi, bronchioles, and alveoli. **Pleural friction rubs** are low-pitched, grating, or creaking lung sounds that occur when inflamed pleural surfaces rub together during respiration.

Assess chest movement. Note whether the chest expands equally on both sides; chest expansion on one side only may indicate serious pulmonary complications, such as a collapsed lung. Look for retraction of the chest wall between the ribs and under the clavicle during inspiration. This can signal late-stage respiratory distress. Be alert for signs and symptoms of **hypoxia** (oxygen deficiency in the cellular tissues) (Box 49.1).

Box 49.1 Signs and Symptoms of Hypoxia

- Apprehension, anxiety, restlessness
- Decreased ability to concentrate
- Disorientation
- Decreased level of consciousness
- Increased fatigue
- Vertigo
- Behavioral changes
- Increased pulse rate; bradycardia as hypoxia advances
- Increased rate and depth of respiration; shallow, slow respirations as hypoxia progresses
- Elevated blood pressure; with continuing oxygen deficiency, decreased blood pressure
- Cardiac dysrhythmias
- Pallor
- Cyanosis (may not be present until hypoxia is severe)
- Clubbing
- Dyspnea

LABORATORY AND DIAGNOSTIC EXAMINATIONS

Diagnostic imaging, laboratory work, and more invasive measures are used to evaluate respiratory status and to identify respiratory conditions. Nurses should be familiar with these tests so they can prepare the patient adequately.

CHEST X-RAY

Sometimes called radiographs, x-rays are an essential diagnostic tool for evaluating disorders of the chest. A chest x-ray allows visualization of the thoracic cavity, lungs, heart, and major thoracic vessels. X-rays show changes in size and location of the pulmonary structures and blood flow and enable identification of lesions, infiltrates, foreign bodies, or fluid. A chest x-ray also shows whether a disorder involves the lung parenchyma (the tissue of an organ, as distinguished from supporting or connective tissue) or the interstitial spaces. Chest x-rays can confirm pneumothorax, pneumonia, pleural effusion, and pulmonary edema.

COMPUTED TOMOGRAPHY

Chest CT Scan

Computed tomography (CT) scans of the lungs take pictures of small layers of pulmonary tissue, usually to identify a pulmonary lesion. These views can be diagonal or cross-sectional, with a scanner rotating at various angles. Although this test is painless and noninvasive, patient teaching is necessary before the procedure to offer explanations and decrease anxiety.

Helical or spiral CT chest scan. *Helical* (also called *spiral* or *volume-averaging*) *CT scanning* is a marked improvement over standard CT scanning. The helical CT scan obtains images continuously. This produces faster and more accurate images than a traditional CT scan. Because the helical CT can scan the abdomen and chest in less than 30 seconds, the entire study can be performed with one breath-hold. Injection or swallowing of the contrast dye helps the organs or tissues show up more clearly.

Pulmonary angiography (pulmonary arteriography). *Pulmonary angiography (pulmonary arteriography)* uses a radiographic contrast material injected into the pulmonary arteries to visualize the pulmonary vasculature. Angiography is used to detect pulmonary embolism (PE) and a variety of congenital and acquired lesions of the pulmonary vessels.

When PE is suspected, typically a CT scan is performed first. If the lung scan is normal, PE is ruled out. If the scan is uncertain, the diagnosis of PE is questionable because pathologic processes (e.g., emphysema, pneumonia) also may cause abnormalities on the lung scan. Definitive diagnosis for PE may require pulmonary angiography.

Ventilation-perfusion scan (V/Q scan). *Ventilation-perfusion (V/Q) scanning* is used primarily to check for a PE. Ventilation *(V)* refers to the air reaching the alveoli; perfusion *(Q)* refers to the blood that reaches the alveoli. A radioisotope is given intravenously for the perfusion portion of the test, and an image of the pulmonary vasculature is obtained. For the ventilation portion of the test, the patient inhales a radioactive gas, and an image of the outlines of the alveoli is obtained. Normal scans show homogeneous radioactivity of both sorts; a high V/Q, however, indicates impaired blood circulation to the alveoli, suggesting the presence of a PE (Medline Plus, 2012).

PULMONARY FUNCTION TESTING

Pulmonary function tests (PFTs) are performed to assess the presence and severity of disease in the large and small airways. PFTs include various procedures to obtain information on lung volume, ventilation, pulmonary spirometry, and gas exchange. Lung volume tests refer to the volume of air that can be exhaled completely and slowly after a maximum inhalation *(vital capacity)*. *Inspiratory capacity* is the largest amount of air that can be inhaled in one breath from the resting expiratory level. *Total lung capacity* is calculated to determine the volume of air in the lung after a maximal inhalation. Ventilation tests evaluate the volume of air inhaled or exhaled in each respiratory cycle. Pulmonary spirometry tests evaluate the amount of air that can be exhaled forcefully after maximum inhalation. These tests require the use of a spirometer.

Determining gas exchange is one of the most important PFTs done to diagnose respiratory diseases. The DLCO (diffusing capacity of the lungs for carbon monoxide) test determines how well oxygen diffusing from the alveoli is taken up by blood in the pulmonary capillary bed. Strangely enough, oxygen is not used in the test; carbon monoxide is used instead of oxygen. Because such a small amount of carbon monoxide is used, the test is not dangerous. After the DLCO test is completed, the patient's rate of oxygen transfer can be determined accurately.

Mediastinoscopy

Mediastinoscopy is a surgical endoscopic procedure in which an incision is created in the suprasternal notch (the base of the neck), allowing the endoscope to be passed into the upper mediastinum. A *biopsy* then is performed, in which a sample of lymph nodes is gathered and subsequently examined for the presence of a tumor. These lymph nodes receive lymphatic drainage from the lungs, so they are valuable in the diagnosis of malignant tumors. Tumors in the mediastinum (e.g., thymoma or lymphoma) also can be biopsied through the mediastinoscope. This procedure is performed in the operating room with the patient under general anesthesia.

Laryngoscopy

Laryngoscopy can be performed for either direct or indirect visualization of the larynx. Indirect laryngoscopy is probably the most common procedure for assessing respiratory difficulties. With the patient awake, a laryngeal mirror is positioned in the mouth for visualization. Direct laryngoscopy with a laryngoscope can be used for biopsy or polyp excision. It requires local or general anesthesia and exposes the vocal cords as the laryngoscope is passed down over the tongue.

Bronchoscopy

Bronchoscopy is performed by passing a bronchoscope into the trachea and bronchi. Using either a rigid bronchoscope or a flexible fiberoptic bronchoscope (the instrument of choice in most cases) allows visualization of the larynx, the trachea, and the bronchi (Fig. 49.7). Diagnostic bronchoscopic examination includes observation of the tracheobronchial tree for (1) abnormalities, (2) tissue biopsy, and (3) collection of secretions for cytologic (cell) or bacteriologic examination. A local anesthetic agent may be used, but an intravenous (IV) general anesthetic agent usually is given. The patient is treated as a surgical patient.

Nursing interventions for the patient after bronchoscopy include (1) keeping the patient on NPO (nothing by mouth) status until the gag reflex returns, usually about 2 hours after the procedure; (2) keeping the patient in a semi-Fowler's position and turning on either side to facilitate removal of secretions (unless the health care provider specifies another position); (3) monitoring the patient for signs of laryngeal edema or laryngospasms, such as stridor or increasing dyspnea; and (4) if lung tissue biopsy is taken, monitoring sputum for signs of hemorrhage (blood-streaked sputum is expected for a few days after biopsy).

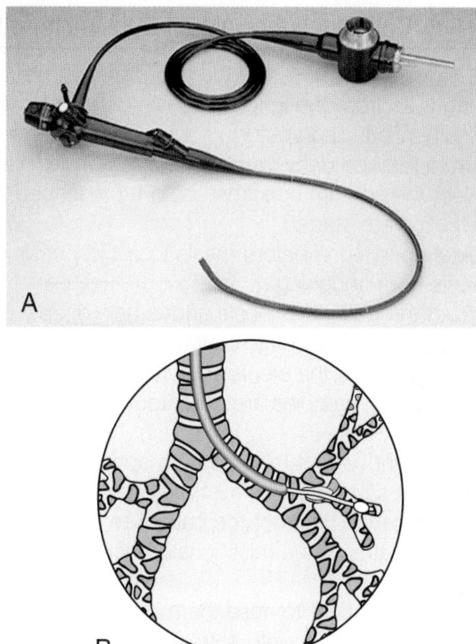

Fig. 49.7 Fiberoptic bronchoscope. A, The transbronchoscopic balloon-tipped catheter and the flexible fiberoptic bronchoscope. B, The catheter is introduced into a small airway and the balloon is inflated with 1.5–2 mL of air to occlude the airway. Bronchial alveolar lavage is performed by injecting and withdrawing 30-mL aliquots of sterile saline solution, gently aspirating after each instillation. Specimens are sent to the laboratory for analysis. (A, Courtesy Olympus America, Inc., Melville, New York. B, Reprinted with permission of the American Thoracic Society. Copyright 2013 American Thoracic Society. Meduri GU, et al: Protected bronchoalveolar lavage, *American Review of Respiratory Disease* 143:855, 1991. Official journal of the American Thoracic Society.)

SPUTUM SPECIMEN

Sputum samples frequently are obtained for microscopic evaluation, such as Gram stain and culture and sensitivity (Box 49.2). For the range of sputum characteristics, see Box 49.3.

CYTOLOGIC STUDIES

Cytologic tests can be performed on any body secretion, such as sputum or pleural fluid, to detect abnormal or malignant cells.

LUNG BIOPSY

Lung biopsy may be done transbronchially or as an open-lung biopsy. The purpose is to obtain tissue, cells, or secretions for evaluation. Transbronchial lung biopsy involves passing a forceps or needle through the bronchoscope to obtain a specimen. Specimens can be cultured or examined for malignant cells. Nursing interventions are the same as for fiberoptic bronchoscopy. Open-lung biopsy is used when pulmonary disease cannot be diagnosed by other procedures. The patient is anesthetized, the chest is opened with a thoracotomy incision, and a biopsy specimen is obtained.

Box 49.2 Guidelines for Sputum Specimen Collection

1. Explain to the patient that the sputum must be brought up from the lungs. Patients who have difficulty producing sputum or who have tenacious sputum may be dehydrated. Encourage fluid intake.
2. Collect the sputum specimen before prescribed antibiotics are started.
3. Collect specimens before meals to avoid possible emesis from coughing.
4. Instruct the patient to inhale and exhale deeply three times, then inhale swiftly, cough forcefully, and expectorate into the sterile sputum container. Usually early morning samples are collected on 3 consecutive days.
5. If the patient cannot raise sputum spontaneously, a hypertonic saline aerosol mist may help produce a good specimen. Instruct the patient to take several normal breaths of the mist, inhale deeply, cough, and expectorate.
6. Instruct the patient to rinse the mouth with water before expectorating into a sterile specimen bottle to decrease sputum contamination.
7. Properly label the sample and send it to the laboratory without delay.
8. Sputum samples also can be obtained indirectly, such as by nasotracheal suctioning with a catheter or by transtracheal aspiration. Take care to ensure that the suction catheters remain sterile. A health care provider's order must be obtained for endotracheal suctioning.

Box 49.3 Range of Sputum Characteristics

COLOR
- Clear
- White
- Yellow
- Green
- Brown
- Red
- Pink tinged
- Streaked with blood

ODOR
- None
- Malodorous

CONSISTENCY
- Frothy
- Watery
- Tenacious

BLOOD
- All the time
- Occasionally
- Early morning

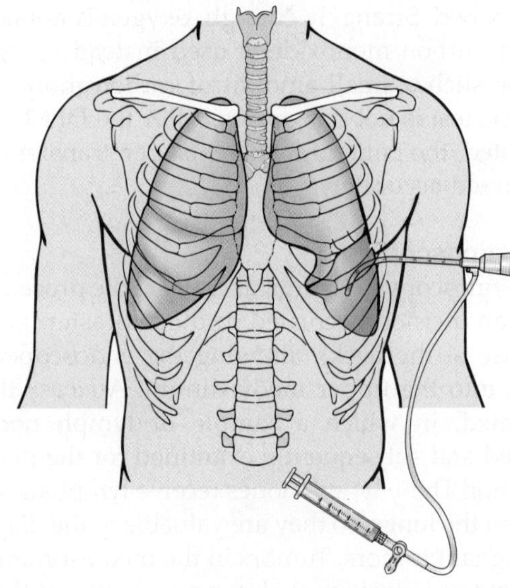

Fig. 49.8 Thoracentesis. The needle has penetrated the fluid-filled pleural space to remove fluid. (From Lewis S, Dirksen SR, Heitkemper MM, et al: *Medical-surgical nursing: Assessment and management of clinical problems,* ed 8, St. Louis, 2011, Mosby.)

THORACENTESIS

In thoracentesis the chest wall is pierced with a needle to withdraw (aspirate) fluid from the pleural space for therapeutic purposes or for the removal of a specimen for biopsy (Fig. 49.8). Diagnostic indications for fluid removal include (1) examining the pleural fluid for specific gravity, white blood cell count, red blood cell count, protein, and glucose and (2) culturing the fluid for pathogens and checking for abnormal or malignant cells. Record the gross appearance of the fluid, the quantity obtained, and the site of the thoracentesis.

Therapeutic indications for thoracentesis include removal of fluid when it is a threat to the patient's safety or comfort and instillation of medication into the pleural space.

Nursing interventions for the patient undergoing thoracentesis include explaining the procedure and obtaining written consent. Try to relieve the patient's anxiety. The procedure usually is carried out in the patient's room. The patient sits on the edge of the bed with the head and arms resting on a pillow placed on an overbed table. If the patient cannot sit up, turn him or her to the unaffected side with the head of the bed elevated 30 degrees.

Monitor vital signs, general appearance, and respiratory status throughout the procedure. Because of the risk of intravascular fluid shift and resultant pulmonary edema, fluid removal is traditionally limited to 1300 mL. After thoracentesis, position the patient on the unaffected side. Label the specimen and send it immediately to the laboratory.

Arterial Blood Gases

Blood gas analysis is essential in diagnosing and monitoring patients with respiratory disorders. The lungs' ability to oxygenate arterial blood adequately is determined by examination of the arterial oxygen tension (PaO_2) and arterial oxygen saturation (SaO_2). Oxygen is carried in the blood in two forms: as oxygen dissolved in the plasma and as oxygen bound to hemoglobin. PaO_2 represents the amount of oxygen dissolved in the plasma and is expressed as millimeters of mercury (mm Hg). *Saturation* (SaO_2) refers to the amount of oxygen bound to hemoglobin binding sites, compared with the amount of oxygen the hemoglobin could carry, and is expressed as a percentage (Woodruff, 2006). For example, if the SaO_2 is 90%, then 90% of the hemoglobin attachment sites for oxygen have oxygen bound to them. Note that oxygen first must dissolve in blood (PaO_2) before it can bind to hemoglobin (SaO_2) (Box 49.4).

The $PaCO_2$ is a measure of the partial pressure of carbon dioxide in the blood. $PaCO_2$ is referred to as the respiratory component in acid-base determination, because this value is controlled primarily by the lungs. As the carbon dioxide level increases, the pH decreases. Therefore the carbon dioxide level and pH are inversely proportional. The $PaCO_2$ level is elevated in primary respiratory acidosis and decreased in primary respiratory alkalosis. Because the lungs compensate for primary metabolic acid-based derangements, $PaCO_2$ levels are affected by metabolic disturbances as well. In metabolic acidosis the lungs attempt to compensate by "blowing off" carbon dioxide to raise the pH. In metabolic alkalosis the lungs attempt to compensate by retaining carbon dioxide to lower the pH.

The bicarbonate ion (HCO_3^-) is a measure of the metabolic (renal) component of the acid-base equilibrium. This ion can be measured directly by the bicarbonate value or indirectly by the carbon dioxide content. As the HCO_3^- level increases, the pH also increases; therefore the relationship of bicarbonate to pH is directly proportional. HCO_3^- is elevated in metabolic alkalosis and decreased in metabolic acidosis. The kidneys also compensate for primary respiratory acid-base derangements. In respiratory acidosis, the kidneys attempt to compensate by reabsorbing increased amounts of HCO_3^-. In respiratory alkalosis the kidneys excrete HCO_3^- in increased amounts in an attempt to lower pH through compensation (Table 49.2).

Arterial blood gas (ABG) testing yields definitive information on the patient's respiratory status and metabolic balance. The procedure is performed at the bedside. A heparinized syringe and needle are used to withdraw 3 to 5 mL of arterial blood, usually from the radial artery. Other possible sites include femoral or brachial arteries. After the sample is obtained, place direct pressure on the puncture site for a minimum of 5 minutes to prevent hematoma formation and blood loss. If the patient is taking anticoagulants, maintain pressure for 20 minutes or longer, until the bleeding stops. Place the capped syringe in a basin of crushed ice and water to preserve the gas and pH levels of the specimen. Send the properly labeled specimen to the laboratory immediately.

Box 49.4 Guidelines for Interpreting Arterial Blood Gas Values

1. Examine each value by itself.
   - Normal arterial blood gas values (ABGs):
   - pH: 7.35–7.45
   - $PaCO_2$: 35–45 mm Hg
   - PaO_2: 80–100 mm Hg
   - HCO_3^-: 21–28 mEq/L
   - SaO_2: 95%
2. Determine whether the pH reflects acidity or alkalinity.
   - pH $\leq$ 7.35 = acidity
   - pH $\geq$ 7.45 = alkalinity
3. Which other value corresponds with that condition?

   NOTE: $PaCO_2$ reflects respiratory factors; HCO_3^- reflects metabolic factors.
   - Carbon dioxide is a potential acid, so carbon dioxide greater than 45 mm Hg reflects acidity.
   - HCO_3^- is a basic (alkaline) substance, so HCO_3^- greater than 28 mEq/L reflects alkalinity.

   Example 1: A patient with acute exacerbation of chronic obstructive pulmonary disease has the following ABGs:
   - pH: 7.42
   - $PaCO_2$: 49 mm Hg
   - PaO_2: 50 mm Hg
   - HCO_3^-: 31 mEq/L
   - SaO_2: 84%

   Because the pH is within the normal range, this is a compensated respiratory problem. The kidneys have increased the amount of bicarbonate they put into the blood to bring the pH to a normal level. The PaO_2 and the SaO_2 are low, indicating hypoxemia.

   Example 2:
   - pH: 7.21
   - $PaCO_2$: 58 mm Hg
   - PaO_2: 70 mm Hg
   - HCO_3^-: 24 mEq/L
   - SaO_2: 84%

   The pH is less than 7.35, indicating acidosis. The $PaCO_2$ is higher than 45 mm Hg, indicating acidosis. The $PaCO_2$ matches the pH, making it a respiratory acidosis. The HCO_3^- is normal, indicating there is no compensation. The PaO_2 and the SaO_2 are low, indicating hypoxemia. The full diagnosis for a patient with these ABG results is uncompensated respiratory acidosis with hypoxemia.

Woodruff D: Take these 6 easy steps to ABG analysis, *Nursing Made Incredibly Easy!* 41:4–7, 2006.

The blood gas values (see Box 49.4) assess the patient's metabolic (acid-base) status by measuring the pH. Carbon dioxide tension is measured by $PaCO_2$ and indicates the patient's ventilation. Oxygen saturation (PaO_2 and SaO_2) also is measured.

PULSE OXIMETRY

Pulse oximetry is a noninvasive way to monitor SaO_2 (saturation of oxygen) for assessment of gas exchange. The system consists of a probe that looks like a large

Table 49.2 Acid-Base Disturbances and Compensatory Mechanisms

ACID-BASE DISTURBANCE	MODE OF COMPENSATION
Respiratory acidosis	Kidneys retain increased amounts of HCO_3^- to increase pH
Respiratory alkalosis	Kidneys excrete increased amounts of HCO_3^- to lower pH
Metabolic acidosis	Lungs "blow off" carbon dioxide to raise pH
Metabolic alkalosis	Lungs retain carbon dioxide to lower pH

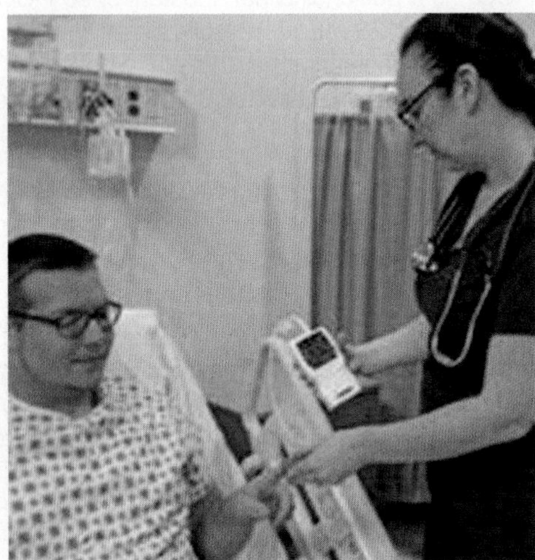

Fig. 49.9 Portable pulse oximeter with spring-tension digit probe displays oxygen saturation and pulse rate. (From Potter PA, Perry AG: *Fundamentals of nursing: Concepts, process, and practice*, ed 8, St. Louis, 2013, Mosby.)

clothespin, which is clipped to a finger, a toe, an earlobe, or the bridge of the nose. The noninvasive probe has a sensor that emits narrow beams of red and infrared light through the tissue and measures the amount of light being absorbed by oxygenated and deoxygenated hemoglobin in pulsating arterial blood. The probe is connected to a computer with a monitor that displays hemoglobin oxygen saturation and pulse rates (Fig. 49.9). A pulse oximeter beeps if the patient's SaO_2 registers outside of the limits set according to the health care provider's order. Pulse oximetry monitoring can be continuous or intermittent.

For decades, health care providers have relied on ABG analysis to evaluate gas exchange and oxygen transport. As valuable as this test is, ABG results reflect a patient's oxygenation status at only one moment in time. Today, pulse oximetry permits continuous, noninvasive monitoring of SaO_2. Oximetry technology allows the nurse to assess changes in arterial saturation as they happen, intervene before hypoxemia (reduced oxygen in the blood) produces obvious and serious signs and symptoms, and evaluate the patient's response to treatment. Pulse oximetry alone does not provide data about PaO_2 and acid-base balance. In addition, pulse oximetry can result in inaccurate results if the area the probe is attached to is cold, if nail polish or artificial nails are present when the fingertip is used, or if the patient's heart rate is irregular. For these reasons thorough assessment of the patient for signs of hypoxia is essential. Arterial blood gas levels may be needed periodically as well.

An SaO_2 of 90% to 100% is needed to replenish tissues adequately with oxygen, with 95% to 100% desired. The ability of hemoglobin to feed oxygen to the tissues weakens significantly when the SaO_2 drops below 85%.

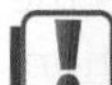 **Safety Alert**

An SaO_2 of Less Than 70% Is Considered Life Threatening

Arterial oxygen saturation can be determined quickly and noninvasively through pulse oximetry. Severe circulatory problems may diminish the accuracy of the reading. If oximetry results seem questionable, the health care provider usually orders ABG tests. A pulse oximeter can detect a change within 6 seconds. To get optimal results, remember these points:

- Do not attach the probe to an extremity that has a blood pressure cuff or arterial catheter in place; these devices reduce blood flow.
- Place the probe over a pulsating vascular bed.
- While the probe is on the patient, protect it from strong light (such as direct sunlight), which can affect the reading.
- Avoid excess patient movement to ensure accuracy.
- Remember that hypothermia, hypotension, and vasoconstriction can affect readings.

DISORDERS OF THE UPPER AIRWAY

EPISTAXIS

Etiology and Pathophysiology

The underlying cause of **epistaxis** (bleeding from the nose) is congestion of the nasal membranes, leading to capillary rupture. This condition frequently is caused by injury and occurs more frequently in men.

Epistaxis can be either a primary disorder or secondary to other conditions. It can be related to menstrual flow in women or to hypertension. Other causes include local irritation of nasal mucosa, such as dryness, chronic infection, trauma (e.g., injury, vigorous nose blowing, or nose picking), topical corticosteroid use, nasal spray abuse, or street drug use. Epistaxis often results if the patient has a disorder that results in prolonged bleeding time or reduction in platelet counts. Bleeding also may be prolonged if the patient takes aspirin or nonsteroidal antiinflammatory drugs (NSAIDs). A major factor in epistaxis is the many capillaries in the nasal passages.

Safety Alert

If the patient has an episode of epistaxis or complains of frequent episodes of epistaxis, check his or her blood pressure!

Clinical Manifestations

The primary observation is bright red blood draining from one or both nostrils. With a severe nasal hemorrhage, adults can lose as much as 1 L of blood per hour, but this rate of loss is not prolonged. Exsanguination (loss of blood to the point at which life can no longer be sustained) from epistaxis is rare.

Assessment

Collection of subjective data includes asking the patient to relate the duration and severity of bleeding and identifying precipitating factors, if possible.

Collection of objective data involves assessing the presence of bleeding from one or both nostrils. If possible, determine whether the bleeding is occurring in the anterior or posterior portion of the nasal passageway. Assess the patient's blood pressure for hypotension, temperature, pulse, respirations, and any evidence of hypovolemic shock. Hypotension is a late sign of shock.

Diagnostic Tests

A hemoglobin and hematocrit determination aids in establishing an estimate of the blood loss. Prothrombin time (PT), international normalized ratio (INR), and partial thromboplastin time (PTT) assist in identifying contributing factors, such as a bleeding tendency and clotting abnormalities. A rhinoscopy may be performed to locate the bleeding site and possible causes and treatment. This procedure involves inserting a lighted nasal speculum into the nasal cavity.

Medical Management

Epistaxis has many possible treatments, including nasal packing with cotton saturated with 1:1000 epinephrine to promote local vasoconstriction. Cautery can be either electrical (burning [cauterizing] the bleeding vessel) or chemical (applying a silver nitrate stick to the site of the bleeding). Posterior packing of the nasal cavity may be needed. A balloon tampon may be done by inserting a Foley-like catheter into the nose and inflating the balloon after it is placed posteriorly. Traction then is placed on the catheter to compress the vessel in the area. Also, some health care providers prescribe antibiotics (penicillin) after the bleeding is controlled to minimize risk of infection.

Nursing Interventions and Patient Teaching

Nursing interventions include keeping the patient calm. Place the patient in a sitting position, leaning forward, or in a reclining position with head and shoulders elevated. Be aware that the patient may vomit if sitting in this position and have an emesis basin ready. Apply direct pressure by pinching the entire soft lower portion of the nose for 10 to 15 minutes. Apply ice compresses to the nose and have the patient suck on ice. Partially insert a small gauze pad into the bleeding nostril, and apply digital pressure if bleeding continues. Monitor for signs and symptoms of hypovolemic shock.

Patient problems and interventions for the patient with epistaxis include but are not limited to the following:

Patient Problem	Nursing Interventions
Compromised Blood Flow to Cerebral and/or Cardiopulmonary Tissue, related to blood loss	Assess vital signs and level of consciousness q 15 min and report any changes Document estimated blood loss
Potential for Aspiration Into Airway, related to bleeding	Elevate head of bed; place patient in Fowler's position with the head forward; encourage patient to let the blood drain from the nose Pinch nostrils; have the patient breathe through the mouth; apply ice compresses over the nose (however, the primary benefit of the application of ice is that it requires the patient to remain still); assist patient in clearing secretions Maintain airway patency Instruct patient to expectorate any blood or clots rather than swallow them, which could cause nausea and vomiting

Instruct the patient (and the family, if possible) not to pick, scratch, or otherwise irritate the nares. To prevent recurrent hemorrhage, warn the patient not to blow the nose vigorously and to avoid dryness of the nose. Instruct the patient and the family regarding the risks of foreign objects inserted in the nose (this is especially important in pediatric patients). Encourage the patient to use a vaporizer and saline or nasal lubricants to keep nasal mucous membranes moist. Advise the patient to avoid using aspirin-containing products or NSAIDs, and teach him or her to sneeze with the mouth open.

Prognosis

With treatment, the prognosis is good.

DEVIATED SEPTUM AND NASAL POLYPS

Etiology and Pathophysiology

Common conditions that cause nasal obstruction include nasal polyps or a deviated septum caused by congenital abnormality or, more likely, injury. The septum deviates from the midline and can obstruct the nasal passageway partially. Nasal polyps are tissue growths on the nasal tissues that frequently are caused by prolonged sinus inflammation; allergies are often the underlying cause.

Clinical Manifestations

The major manifestations of nasal septal deviations and polyps are **stertorous** (characterized by a harsh snoring sound) respirations, dyspnea, and sometimes postnasal drip.

Assessment

Collection of subjective data includes establishing the presence of previous injuries or infections, allergies, and sinus congestion. The patient complains of dyspnea.

Collection of objective data involves identifying the condition and its location. Note the rate and character of the patient's respirations.

Diagnostic Tests

Sinus radiographic studies depict the presence of shadowy sinuses when nasal polyps are present. A shift of the nasal septum is evident with a septal defect. A deviated septum also may be seen on visual examination.

Medical Management

These conditions frequently require surgical correction. Nasoseptoplasty is the operation of choice to reconstruct, align, and straighten the deviated nasal septum. A nasal polypectomy is performed to remove the polyps. Actions include nasal packing to control bleeding for 24 hours, and then maintaining nasal mucosa hydration with nasal irrigation of saline or application of a light layer of petroleum jelly to the external nares to prevent drying. Medications include (1) corticosteroids (prednisone), which cause polyps to decrease or disappear; and (2) antihistamines for allergy signs and symptoms and to decrease congestion in septal deviations and polyps. Antibiotic agents (penicillin) may be used in both conditions to prevent infection. Analgesics (acetaminophen [Tylenol]) may be given to relieve the headache that occurs with septal deviation.

Nursing Interventions and Patient Teaching

Nursing interventions generally are aimed at maintaining airway patency and preventing infection. Postoperative interventions for nasal surgery include monitoring closely for infection or hemorrhage and maintaining patient comfort.

Patient problems and interventions for the patient with deviated septum or nasal polyps include but are not limited to the following:

Patient Problem	Nursing Interventions
Inability to Clear Airway, related to nasal exudates	Document patient's ability to clear secretions, and note respiratory status Elevate head of bed, and apply ice compresses to the nose to decrease edema, discoloration, discomfort, and bleeding Change nasal drip pad as needed, documenting color, consistency, and amount of exudates
Potential for Injury, related to trauma to bleeding site associated with vigorous nose blowing	Assess and report exudates (as stated above) Instruct patient against blowing nose in immediate postoperative period, because this could increase bleeding, edema, and ecchymosis

Instruct the patient to contact the health care provider if bleeding or signs of infection develops. The patient should use nasal sprays and drops judiciously because of the possible rebound effect on nasal mucous membranes. Remind the patient to avoid nose blowing, vigorous coughing, or Valsalva's maneuver (holding the breath and bearing down as if straining during a bowel movement) for 2 days postoperatively. Instruct the patient that facial ecchymosis and edema may persist for several days after surgery.

Prognosis

With surgical correction, the prognosis is excellent.

ANTIGEN-ANTIBODY ALLERGIC RHINITIS AND ALLERGIC CONJUNCTIVITIS (HAY FEVER)

Etiology and Pathophysiology

Allergic rhinitis and allergic conjunctivitis (hay fever) are atopic allergic conditions that result from antigen-antibody reactions in the nasal membranes, nasopharynx, and conjunctiva from inhaled or contact allergens. Many infants, children, and adults have these seasonal or perennial conditions, which often result in absences from school and work.

During the antigen-antibody reaction of rhinitis and conjunctivitis, ciliary action slows; mucosal gland secretion increases; leukocyte (eosinophil) infiltration occurs; and, because of increased capillary permeability and vasodilation, local tissue edema results. Common allergens are tree, grass, and weed pollens; mold spores; fungi; house dusts; mites; and animal dander. Some foods, drugs, and insect stings also may cause these reactions.

Clinical Manifestations

Acute ocular manifestations include edema, photophobia, excessive tearing, blurring of vision, and pruritus. Individuals with rhinitis complain of excessive secretions or inability to breathe through the nose because of congestion and/or edema. Otitis media symptoms can occur if the eustachian tubes are occluded. These symptoms occur more in childhood, with the individual complaining of ear fullness, ear popping, or decreased hearing.

Assessment

The initial complaints of seasonal rhinitis and conjunctivitis include severe sneezing, congestion, pruritus, and lacrimation (watery eyes). Cough, epistaxis, and headache also may occur. More chronic signs and symptoms include headache, severe nasal congestion, postnasal drip, and cough. If these are not treated, chronic sufferers eventually develop secondary infections, such as otitis media, bronchitis, sinusitis, and pneumonia.

Diagnostic Tests

In allergic rhinitis, the mucosa of the turbinates is usually pale because of venous engorgement, which is in contrast to the erythema of viral rhinitis.

Skin testing can be done in a health care provider's office. A site, usually an adult's forearm or a child's back, is cleaned with alcohol, and the nurse draws small marks on the skin with a special pen. Next to each mark the nurse uses a lancet to prick the skin with various allergens. A new lancet is used for each allergen. Some allergens react quickly, whereas others may take up to 15 minutes. If an allergic reaction is present, the patient has a raised, red, itchy bump, or *wheal*, that may look like a mosquito bite. The nurse then measures the size of the wheal and records the results.

The serum radioallergosorbent test, or RAST, is done by drawing blood and then mixing the blood with various allergens. This procedure gives definitive diagnosis of allergies by the increases in allergen-specific immunoglobulin E (IgE) (National Library of Medicine, 2012).

Medical Management

Treatment goals are to relieve signs and symptoms and prevent infections and other complaints, such as malaise, extreme fatigue, and severe headaches. Avoiding the allergen is effective. Perennial use of antihistamines, intranasal corticosteroids, and leukotriene receptor antagonists such as zafirlukast (Accolate) or montelukast (Singulair) is recommended. Changing from one antihistamine to another seasonally may help impede tolerance to any one medication.

Decongestants may be added and used intermittently for 3 to 5 days if congestion occurs. Common over-the-counter decongestants—such as phenylephrine, pseudoephedrine, chlorpheniramine, and phenylpropanolamine—are contained in familiar products such as Actifed, Triaminic, and Robitussin. These products may produce a "rebound" effect, causing the patient to feel more uncomfortable and congested.

Lodoxamide (Alomide) four times a day is the recommended treatment for mild to moderately severe allergic conjunctivitis.

Although long-term, consistent use of topical or nasal corticosteroids once was considered appropriate treatment, they are no longer recommended because of the tolerance that is built up with continuous use. Medications included in this category are beclomethasone (Beconase), dexamethasone, flunisolide, fluticasone (Flonase), and budesonide (Rhinocort).

Pressure headaches may require analgesics until signs and symptoms are relieved. Hot packs over facial sinuses offer relief if the headache is related to sinus congestion.

Nursing Interventions and Patient Teaching

These illnesses are self-limiting, so focus on health promotion and maintenance teaching to provide for self-care management. Include ways to avoid allergens, self-care management through symptom control, and medication action and usage.

OBSTRUCTIVE SLEEP APNEA

Etiology and Pathophysiology

Obstructive sleep apnea (OSA) is characterized by partial or complete upper airway obstruction during sleep, causing apnea and hypopnea. *Apnea* is the cessation of spontaneous respirations; *hypopnea* is abnormally shallow and slow respirations. Airflow obstruction occurs when the tongue and the soft palate fall backward and partially or completely obstruct the pharynx. The obstruction may last from 15 to 90 seconds. During the apneic period, the patient experiences severe hypoxemia (decreased PaO_2) and hypercapnia (increased $PaCO_2$). These changes are ventilatory stimulants and cause the patient to awaken partially. The patient has a generalized startle response, snorts, and gasps, which cause the tongue and soft palate to move forward and the airway to open. Apnea and arousal cycles occur repeatedly, as many as 200 to 400 times during 6 to 8 hours of sleep.

Sleep apnea occurs in an estimated 18 million adults in the United States, but as many as 90% of them are undiagnosed (American Association for Respiratory Care, 2017). Often patients are unaware of sleep apnea until pulmonary edema develops or when the patient needs general anesthesia, which can cause a serious complication. General anesthesia suppresses upper airway activity and allows the airway to close. Anesthesia may increase the number of episodes and the duration of episodes, thereby decreasing arterial oxygenation. Anesthesia inhibits the arousals that occur during sleep, making it harder to bring the patient out of anesthesia.

Clinical Manifestations and Assessment

Clinical manifestations of sleep apnea include frequent awakening at night, insomnia, excessive daytime sleepiness, and witnessed apneic episodes. The patient's bed partner may complain about loud snoring, sometimes so loud that both people cannot sleep in the same room. Other symptoms include morning headaches (from hypercapnia, which causes vasodilation of cerebral blood vessels), personality changes, and irritability. Systemic hypertension, cardiac dysrhythmias, right-sided heart failure from pulmonary hypertension caused by nocturnal hypoxemia, and stroke are serious complications that may occur.

Symptoms of sleep apnea alter many aspects of a patient's lifestyle. With chronic sleep loss, the patient may have diminished ability to concentrate, impaired memory, failure to accomplish daily tasks, and interpersonal difficulties. Men may experience impotence. Driving accidents are more common in habitually sleepy people. Family life and the patient's ability to maintain employment also often are compromised. As a result, the patient may experience severe depression. Risk factors for OSA include the following (Mayo Clinic, 2018b):

- *Male gender:* About twice as many men as women have OSA.
- *Older age:* Although younger patients can develop OSA, the incidence increases with age over 60 years, probably because of weight gain and loss of pharyngeal muscle strength.
- *Obesity:* An obese person's pharynx may be infiltrated with fat, and the tongue and soft palate may be enlarged, crowding the air passages. An obese individual also may have a short, thick neck increasing susceptibility to obstruction.
- *Nasal conditions:* Nasal allergies, polyps, or septal deviation decrease the diameter of the pharynx.
- *Receding chin:* A person with a receding chin may not have enough room in the pharynx for the tongue, thus contributing to obstruction.
- *Pharyngeal structural abnormalities:* A person with OSA may have enlarged tonsils, an elongated uvula, an especially long tongue, or a soft palate that rests on the base of the tongue. Any of these structural abnormalities can impinge on the airway.

Appropriate referral should be made if problems are identified. Cessation of breathing reported by the bed partner is usually a source of great anxiety because of fear that breathing may not resume.

Diagnostic Tests

Diagnosis of sleep apnea is made during sleep with the use of polysomnography. Electrodes are placed on the patient's scalp, mandibular area, and lateral area of the eyelids. A nasal cannula measures airflow, and pulse oximetry measures SpO_2 (National Heart, Lung, and Blood Institute, 2012). The patient's chest and abdominal movements, oral airflow, nasal airflow, SpO_2, ocular movement, muscle activity, brain activity, and heart rate and rhythm are monitored, and time in each sleep stage is determined. A diagnosis of sleep apnea requires documentation of multiple episodes of apnea (no airflow with respiratory effort) or hypopnea (airflow diminished 30% to 50% with respiratory effort). Polysomnography may be carried out in a sleep laboratory, or the patient may be taught to attach monitoring leads for a home sleep study.

Medical Management and Nursing Interventions

Mild sleep apnea may respond to simple measures. Instruct the patient to avoid sedatives and alcoholic beverages for 3 to 4 hours before sleep. Referral to a weight loss program may help, because excessive weight exacerbates symptoms. Symptoms resolve in half of the patients with OSA who use an oral appliance during sleep that brings the mandible and tongue forward to enlarge the airway space, thereby preventing airway occlusion. Some individuals find a support group beneficial so that they can express concerns and feelings and discuss strategies for resolving problems.

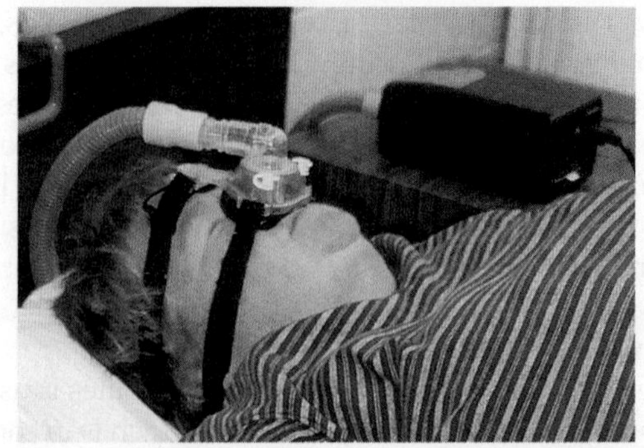

Fig. 49.10 Nasal continuous positive airway pressure (nCPAP). The patient applies a nasal mask attached to a blower to maintain positive pressure.

In patients with more severe symptoms, nasal continuous positive airway pressure (nCPAP) may be used. With nCPAP the patient applies a nasal mask that is attached to a high-flow blower (Fig. 49.10). The blower is adjusted to maintain sufficient positive pressure (5 to 15 cm H_2O) in the airway during inspiration and expiration to prevent airway collapse. Some patients cannot adjust to exhaling against the high pressure. A technologically more sophisticated therapy, bilevel positive airway pressure (BiPAP), capable of delivering higher pressure during inspiration (when the airway is most likely to be occluded) and lower pressure during expiration, may be helpful and is better tolerated. Although CPAP is highly effective, compliance is poor even if symptoms of sleep apnea are relieved.

UPPER AIRWAY OBSTRUCTION

Etiology and Pathophysiology

Upper airway obstruction is precipitated by a recent respiratory event, such as traumatic injury to the airway or surrounding tissues. Common airway obstructions include choking on food; dentures; aspiration (inhalation) of vomitus or secretions; and, the most common airway obstruction in an unconscious person, the tongue.

Altered physiology includes any condition that could produce airway obstruction, such as laryngeal spasm caused by tetany resulting from hypocalcemia. Another cause may be laryngeal edema caused by injury.

Clinical Manifestations

The main signs are stertorous respirations, altered respiratory rate and character, and apneic periods. Severe obstructions are accompanied by cyanosis, choking, and difficulty in breathing. Behavioral signs of upper airway obstruction include agitation, changes in level of consciousness, and confusion.

Assessment

Subjective data are limited because a patient is unable to talk when the airway is obstructed. The nurse therefore must make a prompt and accurate assessment of objective data.

Collection of objective data includes prompt assessment for the classic sign of choking, in which the patient places a hand over his or her throat. Also monitor for signs of hypoxia (an inadequate, reduced tension of cellular oxygen) (see Box 49.1), **cyanosis** (slightly bluish, grayish, slatelike, or dark purple discoloration of the skin resulting from excessive amounts of deoxygenated hemoglobin in the blood), stertorous respirations, and wheezing or stridor (harsh, high-pitched sounds during respiration, caused by obstruction). As hypoxia progresses, the respiratory centers in the brain (medulla oblongata and pons) are depressed, resulting in bradycardia and shallow, slow respirations.

Diagnostic Tests

This is a medical emergency; the focus is on prompt management of the condition. This condition is diagnosed by prompt and accurate assessment. Foreign bodies may be identified by radiographic studies.

Medical Management

The patient may require abdominal thrusts (Heimlich maneuver) or an emergency tracheostomy to remove the obstruction. Depending on the cause of the obstruction, an artificial airway may be inserted to maintain patency. A pharyngeal, endotracheal, or tracheal artificial airway may be used.

Nursing Interventions and Patient Teaching

The most immediate nursing intervention is to open the airway and restore patency. This may be accomplished by properly repositioning the patient's head and neck, or it may require further maneuvers. The head-tilt/chin-lift technique recommended by the American Heart Association minimizes further damage in the presence of a suspected cervical neck fracture. With a foreign body airway obstruction, the Heimlich maneuver is used.

Patient problems and interventions for the patient with an airway obstruction include but are not limited to the following:

Patient Problem	Nursing Interventions
Inability to Clear Airway, related to obstruction in airway	Reestablish and maintain secure airway Administer oxygen as ordered Suction as needed and assess patient's ability to mobilize secretions Monitor vital signs and breath sounds closely
Potential for Aspiration Into Airway, related to partial airway obstruction	Monitor respiratory rate, rhythm, and effort Assess patient's ability to swallow secretions by elevating the head of the bed Assess and document breath sounds Facilitate optimal airway and functional swallowing by elevating head of bed Note amount, color, and characteristics of secretions Suction as needed

The goal of education is prevention. Teach the patient and the family how to assess for airway patency. Describe appropriate use of the Heimlich maneuver. Explain the rationale for all treatments and procedures.

Prognosis

With immediate medical and nursing intervention, the prognosis is good; without emergency intervention, the condition is life threatening.

CANCER OF THE LARYNX

Etiology and Pathophysiology

The American Cancer Society (2018) estimated that about 13,150 new cases of laryngeal cancer (10,490 in men and 2660 in women) and about 3710 deaths (2970 men and 740 women) resulting from this disease would occur in 2018. The American Cancer Society has found a decrease in the rate of occurrence of new cases since 2009.

Laryngeal cancers occur most often in people older than age 65. The incidence appears to be correlated to prolonged tobacco use (cigarettes, pipes, cigars, chewing tobacco, smokeless tobacco) and heavy alcohol use, chronic laryngitis, vocal abuse, gastroesophageal reflux disease, and family history. Because of the increase in the number of women who are heavy smokers, their incidence of carcinoma of the larynx is increasing.

Laryngeal cancer limited to the true vocal cords is slow-growing because of decreased lymphatic supply; however, elsewhere in the larynx there is an abundance of lymph tissue, and cancer in these tissues spreads rapidly and metastasizes early to the deep lymph nodes of the neck.

Clinical Manifestations

Progressive or persistent hoarseness is an early sign. Any person who is hoarse longer than 2 weeks should seek medical treatment. Signs of metastasis to other areas include pain in the larynx radiating to the ear, difficulty in swallowing (dysphagia), a feeling of a lump in the throat, and enlarged cervical lymph nodes.

Assessment

Collection of subjective data includes assessing the onset and duration of symptoms. Complaints of referred pain to the ear (otalgia) and difficulty breathing (dyspnea) or swallowing should be noted.

Collection of objective data includes examining sputum for blood (*hemoptysis,* or blood expectorated from the respiratory tract).

Diagnostic Tests

Visual examination of the larynx by direct laryngoscopy, with a fiberoptic scope, is done to determine the presence of laryngeal cancer. Other diagnostic tests to detect local and regional spread of laryngeal cancer include CT scan, magnetic resonance imaging (MRI), and positron emission tomography (PET). The patient also may have a chest x-ray study and a CT scan to determine whether there is lung or liver metastasis (American Cancer Society, n.d.). A health history helps in making the diagnosis, and a biopsy and microscopic study of the lesion are definitive.

Medical Management

Treatment is determined by the extent of tumor growth. If the tumor is confined to the true vocal cord without limitation of cord movement, then radiation therapy is the best course of treatment. Surgical intervention is considered when extension of the tumor becomes affixed to one of the cords or extends upward or downward from the larynx; surgical options include a total or partial laryngectomy or a radical neck dissection. A partial laryngectomy is done to remove the diseased vocal cord and possibly a portion of thyroid cartilage. This requires placement of a temporary tracheostomy, which is closed when the edema has decreased. A total laryngectomy is performed when the cancer of the larynx is advanced; this requires placement of a permanent tracheostomy. Because the patient can no longer breathe through the nose, usually the sense of smell is lost and the sense of taste is affected. The voice is also absent once the larynx is removed. There is no connection between the patient's mouth and trachea.

A radical neck dissection to remove cervical lymph nodes is done often in conjunction with a total laryngectomy in patients who have a high risk of metastasis to the neck from carcinoma of the larynx. This surgery entails removal of the submandibular salivary gland, the sternocleidomastoid muscle, the spinal accessory nerve, and the internal jugular vein, which results in one-sided shoulder droop. This surgery results in a very large tracheostomy opening, and no tracheostomy tube is used. The opening narrows as the patient heals from chemotherapy.

Chemotherapy using cisplatin and 5-fluorouracil (5-FU) before and after surgery or radiation has achieved a positive response in many cases (American Cancer Society, n.d.).

Nursing Interventions and Patient Teaching

If a tracheostomy is created, then airway maintenance through proper suctioning techniques is important. Assess skin integrity surrounding the tracheal opening; be alert for signs of infection.

Monitor intake and output (I&O) balance and assist with tube feedings as ordered. Explain to the patient that the tube feedings are temporary and that normal eating may begin again when healing occurs in a few weeks. Weigh the patient daily and assess hydration status to determine the need for additional fluids; note skin turgor and observe for diarrhea.

Because of neck and facial disfigurement and loss of voice, a thorough psychosocial assessment and resultant interventions are beneficial. Encourage communication through writing and facial and hand gestures. Often no one can reassure a patient that speech can be regained as well as a fellow patient who has undergone the same surgical intervention. Many cities have a Lost Chord Club or a New Voice Club, whose members are willing to visit hospitalized patients. A speech therapist should meet with the patient after a total laryngectomy to discuss voice restoration options, including a voice prosthesis, esophageal speech, and an electrolarynx.

Patient problems and interventions for the patient with a tracheostomy include but are not limited to the following:

Patient Problem	Nursing Interventions
Inability to Clear Airway, related to secretions or obstruction	Suction secretions as needed Provide tracheostomy care according to protocol; ensure the availability of emergency equipment (oxygen and tracheostomy tray) Offer small, frequent feedings, and give liquid or pureed food as tolerated to avoid choking Teach patient stoma protection Assess respiratory rate and characteristics q 1–2 hr Auscultate lung sounds, monitor SaO_2 q 4 hr Elevate head of bed 30 degrees or higher Turn patient and encourage coughing and deep breathing q 2–4 hr Provide constant humidity Suction tracheostomy tube as needed, using aseptic technique; instruct patient to inhale as catheter is advanced Clean inner cannula of tracheostomy tube q 2–4 hr and as needed, using a solution of ½ normal saline and ½ hydrogen peroxide

Patient Problem	Nursing Interventions
Compromised Verbal Communication	Provide patient with implements for communication, including pencil, paper, Magic Slate, picture books, or electronic voice device Anesthesia interferes with the patient's memory, so providing a notebook for the family to include relevant events can help orient the patient Keep call signal by patient's hand at all times If possible, ask patient questions that require only a yes or no response to avoid fatigue and frustration Refer patient to local support groups and the local chapter of the American Cancer Society Assist with speech rehabilitation Review instructions about esophageal and electroesophageal speech Reinforce need for regular follow-up with speech pathologist and surgeon after discharge

Explain techniques of airway maintenance, such as oxygen usage, deep breathing, and coughing. Discuss the importance of dietary management in relationship to airway maintenance. Encourage optimal fluid intake for the patient: an uncovered tracheostomy can dehydrate the patient. Promote optimal communication through speech rehabilitation and community support groups.

Prognosis

If the tumor is limited to the true cord, the cure rate is 80% to 90% for stage I, decreasing to 44% at stage IV. The prognosis in primary supraglottic and subglottic cancer is poorer. The 5-year survival rate is 65% for stage I, decreasing to 32% for stage IV (American Cancer Society, 2018).

RESPIRATORY INFECTIONS

ACUTE RHINITIS

Etiology and Pathophysiology

Acute rhinitis (or acute **coryza**), known as the *common cold,* is an inflammatory condition of the mucous membranes of the nose and accessory sinuses. It typically is characterized by edema of the nasal mucous membrane. The common cold usually is caused by one or more viruses; however, it may become complicated by a bacterial infection. Signs and symptoms usually are evident within 24 to 48 hours after exposure. Sinus congestion causes increased sinus drainage, leading to postnasal drip. The postnasal drip causes throat irritation, headache, and earache. Most people with colds contaminate their hands when coughing or sneezing, thus contaminating everything they touch. Others become infected when touching the telephone, computer, or anything else that has been touched by the person with a cold. Also, many colds are believed to be spread by shaking hands with a person who has a cold.

Clinical Manifestations

An increased amount of thin, serous nasal exudate and a productive cough are two of the most common signs. Sore throat and fever are often present. If the infection remains uncomplicated, it generally subsides in a week. In addition, the patient may report aches, pains, fatigue, and loss of appetite.

Assessment

Subjective data include the patient's complaints of sore throat, dyspnea, and congestion of varying duration.

Collection of objective data includes noting the color and consistency of the nasal exudate. A visual examination of the throat may reveal erythema, edema, and local irritation. Also document the presence and duration of fever.

Diagnostic Tests

Throat and sputum cultures indicate the presence and nature of microorganisms.

Medical Management

Medical management is aimed at accurate diagnosis and prevention of complications. No specific treatment is available for the common cold. Among the medications used are (1) aspirin or acetaminophen for analgesia and reduction of temperature (aspirin is not used in infants, children, and adolescents because of the danger of developing Reye's syndrome); and either (2) a cough suppressant for a dry, nonproductive cough or (3) an expectorant to help dislodge mucus for a productive cough. If a secondary bacterial infection is confirmed, an antibiotic agent (e.g., erythromycin) is prescribed (see the Complementary and Alternative Therapies box).

Nursing Interventions and Patient Teaching

Nursing interventions are aimed at promoting comfort. Such measures include encouraging fluids and applying warm, moist packs to sinuses.

Patient problems and interventions for the patient with acute rhinitis include but are not limited to the following:

Patient Problem	Nursing Interventions
Inability to Clear Airway, related to nasal exudates	Encourage fluids to liquefy secretions and aid in their expectoration Use vaporizer to moisten mucous membranes and prevent further irritation

Continued

Patient Problem	Nursing Interventions
Willingness for Improved Health Management	Remind patient and family of health maintenance behaviors to decrease risk of illness, such as adequate fluid and nutritional management and sufficient rest Teach importance of hygiene measures to decrease spread of infection

Complementary and Alternative Therapies

Respiratory Disorders

- Herbal medicines for respiratory problems include remedies for nasal discharge and congestion, cough, sore throat, fever and headache, and immunostimulant effects. Ephedra *(Ephedra sinica, Ephedra vulgaris)* is a stimulant and is illegal in some areas. Expectorants include anise *(Pimpinella anisum)*, coltsfoot *(Tussilago farfara)*, and horehound *(Marrubium vulgare)*. Coltsfoot and horehound also are believed to have antitussive action.
- Sore throat remedies include mint (*Mentha piperita* [peppermint], *Mentha spicata* [spearmint]), and slippery elm *(Ulmus rubra)*. Remedies for the fever and headache that may accompany colds and influenza include boneset *(Eupatorium perfoliatum)*, feverfew *(Tanacetum parthenium)*, and willow *(Salix purpurea, S. fragilis, S. daphnoides)*.
- Stimulants of the immune system, believed to help ward off colds and flu, include echinacea *(Echinacea angustifolia, E. pallida, E. purpurea)* and goldenseal *(Hydrastis canadensis)*.
- Some interventions that contribute to comfort in patients experiencing dyspnea include the following:
  - Breathing exercises
  - Relaxation therapy
  - Massage
  - Acupuncture
  - Hypnosis
  - Visualization
- Some people believe that reflexology helps relieve congestion.
- Facial massage with diluted aromatic oils is believed by some to open occluded sinuses and relieve congestion. These essential oils include lavender, eucalyptus, peppermint, and tea tree oil.

Teach the patient the correct handwashing technique and proper disposal of tissues used for nasal secretions. Instruct the patient to limit exposure to others during the first 48 hours and to check his or her temperature every 4 hours.

A small ceramic pot, called a neti pot, is used to flush out the nasal passages with a saltwater solution—a process known as nasal irrigation. Some patients do not tolerate neti pot irrigations, but for those who do, the result is thinner mucus that drains more easily and less congestion.

Prognosis

Signs and symptoms resolve in 2 to 10 days. Even though the common cold does not cause death, its economic importance is vast, because it is the greatest cause of absenteeism in industry and schools.

ACUTE FOLLICULAR TONSILLITIS

Etiology and Pathophysiology

Acute follicular tonsillitis can be an acute inflammation of the tonsils. It is the result of an airborne or foodborne bacterial infection, often streptococci. Less frequently, it also often may be viral. If it is caused by group A beta-hemolytic streptococci, sequelae such as rheumatic fever, carditis, and nephritis must be considered. It appears to be most common in school-age children. Signs and symptoms of tonsillitis include sore throat, fever, chills, and anorexia. The tonsils become enlarged and often contain purulent exudate.

Clinical Manifestations

Acute follicular tonsillitis is manifest clinically with enlarged, tender cervical lymph nodes. Fever may be present with chills, general muscle aching, and malaise. Laboratory data reveal an elevated white blood cell count.

Assessment

Collection of subjective data includes monitoring the severity of throat pain and the possibility of referred pain to the ears. Note headache or joint pain.

Collection of objective data includes a visual examination that shows increased throat secretions and enlarged, erythematous tonsils.

Diagnostic Tests

Throat cultures identify the causative microorganism, most commonly beta-hemolytic streptococci. A complete blood count (CBC) is done to determine whether the white blood cell count is elevated. Commonly, the abnormal white blood cell count is 10,000 to 20,000/mm^3.

Medical Management

If antibiotics to which the offending organism is sensitive are administered early, infection subsides. An elective tonsillectomy and adenoidectomy (T&A), in which the tonsils and adenoids are excised surgically, is performed in people who have recurrent attacks of tonsillitis. The procedure usually is performed from 4 to 6 weeks after an acute attack has subsided. Either general or local anesthesia is used. Post-T&A hemostasis (i.e., the stoppage of bleeding) is paramount, because the patient can lose a large amount of blood through hemorrhage without demonstrating any signs of bleeding. The health care provider may be able to control minor postoperative bleeding by applying a sponge soaked in a solution of epinephrine to the site. The patient who is bleeding excessively often is returned to the operating room for surgical treatment to stop the hemorrhage.

Medications used in tonsillitis include analgesics and antipyretics (e.g., acetaminophen) and antibiotic agents (e.g., penicillin). Warm saline gargles are also beneficial.

Nursing Interventions and Patient Teaching

One of the primary nursing goals for acute tonsillitis is to provide meticulous oral care, which promotes comfort and assists in combating infection. Observe and report if the patient swallows frequently, because this is often a subtle but reliable indication of excessive bleeding.

Postoperative care for tonsillectomy includes maintaining IV fluids until the nausea subsides, at which time the patient may begin drinking ice-cold clear liquids. The diet is advanced to custard and ice cream and then to a normal diet as soon as possible. Spicy foods should be avoided because they often irritate the throat after surgery. Hot liquids and food are avoided because these cause vasodilation, leading to bleeding. Apply an ice collar to the neck for comfort and to reduce bleeding by vasoconstriction. Monitor vital signs to assess for hemorrhage, postoperative fever, or other complications. Comfort measures are important, and emotional support is essential.

Patient problems and interventions for the patient with acute follicular tonsillitis include but are not limited to the following:

Patient Problem	Nursing Interventions
Discomfort, related to inflammation and irritation of the pharynx	Assess degree of pain and need for analgesics Document effectiveness of medication and offer analgesic as ordered Maintain bed rest and promote rest Offer warm saline gargles, ice chips, and ice collar as needed
Potential for Inadequate Fluid Volume, related to inability to maintain usual oral intake because of painful swallowing	Assess hydration status by noting mucous membranes, skin turgor, and urinary output Encourage ice pops, ice chips, and increased oral intake; cold liquids, sherbet, and ice cream are best tolerated; carbonated drinks may be taken if patient tolerates; avoid offering citrus juices because they may burn the throat
Potential for Aspiration Into Airway, related to postoperative bleeding	Maintain patent airway; keep patient lying on side as much as possible to prevent aspiration Observe for vomiting of dark brown fluid; patient may have "swallowed" blood during surgery Watch for frequent swallowing, which may indicate bleeding; check frequently with flashlight to see if blood is trickling down posterior pharynx

Instruct the patient (or the family for a child) that the patient should complete the entire course of the prescribed antibiotic. If the patient had surgery (T&A), offer dietary instruction regarding appropriate foods and liquids. Advise the patient to avoid attempting to clear the throat immediately after surgery (may initiate bleeding) and to avoid coughing, sneezing, or vigorous nose blowing for 1 to 2 weeks. Most surgeons no longer prescribe aspirin for pain after tonsillectomy, because it increases the tendency to bleed; acetaminophen or another aspirin substitute usually is ordered. Analgesics usually are given orally in liquid form. Remind the patient to avoid overexertion, and make certain that the patient and the family know how to reach the health care provider in case of increased pain, fever, or bleeding.

Prognosis

Tonsillitis is usually self-limiting but may have serious complications, such as sinusitis, otitis media, mastoiditis, rheumatic fever, nephritis, or peritonsillar abscess.

LARYNGITIS

Etiology and Pathophysiology

Laryngitis often occurs secondary to other respiratory infections. Laryngeal inflammation is a common disorder that can be either chronic or acute. Acute laryngitis may cause severe respiratory distress in children younger than 5 years of age because the relatively small larynx is subject to spasm when irritated or infected and readily becomes partially or totally obstructed.

Acute laryngitis often accompanies viral or bacterial infections. Other causes include excessive use of the voice or inhalation of irritating fumes. Chronic laryngitis usually is associated with inflammation of the laryngeal mucosa or edematous vocal cords.

Clinical Manifestations

Laryngitis often produces hoarseness to some degree, or even complete voice loss. The throat feels scratchy and irritated, and the patient may have a persistent cough.

Assessment

Subjective data include the patient reporting progressive hoarseness and a cough that may be productive or may be dry and nonproductive. Attempt to identify any precipitating factors such as excessive voice use or exposure to inhaled irritants.

Collection of objective data includes evaluating the patient's voice quality and the characteristics (color, consistency, and amount) of sputum produced.

Diagnostic Tests

Laryngoscopy reveals abnormalities (edema, drainage) of vocal cords and erythematous laryngeal mucosa.

Medical Management

If the laryngitis is due to a virus, there is no specific therapy; if it is bacterial, medications include antibiotics (such as erythromycin or levofloxacin [Levaquin]). Analgesics or antipyretics for comfort, antitussives to relieve cough (such as promethazine with codeine), and throat lozenges to promote comfort and decrease irritation are useful.

Nursing Interventions and Patient Teaching

General interventions include use of warm or cool mist inhalation via a vaporizer. Encourage the patient to rest the voice by limiting verbal communication.

Patient problems and interventions for the patient with laryngitis include but are not limited to the following:

Patient Problem	Nursing Interventions
Discomfort, related to pharyngeal irritation	Assess level of pain, and offer medications to promote comfort Use steam inhalation as ordered Instruct patient on the importance of resting the voice
Compromised Verbal Communication, related to edematous vocal cords	Instruct patient on the importance of resting the voice Provide other means for communication (written word, gestures) Anticipate patient's needs whenever possible

If the patient receives antibiotic agents, instruct him or her to finish the entire prescribed course. Remind the patient of the need to limit use of the voice. Encourage patients who are smokers to quit and to limit exposure to irritating fumes.

Prognosis

The prognosis is good in adults. In the infant and the young child, respiratory edema can result in respiratory distress.

PHARYNGITIS

Etiology and Pathophysiology

Pharyngitis may be either chronic or acute. It is the most common throat inflammation and frequently accompanies the common cold. Pharyngitis is usually viral but can be caused by beta-hemolytic streptococci, staphylococci, or other bacteria. There is increased evidence of gonococcal pharyngitis caused by the gram-negative diplococcus *Neisseria gonorrhoeae*. A severe form of acute pharyngitis often is referred to as *strep throat* because the *Streptococcus* organism is commonly the cause. This disorder is contagious for 2 or 3 days after the onset of signs and symptoms.

Clinical Manifestations

Pharyngitis is manifest clinically by a dry cough, tender tonsils, and enlarged cervical lymph glands. The throat appears erythematous, and soreness may range from slight scratchiness to severe pain with difficulty in swallowing.

Assessment

Subjective data include any reported pharyngeal discomfort, fever, or difficulty in swallowing.

Collection of objective data includes palpating for enlarged, edematous glands and associated tenderness and noting elevated temperature.

Diagnostic Tests

A rapid strep screen test is performed to determine the presence of beta-hemolytic streptococci. This is only a preliminary diagnosis. A culture is obtained at the same time in case the rapid strep screen yields a false-negative result. Obtain a specimen from the pharynx and make sure the swab does not touch the tongue or gums during insertion. The patient often gags if the specimen is obtained correctly.

Medical Management

Commonly ordered medications include antibiotics, such as penicillin or erythromycin, to (1) treat severe infections or (2) prevent superimposed infections, particularly in people who have a history of rheumatic fever or bacterial endocarditis. Analgesics and antipyretics, such as acetaminophen, are used to promote comfort.

Nursing Interventions and Patient Teaching

Offer saline throat rinses or gargles and encourage oral intake. Emphasize the importance of adequate rest and use of a vaporizer to increase humidity.

Patient problems and interventions for the patient with pharyngitis include but are not limited to the following:

Patient Problem	Nursing Interventions
Compromised Oral Mucous Membrane, related to edema	Provide warm saline gargles to promote comfort Assess level of pain and provide medications as ordered Encourage oral intake of fluids Offer frequent oral care
Potential for Inadequate Fluid Volume, related to decreased oral intake as a result of painful swallowing	Observe and record patient's hydration status Monitor I&O and patient's temperature Maintain IV therapy if indicated

Perform and document medication teaching, including the importance of completing the entire prescribed course of antibiotics and any side effects of medications. Instruct the patient to avoid exposure to inhaled irritants and to apply preventive measures, such as using a vaporizer and maintaining adequate fluid intake.

Prognosis

Signs and symptoms usually resolve in 4 to 6 days unless secondary complications develop.

SINUSITIS

Etiology and Pathophysiology

Sinusitis can be chronic or acute, involving any sinus area, such as the maxillary or frontal sinuses. This infection can be either viral or bacterial and often is a complication of pneumonia or nasal polyps. The underlying pathophysiology begins with an upper respiratory tract infection that leads to a sinus infection.

Clinical Manifestations

The patient with sinusitis often complains of a constant, severe headache with pain and tenderness in the particular sinus region and often has purulent exudate.

Assessment

Subjective data include patient reporting decreased appetite or nausea. The patient also may complain of generalized malaise, headache, diminished sense of smell, and increased pain in the sinus region when bending forward or when gentle pressure is applied over the infected sinus region.

Collection of objective data involves assessing vital signs, particularly temperature, and also assessing the character and amount of drainage. Headache, facial pain (with and/or without palpation), thick nasal secretions, congestion, edema of the eyelids, fatigue, and elevated temperature are common symptoms.

Diagnostic Tests

Sinus radiographic studies frequently are done to depict cloudy or fluid-filled sinus cavities. A simple way to diagnose sinusitis is with transillumination. This procedure involves shining a light in the mouth with the lips closed around it; infected sinuses look dark, whereas normal sinuses transilluminate. To confirm the diagnosis, a sinus CT scan may be performed.

Medical Management

Nasal windows or other surgical incisions can be created to allow better drainage and removal of diseased mucosal tissue. A common surgical procedure to relieve chronic maxillary sinusitis, the Caldwell-Luc operation (or radical antrum operation), involves making an incision between the gum and upper lip, allowing access to the floor of the maxillary sinus. This is followed by removal of a small piece of maxillary bone. This opening allows the infected maxillary sinus to drain.

Medications used to treat sinusitis include the following:

- *Saline nasal irrigation:* A saline solution is sprayed into the nose to rinse the nasal passages.
- *Nasal corticosteroids:* These nasal sprays help prevent and treat inflammation. Examples include fluticasone (Flonase), budesonide (Rhinocort Aqua), triamcinolone (Nasacort AQ), mometasone (Nasonex), and beclomethasone (Beconase AQ).
- *Oral or injected corticosteroids:* These medications are used to relieve inflammation from severe sinusitis, especially if the patient also has nasal polyps. Examples include prednisone and methylprednisolone. Oral corticosteroids can cause serious side effects when used long term, so they are used only to treat severe symptoms.
- *Decongestants:* These medications are available as over-the-counter (OTC) and prescription liquids, tablets, and nasal sprays. Examples of OTC oral decongestants include Sudafed and Actifed. An example of an OTC nasal spray is oxymetazoline (Afrin). These medications generally are taken for a few days at most; otherwise they can cause the return of more severe congestion (rebound congestion).
- *Over-the-counter pain relievers:* Over-the-counter pain relievers include aspirin, acetaminophen (Tylenol, others), and ibuprofen (Advil, Motrin IB, others). Because of the risk of Reye's syndrome—a potentially life-threatening illness—never give aspirin to anyone younger than age 18 years.
- *Antibiotics:* Antibiotics are prescribed only if the health care provider determines that the cause of the sinusitis is bacterial.

Nursing Interventions and Patient Teaching

Steam inhalation and warm, moist packs facilitate drainage and promote comfort.

Neti pots have been used for irrigation of the sinus cavities, using a salt and warm water solution. Care must be taken when making your own solution. Using filtered water or distilled water is recommended by the Centers for Disease Control and Prevention (CDC).

Patient problems and interventions for the patient with sinusitis include but are not limited to the following:

Patient Problem	Nursing Interventions
Inability to Maintain Adequate Breathing Pattern, related to nasal congestion	Assess respiratory status frequently, noting any changes; mouth breathing may be necessary because of nasal airway and sinus discomfort
Discomfort, related to sinus congestion	Document comfort level Assess need for analgesics and document patient response Elevate head of bed to promote drainage of secretions Apply warm, moist packs four times a day to promote secretion drainage and provide relief

The aim of patient education is to prevent recurrence or complications of sinus infection. Instruct the patient to be alert to signs and symptoms of sinusitis so that early treatment can be obtained.

Prognosis

Prognosis for uncomplicated sinusitis is good; complications include cavernous sinus thrombosis and spread of infection to bone, brain, or meninges, which can result in meningitis, osteomyelitis, or septicemia.

DISORDERS OF THE LOWER AIRWAY

ACUTE BRONCHITIS

Etiology and Pathophysiology

Usually acute bronchitis is secondary to an upper respiratory tract infection, but it can be related to exposure to inhaled irritants. Inflammation of the trachea and bronchial tree causes congestion of the mucous membranes, which results in retention of tenacious secretions. These secretions can become a culture medium for bacterial growth.

Clinical Manifestations

Acute bronchitis manifests itself with symptoms such as a productive cough, diffuse rhonchi and wheezes, dyspnea, chest pain, and low-grade fever. Generalized malaise and headache are also common symptoms.

Assessment

Subjective data include the patient's complaints of feeling poorly and experiencing headache and aching tightness in the chest.

Collection of objective data includes monitoring vital signs frequently, checking breath sounds, and noting the presence of wheezes or basilar crackles.

Diagnostic Tests

The usual diagnostic aids include a chest radiographic examination to ensure clear lung fields and a sputum specimen to determine the presence of associated bacterial infections.

Medical Management

A quick recovery is promoted by preventing further infectious complications. The health care provider may order sputum cultures periodically to ensure that there is no secondary infection.

Medication regimens include cough suppressants such as codeine and dextromethorphan (Pertussin), antipyretics (acetaminophen), and bronchodilators (albuterol [Ventolin, Proventil]). Antibiotics such as ampicillin may be ordered to combat or prevent an infectious process.

Nursing Interventions and Patient Teaching

The goal of nursing interventions is to facilitate recovery and prevent secondary infections. Such actions include placing the patient on bed rest to conserve energy, using a vaporizer to add humidity to inhaled air, and increasing fluid intake.

Patient problems and interventions for the patient with acute bronchitis include but are not limited to the following:

Patient Problem	Nursing Interventions
Potential for Infection, related to retained pulmonary secretions	Assess for signs and symptoms of infection: fever, dyspnea, mucopurulent (yellow-green) sputum, and amount of sputum production Administer antipyretics and antibiotics as ordered
Inability to Clear Airway, related to tenacious pulmonary secretions	Assess patient's ability to move secretions; also note any increase in retained pulmonary secretions Facilitate airway clearance by elevating head of bed and liquefying secretions by use of humidifier and adequate fluid intake (3000–4000 mL/day) Suction as needed When offering fluids, avoid dairy products, which tend to produce more tenacious secretions

Instruct the patient in measures that prevent exacerbation or recurrence of infection. Such measures include increasing oral fluid intake, incorporating rest periods between activities, and recognizing the signs that may indicate worsening infection (purulent sputum and increased dyspnea). Emphasize the importance of adhering to the prescribed medication regimen and using analgesics and antipyretics to reduce fever and malaise. Advise the patient to limit exposure to others reduce potential transmission of the infection. Avoid irritants such as smoking or fumes.

Prognosis

The prognosis for acute bronchitis is good.

LEGIONNAIRES' DISEASE

Etiology and Pathophysiology

The causative microorganism of legionnaires' disease is *Legionella pneumophila,* first identified in 1976 when it caused a pneumonia outbreak at a convention of the American Legion in Philadelphia. *L. pneumophila* is a gram-negative bacillus not previously recognized as an agent of human disease. This organism thrives in water reservoirs, such as in air conditioners, humidifiers, and whirlpool spas. It is transmitted through airborne routes. The *Legionella* microbe can progress in two different forms: influenza or legionnaires' disease. The latter characteristically results in life-threatening pneumonia that causes lung consolidation and alveolar necrosis. The disease progresses rapidly (less than 1 week) and can result in respiratory failure, renal failure, bacteremic shock, and ultimately death.

Clinical Manifestations

Clinical manifestations include significantly elevated temperature, headache, nonproductive cough, diarrhea, and general malaise.

Assessment

Collection of subjective data includes noting the patient's complaints of dyspnea, headache, and chest pain on inspiration.

Objective data include many significant signs associated with this infectious process. A significantly elevated temperature (102° to 105°F [38.8° to 40.5°C]) bears close watching and may require immediate interventions. The patient also has a nonproductive cough with difficult and rapid breathing. Auscultation of lungs reveals crackles or wheezes. Because of the high fever and extreme respiratory effort, tachycardia and signs of shock may be present. Hematuria may develop, indicative of renal impairment.

Diagnostic Tests

Urine testing is relatively inexpensive and may be used to confirm the diagnosis. Additional diagnostic tests may include blood, sputum, or pulmonary tissue or fluid cultures (CDC, 2017b).

Medical Management

To control and compensate for impaired and ineffective respiratory function, the patient with legionnaires' disease needs oxygen therapy, possibly even mechanical ventilation. The patient placed on mechanical ventilation requires intubation via the mouth or nose, or directly via a tracheostomy tube. Close observation for disease progression is required. The patient needs adequate IV fluid therapy to maintain hydration and electrolyte status and may require temporary renal dialysis because of acute kidney failure.

Antibiotic agents (erythromycin) are given intravenously early in the disease and then orally for a prolonged period to treat the infection. Rifampin is also beneficial. Antipyretics are administered to reduce the patient's temperature. The patient also may require vasopressors (dopamine or dobutamine) and analgesics to treat shock and promote comfort.

Nursing Interventions and Patient Teaching

Maintain the patient on bed rest, with the head of the bed elevated at least 30 degrees for ease of respiratory effort, and monitor I&O.

Patient problems and interventions for the patient with legionnaires' disease include but are not limited to the following:

Patient Problem	Nursing Interventions
Compromised Blood Flow to Cardiopulmonary or Renal Tissue, related to lack of oxygen	Monitor and report signs and symptoms of impending shock (decreased blood pressure and increased pulse) Administer vasopressor drugs as ordered Maintain hydration status and urinary output Assess changes in level of consciousness Assist with acute hemodialysis if indicated
Inability to Maintain Adequate Breathing Pattern, related to respiratory failure	Assess signs and symptoms of respiratory failure Note respiratory rate, rhythm, and effort Be alert for cyanosis and dyspnea Assist with oxygen therapy or mechanical ventilation as ordered Facilitate optimal ventilation; place patient in semi-Fowler's position if tolerated; suction as needed Have patient cough and deep breathe q 2 hr if able Identify associated factors, such as ineffective airway clearance, pain, and altered level of consciousness

Because of the many alarming actions necessary to treat this disease and its complications, patient and family education is important. Instruct the patient and family on the purpose of respiratory support (oxygen therapy or ventilator assistance) and how to use these procedures for the greatest benefit. Before their implementation, explain all procedures, including the purpose of hemodialysis and why it is required. Stress the importance of controlling the patient's temperature and fluid and electrolyte status. Offer emotional support to the patient and the family as needed.

Prognosis

Usually the disease is self-limiting, but legionnaires' disease can be severe and fatal. The mortality rate is 1 out of 10 patients with the infection (CDC, 2017b).

SEVERE ACUTE RESPIRATORY SYNDROME

Etiology and Pathophysiology

Severe acute respiratory syndrome (SARS) is an infection caused by a coronavirus. The virus spreads by close contact between people, most likely via droplets in the air. It is possible that SARS also may be spread by touching contaminated objects. According to the CDC, there have been no reported cases of SARS since 2004 (CDC, 2013).

Clinical Manifestations

In general, SARS begins with a fever greater than 100.4°F (38°C). Other manifestations may include headache, an overall feeling of discomfort, and muscle aches. Some people also experience mild respiratory symptoms. After 2 to 7 days, SARS patients may develop a dry cough and shortness of breath, difficulty breathing, or hypoxia. About 20% of patients with SARS need intubation and mechanical ventilation (American Lung Association, n.d.e).

Diagnostic Tests

A chest radiograph typically is ordered. In the early stages of SARS, the chest radiograph may be normal. In some patients a chest radiograph may later reveal some interstitial infiltrates that progress to a patchy appearance.

In later stages, a SARS diagnosis can be based on detection of serum antibodies made in response to the SARS coronavirus (SARS-CoV) or positive tissue cultures. Blood specimens for laboratory tests, nasopharyngeal and oropharyngeal swabs, and nasopharyngeal aspirate are obtained. Bronchoalveolar lavage may be used to obtain secretions from the lower respiratory tract. Reverse transcription-polymerase chain reaction tests may be done on serum, stool, and nasal secretions.

Initially, the patient's white blood cell count is normal or low. In about 50% of cases, platelet counts are 50,000 to 150,000/mm^3 (normal range, 150,000 to 400,000/mm^3). Early in the respiratory phase, creatine phosphokinase levels may be as high as 3000 units/L (normal, 5 to 200 units/L) (CDC, 2013).

Additional criteria to establish a diagnosis of SARS include travel within 10 days of symptom onset to an area with current community transmission of SARS—in the recent past, these areas included mainland China (particularly Beijing), Hong Kong, Vietnam, Singapore, Taiwan, and Toronto—or close contact within 10 days of symptom onset with a person suspected of having SARS (CDC, 2013).

Medical Management

Because the disease is severe, treatment is started based on symptoms before the cause of the illness is confirmed. First, people who are suspected of having SARS are placed in respiratory isolation, including use of an appropriate disposable particulate respirator mask to protect other patients and health care workers. Although no definitive treatment exists, antiviral medications (such as ribavirin) and corticosteroids may be given. Antibiotics do not help with SARS (because it is believed to be caused by a virus), but they may be used when the patient also has a bacterial infection.

Nursing Interventions and Patient Teaching

The infection control nurse must notify the local public health department. Respiratory isolation with meticulous hand hygiene is carried out to prevent the spread of SARS. When the patient's respiratory status returns to baseline, he or she is discharged home. The patient can go out in public and return to work 10 days after the fever has resolved and respiratory symptoms are improving or absent (CDC, 2013).

Prognosis

About 80% to 90% of infected people start to recover after 6 to 7 days. However, 10% to 20% develop severe breathing problems and may need mechanical ventilation. The risk of death is higher for this group and appears to be linked to preexisting health conditions. Risk factors associated with poor outcomes include older age (over 65), comorbid conditions such as diabetes, chronic hepatitis B and chronic obstructive pulmonary disease (COPD), atypical symptoms, and renal failure (Medline Plus, 2013).

ANTHRAX

Etiology and Pathophysiology

Anthrax is an infectious disease caused by the spore-forming bacterium *Bacillus anthracis.* In nature, anthrax most commonly infects wild and domestic hoofed animals. It is spread through direct contact with the bacteria and its spores—dormant, encapsulated bacteria that become active when they enter a living host.

In humans, anthrax gains a foothold when spores enter the body via the skin, intestines, or lungs. It is not contagious by person-to-person contact, so treating family members and others in contact with an infected person is not recommended unless they were exposed to the same source of the spores that caused the infection.

Three types of anthrax. Anthrax symptoms depend on the initial site of infection. The three types of anthrax are as follows:

1. *Cutaneous anthrax,* the most common type, occurs after bacteria or spores enter the skin through a cut or abrasion. Within several days of exposure, a pruritic reddened macule or papule develops, followed by vesicle formation. The lesion resembles an insect bite at first, until black eschar (dead, sloughing tissue) appears at the center of the lesion, and the site becomes edematous. Although a patient may develop bacteremia if the organism enters his or her bloodstream, cutaneous anthrax is rarely fatal if it is treated with antibiotics.
2. *Gastrointestinal anthrax,* the least common type, occurs after ingestion of the organism in contaminated, undercooked food. Spores can germinate in the mouth, the esophagus, the stomach, or the small and large intestines, causing ulcers. Inflammation of the gastrointestinal tract can cause nausea, vomiting,

fever, abdominal pain, and diarrhea. Unless treated early, a patient may die from sepsis.

3. *Inhalational anthrax,* seen in global germ warfare, is the most deadly type. It develops when spores are inhaled deeply into the lungs. Immune cells sent to fight the lung infection carry some bacteria back to the lymph system, which spreads the infection to other organs.

Initial symptoms of inhalational anthrax resemble those of the common cold or influenza, except that the patient usually does not develop an increased amount of thin, clear nasal exudate. Subsequent breathing problems may be mistaken for pneumonia, delaying diagnosis. Other severe symptoms, including hemorrhage, tissue necrosis, and lymphedema, are caused by bacterial toxins. Death usually results from blood loss and shock.

Diagnostic Tests

Initial testing for anthrax traditionally begins by ruling out other potential conditions. A chest x-ray helps differentiate inhalational anthrax from pneumonia. A widening mediastinum from lymphadenopathy is characteristic of inhalational anthrax infection; infiltrates characterize pneumonia.

Additional diagnostic tests for anthrax include blood and sputum cultures and lumbar punctures. When managing patients with symptoms consistent with inhalational anthrax, use standard precautions to obtain specimens for a blood smear and culture. A nasal swab is not recommended to diagnose anthrax infection. For a patient suspected of having cutaneous anthrax, obtain a culture specimen from the lesion's vesicular fluid. Obtain a stool specimen for culture if intestinal anthrax is suspected.

Medical Management

Antibiotic treatment is indicated for anyone diagnosed with anthrax or exposed to anthrax spores. For children and adults, ciprofloxacin (Cipro) has been considered the treatment of choice for all three forms of anthrax because of concerns that genetically engineered anthrax strains may resist older antibiotics. Most anthrax strains are susceptible to many other antibiotics, including penicillin and doxycycline (Vibramycin). A 60-day therapy is prescribed. Because of concerns about drug resistance, health experts in the United States have urged health care providers to avoid prescribing antibiotics indiscriminantly because of the danger of antimicrobial resistance (Mayo Clinic, 2017a).

The CDC recommends a 60-day course of therapy to ensure eradication of inactive spores and bacteria. An alternative treatment for postexposure prophylaxis is 30 days of antibiotics and three doses of the anthrax vaccine, if it is available. (The anthrax vaccine currently is not recommended for the general public in the absence of anthrax exposure.) Consult the US Food and Drug Administration (FDA) and CDC websites for prescribing information for children and other treatment updates (CDC, 2017a).

TUBERCULOSIS

Etiology and Pathophysiology

In 1882 Robert Koch identified the tubercle bacillus *(Mycobacterium tuberculosis)* as the causative agent for tuberculosis (TB). TB is a chronic pulmonary and extrapulmonary (outside of the lung) infectious disease acquired by inhalation of a dried droplet nucleus containing a tubercle bacillus, coughed or sneezed into the air by a person whose sputum contains **virulent** (capable of producing disease) tubercle bacilli, and inhaled into the alveolar structure of the lung. It is characterized by stages of early infection (frequently asymptomatic), latency, and a potential for recurrent postprimary disease. It most commonly affects the respiratory system, but other parts of the body such as the gastrointestinal and genitourinary tracts, bones, joints, nervous system, lymph nodes, and skin may become infected (see the Cultural Considerations box).

Cultural Considerations

Tuberculosis

- Tuberculosis (TB) in the United States tends to be a disease of the older population, urban poor, minority groups, and patients with acquired immunodeficiency syndrome. All new admittances to nursing homes require a two-step TB test. Homeless patients admitted to the hospital also require a TB test. A total of 9557 TB cases (a rate of 3.0 cases per 100,000 persons) were reported in the United States in 2015 (CDC, 2016b).
- At all ages the incidence of tuberculosis among nonwhites is at least twice that of whites.
- TB is one of the top 10 causes of death worldwide (WHO, 2018).
- Ending the TB epidemic by 2030 is among the health targets of the newly adopted Sustainable Development Goals (WHO, 2018).
- Six countries account for 60% of the total, with India leading the count, followed by Indonesia, China, Nigeria, Pakistan, and South Africa (WHO, 2018).

It is important to differentiate *infection* with TB from *active disease.* Although infection always precedes the development of active disease, only about 10% of infections progress to active disease. TB infection is characterized by mycobacteria in the tissue of a host who is free of clinical signs and symptoms and who demonstrates the presence of antibodies against mycobacteria. TB disease is manifest as pathologic and functional signs and symptoms indicating destructive activity of mycobacteria in host tissue.

In the lung, pulmonary macrophages ingest TB bacteria. Macrophages engulf the organisms, but do not kill them. Instead they surround them and wall them off in tiny, hard capsules called *tubercles.* Macrophages activate lymphocytes, and within 2 to 10 weeks, activated lymphocytes usually control the initial infection in the lung and nonpulmonary sites. Nonmultiplying tubercle bacilli can survive more than 50 years in human tissue.

Most people who become infected with the TB organism do not progress to the active disease stage. They remain asymptomatic and noninfectious. They have a positive tuberculin skin test, and chest radiographs are negative. These people still retain a lifelong risk of developing reactivation of TB if the immune system is compromised.

A common misconception about TB is that it is transmitted easily. In fact, most people exposed to TB do not become infected. The body's first line of defense, the upper airway, prevents most inhaled TB organisms from ever reaching the lungs. If the inhaled particles are small enough, the organisms can survive in the upper respiratory tract, reach the alveoli, and establish infection. Less commonly, transmission may occur by ingestion or by invasion of the skin or mucous membranes.

TB had been epidemic in the Western world. With the introduction of pharmacologic management in the late 1940s and early 1950s, the prevalence of TB decreased dramatically. TB had been responsible for one-third of the deaths of the young adults in Europe. After Koch's discovery, improvement in living conditions, sanitation, and the development of effective drug therapy and treatment brought about a steady decline in mortality attributable to TB. Shortly after the centennial of Koch's work, eradication of the disease in the United States by the year 2010 was considered a realistic goal.

TB has been particularly prevalent among people infected with human immunodeficiency virus (HIV). The status of the host's immune system is the major determinant for the development of active TB. The disease occurs most often in individuals with incompetent immune systems, such as HIV-infected people, older adults, people receiving immunosuppressive therapy, and the malnourished.

Hospitals are a high-risk setting for TB transmission, and health care workers are at high occupational risk for TB infection. Until recently the vulnerability of hospital workers to TB infection had not been emphasized. This complacency is changing with the wide publicity accompanying the increase in TB (Box 49.5).

Clinical Manifestations

The clinical manifestations are insidious. Generally patients have fever, weight loss, weakness, and a productive cough. Later in the disease, daily recurring fever with chills, night sweats, and hemoptysis is seen.

Assessment

Subjective data include the patient reporting loss of muscle strength and weight loss.

Box 49.5 High-Risk Groups to Screen for Tuberculosis

- People infected with human immunodeficiency virus
- Close contacts (especially children and adolescents) of people with active infectious tuberculosis (TB)
- People with conditions that increase the risk of active TB after infection, such as silicosis, diabetes, chronic renal failure, history of gastrectomy, weight 10% below ideal body weight, prolonged corticosteroid or other immunosuppressive therapy, some hematologic disorders (e.g., leukemia and lymphomas), and other malignancies
- People born in countries with a high prevalence of TB
- Substance abusers, such as alcoholics, intravenous drug users, and cocaine or crack users
- Residents of long-term care facilities, nursing homes, prisons, mental institutions, homeless shelters, and other congregate housing settings
- Medically underserved low-income populations, including racial and ethnic minorities, homeless people, and migrant workers
- Health care workers and others who provide services to any high-risk group

Collection of objective data includes evaluating and recording the amount, color, and characteristics of sputum produced.

Diagnostic Tests

Diagnostic evaluation includes the tuberculin skin test (Mantoux), using purified protein derivative (PPD), to identify people infected with the TB organism. A positive reaction indicates infection 2 to 10 weeks after exposure to the tubercle bacillus. To read the test 48 to 72 hours later, measure and record the subsequent induration (an area of hardened tissue); do not measure the erythema (redness). A negative reaction is less than 5 mm. If the patient is infected with TB (whether active or dormant), lymphocytes recognize the PPD antigen in the skin test and cause a local indurated reaction. Generally, the larger the reaction, the greater the likelihood that the person is infected with the TB organism, unless of course the person has had a false-positive result in the past and does not have an active infection. However, a negative reaction does not rule out infection. An infected person whose immune system has been weakened by disease, drugs, or old age may have a limited or negative reaction. If the test is negative and the health care provider strongly suspects TB, a "second-strength" or two-step tuberculin test can be used. If this test is negative, the patient does not have TB.

Other diagnostic tests used to confirm the diagnosis of pulmonary TB are chest radiograph and evaluation of sputum specimens for mycobacterial organisms. Sputum specimens can be smeared, stained, and screened rapidly for the presence of acid-fast organisms, the definitive test for TB. Mycobacteria are one of the few organisms that are characteristically acid fast. Three positive acid-fast smears constitute a presumptive diagnosis of TB and indicate the need for treatment. The diagnosis of TB is confirmed if tubercle bacilli grow in culture, a process that may take 6 to 8 weeks.

QuantiFERON-TB Gold test. In May 2005 the FDA approved a blood test to aid in the diagnosis of latent TB. This blood test, the QuantiFERON-TB Gold (QFT-G), is more specific for *Mycobacterium* tubercle bacillus than the PPD skin test (WHO, 2011). The advantages of QFT-G are greater specificity and results 24 hours after blood is collected. The PPD skin test requires a 2- to 3-day wait and a return visit to the health care provider. Sputum smears and cultures are still done, but the QFT-G offers a quick and reliable diagnosis for the patient and health care provider.

All patients diagnosed with TB must be reported to the public health personnel for appropriate investigation and follow-up care (WHO, 2018).

Medical Management

Drug therapy is the mainstay of TB treatment. Infectiousness declines rapidly once drug therapy is initiated, even before sputum smears become negative. Cough frequently also declines with drug therapy.

Isolation is indicated for patients with pulmonary TB who have a positive sputum smear or a chest radiograph that strongly suggests current (active) TB. Laryngeal TB also is included in this isolation category. In general, infants and young children with pulmonary TB do not require isolation precautions because they rarely cough and their bronchial secretions contain few acid-fast bacilli (AFB), compared with adults with pulmonary TB. If there is a question of infectiousness in the adult patient with TB, hospitalized patients usually remain in respiratory isolation during their hospital stay.

Compared with most other infectious diseases, treatment for TB is lengthy, typically 6 to 9 months, and sometimes longer for extrapulmonary disease. If treatment is not continued for a long time, some of the TB organisms survive, and the patient is at risk for a relapse.

Treatment now involves multiple drugs to which the organisms are susceptible. If only one drug is given, the mycobacteria may become resistant to it. Treatment usually consists of a combination of at least four drugs, each of which helps prevent the emergence of organisms resistant to the others, thus increasing the therapeutic effectiveness. A series of medications that are often used to treat TB include isoniazid, rifampin, and pyrazinamide. Streptomycin or ethambutol is also used in the regimen. Pyrazinamide is associated with uric acid elevations. Patients prescribed this medication will require both baseline and follow up serum levels of uric acid. Patients having a history of gout may not be eligible to take this medication (Hercine et al., 2017). In the event the disease becomes resistant to the prescribed first line therapy the second-line medications will be implemented. Second-line drugs are ethionamide, *para*-aminosalicylate sodium (PAS), cycloserine, capreomycin, kanamycin, amikacin, levofloxacin, ofloxacin, and ciprofloxacin (Table 49.3).

Table 49.3 Medications for Respiratory Disorders

GENERIC NAME (TRADE NAME)	ACTION	SIDE EFFECTS	NURSING IMPLICATIONS
acetylcysteine	Mucolytic agent; also used as antidote in acetaminophen overdose	Nausea, vomiting, rhinorrhea, mucorrhea, bronchospasm	Store product in refrigerator. Bad taste may be masked by mixing with soft drink when using as antidote.
aminophylline	See entry for theophylline	See entry for theophylline	See entry for theophylline.
azatadine; also available in numerous combination allergy and cold preparations	Antihistamine; blocks allergic response through histamine receptor blockade	Drowsiness, confusion, dry mouth, constipation, urinary retention, blurred vision, increased viscosity of respiratory secretions	Avoid use with alcohol or other CNS depressants. Avoid driving and other hazardous activities.
Short-acting beta$_2$-receptor agonists: albuterol (Proventil, Ventolin), others	Beta$_2$-receptor agonists; cause bronchodilation, smooth muscle relaxation	Common: Anxiety, headache, insomnia, dizziness, restlessness, tachycardia Rare: Cardiac palpitations, angina or chest pain, cardiac dysrhythmias	Use with caution in cardiac disease. Teach patient that paradoxic bronchospasm may occur, and if so to stop drug immediately and call health care provider. Teach proper use of metered dose inhaler to achieve an appropriate therapeutic response.

Continued

Table 49.3 Medications for Respiratory Disorders—cont'd

GENERIC NAME (TRADE NAME)	ACTION	SIDE EFFECTS	NURSING IMPLICATIONS
Long-acting beta$_2$-receptor agonists: salmeterol (Serevent)	Causes bronchodilation; used in prevention of exercise-induced asthma	Tremors, anxiety, insomnia, headache, stimulation, tachycardia, dry mouth, bronchospasm	Avoid use of OTC medications; overstimulation may occur. Use with caution in cardiac disorders, hyperthyroidism, hypertension, and narrow-angle glaucoma.
Corticosteroids: prednisone, methylprednisolone (Medrol), hydrocortisone (Cortef)	Antiinflammatory agents	Short-term: Sodium and water retention, hypokalemia, hyperglycemia, euphoria	Do not discontinue medication abruptly; dosage must be tapered slowly. Have patient carry identification signaling steroid use. Take with food or milk to minimize stomach upset.
fluticasone (Flovent) (inhaled corticosteroid)		Long-term: Osteoporosis, increased susceptibility to infection, poor wound healing, bruising, thinning of skin, Cushingoid weight distribution, cataracts, glaucoma, peptic ulcer disease, myopathy, muscle weakness, suppression of endogenous glucocorticoid production	
epinephrine (Adrenalin, others)	Beta$_1$- and beta$_2$-receptor agonist; causes bronchodilation and cardiac stimulation; alpha$_1$-agonist activity may cause vasoconstriction	Tachycardia, palpitations, angina, chest pain, myocardial infarction, cardiac dysrhythmias, hypertension, restlessness, agitation, anxiety	Use with extreme caution in cardiac disease; do not use in conjunction with OTC cough or cold preparations; do not use discolored preparations.
ethambutol (Myambutol)	Antitubercular agent	Optic neuritis, blurred vision or decreased visual acuity, hyperuricemia, exacerbation of gout, drowsiness, confusion, GI effects, hepatotoxicity, thrombocytopenia	Patient should have baseline visual examination at start of therapy. Emphasize that long-term therapy is required for cure.
isoniazid (INH) (others)	Antitubercular agent	Peripheral neuropathy, hepatotoxicity, SLE-like syndrome, hyperglycemia, bone marrow suppression	Monitor liver function. Emphasize that long-term therapy is required. Instruct patient to report numbness or tingling of extremities.
Leukotriene modifiers; leukotriene receptor antagonists (zafirlukast [Accolate] montelukast [Singulair]); leukotriene synthesis inhibitors (zileuton [Zyflo])	Interferes with the synthesis, or blocks the action, of leukotrienes, causing both bronchodilator and antiinflammatory effects; for long-term treatment of asthma	Zafirlukast: Hepatic dysfunction, systemic eosinophilia, headache, infection, nausea, asthenia (abnormal weakness), abdominal pain Montelukast: Tiredness, fever, abdominal pain, dizziness Zileuton: Headache, abdominal pain, asthenia, dyspepsia	Monitor for eosinophilia, worsening pulmonary symptoms, cardiac complications, and neuropathy. Administer after meals for GI symptoms.
oxymetazoline (Afrin, others)	Vasoconstrictor, used for nasal congestion	Local nasal irritation, dryness, rebound congestion	Do not use for more than 4 consecutive days to minimize rebound congestion.

Table 49.3 **Medications for Respiratory Disorders—cont'd**

GENERIC NAME (TRADE NAME)	ACTION	SIDE EFFECTS	NURSING IMPLICATIONS
para-aminosalicylate sodium (PAS)	Antitubercular agent	Nausea, vomiting, diarrhea, abdominal pain, hypersensitivity reactions, hepatotoxicity, leukopenia, thrombocytopenia	Take with food. Discard if discolored. Use with caution in peptic ulcer disease or congestive heart failure. Emphasize that long-term therapy is required.
Potassium iodide (many; also available in numerous combination preparations)	Expectorant, mucokinetic agent	Hypersensitivity, rash, metallic taste, burning in mouth or throat, GI irritation, headache, parotitis, hyperkalemia	Should not be used by pregnant women. Mix with fruit juice to mask taste.
pyrazinamide (pms-Pyrazinamide)	Antitubercular agent	Hyperuricemia, exacerbation of gout, hepatotoxicity	Monitor liver function tests and serum uric acid levels. Instruct patient not to use alcohol. Emphasize that long-term therapy is required.
rifampin (Rifadin, Rimactane)	Antitubercular agent	Flulike syndrome, hematopoietic reactions, hepatotoxicity, rash, red-orange coloration of body fluids, shortness of breath, heartburn, sore mouth and tongue, dizziness, confusion	Give on empty stomach; emphasize that long-term therapy is required. May accelerate metabolism of other drugs, including theophylline, oral contraceptives, and warfarin. Instruct patient that body fluids may be discolored; may cause permanent staining of soft contact lenses.
rifapentine (Priftin)	Antitubercular agent	Hepatotoxicity, hyperuricemia, neutropenia, pyuria, proteinuria, rash, anemia, leukopenia, arthralgias, nausea, vomiting, dyspepsia, pseudomembranous colitis	Monitor liver function tests and serum uric acid. Monitor WBC count. Tell the patient that rifapentine may produce red-orange discoloration of body tissues or fluids (e.g., skin, teeth, tongue, urine, feces, saliva, sputum, tears, cerebrospinal fluid). Emphasize importance of not missing any doses.
theophylline (aminophylline is a salt of theophylline)	Bronchodilator	Anxiety, restlessness, insomnia, headache, seizures, tachycardia, cardiac dysrhythmias, nausea, epigastric pain, hematemesis, gastroesophageal reflux, tachypnea	Do not crush sustained-release preparations; contents of pellet-containing capsules may be sprinkled over food. Avoid caffeine; use with caution in peptic ulcer disease or cardiac dysrhythmias. Metabolism is affected by other medications (erythromycin, ciprofloxacin, cimetidine, rifampin); monitor serum concentrations.

GI, Gastrointestinal; *OTC,* over-the-counter; *SLE,* systemic lupus erythematosus; *WBC,* white blood cell.

Monitoring patients with TB is critical; failure to complete prescribed medication treatment is a major factor in the emergence of multidrug resistance and treatment failures (American Lung Association, n.d.d). To ensure compliance and to help prevent the development of drug-resistant strains of the tubercle bacillus, in some cases the health care worker may need to watch the patient take the medications; this is referred to as *directly observed therapy*.

Nursing Interventions and Patient Teaching

If TB is suspected, immediately ask permission to place the patient under AFB isolation precautions. These precautions include the use of isolation rooms with negative air pressure so that air flows into, rather than out of, the room. Keep doors and windows closed to maintain airflow control. Room air should be exhausted directly to the outside and not recirculated to other rooms. Also included in AFB isolation precautions is the use of high-efficiency particulate respiration masks (because AFB particles pass through standard masks). Although TB is not transmitted easily, it is transmitted more easily in closed spaces and in areas with poor ventilation and no environmental controls.

Perhaps the simplest, most effective technique for stopping TB at the source is kindly insisting that patients cover their noses and mouths when coughing or sneezing. The CDC recommends the following for coughing:

- *Cover your mouth and nose* with a tissue when you cough or sneeze.
- Put your used tissue in a waste basket.
- If you do not have a tissue, cough or sneeze into your upper sleeve, not your hands.
- Remember to *wash your hands* after coughing or sneezing (CDC, 2016c).

To help the patient comply with the prescribed medication regimen, develop a supportive relationship. Nursing interventions focus on preventing complications and illness transmission.

Patient problems and interventions for the patient with TB include but are not limited to the following:

Patient Problem	Nursing Interventions
Inability to Maintain Adequate Breathing Pattern, related to pulmonary infection process	Monitor breathing for evidence of dyspnea or signs and symptoms of pneumothorax Evaluate degree of respiratory effort and assist as needed Assess expectorated sputum for hemoptysis Help immobile patient to turn, cough, and deep breathe q 2–4 hr to prevent pooling of secretions
Potential for Infection (patient contacts), related to viable M. tuberculosis *in respiratory secretions*	Obtain specimen for culture (incorrect collection and handling may destroy or contaminate specimen, thus interfering with diagnostic results) Employ AFB isolation until antimicrobial therapy is initiated successfully for sputum-positive patients, to prevent transmission of organisms Employ drainage and secretion precautions until wounds from patient with extrapulmonary TB stop draining, to prevent transmission of organism Instruct the patient to cough and sneeze into tissue and properly dispose of it to prevent organism transmission

Teach the patient techniques of proper disposal and handwashing related to coughing and sneezing. These measures decrease the spread of infection. Explain the importance of adhering to the medication regimen as ordered, complying with prolonged treatment (possibly 6 months or longer), and completing the regimen to avoid multidrug-resistant TB strains. Instruct the patient on medication, dosage, frequency, and possible side effects. Emphasize the need to report hemoptysis, dyspnea, vertigo, or chest pain. Remind the patient to maintain adequate fluid and nutritional intake. Patients with TB need follow-up appointments with their health care provider or their county Health Department to ensure that they are indeed taking the medications and to discuss any side effects they may be experiencing.

Prognosis

Active TB requires a long course of drug ingestion—6 to 9 months minimum, and often longer—to stop the disease. The length of treatment leads some patient to become noncompliant with therapy. Numerous drug-resistant TB cases have been reported in HIV-infected people (CDC, 2016a). Between 2000 and 2016, an estimated 53 million lives were saved through TB diagnosis and treatment (WHO, 2018).

PNEUMONIA

Etiology and Pathophysiology

Pneumonia is an inflammatory process of the respiratory bronchioles and the alveolar spaces that is caused by an infection. It also may be caused by oversedation, inadequate ventilation, or aspiration.

Pneumonia can occur in any season but is most common during winter and early spring. People of all ages are susceptible, but pneumonia is more common among infants and older adults. Pneumonia often is caused by aspiration of infected materials into the distal bronchioles and alveoli. High-risk people include those whose normal respiratory defense mechanisms are damaged or altered (those with COPD, influenza, or tracheostomy and those who have recently had anesthesia); people who have a disease affecting the antibody response; people with alcoholism, in whom there is increased danger of aspiration; and people with delayed white blood cell response to infection. Increasingly, nosocomial (hospital-acquired) pneumonia is a cause of morbidity and mortality (see the Health Promotion box).

Pneumonia is a communicable disease; the mode of transmission depends on the infecting organism. Pneumonia is classified according to the offending organism rather than the anatomic location (lobar or bronchial), as was the practice in the past. Pneumonia can be caused by bacteria, viruses, mycoplasma, fungi, and chemicals. Currently, about half of pneumonia cases are caused by bacteria and half by virus. Up to 96% of bacterial pneumonia is caused by four organisms: *Streptococcus pneumoniae* (pneumococcal), hemolytic *Streptococcus* type A, *Staphylococcus aureus,* and *Haemophilus influenzae* type B. Nonbacterial or atypical pneumonia is caused by *Mycoplasma pneumoniae, L. pneumophila* (legionnaires' disease), and *Pneumocystis jiroveci* (formerly *carinii*) pneumonia.

Aspiration pneumonia is frequently called *necrotizing pneumonia* because of the pathologic changes in the lungs. Aspiration pneumonia occurs most commonly as a result of aspiration of vomitus when the patient is in an altered state of consciousness because of a seizure, drugs, alcohol, anesthesia, acute infection, or shock. Aspiration pneumonia may be acquired through foreign body aspiration, such as food or fluids, especially if the person has dysphagia, or may follow aspiration of toxic materials, such as gasoline or kerosene.

The causative agents of bacterial aspiration pneumonia include *S. aureus, Escherichia coli, Klebsiella pneumoniae, Pseudomonas aeruginosa,* and *Proteus* species.

The pathophysiology of pneumonia depends on the causative agent. Bacterial pneumonia is marked by an alveolar suppurative (process of pus formation) exudate with consolidation of infection. Mycoplasmal and viral pneumonia produce interstitial inflammation with no consolidation or exudate. Fungal and mycobacterial pneumonias are marked by patchy distribution that may undergo necrosis with the development of cavities. Aspiration pneumonia is manifest with various physiologic responses depending on the pH of the aspirated substance.

An overview of the pathophysiology is as follows: (1) pulmonary cilia cannot remove accumulating secretions from the respiratory tract; (2) these retained secretions then become infected; (3) inflammation of some part of the respiratory tract develops, leading to a localized edema; and (4) this causes decreased oxygen–carbon dioxide exchange. This process can begin in the bronchi or in the lobe of one lung, and it can become more extensive.

Health Promotion

Pneumonia

- A number of nursing interventions can help prevent the occurrence of, as well as the morbidity associated with, pneumonia.
- Teach the patient to practice good health habits, such as proper diet and hygiene, adequate rest, and regular exercise, to maintain the natural resistance to infecting organisms.
- Encourage the individual at risk for pneumonia (e.g., the chronically ill, older adult) to obtain influenza and pneumococcal vaccines.
- In the hospital, identify the patient at risk and take measures to prevent the development of pneumonia.
- Place the patient with altered consciousness in positions that will prevent or minimize the risk of aspiration (e.g., side lying, upright). Turn and reposition the patient at least every 2 hours to facilitate adequate lung expansion and to discourage pooling of secretions.
- The patient who has difficulty swallowing (e.g., stroke patient) needs assistance in eating, drinking, and taking medication to prevent aspiration.
- The patient who recently has had surgery and others who are immobile need assistance with turning and deep-breathing measures at frequent intervals and use of incentive spirometer.
- Aspiration pneumonia can occur as a result of nasogastric tube feedings. Always check for correct placement and keep the head of the bed elevated to 30 degrees.
- Be careful to avoid overmedication with opioids or sedatives, which can cause a depressed cough reflex and accumulation of fluid in the lungs.
- Before providing food or fluids, ensure the gag reflex has returned to the patient who had local anesthesia to the throat.
- Practice strict medical asepsis and adherence to infection control guidelines to reduce the incidence of nosocomial infections. Health care providers should wash their hands each time before they provide care to a patient. Comply with current Centers for Disease Control and Prevention (CDC) hand hygiene guidelines.
- The CDC (2017c) suggests vaccination with the pneumococcal conjugate vaccine for all babies and children younger than 2 years old, all adults 65 years or older, and people 2 through 64 years old with certain medical conditions. Pneumococcal polysaccharide vaccine is recommended for all adults 65 years or older, people 2 through 64 years old who are at increased risk for disease because of certain medical conditions, and adults 19 through 64 years old who smoke cigarettes.

Lifespan Considerations

Older Adults

Respiratory Disorders

- Signs and symptoms of pneumonia are often atypical in older adults. Fever, cough, and purulent sputum may be absent. Generalized signs and symptoms such as lethargy, disorientation, dyspnea, tachypnea, chills, chest pain, and vomiting, as well as an unexpected exacerbation of coexisting conditions, should be viewed with suspicion because they may indicate pneumonia in the older adult.
- Adequate hydration is important for the older person with pneumonia. It helps liquefy secretions and promotes expectoration.
- Many older adults have difficulty expectorating. This slows resolution of congestion and increases the difficulty of obtaining sputum specimens. Because deep breathing and coughing are difficult, the older person may require suctioning to remove respiratory secretions. Perform this with caution, because too-frequent suctioning can stimulate increased production of secretions.
- Older adults, particularly those living in an institution, should have routine skin tests for tuberculosis. Many older adults were exposed to tuberculosis during their childhood and have positive results on skin tests. These individuals should receive routine chest radiographic studies. Older adults who have a history of inactive tuberculosis should be watched for recurrence of active tuberculosis. Signs and symptoms are often vague and include loss of appetite and weight loss.
- Closely watch older immigrants and immunosuppressed older adults for drug-resistant strains of tuberculosis.
- Provided that there is no serious disease of the respiratory tract, the older person is generally able to maintain adequate ventilation and oxygenation. However, changes of aging do have an effect on respiratory function.
- Drier mucous membranes and decreased number of cilia affect the older individual's ability to humidify inhaled air and trap debris. This increases the risk for inflammation and irritation of the upper respiratory tract.
- Kyphosis and calcification of costal cartilage are common changes. These restrict expansion of the thoracic cavity and lead to a barrel-chested appearance.
- Intercostal muscles and the diaphragm lose elasticity, resulting in a decreased ability to breathe deeply and cough.
- The elasticity of airways and alveoli decreases, alveoli thicken, and pulmonary blood flow decreases, resulting in an increased risk for impaired gas exchange.
- Years of exposure to air pollution, smoke, and mechanical irritants increase the risk for respiratory disease in older adults, particularly those who have emphysema or chronic bronchitis.
- Inactivity and immobility increase the risk of stasis pooling of respiratory secretions. This increases the risk of pneumonia.
- Neurologic damage as a result of strokes, Parkinson's disease, and other conditions is increasingly common in the older adult. Any neurologic disorder that decreases the gag or swallow reflexes increases the risk of aspiration of fluids and food, with resultant trauma to the respiratory tract.
- Cor pulmonale with right-sided heart failure, as well as left-sided heart failure with pulmonary congestion, are common complications of chronic obstructive pulmonary disease in the older adult.

Clinical Manifestations

Many significant signs and symptoms are seen in pneumonia. A productive cough is common; color and consistency of sputum vary depending on the type of pneumonia present. Severe chills, elevated temperature, and increased heart and respiratory rates may accompany the painful, productive cough (see the Lifespan Considerations box).

Clinical manifestations depend on the type of pneumonia:

- *Streptococcal (pneumococcal):* Sudden onset; chest pain; chills; fever; headache; cough; rust-colored sputum; crackles and possibly friction rub; hypoxemia as blood is shunted away from area of consolidation; cyanosis; area of consolidation visible on chest radiograph; sputum culture needed to determine causative agent
- *Staphylococcal:* Many of the same signs as streptococcal; sputum copious and salmon-colored
- *Klebsiella:* Many of the same signs and symptoms as streptococcal; onset more gradual; more bronchopneumonia (inflammation of the terminal bronchioles and alveoli) visible on chest radiograph; if treatment is delayed beyond the second day after onset, the patient becomes critically ill and the mortality rate is high
- *Haemophilus:* Commonly follows upper respiratory tract infection; low-grade fever; croupy cough; malaise; arthralgias; yellow or green sputum
- *Mycoplasmal:* Gradual onset; headache; fever; malaise; chills; cough severe and nonproductive; decreased breath sounds and crackles; chest radiograph clear; white blood cell count normal
- *Viral:* Signs and symptoms generally mild; cold symptoms; headache; anorexia; myalgia (tenderness or pain in muscles); irritating cough that produces mucopurulent or bloody sputum; bronchopneumonic type of infiltration on chest radiograph; white blood cell count usually normal; rise in antibody titers

Assessment

Subjective data include the patient's description of the onset and duration of cough. The patient may complain of fever and night sweats.

Collection of objective data includes checking the level of consciousness and vital signs, especially temperature and respirations, every 2 hours or as ordered. Note the color, consistency, and amount of sputum produced. Inspect the thorax to determine the patient's use of accessory muscles (abdominal or intercostal) in respiratory effort, and note any cyanosis or dyspnea. Perform auscultation; the patient will have crackles on inspiration and possibly a pleural effusion.

Diagnostic Tests

Blood and sputum cultures help identify organisms. Collect sputum for culture and sensitivity before starting antibiotic therapy. Chest radiographic studies reveal changes in density, primarily in the lower lobes. The white blood cell count is normal or even low in viral or mycoplasmal pneumonia, whereas it is elevated in bacterial pneumonia. Leukocytosis is found in the majority of patients with bacterial pneumonia, usually with a white blood cell count greater than $15,000/mm^3$. PFTs may be done to determine whether lung volume is decreased, and ABG values are determined to identify altered gas exchange. Pulse oximetry is ordered to monitor oxygen saturation of arterial blood levels. Oximetry is invaluable for rapid and continuous assessment of oxygen needs.

Medical Management

If pus accumulates in the pleural space **(empyema)**, the health care provider inserts a chest tube for drainage. The health care provider also prescribes oxygen therapy and physiotherapy (chest percussion and postural drainage). Encourage patients to cough and breathe deeply to maximize ventilatory capabilities.

Commonly prescribed medications include antibiotics (penicillin, erythromycin, cephalosporin, and tetracycline), depending on the causative organism and sensitivity. With prompt treatment and correct antibiotic therapy, patients with bacterial or mycoplasma pneumonia usually respond to therapy fairly quickly. Currently, viral pneumonia has no definitive treatment. Analgesics and antipyretics (acetaminophen or aspirin), expectorants, and bronchodilators often are prescribed. Humidification with a humidifier or nebulizer, if secretions are tenacious and copious, is useful. Oxygenation is prescribed if the patient has an oxygen saturation of less than 90% to 92%.

A vaccine is now available for the most common and important bacterial pneumonia, that is, streptococcal (or pneumococcal) pneumonia. The pneumococcal vaccine is indicated primarily for the individual considered at risk who (1) has chronic illnesses such as lung and heart disease and diabetes mellitus, (2) is recovering from a severe illness, (3) is 65 years of age or older, or (4) is in a nursing home or other long-term care facility. This is particularly important because the rate of drug-resistant streptococcal pneumonia is increasing. The vaccine is 50% to 80% effective in preventing pneumococcal disease. The current recommendation is that pneumococcal vaccine is good for the person's lifetime. However, in the immunosuppressed individual or the older adult at risk for development of fatal pneumococcal infection, revaccination should be considered every 5 years. When given in different arms, the influenza vaccine and the pneumococcal vaccine may be administered at the same time.

Nursing Interventions and Patient Teaching

Nursing strategies are aimed at helping the patient conserve energy. Allow rest periods and facilitate optimal air exchange by placing the patient in a high Fowler's position. Place the patient on the side with the "good lung down." This position benefits those with unilateral pulmonary disease, including unilateral pneumonia. In pneumonia and many other pulmonary problems, PaO_2 rises when the healthy lung is dependent (or "good lung down"). When the unimpaired lung is down, this better ventilated lung also is perfused much better. Studies have revealed that hypoxia worsened when patients were placed on their back or side with the affected (sick) lung down.

Assess the patient's ability to move secretions. If the patient is unable to expectorate secretions, assist with appropriate measures (such as coughing, positioning, suctioning, and liquefying secretions). Promptly administer bronchodilators, mucolytics, and expectorants as prescribed to dilate bronchioles and remove secretions. Carefully and frequently auscultate the chest for quality of breath sounds and adventitious sounds. Note cough and sputum characteristics and document. Provide hydration to liquefy secretions and replace fluids. Fluid intake of at least 3 L/day is important in the supportive treatment of pneumonia. If oral intake cannot be maintained, IV administration of fluids and electrolytes may be necessary for the acutely ill patient. Fluid intake must be individualized for patients with heart failure.

An intake of at least 1500 calories/day should be maintained to provide energy for the patient's increased metabolic processes. Small, frequent meals are better tolerated by the dyspneic patient.

Patient problems and interventions for the patient with pneumonia include but are not limited to the following:

Patient Problem	Nursing Interventions
Inability to Maintain Adequate Breathing Pattern, related to inflammatory process and pleuritic pain	Assess ventilation, including breathing rate, rhythm, and depth; chest expansion; and presence of respiratory distress such as dyspnea, shortness of breath, nasal flaring, pursed-lip breathing, or prolonged expiratory phase and use of accessory muscles

Continued

Patient Problem	Nursing Interventions
	Auscultate lungs for crackles, wheezes, and pleural friction rub Identify contributing factors such as airway clearance or obstruction problem or weakness Encourage increased fluid intake to 3 L/day, unless contraindicated, to liquefy secretions for easier expectoration Maintain patient in position that facilitates ventilation (head of bed in semi-Fowler's position or sitting and leaning forward on overbed table)
Inefficient Oxygenation, related to alveolar-capillary membrane changes secondary to inflammation	Assess patient to identify signs (e.g., restlessness, disorientation, and irritability) that may indicate the body's response to altered blood gas states (hypoemia) If necessary and with health care provider consultation, administer oxygen by nasal cannula or Venturi mask to maintain oxygen saturations above 90% Carefully monitor body temperature, which may fluctuate because of alterations in metabolism or infection

Teach the patient and the family about (1) deep-breathing and coughing techniques and the use of an incentive spirometer; (2) the importance of handwashing to prevent the spread of the disease; (3) prescribed medications such as antibiotics, including the purpose, action, dosage, frequency of administration, and side effects; (4) the specific type of pneumonia the patient has, treatment, anticipated response, possible complications, and probable disease duration; (5) the importance of consuming large quantities of fluid; except in the patient with pulmonary edema, congestive heart failure, and/or renal failure; (6) adaptive exercise and rest techniques; and (7) the availability of pneumococcal vaccine. Also inform the patient about changes in health status that must be reported to the health care provider. These include a change in sputum characteristics or color, decreased activity tolerance, fever despite the antibiotics, increasing chest pain, or a feeling that things are not getting better.

Prognosis

Improvement occurs in 48 to 72 hours with appropriate antibiotics in uncomplicated cases (Mayo Clinic, 2013). The disease usually resolves within 2 to 3 weeks with proper treatment. However, pneumonia is the most common cause of death from infectious disease in North America. It is also the major cause of disease and death in critically ill or older adult patients. The number of deaths from pneumonia in the United States is 50,622 (CDC, 2017c). Even with treatment with new antimicrobial agents, pneumonia and influenza still remain the eighth leading cause of death in the United States (CDC, 2017c).

PLEURISY

Etiology and Pathophysiology

Pleurisy is an inflammation of the visceral and parietal pleura. Pleurisy can be caused by either a bacterial or viral infection. The underlying physiologic change is an inflammation of any portion of the pleura. It may occur spontaneously but more frequently is a complication of pneumonia; pulmonary infarctions; viral infections; trauma to the chest, ribs, or intercostal muscles; or early stages of TB or lung tumor.

Clinical Manifestations

One of the first symptoms of pleurisy may be a severe inspiratory pain, often radiating to the shoulder or abdomen of the affected side. The pain is caused by stretching of the inflamed pleura. If pleural effusion develops, pain subsides and fever and dry cough occur. Other signs and symptoms include dyspnea, cough, and elevated temperature.

Assessment

Subjective data include the patient's complaint of chest pain on inspiration. The patient also may report an elevated temperature.

Collection of objective data includes assessment of the inspiratory pain, noting its radiation points. Monitor vital signs, especially temperature, every 2 to 4 hours. Monitor and document respiratory rate and rhythm, including dyspnea. On auscultation of the lungs, a pleural friction rub is heard.

Diagnostic Tests

The presence of a pleural friction rub may be considered diagnostic. Chest radiographic examination is of limited value in diagnosing pleurisy unless pleural effusion is present and fluid accumulates.

Medical Management

The health care provider may inject an anesthetic around the vertebrae to block the intercostal nerves, thus relieving pain. Prescribed medications may include antibiotics (penicillin) to combat the infection and analgesics to decrease pain when the patient takes deep breaths and coughs. Antipyretics (acetaminophen) are used for fever. Oxygen may be administered.

Nursing Interventions and Patient Teaching

Position the patient comfortably on the affected side to splint the chest, and apply heat to the area.

Patient problems and interventions for the patient with pleurisy include but are not limited to the following:

Patient Problem	Nursing Interventions
Discomfort, related to stretching of the pulmonary pleura as a result of fluid accumulation	Assess patient's pain level and need for analgesics; administer as needed, documenting effectiveness Assist with splinting affected side when patient coughs and takes deep breaths
Inefficient Oxygenation, related to pain on inspiration and expiration	Assess patient's level of consciousness, noting any increase in restlessness or disorientation, which may indicate ineffective breathing Auscultate lungs for wheezes, crackles, and pleural friction rub Reposition patient q 2 hr to prevent pooling of secretions and to promote optimal lung expansion Elevate head of bed to facilitate optimal ventilation

Instruct the patient to be alert to signs and symptoms of exacerbation: purulent sputum production, further increase in temperature, and increased pain. Teach the patient to cough effectively every 2 hours and to splint the affected side.

Prognosis

The prognosis is usually excellent. Complications such as atelectasis (collapsed lung caused by airway blockage) or secondary infection such as pneumonia may develop.

PLEURAL EFFUSION/EMPYEMA

Etiology and Pathophysiology

Once the pleural lining is inflamed (as in pleurisy), fluid can accumulate in the pleural space. This accumulation of fluid is known as *pleural effusion*. Pleural effusion is rarely a disease by itself but occurs as a secondary problem when the physiologic pressure in the lungs and pleurae is disturbed. If the fluid becomes infected, it is called *empyema,* which is the accumulation of pus in a body cavity, especially the pleural space.

Pleural effusions happen when the normal flow of pleural fluid through the pleural space is disrupted, often leading to pleural empyema. Empyema may be acute or chronic. In acute empyema the affected area is inflamed with a thin layer of fluid. If this goes untreated, the fluid thickens and the pleura becomes scarred and fibrosed, losing its elasticity.

Clinical Manifestations

Pleural effusion generally is associated with other disease processes, such as pancreatitis, cirrhosis of the liver, pulmonary edema, congestive heart failure, kidney disease, or carcinoma involving altered capillary permeability. Empyema usually is seen as a result of bacterial infection, as in pneumonia, TB, or blunt chest trauma. The patient may have a persistent fever in spite of receiving antibiotics.

Assessment

Subjective data include patient complaints of dyspnea and air hunger. The patient also may report fear and anxiety related to decreased levels of oxygen.

Collection of objective data in pleural effusion and empyema includes assessment of signs and symptoms of respiratory distress, such as nasal flaring, tachypnea, and decreased breath sounds. Assess breath sounds and vital signs, especially temperature, frequently.

Diagnostic Tests

Effusions, or pleural fluid, will be evident on chest radiographic examination. Often a thoracentesis (needle inserted into the pleural space to aspirate excess fluid) is done to obtain a specimen for culture to identify the causative agent and to relieve dyspnea and discomfort.

Medical Management

Usually this condition requires a thoracentesis to remove fluid from the pleural space. A possible danger from this procedure is removing fluid too rapidly; less than 1300 to 1500 mL at one time is recommended.

A chest tube or tubes may be inserted for continuous drainage of fluid, blood, or air from the pleural cavity and for medication instillation. The tubes are sutured in place and covered with a sterile dressing. To prevent the lung from collapsing, a closed drainage system is used, which maintains the lung cavity's normal negative pressure. Under normal conditions, intrapleural pressure is below atmospheric pressure (approximately 4 to 5 cm H_2O below atmospheric pressure during expiration and approximately 8 to 10 cm H_2O below atmospheric pressure during inspiration). If intrapleural pressure becomes equal to atmospheric pressure, the lungs will collapse. The chest tubes and attached closed drainage system restore normal intrapleural pressure and facilitate expansion of the lung.

With this procedure one or, more commonly, two thoracotomy tubes are inserted into the pleural space and are attached to a closed-drainage, water-seal system. One catheter is inserted through a stab wound in the anterior chest wall; this is referred to as the *anterior tube.* It removes air from the pleural space. The second tube, the *posterior tube,* is inserted through a stab wound in the posterior chest. It is primarily for the drainage of serosanguineous fluid or purulent exudate. The posterior (lower) tube may be larger in diameter than the anterior (upper) tube to prevent it from becoming occluded with exudate or clots (Fig. 49.11). Chest tubes connect to a pleural drainage system with a water-seal to reestablish negative pressure in the thoracic cavity.

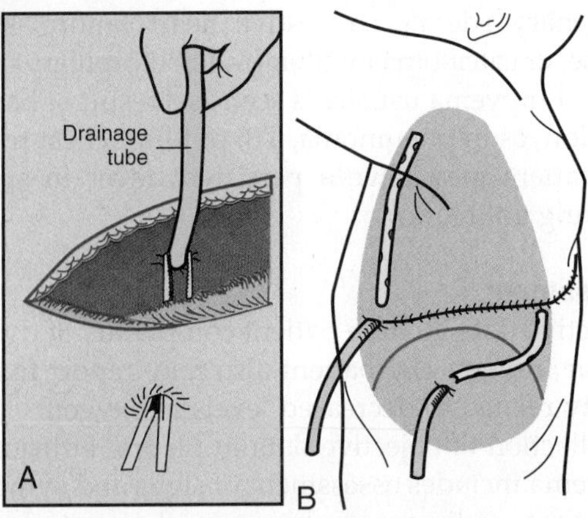

Fig. 49.11 A, Drainage tube inserted into pleural space. B, Note that anterior and posterior tubes are placed well into the pleural space.

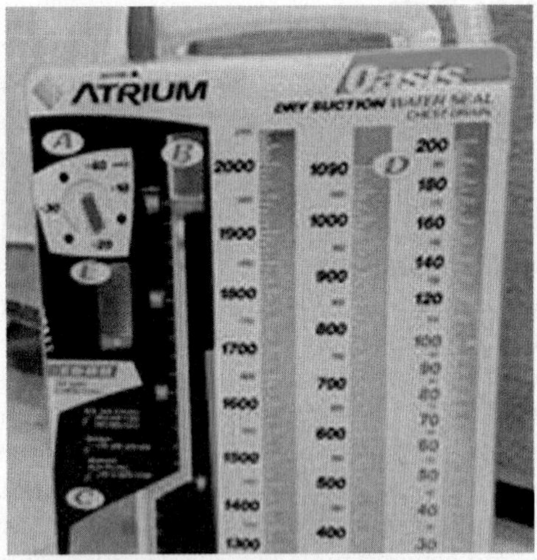

Fig. 49.12 Pleur-Evac, Teleflex's disposable, commercial chest drainage system. (From Potter PA, Perry AG: *Fundamentals of nursing*, ed 7, St. Louis, 2009, Mosby.)

Suction applied to the drainage system may be ordered by the health care provider (Fig. 49.12).

Nursing Interventions and Patient Teaching

General nursing measures include placing the patient on bed rest. If the patient is receiving oxygen therapy, provide frequent oral care to keep mucous membranes moist. Also encourage effective coughing and deep-breathing techniques and respiratory treatments. If the patient has had a thoracentesis, apply a large sterile dressing and assess it for drainage, noting the color and amount.

Ensure that patency of the chest tube system is maintained so that it can drain fluid adequately. Areas of concern are the following:

- *Proper system function:* Ensure that the water in the water-seal chamber fluctuates when suction is applied. There should not be any bubbling in the water seal, because this indicates an air leak.
- *Potential atelectasis resulting from hypoventilation:* Assess for increased dyspnea; check chest radiographic studies frequently to compare degree of lung consolidation.
- *Increased air in the pleural space:* Note any air leaks in the system; ensure tubing is secure and remains patent.
- *Infection:* Note any increase in white blood cells, elevated temperature, and presence of purulent drainage.

A patient with a chest tube in place usually is positioned on the unaffected side to keep the tube from becoming kinked; however, the patient may assume any position of comfort in bed. There is no contraindication to ambulation with a chest tube in place, as long as the water-seal bottle remains below the level of the chest. Never elevate the drainage system to the level of the patient's chest, because this would cause fluid to drain back into the pleural cavity. Facilitate coughing and deep-breathing procedures at least every 2 hours and auscultate breath sounds frequently. Document the amount and characteristics of pleural fluid drainage by marking the drainage level on the container at the end of each shift, along with the date and the hour (Box 49.6). Prevent a chest tube from being removed accidentally by paying careful attention to securing connections and positioning drainage tubes. Be careful to keep tubing as straight as possible and coiled loosely. Do not let the patient lie on it. Tubing never should be placed over the side rails. Administer antibiotic agents as ordered.

Patient problems and interventions for the patient with pleural effusion or empyema include but are not limited to the following:

Patient Problem	Nursing Interventions
Inefficient Oxygenation, related to ineffective breathing pattern	Assess for changes in level of consciousness, such as disorientation, restlessness, or irritability, because these may indicate increasing hypoxia as a result of ineffective breathing Monitor ABGs and pulse oximetry Encourage coughing and deep breathing to remove secretions and facilitate lung expansion Reposition patient q 2 hr to prevent pooling of secretions Assess for atelectasis
Inability to Feed, Dress, and/or Bathe Self	Assess patient's ability to care for self, and assist when needed Encourage increasing activity level when fever is reduced

Explain all procedures before their implementation. Prepare the patient emotionally for chest tube insertion. Teach the patient and the family about this condition

Box 49.6 Guidelines for Care of Patient With Chest Tubes and Water-Seal Drainage

- Keep all tubing as straight as possible and coiled loosely below chest level. Do not let the patient lie on it.
- Keep all connections between chest tubes, drainage tubing, and the drainage collector tight, and apply tape at connections.
- Keep the water-seal and suction control chamber at the appropriate water levels by adding sterile water as needed, because water loss by evaporation may occur.
- Mark the time measurement and the fluid level with a black marker pen on the drainage chamber according to the prescribed orders. Marking intervals may range from every hour to every 8 hours. Any change in the quantity or characteristics of drainage (e.g., clear yellow to serosanguineous) should be reported to the health care provider and recorded. Record output on chart.
- Observe for air bubbling in the water-seal chamber and fluctuations (tidaling). If no tidaling is observed (rising with inspiration and falling with expiration in the spontaneously breathing patient; the opposite occurs during positive-pressure mechanical ventilation), the drainage system is occluded or the lungs are reexpanded. If bubbling increases, there may be an air leak.
- Bubbling in the water seal may occur intermittently. When bubbling is continuous and constant, the source of the air leak may be determined by momentarily clamping the tubing at successively distal points away from the patient until the bubbling ceases. Retaping tubing connections or replacing the drainage apparatus may be necessary to correct the air leak.
- Monitor the patient's clinical status. Take vital signs frequently, auscultate lungs, and observe the chest wall for any abnormal chest movements.
- Never elevate the drainage system to the level of the patient's chest, because this will cause fluid to drain back into the pleural space. Secure the drainage system to the metal drainage stand or racks. Do not empty the drainage chamber unless it is in danger of overflowing.
- Encourage the patient to breathe deeply periodically to facilitate lung expansion, and encourage range-of-motion exercises to the shoulder on the affected side.
- Check the position of the chest drainage system. If it is overturned and the water seal is disrupted, return the system to an upright position and encourage the patient to take a few deep breaths, followed by forced exhalations and cough maneuvers.
- Do not strip or milk chest tubes routinely because this increases pleural pressures.
- If the drainage system breaks, place the distal end of the chest tubing connection in a sterile water container at a 2-cm level as an emergency water seal.
- Chest tubes are not clamped routinely. Clamps with rubber protection are kept at the bedside for special procedures such as changing the chest drainage system and assessment before removal of chest tubes.

and the healing process. Instruct the patient on effective coughing and deep-breathing techniques.

Prognosis

The prognosis is variable, depending on the patient's overall health status.

ATELECTASIS

Etiology and Pathophysiology

Atelectasis (the collapse of alveoli, preventing the respiratory exchange of carbon dioxide and oxygen) occurs from occlusion of air (blockage) to a portion of the lung. Atelectasis is a common postoperative complication from a mucous plug resulting from shallow breathing, which interferes with coughing and effective clearance of secretions. All or part of the lung collapses, usually as a result of **hypoventilation** (the condition in which the amount of air that enters the alveoli and takes part in gas exchange is not adequate for the body's metabolic needs), which then leads to bronchial obstruction caused by mucus accumulation. Accumulation of secretions, a foreign body, or a tenacious plug of mucus may occlude a bronchus completely, closing off all air to a portion of the patient's lung. Atelectasis also can result from obstruction of the airway by aspiration of a foreign body or compression of lung tissue caused by emphysema, pneumothorax, or tumor.

The altered physiology depends on the site and degree of occlusion. If the mainstem bronchus is obstructed, severe ventilatory compromise occurs. When a small bronchiole becomes obstructed, as with secretion accumulation, fewer signs and symptoms are seen, because the respiratory system tries to compensate. However, in either case, atelectasis can lead to stasis pneumonia (because the retained secretions are rich in nutrients for the growth of bacteria) and lung damage.

Clinical Manifestations

The patient displays dyspnea, **tachypnea** (an abnormally rapid rate of breathing), pleural friction rub, restlessness, hypertension, and elevated temperature.

Assessment

Subjective data include patient complaints of severe shortness of breath (dyspnea) requiring much effort, which results in fatigue. The patient also may verbalize a feeling of air hunger and resulting anxiety.

Objective data include decreased breath sounds and crackles on auscultation. Assess vital signs frequently because tachycardia and hypertension are present at first, followed by hypotension and bradycardia. Note respiration rate and amount of effort required for breathing. The patient may exhibit altered levels of consciousness caused by hypoxia.

Diagnostic Tests

Serial chest radiographic studies (repeated radiographic examinations of the same area, done for comparison) demonstrate atelectatic changes. A chest CT scan can detect compression in the airway and also may reveal the underlying pathologic condition contributing to the problem. ABGs reveal a PaO_2 of less than 80 mm Hg initially; this generally improves within the first 24 hours. Pulse oximetry reveals oxygen saturation levels below 90%. $PaCO_2$ is normal or low because of hypoventilation. Bronchoscopy with a flexible fiberoptic bronchoscope may reveal a bronchial obstruction; this procedure also can be used to remove a mucous plug or retained secretions.

Medical Management

Maintenance of ventilation by intubation often is required. Incentive spirometry 10 times every hour while the patient is awake helps provide visual feedback of respiratory effort. Respiratory therapy with oxygen is ordered. Chest physiotherapy with postural drainage is administered. The patient may require suctioning, encouragement to cough, and vigorous respiratory and physical therapy if a mechanical obstruction is present. Prescribed medications may include bronchodilators (e.g., albuterol) to facilitate secretion removal, antibiotics to prevent infection, and mucolytic agents (e.g., acetylcysteine) to reduce the viscosity of secretions. A bronchoscope can be used to remove a thick, tenacious secretion or a mucous plug.

Nursing Interventions and Patient Teaching

Postoperatively, remind patients to cough, breathe deeply, use their incentive spirometer, and change positions every 1 to 2 hours. Effective coughing is essential in mobilizing secretions. If secretions are present in the respiratory passages, deep breathing and use of the incentive spirometer often move them up to stimulate the cough reflex, and then they can be expectorated. Administer analgesics to relieve pain and increase the patient's ability to carry out respiratory exercises and to clear airway passages. Provide emotional support. Encourage early ambulation.

Patient problems and interventions for the patient with atelectasis include but are not limited to the following:

Patient Problem	Nursing Interventions
Inability to Clear Airway, related to inability to clear secretions	Assess patient's ability to move secretions, and assist if needed Encourage use of incentive spirometer 10 times q hr while awake Encourage coughing and deep breathing q 1–2 hr while awake Encourage adequate hydration to liquefy secretions Auscultate breath sounds frequently, documenting and reporting any changes Assess color, consistency, and amount of secretions removed via either coughing or suction
Impaired Coping, related to invasive medical regimen	Assess the patient's ability to comply with the prescribed regimen and to cooperate with caregivers Identify patient's emotional support systems

Instruct the patient on proper techniques for effective coughing, deep breathing, and other measures to facilitate optimal air exchange, such as increasing movement and changing position. Medication teaching should address the rationale and side effects of prescribed medications.

Prognosis

The prognosis depends on the patient's age and any preexisting illness.

PNEUMOTHORAX

Etiology and Pathophysiology

Pneumothorax, like atelectasis, is a collapsed lung; but it is due to a collection of air or other gas in the pleural space, causing the lung to collapse. It can be secondary to a ruptured bleb on the lung surface (as in emphysema) or a severe coughing episode. It can be caused by a penetrating chest injury that punctures the pleural lining, fractured ribs, or injury to the pleura from insertion of a subclavian catheter. A spontaneous pneumothorax also may occur suddenly without any apparent cause (Fig. 49.13).

When the pleural space is penetrated, air enters, thus interrupting the normal negative pressure. Consequently the lung cannot remain fully inflated.

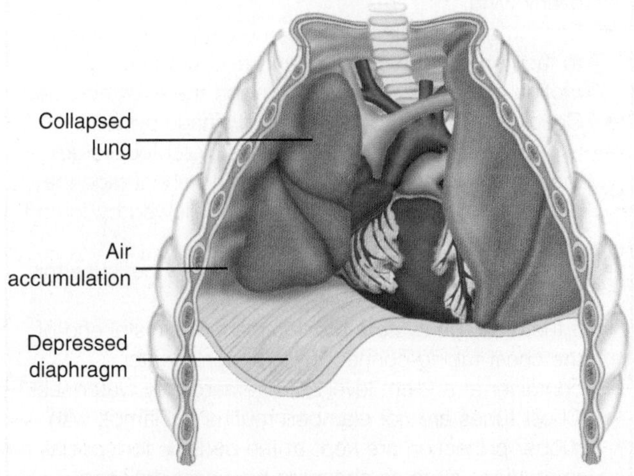

Fig. 49.13 Pneumothorax (complete collapse of the right lung). (From Seidel HM, Ball JW, Dains JE, et al: *Mosby's guide to physical examination*, ed 7, St. Louis, 2011, Mosby.)

Clinical Manifestations

The patient may have had a recent chest injury. He or she will have decreased breath sounds on the affected side and a sudden, sharp, pleuritic chest pain with dyspnea. The patient may be diaphoretic (perspiring) and exhibit an increased heart rate, tachypnea, and dyspnea. Normal chest movements on the affected side cease. With a pneumothorax resulting from penetrating injury, a sucking sound is heard on inspiration.

As intrathoracic pressure increases in the pleural space, the lung collapses. Because lung tissue no longer expands, the mediastinum may shift to the unaffected side (mediastinal shift), which subsequently is compressed. As the intrathoracic pressure increases, cardiac output is altered because of decreased venous return and compression of the great vessels.

Assessment

Collection of subjective data includes reporting a precipitating respiratory condition, such as COPD, a recent penetrating chest injury, or severe coughing episode. The patient may complain of chest pain, shortness of breath of sudden onset, and feelings of anxiety associated with air hunger.

Collection of objective data involves taking frequent vital signs, noting any change in respiratory and cardiac rate and rhythm. A small pneumothorax usually manifests with mild tachycardia and dyspnea. A larger pneumothorax causes respiratory distress, including rapid shallow respirations, air hunger, dyspnea, and oxygen desaturation. Hemoptysis and cough may be present in some cases of pneumothorax, but this is not always present. Findings on auscultation are bilaterally unequal breath sounds, with no breath sounds over the affected area. Note color, characteristics, and amount of sputum.

Diagnostic Tests

Chest radiographic examination shows the presence of pneumothorax. ABGs show a decrease in pH and PaO_2, with an increased $PaCO_2$.

Medical Management

Cutting through the chest wall (a thoracotomy) may be needed, with insertion of a chest tube. The chest tube is inserted in the fifth or sixth intercostal space, under the patient's arm (i.e., at the midaxillary line). The chest tube is attached to a water-seal drainage system (see Figs. 49.11 and 49.12). The patient will require a follow-up chest x-ray to determine correct placement of the chest tube.

Another approach to correcting a pneumothorax is the use of a Heimlich valve, which typically is applied as a stopgap measure until chest tube therapy can be started. The one-way valve attaches to a catheter and is inserted into the chest. As the patient exhales, air and fluid drain through the valve into a plastic bag. When the patient inhales, however, the flexible tubing in the valve collapses, preventing secretions and air from reentering the pleura.

Nursing Interventions and Patient Teaching

General measures include maintaining airway patency and providing adequate oxygenation. Assess and document patency of the chest tube system, keeping it free from kinks. Note the color and amount of drainage and assess integrity of the drainage system. Monitor blood pressure and place the patient in a high Fowler's position to promote airway clearance and lung expansion. Control pain by administering appropriate analgesics, but medications should be avoided if they cause respiratory depression. Demerol (meperidine), Dilaudid (hydromorphone), and acetaminophen with hydrocodone may be avoided.

Patient problems and interventions for the patient with pneumothorax include but are not limited to the following:

Patient Problem	Nursing Interventions
Inability to Maintain Adequate Breathing Pattern, related to nonfunctioning lung	Assess respiratory rate and rhythm, and note any signs of respiratory distress, such as dyspnea, use of accessory muscles, nasal flaring, and anxiety Provide chest tube care, maintaining secure placement Facilitate ventilation by elevating head of bed, and administer oxygen as ordered Suction as needed to remove secretions Encourage adaptive breathing techniques to decrease respiratory effort Encourage rest periods interspersed with activities
Discomfort, related to feeling of air hunger	Assess patient's feelings of fear related to health concerns and feeling of air hunger Identify positive coping methods, and support their use Determine support systems available to patient

Explain the rationale for treatments (oxygen therapy and chest tube drainage) before their implementation. Reinforce effective breathing techniques and the need for ongoing medical care. Instruct the patient to limit exposure to people who may have infections, such as upper respiratory tract infection or influenza. Advise the patient not to smoke but to drink plenty of fluids, to avoid fatigue and strenuous activity, and to report any signs and symptoms of recurrence (e.g., chest pain, difficulty breathing, or fever) to the health care provider.

Prognosis

The lung usually reexpands within several days. The health care provider removes the chest tube when a chest radiograph shows that the lungs are expanded completely. An occlusive dressing is placed over the chest area where the tube was removed, with a gauze pad taped in place to prevent air from reentering the pleural cavity. After removal of the chest tube, check the chest area for drainage and listen for complaints of pain by the patient. Monitor for shortness of breath, which would mean that air is once again entering the chest cavity.

CANCER OF THE LUNG

Etiology and Pathophysiology

The incidence of lung cancer has been increasing steadily over the past 50 years in men and women. In 1987 cancer of the lung surpassed breast cancer to become the number one cancer killer of women. Responsible for 27% of all cancer deaths, lung cancer is now the leading cause of death from cancer in men and women. The American Cancer Society estimates that about 222,500 new cases of lung cancer (116,990 in men and 105,510 in women) and about 155,870 deaths from lung cancer (84,590 in men and 71,280 in women) will occur in 2017 (American Cancer Society, 2017).

Lung tumors may be primary tumors or may result from metastasis anywhere in the body; metastasis from the colon and kidney is common. Metastasis to the lungs may be discovered before the primary lesion is known, and sometimes the location of the primary lesion is not determined during the person's life. The majority of lung tumors are linked to cigarette smoking. A history of smoking, especially for 20 years or more, is considered to be a prime risk factor. The more cigarettes someone smokes each day, the higher the risk. "Passive smoking" (breathing in sidestream smoke) is qualitatively similar to mainstream smoking; involuntary (secondhand) smoking poses a risk for the development of lung cancer in nonsmokers. Occupational exposure, such as to asbestos, radon, and uranium, is also a risk factor. It is suspected that air pollutants may increase risk. Most people who develop the disease are older than 50 years of age.

Many studies suggest the importance of certain antioxidant vitamins, especially vitamins A and E, to reduce the risk of developing lung cancer. Studies report that an increased intake of fruits and vegetables can lower the risk for lung cancer development. Beta-carotene supplements have been shown to raise the risk of lung cancer in smokers. No changes to the rate of risk for nonsmokers has been demonstrated (National Cancer Institute, 2012).

The mortality of people with lung cancer depends primarily on the specific type of cancer and the size of the tumor when detected. Lung cancer is classified by microscopic study of the tumor. Treatment is based on the type and extent of the disease, using two major classifications. Small cell lung cancer (SCLC) (oat cell cancer) constitutes about 10% to 15% of lung cancers. This type of lung cancer tends to spread quickly; non-small lung cancer (NSCLC) is the most common type of lung cancer, comprising 85% of all lung cancers. Squamous cell, adenocarcinoma, and large cell carcinoma make up this group of lung cancer; lung carcinoid tumors make up less than 5% of lung cancers. They also are called neuroendocrine tumors, and they tend to grow slowly and seldom spread (American Cancer Society, 2017).

Clinical Manifestations

Lung cancer is insidious, because it is usually asymptomatic in the early stages. If the lesion is located peripherally, it produces few symptoms and may not be discovered until visualized on a routine chest radiographic examination. If the peripheral lesion perforates the pleural space, pleural effusion and severe pain occur. Central lesions originate from a larger branch of the bronchial tree. These lesions cause obstruction and erosion of the bronchus. Signs and symptoms are cough, hemoptysis, dyspnea, fever, and chills. Auscultation may reveal wheezing on the affected side. Phrenic nerve involvement causes paralysis of the diaphragm.

As the disease progresses, metastasis may occur, along with weight loss, fatigue, decreased stamina, and changes in functional status. Pain is unlikely, unless the tumor is pressing on a nerve or the cancer has spread to the bones. Primary lung tumors usually metastasize to the liver or to nearby structures, such as the esophagus, the pericardium, skeletal bone, and the brain.

Assessment

Subjective data include the patient's complaints of a chronic cough and of hoarseness. The patient also may report weight loss and extreme fatigue. Interview the patient regarding a family history, especially a history of cigarette smoking and of exposure to occupational irritants.

Collection of objective data includes assessing the cough, noting color (especially blood streaks) and consistency of sputum, as well as frequency, duration, and precipitating factors. Also assess the characteristics of the cough (moist, dry, hacking) and effect of body position and identify with the patient what, if anything, helps to relieve the cough. Auscultate the lungs to determine if unilateral wheezing or crackles are present. Invasion of the superior vena cava causes edema of the neck and face and is called *superior vena cava syndrome.*

Diagnostic Tests

Initially, imaging studies such as x-rays and spiral CT scans of the chest are used to identify the location and size of the tumor. MRI may be used along with or instead of spiral CT scans and endobronchial ultrasound. PET may be used to differentiate between malignant and benign lung masses. When the lesion is on the lung periphery, the health care provider can obtain specimens via percutaneous fine-needle aspiration guided by fluoroscopy or CT. Bronchoscopy with biopsy or brushings for cytologic findings indicates the presence of malignant cells (MD Anderson Cancer Center, 2013). A mediastinoscopy may be done to determine whether the tumor has spread to the lymph nodes. A scalene lymph node biopsy also may be done to identify metastasis. In this procedure, lymph node tissue is excised from supraclavicular lymph nodes in the neck, close to the scalene muscles.

Medical Management

The treatment of lung cancer depends on the type and stage. Unfortunately, most patients are not diagnosed early enough for curative surgical intervention. It is estimated that one-third of patients are inoperable when first seen because of the advanced stage of the disease, and that another one-third are found to be inoperable on exploratory thoracotomy. One in twenty patients has only a single tumor; patients with single tumors typically have the best surgical outcomes. The more advanced the stage of lung cancer, the less probable it is that surgery is a viable option (American Cancer Society, n.d.). A pneumonectomy is the most common surgical treatment. This consists of removing the entire lung. Because there is no lung left to require reexpansion, drainage tubes are usually not necessary. The fluid remaining in that area consolidates eventually, which helps prevent a mediastinal shift. A lobectomy is performed when one lobe is involved rather than the entire lung. If only a portion of a lobe of a lung is involved, a segmental resection is done. Lobectomy and segmental resection require chest tube insertion with water-seal drainage to facilitate lung reexpansion (see Figs. 49.11 and 49.12). Video-assisted thoracoscopic surgery allows surgeons to remove tumors through a small keyhole incision in the chest cavity.

Radiation therapy and chemotherapy often are done in conjunction with surgery to enhance recovery for NSCLC. The oral drug gefitinib (Iressa) has been approved as monotherapy in patients with locally advanced or metastatic NSCLC after failure of first-line treatment with platinum-based and docetaxel chemotherapies (see the Home Care Considerations box). In small cell lung carcinoma (SCLC), chemotherapy alone or combined with radiation has replaced surgery as the treatment of choice because, regardless of staging, SCLC is considered to be metastatic at diagnosis. A large percentage of these patients experience remission; in a few cases the remission has been long lasting. At present about one-third of the patients who have surgery experience tumor spread.

Among the promising biologic response modifiers are interferon-alpha, interleukin-2, interleukin-4, tumor necrosis factor, and monoclonal antibodies. The latter are being investigated alone and in combination with radioisotopes, toxins, and standard chemotherapeutic drugs to see if they can identify and destroy cancer cells with specific antigens (American Cancer Society, n.d.).

Home Care Considerations

Lung Cancer

- If the patient with lung cancer smokes, teach her or him that stopping smoking can improve pulmonary function, minimize postoperative complications, decrease the risk of pneumonia, and improve appetite during treatment.
- The patient who has had a surgical resection of the lung with intent to cure should be followed up carefully after discharge for manifestations of metastasis.
- Instruct the patient and the family to contact the health care provider if symptoms such as hemoptysis, dysphagia, chest pain, and hoarseness develop.
- For many individuals who have lung cancer, little can be done to significantly prolong their lives.
- Many people with lung cancer require palliative and hospice care. Encourage the patient and his or her family to adjust their expectations and adapt their goals from controlling disease to improving symptom relief.
- Radiation therapy and chemotherapy can provide palliative relief from distressing symptoms.
- Constant pain usually becomes a major problem, requiring measures to relieve pain.

Nursing Interventions and Patient Teaching

Whether treatment offers comfort or cure, the patient needs comprehensive nursing interventions. From patient education to symptom management to emotional support, nursing care can improve the quality of life and help the patient and the family cope with a frightening diagnosis. Nursing interventions often are directed at postsurgical interventions, including facilitating recovery and preventing complications by promoting effective airway clearance through frequent repositioning, coughing, and deep breathing.

Encourage the use of incentive spirometry. Explain the importance of changing position (to prevent atelectasis) and exercising the legs and feet (to prevent deep vein thrombosis [DVT]). Administer supplemental oxygen and monitor oxygen saturation levels. If a patient has chest tubes to water-seal drainage system, assess for patency, and record the amount, color, and consistency of drainage. Carefully assess lung sounds and record findings. Assess vital signs frequently. After checking routine postoperative vital signs, check the patient every 2 hours until he or she is stable, and then every 4 hours.

Prescribed medications are primarily antineoplastic agents to prevent or reduce tumor growth. Medications are also given for symptomatic relief: opioid analgesics for pain control, antipyretics for fever, and antiemetics for nausea.

Patient problems and interventions for the patient with lung cancer include but are not limited to the following:

Patient Problem	Nursing Interventions
Inability to Clear Airway, related to lung surgery	Facilitate optimal breathing by placing patient in a sitting position Assist with position changes frequently Promote coughing and deep breathing, providing necessary splinting Encourage early ambulation to mobilize secretions Encourage use of an incentive spirometer
Fearfulness, related to cancer, treatment, and prognosis	Monitor changes in communication patterns with others Monitor expression of feelings, such as worthlessness, anxiety, powerlessness, abandonment, or exhaustion Listen and accept expressions of anger without taking it personally Encourage patient to identify problem, redefine the situation, obtain needed information, generate alternatives, and focus on solutions

Teach the patient effective coughing techniques. Instruct the patient and the family regarding nutritional needs and the importance of maintaining physical mobility. If the patient smokes, encourage him or her to quit; encourage family members to stop also. Encourage the patient to eat a diet high in protein and calories. Instruct the patient and the family regarding signs and symptoms that could indicate recurrence of metastasis, such as fatigue, weight loss, increased coughing or hemoptysis, central nervous system changes, and arm or shoulder pain. Identify resources in the community, such as the American Cancer Society and the American Lung Association, that can assist the patient and the family with information, support groups, and equipment needed.

Prognosis

According to the American Lung Association the 5-year survival rate after diagnosis is 17.7% (American Lung Association, n.d.c). For cancers diagnosed while still localized in the lung, the 5-year survival rate raises to 55%. Unfortunately, only about 16% of lung cancer cases are diagnosed at an early stage. For distant tumors (spread to other organs), the 5-year survival rate drops to 4%.

PULMONARY EDEMA

Etiology and Pathophysiology

Pulmonary edema is an accumulation of serous fluid in interstitial lung tissue and alveoli. Some causes include (Mayo Clinic, 2014):

- Coronary artery disease
  - As diseased vessels prevent effective circulation through the heart, blood begins backing up to the lungs. Fluid then begins passing through the capillary walls into the lung tissue and alveoli.
- Cardiomyopathy, resulting in left ventricular failure
  - This decreases the heart's ability to circulate blood throughout the body.
- Rapid administration of IV fluids (packed red blood cells, plasma, or fluids)
- Altered capillary permeability of lungs: inhaled toxins, inflammation (e.g., pneumonia), severe hypoxia, near-drowning
- Pulmonary embolism, result on blockage of circulations through the lungs
- Opioid overdose causing depressed respirations
- Acute pulmonary edema found in patients with sleep apnea can be the initial feature in the diagnosis of sleep apnea

Cardiogenic pulmonary edema usually accompanies underlying cardiac disease in which the failure of the left ventricle causes pooling of fluid, which backs up into the left atrium and into the pulmonary veins and capillaries. The most common cause of pulmonary edema is increased capillary pressure from left ventricular failure. Because the pulmonary capillary pressure exceeds the intravascular pressure, serous fluid is forced rapidly into the alveoli. Fluid rapidly reaches the bronchioles and bronchi, and patients begin to drown in their own secretions. As oxygen decreases, the person shows signs of severe respiratory distress. Pulmonary edema is acute and extensive and may lead to death unless treated immediately.

Clinical Manifestations

The primary signs and symptoms of pulmonary edema are dyspnea and related breathing disturbances. Labored respirations; tachypnea; tachycardia; cyanosis; and, especially, pink (or blood-tinged), frothy sputum are the most obvious signs. The patient also may exhibit restlessness or agitation because of the altered tissue perfusion and resulting hypoxia and respiratory failure.

Assessment

Subjective data include the patient's complaints of severe dyspnea and a feeling of impending death.

Collection of objective data involves assessing for signs of respiratory distress, including nasal flaring and sternal retractions with inspiration; rapid, stertorous respirations; hypertension; tachycardia; restlessness; and disorientation. On auscultation the nurse will most likely hear wheezing and crackles. The patient may have a sudden weight gain because of fluid retention; decreased urinary output as a result of retained fluid in the pulmonary vasculature; and a productive cough of frothy, pink sputum.

Diagnostic Tests

Chest radiographic examination reveals fluid infiltrates, indicating alveolar edema, increased pleural space fluid (pleural effusion), and enlarged heart (cardiomegaly). ABGs are altered, with varying PaO_2 and $PaCO_2$ levels. The patient may have respiratory alkalosis or acidosis. Sputum cultures are done periodically to rule out a bronchopulmonary infection.

Medical Management

The health care provider orders oxygen therapy and may intubate the patient for adequate ventilation support. Medications include diuretics to reduce alveolar and systemic edema by increasing urinary output (furosemide [Lasix]). Patients also are given an opioid analgesic, usually morphine sulfate, to decrease the respiratory rate; lower the anxiety level; reduce venous return; and dilate the pulmonary and systemic blood vessels, thus improving the exchange of gases. IV nitroprusside (Nipride) is a potent vasodilator that improves myocardial contraction and reduces pulmonary congestion. Because of its effects on the vascular system, it is the drug of choice for the patient with pulmonary edema. Medications for the treatment of heart failure are used to address underlying cardiac conditions.

Nursing Interventions and Patient Teaching

An important nursing measure is accurate assessment and documentation to identify changes in the patient's condition. This includes assessment of respiratory status and frequent monitoring of cardiac status, I&O, vital signs, ABGs, pulse oximetry, and electrolyte values. Maintain oxygenation therapy as ordered—commonly delivered by Venturi mask at 40% to 70% concentration. Mechanical ventilation may be required; in this case provide the intubated patient with oral and tracheostomy care according to protocol. Facilitate optimal air exchange by placing the patient in a high Fowler's position. Maintain a patent IV line (saline block) for administering prescribed IV medications. IV fluids usually are withheld to prevent adding even more fluid to the overloaded patient.

Patient problems and interventions for the patient with pulmonary edema include but are not limited to the following:

Patient Problem	Nursing Interventions
Inefficient Oxygenation, related to excess fluid in pulmonary vessels interfering with oxygen diffusion	Be alert for any signs indicating altered ventilation, such as restlessness, irritability, disorientation, or apprehension Monitor ABGs and notify health care provider of any change Frequently monitor vital signs, including cardiac rhythm Administer oxygen therapy as ordered and document patient response Administer diuretics, bronchodilators, morphine sulfate, cardiotonic glycosides, and other medications as ordered
Fluid Volume Overload, related to altered tissue permeability	Assess indicators of patient's fluid volume status, such as breath sounds and skin turgor Monitor I&O accurately Monitor electrolyte values closely, and notify health care provider of alterations Administer diuretics as ordered, and note patient response Weigh patient daily on same scale at same time of day with same amount of bed linen and patient clothing Provide low-sodium diet to prevent excess fluid retention

Teach the patient effective breathing techniques. Inform the patient and the family about actions, side effects, and dosage of prescribed medications. Instruct the patient and the family about a low-sodium diet and refer them to a dietitian for follow-up. Emphasize the signs and symptoms to observe that would indicate an alteration in health, such as a productive cough (noting the color and characteristics of sputum), activity intolerance, or dyspnea.

Prognosis

The prognosis for acute pulmonary edema is guarded; it may lead to death unless treated rapidly. The health care provider normally orders oxygen therapy at a lower dose, 2 to 3 L/minute, via mask. A nasal cannula may be used, if the patient will leave it in place and the oxygen saturation stays above 90%.

PULMONARY EMBOLISM

Etiology and Pathophysiology

The most common pulmonary perfusion abnormality, pulmonary **embolism** (PE), is caused by the passage of a foreign substance (blood clot, fat, air, tumor tissue, or amniotic fluid) into the pulmonary artery or its branches, with resulting obstruction of the blood supply to lung tissue and subsequent collapse. PE usually occurs in patients identified to be at risk, such as those with prior thrombophlebitis; those who have recently had surgery, been pregnant, or given birth; women who are taking contraceptives on a long-term basis; and those with a history of congestive heart failure, obesity, or immobilization from fracture. Immobilization appears to be a key consideration.

Venous stasis, venous wall injury, and increased coagulability of blood cause the formation of a venous thrombus. The thrombus (usually in the deep veins of the lower extremities) dislodges and travels through the venous circulation; it passes through the right side of the heart and enters the pulmonary artery, where it becomes lodged. NOTE: A thrombus that breaks loose and travels elsewhere in the body is referred to as an embolus.

Once an embolus obstructs pulmonary blood flow, a V/Q mismatch develops: an area of lung is ventilated but not perfused (for review, see the description of V/Q scans in the earlier section "Laboratory and Diagnostic Examinations"). The obstruction hinders oxygenation of the blood. Atelectasis develops, and pulmonary vascular resistance increases. Arterial hypoxia is the result.

Clinical Manifestations

The classic signs and symptoms of a PE are dyspnea, hemoptysis, and chest pain. Unfortunately, not all patients have all the classic symptoms. This can make diagnosis difficult. A PE may be manifest by a sudden, sharp, constant, nonradiating, pleuritic chest pain that worsens with inspiration. The impairment of gas exchange may result in the patient experiencing acute dyspnea. The respiratory rate is rapid. In small areas of infarction, presenting signs and symptoms include a small amount of hemoptysis, pleuritic chest pain, elevated temperature, and increased white blood cell count. In large areas of infarction, symptoms include hypoxia, hemoptysis, hypotension, tachycardia, diaphoresis, and tachypnea. Regional bronchoconstriction, atelectasis, and pulmonary edema develop, along with decreased surfactant production. Lung sounds are diminished, and wheezes may be present.

Assessment

Subjective data include the patient's report of dyspnea (presence and degree) and pleuritic chest pain. The patient may complain of a sense of impending doom. Nursing assessment also includes identifying associated risk factors.

Collection of objective data involves assessing for pleuritic pain and noting the nature of the patient's cough. Also assess breath sounds and vital signs, and be alert for tachycardia, hypotension, and tachypnea. Auscultation reveals crackles, decreased breath sounds over the affected area, and a pleural friction rub. In assessing the patient's psychological response, document the presence and degree of anxiety, which often is associated with air hunger. Other objective data may include hemoptysis, elevated temperature, increased white blood cell count, and diaphoresis.

Diagnostic Tests

ABGs are altered significantly, indicating hypoxia. The pH remains normal unless respiratory alkalosis develops early from hyperventilation as respiratory drive diminishes. Respiratory acidosis with hypoxemia often follows.

Initially, the chest radiograph is normal. After 24 hours the radiograph may reveal small infiltrates secondary to atelectasis. Chest radiographic examination also shows an enlarged main pulmonary artery. In most cases of PE, the chest radiograph is normal and is useful only to rule out pulmonary edema or pneumothorax.

A helical (or spiral) CT scan of the lung to visualize the pulmonary vasculature is ordered. This noninvasive scan can be performed in a few seconds and is replacing the V/Q scan, although the V/Q scan still is used in smaller facilities where spiral CT is not available. If the V/Q scan result, that is, the V/Q ratio, is intermediate or low, but the health care provider still suspects a PE based on the patient's signs, symptoms, and risk factors, he or she may order a pulmonary angiogram.

The pulmonary angiogram is considered a leading test for the detection of PE because it provides a direct anatomic view of the pulmonary vessels to assess perfusion defects. ABG analysis is important, as is a D-dimer serum test. D-dimer is a product of fibrin degradation (a change to a less complex form). When a thrombus or embolus is present, plasma D-dimer concentrations are usually greater than 1591 ng/mL. The normal range for D-dimer is 68 to 494 ng/L. If the D-dimer levels are elevated, a venous ultrasound is indicated to look for a DVT. Positive results from venous ultrasound are helpful in diagnosing DVT.

Medical Management

When multiple PEs are present, an umbrella filter may be placed in the inferior vena cava to retain the emboli, preventing their migration to other parts of the body.

The health care provider prescribes anticoagulant therapy, for example, oral warfarin (Coumadin) or subcutaneous low-molecular-weight heparin (enoxaparin sodium [Lovenox]) or dalteparin [Fragmin]), to prevent clot formation. Initially heparin may be administered intravenously by a continuous pump infusion.

Heparin does not dissolve an existing thrombus; its role is to keep it from enlarging and to prevent more thrombi from forming while the body's natural fibrinolytic mechanism lyses (destroys) the existing clot. The effectiveness of heparin is determined by monitoring PTT values, which should be maintained at 1½ to 2 times the control (or normal) values. In the event of overheparinization resulting in profound bleeding, the treatment is IV administration of protamine sulfate.

Heparin therapy is tapered gradually (it may take several days). Oral anticoagulation (warfarin) then is initiated. The patient takes warfarin for up to 1 year. The effectiveness of warfarin therapy is determined by monitoring PT and INR values, with the goal being 1¼ to 1½ times the control (or normal) values. Vitamin K reverses the effects of warfarin. Fresh frozen plasma may be required in cases of severe bleeding.

A massive PE must be dissolved by administering thrombolytics such as the tissue plasminogen activator alteplase (Activase).

Nursing Interventions and Patient Teaching

General nursing interventions include applying antiembolism stockings (e.g., TED [thromboembolism-deterrent] stockings) and elevating the lower extremities. Check peripheral pulses and frequently measure bilateral calf circumference to monitor for occlusion caused by a clot. Slightly elevate the head of the bed, and administer oxygen by mask or nasal cannula to facilitate optimal gas exchange. Promote lung expansion by encouraging the patient to cough and breathe deeply.

Related nursing interventions include assessing for signs of bleeding: epistaxis, hemoptysis, bleeding from gums or rectum, and ecchymosis. Keep the patient adequately hydrated; place the patient on bed rest for the first few days, and gradually increase activity.

Patient problems and interventions for the patient with PE include but are not limited to the following:

Patient Problem	Nursing Interventions
Inefficient Oxygenation, related to alteration in pulmonary vasculature	Assess sensorium and vital signs q 2 hr or as needed, noting any changes indicative of altered oxygenation or ventilation
	Elevate head of bed 30 degrees to improve ventilation
	Administer oxygen as ordered
	Monitor ABGs frequently, reporting any increase or decrease in $PaCO_2$ and PaO_2 of more than 10 mm Hg
Compromised Blood Flow to Tissue, related to risk of prolonged bleeding or hemorrhage secondary to anticoagulation therapy	Monitor vital signs for indicators of profuse bleeding or hemorrhage resulting from anticoagulant therapy: hypotension, tachycardia, and tachypnea
	At least once a shift, check stool, urine, sputum, and vomitus for occult blood, using agency-approved method for testing
	At least once a shift, inspect wounds, oral mucous membranes, any entry site of an invasive procedure, and nares for evidence of bleeding
	To prevent hematoma formation, avoid giving intramuscular injection unless it is unavoidable
	Teach patient the necessity of using sponge-tipped applicators and mouthwash for oral care to minimize the risk of gum bleeding
	Instruct patient to shave with an electric rather than a bladed razor

Medication teaching regarding long-term anticoagulant therapy is a major nursing concern. Patients with recurrent emboli are treated indefinitely; typical anticoagulant therapy continues for at least 3 to 6 months. Oral anticoagulation often becomes a lifelong regimen that bears close monitoring. Assess the patient's present knowledge base and expand on it. Preventive measures are also important, especially in the postoperative period. Teach the patient techniques to reduce venous pooling (which could precipitate thrombophlebitis), such as changing positions and wearing nonrestrictive clothing. Tell the patient to avoid crossing the legs while sitting or lying down and to avoid standing in one place for a prolonged period, because these activities increase venous pooling. Teach the rationale and application procedure for TED hose. Explain that the patient should put them on in the morning before getting out of bed. Instruct the patient and the family about signs and symptoms of PE to report to the health care provider, such as chest pain, dyspnea, and blood-tinged sputum or blood in the urine, which could result from anticoagulant therapy.

Prognosis

Early diagnosis and appropriate treatment reduce mortality to 2% to 8%. Untreated PE carries a 30% mortality rate. It is one of the most common causes of preventable death in hospitalized patients (National Heart, Lung, and Blood Institute, 2011). Although most PEs resolve completely and leave no residual deficits, some patients may be left with chronic pulmonary hypertension.

ACUTE RESPIRATORY DISTRESS SYNDROME

Etiology and Pathophysiology

Acute respiratory distress syndrome (ARDS) is not a disease but a complication that occurs as a result of other disease processes. ARDS has many causes, which result from either a direct or an indirect pulmonary injury. Possible causes include viral or bacterial pneumonia, chest trauma, pulmonary contusion, aspiration, inhalation injury, near-drowning, fat emboli, sepsis, or any type of shock. Drug overdoses, renal failure, and pancreatitis also are known causative factors, as are COPD, neuromuscular defects with Guillain-Barré syndrome, and myasthenia gravis. Among these, sepsis is the most common precursor of ARDS.

Regardless of the cause of ARDS, the body's response follows a similar sequence. The surface of the alveolar capillary membrane is altered, causing increased permeability, which then allows fluid to leak into the interstitial spaces and alveoli. This creates pulmonary edema and hypoxia. The alveoli lose their elasticity and collapse, which causes the blood to be shunted through the impaired alveoli, interfering with oxygen transport. The damaged capillaries allow plasma and red blood cells to leak out, resulting in hemorrhage. ARDS is characterized by pulmonary artery hypertension, which results from vasoconstriction.

Clinical Manifestations

ARDS manifests 12 to 24 hours after injury, resulting in lung tissue damage or hypovolemic shock; 5 to 10 days after sepsis development, the patient experiences respiratory distress with altered breath sounds. There may be altered sensorium as a result of elevated $PaCO_2$ and decreased PaO_2. Additional signs include tachycardia, hypotension, and decreased urinary output.

Assessment

Subjective data include background information and a history of the present illness (obtained from family members, because the patient is usually too ill to give details).

Collection of objective data involves being an astute observer of any change in the patient's condition, no matter how small or gradual. Make an accurate and thorough initial assessment so that such changes are recognized quickly. Initial assessment includes identifying and documenting respiratory rate, rhythm, and effort. Note signs of dyspnea, such as nasal flaring, sternal and subclavicular retractions, or cyanosis. Auscultate the lungs and document the presence of crackles or wheezing. Closely observe vital signs. Frequent assessment of the level of consciousness, with particular attention to increased restlessness or lethargy, is necessary.

Diagnostic Tests

PFTs are done to determine the ease or difficulty with which oxygen crosses the alveolar capillary membrane. ABGs show definitive changes: PaO_2 is decreased (less than 70 mm Hg), $PaCO_2$ is increased (greater than 35 mm Hg), and HCO_3^- is decreased (less than 22 mEq/L). Initially, HCO_3^- increases to buffer the elevated $PaCO_2$ level, thereby maintaining pH in the normal range. The pH is elevated initially but steadily decreases as the patient's condition deteriorates. A chest radiographic examination depicts thickened bronchial margins and possibly diffuse infiltrates.

Medical Management

The medical plan focuses on supportive treatment by maintaining adequate oxygenation and treating the cause: drug overdose, infections, or inhaled toxins. Medications commonly used to treat associated conditions include corticosteroids, antibiotics, vasodilators such as nitroprusside, bronchodilators, mucolytics, and diuretics to treat pulmonary edema, aiding in restoring lung tissue to its normal structure and function. Morphine sulfate commonly is given to sedate restless patients and to decrease the respiratory rate. When the patient is intubated and ventilator dependent, a neurologic blocking agent, such as pancuronium, may be administered to suppress the patient's own respiratory effort, relying instead on controlled ventilator assistance. Positive end-expiratory pressure is the most important ventilator treatment component for the patient with ARDS (Mayo Clinic, 2018a). Other medications may include cardiotonic glycosides (digoxin) to enhance cardiac function.

An experimental treatment involves the administration of nitric oxide gas, which, when inhaled, causes local vasodilation and maximizes perfusion in ventilated areas of the lungs, often significantly improving oxygenation. Nitric oxide usually is administered via a face mask; if the patient is ventilator dependent, however, the ventilator is the mode of delivery.

Nursing Interventions and Patient Teaching

The goal of nursing interventions is to provide adequate oxygenation and ventilation and to treat the multisystem responses caused by ARDS. Nurses must be knowledgeable about mechanical ventilator settings and effects. Care for intubated patients includes suctioning, providing oral care, and assessing for signs of inadequate ventilation. Closely monitor ABGs and pulse oximetry and report any changes.

To improve gas exchange, frequently reposition the patient from side to side, thus preventing one region of the lung from being in a dependent position for prolonged periods (Koenig, 1990). Studies suggest some people with ARDS demonstrate a marked improvement in PaO_2 when turned from the supine to prone position. Not all patients respond to prone positioning (Koenig, 1990). Furthermore, an accurate, ongoing assessment of cardiac function is important. Be alert for and document any rate or rhythm changes. The registered nurse notifies the health care provider of any changes.

Assess vital signs and identify elevated temperatures so that cultures can be obtained to treat infections.

Patient problems and interventions for the patient with ARDS include but are not limited to the following:

Patient Problem	Nursing Interventions
Inefficient Oxygenation, related to tachypnea	Monitor ABGs and report any changes

Patient Problem	Nursing Interventions
	Address any factors that would contribute to restlessness and anxiety because they increase the body's oxygen demand and exacerbate the patient's already serious condition Administer oxygen as ordered, assessing and recording patient response Monitor electrocardiogram (ECG) changes Report any changes in vital signs and any change in patient's response, no matter how small or gradual
Inability to Maintain Adequate Breathing Pattern, related to respiratory distress	Assess respiratory rate, rhythm, and effort, being alert to signs of dyspnea Facilitate optimal ventilation by proper positioning Maintain airway patency by encouraging frequent coughing and deep breathing, if able, or suctioning as needed

Teach the patient effective breathing techniques, emphasizing the importance of frequent position changes, coughing, and deep breathing. If the patient is intubated, explain all procedures before their implementation and explain the importance of working with the ventilator and not trying to breathe independently. Reassure the patient that the ventilator will breathe for him or her and that those breaths will be more effective than his or her own. Explain to the patient and the family the importance of using rest and activity appropriately. Also explain the purpose and side effects of all medications.

Prognosis

ARDS affects an estimated 150,000 to 200,000 people each year. The complications that may arise from the condition include pneumothorax, lung scarring, infections, and blood clots. The disorder is associated with mortality rates of 40% with severe ARDS when trauma is the cause and 55% to 70% when the condition is associated with sepsis.

CHRONIC OBSTRUCTIVE PULMONARY DISEASE

COPD is a progressive and irreversible condition characterized by diminished inspiratory and expiratory capacity of the lungs. It is a chronic respiratory condition that obstructs the flow of air to or from the patient's bronchioles (Fig. 49.14). COPD includes emphysema and chronic bronchitis. These diseases are characterized by chronic airflow limitation.

EMPHYSEMA

Etiology and Pathophysiology

Emphysema symptoms usually develop when the patient is in his or her 40s, with disability increasing by age 50 to 60. This condition is characterized by changes in the alveolar walls and capillaries: thus emphysema is primarily an *alveolar disease* (see Fig. 49.14C).

Emphysema is an abnormal, permanent enlargement of the alveoli distal to the terminal bronchioles, accompanied by destruction of their walls. There is usually an overlap between chronic bronchitis and emphysema. The bronchi, bronchioles, and alveoli become inflamed as a result of chronic irritation. Because of bronchiole lumen narrowing, air becomes trapped in the alveoli during expiration, causing alveolar distention (Fig. 49.15). The alveoli then rupture and scar, losing their elasticity. Oxygen in the arterial blood decreases and carbon dioxide increases.

This process is worsened by cigarette smoking and other inhaled irritants. There is a lag of 30 to 35 years, on average, between taking up smoking and the onset of signs and symptoms. Cigarette smoking is by far the most common cause of emphysema and chronic bronchitis; 90% of COPD cases are caused by smoking, whereas as few as 25% of nonsmokers develop the disorder. This suggests that genetic susceptibility may

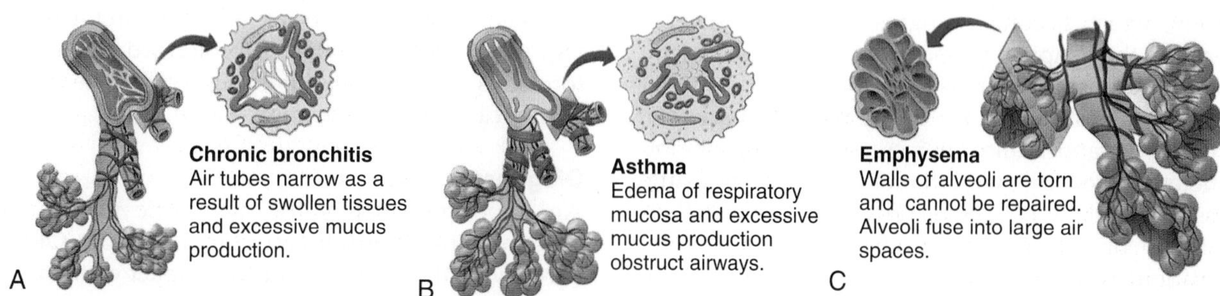
Chronic bronchitis
Air tubes narrow as a result of swollen tissues and excessive mucus production.
A
Asthma
Edema of respiratory mucosa and excessive mucus production obstruct airways.
B
Emphysema
Walls of alveoli are torn and cannot be repaired. Alveoli fuse into large air spaces.
C

Fig. 49.14 Disorders of the airways in patients with chronic bronchitis, asthma, and emphysema. A, *Chronic bronchitis:* Excessive amounts of mucus accumulate in the airways, obstructing airflow and impairing ciliary function. B, *Asthma:* Bronchial smooth muscle constricts in response to irritants, resulting in airflow obstruction and wheezing. C, *Emphysema:* Alveoli become overinflated and destructive changes occur in alveolar walls. (From Lewis SL, Collier IC, Heitkemper MM: *Medical-surgical nursing: Assessment and management of clinical problems,* ed 4, St. Louis, 1996, Mosby.)

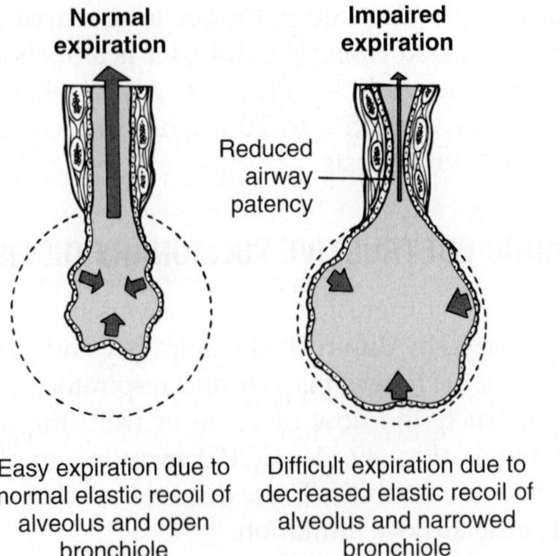

Fig. 49.15 Mechanisms of air trapping in emphysema. Damaged or destroyed alveolar walls no longer support and hold airways open. Alveoli lose their property of passive elastic recoil. Both of these factors contribute to collapse during expiration. (From McCance KL, Huether SE: *Pathophysiology: The biologic basis for disease in adults and children*, ed 5, St. Louis, 2006, Mosby.)

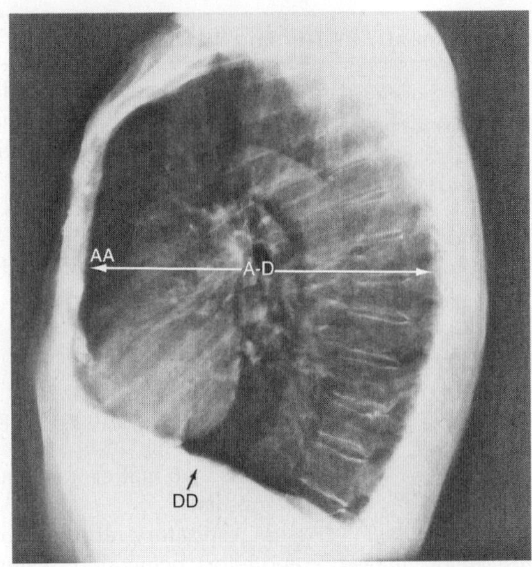

Fig. 49.16 Barrel chest. Hyperinflation is manifested by *AA*, increased anterior air space; *DD*, depressed diaphragm; and *A-D*, increased anteroposterior dimension. (From Heuer AJ, Scanlan CL: *Wilkins' clinical assessment in respiratory care*, ed 8, St. Louis, 2018, Elsevier.)

play a role in the risk for COPD (American Lung Association, n.d.a). Risk factors for emphysema are the same as for chronic bronchitis, with one addition: heredity. An inherited form of emphysema is caused by a deficiency of alpha$_1$-antitrypsin (ATT), a lung-protective protein produced by the liver, which acts predominantly by inhibiting neutrophil elastase in the lungs. ATT deficiency accounts for less than 1% of emphysema in the United States.

The patient with emphysema is disabled because all available energy must be used for breathing. COPD can lead to **cor pulmonale,** an abnormal cardiac condition characterized by hypertrophy of the right ventricle of the heart as a result of hypertension of the pulmonary circulation. Cor pulmonale results in edema in the lower extremities and in the sacral and perineal areas, distended neck veins, and enlargement of the liver with ascites. Cor pulmonale is a late complication of emphysema.

Clinical Manifestations

The primary symptom of emphysema is dyspnea on exertion, which becomes progressively more severe. Over time the dyspnea worsens and becomes present even at rest. Initially there is little sputum production, but later it becomes copious. Many patients assume a barrel-chested appearance (an increased anteroposterior diameter caused by overinflation) and begin using accessory muscles for breathing (Fig. 49.16). Spontaneous pursed-lip breathing and chronic weight loss with emaciation ensue.

Assessment

Subjective data include a history of onset of symptoms. Note the duration and intensity of dyspnea, cough, and sputum production (documenting color and amount). Also determine the patient's reported history of smoking and exposure to inhalants and the family history of respiratory disorders.

Collection of objective data includes assessment of presenting signs, such as tachycardia, tachypnea, orthopnea, peripheral cyanosis, clubbing of fingers, and a barrel chest. The most outstanding feature of clubbing is a lateral and longitudinal curvature of the nails accompanied by soft tissue enlargement, presenting a bulbous (bulb-shaped), shiny appearance. A barrel chest, which occurs late in the disease, is more difficult to distinguish. Have the patient sit so that the health care provider will have a lateral view of the patient; this makes the assessment of a barrel chest easier. Hypoxemia (especially during exercise) may be present, but hypercapnia does not develop until late in the disease. The patient with COPD often begins to exhibit weight loss. The patient is in a hypermetabolic state with increased energy requirements that are due partly to the increased work of breathing. A therapeutic posture for the patient with COPD is the tripod position (leaning forward with the head forward and the arms resting on the patient's legs or a table). Expiration is prolonged as the patient forces his or her breath out through obstructed airways (American Lung Association, n.d.a).

Diagnostic Tests

An important goal of the diagnostic workup is to determine the major disease component of COPD, the severity of the disease, and the impact of the disease on the patient's quality of life. A history and physical examination are extremely important.

PFTs measure total lung capacity, which is decreased with COPD. Residual volume is increased, as are compliance and airway resistance. Ventilatory response is decreased. Pulse oximetry is useful in assessing oxygen saturation in arterial blood.

ABGs usually are assessed in the severe stages and are monitored in hospitalized patients with acute exacerbations. ABGs reveal respiratory acidosis. A chest radiographic examination shows hyperinflation of the lungs, widened intercostal spaces, and flattened diaphragm with increased anteroposterior diameter (barrel chest). Hematologic studies determine whether the patient is positive for AAT deficiency (a deficiency that causes airway abnormalities, resulting in emphysema); this is present in an inherited form of emphysema. CBC reveals elevated erythrocytes and hemoglobin and hematocrit levels (secondary polycythemia, as a compensatory response to chronic hypoxia). This is also a late manifestation of emphysema.

Medical Management

The medical plan includes long-term management with home oxygen therapy and chest physiotherapy as needed. In an acute exacerbation the patient may require mechanical ventilation.

Prescribed medications include bronchodilators such as beta-adrenergic agonists (e.g., short-acting albuterol and long-acting inhaled salmeterol [Serevent]) or theophylline. Anticholinergics such as ipratropium (Atrovent) are also effective bronchodilators. Bronchodilators enlarge the bronchioles for greater oxygenation and ease of secretion clearance, and corticosteroids decrease pulmonary inflammation and obstruction. Corticosteroids usually are prescribed only during an acute exacerbation because of the many side effects seen in long-term steroid therapy. Antibiotics frequently are ordered to reduce the risk of infection related to retained pulmonary secretions. Diuretics assist with fluid removal. Pulmonary therapy can help mobilize secretions and improve oxygenation.

Many health care providers prescribe pulmonary rehabilitation therapy that includes aerobic exercise such as walking. Prescribed exercise training improves aerobic capacity, endurance, and strength; improves and maintains functional performance in everyday life; and reduces breathlessness and fatigue during exertion.

During an acute exacerbation, severe dyspnea can produce considerable anxiety, restlessness, or irritability. Carefully monitor the patient with COPD because of the increased risk for respiratory failure from central nervous system depressants. Careful evaluation for hypoxemia is necessary before a central nervous system depressant is prescribed.

Nursing Interventions and Patient Teaching

Nursing interventions are directed toward decreasing the patient's anxiety and promoting optimal air exchange. Such measures include elevating the head of the bed and administering low-flow oxygen (1 to 2 L by nasal cannula) as ordered. This is extremely important for patients with COPD because a higher flow of oxygen delivery can be dangerous, because it diminishes the responsiveness of the brain's respiratory (regulatory) center, leading to decreased respiratory drive and respiratory failure. Avoid use of respiratory depressants to ensure adequate alveolar ventilation. Assist with chest physiotherapy, which includes percussion, vibration, and postural drainage. All three techniques help loosen secretions to be expectorated; sometimes it takes several hours after chest physiotherapy before the patient can expectorate loosened secretions. Increasing oral intake of fluids liquefies secretions, thus aiding in their removal. In addition, the use of a humidifier enhances this process. Allow sufficient rest periods and assist the patient in activities of daily living to prevent a decrease in oxygen saturation levels.

Assist the patient in maintaining nutritional intake by advising rest for 30 minutes before eating. This conserves energy and decreases dyspnea. The patient with emphysema has a markedly increased need for protein and calories to maintain an adequate nutritional status. A high-protein, high-calorie diet should be divided into five or six small meals a day. Oral fluid intake should be 2 to 3 L/day unless contraindicated (e.g., because of congestive heart failure). Instruct the patient to drink fluids between meals, rather than with meals, to reduce gastric distention and pressure on the diaphragm. Perform frequent oral hygiene to freshen the patient's mouth after coughing exercises and before meals.

Cessation of cigarette smoking in the early stages is probably the most significant factor in slowing the progression of the disease and improving pulmonary function. Use of nicotine replacement therapy or medications to assist with smoking cessation may be required. These therapies should be combined with other modalities such as support groups, education materials, and behavior modification programs.

The patient with COPD should receive an influenza virus vaccine yearly and a pneumococcal revaccination every 5 years.

Patient problems and interventions for the patient with emphysema include but are not limited to the following:

Patient Problem	Nursing Interventions
Inability to Clear Airway, related to narrowed bronchioles	Assess patient's ability to mobilize secretions, intervening as needed Encourage coughing and deep breathing, frequent position changes, and increased oral intake (up to 2–3 L/day) Elevate head of bed; suction as needed Assist with respiratory treatments Auscultate lungs, and report any changes in lung sounds

Continued

Patient Problem	Nursing Interventions
Inability to Tolerate Activity, related to imbalance between oxygen supply and demand, secondary to inefficient work of breathing	Organize care so that periods of activity are interspersed with at least 90 min of undisturbed rest Assist patient with active range-of-motion exercises to build stamina and prevent complications of decreased mobility Monitor patient's respiratory response to activity. Activity intolerance is indicated by excessively increased respiratory rate (e.g., increased more than 10 breaths/min above patient's baseline) and depth, dyspnea, and use of accessory muscles of respiration

Instruct the patient and the family on (1) the importance of not smoking and of reducing exposure to other inhaled irritants, (2) effective breathing techniques (such as pursed-lip breathing), and (3) relaxation exercises for anxiety control. Teach the patient about the dangers of increased oxygen intake for a patient dependent on hypoxic drive (stimulation of respiration by low PaO_2) for ventilation. Also teach the patient and the family how to prevent infection and symptoms that should be reported to the health care provider (see the Home Care Considerations box, the Communication box, and Nursing Care Plan 49.1).

Prognosis

Emphysema is usually irreversible. There are numerous complications associated with the condition. They include right-sided heart failure, frequent pulmonary infections, cardiac arrhythmias, pneumonia, and pneumothorax. COPD is the third leading cause of death in the United States. COPD affects about 16 million Americans with about 120,000 deaths each year (NIH, 2017).

CHRONIC BRONCHITIS

Etiology and Pathophysiology

Chronic bronchitis is characterized by a recurrent or chronic productive cough for a minimum of 3 months/year for at least 2 years. It is caused by physical or chemical irritants and recurrent lung infections. Cigarette smoking is by far the most common cause of chronic bronchitis. Workers exposed to dust, such as coal miners and grain handlers, also are at higher risk. The underlying process is an impairment of cilia, so they can no longer move secretions. Mucous gland hypertrophy causes hypersecretion, altering cilia function (see Fig. 49.14A). Excessive mucus is trapped in edematous airways, obstructing airflow. The lining of the bronchial tubes becomes inflamed and eventually scarred. The patient cannot clear tenacious mucus, and

Home Care Considerations

Chronic Oxygen Therapy at Home

- Improved prognosis has been noted in patients with chronic obstructive pulmonary disease who receive nocturnal or continuous oxygen to treat hypoxemia.
- The longer the continuous daily use of oxygen is maintained, the greater the improvement.
- Periodic reevaluations are necessary for the patient who is using chronic supplemental oxygen in the home.
- Home oxygen systems usually are rented from a company that sends a respiratory therapist or pulmonary nurse specialist to the patient's home.
- The therapist teaches the patient how to use the oxygen system, how to care for it, and how to recognize when the supply is running low and needs to be reordered.
- Post "No smoking" warning signs where they can be seen in the home.
- Do not use electric razors, portable radios, open flames, wool blankets, petroleum-based products, or mineral oils in the area where oxygen is in use.
- Do not allow smoking in the home.

Communication

Mr. O., a 91-year-old, lives at home with his wife of 38 years. He was admitted to the hospital with an acute **exacerbation** (an increase in the seriousness of a disease or disorder as marked by greater intensity in the signs or symptoms) of emphysema. Mr. O. has a 24-year history of emphysema, with progression of signs and symptoms, including exertional dyspnea, expectoration of copious amounts of tenacious mucus, fatigue, and fear of suffocation.

Patient: Will it always be like this? I'm so short of air.

Nurse: Tell me how you are feeling.

Patient: I'm not afraid of dying, but it's the constant struggle to breathe.

Nurse: (gently touches Mr. Oden's arm) Try taking slow, deep breaths.

Patient: Sometimes I can't even get to the bathroom and do my business—much less help my wife with the dishes or even putter in the yard like I enjoy doing.

Nurse: Have you talked with your wife about your feelings?

Patient: I have to be good to my wife. I want to have something left to give her.

Nurse: I think sharing your feelings with your wife is a good thing to do.

Patient: Just having you listen to my concerns has been helpful. I feel like my breathing is getting a little better now.

Nurse: Yes, I can see that. I am going to let you rest now and will check on you soon.

it becomes a medium for bacteria and infection. This increased airway resistance leads to bronchospasm. The condition results in altered oxygen–carbon dioxide exchange, hypoxia (an inadequate, reduced tension of cellular oxygen), and **hypercapnia** (greater

 Nursing Care Plan 49.1 **The Patient With Emphysema**

Mr. O. is a 91-year-old patient admitted with an exacerbation of chronic obstructive pulmonary disease (COPD). His respirations are 32 breaths/min and labored. He has nasal flaring, and his nailbeds are cyanotic. He has a barrel chest and digital clubbing. He states he has a productive cough and "can't get my air." It is noted he expectorates tenacious yellow mucus. He appears anxious during the assessment.

PATIENT PROBLEM

Inability to Clear Airway, related to tenacious secretions and expiratory airflow obstruction

Patient Goals and Expected Outcomes	Nursing Interventions	Evaluation
Patient will maintain patent airway as evidenced by decreased wheezes, tachypnea, dyspnea, and arterial blood gas (ABG) values within limits (for this patient)	Assess lung sounds q 2–4 hr. Encourage turning, coughing, and deep breathing q 2–4 hr. Suction as needed. Explain all medications used in inhalation therapy and assist with treatment. Monitor effectiveness. Ensure hydration: oral intake of 2–3 L/day to liquefy secretions for easier expectoration.	Patient's respiratory status remains within baseline for this patient. Patient has normal breath sounds on auscultation. Patient is able to expectorate sputum without difficulty.

PATIENT PROBLEM

Inability to Maintain Adequate Breathing Pattern, related to decreased lung expansion secondary to chronic airflow limitations

Patient Goals and Expected Outcomes	Nursing Interventions	Evaluation
After treatment intervention, patient's breathing pattern will improve as evidenced by patient maintaining respiratory rate within 5 breaths/min of baseline Patient will demonstrate relaxed appearance	Assess for indicators of respiratory distress (agitation, restlessness, decreased level of consciousness, and use of accessory muscles of respiration). Auscultate breath sounds; report a decrease in breath sounds or an increase in adventitious breath sounds. Instruct patient in the use of pursed-lip breathing, which provides internal stability to the airways and may prevent airway collapse during expiration. Administer bronchodilator therapy as prescribed. Monitor patient's response to prescribed oxygen therapy. Be aware that high concentrations of oxygen can depress the respiratory drive in individuals with chronic carbon dioxide retention. Avoid use of respiratory depressants to ensure adequate alveolar ventilation.	Patient's arterial blood gases are within normal values. Patient has absence of adventitious breath sounds. Patient is sleeping for 5–6 hr without respiratory distress.

CRITICAL THINKING QUESTIONS

1. Mr. O. turns on his call light and states, "I'm unable to get my air." The nurse notes subclavicular retractions and a respiratory rate of 36 breaths/min. His oxygen is flowing at 1 L/min via nasal cannula. What nursing interventions would decrease his dyspnea?
2. While the nurse is performing an assessment on Mr. O., he states, "I'm so tired of fighting to breathe that I wish I could just go to sleep and never wake up." What is an appropriate response?
3. When performing the assessment, the nurse notes the following: temperature is 102°F (38.8°C), pulse rate is 110 bpm, and the respiratory rate is 44 breaths/min. What risk factors are increased as a result of Mr. O.'s COPD?

than normal amounts of carbon dioxide in the blood).

Clinical Manifestations

Primary signs include a productive cough, most pronounced in the mornings (this often is overlooked by cigarette smokers). The patient also has increased dyspnea and use of accessory muscles. A complication of chronic bronchitis is cor pulmonale, which is hypertrophy of the right side of the heart resulting from pulmonary hypertension. Cyanosis develops, often accompanied by right ventricular failure. The patient with chronic bronchitis often has a characteristic reddish blue skin (resulting from chronic hypoxia, which stimulates erythropoiesis, thus resulting in polycythemia, cyanosis, and dependent edema).

Assessment

Subjective data include a detailed history of smoking or exposure to irritants and family history of respiratory disorders. Also determine the patient's current medication and treatment regimen.

Collection of objective data includes assessing the patient's productive cough, noting characteristics and amount of sputum. Assess the severity of dyspnea and presence of wheezing, and note the patient's level of restlessness. Obtain vital signs. Assess degree of tachycardia and tachypnea. Record any temperature elevation.

Diagnostic Tests

Chest radiographs taken early in the disease may not show abnormalities; later in the disease they will. An ECG may be normal or show signs indicative of right ventricular failure. An echocardiogram can be used to evaluate right and left ventricular function.

A CBC shows increased erythrocytes, hemoglobin, hematocrit, and white blood cell count. Polycythemia develops as a result of increased production of red blood cells as the body attempts to compensate for chronic hypoxemia. Hemoglobin concentrations may reach 20 g/dL or more. ABG values reveal respiratory acidosis, hypoxia, and hypercapnia. Pulse oximetry is valuable to assess oxygen saturation levels in arterial blood. PFTs reveal airflow limitation on expiration, increased airway resistance and residual volume, and often electrolyte abnormalities. Monitor oximetry levels on all patients with hypoxia.

Medical Management

The medical plan is aimed at slowing the disease progression and facilitating optimal air exchange by reducing spasms and secretions.

Three main classes of bronchodilators typically are used to treat COPD. To reverse bronchospasm, the health care provider may order beta-adrenergic agonists such as short-acting albuterol and long-acting salmeterol. Both theophylline as well as anticholinergic medications such as ipratropium are effective bronchodilators. Corticosteroids are helpful in reducing airway inflammation. Long-term use of systemic steroids can lead to many adverse reactions, including osteoporosis, diabetes, and eye problems. Inhaled steroids have fewer systemic effects and are preferred. Mucolytics such as guaifenesin to break up tenacious mucus may be helpful. Antibiotic agents (erythromycin) are commonly ordered.

Nursing Interventions and Patient Teaching

Provide adequate hydration to liquefy secretions and aid in their removal. Suction the patient as needed, and provide low-flow oxygen to maintain SaO_2 above 90%. Offer frequent oral hygiene and provide rest periods. The nutritional needs are similar to those of the patient with emphysema.

Patient problems and interventions for the patient with chronic bronchitis include but are not limited to the following:

Patient Problem	Nursing Interventions
Inability to Maintain Adequate Breathing Pattern, related to retained pulmonary secretions	Assess degree of dyspnea, noting nasal flaring, sternal retractions, and pursed-lip breathing Instruct on effective breathing techniques Suction as needed
Lethargy or Malaise, related to increased respiratory effort	Assess degree of fatigue, and use problem-solving techniques with patient to explore ways to decrease fatigue Provide treatments in calm, unhurried manner Identify support systems and provide referrals if needed Encourage adequate periods of rest

Teach the patient effective breathing techniques, and instruct the patient and the family on avoidance of infection exposure. Instruct the patient to notify the health care provider at the first sign of a respiratory infection. Usually the best indication of such an infection is a change in the color, consistency, or amount of sputum. Provide medication teaching, including action, rationale, and side effects. Stress the importance of increasing fluid intake, unless contraindicated. Encourage the patient and the family not to smoke. Provide information concerning smoking cessation programs.

Prognosis

Chronic bronchitis is usually irreversible. COPD is the fourth leading cause of death in the United States. The chronic nature of the condition often leads to debilitating damage to the lung tissues and impacts the overall quality of life.

ASTHMA

Etiology and Pathophysiology

Asthma is a broad clinical syndrome and an airway pathologic condition. It involves episodic increased tracheal and bronchial responsiveness to various stimuli, resulting in widespread narrowing of the airways. Asthma usually improves either spontaneously or with treatment. It is classified as extrinsic or intrinsic. **Extrinsic** means it is caused by external factors, such as environmental allergens (e.g., pollen, dust, feathers, animal dander, foods); **intrinsic** asthma is from internal causes, not fully understood but often triggered by respiratory tract infection. Recurrence of attacks is influenced strongly by secondary factors, by mental or physical fatigue, and by emotional factors.

Asthma can result from an altered immune response or increased airway resistance and altered air exchange. Gastroesophageal reflux disease (GERD) can trigger an asthma attack (Mayo Clinic, 2017b). The actual course of GERD resulting in an asthma attack is unknown, but it is assumed that the gastric acid reflux in the esophagus is aspirated into the lungs, resulting in vagal stimulation and bronchoconstriction (Dartmouth-Hitchcock Norris Cotton Cancer Center, 2013). An acute asthma attack may be caused by an antigen-antibody reaction in which histamine is released. There are three mechanisms involved (see Fig. 49.14B):

- Recurrent, reversible obstruction of airflow in the bronchioles and smaller bronchi secondary to bronchospasm. The muscles around the bronchioles tighten and narrow the air passages.
- Increased capillary permeability resulting in edema of mucous membranes with increased narrowing of airways and increased mucus secretion.
- An acute inflammatory response by mast cells in the lungs, caused by exposure to an asthma trigger. These cells release histamine and other inflammatory agents. Systemic immune system cells release substances that cause circulating inflammatory cells to migrate to the lungs.

Clinical Manifestations

Mild asthma is manifested by dyspnea on exertion and wheezing. Symptoms usually are controlled by medications. An acute asthma attack usually occurs at night and includes tachypnea, tachycardia, diaphoresis, chest tightness, cough, expiratory wheezing, use of accessory muscles, and nasal flaring. The wheezing sound characteristic of asthma is caused by air forcing its way through the narrowed bronchioles and by vibrating mucus. The patient also has increased anxiety; diaphoresis; and a productive cough of copious, thick mucus. Asthma can be triggered by external factors (e.g., dust, mold, or lint) or precipitated intrinsically by a respiratory tract infection or exercise.

Status asthmaticus is a severe, unrelenting, life-threatening attack that fails to respond to usual treatment and places the patient at risk for respiratory failure. Symptoms of an acute attack are present, and the trapped air leads to exhaustion and ultimately respiratory failure.

Assessment

Subjective data include complaints of anxiety, fear of suffocation, breathlessness, chest tightness, and cough, particularly at night and in the early morning (National Heart, Lung, and Blood Institute, 2012).

Collection of objective data includes assessing for signs of hypoxia, which may include restlessness, inappropriate behavior, increased pulse and blood pressure, and tachypnea. The patient may assume a "hunched forward" position to get more air. Auscultate the lungs for inspiratory and expiratory wheezing as well as expectoration of mucus.

Diagnostic Tests

Pulmonary function tests are performed to assess respiratory capacity. The spirometry test is performed to assess the amount of air that is exhaled during the expiratory phase of the respiratory process. Peak flow testing is used to determine the force exerted by the lungs with breathing. Normal values for these tests vary, depending on the patient's age, weight, and sex. In an acute asthma episode the patient cannot perform a complete pulmonary function study, but the nurse can check the peak expiratory flow rate. ABGs may be ordered during an acute exacerbation of asthma. Pulse oximetry is used to monitor the patient's SaO_2.

Obtain a sputum culture from the patient to rule out any secondary infection. CBC and differential reveal an increased eosinophil count, which is indicative of an allergic response. If the patient has been taking theophylline, draw a blood sample to determine whether the prescribed dosage is maintained at a therapeutic level; the acceptable therapeutic range is 10 to 20 mcg/mL. This also reduces the risk of complications as a result of toxicity.

Medical Management

Medication management of asthma can be placed in two categories: maintenance therapy and acute (or rescue) therapy. *Maintenance therapy* prevents and minimizes symptoms; the medications are taken on a regular basis. These include the long-acting $beta_2$-agonist salmeterol and formoterol (Foradil), which are used prophylactically only; inhaled corticosteroids, such as fluticasone; cromolyn; and theophylline. A combination of fluticasone and salmeterol (Advair Diskus) sometimes is prescribed also.

A group of drugs called *leukotriene modifiers* is now available for the prophylaxis and chronic treatment of asthma. Leukotrienes are chemicals present in the body that are powerful bronchoconstrictors and vasodilators; some also cause airway edema and inflammation, thus contributing to the symptoms of asthma. The two types of leukotriene modifiers are leukotriene receptor antagonists (zafirlukast, montelukast) and leukotriene synthesis inhibitors (zileuton [Zyflo]). These drugs interfere with the synthesis, or block the action, of leukotrienes. A major advantage is that they have bronchodilator and antiinflammatory effects. These drugs are not recommended as the only treatment for persistent asthma. A broad range of patients, with mild to severe asthma, can benefit from leukotriene modifiers. Leukotriene modifiers are not indicated for use in the reversal of bronchospasms in acute asthma attacks. They are indicated for the chronic treatment of asthma (see Table 49.3).

Acute (or *rescue*) *therapy* works immediately to relieve the symptoms of an asthma attack. The drugs involved include short-acting inhaled $beta_2$-agonist albuterol and pirbuterol taken by means of a metered dose inhaler using spacer devices or by a nebulizer; oral or IV corticosteroids; and epinephrine. One study has shown that inhaled corticosteroids, given with short-acting $beta_2$-agonists, may be better and faster than IV corticosteroids at treating an acute exacerbation (National Heart, Lung, and Blood Institute, 2012). Short-acting beta$_2$-agonists quickly relax the muscles around the airway and are the most effective drugs for relieving acute bronchospasms (see Table 49.3). Epinephrine, given subcutaneously or intramuscularly, may be considered in an emergency when symptoms have not been relieved by the use of a beta$_2$-agonist. Epinephrine acts as a bronchodilator. Although the value of administering aminophylline in the treatment of acute asthma has been questioned, IV aminophylline may be considered if the asthma is severe or there is minimal or no response to short-acting inhaled beta$_2$-agonists.

In acute asthma, oxygen therapy should be started immediately and its administration monitored by pulse oximetry and, in severe cases, by measurement of ABGs.

Using a peak flowmeter can help the patient manage asthma. This device measures the peak expiratory flow rate—the flow of air in a forced exhalation in liters per minute, which is a good indicator of lung function. Peak flow monitoring measures how well air moves out of the lungs when blown out as hard and fast as possible. Peak flow measurement can help the patient detect early signs of asthma episodes before symptoms occur. Normal peak flow is 80% to 100% of the value predicted for the patient based on height, weight, age, and sex. Severe, persistent asthma is characterized by a peak flow of less than 60% of the predicted value. A severe, life-threatening exacerbation of asthma is characterized by a peak flow of less than 50% of the patient's predicted value.

Once the acute event is over, the medical plan includes identifying precipitating factors and promoting optimal health. Elimination of allergens or countermeasures, such as desensitization or hyposensitization, are desirable.

Nursing Interventions and Patient Teaching

Nursing interventions include administering prescribed medications and ensuring adequate fluid intake and optimal ventilation. To accomplish these goals, incorporate rest periods into activities and interventions; elevate the head of the bed; teach effective breathing techniques, such as pursed-lip breathing and correct use of the peak flowmeter; and provide oxygen therapy as ordered. Monitor vital signs and electrolytes. Kind and empathic emotional support is vital.

Patient problems and interventions for the patient with asthma include but are not limited to the following:

Patient Problem	Nursing Interventions
Inability to Maintain Adequate Breathing Pattern, related to narrowed airway	Assess ventilation, and be alert for signs of increasing dyspnea, such as using accessory muscles, nasal flaring, pursed-lip breathing, or prolonged expiration Maintain position to facilitate ventilation Administer prescribed medications Assist with administration of respiratory treatments Provide care in calm, unhurried manner Attempt to minimize exposure to dust and other irritants by maintaining clean environment and use of humidifier Maintain adequate hydration
Impaired Health Maintenance, related to possible allergens in the home	Implement mutual problem solving to explore with patient and family what stimulants may be in home environment, such as allergens Facilitate allergy testing if needed Teach the patient and the family importance of avoiding exposure to known irritants

Educate the patient and the family to identify signs and symptoms and recognize asthma "triggers" and avoid them or lessen their effects to prevent recurrent attacks. Instruct the patient on relaxation techniques to manage anxiety. Stress the importance of health maintenance measures, such as adequate fluid intake and effective breathing techniques. Teach the patient to take prescribed medications correctly and on time, to monitor peak flowmeter results to recognize the early signs of an asthma attack and begin treatment immediately, and to follow the program treatment steps during an attack. The goal is to provide good control of symptoms with the least possible medication.

Prognosis

The diagnosis of asthma can have a profound impact on the patient's quality of life. Some patients are unable to participate in activities they enjoy. Sleep may be impaired by the presentation of nighttime attacks. There can be permanent damage to the lungs as well as a nagging and persistent cough. Ongoing breathing problems can require the use of breathing machines. Although the incidence of asthma has increased steadily, the mortality and morbidity rates currently are decreasing. Current statistics from the CDC indicate 3518 deaths per year from asthma (CDC, 2018), which is disheartening, because treatment and education can reduce or eliminate asthma attacks. If status asthmaticus is not reversed, death will ensue.

BRONCHIECTASIS

Etiology and Pathophysiology

Bronchiectasis is a disease characterized by abnormal permanent dilation of one or more large bronchi. This dilation eventually destroys muscular elements and bronchial elastic fibers that support the bronchial wall. Pulmonary muscle tone is lost gradually after one or, more often, repeated pulmonary infections in children and adults. Because of the disease, it is much more difficult to clear mucus from the lungs, and the lungs experience decreased expiratory airflow.

This condition is usually secondary to failure of normal lung tissue defenses (as caused by cystic fibrosis, foreign body, or tumor). It occurs as a complication of a recurrent inflammation and infection process that gradually alters the pulmonary structures.

Clinical Manifestations

Signs and symptoms occur after a respiratory tract infection. The late signs and symptoms usually seen are dyspnea, cyanosis, and clubbing of fingers. The patient has paroxysms of coughing when arising in the morning and when lying down. This severe coughing produces copious amounts of foul-smelling sputum. Fatigue, weakness, and a loss of appetite also are noted.

Assessment

Subjective data include the patient's report of difficulty breathing, weight loss, and fever.

Objective data include fine crackles and wheezes in the lower lobes on auscultation. The patient exhibits a prolonged expiratory phase and increased dyspnea. Hemoptysis is seen in 50% of the patients.

Diagnostic Tests

Chest radiographic examination is essentially normal, but inflammation and mediastinal shift may result from overinflation of specific lobes. High-resolution CT scan of the chest is the gold standard for diagnosing bronchiectasis. Sputum cultures can rule out a bacterial infection. PFTs show a decreased forced expiratory volume.

Medical Management

Medical management of bronchiectasis involves treatment of exacerbations with antibiotics, bronchodilators, and expectorants. A sputum culture is preferable before treatment with antibiotics, but if a culture is not obtainable, an antibiotic is still prescribed (American Lung Association, n.d.b).

Oxygen may be ordered at low-flow volume. Hydration and chest physiotherapy also are included in the plan of care. If a patient does not respond to more conservative treatment modalities, he or she may benefit from a lobectomy.

Nursing Interventions and Patient Teaching

General nursing interventions include using a cool mist vaporizer to provide humidity and increasing oral intake of fluids to aid in secretion removal. Assess vital signs and lung sounds every 2 to 4 hours. Suction the patient as needed and provide assistance in turning, coughing, and deep breathing every 2 hours. Assist with chest physiotherapy.

Patient problems and interventions for the patient with bronchiectasis include but are not limited to the following:

Patient Problem	Nursing Interventions
Inability to Clear Airway, related to retained pulmonary secretions	Assess patient's ability to mobilize secretions, assisting as needed Encourage postural drainage and coughing; suction if needed Encourage frequent position changes to facilitate secretion mobility and removal Maintain adequate hydration Administer mucolytic agents as ordered, and note patient response
Compromised Physical Mobility, related to decreased exercise tolerance	Assess patient's activity tolerance, and promote adaptive techniques, such as incorporating rest periods into activities Promote a gradual increase in activity, noting patient tolerance Problem solve with patient and family to identify methods of energy conservation and ways to integrate them into lifestyle

Teach the patient and the family environmental awareness (avoidance of smoke, fumes, and irritating inhalants). Discourage smoking, and advise the patient on appropriate rest and exercise practices. Perform medication teaching, including dosage, rationale, and side effects. Instruct the patient and the family about signs and symptoms of a secondary infection, and make sure the patient knows how to reach the health care provider after discharge.

Prognosis

Bronchiectasis is a chronic disease. Surgical removal of a portion of the patient's lung is the only cure. Complications may include cor pulmonale, hypoxia, and recurrent respiratory infections.

NURSING PROCESS FOR THE PATIENT WITH A RESPIRATORY DISORDER

The role of the licensed practical nurse/licensed vocational nurse (LPN/LVN) in the nursing process as stated is that the LPN/LVN will:

- Participate in planning care for patients based on patient needs
- Review patient's care plan and recommend revisions as needed

- Review and follow defined prioritization for patient care
- Use clinical pathways, care maps, or care plans to guide and review patient care

◆ ASSESSMENT

When a patient is admitted with a respiratory disorder, a thorough, immediate, and accurate nursing assessment is an essential first step. The assessment should include the patient's level of consciousness, vital signs, lung sounds (crackles, wheezes, pleural friction rub), and oximetry level. Ask if the patient has shortness of breath, dyspnea on exertion, or cough. If the patient has a cough, ask whether it is productive or nonproductive and the amount and the color of the sputum expectorated. Observe the patient's facial expressions and for signs of respiratory distress such as flaring nostrils, substernal or clavicular retractions, asymmetric chest wall expansion, and abdominal breathing.

◆ PATIENT PROBLEM

Assist in the development of nursing diagnoses. Patient problems specific to the patient with a respiratory disorder include but are not limited to the following:

- *Anxiousness*
- *Inability to Clear Airway*
- *Inability to Maintain Adequate Breathing Pattern*
- *Inability to Tolerate Activity*
- *Inefficient Oxygenation*
- *Insufficient Nutrition*

◆ EXPECTED OUTCOMES AND PLANNING

The overall goals are that the patient with a respiratory disorder will have (1) effective breathing patterns, (2) adequate airway clearance, (3) adequate oxygenation of tissues, and (4) a realistic attitude toward compliance to treatment. The care plan may include the following goals:

Goal 1: Patient will achieve improved activity tolerance.
Outcome: Patient reports lessened dyspnea with exercise.
Goal 2: Patient will maintain a patent airway.
Outcome: Patient clears airway by coughing.

◆ IMPLEMENTATION

Maintaining the patient's optimal health is important in reducing respiratory symptoms. Nursing interventions may include improving the patient's activity tolerance. This enables the patient to perform activities of daily living while not increasing dyspnea.

◆ EVALUATION

Evaluate the expected outcomes and determine their effectiveness. Notify the health care provider if the patient's respiratory status does not improve immediately. Examples of goals and evaluative measures are as follows:

Goal 1: Patient will achieve improved activity tolerance.
Evaluative measure: Assess patient's exercise tolerance.
Goal 2: Patient will maintain a patent airway.
Evaluative measure: Auscultate lungs after hearing patient cough.

Get Ready for the NCLEX® Examination!

Key Points

- The primary function of the respiratory system is to exchange oxygen and carbon dioxide at the alveolar-capillary level.
- The most important structure of the respiratory system is the alveolus, where oxygen and carbon dioxide exchange occurs.
- The combination of one inspiration plus one expiration equals one respiration.
- For breathing to occur, pressure changes must take place within the thoracic cavity.
- The lungs' ability to expand and contract depends on musculoskeletal and neurologic functions, as well as physiologic conditions affecting the respiratory system.
- When air is inhaled, it is warmed, moistened, and filtered to prepare it for use by the body.
- Activity tolerance frequently is altered as a result of decreased oxygenation-ventilation.
- Anxiety can exacerbate pulmonary disorders, increasing the body's need for oxygen.
- Breathing exercises can improve ventilation.
- Effective breathing techniques include elevating the head and chest to maintain airway patency; deep breathing and coughing exercises to facilitate lung expansion; and pursed-lip breathing to decrease the effort of breathing.
- Adequate fluid intake and humidity help moisten secretions, thus aiding in their clearance.
- A thorough psychosocial assessment and resultant interventions are necessary for the patient with a laryngectomy because of loss of voice and neck and facial disfigurement.
- In May 2005 the FDA approved a new version of a blood test to aid in diagnosing latent TB infection and active TB. It is called QuantiFERON-TB Gold (QFT-G), and it can be used in place of the traditional PPD skin test. The QFT-G may detect TB with greater specificity than the PPD test.
- SARS is a serious acute respiratory infection caused by a coronavirus.
- People who are suspected of having SARS should be placed in respiratory isolation, including use of an appropriate disposable particulate respirator, to protect other patients and health care workers.

- Clinical manifestations of sleep apnea include frequent awakening at night, insomnia, excessive daytime sleepiness, witnessed apneic episodes, morning headaches, personality changes, and irritability.
- Chest drainage serves a twofold purpose: (1) it drains air, blood, or fluid from the pleural space; and (2) restores negative pressure. It requires a water seal to prevent air from reentering the pleural space.
- Techniques used in chest physiotherapy include percussion, vibration, and postural drainage.
- Nursing interventions after thoracic surgery that assist in preventing complications by promoting effective airway clearance are (1) frequent repositioning, (2) coughing, and (3) deep breathing.
- Studies have revealed that hypoxia worsens when patients are placed on their backs or sides with the affected (sick) lung down.
- Low-flow oxygen therapy is required for patients with COPD because higher oxygen concentrations depress the body's own respiratory regulatory centers.
- Hospitals are a high-risk setting for TB transmission, and health care workers are at high occupational risk for TB infection.
- Because PE impairs gas exchange, its hallmark is acute, unexplained dyspnea with abrupt, constant, nonradiating pain that worsens with inspiration.
- Patients with respiratory disorders must reduce exposure to infection, which increases the body's oxygen demands.
- COPD disorders include emphysema, chronic bronchitis, asthma, and bronchiectasis.
- Transmission of TB is primarily by inhalation of minute droplet nuclei (each containing a single tubercle bacillus) coughed or sneezed by a person whose sputum contains tubercle bacilli.
- Pulse oximetry is a noninvasive method providing continuing monitoring of SaO_2 (saturation of oxygen).

Additional Learning Resources

SG Go to your Study Guide for additional learning activities to help you master this chapter content.

evolve Be sure to visit the Evolve site at *http://evolve.elsevier.com/Cooper/foundationsadult/* for additional online resources.

Review Questions for the NCLEX® Examination

1. When are rapid and deeper respirations stimulated by the respiratory center of the brain?
   1. When oxygen saturation levels are greater than 90%
   2. When carbon dioxide levels increase
   3. When the alveoli contract
   4. When the diaphragm contracts and lowers its dome
2. What is the most appropriate nursing intervention for a patient requiring finger probe pulse oximetry?
   1. Apply a sensor probe over a finger and cover lightly with gauze to prevent skin breakdown.
   2. Set alarms on the oximeter to at least 100%.
   3. Identify if the patient has had a recent diagnostic test using intravenous dye.
   4. Remove the sensor between oxygen saturation readings.
3. The walls of the thoracic cavity are lined with a serous membrane composed of tough endothelial cells; what is this membrane called?
   1. Visceral pleura
   2. Apneustic serosa
   3. Pneumotaxic serosa
   4. Parietal pleura
4. A patient is diagnosed with chronic bronchitis. He is very dyspneic and must sit up to breathe. What is the name of this abnormal condition, in which there is discomfort in breathing in any but an erect sitting position?
   1. Orthopnea
   2. Dyspnea
   3. Orthopsia
   4. Cheyne-Stokes
5. A patient is being evaluated to rule out pulmonary tuberculosis (TB). Which finding is most closely associated with TB?
   1. Leg cramps
   2. Night sweats
   3. Skin discoloration
   4. Green-colored sputum
6. The health care workers caring for a patient with active TB are instructed in methods of protecting themselves from contracting TB. What does the Centers for Disease Control and Prevention currently recommend for health care workers who care for TB-infected patients?
   1. Ask the patient to wear a mask while in isolation.
   2. Wear a surgical mask.
   3. Wear a small-micron, fitted filtration mask.
   4. Receive the BCG vaccine.
7. The health care provider ordered a blood culture and sputum specimen for a patient who has pneumonia. When should the nurse collect these specimens? *(Select all that apply.)*
   1. After initiation of antibiotic therapy
   2. The morning after admission
   3. Before initiation of antibiotic therapy
   4. At the first sign of elevated temperature
   5. After the patient has had breakfast
8. A patient has just returned to her room after a bronchoscopy. No food or fluids shall be given after the examination until which event has occurred?
   1. There is a total absence of blood-streaked sputum.
   2. The head nurse gives the order.
   3. The patient's gag reflex returns.
   4. The patient is up and about and steady on her feet.
9. A second-day postoperative patient is recovering from thoracic surgery. Which therapeutic nursing intervention would the nurse carry out first?
   1. Help the patient cough and deep breathe by splinting the anterior and posterior chest
   2. Splint the anterior chest for coughing
   3. Place the patient in a supine position
   4. Allow the patient to sleep uninterrupted for 8 hours

10. Which patient problem for a client with an acute asthma attack has the highest priority?
    1. *Anxiousness, related to difficulty in breathing*
    2. *Inability to Clear Airway, related to bronchoconstriction and increased mucus production*.
    3. *Inability to Maintain Adequate Breathing Pattern, related to anxiety*
    4. *Impaired Health Maintenance, related to lack of knowledge about attack triggers and appropriate use of medications*
11. A patient had a laryngectomy because of cancer of the larynx. Discharge instructions are given to the patient and his family. Which response, by written communication from the patient or verbal response by the family, indicates that the instructions need to be clarified?
    1. Report swelling, pain, or excessive drainage.
    2. The suctioning at home must be a clean procedure, not sterile.
    3. Cleanse skin around stoma twice daily (bid), using hydrogen peroxide; rinse with water; pat dry.
    4. It is acceptable to take over-the-counter medications now that the condition is stable.
12. Where do most pulmonary embolisms (PEs) originate?
    1. Deep vein thrombosis (DVT)
    2. Ventilation/perfusion (V/Q) mismatch
    3. Increased pulmonary vascular resistance
    4. Right-sided heart failure
13. Which health promotion activities planned by a nurse working with a group of community-dwelling senior citizens would be most likely to prevent influenza and pneumonia? *(Select all that apply.)*
    1. Indoor exercise programs during the winter months
    2. Influenza vaccine clinics at the senior citizen centers
    3. Teaching effective handwashing
    4. Advising seniors to avoid crowds
    5. Encouraging seniors not to visit with children
14. A patient was seen in a clinic for an episode of epistaxis, which was controlled by placement of anterior nasal packing. During discharge teaching, what instructions will the nurse discuss with the patient?
    1. Avoid vigorous nose blowing and strenuous activity.
    2. Use aspirin or aspirin-containing compounds for pain relief.
    3. Apply ice compresses to the nose every 4 hours for the first 48 hours.
    4. Leave the packing in place for 7 to 10 days until it is removed by the health care provider.
15. How is TB spread?
    1. Contact with clothing, bedding, or food
    2. Eating from utensils used by an infected person
    3. Inhaling the TB bacteria after a person with TB coughs, speaks, or sneezes
    4. Talking with an individual with TB
16. A patient with TB has a patient problem statement of *Noncooperation or Nonconformity*. What does the nurse recognize as the most common etiologic factor?
    1. Fatigue and lack of energy to manage self-care
    2. Lack of knowledge about how the disease is transmitted
    3. Little or no motivation to adhere to a long-term drug regimen
    4. Feelings of shame and the response to the social stigma associated with TB
17. To obtain optimal results from pulse oximetry, which statements are correct? *(Select all that apply.)*
    1. Do not attach the transducer to an extremity that has a blood pressure cuff in place.
    2. While the probe is in place, protect it from decreased light, which can affect the reading.
    3. Place the probe over a pulsating vascular bed.
    4. Hypothermia, hypotension, and vasoconstriction can affect readings.
    5. Reduced body temperature will affect readings.
18. *Inability to Clear Airway, related to tracheobronchial obstruction or secretions*, is a problem statement for a patient with COPD. Which nursing interventions are correct? *(Select all that apply.)*
    1. Offer small, frequent, high-calorie, high-protein feedings.
    2. Encourage generous fluid intake.
    3. Restrict fluid intake to decrease congestion.
    4. Have the patient turn and cough every 2 hours.
    5. Teach effective coughing technique.
19. *Inability to Maintain Adequate Breathing Pattern, related to decreased lung expansion during an acute attack of asthma,* is an appropriate patient problem statement. Which nursing interventions are correct? *(Select all that apply.)*
    1. Place patient in a supine position.
    2. Administer oxygen therapy as ordered.
    3. Remain with patient during acute attack to decrease fear and anxiety.
    4. Incorporate rest periods into activities and interventions.
    5. Maintain semi-Fowler's position to facilitate ventilation.
20. What does the patient with respiratory acidosis demonstrate? *(Select all that apply.)*
    1. Disorientation
    2. pH less than 7.35
    3. pH more than 7.44
    4. Rapid respirations
    5. Slow deep respirations
21. Patient teaching after a tonsillectomy and adenoidectomy would include which instruction(s)? *(Select all that apply.)*
    1. Avoid attempting to clear the throat, coughing, and sneezing.
    2. Avoid vigorous nose blowing for 1 to 2 weeks.
    3. Resume foods and fluids as tolerated.
    4. Take aspirin, gr 10 (10 grains), every 4 hours.
    5. Notify the health care provider in case of increased pain, fever, or bleeding.

22. If the patient has an epistaxis, what is the correct nursing intervention(s)? *(Select all that apply.)*
1. Place the patient in Fowler's position with the head forward.
2. Place the patient in Fowler's position with the head extended.
3. Compress the nostrils tightly below the bone and hold for 10 minutes or longer.
4. Place ice compresses over the nose.
5. Encourage slow, deep breathing through the mouth.

23. In pulmonary edema, what is often included in medical management? *(Select all that apply.)*
1. IV infusion fluid bolus
2. Furosemide (Lasix) IV
3. Oxygen therapy
4. Orthopneic position
5. Morphine sulfate to decrease respiratory rate

24. An appropriate problem statement for a patient with pulmonary edema is *Fluid Volume Overload, related to altered tissue permeability*. Which nursing intervention(s) for this patient problem statement are correct? *(Select all that apply.)*
1. Assess indicators of patient's fluid volume status, such as breath sounds; skin turgor; and pedal, sacral, and periorbital edema.
2. Monitor intake and output accurately.
3. Administer diuretics as ordered.
4. Weigh daily.
5. Provide regular diet with normal sodium intake.

25. The nurse should educate the patient in the proper techniques to use for the collection of a sputum specimen. Which guideline(s) are correct? *(Select all that apply.)*
1. Explain to the patient the need to bring the sputum up from the lungs.
2. Encourage fluid intake.
3. Collect specimens after meals, when patient feels stronger.
4. Notify staff as soon as specimen is collected so that it can be sent to the laboratory without delay.
5. Place sputum specimen in sterile container.

26. Medical management and nursing interventions for the patient with pulmonary embolism usually include: *(Select all that apply.)*
1. bed rest.
2. administration of intravenous heparin per protocol.
3. semi-Fowler's position.
4. administration of vitamin K subcutaneously.
5. oxygen by mask or nasal cannula.

50 Care of the Patient With a Urinary Disorder

http://evolve.elsevier.com/Cooper/foundationsadult/

Objectives

Anatomy and Physiology

1. Describe the structures of the urinary system, including functions.
2. List the three processes involved in urine formation.
3. Name three hormones and their influence on nephron function.
4. Compare the normal components of urine with the abnormal components.

Medical-Surgical

5. Identify the effects of aging on urinary system function.
6. Describe the changes in body image created when the patient experiences an alteration in urinary function.
7. Incorporate pharmacotherapeutic and nutritional considerations into the nursing care plan of the patient with a urinary disorder.
8. Prioritize the special needs of the patient with urinary dysfunction.
9. Describe the alterations in kidney function associated with disorders of the urinary tract.
10. Address patient concerns in teaching about altered sexuality secondary to urinary disorders and treatments.
11. Investigate community resources for support for the patient and significant others as they face lifestyle changes from chronic urinary disorders and treatments.
12. Select patient problem statements related to alterations in urinary function.

Key Terms

anasarca (ăn-ă-SĂR-kă, p. 1682)
anuria (ă-NŪ-rē-ă, p. 1657)
asthenia (ăs-THĒ-nē-ă, p. 1665)
azotemia (ă-zō-TĒ-mē-ă, p. 1669)
bacteriuria (băk-tēr-ē-Ū-rē-ŭh, p. 1665)
costovertebral angle (CVA) (kŏs-tŏ-VĔR-tĕ-brăl ĂNG-gŭl, p. 1669)
cytologic evaluation (sī-tŏ-LŎJ-ĭk ĕ-văl-ū-Ā-shŭn, p. 1676)
dialysis (dī-ĂL-ĭ-sĭs, p. 1687)
dysuria (dĭs-Ū-rē-ă, p. 1655)
hematuria (hĕm-ă-TŪ-rē-ă, p. 1651)
hydronephrosis (hī-drō-nĕ-FRŌ-sĭs, p. 1671)
ileal conduit (ĭl-ē-ăl KŎN-dū-ĭt, p. 1693)
Kegel exercises (p. 1661)
micturition (mĭk-tū-RĬSH-ŭn, p. 1671)
nephrotoxins (nĕf-rō-TŎK-sĭnz, p. 1694)
nocturia (nŏk-TŪ-rē-ă, p. 1665)
oliguria (ŏl-ĭ-GŪ-rē-ă, p. 1676)
pessary (p. 1663)
prostatodynia (prŏs-tĕ-tō-DĪN-ē-ă, p. 1668)
pyuria (pĭ-Ū-rē-ă, p. 1665)
renal colic (p. 1670)
residual urine (rĕ-ZĬ-dū-ăl Ū-rĭn, p. 1659)
urinary retention (rē-TĔN-shŭn, p. 1661)
urolithiasis (ū-rō-lĭ-THĪ-ă-sĭs, p. 1672)

ANATOMY AND PHYSIOLOGY OF THE URINARY SYSTEM

Each day, the cells throughout the body metabolize ingested nutrients. This process provides energy for the body and produces waste products. As proteins break down, nitrogenous waste—urea, ammonia, and *creatinine* (a nitrogenous compound produced by metabolic processes in the body)—is produced. The urinary system is largely responsible for maintenance of homeostasis in the body. The primary function of the kidneys is excretion of these waste products. The kidneys also assist in regulating the body's water, electrolytes, secretion of erythropoietin (which stimulates red blood cell production), and acid-base balance.

The urinary system consists of two kidneys, two ureters, the bladder, and the urethra. The kidneys remove waste, excess water, and electrolytes from the blood and concentrate them into urine. The ureters transport urine from the kidneys to the bladder. The bladder collects and stores urine. The urethra transports urine from the bladder to the outside of the body during elimination (Fig. 50.1). This chapter explores the filtering process of the kidneys, the composition of urine, and the how urine is removed from the body.

KIDNEYS

The kidneys lie behind the parietal peritoneum (retroperitoneal), just below the diaphragm, on each side of the vertebral column. Kidneys are dark red, bean-shaped

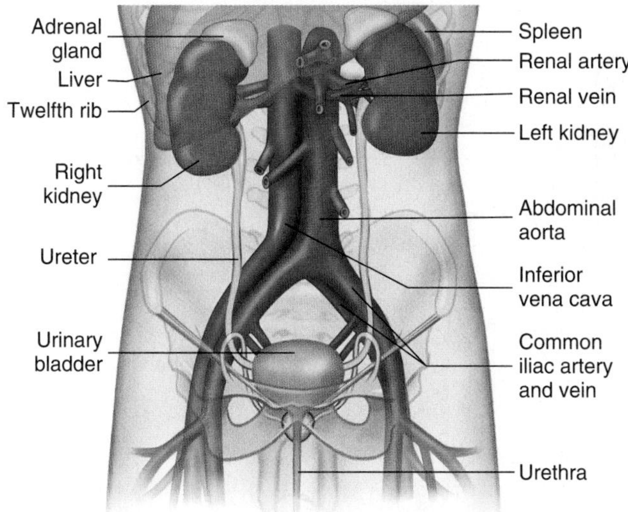

Fig. 50.1 Location of urinary system organs. (From Patton KT, Thibodeau GA: *Anatomy and physiology*, ed 8, St. Louis, 2013, Mosby.)

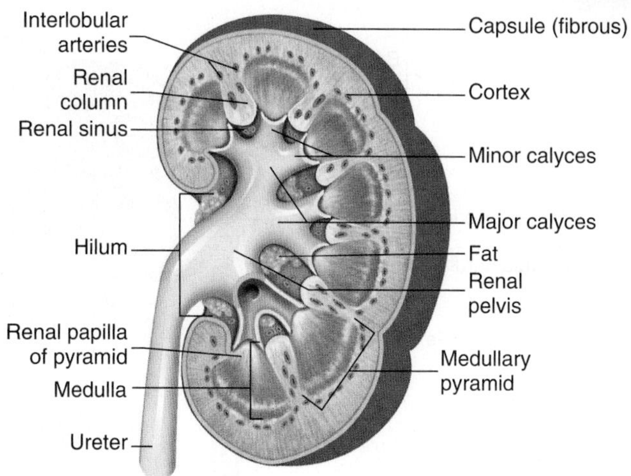

Fig. 50.2 Coronal section of the kidney. (From Patton KT, Thibodeau GA: *Anatomy and physiology*, ed 8, St. Louis, 2013, Mosby.)

organs that are 4 to 5 inches (10 to 12 cm) long, 2 to 3 inches (5 to 7.5 cm) wide, and about 1 inch (2.5 cm) thick. Because of the position of the liver, the right kidney lies slightly lower than the left. The kidneys are surrounded and anchored in place by a layer of adipose tissue. Near the center of each kidney's medial border is a notch or indentation called the *hilus,* where the renal artery enters and the renal vein and the ureter exit the kidney.

The adrenal glands, a part of the endocrine system, sit near the top of each kidney. The adrenal glands secrete hormones that help control blood pressure and heart rate, among other functions. The primary substance secreted by the adrenal cortex is a mineralocorticoid hormone called aldosterone. The level of potassium concentration in the plasma is the primary regulator of aldosterone. Changes evoked through the adrenal glands produce changes in kidney function (see Chapter 51).

Gross Anatomic Structure

The outer covering of the kidney is a strong layer of connective tissue called the *renal capsule.* Directly beneath the renal capsule is the renal *cortex.* It contains 1.25 million renal tubules, which are part of the microscopic filtration system. Immediately beneath the cortex is the *medulla,* which is a darker color. The medulla contains the triangular *pyramids.* Continuing inward, the narrow points of the pyramids *(papillae)* empty urine into the calyces. The *calyces* (singular, *calyx*) are cuplike extensions of the renal pelvis that guide urine into the main part of the renal pelvis. The *renal pelvis* is an expansion of the upper end of the ureter; the ureter in turn drains the finished product, urine, into the bladder (Fig. 50.2).

Microscopic Structure

Nephron. Each kidney contains more than 1 million nephrons. The *nephron* resembles a microscopic funnel with a long stem and two convoluted sections (Fig. 50.3). It filters the blood and processes the urine by: (1) controlling body fluid levels by selectively removing or retaining water, (2) helping to regulate the pH of the blood, and (3) removing toxic waste from the blood. Approximately 60 times a day, the body's entire volume of blood is filtered through the kidneys.

A nephron has two main structures: the renal corpuscle and renal tubule. The renal corpuscle is a tightly bound network of capillaries called *glomeruli* (singular, *glomerulus*) that are held inside a cuplike structure, the *Bowman's capsule.* The renal arteries (right and left) branch off the abdominal aorta and enter each kidney at the hilus. The renal arteries continue branching inside the kidney until blood is delivered to the glomerulus by an afferent arteriole. The filtered blood leaves the glomerulus through an efferent arteriole and flows to a peritubular capillary. The cleansed blood finally reaches the renal veins and flows into the inferior vena cava.

The renal tubule becomes tightly coiled (at the proximal convoluted tubule), makes a sudden straight drop, and curves back upward like a hairpin (at Henle's loop, or nephron loop) and becomes tightly coiled again (at the distal convoluted tubule). The convoluted tubule terminates at the collecting tubule or duct. Several collecting ducts unite in a pyramid and open at the papilla to empty urine into the associated calyx.

The juxtaglomerular apparatus is a microscopic structure in the kidney that regulates the function of each nephron. The juxtaglomerular apparatus is named for its proximity to the glomerulus; it is found between the vascular pole of the renal corpuscle and the returning distal convoluted tubule of the same nephron. This location is critical to its function in regulating renal blood flow and the glomerular filtration rate. The juxtaglomerular apparatus is where the afferent arterioles come into direct contact with the distal convoluted tubule. The juxtaglomerular apparatus regulates systemic blood pressure and filtrate formation.

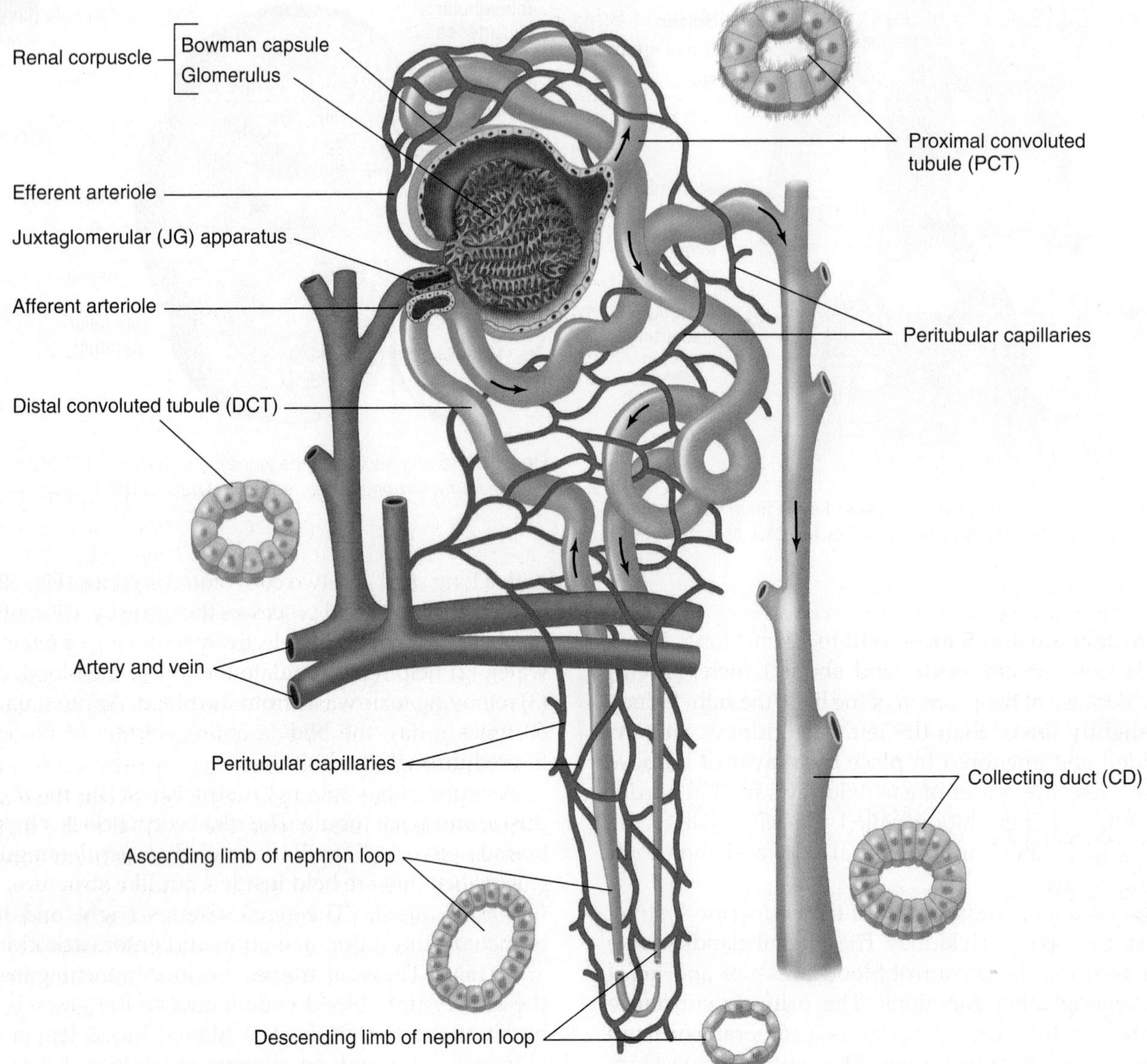

Fig. 50.3 The nephron unit. Cross-sections from the four segments of the renal tubule are shown. The differences in appearance in tubular cells seen in a cross-section reflect the differing functions of each nephron segment. (From Thibodeau GA, Patton KT: *Structure and function of the body*, ed 14, St. Louis, 2012, Mosby.)

The specialized cells of the afferent arteriole at this region are called *juxtaglomerular cells*. These cells contain the enzyme renin and sense blood pressure.

The specialized cells of the distal convoluted tubule at the point of contact with the afferent arteriole are the macula densa cells. These cells sense changes in the solute concentration and flow rate of the filtrate.

When systemic blood pressure decreases, the juxtaglomerular cells have a decreased stretch, which leads to their release of renin. Renin release activates the renin-angiotensin mechanism, which ultimately leads to increased blood pressure.

Reabsorption begins as soon as the filtrate reaches the tubule system. The filtrate contains important products needed by the body: water, glucose, and ions are absorbed. In fact, 99% of the filtrate returns to the body (see Fig. 50.3).

In summary, the three phases of urine formation (Table 50.1) and location of the processes are as follows:

1. *Filtration* of water and blood products occurs in the glomerulus of Bowman's capsule.
2. *Reabsorption* of water, glucose, and necessary ions back into the blood occurs primarily in the proximal convoluted tubules, Henle's loop, and the distal convoluted tubules.
3. *Secretion* of certain ions, nitrogenous waste products, and drugs occurs primarily in the distal convoluted tubule. This process is the reverse of reabsorption; the substances move from the blood to the filtrate.

Hormonal influence on nephron function. When the body experiences increased fluid loss through hemorrhage, diaphoresis, vomiting, diarrhea, or other means, the blood pressure drops. These events decrease the amount of filtrate produced by the kidneys. The posterior

Table 50.1 Functions of the Parts of the Nephron in Urine Formation

PART OF NEPHRON	PROCESS IN URINE FORMATION	SUBSTANCES MOVED AND DIRECTION OF MOVEMENT
Glomerulus	Filtration	Water and solutes (sodium and other ions, nitrogenous wastes [urea, uric acid, creatinine], glucose, and other nutrients) filter through the glomeruli into Bowman's capsule
Proximal convoluted tubule	Reabsorption	Water and solutes
Loop of Henle	Reabsorption	Sodium and chloride ions
Distal convoluted and collecting tubules	Reabsorption Secretion	Water, sodium and other ions Ammonia, potassium ions, urea, uric acid, creatinine, hydrogen ions, and some drugs

Box 50.1 Major Functions of the Kidneys

Urine formation: Glomerular filtration, tubular reabsorption, and secretion; 1000 to 2000 mL of urine formed each day

Fluid and electrolyte control: Maintain correct balance of fluid and electrolytes within a normal range by excretion, secretion, and reabsorption

Acid-base balance: Maintain pH of blood (7.35 to 7.45) at normal range by directly excreting hydrogen ions and forming bicarbonate for buffering

Excretion of waste products: Direct removal of metabolic waste products contained in the glomerular filtrate

Blood pressure regulation: Regulation of blood pressure by controlling the circulating volume and renin secretion

Red blood cell (RBC) production: Secretion of erythropoietin, which stimulates bone marrow to produce RBCs

Regulation of calcium-phosphate metabolism: Regulation of vitamin D activation

pituitary gland releases antidiuretic hormone (ADH). ADH causes the cells of the distal convoluted tubules to increase their rate of water reabsorption. This action returns the water to the bloodstream, which raises the blood pressure to a more normal level and causes the urine to become concentrated. See Box 50.1 for major functions of kidneys.

URINE COMPOSITION AND CHARACTERISTICS

The word *urine* comes from one of its components, uric acid. Each day, the body forms 1000 to 2000 mL of urine; this amount is influenced by several factors, including mental and physical health, oral intake, and blood pressure. Urine is 95% water; the remainder is nitrogenous waste and salts. It is usually a transparent yellow with a characteristic odor. Normal urine is yellow because of urochrome, a pigment resulting from the body's destruction of hemoglobin. Urine is slightly acidic, with a pH of 4.6 to 8 and a specific gravity of 1.003 to 1.030. Healthy urine is sterile, but at room temperature it rapidly decomposes and smells like ammonia as a result of the breakdown of urea.

URINE ABNORMALITIES

A urinalysis, which examines the physical, chemical, and microscopic properties of urine, can provide important diagnostic information. If the body's homeostasis has been compromised, certain substances may spill into the urine. Some of the more common substances include the following:

- *Albumin* in the urine (albuminuria) indicates possible renal disease, increased blood pressure, or toxicity of the kidney cells from heavy metals.
- *Glucose* (sugar) in the urine (glycosuria) most often indicates a high blood glucose level. When the blood glucose level rises above the renal threshold (the point at which the renal tubules can no longer reabsorb), the glucose spills into the urine.
- *Erythrocytes* in the urine **(hematuria)** may indicate infection, tumors, or renal disease. Occasionally an individual may have a renal calculus (kidney stone; plural, *calculi*), and irritation produces hematuria.
- *Ketone bodies* in the urine are called *ketoaciduria* (or ketonuria). It occurs when too many fatty acids are oxidized. This condition is seen with diabetes mellitus, starvation, or any other metabolic condition in which fats are catabolized rapidly.
- *Leukocytes* (white blood cells [WBCs]) are found in urine when there is an infection in the urinary tract.

URETERS

Once the urine has been formed in the nephrons, it passes to the paired ureters. Ureters are extensions of the renal pelvis and extend downward 10 to 12 inches (25 to 30 cm) to the lower part of the urinary bladder. As the ureters leave the kidneys, they remain in the retroperitoneal space and pass under the urinary bladder before entering it. As the ureters enter the bladder (at the ureterovesical junction), internal mucous membrane folds act as a valve to prevent backflow of urine.

URINARY BLADDER

The urinary bladder (Fig. 50.4) is a temporary storage pouch for urine. It is composed of collapsible muscle and is located anterior to the small intestine and posterior to the symphysis pubis (where the right and left pelvic

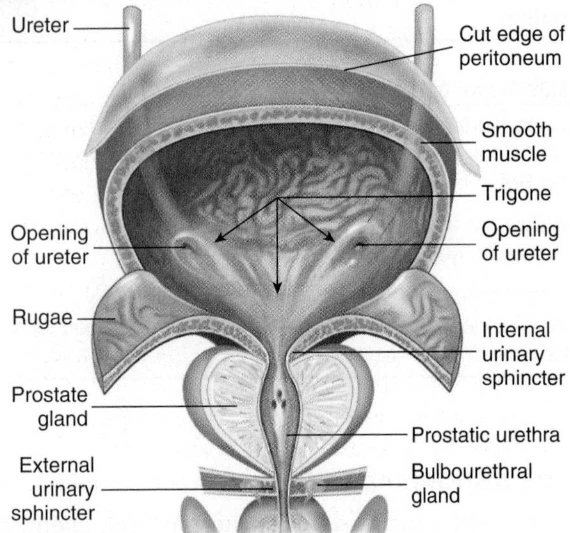

Fig. 50.4 The male urinary bladder, cut to show the interior. Note how the prostate gland surrounds the urethra as it exits the bladder. (From Thibodeau GA, Patton KT: *Structure and function of the body*, ed 14, St. Louis, 2012, Mosby.)

bones join, just above the penis in men, and just above the vulva in women). As the bladder fills with urine, it rises into the abdominal cavity and can be palpated. The bladder can hold 750 to 1000 mL of urine. When the bladder contains approximately 250 mL of urine, the individual has a conscious desire to urinate. This is because the stretch receptors become activated and a message is sent to the spinal cord. A moderately full bladder holds 450 mL (1 pint) of urine.

Two sphincters control the release of urine. The internal sphincter, located at the bladder neck, is composed of involuntary muscle. As the bladder becomes full, the stretch receptors cause contractions, pushing the urine past the internal sphincter. The urine then presses on the external sphincter, which is composed of skeletal or voluntary muscle at the terminus of the urethra.

URETHRA

The *urethra* is the terminal portion of the urinary system. It is a small tube that carries urine by peristalsis from the bladder out of its external opening, the *urinary meatus*. In females it is embedded in the anterior wall of the vagina vestibule and exits between the clitoris and the vaginal opening. The female urethra is approximately ¼ inch in diameter and 1½ inches long. In males the urethra is approximately 8 inches long, passing through the prostate gland and extending the length of the glans penis. In the male the urethra serves two functions: as a passageway for urine and semen.

EFFECTS OF NORMAL AGING ON THE URINARY SYSTEM

With aging the kidneys lose part of their normal functioning capacity. By age 70 the filtering mechanism is only 50% as efficient as at age 40. This occurs because of decreased blood supply and loss of nephrons.

In the aging woman the bladder loses tone and the perineal muscles may relax, resulting in stress incontinence. In the aging man the prostate gland may become enlarged, leading to constriction of the urethra. Incomplete emptying of the bladder in men and women increases the possibility of urinary tract infection (UTI) (see the Lifespan Considerations box).

Lifespan Considerations

Older Adults

Urinary Disorders

- Urinary frequency, urgency, nocturia (excessive urination at night), retention, and incontinence are common with aging. These occur because of weakened musculature in the bladder and urethra, diminished neurologic sensation combined with decreased bladder capacity, and the effects of medications such as diuretics.
- Urinary incontinence can lead to a loss of self-esteem and result in decreased participation in social activities.
- Older women are at risk for stress incontinence because of hormonal changes and weakened pelvic musculature.
- Older men are at risk for urinary retention because of prostatic hypertrophy.
- Urinary tract infections in older adults often are associated with invasive procedures such as catheterization, diabetes mellitus, and neurologic disorders.
- Inadequate fluid intake, immobility, and conditions that lead to urinary stasis increase the risk of infection in the older adult.
- Frequent toileting and meticulous skin care can reduce the risk of skin impairment secondary to urinary incontinence.

LABORATORY AND DIAGNOSTIC EXAMINATIONS

Diagnostic tests for urinary tract conditions include laboratory tests, diagnostic imaging, and endoscopic procedures. Nursing responsibilities vary according to the studies performed. Be aware of specific patient variables that may influence test results: state of hydration, nutritional status, or trauma (see the Cultural Considerations box). Prepare patients for diagnostic testing by briefly describing the purpose of the procedure and what the patient can expect to happen.

URINALYSIS

The most common urinary diagnostic study is the urinalysis. Table 50.2 describes normal and abnormal constituents in the urine and possible factors that influence test results. A urinalysis may be done during assessments of other body systems because of the role of the kidneys in maintaining homeostasis. Urine culture and sensitivity may be done to confirm suspected infections, to identify causative organisms, and to determine appropriate antimicrobial therapy. Cultures also are obtained for periodic screening of urine when the threat of a UTI

Table 50.2 Urinalysis

CONSTITUENT	NORMAL RANGE	INFLUENCING FACTORS
Color	Pale yellow to amber	Diabetes insipidus, biliary obstruction, medications, diet
Turbidity	Clear to slightly cloudy	Phosphates, white blood cells, bacteria
Odor	Mildly aromatic	Medication, bacteria, diet
pH	4.6–8	Stale specimen, food intake, infection, homeostatic imbalance
Specific gravity	1.003–1.030	State of hydration, medications
Glucose	Negative	Diabetes mellitus, medications, diet
Protein	Negative	Renal disease, muscle exertion, dehydration
Bilirubin	Negative	Liver disease with obstruction or damage, medications
Hemoglobin	Negative	Trauma, renal disease
Ketones	Negative	Diabetes mellitus, diet, medications
Red blood cells	Up to 2 per LPF	Renal or bladder disease, trauma, medications
White blood cells	0–4 per LPF	Renal disease, urinary tract infection
Casts	Rare	Renal disease
Bacteria	Negative	Urinary tract infection

LPF, Low-power field.

Cultural Considerations

Urinary Disorders

A cultural assessment reflects a dynamic process in which the health care team seeks to gain insights concerning the patient's understanding of the meaning of care, health, and well-being. Integral components of a cultural assessment include communication, time orientation, personal space, pain, religious beliefs, taboos, customs, dietary practices, health practices, family roles, and views of death.

Professional discussion of urinary problems requires sensitivity because of the association of the urinary system with the reproductive system and the associated cultural taboos surrounding sexuality. Often the patient's self-image and sexual performance are affected by altered urinary function. Be sensitive to the patient's feelings, guiding the interview to ensure accurate assessment while maintaining the patient's dignity.

persists. Various reagent strips to test urine for abnormal substances are a quick reference that can be used in a clinical setting or at home. Common substances measured to monitor kidney function include total urine protein, creatinine, urea, uric acid levels, and catecholamines. Low levels of protein in the urine are normal. Elevated levels may be noted temporarily with illness. Chronically elevated levels are seen in renal damage and cardiac disease. Creatinine level abnormalities are nonspecific but may be noted with a variety of conditions, including kidney failure, urinary obstruction, and infection. Uric acid results from the breakdown of purines. Low levels may be tied to alcohol use and glomerulonephritis. Catecholamines are made by nervous tissue and the adrenal glands. Their levels may be elevated with the ingestion of many medications, including tricyclic antidepressants and amphetamines. Levels are reduced with monoamine oxidase (MAO) inhibitors and salicylates. Elevated levels may be associated with metastatic cancers, bone marrow disorders, and gout.

Urinalysis is performed on a sample obtained using clean-catch technique or by catheterization. A sterile urine specimen can be obtained either by inserting a straight catheter into the urinary bladder and removing urine or by obtaining a specimen via the catheter port of an indwelling catheter, using sterile technique. Because the kidneys excrete substances in varying amounts and rates during a 24-hour period, a 24-hour urine sample may be collected. Discard the first voiding and note the time at the beginning of the 24-hour urine collection. For the next 24 hours all urine is collected and placed in a special laboratory container that is opaque to prevent light damage to substances in the urine. The collection container is stored on ice during the collection period.

URINE SPECIFIC GRAVITY

To determine the specific gravity of urine, the density of a urine sample is compared with that of water. It is only an approximation of the concentration of particles (i.e., solutes) in urine but does indicate a patient's hydration status and gives information about the kidneys' ability to concentrate urine. Urine specific gravity is decreased by high fluid intake, reduced renal concentrating ability, diabetes insipidus (an endocrine disorder in which the kidneys are unable to conserve water when they purify blood), and diuretic use. It is increased in dehydration because of fever, diaphoresis, vomiting, diarrhea, and medical conditions such as diabetic ketoacidosis or hyperglycemic hyperosmolar nonketotic coma (complications of diabetes mellitus in which the kidneys are unable to excrete the high amounts of glucose in the blood) and inappropriate secretion of ADH. The normal value ranges between 1.005 and 1.030, with the lower values suggesting more dilute urine (Medscape, 2014).

BLOOD (SERUM) UREA NITROGEN

Blood urea nitrogen (BUN) is a laboratory test used to determine the kidneys' ability to rid the blood of nonprotein nitrogenous (NPN) waste and urea, which result from protein breakdown (catabolism). The test may be performed to assess the overall function of the kidneys, to monitor the progression of kidney disease, or to evaluate the effectiveness of prescribed therapies. The acceptable serum range for BUN is 10 to 20 mg/dL. For a more accurate test result, the patient should receive nothing by mouth (NPO) for 8 hours before blood sampling (WebMD, 2010). In addition to renal disease, elevated levels are associated with dehydration, heart disease, and a diet high in protein. If the BUN is elevated, institute preventive nursing measures to protect the patient from possible disorientation or seizures.

BLOOD (SERUM) CREATININE

Creatinine is a catabolic product of creatine, which is used in skeletal muscle contraction. The daily production of creatine, and subsequently creatinine, depends on muscle mass, which fluctuates little. Creatinine, as with BUN, is excreted entirely by the kidneys and is therefore directly proportional to renal excretory function. Thus, with normal renal excretory function, the serum creatinine level should remain constant and normal. Elevated levels may be caused by nonrenal factors such as dehydration, preeclampsia, and muscular dystrophy. Levels may be elevated as a result of renal causes, including acute tubular necrosis, glomerulonephritis (inflammation of the glomeruli), pyelonephritis (typically a bacterial infection of the kidneys and upper urinary tract), reduced kidney function, and renal failure. Lower levels may be noted with myasthenia gravis and late-stage muscular dystrophy.

The serum creatinine test, as with BUN, is used to diagnose impaired kidney function. However, unlike BUN, the creatinine level is affected little by dehydration, malnutrition, or hepatic function. The creatinine level is interpreted in conjunction with the BUN. The acceptable serum creatinine range is 0.6 to 1. mg/dL (female) and 0.7 to 1.3 mg/dL (male). The level in women is lower because they usually have less muscle mass (National Library of Medicine, 2017a).

CREATININE CLEARANCE

Creatinine, an NPN substance, is present in the blood and urine. Creatinine is generated during muscle contraction and then excreted by glomerular filtration. Levels are related directly to muscle mass and usually are measured for a 24-hour period. During the testing period, the patient avoids excessive physical activity. A fasting blood sample is drawn at the onset of testing and another at the conclusion. Discard the initial urine specimen and start the 24-hour timing at that point. Collect all urine in the 24-hour period, because any deviation will alter test results. An elevated serum level with a decline in urine level indicates renal disease. Normal ranges are as follows: *serum,* 0.6 to 1.1 mg/dL (female), 0.7 to 1.3 mg/dL (male); *urine,* 88 to 128 mL/min (female), 97 to 137 mL/min (male) (National Library of Medicine, 2017b).

PROSTATE-SPECIFIC ANTIGEN

Prostate-specific antigen (PSA) is an organ-specific glycoprotein produced by normal prostatic tissue. Measurement of PSA has almost replaced that of prostatic acid phosphatase because it is a more accurate test. The normal range is less than 4 ng/mL. Older men normally have levels higher than those of younger men. It may be used to evaluate the prostate health of men being treated for cancer or as a diagnostic screening. Elevated levels may result from prostate cancer, inflammation or infection, urinary tract infection, or recent cystoscopy or prostatic biopsies. The test is not a specific determination of the presence of prostate cancer. Elevations in levels warrant additional studies.

URINE OSMOLALITY

Assessment of urine *osmolality,* which directly determines the number of particles (i.e., solute) per volume of water (i.e., solvent), is sometimes more informative than urine specific gravity but is a more difficult test to perform. Plasma osmolality may be determined in conjunction with the urine sampling when pituitary disorders are suspected. Results provide information on the concentrating ability of the kidneys.

KIDNEY-URETER-BLADDER RADIOGRAPHY

A kidney-ureter-bladder (KUB) radiograph assesses the general status of the abdomen and the size, structure, and position of the urinary tract structures. No special preparation is necessary. Explain to the patient that the procedure involves changing position on the radiography table, which may be uncomfortably firm. Abnormal findings related to the urinary system may indicate tumors, calculi, glomerulonephritis, cysts, and other conditions.

INTRAVENOUS PYELOGRAPHY OR INTRAVENOUS UROGRAPHY

Intravenous pyelography (IVP), also called intravenous urography (IVU), evaluates structures of the urinary tract, filling of the renal pelvis with urine, and transport of urine via the ureters to the bladder. Before performing this procedure, it is critical to determine whether the patient has an allergy to iodine (or iodine-containing foods such as iodized salt, saltwater fish, seaweed products, or vegetables grown in iodine-rich soils), because iodine is the basis of the radiopaque dye injected into the patient's vein for this and other radiologic examinations. If the patient is allergic to iodine, the health care provider may order administration of a corticosteroid or an antihistamine before testing or, alternatively, may order ultrasonography.

Because kidneys and ureters are positioned in the retroperitoneal space, gas and stool in the intestines interfere with radiographic visualization. Preparation usually includes eating a light evening meal, taking a non–gas-forming laxative, and remaining NPO for 8 hours before the test. If additional tests using barium-based studies are planned, the IVP is scheduled first. When the dye is injected, the patient experiences a warm, flushing sensation and a metallic taste. During the procedure, monitor vital signs frequently. Radiographs are taken at various intervals to monitor movement of the dye. Abnormal findings may indicate structural deviations, hydronephrosis (kidney swelling), calculi within the urinary tract, polycystic renal (kidney) disease (PKD), tumors, and other conditions.

RETROGRADE PYELOGRAPHY

Retrograde pyelography involves examination of the lower urinary tract with a cystoscope under aseptic conditions. The urologist injects radiopaque dye directly into the ureters to visualize the upper urinary tract. Urine samples can be obtained directly from the renal pelvis. Additional retrograde studies include the following:

- *Retrograde cystography:* Radiopaque dye is injected through an indwelling catheter into the urinary bladder to evaluate its structure or to determine the cause of recurrent infections.
- *Retrograde urethrography:* A catheter is inserted and dye injected as in retrograde cystography to assess the status of the urethral structure.

VOIDING CYSTOURETHROGRAPHY

Voiding cystourethrography is used in conjunction with other diagnostic studies to detect abnormalities of the urinary bladder and the urethra. Preparation includes administering an enema before the test. An indwelling catheter is inserted into the urinary bladder, and dye is injected to outline the lower urinary tract. Radiographs are taken, and the catheter is then removed. The patient is asked to void while radiographs are being taken. Some patients experience embarrassment or anxiety related to the procedure and should be given the opportunity to express their feelings. Structural abnormalities, diverticula, and reflux into the ureter may be detected.

ENDOSCOPIC PROCEDURES

Endoscopic procedures are visual examinations of hollow organs, done with a scope (typically a flexible tube equipped with a light and camera). Because of the invasive nature of the procedure, a signed written consent is necessary. The procedure may be done in the surgical suite; if so, the patient requires preoperative preparation (see Chapter 42). The procedure is performed by a urologist.

Cystoscopy is a visual examination done to inspect, treat, or diagnose disorders of the urinary bladder and proximal structures. As with all medical procedures, patient preparation includes a description of what is going to happen. Usually the procedure is carried out with a local anesthetic after the patient has been sedated. Patient safety is paramount when the patient is sedated. The patient is placed in a lithotomy position (i.e., supine, with the legs spread apart and the feet in stirrups) for the procedure, which may produce embarrassment and anxiety. The thought of a scope being inserted while the patient is awake may intensify these feelings. Provide an opportunity for the patient to verbalize feelings.

The scope is inserted under aseptic conditions after a local anesthetic has been instilled into the urethra. The patient experiences a feeling of pressure as the scope enters. Continuous fluid irrigation of the bladder is necessary to facilitate visualization. Care after the procedure includes hydration to dilute the urine. Monitor the first voiding after the procedure, assessing time, amount, color, and any **dysuria** (painful or difficult urination). The first voiding is occasionally blood tinged because of the trauma of the procedure.

The urologist can perform a brush biopsy via a ureteral catheter during a cystoscopy. A nylon brush is inserted through the catheter to obtain specimens from the renal pelvis or calyces. Nephroscopy (renal endoscopy) done via the percutaneous route (i.e., through the skin) provides direct visualization of the upper urinary structures. The urologist can obtain biopsy or urine specimens or remove calculi.

RENAL ANGIOGRAPHY

The use of renal angiography helps to evaluate blood supply to the kidneys, assesses masses, and detects possible complications after kidney transplantation. Withhold oral intake the night before the procedure. The procedure requires passing a small catheter into an artery (usually the femoral artery) to provide a port for the injection of radiopaque dye. Therefore, when the procedure is completed, the patient must lie flat in bed for several hours to minimize the risk of bleeding. Assess the puncture site for bleeding or hematoma, and maintain the pressure dressing at the site. Assess the circulatory status of the involved extremity every 15 minutes for 1 hour and then every 2 hours for 24 hours.

RENAL VENOGRAPHY

Renal venography provides information about the kidneys' venous drainage. The catheter through which a radiopaque dye is injected is inserted into the femoral vein. Care after the procedure includes assessment of vital signs. Monitor the patient for bleeding at the puncture site. Assess for bruising and swelling at the site. Assess pulses distal to the puncture site. Potential complications after the procedure include allergic reaction to the dye, bleeding, clots, or injury to the vein.

COMPUTED TOMOGRAPHY

A computed tomography (CT) scan differentiates masses in the kidney. Images are obtained by a computer-controlled scanner. A radiopaque dye may be injected to enhance the images. Serum urea and creatinine levels are obtained before use of radiopaque dye. The dye is not used if inadequate kidney function is noted. Inform the patient that the table on which he or she is placed and the machine "taking pictures" will move at intervals and that it is important to lie still. The CT body-scanning unit takes multiple cross-sectional pictures at several different sites, creating a three-dimensional map of the renal structure. The adrenal glands, the bladder, and the prostate also may be visualized.

MAGNETIC RESONANCE IMAGING

Magnetic resonance imaging (MRI) uses nuclear magnetic resonance as its source of energy to obtain a visual assessment of body tissues. The patient requires no special preparation other than removal of all metal objects that may be attracted by the magnet. Patients with metal prostheses (such as heart valves, orthopedic screws, or cardiac pacemakers) cannot undergo MRI.

Emphasize that the examination area will be confining and that a repetitive "pounding" sound will be heard (somewhat like the sound of a muffled jackhammer). MRI can be used to diagnose pathologic conditions of the renal system.

RENAL SCAN

A radionuclide tracer substance that will be taken up by renal tubular cells or excreted by the glomerular filtrate is injected intravenously. A series of computer-generated images then is made. The scan provides data related to functional parenchyma (the essential parts of an organ that are concerned with its function). No special patient preparation is needed. Check facility policy concerning the disposal of the patient's urine for the first 24 hours. Pregnant nurses should refrain from caring for patients administered radioactive substances.

ULTRASONOGRAPHY

Ultrasonography is a diagnostic tool that uses the reflection of sound waves to produce images of deep body structures. Inform the patient that a conducting jelly will be applied on the skin over the area to be studied; this improves the transmission of sound waves. The sound waves are high frequency and inaudible to the human ear; the waves are converted into electrical impulses that are photographed for study.

Ultrasonography can visualize size, shape, and position of the kidney and delineate any irregularities in structure. Deviations from normal findings may indicate tumors, congenital anomalies, cysts, or obstructions. No special patient preparation is necessary.

TRANSRECTAL ULTRASOUND

Transrectal ultrasound instrumentation of the prostate gland provides clear images of prostatic tumors that otherwise may go undiagnosed. Transrectal ultrasound–guided biopsy is performed to obtain samples of prostatic tissue from various areas with minimal discomfort to the patient.

RENAL BIOPSY

The kidney can be biopsied by an open procedure similar to other surgical procedures on the kidney or by the less invasive method of needle biopsy, also called a *percutaneous biopsy*. Inform the patient that he or she may experience pain during the procedure and should follow instructions, such as holding the breath. Bed rest is important for 24 hours after the procedure. Mobility is restricted to bathroom privileges for the next 24 hours, and gradual resumption of activities is allowed after 48 to 72 hours. Potential complications associated with the procedure include infection, damage to the kidney, and bleeding. Teach the patient to report signs of complications including temperature elevations, unrelieved pain, and difficulty voiding.

URODYNAMIC STUDIES

Urodynamic studies are indicated when neurologic disease is thought to be the underlying cause of incontinence. These studies evaluate the activity level of the urinary bladder muscle (detrusor). This may cause the patient to be embarrassed and somewhat uncomfortable. A simple urodynamic study is cystometrography, in which a catheter is inserted into the bladder and then connected to a cystometer, which measures bladder capacity and pressure. The examiner asks the patient about sensations of heat, cold, and urge to void and instructs the patient at times to void and change position.

Cholinergic and anticholinergic medications may be administered during urodynamic studies to determine their effects on bladder function. A cholinergic drug, such as bethanechol (Urecholine), stimulates an atonic bladder; an anticholinergic drug, such as atropine, brings an overactive bladder to a more normal level or function.

Associated testing includes rectal electromyography, which involves placement of an electrode into the anal sphincter; and a urethral pressure profile, in which a special catheter connected to a transducer evaluates urethral pressures.

MEDICATION CONSIDERATIONS

The kidneys filter a wide range of water-soluble products from the blood, including medications. The kidneys' ability to remove certain medications from the blood may be affected by various conditions, such as renal disease, changes in the urine pH, and age. Patients with renal disease are given smaller doses of medications to minimize further damage or drug toxicity. Alteration in urinary pH affects the absorption rate of certain medications. Older patients may have decreased physiologic functioning, diminishing the kidneys' capacity to excrete drugs. Diminished kidney function interferes with the filtration of water-soluble medications.

The medications included in this discussion are representative of those that directly affect kidney function or are used to treat urinary disorders.

DIURETICS TO ENHANCE URINARY OUTPUT

Diuretics enhance urinary output by increasing the filtration of sodium, chloride, and water at various sites in the kidney. Diuretics are used in the management of a variety of disorders, such as heart failure and hypertension. Diuretics are classified by chemical structure and by the site and type of action in the kidney.

Thiazide Diuretics

Thiazide diuretics such as chlorothiazide (Diuril) act at the distal convoluted tubule to impair sodium and chloride reabsorption, leading to excretion of electrolytes and water. In addition to their intended effects, thiazide diuretics can cause hypokalemia (extreme potassium depletion in blood), hyponatremia (decreased sodium concentration in blood), and/or hypercalcemia (excessive amounts of calcium in blood). Hypochloremic alkalosis occurs from a deficiency of chloride. The primary indication for use is to manage systemic edema and control mild to moderate hypertension. It may take a month to achieve the full antihypertensive effect. Chlorothiazide is contraindicated in **anuria** (urinary output of less than 100 mL/day).

Loop (or High-Ceiling) Diuretics

Loop, or *high-ceiling, diuretics* such as furosemide (Lasix) act primarily in the ascending loop of Henle to inhibit tubular reabsorption of sodium and chloride. This group is the most potent of all diuretics and may lead to significant electrolyte depletion. These diuretics are effective for use in patients with impaired kidney function.

In addition to their intended effects, loop diuretics can cause hypokalemia, hypochloremia, hyponatremia, hypocalcemia (abnormally low blood calcium), and/or hypomagnesemia (decreased magnesium in the blood). Their effect on the acid-base balance can lead to the development of hypochloremic alkalosis. Furosemide is used in nephrotic syndrome, heart failure, and pulmonary edema. Side effects are those associated with rapid fluid loss: vertigo, hypotension, and possible circulatory collapse.

Potassium-Sparing Diuretics

Potassium-sparing diuretics act on the distal convoluted tubule to inhibit sodium reabsorption and potassium secretion. Potassium-sparing diuretics decrease the sodium-potassium exchange. Although the actions of these medications vary, they all conserve potassium that usually is lost with sodium in diuresis. However, because they are weak, they usually are used in combination with other diuretics. Potassium-sparing diuretics are contraindicated in patients with hyperkalemia because further retention of potassium could cause a fatal cardiac dysrhythmia. There are two types of potassium-sparing diuretics: aldosterone antagonists and nonaldosterone antagonists. (Note: Cells function and communicate with each other by means of receptors on their surface. Natural ligands bind to these receptors and cause something specific to happen: each receptor type binds to a particular ligand. *Agonists* and *antagonists* are drugs that mimic a receptor's natural ligand, but with opposite effects: an antagonist prevents a particular cell response, and an agonist usually prolongs that response.)

The aldosterone antagonist spironolactone (Aldactone) blocks aldosterone in the distal tubule to promote potassium uptake in exchange for sodium secretion. Although it can be used in combination with other diuretics, primarily in the treatment of hypertension and edema, spironolactone is used most frequently for its potassium-sparing quality.

The nonaldosterone antagonist triamterene (Dyrenium) directly reduces ion transportation in the distal tubule, although it has little diuretic effect. Triamterene is used instead to help limit the potassium-wasting effect of other diuretics.

Osmotic Diuretics

Osmotic diuretics act at the proximal convoluted tubule to increase plasma osmotic pressure, causing redistribution of fluid toward the circulatory vessels. Osmotic diuretics are used to manage edema, promote systemic diuresis in cerebral edema, decrease intraocular pressure, and improve kidney function in acute renal failure (ARF). In ARF, osmotics are used to prevent irreversible failure, but they are contraindicated in advanced stages of renal failure.

An example of an osmotic diuretic is mannitol (Osmitrol). It increases the osmolarity of glomerular filtrate; decreases reabsorption of water electrolytes; and increases urinary output, sodium excretion, and chloride excretion, while exerting only a minimal effect on the acid-base balance. Mannitol is used to prevent or treat the oliguric phase of ARF, promote systemic diuresis in cerebral edema, and decrease intraocular pressure. Careful assessment of the cardiovascular system before administering mannitol is essential because of the high risk of inducing heart failure. Avoid extravasation (escape of the medication from the blood vessel into the tissues), which may lead to tissue irritation or necrosis.

Carbonic Anhydrase Inhibitor Diuretics

The enzyme carbonic anhydrase (present in red blood cells) converts water and carbon dioxide to bicarbonate, helping to maintain the acid-base balance in the blood. In the proximal convoluted tubules of the kidneys, acetazolamide (Diamox) inhibits this enzyme, which leads to diuresis; therefore acetazolamide is called a *carbonic anhydrase inhibitor diuretic*. It has limited usefulness as a diuretic and is used to lower intraocular pressure.

Nursing Interventions

Because patients receiving diuretics often have complicated disease conditions such as heart failure and pulmonary edema, monitor for signs and symptoms of fluid overload: changes in pulse rate, respirations, cardiac sounds, and lung fields. Record daily morning weights for the patient receiving diuretics. Keep accurate intake and output (I&O) records, and document blood pressure, pulse, and respirations four times a day for the patient on diuretic therapy. Assess BUN, serum electrolytes, and urine as ordered. When instructing the patient and the family about diet, include a warning to avoid overuse of salt in cooking or as a table additive. Several salt substitutes are currently on the market; however, the long-term effects of those potassium preparations are not known and could complicate the renal patient's condition further. The use of most diuretics, with the exception of the potassium-sparing diuretics, requires adding daily potassium sources (e.g., baked potatoes, raw bananas, apricots, or navel oranges). In some cases the health care provider orders potassium supplements to be taken with the diuretic.

When a diuretic is effective, the serum concentration of other medications may increase as a result. Carefully monitor this potentiating effect to prevent toxicity from other medications. For example, as diuretics effectively decrease the volume of extracellular fluid, the serum level of digoxin may increase proportionately, resulting in digitoxicity. Special care is required in the selection and management of diuretics in the treatment of children, adolescents, and older adults.

MEDICATIONS FOR URINARY TRACT INFECTIONS

Certain antimicrobial agents are administered primarily to treat infections within the urinary tract. Culture and sensitivity testing are used to aid in the selection of the medication that will eradicate the identified pathogen. Urinary antiseptics inhibit bacterial growth and are used to prevent and treat urethritis and cystitis. The health history should include factors such as pregnancy and allergies to ensure the correct medications for the individual are selected.

Medications used to manage urinary tract infections include several categories of medications. Representatives from classes frequently used are listed below.

Quinolones

In the past the quinolone nalidixic acid frequently was used to treat UTIs caused by gram-negative microbes (e.g., *Escherichia coli* and *Proteus mirabilis*). There were problems with the absorption rate of the medication and limited activity. Newer agents, the fluoroquinolones, include ciprofloxacin, which has gram-negative bacteria, and levofloxacin and norfloxacin, which work against gram-positive and gram-negative bacteria (e.g., *E. coli, P. mirabilis, Pseudomonas* organisms, *Staphylococcus aureus,* and *Staphylococcus epidermidis*). It is used in the treatment of UTIs, gonorrhea, and gonococcal urethritis. It is administered with a full glass of water 1 hour before or 2 hours after meals or with antacids.

The common side effects are headaches, nausea, vomiting, and diarrhea.

Nitrofurantoin

Nitrofurantoin (Macrodantin, Macrobid) is effective against gram-positive and gram-negative microbes (e.g., *Streptococcus faecalis, E. coli,* and *P. mirabilis*) in the urinary tract. Common side effects are loss of appetite, nausea, and vomiting.

Methenamine

Methenamine hippurate (Mandelamine) suppresses fungi and gram-negative and gram-positive organisms (e.g., *E. coli,* staphylococci, and enterococci). Acidification of the urine by means of an acid-ash diet (such as a diet high in meat, whole grains, eggs, cheese, cranberries, prunes, and plums) or other acidifiers to a pH of less than 5.5 is necessary for effective action. Methenamine mandelate is used for patients with chronic, recurrent UTIs as a preventive measure after antibiotics have cleared the infection. Although side effects are rare, they include nausea, vomiting, skin rash, and urticaria (hives).

NURSING INTERVENTIONS

Before administering antibiotics for UTIs, be certain to check all medications the patient is using for potential negative drug interactions. Instruct the patient to complete the full course of the medication, even though the symptoms may subside quickly. Hydrate the patient to produce a daily urinary output of 2000 mL, unless contraindicated. When indicated, teach the patient to consume an acid-ash diet to help maintain a urine pH of 5.5. Soothe skin irritations with cornstarch or a bath of bicarbonate of soda or dilute vinegar. Report continuing signs of infection.

Monitor the patient receiving nitrofurantoin for signs of allergic response such as erythema, chills, fever, and dyspnea. If these signs or symptoms develop, discontinue the medication and notify the health care provider (trial doses of this medication may be used to detect a possible allergic reaction before administering the full dose).

NUTRITIONAL CONSIDERATIONS

The nutritional needs of the patient with a urinary tract disorder vary with each disease process. Some general guidelines include provision of food choices and number of servings as recommended by the US Department of Agriculture's MyPlate nutrition planning tool and a daily intake of 2000 mL of water, unless contraindicated. Unique nutritional requirements are discussed with each disorder. Box 50.2 gives an example of dietary modifications to prevent urolithiasis (calculi or stones formed anywhere in the urinary system). Patients with other systemic diseases, such as diabetes mellitus, require strict adherence to those restrictions as well.

MAINTAINING ADEQUATE URINARY DRAINAGE

Urine clears the body of waste materials and helps balance electrolytes. Conditions that interfere with urinary drainage may create a health crisis. Therefore it is important to reestablish urine flow as soon as possible to prevent the buildup of toxins in the bloodstream. Patients at risk for difficulty with urine elimination include those who have undergone surgical procedures of the bladder, the prostate, or the vagina; patients with primary urologic problems, such as urethral stricture (an abnormal narrowing of the urethra); and those who are critically ill with multisystem problems.

Urinary catheters are used to maintain urine flow, to divert urine flow to facilitate healing postoperatively, to introduce medications by irrigation, and to dilate or prevent narrowing of some portion of the urinary tract. Catheters may be used for intermittent or continuous urinary drainage. Urinary catheters may be introduced into the bladder, the ureter, or the kidney. The type and size of urinary catheter are determined by where it is to be placed and by the cause of the urinary tract problem. Catheter size is measured by the French (Fr) system: 1 French (1 Fr) equals a diameter of 0.3 mm. Urethral catheters range from 14 Fr to 24 Fr for adult patients. Ureteral catheters are usually 4 Fr to 6 Fr. The health care provider always inserts ureteral catheters, whereas the nurse usually inserts indwelling urethral catheters.

TYPES OF CATHETERS

Catheter type varies by purpose (Fig. 50.5). The *coudé catheter* has a tapered tip and is selected for ease of insertion when enlargement of the prostate gland is suspected. The coudé catheter is less traumatic during insertion because it is stiffer and more easily controlled than the straight-tip catheter. The material used results in a reduced level of tissue irritation and encrustation when used for extended periods (Medline, 2017). The *Foley catheter* has a balloon near its tip that may be inflated after insertion, holding the catheter in the urinary bladder for continuous drainage. *Malecot* and *de Pezzer,* or *mushroom, catheters* are used to drain urine from the renal pelvis of the kidney. The *Robinson catheter* has multiple openings in its tip to facilitate intermittent drainage. *Ureteral catheters* are long and slender to pass into the ureters. The *whistle-tip catheter* has a slanted, larger orifice at its tip to be used if there is blood in the urine. The *cystostomy, vesicostomy,* or *suprapubic catheter* is introduced by the health care provider through the abdominal wall above the symphysis pubis. This catheter diverts urine flow from the urethra as needed to treat injury to the bony pelvis, the urinary tract, or surrounding organs; strictures; or obstruction. The catheter is inserted via surgical incision or puncture of the abdominal and bladder walls with a trocar (a sharp-pointed instrument). The catheter is connected to a sterile closed drainage system and secured to avoid accidental removal; the wound is covered with a sterile dressing. When the lower urinary tract has healed, the patient's ability to void is tested by clamping the catheter so that the patient can try to void naturally. When the measured **residual urine** (the amount left in the bladder after urination) is consistently less than 50 mL, the catheter usually is removed and a sterile dressing is placed over the wound.

An *external (Texas or condom) catheter* is not actually a catheter but rather a drainage system connected to the external male genitalia. This noninvasive appliance is used for the incontinent male to minimize skin irritation from urine and to reduce risk of infection from an indwelling catheter. The appliance is removed daily for cleansing and inspection of the skin. Use of the external catheter allows the patient to have a more normal lifestyle.

An external catheter has been developed for women who are experiencing incontinence. The device places a wick between the labia and the gluteus. This is then attached to a low suction which pulls the urine away. The wick is changed two to three times per day or when soiled (Purewick.com, n.d.).

Box 50.2 Acid-Ash and Alkaline-Ash Foods

ACID-ASH FOODS[a]

- Meat, whole grains, eggs, cheese, cranberries, prunes, and plums

ALKALINE-ASH FOODS

- Milk, vegetables, fruits (except cranberries, prunes, and plums)

[a]Acid-ash diets should be supplemented with vitamins C and A and with folic acid.

NURSING INTERVENTIONS AND PATIENT TEACHING

Problems of the urinary tract may be indicative of a primary disorder or may be one of multiple symptoms

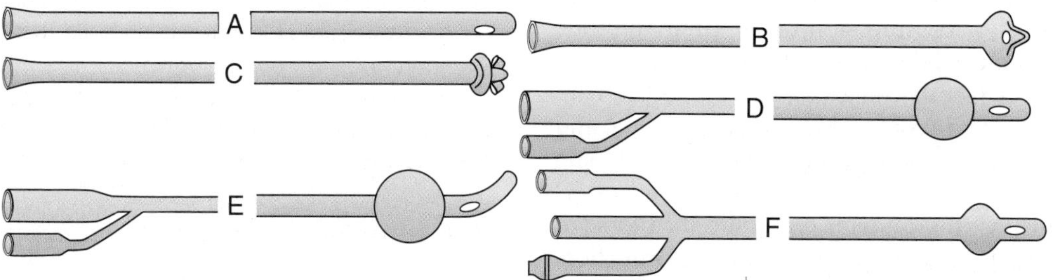

Fig. 50.5 Commonly used catheters. A, Simple urethral catheter. B, Mushroom or de Pezzer (can be used for suprapubic catheterization). C, Winged-tip or Malecot. D, Indwelling with inflated balloon. E, Indwelling with coudé tip. F, Three-way indwelling (the third lumen is used for irrigation of the bladder). (From Lewis SL, Heitkemper MM, Dirksen SR, et al: *Medical-surgical nursing: Assessment and management of clinical problems,* ed 7, St. Louis, 2007, Mosby.)

of complex, chronic disease. Therefore it is important to assess urinary elimination at the time of admission. Because of embarrassment and sociocultural taboos, some patients may be reluctant to share information with the nurse. Often the medical system intensifies this discomfort by repeatedly asking the patient to describe the problem to staff in the laboratory, radiology department, and other departments. Discretion during the admission interview and health assessment with strict adherence to Health Insurance Portability and Accountability Act standards enhance patient privacy and comfort.

Nursing interventions for the patient with a urinary drainage system involve considerations to prevent and detect infection and trauma:

1. Follow aseptic technique to avoid introducing microorganisms from the environment. Never rest the collecting bag on the floor.
2. Record I&O. For precision monitoring, such as hourly urinary output, add a urometer to the drainage system. If urinary output falls below 50 mL/h, check the drainage system for proper placement and function before contacting the health care provider.
3. Adequately hydrate the patient to flush the urinary tract.
4. Do not open the drainage system after it is in place except to irrigate the catheter, and then only with health care provider orders. It is important to maintain a closed system to prevent UTIs.
5. Perform catheter care twice daily and as needed, using standard precautions. Each institution has a specific protocol for catheter care. Cleanse the perineum (the region between the thighs, from the anus to the scrotum [in males] or vulva [in females]) with mild soap and warm water, from the front to the back; rinse well; and pat dry. At times an antiseptic solution or ointment may be ordered for use at the catheter incision site.
6. Check the drainage system daily for leaks.
7. Avoid placement of the urinary drainage bag above the level of the catheter insertion, which would cause urine to reenter the drainage system and contaminate the urinary tract.
8. Prevent tension on the system or backflow of urine while transferring the patient.
9. Ambulate the patient if possible to facilitate urine flow. If the patient's activity must be restricted, turn and reposition every 1½ hours.
10. Avoid kinks or compression of the drainage tube that may cause pooling of the urine within the urinary tract. Gently coil excess tubing, secure with a clamp or pin to avoid dislodging the catheter, and release the tubing before transferring or repositioning the patient.
11. Gently inspect the catheter entry site for blood or exudate that may indicate trauma or infection. Observe the color and composition of the urine for blood or sediment. During drainage of the collection bag, note the presence of odor that is not consistent with the normal smell of urine.
12. Collect specimens from the catheter by cleansing the drainage port with alcohol and then withdrawing the urine with a sterile adapter and a sterile 10-mL syringe, using standard precautions. Send the urine specimen immediately to the laboratory.
13. Report and record assessment findings and interventions initiated.

After the urinary catheter is removed, the patient may experience difficulty voiding until bladder tone and sensation return. If the patient complains of urinary retention, stimulate urination by running water, placing the patient's hands in water, or pouring water over the perineum. With the last method, subtract the amount of water used in calculating the correct amount voided. If the patient's condition permits, a woman can sit on a bathroom stool or commode, and a male can stand, to void.

The patient may experience some dribbling of urine after voiding as a result of dilation of the sphincter from the catheter. Record the time, amount, and color of the urinary output. Nursing care for patients who have had their indwelling catheter removed includes assessment of the volume voided, review of intake with consideration to output, and bladder palpation to ensure urinary retention is not occurring.

Patient problem statements and interventions for the patient with a urinary catheter include but are not limited to the following:

Patient Problem	Nursing Interventions
Potential for Trauma, related to insertion and maintenance of the catheter	Maintain sterile technique during insertion Use smallest size catheter possible Lubricate catheter Secure catheter to leg, as appropriate Provide adequate fluids Administer urinary analgesic as ordered Allow enough slack in tubing for patient to move about freely while in bed Inspect insertion site to determine whether area is clean and without signs of possible infection or bleeding
Potential for Infection, related to invasive use of catheter	Use aseptic technique and meticulous catheter care Maintain closed urinary drainage system Avoid placement of drainage bag above level of catheter insertion (meatus) Avoid reflux of urine Encourage adequate fluid intake Administer antimicrobials as ordered Monitor patient's temperature and the color, odor, and clarity of urine

Instruct the patient about proper transfer from bed, chair, or stretcher and the principles of catheter care. Encourage fluid intake to flush the urinary system.

Self-Catheterization

Self-catheterization may be the intervention of choice for the patient who experiences spinal cord injury or other neurologic disorders that interfere with urinary elimination. Intermittent self-catheterization promotes independent function. At home there is less risk of cross-contamination than in the hospital, so the catheterization procedure can be modified safely as a clean technique. Nevertheless, instruct the patient in the use of strict surgical asepsis in the hospital because of the risk of infection there. Emphasize the need for the patient to be alert for signs and symptoms of infection and to undergo periodic evaluations by the health care provider. Follow institutional guidelines for catheter insertion.

Bladder Training

Bladder training involves developing the muscles of the perineum to improve voluntary control over voiding; bladder training may be modified for different problems. In preparation for removal of a urethral catheter, the health care provider may order a clamp-unclamp routine to improve bladder tone. This method was once widely used but is now less common. A patient with stress incontinence can learn to control leakage by performing **Kegel exercises,** or *pubococcygeal exercises,* that tighten the muscles of the perineal floor. The patient can develop awareness of the appropriate muscle group by trying to stop the flow of urine during voiding. Once the patient has identified the correct muscles and the feeling of their contraction, direct her to tighten the muscles of the perineum, hold that tension for 10 seconds, and then relax for 10 seconds. The exercises should be done initially in groups of 10, building to groups of 20, four times a day. Because muscle control develops gradually, it may take 4 to 6 weeks to learn to control leakage.

For habit training, establish a voiding schedule. Monitor the patient's voiding for a few days to identify patterns, or schedule voiding times to correlate with the patient's activities. Typical voiding times are on arising, before each meal, and at bedtime. Help the patient void as scheduled. After a few days, evaluate whether the scheduled voiding pattern keeps the patient continent. Modify the schedule until continence is established. Fluid intake and medications may influence voiding patterns (e.g., the patient may need to void 30 minutes after ingesting coffee or furosemide in response to the diuretic effect). Reduction of fluid intake before bedtime may help keep the patient dry during sleep.

PROGNOSIS

The outcome for patients with urinary disorders depends on many variables: age, preexisting health conditions, general health status, complications, compliance, and available family and community support.

DISORDERS OF THE URINARY SYSTEM

ALTERATIONS IN VOIDING PATTERNS

URINARY RETENTION

Etiology and Pathophysiology

Urinary retention is the inability to void even with an urge to void. The patient may not be able to empty the bladder, creating urinary stasis and increasing the possibility of infection. Bladder capacity may be exceeded, and the urine may overflow the bladder, causing incontinence. The condition may be acute or chronic. Individuals experiencing acute urinary retention may be completely unable to void despite having a full bladder. Chronic retention is characterized by a sense of the need to void but being unable to completely empty the bladder (Cleveland Clinic, 2014).

Urinary retention has a variety of causes that may be classified as obstructive, infectious/inflammatory, pharmacologic, neurologic, or other. Obstructions may include calculi or tumor. Infectious/inflammatory processes include urinary tract infections and pyelonephritis. Medications implicated in urinary retention include antiarrhythmics such as disopyramide (Norpace); antihistamines such as fexofenadine (Allegra) and diphenhydramine (Benadryl); antispasmodics/anticholinergics including oxybutynin; and tricyclic antidepressants including imipramine (Tofranil) and amitriptyline (NIDDK, 2014). Damage to the nerves controlling bladder emptying may be the result of spinal cord injury, stroke, or postoperative complications resulting in interference with the sphincter muscles. Other potential causes may include childbirth or other trauma.

Clinical Manifestations

The signs and symptoms of urinary retention are sometimes vague and easily overlooked. The bladder becomes increasingly distended and may be palpated above the symphysis pubis. Urinary retention may cause the patient considerable discomfort and anxiety.

Assessment

Subjective data include patient complaints of frequency with or without symptoms of burning, urgency, nocturia, and occasionally acute discomfort. Initial symptoms may not seem to be associated directly with urinary retention.

Collection of objective data includes assessing urinary bladder distention (palpable ovoid [egg-shaped] bladder arising suprapubically). The patient may void frequently, void small amounts, and have episodes of incontinence. Patients with diminished sensorium, as from spinal cord injury or organic brain disorder, may be restless and irritable without direct complaints about difficulty voiding.

Medical Management

Diagnostic studies used to confirm diagnosis and potential causes include laboratory studies such as urinalysis, serum blood urea nitrogen, and prostate-specific antigen and imaging studies including renal, bladder, and pelvic ultrasonography, and CT of the abdomen and pelvis.

Mechanical methods, such as the use of urinary catheters or the surgical release of obstructions, may be needed to treat urinary retention. Administer urinary analgesics and antispasmodics as prescribed to enhance patient relaxation and comfort. Continued medical treatments focus on alleviating the underlying cause.

Nursing Interventions

The primary goal of nursing interventions is the reinstitution of normal voiding patterns. Regardless of the pathologic findings and medical intervention, help the patient achieve adequate voiding by providing a private, relaxed environment. Bladder training approaches may assist the patient in emptying the bladder. Warm showers or sitz baths may promote relaxation of the abdominal, gluteal, and sphincter muscles. Provide warm beverages to help the patient relax. If possible, permit the patient whatever position is preferred for voiding: for women, sitting on a commode or bathroom stool is best; for men, standing may be more natural.

When continence is established, the patient may be catheterized intermittently to determine whether the bladder is emptying. Allow the patient to void and measure the amount. Catheterize the patient immediately after the voiding and measure the amount retained in the bladder; this is *residual urine* and should be less than 50 mL. If the underlying pathologic condition remains unchanged, this patient may be at risk for again developing retention. Urinary retention also can be the root cause of repeated urinary tract infections. Teach the patient or primary caretaker to observe for signs and symptoms of urinary retention and to notify the health care provider immediately if they return.

A patient problem statement and interventions for the patient with urinary retention include but are not limited to the following:

Patient Problem	Nursing Interventions
Retaining Urine or Inability to Urinate, related to: • Sensory or motor impairment • Neuromuscular impairment • Mechanical trauma	Establish urinary drainage Develop a voiding schedule Teach the patient Kegel exercises Assist with skin care Suggest use of protective clothing Engage patient in social activities Teach importance of adequate fluid intake Ensure that patient verbalizes an understanding of factors that alter urinary pattern

URINARY INCONTINENCE

Urinary incontinence (UI) refers to the loss of bladder control. It may range from leaking to full loss of the bladder's contents. An estimated 20 million Americans are affected by urinary continence; 85% of that total are women. Underreporting is likely, given the potential embarrassment related to the condition (Mayo Clinic, n.d.).

Etiology and Pathophysiology

UI is the involuntary loss of urine from the bladder. The patient may be totally incontinent, have dribbling, or experience leakage while lifting or sneezing (stress incontinence). Incontinence may arise as a complication of many disorders, such as UTI, loss of sphincter control, or sudden change of pressure within the abdomen. Incontinence may be permanent, as with spinal cord trauma, or temporary, as with pregnancy. Women with weakened structures of the pelvic floor are prone to stress incontinence. Although incontinence may occur at any age, loss of control of urination is a particular problem for older adults.

Physical exertion such as heavy lifting, jobs that require long periods of standing, and high-impact sports may increase an individual's risk for UI. UI may also result from physiologic conditions such as obesity, chronic lung disease, smoking, pelvic floor injury, and surgery. Lack of estrogen in postmenopausal women contributes to atrophy of the vaginal and urethral walls with subsequent loss of muscle tone that may result in postvoiding urine retention and possible prolapse of the bladder.

There are various types of incontinence, which are classified according to their causes. Types of incontinence include the following (Mayo Clinic, 2017):

- *Stress incontinence:* Results from the pressure or stressors on the bladder sphincter by events such as sneezing or heavy lifting
- *Urge incontinence:* Feelings of an urgency to void followed by incontinence. It is associated with conditions such as Parkinson's disease and Alzheimer's disease
- *Overflow incontinence:* Repeated inability to fully empty the bladder results in an overly full bladder, which leaks out unexpectedly
- *Mixed incontinence:* A mixture of stress and urge incontinence
- *Functional incontinence:* The influence of mental and physical impairments resulting in an inability to make it to the toilet in time to void

Clinical Manifestations

The cardinal sign of UI is the involuntary loss of urine, which may or may not be the primary reason the patient seeks treatment.

Assessment

Subjective data include information concerning the patient's inability to control the urine. Determine factors related to the episodes of incontinence. Review voiding patterns and behaviors.

Collection of objective data requires alertness for clues that the patient is experiencing difficulty controlling the flow of urine. Follow the assessment guidelines to clarify the patient's complaints. Although more common in women, UI is a common symptom for men who have benign prostatic hypertrophy (BPH) and should be included in the assessment.

Medical Management

The management of incontinence depends on the underlying cause. If the problem arises from a disorder within the neck of the bladder, surgical repair may be necessary. Incontinence related to sphincter or urethral weakness may be treated by infecting bulking materials into the tissue surrounding the urethra. This offers support and keeps it closed preventing loss of urine. Botulinum toxin type A (Botox) may be used to manage overactive bladder. The medication is injected into the bladder muscle. Temporary or permanent urinary diversion by an indwelling catheter may be indicated. A nerve stimulator may be implanted to emit an electrical stimulus to the nerves of the bladder. This is implanted under the skin in the buttock, providing access to the sacral nerves.

The **pessary** is a device that can be inserted into the vagina to support the bladder and to reduce pressure on the bladder from the uterus in cases of prolapse (Fig. 50.6). This option is beneficial to those patients who are not candidates for surgery or pharmacologic management. It also may be the first line of treatment before more aggressive management approaches are attempted.

Management of stress incontinence should include behavior modification, pelvic floor muscle therapies (Kegel exercises), medications, and mechanical devices before resorting to surgical procedures. If these strategies are not effective, surgical interventions offer other treatment options. One procedure is the transvaginal tape sling procedure. The surgeon passes a permanent polypropylene mesh tape, covered by a protective plastic sheath with stainless steel needles attached at each end, through a small incision in the anterior vaginal wall. The U-shaped sling supports the urethra during stress and increased intraabdominal pressure during routine activities. This procedure is not without difficulties. Careful patient teaching is important before any surgical treatment.

Estrogen replacement for the treatment of UI is controversial, and its reported effectiveness varies. Topical administration of prednisone and estrogen may help restore turgor and elasticity of the vaginal submucosa. Transdermal oxybutynin (Oxytrol) is effective in reducing the symptoms of an overactive bladder with few side effects. A new self-catheterization system, the Self-Cath Closed System, is available for patients who must maintain intermittent self-catheterization. It is designed for patient convenience and minimization of bacterial contamination. An artificial urinary sphincter is a surgical option to reestablish continence, although there is controversy over its use.

Nursing Interventions

The incontinent patient may reduce fluid intake to decrease voiding, but without adequate fluids, urine may become more concentrated, irritating the bladder mucosa and increasing the urge to urinate. Therapeutic dietary modifications to assist in the management of urinary incontinence include avoidance of alcohol, caffeine, and spicy foods, which may be sources of bladder irritation, resulting in urgency and ultimately incontinence. Discuss timing of intake to avoid late hours just before retiring. Bladder training exercises may be implemented to improve the tone of the perineal muscles (Mayo Clinic, 2017). For the female patient, Kegel exercises are helpful; 10 repetitions, 5 to 10 times a day is suggested to improve muscle tone. Establish a 2-hour schedule for the patient to go to the bathroom. Once continence has been achieved, the goal may be raised to 3 hours.

Incontinence pads of various absorbencies are available in most grocery stores and pharmacies. They can increase the patient's confidence to participate in social activities. Use of protective undergarments may help keep the patient and the patient's clothing dry.

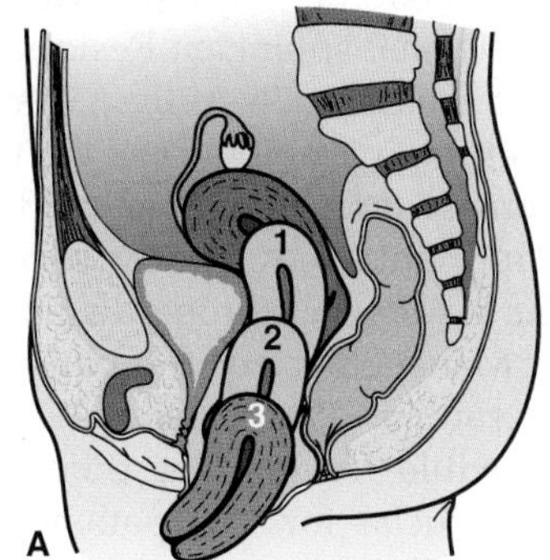

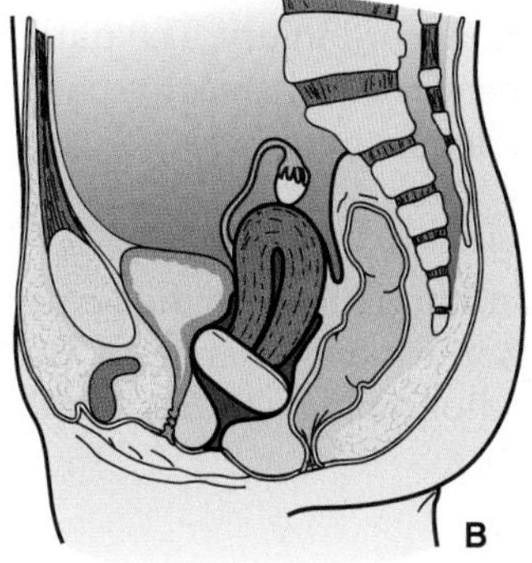

Fig. 50.6 A, Uterine prolapse. B, Donut pessary in place to correct uterine prolapse. (From Phillips NF: *Berry & Kohn's operating room technique,* ed 12, St. Louis, 2013, Mosby.)

Many patients who are incontinent have low self-esteem. Be supportive by listening, encouraging the patient to express feelings, and providing kind reassurances. Never scold the patient.

NEUROGENIC BLADDER

Etiology and Pathophysiology

Neurogenic bladder means the loss of voluntary voiding control, resulting in urinary retention or incontinence. Neurogenic bladder is caused by a lesion of the nervous system that interferes with normal nerve conduction to the urinary bladder. The lesion may be caused by a congenital anomaly (e.g., spina bifida), a neurologic disease (e.g., multiple sclerosis), or trauma (as in spinal cord injury). The two types of neurogenic bladder are *spastic* and *flaccid*.

Spastic (reflex or automatic) bladder is caused by an upper motor neuron lesion (above the voiding reflex arc) that results in a loss of the urge to void and a loss of motor control. The bladder wall atrophies, decreasing bladder capacity. Urine is released on reflex, with little or no conscious control.

A flaccid (atonic, nonreflex) bladder, caused by a lower motor neuron lesion (below the voiding reflex arc), continues to fill and distend, with pooling of urine and incomplete emptying. Because of the accompanying loss of sensation, the patient may not experience discomfort that would indicate retention.

Clinical Manifestations

Identification of the disease process is the first step in assessing the potential problem of neurogenic bladder. Prevention of complications is a major concern; infection occurs from urinary stasis and repeated catheterization. Retention of urine may lead to backup of urine (reflux) into the upper urinary tract and to distention of structures of the urinary tract.

Assessment

Subjective data include patient complaints of diaphoresis, flushing, and nausea before reflex incontinence, or infrequent voiding.

Collection of objective data involves investigating the urinary status of the patient at risk for neurogenic bladder; this includes patients with a congenital anomaly, a neurologic disease, or a spinal cord injury. The patient with a spastic bladder experiences UI, whereas the patient with a flaccid bladder describes infrequent voiding.

Diagnostic Tests

To assess the type and extent of damage to the urinary tract, chemistry studies monitor any change in BUN and creatinine levels. Radiographic studies outline structural changes that occur.

Medical Management

Closely monitor patients identified as at risk for neurogenic bladder. Assess urinary function early in the course of treatment, and give antibiotics to treat signs of infection. The patient is aided by the use of parasympathomimetic medication (e.g., bethanechol) to increase the bladder's contractility. The patient may need to use intermittent self-catheterization or a urinary collection system if continence is not achieved.

Sacral nerve modulation (sacral neuromodulation) and stimulation. Electronic devices to modulate nerve impulses are used experimentally and in clinical practice for treating various bladder problems: urinary frequency, urgency, incontinence, chronic pain, and interstitial cystitis (IC).

Sacral nerve stimulation for urinary urge incontinence involves the use of a permanently implantable electrical stimulation device to change neuronal activity in the sacral efferent and afferent nerves to reduce urinary urge incontinence. The InterStim device, marketed by Medtronic Inc., delivers continuous low-level electrical impulses to the bladder and urethral sphincters via the sacral nerves. It corrects UI by modulating the neural reflexes, reducing stimulation to an overactive bladder, or by boosting stimulation to an underactive one. The mode of action of the impulses is unknown.

Four electrodes are connected to a battery-operated generator. The wire is inserted into the sacral foramen through a 2-cm incision. The end of the wire is tunneled across subcutaneous tissue, exits on the patient's back, and is connected to a temporary generator attached to the outside of the body. The patient tests this temporary implant for 1 to 2 weeks. If the patient achieves 50% continence, a permanent implant is put in place.

Nursing Interventions and Patient Teaching

The management goal for the patient with neurogenic bladder is to establish urinary elimination and prevent complications. Because neurologic function is disturbed, it may not be possible to reinstate normal voiding. The patient with a spastic bladder may be placed on a bladder training program, with self-stimulation used every 2 hours to empty the bladder: The patient tries to initiate voiding using bladder compressions by applying pressure to the abdomen suprapubically or by digital stimulation of the anal sphincter. Residual urine is measured then by catheterization. As the patient becomes more proficient in emptying the bladder, the time between catheterizations is increased until voiding is independent. It is important to educate the patient to be alert for signs of the bladder becoming distended.

Management of the patient with a flaccid bladder is similar. Place the patient on a 2-hour voiding schedule for bladder training. Issues of self-esteem are crucial for this patient to remain in social settings. Provide a supportive, sensitive environment for the patient to discuss ways to adapt to an altered self-image.

INFLAMMATORY AND INFECTIOUS DISORDERS OF THE URINARY SYSTEM

URINARY TRACT INFECTIONS

A UTI is caused by the multiplication of microorganisms in any urinary system structure. Infections may result from bacteria, viruses, or fungi. **Bacteriuria** (bacteria in the urine) is the most common of all nosocomial (hospital-acquired) infections. *Escherichia coli* is the most common pathogen. Risk factors associated with UTIs include instrumentation (catheterization, surgical manipulation, and invasive diagnostic testing such as a cystoscopy), diaphragm use, condom use, and conditions causing urinary stasis or retention. Immobility, sensory impairment, and multiple organ impairment may increase the chances of infection in older adults. Women are more susceptible to UTIs than men because the urethra is short and proximal to the vagina and rectum.

Etiology and Pathophysiology

UTIs are caused by pathogens that enter the urinary tract and may or may not cause symptoms. Normally the flushing of the urinary tract with urine is sufficient to wash away pathogens. However, some conditions interfere with this process; urinary obstruction, neurogenic bladder, ureterovesical or urethrovesical reflux, sexual intercourse, and catheterization may introduce bacteria into the urinary system. Many chronic health problems predispose the patient to a UTI: diabetes mellitus, multiple sclerosis, spinal cord injuries, hypertension, and renal diseases.

Changes in urinary tract homeostasis allow the concentration of bacteria and increase the risk of infection. The patient with a compromised immune system does not seem to be predisposed to UTI infections, but once the infection is established, that patient has difficulty recovering. Infections of the lower urinary tract increase the risk of infection of the upper urinary tract, especially if untreated.

Gram-negative microorganisms that commonly infect the urinary tract (e.g., *E. coli* and *Klebsiella, Proteus,* or *Pseudomonas* organisms) are usually from the gastrointestinal tract and ascend through the urinary meatus. Normally the body's defenses keep infections in check and clear them from the system before signs and symptoms appear. If there is incomplete emptying of the bladder or reflux of urine, the retained urine supports growth of bacteria.

Clinical Manifestations

The common signs and symptoms associated with UTI are urgency, frequency, burning on urination, and hematuria that is microscopic to gross (visible without the aid of a microscope). UTIs are identified by the location of the infection: urethritis (urethra), cystitis (urinary bladder), pyelonephritis (kidney), and prostatitis (prostate gland). Infections of the bladder are said to be *lower* UTIs, whereas infections of the kidneys are *upper* UTIs.

Assessment

Subjective data include patient complaints of pain or burning on urination, urgency, frequency, and **nocturia** (excessive urination at night). The patient also may have related **asthenia** (a general feeling of tiredness and listlessness). Abdominal discomfort, perineal pain, or back pain may be present, depending on the extent of the disease process and site of infection.

Collection of objective data involves palpation of the lower abdomen, which may produce discomfort over the urinary bladder. Urine may be cloudy or blood tinged.

Diagnostic Tests

Urine culture and bacteriologic tests confirm the diagnosis. For patients with recurrent UTIs or systemic disease, more detailed urologic studies, such as an IVP and a voiding cystogram, are completed to assess the extent of involvement and damage to the structures of the urinary tract. Microscopic inspection of the urine often reveals bacteria, *hematuria* (blood in the urine), and **pyuria** (pus in the urine). Prostatitis is confirmed by patient history and culture of prostatic fluid or tissue.

Medical Management

The goal of medical management is to eliminate bacteria from the urinary tract, thereby relieving symptoms, preventing damage to renal structures, and preventing spread of infection to other body systems. The primary care provider prescribes antiinfective medications. Medications to treat uncomplicated urinary tract infections often include a 3-day regimen of sulfamethoxazole-trimethoprim (Bactrim, Septra) or ciprofloxacin (Cipro). Longer therapies for 7 to 10 days of amoxicillin or ampicillin, nitrofurantoin (Furadantin, Macrodantin), and levofloxacin (Levaquin) also may be prescribed. Most patients report symptom relief in 24 to 48 hours (New York Times, 2017). It is important to instruct patients to complete the full prescribed therapy to aid in the prevention of recurrence. Many patients experience significant discomfort with voiding until the antiinfectives begin to take effect. Phenazopyridine, an over the counter medication, may be encouraged to manage the discomfort. Its use should be limited to 2 days. It will turn the urine's color to a bright orange.

Some individuals experience recurrent infections. They may be placed on longer-term prophylactic antibiotic therapies for an additional 6 months. If the infection is complicated by obstruction, that obstruction should be removed. For neurogenic bladder or other retention, intermittent catheterization permits urinary drainage (see the Complementary and Alternative Therapies box).

Nursing Interventions

Nursing interventions should be supportive, with patient education for adequate hydration and hygiene. Because these infections tend to recur or persist, patient education

Complementary and Alternative Therapies

Urinary Disorders

- Cranberry (Cranberry Plus, Ultra Cranberry) has been used to manage urinary tract infections (UTIs), particularly in women prone to recurrent infection. Studies supporting its use are limited. It also has been used to treat acute UTI. Monitor patients for lack of therapeutic effect.
- Echinacea stimulates the immune system and treats UTI. Patients with human immunodeficiency virus infections, including acquired immunodeficiency syndrome, tuberculosis, collagen disease, multiple sclerosis, or other autoimmune disease, should avoid its use. Echinacea should not be used in place of antibiotic therapy.
- Sea holly *(Eryngium campestre)*, specifically the above-ground plant parts, have a mild diuretic effect. The roots have an antispasmodic effect. The above-ground parts are used in UTI and prostatitis; the roots are used to treat kidney and bladder calculi, renal colic, kidney and urinary tract inflammation, and urinary retention.
- Nettle *(Urtica dioica)* currently is being investigated as an irrigation for the urinary tract and to treat benign prostatic hypertrophy. Patients with fluid retention caused by reduced cardiac or renal activity should not use this herb.
- Some believe that acupuncture applied to the abdominal meridian may help relieve cystitis.
- Some advocate massage with diluted rosemary, juniper, or lavender to aid in relieving pain associated with cystitis.

must include early detection. Comfort measures include a regimen of antiinfective agents, urinary analgesics (e.g., phenazopyridine), adequate fluid intake, and perineal care. If treatment is effective, the patient should receive relief quickly. Infection may spread from the urinary system to other parts of the body. *Urosepsis* is septic poisoning resulting from retention and absorption of urinary products in the tissues.

Because of the high incidence of nosocomial UTIs, it is important that regular staff in service periodically review the basic procedures for catheter insertion and maintenance. Patient education for those who practice self-catheterization should include return demonstration to evaluate the success of maintaining clean technique.

URETHRITIS

Etiology and Pathophysiology

Urethritis, inflammation of the urethra, is classified by the presence or absence of gonorrhea. Nongonorrheal urethritis is called *nonspecific urethritis (NSU)*. NSU may be caused by bacteria such as *Chlamydia* or by the protozoan *Trichomonas*. Viral causes include herpes simplex virus. Sensitivity to contraceptive spermicides also may result in urethritis. Bacteria are normally present in the urethra but do not cause problems unless the integrity of the mucous membrane or tissues is interrupted, as when a catheter is in place or trauma has occurred.

Clinical Manifestations

The clinical manifestations include inflammation of the urethra with pus formation in the mucus-forming glands within the urethral lining. With gonorrheal urethritis, acute infection of the mucous membrane of the urethra causes a purulent exudate from the meatus; the patient feels discomfort, frequency, and burning on urination.

Assessment

Subjective data vary: the patient may be asymptomatic or may complain of dysuria, urethral pruritus, and urethral discharge. Women may complain of vaginal discharge or vulvar irritation.

Collection of objective data includes light palpation of the lower abdomen, which may produce discomfort over the urinary bladder. Inspection of the urethra may reveal purulent exudates or inflammation. Culture and sensitivity tests may be ordered (to identify the microorganism and the antibiotics to which it is sensitive, respectively); follow the institution's procedure.

Diagnostic Tests

Diagnostic tests usually are limited to a Gram stain of the exudate to identify the pathogen.

Medical Management

The first step in medical management is prevention of injury to the urethra during catheterization or sexual intercourse. Treatment is based on identifying and treating the cause and providing symptomatic relief. Drugs that may be prescribed are sulfamethoxazole-trimethoprim (Bactrim, Septra), metronidazole (Flagyl), clotrimazole (Mycelex), and nystatin. Comfort measures include antibiotics, adequate fluid intake to flush the system, warm sitz baths, and special care of the perineum using clean technique.

Patients with continuous catheter drainage may use a traditional bedside bag or a leg bag. Some patients may opt to utilize a bag worn around the waist. This allows for increased privacy, improved ambulation and has a lessened impact on the activities of daily living as the bag is not outwardly obvious. The 1000 mL capacity and the antireflux valve allow the device to be work continuously (healthykin.com, n.d.).

Nursing Interventions

Nursing interventions focus on patient education: avoid sexual activity until the infection clears; take all medications, especially antibiotics, to ensure the infection is resolved; and use condoms for protection from reinfection. Instruct patients with sexually transmitted urethritis to refer their sexual partners for evaluation and testing if they had sexual contact in the 60 days preceding onset of the patient's symptoms or diagnosis.

CYSTITIS

Etiology and Pathophysiology

Cystitis is an inflammation of the wall of the urinary bladder, usually caused by urethrovesical reflux, introduction of a catheter or similar instrument, or contamination from feces. The most common microorganism causing acute cystitis is *E. coli*. Cystitis is most common in women because of the ease of entrance of pathogens through the short urethra, even during voiding. Conflicting data exist about the role of bubble baths, clothing, and hygiene in increasing the risk of cystitis in women. Cystitis in men usually occurs secondary to another infection, such as prostatitis or epididymitis (see the Patient Teaching box).

 **Patient Teaching**

Cystitis

- Teach the patient to cleanse the perineal area from front to back to prevent contamination by spread of pathogens (especially *E. coli*) from the rectum to the short urethra.
- Encourage drinking 2000 mL of liquids per day unless contraindicated.
- Instruct the patient to take all prescribed medications even though symptoms may subside quickly.
- Remind the patient to empty the bladder as soon after intercourse as possible.
- If UTIs are associated with intercourse, recommend cleansing the genitalia with soap and water before having sexual relations.
- Encourage showers instead of tub baths.
- Limit the use of bubble baths.
- Instruct the patient about early detection and testing with a urine test strip such as the Chemstrip 2 LN.

Clinical Manifestations

The common signs and symptoms associated with cystitis are dysuria, urinary frequency, and pyuria.

Assessment

Collection of subjective data includes assessment of the lower abdomen, which may produce discomfort over the urinary bladder. Patient complaints include burning on urination, dysuria, frequency, urgency, and nocturia. The urine may be cloudy, strong-smelling, or reflect hematuria. A low-grade fever also may be present (Mayo Clinic, 2012).

Collection of objective data includes a clean-catch or catheterized urinalysis with culture and sensitivity tests to aid in confirming the diagnosis and in determining the appropriate treatment.

Diagnostic Tests

Microscopic inspection of the urine often reveals bacteria and hematuria. A voiding cystogram may be used to identify reflux of urine into the bladder. Diagnosis is confirmed by a clean-catch, midstream urinalysis that reveals a bacterial count greater than 100,000 organisms/mL.

Medical Management

For cystitis without the complications of obstruction or other underlying pathologic conditions, medical management consists of short-term therapy with an antiinfective agent. If the treatment is effective, the patient should receive relief quickly. A repeat urinalysis 1 to 3 days after initiation of the medication confirms the effectiveness of the intervention.

Nursing Interventions and Patient Teaching

Nursing interventions focus on teaching that these infections tend to recur by either reinfection or persistent infection. Encourage the patient to drink 2000 mL of fluid per day. Record accurate I&O. Include early detection in the teaching. Long-term prophylaxis with low doses of medication may be necessary. A simple urine test, for example, the Chemstrip 2 LN, allows the patient to test the urine at the first sign of infection and to call the health care provider for a prescription.

Prognosis

Successful treatment depends on the patient's ability to adequately flush the urinary tract and complete the course of antibiotics prescribed.

INTERSTITIAL CYSTITIS

Etiology and Pathophysiology

Interstitial cystitis (IC) is a chronic pelvic pain disorder with recurring discomfort or pain in the urinary bladder and surrounding region. Up to an estimated 8 million Americans have interstitial cystitis. It can affect any age and gender, but it most commonly strikes women at age 30 to 40 years. The pathophysiology is unknown. Bacterial infection does not trigger it. It seems to be caused by a breech in the bladder's protective mucosal lining that allows urine to seep through to the bladder wall, resulting in pain, inflammation, and small vessel bleeding. The bladder wall is infiltrated by inflammatory cells, resulting in ulceration and scarring of the mucosa, spasm of the detrusor muscle, hematuria, urgency, frequency, and pain on urination (PubMed, 2012).

Diagnosing the condition may be challenging. It is often mistaken for a urinary tract infection, prostatitis, or overactive bladder. The diagnostic workup involves eliminating other potential causes. The absence of bacteria in the urinalysis or a negative urine culture supports the diagnosis.

ADLs and personal relationships may be disrupted by voiding patterns; some patients report voiding 60 times a day.

Clinical Manifestations

The common signs and symptoms associated with IC are similar to those of cystitis: dysuria, urinary frequency, and microscopic bleeding. IC is characterized by urinary frequency, urgency, suprapubic pain, and dyspareunia (abnormal pain during sexual intercourse); it often is associated with fibromyalgia and irritable bowel syndrome. Autoimmune, allergic, and infectious causes are being studied.

Assessment

Subjective data include complaints of discomfort over the urinary bladder, dysuria, frequency, urgency, and nocturia.

Collection of objective data includes assessment of the lower abdomen, which may produce discomfort over the urinary bladder and the lower quadrants of the abdomen. A clean-catch midstream sample for urinalysis is used to rule out infection. Cystoscopy and tissue biopsy are used to establish a differential diagnosis.

Medical Management

IC is difficult to treat. Pharmacologic therapies are geared at symptom management. Antihistamines such as hydroxyzine pamoate (Vistaril) help reduce urinary frequency. Amitriptyline and nortriptyline are two antidepressants that reduce the burning pain and frequency of urination. The only oral medication approved by the US Food and Drug Administration to treat the pain or discomfort of IC is pentosan polysulfate sodium. It improves the bladder's protective mucosal layer and relieves the pain of IC by decreasing the irritating effects of urine on the bladder wall. More invasive medication therapies may include dimethyl sulfoxide (DMA), heparin, or lidocaine instillation directly into the bladder. Nonpharmacologic management strategies include biofeedback and physical therapy to manage spasms of the pelvic floor. Dietary therapies also have received some attention. Patients may benefit from diets that avoid foods and beverages known to cause bladder irritation. These foods include aged cheeses, alcohol, artificial sweeteners, chocolate, citrus juices, onions, soy, caffeine, and tomatoes.

Relief of symptoms takes time: it may be 4 weeks to 3 months before significant improvement occurs. For immediate relief, a brief course of opioid analgesics may be prescribed.

Surgical interventions include studies of the effect of sacral nerve root stimulation via implantation of electrodes; cystectomy, with the creation of a urostomy; and urinary diversion. Some patients continue to experience pain even after surgery.

Nursing Interventions and Patient Teaching

Nursing interventions focus on pain control and comfort measures. Because all medications have side effects, patients must consult their health care provider before taking any prescription or over-the-counter medication. Pelvic floor exercise may help decrease urgency and nocturia. Patients may be asked to keep a daily bladder diary; this information can be used to make treatment decisions.

Teach the patient about dietary choices. A complete IC diet, self-management strategies, and other nonmedical management tools are available from the Interstitial Cystitis Association.

IC often is associated with a reduced quality of life. Embarrassment, pain, and inability to manage elimination may lead to withdrawal from business, social, and intimate relationships. The patient and significant others need psychosocial support to face an uncertain outcome.

Prognosis

Only about half of patients with IC recover fully. Until researchers find a cause and an effective treatment, symptoms continue.

PROSTATITIS

Etiology and Pathophysiology

Prostatitis, defined as inflammation and/or infection of the prostate gland, is a group of diseases. Bacterial prostatitis is caused by infectious organisms such as *Pseudomonas* organisms and *S. faecalis* traveling up the urethra. Nonbacterial prostatitis may result from a variety of conditions related to occlusion of the urethra, such as enlargement of the prostate gland.

Prostatodynia (pain in the prostate gland) manifests with neither inflammation nor infection but demonstrates the other symptoms typical of prostatitis.

Clinical Manifestations

The signs and symptoms vary in number and intensity. The patient may experience fever; chills; malaise; arthralgia; myalgia; perineal prostatic pain; dysuria; obstructive urinary tract symptoms, including frequency, urgency, dysuria, nocturia, hesitancy, weak stream, and incomplete voiding; low back pain; low abdominal pain; spontaneous urethral discharge; ejaculatory pain; and erectile dysfunction. Chronic bacterial prostatitis may be asymptomatic. Edema of the prostate gland may serve as an obstruction, causing urinary retention as a complication to the prostatitis. Pooling of urine also may foster stone formation. Other complications are epididymitis, pyelonephritis, and bacteremia (the presence of bacteria in the blood). The patient may be asymptomatic, but the symptoms of acute bacterial prostatitis are often the same as those of UTI, with pain in the low back, perineum, or rectum. The condition may become chronic.

Diagnostic Tests

Diagnosis is confirmed by patient history and culture of prostatic fluid or tissue. The expressed prostatic secretion (EPS) is considered useful in the diagnosis of prostatitis. EPS is obtained using a premassage and postmassage test. The patient is asked to void into a specimen cup just before and just after a vigorous prostate massage. Prostatic massage (for EPS) should be avoided if acute bacterial prostatitis is suspected, because compression is extremely painful and increases the risk of bacterial spread. Transabdominal ultrasound, MRI, or CT scan may be included in the diagnostic workup. A urinalysis and urine culture, WBC count, and blood cultures also may be performed.

Assessment

Subjective data include complaints of chills and low back and perineal pain. Chronic bacterial prostatitis causes dysuria; urgency; frequency; nocturia; and pain in the lower abdomen or back, perineum, or genitalia.

Collection of objective data involves assessing for elevated temperature and rectal palpation of the prostate gland by the health care provider, which may reveal it to be firm, edematous, and tender.

Medical Management

If the condition is infectious, management focuses on control of the infection and prevention of the complications of abscess formation or bacteremia. Patients with acute prostatitis who have a high fever or other signs consistent with impending sepsis will be hospitalized and prescribed intravenous antibiotics. Patients who are more stable are managed from home. Antibiotics commonly used for acute and chronic bacterial prostatitis include trimethoprim-sulfamethoxazole or fluoroquinolone. The course of therapy ranges from 2 to 4 weeks. Doxycycline or tetracycline may be prescribed for patients with multiple sex partners. Additional pharmacologic needs may include antipyretics, urinary analgesics, analgesics, and stool softeners. Antiinflammatories are the most common agents used for pain control in prostatitis, but these provide only moderate pain relief. Opioid analgesics can be given, but cautiously, because this pain can be chronic. The pain resolves as the infection is treated.

Patients with chronic bacterial prostatitis are given oral antibiotic therapy for 4 to 16 weeks.

Nursing Interventions and Patient Teaching

Comfort measures used are analgesics, sitz baths, and stool softeners to reduce pain, edema, spasm, and straining pressure in the pelvis. Education is needed concerning the medication regimen.

Warn the patient with acute prostatitis to avoid sexual arousal and intercourse so that the prostate can rest; however, intercourse may be beneficial in the treatment of chronic prostatitis. Follow-up with the health care provider is crucial because of the likelihood that the disorder will become chronic.

Prognosis

Prostatitis is difficult to cure and requires long periods of antibiotic treatment. Stress the importance of taking all the antibiotics prescribed, even after the initial symptoms have subsided.

PYELONEPHRITIS

Etiology and Pathophysiology

Pyelonephritis is an inflammation of the structures of the kidney—the renal pelvis, renal tubules, and interstitial tissue. Pyelonephritis almost always is caused by *E. coli*. The kidney becomes edematous and inflamed, and the blood vessels are congested. The urine may be cloudy and contain pus (pyuria), mucus, and blood. Small abscesses may form in the kidney.

Pyelonephritis usually is seen in association with pregnancy; chronic health problems such as diabetes mellitus, or polycystic or hypertensive renal disease; insult to the urinary tract from catheterization; or infection, obstruction, or trauma. Careful management of these disorders is important to prevent pyelonephritis.

Clinical Manifestations

Acute pyelonephritis may be unilateral or bilateral, causing chills, fever, prostration, and flank pain. Repeated episodes of pyelonephritis lead to a chronic disease pattern, with atrophy of the kidney as the nephrons are destroyed. **Azotemia** (the retention of excessive amounts of nitrogenous compounds in the blood) develops if enough nephrons are nonfunctional.

Assessment

Subjective data in acute pyelonephritis include a patient who is acutely ill, with malaise and pain in the **costovertebral angle (CVA)** (the angle formed on either side of the patient's back by the twelfth rib and spinal column; the patient's kidneys lie just under the CVA). CVA tenderness to percussion is a common finding in pyelonephritis. In the chronic phase the patient may show unremarkable symptoms, such as nausea and general malaise.

Collection of objective data includes assessing the patient for signs of infection: elevated temperature, vomiting, and chills. The chronic disease results in systemic signs: elevated blood pressure and gastrointestinal irritation such as vomiting and diarrhea.

Diagnostic Tests

Diagnosis is confirmed by the presence of bacteria and pus in the urine, varying degrees of hematuria, WBCs and WBC casts in the urine (indicating involvement of the renal parenchyma), and leukocytosis. A clean-catch or catheterized urinalysis with culture and sensitivity tests identifies the pathogen and determines appropriate antimicrobial therapy. To prevent spread of infection in the early stages of acute pyelonephritis, imaging examinations, such as an intravenous pyelogram (IVP) or CT scan requiring injection of contrast materials, usually are not performed. Ultrasound of the urinary system often is done to identify anatomic abnormalities such as renal abscesses, obstructing calculus, or hydronephrosis. BUN and creatinine levels of the blood and urine may be assessed to monitor kidney function.

Medical Management

The patient with mild signs and symptoms may be treated on an outpatient basis with antibiotics for 14 to 21 days. Parenteral (intravenous) antibiotics often are given initially in the hospital to establish high serum and urinary medication levels. When initial treatment resolves the acute symptoms and the patient can tolerate oral fluids and medications, he or she may be discharged on a regimen of oral antibiotics for an additional 14 to 21 days. Antibiotics are selected according to results of urine culture and sensitivity tests and may include broad-spectrum medications such as ampicillin or vancomycin combined with an aminoglycoside (e.g., tobramycin, gentamicin); other treatment options include trimethoprim-sulfamethoxazole and fluoroquinolones, such as ciprofloxacin and ofloxacin.

Adequate fluids (at least eight 8-ounce glasses per day) are encouraged. Urinary analgesics such as phenazopyridine are helpful. Follow-up urine culture is indicated.

Nursing Interventions and Patient Teaching

Patient problems and interventions for the patient with pyelonephritis include but are not limited to the following:

Patient Problem	Nursing Interventions
Potential for Infection, related to bacteria in the urinary tract	Monitor urine character and odor Encourage oral fluids Instruct patient to void when he or she feels the urge Encourage perineal hygiene
Willingness for Improved Health Management, related to desire for prevention of further renal disease	Assess knowledge level concerning measures to prevent recurrence of symptoms Discuss personal health habits (diet, exercise) Discuss treatment plan with patient and family

Teach the patient to identify the signs and symptoms of infection: elevated temperature, flank pain, chills, fever, nausea and vomiting, urgency, fatigue, and general malaise. Also teach the patient indications, dose, length of course, and side effects of the medications. Emphasize the importance of follow-up care with the health care provider on a routine basis and when signs of infection arise.

Prognosis

Prognosis depends on early detection and successful treatment. Baseline assessment for every patient must include urinary assessment, because pyelonephritis can occur as a primary or secondary disorder (a condition resulting from complications of another disorder).

OBSTRUCTIVE DISORDERS OF THE URINARY TRACT

URINARY OBSTRUCTION

Etiology and Pathophysiology

Obstruction at any point within the urinary tract can affect function adversely and alter structure. Causes of obstruction include strictures, kinks, cysts, tumors, calculi, and prostatic hypertrophy. Obstruction may lead to alterations in blood chemistry; infection, which thrives as a result of urine stasis; ischemia resulting from compression; or atrophy of renal tissue.

Clinical Manifestations

The patient may be unaware of any problems at first if the obstruction is partial, allowing urine to drain and kidney function to remain within normal limits. With prostatic hypertrophy the obstructive process may be so gradual that the patient ignores the vague symptom of dull flank pain and seeks medical attention only when urination becomes acutely difficult. Acute pain occurs as the musculature is stretched by increasing pressure from urine accumulation and as muscular contractions increase to try to move urine past the obstruction. This acute pain is called **renal colic** and is a classic symptom of renal calculi.

Assessment

Subjective data include the patient's cardinal complaint of a sensation of needing to void but only being able to void small amounts. Pain may range from dull flank pain to acute, incapacitating pain. Nausea often accompanies acute pain.

Collection of objective data includes noting on physical assessment whether the bladder is palpable suprapubically because of urine retention. The affected kidney also may be palpable. Retention with overflow occurs when the patient is unable to completely empty the urinary bladder and it quickly refills, causing the urge to void again. Assess time and amount of voidings.

Diagnostic Tests

As a quick evaluation, the health care provider may order a KUB radiograph. Renal ultrasonography or IVP provides definitive information about structural changes. Other diagnostic tests may include visual examinations with the aid of endoscopy and a blood chemistry profile.

Medical Management

Initial intervention is aimed at establishing urine drainage and relieving discomfort. Conservative measures include inserting an indwelling catheter and administering an analgesic (usually opioid) and an anticholinergic agent (atropine) to decrease smooth muscle motility. It may be necessary to establish urine drainage surgically by inserting a catheter directly into the bladder through the abdominal wall (suprapubic cystostomy), into a ureter (ureterostomy), or into the kidney (nephrostomy).

Surgical correction of an obstruction in the urinary system may involve a tube, called a *stent*. Stent insertion is used for patients who are poor operative risks. A meshlike tube or coil-shaped device is inserted through an endoscope into the ureter. The stent holds the tubular structure open to facilitate drainage. Stents may be permanent or temporary. Closely monitor the patient for signs of infection, obstruction, and pain.

Nursing Interventions

After surgery, observe the patient for hemorrhage, provide aseptic care of the surgical site, and provide a safe environment to prevent injury and infection.

Prognosis

The prognosis varies, depending on the cause of the obstruction. If surgical correction is successful, the prognosis is excellent.

HYDRONEPHROSIS

Etiology and Pathophysiology

Hydronephrosis (dilation of the renal pelvis and calyces) may be congenital or may develop at any time. It can occur unilaterally or bilaterally. Hydronephrosis is caused by obstructions in the lower urinary tract, the ureters, or the kidneys. The location of the obstruction determines whether one or both kidneys are affected. Potential causes may include renal calculi, tumors, strictures, vesicoureteric reflux, and scarring (Fig. 50.7).

An obstruction generates pressure from accumulated urine that cannot flow past it. This pressure may cause functional and anatomic damage to the renal system. The renal pelvis and ureters dilate and hypertrophy. This pressure, if prolonged, causes fibrosis and loss of function in affected nephrons. If the condition is left untreated, the kidney may be destroyed.

Clinical Manifestations

Hydronephrosis can occur without any symptoms as long as kidney function is adequate and urine can drain.

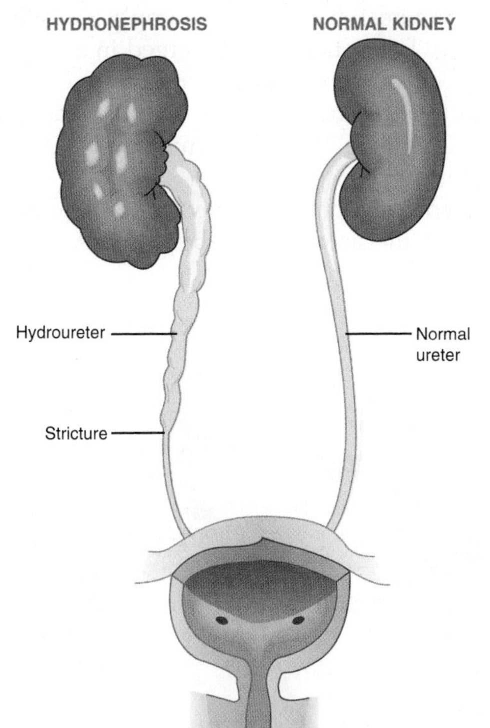

Fig. 50.7 Hydronephrosis. (From Adams AP, Proctor DB: *Kinn's medical assistant: An applied learning approach*, ed 11, St. Louis, 2011, Saunders.)

The amount of pain is proportional to the rate of stretching of urinary tract structures. Slowly developing hydronephrosis may cause only a dull flank pain, whereas a sudden occlusion of the ureter, such as from a calculus, causes a severe stabbing (colicky) pain in the flank. Nausea and vomiting, which often accompany hydronephrosis, are a reflex reaction to the pain and usually subside when the pain is controlled.

Assessment

Subjective data include patient reports of pain, including location, intensity, and character, and nausea. Discuss the patient's voiding pattern: frequency, difficulty starting a stream of urine, dribbling at the end of **micturition** (voiding), nocturia, and burning on urination. Note any history of obstructive disorders.

Collection of objective data includes assessing the patient suspected of having hydronephrosis for vomiting, hematuria, urinary output, edema, a palpable mass in the abdomen, bladder distention (detected on palpation), and tenderness over the kidneys or bladder.

Diagnostic Tests

Urinalysis and serum kidney function studies that include measurement of urea and creatinine are obtained. Cystoscopy may be performed with or without retrograde pyelogram. Radiographic examinations may include IVP or IVU, KUB radiograph, CT scan, or ultrasound evaluation. Sometimes a renal biopsy is performed.

Medical Management

Management is usually conservative if the condition is not severe. Surgery relieves the obstruction and preserves kidney function. If the kidney is severely damaged, a nephrectomy may be necessary. If infection is present, antiinfective medications are administered: penicillin in combination with sulfamethoxazole-trimethoprim (Bactrim). Opioids, such as morphine and meperidine, in combination with antispasmodic drugs, such as propantheline and belladonna preparations, are usually necessary to relieve severe, colicky pain.

Nursing Interventions and Patient Teaching

Nursing interventions for the patient with hydronephrosis include administering medications as ordered, monitoring I&O, observing for signs and symptoms of infection, and monitoring vital signs. Encourage the patient to take fluids, and assess the patient for pain. Keep any drainage tubes open and anchored to avoid inadvertent displacement. If a catheter is present, provide catheter care. If surgery has been performed, observe the dressing because drainage of urine may continue for some time. Keep the area clean and dry to avoid excoriation of the skin. Explain all procedures to the patient and the family.

Patient teaching includes explaining the abnormality and the signs and symptoms of infection or obstruction. Describe measures to prevent infection, such as adequate fluid intake, perineal hygiene daily with mild soap and water (drying thoroughly), and regular emptying of the bladder.

Prognosis

Prognosis depends on the degree of urinary system destruction and the need for surgical intervention.

UROLITHIASIS

Urolithiasis (formation of urinary calculi) can develop in any area of the urinary tract. *Urolithiasis* is a general term that encompasses all urinary calculi, but specific names also are used to indicate where they are located or formed: *nephrolithiasis* (formation of a kidney stone, or *nephrolith*), *ureterolithiasis* (formation of a stone in the ureter, or *ureterolith*), and *cystolithiasis* (a bladder stone, or *cystolith*). Another descriptive term is *lithogenesis* (the formation of stones).

Etiology and Pathophysiology

Urolithiasis occurs when minerals precipitate out of solution and adhere, forming stones that vary in size and shape. The event that initiates stone formation remains unknown. Factors predisposing individuals to urolithiasis include immobility, obesity, family history, male gender, hyperparathyroidism (in which calcium leaves the bones and accumulates in the bloodstream), or recurrent UTIs. Dietary influences may contribute to stone development. Chronic use of medications such as diuretics, calcium-based antacids, and topiramate are linked to stone formation. Thorough assessment and analysis of the composition of the stones guide medical and nursing management.

Clinical Manifestations

Symptoms depend on the stones' size and degree of mobility. The patient with renal colic seeks care immediately, whereas a person with a less mobile stone may not seek assistance until signs of infection or hydronephrosis occur.

Assessment

Subjective data include the patient with mobile calculi complaining of intractable pain (pain that is unrelieved by ordinary medical measures and usually is accompanied by nausea and vomiting). The patient describes the pain as starting in the flank and radiating into the groin, the genitalia, and the inner thigh. The patient with a less mobile stone may develop signs and symptoms associated with UTI secondary to hydronephrosis.

Collection of objective data includes assessing for hematuria and vomiting.

Diagnostic Tests

Diagnostic tests include KUB and IVP or IVU radiography, ultrasound, cystoscopy, and urinalysis. Other tests may be ordered to determine stone content, presence of infection, and alterations in blood chemistry that influence stone formation. Twenty-four–hour urine examination may detect abnormal excretion of calcium oxalate, phosphorus, or uric acid.

Medical Management

Stone removal and pain management are the primary goals of treatment. Antiinfective agents may be administered to treat infection or prophylactically. If stones are not passed, invasive techniques may be indicated (Fig. 50.8). Stones in the lower tract can be removed by cystoscopy with stone manipulation or by surgical incision. Terminology describes the location: ureterolithotomy, pyelolithotomy, and nephrolithotomy. Chemolytic agents, either alkylating or acidifying agents, may be instilled to dissolve stones.

Extracorporeal shock wave lithotripsy is an alternative to surgery. The patient is submerged in a special tank of water, and ultrasonic shock waves are used to pulverize the stone. Urine must still be strained, even if a catheter is in place. Renal colic may occur as the patient passes the stone fragments.

Percutaneous nephrolithotomy may be used to manage larger stones that are not able to be passed. A nephroscope

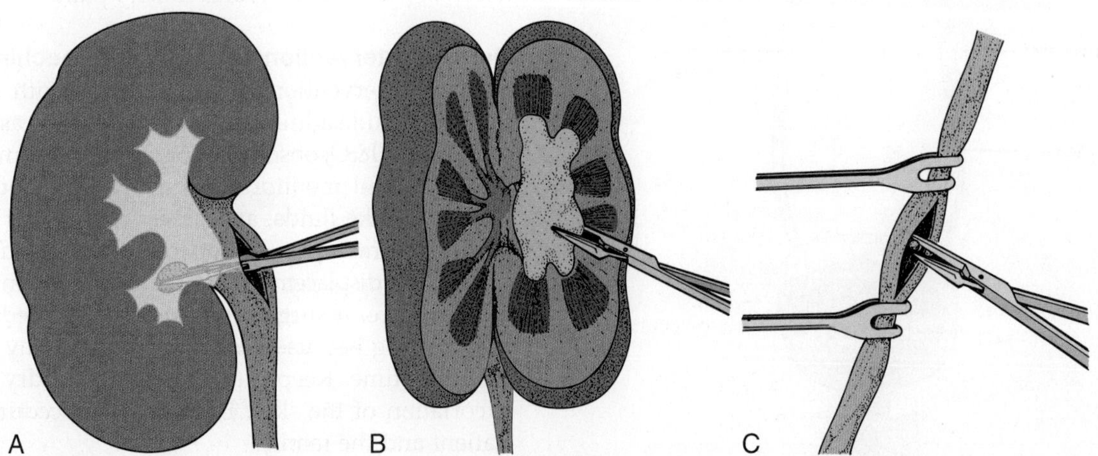

Fig. 50.8 Location and methods of removing renal calculi from upper urinary tract. A, Pyelolithotomy, removal of stone through renal pelvis. B, Nephrolithotomy, removal of staghorn calculus from renal parenchyma (kidney split). C, Ureterolithotomy, removal of stone from ureter. (From Beare PG, Myers JL: *Adult health nursing*, ed 3, St. Louis, 1998, Mosby.)

allows the stone to be visualized and removed through a small incision directly into the kidney through the back. Then, a small rubber catheter is placed into the kidney and the stone is removed. If the stone is large, it may be broken down using lasers before removal.

Long-term management may include dietary adjustments to alter urine pH or to decrease the availability of certain substances that cause stone formation. Moderate reduction of foods containing calcium, phosphorus, and purine may help when stones are caused by metabolic abnormalities. Foods to avoid include cheese, greens, whole grains, carbonated beverages, nuts, chocolate, shellfish, and organ meat. Daily fluid intake of 2000 mL (unless clinically contraindicated) helps cleanse the urinary tract. Additional dietary modifications may be implemented based upon the composition of the stones being experienced.

Drug therapy depends on stone composition. To prevent calcium stone formation, sodium cellulose phosphate is taken; it binds with ingested calcium and prevents its absorption. Aluminum hydroxide gel binds with excess phosphorus, allowing intestinal excretion rather than urinary excretion; and allopurinol (Zyloprim) reduces serum urate levels, thereby facilitating reabsorption of urate crystals.

Nursing Interventions and Patient Teaching

Physical activity and hydration facilitate stone passage. The patient may require opioid medications to manage the pain. If analgesics are given, provide assistance with ambulation. If the patient is unable to tolerate sufficient oral intake, intravenous fluids may be prescribed. All urine is strained. Any stones or "gravel" noted must be sent to the laboratory for analysis. Assess urine for possible hematuria. Monitor BUN and creatinine for indications of continuing urinary tract obstruction.

Patient problems and interventions for the patient with urolithiasis include but are not limited to the following:

Patient Problem	Nursing Interventions
Potential for Infection, related to bacteria in the urinary tract	Monitor urine character and odor Encourage oral fluids Instruct the patient to void when urge is felt Encourage perineal hygiene Encourage fluid intake
Willingness for Improved Health Management, related to desire for prevention of further renal disease	Assess knowledge level concerning measures to prevent recurrence of symptoms Discuss personal health habits (diet, exercise) Discuss treatment plan with patient and family

Discuss the prescribed diet, including fluid intake, and home medications (their purpose, dosage, refills, and side effects). The patient should avoid inactivity by walking frequently. Emphasize the need for follow-up with the health care provider, including keeping scheduled appointments and reporting difficulty with urination.

Although opinions vary greatly as to benefits of dietary restrictions, the nurse may be responsible for clarifying diet instructions. Encourage a fluid intake of at least 2000 mL in 24 hours, unless contraindicated. People who tend to form calcium stones may need to curtail their intake of dietary calcium (dairy products, antacids) to within minimum recommended dietary allowance guidelines. New research on the impact of diet on the development of calcium oxalate kidney stones concludes that restricting consumption of animal protein and salt in combination with normal calcium intake reduces the risk of kidney stones better than the traditional low-calcium diet.

Prognosis

Prognosis is related to the location of the stone and the extent of invasive procedures necessary to remove the stone. A certain population, categorized as "stone formers," is at risk for recurrence.

TUMORS OF THE URINARY SYSTEM

RENAL TUMORS

Etiology and Pathophysiology

The majority of renal tumors are malignant adenocarcinomas, also known as renal cell carcinomas, that develop unilaterally and are often large when first detected. Renal cell carcinoma as a primary malignant tumor appears to arise from cells of the proximal convoluted tubules. This is the eighth most common cancer, accounting for nearly 4% of all cancers in adults, with a median age at diagnosis of 64 years. Renal cancer is seen more in men than women. Populations who are affected more frequently include African American, American Indians, and Native Alaskans. Twice as many men as women are diagnosed with renal cancer (SEER, n.d.).

Risk factors include a history of dialysis (filtration of the blood to remove excess water and waste products), family history, hypertension, horseshoe kidney (a developmental anomaly in which the kidneys are fused together), polycystic kidney disease, and smoking. The strongest risk factors appear to be genetic; multifocal renal adenocarcinomas have a hereditary basis, which is being studied intensively. Several multiorgan syndromes are associated with a high risk for renal malignancies; the most prominent is von Hippel–Lindau disease, an autosomal dominant hereditary disease.

Because of the isolated anatomic location of the kidney, renal adenocarcinomas can grow large while remaining clinically silent. Most demonstrate a characteristic hypervascularity. Renal adenocarcinomas tend to grow intravascularly, within the renal vein and into the inferior vena cava. These tumor thrombi may extend as far as the right atrium, presenting a unique surgical challenge. Although essentially every organ can be affected, the most common sites of metastases are the lungs, adrenal glands, liver, and bones.

Clinical Manifestations

The historic sign-and-symptom triad of renal adenocarcinoma is hematuria, flank pain, and a flank mass. Most cases with these symptoms are advanced and incurable. Other common signs and symptoms are hypercalcemia, fever, anemia, weakness, and erythrocytosis. Gross hematuria is rarely a sign of renal adenocarcinoma until the malignancy is advanced. Check the patient's home medications for anticoagulant therapy, because this may be the cause of hematuria.

Assessment

Subjective data include a patient history of blood in the urine, which "comes and goes." When the bleeding occurs, there is usually no associated pain. In advanced stages of the illness, the patient experiences weight loss, fatigue, and dull flank pain.

Collection of objective data involves a physical assessment that reveals a mass in the patient's flank in the advanced stages of the illness. Hematuria and signs related to systemic metastasis may be obvious.

Diagnostic Tests

Localized adenocarcinoma may be diagnosed in patients who have no signs and symptoms specifically related to the tumor; these tumors often are discovered incidentally during evaluation of other complaints. Patients with gross hematuria should be assessed by a urologist. A cystoscopy followed by an IVP with tomography should be performed.

The majority of solid masses are malignant and require definitive evaluation and treatment. Percutaneous biopsy of a solid renal mass rarely is done because it is unlikely to change the future treatment unless there is evidence of advanced disease. A CT (with or without contrast), a chest x-ray, and, in some cases, a bone scan are used to stage renal adenocarcinoma.

Medical Management

Because renal adenocarcinoma is relatively radioresistant, radiation therapy has little or no role in its treatment. Surgery is the sole intervention capable of cure. The standard procedure is radical nephrectomy along with removal of adjacent lymph nodes and tissue. In the patient with renal insufficiency or a solitary kidney, partial nephrectomy (a far more complex procedure) may be indicated.

Nursing Interventions and Patient Teaching

Care of the patient with surgery of the urinary tract is addressed later in this chapter.

Patient problems and interventions for the patient with renal tumors include but are not limited to the following:

Patient Problem	Nursing Interventions
Impaired Coping, related to powerlessness	Encourage patient to express feelings Assist patient in identifying personal strengths and coping skills Actively listen Support realistic hope; answer questions honestly
Impaired Decision-Making Ability, with verbalized uncertainty about choice to have renal surgery	Assess patient's capacity to make decisions Assess knowledge of procedure Review outline of surgical procedure and what nursing interventions the patient and significant others can expect postoperatively
Compromised Physical Mobility, related to pain and discomfort	Plan activities when pain control is greatest Encourage active or passive range-of-motion exercises Assess need for assistive devices

Instruct the patient about community resources, support groups, and home health care. Emphasize the importance of follow-up care, including following discharge instructions and keeping return appointment.

Prognosis

Survival rates are tied closely to the staging of cancer at the time of diagnosis. Stage I has a 5-year survival rate of 81%. Stage IV has a survival rate of only 8%. The natural history of renal adenocarcinoma is far more unpredictable than that of most solid tumors. Disease may recur more than 15 years after removal of the original primary lesion. Metastatic disease has a poor prognosis and is rarely curable. Metastatic recurrence at a remotely distant time is not uncommon.

RENAL CYSTS

Etiology and Pathophysiology

Renal cysts are round, fluid-filled sacs on the kidneys. Cysts increase in frequency with aging. Many cysts initially are observed during imaging diagnostic testing. Cysts must be evaluated to distinguish them from more causes of cystic disease such as renal cell carcinoma (Merck, 2013). Renal cell carcinoma is typically irregular or multiloculated with irregular walls and areas of unclear demarcation.

Patients with renal cysts have a higher incidence of renal carcinoma. Some health care providers periodically screen patients with cysts for renal carcinoma, using ultrasonography or CT.

Multiple cysts are most common in patients with chronic renal failure, especially those undergoing hemodialysis. The cause is unknown, but the cysts may be due to compensatory hyperplasia of residually functioning nephrons. A criterion for diagnosis is more than four cysts in each kidney on ultrasonography or CT.

The most significant problems arise with *polycystic kidney disease (PKD)*. PKD is a genetic disorder characterized by the growth of numerous fluid-filled cysts, which can slowly replace much of the kidney. A patient with long-standing renal insufficiency or a dialysis patient may develop polycystic disease. Kidney function is compromised by the pressure of the cysts on renal structures, secondary infections, and tissue scarring caused by rupture of the cysts. The patient may progress to end-stage renal disease (ESRD).

Clinical Manifestations

Signs and symptoms are influenced by the degree of renal structure involvement. The most common site is the collecting ducts, which fill with urine and/or blood. As the disease progresses, fewer nephrons are available to maintain normal kidney function.

The Bosniak renal cyst classification system classifies lesions according to their character. Class I lesions are simple, benign cysts and do not warrant further workup. Class II lesions are minimally complicated with some features that cause concern. They have smooth, sharp margins; are thicker; and require follow-up scanning. Class III lesions have irregular and thickened walls and multiloculated cysts; they require surgical exploration. Class IV lesions show nonuniform wall thickening and irregular margins; they contain solid components visible on CT. These lesions are clearly malignant, and a total nephrectomy is warranted.

Assessment

Subjective data include the most common symptoms of abdominal and flank pain, followed by headache, gastrointestinal complaints, voiding disturbances, and a history of recurrent UTIs.

Collection of objective data involves observation for systemic changes. Closely monitor blood pressure, which usually is elevated, and hematuria. Document patient complaints and response to intervention.

Diagnostic Tests

Diagnosis is established by family history, physical examination, intravenous pyelogram, and imaging of cysts on radiographic examination or sonography. Blood chemistry results, such as urea and creatinine levels, are used to monitor the level of kidney function.

Medical Management

PKD has no specific treatment. Medical treatment is aimed at relief of pain and other symptoms. Heat and analgesics may relieve some of the discomfort caused by the enlarging kidneys. If the patient bleeds, discontinue heat and place the patient on bed rest. Hypertension is treated vigorously with antihypertensive agents, diuretics, and fluid and dietary modifications. Because infections are common, antibiotics often are prescribed. As the disease progresses, dialysis or kidney transplantation may be required.

Nursing Interventions

Individual complaints and the severity of the disease process influence nursing interventions. Provide information to patients and family members about the availability of genetic counseling. Emphasize the need to report any changes in health status to the health care provider.

Prognosis

The prognosis is favorable with a single cyst but guarded with polycystic disease because of its chronic nature.

TUMORS OF THE URINARY BLADDER

Etiology and Pathophysiology

The bladder is the most common site of cancer in the urinary tract. A bladder tumor is an excess growth of cells that line the inside of the bladder, in many cases because the cells were exposed to certain chemicals. Tumors of the urinary bladder range from benign papillomas to invasive carcinomas. Papillomas have the potential to become cancerous and are removed when detected. Benign tumors of the kidney can be problematic and traditionally are removed.

A review of the statistics for bladder cancer over the past two decades shows minimal changes with regard to incidence and mortality rates for most populations. Bladder cancer is four times more common in men than women. Declines in mortality rates for bladder cancer can be found in women and African Americans. There are racial differences with regard to diagnosis. Twice as many whites as African Americans or Hispanic Americans are diagnosed. Risk factors include smoking, a family history of bladder cancer, and occupational exposures to chemicals in paint, dye, and petroleum products. The incidence of bladder cancer increases with aging. The average age at diagnosis is 73 years.

Several types of carcinoma arise on the bladder surface. The most common type diagnosed in North America is transitional cell carcinoma (TCC), which can occur anywhere in the urinary tract but usually is found in the urinary bladder. TCC involves development of a papillary tumor that projects into the bladder lumen and, if untreated, continues into the bladder muscle, where it can metastasize.

Clinical Manifestations

The patient may delay seeking medical attention because the primary sign of bladder cancer is painless, intermittent hematuria.

Assessment

Subjective data include symptoms such as changes in voiding patterns, signs of urinary obstruction, or renal failure, depending on the extent of the disease process.

Collection of objective data includes assessing the patient's understanding of his or her current health status, which aids in planning teaching interventions. Accurately document the time and amount of voiding, including a urine description.

Diagnostic Tests

Diagnosing bladder cancer often begins with a urinalysis and culture. This identifies abnormalities in the urine such as blood or infection. Urine tumor marker testing may be completed. This allows the urine to be assessed for particles secreted by bladder cancer cells. The next level of diagnostic testing includes a urine **cytologic evaluation** (study of cells) and/or one of several available bladder cancer markers. Bladder biopsies are needed to confirm a diagnosis.

Bladder cancer tumors are staged most commonly according to the system developed by the American Joint Committee on Cancer. The stage of the tumor is the most important indicator of prognosis and overall survival for patients with invasive tumors. Staging is an assessment of how far the tumor has spread.

Medical Management

Local disease may be treated by fulguration (also called electrocautery): removing the tissue by burning it away with the tip of an electrically heated electrode. Laser treatment, instillation of chemotherapy agents, or radiation therapy also may be used. Closely monitor these patients with cytologic studies and cystoscopy, because the recurrence rate is as high as 60%. A partial or total cystectomy may be performed to remove invasive lesions. With complete removal of the urinary bladder, urinary diversion or a neobladder (i.e., a new bladder created from intestinal tissue) is necessary. (See the section "Urinary Diversion" regarding ileal conduits and sigmoid conduits.)

Nursing Interventions and Patient Teaching

Care of the patient with bladder cancer is influenced by the extent of the disease process, medical treatment, coincidental illness, and the patient's response to treatment. Observe voiding patterns and urine characteristics to monitor response to these therapies. Provide teaching and support so that the patient can return to optimum performance of ADLs. Emphasize the importance of follow-up care for the patient with papillomas.

Prognosis

The prognosis is related directly to the extent of the disease process when diagnosed. Another important aspect in recovery is the patient's adaptability to any changes in urinary elimination as a result of treatment.

CONDITIONS AFFECTING THE PROSTATE GLAND

BENIGN PROSTATIC HYPERTROPHY

Etiology and Pathophysiology

The prostate gland encircles the male urethra at the base of the urinary bladder. It secretes an alkaline fluid that helps neutralize seminal fluid and increases sperm motility. BPH, enlargement of the prostate gland, is common in men older than 50 years of age. The cause is unclear but may be influenced by hormonal changes. The prostate enlarges, exerting pressure on the urethra and vesicle neck of the urinary bladder, which prevents complete emptying.

Clinical Manifestations

The patient has symptoms associated with urinary obstruction. Other clinical manifestations include complications of urinary obstruction, such as UTI, hematuria, **oliguria** (decreased urinary output), and signs of renal insufficiency.

Assessment

Subjective data include the patient describing urination as painful, and the urine stream as difficult to start and to slow, with complaints of frequency and nocturia. Collectively, these symptoms may be referred to as *prostatism* (any condition of the prostate gland that causes retention of urine in the bladder).

Collection of objective data involves eliciting information about voiding patterns to aid in determining the severity of the obstruction.

Diagnostic Tests

On rectal examination the health care provider may palpate the enlarged prostate gland, which has an elastic consistency. The hypertrophied prostate is enlarged symmetrically with a uniform, boggy presentation. Severity of the process can be determined by detecting alterations in blood chemistry, by measuring residual urine, or by cystoscopy or IVP. Cytologic evaluation determines whether the process is benign or malignant.

Medical Management

Treatment is based on the degree of occlusion and on signs and symptoms. Pharmacologic agents include alpha blockers, which improve the ability to urinate by relaxing the bladder neck and the fibers of the prostate. These medications elicit improved voiding in only a few days. Examples include terazosin, doxazosin (Cardura), and tamsulosin (Flomax). To shrink the prostate 5-alpha-reductase inhibitors are prescribed. Medications in this group include finasteride (Proscar) and dutasteride (Avodart). The 5-alpha-reductase inhibitors take weeks or months before changes in condition are noted. The two therapies may be combined to manage the condition.

Pharmacologic options are investigated first. If the condition worsens, surgery may be necessary.

Deciding which treatment intervention to choose is difficult. Transurethral resection of the prostate (TURP) still is considered the standard for surgical intervention. The newer, less invasive treatments still are being evaluated. In general, these treatments are considered to cause less morbidity, but the results are not considered as effective or long-lasting as those of TURP.

Transurethral microwave thermotherapy. Transurethral microwave thermotherapy (TUMT) is one of various procedures used for the treatment of lower urinary tract symptoms resulting from BPH. TUMT involves the insertion of a specially designed urinary catheter into the bladder, allowing a microwave antenna to be positioned within the prostate; there it heats and destroys hyperplastic prostate tissue. The goal of TUMT is to provide a one-time treatment. Candidates for TUMT include persons with moderate-to-severe voiding symptoms resulting from BPH: those with side effects to medical therapy, those in whom medical therapy has failed, and those who choose not to be treated medically. There are many exclusions to the use of TUMT, so all patients require a thorough history and physical examination.

Patients should return to the clinic for follow-up. If a catheter is placed, it can be removed at home or in the clinic. Instruct patients to watch for an inability to void, painful voiding, high fevers, abdominal pain, or other problems. Posttreatment convalescence is relatively rapid, with most patients able to void and recover in less than 5 days at home.

Transurethral needle ablation. Transurethral needle ablation (TUNA) of the prostate is another procedure used to treat BPH. It is performed by placing interstitial radiofrequency needles through the urethra and into the lateral lobes of the prostate, causing heat-induced coagulation necrosis. The tissue is heated to 230°F (110°C) for approximately 3 minutes per lesion. A coagulation defect is created. A comprehensive history and physical examination are necessary to determine the benefits of using this procedure. Urethrocystoscopy may be indicated to help select the optimal form of therapy.

Photoselective vaporization of the prostate. Photoselective vaporization of the prostate (PVP), using a GreenLight laser, is another option for the treatment of BPH. PVP is a safe alternative for patients who are seriously ill, are taking anticoagulants, or have unfavorable anatomy (i.e., a large prostate). The technique employs a laser beam, which emits a visible green light at a wavelength that has shallow tissue penetration and is absorbed selectively by blood. A urologist delivers the laser's energy by way of a thin fiber inserted into the urethra through a 23-Fr continuous-flow cystoscope. The GreenLight laser vaporizes the prostate tissue.

Nursing Interventions

Initial management is aimed at relieving the obstruction, usually by insertion of a Foley catheter. Take care to avoid rapid decompression of the bladder to prevent rupture of mucosal blood vessels. Usually no more than 1000 mL of urine should be removed from a distended bladder initially. Follow the health care provider's orders for the individual patient.

Prostatectomy (removal of the prostate gland) is indicated to relieve or prevent further obstruction of the urethra. The health care provider chooses the surgical approach for the prostatectomy after thorough appraisal of the patient. Preoperatively, the health care provider may order an enema to reduce the possibility of the patient's straining to defecate after surgery, which could cause bleeding. Other preoperative preparations are standard, as noted in Chapter 42. A prostatectomy may be done using any of four surgical techniques (Box 50.3 and Fig. 50.9).

With BPH, TURP is the resection most often chosen because it is less invasive and less stressful for the patient, especially the older patient or the patient with coincidental illness. The tissue is removed through the urethra. With this procedure the outer capsule of the prostate gland is left in place, maintaining the continuity between the bladder and the lower urethra (see Fig. 50.9A). Care of this patient centers on observing urine characteristics and maintaining patency of the Foley catheter.

The patient who has a TURP may have continuous closed bladder irrigation or intermittent irrigation to prevent occlusion of the catheter with blood clots, which would cause bladder spasms. Inform the patient and the family that hematuria is expected after prostatic surgery. Monitor vital signs and urine color every 2 hours for the first 24 hours to detect early signs of complications. With continuous bladder irrigation the urine will be light red to pink, and with intermittent irrigation the urine will be a clear, cherry red. Continuous

Box 50.3 Four Prostatectomy Techniques

1. *Transurethral prostatectomy* involves approaching the gland through the penis and bladder, using a resectoscope, a surgical instrument with an electric cutting wire for resection and cautery to resect the lobes away from the capsule (see Fig. 50.9A).
2. *Suprapubic prostatectomy* is accomplished by an incision through the abdomen; the bladder is opened, and the gland is removed from above with the finger (see Fig. 50.9B).
3. *Radical perineal prostatectomy* requires an incision through the perineum between the scrotum and the rectum (see Fig. 50.9C).
4. *Retropubic prostatectomy* requires a low abdominal incision, but the bladder is not opened. The gland is removed by making an incision into the capsule encasing the prostate gland (see Fig. 50.9D).

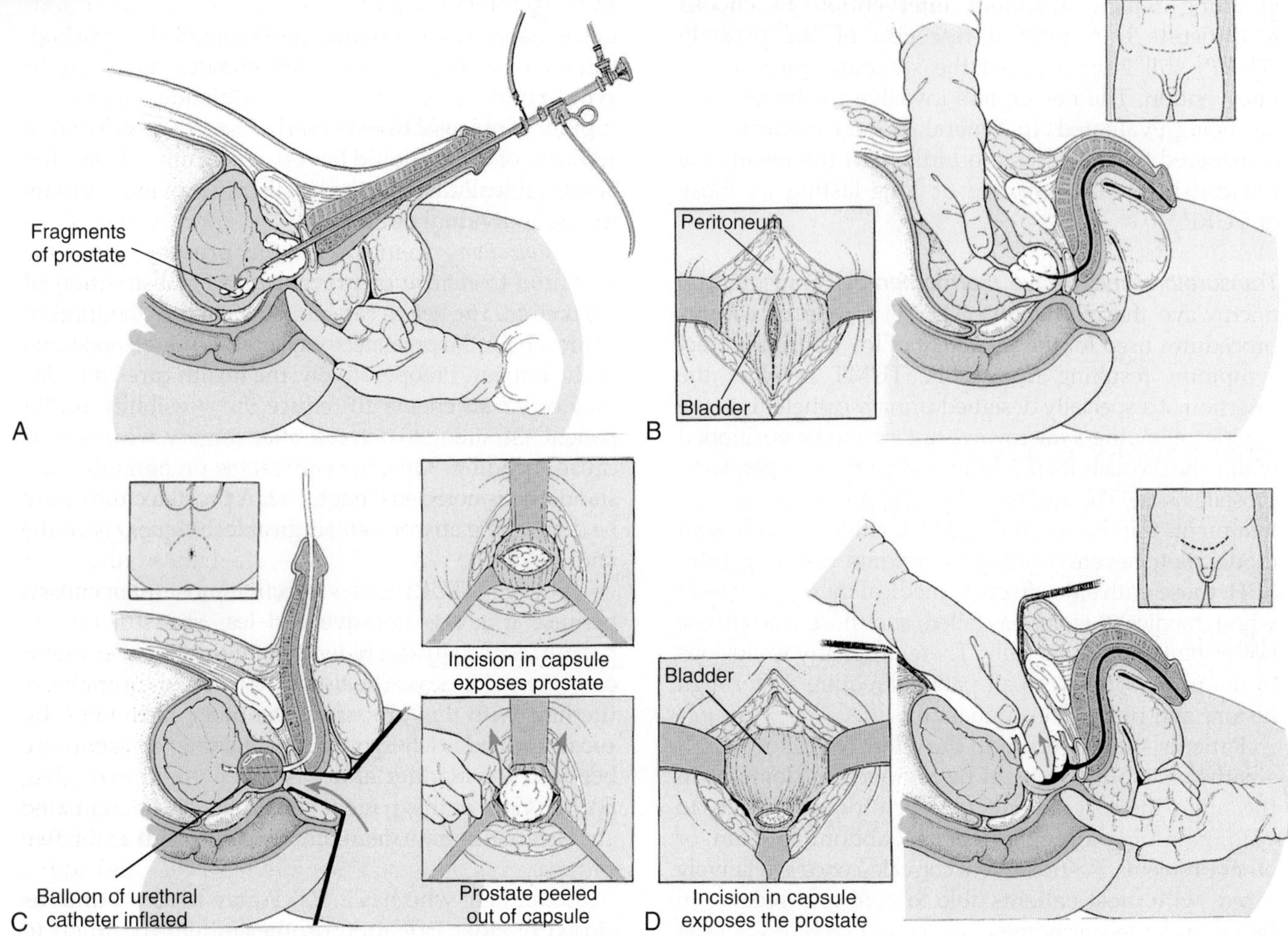

Fig. 50.9 Four types of prostatectomies. A, Transurethral resection of prostate gland by means of resectoscope. Note the enlarged prostate gland surrounding the urethra and the tiny pieces of prostatic tissue that have been cut away. B, Suprapubic. C, Radical perineal. D, Retropubic prostatectomy.

irrigation is achieved with a three-way catheter (one lumen for irrigation fluid, one for urine drainage, and one to the retention balloon) or by using two catheters (Foley and suprapubic—one for irrigation fluid and one for urine drainage). The irrigant is an isotonic solution. To determine urinary output, subtract the amount of irrigation fluid used from the Foley catheter output. This is reported as "actual urinary output." Check catheter drainage tubes frequently for kinks that would occlude urine flow and cause bladder spasms. Advise the patient not to try to void around the catheter because this contributes to bladder spasms. Hemorrhage is always a possibility. Belladonna and opium rectal suppositories are helpful to relieve bladder spasms but are not used in the retropubic approach because rectal stimulation is contraindicated.

Institute routine postoperative care. Have the patient avoid prolonged sitting because the increased intra-abdominal pressure may cause the operative site to bleed. Remove the catheter when the urine becomes clear. Inform the patient that initially he may experience frequency, voiding small amounts with some dribbling. Instruct him to void with the first urge to prevent increased bladder pressure against the operative site.

Some health care providers may request that samples of the most recent voiding be saved for assessment. Record the time, the amount, and the color of each voiding.

A suprapubic or abdominal approach requires dressing observations and changes. When a suprapubic catheter is present, observe it for unobstructed flow and color of the urine and monitor it for total output (see the Patient Teaching box).

Prognosis

Prognosis is favorable without residual effects. Problems with urine dribbling vary.

CANCER OF THE PROSTATE

Etiology and Pathophysiology

Prostatic cancer is common in men older than 50 years of age. This insidious cancer usually starts as a nodule on the posterior portion of the prostate without noticeable symptoms. When the tumor causes urinary symptoms, the cancer is in advanced stages. At this point, metastasis

 Patient Teaching

Postprostatectomy

ACTIVITY

- Light activity for 48 hours to avoid postoperative bleeding.
- Do not drive for 48 hours.
- No sexual activity for 2 weeks or as directed by health care provider.
- Avoid constipation. Maintain oral fluid intake and a diet high in fiber and roughage.
- Report signs of urinary track infection such as burning with urination.
- Do not take aspirin or other anticoagulant medications.
- Follow prescribed medication therapies as directed.

MANAGING URINARY INCONTINENCE

- It usually takes several weeks to achieve urinary continence. Continence may improve for up to 12 months.
- Maintain oral fluids between 2000 and 3000 mL/day (unless contraindicated).

ERECTILE DYSFUNCTION

- Sexual counseling and treatment options may be necessary if erectile dysfunction becomes a chronic or permanent problem.

INDWELLING CATHETER

- If the patient goes home with an indwelling catheter, send instructions for catheter care and local stores where supplies can be purchased.

is common; frequent sites are the pelvic lymph nodes and bone. Regular rectal examinations and PSA measurement to detect abnormalities of the prostate gland lead to early treatment and an increased survival rate.

Clinical Manifestations

The patient has signs and symptoms related to urinary obstruction. Other signs and symptoms are determined by the presence or degree of metastasis.

Assessment

Collection of subjective data involves understanding that the patient with prostatic cancer may have no symptoms until the disease is advanced. The patient may seek medical intervention for BPH, which often accompanies prostate cancer, or when he experiences back pain or sciatica from metastatic changes in the bony pelvis. The patient may complain of dysuria, frequency, and nocturia.

Objective data include metastatic changes in the lymph glands of the pelvis and in the bones of the lower spine, the pelvis, and the hips with associated signs. Hematuria may or may not be present, depending on the stage of the malignancy.

Diagnostic Tests

On rectal examination by the health care provider, the involved area of the prostate gland feels firm and fixed with hardened nodules typically in the posterior lobe of the gland. Definitive diagnosis is made by cytologic examination. Prostate cells can be obtained by needle aspiration.

Men should consider a yearly PSA and digital rectal examination starting at age 50 or at age 45 if at high risk (African Americans or men with a father or brother diagnosed with prostate cancer at an early age). Prostate specific antigen (PSA) test is increasing greatly the odds of early diagnosis. PSA, normally secreted and disposed of by the prostate, increases in the bloodstream in cancer of the prostate as well as in the harmless condition of BPH. The normal PSA level is 0 to 4 ng/mL. It is important to monitor even a slight increase in PSA levels. Elevated PSA levels mean further diagnostic evaluation is needed. When PSA levels are high but a digital examination is normal, transrectal ultrasound is proving increasingly helpful in detecting cancer of the prostate gland too small to be palpated rectally. Other tests, such as a bone scan and serum alkaline phosphatase, are performed to assess the degree of metastasis.

The Gleason grading system is the most widely used system for grading prostate cancer. Based on microscopic identification of glandular differentiation in tumor cells, tumors are graded from 1 to 5. Grade 1 represents the most well differentiated (most like the original cells), and grade 5 represents the most poorly differentiated (undifferentiated). Gleason grades are given to the two most commonly occurring patterns of cells and added together. The Gleason score, a number from 2 to 10, is used to predict how quickly the cancer will progress. A score of 2 to 4 indicates a slow-growing tumor. Grades 5 to 7 are associated with a more aggressive tumor (Prostate Cancer Treatment Guide, n.d.).

Medical Management

Treatment is based on the stage of the cancer—whether it has spread beyond the wall of the prostate, and to what extent—and the patient's age. In an older man with an estimated remaining lifespan of 5 to 10 years, controlling the disease with radiation or hormone therapy may be enough. In many cases, particularly in men older than 70 years of age, prostate cancer grows slowly, and hormone therapy can hold the disease at bay for several years.

Localized prostate cancer can be cured by radiation therapy or surgery. A treatment in which radioactive seed implants are placed directly in the prostate gland while sparing the surrounding tissue (rectum and bladder) is called *brachytherapy*. The seeds are placed accurately with a needle through a grid template guided by transrectal ultrasound. Brachytherapy is a convenient, one-time outpatient procedure, whereas external radiation can take 5 to 6 weeks (Cheuck, 2017). The seeds remain in the body, but their radioactivity declines over a period of months. Patients are advised to refrain from having children (or adults) sit in their lap and to avoid intercourse during the first 2 months after therapy.

Radiation therapy also is used in an attempt to destroy cancer cells and shrink the prostate when the cancer has spread to just outside the gland.

The operation to remove the prostate is a radical prostatectomy. Radical prostatectomy by the perineal approach is used in patients in the early stages of clinical disease and is considered one of the most effective ways of eradicating the tumor. This procedure involves removing the entire prostate, including the true prostatic capsule, seminal vesicles, and a portion of the bladder neck. The remaining portion of the bladder neck is reanastomosed (reconnected) to the urethra. The retropubic approach is often the first choice because it provides access to the pelvic lymph nodes (pelvic lymphadenectomy) and affords more urinary control and less stricture formation. A third, nerve-sparing prostatectomy procedure uses a retropubic and perineal approach to try to prevent impotence and reduce the likelihood of UI.

The three goals of a radical prostatectomy are (1) removal of the entire tumor, (2) preservation of urine control, and (3) maintenance of sexual function. Extent of sexual function may not be known for 6 to 12 months postoperatively. The patient needs emotional support related to the cancer and the possibility of impotence after surgery. Preoperative teaching should include an opportunity for the patient and his partner to discuss treatment options and mortality rate.

When the capsule of the prostate gland is removed, as with the perineal approach, the bladder and the lower urethra are no longer connected. The area where these two structures are reconnected usually is supported by placement of a Foley catheter. Extreme care must be taken to avoid placing tension on the catheter, which would disturb the surgical area. The catheter remains in place for several postoperative days.

Prostate cancer cells typically grow in response to testosterone making hormone deprivation therapy a potential method of treatment for cases of advanced prostatic cancer. The therapy alters tumor growth by blocking testosterone production. Hormone deprivation therapy can involve other hormones and drugs as well: estrogen, gonadotropin-releasing hormone analogues, antiandrogens, and luteinizing hormone–releasing hormone (LHRH) drugs:

- *LHRH agonists* act indirectly by causing an initial surge in luteinizing hormone and testosterone, rapidly followed by a decline in testosterone level similar to that achieved by castration. The primary forms of LHRH agonists are leuprolide (Lupron) and goserelin (Zoladex).
- *LHRH antagonists* act more directly, stopping the production of testosterone in the testes.

Degarelix (Firmagon) is a second-generation LHRH antagonist. Alternatives to LHRH drugs include oral nonsteroidal antiandrogens, including bicalutamide (Casodex), flutamide, and nilutamide (Nilandron) (NCI, 2014). Palliative therapy for patients with metastatic disease also may include orchiectomy (removal of the testes). Bilateral orchiectomy eliminates 95% of testosterone production, a step that is useful in managing metastatic disease. The patient may receive relief from such symptoms as pain or obstruction but may experience feminization, increased incidence of cardiac disease, thrombophlebitis, pulmonary embolus, and stroke. Additional therapies are instituted to treat these side effects.

Radiation therapy may be used in advanced stages of the illness as primary or palliative treatment. Management of disseminated disease with cytotoxic drugs has been marginally successful.

Because a cure for cancer of the prostate is possible only when the tumor is discovered early, it is important to teach all male patients older than the age of 40 to have annual or biannual rectal examinations and yearly PSA serum level determinations.

Nursing Interventions and Patient Teaching

Postoperative nursing management for prostatectomy is similar to that for perineal surgery, with special attention to maintenance of bowel and bladder function while keeping the surgical wound clean and avoiding pressure on the perineum and wound. Adequate fluid intake, modification of dietary selections, and perineal exercises may be used to promote regulation of bowel and bladder function. Take extreme care to prevent further trauma to the perineum; one unintended sequela of prostatectomy is fistula formation, in which a channel forms between the urethra and rectum. Rectal temperature-taking, enemas, and use of rectal tubes therefore are forbidden. Also take care not to place tension on the Foley catheter, which would disturb the surgical area. Observe the color of the urine for signs of bleeding. The patient will also have a tissue drain inserted during surgery to promote drainage from the wound in the perineum. Initially there may be a small amount of urine from the drain, but this should cease in 1 or 2 days. Follow surgical asepsis during dressing changes. Irrigation of the perineum may be ordered to cleanse the wound and soothe the patient. Administer comfort measures and analgesics as ordered for pain control in the lower back, pelvis, upper thighs, and operative site.

Patient problems and interventions for the patient undergoing prostate surgery include but are not limited to the following:

Patient Problem	Nursing Interventions
Potential for Inadequate Fluid Volume, related to hemorrhage or decreased fluid intake	Monitor signs and symptoms of fluid deficit (decreasing or increasing blood pressure, dyspnea) Observe catheter for urine color and amount Avoid manipulation of rectum by thermometer or rectal tube

Patient Problem	Nursing Interventions
Impaired Sexual Expression, related to surgical trauma and altered body function	Encourage verbalization of sexual concerns Provide privacy with significant others to discuss concerns Inform health care provider of patient concerns Explore professional resources (clergy, sexual counselors)

Because UI may occur postoperatively, teach the patient how to keep himself clean. He may need to discuss feelings of depression about his altered body function. Modifying lifestyle and maintaining confidence are important for his return to preillness function. Discuss alternative expressions of sexuality, the value of sexual counseling, and the possibility of recovering some or all sexual function after the treatment is completed.

Emphasize the need for adequate fluid intake, exercise, and rest. Instruct the patient regarding pain-relieving measures such as exercise, warmth, and medication. Discuss new pharmacologic agents that act as adjuvants in the treatment of cancer and for pain relief during the postoperative recovery period.

Prognosis

The patient's prognosis is correlated directly to the extent of the disease process when diagnosed. Grading of the tumor (well, moderately, or poorly differentiated) correlates with the prognosis; the more poorly differentiated the tumor, the poorer the prognosis. Under the Gleason system discussed previously, a low score of 2 through 4 is good; a high score of 7 through 10 is not. The treatment goal for the localized disease process is a cure; palliation is used for the extended disease process.

DISORDERS OF THE URINARY TRACT

URETHRAL STRICTURES

Etiology and Pathophysiology

A *urethral stricture* is a narrowing of the lumen of the urethra that interferes with urine flow. Narrowing may be congenital or acquired. Acquired strictures may be caused by chronic infection, trauma, or tumor or occur as a complication of radiation treatment of the pelvis.

Clinical Manifestations

Signs and symptoms include dysuria, weak stream, splaying (spreading out) of the urine stream, nocturia, and increasing pain with bladder distention. In the presence of infection, fever and malaise may be apparent.

Assessment

Subjective data include patient complaints of difficulty initiating the urine stream and the stream seeming to splay more than usual or even seeming to "fork."

Collection of objective data includes assessing for signs that may indicate an infectious process and for information indicating the extent of the stricture and possible presence of an obstruction.

Diagnostic Tests

Diagnosis can be confirmed by a voiding cystourethrogram, which demonstrates stricture. Additional diagnostic studies help evaluate damage caused by the obstruction.

Medical Management

Correction of the stricture may be achieved by dilation with metal sounds (instruments designed to dilate the urethra) or surgical release (internal urethrotomy).

Nursing Interventions

Care includes adequate hydration to decrease discomfort when voiding and monitoring urinary output. Mild analgesics should relieve discomfort. Sitz baths may encourage voiding. Reconstruction of the urethra (urethroplasty) may require temporary urinary diversion. After the procedure a splinting catheter supports the suture line. Take care not to place tension on the catheter.

Prognosis

The prognosis after surgical correction or dilation is favorable.

URINARY TRACT TRAUMA

Etiology and Pathophysiology

Assess any patient with a history of traumatic injury for possible involvement of the urinary tract. Such injuries may include contusions or rupture of the urinary structures. Also observe a patient who has undergone abdominal surgery for possible incidental injury sustained during the operation. Traumatic invasion of the urinary tract may be evident in open wounds to the lower abdomen, such as gunshot or stab wounds. Trauma to the bladder can occur from a fractured pelvis. Contusion or laceration of the urethra may lead to urethral stricture and possible impotence in men secondary to soft tissue, blood vessel, and nerve damage.

Clinical Manifestations

Monitor urinary output hourly for amount and color. Report any evidence of hematuria. Assess the patient for abdominal pain and tenderness, which may indicate internal hemorrhage, peritonitis, or seepage of urine into the tissues.

Assessment

Collection of subjective data involves understanding that the trauma patient may be unable to relate any symptoms that would aid in the assessment of urinary tract involvement. If the patient can respond, asking about signs of hematuria is extremely important.

Collection of objective data includes a comprehensive assessment of the trauma patient, reviewing all body systems. Assessment related to the urinary tract includes hourly measurement of I&O; observation of urine character or difficulty voiding; evaluation of complaints of abdominal, flank, or referred shoulder pain; and evaluation of abdominal distention and girth.

Diagnostic Tests

Diagnosis of traumatic involvement of the urinary tract may be aided by KUB radiography, IVP, urinalysis, excretory urography, and cystoscopy.

Medical Management

Surgical intervention is necessary for correction of tears or rupture of the urinary tract to reinstate urine flow. If damage is severe, removal of a kidney or the bladder may be necessary with the creation of urinary diversion, as discussed later in this chapter. Management of possible hemorrhage and prevention of infection are necessary before and after surgery.

Nursing Interventions

Document and report all findings.

Prognosis

The prognosis depends on the extent and location of the trauma.

IMMUNOLOGIC DISORDERS OF THE KIDNEY

NEPHROTIC SYNDROME

Etiology and Pathophysiology

Nephrotic syndrome (nephrosis) is a disorder characterized by marked proteinuria, hyperlipidemia, hypoalbuminemia, and edema. Several events may precipitate nephrotic syndrome; the primary form of nephrosis occurs in the absence of glomerulonephritis or systemic disease, with the inciting event being an upper respiratory tract infection or allergic reaction.

The most common sign is excess fluid in the body. This may take several forms: periorbital edema (around the eyes), characteristically in the morning; pitting edema over the legs; fluid in the pleural cavity (pleural effusion); or fluid in the peritoneal cavity (ascites).

In nephrotic syndrome, the glomeruli become damaged because of inflammation so that small proteins, such as albumins, immunoglobulins, and antithrombin, can pass through the kidneys into the urine. Physiologic changes in the glomeruli interfere with selective permeability. Blood protein is allowed to pass into the urine (proteinuria), causing a loss of serum protein (hypoalbuminemia). This decreases serum osmotic pressure, thus allowing fluid to seep into interstitial spaces, and edema occurs.

Immune responses, humoral and cellular, are altered in the patient with nephrotic syndrome; as a result, infection is an important cause of morbidity and mortality.

Clinical Manifestations

The patient has severe generalized edema (**anasarca**). Weight loss is evident. When questioned about his or her diet, the patient reports anorexia. Activity intolerance and fatigue are reported. Urine is foamy.

Assessment

Subjective data include patient complaints of loss of interest in eating, constant fatigue, foamy urine from the presence of protein, and decreased urinary output (oliguria), less than 500 mL in 24 hours.

Collection of objective data includes assessing the degree of fluid retention by monitoring daily weight, I&O, respiratory effort, and level of consciousness. The patient may relate problems with "swelling" of the face, hands, and feet. Assess skin integrity to determine special needs. Assess lung fields for the presence of crackles indicating fluid buildup. Assess for neck vein distention.

Diagnostic Tests

Blood chemistry findings include hypoalbuminemia and hyperlipidemia. The urinalysis reveals protein in the urine. A 24-hour urine collection is included in the diagnostic workup. Renal biopsy provides identification of the type and extent of tissue change. Other diagnostic testing is performed to identify the specific underlying cause.

Medical Management

Medical management depends on the extent of tissue involvement and may include the use of corticosteroids (prednisone); antineoplastic agents for immunosuppressive effect; loop diuretics; and a low-sodium, high-protein diet for therapeutic management of edema. Hypoproteinemia may be treated with normal serum albumin and protein-rich nutrition replacement therapy.

Nursing Interventions and Patient Teaching

Nursing interventions include monitoring fluid balance. Daily weight should be determined. The abdominal girth should be measured daily for changes. I&O should be recorded along with characteristics of urine passed. Other nursing interventions include maintaining bed rest in the presence of extreme edema (recumbent position may initiate diuresis) and assessing for electrolyte imbalance. Skin care is important, as is a gradual increase in activity as the edema is resolved.

Diet includes protein replacement, using foods that provide high biologic value (meat, fish, poultry, cheese, eggs) and restriction of sodium to decrease edema. Blood pressure often is elevated and should be monitored closely for changes.

As the patient begins to convalesce, the teaching plan includes the medication regimen (type, dosage, side effects, and need to finish all prescriptions), nutrition (high protein, low sodium), self-assessment of fluid status (monitor weight, presence of edema), awareness of signs and symptoms indicating a need for medical attention (increase in edema, fatigue, headache, infection), and the need for follow-up care.

Prognosis

In approximately 25% of children and 50% to 75% of adults who develop nephrosis, the disease progresses to renal failure within 5 years. Other patients (particularly children) may have remissions or chronic nephrotic syndrome. Aside from treating the underlying illness, little can be done to prevent a recurrence of nephrosis.

NEPHRITIS

Nephritis encompasses renal disorders characterized by inflammation of the kidney—involving the glomeruli, tubules, or interstitial tissue—and abnormal function. Included in this group of disorders is acute and chronic glomerulonephritis.

Acute Glomerulonephritis

Etiology and pathophysiology. The health history commonly reveals that the onset of acute glomerulonephritis was preceded by an infection, such as a sore throat or skin infection (most commonly beta-hemolytic streptococci) 2 to 3 weeks earlier, or other preexisting multisystem diseases, such as systemic lupus erythematosus. The infectious disease process triggers an immune response that results in inflammation of glomeruli that allows excretion of red blood cells and protein in the urine. This condition is common in children and young adults.

Clinical manifestations. Often family members first note that the individual has "swelling" of the face, especially around the eyes. Some patients may be acutely ill with a multitude of symptoms, whereas others may be diagnosed on routine examination with only vague symptoms.

Assessment. Subjective data include symptoms indicative of anorexia, nocturia, malaise, and exertional dyspnea.

Collection of objective data includes assessment of skin integrity and general condition of skin; the presence and degree of edema with associated difficulty in breathing on exertion, when recumbent, or as evidenced by changes in lung and heart sounds (unusual heart sounds, crackles over lung fields, distention of neck veins); hematuria with changes in urine color from "cola" to frankly sanguineous; or changes in voiding, a decrease in amount of urinary output, or dysuria.

Diagnostic tests. Diagnostic tests reveal elevation of BUN, serum creatinine, potassium, erythrocyte sedimentation rate, and antistreptolysin-O titer. Urinalysis shows red blood cells, casts, and/or protein.

Medical management. Medical management includes treatment of primary symptoms while preventing complications to cerebral and cardiac function. Serum electrolyte levels (sodium and potassium) may indicate a need to adjust dietary intake of sodium and potassium. Level of consciousness should be monitored when the BUN is elevated. Bed rest and fluid intake adjustments are guided by urinary output until diuresis is adequate.

A prophylactic antimicrobial agent, such as penicillin, may be administered for several months after the acute phase of the illness to protect against recurrence of infection. Diuretics may be prescribed to control fluid retention and antihypertensives to reduce blood pressure.

Nursing interventions and patient teaching. Nursing interventions are guided by individual patient needs, focusing on control of symptoms and prevention of complications. Dietary intake includes protein restrictions (to decrease blood urea levels), with carbohydrates providing a source of energy.

Monitor I&O and vital signs. Determine the level of activity based on the degree of edema, hypertension, proteinuria, and hematuria, because excessive activity may increase these signs (see the Health Promotion box).

 Health Promotion

The Patient With Nephritis

ACTIVITY

- Keep patient on bed rest until edema and blood pressure are reduced.
- Encourage quiet diversional activities.
- Ambulate gradually with assistance.
- Space out activities to lessen fatigue.

FLUID BALANCE MAINTENANCE

- Implement dietary restrictions.
- Monitor intake and output.
- Document reactions to medication.

DIET THERAPY

- Restrict protein to decrease nitrogenous wastes.
- Restrict sodium to prevent further fluid retention.
- Increase calories for energy source.

DRUG THERAPY

- Prophylactic antibiotics
- Antihypertensives
- Diuretics
- Drug interactions, side effects to expect and report

HEALTH MAINTENANCE

- Recovery may be extended.
- Health care provider will monitor urine for albumin and red blood cells (RBCs).
- Teach early signs of fluid retention.
- Signs and symptoms may resolve and then become worse.
- Normal activities may be resumed after urine is free of albumin and RBCs for 1 month, although the patient is not considered cured until the urine is free of albumin and RBCs for 6 months.
- Report hematuria, headache, edema.

Because glomerulonephritis is long term, patient teaching is important. Proteinuria and hematuria may exist microscopically even when other symptoms subside. Although possibly fatigued, these patients usually feel well; therefore they often must be convinced of the need to continue prescribed treatment and to return for follow-up care. Explain the nature of the illness and the effect of diet and fluids on fluid balance and sodium retention. Teach about prescribed sodium and fluid restrictions (provide written information regarding sodium content of foods, as necessary). Include information about protein restrictions and carbohydrate sources. Also discuss the medication regimen (dose, frequency, side effects, need to continue per health care provider instructions). Stress the need to pace activities with rest if fatigued; to avoid trauma and infection (which may exacerbate the illness); and to obtain follow-up health care. Teach the patient about the signs and symptoms indicating the need for medical attention (hematuria, headache, edema, hypertension).

Prognosis. The prognosis for patients with acute poststreptococcal glomerulonephritis is generally good; however, some patients develop chronic glomerulonephritis and ESRD, requiring dialysis or kidney transplantation.

Chronic Glomerulonephritis

Etiology and pathophysiology. With chronic glomerulonephritis there is usually no indication of an inciting event. Occasionally the patient with acute glomerulonephritis progresses to a chronic phase. Because other chronic illnesses (e.g., diabetes mellitus or systemic lupus erythematosus) may mask the symptoms of renal degeneration, many patients do not seek medical attention until kidney function is compromised. Chronic glomerulonephritis is characterized by slow, progressive destruction of glomeruli with related loss of function. The kidneys atrophy (actually decrease in size).

Clinical manifestations. Signs and symptoms may include malaise, morning headaches, dyspnea with exertion, visual and digestive disturbances, edema, and fatigue. Physical findings include hypertension, anemia, proteinuria, anasarca, and cardiac and cerebral manifestations.

Assessment. Subjective data include patient complaints of fatigue and a decreased ability to perform ADLs as a result of dyspnea and decreasing ability to concentrate. Investigate complaints of morning headaches (their location, pattern, and character), and note the presence of any visual disturbance.

Collection of objective data includes clarifying outward manifestations of the headache and respiratory effort that may interfere with daily task performance. Assess mental functioning, irritability, slurred speech, ataxia, or tremors. Carefully assess and document the degree of edema, noting specific location and response to pressure by pressing the fingers into the edematous area and observing for pitting. Note skin color, ecchymoses (irregularly formed hemorrhagic areas of the skin) or rash, dry skin, and scratching. Observe urine color and amount. Monitor vital signs, including a chest assessment for cardiac and pulmonary signs of fluid retention: unusual heart sounds, crackles over lung fields, and distention of neck veins.

Diagnostic tests. Early disease shows albumin and red blood cells in the urine, although kidney function test results are within normal limits. With advanced destruction of nephrons, the specific gravity becomes fixed and blood levels of NPN wastes (creatinine and urea) increase. Creatinine clearance may be as low as 5 to 10 mL/min, compared with the normal range of 107 to 139 mL/min in men and 87 to 107 mL/min in women.

Medical management. Medical management includes control of secondary side effects as discussed for acute glomerulonephritis, with renal dialysis and possible kidney transplantation to provide elimination of wastes from the body.

Nursing interventions and patient teaching. Nursing interventions for the patient with chronic glomerulonephritis represent a special challenge. This patient already has had major damage to the kidney filtration system. It is crucial that the patient's condition not be further compromised by infection or other complications. Monitor changes in vital signs and diagnostic tests to aid in choosing proper nursing interventions. Interventions parallel those noted with nephrotic syndrome and acute glomerulonephritis. Chronic glomerulonephritis may progress to ESRD, necessitating related nursing interventions (see the Health Promotion box: The Patient With Nephritis).

Patient problems and interventions for the patient with chronic glomerulonephritis include but are not limited to the following:

Patient Problem	Nursing Interventions
Fluid Volume Overload, related to decreased urinary output	Assess the patient's understanding of therapeutic interventions Note I&O q hr (or more often) Monitor signs and symptoms of fluid excess (weight gain, hypertension, edema, dyspnea) Provide ice chips for thirst with prescribed diet Monitor and report abnormal laboratory results
Inability to Tolerate Activity, related to kidney dysfunction	Assess level of activity tolerance Encourage patient to report activities that increase fatigue Plan activities to minimize fatigue

Patient teaching focuses on preventive health maintenance, emphasizing a health-promoting lifestyle, with prevention and early treatment of infections.

Prognosis. Some people with minimal impairment in kidney function continue to feel well and show little progression of disease. With other patients the progression of renal deterioration may be slow but steady and end in renal failure. In still others the disease progresses rapidly.

RENAL FAILURE

Renal failure is characterized by the kidneys' inability to remove wastes, concentrate urine, and conserve or eliminate electrolytes. Diabetes mellitus is the most common cause of renal failure, accounting for more than 40% of new cases. Other predisposing concurrent illnesses include burns, trauma, heart failure, volume depletion, and renal disease. Nursing interventions to prevent the development of renal failure include providing adequate hydration, preventing infections, monitoring for signs and symptoms of shock, and teaching drug side effects to report immediately.

ACUTE RENAL FAILURE

Etiology and Pathophysiology

Kidney function may be altered by interference with the kidneys' ability to be selective in filtering blood or by an actual decrease in blood flow to the kidneys. ARF can be caused by many medical conditions, such as hemorrhage, trauma, infection, and decreased cardiac output. Certain medications also may be nephrotoxic. These include medications such as analgesics (acetaminophen and aspirin), antihistamines (including diphenhydramine), and antimicrobials (penicillin and cephalosporin).

The course of ARF is divided into phases. In the *oliguric phase,* BUN and serum creatinine levels rise while urinary output decreases to less than 400 mL in 24 hours. The oliguric phase may last from several days to 4 weeks to several months. Some patients may experience the nonoliguric form, usually caused by nephrotoxic antibiotics, in which urinary output may exceed 2 L in 24 hours. In the *diuretic phase,* blood chemistry levels begin to return to normal and urinary output increases to 1 to 2 L in 24 hours. The diuretic phase usually lasts 1 to 3 weeks. Return to normal or near-normal function occurs in the *recovery phase*. Recovery begins as the glomerular filtration rate rises. Recovery can take up to 1 year.

Clinical Manifestations

The patient may experience anorexia, nausea, vomiting, edema, and associated signs and symptoms of diminished kidney function.

Assessment

Subjective data include patient reports of lethargy, loss of appetite, nausea, and headache.

Objective data involve physical findings of progression of the disease process. Assess for dry mucous membranes, poor skin turgor, urinary output of less than 400 mL in 24 hours, vomiting, diarrhea, and anasarca. Note skin color changes. Monitor daily weight and changes in body mass. Assessment findings may include central nervous system manifestations of drowsiness, muscle twitching, and seizures.

Diagnostic Tests

Physical assessment, history, and elevated blood chemistry tests such as BUN and creatinine (azotemia) confirm the diagnosis. After the patient is stabilized, further studies may be done to assess for residual damage.

Medical Management

Measures include administration of fluids and osmotic preparations to prevent decreased renal perfusion, manage fluid volume, and treat electrolyte imbalances. Renal dialysis may be necessary to manage systemic fluid shifts, especially cardiac and respiratory, and may be effective in removing some nephrotoxins.

Diet should be protein sparing, high in carbohydrates, and low in potassium and sodium. Drug therapy may include diuretics to increase urinary output (e.g., furosemide, hydrochlorothiazide). Potassium-lowering agents are used to remove potassium through the gastrointestinal tract; sodium polystyrene sulfonate is administered orally, per nasogastric tube, or as a retention enema. Antibiotics that are not dependent on kidney excretion are used to eradicate or prevent infection. Whatever combination of drug therapy is used, dosage and administration times require adjustment according to the level of kidney function.

Nursing Interventions and Patient Teaching

Accurately document urinary output to identify the level of kidney function. Azotemia may be revealed by blood chemistry studies. Observe the patient with azotemia for changes in level of consciousness. Closely monitor fluid status, vital signs, and response to therapies. Frequent skin care with tepid water to remove urea crystals is comforting. Dialysis presents special nursing challenges, discussed later in this chapter.

Teaching includes identifying preventable environmental or health factors contributing to the illness (such as hypertension, nephrotoxic drugs). Teach the patient about activity restrictions, dietary restrictions, and the medication regimen. Provide nutritional support with specialized enteral formulas, which may contain essential amino acids and minerals, in addition to replacement of electrolytes (especially sodium to match insensible loss) and provision of caloric needs. Make a nutritional assessment with appropriate modifications daily.

Stress the need to report signs and symptoms of infection and of returning renal failure to the health care provider. Emphasize the need for ongoing follow-up care.

Prognosis

Recovery from an episode of ARF depends on the underlying illness, the patient's condition, and careful supportive management given during the period of kidney shutdown. The leading cause of death is infection, such as that of the urinary tract, lungs, and peritoneum. Mortality from fluid overload and acidosis has been reduced as a result of dialysis and other forms of therapy. Patients who survive the acute episode of tubular insufficiency have a chance of recovering kidney function. Although renal tissue may regenerate more completely after toxic injury than ischemia, both forms usually show a return to normal or near-normal kidney function.

For those in whom ARF has been caused by glomerular disease or severe infection of renal tissue, the prognosis may not be as favorable. Return of kidney function is determined by the extent of scarring and destruction of functional renal tissue that has occurred during the acute episode of renal failure.

CHRONIC RENAL FAILURE (END-STAGE RENAL DISEASE)

Etiology and Pathophysiology

Chronic renal failure, or ESRD, exists when the kidneys are unable to regain normal function. ESRD develops slowly over an extended period as a result of renal disease or other disease processes that compromise renal blood perfusion. As much as 80% of nephrons may be severely impaired before loss of kidney function is detected. The most common causes of ESRD are pyelonephritis, chronic glomerulonephritis, glomerulosclerosis, chronic urinary obstruction, severe hypertension, diabetes mellitus, gout, and PKD. Whatever the cause, dialysis or kidney transplantation is needed to maintain life.

ESRD represents a significant health problem worldwide. The number of patients diagnosed with ESRD has increased by 57%. There are currently more than 615,000 patients being treated for ESRD in the United States. In 2011 more than 92,000 people died from ESRD (National Kidney Foundation, 2013). ESRD also may cause a financial crisis for patients and their families. For some, the government actively helps defray costs through the Medicare program.

Clinical Manifestations

The onset of signs and symptoms may be so gradual and the signs and symptoms so vague that the patient is unable to identify when the problems started. When questioned, the patient may be able to relate occurrences that seemed insignificant at the time. The clinical picture is usually unique to the individual. Common symptoms include headache; lethargy; asthenia (decreased strength or energy); anorexia; pruritus; elimination changes; anuria; muscle cramps or twitching; impotence; characteristic dusky yellow-tan or gray skin color from retained urochrome pigments; and signs and symptoms characteristic of central nervous system involvement, such as disorientation and mental lapses.

Other associated conditions are responsible for many of the symptoms. Azotemia develops as excessive amounts of nitrogenous compounds build up in the blood. Anemia occurs when the production of renal erythropoietin is decreased as a result of loss of kidney function. Acidosis, hypertension, and glucose intolerance may occur as a result of the insult to homeostasis.

Assessment

Subjective data include patient complaints of joint pain and edema; severe headaches; nausea; anorexia; intermittent chest pain; weakness; and in particular, fatigue, intractable singultus (hiccups), decreased libido, menstrual irregularities, and impaired concentration. The clinical consequences of renal failure are far-reaching, affecting nearly every body system.

Collection of objective data involves a nursing assessment that may yield unremarkable results, except for signs and symptoms that support the patient complaints. Uremic encephalopathy affects the central nervous system. Usually the first sign is a reduction in alertness and awareness. The patient exhibits Kussmaul's respirations (abnormally deep, very rapid sighing respirations), and coma develops. The accumulation of urates results in halitosis with a urine odor and "uremic frost" on the skin in the form of a white powder.

Diagnostic Tests

Diagnosis of ESRD is confirmed by elevated BUN of at least 50 mg/dL and serum creatinine levels greater than 5 mg/dL, electrolyte imbalance (including decreased bicarbonate and magnesium and increased potassium, sodium, and phosphate), and other indicators related to the underlying cause. Kidney function studies assess the degree of damage or level of kidney function.

Medical Management

Medical management is instituted to conserve kidney function as long as possible. Renal dialysis is initiated when necessary, and the patient may be prepared for kidney transplantation. Drug therapy may include anticonvulsants to control seizure activity (phenytoin [Dilantin], diazepam [Valium]), antianemics, vitamin supplements to counteract nutritional deficiencies, antiemetics (prochlorperazine), antipruritics (cyproheptadine), and biologic response modifiers to stimulate red cell production (epoetin alfa [Epogen, EPO]) to treat anemia caused by a reduced production of erythropoietin. Iron deficiency anemia must be treated with ferrous sulfate orally or with iron dextran (DexFerrum by Z-track intramuscular injection) before epoetin alfa will be effective.

Nursing Interventions and Patient Teaching

Nursing interventions focus on restoring homeostasis. Measures to control fluid and electrolyte balance vary greatly, according to individual patient needs. Nutritional therapy is aimed at preserving protein stores and preventing production of additional protein waste products that the kidney would have to clear. Patients on dialysis often need 8 to 10 g of protein daily.

The diet is high in calories from carbohydrates and fats from polyunsaturated sources (to maintain weight and spare protein), at least 2500 to 3000 calories daily. Other dietary restrictions are related to the patient's degree of acidosis. Potassium is retained, so foods high in potassium are restricted. Sodium is controlled at a level sufficient to replace sodium loss without causing fluid retention.

Nursing interventions for ARF also are instituted for ESRD. Provide emotional support for the patient who faces role changes and invasive treatments such as dialysis or kidney transplantation. As discussed in the Health Promotion box, fluid balance is of prime importance. The patient may have fluid equal to the amount excreted in the urine plus about 300 to 600 mL to compensate for *insensible* (imperceptible) *fluid loss* (fluid lost through the lungs, perspiration, and feces). Salt substitutes are not advised because most contain potassium. If seizure activity occurs, institute safety measures to protect the patient (Nursing Care Plan 50.1).

Patient teaching should emphasize food exchanges and fluid intake within restrictions prescribed for that patient. Encourage the patient to increase activity as tolerated; maintain impeccable skin care; prevent infection and injury; and develop coping behaviors to adapt to lifestyle changes for patient, family, and caregiver.

Health Promotion

The Patient With Renal Failure

FLUID AND ELECTROLYTE BALANCE

- Assess intake and output (hourly if indicated).
- Weigh daily (same time, same clothing, same scale).
- Assess overt (open to view) signs of hydration status: edema, turgor.
- Assess covert (hidden) signs of hydration status: breath sounds, laboratory studies, and so on.

NUTRITION

- Provide prescribed diet.
- Guide patient food selection.
- Plan fluid intake per shift within prescribed limits and according to patient preference.
- Reinforce diet instructions as indicated.

COMFORT AND SAFETY

- Provide quiet environment (sound and lighting).
- Space nursing interventions to conserve patient energy.
- Medicate as needed for comfort.
- Provide skin care to alleviate discomfort from pruritus.
- Provide mouth care as needed.
- Maintain asepsis during procedures.
- Prevent exposure to pathogens.

COPING BEHAVIORS

- Listen (to patient and significant others).
- Refer to pastoral care or religious support group.
- Provide private times with significant others.
- Offer interview with social services.

DOCUMENTATION AND REPORTING

- Document all relevant findings.
- Maintain open communications with supervisory staff.
- Adjust nursing care plan as indicated to meet changing patient needs.
- Maintain dietary restrictions: food exchange, measuring fluids, food diary.
- Take health promotion–illness prevention measures.

CARE OF THE PATIENT REQUIRING DIALYSIS

Dialysis is a medical procedure for the removal of certain elements from the blood; the process is based on differences in the rate of diffusion of these elements through an external semipermeable membrane or, in the case of peritoneal dialysis, through the peritoneal membrane. Dialysis mimics kidney function, helping to restore balance when normal kidney function is interrupted temporarily or permanently. Dialysis involves the *diffusion* of wastes, drugs, and/or excess electrolytes and *osmosis* of water across a semipermeable membrane into a dialysate fluid that is prescribed to meet individual needs. Dialysis is achieved by the process of hemodialysis or peritoneal dialysis.

HEMODIALYSIS

Hemodialysis is used for patients with acute or irreversible renal failure and fluid and electrolyte imbalances. Hemodialysis requires access to the patient's circulatory system to route blood through the artificial kidney (dialyzer) for removal of wastes, fluids, and electrolytes; the blood is then returned to the patient's body. Box 50.4 lists nursing intervention guidelines. Temporary methods include subclavian or femoral catheters or an external shunt placed in the nondominant forearm (Fig. 50.10A). In ESRD, access can be achieved by constructing a direct arteriovenous (AV) fistula (surgically connecting an artery to a vein) or a graft (placing a synthetic tubelike material between an artery and a vein) (see Fig. 50.10B). The AV fistula is preferred for permanent access because synthetic grafts frequently become clotted with blood ("clotting off"). Hemodialysis usually is scheduled three times a week for 3 to 6 hours. Patients can be maintained on dialysis therapy indefinitely or while waiting for kidney transplantation. Hemodialysis while managing the condition does not cure or reverse it.

There are complications of hemodialysis. Cardiovascular complications include heart failure, stroke, angina and peripheral vascular disease. The leading cause of disease of patients on hemodialysis is cardiovascular disease. Additional complications related to rapid changes in fluid and electrolyte levels include hypotension, muscle cramping, dysrhythmias, headaches, nausea, and vomiting (Hinkle and Cheever, 2017).

In a comparative study of the use of daily versus traditional hemodialysis on alternative days, researchers found that more frequent hemodialysis decreased the risk of fatal nonrenal complications of ARF (Schiffl et al, 2002).

Nursing Care Plan 50.1 The Patient With End-Stage Renal Disease

Mr. J., a 37-year-old high school basketball coach, visited his family health care provider with complaints of weight gain, decreasing strength, increasing inability to concentrate, and morning headaches. Physical examination revealed severe hypertension, yellow-gray skin color, and pale mucous membranes. After diagnostic studies reveal chronic glomerulonephritis with end-stage renal disease (ESRD), Mr. J. is admitted to the hospital to stabilize his condition.

PATIENT PROBLEM

Fluid Volume Overload, related to compromised renal regulatory mechanism, as evidenced by systemic edema

Patient Goals and Expected Outcomes	Nursing Interventions	Evaluation
The patient will be able to reduce fluid to precrisis level	Record baseline assessment data. Create chart for patient to monitor: • Daily weight • Intake and output • Edema	Patient is able to complete daily self-monitoring with 1-lb weight loss daily.
The patient will modify diet to exclude foods and fluids that foster sodium, potassium, and water retention	Teach nutritional guidelines for dietary and fluid parameters with scheduling. Evaluate daily or as needed for systemic edema: girth, skin turgor, respiratory rate and quality. Monitor for manifestations of electrolyte imbalance. Teach patient and significant other about the type, cause, and treatment for fluid and electrolyte imbalance, as appropriate.	Patient can order daily diet and fluids within prescribed parameters.

PATIENT PROBLEM

Helplessness, related to sudden onset of life-altering illness as evidenced by patient statements: "I've always tried to take care of myself—look where it got me. Nowhere! Now I have to face my own death!"

Patient Goals and Expected Outcomes	Nursing Interventions	Evaluation
The patient will be empowered to assist in planning own care and in goal achievement	Provide support for the patient. Explain plans and procedures before scheduled times, according to patient's ability to understand. Negotiate with patient when changes are necessary. Accept patient's expression of self and values. Include significant other in planning for the patient's maximum role in self-management. Communicate unique patient planning arrangements for continuity with all treatment team members.	Patient voices a sense that the staff is sensitive to his needs. Patient seems able to plan modifications in work and home schedules to accommodate health needs.

PATIENT PROBLEM

Insufficient Knowledge, related to health education and home maintenance for ESRD

Patient Goals and Expected Outcomes	Nursing Interventions	Evaluation
The patient will describe the fundamental characteristics of ESRD and treatment options	Assess the amount and depth of the patient's information about ESRD. Collaborate with health care provider and treatment team in individualizing established institutional protocol for care of the patient with ESRD: 1. What happens when kidneys fail? 2. Treatment options include hemodialysis, peritoneal dialysis, and kidney transplantation 3. Inpatient versus outpatient care 4. Financing treatment 5. Teaching aids 6. Organizations that can help Plan time to listen to the patient's and family's concerns and fears. Allow time for questions and answers and teaching reinforcement each day. Arrange (with patient's permission) opportunity for patient and family to meet with a patient or family that is positively adapting to ESRD. Be consistent in scheduling treatments with primary health care providers. Participate in end-of-life planning, when and if appropriate.	Patient can correctly answer basic questions about treatment options. Patient can correctly answer questions from teaching and is open to pose new questions.

Nursing Care Plan 50.1 The Patient With End-Stage Renal Disease—cont'd

CRITICAL THINKING QUESTIONS

1. Mr. J. complains of loss of appetite and limited food choices. What would be some helpful suggestions to improve his nutritional status?
2. Mr. J. established a therapeutic nurse-patient relationship with the nurse and confided that he is having marital problems partly because of his inability to have a satisfactory sexual relationship with his wife. What would be an appropriate response?
3. The nurse notes Mr. J.'s lack of interest in his therapeutic regimen of diet, medications, and fluid restrictions. He states, "What's the use? I will never be well again." What would be some therapeutic interventions?

Medical Management

Medical management includes continuation of previously instituted therapies. Closely monitor blood levels of drugs excreted by the kidney to maintain therapeutic levels and prevent toxic accumulations. Dose adjustments are affected by the glomerular filtration rate, dialysis, vomiting, and doses missed during hospital treatments. Medication may include antihypertensives, cardiac glycosides, antibiotics, and antidysrhythmics. Instruct the patient not to take over-the-counter medications without consulting the health care provider.

Nursing Interventions

Nursing interventions are dictated by individual patient conditions, including other acute or chronic problems. Most patients are dialyzed on an outpatient basis. (General nursing intervention guidelines are noted in Box 50.4 and Nursing Care Plan 50.1.) Psychosocial aspects of care for patients receiving dialysis are illustrated in the Communication box.

Nurses have a key responsibility for maintaining access sites and preventing or managing infection. Use a structured teaching program, with individualized patient teaching strategies to accommodate culture and knowledge level.

PERITONEAL DIALYSIS

Peritoneal dialysis can be performed with a minimum of equipment and by an ambulatory patient. Unlike hemodialysis, peritoneal dialysis is performed four times a day, 7 days a week. One exchange cycle usually requires 30 to 40 minutes. The principle of osmosis and diffusion through a semipermeable membrane is the same as in hemodialysis, but the peritoneal membrane lining the peritoneum is used as the semipermeable membrane instead of an artificial kidney. Peritoneal dialysis is contraindicated for patients with systemic inflammatory disease, previous abdominal surgery, and chronic back pain, among other conditions.

To facilitate peritoneal dialysis, the health care provider places a catheter into the peritoneal space under aseptic conditions (Fig. 50.11). The dialyzing fluid is instilled for a predetermined period; this fluid draws waste from blood vessels in the peritoneal lining and then is drained and replaced. The patient with ESRD may be maintained on peritoneal dialysis, continuous ambulatory peritoneal dialysis (CAPD), or continuous cycle peritoneal dialysis (CCPD). Nocturnal intermittent peritoneal dialysis can be done three to five times per week for 10 to 12 hours. The patient is taught how to do the dialysis, which allows for more freedom. Although hemodialysis also can be done at home using strict

Box 50.4 Nursing Intervention Guidelines for the Patient Undergoing Hemodialysis

PATIENT TEACHING

- Reinforce explanation of dialysis procedure.
- Inform of community resources.
- Explain dietary restrictions.
- Teach about self-care and provide general information.

MONITORING DURING DIALYSIS

- Maintain asepsis and universal precautions.
- Weigh before and after treatment.
- Obtain vital signs every 30 to 60 minutes (take blood pressure in arm without fistula).
- Maintain orientation (thought processes may be altered).
- Assess for hemorrhage resulting from heparin use during dialysis.
- Monitor equipment (interruption of procedure).

ACTIVITY

- Provide diversions (reading, television, sleep).
- Ensure patient comfort (reclining, sitting, lying).
- Monitor dietary intake (may be hungry or nauseated).

CARE AFTER DIALYSIS OR BETWEEN TREATMENTS

- Schedule fluid intake within restrictions.
- Monitor for signs of fluid and electrolyte imbalance.
- Assess the access site for signs of infection, adequate circulation.
- Post signs regarding location of access site; do not take blood pressure or perform a venipuncture on arm with access site.
- Auscultate arteriovenous fistula for bruit (adventitious sound of venous or arterial origin heard on auscultation); palpate arteriovenous fistula for thrill (abnormal tremor).
- Assess, document, and report changes in general status.
- Provide skin care: bathe with tepid water to remove urea deposits.

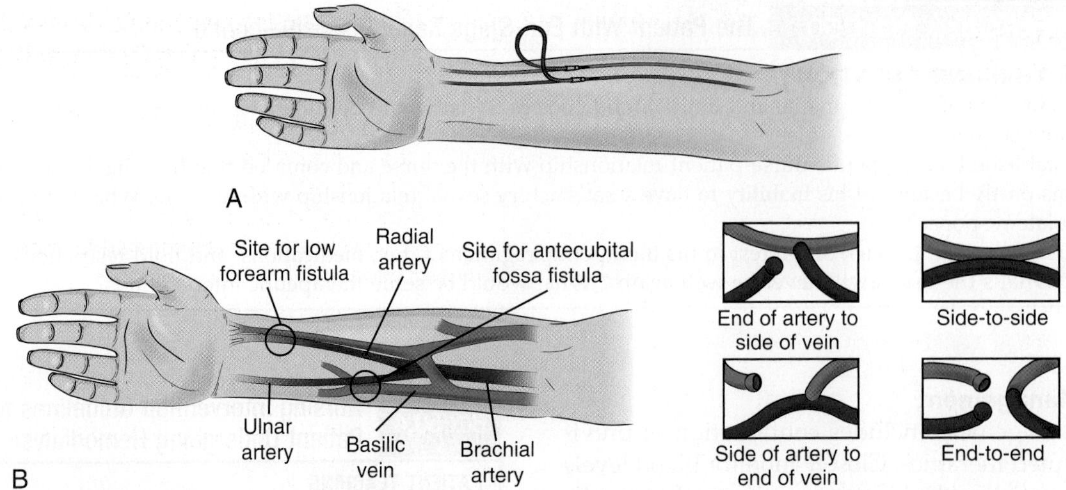

Fig. 50.10 A, External arteriovenous shunt. B, Internal arteriovenous fistula. Types of fistula construction.

aseptic technique, it is much more expensive and confining than CAPD.

Nursing Interventions

Common complications associated with peritoneal dialysis guide nursing interventions. Hypotension may occur with excessive sodium and fluid removal. Peritonitis may arise from sepsis. Pain and hemorrhage may accompany instillation of the dialysate. Box 50.5 lists nursing intervention guidelines for peritoneal dialysis.

Patient problems and interventions for the patient undergoing dialysis include but are not limited to the following:

Patient Problem	Nursing Interventions
Impaired Role Functioning, related to: • Chronic illness • Treatment side effects	Encourage verbalization of self-concept Assist in identifying personal strengths Assist patient and significant others with clarifying expected roles and those that must be relinquished or altered Support grief work if loss of role has occurred
Compromised Blood Flow to Tissue, Peripheral, related to: • Risk of disconnection • Clotting of vascular access	Avoid taking blood pressure and performing venipuncture in arm with fistula or graft Auscultate for bruits Observe access site for skin color and condition After dialysis, inspect needle puncture sites for bleeding

Prognosis

The patient with effective medical management can be maintained indefinitely on dialysis.

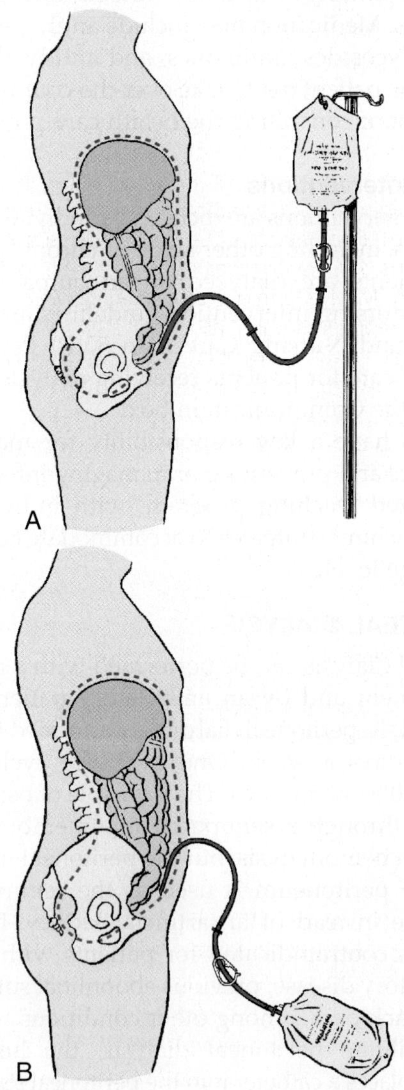

Fig. 50.11 Peritoneal dialysis. A, Inflow. B, Outflow. (From Tucker S, Canobbio MM, Paquette EV, et al: *Patient care standards: Collaborative practice planning guides*, ed 6, St. Louis, 1996, Mosby.)

Communication

Psychosocial Aspects of Care for Patients Receiving Dialysis

Mr. J., a student nurse, enters Mr. K.'s room to complete the initial morning assessment and finds him crying while struggling to get out of bed.

Nurse: Mr. K., what's wrong? (general lead, allows patient to describe)

Patient: Oh, nothing!

Nurse: (therapeutic silence, remains attentive, gives time)

Patient: Nothing is going right. I might as well be dead.

Nurse: What's wrong? (general lead, patient did not answer, encourages description)

Patient: I was trying to get up to take a shower, but I'm so weak I can't get myself out of bed.

Nurse: That must be frustrating. (voicing the implied)

Patient: That's an understatement! Look at me! I'm 37 years old—I should be in my prime but instead I'm gaining weight. I can't do my job because I can't concentrate. How am I supposed to feel?

Nurse: It must be frightening to experience all these changes. It would be understandable for you to be scared. (validating feelings)

Patient: I am scared! What if I never get better? I read this article about someone younger than I am who had the same thing, and he died when he had to go on dialysis.

Nurse: What do you think will happen to you? (general lead, encourages description without prescribing response)

Patient: Well, I don't know. The doctor keeps avoiding my questions and I see myself being less able to do anything. Maybe I am afraid—afraid of dying.

Nurse: (therapeutic silence, allows time for reflection)

Patient: Well, I never thought I'd say that—being afraid to die. It doesn't seem so frightening to say. I guess I didn't trust myself to be honest with myself or anyone else.

Nurse: Being honest with yourself is an important step to understanding. (pause) It seems, too, that you may not have accurate information about your illness. Let's plan to talk with your doctor about what you can reasonably expect—things you will be able to do, limitations, and things that you can do to enhance your physical and emotional health. (summarizing and goal setting for individualized patient teaching and discharge planning)

Patient: That sounds great, Mr. J. I really do want to do whatever I can to improve my chances of a better life. Would you help me get up to shower?

SURGICAL PROCEDURES FOR URINARY DYSFUNCTION

If damage to the urinary system cannot be corrected by medical management, surgical intervention may be necessary for temporary or permanent resection of the affected organ, such as when kidney function is lost. Dialysis is a viable management alternative, but a kidney transplant is preferable. The patient may require a kidney from a live or cadaver donor to replace the damaged kidney. Common surgical interventions and nursing intervention priorities are listed in Table 50.3. Preoperative and intraoperative management measures are the same as for major abdominal surgery with general anesthesia (see Chapter 42). Suggested patient problem statements include those for abdominal surgery.

Box 50.5 Nursing Intervention Guidelines for the Patient Undergoing Peritoneal Dialysis

PATIENT TEACHING

- Explanation of procedure
- Signs of complications
- Diet or fluid restrictions
- Medication (schedule in relation to dialysis time)
- Dialysate kept at body temperature to lessen discomfort

MONITORING DURING DIALYSIS

- Weight before and after procedure
- Hemorrhage (smoky, pink, or red-tinged dialysate)
- Type of dialysate (tailored to patient needs)
- Amount and timing of dialysate instillation
- Vital signs

CARE BETWEEN DIALYSES

- Signs of peritonitis (pain, fever, cloudy fluid)
- Strict aseptic care of catheter site
- Weigh daily

NEPHRECTOMY

Nephrectomy is the surgical removal of the kidney, either a small portion or the entire organ and surrounding tissues. In partial nephrectomy, only the diseased or infected portion of the kidney is removed. Radical nephrectomy involves removing the entire kidney, a section of the ureter, the adrenal gland, and the fatty tissue surrounding the kidney.

Postoperative management for surgical removal of the kidney is based on the prevention and detection of hemorrhage by monitoring vital signs, especially pulse and blood pressure; observation for restlessness and for gastrointestinal complications of nausea, vomiting, and abdominal distention; and establishment of adequate urinary drainage. Record I&O. If the thoracic cavity is opened during surgery, the patient will have chest tubes (see Chapter 49). Pain may compromise respiratory efficiency. Administer analgesics as ordered to facilitate lung expansion and the patient's activity level. Reposition the patient every 2 hours and ambulate as ordered. Change dressings according to the health care provider's order, and record the amount and color of any drainage. Maintain close surveillance on the function of the remaining kidney.

Patient Teaching

Instruct the patient to avoid heavy lifting, drink 2000 mL of fluid each day (unless contraindicated), monitor output, avoid consumption of alcohol, and avoid respiratory tract infections and hazardous activities that could damage the remaining kidney.

Prognosis

Complete recovery from nephrectomy is expected in the absence of any complication.

Table 50.3 Surgical Procedures for Urinary Dysfunction

SURGICAL INTERVENTION	NURSING INTERVENTION PRIORITIES
Nephrostomy: Surgical procedure in which an incision is made on the patient's flank so that a catheter can be inserted into the renal pelvis for drainage	Meticulous skin care, assessment for hemorrhage, accurate intake and output (I&O)
Nephrectomy: Surgical removal of the kidney	Assessment for hemorrhage, promotion of respiratory effort, accurate I&O
Cystectomy: Surgical removal of the bladder	Promotion of urinary drainage via ileal conduit, I&O
Ureterosigmoidostomy: Surgical procedure in which a ureter is implanted in the sigmoid colon of the intestinal tract	Meticulous skin care, monitoring of electrolyte imbalance, assessment of signs and symptoms of infection
Cutaneous ureterostomy: Surgical implantation of the terminal ends of the ureter under the skin	Meticulous skin care, assessment of urinary obstruction, accurate I&O

NEPHROSTOMY

A nephrostomy is an incision created between the kidney and the skin to drain urine directly from the renal pelvis. A nephrostomy is performed when an occlusion keeps urine from passing from the kidney, through the ureter, and into the urinary bladder. Without a way for urine to drain, pressure would rise within the urinary system and damage the kidneys. The most common cause of obstruction is cancer. This procedure also can be used to remove kidney stones.

Catheters are used to drain the wound. Take care to prevent obstruction of the catheters with blood clots postoperatively. Measure and record the amount and nature of drainage from the catheters, and change dressings frequently, keeping the skin clean by surgical asepsis. Turn the patient to position on the affected side as ordered to facilitate drainage and assist in respiratory ventilation. Never clamp a nephrostomy catheter (tube); acute pyelonephritis may result. If ordered by the health care provider, irrigate a nephrostomy catheter, using strict aseptic technique. Gentle instillation of no more than 5 mL of sterile saline solution at one time prevents renal damage.

KIDNEY TRANSPLANTATION

Kidney transplantation is performed as an intervention in irreversible renal failure. The donor kidney surgically is placed retroperitoneally in the iliac fossa. The nonfunctioning kidney is typically not removed. The donor renal artery is anastomosed to the recipient's internal or external iliac artery and the donor renal vein to the recipient's iliac vein. Usually, the kidney begins to function immediately.

Selection of a transplant recipient is based on careful evaluation of the patient's medical, immunologic, and psychosocial status. Usually a recipient is younger than age 70, has an estimated life expectancy of 2 years or more, and is expected to have improved quality of life after transplantation. Through conservative management and dialysis, the patient's state is as nontoxic as possible. Preoperative nursing intervention is complicated by the patient's fear and anxiety about transplantation and about possible rejection of the implanted organ. The patient is dialyzed until surgery can be completed satisfactorily. In surgery the nonfunctioning kidney remains in place and the donor kidney is positioned in the iliac fossa anterior to the crest of the ileum. The ureter is anastomosed into either the patient's ureter or bladder (Fig. 50.12). However, bilateral nephrectomy may be performed before the transplantation procedure for persistent or active bacterial pyelonephritis, uncontrolled renin-mediated hypertension, polycystic kidneys, or rapidly progressive glomerulonephritis.

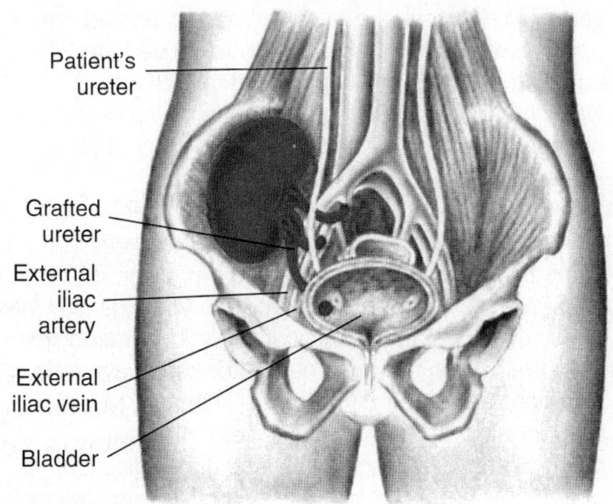

Fig. 50.12 Kidney transplantation. (From Belcher AE: *Cancer nursing*, St. Louis, 1992, Mosby.)

Postoperatively, assess the patient for signs of rejection and infection: apprehension, generalized edema, fever, increased blood pressure, oliguria, edema, and tenderness over the graft site. An immunosuppressive agent, such as cyclosporine, is used alone or in conjunction with steroids. Cyclosporine is considered an effective drug in suppressing the immune system's efforts to reject tissue while leaving the recipient sufficient immune activity to combat infection. Mycophenolate (CellCept) and tacrolimus (Prograf) are drugs used to prevent rejection of kidney transplants; they are used in combination with corticosteroids. Immunosuppressive therapy increases the risk for infection and possible steroid-induced bleeding. Teaching the patient about the medications prescribed to prevent rejection is key to the patient's successful recovery.

Patient Teaching

Postoperative care includes special assessment of kidney function and electrolyte balance. The function of the transplanted kidney is the primary concern after surgery. Home follow-up becomes a life pattern for the transplantation patient. Patient education is extensive: diet, fluids, daily weights, strict I&O measurements, prevention of infection, and avoidance of activities that may compromise the integrity of the urinary tract. Community support groups, sponsored by the American Association of Kidney Patients, help the patient and the family adapt to living with dialysis and transplantation. The National Kidney Foundation has a written protocol for the procurement of organs for donation.

Prognosis

Success of kidney transplantation parallels the individual patient's general health status and compliance with the treatment plan. Transplantation offers the only possibility of return to a normal lifestyle for the patient with ESRD. Successful kidney transplantation prolongs and markedly improves quality of life, freeing the patient from the restrictions of dialysis.

URINARY DIVERSION

Several types of procedures are used to divert the flow of urine when required for treatment of bladder cancer, invasive cervical cancer, neurogenic bladder, and congenital anomalies. Often a cystectomy (the surgical removal of the bladder) is performed.

The cystectomy patient presents a unique challenge because of the need to create an artificial port for urine elimination. The most common urinary diversion procedure is the **ileal conduit** (Bricker's procedure or ileal loop); the ureters are implanted into a loop of the ileum that is isolated and brought to the surface of the abdominal wall (Fig. 50.13). On occasion, a segment of the sigmoid colon is isolated and used instead of the ileum to form a sigmoid conduit. Bowel function is maintained with anastomosis of the remaining intestine. A drainage bag (urostomy bag or appliance) is fitted over the stoma to contain the constant drainage of urine. Continuous urine drainage prevents increased pressure within the conduit that would cause backflow to the kidneys, compromise the circulatory integrity of the conduit, or rupture the surgical anastomosis. Decreased urinary output and low abdominal pain may signal the onset of such problems. Complications of this procedure are wound infection, dehiscence (unintended wound opening), urinary leakage, ureteral obstruction, small bowel obstruction, stomal gangrene or atrophy, pyelonephritis, renal calculi, and compromised respiratory status secondary to incisional pain.

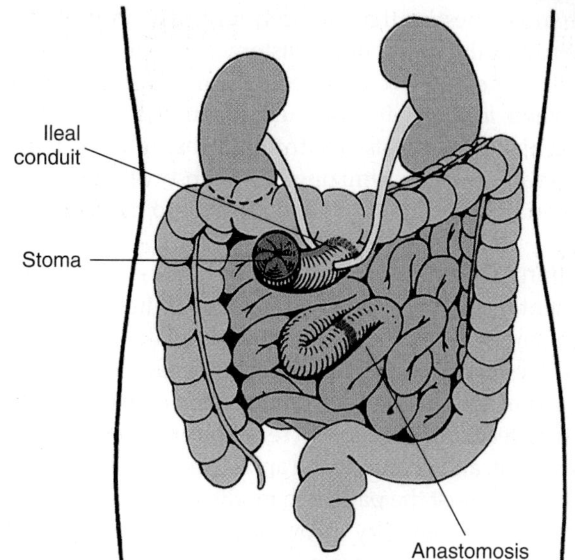

Fig. 50.13 Ileal conduit or ileal loop.

Postoperatively, measure urine flow hourly. Report output less than 30 mL/h to the health care provider immediately. A healthy stoma appears moist and pink and may even bleed slightly. Inspect the skin around the stoma daily for signs of bleeding, excoriation, and infection. Mucus is present in the urine from the intestinal secretions. The patient should ingest large quantities of water to flush the ileal conduit. Any odor of urine about the patient may indicate an infection or leak of urine from the drainage bag. Early signs of urinary leakage (indicating a leak in an anastomosis) include increased abdominal girth; fever; and drainage through the incision, tubes, or drains. Ureteral separation from the conduit may cause urine to seep into the peritoneal cavity; observe the patient for signs and symptoms of peritonitis such as fever, abdominal pain and rigidity, and absence of bowel sounds.

Care of the patient with an ileal conduit is a nursing challenge because of the continuous drainage of urine through the stoma.

To change the urostomy bag, remove and drain it. Cleanse the skin with water, and apply the new appliance as outlined in the institution's standards of care. When the peristomal skin is healed, the bag is emptied at 2- to 3-hour intervals. At night a straight drainage tube is connected to a drainage bag. A permanent urostomy bag can be left in place for 4 to 7 days if it remains sealed. Recommend that the patient have two bags so that one can be worn while the other is washed. Some patients prefer to use disposable bags. Odor is controlled by using deodorant drops or tablets in the urostomy bag; avoiding odor-producing foods, such as beans, onions, cabbage, asparagus, high-fiber wheat, simple sugars, and milk in the lactose-intolerant patient; and cleansing the urostomy bag with a vinegar-and-water rinse and thoroughly drying.

The *continent ileal urinary reservoir,* or *Kock pouch,* is created by implantation of the ureters into a segment of the small intestine that has been surgically removed from the rest of the bowel and anastomosed to the abdominal wall. Urine flow is controlled by a nipple-like valve that prevents leakage. To drain urine from the reservoir, the patient inserts a catheter through the valve at regular intervals, thus minimizing the reabsorption of waste materials from the urine and reflux into the ureters.

Patient Teaching

Patient teaching centers on the tasks of lifestyle adaptation: care of the stoma, nutrition, fluid intake, maintenance of self-esteem in light of altered body image, modification of sexual activities, and early detection of complications. Patient teaching begins with selecting an appliance, sizing the stoma, and changing the appliances. The home health nurse can assist the patient in modifying care in the home environment and by providing support during this stressful adjustment period (see the Home Care Considerations box).

 Home Care Considerations

Urinary Diversion Warning Signs

Provide the patient and significant others with the following list of warning signs and symptoms that, if they occur at home, should be reported to the health care provider:

- Keep this list handy and call the health care provider (phone number: ___-___-____) if you notice any of the following signs or symptoms:
  - Decrease in urinary output
  - Change in urine color: bloody, cloudy
  - Fever greater than 101°F
  - Change in appearance of stoma: pale color, swelling, "drawing in" of stoma
  - Skin changes around stoma: redness, burning, breakdown
  - General feeling of weakness
  - Nausea and vomiting
  - Abdominal distention or pain
  - Any other health changes that are new or worse

Prognosis

Although the patient may recover fully without recurrence, the day-to-day challenges of managing a urinary diversion are permanent.

NURSING PROCESS FOR THE PATIENT WITH A URINARY DISORDER

The role of the licensed practical nurse/licensed vocational nurse (LPN/LVN) in the nursing process as stated is that the LPN/LVN will:

- Participate in planning care for patients based on patient needs
- Review patient's care plan and recommend revisions as needed
- Review and follow defined prioritization for patient care
- Use clinical pathways, care maps, or care plans to guide and review patient care

ASSESSMENT

Assessment of the urinary tract is included in baseline data for all patients. The assessment includes subjective data: the patient's description of urination patterns and associated sensations, such as complaints of burning or pain on urination or difficulty maintaining the urine stream. Supplement subjective data with objective data by assessing for signs of fluid overload or depletion. The skin provides easily assessed clues about the patient's state of hydration. For example, dryness and pruritus (itching) can occur as a result of electrolyte imbalance or the buildup of waste products.

Pay careful attention to assessment of high-risk populations. Urinary disorders are associated with systemic malformations and structural anomalies in newborns. Pediatric patients, especially girls, are susceptible to urinary tract infections because of their short urethra. Geriatric patients may experience weakened musculature and sphincter tone, with resultant difficulty in bladder control. In male patients, enlargement of the prostate gland may interfere with initiating and maintaining an adequate urine stream.

Occupational and environmental factors also contribute to the development of renal disease. **Nephrotoxins** are substances with specific destructive properties for the kidneys. Sources include industrial exposure to heavy metals, such as lead and mercury, and medical treatment with cisplatin, aminoglycoside antibiotics (gentamicin or kanamycin), nonsteroidal antiinflammatory drugs, or radiopaque contrast media.

Other vulnerable populations include patients experiencing systemic changes from altered health states, such as pregnancy, diabetes mellitus, or hypertension. Most susceptible are those with conditions that directly compromise kidney function: trauma, fluid depletion or retention, and active or suspected renal disease.

PATIENT PROBLEM

The nurse assists in the development of patient problem statements. Patient problem statements for the patient with a urinary disorder include but are not limited to the following:

- *Alteration in Urinary Elimination*
- *Compromised Blood Flow to Tissue: Renal*
- *Fluid Volume Overload*
- *Impaired Sexual Expression*
- *Insufficient Knowledge*
- *Potential for Inadequate Fluid Volume*
- *Potential for Infection*
- *Recent Onset of Pain; Prolonged Pain*

EXPECTED OUTCOMES AND PLANNING

For the patient with a urinary disorder, the nursing care priority is the short-term goal of reestablishing urinary flow and kidney function. Long-term planning for the patient and the family or significant other focuses on prevention of complications and quick response to recurrent problems. Goals are individualized for each patient and are modified to adapt to the patient's changing health status and urinary elimination management. The care plan may include the following goals and outcomes:

Goal 1: The patient will achieve control of the elimination of urine.

Outcome: Patient reports effective management of normal patterns of urination.

Goal 2: The patient will practice proper protocol such as drinking adequate fluids and correct methods of perineal cleansing for the female to prevent UTI.

Outcome: Patient reports no signs or symptoms of recurrent urinary difficulty.

◆ IMPLEMENTATION

Assist the patient in bladder training to promote normal patterns of urination. Educate the patient in the importance of drinking 2 to 3 L of water daily (unless contraindicated). Teach the female patient the importance of cleansing from anterior to posterior in the perineal area after a bowel movement to prevent contamination of the urethra with *E. coli*.

◆ EVALUATION

Evaluation of urinary status is determined by success in attaining expected outcomes. Monitoring urinary output and character is continual. Because some urinary disorders become chronic, patient involvement in the prevention of complications is vital. Avoidance of risk factors and early detection of symptoms are essential to limit damage to the urinary tract. Examples of goals and evaluative measures are as follows:

Goal 1: The patient will experience normal patterns of urinary elimination.

Evaluative measure: Patient reports return to own normal voiding.

Goal 2: The patient will monitor self for early signs and symptoms of recurrent UTI.

Evaluative measure: Patient can answer questions correctly about signs and symptoms and appropriate measures to take for treatment.

Get Ready for the NCLEX® Examination!

Key Points

- The kidneys lie retroperitoneally, just below the diaphragm.
- The functioning unit of the kidney is the nephron.
- The kidneys rid the body of wastes and excess electrolytes, maintain water and electrolyte balance, and maintain acid-base balance.
- Kidney function is achieved by the processes of filtration, secretion, and reabsorption.
- Assessment of the urinary tract is included in baseline data for all patients.
- The subject of urinary problems is an embarrassing topic for many patients. Be sensitive to the patient's feelings and be supportive.
- Aging may have a negative influence on urinary function, but many problems can be corrected.
- Hydration status is monitored by assessing weight daily, I&O, laboratory studies, skin and mucous membranes, and level of consciousness.
- A large percentage of nosocomial infections involve the urinary tract.
- Proper care of urinary catheters decreases the chance of UTIs.
- Surgical intervention may be indicated for urinary dysfunction that cannot be corrected by medical management.
- Dialysis, which mimics kidney function, may be used temporarily or as a long-term therapy.
- Dietary, fluid, and medication modifications may be necessary for the patient with urinary dysfunction.
- Sacral nerve stimulation for urinary urge incontinence is conducted with a permanently implanted electrical stimulation device that changes neuronal activity in the sacral efferent and afferent nerves.

Additional Learning Resources

SG Go to your Study Guide for additional learning activities to help you master this chapter content.

evolve Be sure to visit the Evolve site at *http://evolve.elsevier.com/Cooper/foundationsadult/* for additional online resources.

Review Questions for the NCLEX® Examination

1. The nurse is reviewing the urinalysis report on an assigned patient. The nurse recognizes which findings to be normal? *(Select all that apply.)*
   1. Turbidity clear
   2. pH 6.0
   3. Glucose negative
   4. Red blood cells, 15 to 20
   5. White blood cells, 1 to 3

2. The nurse is caring for a patient who has just had a renal angiography performed. What is the priority assessment?
   1. Blood pressure
   2. Respiratory effort
   3. Puncture site
   4. Urinary output

3. The nursing care plan includes teaching a patient Kegel exercises. The nurse teaches the patient to alternately tighten and relax which group of muscles?
   1. Perineal floor
   2. Pubococcygeal
   3. Abdominis rectus
   4. Detrusor
4. The health care provider has talked to a patient and his wife about the treatment plan for his bladder cancer. Later, the patient tells the nurse he does not understand what the health care provider is going to do. What is the most appropriate initial response by the nurse?
   1. "Okay. I'll explain it to you again."
   2. "Make a list of questions for the doctor."
   3. "Try not to think about the treatment."
   4. "Tell me what you know about the treatment."
5. Which activity would be most harmful for the incontinent patient?
   1. Restricting fluid intake
   2. Drinking only water
   3. Fluid intake of 2000 mL/day
   4. Restricting acidic fruit juice intake
6. The nurse is reviewing the culture and sensitivity reports for a patient being treated for pyelonephritis. What pathogen will most likely be identified as the infecting agent?
   1. *Candida albicans*
   2. *Klebsiella*
   3. *Escherichia coli*
   4. *Pseudomonas*
7. Which factor will most likely promote patient compliance with the prescribed treatment plan?
   1. A set time schedule to follow
   2. Data on success rates
   3. Written information about the plan
   4. An active role in the planning
8. When scheduling the administration of furosemide (Lasix), it would be in a patient's best interest to schedule the medication to be given what time?
   1. 09:00
   2. 12:00
   3. 21:00
   4. 24:00
9. In discussing dietary needs with a patient with ESRD, the nurse indicates that potassium-rich foods should be limited in the diet. Which selections should be limited? *(Select all that apply.)*
   1. Baked potatoes
   2. Bananas
   3. Apricots
   4. Apples
   5. Pine nuts
10. Phenazopyridine hydrochloride (Pyridium) has been prescribed for a patient. What information should be provided to the patient about this medication? *(Select all that apply.)*
    1. "This medication will result in experiencing reduced bladder discomfort."
    2. "Decrease in burning sensation will be experienced as a result of this medication therapy."
    3. "This medication will result in an increased urinary output."
    4. "The urine will have an orange hue as a result of this medication."
    5. "This medication should be taken during the entire 7-day period of treatment with the antibiotics prescribed."
11. When calculating actual urinary output during continuous bladder irrigations, the nurse would:
    1. Measure and record all fluid output in the drainage bag
    2. Measure the total output and deduct the amount of irrigation solution used
    3. Add the total of all intravenous and irrigation solutions and deduct output
    4. Measure total output and deduct the total intravenous solutions
12. What statement by a patient indicates the need for further teaching before renal angiography?
    1. "I will miss having breakfast."
    2. "I know the nurse will be checking my pulse after the test."
    3. "I'm glad I don't have to stay in bed after the test."
    4. "I had a test similar to this 3 years ago."
13. The nurse performs a catheterization immediately after a patient voids and obtains 30 mL of residual urine. What action by the nurse should be taken next?
    1. Document the procedure with outcome data.
    2. Continue the catheterization routine after each voiding.
    3. Restrict fluid intake after dinner.
    4. Immediately notify the health care provider of the results.
14. Which goal would have priority in planning care of the aging patient with urinary incontinence?
    1. Recognizes the urge to void
    2. Mobility necessary for toileting independently
    3. Episodes of incontinence decrease
    4. Drinks a minimum of 2000 mL of fluid per day
15. What is the goal for peritoneal dialysis?
    1. Removal of toxins and metabolic waste
    2. Production of rapid fluid shifts
    3. Increased clearance of dialysate flow
    4. Restoration of normal kidney function
16. The nurse is caring for a patient during the postoperative period after an arteriovenous shunt has been placed. What is the most important action to be taken?
    1. Secure the shunt with an elastic bandage.
    2. Notify the health care provider if a bruit or thrill is present.
    3. Change the shunt if clotting occurs.
    4. Use strict surgical asepsis for dressing changes.

17. What is the primary function of the kidney?
1. Regulation of enzymes
2. Filtration of water and blood products
3. Collection of urine from the body
4. Control of the adrenal glands

18. The priority short-term goal for disorders of the urinary system is:
1. Patient confidentiality
2. Privacy
3. Education for patient and family
4. Normal patterns of urinary elimination

19. The nurse making rounds discovers that there is no urine drainage from a postoperative patient's Foley catheter. What action by the nurse should be performed first?
1. Ensure patency.
2. Irrigate until clear.
3. Call the health care provider.
4. Insert larger lumen catheter.

20. Which problem constitutes a medical emergency?
1. Anuria
2. Polyuria
3. Dysuria
4. Dyspnea

21. The most common cause of renal failure is:
1. Trauma
2. Diabetes mellitus
3. Cancer
4. Heart failure

22. What clinical findings in the oliguric phase of acute renal failure will be noted?
1. BUN levels rise.
2. Urinary output decreases.
3. Signs of impending shock are present.
4. Blood flow to the kidneys increases.
5. Creatinine levels decrease.

23. What are correct patient teachings for a patient with cystitis? *(Select all that apply.)*
1. Teach the patient to drink apple juice to treat and prevent UTIs.
2. Teach the female patient to cleanse the perineal area from anterior to posterior to prevent rectal *E. coli* contamination of the urethra.
3. Encourage the patient to drink 2000 mL of fluid per day, unless contraindicated.
4. Instruct the patient that it is acceptable to stop taking prescribed medications when symptoms subside.
5. Instruct the patient to void as soon after sexual intercourse as possible.

24. The nurse is reviewing the health history of a patient suspected of having renal calculi. What factors in the patient's history increase the patient's risk for developing the condition? *(Select all that apply.)*
1. Stasis of urine caused by obstruction
2. Infections of urinary tract
3. Hypoparathyroidism
4. Diabetes mellitus
5. Immobility

25. The collection of subjective and objective data for a patient with acute glomerulonephritis could include which symptoms? *(Select all that apply.)*
1. Periorbital edema
2. Anorexia
3. Hypotension
4. Frankly sanguineous urine
5. Headaches

26. Careful preparation of a patient for an IVP is necessary. What nursing interventions would be included in the preparation? *(Select all that apply.)*
1. NPO for about 8 hours before examination
2. Ascertaining whether patient has allergy to magnesium
3. Giving prescribed bowel prep
4. Instructing patient concerning IVP
5. Discussing the anesthesia needed for the procedure

27. A patient diagnosed with ESRD is treated with conservative management, including erythropoietin injections. After teaching the patient about management of ESRD, the nurse determines teaching has been effective when the patient makes which statement?
1. "I will measure my urinary output each day to help calculate the amount I can drink."
2. "I need to take the erythropoietin to boost my immune system and help prevent infection."
3. "I need to try to get more protein from dairy products."
4. "I will try to increase my intake of fruits and vegetables."

28. As the nurse reviews a diet plan with a patient with diabetes mellitus and renal insufficiency, the patient states that with diabetes and renal failure there is nothing that is good to eat. The patient says, "I am going to eat what I want; I'm going to die anyway!" What is the best patient problem statement for this patient?
1. *Insufficient Nutrition, related to knowledge deficit about appropriate diet*
2. *Potential for Noncompliance or Nonconformity, related to feelings of anger*
3. *Grief, related to actual and perceived losses*
4. *Potential for Impaired Health Maintenance, related to complexity of therapeutic regimen*

29. The nurse has instructed a patient who is receiving hemodialysis about dietary management. Which diet choices by the patient indicate that the teaching has been successful?
1. Scrambled eggs, English muffin, and apple juice
2. Cheese sandwich, tomato soup, and cranberry juice
3. Split-pea soup, whole-wheat toast, and nonfat milk
4. Oatmeal with cream, half a banana, and herbal tea

51 Care of the Patient With an Endocrine Disorder

http://evolve.elsevier.com/Cooper/foundationsadult/

Objectives

Anatomy and Physiology

1. List and describe the endocrine glands and their hormones.
2. Define *negative feedback*.
3. Explain the action of hormones on their target organs.
4. Describe how the hypothalamus controls the anterior and posterior lobes of the pituitary gland.

Medical-Surgical

5. Discuss the etiology and pathophysiology, clinical manifestations, assessment, diagnostic tests, medical management, nursing interventions, patient teaching, and prognosis for patients with acromegaly, gigantism, dwarfism, diabetes insipidus, syndrome of inappropriate antidiuretic hormone, hyperthyroidism, hypothyroidism, goiter, thyroid cancer, hyperparathyroidism, hypoparathyroidism, Cushing's syndrome, and Addison's disease.
6. Explain how to test for Chvostek's sign, Trousseau's sign, and carpopedal spasms.
7. List two significant complications that may occur after thyroidectomy.
8. Describe the etiology and pathophysiology, clinical manifestations, assessment, diagnostic tests, medical management, nursing interventions, patient teaching, and prognosis for the patient with diabetes mellitus.
9. Differentiate between the signs and symptoms of hyperglycemia and hypoglycemia.
10. Differentiate among the signs and symptoms of diabetic ketoacidosis, hyperglycemic hyperosmolar nonketotic coma, and hypoglycemic reaction.
11. Explain the roles of nutrition, exercise, and medication in the control of diabetes mellitus.
12. Discuss how the various classes of oral hypoglycemic medications work to improve the mechanisms by which insulin and glucose are produced and used by the body.
13. Discuss the various insulin types and their characteristics.
14. Describe the correct way to draw up and administer insulin.
15. Discuss the acute and long-term complications of diabetes mellitus.

Key Terms

Chvostek's sign (KHVŎS-tĕks sīn, p. 1712)
Circadian rhythm (sĕr Kā dē ăn Rĭ thĕm, p. 1702)
dysphagia (dĭs-FĀ-jē-ă, p. 1711)
endocrinologist (ĕn-dō-krĭ-NŎL-ŏ-jĭst, p. 1705)
glycosuria (glī-kōs-Ū-rē-ă, p. 1725)
hirsutism (HĔR-sūt-ĭszm, p. 1719)
hyperglycemia (hī-pĕr-glī-SĒ-mē-ă, p. 1725)
hypocalcemia (hī-pō-kăl-SĒ-mē-ă, p. 1701)
hypoglycemia (hī-pō-glī-SĒ-mē-ă, p. 1731)
hypokalemia (hī-pō-kă-LĒ-mē-ă, p. 1719)
idiopathic hyperplasia (ĭd-ē-ō-PĂTH-ĭk hī-pĕr-PLĀ-zhă, p. 1702)
ketoacidosis (kē-tō-ă-sĭ-DŌ-sĭs, p. 1725)
ketone bodies (KĒ-tōn BŎD-ēz, p. 1725)
lipohypertrophy (lĭp-ō-HĪ-pĕr-trŏ-fē, p. 1731)
neuropathy (nū-RŎP-ĕ-thē, p. 1734)
polydipsia (pŏl-ē-DĬP-sē-ă, p. 1706)
polyphagia (pŏl-ē-FĀ-jă, p. 1725)
polyuria (pŏl-ē-Ū-rē-ă, p. 1706)
Trousseau's sign (trū-SŌZ sīn, p. 1712)
turgor (TŬR-gŏr, p. 1707)
type 1 diabetes mellitus (tīp 1 dī-ă-BĒ-tēz MĔL-ĭ-tŭs, p. 1724)
type 2 diabetes mellitus (tīp 2 dī-ă-BĒ-tēz MĔL-ĭ-tŭs, p. 1740)

ANATOMY AND PHYSIOLOGY OF THE ENDOCRINE SYSTEM

ENDOCRINE GLANDS AND HORMONES

A *gland* is a specialized organ devised from a group of epithelial cells that form tissues that work together to produce and secrete hormones, enzymes, and other components that help regulate the body. There are two different types of glands, and each one regulates a reciprocal system. The *exocrine glands* secrete fluid products called enzymes. The enzymes are transported through a series of ducts and/or channels. The primary purpose of the exocrine ducts and channels is to move substances into the body or outside the body. The exocrine gland is responsible for the digestive system (gastric enzymes and saliva) as well as the sweat glands. The exocrine gland secretions are protective and functional.

Endocrine glands are ductless and release hormones directly into the bloodstream. The hormones control regulatory function such as cellular metabolism, human growth, fluid and electrolyte balance, and finally the production of energy. Endocrine and exocrine glands control homeostasis (constant balance) by communicating with other organs and tissues while regulating their assigned bodily functions. *Hormones* are chemical messengers that travel through the bloodstream to their target organs and work closely with the nervous system. Metabolic changes occur in response to the actions of hormones.

The slightest change in hormonal levels can disrupt the metabolic balance of the entire body. Hormones can increase or decrease a normal body process by affecting a target organ, and the actions are known to be interrelated. Interrelatedness refers to a fluctuation in a single hormone, which can affect significantly the actions of other hormones. The endocrine glands (Fig. 51.1) have a generalized effect on the patient's metabolism, growth, development, reproduction, and many other bodily activities such as temperature, fluid balance, and emotional responses as seen in the fight-or-flight response.

The amount of hormone released is controlled by *negative feedback inhibition.* The negative feedback inhibition process occurs when a gland releases a primary hormone, which stimulates target cells to release a secondary hormone; the gland slows the release of the primary hormone as it senses the rise of the secondary hormone. Information is exchanged constantly via the bloodstream between target organs and endocrine glands, which is described specifically later in this chapter.

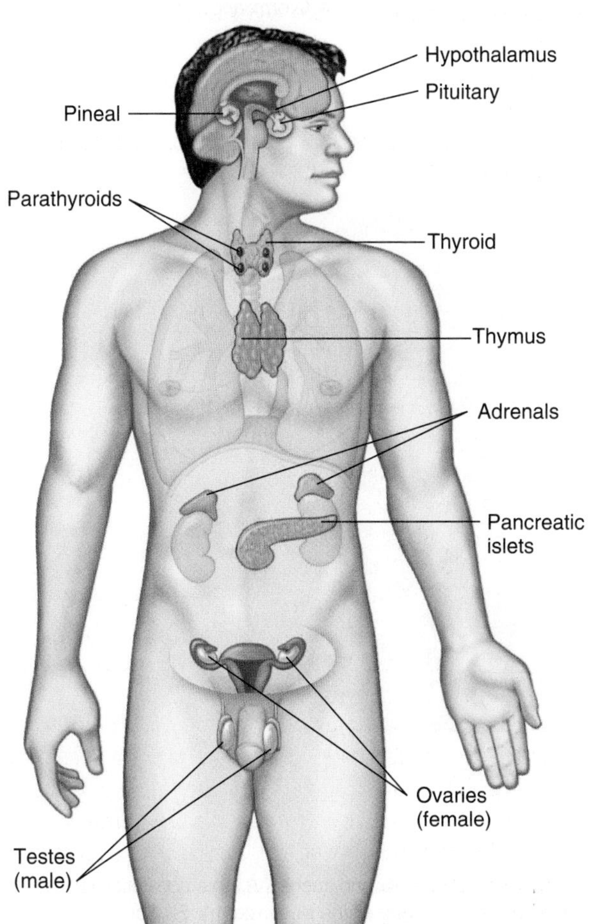

Fig. 51.1 Location of the endocrine glands in women and men. The thymus gland is shown at maximal size at puberty. (From Patton KT, Thibodeau GA: *Anatomy and physiology,* ed 8, St. Louis, 2013, Mosby.)

Pituitary Gland

The pea-sized *pituitary gland* (hypophysis) is one of the most powerful glands in the body. It has been called the "master gland" because, through negative feedback, it controls the other endocrine glands (Gonzalez-Iglesias and Freeman, 2013). This gland is located beneath the hypothalamus of the brain in a cranial cavity in a small, saddle-like depression in the sphenoid bone. It is divided into two segments: the *anterior pituitary* (adenohypophysis) and the *posterior pituitary* (neurohypophysis). Each segment produces specialized hormones for specific targeted responses. The hypothalamus produces the hormones of the posterior pituitary and releases the hormones for storage in the posterior pituitary gland. The hormones are released from the posterior pituitary as a result of nerve impulses received from the hypothalamus.

Anterior pituitary gland. Six major hormones are secreted by the anterior pituitary gland:

1. Somatotropin, or growth hormone (GH)
2. Adrenocorticotropic hormone (ACTH)
3. Thyroid-stimulating hormone (TSH)
4. and 5. Gonadotropic hormones: Follicle-stimulating hormone (FSH) and luteinizing hormone (LH)
6. Prolactin (PRL)

The first five hormones in the list are known as *tropic* hormones. Tropic hormones are defined as ones that stimulate the activity of another endocrine gland. Prolactin is a nontropic hormone and has a direct effect on the mammary glands, which in return are stimulated to *produce* milk. These hormones and their functions are shown in Fig. 51.2.

Posterior pituitary gland. *Oxytocin* and the *antidiuretic hormone* (ADH) are the only two hormones stored in the posterior pituitary and released by the posterior pituitary when the hypothalamus is stimulated (see Fig. 51.2). Oxytocin promotes the *release* of milk and stimulates uterine contractions during labor. ADH, also called *vasopressin,* causes the kidneys to conserve water by decreasing the amount of urine produced. ADH/vasopressin also causes constriction of the arterioles in the body, producing a systemic pressor effect, which results in increased blood pressure.

Thyroid Gland

The *thyroid gland* is butterfly shaped, with one lobe lying on either side of the trachea just below the larynx (Fig. 51.3). The lobes are connected by the *isthmus*. The thyroid gland is very vascular and receives approximately 80 to 120 mL of blood per minute.

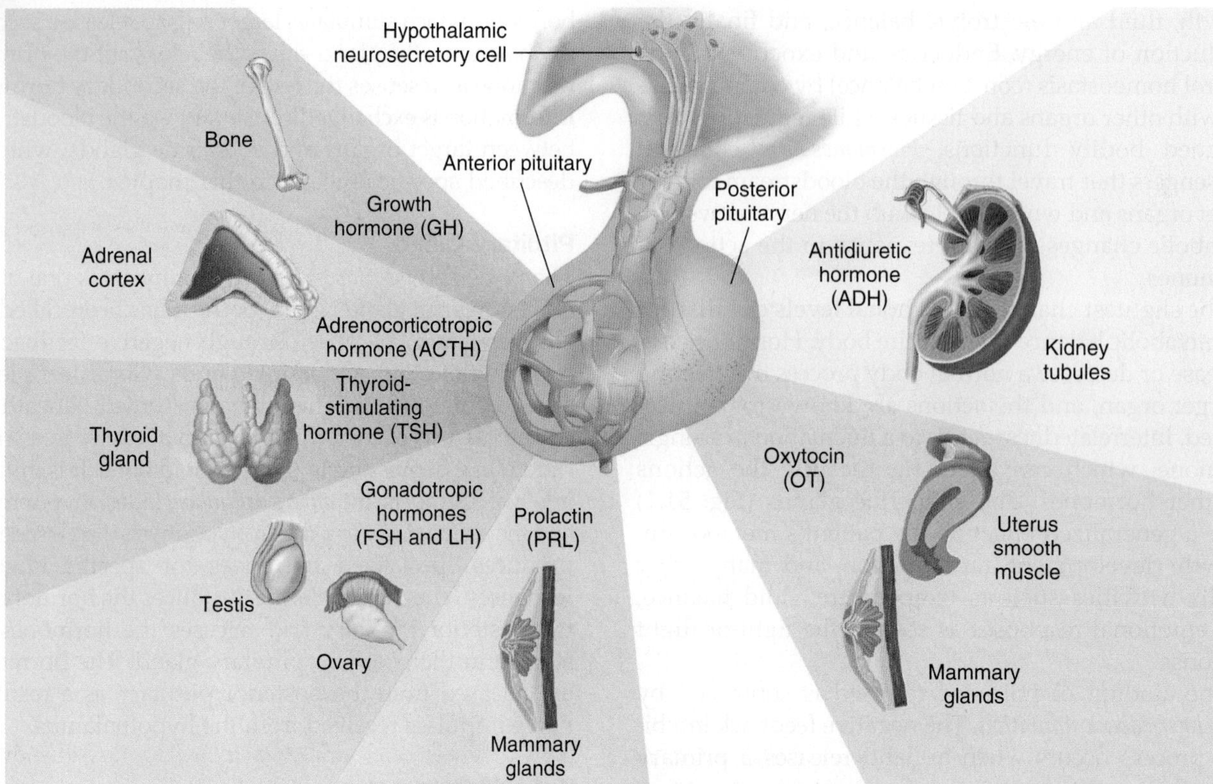

Fig. 51.2 Pituitary hormones. Shown are the principal anterior and posterior pituitary hormones and their target organs. *FSH,* Follicle-stimulating hormone; *LH,* luteinizing hormone. (From Patton KT, Thibodeau GA: *Anatomy and physiology,* ed 8, St. Louis, 2013, Mosby.)

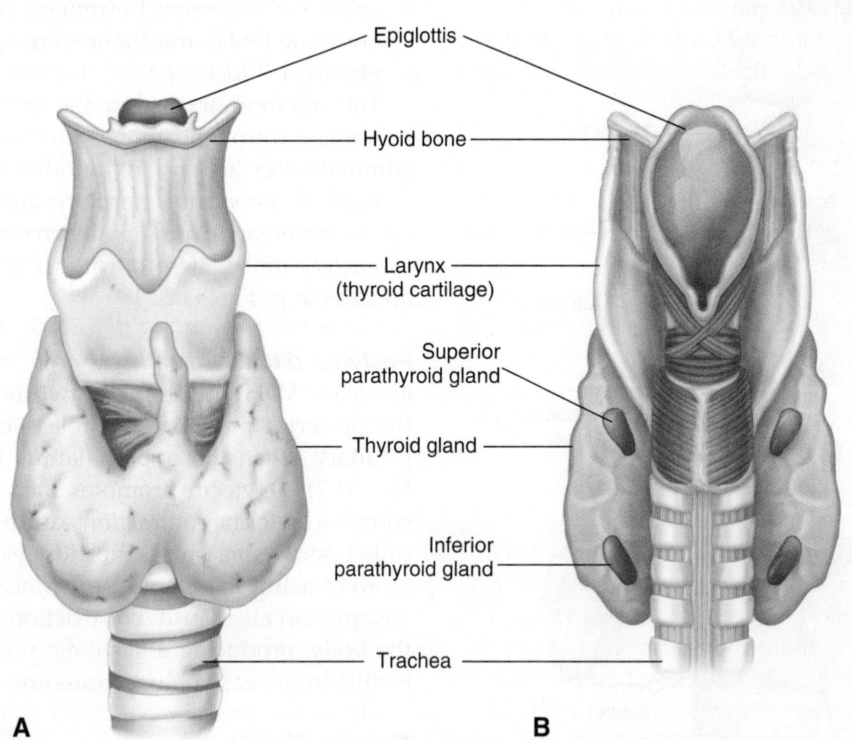

Fig. 51.3 Thyroid and parathyroid glands. Note their relations to each other and to the larynx and trachea. A, Anteroposterior view. B, Posteroanterior view. (From Thibodeau GA, Patton KT: *Structure and function of the body,* ed 14, St. Louis, 2012, Mosby.)

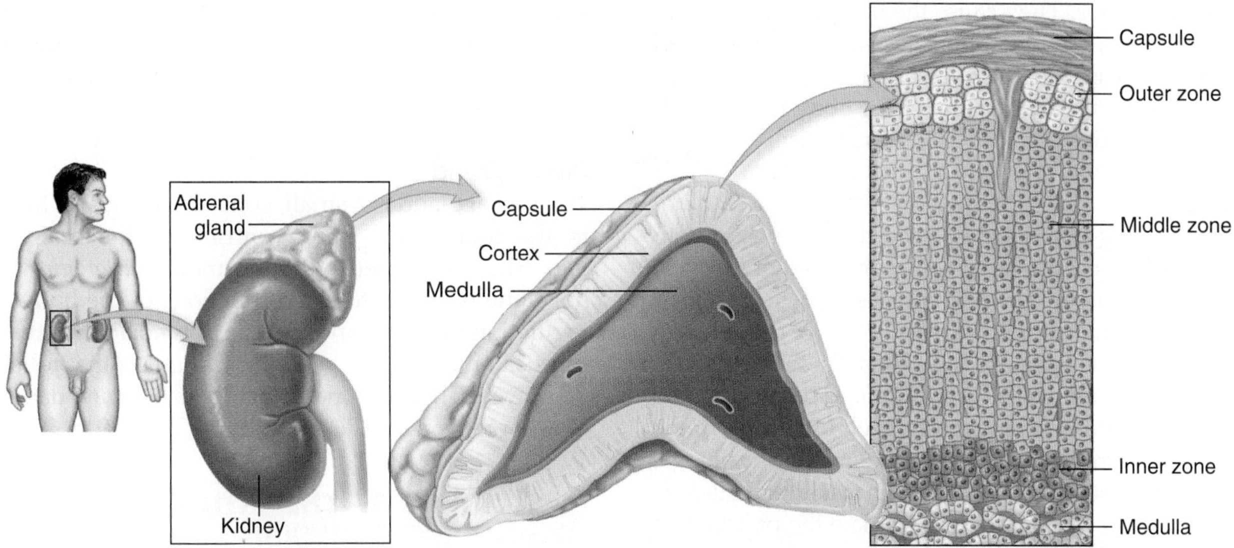

Fig. 51.4 Structure of the adrenal gland. The outer zone (zona glomerulosa) of the cortex secretes abundant amounts of glucocorticoids, chiefly aldosterone. The middle zone (zona fasciculata) secretes glucocorticoids, primarily cortisol, as well as small amounts of sex hormone. The inner zone (zona reticularis) secretes sex hormones. A portion of the medulla is visible at the bottom of the illustration. (From Patton KT, Thibodeau GA, Douglas MM: *Essentials of anatomy and physiology*, ed 1, St. Louis, 2012, Mosby.)

The thyroid gland secretes two main hormones: *triiodothyronine* (T_3) and *thyroxine* (T_4). Adequate oral intake of iodine is necessary for the formation of thyroid hormones. These two specific hormones regulate three functions: (1) growth and development, (2) metabolism, and (3) activity of the nervous system. Their function is controlled by the release of TSH from the pituitary gland.

Calcitonin is the third hormone released by the thyroid gland. It decreases blood calcium levels by causing calcium to be stored in the bones.

Parathyroid Glands

The four parathyroid glands are located on the posterior surface of the thyroid gland (see Fig. 51.3) and secrete *parathyroid hormone* (PTH, parathormone). As an antagonist to calcitonin from the thyroid, PTH tends to increase the concentration of calcium in the blood. It also regulates the amount of phosphorus in the blood.

The delicate balance of calcium in the blood is extremely important for normal body function. When calcium blood levels are low (**hypocalcemia**), the nerve cells become excited and stimulate the muscles with too many impulses, resulting in spasms *(tetany)*. Hypocalcemia also slows the heart rate, causing cardiac irritability and heart failure (Marks, 2003). When blood calcium levels are abnormally high (hypercalcemia), heart function becomes impaired and can result in death if not treated. Under the influence of PTH, two changes occur in the kidneys: increasing the reabsorption of calcium and magnesium from the kidney tubules and accelerating the elimination of phosphorus in the urine.

Adrenal Glands

The two adrenal glands (suprarenal glands) are small, yellow masses that sit on top of the kidneys. Both glands contain the adrenal cortex (outer section) and the adrenal medulla (inner section) (Fig. 51.4).

Adrenal cortex. The adrenal cortex is divided into three separate layers. Each layer secretes a particular hormone, called a *steroid:*

- *Mineralocorticoids* are secreted by the outer zone (zona glomerulosa): These are involved primarily in water and electrolyte balance (homeostasis) and indirectly manage blood pressure. Aldosterone, the principal mineralocorticoid, regulates sodium and potassium levels by affecting the renal tubules. It decreases the level of potassium and increases the level of sodium in the bloodstream. The retention of sodium causes retention of water, which leads to an increase in blood volume and blood pressure.
- *Glucocorticoids* are secreted by the middle zone (zona fasciculata). The most important of these is cortisol, which is involved in glucose metabolism and provides extra reserve energy in times of stress. Glucocorticoids also exhibit antiinflammatory properties.
- *Sex hormones* are secreted by the inner zone (zona reticularis): Androgen hormones are the primary hormones secreted and are needed early for the development of the male reproductive system and then create the testosterone hormone, which is stored and secreted in the male testes, and estrogen hormone in females. In the adult, the adrenal glands release a relatively small amount of these hormones, which have an insignificant impact on the system.

Adrenal medulla. The cells composing the adrenal medulla arise from the same type of cells as the sympathetic nervous system. Two hormones are released during times of stress: (1) *epinephrine* (adrenaline) and

(2) *norepinephrine*. They cause the heart rate and blood pressure to increase, the blood vessels to constrict, and the liver to release glucose reserves for immediate energy. This is a systemic preparation of the body for a "fight-or-flight" response needed in times of crisis.

Pancreas

The pancreas is an elongated gland that lies posterior to the stomach. It is an active organ, composed of exocrine and endocrine tissue. The endocrine tissue of the pancreas contains more than a million tiny clusters of cells known collectively as the islets of Langerhans. These cells secrete two major hormones. The first, *insulin,* is secreted by the *beta cells* in response to increased levels of glucose in the blood. The secretion pattern of insulin is a physiologic example of negative feedback between insulin and glucose. Elevated blood glucose levels stimulate the pancreas to secrete insulin. The stimulus for insulin secretion decreases as blood glucose levels decrease. The homeostatic mechanism is considered negative feedback because it reverses the change in blood glucose level. The second pancreatic hormone is *glucagon*. Glucagon is secreted by *alpha cells* in response to decreased levels of glucose in the blood. Insulin and glucagon play a major role in carbohydrate, fat, and protein metabolism.

Female Sex Glands

Deep in the lower abdominal region, lying to the left and right of the uterus, are two almond-shaped *ovaries,* the major female sex glands. At puberty the ovaries begin producing two hormones: *estrogen* (responsible for the development of secondary sex characteristics, such as axillary hair and pubic hair, and for maturation of the reproductive organs) and *progesterone*. Progesterone continues the preparation of the reproductive organs that was initiated by estrogen. (See Chapter 52 for more information.)

The *placenta* is a temporary endocrine gland that forms and functions during pregnancy. During this time the ovaries become inactive, and the placenta releases the estrogen and progesterone needed to maintain the pregnancy. (For a more in-depth discussion, see Chapter 52.)

Male Sex Glands

Suspended outside the body in the *scrotum,* a saclike structure, are the two oval sex glands called the *testes*. They release the hormone *testosterone,* which is responsible for the development of the male secondary sex characteristics, including axillary, pubic, and facial hair; maturation of the reproductive organs; deepening of the voice; and development of muscle and bone mass. Testosterone is necessary for sperm formation.

Thymus Gland

The thymus gland lies in the upper thorax, posterior to the sternum (see Fig. 51.1). It produces the hormone *thymosin,* which plays an active role in the immune system. T lymphocytes (a type of white blood cell) are stimulated to carry out immune reactions to certain types of antigens. The thymus gland programs this information into the T lymphocytes in utero and during the first few months of life.

Pineal Gland

The pineal gland is a small, cone-shaped gland located in the roof of the third ventricle of the brain (see Fig. 51.1). It secretes the hormone *melatonin*. This hormone is linked to sleep functions of the body and regulation of circadian rhythms. **Circadian rhythms** are physical, mental, and behavioral changes that follow a daily cycle. They respond primarily to light and darkness in an organism's environment (NIGMS, 2018).

DISORDERS OF THE PITUITARY GLAND (HYPOPHYSIS)

ACROMEGALY

Etiology and Pathophysiology

An overproduction of somatotropin (growth hormone [GH]) after the onset of puberty causes *acromegaly,* a condition that affects an estimated 6 people per 100,000 (NIDDKS, 2012). The cause may be either (1) **idiopathic hyperplasia** (an increase in the number of cells, without a known cause) of the anterior lobe of the pituitary gland or (2) tumor growth. Unfortunately, growth changes that occur in acromegaly are irreversible, even with adequate medical or surgical intervention.

Clinical Manifestations

Manifestations of acromegaly begin gradually, usually in the third or fourth decade of life. Typically an average of 7 to 9 years passes between the initial onset of signs and symptoms and final diagnosis. The subsequent overabundance of somatotropin (or GH) produces many changes throughout the patient's body, including enlarged cranium and lower jaw, separated and maloccluded teeth, bulging forehead, bulbous nose, thick lips, enlarged tongue, and generalized coarsening of the facial features (Fig. 51.5). Enlargement of the tongue results in speech difficulties, and the voice deepens as a result of hypertrophy of the vocal cords. The hands and feet grow larger; the fingertips develop a tufted or clubbed appearance. There is enlargement of the heart, liver, and spleen. Muscle weakness usually develops. Joints may hypertrophy and become painful and stiff. Male patients may become impotent, and female patients may develop a deepened voice, increased facial hair, and amenorrhea (lack of menstrual cycles). If a tumor is present, pressure on the optic nerve may cause partial or complete blindness. Visual disturbances are often a first sign of acromegaly. Severe headaches are common.

Assessment

Subjective data include headaches or visual disturbances and painful, stiff joints. Evaluate muscle weakness and

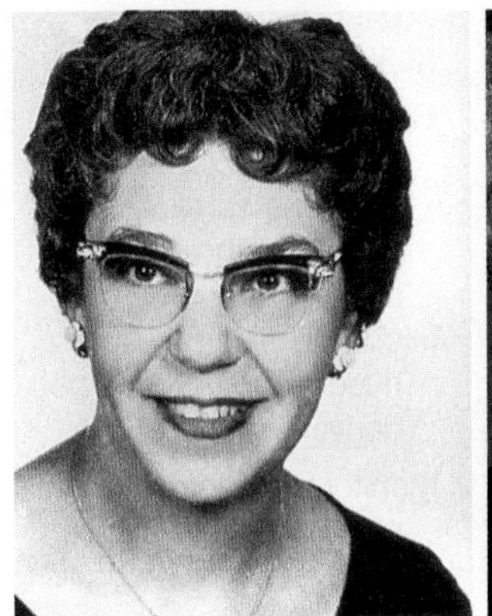
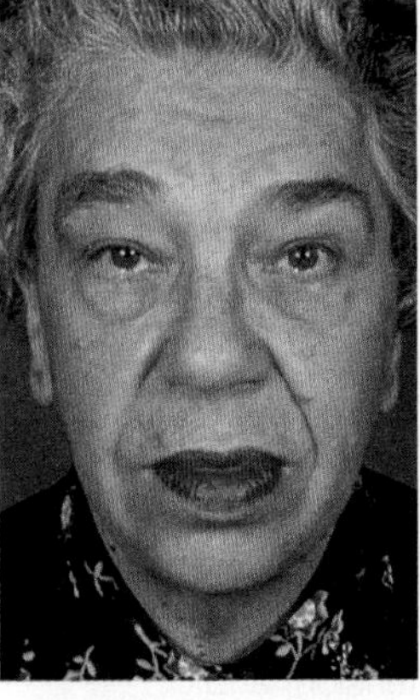

Fig. 51.5 *Left,* A patient's face before she developed a pituitary tumor. *Right,* The same patient, years later; her face shows the coarse features typical of acromegaly. (Courtesy the Group for Research in Pathology Education.)

its effect on the patient's ability to perform activities. Encourage patients to share their emotional responses to sexual problems (such as impotence in men and masculinization in women). Particular attention should be paid to the emotional distress associated with the physical changes during the progression of acromegaly.

Collection of objective data includes ongoing assessment of bone enlargement and joint involvement, as evidenced by gait changes and decreasing ability to perform activities. Changes in vital signs that may herald the onset of early heart failure include dyspnea, tachycardia, weak pulse, and hypotension. The patient's fluid volume status should be assessed with each interaction. After surgical removal of the pituitary tumor, the patient is at risk for diabetes insipidus. If the posterior pituitary gland was damaged during surgery, it may cause a lack of ADH, resulting in diabetes insipidus. Diabetes insipidus is a condition in which the kidneys do not conserve water properly and is discussed more in depth in this chapter. Hypertension, heart failure, and cardiomyopathy are possible complications secondary to enlargement of the heart and other organs.

Diagnostic Tests

Diagnosis of acromegaly is based on the history and clinical manifestations, computed tomography (CT) scan, magnetic resonance imaging (MRI), and cranial radiographic evaluation. A complete ophthalmologic examination, including visual fields, usually is performed because a large tumor of the pituitary gland potentially causes pressure on the optic nerves or optic chiasm (where the optic nerves cross, just in front of the pituitary gland). Laboratory tests confirm elevated levels of serum GH and plasma insulin-like growth factor-1. The definitive test for acromegaly is the growth hormone suppression test (Mayo Clinic, 2018a). The GH concentration normally falls during this challenge test, but in acromegaly these levels do not fall. Note: Restrict the patient's oral intake for 10 to 12 hours before this test (NLM, 2018).

Medical Management

Medical treatments include dopamine agonists such as cabergoline and somatostatin analogues (which inhibit GH), such as octreotide (Sandostatin, Sandostatin LAR Depot) (Table 51.1), especially in patients who are not candidates for surgery or radiation therapy. These drugs are used in an attempt to suppress GH secretion. Surgical treatment to remove pituitary tumors associated with acromegaly is accomplished with the transsphenoidal removal of tumor tissue. The goal of transsphenoidal surgery is to remove only the tumor that is causing GH secretion. Irradiation procedures using proton beam therapy have been used to destroy GH-secreting tumors. Proton beam treatment uses very low doses of radiation and therefore is much less destructive to adjacent tissues, such as the hypothalamus and temporal lobes, than conventional radiation therapy. This procedure is known as the *gamma knife radiosurgery.*

Nursing Interventions and Patient Teaching

Nursing interventions are primarily supportive and are geared toward relieving the discomforts of the patient. Muscle weakness, joint pain, and stiffness warrant assessment of the ability to perform activities of daily living (ADLs). Joint pain/discomfort should be assessed frequently. Headache may impair the patient's ability to socialize and also may impede education and employment. Worsening headaches may indicate tumor progression. Jaw muscles and the temporomandibular joint may be involved. The diet should be soft and easy to chew. Encourage the patient to chew thoroughly, and allow adequate time during meals, assisting when necessary. Nonopioid analgesics may be given for pain relief. Visual impairment may increase the risk of injury for these patients, so take care to prevent them from stumbling into furniture or dropping objects.

As the body changes, the patient may develop problems with self-esteem and may feel physically unattractive. The patient may have difficulty communicating with significant others, which can disrupt individual or family coping methods. Other complications of acromegaly are related to enlargement of the liver, spleen, and heart. Cardiac dysrhythmias may develop, and the patient may experience heart failure. Abdominal girth may increase as a result of weight gain and inactivity, and respiratory difficulty may occur.

A patient problem and interventions for the patient with acromegaly include but are not limited to the following:

Patient Problem	Nursing Interventions
Distorted Body Image, related to physical manifestations of the condition (may include enlargement of hands, feet, tongue, jaw, and soft tissue)	Convey respect and nonjudgmental acceptance of patient as a person Help the patient set achievable short-term goals

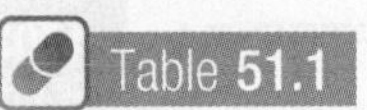 Table 51.1 **Medications for Endocrine Disorders**

GENERIC NAME (TRADE NAME)	ACTION	SIDE EFFECTS	NURSING IMPLICATIONS
bromocriptine (Parlodel)	Inhibits prolactin secretion; lowers serum levels of growth hormone, dopamine receptor agonist	Nausea, headache, dizziness, abdominal cramping, orthostatic hypotension	Give with meals to prevent GI effects; change positions carefully to prevent orthostatic hypotension; contraindicated with hypersensitivity to ergot derivatives
Calcium salts (gluconate, lactate, chloride gluceptate)	Calcium electrolyte replacement	Hypercalcemia, phlebitis, necrosis, and burning at IV site; bradycardia, hypotension, and dysrhythmias with rapid IV administration	Monitor cardiac status and blood pressure and for extravasation when giving intravenously
fludrocortisone	Adrenal corticosteroid with mineralocorticoid activity; promotes sodium and water retention	Hypertension, edema, sweating, rash, hypokalemia	Monitor for hypokalemia and fluid retention or depletion; do not discontinue abruptly; patient should carry identification signaling use
levothyroxine (Synthroid, Levothroid) liothyronine (Cytomel) liotrix (Thyrolar) thyroid (Thyrar, Armour Thyroid)	Thyroid hormone replacement	Most side effects are due to therapeutic overdose; include anxiety, insomnia, headache, hypertension, tremors, angina, dysrhythmias, tachycardia, menstrual irregularities, nervousness, irritability, nausea, diarrhea, appetite changes, leg cramps	Give in morning to minimize insomnia; use caution in older adults or patients with coronary artery disease; monitor for signs of overdose; do not switch brands unless instructed
mitotane (Lysodren)	Adrenal cytotoxic agent; reduces production of adrenal steroids	Anorexia, nausea, vomiting, diarrhea, lethargy, somnolence, vertigo, rash	Tell patient to use contraception; instruct patient to use caution when driving or performing tasks requiring alertness; monitor for dehydration
potassium iodide (SSKI)	Blocks release of thyroid hormone in thyroid storm and hyperthyroidism; also used as an expectorant	Hypersensitivity reactions, rash, metallic taste, burning in mouth or throat, GI irritation, headache, parotitis, hyperkalemia	Do not use in pregnant women; mix with fruit juice to mask taste
Somatostatin analogues: octreotide (Sandostatin)	Inhibits growth hormone secretion; suppresses secretion of serotonin, gastroenteropancreatic peptides; enhances fluid and electrolyte absorption from the GI tract; used to treat carcinoid tumors, VIPomas,[a] and high-output fistulas[b]	Nausea, diarrhea, abdominal pain, headache, injection site discomfort, hyperglycemia, hypoglycemia	SubQ route of administration is preferred but also may be given IV
Antidiuretic hormone: vasopressin (Pitressin)	Synthetic pituitary hormone with antidiuretic effects on the kidney (used to treat diabetes insipidus); also a potent vasoconstrictor (used to treat bleeding esophageal varices)	Nasal irritation and congestion with nasal preparations; hypertension; ischemia of heart, mesenteric organs, and kidneys; angina; myocardial infarction; water retention; hyponatremia	Use with caution in older adults or patients with coronary artery disease or heart failure; discontinue if chest pain develops; monitor urinary output and serum sodium

[a]VIPomas are neuroendocrine tumors of the pancreas that secrete vasoactive intestinal polypeptide (VIP) autonomously.
[b]A *fistula* is an abnormal passage from an internal organ through the skin to the outside of the body, and through which internal secretions and water pass. They often are triggered by surgery. A high-output fistula produces 500 mL/day or more.
GI, Gastrointestinal; *IV*, intravenous; *subQ*, subcutaneous.

The patient should remain under the supervision of a health care provider so that any complications can be diagnosed promptly and adequately treated. Teach the patient exercises that can be performed at home, such as active range-of-motion of joints of the extremities and of the neck, to help prevent muscle atrophy and loss of movement.

Prognosis

Even with adequate medical or surgical treatment, the physical changes are irreversible, and the patient is prone to developing complications such as diabetes, heart failure, hypertension, osteoarthritis, colon polyps, sleep apnea, and vision loss (Mayo Clinic, 2018a).

GIGANTISM

Etiology and Pathophysiology

Gigantism usually results from an oversecretion of GH before the onset of puberty, as a result of hyperplasia of the anterior pituitary. The hyperplastic tissue may develop into a tumor. Another possible cause is a defect in the hypothalamus that directs the anterior pituitary to release excessive amounts of GH.

Clinical Manifestations

When overproduction of GH occurs in a child before the epiphyses (growth plates at each end of the bones) close, there is an overgrowth of the long bones. This causes the individual to grow abnormally tall and have increased muscle and visceral development. Weight increases, but body proportions are usually normal. Despite their size, these patients are usually weak. Other kinds of gigantism may be caused by certain genetic disorders or by disturbances in sex hormone production. Once identified, these children should be referred for further medical evaluation and follow-up.

Assessment

Collection of subjective data includes assessment of the patient's understanding of the disease process and his or her ability to verbalize emotional responses.

Collection of objective data requires frequent measurement of height. Assess the patient's use of adaptive coping measures and family interactions.

Diagnostic Tests

A GH suppression test may be done to evaluate GH levels (Mayo Clinic, 2018a). In the patient with gigantism, baseline levels of GH are high. Blood levels of GH also are evaluated for diagnosis of gigantism.

Medical Management

Medical management of children with gigantism may include surgical removal of tumor tissue or irradiation of the anterior pituitary gland, with subsequent replacement of pituitary hormones as indicated. The health care provider then observes the child for the development of related complications, such as hypertension, heart failure, osteoporosis, thickened bones, and delayed sexual development.

Nursing Interventions and Patient Teaching

Nursing interventions primarily include early identification of children who are experiencing increased growth rates compared with other children their age. The child's height is recorded at each visit to the primary health care provider, and a deviation of two or more percentile levels from the median should be reported. The condition causes potential problems with self-image, especially if the child is a preteen who is a great deal taller than peers. Girls usually experience more emotional trauma in this situation than boys do. Be understanding and compassionate regarding the emotional and physical aspects of being taller than their peers.

Early diagnosis of these patients is essential, because proper medical management can hinder the height a child will reach. Stress to the parents the importance of regular visits to the pediatrician or pediatric **endocrinologist** (a health care provider who specializes in endocrinology).

Prognosis

With new medical and surgical advances, the expected life span of these patients is longer than it was previously. However, their life expectancy is still less than that of the average individual, primarily because of cardiovascular and joint disorders.

DWARFISM

Etiology and Pathophysiology

There are differing types of dwarfism or short stature. The condition may be caused by genetic mutations; GH deficiency; and other, unknown causes. Individuals affected by hypopituitarism are in the minority of cases. *Hypopituitary dwarfism* is a condition caused by deficiency in GH. Most cases are idiopathic, but a small number can be attributed to an autosomal recessive trait. In some cases the patients also lack ACTH, TSH, and the gonadotropins.

Clinical Manifestations

Short stature is the most obvious clue to a potential deficiency in growth hormone. These patients are usually well proportioned and well nourished but appear younger than their chronologic age. If a child's height is below the third percentile, there is cause for follow-up. They may have problems with dentition as the permanent teeth erupt, because the jaws are underdeveloped (Mayo Clinic, 2018b). Sexual development is usually normal but delayed. Many people with hypopituitary dwarfism are able to reproduce offspring of average height, unless there is an accompanying deficiency in gonadotropins. Because only a small number of children with short stature or delayed growth have dwarfism, a thorough diagnostic workup is crucial.

Assessment

Subjective data include the patient's understanding of the disease process and emotional responses to it. A family history of dwarfism may reveal previously successful coping strategies. Encourage the patient to verbalize feelings. Affected children typically have normal intelligence. The child's history usually reveals a normal birth weight. It is important to determine when the child's growth retardation first was noted.

Collection of objective data includes regular measurement of height and weight to determine responses to GH and other hormones that may be administered. Review birth weight and length. Compare current height and weight with standard growth charts, and compare the child's growth pattern with that of siblings and other relatives at a comparable age.

Diagnostic Tests

Diagnostic tests include radiographic evaluation of the skull and skeleton. There is a review of differences between the patient's bone age and chronological age. Significant differences may signal a growth problem. MRI or a CT scan will be used to rule out a pituitary tumor. Definitive diagnosis is based on decreased plasma levels of GH. NOTE: Restrict the patient's oral intake after midnight for this test. Additional genetic testing may be indicated to distinguish specific types of dwarfism and to help in future family planning decisions (Mayo Clinic, 2018b).

Medical Management

Medical treatment involves replacement of GH by injection and the addition of other hormones as needed to correct deficiencies. If a tumor is the cause of dwarfism, surgery usually is indicated. Nurses should be aware that replacement of GH by injection is expensive and may prevent uninsured or underinsured parents from pursuing this treatment option.

Nursing Interventions and Patient Teaching

Exercise particular care to identify children with growth problems. The health care provider correlates the onset of growth retardation with symptoms of headache, visual disturbances, or behavior changes that may indicate a tumor, so be alert for these symptoms. Avoid making the parents feel guilty about any delay in seeking medical attention for their child.

Encourage the child to wear age-appropriate clothing and engage in activities with peers, because significant problems with self-esteem can occur in dwarfism. Emphasize the child's abilities and strengths instead of his or her physical size. Ensuring that older children and young adults have clothing that is consistent with their peers, fashionable, and age appropriate contributes to their emotional well-being.

Prognosis

Most of these patients lead fairly average lives, and many become parents of average-height children. Complications experienced are often of the musculoskeletal and cardiovascular systems. The lifespan of a patient with dwarfism is typically normal, depending on the management of complications.

DIABETES INSIPIDUS

Etiology and Pathophysiology

Diabetes insipidus is a metabolic disorder of the pituitary gland. Diabetes insipidus develops when there is a decrease in production of ADH from the posterior pituitary or the action of ADH is diminished. The condition may be transient or permanent. A decrease in ADH causes increased urinary output, which in turn results in dehydration and increased plasma osmolality—that is, a state of imbalance between the electrolyte and fluid components of the plasma.

The condition may be either primary as a result of a deficiency of ADH or secondary due to intracranial tumor, aneurysm, head injury of infectious process such as encephalitis or meningitis.

Clinical Manifestations

Diabetes insipidus is characterized by significant **polyuria** (excretion of an abnormally large quantity of urine) and intense **polydipsia** (excessive thirst). The urine is very dilute, looking pale and clear like water. Associated urine specific gravity (the density of urine compared with that of water) is 1.001 to 1.005 (the normal range is 1.003 to 1.030). Normal urinary output is 1.5 L/24 h; patients with diabetes insipidus may have a urinary output exceeding 1 to 1.5 L/h or 5 to 20 L/24 h. The patient craves fluids and may drink 4 to 20 L of fluid daily yet still becomes severely dehydrated and has increased levels of sodium in the blood (hypernatremia) because of excess urine output. These patients continue to produce copious quantities of urine when unconscious after surgery or head trauma; if not prevented, diabetes insipidus under these circumstances can lead to hypovolemic shock (failure to adequately perfuse vital organs as a result of insufficient blood volume). Manifestations of this complication include changes in level of consciousness, tachycardia, tachypnea, and hypotension. Hypovolemic shock usually follows trauma and consequent blood loss; in these cases the body increases its release of ADH in an effort to maintain blood volume; in diabetes insipidus–related hypovolemic shock, urinary output remains high rather than decreases.

Assessment

Subjective data include the patient's understanding of the relationship of symptoms (such as thirst and polyuria) to the underlying cause. The patient should be able to state the importance of not restricting oral fluids. Assess the severity of thirst. The patient may be embarrassed about the constant need to drink and then empty the bladder and voluntarily may restrict social contacts and work activities. The patient is weak, tired, and lethargic. Assessment of the patient should include symptoms indicating an electrolyte imbalance.

Collection of objective data includes assessment of skin **turgor** (the normal resiliency of the skin) and color and specific gravity of the urine and vital signs. Carefully monitor intake and output (I&O). The skin is dry, turgor is poor, and body weight is lost. Constipation may occur from lack of fluid in the bowel. Weigh the patient daily in the early morning, before breakfast. Determine whether the patient has nocturia, because this may interrupt sleep patterns.

Diagnostic Tests

Diagnosis is based on clinical manifestations, urine specific gravity, and urine ADH measurement. The urine specific gravity often drops below 1.003, and the serum sodium level increases to more than 145 mEq/L (normal serum sodium level is 135 to 145 mEq/L). Because of hemoconcentration the serum osmolality may be greater than 300 mOsm/kg (normal is 280 to 300 mOsm/kg). The fluid deprivation (water deprivation) test may be ordered to determine how well the pituitary is producing ADH and to help rule out other causes. This test involves withholding fluids for a period of up to 12 hours. During the testing period, urine specific gravity and serum osmolality frequently are measured, as well as orthostatic vital signs. Beginning and ending weights also are obtained for comparison. A CT scan and radiographic evaluation of the sella turcica (the "Turkish saddle"–shaped depression in the sphenoid bone that houses the pituitary gland) may be done to help evaluate the pituitary structures.

Medical Management

Medical treatment involves intravenous (IV), subcutaneous, intranasal, or oral administration of synthetic ADH preparations in the form of desmopressin acetate (1-deamino-8-D-arginine vasopressin, or DDAVP). Coffee, tea, and other beverages containing caffeine usually are eliminated from the diet because of their possible diuretic effect. If the patient cannot match the urinary losses through oral intake, he or she is at risk for dehydration and severe hypernatremia. IV fluids of hypotonic saline or dextrose 5% in water are needed.

Nursing Interventions and Patient Teaching

Specific nursing interventions are aimed at protecting the patient from injury. The patient likely is fatigued from frequent ambulation to the bathroom to void and impaired sleep pattern. The patient may be at risk for injury or falls secondary to fatigue, exhaustion, and electrolyte imbalances. Carefully monitor the patient's I&O and document. Assess skin turgor frequently, along with the condition of oral mucous membranes. Weigh the patient and record I&O daily. Do not limit oral fluids in an effort to reduce urinary output.

A patient problem and interventions for the patient with diabetes insipidus include but are not limited to the following:

Patient Problem	Nursing Interventions
Potential for Inadequate Fluid Volume, related to excessive urine production	Assess for signs and symptoms of dehydration (dry oral mucous membranes, poor skin turgor, soft eyeballs, lowered blood pressure, rapid pulse) Monitor electrolyte status carefully Measure I&O

Instruct the patient to wear some form of medical alert identification, such as a necklace or bracelet, stating the potential for and diagnosis of diabetes insipidus. Stress that the patient must remain under medical supervision for monitoring of the metabolic state, because the condition may worsen with time.

Prognosis

The prognosis depends on the cause. Patients who survive usually are dependent on medication for the rest of their lives. With proper treatment, most patients can expect to live a relatively normal life.

SYNDROME OF INAPPROPRIATE ANTIDIURETIC HORMONE

Syndrome of inappropriate ADH (SIADH) occurs when the pituitary gland releases too much ADH. In response to ADH, the kidneys reabsorb more water, decreasing urinary output and expanding the body's fluid volume. The patient experiences hyponatremia (low sodium), hemodilution, and fluid overload without peripheral edema.

Etiology and Pathophysiology

ADH regulates the body's water balance. Synthesized in the hypothalamus, ADH is stored in the posterior pituitary gland. When released into the circulation, it acts on the kidneys' distal tubules and collecting ducts, increasing their permeability to water. This decreases urine volume, because more water is reabsorbed and returned to the circulation, which increases blood volume.

When the body's system of checks and balances malfunctions—whether from a tumor, medication, unrelated disease process, or some other cause—ADH may be released continuously, causing SIADH, which occurs more commonly in older adults.

ADH is released in response to stress. Be alert to patients who have the following risk factors and who are also in pain or undergoing stressful procedures:

- Medications, including anesthetics, opiates, barbiturates, thiazide diuretics, and oral hypoglycemics
- Malignancies (the most common cause of SIADH; cancerous cells are capable of producing, storing, and releasing ADH)

- Nonmalignant pulmonary diseases, including chronic obstructive pulmonary disease, tuberculosis, lung abscesses, and pneumonia
- Nervous system disorders, including head trauma, cerebral vascular accident, encephalitis, meningitis, and Guillain-Barré syndrome
- Miscellaneous causes, including lupus erythematous, adrenal insufficiency, and thyroid and parathyroid deficiencies

Clinical Manifestations

Clinically, SIADH is characterized by hyponatremia and water retention that progresses to water intoxication. The severity of the patient's condition is linked primarily to the sodium levels and the location of fluid accumulation. Most signs and symptoms appear when serum sodium levels fall below 125 mEq/L. Signs and symptoms include nausea, vomiting, irritability, confusion, tremors, seizures, stupor, coma, and pathologic reflexes.

Assessment

Subjective data include vague complaints. Hyponatremia triggers the earliest symptoms, which are nonspecific and could indicate other disorders. Assess for complaints or reports of cramping, anorexia, nausea, and headaches.

Collection of objective data includes assessment for hyponatremia. Fluid intake exceeds urinary output. The patient does not develop peripheral edema, because excess fluid is accumulating in the vascular system, not in the interstitial spaces; therefore weight gain is not always noted with SIADH.

As water intoxication progresses and the patient's serum becomes more hypotonic, brain cells expand (become edematous), and therefore the later signs of SIADH are neurologic. The patient becomes progressively lethargic, with marked personality changes. The patient has seizures, and the deep tendon reflexes diminish or disappear altogether.

All electrolyte levels should be monitored and the patient assessed often for signs and symptoms of increases and decreases in electrolytes, either from the disease process or the implementing of treatments for correction.

Diagnostic Tests

The diagnosis of SIADH is made by simultaneous measurements of urine and serum osmolality. Serum osmolality is less than 280 mmol/kg (normal is 285 to 295 mOsm/kg). Laboratory tests show hyponatremia (sodium less than 134 mEq/L). The serum is diluted and the urine is concentrated. Urine specific gravity is greater than 1.032, and urine sodium is elevated because of concentration.

Medical Management

The health care provider orders fluid restriction, initially 800 to 1000 mL/day. However, with severe hyponatremia fluids may be restricted to 500 mL/day. Daily fluid intake should equal fluid output. If fluid restriction is adequate, tests show a gradual increase in serum sodium along with a decrease in body weight.

A hypertonic saline solution (3% to 5%) may be ordered via IV infusion pump at a very slow rate to avoid too rapid a rise in sodium. This is necessary to correct sodium imbalance and to pull water out of edematous brain cells.

The health care provider may order medications such as demeclocycline, a tetracycline derivative, at a dosage of 300 mg orally four times daily. The health care provider also may prescribe lithium carbonate. Both drugs interfere with the antidiuretic action of ADH and cause polyuria. Diuretics such as furosemide (Lasix)—40 to 80 mg/day orally in divided doses or 20 to 40 mg IV daily—may be prescribed, to eliminate excess fluid, but only if the serum sodium is at least 125 mEq/L, or the drug may promote more loss of sodium. Taking furosemide increases losses of potassium, magnesium, and calcium; supplements may be needed.

Treatment also must be directed at eliminating the underlying problem. Surgical resection, radiation, or chemotherapy may be indicated for malignant neoplasms. If the causative factor is a medication, it is discontinued.

Monitoring the patient for signs and symptoms of further electrolyte imbalances is a priority nursing assessment. I&O should be monitored to ensure there is no significant fluid overload or signs of dehydration.

Nursing Interventions and Patient Teaching

The goals of nursing care are focused on assessment of the condition with documentation and reporting of changes. Timing of the assessment frequency is based on the patient's condition. Perform a neurologic examination and assess the patient's hydration status frequently. Auscultate lung sounds; crackles indicate fluid overload. Monitor the patient's oxygen saturation frequently. Carefully observe serum electrolytes, urine sodium, and urine specific gravity, because overcorrection can cause hypernatremia. Weigh the patient daily and closely monitor I&O; output is the primary guide to regulating fluid intake.

Restriction of fluid intake prevents fluid overload. Provide and frequently reinforce education. Solicit patient input in scheduling fluid allotments and types of fluids. Patients on diuretic therapy may require supplementation of sodium and potassium. Instruct patients to avoid foods high in sodium content, which may promote thirstiness.

Use simple explanations when detailing the plan of care, because anxiety can aggravate SIADH. If the patient reports nausea, obtain an order for an antiemetic before administration.

Patient problems and interventions for the patient with SIADH include but are not limited to the following:

Patient Problem	Nursing Interventions
Fluid Volume Overload, related to decreased urinary output	Obtain daily weight, same scales, same time Assess and record I&O Monitor laboratory results Administer medications as ordered Maintain dietary and fluid restrictions (fluids should be high in sodium; avoid salty foods) Monitor IV infusions (such as 3%–5% sodium chloride over several hours)
Potential for Compromised Oral Mucous Membranes, related to fluid restrictions of 500 mL/day	Provide frequent oral care; avoid alcohol-based mouthwashes Allow patient to choose fluids and to divide the allotted amount (such as half in morning, one third in evening, and the remainder at night)

Patient teaching should be an ongoing part of nursing care. Be certain the patient understands the treatment plan, the rationale behind it, and the expected outcome. Provide information about signs and symptoms of SIADH, and tell the patient to alert the health care provider if any changes are noted. SIADH can recur after discharge.

Prognosis

SIADH resulting from an adverse reaction to medication, or secondary to a head trauma, is self-limiting. The ability to manage metabolic conditions determines the chronicity of the disease. SIADH is potentially dangerous but treatable. Early diagnosis and medical management improve the prognosis.

DISORDERS OF THE THYROID AND PARATHYROID GLANDS

HYPERTHYROIDISM

Etiology and Pathophysiology

Hyperthyroidism—also called *Graves' disease,* exophthalmic goiter, and thyrotoxicosis—is a condition in which there is increased activity of the thyroid gland, with overproduction of the thyroid hormones T_3 and T_4, resulting in an exaggeration of metabolic processes. Graves' disease (the most common cause of hyperthyroidism) occurs most frequently in women in the 20- to 40-year-old age group. Two percent of the female population is affected by Graves' disease, compared with 0.2% of the male population. Graves' disease is an autoimmune disorder of unknown cause.

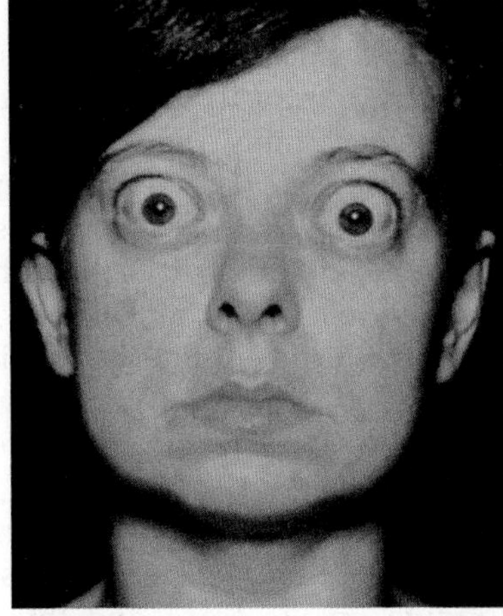

Fig. 51.6 Exophthalmos of Graves' disease. (From Seidel HM, Ball JW, Dains JE, et al: *Mosby's guide to physical examination,* ed 5, St. Louis, 2003, Mosby.)

Clinical Manifestations

Clinical manifestations are numerous and varied, from mild to severe. The patient usually has visible edema of the anterior portion of the neck as a result of enlargement of the thyroid. In severe cases, exophthalmos (bulging of the eyeballs) may occur, usually attributable to periorbital edema (Fig. 51.6). The classic finding of exophthalmos occurs in 20% to 40% of patients with Graves' disease. Exophthalmos is when the eyeballs are forced outward, resulting in incomplete closure of the eyelids; the exposed corneas become dry with subsequent development of corneal ulcers and loss of vision.

Assessment

Subjective data include the patient's description of an inability to concentrate and memory loss. The patient may complain of dysphagia or may be hoarse. There is usually weight loss, even with a voracious appetite. The patient reports feeling nervous, jittery, and excitable and may experience insomnia. Assess the patient for complaints of "heart palpitations" or other cardiac concerns, such as shortness of breath. These patients are emotionally labile and may overreact to stressful situations.

Objective data include changes in vital signs. The pulse is usually rapid, blood pressure is elevated, with cardiac arrhythmias noted. A bruit may be auscultated over the thyroid. The skin is warm and flushed, and the hair becomes fine and brittle. Female patients may cease to menstruate. Elevated body temperature may be accompanied by intolerance to heat, with profuse diaphoresis. The patient may have an increase in bowel movements. Note tremors of the hands. Behavior changes may include hyperactivity and clumsiness. Daily weighing usually shows weight loss.

Diagnostic Tests

The thyroid is controlled by the hypothalamus. Under normal conditions the thyroid secretes T_3 and T_4 in response to TSH released by the pituitary. As the T_3 and T_4 levels in the blood increase, the pituitary stops secreting TSH—an example of the negative feedback loop described earlier in this chapter.

If the thyroid becomes impaired, its hormone secretion may not respond normally to TSH. It may secrete too much (hyperthyroidism) or too little (hypothyroidism) T_3 and T_4. Hyperthyroidism is confirmed by a decrease in TSH level (because the overactive thyroid is releasing high amounts of T_3 and T_4, which exert negative feedback on the pituitary gland, causing it to stop secreting TSH) and an elevation of the level of free T_4 (FT_4). Total T_3 and T_4 levels may be evaluated but are not as helpful in the diagnosis. Additional diagnostic tests include radioactive iodine uptake scans and thyroid scans, typically performed in an outpatient setting (Box 51.1).

Box 51.1 Diagnostic Tests for Hyperthyroidism

- *T_3 (serum triiodothyronine):* Measures the T_3 level in the blood. The normal level is 65 to 195 ng/dL. As with serum thyroxine (T_4), the serum T_3 level provides an accurate measurement of thyroid function. T_3 is less stable than T_4; an elevated T_3 determination is clinically important in the patient who has a normal T_4 level but has all the signs and symptoms of hyperthyroidism. In this patient the test may identify T_3 thyrotoxicosis.
- *T_4 (serum thyroxine):* Measures the T_4 level in the blood. The normal level is 5 to 12 mcg/dL. Some medications such as oral contraceptives, steroids, estrogens, and sulfonamides may be withheld for several hours before the T_3 and T_4 tests, but food and fluids are not withheld. Elevated levels of these tests usually indicate hyperthyroidism.
- *Free T_4 (FT_4):* Measures the active component of total T_4. Normal values are 1 to 3.5 ng/dL. Because this level remains constant, this is considered a better indication of function than T_4 and is useful in diagnosing hyperthyroidism and hypothyroidism. High FT_4 suggests hyperthyroidism; low FT_4 suggests hypothyroidism.
- *Thyroid-stimulating hormone (TSH):* Measures the level of TSH. Normal values are 0.3 to 5.4 mcg/mL. This is considered the most sensitive method for evaluating thyroid disease. It is generally recommended as the first diagnostic test for thyroid dysfunction. TSH is suppressed in hyperthyroidism and elevated in hypothyroidism.
- *Radioactive iodine uptake (RAIU) test:* Radioactive iodine, ^{131}I, is given by mouth to the fasting patient. After 2, 6, and 24 hours, a scintillation camera is held over the thyroid to measure how much of the isotope has been removed from the bloodstream. A hyperactive thyroid may remove 35% to 95% of the drug. This test may be affected by prior ingestion of iodine-containing substances or foods. A signed consent form is required for this test. Also note any allergy to iodine on the request form, along with medications currently being taken. No radiation precautions are necessary, except to ensure that pregnant health care professionals do not come in close contact with the patient.
- *Thyroid scan:* ^{131}I is given to the patient either orally or intravenously. If an intravenous dose is given, the scan may be done in 30 to 60 minutes. A scintillation camera positioned over the patient's thyroid sends images that are received on an oscilloscope and may be printed out on special paper. A signed consent form is required for this test. No radiation precautions are necessary.

Medical Management

Ablation therapy using radioactive iodine is the gold standard for treating hyperthyroidism. The goal is to destroy enough of the hypertrophied thyroid tissue to produce a normally functioning thyroid gland. Dosing is patient specific and often results in the development of hypothyroidism. The therapeutic dose of radioactive iodine is low, so no radiation safety precautions are necessary, with the exception of danger to pregnant women providing care.

Medical management for hyperthyroidism may include daily administration of drugs that block the production of thyroid hormones, such as propylthiouracil (PTU) or methimazole (Tapazole) (Table 51.2). The patient usually begins to notice a decrease in symptoms within 6 to 8 weeks after starting drug therapy. This may be followed after the acute stage by ablation therapy using a therapeutic dose of radioactive iodine ($Na^{131}I$ or $Na^{125}I$), based on the patient's age, clinical manifestations, and estimated weight of the thyroid.

Because of the possible development of hypothyroidism after this treatment, the patient must have adequate follow-up medical supervision. If a patient develops hypothyroidism after treatment, levothyroxine therapy will be needed. NOTE: ^{131}I is not a radiation hazard to the nonpregnant patient but absolutely is contraindicated during pregnancy. Pregnant health care professionals should not care for this patient for several days after treatment.

Surgery has fallen out of favor because of possible serious complications, such as hemorrhage, hypoparathyroidism, and vocal cord paralysis. Surgery still may be indicated for patients who cannot tolerate antithyroid drugs, are not good candidates for radioactive iodine therapy, have a possible malignancy, or have large goiters causing tracheal compression.

Surgical treatment for hyperthyroidism is subtotal thyroidectomy, a procedure in which approximately five-sixths of the thyroid is removed. If too much tissue is taken, the gland will not regenerate after surgery, and hypothyroidism will result. Surgery usually is delayed, if possible, until the patient is in a normal thyroid (euthyroid) state because of the risk of excessive bleeding during thyroidectomy and postoperative thyroid crisis.

Patients with mild hyperthyroidism are admitted rarely to the acute care hospital. They are treated by

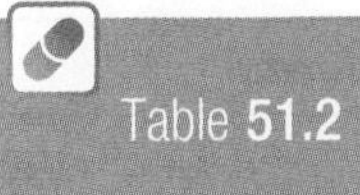

Table 51.2 **Medications Commonly Used to Treat Hyperthyroidism and Hypothyroidism**

MEDICATIONS	COMMON SIDE EFFECTS
Hyperthyroidism	
Iodine or iodine products (potassium or sodium iodide with strong iodine solution, potassium iodide, Lugol's solution)	Nausea, vomiting, diarrhea, abdominal pain
Radioactive iodine (^{131}I or ^{125}I)	Sore throat, edema or pain in neck, temporary loss of taste, nausea, vomiting, painful salivary glands
methimazole (Tapazole), propylthiouracil (PTU)	Rash or pruritus, vertigo, nausea, vomiting, loss of taste, paresthesias, abdominal pain
Hypothyroidism	
levothyroxine (Synthroid, Eltroxin, Levo-T, Unithroid) liothyronine (Cytomel) liotrix (Thyrolar) thyroid (Armour Thyroid, Thyrar)	Nervousness, irritability, tremors, insomnia, tachycardia, hypertension, palpitations, cardiac dysrhythmias, vomiting, diarrhea, nausea, appetite changes, weight loss, menstrual irregularities, leg cramps, fever

the health care provider in an office or clinic setting. However, the hospital nurse may come in contact with the hyperthyroid patient admitted for a different condition and also may care for these patients before and after thyroidectomy.

Nursing Interventions and Patient Teaching

The hyperthyroid patient needs more nutrients because of increased metabolism. Diet therapy usually consists of food high in protein. Increased vitamins (especially the B vitamins), minerals, and carbohydrates also are indicated. Losses in bone density may be attributed to hyperthyroidism. Supplementation with calcium and vitamin D is indicated to avoid the development of osteoporosis. Offer between-meal snacks. Food should be soft and easily swallowed if the patient has **dysphagia** (difficulty swallowing). Coffee, tea, and colas should be avoided because of their stimulant effect.

Preoperative teaching is extremely important for the patient who is scheduled for a thyroidectomy. Keep the environment as stable as possible to prevent increased stimulation. Include instructions on how to properly support the head while turning in bed or rising to a sitting or standing position. The nurse (or patient) places both hands behind the head and maintains anatomic position while the rest of the body is being moved. Also teach the patient to deep breathe. The health care provider determines whether postoperative coughing is allowed, because it strains the suture line. Inform the patient that a period of "voice rest" may be enforced for 48 hours postoperatively and that pencil and paper will be provided for writing notes instead of talking. Do voice checks every 2 to 4 hours, as ordered by the health care provider, to rule out damage to the laryngeal nerve resulting in inability to speak. Ask the patient to say "ah" and check for excessive hoarseness or voice change. Slight hoarseness is expected and should not cause alarm. Damage to the laryngeal nerve during surgery occurs in approximately 12.4% of cases, but the damage is not always permanent.

Postoperative management includes keeping the patient in a semi-Fowler's position, to decrease edema at the operative site and to enhance respiratory status, with pillows supporting the head and shoulders. Caution the patient to avoid hyperextending the head to prevent excess tension on the incision, which usually is made in a horizontal crease in the anterior neck. Have a suction apparatus and tracheotomy tray available for emergency use. A cool-mist humidifier at the bedside may help soothe the throat and prevent coughing. Check vital signs frequently, with special attention paid to the rate and depth of respirations and observations for any dyspnea (shortness of breath or difficulty breathing) related to edema in the operative site. Before giving any liquid orally, be sure the swallowing and cough reflexes have returned. Be alert for signs of internal or external bleeding; early signs of internal bleeding include restlessness, apprehension, increased pulse rate, decreased blood pressure, and a feeling of fullness in the neck. Later, cyanosis may develop, signaling an obstructed airway; provide for adequate airway management and notify the surgeon immediately. Inspect the dressing on the neck frequently for obvious external bleeding. Also check for bleeding at the sides and back of the neck and on top of the patient's shoulders, because oozing blood may pool there as a result of gravity. Most surgeons allow a dressing to be reinforced as needed and loosened slightly if the patient complains that it is too tight.

Postoperatively, the diet initially consists of clear, cool liquids, progressing to soft food as tolerated. This is followed by a regular diet as soon as possible to help the patient regain lost weight and correct any nutritional deficiencies.

Another significant postoperative complication after thyroidectomy is tetany. One possible cause of tetany is the inadvertent removal of one or more of the parathyroid glands during surgery. Another is edema in the operative area, which occludes release of PTH into the bloodstream, resulting in a low serum calcium level (normal serum calcium is 9.0 to 10.5 mg/dL). The symptoms include numbness and tingling in the fingertips and toes and around the mouth. The patient also may have *carpopedal spasms* (muscle spasms in the wrists and feet) and increased pulse, respirations, and blood pressure, accompanied by anxiety and agitation.

Laryngeal spasm and stridor may occur. **Chvostek's sign** is a clinical sign of abnormal spasm of the facial muscles when elicited by light taps on the facial nerve, which is located at the angle of the jaw. This is seen in patients who are experiencing hypocalcemia. **Trousseau's sign** assesses for latent tetany, which is a carpal spasm that is induced by inflating a sphygmomanometer cuff on the upper arm to a pressure exceeding systolic blood pressure for 3 minutes; a positive result may be seen in hypocalcemia and hypomagnesemia. If untreated, the condition may progress to convulsions or lethal cardiac dysrhythmias. Emergency treatment of tetany is the intravenous administration of calcium gluconate, which always should be available postoperatively.

The other serious complication after thyroidectomy is thyroid crisis, or thyroid storm. Fortunately, it occurs rarely and usually can be attributed to manipulation of the thyroid during surgery, which causes the release of large amounts of thyroid hormones into the bloodstream. If thyroid crisis occurs, it usually does so within the first 12 hours postoperatively. In thyroid crisis, all the signs and symptoms of hyperthyroidism are exaggerated. In addition, the patient may develop nausea, vomiting, severe tachycardia, severe hypertension, and occasionally hyperthermia up to 106°F (41°C). Extreme restlessness, cardiac dysrhythmia, and delirium also may occur. The patient may develop heart failure as evidenced by decreased cardiac output secondary to cardiac strain and tachycardia. Diagnostic tests indicate increased FT_4 and decreased TSH.

The three goals of thyroid storm management are (1) to induce a normal thyroid state, (2) prevent cardiovascular collapse, and (3) prevent excessive hyperthermia. Emergency treatment of thyroid crisis includes administration of IV fluids, sodium iodide, corticosteroids, antipyretics, an antithyroid drug (such as PTU or methimazole), and oxygen as needed. Prompt, adequate treatment usually results in dramatic improvement within 12 to 24 hours.

Patient problems and interventions for the patient having a thyroidectomy include but are not limited to the following:

Patient Problem	Nursing Interventions
Preoperative	
Potential for Elevated Body Temperature, related to increased metabolism	Assess body temperature at regular intervals Regulate environment (room temperature, linens, clothing) to help keep patient comfortable Administer acetaminophen as prescribed
Insufficient Nutrition, related to increased metabolism	Encourage patient to eat prescribed diet and avoid caffeine Assess daily weight and food intake
Postoperative	
Compromised Swallowing Ability, related to postoperative edema	Ensure swallowing and cough reflexes are present before oral intake Encourage patient to drink slowly and chew food thoroughly
Potential for Inability to Maintain Adequate Breathing Pattern, related to: • Postoperative edema • Pain	Monitor rate and depth of respirations Assess breath sounds and skin color Encourage slow, deep breaths at least hourly Position patient to maximize respiratory effort

Patient education after thyroidectomy includes stressing the importance of follow-up medical supervision. Thyroid function tests are done periodically to access thyroid hormone levels. Before discharge, teach the patient proper care of the incision site and symptoms that may indicate development of an infection, in which case he or she should notify the surgeon immediately. Discuss with the patient the need for a high-calorie, high-protein, high-carbohydrate diet until weight is stable.

Prognosis

With adequate, appropriate medical or surgical treatment, these patients usually have a normal life expectancy. However, exophthalmos, if present, may remain to a lesser degree in some patients.

HYPOTHYROIDISM

Etiology and Pathophysiology

Hypothyroidism is one of the most common medical disorders in the United States. It occurs most often in women 30 to 60 years of age and is more common in older adults than previously thought. Hypothyroidism occurs when the thyroid fails to secrete sufficient hormones, slowing all of the body's metabolic processes. Causes include an autoimmune response, radiation therapy, pituitary disorders, or iodine deficiency. It sometimes results from medical or surgical treatment of hyperthyroidism (Mayo Clinic, 2012a). *Myxedema* denotes severe hypothyroidism in adults. It is characterized by edema of the hands, face, feet, and periorbital tissues. Congenital hypothyroidism is called *cretinism* and is estimated to occur in 1 of every 4000 births (Daniel and Postellon, 2013). All infants in the United States are screened for decreased thyroid function at birth.

Clinical Manifestations

Clinical manifestations range from mild to severe and depend on the degree of thyroid hormone deficiency present. All the body's metabolic processes slow, resulting in decreased production of body heat, intolerance to cold, and weight gain. Atherosclerotic changes may result in coronary artery disease. Hypothyroidism may have adverse effects on the heart, with decreased cardiac output and contractility; the patient experiences decreased exercise tolerance and dyspnea on exertion. Early signs are weight gain, difficulty concentrating, constipation, and fluid/weight gain. Late signs include mood swings, infertility (in women), acute fatigue syndrome, and depression.

Assessment

Subjective data include the patient's mental and emotional status, which may include depression, paranoia, impaired memory, and general slowing of thought processes. Speech and hearing may be deficient. The patient is lethargic, forgetful, and irritable. Because of the body's slowed metabolism, cold intolerance, anorexia, and constipation may develop. Both sexes may experience decreased libido and reproductive difficulty. Assess the patient's adaptive coping methods.

Collection of objective data includes assessment of the skin and hair. The hair thins and may fall out; the skin becomes thickened and dry. Facial features may enlarge to give the patient an edematous appearance with a masklike facial expression. The voice is characteristically low and hoarse. Decreased metabolism usually causes bradycardia, decreased blood pressure and respirations, and exercise intolerance. The patient has decreased ability to perform activities because of weakness, clumsiness, and ataxia. Assess the respiratory rate after administration of any central nervous system depressant. Evaluate the abdomen for distention, because *myxedema ileus* (intestinal obstruction) may occur. Menorrhagia (excessive menstrual flow) is a frequent complaint of women with hypothyroidism. Also, inhibition of ovulation with subsequent infertility may occur.

Diagnostic Tests

Diagnosis of hypothyroidism is based on the physical examination and history and on appropriate laboratory tests, such as TSH, T_3, T_4, and FT_4 levels. Low levels of T_3, T_4, and FT_4 are the underlying stimuli for TSH secretion. Therefore a compensatory elevation of TSH occurs in patients with primary hypothyroid states, and low levels of T_3, T_4, and FT_4 are present. Subclinical cases may go undiagnosed for years, so be aware of subtle clues while interviewing and caring for the patient.

Medical Management

Hypothyroidism is treated with hormone replacement therapy using desiccated animal thyroid (Armour thyroid), T_4, or synthetic products such as levothyroxine (Levothroid, Synthroid, Levo-T) (see Table 51.2). Synthetic products typically are preferred over biologic agents to treat hypothyroidism. The drugs usually are given in the morning to enhance nutrient metabolism of ingested food during the daily meals. Teach the patient to take levothyroxine on an empty stomach. The patient initially is given a small dose, with increases as necessary until the desired effect is achieved. A maintenance dosage then is established. Early in treatment, the hormone level should be monitored about every 6 to 8 weeks until the patient's TSH level is normal and then tested at least annually. Watch the patient for adverse effects of drug therapy, which mimic the signs and symptoms of hyperthyroidism. There is usually a dramatic change in the patient after replacement therapy begins. Lifelong thyroid replacement therapy usually is required, as well as laboratory monitoring of T_3, T_4, and TSH levels to adjust the dosage and minimize the effects of hypothyroidism or hyperthyroidism as a result of a too-high dosage.

Nursing Interventions and Patient Teaching

Nursing interventions for the hospitalized patient with severe hypothyroidism center mainly on symptomatic relief. Keep the room at least 70° to 74°F (21° to 23°C), and be certain the patient does not become chilled during bathing or other procedures. Allow extra time for physical care so that the patient does not feel rushed. Keep accurate records of bowel elimination, because constipation may be severe. Stool softeners and bulk laxatives may be ordered. Provide a high-protein, high-fiber, low-calorie diet, and encourage increased fluid intake. The patient should avoid concentrated carbohydrates, such as sweets, to help prevent excessive weight gain. Watch for chest pain or dyspnea accompanied by changes in the rate or rhythm of the heart; this may indicate cardiac involvement. Caution the patient to not stop taking the thyroid hormone without consulting a health care provider. This medication must be taken for the rest of the patient's life. Because most patients with hypothyroidism are more susceptible to the effects of sedatives, hypnotics, and anesthetics, be alert for possible adverse effects if these agents are given.

Teach the patient to take the thyroid hormone on a consistent schedule, typically in the morning on an empty stomach. Taking the medication with food, vitamins, and minerals can impair absorption. In addition, the patient should inform the health care provider if the diet typically contains soybean flour, cottonseed oil, or walnuts, which can impair absorption.

Patient problems and interventions for the patient with hypothyroidism include but are not limited to the following:

Patient Problem	Nursing Interventions
Insufficient Cardiac Output, related to decreased metabolism	Assess pulse, blood pressure, skin color, and temperature Schedule nursing activities around patient's activity cycle, with rest periods as needed to conserve energy

Continued

Patient Problem	Nursing Interventions
Infrequent or Difficult Bowel Elimination, related to decreased peristaltic action	Assess frequency and character of stools Encourage increased intake of oral fluids and high-fiber foods

Regular checkups are essential because the drug dosage may have to be adjusted periodically. The patient and significant other should understand the desired effects and major adverse effects of the medication. Instruct the patient to eat well-balanced meals of high-fiber foods, such as fruits, vegetables, and whole-grain cereals and breads. The patient also needs an adequate intake of iodine, found in foods such as saltwater fish, milk, and eggs. Increased fluid intake helps prevent constipation. Tell the patient and the family that mental and physical slowness may still be present but should improve with thyroid replacement therapy.

Prognosis

Most patients with hypothyroidism do well with proper medical supervision, although they probably will have to take medication for the rest of their lives. In children, when T_4 replacement begins before epiphyseal fusion, the chance for normal growth is improved greatly.

SIMPLE (COLLOID) GOITER

Etiology and Pathophysiology

A simple, or colloid, goiter develops when the thyroid gland enlarges in response to low iodine levels in the bloodstream or when it is unable to use iodine properly. When the blood level of T_3 is too low to signal the pituitary to decrease TSH secretion, the thyroid gland responds by increasing the formation of thyroglobulin (colloid), which accumulates in the thyroid follicles and causes the gland to enlarge (Fig. 51.7). Most cases of simple goiter can be attributed to insufficient dietary intake of iodine, leading to this overgrowth of thyroid tissue.

Clinical Manifestations

The patient usually has no manifestations of overt thyroid dysfunction, and the diagnosis is based on the patient's physical appearance.

Assessment

Subjective data include the patient's emotional response to the unsightly enlargement of the thyroid. Encourage the patient to talk about his or her feelings. The patient may complain only of symptoms of dysphagia, hoarseness, or dyspnea related to the pressure of the enlarged gland against the esophagus and trachea. Dysphagia may make it difficult to eat and drink adequate amounts. Assess the patient for increasing dyspnea. Determine the patient's understanding of the need for medication, diet therapy, and medical follow-up.

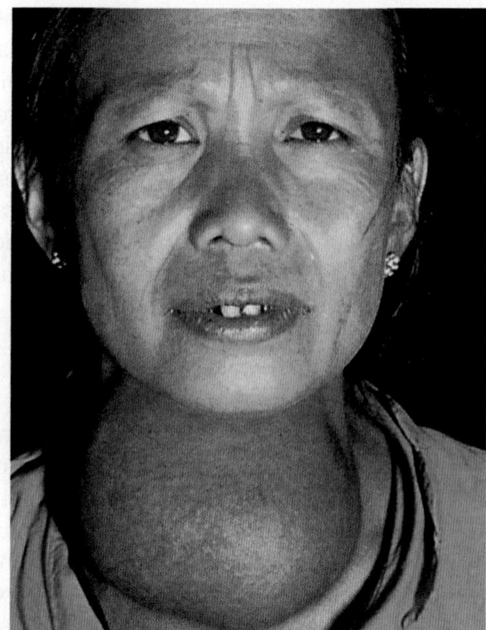

Fig. 51.7 Simple goiter. (Courtesy L.V. Bergman & Associates, Inc., Cold Spring, New York.)

Collection of objective data includes assessment of increased goiter size, voice changes, and adequacy of food and fluid intake.

Diagnostic Testing

Diagnostic testing includes a thyroid scan or an ultrasound of the thyroid gland to determine function and structure. Serum tests to evaluate T_3, T_4, and TSH levels also are completed.

Medical Management

The thyroid may be only slightly enlarged, or it may be so enlarged that surgery is necessary to improve respiration or swallowing. Surgery also is performed sometimes for cosmetic effect, because this type of goiter can be unsightly and damage the patient's self-image and self-esteem. Lugol's solution is one antihyperthyroid agent used in conjunction with other antihyperthyroid medications, to decrease or shrink the thyroid gland, typically before surgery. It also is used in cases in which surgical removal of the thyroid gland is not feasible or must be delayed (NLM, 2013).

If thyroidectomy is completed, most of the gland is removed. Medical treatment consists of oral administration of potassium iodide and foods high in iodine (such as seafood, seaweed, dairy, grains, iodized salt, and eggs) (Office of Dietary Supplements, n.d.).

Nursing Interventions and Patient Teaching

Nursing interventions after thyroidectomy (previously discussed) are aimed at prevention of complications such as bleeding, tetany, and thyroid crisis.

Patient problems and interventions for the patient with simple (colloid) goiter include but are not limited to the following:

Patient Problem	Nursing Interventions
Potential for Noncooperation or Nonconformity	Provide opportunities for patient to express feelings about treatment plan Correct misconceptions and reinforce previous medical instruction Stress importance of taking prescribed medications, having regular checkups, and avoiding any identified goitrogenic foods
Potential for Distorted Body Image, related to altered physical appearance	Develop open and trusting relationship so that the patient will express his or her feelings Discuss ways to disguise thyroid enlargement (scarves, high collars) Encourage and offer support groups for patients with similar situations

Stress the importance of adequate dietary intake of iodine by the patient. Medical supervision is recommended at regular intervals.

Prognosis

Most patients can expect to live a normal life after adequate treatment of goiter. If the thyroid becomes inactive, a diagnosis of hypothyroidism is made, and the patient is treated with conventional replacement therapy medications.

CANCER OF THE THYROID

Etiology and Pathophysiology

Cancer of the thyroid is a relatively rare malignancy, affecting approximately 25 per 1 million people in the United States each year. Risk factors include diets low in iodine (not common in the United States) and radiation exposure; women in their 40s and 50s are at greater risk as well. In the late 1940s and up into the 1960s, radiation was used more frequently than it is today for medical procedures. At one time, radiation was used to treat acne, enlarged thymus tissue, and tonsils/adenoids in children and teens (American Cancer Society [ACS], 2013). Cancer of the thyroid occurs more frequently in females and in whites. The incidence rises as age increases (Norman, 2012). About 75% of malignancies of the thyroid are papillary, well-differentiated adenocarcinomas, a type of cancer that grows slowly, usually is contained, and does not spread beyond the adjacent lymph nodes. Cure rates after thyroidectomy in these cases are excellent. Other cancers, follicular and anaplastic, are rarer and have extremely low cure rates.

Clinical Manifestations

The principal clinical manifestation of thyroid cancer is a firm, fixed, small, rounded, painless mass or *nodule* that is felt during palpation of the gland. Only in rare instances are the symptoms of hyperthyroidism seen.

Assessment

Subjective data include the patient's use of adaptive coping methods to deal with the diagnosis. Also observe the support system provided by the patient's significant others. Assess the patient's understanding of the importance of medical follow-up, and for reports of trouble breathing, hoarseness, or difficulty in swallowing.

Objective data include progressive enlargement of the tumor area preoperatively, response to ^{131}I therapy, and skin involvement in the neck and torso after radiation therapy. Assess for trachea and vocal cord involvement as well.

Diagnostic Tests

Papillary thyroid cancer is suspected when a thyroid scan shows a "cold" nodule, indicating decreased uptake of ^{131}I. Benign adenomas and follicular cancers usually are visualized as "hot" nodules because of their increased uptake of the isotope. Thyroid function tests usually yield normal results. The health care provider uses ultrasound and CT scans of the thyroid to further investigate the thyroid and surrounding tissue. If the parathyroid gland is involved, the serum calcium level may be elevated as well. To confirm the diagnosis, a thyroid needle biopsy may be completed, but only by a skilled health care provider to avoid seeding of adjacent tissues. Metastasis could result, with the prognosis becoming much more grave.

Medical Management

Treatment of thyroid cancer is a total thyroidectomy, with subsequent lifelong thyroid hormone replacement therapy. If metastasis is present at the time of the initial surgery, a radical neck dissection may be performed. In addition, radiation therapy, chemotherapy, and administration of radioactive ^{131}I may be done.

Nursing Interventions and Patient Teaching

Nursing interventions are like those for the patient who has undergone thyroidectomy (see the previous section, "Hyperthyroidism"). As with a thyroidectomy for noncancerous lesions, the major postoperative complications are respiratory distress, recurrent laryngeal damage, hemorrhage, and hypoparathyroidism. Assess the patient's oxygen saturation, voice tone and presence, and surgical site and monitor for signs and symptoms of hypothyroidism and hypoparathyroidism, including serum calcium levels. Assess the posterior neck area as well. The drainage from the incision may pool at the posterior neck and not be obvious from the anterior view.

Patient problems and interventions for the patient with cancer of the thyroid include but are not limited to the following:

Patient Problem	Nursing Interventions
Anxiousness, related to situational crisis	Encourage patient to discuss feelings about upcoming surgery Monitor level of anxiety Maintain a calm environment; try to decrease stressors
Potential for Injury, related to increased metabolic action of thyroid hormone and decreased calcium serum levels	Monitor for signs and symptoms of decreased calcium (muscle spasms, irritability, tetany, and cardiac dysrhythmias) Monitor for signs and symptoms of hyperthyroidism and hypothyroidism (changes in vital signs, temperature intolerance, tremors or changes in sleep pattern)
Inadequate Fluid Volume, related to postoperative hemorrhage	Monitor incision and posterior neck for increased drainage Maintain accurate record of intake and output Monitor vital signs for changes such as increased pulse

Stress the importance of proper medical follow-up to monitor thyroid hormone replacement therapy and to help ensure prompt diagnosis of any metastatic lesions. Before discharge from the hospital, teach the patient proper care of the surgical incision. Include teaching on the possibility of surgically induced hypothyroidism (depending on the amount of thyroid gland removed), including the need to take thyroid replacement therapy correctly, and signs and symptoms of hyperthyroidism (if the dosage is too high).

Prognosis

The prognosis after treatment for thyroid cancer depends on the type of tumor. For papillary carcinoma the prognosis is excellent, and the 5-year survival rate for stages I and II is nearly 100%. For stages III and IV the rate is 93% and 51%, respectively; for follicular and anaplastic carcinomas, the prognosis is much less favorable (ACS, 2013).

HYPERPARATHYROIDISM

Etiology and Pathophysiology

Hyperparathyroidism involves overactivity of the parathyroid glands, with increased production of PTH. The cause of this condition may be a primary hypertrophy of one or more of the tiny parathyroid glands, usually in the form of an adenoma (benign growths that may evolve into adenocarcinomas). It also may result from chronic renal failure, pyelonephritis, or glomerulonephritis. Parathyroid carcinoma may in rare cases result in hyperparathyroidism with rapid progress and a grave prognosis. Hyperparathyroidism usually occurs in adults between 30 and 70 years of age, and it occurs twice as often in women. Risk factors include postmenopausal status, prolonged or severe calcium or vitamin D deficiency, lithium use, and radiation to the neck (Mayo Clinic, 2011a).

Clinical Manifestations

The primary clinical manifestation is hypercalcemia. This occurs as calcium leaves the bones and accumulates in the bloodstream. As a result, the bones become demineralized, causing skeletal pain, pain on weight-bearing, and pathologic fractures (fractures that result from slight or no trauma to diseased bone). The first presentation of the illness may be a patient seen for a fractured bone that is unrelated to trauma. The high level of calcium in the blood may lead to the formation of kidney stones.

Assessment

Collection of subjective data includes assessment of the severity of skeletal pain, the degree of muscle weakness, and the effectiveness of analgesics. It is important to determine nursing measures that contribute to the patient's comfort and mobility. As neuromuscular function decreases, the patient has generalized fatigue, drowsiness, apathy, nausea, and anorexia; assess the degree of anorexia and nausea. There may be constipation, personality changes, disorientation, and even paranoia. Renal colic and dull back pain may indicate calculus (kidney stone) formation.

Collection of objective data includes careful observation for any skeletal deformity or abnormal movement of bone that may indicate a pathologic fracture. Observe the urine for quantity and the presence of hematuria and stones. There may be vomiting and weight loss. Hypertension and cardiac dysrhythmias may present significant problems. Changes in the serum calcium level may cause bradycardia and other cardiac irregularities. The level of consciousness may decrease to the level of stupor or coma.

Diagnostic Tests

Radiographic examination may reveal skeletal decalcification. Blood PTH levels are increased, as are alkaline phosphate levels. The patient should receive nothing by mouth for 8 to 12 hours before these tests. The serum calcium level is elevated, whereas the serum phosphorus level is decreased. Bone density measurements also may be used to detect bone loss. Imaging, such as MRI, CT, and ultrasound, may be used to localize the adenoma. A sestamibi parathyroid scan is useful in determining the location of a parathyroid tumor. In this diagnostic test, a radioactive dye is injected into the patient's vein and the parathyroid gland absorbs the agent, which is then detectable on imaging (Alkhalili et al, 2015). The primary health care provider also may request 24-hour urine collection to determine calcium levels. An elevated urine calcium level is indicative of increased parathyroid hormone levels (NLM, 2011). A differential diagnosis should be made to rule out multiple myeloma, Cushing's syndrome, vitamin D excess, and other causes of hypercalcemia.

Medical Management

Treatment for hyperparathyroidism will be based upon the level of hormone elevation. If the levels are only mildly elevated and renal function is normal the medical management may be conservative and consist of close monitoring of parathyroid hormone levels.

Surgical removal of the abnormal tissue is the most common plan for condition management.

Nursing Interventions and Patient Teaching

Preoperative nursing interventions include helping restore fluid and electrolyte balance by encouraging increased oral fluid intake and by carefully monitoring IV fluid therapy. Monitor the patient's I&O, because diuretics may be used to encourage elimination of serum calcium. Furosemide is the diuretic of choice. Thiazide diuretics are not used, because they decrease renal excretion of calcium and thus increase the hypercalcemic state. Urine may be strained if the patient exhibits signs of kidney calculi. Daily serum calcium levels may be ordered. The diet should be low in calcium, eliminating milk and other dairy products. Antacids are high in calcium and should not be used. Accurately assess the patient's pain and administer prescribed analgesics as needed. Postoperatively, care for the patient in the same manner as after a thyroidectomy, with careful monitoring of I&O. These patients commonly retain fluid in the tissues after surgery and often have decreased urinary output. It is important to avoid overhydration at this point. Assess the patient frequently for signs of hypocalcemia, such as tetany, cardiac dysrhythmias, and carpopedal spasms (i.e., spasms of the hands or feet). If tetany does occur, it is treated with calcium gluconate intravenously.

Patient problems and interventions for the patient with hyperparathyroidism include but are not limited to the following:

Patient Problem	Nursing Interventions
Inability to Tolerate Activity, related to neuromuscular dysfunction	Help patient identify factors that increase or decrease activity tolerance and to eliminate or reduce painful, fatiguing activities Encourage patient to follow prescribed individualized activity or exercise program
Recent onset of pain, related to hormonal imbalances and physiologic variables	Assess factors that cause or worsen pain, and help patient adjust body mechanics or activity
Renal colic, related to physiologic variables	Encourage adequate fluid intake while assessing cardiac and urinary output

Teach the patient the principles of good body mechanics to prevent pathologic fractures during ambulation. Reassure the patient that bone pain should decrease gradually as electrolyte balance is restored and the condition is alleviated. Encourage the patient to participate in mild exercise as prescribed by the health care provider to regain muscle strength and promote bone health. Encourage the patient to consume plenty of water, monitor the amount of dietary calcium and vitamin D, and avoid smoking. Teach the patient that certain medications such as some diuretics and lithium can elevate the serum calcium level. Evaluate the home environment and develop a plan of changes necessary to prevent accidents, such as eliminating tripping hazards.

Prognosis

With proper medical or surgical treatment, the patient can maintain an average life expectancy. In patients with parathyroid carcinoma, the prognosis is grave.

HYPOPARATHYROIDISM

Etiology and Pathophysiology

Hypoparathyroidism occurs when there is decreased PTH, resulting in decreased levels of serum calcium. Idiopathic hypoparathyroidism is a rare condition, thought to be either autoimmune or familial in origin. The most common cause is the inadvertent removal or destruction of one or more of the tiny parathyroid glands during thyroidectomy. Other causes include previous radiation treatments to the neck area, an overdose of vitamin D or calcium, cancer (lymphoma or multiple myeloma), and a low magnesium level.

Clinical Manifestations

Decreased PTH levels in the bloodstream cause an increased serum phosphorus level and a decreased serum calcium level, resulting in neuromuscular hyperexcitability, involuntary and uncontrollable muscle spasms, and hypocalcemic tetany. Severe hypocalcemia may result in laryngeal spasm, stridor, cyanosis, and an increased possibility of asphyxia. Some patients have calcification of the basal ganglia in the brain, causing a parkinsonian syndrome with bizarre posturing and spastic movements.

Assessment

Collection of subjective data includes assessment of neuromuscular activity for symptoms such as dysphagia and numbness or tingling of the lips, fingertips, and occasionally feet and increased muscle tension leading to paresthesia (burning or prickling sensations) and stiffness. The patient may feel anxious, irritable, or depressed. The patient may experience headaches and nausea. Abdominal or flank pain may occur if a renal calculus attempts to pass down the ureter into the bladder. Assess the effectiveness of narcotics used to relieve renal colic.

Objective data include a positive Chvostek's sign or Trousseau's sign. If laryngeal spasm and stridor occur, cyanosis may appear. Cardiac output may decrease as a result of hypocalcemia, and the patient may develop dysrhythmias. Tetanic spasms of the extremities may be observed. The magnesium level should be monitored closely.

Diagnostic Tests

Diagnostic laboratory studies confirm the decreased serum calcium and PTH with increased urinary calcium, and increased serum phosphorus with decreased urinary phosphorus. Rule out other possible causes of hypocalcemia, such as vitamin D deficiency, kidney failure, and acute pancreatitis. Additional diagnostic testing includes electrocardiography, x-rays, and bone density scans.

Medical Management

The immediate treatment of hypoparathyroid tetany is IV administration of calcium gluconate or calcium chloride (10%). This drug irritates the vessel wall and always should be given slowly, at a rate not to exceed 1 mL/min. The patient may complain of a hot feeling of the skin or tongue. If given too rapidly, IV calcium can precipitate hypotension, serious cardiac dysrhythmias, or cardiac arrest. Thus electrocardiographic monitoring is indicated when administering calcium. Take care that none of the drug escapes the vein (extravasates) and moves into the tissues, because sloughing may occur. After the initial IV dose, calcium may be continued in a slow IV infusion until tetany is controlled; then it is given orally. Vitamin D usually also is given orally to increase the absorption and blood level of calcium.

Nursing Interventions and Patient Teaching

Monitor any patient receiving calcium, especially intravenously, for signs of hypercalcemia. The most common clinical manifestations of this are vomiting, disorientation, anorexia, abdominal pain, and weakness. Assess the patient for respiratory distress; renal involvement; and adverse reactions to calcium therapy, such as bradycardia, syncope, and hypotension. Use calcium cautiously in digitalized patients, because it may cause digitalis toxicity. Cimetidine (Tagamet) interferes with normal parathyroid functioning and should be used carefully in these patients. Vitamin D supplements are prescribed to improve the absorption of calcium in the intestinal tract and improve bone resorption in patients with chronic and resistant hypocalcemia. Calcitroil (Rocaltrol) is the preferred medication (NLM, 2010). The diet should contain foods high in calcium, such as low-fat dairy products, dark green vegetables, soybeans, tofu, and canned fish with the bones included. Offer high-calcium snacks. Patients should be encouraged to consume adequate amounts of calcium (1200 mg/day in divided doses for adults) via their diet. If this is not likely, calcium supplements should be considered. A diet low in phosphorus is also important. Foods low in phosphorus include soy milk, white rice, jam, honey, lemon-lime soda, cucumbers, lettuce, peppers, tomatoes, and non-organ meats.

A patient problem and interventions for the patient with hypoparathyroidism include but are not limited to the following:

Patient Problem	Nursing Interventions
Potential for Injury, related to postoperative hypocalcemia	Assess for signs and symptoms of hypocalcemia (muscle spasms, laryngeal stridor, convulsion) Calcium therapy if needed

Teach the patient the early symptoms of hypocalcemia, with instructions to notify the nurse or health care provider if they occur. Draw blood levels of calcium and phosphorus periodically while the patient is hospitalized. Teach the patient to monitor the pulse for changes, maintain fluid balance, and use calcium supplements at home. Stress the need for lifelong treatment and follow-up care, including monitoring calcium levels three or four times a year.

Prognosis

For most patients, treatment keeps the symptoms under control, and those affected have a normal life expectancy.

DISORDERS OF THE ADRENAL GLANDS

ADRENAL HYPERFUNCTION (CUSHING'S SYNDROME)

Etiology and Pathophysiology

Cushing's syndrome is a spectrum of clinical abnormalities caused by excess corticosteroids, particularly glucocorticoids. This syndrome may be caused by hyperplasia of adrenal tissue resulting from overstimulation by the pituitary hormone ACTH, by a tumor of the adrenal cortex, by ACTH-secreting neoplasms outside the pituitary (such as small-cell carcinoma of the lung), and by prolonged administration of high doses of corticosteroids. The body's protective feedback mechanism fails, resulting in excess secretion of the adrenal hormones: glucocorticoids, mineralocorticoids, and sex hormones.

Clinical Manifestations

This overabundance of corticosteroids produces the signs and symptoms commonly associated with Cushing's syndrome, including moon face and buffalo hump.

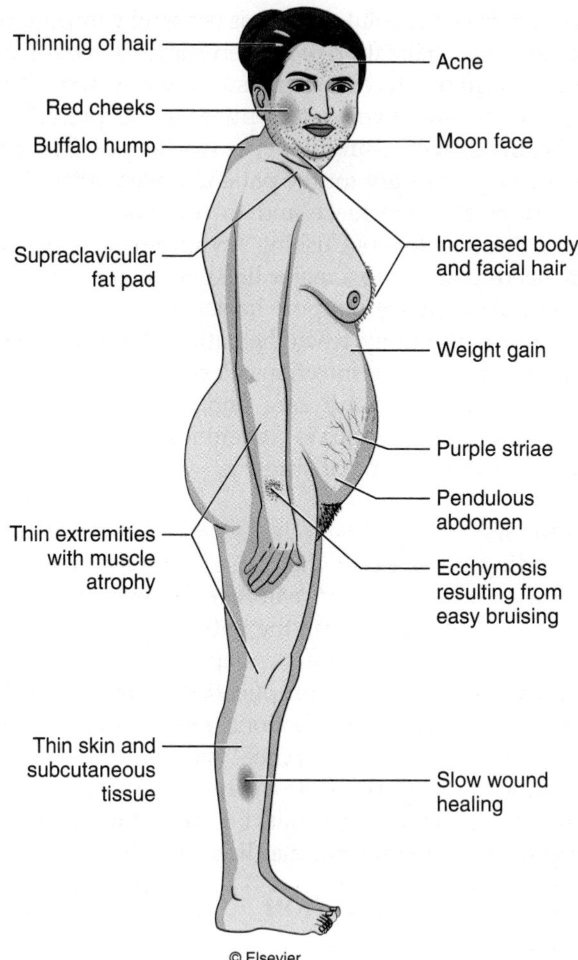

Fig. 51.8 Common characteristics of Cushing's syndrome.

Weight gain, the most common feature, results from accumulation of adipose tissue in the trunk, face, and cervical spine area (Fig. 51.8). The arms and legs become thin as a result of muscle wasting. **Hypokalemia** (low potassium) is usually present. Hyperglycemia occurs because of glucose intolerance (associated with cortisol-induced insulin resistance) and increased glucose release by the liver. The patient usually has protein in the urine and increased urinary calcium excretion, which may lead to the development of renal calculi. Osteoporosis results from abnormal calcium absorption, and kyphosis (excessive curvature of the thoracic vertebra, or hunchback) may develop. The patient is susceptible to infections, but the symptoms may be masked and the infection not detected until it is life threatening.

Assessment

Collection of subjective data includes assessment of the patient's ability to concentrate. The patient may have mood disturbances such as irritability, anxiety, euphoria, insomnia, irrationality, and occasionally psychosis. Depression is common, and the possibility of suicide is an ever-present concern. Depression is also apparent in patients with other endocrine disorders such as diabetes and hypothyroidism. When assessing the endocrine system, include an assessment of psychological demeanor. Be alert to subtle changes in the patient's affect, and take precautions to prevent the patient from inflicting self-harm. Patients of both sexes may experience loss of libido and alterations in self-esteem with concerns about sexual dysfunction. Encourage the patient to verbalize concerns about altered body image. Severe backache is often present and may signal a compression fracture of a vertebral body. Assess the severity of back pain and nursing measures that contribute to the patient's comfort. Appetite usually increases. Ensure that the patient understands the dietary restrictions (low sodium, controlled calories and carbohydrates with increased potassium) and the importance of medical follow-up.

Collection of objective data includes observation of the skin for ecchymoses and petechiae. The skin becomes thin and fragile, and wound healing is delayed. The patient may have weight gain and abdominal enlargement, with development of *striae* (a streak or linear scar that often results from stretching of the skin); this increased girth may contribute to difficulty with mobility. Monitor the patient's weight, because peripheral edema and associated hypertension are common. Impaired carbohydrate metabolism results in hyperglycemia. Women may experience **hirsutism** (excessive body hair in a masculine distribution), menstrual irregularities, and deepening of the voice. Elevated body temperature may indicate an undetected infection.

Diagnostic Tests

Diagnosis usually is based on the patient's clinical appearance and laboratory test results. Plasma cortisol levels usually are elevated. Plasma ACTH levels may be increased or decreased, depending on the location of the tumor. Skull radiographic evaluation may detect erosion of the sella turcica in the presence of a pituitary tumor. Adrenal angiography aids in diagnosing an adrenal tumor. A 24-hour urine test for 17-ketosteroids and 17-hydroxysteroids shows increased levels. Blood glucose determination for hyperglycemia and urinalysis for glycosuria are other diagnostic tests associated with but not diagnostic of Cushing's syndrome. An abdominal CT scan, MRI, and ultrasound may help localize an abdominal tumor.

Medical Management

Treatment is directed toward the causative factor. If an adrenal tumor is present, adrenalectomy usually is indicated for its removal. Pituitary tumors may be irradiated or removed surgically by transsphenoidal microsurgery. If the patient is unable to undergo surgery because of inoperable cancer elsewhere in the body or another preexisting condition, mitotane (Lysodren) therapy may be used. Mitotane alters the metabolism of cortisol in the periphery (in this case "peripheral metabolism" means elsewhere than in the adrenal gland), decreases the plasma corticosteroid level, and suppresses cortisol production—essentially providing a "medical adrenalectomy." This cytotoxic agent damages the adrenal glands and is given for at least 3 months, during which time the patient must be monitored for symptoms of hepatotoxicity, such as jaundice, gastrointestinal upset, and pruritus. The diet should be low in sodium to help decrease edema. Reduced calories and carbohydrates help control hyperglycemia, and foods high in potassium help correct hypokalemia. If Cushing's syndrome has developed during the course of prolonged administration of corticosteroids (e.g., prednisone), one or more of the following alternatives may be tried: (1) gradually discontinuing corticosteroid therapy, (2) reducing the corticosteroid dosage, or (3) converting to an alternate-day regimen. Gradually tapering the corticosteroid is necessary to avoid potentially life-threatening adrenal insufficiency.

Nursing Interventions and Patient Teaching

Important nursing interventions include gentle handling to prevent skin impairment or excessive ecchymosis and frequent assessment for erythema, edema, or early signs of infection. Encourage the patient to turn frequently and ambulate as tolerated to eliminate undue pressure on bony prominences. Elbow and heel protectors and a pressure-reducing mattress or pad may help prevent decubitus ulcers in the bedridden patient. Encourage the patient to participate as fully as possible in typical ADLs, interspersing personal hygiene tasks with rest periods to prevent overtiring.

Patient problems and interventions for the patient with Cushing's syndrome include but are not limited to the following:

Patient Problem	Nursing Interventions
Insufficient Knowledge, related to therapeutic regimen	Assess patient's understanding of prescribed medication and diet Encourage patient to wear a medical alert bracelet or necklace, and to carry a wallet identification card
Inability to Tolerate Activity, related to weakness and immobility	Assess patient's current activity tolerance, and identify priorities for energy expenditures Plan activity and rest periods with patient
Potential for Infection, related to: • Suppression of immune system • Lowered resistance to stress	Monitor patient for complaints of pain, purulent exudates, or decrease in function because the usual signs and symptoms of inflammation, such as fever and erythema, may not be present (Lewis et al, 2011) Practice meticulous handwashing before caring for patient

The patient's mental attitude is extremely important. Encourage verbalization of concerns and watch for the development of depression and suicidal thoughts. Help the patient understand the purpose of prescribed medications, such as mitotane, as well as possible side effects. It is important for the patient to wear a medical-alert bracelet or necklace and to carry a wallet card stating the diagnosis of Cushing's syndrome. The patient may need to adjust to a major lifestyle change, and the aid of a community support liaison may be enlisted. Before adrenalectomy, teach the patient the importance of avoiding stress and infections. Postoperative teaching includes proper wound care and the symptoms of Addison's disease, which is sometimes an unavoidable sequela after this type of surgery.

Prognosis

Depending on whether the cause of the disease was benign or malignant and whether the treatment was successful or unsuccessful, the patient with Cushing's syndrome can expect to have major lifestyle changes, possibly with many complications (osteoporosis, hypertension, frequent infections, loss of muscle mass and strength, and interference with other hormone levels). Life expectancy for a patient with Cushing's syndrome is shortened, in part because of the multiple complications noted with the disease.

ADRENAL HYPOFUNCTION (ADDISON'S DISEASE)

Etiology and Pathophysiology

Adrenocortical insufficiency occurs when the adrenal glands do not secrete adequate amounts of glucocorticoids, mineralocorticoids, and androgens. It initially may be seen as Addison's disease, a rare primary condition; or it may result from adrenalectomy, pituitary hypofunction, or longstanding steroid therapy. The most common cause of Addison's disease is an autoimmune response: adrenal tissue is destroyed by antibodies against the patient's own adrenal cortex. Addison's disease can result from idiopathic adrenal atrophy or cancer of the adrenal cortex. Tuberculosis causes Addison's disease worldwide, and tuberculosis is on the rise. Other causes include infarction, fungal infections (e.g., histoplasmosis), acquired immunodeficiency syndrome, and metastatic cancer. Deficiencies in aldosterone and cortisol produce disturbances of the metabolism of carbohydrates, fats, and proteins, as well as sodium, potassium, and water. This results in electrolyte and fluid imbalance, dehydration, water loss, and hypovolemia (decreased plasma volume). Adrenal insufficiency most often occurs in adults younger than 60 years of age and affects both genders equally.

Clinical Manifestations

Because manifestations are usually not evident until 90% of the adrenal cortex is destroyed, the disease often is advanced before it is diagnosed. Clinical manifestations are related directly to imbalances in adrenal hormones, nutrients, and electrolytes.

Assessment

Subjective data include progressive weakness, fatigue, nausea, anorexia, and craving for salt. Orthostatic hypotension (or postural hypotension; a sudden drop in blood pressure provoked by standing up) may be associated with vertigo, weakness, and syncope, resulting in reluctance to attempt normal activities. The patient may complain of severe headache, disorientation, abdominal pain, or general joint and muscle pain, which could represent early symptoms of addisonian crisis (see below). This patient tolerates stress poorly and feels anxious and apprehensive. It is important to assess emotional status and allow the patient to share feelings about his or her altered self-image. Also assess the patient's overall understanding of the disease process and the importance of medical treatment and follow-up.

Collection of objective data includes observation of changes in the color of the mucous membranes and the skin. Skin hyperpigmentation, a common feature, is seen primarily in sun-exposed areas of the body; at pressure points; over joints; and in creases, especially in palmar creases. The patient usually loses weight, often with vomiting and diarrhea. Hypoglycemia may contribute to fatigue; assess the patient's ability to perform ADLs. An abnormally low or abnormally high body temperature, orthostatic hypotension, hyponatremia, and hyperkalemia are signs of impending *addisonian crisis,* a life-threatening emergency caused by insufficient adrenocortical hormones or a sudden sharp decrease in these hormones. Precipitating factors that can trigger an addisonian crisis are stress-producing situations such as infections, surgery, trauma, hemorrhage, psychological stress, sudden withdrawal of corticosteroid hormone replacement therapy, after adrenal surgery, or sudden pituitary gland destruction (Mayo Clinic, 2012b). See Table 51.3 for a comparison of Cushing's syndrome and Addison's disease.

Diagnostic Tests

Laboratory studies show decreased serum sodium, increased serum potassium, and decreased serum glucose (Mayo Clinic, 2012b). Serum levels of cortisol, ACTH, and antibodies also are monitored. Fasting plasma cortisol levels and aldosterone levels are low with an ACTH stimulation test. The ACTH simulation test involves obtaining cortisol levels before and after injections of synthetic ACTH. A glucose tolerance test may yield abnormal results. Insulin and cortisol levels also are measured before and after the injection of insulin to monitor for increases and decreases. A CT and MRI of the abdomen may be indicated to assess the status of the adrenal glands. A CT scan and MRI of the pituitary gland also indicate the cause of the disease.

Medical Management

Medical treatment involves the prompt restoration of fluid and electrolyte balance and replacement of the deficient adrenal hormones. The most common form of replacement therapy is hydrocortisone, which has mineralocorticoid and glucocorticoid properties. Glucocorticoid dosage must be increased during times of physiologic stress to prevent addisonian crisis. Fludrocortisone (Florinef) (a mineralocorticoid) also is administered. The diet should be high in sodium and low in potassium.

Treatment for the life-threatening emergency of an addisonian crisis includes management of shock, high-dose hydrocortisone replacement therapy, and large volumes of 0.9% saline and 5% dextrose solutions to improve electrolyte imbalances and reverse hypotension.

Table 51.3 Nursing Assessment of Patients With Cushing's Syndrome or Addison's Disease

AREA OF ASSESSMENT	CLINICAL MANIFESTATIONS IN CUSHING'S SYNDROME	CLINICAL MANIFESTATIONS IN ADDISON'S DISEASE
Cardiovascular	Mild to moderate hypertension	Postural hypotension, vertigo, syncope
Neurologic	Impaired memory and concentration, insomnia, irritability	Lethargy, headache
Musculoskeletal	Muscle weakness, muscle wasting in extremities, back and rib pain, kyphosis	Muscle weakness, fatigue, muscle aches, muscle wasting
Integumentary	Thin skin, red cheeks, acne, frequent petechiae and ecchymoses, increased body and facial hair, poor wound healing	Hyperpigmentation, decreased body hair
Self-care and self-concept	Tires easily; insomnia, malaise, negative feelings regarding changes in body	Tires easily; profound weakness, lack of interest in usual activities and relationships
Nutrition and fluid balance	Increased appetite, moderate weight gain, edema, buffalo hump, moon face, obesity of trunk, hyperglycemia; need for decreased salt intake, reduced calories and carbohydrate intake, increased potassium intake	Nausea and vomiting, fluid and electrolyte imbalance, dehydration, weight loss, hypoglycemia; need for increased salt and decreased potassium intake

Nursing Interventions and Patient Teaching

Carefully assess the patient's circulatory status, keep accurate I&O records, and record daily weight. Check skin turgor and offer fluids frequently. Monitor vital signs at regular intervals, paying attention to temperature and blood pressure. Also monitor the patient for response to prescribed steroid drugs, and promptly report any adverse effects to the health care provider. Keep the environment as free from stress as possible. Visitors and hospital personnel should be screened for infectious disease and excluded from the patient's room. Protect the patient from injury and advise the patient to rise slowly from a sitting or lying position if orthostatic hypotension is a concern. Continually assess the patient for signs of developing adrenal (addisonian) crisis, manifested by a sudden, severe drop in blood pressure; nausea and vomiting; an extremely high temperature; and cyanosis, progressing to vasomotor collapse and possibly death. The patient should carry an emergency kit at all times with 100 mg of IM hydrocortisone, syringes, and instructions for use (Mayo Clinic, 2012b). Teach the patient and significant others to give an IM injection in case replacement therapy cannot be taken orally. Also advise the patient to consult with the health care provider to adjust (increase) medication doses during periods of physical or emotional stress. Patient education is imperative for long-term compliance in the management of Addison's disease.

Patient problems and interventions for the patient with Addison's disease include but are not limited to the following:

Patient Problem	Nursing Interventions
Potential for Infection, related to altered metabolic processes	Assess environment for stressors Screen visitors and personnel for contagious disease Monitor temperature routinely Stress the importance of taking prescribed medications
Potential for Injury, related to decrease in blood pressure on rising	Monitor vital signs (blood pressure and pulse) and for dizziness when rising Assist patient when rising, using a gait belt to prevent falls

Before discharge from the hospital, teach the patient the importance of adhering to the prescribed drug therapy; having regular medical checkups; and immediately reporting all illnesses, even a cold, to the health care provider. Emphasize that stress is one of the major precipitating factors in addisonian crisis, and encourage the patient to minimize stress through cognitive behavior therapy, relaxation therapy, biofeedback, and mental imagery. Other conditions to avoid include overexertion, diarrhea, infection, decreased intake of salt, exposure to cold, and surgery. The patient must wear a medical alert bracelet and carry a wallet card stating that the patient has Addison's disease so that appropriate therapy can be initiated in case of trauma, accident, or crisis.

Prognosis

With long-term steroid therapy, adequate medical care, and follow-up, this patient has a fair prognosis.

PHEOCHROMOCYTOMA

Etiology and Pathophysiology

A *pheochromocytoma* is a rare tumor of the adrenal medulla that causes excessive secretion of a catecholamine (epinephrine and/or norepinephrine). These tumors occur most often in adults between 20 and 60 years of age and are almost always benign; only about 10% are malignant. The secretion of excessive catecholamine results in severe hypertension.

Clinical Manifestations

Pheochromocytoma results in severe hypertension because of sympathetic nervous system stimulation. Other classic clinical signs and symptoms include anxiety, severe headache, diaphoresis, tachycardia, feelings of extreme fright, and unexplained abdominal pain (Mayo Clinic, 2011b). Hypertensive crisis may occur, during which the blood pressure may fluctuate widely, sometimes as high as 300/175 mm Hg. Signs and symptoms may be triggered by an identifiable factor, such as overexertion or emotional trauma, or they may occur for no apparent reason. Extreme hypertension may result in stroke, kidney damage, and retinopathy. Cardiac damage may occur, resulting in heart failure.

Assessment

Subjective data during a hypertensive crisis include severe headache and palpitations. The patient may feel nervous, dizzy, and dyspneic and may experience paresthesia, nausea, and intolerance to heat. Anxiety is common, and the patient may have trouble sleeping. Question the patient about the occurrence of symptoms in relation to identifiable factors, such as excess stress or overexertion, and identify the coping methods used.

Collection of objective data includes frequent measurement of blood pressure and respiratory rate for increases and of pulse for tachycardia. The patient may have tremors, diaphoresis, dilated pupils, glycosuria, and hyperglycemia. Assess responses to prescribed medications.

Diagnostic Tests

The measurement of urinary metanephrines (catecholamine metabolites), usually performed as a 24-hour urine collection, is the simplest and most reliable test. Values are elevated in at least 90% of those with pheochromocytoma. Vanillylmandelic acid (VMA) also may be measured in a 24-hour urine sample. However, this test has more false negatives than that for urine metanephrines. Plasma catecholamines also are elevated. It is preferable to measure serum catecholamines during an "attack." A CT scan and MRI of the adrenal glands may help in locating the tumor.

Medical Management

Treatment is usually the surgical removal of the tumor. Surgery is more common via laparoscopic adrenalectomy than open abdominal incision. Preoperatively, the patient may be given calcium channel blockers such as nicardipine (Cardene) or alpha-adrenergic blocking agents such as phentolamine mesylate or phenoxybenzamine hydrochloride (Dibenzyline) in an effort to control hypertension. Beta blockers (e.g., propranolol [Inderal]) to decrease tachycardia and other dysrhythmias also are used (Mayo Clinic, 2011b). Metyrosine (Demser) may be given to help inhibit catecholamine production, and the drug must be continued on a long-term basis if the tumor is inoperable.

Nursing Interventions and Patient Teaching

Postoperative care is carried out in the same manner as for any major abdominal surgery, with the following special concerns. If the patient has undergone adrenalectomy, large amounts of hydrocortisone will be given. Watch carefully for fluctuations in blood pressure caused by adrenal manipulation during surgery, with subsequent release of epinephrine and norepinephrine. These fluctuations may be severe and life threatening if cardiovascular collapse occurs. The patient should avoid excess stress and must be allowed adequate time to rest; give sedatives to ensure this. Keep a careful I&O record and monitor IV infusions carefully. Vasopressors and corticosteroids may be given. The diet should be free from stimulants, such as coffee, tea, and soft drinks containing caffeine.

Patient problems and interventions for the patient with pheochromocytoma include but are not limited to the following:

Patient Problem	Nursing Interventions
Compromised Blood Flow to Tissue (Cardiopulmonary, Renal), related to hypertension	Monitor blood pressure and pulse and record I&O Eliminate smoking and caffeine-containing beverages
Inability to Tolerate Activity, related to hypertension	Assist with gradual position changes from lying to sitting or standing Limit activity, as needed, to prevent increased hypertension

Follow-up 24-hour urine tests (for catecholamine metabolites or VMA) may determine when the levels have returned to normal. The patient then is considered cured and may resume normal activities. If the tumor is inoperable, the patient remains under lifelong medical supervision. Stress the importance of compliance with prescribed treatment. The patient should wear medical-alert identification and carry a wallet card. Teach the patient self-monitoring of blood pressure and when to call the health care provider if elevation occurs.

Prognosis

If undiagnosed and untreated, pheochromocytoma may lead to diabetes mellitus, cardiomyopathy, and death. The prognosis after successful removal of the causative tumor is good; for an inoperable tumor, the prognosis depends on adequate medical management of hypertension.

DISORDERS OF THE PANCREAS

DIABETES MELLITUS

Diabetes mellitus (DM) is a systemic metabolic disorder that involves improper metabolism of carbohydrates, fats, and proteins. It is centered on the body's use of insulin, a protein that allows the body's cells to absorb glucose from the bloodstream. DM is a chronic multisystem disease related to a decrease or absolute lack of insulin production by the beta cells of the islets of Langerhans in the pancreas or by impaired insulin use, or both. In patients who do not have DM, the beta cells are stimulated by increased blood glucose levels. Insulin secretion reaches peak levels about 30 minutes after meals and returns to normal in 2 to 3 hours. Between meals or during a period of fasting, insulin levels remain low, and the body uses its supply of stored glucose and amino acids to provide energy for the tissues. The beta cells of the pancreas continuously release insulin into the bloodstream in small amounts. A larger quantity (i.e., a *bolus*) of insulin is released after the intake of food. The average amount of insulin secreted by the beta cells of the pancreas in an adult is 40 to 50 units every 24 hours. The release of insulin in this systematic manner results in the body maintaining a normal blood glucose level between 70 and 100 mg/dL. In patients with DM, the body's insulin supply is either absent or deficient, or target cells resist the action of insulin. There are several types of DM, but in each type, hyperglycemia is the principal clinical manifestation.

There are two main types of DM: *type 1* and *type 2*. Type 1 formerly was called juvenile diabetes, juvenile-onset diabetes, or insulin-dependent DM. Type 2 formerly was called adult-onset diabetes, maturity-onset diabetes, or non–insulin-dependent DM. Because type 2 DM is becoming more common in children, and because some people with type 2 DM use insulin, these terms are no longer appropriate. Other patients with DM have conditions such as pancreatitis, genetic syndromes, malnutrition, chemical- or drug-induced disease, and pregnancy. Type 1 and type 2 DM have some distinct differences (Table 51.4). In type 1 an autoimmune disease (probably stimulated by a virus) eventually results in destruction of beta cells in the pancreatic islets and results in deficient insulin *production;* the patient retains normal sensitivity to insulin action. Within 5 years of diagnosis, all of the patient's beta cells have been destroyed and no insulin is produced. In type 2 DM the main problem is an abnormal resistance to insulin *action*.

Table 51.4 Comparison of Type 1 and Type 2 Diabetes Mellitus

FACTOR	TYPE 1	TYPE 2
Age at onset	Usually 30 yr or younger but can occur at any age	Usually age 35 yr or older but can occur at any age Incidence is increasing in children
Body weight	Normal or underweight	80% are overweight
Symptoms at onset	Sudden; polyphagia, polydipsia, polyuria, weight loss, weakness, fatigue; glycosuria, hyperglycemia; acidosis, progressing to DKA	Gradual; may be asymptomatic at onset; later, may develop signs and symptoms of type 1 DM; others include slow wound healing, blurred vision, pruritus, boils or other skin infections; vaginal infections in women
Treatment	Diet, exercise, and insulin; may add subcutaneous insulin-enhancing drug (pramlintide [Symlin])	Diet and exercise; or diet, exercise, and oral hypoglycemic agents; or diet, exercise, oral hypoglycemic agents, and insulin during times of illness or stress; may add a subcutaneous insulin-enhancing agent such as exenatide (Byetta) or pramlintide
Incidence of complications	Frequent	Frequent
Psychosocial and sexual concerns	Irritability; disturbed body image; mood swings, depression; menstrual irregularities; decreased libido	Disturbed body image; amenorrhea; decreased libido; poor tolerance to stress

DKA, Diabetic ketoacidosis.

Regardless of the type of DM, all of these patients have impaired glucose tolerance. Only 5% to 10% of all people with DM have type 1. About 90% of people with DM in the United States have type 2, with a high incidence among African Americans, Hispanic Americans, and Native Americans, especially members of the Pima tribe. The American Diabetes Association (ADA) estimates that as many as 20.8 million Americans (7% of the population) have DM, and 41 million more people have prediabetes.

CAUSES AND COMPLICATIONS OF DIABETES MELLITUS

The exact cause of both types of DM is unknown. A number of factors contribute to its development: genetic predisposition, viruses (such as coxsackievirus B, rubella, and mumps), the aging process, diet and lifestyle, and ethnicity. Obesity is believed to be a major factor. The T lymphocytes may play a role in the autoimmune destruction of pancreatic insulin-producing cells.

Complications of DM are as follows: blindness (retinopathy); renal failure (nephropathy); amputation of a lower extremity because of infection and decreased circulation; and cardiovascular complications including heart disease, hypertension, and stroke. Neuropathy is a common complication found in patients with DM and includes painful feet and fingers, loss of sensation, and risk of injury because of loss of sensation (falls, burns, tissue infection). The patient with elevated serum glucose is at risk for infection (1) because the increased amount of glucose is a food source for pathogens, and (2) because of circulatory and neurovascular complications. The patient should be taught that complications from DM can be decreased significantly by properly maintaining the blood glucose level (60 to 99 mg/dL) and the hemoglobin A_{1c} (HbA_{1c}) level (less than 5% to 6%).

TYPE 1 DIABETES MELLITUS

Etiology

Type 1 DM results from progressive destruction of beta cell function in the pancreas as a result of an autoimmune process in a susceptible individual. The pancreatic islets of Langerhans cell antibodies and insulin autoantibodies cause an 80% to 90% reduction in beta cells before hyperglycemia and symptoms occur. Type 1 DM is characterized by autoimmune beta cell destruction, which is attributed to a genetic predisposition. Genetics plus infection with one or more viral agents and possibly chemical agents are believed to cause type 1 DM. It is not known whether these are the only factors involved.

The onset and progression of hyperglycemic signs and symptoms are usually more rapid and acute in type 1 DM than in type 2. Type 1 DM may occur at any age, but signs and symptoms usually appear before 30 years of age. The patient is usually thin. The patient is often hyperglycemic, with urine that is strongly positive for ketones (signs that fat is being used for energy instead of glucose because of a shortage of insulin), and depends on insulin therapy to prevent ketoacidosis (an abnormal buildup of acidic ketones in the blood) and to sustain life. Because they do not produce adequate amounts of endogenous insulin (i.e., insulin produced by the body), patients with type 1 DM must take regular injections of exogenous insulin (i.e., synthetic insulin) or they will die. Typically, a patient with type 1 DM is healthy with the exception of the lack of insulin produced by the pancreas. In comparison, a patient with type 2 DM often has a history of hypertension, obesity, dyslipidemia, hypercholesterolemia, and cardiovascular risk (myocardial infarction, stroke) before DM is diagnosed.

In prediabetes, *insulin resistance*—the lessening response of the body to the production of insulin by the pancreas—often occurs. In the patient with insulin resistance, the serum glucose level may be normal, but the pancreas is working overtime to maintain that normal level. Excessive amounts of insulin are secreted by the pancreas to get a little bit of glucose control. The patient with insulin resistance should have the insulin level monitored in addition to the serum glucose level. The patient is treated with oral hyperglycemic agents and instructed to lose weight (if obese); dietary management is similar to that of the patient with DM. The goal in insulin resistance is to maintain normal insulin and glucose levels and to avoid the onset of DM. This is accomplished by diet, exercise, and medications if needed.

In type 1 DM there is no insulin resistance; there is an absence of insulin production. It is diagnosed when the patient's pancreas does not produce insulin. Insulin then must be obtained through exogenous sources and administered mainly via the subcutaneous route (via insulin pump or injections). In serious situations, short-acting regular insulin can be administered via the intravenous (IV) route. People with type 1 DM are often healthy with the exception of the lack of insulin production. Although patients with type 1 DM are at risk for the typical complications of poor glucose control, they often do not have the history of high cholesterol, obesity, and high blood pressure that is noted with type 2 DM. Goals for treatment are to maintain a normal blood glucose level (60 to 99 mg/dL) via insulin administration, diet, and exercise. Clinical manifestations include the three *polys:* polydipsia (abnormal thirst partially because of the high glucose content of the blood and the kidney's attempt to dilute it), polyuria (frequent urination in response to the kidney's need to dilute and increase fluid intake), and **polyphagia** (increased food intake). Despite the increased consumption of food, the patient with type 1 DM typically loses weight because the body burns fat and protein instead of glucose for energy. Although there is plenty of glucose in the bloodstream, the body is unable to use it because there is no insulin available to move it into the cells. However, when the patient exercises, the muscles use glucose even if insulin is not available, which is why exercise is so important for maintaining the glucose level.

Pathophysiology

In normal metabolism the end products of digestion (glucose, fatty acids and glycerol, and amino acids) are absorbed into the venous circulation and carried to the liver, where they may be used immediately or stored for later use. The liver can change glycerol and fatty acids into glucose, and glucose into triglycerides, as needed. When glucose is not available as fuel or cannot be used, the liver changes fatty acids into **ketone bodies**. There are three types of ketones: beta-hydroxybutyric acid, acetoacetic acid, and acetone. The ketones serve as fuel for the muscles and as an energy source for the brain. Free glucose in the bloodstream always can be used by the brain and kidney, because these tissues do not need insulin to move glucose molecules into brain cells or glomeruli.

Glucose also is stored in the form of glycogen in the liver. Glycogen can be changed back into glucose as needed by the body for energy. In the patient with DM, lack of proper amounts of insulin or its poor utilization impairs the use of glucose by the body. The excess glucose accumulates in the bloodstream, and **hyperglycemia** (greater than normal amounts of glucose in the blood) results.

To rid the body of this abnormal amount of glucose, the kidneys excrete it in the urine. This is called **glycosuria** (abnormal presence of a sugar, especially glucose, in the urine), a condition that necessitates an extra amount of water for proper dilution of the urine. The patient thus develops polyuria and also polydipsia. Often the patient is unable to drink enough fluid to compensate for polyuria and may become dehydrated.

Even though abundant glucose is available in the bloodstream, the body tissues cannot use it without the help of insulin. Thus the cells are not nourished properly, and *polyphagia* (increased hunger and consumption of food) develops. Despite increased intake, the body is unable to metabolize the food, and the patient loses weight. Because carbohydrates cannot be used properly, proteins and fats are broken down and ketone bodies are used excessively for heat and energy. Ketone bodies are acid substances, so the patient may develop acidosis. *Diabetic* **ketoacidosis** (DKA) (acidosis accompanied by an accumulation of ketones in the blood), formerly called *diabetic coma,* may develop and the patient could die. DKA is a severe metabolic disturbance caused by an acute insulin deficiency, decreased peripheral glucose use, increased fat mobilization, and ketogenesis.

Clinical Manifestations

The hallmark symptoms of type 1 DM include the three classic *polys*: polyuria, polydipsia, and polyphagia. As ketone bodies accumulate in the bloodstream, imbalances of sodium, potassium, and bicarbonate result.

Assessment

Subjective data include hunger, thirst, and nausea. In addition to frequent, copious urination, the patient may complain of nocturia, weakness, and fatigue. The patient may have blurred vision, the appearance of halos around lights, and headache. Symptoms such as cold extremities, cramping pain in the calves and feet during exercise or walking, decreased sensation to pain and temperature in the feet, and numbness and tingling of the lower extremities may occur. Symptoms of delayed stomach emptying such as nausea, vomiting, and early satiety (feeling of being full after eating) may develop. Male patients may become impotent. The patient may verbalize negative feelings about his or her body and the ability to cope with the illness. Assess coping methods and knowledge about the disease process. Misunderstandings and lack of interest may result in inadequate skills—such as diet planning, injections, and exercise programs—to manage the necessary diabetic lifestyle. Assess the patient's understanding of the importance of adhering to prescribed medical treatment and obtaining adequate follow-up.

Collection of objective data includes assessment of the skin, because slow wound healing, furuncles, carbuncles, and ulcerations are common. Women with DM may have frequent urinary tract and vaginal infections, and vaginal discharge is often bothersome. In patients with type 1 DM, weight loss and muscle wasting may be seen. The skin on the lower extremities may appear shiny and thin, with less hair present. The legs and feet may feel cold to the touch, and there may be ulcerated areas. Gangrene of the toes is a dreaded sign. Assess the patient's ability to perform blood glucose testing and proper injection of insulin.

Diagnostic Tests

Diagnosis of DM is made based on clinical manifestations plus the patient's history and laboratory findings. The patient with a random blood glucose level greater than 200 mg/dL, a fasting plasma glucose level greater than 126 mg/dL, or a glucose 2-hour post-load level greater than 200 mg/dL should be evaluated further. Blood tests commonly performed include those listed in Box 51.2. Measurement of the patient's glycosylated hemoglobin (HbA_{1c}) permits the health care provider to see an average of glucose levels over the past 120 days. The average life span of a red blood cell is approximately 120 days. When the amount of glucose attached to the red blood cells is measured, the results indicate an average glucose level for the past 120 days (3 months). HbA_{1c} is ideal for monitoring long-term compliance and regulating the blood glucose level. This benefits patient education and management because a one-time measurement of the blood glucose level shows only that day's management and may not reflect past glucose production.

The ADA recommends self-monitoring of blood glucose (SMBG) instead of urine testing in any patient with DM. Blood from a finger-stick is placed on a reagent strip, and a result is available for the patient in less than a minute. SMBG is the monitoring tool of choice because it provides an accurate picture of current blood glucose levels (Fig. 51.9).

The frequency of monitoring depends on the glycemic goals the patient and health care provider set and the intensity of the treatment regimen. The patient receiving two or more injections of insulin per day may want to test before meals and at bedtime every day. If glycemic control is relatively stable, the patient may elect to test

Box 51.2 Diagnostic Test for Diabetes Mellitus

- *Fasting blood glucose (FBG):* After an 8-hour fast, blood is drawn. Normal is 60 to 100 mg/dL of venous blood; 126 mg/dL or greater is considered abnormal.
- *Oral glucose tolerance test (OGTT):* A blood sample is taken, and then, after the patient drinks fluid containing a known amount of glucose, the blood is sampled periodically for the next 3 hours. An OGTT is usually not necessary for patients showing overt signs and symptoms of hyperglycemia, polyuria, polydipsia, and polyphagia, together with FBG levels of 126 mg/dL or greater. However, whenever an OGTT is performed, the accuracy depends on adequate patient preparation and attention to the many factors that may influence the outcome of the test.
- *Serum insulin:* Insulin is absent in type 1 diabetes mellitus (DM); normal to high in type 2 DM.
- *Postprandial (after a meal) blood glucose (PPBG):* Give a fasting patient a measured amount of carbohydrate solution orally, or have the patient eat a measured amount of foods containing carbohydrates, fats, and proteins. Draw a blood sample 2 hours after completion of the meal. Elevated plasma glucose (more than 160 mg/dL) may indicate the presence of DM.
- *Patient self-monitoring of blood glucose (SMBG):* A blood sample is obtained by the finger-stick method, by either the patient or the nurse, and tested with a blood glucose–monitoring device.
- *Glycosylated hemoglobin (HbA_{1c}):* This blood test measures the amount of glucose that has become incorporated into the hemoglobin within an erythrocyte; these levels are reported as a percentage of the total hemoglobin. Because glycosylation occurs constantly during the 120-day lifespan of the erythrocyte, this test reveals the effectiveness of diabetes therapy for the preceding 8 to 12 weeks. Glycosylated hemoglobin levels remain more stable than plasma glucose levels and are evaluated by venipuncture every 6 to 8 weeks. Normal HbA_{1c} is approximately 4% to 6% of the total. There is an urgent need to reduce HbA_{1c} values to below 7% to reduce complications. A result greater than 8% represents an average blood glucose level of approximately 200 mg/dL and signals a need for changes in treatment.
- *C-peptide test:* The production of insulin by beta cells of the pancreas begins with proinsulin, which consists of an A chain and a B chain connected by an amino acid chain called the C-peptide. The C-peptide is removed, allowing the A and B chains to fold and cleave together, creating the structure of insulin. The C-peptide remnant then is secreted into the bloodstream by the pancreas along with insulin. A patient's C-peptide level indicates whether any insulin is being produced. A newly diagnosed patient with DM often uses this test to determine whether he or she has type 1 or type 2 DM. Normal values are 0.5 to 2 ng/mL. The patient with type 1 diabetes is unable to produce insulin and therefore has decreased levels of C-peptide; C-peptide levels in patients with type 2 DM are normal or higher than normal.

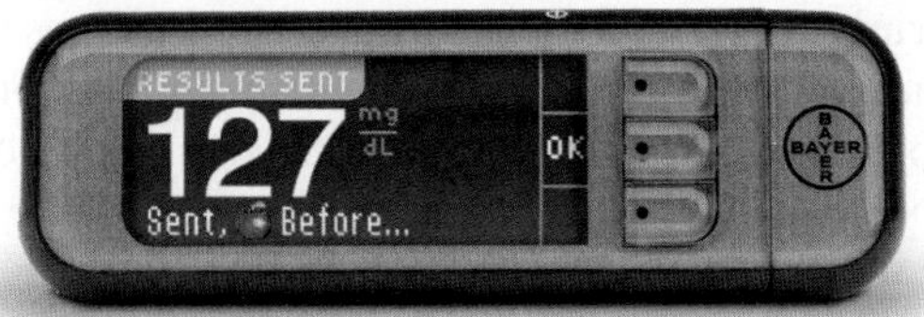

Fig. 51.9 Glucose sensor for self-monitoring of blood glucose. CONTOUR NEXT LINK blood glucose meter from Bayer sends results wirelessly to the insulin pump. (Copyright Bayer HealthCare Medical Care, Whippany, New Jersey.)

two or more times a day on certain days of the week. Testing usually takes place before meals, but it can occur any time the patient needs to know the way a factor, such as stress, is affecting the blood glucose level. How often SMBG results are recorded to guide therapy decisions should be determined jointly by the health care provider and the patient.

The technology used for SMBG changes rapidly, with newer and more convenient systems being introduced every year. Blood glucose monitoring based on noninvasive spectroscopy—in which a laser light is shone on the skin of the forearm or between finger and thumb—is being researched. Implantable sensors for continuous glucose monitoring also are being tested.

Urine testing for ketonuria is a valuable aid in determining the advent of DKA and is recommended for every patient with type 1 DM when the patient is experiencing hyperglycemia or acute illness.

Medical Management

Medical treatment for DM, regardless of type, consists of education, monitoring, meal planning, and exercise. Pharmacologic therapies also may be required to maintain a healthy serum glucose level. The overall goal is to assist people with DM to make changes in nutrition and exercise habits that lead to improved metabolic control. Additional goals include the following:

- Maintaining as near-normal blood glucose levels as possible by balancing food intake with insulin or oral glucose-lowering medications and activity levels. By maintaining near normal glucose levels (60 to 99 mg/dL), the patient greatly reduces the risk of complications.
- Losing weight, especially in the case of a patient with type 2 DM who is overweight.
- Achieving optimal serum lipid levels.
- Consuming adequate calories for maintaining or attaining reasonable weight. Reasonable weight is defined as the weight the patient and health care provider decide is achievable and maintainable in the short term and the long term. This may not be the same as the usually defined desirable or ideal body weight. Adequate nutrition also means maintaining normal growth and development rates for children and adolescents and meeting increased metabolic needs during pregnancy, lactation, and recovery from illnesses.
- Preventing and treating acute complications such as hypoglycemia and long-term complications such as renal disease, neuropathy, hypertension, and cardiovascular disease.
- Improving overall health through optimal nutrition. The US Department of Agriculture's MyPlate food planning tool summarizes nutritional guidelines and nutrient needs for all healthy Americans and can be used by the patient with DM.

Diet. Nutritional therapy for the patient with DM is aimed at helping to achieve a normal blood glucose level of less than 126 mg/dL, an HbA_{1c} of 4% to 6%, and attaining or maintaining a reasonable body weight, while ensuring proper growth and body maintenance. Nutritional therapy is the cornerstone of care for the person with DM. A nutritionally adequate meal plan ideally should have a reduction in the total amount of fat, especially saturated fat, to lessen the risk of stroke and heart attack. Enlist the services of a dietitian for each newly diagnosed patient with DM. The menu must be individualized, taking into consideration the patient's age, weight, activity level, lifestyle, ethnic background, and food preferences. Assess the patient's ability to select and pay for groceries, prepare food, and properly store leftovers to ensure that he or she can follow dietary instructions after discharge. If the patient is living with family, teach the person who plans and prepares the meals how to accommodate the patient's dietary needs in the family menus. Dietary treatment, also called *medical nutrition therapy for diabetes,* involves individualized meal plans. Diets are based on ADA recommendations, and patients may obtain additional information and menus from that organization at no cost.

Traditional *quantitative* diabetic diets involved following a recommended diet of 45% to 50% of total kilocalories from carbohydrates, 10% to 20% of total kilocalories from proteins, and no more than 30% of total kilocalories from fats. In recent years the rigid rules on carbohydrates have softened. Now the emphasis is on the total amount of carbohydrates consumed, rather than on the type. Once it was believed that a simple carbohydrate (sugar) would drive up blood glucose levels, so patients were advised to consume only complex carbohydrates. This has proven inaccurate, however, because (1) some complex carbohydrates (rice, potatoes, and bread) produce a glycemic response similar to that caused by sucrose (table sugar), and (2) milk and fruit have less effect on blood glucose than most starches. As a result, sugars and complex carbohydrates are counted together as total carbohydrates.

Different carbohydrate foods affect the blood glucose level in different ways; this varying effect is termed the *glycemic index.* Therefore emphasis may be placed not only on the amount of carbohydrate eaten but also on the glycemic index of those foods.

The *qualitative* diabetic diet is unmeasured and more unrestricted, stressing moderation when selecting foods from the MyPlate food planning tool and reducing the use of simple carbohydrates, saturated fats, and alcohol. This diet may be used for the patient whose blood glucose levels are not extremely high, for the pediatric patient, or for the patient who does not adhere to the ADA diet.

Insulin-dependent patients usually have mid-afternoon and bedtime snacks in addition to their regular three meals a day. It is important to distribute food intake evenly throughout the day, taking insulin dosage and exercise into consideration. The patient who plans to engage in strenuous exercise should be advised by the health care provider on dietary changes needed before, during, and after exercise, because exercise increases the absorption rate of insulin, thereby enabling muscles to use glucose more effectively.

Exercise. The patient with DM should exercise regularly under the direction of the primary health care provider. The health care provider helps determine the best type of exercise for each patient. Exercise is beneficial not only because it aids in promoting proper use of glucose but also because it is important to the overall functioning of the cardiovascular system, leads to weight loss, and increases the patient's feeling of well-being. Of all the therapies available for treating type 2 DM, exercise is probably the least expensive and most cost effective. Exercise can reduce insulin resistance and increase glucose uptake for as long as 72 hours; it also reduces blood pressure and lipid levels. However, it can carry some risks, including hypoglycemia. Patients should have a complete physical examination before beginning a rigorous exercise program. Like medication, exercise can be adjusted to improve blood glucose control. With exercise, motivation is more important than facts and information. General guidelines are available, and the patient should be encouraged to discuss specific plans with the health care provider. If the patient's glucose is less than 100 mg/dL, a carbohydrate snack is necessary before beginning to exercise. If the glucose measures above 250 mg/dL, the patient may experience excess ketones (and therefore ketoacidosis) during exercise and should consult the health care provider before exercising. Educate the patient to maintain a consistent, health care provider–approved level of exercise and to avoid sudden increases or decreases in exercise pattern.

Stress of acute illness and surgery. Emotional and physical stress can increase the blood glucose level and result in hyperglycemia. However, it is impossible to avoid stress in life situations such as a death in the family, job, interviews, and final examinations. These situations may require extra insulin to avoid hyperglycemia.

Common stress-evoking situations include acute illness, pregnancy, and the controlled stress of surgery. The patient with DM who has a minor illness such as a cold or the flu should continue drug therapy and food intake. A carbohydrate liquid substitution such as regular soft drinks, gelatin dessert, or beverages such as Gatorade may be necessary. The patient should understand that food intake is important during this time, because the body requires extra energy to deal with the stress of the illness.

Blood glucose monitoring should be done every 1 to 2 awake hours by either the patient or a person who can assume responsibility for care during the illness. Urinary output and the presence and degree of ketonuria should be monitored, particularly when fever is present. Increase fluid intake to prevent dehydration, with a minimum of 4 ounces per hour for an adult.

Instruct the patient to contact the health care provider when the blood glucose level exceeds 250 mg/dL; in such cases, fever, ketonuria, and nausea and vomiting may occur. The health care provider should supervise the necessary adjustments in the treatment regimen during times of stress. Eventually the well-informed patient will be able to make most adjustments independently based on experience.

Surgery is a controlled stress, and adjustments in the DM regimen can be planned to ensure glycemic control. The patient is given IV fluids and insulin immediately before, during, and after surgery when there is no oral intake. For the patient with type 2 DM who takes oral antidiabetic medications, usually the drugs are discontinued 48 hours before surgery, and the patient is treated with insulin during the surgical period. Explain to the patient that this is a temporary measure, not a worsening of DM. Treatment with short-acting or rapid-acting insulin allows more accurate control and adjustment in patient treatment.

Medications. Insulin and oral hypoglycemic drugs are the drugs of choice for patients with DM. Insulin administration is necessary for all patients with type 1 DM.

Insulin. In the past, insulin was obtained from the pancreas of cows and pigs. Currently only biosynthetic insulin is used. Biosynthetic insulin is produced by genetically altered common bacteria or yeast, using deoxyribonucleic acid (DNA) technology. This insulin exhibits chemical and biologic properties identical to those of human insulin produced by human beta cells in the pancreas (Fig. 51.10). Insulin is a peptide hormone and is absorbed most commonly into the patient's bloodstream. Insulin is given subcutaneously, although IV administration of regular insulin can be done when immediate onset of action is desired. IV regular insulin is mixed in normal saline solution (0.9% sodium chloride). The amount of solution depends on the institution's protocol.

Insulins differ regarding onset, peak, action, and duration (Table 51.5). The specific preparation of each type of insulin is matched with the patient's diet and activity. By adding zinc, acetate buffers, and protamine to insulin in various ways, the onset of activity, peak, and duration times can be manipulated. Different combinations of these insulins can be used to tailor treatment to the patient's specific pattern of blood glucose levels.

Formulas are classified as follows:

Rapid-acting: Lispro (Humalog); aspart (NovoLog); glulisine (Apidra)

Short-acting: Regular insulin (Humulin R, Novolin R, ReliOn R)

Intermediate-acting: NPH insulin (Humulin N, Novolin N, and ReliOn N)

Long-acting: Glargine (Lantus), detemir (Levemir)

Glargine is used once a day at bedtime and works around the clock for 24 hours. It is a "peakless" insulin that provides a continuous insulin level similar to the slow, steady (basal) secretions of insulin from a normal pancreas. Glargine must not be mixed in the same syringe with other insulins, because it will interfere with their action (Fig. 51.11).

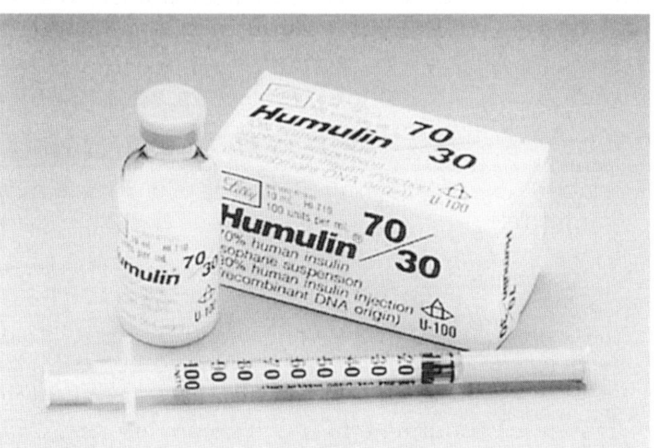

Fig. 51.10 Humulin 70/30 (70% human insulin isophane suspension and 30% human insulin injection [recombinant DNA origin]), containing 100 units of insulin per milliliter (U-100). Humulin is NPH (neutral protamine Hagedorn) insulin. Also shown is a disposable U-100 insulin syringe.

If hyperglycemia occurs, elevated blood glucose is covered with sliding-scale regular insulin. Premixed combinations are 70/30 (70% NPH insulin and 30% regular insulin; trade names Humulin 70/30 [see Fig. 51.10] and Novolin 70/30) and 50/50 (50% NPH insulin and 50% regular insulin; trade name Humulin 50/50). Recently, two more combinations have become available: 75/25 insulin lispro (75% lispro protamine [intermediate-acting] and 25% lispro [rapid-acting]; trade name Humalog mix 75/25) and 70/30 insulin aspart (70% aspart protamine [intermediate-acting] and 30% aspart [rapid-acting]; trade name NovoLog mix 70/30). The premixed insulins are most helpful for those with stable insulin needs. Timing of insulin action to match food intake can be a challenge, and it tends to be more difficult for people with type 1 DM because their only source of insulin is by injection. Regular insulin is prescribed when a rapid onset of glucose-lowering action is needed, such as before meals and during periods of acute illness, surgery, or stress. Only regular insulin can be administered intravenously; thus it is used in emergencies.

A human insulin formula, called insulin lispro, begins to take effect in less than half the time of regular, short-acting insulin. Older insulin products must be taken subcutaneously 30 to 60 minutes before a meal; the

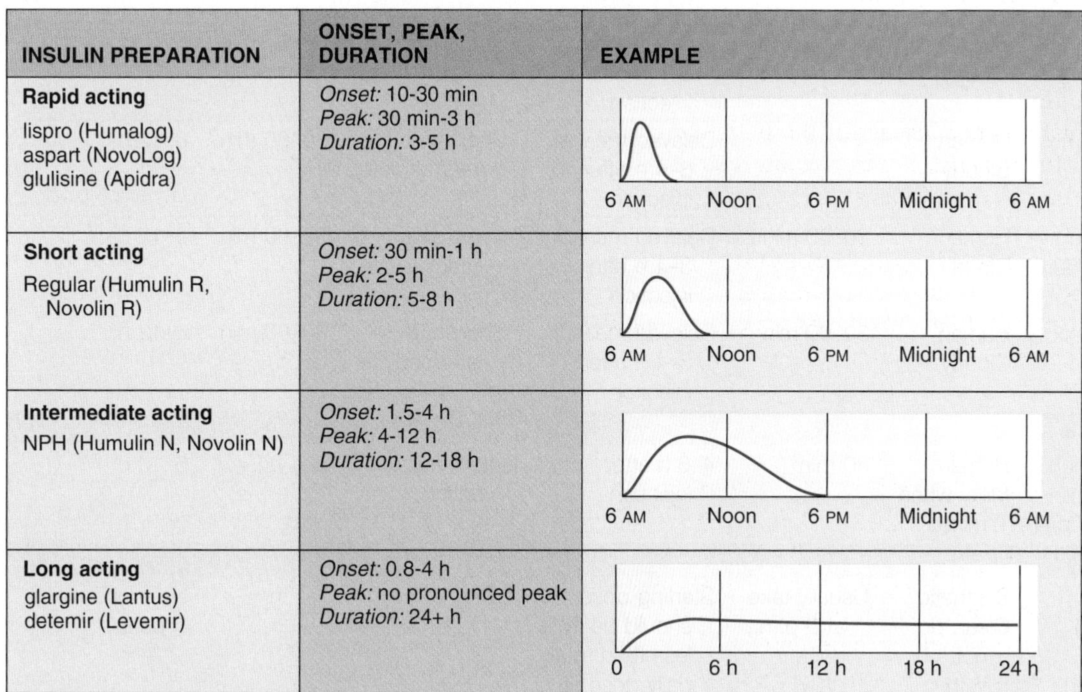

INSULIN PREPARATION	ONSET, PEAK, DURATION	EXAMPLE
Rapid acting lispro (Humalog) aspart (NovoLog) glulisine (Apidra)	*Onset:* 10-30 min *Peak:* 30 min-3 h *Duration:* 3-5 h	6 AM Noon 6 PM Midnight 6 AM
Short acting Regular (Humulin R, Novolin R)	*Onset:* 30 min-1 h *Peak:* 2-5 h *Duration:* 5-8 h	6 AM Noon 6 PM Midnight 6 AM
Intermediate acting NPH (Humulin N, Novolin N)	*Onset:* 1.5-4 h *Peak:* 4-12 h *Duration:* 12-18 h	6 AM Noon 6 PM Midnight 6 AM
Long acting glargine (Lantus) detemir (Levemir)	*Onset:* 0.8-4 h *Peak:* no pronounced peak *Duration:* 24+ h	0 6 h 12 h 18 h 24 h

Fig. 51.11 Commercially available insulin preparations, including onset, peak, and duration of action. (From Lewis SL, Heitkemper MM, Dirksen SR, et al: *Medical-surgical nursing: Assessment and management of clinical problems*, ed 9, St. Louis, 2014, Mosby.)

Table 51.5 **Types of Insulin and Their Use**

TYPE OF INSULIN	SOURCE AND COLOR	INJECTION TIME (BEFORE MEAL)	RISK TIME FOR HYPOGLYCEMIC REACTION	ACTION	ONSET OF ACTION	PEAK ACTION	DURATION
Rapid Acting							
lispro (Humalog)	Human Clear	5–15 min	No meal within 30 min	Rapid	15–30 min	1–2 h	3–4 h
aspart (NovoLog)	Human Clear	5–15 min	No meal within 30 min	Rapid	15–30 min	1–3 h	3–5 h
glulisine (Apidra)	Human Clear	5–15 min	No meal within 30 min	Rapid	15–30 min	1–3 h	3–5 h
Short Acting							
Regular Humulin R Novolin R ReliOn R	Human Clear	30 min	Delayed meal or 3–4 h after injection	Short	30–60 min	2–4 h	6–8 h
Mixed							
NovoLog Mix 70/30 (neutral protamine aspart and aspart)	Human Cloudy	15 min	No meal within 30 min	Rapid and intermediate	15–30 min	2–10 h	12–16 h
Humalog mix 75/25 (neutral protamine lispro and lispro)	Human Cloudy	15 min	No meal within 30 min	Rapid and intermediate	15–30 min	2–10 h	12–16 h
NPH/regular mix 70/30 Humulin mix 70/30	Human Cloudy	30–60 min	Delayed meal or 3–4 h after injection	Short and intermediate	30–60 min	6–12 h	18–24 h
Novolin mix 70/30	Human Cloudy	30–60 min	Delayed meal or 3–4 h after injection	Short and intermediate	30–60 min	6–12 h	18–24 h
ReliOn N mix 70/30	Human Cloudy		Delayed meal or 3–4 h after injection	Short and intermediate	30–60 min	6–12 h	18–24 h
NPH/Regular Mix 50/50	Human Cloudy	30–60 min	Delayed meal or 3–4 h after injection	Short and intermediate	30–60 min	6–12 h	18–24 h
Humulin mix 50/50	Human Cloudy	30–60 min	Delayed meal or 3–4 h after injection	Short and intermediate	30–60 min	6–12 h	18–24 h
Intermediate Acting							
NPH Humulin N, Novolin N, ReliOn N	Human Milky when mixed	30 min	4–6 h after injection	Intermediate acting	2–4 h	6–10 h	12–16 h
Long Acting							
glargine (Lantus) detemir (Levemir)	Synthetic Clear; do not mix with others	Usually take at 9 p.m., once daily[a]	Starting dose should be 20% less than total daily dose of NPH	Long lasting	1–2 h	No pronounced peak	24 h[b]

[a]May take at other times.
[b]For patients with type 1 diabetes, once or twice daily; for patients with type 2 diabetes, once daily.
From Lewis SM, Heitkemper MM, Dirksen SR, et al: *Medical-surgical nursing: Assessment and management of clinical problems,* ed 7, St. Louis, 2007, Mosby.

newer lispro formula can be injected 15 minutes before a meal. This timing more closely mimics the body's own hormone activity. Lispro brings the most benefit to people with type 1 DM who take short-acting insulin before meals combined with a longer-acting insulin once or twice a day. Two additional rapid-acting insulins, aspart (NovoLog) and glulisine (Apidra), with similar onset of action as lispro (Humalog), also are used. Insulins are used commonly in combination to mimic normal pancreatic insulin secretion.

When giving insulin, be careful to inject only into the *subcutaneous tissue* (between the fat and muscle layers), avoiding depositing the medication directly into the fat or muscle. Insulin administration requires the appropriate syringe. Most commercial insulin is available as U-100, indicating that each milliliter contains 100 units of insulin. U-100 insulin must be used with a U-100–marked syringe. For a user taking smaller doses of insulin, insulin syringes marked for 25, 30, or 50 units are available for use with U-100 insulins. One important distinction is that the 100-unit syringe is marked in 2-unit increments, whereas the 50- and 30-unit syringes are marked in 1-unit increments. Be certain that the patient gets the correct size of syringe and does not switch syringes, thus avoiding serious dosing errors. The Joint Commission now recommends using *units* instead of the abbreviation *U* on medication orders and medication administration records to decrease errors in dosing.

Insulin pens are another popular method of administering insulin. The pen serves the same function as a needle and syringe but is compact and portable, thus making it more convenient. Insulin pens are handy in that they contain all the necessary parts in one piece, but the user must also attach a needle and discard it after each use (Fig. 51.12). The units to be delivered are magnified on the pen, allowing more accurate dosing for the patient with visual impairment.

Needles are very fine, usually 25 to 32 gauge, so that they are as atraumatic to the tissue as possible. An open bottle of insulin currently being used does not have to

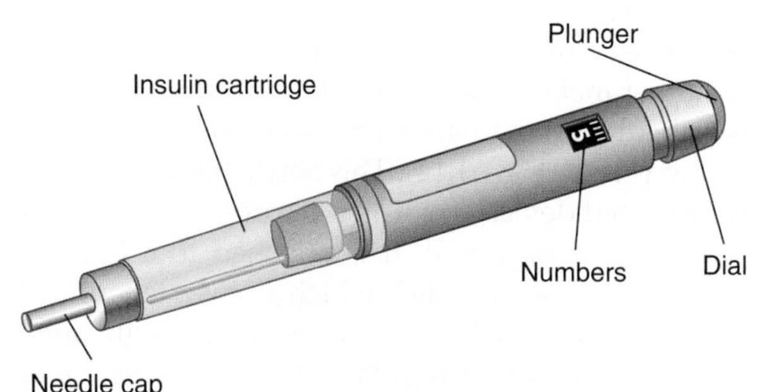

Fig. 51.12 A NovoPen insulin pen. (From Lewis SL, Heitkemper MM, Dirksen SR, et al: *Medical-surgical nursing: Assessment and management of clinical problems*, ed 9, St. Louis, 2014, Mosby.)

be refrigerated. In fact, it is now believed that insulin should be administered at room temperature, not straight from the refrigerator, to help prevent insulin **lipohypertrophy** (a subcutaneous skin disorder in which a firm lump under the skin develops after long-term subcutaneous insulin injections). Lipohypertrophy can impede insulin absorption. Extra bottles are stored in the refrigerator. Box 51.3 offers guidelines for preparation of a dose of insulin, one or two types at a time.

Patients who self-inject insulin at home may want to have a family member oversee the procedure. Nurses administering insulin injections always must have another licensed person check and document the dose drawn up in the syringe to prevent medication errors. The patient with DM ideally should be taught self-injection technique before discharge from the hospital. However, some patients are unable to perform this because of physical problems, intellectual incapacity, visual disturbances, or age. In these cases, family members or others must administer the injections. Before discharge, either the patient or the significant other, or both, must display the ability to correctly draw up and inject insulin.

In a newly diagnosed patient, regular or rapid-acting insulin may be injected before each meal. After reasonable control of hyperglycemia is achieved, the dosage schedule may be changed to once a day, in the morning before breakfast, with the type of insulin being intermediate or long acting (see Fig. 51.11 and Table 51.5 for types of insulin). Sometimes patients with DM take two divided doses of insulin, one before breakfast and one before the evening meal. Be alert for signs of **hypoglycemia** (low blood glucose) at the peak of action of whatever type of insulin the patient is receiving. Instruct the patient to notify a member of the nursing staff if any of the following signs of hypoglycemic (insulin) reaction occur: faintness, sudden weakness, excessive perspiration, irritability, hunger, palpitations, trembling, or drowsiness. Sometimes hypoglycemia signs and symptoms mimic a stroke, and a blood glucose level must be obtained immediately (Walker, 2011).

After appropriate blood glucose testing, the patient chooses an injection site. The subcutaneous pocket is the desired layer into which insulin should be injected. Insulin should not be injected into the muscle, because it enters the bloodstream too quickly and could cause hypoglycemia. Site selection is crucial, as is site rotation. The patient may choose sites on the abdomen (except for 2 inches [5 cm] around the navel), the upper arms, the anterior or lateral aspects of the thighs, and the hips or buttocks. The abdomen provides the fastest, least variable absorption, followed by the arms, thighs, and buttocks (Fig. 51.13). Patients may find it easier to keep track of their injection sites by recording each injection on a numbered chart.

Because of differing anatomic absorption rates of insulin, it currently is recommended that injections be given in all the available areas in a site, such as the

Box 51.3 Preparation of Insulin

1. Thoroughly wash hands with warm water and soap. Bring the insulin to room temperature; an injection of cold insulin can be painful.
2. Assemble all equipment needed, such as a properly calibrated insulin syringe with a prefitted needle, alcohol swab, and insulin.
3. Turn the insulin vial onto its side and gently rotate between the hands several times to be certain it is mixed. The precipitate should be blended evenly. This is not necessary with regular insulin because it has no precipitate. Never shake insulin vigorously because this creates air bubbles.
4. Clean the rubber stopper on the vial with an alcohol swab.
5. Remove the needle cover and draw in the same amount of air as units of insulin to be injected.
6. Insert the needle through the rubber stopper of the vial and then inject the air. Invert the bottle with the syringe unit attached, making sure the tip of the needle is below the level of the insulin so that air will not be drawn into the syringe.
7. Pull back slowly on the plunger, a few units past the desired dose of insulin.
8. Inspect for air bubbles in the syringe; if any are seen, gently tap the barrel until they rise to the top, then push back into the vial with the plunger to the level of the desired dose of insulin.
9. Holding on to the barrel and plunger, remove the syringe unit and put the needle cover back on. Always check an insulin dose with a second licensed nurse. Proceed with the injection procedure.

TWO INSULINS

1. Follow Steps 1 through 5 above.
2. Insert the desired amount of air into the vial of the longer-acting insulin first. Do not mix insulin glargine (Lantus) or detemir (Levemir) with any other insulin or solution.
3. Inject the desired amount of air into the shorter-acting insulin vial; leave the syringe unit in this vial; invert, and proceed through Steps 6 through 9, but do not inject yet. Set the vial of shorter-acting insulin out of reach to prevent accidental reuse.
4. Insert the needle into the vial of longer-acting insulin, being careful to hold on to the plunger so that none of the insulin in the syringe enters that vial.
5. Slowly pull the plunger to the level of the combined total of both types of insulin desired (such as regular 10 units, NPH 30 units, totaling 40 units). Do not pull extra units into the syringe. Take special care not to get any air bubbles into the syringe because they will displace some of the insulin and make the dose incorrect. If this happens, discard the whole syringe and start all over again. Check the insulin dose with a second licensed nurse.
6. If the dose is correct, proceed with the injection procedure.

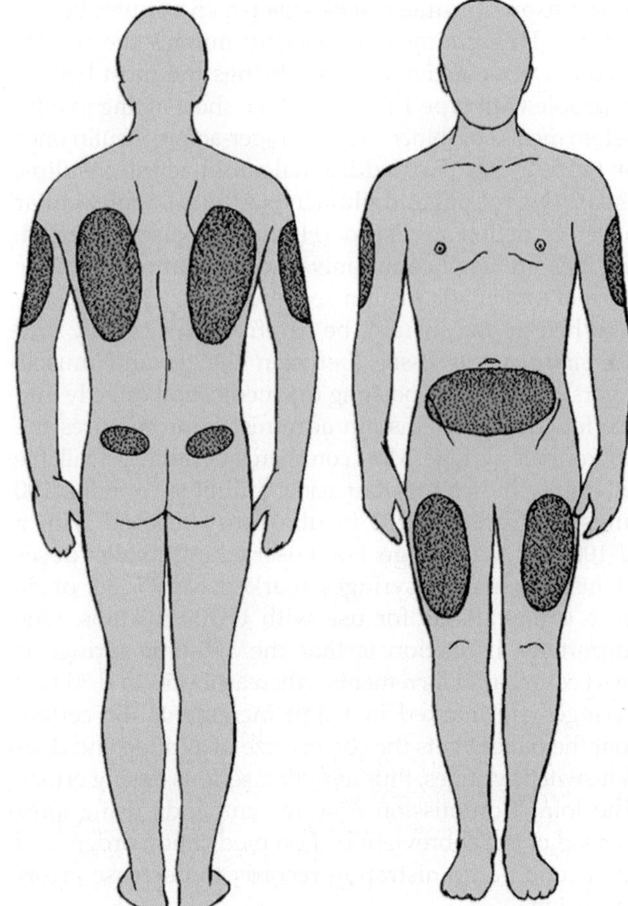

Fig. 51.13 Rotation of sites for insulin injections. (From Potter PA, Perry AG, Stockert PA, et al: *Fundamentals of nursing*, ed 8, St. Louis, 2013, Mosby.)

thigh, before moving to another site. In this way the patient with DM may take eight or more injections, spaced 1 to 1½ inches (2.54 to 3.81 cm) apart, and allow the tissues in other sites to recover more fully before being used again. This technique helps prevent lipohypertrophy, a condition that can lead to unsightly lumps under the skin and a decrease in insulin absorption. The technique for insulin injection is described in Box 51.4.

Several new delivery systems are available for patients who find injections emotionally and physically uncomfortable. These include automatic injectors, the jet stream (needleless) injector, the Insuflon indwelling insulin delivery service, and the button infuser.

Another method of insulin administration is continuous subcutaneous insulin infusion using an external infusion pump (Fig. 51.14). This small, battery-powered computerized device is worn on the user's body, usually in a pocket or on a belt. It is attached to a thin tube with a needle on the end, which is inserted into the subcutaneous tissue. A continuous, or basal, rate of rapid- or short-acting regular insulin delivery can be programmed, with bolus doses administered as needed. The insulin pump is as close a substitute as available to a healthy, working pancreas. It mimics the pancreas

Box 51.4 Technique for Insulin Injection

1. Follow the Steps in Box 51.3 to prepare the insulin dose.
2. Don disposable gloves.
3. Clean the injection site with an alcohol swab, using a circular motion. Allow the alcohol to dry. Place the swab between the last two fingers of the hand not used to inject the insulin.
4. Pick up the syringe and remove the needle cover and lay it aside. Hold the syringe like a dart.
5. Using the other hand, gently pinch up at least a 2-inch (5.1 cm) fold of tissue (not just the skin).
6. Quickly insert the needle into the top of the fold, entering the subcutaneous tissue. The needle should be inserted at a 90-degree angle unless the patient is very thin and has little subcutaneous tissue. In that case the angle may be reduced by up to 45 degrees to avoid intramuscular injection.
7. Release the skinfold and use that hand to steady the barrel of the syringe.
8. Inject the insulin slowly.
9. Place the alcohol swab against the needle hub, at the injection site, and pull the syringe unit straight out in one swift motion. Do not massage the site.
10. Carefully place the entire unit, uncapped, into the sharps container provided.
11. Record the injection site and insulin dose on a chart, computer, or other documentation sheet. Include the second licensed nurse who witnessed the insulin dose during preparation; ask this nurse to witness the dose given. Store insulin and other supplies properly.
12. When instructing a patient to self-inject insulin, use the following guidelines (if appropriate):
    - Aspiration is not necessary before injection.
    - The injection site does not have to be cleansed with alcohol.

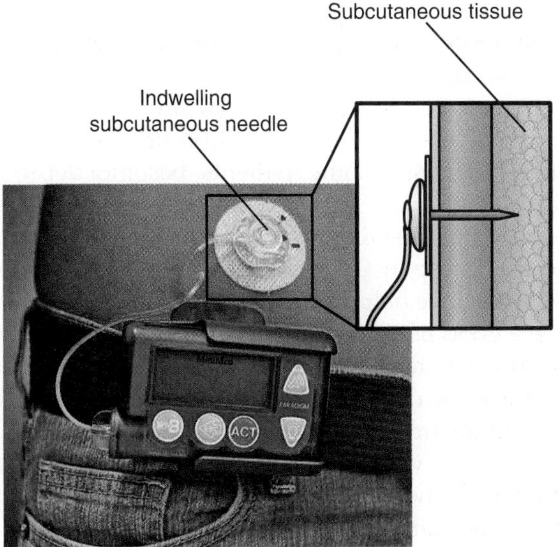

Fig. 51.14 Medtronic MiniMed insulin pump. (Modified from Lewis SL, Heitkemper MM, Dirksen SR, et al: *Medical-surgical nursing: Assessment and management of clinical problems,* ed 7, St. Louis, 2007, Mosby.)

by releasing small amounts of rapid-acting insulin every few minutes. Buffered regular insulin may be substituted in patients unable to use rapid-acting insulin to improve postprandial blood glucose levels and long-term glucose control. The basal rate is designed to keep the blood glucose level steady between meals and during sleep. When food is eaten, the pump is programmed (at the touch of a button) to deliver a larger quantity (bolus) of insulin right away to cover the carbohydrate in the meal. The bolus can also be adjusted on the basis of blood glucose level and planned physical activity. For carefully selected and properly educated patients, the pump offers improved flexibility in lifestyle, improved control of blood glucose and glycosylated hemoglobin (HbA_{1c}) levels (see Box 51.2), and freedom from multiple daily injections. Some disassembled insulin pump models can even be worn during bathing or while swimming. The insertion site is usually the abdomen, but the buttocks, thighs, arms, and sections of the back may be used, with the insertion site covered by a clear occlusive dressing, which usually is changed every other day.

Other treatments. Pramlintide (Symlin) is a subcutaneous agent that acts as an adjunct to insulin therapy, not a replacement for it. It decreases gastric emptying, glucagon secretion, and glucose output from the liver and increases satiety.

Another drug that may be used to treat hypoglycemic reactions in DM is glucagon, a hormone normally secreted by the alpha cells of the pancreas. It stimulates the liver to change stored glycogen into glucose, which then is released into the bloodstream. Glucagon is available in a purified, crystallized form for reconstruction and subcutaneous, IM, or IV administration in the event of loss of consciousness as a result of hypoglycemic reaction. The usual dose is 0.5 mg to 1 mg for adults, with smaller doses for children. Some form of oral protein and carbohydrate, such as milk and crackers, should be given after the patient regains consciousness. Many people with DM carry a commercially prepared kit containing glucagon and concentrated carbohydrate such as candy or glucose gel (see the Complementary and Alternative Therapies box).

Selected patients with type 1 DM now have the option of a pancreas transplant. Usually a pancreas transplant is performed on a patient with DM who has end-stage renal disease and has already had a kidney transplant or will have one in the near future. Kidney and pancreas transplants usually are done at the same time. Patients who undergo kidney and pancreas transplantation must have lifelong immunosuppression therapy to prevent rejection of the transplants.

Nursing Interventions and Patient Teaching

People with DM may be hospitalized as a direct result of their disease process, or they may have a different primary diagnosis.

Complementary and Alternative Therapies

Endocrine Disorders

- Herbal medicines used in the treatment of type 2 DM include aloe vera juice, beans (*Phaseolus* species), bitter gourd, karela *(Momordica charantia)*, black tea *(Camellia sinensis)*, fenugreek *(Trigonella foenum-graecum)*, gurmar *(Gymnema sylvestre)*, macadamia nut, and Madagascar periwinkle *(Catharanthus roseus)*. Effects of these herbs include lowering of blood pressure (fenugreek), boosting of insulin production (gurmar), and increased use of available insulin (black tea).
- Kelp *(Fucus vesiculosus)* may help with weight loss in hypothyroid disorders. Milk thistle *(Silybum marianum)* is used for treatment and prophylaxis of chronic hepatotoxicity, inflammatory liver disorders, and certain types of cirrhosis.
- Yoga may help the patient with DM with diet control and may improve pancreatic function.

The daily routine for the patient with DM includes accurate monitoring of blood glucose levels, either by finger-stick specimens or by laboratory testing. Careful attention to diet is important; note the amount of food eaten at each meal and record it accurately.

If the patient with type 1 DM is ill, nauseated, or cannot eat for any reason (such as NPO [nothing by mouth] status), consult with the health care provider. Physiologic and psychological stress raises the patient's blood glucose level. Do not withhold insulin in a patient with type 1 DM without consulting the health care provider or reviewing the written orders for hypoglycemic episodes. Without insulin to promote glucose to enter the cells, the body must seek an alternative source for energy. Fats and protein are used. When these cells break down, ketones are formed. Accumulation of ketones results in ketosis and acidosis. If this situation is not corrected, the patient may develop DKA.

Often the primary health care provider recommends providing Popsicles or apple juice, which can compensate for a decrease in calories when a regular diet cannot be consumed. If the patient does not like the types of food on the meal tray, arrange for a dietitian to consult.

Good skin care is essential for the person with DM, because poor circulation can lead to the development of skin problems. Compromised skin integrity makes a patient with DM more susceptible to infection. In DM, elevated glycosylated hemoglobin in the red blood cells impedes the release of oxygen to the tissues. Elevated blood glucose levels also make some pathogens thrive and proliferate. Vascular changes decrease blood, oxygen, and nutrient supply to the tissues and affect the supply of white blood cells in the area, because if white blood cells do not function properly, phagocytosis is defective.

Report to the health care provider any abnormalities such as cuts, scratches, or lesions anywhere on the body, and treat them before infection develops. Special foot care is crucial for the patient with DM, because poor circulation and decreased nerve sensation or **neuropathy** (any abnormal condition characterized by inflammation and degeneration of the peripheral nerves) increase the danger of ulcers or other abnormal lesions developing into gangrene. The patient should be instructed to use a mirror for inspection of the feet if mobility is impeded, or to have a family member or friend inspect the feet on a daily basis. Many patients seek the services of a podiatrist for their foot care. The patient should wash the feet thoroughly with soap and water every day; dry them thoroughly; and inspect them carefully for cracks, blisters, or foreign objects, paying special attention to the area between the toes. Foot soaks or powders are not recommended. The patient should wear clean socks daily and avoid tight garters. The toenails should be clipped straight across so that the edges do not become ingrown. Never trim the toenails of a patient with DM without a health care provider's written order. Do not put hot water bottles or heating pads on the feet, because burns may occur and may not be felt. The patient should wear sturdy, properly fitting shoes, preferably with wide toe boxes or molded shoes that are less constrictive. Medicare now reimburses patients with DM who have certain conditions for the cost of specially molded shoes. The patient should not go barefoot at any time. Notify the health care provider immediately of any injury to the toes or feet (see the Health Promotion box).

The patient with DM is encouraged to have eye examinations every 6 to 12 months to allow for early diagnosis and intervention of diabetes-related vision concerns such as retinopathy.

Carefully watch the patient who is receiving insulin for development of hypoglycemia, especially when the particular kind of insulin being injected is at its peak of action. Hypoglycemia is seen less frequently in patients receiving oral hypoglycemic medication, but it can occur.

The emotional aspects of DM are numerous, and many patients experience a period of denial after the initial diagnosis. Some patients become depressed. Because this disease affects all age groups, nursing interventions are tailored to fit the needs of each patient (see the Lifespan Considerations box). Patients with DM must have help in working through their feelings, so be a good listener and supportive. The patient who does not satisfactorily resolve any major problems in accepting the diagnosis of DM may be noncompliant with the treatment plan.

The nurse who supervises the patient in a home setting must encourage the patient to take the prescribed medication faithfully, eat the right kinds of food, test blood or urine correctly, and exercise regularly. If a family member is responsible for the patient's care, ensure that the caregiver is functioning adequately in this role. Some patients live alone and do well caring

Health Promotion

Foot Care for the Patient With Diabetes Mellitus

- Wash feet daily with a mild soap and *warm* water. Test water temperature with hands first.
- Pat feet dry gently, especially between toes.
- Examine feet daily for cuts, blisters, edema, erythema, and tender areas. If patient's eyesight is poor, have others inspect feet.
- Use lanolin on feet to prevent skin from drying and cracking. Do not apply between toes.
- Use mild foot powder on feet if perspiring.
- Do not use commercial remedies to remove calluses or corns.
- Cleanse cuts with *warm* water and mild soap, covering with clean dressing. Do not use iodine, rubbing alcohol, or strong adhesives.
- Report skin infections or nonhealing lesions to health care provider immediately.
- Cut toenails even with rounded contour of toes. Do not cut down corners. The best time to trim nails is after a shower or bath.
- Separate overlapping toes with cotton or lamb's wool.
- Avoid open-toe, open-heel, and high-heel shoes. Leather shoes are preferred to plastic ones. Wear slippers with soles. Do not go barefoot. Shake out shoes before putting on.
- Wear clean, absorbent cotton socks. Colored socks must be colorfast.
- Do not wear clothing that constricts circulation.
- Do not use hot water bottles or heating pads to warm feet. Wear socks for warmth.
- Guard against frostbite.
- Exercise feet daily either by walking or by flexing and extending feet in suspended position. Avoid prolonged sitting, standing, and crossing of legs.

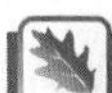

Lifespan Considerations

Older Adults

Endocrine Disorders

- DM is more prevalent in older adults. A major reason for this is that the process of aging involves insulin resistance and glucose intolerance, which are believed to be precursors to type 2 DM.
- The classic signs and symptoms of DM may not be obvious in older adults.
- Dietary management may be complicated by a variety of functional, social, economic, and financial factors.
- Hormone supplements must be administered with caution.
- Older adult patients with DM are at increased risk for infection and should be counseled to receive proper immunizations and seek regular medical attention for even minor symptoms. The older adult often has difficulty in managing DM.
- Some symptoms of hypothyroidism in the older adult are similar to those in a younger person but are more likely to be overlooked because the symptoms—fatigue, mental impairment, sluggishness, and constipation—often are attributed solely to aging. The older person with hypothyroidism has symptoms unique to the age set, including more disturbances of the central nervous system, such as syncope, convulsions, dementia, and coma. There is often pitting edema and deafness.
- The older patient with hyperthyroidism frequently has manifestations related only to the cardiovascular system, such as palpitations, angina, atrial fibrillation, and breathlessness. Signs and symptoms often attributed to "aging" actually may indicate an endocrine problem.

for themselves, with occasional visits from a home health or public health nurse. Others who have visual disturbances, circulatory problems, or other conditions may need daily visits and more actual nursing intervention, such as help with hygiene, meals, and insulin injections (Nursing Care Plan 51.1).

Acute complications. One of the acute complications of DM is coma, which may be attributed to three different causes. The first type of coma can occur during DKA, which results from inadequate amounts of insulin or from inadequate insulin use. The second type, hyperglycemic hyperosmolar nonketotic coma (HHNC), involves no acidosis or ketonemia (excessive levels of ketone bodies in the blood) but results from excess glucose, diuresis, and dehydration without adequate fluid replacement. The third type may occur during a hypoglycemic reaction, which results from an excess amount of insulin without an adequate amount of glucose present. These three complications are compared and contrasted in Table 51.6. (See also the Safety Alert boxes: Emergency Care for Hypoglycemic Reaction and Emergency Care for Hyperglycemic Reaction.)

Another acute complication faced by the patient with DM is the development of infections of any kind. Hyperglycemia and ketonemia hinder the phagocytic action of leukocytes. An infection therefore may become more severe and last longer, with poor wound healing taking place. Infection increases the possibility of DKA and makes it harder to control the disease. Patients with DM often are hospitalized for treatment of infections that may be handled on an outpatient basis for the nondiabetic patient.

Chronic complications. Primary chronic complications associated with DM are those of end-organ disease, which results from damage to blood vessels (angiopathy) secondary to chronic hyperglycemia. Chronic complications of DM include blindness, cardiovascular problems, and renal failure (Fig. 51.15).

DM causes more cases of blindness in the United States than any other disease. Diabetic retinopathy involves progressive changes in the microcirculation of the retina, resulting in hemorrhages, scar tissue formation, and various degrees of retinal detachment. Surgical

Nursing Care Plan 51.1 The Patient With Diabetes Mellitus

Ms. T. is an obese, 52-year-old, married patient with type 2 diabetes mellitus (DM) diagnosed 3 years ago. She was referred to a short-term ambulatory diabetes education program by her health care provider for instruction on insulin administration because she has not achieved blood glucose control with dietary measures.

Objective data included blood glucose 220 mg/dL, weight 200 pounds, and blood pressure 134/84 mm Hg. Collaborative nursing actions include teaching Ms. T. measures that will help her control blood glucose (insulin, diet, and exercise) and how to detect, prevent, and treat hypoglycemic reactions. The nurse reported Ms. T.'s work schedule to the health care provider and asked for insulin dosage alterations on weekends. The health care provider was unaware of her work schedule and stated that blood glucose control could not be optimum with this schedule.

PATIENT PROBLEM

Insufficient Knowledge: Self-injections, Self-Monitoring of Blood Glucose (SMBG), related to lack of exposure

Patient Goals and Expected Outcomes	Nursing Interventions	Evaluation
Patient will independently self-administer insulin Patient will perform SMBG accurately Patient will use measurements obtained by SMBG to achieve blood glucose less than 126 mg/dL Patient will be able to detect and treat hypoglycemia	Support patient as necessary to self-inject insulin. Observe patient's skill in SMBG; correct as necessary. Review with patient the effect of activity, dietary intake, and insulin on blood glucose. Instruct patient on frequency and timing of SMBG. Review with patient signs and symptoms and treatment measures. Refer to dietitian for modification of diet necessary with insulin and for verification of diet knowledge.	Patient demonstrates safety in drawing up and self-administering insulin. Patient demonstrates accuracy in SMBG. Patient can verbalize the effect of activity, diet, and insulin on blood glucose. Patient can recite signs and symptoms of hypoglycemia and the correct immediate treatment to pursue.

PATIENT PROBLEM

Compromised Maintenance of Health, related to ineffective coping skills

Patient Goals and Expected Outcomes	Nursing Interventions	Evaluation
Patient will state at least one change that will improve blood glucose control	Teach patient effects of stress, lack of exercise, and activity pattern on blood glucose level. Explore with patient willingness and ability to change behaviors: sleep activity, coping, and exercise. Engage patient in mutual problem solving; refrain from prescribing. Explore sources for long-term support in learning more effective coping skills; suggest support groups: • For patients with DM • For weight loss and maintaining weight loss • Available at work in health service program	Patient has enrolled in an exercise and weight reduction program to assist in achieving a reasonable weight and beneficial exercise.

CRITICAL THINKING QUESTIONS

1. Ms. T. received Humalog mix 75/25, 25 units subcutaneously at 7:30 a.m. She followed the American Diabetes Association diet for her breakfast and lunch selections. At 3:00 p.m. she complains of being hungry, nervous, and tremulous. What are the immediate nursing interventions?
2. Ms. T. states, "I need to lose about 40 pounds, and I'm considering joining a weight reduction club." What would be some helpful suggestions by the nurse?
3. In discharge planning, the nurse notes that Ms. T. has poorly fitting shoes. What would be some important discharge patient teaching for foot care?

techniques such as laser beam coagulation of retinal vessels may improve vision for selected patients with early diagnosis. The risk for the development of glaucoma is 40% greater in the patient with DM. Longevity of the disease and aging are key factors in the development of the condition (American Diabetes Association [ADA], 2013). Cataract development is 60% greater in the patient with DM.

Vascular changes in patients with DM, especially capillary changes, contribute to the development of renal sclerosis, often progressing to end-stage renal disease. Approximately 45% of patients with DM must undergo either peritoneal dialysis or hemodialysis as a result. DM contributes to accelerated atherosclerotic changes in the blood vessels, resulting in myocardial infarction, stroke, and gangrene in the lower extremities.

Nervous system manifestations (diabetic neuropathy) are seen commonly, which cause pain and decreased sensation in the extremities and contribute to the development of diabetic gangrene. Symptoms include

Table 51.6 Comparison of Types of Diabetic Coma

ASSESSMENT	HYPERGLYCEMIC REACTION, DIABETIC KETOACIDOSIS	HYPOGLYCEMIC REACTION	HYPERGLYCEMIC HYPEROSMOLAR NONKETOTIC COMA
Type of diabetes	Type 1	Type 1 or type 2	Type 2
Cause	Inadequate insulin	Too much insulin or oral hypoglycemic agent	Inadequate insulin or oral hypoglycemic agent
Patient history	Omitted or insufficient dose of insulin, physical or emotional stress, gastrointestinal upsets, dietary noncompliance	Reduced food intake, delayed meal, too much exercise	Reduced fluid or food intake with increased urinary output, resulting in severe dehydration
Onset of symptoms	Hours to days	Minutes to hours	Days
Previous diagnosis of having diabetes	Almost always	Yes; on medication	Usually type 2 DM, on hypoglycemic agent
Age of patient	Usually younger patient	Usually younger patient	Usually older adult patient
Appearance of skin	Hot, dry, flushed	Cool, moist	Hot, dry; body temperature elevated
Breath	Fruity (from ketones)	Normal	Normal
Mucous membranes	Dry	Moist	Very dry
Respirations	Deep; may have Kussmaul's respirations (air hunger) as a result of metabolic acidosis	Rapid, shallow	Normal
Neurosensory	Drowsiness to coma	Irritability, tremors, impaired consciousness, personality changes; may lose consciousness	Lethargy, decreased consciousness; may lose consciousness
Blood pressure	Low	Normal	Decreased
Glycosuria and ketonuria	Present	Absent	Glycosuria present; no ketonuria
Polyuria and polydipsia	Present	Absent	Present
Hunger	Absent; may have nausea and vomiting	Present; may be nauseated	Absent
Blood glucose level	Usually 300–800 mg/dL	Usually <50 mg/dL	600–2000 mg/dL; serum osmolality greatly increased
Emergency treatment	Insulin, usually regular	Glucose (oral or IV) or glucagon (subQ, IM, or IV)	Large amounts of intravenous fluids; regular insulin

GI, Gastrointestinal; *IM,* intramuscular; *IV,* intravenous; *subQ,* subcutaneous.

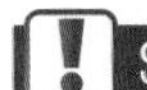
Safety Alert

Emergency Care for Hypoglycemic Reaction

IMMEDIATE TREATMENT: IF CONSCIOUS

- Give patient 15 to 20 g of quick-acting carbohydrate in some form, such as 4 to 6 oz of orange juice or a regular soft drink (not a diet drink); half of a candy bar; commercially prepared concentrated glucose tablets or glucose paste; one tube of icing gel (small); 1 TBS of sugar or honey; six jelly beans or gumdrops; five or six pieces of hard candy or other roll candy; four animal crackers; or one granola bar. Offer another 5 to 20 g of quick-acting carbohydrate in 15 minutes if no relief is obtained.
- Give patient additional food, a longer-acting carbohydrate (e.g., slice of bread, crackers with peanut butter), after symptoms subside to maintain glucose level after the quick-acting (simple) carbohydrate has been metabolized.

IMMEDIATE TREATMENT: IF UNCONSCIOUS

- Administer glucose gel tube (follow package instructions) between the cheek and gums (in the buccal space).
- Give Glucagon injection (follow package and healthcare provider instructions for dosage and location).
- Administer IV bolus of 20–50 mL of dextrose 50% in water. (ADA, 2015)

NURSING INTERVENTIONS DURING AND AFTER HYPOGLYCEMIC EPISODE

- Stay with the patient; check vital signs and do finger-stick blood glucose levels.
- Monitor for worsening of condition or relief of symptoms.
- If patient becomes unconscious, administer glucagon buccally, subcutaneously, intramuscularly, or intravenously.
- Be certain patient ingests food such as milk, six crackers with peanut butter, or one slice of cheese and six crackers after symptoms end (if able).
- Observe closely for 1 to 2 hours after cessation of symptoms.
- Notify health care provider about the hypoglycemic reaction.
- Assess reason the reaction may have occurred.

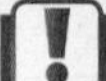

Safety Alert

Emergency Care for Hyperglycemic Reaction (Diabetic Ketoacidosis)

USUAL TREATMENT DURING ACUTE STAGE

The nurse would expect the following orders from the health care provider:

- Start an intravenous (IV) line, using a large-gauge IV catheter, and begin fluid replacement, usually with normal saline (0.9% sodium chloride) at 1 L/h, until blood pressure is stabilized and urinary output is 30 to 60 mL/h. When blood glucose levels approach 250 mg/dL, add 5% dextrose to the fluid regimen to prevent hypoglycemia.
- Give regular insulin (the only kind that can be given intravenously) as a piggyback infusion, using 100 units of regular insulin in 500 mL of normal saline. Administer the infusion with a pump controller. Adjust the infusion rate to obtain and maintain desired blood glucose levels.
- Determine blood glucose level hourly (self-monitoring of blood glucose [SMBG] method or venous sample).
- Provide IV replacement of potassium to help move insulin into cells; monitor serum potassium.
- Monitor arterial blood gas (ABG) values specifically for acidosis.
- Administer oxygen via nasal cannula or nonrebreather mask to maintain oxygen saturation at 95% or greater.
- Monitor cardiac status, with central venous pressure and Swan-Ganz monitoring if available.
- Insert Foley catheter and monitor intake and output (I&O) hourly.
- Assess vital signs and neurologic status.

NURSING INTERVENTIONS DURING AND AFTER DIABETIC KETOACIDOSIS

- Keep airway open (patent).
- Maintain patent IV infusion at prescribed rate.
- Keep accurate I&O record.
- Do accurate blood testing for glucose and urine testing for acetone.
- Monitor vital signs frequently, and assess cardiac status on monitor.
- Assess breath sounds for fluid overload.
- Assess level of consciousness frequently, and perform neurologic checks as ordered.
- Assess the cause of diabetic ketoacidosis.

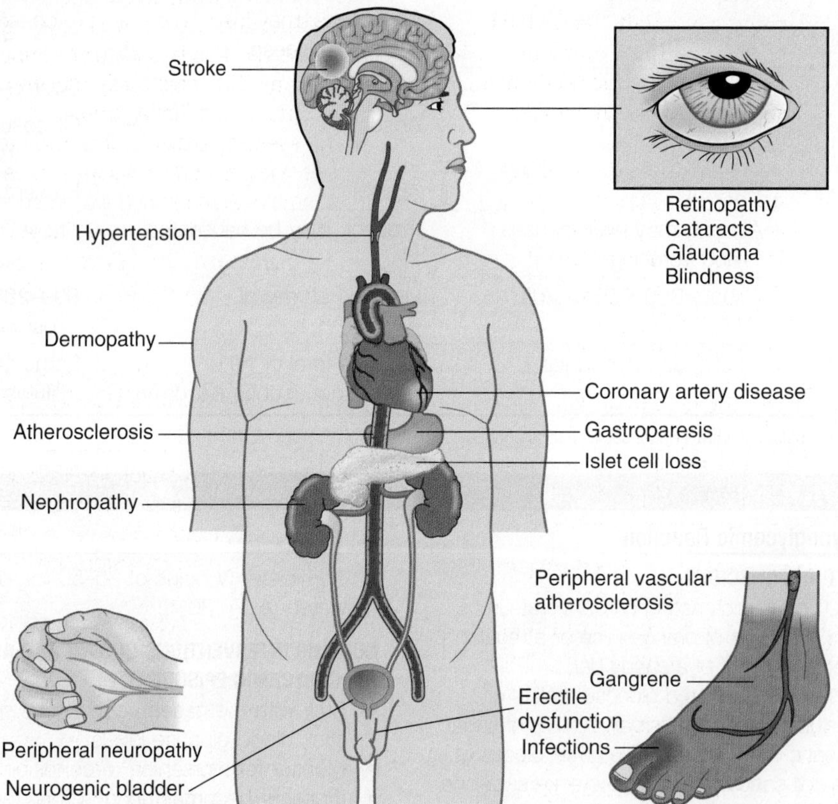

Fig. 51.15 Long-term complications of diabetes mellitus. (From Lewis SL, Heitkemper MM, Dirksen SR, et al: *Medical-surgical nursing: Assessment and management of clinical problems*, ed 9, St. Louis, 2014, Mosby.)

pain and paresthesia. The pain—described as burning, cramping, itching, or crushing—is usually worse at night and may occur only at that time. Complete or partial loss of sensitivity to touch and temperature is common. Foot injury and ulcerations may occur without the patient ever feeling pain. At times the skin becomes so sensitive (hyperesthesia) that even light pressure from bed sheets cannot be tolerated.

As many as 50% of men with DM experience problems with impotence and erectile dysfunction (Bryant, 2004). Reports of prevalence of impotence among men with DM vary from 30% to 60%. Impotence associated with

DM is believed to result from damage to the sacral parasympathetic nerves. Patients of either gender may have orthostatic hypotension and bladder or bowel dysfunction.

Neuropathy affecting the autonomic nervous system also may result in gastropathy, a delayed gastric emptying that can produce anorexia, nausea, vomiting, early satiety, and a persistent feeling of fullness. These problems previously were referred to as *gastroparesis,* a term now reserved for the condition in which the stomach is severely affected and is very slow to empty solid foods. Metoclopramide (Reglan) stimulates gastric emptying and has been used in the treatment of gastroparesis.

Patient problems and interventions for the patient with DM include but are not limited to the following:

Patient Problem	Nursing Interventions
Impaired health maintenance, related to health beliefs	Instruct in proper self-injection of insulin; have patient perform return demonstration Reinforce instructions regarding availability of glucose and glycogen sources Remove potentially hazardous objects from environment
Potential for compromised maintenance of health	Establish therapeutic relationship so that patient can express negative feelings Correct misconceptions about treatment regimen Assist patient in setting long-term goals for lifetime optimal disease management Involve significant others when possible, and encourage communication between them and the patient Refer patient to appropriate agencies and services (local support groups, ADA)

Education for the person with DM has many important aspects, including the proper administration of insulin or oral hypoglycemic medications and their side effects; the signs and symptoms of hyperglycemia and hypoglycemia; methods of testing blood glucose levels and of urine testing for acetone; planning and preparing the prescribed diet; and personal hygiene, emphasizing skin and foot care. Stress the interrelationships of diet, medication, and exercise. Instruct the patient to visit the dentist regularly and an ophthalmologist annually. Because infections and illnesses of any kind could result in loss of diabetic control, instruct the patient to notify the health care provider at the first sign of any illness. Special plans for travel include taking extra insulin vials and syringes, carrying food and some form of concentrated carbohydrate, and arranging for SMBG or urine testing. Provisions for adequate rest time must be made, because exhaustion can lead to changes in the overall condition.

Before discharge from the hospital, the patient should verbalize an understanding of how to prevent complications and display an interest in maintaining optimal wellness (see the Cultural Considerations box). Stress the importance of regular medical checkups. The social aspects of DM cannot be ignored. Patients need to learn about lifestyle adjustment and should wear a medical alert bracelet or necklace, and carry medical information wallet cards at all times. Decisions such as whether to attempt pregnancy should be considered thoroughly by women with DM. Above all, the patient must accept the responsibility for self-care and recognize that making the right choices can affect life expectancy and quality. A current trend is for hospitals to employ a diabetes nurse specialist to develop and implement patient and staff education (see the Home Care Considerations box).

Cultural Considerations

Chronic Conditions

- When caring for a patient with a chronic condition, the health care team should identify the patient's cultural background, values, and beliefs to identify appropriate regimens. This is particularly important in a condition such as DM, which may require major lifestyle changes for successful management.
- In assessing patients, it is important to consider the best way to communicate across cultures. For example, Asian and Mexican cultures consider asking a direct question and expecting a direct answer to be ill mannered and rude. Phrasing questions in a more indirect way fosters more effective communication.

Home Care Considerations

Diabetes Mellitus

- Most of the education for the patient with DM is provided outside of the hospital environment.
- Frequently, older adults have difficulty with mobility and changes in vision that may hamper the drawing up of insulin.
- Often there is missing information as to why control cannot be obtained; that missing link may be found during a home visit.
- DM caregivers and home care agencies often team up to provide specific care for the older adult.
- Home care personnel network with other community resources to improve the older adult's quality of life or help deal with economic issues.
- Diabetic management should include education in the following:
    - Motivation
    - Self-monitoring of blood glucose
    - Exercise
    - Nutrition therapy
    - Medications
    - Written treatment plan

Prognosis

Although the life expectancy for the person with DM usually is decreased, current research and recent advances have led to hope for a much better prognosis. Early diagnosis and prompt, accurate treatment are essential in promoting longevity. Quality of life has been enhanced by better ways to control hyperglycemia and by earlier recognition of developing complications. Life expectancy and quality of life are related directly to glycemic control.

TYPE 2 DIABETES MELLITUS

Etiology

Type 2 diabetes mellitus usually occurs in people who are older than 35 years of age, with about half of the people diagnosed being older than 55 at diagnosis. About 80% to 90% of patients with type 2 DM are overweight at the time of diagnosis. Type 2 DM often is diagnosed after the patient has suffered from high cholesterol, high blood pressure, obesity, and insulin resistance for some time. These disorders further complicate the type 2 patient's prognosis in terms of cardiovascular and neurologic risk factors. Most newly diagnosed patients with type 2 DM have had the disease for as long as 10 years without treatment and therefore have been at risk for serious complications before diagnosis.

Pathophysiology

The pathophysiologic factors that have been identified in type 2 DM include (1) decreased tissue (e.g., fat, muscle) responsiveness to insulin as a result of receptor or postreceptor defects; (2) overproduction of insulin early in the disease, but eventual decreased secretion of insulin (the result of beta cell exhaustion); and (3) abnormal hepatic glucose regulation. These factors result in what is often referred to as *peripheral insulin resistance*. This resistance stimulates increased insulin production as a compensatory response, which also may predispose the patient to weight gain.

Clinical Manifestations

Patients with type 2 DM have few classic symptoms. The patient is usually not prone to ketoacidosis except during periods of stress. The patient may be asymptomatic in the early stages of the disease but later may complain of symptoms associated with type 1, plus many others. These patients may not seek medical care until a severe complication such as kidney involvement, retinopathy, impotence, neuropathy, or gangrene occurs.

Assessment

The assessments for type 2 DM are similar to those of type 1. However, rather than weight loss and muscle wasting, most of these patients remain obese.

Diagnostic Tests

The diagnostic tests for type 2 DM are similar to those for type 1.

Medical Management

Patients with type 2 DM are encouraged to manage their disease with diet (control of carbohydrates and calories) as well as exercise. If cardiovascular disease is a concern, education to modify the diet is vital. The patient needs instruction in managing appropriate carbohydrates, calories, sodium (if hypertensive), fat, and cholesterol (if at risk for cardiovascular disease) and maintaining a healthy weight. Weight loss for the obese patient with type 2 DM tends to reverse this problem. Oral hypoglycemic agents are considered when the patient is unable to maintain normal glucose levels with the above-described lifestyle changes. In some cases, insulin is added to the treatment regimen to further control the disorder. These medications increase insulin production, improve cell receptor binding, regulate hepatic glucose production, and delay carbohydrate absorption from the small intestine.

When a patient with type 2 DM is hospitalized or otherwise experiences decreased mobility, medications (such as steroids), infection, and stress, the blood glucose levels often rise. The patient may require insulin to further manage blood glucose levels.

Oral hypoglycemics. *Oral hypoglycemic medications* are compounds used to treat type 2 DM, each having a different mechanism of action. Oral hypoglycemic agents are not oral insulin or a substitute for insulin. The patient must have some functioning insulin production for oral hypoglycemics to be effective.

Five classes of oral drugs—sulfonylureas, meglitinides, alpha-glucosidase inhibitors, thiazolidinediones, and biguanide—are available for patients whose insulin production or use is inadequate because of type 2 DM (Table 51.7):

- *Sulfonylureas:* Sulfonylureas have blood glucose–lowering effects. They stimulate the pancreas to release insulin. A second generation of sulfonylureas, approved for use in the United States, includes glipizide (Glucotrol XL), glyburide (Diabeta, Glynase), and glimepiride (Amaryl). They are more potent than previous drugs and do not require renal excretion.
- *Meglitinides:* Meglitinides are a class of oral hypoglycemics that stimulate increased insulin release in the pancreas; they include repaglinide (Prandin) and nateglinide (Starlix).
- *Alpha-glucosidase inhibitors:* Alpha-glucosidase inhibitors are another class of oral hypoglycemics; they lower blood glucose by delaying carbohydrate absorption from the small intestine. This drug class includes acarbose (Precose) and miglitol (Glyset). The best way to gauge the effectiveness of therapy with acarbose and miglitol is to monitor the patient's 2-hour postprandial blood glucose level.
- *Thiazolidinediones:* Thiazolidinediones are a class of oral hypoglycemic medications that lower blood glucose by increasing insulin sensitivity at the insulin receptor sites on the cells. The two drugs currently

Table 51.7 Five Classes of Oral Hypoglycemics

GENERIC NAME (TRADE NAME)	ACTION
Sulfonylureas	
glimepiride (Amaryl) glipizide (Glucotrol, Glucotrol XL) glyburide (Diabeta, Glynase)	Insulin secretagogues (i.e., chemicals triggering insulin release) primarily stimulate beta cells of the pancreas to release insulin, particularly in the early course of type 2 DM. Sulfonylureas increase the sensitivity to insulin at receptor sites.
Meglitinides	
nateglinide (Starlix) repaglinide (Prandin)	Insulin secretagogues, like the sulfonylureas, stimulate beta cells in the pancreas to increase insulin release. Their effects, which are glucose dependent, decrease when the patient's blood glucose level decreases. Requires functioning pancreatic beta cells.
Biguanides	
metformin (Glucophage, Glucophage XR, fotamet, Riomet)	Metformin works primarily by reducing hepatic glucose production and lowers fasting blood glucose levels. It also enhances tissue response to insulin and improves glucose transport into the cells.
Alpha-Glucosidase Inhibitors	
acarbose (Precose) miglitol (Glyset)	Alpha-glucosidase inhibitors compete with intestinal enzymes to digest carbohydrates. They delay carbohydrate absorption from the small intestine.
Thiazolidinediones	
pioglitazone (Actos) rosiglitazone (Avandia)	Thiazolidinediones increase insulin sensitivity at insulin receptor sites on the cells. They are most appropriate for adults whose bodies produce insulin but cannot use it because of inadequate or ineffective insulin receptor sites.

Data from Funnel MM, Barlage DL: Managing diabetes with "Agent Oral." *Nursing* 2004;34(3):36–40.

Table 51.8 Insulin-Enhancing Drugs

GENERIC NAME (TRADE NAME)	ACTION
pramlintide (Symlin); administered subQ	A synthetic form of amylin, a pancreatic hormone that slows gastric emptying and suppresses the release of glucagon and the formation of glycogen in the liver. Used as an adjunct to insulin therapy in patients with type 1 or type 2 DM. It carries a black box warning because of its potential to cause severe hypoglycemia within 3 h of administration.
exenatide (Byetta); administered subQ	Incretin mimetics. Designed for use in patients with type 2 DM. Incretins are gut hormones that promote insulin secretion during a meal, suppress glucagon release, and delay gastric emptying, which effectively reduces postprandial blood glucose level. It is not indicated for use with insulin.

Data from Bass A, Will T, Todd M, et al: The latest tools for patients with diabetes. *RN* 70(6):39–43, 2007.

available in this class are rosiglitazone (Avandia) (see Table 51.7) and pioglitazone (Actos). They are most appropriate for adults whose bodies produce insulin but cannot use it because of inadequate or ineffective insulin receptor sites.

- *Biguanides:* Metformin (Glucophage) is a *biguanide* glucose-lowering agent. It works primarily by reducing hepatic glucose production and lowers fasting blood glucose levels. It also enhances the tissue response to insulin and improves glucose transport into cells. Metformin usually does not promote weight gain and may help improve lipid levels. Metformin is used widely by itself and in combination with a sulfonylurea. Combined glyburide-metformin (Glucovance) is another oral hypoglycemic agent that may be prescribed.

Once an oral drug becomes ineffective, simple substitution rarely works. But combination therapy can be highly effective. For example, oral drugs from two or more classes may be combined, or an oral drug may be combined with a bedtime dose of NPH or glargine insulin or detemir. Metformin and insulin are chosen commonly for combination therapy with sulfonylureas (Funnel and Barlage, 2004).

Other treatments. In addition to pramlintide (Symlin), exenatide (Byetta) can be used as an adjunct to insulin therapy for type 2 DM. It stimulates release of insulin from the pancreatic beta cells, decreases glucagon secretion, increases satiety, and decreases gastric emptying (Table 51.8). However, the US Food and Drug

Administration (2009) warns that it may increase the risk for kidney problems; labeling changes include dosing cautions and contraindications in patients with renal impairment.

GESTATIONAL DIABETES

Etiology

Risk factors for gestational diabetes include age over 25 years, family or personal history of diabetes or prediabetes, excess weight (body mass index >30), and nonwhite race. Complications include increased birth weight of baby (typically more than 9 lb [4.1 kg]), preterm delivery with respiratory distress syndrome, hypoglycemia in the infant after delivery, and risk for the mother to develop type 2 DM late in life (Mayo Clinic, 2017).

Clinical Manifestations

Signs and symptoms of gestational diabetes are consistent with type 2 DM.

Assessment

The health care provider checks for gestational diabetes during the pregnant patient's prenatal visits, especially during the last half of the pregnancy.

Medical Management

The goal of therapy is to maintain a normal glucose level during pregnancy, using insulin, diet, and exercise as deemed appropriate by the health care provider. By maintaining normal glucose levels during pregnancy, the patient can decrease the risk of complications significantly.

❖ NURSING PROCESS FOR THE PATIENT WITH AN ENDOCRINE DISORDER

The role of the licensed practical nurse/licensed vocational nurse (LPN/LVN) in the nursing process as stated is that the LPN/LVN will do the following:

- Participate in planning care for patients based on patient needs
- Review patient's care plans and recommend revisions as needed
- Review and follow defined prioritization for patient care
- Use clinical pathways, care maps, or care plans to guide and review patient care

◆ ASSESSMENT

Hormones affect every body tissue and system, causing diverse signs and symptoms of endocrine dysfunction. Endocrine disorders may have nonspecific or specific clinical manifestations. Some specific signs of endocrine dysfunction are the classic "*polys*" (polyuria, polydipsia, and polyphagia) in DM and exophthalmos in hyperthyroidism. Specific signs make the assessment easier, whereas nonspecific signs and symptoms, such as tachycardia, fatigue, and depression, are more problematic.

◆ PATIENT PROBLEM

Patient problems are determined from careful examination of patient data. Patient problem statements for the patient with an endocrine disorder may include but are not limited to the following:

- *Compromised Maintenance of Health*
- *Distorted Body Image*
- *Impaired Coping*
- *Impaired Neurovascular Function*
- *Impaired Sexual Function*
- *Inability to Tolerate Activity*
- *Insufficient Knowledge*
- *Insufficient Nutrition*
- *Noncooperation or Nonconformity*
- *Potential for Impaired Self-Esteem due to Current Situation*
- *Potential for Inadequate Fluid Volume*
- *Potential for Infection*
- *Potential for Injury*

◆ EXPECTED OUTCOMES AND PLANNING

The plan for management of patients with endocrine disorders must center on education to enable patients to understand their disorders, develop a healthy lifestyle, and prevent complications of their disease.

The care plan focuses on accomplishing individual goals and outcomes that relate to the identified patient problems. Examples of these include the following:

Goal 1: Patient will demonstrate safety in self-injections of insulin.

Evaluation: Patient independently administers insulin injection safely and accurately.

Goal 2: Patient will demonstrate SMBG.

Evaluation: Patient performs SMBG accurately.

◆ IMPLEMENTATION

A major nursing responsibility is to help patients gain self-management skills for their chronic endocrine disorder through teaching and counseling. Self-management skills are probably the major factor in controlling the health problem and maintaining an optimal quality of life. Self-management skills are implemented through education in the disease process, the management of medications, the management of nutrition, and the role of exercise; SMBG; hygiene; the prevention of complications; and assistance with psychological adjustment.

◆ EVALUATION

During and after patient educational teaching on self-management skills, assist in evaluating the success of the teaching by noting patient progress, based on stated goals and outcomes. For example, when the patient performs SMBG, observe the patient's skill, correct him or her as necessary, and evaluate the patient's technique to ensure accuracy. When patients are unable to meet expected outcomes, be ready to revise the care plan to promote success.

Get Ready for the NCLEX® Examination!

Key Points

- Endocrine glands are ductless glands that release chemicals (hormones) into the bloodstream to regulate body activities.
- The pituitary gland, located in the brain, is the master gland of the endocrine system.
- Hormones have a generalized effect on metabolism, growth and development, and reproduction.
- Endocrine glands regulate themselves by a series of negative feedback messages.
- Hormones secreted by the endocrine glands affect tissues of the entire body, and an imbalance in their levels may contribute to pathologic changes in many different systems.
- Acromegaly and gigantism, disorders of the pituitary gland, result in growth changes that may have a negative effect on the patient's self-image and self-esteem.
- Diabetes insipidus is a disorder of the posterior pituitary and must not be confused with diabetes mellitus, a disorder of the pancreas.
- Clinically, SIADH is characterized by hyponatremia and water retention that progresses to water intoxication.
- When caring for the patient with hyperthyroidism, provide for adequate rest periods and be sure that fluid and food intake meet the patient's nutritional needs.
- The emotions of the patient with hyperthyroidism are labile, so try to eliminate sources of stress from the environment, to help prevent emotional trauma.
- ^{131}I should not be administered to a pregnant patient because of risk to the fetus; nurses who are pregnant should not care for these patients.
- The thyroidectomy patient faces three life-threatening postoperative complications: hemorrhage, tetany, and thyroid crisis.
- The patient with hypothyroidism may experience sluggish mental and physical functioning, so be patient and allow adequate time for nursing routines.
- The prognosis for papillary adenocarcinoma of the thyroid is excellent because few of these tumors metastasize.
- When administering IV calcium chloride to any patient, be careful that none of the drug extravasates because tissue sloughing may result.
- The extreme hypertension often seen in patients with pheochromocytoma may result in cerebrovascular accident.
- Depression is common in patients who suffer from Cushing's syndrome; be alert for suicidal thoughts and suicide attempts.
- The four main facets of medical treatment for the patient with DM are diet, SMBG, exercise, and medication.
- Type 1 DM usually is diagnosed first in people younger than 30 years of age; type 2 DM is found more commonly after age 35, and the incidence increases with age.
- As insulin resistance progresses, the pancreas secretes greater amounts of insulin to compensate. This in turn leads to progressive beta cell failure and a lessening of insulin production. Both beta cell dysfunction and insulin resistance are required for the development of hyperglycemia, the central metabolic characteristic of type 2 DM.
- The older person with diabetes may have a high blood glucose level before excreting any into the urine because of an increased renal threshold for glucose.
- The diabetic diet must be individualized, taking into consideration many factors, such as age, lifestyle, food preferences, and the ability to cook and store food.
- The person with type 1 DM must have access to a source of quick glucose at all times, in the event of a hypoglycemic reaction.
- Become familiar with the clinical manifestations of DKA, HHNC, and hypoglycemic reaction to properly assess diabetic patients, respond therapeutically, and educate them in self-care.
- Observe patients on insulin therapy and oral hypoglycemic medications during the time of peak action of the medication, and initiate treatment promptly if hypoglycemia develops.
- The nurse must be knowledgeable about various insulin types and characteristics.
- Two new insulin-enhancing drugs given subcutaneously are pramlintide and exenatide.
- There are five classes of oral hypoglycemic drugs: sulfonylureas, meglitinides, biguanides, alpha-glucosidase inhibitors, and thiazolidinediones.
- DKA can result in seizures, brain damage, or death for the patient with type 1 DM.

Additional Learning Resources

SG Go to your Study Guide for additional learning activities to help you master this chapter content.

evolve Be sure to visit the Evolve site at *http://evolve.elsevier.com/Cooper/foundationsadult/* for additional online resources.

Review Questions for the NCLEX® Examination

1. Which hormones are responsible for "fight or flight"?
   1. Estrogen and testosterone
   2. FSH and LH
   3. Epinephrine and norepinephrine
   4. Calcitonin and parathyroid hormone
2. Which hormones are responsible for blood calcium levels?
   1. Calcitonin and parathyroid hormone
   2. Estrogen and progesterone
   3. Melatonin and follicle-stimulating hormone (FSH)
   4. Thyroxine and parathyroid hormone
3. What is the master gland of the body?
   1. Thyroid gland
   2. Adrenal gland
   3. Pineal gland
   4. Pituitary gland

4. Early in the day, a patient had a subtotal thyroidectomy. During evening rounds, you assess the patient, who now has nausea, a temperature of 105°F (40.5°C), tachycardia, and extreme restlessness. What is the most likely cause of these signs?
   1. Diabetic ketoacidosis
   2. Thyroid crisis
   3. Hypoglycemia
   4. Tetany
5. The nurse is caring for a patient recovering from a total thyroidectomy. The first night the patient experiences signs and symptoms of postoperative tetany. Which medication should the nurse anticipate will be ordered by the health care provider?
   1. Sodium iodide PO
   2. Potassium chloride IV
   3. Magnesium sulfate IM
   4. Calcium gluconate IV
6. The nurse is caring for a patient who had cranial surgery to remove a pituitary tumor 3 days ago, leaving the patient with partial left hemiparesis and diabetes insipidus. Which patient problem is of the greatest priority postoperatively?
   1. *Potential for Inadequate Fluid Volume, related to excessive loss via the urinary system*
   2. *Despair, related to development of chronic illness (hemiparesis and diabetes insipidus)*
   3. *Potential for Compromised Oral Mucous Membranes, related to dehydration*
   4. *Potential for Impaired Family Coping, related to chronic illness*
7. A male patient has hypoglycemia. To control hypoglycemic episodes, the nurse should recommend which of the following?
   1. Increasing saturated fat intake and fasting in the afternoon
   2. Increasing intake of vitamins B and D and taking iron supplements
   3. Eating a candy bar if light-headedness occurs
   4. Consuming a low-carbohydrate, high-protein diet and avoiding fasting
8. The nurse is assessing a postoperative thyroidectomy patient for damage to the laryngeal nerve. Which is most likely to suggest that damage may have occurred?
   1. The patient complains of a slight sore throat.
   2. The patient's voice tone has changed slightly.
   3. The patient is unable to swallow fluids.
   4. The patient is becoming increasingly hoarse.
9. The nurse is reviewing the plan of care for a patient newly diagnosed with type 1 diabetes mellitus. Which is the greatest priority in the care plan?
   1. Teach the patient the effect of diet, exercise, and insulin on the blood glucose level.
   2. Refer the patient to the hospital dietitian for education about dietary needs.
   3. Instruct the patient on SMBG, observe return demonstrations, and correct the technique as needed.
   4. Review with the patient the desired effects of his medication, as well as possible side effects.
10. The nurse is educating a patient who has had type 1 diabetes for the past year. Which statement demonstrates his need for additional teaching?
   1. "If I want to lose weight, all I have to do is increase my dose of insulin."
   2. "I can have an occasional beer if it's calculated into my diet."
   3. "I will maintain better control of my blood sugar if I eat regular meals."
   4. "It is important that I eat properly, exercise regularly, and take my insulin injections."
11. The nurse is caring for a patient diagnosed with Addison's disease (adrenal hypofunction). The nurse's assessment reveals postural hypotension, fatigue, nausea, vomiting, and poor skin turgor. Which of these patient problems is of greatest priority at this time?
   1. *Potential for Infection*
   2. *Potential for Inability to Regulate Body Temperature*
   3. *Pain*
   4. *Potential for Inadequate Fluid Volume*
12. The nurse is caring for a patient who states the health care provider is prescribing an insulin that "takes effect in less than half the time of regular (short-acting) insulin." The nurse is aware that this patient has been prescribed which type of insulin?
   1. Humulin R, Novolin R
   2. Lispro (Humalog), aspart (NovoLog)
   3. Humulin N, Novolin N
   4. Humulin 70/30, Novolin 70/30
13. The nurse is aware that the polydipsia and polyuria experienced by a patient with poorly controlled diabetes are caused primarily by which of the following?
   1. The release of ketones from cells during fat metabolism
   2. Fluid shifts resulting from the osmotic effect of hyperglycemia
   3. Damage to the kidneys from exposure to high levels of glucose
   4. Changes in RBCs resulting from attachment of excessive glucose to hemoglobin
14. The nurse is planning care for an elderly patient with type 2 diabetes admitted to the hospital with pneumonia. What should the nurse understand about this patient?
   1. Must receive insulin therapy to prevent the development of ketoacidosis
   2. Has islet cell antibodies that have destroyed the ability of the pancreas to produce insulin
   3. Has minimal or absent endogenous insulin secretion and requires daily insulin injections
   4. May have sufficient endogenous insulin to prevent ketosis but is at risk for development of hyperosmolar coma
15. Which is an appropriate instruction for the patient with diabetes related to care of the feet?
   1. Use heat to increase blood supply.
   2. Avoid softening lotions and creams.
   3. Inspect all surfaces of the feet daily.
   4. Use iodine to disinfect cuts and abrasions.

16. The nurse is conducting a class for patients with diabetes in the community. What information should the nurse include in the educational plan? *(Select all that apply.)*
    1. Regular insulin (Humulin R) has an onset of action of 30 minutes to 1 hour.
    2. Lispro (Humalog) has an onset of action of 15 minutes.
    3. NPH (Humulin N) has an onset of action of 2 hours.
    4. Glargine (Lantus) has an onset of action of 6 to 10 hours.
    5. Lantus has a peak of 8 to 10 hours.
17. In the syndrome of inappropriate antidiuretic hormone (SIADH), what best describes the body's secretions?
    1. Too much antidiuretic hormone
    2. Too little antidiuretic hormone
    3. Too much diuretic hormone
    4. Too little diuretic hormone
18. The nurse is aware that SIADH is characterized by which clinical characteristics? *(Select all that apply.)*
    1. Peripheral edema
    2. Hyponatremia
    3. Water retention
    4. Brain cells becoming edematous
    5. Intake equal to output
19. The nurse is providing care to a patient with SIADH. What can most likely be anticipated to be included in the health care provider's orders?
    1. Increased fluid intake to 3000 mL/day
    2. Fluid restriction to 800 to 1000 mL/day
    3. Discontinue the ordered diuretics
    4. Antiemetics for complaints of nausea
20. The nurse is reviewing the plan of care for a patient with syndrome of inappropriate antidiuretic hormone (SIADH). What would nurse would include in the interventions? *(Select all that apply.)*
    1. Daily weight
    2. I&O
    3. Fluid restriction
    4. Foods high in sodium
    5. Assessment for abdominal sounds
21. The nurse is teaching a diabetic education class in the community. What information should the nurse include in the educational plan?
    1. Exercise leads to a decreased need for insulin.
    2. Insulin should be adjusted on the basis of the amount of protein ingested at each meal.
    3. During illness, the patient should avoid all insulin injections.
    4. Slow-healing wounds are expected and do not have to be reported to the health care provider.
22. What is an appropriate nursing intervention for a patient admitted into the hospital with signs and symptoms of diabetic ketoacidosis?
    1. Obtain blood glucose immediately.
    2. Administer NPH insulin intravenously.
    3. Give intravenous glucagon.
    4. Take vital signs every 4 hours.
23. Which is a principal clinical manifestation in the patient with pheochromocytoma?
    1. Darkly pigmented skin and mucous membranes
    2. Moonface and buffalo hump
    3. Severe hypertension
    4. Carpopedal spasms

52 Care of the Patient With a Reproductive Disorder

http://evolve.elsevier.com/Cooper/foundationsadult/

Objectives

Anatomy and Physiology

1. List and describe the functions of the organs of the male and female reproductive tracts.
2. Discuss menstruation and the hormones necessary for a complete menstrual cycle.

Medical-Surgical

3. Discuss the impact of illness on the patient's sexuality.
4. Discuss nursing interventions for the patient undergoing diagnostic studies related to the reproductive system.
5. Discuss the importance of the Papanicolaou test in early detection of cervical cancer and mammography as a screening procedure for breast cancer.
6. List nursing interventions for patients with menstrual disturbances.
7. Discuss the etiology and pathophysiology, clinical manifestations, assessment, diagnostic tests, medical management, nursing interventions, patient teaching, and prognosis for infections of the female reproductive tract.
8. Discuss four important points to be addressed in discharge planning for the patient with pelvic inflammatory disease.
9. List four patient problems pertinent to the patient with endometriosis.
10. Identify the clinical manifestations of a vaginal fistula.
11. Describe the common problems with cystocele and rectocele and the related medical management and nursing interventions.
12. Discuss the etiology and pathophysiology, clinical manifestations, assessment, diagnostic tests, medical management, nursing interventions, patient teaching, and prognosis for cancers of the female reproductive system.
13. Identify four patient problems pertinent to ovarian cancer.
14. Describe the preoperative and postoperative nursing interventions for the patient requiring major surgery of the female reproductive system.
15. Describe six important points to emphasize in teaching breast self-examination.
16. Compare four surgical approaches for cancer of the breast.
17. Discuss adjuvant therapies for breast cancer.
18. Discuss nursing interventions for the patient who has had a modified radical mastectomy.
19. List several discharge planning instructions for the patient who has undergone a modified radical mastectomy.
20. Discuss the etiology and pathophysiology, clinical manifestations, assessment, diagnostic tests, medical management, nursing interventions, patient teaching, and prognosis for inflammatory disorders of the male reproductive system.
21. Distinguish between hydrocele and varicocele.
22. Discuss the importance of monthly testicular self-examination beginning at 15 years of age.
23. Discuss patient education related to prevention of sexually transmitted infections.

Key Terms

amenorrhea (ă-mĕn-ŏ-RĒ-ă, p. 1759)
candidiasis (kăn-dĭ-DĪ-ă-sĭs, p. 1805)
carcinoma in situ (kăr-sĭ-NŌ-mă ĭn SĪ-tū, p. 1779)
chancre (SHĂNG-kĕr, p. 1803)
Chlamydia trachomatis (klă-MĬD-ē-ă tră-KŌ-mă-tĭs, p. 1805)
circumcision (sĭr-kŭm-SĬZH-ŭn, p. 1748)
climacteric (klī-MĂK-tĕr-ĭk, p. 1765)
colporrhaphy (kŏl-PŎR-ă-fē, p. 1777)
colposcopy (kŏl-PŎS-kŏ-pē, p. 1754)
cryptorchidism (krĭp-TŎR-kĭ-dĭz-ĕm, p. 1799)
culdoscopy (kŭl-DŎS-kŏ-pē, p. 1755)
curettage (kū-rĕ-TĂHZH, p. 1756)
dysmenorrhea (dĭs-mĕn-ō-RĒ-ă, p. 1760)
endometriosis (ĕn-dō-mē-trē-Ō-sĭs, p. 1774)
epididymitis (ĕp-ĭ-dĭd-ĕ-MĪ-tĭs, p. 1797)
fistula (FĬS-tū-lă, p. 1775)
introitus (ĭn-TRŌ-ĭ-tŭs, p. 1750)
laparoscopy (lă-pă-RŎS-kō-pē, p. 1755)
mammography (măm-MŎG-ră-fē, p. 1757)
menorrhagia (mĕn-ō-RĀ-jă, p. 1763)
metrorrhagia (mĕ-trō-RĀ-jă, p. 1763)
panhysterosalpingo-oophorectomy (păn-HĬS-tĕr-ō-SĂL-pĭng-gō-ūf-ō-RĔK-tō-mē, p. 1783)
Papanicolaou test (Pap smear) (pă-pĕ-NĬ-kō-lō tĕst, smēr, p. 1755)
perimenopause (p. 1765)
phimosis (fĭ-MŌ-sĭs, p. 1798)
procidentia (prō-sĭ-DĔN-shă, p. 1776)
sentinel lymph node mapping (SĔN-tĭ-nĕl lĭmf nōd MĂP-ĭng, p. 1788)
trichomoniasis (trĭk-ō-mō-NĪ-ă-sĭs, p. 1804)

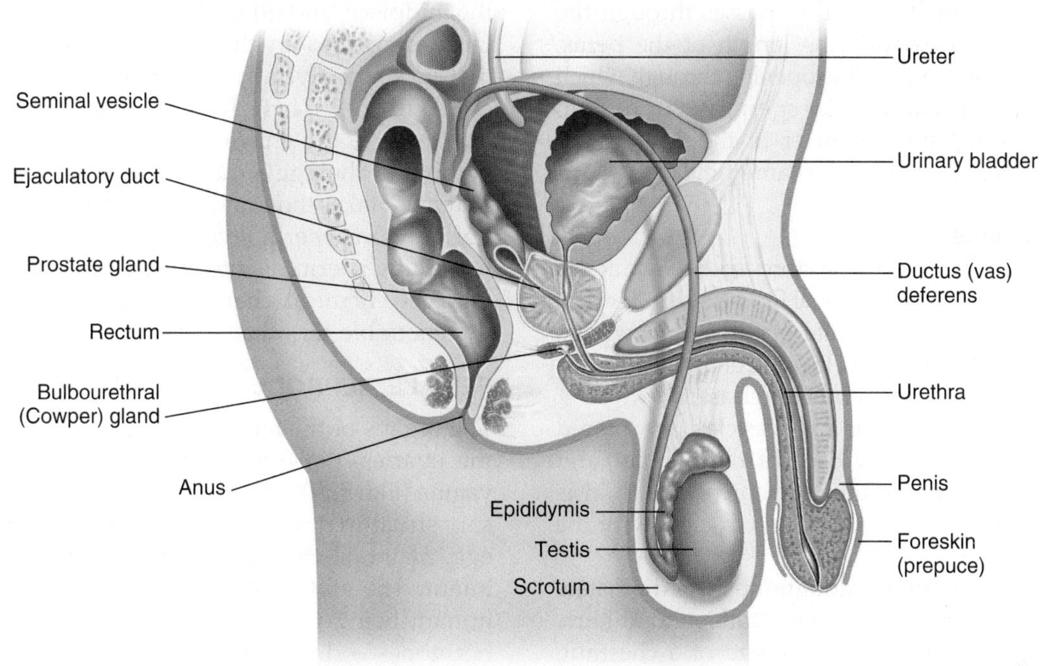

Fig. 52.1 Longitudinal section of the male pelvis, showing the location of the male reproductive organs. (From Patton KT, Thibodeau GA, Douglas MM: *Essentials of anatomy and physiology,* St. Louis, 2012, Mosby.)

The period of life from conception through birth is made possible through the dynamics of the normally functioning male and female reproductive systems. Reproduction of like individuals is necessary for the continuation of the species. The male and female sex glands *(gonads)* produce the gametes *(sperm, ova)* that unite to form a fertilized egg *(zygote),* the beginning of a new life.

ANATOMY AND PHYSIOLOGY OF THE REPRODUCTIVE SYSTEM

MALE REPRODUCTIVE SYSTEM

The organs of the male reproductive system include the testes, the ductal system, the accessory glands, and the penis (Fig. 52.1). These structures have various functions: (1) producing and storing sperm, (2) depositing sperm for fertilization, and (3) developing the male secondary sex characteristics.

Testes (Testicles)

The two oval testes (or testicles; the male gonads in animals) are enclosed in the *scrotum,* a saclike structure that lies suspended from the exterior abdominal wall. This position keeps the temperature in the testes below normal body temperature, which is necessary for viable sperm production and storage. Each testis contains one to three coiled *seminiferous tubules,* which produce the sperm cells. After puberty, millions of sperm cells are produced daily. The testes also produce the hormone *testosterone.* Testosterone is responsible for the development of male secondary sex characteristics.

Ductal System

Epididymis. Sperm produced in the seminiferous tubules immediately travel through a network of testicular ducts called the *rete testis.* These passageways contain cilia that sweep sperm out of the testes into the *epididymis,* a tightly coiled tube structure that lies superior to the testes and extends posteriorly. The smooth muscles within the walls of the epididymis contract in response to sexual stimulation. This forces the sperm to the ductus deferens.

Ductus deferens (vas deferens). The ductus deferens (also called the vas deferens) is approximately 18 inches (46 cm) long and rises along the posterior wall of the testes. As it moves upward, it passes through the inguinal canal into the pelvic cavity, loops over the urinary bladder, and joins with the ejaculatory duct. The ductus deferens and its accompanying nerves and blood vessels are enclosed in a connective tissue sheath called the *spermatic cord.* If a man chooses to be sterilized for birth control, it is a simple procedure to make small slits on either side of the scrotum and sever the ductus deferens. This procedure is called a *vasectomy.* It renders the man sterile because sperm can no longer be expelled.

Ejaculatory duct and urethra. Behind the urinary bladder, the ejaculatory duct connects the ductus deferens and seminal vesicle with the prostatic portion of the urethra. The ejaculatory duct is only 1 inch (2.5 cm) long. It unites with the urethra to pass through the prostate gland. Each of the two ejaculatory ducts empties into the prostatic urethra. The urethra passes through the prostate gland and extends the length of the penis, ending at the *urinary meatus* (the opening through which urine passes). The urethra carries sperm and urine, but, because of the urethral sphincter at the base of the bladder, it does not do so at the same time.

Accessory Glands

The ductal system transports and stores sperm. The accessory glands, which produce seminal fluid (semen), include the seminal vesicles, the prostate gland, and Cowper's glands. With each ejaculation (2 to 5 mL of fluid), approximately 200 to 500 million sperm are released.

- *Seminal vesicles:* The seminal vesicles are paired structures that lie at the base of the bladder and produce 60% of the volume of semen. The fluid is released into the ejaculatory ducts to meet with the sperm.
- *Prostate gland:* The single, doughnut-shaped prostate gland surrounds the neck of the bladder and urethra. It is a firm structure, about the size of a chestnut, composed of muscular and glandular tissue. The prostate secretes alkaline fluid that contributes to the motility of sperm. Smooth muscle of the prostate contracts during ejaculation, expelling semen along the urethra. The ejaculatory duct passes obliquely through the posterior part of the gland. The prostate gland often hypertrophies with age, expanding to surround the urethra and making voiding difficult.
- *Cowper's glands:* Cowper's glands are two pea-sized glands under the male urethra. They correspond to Bartholin's glands in women and provide lubrication during sexual intercourse.

Urethra and Penis

The male urethra has two purposes: conveying urine from the bladder and carrying sperm to the outside. The cylindrical penis is the organ of copulation. The shaft of the penis ends with an enlarged tip called the *glans penis.* The skin covering the penis, called the *prepuce,* or *foreskin,* lies in folds around the glans. This excess tissue sometimes is removed in a surgical procedure called **circumcision** to prevent phimosis (tightness of the prepuce of the penis that prevents retraction of the foreskin over the glans).

Three masses of erectile tissue, the *corpus spongiosum* and two *corpora cavernosa,* contain numerous sinuses that fill the shaft of the penis. With sexual stimulation the sinuses fill with blood, causing the penis to become erect. Sexual stimulation concludes with ejaculation, which is brought about by peristalsis of the reproductive ducts and contraction of the prostate gland. After ejaculation, the penis returns to a flaccid state.

Sperm

Spermatogenesis (the process of developing spermatozoa) begins at puberty and continues throughout life. Mature sperm consist of three distinct parts: (1) the head; (2) the midpiece; and (3) the tail, which propels the sperm. Once deposited in the female reproductive system, mature sperm live approximately 48 hours (or in some cases up to 5 days). If they come in contact with a mature egg, the enzyme on the head of each sperm bombards the egg in an attempt to break down its coating. It takes thousands of sperm to break the coating, but only one sperm enters and fertilizes the egg. The remaining sperm disintegrate. Once fertilization takes place, a chemical change occurs, making the ovum impenetrable for other sperm.

FEMALE REPRODUCTIVE SYSTEM

The organs of the female reproductive system include the ovaries, the uterus, the fallopian tubes, and the vagina (Fig. 52.2). These organs, along with a few accessory structures, produce the ovum, house the fertilized egg, maintain the embryo, and nurture the newborn infant. The ability to conceive and nurture this new human being requires the intricate balance of many hormones and the menstrual cycle.

Ovaries

The paired ovaries (the female gonads in animals) are the size and shape of almonds. They are located bilateral to the uterus and immediately inferior to the fallopian fimbriae. Each ovary contains 30,000 to 40,000 microscopic ovarian follicles. At puberty they release progesterone and the female sex hormone *estrogen,* and they release a mature egg during the menstrual cycle.

Fallopian Tubes (Oviducts)

The fallopian tubes are a pair of ducts opening at one end into the *fundus* (upper portion of the uterus) and at the other end into the peritoneal cavity, over the ovary. They are approximately 4 inches (10 cm) long with the fimbriae at the distal ends. The entire inner surface of the tubes is lined with cilia. When the mature (or graafian) follicle in the ovary ruptures and releases the mature ovum, the fimbriae sweep the ovum into the fallopian tube. Fertilization takes place in the outer third of this tube, and the fertilized ovum *(zygote)* is moved through the tube by a combination of muscular peristaltic movements and the sweeping action of the cilia. If the mature ovum is not fertilized, it disintegrates.

Uterus

The uterus is shaped like an inverted pear and measures 3 inches long by 2 inches wide (7.5 × 2.5 cm) in the nonpregnant state (Fig. 52.3). It is located between the urinary bladder and the rectum and consists of three layers of tissue: (1) the *endometrium,* or inner layer; (2) the *myometrium,* or middle layer; and (3) the *perimetrium,* or outer layer. The uterus is divided into three major portions (see Fig. 52.3). The *fundus* (upper, rounded portion) is the insertion site of the fallopian tubes. The larger midsection is the *corpus* (body). The smaller,

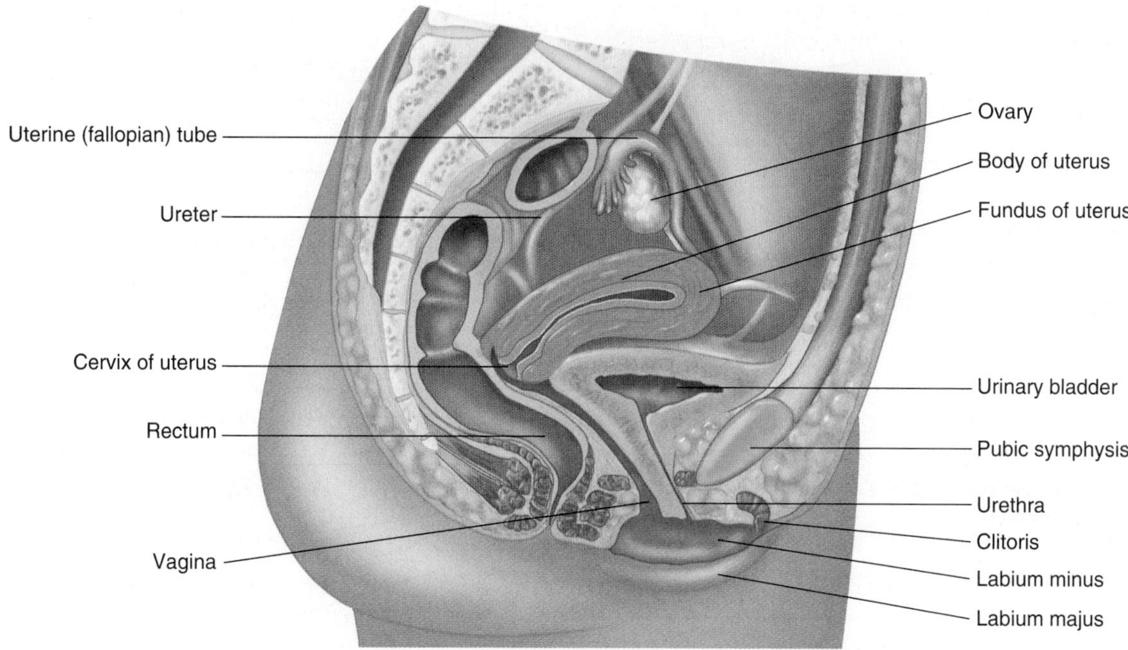

Fig. 52.2 Longitudinal section of the female pelvis, showing the location of the female reproductive organs. (From Thibodeau GA, Patton KT: *Structure and function of the body,* ed 14, St. Louis, 2012, Mosby.)

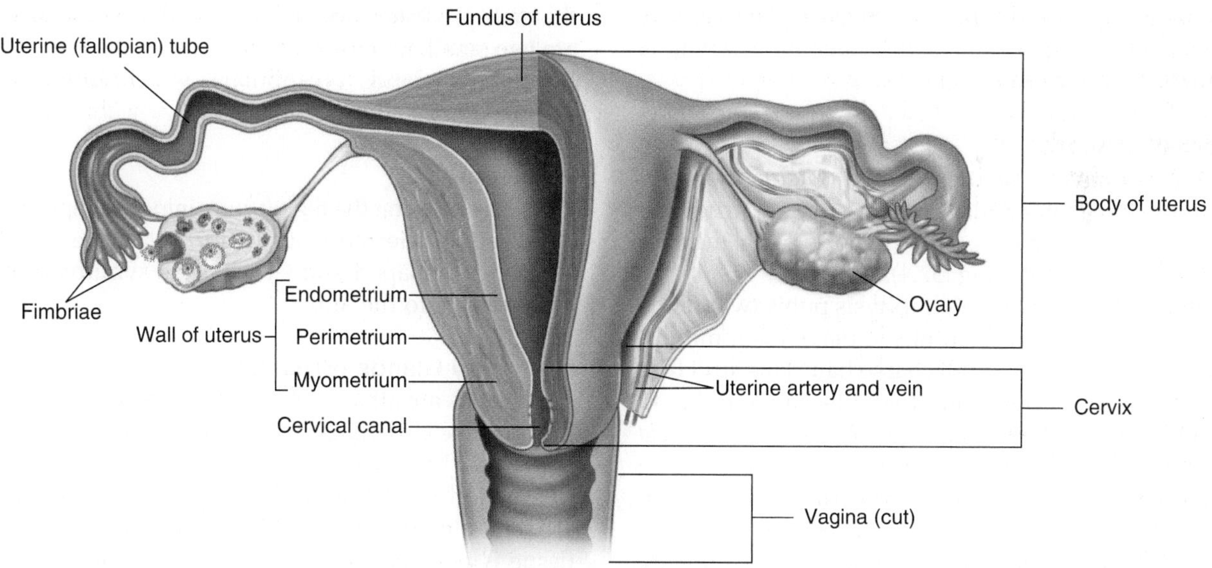

Fig. 52.3 Sectioned view of the uterus, showing its relationship to the ovaries and the vagina. (From Patton KT, Thibodeau GA: *The human body in health and disease,* ed 6, St. Louis, 2014, Mosby.)

narrower lower portion of the uterus is the *cervix,* part of which descends into the vaginal vault.

Vagina

The vagina is a thin-walled, muscular, tubelike structure of the female genitalia, approximately 3 inches (7.5 cm) long. It is located between the urinary bladder and the rectum. The superior portion articulates with the cervix of the uterus; the inferior portion opens to the outside of the body. The vagina is lined with a mucous membrane, responsible for lubrication during sexual activity. The walls of the vagina normally lie in folds called *rugae.* This enables the vagina to stretch to receive the penis during intercourse and to allow passage of the infant during birth.

The external opening of the vagina is covered by a fold of mucous membrane, skin, and fibrous tissue called the *hymen.* For centuries, some cultures considered the

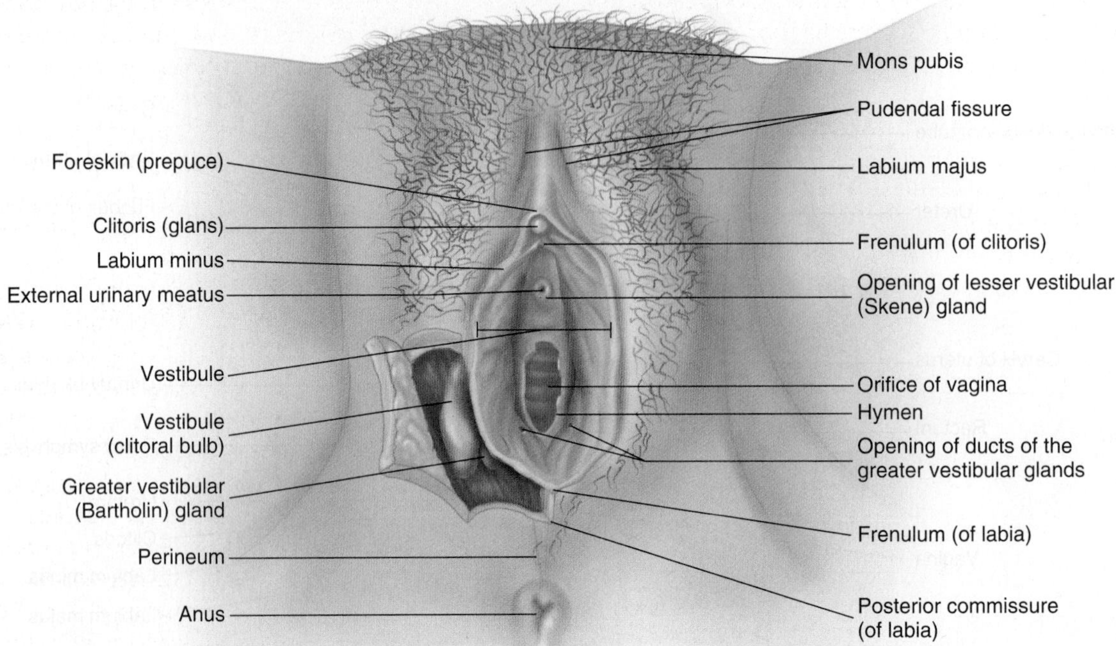

Fig. 52.4 External female genitalia (vulva). (From Patton KT, Thibodeau GA: *The human body in health and disease,* ed 6, St. Louis, 2014, Mosby.)

hymen a symbol of virginity, but it is now known that rigorous exercise or the insertion of a tampon may tear the hymen. If the hymen does remain intact, it is ruptured by *coitus* (intercourse).

External Genitalia

The reproductive structures located outside the body are the external genitalia, or *vulva*. These structures include the mons pubis, labia majora, labia minora, clitoris, and vestibule (Fig. 52.4).

Located superior to the symphysis pubis (where the iliac bones join at the front of the pelvis) is a mound of fatty tissue, covered with coarse hair. This structure is the *mons pubis.* Extending from the mons pubis to the perineal floor are two large folds called the *labia majora* (Latin, meaning "large lips"; singular, *labium majus*). These protect the inner structures and contain sensory nerve endings and an assortment of sebaceous (oil) glands and sudoriferous (sweat) glands. Directly under the labia majora lie the labia minora ("small lips"; singular, *labium minus*). These are smaller folds of tissue, devoid of hair, that merge anteriorly to form the prepuce of the clitoris. The *clitoris* is comparable to the male penis and is composed of erectile tissue that becomes engorged with blood during sexual stimulation.

The space enclosing the structures located beneath the labia minora is called the *vestibule*. It contains the clitoris, the urinary meatus, the hymen, and the vaginal opening **(introitus).**

Accessory Glands

Bilateral to the urinary meatus lie the paraurethral, or Skene's, glands, the largest glands opening into the urethra. These glands secrete mucus and are similar to the male prostate gland. Bilateral to the vaginal opening are two small, mucus-secreting glands called the greater Bartholin's glands (vestibular), which lubricate the vagina for sexual intercourse.

Perineum

The area enclosing the region containing the reproductive structures is referred to as the *perineum*. The perineum is diamond shaped and starts at the symphysis pubis and extends to the anus.

Mammary Glands (Breasts)

The breasts are attached to the pectoral (chest) muscles. Breast tissue is identifiable in both sexes. During puberty, the female breasts change their size, shape, and ability to function. Each breast contains 15 to 20 lobes, which are separated by adipose tissue. The amount of adipose tissue is responsible for the size of the breast. Within each lobe are many lobules that contain milk-producing cells; these lobules lead directly to the lactiferous ducts that empty into the nipple (Fig. 52.5).

The nipple is composed of smooth muscle that allows it to become erect. The dark pink or brown tissue surrounding the nipple is called the *areola*. Milk production does not start until a woman gives birth. At this time, under the influence of prolactin, the milk is formed. The hormone oxytocin allows milk to be released.

Menstrual Cycle

Menarche, the first menstrual cycle, usually begins at approximately 12 years of age. Each month, for the next 30 to 40 years, an ovum matures and is released about

14 days before the next menstrual flow, which occurs on average every 28 days. If fertilization occurs, menstrual cycling subsides and the body adapts to the developing fetus.

The menstrual cycle is divided into three phases: (1) menstrual, (2) preovulatory, and (3) postovulatory. This discussion uses the example of a 28-day cycle. On days 1 through 5 of the cycle (the menstrual phase), the endometrium sloughs off, accompanied by 1 to 2 ounces (30 to 60 mL) of blood loss. The anterior pituitary gland begins to release follicle-stimulating hormone (FSH); as the level of FSH increases, the egg matures within the graafian follicle (a pocket or envelope-shaped structure where the ovaries prepare the ovum; Fig. 52.6). From days 6 through 13 (preovulatory phase), estrogen is released from the maturing graafian follicle. This estrogen causes vascularization of the uterine lining. On day 14, the anterior pituitary gland releases luteinizing hormone (LH), which causes the rupture of the graafian follicle and release of the mature ovum. The finger-like projections of the fallopian tubes (fimbriae) sweep the ovum into the fallopian tube. Once this mature ovum has been expelled, the follicle is transformed into a glandular mass called the *corpus luteum*. During days 15 through 28 (postovulatory phase), the developing corpus luteum releases estrogen and progesterone. If pregnancy occurs, the corpus luteum continues to release estrogen and progesterone to maintain the uterine lining until the placenta is formed, which then takes over the job of hormonal release. If pregnancy does not occur, the corpus luteum lasts 8 days and then disintegrates. Normally the corpus luteum shrinks and is replaced by scar tissue called *corpus albicans*. At this point the hormone level decreases over several days, and menstruation starts again.

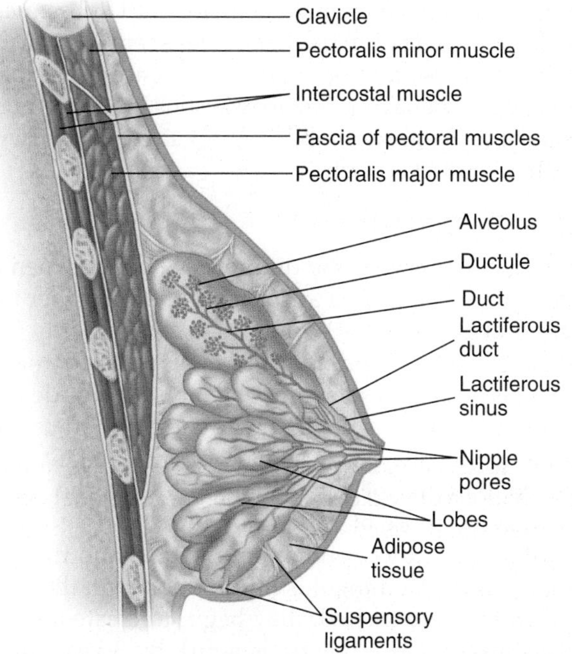

Fig. 52.5 Lateral view of the breast (sagittal section). The breast is fixed to the overlying skin and the pectoralis muscles by the suspensory ligaments of Cooper. Each lobule of secretory tissue is drained by a lactiferous duct that opens through the nipple. (From Patton KT, Thibodeau GA, Douglas MM: *Essentials of anatomy and physiology*, St. Louis, 2012, Mosby.)

EFFECTS OF NORMAL AGING ON THE REPRODUCTIVE SYSTEM

Menopause usually occurs in women between 42 and 58 years of age. The average age is 51. Whether it occurs earlier or later, menopause should not be considered abnormal. Cigarette smoking, family history, living at high altitudes, and surgical intervention or other disease management interventions are associated with early menopause. During menopause the menstrual flow ceases and hormone levels decrease. A woman may experience "hot flashes" (sudden warm feelings), which

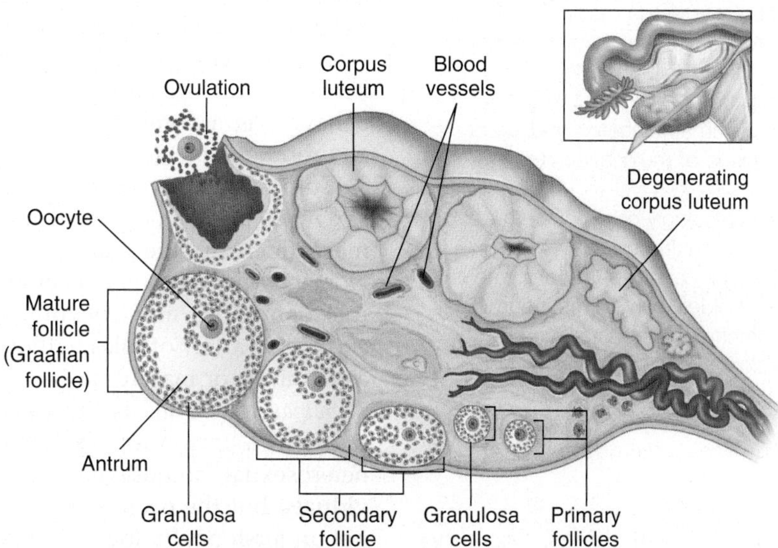

Fig. 52.6 Mammalian ovary showing successive stages of ovarian follicle and ovum development. (From Patton KT, Thibodeau GA: *Anthony's textbook of anatomy and physiology*, ed 20, St. Louis, 2013, Mosby.)

are caused by the decrease in estrogen production. Changes also occur in the reproductive organs. The vagina loses some of its elasticity, and the breasts and vulva lose some adipose tissue, resulting in decreased tissue turgor. The bones also may become brittle and prone to osteoporosis.

Hormonal changes in men are more subtle. The impact of declining hormone levels are noted but not with the same emphasis as in women. Sperm production decreases but does not cease. In later years, testosterone production decreases but not dramatically.

Basically, as long as the older individual is healthy, nothing in the aging process prohibits normal sexual function (see the Lifespan Considerations box).

Lifespan Considerations

Older Adults

Reproductive Disorders

WOMEN

- Many older women are reluctant to seek medical care for problems of the reproductive system. This may be related to cultural factors, embarrassment, or lack of knowledge. Routine gynecologic examination should continue as part of the overall physical examination, even after menopause.
- Certain forms of cancer of the reproductive tract are more common with aging. Any vaginal bleeding should be reported promptly to the health care provider, as should pelvic pain, pruritus, or skin lesions in the genital region.
- Decreased levels of estrogen and systemic diseases, such as diabetes, predispose older women to vaginitis.
- Breast cancer risk increases after 40 years of age. Breast examination should continue throughout the lifespan. The American Cancer Society (ACS) recommends an annual mammogram for women starting between ages 40 and 44 years. From age 55 women in consultation with their physician may opt to have mammograms annually or every other year (ACS, 2017a).

MEN

- Decreased production of testosterone results in changes in the male reproductive system, but the ability to procreate can continue into the eighth decade. Sexual interest often continues late in life.
- Chronic health problems, such as diabetes mellitus or hypertension, and many kinds of medication result in impotence in older men.
- Prostate enlargement is increasingly common with each decade after 40 years of age. Although this enlargement is usually benign, cancer of the prostate is a serious condition seen in older men. Ultrasonography of the prostate, when combined with rectal examination and prostate-specific antigen testing, is particularly useful in diagnosing prostate cancer.

HUMAN SEXUALITY

Sexuality and sex are two different things. *Sexuality* often is described as the sense of being a woman or a man. It has biologic, psychological, social, and ethical dimensions. Sexuality influences life experiences, and sexuality is influenced by life experiences. The term *sex* has a more limited meaning. It usually describes the biologic aspects of sexuality such as genital sexual activity. Sex may be used for pleasure or reproduction. As a result of life's changes or by personal choice, sexual activity may be absent from a person's life for brief or prolonged periods. Some persons may choose to remain celibate.

The process by which people come to know themselves as women or men is not clearly understood. Being born with female or male genitalia and subsequently learning female or male social roles seem to be factors, although these do not explain differences in sexuality and sexual behavior. Such variations are more understandable if you remember that sexuality is intertwined with all aspects of self.

SEXUAL IDENTITY

Biologic identity, or the differences between men and women, is established at conception and further influenced at puberty by hormones. *Gender identity* is the sense of being feminine or masculine. As soon as the infant is born (and sometimes before), the outside world labels the child as a girl or boy. Adults adjust their behavior to relate to a female or male infant. These varied patterns of interaction influence the infant's developing sense of gender identity.

Children explore and seek to understand their own bodies. By combining this information with the way in which they are treated, they begin to create an image of themselves as a boy or as a girl. By 3 years of age, children are aware that they will remain boys or girls and that no outward change in their appearance will alter this. This understanding is part of the development of self-concept.

Gender role is the manner in which a person acts as a woman or man. Many believe that society influences female and male behavior and is thus the primary source of femaleness or maleness. Because society encourages certain behaviors according to one's gender, differences between individuals' sexual behaviors develop. Sexual behavior is a combined interaction of biologic and environmental factors.

Cultural factors can be key ingredients in defining sex roles. Some cultures dictate roles as feminine or masculine (e.g., the man is the breadwinner, and the woman is the caregiver). Other groups have more flexible role definitions and encourage men and women to explore a variety of roles without labeling the behavior as feminine or masculine.

Sexual orientation is the clear and persistent erotic desire of a person for one sex or the other. There are heterosexual, homosexual, lesbian, and bisexual individuals, but the origins of sexual orientation are still not understood. Biologic theorists describe orientation in genetic terms, meaning it is determined at conception. Psychological theorists attribute orientation to early learning experiences, believing that cognitive processes are the determining factor. Other theorists state that genetics and environment play roles in the development of sexual preference.

For some people the inward sense of sexual identity does not match their biologic body. These people are known as *transgendered*. Researchers do not clearly understand how this mismatch occurs. Transgendered people do not see their sexual identity as a choice; it is a clear and persistent orientation dating back to early childhood. In contrast, most homosexual men and women define themselves as satisfied with their gender and social roles; they simply have a persistent sexual attraction to members of the same sex.

A *transvestite* is most often a heterosexual man who periodically dresses like a woman; however, a transvestite may be a homosexual. Cross-dressing usually is done in private and kept secret even from those who are closest to him.

Because sexuality is linked to every aspect of living, any sexual choice involves personal, family, cultural, religious, and social standards of conduct. Ideas about ethical sexual conduct and emotions related to sexuality form the basis for sexual decision making. The range of attitudes about sexuality extends from a traditional view of sex only within marriage to a point of view that allows individuals to determine what is right. Sexual choices that overstep a person's ethical standard may result in internal conflicts.

Some people may judge sexual decisions as moral or immoral solely on the basis of religious standards; others view any private sexual act between consenting adults as moral. People will always have differing beliefs about sexual ethics. The debate over sexuality-related issues such as abortion, contraception, sex education, sexual variations, and premarital or extramarital intercourse will continue. Maintain a nonjudgmental attitude while caring for all patients.

TAKING A SEXUAL HISTORY

Because overall wellness includes sexual health, sexuality should be a part of the health care program. Yet health care services do not always include sexual assessment and interventions. The area of sexuality can be an emotional one for nurses and patients.

Giving patients information about sexuality does not imply agreement with specific beliefs. Patients need accurate, honest information about the effects of illness on sexuality and the ways that sexuality contributes to health and wellness. Provide this information without influencing patient choices. Professional behavior must guarantee that patients receive the best health care possible without diminishing their self-worth. Promotion of self-education and honest examination of sexual beliefs and values can help in reducing sexual bias.

Although there is no single approach to taking a sexual history, certain principles make it more comfortable for you and for the patient (Box 52.1):

Box 52.1 Requirements for Taking a Sexual History

- Provision of privacy—a closed room
- An atmosphere of trust—ensure confidentiality
- Nurses' comfort with their own sexuality
- Nonjudgmental approach

HEALTH PROMOTION

Factors That Can Interfere With the Promotion of Sexual Health

- Lack of information
- Conflicting values system (attitudes and beliefs)
- Anxiety: Are specific attitudes, feelings, and actions "normal"?
- Guilt
- Lack of comfort with sexuality
- Invasion of privacy
- Lack of regard for hospitalized patient's need for time alone with significant other
- Manner in which the patient is touched
- Fear of being judged
- Lack of understanding of the effects of illness and treatment on sexual functioning

Box 52.2 Brief Sexual History

- Has your (illness, pregnancy, hospitalization) interfered with your being a (husband, wife, significant other, father, mother)?
- Has your (abortion, heart attack) changed the way you see yourself as a (woman, man)?
- Has your (colostomy, mastectomy, hysterectomy) changed your ability to function sexually (or altered your sex life)?

- Obtain the sexual history early in the nurse-patient relationship, which indicates permission for patients to discuss sexual concerns. Traumatic situations such as those in which a rape or assault has taken place require a slower progression in data collection.
- Avoid overreacting or underreacting to a patient's comments; this aids in truthful data collection.
- Use language that the patient understands; you and the patient may need to define terms to ensure accurate data gathering.
- Move from the less sensitive to the more sensitive areas. This promotes a certain comfort level between you and the patient.
- At the end of the sexual history, ask if the patient has additional questions or concerns.

A brief sexual history assessment can be made and included in the nursing history through the use of three questions (Box 52.2). The questions may be adapted to address illness, hospitalization, life events, or any other relevant matter that influences or interferes with sexual health. The questions also may be adjusted to find out what the patient expects to happen as a result of procedures, medications, or surgery. Often you do not need to ask the last two questions, because many patients voice their concerns about masculinity, femininity, and sexual functioning without further encouragement.

Nurses may intervene in sexual problems among patient populations through four strategies: (1) educating patient groups likely to have sexual concerns, (2) providing anticipatory guidance throughout the life cycle, (3) promoting a milieu conducive to sexual health, and (4) validating normalcy about sexual concerns.

ILLNESS AND SEXUALITY

Illness may change a patient's self-concept and result in an inability to function sexually. Medications, stress, fatigue, and depression also affect sexual functioning. Alcohol abuse can lead to a reduced sex drive and inadequate sexual functioning.

Changes in libido (sexual interest), desire, or ability fluctuate during an individual's life. A variety of factors can affect sexual libido. Health status has a strong influence on sexual interest and desire. Lack of interest or desire for sexual activity often occurs when patients are preoccupied with symptoms of illness. The sexual symptoms often disappear as patients recover from the acute phase of illness and resume sexual activity. Some illnesses—such as diabetes mellitus, end-stage renal disease, prostate cancer, certain types of prostate surgery, spinal cord injuries, and heart disease—may cause patients concern or may result in actual inability to function sexually.

Changes in the nervous system, circulatory system, or genital organs may lead to sexual health problems. Spinal cord injuries can interrupt the peripheral nerves and spinal cord reflexes that involve sexual responses. This can affect the ability to achieve orgasm. Some men and women who have spinal cord injuries have reported having satisfying orgasms in spite of denervation of pelvic structures (University of Miami/Jackson Memorial Medical Center, 2009).

An estimated 50% of men with diabetes mellitus are affected by sexual dysfunction at some point in the course of their disease. Chronic lack of glycemic control is associated with damage to vessels that serve the sex organs, resulting in an inability to achieve or maintain an erection. Sexual counseling is important to (1) provide accurate information about the sexual aspects of the disorder, (2) dispel the patient's incorrect assumptions and expectations, and (3) give advice to improve the patient's sexual self-esteem and dispel the guilt frequently found in both partners.

A mastectomy results in physical and emotional trauma. In addition to the resultant disfigurement, a patient must also grapple with the emotional implications of the cancer diagnosis and the impact of the physical changes on her relationship with her spouse or significant other. Problems that arise with pelvic irradiation for cancer of the cervix are much harder to treat than those of mastectomy; the entire physiology of the vagina is altered by the radiation, causing a true loss of function. With a mastectomy the only function lost is the ability to nurse an infant. The goal for the patient and her partner is to face the issue in a straightforward manner, acknowledging the diagnosis and discussing their true feelings. If feelings are repressed rather than shared, the patient and her significant other may suffer. Therapeutic counseling before surgery can aid the patient's and partner's acceptance and recovery after surgery.

LABORATORY AND DIAGNOSTIC EXAMINATIONS

DIAGNOSTIC TESTS FOR WOMEN

A health care provider performs the pelvic examination, which involves visualization and palpation of the vulva, the perineum, the vagina, the cervix, the ovaries, and the uterine surfaces. During the pelvic examination, specimens frequently are obtained for diagnostic purposes. The bimanual pelvic examination progresses from the visualization and palpation of the external genital organs for edema and irritations to an inspection for abnormalities of the internal organs. To visualize the cervix and vaginal mucosa a vaginal speculum (an instrument used to enlarge the vaginal opening) is inserted. The health care provider may perform a rectovaginal examination to evaluate abnormalities or problems of the rectal area and the posterior internal organs (Box 52.3).

Colposcopy

Colposcopy (*colpo*, vagina or vaginal; and *scopy*, observation) provides direct visualization of the cervix and vagina. Douching or having intercourse within 24 hours of the examination is not recommended. These activities may mask abnormal cells and reduce the specimens available for collection. Prepare the patient for a pelvic examination and explain the purpose of the procedure. Encourage the patient to void or have a bowel movement if needed. In the procedure, a speculum is inserted into the vagina. The vaginal walls may be swabbed with an iodine or vinegar solution to remove surface mucus to improve visualization. A colposcope (a microscope adapted to visualize the vaginal walls and cervix) is inserted for inspection of the area. Tissue color, the presence of growths and lesions, and vascular condition

Box 52.3 Endoscopic Procedures for Visualization of Pelvic Organs

- *Colposcopy:* Visualization of vagina and cervix under low-power magnification
- *Culdoscopy:* Insertion of a culdoscope through posterior vaginal vault into Douglas's cul-de-sac for visualization of fallopian tubes and ovaries
- *Laparoscopy:* Insertion of a laparoscope (with patient under general anesthesia) through small incision in abdominal wall (inferior margin of umbilicus), then insufflation of abdomen with carbon dioxide; permits visualization of all pelvic organs

are observed and specimens obtained as necessary. The procedure usually is not performed during menstruation (Mayo Clinic, 2018a).

Culdoscopy

Culdoscopy (*cul-de-sac;* and *scopy,* observation) is a diagnostic procedure that provides visualization of the uterus and uterine appendages (i.e., the ovaries and fallopian tubes). Before the procedure, prepare the patient for the vaginal operation with preoperative instructions. The patient is given a local, spinal, or general anesthetic. After the anesthetic is administered, the patient is assisted to a knee-chest position. The culdoscope (a thin, hollow endoscope with a camera at the end) is passed through the posterior vaginal wall. The area is examined for tumors, cysts, and endometriosis. During the procedure, *conization* (removal of eroded or infected tissue) may be done. A culdoscopy generally is performed on an outpatient basis. After the operation, assess for bleeding, assess vital signs, and monitor voiding.

Laparoscopy

Laparoscopy (examination of the abdominal cavity with a laparoscope, inserted through a small incision made beneath the umbilicus) provides direct visualization of the uterus and its appendages. Preparation of the patient includes insertion of a Foley catheter to maintain bladder decompression for an open view. The procedure is done with a general anesthetic. Carbon dioxide may be introduced to distend the abdomen for easier visualization. If a biopsy is to be done or organs are to be manipulated, a second incision may be made in the lower abdomen to allow for instrument insertion. The ovaries and fallopian tubes are observed for masses, ectopic pregnancy, adhesions, and pelvic inflammatory disease (PID). Tubal ligations may be done using this procedure. Instruct the patient of the probability of shoulder pain afterward because of carbon dioxide introduced into the abdomen.

Papanicolaou Test (Pap Smear)

The **Papanicolaou test (Pap smear)** is a simple way to detect cervical cancer in women. In this procedure, a speculum is used to widen the vagina, allowing access to the cervix. Exfoliative (i.e., peeling) and sloughed-off tissue or cells are collected from the cervix, stained, and examined.

In traditional Pap smears, the cells are spread on a glass slide and then sprayed with a fixative and sent to the laboratory for analysis. In the newer Pap tests, such as Sure Path and ThinPrep Pap test, cell specimens are obtained and then rinsed in a liquid solution. Some studies support them as being more effective in the diagnosis of cancer. The specimens must be labeled with the date, time of the last menstrual period, and whether the woman is taking estrogen or birth control pills. Instruct patients not to douche, use tampons or vaginal medications, or have sexual intercourse for at least 24 hours before the examination. Collect careful menstrual and gynecologic history.

The American Cancer Society highly recommends that every woman begin annual Pap tests within 3 years of becoming sexually active or no later than 21 years of age. Women should be tested every year (regular Pap smear) or every 3 years (ThinPrep Pap test). Women age 30 years or older may choose to have Pap screening every 3 years or, if combined with HPV screening, every 5 years instead of annually. Women age 65 years or older who have had screening over the past 10 years with normal findings may decide to stop having cervical screenings. Also, women who have had a hysterectomy may stop having cervical cancer screenings (unless their surgery was done as a treatment for cervical cancer or precancerous cells [ACS, 2016a]).

The health care provider may recommend more frequent testing for women with a history of multiple sexual partners or sexually transmitted infections (STIs), a family history of cervical cancer, or those whose mothers used diethylstilbestrol during pregnancy.

Table 52.1 provides a comparison of interpretation classifications of the cytologic findings and treatment recommendations. The Bethesda system is preferred because it allows better communication between the cytologist and the clinician. The Bethesda system evaluates the adequacy of the sample (i.e., whether or not it is satisfactory for interpretation) and provides a general classification of normal or abnormal findings and a descriptive diagnosis of the Pap smear. Although the classification system used may vary, clinicians agree it is important to monitor Pap smears and ensure proper follow-up, including treatment of vaginal infections and colposcopy if necessary.

Pap tests have long been used to look for cervical cancer and precancerous cells. Nearly all cases of cervical cancer can be attributed to high-risk types of human papillomavirus (HPV). Twelve types of HPV have been identified as being high risk. There are several tests available that can identify the presence of HPV. Most tests identify the DNA of those HPV types deemed as high risk for causing cervical cancer.

Biopsy

Biopsies are procedures in which samples of tissue are taken for evaluation to confirm or locate a lesion. Tissue is aspirated by special needles or removed by forceps or through an incision.

A breast biopsy is performed to differentiate between benign or malignant conditions of the breast. Breast biopsy is indicated for patients with palpable masses; suspicious areas appearing on mammography; and persistent, encrusted, purulent, inflamed, or sanguineous discharge from the nipples. The procedure may remove all or a portion of the suspicious growth. If the mass is palpable, the procedure is typically done on an outpatient basis.

Table 52.1 Pap Test Interpretation, Classifications, and Action

INTERPRETATION	NUMERICAL SYSTEM	DYSPLASIA CYTOLOGIC CLASSIFICATION	CIN CLASSIFICATION	BETHESDA SYSTEM[a]	ACTION
Negative (normal)	Class I	Negative squamous metaplasia	No designation	Negative (normal)	Repeat annually
Probably negative, may indicate infection	Class II	Atypical squamous cells	No designation	Infection Atypical squamous cells Reactive changes	Treat infection, repeat Pap
Suspicious, but not conclusive for malignancy	Class III	Mild dysplasia Moderate dysplasia	CIN I CIN II	Low-grade squamous intraepithelial lesion[b]	Treat infection, repeat Pap in 8–12 wk; colposcopy
More suspicious, strongly suggestive of malignancy	Class IV	Severe dysplasia Carcinoma in situ	CIN III	High-grade squamous intraepithelial lesion[b]	Colposcopy, biopsy, treatment
Conclusive for malignancy	Class V	Invasive carcinoma	Invasive carcinoma	Invasive squamous cell carcinoma	Colposcopy, biopsy, conization, treat by hysterectomy

CIN, Cervical intraepithelial neoplasia.
[a]The Bethesda system is the preferred system.
[b]The Bethesda Working Group suggests that "these two new terms encompass the spectrum of terms currently used to delineate the squamous cell precursors to invasive squamous carcinoma, including the grades of CIN, the degree of dysplasia, and carcinoma in situ."

Various techniques may be employed. The biopsy may be performed by fine needle aspiration (FNA); stereotactic or ultrasound-guided core needle biopsy, under local anesthetic; or surgical biopsy, with general or local anesthetic:

- *Fine needle aspiration:* In FNA, fluid is aspirated from a palpable breast mass and expelled into a specimen bottle. Pressure is placed on the site to stop the bleeding, and an adhesive bandage is applied. FNA may or may not require a local anesthetic, and typically is done in the health care provider's office.
- *Stereotactic or ultrasound-guided core needle biopsy:* Core needle biopsy is a reliable diagnostic technique to obtain a breast biopsy if an abnormal mass is seen on the mammogram. The skin is anesthetized, and a small incision is made. Under the guidance of ultrasound or stereotactic imaging, a biopsy gun is used to fire the core needle into the lesion to remove a sample of the mass. Compared with an open surgical biopsy, this procedure produces less scarring, requires only local anesthesia, is less expensive, and is done on an outpatient basis. Patients must be advised to stop aspirin or blood thinning products and to avoid talcum powder and deodorant the day of the procedure (Guenin, 2017).
- *Open surgical biopsy:* In an open surgical biopsy, an excisional biopsy usually is performed in a portion of the breast to expose the lesion and then remove the entire mass. Specimens of selected tissue may be frozen and stained for rapid diagnosis. The wound is sutured and a bandage applied. The incision site is monitored for bleeding, tenderness, and erythema (Johns Hopkins, n.d.).

A cervical biopsy is done to evaluate cervical lesions and to diagnose cervical cancer. The biopsy generally is done without anesthesia. A colposcope is inserted through the vaginal speculum for direct visualization, the cervical site is selected and cleansed, and tissue is removed. The area then is packed with gauze or a tampon to check the blood flow.

An endometrial biopsy is performed to collect tissue for diagnosis of endometrial cancer and analysis for infertility studies. The procedure generally is performed at the time of menstruation, when the cervix is dilated and cells are obtained more easily. The cervix is anesthetized locally, a curette (a spoon-shaped instrument used to obtain samples from the wall of a cavity) is inserted, and tissue is obtained from selected sites of the endometrium.

Other Diagnostic Studies

Conization of the cervix is used to remove eroded or infected tissue or to confirm cervical cancer. A cone-shaped section is removed when the mass is confined to the epithelial tissue. After surgery the area is packed with gauze to control bleeding. The patient is observed for bleeding and generally discharged from the hospital the same day.

Dilation and **curettage** (D&C) (*curettage* is the scraping of material from the wall of a cavity or other surface; performed to remove tumors or other abnormal tissue for microscopic study) is a procedure used to obtain tissue for biopsy, to correct cervical stricture, and to treat dysmenorrhea. The patient is placed under general anesthesia, the cervix is dilated, and the uterine walls are scraped with a curette. Packing may be inserted for hemostasis, and a perineal pad is applied for absorption of drainage. After vaginal packing is removed, instruct the patient to monitor for excessive vaginal bleeding or malodorous drainage.

Cultures and smears are collected to examine and identify infectious processes, abnormal cells, and hormonal changes of the reproductive tissue. Specimens collected for smears are prepared by spreading ("smearing") the collected cells on a glass slide and covering the sample with a second slide or spraying it with a fixative. Specimens are handled aseptically, with care taken to avoid the transfer and spread of organisms. Cultures are taken from exudates of the breast, the vagina, rectum, and urethra. STIs and mastitis are diagnosed by isolation of the causative organisms. Treatment is prescribed according to the results of the culture.

Schiller's iodine test is used for the early detection of cancer cells and to guide the health care provider in doing a biopsy. An iodine preparation is applied to the cervix, and in its presence glycogen, which is present in normal cells, stains brown. Abnormal or immature cells do not absorb the stain. Unstained areas may be biopsied. This method of detection is valuable but not entirely reliable, because normal cells sometimes lack glycogen and malignant tissue sometimes contains glycogen. After the procedure the patient should wear a perineal pad to avoid stains on the clothing.

Radiographic examinations are performed to detect abnormal tissue, locate abnormal structures, and confirm the patency of ducts.

Hysterograms and hysterosalpingograms (images of the uterus and of the uterus and fallopian tubes, respectively) (Fig. 52.7) are taken to confirm (1) tubal abnormalities (adhesions and occlusions), (2) the presence of foreign bodies, (3) congenital malformations and leiomyomas (fibroids; noncancerous uterine growths), and (4) traumatic injuries. The patient is placed in the lithotomy position. A speculum is inserted into the vagina, a cannula is inserted through the speculum into the cervical cavity, and a contrast medium is injected through the cannula. As the contrast medium progresses through the cavity, the uterus and fallopian tubes are viewed with a fluoroscope and films are taken.

Mammography is radiography of the soft tissue of the breast, done to allow identification of various benign and neoplastic processes, especially those not palpable on physical examination. Digital mammography is a newer technique that allows a clearer, more accurate image; it involves digitally coding x-ray images into a computer (traditional mammography images are captured on a film cassette). Digital images may be manipulated by the health care provider to enhance elements of concern found in the image. In addition, digital mammography is a more rapid assessment and reporting system. It is believed that the average breast tumor is present for 9 years before it is palpable; therefore the ACS recommends that mammography begin annually between the ages of 40 and 44 years (2017a).

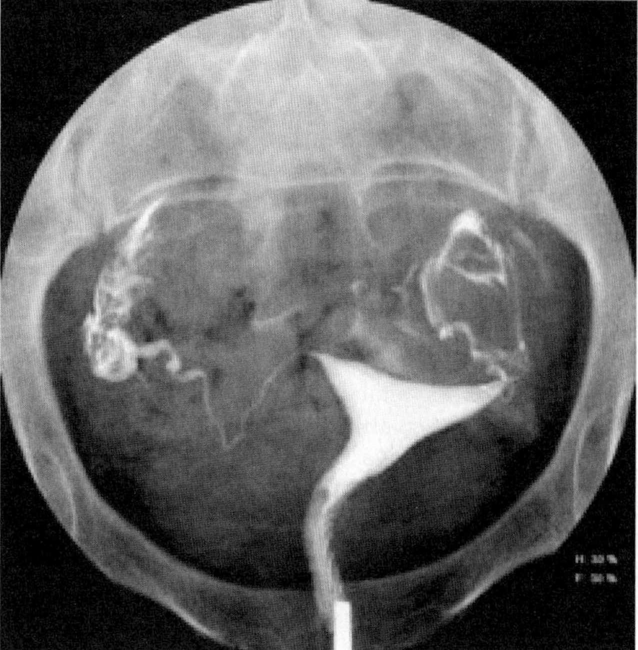

Fig. 52.7 Normal hysterosalpingogram in a young woman with primary infertility. The metal cannula within the external os is seen at the bottom of the figure. The uterine cavity and both fallopian tubes are normal in appearance. There is contrast spilling from both tubes into the pelvic peritoneal cavity, a normal finding.

When the mammography procedure is scheduled, advise the patient to refrain from using body powders, deodorants, and ointments on the breast areas, because this could cause false-positive results. Before the procedure give the patient a gown and ask her to remove jewelry and upper garments. The technician asks the patient to sit or stand in an upright position and rest one breast on the radiographic table. A compressor is placed on the breast, and the patient is asked to hold her breath as an anterior view is taken. The machine is rotated, the breast is again compressed, and a lateral view is taken. This procedure is repeated on the other breast. The patient may be asked to remain until the radiographic films are read.

Because of the greater density of breast tissue, mammography is less sensitive in younger women, which may result in more false-negative results. About 10% to 15% of all breast cancers can be detected only by palpation; they cannot be seen on mammography. Even if mammogram findings are unremarkable, all suspicious masses should be biopsied.

Women with a positive family history for breast cancer should be evaluated by mammography accompanied by magnetic resonance imaging (MRI). This testing is recommended for women with a 20% or greater chance for the development of breast cancer in their lifetimes. An MRI is not recommended as a routine screening for all eligible women because of its high cost and greater risk of false positives as compared with mammograms.

Ultrasound is used for further exploration after an examination or mammography reveals a suspicious finding. It is a helpful diagnostic tool to differentiate a benign tumor from a malignant tumor. It is useful in women who have dense breasts with fibrocystic changes. Unlike a mammogram, ultrasound will not detect microcalcifications, which are often the precursors of breast cancer.

In pelvic ultrasonography, high-frequency sound waves are passed into the area to be examined, and images are viewed on a screen; this is similar to a radiographic film. Ultrasound is useful in detecting foreign bodies (such as intrauterine contraceptive devices [IUDs]), distinguishing between cystic and solid tumor bodies, evaluating fetal growth and viability, detecting fetal abnormalities, and detecting ectopic pregnancy. In general, it is noninvasive, safe, and painless. Encourage the patient to drink fluids beforehand. Explain that a full bladder is essential to the accuracy of the test.

Tubal insufflation (Rubin's test) involves transuterine insufflation of the fallopian tubes with carbon dioxide (*insufflation* is the blowing of gas, in this case carbon dioxide, into a body cavity). The procedure enables evaluation of the patency of the fallopian tubes and may be part of a fertility study. Tubal insufflation takes approximately 30 minutes and usually is performed on an outpatient basis. If the tubes are open, the gas enters the abdominal cavity. A high-pitched bubbling is heard through the abdominal wall with a stethoscope as the gas escapes from the tubes. The patient may complain of shoulder pain from diaphragmatic irritation. In this case a radiographic film shows free gas under the diaphragm. If the tubes are occluded, gas cannot pass from the tubes, and the patient will not report pain.

All pregnancy tests, regardless of method, are based on detection of human chorionic gonadotropin (hCG), which is secreted into the urine after fertilization of the ovum. Regardless of method, it is important to know that the tests do not indicate whether the pregnancy is normal. In addition, false-positive results may occur.

Serum CA-125 is a tumor antigen associated with ovarian cancer; it is positive in 80% of such cases. CA-125 antigen levels in the blood decrease as cancer cells decrease. CA-125 has been touted as a way to detect primary ovarian cancer, but unfortunately it does not do so. CA-125 is useful mainly to signal a recurrence of ovarian cancer and to monitor the response to chemotherapy treatment. If chemotherapy causes a progressive decline in CA-125, it is an accurate indicator of a good response and is a good prognostic sign. Other conditions—such as endometriosis, PID, pregnancy, gynecologic cancers, and cancer of the pancreas—may result in an elevation of serum CA-125.

DIAGNOSTIC TESTS FOR MEN

Testicular Biopsy

Testicular biopsy is a means to detect abnormal cells and the presence of sperm. The testing can be done by aspiration or through an incision. The anesthetic used depends on the technique. Postbiopsy care measures consist of scrotal support, ice pack, and analgesic medications. Warm sitz baths for edema also may be helpful. Instruct the patient to call the health care provider if bleeding or elevated temperature occurs.

Semen Analysis

Semen analysis is often one of the first tests performed on the male when evaluating fertility. Other indications include substantiating the effectiveness of a vasectomy, detecting a specimen on a suspected rape victim, and ruling out or determining paternity. Semen can be collected for testing by manual stimulation, coitus interruptus, or the use of a condom.

Prostatic Smears

Prostatic smears are obtained to detect and identify microorganisms, tumor cells, and even tuberculosis in the prostate. The health care provider massages the prostate by way of the rectum, and the patient voids into a sterile container that has been prepared with additive preservative. The specimen is collected and a smear is prepared in the laboratory.

Cystoscopy

In cystoscopy a man's prostate and bladder can be examined by passing a lighted cystoscope (a specially adapted endoscope) through the urethra to the bladder (Mayo Clinic, n.d.) (Fig. 52.8). Before the procedure, obtain a signed consent form and educate the patient about the procedure. The procedure may be performed with sedation or anesthesia. A numbing gel may be applied to the urethra to aid in the passage of the scope. After the cystoscopy the patient may have pink-tinged urine, and greater frequency and burning on urination. Baths may be restricted by some physicians. Warm compresses can be used to promote comfort when held at the urinary opening. Cystoscopy can be done for men and women to detect bladder infections and tumors.

Other Diagnostic Studies

Other diagnostic studies for men include the rectal digital examination and the test for prostate-specific antigen

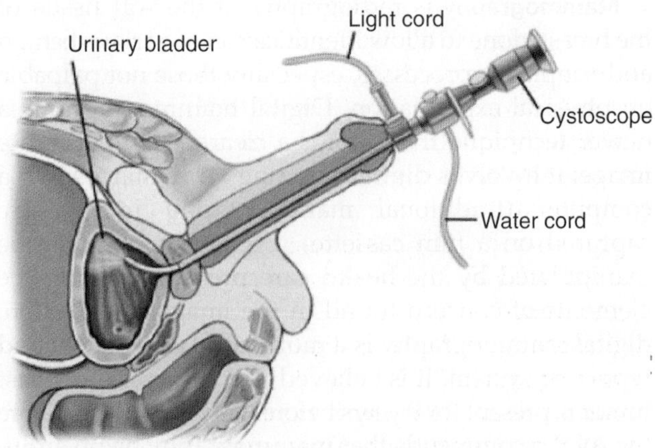

Fig. 52.8 Cystoscopy.

(PSA), a highly sensitive blood test. PSA, which normally is secreted and disposed of by the prostate, shows up in the bloodstream in cancer of the prostate and in a harmless condition called benign prostatic hyperplasia or prostate enlargement. The normal PSA level is less than 4 ng/mL. Elevated PSA levels in the bloodstream mean something must be checked. Even a slight increase in PSA level must be monitored closely; referral to a urologist for a biopsy is recommended. Still another study is the alkaline phosphatase (ALP) test. The normal ALP level is 35 to 142 units/L for men and 25 to 125 units/L for women. These specific tests are useful in diagnosing benign prostatic hyperplasia, prostatic cancer, bone metastasis in prostatic cancer, and other disease conditions.

THE REPRODUCTIVE CYCLE

Menarche, the beginning of menses, designates the first menstrual cycle. Menarche occurs in late puberty and indicates that the body is capable of supporting pregnancy. Menarche traditionally occurs approximately 2 to 2½ years after breast development. The age ranges from as young as 8 to as old as 15 years. The average age of onset is 12 years. If a girl has not started menstruation by age 15 years, or if it has been longer than 3 years since breast development, a health care provider should be consulted. The length of the menstrual cycle varies from 24 to 32 days; the average cycle lasts 28 days. Day 1 of the menstrual cycle is the day that blood flow (called the *menstrual period*) begins. The flow lasts from 1 to 8 days; the average is 3 to 5 days. The amount of flow ranges from 10 to 75 mL; the average is 35 mL per cycle.

Help patients maintain their reproductive and sexual health by instructing or counseling women about personal hygiene. Personal cleanliness is a health habit that should be promoted for all patients and implemented in each care plan. Cleanliness is especially important during menstruation (see the Health Promotion box).

DISTURBANCES OF MENSTRUATION

Because of the relationship between the menstrual cycle and the body's mechanisms of hormonal secretion, a decrease or increase in activity of the hormonal glands can disturb menstruation. The most common disturbances include the following:

- *Amenorrhea:* Absence of menstrual flow
- *Dysmenorrhea:* Painful menstruation
- *Dysfunctional uterine bleeding (DUB):* Abnormal uterine bleeding
- *Menorrhagia:* Bleeding that is excessive in amount and duration
- *Metrorrhagia:* Bleeding between menstrual periods

Another disturbance of the menstrual cycle is premenstrual syndrome (PMS), which is discussed later.

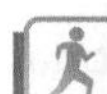

Health Promotion

Health Teaching for Menstruation

KNOWLEDGE OF THE PHYSIOLOGIC PROCESS

- Factors that may alter the menstrual cycle: stress, fatigue, exercise, acute or chronic illness, changes in climate or working hours, and pregnancy

PERSONAL HYGIENE

- Wear pads during early period of heavy flow.
- Change tampons frequently to decrease risk of toxic shock syndrome.
- Consult health care provider if tampon use frequently causes discomfort.
- Take a daily shower for comfort; warm baths may relieve slight pelvic discomfort.
- Keep perineal area clean and dry; cleanse from anterior to posterior.
- Wear cotton underwear; remember that nylon pantyhose and tight-fitting slacks retain moisture and should not be worn for extended periods.
- Feminine hygiene products, such as vaginal sprays and suppositories, may contribute to a feeling of cleanliness.
- A daily douche is not recommended because it changes the protective bacterial flora of the vagina and predisposes the woman to infection.

EXERCISE

- Exercise is not contraindicated and may help prevent discomfort.
- Modify exercise if fatigue occurs.

DIET

- Restrict salt intake if fluid retention is present.
- Consult a health care provider if fluid retention persists after menstruation.

DISCOMFORT

- For mild discomfort, take aspirin, acetaminophen (Tylenol), or ibuprofen (Motrin); apply warmth; and rest.
- For prolonged, severe discomfort, consult a health care provider.

Suggested nursing diagnoses are anxiety, ineffective coping, fear, pain, deficient knowledge, and low self-esteem. Nursing interventions are based on specific behaviors, symptoms, and treatments.

AMENORRHEA

Amenorrhea (absence of menstrual flow) is normal before puberty, after menopause, during pregnancy, and sometimes during lactation. Menstrual flow also may be absent or suppressed as a result of hormonal abnormalities or surgical interventions such as a hysterectomy (surgical removal of the uterus).

Etiology and Pathophysiology

Amenorrhea is classified as *primary* when menarche has not occurred by the age of 17 to 18 years. The other changes associated with puberty may or may not have taken place. This may be the result of hormonal imbalances or genetic disorders. Potential structural causes include congenital defects such as an imperforate hymen, blockages or narrowing of the cervix, missing uterus or vagina, or a vaginal septum. *Secondary amenorrhea* means menarche has occurred but flow has ceased for at least 6 months. This diagnosis excludes those women who are pregnant, breast-feeding, or menopausal. Secondary amenorrhea may be due to frequent, vigorous exercise, as in female athletes; low body fat; anxiety or an emotional disorder such as depression; pituitary tumors; hyperactive thyroid gland; polycystic ovarian syndrome (PCOS); and medications such as oral and injectable contraceptives. Hormone levels may be altered significantly by antihypertensives and antidepressive medications resulting in amenorrhea. Estrogen producing cells and eggs within the ovaries can be killed by chemotherapy also resulting in amenorrhea.

Although the primary manifestation is the absence of menstruation, there may be other symptoms present. Weight gain or loss may be reported. Additional changes that may signal hormonal imbalances include breast discharge, vaginal dryness, increased hair growth, changes in breast size, and voice changes.

Assessment

Early diagnosis and prompt management are necessary to prevent more serious reproductive and genital problems. Discussions concerning the presence or absence of menstruation should be included in the health teaching provided to girls and their parents about the progression of puberty and the onset of menses. Urge the sexually active woman to see a health care provider as soon as a menstrual period is missed. Women who suspect their amenorrhea is caused by menopause can be examined by a health care provider to confirm this.

Assess emotional or behavioral factors that may influence the menstrual cycle. A menstrual history includes a discussion of the number of menstrual periods, characteristics of prior periods, and any experience with amenorrhea. A review of medication and drug use history also is needed.

Diagnostic Tests

Confirming the absence of pregnancy is the first step. Beyond the preliminary workup and when pregnancy is not a possibility, the diagnostic study for primary and secondary amenorrhea is the same. This includes a pelvic examination. The pelvic examination determines the presence of structural abnormalities or the presence of growths. Serum studies review hormone levels including estradiol, follicle-stimulating hormone (FSH), prolactin, testosterone, and thyroid-stimulating hormone (TSH). An examination of internal structure may include a computed tomography (CT) scan, MRI, ultrasound, or hysterosalpingogram. Genetic testing also may be indicated.

Medical Management

Treatment is based on the underlying cause and must be determined on an individual basis. Hormonal therapy may be needed.

Nursing Interventions and Patient Teaching

A patient problem and interventions for women with amenorrhea include but are not limited to the following:

Patient Problem	Nursing Interventions
Anxiousness, related to loss of menstrual cycles	Acknowledge patient's feelings and provide emotional support Refer for counseling as necessary Explain diagnostic procedures Provide information, privacy, and consultation as indicated for sexual concerns

Encourage patients to comply with treatment, and emphasize the importance of follow-up visits with the health care provider for treatment, therapy, and evaluation of treatment efficacy.

DYSMENORRHEA

Dysmenorrhea is uterine pain with menstruation, commonly called "menstrual cramps." Primary dysmenorrhea that is not associated with pelvic disorders usually develops when ovulatory function is established (before 20 years of age) and there is no underlying organic disease. Often it disappears or declines after pregnancy or by the time a woman is in her late 20s. The discomfort usually begins at the time of menstruation or in the 1 to 2 days preceding (Cleveland Clinic, 2014). Secondary dysmenorrhea is painful menstruation in women who have normal periods. The cause is linked to disorders of the reproductive tract. Potential causes include fibroid tumors, endometriosis, pelvic inflammatory disease (PID), sexually transmitted infections (STIs), and premenstrual syndrome (PMS). Stress and anxiety are also related causes.

Dysmenorrhea is the greatest single cause of absenteeism among girls in school and women in the workplace. It is one of the most common health problems for which women seek treatment.

Etiology and Pathophysiology

The leading risk factors for dysmenorrhea are age (<20 years) and nulliparity (the condition of never having given birth). Other risk factors may include heavy periods, anxiety/depression, smoking, and attempts to lose weight. The causes of dysmenorrhea can be related to endocrine imbalance; an increase in prostaglandin secretions; or chronic illnesses, fatigue, and anemia. A recent theory proposes that dysmenorrhea may be caused by hypercontractility of the uterus resulting from higher-than-normal levels of prostaglandins. Conditions that cause general debilitation, such as inadequate diet and exercise, anemia, and fatigue, often are related to dysmenorrhea.

Assessment

Many women have systemic symptoms of breast tenderness, abdominal distention, nausea and vomiting, headache, vertigo, palpitations, and excessive perspiration. Assess the woman for colicky and cyclic pain and, infrequently, dull pain in the lower pelvis that radiates toward the perineum and back. This pain may be experienced 24 to 48 hours before menses or at the onset of menses. The family history is important, because dysmenorrhea has been reported to be significantly more common among mothers and sisters of women with dysmenorrhea. Secondary dysmenorrhea is suspected if the symptoms begin after 20 years of age. It has been described as a steady or cramping pain and may be specific to the site of pelvic disorder.

Diagnostic Tests

Diagnostic studies include a complete blood count and cultures to check for the presence of STIs. A pelvic examination is performed to assess for structural abnormalities. Ultrasonography can be used to assess contents of the abdominal or pelvic cavity. Surgical diagnostics may involve a laparoscopy to visualize the reproductive and abdominal organs or structures. Hysterosalpingography or a D&C may be employed as well.

Medical Management

Treatment of secondary dysmenorrhea is aimed at the cause. Surgical and medication intervention may be appropriate, depending on the severity and underlying causes of dysmenorrhea.

Interventions that are helpful in the management of dysmenorrhea not related to organic causes include a nutritious diet rich in complex carbohydrates. High fiber intake also is recommended. Intake of caffeine, sugar, and alcohol should be limited. During episodes of dysmenorrhea drinking warm beverages and eating small, frequent meals is helpful. Local applications of heat and warm showers are helpful. Mild analgesics are prescribed. Medications for dysmenorrhea include over-the-counter prostaglandin inhibitors, such as ibuprofen (Motrin, Advil), celecoxib (Celebrex), and naproxen sodium (Anaprox). Oral contraceptives may be used to suppress ovulation by inhibiting prostaglandin levels (Table 52.2). Supplementation with vitamin

Table 52.2 Medications for Reproductive Disorders

GENERIC NAME (TRADE NAME)	ACTION	SIDE EFFECTS	NURSING IMPLICATIONS
acyclovir ointment (Zovirax)	Antiviral agent, interferes with DNA synthesis needed for viral replication	Mild pain with transient burning; stinging, pruritus, rash, vulvitis	Apply ointment q 3 hr or six times daily around the clock; cover all lesions; use gloves for self-protection when applying
clotrimazole (Mycelex)	Interferes with fungal DNA replication; binds sterols in fungal cell membrane	Rash, urticaria, stinging, burning, peeling, blistering skin fissures, abdominal cramps, bloating, urinary frequency	Watch for allergic reactions; note therapeutic response (decrease in size and number of lesions); use gloves for application; can be used through menstrual cycle; avoid use of other vaginal creams or suppositories during therapy
conjugated equine estrogen (Premarin)	Affects release of gonadotropins; inhibits ovulation; is involved in adequate calcium use in bone structure	Nausea, peripheral edema, enlargement of breasts, breast tenderness, anorexia, vomiting, diarrhea, headache, thrombophlebitis, dizziness, depression	Notify health care provider of weight gain of ≥5 lb/wk (11 kg/wk) (patient may need diuretic); monitor BP; check liver function test; check Homans' sign for possible clots; give IV product slowly to prevent flushing
danazol	Synthetic androgen, causes atrophy of endometrial tissue; decreases FSH and LH, which leads to amenorrhea and anovulation	Fluid retention, virilization, androgenic effects, weight gain, amenorrhea, dizziness, headache, rashes, hepatic impairment	Check weight; monitor I&O; check for edema; give with food or milk to decrease gastrointestinal upset

Continued

Table 52.2 Medications for Reproductive Disorders—cont'd

GENERIC NAME (TRADE NAME)	ACTION	SIDE EFFECTS	NURSING IMPLICATIONS
estradiol transdermal system	Same as conjugated equine estrogen	Same as conjugated equine estrogen	Same as conjugated equine estrogen
fluconazole (Diflucan)	Used to treat or prevent fungal infections	Nausea, stomach pain, diarrhea, headache, dizziness	Take medication with a full glass of water
medroxyprogesterone acetate (Provera, Depo-Provera)	Inhibits secretion of pituitary gonadotropins, which acts to prevent follicular maturation and ovulation; stimulates growth of mammary tissue	Irregular bleeding, breast tenderness, masculinization of fetus, edema, cholestatic jaundice, thrombophlebitis, anorexia, acne, mental depression, weight gain or loss	Notify health care provider of weight gain of ≥5 lb/wk; monitor BP at beginning of treatment and periodically thereafter; check liver function test; discontinue if patient is pregnant
metronidazole (Flagyl)	Direct-acting amebicide-trichomonacide; binds, degrades DNA in infecting organism	Rash, headache, dizziness, fatigue, convulsions, blurred vision, nausea, vomiting, diarrhea, pseudomembranous colitis, albuminuria, neurotoxicity, metallic taste, disulfiram-type reaction with alcohol	Watch for allergic reactions and superinfection; check stool for parasites; give oral form with food; watch for vision problems; tell patient not to drink alcohol during therapy
miconazole nitrate (Monistat-3, Monistat-7)	Same as clotrimazole	Vulvovaginal burning, itching, pelvic cramps, rash, urticaria, stinging, burning, contact dermatitis	Same as clotrimazole
nystatin	Same as clotrimazole	Rash, urticaria, stinging, burning	Same as clotrimazole
Oral contraceptives: estrogen-progesterone combinations (Ortho-Novum)	Inhibits ovulation by suppressing gonadotropins, FSH, and LH; alters genital tract to inhibit sperm penetration and inhibit implantation	Nausea, cramps, diarrhea, appetite change, acne, rash, increased BP, thrombophlebitis, edema, dysmenorrhea, bleeding irregularities, depression, fatigue, breast changes, cholestatic jaundice, optic neuritis	Monitor glucose, thyroid function, and liver function tests; check Homans' sign for clot detection; monitor BP; discontinue if patient is pregnant
terconazole	Same as clotrimazole	Vulvovaginal burning, itching, pelvic cramps, rash, urticaria, stinging, burning	Same as clotrimazole
testosterone cypionate (Andro-Cyp)	Increases weight by building body tissue; increases potassium, phosphorus, chloride, and nitrogen levels; increases bone development	Acne, flushing, gynecomastia, edema, hypercalcemia, nausea, cholestatic hepatitis, aggressive behavior, headache, anxiety, mental depression, androgenic and anabolic activity	Check weight daily; monitor BP; monitor growth rate in children; check electrolyte (potassium-sodium, chloride, calcium) and cholesterol levels; monitor liver function test
tioconazole ointment (Vagistat-1)	Same as miconazole but two to eight times more potent	Vulvovaginal burning, itching, soreness, swelling	Same as clotrimazole

Table 52.2 Medications for Reproductive Disorders—cont'd

GENERIC NAME (TRADE NAME)	ACTION	SIDE EFFECTS	NURSING IMPLICATIONS
topical amphotericin B	Binds to ergosterol, altering cell membrane permeability in susceptible fungi	Urticaria, stinging, burning, dry skin, pruritus, contact dermatitis, staining of nail lesions	Cover lesions completely after cleansing and drying well; use gloves to prevent further infection; watch for allergic reactions; tell patient that it may discolor skin and clothing
topical nystatin	Interferes with fungal DNA replication; causes fungal cell membrane permeability	Rash, stinging, burning, urticaria, nausea, vomiting, anorexia, diarrhea	Watch for allergic reaction; use gloves for topical application; for vaginal preparation, tell patient that she may need protective perineal pads

BP, Blood pressure; *DNA*, deoxyribonucleic acid; *FSH*, follicle-stimulating hormone; *I&O*, intake and output; *IV*, intravenous; *LH*, luteinizing hormone.

B_6, calcium, and magnesium also has been used to manage dysmenorrhea with some success. Walking and weight loss for the overweight are helpful. Aerobic exercise is most beneficial (Osayande and Mehulic, 2014).

Nursing Interventions and Patient Teaching

A patient problem and interventions for women with dysmenorrhea include but are not limited to the following:

Patient Problem	Nursing Interventions
Insufficient Knowledge, related to disease process and treatment	Present information on disease process, procedures to be performed, medications, and treatments Prepare for informational question-and-answer sessions according to patient needs Teach procedures patient must know how to perform Obtain feedback Be certain learning has taken place; reinforce teaching as needed Develop a trusting relationship Involve patient in care

Encourage a positive attitude and instruct women to maintain good posture, exercise, and practice good nutrition.

ABNORMAL UTERINE BLEEDING (MENORRHAGIA AND METRORRHAGIA)

Abnormal uterine bleeding may take many forms, including menorrhagia and metrorrhagia.

Menorrhagia is excessive bleeding at the time of regular menstrual flow. The excessive bleeding can be characterized as increased in duration (more than 7 days), increased in amount (more than 80 mL), or both. Potential causes may involve uterine growths or tumors, cancer of the uterus, hormonal imbalance, pelvic inflammatory disease, medications such as aspirin, and disorders of coagulation. In younger women it may be attributed to hormonal or endocrine disturbances, but in older women it usually indicates inflammatory disturbances or uterine tumors. Uterine fibroids (also called *leiomyomas*) and endometrial polyps are common causes of menorrhagia in women in their 30s and 40s. Emotional or psychological problems may also affect uterine bleeding. The severity of menorrhagia usually is estimated in terms of the number of pads or tampons used in excess of those used for regular menstrual flow.

Metrorrhagia is the appearance of uterine bleeding between regular menstrual periods or after menopause. It merits early diagnosis and treatment because it may indicate cancer or benign tumors of the uterus and ovaries. Endometrial cancer must be considered for postmenopausal women experiencing spotting.

The diagnostic process begins with a complete health history and review of the symptoms being reported. Focus should be on the past menstrual history. This should include length of periods and characteristics of the bleeding. The age at menarche should be recorded as well. Medication history should include the use of oral contraceptives and the ingestion of prescription and over-the-counter medications. Review the patient's obstetric history. The sexual history should include partners, onset of regular sexual activity, and any past or present STIs.

Diagnostic evaluation includes a Pap smear and routine speculum and pelvic examination. Laboratory testing includes blood tests and may include thyroid function assessments, hormone levels, pregnancy testing, and complete blood count studies. Endometrial biopsy and ultrasonography also are used to diagnose gynecologic causes of menorrhagia and metrorrhagia. Endometrial ablation done by laser or electrosurgical technique has been successful with many patients with menorrhagia.

Nursing interventions for the woman who is experiencing bleeding abnormalities include assessment of bleeding and pain and review of the patient's concerns and feelings. The woman should be asked to keep a log of her menstrual and bleeding history. Recording the dates, type, and characteristics of the bleeding, and the number of pads or tampons used, is important.

Women of all ages need to be educated about the importance of follow-up care when abnormal uterine bleeding is detected initially. Menopausal women may believe that the return of bleeding is normal or a reoccurrence of menstruation. Vaginal bleeding in postmenopausal women is never normal. Education and assessment of women in this age group should include this vital health teaching.

PREMENSTRUAL SYNDROME

An estimated 75% of women experience PMS at some point during their childbearing years. It differs from dysmenorrhea because it has no relation to ovulation.

Etiology and Pathophysiology

The etiology and pathophysiology are not well understood. An exact cause for the condition is not known. There are many theories but the most common links PMS to neuroendocrine events occurring within the anterior pituitary gland. A loss of intravascular fluid into the body tissues causes water retention, bloating, and weight gain. PMS is thought to have a biologic trigger with compounding psychosocial issues. Some women have a genetic predisposition to PMS. Other proposed causes of PMS include estrogen and progesterone imbalances and nutritional deficiencies of pyridoxine (vitamin B_6) or magnesium. Risk factors for premenstrual syndrome include the following:

- Age 25 to 40 years, with symptoms worsening as menopause nears
- Diet high in sugar
- Personal or family history of depression
- History of postpartum depression (Winchester Hospital, 2016)

Premenstrual dysphoric disorder (PMD-D) is the term applied to a type of PMS that includes a severe mood disorder. PMD-D has similar symptomology but demonstrates an excessive response in one or more of the following: sadness or hopelessness; anxiety or tension; extreme moodiness; marked irritability or anger (USDHHS, 2018).

PMS occurs 7 to 10 days before the menstrual period and usually subsides within 1 to 2 days after the onset of the menstrual flow.

Clinical Manifestations

Symptoms are multiple and vary among individuals. Behavioral symptoms include anxiety, mood swings, irritability, lethargy (inactivity), fatigue, sleep disturbances, and depression. Women may report difficulty concentrating or forgetfulness. Physical symptoms—such as headache, vertigo, backache, breast tenderness, abdominal distention, acne, paresthesia (burning or tingling) of hands and feet, and allergies—appear or may become worse. Many symptoms appear alone or in combination with other symptoms. Some women accept the symptoms as being normal and seek medical help only after the symptoms become severe or begin to affect their family processes and interactions with others.

Assessment

Subjective data are specific symptoms experienced by each woman. Ask each patient to maintain a log for three consecutive menstrual cycles and to note symptoms and activities that relate to the menstrual period. The collected information can be analyzed and symptoms treated accordingly.

Objective data pertinent to the syndrome include the inability to perform activities of daily living (ADLs) in the multiple roles of wife, mother, and career person.

Diagnostic Tests

PMS is diagnosed only after eliminating other possible causes for the symptoms. A focused health history and a physical examination are done to identify any underlying conditions, such as thyroid dysfunction, uterine fibroids, or depression that may account for the symptoms. No definitive diagnostic test is available for PMS.

Patients may be asked to keep a journal of their symptoms for two or three menstrual cycles (USDHHS, 2018). Tests include evaluation of estrogen and progesterone levels to rule out hormonal imbalances and determination of glucose levels; low levels may lead to irritability.

Medical Management

PMS has no single treatment and no specific medication. Some health care providers prescribe analgesics such as aspirin, ibuprofen, or other NSAIDs. To manage fluid retention and bloating hydration by drinking water and juice is recommended. Diuretics may be prescribed. Dietary management includes limiting sugar and sodium and increasing consumption of whole grains and fiber. Caffeine should be sharply limited or eliminated. Small, frequent meals are recommended. Supplements of vitamin B_6, calcium, and magnesium may be administered as prescribed. Alcohol and smoking should be discontinued. Encourage regular exercise three or four times a week for 30 minutes, especially during the premenstrual interval. Exercise results in release of endorphins, leading to mood elevation. Techniques for stress reduction include yoga, meditation, imagery, and biofeedback training. Because fatigue may exaggerate PMS symptoms, adequate rest, sleep, and relaxation are helpful. Buspirone taken during the luteal phase of the menstrual cycle has helped some women manage the anxiety. Women with PMD-D may benefit from antidepressants, including fluoxetine (Prozac, Sarafem) and tricyclic antidepressants such as amitriptyline (Elavil). Selective serotonin reuptake inhibitors (SSRIs) such as sertraline (Zoloft) have provided significant relief to women with severe PMS (USDHHS, 2018).

Nursing Interventions and Patient Teaching

A patient problem and interventions for the woman with PMS include but are not limited to the following:

Patient Problem	Nursing Interventions
Anxiousness, related to PMS	Encourage verbalization of feelings Acknowledge existence of syndrome and its symptoms Encourage patient to keep a menstrual symptom diary to document the cycle and nature of the symptoms Encourage patient to plan activities during the symptom-free part of her cycle Administer supplements of vitamin B_6, calcium, and magnesium as prescribed Encourage attending self-help groups and reading self-help literature; group support tends to reduce stress Provide emotional support in a nonjudgmental and caring manner Assist in identifying possible sources of anxiety and coping mechanisms

The patient should take responsibility for following a dietary plan of eating small meals and restricting or eliminating sugar, alcohol, caffeine, and nicotine; this may minimize the symptoms of PMS or PMD-D.

MENOPAUSE

The **climacteric** is the phase of the aging process of women and men who are making a transition from a reproductive phase to a nonreproductive stage of life. The female climacteric is called *menopause*. This term refers to the normal cessation of menses. Menopause may be hormonal, surgical, or pharmacologic. Hormonal menopause occurs in middle adulthood and marks the onset of physical changes, a decrease in hormone secretion, and the cessation of ovulation and menses. Surgical menopause results from the loss of hormone production after surgical intervention involving removal of the ovaries (bilateral salpingo-oophorectomy). Medication therapies can result in the onset of menopausal signs and symptoms. Medications to manage fibroid tumors include gonadotropin-releasing hormone (GnRH) agonists (e.g., Lupron and Synarel). This class of medication causes levels of estrogen and progesterone to fall, resulting in a menopausal state.

Perimenopause is experienced by most women as they near the middle adulthood years. During this period the level of estrogen produced begins to fall. This may begin as early as the early to mid-30s. Perimenopause (state of transition to menopause) may last for several years, with an average of 4 years. This stage lasts until the ovaries no longer produce estrogen and the woman has had a full year without a menstrual period.

Etiology and Pathophysiology

Menopause is the normal decline of ovarian function resulting from the aging process. Menopause begins in most women between 42 and 58 years of age (the average age being 51) and is characterized by infrequent ovulation, decreased menstrual function, and eventual cessation of the menstrual flow. Factors that have been linked to an earlier age at menopause include higher body mass index; cigarette smoking; and racial, ethnic, and socioeconomic factors.

Menopause may be induced artificially by such procedures as irradiation of the ovaries or surgical removal of both ovaries. Both cause menopause with all its physiologic changes, whereas ovaries left intact after a hysterectomy continue to function provided the woman has not yet reached the age of the climacteric. Menopause also may occur earlier because of illness, side effects of chemotherapy, or drugs.

Decline in ovarian function produces a variety of symptoms, including a decrease in the frequency, amount, and duration of the menstrual flow; spotting; amenorrhea; and polymenorrhea (increased number of menstrual periods). Symptoms can last from a few months to several years before menstruation ceases permanently. Menopause is not considered complete until 1 year after the last menstrual period.

Clinical Manifestations

Physical changes that occur in the body generally do not develop until after permanent cessation of menstruation. Changes in the reproductive system include shrinkage of vulval structures, atrophic vulvitis, shortening of the vagina, and dryness of the vaginal wall. A relaxation of supporting pelvic structures results from the decrease in estrogen. Cystitis and urinary frequency and urgency may appear as a result of changes in the urinary system. There is loss of skin turgor and elasticity; increased subcutaneous fat; decreased breast tissue; and thinning of hair of the axilla, the head, and the pubis. About 25% of postmenopausal women develop osteoporosis.

Assessment

Subjective data include a family history. Determine whether family members and significant others are aware of the transition and whether they are supportive. Note emotional illness, if present. Hot flashes caused by glandular imbalances may become prominent. Other symptoms may include fatigue, vertigo, headache, nausea, dyspareunia (painful intercourse), palpitations, and chest and neck pain. Some experience a feeling of being unwanted, and some may fear growing old; both feelings could cause depression.

Collection of objective data includes an awareness that some patients may display frequent crying spells or outbursts of anger. Explore the use of contraceptives. Assess frequency, amount, and duration of the menstrual flow. Diaphoresis, weight gain, vomiting, and tachycardia may occur.

Diagnostic Tests

Tests include analysis of hormonal levels. Other diagnostic testing may be indicated by specific symptoms. Some examinations are performed to rule out conditions such as cancer.

Medical Management

The status of hormone replacement therapy (HRT) for postmenopausal women has been a source of study and discussion. Hormone replacement is used in menopausal women to help with some of the troubling manifestations associated with the loss of estrogen. Symptoms improved by the use of HRT include hot flashes, night sweats, and vaginal dryness. Therapies are also beneficial to maintaining bone density. Despite these positive findings there are risk factors for some women for the development of heart disease, stroke, and blood clots. Side effects of HRT include breast tenderness, cramping, bloating, and vaginal spotting. A change in dosage or type of prescribed therapies may help in the management of side effects. At present, the US Food and Drug Administration (FDA) recommends that women with moderate to severe symptoms of menopause be prescribed the lowest effective dose possible for the shortest duration possible. Women who still have their uterus are prescribed replacement estrogen and progesterone. If the woman has her uterus and progesterone is not included in the replacement therapy, there is an increased risk of endometrial cancer. Estrogen therapy is also used for women who no longer have a uterus (i.e., who have undergone a hysterectomy).

Nurses are in a good position to apprise their patients of the benefits, risks, and appropriate uses of HRT. HRT is used for short-term treatment of moderate to severe symptoms of menopause, such as hot flashes, night sweats, and vaginal dryness. At present, no data indicate how long HRT can be taken without the risk of cardiovascular or other adverse effects, and it is not known whether lower dosages lessen the risk of complications. In women with moderate to severe menopausal symptoms, it is assumed that risk can be minimized by providing HRT only until the severe symptoms disappear and using the lowest effective dosage. HRTs may be administered in a number of ways, including orally or by transdermal patch, gels, subcutaneous implants, creams, injections, and suppositories. Low-dose alternatives in HRT include low-dose PREMPRO, containing either 0.45 mg of conjugated estrogens and 1.5 mg of medroxyprogesterone, or 0.3 mg of conjugated estrogens and 1.5 mg of medroxyprogesterone; or low-dose intravaginal estrogen products, such as estrogen topical vaginal cream (Premarin vaginal cream or Estrace) and low-dose vaginal rings. Because of the later diagnosis of breast cancer and colon cancer in women receiving combination HRT, closely scrutinize any abnormal mammogram and screen for colon cancer as part of the follow-up.

Most health care providers recommend calcium and vitamin D supplements, which are available in many forms; the generic calcium carbonate products are the most cost effective.

Herbals and dietary modification are also useful in the management of menopause-related symptoms. Phytoestrogens are compounds that mimic estrogen in structure. They are found in yams, sesame seeds, and tofu (National Institute on Aging, 2017).

SSRIs, including the antidepressants paroxetine (Paxil), fluoxetine, and venlafaxine (Effexor), are an effective alternative to HRT in reducing hot flashes, even if the user is not depressed. Also known to relieve hot flashes are clonidine (Catapres), an antihypertensive drug, and gabapentin (Neurontin), an antiseizure drug (Mayo Clinic, 2018b).

Nonhormonal therapy. To relieve menopausal symptoms without the risks of HRT, several methods to decrease heat produced by the body and promote heat loss have been recommended. Reducing intake of caffeine and alcohol lowers the production of body heat. Suggestions to promote heat loss at night when hot flashes interfere with sleep include increasing air circulation, using light covers and loose-fitting clothing, and placing cool cloths on flushed areas.

Nursing Interventions and Patient Teaching

Education regarding menopause should occur before its onset. Many women appreciate opportunities to discuss menopause. Set up an exercise program that includes movement and weight bearing to slow bone loss and modify coronary artery disease risk factors. Walking is an excellent weight-bearing exercise. Other exercises include bicycling, stationary cycling, and aerobic dancing three or four times per week.

Patient problems and interventions for the menopausal patient include but are not limited to the following:

Patient Problem	Nursing Interventions
Impaired Self-Esteem due to Current Situation, related to concerns about femininity, sexuality, and aging	Encourage patient and significant others to verbalize concerns Assess knowledge of menopause Provide education related to menopause Refer patient to couple, family, and sex therapy as appropriate Provide understanding and support

Patient Problem	Nursing Interventions
Insufficient Knowledge, Regarding Patient's Physiologic and Psychological Changes, related to menopause	Explain the process of climacteric and menopause, at a level the patient can understand Explain importance of keeping fit, eating a well-balanced diet, getting adequate rest and sleep, avoiding stress and fatigue, and continuing contraception until contraindicated by health care provider If estrogen replacement therapy is ordered, inform patient about side effects Instruct patient to report any vaginal bleeding occurring 6 months or more after last menstrual period Inform patient of the availability of water-soluble lubricants if needed before coitus

For patient teaching, emphasize that the climacteric is normal and self-limiting and that menopause is not the end of the patient's sex life. A nutritious diet and weight control improve physical condition, and an exercise program promotes vitality. Interest and participation in various activities help decrease anxiety and tension. Skin creams and lotions can be used to prevent drying, pruritus, and cracking skin. Encourage the woman to perform breast self-examination (BSE) monthly and to monitor calcium intake. Contraceptives should be used for 1 year after the last menstrual period. The patient can obtain a prescription for the treatment of pruritus or burning of the vulva. Women can practice Kegel exercises regularly to strengthen pelvic muscles (see the Health Promotion box). A water-soluble lubricant, such as K-Y jelly, can be used to prevent dyspareunia. Explain the side effects of any medications or hormonal therapy. Emphasize that an annual physical examination is important for maintaining good health.

 Health Promotion

Kegel Exercises

Kegel exercises are performed to help strengthen and tighten muscles that support the pelvic organs. These muscles (pelvic floor) are used to stop the flow of urine. To perform Kegel exercises while standing or sitting, tighten the pelvic floor muscles as hard as you can. Hold for 5 seconds, then release. Repeat at least 10 times. This exercise can be done as many as 40 to 50 times each day.

MALE CLIMACTERIC

Etiology and Pathophysiology

The climacteric is less pronounced in men and often may not even be apparent. The appearance of the climacteric phase is gradual and occurs between 55 and 70 years of age. There is a gradual decrease of testosterone levels and seminal fluid production. The impact is largely psychological, possibly because of the recognition of some reduction of sexual activity and interests.

Clinical Manifestations

Manifestations are mostly physiologic changes. Erections require more time and are not as full or firm. The prostate gland enlarges, and secretions diminish; seminal fluid decreases. The physical changes occur as the man grows older, and the most noticeable signs are loss or thinning of hair from the head, chest, axillae, and pubis. There may be some flushing and chilling. Muscle tone is decreased.

Assessment

Collection of subjective data reveals that the man is generally at the peak of his career or possibly considering retirement. He interprets his decreased sexual needs as a loss of productivity and sexual power. Therefore the assessment should invite verbalization of emotions with coping mechanisms.

Collection of objective data includes assessment of behaviors that may be causing the man stress and concern. Ask him to explore changes he has noted regarding his lifestyle and feelings of loss of self-worth.

Diagnostic Tests

Diagnostic tests include a complete physical examination to rule out abnormalities of structure and function. Hormone level assessments provide information about potential imbalances.

Nursing Interventions and Patient Teaching

A patient problem and interventions for men experiencing male climacteric include but are not limited to the following:

Patient Problem	Nursing Interventions
Impaired Coping, related to situational crisis (climacteric)	Show understanding and concern Assist patient in identifying how the problem affects his life and future, his family, and significant others Encourage patient to talk about factors that could be influencing the way he sees the problem Assist patient in identifying strengths and coping skills and the nature and strength of situational support Collect data about current and potential sources of support Assist patient in planning alternative solutions Give positive reinforcement

Inform the patient that the climacteric is normal. Encourage the patient to verbalize his fears and to seek counseling if stress increases.

ERECTILE DYSFUNCTION

Erectile dysfunction (ED) is a man's inability to attain or maintain an erect penis that allows satisfactory sexual performance. In the past the condition was referred to as *impotence*. ED has largely replaced this terminology. ED may arise from a variety of causes:

- *Psychological causes:* ED may have a psychological basis, including stress, depression, and other mental conditions.
- *Organic causes:*
  - Anatomic anomalies may result in a physical defect in the genital structures
  - Atonic ED: Conditions associated with atonic ED include advanced syphilis; congenital spinal cord anomalies, such as spina bifida; spinal cord tumors; amyotrophic lateral sclerosis (Lou Gehrig's disease); multiple sclerosis; and cord compression caused by a herniated disk
  - Surgical interventions, such as radical prostatectomy, often lead to ED
  - Low testosterone levels
  - Hypertension
  - Substance use/abuse

ED potentially can interfere with a man's self-esteem, relationships, confidence, and sense of well-being. The prevalence alone makes ED a significant condition. An estimated 30 million men in the United States experience ED. The rate of incidence increases with aging, with approximately 4% of men in their 50s affected by ED. This rate increases to 17% during the seventh decade of life. Among men in their 70s, the rate of incidence of ED nears 50%. ED in younger men may result from substance abuse, including alcohol or recreational drugs. Medical conditions associated with ED are diabetes mellitus, hypertension, renal disorders, cancer, coronary artery bypass surgery, and organ transplants. Understand ED by developing a broad understanding of the factors that contribute to the condition.

ED can result when the physiology of the erection faces interference. Stimulation sends impulses to the brain and to the corpora cavernosa of the penis. This results in its relaxation and allows blood to enter and fill the spaces. Pressure in the corpora cavernosa causes the penis to expand and harden. Many disorders have the ability to interfere with this process, thus causing ED (National Kidney and Urologic Diseases Information Clearinghouse, 2015).

Medical Management

Review of the patient's history is the first step. The information collected should include a detailed sexual history, medication and drug use, and past and current medical conditions. Medical treatment is based on careful assessment of the causative factors. It is known that medications such as antihypertensives, antidepressants, antihyperlipidemics, diuretics, drugs for Parkinson's disease, marijuana, cocaine, antianxiety agents, and some cardiac agents may cause ED. Illicit or abused substances such as alcohol, cocaine, and nicotine also are known to cause ED. Disease conditions, such as diabetes mellitus or end-stage renal, heart, and chronic obstructive pulmonary disease, also may be causative factors.

A drug named sildenafil citrate (Viagra) is prescribed as an oral therapy for ED. The physiologic mechanism of erection of the penis involves release of nitric oxide in the corpus cavernosum during sexual stimulation. The drug enhances smooth muscle relaxation and the inflow of blood in the corpus cavernosum, thus allowing erection to occur. For most patients, the recommended dose is 50 mg taken as needed approximately 1 hour before engaging in sexual activity. However, sildenafil may be taken from 30 minutes to 4 hours before sexual activity. Sildenafil has been shown to potentiate the hypotensive effects of nitrates; therefore its administration to patients who are using nitrates (either regularly or intermittently) in any form is contraindicated. Tadalafil (Cialis) is another antiimpotence agent for ED contraindicated for concurrent use with nitrates, nitric oxide, or alpha-adrenergic blockers. It should not be used in patients who have unstable angina, a recent history of stroke, life-threatening heart failure, uncontrolled hypertension, or myocardial infarction within 90 days. For most patients, the recommended dose is 10 mg before sexual activity (range, 5 to 20 mg; not to exceed one dose in 24 hours). A third antiimpotence agent is vardenafil (Levitra), 10 mg, taken 1 hour before sexual activity (range, 5 to 20 mg; no more than once daily). This drug is not to be used with nitrates because of the potential for an unsafe decrease in blood pressure, which could result in myocardial infarction or stroke. The side effects of all three medications are similar and include headache, hypotension, and dyspepsia (Spratto, 2012). Medications alone will not result in an erection. Sexual stimulation is needed.

Management also may include penile injections. Alprostadil and phentolamine are used for this purpose. The patient can self-inject the medication into the side or the base of the penis. The medications typically provide an erection that can last 20 to 40 minutes.

Mechanical devices are available for the patient with ED. The least invasive means may be the use of a vacuum pump device. The vacuum is placed over the penis and suction is applied by a hand-generated or battery-operated means. Once the erection occurs a ring, is placed over the base of the penis to maintain it (Mayo Clinic, 2018c). Surgical implantation of a penile prosthesis may be performed as a same-day procedure or may require hospitalization for 5 or more days, depending on the patient and the device used (Fig. 52.9).

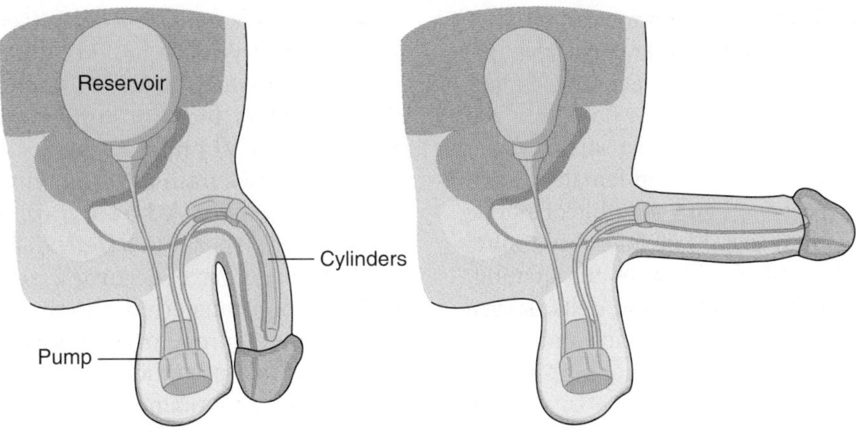

Fig. 52.9 The Scott inflatable prosthesis has erect and flaccid positions designed to mimic normal erectile function. (From Beare PG, Myers JL: *Adult health nursing*, ed 3, St. Louis, 1998, Mosby.)

Nursing Interventions and Patient Teaching

The nurse is responsible for teaching the patient to administer prescribed medications and to watch for side effects. For patients who have received penile implants, inform the patient about signs and symptoms of infection of the implant, including tenderness of the penis, fever, dysuria, and signs of urinary tract infection. Tell the patient to seek medical attention promptly if infection occurs.

INFERTILITY

Etiology and Pathophysiology

Infertility is defined as the inability to conceive after 1 year of sexual intercourse without birth control measures. If the woman is over the age of 35, the time period is reduced to 6 months. Primary infertility refers to couples who have never conceived (NIH, 2017). Secondary infertility refers to couples who have conceived but are now unable to do so. An estimated 10% to 15% of couples are infertile (Puscheck, 2016).

A woman's age has a significant bearing on her ability to conceive. Women are most fertile between 20 and 29 years of age. After age 35 fertility begins to decline (National Library of Medicine, 2013). As the woman approaches menopause fertility is minimal. A man's fertility does not dramatically decrease with aging.

The inability to conceive may be attributed to the woman or the man; in some cases both have factors resulting in infertility. Statistically, the causes are relatively evenly spread between the partners, with approximately one-third of the causes linked to the woman, the man, and to both combined (Mayo Clinic, 2018d).

Damage to sperm production, longevity, or sperm motility issues are the leading causes of male-related infertility. The sperm count may be diminished or absent. Structural abnormalities and low motility may account for infertility. Abnormally shaped sperm cannot penetrate and fertilize the ovum. Excessive heat exposure of the testicles associated with undescended testicles and hot tubs are implicated with male-based infertility. Inability to travel to the fallopian tubes as a result of poor motility will prevent conception as well. Additional male-related causes include hormonal imbalances, anatomic abnormalities, and genetic defects (Mayo Clinic, 2015). Lifestyle and other health-related behaviors also may affect male fertility. The use of alcohol and drugs, smoking, exposure to environmental toxins, and some medications may result in reduced or absent fertility. Illness such as cancer and the related treatments may render a man infertile.

Female-related causes of infertility include ovulatory issues, hormonal imbalances, and structural abnormalities. Ovulation-related disorders compromise the majority of female-related cases of infertility. Women who do not experience ovulatory menstrual cycles will not conceive. Hormonal imbalances can be linked to problematic levels of estrogen, progesterone, and FSH. These hormones are responsible for the maturation and release of the ovum from the ovaries as well as preparation of the uterus for implantation of the fertilized egg. Structural abnormalities may include scarring from sexually transmitted infections or endometriosis, abnormalities in the shape and size of the uterus, the presence of uterine fibroid tumors, and blockages in the fallopian tubes. Lifestyle factors that may play a part in a woman's fertility include increasing age, smoking, excessive alcohol use, athletic training, obesity, or being underweight.

Assessment

Collection of subjective and objective data includes physical examination and health histories for both partners to make the infertility assessment and prepare a treatment plan.

Diagnostic Tests

Specific testing is necessary to rule out systemic diseases such as diabetes mellitus, neoplasms, hepatic and renal diseases, and viral conditions. Genetic defects and disorders of the testes are explored. Diagnostic testing can produce a great deal of anxiety and stress. This testing may continue for fairly long periods with or without favorable results. Infertility testing can be expensive and may not be covered by some insurance carriers. Male testing is somewhat simpler and usually less expensive than female testing. If there is reason to suspect the man is infertile or sterile, it is appropriate to test him first. Male infertility testing includes semen analysis, which measures the quantity and quality of semen, volume of sperm cells, sperm motility, and sperm density; and endocrine imbalance testing, which explores possible disruption of the pituitary gonadotropins and testosterone production.

Female testing focuses on the ovulation process and function of the reproductive organs. Testing commonly includes (1) assessment of ovulatory functioning; (2) endometrial biopsy, which confirms ovulation and endometrial cyclic changes; and (3) hysterosalpingography and hysterography to assess the position and alignment of the reproductive organs.

Male and female interaction studies include (1) Huhner's test, which examines the cervical mucus for motile sperm cells after intercourse, at mid-menstrual cycle; (2) immunologic or immunoglobulin (antibody) testing for detection of spermicidal antibodies in the woman's serum; and (3) testing the man and woman for normalcy of their sex chromosomes.

Medical Management

The management of infertility problems depends on the cause. If infertility is secondary to an alteration in ovarian function, supplemental hormone therapy may be attempted to restore and maintain ovulation. Drugs used to induce ovulation include clomiphene citrate (Clomid) and bromocriptine (Parlodel). These drugs increase the risk for multiple births. Structural abnormalities may be investigated for surgical correction. Fibroid tumors and scar tissue may be candidates for surgery. Hormonal imbalances also may be treated pharmacologically. Progesterone may be administered by an injection or vaginal gel/jelly. If pregnancy results, it may also be continued until 10 to 12 weeks' gestation, when the placenta will be functioning and can take over the hormone production.

Poor cervical mucus may be a result of chronic cervicitis or inadequate estrogenic stimulation. Careful cauterization of the cervix may eradicate the chronic cervicitis, and the administration of estrogens can improve the quantity and quality of the cervical mucus.

Improving the patient's general health may help, especially when a debilitating or chronic illness is present. Eliminating or reducing psychological stress can improve the emotional climate, making it more conducive to achieving a pregnancy. Education of the couple regarding the probable time of ovulation and appropriate coital technique also may be indicated. Timing of sexual intercourse to the days preceding and at ovulation is best.

When a couple has not succeeded in conceiving even with infertility management, another option is intrauterine insemination with the partner's or a donor's sperm. If this technique does not succeed, in vitro fertilization (IVF) may be used. IVF is the removal of mature oocytes from the woman's ovarian follicles via laparoscopy, followed by fertilization of the ova with the partner's sperm in a Petri dish. When fertilization and cleavage have occurred, some of the resulting embryos are transferred into the woman's uterus. The procedure requires 2 or 3 days to complete and is used in cases of fallopian tube obstruction, decreased sperm count, and unexplained infertility. IVF is costly and emotionally stressful, but it has become an accepted therapy for infertile couples.

Assisted reproductive technologies (ARTs) have developed rapidly since the first IVF baby was born in 1978. ARTs include IVF, gamete intrafallopian transfer (GIFT), zygote intrafallopian transfer (ZIFT), cryopreserved embryo transfer (CPE), and donor oocyte programs. Current research could lead to a rapid expansion of these techniques. With the increased knowledge of freezing techniques for embryos (CPE), couples will have increased pregnancy potential. Researchers also are investigating the replication of normal tubal secretions. This tubal factor is important because the pregnancy rate is higher with GIFT and ZIFT than with IVF. Finally, the development of embryo biopsy and genetic engineering may allow for preconception techniques for those couples with identified genetic abnormalities. It also raises the possibility of gender selection. Thus noncoital reproduction poses many ethical, legal, and social concerns. All decisions related to infertility are influenced by the couple's age, their wishes, and the length of time they have been attempting to conceive.

Nursing Interventions and Patient Teaching

The nurse has a responsibility to teach and provide emotional support throughout the infertility testing and treatment period. Feelings of anger, frustration, sadness, and helplessness between partners and between the couple and health care providers may increase as more tests are performed. Infertility can generate great tension in a marriage as the couple exhausts their financial and emotional resources. Few insurance carriers cover the cost of infertility testing or the therapeutic measures associated with infertility. Shame and guilt may arise when other people become involved in such an intimate area of a relationship.

Recognizing and dealing with the psychological and emotional factors that surface can assist the couple in coping with the situation. Encourage couples to participate in a support group for infertile couples and in individual therapy. Continue providing information and emotional support as therapeutic measures are attempted. Give couples ample opportunity to plan what is financially realistic. IVF treatments can cost $10,000 to 15,000 per cycle in the United States (IHR, 2018).

Prognosis

The condition causing the infertility and the age of the woman are the primary deciding factors determining the outcome of infertility treatments. Women over age 40 have reduced chances of achieving pregnancy. An estimated 50% of couples who undergo diagnostic testing and treatments for fertility are able to conceive.

INFLAMMATORY AND INFECTIOUS DISORDERS OF THE FEMALE REPRODUCTIVE TRACT

Infections of the female reproductive tract are found most commonly in the vagina, the cervix, the fallopian tubes, and their adjacent areas. The vagina is lubricated and protected by normal flora, an acidic pH, and secretions from the vaginal and cervical cells.

A number of organisms can cause vaginal infections. Vaginal infections may be caused by bacteria, fungi, or viruses. Infections are more likely to occur when the flora and the acidity of the vagina are disturbed by medications (e.g., birth control pills, antibiotics), stress, malnutrition, douching, aging, and disease. Health-related concerns may include diabetes mellitus and pregnancy.

Organisms often are introduced from external sources by way of unclean douche nozzles, poor hygiene, inadequate handwashing, neglected nail care, soiled clothing, and intercourse. Vaginal infections can be transmitted sexually and will return unless both partners are treated.

SIMPLE VAGINITIS

Etiology and Pathophysiology

Vaginitis is a common vaginal infection. The cause of the condition may be bacterial or inflammatory. *Escherichia coli,* an organism found in feces and the rectum, is a common cause. Other potential pathogens include staphylococcal and streptococcal organisms; *Trichomonas vaginalis* (a flagellated protozoan); *Candida albicans* (a yeastlike fungus); and *Gardnerella vaginalis,* a coccobacillus.

Vaginitis is an inflammation of the vagina. If the patient changes perineal pads or tampons infrequently, the vaginal tract and inner groin become irritated. This creates a medium suitable for organism growth. Examination of the vaginal walls will show a profuse foamy (bubbly) exudate if the vaginitis is caused by *T. vaginalis*. If *C. albicans* is the causative agent, a thick, cheeselike discharge results. Bacterial vaginitis produces a malodorous milky discharge.

Clinical Manifestations

The exudate in vaginitis is yellow, white, or grayish white; curdlike; and generally accompanied by pruritus, burning, and edema of the surrounding tissue. Voiding and defecation generally intensify the symptoms.

Assessment

Subjective data include menstrual history, age at menarche, length of cycles, duration and nature of flow, dysfunctions, birth control methods, medications taken, family history of diabetes mellitus, previous vaginal infections, and STIs. Ask about sexual practices and signs of infection in the sex partner. Dysuria may occur as a consequence of local irritation of the urinary meatus.

Collection of objective data includes observation for excoriations of the skin caused by scratching, in which case secondary infection may result. Observe the specific type of exudate.

Diagnostic Tests

Diagnostic tests include direct visual examination of the vagina, culture of the organism, and bimanual examination to assess for inflammation of the vagina and its surrounding tissues.

Medical Management

Vaginal infection can be treated by a variety of methods. The major goals of treatment are to (1) cure the infection, (2) prevent reinfection, (3) prevent complications, and (4) prevent infection of the sexual partner(s). Douching frequently is prescribed for treatment, as are local applications of vaginal suppositories, ointments, and creams. Advise the patient to use the medication at bedtime and to remain recumbent for more than 30 minutes after insertion to allow absorption and to prevent loss of any medication from the vagina. The patient may require oral medications appropriate to the infecting organism. During treatment the patient should refrain from intercourse or request that her partner use a condom (see Table 52.2).

Nursing Interventions and Patient Teaching

Advise the patient of the importance of hand washing before and after vaginal application of medications. Heat may be applied in the form of douches, perineal irrigations, or sitz baths. Douching too frequently can alter normal vaginal flora. Discourage douching unless specifically prescribed by the health care provider.

Most patients with vaginal infections are directed to abstain from sexual intercourse during treatment. The male partner's use of a condom until the symptoms of infection disappear may be advised. Also inform the patient that her sexual partner(s) should be treated.

Prognosis

With proper treatment, the prognosis is good.

SENILE VAGINITIS OR ATROPHIC VAGINITIS

Low estrogen levels cause the vulva and vagina to thin and atrophy, becoming more susceptible to bacterial invasion. The subsequent exudate causes pruritus, edema, and skin irritations. Although the condition is seen most commonly after menopause, it may be experienced by any patient whose condition is associated with reductions in estrogen levels. Estrogen, vaginal suppositories, and ointments may be prescribed (Mayo Clinic, 2018e).

CERVICITIS

Cervicitis is the inflammation of the cervix. It may be caused by various causes but is linked most commonly to sexually transmitted infections such as chlamydia, gonorrhea, herpesvirus, human papillomavirus, and trichomoniasis. Bacteria including *Staphylococcus* and *Streptococcus* can cause cervicitis. Other potential causes may include cervical caps, diaphragms, or pessary devices. Allergic reactions to condoms, douches, or spermicides also may be implicated. Risk-increasing behaviors include multiple sexual partners, a history of sexually transmitted infections, and sexual intercourse at an early age. Therapy is specific to the causative organisms. Symptoms are dyspareunia (painful intercourse); vaginal pain; pelvic heaviness; abnormal vaginal bleeding; and a gray, white, or yellow vaginal discharge. If cervicitis remains untreated, the tissues are continually irritated and the infection may spread to other pelvic organs. Personal hygiene and frequent warm tub baths can minimize odor and discomfort. Local applications of vaginal suppositories, ointments, and creams usually are prescribed. Drug therapy also includes azithromycin (Zithromax), 1 g orally as a single dose, or doxycycline (Vibramycin), 100 mg orally twice a day for 7 days; the partner is treated with the same drugs (Ollendorf, 2017). More advanced conditions may require more invasive therapies such as cryosurgery, electrocauterization, and laser therapy.

PELVIC INFLAMMATORY DISEASE

PID is any acute, subacute, recurrent, or chronic infection that may involve the cervix (cervicitis), uterus (endometritis), fallopian tubes (salpingitis), or ovaries (oophoritis) and may extend to the connective tissues lying between the layers of the broad ligaments (folds of peritoneum supporting the uterus).

Etiology and Pathophysiology

The most common causative organisms are *Neisseria gonorrhoeae,* streptococci, staphylococci, chlamydiae, and tubercle bacilli. PID can follow the insertion of a biopsy curette or an irrigation catheter, abortion, pelvic surgery, sexual intercourse, or pregnancy. The condition may occur with or without gonorrheal infection and may be mild or severe.

When conditions or procedures alter or destroy the cervical mucus, bacteria ascend into the uterine cavity. Pelvic examination and movement of the reproductive organs become painful. PID is serious because it may cause adhesions and sterility. Sexually active women with more than one partner are at increased risk for PID.

Clinical Manifestations

Signs and symptoms are temperature elevation, chills, severe abdominal pain, malaise, nausea and vomiting, and malodorous purulent vaginal exudate.

Assessment

Subjective data relate to the severity of the disorder, pain, time of onset, and frequency (primary infection or continuous reinfection). Sexual history, pelvic examinations, and pelvic procedures are important because they may reveal the origin of the pathogen. The patient may complain of lower abdominal and pelvic pain, dysmenorrhea, dysuria, and vulvar pruritus.

Objective data include the patient's knowledge, level of discomfort, and coping mechanisms. Assess the patient for fever and chills and the amount and characteristics of vaginal discharge. The vaginal discharge is purulent to thin and mucoid.

Diagnostic Tests

Diagnostic tests include Gram stains of secretions from the endocervix, urethra, and rectum. Culture and sensitivity testing identifies organisms and is helpful in selecting antibiotics for treatment. Ultrasound or magnetic resonance imaging (MRI) may be used to visualize the pelvic cavity. Vaginal ultrasonic examinations can aid in diagnosing abscesses and monitoring the treatment and healing process. Laparoscopic visualization of the pelvic inflammation may be necessary to confirm the extent of infection. Laboratory testing includes leukocyte count, C-reactive protein rates, and erythrocyte sedimentation rate, which are elevated.

Medical Management

The goal of treatment is to control and eradicate the infection by preventing it from spreading to other body systems. Treatment includes systemic antibiotics administered intravenously or intramuscularly. The antibiotics of choice are usually cefoxitin (Mefoxin) and doxycycline to provide thorough coverage against the responsible pathogens. Intercourse must be avoided for the entire time of treatment. The patient's partner(s) must be examined and treated as well. Pain control, rest, and adequate fluid intake are essential to the care. A corticosteroid often is added to the antibiotic treatment to aid in more rapid recovery and improvement in maintaining fertility.

Nursing Interventions and Patient Teaching

The patient usually is hospitalized to isolate the organism and plan treatment. Inform the patient and those assisting with the patient's care of all specific precautions and observe standard precautions. Use goggles if any splashing is likely. Nursing interventions include (1) assessing pain and administering prescribed analgesics as needed; (2) monitoring vital signs and progress of treatment; (3) providing fluids to avoid dehydration; (4) performing palliative measures for comfort such as bathing, changing of perineal pads, personal hygiene, and warm douches; (5) providing patient support with a positive, nonjudgmental attitude; and (6) positioning the patient in Fowler's position to facilitate drainage.

Patient problems and interventions for the patient with PID include but are not limited to the following:

Patient Problem	Nursing Interventions
Recent Onset of Pain	Manage pain with analgesics as ordered; assess effectiveness of pain-relief measures Provide comfort measures
Impaired Health Maintenance, related to insufficient knowledge of condition and complications	Teach patient about the significance of PID and the importance of complying with medication therapy

Education of the patient should include the following:

- Discussion about the signs and symptoms to report to the health care provider
- Medication therapy
- Personal hygiene practices to reduce infection (hand washing and avoidance of tampons)

Prognosis

PID can lead to complications such as adhesions and strictures of the fallopian tubes as a result of scarring. Ectopic pregnancy risk is elevated. Infertility may result. Early diagnosis and treatment will reduce the potential for complications.

TOXIC SHOCK SYNDROME

Etiology and Pathophysiology

Toxic shock syndrome (TSS) is an acute bacterial infection caused by *Staphylococcus aureus*. It usually occurs in women who are menstruating and using tampons (particularly superabsorbent tampons). If the tampon is left in place too long, the bacteria may proliferate and release toxins into the bloodstream, causing TSS. Women at the greatest risk are those who insert tampons with their fingers instead of with inserters, women with chronic vaginal infections, and women with genital herpes. TSS can also occur in nonmenstruating women. Additional risk factors include recent childbirth, surgery, and internal medical packing (National Library of Medicine, 2018a).

Clinical Manifestations

Often the patient has flulike symptoms for the first 24 hours. Between days 2 and 4 of the menstrual period, the patient may have an elevated temperature (up to 102°F [39°C]), vomiting, dizziness, headache, diarrhea, myalgia, hypotension, and signs suggesting the onset of septic shock. Sore throat, headache, and a red macular palmar or diffuse rash followed by desquamation of the skin, hands, and feet may develop; urinary output is decreased, and the blood urea nitrogen (BUN) level is elevated. Disorientation may occur from dehydration and the release of toxins. Pulmonary edema and inflammation of mucous membranes may occur.

Assessment

Collection of subjective data includes determining whether the patient recently has used tampons and how long she used a single tampon before changing it. Obtain information about myalgia, sore throat, headache, and fatigue.

Collection of objective data includes assessing for edema. Assess the palms and soles for an erythematous rash. Desquamation and sloughing occur within 1 to 2 weeks after the rash. Note the patient's level of consciousness. Hypotension is a sign of TSS, as are nonpurulent inflammation of the conjunctiva and hyperemia of the oropharynx and vagina.

Diagnostic Tests

There is no definitive test for TSS. However, cervical-vaginal isolates of *S. aureus* are present 90% of the time. Blood tests demonstrate leukocytosis; thrombocytopenia; and elevated levels of bilirubin, BUN, creatinine, serum glutamic-pyruvic transaminase (alanine aminotransferase), serum glutamic-oxaloacetic transaminase (aspartate aminotransferase), and creatine phosphokinase. Blood and urine cultures should be taken along with throat cultures when appropriate.

Medical Management

Treatment of TSS varies because of the range in types and severity of symptoms. Antibiotic therapy is given according to the results of culture and sensitivity tests. Parenteral therapy is given to maintain proper fluid balance. Laboratory data are evaluated for electrolyte imbalance caused by vomiting and diarrhea, elevated BUN suggesting renal involvement, and elevated enzymes suggesting liver dysfunction.

Nursing Interventions and Patient Teaching

When the patient is hospitalized, bed rest is prescribed and antibiotics are administered. Closely monitor vital signs and fluid status. If there is respiratory distress, oxygen therapy is instituted.

A patient problem and interventions for the patient with TSS include but are not limited to the following:

Patient Problem	Nursing Interventions
Inadequate Fluid Volume, related to vomiting and diarrhea	Monitor amount, frequency, and characteristics of vomitus and diarrhea Assess tissue turgor for evidence of dehydration Assess patient for dry mucous membranes, and monitor parenteral fluids; give fluids and electrolytes as ordered Monitor intake and output (I&O)

Because the use of tampons during menstruation has been linked to TSS, advise patients not to use superabsorbent tampons. If tampons are used, they should be alternated with the use of pads. Before it is used, a tampon should be inspected for flaws and discarded if any are noted. Tampons should be changed frequently (every 4 hours) and should be inserted carefully to avoid abrasions. Patients who have had TSS should not use tampons. Instruct the patient to wash her hands thoroughly before inserting a tampon. Advise women who are menstruating and develop a sudden high fever accompanied by vomiting and diarrhea to seek immediate medical attention. If the woman is wearing a tampon, she should remove it immediately.

Prognosis

TSS is a rare and sometimes fatal disease. The effect of the toxin on the liver, kidneys, and circulatory system makes this a potentially life-threatening condition. The prognosis depends on the severity of the disease and how quickly therapeutic measures are instituted to combat shock and renal failure, if present.

DISORDERS OF THE FEMALE REPRODUCTIVE SYSTEM

ENDOMETRIOSIS

Etiology and Pathophysiology

Endometriosis is a condition in which endometrial tissue appears outside the endometrial cavity. Endometrial tissue can be found on the ovaries, the fallopian tubes, and the uterus; within the abdominal cavity (the uterovesical peritoneum); and in the vagina (Fig. 52.10). Tissue is believed to spread through the lymphatic circulation, by menstrual backflow to the fallopian tubes and pelvic cavity, or through congenital displacement of the endometrial cells. The condition is believed to affect 40% to 60% of women who experience painful menstrual periods (National Library of Medicine, 2017).

The tissue responds to the normal monthly hormonal stimulation of the ovaries. The displaced tissue bleeds each month and forms an endometrial crust, which causes the development of an endometrial cyst. This cyst may rupture and cause further reproduction of tissue.

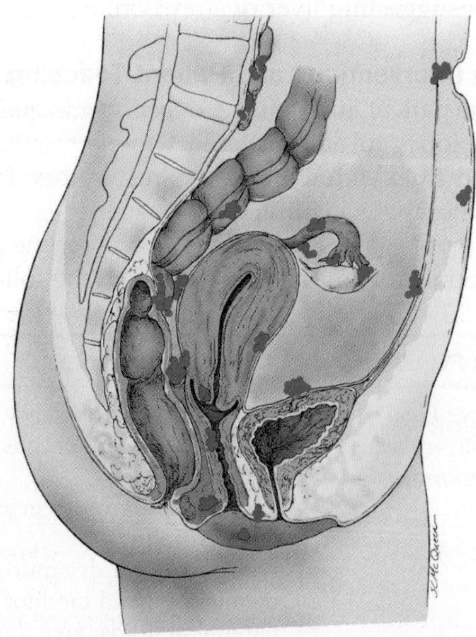

Fig. 52.10 Common sites of endometriosis. (From Lentz GM, Lobo RA, Gershenson DA, et al, editors: *Comprehensive gynecology*, ed 6, Philadelphia, 2013, Mosby.)

Clinical Manifestations

Dysmenorrhea is the most common complaint. Lower abdominal and pelvic pain with or without pain in the rectum, that may be unilateral or bilateral and may radiate to the lower back, legs, and groin, also is reported. Dyspareunia also is experienced frequently. Symptoms are more acute during menstruation and subside after menstruation. Some evidence indicates that women have a greater chance (about seven times greater) of developing endometriosis if a sister or mother has it. The highest incidence of endometriosis is among white women 25 to 35 years of age who are in the higher socioeconomic classes and who postpone childbearing until the later reproductive years. Women who have not conceived or lactated are at greater risk.

Assessment

Subjective data include a history of the patient's symptoms, including pelvic pain with menstruation, aching, cramping, a bearing-down sensation in the pelvis, or lower back dyspareunia. The type of pain may indicate cysts that are about to rupture or infected tissue. The patient may reveal a history of menstrual irregularities such as amenorrhea.

Collection of objective data involves noting signs such as abnormal uterine bleeding, which appear 5 to 7 days before menses and last 2 or 3 days. Signs also may include infertility.

Diagnostic Tests

Ultrasound may be performed to identify cysts and large areas of endometrial tissue outside of the uterus. Laparoscopy with a biopsy of the lesions may confirm the diagnosis. Regular pelvic examinations are recommended to monitor progression.

Medical Management

Medical treatment consists of high-dose antiovulatory medications to inhibit ovulation and induce a state physiologically similar to pregnancy, thus suppressing menstruation. Synthetic androgens such as danazol or a gonadotropin-releasing hormone agonist (e.g., leuprolide [Lupron]) may be prescribed to arrest proliferation of the endometrium and prevent ovulation, producing atrophy of the displaced endometrium. Unfortunately, the symptoms and progression of the disease return once the medications are discontinued. On occasion, endometriosis spontaneously disappears. It is believed that an interruption of the menstrual cycle slows the progress of the disorder. Some women who become pregnant are asymptomatic after pregnancy. When involvement is severe, surgery may be necessary. A laparoscopy may be performed to remove endometrial implants and adhesions. Lasers may be used to vaporize the small implants of endometrial tissue. Advanced cases of endometriosis may require a more drastic action, such as hysterectomy (removal of the uterus), oophorectomy (removal of the ovaries), and salpingectomy (removal of the fallopian tubes).

Nursing Interventions and Patient Teaching

Reinforce the health care provider's explanation of the expected results of treatment; instruct the patient regarding the dosage, frequency, and side effects of prescribed medications; and emphasize the importance of regular checkups and of reporting abnormal vaginal bleeding. Also encourage the patient to verbalize her concerns, and assist the patient with comfort measures. Managing the discomforts associated with endometriosis may include the use of heating pads. Some patients report success with the use of acupuncture, TENS (transcutaneous electrical nerve stimulation), and yoga. Eating a balanced diet and regular physical activity are also helpful.

Patient problems and interventions for the patient with endometriosis include but are not limited to the following:

Patient Problem	Nursing Interventions
Pain, related to displaced endometrial tissue	Institute comfort measures to cope with pain, such as medications and warm compresses to abdomen Maintain bed rest when pain is most severe
Impaired Sexual Function, related to painful intercourse or infertility	Emphasize importance of communicating fears and concerns that lead to anxiety

Prognosis

Approximately half of the women with endometriosis are infertile. Delaying childbearing by women with endometriosis is not recommended because worsening of the condition may result in a loss of fertility. Pregnancy and menopause stop the progression of the condition.

VAGINAL FISTULA

Etiology and Pathophysiology

A **fistula** is defined as an abnormal opening between two organs. Vaginal fistulas are caused by an ulcerating process resulting from cancer, radiation, weakening of tissue by pregnancies, and surgical interventions. Vaginal fistulas are named for the organs involved (Fig. 52.11). For example, a urethrovaginal fistula is an opening between the urethra and the vagina; a vesicovaginal fistula is an opening between the bladder and the vagina; and a rectovaginal fistula is an opening between the rectum and the vagina.

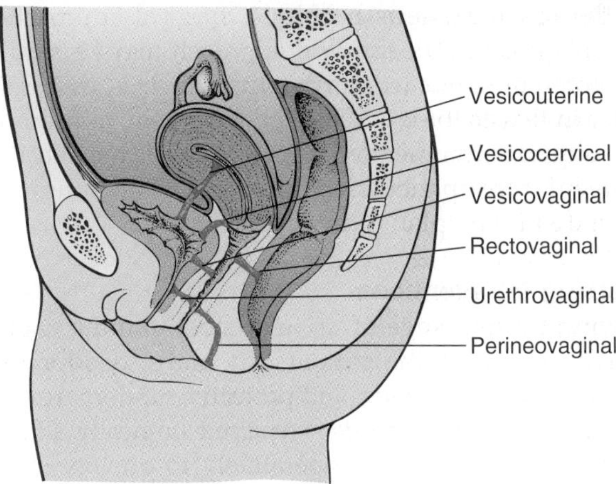

Fig. 52.11 Types of fistulas that may develop in the vagina and the uterus. (From Stenchever MA, Droegemueller W, Herbst AL, et al: *Comprehensive gynecology*, ed 3, St. Louis, 1998, Mosby.)

Clinical Manifestations

Fistulas are recognized by their exudate, which has a distinct odor of urine or feces. In general, a bladder infection is present. The vesicovaginal fistula causes a constant trickling of urine into the vagina; a rectovaginal fistula allows feces and flatus to enter the vagina.

Assessment

Subjective data include the patient's understanding of the exudate that occurs and of any causative factors. The patient reports the presence of urine or feces from the vagina.

Collection of objective data includes noting any behaviors that indicate stress, anxiety, and pain. The patient may express feelings of decreased self-esteem because of the condition. Observe for urine or feces on the perineal pad.

Diagnostic Tests

Diagnostic testing includes a methylene blue instillation in the bladder, and an intravenous (IV) pyelogram or cystoscopy to assist in locating the fistula. Pelvic examination is performed.

Medical Management

Smaller fistulas may be managed conservatively. The vesicovaginal fistula may be managed by transvesical or transvaginal application of a fibrin glue sealant, which is applied to close the fistula. Success has been limited but it provides a nonsurgical option for repair (Kumar et al, 2007). Larger fistulas may require surgical intervention accompanied by urinary or bowel diversion.

If the organ tissue is healthy, a surgical approach is recommended. The surgical approach may be similar to anteroposterior colporrhaphy, which is discussed later in this chapter. A diet high in protein, to promote healing, is recommended. Dietary fiber is beneficial to prevent constipation and straining. Antibiotics are included in the plan of treatment.

Nursing Interventions

Soiling from leakage of urine or stool into the vagina is disturbing for the patient. Sitz baths, deodorizing douches, perineal pads, and protective undergarments are necessary. If the fistula is repaired surgically, a Foley catheter is inserted postoperatively to prevent strain on the suture line by a full bladder.

Patient problems and interventions for the patient with vaginal fistula include but are not limited to the following:

Patient Problem	Nursing Interventions
Compromised Skin Integrity, related to exudates	Teach how to care for the skin with douches, creams, and sitz baths
Impaired Sexual Function, related to pain during sexual activity	Offer support and understanding of distress concerning sexual activities and self-esteem

Prognosis

Vaginal fistulas may close spontaneously but frequently must be repaired surgically. If so, 4 to 6 months are required for the inflammation to subside before surgery can be attempted.

RELAXED PELVIC MUSCLES

The most common problems resulting from relaxed pelvic muscles are as follows:

- *Displaced uterus:* A uterus that has moved away from its normal position
- *Prolapsed uterus:* A uterus that has protruded into the vaginal canal, or beyond the vaginal opening (*procidentia*)
- *Cystocele:* A bladder that has protruded into the vagina
- *Urethrocele:* A urethra that has protruded into the vagina
- *Rectocele:* A rectum that has protruded into the vagina
- *Enterocele:* A small bowel that has protruded into the vagina

Displaced Uterus

A displaced uterus is usually congenital but may be caused by childbirth. Normally the uterus lies with the cervix at a right angle to the long axis of the vagina, and the body of the uterus is angled forward (see Fig. 52.2). The terms *retroversion* and *retroflexion* describe ways in which the uterus may be displaced: the retroverted uterus is aligned with the vagina and points toward the sacrum; the retroflexed uterus is flexed even farther backward. The patient with a displaced uterus has backache, muscle strain, leukorrhea (a whitish-colored discharge from the vagina), and heaviness in the pelvic area. The patient also tires easily. Treatment consists of a *pessary* (a rubber or plastic doughnut-shaped ring placed in the vagina, to help prop up the uterus) and possibly uterine suspension (a surgical procedure in which the uterus is repositioned).

Uterine Prolapse

Etiology and pathophysiology. Prolapse of the uterus is considered mild if the cervix drops to the lower vaginal segment. Moderate prolapses present with the cervix being visible at the vaginal opening. A severe prolapse, also termed a **procidentia,** results when the entire cervix protrudes through the vaginal opening (Fig. 52.12). Obstetric trauma, overstretching of the uterine muscle support system, multiple births, coughing, straining, the aging process, and lifting heavy objects contribute to uterine prolapse. Estrogen losses after menopause also are implicated in the condition.

Clinical manifestations. The patient complains of a feeling of "something coming down." She may have dyspareunia, a dragging or heavy feeling in the pelvis, backache, and bowel or bladder problems if cystocele or rectocele is also present. Stress incontinence is a common and troubling problem.

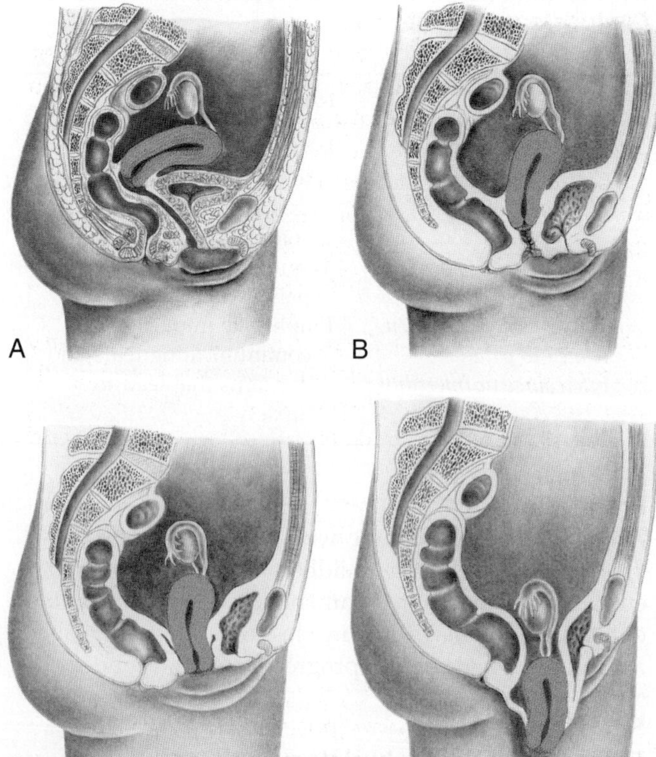

Fig. 52.12 Uterine prolapse. A, Normal uterus. B, First-degree prolapse of the uterus. C, Second-degree prolapse of the uterus. D, Third-degree prolapse of the uterus (procidentia). (From Seidel HM, Ball JW, Dains JE, et al: *Mosby's guide to physical examination,* ed 7, St. Louis, 2011, Mosby.)

Medical management. Treatment is not undertaken unless the condition begins to trouble the patient or the uterus drops into the opening of the vagina. The type of surgical procedure will be determined by the degree of prolapse, plans for future pregnancies, the woman's age and overall health, and the woman's desire to maintain vaginal function. Surgery generally involves a vaginal hysterectomy (i.e., removal of the uterus through the vagina) with anterior and posterior repair of the vagina and underlying fascia (Mayo Clinic, 2018f). It is also called an anteroposterior **colporrhaphy** (suture of the vagina) (also referred to as anterior posterior colporrhaphy or A&P repair).

When surgery is contraindicated, pessaries are used to provide uterine support. Before insertion of the vaginal pessary, the uterus is replaced manually in its normal position. Once inserted, the pessary holds the cervix in a posterior (anteflexed) position. When the pessary is properly placed, the woman is unaware of its presence and has no difficulty voiding or having intercourse. A variety of pessaries are available for the differing levels of prolapse. Every 3 to 4 months the pessary is cleaned and replaced by the woman, if possible, or by her health care provider. The vaginal walls should be assessed for signs of irritation. Pessaries that are unattended for long periods are associated with erosion, fistulas, and an increased incidence of vaginal carcinoma. Potential side effects of pessaries include foul-smelling discharge, vaginal ulcerations, and difficulty with normal sexual activity.

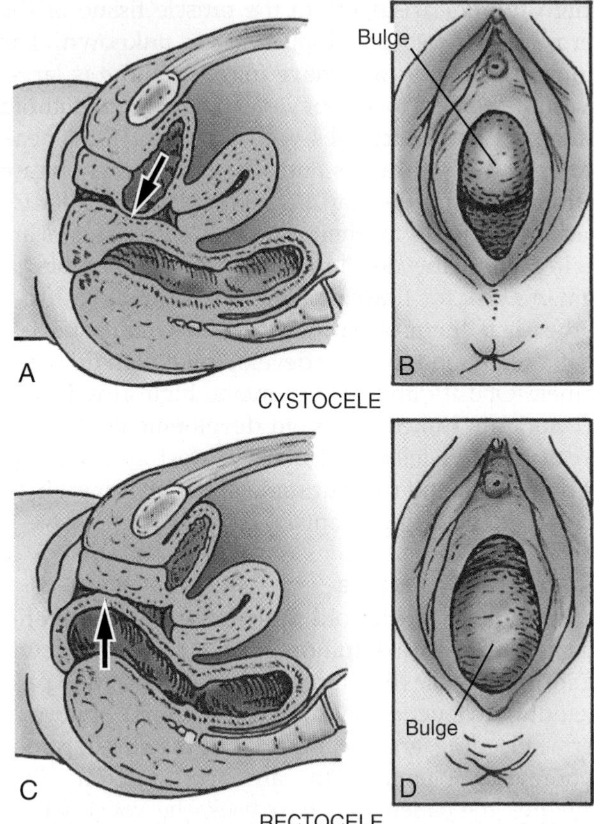

Fig. 52.13 A and B, Cystocele. C and D, Rectocele. (From Black JM, Hawks JH: *Medical-surgical nursing: Clinical management for positive outcomes,* ed 8, St. Louis, 2009, Mosby.)

Cystocele and Rectocele

Etiology and pathophysiology. When the tissue, muscles, and ligaments that support the uterus and perineum have been stretched and weakened by childbearing, multiple births, or cervical tears, the organs gradually move into other positions. Relaxation of the tissues, muscles, and ligaments of the bladder may cause a displacement of the bladder into the vagina. This is referred to as a *cystocele* (Fig. 52.13A and B).

Clinical manifestations. Clinical symptoms are urinary urgency, frequency, and incontinence; fatigue; and pelvic pressure. A large cystocele prevents complete emptying of the bladder, which leads to bacterial growth and infection.

Relaxation of the supporting tissues to the rectum causes the rectum to move toward the posterior vaginal wall and form a rectocele (Fig. 52.13C and D). The rectocele causes constipation, rectal pressure, heaviness, and hemorrhoids.

Medical management. Cystocele and rectocele are corrected through anteroposterior colporrhaphy, a surgical repair involving shortening of the muscles that support the bladder and repair of the rectocele.

Nursing interventions and patient teaching. An important aspect of preoperative care for colporrhaphy is ensuring as clean an operative area as possible. Patients may be given a cathartic followed by enemas to be sure the bowel is completely empty. A liquid diet for 48 hours before surgery helps keep the bowel empty. A cleansing vaginal douche is given the evening before and the morning of surgery. Postoperative care includes checking vital signs and observing for hemorrhage. A Foley catheter usually is inserted into the bladder to keep it empty and to prevent pressure on sutures. Stool softeners often are prescribed. Small to scant amounts of vaginal bleeding will be noted.

Encourage early ambulation. Advise the patient against standing for long periods or lifting heavy objects. Coitus must be avoided until healing occurs, usually after about 6 weeks.

Prognosis. Surgical intervention to treat a cystocele and rectocele may result in complications such as infection, bladder injury causing urinary retention or urinary incontinence, or fistula development. An estimated 20% of women who undergo surgical correction experience reoccurrence of the prolapse.

LEIOMYOMAS OF THE UTERUS

Etiology and Pathophysiology

Leiomyomas (fibroids, myomas) are the most common benign tumors of the female genital tract. Fibroids are benign tumors arising from the muscle tissue of the uterus. The cause of leiomyomas is unknown. The number of women who have fibroid tumors is large. An estimated 20% to 80% of women have them. Fibroid tumor incidence increases with age, with their peak incidence during the 30s and 40s. During menopause the tumors shrink, as they are dependent on the body's ovarian hormones for their growth. Genetic factors are implicated in the development of fibroid tumors. A woman's risk for fibroids is increased threefold if her mother had them. African American women have a greater likelihood for their development than do white women. Obesity and dietary intake high in red meat and pork are linked to fibroid development. The size and number of leiomyomas vary. Most are found in the body of the uterus, but some occur in the cervix or involve the broad ligaments.

Clinical Manifestations

Some women with fibroid tumors are asymptomatic. Increasing pressure of tumors on the uterus and pelvic organs may cause discomfort. These may include pain (including dysmenorrhea and dyspareunia), abnormal uterine bleeding, and menorrhagia. If the fibroid tumor becomes large enough to cause pressure on other structures, the patient may have backache, constipation, and urinary symptoms.

Assessment

Collection of subjective data includes asking the patient about pain with menstruation or abnormally heavy menstrual flow. Have the patient describe her symptoms, which may include pelvic fullness or heaviness, constipation, urinary frequency or urgency, and menorrhagia.

Collection of objective data includes assessing the patient for excessively heavy discharge of blood by observing the number and saturation of perineal pads.

Diagnostic Tests

Initially a pelvic examination will be performed. The health care provider may be able to palpate the tumors during the bimanual examination. Diagnostic tests to confirm the presence of fibroid tumors may include pelvic ultrasonography, MRI, x-rays, and a CT scan. More invasive studies include the hysterosalpingogram. Surgical intervention such as a laparoscopy or hysteroscopy may be used to visualize fibroid tumors.

Medical Management

The treatment of fibroid tumors depends on the patient's symptoms, her age and how close to menopause she is, and whether she desires more children. Conservative nonsurgical management will be implemented if the tumors are not causing too-significant levels of discomfort. Pain management may include ibuprofen or acetaminophen. Women who experience heavy menstrual bleeding may require iron supplementation. Dysmenorrhea may be managed with low-dose oral contraceptives.

Myomectomy (removal of uterine myomas while leaving the uterus in place) is the procedure of choice for women hoping to maintain fertility. If during the surgery there is severe bleeding or an obstruction is found, a hysterectomy may still be necessary. Before surgical intervention medications may be prescribed to shrink the tumors. A gonadotropin-releasing hormone agonist (GnRHa) may be administered by injection or nasal spray, or implanted. The GnRHa places the woman in a medication-induced form of menopause. Side effects of the drug therapy include hot flashes, depression, reduced libido, and joint pain.

A hysterectomy is performed if the fibroids cause excessive vaginal bleeding or if the woman has no desire to maintain fertility. The hysterectomy is limited to removal of the uterus. The ovaries are preserved in the absence of other anomalies.

An increasingly used alternative treatment for uterine fibroids is uterine artery embolization. This procedure consists of injecting embolic material (small plastic or gelatin beads) into the uterine artery, which carries the material to the fibroid branches and thus occludes the arteries supplying blood to the tumor. Deprived of oxygen and nutrients, the tumor shrinks over time and symptoms diminish.

Six months after uterine artery embolization, fibroids are typically about 50% smaller in most women, and in 80% to 90% of women the symptoms are considerably decreased or gone. About 5% of patients experience complications from the procedure, such as infection or permanent cessation of menstrual periods.

Nursing Interventions and Patient Teaching

Preoperative and postoperative nursing interventions are like those discussed for a patient who undergoes a hysterectomy. Reinforce the health care provider's explanation of the treatment plan—either a total hysterectomy or pelvic examination at regular intervals to monitor the status of the fibroid tumor. Instruct the patient about the dosage, frequency, and possible side effects of prescribed medications. Tell the patient with menorrhagia to include adequate iron in her diet to prevent iron deficiency anemia from the extra blood loss. Stress the importance of regular checkups to monitor the status of the fibroid tumor, and encourage the patient to express her feelings and assist her with coping mechanisms.

A patient problem and interventions for the patient with fibroid tumors include but are not limited to the following:

Patient Problem	Nursing Interventions
Pain, related to fibroid tumors	Assess pain location, onset, and duration Administer analgesics as ordered. Provide comfort measures as needed

Prognosis

Fibroid tumors of the uterus tend to diminish and disappear spontaneously with menopause. They rarely become malignant. Infertility may result from a myoma that obstructs or distorts the uterus or fallopian tubes. Myomas in the body of the uterus may cause spontaneous abortions; those near the cervical opening may make the delivery of a fetus difficult and may contribute to postpartum hemorrhage.

OVARIAN CYSTS

Etiology and Pathophysiology

Ovarian cysts are benign tumors that arise from dermoid cells of the ovary or from a cystic corpus luteum or graafian follicle.

Clinical Manifestations

Ovarian cysts enlarge and are palpable on examination. They may cause no symptoms, or they may result in a disturbance of menstruation, a feeling of heaviness, and slight vaginal bleeding. Some individuals report sharp abdominal pain that may subside with rupture of the cyst.

Medical Management

The cysts may be removed by ovarian cystectomy. Often ovarian cysts are not removed if the patient is not experiencing debilitating symptoms.

Nursing Interventions

If surgery is performed, nursing interventions are similar to those for the patient undergoing an abdominal hysterectomy (i.e., removal of the uterus through an abdominal incision).

Prognosis

The prognosis is good; ovarian cysts do not become malignant.

CANCER OF THE FEMALE REPRODUCTIVE TRACT

Cancer is the second most common cause of death in women, and malignant tumors of the reproductive tract represent a significant portion of the total number of deaths from cancer (see the Cultural Considerations box).

Cervical cancer often affects women in their reproductive years. The cancer can be detected in its early stages with a diagnostic Pap test. Endometrial cancer is primarily a disease of women older than 50 years of age, but the incidence among younger women is increasing. Most cases of ovarian cancer occur in women older than 50, but malignant neoplasms of the ovaries may occur at any age. Ovarian cancer is largely "silent," that is, symptom free, until late in its progression, resulting in a relatively poor prognosis.

Cultural Considerations

Cancer of Female Reproductive System

- Ovarian cancer is seen more frequently among white women than among African American women.
- Japanese women have a low incidence of ovarian cancer. However, second- and third-generation Japanese women in the United States have much higher rates, similar to those of white women born in the United States. Dietary practices may explain this difference.
- Endometrial cancer occurs more frequently among white women than among African American women.
- The 5-year survival rate for endometrial cancer (all stages combined) is 80% for white women and 55% for African American women.
- Cervical cancer has a higher incidence among Hispanic, African American, and Native American women than among white women. The mortality rate for cervical cancer is more than twice as high among African American women as among white women.
- Jewish American women have a low incidence of cervical cancer.

CANCER OF THE CERVIX

Cancer of the cervix is a neoplasm that can be detected in the early, curable stage by a Pap test. The rate of cervical cancer has declined over the past few decades. This decline is attributed to annual Pap testing by women. Cancer of the cervix is usually a squamous cell carcinoma. An estimated 11,955 cases of cervical cancer were diagnosed in 2013. An estimated 4217 cervical cancer deaths occurred in 2013 (CDC, 2017a). The 5-year relative survival rate for localized stage IA cervical cancer was 93% (ACS, 2017b).

Etiology and Pathophysiology

Women who become sexually active in their teens are at an increased risk for cancer of the cervix, as are those who have had multiple sexual partners, had partners who had multiple sexual partners, and are of lower socioeconomic status. Cervical cancer risk is closely linked to sexual behavior, to STIs with several strains of HPV, and to smoking. Women who smoke have a 50% higher risk of developing cervical cancer than nonsmokers. Chronic infections and erosions of the cervix are most likely significant in the development of cancer.

Carcinoma in situ, including that of the cervix, is a term used to describe a preinvasive, asymptomatic carcinoma that can be diagnosed only by microscopic examination. Once diagnosed, it can be treated early without radical surgery. Carcinoma in situ of the cervix is 100% curable.

Clinical Manifestations

Cervical cancer is typically silent in the early stages and offers few symptoms. The two primary symptoms are leukorrhea and irregular vaginal bleeding or spotting between menses. Bleeding often occurs after coitus or after menopause. Bleeding is slight at first but increases as the disease progresses. The vaginal exudate becomes watery and then increases and becomes dark and bloody, with an offensive odor caused by necrosis (death of tissue) and infection of the tumor mass. As the cancer progresses, the bleeding may become constant and may increase in amount. With advanced stages the patient has severe pain in the back, upper thighs, and legs.

Assessment

Subjective data in the early stages of cancer of the cervix are not available, because the woman has no symptoms. If the tumor becomes more invasive, the patient experiences back and leg pain, weight loss, and malaise. Urge women to have regular health appraisals and pelvic examinations so that cancer of the cervix can be detected in its earliest stages.

Collection of objective data includes observing the sanitary pads for abnormal vaginal discharge. The vaginal exudate may be watery to dark red and malodorous. Note the number and saturation of the perineal pads. If the tumor becomes more invasive, assess the patient for anemia, fever, and lymphedema.

Diagnostic Tests

Cervical cancer is diagnosed with the following tests: (1) Pap test; (2) physical examination; (3) colposcopy and cervical biopsy; and (4) additional diagnostic studies, such as a computed tomography (CT) scan, chest radiographic evaluation, IV pyelogram, cystoscopy, sigmoidoscopy, or liver function studies to determine the extent of invasion. The ACS recommends that cervical cancer screening begin approximately 3 years after a woman begins having vaginal intercourse, but no later than 21 years of age. Traditional Pap tests are less than 100% accurate in screening for cervical cell abnormalities, and false-positive and false-negative results do occur. A newer, liquid-based technique can reduce the number of inaccurate Pap tests results.

Medical Management

Gardasil is a vaccine that reduces the incidence of cervical cancer resulting from infection with HPV types 6, 11, 16, and 18. The vaccine is administered to men and women. Vaccination is recommended to begin between ages 11 and 12 years. To be effective, the vaccine should be given before a person becomes sexually active. The goal of these vaccines is to reduce the incidence of HPV-related genital disease, including precancerous cervical lesions and cervical cancer. Three injections are given over 6 months. The second dose is given 2 months after the first dose and the third dose 6 months after the first dose. Vaccination also is recommended for female adolescents, 13 to 18 years of age, to catch up on a missed vaccine or to complete the vaccination series (CDC, 2016a).

Cervarix is a three-dose vaccine to prevent cervical cancer; cervical intraepithelial neoplasia (CIN) grades 1, 2, or worse; and adenocarcinoma in situ. It was approved by the FDA in 2009 for girls and young women 10 to 25 years old and is undergoing pediatric testing for use in 9-year-old girls. Cervarix is effective against HPV types 16 and 18, but it does not offer coverage against all the other types of HPV infection, nor is it effective after exposure to HPV (FDA, 2018).

Carcinoma in situ is treated by removal of the affected area. A variety of techniques can be used, including electrocautery, cryosurgery (use of subfreezing temperature to destroy tissue), laser, conization, and hysterectomy. Conization is the surgical removal of a cone-shaped section of the cervix and is particularly useful in preserving childbearing function.

Early cervical carcinoma can be treated with a hysterectomy or intracavitary radiation (see Chapter 57).

A radical hysterectomy with pelvic lymph node dissection may be required for more extensive lesions. Invasive cervical cancers generally are treated by surgery, radiation, or both, as well as chemotherapy (cisplatin-based) in some cases. Radiation may be external or internal (e.g., cesium, radium). Brachytherapy is a form of radiation therapy in which the source of radiation is implanted in the cervix. The patient is hospitalized for 48 hours for treatment. The treatment plan is tailored to each patient, based on the extent of the disease.

Nursing Interventions and Patient Teaching

Nursing interventions should include verbal reassurance and support. In advanced cervical cancer, position the patient comfortably; change her position slowly; maintain her body alignment; provide pain relief measures; change the patient's dressings and sanitary pads often; and assess color, odor, and amount of drainage. Assess the skin for impairment. See the section "Abdominal Hysterectomy" for a description of nursing interventions for a patient undergoing a hysterectomy.

Patient problems and interventions for the patient with cancer of the cervix include but are not limited to the following:

Patient Problem	Nursing Interventions
Alteration in urinary elimination, related to postsurgical sensorimotor impairment	Connect indwelling catheter to closed gravity drainage Give meticulous catheter care as indicated Record color and amount of urinary output Promote micturition at regular intervals when catheter is removed Catheterize for residual urine as ordered

Patient Problem	Nursing Interventions
Potential for Impaired Self-Esteem due to Current Situation, related to body image change and value of reproductive organs	Encourage discussion with significant others Relate importance of communicating anything that causes anxiety Reinforce correct information to correct any misconceptions
Compromised Blood Flow to Peripheral Tissue, related to: • Pelvic surgery • Thrombophlebitis	Ensure that bed is not elevated in the knee gatch position Assess proper placement of antiembolism stockings q 4 hr as ordered Assist in passive and active leg exercises every shift Encourage ambulation Assess legs for erythema, increased tenderness, and severe cramping every shift

The key to preventing cervical cancer and treating it in the early stages is education. Educate and encourage patients to be responsible for their health by having a yearly Pap test. Education about the HPV vaccine for females is very important. Encourage patients to seek prompt medical assistance for any abnormal vaginal exudate.

Prognosis

The prognosis is good if the cancer is treated in the early stages. It usually takes 2 to 10 years for squamous cell carcinoma to become invasive beyond the basement membrane and metastasize. Therefore early diagnosis and treatment are vital.

CANCER OF THE ENDOMETRIUM

Etiology and Pathophysiology

Cancer of the endometrium usually affects postmenopausal women. In 2018 an estimated 62,230 women will be diagnosed with endometrial cancer. Approximately 11,350 will succumb to the disease (ACS, 2018a). Endometrial cancer is usually an adenocarcinoma (a tumor originating from glandular epithelial cells). The tumor is more likely to be localized but may spread to the cervix, bladder, rectum, and surrounding lymph nodes. It is the most common malignancy of the female genital tract. Women at increased risk are those with a history of irregular menstruation, difficulties during menopause, obesity, hypertension, or diabetes mellitus; those who have not had children; and those with a family history of uterine cancer. Obesity is a risk factor because adipose cells store estrogen. Women who used estrogen replacement therapy to treat menopausal symptoms are more likely to develop endometrial cancer. Progesterone plus estrogen replacement therapy (HRT) may largely offset the increased risk related to using only estrogen. Also at increased risk for developing endometrial cancer are women at high risk for developing breast cancer as well as those in an advanced stage of breast cancer who are taking tamoxifen, an antiestrogen drug that blocks estrogen receptors.

Carcinoma in situ is slow growing. Invasion and metastasis occur later, with expansion to the cervix and the myometrium and ultimately to the vagina, the pelvis, and the lungs.

Clinical Manifestations

Abnormal bleeding is seen in 90% of women diagnosed with endometrial cancer. This may include vaginal bleeding post menopause or bleeding between menstrual periods. Approximately 10% will experience an abnormal nonbloody vaginal discharge (ACS, 2016).

Assessment

Collection of subjective data includes assisting the patient in identifying and reporting changes in reproductive or sexual health. The patient may report abdominal pressure, pain, and pelvic fullness. The patient will have a history of postmenopausal bleeding and leukorrhea. Pelvic and back pain and postcoital bleeding are late signs and symptoms.

Collection of objective data includes observing the color and amount of vaginal exudate on perineal pads. Assess the patient for enlarged lymph nodes.

Diagnostic Tests

Pelvic and rectal examination and endometrial biopsy are used to diagnose cancer of the endometrium. Any report of abnormal or unexpected bleeding in a postmenopausal woman requires a tissue sample to exclude endometrial cancer. The National Cancer Institute (NCI, 2018) reports that screening of asymptomatic or low-risk women by means of an endometrial biopsy is not encouraged. The Pap test is not a reliable diagnostic tool for endometrial cancer, but it can rule out cervical cancer.

Medical Management

Treatment of cancer of the endometrium depends on the stage of the tumor and the woman's health. Surgery, radiation, or chemotherapy may be used to remove the tumor and to treat metastasis. For early cancer of the endometrium, total abdominal hysterectomy with bilateral salpingo-oophorectomy (TAH-BSO) is done. The hysterectomy is performed abdominally as opposed to vaginally to allow the surgeon the ability to view the inside of the abdominal and pelvic cavities to assess for potential areas of concern and metastasis. Intracavitary radiation followed by a TAH-BSO may be done for the early stage of endometrial cancer (stage I). Patients with stage II disease may receive pelvic irradiation to shrink the tumor and to help prevent spread. Afterward the patient undergoes a hysterectomy. Patients with stages III and IV disease are uncommon, and treatment is based on the extent of the disease.

Nursing Interventions and Patient Teaching

See the section "Abdominal Hysterectomy," later in this chapter, for a description of nursing interventions for the patient undergoing a hysterectomy; also see Chapter 57 for care of the patient through intracavitary radiation.

Health teaching and follow-up after discharge should emphasize the need for regular physical examination by the health care provider and the importance of compliance with the prescribed treatment plan.

Prognosis

Cancer of the endometrium is primarily a slow-growing adenocarcinoma. Metastasis occurs late, and the sign of irregular vaginal bleeding often appears early enough to allow for cure of the disease. Approximately 66.7% of endometrial cancer patients are diagnosed when the disease is localized without spread to other parts of the body. The 5-year survival rate for this group of patients is 95%. The populations who are diagnosed once the disease has spread to nearby regions (21%) or metastasized (9%) experience a lessened rate of survival at the 5-year point of 69% and 16%, respectively (ACS Cancer Statistics Center, 2017c). For those women whose cancer has spread, the rate is reduced significantly—only 25% at 5 years (NLM, 2018b).

CANCER OF THE OVARY

Etiology and Pathophysiology

Ovarian cancer, the fifth most common cause of cancer death in women, is the leading cause of gynecologic death in the United States, following cancer of the uterine corpus. Risk for ovarian cancer increases with age. More than half are over the age of 63 years when diagnosed (cancer.org, 2017).

The ACS (2018b) estimated that in 2017, 22,440 women would be diagnosed with ovarian cancer and nearly 14,080 would die of the disease.

In the early stages the tumors are asymptomatic; when detected, they usually have spread to other pelvic organs. Nothing alters the magnitude of risk for ovarian cancer more than genetics. Hereditary ovarian cancer accounts for 5% to 10% of ovarian cancers. In general, the closer the relative with ovarian cancer and the younger the relative at diagnosis, the higher the risk is. Women at increased risk are those who are infertile, anovulatory, nulliparous, and habitual aborters. Because they reduce the number of ovulatory cycles, thus reducing exposure to estrogen, the following practices can reduce the risk of ovarian cancer: oral contraceptive use (greater than 5 years), multiple pregnancies, breastfeeding, and early age of first birth. Other risk factors include a high-fat diet and exposure to industrial chemicals such as asbestos and talc. Ovarian cancer commonly spreads by peritoneal seeding of the cancer cells. Common sites of metastasis are the peritoneum (the membrane that lines the abdominal cavity), the omentum (peritoneal folds that connect the organs to one another or to the abdominal wall), and bowel surfaces.

Clinical Manifestations

In the early stages the symptoms may cause vague abdominal discomfort, flatulence, mild gastric disturbances, pressure, bloating, cramps, sense of pelvic heaviness, feeling of fullness, and change in bowel habits. Pain is not an early symptom. As the tumor progresses, abdominal girth enlarges from ascites (accumulation of fluid in the peritoneal cavity), and there is flatulence with distention. Other symptoms may include urinary frequency, nausea, vomiting, constipation, menstrual irregularities, and weight loss. A challenge of ovarian cancer management is the fact that it often is caught after the disease has spread. The symptoms usually include bloating, pelvic or abdominal pain, urinary disturbances, difficulty eating, or feelings of fullness. These symptoms are attributed easily to other benign disorders. Women who experiences these symptoms are encouraged to seek prompt care with their health care provider. Women are strongly advised to see their gynecologist if they experience any of these symptoms almost daily for more than a few weeks.

Assessment

Collection of subjective data requires an awareness that cancer of the ovary is difficult to detect. The patient reports symptoms of abdominal discomfort, bloating, fullness, gastric disturbances (nausea, constipation), and urinary frequency.

Collection of objective data includes observing any increase in abdominal girth. The patient may void at frequent intervals because of pressure on the bladder. The patient may be dyspneic because of ascites and pressure on the diaphragm.

Diagnostic Tests

Although detecting ovarian cancer early is difficult, an annual bimanual pelvic examination may help to identify pelvic masses. Because the ovaries are movable and therefore harder to assess, screening for ovarian tumors requires a thorough examination, including bimanual and rectovaginal examination. Postmenopause palpable ovary syndrome (a palpable ovary in a woman 3 to 5 years past menopause) may indicate an early tumor. CT scan of the pelvis and abdomen is indicated if an ovarian mass is palpable. Definitive diagnosis of ovarian cancer usually is established by a tumor biopsy at the time of exploratory laparotomy, when staging and tumor debulking take place.

Ovarian cancer is diagnosed by palpation of a pelvic mass, aspiration of ascitic fluid, and detection of cancer cells in the fluid. A blood test to determine CA-125 is used to identify women with ovarian cancer. High levels of CA-125 are found in the blood of 80% of women with epithelial ovarian cancer. However, although the antigen test can help evaluate a woman's response to cancer treatment, it is controversial as an independent screening tool. Because of the test's lack of specificity and sensitivity, false-positive and false-negative results can occur. Many benign conditions, including endometriosis and fibroid tumors, can raise CA-125 levels above normal.

Vaginal ultrasonography, which also lacks specificity and sensitivity, may be used with pelvic examination and CA-125 antigen testing to monitor a woman at increased risk.

Medical Management

Treatment often involves surgery alone or in conjunction with radiation or chemotherapy. Treatment depends on the stage of ovarian cancer (see Chapter 57). Surgery may be a TAH-BSO and omentectomy (excision of portions of the peritoneal folds). In some very early tumors, only the involved ovary is removed, especially in young women who wish to have children. Targeted therapy also may be employed. This type of therapy uses drugs or other substances such as antibodies to attack the cancer cells but not damage the normal cells.

Nursing Interventions

Nursing interventions for any patient with ovarian cancer include management similar to that for patients undergoing abdominal hysterectomy and receiving chemotherapy and external radiation (see Chapter 57). Because ovarian cancer is generally at an advanced stage when diagnosed, despite the woman's feeling well, support and encouragement to comply with the treatment regimen are important nursing interventions. As the disease progresses, become involved in activities to increase the patient's comfort.

Patient problems and interventions for the patient with cancer of the ovaries include but are not limited to the following:

Patient Problem	Nursing Interventions
Fearfulness, related to diagnosis of cancer	Assist patient with recognizing and clarifying fears and with developing coping strategies for those fears Be an active listener
Impaired Self-Esteem due to Current Situation, related to body image change and value of reproductive organs	Encourage patient's comments and questions about condition Encourage discussion with significant others Provide factual information to correct any misconceptions

Prognosis

More than 75% of women with ovarian cancer are diagnosed with advanced disease. The 5-year survival rate for all stages is 47%. If diagnosed early and treated while the disease is localized, the 5-year survival rate is 92%. Relative survival rates for more advanced disease are 71% for regional disease and 31% for disease that has spread to distant sites (ACS Cancer Statistics Center, 2018b).

HYSTERECTOMY

A hysterectomy involves removal of the uterus; the cervix, fallopian tubes, ovaries, and other structures may also be removed. This procedure may be done for many conditions, including dysfunctional uterine bleeding, endometriosis, malignant and nonmalignant tumors of the uterus and cervix, and disorders of pelvic relaxation and uterine prolapse.

Various terms are used to describe removal of the uterus:

- *Subtotal hysterectomy:* A subtotal hysterectomy involves removal only of the uterus, either vaginally, abdominally, or laparoscopically. The cervix remains intact and the vagina retains its usual length. Intercourse is possible even though childbearing is not; leaving the cervical stump in place may play a role in a woman's sexual pleasure and orgasm. Estrogens are still released because the ovaries are still present. Menopause occurs naturally.
- *Total hysterectomy:* A total hysterectomy involves removal of the uterus and cervix, either vaginally, abdominally, or laparoscopically. The vagina remains intact, but somewhat shortened; intercourse is possible even though childbearing is not. Estrogens are still released because the ovaries are still present. Menopause occurs naturally.
- *Total abdominal/laparoscopic hysterectomy with bilateral salpingo-oophorectomy (TAH-BSO/TLH-BSO):* Total abdominal/laparoscopic hysterectomy with bilateral salpingo-oophorectomy involves removal of the uterus, fallopian tubes, and ovaries; this is done abdominally (TAH-BSO) or laparoscopically (TLH-BSO). It is sometimes called a **panhysterosalpingo-oophorectomy.** Because the ovaries are removed, menopause is induced.
- *Radical hysterectomy:* A radical hysterectomy also includes removal of the pelvic lymph nodes; this is done abdominally. Because the ovaries are removed, menopause is induced.

VAGINAL HYSTERECTOMY

A vaginal hysterectomy is typically done for a prolapsed uterus. In this procedure the patient is placed in the lithotomy position, and the uterus is removed through the vagina. The vaginal route is not used as often as the abdominal approach; there are, however, clear advantages to the vaginal approach. Patients who are poor candidates for abdominal surgery or prolonged anesthesia may benefit from this option. The procedure is less expensive and requires a reduced period of hospitalization. A vaginal hysterectomy does not require an abdominal incision, which facilitates recovery. Postoperative discomfort is less than with the abdominal approach. There is a reduced risk for the development of complications. The most important disadvantage of the vaginal route is the necessarily limited view of the operative field for visualizing intrapelvic and intra-abdominal organs. Vaginal hysterectomy is not used in cases of large uterine fibroids, enlarged uterine size, or suspicions of malignancy.

ABDOMINAL HYSTERECTOMY

An abdominal hysterectomy is preferred when there is a need to explore the pelvic cavity and when the fallopian tubes and ovaries are to be removed. The laparoscopic hysterectomy may be performed when there is no need to have a more extensive visualization of the pelvic or abdominal cavities.

Nursing Interventions

Preoperative interventions. When the health care provider has explained the surgery to the patient, reinforce the explanation and answer any questions. Encourage verbalization of fears. Provide additional preoperative instructions to help the woman prepare for postoperative recovery. Instruct the patient how to turn, cough, and deep breathe.

Before a vaginal or abdominal hysterectomy, the colon is emptied to prevent postoperative distention. The patient may be on a low-residue diet for several days preoperatively. Enemas may be given the evening before surgery. An indwelling catheter is placed to decompress the bladder, to prevent trauma during surgery. The catheter normally is removed the day after surgery. An antiseptic vaginal douche may be ordered to decrease microbial invasion of the surgical site.

Surgical preparation of the skin on the abdomen, the pelvis, and the perineum often is performed in surgery. The patient signs a consent form, and oral intake after midnight is restricted. On occasion, ureteral stents are placed in the ureters for identification and to prevent possible trauma to the ureters during surgery.

Postoperative interventions. Nursing interventions after surgery focus on monitoring and recording patient status, preventing complications, and reporting concerns to the surgeon. The postoperative nursing assessment is performed at least every 4 hours during the first day after surgery. Lung fields are assessed. The patient is assisted to turn, cough, and deep breathe every 2 hours. Instruct the patient to splint the abdomen as needed. Incentive spirometry to encourage deep breathing is often prescribed during waking hours. Vital signs are assessed and compared with the preoperative baselines. Oxygen saturation levels are assessed. The urinary catheter is assessed to ensure patency (i.e., that it is unblocked). The amount of urine also must be recorded. Output less than 30 mL/h must be reported. The incidence of urinary retention after a hysterectomy is greater than after any other type of surgery, because some trauma to the bladder is unavoidable. The abdomen is assessed for distension and bowel sounds. As the postoperative period progresses assess for passage of flatus. The lower extremities are evaluated for redness or tenderness. Early ambulation is initiated to promote bowel activity and prevention of venous thrombus. When bowel sounds have returned and flatus is being expelled, the patient is allowed liquids by mouth and a gradual return to solid foods.

Patients undergoing pelvic surgery are susceptible to venous stasis and thrombophlebitis because of trauma to blood vessels. The patient usually is permitted out of bed on the first postoperative day. Encourage the patient to sit on the side of the bed and dangle her legs before standing and walking, to avoid postural hypotension. Encourage the patient to cough, deep breathe, and use an incentive spirometer to prevent postoperative pneumonia and atelectasis. Antiembolism stockings may be used to prevent thrombus or embolus formation, and the legs should be exercised frequently when the patient is in bed. Many health care providers prescribe intermittent pneumonic compression cuffs for the calves to prevent venous stasis, deep-vein thrombosis, and pulmonary embolism. The patient should avoid bending her knees. This could cause pooling of blood in the pelvic cavity, resulting in stasis in the lower extremities. The patient at risk for thromboembolic disease may receive low-dose heparin or low molecular weight enoxaparin (Lovenox) to prevent thrombus formation.

Analgesics such as morphine may be ordered for relief of pain. Slight vaginal drainage may occur for several days. Report any unusual bleeding to the health care provider. Observe the abdominal dressing on the patient with an abdominal hysterectomy for evidence of hemorrhage. Use surgical asepsis for the dressing change. The patient usually receives IV feedings for the first postoperative day. Carefully monitor the rate of flow and the condition of the IV site.

Patient problems and interventions for the patient who has had a hysterectomy include but are not limited to the following:

Patient Problem	Nursing Interventions
Prolonged Pain, related to metastatic process	Monitor and document pain characteristics Administer prescribed analgesics q 3-4 hr to control pain Provide environment conducive to comfort and rest
Fluid Volume Overload, related to ascites	Monitor IV fluids Maintain accurate I&O Weigh patient daily Observe for signs of edema Measure abdominal girth daily

Patient Problem	Nursing Interventions
Impaired Family Coping, related to poor prognosis	Assess present coping abilities Encourage and allow time for verbalization of feelings Support patient's coping strengths, and discuss alternative coping measures Involve patient and significant others in nursing interventions and procedures

Patient Teaching

Before discharge, the health care provider explains to the woman and her partner that they should not have sexual intercourse for 4 to 6 weeks after surgery. With an abdominal incision, there may be further restrictions on heavy lifting (nothing greater than 10 pounds), walking up and down stairs, and prolonged riding in the car. Riding in the car may cause pelvic pooling and development of a thrombus in the legs.

Inform the patient that vaginal drainage is normal for about 2 to 4 weeks after an abdominal hysterectomy. Advise her to avoid wearing any tight clothing such as a girdle or knee-high hose, which may constrict circulation to the surgical site and cause venous stasis.

Several signs and symptoms of infection should be reported to the health care provider if they occur: (1) erythema, edema, exudate, or increased tenderness along the surgical incision; (2) increased malodorous vaginal exudate; (3) a temperature of 101°F (38.3°C) or more; and (4) any problems with urinating, such as difficulty in starting to void, voiding too often, voiding small amounts, or a burning sensation while urinating (indicative of a bladder infection).

DISORDERS OF THE FEMALE BREAST

FIBROCYSTIC BREAST CONDITION

Etiology and Pathophysiology

Fibrocystic breast condition involves benign tumors of the breasts. It usually occurs in women 30 to 50 years of age and is rare in postmenopausal women. This suggests that the occurrence is related to ovarian activity.

The cysts are characterized by numerous cellular changes, with an abnormal amount of epithelial hyperplasia and cystic formation within the mammary ducts. The cysts rarely become malignant, but the risk of breast cancer does increase for women who have fibrocystic breast condition; therefore the cysts are monitored carefully.

Clinical Manifestations

Cystic lesions are often bilateral and multiple. The cysts are soft, well differentiated, tender, and freely movable. The lumpiness and tenderness are more apparent before menses.

Diagnostic Tests

The disorder is diagnosed by mammography or ultrasound and confirmed by biopsy. As a therapeutic measure, the cyst is aspirated by needle and syringe to empty the secretions, and the fluid is sent to the laboratory for cytologic examination to rule out a malignancy. Aspiration produces a turbid, nonhemorrhagic fluid that is yellow, greenish, or brownish.

Medical Management

When a cyst recurs in the same area and repeated aspirations are ineffective, surgical excision of the cyst may be done.

Conservative treatment is the usual approach to fibrocystic breast condition. The usefulness of eliminating methylxanthines (in coffee, tea, and cola) from the diet is still controversial, but it is the least expensive therapy. Many women have reported decreased symptoms after altering their diet, even though findings by palpation and mammogram were not significantly changed. Danazol may be prescribed to inhibit FSH and LH production, thereby decreasing ovarian production of estrogen. Danazol may cause weight gain, hot flashes, menstrual irregularities, hirsutism, and deepening of the voice. Vitamin E also may be prescribed, but its efficacy has not been proven.

Nursing Interventions and Patient Teaching

Instruct the patient to perform breast self-examination (BSE) 1 week after menses, to recognize the presence of cysts, and to note any changes.

ACUTE MASTITIS

Acute mastitis is an acute bacterial infection of the breast tissue, usually caused by *S. aureus* or streptococci. It is observed most often during lactation and late pregnancy. The infection may result from a clogged milk duct, inadequate cleanliness of the breasts, a nipple fissure, or infection in the infant. The breasts are tender, inflamed, and engorged, obstructing the milk flow.

Treatment involves application of warm packs, support of the area with a well-fitting brassiere (which also supplies comfort), and systemic treatment with antibiotics. Women who are breast-feeding are permitted to continue with nursing because this promotes emptying of the inflamed ducts and reduce the incidence of milk stasis.

CHRONIC MASTITIS

Chronic mastitis tends to develop in women between 30 and 50 years of age and is more common in those who have had children, have had difficulty with inverted and cracked nipples, and have had problems nursing their infants. A traumatic blow to the breasts causes the fat to necrose in the area and form abscesses. Increased fibrosis of the tissue causes cysts to form. The cysts are tender, painful, and palpable on examination. The disorder is generally unilateral and benign and most frequently occurs in obese women. Treatment is the same as for acute mastitis.

CANCER OF THE BREAST

Breast cancer is the second most common malignancy (after lung cancer) affecting women in the United States: approximately one of every eight American women will develop breast cancer during her lifetime. In contrast, the incidence of breast cancer in men is rare. It is predicted that in 2018 fewer than 3000 men will will be diagnosed with invasive breast cancer. This is significantly less than the more than 266,000 cases that will impact women in the same time period (ACS, 2018c; Breastcancer.org, 2018).

Women over 60 years of age have twice the incidence of breast cancer as women ages 45 to 60. In women older than 55, 50% more patients have metastatic disease at presentation than do younger women. Vital to the process of detection are monthly BSEs, breast imaging with digital mammography and MRI or ultrasound to differentiate a cyst from a lesion and to detect small tumors before they can be palpated, and periodic breast examinations by a health care provider.

Etiology and Pathophysiology

The cause of breast cancer is unknown. The high incidence in women implies a hormonal cause (Box 52.4).

The primary risk factors are female gender, age greater than 50 years, North American or Northern European descent, a personal history of breast cancer, atypical hyperplasia or carcinoma in situ, two or more first-degree relatives with the disease, and a first-degree relative with bilateral premenopausal breast cancer. Other risk factors include early menarche, a first pregnancy after age 30, natural menopause after age 55, and one or more breast cancer genes. The inherited susceptibility genes, *BRCA1* and *BRCA2,* account for approximately 2% to 7% of all cases and confer an increased lifetime risk in these women (CDC, 2018). Findings suggest that prophylactic removal of the breasts and/or ovaries in *BRCA1* and *BRCA2* carriers decreases the risk of breast cancer considerably, although not all women who choose this surgery would have developed cancer. Women who consider this option should have an opportunity for counseling before reaching a decision. Some research studies assessing the relationship between survival rates and obesity have found some evidence showing that obese women have a lessened survival rate for breast cancer. Current data indicate that tamoxifen and raloxifene decrease breast cancer risk in women who are at increased risk. With the exception of advancing age and being female, however, most women who develop breast cancer do not have any risk factors for the disease. That is why it is so important to encourage even healthy women to undergo screening examinations.

Breast cancer is usually an adenocarcinoma, arising from the epithelium and developing in the lactiferous ducts; it infiltrates the parenchyma (the functioning tissue of an organ other than the supporting or connective tissue). The cancer occurs most often in women who have not given birth or breast-fed a child. It occurs most often in the upper outer quadrant of the breast because this is the location of most of the glandular tissue. A slow-growing breast cancer may take up to 10 or more years to become palpable, or to reach the size of a small pea. Slow-growing lesions often are associated with a lower mortality rate. When referring to estimated growth rate of breast cancer, the term *doubling time* indicates the time it takes malignant cells to double in number. Assuming that the doubling is constant and that the neoplasm originates in one cell, a carcinoma with a doubling time of 100 days may not reach clinically detectable size (1 cm) for 8 years. Rapid-growing cancers have a much shorter preclinical course and a greater tendency to metastasize to regional nodes or more distant sites by the time a breast mass is discovered. In breast cancer, metastasis occurs via the lymphatic system and bloodstream (Fig. 52.14). The most common sites for metastasis are, in order, the bones, lungs, pleura, other breast sites, central nervous system, and liver.

Box 52.4 Predisposing Factors for Women at High Risk for Breast Cancer

- *Gender:* Being female introduces a high risk.
- *Age:* Higher incidence occurs among women over 40 years of age and in the postmenopausal phase of life. After age 60 the incidence increases dramatically.
- *Race:* White women, in the middle or upper socioeconomic class, are at higher risk.
- *Genetics:* The inherited susceptibility genes *BRCA1* and *BRCA2* account for approximately 5% of all cases and confer a lifetime risk in these women, ranging from 35% to 85%.
- *Family history:* This is especially important if a diagnosed family member had ovarian cancer, was premenopausal, had bilateral breast cancer, or is a first-degree relative (mother, sister, daughter).
- *Parity (total number of pregnancies):* Risk is decreased for women who gave birth before reaching 18 years of age; it is increased for women who are not sexually active, infertile women, and women who became pregnant for the first time after 30 years of age.
- *Menopause:* Menopause after 55 years of age increases the risk.
- *Obesity:* Weight gain and obesity after menopause increase the risk.
- *Other cancer:* Risk is increased for women diagnosed with some other form of cancer, such as endometrial, ovarian, or colon cancer; if cancer has appeared in one breast, it is more likely to occur in the other breast.

Clinical Manifestations

Breast cancer is detected as a lump or mammographic abnormality in the breast. Breast tumors are usually small, solitary, irregularly shaped, firm, nontender, and nonmobile. There may be a change in skin color, feelings

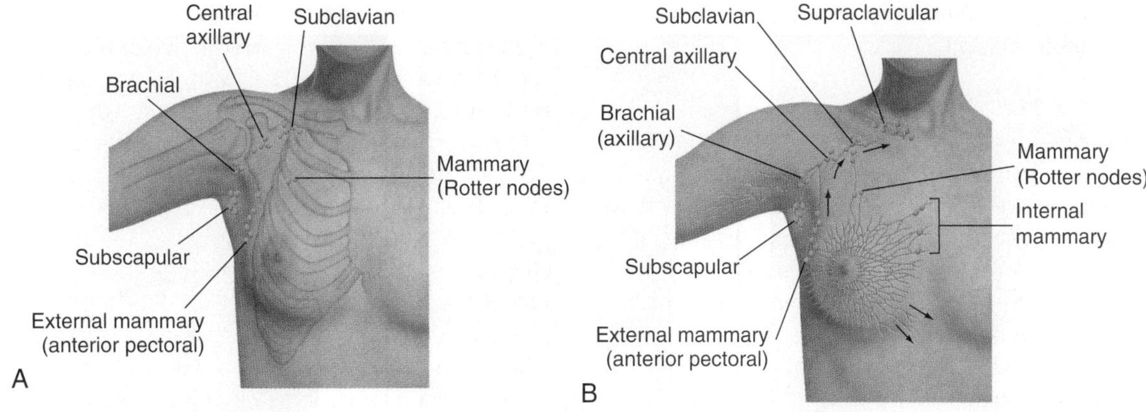

Fig. 52.14 A, Lymph nodes of the axilla. B, Lymphatic drainage of the breast. (From Seidel HM, Ball JW, Dains JE, et al: *Mosby's guide to physical examination,* ed 7, St. Louis, 2011, Mosby.)

of tenderness, puckering or dimpling of tissue (peau d'orange—skin with the appearance and texture of an orange peel), nipple discharge, retraction of the nipple, and axillary tenderness.

Women should perform BSEs monthly, preferably 1 week after menses. Postmenopausal women should perform a BSE on the same day each month (Fig. 52.15). If there are questionable findings, the patient should immediately contact her health care provider (see the Patient Teaching box).

Patient Teaching

Breast Self-Examination

- The majority of breast lumps are not cancer.
- Cancerous breast lesions are treatable.
- Breasts should be examined by premenopausal women each month, 7 or 8 days after conclusion of the menstrual period when they are least congested, and by postmenopausal women on the same day of each month.
- Visual inspection and palpation should be done.
- Visual inspection should be done when the woman is stripped to the waist and looking in a mirror, using the following arm positions: (1) arms at rest at sides, (2) hands on hips and pressed into hips, (3) contracting chest muscles, (4) hands over the head (torso in upright position), and (5) hands over the head (torso leaning forward).
- Palpation may be done in the shower, where the soap and water help the hands glide over the skin. However, examination of large breasts and axillae is better done in a supine position rather than while standing.
- The entire breast should be examined in a systematic way, moving clockwise, with a circular motion, or moving back and forth. Always include the axillae in the examination.
- Do not forget specific examination of the nipple, through compression for discharge, and the areola, through palpation.
- Report any changes to the health care provider.

Diagnostic Tests

The essential factors in the early detection of breast cancer are the regular performance of BSE, regular clinical breast examination (CBE), and routine mammography. The frequency of these examinations is determined by the woman's age, the presence of significant risk factors, and her medical history. Current guidelines accepted by the ACS regarding breast surveillance practices include the following:

- Monthly BSE starting at 20 years of age.
- Physical examinations of the breast by a trained health professional; CBE every 3 years between 20 and 40 years of age and every year for women 40 and older.
- Screening mammography annually beginning between 40 and 44 years of age. If a first-degree family member has a history of breast cancer, a screening mammogram is recommended at 35 years.
- MRI screening combined with mammograms for women with a significant family history or genetic tendencies (Breastcancer.org, 2016a).

Guidelines from the US Preventive Services Task Force established in 2009 recommend the following: (1) women age 40 to 49 should not receive routine screening mammography for breast cancer, but these women should decide for themselves when to begin mammography after weighing the risks and benefits; (2) women age 50 to 74 should receive screening mammography every 2 years (instead of annually); (3) routine breast self-examination (BSE) should no longer be taught. The Task Force states that this is not a recommendation against mammography for women in their 40s and BSE, but that there is not enough evidence to prove that women benefit from them.

Several techniques can be used to screen for breast disease or to diagnose a suspicious physical finding. Mammography is a radiographic technique used to visualize the internal structure of the breast. Mammography can detect tumors that cannot be felt by palpation. The minimum size detectable by physical examination is 1 cm. It takes 10 or more years to grow a tumor this size. Mammography can detect masses of

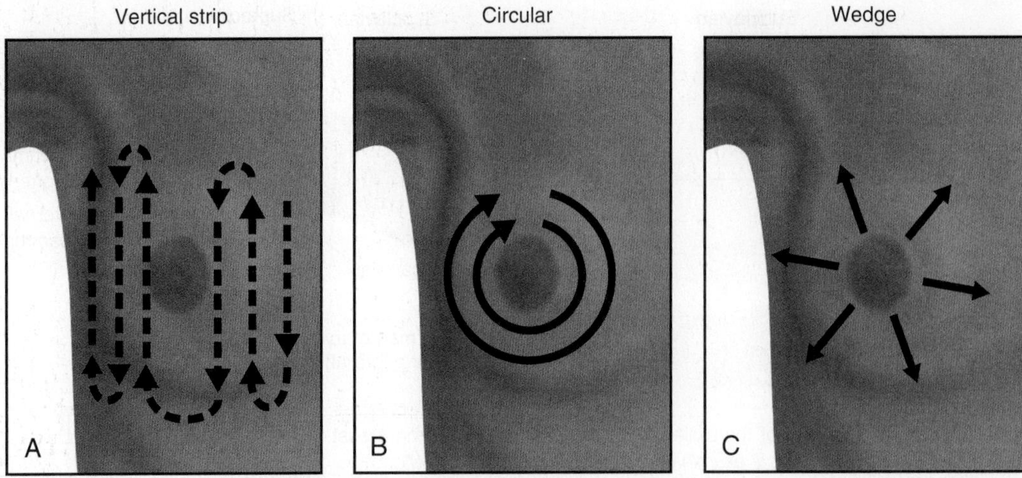

Fig. 52.15 Methods for palpation. A, Back and forth. B, Concentric circles. C, Palpation out from the center in wedge sections. (From Seidel HM, Ball JW, Dains JE, et al: *Mosby's guide to physical examination*, ed 7, St. Louis, 2011, Mosby.)

0.5 cm. Because tumors usually metastasize late in the preclinical course, earlier detection by mammography may prevent metastasis of smaller lesions.

Comparative mammography may show early cancer tissue changes. The diagnostic accuracy of mammography in combination with physical examination has significantly improved early and accurate detection of breast malignancies. In younger women, mammography is less sensitive because of the greater density of breast tissue, resulting in more false-negative results. Mammography will not reveal 10% to 25% of breast cancers. Masses should be biopsied, even if mammogram findings are unremarkable.

Definitive diagnosis of a mass can be made only by means of histologic examination of biopsied tissues. Biopsy techniques may include either fine needle aspiration (FNA) biopsy and cytologic examination or core-cutting needle biopsy, excisional biopsy, and incisional biopsy. Even if the lesion is nonpalpable, an FNA biopsy can be used. FNA and cytologic evaluation should be done only if an experienced cytologist is available, and all lesions read as negative are followed up by a more definitive biopsy procedure. If the aspirated specimen is positive for malignancy, the patient can be given this information at the same visit and begin learning about treatment issues.

Improved imaging techniques have reduced the radiation exposure that accompanies mammography to insignificant levels. Therefore the benefits of mammography outweigh the risks from radiation exposure. Ultrasound (echogram, sonogram) also can be used to differentiate a benign cyst (fluid filled) from a malignant mass (solid). An ultrasound will not detect microcalcifications, which are often the only indicators of very small tumors.

Other methods used to help diagnose and stage breast cancer include MRI and positron emission tomography (PET). MRI and PET scans are used to help differentiate between malignant and benign disease in select patients.

A relatively new diagnostic tool used before therapeutic surgery is **sentinel lymph node mapping,** which identifies the first lymph node most likely to drain the cancerous cells. During this procedure a radioactive substance is injected around the breast biopsy site. The patient is then sent to the operating room, where a blue dye is injected as well. The area then is monitored to see which nodes take up the substances. The node that "lights up," containing the most radioactivity and blue dye, is considered the sentinel node and the one most likely to contain cancer cells. The identified node and at least two other nodes then are biopsied to see if they contain tumor cells. If they do not, it is likely that the more distant axillary nodes are cancer free. The nodes can be left intact, reducing the threat of complications such as edema, infection, pain, and loss of function of the arm. Sentinel lymph node dissection has been associated with lower morbidity rates and greater accuracy compared with complete axillary node dissection. National clinical research trials are evaluating whether standard lymph node dissection can be avoided if sentinel lymph node dissection is performed. If one or more sentinel lymph nodes are positive for malignant cells, an axillary lymph node dissection generally is recommended (NCI, 2011).

Axillary lymph node involvement is one of the most important prognostic factors in early stage breast cancer. Metastasis in axillary nodes can be determined by pathologic examination of as few as 6 to 10 nodes. The more nodes involved means the greater the risk of recurrence. Patients with four or more positive nodes have the greatest risk of recurrence. During examination, the lymph nodes can provide prognostic information that helps further determine treatment (chemotherapy, hormone therapy, or both).

Another diagnostic test useful for determining prognosis and treatment is estrogen and progesterone receptor status. Receptor-positive tumors commonly (1) show evidence of being well differentiated (see Chapter 57, Box 57.2), (2) have a more normal DNA content and low proliferation, (3) have a lower chance for recurrence, and (4) are hormone dependent and responsive to hormonal therapy. Receptor-negative tumors (1) are often poorly differentiated, (2) have a high incidence of abnormal DNA content and high proliferation, (3) frequently recur, and (4) are usually unresponsive to hormonal therapy (komen.org, 2018a).

Medical Management

The intervention for treatment of breast cancer depends on the tumor stage, the patient's age and health, the hormonal status, and the presence of estrogen receptors in the tumor. Radiation, chemotherapy, and surgery alone or in combination are the most common modes of treatment for breast cancer (see Chapter 57).

Staging. After breast surgery and axillary dissection, the staging process is completed. Axillary lymph node dissection or sentinel lymph node mapping usually is performed regardless of the treatment option selected. Examination of nodes provides the most powerful prognostic data currently available. Also, removal of axillary nodes is highly effective in preventing axillary recurrence, aids in decision making regarding adjuvant chemotherapy or hormonal therapy, and eliminates the need for axillary nodal radiation. Radiation of the axilla is equally effective in decreasing the incidence of axillary recurrence (see Fig. 52.14).

The most widely accepted staging method for breast cancer is the American Joint Committee on Cancer's TNM system. This system uses tumor size (T), nodal involvement and size (N), and presence of metastasis (M) to determine the stage of disease (Box 52.5).

Surgical intervention. Surgery plays a vital role in the management of breast cancer. Tissue biopsy, inspection and biopsy of lymph nodes in the axillary areas, radiologic examinations, and laboratory reports aid in making the decision to perform surgery.

Because estrogen can affect a tumor's invasive ability, it is suggested that premenopausal women be operated on during the menstrual phase, when estrogen levels are lower or opposed by progesterone.

Several surgical options are available for the removal of a breast carcinoma. In breast conservation surgery (termed *lumpectomy*), which conserves the breast, a circumscribed area is removed along with the tumor. This surgery is usually done when the tumor is small and located on the peripheral area of the breast. The breast contour and muscle support are preserved if possible. Axillary nodes often are removed in these breast-sparing procedures as well. Contraindications to lumpectomy or excisional biopsy include two or more separate tumors in separate quadrants of the breast, diffuse microcalcifications, a history of previous radiation to the region, a large tumor-to-breast ratio, a history of collagen vascular disease, large breasts, and a tumor located underneath the nipple.

One of the main advantages of breast conservation surgery and radiation is that it preserves the breast, including the nipple. The goal of the combined surgery

Box 52.5 TNM System for Staging Breast Cancer

Breast cancer is staged using the TNM (tumor, node, metastasis) system, which categorizes the disease by tumor size and spread, lymph node involvement, and metastasis. The TNM system, which was developed by the American Joint Committee on Cancer and revised in 2003, works this way:

- *Tumor:* A number from 0 to 4 indicates the tumor's size and whether it has spread to nearby tissue (if it has not, this indicates a carcinoma in situ). Higher numbers indicate a larger tumor or wider spread. For example, a tumor labeled T1 is 2 cm or smaller; T4 indicates a tumor of any size that has spread to the chest wall or the skin.
- *Nodes:* A number from 0 to 3 indicates whether the cancer has spread to surrounding lymph nodes and, if so, the number of nodes that are affected. For example, N1 indicates a spread to one, two, or three lymph nodes under the arm on the same side as the breast cancer.
- *Metastasis:* M0 means the cancer has not spread to distant organs; M1 means the cancer has metastasized to other organs.

All of this information is combined to determine an overall stage of 0 to IV.

- *Stage 0:* Refers to carcinoma in situ, in which the tumor is confined to the milk duct or the lobule, no lymph nodes have been affected, and no metastasis has occurred.
- *Stage I:* The tumor is 2 cm or smaller. Lymph nodes are negative. There is no distant cancer spread.
- *Stage IIA:* The tumor is 5 cm or smaller. It may have spread to one, two, or three axillary nodes. There is no distant cancer spread.
- *Stage IIB:* The tumor can be larger than 5 cm. Up to three lymph nodes may be involved, but there is no metastasis to other organs.
- *Stage IIIA:* The tumor may be more than 5 cm and has spread to more than 3 but fewer than 10 lymph nodes. No distant organs are involved.
- *Stage IIIB:* The tumor, regardless of size, has spread to the chest wall or the skin. There is lymph node involvement but no distant metastasis.
- *Stage IIIC:* Refers to any size tumor, including one that has spread to the chest wall or the skin. There is involvement of 10 or more lymph nodes, but no distant metastasis.
- *Stage IV:* The tumor can be any size. There is nodal involvement and metastasis to distant organs.

Data from American Cancer Society: Breast cancer stages, 2017. Available at https://www.cancer.org/cancer/breast-cancer/understanding-a-breast-cancer-diagnosis/stages-of-breast-cancer.html and from Lewis SL, Dirksen SR, Heitkemper MM, et al: *Medical-surgical nursing: Assessment and management of clinical problems*, ed 9, St. Louis, 2014, Mosby.

and radiation is to maximize the benefits of cancer treatment and cosmetic outcome while minimizing risks. Disadvantages of this surgery plus radiation include the increased cost over surgery alone and the possible side effects of radiation. Lumpectomy is followed by 6 weeks of radiation.

A simple mastectomy involves removal of the entire breast. The skin flap is retained to cover the incised area. Pectoralis major and pectoralis minor muscles are left intact. The patient has the option of breast reconstruction.

A modified radical mastectomy may be performed if the tumor is 4 cm or larger, if it is invasive, or if the patient and health care provider decide this procedure is in the patient's best interest. In this operation all breast tissue, overlying skin, nipple, and pectoralis minor muscles are removed, as are samples of axillary lymph nodes and fascia under the breast. The pectoralis major muscle remains intact. The patient has the option of breast reconstruction, which can be performed immediately after the mastectomy or can be delayed until postoperative recovery is complete (about 6 months).

Most women diagnosed with early stage breast cancer (tumors less than 5 cm) are candidates for either lumpectomy and radiation or modified radical mastectomy. Overall 10-year survival with lumpectomy and radiation is about the same as with modified radical mastectomy (komen.org, 2018b).

Adjuvant therapies

Radiation therapy. Depending on the tumor's size, regional spread, and aggressiveness, radiation therapy often is prescribed. Radiation therapy may be used for breast cancer (1) as the primary therapy to destroy the tumor or as a companion to surgery to prevent local recurrence, (2) to shrink a large tumor to operable size, and (3) as palliative treatment for the pain caused by local recurrence and metastasis. Lumpectomy is almost always followed by radiation. Radiation therapy is usually started 2 to 3 weeks after surgery, when the wound is completely healed and the patient can comfortably raise her arm over her head. Contraindications include a diagnosis of breast cancer during the first or second trimester of pregnancy, delayed wound healing, collagen vascular disease, and previous radiation to the same breast.

In external beam radiation, the radiation procedure uses an external beam of high-energy protons. The treatments are usually done 5 days a week for 5 to 6 weeks. Adverse effects include fatigue and skin reactions such as erythema, pruritus, dryness, infection, and pain. The skin literally has a burned appearance.

Internal radiation, also known as implant radiation or brachytherapy, is a new procedure that is an alternative to traditional radiation treatment for early stage breast cancer. The technique uses a balloon catheter to insert radioactive seeds into the breast after the tumor is removed (at the time of the lumpectomy or shortly thereafter into the tumor resection cavity). The seeds deliver a high dose of concentrated radiation directly to the site where the cancer is most likely to recur.

Chemotherapy. Patients who require postsurgical chemotherapy—typically those with lymph node involvement or metastasis to distant organs—receive antineoplastic medications, hormones, a monoclonal antibody, or a combination of these medications. Regimens for node-negative disease (i.e., cancer that has not spread to the lymph nodes) include cyclophosphamide, methotrexate, and 5-fluorouracil (Efudex), referred to as CMF; cyclophosphamide, doxorubicin, and 5-fluorouracil, or CAF; or doxorubicin and cyclophosphamide, commonly called AC. For those with node-positive disease, the regimens include CAF, AC followed by paclitaxel, doxorubicin followed by CMF, and CMF.

The most common adverse effects of traditional antineoplastic drugs are bone marrow suppression (which causes anemia, thrombocytopenia, and leukopenia), nausea and vomiting, alopecia, weight gain, mucositis, and fatigue. Agents such as filgrastim (Neupogen), which raise leukocyte counts, can combat the threat of infection that accompanies bone marrow suppression. Epoetin alfa (Procrit) is helpful in raising erythrocyte counts to help correct anemia. Other drugs typically ordered for chemotherapy patients are phenothiazines, such as prochlorperazine, and serotonin antagonists such as granisetron and ondansetron (Zofran). These drugs prevent or lessen nausea and vomiting.

Hormonal therapy. Estrogen can promote the growth of breast cancer cells if the cells are estrogen receptor positive. Hormonal therapy removes or blocks the source of estrogen, thus promoting tumor regression.

Two advances have increased the use of hormonal therapy in breast cancer. First, hormone receptor assays, which are reliable diagnostic tests, have been developed to identify women who are likely to respond to hormonal therapy. The tumor's estrogen and progesterone receptor status can be determined. These assays can predict whether hormonal therapy is a treatment option for women with breast cancer, either at the time of initial therapy or if the cancer recurs. Second, drugs have been developed that can inactivate the hormone-secreting glands as effectively as surgery or radiation. Premenopausal and perimenopausal women are more likely to have tumors that are not hormone dependent, whereas women who are postmenopausal are more likely to have hormone-dependent tumors. Chances of tumor regression are significantly greater in women whose tumors contain estrogen and progesterone receptors.

Estrogen deprivation can occur by destroying the ovaries by surgery, radiation, or drug therapy. Hormonal therapy can block or destroy the estrogen receptors. Hormonal therapy is used to treat recurrent or metastatic cancer but also may be used as an adjuvant to primary treatment.

Tamoxifen is the hormonal agent of choice in postmenopausal, estrogen receptor–positive women with or without lymph node involvement. Tamoxifen, an antiestrogen drug, blocks the estrogen receptor sites of malignant cells and thus inhibits the growth-stimulating effects of estrogen. It is commonly used in advanced and early stage breast cancer to prevent or treat recurrent disease. Tamoxifen also may be used to prevent breast cancer in high-risk individuals. Side effects of tamoxifen are minimal but include hot flashes, nausea, vomiting, vaginal discharge, and other effects commonly associated with decreased estrogen. It also increases the risk of blood clots, cataracts, and endometrial cancer in postmenopausal women. Tamoxifen is not used in women desiring continued fertility.

Toremifene (Fareston), an antiestrogen agent similar to tamoxifen, is indicated as first-line treatment for metastatic breast cancer in postmenopausal women with estrogen receptor–positive or estrogen receptor–unknown tumors. Fulvestrant (Faslodex) may be given to women with advanced breast cancer who no longer respond to tamoxifen. This drug slows cancer progression by destroying estrogen receptors in the breast cancer cells. Fulvestrant is given intramuscularly on a monthly basis.

Aromatase inhibitor drugs, which interfere with the enzyme that synthesizes endogenous estrogen, are used to treat advanced breast cancer in postmenopausal women with disease progression. These drugs include anastrozole (Arimidex), letrozole (Femara), exemestane (Aromasin), and aminoglutethimide (Cytadren).

Research has shown that letrozole reduced the risk of recurrence of breast cancer and lengthens the period before reoccurrence in those who ultimately experienced a return of the disease (Breastcancer.org, 2017). Letrozole, previously approved by the FDA for advanced breast cancer, offers an option for extending treatment of early-stage disease. Letrozole, like tamoxifen, works by interfering with the hormone estrogen, which feeds breast cancer cells. Tamoxifen blocks estrogen receptors on the cells, whereas letrozole inhibits the creation of estrogen.

Bisphosphonates, such as pamidronate sodium (Aredia), are being used to delay bone metastases and reduce the occurrence of skeletal problems in patients with advanced breast cancer (www.cancereffects.com, 2013). The loss of bone also may be reduced with the use of bisphosphonates (clodronate, risedronate, ibandronate, zoledronate). Raloxifene (Evista), used to prevent bone loss, may also reduce the risk of breast cancer without stimulating endometrial growth. Raloxifene acts as an estrogen antagonist at the hormone-sensitive tissues of breast cancer and bone. Additional drugs that may be used to suppress hormone-dependent tumors include megestrol, diethylstilbestrol, and fluoxymesterone (Breastcancer.org, 2016b).

Monoclonal antibody therapy. Another drug treatment for breast cancer is the monoclonal antibody trastuzumab (Herceptin). It is used to treat metastatic breast cancer in women who overexpress (i.e., have an excess amount of) a breast cancer cell antigen called HER2. Up to 30% of patients fall into this category.

Ovarian ablation. Another promising treatment option is ovarian ablation by means of a bilateral oophorectomy, which is used in combination with tamoxifen for metastatic disease.

Bone marrow and stem cell transplantation. Autologous (i.e., originating within self) bone marrow or stem cell transplantation combined with high-dose chemotherapy has been used to treat patients with advanced metastatic breast cancer. In this technique, patients donate their own bone marrow or peripheral blood, from which stem cells are harvested. They then receive high doses of chemotherapy, which causes bone marrow suppression. The patient subsequently undergoes autologous bone marrow or stem cell transplantation to reconstitute or "rescue" their hematopoietic (i.e., blood-forming) system to start producing blood cells.

Nursing Interventions

The health care provider discusses with the patient and the family the rationale for the specific surgical approach and the manner of coping with the cosmetic effects of and psychological response to the surgery. Patients will have questions about possible alternatives to standard or modified mastectomy.

The patient may be confused with so many options for therapy and surgical interventions. During this time, play an active role as listener, reinforce information provided by the health care provider, and encourage the patient to verbalize her concerns and recognize her feelings about the surgery. The emotional preparation of the patient may be more important than the physical preparation. Often she undergoes anticipatory grieving for the loss of a body part.

Preoperative preparation involves the patient, support group, and nursing staff so that progressive care can run continuously from admission through surgery, recovery, and the postoperative period. The initial admission assessment provides data that are helpful for the nurse and patient in planning care. Nursing diagnoses can be developed and a care plan individualized according to the patient's needs (Nursing Care Plan 52.1).

Assess and identify members of the patient's support system to know their strengths and concerns about the pending treatment and interventions. Support does not always need to come from the immediate family and close friends. Outside support and resources can come from co-workers, religious groups, oncology clinicians, psychologists, and Reach to Recovery support groups. It is important to openly discuss the patient's fears; establishing a therapeutic relationship with the patient and family enables this to happen.

Reach to Recovery volunteers are a source of information, encouragement, and support for women with breast cancer. The organization is based on the premise that rehabilitation for the cancer patient should include

Nursing Care Plan 52.1 The Patient Undergoing Modified Radical Mastectomy

Ms. C., age 52, was diagnosed with ductal cell carcinoma of the left breast. She has undergone a left modified radical mastectomy.

PATIENT PROBLEM

Fearfulness, related to the cancer diagnosis and surgical intervention

Patient Goals and Expected Outcomes	Nursing Interventions	Evaluation
Patient will be able to state fears Patient will state she has made improvement in coping	Encourage patient to talk about specific fears and feelings about each fear. Provide a calm, supportive environment. Provide information on coping mechanisms. Encourage consultation with resource persons (psychologist, clergy, nurse specialist, Reach to Recovery). Use support of family and significant others. Encourage use of comfort measures, such as music. Encourage patient's comments and questions about surgery and postoperative care.	Patient verbalizes fear, has support of significant others, and expresses confidence in ability to cope.

PATIENT PROBLEM

Potential for Infection, related to surgical incision and presence of drain

Patient Goals and Expected Outcomes	Nursing Interventions	Evaluation
Skin will remain free of signs and symptoms of infection Vital signs and white blood cell (WBC) value will be maintained within normal limits	Assess skin integrity. Instruct patient on signs and symptoms of infection. Assess and report abnormal vital signs and elevated WBC count; skin changes; and comfort level. Observe and record amount of exudate. Check drainage tubing for patency. Instruct patient to examine remaining breast every month. Caution patient to avoid injections, vaccinations, taking of blood pressure, taking of blood samples, or insertion of intravenous line in affected area.	Incision has no erythema or purulent drainage. Temperature remains within normal range. WBC count remains normal.

PATIENT PROBLEM

Distorted Body Image, related to loss of breast through modified radical mastectomy

Patient Goals and Expected Outcomes	Nursing Interventions	Evaluation
Patient will verbalize acceptance of altered body image as evidenced by absence of weeping, irritability, or verbalization of discomfort with present body; and by the attempting of difficult physical or mental tasks despite limitations Patient will demonstrate interest in her personal appearance Patient will verbalize plans to resume former activities	Encourage patient's comments and questions about surgery, progress, and prognosis. Encourage patient to discuss change in her body with husband or significant other. Reinforce correct information, and provide factual information to correct any misconceptions. Relate importance of communicating anything that causes anxiety. Encourage patient to verbalize and explore feelings regarding impact missing body part might have on patient's functioning as a sexual partner and in activities of daily living. Encourage patient to continue activities associated with femininity, such as fixing hair, using makeup, and wearing own apparel. Encourage patient to look at and touch the changed body part when she is ready. Encourage use of rehabilitation services (Reach to Recovery, Wellness Community).	Patient verbalizes feelings about surgery and change in body image; indicates beginning resolution of negative feelings toward self; and begins to accept altered body image.

CRITICAL THINKING QUESTIONS

1. Ms. C. confides in her nurse that she feels ugly and unattractive and she refuses to look at her incision. What would be a helpful approach by the nurse?
2. In assessing Ms. C., the nurse notes her holding her left arm guardedly in an adducted position. She does not use it for activities of daily living. What should effective patient teaching include?
3. What should be included in discharge teaching for Ms. C. to prevent trauma and infection of her left arm?

communication with and support from another who was in a similar situation and learned to cope and resume her normal activities.

Nursing interventions for patients who undergo modified radical mastectomy include monitoring vital signs and observing for symptoms of shock or hemorrhage, because many large blood vessels are involved in the procedure. Drains such as a Jackson-Pratt, Davol, or Hemovac drain may be placed in the axilla to facilitate drainage and to prevent formation of a hematoma. Postoperative dressings are usually constrictive and bulky and may tend to impede respiratory effort and cause pain and discomfort. Assess for excessive exudates on the dressing and in the axillary region. Place a smaller, less bulky dressing over the incisional site for the first postoperative day. When the vital signs are stable, place the patient in a 45-degree Fowler's position to promote drainage. Change the position frequently, and encourage deep breathing and coughing.

Some patients may experience incisional pain for several days after surgery and when doing arm exercises. They may complain of numbness and referred pain in the arm of the operative area. The pain radiates to the shoulder and back because of the severance of the peripheral nerves. Most of the nerves regenerate, but there are cases of residual numbness.

No matter what type of surgery the patient has, pain management and wound care are priorities. Typically a patient has a patient-controlled analgesia pump with morphine for 12 to 24 hours. She then receives oral analgesics as needed.

Box 52.6 Hand and Arm Care After Breast Surgery

PREVENTION OF INFECTION
- Wear gloves when cleaning with harsh detergent.
- Wear gloves when gardening.
- Avoid injections, vaccinations, and venipuncture in involved arm.
- Use cuticle remover rather than cutting cuticles.
- Sew with a thimble.
- Avoid chapped hands; use lanolin cream daily.
- Take care when using equipment that might cut, scrape, or abrade.
- Shave underarms with an electric razor.
- Avoid insect bites; use insect repellent.

PREVENTION OF CONSTRICTING CIRCULATION
- Do not take blood pressure in involved arm.
- Wear loose clothing; avoid tight bra straps or tight sleeves.
- Wear watch or jewelry on uninvolved arm.
- Carry purse on uninvolved arm or shoulder.
- Prevent drag or pull:
  - Carry heavy packages on uninvolved arm.
  - Avoid motions that increase centrifugal force.

PREVENTION OF BURNS
- Wear padded mitts to reach into oven; use potholders.
- Prevent sunburn; use sunscreens with SPF of 15; cover arms during prolonged exposure.
- Immediately report any signs of erythema, edema, warmth, or pain.

Patient Teaching

The patient must deep breathe and cough to prevent postoperative atelectasis.

Health care providers differ in opinion about the best position for the affected arm. Some health care providers place the arm in the dressing and place it in a sling for a couple of days postoperatively. Some health care providers prefer to avoid slings. If the arm is not restricted by dressings, it may be elevated on a pillow with the hand and wrist higher than the elbow and the elbow higher than the shoulder joint. This facilitates the flow of fluids through the lymph and venous routes and prevent lymphedema (accumulation of lymph in soft tissues).

Usually the patient is allowed to ambulate on the first postoperative day. She needs assistance in moving out of bed as she learns to maintain balance because of breast removal and bulky dressings.

Instruct the patient not to have any procedures involving the arm on the affected side—blood pressure readings, injections, IV infusion of fluids, or the drawing of blood, which may cause edema or infection. She also needs to guard against infections from burns, needle pricks (sewing), and gardening injuries because defense mechanisms are lessened by the removal of lymph nodes. Removing lymph nodes and channels increases the risk of developing lymphedema, even years after surgery. Referral to physical therapy may be indicated to control lymphedema if it develops. An exercise regimen, built up gradually, can help decrease lymphedema. However, exercise should not be started until the incision has healed completely, which takes up to 2 weeks, or at the health care provider's discretion. Tell the patient to avoid lifting heavy objects with the affected arm for 6 to 8 weeks. Instruct her to avoid sleeping on the involved arm. Clothing on the affected arm should be nonconstricting. Bracelets and watches should be worn on the unaffected arm (Box 52.6).

The longer the edema persists, the more difficult it is to manage. Diuretics and low-sodium diets often are prescribed. If the edema persists, an elastic stockinette is measured for precise fit to avoid venous flow constriction. The sleeve is applied from the wrist to the shoulder and worn when the patient is out of bed. When the patient is sleeping, position the arm to aid venous flow. If the lymphedema is severe, the health care provider may order a knit compression sleeve (Jobst extremity therapy) to manage the condition. A pneumomassage sleeve with automatic inflation and deflation can be placed on the arm. The compression pump is strictly contraindicated when there is evidence of acute phlebitis, perivascular lymphangitis, or cellulitis.

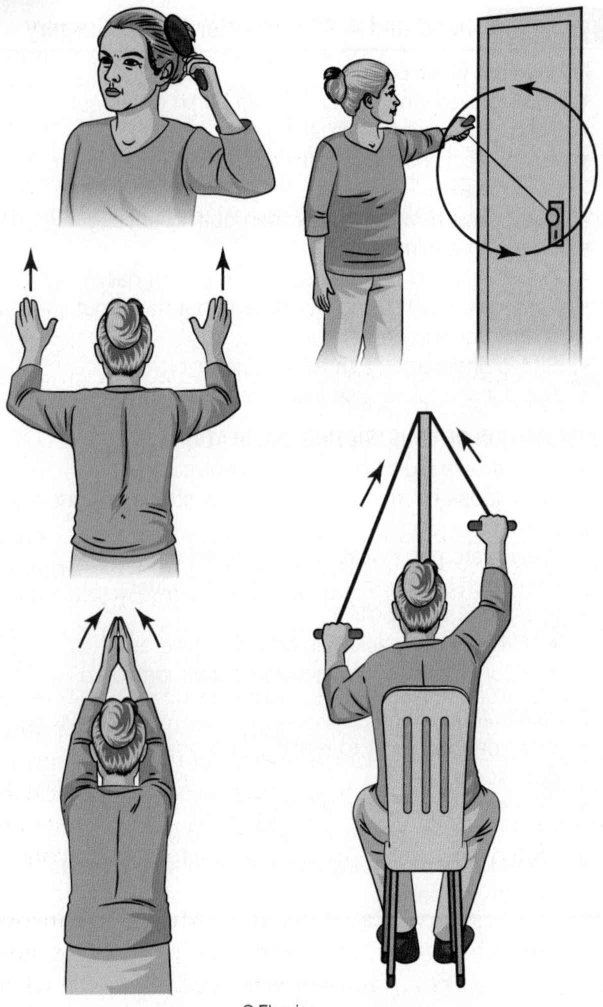

Fig. 52.16 Exercises after mastectomy.

Isometric exercises are helpful for increasing the circulation and developing the collateral lymph system. The patient can open and clench fingers and squeeze a rubber ball in the first few postoperative days. This activity provides extension and flexion of the wrist and elbow; it is equivalent to sewing, knitting, typing, and playing piano when at home.

Preventing muscle contractures. Specific exercises may be ordered to restore the muscle strength and full range of motion of the affected area. Gentle exercises started early in the postoperative course help to decrease muscle tension and to regain muscle function more quickly. The nurse or the therapist should instruct the patient and encourage the continuation of the exercises on discharge. Many of the exercises may be incorporated into ADLs as they are resumed (Fig. 52.16 and Box 52.7). Exercising can be painful, but the patient can meet the challenge with the encouragement of a support group.

Body image acceptance. After losing a breast, many patients experience grief over the loss of a body part. This acute grief is like a crisis and may last 4 to 6 weeks or longer. Grief makes the fact of loss real, and the process is essential for personal adaptation to the loss. Assist the patient in finding helpful coping mechanisms.

Initial coping mechanisms often begin to lose effectiveness at about 3 months, and a period of depression ensues. Provide anticipatory guidance for this eventuality. Special nursing interventions, in terms of psychological support and self-care education, are necessary if the cancer recurs. Participation in a cancer support group is important and has been found to have a clinically significant impact on survival.

When deep-breathing exercises are started immediately after surgery and the patient splints the area and exercises her arm, she will recognize the absence of the breast through touch. Dressing changes and incision cleansing with patient involvement make the absence real. Being involved and responsible for the dressing and incision allows a more personal approach to the patient. At this time, the nurse's support is important. Provide a mirror, or seat the patient in front of a mirror so that she can see the operative site being cleansed and dressed. Be

Box 52.7 Postmastectomy Arm Exercises

CLIMBING THE WALL

1. Stand facing wall with toes 6 to 12 inches from wall.
2. Bend elbows and place palms of hands against wall at shoulder level.
3. Move both hands parallel to each other up the wall as far as possible until incisional pull or pain occurs.
4. Move both hands down to starting position.
5. Goal is complete extension with elbows straight.
6. Activities that use the same action include reaching top shelves, hanging out clothes, washing windows, hanging curtains, and setting hair.

ELBOW PULL-IN

1. Extend arms sideways to shoulder level.
2. Clasp hands behind neck.
3. Pull elbows forward until they touch.
4. Return to position 2.
5. Unclasp hands and extend arms sideways at shoulder level.
6. Lower arms to side.

BACK SCRATCH

1. Place hand of unoperated side on hip for balance.
2. Bend elbow of affected arm, placing back of hand on small of back.
3. Work hand up the back slowly until fingers reach opposite shoulder blade.
4. Lower arm and straighten both arms.

ROPE PULL

1. Attach a rope over a shower rod, a hook, or the top of an open door.
2. Sit on a chair (with door between legs if using a door) and grasp each end of rope.
3. Alternately pull on each end, raising affected arm to a point of incisional pull or pain. (The goal is to raise the affected arm almost directly overhead.)

sensitive to the patient and be alert for signs of readiness to become involved in care and accept the loss of the body part. The incisional area may be erythematous and edematous, but the discoloration gradually lessens and the site becomes more comfortable. Encourage her to massage in cocoa butter or a cream to make the incisional line softer. Advise the patient that it takes time to accept the loss and to heal emotionally and physically.

Prosthesis. A breast prosthesis should not be worn unless authorized by the health care provider. Many breast forms are available. Forms are made of gels, molded silicone, and saline solution. Most forms are covered with soft fabric, are lightweight, and feel like breast tissue. There is a shape for each type of breast, because each body is different and each surgery is different. Forms have been developed that can be fitted for a right or left breast, slanted for the breast that was slanted, or formed with an outer curve that simulates the extension of a full breast under the axilla and upward on the chest. It is advisable to have a skilled fitter from a reliable company fit the prosthesis.

A well-fitted brassiere is essential before choosing the shape form. If the woman is active, she may desire a pocket or restraining cup. Some forms can be worn against the skin with no underpadding or bra cups. Most forms can be washed with water and mild detergent to keep them clean and supple. Many prostheses are waterproof and can be worn swimming; when wet, they do not "weigh down" the wearer.

When the patient is being fitted with a prosthesis, the best assurance that the fit is right is when each of the following is observed:

- The brassiere fits snugly around the rib cage.
- The prosthesis fills the bottom of the bra cup.
- The prosthesis projects the same as the remaining breast, with form bulk and nipples in position.
- The breasts are separated when the bra is centered.
- The top of the bra cup is filled and appears like the other breast.

Breast Reconstruction

The patient whose disease is limited to the breast may benefit from reconstructive surgery. The benefits of breast reconstruction include avoidance of an external prosthesis that has potential for slipping, greater choice of clothing (including lower necklines), and loss of self-consciousness about appearance. For many women, breast reconstruction is beneficial in improving self-esteem. Breast reconstruction can provide many women with a renewed sense of wholeness and a return to a normal state. The most important indicators for reconstruction are the patient's motivation and desire for the procedure. The primary determinant for the procedure is the patient's clinical status. Goals for reconstruction are to select the simplest type that meets the patient's needs and expectations and to match the opposite breast in size, shape, and contour.

Breast reconstruction can be performed immediately after surgery or at a later time. An increasing number of women are electing immediate reconstruction; this may prolong the initial hospitalization but eliminates the need for a second hospitalization and contributes to self-esteem. Others wait until they have completed adjuvant chemotherapy or radiation to be certain the area is disease free.

Breast implant. If the remaining skin is sufficient to cover an implant, surgery may consist of placing a permanent silicone implant under the pectoralis muscle. Possible complications of silicone implants include infection, deflation, a false mammography result, and silicone leaks.

Some researchers have suggested that the silicone filling or the implant covering can lead to autoimmune or connective tissue disease. Although most surgeries have not resulted in complications, differing opinions regarding the safety of breast implants led the FDA (2004) to issue some recommendations in early 1992. Breast implants were permitted after breast cancer surgery because of the offsetting positive contribution to recovery, but a moratorium was imposed on silicone implants solely for cosmetic purposes until data establishing safety could be provided. Many implants are now filled with saline or dextran instead of silicone.

Musculocutaneous flap procedure. Musculocutaneous flap surgery has made reconstruction possible for most patients who have undergone mastectomy, even when the pectoralis muscles have been removed or when nerve damage has resulted in muscle atrophy. The flap receives its blood supply from muscle, and also from the overlying layer of skin. At the same time that this procedure is performed, a silicone or saline breast implant may be inserted; if enough tissue is available, no implant is needed.

Musculocutaneous flaps most often are taken from the back (latissimus dorsi muscle) or the abdomen (transverse rectus abdominis muscle). When the latissimus dorsi musculocutaneous flap is used for reconstruction, a block of skin and muscle from the patient's back is used to replace tissue removed during mastectomy (Fig. 52.17E). The transverse rectus abdominis musculocutaneous (TRAM) flap is the most frequently used flap operation for breast reconstruction. The rectus abdominis muscles are paired, flat muscles running from the rib cage down to the pubic bone. Arteries inside the muscle branch at many levels, and these branches supply blood to the fat and skin across a large expanse of the abdomen. In the TRAM technique, the surgeon elevates a large block of tissue from the lower abdominal area, but leaves it attached to the rectus muscle (see Fig. 52.17A to D). This tissue then is tunneled under the skin or detached and placed as a "free flap" at the site of the breast reconstruction. The tissue is trimmed and shaped to form a breast mound similar

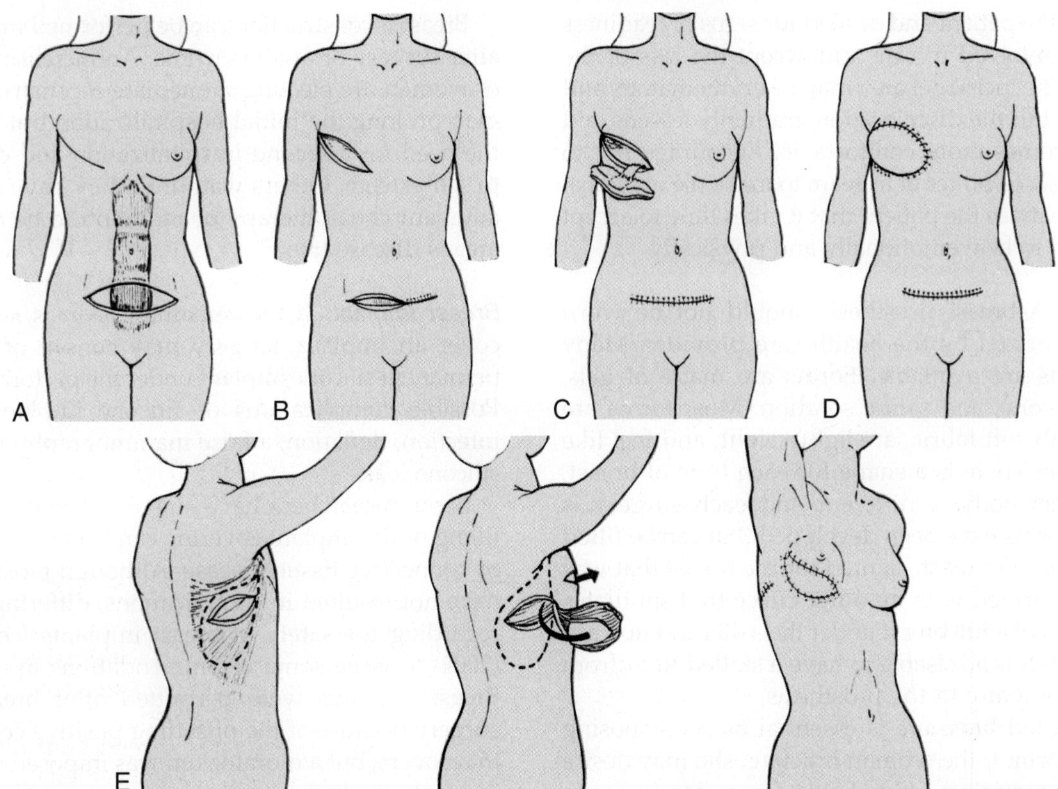

Fig. 52.17 Transverse rectus abdominis musculocutaneous (TRAM) flap. A, Pedicle TRAM flap procedure is planned. B, The abdominal tissue, still attached to the rectus muscle, nerve, and blood supply, is moved through a tunnel beneath the skin, from the abdomen to the chest. C, The flap is trimmed to shape the breast. The lower abdominal incision is closed. D, Nipple and areola are reconstructed after the breast has healed. E, In the latissimus dorsi musculocutaneous flap, a block of skin and muscle from the patient's back is used to replace tissue removed during mastectomy. (From Belcher AE: *Cancer nursing*, St. Louis, 1992, Mosby.)

to that of the opposite breast. An implant may be used in addition to the flap to achieve symmetry. The abdominal incision is closed in a fashion similar to that of an abdominal hysterectomy or a "tummy tuck." This surgical procedure can last 2 to 8 hours, with recovery taking 4 to 6 weeks. Complications include bleeding, hernia, and infection (breastcancer.org, 2015).

Nipple reconstruction usually is performed as a separate procedure after the breast reconstruction has been completed. Nipple construction is generally from available tissue at the site or harvested tissue from the opposite breast. New techniques allow the nipple to be created from tissue and subcutaneous tissue of the breast mound. Areola reconstruction is provided by obtaining pigmented skin from the upper thigh or by using skin from the lateral chest area. Newer procedures may employ a sutured tuck to create a nipple and using a tattoo for the areola.

Prognosis

The 5-year relative survival rate for localized breast cancer is close to 100%. Survival rate for stage II at 5 years is about 93% and 72% for stage III. Once the cancer is metastatic the rate of survival drops to a 5-year rate of survival at 22% (ACS, 2017d). Breast cancer ranks second among cancer deaths in women. The most

Home Care Considerations

Cancer of the Breast

- Explain the follow-up routine to the patient and emphasize the importance of beginning and continuing breast self-examination and annual mammography.
- Symptoms that should be reported to the health care provider include new back pain, weakness, constipation, shortness of breath, and confusion.
- If adjuvant therapy is to be used, give the woman specific instructions about appointment times and treatment locations.
- If applicable, stress the importance of wearing a well-fitting prosthesis. The return of a normal external appearance is important to most women.
- Often the husband, sexual partner, or family member may need assistance in dealing with his or her emotional reactions to the diagnosis and surgery for him or her to effectively support the patient.
- If difficulty in adjustment or other problems develop, counseling may be necessary for women with breast cancer to deal with the emotional component of a modified radical mastectomy and the diagnosis of cancer.

important prognostic factor is the stage of the disease and nodal involvement. Even having one to three nodes involved carries a 50% to 60% risk for metastatic recurrence (see Box 52.6 and the Home Care Considerations box: Cancer of the Breast).

INFLAMMATORY AND INFECTIOUS DISORDERS OF THE MALE REPRODUCTIVE SYSTEM

PROSTATITIS

Etiology and Pathophysiology

Prostatitis refers to inflammation or infection of the prostate gland. The condition may be acute or chronic. The cause is most commonly bacterial. There are, however, cases of nonbacterial prostatitis. Causative organisms in bacterial prostatitis include *E. coli, Klebsiella, Proteus, Pseudomonas, Streptococcus, N. gonorrhoeae,* and *Chlamydia trachomatis.*

Clinical Manifestations

The clinical manifestations of acute prostatitis include chills, fever, prostate pain and tenderness, and arthralgias. Specific urinary symptoms may include dysuria, frequency, nocturia, weak stream, and hesitancy. An exacerbation of chronic prostatitis often has a slower onset of symptoms. Symptoms of the chronic condition are not typically systemic and often include dysuria and recurrent urinary tract infections. The patient also may have acute urinary retention caused by prostatic edema. On palpation, the gland is tender, edematous, and firm. In chronic prostatitis, many patients may appear asymptomatic, but generally the symptoms are the same as in the acute phase but less intense.

Diagnostic Tests

Diagnosis is based on culture and sensitivity tests of the urethra, prostatic fluid, and urine for organism identification and appropriate antibiotic therapy. Prostatic fluid is collected by prostate massage and expression of fluid. The pH of the fluid generally is elevated. A rectal examination done by the health care provider reveals gland tenderness and edema.

Medical Management

Medical management includes antibiotic therapy such as ofloxacin, ciprofloxacin (Cipro), and sulfamethoxazole-trimethoprim (Bactrim). For patients who have multiple sex partners, doxycycline may be ordered. Oral antibiotics are given for up to 4 weeks for patients with acute prostatitis and for 4 to 16 weeks for chronic prostatitis. The most common medications used for pain control are antiinflammatory agents. Opioids should be used carefully because of the chronic nature of the pain. Periodic digital massage of the prostate by the health care provider to increase the flow of infected prostatic secretions may be performed. Heat may be applied using sitz baths.

Nursing Interventions

Nursing interventions primarily focus on symptoms and include (1) a full explanation of antibiotic therapy and the need for compliance with treatment, which may be lengthy in chronic prostatitis; (2) supportive care such as bed rest to relieve strain and pain of the perineum and suprapubic area, sitz baths to promote muscle relaxation, and stool softeners to prevent straining on defecation; (3) monitoring of I&O; (4) bladder drainage with suprapubic catheterization if acute urinary retention develops into acute prostatitis (in acute prostatitis, passage of a catheter through an inflamed urethra is contraindicated); and (5) encouragement of follow-up for evaluation of the inflammation.

Patient problems and interventions for the patient with prostatitis include but are not limited to the following:

Patient Problem	Nursing Interventions
Recent Onset of Pain, related to disease process	Assess type and location of pain; provide analgesics as ordered Encourage bed rest to promote comfort Provide nonpharmacologic comfort measures: • Assist patient with assuming comfortable position • Provide diversional activity • Provide a restful environment Instruct patient on necessity of taking prescribed antibiotics and following orders for activity level
Potential for Impaired Self-Esteem due to Current Situation, related to: • Fear of impotence • Embarrassment	Encourage patient to express feelings Actively listen Encourage adaptive coping behaviors

Prognosis

Recurrent episodes of acute prostatitis may cause fibrotic tissue to form; such fibrosis causes a hardening of the prostate gland that initially may be confused with carcinoma. With treatment, the prognosis for bacterial prostatitis is favorable.

EPIDIDYMITIS

Etiology and Pathophysiology

Epididymitis is an infection of the cordlike excretory duct of the testicle, usually secondary to an infectious process (sexually or nonsexually transmitted). It is one of the common infections of the male reproductive tract. The infection often travels to the epididymis from the urethra. The causative organisms include *S. aureus, E. coli,* streptococci, chlamydia, and *N. gonorrhoeae.* The inflammation is associated with urethral strictures, cystitis, and prostatitis.

Symptoms can occur after trauma to the genital area, after instrumentation of the urethra and cystoscopy, and after physical exertion or prolonged sexual activity. Risk factors include being uncircumcised, recent surgery involving the urinary tract, structural issues, regular use of a urethral catheter, and unprotected sexual intercourse with multiple partners.

Clinical Manifestations

Severe pain appears suddenly in the scrotum and radiates along the spermatic tube. Additional sites for pain can include the groin, pelvic region, and lower abdomen. Testicular pain worsens with bowel movements. Edema appears and the patient develops a "duck walk" or "waddling gait" because of the sensitivity and pain that walking stimulates. The scrotal area becomes tender. Pyuria (pus in urine) or blood in the semen may be noted. Chills and fever are noted. The physical examination reveals swelling and tenderness at the affected testicle. Lymph nodes may be enlarged.

Diagnostic Tests

Diagnostic testing includes urinalysis and a complete blood cell count. The epididymis is massaged by the health care provider, and a fluid expression specimen is sent to the laboratory. The patient also may be tested for gonorrhea and chlamydia.

Medical Management

Medical management includes a regimen of bed rest and support of the scrotum. The use of antibiotics is important for both partners, if the transmission is through sexual contact. Apply cold for relief of edema and discomfort, and administer the appropriate antibiotic. If abscess formation occurs, incision and drainage of the scrotum may be required. Antiinflammatory medications may be included in the treatment plan.

Nursing Interventions

Nursing interventions for patients with epididymitis include (1) bed rest during the acute phase of illness; (2) support of the testicular area, with scrotal support by elevation of the scrotum on a folded towel during bed rest and athletic support when ambulatory; (3) ice compresses to the area in the initial phase to hasten recovery; (4) explanation of the need for compliance with antibiotic therapy until all signs of inflammation have disappeared; and (5) advice to refrain from sexual intercourse during the acute phase.

Prognosis

Promptly treated, epididymitis can be resolved. The infection can be bilateral and may recur. Bilateral epididymitis can cause sterility. Untreated epididymitis leads to necrosis of testicular tissue. Abscesses and fistulas can form, and septicemia can develop, which can be fatal.

DISORDERS OF MALE GENITAL ORGANS

PHIMOSIS AND PARAPHIMOSIS

Etiology and Pathophysiology

Phimosis is a condition in which the prepuce (foreskin) is too small to allow it to be retracted over the glans penis. Phimosis is often congenital but may be a result of adhesions caused by local inflammation or disease and poor hygiene. The condition is rarely severe enough to obstruct the flow of urine but may contribute to local infection because it does not permit adequate cleansing.

Paraphimosis is an inability to return the retracted foreskin over the glans of the penis as a result of edema. If the foreskin is not placed back in the forward position, an ulcer can develop. Paraphimosis can occur when the foreskin remains contracted during perineal cleansing, use of a urinary catheter, or intercourse.

Medical Management

Circumcision may be performed to manage either condition. Paraphimosis is a urologic emergency requiring prompt intervention. Manual reduction is the first line of treatment attempted. It requires that the glans be pushed back and the foreskin returned to its original location. Chilling the penis with ice for a few minutes before this procedure may aid in reduction of the inflammation. A puncture method also may be used. This procedure engages the use of needles to puncture the foreskin to allow trapped fluid to escape. A tourniquet can be applied to the penis and needles used to aspirate blood from the glans in an attempt to reduce volume and allow for subsequent manual reduction. If none of the manual retraction methods are successful, the swollen foreskin may be incised surgically to allow for the glans to be freed and circulation restored.

Nursing Interventions

Assessment of the degree of swelling and management of discomfort are priorities for the nurse. Care of the patient experiencing either phimosis or paraphimosis also includes education and emotional support. After a circumcision a sterile petrolatum gauze dressing is applied and changed after each voiding. Regardless of the management of the condition, aftercare includes assessment of bleeding and urinary output.

HYDROCELE

Etiology and Pathophysiology

A *hydrocele* is an accumulation of fluid between the two layers of the *tunica vaginalis,* a membrane covering the testicle. The scrotum slowly enlarges as the fluid accumulates. Distinguishing a hydrocele from a cancerous testicular mass is fairly simple: when a strong light is directed from a point behind the scrotum (transillumination), the light passes through if the swelling is a hydrocele; if the swelling is a solid mass the light does not pass through. Pain occurs if the hydrocele develops suddenly. Most hydroceles occur in men older than 21 years of age, but they can occur in infants and children. A hydrocele also may develop as a result of trauma in the area, orchitis (inflammation of the testes), or epididymitis.

Medical Management

No treatment is indicated unless the swelling becomes large and uncomfortable, in which case treatment includes aspiration of fluid from the sac or surgical removal of the sac to avoid constriction of the circulation of the testicles. After aspiration the pain is relieved and the scrotum can be examined more easily.

Nursing Interventions

Nursing interventions consist of maintaining bed rest, scrotal support with elevation, ice to edematous areas, and frequent changes of dressings to avoid skin impairment.

Prognosis

With treatment, the prognosis is good.

VARICOCELE

Varicocele occurs when veins within the scrotum become dilated, usually after internal spermatic vein reflux. Obstruction and malfunctioning of the veins cause engorgement and elongation, preventing adequate drainage of blood from the testis. Symptoms include a "pulling" sensation that causes a dull aching and pain accompanied by edema of the scrotal area. Treatment involves sealing off the problem vein, either by ligation (tying it off) or by embolization (essentially plugging the vein, using a chemical agent or device); blood flow then is redirected into other, normal veins. Complications that may result from the condition include infertility (probably the result of increased testicular temperature) and shrinkage of the testicles. Nursing interventions after treatment include bed rest with scrotal support, ice on the incisional site, and medication for discomfort as ordered.

Ligation of the internal spermatic vein in the treatment of varicocele has been shown to improve semen quality.

CANCER OF THE MALE REPRODUCTIVE TRACT

The more common tumors of the male reproductive tract involve the testis, the prostate gland, and the penis. Most tumors of the male reproductive system are malignant (see Chapter 50).

CANCER OF THE TESTIS (TESTICULAR CANCER)

Etiology and Pathophysiology

Testicular cancer is relatively uncommon. It is the most common cancer in men ages 15 to 35 years of age. It is estimated that in 2017 about 8850 cases will be diagnosed. The risk for developing testicular cancer is only about 1 in 263 (ACS, 2018d). Risk factors for the development of this form of cancer include abnormal testicular development and **cryptorchidism** (failure of testes to descend into the scrotum). The condition is seen more in white men than in African American or Asian American men. Most testicular cancers develop from embryonic germ cells. The two types of germ cell cancers are seminomas and nonseminomas. Seminomas are the most common and the least aggressive; nonseminoma testicular germ cell tumors are rare and very aggressive.

Clinical Manifestations

Testicular cancer may have a slow or rapid onset, depending on the type of tumor. The signs and symptoms of early disease include an enlarged scrotum and a firm, nontender, painless, smooth mass in the testicular area. Some patients complain of a dull ache or heavy sensation in the lower abdomen, perianal area, or scrotum. Acute pain is the presenting symptom in about 10% of patients. Some men may display gynecomastia (excessive breast tissue development).

Diagnostic Tests

Palpation of the scrotal contents is the first step in diagnosing testicular cancer. A cancerous mass is firm and does not transilluminate. Ultrasound of the testes is indicated when testicular cancer is suspected (e.g., a palpable mass) or persistent or painful testicular edema is present. If a testicular neoplasm is suspected, obtain blood to determine the serum levels of alpha-fetoprotein, lactate dehydrogenase, and hCG. A chest radiograph and CT scan of the abdomen and pelvis are obtained to detect metastasis.

Medical Management

Radical inguinal orchiectomy is usually the treatment of choice. This is the removal of the testis, epididymis, a portion of the gonadal lymphatics, and their blood supply. The remaining testis provides enough testosterone to maintain the man's sexual characteristics. He may, however, have a lower sperm count and decreased sperm mobility. Surgery generally is followed by radiation or chemotherapy. Often a retroperitoneal lymph node dissection is performed to remove affected nodes and assist in determining the tumor stage. Staging a testicular tumor helps determine treatment.

Nursing Interventions and Patient Teaching

The most important aspect of care of patients who have or are at risk for a tumor of the testis is early detection by testicular self-examination (TSE). Young men should be taught to perform TSE monthly, beginning at puberty. Video media and illustrations are available as teaching aids and ideally should be introduced during high school or college physical education classes. Information about TSE is available on the ACS website and other websites. The examination takes 3 minutes and should be done monthly. The best time to perform a TSE is after a warm

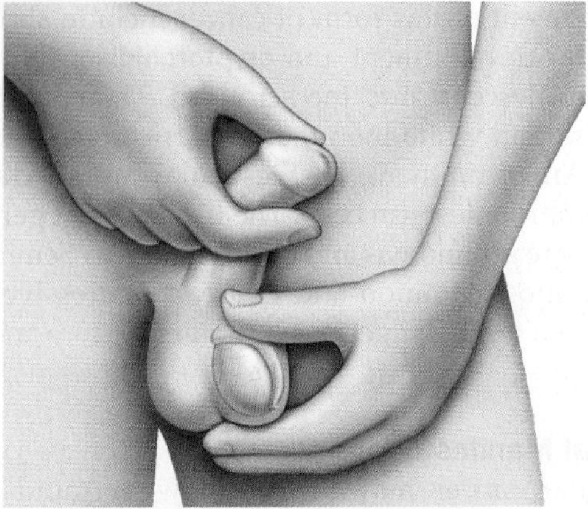

Fig. 52.18 Testicular self-examination. (From Harkreader H, Hogan MA: *Fundamentals of nursing: Caring and clinical judgment*, ed 3, St. Louis, 2007, Saunders.)

shower, when the scrotal skin is relaxed. The scrotum is checked for color, contour, and skin breaks. The left side is usually longer because the left testicle is suspended from a longer spermatic cord. Each testicle is palpated gently by grasping the scrotum in the center with the thumb and index finger (see the Patient Teaching box and Fig. 52.18). Normal testicles are firm but somewhat resilient, smooth, and mobile. If a testicle is indurated (hardened), carcinoma is suspected.

Prognosis

With the advent of tumor markers (which indicate the presence of disease and enable the health care provider to monitor its response to treatment), early detection, refined surgery, and effective chemotherapy are heralded as keys to the increases in survival rates. The survival rate is higher than 95% for those patients with cancer diagnosed and treated in the early stages. Testicular cancer metastasis occurs most commonly to the abdomen, lungs, the retroperitoneal region, and spine (ACS, 2018e).

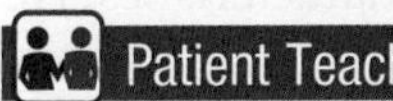 Patient Teaching

Testicular Self-Examination

- Examine the scrotum once a month.
- Perform testicular self-examination after a bath or shower, when the scrotum is warm and most relaxed.
- Grasp the testis with both hands and palpate gently between the thumb and index finger. The testis should feel smooth and egg shaped and be firm to the touch.
- The epididymis, found behind the testis, should feel like a soft tube (see Figs. 52.1 and 52.18).

CANCER OF THE PENIS

Etiology and Pathophysiology

Cancer of the penis is rare. It generally appears in men older than 50 years of age. Men who have not been circumcised, have not maintained good personal hygiene, or have had STIs are at risk.

Clinical Manifestations

The tumor is painless, and a wartlike growth or ulceration on the glans under the prepuce is present. It is common for metastasis to occur to the inguinal nodes and adjacent organs.

DIAGNOSTIC TESTS

Biopsy confirms the diagnosis.

Medical Management

Surgical intervention requires removal of as little tissue as possible, but it may be necessary to do a partial or total amputation of the penis and to remove the adjacent tissue and inguinal lymph nodes. When metastasis involves the bladder and rectum, more radical surgery may be needed, and outlets for urinary or fecal elimination are provided by creating an ileal conduit and a colostomy. The surgeon may place a suprapubic catheter into the bladder to drain the urine.

Nursing Interventions

Nursing interventions include providing emotional support. If amputation of the penis is required, the patient faces the psychological trauma associated with the loss of sexuality and the ability to urinate naturally. Monitor urinary output by suprapubic catheter or, if an ileal conduit was constructed, monitor urine in the urostomy bag. Elevation of the scrotum controls edema. Provide comfort measures to control pain.

SEXUALLY TRANSMITTED INFECTIONS

Today, despite sweeping advances in the diagnosis and treatment of communicable diseases, the incidence of infections transmitted through intimate or sexual activities continues to increase worldwide. Sexually transmitted infections (STIs) previously were called *sexually transmitted diseases* or *venereal diseases*. These infections usually are transmitted during intimate sexual contact. They may have other routes of transmission (e.g., from an infected mother to her newborn), occur with or without symptoms, and have long periods of asymptomatic infectivity.

Any sexually active person may be at risk for an STI. People who have frequent sexual contact with multiple partners and who engage in unprotected sexual activity are at increased risk. Commonly, those most at risk are young, single, urban, poor, male, and homosexual. Some STIs can be managed but cannot be cured. Other STIs such as herpes simplex and human papillomavirus may persist without obvious outward symptoms and place unsuspecting individuals at risk. Collection of data to assess risk for STIs is an important role of the nurse (Table 52.3).

Despite the physical and emotional discomfort, the possibility of long-term disability (infertility, chronic infectivity), and advances in diagnosis and treatment that sharply decrease the period of infectivity, STIs

Table 52.3 Assessment of Risk Factors for Sexually Transmitted Infections Using the 5 Ps

5 Ps	QUESTIONS TO ASK
Past STIs	Have you ever had an STI in the past?
Partners	Have you had sex with men, women, or both? In the past 6 months how many people have you had sex with? Have any of your partners in the past 12 months had sex with other partners while they were in a relationship with you?
Practices	Do you have… • Vaginal sex? • Oral sex? • Anal sex? Have you used needles to shoot/inject drugs?
Prevention	What do you do to prevent STIs and HIV? Tell me about your use of condoms with your most recent partner.
Pregnancy	How would it be if you got pregnant now? What are you doing to prevent pregnancy?

HIV, Human immunodeficiency virus; *STI*, sexually transmitted infection.
Modified from the California Department of Public Health: *Sexual risk assessment and risk factors for sexually transmitted diseases*, 2011. Retrieved from *www.cdph.ca.gov/pubsforms/Guidelines/Documents/CA-STD-Sexual-risk-assessment-and-STD-risk-factors.pdf*.

continue to be among the world's most common communicable diseases. Four main factors are responsible: (1) unprotected sex, (2) antibiotic resistance, (3) treatment delay, and (4) sexual behavior patterns and permissiveness. The following is a discussion of some of the more commonly diagnosed STIs (see the Safety Alert box).

GENITAL HERPES

Etiology and Pathophysiology

Genital herpes, caused by herpes simplex virus (HSV), is an infectious viral disease characterized by recurrent episodes of acute, painful, erythematous, vesicular eruptions (blisters) on or in the genitalia or rectum. The two closely related forms are designated types 1 and 2. Most people are infected in infancy with type 1 during feeding or kissing by adults. HSV type 2 is usually acquired sexually, in the genital or anal regions, after puberty commences. Among individuals 14 to 49 years of age, an estimated one in six has genital herpes.

Clinical Manifestations

Signs include the appearance of fluid-filled vesicles 2 days to 2 weeks after exposure. In women the vesicles usually occur on the cervix, which is considered the primary site but also may be seen on the labia, rectum, vulva, vagina, and skin. In men vesicles are found on the glans penis, foreskin, and penile shaft (Fig. 52.19). Other lesions may appear on the mouth and anus.

! Safety Alert

Sexually Transmitted Infections

- Teach "safe" sex practices including abstinence, monogamy with an uninfected partner, avoidance of certain high-risk sexual practices, and use of condoms and other barriers to limit contact with potentially infectious body fluids or lesions.
- All sexually active women should be screened for cervical cancer. Women with a history of STIs are at greater risk for cervical cancer than women without this history.
- Inform patients of the new HPV vaccine for girls and boys beginning at ages 11 to 12 years to prevent HPV infection and the precancerous changes that lead to cervical cancer.
- Instruct patients in hygiene measures, such as washing and urinating after intercourse to rid the body of causative organisms.
- Explain the importance of taking all antibiotics as prescribed. Symptoms often improve after 1 or 2 days of therapy, but organisms may still be present.
- Teach patients about the need for treatment of sexual partners with antibiotics to prevent transmission of disease.
- Instruct patients to abstain from sexual intercourse during treatment and to use condoms when sexual activity is resumed, to prevent spread of infection and reinfection.
- Explain the importance of follow-up examination and reculture at least once after treatment (if appropriate) to confirm complete cure and to prevent relapse.
- Allow patients and partners to verbalize concerns to clarify areas that need explanation.
- Instruct patients about symptoms of complications and the need to report problems to ensure proper follow-up and early treatment of reinfection.
- Explain precautions to take, such as being monogamous; asking potential partners about sexual history; avoiding sex with partners who use IV drugs or who have visible oral, inguinal, genital, perineal, or anal lesions; using condoms; and voiding and washing genitalia after coitus to reduce the occurrence of reinfection.
- Inform patients regarding their state of infectivity to prevent a false sense of security, which may result in careless sexual practices and poor personal hygiene.

Vesicles may rupture and develop into shallow, painful ulcers; they are erythematous with marked edema and tenderness. Lymph nodes may become involved. Initial lesions last from 3 to 10 days, and recurrent lesions have a duration of 7 to 10 days. The primary infection may be accompanied by fever; malaise; myalgia; dysuria; and, in women, leukorrhea. Urination may be painful, the result of urine contacting active lesions.

After the initial outbreak has subsided the virus lies dormant in the body. It may be triggered by illness, fatigue, injury, or stress in the individual. Recurrent outbreaks are typically less painful and shorter in

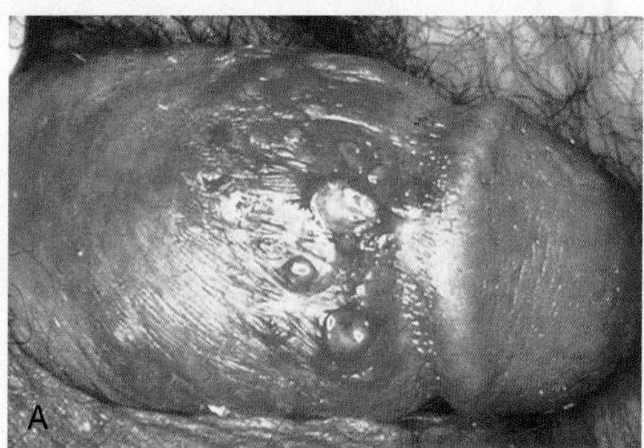

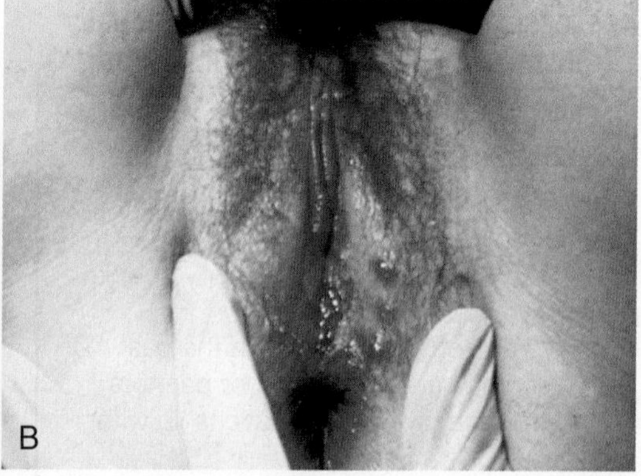

Fig. 52.19 Herpes simplex virus type 2 in male and female patients. Vesicular lesions on A, penis and B, perineum. (From Beare PG, Myers JL: *Adult health nursing*, ed 3, St. Louis, 1998, Mosby.)

duration. The frequency of subsequent outbreaks is individualized, with some people never having an outbreak and others experiencing them frequently.

Diagnostic Tests

Diagnosis is based on the physical examination and the patient history. The diagnosis is confirmed by the appearance of the virus on tissue cultures. Cultures are more frequently positive when the lesions are from a primary infection versus recurrent infections. Asymptomatic disease may be identified by serologic testing.

Medical Management

The skin lesions of genital herpes heal spontaneously unless secondary infection occurs. Encourage symptomatic treatment such as practicing good genital hygiene and wearing loose-fitting cotton undergarments. The lesions should be kept clean and dry. Frequent sitz baths may soothe the area and reduce inflammation. Pain may require a local anesthetic such as lidocaine (Xylocaine) or systemic analgesics such as codeine and aspirin. Advise patients to abstain from sexual contact while lesions are present. Transmission of the virus has been documented in the absence of symptoms, making the practice of safe sex necessary at all times.

Antiviral medications can be prescribed to manage the initial outbreak, subsequent outbreaks, or as a suppressive therapy to prevent outbreaks in the future. Treatment regimens of antiviral medications may include acyclovir (Zovirax), valacyclovir (Valtrex) and famciclovir. These medications do not cure the disease but reduce the severity of symptoms and shorten the duration of the outbreak. Therapy for the initial outbreak often is prescribed for 7 to 10 days. Subsequent outbreaks are managed with a 5-day course of therapy. Suppressive therapy requires that the individual take the daily medications to lessen outbreaks over time. Continued use of oral acyclovir for up to 5 years is safe and effective, but it should be interrupted after 1 year to assess the patient's episode recurrence rate. Adverse reactions to acyclovir are mild and include headache, occasional nausea and vomiting, and diarrhea. The safety of systemic acyclovir for the treatment of pregnant women has not been established. Acyclovir ointment appears to be of no clinical benefit in the treatment of recurrent lesions, either in speed of healing or in resolution of pain. IV acyclovir is reserved for severe or life-threatening infections in which hospitalization is required for the treatment of central nervous system infections (meningitis) or pneumonitis. Nephrotoxicity has been observed with high-dose IV use.

Nursing Interventions and Patient Teaching

Advise the patient to keep genital lesions clean and dry. Hands should be washed thoroughly after touching a lesion. Loose, absorbent underclothing is usually more comfortable than close-fitting clothing. Sitz baths decrease lesional discomfort and enhance urinary and bowel elimination. Teach the patient that sexual intercourse during the active lesion phase increases the risk of transmission and also may be painful. Patients should inform future sexual partners and health care providers of recurring or latent infections. Sexual transmission of HSV has been documented during asymptomatic periods; encourage the use of barrier methods, especially condoms. Inform the patient about the role of stress, poor nutrition, and insufficient rest in recurrences of signs and symptoms. Female patients need a yearly Pap test and should inform their health care provider in the event of pregnancy so that the disease can be monitored closely; there is a possibility of spontaneous abortion. Provide the patient with nonjudgmental support and with the contact number of the local herpes support group if one exists.

Prognosis

Genital herpes is a recurrent disease with no cure.

SYPHILIS

Etiology and Pathophysiology

The coiled spirochete *Treponema pallidum* causes syphilis. In 2015 there were 23,872 new cases of syphilis reported. An increase in syphilis rates since the early 2000s has been noted. In 2007 the total number of cases was 11,466.

The rates of primary syphilis in men who have sex with men is high, accounting for 82% of cases (CDC, 2017b).

Syphilis is the third most frequently reported communicable disease in the United States, exceeded only by varicella (chickenpox) and gonorrhea. Transmission occurs primarily through sexual contact during the primary, secondary, and latent stages of the disease. In addition to sexual contact, syphilis may be spread through contact with infectious lesions and sharing of needles among drug addicts. Prenatal infection from the mother to the fetus is possible. The organism thrives in the warm parts of the body and can be destroyed by soap and water. The spirochete penetrates intact skin and openings in the mucous membranes of the genital organs, rectum, and mouth.

Clinical Manifestations

Syphilis has four stages—primary, secondary, latent, and tertiary—each with its peculiar signs and symptoms. The signs and symptoms of syphilis include the clean-based **chancre** (painless erosion or papule that ulcerates superficially with a scooped-out appearance) of primary syphilis to the skin rashes of secondary syphilis. Moist, raised, gray to pink lesions of the genital or perirectal skin; enlarged lymph nodes; fever; fatigue; or infections of the eyes, bones, liver, or meninges may occur. In the late stages of syphilis, dementia, pain or loss of sensation in the legs, and destruction of the aorta occur. Destructive inflammatory masses can appear in any organ. In tertiary or late-stage syphilis the heart and blood vessels (cardiovascular syphilis) and the central nervous system (neurosyphilis) frequently are involved. Spinal cord degeneration, partial paralysis, and various psychoses may result.

Diagnostic Tests

Diagnostic tests include the Venereal Disease Research Laboratory (VDRL) slide test and rapid plasma reagin (RPR) test. All patients should be checked for gonorrhea as well.

Medical Management

Therapeutic management of syphilis is aimed at eradication of all syphilitic organisms. However, treatment cannot reverse damage that is already present in the late stage of the disease. Parenteral benzylpenicillin (penicillin G) remains the treatment of choice for all stages of syphilis. In patients who have an allergy to penicillin tetracycline, erythromycin, and ceftriaxone are prescribed. All stages of syphilis should be treated.

Appropriate antibiotic treatment of maternal syphilis before the 18th week of pregnancy prevents infection of the fetus. Appropriate treatment after 18 weeks of pregnancy cures mother and fetus, because the antibiotics can cross the placental barrier. Treatment administered in the second half of pregnancy may pose a risk of premature labor. Some authorities recommend hospitalization and fetal monitoring of women at 20 weeks of gestation or later.

Carefully monitor all patients with neurosyphilis by periodic serologic testing, clinical evaluation at 6-month intervals, and repeated cerebrospinal fluid examinations for at least 3 years. Specific therapeutic management is based on the specific symptoms.

Nursing Interventions

In addition to routine interventions for patients with STIs, monitor for drug reaction to penicillin, stress good handwashing technique, encourage follow-up visits with the health care provider, and inform the patient that he or she should absolutely not engage in sexual intercourse until cured.

Prognosis

Syphilis infection must be treated at the earliest stage possible. Patients treated in the primary and secondary stages have the highest potential positive outcome. Although syphilis can be cured in late stages, damage to the body is more difficult to manage. As the disease progresses physiologic damage may result. Advanced stages of syphilis may result in the formation of gummas (bumps on the skin, bones, or body organs), neurologic damage, and cardiovascular illness. About 20% of patients with tertiary syphilis who are not treated die of the condition. Untreated syphilis advances from the primary stage to the secondary stage, latent stage, and eventually the tertiary stage.

GONORRHEA

Etiology and Pathophysiology

Gonorrhea is caused by *Neisseria gonorrhoeae,* a gram-negative diplococcoid bacterium, and almost exclusively follows sexual contact. It may be referred to as "the clap" or "the drip." It is the second most commonly reported STI in the United States (chlamydial infections are the most commonly reported). Gonorrhea rates remained stable from 1997 to 2000 after a 74% decline from 1975 to 1997. Since that time the rate of gonorrhea infections has sharply risen. The Centers for Disease Control and Prevention estimate that 820,000 people are infected annually, but only half are diagnosed and reported. Nearly 400,000 cases were reported in 2015 (CDC, 2016b). The highest incidence of gonorrhea occurs in adolescents and young adults of all racial and ethnic groups. African Americans are also a high-risk population. Gonorrhea is primarily an infection of the genital or rectal mucosa but is not limited to the genital organs; it can infect the mouth and throat through oral sex with an infected partner. It also may infect the eyes.

Clinical Manifestations

Some infected men may be asymptomatic after the incubation period. Typically within 2 to 5 days of exposure, symptoms develop. Signs and symptoms of urethritis, dysuria, infection with a profuse purulent discharge, and edema of the affected area are most common. A common sensation experienced by infected symptomatic individuals is that of "peeing razor blades." Most women remain asymptomatic but may show a greenish yellow discharge from the cervix. Other female signs and symptoms, depending on the infection site, are urinary frequency, purulent discharge from the urethra, pruritus, burning and pain of the vulva, vaginal engorgement and erythema, abdominal pain and distention, muscular rigidity, and tenderness. As the infection spreads, nausea, vomiting, fever, and tachycardia may develop. Other signs and symptoms are pharyngitis, tonsillitis, rectal burning, and purulent rectal discharge.

Diagnostic Tests

Diagnosis is determined by cultures from the site of infection to isolate and identify the organism. Cultures of the discharge or secretion can provide a definitive diagnosis after incubation for 24 to 48 hours. An important concern in the treatment for gonorrhea is coexisting chlamydial infection (see the section "Chlamydia" for more information). Chlamydia has been documented in up to 45% of gonorrhea cases. It is important to test for syphilis as well.

Medical Management

A history of sexual contact with a partner known to have gonorrhea is considered good evidence for the infection. Because of the short incubation period and high infectivity, treatment is instituted without awaiting culture results, even in the absence of signs or symptoms. Treatment of gonorrhea in the early stage is curative. Traditionally, the drug of choice for gonorrheal therapy was penicillin, but changes have been made because of (1) a rapid increase in the number of cases of gonorrhea caused by resistant strains of *N. gonorrhoeae* and (2) coexisting chlamydial infection.

There is no clinical distinction between infections caused by resistant or sensitive strains of *N. gonorrhoeae*. As a result, ceftriaxone, a penicillinase-resistant cephalosporin, has become part of the treatment plan. The most common treatment for gonorrhea is a single IM dose of ceftriaxone. Cefixime (Suprax) given orally one time is also effective. Other medications that may be used in the treatment of gonorrhea are ciprofloxacin, ofloxacin, and levofloxacin. The high frequency of coexisting chlamydial and gonococcal infections has led to the addition of doxycycline or tetracycline to the treatment plan. The expense of diagnosing chlamydial infection and the sequelae make this strategy cost effective. Patients with co-incubating syphilis are likely to be cured by the same drugs.

All sexual contacts of patients with gonorrhea must be treated to prevent reinfection after resumption of sexual relations. The "ping-pong" effect of reexposure, treatment, and reinfection will cease only when infected partners are treated simultaneously. In addition, advise the patient to abstain from sexual intercourse and alcohol for 2 to 4 weeks. Sexual intercourse allows the infection to spread and can retard complete healing as a result of vascular congestion. Alcohol irritates the healing urethral walls. Caution men against squeezing the penis to look for further discharge. Follow-up examination and reculture should be done at least once after treatment, usually in 4 to 7 days. Treat relapse, reinfection, and complications appropriately.

Be alert to changes in CDC recommendations. Report the disease to infection control authorities as required by the local health agency.

Nursing Interventions and Patient Teaching

Advise patients that loose, absorbent underclothes, changed frequently after perineal or penile cleansing, enhance comfort. Sitz baths decrease lower abdominal discomfort and dysuria. Obtain laboratory specimens as ordered. Discuss alternative methods of birth control as appropriate. Encourage notification of present and past sexual partners of the diagnosis and stress the need for them to promptly seek medical care. Inform the patients that sterility may occur as a result of gonorrhea.

Prognosis

With treatment, gonorrhea is curable. The inflammation may clear up without serious results, or it may become chronic and produce urethral stricture. Complications include prostatitis, epididymitis, orchitis, arthritis, and endocarditis. It can result in sterility and pelvic inflammatory disease in the female. No case of acute gonorrhea in the female should be considered cured until three consecutive negative smears of the cervix and Bartholin's and Skene's glands are obtained. The main cause of infections identified after completed treatment is reinfection, not treatment failure.

TRICHOMONIASIS

Etiology and Pathophysiology

Trichomoniasis is an STI caused by the protozoan *Trichomonas vaginalis*. In the United States, an estimated 3.7 million people are infected (CDC, 2017c). The incubation period is 4 to 28 days. Trichomoniasis usually is transmitted by sexual intercourse. On occasion, a newborn develops an infection from an infected mother. *T. vaginalis* thrives when the vaginal mucosa is more alkaline than normal. Frequent douching and use of oral contraceptives and antibiotics raise the normal pH of the vagina, making women more vulnerable to trichomoniasis.

Clinical Manifestations

Most men and approximately 70% of women are asymptomatic. The male signs and symptoms are mild to severe transient urethritis, dysuria, frequent urination, pruritus, and purulent exudate. In women, signs and symptoms include profuse, frothy, gray, green, or yellow malodorous discharge; pruritus; edema; tenderness of vagina; dysuria; frequency of urination; spotting; menorrhagia; and dysmenorrhea. Signs and symptoms may persist for a week to several months and may be more pronounced after menstruation or during pregnancy.

Diagnostic Tests

Diagnosis is based on microscopic examination of a vaginal discharge sample that identifies *T. vaginalis*.

Medical Management

Treatment for men and women is oral metronidazole (Flagyl) in small doses for 7 days or a single large dose. The patient should avoid alcoholic beverages, because alcohol can cause reactions such as disorientation, headache, cramps, vomiting, and possibly convulsions. Metronidazole can cause the urine to turn dark brown (see Table 52.2).

Nursing Interventions and Patient Teaching

Advise the patient to avoid alcohol during treatment; inform patients that their urine may turn dark orange or brown; and counsel patients to avoid douches, sprays, and powders during treatment. Teach the patient how to disinfect douche nozzles, applicators, diaphragms, and the toilet area. Encourage the patient to wear loose-fitting clothing and cotton underwear, to schedule follow-up visits with the health care provider, and to contact sexual partners so that they can get treatment.

Prognosis

With treatment, trichomoniasis is curable. Reinfection is common if sexual partners are not treated simultaneously. Chronic infection may develop in untreated cases.

CANDIDIASIS

Etiology and Pathophysiology

Candidiasis (thrush) is a mild fungal infection that appears in men and women. Candidal infections usually are caused by *C. albicans* and *Candida tropicalis*. The fungi are a part of the normal flora of the gastrointestinal tract, mouth, vagina, and skin. The infection often occurs when the glucose level rises from diabetes mellitus or when resistance is lowered from diseases such as carcinoma. Radiation, immunosuppressant drugs, hyperalimentation (IV feeding), antibiotic therapy, and oral contraceptives may predispose individuals to candidiasis. Infected men and women display signs of scaly skin; erythematous rash; and occasional exudates that appear under the breasts, between the fingers, and in the axillae, groin, and umbilicus.

Clinical Manifestations

If the mother is infected, a newborn can contract thrush during delivery. The infant may display a diaper rash. The infant's nails become edematous and have a darkened, erythematous nail base with purulent exudate. Thrush may appear on the mucous membranes of the infant's mouth as pearly, bluish white "milk-curd" lesions and cause edema and engorgement. The infant may have an edematous tongue that can cause respiratory distress. Poor feeding may be noted. The adult female patient may have a cheesy, tenacious white vaginal discharge accompanied by pruritus and an inflamed vulva and vagina. The adult male patient has signs of an infected penis with purulent exudate. Systemic infections are indicated by chills, fevers, and general malaise.

Diagnostic Tests

Diagnosis is based on evidence of a *Candida* species on a Gram stain of specimens collected from scraping of the vagina and penis, from pus, and from exudate from the mouth.

Medical Management

Treatment consists of managing any underlying condition, such as controlling diabetes mellitus, and discontinuing antibiotics and oral contraceptives. Nystatin is effective for superficial candidiasis; topical amphotericin B is effective for skin and nail infections.

Nursing Interventions and Patient Teaching

Emphasize the use of prescribed ointments, sprays, and creams as indicated for each part of the body affected. Teaching includes the method for inserting vaginal suppositories (to be inserted high into the vagina when in a dorsal recumbent position) and remaining on the back for 30 minutes to allow suppository absorption. Patients should encourage sexual partners to have an examination and treatment. Teach good handwashing techniques to avoid reinfection or the transfer of the fungi. Encourage pregnant women to accept treatment to prevent infection of the newborn at the time of delivery.

Prognosis

Candidiasis is curable with the use of the prescribed treatment.

CHLAMYDIA

Etiology and Pathophysiology

Chlamydia trachomatis, a gram-negative, intracellular bacterium, causes several common STIs. Cervicitis and urethritis are most common, but like gonococci, chlamydial organisms also cause epididymitis in men and salpingitis in women. Chlamydial infections are the most commonly occurring STI in the United States. They are responsible for about 20% to 30% of diagnosed PID cases. In 2014 there were more than 1,400,000 cases of chlamydial infections reported in the United States (CDC, 2015). It is estimated that about 11,000 women each year become involuntarily sterilized and 36,000 suffer ectopic pregnancies as a result of this organism. The incidence of chlamydia is highest in young, promiscuous, indigent, unmarried women who live in the inner city and in those who have a prior history of STIs. Increases in chlamydia rates are more likely a result of better screening and use of more sensitive tests, rather than an increase in the total burden of the disease in the United States (CDC, 2015). Chlamydia can be transmitted during vaginal, anal, or oral sex.

Although men and women may have asymptomatic infection, women are more likely to be asymptomatic carriers even with deep pelvic infections, such as infection of the fallopian tubes and PID.

Clinical Manifestations

In men, signs and symptoms may include a scanty white or clear exudate, burning or pruritus around the urethral meatus, urinary frequency, and mild dysuria. Signs and symptoms of cervicitis in women may include one or more of the following: (1) vaginal pruritus or burning, (2) dull pelvic pain, (3) low-grade fever, (4) vaginal discharge, and (5) irregular bleeding. Symptoms of chlamydia may be absent or cause minor discomfort; therefore it has been called a silent disease. Females may develop a PID, which can result in infertility. For this reason the CDC (2017d) recommends that all females younger than 25 years of age be screened routinely for chlamydia at their annual gynecologic examination. The CDC further advises annual screening of all women older than 25 years of age with one or more risk factors for the disease (CDC, 2017d).

Diagnostic Tests

The direct fluorescent antibody test provides a ready basis for diagnosis. However, this test is less specific than a culture and may produce false-positive results. Culturing for chlamydial organisms should be done if the laboratory facilities are available. New techniques using nucleic acid amplification promise to surpass culture as the gold standard of chlamydial testing. Treatment can be initiated promptly, based on a confirmed diagnosis.

Medical Management

Chlamydial infections respond to treatment with tetracycline, doxycycline, azithromycin, or ofloxacin. For tetracycline, the dosage is 500 mg orally four times a day for at least 7 days. For doxycycline, the dosage is 100 mg two times a day. For ofloxacin, the dosage is 300 mg twice a day. Azithromycin (1 g in a single dose) offers the advantage of ease of administration, but safety for patients younger than 15 years of age has not been established. Alternative regimens include erythromycin, ofloxacin, and levofloxacin. Erythromycin is the drug of choice for use in pregnant patients. If this treatment is not tolerated, amoxicillin is an alternative. Follow-up care includes advising the patient to return if symptoms persist or recur, treating sexual partners, and encouraging the use of condoms during all sexual contact.

Because chlamydial infections are closely associated with gonococcal infections, both infections usually are treated concurrently, even without diagnostic evidence.

Nursing Interventions and Patient Teaching

Patients' physical symptoms often are complicated by their emotional responses to STIs. Depression, anger, fear, and guilt must be addressed if education and treatment are to be effective. Outcome also is influenced by educational and income levels, primary language, health insurance coverage, and support network. Patient education focuses on prevention (Box 52.8).

Box 52.8 Prevention of Sexually Transmitted Infections

- Reduce the number of sexual partners, preferably to one person.
- Avoid contact with individuals known to be infected or who are at risk of infection.
- Avoid contact with the genital area if signs and symptoms develop.
- Wash the hands and the genital-rectal area before and immediately after having intercourse.
- Pay special attention to washing the foreskin.
- An antiseptic mouthwash or gargle with hydrogen peroxide (1 part peroxide to 3 parts of water) may slightly reduce the risk of oropharyngeal sexually transmitted infection (STI).
- Use barrier (condom) contraceptives with new partners.
- Use a water-based lubricant as opposed to an oil-based lubricant.
- Void after intercourse.
- Avoid excess douching.
- If an STI infection is suspected, seek medical help immediately.
- Individuals with multiple sexual partners should have an STI examination twice a year or more if needed.

Prognosis

With treatment, chlamydial infection is curable. Reinfection occurs if sexual partners are not treated simultaneously. Chlamydial infections can be transmitted to infants during delivery, causing conjunctivitis and pneumonia. Poorly treated or untreated chlamydial infection can result in ectopic pregnancy or infertility.

ACQUIRED IMMUNODEFICIENCY SYNDROME

Acquired immunodeficiency syndrome (AIDS) is the ultimately fatal, advanced stage of infection with the retroviral human immunodeficiency virus (HIV), which gradually destroys the cell-mediated immune system. For a more detailed discussion on this infection, see Chapter 56.

FAMILY PLANNING

Advances in drug therapy and family planning technology have made a range of options available for individuals wishing to prevent or plan conception. Birth control planning involves moral, religious, cultural, and personal values; be sensitive to these factors when discussing birth control with patients.

Numerous types of birth control procedures or devices can be employed. The selection of a method should be

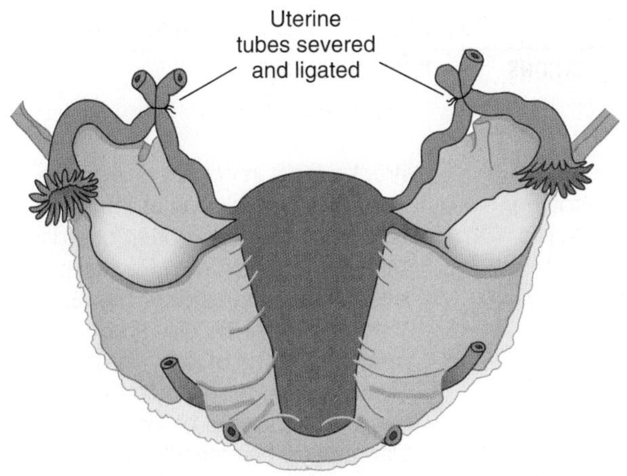

Fig. 52.20 Tubal ligation. Oviduct is severed and ligated. (From Lowdermilk DL, Perry SE, Cashion K, Alden KR: *Maternity and women's health care,* ed 10, St. Louis, 2012, Mosby.)

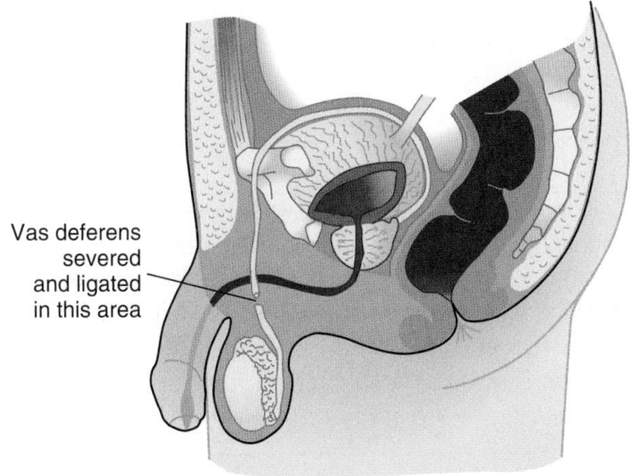

Fig. 52.21 Vasectomy. Sperm duct is severed and ligated. (From Lowdermilk DL, Perry SE, Cashion K, Alden KR: *Maternity and women's health care,* ed 10, St. Louis, 2012, Mosby.)

based on the patient's health, effectiveness of the method, cost, lifestyle, ease of use, and age and parity (total number of pregnancies) of the patient. The patient's willingness to comply with use and the couple's preference are two additional factors taken into consideration when selecting a method of contraception. Reinforce the information given by the health care provider and encourage patients to seek more information, directing them to the source.

Contraceptive methods and products can be categorized as surgical (Figs. 52.20 and 52.21), hormonal, barrier, and behavioral (Table 52.4).

NURSING PROCESS FOR THE PATIENT WITH A REPRODUCTIVE DISORDER

The role of the licensed practical nurse/licensed vocational nurse (LPN/LVN) in the nursing process as stated is that the LPN/LVN will do the following:

- Participate in planning care for patients, based on patient needs
- Review patient's care plan and recommend revisions as needed
- Review and follow defined prioritization for patient care
- Use clinical pathways, care maps, or care plans to guide and review patient care

ASSESSMENT

People with reproductive disorders require skilled assessment by the nurse and the health care provider. Assessment occurs through observation of the patient during the patient health history and while doing baseline and continuing assessment of the patient's objective and subjective data.

Health history data should be relevant to the patient's developmental age. Information about reproductive health and sexuality can form a large portion of the collected data. This history is as important as the physical and emotional data in determining appropriate patient problems and interventions. Data collected about sexual health, sexual relations, birth control methods, STIs, and the use of chemical substances provide an opportunity to clarify any misconceptions or myths revealed during history taking.

Data Collection for Women

Data collection for adolescent and adult women focuses on the reproductive tract and the menstrual, gynecologic, and obstetric history.

The menstrual history encompasses menarche (onset of menstrual flow) through the climacteric (cessation of menstrual cycle), including (1) age of onset; (2) date of last menstrual flow; (3) usual amount and volume of flow (number of pads used per day); (4) presence of dysmenorrhea (painful menstruation), menorrhagia (excessive flow), amenorrhea (absence of flow), or metrorrhagia (excessive spotting between cycles); and (5) other difficulties during menses.

The gynecologic assessment includes data on (1) vaginal discharge (odor, color, frequency, and duration), (2) vaginal pruritus (itching), (3) vaginal irritation with coital activity, (4) date and results of the last Pap test, (5) birth control methods or kinds of contraceptives used, and (6) any family history of cancer of the reproductive system.

If the patient has conceived, information should be collected as to gravidity (number of pregnancies), parity (number of births), abortions, miscarriages, and stillbirths.

Assessment of the breast includes (1) tenderness of the breast areas; (2) pain; (3) masses in any specific areas; (4) presence of nipple discharge; (5) knowledge and frequency of BSE; and (6) date and results of last mammogram, if applicable.

Data Collection for Men

The data collected from the male adolescent and the adult man include (1) urologic history of voiding

Table 52.4 Methods of Birth Control

DESCRIPTION	SIDE EFFECTS AND COMPLICATIONS	PATIENT EDUCATION
Temporary Methods		
Combined		
Combination pill contains estrogen and progesterone (standard and low dose). Usually taken on 5th through 25th day of each cycle. Prevents ovulation; causes changes in endometrium; causes alterations in cervical mucus and tubal transport. Simple and unobtrusive in use. 99% effective. Failure from irregular or incorrect use.	*Side effects:* Weight gain, nausea and vomiting, spotting and breakthrough bleeding, postpill amenorrhea, breast tenderness, headache, melasma, irritability, nervousness, depression, and decreased libido. *Complications:* Benign liver tumors, gallstones, myocardial infarction, thromboembolism, stroke (smokers over age 35 yr at higher risk). *Contraindications:* History of cardiovascular or liver disease, hypertension, breast or pelvic cancer; use caution with diabetes mellitus, sickle cell anemia. Provides no protection against HIV transmission.	Instruct patient in correct use of pills. Tell patient to take pill at the same time each day; if forgotten one day, take two the next day. Review side effects and contraindications. Explain that the patient should report cramps, edema of legs, chest pain. Discuss need for periodic (q 6–12 mo) checkup of weight, BP, Pap smear, hematocrit. Review danger signs of drug. Take drug history; ask about use of phenytoin, phenobarbital, antibiotic (ampicillin), which decrease contraceptive action. Inform patient that method is usually not recommended for women over age 35. Discourage smoking.
Morning-after pill, also called Plan B (norgestrel and ethinyl estradiol), contains ethinyl estradiol 50 mcg and norgestrel 500 mg. Another use of combined hormonal contraception. 98.4% effective. Creates hostile uterine lining and alters tubal transport.	Nausea for 1–2 days. Does not prevent an ectopic pregnancy. Patient is at risk for usual hormonal complications of abdominal pain, chest pain, cough, shortness of breath, headache, dizziness, weakness, leg pain.	Take two Ovral within 72 h of coitus. Repeat if vomiting occurs. Take second dose 12 h later. Menses should begin within 2–3 wk. Start an ongoing method of contraception immediately after menses.
Progestin Only		
Progestin-only pills (POPs or Minipills) are taken daily, with no pill-free days. Preferred for women who are breast-feeding. Does not suppress lactation. Inhibits ovulation. Thickens cervical mucus. Alters uterine lining. Lower cardiovascular risk than combined pills.	Menstrual changes, breakthrough bleeding, prolonged cycles or amenorrhea. Increase incidence of functional cysts of the ovary, ectopic pregnancy.	Use alternative contraception when starting POPs or if pill is missed. Take pill at same time every day. Keep record of menses and undergo pregnancy testing if 2 wk late.
Medroxyprogesterone (Depo-Provera, DMPA) is a progestin-only drug given by injection q 3 mo. A private, convenient, and highly effective method. Efficacy similar to that of surgical sterilization.	May cause amenorrhea, headaches, bloating, and weight gain. Return of fertility may be delayed for several months after discontinuation.	Return q 3 mo for injection. Discontinue method for several months before planning to conceive.
Implanon is a thin, flexible rod containing 68 mg of etonogestrel that is inserted subdermally. The device provides contraceptive protection for up to 3 yr.	Changes in menstruation patterns, breast tenderness, and weight gain.	Removal must be completed by a trained health care provider. Review patient history, as contraindications include a history of thrombolytic disease, liver disease, and undiagnosed vaginal bleeding.

Table 52.4 Methods of Birth Control—cont'd

DESCRIPTION	SIDE EFFECTS AND COMPLICATIONS	PATIENT EDUCATION
Barrier Methods		
Diaphragms are dome-shaped latex caps with a flexible metal ring (varies in size) covering the cervix. Inner surface is coated with spermicide before insertion. Provides mechanical barrier to sperm. Available by prescription, fitted by professional. Continuing motivation to use is necessary. 87% effective. Failure from improper fitting or placement of device.	Allergy to latex or spermicide.	Demonstrate how to hold, insert, and remove device, using model. Allow for insertion and removal practice sessions. Advise patient that insertion may be done just prior to coitus, but removal should be 6–8 h after coitus. Tell patient to empty bowel and bladder before insertion. Give instructions for cleansing and storing, checking for holes or deterioration. Advise patient that diaphragm must be refitted after pregnancy, weight loss, or weight gain. Advise patient that its use is not suitable if severe pelvic relaxation is present.
Cervical caps are rubber thimble-shaped shields covering cervix, held in place by suction. Spermicide in inner surface provides mechanical barrier to sperm. Fitted by professional. Effectiveness similar to that of diaphragm. Failure from dislodgment and improper fit.	Allergy to rubber; or spermicide, possible cervical irritation or erosion from suction.	Provide sufficient time for practice with insertion and removal (more time than for diaphragm). Give instructions for cleaning, storing, and inspecting for damage. Inform patient that it can be used with abnormalities of vaginal canal but not with cervical inconsistencies or PID.
Condoms *Male:* Thin rubber sheath fitting over erect penis, providing mechanical barrier to sperm. Simple method to use. No prescription necessary. 85% effective. Failure from tearing or slipping during coitus. Used with spermicide. Affords some protection against STIs and HIV transmission.	Possible allergy to rubber or latex; possible decrease in sensation and interference with foreplay.	Advise patient to roll sheath along entire penis, leaving slack at end to receive semen. Inform patient that sharp objects (fingernails) may tear the condom. Tell patient to hold sheath in place when penis is withdrawn to prevent emptying of sperm in or near vagina.
Female: Double-ring system fitted into the vagina up to 8 h before intercourse. No prescription necessary. Affords protection against HIV, cytomegalovirus, and hepatitis B.	No significant side effects; generally acceptable to couple.	Discuss insertion, lubrication, and method of removal. More expensive than male condoms.
Other Methods		
Intrauterine devices (IUDs) are inserted into uterus; they are flexible objects made of plastic or copper wire (nonmedicated or medicated with substance to alter uterine environment), usually with attached string that protrudes into vagina. Contraception probably provided by inflammatory response in endometrium, preventing implantation. After insertion, no additional equipment necessary. 97% to 99% effective. Failure mainly from undetected expulsion. Most common type used today is Progestasert (contains progestins).	Increased menstrual flow, intramenstrual bleeding, and cramping, especially during early months of use. Possible complications include ectopic pregnancy, pelvic infection, perforation of uterus, infertility. Undetected expulsion of IUD may result in pregnancy.	Discuss techniques and experience of insertion and removal. Inform patient that insertion may be more difficult and expulsion and complications greater in nulliparous patients. Instruct patient to check for string in vagina after each period; report to health care provider if unable to locate. Discuss need for annual pelvic examination and Pap test.

Continued

Table 52.4 Methods of Birth Control—cont'd

DESCRIPTION	SIDE EFFECTS AND COMPLICATIONS	PATIENT EDUCATION
Rhythm method requires periodic abstinence during fertile portion of menstrual cycle. Requires strong motivation, self-control. Complies with all religious doctrines. 60% to 65% effective. Failure from difficulty in determining precise day of ovulation, irregularity of menses.	Inaccurate or incomplete knowledge of menstrual cycle.	Discuss methods to establish baseline menstrual patterns and identify ovulation. Give instructions in use of calendar or basal body temperature method to determine ovulation and fertile period.
Permanent		
Tubal sterilization includes a variety of abdominal and vaginal surgical procedures (laparotomy, laparoscopy, culdoscopy) that permanently prevent sperm and ovum from meeting. Crushing, ligating, clipping, or plugging of fallopian tubes (potentially reversible procedure). Nearly 100% (99.96%) effective. Failure due to recanalization of fallopian tubes, erroneous ligation (see Fig. 52.20).	Bowel injury, hemorrhage, or infection.	Determine whether temporary contraceptives were used and reason for patient's dissatisfaction. Counsel regarding effects of procedure on physiology and sexual performance. Assist in obtaining written informed consent for procedure. Inform patient that procedure may require short-term hospitalization or can be done on outpatient basis.
Hysterectomy is surgical removal of uterus. 100% effective.	Bladder infection, vascular disorders, infection, hemorrhage, pain, psychological adjustment.	Assess or counsel regarding understanding of extent of surgery, altered physiology, complications, and sexual performance. Hysterectomy only performed for reasons other than contraception; sterility is secondary benefit when desired.
Vasectomy is bilateral surgical ligation and resection of ductus deferens.	Hematoma, edema, psychological adjustment (see Fig. 52.21).	Inform patient that procedure is usually done as outpatient procedure and takes 15 to 30 min. Tell patient that alternative form of contraception is needed until no sperm are seen on examination. Explain that procedure does not affect masculinity.

BP, Blood pressure; *HIV*, human immunodeficiency virus; *PID*, pelvic inflammatory disease; *STI*, sexually transmitted infection.
Modified from Lewis SL, Heitkemper MM, Dirksen SR, et al: *Medical-surgical nursing: Assessment and management of clinical problems*, ed 7, St. Louis, 2007, Mosby.

difficulties and any discharge from the penis; (2) characteristics of the urine (odor, color, amount, and frequency); (3) information on prostate and testicular problems; (4) frequency of PSA testing, if applicable; (5) masses or lesions on genitalia; (6) frequency of TSE; (7) frequency of professional testicular examination; (8) measures to prevent infections; and (9) birth control method. In addition, note concerns about sexual health voiced by the patient.

◆ PATIENT PROBLEM

Possible patient problems for the patient with a reproductive disorder include but are not limited to the following:

- *Alteration in Urinary Elimination*
- *Anxiousness*
- *Compromised Blood Flow to Tissue*
- *Compromised Skin Integrity*
- *Distorted Body Image*
- *Fearfulness*
- *Impaired Coping*
- *Impaired Health Maintenance*
- *Impaired Self-Esteem due to Current Situation*
- *Impaired Sexual Function*
- *Insufficient Fluid Volume*
- *Insufficient Knowledge*
- *Potential for Infection*
- *Prolonged Low Self-Esteem*
- *Prolonged Pain*
- *Recent Onset of Pain*

◆ EXPECTED OUTCOMES AND PLANNING

Planning is a category of nursing behaviors in which patient-centered goals are established and strategies designed to achieve the goals and outcomes that relate to the identified patient problem (Table 52.5).

Table 52.5 Planning and Setting Goals for the Patient With a Reproductive Disorder

PATIENT PROBLEM	GOAL	OUTCOME
Impaired Coping, related to fear of positive diagnosis of breast cancer	Patient will attend cancer support group weekly.	Patient expresses fears of unfavorable outcome.
Insufficient Knowledge, regarding postoperative care at home after modified radical mastectomy	Patient will state four postoperative risks before discharge.	Patient verbalizes signs and symptoms of infection. Patient demonstrates exercises for affected arm. Patient verbalizes need to avoid injections and taking of blood or blood pressure in affected arm. Patient verbalizes need to examine remaining breast once a month.

Complementary and Alternative Therapies

Male and Female Reproductive Disorders

MALE REPRODUCTIVE SYSTEM
- Yohimbine *(Pausinystalia yohimbe)* for erectile dysfunction and impotence

FEMALE REPRODUCTIVE SYSTEM
- Biofeedback, therapeutic touch, and acupuncture for primary dysmenorrhea
- Black cohosh *(Cimicifuga racemosa)* for menstrual irregularity, premenstrual syndrome (PMS), and menopausal problems
- Chamomile *(Matricaria recutita, Chamaemelum nobile)* for menstrual cramps
- Chaste tree *(Vitex agnus-castus)* for PMS
- Evening primrose *(Oenothera biennis)* for PMS
- Feverfew *(Tanacetum parthenium)* for menstrual problems
- Sage *(Salvia officinalis)* for menstrual irregularity
- Soybeans and other legumes for their phytoestrogens that may help prevent breast cancer

Modified from Black JM, Hawks HJ: *Medical-surgical nursing: Clinical management for positive outcomes*, ed 8, Philadelphia, 2009, Saunders.

◆ IMPLEMENTATION

The implementation step for the patient with a reproductive disorder is the action-oriented phase of the nursing process, in which the nurse initiates and carries out the objectives of the nursing care plan. See the Complementary and Alternative Therapies box for additional treatment methods.

◆ EVALUATION

Examples of goals and their corresponding evaluative measures include the following:

Goal 1: Patient will be able to cope effectively.

Evaluative measure: Patient verbalizes fears and identifies two strategies for dealing with fear, such as questioning for clarification and relaxation breathing technique.

Goal 2: Patient will have adequate knowledge regarding postoperative care at home after modified radical mastectomy.

Evaluative measures: Patient states signs and symptoms of wound infection; lists proper arm exercises; verbalizes the need for BSE once per month; and states the need to avoid blood pressure checks, injections, and blood draws in affected arm.

Get Ready for the NCLEX® Examination!

Key Points

- Sperm are produced in the seminiferous tubules and stored in the epididymis.
- Testosterone, the male sex hormone, is responsible for male secondary sex characteristics.
- Seminal fluid is produced in the seminal vesicles, prostate gland, and Cowper's glands.
- The male urethra serves the twofold purpose of conveying urine from the bladder and carrying the reproductive cells and secretions to the outside.
- The uterus consists of three layers of tissue: (1) endometrium, the inner layer; (2) myometrium, the middle layer; and (3) perimetrium, the outer layer.
- In the ovulating female, an egg matures each month in the graafian follicle, which is located in the ovary.
- The menstrual cycle prepares the uterus and causes ovulation to occur each month.
- Because of the relationship between the menstrual cycle and the body's mechanisms of hormonal secretion, a decrease or increase in the activity of the hormonal glands can disturb menstruation.

- Early diagnosis and prompt management are necessary to prevent serious reproductive and genital problems.
- Health teaching for patients with menstrual disturbances includes a knowledge of the physiologic process, factors that alter menstruation, personal hygiene, exercise, diet, and pain management.
- Discharge planning is vital to prevent reinfection after PID.
- Pregnancy is encouraged in the patient with endometriosis, because it will slow the progress of the disorder; infertility is a complication as the condition continues.
- Menarche, the first menstrual cycle, usually begins around the age of 12 years.
- Serum CA-125 assessment is useful mainly to signal a recurrence of ovarian cancer and in monitoring the response to treatment.
- PSA is a highly sensitive blood test that is elevated in cancer of the prostate and in benign prostatic hyperplasia.
- There is no definitive test for TSS. However, cervical-vaginal isolates of *Staphylococcus aureus* are present 90% of the time with TSS.
- Vaginal fistulas are caused by an ulcerating process resulting from cancer, radiation, weakening of tissue from pregnancies, or surgical interventions.
- Correction of cystocele and rectocele is a surgical repair involving shortening of the muscles that support the bladder and repair of the rectocele. This is known as anteroposterior colporrhaphy.
- Screening tests for cervical abnormalities include routine Pap smears (a newer, liquid-based Pap test is recommended) and testing for HPV.
- Vaccines are now available that reduce the incidence of cervical cancer resulting from infection with HPV (types 6, 11, 16, 18).
- A panhysterosalpingo-oophorectomy involves removal of the uterus, fallopian tubes, and ovaries.
- In patients with breast cancer an axillary lymph node dissection usually is performed regardless of treatment options available. Examination of nodes provides the most powerful prognostic data currently available.
- A relatively new diagnostic tool used before therapeutic surgery for breast cancer is sentinel lymph node mapping, which identifies the first lymph node most likely to drain the cancerous cells.
- Overall 10-year survival with lumpectomy and radiation is about the same as with modified radical mastectomy.
- After losing a breast, many patients experience acute grief that may last 4 to 6 weeks or longer. Grief makes the fact of loss real.
- Caution patients who have undergone a modified radical mastectomy to avoid injections, vaccinations, taking of blood pressure or blood samples, or insertion of IV line in the affected arm.
- Phimosis is a condition in which the prepuce is too small to retract over the glans penis.
- Young men should be taught to perform TSE monthly beginning at 15 years of age for detection of testicular carcinoma.
- Oral acyclovir is prescribed for primary genital herpes to shorten the duration of healing and to suppress 75% of recurrence with daily use.
- Parenteral penicillin remains the treatment of choice for all stages of syphilis. All stages of syphilis should be treated.
- Because of penicillin-resistant strains of *N. gonorrhoeae,* penicillin, the former drug of choice for treatment of gonorrhea, has been changed to ceftriaxone.
- Chlamydial infections respond to treatment with tetracycline, doxycycline, azithromycin, or ofloxacin. Erythromycin is the drug of choice for use in pregnant patients.

Additional Learning Resources

SG Go to your Study Guide for additional learning activities to help you master this chapter content.

evolve Be sure to visit the Evolve site at *http://evolve.elsevier.com/Cooper/foundationsadult/* for additional online resources.

Review Questions for the NCLEX® Examination

1. A patient visits her health care provider because of an increase in her abdominal girth and dyspnea during the past month as a result of pressure on her diaphragm. She is diagnosed as having ovarian cancer. The cause for these manifestations can be explained by what physiologic occurrence?
   1. Development of ascites
   2. Metastasis to the bowel
   3. Dilation of the alveoli
   4. Bladder distention
2. The nurse is discussing breast self-examination with a 30-year-old premenopausal patient. When should the nurse advise is the best time for the patient to perform her monthly self-examination of the breasts?
   1. During her menstruation
   2. 7 to 8 days after conclusion of the menstrual period
   3. The same day each month
   4. The 26th day of the menstrual cycle
3. A 52-year-old patient has ductal cell carcinoma of the left breast. After a modified radical mastectomy, a Davol drain is placed in the left axillary region. What is the primary purpose of this drain?
   1. To control numbness of her left incisional site
   2. To improve her ability to perform range-of-motion exercises on her affected side
   3. To facilitate drainage and to prevent formation of a hematoma
   4. To prevent postoperative phlebitis in her affected arm

4. A 35-year-old patient has undergone a vasectomy. Teaching for this patient should include what information? *(Select all that apply.)*
   1. The procedure is reversible if he later changes his mind.
   2. He should abstain from sexual intercourse until the incision is completely healed.
   3. He should apply warm compresses to the scrotum four times a day.
   4. He should return to the health care provider at regular intervals for sperm counts.
   5. Contraceptive use is indicated in the initial weeks after the procedure.
5. A 44-year-old patient is admitted for an abdominal hysterectomy. She is instructed that she will have a Foley catheter in place postoperatively. She asks the nurse how many days she will have the catheter in place. What is the best response by the nurse?
   1. "The indwelling catheter will probably remain in place for 1 week."
   2. "The indwelling catheter will be removed after you are fully awake from the anesthesia."
   3. "The indwelling catheter will generally be removed on the first postoperative day."
   4. "The indwelling catheter will remain in place for a few days postdischarge."
6. A 60-year-old patient underwent a vaginal hysterectomy for a prolapsed uterus. The nurse is aware that patients undergoing pelvic surgery are more susceptible to what postoperative complications? *(Select all that apply.)*
   1. Wound dehiscence
   2. Postoperative loss of libido
   3. Urinary retention
   4. Venous stasis
   5. Thrombophlebitis
7. A 49-year-old obese patient with diabetes has had a total abdominal hysterectomy. On the second postoperative day, the patient complains of increased pain in the operative site. She states, "It feels like something suddenly popped." With the symptoms presented, it would be likely that when the nurse removes the abdominal dressing she may note what occurrence?
   1. The wound has a purulent exudate.
   2. Dehiscence has occurred.
   3. The wound is indurated and tender.
   4. The wound is well approximated.
8. A 20-year-old patient goes to the health care provider's office with vaginal pruritus, burning, dull pelvic pain, and purulent vaginal discharge. A diagnostic test reveals she has chlamydia. What nursing interventions would best promote a successful patient outcome? *(Select all that apply.)*
   1. Encourage her to have her sexual partner(s) seek medical care as soon as possible to avoid reinfection of the patient.
   2. Recommend she abstain from sexual contact while lesions are present.
   3. Provide social and emotional support because the edematous, draining lymph nodes may be disturbing to the patient's self-image.
   4. Educate the patient that the causative organism is a spirochete that gains entrance into the body during intercourse.
   5. Discuss means to prevent future exposures to this infection.
9. A 23-year-old man is diagnosed with gonorrhea. Because of statements made in his patient interview, the nurse has established a patient problem of *Nonconformity*. Which is the most effective way to overcome *Nonconformity* for this patient?
   1. Telephone follow-up
   2. Case finding
   3. Single-dose treatment of ceftriaxone (Rocephin) IM
   4. Extensive patient education program
10. The nurse is teaching a group of teenagers about contraception and sexually transmitted infections (STIs). The nurse asks the students if they know which is the most prevalent STI. Which response by the participants is correct?
    1. Syphilis
    2. Chlamydial infection
    3. Gonorrhea
    4. Genital herpes
11. A 73-year-old patient comes to the health care provider's office with a complaint of constant seepage of feces from her vagina, causing her embarrassment because of soilage and odor. These manifestations are most consistent with what condition?
    1. Rectovaginal fistula
    2. Vesicovaginal fistula
    3. Urethrovaginal fistula
    4. Rectocele
12. The American Cancer Society recommends that women have an annual screening mammography beginning at what age?
    1. 21 years
    2. 35 years
    3. 40 years
    4. 52 years
13. The first lymph node most likely to drain the cancerous site in a patient with breast cancer is known as the:
    1. axillary node.
    2. contaminated node.
    3. primary node.
    4. sentinel node.

14. While discussing breast cancer with a group of women, what should the nurse stress as the greatest risk factor for breast cancer?
1. Being a woman over the age of 50 years
2. Experiencing menstruation for 40 years or more
3. Using estrogen replacement therapy during menopause
4. Having a paternal grandmother with postmenopausal breast cancer

15. A patient diagnosed with breast cancer has been offered the treatment choice of breast conservation surgery with radiation or a modified radical mastectomy. Which statement by the patient concerning the lumpectomy with radiation indicates understanding of the procedure?
1. "It preserves the normal appearance and sensitivity of the breast."
2. "It provides a shorter treatment period with fewer long-term complications."
3. "It has about the same 10-year survival rate as the modified radical mastectomy."
4. "It has a much higher survival rate than the modified radical mastectomy."

16. The nurse is educating a patient who has undergone a modified radical mastectomy in ways to prevent lymphedema. What should the nurse include in the information provided? *(Select all that apply.)*
1. Use a sling for the first 2 weeks after the procedure.
2. Expose the arm to sunlight to increase circulation.
3. Wrap the arm with elastic bandages during the night.
4. Avoid unnecessary trauma (e.g., venipuncture, blood pressure) to the arm on the operative side.
5. Elevate the hand and arm above the level of the chest.

17. The nurse plans early and frequent ambulation for a patient who has undergone an abdominal hysterectomy to: *(Select all that apply.)*
1. prevent urinary retention.
2. prevent deep-vein thrombosis.
3. relieve abdominal distention.
4. maintain a sense of normalcy.
5. reduce postoperative nausea.

18. On the second postoperative day, a 63-year-old patient who underwent an abdominal hysterectomy complains of gas pains and abdominal distention. The patient has not had a bowel movement since surgery. Which nursing intervention will best stimulate peristalsis and relieve distention?
1. Offering carbonated beverages
2. Encouraging ambulation at least four times daily
3. Administering a 1000-mL soapsuds enema
4. Applying an abdominal binder

19. A 40-year-old patient has a history of multiple births in the past 15 years. Her health care provider is concerned she has a cystocele. What manifestations provide support to the diagnosis?
1. Rectal pressure
2. Dysmenorrhea
3. Hemorrhoids
4. Urinary frequency

20. The nurse is assisting the health care provider with a Pap test. What condition will be diagnosed by this diagnostic study?
1. Cervical cancer
2. Breast cancer
3. Pelvic inflammatory disease
4. Ovarian cancer

21. A patient has reported to the emergency department. The health care provider suspects toxic shock syndrome. What manifestations confirm this suspicion? *(Select all that apply.)*
1. Sudden high fever
2. Vaginal hemorrhage
3. Diarrhea
4. Sudden hypertension
5. Headache

22. Lower abdominal and lower back pain that increases in severity during menstruation may signal which condition?
1. Cervical polyp
2. Ovarian tumor
3. Endometriosis
4. Uterine cancer

23. The nurse is reviewing the health history of an assigned patient. The patient was treated for pelvic inflammatory disease. What conditions may be noted in the patient's history as a result of the condition? *(Select all that apply.)*
1. Vaginal discharge
2. Infertility
3. Hemorrhage
4. Dyspareunia
5. Dysmenorrhea

24. Which woman is most likely to develop toxic shock syndrome?
1. The woman with multiple sexual contacts
2. The woman who inserts tampons with her fingers
3. The woman with untreated chronic PID
4. The woman who has undergone multiple abortions

25. A patient is scheduled to have a Pap smear. The nurse can provide correct information about preparing for the examination by including what information?
1. Use a mild vinegar douche the night before the test.
2. Abstain from intercourse 24 hours before the test.
3. Take a warm tub bath the night before the test.
4. Save a first-voided morning urine specimen.

26. A patient's husband tells the nurse that his wife, who has been diagnosed with inoperable ovarian cancer, is talking about dying and her fear of death. He asks the nurse for suggestions to help his wife. Which response by the nurse would be most helpful?
1. "Your wife will probably die of another disease before she dies of ovarian cancer."
2. "Talk of death is normal at this time, but will diminish in the future."
3. "Your wife is expressing acceptance of the need for hospice care."
4. "It is perfectly normal to want to talk about death. It is most helpful to support her by listening."

Care of the Patient With a Sensory Disorder

53

http://evolve.elsevier.com/Cooper/foundationsadult/

Objectives

Anatomy and Physiology

1. Describe structures and functions of the visual and auditory systems.
2. Explain normal vision and hearing physiologic processes.
3. Differentiate between abnormal and normal physical assessments of the visual and auditory systems.

Medical-Surgical

4. Describe two age-related changes and assessment findings in the visual and auditory systems.
5. Discuss the refractory errors of astigmatism, strabismus, myopia, and hyperopia, including etiology, pathophysiology, clinical manifestations, assessment, diagnostic tests, medical management, nursing interventions, and patient teaching.
6. Describe inflammatory conditions of the eye, including etiology, pathophysiology, clinical manifestations, assessment, diagnostic tests, medical management, nursing interventions, patient teaching, and prognoses.
7. Discuss Sjögren syndrome, ectropion, and entropion, including etiology, pathophysiology, clinical manifestations, diagnostic tests, medical management, nursing interventions, and prognosis.
8. Compare and contrast the nature of cataracts, diabetic retinopathy, macular degeneration, retinal detachment, and glaucoma, including the etiology, pathophysiology, clinical manifestations, assessment, diagnostic tests, medical management, nursing interventions, patient teaching, and prognoses.
9. Discuss corneal injuries, including etiology, pathophysiology, clinical manifestations, assessment, diagnostic tests, medical management, nursing interventions, patient teaching, and prognoses.
10. Describe the various surgeries of the eye, including the nursing interventions and prognoses.
11. Differentiate between conductive and sensorineural hearing loss.
12. Describe the appropriate care of the hearing aid.
13. List tips for communicating with people with visual and hearing impairments.
14. Identify communication resources for people with visual and/or hearing impairment.
15. Describe inflammatory and infectious and noninfectious disorders of the ear, including etiology, pathophysiology, clinical manifestations, assessment, diagnostic tests, medical management, nursing interventions, patient teaching, and prognoses.
16. Describe the various surgeries of the ear, including the nursing interventions, patient teaching, and prognoses.

Key Terms

astigmatism (ă-STĬG-mă-tĭsm, p. 1822)
audiometry (ăw-dē-ŎM-ĕ-trē, p. 1845)
automated perimetry test (ĂW-tō-māt-ĕd pĕr-Ĭ-mĕt-rē, p. 1819)
cataract (KĂT-ă-răkt, p. 1828)
conjunctivitis (kŏn-jŭnk-tĭ-VĪ-tĭs, p. 1825)
cryotherapy (krī-ō-THĔR-ă-pē, p. 1832)
diabetic retinopathy (dī-ă-BĔT-ĭk rĕ-tĭn-NŎP-ă-thē, p. 1831)
enucleation (ē-nū-klē-Ā-shŭn, p. 1841)
glaucoma (glăw-KŌ-mă, p. 1835)
Goldmann tonometry (GŌLD-măn tōn-Ŏ-mĕt-rē, p. 1819)
hyperopia (hī-pĕr-Ō-pē-ă, p. 1822)
keratitis (kĕr-ă-TĪ-tĭs, p. 1826)
keratoplasty (kĕr-ă-tŏ-PLĂS-tē, p. 1841)
keratotomy (kĕ-ră-TŎT-ŏ-mē, p. 1823)
labyrinthitis (lăb-ĭ-rĭnth-Ī-tĭs, p. 1852)
mastoiditis (măs-tŏy-DĪ-tĭs, p. 1851)
miotics (mī-ŎT-ĭks, p. 1836)
mydriatics (mĭd-rē-ĂT-ĭks, p. 1819)
myopia (mī-Ō-pē-ă, p. 1822)
myringotomy (mĭr-ĭn-GŎT-ŏ-mē, p. 1850)
photocoagulation (fō-tō-kō-ăg-yū-LĀ-shŭn, p. 1832)
refraction (rē-FRĂK-shŭn, p. 1819)
retinal detachment (RĔ-tĭ-năl dē-TĂCH-mĕnt, p. 1833)
Sjögren syndrome (SHĔR-grĕn SĪN-drōm, p. 1827)
Snellen test (SNĔL-ĕn tĕst, p. 1819)
stapedectomy (stā-pĕ-DĔK-tŏ-mē, p. 1856)
strabismus (stră-BĬZ-mŭs, p. 1822)
tinnitus (TĬ-nĭ-tĭs, p. 1850)
tympanoplasty (tĭm-pă-nō-PLĂS-tē, p. 1857)
umami (p. 1858)
vertigo (VĔR-tĭ-gō, p. 1846)
vitrectomy (vĭ-TRĔK-tŏ-mē, p. 1842)

ANATOMIC STRUCTURES AND PHYSIOLOGIC FUNCTIONS OF THE VISUAL SYSTEM

ANATOMY OF THE EYE

The primary sensory system of the human body is the visual system. The visual system consists of highly sensitive tissues and structures that surround the eye and the many layered tunics of the globe (eyeball) that protect and control the refractory media and visual pathways. The eyes are 1-inch (2.5 cm) spherical structures that contain 70% of the sensory receptors of the body. The optic tracts contain more than 1 million nerve fibers that carry messages from the eyes to the brain, where they are interpreted. Only a small portion of each eye is visible externally; the remainder is enclosed in the *orbit*. The orbits consist of orbital bones of the face and cushioned in layers of fat. The orbital bones include the frontal, zygomatic, ethmoid, sphenoid, and lacrimal.

STRUCTURE OF THE EYE

External Structures of the Eye

The external structures of the eye include the eyebrows, eyelashes, lids, and the lacrimal apparatus. The primary function of the external structures is of a protective capacity. In addition to protection, three pairs of extraocular muscles control each eye. The extraocular paired muscles consist of (1) superior and inferior rectus muscles, (2) medial and lateral rectus muscles, and (3) superior and inferior oblique muscles. The extraocular muscles control eye movement via cranial nerves III (ocular nerve), IV (trochlear nerve), and VI (abducens nerve).

The *lacrimal apparatus* (Fig. 53.1) manufactures and drains tears to keep the eye moist and to sweep away debris that may enter the eye. Tears are composed of a watery secretion that contains salt, mucus, and a bactericidal enzyme, *lysozyme*. The lacrimal glands are located superior and lateral to each eye. Blinking causes tears to flow medially to the lacrimal ducts, which empty into the nasolacrimal ducts and drain into the nasal cavity.

The *conjunctiva* is a thin, transparent mucous membrane that lines the inner aspect of the eyelids and the anterior surface of the eye to the edge of the cornea. The lower conjunctival sac is where eyedrops and eye ointment medication usually are administered.

Internal Structures of the Eye

The eye is composed of three layers, or tunics (Fig. 53.2). The outermost layer of the eye is the fibrous tunic; it is composed of the sclera and the cornea. The *sclera* is a thick, white, opaque structure composed of collagen fibers meshed together and is known as the white of the eye. The sclera gives shape to the eye and, because of its toughness, protects the intraocular structures.

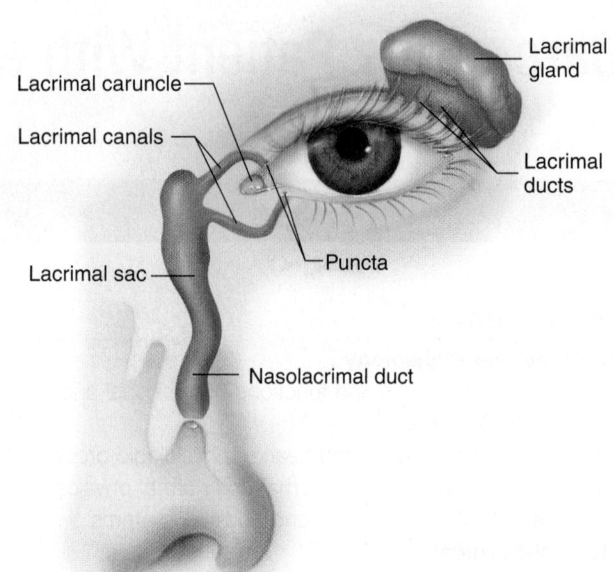

Fig. 53.1 Lacrimal apparatus. (From Patton KT, Thibodeau GA: *Anatomy and physiology*, ed 10, St. Louis, 2019, Elsevier.)

The *cornea* is the central anterior portion of the sclera. It is a transparent clear layer that covers the iris, which is the colored portion of the eye. The cornea allows light rays to enter the inner portion of the eye and is the first part of the eye that refracts (bends) light rays. The cornea is a dense layer that is uniform in thickness, nonvascular, and projects like a dome beyond the sclera. The cornea is one of the most highly developed, sensitive tissues in the body and is innervated by cranial nerve V (trigeminal nerve). The avascular cornea obtains oxygen primarily through absorption from the tear film layer that bathes the epithelium. A small amount of oxygen is obtained from the *aqueous humor* (watery fluid in front of the lens in the anterior chamber of the eye) through the endothelial layers. The degree of corneal curvature varies in each individual and progressively changes as the patient ages. The curvature is more pronounced in youth and changes to a more flattened curve in advancing age.

The junction of the sclera and cornea is called the *canal of Schlemm*. This tiny venous sinus, at the angle of the anterior chamber of the eye, drains the aqueous humor and funnels it into the bloodstream. This helps control intraocular pressure (IOP, the pressure within the eye).

The middle layer of the eye is the *vascular tunic*. It includes the choroid, the ciliary body, and the iris. The posterior portion of the vascular tunic is the *choroid*, which is a thin, dark brown membrane that lines most of the internal area of the sclera. It is extremely vascular and supplies nutrients to the retina. The anterior portion of the vascular tunic forms the ciliary body, which is an intrinsic muscular ring that holds the lens in place and changes its shape for near or distant vision. The

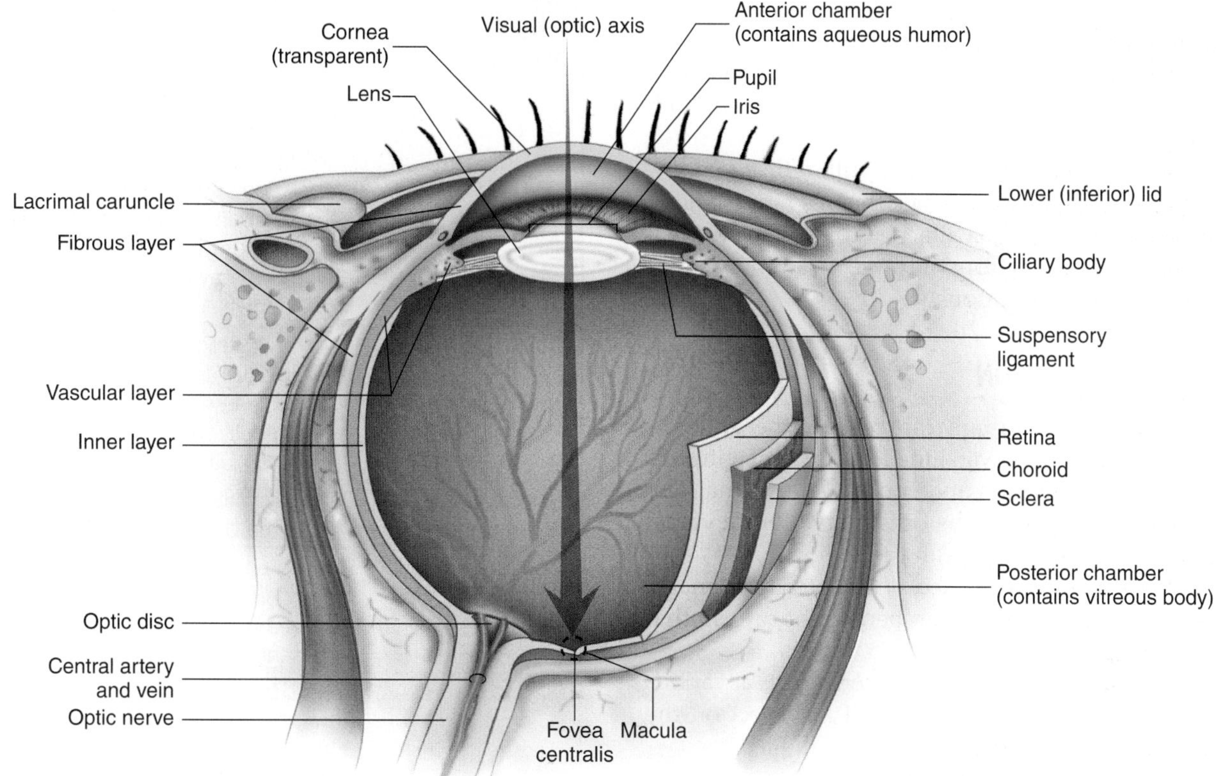

Fig. 53.2 Horizontal section through the eyeball. The eye is viewed from above. (From Patton KT, Thibodeau GA: *Anatomy and physiology*, ed 10, St. Louis, 2019, Elsevier.)

ciliary body also attaches to the *iris,* which is the pigmented part of the eye. The iris is a flat muscular ring located between the cornea and the lens and contains a round opening in the center, which is known as the *pupil.* The muscular ring of the iris surrounds the pupil to constrict and dilate according to light levels, much like a camera shutter. In darker light, the pupil dilates open to allow an increase of light to enter, and in brighter light the pupil constricts and becomes smaller to allow less light into the eye. Two sets of smooth muscles control the iris, which in turn controls the size of the pupil. In bright light, the circular muscle fibers of the iris contract and the pupil constricts; in dim light, the radial muscles contract and the pupil dilates. Pupillary constriction is a reflex that protects the retina from intense light and permits clearer, acute near vision.

The innermost tunic of the eye is the *retina.* The retina comprises nervous tissue membranes that receive images of external objects and transmits impulses through the optic nerve to the brain. The rods and cones are scattered throughout the retina except where the optic nerve exits the eye. The area where the retinal nerve fibers collect to form the optic nerve is known as the *optic disc;* this area is also called the *blind spot,* because of its lack of photoreceptors. Rods are receptors for vision in dim light and are unable to perceive color. The rods are located primarily in the periphery of the retina and are responsible for peripheral vision. Cones, which are located more centrally in the retina, require bright light to perceive color. The cones are divided into three types, which are each sensitive to a different color: red, green, or blue. Rod and cone cells respond to light by way of photopsin, a photosensitive pigment, at their tips. The body requires vitamin A to synthesize photopsin.

Located in the center of the retina is the *fovea centralis,* a pinpoint depression composed only of densely packed cone cells. The fovea centralis contains the greatest concentration of cones of any area in the retina. This area of the retina provides the sharpest visual acuity and most acute color vision. Surrounding the fovea is the *macula,* an area of less than 1 mm^2 that has a high concentration of cones and is relatively free of blood vessels. The absence of the three types of cones causes color blindness, which is an inherited condition found primarily in males.

CHAMBERS OF THE EYE

The eye is divided into anterior and posterior chambers by the *crystalline lens,* a transparent, colorless structure that is biconvex, enclosed in a capsule, and held in place just behind the pupil by the suspensory ligament. The crystalline lens focuses light rays so that they form a perfect image on the retina. Anterior to the crystalline lens is the anterior chamber, which is filled with *aqueous humor,* a clear, watery fluid similar to blood plasma.

The ciliary bodies of the choroid constantly secrete, drain, and replace aqueous humor to maintain normal intraocular pressure. Aqueous humor also helps maintain the eye's shape, keeps the retina attached to the choroid, and refracts light.

The posterior chamber is filled with *vitreous humor*, a transparent, jellylike substance that also gives shape to the eye, keeps the retina attached to the choroid, and refracts light. It differs from the aqueous humor in that it is not replaced continuously.

PHYSIOLOGY OF VISION

Light must travel through the cornea, the aqueous humor, the pupil, the crystalline lens, and the vitreous humor to reach the rods and cones of the retina. The image is transported via the optic nerve to the visual center of the cerebral cortex in the brain.

Four basic processes are necessary to form an image:

1. *Refraction:* The eye is able to bend light rays so that the rays fall onto the retina.
2. *Accommodation:* The eye can focus on objects at various distances. It focuses the image of an object on the retina by changing the curvature of the lens.
3. *Constriction:* The size of the pupil, which is controlled by the dilator and constrictor muscles of the iris, regulates the amount of light entering the eye.
4. *Convergence:* Medial movement of both eyes allows light rays from an object to hit the same point on both retinas.

NURSING CONSIDERATIONS FOR CARE OF THE PATIENT WITH COMMON EYE COMPLICATIONS

In caring for the patient with an eye disorder, review the following items:

- Eye pain, pruritus, photophobia, excessive tearing, dryness, floaters (dark to semitransparent spots in the visual field), light flashes, scotomas (diminished vision in a defined area of the visual field), halos around lights, diplopia (double vision), discharge, visual changes such as depth perception and peripheral vision changes, blind spots, or fading color vision
- Headaches
- Nystagmus (involuntary, rhythmic movements of the eyes)
- History of allergies
- Current medications, over the counter and prescription
- Side effects of any medications
- Use of visual assistive devices (glasses, contact lenses, or magnifying glasses)
- Adequacy of current eyewear prescription
- Personal habits related to care of eyewear
- Any previous eye injuries or surgeries

After gathering the information and reporting it to the health care provider, provide assistance with the eye examination. The results of the initial examination are compared with normal findings (Table 53.1).

Table 53.1 Normal Findings of the Adult Eye

AREA EXAMINED	FINDINGS
Eyelid	Blink reflex to light or touch intact. Lid margins just above the corneal borders
Eyeball	Eyeball does not protrude beyond the supraorbital ridge of the frontal bone. The eyeball is usually moist; moisture may be diminished in the older adult
Conjunctiva	Palpebral (eyelid): Pink, uniform blood vessels without discharge Bulbar: Clear, tiny red vessels; in the older adult, the bulbar conjunctiva may lose luster
Sclera	Generally white; may have yellow-tan dots in a dark-skinned individual
Cornea	Transparent, smooth, convex. In the older adult, a gray ring around the cornea (arcus senilis) may be present as a result of lipid deposits
Iris	Round, intact, bilateral coloration. In the older adult, color may be paler and shape less regular
Pupil	Equal, round, reactive to light and accommodation. Response to light is equal bilaterally. In the older adult, constriction response may be slower
Internal eye (including retina, vessels, and optic disc)	Retina is intact. Vessel structure is intact and bilaterally similar in pattern. Optic disc has well-defined border
Visual Acuity	
Distant vision	20/20 (able to read line 11 of eye chart at a distance of 20 ft)
Near vision	Able to read newspaper print at 14 inches
Peripheral vision	Side vision 90 degrees from central visual axis; upward 50 degrees; downward 70 degrees
Eye movement	Coordinated eye movement bilaterally
Color perception	Able to properly identify colors of major groups: red, blue, and green

LABORATORY AND DIAGNOSTIC EXAMINATIONS

After the review of the medical history and any complaints, an initial eye examination is performed. The goals of the examination are to evaluate visual acuity, visual fields, refraction, peripheral vision, and overall health of the eye and supportive structures. Additional diagnostic testing may be performed to assess for disorders or to determine progression of disease.

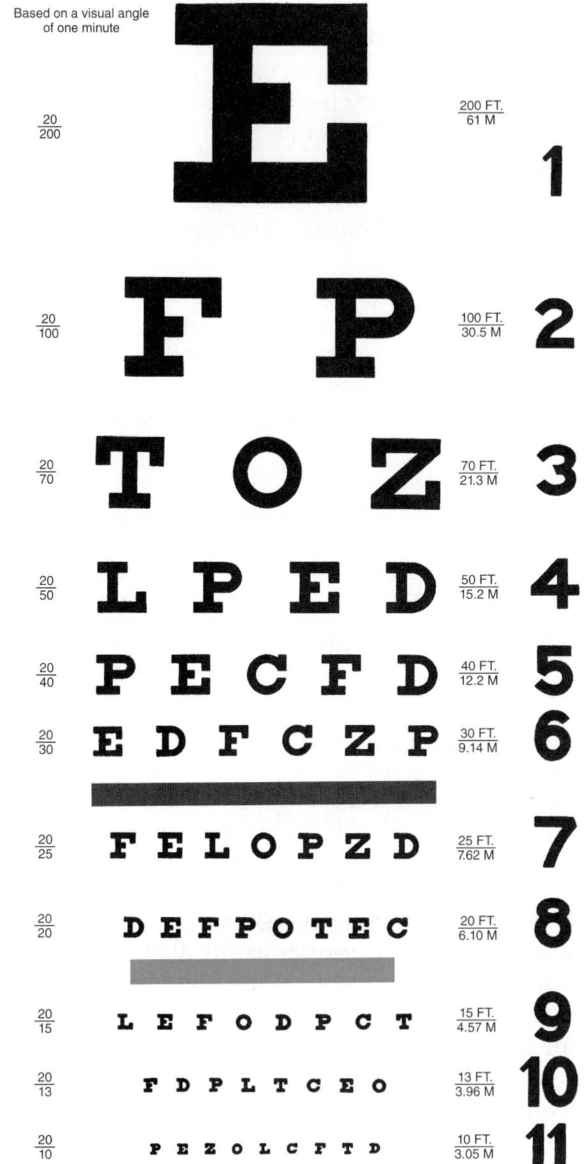

Fig. 53.3 Snellen chart. (From Patton KT, Thibodeau GA: *Laboratory manual for anatomy and physiology*, ed 10, St. Louis, 2019, Elsevier.)

The most commonly performed examination is the **Snellen test,** which assesses visual acuity. The patient is placed 20 feet from the Snellen chart and asked to read lines (Fig. 53.3). The degree of vision is evaluated and the patient's acuity is assigned. Vision said to be 20/20 indicates that the individual has normal vision and can read at 20 feet the prescribed line. Vision identified as 20/40 indicates the patient can read at 40 feet what the normal eye can see at 20 feet. The chart is modified for children by using shapes or pictures.

Refraction refers to the bending of light rays as they enter the retina. An inability of the eye to accommodate the images seen is known as refractive errors. Refractive errors are diagnosed by asking the patient to sit with his or her chin resting on a supportive bar and looking into a device. The patient then is asked to read a chart 20 feet away, using a variety of lenses. As the lenses are changed, the patient is asked to evaluate the clarity of the information viewed. The result will determine the degree of visual acuity. Potential diagnoses of visual disorders include hyperopia, myopia, astigmatism, and presbyopia (Table 53.2).

Visual field assessment is key in the evaluation of vision. There are six visual fields. The examination identifies the loss or deterioration of any field. Sitting straight in front of the patient, the examiner reviews the patient's ability to see items as they are moved into the field of vision. The **automated perimetry test** places the patient in front of a computer-like device and asks him or her to stare at a screen and to press a button when flashes of light enter the field of vision (National Library of Medicine, 2013a).

The Amsler grid assesses for disturbances in central vision. It is used to evaluate the health of the macula, identifying conditions such as macular degeneration. Black grid markings are superimposed on a white background. A centralized black dot is used as the point of reference. The patient is asked to view the grid, concentrating on the dot, and report areas of distortion (Fig. 53.4).

The *slit lamp examination* uses magnification devices to view the eyelids, sclera, iris, conjunctiva, and cornea (National Library of Medicine, 2013b). A slit lamp also can help evaluate intraocular pressure by tonometry to detect glaucoma. Dilating drops (**mydriatics**) may be used to evaluate internal surfaces and will cause photosensitivity for a few hours after the examination. Conditions that may be diagnosed by this technique include cataracts, corneal injury, macular degeneration, and disorders of the retina, including detachment, vessel occlusion, and retinitis pigmentosa.

Retinal blood flow may be evaluated by *fluorescein angiography.* Dye is injected into vessels of the arm or hand. This is an invasive procedure requiring the patient's consent. The patient should be instructed that urine could be darkened or possibly orange for a few days after the test. Assess for allergies to seafood or iodine because this also may cause sensitivity to the dye used in the examination. Conditions that may be diagnosed by this test include retinal detachment, retinopathy, tumors, and macular degeneration (National Library of Medicine, 2018).

Today the measurement of intraocular pressure *(tonometry)* is done most commonly by puffing air onto the surface of the open eye (National Library of Medicine, 2012). The eye pressure is measured by evaluating how the light reflections change as the air hits the eye (Fig. 53.5). A more invasive study is **Goldmann tonometry,** in which the eye is numbed and a cone-shaped device is used to depress the eyeball gently to assess for internal pressure.

Table 53.2 Common Refractory Errors

DESCRIPTION	ETIOLOGY AND PATHOPHYSIOLOGY	CLINICAL MANIFESTATIONS
Astigmatism: Defect in the curvature of the eyeball surface	May be hereditary or a muscular deficit Occurs when light rays cannot be focused clearly on a point on the retina because of an abnormal curvature of the cornea	Blurring of vision Difficulty focusing Complaints of eye discomfort
Esotropia: A form of strabismus in which one or both eyes turn in the direction of the nose	The eyes are unable to simultaneously fix on an object	Difficulty following objects visually
Exotropia: A form of strabismus in which one or both eyes turn outward, away from the nose		Only one eye focuses or is able to track a moving object
Hyperopia: Condition of farsightedness	May result from error of refraction in which rays of light entering the eye are brought into focus behind the retina	Inability to see objects at close range
Myopia: Condition of nearsightedness	Elongation of the eyeball or an error in refraction so that parallel rays are focused in front of the retina	Inability to see objects at a distance
Strabismus: Inability of the eyes to focus in the same direction; commonly referred to as being *cross-eyed*	May result from neurologic or muscular dysfunction, or may be inherited	The positions of the eyeballs are not symmetric

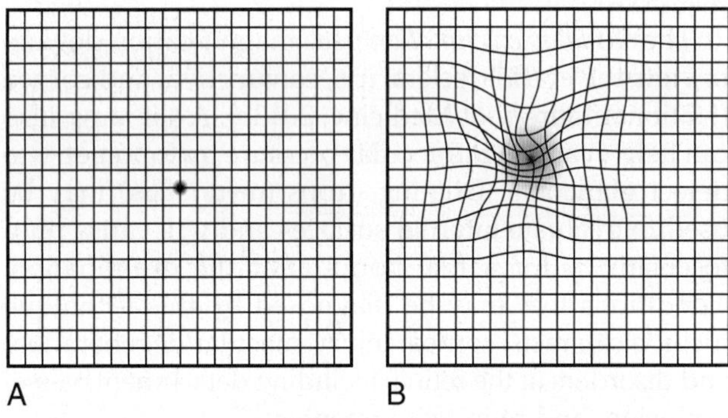

Fig. 53.4 Amsler grid. (From Miller RG, Ashar BH, Sisson SD: *The Johns Hopkins internal medicine board review: 2010–2011,* ed 3, Philadelphia, 2010, Mosby.)

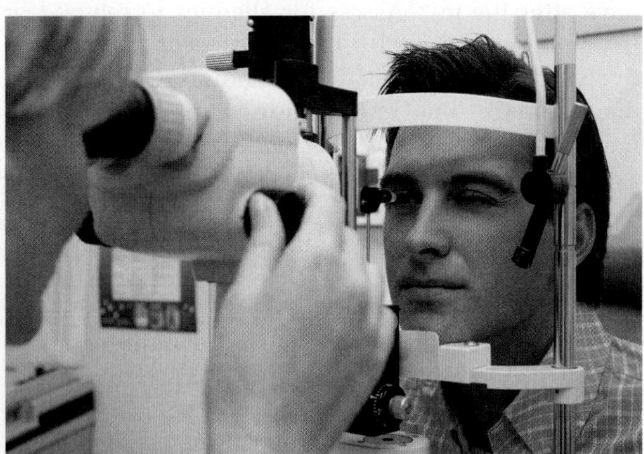

Fig. 53.5 Measurement of internal eye pressure by tonometry (Copyright 1999–2012 Thinkstock. All rights reserved.)

DISORDERS OF THE EYE

BLINDNESS AND NEAR BLINDNESS

Etiology and Pathophysiology

Blindness is a loss of visual acuity that ranges from partial to total loss of sight. Total blindness is defined as no light perception and no usable vision. Functional blindness is present when the patient has some light perception but no usable vision. It may be congenital or acquired.

The Centers for Disease Control and Prevention estimates that in the United States approximately 3.4 million people are blind or visually impaired (Centers for Disease Control and Prevention, 2009). The estimates for patients with visual problems and potentially blinding diseases range from 21 to 80 million people in the United States. *Legal blindness* refers to individuals with a maximum visual acuity of 20/200 with corrective eyewear and/or visual field sight capacity reduced to 20 degrees (the normal visual field range is 180 degrees).

Categories have been established to help determine the exact extent of vision loss and what assistive measures are appropriate for the individual. These categories range from low vision loss (20/70 to 20/200) to three categories of blindness (20/400, 20/1200, and no light perception).

Congenital blindness results from various birth defects. Acquired blindness in adults occurs as a result of disorders such as diabetic retinopathy, glaucoma, cataracts, retinal degeneration, infections, tumors, and acute trauma.

Clinical Manifestations

The degree of vision loss depends on the extent of trauma or disease. Symptoms may include diplopia (double vision), blurred vision, pain, and presence of floaters or flashes of light in the visual field, light sensitivity, and burning of the eyes. Additional physical manifestations of the visually impaired patient may include loss of peripheral vision; halos (described as rainbow colors seen around lights); a sense of increased orbital pressure; bulging of the eye(s); and any difference in the appearance of an eye structure, such as the pupil.

The wide variety of emotions associated with blindness range from fear, anxiety, disorientation, depression, helplessness, and hopelessness to acceptance. The patient may experience poor interpersonal communication skills and coping mechanisms. Because self-care skills may be impaired, an individual who is blind may prefer isolation, causing additional physical and emotional difficulties.

Assessment

Subjective data may include patient reports of blurred vision, diplopia, loss of visual fields, halos, or increased pressure as early symptoms of eye disorders. It is important for the health care provider to determine the onset, severity, and duration of symptoms or pain, as well as any factors that relieve them.

Objective data may include a functional vision assessment (FVA). According to the American Foundation for the Blind (2018), an FVA investigates visual functionality for near task (closer than 16 inches [0.4 m]), intermediate task (16 inches to 3 feet [0.4 to 0.9 m]), and then a distance task (more than 3 feet). The assessment also includes visual acuity, visual field, contrast sensitivity and color vision. It is also important to note the patient's compensation measures, such as use of a magnifying glass, as well as the effectiveness of the patient's current use of assistive eyewear.

Medical Management

Corrective eyewear is the first method of medical management for a partially sighted patient. If the visual defect results from an inflammatory disorder, medication appropriate to the causative agent is prescribed.

Additional assistive devices for a visually impaired patient include canes, guide dogs, magnifying systems, computers, and telescopic lenses. An eye specialist should evaluate the patient to determine which devices are best suited for the level of vision loss. Some of the more technologically complex devices are expensive and may not be covered by insurance.

Canes are the most frequently used devices for the partially or totally blind person. They are lightweight and portable and allow the patient simple maneuvering. The drawback is that canes usually do not help in detecting overhead objects. Guide dogs can be helpful in this respect; they allow the person who is visually impaired increased mobility that otherwise would be difficult to achieve independently. Trained guide dogs steer the patient away from obstacles and assist the patient to move through crowds. The guide dog is trained to detect curbs, stairs, and elevations that may cause the patient to fall or stumble.

The patient requires instruction on ambulatory safety before using ambulatory aids or assistants. Advise the patient to walk slowly; obtain verbal clues from the walking companion, if present; and touch objects or borders with the tip of the cane to determine the boundaries of obstructions. The walking companion should precede the patient by about 1 foot, with the patient's hand on the companion's elbow for security (Fig. 53.6). Describe the surroundings when assisting the patient with visual impairment in new surroundings.

Surgical correction of the visual defect may provide improved eyesight. Laser surgeries provide excellent results in selected cases. Corneal transplants can restore vision in patients with corneal damage.

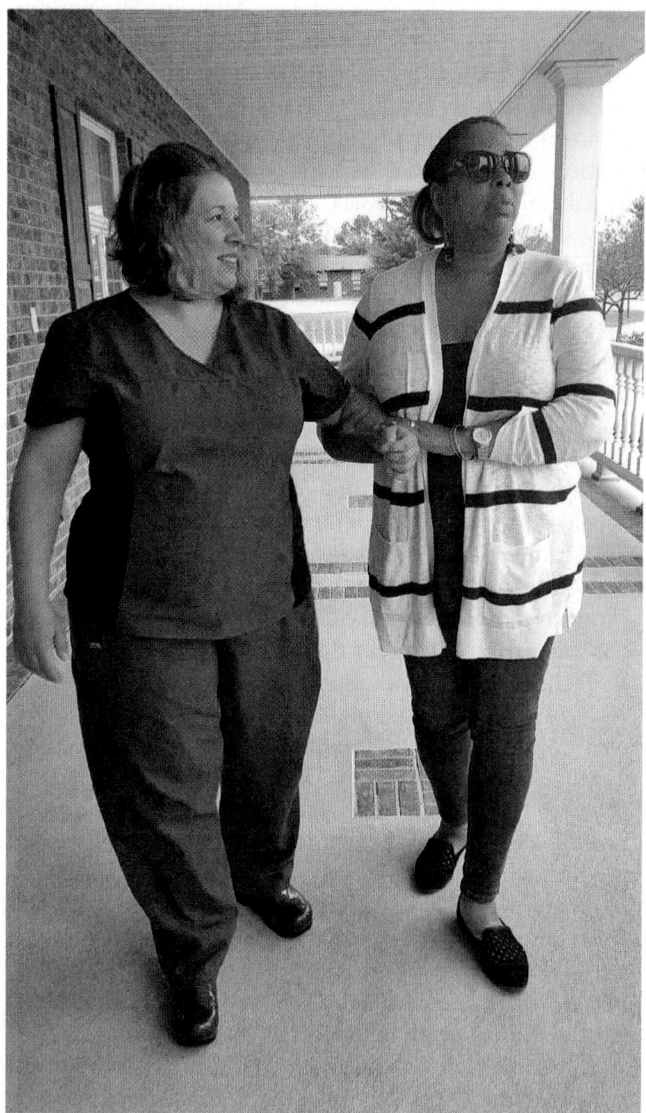

Fig. 53.6 Sighted-guide technique. The walking companion serves as the sighted guide, walking slightly ahead of the patient with the patient holding the back of the companion's arm.

Box 53.1 Guidelines for Communicating With People Who Are Visually Impaired

- Announce your presence when entering the room.
- Talk in a normal tone of voice.
- Do not try to avoid common phrases in speech, such as "See what I mean?"
- Introduce yourself with each contact (unless well known to the person).
- Explain any activity occurring in the room.
- Announce when you are leaving the room so that the blind person is not put in the position of talking to someone who is no longer there.

Nursing Interventions and Patient Teaching

Understand that the complications of loss of vision or blindness could result in physical and emotional manifestations by the patient. Assess the patient's ability to perform self-care and provide assistance with activities of daily living (ADLs) as needed. Allowing the patient adequate time to assist in self-care helps foster independence and promotes the confidence of the patient to perform daily activities. Nursing interventions for patients with visual impairments must include consideration of emotional aspects, including appropriate communication (Box 53.1).

Vision loss affects not only the patient but also family, friends, and the community. Individuals have different coping mechanisms; consider this when caring for the visually impaired patient. Be aware of the services and devices available for the patient with a visual impairment and make appropriate referrals. Over time, with treatment and rehabilitation, the patient with visual impairment can develop the skills necessary to become independent in daily life. The primary resource for services for the patient who is legally blind is the local government; each state has a department for rehabilitation of the blind. The American Foundation for the Blind (www.afb.org) also lists agencies to assist and educate the patient with visual impairment.

Technological advances such as computers with voice recognition enable the patient to read, use the Internet, and communicate with others. Optical scanners can capture images and, by recognizing the written text, convert the images into identifiable characters and words. These then are recorded and played back, using a voice synthesizer. The information also can be saved as printed braille. Braille allows the patient to read, function effectively in the environment with signage, and enjoy an improved quality of living. Braille writers use advanced touch keyboards to record data for the production of written materials for the blind. Braille readers provide technology that allows for use of mobile phones and talking clocks (Chin, n.d.). Using a guide dog and a cane facilitates further independence. The nurse is responsible for patient education, providing assistance, counseling, and preventing complications for the patient with visual impairment. A comprehensive approach to care can help the patient with visual impairment successfully adjust to home, work, and society.

Patient problems and interventions for the patient with visual impairment include but are not limited to the following:

Patient Problem	Nursing Interventions
Fearfulness, related to visual loss or impairment	Determine the patient's level of fear Actively listen to the patient's concerns/fears and assist with addressing the issues with the appropriate resources
Potential for Injury, related to new/unfamiliar environment	Orient the patient to the new environment Use therapeutic touch Avoid loud sounds that may startle the patient Use protective and assistive devices, such as side rails and canes Alter surroundings to create a safe environment (e.g., clear walkways, remove throw rugs)

REFRACTORY ERRORS

An abnormally shaped eye and/or cornea may lead to refractive errors. These disorders result in blurred images because the eye is unable to bend the light from objects as they are viewed. Errors of refraction are treated with corrective lenses or by surgical intervention. Refractory errors can be progressive, requiring changes in the prescription for correction (see Table 53.2).

Common refractory errors (**astigmatism, strabismus, myopia**, and **hyperopia**) are described in Table 53.2.

MYOPIA

See Table 53.2.

Diagnostic Tests

Diagnosis of myopia commonly follows a visit to the health care practitioner because of the patient's inability to see distant objects clearly. After routine examinations by an optometrist the patient is assessed for corrective lenses or corrective refractory surgery.

Medical Management

The majority of patients are prescribed corrective eyeglasses or contact lenses. Patients who are unable or unwilling to wear corrective eyewear for occupational or cosmetic reasons may elect to seek surgical correction.

Surgical Management

Refractory surgery, such as reshaping the corneal curvature, is effective in treating the underlying complications causing visual problems. Myopia is the refractive error most commonly corrected by laser surgery. Patients are selected on the basis of the degree of myopia; the shape of the cornea; and the absence of medical conditions such as severe diabetes, glaucoma, or pregnancy. The usual age for correction is between 20 and 60 years. Radial keratotomy (RK), photorefractive keratectomy (PRK), laser-assisted in situ keratomileusis (LASIK), laser thermal keratoplasty (LTK), and conductive keratoplasty (CK) surgeries are procedures used to correct myopia and markedly improve vision.

Radial **keratotomy** (RK) is a technique in which the surgeon makes partial-thickness radial incisions in the patient's cornea, leaving an uncut optical zone in the center. The patient must evaluate the risk of serious complications, such as operative infection and corneal scarring, when considering this procedure.

Photorefractive keratectomy (PRK) involves the use of an excimer laser (a type of ultraviolet laser) to reshape the central corneal surface. It is used primarily to correct myopia but also is used for hyperopia and astigmatism. Evidence suggests that final visual acuity with this procedure is more predictable than with radial keratotomy, at least in the short term.

Laser-assisted in situ keratomileusis (LASIK) is a procedure in which first a corneal flap is folded back and then an excimer laser removes some of the internal layers of the cornea. Afterward, the flap is returned to its normal position and allowed to heal in place. Evidence supports claims that LASIK creates earlier visual stability in patients with a high degree of myopia than with PRK. Unlike RK, PRK and LASIK procedures affect the central zone of the cornea (Lewis et al, 2007).

Intracorneal implants, known as Intacs, are microthin rings implanted through incisions in the side of the cornea (Fig. 53.7). The corneal rings reshape the curvature of the cornea to improve visual acuity. Intacs are used for the patient who has keratoconus, a progressive disease in which the cornea thins. The Intac rings can be removed if necessary, and the effects on refractive error then are reversed completely (US Food and Drug Administration, 2012).

Nursing Interventions and Patient Teaching

The patient undergoing corrective surgery will leave the hospital or clinic shortly after surgery. An eye patch is placed on the operative site until the next morning. The patient can be up and around at home, but because of visual limitations he or she may need some assistance.

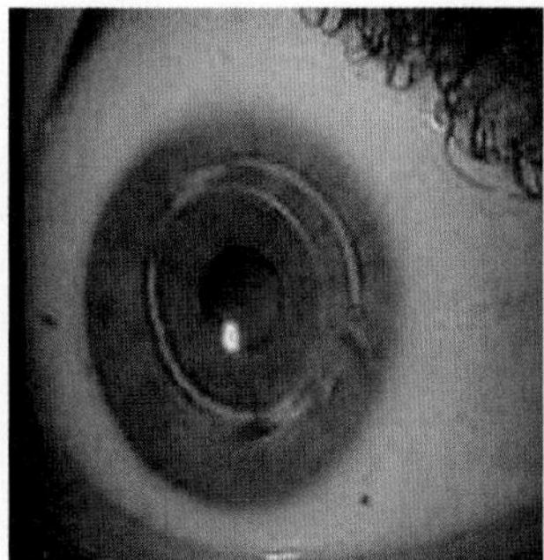
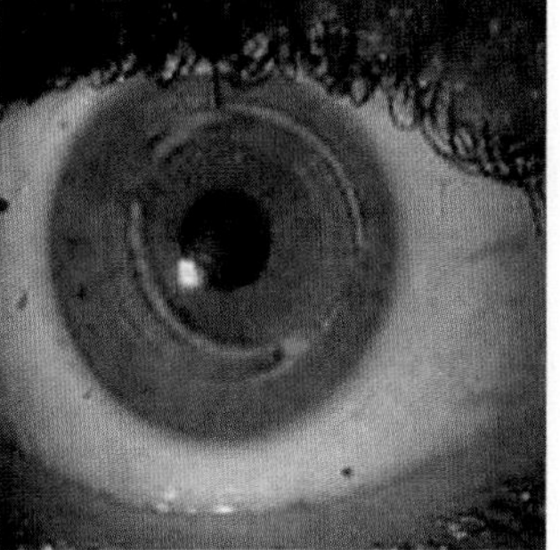

Fig. 53.7 Intacs. (From Kymionis GD, Siganos CS, Tsiklis NS, et al: Long-term follow-up of Intacs in keratoconus. *Am J Ophthalmol* 2007;143:236–244.)

The patient may be photosensitive and complain of blurred vision initially, but his or her vision should improve quickly. The health care provider will schedule the patient for a follow-up examination the day after the surgery. Postoperative visual checkups are scheduled at 1 week and then monthly for 6 months. Patient problems and interventions for the patient with myopia are the same as for astigmatism and strabismus errors.

Instruct the patient preoperatively to stop wearing contact lenses 1 to 2 weeks before the surgical evaluation; contacts change the shape of the cornea and may alter the evaluation. Encourage rest the first day postoperatively. Inform the patient to notify the health care professional if pain persists after the first day of surgery. Educate the patient about the complications and symptoms that could occur postoperatively, including dry eyes, pain, photophobia, burning, itching, and infection. Inform the patient of the evaluation schedule for testing their functional vision in the postoperative period. Advise patients that postoperative visual acuity is not always 20/20 without glasses. The goals of operative interventions are to improve visual acuity. As a result of a slightly dilated pupil, the patient may experience a glare or halos from lights, which may require wearing glasses for night driving.

HYPEROPIA

Hyperopia is described in Table 53.2.

Diagnostic Tests

Common tests used in the diagnosis of hyperopia include ophthalmoscopy, retinoscopy, visual acuity tests, and refraction tests.

Medical Management

The primary treatment for farsightedness is corrective eyewear, either contact lenses or glasses. Some individuals may choose to self-treat these changes with over-the-counter eye wear until visual changes necessitate consultation with the eye care professional.

Nursing Interventions and Patient Teaching

Emphasize the importance of proper care of contact lenses (see the Health Promotion box). Eyeglasses should properly fit the bridge of the nose to eliminate slippage and an uneven level of each lens.

A patient problem and interventions for the patient with hyperopia include but are not limited to the following:

Patient Problem	Nursing Interventions
Insufficient Knowledge, related to lack of experience with corrective eyewear	Answer all questions the patient may have regarding eyewear maintenance Obtain literature on lens care Encourage follow up with the eye health care provider as directed

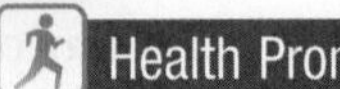

Health Promotion

Contact Lens Care

DO

- Wash and rinse hands thoroughly before handling contact lenses.
- Keep fingernails short and clean.
- Remove lenses from their storage case one at a time and place on the eye.
- Use the lens placement technique learned from eye care specialist.
- Use proper lens care products and clean the lenses as directed by the manufacturer. If using daily wear contacts, dispose of on a daily basis.
- Keep the lens storage kit clean.
- Wear lenses daily and follow the prescribed wearing schedule.
- Remove a lens if it becomes uncomfortable.
- Dispose of lenses if an eye infection occurs.
- Avoid potential corneal abrasions.
- Report any signs of photophobia, dryness, excessive burning, or tearing.
- Keep regular appointments with the eye care specialist.

DO NOT

- Use soaps that contain cream or perfume for cleansing lenses.
- Let fingernails touch lenses.
- Mix up lenses.
- Exceed prescribed wearing time.
- Use saliva to wet lenses.
- Use homemade saline solution or tap water to wet or clean lenses.
- Borrow lens cases or solution from others.

Nursing Interventions and Patient Teaching

The hospitalized patient wearing corrective eyewear requires daily assistance in cleaning and maintaining the eyewear. Eyeglass lenses should be cleaned daily with a clean, soft, dry cloth; check with the patient for special care instructions before cleaning. Check screw fittings to make sure they are secure. Contact lenses are cared for according to the manufacturer's directions. When not in use, place the lenses in a storage case. Take safety precautions when corrective eyewear is not worn.

A patient problem and interventions for the patient with astigmatism, strabismus, myopia, and hyperopia include but are not limited to the following:

Patient Problem	Nursing Interventions
Potential for Injury, related to visual changes	Provide adequate lighting in the environment Orient patient to the environment Remove small, movable objects from the path of the visually impaired patient

Encourage the patient to see an optometrist or ophthalmologist yearly to keep the eyewear prescription current. Instruct the patient on the use and care of eyewear; complications may result if the patient does not follow use and care instructions.

INFLAMMATORY AND INFECTIOUS DISORDERS OF THE EYE

HORDEOLUM, CHALAZION, AND BLEPHARITIS

The most common infections and inflammatory disorders of the eyelid are listed in Table 53.3 (Fig. 53.8).

Table 53.3 Common Infections and Inflammatory Disorders of the Eyelid

DESCRIPTION	ETIOLOGY AND PATHOPHYSIOLOGY	CLINICAL MANIFESTATIONS
Blepharitis: Inflammation of eyelid margins usually involving portion of the eyelid where the lashes grow	*Ulcerative:* Caused by bacterial infection, usually staphylococcal organisms *Nonulcerative:* Caused by psoriasis, seborrhea, or allergic response	Pruritus, erythema of eyelid, eyelid pain, photophobia Excessive tearing Matting during periods of extended closure such as sleep
Chalazion: Inflammatory cyst on the meibomian gland at the eyelid margin	Most often results from blockage of an oil gland in the eyelid May be the result of complications with a hordeolum (stye) Less frequently may be caused by infection	Discomfort, mass on eyelid, edema, visual disturbance Pressure may be felt as eyelid closes over cornea
Hordeolum: Acute infection of eyelid margin or sebaceous glands of the eyelashes; also called a *stye*	Frequently caused by staphylococcal organisms One or more pustules may form	Abscess localized to base of eyelashes, with edema of lid Warmth and redness Tenderness and pain that may diminish after pustule ruptures Tearing of eye Blurred vision Patient reports feelings of scratching sensation in the eye

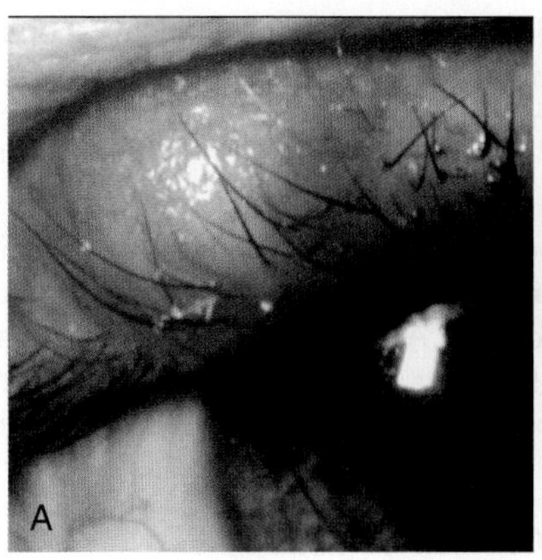

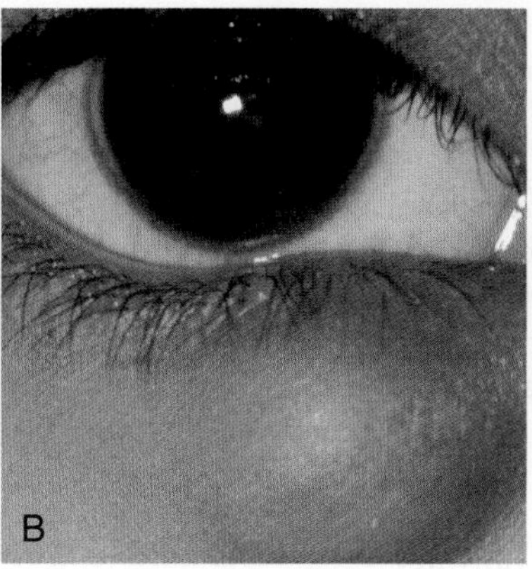

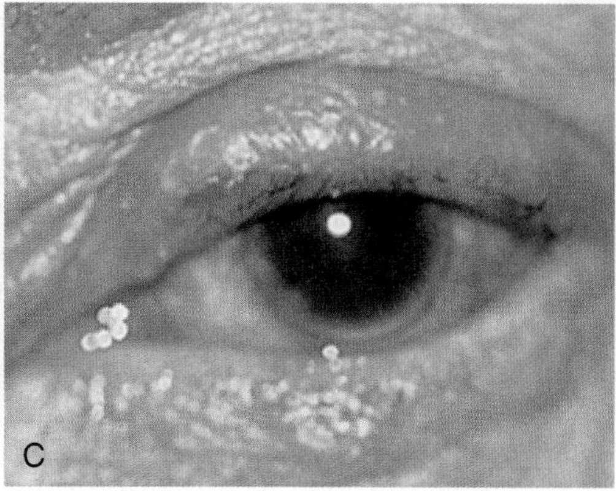

Fig. 53.8 A, Hordeolum. B, Chalazion. C, Blepharitis. (A and B, from Kanski JJ: *Signs in ophthalmology: Causes and differential diagnoses,* London, 2010, Mosby. C, from Kanski JJ: *Clinical ophthalmology: A test yourself atlas*, ed 2, New York, 2002, Butterworth-Heinemann.)

Diagnostic Tests

Assess for the presence of visual disturbances. Diagnosis of the condition begins with assessment of the eyelid margin. Characteristics of the inflammation and the presence of drainage are noted. Culture and sensitivity tests of any drainage may be ordered.

Medical Management

The health care provider may prescribe antiinfective agents (cephalexin and erythromycin) and may perform localized incision and drainage of a cyst or stye with the patient under local anesthesia. Warm normal saline (0.90% NaCl) compresses are ordered for 10 to 20 minutes two to four times a day. Lid scrubs using no-tear baby shampoo may be ordered. Topical therapies are normally sufficient to manage the conditions. Recurrent or complicated infections may require oral or systemic antibiotic therapies.

Nursing Interventions and Patient Teaching

A primary objective of nursing care for the patient with an infectious or inflammatory process of the lids is prevention of the spread of infection. Hand hygiene is essential before contact with the eye. Discuss taking care with the application of warm compresses to ensure the skin is not injured. Gentle massage of the affected area may be prescribed. Provide accompanying teaching about this procedure.

Caution the patient to avoid irritating scents, fumes, or smokes, which may cause rubbing of the eyes, leading to further infection. Discourage the use of eye makeup until all inflammation subsides. Eye makeup should be replaced after an eye infection, and every 3 to 6 months thereafter, because of the potential for the makeup to harbor bacteria.

Prognosis

Some cases may resolve without treatment in 1 to 2 weeks. In the majority of patients the inflammatory and infectious phases of these conditions respond favorably to topical antimicrobials. Surgical incision and drainage of cystlike formations result in minimal complications and are of low risk to the patient.

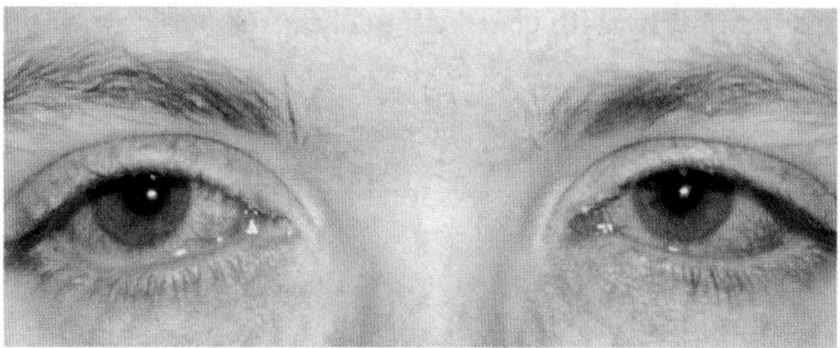

Fig. 53.9 Conjunctivitis. (From Palay DA, Krachmer JH: *Primary care ophthalmology*, ed 2, Philadelphia, 2005, Mosby.)

INFLAMMATION OF THE CONJUNCTIVA

Etiology and Pathophysiology

Conjunctivitis is a common disorder of the eye. It is responsible for 30% of all reported eye disorders. It involves an inflammation of the conjunctiva. Causes may be bacterial or viral infections, allergies, or environmental factors. It is commonly called *pinkeye*. Although this typically occurs initially in one eye, it spreads rapidly to the unaffected eye (Fig. 53.9).

The hands usually transmit acute bacterial conjunctivitis after direct contact with a contaminated object. Pneumococcal, staphylococcal, streptococcal, gonococcal, and chlamydial organisms and *Haemophilus influenzae* are the major causative bacterial agents. The eye is an excellent medium for bacterial growth because of the moisture, warmth, and extensive vascularization of the eye. The disease is usually self-limiting, leaving no permanent impairment. Trachoma, a highly contagious form of conjunctivitis, is caused by a strain of *Chlamydia trachomatis*. Transmission is by direct contact with an ocular discharge. It is rare in the United States but is a major cause of blindness in Asian and Mediterranean countries.

Viruses of the respiratory tract may, in addition to causing a cold, lead to a secondary infection of the eye. The two most common viral agents are adenovirus and type 1 herpes simplex virus (HSV). Like bacterial conjunctivitis, viral conjunctivitis is highly contagious.

Clinical Manifestations

Contamination leads to an inflammatory process that produces erythema of the conjunctiva, edema of the lid, and a mucopurulent crusting discharge on the lids and cornea. If untreated, this infection leaves the eyelid scarred with granulations that invade the cornea, resulting in loss of vision.

Assessment

Subjective data include reports of pruritus, burning, and excessive tearing. During allergy seasons and exposures to environmental irritants these complaints may be increased.

Objective data include observing eyes that are erythematous with edema of the lid. Also look for dried exudate.

Diagnostic Tests

The conjunctiva is tested for bacteria and stained for microscopic examination.

Medical Management

Medical treatment is similar to that for blepharitis.

Nursing Interventions and Patient Teaching

The lid and lashes are cleansed of exudate with normal saline. Warm compresses are applied two to four times a day. When allergies are present, cold saline compresses may be ordered to control edema and pruritus. Eye irrigations with normal saline or lactated Ringer's solution may be prescribed to remove secretions. Administer topical antibiotics and adrenocortical steroid medications as ordered. Eye pads are contraindicated because they enhance bacterial growth.

A patient problem and interventions for the patient with conjunctivitis include but are not limited to the following:

Patient Problem	Nursing Interventions
Pain, related to inflammatory process	Apply warm or cold compresses Administer prescribed eye medications; ensure proper instillation of eyedrops and ointments; administer eye irrigation as prescribed Administer analgesics as ordered

Instruct patients and their family to avoid contact with infected eyes or soiled materials when an infection is present. Patients with infection should use individual washcloths and towels, separate from the rest of their family. Tell patients to wash their hands if contact is made with the eyes and before any treatments. Teach patients the steps to perform prescribed treatments such as irrigations, application of compresses, and medication administration; evaluate their ability to perform these steps before leaving the care of the nurse. Patients should avoid noxious fumes or smoke and should not wear contact lenses during the treatment period.

Prognosis

Conjunctivitis responds successfully to topical antimicrobials. Patient teaching reduces the risk of continued exposure and reinfection. Although highly contagious, the disease is self-limiting, leaving no chance of permanent visual impairment unless a chronic condition develops.

INFLAMMATION OF THE CORNEA

Etiology and Pathophysiology

Keratitis, an inflammation of the cornea, may result from injury; irritants; allergies; bacterial infections, including syphilis; viral infections such as HSV and varicella-zoster virus; fungal infections including *Candida*; and some nervous disorders. It may be superficial and involve the epithelial layer only or may invade the subepithelial layer and the endothelial membrane. The layers of the eye are innervated, and thus, inflammation causes acute pain. Ulcers may form in the membrane layers, resulting in scattered scarring of the corneal surface.

Pseudomonas, staphylococci, streptococci, and *Haemophilus* organisms are the most common bacterial causes of keratitis. The viral agent most often responsible for corneal inflammation is herpes simplex virus (HSV). HSV keratitis is a growing problem, especially in immunocompromised patients. Keratitis can be triggered by stress, illness, and exposure to ultraviolet (UV) light. The condition may be associated with the use of ophthalmologic steroid medications. Overuse or abuse of topical steroids may injure epithelial cells.

Another form of keratitis is acanthamoebic keratitis, which is caused by amebic parasites. The *Acanthamoeba* organism is found in the soil, airborne dust, fresh water, and the noses and throats of healthy humans. This organism is often resistant to antimicrobial agents. Contact lens wearers are more susceptible because traditional cleaning agents for lenses include rinsing with clean or distilled water. People who swim frequently are at greater risk because the organism is not killed by usual methods of disinfection, such as chlorine.

Clinical Manifestations

Severe eye pain is the most common symptom that differentiates this disease from other inflammatory eye diseases. If uncontrolled, keratitis may result in blepharospasms (involuntary blinking or spasms of the eyelid) and vision loss. Other symptoms include photophobia, tearing, edema, and visual disturbances.

Assessment

Subjective data include the duration and severity of the pain, the extent of light sensitivity (photophobia), and any vision loss.

Objective data include assessing the patient for facial grimacing, lacrimation, and photophobia.

Diagnostic Tests

Depending on the causative agent, a variety of diagnostic tests may be ordered, including culture and sensitivity tests, and fluorescein-gram staining. Gram-positive bacteria appear yellow and gram-negative bacteria appear green during the staining process (Ciancaglini, Fazil, and Sforza, 2004). Ophthalmoscopic examination also is performed.

Medical Management

Medical management includes topical antibiotic therapy. Systemic antibiotics may be prescribed for severe cases. Cycloplegic-mydriatic drugs paralyze the ocular muscles of accommodation and dilate the pupil. For viral keratitis, therapy includes corneal débridement followed by topical therapy with vidarabine or trifluridine (Viroptic) for 2 to 3 weeks. Corticosteroids are *contraindicated* because they contribute to a longer course, possible deeper ulceration of the cornea, and systemic complications. Drug therapy also may include antiviral therapy such as acyclovir (Zovirax). Analgesics are used to control pain associated with acute inflammation. Pressure dressings may be ordered to relax the eye muscle and decrease discomfort. These dressings often are applied to both eyes because the eyes move together. Warm or cold compresses two to four times daily are prescribed for symptomatic relief. Epithelial débridement of loose tissue may be performed. Surgical management involves a corneal transplant, known as *keratoplasty*.

Nursing Interventions and Patient Teaching

Nursing interventions for keratitis include control of pain, safety, and prevention of complications. Nursing diagnoses and interventions for the patient with keratitis are the same as for conjunctivitis. Provide information on self-care of a corneal abrasion. Also teach the patient to wash hands before instilling medication and to prevent infection by not rubbing the eyes. Instruct the patient to note any change in discharge or increase in pain and to notify the health care practitioner immediately.

Prognosis

Topical antibiotic, antiviral, or antifungal eyedrops, when started promptly after diagnosis by culture, result in rapid healing and minimal visual impairment. Chronic keratitis may develop if treatment is delayed. Infection of the cornea can produce corneal ulcer and vision loss as a result of opaque scarring. Keratoplasty then may be indicated.

NONINFECTIOUS DISORDERS OF THE EYE

DRY EYE DISORDERS

Etiology and Pathology

Complaints of dry eye, caused by a variety of ocular disorders, are characterized by decreased tear secretion or increased tear film evaporation. Keratoconjunctivitis sicca (dry eye) is caused by lacrimal gland dysfunction, usually the result of an autoimmune reaction. If the patient with keratoconjunctivitis sicca has associated dry mouth, the patient may have primary **Sjögren syndrome** (an immunologic disorder characterized by deficient fluid production by the lacrimal, salivary, and other glands, resulting in abnormal dryness of the mouth, eyes, and other mucous membranes) (NLM, 2016a). Secondary Sjögren syndrome occurs in the presence of other systemic conditions such as rheumatoid arthritis, scleroderma, or systemic lupus erythematosus.

Risk factors for the development of dry eyes include female gender and advancing age. Most cases occur in individuals older than age 50 years. Medications associated with the development of the condition include antihistamines, nasal decongestants, tranquilizers, oral contraceptives, and antidepressants. Dietary factors may be implicated. Diets that are low in Vitamin A and Omega 3 fatty acids are seen in individuals with dry eyes. The development of dry eye conditions may be noted after refractive eye treatment surgeries. In these patients the condition may be time limited.

Clinical Manifestations

The eyes may appear reddened or contain stringy mucus. A variety of subjective complaints may be reported. Patients experience photosensitivity, eye fatigue, and blurred vision. These complaints may result in difficulty using computer aids and reading. The patient complains of a sandy or gritty sensation that typically worsens during the day and is better in the morning after eye closure with sleep.

Diagnostic Tests

The definitive test for dry eye, a noninfectious disorder of the lacrimal gland, is *Schirmer's test*. Schirmer's test involves the placement of filter paper in the lower lid of the eye. After 5 minutes the paper is removed and the moisture on the paper is evaluated. Normal results are 10 to 15 mm of wet paper. Fluorescein drops also are administered to assess the structural integrity of the cornea and the ability of tears to flow across the eye and through the lacrimal duct to the nose. Results of the fluorescein-staining test for excessive tear disorder are considered normal if the dye disappears from the lacrimal cul-de-sac within 1 minute.

Medical Management

Medical management for dry eye includes artificial tear replacement. Many nonprescription products are available. They should be used sparingly because preservatives in the drops or overuse can cause further irritation. Preservative-free drops are available and will not result in irritation after long-term use (American Optometric Association, 2018). Cyclosporine, an immunosuppressant agent, is a prescription medication available to manage dry eye. It can increase tear production and reduce inflammation. It may take 3 to 6 months for the medication to provide noticeable improvement in the condition. Short-term corticosteroid drops may be prescribed to reduce inflammation in severe cases. Punctal plugs (temporary or permanent) may be inserted to close the tear ducts and keep the tears in the eyes longer.

Patients taking medications associated with the development of dry eye may have their prescriptions changed to medications that are less drying. If an infection accompanies the dry eye syndrome, antibiotic therapy may be prescribed. Eliminate as many environmental irritants as possible. High-efficiency particulate absorption (HEPA) filters are available to control pollen and dust levels in the home environment. If contact lenses cause local irritation and dry eye, a change in the prescription, type of lens, contact solution, or the addition of rewetting drops may be advised. Moderate to severe dry eyes may be managed by the daily insertion of hydroxypropyl cellulose (Lacrisert) in the lower eyelid. It dissolves and provides the needed lubrication (Mayo Clinic, 2015).

Surgical repair of an injured punctal sac by correctly aligning the eyelid margin or by probing an obstructed punctum (opening to the tear duct) is the recommended method of treatment to allow for tear absorption.

Nursing Interventions and Patient Teaching

The appropriate patient problem is *Pain, related to lack of natural eye moisture*. Interventions are similar to those for conjunctivitis. Instruct the patient on instilling eye medications, practicing appropriate hand and eye hygiene, and avoiding irritants.

Prognosis

Eyedrops alleviate the majority of symptoms caused by dry eye. Control of medical conditions minimizes discomfort and complications. Surgical repair of the punctal sac is a safe procedure and has a good prognosis.

ECTROPION AND ENTROPION

Etiology and Pathophysiology

Ectropion and entropion are two noninfectious disorders of the eyelid, causing an abnormal turning of the eyelid margins.

Ectropion is the outward turning of the eyelid margin. In the older patient it is common for the orbicularis oculi muscle to be relaxed. Paralytic ectropion occurs when orbicularis muscle function is disturbed, as with Bell's palsy. Other causes of ectropion are birth defects, eyelid laceration, and burns of the conjunctival tissue.

Entropion is an inward turning of the eyelid. The lower eyelid margin is the most frequently involved. Entropion causes include atrophy of the eyelid tissue, spasms of the orbicularis oculi muscle, or scarring of the tarsal plate (dense connective tissue that stiffens the eyelid) caused by congenital conditions or eye trauma. Varying degrees of atonia commonly exist in the older adult orbicularis oculi.

Clinical Manifestations

Ectropion and entropion are characterized by abnormal positions of the eyelid, with tearing and corneal dryness. Redness of the sclera also may be present.

Assessment

Collection of subjective data includes noting the degree of vision loss and determining tear loss and dryness of the cornea.

Collection of objective data includes observing the extent to which the patient can perform ADLs and the presence of any eyelid margin inflammation.

Diagnostic Tests

The health care practitioner diagnoses these conditions after a visual and ophthalmologic examination.

Medical Management

Medical intervention consists of topical medications to reduce conjunctival and corneal inflammation or drying. Surgery is the preferred treatment. Resection of the tarsal plate, removal of the scarred tissue, or tightening of the orbicularis oculi muscle is the recommended treatment for permanent repair.

Nursing Interventions and Patient Teaching

Interventions for ectropion and entropion involve monitoring the medical treatment and reporting its progress. A patient problem statement for the patient with ectropion or entropion is *Impaired Sensory Awareness, related to edema and exudate*. Interventions include assistance in self-care activities, safety measures, observation for infection and inflammation, and medication and dressing treatments as prescribed.

Prognosis

Early diagnosis and treatment of eyelid disorders reduce the risk of conjunctival and corneal inflammation and scarring. Monitoring treatment reduces the need for surgical intervention and minimizes visual disturbances.

DISORDERS OF THE LENS

CATARACTS

Etiology and Pathophysiology

A **cataract** is a crystalline opacity or clouding of the lens (Fig. 53.10). The patient may have a cataract in one or both eyes. If they are present in both eyes, one cataract may affect vision more than the other. In the aging patient, opacification of the lens gradually occurs. About 50% of seniors between 65 and 74 years old have some degree of cataract formation. After 75 years of age, the percentage rises to about 70%. Cataract removal is the most common surgical procedure for people greater than 65 years of age. When a cataract develops, the lens becomes foggy, decreasing visual acuity, and if a large enough portion of the lens becomes opaque, light cannot reach the retina.

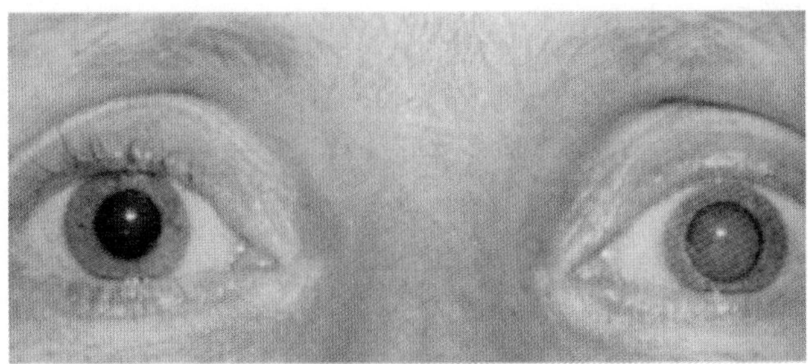

Fig. 53.10 Cataract in subject's left eye. (From Swartz MH: *Textbook of physical diagnosis*, ed 4, Philadelphia, 2002, Saunders.)

Cataracts may be congenital (e.g., a result of exposure to maternal rubella) or acquired from systemic disease, trauma, toxins (e.g., radiation or UV light exposure, certain drugs such as systemic corticosteroids or long-term topical corticosteroids), and intraocular inflammation. Most cataracts are age related (senile cataracts). Systemic disorders associated with the development of cataracts include diabetes mellitus and hypertension. Smoking has been linked with the development of cataracts. Numerous factors contribute to cataract development. In senile cataract formation, it appears that altered metabolic processes within the lens cause an accumulation of water and alterations in the fiber structure. These changes affect lens transparency, causing vision changes.

Clinical Manifestations

Cataract symptoms are painless but include blurred vision, difficulty reading fine print, diplopia, photosensitivity, glare (the sense that normal light is too bright), abnormal color perception, and difficulty driving at night. Glare is due to light scatter caused by the lens opacities, and it may be significantly worse at night when the pupil dilates. The visual decline is gradual, and the rate of cataract development varies from patient to patient. The opacity can be seen in the center of the lens (see Fig. 53.10).

Assessment

Subjective data include blurred vision, often the first symptom expressed by the patient. Note any subjective complaints, such as "hazy" or "fuzzy" vision or abnormal color perception.

The gathering of objective data involves observing the patient for difficulty in reading, such as noting whether the patient brings a newspaper close to the eyes. Also note sensitivity to light.

Diagnostic Tests

Diagnosis is based on decreased visual acuity or other complaints of visual dysfunction. The opacity is directly observable by ophthalmoscope or slit-lamp microscopic examination. A totally opaque lens creates the appearance of a white pupil (see Fig. 53.10).

Medical Management

Monitor the patient for changes in vision associated with increasing cataract size. For many patients, the diagnosis is made long before they actually decide to have surgery. Often, changing the patient's eyewear prescription can improve the visual acuity, at least temporarily. If glare makes it difficult to drive at night, the patient may drive only during daylight hours and have a family member drive at night. When palliative measures no longer provide an acceptable level of visual function, the patient is an appropriate candidate for surgery. Surgery is the only definitive method of treatment and can be performed at any age. It can be done using a local or topical anesthetic, or under general anesthesia.

There are two surgical methods to improve vision: intracapsular and extracapsular extraction. Intracapsular extraction surgery involves removing the lens and its entire capsule. Although some surgeons still perform intracapsular extraction (and it may be necessary in instances of trauma), the intracapsular technique has been largely replaced by extracapsular extraction. In the extracapsular extraction method, the anterior capsule is opened and the lens nucleus and cortex are removed, leaving the remaining capsular bag intact. Healing is rapid with this method.

Phacoemulsification is the most common type of extracapsular cataract extraction. This technique uses ultrasound to break up and remove the cataract through a small incision, thereby reducing the healing time and decreasing the chance of complications.

During surgery the physician implants a synthetic intraocular lens in the posterior chamber behind the iris. At the end of the procedure, the patient receives injections of subconjunctival corticosteroid and antibiotics. Then an antibiotic and corticosteroid ointment are applied, and the patient's eye is covered with a patch and protective shield. The patch usually is worn overnight and removed during the first postoperative visit. Antibiotic and corticosteroid therapies continue for 1 to 2 weeks after surgery. The patient is encouraged to wear protective eyewear at night. During the day the patient wears protected goggle-type sunglasses. Many refractive errors are corrected with the surgery. A patient who wore prescriptive eyewear before surgery may no longer need it. Even a patient needing prescription eyewear after surgery will likely have changes in the prescription.

Nursing Interventions and Patient Teaching

Preoperative and postoperative nursing care is a primary nursing responsibility (Nursing Care Plan 53.1). Cataract symptoms usually develop slowly and can be detected easily. Encourage patients to have annual eye examinations. Surgery provides about a 90% success rate in achieving acceptable levels of vision. Unless complications occur, the patient is usually ready to go home within a few hours after the surgery, as soon as the effects of sedation have worn off. Postoperative medications usually include antibiotic and corticosteroid

Nursing Care Plan 53.1 The Patient With Cataracts

Ms. J. is an 82-year-old who lives alone. She has developed bilateral cataracts and is admitted to same-day surgery for a right cataract extracapsular procedure with intraocular lens implantation.

PATIENT PROBLEM

Potential for Injury, related to altered visual acuity

Patient Goals and Expected Outcomes	Nursing Interventions	Evaluation
Patient will not have any evidence of injury Patient will have a safe environment in which she will avoid injury	**PREOPERATIVE** Instill eyedrops as prescribed, wearing clean latex or vinyl gloves. Administer preoperative medications or sedatives as ordered. Explain which postoperative procedures to expect, such as patches and eyedrops. **POSTOPERATIVE** Instill mydriatic-cycloplegic and corticosteroid eyedrops as prescribed while wearing clean latex or vinyl gloves. Instruct patient to avoid moving head suddenly, heavy lifting, bending over, coughing, sneezing, vomiting, and straining with elimination, which cause increased intraocular pressure. Keep eye patch or shield in position during specified hours. Instruct patient to avoid lying on the side of the affected eye on the night after surgery. Remove environmental barriers to ensure safety. Keep side rails up at all times. Plan all care with patient: Explain what will happen and when. Visit often and announce yourself on entering the room. Assist with deep-breathing exercises q 1-2 hr while awake. Check with health care practitioner for any special positioning or precautions. (If turned, position patient on the unaffected side.) Elevate head of bed 30 degrees as ordered. Assist with and teach active and passive range-of-motion exercises q 4 hr. Provide increased activities and ambulation as ordered; assist as needed. Teach self-care activities, and assist as needed. Instruct family to remove unnecessary furniture and pick up objects that may be blocking pathways. Instruct patient that cataract surgery does not correct nearsightedness or farsightedness. Corrective lenses are still needed for these problems after surgery.	Patient experienced no injuries during the preoperative and immediate postoperative phase. Patient understands and demonstrates injury prevention measures in the home.

PATIENT PROBLEM

Anxiousness/Fearfulness, related to visual impairment

Patient Goals and Expected Outcomes	Nursing Intervention	Evaluation
Patient will voice decreased anxiety and fear	Observe level of patient and family anxiety. Note patient's coping mechanism related to vision loss. Encourage patient and family to vent feelings and concerns. Support patient and family's positive actions toward adapting to visual limitations.	Patient and family display trust and security after venting feelings.

CRITICAL THINKING QUESTIONS

1. Ms. J. puts her call light on and tells the nurse that she has severe pain and pressure in her right eye. What should be the initial response by the nurse?
2. What should be included in Ms. J.'s discharge planning to minimize the risk of injury to her operative eye?
3. In visiting with Ms. J., the nurse learns that Ms. J. enjoys embroidery and knitting. Ms. J. states that she is looking forward to resuming her handiwork. What should be included as appropriate patient teaching?

drops to prevent infection and decrease the postoperative inflammatory response. The ophthalmologist instructs the patient to avoid activities that increase IOP, such as bending, stooping, coughing, or lifting. Ophthalmologists also may recommend using an eye shield over the operative eye at night for protection. Discuss safety measures appropriate to vision alterations, and instruct the patient to notify the health care practitioner of any complications, such as pain, erythema, drainage, or sudden visual changes. If sudden pain occurs, call the health care practitioner (see the Communication box and the Patient Teaching box).

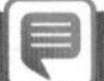 Communication

Nursing-Patient Dialogue Regarding Postoperative Eye Surgery

Mrs. B., a 71-year-old patient, has been experiencing decreasing vision for the past 5 years. She seeks medical attention and is told that surgery is required to correct her condition. While talking to the patient, the nurse senses her reluctance to comply with postoperative treatment.

Patient: I'm too old to go through all the routines that the doctor wants me to. It involves too much.

Nurse: I know that surgery is a concern for you. You must have many emotions right now. It's understandable that you have concerns about your recovery.

Patient: There's so much to think about and remember.

Nurse: The doctor and our staff are here to help make your recovery as easy as possible for you. Can you tell me what bothers you the most?

Patient: What if I go home and fall? I could reinjure my eye or break something, like my hip.

Nurse: There are several things that you and your family can do to prevent any injury during your recovery. The nursing staff will provide education to you both before and after surgery to assist you with care after discharge.

Prognosis

Gradual loss of lens transparency increases the risk of injury because of vision loss. Carefully monitor patients for degeneration of the lens. The condition may be accompanied by secondary glaucoma, which further reduces visual acuity. Surgical intervention is advised to improve vision. Postoperative complications of cataract surgery are uncommon, but may include infection, hemorrhage, inflammation, glaucoma, and retinal detachment (Mayo Clinic, 2010). Complications may recur years after cataract surgery and should be reported to the ophthalmologist.

DISORDERS OF THE RETINA

DIABETIC RETINOPATHY

Etiology and Pathophysiology

Diabetic retinopathy is a disorder of retinal blood vessels characterized by capillary microaneurysms, hemorrhage, exudates, and the formation of new vessels and connective tissue. Patients may present to their health care provider with visual alterations, which may lead to the initial diagnosis of diabetes mellitus. After 15 years with diabetes mellitus, nearly all patients with type 1 diabetes and 80% with type 2 diabetes have some degree of retinal disease accompanied by nephropathy. The incidence of diabetic retinopathy greatly increases in relation to how long the patient has diabetes mellitus and how well his or her blood glucose levels are controlled. The disorder occurs more frequently in patients with longstanding, poorly controlled diabetes mellitus (see the Cultural Considerations box).

The initial stage of diabetic retinopathy may last several years. The earliest and most treatable stages

 Patient Teaching

After Eye Surgery

- Discuss proper hand hygiene, which includes washing hands before and after caring for eyes, including the application of medications and dressing changes.
- Review signs and symptoms to report to the health care provider.
- Shaving, bathing, and washing of the face are permitted, but the patient must avoid excess water exposure and wetting of the area near the eyes.
- Shampoos and soaps must be used with caution near the eyes.
- Avoid the use of cosmetics for up to 4 weeks or as prescribed by the health care provider.
- Discuss personal hygiene.
- Normal symptoms include slight redness, mild watering, mild irritation, glare, and slight ptosis (drooping) of the upper eyelid. These symptoms may remain for 6 to 8 weeks after the operation.
- Abnormal symptoms include sudden onset of extreme pain, trauma or injury, decreased visual acuity, floaters, flashes of light, purulent drainage, or bleeding.
- Teach the patient postoperative restrictions on head positioning, bending, coughing, and the Valsalva maneuver to optimize visual outcomes and to prevent increased intraocular pressure (IOP).
- Postoperative restrictions include limitations on lifting, driving, and sexual relations for a period specified by the health care provider.
- Teach the prescribed medication therapies. Allow the patient to provide a return demonstration. Observe the use of aseptic technique.
- Instruct the patient to monitor pain and to take the prescribed medication for pain as directed and to report pain symptoms not relieved by medications.
- Make a follow-up appointment and provide a written appointment card for the patient.

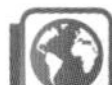 Cultural Considerations

Incidence of Hearing and Visual Problems

- Caucasians have a higher incidence of hearing impairment than African Americans or Asian Americans.
- The incidence and severity of glaucoma are greater among African Americans than among Caucasians.
- Hispanics have an increased incidence of diabetic retinopathy.
- Native Americans have an increased incidence of otitis media when compared with whites.
- Whites have a higher incidence of macular degeneration than Hispanics, African Americans, and Asian Americans.
- Inuits are susceptible to primary closed-angle glaucoma, resulting from a thicker lens and a shallow chamber angle.
- Native Americans and African Americans have a higher incidence of astigmatism than whites.

often produce no changes in vision. Because of this, the patient with diabetes must have regular dilated eye examinations by an ophthalmologist or optometrist for early detection and treatment. As the disease progresses, the blood vessels in the retina begin to widen and become tortuous. Microaneurysms then develop at the periphery, and small hemorrhages develop. These may disappear, but they leave in their place scars that can decrease vision. Increased capillary permeability causes protein exudate.

New blood vessels form on the retina and into the vitreous body as the disease progresses. These new vessels rupture, causing decreased vision. Some of the blood may be reabsorbed, which improves vision until another hemorrhage occurs. With progressive hemorrhages, the patient may have significant vision loss over time. Vitreous contraction and full retinal detachment can occur as the vessels and surrounding tissue become more fibrous and less flexible.

Clinical Manifestations

Symptoms include microaneurysms, which can be identified only by ophthalmoscopy in the initial stage. In the advanced stages, the patient has progressive vision loss and the presence of "floaters," which are minute products of the hemorrhage.

Assessment

Collection of subjective data includes assessment of the duration of the disease and how well the diabetes mellitus is controlled. Patients may have varying degrees of vision loss, from decreased vision to complete blindness. Assess each patient's knowledge of therapy and treatments.

Collection of objective data involves noting that in the early stages there are no symptoms; as the disease progresses, vision becomes diminished.

Diagnostic Tests

Indirect ophthalmoscopy shows dilated and tortuous vessels and narrowing or obliteration of the arteries. Opacities, hemorrhages, and microaneurysms can be visualized. Slit-lamp examination magnifies the lesions.

Medical Management

Surgical intervention includes early photocoagulation (see "Photocoagulation," below), cryotherapy (cryopexy), and/or vitrectomy (see "Vitrectomy" discussions). **Photocoagulation** uses a laser beam to destroy new blood vessels, seal leaking vessels, and help prevent retinal edema. A vitrectomy or cryotherapy may be performed when photocoagulation is not possible. A topical anesthetic is used in **cryotherapy** so that the probe can be placed directly on the surface of the eye to deliver therapy. When the probe is located properly on the eye, the tip of the probe creates a frozen area that extends through the external tissue, and reaches a specific point on the retina. Vascular endothelial growth factor (VEGF) inhibitors may be injected into the retina. These medications work to stop the growth of the new blood vessels (Mayo Clinic, 2018).

Nursing Interventions and Patient Teaching

A patient problem and interventions for the patient with diabetic retinopathy include but are not limited to the following:

Patient Problem	Nursing Interventions
Insufficient Knowledge, related to unfamiliarity with therapeutic procedure	Determine patient's knowledge of purpose and procedures of photocoagulation, cryotherapy, or vitrectomy

Home care after surgery for the patient with diabetic retinopathy is the same as for any eye surgery.

Prognosis

The best treatment of diabetic retinopathy is early detection. Frequent eye examinations reduce the complication of vision loss, and modern laser technology is highly effective in reducing further damage to the retina and improving vision.

AGE-RELATED MACULAR DEGENERATION

Etiology and Pathophysiology

Age-related macular degeneration (ARMD) of the retina is characterized by slow, progressive loss of central and near vision. ARMD is the most common cause of vision loss in people older than 60 years. There is evidence of a genetic component of ARMD, and a positive family history for ARMD is a major risk factor. Additional risk factors include long-term exposure to UV light, hyperopia, cigarette smoking, gender (female), obesity, race, and light-colored eyes. Nutrition may play a role in the progression of ARMD. Dietary supplementation with vitamin C, vitamin E, vitamin A (beta-carotene), copper, and zinc slows the development of advancing ARMD; however, it does not seem to have any effect on people with minimal ARMD.

There are two types of macular degeneration. The first is known as the *wet type* (also called *neovascular macular degeneration*). This is characterized by sudden new vessel growth in the macular region. The macula becomes displaced and scarring occurs. Because scarred cells no longer register light, vision loss is irreversible. Wet macular degeneration accounts for 10% of cases.

The second, known as the *dry type* (also called *nonexudative* or *nonneovascular macular degeneration*), occurs in 90% of cases. It is caused by degenerative changes, including lipid deposits. These are followed by slow atrophy of the macular region, including the retina. People with dry ARMD notice that reading and other close-vision tasks become more difficult. In this form, the macular cells have wasted or atrophied, resulting in decreased function. The patient may report, "Sometimes I see the image and sometimes it sort of blinks at me, like I have a short circuit."

Clinical Manifestations

The hallmark of ARMD is the appearance of drusen in the fundus (the interior surface of the eye), found on ophthalmoscopic evaluation. Drusen are yellowish exudates found beneath the retinal pigment epithelium and represent localized or diffuse deposits of extracellular debris. The main symptom of macular degeneration is gradual and variable bilateral loss of *central vision*. One eye may have a greater loss than the other and color perception also may be affected.

Assessment

The collection of subjective data includes asking the patient if he or she has noticed difficulty in distinguishing colors correctly. Assess for visual disturbances and coping mechanisms related to the loss of vision. Macular degeneration develops differently in each person, and therefore the symptoms may vary. However, some of the most common symptoms include (1) a gradual loss of ability to see objects clearly; (2) distorted vision, with objects appearing to be the wrong size or shape or straight lines appearing wavy or crooked; (3) gradual loss of clear color vision; (4) scotomas (blind spots in the visual field); and (5) a dark or empty area appearing in the center of vision.

The collection of objective data includes noting the degree to which the patient can centrally view objects.

Diagnostic Tests

Ophthalmoscopy is used to detect opacity, hemorrhage, and new blood vessel formation. The examiner looks for retinal detachment, drusen, and other fundus changes associated with ARMD, and any other abnormalities. Using an Amsler grid test may help define the involved areas. Fluorescein angiography is used to assess for the presence of leaking blood vessels and to confirm diagnosis.

Medical Management

Medications can be used to stop the growth of new blood vessels. Bevacizumab (Avastin) and pegaptanib (Macugen) are injected directly into the eye. Antibiotic drops may be prescribed to accompany the injections in an effort to prevent infection. Photodynamic therapy is a treatment for wet ARMD. This treatment uses intravenous verteporfin (Visudyne) and a "cold" laser. Verteporfin becomes active when exposed to the "cold" laser light wave. This procedure causes deconstruction of abnormal blood vessels but does not cause permanent damage to the retinal pigment epithelium and photoreceptor cells. The specific guidelines for use of this therapy in patients with wet ARMD are very strict, and only about 10% of patients are eligible for treatment. After delivery of this therapy the patient must understand that caution should be used to avoid direct exposure to sunlight and other intense forms of light for 5 days after treatment. Destruction of abnormal vessels may be performed with laser beam therapy. It has limited use. At present, there is no treatment for dry macular degeneration.

Unfortunately, central vision damaged by macular degeneration cannot be restored. However, because macular degeneration does not damage peripheral vision, low vision aids such as telescopic and microscopic special lenses, magnifying glasses, and electronic magnifiers for close work can be prescribed to help make the most of remaining vision. Often, with adaptation, people can cope well and continue to do most things they were accustomed to doing. High-dose nutritional supplements of zinc, beta-carotene, and vitamins C and E have been shown to reduce the risk of progression to advanced ARMD by 25% (National Eye Institute, National Institutes of Health, 2008). A diet rich in fruits and dark green, leafy vegetables is also recommended (Krishnadev, Meleth, and Chew, 2010).

Nursing Interventions and Patient Teaching

The patient needs patience and understanding to cope with the continuing loss of sight. Help the patient through the process of accepting loss of sight. Maintaining safety is important because only peripheral vision exists.

A patient problem and interventions for the patient with macular degeneration include but are not limited to the following:

Patient Problem	Nursing Interventions
Impaired Sensory Awareness, related to disease process	Note the extent of visual loss and the level of ability to perform ADLs; assist the patient in developing ways to perform these activities Determine the patient's support systems and solicit help if available

Instruct the patients about the disease process, stressing that peripheral vision will be maintained. Provide ways for the patient to maintain as much independence as possible, and help family and friends determine the areas in which to assist.

Prognosis

Early diagnosis of macular degeneration is critical to prevent blindness. Watchful waiting is the only approach to dry macular degeneration. Ophthalmic laser surgery is of limited benefit because of the gradual and progressive course of the disorder. Photocoagulation is preventive, not curative.

RETINAL DETACHMENT

Etiology and Pathophysiology

Retinal detachment is a separation of the retina from the choroid in the posterior area of the eye (Fig. 53.11). This usually results from a hole in the retina that allows vitreous humor to leak between the choroid and the retina. The immediate cause may be severe trauma to

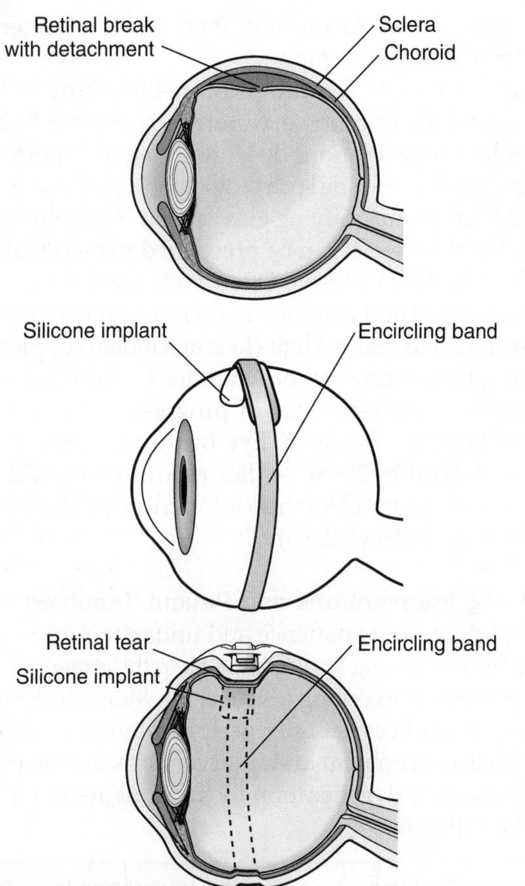

Fig. 53.11 Retinal break with detachment. Surgical repair by scleral buckling technique. (From Lewis SL, Bucher L, Heitkemper MM, et al: *Medical-surgical nursing: Assessment and management of clinical problems*, ed 10, St. Louis, 2017, Mosby.)

the eye, such as a contusion or a penetrating wound. In most cases, however, retinal detachment is the result of internal changes related to aging and sometimes inflammation of the eye. Retinal detachment also may occur in debilitated patients when there is sudden, severe physical exertion. As the detachment progresses, it interrupts the transmission of visual images from the retina to the optic nerve. The result is a progressive loss of vision to complete blindness.

Clinical Manifestations

Symptoms include a sudden or gradual development of flashes of light, followed by floating spots, a "cobweb," a "hairnet," and loss of a specific field of vision. As the detachment progresses, patients may describe an enlarging dark spot in their visual field. Patients have described this as having a curtain or shade being drawn over their eye. This dark area may occur in any of the visual fields but typically begins in the peripheral visual field. The dark area may progress to include the entire visual field if the retinal detachment includes the entire retina.

Assessment

Subjective data include patient complaints of flashing lights unilaterally and floaters. Progressive vision restriction occurs in one area. If the tear is acute and extensive, the patient describes a sensation like a curtain being drawn across the eye. This is a painless condition, because the retina does not contain sensory nerves that relay sensations of pain.

Collection of objective data includes observing the patient for the ability to perform ADLs. Also assess the level of anxiety associated with coping.

Diagnostic Tests

Visual acuity measurements should be the first diagnostic procedure with any complaint of vision loss. Indirect and direct ophthalmoscopy are used to detect pallor of the retina and detachment. The gonioscopy is used to provide a view of the anterior chamber of the eye. It provides a magnified view of any retinal lesions. Slit-lamp examination magnifies the lesions. Ultrasound may be useful to identify a retinal detachment if the retina cannot be visualized directly (e.g., when the cornea, lens, or vitreous humor is hazy or opaque).

Medical Management

The treatment of choice is early corrective intervention. The typical time frame for retinal repair depends on the involvement of the macula. If the macula remains intact and the patient's central vision remains, then repair typically is done within 24 to 48 hours. If the macula is detached, the patient will have decreased central vision and the time frame for repair will be within 7 to 10 days. One of five procedures may be performed:

- *Laser photocoagulation* burns localized tears or breaks in the posterior portion of the eye, eventually sealing the tear or break.
- *Cryotherapy* freezes the borders of a retinal hole with a frozen-tipped probe. The probe is applied to the scleral surface directly over the retinal tear. The tear seals when the resultant inflammatory process produces scarring.
- *Electrodiathermy* burns a retinal break, using an ultrasonic probe. The probe is applied to the scleral surface directly over the retinal break. Sealing occurs from the resultant inflammatory and scarring process.
- *Scleral buckling* is an extraocular surgical procedure that involves indenting the globe of the eye so that the retinal pigment epithelium, choroid, and sclera move toward the detached retina. This not only helps seal retinal breaks but also helps relieve inward traction on the retina. The retinal surgeon sutures a silicone implant against the sclera, causing the sclera to buckle inward. The surgeon may place an encircling band over the implant if there are multiple retinal breaks, if the surgeon cannot locate suspected break(s), or if there is widespread inward traction on the retina (see Fig. 53.11). If present, subretinal fluid may be drained by inserting a small-gauge needle to facilitate contact between the retina and the buckled sclera. Scleral buckling usually is accomplished with the patient under local anesthesia. The patient may be

discharged on the first postoperative day, or scleral buckling surgery may be performed as an outpatient procedure.

- *Pneumatic* (pertaining to air or gas) *retinopexy* is an intraocular procedure that involves the injection of a gas into the vitreous cavity to form a temporary bubble that closes retinal breaks and places pressure on the separated retinal layers. This bubble is temporary and is combined with laser photocoagulation or cryotherapy treatment. For several weeks after therapy, the patient must position his or her head in a forward position so that the bubble remains in contact with the retinal break.

Nursing Interventions and Patient Teaching

Postprocedure management includes cycloplegic, mydriatic, and antiinfective eyedrops. Eye patches are applied over only the operative eye or both eyes, allowing the eyes to rest for 1 or 2 days. Safety measures are essential because the eyes are patched. Depending on the procedure, how the patient's head may be positioned postoperatively may vary. If air is injected into the vitreous, the head is positioned with the unaffected eye upward and the patient lying on the abdomen or sitting forward for 4 to 5 days. Dark glasses are prescribed after removal of the eye patches to decrease the discomfort of *photophobia*. A patient problem and interventions for the patient with retinal detachment include but are not limited to the following:

Patient Problem	Nursing Interventions
Anxiousness, related to visual alterations	Allow the patient the opportunity to discuss feelings and fears about the possible loss of vision Answer questions honestly and educate the patient if misunderstandings still exist Provide a rationale for restrictions of activities and for procedures

Discuss with the patient temporary restrictions of physical activity after therapy (see the Patient Teaching box).

Patient Teaching

Retinal Detachment

- Refrain from strenuous physical activity, heavy lifting, or high-risk activities to reduce the risk of traumatic injury to the eye.
- Check with the health care provider about shampooing hair. Prevent getting shampoo or soap in the affected eye.
- Use correct techniques for administration of eye medications as discussed earlier in the chapter.
- Report to the ophthalmologist any signs of further detachment (flashes of light, increase in floaters, blurred vision).
- Report for medical follow-up visits as instructed.

Prognosis

Retinal detachment requires immediate treatment. Reattachment is successful in 90% of cases; the degree of sight restoration depends on the extent and duration of separation. Maximum vision is achieved within 3 months after surgery. Unless replaced, a detached retina slowly dies after several years. Blindness from retinal detachment is irreversible.

GLAUCOMA AND CORNEAL INJURIES

GLAUCOMA

Etiology and Pathophysiology

Glaucoma is not one disease but rather a group of disorders characterized by (1) increased intraocular pressure (IOP) because of obstruction of the outflow of aqueous humor, (2) optic nerve atrophy, and (3) progressive loss of peripheral vision (Fig. 53.12). Glaucoma is found in people who are middle aged and older. Approximately 9% to 12% of all blindness in the United States results from glaucoma (Glaucoma Research

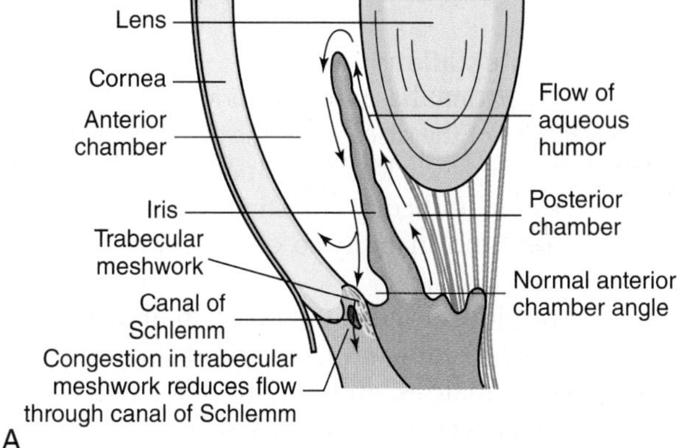

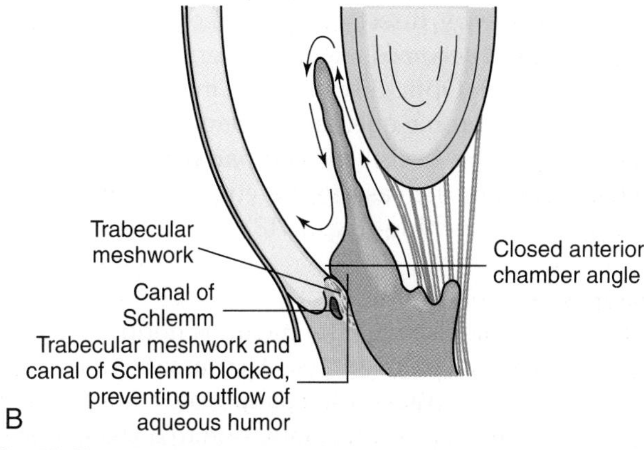

Fig. 53.12 A, Primary open-angle glaucoma (POAG). Congestion in the trabecular meshwork reduces the outflow of aqueous humor. B, Acute angle-closure glaucoma (AACG). The angle between the iris and the anterior chamber narrows, obstructing the outflow of aqueous humor. (From Havener WH: *Synopsis of ophthalmology*, St. Louis, 1997, Mosby.)

Foundation, 2017). One in 50 whites is affected, whereas 1 in 10 African Americans will develop glaucoma. It is seldom seen in people younger than 35 years of age but may occur in infancy.

Open-angle glaucoma, also known as *primary open-angle glaucoma (POAG),* represents 90% of the cases of primary glaucoma. In POAG the outflow of aqueous humor is decreased in the trabecular meshwork. In essence, the drainage channels become occluded, like a clogged kitchen sink. The course of the disease is slowly progressive and results from degenerative changes; often this occurs bilaterally.

Closed-angle glaucoma, also known as *acute angle-closure glaucoma (AACG),* occurs if there is an abrupt angle change of the iris, causing rapid vision loss and dramatic symptoms. This type of glaucoma represents 10% of the total number of glaucoma cases in the United States. Medication therapies for conditions such as depression, allergies, and Parkinson's disease may be implicated in the development of AACG. Corticosteroids, topical anticholinergics, tricyclic antidepressants, MAO (monoamine oxidase) inhibitors, antihistamines, and antipsychotic medications may be linked to glaucoma development and are used with caution and only under the close direction of the health care provider in the patient with a diagnosis of glaucoma (Rhee, 2012).

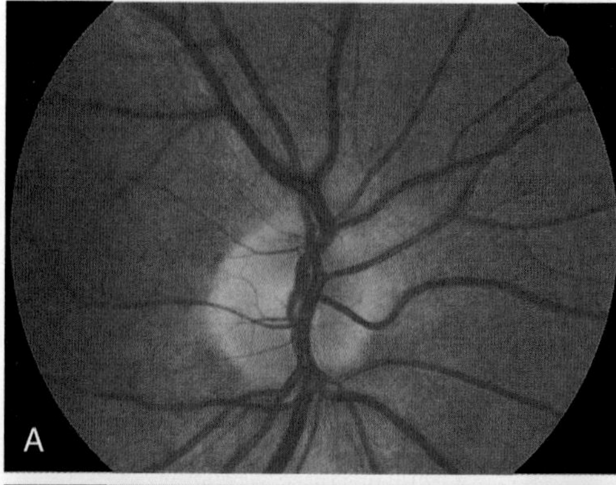

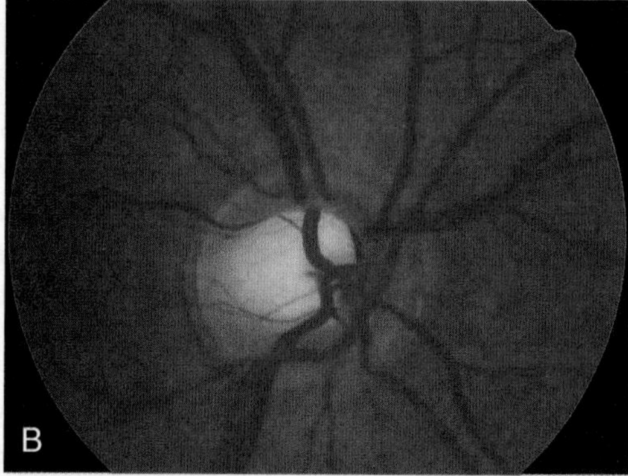

Fig. 53.13 A, In the normal eye, the optic disc is pink with little cupping. B, In the glaucomatous eye, the optic disc is bleached and optic cupping is present. (Note the appearance of the retinal vessels, which travel over the edge of the optic cup and appear to dip into it.) (From Lewis SL, Bucher L, Heitkemper MM, et al: *Medical-surgical nursing: Assessment and management of clinical problems,* ed 10, St. Louis, 2017, Mosby.)

Clinical Manifestations

In POAG the patient has no signs or symptoms during the early stages of the disease. As the symptoms become apparent, they include loss of peripheral vision (tunnel vision), eye pain, difficulty adjusting to darkness, halos around lights, and inability to detect colors. The IOP is elevated.

AACG produces excruciating pain in or around the eye, decreased vision, and nausea and vomiting. The sclera is erythematous, and the pupil is enlarged and fixed. The patient sees colored halos around lights and has an acute increase in IOP.

Optic disc cupping occurs as glaucoma progresses. This is visible by direct or indirect ophthalmoscopy. The optic disc becomes wider, deeper, and paler (light gray or white). Optic disc cupping may be one of the first signs of chronic open-angle glaucoma. Optic disc photographs are useful for comparison over time to demonstrate an increase in the cup-to-disc ratio and progressive blanching (Fig. 53.13).

Assessment

Collection of subjective data includes noting the time of day that eye pain occurs. Also assess frequency, intensity, and duration of the pain. Note complaints of peripheral vision loss, maladaptation to darkness, and halos seen around lights. Determine the severity of headaches and the presence of nausea and vomiting.

Collection of objective data includes noting a need for frequent eyeglass prescription changes. Elevated IOP is also present.

Diagnostic Tests

Tonometry is used to determine intraocular pressure (see Fig. 53.5). A patient with glaucoma tests above the normal range of 10 to 22 mm Hg. Intraocular pressure is usually between 22 and 32 mm Hg in POAG. IOP may be 50 mm Hg or higher in AACG. Visual field studies show a decline in the patient's peripheral vision. Optic disc cupping occurs as glaucoma progresses and will lead to optic nerve damage over time.

Medical Management

Keeping the intraocular pressure low enough to prevent the patient from developing optic nerve damage is the primary focus of glaucoma therapy.

POAG is treated medically by the use of beta blockers, **miotics** (agents that cause the pupil to constrict), and carbonic anhydrase inhibitors (Table 53.4). A beta blocker, such as betaxolol hydrochloride (Betoptic), reduces IOP. Miotics, such as pilocarpine, constrict the pupil and draw the iris away from the cornea, allowing aqueous humor to drain out of the canal of Schlemm (see Fig. 53.12). Carbonic anhydrase inhibitors, such as acetazolamide (Diamox), decrease the production of aqueous humor, which results in lower intraocular pressures. Surgery, which consists of a trabeculectomy or laser trabeculoplasty, is done when medications alone fail to

Table 53.4 **Medications for Eye Disorders**

GENERIC NAME (TRADE NAME)	ACTION AND USE	SIDE EFFECTS	NURSING IMPLICATIONS
acetazolamide (Diamox)	Lowers intraocular pressure; used for open-angle glaucoma	Diarrhea, weakness, discomfort, urinary frequency, loss of appetite, nausea, vomiting, numbness in hands; contraindicated with severe renal, hepatic, or adrenocortical impairment	Know pregnancy and lactation cautions; give with food; in diabetes, it may increase blood and urine glucose levels; caution patient about drowsiness; monitor intake and output (I&O) and weight daily
betaxolol hydrochloride (Betoptic)	Beta-adrenergic blocking agent that reduces formation of aqueous humor; used for open-angle glaucoma	Insomnia, irritation of eyelids, stinging on instillation, occasional tears, photophobia, systemic effects include possible disorientation, bradycardia, weakness, dyspnea	Know pregnancy cautions; do not touch dropper on eye; keep container tightly closed; determine intraocular pressure 4 wk after treatment; use cautiously in patients with history of heart failure or with diabetes mellitus
cyclopentolate hydrochloride (Cyclogyl)	Anticholinergic drug that produces dilation of pupil and temporary paralysis of ciliary muscles; used in glaucoma; a diagnostic agent for angle-closure glaucomas	Ataxia, behavioral disturbances, tachycardia, disorientation, fever	Prevent contamination of dropper; warn patient of increased sensitivity to light and suggest sunglasses; contraindicated in angle closure glaucoma; use cautiously in older adults
dexamethasone	Decreases inflammation	Local irritation, retardation of corneal healing, blurred vision, eye pain, secondary eye infection	It may mask infection; use only for short term in children; tell patient not to wear contact lens during treatment; shake bottle before using; check with health care practitioner before using for future eye conditions; check with health care practitioner if condition does not improve in 5–7 days
gentamicin sulfate	Bactericidal antibiotic; used for treatment of blepharitis and conjunctivitis	Pruritus, erythema, edema, ocular discomfort, blurred vision (may occur for a few minutes after application)	Comply with full course of therapy; if no improvement occurs after a few days, check with health care practitioner
mannitol (Osmitrol)	Osmotic diuretic that reduces intraocular pressure; used for glaucoma	Fluid and electrolyte imbalance, chest pain, tachycardia, chills and fever, difficult urination	Administer by intravenous infusion; know pregnancy caution; duration of action is 1–3 h; monitor vital signs at least hourly and I&O, weight, and potassium levels daily
pilocarpine hydrochloride (Isopto Carpine)	Reduces intraocular pressure; used for open-angle glaucoma	Muscle tremors, nausea and vomiting, dyspnea, wheezing, bronchial spasms, local irritation	Encourage patient to have periodic intraocular pressure determinations; monitor for blurred vision or changes in vision; use cautiously in bronchial asthma and hypertension; apply light finger pressure on lacrimal sac 1 min after instillation of drops
polyvinyl alcohol (Liquifilm Forte)	Tearlike lubricant; used for dry eyes and eye irritations	Headache, burning, blurred vision, eye pain	Teach patient to instill; to avoid contamination of solution, warn patient not to touch tip of container to eye

Continued

Table 53.4 Medications for Eye Disorders—cont'd

GENERIC NAME (TRADE NAME)	ACTION AND USE	SIDE EFFECTS	NURSING IMPLICATIONS
sulfacetamide sodium	Broad-spectrum bacteriostatic antiinfective agent used in the treatment of ocular infections (conjunctivitis, corneal ulcers, trachoma, and chlamydial infections)	Pruritus, edema, erythema, other eye irritations	It is contraindicated in those with sulfonamide hypersensitivity; purulent exudate may inactivate drug; do not use silver preparations concurrently; encourage patient to comply with full course of treatment; store properly; discard solution if it discolors; warn patient to avoid sharing washcloths and towels with family members
timolol maleate (Timoptic)	Beta-adrenergic blocking agent that reduces aqueous humor formation; used for open-angle glaucoma and hypertension; used with caution for patients who have heart conditions	Ocular sensitivity, severe irritation of eye or eyelid, systemic effects include cardiac failure, chest pain, disorientation, diarrhea, dizziness, exacerbation of asthma	It may mask hypoglycemia; measure intraocular pressure after 4 wk of treatment; avoid abrupt cessation; use cautiously in patients with bronchial asthma and heart conditions; know pregnancy and breastfeeding cautions; keep container tightly closed

control intraocular pressure. *Trabeculectomy* is the removal of corneoscleral tissue, usually the canal of Schlemm and trabecular meshwork. This produces an increase in the outflow of aqueous humor. Laser trabeculoplasty produces openings in the trabecular meshwork.

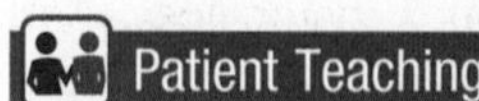

Patient Teaching

Glaucoma

- Regular medical and ophthalmic care is required for the rest of the patient's life.
- Eyedrops *must* be continued as long as prescribed even in the absence of symptoms; typically treatment is lifelong.
- Blurred vision decreases with prolonged use.
- Avoid driving for 1 to 2 hours after administration of miotics.
- To prevent complications:
  - Press lacrimal duct for 1 minute after eyedrop application to prevent rapid systemic absorption.
  - Keep reserve bottles of eyedrops at home.
  - Carry eyedrops when away from home.
  - Carry a card listing glaucoma as a diagnosis and the eyedrop solution prescribed.
  - There is no apparent relationship between vascular hypertension and ocular hypertension.
  - Report any reappearance of symptoms immediately to the health care provider.
  - If admitted to the hospital, alert the staff of the continued need for prescribed eyedrops.
  - Avoid the use of mydriatic or cycloplegic drugs (e.g., atropine) that dilate the pupils.

Medical marijuana use has become an increasingly popular option for reducing the intraocular pressures associated with glaucoma. However, the effects of marijuana decrease IOP only for short time periods, typically 3 to 4 hours. For the patient to receive the benefits of consistently decreased IOPs with medical marijuana, the patient would have to consume the treatment six to eight times a day. Using medical marijuana at such a high frequency may leave the patient too impaired to lead an active lifestyle. The patient should be urged to consult with his or her health care provider concerning the use of both prescription and over-the-counter medications to avoid drug-related increases in IOP.

AACG is treated medically with osmotic diuretics, such as mannitol, carbonic anhydrase inhibitors, and miotics. Surgical treatments include peripheral iridectomy or iridotomy. Peripheral iridectomy is the surgical removal of part of the iris. The procedure is performed with the patient under local anesthesia. This procedure often restores drainage of the aqueous humor. Iridotomy is an incision into the iris of the eye to create an opening for aqueous flow; this is done under local or general anesthesia. Postoperatively, observe the patient for signs and symptoms of local hemorrhage, excessive or uncontrolled pain, and signs of excessive drainage from the eye.

Nursing Interventions and Patient Teaching

Nursing interventions involve protecting the patient's safety, monitoring compliance with therapy, and reinforcing discharge instructions. Depending on the practice setting, educate individual patients and families, groups of patients, or entire communities about the risks of glaucoma. In teaching, identify the increased incidence of glaucoma that occurs with age and the need for regular comprehensive ophthalmic examinations. Stress the importance of early detection and treatment in preventing long-term visual impairment. The current recommendation is for an ophthalmologic examination every 2 to 4 years for people between 40 and 64 years of age, and every 1 to 2 years for people 65 years of age or older. African Americans in every age group should have more frequent examinations because of the increased incidence and more aggressive nature of glaucoma in this patient population.

Glaucoma is a chronic condition requiring close observation for changes in condition. Follow-up care is needed to ensure that visual loss does not take place. The prescribed therapeutic regimen must be presented clearly to the patient and significant other(s). The implications of nonadherence must be addressed (see the Patient Teaching box for glaucoma). Information to be provided includes medication therapies, follow-up care, and signs and symptoms to report. Teach the patient about the purpose, frequency, and technique for administering prescribed medications. In addition to verbal instructions, give all patients written instructions that contain the information provided.

Prognosis

Today's method of medical and surgical management provides the patient with an excellent prognosis for a full recovery. Complications are few if care is obtained early in the course of the condition. When the patient ignores glaucoma or is noncompliant with therapy, blindness may occur. Regular eye examinations are required to detect and monitor for increased intraocular pressure. In general, once damage has occurred, the condition is irreversible. Surgery and medication can help lessen the complications from glaucoma.

CORNEAL INJURIES

Etiology and Pathophysiology

The cornea is composed of five layers of tissue and is uniform in nature. The cornea is nonvascular; therefore no bleeding occurs from injury unless subcorneal structures are involved. The cornea is kept moist by tear production and is protected from daily insult by the eyelid. Any wound to the cornea can decrease the level of transparency, through scar formation.

Corneal injuries include the following:

- Foreign bodies
- Burns: chemical or thermal
- Abrasions and lacerations
- Penetrating wounds

Foreign bodies are the most common cause of corneal injury. Dust particles, propellants, and eyelashes may lodge in the conjunctiva or cornea. Blinking and tearing help to clear the irritant, but further irritation may occur from the upper lid, closing and moving the foreign body into deeper layers or over a wider area of the cornea.

Burns occur in the home and workplace. When burns affect the eye, it is a medical emergency. Burns are classified as chemical burns or thermal burns. Depending on what has caused a burn, the damage may be superficial or deep; regardless, it is essential to seek immediate emergency care after an exposure. Chemical irritants such as acids, alkalis, and metal flashes from acetylene blowtorches cause significant pain, depending on the depth of chemical erosion.

Abrasions and lacerations are usually superficial scratches caused by fingernails or clothing. They may be painful, depending on the depth of the abrasion.

Penetrating wounds are the most serious corneal injuries. Eye structures may be injured permanently, resulting in total blindness. Infection may result from the introduction of microorganisms on the penetrating object.

Clinical Manifestations

Foreign bodies produce pain when the eye moves or the eyelid moves over the eye during blinking. Excessive tearing, erythema of the conjunctiva, and pruritus may occur. Acute pain and burning are the primary symptoms with any topical (surface) burn to the eye. Abrasions and lacerations produce mild to severe pain, depending on the depth of corneal involvement. The pain may be transitory and slight, or spasmodic and deep. Penetrating wounds result in varying degrees of pain. If underlying structures are involved, pain may be absent because the nerves have been severed.

Assessment

Foreign bodies. Subjective data include the time and type of exposure or injury. Assess the patient for the degree and severity of eye pain and vision loss. Ask about any first aid treatment provided. Objective data include observation of the foreign body and extent of damage. When the intracapsular area has been penetrated, fluids leak from the affected eye.

Burns. Subjective data include the degree of pain. It is important to assess the type of burn, thermal or chemical; the type of chemical exposure that caused the burn; and any first aid treatment that has been provided. Visual losses will be determined after examination by the health care professional.

Collection of objective data includes noting the extent of the burn in and around the eye, including eyelashes and eyebrows, and assessing the general condition of the eye and surrounding structures.

Abrasions and lacerations. Subjective data include the degree of pain after the incident and how the injury occurred. Note treatments used at the time of injury.

Collection of objective data includes assessing the degree of damage to the eye and surrounding structures and noting any vision loss.

Penetrating wounds. Subjective data include the duration of exposure and causative factors related to the injury. Assess the presence and severity of pain. Determine whether any first aid treatment was given.

Objective data include the type and size of the penetrating object. Note any fluid leakage from the eye and damage to surrounding structures.

Diagnostic Tests

Tests include visual and ophthalmoscopic examination, fluorescein staining, peripheral vision tests, and slit-lamp examination.

Medical Management

Foreign bodies are treated medically with a flush of normal saline when the object is near the sclera and conjunctiva; it then can be removed by a clean swab or tissue. Cotton is not used, because it may scratch the cornea. If the object is not flushed away easily, the individual must see an ophthalmologist to have the object removed. Antibiotic topical eye ointments are ordered.

Burns are treated medically with a 20-minute or longer normal saline flush immediately after burn exposure; this helps to prevent scar formation and subsequent loss of vision. Separate the eyelids while flushing the affected eye to ensure maximum irrigation. Thermal or chemical burns of the eye and surrounding eye structures are an emergency problem and require immediate medical treatment and examination by an ophthalmologist. After examination by an ophthalmologist, the patient with an eye burn may be prescribed topical antimicrobial medications.

Abrasions and lacerations of the eye are cleaned medically or flushed with a normal saline (0.9 NaCl) solution by the health care professional. Antibiotic therapy, usually topical, may be prescribed after injury (see the Safety Alert box).

Seek medical assistance immediately for eye injuries, burns, and foreign bodies that remain in the eye. Immediately after a penetrating wound injury, both eyes should be covered while the patient is transported to the hospital. Both eyes work in synchrony, so covering the unaffected eye prevents it from involuntarily moving with the other eye. A shield reduces further injury but must not touch the foreign object. A Styrofoam cup provides adequate coverage and is usually readily available. The foreign object should not be removed except by the ophthalmologist or surgeon after examination.

Nursing Interventions and Patient Teaching

Nursing interventions for foreign bodies include assisting with the required irrigation of the eye. For burns, assist with the flushing process and providing eye medications as ordered. For abrasions and lacerations, assist with cleaning the eye as ordered and providing general first aid.

When a patient has a penetrating wound, note whether the pupil on the affected side has become irregular in size. This results when the iris of the affected eye moves to occlude the wound area. Infection potential is high; therefore topical and systemic antibiotics are ordered. If the wound is small, there may not be a need for surgical intervention. If the wound is large or deep, enucleation of the eye may be necessary.

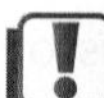
Safety Alert

Eye Safety Measures

- Do not rinse eyes with unprescribed solutions.
- Discard any ophthalmic solution that is cloudy, discolored, contains particles, or that has been open for longer than 3 months.
- Do not self-treat an eye inflammation with a medication prescribed for a previous eye disorder.
- To avoid eye strain:
  - Use a good light for reading or doing work that requires careful visual focus.
  - When reading or focusing eyes for long periods, look at distant objects for a few minutes at repeated intervals to rest eyes.
- Avoid rubbing the eyes.
- Wash hands before and after touching the eyes.
- Wear safety glasses when engaging in activities that could injure the eyes. If injury occurs, seek immediate medical attention.
- Wear dark glasses for prolonged exposure to bright light (prolonged daylight exposure, activities in the snow, or on the water).
- Flush eyes immediately for 15 to 20 minutes or longer with cool water when any irritating substances are introduced. The Morgan lens traditionally is used to flush the eye in emergency cases (Fig. 53.14).
- Do not attempt to remove foreign bodies from the cornea; cover the eye with an eye shield (e.g., Styrofoam cup) to prevent excessive movement or touching of the eye. Seek medical attention immediately.
- If a speck of dust blows into the eye, pull the upper lid over the lower lid and let the tears wash the speck to the inner canthus (corner of the eye) or lower lid, where it may be removed safely. Irrigate the eye with cool tap water, if necessary.
- Eye makeup should be replaced every 3 months and with every eye infection to prevent the growth of bacteria or reinfection.
- Never share eye makeup, and when sampling makeup in stores use only fresh applicators and samples that have not been contaminated by multiple users. (The safest choice is to avoid store samples altogether.)

Effective and immediate therapy is crucial for any eye injury. If treatment is interrupted, ineffective, or not sustained, permanent eye damage will occur. The most frequent complications include infection, vision disturbances, and blindness. A patient problem for the patient with an eye injury will be *Recent Onset of Pain, related to inflammatory processes secondary to trauma or injury*. (See the preceding discussion on conjunctivitis.)

Ensure that the patient can apply ointments and dressings, if ordered. Instruct the patient in the use of other therapy devices, such as warm or cool compresses as needed. Teach proper handwashing techniques. The patient should wear dark sunglasses if cycloplegic or mydriatic eyedrops are used. Instruct the patient to avoid future exposures to chemical or environmental hazards. Ensure that the patient understands the discharge instructions, including the need for follow-up

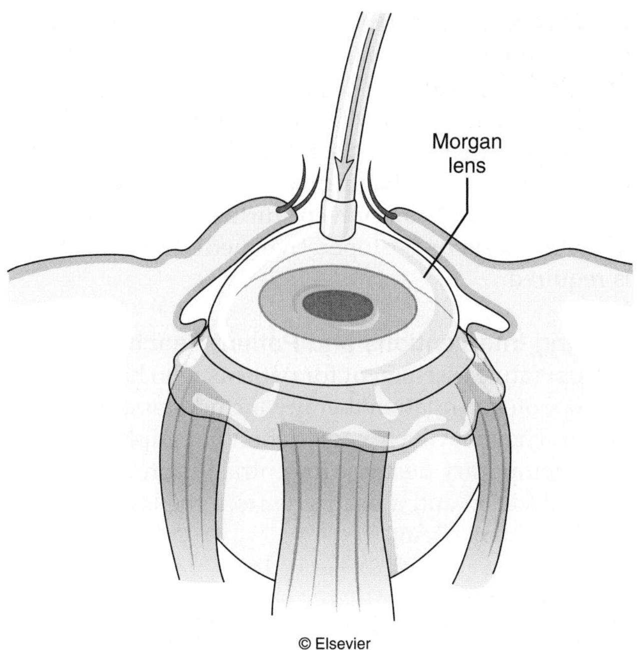

Fig. 53.14 The Morgan lens used to flush the eye in an emergency.

provider visits and symptoms to report. Determine the patient's knowledge about therapy, treatment, and the patient's ability to perform the necessary steps to care for his or her injury.

Prognosis

Immediate and appropriate treatment reduces the severity and complications of eye injuries. Superficial corneal abrasions usually heal without incident. Deeper abrasions or burns may result in permanent visual loss because of scarring.

SURGERIES OF THE EYE

ENUCLEATION

Enucleation of the eye is the surgical removal of the eyeball. It is often necessary after severe eye trauma but may be done because of other complications, such as malignant tumors. During the enucleation, an implant is inserted into the eye socket; this will allow the patient to have a prosthetic eye fitted and placed once the surgical wound has healed.

Nursing Interventions and Patient Teaching

The loss of an eye is extremely traumatic for the patient. Electing to have the procedure performed presents the patient with a difficult decision. The patient normally grieves the loss of the eye. The enucleation results in a life-altering change in appearance. There are concerns related to functionality, lost vision, and social implications (i.e., how others will perceive the patient). Priorities for care by the nurse include emotional support, open communication, and honest provision of information. Other nursing responsibilities include facilitating a therapeutic dialogue between the health care provider and the patient regarding the exact nature of the surgery and the expected course of therapy after the enucleation.

Postoperatively, apply a pressure dressing over the socket of the eye to control hemorrhage. Observe the dressing at least every hour for the first 24 hours. The recovery period includes a protective eye patch that will be worn for days to weeks after surgery. Ask the patient about any pain on the affected side of the head or any headache, which may indicate hemorrhage or infection. Report these findings to the health care provider immediately. Avoid routine postoperative procedures of coughing and turning onto the affected side to prevent sutures from dislodging or hemorrhage. The wound is healed adequately approximately 6 weeks after enucleation. An ocularist creates a prosthetic eye that fits the orbital socket and is designed to match the remaining eye. The patient must be educated in how to remove, cleanse, and insert the prosthesis carefully. Continued monitoring of the socket is necessary to ensure proper fit of the prosthesis, because changes, including atrophy of the socket, may occur.

KERATOPLASTY (CORNEAL TRANSPLANT)

Keratoplasty is the removal of the full thickness of the patient's cornea followed by surgical implantation of a cornea from a human donor. It is done to replace a damaged cornea resulting from trauma, ulceration, or congenital deformities. Keratoplasty is performed with the patient under local or general anesthesia. The transplanted tissue is sutured into place to maintain graft alignment and a watertight wound.

Approximately 40,000 corneal transplants are performed in the United States each year. Improved methods of tissue procurement and preservation, refined surgical techniques, postoperative topical corticosteroids, and careful follow up have decreased graft rejection. Immunosuppressants, medications that suppress the immune system and prevent rejection (e.g., cyclosporine), may be ordered postoperatively.

Corneal grafts usually are taken from the organ donor within 4 hours of death. An ideal donor is between 25 and 35 years of age who died from traumatic injury or an acute disease process. The corneas of people with chronic or communicable diseases—such as hepatitis, acquired immunodeficiency syndrome, or cancer—are not appropriate for transplantation. The eye bank will test donors for human immunodeficiency virus and hepatitis B and C. The donor's eye should have normal light perception and projection. The donor's tissue is best used within 5 days after removal.

Responsibilities of the nurse in a potential organ donation case are to notify the appropriate supervisory personnel and other agencies as directed by policy.

Nursing Interventions and Patient Teaching

Before surgery, encourage the patient to ask questions and express concerns related to the surgery. Teach the patient about the use of protective eyeglasses if a dilation-causing eye medication is to be used. Clean and prepare the surgical areas as ordered, usually with an antiseptic solution. Preoperative patient teaching includes deep breathing and turning to reduce any complications associated with surgery. Coughing is discouraged, because damage can occur to the surgical site. Maintain dietary restrictions, if ordered, and administer prescribed medications.

After surgery, ensure that correct postoperative positioning is maintained; the patient usually is positioned on the back or on the nonoperative side. The health care provider should provide specific orders for activity limitations and care of the surgical site postoperatively. Use safety measures, including adequate lighting, clear paths, and orientation to unfamiliar environments, until the patient is able to ambulate safely. Prevent injuries by providing safety devices and orienting the patient to each new environment in the postoperative period. Anyone coming into the room should announce his or her presence. The patient should avoid bending, lifting, and straining for approximately 1 month to prevent increases in intraocular pressure or suture tension.

Reinforce the scheduled postoperative visits with the eye surgeon and other eye health care providers. Report any severe or progressive pain to the surgeon immediately, as well as any complaints of erythema, loss of vision, or photophobia that would occur with corneal rejection. Administer systemic and ophthalmic medications as prescribed. Maintain strict surgical asepsis during dressing changes. Staff, the patient, and the family must wash hands thoroughly before any contact with the eye area. Instruct the patient to avoid the use of irritants, including fragrant powders, perfumes, or eye makeup that may cause irritation, sneezing, or coughing and subsequent displacement of sutures. The patient should not rub the eye area to avoid contaminating the site or displacing sutures. Assess the patient's diversion activities; television usually is permitted, but reading is limited because the side-to-side movement of the eyes may loosen the sutures. If an eye patch or metal eyecup shield is ordered, demonstrate how to use and care for the device. The eye patch is applied snugly to inhibit the blink reflex and allow the eye to rest. The metal eye shield is used at night to protect the eye from trauma. Obtain discharge instructions from the health care provider regarding use of protective eyewear.

Prognosis

Because the cornea is avascular, healing is slow, and the incidence of infection is increased. Rejection of the donor tissue may occur. Teaching the patient and family to recognize the signs and symptoms of rejection is an essential part of the discharge planning.

PHOTOCOAGULATION

Photocoagulation is a nonsurgical procedure usually performed on an outpatient basis. A small, intense beam of light is directed into a small spot on the retina. The light converts to heat energy, and coagulation of tissue protein occurs. The structures of the eye remain undisturbed and only the sealing of leaks and destruction of offending tissue occur. The procedure is used to manage conditions such as ARMD and diabetic retinopathy.

Photocoagulation is useful in diabetic retinopathy to cauterize hemorrhaging vessels. It cannot increase visual acuity but can prevent further loss. Usually no hospitalization or postoperative medical management is required.

Nursing Interventions and Patient Teaching

Postoperative assessment for patients who have undergone photocoagulation therapy includes assessment of vision. They may have constriction of peripheral fields and a temporary decrease in central vision. A decrease in night vision and a headache from the laser's bright light also may occur.

Prognosis

Photocoagulation is used to prevent eye damage and is not curative. Minimal destruction of tissue occurs with photocoagulation. The procedure is nonsurgical; therefore infection risk is minimal.

VITRECTOMY

A **vitrectomy** is the removal of excess vitreous fluid caused by hemorrhage and replacement with normal saline. The procedure allows for the removal of any existing scar tissue. The procedure is done to manage eye conditions such as retinal detachment, macular holes, and vitreous hemorrhage.

Postoperative management includes the application of topical eye medication for 4 to 6 weeks. Analgesics are prescribed for postoperative pain management. A pressure patch for the operative eye is placed immediately after surgery. Cold compresses may be used to reduce inflammation.

Nursing Interventions and Patient Teaching

The patient is required to lay on his or her abdomen or to sit forward, resting the nonoperative side of the head on a table, to allow air that is in the eye to float against the retina. This position is maintained for 4 to 5 days.

Dark glasses are prescribed postoperatively to decrease the discomfort of photophobia. Postoperative care includes assessing the eye patch; applying cold packs; monitoring vital signs, especially for fever; and assessing the dressing for bleeding.

ANATOMY AND PHYSIOLOGY OF THE EAR

The external ear *(pinna,* or *auricle)* reveals only a portion of the complex organ of hearing. Within the ear are many structures that enable hearing and interpretation of sound and assist in maintaining equilibrium (balance). Anatomically, from the external structures to the internal structures, the ear has three distinct divisions: the external ear, the middle ear, and the inner ear (Fig.

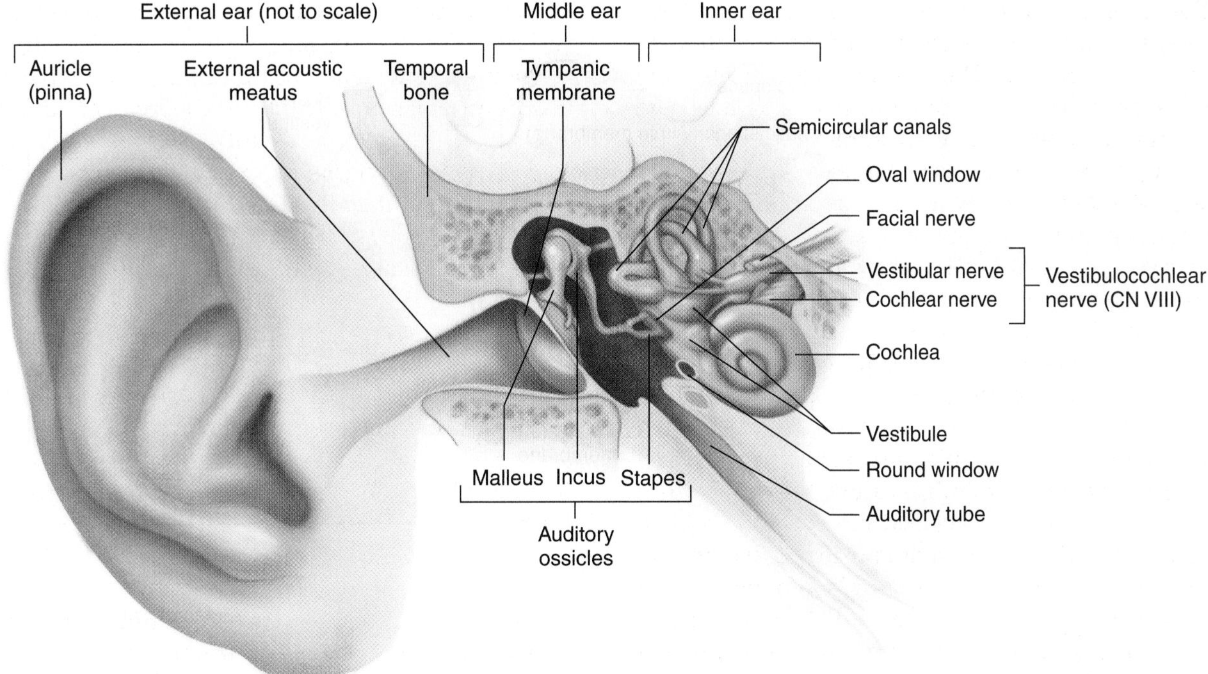

Fig. 53.15 External, middle, and inner ear (not to scale). (From Patton KT, Thibodeau GA: *The human body in health and disease*, ed 7, St. Louis, 2018, Elsevier.)

53.15). The external ear and the middle ear deal exclusively with sound waves, whereas the inner ear deals with sound waves and equilibrium.

EXTERNAL EAR

The external ear is composed of the auricle (pinna) and the external auditory canal. The canal is shaped like a small, curved tube (about 1 inch [2.5 cm] in length). It extends into the temporal bone, ending at the *tympanic membrane*—a thin, semitransparent membrane. The tympanic membrane separates the external ear from the middle ear and transmits sound vibrations to the internal ear by means of the auditory ossicles. The external ear is designed to collect sound waves and channel them to the middle ear. The upper part of the pinna is composed of elastic cartilage, whereas the lower part, the lobe, is mainly fleshy tissue. The whole structure is attached to the skull by ligaments and muscles.

The walls of the external auditory canal are composed of cartilage-lined bone. The external auditory canal contains cilia (fine hairs) and specialized sebaceous glands called *ceruminous glands* that secrete cerumen (earwax). Together the cilia and cerumen protect the lining and inner ear from foreign bodies and potential sources of obstruction or infection.

MIDDLE EAR

The middle ear, or tympanic cavity, is a small, air-filled chamber located within the temporal bone. The *eustachian tube,* or auditory tube, is lined with a mucous membrane that joins the nasopharynx and the middle-ear cavity. During swallowing or yawning, the tube allows air to enter the middle ear, which equalizes the air pressure on either side of the tympanic membrane. Because the pharynx, the eustachian tube, and the middle ear are covered with a continuous mucous membrane, bacteria and viruses can travel easily from the throat to the middle ear. This often is seen in young children, in whom the eustachian tube is more level, making drainage difficult. The posterior wall of the middle ear opens into the mastoid process, an area filled with air spaces, which also aids in equalizing air pressure. Infection of the middle ear, if untreated, can spread to the mastoid process.

Extending along the middle-ear chamber are three small bones (ossicles) that carry sound waves from the external ear to the inner ear. These ossicles are named according to their shape: the *malleus* (hammer), the *incus* (anvil), and the *stapes* (stirrup). The internal surface of the tympanic membrane is connected to the first of these three bones, the malleus. The malleus transfers sound waves to the incus, which in turn transfers them to the stapes. The stapes pushes against the oval window, a small membrane that marks the beginning of the inner ear. When sound waves cause the tympanic membrane to vibrate, that vibration is transmitted and amplified by the ear ossicles as it passes through the middle ear. Movement of the stapes against the oval window causes movement of fluid in the inner ear.

INNER EAR

The *labyrinth* is a series of canals making up the inner ear (Fig. 53.16). Structurally, it consists of the bony

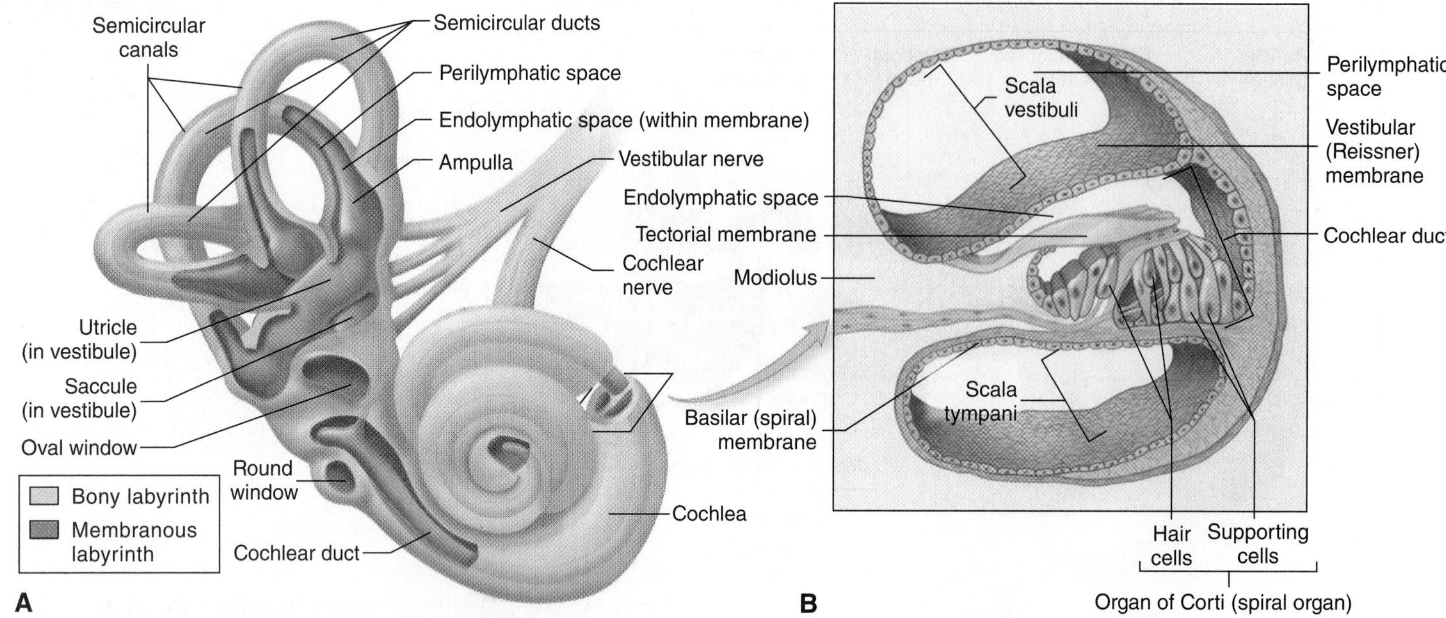

Fig. 53.16 The inner ear. A, The bony labyrinth is the hard outer wall of the entire inner ear and includes semicircular canals, the vestibule, and the cochlea. Within the bony labyrinth is the membranous labyrinth *(purple)*, which is surrounded by perilymph and filled with endolymph. Each ampulla in the vestibule contains a crista ampullaris that detects changes in head position and sends sensory impulses through the vestibular nerve to the brain. B, A section of the membranous cochlea. Hair cells in the organ of Corti detect sound and send the information through the cochlear nerve. Then vestibular and cochlear nerves join to form the eighth cranial nerve. (From Patton KT, Thibodeau GA: *The human body in health and disease*, ed 7, St. Louis, 2018, Elsevier.)

labyrinth, which is filled with a fluid called *perilymph.* The bony labyrinth has three subdivisions called the *semicircular canal* (associated with the sense of balance), the *vestibule,* and the *cochlea.* The membranous labyrinth is a series of sacs and tubes that contain a thicker fluid called *endolymph.* Endolymph and perilymph conduct sound waves through the inner-ear system.

The cochlea resembles a snail's shell and contains the *organ of Corti,* known as the organ of hearing. It contains many fine hair cell receptors, which respond to sound waves by stimulating the cochlear nerve (a branch of the eighth cranial nerve—the vestibulocochlear, or acoustic nerve), which transmits the message to the brain. These hair cells may become damaged over time from noise pollution (i.e., high-intensity sounds such as those produced by jet engines, factory equipment, and rock bands). Once these cells are damaged or destroyed, hearing becomes permanently impaired.

Deeper in the inner ear, past the cochlea, lies an oval central portion of the bony labyrinth known as the *vestibule.* The vestibule contains receptors that respond to gravity and provides information on which way is up and which way is down, enabling an individual to remain in an upright position. Extending upward from the vestibule are three semicircular canals responsible for maintaining balance and equilibrium. These canals contain sensory hair cells and endolymph. The motion of the endolymph stimulates the hair cells, which in turn stimulate the receptors to send the message to the brain for interpretation (see Fig. 53.16).

NURSING CONSIDERATIONS FOR CARE OF THE PATIENT WITH AN EAR DISORDER

Once the history and general assessment have been completed, focus on assessment of the ear. Additional information would include the following:

- Occurrence of ear drainage, tinnitus, vertigo, cerumen buildup, pressures, pain, and pruritus
- Other medical diagnoses that may affect hearing
- Family history
- Exposure to loud noises
- Behavioral clues indicating hearing loss (Box 53.2)
- History of medications use, specifically those known to be ototoxic
- Current medications for an ear disorder
- Side effects of medications, if any
- Associated speech pattern abnormalities
- Use of assistive hearing devices
- Use of home remedies that cause ear trauma

Communicate the gathered data to the appropriate personnel and document the findings in the patient record. The next step in the assessment process is to prepare the patient for the initial otoscopic diagnostic evaluation.

Box 53.2 Behavioral Clues Indicating Hearing Loss

Any adult who:

- Is irritable, hostile, and hypersensitive in interpersonal relations
- Has difficulty hearing upper-frequency consonants
- Complains about people mumbling
- Turns up volume on television and radio
- Asks for frequent repetition and answers questions inappropriately
- Loses sense of humor, becomes grim
- Leans forward to hear better; face becomes serious and strained
- Shuns large- and small-group audience situations
- May appear aloof and uninterested
- Complains of ringing in the ears
- Has an unusually soft or loud voice
- Repeatedly asks, "What did you say?"

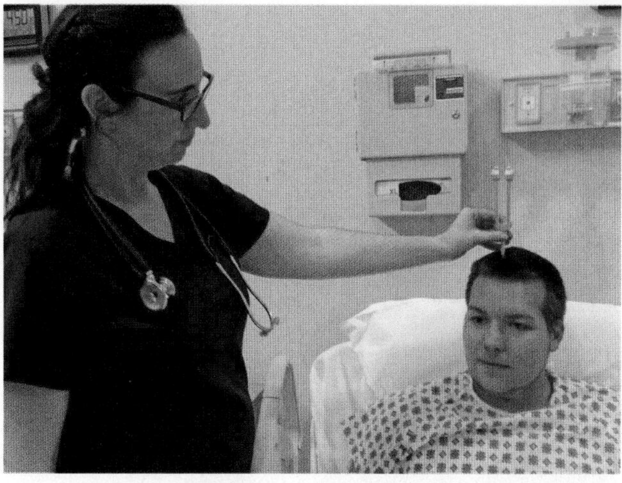

Fig. 53.17 The Weber tuning fork test.

LABORATORY AND DIAGNOSTIC EXAMINATIONS

OTOSCOPY

With an otoscope the examiner can visualize the external auditory canal and the tympanic membrane. Normally the tympanic membrane is disk shaped and pearl pale pink. Otoscopy is the initial examination of the ear, performed before other testing. One of the nurse's responsibilities is to explain to the patient the purpose and procedure. Reassure the patient that otoscopy is a painless test requiring only about 1 to 2 minutes, with slight pulling of the ear upward and backward for an adult and down and back for a child.

WHISPERED VOICE TEST

General screening regarding the patient's ability to hear can occur with tests using the whispered and spoken voice. The examiner stands 12 to 24 inches (30 to 60 cm) to the side of the patient and speaks simple one- and two-syllable words in a low whisper. The patient is asked to repeat the words or information given. The examiner increases volume until the patient responds appropriately. Test each ear, with the patient covering the other ear. An accuracy of 50% is considered normal.

TUNING FORK TESTS

The two most common tests using tuning forks are the Weber test and the Rinne test. These tests are used to determine hearing loss and collect data related to the type of loss.

- *Weber test:* The *Weber test* is a method of assessing auditory acuity, especially useful in determining whether defective hearing in an ear is a conductive loss caused by a middle-ear problem or a sensorineural loss, resulting from a disorder in the inner ear or auditory nerve system. The test is performed by placing the stem of a vibrating tuning fork in the center of the patient's forehead or on the maxillary incisors. The sound is equally loud in both ears if hearing is normal. If the person has a sensorineural loss in one ear, the unaffected ear perceives the sound as louder. When conductive hearing loss is present, the sound is louder in the affected ear. The patient does not hear ordinary background noise conducted through the air and receives only vibrations by bone conduction (Fig. 53.17).
- *Rinne test:* The *Rinne test* is a method of distinguishing conductive from sensorineural hearing loss. The test is performed with tuning forks placed ½ inch (1.25 cm) from the external auditory meatus and the vibrating stem placed over the mastoid bone. While one ear is tested, the other is masked (Fig. 53.18). In sensorineural loss the sound is heard longer by air conduction, whereas in conductive hearing loss the sound is heard longer by bone conduction.

Nursing responsibility in the Weber test and the Rinne test includes explanation of the purpose and procedure of the tests. Stress that the patient needs to concentrate and use hand signals to indicate the ear in which the sound is heard in the Weber test and when it is no longer heard in the Rinne test. These tests can be performed in a few minutes and are painless and noninvasive measures.

AUDIOMETRIC TESTING

Audiometry is a test of hearing acuity. Audiometry is beneficial as a diagnostic test for determining the degree and type of hearing loss and as a screening test for hearing acuity. Various audiometric tests determine the lowest intensity of sound at which an individual can perceive auditory stimulus (hearing threshold), hear different frequencies, and distinguish different speech tones.

Nursing responsibilities include explaining the purpose and procedure of each test and reviewing any required responses by the patient.

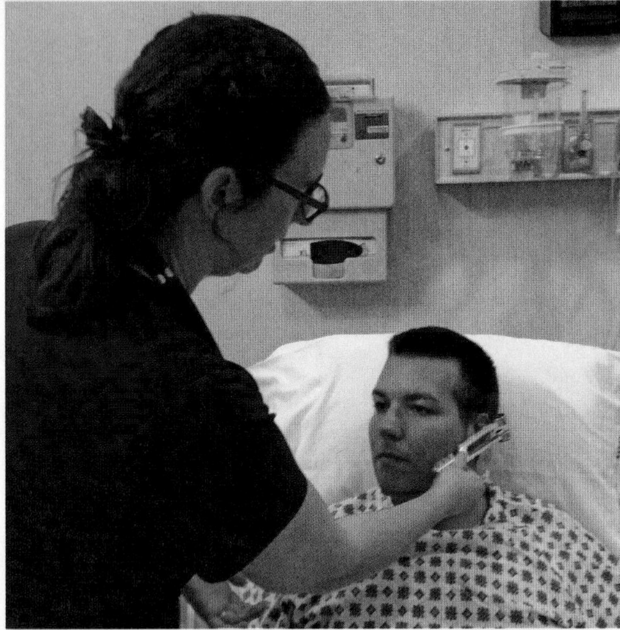

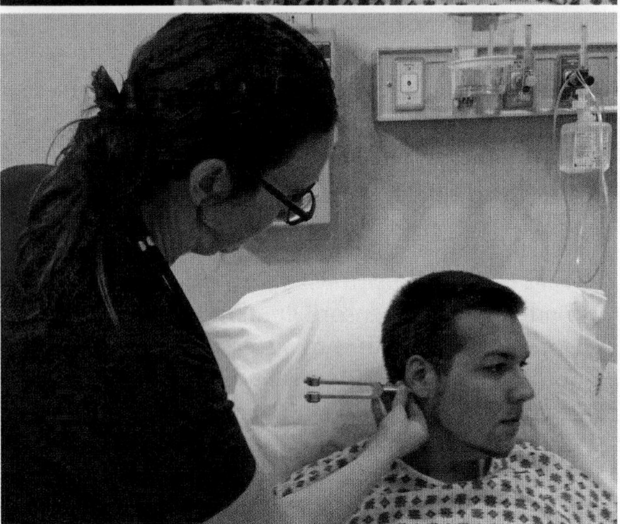

Fig. 53.18 The Rinne tuning fork test.

VESTIBULAR TESTING

The auditory and vestibular (balance and equilibrium) systems are closely related. Appropriate diagnosis depends on close observation of the patient's signs and symptoms to ascertain if they are related to balance or hearing loss. Ask the patient to describe the signs and symptoms that he or she is experiencing in accurate detail through the interview portion of the history.

Problems of the vestibular system may manifest as nystagmus or vertigo. *Nystagmus* is involuntary, rhythmic movements of the eye. The movements may be horizontal, vertical, rotary, or mixed (*Mosby's Dictionary of Medicine, Nursing, & Health Professions*, 2013). The sensation that the person or objects are moving or spinning is referred to as **vertigo.** Moving the head in any direction further heightens this feeling of vertigo. The Romberg and past-point tests are used for patients complaining of dizziness or disequilibrium.

- *Romberg test:* The *Romberg test* measures the patient's ability to perform specific tasks with eyes open and then with eyes closed. The normal response is to maintain balance throughout the entire test. An abnormal response (in which the patient loses balance when standing erect, feet together, eyes closed) indicates loss of the sense of position.
- *Past-point testing:* In past-point testing, the patient's ability to place a finger accurately on a selected point on the body is measured. Inability to correctly perform the test indicates a lack of coordination in voluntary movements.

Explain the purpose and procedure of each test. Institute safety measures to prevent patient injury during the Romberg test if the patient cannot maintain balance.

DISORDERS OF THE EAR

LOSS OF HEARING (DEAFNESS)

Hearing impairment is a state of decreased auditory acuity that ranges from partial to complete hearing loss. It is the most common disability in the United States affecting 28 million people. Among people older than 65 years of age, it is the third most common chronic condition. The quality of life for one-third of the adults in the United States between 65 and 75 years of age is decreased because of hearing impairments. Recognition, diagnosis, and early treatment may help prevent further impairment and damage.

The implications of hearing loss are great. Hearing is needed to develop speech and conceptual ability; thus hearing loss may affect personality development when the hearing impairment is severe and congenital. This may have implications for the person's education and socialization. As hearing loss increases, the person may withdraw socially because of the inability to understand and be understood; this could lead to isolation and depression (see the Health Promotion box).

Types of Hearing Loss

There are six types of hearing loss: conductive, sensorineural, mixed, congenital, functional (psychogenic), and central.

- In *conductive hearing loss,* sound is inadequately conducted through the external or middle ear to the sensorineural apparatus of the inner ear. Common causes are buildup of cerumen and otitis media with effusion. Other conditions that may result in conductive hearing loss are foreign bodies, otosclerosis, and stenosis of the external auditory canal. Sensitivity to sound is diminished, but clarity or interpretation of sound is not changed. Increased volume or amplification compensates for the conductive loss; therefore a hearing aid may be helpful.
- In *sensorineural hearing loss,* sound is conducted through the external and middle ear in the normal

Health Promotion

Facilitating Communication for People With Impaired Hearing

- If the patient wears a hearing aid, make certain it is in place, turned on, and functioning properly.
- Get the person's attention by raising an arm or hand.
- Ask permission to turn off the television or radio or turn down the volume.
- Ensure adequate lighting so that the patient will be able to understand or lip-read.
- Face the person when speaking.
- Lip-reading is a skill that not all hearing impaired are capable of achieving. Do not assume all people who are hearing impaired can lip-read.
- Speak clearly, but do not over accentuate words.
- Speak in a normal tone; do not shout or raise the pitch of voice. Shouting overuses normal speaking movements and may cause distortion in the sound that may be too loud for the person with sensorineural damage. If the person has conductive loss only, sometimes making the voice louder without shouting is helpful.
- If the person does not seem to understand what is said, express it differently. Some words are difficult to distinguish by lip-reading, such as *white* and *red*.
- Move closer to the person and toward the better ear if the person does not hear you.
- Write out proper names or any statement that you are not sure was understood.
- Do not eat, drink, chew gum, or cover your mouth when talking to a person with limited hearing.
- Observe for inattention that may indicate tiredness or lack of understanding.
- Use phrases rather than one-word answers to convey meaning. State the major topic of the discussion first and then give details.
- Do not show annoyance by careless facial expression. People who are hard of hearing depend more on visual clues for acceptance.
- Encourage the use of a hearing aid if the person has one; allow the person to adjust it before speaking.
- If in a group, repeat important statements and avoid asides to others in the group.
- Do not avoid conversation with a person who has hearing loss.

way, but a defect in the inner ear results in its distortion, making discrimination difficult. Trauma, infectious processes, presbycusis, congenital conditions, and exposure to ototoxic drugs may cause this type of hearing loss. Destruction of the cochlear hair by intense noise also may cause sensorineural hearing loss. Amplifying sound with a hearing aid may help some people with this type of loss. However, many people have intolerance to loud noise and are not helped by a hearing aid.

- *Mixed hearing loss* is combined conductive and sensorineural hearing loss.
- *Congenital hearing loss* is present from birth or early infancy. It can be caused by anoxic injury (brain injury resulting from oxygen deprivation) or trauma during delivery, Rh factor incompatibility, or the mother's exposure during pregnancy to syphilis or rubella, or the use of ototoxic drugs.
- *Functional hearing loss* has no organic cause. It also is known as *psychogenic* or *nonorganic hearing loss*. Functional hearing loss may be caused by an emotional or psychological factor.
- *Central hearing loss* occurs when the brain's auditory pathways are damaged, as in a stroke or a tumor.

Clinical Manifestations

Clinical manifestations vary, depending on the degree of hearing loss. Symptoms range from subtle clues, such as requests for repeating information, to more obvious signs of nonresponsiveness.

Assessment

Collection of subjective data includes noting the onset and progression of the condition, deficit in one or both ears, family history, history of head trauma, mental status changes, exposure to noise, current medications, visual or speech disorders, and any other ear symptoms.

Objective data must include an assessment of behavioral clues that indicate a hearing difficulty (see Box 53.2).

Diagnostic Tests

Conductive hearing loss produces lateralization of sound to the deaf ear in the Weber test. Results of the Rinne test show that sounds transmitted through bone conduction are heard longer than, or at least as long as, sounds transmitted through air conduction.

Sensorineural hearing loss produces lateralization of sound to the better ear in the Weber test. Results of the Rinne test show that air-conducted sounds are heard longer than bone-conducted sounds, but not twice as long.

Audiometric testing determines the type of hearing loss and the degree of impairment.

Medical Management

Medical management depends on the type of impairment. Surgical procedures may be required. Hearing aids or cochlear implants may be used when appropriate. Cochlear implantation is performed in individuals with profound bilateral sensorineural hearing loss who receive no measurable assistance from hearing aids (see "Cochlear Implant," below, and Fig. 53.19).

Nursing Interventions and Patient Teaching

Patients with partial hearing loss may benefit from a hearing aid. Help the patient care for the hearing aid as detailed in Box 53.3.

The hearing aid can be useful only if it is worn. Factors leading to nonuse may include the patient's perception of the hearing aid as a sign of disability. Also, the magnification of sound may cause discomfort for the patient. Therefore ensure that the hearing aid is used and works properly.

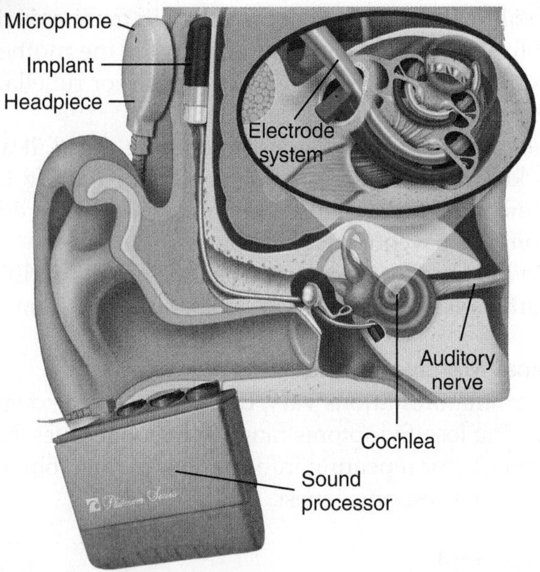

Fig. 53.19 Cochlear implant. (Lemmi FO, Lemmi CAE: *Physical assessment findings CD-ROM*, Philadelphia, 2000, Saunders.)

Box 53.3 Care of the Hearing Aid

DO

- Handle with care.
- Wash the ear mold or plug daily in mild soap and water.
- Dry the ear mold or plug thoroughly before reconnecting it to the receiver.
- Always keep extra batteries and cord available.
- When the hearing aid is not in use, turn the aid off and open the battery compartment.
- If the hearing aid whistles, reinsert the ear mold.
- If a hearing aid fails to work:
  - Check the on-off switch.
  - Inspect the ear mold for cleanliness.
  - Examine the battery for tightness of fit.
  - Examine the cord plug for tightness of insertion.
  - Examine the cord for breaks.
  - Replace the battery or cord.
  - Check for cracks in the tubing or ear mold.
  - Check to see that the ear mold and hearing aid are inserted in the correct ear.
  - Check that the ear mold or hearing aid is properly inserted.
  - Check that the volume control wheel is turned up to an appropriate setting.

DO NOT

- Put the hearing aid on a heated surface.
- Wash the hearing aid.
- Drop the hearing aid.
- Wear the hearing aid in the bath or shower.
- Wear the hearing aid overnight.
- Ignore a hearing aid that is "whistling."
- Use in contact with cream, oil, or hair spray when the hearing aid is on.

Patient problems and interventions for the patient with hearing loss include but are not limited to the following:

Patient Problem	Nursing Interventions
Impaired Sensory Awareness, related to disease process	Facilitate communication with the patient by following the interventions provided in the Health Promotion box for people with impaired hearing
Social Seclusion, related to loss of hearing	Assess factors that contribute to social isolation Identify support systems for patient Identify patient concerns Establish effective communication

Patient Teaching

Assist the patient in learning to care for a hearing aid, if prescribed (see Box 53.3). Advise the patient to request that others speak slowly or more clearly and repeat if necessary.

Prognosis

Surgical repair of the injured structures increases the likelihood of restoring partial or complete hearing, especially when implants are used. Complications of surgery are rare. Technical advances also have improved the quality of hearing. Microtechnology has reduced the size of hearing aids so that they are almost undetectable.

INFLAMMATORY AND INFECTIOUS DISORDERS OF THE EAR

EXTERNAL OTITIS

Etiology and Pathophysiology

External otitis, or otitis externa, is an inflammation or infection of the external canal or the auricle of the external ear. It is sometimes called *swimmer's ear.* External otitis may be acute or chronic.

Allergies, bacteria, fungi, viruses, or trauma may cause external otitis. Common sources of allergic reactions can stem from nickel or chromium in earrings, chemicals in hair sprays, cosmetics, hearing aids, or medications (especially sulfonamides and neomycin). Common bacterial agents are *Staphylococcus aureus, Pseudomonas aeruginosa,* and *Streptococcus pyogenes.* Viruses including herpes simplex virus and varicella-zoster virus, and fungi such as *Aspergillus* and *Candida,* can be a source of chronic infection and may be difficult to treat. The external ear also may be affected by skin disorders including eczema, psoriasis, and seborrheic dermatitis. External otitis is more prevalent during hot, humid weather. Excessive swimming in hot, humid weather may wash out the protective cerumen and lead to secondary infection.

Trauma from cleaning or scratching the ear canal with a foreign object (such as a cotton swab, bobby pin, or finger) may result in irritation and possible introduction of infectious organisms into the ear.

Cerumen in the older adult becomes dry and hard, making it difficult to remove adequately. As a result, the cerumen may become impacted, causing discomfort and decreased hearing. Certain activities allow moisture to become trapped in the ear, creating a medium for infection; these include using earphones, hearing aids, earplugs, earmuffs, and stethoscopes.

Malignant external otitis is a rare, lethal condition caused by *Pseudomonas* organisms, occurring mostly in patients with diabetes. It is a bone-destroying infection that quickly involves all surrounding ear structures.

Clinical Manifestations

The acute inflammatory or infectious process produces pain with movement of the auricle or chewing, and often the entire side of the head aches. Erythema, scaling, pruritus, edema, watery discharge, and crusting of the external ear may occur. Drainage may be purulent or serosanguineous. If the *Pseudomonas* organism is the cause of the infection, the drainage is green and has a distinct odor. Dizziness and decreased hearing also may be present if edema occludes the ear canal. With chronic external otitis there is usually pruritus and drainage but no pain with movement of the auricle.

Assessment

Collection of subjective data includes determining the onset, duration, and severity of pain, which is crucial to the assessment of inflammatory disease of the ear. An early indication of inflammation or infection of the ear is the complaint of ear pain accompanied by the patient gently pulling on the pinna. Ask the patient about any home remedies used to treat infections. Also assess knowledge of preventive measures.

Collection of objective data includes noting discharge amount, color, and odor, which may be watery or yellow with a pungent odor. Discharge from a fungal infection is black. The patient may have a partial loss of hearing or feel like the ear is occluded if the ear canal is edematous or is obstructed by adenoids (small clumps of lymphoid tissue in the back of the throat). Palpation of the external ear or pulling the pinna gently to examine the ear may produce pain.

Diagnostic Tests

Obtain a culture of exudates to identify bacterial, viral, or fungal organisms.

Medical Management

Oral analgesics may be used if the pain is severe. Corticosteroids (1% hydrocortisone) may be used to reduce edema to allow antibiotics to penetrate. Antimicrobial agents such as antibiotic or antifungal eardrops may be used to treat infections. The most commonly used contain neomycin (0.5%) or polymyxin B (10,000 units/mL). Systemic antibiotics are used only if the infection is severe. The specific antibiotic used depends on the results of the culture.

Nursing Interventions and Patient Teaching

Carefully clean the ear canal. Heat may be applied to the external ear for pain relief. Implement an adequate method of communication. Instill eardrops as prescribed.

A patient problem and interventions for the patient with external otitis include but are not limited to the following:

Patient Problem	Nursing Interventions
Pain, related to inflammatory process	Apply warm compresses as ordered Administer prescribed analgesics and instill ordered ear medications

Ensure that the patient has the information needed to prevent further infection and can adequately care for the infected ear at home.

Prognosis

External otitis responds favorably to topical antibiotic and corticosteroid eardrops. Systemic antibiotics rarely are required unless cellulitis is present. Acute external otitis may become a chronic problem. If the infection remains untreated and enters the brain, death can occur. The rare malignant external otitis media has a mortality rate of 50% to 75% unless the condition is treated.

ACUTE OTITIS MEDIA

Etiology and Pathophysiology

Acute otitis media, an inflammation or infection of the middle ear, is the most common disorder of the middle ear. Acute otitis media most often is caused by *Haemophilus influenzae* or *Streptococcus pneumoniae.* Gram-negative bacteria, such as *Proteus, Klebsiella,* and *Pseudomonas* organisms, usually cause chronic otitis media; however, additional sources of infection include allergies, exposure to cigarette smoke, mycoplasma, and several viruses.

Otitis media occurs more frequently in children, especially at 6 to 36 months of age, and in the winter and early spring. Children's shorter and straighter eustachian tubes provide easier access of the organisms from the nasopharynx to travel to the middle ear. The patient usually has had a recent upper respiratory tract infection that ascends via the eustachian tube and involves the lining of the entire middle ear. Typically, only one ear is affected.

Viral infections frequently cause a serous otitis media. Retraction of the tympanic membrane occurs with a buildup of sterile serous exudate. If there is a secondary bacterial infection, purulent exudate collects behind the tympanic membrane, causing it to bulge. This is called *purulent otitis media.*

Clinical Manifestations

The patient experiences a sense of fullness in the ear and also has severe, deep throbbing pain behind the tympanic membrane. This severe pain may disappear if the tympanic membrane ruptures. Hearing loss, **tinnitus** (a subjective noise sensation heard in one or both ears; ringing or tinkling sounds in the ear), and fever also may be present.

Assessment

Subjective data are the same as for external otitis. Objective data are the same as for external otitis, with the exception of noting pain on palpation of the external ear.

Diagnostic Tests

A culture of the purulent drainage is obtained to identify the causative organisms.

Medical Management

Antibiotic therapy is still the most common form of treating otitis media, and it may be based on results of the culture. Analgesics are prescribed for severe pain, as well as nasal decongestants. Sedatives may be prescribed for children to provide rest and pain relief in combination with local heat (Table 53.5).

Needle aspiration of secretions collected behind the tympanic membrane may be necessary. **Myringotomy**—a

Table 53.5 Medications for Ear Disorders

GENERIC NAME (TRADE NAME)	ACTION AND USE	SIDE EFFECTS	NURSING IMPLICATIONS
acetic acid (VoSol hydrochloride otic)	Antibacterial, antifungal, astringent; used for superficial infections of external auditory canal	Contact dermatitis, transient stinging	Clean ear first; use cotton plug for first 24 h; contact health care practitioner if condition worsens or no improvement occurs after 5–7 days; do not wash dropper—doing so may dilute medication
amoxicillin trihydrate (Amoxil)	Systemic penicillin antibiotic used in acute otitis media	Anaphylaxis, skin rash, diarrhea	Use caution during pregnancy and lactation; take for full treatment period; consult with health care practitioner if no improvement occurs in a few days; take on full or empty stomach; check with health care practitioner about treating diarrhea; do not give if patient has penicillin or cephalosporin allergy
antipyrine and benzocaine (Auralgan)	Analgesic; local anesthetic; used for otitis media; adjunct to cerumen removal	Contact dermatitis	Use caution during pregnancy and lactation; date bottle and discard after 6 mo from first use; do not use if eardrums are perforated; warm the bottle; position patient on side and fill ear canal; use cotton plug; wash dropper before replacing in bottle
carbamide peroxide (Debrox)	Cerumen removal	Contact dermatitis	Do not use if eardrum is perforated or if there is ear discharge; not recommended for children; avoid eyes; reevaluate if edema, erythema, or pain persists; use proper administration technique by allowing drops to enter ear canal; do not touch tip of dropper
cefaclor (Ceclor)	Second-generation cephalosporin used to treat amoxicillin-resistant otitis media	Anaphylaxis, skin rash, joint pain; fever, diarrhea, abdominal cramping	Store suspension in refrigerator; give full course of therapy; tell patient not to use alcohol; give on full or empty stomach; do not give if patient has penicillin or cephalosporin allergies
colistin, neomycin, hydrocortisone, and thonzonium (Coly-Mycin S Otic)	Antibiotic-steroid-detergent used for susceptible disease of external auditory canal, mastoidectomy, and otitis media fenestration	Ototoxicity with prolonged use; contact dermatitis; hypersensitivity, including pruritus, skin rash, erythema, and edema	Do not heat bottle above body temperature; with herpes simplex, do not use if patient is infected; do not use if eardrum is perforated; use for 10 days only; keep dropper from touching skin; check with health care practitioner if signs and symptoms worsen or do not improve after 1 wk; shake well before using; use cotton plug to keep moist; change plug daily

Table 53.5 Medications for Ear Disorders—cont'd

GENERIC NAME (TRADE NAME)	ACTION AND USE	SIDE EFFECTS	NURSING IMPLICATIONS
dimenhydrinate (Dramamine)	Anticholinergic antihistamine used in treatment of vertigo	Blurred vision, drowsiness, shortness of breath, painful urination, disorientation	Antihistamines may inhibit lactation; give no CNS depressants; give with food or milk; use caution during pregnancy in early months
meclizine hydrochloride (Antivert)	Anticholinergic antihistamine that acts as antiemetic, antivertigo agent; treatment and prophylaxis; possibly effective for diseases affecting vestibular system	Drowsiness, blurred vision, dry mouth	Use caution during pregnancy and breastfeeding; give with food, water, or milk; tell patient to avoid alcohol and central nervous system (CNS) depressants; not recommended for children under 12 yr
polymyxin B, neomycin, bacitracin, and hydrocortisone (Cortisporin)	Antibiotic and steroid used in the same way as Coly-Mycin S; used to treat swimmer's ear	Ototoxicity with prolonged use, contact dermatitis, pruritus, erythema, edema	Use caution during pregnancy and lactation; do not use if eardrum is perforated; keep dropper from touching skin; shake well before using; use cotton plug to keep moist; change plug daily
triethanolamine polypeptide oleate (Cerumenex)	Cerumen removal	Contact dermatitis	Fill ear canal; insert cotton plug after 15–30 min; irrigate ear canal with warm water
trimethoprim-sulfamethoxazole (Bactrim)	Systemic antibacterial; used for acute otitis media; no sulfonamide allergy	Fever, itching, skin rash, photosensitivity, dizziness	Not recommended during lactation or pregnancy; emphasize importance of proper dental care; blood glucose levels may be affected in patients using oral antidiabetic agents; maintain adequate fluid intake; advise patient to avoid sun exposure; complete treatment; with pediatric suspension, shake well

surgical incision of the tympanic membrane to relieve pressure and release purulent exudate from the middle ear—may be required to prevent spontaneous rupture. A tympanostomy tube may be placed for short- or long-term use. Prompt treatment of an episode of acute otitis media generally prevents spontaneous perforation of the tympanic membrane.

Nursing Interventions and Patient Teaching

Inner-ear pressure may cause discomfort, requiring an analgesic. Sedatives may be ordered for young children. Hearing loss also may occur, which means that clear, effective communication with the patient is essential. Alert parents of young patients to this fact and enlist their help in monitoring the level of loss.

Chronic otitis media caused by repeated attacks of acute otitis media may result in a permanent perforation of the tympanic membrane. The result is a slight to moderate conductive hearing loss.

A growth called *cholesteatoma* (a mass of epithelial cells and cholesterol in the middle ear) occurs when a tympanic membrane perforation allows keratinizing squamous epithelium of the external auditory canal to enter and grow in the middle ear. Enlargement is slow, but the mass can expand into the mastoid antrum and destroy adjacent structures. Unless removed surgically, a cholesteatoma can cause extensive damage to the structures of the middle ear; erode the bony protection of the facial nerve; create a labyrinthine fistula; or even invade the dura, threatening the brain.

Mastoiditis, an infection of one of the mastoid bones, may develop as an extension of a middle-ear infection that was left untreated or inadequately treated. Immediately report signs of mastoiditis, including earache, fever, headache, malaise, and large amounts of purulent exudate.

A patient problem and interventions for the patient with otitis media include but are not limited to the following:

Patient Problem	Nursing Interventions
Compromised Skin Integrity, related to edema and exudates	Note and report any purulent outer ear exudates Keep ear clean and dry; use sterile cotton to absorb drainage, if ordered Monitor temperature and report changes

Ensure that the patient and parents (if appropriate) are aware of the necessity to complete the entire course of antibiotic therapy. Children are fed upright to prevent nasopharyngeal flora from entering the eustachian tube. Instruct the patient to blow the nose gently, not forcefully. If a myringotomy has been performed, instruct the patient or the parents to change the cotton in the outer ear at least twice a day (see the Patient Teaching box).

 Patient Teaching

Ear Infection

PREVENTION OF FURTHER INFECTION
- Protect the ear canals during showers (earplugs may be used to keep water out of the ears).
- Avoid swimming during active infection or after an eardrum has been perforated; avoid swimming in contaminated water.
- Continue antibiotic therapy for the prescribed number of days, even when symptoms disappear.
- Get adequate and early treatment of upper respiratory tract infections and allergic conditions.

CARE OF INFECTED EAR
- Use correct eardrop insertion or ear irrigations, as prescribed.
- Wash hands before and after medication administration to prevent secondary infection.
- Keep external ear clean and dry to protect skin from drainage.

SIGNS REQUIRING MEDICAL ATTENTION
- Fever
- Return of ear pain or purulent discharge

Prognosis

Middle-ear infections usually resolve completely with antibiotic therapy. Since the advent of treatment with antibiotics, the incidence of severe and prolonged infections of the middle ear has been reduced greatly. Chronic or untreated otitis media may lead to sound transmission hearing loss, which is successfully treated by tympanoplasty.

Mastoiditis is difficult to treat and may require intravenous antibiotic therapy for several days. Because children are affected most often, immediate treatment of the infection is crucial. Residual hearing loss may follow the infection. If early decalcification is present, intense antibiotic therapy and myringotomy usually can cure mastoiditis; if it has progressed to further destruction, simple mastoidectomy is necessary.

LABYRINTHITIS

Etiology and Pathophysiology

Labyrinthitis is an inflammation of the labyrinthine canals of the inner ear. Labyrinthitis is the most common cause of vertigo. A common cause is a viral upper respiratory tract infection that spreads into the inner ear; other causes include certain drugs and foods. The vestibular portion of the inner ear may be destroyed by streptomycin. Exposure to tobacco and alcohol also may be causative factors. A rarer form of labyrinthitis is caused by bacteria, which usually is associated with middle-ear and mastoid infections. Since the advent of antibiotics, bacterial labyrinthitis occurs infrequently.

Clinical Manifestations

Severe and sudden vertigo is the most common symptom of labyrinthitis. Other symptoms include nausea and vomiting, nystagmus, photophobia, headache, and ataxic gait.

Assessment

Subjective data include the frequency and duration of the vertigo and any safety measures taken by the patient during an attack. Assess other symptoms such as hearing ability, tinnitus, and nausea. Because fear is associated with the attacks, explore the patient's feelings.

Objective data include noting vomiting and any signs of nystagmus and laterality (favoring either the right or left side of the body). Assess the coloration and moistness of the skin to determine the extent of autonomic response (changes in heart rate, blood pressure, and respirations).

Diagnostic Tests

Electronystagmography, done to record involuntary movements of the eye, may show diminished or absent nystagmus with stimulation. Audiometric testing shows low-tone sensorineural hearing loss.

Medical Management

Labyrinthitis has no specific treatment. Usually antibiotics and dimenhydrinate (Dramamine) or meclizine (Antivert) for vertigo are prescribed. If nausea and vomiting persist, administer parenteral fluids.

Nursing Interventions and Patient Teaching

Note the frequency and degree of vertigo. Administer antibiotics and medications and assess fluid intake to ensure that dehydration does not occur.

Patient problems and interventions for the patient with labyrinthitis include but are not limited to the following:

Patient Problem	Nursing Interventions
Potential for Injury, related to altered sensory perception (vertigo)	Keep side rails up Note presence of vertigo before patient ambulates Supervise ambulation Caution the patient not to attempt ambulation alone and to call for assistance
Fearfulness, related to altered sensory perception (vertigo)	Explore patient's feelings about attack Teach patient concerning actions during an attack (see the Patient Teaching box) Reinforce health care practitioner's treatment orders

Instruct the patient about vertigo and how it is treated (see the Patient Teaching box).

Patient Teaching

Vertigo

- Nature of the disorder
- Physiologic basis for the vertigo
- Avoidance of any known precipitating factors
- Rationale for a low-salt diet
- Actions to take during an attack
  - Lie down immediately, and call for help if necessary at the first signs of an attack.
  - If driving when an attack occurs, pull over immediately to the curb.
  - Lie immobile and hold head in one position until vertigo lessens.
  - Ask for assistance when ambulating if dizzy.
- Take prescribed medications as instructed even if no recent attacks have occurred; check with the health care provider before discontinuing any medication.
- Seek medical attention for changes in symptoms or in the nature of attacks.

OBSTRUCTIONS OF THE EAR

Etiology and Pathophysiology

Ear canal obstruction usually is caused by impaction or excessive secretion of cerumen or by foreign bodies, including insects. Children often place beans, beads, pebbles, and small toys in their ears. Usually those objects are found on routine examination. Obstruction by cerumen can be caused when excessive amounts are produced by overactive glands or from impaction of cerumen in narrow or tortuous ear canals.

Clinical Manifestations

Obstruction may cause the ear to feel occluded. The patient may have tinnitus or buzzing, pain in the ear, and hearing loss.

Assessment

Collection of subjective data includes interviewing the patient about any possible foreign bodies being introduced into the ear and any home remedies used to remove the object. If the patient is a child, determine risk factors related to ear obstructions, such as beads or nuts.

Collection of objective data involves noting any presence of a foreign body in the external ear canal. Observe children for tugging of the pinna.

Diagnostic Tests

Otoscopic examination provides visualization of the possible causes of the obstruction.

Medical Management

Medical management includes removal of cerumen by irrigation or cerumen spoon. Remove foreign objects with forceps, if possible. Smother insects with drops of an oily substance and remove them with forceps. Medications, such as carbamide peroxide 6.5%, may be used to soften cerumen. Surgical removal of the foreign object may be necessary.

Nursing Interventions and Patient Teaching

Assist with the irrigation of the ear. Instill medications into the ear as ordered.

A patient problem and interventions for the patient with obstructions of the ear include but are not limited to the following:

Patient Problem	Nursing Interventions
Impaired Sensory Awareness, related to presence of foreign body causing obstruction	Note the presence and amount of hearing impairment and tinnitus Assure the patient (or parents) that once the obstruction is removed, any hearing loss or tinnitus should disappear

Inform the patient and parents about the danger of placing objects in the ears. Also reinforce the method for preventing cerumen obstruction by instilling prescribed drops at night. This is followed by hydrogen peroxide in the morning and cleaning with a soft cotton wick.

Prognosis

Ear canal obstructions caused by cerumen and foreign bodies resolve completely with treatment. Vertigo may be experienced temporarily until the ear canal dries. The older adult may become disoriented from the cerumen impaction and temporary loss of hearing.

NONINFECTIOUS DISORDERS OF THE EAR

OTOSCLEROSIS

Etiology and Pathophysiology

Otosclerosis is a condition characterized by chronic progressive deafness caused by the formation of spongy bone, especially around the oval window, with resulting ankylosis (stiffening, immobility) of the stapes. In otosclerosis, formation of new bone in adolescence or early adulthood progresses slowly. Gradually, normal bone in the otic capsule is replaced by highly vascular otosclerotic bone. This replacement bone is described as *spongy*. Calcification of the area follows, and fixation of the footplate of the stapes in the oval window causes tinnitus and then deafness.

Otosclerosis is an autosomal dominant genetic disease. Women are affected twice as often as men. Otosclerosis is bilateral in about 80% of patients. Frequently, pregnancy triggers a rapid onset of this condition. Previous ear infections are not believed to be related to otosclerosis.

Clinical Manifestations

The patient with otosclerosis experiences slowly progressive conductive hearing loss and low- to medium-pitched tinnitus. The deafness usually is noted first between the ages of 11 and 20 years.

Assessment

Subjective data include the degree and progression of hearing loss or tinnitus and mild dizziness to vertigo. Assess family history for the disease.

Objective data include assessment of behavioral clues related to hearing loss (see Box 53.2).

Diagnostic Tests

Otoscopy reveals a normal eardrum. A pink blush called *Schwartz sign* may be seen through the eardrum; this indicates a high degree of vascularity in active otosclerotic bone. The result of the Rinne test shows that sounds transmitted by bone conduction last longer than those transmitted by air conduction in the affected ear. Weber test results are the opposite of those for normal hearing. The Weber test and audiometric testing show a lateralization of sound, more to the affected ear. Audiometric testing may show minimal to total hearing loss. Tympanometry may reveal evidence of stiffness in the sound conduction system. Hearing loss ranges from mild in the early stages to total loss in the later stages.

Medical Management

Supplements such as fluoride, vitamin D, and calcium carbonate are sometimes used to attempt to stabilize the hearing loss that results from otosclerosis. It is believed that these supplements can slow hearing loss by preventing further bone resorption and promoting calcification of bony lesions. Hearing aids may be effective because there is normal inner ear function. Surgical treatment by stapedectomy restores this conductive hearing loss. The ear with greater hearing loss typically is repaired first.

Nursing Interventions and Patient Teaching

Patient problems and interventions of otosclerosis are specific to post-stapedectomy care. See the Patient Teaching box "After Ear Surgery" for relevant discussion.

Prognosis

Patients report varying degrees of success with hearing after stapedectomy surgery. For some patients, stapedectomy is successful in permanently restoring hearing. A hearing aid may further enhance sound conduction to more normal levels.

MÉNIÈRE'S DISEASE

Etiology and Pathophysiology

Ménière's disease is a chronic disease of the inner ear characterized by recurrent episodes of vertigo, progressive unilateral nerve deafness, and tinnitus. Ménière's disease is most common in women between 30 and 60 years of age. Risk factors include recent viral infection, stress, alcohol use, family history and allergies. There is no identified specific causation but the condition is likely tied to a series of factors.

There is an increase in endolymph fluid, either from increased production or decreased absorption. This causes increased pressure in the inner-ear labyrinth. Attacks of severe vertigo, tinnitus, and progressive deafness result from this increased pressure. Usually one ear only is involved.

Clinical Manifestations

The patient experiences recurrent episodes of vertigo with associated nausea, vomiting, diaphoresis, tinnitus, and nystagmus. A sense of fullness in the ear and hearing loss may be present. These attacks last from a few minutes to several hours. Attacks may occur several times a year. Sudden movements often aggravate the symptoms.

Assessment

Collection of subjective data includes noting the frequency and severity of the vertigo attack. The patient may complain of tinnitus. Note the patient's history and knowledge of the disorder and circumstances that precipitate an attack. Assess actions taken by the patient during an attack and the degree of relief those actions provide.

Collection of objective data includes determining unilateral or bilateral hearing loss. Observe the patient for associated signs during an attack.

Diagnostic Tests

To confirm a diagnosis two or more episodes must be documented, accompanied by positive findings from other diagnostic tests. Diagnostic tests such as magnetic resonance imaging (MRI) or computed tomography (CT) often are ordered to rule out central nervous system disease. An audiogram demonstrates mild low-frequency sensorineural hearing loss. Tuning fork tests show a sensorineural deficit. Vestibular testing shows lack of balance.

Medical Management

There is no specific therapy for Ménière's disease. Fluid restriction, diuretics, and a low-salt diet are prescribed in an attempt to decrease fluid pressure. Advise the patient to avoid caffeine and nicotine.

Dimenhydrinate, meclizine, diazepam (Valium), diphenhydramine (Benadryl), and fentanyl with droperidol may be prescribed for use between attacks to reduce the vertigo. In acute attacks the medications may be given intravenously. Atropine also is given for its anticholinergic effect during these acute attacks.

For preservation of hearing, surgical procedures may be performed. Approximately 5% to 10% of patients with Ménière's disease require surgery. Surgical intervention may involve destruction of the labyrinth, insertion of drainage tubes into the subarachnoid space, or dissection

Table 53.6 Surgery for Ménière's Disease

TYPE	DESCRIPTION	RESIDUAL	POSTOPERATIVE NURSING INTERVENTIONS
Surgical destruction of labyrinth	Extraction of membranous labyrinth by suction; access to inner ear through external canal (stapes and incus removed)	Destroys remaining hearing	Keep patient on bed rest and NPO until vertigo subsides in 1–3 days Avoid sudden movement of head for 1–2 wk Take action to prevent falls from unsteadiness for 1–3 wk
Endolymphatic subarachnoid shunt	Insertion of drain tube from endolymphatic sac into subarachnoid space; access through mastoid	Preserves hearing in 60%–70% of patients	Monitor for vertigo (rare)
Cryosurgery	Application of intense cold to lateral semicircular canals to decrease sensitivity or to create an otic-periotic shunt; access through mastoid	Preserves hearing in 80% of patients	Monitor for dizziness for 2 days Take action to prevent falls from unsteadiness for 2–3 wk
Vestibular nerve section	Dissection of cranial nerve VIII (vestibular portion); access through mastoid or by cranial drilling over roof of internal auditory canal	Preserves hearing in 90% of patients	Same as for surgical destruction of labyrinth

NPO, Nothing by mouth.

of cranial nerve VIII (vestibular portion). These surgeries are relatively successful, with the preservation of hearing reported in 60% to 90% of patients. Postoperative care involves bed rest for the first 1 to 3 days, avoidance of sudden head movements for 1 to 2 weeks, and the implementation of safety precautions to avoid falls related to dizziness (Table 53.6).

Nursing Interventions and Patient Teaching

Maintain the prescribed low-salt diet and administer diuretics as ordered. Acute vertigo is treated symptomatically with bed rest, sedation, and antiemetics or with medications for motion sickness. Nursing interventions are planned to minimize vertigo and provide for patient safety. During an acute attack keep the patient in a quiet, darkened room in a comfortable position. The patient may have some auditory deficit, which requires alternative methods of communication. If the patient's tinnitus becomes distressing, an increase in background noise, such as music, may provide relief. Fluorescent or flickering lights or watching television may exacerbate symptoms and should be avoided. Have an emesis basin available because vomiting is common.

Patient problems and interventions for the patient with Ménière's disease include but are not limited to the following:

Patient Problem	Nursing Interventions
Potential for Injury, related to sensory-perceptual alterations (vertigo)	Keep side rails up Assist with ambulation and instruct the patient to call for assistance before attempting to ambulate Have the patient sit or lie down when vertigo occurs Have the patient move slowly and avoid turning the head suddenly Administer medications as prescribed Position patient on unaffected side Stand in front of patient to prevent head turning Avoid bright or glaring lights around patient Place all needed supplies so that patient does not have to turn head
Social Seclusion, related to unpredictable vertigo attacks	Assess factors that contribute to social isolation Assess feelings of loneliness and abandonment Identify support systems for patient Identify patient concerns Establish effective communication

Provide information about a low-salt diet and the taking of diuretics. Warn the patient to avoid reading when vertigo or tinnitus is present. Instruct the patient to avoid smoking to prevent vasoconstriction. The patient should learn to identify precipitating factors and the proper actions to take when an attack occurs: (1) sit or lie down immediately; (2) if driving, stop the car and

 Nursing Care Plan 53.2 **The Patient With Ménière's Disease**

Ms. L. is a 66-year-old patient admitted with Ménière's disease. She complains of severe dizziness, nausea, vomiting, ringing in the ears, hearing loss, and an unsteady gait. She is accompanied by her husband of 35 years.

PATIENT PROBLEM

Anxiousness, related to effect of disorder

Patient Goals and Expected Outcomes	Nursing Interventions	Evaluation
Patient will voice and demonstrate decreased signs and symptoms of anxiety Patient will control her anxiety level	Encourage patient to explore concerns about decreased hearing and effects of vertigo attacks and to take action in relation to the concerns. Explore patient's knowledge of the disorder and correct misunderstandings. Educate patient on strategies that can give her back some control over her life. Suggest keeping an emesis basin, a pillow, a blanket, a cell phone, and a large sign with the words "HELP, POLICE" in the car in case of a sudden Ménière's attack. Encourage realistic hope about expected hearing ability as described by health care practitioner. Refer patient to necessary support services, such as social worker or audiologist. Refer patient for more information to Vestibular Disorders Association (VEDA).	Patient states that level of anxiety has decreased.

PATIENT PROBLEM

Potential for Injury, related to vestibular auditory alterations

Patient Goals and Expected Outcomes	Nursing Interventions	Evaluation
Patient will describe actions to avoid vertigo Patient will remain free of injury Patient will remain safe from falls	Help patient identify avoidable actions that precipitate vertigo attacks. Encourage patient to move slowly and not turn head suddenly when vertigo is present. If tinnitus is distressing, increase background noises, such as music. If hearing is decreased: • Use measures to facilitate communication with hearing impaired. • Carry wax earplugs; even after losing some hearing, ears are often sensitive to loud noises, which can trigger vertigo. • Refer patient to audiologist, if appropriate. Keep side rails up when patient with vertigo is in bed. Assist with ambulation as needed. Encourage patient to sit or lie down and to remain immobile if signs of dizziness occur. Teach patient to stop car at side of road immediately at first signs of dizziness while driving.	Patient avoids physical environment that could cause injury. Patient does not manifest evidence of injury.

CRITICAL THINKING QUESTIONS

1. Ms. L. states that she would prefer going to the bathroom without the assistance of a nurse. What is an appropriate response by the nurse?
2. Ms. L. tells the nurse that she is depressed because of her unpleasant symptoms and wonders if she will ever feel well again. What would be a therapeutic reply?
3. The nurse notes an unpleasant odor from Ms. L.; her hair is unkempt, and she has poor oral hygiene. The nurse is preparing to give her a warm, therapeutic bed bath. Ms. L. states, "I feel too dizzy to take a bath." What nursing interventions would help promote personal hygiene and patient compliance?

pull over to the side of the road; and (3) keep medication available at all times (Nursing Care Plan 53.2).

Prognosis

Approximately 75% to 85% of patients experience improvement with medical management and supportive therapy. The remaining patients may, in time, require surgical intervention. Usually attacks occur several times yearly, until the disease either resolves itself or progresses to complete deafness in the affected ear.

SURGERIES OF THE EAR

STAPEDECTOMY

Stapedectomy is the removal of the stapes of the middle ear and insertion of a graft and prosthesis, performed to restore hearing in cases of otosclerosis. The stapes that has become fixed is replaced so that vibrations can again transmit sound waves through the oval window to the fluid of the inner ear.

Using a local anesthetic and an operating microscope for visualization, the surgeon removes the stapes and covers the opening into the inner ear with a graft of body tissue. One end of a small plastic tube or piece of stainless steel wire is attached to the graft, while the other end is attached to the two remaining bones of the middle ear, the malleus and the incus.

Nursing Interventions and Patient Teaching

Postoperative management consists of external ear packing to ensure healing; the packing is left in place for 5 or 6 days. Depending on the health care provider's preference, the patient remains in bed for approximately 24 hours and resumes activity gradually. Keep the patient flat with the operative side facing upward to maintain the position of the prosthesis and graft; make certain that the patient is not turned. Headache, nausea, vomiting, and dizziness are expected early in the postoperative period as a result of stimulation of the labyrinth intraoperatively. The patient's hearing does not improve until the edema subsides and the packing is removed by the health care provider (see the Patient Teaching box).

Patient Teaching

After Ear Surgery

- Change cotton in ear daily as prescribed.
- Open mouth when sneezing or coughing and blow nose gently one side at a time for 1 week (to prevent increased ear pressure and infection).
- Keep ear dry for 6 weeks (to prevent infection).
- Do not wash hair for 1 week.
- Protect ear when outdoors, using two pieces of cotton.
- Protect ear with shower cap when bathing.
- Wear ear protection as necessary to prevent exposure to loud noises.
- Follow activity guidelines:
  - No physical activity for 1 week
  - No exercises or active sports for 3 weeks
  - Return to work in 1 week (3 weeks for strenuous work).
  - Avoid exposure to people with upper respiratory tract infections.
  - Avoid airplane flights for at least 1 week (to prevent effects of pressure changes).

Possible complications of the stapedectomy include infection of the external, middle, or inner ear. Displacement or rejection of the prosthesis or graft may occur, or perilymph fluid may leak around the prosthesis into the middle ear, causing tinnitus and vertigo.

Prognosis

During surgery the patient often reports an immediate improvement in hearing in the operative ear. Because of the accumulation of blood and fluid in the middle ear, the hearing level decreases postoperatively but does return to near-normal levels. After stapedectomy, 90% of patients experience an improvement in hearing, in many instances to near-normal levels.

TYMPANOPLASTY

Tympanoplasty is any of several operative procedures on the eardrum or ossicles of the middle ear to restore or improve hearing in patients with conductive hearing loss. These operations may be used to repair a perforated eardrum, for otosclerosis, or for dislocation or necrosis of a small bone of the middle ear.

Nursing Interventions

Postoperative management consists of bed rest until the next morning. Elevate the head of the bed 40 degrees, and keep the operative side facing upward. Medications include opioid analgesics, otic and oral antibiotics, and meclizine for vertigo.

After the operation, monitor and report the presence of bleeding; the amount, color, and consistency of drainage; and temperature. Note complaints of vertigo when the patient is getting out of bed; with sudden movements, nausea and vertigo may occur. Possible complications include infection and displacement of the graft.

Patient problems and interventions for the patient after a tympanoplasty include but are not limited to the following:

Patient Problem	Nursing Interventions
Compromised Physical Mobility, related to surgical procedure	Note patient's ability to comply with bed rest order Keep the patient's operative side up; do not allow the patient to be turned
Potential for Inability to Tolerate Activity, related to pain and vertigo	Keep side rails up When movement is allowed, begin gradually Administer prescribed medications for pain and vertigo as needed Assist with ambulation to prevent injury

Prognosis

Hearing will improve if there is no involvement of the ossicles.

MYRINGOTOMY

Myringotomy, also called *tympanotomy*, is a surgical incision of the eardrum. It is performed to relieve pressure and to release purulent exudate from the middle ear. The procedure is done with the patient under either local or general anesthesia. A myringotomy may be performed in one of two ways: (1) using a myringotomy knife, the surgeon makes a curved incision in the drumhead; or (2) a heated wire loop is touched for about 1 second to the drumhead, producing a 2-mm hole.

Nursing Interventions and Patient Teaching

Purulent exudate and fluid may drain immediately, requiring suctioning. Cotton placed in the ear absorbs drainage, which may continue for several days. Change the cotton frequently to avoid recontamination of the surgical area. The incision usually heals quickly with little scarring. Hearing usually is not disrupted.

Medications commonly used are tetracycline (Achromycin V) and polymyxin B (Neosporin) eardrops as antiinfective agents. Tylenol with codeine may be used for pain. Monitor for signs of bleeding and report any occurrence. Note incisional pain or hearing impairment.

Patient teaching involves providing the information in the Patient Teaching box "After Ear Surgery" and ensuring that the patient understands.

Prognosis

Once pressure is relieved, hearing is restored to more normal levels unless scarring is present.

COCHLEAR IMPLANT

The cochlear implant is a hearing device for the profoundly deaf. The system consists of a surgically implanted induction coil beneath the skin behind the ear and an electrode wire placed in the cochlea (see Fig. 53.19). The implanted parts interface with an externally worn speech processor. The system stimulates auditory nerve fibers by an electric current so that signals reach the brainstem's auditory nuclei and ultimately the auditory cortex. The implant is intended for the patient whose sensorineural hearing loss is either congenital or acquired. A small computer changes the spoken words into electrical impulses that are transmitted to the implanted cochlear coil. The ideal candidate is one who became deaf after acquiring speech and language. The adult who was born deaf or became deaf before learning to speak may be considered a candidate for a cochlear implant if she or he has followed an aural-oral educational approach.

The implant offers the profoundly deaf the ability to hear environmental sounds, including speech, at comfortable loudness levels. Multichannel cochlear implants also aid in speech production. Extensive training and rehabilitation are essential to receive maximum benefit from these implants. The positive aspects of a cochlear implant include providing sound to the person who heard none, improving the sense of security, and decreasing the feelings of isolation. With continued research, the cochlear implant may offer the possibility of hearing rehabilitation for a wider range of hearing-impaired individuals.

The deaf community is concerned with cultural pride. They believe that life without hearing is healthy and functional and that deafness is not a disease that must be cured. The National Association of the Deaf originally opposed the use of cochlear implants; it now endorses their use, stating, "cochlear implantation is a technology that represents a tool to be used in some forms of communication, and not a cure for deafness" (Munson, 2006).

OTHER SPECIAL SENSES

TASTE AND SMELL

The tongue of the average adult contains approximately 10,000 taste buds; some also are located on the inner aspect of the cheeks. It was once believed that there were specific receptors in specific locations on the tongue that were able to detect the individual taste sensations. This is no longer believed to be true. Traditionally there were four identified taste sensations. This has been expanded to include a fifth taste. Research is ongoing relating to the discovery of other potential tastes such as fat (NLM, 2016).

1. *Sweet:* Respond to sugar and other sweet substances
2. *Sour:* Respond to acid content of foods
3. *Salty:* Respond to metal ions within foods
4. *Bitter:* Respond to alkaline or basic ions within foods
5. ***Umami*** *(Savory):* Respond to flavors similar to meat broth. Amino acids glutamic acid or aspartic acid are responsible for this flavor profile.

The receptors for the sense of smell (olfactory receptors) are located in the roof, or the upper part, of the nasal cavity. On inhalation, an odor comes in contact with the olfactory receptors and the message is sent to the brain. Certain odors are remembered for a long time and stimulate certain memories. The body is not able to regenerate olfactory cells; once they are damaged, the sense of smell is impaired permanently.

TOUCH

The receptors for touch *(tactile receptors)* are located throughout the integumentary system. They respond to touch, pressure, and vibration.

POSITION AND MOVEMENT

Proprioception (sense of position) maintains the proper position of the body. *Proprioceptors* include any sensory nerve ending—such as those located in muscles, tendons, and joints—that responds to stimuli originating from within the body regarding movement and spatial position. The proprioceptors work in conjunction with the semicircular canals and the vestibule of the inner ear to maintain proper coordination. These systems work in conjunction to orchestrate the body's movements in running, walking, dancing, and many other activities. Once the proprioceptors receive information from the environment, they send it to the cerebellum for interpretation. Proprioceptors enable one to sense the position of the different parts of the body and to be aware of the movement of each.

EFFECTS OF NORMAL AGING ON THE SENSORY SYSTEM

As an individual ages, the crystalline lens of the eye hardens and becomes too large for the eye muscles, thus causing a loss of accommodation. This often results in a need for bifocals or trifocals. The crystalline lens loses some of its transparency and becomes more opaque, and glare begins to become a problem. The lens proteins are vulnerable to biochemical changes and exposure to UV light, resulting in cataract development. Hypertension and atherosclerosis lead to retinal vascular changes. Age-related macular degeneration (ARMD) also contributes to impaired vision. The pupils become smaller and decrease the amount of light that reaches the retina, resulting in a need for brighter lighting for reading.

Impaired hearing can result from age-related changes in the auditory system. A condition called *presbycusis,* a hearing deficit secondary to aging, can occur from numerous sources such as noise, vascular or systemic diseases, poor nutrition, ototoxic drugs, and pollution. These exposures occurring over the lifespan can damage the delicate hair cells of the organ of Corti, cause calcification of the ossicles of the middle ear, and interfere with sound conduction. Tinnitus (ringing in the ear) also may occur secondary to the aging process and prolonged exposure to loud noises.

Visual and hearing losses in the older adult can result in physical and psychosocial problems. Early detection of visual and hearing changes may enable the patient to maintain an active and productive lifestyle. The remaining senses undergo slight changes, including decreases in their reaction or threshold times, which results in slower responses or diminished sensation.

NURSING PROCESS FOR THE PATIENT WITH A VISUAL OR AUDITORY DISORDER

The role of the licensed practical nurse/licensed vocational nurse (LPN/LVN) in the nursing process as stated is that the LPN/LVN will:

- Participate in planning care for patients based on patient needs
- Review patient's care plan and recommend revisions as needed
- Review and follow defined prioritization for patient care
- Use clinical pathways, care maps, or care plans to guide and review patient care

ASSESSMENT

The complexity of the assessment for eye and ear disorders depends on the patient's disease or problem. Subjective data for eye and ear disorders include the following:

- Health history, including any acute or chronic disease
- History of current complaint
- Medications, including prescription, over-the-counter, and home remedies or folk medicines
- Surgery and other treatments

Collection of objective data includes external and internal assessment of the eye and ear. Use inspection and palpation to assess the external components of the eye and ear, noting any abnormalities. Review results of the internal examination of the eye and ear by the primary care provider. Note results of diagnostic tests. Because seeing and hearing are necessary for safety, communication, self-care, and psychosocial interaction, assess these areas as well.

PATIENT PROBLEM

Nursing assessment identifies the patient's needs. Care is based on the patient problems that have been identified. Possible patient problems include the following:

- *Anxiousness*
- *Compromised Maintenance of Health*
- *Compromised Social Interaction*
- *Fearfulness*
- *Impaired Health Maintenance*
- *Impaired Self-care (specify)*
- *Impaired Sensory Awareness*
- *Lonesomeness*
- *Potential for Injury*
- *Social Seclusion*

EXPECTED OUTCOMES AND PLANNING

Impairment of vision or hearing requires a major adjustment in the life of an individual. The patient must adjust to the loss and changes in lifestyle, whether the loss is permanent or temporary. The care plan focuses on achieving specific goals and outcomes that relate to the identified patient problems. Examples of these include the following:

Goal 1: Patient will remain free of injury.

Outcome: Patient and family inspect environment for potential hazards related to loss of vision or hearing.

Goal 2: Patient will remain socially active.

Outcome: Patient displays interest in social and recreational activities.

IMPLEMENTATION

Measures used in the care of a patient with vision or hearing loss center around helping the patient remain physically and emotionally safe and secure and ensuring that the patient's needs are communicated and met while adjusting to the loss. Nursing interventions include promoting safety, assisting with ADLs, facilitating communication, and encouraging diversional activity. Also assess readiness to learn and teach health promotion practices (see the Patient Teaching boxes throughout this chapter). Consider the patient's culture, beliefs, values, and habits and the special needs of the older adult.

EVALUATION

Systematic evaluation requires determining whether expected outcomes have been met. Refer to the goals and outcomes identified when assisting in planning care and evaluating the achievement of the goals.

Examples of goals and their evaluative measures include the following:

Goal 1: Patient will remain free of injury.

Evaluative measure: Ask patient and family to describe what environmental changes must be made to ensure safety.

Goal 2: Patient will remain socially active.

Evaluative measure: Observe patient participating in social activities.

Get Ready for the NCLEX® Examination!

Key Points

- The five major senses are taste, touch, smell, sight, and hearing.
- The accessory structures of the eye are the eyebrows, eyelids, eyelashes, and the lacrimal apparatus.
- The three tunics of the eye are the fibrous tunic (sclera), the vascular tunic (choroid), and the retina.
- The two chambers of the eye are the anterior chamber, which contains aqueous humor, and the posterior chamber, which contains vitreous humor.
- Image formation at the retina requires four basic processes: refraction, accommodation, constriction, and convergence.
- The photoreceptors of the retina are the rods and cones. The rods control vision in dim light, and the cones control vision in bright light. The cones are also responsible for color vision.
- Light entering the eye must travel through the cornea, the aqueous humor, the pupil, the crystalline lens, the vitreous humor, and finally the retina.
- The ear is divided into external, middle, and inner ears.
- The external ear flap is called the pinna (auricle); it extends into the external ear canal.
- The middle ear contains the ossicles and the entrance of the eustachian tube and ends with the tympanic membrane.
- The inner ear contains the vestibule, the cochlea, and the semicircular canals.
- The organ of Corti is the organ of hearing; it is located within the cochlea.
- The semicircular canals are responsible for the sense of balance and equilibrium.
- The taste buds differentiate four basic tastes: sweet, sour, salty, bitter, and umami (savory).
- Normal aging causes decreased hearing and sight as a result of normal changes of the structures.
- Individuals who have chronic disease or are older than 40 should be examined yearly to detect eye abnormalities or to prescribe changes in therapy.
- Refractory errors include hyperopia, presbyopia, and astigmatism.
- Ranges of 20/20 to 20/40 vision are considered normal, whereas 20/200 with correction is defined as legal blindness.
- ARMD is divided into two classic forms: dry and wet. In dry ARMD, which accounts for 90% of patients with ARMD, the macular cells have wasted or atrophied. Wet ARMD is characterized by the development of abnormal blood vessels in or near the macula.
- Cataracts are opaque areas in the lens and may be removed by intracapsular or extracapsular extraction.
- Glaucoma is not one disease but rather a group of disorders characterized by (1) increased IOP and the consequences of elevated pressure, (2) optic nerve atrophy, and (3) peripheral visual field loss.
- Loss of hearing may result from cerumen buildup, infection, trauma, or use of ototoxic drugs, or it may be a congenital condition.
- Conductive hearing loss is a decrease in amplification, whereas sensorineural hearing loss is interference within the inner ear and nerve conduction.
- Prevention of serious complications of ear disorders, such as infections, mastoiditis, and brain abscess, requires early detection and treatment.
- *Potential for Injury* is the primary patient problem for the patient experiencing vertigo, which occurs in labyrinthitis and Ménière's disease.
- An essential communication tip for speaking to the hearing impaired is to face the patient and to speak clearly without shouting.
- A cochlear implant is a hearing device for the profoundly deaf. The implanted device is intended for the patient with sensorineural hearing loss.

Additional Learning Resources

SG Go to your Study Guide for additional learning activities to help you master this chapter content.

evolve Be sure to visit the Evolve site at *http://evolve.elsevier.com/Cooper/foundationsadult/* for additional online resources.

Review Questions for the NCLEX® Examination

1. A patient is to have a laser treatment to cauterize hemorrhaging vessels caused by diabetic retinopathy. The patient asks the nurse what this procedure is called. Which response by the nurse is correct?
   1. Enucleation
   2. Scleral buckle
   3. Photocoagulation
   4. Trabeculoplasty
2. The parents want to know more about their child's conductive hearing loss. Which is the best explanation by the nurse?
   1. "Sound is delivered through the external and middle ear, but a defect in the inner ear results in distortion of sound."
   2. "Sound is inadequately delivered through the external or middle ear to the inner ear."
   3. "There is no organic cause, but a functional problem exists."
   4. "The brain's auditory pathways are damaged."

3. A patient has impaired hearing. Which action by the nurse would best facilitate communication?
  1. Face the patient when speaking.
  2. Overaccentuate words to make the communication more effective.
  3. Shout to allow the patient to hear.
  4. Use one-word phrases when speaking.

4. A patient tells the nurse he has dizziness. He states that the health care provider used another term. What term did the health care provider most likely use?
  1. Tinnitus
  2. Labyrinthitis
  3. Sensorineural
  4. Vertigo

5. A patient is diagnosed with an inner ear problem. For what symptom should the nurse monitor the patient closely?
  1. Echoing
  2. Intense pain
  3. Vertigo
  4. Loss of hearing

6. The nurse is evaluating a patient's eye as it adjusts to seeing objects at various distances. When documenting, how should the nurse identify this test?
  1. PERRLA
  2. Refraction
  3. Focusing
  4. Accommodation

7. A patient is suspected of having a retinal detachment. What signs/symptoms will provide support to this diagnosis? *(Select all that apply.)*
  1. "I have tunnel vision."
  2. "I am having a lot of pain in my eye."
  3. "It feels like I'm looking through cobwebs."
  4. "I see specks floating around the edges of my vision."
  5. "I feel like someone pulled a curtain over my eye."

8. Which of the following would be most hazardous in the home of a patient who is visually impaired?
  1. Area rugs
  2. Room carpeting
  3. Tile floor
  4. Concrete flooring

9. A patient arrives in the emergency room after an accident that resulted in a piece of metal penetrating the eye. What nursing action should be taken initially on the patient's arrival at the hospital?
  1. Apply a cool compress immediately.
  2. Lightly cover both eyes with an eye shield.
  3. Attempt to gently remove the object.
  4. Irrigate the eye with tap water.

10. A patient has just had cataract surgery. What information should the nurse include in the discharge instructions? *(Select all that apply.)*
  1. Wear an eye shield at night on the operative eye.
  2. Avoid bending, stooping, coughing, or lifting.
  3. Instill prescribed eyedrops into the conjunctival sac.
  4. Take an analgesic every 4 hours.
  5. Avoid lying on the affected eye for 2 weeks after surgery.

11. Which assessment finding would indicate a need for possible glaucoma testing? *(Select all that apply.)*
  1. Presence of "floaters"
  2. Halos around lights
  3. Progressive loss of peripheral vision
  4. Pruritus and erythema of the conjunctiva
  5. Lack of ability to adapt to darkness

12. While communicating with a patient, you notice a possible hearing deficit in one ear. Which nursing intervention would be appropriate?
  1. Shout in the affected ear.
  2. Speak clearly and in a slightly louder voice toward the patient's face.
  3. Plug the affected ear and shout in the unaffected ear.
  4. Speak more softly than usual in the affected ear.

13. The nurse is admitting an adult patient to a walk-in clinic. The patient complains of recent hearing loss. What does the nurse anticipate as the most probable cause of this patient's hearing loss?
  1. Cerumen buildup
  2. Ossification of the pinna
  3. Low batteries in the hearing aid
  4. Fluid in the ear

14. A 71-year-old patient complains of being severely dizzy. What instruction should the nurse give the patient?
  1. Avoid sudden movements.
  2. Avoid noises.
  3. Increase fluid intake.
  4. Lie on the affected side.

15. A patient who has been blind for the past 10 years is hospitalized with heart failure. What intervention should the nurse include in the plan of care?
  1. Keep all personal care items at a distance so that he won't bump into them.
  2. Schedule a consultation with an occupational therapist to teach activities of daily living.
  3. All personnel announce themselves when entering and leaving the room.
  4. Initiate a referral to the Department of Health and Human Services.

16. A patient has a family history of cataracts. He asks what early symptoms he should watch for that would alert him to the development of cataracts. What is the nurse's best response?
  1. Pain in the eyes
  2. Blurred vision
  3. Loss of peripheral vision
  4. Dry eyes

17. A patient is scheduled for a stapedectomy. What postoperative instructions should the nurse include in patient teaching? *(Select all that apply.)*
  1. Change cotton in external ear canal hourly.
  2. Gently blow through both nares simultaneously.
  3. Teach the patient to open the mouth when sneezing or coughing.
  4. Limit exercise or active sports for 3 weeks.
  5. Avoid exposure to people with upper respiratory tract infections.

18. A 15-year-old hearing-impaired patient is having problems communicating with the staff. Which behavior would improve communication? *(Select all that apply.)*
1. Overaccentuating words
2. Facing the patient when speaking
3. Speaking in conversational tones
4. Asking permission to turn off the television or radio
5. Using written communication for most interactions

19. The nurse is caring for a patient with vertigo. What is the nurse's priority concern when caring for this patient?
1. Safety
2. Comfort
3. Hygiene
4. Quiet

20. While cleaning the garage, a patient splashed a chemical in his eyes. What is the initial action after the chemical burn?
1. Transport to an emergency facility immediately.
2. Cover the eyes with sterile gauze.
3. Lubricate eye with petroleum-based jelly.
4. Irrigate the eye with water for 20 minutes.

21. A patient visits the health care provider to have her vision tested using the Snellen eye chart. What instruction should the nurse provide to the patient?
1. Use both eyes to read the chart.
2. Read the chart from right to left.
3. Cover one eye while testing the other.
4. Use either eye because they will be the same.

22. A 78-year-old patient comes into the clinic complaining of progressive loss of vision in the center of the visual field. The nurse is aware that the patient is most likely experiencing symptoms of which disorder?
1. Macular degeneration
2. Primary open-angle glaucoma
3. Color blindness
4. Retinal degeneration

23. After cataract surgery a patient complains of sudden sharp pain in the operative eye. What is the most appropriate nursing action?
1. Remove the metal eye shield to relieve pressure.
2. Call the surgeon.
3. Administer an analgesic.
4. Document complaint of pain on chart.

24. A patient is asked to sign a surgical consent for treatment of otosclerosis. Which statement indicates correct understanding of the procedure?
1. "It involves surgical repair of the external ear."
2. "It means cutting the nerve in my ear."
3. "It cleans the ear canal of wax."
4. "It will help me hear sounds again."

25. The nurse receives medication orders for a patient with open-angle glaucoma. Which medication order does the nurse anticipate?
1. Atropine, cyclopentolate hydrochloride
2. Betoptic, pilocarpine hydrochloride
3. Dexamethasone, Liquifilm
4. Mannitol, Cyclogyl

Care of the Patient With a Neurologic Disorder

54

http://evolve.elsevier.com/Cooper/foundationsadult/

Objectives

Anatomy and Physiology

1. Name the two structural divisions of the nervous system and give the functions of each.
2. List the parts of the neuron, and describe the function of each part.
3. Explain the anatomic location and functions of the cerebrum, the brainstem, the cerebellum, the spinal cord, the peripheral nerves, and cerebrospinal fluid.
4. Discuss the parts of the peripheral nervous system and how the system works with the central nervous system.
5. List the 12 cranial nerves and the areas they serve.

Medical-Surgical

6. List physiologic changes that occur with aging in the nervous system.
7. Explain the importance of prevention in problems of the nervous system, and give several examples of prevention.
8. Identify the significant subjective and objective data related to the nervous system that should be obtained from a patient during assessment.
9. Differentiate between normal and common abnormal findings of a physical assessment of the nervous system.
10. Discuss the Glasgow Coma Scale.
11. List common laboratory and diagnostic examinations for evaluation of neurologic disorders.
12. List five signs and symptoms of increased intracranial pressure, why they occur, and nursing interventions that decrease intracranial pressure.
13. Discuss various neurologic disturbances in motor function and sensory-perceptual function.
14. List four classifications of seizures, their characteristics, clinical signs, aura, and postictal period.
15. Give examples of six degenerative neurologic diseases and explain the etiology, pathophysiology, clinical manifestations, assessment, diagnostic tests, medical management, nursing interventions, and prognosis for each.
16. Discuss the etiology, pathophysiology, clinical manifestations of stroke and the assessment, diagnostic tests, medical management, nursing interventions, and prognosis for a stroke patient.
17. Differentiate between trigeminal neuralgia and Bell's palsy.
18. Discuss the etiology, pathophysiology, clinical manifestations, assessment, diagnostic tests, medical management, nursing interventions, and prognosis for GBS, meningitis, encephalitis, and AIDS.
19. Explain the mechanism of injury to the brain that occurs with a stroke and traumatic brain injury.
20. Discuss the etiology, pathophysiology, clinical manifestations, assessment, diagnostic tests, medical management, nursing interventions, and prognosis for intracranial tumors, brain trauma, and spinal trauma.

Key Terms

agnosia (ăg-NŌ-zhă, p. 1886)
aneurysm (ĂN-ūr-ĭ-zĭm, p. 1905)
aphasia (ă-FĀ-zē-ă, p. 1872)
apraxia (ă-PRĂK-sē-ă, p. 1899)
ataxia (ă-TĂK-sē-ă, p. 1891)
aura (ĂW-ră, p. 1877)
bradykinesia (brā-dē-kĭ-NĒ-zē-ă, p. 1893)
deep brain stimulation (DBS) (p. 1895)
diplopia (dĭp-LŌ-pē-ă, p. 1880)
dysarthria (dĭs-ĂHR-thrē-ă, p. 1873)
dysphagia (dĭs-FĀ-jē-ă, p. 1883)
flaccid (FLĂK-sĭd, p. 1873)
Glasgow Coma Scale (GLĂS-gō KŌ-mă SKAL, p. 1871)
global cognitive dysfunction (GLŌ-băl KŎG-nĭ-tĭv dĭs-FŬNK-shŭn, p. 1915)
Guillain-Barré syndrome (GBS) (GĒ-yăn bă-RĀ, p. 1912)
hemianopia (hĕm-ē-ă-NŌ-pē-ă, p. 1873)
hemiplegia (hĕm-ē-PLĒ-jă, p. 1884)
hyperreflexia (hī-pĕr-rē-FLĔK-sē-ă, p. 1919)
neoplasm (p. 1916)
nystagmus (nĭs-TĂG-mŭs, p. 1891)
paresis (pă-RĒ-sĭs, p. 1873)
postictal period (pōst-ĬK-tăl PĒ-rē-ŏd, p. 1887)
proprioception (prō-prē-ō-SĔP-shŭn, p. 1873)
spastic (SPĂS-tĭk, p. 1873)
stroke (strōk, p. 1903)
unilateral neglect (ū-nĭ-LĂT-ĕr-ăl nĕ-GLĔCT, p. 1873)

ANATOMY AND PHYSIOLOGY OF THE NEUROLOGIC SYSTEM

The nervous system is responsible for communication and control within the body. It interprets or processes the information received and sends it to the appropriate area of the brain or spinal cord, where the response is generated. The nervous system is the body's link with the environment. It works in conjunction with the endocrine system to maintain the body's homeostasis. The nervous system reacts in split seconds, whereas the hormones secreted by the endocrine glands work more slowly in initiating a response. The clinical picture for the patient with neurologic problems is often complex. Understanding these conditions requires knowledge of the anatomy and physiology of the nervous system.

STRUCTURAL DIVISIONS

The nervous system has two main structural divisions, the central nervous system and the peripheral nervous system:

- *Central nervous system:* The central nervous system (CNS) is made up of the brain and the spinal cord. It occupies a medial position in the body and is responsible for interpreting incoming sensory information and issuing instructions based on past experiences.
- *Peripheral nervous system:* The peripheral nervous system includes all the nerves that lie outside the CNS.

The peripheral nervous system contains two main divisions: the somatic nervous system and the autonomic nervous system:

- *Somatic nervous system:* The somatic nervous system sends messages to the CNS via sensory (or afferent) neurons and from the CNS to the skeletal muscles (voluntary muscles) via motor (or efferent) neurons.
- *Autonomic nervous system:* The autonomic system transmits messages from the CNS to the smooth muscle, the cardiac muscle, and certain glands. The autonomic system is sometimes called the *involuntary nervous system* because its action takes place without conscious control. It has two divisions: the sympathetic and parasympathetic.

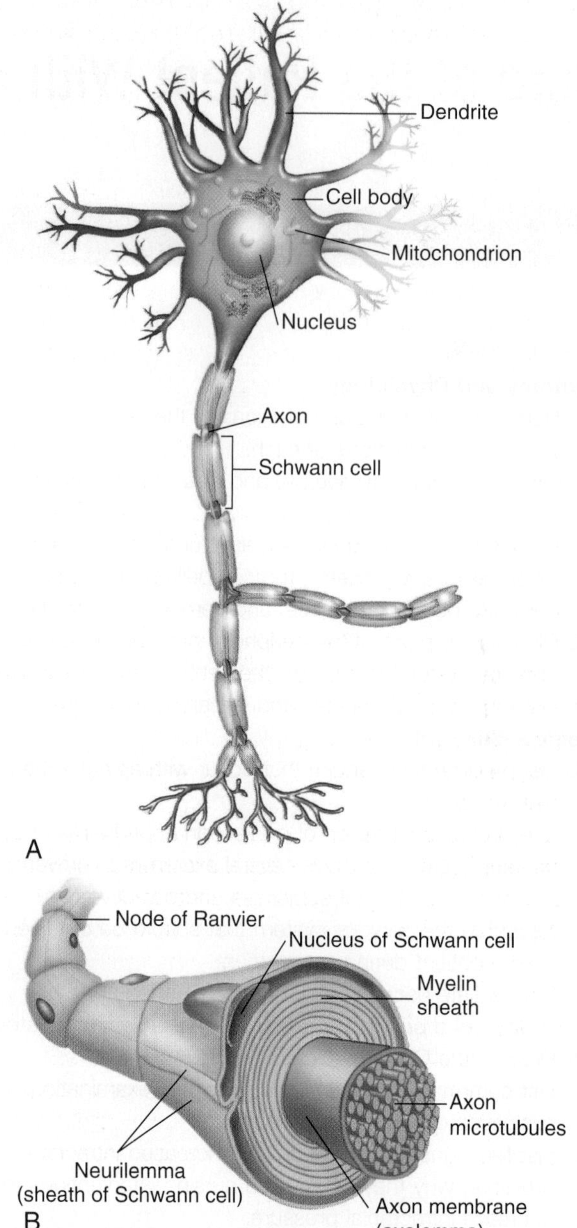

Fig. 54.1 A, Diagram of a typical neuron showing dendrites, cell body, and axon. B, Cross-section of a myelinated axon, showing the concentric, myelinated layers of the Schwann cell. (From Patton KT, Thibodeau GA: *The human body in health and disease*, ed 7, St. Louis, 2018, Elsevier.)

CELLS OF THE NERVOUS SYSTEM

Two broad categories of cells exist within the nervous system. The neurons occupy the first category. Their role as transmitter is to carry messages to and from the brain and spinal cord (Fig. 54.1). The neuroglia or glial cells represent the second category; they support and protect the neurons while producing cerebrospinal fluid (CSF), which continuously bathes the structures of the CNS.

Neuron

A *neuron* (nerve cell) is the basic cell of the nervous system. It is a separate unit composed of three main structures: the cell body, the axon, and the dendrites. The cell body contains a nucleus surrounded by cytoplasm. The axon is the cylindric extension of a nerve cell that conducts impulses away from the neuron cell body. The dendrites are branching structures that extend from the cell body and receive impulses. Between each neuron is a gap (space) called the *synapse,* defined as the region surrounding the point of contact between two neurons or between a neuron and an effector organ, and across which nerve impulses are transmitted through the action of a neurotransmitter.

All neurons are governed by the "all-or-none law," which means there is never a partial transmission of a message; the impulse is either strong enough to elicit a response or too weak to generate the message.

Neuromuscular Junction

The area of contact between the ends of a large myelinated nerve fiber and a fiber of skeletal muscle is called the *neuromuscular junction*. The body's nervous system connects with the muscular system via these areas of contact. Neurotransmitters act to make certain that the neurologic impulse passes from the nerve to the muscle.

Neurotransmitters

Numerous chemicals called *neurotransmitters* modify or result in the transmission of impulses between synapses and at neuromuscular junctions. The best-known neurotransmitters are acetylcholine, norepinephrine, dopamine, and serotonin.

- *Acetylcholine* plays a role in nerve impulse transmission; it spills into the synapse area and speeds the transmission of the impulse. The enzyme cholinesterase then is released to deactivate the acetylcholine once the message or impulse has been sent. This happens rapidly and continuously as each impulse is relayed.
- *Norepinephrine* has an effect on maintaining arousal (awakening from a deep sleep), dreaming, and regulation of mood (e.g., happiness, sadness).
- *Dopamine* affects primarily motor function; it is involved in gross subconscious movements of the skeletal muscles. It also plays a role in emotional responses. A person with Parkinson's disease has decreased dopamine levels and suffers involuntary, trembling muscle movements, or *tremors*.
- *Serotonin* induces sleep, affects sensory perception, controls temperature, and has a role in control of mood.

Neuron Coverings

Many neuron fibers (axons and dendrites) (see Fig. 54.1) are covered with a white, waxy, fatty material called *myelin*. Myelin increases the rate of transmission of impulses and protects and insulates the fibers. Axons leaving the CNS are wrapped in layers of myelin with indentations called the *nodes of Ranvier*. These nodes further increase the rate of transmission because the impulse can jump from node to node.

In the peripheral nervous system the myelin is produced by Schwann cells (see Fig. 54.1). The outer membrane of the Schwann cells gives rise to another layer called the neurilemma. The neurilemma is important because it helps regenerate injured axons. Thus regeneration of nerve cells occurs only in the peripheral nervous system. Cells damaged in the CNS result in permanent damage (paralysis) because they do not have a neurilemma and are not able to regenerate.

CENTRAL NERVOUS SYSTEM

The CNS is composed of the brain and the spinal cord and represents one of the two main divisions of the nervous system. It functions somewhat like a computer but is much more complex. The cranium protects the brain, and the vertebral column protects the spinal cord.

Brain

Specialized cells in the brain's mass of convoluted, soft, gray or white tissue coordinate and regulate the functions of the CNS. The brain is one of the largest organs in the body, weighing approximately 3 pounds (1.4 kg). It is divided into four principal parts: the cerebrum, the diencephalon, the cerebellum, and the brainstem.

Cerebrum. The cerebrum is the largest part of the brain (Fig. 54.2). It is divided into left and right hemispheres. The outer portion of the cerebrum is composed of gray matter and is called the *cerebral cortex*. It is arranged in folds, called *gyri* (convolutions); the grooves are called *sulci* (fissures). The connecting structure or bridge is called the *corpus callosum*. Two deep sulci subdivide the two hemispheres into four lobes that are named for the bones lying over them: the frontal lobe, the parietal lobe, the temporal lobe, and the occipital lobe. Each hemisphere of the cerebrum controls initiation of movement on the opposite side of the body. The functions of the cerebrum are multiple and complex. Specific areas of the cerebral cortex are associated with specific functions (Fig. 54.3 and Box 54.1).

Basal nuclei. The basal nuclei (formerly referred to as the basal ganglia) are additional islands of gray matter buried deep within the two cerebral hemispheres. They control automatic movement of the body as well as posture. This portion of the cerebrum regulates voluntary motor function, including the muscle contractions associated with walking and maintaining posture. The basal nuclei also are involved with thinking and learning (National Library of Medicine [NLM], 2018a).

Diencephalon. The diencephalon often is called the *interbrain*. It lies beneath the cerebrum and contains the thalamus and the hypothalamus. The thalamus serves as a relay station on the way to the cerebral cortex for some sensory impulses; it interprets other sensory messages, such as pain, light touch, and pressure. The hypothalamus, which lies beneath the thalamus, plays a vital role in the control of body temperature; fluid balance; appetite; sleep; and certain emotions, such as fear, pleasure, and pain. The sympathetic and parasympathetic divisions of the autonomic system are under the control of the hypothalamus, as is the pituitary gland. Thus the hypothalamus influences the heartbeat, the contraction and relaxation of the walls of the blood vessels, hormone secretion, and other vital body functions (see Fig. 54.2).

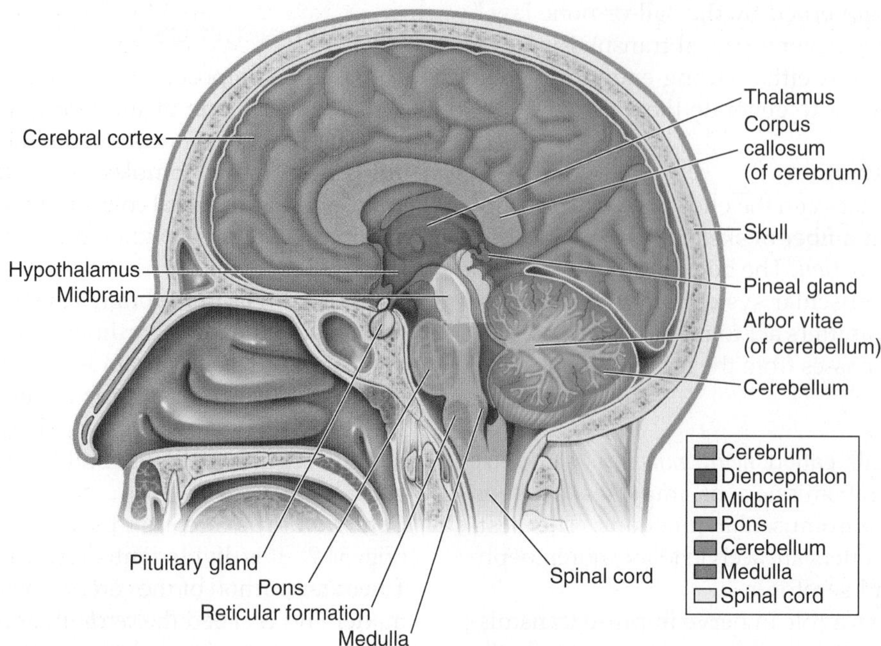

Fig. 54.2 Sagittal section of the brain. (From Patton KT, Thibodeau GA: *The human body in health and disease,* ed 7, St. Louis, 2018, Elsevier.)

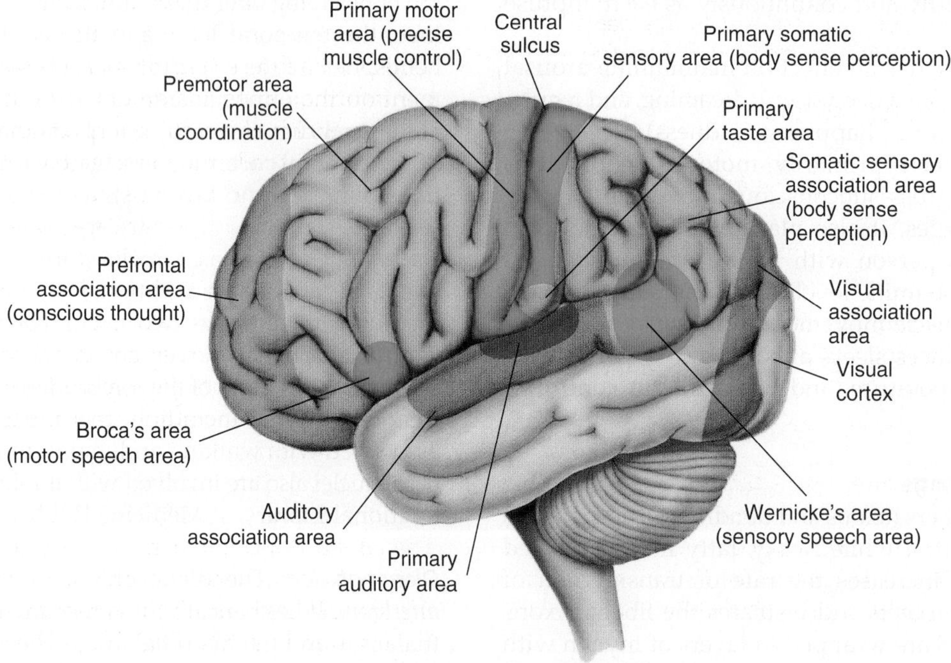

Fig. 54.3 Cerebral cortex. (From Patton KT, Thibodeau GA: *The human body in health and disease,* ed 7, St. Louis, 2018, Elsevier.)

Cerebellum. The cerebellum lies posterior and inferior to the cerebrum and is the second largest portion of the brain. It contains two hemispheres with a convoluted surface much like the cerebrum. It is mainly responsible for coordination of voluntary movement and maintenance of balance, equilibrium, and muscle tone (a muscle's baseline degree of tension). It coordinates and smooths movement (e.g., the complex and quick coordination of many different muscles needed in playing the piano, swimming, or juggling). It is like the automatic pilot on an airplane in that it adjusts and corrects voluntary movement but operates entirely below the conscious level. Sensory messages from the semicircular canals in the inner ear send their messages to the cerebellum (see Fig. 54.2).

Brainstem. The brainstem is located at the base of the brain and contains the *midbrain,* the *pons,* and

Box 54.1 Functions of the Cerebrum

FRONTAL LOBE
- Written speech: Ability to write
- Motor speech, Broca's area: Ability to speak. Motor speech is mediated in Broca's area in the frontal lobe. When an injury to Broca's area (or the hemisphere in general) occurs, expressive aphasia can result and the patient will not be able to speak. The patient can produce only a garbled sound but can understand language and knows what he or she wants to say.
- Motor ability: Movements of body. The left side of the brain controls the right side of the body, and the right side of the brain controls the left side of the body.
- Intellectualization: The ability to form concepts, personality, emotion, behavior
- Judgment formation

PARIETAL LOBE
- Interpretation of sensory impulses from the skin, such as touch, pain, and temperature
- Recognition of body parts
- Determination of left from right
- Determination of shapes, sizes, and distances

TEMPORAL LOBE
- Wernicke's area: Language comprehension. When Wernicke's area is damaged in the person's dominant hemisphere, receptive aphasia results. The person hears sound, but it has no meaning, like hearing a foreign language.
- Integration of auditory stimuli

OCCIPITAL LOBE
- Interpretation of visual impulses from the retina

the *medulla oblongata* (see Fig. 54.2). These structures connect the spinal cord and the cerebrum. The brainstem carries all nerve fibers between the spinal cord and the cerebrum.

Midbrain. The midbrain forms the superior portion of the brainstem. It merges into the thalamus and the hypothalamus. It is responsible for motor movement, relay of impulses, and auditory and visual reflexes. It is the origin of cranial nerves III and IV.

Pons. The pons connects the midbrain to the medulla oblongata; the word *pons* means "bridge." It is the origin of cranial nerves V through VIII. The pons is composed of myelinated nerve fibers and is responsible for sending impulses to the structures that are inferior and superior to it. It also contains a respiratory center that complements respiratory centers located in the medulla.

Medulla oblongata. The medulla oblongata is the distal portion of the brainstem. It is the origin of cranial nerves IX and XII. The medulla controls heartbeat, rhythm of breathing, swallowing, coughing, sneezing, vomiting, and hiccups *(singultus)*. A vasomotor center regulates the diameter of the blood vessels, which aids in the control of blood pressure.

Coverings of the brain and the spinal cord. The brain and the spinal cord are surrounded by three protective coverings called the *meninges:* (1) the dura mater, the outermost layer; (2) the arachnoid membrane, the second layer; and (3) the pia mater, the innermost layer, which provides oxygen and nourishment to the nervous tissue. These layers also bathe the spinal cord and the brain in CSF.

Ventricles. The four ventricles are spaces or cavities located in the brain. The CSF, which is clear and resembles plasma, flows into the subarachnoid spaces around the brain and the spinal cord and cushions them. It contains protein, glucose, urea, and salts; it also contains certain substances that form a protective barrier (the blood-brain barrier) that prevents harmful substances from entering the brain and the spinal cord.

Spinal Cord

The spinal cord is a 17- to 18-inch cord that extends from the brainstem to the second lumbar vertebra. It has two main functions: conducting impulses to and from the brain and serving as a center for reflex actions such as a knee jerk (Fig. 54.4). A sensory neuron sends the information to the spinal cord, a central neuron (located within the cord) interprets the impulse, and a motoneuron sends the message back to the muscle or organ involved. Thus a message is sent, interpreted, and acted on without traveling to the brain.

Peripheral Nervous System

The *peripheral nervous system* is made up of the motor nerves, the sensory nerves, and ganglia outside the brain and the spinal cord. It is composed of 31 pairs of spinal nerves, 12 pairs of cranial nerves, and the autonomic nervous system.

Spinal Nerves

The 31 pairs of spinal nerves are all mixed nerves. This means that they transmit sensory information to the spinal cord through afferent neurons and motor information from the CNS to the various areas of the body through efferent neurons. The spinal nerves are named according to the corresponding vertebra (e.g., *C1* for cervical spinal nerve 1, and *C2* for cervical spinal nerve 2).

Cranial Nerves

There are 12 pairs of cranial nerves, which attach to the posterior surface of the brain, mainly the brainstem. Eleven of the pairs conduct impulses between the head, the neck, and the brain; the vagus nerve (cranial nerve X) also serves organs in the thoracic and abdominal cavities (Fig. 54.5). Table 54.1 lists the cranial nerves, their impulses, and functions.

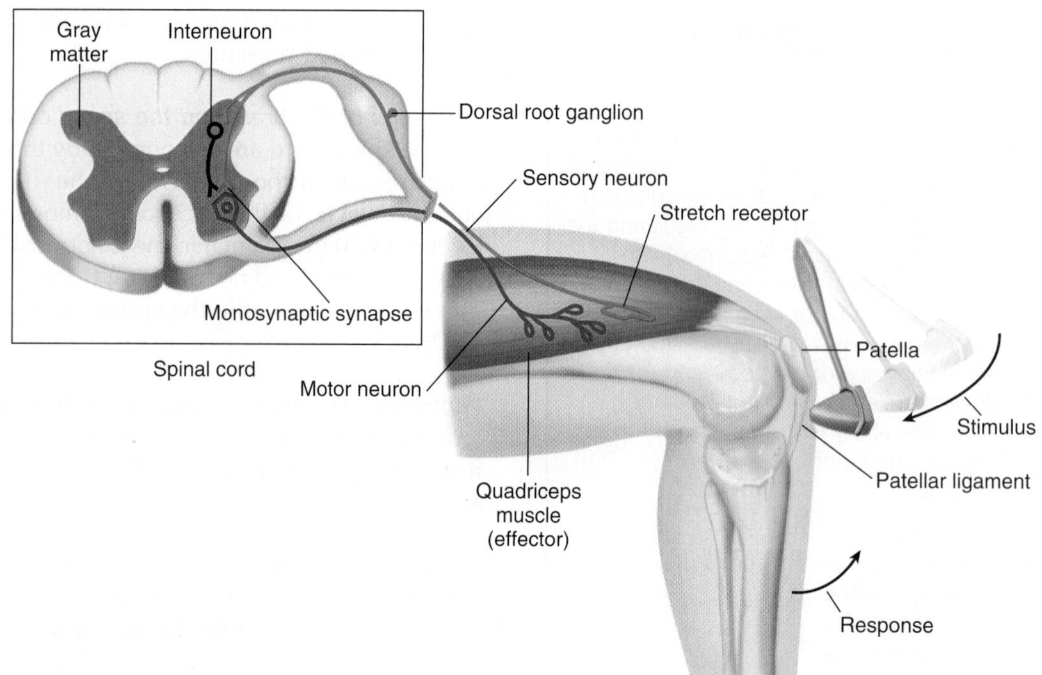

Fig. 54.4 Neural pathway involved in the patellar reflex. (From Patton KT, Thibodeau GA: *The human body in health and disease,* ed 7, St. Louis, 2018, Elsevier.)

Table 54.1 Cranial Nerves

NERVE[a]	CONDUCTS IMPULSES	FUNCTIONS
I: Olfactory	From nose to brain	Sense of smell
II: Optic	From eye to brain	Vision
III: Oculomotor	From brain to eye muscles	Eye movements, extraocular muscles, pupillary control (pupillary constriction)
IV: Trochlear	From brain to external eye muscles	Down and inward movement of eye
V: Trigeminal Ophthalmic branch Maxillary branch Mandibular branch	From skin and mucous membranes of head to brain; from teeth to brain; from brain to chewing muscles	Sensations of face, scalp, and teeth; chewing movements
VI: Abducens	From brain to external eye muscles	Outward movement of eye
VII: Facial	From taste buds of tongue to brain; from brain to facial muscles	Sense of taste on anterior two-thirds of tongue; contraction of muscles of facial expression
VIII: Acoustic (vestibulocochlear)	From ear to brain	Hearing; sense of balance (equilibrium)
IX: Glossopharyngeal	From throat and taste buds of tongue to brain; from brain to throat muscles and salivary glands	Sensations of throat, taste, swallowing movements, gag reflex, sense of taste on posterior one third of tongue, secretion of saliva
X: Vagus	From throat, larynx, and organs in thoracic and abdominal cavities to brain; from brain to muscles of throat and to organs in thoracic and abdominal cavities	Sensations of throat, larynx, and thoracic and abdominal organs; swallowing, voice production, slowing of heartbeat, acceleration of peristalsis
XI: Spinal accessory	From brain to certain shoulder and neck muscles	Shoulder movements (trapezius muscle) and turning movements of head (sternocleidomastoid muscles)
XII: Hypoglossal	From brain to muscles of tongue	Tongue movements

[a]The first letter of the words in the following sentence are the first letters of the names of cranial nerves: "On Old Olympus's Towering Tops A Finn And German Viewed Some Hops." Many generations of students have used this or a similar mnemonic to help them remember the names of cranial nerves.

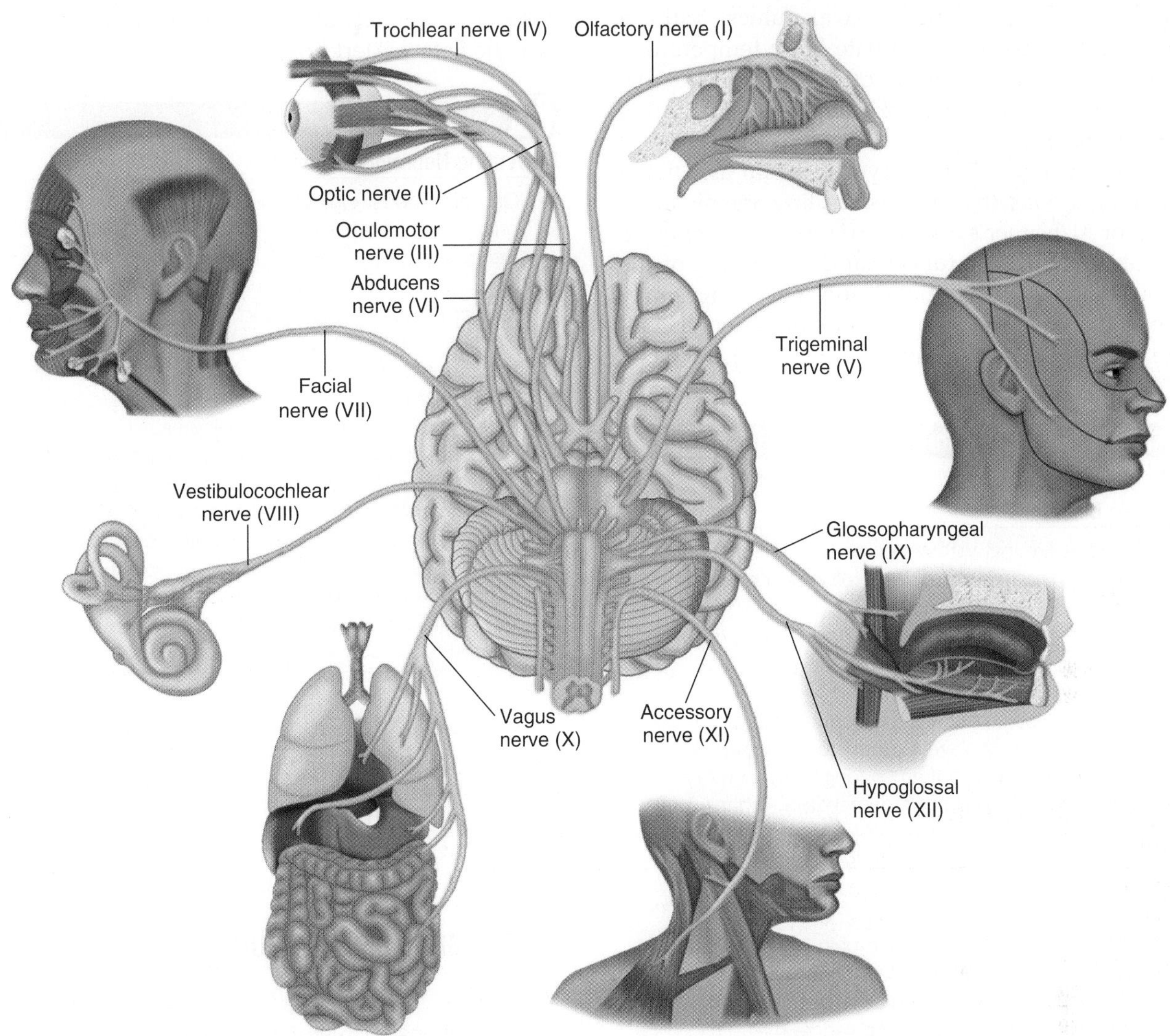

Fig. 54.5 Cranial nerves. (From Patton KT, Thibodeau GA: *The human body in health and disease,* ed 7, St. Louis, 2018, Elsevier.)

Autonomic Nervous System

The autonomic nervous system controls the activities of the smooth muscle, the cardiac muscle, and all glands. The autonomic nervous system is not a separate nervous system but a subdivision of the peripheral nervous system.

It is misleading to think of this system as the automatic system, although most activity is performed on an unconscious level. Its primary function is to maintain internal homeostasis; for example, it strives to maintain a normal heartbeat, a constant body temperature, and a normal respiratory pattern.

To maintain this homeostasis, the autonomic system has two divisions: the *sympathetic nervous system* and the *parasympathetic nervous system.* These two divisions are antagonistic: one slows an action, and the other accelerates the action. These systems function simultaneously, but they are able to dominate each other as the need arises. In times of stress the sympathetic system takes over to prepare the body for "fight or flight." Heartbeat accelerates, blood pressure rises, and adrenal glands increase their secretions. To calm the body after a crisis, the parasympathetic system becomes dominant, slowing the heartbeat and decreasing the blood pressure and adrenal hormone output.

EFFECTS OF NORMAL AGING ON THE NERVOUS SYSTEM

The effects of aging on the nervous system are variable. The changes that occur include a loss of brain weight and a substantial loss of neurons (1% per year after age 50); the cortex loses cells faster than the brainstem. The remaining cells undergo structural changes. Aging also brings about a general decline in interconnections of dendrites, a reduction in cerebral blood flow, and a decrease in brain metabolism and oxygen use. The neurons may contain senile plaques, neurofibrillary tangles, and the age pigment lipofuscin. Older adults often have an altered sleep-to-wakefulness ratio, a decrease in the ability to regulate body temperature, and a decrease in the velocity of nerve impulses. The blood supply to the spinal cord is decreased, resulting in slower reflexes.

Normal changes in the nervous system associated with aging are *not* the same as senility, organic brain disease, or Alzheimer's disease (AD). Many older people reach old age with no functional deterioration of the nervous system. However, these normal changes may make care or rehabilitation of the older patient a challenge (see the Lifespan Considerations box).

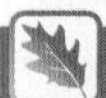

Lifespan Considerations

Older Adults

Neurologic Disorder

- As neurons are lost with aging, neurologic function deteriorates, resulting in slowed reflex and reaction time.
- Tremors that increase with fatigue are common.
- The sense of touch and fine motor coordination diminish with aging.
- Most older people possess the ability to learn, but the speed of learning is slowed. Short-term memory is affected more by aging than by long-term memory.
- The incidence of physiologic dementia or organic brain syndrome—including Alzheimer's disease, Pick's disease, and multiinfarct dementia—increases with age.
- The incidence of stroke increases with age. Nerve irritation from arthritis, joint injuries, or spinal cord compression can cause chronic pain or weakness.
- Dementia is not a normal consequence of aging but may be a result of many reversible conditions, including anemia, fluid and electrolyte imbalance, malnutrition, hypothyroidism, metabolic disturbances, drug toxicity, a drug reaction or idiosyncrasy, and hypotension.

PREVENTION OF NEUROLOGIC PROBLEMS

Many conditions of the nervous system have no known cause. Other neurologic problems can be prevented or their effects reduced by modifying lifestyle factors. Neurovascular diseases are in part associated with defined risk factors. These risk factors are the same factors that increase the risk of cardiac disease, including high blood pressure, high blood cholesterol levels, cigarette smoking, obesity, stress, and lack of exercise.

Prevention of neurologic problems resulting from trauma is a major challenge. These injuries include spinal cord injury and head injury, which occur frequently in young people. Patient teaching on avoiding such injuries should include avoidance of drug and alcohol use, safe use of motor vehicles (e.g., using automobile seatbelts; wearing helmets with bicycles, motorcycles, and snowmobiles), safe swimming practices (e.g., not diving into shallow water), safe handling and storage of firearms, use of hardhats in dangerous construction areas, and use of protective gear as needed for sports (see the Safety Alert box).

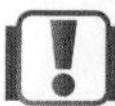

Safety Alert

Preventing Neurologic Injuries

- One of the best ways to prevent head injuries is to prevent car and motorcycle accidents.
- Become active in campaigns that promote safe driving. Speak to driver's education classes regarding the danger of unsafe driving and driving after drinking alcohol or taking drugs.
- The use of seatbelts in cars and the use of helmets for riding on motorcycles are the most effective measures for increasing survival after accidents.
- Individual states have legislation requiring the use of automobile safety devices for children and adults.
- Recommend wearing protective helmets when engaging in potentially risky activities such as bike riding, horseback riding, and motorcycling.
- Encourage swimmers of all ages to refrain from diving into shallow water or areas in which water depth is unknown.

Neurologic diseases, such as meningitis or brain abscess, that occur as a result of infection sometimes can be prevented by prompt treatment of ear and sinus infections. Health teaching concerning immunizations to prevent diseases such as meningitis can reduce neurologic health concerns.

ASSESSMENT OF THE NEUROLOGIC SYSTEM

HISTORY

A comprehensive history is essential for diagnosing neurologic disease. This includes specifics about symptoms experienced and the patient's understanding and perception of what is happening. Obtaining information from family members or significant others also may be helpful. Follow the same format routinely to make certain information is complete.

For patients with suspected neurologic conditions, the presence of many symptoms or subjective data may be significant. These include the following:

- Headaches, especially those that first occur after middle age or those that change in character (e.g., headaches that are worse in the morning or awaken a person from sleep)
- Clumsiness or loss of function in an extremity
- Change in visual acuity
- Any new or worsened seizure activity
- Numbness or tingling in one or more extremities
- Pain in an extremity or other part of the body
- Personality changes or mood swings
- Extreme fatigue or tiredness

MENTAL STATUS

Assessment of the neurologic patient's mental status generally includes orientation (person, place, time, and purpose), mood and behavior, general knowledge (such as the names of US presidents), and short- and long-term memory. The patient's attention span and ability to concentrate also may be assessed.

Document the mental status in specific terms. Record as much information as possible to highlight the patient's status. For example, it is better to note "oriented to name, date, hospital, and purpose" than to note simply "oriented." Record actual statements made by the patient. Vary orientation questions to limit patients' ability to answer correctly simply because they have learned the right answers through repetition.

Level of Consciousness

Level of consciousness (LOC) is the earliest and most sensitive indicator of the patient's neurologic status. Changes in LOC are a result of impaired cerebral blood flow, which deprives the cells of the cerebral cortex and the reticular activating system (RAS) of oxygen. The RAS, located in the brainstem, is a functional system essential for wakefulness, attention, concentration, and introspection (*Mosby's Dictionary of Medicine, Nursing, & Health Professions,* 2017). A decreasing LOC is the earliest sign of increased intracranial pressure (ICP). LOC has two components: *arousal* (or wakefulness) and *awareness*. Wakefulness is the most fundamental part of LOC. If the patient can open his or her eyes spontaneously, in response to voice or to pain, the wakefulness center in the brainstem is still functioning. Awareness, a higher function controlled by the RAS, is the ability to interact with and interpret the environment. Awareness has four components, which are assessed as follows:

1. *Orientation:* Ask questions to determine the patient's orientation to person, place, time, and purpose.
2. *Memory:* Assess short-term memory; do not ask yes or no questions.
3. *Calculation:* Ask a simple math problem (e.g., "If you had $2 and your apple costs $1.25, how many quarters would you get back?").
4. *Fund of knowledge:* Ask the patient to name the president and to tell you what's on the national news.

Restlessness, disorientation, and lethargy may be seen first. Record observations in terms of behavior and signs—not labels such as "disoriented." Table 54.2 shows one method of classifying LOC.

Glasgow Coma Scale

The **Glasgow Coma Scale** (Table 54.3) is a quick, practical, and standardized system for assessing the degree of consciousness impairment in the critically ill and for predicting the duration and ultimate outcome of coma, particularly with head injuries. A patient's score on the Glasgow Coma Scale can change, along with the patient's health continuum. The Glasgow Coma Scale consists of a three-part neurologic assessment: eye opening, best motor response, and best verbal response.

Table 54.2 Levels of Consciousness

LEVEL	DESCRIPTION
Alert	Responds appropriately to auditory, tactile, and visual stimuli
Disorientation	Disoriented; unable to follow simple commands; thinking slowed; inattentive, flat affect
Stupor	Responds to verbal commands with moaning or groaning, if at all; seems unaware of the surroundings
Semicomatose	Is in an impaired state of consciousness, characterized by stupor, from which a patient can be aroused only by energetic stimulation
Comatose	Unable to respond to painful stimuli; corneal and pupillary reflexes are absent Cannot swallow or cough Is incontinent of urine and feces Electroencephalogram pattern demonstrates decreased or absent neuronal activity

Table 54.3 Glasgow Coma Scale: Measurement of Level of Consciousness[a]

CATEGORY OF RESPONSE	RESPONSE	SCORE
Eye-opening response	Spontaneous—open with blinking at baseline	4
	To verbal stimuli, command, speech	3
	To pressure (not applied to face)	2
	No response	1
Verbal response	Oriented	5
	Confused conversation, but able to answer questions	4
	words	3
	sounds	2
	No response	1
Motor response	Obeys commands for movement	6
	Purposeful movement to painful stimulus	5
	Withdraws in response to pain	4
	Flexion in response to pain (decorticate posturing)	3
	Extension response in response to pain (decerebrate posturing)	2
	No response	1

[a]The Glasgow Coma Scale provides a score ranging from 3 to 15; patients with scores of 3 to 8 are usually said to be in a coma. The total score is the sum of the scores in the three categories.
Modified from The Glasgow Structured Approach to Assessment of the Glasgow Coma Scale: What's new? n.d. Retrieved from *http://www.glasgowcomascale.org/whats-new*.

The stronger the stimulus needed to obtain a response is, the lower the patient's score. The number values assigned to each part of the scale are added to yield an objective score. The score for a patient who is not neurologically impaired is 15; the lowest possible score is 3. In general, any score of 8 or less commonly is accepted as a definition of coma. The scale has a high degree of consistency even when used by staff of varied experience. There are some factors that may interfere with the outcomes of the scale. These are grouped into three categories: preexisting factors, effects of current treatments, and effects of other injuries or lesions. Language and cultural differences may act as barriers for the assessment. A hearing or intellectual deficit may result in impaired responses. Treatments such as pain medications or sedatives may influence the ability of the patient to appropriately respond. Coexisting conditions such as spinal trauma may result in altered findings (Glasgow Coma Scale, 2014).

FOUR Score Coma Scale

In response to criticisms of the Glasgow Coma Scale, the FOUR (Full Outline of UnResponsiveness) score coma scale was developed. This scale is used to assess patients with neurologic conditions that affect cognitive function such as stroke, craniotomy, and traumatic brain injury. It has been heralded as a more user-friendly system to evaluate the neurologic status of patients. It also allows for improved evaluation of intubated patients, unlike the Glasgow Coma Scale. There are four categories: eye response, motor response, brainstem reflexes, and respiration pattern (Table 54.4). Each component is graded on a scale of 0 (worst response) to 4 (best response). The scores are not totaled; therefore there is not a *sum* score in this scale.

The FOUR score coma scale may be used as an alternative or complementary grading scale, along with the Glasgow Coma Scale (Jalali and Rezaei, 2014). The Glasgow Coma Scale and FOUR score usually are implemented in the intensive care unit and or emergency department.

Table 54.4 FOUR Score Coma Scale

CATEGORY OF RESPONSE	RESPONSE	SCORE
Eye response (E)	Eyelids open or opened, tracking, or blinking to command	4
	Eyelids open but not tracking	3
	Eyelids closed, open to loud noise, not tracking	2
	Eyelids closed, open to pain, not tracking	1
	Eyelids remain closed with pain	0
Brainstem reflexes (B)	Pupil and corneal reflexes present	4
	One pupil wide and fixed	3
	Corneal or pupillary reflexes absent	2
	Corneal and pupillary reflexes absent	1
	Absent pupil, corneal, and cough reflexes	0
Motor response (M)	Thumbs up, fist or peace sign, to command	4
	Localizing to pain	3
	Flexion response to pain	2
	Extensor posturing	1
	No response to pain or generalized myoclonus status epilepticus	0
Respiration (R)	Not intubated, regular breathing pattern	4
	Not intubated, Cheyne-Stokes breathing pattern	3
	Not intubated, irregular breathing pattern	2
	Breathes above ventilator rate	1
	Breathes at ventilator rate or apnea	0

From Wijdicks EJ, Bamlet WR, Maramattom BV, et al: Validation of a new coma scale: The FOUR score, *Ann Neurol* 2005;58(4):585–593.

LANGUAGE AND SPEECH

It is important to assess the language and speech capability of the neurologic patient (see Box 54.1 and Fig. 54.3). Speech is a function of the dominant hemisphere, which is on the left side of the brain for all right-handed people and most left-handed people.

Aphasia

Aphasia is an abnormal neurologic condition in which the language function is defective or absent because of an injury to certain areas of the cerebral cortex. This most commonly involves Broca's area in the frontal lobe and Wernicke's area in the posterior part of the temporal lobe.

Aphasia can affect all areas of language, including speech, reading, writing, and understanding. Aphasia can manifest in various ways; some of its subdivisions are as follows:

- *Sensory aphasia,* or *receptive aphasia:* Inability to comprehend the spoken word or written word. Wernicke's area in the temporal lobe is associated with language comprehension. Pathologic conditions in this area result in receptive aphasia.
- *Motor aphasia:* Inability to speak or write, using symbols of speech (also called *expressive aphasia*). Broca's area in the frontal lobe mediates motor speech. Pathologic conditions in this area result in expressive aphasia.
- *Global aphasia:* Inability to understand the spoken word or to speak. Pathologic conditions in Broca's and Wernicke's areas result in global aphasia.
- *Anomic aphasia:* A form of aphasia characterized by the inability to name objects.

Dysarthria

Dysarthria is difficult, poorly articulated speech that usually results from interference in control over the muscles of speech. The general cause is damage to a central or peripheral nerve.

CRANIAL NERVES

Assessment of cranial nerve function is another important part of the neurologic assessment (see Fig. 54.5). The 12 pairs of nerves emerge from the cranial cavity through openings in the skull (see Table 54.1 for specifics of cranial nerve classification and assessment). The cranial nerves are tested in the following ways:

I (olfactory): Identification of common odors
II (optic): Testing of visual acuity and visual fields
III (oculomotor): Testing of ability of eyes to move together in all directions; testing pupillary response
IV (trochlear): Tested with oculomotor; testing eye movements
V (trigeminal): Jaw strength and sensation of face; corneal reflex
VI (abducens): Tested with oculomotor; testing eye movements
VII (facial): Ability of face to move in symmetry, identification of tastes
VIII (acoustic, or *vestibulocochlear):* Testing of hearing through whisper or other means and checking equilibrium and balance
IX (glossopharyngeal): Identification of tastes
X (vagus): Gag reflex, movement of uvula and soft palate
XI (spinal accessory): Shoulder and neck movement
XII (hypoglossal): Tongue motion

MOTOR FUNCTION

Evaluation of the neurologic patient's motor status detects abnormalities in the normal functioning of nerves and muscles. Motor function disturbances are the most commonly encountered neurologic symptom. In general, the motor status examination includes gait and stance, muscle tone, coordination, involuntary movements, and the muscle stretch reflexes.

Reflexes that usually are tested include biceps, triceps, brachioradialis, quadriceps, gastrocnemius, and soleus muscles. The examiner taps briskly over the muscle with a reflex hammer. The response is noted and graded on a scale, usually from 0 to 4+, with 4+ being hyperreflexic. The most important feature of any reflex pattern is not the absolute value on the scale but the comparison of one side of the body with the other. Stick figures are used commonly to record the bilateral values.

Damage to the nervous system often causes a serious problem in mobility. A complete loss of function is called *paralysis;* a partial loss of function is called **paresis.**

Injury or disease of motoneurons causes alterations in muscle strength, tone, and reflex activity. The specific signs and symptoms vary according to whether the lesion involves the upper motoneurons or lower motoneurons:

Lower motoneuron dysfunction: Muscles may be **flaccid** (weak, soft, and flabby and lacking normal muscle tone), with weak or absent deep tendon reflexes; muscle atrophy may occur; *fasciculations* (small, rapid muscle twitches) may occur and are localized, spontaneous, and involuntary.

Upper motoneuron dysfunction: Muscles may be **spastic** (prone to spasms, i.e., involuntary, sudden movements or muscular contractions), with increased reflexes (hyperreflexia). *Clonus* (alternating contractions and partial relaxation of a muscle, initiated by muscle stretching) may occur.

SENSORY AND PERCEPTUAL STATUS

The sensory examination is the most difficult part of the neurologic evaluation. Specific alterations in sensation that should be assessed include pain; touch; temperature; and **proprioception,** the body's sense, based on internal stimuli, of its own position and limb movements. This sensation enables one to know the position of the body without looking at it and to recognize objects by the sense of touch.

The sensory evaluation may reveal conditions of which the patient is unaware. An example is **unilateral neglect,** a condition in which an individual is perceptually unaware of and inattentive to one side of the body. Another perceptual problem is **hemianopia,** which is characterized by defective vision or blindness in half of the visual field.

In most clinical settings it is usually not feasible or necessary to complete the total neurologic examination during shift-to-shift assessments of the patient. However, in many settings, such as intensive care units, the neurologic checks may be done as frequently as every 15 minutes. The most important factors include orientation, LOC, bilateral muscle strength, speech, involuntary movements, ability to follow commands, and any abnormal posturing.

LABORATORY AND DIAGNOSTIC EXAMINATIONS

BLOOD AND URINE TESTS

Assessment of the neurologically impaired patient includes a variety of blood and urine tests. A culture of the urine may rule out infection involving the urinary tract. Other urine testing may indicate the presence of diabetes insipidus. Urine drug screens may be done to rule out drug use as a cause of lethargy or to identify specific drugs ingested.

Arterial blood gas (ABG) values are an important diagnostic tool for monitoring the oxygen and carbon dioxide content of the blood. These gas levels may be altered with neurologic diseases such as Guillain-Barré syndrome (GBS), which may affect breathing patterns. Routine blood tests may help narrow the diagnosis of a neurologic disorder.

CEREBROSPINAL FLUID

Examination of the CSF can yield information about many neurologic conditions. CSF normally contains up to 10 lymphocytes per milliliter. An increase in the number of lymphocytes may indicate a bacterial, fungal, or viral infection. Low levels of CSF glucose may occur with bacterial and fungal infections such as meningitis. In the case of meningitis, a culture or smear examination is done to determine the causative organism. Spinal fluid protein is elevated when a degenerative disease or a brain tumor is present. Blood in the spinal fluid may indicate hemorrhage somewhere in the brain or spinal cord. A protein electrophoresis evaluation may give evidence of neurologic diseases such as multiple sclerosis (MS).

Lumbar Puncture

A lumbar puncture is often a part of the diagnostic workup for the patient who may have a neurologic problem. It is contraindicated in patients who may have increased ICP because the withdrawal of fluid may cause the medulla oblongata to protrude downward (herniate) into the opening at the base of the skull (the foramen magnum).

A lumbar puncture is done to obtain CSF for examination, to relieve pressure, or to introduce dye or medication. It is a common procedure, done in the patient's room or in the diagnostic imaging department. The procedure takes approximately 30 minutes.

The patient usually is positioned on the side with the knee and head flexed at an acute angle. This allows for maximal lumbar flexion and separation of the interspinous spaces. After anesthetizing the area with a local anesthetic, the health care provider inserts a hollow needle into the space between the lumbar vertebrae (often between L4 and L5, called the L4-L5 interspace), below where the spinal cord ends. The patient may feel slight pain and pressure as the dura is entered. The stylet within the hollow needle is removed to allow for collection and analysis of spinal fluid. A manometer attached to the needle is used to measure the CSF pressure. The first specimen of spinal fluid may contain blood from slight bleeding at the site of the puncture. This specimen should not be sent for cell count.

After the procedure, the patient should lie flat in bed for several hours. Assess the site of the puncture for any leakage, as evidenced by moisture on the bandage or around the puncture site. Assess for pain, numbness, and tingling in the extremities after the procedure. Back and leg pain may be experienced but should not be persistent. Acetaminophen may be given to manage minor discomfort. Approximately 40% of patients develop mild postprocedure headaches, believed to be caused by puncture of the dura during the procedure or with withdrawal of the needle, resulting in leakage of cerebrospinal fluid. Headaches may begin within hours of the procedure. Some do not begin until more than 24 hours later. Nausea and vomiting may accompany the headaches. Options to manage the headache include bed rest, analgesics, rehydration, and ice applied to the head. Opioids are usually not helpful. Approximately 85% of headaches are managed successfully with conservative interventions. A blood patch may be performed to provide relief for severe and lingering headaches (NLM, 2018b). This procedure involves the withdrawal of 20 to 30 mL of blood from a large vein, most commonly in the arm. The blood then is reinjected into the epidural space. The rationale behind the intervention is to provide a blood plug at the site of the dura's puncture to stop the leakage of spinal fluid.

OTHER TESTS

Routine radiographs of the head and vertebral column are useful for ruling out fractures of the skull and cervical vertebrae. Computed tomography (CT) scanning has reduced the use of skull radiography.

Computed Tomography Scan

The purpose of the CT scan, also called the *CAT scan*, is to detect pathologic conditions of the cerebrum and spinal cord, using a technique of scanning without radioisotopes. No special physical preparation is required for the test. A CT scan takes 20 to 30 minutes if done without contrast medium and about 60 minutes with contrast. If the use of contrast medium is anticipated, document and report to the health care provider any history of allergy to iodine and seafood, because iodine is present in the contrast medium. If contrast medium is employed, the patient may be NPO for 4 to 6 hours before the testing begins. The procedure is painless, except for the slight discomfort when an intravenous (IV) line is started for injection of the contrast dye. There may be a brief metallic taste and flushing sensation as the medium is infused. The patient also may feel some discomfort from being required to lie still and may experience a sense of claustrophobia by being held in a small space.

During the procedure the patient lies face up (supine) with the head positioned within a rubber head holder to prevent air gaps between the machine and the scalp. The head is scanned in two planes simultaneously and at various angles. Each image that appears represents a specific layer of brain tissue. The computer displays a printout that indicates areas of increased density (e.g., tumors or thrombi).

Brain Scan

Like the CT scan, the purpose of a brain scan is to detect pathologic conditions of the cerebrum. It requires the use of radioactive isotopes and a scanner. No special physical preparation is required. The procedure takes approximately 45 minutes for the actual scan. The patient is injected with a radioisotope and then lies still while a scanner passes over the brain area. Concentrated areas of uptake are reflected. There are generally no adverse effects from the procedure and only minimal discomfort associated with the IV administration of the radioactive isotopes. Brain scans are being used less frequently than in the past because of the excellent results obtained from CT scans and magnetic resonance imaging (MRI).

Magnetic Resonance Imaging

MRI uses magnetic forces to image body structures. It is used to detect pathologic conditions of the cerebrum and the spinal cord and in the detection of stroke, MS, tumors, trauma, herniation, and seizure. Because MRI yields greater contrast in the images of soft tissue structures than does the CT scan, it is the diagnostic test of choice for many neurologic diseases. Advances in MRI techniques include diffusion-weighted imaging and magnetic resonance spectroscopy. Because MRI involves a magnetic force, watches, credit cards, and any metal from the clothing must be removed before entering the scanning room. Ask the patient about the presence of any metal in the body that would preclude the use of MRI, such as orthopedic appliances, aneurysm clips, and pacemakers.

During the procedure the patient lies supine with the head positioned in a head holder. The test takes 45 to 60 minutes. The procedure is painless, except for the discomfort from lying still and possible feelings of claustrophobia when a "closed MRI" is performed. Warn the patient that the machine makes various loud noises during the scanning procedure.

Magnetic Resonance Angiography

Magnetic resonance angiography (MRA) uses differential radio waves and magnetic field signals to visualize flowing blood to evaluate extracranial and intracranial blood vessels. It is a noninvasive procedure for viewing possible occlusions in arteries. It provides anatomic and hemodynamic information. It can be used in conjunction with contrast media (contrast-enhanced MRA). MRA rapidly is replacing cerebral angiography in diagnosing cerebrovascular diseases. MRA has been useful to evaluate the cervical carotid artery and large-caliber intracranial arterial and venous structures.

Positron Emission Tomography Scan

Another evaluative measure that is similar to CT and MRI scans is the positron emission tomography (PET) scan. In this procedure the patient receives an injection of deoxyglucose combined with radioactive fluorine. The area in question is scanned, and a color composite picture is obtained. Shades of color indicate the level of glucose metabolism, with abnormal levels suggestive of a pathologic state. PET scanning provides a noninvasive means of determining biochemical processes that occur in the brain. It is being used increasingly to monitor patients who have had a stroke or who have AD, Huntington's disease, tumors, epilepsy, and Parkinson's disease. As with the CT scan, discomfort is minimal. Inform the patient of the need to lie still for the duration of the scan, which is usually about 45 minutes.

Electroencephalogram

The electroencephalogram (EEG) provides evidence of focal or generalized disturbances of brain function by measuring the electrical activity of the brain. Among the cerebral disorders assessed by EEG are epilepsy, mass lesions (e.g., tumors, abscess, hematoma), cerebrovascular lesions, and brain injury. The test requires no special preparation, but encourage the patient to be quiet and rest before the procedure. An exception is a sleep-deprived EEG, during which the patient is kept awake the night before the test; the EEG usually is done first thing in the morning. An EEG usually takes about 1 hour to complete. The patient's hair and scalp should be clean. The electrodes are secured to the scalp with a gluelike substance called collodion, in a set pattern to cover all scalp areas. An EEG is painless.

The basic resting rhythm of the EEG is affected by opening the eyes or altering attention. Recordings sometimes are made while the patient is asleep or sleep deprived, when the seizure threshold may be lowered. Comparisons are made of different patterns of the recordings. After the test, allow the patient to rest. Assist the patient if necessary in washing the hair and removing the collodion from the scalp.

Myelogram

A myelogram commonly is used to identify lesions in the intradural or extradural compartments of the spinal canal by observing the flow of radiopaque dye through the subarachnoid space. The most common lesion for which this test is used is a herniated or protruding intervertebral disk. Other lesions include spinal tumors, adhesions, bony deformations, and arteriovenous malformations. Before the procedure, assess and document the patient's baselines of lower extremity strength and sensation. Tell the patient that the procedure takes about 2 hours, it may involve slight discomfort as the dura is entered, and he or she may be asked to assume a variety of positions during the procedure.

Water-soluble iodine dyes such as iopamidol (Isovue) commonly are used because they are absorbed into the bloodstream and excreted by the kidneys. Preparation for this procedure is the same as for lumbar puncture. Before the dye is injected, ask the patient whether he or she has any allergies and specifically about any anaphylactic or hypotensive episodes related to other dyes. The patient usually is positioned on the side with both knees and the head flexed at an acute angle to allow maximal flexion of the lumbar area for ease in performing the lumbar puncture. After the puncture is performed, the inner stylet is removed to allow drainage of CSF, measurement of pressure, and collection of specimens. The dye is instilled and the needle is removed. The patient then is turned to various positions so that the spinal cord can be visualized while fluoroscopic and radiopaque films are taken. The patient usually undergoes a CT scan 4 to 6 hours after a myelogram.

After the procedure, observe the puncture site for any leakage of CSF, and assess the strength and sensation of the lower extremities. Headache is fairly common. It may be accompanied by nausea and occasionally by vomiting. The patient should lie flat in bed for a few hours.

Angiogram

The angiogram (cerebral arteriography) is a procedure used to visualize the cerebral arterial system by injecting radiopaque material. It allows detection of arterial aneurysms, vessel anomalies, ruptured vessels, and displacement of vessels by tumors or masses.

Before the procedure the patient usually is given clear liquids, although in some institutions all oral intake is restricted. Assess the patient for any allergy to iodine, because the dye contains iodine. If the femoral approach (through the leg) is to be used, mark the locations of the pedal pulse in both feet. If the carotid artery is used, measure the neck circumference as part of the baseline data. Immediately before the procedure, measure baseline vital signs and pulses and perform a neurologic check.

The test takes approximately 2 to 3 hours. The patient may become uncomfortable lying still for that length of time. When the dye is injected, most patients complain of feeling extremely hot, feeling flushed, and experiencing a metallic taste. The patient is positioned supine on the radiograph table. A local anesthetic agent is used to anesthetize the area of the puncture site. The catheter is introduced through the skin (percutaneously) and introduced into the relevant vessels. At times the catheter may be inserted directly into the carotid or vertebral arteries. After all injections are done, the catheter is withdrawn and pressure is applied to the puncture site for at least 15 minutes.

After the procedure, bed rest is ordered, usually for 4 to 6 hours. Check vital signs and perform a neurologic check frequently (at times as often as every 15 minutes). Assess the puncture site frequently for the presence of a hematoma. With a femoral stick (i.e., when the puncture site is in the femoral artery), check the pulses distal to the site for evidence of arterial occlusion. With a carotid stick, assess whether the patient has any difficulty breathing or swallowing or an increase in the girth of the neck.

The patient undergoing this procedure is at risk for cerebrovascular accident and increased ICP. Promptly report any change in LOC or in other parts of the neurologic assessment.

MRA is replacing cerebral arteriography rapidly in many facilities.

Carotid Duplex

A carotid duplex study uses combined ultrasound and pulsed Doppler technology. A technician places a probe on the skin over the carotid artery and slowly moves the probe along the course of the common carotid to the bifurcation of the external and internal carotid arteries. The ultrasound signal emitted from the probe reflects off the moving blood cells within the vessel. The frequency of the reflected signal corresponds to the blood velocity. This response is amplified and is registered on a graphic record and also as sound. The graphic record registers blood velocity. Increased blood flow velocity can indicate stenosis of a vessel. Carotid duplex scanning is a noninvasive study that evaluates carotid occlusive disease. This study often is ordered when a patient has had a transient ischemic attack (TIA).

Electromyogram

An electromyogram (EMG) measures the contraction of a muscle in response to electrical stimulation. It provides evidence of lower motor neuron disease; primary muscle disease; and defects in the transmission of electrical impulses at the neuromuscular junction, such as in myasthenia gravis. There is no special preparation for the test. The test takes approximately 45 minutes for one muscle study. Inform the patient that it is uncomfortable when the electrode is inserted into the muscle and when the electrical current is used. The muscle may ache for a short time after the procedure.

During the test an electrode is inserted into selected skeletal muscles. An electric current is passed through the electrode, and the machine graphs the variations of muscle potentials (voltage). After the procedure, assess the patient for signs of bleeding at the site of the electrode insertion. The patient may need an analgesic for discomfort and a rest period.

Echoencephalogram

An echoencephalogram uses ultrasound to depict intracranial structures of the brain. It is especially helpful in detecting ventricular dilation and a major shift of midline structures in the brain as a result of an expanding lesion. The preparation of the patient, the actual procedure, and aftercare are similar to those of the brain scan.

COMMON DISORDERS OF THE NEUROLOGIC SYSTEM

HEADACHES

Etiology and Pathophysiology

Headache is a common neurologic complaint; its significance and its causes vary. The source of recurring headache should be determined through careful physical examination with appropriate neurologic assessment.

The exact mechanism of head pain is not known. Although the skull and brain tissues are not able to feel sensory pain, pain arises from the scalp, its blood vessels and muscles, and the dura mater and its venous sinuses. Pain also arises from the blood vessels at the base of the brain and from cervical cranial nerves. Blood vessels may dilate and become congested with blood.

Headaches can be classified as vascular, tension, and traction-inflammatory:

- *Vascular headaches* include migraine, cluster, and hypertensive headaches.
- *Tension headaches* may arise from psychological problems related to tension or stress, or from medical problems such as cervical arthritis.
- *Traction-inflammatory headaches* include those caused by infection, intracranial or extracranial causes, and temporal arteritis.

The exact cause of migraine headaches is unknown. It is theorized that changes in blood flow in the brain and surrounding tissues may contribute to the headaches. Abnormal metabolism of serotonin, a vasoactive neurotransmitter found in platelets and cells of the brain, plays a major role. Migraine headaches are three times more common in women than men (NLM, 2014). There is often a familial link. The age of onset is traditionally between 10 and 45 years.

Patients with migraine often report experiencing an **aura** (prodromal signs that occur before the headache). Auras most often are reported to occur in the half-hour preceding the attack but may occur up to 24 hours before the onset of pain. Each patient's aura is individualized but commonly includes visual field defects; unusual smells or sounds; disorientation; paresthesias; and, in rare cases, paralysis of a part of the body. Migraine headache pain is described classically as throbbing and pounding. It is often worse on one side of the head. Additional symptoms experienced during the headache include nausea, vomiting, sensitivity to light, chilliness, fatigue, irritability, diaphoresis, edema, and other signs of autonomic dysfunction. Migraine headaches may be triggered by a series of factors.

Assessment

Subjective data include the patient's understanding of the headache, possible causes, and any precipitating factors. Determine what measures relieve the symptoms and the location, frequency, pattern, and character of the pain. This includes the site of return of the headache, time of day, and intervals between headaches. Also assess the initial onset of the headache, any symptoms that occur before the headache or associated symptoms, the presence of allergies, and any family history of similar headache patterns.

Objective data include any behaviors indicating stress, anxiety, or pain. Changes in the ability to carry out activities of daily living (ADLs), an abnormally raised body temperature, and sinus drainage may be important. Also document abnormalities noted during the physical examination.

Diagnostic Tests

It is important to evaluate headaches that are not transient. Usual testing includes a neurologic examination, a CT scan (MRI or PET scan also may be done), a brain scan, skull radiographs, and a lumbar puncture. However, a lumbar puncture is not done if there is evidence of increased ICP or if a brain tumor is suspected, because quick reduction of pressure produced by removal of the spinal fluid may cause brain herniation. In these situations, a CT scan is done first.

Medical Management

Dietary counseling. Some foods may cause or worsen headaches. These include foods containing tyramine, nitrites, or glutamates (e.g., monosodium glutamate [MSG], often used in the preparation of Chinese foods and processed meats). Tyramine is an amino acid that helps to control blood pressure. It is found in foods including aged cheeses (cheddar and Swiss), cured meats, fermented cabbage (sauerkraut), and soy and fish sauces. Nitrites are present in curing substances used in the preparation of meats such as bologna, ham, hot dogs, and bacon. Other substances that may provoke headaches include vinegar, chocolate, yogurt, alcohol, fermented or marinated foods, and caffeine. Patients may not realize how often they are ingesting potential headache triggers; instructing them to keep a food diary is helpful.

Psychotherapy. Patients with headaches may respond to psychotherapy. This does not mean that the headache pain is not physiologic, but counseling can help the patient develop awareness of stress factors and deal with the pain. The patient may need help expressing feelings about intractable headache pain.

Medications. Medications often are used to treat headaches.

Migraine headaches. Mild migraine episodes may be managed with over-the-counter medications. Acetylsalicylic acid (aspirin), acetaminophen, or ibuprofen may be used. Using these medications more than 3 days per week can cause rebound headaches. For moderate to severe headaches, the triptans have become the first line of the therapy. Triptans are thought to act on receptors in the extracerebral, intracranial vessels that become dilated during a migraine attack. Stimulating these receptors constricts cranial vessels, inhibits neuropeptide release, and reduces nerve impulse transmission along trigeminal pain pathways. Triptans commonly prescribed include eletriptan (Relpax), the seventh triptan to be marketed for treatment of migraine, joining almotriptan (Axert), frovatriptan (Frova), naratriptan (Amerge), rizatriptan (Maxalt), sumatriptan (Imitrex), and zolmitriptan (Zomig). Classified as selective serotonin receptor agonists, these drugs are indicated to treat acute migraine (with or without aura) in adults. In addition to relieving headache pain, the triptans also relieve the nausea, vomiting, and photophobia associated with an acute migraine attack.

Ergotamine preparations manage migraine headache pain by preventing the blood vessels in the brain from expanding and causing headaches. Ergotamine is combined with caffeine and the compounds are taken orally. They are most effective when taken at the first sign of migraine pain.

Another approach for managing migraine headaches is to prevent them by taking medications before the onset of pain. The decision to do this is based on the severity and frequency of headache pain. Topiramate (Topamax) taken daily has been an effective therapy for migraine prevention in adults. Other preventive drugs for migraine headaches include beta-adrenergic blockers (e.g., propranolol [Inderal], atenolol [Tenormin]), tricyclic antidepressants (e.g., amitriptyline), selective serotonin reuptake inhibitors (e.g., fluoxetine [Prozac]), calcium channel blockers (e.g., verapamil), divalproex (Depakote), clonidine (Catapres), and thiazide diuretics.

Cluster headaches. Cluster headaches are named for the pattern with which they occur. These headaches occur almost daily for a period of time and then subside. They return and occur again, regularly. The period of attack may be a week to a year. The period of remission may be a month or longer. The exact cause is unknown, although theories support a sudden release of histamine or serotonin by the body. The pain of cluster headaches is usually one sided and is described as *burning, sharp,* and *steady*. It may be accompanied by watering of the eyes (tearing) and nasal stuffiness. Their onset is sudden and they often occur at the same time of day. Cluster headaches occur more commonly in men. They affect adolescents and middle-aged adults. Like migraine headaches, there are familial tendencies. The triggering factors for cluster headaches are similar to those of migraine headaches but also include exertion, heat, and high altitudes (NLM, 2018).

Diagnosis of cluster headaches usually is based on the presentation of symptoms. If the health care provider is present during an attack, Horner's syndrome frequently is noted. This is the presentation of a small pupil or eyelid drooping on one side. These signs are not present in the absence of the headache. Other testing, such as MRI, may be performed to rule out other causes.

Because the pain associated with vascular cluster headaches is often severe, opioid analgesics, sometimes given intramuscularly, are used. Sumatriptan (Imitrex) may be prescribed to manage the headaches. Prednisone therapy may be initiated. During this type of intervention, the patient begins with a high dose of the steroid and then the doses gradually are reduced over time. Dihydroergotamine (DHE) may be injected and can stop pain within 5 minutes. It cannot be taken in conjunction with sumatriptan. Patients with cluster headaches usually feel fine between attacks, so no analgesic is needed during these times.

Tension headaches. Nonopioid analgesics often are used to treat tension headaches. These include acetaminophen, ibuprofen, and aspirin. Opioids are avoided because these drugs are often subject to abuse; it is much better to counsel patients to develop other ways to relieve tension headaches.

Nursing Interventions and Patient Teaching

Because stress and emotional upsets may precipitate some headaches and worsen others, the patient requires relaxation and rest. Help the patient with relaxation techniques, planned sleeping hours, and regular rest periods. Alcohol should not be used to relieve tension because it may become addicting and has been found to be a significant cause of cluster headaches. Regular physical exercise also may help prevent headaches, especially those caused by tension.

If a patient is suffering from a severe headache, plan nursing interventions so that only essential activities take place. Plan interventions so that the patient has adequate time to rest.

Comfort measures. Other treatments that may help a patient with a headache include cold packs applied to the forehead or base of the skull and pressure applied to the temporal arteries. People with migraine headaches are usually most comfortable lying in a dark, quiet room.

Identifying triggering factors. Triggering factors associated with severe and recurring headaches may include fatigue, alcohol, stress, seasonal climate changes, hunger, allergies, and menstruation. Help the patient identify these factors, if necessary, through ongoing observation or assessment of the patient's personality, habits, ADLs, career plans, work habits, family relationships, coping mechanisms, and relaxation activities. The patient may keep a diary or journal to help collect this information.

Patient problems and interventions for the patient with headache include but are not limited to the following:

Patient Problem	Nursing Interventions
Anxiousness, related to pain	Provide quiet environment Encourage verbalization of concerns Provide diversional activities
Recent Onset of Pain or Prolonged Pain, related to disease process	Administer prescribed medications Provide comfort measures Maintain nonstressful environment Encourage pain reduction techniques as appropriate: rocking movements, external warmth, breathing patterns

Teaching is an important part of the nursing intervention for the patient with headaches. Topics include (1) avoidance of factors that trigger headaches; (2) relaxation techniques, including biofeedback; (3) maintenance of regular sleep patterns; (4) medications to be used (including dosage, actions, and side effects); and (5) the importance of follow-up care.

Prognosis

With proper treatment the person with headaches can expect to live a normal life. Changes in lifestyle may have to occur, especially during acute episodes of headache pain. The person may have to adjust to periodic headaches and rest until the headache resolves. Chronic headaches have a broad-reaching impact on the patient and family with regard to emotional well-being, physical impairment, and employment. Ninety percent of migraine patients are unable to function normally when a headache occurs. An estimated 25% of individuals who experience migraines have missed a day of work in the past 3 months. There are many types of headaches. For additional information, visit the National Headache Foundation website *(https://headaches.org)*.

NEUROPATHIC PAIN

Etiology, Pathophysiology, and Clinical Manifestations

Neuropathic pain refers to pain originating from the peripheral or central nervous system caused by direct stimulation of the myelinated nervous tissue. It is characterized as a tingling or burning pain in areas of sensory loss. Neuropathic pain may result from postherpetic neuralgia, diabetic neuropathies, and trigeminal neuralgia; phantom limb pain is now considered a neuropathic pain. Patients may have disabling pain, caused by a disorder either within the nervous system or at a distant part of the body. Neuropathic pain may arise from lesions involving the peripheral cutaneous nerves, the sensory nerve roots, the thalamus, and the central pain tract (lateral spinothalamic tract) at some level. Each produces characteristic pain. Pain receptors are not adaptable—they are specific for pain only—and pain impulses continue at the same rate as long as the stimulus is present. Pain receptors can be activated by cellular damage, certain chemicals such as histamine, heat, ischemia, muscle spasm, and sensations of cold and pruritus that go beyond a specific level of intensity.

Pain that is described as unbearable and does not respond to treatment is classified as *intractable*. It is chronic and often debilitating and may prevent the patient from functioning in everyday life.

Assessment

The perception of pain is highly subjective. Pain may vary from mild to excruciating. Subjective data include the patient's understanding of the pain; any precipitating factors; and measures that relieve stress, including medication. The site, frequency, and nature of the pain are important, as is the patient's usual coping patterns when under stress. Encourage the patient to use a pain scale to express the level of pain experienced. Associated symptoms and measures that make the pain worse are important subjective data.

Objective data may be limited when assessing neuropathic pain. Objective factors to assess are behavioral signs indicating pain or stress, a change in the ability to carry out ADLs, muscle weakness or wasting, vasomotor responses (such as flushing), abnormalities of spinal reflexes, and abnormalities noted during the sensory examination.

Diagnostic Tests

Diagnostic tests for the patient in pain may include electrical stimulation, used to define the pain to a greater degree. Psychological testing may be part of the workup. If back or neck pain is present, a myelogram usually is performed.

Medical Management

Nonsurgical methods of pain control. Neuropathic pain sometimes responds to other methods of pain control. These include transcutaneous electrical nerve stimulation and spinal cord stimulation. Both techniques use electrodes applied near the site of pain, or on or around the spine. The stimulator modifies the sensory input by blocking or changing the painful sensation with a stimulus that is perceived to be less or not at all painful. Acupuncture also is used to treat patients with neuropathic pain.

Nerve block. A nerve block is used to control intractable pain. It involves injecting a local anesthetic, alcohol, or phenol close enough to a nerve to block the conduction of impulses. Sources of pain often treated with a nerve block include trigeminal neuralgia, cancer, and peripheral vascular disease. The effect lasts from several months to several years. Pain and spasticity also may be controlled by means of an epidural catheter. Medication usually is administered continuously.

Medications. Medications often are used to treat patients with neuropathic pain. Anticonvulsant medications such as gabapentin (Neurontin) and carbamazepine (Tegretol) are often useful. Other medications include nonopioid analgesics such as acetaminophen, nonsteroidal anti-inflammatory drugs, and acetylsalicylic acid. Opioids do not appear as helpful for neuropathic pain, although they sometimes are used. Antidepressants—such as amitriptyline, doxepin, imipramine, and nortriptyline (Pamelor)—appear to be effective in treating neuropathic pain. The emphasis should be on helping the patient learn various other measures to control the pain.

Surgical methods of pain control. When intractable pain does not respond to more conservative measures, surgery may be necessary to reduce or eliminate the pain.

Nursing Interventions and Patient Teaching

Comfort measures. A patient with neuropathic pain may be uncomfortable and should be assisted to assume a position of comfort. For example, the patient with back pain should avoid movements that cause direct or indirect movement of the spinal cord. The patient may find lying in a supine position uncomfortable. Help the patient find a comfortable position and, if necessary, actively assist the patient in turning or moving. Straining when having a bowel movement can intensify pain, and a stool softener may be needed. Offer prune juice and a high-fiber diet and encourage the patient to drink up to 2000 mL/day or more of fluids.

Promotion of rest and relaxation. As with headache, stress and emotional upsets may precipitate or exacerbate neuropathic pain. Facilitate rest and relaxation, with planned sleeping hours and rest periods as needed.

Some patients with pain, especially intractable pain, may respond well to psychotherapy. This does not mean that the pain does not have a physiologic basis, but counseling can help the patient develop awareness of what makes the pain worse and how to cope with the discomfort.

Patient problems and interventions for the patient with neuropathic pain are the same as those listed previously for headache, with the addition of but not limited to the following:

Patient Problem	Nursing Interventions
Risk for Contractures or Muscle Atrophy, related to lack of use of a body part as a result of pain	Explain need for a regular exercise program to maintain joint mobility; provide range-of-motion (ROM) exercises to all body joints q 2–4 hr Be positive and reassuring in approach
Inability to Feed, Bathe, Dress, or Toilet Self, related to pain	Assist with basic ADL needs as necessary, but encourage patient to participate as much as possible Provide sufficient time for ADLs Facilitate use of self-help devices as needed Provide for total hygiene as indicated

Teaching the patient with neuropathic pain is an important nursing intervention. Include the factors taught to the patient with headache, and help the patient become aware of physical methods such as positioning the body to increase comfort and structuring the home and work setting to minimize stress.

Prognosis

As with headache pain, neuropathic pain can in most cases be treated adequately. Lifestyle changes may be helpful in allowing the person to have a better quality of life.

INCREASED INTRACRANIAL PRESSURE

Etiology, Pathophysiology, and Clinical Manifestations

Increased ICP is a complex grouping of events that occurs because of multiple neurologic conditions. It often occurs suddenly, progresses rapidly, and requires surgical intervention. It is a potential complication in many neurologic conditions and rapidly can lead to death if not treated and reversed.

Increased ICP occurs in patients with acute neurologic conditions such as a brain tumor, hemorrhage, anoxic brain injury, and toxic or viral encephalopathies; it most commonly is associated with head injury. The Monro-Kellie doctrine states that the volume of the contents of the cranium (brain tissue, cerebrospinal fluid, and blood) is constant. An increase in any constituent must be accompanied by a decrease in one of the others or else increased ICP will result. This is because the cranial vault is rigid and nonexpandable, that is, it does not allow for increases. Pressure may build up slowly over weeks or rapidly, depending on the cause. Usually one side of the brain is more involved, but both sides of the brain eventually become involved.

As the pressure increases within the cranial cavity, it is first compensated for by venous compression and CSF displacement. As the pressure continues to rise, the cerebral blood flow decreases and inadequate perfusion of the brain occurs. This inadequate perfusion starts a vicious cycle in which the carbon dioxide concentration in the blood ($PaCO_2$) increases, and the oxygen concentration (PaO_2) and pH decrease. These changes cause vasodilation and cerebral edema. The edema further increases the ICP, which causes increased compression of neural tissue and an even greater increase in ICP.

When the pressure buildup is greater than the brain's ability to compensate, pressure is exerted on surrounding structures where the pressure is lower. This movement of pressure is called *supratentorial shift* and can result in herniation. As a result of herniation of the brain, the brainstem is compressed at various levels, which in turn compresses the vasomotor center, the posterior cerebral artery, the oculomotor nerve, the corticospinal nerve pathway, and the fibers of the ascending RAS. The life-sustaining mechanisms of consciousness, blood pressure, pulse, respiration, and temperature regulation become impaired. A rise in systolic pressure and an unchanged diastolic pressure, resulting in a widening pulse pressure, bradycardia, and abnormal respiration, are late signs of increased ICP and indicate that the brain is about to herniate.

Assessment

Increased ICP must be detected early while it is still reversible. The ability to make accurate observations, interpret observations intelligently, and record observations carefully is most important for the nurse working with patients with increased ICP.

Subjective data for a diagnosis of increased ICP include the patient's understanding of the condition, any visual changes such as **diplopia** (double vision), a change in the patient's personality, and a change in the ability to think. The diplopia usually results from paralysis or weakness of one of the muscles that control eye movement. It often occurs fairly early in the process. Nausea or pain, especially headache, is also important.

The headache is thought to result from venous congestion and tension in the intracranial blood vessels as the cerebral pressure rises. Headache that occurs with increased ICP usually increases in intensity with coughing, straining at stool, or stooping. It is usually present in the early morning and may awaken the patient from sleep.

Objective data include a change in LOC, which is the earliest sign of increased ICP. During assessment, it takes more stimulation to get the same response from the patient. Manifestations of a change in LOC include disorientation, restlessness, and lethargy. Record observations in terms of behaviors and signs and symptoms; not in terms of labels. Pupillary signs also may change with increased ICP. Pupillary responses are controlled by cranial nerve III (the oculomotor nerve). The pupils usually change on the same side as the lesion. The first and most subtle clue to trouble is that the pupil reacts, but sluggishly. As the brain herniates, the nerve is compressed—with the top part of the nerve being affected first. The *ipsilateral* pupil (when the lesion is in one hemisphere) remains dilated and is incapable of constricting. The pupil appears larger than that of the affected side and does not react to light. As the ICP increases and both halves of the brain become affected, bilateral pupil dilation and fixation occur. Dilating pupils that respond slowly to light are a sign of impending herniation. A pupil that is fixed and dilated, sometimes called a *blown pupil,* is an ominous sign that *must* be reported to the health care provider immediately (Fig. 54.6).

Changes in the blood pressure and pulse are seen with increasing ICP. Herniation causes ischemia of the vasomotor center, which excites the vasoconstrictor fibers, causing the systolic blood pressure to rise. If the ICP continues to increase, widening pulse pressure (i.e., increasing systolic pressure and decreasing diastolic pressure) occurs.

Pressure in the vasomotor center also increases the transmission of parasympathetic impulses through the vagus nerve to the heart, causing a slowing of the pulse. Widened pulse pressure, increased systolic blood pressure, deepening, irregular respirations and bradycardia are together called *Cushing's response.* It is considered an important diagnostic sign of late-stage brain herniation.

Brain herniation produces respiratory problems that are variable and related to the level of the brainstem compression or failure. The breathing pattern may be deep and stertorous (snorelike) or periodic (Cheyne-Stokes respiration). *Ataxic* breathing also may occur; this is an irregular and unpredictable breathing pattern with random, shallow, and deep breaths and occasional pauses. It is seen in patients with medulla oblongata damage. As ICP increases to fatal levels, respiratory paralysis occurs.

Failure of the thermoregulatory center because of compression occurs later with increased ICP. It results in high, uncontrolled temperatures. This hyperthermia increases the metabolism of brain tissue.

Compression of the upper motoneuron pathway (corticospinal tract) interrupts transmission of impulses to the lower motoneurons, and progressive muscle weakness occurs. Babinski's reflex, hyperreflexia, and rigidity are additional signs of decreased motor function. Seizures may occur. Herniation of the upper part of the brainstem may produce characteristic posturing when the patient is stimulated (Fig. 54.7). The worsening of motor problems is significant, because it means that the ICP is continuing to increase.

Vomiting and singultus (hiccups) are two objective signs of increased ICP. The vomiting is often projectile and usually not preceded by nausea; this is called *unexpected vomiting.* Singultus is caused by compression of the vagus nerve (cranial nerve X) as brainstem herniation occurs.

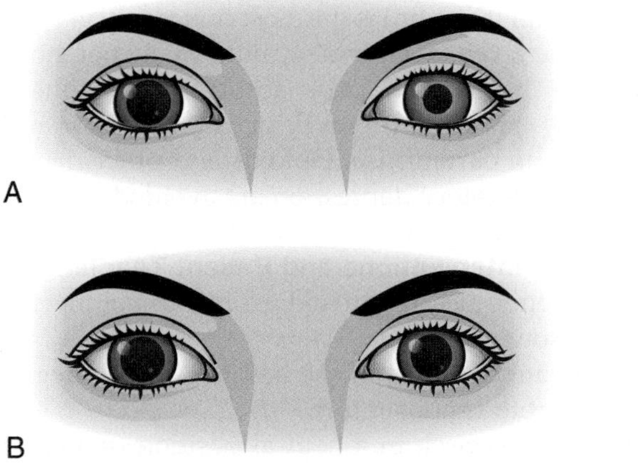

Fig. 54.6 A, Unequal pupils, also called *anisocoria.* B, Dilated and fixed pupils, indicative of severe neurologic deficit.

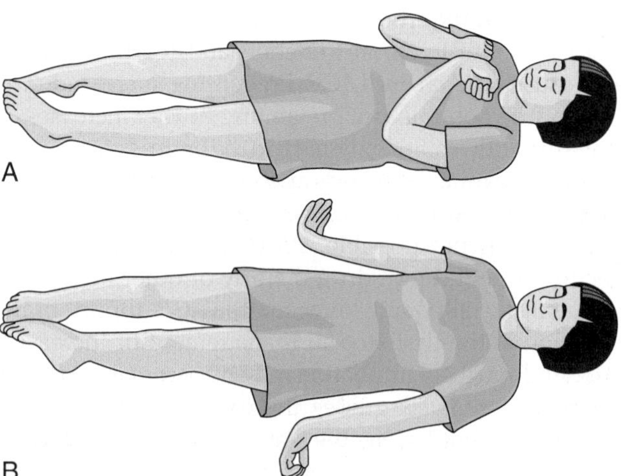

Fig. 54.7 Decorticate and decerebrate responses. A, Decorticate response is characterized by flexion of the arms, wrists, and fingers with adduction of the upper extremities, and extension, internal rotation, and plantar flexion of the lower extremities. B, Decerebrate response: All four extremities are in rigid extension, with hyperpronation of the forearms and plantar extension of the feet. (From Ignatavicius DD, Workman ML, Blair M, et al: *Medical-surgical nursing: Patient-centered collaborative care,* ed 8, St. Louis, 2016, Elsevier.)

One last objective sign is papilledema, which is detected with the use of an ophthalmoscope (usually by the health care provider). As ICP increases, the pressure is transmitted to the eyes through the CSF and to the optic disc at the back of the eye. As the optic disc becomes edematous, the retina also is compressed. The damaged retina cannot detect light rays. Visual acuity is lessened as the blind spot enlarges. *Papilledema* is also called a *choked disc.*

Diagnostic Tests

Diagnostic studies are aimed at identifying the presence and the underlying cause of increased ICP. The diagnosis of increased ICP is made by CT or MRI, which can show actual structural herniation and shifting of the brain. Because of CT and MRI, the diagnosis of increased ICP has been revolutionized completely and the therapeutic options greatly increased (Lewis et al, 2007).

Most of the time, acute increased ICP is a medical emergency, and diagnostic tests must be done quickly. Other tests include ICP measurement, EEG, cerebral angiography, transcranial Doppler studies, and PET. In general, lumbar puncture is not performed when increased ICP is suspected because of the possibility of cerebral herniation from the sudden release of the pressure in the skull from the area above the lumbar puncture. This can lead to pressure on cardiac and respiratory centers in the brainstem and potentially death (Pappu and Khraishi, 2016).

In postoperative or critically ill patients, internal measuring devices are used to diagnose increased ICP. One of the most common measuring devices requires the placement of a hollow screw through the skull into the subarachnoid space. The device is connected to a transducer and oscilloscope for continuous monitoring. Waveforms are produced that indicate the ICP.

Medical Management

The goals of treatment are to identify and treat the underlying cause of increased ICP. Preventing increased ICP may not be possible, but preventing further increases in pressure with resulting damage to the brain is crucial. The medical treatment depends on the cause of the pressure. For example, surgery may be done to remove a tumor. If surgery is not possible, efforts are made to reduce the pressure through drug therapy or other measures.

Ensuring adequate oxygenation to support brain function is the first step in management of increased ICP. Endotracheal intubation may be necessary. Arterial blood gas analysis guides the oxygen therapy. With controlled ventilation, the $PaCO_2$ can be lowered to below normal, which causes a slightly alkalotic pH. The decrease in $PaCO_2$ and the increase in pH will decrease vasodilation and decrease ICP. The goal is to maintain the PaO_2 at 100 mm Hg.

Mechanical decompression. Rapidly rising ICP can be relieved by mechanical decompression. This may include a craniotomy, in which a bone flap is removed and then replaced, or a craniectomy, in which a bone flap is removed and not replaced. Other means of decompression include drainage of the ventricles or of any subdural hematoma.

Internal monitoring devices are being used more frequently to diagnose and monitor increased ICP. Three basic monitoring systems are used: the ventricular catheter, the subarachnoid bolt or screw, and the epidural sensor. These monitoring devices detect pressure waves that can be used to indicate the status of ICP.

Medications. Three types of medications usually are administered to patients with increased ICP: osmotic diuretics, corticosteroids, and anticonvulsants. Osmotic diuretics also are called hyperosmolar drugs. They draw water from the edematous brain tissue. An example of this type of medication is mannitol. It begins to reduce increased ICP within 15 minutes, and its effects last for 5 to 6 hours. Loop diuretics such as furosemide (Lasix), bumetanide (Bumex), and ethacrynic acid (Edecrin) also may be used in the management of increased ICP. Continuous midazolam and atracurium besylate infusions also are used.

Traditionally, health care providers have prescribed the corticosteroid dexamethasone. There are studies that demonstrate that corticosteroids may have limited value in managing head-injured patients. The use of corticosteroids in the care of head-injured patients was once standard. Studies have shown that patients managed with corticosteroid therapies reflect a higher mortality rate. Today, corticosteroids are not standard in the plan of care. However, those patients receiving this medication warrant close assessment of their blood glucose levels. Steroids can affect carbohydrate metabolism and glucose utilization and result in elevated blood glucose levels.

To prevent gastrointestinal ulcers and bleeding, patients receiving corticosteroids concurrently should be given antacids, histamine receptor blockers (e.g., cimetidine [Tagamet], ranitidine [Zantac]), or proton pump inhibitors (e.g., omeprazole [Prilosec], pantoprazole [Protonix, Protonix IV]).

Anticonvulsants are given to prevent seizures. Phenytoin (Dilantin) is the most commonly given drug. It can be given intravenously but usually not intramuscularly because of poor absorption. Fosphenytoin (Cerebyx) is a short-term IV or intramuscular anticonvulsant in current use. Opioids and other drugs that cause respiratory depression are avoided.

Nursing Interventions and Patient Teaching

Therapeutic measures to reduce venous volume include the following:

- Elevate the head of the bed to 30 to 45 degrees to promote venous return.
- Place the neck in a neutral position (not flexed or extended) to promote venous drainage.

- Position the patient to avoid flexion of the hips, the waist, and the neck and rotation of the head, especially to the right. Avoid extreme hip flexion because this position causes an increase in intraabdominal and intrathoracic pressures, which can produce a rise in ICP.
- Instruct the patient to avoid isometric or resistive exercises.
- Restrict fluid intake.
- Implement measures to help the patient avoid the Valsalva maneuver (any forced expiratory effort against a closed airway, such as straining during bowel movement). Avoid enemas and laxatives if possible.
- Have a Foley catheter in place if the patient is not alert because of the large amount of urine that is produced.
- Perform suctioning only as necessary and for no longer than 10 seconds, with administration of 100% oxygen before and after to prevent decreases in the PaO_2.
- Administer oxygen via mask or cannula to improve cerebral perfusion.
- Use a hypothermia blanket to control body temperature (increased body temperature increases brain damage).

Patient problems and interventions for the patient with increased ICP may include but are not limited to the following:

Patient Problem	Nursing Interventions
Inability to Maintain Adequate Breathing Pattern, related to neuromuscular impairment	Maintain patent airway; avoid flexion of neck Administer oxygen and humidification as ordered Provide oral nasopharyngeal airway as indicated for managing secretions; suction oropharynx as needed
Potential for Injury, related to physiologic effects of sustained ICP elevation	Elevate head of bed to 30 degrees Maintain body position; avoid semiprone or prone position Avoid compression of neck veins Check blood pressure, pulse, and respiration q 30 min Perform neurologic check q 30 min using Glasgow Coma Scale; report any findings below 8 to health care provider

The patient with increased ICP is often unresponsive. Share information about procedures that are being done with the patient and the family. This may help both to be as cooperative as possible.

Prognosis

The prognosis for the patient with increased ICP depends on the cause and the speed with which it is treated. The nurse assumes an important role in monitoring the patient for signs and symptoms of increased pressure. After herniation of the brain has begun as a result of pressure, there is little chance for complete reversal without significant brain damage.

DISTURBANCES IN MUSCLE TONE AND MOTOR FUNCTION

Etiology and Pathophysiology

Motor function disturbances are the most commonly encountered neurologic signs and symptoms. Damage to the nervous system often causes serious problems in mobility. An example of this is the patient with cerebral palsy.

Clinical Manifestations

Injury or disease of motoneurons results in alterations of muscle strength, tone, and reflex activity. Muscle tone may be described as *flaccid* (weak, soft, flabby, and lacking normal muscle tone) or *hyperreflexic* (excessive reflex responses). The specific clinical manifestations differ according to the location of the neurologic lesion.

Assessment

Subjective data for patients with motor problems include the patient's understanding of the problem and possible causes. Ask about the initial onset of the symptoms; measures that improve symptoms; and the presence of clumsiness, incoordination, or abnormal sensation. If the lesion occurs suddenly, as in traumatic spinal cord injury, subjective symptoms may be minimal. If the motor deficit develops slowly, subjective symptoms may be so subtle that they are at first ignored.

Objective data include coordination, muscle strength, muscle tone, and muscle atrophy. Reflexes often are checked, as well as the presence of clonus or fasciculations and the ability to move muscles. Any abnormal gait is significant, as is a change in the ability to carry out ADLs.

Diagnostic Tests

One of the most common procedures for detecting pathologic conditions of muscle is the EMG. It detects the various types of electrical activity and abnormal patterns that may appear in resting muscle in the presence of disease.

Medical Management

Patients with motor problems may have spasticity. Muscle relaxants may be used to decrease tone and involuntary movements. Some commonly prescribed medications include baclofen (Lioresal), dantrolene (Dantrium), and diazepam (Valium). Baclofen has been used intrathecally to reduce spasticity. Common side effects of these drugs include drowsiness and vertigo. These side effects are increased by the use of alcohol or other depressants.

Some patients may have severe swallowing difficulty **(dysphagia).** This commonly results from obstructive or motor disorders of the esophagus and often is associated with neurologic problems. The patient with dysphagia often requires prefeeding and feeding exercises.

Some patients are at severe risk for aspiration. These patients may undergo videofluoroscopy with barium to determine which muscles are not working right and which types of food are safest. The procedure requires the patient to swallow a small amount of liquid or semisolid food, mixed with barium, while a fluoroscopic examination is being done.

For patients with paralysis, the eye on the affected side of the body may have to be protected if the lid remains open and there is no blink reflex. The patient is at high risk for corneal scratches or irritation. Irrigation with a physiologic solution of sodium chloride may be used, followed by eyedrops. An eye pad may be used to keep the eye closed, although an eye shield is preferable.

Nursing Interventions

Safety needs. Patients with paralysis have significant safety needs. This includes protection from falling, including the use of side rails when the patient is in bed and a chair restraint when the patient is in a chair, especially if balance cannot be maintained. If the patient also has a sensory problem, which often accompanies paralysis, he or she may not realize when part of the body is in danger. For example, a patient with a stroke may not be aware that a hemiplegic arm is hanging over the side of the wheelchair.

The eye on the affected side of the body should be cleaned and assessed for signs of infection on a regular basis, usually three times a day or more. Also inspect affected body parts for injury.

Regularly inspect the skin over bony prominences for signs of pressure. Paralyzed people are at risk for skin impairment, so teach them to turn themselves in bed and to reposition themselves in the bed or chair independently, if possible. If the patient is unable to turn independently, carry out this function. Usually the patient is turned from one side to another or from one side to the back to the other side. Repositioning also includes weight shifts, done by the patient or by staff. These weight shifts may include controlled leaning from one side to another or chair push-ups. If the patient is not able to do the activity, have him or her take responsibility for reminding staff when it is time to do weight shifting.

Inspect paralyzed or weakened areas at least daily for any signs of skin impairment. A mirror often is used to help the patient assess the skin so that he or she is not as dependent on staff or family.

Activity needs. The extremities of a person who has an acute motor problem may be flaccid at first. Spasticity of muscles develops gradually. The joints then become flexed and fixed in useless, deformed positions unless preventive measures are taken.

Carefully place the extremities in a normal anatomic position to prevent deformity. Counterpositioning may be helpful. In **hemiplegia** (paralysis of one side of the body) the affected upper extremity is pulled inward at the shoulder joint and the wrist drops; in the lower extremity the knee flexes and the foot drops. In counterpositioning, the patient is placed so that the shoulder and upper arm are in abduction, the elbow is flexed, the wrist is dorsiflexed (i.e., the hand is bent upward, toward the top of the wrist), the knee is in neutral position, and the foot is dorsiflexed (i.e., pulled up toward the knee). If the person is supine, place a pillow between the upper arm and the body to hold the arm in abduction. Physical therapists and occupational therapists can provide splints and braces that can aid in positioning (Fig. 54.8).

Footboards may be used to prevent footdrop, although some believe that these contribute to increased spasticity and should not be used routinely for patients who have muscle spasms. High-top tennis shoes or other devices, such as splints or braces, can help prevent footdrop, if therapy is initiated early. In some hospitals, casts are applied to patients' lower extremities to prevent footdrop or to reverse contractures. The presence of the cast impedes spasticity.

The prone position is excellent for patients who are able to tolerate it. Not only does this position decrease the chance of skin impairment but it also causes extension of the hip, the knee joints, and the ankles by means of gravity. A pillow placed under the chest may help patients comfortably assume this position.

Positioning of the paralyzed person is extremely important. Complications such as footdrop and flexion contractures of the knee seriously limit mobility. As a result, the level of self-care and independence is diminished. Most joint deformities in a paralyzed person are preventable with early and continuing nursing interventions.

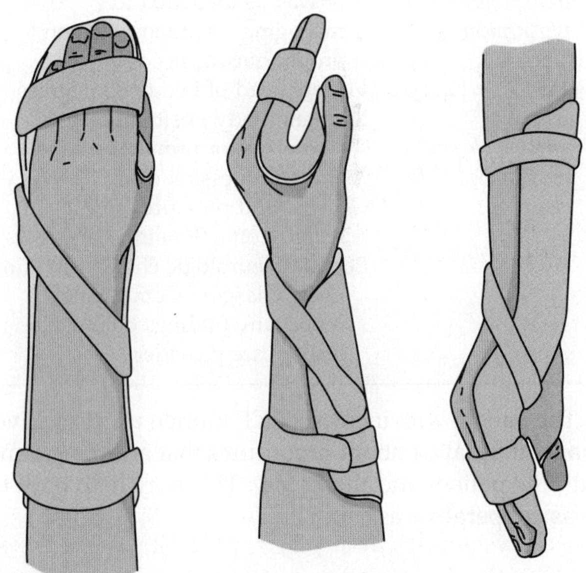

Fig. 54.8 Volar resting splint provides support to wrist, thumb, and fingers of patient after a cerebrovascular accident (stroke), maintaining them in a position of extension. (From Black JM, Hawks JH: *Medical-surgical nursing: Clinical management for positive outcomes*, ed 8, St. Louis, 2009, Saunders.)

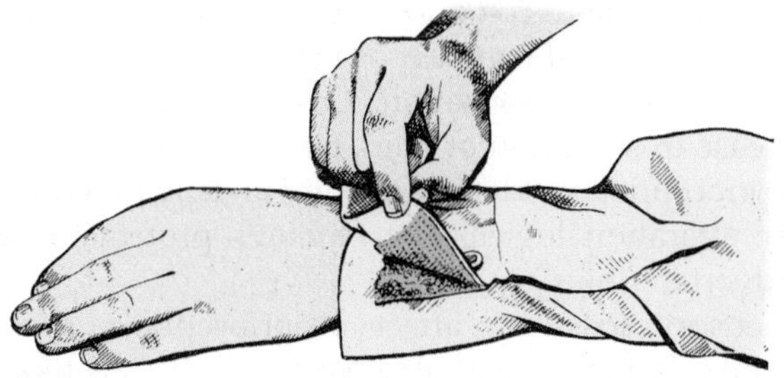

Fig. 54.9 Velcro shirtsleeve to facilitate closure. (From Hoemann SP: *Rehabilitation nursing: Process and application*, ed 2, St. Louis, 1996, Mosby.)

In addition to positioning, interventions for the person with paralysis include ROM exercises to all joints. These may be passive (carried out by the nurse) or active (carried out by the patient). Passive ROM is indicated at least three times daily for all joints that the patient cannot voluntarily move.

Nutritional needs. Patience and persistence are often necessary in giving food and fluids to the patient with hemiplegia. Aspiration can occur and is related to loss of pharyngeal sensation, loss of oropharyngeal motor control, and decreased LOC. Consider consultation with a speech and language pathologist for a swallowing evaluation and recommendations for treatment (American Speech-Language-Hearing Association, n.d.). Important nursing measures include avoiding foods that cause choking, checking the affected side of the mouth for accumulation of food and resultant poor hygiene, not mixing liquids and solid foods, and encouraging the patient to take small bites. Adding a thickening agent (such as Thick-It) to liquids often helps prevent choking. If the patient has dentures, they should be worn. The patient should sit at a 90-degree angle with the head up and chin slightly tucked. The head should not be extended; encourage the patient to tip the head toward the unaffected side while swallowing. Avoid straws. Assistive devices for feeding include utensils with universal cuffs, covered plastic cups, scoop dishes, and plate guards. These enable the patient to be less dependent on the staff, and they are available through therapists in most hospitals.

Activities of daily living. During the acute rehabilitative phases of a motor problem, teach patients with paralysis how to carry out ADLs to the extent that they are able. A variety of devices are available to assist with dressing and grooming (Figs. 54.9 and 54.10). The occupational therapist becomes involved in many of these activities, including homemaking. Stress the concept of the rehabilitative team in managing these patients. Teach the patient to compensate for weakness or paralysis. Give the patient the time to do activities on his or her own if able. It is often easier and faster to do things for the patient, but this defeats the purpose of rehabilitation.

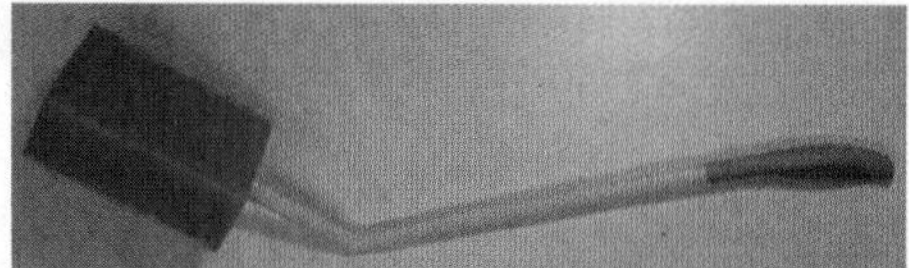

Fig. 54.10 Long-handled bath sponge. (From Sorrentino SA, Remmert LN: *Mosby's textbook for nursing assistants*, ed 8, St. Louis, 2012, Saunders.)

Psychological adjustments. The person with paralysis may need assistance in adjusting to body changes. The loss of the ability to function independently is traumatic, and the patient may have fears of rejection, loss of self-esteem, and concerns about the future. A grief reaction similar to that described for a death may occur. The patient may relate to the paralyzed part of the body as though it were not a part of him or her and may have nicknames for the body part. To help the patient cope with the loss of function and change in body image, praise the patient for achievements, encourage expression of fears and grief, and help him or her see that there is life after disability. It may be helpful to arrange a visit by someone with the same disability who has been rehabilitated successfully.

Patient problems and interventions for the patient with alterations in muscle tone and motor function include but are not limited to the following:

Patient Problem	Nursing Interventions
Compromised Physical Mobility, related to neuromuscular impairment	Perform active or passive ROM exercise q 4 hr, to all extremities, neck, hands, fingers, wrists, elbows, and knees Provide physical therapy as ordered (massage and stretching exercises) Maintain planned rest periods Encourage ambulation to tolerance Arrange for necessary assistive devices for home care needs
Risk for Contractures or Muscle Atrophy, related to impaired functioning of body part	Perform hand, finger, and foot exercises; assist in active and passive ROM exercises q 2-4 hr Assist patient with using supportive devices as indicated (overhead trapeze, braces, walker, cane) Encourage use of involved side when possible Instruct patient to use unaffected extremity to support weaker side (e.g., lift involved left leg with right leg or lift involved left arm with right arm) Turn q 2 hr

Patient Teaching

Teaching is an extremely important part of caring for the person with motor problems. Appropriate teaching activities include safety needs, skin care, activity (ROM

Health Promotion

The Patient With a Neurologic Disorder

- *Nutritional-metabolic pattern:* Neurologic problems can result in inadequate nutrition. Problems related to chewing, swallowing, facial nerve paralysis, and muscle coordination could make it difficult for the patient to ingest adequate nutrients.
- *Elimination pattern:* Bowel and bladder problems often are associated with neurologic problems, such as stroke, head injury, spinal cord injury, multiple sclerosis, and dementia. It is important to determine whether the bowel or bladder problem was present before the neurologic event to plan appropriate interventions.
- *Activity-exercise pattern:* Many neurologic disorders can cause problems in the patient's mobility, strength, and coordination. These problems can change the patient's usual activity and exercise patterns.
- *Sleep-rest pattern:* Sleep can be disrupted by many neurologically related factors. Discomfort from pain and inability to move and change to a position of comfort because of muscle weakness and paralysis could interfere with sound sleep.
- *Cognitive-perceptual pattern:* Because the nervous system controls cognition and sensory integration, many neurologic disorders affect these functions. Assess memory, language, calculation ability, problem-solving ability, insight, and judgment.
- *Self-perception–self-concept pattern:* Neurologic disease can alter drastically control over one's life and create dependency on others for daily needs.
- *Role-relationship pattern:* Ask the patient if neurologic problems have led to changes in roles, such as spouse, parent, or breadwinner. These changes can affect dramatically the patient and significant others.
- *Sexuality-reproductive pattern:* Assess the ability to participate in sexual activity, because many nervous system disorders can affect sexual response.
- *Coping–stress tolerance pattern:* The physical sequelae of a neurologic problem can seriously strain a patient's ability to cope. Often the problem is chronic and may require the patient to learn new coping skills.
- *Value-belief pattern:* Many neurologic problems have serious, long-term, life-changing effects. These effects can strain the patient's belief system and should be assessed.

and positioning), medications (dosage, action, times, and side effects), good nutrition, ADLs, bowel and bladder care, and follow-up care. Written instructions reinforce teaching and give the patient something to refer to at home (see the Health Promotion box). Prepare family members to assume some of the care for the patient.

DISTURBED SENSORY AND PERCEPTUAL FUNCTION

Etiology and Pathophysiology

The presence of a lesion anywhere within the sensory system pathway, from the receptor to the sensory cortex, alters the transmission or perception of sensory information. The parietal cortex is of major importance in the interpretation of sensation. Loss of, decrease in, or increase in sensation of pain, temperature, touch, and proprioception results in difficulty in daily functioning. Any alteration lessens the patient's protection from inadvertent injury.

Sensory loss can affect proprioception, that is, the body's innate spatial sense. **Agnosia** is a total or partial loss, as a result of organic brain damage, of the ability to recognize familiar objects by sight, touch, or hearing or to recognize familiar people through sensory stimuli.

Assessment

Subjective data include the patient's understanding of the sensory disturbance, measures that relieve symptoms (including medications), and symptoms that occur with the sensory problem. An example is the person who experiences weakness of a hand and at the same time feels numbness and tingling. Collect information on the onset of the sensory problem and the specific site in the body.

Collection of objective data includes noting the patient's ability to perform purposeful movements or to recognize familiar objects.

Medical Management

Medical management will be determined by the underlying cause of the alteration in muscle tone and motor function.

Nursing Interventions and Patient Teaching

The most important nursing intervention for the patient with sensory dysfunction is to teach the patient protective measures. This includes helping the patient learn to inspect parts of the body that have no feeling, or to protect sensitive body parts from the discomfort of linen rubbing over them. If a patient has a deficit in one sense, he or she should learn to compensate with another (e.g., the patient who learns to lip-read because of a hearing deficit; the patient with hemianopia who is taught to scan the printed page).

Patient problems and interventions for the patient with a sensory or perceptual problem are the same as those for the patient with a motor problem, with the addition of but not limited to the following:

Patient Problem	Nursing Interventions
Potential for Injury, related to sensory or perceptual disturbances	Maintain safe environment Teach patient to protect body parts that have decreased sensation Teach patient to inspect body parts for possible injury Protect patient from sustaining injury from hot liquid or heating pads

The teaching for a patient with a sensory deficit is essentially the same as that for the patient with a motor deficit.

OTHER DISORDERS OF THE NEUROLOGIC SYSTEM

Functioning of the neurologic system can be interrupted for a variety of reasons. These include conduction abnormalities, degenerative diseases, vascular problems, infection, tumors, trauma, and cranial and peripheral nerve disorders. Selected disorders in each area are discussed.

CONDUCTION ABNORMALITIES

EPILEPSY OR SEIZURES

Etiology and Pathophysiology

Seizure activity is the result of abnormal electrical activity within the brain. There are several conditions that may cause seizures. These include severe elevations in body temperature, drug use, electrolyte imbalance, brain tumors, brain infection, and epilepsy. Not all individuals experiencing seizure activity have epilepsy.

Epilepsy is a group of neurologic disorders characterized by recurrent episodes that may include convulsive seizure, sensory disturbances, abnormal behavior, and changes in LOC.

Cases of epilepsy have been recorded throughout history. Seizures occur in all races and affect men and women equally. There are no apparent geographic boundaries. In the United States approximately 3.4 million people suffer from active epilepsy, with 150,000 new cases being diagnosed each year (Epilepsy Foundation, 2014). The incidence rates are higher in the first year of life, decline through childhood and adolescence, plateau in middle age, and rise sharply again among older adults.

Clinical Manifestations

Seizures can be classified according to the features of the attack. The types include generalized tonic-clonic (grand mal), absence (petit mal), psychomotor (automatisms), jacksonian (focal), and miscellaneous (myoclonic and akinetic) seizures (Table 54.5).

Epilepsy is associated with paroxysmal, uncontrolled electrical discharges in the neurons of the brain that result in the sudden, violent, involuntary contraction of a group of muscles. The patterns or forms of seizures vary and depend on the area of the brain from which the seizure arises. The excessive neuronal discharges may result in a tonic convulsion, with alternate contraction and relaxation of opposing muscle groups. This gives the characteristic tonic-clonic jerking movements of the body. Seizures are followed by a rest period of variable length, called the **postictal period** (after a seizure). During this period the patient usually feels groggy and acts disoriented. Complaints of headache and muscle aches are common. Usually the patient sleeps after a seizure and may experience amnesia for the event.

When recurrent, generalized seizure activity occurs at such frequency that full consciousness is not regained between seizures, it is called *status epilepticus*. This is a medical emergency and requires medical and nursing interventions. Repeated seizures cause the brain to use more energy than can be supplied; the neurons become exhausted and cease to function, which may result in permanent brain damage or death. The most common cause of status epilepticus is sudden withdrawal of anticonvulsant medications. The nursing interventions always involve ensuring that there is a patent airway and protecting the patient from injury. Medications to stop the seizure activity may be given in high doses that render the patient unconscious. The nurse must then assume total care of the patient's needs. Insert a Foley catheter and an IV line. Intubate the patient if necessary for ventilatory support. Protect the skin from injury. Take care with safety reminder devices such as bed check monitoring systems if the patient is awake and active so that they do not cause injury if the patient begins to have a seizure.

Assessment

Subjective data include the patient's awareness of the disorder and any precipitating factors. Assess whether an aura preceded the seizure. An aura occurs in about 50% of all patients with generalized tonic-clonic seizures. *Aura* is a sensation (such as of light or warmth) or emotion (such as fear) that may precede an attack of migraine or an epileptic seizure. An epileptic aura may be psychic, or it may be sensory with olfactory, visual, auditory, or taste hallucinations. The exact character of the aura varies from person to person. Awareness of an aura warns the person of the impending seizure and allows him or her to seek safety and privacy.

Objective data include the number of seizures occurring within a specific time, the character of the seizure, and any behaviors noted and injuries suffered. Describe the seizure as completely as possible, including duration, the patient's movements, whether the patient was incontinent, any cries or sounds that were made, and the level of alertness.

Diagnostic Testing

Diagnostic testing includes blood tests to assess for the presence of infection or chemical imbalances. A diagnosis of epilepsy cannot be made on the basis of a single seizure; epilepsy is a condition characterized by recurrent seizure activity. CT and MRI are performed to assess for the presence of lesions or to identify the location of seizure activity. PET scans may be used to pinpoint brain abnormalities. The most common test used to evaluate seizures is the EEG. It allows a specific diagnosis of the seizure.

Table 54.5 Characteristics of Seizures

INCIDENCE	CHARACTERISTICS	CLINICAL SIGNS	AURA	POSTICTAL PERIOD
Generalized Tonic-Clonic (Formerly Called Grand Mal)				
Most common	Generalized; characterized by loss of consciousness and falling to the floor or ground if patient is upright, followed by stiffening of the body (tonic phase) for 10–20 s and subsequent jerking of the extremities (clonic phase) for another 30–40 s	Aura Cry Loss of consciousness Flashing lights or smells Partial loss of vision Fall Tonic-clonic movements Incontinence, cyanosis, excessive salivation, tongue or cheek biting	Yes	Yes Need for 1–2 h of sleep Headache, muscle soreness commonly felt May not feel normal for several hours or days after a seizure No memory of a seizure
Absence (Formerly Called Petit Mal)				
Occurs during childhood and adolescence Frequency decreases as child gets older Rarely continues beyond adolescence	Sudden impairment in or loss of consciousness with little or no tonic-clonic movement Occurs without warning Has tendency to appear a few hours after arising or when person is quiet	Sudden vacant facial expression with eyes focused straight ahead (staring spell) that lasts only a few seconds All motor activity ceases except perhaps for slight symmetric twitching about eyelids Possible loss of muscle tone May have an extremely brief loss of consciousness	No	No
Psychomotor (Automatisms; Also Called Partial Seizures)				
Occur at any age	Sudden change in awareness associated with complex distortion of feeling and thinking and partially coordinated motor activity Longer than absence seizures	Behaves as if partially conscious; may continue an activity that was initiated before the seizure, such as counting out change or picking items from a grocery shelf, but after the seizure does not remember the activity Often appears intoxicated Complex hallucinations or illusions May do antisocial things, such as exposing self or carrying out violent acts Autonomic complaints, such as shivering, lip smacking, repetitive movements that may not be appropriate Urinary incontinence	Yes	Yes Confusion Amnesia Need for sleep
Jacksonian-Focal (Local or Partial)				
Occur almost entirely in patients with structural brain disease	Depends on site of focus May or may not be progressive	Commonly begin in hand, foot, or face with numbness and tingling May end in tonic-clonic seizure	Yes	Yes
Myoclonic				
May antedate tonic-clonic by months or years	May be very mild or may have rapid, forceful movements	Sudden, excess jerk of the body or extremities; may be forceful enough to hurl the person to the floor or ground Brief seizures that may occur in clusters No loss of consciousness	No	No
Akinetic				
Not common	Peculiar generalized tonelessness	Falls in flaccid state Unconscious for a minute or two	Rarely	No

Table 54.6 **Medications for Preventing and Controlling Seizures**

GENERIC NAME (TRADE NAME)	USE RELATED TO SEIZURE TYPE	TOXIC EFFECTS
carbamazepine (Tegretol)	Generalized tonic-clonic, psychomotor	Rash, drowsiness, ataxia
clonazepam (Klonopin)	Absence seizures, akinetic, myoclonic, generalized tonic-clonic seizures	Drowsiness, ataxia, hypotension, respiratory depression
diazepam (Valium)	Generalized tonic-clonic and status epilepticus, mixed	Drowsiness, ataxia
divalproex (Depakote)	Generalized tonic-clonic and myoclonic seizures	Sedation, drowsiness, behavior changes, visual disturbances, hepatic failure
ethosuximide (Zarontin)	Absence seizures, psychomotor, myoclonic, akinetic	Drowsiness, nausea, agranulocytosis
felbamate (Felbatol)	Seizures in children, generalized tonic-clonic seizures in adults; may be used to treat patients whose seizure disorders are refractory to other drugs	Irritability, insomnia, anorexia, nausea, headache; can cause aplastic anemia and hepatic failure
fosphenytoin sodium (Cerebyx)	Short-term parenteral (IV or IM) in acute generalized tonic-clonic seizures; used for status epilepticus and for preventing and treating seizures during neurosurgery	Dizziness, paresthesia, tinnitus, pruritus, headache, somnolence, ataxia, muscular incoordination, nystagmus, double vision, slurred speech, nausea, vomiting, and hypotension
gabapentin (Neurontin)	Focal, generalized tonic-clonic in adults	Somnolence, fatigue, ataxia, dizziness, anorexia
lamotrigine (Lamictal)	Focal, generalized tonic-clonic in adults	Rash, dizziness, tremor, ataxia, diplopia, headache, gastrointestinal upset, Stevens-Johnson syndrome (rare)
mephenytoin	Tonic-clonic, focal, psychomotor	Ataxia, nystagmus, pancytopenia, rash
oxcarbazepine (Trileptal)	Generalized tonic-clonic and partial seizures	Feeling abnormal, headache, dizziness, vertigo, anxiety, blurred vision
phenobarbital (Luminal)	Generalized tonic-clonic, focal, psychomotor	Drowsiness, rash
phenytoin sodium (Dilantin)	Generalized tonic-clonic, focal, psychomotor	Ataxia, vomiting, nystagmus, drowsiness, rash, fever, gum hypertrophy, lymphadenopathy
primidone (Mysoline)	Generalized tonic-clonic, focal, psychomotor	Drowsiness, ataxia
topiramate (Topamax), tiagabine (Gabitril), levetiracetam (Keppra), zonisamide (Zonegran)	Indicated for partial seizures and for secondary generalized seizures; currently used as adjunctive therapy	Topiramate: Somnolence, dizziness, ataxia, speech disorders and related speech problems, difficulty with memory, paresthesia, diplopia Tiagabine: Dizziness, lightheadedness, asthenia (lack of energy), somnolence, nausea, nervousness, irritability, tremor, thinking abnormally, difficulty with concentration or attention
trimethadione (Tridione)	Absence seizures	Rash, photophobia, agranulocytosis, nephrosis
valproic acid (Depakene)	Absence seizures	Nausea, vomiting, indigestion, sedation, emotional disturbance, weakness, altered blood coagulation

IM, Intramuscular; *IV*, intravenous.

Medical Management

Medications. In 70% of patients, seizure disorders are controlled by one or more antiseizure drugs (Table 54.6). Therapy is aimed at preventing seizures because cure is not possible. Drugs generally act by stabilizing nerve cell membranes and preventing spread of the epileptic discharge. The choice of medication depends on the type of seizure. Failure to take the prescribed medication or an adequate dose is often the cause of treatment failure. Blood levels may be checked to determine the therapeutic level of the medications taken. The primary goal of antiseizure drug therapy is to obtain maximum seizure control with minimum toxic side effects.

Surgical therapy. Pharmacologic therapies to control seizure activity are not possible for some patients with epilepsy. They may be considered candidates for surgical intervention. Surgery to manage seizure activity may include removal of the small area of the brain that is experiencing the misfiring and causing the seizures. This is called a *resection*. The connective tissue between the two hemispheres of the brain also may be severed in some cases (Mayo Clinic, 2018a).

Activities of daily living. Until seizures are controlled, patients should avoid activities such as driving a car, operating machinery, or swimming. Maintaining adequate rest and good nutrition is also important. Alcohol use should be avoided. If the patient is receiving long-term phenytoin therapy, good hygiene practices for the mouth and teeth are important because of the side effect of edematous and enlarged gums (gingival hyperplasia). The patient should wear a medical-alert bracelet or tag (see the Patient Teaching box).

 Patient Teaching

The Patient With Seizures

- Explain the need for the patient to continue taking medications even when seizure activity has stopped.
- Teach the patient about medications prescribed, including expected results, time and dosage, and side effects.
- Inform the patient that medical-alert bracelets, necklaces, and identification cards are available. The use of these medical identification tags is optional. Some patients have found them beneficial, but others prefer not to be identified as having a seizure disorder.
- Caution the patient to avoid the use of alcohol if taking antiseizure medications.
- Explain the need for good oral hygiene for people taking phenytoin (Dilantin) (a side effect is gingival hyperplasia).
- Stress the importance of adequate rest and a balanced diet.
- Educate about available community resources.
- Explain restrictions concerning driving.
- Explain the importance of follow-up care.
- A tonic-clonic seizure can be treated with first aid; it is not necessary to send the patient to the hospital (or to call an ambulance) after a single seizure unless the seizure is prolonged, another seizure immediately follows, or extensive injury has occurred.
- In the event of an acute seizure, protect the patient from injury. This involves supporting and/or protecting the head, turning the patient to one side, loosening any constricting garments, and, if the patient is seated, easing him or her onto the floor.

Nursing Interventions and Patient Teaching

Care during a seizure. The primary goals of the nurse and the family caring for a patient having a seizure are protection from aspiration and injury and observation and recording of the seizure activity. Never leave the patient alone. If the patient is sitting or standing, lower him or her to the floor in an area away from furniture and equipment. Support and protect the head; if possible, turn the head to the side to maintain the airway. Loosen restrictive clothing around the neck if possible. Do not try to restrain the patient during the seizure. Do *not* try to pry open the jaw to insert a padded tongue blade. No objects should be placed in the mouth. After the seizure the patient may require suctioning and oxygen. Padded side rails may be used, especially if seizures often occur during sleep.

When a seizure occurs, carefully observe and record details of the event because the diagnosis and subsequent treatment often rest solely on the seizure description. Note all aspects of the seizure: What events preceded the seizure? When did the seizure occur? How long did each phase (aural [if any], ictal, postictal) last? What occurred during each phase?

Patient problems and interventions for the patient with seizures may include but are not limited to the following:

Patient Problem	Nursing Interventions
Inability to Clear Airway, related to mucus accumulation in oropharyngeal area during seizure	Place patient in side-lying position to prevent aspiration and ensure airway patency Suction secretions as needed
Potential for Injury, related to rapid onset of altered state of consciousness and seizure activity	If patient is out of bed during seizure activity, assist to the floor and remove objects that may harm him or her Provide privacy Maintain patent airway After the seizure, inform patient of seizure and reorient if necessary

Prognosis

Seizure disorders can affect a patient's emotional, economic, and social well-being. Society's attitude has improved, but epilepsy still carries a social stigma. Most states have legal sanctions against driving if one has epilepsy. The inability to maintain a driver's license can affect one's lifestyle negatively.

The majority of patients with seizures are able to control them with medications and can lead a fairly normal life. With most seizure disorders, the number and intensity of seizures stay constant. For patients who experience a first seizure as a result of a brain tumor or another brain pathologic condition, the prognosis is more uncertain.

DEGENERATIVE DISEASES

The term *degenerative diseases* refers to neurologic disorders in which there is a premature aging of nerve cells, which is caused by suspected metabolic disturbance or for which the cause is unknown. Six diseases are discussed: multiple sclerosis (MS), Parkinson's disease, Alzheimer's disease (AD), myasthenia gravis (MG), amyotrophic lateral sclerosis (ALS), and Huntington's disease.

MULTIPLE SCLEROSIS

Etiology and Pathophysiology

MS is a chronic, progressive, degenerative neurologic disease that affects many people. The cause is unknown, although genetics have been implicated, because there is a higher rate of the disease among relatives. Patients with the first signs and symptoms of MS have a proliferation of a certain type of immune cell called *gamma delta T cells* in their spinal fluid. These cells are not found in patients who have had the disease for a long time. T cells, the "field commanders" of the immune system, usually defend the body from outside attackers. In MS, however, something goes wrong and induces the T cells to attack the body. Myelin damage occurs. The beginning mechanism may be a viral infection early in life that becomes apparent as an immune process later in life. A defective immune response also seems to have an important role in the pathology of MS.

The onset of signs and symptoms is usually between 15 and 50 years of age. Women are affected more often than men. The highest number of people with MS live in the Great Lakes area, the Pacific Northwest, and the North Atlantic states. MS is five times more prevalent in temperate climates between 45 and 66 degrees of latitude.

Multiple foci of *demyelination* are distributed randomly in the white matter of the brainstem, the spinal cord, optic nerves, and the cerebrum. During the demyelination process, the myelin sheath and the sheath cells are destroyed, causing an interruption or distortion of the nerve impulse so that it is slowed or blocked (Fig. 54.11). Areas of degeneration show evidence of partial healing, which explains the transitory nature of early signs and symptoms.

Clinical Manifestations

The onset is often insidious and gradual, with vague symptoms that occur intermittently over months or years, and thus the disease may not be diagnosed until long after the onset of the first symptom. Because of the wide distribution of areas of degeneration, the variety of signs and symptoms in MS is greater than in other neurologic diseases. These include visual problems, urinary incontinence, fatigue, weakness or incoordination of an extremity, sexual problems such as impotence in men, and swallowing difficulties. The majority of people have early remissions that may last for a year or more. The disease is characterized by chronic, progressive deterioration in some people and by remissions and exacerbations in others. Exacerbations may be related to fatigue, chilling, or emotional disturbances. With repeated exacerbations, progressive scarring of the myelin sheath occurs, and the overall trend is progressive deterioration in neurologic function.

Assessment

Subjective data include the patient's understanding of the disease. Eye problems such as diplopia, scotoma (partial loss of vision), and blindness may be present. The patient also may talk about weakness or numbness of a part of the body, fatigue, emotional instability, bowel and bladder problems, vertigo, or loss of joint sensation. Involvement of the cerebellum can result in **ataxia** (impaired ability to coordinate movement) and tremor. In men, impotence is significant. Pain is not a common symptom.

Objective data include documented abnormalities in neurologic testing; these may include **nystagmus** (involuntary, rhythmic movements of the eye; the oscillations may be horizontal, vertical, rotary, or mixed); muscle weakness and spasms; changes in coordination; or a spastic, ataxic gait. Cerebellar signs include ataxia, dysarthria, and dysphagia. There may be evidence of behavior changes such as euphoria, emotional lability, or mild depression. Urinary incontinence and intention tremors of the upper extremities may be present.

Diagnostic Tests

MS has no definitive diagnostic test; diagnosis is based primarily on history and clinical manifestations and the presence of multiple lesions over time as measured

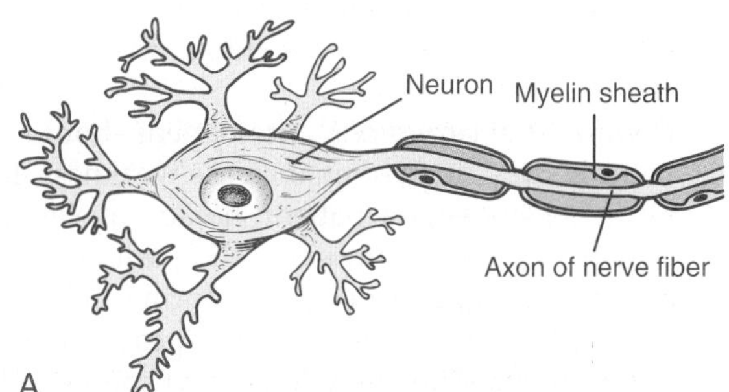

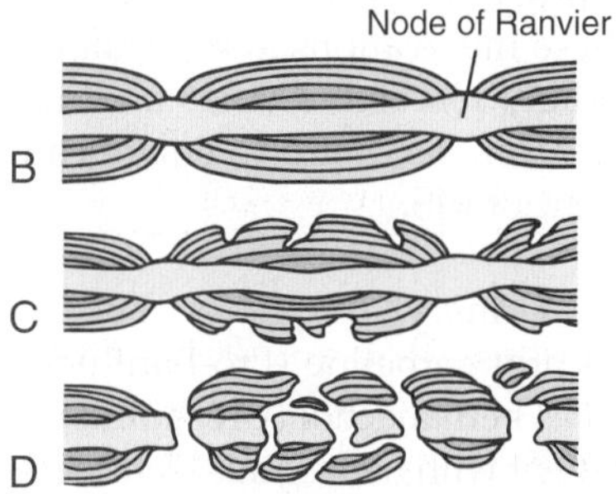

Fig. 54.11 Pathogenesis of multiple sclerosis. A, Normal nerve cell with myelin sheath. B, Normal axon. C, Myelin breakdown. D, Myelin totally disrupted; axon not functioning. (From Lewis SL, Heitkemper MM, Dirksen SR, et al: *Medical-surgical nursing: Assessment and management of clinical problems*, ed 9, St. Louis, 2014, Mosby.)

by MRI. Examination of the CSF in patients with MS may show elevated gamma globulin, a proliferation of gamma delta T cells in the initial phase, and an increased number of lymphocytes and monocytes. A CT scan may show enlargement of the cerebral ventricles. MRI scanning has been helpful in diagnosing MS over time in the presence of multiple lesions; sclerotic plaques as small as 3 to 4 mm in diameter can be detected.

Medical Management

Medications. No specific treatment exists for MS, although many different remedies have been tried. Symptoms are controlled with the use of adrenocorticotropic hormone (ACTH) and corticosteroids such as prednisone (Deltasone) or dexamethasone. These may be given orally, intramuscularly, or intravenously. The effects of ACTH and the steroids on the demyelinating process are unknown, although they probably help by reducing edema and acute inflammation at the site of demyelination. If steroids are used in high doses at the start of an exacerbation, the episode seems to resolve more rapidly. However, these drugs do not affect the ultimate outcome or degree of residual neurologic impairment from the exacerbation. If spasticity is a problem, drugs such as diazepam, dantrolene, and baclofen may help prevent or decrease the spasms. Immunomodulating drugs modify the disease process. Interferon beta-1b (Betaseron), given subcutaneously every other day, is indicated for use in ambulatory patients with relapsing-remitting MS to reduce the frequency of clinical exacerbations. Interferon beta-1a (Avonex) is similar to interferon beta-1b in efficacy and is used in similar patient groups with MS. It is given intramuscularly once a week. Another formulation of interferon beta-1a, Rebif, is administered subcutaneously three times weekly. Glatiramer acetate (Copaxone) is used in relapsing-remitting MS. Glatiramer is not an interferon, but it is believed to help patients with MS by interrupting the inflammatory cycle and preventing the body's immune system from attacking the myelin coating that protects the nerve fibers. It is given subcutaneously daily. Mitoxantrone is a drug for the treatment of primary-progressive and progressive-relapsing MS. It is an immunosuppressant drug that reduces B and T lymphocytes. It is given intravenously monthly. Cardiac assessment and follow-up are needed because these medications may result in cardiac compromise. Many research studies are being conducted in the search for more effective medications to use in the treatment of MS.

Elimination. Urinary frequency and urgency may respond to propantheline (Pro-Banthine). Cholinergic drugs such as bethanechol (Urecholine) sometimes can help the patient with neurogenic bladder (loss of bladder control because of nervous system damage) by exerting a direct antispasmodic effect on smooth muscles. Because urinary tract infections are a major problem in MS, some patients are given prophylactic doses of medications such as trimethoprim-sulfamethoxazole (Bactrim, Septra) or nitrofurantoin (Macrodantin). Cystometric studies, done to evaluate bladder function, can help define the specific bladder problem. Some patients may need to be taught self-catheterization.

Encourage the patient to drink adequate fluids (at least 2000 mL/day). If the patient suffers from constipation, a stool softener such as docusate sodium (Colace) may be used, as well as prune juice.

Nursing Interventions

Nutrition. A well-balanced diet with high-fiber foods and adequate fluids is important. Although there is no standard prescribed diet, a high-protein diet with supplemental vitamins often is recommended. Obesity makes it more difficult for the patient to meet daily needs and maintain mobility. The patient who is obese should be referred to a dietitian and be placed on a calorie-restricted diet that will help the patient lose weight slowly, while receiving adequate nutrition.

Skin care. Teach the patient with MS and/or the caregiver frequent turning to avoid skin impairment. Devices to relieve pressure, such as air mattresses, may be helpful. Because of sensory involvement, the patient may not feel discomfort that signals the need to change position.

Activity. Encourage patients with MS to exercise regularly but not to the point of fatigue. Physical therapy sometimes improves neurologic dysfunction. Exercise also helps daily functioning for patients with MS not experiencing an exacerbation. Exercise decreases spasticity, increases coordination, and retrains unaffected muscles to substitute for impaired ones. Water exercise is an especially beneficial type of physical therapy.

Daily rest periods may be helpful. During an acute exacerbation, patients often are kept as quiet as possible; this includes bed rest.

One side of the body often is more affected than the other. The patient must learn to stabilize the gait by leaning toward the less involved side. If the foot slaps forward while the patient is walking, teach him or her to put the foot down in a pronounced fashion and roll the weight forward on the side of the foot.

Control of environment. The patient should avoid hot baths because they often increase weakness. If summer travel is planned, the patient should travel in the coolest part of the day. If possible, the patient should be in air-conditioned surroundings during the summer.

People with MS do best in a peaceful and relaxed environment. They may have slow speech and be slow to respond. Sudden explosive emotional outbursts of crying or laughing also occur. The patient and family need support in dealing with this behavior.

Patient problems and interventions for the patient with MS may include but are not limited to the following:

Patient Problem	Nursing Interventions
Potential for Helplessness, related to physical limitations imposed by progressive physical deterioration, loss of body control, and threat to physical integrity	Provide emotional support, thorough explanations, and reassurance Be alert to emotional changes and mood swings Encourage the patient's participation and expression of needs and feelings Maintain planned rest periods Encourage self-care as indicated Provide physical care as indicated
Inability to Bathe, Feed, Toilet Self, related to limitations in physical mobility imposed by disease process	Administer oral hygiene as needed Assist with or provide physical hygiene as indicated by physical ability Maintain appropriate bathing temperatures Administer oral hygiene q 4 hr and as needed Catheterize intermittently as indicated; teach self-catheterization when possible Plan bladder dysfunction program as appropriate for spasticity or flaccidity Institute bowel control program (establish regular bowel routine, avoid constipation) Assist in dressing and grooming as indicated Provide nutritious, attractive meals

Patient Teaching

Teaching is important for the patient with MS and significant others. In late stages of the disease, the care functions usually are assumed by someone other than the patient. Important points include those for the patient with motor and sensory problems. In addition, stress the importance of spacing activities and avoiding temperature extremes and the potential for emotional lability. Make certain that the patient or the family has the address of the nearest MS society or support group.

Prognosis

The prognosis is variable. Some patients have MS for many years with few deficits, whereas other patients quickly become debilitated. The patient's ability to conserve energy and avoid stress may help prevent exacerbations. Exacerbations are treated and may resolve. The average life expectancy after the onset of symptoms is more than 25 years.

PARKINSON'S DISEASE

Etiology and Pathophysiology

Parkinsonism is a syndrome that consists of a slowing down in the initiation and execution of movement **(bradykinesia),** increased muscle tone (rigidity), tremor, and impaired postural reflexes. Parkinson's disease, a form of parkinsonism, is named after James Parkinson, who, in 1817, wrote a classic essay on "shaking palsy," a disease whose cause is still unknown today. Many other disorders resemble this disease, but their causes are known. These include drug-induced parkinsonism, postencephalitic parkinsonism, and arteriosclerotic parkinsonism. The pathophysiology of these disorders, with the exception of drug-induced parkinsonism, is the same. Damage or loss of the dopamine-producing cells of the substantia nigra in the midbrain leads to depletion, in the basal ganglia, of dopamine that influences the initiation, modulation, and completion of movement and regulates unconscious autonomic movements. In cases of drug-induced parkinsonism, the dopamine receptors in the brain are blocked.

According to the American Parkinson Disease Association, Parkinson's disease affects more than 1 million people in the United States. Symptoms commonly occur after 50 years of age. Peak onset of Parkinson's disease is in the 60s. The average age of the patient with Parkinson's disease is 65 years. There is an apparent genetic cause but no known cure. The disease rarely occurs in African Americans. Parkinson's disease is more common in men by a ratio of 3:2.

Parkinsonism has many causes. Encephalitis lethargica, or type A encephalitis, has been associated clearly with the onset of parkinsonism. However, the incidence of postencephalitic parkinsonism has dwindled since the 1920s, when there was a large outbreak of this infectious illness. Parkinsonian-like symptoms have occurred after intoxication with a variety of chemicals, including carbon monoxide and manganese (among copper miners) and a product of meperidine-analog synthesis. Drug-induced parkinsonism can follow therapy with selected antipsychotic medications such as phenothiazine and risperidone antiemetics including metoclopramide (Reglan), calcium channel blockers such as flunarizine, and some stimulants such as cocaine and amphetamines (Parkinson's Foundation, n.d.a).

Although patients with cerebrovascular disease may have parkinsonian-like symptoms, there is little evidence that parkinsonism is caused by arteriosclerosis. Distinguishing arteriosclerosis from true Parkinson's disease is important for prognostic purposes. Patients with arteriosclerosis do not respond as well to treatment and are more likely to experience side effects of drug therapy. Most patients with parkinsonism have the degenerative or idiopathic form, for which the term *Parkinson's disease* usually is reserved.

Other factors linked to Parkinson's disease include reduced estrogen levels and exposure to pesticides,

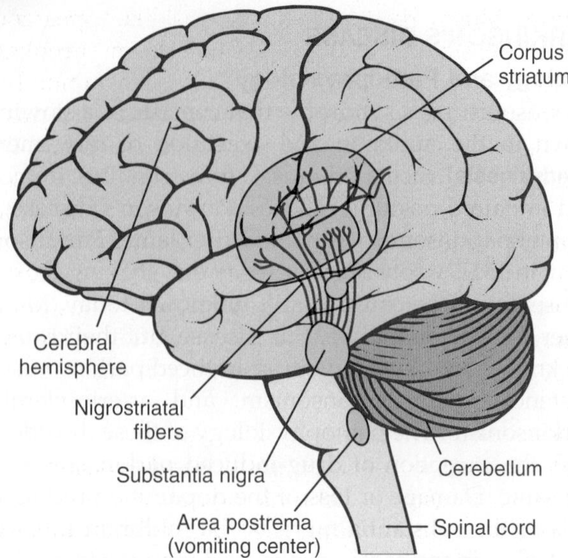

Fig. 54.12 Nigrostriatal disorders produce parkinsonism. Left-sided view of the human brain showing the substantia nigra and the corpus striatum *(shaded area)* lying deep within the cerebral hemisphere. Nerve fibers extend upward from the substantia nigra, divide into many branches, and carry dopamine to all regions of the corpus striatum. (From Lewis SL, Heitkemper MM, Dirksen SR, et al: *Medical-surgical nursing: Assessment and management of clinical problems*, ed 9, St. Louis, 2014, Mosby.)

herbicides, industrial chemicals, and metals such as manganese (Parkinson's Foundation, n.d.b).

The pathology of Parkinson's disease is associated with degeneration of the dopamine-producing neurons in the substantia nigra of the midbrain, which in turn disrupts the normal balance between dopamine and acetylcholine in the basal ganglia (Fig. 54.12). Major signs and symptoms, such as tremors, muscle rigidity, slowed movements, and impaired balance and coordination, occur when approximately 60% to 80% of dopamine-producing cells have been destroyed. It is believed that there is normally a balance between acetylcholine and dopamine in the basal ganglia. Any shift in the balance of activity (an increase in acetylcholine or a decrease in dopamine) seems to lead to parkinsonian-like symptoms. Dopamine is a neurotransmitter that is essential for normal functioning of the extrapyramidal motor system, including control of posture, support, and voluntary motion. In Parkinson's disease the levels of dopamine-synthesizing enzymes and metabolites are reduced, and postmortem analysis of cross-sections of the midbrain shows loss of the normal melanin pigment in the substantia nigra and loss of neurons. In addition, deficient amounts of gamma-aminobutyric acid, serotonin, and norepinephrine have been found in basal ganglia and in the substantia nigra.

Clinical Manifestations

The onset of Parkinson's disease is gradual and insidious, with a gradual progression and a prolonged course. In the beginning stages, only a mild tremor, handwriting changes, a slight limp, or a decreased arm swing may be evident. Later in the disease the patient may have

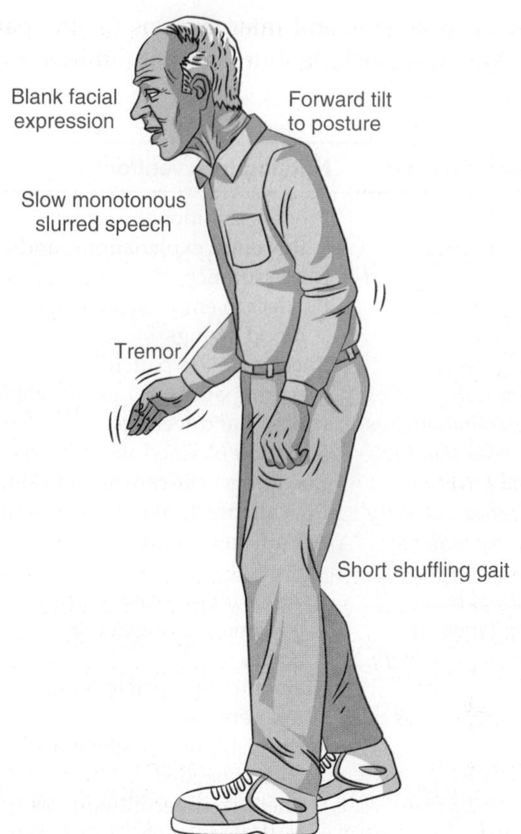

Fig. 54.13 Characteristic appearance of a patient with Parkinson's disease.

a shuffling, propulsive gait with arms flexed and loss of postural reflexes (Fig. 54.13). Some patients may have a slight change in speech patterns. None of these alone is sufficient evidence for a diagnosis of the disease.

Because Parkinson's disease has no specific diagnostic test, the diagnosis is based solely on the history, a thorough neurologic examination, and clinical features. A firm diagnosis can be made only when the patient has at least two signs of the classic triad: tremor, rigidity, and bradykinesia (slow or retarded movement). In the early stage of the disease there are subtle changes in cognitive function that can progress to dementia. The ultimate confirmation of Parkinson's disease is a positive response to a low-dose trial of an antiparkinsonian medication, such as carbidopa-levodopa (Sinemet).

Tremor. Tremor, often the first sign, may be minimal initially, so the patient is the only one who notices it. This tremor can affect handwriting, causing it to trail off, particularly toward the ends of words. Parkinsonian tremor is more prominent at rest but disappears when the patient moves; it is aggravated by emotional stress or increased concentration. The hand tremor is described as "pill rolling" because the thumb and forefinger appear to move in a rotary fashion, as if rolling a pill, coin, or other small object. Tremor can involve the hands, diaphragm, tongue, lips, and jaw but rarely causes shaking of the head. Eventually tremors can become so pronounced that the patient cannot hold a newspaper steady enough to read or make a call on a push-button telephone. Unfortunately, in many people a benign essential tremor has been diagnosed mistakenly as Parkinson's disease. Essential tremor occurs during voluntary movement, has a more rapid frequency than parkinsonian tremor, and is often familial.

Rigidity. Rigidity, the second sign of the triad, is the increased resistance to passive motion when the limbs are moved through their range of motion. Parkinsonian rigidity is typified by a jerky quality when the joint is moved, like intermittent catches in the movement of a cogwheel. This is termed *cogwheel rigidity.* The rigidity is caused by sustained muscle contraction and consequently elicits a complaint of muscle soreness; fatigue and achiness; or pain in the head, the upper body, the spine, or the legs. Another consequence of rigidity is slowness of movement, because it inhibits the alternating contraction and relaxation of opposing muscle groups (e.g., the biceps and triceps). Simple movements such as tying shoes and rising from a chair become a challenge.

Bradykinesia. Bradykinesia is particularly evident in the loss of automatic movements, which is secondary to physical and chemical alteration of the basal ganglia and related structures in the extrapyramidal portion of the CNS. In the unaffected patient, automatic movements are involuntary and occur subconsciously. They include blinking the eyelids, swinging the arms while walking, swallowing saliva, expressing oneself with facial and hand movements, and making minor postural adjustment. The patient with Parkinson's disease does not execute these movements and lacks spontaneous activity. This accounts for the stooped posture, masked face (deadpan expression), drooling, and shuffling gait (festination) that is characteristic of a person with this disease (see Fig. 54.13). The voice softens and loses modulation too, further contributing to communication problems. There may be evidence of bradykinesia in the patient's handwriting. The words become tiny and different from earlier handwriting samples. This is referred to as micrographia (Potgieser et al, 2015). The patient often has a shuffling, propulsive gait that he or she is unable to stop until meeting an obstruction. In addition, there is difficulty initiating movement. Movements such as getting out of a chair cannot be executed unless they are willed consciously.

Assessment

Parkinson's disease starts with subtle symptoms and progresses slowly. Subjective data include fatigue, incoordination, judgment defects, emotional instability, anxiety, depression, and heat intolerance. Assess the patient's understanding of the disease.

Objective data include tremor, which is the outstanding sign of the disease. This has been described as a pill-rolling motion of the fingers or a resting tremor. Bradykinesia is present with rigidity and loss of postural reflexes. Muscle rigidity leads to a masklike appearance of the face; slowed, monotonous speech; and drooling. Dysphagia, or difficulty swallowing, is a common late complication of neurologic degeneration, which poses the risk of choking and aspiration pneumonia. The patient may be constipated. There may be a scaly, erythematous rash, particularly near the ears and eyebrows and in the scalp and nasolabial folds. Moist, oily skin is usually noted. Postural hypotension is prevalent and may be caused by failure of the arterial baroreceptors located in the aortic arch and the internal carotid arteries (Parkinson's Foundation, n.d.).

Diagnostic Tests

Parkinson's disease has no definitive diagnostic tests. If there is a history of chronic dementia, the CT scan may show cerebral atrophy. The EEG may show minimal slowing, and the upper gastrointestinal evaluation may show decreased motility.

Medical Management

Medications. Treatment for Parkinson's disease is based on easing the signs and symptoms of the disease. Several different drugs have had a dramatic effect on the course of the disease: trihexyphenidyl hydrochloride, benztropine mesylate (Cogentin), levodopa (the most commonly prescribed medication for Parkinson's disease), amantadine hydrochloride (Symmetrel), carbidopa-levodopa (for 35 years, the gold standard of therapy), selegiline hydrochloride (Eldepryl), ropinirole (Requip), tolcapone (Tasmar), pramipexole (Mirapex), pergolide, rasagiline (Azilect), and rotigotine (Neupro).

After prolonged treatment with some of the drugs, side effects such as dyskinesia (abnormal, involuntary muscle movements) may occur and the medication's effectiveness may decrease. Hospitalization may be helpful, during which time all drugs are withdrawn for a time. This is called a *drug holiday.* The medications then are restarted, and often smaller doses produce favorable results. Complications such as aspiration can occur during this time because withdrawal of the drugs causes immobility and rigidity (Table 54.7). To combat these problems, newer drug classes have been developed.

Surgery. Surgery that involves destroying portions of the brain that control the rigidity or tremor—so-called ablation surgery—has been used for Parkinson's disease for more than 50 years. However, it has been replaced by **deep brain stimulation (DBS).** DBS involves placing an electrode in the thalamus, globus pallidus, or subthalamic nucleus and connecting it to a generator placed in the upper chest (like a pacemaker). The device is programmed to deliver a specific current to the targeted brain location. DBS can be adjusted to control symptoms and is reversible (the device can be removed). The procedure is nonablative and relatively safe and can improve dyskinesia (impaired ability to execute voluntary movements), gait, rigidity, and tremors.

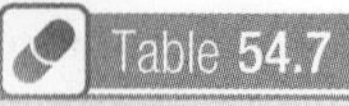

Table 54.7 Medications for Disorders of the Neurologic System

GENERIC NAME (TRADE NAME)	ACTION AND USE	SIDE EFFECTS	NURSING IMPLICATIONS
amantadine hydrochloride	Treats some cases of Parkinson's disease and drug-induced extrapyramidal reactions, although its action in treatment of Parkinson's disease is unknown	Nausea, vomiting, vision changes, dysrhythmias, disorientation, orthostatic hypotension, depression, fatigue	Tell patient to drink no alcohol; administer no CNS depressants; know pregnancy cautions; tell patient not to cease taking medication without conferring with health care provider and not to deviate from prescribed dosage; for best absorption, instruct patient to take after meals; if orthostatic hypotension occurs, instruct patient not to stand or change positions too quickly
baclofen (Lioresal)	Reduces transmission of impulses from spinal cord to skeletal muscles; is antispasticity agent for treatment of spinal spasticity resulting from multiple sclerosis or spinal cord injury	Drowsiness, dizziness, disorientation, lightheadedness, hypotension, urinary frequency, possible increase in blood glucose level	Be aware of pregnancy cautions; give oral form with meals or milk to prevent gastrointestinal distress; watch for increased incidence of seizures in patients with epilepsy; tell patient to avoid activities that require alertness until CNS effects of drugs are known
benztropine mesylate (Cogentin)	Blocks central cholinergic receptors, helping to balance cholinergic activity in basal ganglia; is indicated in treatment of mild cases of Parkinson's disease and control of extrapyramidal reactions	Dizziness, drowsiness, depression, orthostatic hypotension, palpitation, tachycardia	Stress importance of following prescribed dosage; discontinue drug slowly; tell patient not to drink alcohol; advise patient of breast-feeding warnings; give with food; tell patient to rise slowly and notify health care provider of severe allergic reactions; do not give with antacids
carbidopa-levodopa (Sinemet)	Increases levels of dopamine and levodopamine; is antiparkinsonian agent; improves modulation of voluntary nerve impulses transmitted to the motor cortex (lower dosage is needed than with single-dose therapy; efficiency may increase 75% when carbidopa and levodopa are used in combination)	Mental depression, mental changes, nausea and vomiting, orthostatic hypotension, dizziness, uncontrollable body movements	Give with food; give only as directed; effectiveness may take months; warn patient of breast-feeding and pregnancy cautions; caution patient about drowsiness and getting up too fast; lying down may affect control of blood glucose and darken urine
donepezil (Aricept)	Improves cholinergic function by inhibiting acetylcholinesterase; anti-Alzheimer's agent; may temporarily lessen some of the dementia associated with Alzheimer's disease, but does not alter the course	Diarrhea, nausea, vomiting, fatigue, headache, ecchymoses, atrial fibrillation, vasodilation	Monitor heart rate (may cause bradycardia); assess cognitive function periodically during therapy; administer in the evening just before bed; may be taken without regard for food
levodopa	Antiparkinsonian agent (mechanism of action is unknown); increases balance between cholinergic and dopaminergic activity to allow more normal body movements and alleviate signs and symptoms	Aggressive behavior, involuntary grimacing, head and body movements, depression, suicidal tendencies, orthostatic hypotension, nausea, vomiting, darkened urine, excessive and inappropriate sexual behavior	Do not give to patients with narrow-angle glaucoma; monitor patients receiving antihypertensive and hypoglycemic agents; advise patient to change positions slowly and dangle legs; protect drug from heat, light, moisture

Table 54.7 **Medications for Disorders of the Neurologic System—cont'd**

GENERIC NAME (TRADE NAME)	ACTION AND USE	SIDE EFFECTS	NURSING IMPLICATIONS
memantine (Namenda)	Believed to act as an *N*-methyl-D-aspartate receptor antagonist to decrease glutamate, which is an excitatory neurotransmitter in the CNS; approved for the treatment of moderate to severe Alzheimer's disease; does not prevent or slow neurodegeneration, but found in clinical studies to slow symptom progression	Dizziness, headache, constipation, hypertension, urinary frequency	Monitor I&O; do not give to patients with severe renal impairment; use cautiously in those with moderate renal impairment; be aware that conditions that increase urine pH, including severe urinary tract infections, lead to decreased excretion and increased serum levels
pyridostigmine bromide (Mestinon)	Inhibits destruction of acetylcholine released from parasympathetic and somatic efferent nerves; causes acetylcholine to accumulate, promoting increased stimulation of receptor; is used in myasthenia gravis and by the oral route for senility associated with Alzheimer's disease	Headache, seizures, bradycardia, hypotension, bronchospasm, increased bronchial secretions	Judging optimum dosage is difficult; monitor and document patient's response after each dose when using for myasthenia gravis; stress importance of taking drug exactly as ordered, on time, and in evenly spaced doses
selegiline hydrochloride (Eldepryl)	Monoamine oxidase (MAO) inhibitor used as treatment adjunct to levodopa and carbidopa-levodopa; may slow Parkinson's disease and need for increased medication; may increase lifespan of people with Parkinson's disease	Severe orthostatic hypotension, increased tremors, chorea, restlessness, grimacing, nausea and vomiting, slow urination, increased sweating, alopecia	Advise patient not to take more than 10 mg/day (there is no evidence that a greater amount improves effectiveness and it may increase adverse reactions); warn patient not to drink alcohol and drink only a little coffee; give with food; tell patient to rise slowly and notify health care provider of side effects; tell patient not to take over-the-counter cold remedies; monitor blood pressure and respirations
tacrine hydrochloride	Acts as reversible cholinesterase inhibitor, used for treatment of mild to moderate dementia of Alzheimer's type	Bradycardia, nausea and vomiting, loose stools, ataxia, CNS disturbance, anorexia, agitation, increased serum transaminase levels, jaundice	Know risk of ulcers; monitor liver enzyme weekly for first 18 wk; increase dosage at 6-wk intervals; do not use NSAIDs concomitantly; be aware that it potentiates theophylline
trihexyphenidyl hydrochloride	Blocks central cholinergic receptors, helping to balance cholinergic activity of basal ganglia; is antidyskinetic and antiparkinsonian; controls some mild cases as an adjunct to more potent drugs; controls extrapyramidal reactions caused by drugs	Skin rash, eye pain, nervousness, headaches, tachycardia, urinary hesitancy, urine retention, dry mouth, disorientation	Do not give antacids or antidiarrheal agents within 1 h of giving medication; give with food; caution patient to rise slowly; use cautiously in patients with narrow-angle glaucoma and hypertension; warn patient to avoid activities that require alertness until CNS effects of drugs are known; tell patient to relieve dry mouth with cool drinks, ice chips, and hard candy

CNS, Central nervous system; *I&O*, intake and output; *NSAIDs*, nonsteroidal antiinflammatory drugs.

This procedure is often reserved for patients who have developed severe side effects to drug therapy or severe motor complications.

Medications are discontinued several days preoperatively so that signs and symptoms will be at their maximum at the time of surgery.

Another treatment approach for Parkinson's disease involves human fetal dopamine cell transplants into the basal ganglia in an attempt to provide viable dopamine-producing cells to the brain.

Nursing Interventions

Activity needs. Pay special attention to posture. Lying on a firm bed without a pillow may help prevent the spine from bending forward. Holding the hands folded behind the back when walking may help keep the spine erect and prevent the arms from falling stiffly at the sides. Problems secondary to bradykinesia can be alleviated by relatively simple measures. Advise patients who tend to "freeze" while walking to consciously think about stepping over imaginary or real lines on the floor, drop rice kernels and step over them, rock from side to side, lift the toes when stepping, and take one step backward and two steps forward. A patient who has difficulty rising from a sitting position can use a chair that gently propels him or her to an upright position. Do not hurry the patient because it will make the bradykinesia worse.

Nutrition. Diet is of major importance to the patient with Parkinson's disease to avoid malnutrition and constipation. Patients with dysphagia and bradykinesia need appetizing foods that can be chewed and swallowed easily. Food should be cut into bite-sized pieces before it is served. Eating six small meals a day may be less exhausting than eating three large meals. Allow ample time for eating to avoid frustration and encourage independence. When the disease is advanced, aspiration is a real concern. Take care during feeding. Unless the disease is well controlled by medication, drooling can be a problem and increases with general excitement. When patients are dressed, garments with generous pockets for an ample supply of tissues help them to be less conspicuous.

Elimination. The patient with Parkinson's disease may feel urgency and hesitancy in voiding. Measures appropriate for the patient with MS also apply to these patients. Chronic constipation may be a real concern. The patient should be on a diet high in fiber and roughage for bulk. Encourage oral fluid intake, and use stool softeners, suppositories, and prune juice if necessary. Mild cathartics such as Milk of Magnesia are used if required.

Patient problems and interventions for the patient with Parkinson's disease are the same as those for the patient with MS, with the addition of but not limited to the following:

Patient Problem	Nursing Interventions
Compromised Physical Mobility, related to: • Rigidity • Bradykinesia • Akinesia	Assist with ambulation to assess degree of impairment and to prevent injury Perform active ROM exercises to all extremities to maintain joint ROM, prevent atrophy, and strengthen muscles Consult physical therapist or occupational therapist for aids to facilitate ADLs and safe ambulation Teach techniques to assist with mobility by instructing patient to step over imaginary line and rock from side to side to initiate leg movements; these techniques help deal with "freezing" (akinesia) while walking
Potential for Aspiration Into Airway, related to disease process	Ensure that, when eating, the patient sits at 90-degree angle with head up and chin slightly tucked, avoiding extending the head Provide soft-solid and thick-liquid diet because these consistencies are swallowed more easily Consult a speech therapist and a dietitian because they can provide specific plans to improve swallowing Encourage patient to take small bites Avoid use of straws

Patient Teaching

Education for the patient with Parkinson's disease should include the importance of taking medications on the prescribed time schedule. Stress the need for good skin care and keeping active so that the patient remains as mobile as possible. Demonstrate proper ambulation and positioning to the patient and to the family if they will be taking care of the patient. Teach proper feeding techniques to reduce the risk of aspiration (see the Patient Problems box).

Prognosis

There is no cure for Parkinson's disease. Parkinson's disease is a chronic degenerative disorder with no acute exacerbations. If the patient takes medication as prescribed, signs and symptoms can be controlled for a long period. The care of the patient with Parkinson's disease may eventually fall to family members and caregivers. The amount of care needed often increases as the disease progresses.

ALZHEIMER'S DISEASE

Etiology and Pathophysiology

AD is a chronic, progressive, degenerative disorder that affects the cells of the brain and causes impaired intellectual functioning. It is a common cause of dementia in the older person and affects men and women in equal numbers. Approximately 5.2 million Americans suffer from AD. It is estimated that 5 million of them are over age 65 years. Alzheimer's may strike people in their 40s and 50s. The cause is unknown, although research has shown a genetic link.

Changes in the brain of patients with AD include plaques in the cortex, neurofibrillary tangles (a tangled mass of nonfunctioning neurons), loss of connections between cells, and cell death (Fig. 54.14). This neuronal damage occurs primarily in the cerebral cortex and causes a decrease in brain size. These changes were first discovered in 1907 by the German neurologist Alois Alzheimer.

Studies have shown that individuals who engage in activities that require information processing (e.g., reading, learning a new language, doing crossword puzzles) have a lower risk of developing AD. Regular physical activity, leisure activities, and educational achievements throughout the lifespan may decrease AD risk (National Institute on Aging, 2017). Antioxidant-containing foods such citrus fruits, dark green vegetables, tomatoes, brown rice, and foods high in beta-carotene (sweet potatoes and carrots) are considered to lower the risk of the development of Alzheimer's disease.

Clinical Manifestations

Traditionally the progression of AD is divided into four stages. Some experts have developed increasingly advanced methods of staging patients with AD into more complex stages numbering up to 7. In this resource, four stages of the condition are highlighted. In the early stage a person with Alzheimer's has relatively mild memory lapses and may have difficulty using the correct word. The attention span is decreased, and there may be disinterest in surroundings. Depression may occur at this time. In the second stage the person has more obvious memory lapses, especially with short-term memory, and usually is disoriented to time. Loss of personal belongings is common, as is confabulating (making up stories) to explain the loss of memory. Patients may lose their ability to recognize familiar faces, places, and objects and may get lost in a familiar environment. Loss of impulse control is common. Behavioral manifestations of AD (e.g., agitation, repetitiveness, wandering, resisting care) result from changes in the brain. A specific type of agitation is termed *sundowning,* in which the patient becomes more confused and agitated in the late afternoon or evening.

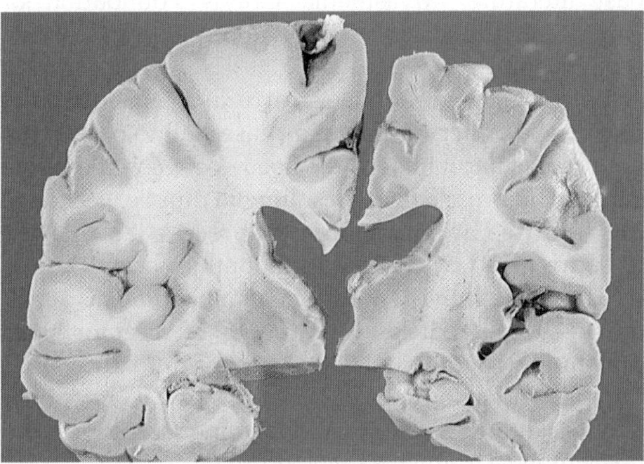

Fig. 54.14 Effects of Alzheimer's disease on the brain. Note the normal brain on the left versus the Alzheimer's brain on the right. (From Lewis SL, Dirksen SR, Heitkemper MM, et al: *Medical-surgical nursing: Assessment and management of clinical problems,* ed 8, St. Louis, 2011, Mosby.)

The AD patient's behavior is neither intentional nor subject to self-control. Some patients develop psychotic manifestations (i.e., delusions, illusions, hallucinations). By the time a person reaches the third stage, he or she has total disorientation to person, place, and time. Motor problems such as **apraxia** (an inability to carry out learned sequential movements on command, perform purposeful acts, or use objects properly), *visual agnosia* (inability to recognize objects by sight), and *dysgraphia* (difficulty communicating via writing) interfere with the ability to carry out daily functions. Wandering is common. In the terminal stage, severe mental and physical deterioration is present. Total incontinence is common.

These stages may have some variations. All people with AD experience a steady deterioration in their physical and mental status, usually lasting 5 to 20 years until death occurs (Box 54.2).

Assessment

Memory loss is the first symptom usually noticed in AD, combined with the inability to carry out normal activities. Other evidence may be agitation or restlessness. It is

Box 54.2 Ten Early Warning Signs of Alzheimer's Disease

1. Memory loss that disrupts daily life
2. Challenges in planning or solving problems
3. Difficulty completing familiar tasks at home, at work, or at leisure
4. Confusion with time or place
5. Trouble understanding visual images and spatial relationships
6. New problems with words in speaking or writing
7. Misplacing things and losing the ability to retrace steps
8. Decreased or poor judgment
9. Withdrawal from work or social activities
10. Changes in mood and personality

important to rule out other conditions such as pernicious anemia, drug reactions, depression, or hormonal imbalances.

Diagnostic Tests

The diagnosis of AD is primarily one of exclusion. AD has no specific diagnostic test. A CT scan, EEG, MRI, and PET may be used to rule out other pathologic conditions. A family history of AD is significant. At times the diagnosis can be confirmed only at the time of autopsy.

Medical Management

The care of the patient with AD can be frustrating for the caregiver and the health care provider because the treatment options are so limited. Often medications make the condition worse. Lorazepam (Ativan) or haloperidol in small doses may be necessary to lessen agitation and unpredictable behavior. Treatment of depression in patients with AD may improve cognitive ability. Depression is treated most often with selective serotonin reuptake inhibitors such as fluoxetine, sertraline (Zoloft), fluvoxamine (Luvox), and citalopram (Celexa). Trazodone, an antidepressant, may help with problems related to sleep but also may cause hypotension. Donepezil (Aricept), rivastigmine (Exelon), and galantamine (Razadyne) may have short-term benefit for mild cognitive impairment. Memantine (Namenda) is the first drug approved for the treatment of moderate to severe AD. Memantine does not prevent or slow neurodegeneration, but it was found in clinical studies to slow symptom progression. Many clinical drug trials are trying to find drugs that manage the signs and symptoms of AD while limiting the rate of disease progression.

Nursing Interventions and Patient Teaching

Nursing interventions are directed toward maintaining adequate nutrition. This can be a challenge because often the patient will not sit still long enough to eat. Providing finger foods and letting the patient eat while walking may help. Frequent feedings with high nutritive value are important. Encourage fluids of at least 2000 mL/day (Nursing Care Plan 54.1).

Safety demands a special mention. Because of memory problems, patients with AD often do dangerous things, such as walking outside while undressed, turning on stoves, wandering away, and setting fires. Measures that the family can take include removing burner controls from the stove at night, double-locking all doors and windows, and keeping the person under constant supervision. Disruptive behavior—including aggressive, agitated behavior—may occur. One frustrating part of the disease is that many patients sleep for only short periods and are awake most of the night.

Most of the time, education is directed at the family, because by the time the condition is diagnosed there is usually serious mental impairment. Help the family set a realistic schedule that also allows them time for rest and relaxation. The family may need to consider placing the patient in a long-term care facility. Put the family in touch with the local support group for AD.

Prognosis

Currently no effective treatment is available to stop the progression of AD, which occurs at a variable rate. The course of the disease can span 5 to 20 years. More than 56% of families report that the disease places a great strain on the family finances. The economic cost of AD in the United States is on average $61,522 annually. Although portions of this cost are absorbed by insurance coverage, large costs are borne by the family (National Institute on Aging, 2015). Ultimately, most patients die from complications such as pneumonia, malnutrition, and dehydration. Special Alzheimer's units and family and nursing approaches may help the patient stay as productive and safe as possible. The burden on the individual, the family, caregivers, and society as a whole is staggering. Support groups for caregivers and family members have been formed throughout the United States to provide an atmosphere of understanding and to give current information about the disease and related topics such as safety and legal, ethical, and financial issues. Nurses often receive personal and professional satisfaction in participating in such support groups.

MYASTHENIA GRAVIS

Etiology and Pathophysiology

MG is an autoimmune disease of the neuromuscular junction, characterized by the fluctuating weakness of certain skeletal muscle groups. MG is an unpredictable neuromuscular disease with lower motoneuron characteristics. MG can occur at any age but most commonly occurs between the ages of 10 and 65 years. Historically, the peak age of onset has been ages 20 to 30, but as the population has begun to age the age of onset is now after age 50. Newer studies have highlighted men being affected more than women, which is a change from past literature (Myasthenia Gravis Foundation of America, 2015). The incidence is about 14 to 20 in every 100,000 population.

With MG, no observable structural change occurs in the muscle or nerve. Nerve impulses fail to pass at the neuromuscular junction (the space between the nerve ending and muscle fiber), resulting in muscle weakness. MG is caused by an autoimmune process. It is thought to be triggered by antibodies that attack acetylcholine receptor sites at the neuromuscular junction. This attack damages and reduces the number of receptor sites, preventing conduction along the normal pathway at normal conduction speeds. Patients with MG have only about one-third as many acetylcholine receptors at the neuromuscular junction as is normal.

About 25% of patients with MG have been found to have a thymoma (a tumor of the thymus), and almost 80% have changes in the cellular structure of the thymus gland.

 Nursing Care Plan 54.1 **The Patient With Alzheimer's Disease**

Ms. A. is a 65-year-old who has been a seamstress. She has a history of progressive memory loss, paranoia, disorientation, and agitation. She was diagnosed as having Alzheimer's disease 2 years ago. Her family kept her at home until 6 months ago, when she was admitted to a long-term care institution. The nursing history indicates that she is incontinent of urine about 50% of the time and expresses a great deal of anxiety, especially around new situations or people. She cries frequently and at times attempts to hit the staff.

PATIENT PROBLEM

Anxiousness, related to cognitive impairments

Patient Goals and Expected Outcomes	Nursing Interventions	Evaluation
Patient will demonstrate decreased anxiety as evidenced by decreased outbursts of agitation or crying, the ability to sleep through most of the night, and cooperation with care	Continue to assess presence of anxiety. Comfort patient when she is crying. Provide simple explanation for all procedures. Use calm, undemanding, unhurried approach. Keep nursing interventions consistent and simple. Assist patient in doing relaxation techniques. Maintain consistency of caregiver when able. Minimize patient's choices in care. Encourage patient to exercise. Offer snack at bedtime.	Patient sleeps 5–6 h per night. Patient remains calm with care. Patient experiences decreased episodes of crying or striking out at others.

PATIENT PROBLEM

Functional Inability to Control Urination, related to condition and cognitive impairment

Patient Goals and Expected Outcomes	Nursing Interventions	Evaluation
Patient will be continent Patient will be free of urinary tract infection	Take patient to bathroom on regular schedule. Encourage adequate fluid intake (at least 2000 mL/day). Determine patient's preference for fluid. Place sign on door indicating "Toilet" or "Bathroom," or with a picture. If patient has urgency, ensure closeness to bathroom. Simplify closures on clothing. Avoid fluids just before bed. Use disposable protective perineal garments (Attends) only as needed.	Patient is free of episodes of incontinence. Patient is free of infection. Patient will void when taken to the bathroom.

CRITICAL THINKING QUESTIONS

1. Ms. A. continually wanders about the long-term care facility. She is unable to sit at the table for an entire meal. She has lost approximately 20 lb in the past 3 months. What are some helpful measures to improve her nutritional status?
2. What are some helpful interventions to help Ms. A. obtain a better sleep pattern?
3. Ms. A. has difficulty in maintaining good personal hygiene. What are some methods for assisting Ms. A. in maintaining personal hygiene?

Clinical Manifestations

MG occurs in ocular and generalized terms. In ocular MG the signs and symptoms include ptosis (eyelid drooping) and diplopia (double vision). In about 15% of cases, MG remains confined to the eye muscles. The generalized variety may vary in presentation, from mild to severe signs and symptoms. The patient may complain initially of ptosis and diplopia. Skeletal weakness involving the muscles of the extremities, the neck, the shoulders, the hands, and the diaphragm; dysarthria; and dysphagia may follow. The vocal cords can become weak, and the voice can sound nasal. As the disease progresses, it affects the trunk and lower limbs, leading to difficulty with walking, sustained sitting, and raising the arms over the head. Usually the distal muscles (those of the lower arms, hands, lower legs, and feet) are not as affected as the proximal muscles (those closer to the center of the body). Muscle weakness may become so severe that the person cannot breathe without mechanical ventilation. Bowel and bladder sphincter weakness occurs with severe loss of muscle control. Exacerbations of the disease may be initiated by upper respiratory tract infections, emotional tension, and menstruation.

Assessment

Subjective data include the patient's understanding of the disease, complaints of weakness or double vision, difficulty chewing or swallowing, and any bowel or bladder incontinence.

Objective data include any documented muscle weakness on neurologic testing. Nasal-sounding speech may be noted; the voice often fades after a long conversation and breath sounds diminish. Note ptosis of the eyelids and weight loss if there are swallowing problems.

Diagnostic Tests

Because of the slow, insidious onset and occurrence of symptoms with stress, MG sometimes is misdiagnosed as hysteria or neurosis. The diagnosis of MG can be made on the basis of history and physical examination. The simplest diagnostic test for MG is to have the patient look upward for 2 to 3 minutes. If the problem is MG, the eyelids will droop so that the person barely can keep the eyes open. The diagnosis can be made partly on the basis of EMG. The IV anticholinesterase test is a reliable diagnostic test. Edrophonium, a short-acting cholinesterase inhibitor, which decreases the amount of cholinesterase at the neuromuscular junction while making acetylcholine available to muscles, is administered intravenously. The patient response is evaluated carefully. Shortly after the administration of IV edrophonium, muscle function improves dramatically in patients who have the illness. Another diagnostic test is serum testing for antibodies to acetylcholine receptors. Acetylcholine receptor antibodies are present in 80% to 90% of patients with generalized myasthenia, and therefore their presence can be used to diagnose the disease.

Medical Management

Medical management includes the use of anticholinesterase drugs such as neostigmine and pyridostigmine (Mestinon). These medications promote nerve impulse transmission and effectively alleviate symptoms. Usually the patient is taught how to adjust the dosage depending on symptoms. Corticosteroids may be used as an adjunct therapy. Immunosuppressive medications, including azathioprine (Imuran), cyclosporine (Sandimmune), and cyclophosphamide, are used because of MG's immune component. Many classes of drugs are contraindicated or must be used with caution in patients with MG; these include anesthetics, antidysrhythmics, antibiotics, quinine, antipsychotics, barbiturates, sedatives, hypnotics, opioids, tranquilizers, and thyroid preparations (Ahmed and Simmons, 2009).

Plasmapheresis separates plasma from blood with a machine called a cell separator, which can be connected to the patient by means of a vascular cannula. This process removes the antibodies produced by the autoimmune response. Plasmapheresis can yield short-term improvement in symptoms and is indicated for patients in crisis or in preparation for surgery, when corticosteroids must be avoided.

Thymectomy is indicated for almost all patients with a thymoma. For some patients without thymoma, thymectomy may result in improvement in symptoms. Excision of the thymus reduces symptoms of MG in many patients. A thymectomy is a complex surgery, and patients with MG are at high risk for complications from anesthesia.

Another treatment option is the administration of IV immune globulin to reduce the production of acetylcholine antibodies. IV immune globulin is used for a severe relapse of MG.

During exacerbations of the disease, and when the respiratory status is compromised, the patient may require intubation and mechanical ventilation. A tracheostomy may be necessary.

Nursing Interventions and Patient Teaching

Respiratory problems typically occur in patients with MG. Upper respiratory tract infections occur because the patient may not have the energy to cough effectively, and pneumonia or airway obstruction may develop. Aspiration often occurs. During acute episodes of the disease, the patient may require hospitalization. Serial determination of vital capacity, minute volumes, and tidal volumes is done to assess the need for respiratory assistance. The patient also may be taught airway-protective techniques during swallowing (e.g., chin tuck, double swallow). Suctioning is done as needed, and if swallowing becomes impaired, a feeding tube may be necessary.

Patient Teaching

Myasthenia Gravis

- Teach the importance of taking medication at the time prescribed and taking it early enough before eating or engaging in activities to obtain maximum relief.
- Explain how to adjust the medication dose to maintain muscle strength.
- Caution about medications to avoid.
- Teach the importance of seeking medical attention at the first sign of an upper respiratory tract infection.
- Explain the importance of eating only when sitting up, to prevent aspiration.
- Caution the patient to avoid crowds in flu and cold season.
- Explain how to adjust to daily activities to allow for leisure activities and rest periods.
- Explain planning to use minimal energy in activities that are essential so that energy may be conserved for activities that the patient enjoys.
- Advise patient to wear a medical-alert bracelet that identifies the patient as having myasthenia gravis.

People with MG may have to change daily patterns of activity. Help the patient and the family plan so that minimal energy is used in activities that are essential to remaining relatively self-sufficient, with energy left for leisure activities. Physical therapy such as ROM exercises may be beneficial for maintaining muscle function.

The patient with MG is usually able to adjust the medication depending on the symptoms. Also, the patient can have much control over preventing respiratory complications. Therefore teaching is important and should include those topics listed in the Patient Teaching box.

Prognosis

MG is a chronic disease. The course is variable with periods of exacerbation and remission. Some cases are mild, but others are severe, with death resulting from respiratory failure. Patients with a thymoma may experience improvement after a thymectomy.

AMYOTROPHIC LATERAL SCLEROSIS

Loss of upper and lower motoneurons is the major pathologic change in ALS, a rare, progressive neurologic disease that usually leads to death in 2 to 6 years. This disease became known as Lou Gehrig's disease when the famous baseball player was stricken with it in 1939. The onset is between 40 and 70 years of age, and two times as many men as women are affected.

For unknown reasons, motoneurons in the brainstem and spinal cord gradually degenerate in ALS. The dead motoneuron cannot produce or transport vital signals to muscle. Consequently, electrical and chemical messages originating in the brain do not reach the muscles to activate them.

The primary symptoms are weakness of the upper extremities (the hands are often affected first), dysarthria, and dysphagia. However, weakness may begin in the legs. Muscle wasting and fasciculations (muscle twitching) result from the denervation of the muscles and lack of stimulation and use. Death usually results from respiratory tract infection secondary to compromised respiratory function.

Unfortunately there is no cure for ALS. A drug called riluzole (Rilutek) slows the progression of ALS. The drug helps protect motoneurons damaged by the disease and can add 3 months or more to a patient's life.

This illness is devastating because the patient remains cognitively intact while wasting away. The challenge of nursing interventions is to guide the patient in the use of moderate-intensity, endurance-type exercises for the trunk and limbs, because this may help reduce ALS spasticity (Mayo Clinic, 2017). Support the patient's cognitive and emotional functions by facilitating communication, providing diversional activities such as reading and human companionship, and helping the patient and the family with advanced care planning and anticipatory grieving related to loss of motor function and ultimate death. Respiratory failure is the greatest cause of death for the patient with ALS. About 30% of patients with ALS live up to 5 years after diagnosis, and 10% to 20% survive for more than 10 years (National Institutes of Health, 2015).

HUNTINGTON'S DISEASE

Huntington's disease is a genetically transmitted autosomal dominant disorder that affects men and women of all races. The offspring of a person with this disease have a 50% risk of inheriting it. The diagnosis often occurs after the affected individual has children. The onset of Huntington's disease is usually between 30 and 50 years of age. In the United States, approximately 25,000 people have Huntington's disease and another 150,000 have a 50/50 chance of developing it.

Diagnosis is based on family history, clinical symptoms, and the detection of the characteristic deoxyribonucleic acid (DNA) pattern from blood samples. People who are asymptomatic but who have a positive family history of Huntington's disease face the dilemma of whether to get tested. If the test is positive, the person will develop Huntington's disease, but at what age and to what extent cannot be determined.

Like Parkinson's disease, the pathology of Huntington's disease involves the basal ganglia and the extrapyramidal motor system. Huntington's disease involves an overactivity of the dopamine pathway. The net effect is an excess of dopamine, which leads to symptoms that are the opposite of those of parkinsonism. The clinical manifestations are characterized by abnormal and excessive involuntary movements (chorea). These are writhing, twisting movements of the face, limbs, and body. The movements get worse as the disease progresses. Facial movements involving speech, chewing, and swallowing are affected and may cause aspiration and malnutrition. The gait deteriorates, and ambulation eventually becomes impossible. Perhaps the most devastating deterioration is in mental functions, which include intellectual decline, emotional lability, and psychotic behavior. Because there is no cure, therapeutic management is palliative. Antipsychotic (e.g., haloperidol), antidepressant (fluoxetine, sertraline), and antichorea (clonazepam [Klonopin]) medications are prescribed and have some effect. However, they do not alter the course of the disease.

The goal of nursing management is to provide the most comfortable environment possible for the patient and the family by maintaining physical safety, treating the physical symptoms, and providing emotional and psychological support. Because of the choreic movements, caloric requirements are as high as 4000 to 5000 calories/day to maintain body weight. As the disease progresses, meeting caloric needs becomes a greater challenge when the patient has difficulty swallowing and holding the head still. Depression and mental deterioration also can compromise nutritional intake. Genetic counseling is important. DNA testing can be done on fetal cells obtained by amniocentesis or chorionic biopsy. Genetic testing can determine whether a person is a carrier. No test is available to predict when symptoms will develop.

This disease presents a great challenge to health care professionals. There is a large risk for depression and suicide in patients diagnosed with Huntington's disease. Death usually occurs 10 to 20 years after the onset of symptoms.

STROKE

Etiology and Pathophysiology

Stroke (cerebrovascular accident) is an abnormal condition of the blood vessels of the brain, characterized by hemorrhage into the brain or the formation of an embolus or thrombus that occludes an artery, resulting in ischemia of the brain tissue normally perfused by the damaged vessels. The term *brain attack* is used increasingly to describe stroke. This term communicates the urgency of recognizing the clinical manifestations of a stroke and treating it as a medical emergency, just as one would with a heart attack.

Prompt medical attention at the first sign of symptoms is needed to reduce disability and death. Stroke is the most common disease of the nervous system. It is estimated that 795,000 people in the United States suffer a stroke annually. It is ranked as the fourth leading cause of death in the United States, with about 140,000 deaths per year (Centers for Disease Control and Prevention [CDC], 2016a). Strokes affect people in all age groups, but most are between 75 and 85 years of age. Strokes leave many people with serious, long-term disability. Of those who survive, 50% to 70% are functionally independent, and 15% to 30% live with permanent disability. Common long-term disabilities include hemiparesis (weakness on one side of the body), inability to walk, complete or partial dependence in ADLs, aphasia, and depression (see the Cultural Considerations box).

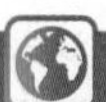

Cultural Considerations

Stroke

A high mortality rate from strokes exists among African Americans, possibly as a result of the high frequency of hypertension, obesity, and diabetes mellitus in this group. Thrombotic strokes are twice as common among African Americans as among whites. Hemorrhagic strokes are three times more common among African Americans than among whites. Hispanics, Native Americans, and Asian Americans have a higher stroke incidence than do whites (CDC, 2016a).

Strokes are classified as ischemic or hemorrhagic, based on the underlying pathophysiologic findings. Ischemic strokes are thrombotic and embolic. These account for 85% of strokes. The remaining 15% are hemorrhagic strokes, which result from bleeding into the brain tissue itself (Fig. 54.15). Many underlying factors also contribute: atherosclerosis, atrial fibrillation, heart disease, hypertension, kidney disease, peripheral vascular disease, and diabetes mellitus. Other risk factors include family history of stroke, obesity, high serum cholesterol, cigarette smoking, stress, cocaine use, and a sedentary lifestyle. Newer low-dose oral contraceptives have lower risks for stroke than early forms of birth control pills, except in those individuals who are hypersensitive and smoke. Hypertension is the single most important modifiable risk factor. Stroke risk can be reduced by up to 42% with appropriate treatment of hypertension. Atrial fibrillation is responsible for about 15% to 20% of all strokes. The risk for stroke in people with diabetes mellitus is four to five times higher than in the general population. Carotid artery stenosis, also called carotid artery disease, is defined as the narrowing of the carotid arteries that supply blood to the brain, usually from plaque buildup (atherosclerosis) in the inner lining of the artery. It is responsible for 80% of the 500,000 TIAs that affect patients annually. Recent studies have reviewed the risk for stroke in women taking hormone replacement therapies. Although the studies indicate that there may be a slight increase in risk, low-dose estrogen therapy in women without significant risk factors is considered safe (Medline Plus, 2016).

Clinical Manifestations

A stroke can affect many body functions, including motor activity, elimination, intellectual function, spatial perception, personality, affect, sensation, and communication.

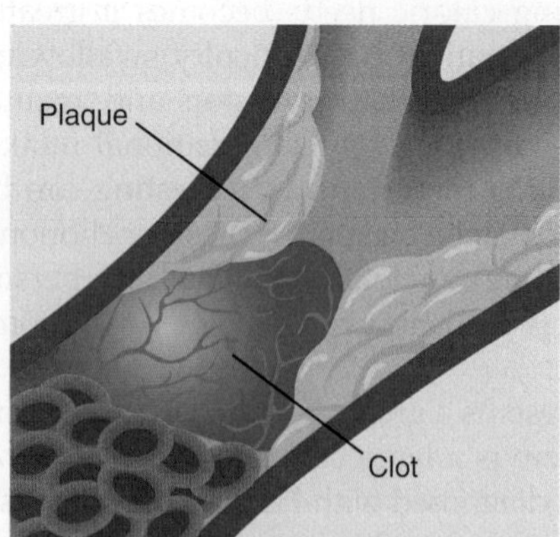

A **Thrombotic stroke.** Cerebral thrombosis is a narrowing of the artery by fatty deposits called *plaque.* Plaque can cause a clot to form, which blocks the passage of blood through the artery.

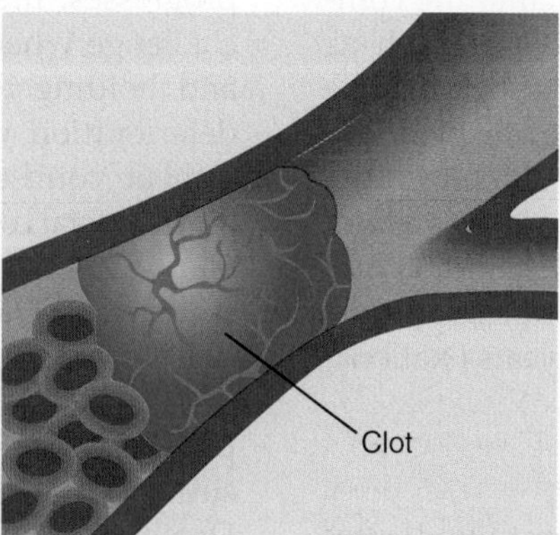

B **Embolic stroke.** An embolus is a blood clot or other debris circulating in the blood. When it reaches an artery in the brain that is too narrow to pass through, it lodges there and blocks the flow of blood.

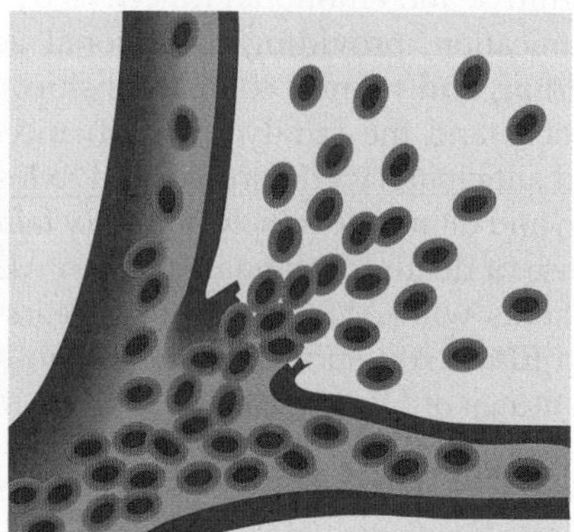

C **Hemorrhagic stroke.** A burst blood vessel may allow blood to seep into and damage brain tissues until clotting shuts off the leak.

Fig. 54.15 Three types of stroke. (From Lewis SL, Bucher, L, Heitkemper MM, et al: *Medical-surgical nursing: Assessment and management of clinical problems,* ed 10, St. Louis, 2017, Elsevier.)

The functions affected are related directly to the artery involved and the area of brain it supplies. Permanent damage can result from a stroke because of anoxia of the brain. The vessel most commonly affected is the middle cerebral artery. The patient may be unconscious and may experience seizures as a result of generalized ischemia and the brain's response to abrupt hypoxia.

Ischemic stroke. Deficient blood flow to the brain from a partial or complete occlusion of an artery results in an ischemic stroke. Ischemic strokes are either *thrombotic* or *embolic* and account for nearly 90% of all strokes (AHA/ASA, 2018).

Thrombotic stroke. Thrombosis is the most common cause of stroke, and the most common cause of cerebral thrombosis is atherosclerosis. Additional disease processes that cause thrombosis are hypertension or diabetes mellitus, both of which accelerate the arteriosclerotic process. Additional risk factors associated with thrombotic strokes include coagulation disorders, polycythemia vera, arteritis, chronic hypoxia, and dehydration. In 30% to 50% of individuals, thrombotic strokes have been preceded by a TIA. Stroke resulting from thrombosis is seen most often in the 60- to 90-year-old age group. Thrombosis occurs in relation to injury of a blood vessel wall and formation of a blood clot. The lumen of the blood vessel becomes narrowed, and if it becomes occluded, infarction occurs. Thrombosis develops readily where atherosclerotic plaques already have narrowed blood vessels. Thrombi usually occur in larger vessels, especially the internal carotid arteries.

Symptoms of this type of stroke tend to occur during sleep or soon after arising. This is thought to result partly because recumbency lowers blood pressure, which can lead to brain ischemia. Postural hypotension also may be a factor. Neurologic signs and symptoms frequently worsen for the first few hours after a stroke and peak in severity within 72 hours as edema increases in the infarcted areas of the brain.

Embolic stroke. Embolism is the second most common cause of stroke. People who have a stroke resulting from embolism are usually younger. The emboli most commonly originate from a thrombus in the endocardial (inside) layer of the heart, often caused by rheumatic heart disease, mitral stenosis and atrial fibrillation, myocardial infarction, infective endocarditis, valvular prostheses, and atrial septal defects. Less common causes of emboli include air, fat from long bone (femur) fractures, amniotic fluid after childbirth, and tumors. The embolus travels upward to the cerebral circulation and lodges where a vessel narrows or bifurcates. They most frequently occur in the midcerebral artery.

Hemorrhagic stroke. Hemorrhagic stroke accounts for approximately 15% of all strokes and results from bleeding into the brain tissue or subarachnoid space. The bleed causes damage by destroying and replacing brain tissue. The peak incidence of aneurysms occurs in people who are 35 to 60 years of age. Women are affected more frequently than men.

An aneurysm is often the cause of hemorrhage. An **aneurysm** is a localized dilation of the wall of a blood vessel usually caused by atherosclerosis and hypertension or, less frequently, by trauma, infection, or a congenital weakness in the vessel wall. It ruptures as a result of a small hole that occurs in a part of the aneurysm. The hemorrhage spreads rapidly, producing localized damage and irritation to the cerebral vessels. The bleeding usually stops when a plug of fibrin platelets is formed. The hemorrhage begins to absorb within 3 weeks. Recurrent rupture is a risk 7 to 10 days after the initial hemorrhage. The patient with intracerebral hemorrhage has no forewarning; has rapid, severe symptoms; and has a poor prognosis for recovery. Fifty percent of patients die soon after the aneurysm. Only about 20% are functionally independent after 6 months.

Transient ischemic attack. *TIA* refers to an episode of cerebrovascular insufficiency with temporary episodes of neurologic dysfunction lasting less than 24 hours and often less than 15 minutes. Most TIAs resolve within 3 hours. TIAs may be caused by microemboli that temporarily occlude the blood flow or by the narrowing of small vessels in the brain. TIAs also often occur in patients with carotid artery stenosis, which causes decreased blood flow to the brain. The most common deficits are contralateral weakness of the lower face, hands, arms, and legs; transient dysphasia; numbness or loss of sensation; temporary loss of vision of one eye; or a sudden inability to speak. Other symptoms may include tinnitus, vertigo, blurred vision, diplopia, eyelid ptosis, and ataxia. Between attacks the neurologic status is normal.

A TIA should be considered a forerunner of a stroke. Testing after a TIA includes a complete laboratory workup, x-rays, ultrasound of the carotid arteries and heart, MRI, CT, and thorough cardiac testing to determine the cause of the TIA. Evaluation must be done to confirm that the signs and symptoms of a TIA are not related to other brain lesions, such as a developing subdural hematoma or an increasing tumor mass. CT of the brain without contrast media is the most important initial diagnostic study.

The major importance of TIAs is that they warn the patient of an underlying pathologic condition. Approximately 40% of patients who experience TIAs will have a stroke in 2 to 5 years. The patient is given medications that prevent platelet aggregation, such as aspirin, ticlopidine, dipyridamole (Persantine), and clopidogrel (Plavix). Aspirin is the most frequently used antiplatelet agent, commonly at a dose of 81 to 325 mg/day. An anticoagulant medication (e.g., oral warfarin [Coumadin]) is the treatment of choice for individuals with atrial fibrillation who have had a TIA.

Surgical interventions for the patient with TIAs from carotid artery disease include carotid endarterectomy (CEA) or percutaneous transluminal angioplasty and stenting.

- *Carotid endarterectomy:* In CEA the atheromatous lesion is removed from the carotid artery to improve blood flow. CEA surgery causes a reduction in stroke and vascular death. This surgery is reserved for patients with occlusions of 70% to 99% of blood flow. The long-term benefit of carotid endarterectomy is based on the severity of the preoperative stenosis. In patients with stenosis of 30% or less, surgery actually increases the risk for an ipsilateral stroke in the first 5 years postoperatively. There has been no proven effect within 5 years when the stenosis is 31% to 40% and only a marginal improvement in patients with 50% to 69% stenosis. However, the greatest benefit occurs when the stenosis is 70% or more (National Institute of Neurological Disorders and Stroke, 2016).
- *Percutaneous transluminal angioplasty:* In percutaneous transluminal angioplasty a balloon is inserted to open a stenosed artery to permit increased blood flow. This procedure is used to treat patients with clinical manifestations related to stenosis in the vertebrobasilar or carotid arteries and their branches. The risk of the angioplasty procedure is the possibility of dislodging emboli, which can travel to the brain or retina.

Assessment

Subjective data include the description of the onset of symptoms; the presence of headache; any sensory deficit, such as numbness or tingling; the inability to think clearly; and visual problems. In the case of a hemorrhage, the headache may be described as sudden and explosive. Assess the patient's ability to understand the condition.

Objective data include hemiparesis or hemiplegia, any change in the LOC, signs of increased ICP, respiratory status, and aphasia. The exact clinical picture varies, depending on the area of the brain affected (Fig. 54.16). A lesion on one side of the brain affects motor function on the opposite (contralateral) side of the body. When the middle cerebral artery is affected, as is most common, the signs and symptoms seen include contralateral paralysis or paresis, contralateral sensory loss, dysphasia or aphasia if the dominant hemisphere is involved, spatial-perceptual problems, changes in judgment and behavior if the nondominant hemisphere is involved, and *contralateral (homonymous) hemianopia* (Fig. 54.17).

In right-handed people and in most left-handed people, the left hemisphere is dominant for language skills. Language disorders affect expression and comprehension of written and spoken words. When a stroke damages the dominant hemisphere of the brain, the patient may experience *aphasia* (total loss of comprehension and use of language). A stroke affecting Broca's areas of the brain (located in the frontal lobe of the brain) results in the person having difficulty with the ability to articulate words *(expressive aphasia)*, but

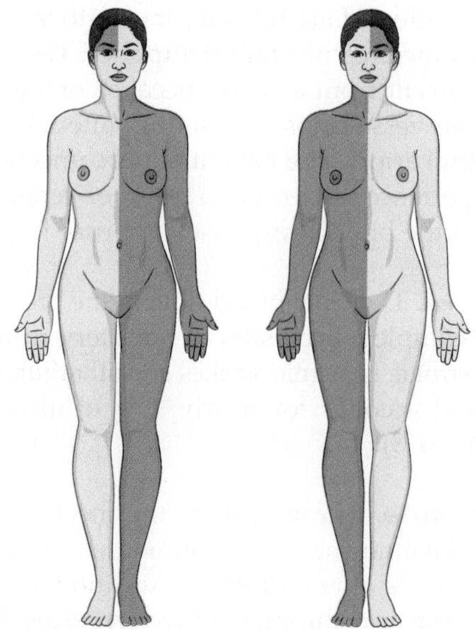

Right brain damage
(Stroke on right side of the brain)
- Paralyzed left side: hemiplegia
- Left-sided neglect
- Spatial-perceptual deficits
- Tends to deny or minimize problems
- Rapid performance, short attention span
- Impulsive, safety problems
- Impaired judgment
- Impaired time concepts

Left brain damage
(Stroke on left side of the brain)
- Paralyzed right side: hemiplegia
- Impaired speech/language aphasias
- Impaired right/left discrimination
- Slow performance, cautious
- Aware of deficits: depression, anxiety
- Impaired comprehension related to language, math

Fig. 54.16 Manifestations of right-sided and left-sided stroke.

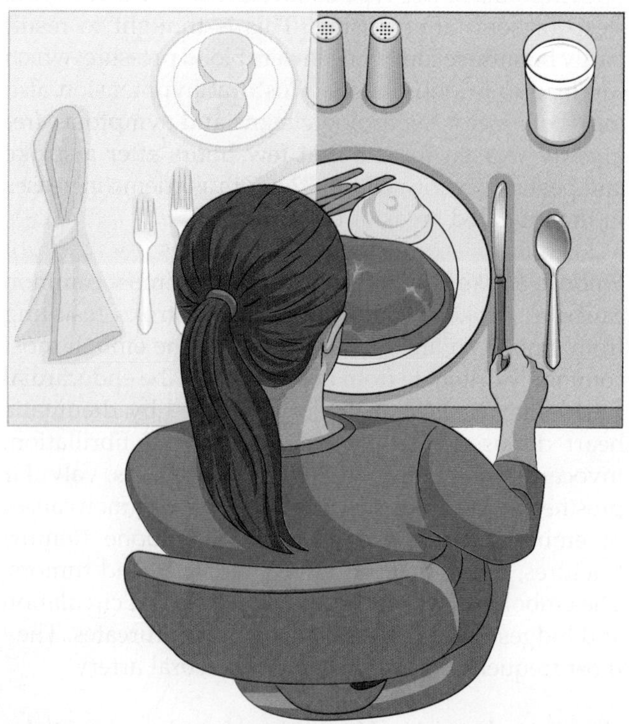

Fig. 54.17 Spatial and perceptual deficits in stroke. Perception of a patient with homonymous hemianopia shows that food on the left side is not seen and thus is ignored.

the ability to make vocal sounds and to understand written and spoken words remains intact (see Fig. 54.3 and Box 54.1). *Receptive aphasia* results when the stroke damages the area of the brain known as Wernicke's area (located in the temporal lobe). Patients with receptive aphasia have difficulty comprehending spoken and written communication.

A stroke patient may experience *dysarthria,* which is difficult or poorly articulated speech. Dysarthria is a result of deficits in the muscular control of speech related to damage that has occurred to the central or peripheral motor nerves (*Mosby's Dictionary of Medicine, Nursing & Health Professions*, 2017). Some stroke patients have a combination of aphasia and dysarthria.

Diagnostic Tests

CT and MRI are the tests most commonly used in the diagnosis of a stroke. The earlier the stroke is diagnosed, the better the chance for recovery from the potential effects. Cardiac testing as well as an EEG will likely be performed during the diagnostic stage. PET also may be useful in assessing the extent of tissue damage by showing the brain's metabolic activity. After TIAs, a cerebral angiogram may be done as well as a Doppler study of the carotid arteries. A cerebral angiogram also allows for a detailed evaluation of the vasculature of the brain.

Medical Management

If the patient has had a hemorrhagic stroke as a result of an aneurysm, surgery may be necessary to prevent a rebleed. The surgery consists of performing a craniotomy; tying off or clipping the aneurysm; and removing the clot to prevent rebleeding into the brain (Fig. 54.18). An aneurysm often causes vasospasm in the brain as blood in the subarachnoid space becomes an irritant. Vasospasm narrows blood vessels in the brain, decreasing perfusion to the areas they supply with blood. It can occur whether or not the patient has surgery. The amount of blood in the subarachnoid space can directly affect the degree of vasospasm. Less invasive than surgery is an endovascular procedure in which a catheter is introduced through a major artery (usually the femoral artery) and guided toward the aneurysm to treat the bleed and prevent the aneurysm from rupturing (AHA/ASA, n.d.).

Vasospasm typically occurs in 30% to 60% of cases between postoperative days 4 and 12. The mortality rate is as high as 50%. If it is not treated rapidly, it can cause cerebral ischemia or cerebral anoxia, leading to severe mental and physical deficits or death. Any patient with subarachnoid hemorrhage should be started on the calcium channel blocker nimodipine (Nimotop) within 96 hours of bleeding and receive it for 21 days to prevent vasospasm.

Research indicates that select patients with *acute ischemic stroke* can benefit from thrombolytics such as tissue plasminogen activator (tPA, alteplase [Activase]), which digests fibrin and fibrinogen and thus lyses the clot. Because tPA is clot specific in its activation of the fibrinolytic system, it is less likely to cause hemorrhage than streptokinase or urokinase. Patients who are treated within 3 hours of the onset of symptoms are at least 30% more likely than patients who do not receive timely treatment to recover with little or no disability after 3 months (AHA/ASA, n.d.). Some patients may be eligible for treatment for up to 4.5 hours depending on condition related factors. Although thrombolysis improves the chances of recovery by up to 30%, only 2% to 3% of ischemic stroke patients receive it because they do not seek treatment soon enough.

Endovascular embolectomy may be performed to remove blood clots inside the brain (and can be done up to 8 hours after acute stroke onset). Using a catheter inserted into the femoral artery physicians may maneuver a device into the brain to manage the clot. Using x-ray assistance the catheter reaches the clot and it is entrapped (Fig. 54.19). Next the balloon catheter is inflated to prevent forward flow temporarily while the blood clot is withdrawn. The clot is enclosed in the balloon catheter and removed from the body. The balloon is deflated and blood flow is restored to the brain. This is an intervention that may be successful for larger clots that are not as responsive to pharmacological attempts to completely dissolve them. This procedure may be used in conjunction with tPA (Mayo Clinic, 2018b).

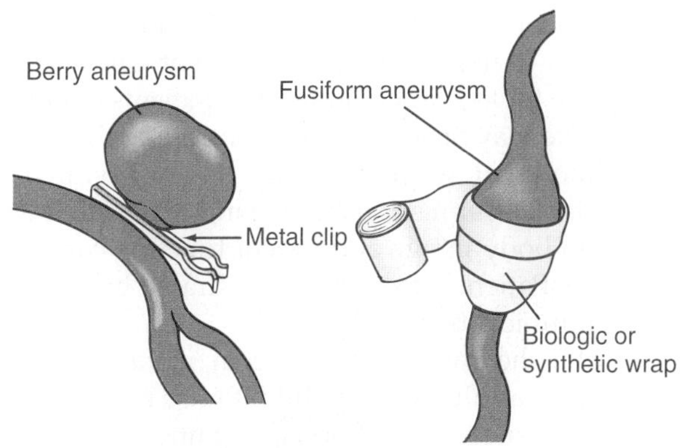

Fig. 54.18 Clipping and wrapping of aneurysms. (From Lewis SL, Heitkemper MM, Dirksen SR, et al: *Medical-surgical nursing: Assessment and management of clinical problems,* ed 9, St. Louis, 2014, Mosby.)

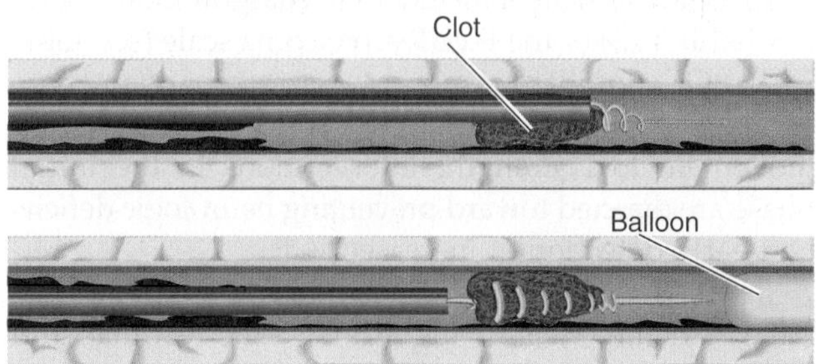

Fig. 54.19 The MERCI retriever is used to remove blood clots in patients who are experiencing ischemic stroke. (From Lewis SL, Heitkemper MM, Dirksen SR, et al: *Medical-surgical nursing: Assessment and management of clinical problems,* ed 9, St. Louis, 2014, Mosby.)

Patients with stroke symptoms need to be triaged, transported, and treated as rapidly as patients experiencing an acute myocardial infarction. In administration of thrombolytic drugs, the single most important factor is timing. Patients are screened carefully before treatment is initiated. This includes blood tests for coagulation disorders, recent history of gastrointestinal bleeding, and a CT or MRI scan to rule out hemorrhagic stroke. In patients with acute ischemic stroke, thrombolytic therapy increases short-term mortality, increases (but not by a statistically significant amount) symptomatic or fatal intracranial hemorrhage, decreases long-term death rate, and decreases dependence in terms of ADLs. The decision to use thrombolytic therapy should be based on a discussion of the risks and benefits with the patient and the family (Cruz-Flores, 2018). Some patients would accept a high risk of death from hemorrhage in an attempt to improve their chances of escaping permanent aphasia or dependency. Others prefer to avoid interventions that carry significant risk. Patients with stroke caused by thrombi and emboli (ischemic strokes) also may be treated with platelet inhibitors and anticoagulants (after the first 24 hours if treated with tPA) to prevent the formation of more clots. Common anticoagulants include heparin, enoxaparin (Lovenox), and warfarin. Platelet inhibitors include aspirin, ticlopidine, clopidogrel, and dipyridamole.

Drugs to reduce ICP, such as dexamethasone, may be given. Suppositories such as bisacodyl (Dulcolax) generally are prescribed to be given daily or every other day. However, some health care providers order stool softeners, laxatives, or enemas.

Fluids may be restricted for the first few days after a stroke in an effort to prevent edema of the brain. The patient is fed IV fluids, or a nasogastric or gastrostomy tube may be inserted and tube feedings begun.

The length of time the patient remains in bed depends on the type of stroke suffered, deficits noted, and the health care provider's judgment regarding early mobilization. Some health care providers prescribe fairly long periods of rest after strokes, whereas others believe in early mobilization—1 or 2 days after the accident occurred.

Nursing Interventions

Carefully monitor the patient's neurologic status. The neurologic assessment includes the Glasgow Coma Scale (see Table 54.3) or the FOUR score coma scale (see Table 54.4), LOC, pupillary responses, assessment of any type of aphasia or dysarthria, vital signs, and extremity movement and strength. Interventions in the initial phase are directed toward preventing neurologic deficits and early detection of increased ICP.

Because nutrition is a concern and the patient may have difficulty swallowing at first, tube feedings and IV fluids may be necessary. See the patient problem statements and accompanying interventions to assist in feeding the patient with dysphagia.

If the patient is responsive after the onset of the stroke, help the patient assume as much self-care as possible. This includes teaching the patient one-handed dressing techniques and one-handed feeding techniques if motor deficits have occurred. It is important to reinforce teaching by other members of the patient's health team.

The patient with a stroke may be incontinent at first. Remove the urinary catheter (if there is one) as soon as possible to prevent urinary tract infection and delayed bladder retraining. Because of the lower incidence of urinary tract infections, an intermittent catheterization program may be used for patients with urinary retention. Place the patient on a bladder training program to assist in regaining continence. This usually includes taking the patient to the bathroom every few hours and encouraging fluids (at least 2000 mL/day), with the majority given between 8 a.m. and 7 p.m. Assess the patient's normal bowel pattern before the stroke and include this in the nursing care plan if possible. If the patient has difficulty with communication, a picture of a bathroom or toilet can be useful.

Return of motor impulses and movement in involved extremities occurs in stages, lasting from hours to months. Recovery also may halt at a specific stage and progress no further. Return of function is significant for functional use of extremities but also increases the possibility of contractures. Appropriate nursing interventions to prevent contractures include passive exercise, active exercise, strength building of the unaffected side, and early ambulation to promote the return of muscle function.

Patients may experience a loss of proprioception with a stroke. Neurologic deficits of apraxia and agnosia (a total or partial loss of the ability to recognize familiar objects or people) also may occur. Assist the patient with activities by repeating directions and demonstrating care. If the patient has hemianopia, which is common, approach the patient from the nonparalyzed side for care. Teach the patient to scan past midline to the side with the deficit. These patients also may fail to recognize that they have a paralyzed side. This is called *unilateral neglect* (described in the section "Sensory and Perceptual Status"). Teach the patient to inspect this side of the body for injury and to protect it from harm. These patients often show poor judgment and may move impulsively or unsafely. Observe for this and take safety precautions if needed until the patient can learn to compensate for this lack of judgment. Patients who have had a stroke may have difficulty controlling their emotions. Emotional responses may be exaggerated or unpredictable. Depression and feelings associated with changes in body image and loss of function can make this worse. Patients also may be frustrated by mobility and communication problems.

To foster the patient's self-esteem, always treat the patient as an adult, not as a child. Praise and reinforce the patient's successful efforts and gains in self-care.

Communication problems. Many stroke patients have speech problems, including dysarthria and aphasia. A speech pathologist evaluates and treats the patient with language disorders. The patient may be frustrated and should be approached in an unhurried manner. Often the patient does much better with communication when not feeling pressured to speak. Giving the patient a communication board may be helpful. The use of computers to assist with communication also may be beneficial. Wait for the patient to communicate, rather than prompting or finishing the sentence before the patient has a chance to find the appropriate word. Inability to articulate does not mean that the patient has decreased cognitive abilities.

Patient problems and interventions for the patient who has had a stroke include but are not limited to the following:

Patient Problem	Nursing Interventions
Compromised verbal communication, related to ischemic injury	Speak slowly and distinctly Ask questions that can be answered by yes or no (or by signals) Try to anticipate patient needs Provide a call signal within reach of the unaffected hand Begin speech therapy as soon as possible Use a communication board when necessary
Insufficient Nutrition, related to impaired ability to swallow	Provide IV fluids and tube feedings as prescribed during the initial period Refer to speech therapist for assessment of swallowing problems Assess ability to swallow before initiating feedings Position patient with head elevated and turned to unaffected side during feedings Provide foods initially that are easier to swallow (soft foods, except for mashed potatoes) Thin liquids are often difficult to swallow and may promote coughing; thicken liquids with a commercially available thickening agent (e.g., Thick-It) Do not use milk products because they tend to increase the viscosity of mucus and increase salivation Use a training cup for fluids as necessary Do not use a straw Inspect mouth for food trapped in cheek pockets Be patient when feeding patient and provide directions for swallowing as needed. Ensure that meals are unrushed and nonstressful Encourage patient to feed self as soon as possible; provide self-help devices as necessary Provide scrupulous oral hygiene after meal because food may collect on the affected side of the mouth

Patient Teaching

Teaching for a patient with a stroke should include techniques to compensate for the deficits suffered as a result of the stroke. In this the nurse functions as part of the rehabilitation team. Begin rehabilitation at the time of admission to the acute care facility. The patient will probably attend occupational and physical therapy and perhaps speech therapy. Depending on the patient's status, the patient's rehabilitation potential, and available resources, the patient may be transferred to a rehabilitation facility or unit.

If the patient is receiving medications (e.g., for hypertension or anticoagulation), teach the patient and the family about side effects and the dosing schedule. Discuss plans for follow-up. Also teach the patient's family techniques to enhance safety and communication. If the patient has a problem with dysphagia, teach the family appropriate communication techniques. Because of the long-term nature of caring for the stroke patient, caregivers are at high risk for stress. Referral to an appropriate stroke support group is needed. Write instructions for the patient or the family to refer to after discharge. Most rehabilitation centers also include therapeutic leaves as a way to test the family's skills and knowledge. Each pass or leave has specific goals; obtain feedback from the family about additional teaching that may be needed. Also educate the family and the patient about perceptual problems associated with stroke and techniques to compensate for these deficits (e.g., writing down instructions for the patient who has trouble carrying out an activity alone).

Prognosis

The prognosis for patients with a stroke depends on the size of the lesion in the brain and the patient's premorbid status. More than 140,000 deaths occur in the United States each year as a result of strokes. Of those who survive, 50% to 70% are functionally independent; however, 15% to 30% have a permanent disability. The most frequent long-term disabilities include hemiparesis, inability to ambulate, aphasia, depression, and complete or partial dependence in ADLs. In the United States the annual cost of stroke was estimated to be more than $34 billion per year (CDC, 2016). With therapy, significant functional gains can be made, even when paralysis or weakness continues. Many patients are able to return home and remain independent after a stroke. With new medical treatment for selected patients, using tPA for thrombolysis or mechanical clot removal, the prognosis is greatly improved.

CRANIAL AND PERIPHERAL NERVE DISORDERS

TRIGEMINAL NEURALGIA

Etiology and Pathophysiology

Trigeminal neuralgia is one specific kind of peripheral nerve problem. It is caused by degeneration of or pressure on the trigeminal nerve (cranial nerve V), and its cause is unknown. It is also called *tic douloureux*. It

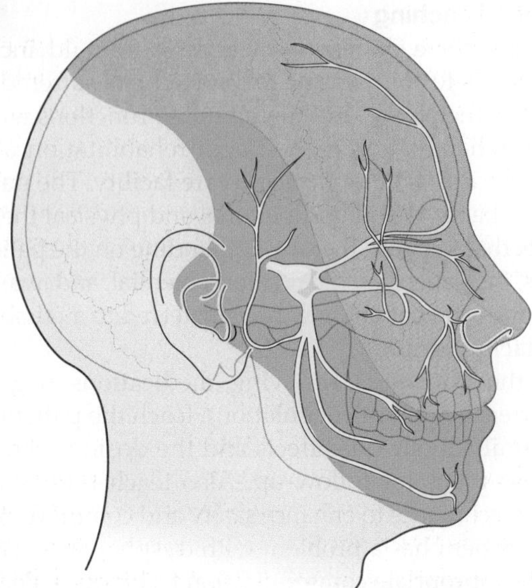

Fig. 54.20 Pathway of trigeminal nerve and facial areas innervated by each of the three main divisions of this nerve.

usually affects people in middle or late adulthood and is slightly more common in women. The pathophysiology is not fully understood.

Clinical Manifestations

Trigeminal neuralgia is characterized by excruciating, knifelike, or lightning-like shock in the lips, upper or lower gums, cheek, forehead, or side of the nose. The pain radiates along one or more of the three divisions of the fifth cranial nerve (Fig. 54.20). The fifth cranial nerve has motor and sensory branches. In trigeminal neuralgia the sensory (or afferent) branches, primarily the maxillary and mandibular branches, are involved. The pain typically extends only to the midline of the face and head because this is the extent of the tissue supplied by the offending nerve. The attacks are usually brief, lasting only seconds to 2 to 3 minutes, and are generally unilateral. Recurrences are unpredictable; they may occur several times a day or weeks or months apart. Areas along the course of the nerve are known as *trigger points,* and the slightest stimulation of these areas may initiate pain. People with trigeminal neuralgia try desperately to avoid triggering them. Precipitating stimuli include chewing, toothbrushing, a hot or cold blast of air on the face, washing the face, yawning, or even talking.

Medical Management

Antiseizure medications such as carbamazepine (Tegretol), phenytoin, valproate, gabapentin, oxcarbazepine (Trileptal), lamotrigine (Lamictal), and topiramate are the drugs used to treat trigeminal neuralgia pain. Antispasmodic, muscle-relaxing agents such as baclofen (Gablofen) may be used alone or in combination with antiseizure medications. Absolute alcohol may be injected into the peripheral branches of the trigeminal nerve and provides relief for weeks to months by damaging the nerves, thus blocking pain signals. Biofeedback, acupuncture, and megavitamins are other therapies used.

Permanent relief of pain often is obtained by surgery, with several different options available. Options for surgical treatment include resecting the sensory root of the trigeminal nerve (traditional surgical method), microvascular decompression, and gammaknife radiosurgery. Discussion between the surgeon and patient, as well as patient risk factors and current condition, determines which surgical approach is the most appropriate.

Nursing Interventions

It is common for patients with trigeminal neuralgia not to have eaten properly for some time, because eating causes pain. They may be undernourished and dehydrated. They may not have washed, shaved, or combed the hair for some time. Oral hygiene often has been neglected. Measures to increase comfort for patients before surgery or for patients being treated nonsurgically are listed in Box 54.3.

Box 54.3 Comfort Measures for Patients With Trigeminal Neuralgia

- Keep room free of drafts; moderate temperature.
- Avoid touching the patient's face.
- Do not urge patients to wash or shave the affected area or to comb the hair during acute attack.
- Stress the importance of hygiene, nutrition, and oral care and convey understanding if previous oral neglect is apparent.
- Provide lukewarm water and soft cloths and cotton saturated with solutions that do not require water for cleaning the face.
- A warm mouthwash or small, soft-bristled toothbrush assists in promoting oral care.
- When analgesia is at its peak, conditions are optimum for instructing in matters of hygiene. Many patients, however, prefer to execute their own care as they fear inadvertent injury at the hands of someone else.
- Avoid hot or cold liquids, which trigger pain.
- Puree food and ensure that it is lukewarm. If necessary, suggest that food be taken through a straw.

Prognosis

The acute pain seldom lasts more than a few seconds or 2 or 3 minutes, but it is excruciating. The onset of pain can occur at any time during the day or night and may recur several times daily for weeks at a time. Some patients have more or less continuous discomfort and sensitivity of the face. Although this condition is considered benign, the severity of the pain and the disruption of lifestyle can result in almost total physical and psychological dysfunction or even suicide. Permanent relief of pain frequently is obtained only by surgery.

BELL'S PALSY (PERIPHERAL FACIAL PARALYSIS)

Etiology and Pathophysiology

Bell's palsy is thought to be caused by an inflammatory process involving the facial nerve (cranial nerve VII), anywhere from the nucleus in the brain to the periphery. Although the exact etiology is not known, there is evidence that reactivated herpes simplex virus (HSV) may be involved in the majority of cases. The reactivation of the HSV causes inflammation, edema, ischemia, and eventual demyelination of the facial nerve, creating pain and disturbances in motor and sensory function. Any of the three branches of the facial nerve may be affected. The disorder can be unilateral or bilateral. It can affect any age group but is more common in the 20- to 60-year-old age range and affects approximately 40,000 people each year (National Institute of Neurological Disorders and Stroke, 2017).

Clinical Manifestations

With Bell's palsy there is usually an abrupt onset of numbness, stiffness, or drawing sensation of the face. Unilateral weakness of the facial muscles usually occurs, resulting in a flaccidity of the affected side of the face with inability to wrinkle the forehead, close the eyelid, pucker the lips, smile, frown, whistle, or retract the mouth on that side. The face appears asymmetric, with drooping mouth and cheek. Other symptoms include loss of taste, altered chewing ability, reduction of saliva on the affected side, pain behind the ear on the affected side, and ringing in the ear or other hearing loss.

Medical Management

Bell's palsy has no specific therapy. Electrical stimulation or warm moist heat along the course of the nerve may help. Stimulation may maintain muscle tone and prevent atrophy. Corticosteroids, especially prednisone, are started immediately, preferably before paralysis is complete. When the patient improves to the point that the corticosteroids are no longer necessary, they should be tapered off over a 2-week period. Because HSV is implicated in approximately 70% of cases of Bell's palsy, treatment with acyclovir (Zovirax), alone or in conjunction with prednisone, is used. Additional antiviral agents to treat HSV, including valacyclovir (Valtrex) and famciclovir, also have been used in the management of Bell's palsy.

Nursing Interventions

Protection of the eye when the eyelid does not close is important. Eye shields used at night help prevent excessive drying and damage to the cornea. Artificial tears may be ordered and should be administered as directed. Massage of the affected areas sometimes is recommended. Active facial exercises may be prescribed for 5 minutes three times a day. These include wrinkling the brow and forehead, closing the eyes, and puffing out the cheeks.

Prognosis

Most patients recover fully within 3 to 6 months, although recovery may take as long as a year. The extent of the nerve damage generally is an indication of how long the recovery process will take. Recovery of taste is the first sign of improvement; if it occurs within the first week, it signals a good chance for full recovery of motor function. Another favorable sign is if paralysis remains incomplete within the first 5 to 7 days. Permanent paralysis occurs only in a few cases, and rarely does the disorder recur.

INFECTION AND INFLAMMATION

Etiology and Pathophysiology

Infection or inflammation commonly interferes with function. Some specific conditions include meningitis, encephalitis, brain abscess, GBS, herpes zoster, neurosyphilis, poliomyelitis, and acquired immunodeficiency syndrome (AIDS). Only GBS, meningitis, encephalitis, brain abscess, and AIDS are discussed in this chapter.

The nervous system may be affected by a variety of organisms and may suffer from toxins of bacteria and viruses. These toxins reach the nervous system from a variety of sources, including adjacent bones, blood, or lymph. Meningitis can occur as a result of an invasive procedure such as surgery.

Assessment

Subjective data include a history of infection, such as an upper respiratory tract infection, and discomfort such as headache or stiff neck. The initial onset of symptoms, difficulty in thinking, and weakness may be important. Assess the patient's understanding of the condition.

Objective data include behavioral signs indicating discomfort or disorientation and an inability to carry out ADLs. Physical assessment may reveal abnormalities; fever, vomiting, abnormal CT results, seizures, altered respiratory patterns, tachycardia, or meningeal irritation. Also assess the patient's LOC and orientation.

Diagnostic Tests

Many infections of the nervous system can be diagnosed by examining the CSF. A CT scan or an EEG also may be done.

Nursing Interventions and Patient Teaching

Patient problems and interventions for the patient with an infection or inflammation are the same as those for the patient who has had a stroke, with the addition of but not limited to the following:

Patient Problem	Nursing Interventions
Elevated Body Temperature, related to inflammatory response to CNS infection	Assess temperature q 2 hr and as needed Provide cooling measures as needed; avoid cooling to point of shivering

Patient Problem	Nursing Interventions
	Administer antipyretics and antibiotics as ordered Monitor parenteral fluids as ordered Control exposure to extremes in temperature Assess temperature, pulse, and respiration q 2 hr as indicated
Recent Onset of Confusion, related to neurophysiologic response to infection	Introduce self to patient and establish rapport to prevent agitation Relate date, time of day, and recent activities Speak in kind tone, using short, simple sentences Maintain a therapeutic environment

Education for the patient with an infection includes teaching about the disease process, the treatments involved, and the expected outcomes. If the patient is seriously ill, the initial teaching involves the family. Other aspects of teaching for motor and sensory problems also may be relevant for the patient with an infection or inflammation, depending on the signs and symptoms demonstrated.

GUILLAIN-BARRÉ SYNDROME (POLYNEURITIS)

Etiology and Pathophysiology

Guillain-Barré syndrome (GBS) is also called *acute inflammatory polyradiculopathy* or *postinfectious polyneuritis*. It is an acute, rapidly progressing, and potentially fatal form of polyneuritis. It results in widespread inflammation and demyelination of the peripheral nervous system. The disease affects people of all ages and is seen equally in men and women and only affects 1 in 100,000 each year. The etiology is unknown, but it is thought to be an autoimmune reaction involving the peripheral nerves, most often after a respiratory or gastrointestinal viral infection. GBS rarely is seen as a result of surgery, viral immunizations, or Epstein-Barr virus (NLM, 2018c).

The peripheral nervous system is composed of 31 pairs of spinal nerves, 12 pairs of cranial nerves, and various plexuses and ganglia. Each nerve cell, or neuron, is composed of several parts, including the axon. Responsible for transmitting nerve impulses, axons are wrapped in segments of insulation called the myelin sheath, which is composed of Schwann cells.

In GBS the antibodies attack the Schwann cells, causing the sheath to break down (a process called *demyelination*) and the uninsulated portion of the nerve to become inflamed. Nerve conduction is interrupted, causing the classic signs of muscle weakness, tingling, and numbness. These signs begin in the legs or feet and work their way upward, perhaps because the signals to and from the legs are most vulnerable because they have to travel the longest distance. The demyelination is self-limiting. Once it stops, the Schwann cells rebuild the lost insulation. Remyelination, and therefore recovery, occurs in reverse; it starts at the top of the body and proceeds downward.

Clinical Manifestations

There is variation in the pattern of the onset of weakness and in the rate of progression of signs and symptoms. The progression may stop at any point. The patient may have difficulty swallowing, breathing, and speaking if cranial nerves VII, IX, and X are involved. Symmetric muscle weakness and lower motoneuron paralysis are present. The paralysis usually starts in the lower extremities and moves upward to include the thorax, the upper extremities, and the face. Respiratory failure may occur if the intercostal muscles are affected. Fluctuating blood pressure may occur as a result of effects on the autonomic nervous system.

Diagnostic Tests

GBS is diagnosed by elimination of other reasons for the signs and symptoms and by the characteristic muscle weakness. A CT scan may be ordered to rule out tumors or stroke. Changes in the respiratory status may aid in the diagnosis. A lumbar puncture is done. CSF in patients with GBS commonly has elevated protein levels. The health care provider may order a nerve conduction velocity study to test for slow impulse transmission. Electromyography and nerve conduction studies are markedly abnormal. A history of a recent infection is considered important.

Medical Management

Once GBS is suspected, hospitalization is essential. The patient's condition can deteriorate rapidly into paralysis that affects the respiratory muscles.

Adrenocortical steroids are used to treat the signs and symptoms of GBS. It also has been found that therapeutic plasmapheresis (the removal of unwanted or pathologic components from the patient's blood serum by means of a continuous-flow separator) in the first 2 weeks of GBS leads to decreased severity and length of symptoms. An alternative to plasmapheresis is IV immune globulin (Sandoglobulin). Patients receiving high-dose immune globulin need to be well hydrated and have adequate renal function.

Patients who develop respiratory failure require mechanical ventilation and may require a tracheostomy. ABG monitoring and pulmonary function tests are used to assess the respiratory status. If the patient has severe paralysis and is expected to have a long recovery period, a gastrostomy tube may be placed to provide adequate nourishment.

Nursing Interventions

Closely monitor respiratory function. If the patient requires mechanical ventilation, be aware that cognition (the mental faculty or process by which knowledge is acquired) is not impaired and that the patient requires reassurance. The patient also may need to be fed intravenously or through a nasogastric tube. Attention to the prevention of complications, such as contractures, pressure ulcers, and loss of ROM, is important to allow complete recovery. Initiate physical therapy early in the course of the disease to prevent contractures. Administer medication to help reduce neuropathic pain, such as gabapentin or a tricyclic antidepressant such as amitriptyline. Assess the patient's vital signs and motor strength frequently. Monitor the patient for signs of hypoxia.

Prognosis

Of the people suffering from GBS, 70% experience a full recovery. After 3 years approximately 30% report residual weakness. Long term weakness is experienced by 15%. Post disease reports of fatigue are common (National Institute of Neurological Disorders and Stroke, 2018). The recovery period may vary from weeks to years. Those not recovering completely have some degree of permanent neurologic deficit. In general, recovery from the disease occurs in the reverse order of how the paralysis or weakness occurred. The level of supportive care received during the acute stage of the illness has a direct correlation to the recovery.

MENINGITIS

Etiology and Pathophysiology

Meningitis is an acute infection of the meninges. It often is caused by one of several bacteria, including pneumococci, meningococci, *Neisseria meningitidis,* staphylococci, streptococci, and *Haemophilus influenzae;* it also can be caused by viral agents. The bacteria cause an inflammatory reaction in the pia mater, with pus accumulation in the arachnoid space, high protein and white blood cell levels in the CSF, and possible injury to nervous tissue.

Meningitis can be classified as bacterial (septic) or viral (aseptic). The incidence of bacterial meningitis is higher in fall and winter, when upper respiratory tract infections are common. Pathologic changes that can occur include hyperemia (excess blood; engorgement) of the meningeal vessels, edema of brain tissue, increased ICP, a generalized inflammatory reaction with exudation of white blood cells into the subarachnoid spaces, and associated hydrocephalus (in infants) caused by exudate occluding the ventricles.

Clinical Manifestations

Two abnormal signs that occur with meningitis are *Kernig's sign* (the inability to extend the legs completely without extreme pain) and *Brudzinski's sign* (flexion of the hip and knee when the neck is flexed). The onset of meningitis is usually sudden and is characterized by severe headache, stiffness of the neck, irritability, malaise, and restlessness. The patient develops nausea and vomiting; delirium; and increased temperature, pulse rate, and respirations.

Diagnostic Tests

A CT of the head is ordered to rule out increased ICP. A lumbar puncture to obtain CSF is performed, unless ICP is increased. The CSF is sent to the laboratory to identify the pathogen responsible for causing the meningitis.

Medical Management

Rapid diagnosis and treatment are crucial in caring for the patient with bacterial meningitis. When meningitis is suspected, cultures are collected and diagnosis is confirmed. Treatment of meningitis includes multiple antibiotics given intravenously over a 2-week period. Medication options include ampicillin, penicillin, vancomycin, piperacillin, and third-generation cephalosporin (usually ceftriaxone [Rocephin] or cefotaxime for treating bacterial meningitis). Corticosteroids (dexamethasone) are given intravenously to decrease ICP. Anticonvulsants are given to prevent seizures. Aseptic (viral) meningitis is treated with supportive therapy, such as maintaining bed rest, ensuring fluid and electrolyte balance, and providing rest and comfort measures. Treatment with antiviral medication is debatable because the disease is usually self-limiting unless encephalitis has developed.

Nursing Interventions

Respiratory isolation is required until the pathogen can no longer be cultured from the nasopharynx. This usually is accomplished after 24 hours of effective antibiotic therapy. Other nursing interventions include the general care given a critically ill patient who may be irritable, disoriented, and unable to take fluids. Dehydration is common, generally requiring IV fluid replacement therapy. Keep the room darkened and noise to a minimum because any increase in sensory stimulation may cause a seizure. If the patient is disoriented, safety precautions should be implemented. Fever must be managed because it increases cerebral edema and the frequency of seizures. Neurologic damage may result from an extremely high temperature over a prolonged time. Acetaminophen may be used to reduce fever. On occasion, patients do not respond to acetaminophen; these patients may require the use of a cooling blanket to lower the body temperature.

Prophylactic antibiotic therapy for family and friends in close contact with a patient with bacterial meningitis may be recommended to destroy the causative bacteria that may have colonized in the nasopharynx.

Some forms of bacterial meningitis can be prevented by vaccination. The pneumococcal vaccine may be given to adults age 65 and older and other high-risk adults. The meningococcal vaccine is effective against *N. meningitidis* and is recommended for patients ages 11 to 12 and a booster given at age 16. If the primary dose was given at age 13 to 15 years the booster can be given at age 16 to 18. If the primary dose was given at age 16 or older, a booster is not necessary. The *H. influenzae* vaccine has significantly decreased meningitis caused by this organism in children (CDC, 2017).

Prognosis

With most cases of meningitis, the prognosis for complete recovery is good. The prognosis depends on the speed with which the infection is diagnosed and antibiotics are administered. With severe cases of meningitis, residual neurologic damage or death may occur.

ENCEPHALITIS

Encephalitis is an acute inflammation of the brain and usually is caused by a virus. Many different viruses have been implicated in encephalitis; some are associated with certain seasons of the year and endemic to certain geographic areas. Epidemic encephalitis is transmitted by ticks and mosquitoes. Nonepidemic encephalitis may occur as a complication of measles, chickenpox, or mumps.

Encephalitis is a serious, sometimes fatal disease. The infection affects 10,000 to 20,000 people in the United States each year. Overall mortality rate ranges from 5% to 20%, with the highest mortality rate in encephalitis caused by HSV and the eastern and Venezuelan equine viruses. Unfortunately, HSV encephalitis is the most common form of viral encephalitis. Cytomegalovirus encephalitis is a common complication in patients with AIDS.

Manifestations resemble those of meningitis, but they have a more gradual onset. They include headache, high fever, seizures, and a change in LOC. Early diagnosis and treatment of viral encephalitis are essential for favorable outcomes. Brain imaging techniques such as MRI and PET, along with viral studies of CSF, allow for earlier detection of viral encephalitis.

Medical management and nursing interventions are symptomatic and supportive. Cerebral edema is a major problem, and diuretics (mannitol) and corticosteroids (dexamethasone) are used to control it. The disease is characterized by diffuse damage to the nerve cells of the brain, perivascular cellular infiltration of glial cells, and increasing cerebral edema. The sequelae of encephalitis include mental deterioration, amnesia, personality changes, and hemiparesis.

Acyclovir and vidarabine are used to treat encephalitis caused by HSV infection. Acyclovir has fewer side effects than vidarabine and is often the preferred treatment. Use of these antiviral agents has been shown to reduce mortality rates from 70% to 30%, although neurologic complications may not be reduced. Long-term symptoms include memory impairment, epilepsy, anosmia, personality changes, behavioral abnormalities, and dysphasia. For maximal benefit, antiviral agents should be started before the onset of coma.

WEST NILE VIRUS

West Nile virus (WNV) has been found commonly in humans and birds and other vertebrates in Africa, Eastern Europe, western Asia, and the Middle East, but it was not documented in the United States until 1999. The virus can infect humans, birds, mosquitoes, horses, and some other animals (CDC, 2018).

The principal route of human infection with WNV is through the bite of an infected female mosquito. Mosquitoes become infected when they feed on infected birds. When the virus is injected into humans by a mosquito, it can multiply and possibly cause illness. The incubation period ranges from 2 to 14 days. The majority (70% to 80%) of people who become infected with the virus do not have any type of illness. Those who develop West Nile fever have flulike manifestations of fever, headache, back pain, myalgia, and anorexia, lasting only a few days and without any long-term health effects. Less than 1% of people infected with WNV develop encephalitis or meningitis. *WNV meningitis* usually is associated with a sudden onset of febrile illness, headache, chills, and neck pain. Patients with *WNV encephalitis* often have fever; headache; altered LOC; disorientation; behavioral and speech disturbances; and other neurologic signs such as hemiparesis, seizures, and coma. Even in areas where the virus is circulating, however, few mosquitoes are infected with the virus. The chances of becoming severely ill from any one mosquito bite are extremely small.

The current standard for diagnosing WNV is by testing blood or CSF with the immunoglobulin M (IgM) antibody capture enzyme-linked immunosorbent assay (ELISA) and immunoglobulin G indirect ELISA. The IgM test may not be positive when symptoms first occur; however, it becomes positive in most infected people within days of symptom onset. Someone recently vaccinated against yellow fever or Japanese encephalitis can also have a positive IgM antibody test result.

WNV cannot be transmitted through casual contact such as touching or kissing a person who has the disease. However, in a small number of cases, the virus has been transmitted through blood transfusion, organ transplantation, breast-feeding, and pregnancy (from mother to fetus).

The risk of becoming infected with WNV can be reduced by applying insect repellent to exposed skin. Choose an insect repellent that contains *N,N*-diethyl-3-methylbenzamide (DEET) and that provides protection for the amount of time to be spent outdoors. Also spray clothing because mosquitoes can bite through thin clothing. Wearing long-sleeved shirts, long pants, and socks while outdoors can reduce the risk. Take special precautions from April to October, the months when mosquitoes are most active.

DEET is the gold standard in currently available over-the-counter insect repellents. DEET was developed in 1946 by the US Army for use by military personnel in insect-infested areas. It has been used worldwide for more than 40 years and has a remarkable safety profile.

Toxic reactions can occur, and they usually are linked to misuse of the product, such as massive exposure resulting from chronic use. Reports of greatest concern involve encephalopathy caused by DEET exposure. Most adverse reactions, though, are less serious, involving eye irritation and inhalation irritation (related to spraying repellent in the eyes or inhaling it).

DEET has been classified as a group D carcinogen (not classifiable as a human carcinogen). For casual use, a 10% to 35% concentration provides adequate protection. The American Academy of Pediatrics recommends limiting DEET repellents to a 30% maximum concentration when used on infants and children. DEET is not recommended for use in children younger than 2 months (CDC, 2008).

Other means of decreasing the mosquito population and thus decreasing the possibility of transmission of the WNV include the following:

- Limit outdoor activities between dusk and dawn.
- Place mosquito netting over infant carriers or strollers when outdoors.
- Use mosquito repellents and wear long-sleeved shirts or pants when exposure is likely.
- Store any containers that may become filled with standing water, such as cans, flowerpots, or trash cans, indoors.
- Install or repair window and door screens so that mosquitoes cannot get indoors.

If WNV infection is confirmed, treatment is supportive, intended to manage symptoms, such as headache, fever, and nausea. In more severe cases, patients may need intensive therapy, often involving hospitalization for IV fluids, airway management, respiratory support, and prevention of secondary infections such as pneumonia. To manage WNV encephalitis, the patient may receive interferon alfa-2b, steroids, antiseizure medications, or osmotic diuretics.

Infected people have a transient viremia, making transmission of the virus via donated blood, organs, or tissue possible, but this is very rare. As with many viruses, contact with the blood of an infected person could lead to transmission of the virus; therefore use the same standard precautions as with all patients.

BRAIN ABSCESS

Brain abscess is an accumulation of pus within the brain tissue that can result from a local or a systemic infection. Direct extension from ear, tooth, mastoid, or sinus infection is the primary cause. Other causes of brain abscess formation include septic venous thrombosis from a pulmonary infection, infective endocarditis, skull fracture, and a nonsterile neurologic procedure. Streptococci and staphylococci are the primary infective organisms.

Clinical manifestations are similar to those of meningitis and encephalitis and include headache and fever. Signs of increased ICP may include drowsiness, confusion, and seizures. Focal symptoms may be present and reflect the local area of the abscess. For example, visual field deficits or psychomotor seizures are common with a temporal lobe abscess, whereas an occipital abscess may be accompanied by visual impairment and hallucinations.

Antimicrobial therapy is the primary treatment for brain abscess. Other manifestations are treated symptomatically. If drug therapy is not effective, the abscess may have to be removed if it is encapsulated. In untreated cases the mortality rate approaches 100%. Seizures occur in approximately 30% of the cases. Nursing interventions are similar to those for management of meningitis or increased ICP.

Other infections of the brain include subdural empyema, osteomyelitis of the cranial bones, epidural abscess, and venous sinus thrombosis after periorbital cellulitis.

ACQUIRED IMMUNODEFICIENCY SYNDROME

Etiology and Pathophysiology

AIDS is a disease that has serious implications for the nervous system: more than 80% of patients with advanced human immunodeficiency virus (HIV) disease have neurologic signs and symptoms. Patients develop neurologic signs and symptoms either from infection with HIV or as a result of associated infections. See Chapter 56 for a discussion of advanced HIV disease (AIDS).

Clinical Manifestations

Patients with AIDS may have AIDS dementia complex (ADC), which originally was known as subacute encephalitis. They may exhibit difficulty concentrating or a recent memory loss, which may progress to a **global cognitive dysfunction** (generalized impairment of intellect, awareness, and judgment). Patients also may experience opportunistic infections such as meningitis, HSV, cytomegalovirus, toxoplasmosis, and cryptococcal meningitis. Primary malignant lymphomas of the CNS also may develop.

Diagnostic Tests

The diagnostic tests used to determine whether a neurologic problem is related to AIDS include serologic studies, analysis of CSF through a lumbar puncture, CT scan, and MRI. At times, a cerebral biopsy may be necessary to make the differential diagnosis.

Medical Management

Treatment of the patient with neurologic problems related to AIDS depends on the infection. Methods of treatment include administration of antiviral, antifungal, and antibacterial agents. Radiation has been used on the affected part of the brain. Experimental therapies, including iron dextran (DexFerrum), have been tried. Dehydration or shock is treated with fluid volume expanders. Seizures are controlled with diazepam, phenytoin, or fosphenytoin. Mortality remains high despite aggressive therapy.

Nursing Interventions

The patient is likely to be disoriented and may need to be reoriented frequently. Safety measures such as padded side rails may be necessary to prevent injury to the patient, who may have seizures. The patient may experience pain and have difficulty sleeping. Administer medications as needed and structure activities to avoid waking the patient. Visual problems also may be associated with the disease; be careful to orient the patient to nursing interventions.

Most patients with AIDS experience depression and a sense of powerlessness about the disease. They may isolate themselves from others. Encourage patients to talk about their fears and concerns, help them find emotional support, and refer them to a support group. Above all, maintain a nonjudgmental attitude, regardless of how the patient contracted the disease.

The patient may be incontinent of bowel and bladder. Encourage an active bowel and bladder program. If the patient has diarrhea, keep the rectal area as clean and dry as possible and administer antidiarrheals if ordered. The patient also may have nausea. Offer foods that the patient likes in small, frequent meals. Tube feedings or total parenteral nutrition may be needed if the patient agrees.

Prognosis

The prognosis for the patient with AIDS is terminal, often within a short time. At present, little can be done to lengthen life substantially. After a patient experiences neurologic complications, AIDS is usually fairly well advanced.

BRAIN TUMORS

Etiology and Pathophysiology

Brain tumors may be primary to the brain or be the result of metastases from another location. There are more than 150 different types of brain tumors. All areas and structures of the brain can be affected. Tumors may be benign or cancerous. The majority of tumors are benign and not primary to the brain. It is estimated that there are more than 700,000 people living with a brain tumor and another 80,000 will be diagnosed in 2018 (American Brain Tumor Association, n.d.). A primary brain tumor, or **neoplasm** (any abnormal benign or malignant mass), originates from the tissues of the brain and forms when changes occur in the genetic structure of normal brain cells (neurons and glial cells). Changes may be caused by a genetic predisposition, an environmental trigger, or both; the causes of most primary brain tumors are unknown. Most benign tumors affect the meninges, whereas most malignant tumors (78%) are gliomas. These tumors develop from the supporting cells of the brain, which are referred to as *glia*. Benign tumors include meningiomas and pituitary adenomas. Metastatic brain tumors occur in an estimated one in four patients with cancer. Brain tumors are named for the tissues from which they arise.

Assessment

Subjective data include the patient's understanding of the diagnosis, changes in personality or judgment, and abnormal sensations or visual problems. The patient may complain of unusual odors with tumors of the temporal lobe. The patient may report difficulty with the ability to think, speak, or articulate words. Patients with brain tumors usually experience headaches as a prominent early symptom. The headache is typically more severe in the morning. Loss of balance and dizziness are common complaints. The patient also may experience paresis (weakness) and vision c hanges.

Objective data include motor strength, gait, the level of alertness and consciousness, and orientation. Assess the pupils for response and equality. In some patients, the initial sign of a brain tumor is new-onset seizures. Seizure activity commonly occurs at some time among patients with brain tumors. Cognitive changes in memory, speech, concentration, and communication are also common. The patient's family may report a change in the patient's personality. Speech impairments, cranial nerve abnormalities, and signs and symptoms of increased ICP are also significant.

Diagnostic Tests

No one procedure is entirely diagnostic of brain tumors, but a CT scan is often the basis for the diagnosis. Other tests that may be performed include the brain scan, MRI, PET scans, and the EEG. Arteriography, as well as a biopsy, also may be done.

Medical Management

The general method of treatment for brain tumors includes surgical removal when feasible, radiation, and chemotherapy. The choice of therapy depends on the tumor type and where it is located. A combination of methods often is used. The blood-brain barrier may limit the effectiveness of chemotherapy when used as adjuvant therapy or to treat tumor recurrence.

Surgery. A surgical opening through the skull is called a *craniotomy.* After removing the bone, the surgeon makes an incision into the meninges and removes the tumor. The removed bone is preserved carefully and may be replaced at the end of surgery if there is no indication of infection or increased ICP. Sometimes the bone cannot be returned; the removal of part of the skull without replacement is called a *craniectomy*. Before the craniotomy/craniectomy a less invasive procedure, a stereotactic biopsy, may be performed to obtain a sample of the tumor tissue. It involves drilling a small hole through the patient's skull, after which the tumor biopsy is obtained.

Brain tumor surgery has become increasingly successful because of computerized devices called *surgical navigation systems.* These systems help pinpoint tumors and guide the neurosurgeon during the surgery. Tumors that once were considered inoperable now can be removed because their location can be mapped accurately by a surgical navigation system.

Nursing Interventions

Preoperative preparation of the patient and the family is important. Specific fears may be related to a permanent change in appearance, dependency, and possible death. A baseline neurologic assessment is important. Explain treatments and procedures, including shaving the hair. Usually hair is shaved in the operating room. Prepare the family for the patient's appearance after surgery.

Postoperative care depends on the patient's condition. Most patients spend one or two nights in an intensive care unit under close nursing observation with frequent neurologic checks. Assess the patient carefully for indications of increased ICP. The patient may have residual motor or sensory problems as a result of the tumor or surgery. A ventriculoperitoneal shunt (i.e., a catheter draining excess fluid from the brain to the abdomen) may be inserted if increased ICP is an issue.

Patient problems and interventions for the patient with a brain tumor are the same as those for the patient who has had a stroke, with the addition of but not limited to the following:

Patient Problem	Nursing Interventions
Impaired Neurovascular Function, Visual, auditory, kinesthetic, tactile, related to compression or displacement of brain tissue	Maintain method of communication Provide for social environment Provide orientation and appropriate level of stimuli
Recent Onset of Confusion, related to: • Altered circulation • Destruction of brain tissue	Protect patient from self-injury Provide soft safety reminder devices as indicated Assist patient in self-care activities Speak in kind tone, using short, simple sentences Give one direction at a time Relate date, time of day, and recent activities Maintain a therapeutic environment Keep equipment and personal possessions in same place Encourage socialization

Prognosis

The outlook for the patient with a brain tumor depends on whether the tumor is benign or malignant and on its size and location. In the past, the diagnosis of a brain tumor had a very high mortality rate within weeks of the diagnosis. Better diagnostic tools and new treatment modalities have increased the lifespan and quality of life for many patients with primary and metastatic brain tumors. The lifespan for many patients diagnosed with a brain tumor is now years rather than weeks.

TRAUMA

Interference with neurologic function can occur as a result of trauma. Parts of the nervous system commonly subjected to trauma include the brain, the spinal cord, and peripheral nerves. Only the first two are discussed in this chapter.

HEAD INJURY

Etiology and Pathophysiology

The term *head trauma* is used primarily to signify craniocerebral trauma, or head injury, which includes an alteration in consciousness, no matter how brief. In the United States, an estimated 1.7 million head injuries occur annually. These injuries account for more than 30% of all injury-related deaths in the United States. Head injury is the second most common cause of neurologic injuries and the major cause of death between ages 1 and 35. Previously, the most common causes of head injury in the United States were motor vehicle collisions and falls. Deaths from motor vehicle collisions and falls have decreased; however, firearm-related head injury death rates have increased. Head injury can result from recreational activities, sports-related trauma, and assaults. There is a noted gender difference. Males in every age group have higher injury rates than women (CDC, 2016b).

Craniocerebral trauma may result in injury to the scalp, skull, and brain tissues. Injuries vary from minor scalp wounds to concussions and open fractures of the skull with severe damage to the brain. The amount of obvious damage is not indicative of the seriousness of the trouble. Effects of severe head injury include cerebral edema, sensory and motor deficits, and increased ICP.

Injuries to the brain can result from direct or indirect trauma to the head. Indirect trauma is caused by tension strains and shearing forces transmitted to the head by stretching the neck. Direct trauma occurs when the head is directly injured. Indirect trauma results in an *acceleration-deceleration* injury, with rotation of the skull and its contents. Bruising or contusion of the occipital and frontal lobes, the brainstem, and the cerebellum may occur.

Clinical Manifestations

Head injuries may be open or closed. Open head injuries result from skull fractures or penetrating wounds. The amount of injury with this type of wound is determined by the velocity, mass, shape, and direction of the impact. A skull fracture (linear, comminuted, depressed, or compound) also may occur. Fractures of the base of the skull are more serious because they are near the medulla.

Closed head injuries include concussions (a violent jarring of the brain against the skull), contusions, and lacerations. Lacerations of the scalp bleed profusely because of the extensive vascularity in the region. Hemorrhage resulting from craniocerebral trauma may occur in the scalp or in the epidural, subdural, intracerebral, and intraventricular areas. Epidural and subdural hematomas require careful and continuous observation. Epidural hematomas resulting from arterial bleeding form as blood collects rapidly between the dura mater and skull. If lethargy or unconsciousness develops after the patient regains consciousness, an epidural hematoma may be suspected and needs immediate treatment.

A subdural hematoma forms as venous blood collects below the dura. Because the bleeding is under venous pressure, subdural hematoma formation is relatively slow. The clot causes pressure on the brain surface and displaces brain tissue. If a patient who has been conscious for several days after head injury loses consciousness or develops neurologic signs and symptoms, suspect a subdural hematoma. Subdural hematomas may be classified as acute, subacute, or chronic.

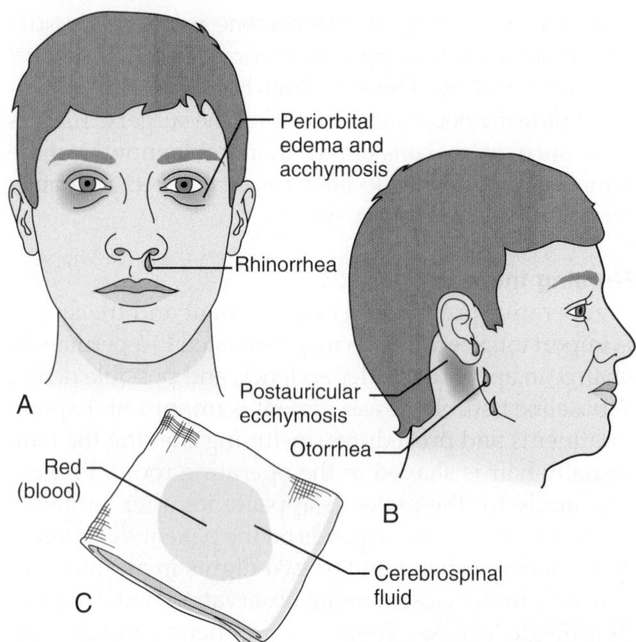

Fig. 54.21 A, "Raccoon eyes" and rhinorrhea (nasal discharge). B, Battle's sign (postauricular ecchymosis) with otorrhea (discharge from the ear). C, Halo or ring sign.

Assessment

Subjective data include the patient's understanding of the injury and the resulting pathologic processes. Determine how the injury happened and whether the patient has headache, nausea, or vomiting. Note abnormal sensations and a history of loss of consciousness and of bleeding from any orifice.

Objective data include the status of the respiratory system, level of alertness and consciousness, and size and reactivity of the pupils; check these frequently. Also assess the patient's orientation, motor status, vital signs, bleeding or vomiting, and abnormal speech patterns. The presence of *Battle's sign* (ecchymosis [a small hemorrhagic spot] behind the ear) usually indicates fracture of a bone of the lower skull (Fig. 54.21).

Diagnostic Tests

CT, MRI, and PET scans are the primary diagnostic imaging examinations in assessing soft tissue injuries.

Medical Management

Immediate care of the patient with a head injury is directed toward lifesaving measures and the maintenance of normal body function until recovery is ensured. It is extremely important to maintain a patent airway and ensure adequate oxygenation. Suctioning may be necessary (but never through the nose because of the possibility of a skull fracture), along with the administration of oxygen. Check ABG levels. Stabilize the cervical spine; assume neck injury with head injury until diagnostic examination proves otherwise.

Medications are used to reduce cerebral edema and increased ICP, which are common problems in patients with head injuries. Medications include mannitol and dexamethasone. Codeine or other analgesics that do not depress the respiratory system are used for pain control. Anticonvulsants may be given to prevent seizures. Take measures to control elevated temperatures, because hyperthermia increases brain metabolism, resulting in brain damage.

Nursing Interventions

Check the patient's ears and nose carefully for signs of blood and serous drainage, which indicate that the meninges are torn and spinal fluid is escaping. *Do not* attempt to clean out the orifice. If there is evidence of drainage from the nose, the patient should not cough, sneeze, or blow the nose. If there is a question about whether the drainage is CSF, a glucose test strip (e.g., Tes-Tape) will show a positive reaction for glucose. Meningitis is a possible complication when communication with the meninges and the nose or ears occurs.

The patient with a head injury often shows a loss of memory and loss of initiative. Behavioral problems associated with a lack of judgment and restlessness also may occur. Restlessness may be caused by the need for a change of position, pain, or the need to empty the bladder. These patients require firm but gentle care, with specific guidelines for what behavior is allowed. Medications to decrease agitation may be needed. It is not helpful to argue with patients, but redirecting their attention may help. Memory aids such as a log book or written schedule can assist with orientation.

The length of convalescence depends on the amount of brain damage and how rapid the recovery is. Many patients with head injury recover physically but have behavioral and psychological problems that make it difficult for them to function independently.

Patient problems and interventions for the patient with a head injury are the same as for the patient who has had a stroke, with the addition of but not limited to the following:

Patient Problem	Nursing Interventions
Compromised Social Interaction, related to cognitive and affective deficits from neurophysiologic trauma	Encourage and support verbalization about feelings, medical conditions, and current treatment; listen nonjudgmentally Build trust through consistency and kept promises Involve patient in care plan Give full attention to patient during verbal interactions and recognize qualities to promote self-esteem

Patient Teaching

A patient with a mild head injury may be seen in the emergency department but not be admitted to the hospital. Teach the patient about observations for complications such as increased drowsiness, nausea, vomiting, worsening headache or stiff neck, seizures, blurred vision, behavioral changes, motor problems, sensory disturbances, or decreased heart rate. Teaching for patients with a head injury who have residual deficits severe enough to require rehabilitation is similar to that needed for patients with motor or sensory problems.

Prognosis

The outcome for a patient with a head injury is often unpredictable. The extent of damage or recovery is not positively correlated with the amount of damage seen in surgery or on CT scan. Even minor head injuries can have residual effects. The person with a head injury is more prone to injuries and problems related to the brain damage (BrainandSpinalCord.org, 2017). Personality changes may result after a head injury. These changes may be short term or permanent. These changes may include depression, mood swings, confusion, anger, and social inappropriateness.

SPINAL CORD TRAUMA

Etiology and Pathophysiology

Spinal cord injury from accidents is a common and increasing cause of serious disability and death. Approximately 10% of traumatic injuries to the nervous system involve the spinal cord. Spinal cord injuries affect males significantly more than women: 80% of injuries involve men. Automobile accidents (38%), falls (30%), violence (13%), and sports (9%) are among the more common causes (National Spinal Cord Injury Statistical Center, 2016).

The soft tissue of the spinal cord is protected by the vertebral column. Injuries to this column include a simple fracture, compressed or wedge fracture, comminuted or burst fracture, or dislocation of the vertebrae (Fig. 54.22). As a result, the cord is often damaged. Severe traumatic lesions of the spinal cord may result in total transection of the spinal cord or tearing of the cord from side to side at a particular level, with a complete loss of spinal cord function. This total transection is also called a *complete cord injury*. With this type of injury, all voluntary movement below the level of the trauma is lost. A partial transection, or *incomplete injury*, of the cord also may occur. Tetraplegic patients (formerly referred to as quadriplegic) are those who sustain injuries to one of the cervical segments of the spinal cord. Paraplegic patients are those whose lesions are confined to the thoracic, lumbar, or sacral segments of the spinal cord. The signs and symptoms of an incomplete spinal injury vary (Table 54.8).

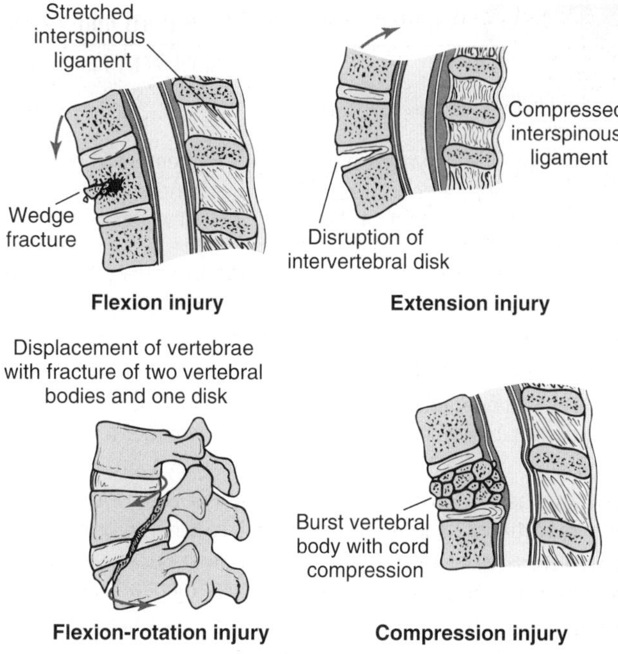

Fig. 54.22 Mechanisms of spinal injury. (From Lewis SL, Heitkemper MM, Dirksen SR, et al: *Medical-surgical nursing: Assessment and management of clinical problems*, ed 7, St. Louis, 2007, Mosby.)

Clinical Manifestations

Initially, in most spinal cord injuries, there is a period of flaccid paralysis and a complete loss of reflexes below the level of trauma. Sensory and autonomic functions are also lost. The loss of systemic sympathetic vasomotor tone may result in vasodilation, increased venous capacity, and hypotension. This is called *areflexia*, or spinal shock, and is temporary. During this time the patient may need temporary respiratory support.

One important complication of spinal cord injury is autonomic dysreflexia or **hyperreflexia,** a neurologic condition characterized by increased reflex actions. It occurs in patients with cord injuries at the sixth thoracic vertebra or higher and most commonly in patients with cervical injuries. Autonomic dysreflexia is an abnormal cardiovascular response to stimulation of the sympathetic

Table 54.8 Functional Level of Spinal Cord Injury and Rehabilitation Potential

LEVEL OF INJURY	MOVEMENT REMAINING	REHABILITATION POTENTIAL
Tetraplegia		
C1-C3 Often fatal injury, vagus nerve domination of heart, respiration, blood vessels, and all organs below injury	Movement in neck and above, loss of innervation to diaphragm, absence of independent respiratory function	Ability to drive electric wheelchair equipped with portable ventilator by using chin control or mouth stick, headrest to stabilize head; computer use with mouth stick, head wand, or noise control; 24-h attendant care, able to instruct others
C4 Vagus nerve domination of heart, respirations, and all vessels and organs below injury	Sensation and movement in neck and above; may be able to breathe without a ventilator	Same as C1-C3
C5 Vagus nerve domination of heart, respirations, and all vessels and organs below injury	Full neck, partial shoulder, back, biceps; gross elbow, inability to roll over or use hands; decreased respiratory reserve	Ability to drive electric wheelchair with mobile hand supports; indoor mobility in manual wheelchair; able to feed self with set-up and adaptive equipment; attendant care 10 h/day
C6 Vagus nerve domination of heart, respirations, and all vessels and organs below injury	Shoulder and upper back abduction and rotation at shoulder, full biceps to elbow flexion, wrist extension, weak grasp of thumb, decreased respiratory reserve	Ability to assist with transfer and perform some self-care; feed self with hand devices; push wheelchair on smooth, flat surface; drive adapted van from wheelchair; independent computer use with adaptive equipment; attendant care 6 h/day
C7-C8 Vagus nerve domination of heart, respirations, and all vessels and organs below injury	All triceps to elbow extension, finger extensors and flexors, good grasp with some decreased strength, decreased respiratory reserve	Ability to transfer self to wheelchair; roll over and sit up in bed; push self on most surfaces; perform most self-care; independent use of wheelchair; ability to drive car with powered hand controls (in some patients); attendant care 0–6 h/day
Paraplegia		
T1-T6 Sympathetic innervation to heart, vagus nerve domination of all vessels and organs below injury	Full innervation of upper extremities, back, essential intrinsic muscles of hand; full strength and dexterity of grasp; decreased trunk stability, decreased respiratory reserve	Full independence in self-care and in wheelchair; ability to drive car with hand controls (in most patients); independent standing in standing frame
T7-T12 Vagus nerve domination only of leg vessels, GI and genitourinary organs	Full, stable thoracic muscles and upper back; functional intercostals, resulting in increased respiratory reserve	Full independent use of wheelchair; ability to stand erect with full leg brace, ambulate on crutches with swing (although gait difficult); inability to climb stairs
L1-L2 Vagus nerve domination of leg vessels	Varying control of legs and pelvis, instability of lower back	Good sitting balance; full use of wheelchair; ambulation with long leg braces
L3-L4 Partial vagus nerve domination of leg vessels, GI and genitourinary organs	Quadriceps and hip flexors, absence of hamstring function, flail ankles	Completely independent ambulation with short leg braces and canes; inability to stand for long periods

GI, Gastrointestinal.

From Lewis SL, Dirksen SR, Heitkemper MM, et al: *Medical-surgical nursing: Assessment and management of clinical problems*, ed 8, St. Louis, 2011, Mosby.

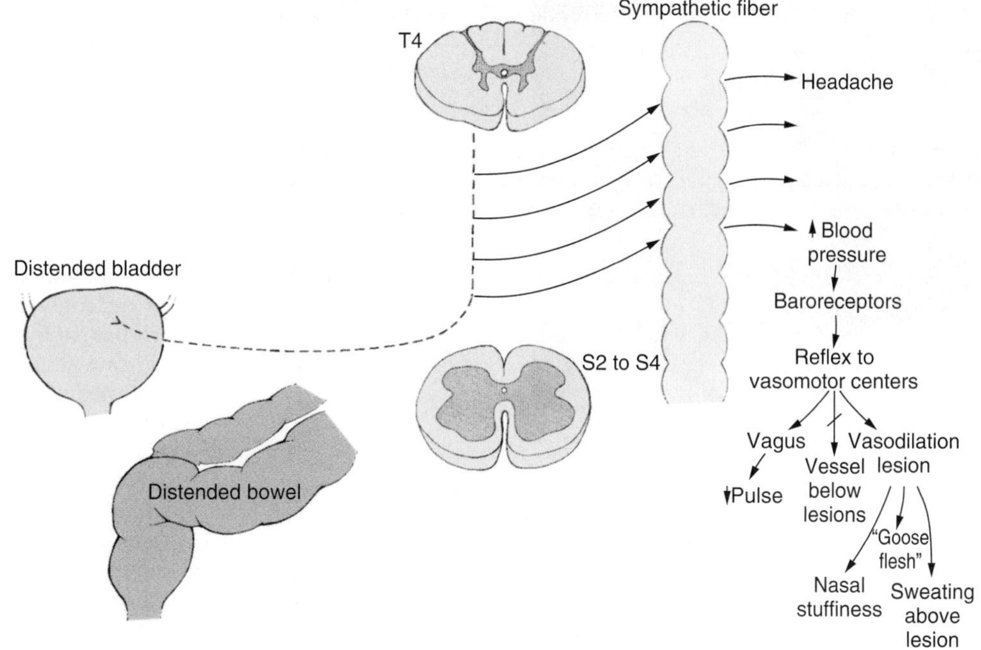

Fig. 54.23 Pictorial diagram of cause of autonomic hyperreflexia (dysreflexia) and results. (From Monahan FD, Sands JK, Neighbors M, et al: *Phipps' medical-surgical nursing: Health and illness perspectives,* ed 8, St. Louis, 2007, Mosby.)

division of the autonomic nervous system; the condition occurs as a result of stimulation of the bladder, large intestine, or other visceral organs (Fig. 54.23). The clinical signs include severe bradycardia, hypertension (systolic blood pressure up to 300 mm Hg), diaphoresis, "goose flesh," flushing (above the level of the lesion), dilated pupils, blurred vision, restlessness, nausea, severe headache, and nasal stuffiness. Patients tend to develop individual signs and symptoms of this condition and are soon able to recognize them. The most common causes of this condition include a distended bladder or a fecal impaction. It is a medical emergency that requires immediate treatment to prevent a stroke, blindness, or death (Box 54.4).

In most cases of spinal cord injury, men experience impotence, decreased sensation, and difficulties with ejaculation. Impaired fertility is common. The experience of orgasm is described as different than before the injury. Women with spinal cord injury are able to continue to perform sexually, although perception of sexual pleasure usually is altered.

Assessment

Subjective data include information about the nature of the injury, any dyspnea, and unusual sensations. The presence of pain, any loss of consciousness, and the absence of sensation on sensory examination are important to assess.

Objective data include the level of alertness and consciousness; orientation; pupil size and reactivity; motor strength; skin integrity; and bowel and bladder status, including distention. Assess for other injuries, such as fractured bones or head injury.

Box 54.4 Emergency Care for Autonomic Dysreflexia or Hyperreflexia

- Unless contraindicated, place patient in sitting position to decrease blood pressure.
- Check patency of catheter for kinking. If catheter is occluded, insert new catheter immediately.
- Check rectum for impaction.
- If it is necessary to remove impaction, use an anesthetic ointment.
- Administer ganglionic blocking agent such as hexamethonium or a vasodilator such as nitroprusside (Nipride) as ordered if conservative measures are not effective.
- Continue monitoring blood pressure.
- Send urine for culture if no other cause is found; urinary tract infection can lead to symptoms of autonomic dysreflexia.

Diagnostic Tests

Radiographs often are taken first to detect any cervical vertebral fracture or displacement. A spinal tap or myelogram also may be done to detect occlusion. A CT scan and MRI may help rule out spinal cord injury.

Medical Management

Immediate care after spinal cord injury is directed toward realignment of the bony column in the presence of fractures or dislocations. This may involve simple immobilization, skeletal traction, or surgery for spinal decompression. Skeletal traction may include Crutchfield tongs (Fig. 54.24), halo traction, or a Stryker or Foster

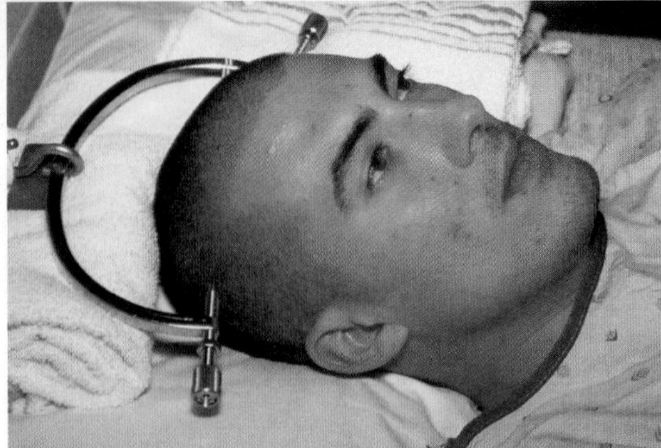

Fig. 54.24 Patient with Crutchfield tongs inserted into skull to hyperextend. (Courtesy Michael S. Clement, MD, Mesa, AZ.)

frame. Bracing may be used for thoracic or lumbar injuries. Often surgical decompression is not performed until after a period of skeletal traction if the injury involves the cervical region. In patients seen within 8 hours of injury, high-dose methylprednisolone is given.

Nursing Interventions and Patient Teaching

Throughout all stages of hospitalization of the patient with a spinal cord injury, nursing and medical interventions are directed toward restoring structural or body integrity. All efforts are taken to ensure that the skin is intact, that contractures do not develop, and that ROM is maintained. Early mobilization is important. When patients, especially those with tetraplegia, begin to sit up, it may be necessary to wrap the legs with thromboembolism stockings to encourage venous return. Slowly increasing the angle of sitting up is essential to prevent hypotension. A recliner wheelchair is usually necessary.

Usually a Foley catheter is inserted initially; later bladder training is started (see Chapter 50). Chronic indwelling catheterization increases the risk of infection. Intermittent catheterization should begin as early as possible. This helps maintain bladder tone and decreases the risk of infection. Encourage fluid intake of more than 2000 mL/day. Encourage cranberry juice to decrease renal calculus (kidney stone) formation.

Patients usually are started on a bowel program early in their hospital stay. At first, bisacodyl suppositories are given at regular intervals (usually every other night). This is followed by digital stimulation to promote peristalsis. The goal is to eliminate the need for suppositories. Other aids to bowel programs are the use of adequate fluids (usually at least 3000 to 4000 mL/day, unless contraindicated), stool softeners, and prune juice.

Patient problems and interventions for the patient with a spinal cord injury are the same as those for the patient with a motor or sensory problem, with the addition of but not limited to the following:

Patient Problem	Nursing Interventions
Impaired Neurovascular Function, related to neurophysiologic trauma to spinal cord above sixth thoracic vertebra	See Box 54.4 for emergency interventions
Alteration in Urinary Elimination, related to sensory-motor impairment	Check carefully for voiding and for distention of bladder Teach patient intermittent self-catheterization if indicated Teach patient Credé's maneuver as indicated Use Foley catheter if indicated; administer meticulous aseptic technique in changing catheters Teach patient signs of infection Encourage patient to have a genitourinary checkup at least yearly Maintain fluid intake of 3000–4000 mL/day unless contraindicated Use adult perineal protector for incontinency, if necessary

Teaching of the patient with a spinal cord injury includes education about autonomic dysreflexia and about sexual functioning after spinal cord injury. Other teaching points are found in the sections of this chapter dealing with the patient with motor or sensory problems.

Prognosis

In cases of complete spinal cord injury, there is almost no chance of return of any function. However, the paraplegic or tetraplegic patient can live a satisfying life with adaptations and assistance. Today, with improved treatment strategies (specifically, intermittent catheterization), even the very young patient with a spinal cord injury can anticipate a long life. The prognosis for life is generally only about 5 years less than for people of the same age without spinal cord injury. Take care to prevent infections, such as urinary tract or respiratory tract infections. In patients with incomplete cord lesions, the amount of function regained is variable and often unpredictable.

NURSING PROCESS FOR THE PATIENT WITH A NEUROLOGIC DISORDER

The role of the licensed practical nurse/licensed vocational nurse (LPN/LVN) in the nursing process as stated is that the LPN/LVN will:

- Participate in planning care for patients based on patient needs

- Review patient's plan of care and recommend revisions as needed
- Review and follow defined prioritization for patient care
- Use clinical pathways, care maps, or care plans to guide and review patient care

◆ ASSESSMENT

People with neurologic deficits require skilled assessment by a nurse and a health care provider. Assessment includes observing the patient during the patient history. Nursing assessment is an ongoing process and should be tailored to meet the patient's needs. For example, hourly neurologic checks will not be as detailed as the initial assessment.

While interviewing the patient, obtain data about subjective complaints, such as pain, dizziness, or vision difficulties. Also assess the ability to speak and reason. Observations may also include vital signs, data about gait, symmetry of body parts, evidence of pain, or seizure activity. During ongoing assessments, data usually are obtained about pupil size, level of alertness, ability to perform motor tasks, changes in LOC, and ability to speak. Because subtle changes in neurologic status often can be the first sign of a complication, be alert for small changes in the neurologic assessment and report these to the proper person.

◆ PATIENT PROBLEM

Nursing assessment helps identify the patient's needs for care and observation. The actual care of the patient then is based on the patient problems that have been identified. Possible patient problems for a patient with a neurologic disorder include but are not limited to the following:

- *Compromised Blood Flow to Tissue*
- *Compromised Physical Mobility*
- *Compromised Swallowing Ability*
- *Compromised Verbal Communication*
- *Grief*
- *Impaired Family Coping*
- *Impaired Neurovascular Dysfunction*
- *Inability to Bathe Self*
- *Inability to Feed Self*
- *Inability to Toilet Self*
- *Insufficient Knowledge*
- *Insufficient Nutrition*
- *Potential for Contractures or Muscle Atrophy*
- *Potential for Falling*
- *Potential for Infection*
- *Prolonged Pain*
- *Recent Onset of Confusion*
- *Recent Onset of Pain*
- *Slow or Delayed Ability to Remember*

◆ EXPECTED OUTCOMES AND PLANNING

The plan for providing neurologic assessment and care should focus on the type of deficit the patient is experiencing and possible complications. Consider a patient's preferences and mental status. The type of care required determines the supplies and equipment needed. Schedule necessary care around tests and procedures and the patient's need for rest.

The care plan focuses on achieving specific goals and outcomes that relate to the identified patient problem. Examples of these include the following:

Goal 1: Patient's cerebral perfusion will be maintained.

Outcome: Patient remains awake, alert, and oriented; coma scale score remains the same or improves.

Goal 2: Patient will maintain optimal nutrition.

Outcome: Patient maintains or attains optimal weight, and laboratory values indicating nutritional health are within normal limits.

◆ IMPLEMENTATION

Nursing interventions for the patient with a neurologic disorder include those that maintain cerebral perfusion and other functioning, as well as those that prevent complications such as skin breakdown, falls, or contractures. Certain principles guide nurses in providing neurologic care:

- The neurologic system is a complex system that produces a wide variety of neurologic signs and symptoms.
- Identical disorders may result in different sets of signs and symptoms in different patients.
- The maintenance of cerebral perfusion is of utmost importance.
- The patient with a neurologic illness is prone to complications.
- Disorders of the nervous system produce physical problems and a wide variety of cognitive difficulties.

While providing care to meet the patient's specific challenges, also assess the patient's readiness to learn. At times the family must receive the primary teaching because the patient is unable to understand. Consider the patient's preferences and background in delivering care. Encourage the patient to be as independent as possible and give appropriate feedback. Preserve the patient's dignity and privacy whenever possible. Also consider the special needs of older patients (see the Lifespan Considerations box in the section "Effects of Normal Aging on the Nervous System").

◆ EVALUATION

Evaluate the success of planned interventions during and after care is given. The process is ongoing and dynamic because the patient's condition often changes. Always be ready to revise the care plan as needed. For example, if a patient has new episodes of confusion after surgery, notify the health care provider, increase safety measures, and assess more frequently.

Ongoing systematic evaluation requires determining whether specific outcomes have been met. The evaluation is specific to measure the goals identified. Examples of goals and their corresponding evaluative measures include the following:

Goal 1: Patient will be free of infection.

Evaluative measure: Assess patient for any signs of infection such as increased temperature, frequency of urination, erythematous incision, elevated white blood cell count, or confusion.

Goal 2: Patient will remain alert and oriented in thought processes.

Evaluative measure: Ask patient to respond to orientation questions. Observe ability to engage in conversation and to carry out care activities.

Get Ready for the NCLEX® Examination!

Key Points

- The nervous system is the body's link with the environment. It allows the interpretation of information and appropriate action.
- The two main structural divisions of the nervous system are the CNS and the peripheral nervous system.
- The CNS is composed of the brain and the spinal cord.
- The peripheral nervous system is composed of the nerve cells lying outside of the CNS. It is divided into the somatic nervous system and the autonomic nervous system.
- A nerve cell is composed of three parts: the dendrites, the cell body, and the axon.
- The brain and the spinal cord are protected by the bony coverings (skull and vertebral column), the CSF, and the three meninges (pia mater, arachnoid mater, and dura mater).
- The cerebrum is the largest part of the brain and contains five major areas: motor, sensory, visual, speech, and auditory. The cerebrum governs the ability to reason and make judgments.
- The diencephalon lies beneath the cerebrum and contains the thalamus and hypothalamus. The thalamus serves as a relay station. The hypothalamus has several roles, such as temperature control, water balance, and appetite.
- The cerebellum is the second largest portion of the brain and is responsible for coordination of skeletal muscles and maintenance of balance and equilibrium.
- The peripheral nervous system is composed of the cranial nerves, the spinal nerves, the somatic nervous system, and the autonomic nervous system.
- The autonomic nervous system contains two subdivisions: the sympathetic nervous system and the parasympathetic nervous system. The sympathetic nervous system speeds things up, and the parasympathetic nervous system slows things down.
- Normal changes of aging are not the same as senility, AD, or organic brain damage.
- The source of prolonged or unusual headaches should be determined through neurologic testing because it may be a symptom of a serious pathologic condition.
- A lumbar puncture should not be done if there is evidence of increased ICP because of the danger of brain herniation.
- Any increase in the volume of one of the contents of the cranium (brain, blood vessels, and CSF) results in increased ICP because the cranial vault is rigid and does not expand.
- Classic signs of increased ICP include restlessness, disorientation, headache, contralateral hemiparesis, an ipsilaterally dilated pupil, and visual changes that include blurring and diplopia.
- Nursing intervention measures can significantly influence ICP.
- Epilepsy is a transitory disturbance in consciousness or in motor, sensory, or autonomic functions with or without loss of consciousness, caused by sudden, excessive, and disorderly electrical discharges of the brain.
- Early signs and symptoms of MS are usually transitory.
- Stroke, or "brain attack," is the most common disease of the nervous system and can be caused by thrombus, embolus, or hemorrhage. The term *brain attack* is used to describe stroke and communicates the urgency of recognizing stroke signs and symptoms and treating their onset as a medical emergency, just as one would with a myocardial infarction.
- The MERCI device, a blood clot remover, can be used for up to 8 hours after acute stroke onset to remove blood clots from arteries deep inside the brain.
- Helpful nursing interventions for the patient with AD include using nonverbal cues or demonstrations as adjuncts to verbal cues, providing few choices, and not hurrying the patient.
- Trigeminal neuralgia (tic douloureux) is characterized by excruciating, burning pain that radiates along one or more of the three divisions of the fifth cranial nerve.
- With Bell's palsy, there is usually an abrupt onset of numbness, a feeling of stiffness, or a drawing sensation of the face.
- Of the people suffering from GBS, 85% regain complete function.
- Approximately 80% of patients with advanced HIV disease (AIDS) have neurologic symptoms that result from infection with HIV itself or from associated complications of the disease.
- Many patients with head injury may recover physically, but they will have behavioral and psychological problems that make it difficult for them to function independently.
- The signs and symptoms of intracranial tumors result from both local and general effects of the tumor.
- Autonomic dysreflexia in the patient with spinal cord injury is a medical emergency that demands quick nursing interventions.
- The first sign of increased ICP may be a declining state of consciousness.

- It is important to document patients' behaviors in terms of what is seen, not what is inferred.
- It is estimated that less than 1% of people infected with WNV will develop encephalitis or meningitis, a more severe form of the disease.

Additional Learning Resources

SG Go to your Study Guide for additional learning activities to help you master this chapter content.

evolve Be sure to visit the Evolve site at *http://evolve.elsevier.com/Cooper/foundationsadult/* for additional online resources.

Review Questions for the NCLEX® Examination

1. A patient is admitted to the hospital with a diagnosis of transient ischemic attack (TIA). The patient asks the nurse to explain to him what a TIA is. Which statement by the nurse is most accurate?
   1. "A TIA is the result of permanent cerebrovascular insufficiency."
   2. "An episode of a TIA may last up to 2 days."
   3. "A TIA is often a precursor to a stroke."
   4. "A TIA generally occurs once and never occurs again."
2. A 35-year-old patient is being seen for complaints of headache, which she has experienced for the past month. Her health care provider wants to rule out a brain tumor. What diagnostic tests will be most helpful in formulating this diagnosis? *(Select all that apply.)*
   1. Brain scan
   2. PET scan
   3. Lumbar puncture
   4. Electroencephalography
   5. MRI
3. A nurse in the emergency department of her community hospital is teaching a group of high school students how to prevent head and spine injuries. What should the nurse include in the presentation? *(Select all that apply.)*
   1. Use helmets for bicycles, motorcycles, and skateboarding.
   2. Use helmets when participating in contact sports.
   3. Never drive or ride with someone under the influence of alcohol or drugs.
   4. Wear seatbelts and shoulder harnesses when driving or riding in a car.
   5. Avoid diving in water less than 6 feet deep.
4. A 70-year-old with back pain is scheduled to have a myelogram in the morning to rule out a pathologic condition of the spine. In preparing him for the procedure, what statement by the nurse is accurate?
   1. "We will be assessing your mental status frequently after the procedure."
   2. "You will need to lie completely supine and still during the procedure."
   3. "You will be able to ambulate immediately after the test."
   4. "We will ask you if you have any numbness or tingling in your legs after the procedure."
5. The nursing assessment of an 80-year-old who has had a stroke found that she had difficulty swallowing. A videofluoroscopy with barium was performed to rule out aspiration. The rehabilitation team in the skilled nursing facility determined that she can eat a soft diet with one-to-one supervision. Which action is important to prevent aspiration?
   1. Tipping the head toward the unaffected side while swallowing
   2. Extending the head during swallowing
   3. Mixing solids and liquids to facilitate swallowing
   4. Encouraging the patient to drink with a straw to make swallowing easier
6. A 12-year-old has a history of generalized tonic-clonic seizures. The nurse educates the patient and his family by including which teaching points?
   1. Most people feel normal immediately after the seizure.
   2. It is important to place a tongue blade in his mouth during the seizure.
   3. The tonic phase of the seizure usually lasts for 3 to 4 minutes.
   4. It is not uncommon to lose consciousness during this type of seizure.
7. A patient was involved in a snowmobile accident. On admission to the emergency department, he is receiving oxygen and is intubated. His Glasgow Coma Scale score is 6. About 10 minutes after arrival, he is noted to have a widened pulse pressure, increased systolic blood pressure, and bradycardia. Which finding indicates to the nurse that late-stage increased ICP is present? *(Select all that apply.)*
   1. Deepening respirations
   2. Supratentorial shift
   3. Cushing's response
   4. Medullary reflex
   5. Shallow respirations
8. A 76-year-old who has had Parkinson's disease for the past 6 years has now been admitted to a long-term care facility. The nurse doing the admission interview and assessment notices which characteristic sign of the disease? *(Select all that apply.)*
   1. Bradykinesia
   2. Increased postural reflexes
   3. Sensory loss
   4. Tremor
   5. Rigidity
9. A 13-year-old student is admitted to the pediatric unit with possible meningitis. The nurse finds that the patient cannot extend her legs completely without experiencing extreme pain. The nurse correctly documents this as which sign?
   1. Brudzinski's sign
   2. Battle's sign
   3. Kernig's sign
   4. Cosgrow's sign

10. A patient is diagnosed with Bell's palsy as indicated by a feeling of stiffness and a drawing sensation of the face. What is important to teach her about the disease?
    1. There is a heightened awareness of taste, so foods must be bland.
    2. There may be an increased sensitivity to sound.
    3. The eye is susceptible to injury if the eyelid does not close.
    4. Drooling from increased saliva on the affected side may occur.
11. The nurse is caring for a patient with a spinal cord injury who displays symptoms of autonomic dysreflexia. What intervention should the nurse implement first?
    1. Sit the patient upright, if permitted.
    2. Check for bladder distention.
    3. Give nitroprusside (Nipride) as ordered.
    4. Assess vital signs.
12. When teaching a patient with Parkinson's disease, which response would indicate the need for further education?
    1. "If I miss an occasional dose of the medication, it doesn't matter much."
    2. "I need to exercise at least some every day."
    3. "I need to be sitting straight up with my chin slightly tucked so I won't choke when I eat or drink."
    4. "I should eat a diet high in fiber and roughage to decrease my constipation."
13. The nurse is caring for a patient who suffered a cervical spinal cord injury. What injury can most likely be anticipated?
    1. Tetraplegia
    2. Hemiplegia
    3. Paraplegia
    4. Paresthesia
14. The nursing care plan for a patient with increased intracranial pressure will include what as the most therapeutic position for the patient?
    1. Keep the head of the bed flat.
    2. Maintain the head of the bed at 30 degrees.
    3. Increase the head of the bed's angle to 30 degrees with patient on left side.
    4. Use a continuous-rotation bed to continuously change patient position.
15. During admission of a patient with a severe head injury to the emergency department, what is the highest priority assessment for the nurse?
    1. Patency of airway
    2. Presence of a neck injury
    3. Neurologic status with the Glasgow Coma Scale
    4. Cerebrospinal fluid leakage from the ears or nose
16. When caring for a patient who has undergone a craniotomy, what is the primary nursing intervention?
    1. Preventing infection
    2. Ensuring patient comfort
    3. Avoiding need for secondary surgery
    4. Preventing increased intracranial pressure
17. A right-handed patient has right-sided hemiplegia and aphasia from a stroke. What is the most likely location of the lesion?
    1. Left frontal lobe
    2. Right brainstem
    3. Motor areas of the right cerebrum
    4. Medial superior area of the temporal lobe
18. A patient experiencing TIAs is scheduled for a carotid endarterectomy. The patient asks the nurse what this procedure is. The nurse correctly responds with which response?
    1. "This procedure promotes cerebral flow to decrease cerebral edema."
    2. "This procedure reduces the brain damage that occurs during a stroke."
    3. "This procedure helps prevent a stroke by removing atherosclerotic plaques obstructing cerebral blood flow."
    4. "This procedure provides a circulatory bypass around thrombotic plaques obstructing cranial circulation."
19. Which sign or symptom of late-stage increased intracranial pressure should the LPN/LVN be aware of? *(Select all that apply.)*
    1. Increase in systolic blood pressure
    2. Widening of pulse pressure
    3. Bradycardia
    4. Unequal pupils that react slowly to light
    5. Tachycardia
20. What nursing interventions should the nurse include in the plan of care for a patient who has had a stroke with right-sided hemiplegia and expressive aphasia? *(Select all that apply.)*
    1. Allow the patient ample time to verbalize his needs.
    2. Encourage self-help behaviors as much as possible, such as feeding.
    3. Monitor the patient's neurologic status once a day.
    4. Perform ROM to affected extremities every shift.
    5. Implement the use of a communication board for the patient to use as needed.
21. The nurse is caring for a patient with myasthenia gravis. The patient asks the nurse about the causes of the disease. Which response by the nurse is correct?
    1. "Myelin sheath breakdown has caused your myasthenia gravis."
    2. "Degeneration of the dopamine-producing neurons in the midbrain most commonly causes the disease."
    3. "Antibodies attacking the acetylcholine receptors, damaging them, and reducing their number is the most likely cause of myasthenia gravis."
    4. "Myasthenia gravis is usually caused by inflammation of cranial nerve VII."

22. A patient who has been experiencing recent seizure activity is preparing to have diagnostic testing performed. The health care provider has explained that the test will provide a graphic recording of the electrical conduction activities of the brain. The patient understands that which test will be performed?
    1. ECG
    2. MRI
    3. PET
    4. EEG
23. A patient has been diagnosed with Bell's palsy. This condition affects which cranial nerve?
    1. Cranial nerve V
    2. Cranial nerve VI
    3. Cranial nerve VII
    4. Cranial nerve VIII
24. When reviewing the medical plan of treatment for a patient with Guillain-Barré syndrome, which therapies are considered to be most therapeutic?
    1. Avonex and Betaseron
    2. Thymectomy and Zarontin
    3. Depakote and Zarontin
    4. Plasmapheresis and intravenous immune globulin
25. Which plan of care is considered beneficial for select patients who have experienced an ischemic stroke?
    1. IV edrophonium in the first 3 hours
    2. Anticholinesterase in the first 3 hours
    3. Thrombolytic such as tPA in the first 3 hours
    4. Intravenous immune globulin in the first 3 hours

55 Care of the Patient With an Immune Disorder

http://evolve.elsevier.com/Cooper/foundationsadult/

Objectives

1. Explain the concepts of immunocompetence, immunodeficiency, and autoimmunity.
2. Differentiate between natural and acquired immunity.
3. Compare and contrast humoral and cell-mediated immunity.
4. Review the mechanisms of immune response.
5. Discuss five factors that influence the development of hypersensitivity.
6. Identify the clinical manifestations of anaphylaxis.
7. Outline the immediate aggressive treatment of systemic anaphylactic reaction.
8. Discuss the two types of latex allergies and recommendations for preventing allergic reactions to latex in the workplace.
9. Discuss selection of blood donors, typing and cross-matching, storage, and administration in preventing transfusion reaction.
10. Explain an immunodeficiency disease.
11. Discuss the cause of autoimmune disorders.
12. Explain plasmapheresis in the treatment of autoimmune diseases.

Key Terms

adaptive immunity (ă-DĂP-tĭv ĭ-MŪ-nĭ-tē, p. 1930)
allergen (ĂL-ĕr-jĕn, p. 1931)
anaphylactic shock (ăn-ĕ-fĭ-lăk-tĭc, p. 1935)
antigen (ĂN-tĭ-jĕn, p. 1930)
attenuated (ă-TĔN-ū-āt-ĕd, p. 1933)
autoimmune (ăw-tō-ĭ-MŪN, p. 1934)
autologous (ăw-TŎL-ŏ-gĕs, p. 1939)
cellular immunity (SĔL-ū-lĕr ĭ-MŪ-nĭ-tē, p. 1931)
humoral immunity (HŪ-mŏr-ĕl ĭ-MŪ-nĭ-tē, p. 1931)
hypersensitivity (hī-pĕr-sĕn-sĭ-TĬV-ĭ-tē, p. 1934)
immunity (ĭ-MŪ-nĭ-tē, p. 1929)
immunization (ĭm-ū-nĭ-ZĀ-shŭn, p. 1931)
immunocompetence (ĭm-ū-nō-KŎM-pĕ-tĕns, p. 1929)
immunodeficiency (ĭm-ū-nō-dĕ-FĬSH-ĕn-sē, p. 1934)
immunogen (ĭm-Ū-nō-jĕn, p. 1931)
immunology (ĭm-ū-NŎL-ŏ-jē, p. 1929)
immunosuppressive (ĭm-ū-nō-sū-PRĔ-sĭv, p. 1939)
immunotherapy (ĭm-ū-nō-THĔR-ă-pē, p. 1933)
innate immunity (ĭ-NĀT ĭ-MŪ-nĭ-tē, p. 1929)
lymphokines (LĬM-fō-kīnz, p. 1930)
plasmapheresis (plăz-mă-fĕ-RĒ-sĭs, p. 1940)
proliferate (prō-lĭf-ĕ-RĀT, p. 1930)

NATURE OF IMMUNITY

The human body exists in an environment of antagonistic forces that constantly are attacking and threatening its integrity. In response to these onslaughts, the body exhibits a wide array of adaptations to protect against external and internal harmful agents. This chapter deals with those mechanisms.

The word *immune* is derived from the Latin word *immunis,* meaning "free from burden." Immunology is an evolving science that essentially deals with the body's ability to distinguish self from nonself. The body makes this distinction through a complex network of highly specialized cells and tissues that are collectively called the *immune system.* The immune system (also called the *host defense system*) is critical to our survival.

The immune system has three main functions (Lewis et al, 2017):

1. To protect the body's internal environment against invading microorganisms by destroying foreign antigens and pathogens, thus preventing the development of infections
2. To maintain homeostasis by removing damaged cells from the circulation, thereby maintaining the body's various cell types in an unchanged and uniform form
3. To serve as a surveillance network for recognizing and guarding against the development and growth of abnormal cells. Abnormal cells (mutations) are being formed constantly in the body but are recognized as abnormal cells and are destroyed

When the immune system responds appropriately to a foreign stimulus, the body's integrity is maintained; this is called *immunocompetence.*

Immunocompetence is the immune system's ability to mobilize and use its antibodies and other responses to stimulation by an antigen. If the immune response is too weak or too vigorous, homeostasis is disrupted, causing a malfunction in the system. This is called *immunoincompetence*. With disruption of the homeostatic balance of the immune system, a number of diseases develop. Examples of inappropriate immune responses can be classified into four categories:

1. Allergies
2. Immunodeficiency
3. Autoimmune disorders
4. Attacks on beneficial foreign tissue

Allergies are caused by hyperactive responses against environmental antigens. This would include medication allergies as well as allergies to allergens such as dust, mold, and pet dander. Immunodeficiency disorders include acquired immunodeficiency syndrome (AIDS), as well as therapy-induced immunodeficiency such as chemotherapeutic agents given for cancer and immunosuppressant medications given to prevent a reaction to organ transplantation. In addition, some individuals are born with immune deficiency disorders, in which the function or development of immune components is impaired (Fernandez, 2018). Autoimmune disorders include systemic lupus erythematosus, celiac disease, thyroid disease, inflammatory bowel disease, type 1 diabetes, multiple sclerosis, myasthenia gravis, psoriasis, rheumatoid arthritis, and many other common diseases. Attacks on beneficial foreign tissue include organ transplant rejection and transfusion reactions.

Immunity is the quality of being insusceptible to or unaffected by a particular disease or condition. Immunity has two major subclassifications: innate (natural) and adaptive (acquired) (Fig. 55.1). Innate immunity is nonspecific, whereas adaptive immunity is specific. The study of the immune system is **immunology.**

INNATE, OR NATURAL, IMMUNITY

The body's first line of defense, **innate immunity,** provides physical, mechanical, and chemical barriers to invading pathogens and protects against the external environment. The innate system includes intact skin and mucous membranes, cilia, stomach acid, tears, saliva, sebaceous glands, and secretions and flora of the intestine and vagina. These organs, tissues, and secretions provide biochemical and physical barriers to disease. The first line of defense provides nonspecific immunity to the individual (Table 55.1).

The nonspecific response of phagocytes, such as neutrophils and macrophages, as well as the response of lymphocytes are also part of innate or natural immunity to disease. Macrophages include any phagocytic cell involved in defense against infection. When organisms pass the epithelial barriers, phagocytes become activated. Phagocytes also migrate through the bloodstream to the tissues for the body's second line of defense against disease. Phagocytes engulf and destroy microorganisms that pass the skin and mucous

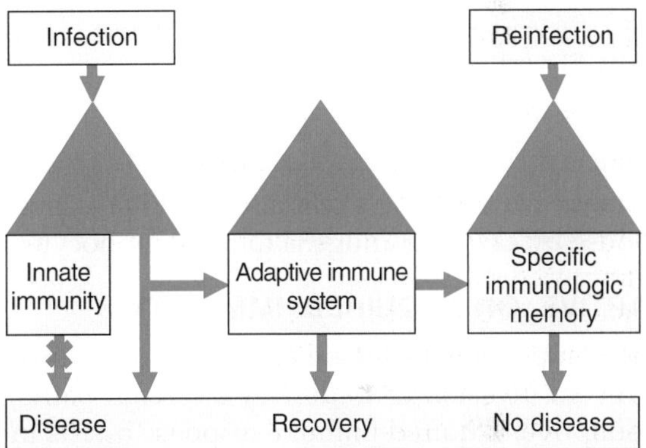

Fig. 55.1 When an infectious agent enters the body, it first encounters elements of the innate immune system. These may be sufficient to prevent disease; if not, a disease will result and the adaptive immune system is activated. The adaptive immune system helps the patient recover from the disease and establishes a specific immunologic memory. When the patient is exposed to the infectious agent a second time, his or her body is able to fight the disease, resulting in no illness developing with this exposure. The individual has acquired immunity to the infectious agent.

Table 55.1 Innate (Natural) and Adaptive (Acquired) Immunity

CHARACTERISTICS	INNATE (NATURAL)	ADAPTIVE (ACQUIRED)
Physical barriers	Physical defense: Skin and mucous membranes Mucous membranes line body cavities such as the mouth and stomach. These cavities secrete chemicals (saliva and hydrochloric acid) that destroy bacteria. Cilia, tears, and flora of the intestine and vagina also provide natural protection	None
Response mechanisms	Nonspecific: Mononuclear phagocytic system; inflammatory response	Specific immune response: Humoral immunity, cellular immunity
Soluble factors	Chemical defense: Lysozyme, complement, acute-phase proteins, interferon	Antibodies, lymphokines
Cells	Phagocytes, natural killer (NK) cells	T cells, B cells
Specificity	None	Present
Memory	None	Present

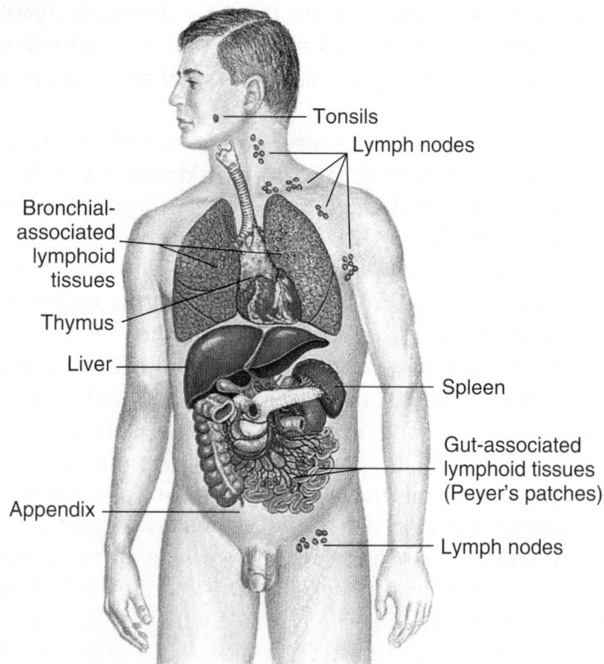

Fig. 55.2 Organization of the immune system. (From Grimes D: *Infectious diseases.* St. Louis, 1991, Mosby.)

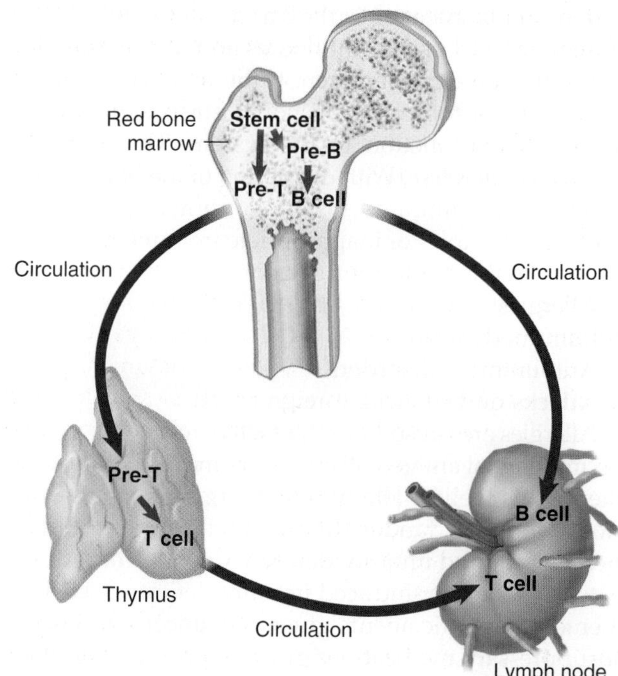

Fig. 55.3 Origin and processing of B and T cells. B and T cells originate in red bone marrow. B cells are processed in the red marrow, whereas T cells are processed in the thymus. Both cell types circulate to other lymph tissues. B cells produce antibodies to destroy specific foreign antigens (humoral immunity). T cells attack and destroy antigens (cell-mediated immunity). (From Patton KT, Thibodeau GA: *Anatomy and physiology,* ed 10, St. Louis, 2019, Elsevier.)

membrane barriers. These cells also assist in the immune response by carrying antigens to the lymphocytes.

ADAPTIVE, OR ACQUIRED, IMMUNITY

If the components of innate or natural immunity fail to prevent invasion or to destroy a foreign pathogen, the adaptive, acquired immune response assists in the battle. This is the body's second line of defense against disease. **Adaptive immunity** provides a specific reaction to each invading antigen and has the unique ability to remember the antigen that caused the attack. The adaptive immune system is composed of highly specialized cells and tissues, including the thymus, the spleen, bone marrow, blood, and lymph (Fig. 55.2). Adaptive immunity includes humoral and cell-mediated immunity. The adaptive immune system's specificity results from the production of antibodies in the cells. Antibodies develop naturally after infection or artificially after vaccinations (Box 55.1).

Box 55.1 Types of Acquired Immunity

ACTIVE	PASSIVE
Natural immunity: Results from exposure to the infectious agent	*Natural immunity:* Results from the passage of maternal antibodies from mother to child
Artificial immunity: Results from immunization or vaccination with an antigen	*Artificial immunity:* Results from the injection of antibodies from other sources

Lymphocytes include the T and B cells (Fig. 55.3) and the large, granular lymphocytes also known as natural killer (or NK) cells. Approximately 70% to 80% of the lymphocytes are T cell lymphocytes. When activated, T cells release compounds called *lymphokines.* **Lymphokines** attract macrophages to the site of infection or inflammation and prepares them for attack. T cells cooperate with the B cells to produce antibodies but do not produce antibodies themselves. T cells are responsible for cell-mediated immunity and protect the body against viruses, bacteria, fungi, and parasites. T cells also provide protection in allografts (transfer of tissue between two genetically dissimilar individuals of the same species) and against malignant cells.

B cells make up approximately 20% to 30% of the lymphocyte population. B cells trigger the production of antibodies and **proliferate** (increase in number) in response to a particular **antigen** (a substance recognized by the body as foreign and that can trigger an immune response). An antigen is usually a protein that causes the formation of an antibody and reacts specifically with that antibody. B cells migrate to the peripheral circulation and tissues and eventually are filtered from the lymph and stored in the lymphoid tissue of the body.

The initial formation of B cells does not require antigen stimulation or any other environmental stimulus. However, B cell proliferation depends on antigen stimulation. B cells are responsible for humoral immunity. B cells produce antibodies and protect against bacteria, viruses, and soluble antigens.

HUMORAL IMMUNITY

Humoral immunity (a form of immunity that responds to antigens) is mediated by the B cells. B cells produce antibodies in response to antigen challenge. On first exposure to a given antigen, a primary humoral response is initiated. This response is generally slow compared with subsequent antigen exposures. When a second exposure occurs, memory B cells cause a quick response, regardless of whether the first exposure was to an antigen or to immunization. **Immunization** is a process by which resistance to an infectious disease is induced or increased.

T lymphocytes can be categorized into T-helper (CD4) and T-suppressor (CD8) cells. T-helper cells coordinate the immune response by activating phagocytes and other T cells, and by stimulating B cells to produce antibodies (National Institute of Allergy and Infectious Diseases, 2008). T-suppressor cells maintain the humoral response at a level appropriate for the stimulus.

Antibodies produced by one's own body are said to provide active immunity. Active immunity develops as the body defends itself from the presence of an active infection or results from immunizations against an antigen. In contrast, temporary, or passive, immunity is provided by antibodies that are formed by one person in response to a specific antigen and administered to another person. Passive immunity can occur as antibodies pass through the placenta or through breast milk. Other examples of passive immunity include antivenom given after a snake bite and immunoglobulin administered after exposure to prevent infection (CDC, 2017).

Even though humoral immunity is mediated by the B cell population, T-helper cells and T-suppressor cells are vital to the immunocompetent person. Immunocompetence is the ability of an immune system to mobilize and deploy its antibodies and other responses after stimulation by an antigen. The number and functions of the T-helper cells and T-suppressor cells help determine the strength and persistence of an immune response. The normal ratio of T-helper cells to T-suppressor cells in the body is 2:1 (Ignatavicius and Workman, 2016). When this ratio is disrupted, autoimmune and immunodeficiency diseases occur. Many factors can weaken the immune response, including the aging process, viruses, radiation, and chemotherapeutic drugs. Anxiety, stress, and loneliness also affect the immune response as does lack of sleep and a lack of key nutrients.

Exposure to antigen and response with antibody may activate either the complement system or an antigen-antibody reaction:

Complement system: One of 25 complex enzyme serum proteins that together compose a system that breaks down bacteria and releases lysosomes to destroy bacteria.

Antigen-antibody reaction: The antigen-antibody reaction results in mast cells releasing histamine, which produces the symptoms of allergy. When symptoms of allergy occur, the antigen is referred to as an **allergen** (a substance that can produce a hypersensitivity reaction in the body but may not be inherently harmful). When immunity results, the antigen is referred to as an **immunogen** (any agent or substance capable of provoking an immune response or producing immunity).

CELLULAR IMMUNITY

Cellular immunity, also called *cell-mediated immunity,* is the mechanism of acquired immunity characterized by the dominant role of T cells. Cell-mediated immunity results when T cells are activated by an antigen. Whole cells become sensitized in a process similar to that which stimulates the B cells to form antibodies. Once these T cells have been sensitized, they are released into the blood and body tissues, where they remain indefinitely. On contact with the antigen to which they are sensitized, they attach to the organism and destroy it. Cellular immunity is involved in resistance to infectious diseases caused by viruses and some bacteria.

Cellular immunity is of primary importance in immunity against pathogens that survive inside cells, including viruses and some bacteria (e.g., *Mycobacterium* organisms), immunity against fungal infections, and tumor immunity. However, cellular immunity also can have negative effects, including rejection of transplanted tissues, contact hypersensitivity reactions, and certain autoimmune diseases (Box 55.2). Hypersensitivity reactions are cell-mediated responses of the body (Box 55.3).

COMPLEMENT SYSTEM

The word *complement* became part of the terminology of immunology at the turn of the 19th century, when researchers recognized that blood plasma contained a substance necessary to complete the destruction of bacteria. The complement system includes approximately 25 serum enzymatic proteins that interact with one another and with other components of the innate (natural) and adaptive (acquired) arms of the immune system. Normally, complement enzymes are inactive in plasma and body fluids. When an antigen and antibody interact, the complement system is activated. The complement system functions in a "step-by-step" series much like the clotting mechanism (see Chapter 47), but with a different purpose (Ignatavicius and Workman, 2016). The complement system can destroy the cell membrane of many bacterial species, and this action attracts phagocytes to the area.

Box 55.2 The Four Rs of the Immune Response

- *Recognize self from nonself:* Normally the body recognizes its own cells and does not produce antibodies to fight those cells; therefore an immune response generally is triggered only in response to agents that the body identifies as foreign. Autoimmune disorders disrupt the ability to differentiate self from nonself, and the immune system attacks the body's own cells as if they were foreign antigens.
- *Respond to nonself invaders:* The immune system responds by producing antibodies that target specific antigens for destruction. New antibodies are produced in response to new antigens. Deficits in the ability to respond may be the result of immunodeficiency disorders.
- *Remember the invader:* The ability to remember antigens that invaded the body in the past allows a quicker response if subsequent invasion by the same antigen occurs.
- *Regulate its action:* Self-regulation allows the immune system to monitor itself by "turning on" when an antigen invades and "turning off" when the invasion has been eradicated. Regulation prevents the destruction of healthy or host tissue. The inability to regulate could result in a chronic inflammation and damage to the host tissue.

GENETIC CONTROL OF IMMUNITY

The genetic role in immunity is currently a subject of intense research. A genetic link exists to well-developed immune systems and poorly developed or compromised immune systems. In addition, researchers are finding that genes responsible for immune function are different in middle age from genes responsible for immune function in early adulthood (Felix et al, 2012).

EFFECTS OF NORMAL AGING ON THE IMMUNE SYSTEM

With advancing age, there is a decline in the immune system (Fagundes et al, 2012; Kalokerinos et al, 2014). Decreased immune function may be responsible for the increased incidence of cancer, infections, and autoimmune disorders seen in older adults (National Library of Medicine [NLM], 2018). Older adults are also more susceptible to infections (such as influenza and pneumonia) from pathogens that they were relatively immunocompetent against earlier in life.

Aging does not affect all aspects of the immune system. The bone marrow is relatively unaffected by increasing age. However, aging has a pronounced effect on the thymus, which decreases in size and activity (Micans, 2017). T and B cells show deficiencies in activation, transit time through the cell cycle, and subsequent differentiation, but the most significant alterations seem to involve T cells (Salam et al, 2013). As thymic output of T cells diminishes, the differentiation of T cells in peripheral lymphoid structures increases. Consequently, there is an accumulation of memory cells rather than new precursor cells responsive to previously unencountered antigens.

Delayed hypersensitivity response, as determined by skin testing with injected antigens, is frequently decreased or absent in older adults. The clinical consequences of a decline in cell-mediated immunity are evident. Older adults have an increased risk of death from cancer (see the Lifespan Considerations box).

Box 55.3 Review of Mechanisms of the Immune Response

- The skin and mucous membranes are natural barriers to infectious agents. When these barriers are crossed, the immune response is triggered in the immunocompetent host.
- The first time an antigen enters the body, the antigen is processed by macrophages and presented to lymphocytes. Responses of B cells to the antigen in humoral immunity require interaction with T-helper cells, which assist B cells to respond to the antigen by proliferating, synthesizing, and secreting the appropriate antibody. Antigens then are neutralized by antibodies or can form immune complexes or be phagocytosed by macrophages or neutrophils.
- Humoral immunity responds to antigens such as bacteria and foreign tissue. Humoral immunity is the result of the development and continuing presence of circulating antibodies in the plasma. Humoral immunity consists of antibody-mediated immunity. *Humoral* means body fluid, and antibodies are proteins found in plasma. Therefore the term *humoral immunity* Cellular immunity is the primary defense against intracellular organisms, including viruses and some bacteria (e.g., mycobacteria).
- In cellular immunity the antigen is processed by macrophages and recognized by T cells. T cells produce lymphokines, which further attract macrophages and neutrophils to the site for phagocytosis, or cytotoxic killer T cells can respond directly.
- Immunodeficiency is an abnormal condition of the immune system in which cellular or humoral immunity is inadequate and resistance to infection is decreased. The immunodeficiency diseases sometimes are classified as B cell (antibody) deficiencies, T cell (cellular) deficiencies, and combined T and B cell deficiencies.
- Hypersensitivity reaction is an inappropriate and excessive response of the immune system to a sensitizing antigen. In hypersensitivity reactions, the antigen is an allergen. Humoral reactions, such as anaphylactic hypersensitivity, are immediate. Cellular reactions are delayed reactions. Examples of delayed reactions include contact dermatitis, tissue transplant rejection, and sarcoidosis (Ignatavicius and Workman, 2016).

Lifespan Considerations

Older Adults

Immune Disorder

- Older adults are at increased risk for inflammation and infections resulting from changes in natural defense mechanisms.
- Pathogens are able to enter through breaks in fragile, dry skin, increasing the risk of skin infections.
- Decreased movement of respiratory secretions increases the risk of respiratory tract infections.
- Decreased production of saliva and gastric secretions increases the risk of gastrointestinal infections.
- Decreased tear production increases the risk of eye inflammation and infections.
- Structural changes in the urinary system that lead to urinary retention or stasis increase the risk of urinary tract infection.
- Signs and symptoms of infection tend to be more subtle than those in younger individuals. Because older adults have decreased body temperature, fever may be more difficult to detect. Changes in behavior such as lethargy, fatigue, disorientation, irritability, and loss of appetite may be early signs of infection.
- Immune system functioning declines with advanced age. Research is continuing.
- The older adult's immune system continues to produce antibodies; therefore immunization for diseases such as pneumonia and influenza is recommended.
- Older adults who have chronic illnesses are generally at increased risk for infection.
- Medications commonly taken by the elderly such as antidepressants, statin drugs for elevated cholesterol, proton pump inhibitors for heartburn, and steroids also can reduce the immune system response.

IMMUNE RESPONSE

There are two ways of helping the body to develop immunity: immunization and **immunotherapy.** The theory behind immunization is that controlled exposure to a disease-producing pathogen develops antibodies while preventing disease. The first immunization is credited to Edward Jenner, who observed that individuals who had had cowpox became immune to the disease. The idea of administering "attenuated [weakened] microbes" developed, and the scientific approach was applied by Louis Pasteur. Vaccines and toxoids are altered, or **attenuated** (the process of weakening the virulence of a disease organism), to reduce their power without affecting their ability to stimulate the production of antibodies. After immunization the immune system mounts a greater response to a second encounter with an antigen. The vaccine, or toxoid, stimulates humoral immunity, which provides protection from disease for months to years.

The Centers for Disease Control and Prevention (2018) recommend the following immunizations for adults with no contraindications:

- Influenza vaccine every year
- Tetanus, diphtheria (Td) vaccine every 10 years; Tetanus, diphtheria, and pertussis (Tdap) once after age 19
- Varicella vaccine: two doses if there is no evidence of immunity to varicella
- Human papilloma vaccination (HPV) for women 19 to 26 years of age; three doses if not previously vaccinated
- Human papilloma vaccination (HPV) for men 19 to 21 years of age; three doses if not previously vaccinated. If having sex with men, vaccine should be given for men ages 19 to 26 years if not previously vaccinated.
- Herpes zoster: two doses adults aged 50 and older
- Measles, mumps, and rubella (MMR): two doses if there is no evidence of immunity
- Pneumococcal 13 (PCV13): one dose
- Pneumococcal 23 (PCV23): one to three doses depending on indication. One dose is required after the age of 65
- Hepatitis A: two to three doses if at risk for hepatitis A for persons 1 year and older
- Hepatitis B—three doses if at risk for hepatitis B available for all age groups
- Meningococcal—one or more doses if at risk for meningitis available beginning at age 11 to 12 years
- *Haemophilus influenza* type B—to one to three doses if at risk for *Haemophilus influenza* type B available for children under the age of 5 years and for older children and adults who have qualifying medical conditions

Immunotherapy is a special treatment of allergic responses wherein the patient receives doses of the offending allergens over a period of 1 to 3 years to develop immunity gradually. Immunotherapy consists of injecting a person with a very diluted antigen (allergen) to which the patient has a type I hypersensitivity. The strength of the dilution is increased weekly until a maintenance dosage is reached. The theory is that immunotherapy assists the individual in building tolerance to the allergen without developing fever or increased signs and symptoms. *Desensitization* is another term used for immunotherapy. It is indicated for patients with clinically significant disease for whom avoidance of the allergen or treatment with medication is inadequate. It is considered safe in properly selected patients but is a lengthy, expensive process with a potential for severe anaphylaxis.

Immunotherapy may be administered during the allergy season, before allergy season, or year-round (perennial). Perennial therapy is most widely accepted because it allows for a higher cumulative dose, which produces a better effect. Perennial therapy usually begins with a very diluted dose of the allergen that is increased progressively each week over the course of up to 18 weeks or more. Immunotherapy is administered subcutaneously. The patient should be observed for at least 20 minutes after administration because a hypersensitivity reaction or anaphylaxis may occur. In the event of anaphylaxis during immunotherapy, the treatment protocol includes the administration of epinephrine chloride given subcutaneously.

Most patients begin immunotherapy at the health care provider's office on a weekly basis. Home administration by the patient or a family member is acceptable once the maintenance level is reached, which often takes 1 to 2 years. Some patients may require immunotherapy for up to 5 years. Interrupted regimens because of illness may place the patient at risk for reaction. Consult the health care provider before administering a dose of diluted allergen if the patient's maintenance immunotherapy was interrupted by illness or other factors.

DISORDERS OF THE IMMUNE SYSTEM

Immune system failure occurs in several ways and expresses itself in mild to severe form. The system can malfunction at many points while attempting to provide the body with protective defense. Failures may be the result of genetic factors, developmental defects, infection, malignancy, injury, drugs, or altered metabolic states.

The severity of altered immune response disorders ranges from mild to chronic to life threatening. The disorders are categorized as follows:

1. **Hypersensitivity** disorder involves allergic response and tissue rejection.
2. **Immunodeficiency** disease involves altered and failed immune response.
3. **Autoimmune** disease involves extensive tissue damage resulting from an immune system that seemingly reverses its function to one of self-destruction.

See Box 55.2 for the four *R*s of the immune response.

HYPERSENSITIVITY DISORDERS

Etiology and Pathophysiology

Hypersensitivity is characterized by an excessive reaction to a particular stimulus. A hypersensitivity reaction is an inappropriate and excessive response of the immune system to a sensitizing antigen. Hypersensitivity disorders arise when harmless substances, such as pollens, danders, foods, and chemicals, are recognized as foreign. The body mounts an immune response in much the same way it does to any foreign protein. The host becomes sensitive after the first exposure and on subsequent exposure exhibits a hypersensitivity reaction. Chronic exposure leads to a chronic allergy response, which ranges from mild to incapacitating signs and symptoms.

Hypersensitivity disorders are believed to be caused by a genetic defect that allows increased production of immunoglobulin E (IgE) with release of histamine and other mediators from mast cells and basophils (Buelow and Routes, 2015). Humoral reactions, mediated by the circulating B lymphocytes, are immediate. Cellular reactions, mediated by the T lymphocytes, are delayed hypersensitivity reactions. Exposure to antigen may occur by inhalation, ingestion, injection, or touch (contact). Signs and symptoms caused by histamine release include vasodilation, edema, bronchoconstriction, mucus secretion, and pruritus. Hypersensitivity reactions may be local (gastrointestinal, skin, respiratory, conjunctival) or systemic (anaphylaxis). The exact mechanism and pathway of these inflammatory responses are not clearly understood.

A combination of interrelated factors increases the severity of symptoms (Box 55.4). Disorders that result from hypersensitivity, which are discussed in other chapters, include urticaria, angioedema, allergic rhinitis, allergic conjunctivitis (hay fever), atopic dermatitis, and asthma. Many cases of asthma are attributed to an allergic response to a specific allergen.

Box 55.4 Factors Influencing Hypersensitivity

- *Host response to allergen:* The more sensitive the individual, the greater the allergic response.
- *Exposure amount:* In general, the more allergen the individual is exposed to, the greater the chance of a severe reaction.
- *Nature of the allergen:* Most allergic reactions are precipitated by complex, high-molecular-weight protein substances.
- *Route of allergen entry:* Most allergens enter the body via gastrointestinal and respiratory routes. Exposure to venoms through bites or stings and injectable medications present a more severe threat of allergic response.
- *Repeated exposure:* In general, the more often the individual is exposed to the allergen, the greater the response.

Assessment

Assessment should involve predominantly the integumentary, gastrointestinal, respiratory, and cardiovascular systems. Be aware of the seasonal nature of the complaints.

Subjective data include pruritus, nausea, and uneasiness.

Objective data include sneezing, excessive nasal secretions, lacrimation, inflamed nasal membranes, skin rash or areas of raised inflammation, diarrhea, cough, wheezes, impaired breathing, and hypotension.

Hypersensitivity illnesses are diagnosed largely through patient history and physical examination. The most important diagnostic tool is a detailed history, including the following:

1. Onset, nature, and progression of signs and symptoms
2. Aggravating and alleviating factors
3. Frequency and duration of signs and symptoms

Assess environmental, household, and occupational factors. Common offenders include pollens, spores, dusts, food, drugs, and insect venoms. Many but not all offenders are seasonal. Signs and symptoms generally vary from mild upper respiratory tract manifestations, such as sneezing and excessive nasal secretions, to watery, itching eyes. Skin signs and symptoms are often eczema-like or urticarial (hives). Diarrhea may be a gastrointestinal complaint in some individuals. More severe signs and symptoms include those of the lower respiratory tract, such as coughing, wheezing, chest discomfort, breathing difficulties, and shock, which could be followed by cardiovascular collapse and respiratory arrest. The complete history assists in an accurate diagnosis (see the Health Promotion box).

Health Promotion

Assessing the Patient With Allergies

- Obtain a comprehensive history that covers family allergies, past and present allergies, and social and environmental factors, especially the physical environment.
- Identify the allergens that may have triggered a reaction.
- Determine the time of year that an allergic reaction occurs as a clue to a seasonal allergen.
- Obtain information about any over-the-counter or prescription medications used to treat allergies.
- In addition to identification of the allergen, find out about the clinical manifestations and course of allergic reaction.
- Ask about pets, trees, and plants on the property; air pollutants; and floor coverings, houseplants, and cooling and heating systems in the home and workplace.
- Have the patient keep a daily or weekly food diary with a description of any untoward reactions.
- Screen for any reaction to medication.
- Review questions about the patient's lifestyle and stress level in connection with allergic symptoms.

The physical examination should include a thorough assessment of the skin, the middle ear, the conjunctiva, the naso-oropharynx, and the lungs.

Diagnostic Tests

Laboratory studies are usually not necessary unless allergic signs and symptoms are severe or last an extended amount of time. A complete blood count with differential to identify the type of white blood cells that are elevated, skin testing, total serum IgE levels, and a specific IgE level for a particular allergen may be ordered. The latter test is called a *radioallergosorbent test* (RAST).

Medical Management

Treatment of hypersensitivity disorders includes the following:

- Symptom management with medications
- Environmental control
- Immunotherapy

The most effective treatment is environmental control, which includes avoidance of the offending allergen. Pollens are seasonal and can be avoided at season peaks with air conditioning and limited time spent outdoors. Mold spores can be reduced by maintaining dry conditions and using air filters. House dust can be controlled by damp dusting, use of air filters, and decreased use of carpet and overstuffed furniture. Most other offending allergens (e.g., food, drugs, chemicals, and stinging insects) should be avoided if possible.

Medications are used to treat and alleviate signs and symptoms. Antihistamines compete with histamine by attaching to the cell surface receptors and blocking histamine release. Antihistamines therefore must be initiated soon after exposure or taken on a regular basis. Drowsiness, mucous membrane dryness, and occasionally central nervous system excitation are side effects of some antihistamines. Examples of these include pseudoephedrine (Actifed), diphenhydramine (Benadryl), chlorpheniramine (Chlor-Trimeton), and brompheniramine (Brovex). Nonsedating antihistamines include cetirizine (Zyrtec), loratadine (Claritin), and fexofenadine (Allegra). The nonsedating antihistamines are more desirable for those who experience drowsiness with antihistamine use (Table 55.2).

Leukotriene inhibitors are agents that significantly reduce symptoms of an allergic reaction caused by the release of leukotrienes from mast cells and basophils. Three are currently available in the United States: montelukast (Singulair) and zafirlukast (Accolate) act as leukotriene receptor blockers, and zileuton (Zyflo) inhibits the production of leukotrienes.

Patient Problems

Patient problems for patients with hypersensitivity include the following:

1. *Potential for Injury, related to exposure to allergen*
2. *Inability to Tolerate Activity, related to malaise*
3. *Potential for Infection, related to inflammation of protective mucous membranes*

Patient Teaching

Patient teaching should revolve around the specific diagnosis. Advise the patient with seasonal allergies to avoid offending allergens and ensure that he or she understands the therapeutic medication plan. Focus on health promotion and health teaching for self-care management (see the Safety Alert box).

ANAPHYLAXIS

Etiology and Pathophysiology

The most severe IgE-mediated allergic reaction is anaphylaxis, or systemic reaction to allergens. Anaphylaxis, or **anaphylactic shock,** is an acute and potentially fatal hypersensitivity (allergic) reaction to an allergen. Allergens that cause anaphylaxis include the following:

- Venoms
- Drugs, such as penicillin and aspirin

Table 55.2 Medications for Hypersensitivity Reactions

GENERIC NAME (TRADE NAME)	ACTION	SIDE EFFECTS	NURSING IMPLICATIONS
dexamethasone	Corticosteroid	Anxiety, nausea, acne, easy bruising, increased appetite	Do not use for extended period; use cautiously with patients with diabetes or peptic ulcers
diphenhydramine (Benadryl)	Antihistamine	Drowsiness, confusion, nasal stuffiness, dry mouth, photosensitivity, urine retention	Use cautiously with central nervous system depressants, including alcohol; tell patient to avoid driving or hazardous activity because of drowsiness
epinephrine (Epinephrine chloride, EpiPen)	Alpha-adrenergic agonist and beta-adrenergic agonist	Nervousness, tremor, headache, hypertension, tachycardia, ventricular fibrillation, stroke	Do not use with monoamine oxidase inhibitor; use cautiously in patients with hyperthyroidism, hypertension, diabetes, and heart disease
fexofenadine (Allegra)	Nonsedating antihistamine	Headache, drowsiness, blurred vision, hypotension, bradycardia, tachycardia, dysrhythmias (rare), urinary retention	Same as for loratadine
flunisolide	Corticosteroid (inhaled)	Headache, transient nasal burning, epistaxis, nausea, vomiting	Not effective for acute episodes; use regularly; teach care and cleaning of inhaler; if symptoms do not improve in 3 wk, consult health care provider
loratadine (Claritin)	Nonsedating antihistamine	Dry mouth, headache, red and irritated eyes	Store in tight container at room temperature. Teach patient and family to avoid driving or other hazardous activities if drowsiness occurs

Safety Alert

Treating the Patient With a Hypersensitivity Reaction

- List all of the patient's allergies on the chart, the nursing care plan, and the medication record.
- After an allergic disorder is diagnosed, therapeutic treatment is aimed at reducing exposure to the offending allergen; treating the symptoms; and, if necessary, desensitizing the person through immunotherapy.
- All health care workers must be prepared for the rare but life-threatening anaphylactic reaction, which requires immediate medical and nursing interventions.
- Instruct the patient to wear a medical alert bracelet listing the particular drug allergy.
- For a patient allergic to insect stings, commercial bee sting kits containing epinephrine and a tourniquet are available. Teach the patient to apply the tourniquet and self-inject the subcutaneous epinephrine. The patient should wear a medical-alert bracelet and carry a bee sting kit whenever he or she goes outdoors.

- Contrast media dyes
- Insect stings (such as bees and wasps)
- Foods such as eggs, shellfish, and peanuts
- Latex
- Vaccines

The hypersensitivity reaction results in a sudden severe vasodilation as a consequence of the release of certain chemical mediators from mast cells. Vasodilation causes an increase in capillary permeability, which causes fluid to seep into the interstitial space from the vascular space.

Clinical Manifestations

In anaphylaxis, the reaction occurs rapidly after exposure, from seconds to a few minutes. A massive release of mediators initiates events in target organs throughout the body. Skin and gastrointestinal signs and symptoms may occur, although respiratory and cardiovascular signs and symptoms predominate. Fatal reactions are associated with a fall in blood pressure, laryngeal edema, and bronchospasm, leading to cardiovascular collapse, myocardial infarction, and respiratory failure. Anaphylactic reactions are classified as mild, moderate, and severe.

Assessment

Early recognition of signs and symptoms and early treatment may prevent severe reactions and even death. In general, the more rapid the onset, the more severe the outcome is. The patient may have a feeling of uneasiness that increases to a sense of severe apprehension, and then a fear of impending death. The skin may or may not be involved. Urticaria, pruritus, and angioedema may be present in mild and moderate anaphylaxis, whereas cyanosis and pallor may be seen in severe reactions. Upper respiratory signs and symptoms range from congestion and sneezing to edema of the lips, the tongue, and the larynx with stridor and occlusion of the upper airways. Lower respiratory signs and symptoms occur soon thereafter and include bronchospasm, wheezing, and severe dyspnea. Gastrointestinal signs and symptoms increase from nausea, vomiting, and diarrhea to dysphagia and involuntary stools. The patient may have cardiovascular signs and symptoms, such as tachycardia and hypotension. Signs and symptoms may worsen, and the patient may display coronary insufficiency, vascular collapse, dysrhythmias, shock, cardiac arrest, respiratory failure, and death.

Medical Management

Immediate aggressive treatment is the goal in anaphylaxis. At the first sign, the prescribed dose of epinephrine 1:1000 is given subcutaneously for mild symptoms. It may be repeated at 5- to 20-minute intervals as prescribed by the health care provider. Epinephrine produces bronchodilation and vasoconstriction and inhibits the further release of chemical mediators of hypersensitivity reactions from mast cells. The effects of epinephrine take only a few minutes. Epinephrine 1:10,000 at 5- to 10-minute intervals may be administered intramuscularly or intravenously for a severe reaction as prescribed by the health care provider. Diphenhydramine 50 to 100 mg may be given intramuscularly or intravenously as indicated for allergic signs and symptoms. If moderate to severe signs and symptoms occur, IV therapy with volume expanders and vasopressor agents such as dopamine (Intropin) may be initiated to prevent vascular collapse, and the patient may be intubated to prevent airway obstruction. Oxygen may be administered by nonrebreather mask. Intubation or a tracheostomy may be required for oxygen delivery if progressive hypoxia exists. Place the patient in a recumbent position, elevate the legs, and keep the patient warm.

Nursing Interventions and Patient Teaching

Nursing interventions begin by assessing respiratory status, including dyspnea, wheezing, and decreased breath sounds. Also assess circulatory status, including dysrhythmias, tachycardia, and hypotension. Monitor vital signs continually. Other assessments include (1) intake and output (I&O); (2) mental status, including anxiety, malaise, confusion, and coma; (3) skin status, including erythema, urticaria, cyanosis, and pallor; and (4) gastrointestinal status, including nausea, vomiting, diarrhea, and incontinence.

The diagnosis most often is made by a history of signs and symptoms. Looking at and listening to the anxious patient should be leading clues in suspecting anaphylaxis. Question the patient about recent exposure to known antigens that cause anaphylaxis (Box 55.5). Most laboratory studies are not beneficial.

A patient problem and interventions for the patient with anaphylaxis include but are not limited to the following:

Patient Problem	Nursing Interventions
Inability to Maintain Adequate Breathing Pattern, related to: • Edema • Bronchospasm • Increased secretions	Maintain airway Administer high-flow oxygen via nonrebreather mask Endotracheal intubation or a tracheostomy will be established for oxygen delivery if progressive hypoxia exists Administer prescribed medications Keep the patient warm Monitor vital signs Suction if necessary Anticipate intubation with severe respiratory distress

Reassure the patient during procedures. After the event, teach the patient about avoidance of the allergen, advise him or her to wear or carry medical alert identification, and teach the patient to prepare and administer epinephrine subcutaneously.

Prognosis

If the signs and symptoms are left untreated, anaphylaxis can lead to death in a relatively short time.

LATEX ALLERGIES

Allergy to latex products has become an increasing problem, affecting patients and health care professionals. The increase in allergic reactions coincided with the sharp increase in glove use after the introduction of universal precautions against infectious diseases in 1992 when the Occupational Safety and Health Administration (OSHA) mandated universal bloodborne pathogen precautions and the use of gloves by health care workers. It is estimated that 8% to 17% of health care workers regularly exposed to latex are sensitized (American Latex Allergy Association, 2018). The more frequent and prolonged the exposure, the greater the likelihood of developing a latex allergy. In addition to gloves, latex-containing products used in health care may include blood pressure cuffs, stethoscopes, tourniquets, IV tubing, syringes, electrode pads, oxygen masks,

Box 55.5 Common Allergens Causing Anaphylaxis

DRUGS	VENOMS	FOODS
Vaccines	Honeybees	Cow's milk
Allergen extracts	Wasps	Peanuts
Enzymes	Hornets	Brazil nuts
Penicillins		Cashew nuts
Sulfonamides		Shellfish
Cephalosporins		Egg albumin
Dextrans		Strawberries
Hormones		Chocolate
Contrast media		Soy
Anesthetic agents		

tracheal tubes, colostomy and ileostomy pouches, urinary catheters, anesthetic masks, and adhesive tape.

Latex proteins can become aerosolized through powder on gloves and can result in serious reactions when inhaled by sensitized individuals; therefore all health care agencies are advised to use powder-free gloves. Certain food proteins are similar to some proteins in rubber; therefore an allergic reaction to latex also may result in an allergic reaction to some foods. Bananas, avocados, kiwi fruit, tomatoes, apples, chestnuts, and melons are common foods to result in an allergy if one is allergic to latex (American College of Asthma, Allergy and Immunology, 2014).

Types of Latex Allergies

Two types of latex allergies that can occur are type IV allergic contact dermatitis and type I allergic reactions. Type IV contact dermatitis is caused by the chemicals used in the manufacturing of latex gloves. It is a delayed reaction that occurs within 6 to 48 hours. Typically the person first has dryness, pruritus, fissuring, and cracking of the skin, followed by erythema, edema, and crusting at 24 to 48 hours. Chronic exposure can lead to thickening and hardening of the skin, scaling, and hyperpigmentation. The dermatitis may extend beyond the area of physical contact with the allergen.

A type I allergic reaction is a response to the natural rubber latex proteins and occurs within minutes of contact with the proteins. These types of allergic reactions can range from skin erythema, urticaria, rhinitis, conjunctivitis, or asthma to full-blown anaphylactic shock. Systemic reactions to latex may result from exposure to protein via various routes, including the skin, mucous membranes, inhalation, or blood.

Nursing Interventions

Identification of patients and health care workers sensitive to latex is crucial in preventing adverse reactions. Collect a thorough health history and history of any allergies, especially for patients with any complaints of latex contact symptoms. However, not all latex-sensitive individuals can be identified, even with a thorough history. Risk factors include long-term exposure to latex products (e.g., health care personnel, individuals who have had multiple surgeries, rubber industry workers) and a history of hay fever, asthma, and allergies to certain foods previously listed.

The National Institute for Occupational Safety and Health (NIOSH) has published recommendations for preventing allergic reactions to latex in the workplace (NIOSH, 2014):

- Non-latex gloves are recommended for tasks that are not likely to involve contacts with infectious materials such as blood (e.g., food preparation, routine housekeeping, and maintenance).
- Workers at high risk of allergic reaction should be screened periodically to detect symptoms early and control or eliminate latex exposure.
- Appropriate work practices should be followed. For example, workers should wash their hands with a mild soap and dry thoroughly after removing latex gloves. Areas contaminated with latex-containing dust should be identified and cleaned, and ventilation filters and vacuum bags used in those areas should be changed frequently.
- Workers should be provided with education programs and training materials about latex allergy.
- Workers showing symptoms of latex allergy should consult a doctor experienced in treating the problem, and workers with a known allergy should avoid latex exposures, wear a medical alert bracelet, and follow their doctor's advice for dealing with allergic reactions.

Use latex precaution protocols for patients identified as having a positive latex allergy test or a history of signs and symptoms related to latex exposure. Many health care facilities have created latex-free product carts that can be used for patients with latex allergies.

TRANSFUSION REACTIONS

Transfusion reactions are hypersensitivity disorders, best illustrated by reactions that occur with mismatched blood. Preventing transfusion reactions requires careful selection of blood donors, followed by careful typing and cross-matching of blood from donor to recipient. Proper storage of blood and adherence to the administration protocol are critical. Blood and blood components must be refrigerated at specific temperatures until a half hour before administration. Blood must be administered within 4 hours of removal from refrigeration, and blood components within 6 hours. Donor and recipient numbers are specific and must be checked thoroughly, and the patient must be identified with an armband. Administer all blood and blood products through microaggregate filters. Monitor for adverse effects.

Transfusion reactions are labeled mild, moderate, and severe. The most severe reactions occur within the first 15 minutes, moderate reactions occur within 30 to 90 minutes, and mild reactions may be delayed to late in the transfusion or hours to several days after transfusion.

Mild transfusion reaction signs and symptoms include dermatitis, diarrhea, fever, chills, urticaria, cough, and orthopnea. Treatment includes (1) stopping the transfusion; (2) notifying the health care provider; and (3) administering saline, steroids, and diuretics as ordered. The health care provider may give instructions to restart the transfusion at a slower rate and to continue to monitor the patient.

Moderate reactions, resulting in fever, chills, urticaria, and wheezing, occur after the first 30 minutes of administration. In the event of a moderate reaction, stop the transfusion, continue with saline, and notify the health care provider. Antihistamines and epinephrine may be ordered. The health care provider will decide whether to continue the transfusion.

Chills seen with mild or moderate transfusion reactions may be caused by the rapid infusion of cold blood, or may be due to a reaction against monocytes, granulocytes, lymphocytes, or leukocytes present in the donated blood.

A severe transfusion reaction often includes fever, chills, pain in the lower back, tightness in the chest, tachycardia, a drop in blood pressure, and blood in the urine. Patients may report a sense of "impending doom." Hemolytic reactions can result in kidney damage requiring dialysis, or death if the transfusion is not stopped as soon as the first signs of a reaction appear.

If a severe reaction occurs, the transfusion is stopped immediately, saline is administered to maintain venous access, and the blood or blood product, along with the tubing, is returned to the laboratory for immediate testing. Further nursing responsibilities after a blood transfusion reaction include (1) following hospital protocol for collecting required blood and urine specimens to assess for hemolysis, (2) filling out a transfusion reaction record, and (3) documenting the transfusion reaction on required facility forms and in the patient's health record.

The best method for preventing transfusion reaction is an **autologous** transfusion (i.e., use of one's own blood) for replacement therapy. The blood can be frozen and stored for as long as 3 years. Usually the blood is stored without being frozen and is given to the person within a few weeks of donation.

DELAYED HYPERSENSITIVITY

Delayed hypersensitivity reactions, occurring 24 to 72 hours after exposure, are mediated by T cells accompanied by release of lymphokines. Delayed reaction contact dermatitis, such as after contact with poison ivy, is one example. Another example is tissue transplant rejection.

Transplant Rejection

Transfer of healthy tissue or organs from a donor to a recipient has been done for many years. The immune process that protects the body from foreign protein is the same process at work in tissue transplant rejection. Knowledge of the function of the immune system has enabled medical experts to find a way to control the rejection process. Now the body is prepared before tissue transplantation to decrease the chances of rejection.

Autografting is the transplantation of tissue from one site to another on the same individual and is generally successful because there is a reduced likelihood of rejection. *Allografting* is the transplantation of tissue between members of the same species. Allografts commonly are used after trauma, especially on full-thickness burns, and in reconstructive surgery. *Isografting* is the transfer of tissue between genetically identical individuals (e.g., identical twins). Because few humans are born with an identical sibling, the allograft is the most common form of tissue transplant.

Antigenic determinants on the cells lead to graft rejection via the immune process. Therefore antigenic determinants in recipient tissue and donor tissue are matched as closely as possible before transplantation. Tissue matching leads to a better chance of success.

Tissue rejection does not occur immediately after transplantation. It takes several days for vascularization to occur. Seven to 10 days after blood supply is adequately established, sensitized lymphocytes may appear in sufficient numbers for sloughing to occur at the site.

Graft rejection is slowed through the use of chemical agents that interfere with the immune response. These chemical agents include corticosteroids, cyclosporine (Neoral, Sandimmune), and azathioprine (Imuran). Administration of these chemical agents is referred to as **immunosuppressive** therapy—the administration of agents that significantly interfere with the immune system's ability to respond to antigenic stimulation.

Infection is a threat to the immunosuppressed patient. Meticulous aseptic technique is required when caring for these individuals. Prophylactic antibiotic therapy may be advisable, and good skin care is necessary. The frequency of bedside visits for staff and family should be limited. Do not allow people with infection near the patient.

IMMUNODEFICIENCY DISORDERS

Immunodeficiency is an abnormal condition of the immune system in which cellular or humoral immunity is inadequate and resistance to infection is decreased. The first evidence of immunodeficiency is an increased susceptibility to infection. The problem can manifest as recurrent or chronic infection. Unusually severe infection with complications or incomplete clearing of an infection also may indicate an underlying immunodeficiency.

When the immune system does not protect the body adequately, an immunodeficient state exists. Immunodeficiency disorders involve an impairment of one or more of the following immune mechanisms:

- Phagocytosis
- Humoral response
- Cell-mediated response
- Complement response
- Combined humoral and cell-mediated deficiency

Immunodeficiency disorders are *primary* if the immune cells are improperly developed or absent, and *secondary* if the deficiency is caused by illnesses or treatment. Primary immunodeficiency disorders are rare and often serious, whereas secondary disorders are more common and may be less severe.

PRIMARY IMMUNODEFICIENCY DISORDERS

The basic categories of primary immunodeficiency disorders include the following:

- Phagocytic defects
- B cell deficiency

- T cell deficiency
- Combined B cell and T cell deficiency

SECONDARY IMMUNODEFICIENCY DISORDERS

Drug-induced immunosuppression is the most common type of secondary immunodeficiency disorder. Immunosuppressive therapy is prescribed for patients to treat a wide variety of chronic diseases, including inflammatory, allergic, hematologic, neoplastic, and autoimmune disorders. Immunosuppressive therapy also is used to prevent rejection of a transplanted organ. Some of these immunosuppressive drugs are cyclosporine, mycophenolate mofetil (CellCept), and azathioprine. Immunosuppression is also a serious side effect of cytotoxic drugs used in cancer chemotherapy. Generalized leukopenia often results, leading to a decreased humoral and cell-mediated response. Therefore secondary infections are common in immunosuppressed patients.

Stress may alter the immune response. This effect involves interrelationships between the nervous, endocrine, and immune systems.

A hypofunctional immune system exists in young children and older adults. Immunoglobulin levels decrease with age and therefore lead to a suppressed humoral immune response in older adults. Thymic involution (i.e., shrinking of the thymus) occurs with aging, along with decreased numbers of T cells. The incidence of malignancies and autoimmune diseases increases with aging and may be related to immunologic deterioration.

Malnutrition also alters cell-mediated immune responses. When protein is deficient over a prolonged period, the thymus gland atrophies and lymphoid tissue decreases. In addition, susceptibility to infections increases.

Radiation destroys lymphocytes either directly or through depletion of stem cells. As the radiation dose is increased, more bone marrow atrophies, leading to severe pancytopenia and severe suppression of immune function.

Surgical removal of lymph nodes, thymus, or spleen can suppress the immune response. Splenectomy in children is especially dangerous and may lead to septicemia from simple respiratory tract infections.

Hodgkin's lymphoma greatly impairs the cell-mediated immune response, and patients may die of severe viral or fungal infections. Viruses, especially rubella, may cause immunodeficiency by direct cytotoxic damage to lymphoid cells. Systemic infections can place such a demand on the immune system that resistance to a secondary or subsequent infection is impaired.

AUTOIMMUNE DISORDERS

Autoimmune disorders entail the development of an immune response (autoantibodies or a cellular immune response) to one's own tissues; thus these disorders are failures of the tolerance to "self." Autoimmune disorders may be described as an immune attack on the self and result from the failure to distinguish "self" protein (self-antigens) from "foreign" protein.

For some unknown reason, immune cells that are normally unresponsive (tolerant to self-antigens) are activated. T cells and B cells can have tolerance to self-antigens. Therefore an alteration in T cells alone or in both B cells and T cells can produce autoantibodies and autosensitized T cells that cause pathophysiologic tissue damage. The particular autoimmune disease depends on which self-antigen is involved.

Autoimmune diseases tend to cluster, so a given person may have more than one autoimmune disease (e.g., rheumatoid arthritis and Addison's disease). The same or related autoimmune diseases may be found in other members of the family. This observation has led to the concept of genetic predisposition to autoimmune disease.

The pathophysiology of autoimmune responses is not clearly understood. Environmental factors, including smoking, viral infections, and low vitamin D levels, have been found to trigger autoimmune diseases in susceptible people (Wein, 2013). In addition, high salt intake may be associated with the autoimmune response (Wein, 2013). Many illnesses are now believed to be in this classification. Included are pernicious anemia, Guillain-Barré syndrome, scleroderma, Sjögren's syndrome, rheumatic fever, rheumatoid arthritis, ulcerative colitis, male infertility, myasthenia gravis, multiple sclerosis, Addison's disease, autoimmune hemolytic anemia, immune thrombocytopenic purpura, type 1 diabetes mellitus, glomerulonephritis, and systemic lupus erythematosus.

PLASMAPHERESIS

Plasmapheresis is the removal of plasma that contains components causing, or thought to cause, disease. When plasma is removed, it is replaced by substitution fluids such as saline or albumin. Therefore the term *plasma exchange* more accurately describes this procedure.

Plasmapheresis has been used to treat autoimmune diseases such as systemic lupus erythematosus, glomerulonephritis, myasthenia gravis, thrombocytopenic purpura, rheumatoid arthritis, and Guillain-Barré syndrome. The rationale is to remove pathologic substances present in plasma. Many disorders for which plasmapheresis is being used are characterized by circulating autoantibodies (usually of the immunoglobulin G [IgG] class) and antigen-antibody complexes. Immunosuppressive therapy prevents recovery of IgG production, and plasmapheresis prevents antibody rebound (in which posttreatment autoimmune antibody concentrations exceed their pretreatment level) that often occurs after immunosuppressive therapy.

In addition to removing antinuclear antibodies (an autoantibody that reacts to nuclear material) and antigen-antibody complexes, plasmapheresis also may remove inflammatory mediators (e.g., complement) that are responsible for tissue damage. In the treatment of systemic lupus erythematosus, plasmapheresis usually is reserved for the patient experiencing an acute attack and who is unresponsive to conventional therapy.

Plasmapheresis involves the removal of whole blood through a needle inserted in one arm and circulation of the blood through a cell separator. The separator divides the blood into plasma and its cellular components by centrifugation or membrane filtration. Plasma, platelets, white blood cells, or red blood cells can be separated selectively. The undesirable component is removed, and the remainder is returned to the patient through a vein in the opposite arm. The plasma is generally replaced with normal saline, lactated Ringer's solution, fresh frozen plasma, plasma protein fractions, or albumin. When blood is removed manually, only 500 mL may be taken at one time. However, with the use of apheresis procedures, more than 4 L of plasma can be pheresed in 2 to 3 hours.

As with administration of other blood products, be aware of side effects associated with plasmapheresis. The most common complications are hypotension and citrate toxicity. Hypotension is usually the result of vasovagal reaction or transient volume changes. Citrate is used as an anticoagulant and may cause hypocalcemia, which may manifest as headache, paresthesias, and dizziness.

Get Ready for the NCLEX® Examination!

Key Points

- The two major forms of immunity are innate (natural) and acquired (adaptive).
- T lymphocytes, B lymphocytes, and macrophages are the three major cell types active in acquired immunity.
- B lymphocytes produce antibodies. T lymphocytes do not produce antibodies but assist the B cells. T lymphocytes release lymphokines.
- Macrophages trap, process, and present antigen to T lymphocytes.
- Autoimmune disorders are failures of the body's tolerance to "self."
- Plasmapheresis is used to treat autoimmune diseases such as systemic lupus erythematosus, glomerulonephritis, myasthenia gravis, thrombocytopenic purpura, rheumatoid arthritis, and Guillain-Barré syndrome.
- Infection is a primary threat to the immunosuppressed patient. Aseptic technique is required when caring for these patients. Good skin care is necessary.
- Careful selection of blood donors and careful typing and cross-matching of blood are important to prevent transfusion reaction.
- Early recognition of signs followed by early treatment may decrease the severity of an allergic reaction.
- The five factors influencing the hypersensitivity response are host response to allergen, exposure amount, nature of the allergen, route of allergen entry, and repeated exposure.
- Two types of latex allergies are type IV allergic contact dermatitis and type I allergic reactions. Type IV is caused by the chemicals used in the manufacturing of latex gloves, whereas the type I allergic reaction is a response to natural rubber latex proteins.

Additional Learning Resources

SG Go to your Study Guide for additional learning activities to help you master this chapter content.

evolve Be sure to visit the Evolve site at *http://evolve.elsevier.com/Cooper/foundationsadult/* for additional online resources.

Review Questions for the NCLEX® Examination

1. Which immune disorder results from a failure to tolerate "self"?
   1. immunodeficiency disorders.
   2. hypersensitivity disorders.
   3. desensitization disorders.
   4. autoimmune disorders.
2. The nurse is caring for a patient who has had a kidney transplant. What should be included in the care of a patient with a suppressed immune system?
   1. Prophylactic antibiotic therapy
   2. Meticulous aseptic technique
   3. Restriction of all visitors
   4. Antineoplastic medication administration
3. Which statements describe innate, or natural, immunity? *(Select all that apply.)*
   1. The body's first line of defense against disease, which protects locally against the external environment
   2. The body's second line of defense against disease, which protects the internal environment
   3. Includes stomach acid, saliva, and secretions/flora of the intestine and vagina
   4. Mediated by B cells to produce antibodies in response to antigenic challenge
   5. Provides an immunity that is specific
   6. Responds with neutrophils, macrophages, and lymphocytes
4. The activation of T cells by antigens indicate which type of immunity is developing? *(Select all that apply.)*
   1. Innate immunity
   2. Adaptive immunity
   3. Humoral immunity
   4. Cellular immunity
5. The nurse is caring for a patient with a history of numerous allergies. What is the most important teaching concept?
   1. Immunotherapy regimen
   2. Avoidance of the allergen
   3. Antihistamine administration
   4. Adrenaline administration

6. Humoral immunity is mediated by which type of cells?
   1. T cells
   2. B cells
   3. Macrophages
   4. Myeloblasts
7. After a bee sting, the patient's face becomes edematous and she begins to wheeze. Based on this assessment, the nurse would be prepared to administer which medication?
   1. Aminophylline
   2. Diphenhydramine
   3. Epinephrine
   4. Diazepam
8. Which is another term for desensitization?
   1. autoimmune disorders.
   2. adaptive immunity.
   3. immunotherapy.
   4. immunodeficiency disease.
9. The nurse gave an intramuscular penicillin injection to a patient. What assessment finding would be most indicative of a systemic anaphylactic response?
   1. Increased blood pressure
   2. Bradycardia
   3. Urticaria
   4. Wheezing
10. A 38-year-old patient is receiving 2 units of packed red blood cells at 125 mL/h. Fifteen minutes after the start of the blood transfusion, the nurse notes the following vital signs: pulse 110 beats/minute, respirations 28 breaths/minute, blood pressure 98/58 mm Hg, and temperature 101°F. The patient is shivering. What is the nurse's initial action?
    1. Slow the infusion rate.
    2. Stop the infusion.
    3. Administer aspirin as ordered for elevated temperature.
    4. Report the findings to the nurse manager.
11. A 72-year-old patient is admitted to the hospital with a diagnosis of immunodeficiency disease. What is the primary nursing goal?
    1. Reduce the risk of the patient developing an infection.
    2. Encourage the patient to provide self-care.
    3. Plan nutritious meals to provide adequate intake.
    4. Encourage the patient to interact with other patients.
12. The patient tells the nurse he is overwhelmed. There is so much he must do to keep his new kidney functioning, and then rejection may still occur. Which patient problem statement is appropriate?
    1. *Impaired Coping*
    2. *Distorted Body Image*
    3. Potential for Unsafe Health Behaviors
    4. *Impaired Self-Esteem due to Current Situation*
13. A patient experienced an anaphylactic reaction to an antibiotic. What are the correct nursing interventions for anaphylaxis? *(Select all that apply.)*
    1. Assess vital signs every 4 hours.
    2. Assess respiratory status frequently.
    3. Maintain patent airway.
    4. Administer epinephrine as ordered.
    5. Monitor vital signs frequently.
14. A patient comes to the clinic for his weekly allergy injection. He missed his appointment the week before because of a family emergency. Which action is appropriate in administering the patient's injection?
    1. Administer the usual dose of the allergen.
    2. Double the dose to account for the missed injection the previous week.
    3. Consult with the health care provider about decreasing the dose for this injection.
    4. Reevaluate the patient's sensitivity to the allergen with a skin test.
15. Type I allergic reaction to latex is a response to the _________ _________ _________.
16. The most common allergens that cause an anaphylactic reaction include: *(Select all that apply.)*
    1. Leafy, green vegetables
    2. Bees, wasps
    3. Shellfish
    4. Peanuts
    5. Oranges
17. Which illnesses are believed to be caused by an autoimmune disorder? *(Select all that apply.)*
    1. Rheumatoid arthritis
    2. Lung cancer
    3. Systemic lupus erythematosus
    4. Guillain-Barré syndrome
    5. Cardiovascular disease
18. The nurse advises a friend who asks the nurse to administer his allergy injections that:
    1. it is illegal for nurses to administer injections outside of a medical setting.
    2. he is qualified to do it if the friend has epinephrine in an injectable syringe provided with his extract.
    3. avoiding the allergens is a more effective way of controlling allergies and allergy shots are not usually effective.
    4. immunotherapy should be administered only in a setting where emergency equipment and drugs are available.
19. A patient is undergoing plasmapheresis for treatment of systemic lupus erythematosus. The nurse correctly recognizes which statement about the procedure? *(Select all that apply.)*
    1. Plasmapheresis will be used to remove the T lymphocytes from the blood that are responsble for producing antinuclear antibodies.
    2. Plasmapharesis will remove normal particles in her blood that are being damaged by autoantibodies.
    3. Plasmapharesis will replace the plasma that contains antinuclear antibodies with a substitute fluid.
    4. Plasma removed during the procedure will be replaced by normal saline.
    5. A side effect of the procedure is hypertension.

Care of the Patient With HIV

56

http://evolve.elsevier.com/Cooper/foundationsadult/

Objectives

1. Describe the agent that causes HIV disease and the history of HIV.
2. Define AIDS by using the current terminology from the Centers for Disease Control and Prevention.
3. Explain the differences between HIV infection, HIV disease, and AIDS.
4. Describe the progression of HIV infection.
5. Discuss how HIV is and is not transmitted.
6. Describe patients who are at risk for HIV infection.
7. Discuss the pathophysiologic features of HIV disease.
8. List signs and symptoms that may be indicative of HIV disease.
9. Discuss the laboratory and diagnostic tests related to HIV disease.
10. Discuss the issues related to HIV antibody testing.
11. Describe the multidisciplinary approach in caring for a patient with HIV disease.
12. List opportunistic infections associated with advanced HIV disease (AIDS).
13. Discuss the nurse's role in assisting the HIV-infected patient with coping, grieving, reducing anxiety, and minimizing social isolation.
14. Discuss the importance of adherence to HIV treatment.
15. Discuss the use of effective prevention strategies in the counseling of patients.
16. Define the nurse's role in the prevention of HIV infection.

Key Terms

acquired immunodeficiency syndrome (AIDS) (ŭ-KWĪRD ĭm-yū-nō-dĕ-FĬSH-ĕn-sē SĬN-drōm, p. 1952)
adherence (ăd-HĔR-ĕns, p. 1964)
CD4⁺ lymphocyte (SĒ DĒ FŌRPLŬS LĬM-fō-sīt, p. 1950)
Centers for Disease Control and Prevention (CDC) (SĔN-tŭrz FŌR dĭz-ĒZ kŭn-TRŌL ĂND prĕ-VĔN-shŭn, p. 1943)
enzyme-linked immunosorbent assay (ELISA) (ĔN-zīm LĬNKD ĭm-ū-nō-ZŎR-bĕnt ĂS-ā, p. 1956)
HIV disease (ĀCH Ī VĒ dĭz-ĒZ, p. 1952)
human immunodeficiency virus (HIV) (HYŪ-mĭn ĭm-yū-nō-dĕ-FĬSH-ĕn-sē VĪ-rŭs, p. 1944)
Kaposi's sarcoma (kă-PŌS-sĕz săr-KŌ-mŭ, p. 1943)
opportunistic (ŏp-pŏr-tū-NĬS-tĭk, p. 1945)
phagocyte (făg-ō-SĪT, p. 1952)
***Pneumocystis jiroveci* pneumonia** (nū-mō-SĬS-tĭs yē-rō-VĔT-zē nū-MŌN-yŭ, p. 1943)
retrovirus (rĕ-trō-VĪ-rŭs, p. 1949)
seroconversion (sĕr-ō-kŏn-VĔR-zhŭn, p. 1948)
seronegative (sĕr-ō-NĔG-ă-tĭv, p. 1956)
seroprevalence (sĕr-ō-PRĔV-ŭ-lŭns, p. 1946)
vertical transmission (VŬR-tĭk-ŭl trănz-MĬSH-ŭn, p. 1947)
viral load (VĪ-rŭl LŌD, p. 1947)
virulent (VĬR-ū-lĕnt, p. 1945)
wasting (WĀST-ĭng, p. 1968)
Western blot (WĔST-ŭrn BLŎT, p. 1956)

NURSING AND THE HISTORY OF HIV DISEASE

As early as 1979, physicians in New York and California were identifying cases of ***Pneumocystis jiroveci*** (formerly *Pneumocystis carinii*) **pneumonia,** an unusual pulmonary disease caused by a fungus that infects primarily people who have suppressed immune systems. The fungus is found commonly in the environment but does not normally affect people who are healthy. During the time when the acquired immunodeficiency syndrome (AIDS) epidemic was at its peak, the majority of people with advanced AIDS developed this lung infection. The use of prophylactic antibiotics significantly has decreased the number of cases of this condition among patients with AIDS (PubMed Health, 2009). Also during the height of the epidemic, physicians noted an increase in the number of people with **Kaposi's sarcoma,** a rare cancer of the skin and mucous membranes characterized by blue, red, or purple raised lesions (Fig. 56.1) that occurred mainly in men of Mediterranean descent. Of interest was that these two diseases were occurring at alarming rates in clusters of young homosexual men whose immune systems were failing. Researchers at the **Centers for Disease Control and Prevention (CDC),** a division of the US Public Health Service that investigates and reports on various diseases, soon learned

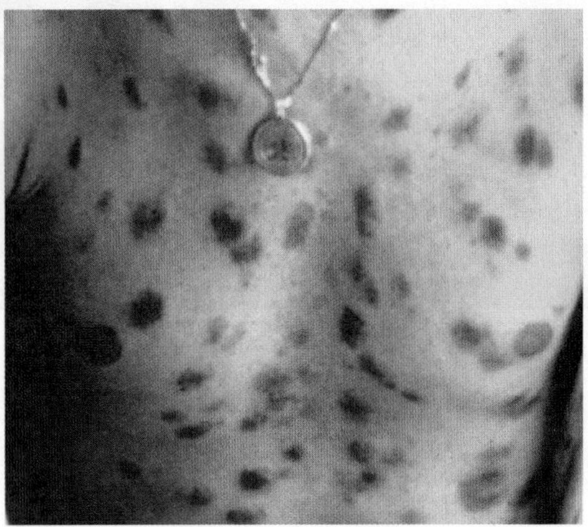

Fig. 56.1 Kaposi's sarcoma. (Courtesy Paul A. Volberding, MD, University of California, San Francisco. US Department of Veterans Affairs.)

that this immune disorder also was affecting people who used injection drugs and patients with hemophilia. Later, the immune disorder also was identified in heterosexual men and women.

The origins of **human immunodeficiency virus (HIV)** remain somewhat obscure, and why HIV gave rise to the AIDS pandemic only in the 20th century has not yet been determined. The earliest case of HIV infection has been dated to 1959. It was identified in the Democratic Republic of Congo through different methods of molecular clock analysis. It also has been estimated that HIV began to radiate from its source in approximately the 1930s (Buonaguro et al, 2007). The escalating pandemic probably resulted from the combination of significant cultural and sociobehavioral changes, the use of nonsterile needles for parenteral injections and vaccinations, and the unintended contamination of products used for medical treatments.

HIV has been recognized as a clinical syndrome since the early 1980s. Several researchers have, however, identified patients who may have fit the CDC's Case Surveillance definition before that time. The unusual and rapid deterioration and death in 1969 of a 15-year-old boy (Robert R.) in St. Louis from aggressive, disseminated Kaposi's sarcoma suggests that his may have been the first confirmed death from HIV infection in the United States (Garry et al, 1988). This patient had no international travel experience, which suggests that other individuals were infected with HIV as well. This also implies that HIV may have existed in some form in the United States since at least the 1960s.

HIV is known as *zoonotic,* an organism that has been able to cross from an animal species to humans. A similar virus (called *simian immunodeficiency virus*) was noted in primates and probably crossed into humans by way of the hunting and consumption of these animals in Africa. Other examples of zoonotic transmission include severe acute respiratory distress syndrome, anthrax, rabies, hantavirus, and West Nile virus (World Health Organization [WHO], 2016a). HIV began to spread in the middle to late 1970s, but because of the long incubation period, the viral epidemic progressed undetected in most countries. When the virus began causing widespread disease in the 1980s, it provoked fear among laypeople and health care providers. It was also a challenging time for health care workers, because they knew they were observing a new pathogen whose route of transmission was not completely understood. In spite of the stigmas and fears that emerged (and still exist to some extent), nurses were at the forefront of providing care to affected patients. Nurses met the challenges of providing and coordinating services, organizing community-based organizations, teaching about prevention, and helping patients deal with a terminal disease.

There are three stages of HIV. Stage 1 is the stage of acute HIV infection. This occurs within 2 to 4 weeks of transmission of the infection and manifests as if the patient had influenza. During this stage, patients are very infectious with elevated numbers of the virus in their blood and some bodily fluids. Stage 2 is known as clinical latency. The patient is often asymptomatic during this stage with low levels of the virus present in their blood. Stage 3 is when the patient develops acquired immunodeficiency syndrome (AIDS). This is the most severe stage of the infection. Patients develop opportunistic infections because their immune systems have been damaged by the HIV infection. Their viral loads are elevated and they are very contagious. Their CD4 count drops to less than 200 cells/mm. They may experience fever, chills, sweating, swollen lymph nodes, weight loss, and weakness (CDC, 2018a).

The CDC (1981) published a notation about some patients with signs and symptoms that later would be attributed to AIDS. The signs and symptoms listed were related to the development of opportunistic infections. Such infections occur when the body's immune system has been weakened. Since that time, AIDS has become known as one of the most challenging infectious diseases of the 20th and 21st centuries. In 1982 the CDC issued a statement that blood and other body fluids may be vehicles for transmitting the disease and that precautions must be used with all blood and body fluids.

The discovery of a second HIV strain was major and alarming, because it was the first clue that HIV could mutate rapidly. This capability for rapid mutation has become the trademark of this virus. It represents an immense challenge for scientists as they search for vaccine strategies. HIV type 1 (HIV-1) is found worldwide and is the prevalent strain in most places, including the United States, Europe, and Central Africa. HIV-1 and HIV type 2 (HIV-2) are spread in the same ways and have similar signs and symptoms. Infection with either of these viral strains also results in opportunistic infections with progression to AIDS. Most people with HIV-1 infection develop profound immunodeficiency and high viral loads, which result in death, but most cases of HIV-2 infection result in long-term nonprogression

(Nayamweya et al, 2013). Patients with HIV-2 tend to progress with higher CD4 counts. The prevalence of HIV-2 infection is confined mostly to West Africa. This is thought to be related to commercial sex trade and immigration. Reports of cases of HIV-2 infections in the United States are rare and can be traced back to the engagement of risky behaviors with people who are from West African countries.

HIV-1 is much more **virulent** (toxic) than HIV-2. People with HIV-2 infection tend to be identified as long-term nonprogressors. Patients infected with HIV-2 develop problems with immunodeficiency more slowly. However, these patients can progress to AIDS with lower viral load levels than patients with HIV-1.

Since the first cases of AIDS were reported in 1981, the CDC has revised the HIV case definition several times in response to improved laboratory and diagnostic methods (CD4$^+$ and viral test results). Diagnostic criteria changes also allow for distinguishing between HIV-1 and HIV-2 infection and early HIV identification (CDC, 2014). The current definition, used by all states and US territories, allows the disease to be monitored consistently for public health purposes. These revisions to the HIV surveillance case definition took into account the advances in diagnostic methods and treatment to provide more accurate information on the numbers of life-threatening illnesses and deaths that are **opportunistic** (caused by normally nonpathogenic organisms in a host whose resistance has been decreased by such disorders as HIV disease) among HIV-infected individuals (CDC, 2016).

It was not until 1987, after the CDC reported three cases of occupationally acquired HIV infection in health care providers, that universal guidelines for blood and body fluid precautions, or *standard precautions,* were developed for the prevention of occupational exposure. These guidelines forever changed the way health care personnel protect themselves and other people from the spread of bloodborne pathogens. That same year, the Association of Nurses in AIDS Care was established to address the needs of individuals with HIV disease and to provide a professional forum for nurses, who often faced discrimination as a result of providing care to HIV-infected patients.

By that time, a broad spectrum of individuals, including children, adults, and people from all socioeconomic groups, were affected by this disorder (see the Lifespan Considerations box). Nurses became instrumental in establishing education and treatment standards, in collaboration with community-based organizations. Today nurses constitute the largest group of health care professionals who care for individuals with HIV disease, which stresses the importance of prevention and influencing policymakers. HIV nursing provides lessons that can be useful in other patient populations as well: the importance of patient education, adherence to medical regimens, prevention, and health-promoting behaviors.

Lifespan Considerations

Older Adults

HIV Disease

- In 2013 people who were 50 years old and older accounted for 42% of all residents of the United States who were living with diagnosed HIV infection (CDC, 2018b).
- Improved treatments and prophylactic medications are contributing to longer lifespans in individuals with HIV disease, which has made the disease chronic.
- Because the immune system's ability to fight infection decreases with age, HIV disease progresses faster and complications increase among older adults with HIV infection.
- Divorced and widowed people are beginning to date again and may be having sex with multiple partners without recognizing their risk for becoming infected with HIV. Age-related changes to women's vaginal tissue may increase their risk for acquiring HIV.

SIGNIFICANCE OF THE PROBLEM

Disease Burden

Throughout the world, HIV is one of the leading causes of death and results in more deaths than does any other disease caused by infection. As of 2015 approximately 36.7 million people were living with HIV infections (WHO, 2016b). In 2015, 1.1 million people died throughout the world as a result of AIDS-related opportunistic infections.

Sub-Saharan Africa has been hit especially hard. This region contains more than 69% of the world's population with HIV but only 12% of the total world population (Henry J. Kaiser Family Foundation, 2013). In 2011, 17.3 million children in that region had lost one or both of their parents to AIDS. Death related to AIDS is associated largely with poor access to prevention and treatment services (Henry J. Kaiser Family Foundation, 2013). Since 2005, the number of people infected with HIV has declined steadily (AVERT, 2018). This decreasing infection rate is thought to be related to increased access to antiretroviral treatments. Managing and treating this disease will remain a challenge for years to come, especially in the sub-Saharan region of Africa.

In the United States approximately 50,000 new cases of HIV are diagnosed each year. More than 1.1 million people in the United States currently are living with HIV (CDC, 2013a). Between 2003 and 2006 the number of new HIV cases in the United States stabilized, but the number of people who were living with the disease increased. At the end of 2013, almost 1.2 million people were infected and living with HIV (AVERT, 2018b).

TRENDS AND MOST AFFECTED POPULATIONS

Beginning in 1996 the use of *highly active antiretroviral therapy* (ART) in people with HIV infection increased greatly in the United States. Since that time, fewer people with HIV infection have developed AIDS. New HIV and AIDS cases affect various racial groups, ethnic groups, geographic areas, and demographic populations; thus this epidemic has affected nonwhite people, women, heterosexuals, and people who use injection drugs. However, people with HIV are living longer (CDC, 2018c).

The CDC reported that the population of men who have sex with other men (MSM) constitutes the biggest proportion of HIV patients, accounting for 78% of the total number of HIV infections in male patients 13 years of age and older (CDC, 2013b). The HIV infection rates among this population decreased from 71% in 1983 to 44% in 1996. Holmberg (1996) predicted that this rate would continue to decrease to approximately 25%. Instead of decreasing, however, the number of new HIV infections in MSM has not continued the anticipated decline. The number of new infections for this population increased from 28,000 in 2009 to 31,000 in 2013. In response the CDC has implemented a system of "High-Impact HIV Prevention" by targeting at-risk populations with efficient and evidence-based interventions (CDC, 2017).

During the first 25 years of this epidemic, the distribution of new cases on the basis of ethnicity and race changed (see the Cultural Considerations box). Disproportionate numbers of Hispanic Americans and African Americans have been infected with HIV. In 2014, although African Americans made up only 12% of the population in the United States, they accounted for 44% of the total number of HIV cases that were diagnosed (CDC, 2018d). African American adults and adolescents are 10 times more likely to receive a diagnosis of AIDS than are white adults and adolescents. The primary risk factor for African American men who developed HIV was sexual contact. In 2014 African American MSM were much more likely than other MSM to be infected with HIV (CDC, 2018d). Another risk factor for African American men is engaging in high-risk heterosexual behavior (CDC, 2013c).

Some African American MSM identify themselves as heterosexuals because of the stigma and homophobia issues. Many African American MSM are secretive about their homosexuality or choose not to identify their sexual orientation. Prevention programs are challenged when people do not identify themselves as engaging in risky behaviors or having increased risk factors.

Initially the face of HIV was predominately homosexual men and people who used injection drugs. Rates of transmission of the disease to women have been startling. Currently, an estimated 19% of HIV sufferers are women (CDC, 2018e). HIV was the leading cause of mortality in African American women between 25 and 34 years of age. African American women are 22 times more likely to be diagnosed with AIDS and 14 times more likely to die from HIV than are white American women (US Department of Health and Human Services, Office of Minority Health, 2016).

Cultural Considerations

HIV Disease

- Since 2000, Hispanic Americans have accounted for 56% of the United States' growth in population. The rate of **seroprevalence** (occurrence of disease within a defined population at one time) is higher among Hispanic Americans than among white Americans, and as a result, HIV prevention education is important. In 2014 Hispanic Americans were only 17% of the total US population, although they represented 24% of new HIV infections (CDC, 2018f).
- Barriers to prevention include difficulty providing care in a nonthreatening environment where health care providers are viewed as authorities.
- Undocumented residents, including Hispanic Americans, are reluctant to seek HIV care because this condition disqualifies them for US legal residency and they fear deportation. In addition, nearly 75% of Hispanic Americans are members of the Catholic church, which historically has been opposed to sex outside marriage, sex between men, and artificial birth control. These beliefs complicate prevention efforts that stress the use of condoms.
- Because of the deportation threat, Hispanic American patients may not share important health information with health care providers.
- In assessment and interventions, nurses should be sensitive to language and cultural differences.
- Nurses should provide a safe, supportive environment for assessment and treatment and should advocate for patients who need treatment, regardless of ability to pay for services or residency status.

Data from *Mosby's dictionary of medicine, nursing and health professions*, ed 9, St. Louis, 2012, Mosby; Bedoya CA, Mimiaga MJ, Beauchamp G, et al: Predictors of HIV transmission risk behavior and seroconversion among Latino men who have sex with men in Project EXPLORE, *AIDS Behav* 2012;16(3):608–617; and Centers for Disease Control and Prevention (CDC): *HIV among Hispanics/Latinos*, 2018f. Retrieved from *http://www.cdc.gov/hiv/group/racialethnic/hispaniclatinos.*

Although Hispanic/Latino Americans account for 17% of the population, they accounted for approximately 25% of new HIV infections in 2014 (CDC, 2018f). Many socioeconomic and cultural factors have contributed to this epidemic and associated prevention challenges in the US Hispanic and Latino communities. For Hispanic men and women, the primary risk factor for developing HIV is sex with men. If current rates continue to trend, the CDC reports that 25% of Hispanic/Latino MSM may be infected with HIV during their life (CDC, 2018f). Rates of other sexually transmitted infections (STIs), including chlamydia, gonorrhea, and syphilis, are also higher among Hispanic Americans than among non-Hispanic white Americans (CDC, 2018f). Transient Hispanic populations often have difficulty receiving access to health care because of social structure, language barriers, and migration patterns (CDC, 2018f). The predicaments caused by poverty limit access to appropriate health care, housing, and HIV prevention. All these factors may increase directly or indirectly risk factors for HIV infection in the Hispanic population.

In 1996 researchers incorrectly predicted that HIV cases would increase among people who use injection drugs (Holmberg, 1996). African American MSM are most affected by HIV (CDC, 2018d). During the past 10 years, the number of new HIV cases diagnosed per year has continued to decline (CDC, 2018g).

As treatment for HIV has advanced, the progression from HIV to stage 3 (AIDS) has slowed, resulting in a decreased mortality rate among people infected with HIV. Data from 1985 to 2012 indicate that, although the number of AIDS cases has remained relatively stable, the death rate has decreased (CDC, n.d.). Advanced treatment options mean that people are living longer after their HIV diagnoses. Unfortunately, in countries where HIV-infected people are without adequate access to health care, HIV infection is still one of the leading causes of death.

TRANSMISSION OF HIV

Despite significant research into the modes of transmission of HIV, considerable fear and misinformation about HIV transmission, perhaps more than for any other disease, still exists. Health care providers and patients must be knowledgeable about modes of transmission and behaviors that put them at risk for HIV infection. Modes of transmission have remained constant throughout the course of the HIV pandemic. Health care providers also need to remember that transmission of HIV occurs through sexual *practices,* not sexual *preferences.*

The patterns in the spread of HIV changed considerably during the first two decades of the epidemic in the United States (Henry J. Kaiser Family Foundation, 2018). Most cases of HIV in the United States are diagnosed in MSM. In the United States, HIV diagnoses that are attributable to injection drug use have fallen significantly since 2005 to 2014. The number of estimated pediatric HIV cases diagnosed each year has declined since 1992. This decline is associated with the increased compliance with universal counseling and testing of pregnant women and the use of antiretroviral therapy (ART) by HIV-infected pregnant women and their newborns (Henry J. Kaiser Family Foundation, 2018).

HIV is an *obligate virus,* which means it must have a host organism to survive. The virus cannot live long outside the human body. HIV transmission depends on the presence of the virus, the infectiousness of the virus, the susceptibility of the uninfected recipient, and any conditions that may increase the recipient's risk for infection. HIV is transmitted from human to human through infected blood, semen, rectal secretions, cervicovaginal secretions, and breast milk (HIV.gov, 2016). If these infected fluids are introduced into an uninfected person, HIV can be transmitted to that person. In addition to the aforementioned body fluids, HIV also is found in pericardial, synovial, cerebrospinal, peritoneal, and amniotic fluids. **Vertical transmission** (transmission from a mother to a fetus) of HIV can occur during pregnancy, during delivery, or through postpartum breast-feeding (transmitted in the breast milk). Conditions that affect the likelihood of infection include the duration and frequency of exposure, the amount of virus inoculated into the recipient, the virulence of the organism, and the recipient's defense capability (immune system). Although HIV has been found in other body fluids such as saliva, urine, tears, and feces, there has been no evidence that these substances are vehicles of transmission, unless the fluids contain visible blood.

HIV generally is transmitted by *behaviors* and not by casual contacts, such as hugging, dry kissing, shaking hands, or sharing food and utensils. HIV is not transmitted by domestic animals or insects; through coughing or sneezing; or through sharing objects such as pencils, computer keyboards, or telephones. The two most common modes of HIV transmission are anal or vaginal intercourse and sharing contaminated injecting drug equipment and paraphernalia (HIV.gov, 2016). Once infected, an individual is capable of transmitting HIV to other people at any time throughout the disease spectrum, even when the infected host appears healthy and has no obvious signs of the infection. In HIV infection, the **viral load** (amount of measurable HIV virions in the blood) peaks quickly after infection and during the later stages of the disease. During these periods, a recipient's unprotected exposure to an infected host increases the likelihood of transmission. However, it is important to remember that HIV can be transmitted during the entire disease spectrum.

SEXUAL TRANSMISSION

Sexual intercourse remains the most common mode of transmission of HIV in the world today and is responsible for the majority of the world's total HIV cases. Sexual activity provides the potential for the exchange of semen, cervicovaginal secretions, and blood. Important risk factors are the presence of HIV in one or both partners and the occurrence of behaviors that put one or both partners at risk for transmission. Some individuals become infected with HIV after a single unprotected sexual encounter, whereas others remain free from infection after hundreds of such encounters.

Although the majority of HIV transmissions in the United States occur among MSM via receptive anal intercourse, heterosexual transmission via anal intercourse is becoming increasingly prevalent. Heterosexual couples may prefer this method of sexual expression or use it because it eliminates the risk of pregnancy. Unfortunately, the most risky sexual activity is unprotected receptive anal intercourse. Because the rectum is generally tighter and the rectal mucosa is less lubricated than the vagina, the rectal mucosa may be torn, providing an excellent portal for the virus to enter the bloodstream.

During any form of sexual intercourse (anal, vaginal, oral), the risk of infection is considerably higher for the receptive partner, although infection can be transmitted to an insertive partner as well. The receptive partner generally has prolonged exposure to semen (HIV.gov, 2016). Other factors that may increase the risk of sexual transmission include ulcerating genital diseases, such as herpes simplex virus (HSV) and syphilis; chancres secondary to STIs; intact (uncircumcised) foreskin; sex that is "forceful or vigorous"; immunosuppression resulting from drug use; and drug use that may lead to high-risk behavior. Infection risk for HIV also can be increased during intercourse when the infected partner has a high viral load (CDC, 2018h). The viral load often is increased in the primary and late stages of infection. Oral-genital transmissions have been reported, and the HIV transmission risk increases if the receiving partner already has an STI that has caused open sores, such as HSV infection.

PARENTERAL EXPOSURE

Injecting Drug Use

HIV may be transmitted by exposure to contaminated blood through the accidental or intentional sharing of injecting equipment and paraphernalia. Such equipment includes syringes, needles, cookers (spoons or bottle caps used for mixing the drug), and filtering equipment (such as cotton balls and rinse water) (CDC, 2018i). People who use injection drugs are the population with the second highest rates of HIV exposure, following MSM (CDC, 2015). Although typically seen in large metropolitan areas, injection drug use occurs in smaller cities and rural areas as well. Such drugs are not limited to illicit drugs; HIV can be transmitted via contaminated equipment used to inject steroids, vitamins, and insulin.

People who use injection drugs confirm needle placement in a vein by drawing back blood into the syringe; the substance is then injected into the vein. Other factors that put people who use illicit injection drugs at risk for HIV include poor nutritional status, poor hygiene, and impaired judgment resulting from mood-altering substances. People who use illicit injection drugs are also less likely to use condoms during sexual intercourse and may engage in sexual activity in exchange for drugs. The long-term effects of illicit injection drug use include increased risk for other diseases, such as hepatitis B, hepatitis C, and other bloodborne illnesses.

Blood and Blood Products

Since 1985, blood banks in the United States have screened all donated blood for HIV-1 antibodies and, since 1992, for HIV-2 antibodies. Blood banks also have implemented procedures to identify blood donors who may be at high risk for infection with HIV. Blood from donors who are deemed to be at high risk or that yields test results positive for HIV is discarded. In addition to HIV, blood currently is screened for human T-lymphotropic virus types 1 and 2 (HTLV-1 and HTLV-2), hepatitis B virus, treponema pallidum (syphilis), West Nile virus, *Trypanosoma cruzi* infection (Chagas disease), and hepatitis C virus (US Food and Drug Administration [FDA], 2013a).

Every year, a small number of blood donations come from donors who are infected with HIV but in whom the HIV antibody was undetected. When a blood donor has not yet undergone **seroconversion** (a change in serologic test results from negative to positive as antibodies develop in reaction to an infection), the current HIV antibody test cannot detect the infection. In the past, there was a 22-day window during which the donor could donate infected blood in which HIV would not be detected by the HIV-1 and HIV-2 antibody test. Since 1995, however, blood also has been screened for HIV-1 p24 antigen. With this addition, this window has been reduced to 16 days. In 1999 the nucleic acid amplification test was introduced; this test detects HIV-1 RNA and has reduced the window to only 11 days. By 2008 only four people were infected with HIV after receiving a blood product transfusion (CDC, 2010). The blood came from three separate donors, and the blood tested negative for HIV with all currently available HIV tests (CDC, 2010). Currently, a person's risk for acquiring HIV through a blood transfusion is estimated to be about 1 per 1.5 million (CDC, 2010). Before 1985, people who received replacement clotting factors for blood coagulation difficulties (e.g., hemophilia) were at increased risk of contracting HIV. Since 1985, a recombinant technique is used to manufacture the clotting factors or the clotting factors are treated with chemicals or heated to kill the HIV.

Occupational Exposure

Almost 25,000 adults who developed AIDS before 2003 were health care workers. This number represents 5% of all AIDS cases among adults who had a known occupation.

The CDC distinguishes between two types of HIV seroconversion. When the infection is "documented," it means that the individual had a documented exposure related to occupation and developed HIV disease. A "possible" infection indicates that the individual worked in a high-risk setting with exposure to blood or other body fluids related to occupation; however, no exposure event was documented.

In the United States through 2008, of the 58 health care workers who were infected with HIV as a result of a documented occupational exposure, 26 (46%) developed AIDS (CDC, 2011). Of all health care workers with HIV, most did not have a documented exposure, and the infection is thought to result from high-risk sexual behavior. No confirmed work-related exposures in health care workers have been reported since 2008.

Most of the health care workers who have been infected with HIV are nurses. The second largest group is laboratory clinicians, and the third largest group is physicians (nonsurgical). Other health care workers with possible exposures included emergency medical technicians, health care aides, housekeepers, and maintenance workers. Most of the infections occurred after a needlestick injury with resulting puncture wound. Exposures are thought to be underreported because such reporting is voluntary. If a health care worker does have a needlestick that results in exposure to a known source of HIV infection, the risk for contracting HIV is low, at approximately 0.3%.

Needlesticks that occur when a health care worker is exposed to patients with known HIV infection are known as *percutaneous exposures.* If the exposure involves a hollow-bore needle filled with blood that had previously been placed in the patient's vein or artery, then the transmission risk of HIV is increased. The transmission risk also is increased if the health care worker suffers a deep injury at the time of the exposure. Scalpels, suture needles, and smaller gauge injection needles also pose a risk for transmission, but that risk is much lower. If only the mucous membranes are exposed during the incident, then the risk for seroconversion is only 0.09%. There is a low risk for seroconverting if the health care worker's skin is not intact and is exposed to blood or body fluids.

Unfortunately, antiretroviral medications used as post-exposure prophylaxis antiretroviral are hepatotoxic. When antiretroviral therapy is given to a health care worker after a documented exposure, it may result in severe hepatitis that may necessitate liver transplantation.

Perinatal (Vertical) Transmission

HIV infection can be transmitted from a mother to her infant during pregnancy, at the time of delivery, or after birth through breast-feeding. It is the most common way for children to be infected with HIV. In the United States, it is estimated that approximately 25% of infected mothers transmit HIV to their infants and that approximately 50% to 70% of the transmissions occur late in utero or during birth. The rate of vertical transmission varies around the world. Factors such as the stage of maternal HIV disease (transmission is more likely to occur during the initial and later stages of infection, when more of the virus is circulating in the mother's blood and body fluids), a decreased $CD4^+$ cell count or high viral load, the presence or absence of STIs, and the mother's nutritional status play a role in vertical transmission. Factors that increase the risk of transmission during delivery include extreme prematurity; lack of health care; gestational complications that lead to extended labor; the mixing of maternal and fetal blood; newborn ingestion of maternal blood, amniotic fluid, or vaginal secretions; skin excoriation in the newborn; and being the first child born in a multiple gestation. HIV-infected mothers are cautioned to use formula in place of breast-feeding because breastmilk is another way to transmit the infection to infants (AIDSinfo, 2018).

Clinical trials have demonstrated that the administration of a combination of antiretroviral medications to pregnant women who are infected with HIV can reduce transmission to approximately 1% of infants. These infants are given HIV medications for 6 weeks after birth to prevent the development of HIV infection in case of exposure.

In addition to drug therapy, substantial advances have been made in understanding the pathophysiology, treatment, and monitoring of HIV infection. These advances have resulted in changes in the standard of care for patients, including pregnant women, with HIV infection. More aggressive combination drug regimens that provide maximal viral suppression are now recommended. Although pregnancy alone is not a reason to defer treatment, the use of anti-HIV drugs during pregnancy requires special consideration. Unfortunately, no long-term data regarding the long-term effects on the fetus exist. Because of this, offering antiretroviral therapy (ART) to HIV-infected women—whether primarily to treat HIV infection or to reduce the likelihood of perinatal transmission—should be accompanied by a discussion of the known and unknown short- and long-term benefits and potential risks. Women who are taking HIV medications during pregnancy are encouraged to enroll in the Antiretroviral Pregnancy Registry (USDHHS, 2018a).

Current recommendations call for routine HIV counseling and voluntary HIV testing of pregnant women and women considering pregnancy. An HIV-infected pregnant woman should be given information to make an informed decision about treatment options. The HIV transmission rates from mother to child have been reduced because of several recommended interventions, including ART, formula feeding, and cesarean section. In developed countries, this number has decreased from 25% (without interventions) to approximately 1% (CDC, 2013d). In countries where ART is not available and mothers continue to breast-feed, the infection rate by age 2 for children born to HIV-infected mothers can be as high as 45% (WHO, 2013a). Infants born to HIV-infected mothers have positive HIV antibody results as long as 15 to 18 months after birth. This finding is caused by maternal antibodies that cross the placenta during gestation and remain in the infant's circulatory system. HIV infection can be diagnosed earlier by means of an HIV viral culture or measuring the amount of HIV RNA or viral load through polymerase chain reaction (PCR) or branched-chain DNA (bDNA) testing.

PATHOPHYSIOLOGY

HIV is classified as a "slow" **retrovirus** or a lentivirus. After infection with these types of viruses, a long time passes before specific signs and symptoms appear. HIV requires cells for replication. The virus takes over the host cell and reproduces viral copies of it. Retroviruses are made of RNA. Most organisms' genetic material is made up of DNA. The retrovirus uses reverse transcriptase, an enzyme, to make its RNA change to DNA. This process allows the virus to be incorporated into the host's genetic material.

HIV can cross over into the host in the dendritic immune cells that are located in the mucosal layer of the vulva, the vagina, the rectum, and the penis. The exterior layer of the dendritic cell passes the virus into the interior portion of the cell. The virus is released into the lymphatic system via tissue or lymph nodes. Then the virus binds to a **$CD4^+$ lymphocyte** (a type of white blood cell; a protein on the surface of cells that normally helps the body's immune system combat disease), by which it can travel farther into the lymphatic system and begin the cycle of infection (AIDSinfo, 2018).

The attachment of the viral particle to the host cell's $CD4^+$ receptor and co-receptor (CCR5 or CXCR4) is the first step in replication of the virus (Fig. 56.2). The HIV virion enters the host cell when the virus binds to the cell. After binding to the cell, co-receptors are needed to continue the fusion process and to enable the viral particle to eject two copies of the virus's RNA. Inside the cell, HIV reverse transcriptase changes the viral RNA into DNA. A full copy of this DNA is created and broken down into smaller, more functional pieces that are moved to the nucleus of the cell. The HIV DNA moves into the nucleus of the cell, where viral integrase helps insert it into the DNA of the host. The inserted virus is called a *provirus.* After activation, the cell makes a new copy of HIV by using viral proteins. Afterward, there is an abnormal amount of immune activation. This perpetuates the progress of the HIV infection because it creates more $CD4^+$ cells that will be under attack by HIV and eventually will exhaust the immune system. The number of $CD8^+$ T cells that are activated at this time is related directly to an increased risk of developing advanced HIV infection, or AIDS. However, the HIV can remain dormant for years if the $CD4^+$ cell remains inactivated. It has been difficult to control HIV completely because of its ability to remain undetected. Patients with HIV are advised to continue taking their antiretroviral medications (AIDSinfo, 2018).

New viral proteins are created when the infected $CD4^+$ cell converts DNA into RNA. This process is called *transcription.* The process relies on the host cell and the viral genetic material. The new RNA is messenger RNA (mRNA), and it is returned from the nucleus back into the cytoplasm. In the cytoplasm, mRNA is used as a template to begin making HIV protein. This process is called *translation.* The protein sequence of the mRNA is changed back into RNA, and this makes up the outer envelope and inner core of HIV. After translation, the genetic materials become smaller and smaller pieces of viral material. The viral protease chunks the genetic products into smaller pieces so that they can infect more $CD4^+$ host cells. This HIV protease is specific to this virus and is targeted by a class of medications called *protease inhibitors* that are used to manage HIV. The envelope's viral proteins are joined together inside the host cell's membrane, with the core proteins, RNA, and enzymes just inside the membrane.

HIV then "buds" by pinching off this cell. One infected $CD4^+$ cell has the ability to make thousands of cell copies quickly. The $CD4^+$ cell dies as a result of this replication process. As time goes on, so many $CD4^+$ cells are destroyed that the immune system becomes dysfunctional and opportunistic infections develop within the host.

INFLUENCES ON VIRAL LOAD AND DISEASE PROGRESSION

HIV replicates quickly after entering the host body. It can produce billions of copies rapidly, which infect $CD4^+$ cells and the lymphatic system (Fig. 56.3). The viral load of the host during the early stage of the infection can be extremely high and increases risk of virus transmission to other people who are exposed. The severity and progression of the infection are related to the host's infection with other STIs, age, and immune response. Basic host immune defenses (cellular and humoral) help limit replication and slow progression of HIV. Unfortunately, these immune responses cannot completely eliminate HIV from the host. The host can continue to appear healthy even when infected with the virus (Table 56.1). Some patients live with the virus for at least 10 years without any treatment and appear healthy. They are referred to as *long-term nonprogressors.*

Many factors can increase HIV disease progression. People who use drugs and engage in high-risk sexual behavior are less likely to employ infection-preventive methods. Poverty, incarceration, immigration status, and co-infection with STIs also can contribute to a person's risk for HIV infection (CDC, 2016). Depression may impair their use of resources to help manage their infection (Kalichman, 2008). Poor coping mechanisms and high levels of emotional stress have a negative effect on HIV disease progression (Ironson and Hayward, 2008; Leserman, 2008; Temoshok et al, 2008).

The virus can make amazing numbers of copies of itself daily (Ho et al, 1995; Wei et al, 1995). HIV contained in blood plasma has a half-life of less than 2 days. While the virus continues to replicate, many millions of $CD4^+$ cells are produced and destroyed each day. The viral load in the patient's blood determines how quickly the $CD4^+$ cells are destroyed.

The HIV viral load in the blood can remain low or difficult to detect for weeks or even months after the initial exposure and infection (Fig. 56.4). When the immune system responds, the viral load decreases quickly as the body effectively contains the infection. Normally, antigens that are deemed foreign intermingle with B cells. At this stage, antibodies are produced. T cells start a cell-based immune response. In the early stages of the infection, the antibodies are able to reduce the viral load. T cells are beckoned to the lymph nodes, where the virus is trapped (see Table 56.1). The virus replicates in the lymph system (nodes, tissue, spleen, and tonsils).

The HIV Life Cycle

HIV medicines in seven drug classes stop HIV at different stages in the HIV life cycle.

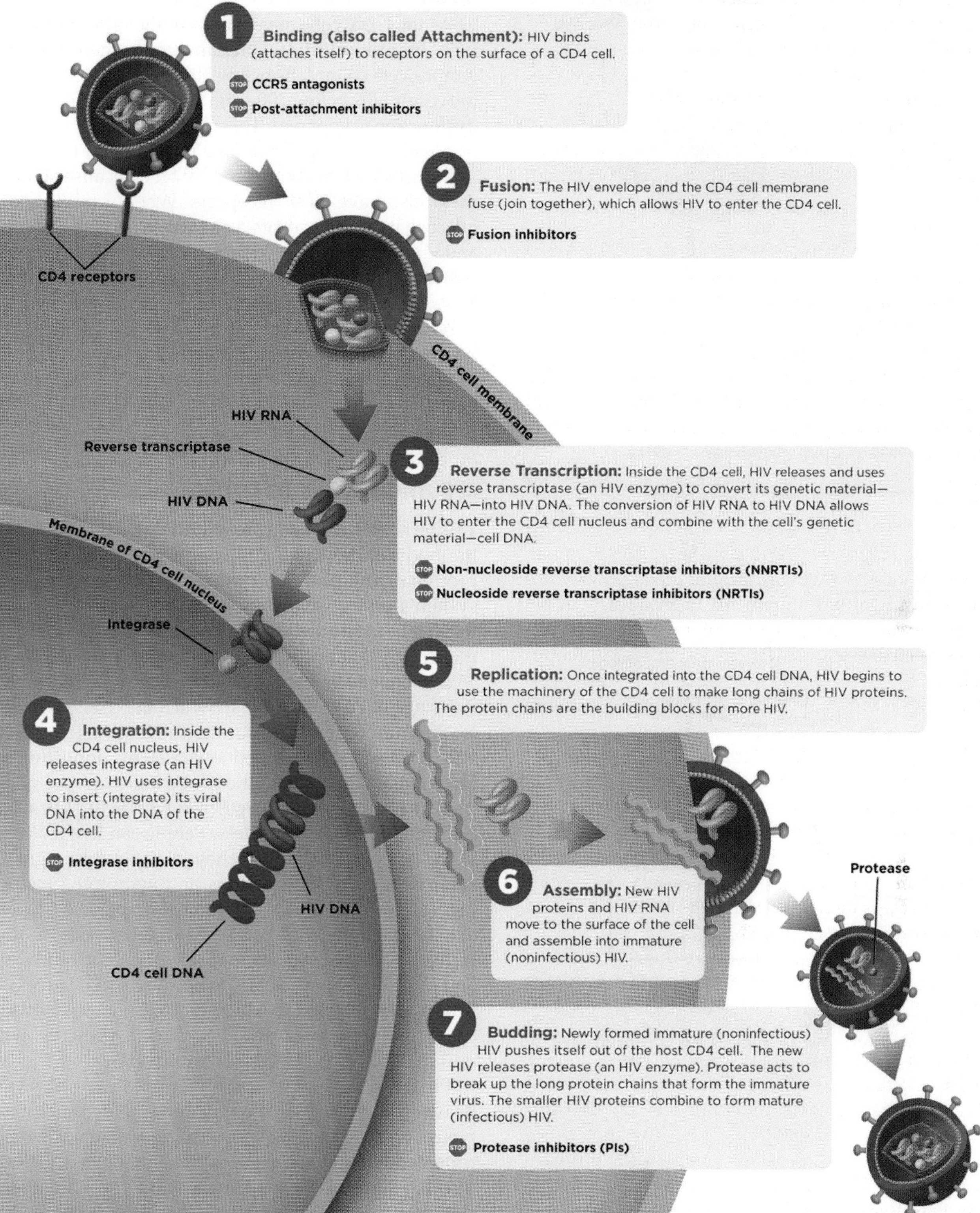

1 Binding (also called Attachment): HIV binds (attaches itself) to receptors on the surface of a CD4 cell.
CCR5 antagonists
Post-attachment inhibitors
2 Fusion: The HIV envelope and the CD4 cell membrane fuse (join together), which allows HIV to enter the CD4 cell.
Fusion inhibitors
CD4 receptors
CD4 cell membrane
HIV RNA
Reverse transcriptase
HIV DNA
3 Reverse Transcription: Inside the CD4 cell, HIV releases and uses reverse transcriptase (an HIV enzyme) to convert its genetic material—HIV RNA—into HIV DNA. The conversion of HIV RNA to HIV DNA allows HIV to enter the CD4 cell nucleus and combine with the cell's genetic material—cell DNA.
Non-nucleoside reverse transcriptase inhibitors (NNRTIs)
Nucleoside reverse transcriptase inhibitors (NRTIs)
Membrane of CD4 cell nucleus
Integrase
5 Replication: Once integrated into the CD4 cell DNA, HIV begins to use the machinery of the CD4 cell to make long chains of HIV proteins. The protein chains are the building blocks for more HIV.
4 Integration: Inside the CD4 cell nucleus, HIV releases integrase (an HIV enzyme). HIV uses integrase to insert (integrate) its viral DNA into the DNA of the CD4 cell.
Integrase inhibitors
HIV DNA
CD4 cell DNA
Protease
6 Assembly: New HIV proteins and HIV RNA move to the surface of the cell and assemble into immature (noninfectious) HIV.
7 Budding: Newly formed immature (noninfectious) HIV pushes itself out of the host CD4 cell. The new HIV releases protease (an HIV enzyme). Protease acts to break up the long protein chains that form the immature virus. The smaller HIV proteins combine to form mature (infectious) HIV.
Protease inhibitors (PIs)

Fig. 56.2 Life cycle of HIV cell.

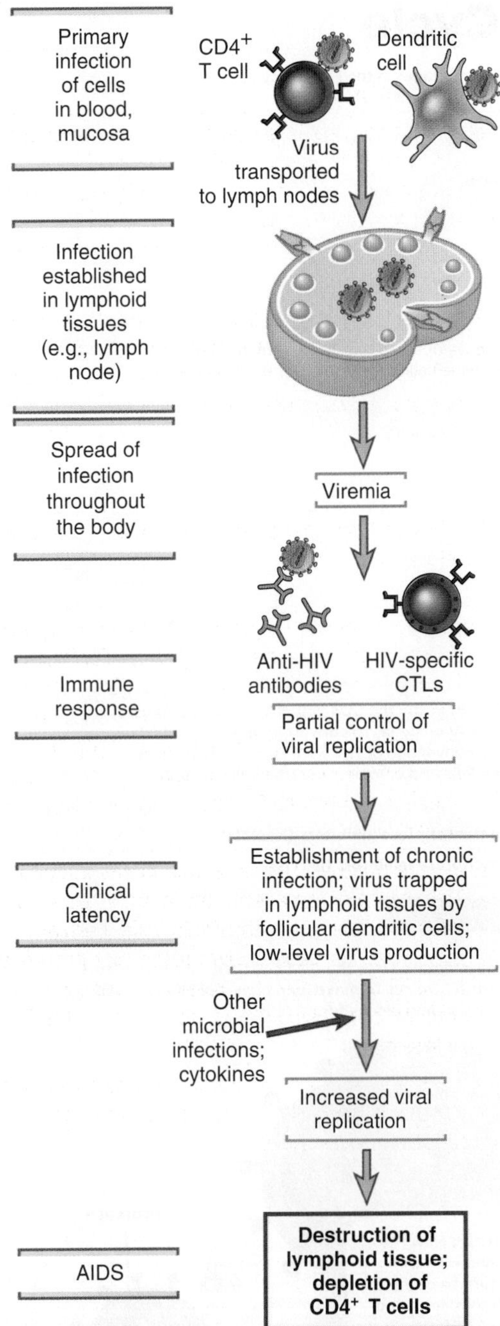

Fig. 56.3 Viral load in the blood and the relationship to $CD4^+$ lymphocyte cell count over the spectrum of human immunodeficiency virus (HIV) disease. *AIDS*, Acquired immunodeficiency syndrome; *CTL*, cytotoxic T lymphocyte. (From Abbas AK, Lichtman AH, Pillai S: *Basic immunology: Functions and disorders of the immune system*, ed 4, St. Louis, 2013, Saunders.)

The lymphatic system carries the infection from one site to another. During this time, the HIV-infected person does not have any signs or symptoms. Over time, the lymphatic system is damaged by the HIV. The virus enters the blood, which increases the rate of disease progression. The body is not able to mount an adequate response to new infections. The immune system damage is apparent on examination of B cell dysfunction, but more important $CD4^+$ cells are destroyed and their levels depleted (see Fig. 56.2).

As the $CD4^+$ cells are destroyed, the immune system fails. Immune dysfunction can occur when the $CD4^+$ lymphocyte count falls below 500/mm^3 of blood. When the count falls below 200/mm^3, severe immune system dysfunction is apparent. This results in the development of possibly fatal opportunistic infections in the host.

Monocytes can be infected by HIV because some of them also have $CD4^+$ receptors. When a monocyte is infected, it can change into a **phagocyte** (a cell that ingests and digests bacteria). When a phagocyte is infected with HIV, it merely works as a factory to create more HIV. An infected phagocyte can rupture as a result of a normal local inflammatory response. When this happens, the HIV is spread even deeper into the body. In this way, the skin, the lungs, bone marrow, the central nervous system, and lymph nodes become directly infected.

SPECTRUM OF HIV INFECTION

The term **HIV disease** (the state in which HIV enters the body under favorable conditions and multiplies, producing injurious effects) encompasses the immune system's progressive dysfunction that is produced by the viral activity within the host. HIV disease replaces the previous term *AIDS-related complex* (ARC) (Table 56.2). **Acquired immunodeficiency syndrome (AIDS)** (the end stage of HIV infection, in which the $CD4^+$ cell count is 200/mm^3 or lower) occurs as the disease progresses and the body is damaged severely by opportunistic infections. At this stage, the host's body can no longer protect itself and is injured (see Fig. 56.3). The $CD4^+$ cell count is 200/mm^3 or less. People can live for years with the infection before they develop any signs or symptoms of HIV. The signs and symptoms include night sweats, weight loss, diarrhea, unexplainable fevers, and fatigue. The viral course of HIV depends on host factors. The host has an increased risk for morbidity and mortality when he or she has inadequate access to health care services, is of lower socioeconomic status, or is under the care of a health care provider with minimal experience in dealing with HIV.

Progression from the early stages to end-stage HIV disease varies greatly. Three patterns have been found: typical progression, long-term nonprogression, and rapid progression. In the typical progression pattern, patients develop signs and symptoms several years after seroconversion. Many do not know they have been infected with HIV and can infect others. In the long-term nonprogression pattern, patients may not develop signs and symptoms even 30 years after seroconversion. The long-term nonprogression pattern is rare; it is thought to be longer because the immune response of affected

Table 56.1 **Types of White Blood Cells and Their Involvement in HIV Disease**

WHITE BLOOD CELL (WBC) TYPE	DESCRIPTION	ROLE IN HIV DISEASE
Neutrophils	Normally constitute 50%–75% of all circulating leukocytes and are capable of phagocytosis Important in the inflammatory response and the first line of defense against infection Short lifespan	Neutropenia (WBC deficiency) commonly occurs in advanced HIV disease. Drug-induced neutropenia is common, especially with drugs used to treat *P. jiroveci* pneumonia, toxoplasmosis, CMV retinitis, or colitis and with NRTIs.
Monocytes, macrophages	Constitute about 3%–7% of all WBCs Involved in the inflammatory response Capable of processing antigens for presentation to T cells Have $CD4^+$ receptors Macrophages: distributed throughout tissue and capable of phagocytosis	Monocytes and macrophages serve as a reservoir for HIV. When activated by stimulation with interferon (inflammatory response), they produce neopterin. Neopterin levels are increased in HIV disease.
Basophils, mast cells	Both: involved in acute inflammation Mast cells: breakdown releases histamine and other factors	In HIV infection, these cells may inhibit leukocyte migration.
T helper cells ($CD4^+$ or T4 cells)	Contain $CD4^+$ receptors Considered the "conductor" of the immune system because of their secretion of cytokines, which control most aspects of the immune response	These cells are the major target of HIV. Progressive infection gradually destroys the available pool of T helper cells so that the overall $CD4^+$ cell count drops. Lower $CD4^+$ cell counts correspond to more immunodeficiency and the onset of opportunistic infections. Infection with HIV can impair T helper cell function without killing the cell.
Cytotoxic T cells or cytotoxic T lymphocytes (CTLs; $CD8^+$ cells)	Contain $CD8^+$ receptors and produce cytokines in a more limited manner than do $CD4^+$ cells Combat viral and bacterial infections and are involved in direct killing of target cells by binding to them and releasing a substance that can perforate the cell membrane	Numbers of these cells increase in HIV infection. This increase represents the cellular response to infection. The strength of this initial cellular response has been shown to predict progression to AIDS (i.e., better cell response implies slower disease progression). Cytotoxic T cells kill T helper cells infected with HIV.
Natural killer (NK) cells	Large granular lymphocytes involved in cell-mediated immune response Able to kill target cells because target cells are coated with antibody that binds to receptors on the surface of NK cells, allowing the NK cell to attach Kill target cells by releasing a substance that triggers lysis (breakdown of cell wall) of cell	Counts and structure of these cells remain normal in patients with HIV infection, but they are functionally defective.
B cells	Produce antibodies specific to an antigen Capable of being stimulated by T helper cells	B cells are involved in the humoral response to HIV infection and produce a variety of antibodies against HIV. They are present throughout the course of HIV disease.

CMV, Cytomegalovirus; *HIV,* human immunodeficiency virus; *NRTI,* nucleoside reverse transcriptase inhibitor; *WBC,* white blood cell.

patients is very intense, so their viral load is lower. Also, there are genetic differences in their receptors (CCR5) on $CD4^+$ lymphocytes that make it difficult for the HIV to attach. This allows their $CD4^+$ and $CD8^+$ cells to be maintained at nearly normal levels.

Approximately 5% of people who are infected with HIV progress rapidly (CDC, 2016). In these patients, HIV infection progresses to an AIDS diagnosis within 3 years. Several common factors are found: their cytotoxic T cells ($CD8^+$ cells) are dysfunctional and unable to contain HIV, the level of virus remains very high throughout the infection, and HIV antibodies are minimal.

The term *acquired immunodeficiency syndrome* has been defined for surveillance and reporting purposes; it is not used alone to characterize serious disease caused by HIV infection (see Table 56.2).

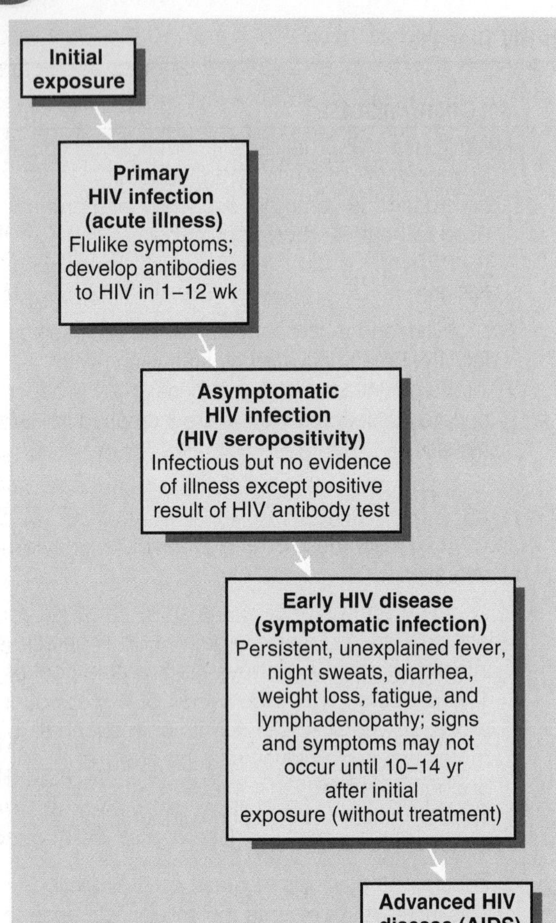

Fig. 56.4 Spectrum of human immunodeficiency virus (HIV) disease and associated signs and symptoms at various stages of the disease process. *AIDS*, Acquired immunodeficiency syndrome.

Table 56.2 Proper Terms Related to HIV and AIDS

MISLEADING PHRASES	MORE ACCURATE PHRASES
High-risk groups	High-risk behaviors
Infection with AIDS	HIV infection
AIDS test	HIV antibody test
AIDS positive	HIV positive
AIDS victim or patient	Person living with HIV or AIDS
AIDS carrier	HIV-infected person

AIDS, Acquired immunodeficiency syndrome; *HIV*, human immunodeficiency virus.

ACUTE RETROVIRAL SYNDROME

Viral replication occurs during the acute infection period. The viral load peaks at millions of copies of virus per milliliter of plasma. The viral load declines right before the appearance of detectable antibodies that can be measured in the blood. The viral set point, or stabilizing of the viral load, is reached 4 to 6 months after exposure. This viral set point is important because some researchers believe it to be a prognostic indicator of long-term survival: that is, the lower the viral set point, the longer the individual will survive with HIV disease. Postexposure prophylaxis (PEP), begun as soon as possible after exposure, may help lower this viral set point. This theory is demonstrated in cases in which health care personnel initiate PEP medications after an exposure and do not undergo seroconversion.

Seroconversion, as defined previously, is the development of antibodies from HIV, which takes place approximately 5 days to 3 months after exposure (generally within 2 to 4 weeks) (AIDSinfo, 2018). This process is accompanied by a flulike or mononucleosis-like syndrome consisting of fever, night sweats, pharyngitis, headache, malaise, arthralgias, myalgias, diarrhea, nausea, and a diffuse rash prominent on the trunk. These symptoms last approximately 1 to 2 weeks, although some symptoms may last for several months. Seroconversion illness occurs in approximately 89% of HIV-infected people. HIV antibodies appear in 95% of people within 3 months of infection, and seroconversion occurs in 99% within 6 months. The viral load during the period of seroconversion is extremely high, with a short-term drop in $CD4^+$ cells. The $CD4^+$ cell level quickly returns to normal as the immune system mounts an attack against the viral infection; as a result, viral loads exist at nearly undetectable levels in the blood. In most people with HIV infection, the acute retroviral illness is mild and may be mistaken for a cold or other minor viral infection (Table 56.3).

Table 56.3 Acute HIV Infection: Frequency of Associated Signs and Symptoms

SIGN OR SYMPTOM	FREQUENCY (%)
Fever	96
Headache	32
Lymphadenopathy	74
Nausea and vomiting	27
Pharyngitis	70
Hepatosplenomegaly	14
Rash	70
Weight loss	13
Myalgia or arthralgia	54
Thrush	12
Diarrhea	32
Neurologic symptoms	12
Oral or genital ulcers	5–20

HIV, Human immunodeficiency virus.
From the Department of Health and Human Services Panel on Antiretroviral Guidelines for Adults and Adolescents. Guidelines for the Use of Antiretroviral Agents in HIV-1 Infected Adults and Adolescents.

EARLY INFECTION

The median time between HIV infection and the development of end-stage HIV disease, or AIDS, in an untreated individual is between 8 and 14 years. This phase of

HIV disease sometimes is called the *asymptomatic phase* because the HIV-infected individual looks and feels healthy. Some individuals have vague symptoms of a viral infection, including fatigue, headaches, low-grade fever, and night sweats. Because many of the symptoms of early infection are nonspecific, a diagnosis of HIV infection may not be made. Consequently, individuals may continue to engage in risky sexual and drug-using behaviors. Although seemingly healthy, the HIV-infected individual can transmit HIV to others. Lack of knowledge of one's HIV antibody status puts one at risk for earlier development of more advanced disease because changes in behaviors, such as those that promote health, are not instituted. Furthermore, if an individual is aware of being infected with the virus, early intervention with antiretroviral medications may prolong the asymptomatic phase and prevent progression to AIDS.

EARLY SYMPTOMATIC DISEASE

The early symptomatic phase of HIV infection occurs when the $CD4^+$ cell count drops below $500/mm^3$. Early symptoms include constitutional problems such as persistent, unexplained fevers; recurrent drenching night sweats; chronic diarrhea; headaches; and fatigue. These signs and symptoms become severe enough to affect activities of daily living. A physical examination may reveal persistent generalized lymphadenopathy; recurrent or localized infections; and neurologic manifestations, such as numbness and tingling or weakness in the extremities (Box 56.1).

One of the most common infections in individuals with early symptomatic disease is oral candidiasis (thrush), a fungal infection that is rare in healthy adults (see Fig. 56.4). Other infections that signal immune dysfunction include varicella-zoster virus (shingles), persistent vaginal candidiasis (yeast infections), and increased frequency of oral or genital HSV outbreaks. Oral hairy leukoplakia, a condition related to the Epstein-Barr virus, and oral thrush are early indicators of HIV disease and prognostic markers for disease progression. Because of this, dental health professionals have a key role in identifying cases of early HIV disease.

Persistent generalized lymphadenopathy is defined as enlargement (≥1 cm) of two or more lymph nodes, located in places other than the inguinal region, that persists for at least 3 months. This condition may be present for many years before AIDS is diagnosed.

Neurologic manifestations of HIV disease occur in more than 90% of individuals who are infected. Neurologic symptoms include peripheral neuropathies, headaches, aseptic meningitis, cranial nerve palsies, and myopathies. These conditions may be caused by the HIV infection or may be side effects related to antiretroviral medications.

Several cofactors may influence a more rapid progression of HIV disease. In very young children and very old adults, the disease progresses more quickly. Concurrent infections such as HSV, cytomegalovirus, or Epstein-Barr virus affect progression. Drug and alcohol use, including smoking, may suppress the immune system. Malnutrition also is known to affect immune function, but further study relative to HIV is needed.

Box 56.1 Signs and Symptoms of HIV Infection

- Abdominal pain
- Chills and fever
- Cough (dry or productive)
- Diarrhea
- Disorientation
- Dyspnea
- Fatigue
- Headache
- Lymphadenopathy (any disorder of the lymph nodes or lymph vessels)
- Malaise
- Muscle or joint pain
- Night sweats
- Oral lesions
- Shortness of breath
- Skin rash
- Sore throat
- Weight loss

HIV, Human immunodeficiency virus.

AIDS

Acquired immunodeficiency syndrome is the term used to describe the end stage, or terminal phase, of the spectrum of HIV infection. The CDC has developed specific diagnostic criteria that must be present to make this diagnosis. These conditions are more likely to occur with severe immunosuppression. As HIV disease progresses, the $CD4^+$ lymphocyte count decreases, and the ratio of $CD4^+$ to $CD8^+$ cells (T helper cells to T suppressor cells), which is normally 2 to 1, gradually shifts, resulting in more $CD8^+$ than $CD4^+$. The amount of virus detectable in the blood increases rapidly and remains high despite pharmacologic interventions. The number of white blood cells also may decline, and the person's reactivity to skin tests, such as purified protein derivative (tuberculin), is decreased or absent. An individual is said to be anergic if no skin response is noted.

Without treatment, people with AIDS can expect to survive approximately 3 years, but this varies greatly. With the advent of more effective antiretroviral and opportunistic disease prophylaxis, the lifespan of an individual infected with HIV is difficult to predict (AIDSinfo, 2018). Morbidity in people with advanced HIV disease also varies widely. Some people are severely ill and die rather quickly, whereas others have only to make minor adjustments in their lifestyle to cope with medical regimens or physical symptoms, such as fatigue or pain. Significant advances in the management of HIV disease have made it resemble a chronic illness. The effects of therapy on mortality have been significant: The number of new AIDS cases reported to the CDC every year has leveled off. This can be attributed to effective prophylaxis for opportunistic infections and to the development of ART.

LABORATORY AND DIAGNOSTIC EXAMINATIONS

Strong evidence shows that early intervention postpones the onset of severe immunosuppression. Encourage individuals at risk for HIV infection to seek HIV antibody testing, and educate them in how to decrease the risk of HIV transmission.

HIV ANTIBODY TESTING

Patients need to understand the implications of an HIV antibody test (Box 56.2):

- The individual's blood is tested for the presence of antibodies to the HIV infection. This is referred to as **enzyme-linked immunosorbent assay (ELISA)** testing. If this screening results in positive findings the blood is tested with a more specific test such as the **Western blot** (CDC, 2014).
- Tests with indeterminate results are repeated at a later date, generally in 4 to 6 weeks. Consistently indeterminate results necessitate the use of a viral culture or the measurement of viral load by means of bDNA measurement, reverse transcriptase–polymerase chain reaction (RT-PCR), or nucleic acid sequence–based amplification (NASBA).
- The series of laboratory tests confirms the presence or absence of antibodies to HIV, but their presence does not mean the person has AIDS. The tests are not diagnostic of AIDS. AIDS is diagnosed according to the 2008 CDC definition.
- A result that is **seronegative** (the state of lacking HIV antibodies as confirmed by blood test) is not an assurance that the individual is free of HIV infection, inasmuch as seroconversion may not yet have occurred.
- A seronegative result does not mean that an individual is free from risk of infection. If an individual continues to engage in risky behaviors, such as unprotected sexual intercourse or use of contaminated needles or drug paraphernalia, transmission may occur (Box 56.3).

Box 56.2 Tests Used to Detect HIV Infection

ANTIBODY DETECTION TESTS

Screening Tests

- Enzyme-linked immunosorbent assay (ELISA) (blood)
- Agglutination assays (blood or clean-catch urine specimen)
- Oral fluid test (swabbing of the cheek and gum)
- Urine screening test

Confirmatory Test

- Western blot
- Indirect immunofluorescent antibody assay
- Radioimmunoprecipitation assay (RIPA)

ANTIGEN DETECTION TESTS (P24 ANTIGEN)

HIV Viral Load Tests/ Nucleic Acid Determination Assays

- Reverse transcriptase–polymerase chain reaction (RT-PCR)
- Branched-chain DNA (bDNA)
- Nucleic acid sequence–based amplification (NASBA)

Viral Culture Method

- HIV culture

Activated Immune Markers

- Neopterin
- β_2-microglobulin
- Absolute $CD4^+$ cell count
- Percentage of $CD4^+$ cells
- Percentage of $CD8^+$ cells
- $CD4^+/CD8^+$ cell ratio

HIV, Human immunodeficiency virus.

$CD4^+$ CELL MONITORING

Monitoring $CD4^+$ cells is one of the laboratory parameters used to track the progression of HIV disease. As the disease progresses, the number of $CD4^+$ cells decreases. The more significant the loss, the more severe the immunosuppression becomes. The $CD4^+$ cell count is the best marker of the immunodeficiency associated with HIV infection. As such, the $CD4^+$ cell count influences making decisions about antiretroviral and prophylactic drug therapy and is used to evaluate specific complaints related to the risk for contracting particular opportunistic infections. For example, *Mycobacterium avium* complex and cytomegalovirus infections are rare in patients with $CD4^+$ cell counts higher than 50/mm^3. *P. jiroveci* pneumonia and cryptococcosis are unusual in patients with $CD4^+$ cell counts higher than 200/mm^3. The $CD4^+$ cell count is not a perfect surrogate marker of immunodeficiency, and factors such as the patient's clinical status always must be taken into account.

The $CD4^+$ cell count reflects the number of $CD4^+$ cells per cubic millimeter (or per microliter) of blood. It does not indicate the total number of $CD4^+$ cells in the body. Millions of new $CD4^+$ cells are produced daily and cleared by normal body processes (unrelated to the virus). The absolute $CD4^+$ cell count can vary greatly in the same individual, depending on the time of day the blood is drawn; which laboratory is used; and the presence of acute illness or other factors, such as alcohol. Therefore continue to use the same laboratory, draw blood at the same time of day, and avoid testing on days when the patient is acutely ill or under abnormal stress. When using the $CD4^+$ cell count to make important treatment decisions, such as initiating prophylaxis for opportunistic infections, collect two separate samples a few weeks apart.

VIRAL LOAD MONITORING

The ability to detect HIV viral load measurements in plasma is a significant advancement in the monitoring of HIV disease. Viral load or burden is a quantitative

Box 56.3 Counseling Before and After HIV Antibody Testing

GENERAL GUIDELINES

- People who are being tested for HIV are commonly fearful of the test results; therefore carry out the following steps:
  - Establish rapport with the patient.
  - Assess the patient's ability to understand counseling.
  - Determine the patient's access to support systems.
- Explain the following benefits of testing:
  - Testing provides an opportunity for education that can decrease the risk of new infections.
  - Infected patients can be referred for early intervention and support programs.
- Discuss the following negative aspects of testing:
  - Breaches of confidentiality have led to discrimination.
  - A positive test result affects all aspects of the patient's life (personal, social, economic) and can raise difficult emotions (anger, anxiety, guilt, thoughts of suicide).

PRETEST COUNSELING

- Determine the patient's risk factors and when the last exposure risk occurred. Individualize counseling according to these parameters.
- Provide education to decrease future risk of exposure.
- Provide education that will help the patient protect sexual and drug-sharing partners.
- Discuss problems related to the delay between infection and an accurate test result:
  - Testing must be repeated at intervals for 6 months after each possible exposure.
  - The patient needs to abstain from further high-risk behaviors during that interval.
  - The patient needs to protect sexual and drug-sharing partners during that interval.
- Discuss the possibility of false-negative test results, which are most likely to occur during the period between infection and seroconversion.
- Provide information regarding the confidentiality of results.
- Explain that a positive test result shows HIV infection, not AIDS.
- Explain that the test result does not establish immunity.
- Assess the patient's support systems; provide telephone numbers and resources as needed.
- Discuss the patient's personally anticipated responses to test results (positive and negative).
- Outline assistance that will be offered if the test result is positive.

POSTTEST COUNSELING

- If the test result is negative, reinforce pretest counseling and prevention education. Remind the patient that test must be repeated at intervals for 6 months after the most recent exposure risk.
- Explain the need to report positive test results to the state health department and CDC.
- Discuss the importance of partner notification.
- If the test result is positive, understand that the patient may be in shock and not hear what is said after receiving that news.
- Provide resources for medical and emotional support, and help the patient get immediate assistance.
- Evaluate the patient's suicide risk, and follow up as needed.
- Determine need to test other people who have had high-risk contact with the patient.
- Discuss retesting to verify results. This tactic provides hope for the patient, but, of more importance, it keeps the patient in touch with health care professionals. While waiting for the second test result, the patient has time to think about and adjust to the possibility of being infected with HIV.
- Encourage optimism:
  - Remind the patient that treatments are available.
  - Review health habits that can improve the immune system.
  - Arrange for patients to speak to HIV-infected people who are willing to share and assist patients with new diagnoses during the transition period.
  - Reinforce that an HIV-positive test result means the patient is infected but does not necessarily mean that the patient has AIDS.

AIDS, Acquired immunodeficiency syndrome; *HIV,* human immunodeficiency virus.
Modified from Bradley-Springer LA, Fendrick R: *HIV instant instructor cards,* El Paso, TX, 1994, Skidmore-Roth; and Consolidated Guidelines on HIV Testing Services: 5Cs: Consent, Confidentiality, Counselling, Correct Results and Connection 2015. Geneva: World Health Organization; 2015 Jul. 3, PRE-TEST AND POST-TEST SERVICES. Available from: *https://www.ncbi.nlm.nih.gov/books/NBK316035.*

measure of HIV viral RNA in the peripheral circulation, or the level of virus in the blood.

Three quantitative assay tests are available to measure viral load levels: NASBA, RT-PCR, and bDNA. Even very small numbers of infected cells can be detected by identifying virions. These tests can be used only to identify HIV. These tests are helpful for identifying HIV in people who have a negative ELISA (antibody) result.

Important characteristics of viral load monitoring include the following:

- In all clinical stages of the illness, HIV virus detection techniques identify measurable amounts of viral RNA copies in the plasma of most HIV-infected individuals.
- Viral load can provide significant information used to predict the course of disease progression, initiate ART, measure the degree of antiretroviral effect achieved, and note the failure of a drug regimen.
- Plasma levels of HIV RNA fall dramatically after effective ART.
- Detection of HIV RNA in plasma does not indicate whether any virus is present in lymphoid or other tissues.

Viral load and $CD4^+$ cell counts are distinct markers that provide different information. Viral load can indicate disease progression and long-term clinical outcome; $CD4^+$ cell measurements can indicate the damage sustained by the immune system (the loss of $CD4^+$ or T cells) and the short-term risk for developing opportunistic infections. Each is an independent predictor of clinical outcome, and in combination they can give a more complete indication of clinical status, treatment response, and prognosis. Coffin (1996) used a metaphor to describe the infected patient without symptoms: as a train rushing along a track, heading for a bridge that has been destroyed. The time the crash will occur is determined by two variables: (1) where the train is at a particular instant ($CD4^+$), and (2) how fast it is going (viral load).

A baseline determination of viral burden is recommended, with subsequent measurements every 3 to 4 months, in conjunction with $CD4^+$ cell monitoring and clinical evaluations such as a history and physical examination. Guidelines continue to be revised as the implications of viral measurement evolve and its interpretation and use become better understood. In the future, opportunistic infection prophylaxis may be based on viral load, as well as on $CD4^+$ cell counts.

RESISTANCE TESTING

Drug resistance to ART can make effective treatment of HIV challenging. In countries with high incomes, 10% to 17% of patients who have never taken HIV medications have mutations that indicate resistance to at least one ART medication (USDHHS, 2017). HIV mutates easily, which makes it hard to treat and contain. After multiple genetic mutations, the replication of HIV is chaotic and disorderly, which makes it more resistant to medication treatment and has prevented the development of an effective vaccine. ART resistance results from a patient's inability to adhere to ART protocols. Assay tests can detect HIV genetic mutations that result in ART resistance. Results of these tests are available in less than a month. A list of ART-resistant mutations has been developed by the International AIDS Society–USA. Phenotyping is available to help estimate how well the specific strain of virus will respond to treatment in people who have been receiving ART for a long time. To perform phenotyping, the patient must have a high viral load (Panel on Antiretroviral Guidelines for Adults and Adolescents, 2018). Genotyping is less expensive to perform, and the results are often available faster than those of phenotyping. Genotyping is recommended for patients who have not received ART (USDHHS, 2017).

During the acute stage of HIV, resistance testing is important for administering appropriate ART to prevent extensive replication of HIV. Some health care providers identify baseline genetic mutations before starting ART. A patient-specific ART regimen can be created to avoid medications that would not work. Patients who are resistant to some ART medications may have cross-resistance issues with other ART medications. Resistant HIV strains are found in people who have undergone ART, as well as in other people who are newly infected and have not received treatment. Resistance to some ART drugs and the ability to transmit resistance to newly infected people are important issues for public health officials who are battling to control and prevent HIV infection.

OTHER LABORATORY PARAMETERS

Hematologic abnormalities are common in HIV infections and may be caused by the HIV, by opportunistic infections, or by drug or radiation therapy. The white blood cell count often is decreased, usually in conjunction with lymphopenia (decreased numbers of lymphocytes). Thrombocytopenia (decreased platelet count) may be caused by antiplatelet antibodies. Anemia is related to the chronic disease process and to HIV invasion of the bone marrow; it is a common adverse effect of antiretroviral agents.

Alterations in liver function tests are not uncommon. Abnormalities may be caused by viral hepatitis, alcohol abuse, opportunistic infections, neoplasms, or medications. Early identification of hepatitis B and hepatitis C viral infections is important, because these infections may follow a more serious course in patients with HIV disease. Patients who are HIV positive are often also seropositive for hepatitis B, inasmuch as infections are bloodborne and sexually transmitted. In addition, about 25% of HIV-infected people in the United States are co-infected with hepatitis C, one of the most significant causes of chronic liver disease.

Syphilis testing is important because syphilis is more complicated and aggressive in HIV infected patients. It is also more difficult to treat with standard therapies and more likely to advance quickly to neurosyphilis. If a person with HIV infection is seropositive for syphilis, assessment and treatment must be performed immediately.

THERAPEUTIC MANAGEMENT

Therapeutic management of HIV-infected patients focuses on monitoring HIV disease progression and immune function, preventing the development of opportunistic diseases, initiating and monitoring ART, detecting and treating opportunistic diseases, managing symptoms, and preventing complications of treatment.

HIV-positive individuals must be linked to various resources, depending on their individual needs. Individuals often deny the infection, neglect their mental and physical health, and continue behaviors that put themselves and other people at risk. Interventions must be sustained and reinforced; the emotional effect of such devastating news ("You are HIV positive") can overshadow any initial information or education provided. Stress safer behaviors and the need for medical and emotional support, such as assistance in family planning, treatment for substance abuse, treatment for STIs, treatment for tuberculosis, and immunizations.

A transdisciplinary care approach is most appropriate for patients with HIV disease because of their complex medical and psychosocial needs. The HIV-infected patient should be the primary member of this team, working along with a physician who specializes in HIV, a social worker, a case manager, a dietitian, and a nurse. Other team members may include a dentist, a primary care provider (physician, osteopath, nurse practitioner, or physician assistant), a mental health worker, a substance abuse counselor, a nontraditional therapist (such as a massage therapist or acupuncturist), and the individual's family and significant other.

PHARMACOLOGIC MANAGEMENT

Opportunistic Diseases Associated With HIV

Probably the most difficult aspect of the medical management of HIV is dealing with the many opportunistic diseases that develop as the immune system degenerates. Although it is usually impossible to totally eradicate opportunistic diseases, the use of ART and prophylactic interventions can control their emergence or progression. However, these regimens must continue throughout the patient's life; otherwise, the disease will return. Advances in the diagnosis and treatment of opportunistic diseases have contributed significantly to increased life expectancy and decreased morbidity. Box 56.4 lists common opportunistic diseases associated with HIV disease.

Box 56.4 Common Opportunistic Diseases Associated With HIV

- Candidiasis of bronchi, trachea, esophagus, or lungs
- Invasive cervical cancer
- Coccidioidomycosis
- Cryptococcosis
- Cryptosporidiosis, chronic intestinal (greater than 1 month's duration)
- Cytomegalovirus (CMV) disease (particularly CMV retinitis)
- Encephalopathy, HIV-related
- Herpes simplex: chronic ulcer(s) (greater than 1 month's duration); or bronchitis, pneumonitis, or esophagitis
- Histoplasmosis
- Isosporiasis, chronic intestinal (greater than 1 month's duration)
- Kaposi's sarcoma
- Lymphoma, multiple forms
- *Mycobacterium avium* complex
- Tuberculosis
- *Pneumocystis carinii* pneumonia
- Pneumonia, recurrent
- Progressive multifocal leukoencephalopathy
- Salmonella septicemia, recurrent
- Toxoplasmosis of brain
- Wasting syndrome resulting from HIV

HIV.gov: *What are opportunistic infections?*, 2017. Retrieved from https://www.aids.gov/hiv-aids-basics/staying-healthy-with-hiv-aids/potential-related-health-problems/opportunistic-infections/.

HIV, Human immunodeficiency virus.

Antiretroviral Therapy

Combination antiretroviral therapy (ART) is an important component in the management of HIV infection (Table 56.4). In 1987 zidovudine was the only medication available to treat patients with HIV disease; since then, the FDA has approved more than 25 antiretroviral medications. Six different classes of ART are used to prevent the viral replication process: integrase strand transfer inhibitors, fusion inhibitors, CCR5 antagonists (also referred to as entry inhibitors), nucleoside reverse transcriptase inhibitors (NRTIs), nonnucleoside reverse transcriptase inhibitors (NNRTIs), and protease inhibitors (PI). Each class of medication interrupts HIV at different stages of the infectious process. Some ART medications are available as a combination of medications so that several medications are combined into one pill that is taken each day, which allows for better patient compliance (HIV.gov, 2017a). In ART, HIV is treated with three or more antiretroviral medications,

Scientists have found that the most effective medication regimen is the use of *cocktails* (generally three or more compounds given together). Medication combinations make it much more difficult for the virus to develop resistance to the drugs. Such intervention also may slow the progression from asymptomatic or mildly symptomatic HIV infection to a more advanced disease. Therapies that can reduce the quantity of circulating virus dramatically in the blood have been developed; in many cases, blood circulating levels become undetectable. It is still possible for one individual to infect another with the virus despite having undetectable viral levels. Protease inhibitors directly reduce the ability of HIV to replicate, or make copies of itself, inside cells. As increasing numbers of therapeutic agents and clinical trial results become available, decisions about ART have become increasingly complex. For now, these combination therapies offer optimism for successful disease management and improvements in the quality and duration of life.

Considerations for ART include the following:

- Previous experience with ART may affect the efficacy of a proposed therapy, because the virus may have

Table 56.4 Pros and Cons of Highly Active Antiretroviral Therapy (ART)

PROs	CONs
• Minimizes chance of emergence of resistant strain of virus • May play a role in the reduction of HIV transmission • Slows disease progression • Improves quality of life	• Can be toxic • Frequent side effects • Complexity of drug and dosing regimens • Difficulty with adherence to regimen (nonadherence can result in treatment failure) • High cost

HIV, Human immunodeficiency virus.

become resistant to medications taken by the patient in the past (e.g., zidovudine, lamivudine).

- Certain combinations of antiretroviral drugs may reverse the resistance to a single drug. Recycling drugs previously taken can sometimes improve viral suppression. Incorrect dosing (timing) or incorrect usage (missed doses) can cause drug resistance.
- Drug incompatibilities, similar side effect profiles, and toxic effects must be considered in the choice of a regimen.
- The patient's commitment to taking medication each day must be considered. Inadequate adherence can lead to drug resistance and, ultimately, to drug failure. This point must be stressed to the patient. Adherence is paramount for survival and success of treatment.

HIV-infected patients should begin taking HIV medications as soon as possible. A provider with expertise in HIV should supervise the care. Treatment should be offered to all patients with early HIV infection, who are pregnant, who have been diagnosed with AIDS or HIV-related coninfections or diseases (AIDSinfo, 2018).

Current HIV treatment is aimed at preventing the immune system damage that results from HIV replication. If HIV replication can be halted, then viral mutation can be prevented, and drug resistance issues can be decreased. ART is aimed at limiting viral loads to undetectable levels. With early ART, the patient's $CD4^+$ cell counts will remain normal for a longer time.

Clinical trials being conducted by the AIDS Clinical Trials Group and the National Institutes of Health in conjunction with universities, pharmaceutical companies, and other agencies may be important considerations for people with HIV disease. Patients may be able to participate in clinical trials or may benefit from the results of such research studies. Benefits include (1) access to new and potentially effective treatments for HIV disease before they are released to the public, (2) the chance to have physician visits and laboratory work paid for by the research study, and (3) the opportunity to be cared for by a health care team with HIV experience (ACGT, n.d.).

Complementary and Alternative Therapies

People with HIV disease often use nontraditional or complementary therapies, such as massage, acupuncture or acupressure, and biofeedback. Some patients use nutritional supplements or herbal remedies with the hope of alleviating the side effects of the disease and the medications. Many patients prefer these therapies because of the limitations or side effects of approved drugs, mistrust of the health care system, easier access, lack of adequate insurance coverage, or the high cost of anti-HIV medications. These alternatives are best used in conjunction with approved therapeutic intervention.

Many patients may consider the use of complementary therapies. Alternative forms of therapy may be beneficial and always should be explored thoroughly. Patients should discuss their use with their health care team. It is important to educate the patient about selective review and use of complementary and alternative therapies. Their potential benefits and risks, along with the associated financial strain, should be evaluated carefully. Patients may need guidance to avoid expensive and particularly dangerous forms of alternative treatments. An open relationship and good communication with the patient build trust, creating a positive atmosphere for addressing difficult issues. They also reinforce the philosophy that the patient is an important participating member of the health care team.

Vaccine Development

Unfortunately, a vaccine for HIV is not yet available; however, clinical trials are under way. It has been difficult to develop a vaccine for HIV because the retrovirus easily mutates, many different viral strains exist, and poor adherence to ART has led to drug resistance issues. However, with greater understanding of the immune response to HIV and more effective ways to administer antigens, an aggressive push to create a vaccine continues. Since the mid-1980s, many initiatives and partnerships among organizations worldwide have attempted to develop a vaccine for HIV. Researchers have taken many approaches: live attenuated vaccinations, live recombinant vaccines, and subunit vaccines (WHO, 2013b). At the time of this publication, a large clinical trial called HVTN 702 is being launched in South Africa to test the effectiveness of an HIV vaccine (SciDevNet, 2016).

NURSING INTERVENTIONS

Establish a comfort level in interacting with people with HIV disease. Patients must be treated in a nonjudgmental, empathetic, and caring manner regardless of their sexual practices or history of drug use. The nurse's attitudes, values, and beliefs should not interfere with the care of a patient with HIV disease. Patients are aware when their caregiver is not comfortable dealing with HIV disease. Knowledge of HIV transmission and competence in standard precautions and body substance isolation will minimize the fear of caring for HIV-infected patients. Boxes 56.5 and 56.6 and Table 56.5 list appropriate nursing assessments, activities, and interventions for HIV infection and disease.

Patient problems and interventions for the patient with HIV disease include but are not limited to the following:

Patient Problem	Nursing Interventions
Potential for Opportunistic Infection	Limit visitors Assess for early onset of infectious processes and unusual cancers Practice good hand hygiene

Patient Problem	Nursing Interventions
Insufficient Knowledge, related to • Health management • Disease process and progression • Prevention of complications • Medications	Provide patient and family teaching concerning diagnosis and health maintenance activities geared toward health promotion
Insufficient nutrition: Less than body requirements	Assess nutritional needs Provide between-meal snacks and supplements as indicated
Inability to Tolerate Activity	Encourage frequent rest periods Cluster care delivery to avoid tiring patient
Potential for Excessive Demand on Primary Caregiver, related to advancing disease in care recipient and inadequate caregiver coping patterns	Assess needs and capabilities of patient and caregiver Assess factors that contribute to caregiver strain Develop supportive and trusting relationship with caregiver Enlist the help of family members, significant others, and friends to assist caregiver Encourage interaction in support groups for caregivers Teach stress reduction techniques to caregiver Encourage caregiver to attend to own personal and health care needs
Frequent, Loose Stools, related to: • Gastrointestinal infections • Malabsorption • Medication side effects	Document quantity, quality, and frequency of stools Monitor intake and output, vital signs, and daily weight Assess for skin impairment Administer antidiarrheals on a routine schedule Encourage increased electrolyte-rich fluid intake (fruit juices, Gatorade, Pedialyte) Encourage high-protein, high-calorie, and low-residue diet

Health care needs can be unpredictable and assessment difficult because of the clinical diversity of HIV infection. HIV disease may necessitate alternating periods of long-term and acute care. The patient may fear isolation from the community or family and friends because of the social stigma associated with HIV disease.

The disease affects primarily young people who are at the most productive time in their lives, a time when they are expected to take control of their lives. For this reason, they often want an active role in the decision-making and planning stages of their care. Patients may experience bouts of serious, debilitating illness and then recover enough to function effectively for an unpredictable amount of time. People with HIV disease often prefer to stay at home as long as possible, and some prefer to die at home. Long-term care in an inpatient setting (e.g., long-term care facility) is not compatible with the social needs of young patients. Prolonged care is expensive. Patients who experience chronic diseases may find their insurance coverage is limited. In addition, the absence of insurance may affect availability and affordability of treatment options. Religious and community-based organization volunteers, such as AIDS project workers, provide support and care services for patients and families. Friends, family, and significant others are also important resources to be considered in the planning of care for the patient with HIV disease.

Health Promotion

Goals for the National HIV Strategy

1. Reduce the number of new HIV infections.
2. Increase access to care and improve health outcomes for people living with HIV.
3. Reduce HIV-related health disparities and health inequities.
4. Achieve a more coordinated national response to the HIV epidemic.

The following are indicators of the progress of this strategy:

- Increase the percentage of people living with HIV who know their serostatus to at least 90%.
- Reduce the number of new diagnoses of HIV by at least 25%.
- Reduce the percentage of young gay and bisexual men who have engaged in HIV-risk behaviors by at least 10%.
- Increase the percentage of newly diagnosed persons linked to HIV medical care within 1 month of their HIV diagnosis to at least 85%.
- Increase the percentage of persons with diagnosed HIV infection who are retained in HIV medical care to at least 90%.
- Increase the percentage of persons with diagnosed HIV infection who are virally suppressed to at least 80%.
- Reduce the percentage of persons in HIV medical care who are homeless to no more than 5%.
- Reduce the death rate among persons with diagnosed HIV infection by at least 33%.
- Reduce disparities in the rate of new diagnoses by at least 15% in the following groups: gay and bisexual men, young black gay and bisexual men, black females, and persons living in the southern United States.
- Increase the percentage of youth and persons who inject drugs with diagnosed HIV infection who are virally suppressed to at least 80%.

[a]From HIV.gov: What is the national HIV/AIDS strategy?, 2017. Retrieved from https://www.aids.gov/federal-resources/national-hiv-aids-strategy/overview/.

Box 56.5 Nursing Assessment of a Patient With HIV Infection

SUBJECTIVE DATA

Important Health Information

Past health history: Route of infection, risk factors, history of hepatitis or other sexually transmitted infections, frequent viral infections, parasitic infections, tuberculosis, alcohol and drug use, foreign travel

Medications: Use of immunosuppressive drugs

Functional Health Patterns

Health perception–health management: Chronic fatigue, malaise, weakness

Nutritional metabolic: Unexplained weight loss; low-grade fevers, night sweats; anorexia, nausea, vomiting; oral lesions, bleeding, ulcerations; abdominal cramping; lesions of lips, mouth, tongue, throat; sensitivity to acidic, salty, or spicy foods; problems with teeth or bleeding gums; difficulty swallowing; skin rashes or color changes, lesions (painful or nonpainful), blisters; nonhealing wounds, pruritus

Elimination: Persistent diarrhea, constipation, painful urination

Activity-exercise: Muscle weakness, difficulty with ambulation; cough, shortness of breath

Cognitive-perceptual: Headaches, stiff neck, chest pain, rectal pain, retrosternal pain; blurred vision, photophobia, loss of vision, diplopia; confusion, forgetfulness, attention deficit, changes in mental status, memory loss; hearing impairment, personality changes, paresthesias; hypersensitivity in feet

Sexuality-reproductive: Lesions on genitalia (internal or external), pruritus, or burning in vagina or on penis; painful sexual intercourse; changes in menstruation; vaginal or penile discharge

OBJECTIVE DATA

General: Vital signs, weight, general status, diaphoresis

Eyes: Exudate, retinal lesions or hemorrhage, papilledema, pupillary response, extraocular muscle movements

Oral: A variety of mouth lesions, including blisters (herpes simplex virus type–1 lesions), white-gray patches (*Candida* organisms), painless white lesions on lateral aspects of tongue (oral hairy leukoplakia), discolorations (Kaposi's sarcoma), gingivitis, tooth decay or loosening

Neck: Enlarged lymph nodes, nuchal rigidity, enlarged thyroid

Throat: Redness or white patchy lesions

Integumentary: Skin integrity and skin turgor; general appearance; lesions, eruptions, discolorations; enlarged lymph nodes, bruises, cyanosis, dryness, delayed wound healing, alopecia

Respiratory: Crackles or rhonchi, dyspnea, cough (productive or nonproductive, color and amount of sputum), wheezing, tachypnea, intercostal retractions, use of accessory muscles

Lymphatic: Generalized lymphadenopathy

Abdominal: Tenderness, masses, enlarged liver or spleen, hyperactive bowel sounds

Genitourinary-rectal: Lesions or discharge, abdominal pain indicative of pelvic inflammatory disease, difficult or painful urination

Neuromuscular: Aphasia, ataxia, lack of coordination, sensory loss, tremors, slurred speech, memory loss, apathy, agitation, social withdrawal or isolation, pain, inappropriate behavior, changes in level of consciousness, depression, seizures, paralysis, coma

HIV, Human immunodeficiency virus.

Box 56.6 Nursing Interventions for the Patient With HIV Infection or HIV Disease

PREVENT INFECTION

- Wash hands frequently, and administer skin lubricants to patient and caregiver to prevent skin breakdown.
- Use a gentle liquid soap.
- Provide for daily showering or basin bath; do not give patient tub bath if rashes are present; avoid extremely hot temperatures.
- Use a separate washcloth for lesions.
- For oral hygiene, provide soft toothbrushes; nonabrasive toothpaste; and mouth rinses with sodium bicarbonate, saline, or lemon and hydrogen peroxide before and after meals and at bedtime.
- Use measures to prevent skin impairment, such as turning sheets, air mattresses.
- Elevate and support areas of edema.
- Observe biopsy sites and intravenous insertion sites daily for signs of infection.
- Change dressings at least every other day; avoid plastic occlusive dressings.
- Prevent exposure to sources of microbes, such as plants or uncooked fresh fruits and vegetables.
- Carry out measures to prevent spread of infection: Use gloves for contact with bodily secretions, double plastic bags to dispose of bodily secretions, bleach and water (1 : 10) solution for cleaning contaminated areas.

MODIFY ALTERATIONS IN BODY TEMPERATURE

- Administer prescribed antibiotics, intravenous fluids, or antipyretics.
- Encourage fluid intake of more than 2500 mL/day.
- Maintain daily intake and output records.
- Weigh patient daily.
- Provide tepid sponge baths and linen changes as necessary.
- Instruct patient in deep-breathing and coughing exercises to prevent atelectasis and additional fever.

PROMOTE GOOD NUTRITION

- Provide instruction for high-calorie, high-protein, high-potassium, low-residue diet.
- Encourage high-calorie, high-potassium snacks.
- Suggest foods that are easy to swallow (gelatin, yogurt, puddings) when dysphagia is present.

Box 56.6 Nursing Interventions for the Patient With HIV Infection or HIV Disease—cont'd

- Advise patient to avoid foods that are spicy or acidic, rare meats, and raw fruits and vegetables.
- Provide oral care before and after meals patient eats.
- Encourage patient to get out of bed and sit up for meals, if possible.
- Avoid odors by aerating room.
- Refer patient and caregiver for appropriate dietary consultations.
- Educate patient and caregiver about food safety and food preparation.

PROMOTE SELF-CARE

- Assess realistic functional ability.
- Plan, supervise, and assist with activities of daily living as necessary.
- Encourage patient to be as active and independent as possible.
- Assist patient with range-of-motion exercise to prevent contractures.
- Provide equipment such as assistive eating devices, walkers, and commodes to promote patient independence.
- To prevent fatigue, pace activities and schedule rest periods.

PROVIDE COUNSELING

- Assess and support patient's coping mechanisms.
- Explore with patient and significant others normality of grief.
- Assist patient and significant others in acknowledging and planning for anticipated losses.
- Provide information as desired and necessary, depending on patient's ability to understand.
- Suggest appropriate religious support.
- Facilitate participation in support groups or individual counseling as appropriate.

HIV, Human immunodeficiency virus.

Table 56.5 Nursing Activities in HIV Disease

LEVELS OF CARE AND GOALS	ASSESSMENT	INTERVENTIONS
Health Care Promotion and Maintenance		
Prevention of HIV infection Early detection of HIV infection	Risk factors: What behavioral, social, physical, emotional, pathologic, and immune factors place patient at risk? Does patient need to be tested?	Educate patient, including knowledge, attitudes, and behaviors, with an emphasis on risk reduction: • Regarding general population (cover general information) • Regarding individual patient (specific to assessed need) Empower patient to take control of prevention measures. Provide HIV-antibody testing with pretest and post-test counseling.
Acute Intervention		
Promotion of health and limitation of disability Successful management of problems caused by HIV infection	Physical health: Is patient experiencing problems? Mental health status: How is the patient coping? Resources: Does the patient have family and social support? Is patient accessing community services? Are money and insurance a problem? Does patient have access to spiritual support?	Provide case management. Educate regarding HIV, the spectrum of infection, options for care, signs and symptoms to watch for. Educate regarding immune enhancement and harm reduction. Establish long-term, trusting relationship with patient, family, and significant others. Refer to needed resources. Provide emotional and spiritual support. Provide care during acute exacerbations: recognition of life-threatening developments, life support, rapid intervention with treatments and medications, patient and family emotional support during crisis, comfort, and hygiene needs. Develop resources for legal needs: discrimination prevention, wills and powers of attorney, child care wishes. Empower patient to identify needs, direct care, seek services.

Continued

Table 56.5 Nursing Activities in HIV Disease—cont'd

LEVELS OF CARE AND GOALS	ASSESSMENT	INTERVENTIONS
Chronic and Home Management		
Maximizing quality of life Resolution of life and death issues	Physical health: Are new symptoms developing? Is patient experiencing drug side effects or interactions? Mental health status: How is patient coping? What adjustments have been made? Finances: Can patient maintain health care and basic standards of living? Family, social, and community supports: Are these supports available? Is patient using supports in an effective manner? Spirituality issues: Does patient desire support from an established religious organization? Are spirituality issues private and personal? What assistance does patient need?	Continue case management. Educate regarding treatment options. Empower patient to continue directing care and to make desires known to family members and significant others. Continue physical care for chronic disease process: treatments, medications, comfort and hygiene needs. Refer to resources that will assist in meeting identified needs. Promote health maintenance measures. Assist with end-of-life issues: resuscitation orders, funeral plans, estate planning, child care continuation.

HIV, Human immunodeficiency virus.

ADHERENCE

Adherence to a prescribed regimen (following a prescribed regimen of therapy or treatment for disease) is paramount to survival and the success of treatment. The nurse is in a unique position to help patients adapt and maintain vigilance in their treatment. Nurses must assist patients to understand that ART is a lifelong undertaking. The ability to incorporate anti-HIV treatment into a lifestyle is affected by multiple factors, including treatment knowledge or misinformation, underlying psychiatric or psychological pathologic conditions, physical status, family and caregiver support, socioeconomic status, culture, fear of side effects, denial, and skills (memory, impaired function) necessary to adhere to a medical regimen.

Patients with a higher level of motivation to take their medications as ordered can have much better outcomes than do patients who are less compliant. Drug resistance to ART can easily develop when even a few doses of medication are missed or taken incorrectly. Compliance rates increase when HIV-infected patients are prescribed one combination ART medication per day and receive positive reinforcement from their health care team members (USDHHS, 2018b).

Strategies that can assist nurses in increasing patient adherence include determining their own level of comfort with regard to HIV, learning to listen, having knowledge about the disease, using therapeutic communication skills, giving the patient and caregivers permission to grieve and feel sad, acknowledging frustration and helplessness, providing a safe environment, and seeking expert assistance as needed. All of these can help patients incorporate this difficult treatment into their lifestyle (Box 56.7).

Box 56.7 Barriers to Adherence

- Caregivers' incomplete knowledge of the demands of patients' lives
- Prejudice
- Insufficient appointment time
- Lack of resources for patients who have doubts or questions
- Negative stereotypes about doctors
- Insufficient multidisciplinary communication

From NAM Publications: *Common barriers to adherence*, 2013.

PALLIATIVE CARE

The World Health Organization (WHO) defines palliative care as helping patients and families deal with possibly fatal illnesses and quality-of-life issues. The focus of palliative care is on preventing and relieving suffering by quickly identifying and treating pain. The goal of palliative care is to improve and maintain quality of life as much as possible by focusing on all physical, spiritual, psychological, social, and existential needs of the patient or the family who is dealing with a terminal illness (WHO, 2013c).

Palliative care is not seen as hastening the dying process or postponing death. Nurses realize that death is a natural process of life, but other people may believe that a patient's death signifies the failure of medicine and loss of hope. Palliative care often is delayed as a result of this false belief. Most hospice programs use a palliative care approach, with the understanding that impending death means a shift from curing to caring. Remember that the goal is to relieve suffering through management of pain and symptoms at *any* point in the patient's disease process.

For patients with HIV disease, it is important for palliative care not only to address the potential chronic debilitating conditions associated with HIV disease but also to address superimposed acute exacerbations of opportunistic infections and related symptoms. Intravenous therapy, blood transfusions, and antibiotic usage may be considered palliative in the end stage of HIV disease, because these interventions help keep the patient comfortable and help maintain quality of life. In AIDS care, short-term aggressive, curative therapy is often important in treating acute infections such as pneumonia, but the overall goal remains palliation.

The complex needs of patients with HIV disease necessitate the services of a multidisciplinary team of physicians, nurses, social workers, pharmacists, dietitians, physical therapists, and clergy. The nurse is the "voice" and advocate for the patient who may or may not be able to communicate his or her treatment desires. Because of this unique role, it is important to be comfortable discussing treatment issues and options with patients, as well as respecting their decisions. Families and significant others of patients with end-stage HIV disease can experience *disenfranchised grief,* which occurs when a loss is not openly acknowledged, publicly mourned, or socially supported (Sherman, 2001). Symptoms such as pain, fatigue, anorexia, fever, shortness of breath, diarrhea, and insomnia are common among people who suffer disenfranchised grief. Become familiar with the causes and interventions necessary to alleviate these symptoms. Remember that symptoms such as pain are a subjective experience and must be treated appropriately until the patient indicates the treatment has worked. Although this phase of life is difficult for the patient and nurse, many nurses express significant satisfaction with these interactions, relationships, and their outcomes.

As the HIV pandemic has changed over time as a result of the use of ART and aggressive approaches to treatment, fewer patients with HIV infection are requiring hospice or palliative care. In some patients, however, HIV is not diagnosed until they are in a later stage of the disease process. These patients may choose palliative or hospice care instead of treatment.

PSYCHOSOCIAL ISSUES

People who have received a diagnosis of HIV infection deal with a complex set of psychosocial issues. Often, they are uncertain, fearful, depressed, and isolated. HIV infection can be treated, but it is incurable and contagious. Many infected people feel isolated and abandoned by friends and family because of the stigma associated with HIV. Like the health care costs associated with many chronic diseases, the expenses involved in treating HIV infection are daunting for many patients.

Nurses and health care providers must be empathetic during contact with patients. Listening is an important skill to help convey compassion. Therapeutic communication skills should be used to enhance rapport with a patient. Help the patient plan and decide about health care options. The patient has the right to be supported even when the decision seems imprudent.

Box 56.8 Psychological Crisis Intervals in the Course of HIV Disease

- Diagnosis of HIV infection
- Viral load testing
- Increases in viral load
- Initiation of antiretroviral therapy
- Signs of treatment failure
- Adding prophylaxis therapies (e.g., for *Pneumocystis jiroveci* pneumonia)
- Occurrence of opportunistic illnesses
- Change in antiretroviral treatment regimen
- Illness or death in support networks
- New treatment advances

HIV, Human immunodeficiency virus.

Assisting With Coping

Individuals who have been exposed to HIV infection but who are without any symptoms or complications live with uncertainty, anxiety, denial, and hopefulness (Box 56.8). The nurse's role in this stage of the disease process is to provide continued education about HIV disease and prevention and to assist in realistic goal setting. Make every effort to include the patient and the support system in planning care. Early in the care process, assess past coping styles and support systems and continually reevaluate these issues. Encourage healthy patterns of coping, such as talk therapy, relaxation, and meditation. Relationships with family, friends, and significant others should be maintained and in fact may become stronger during the HIV crisis. However, prior family conflicts may worsen as a result of the stress of the illness. Families with poor communication skills are at particular risk for this outcome.

As HIV disease progresses through the clinical complications of infections and cancers, patients experience multiple losses, including the loss of energy; a self-care deficit that necessitates assistance with activities of daily living; and the loss of independence, employment, finances, and hope. The reality of death emerges. Nursing interventions should focus on a philosophy of facing life one day at a time and living each day to its fullest. This may be a time for strengthening personal and spiritual relationships and resolving any conflicts.

Anxiety and depression can become chronic, ultimately interfering with daily functioning, relationships, communication, and even the ability to make simple decisions. Although anxiety and depression are normal when a patient is dealing with a significant health care threat, refer patients to mental health professionals for possible pharmacologic or verbal counseling when these feelings affect daily functioning for more than 2 weeks.

Patients with HIV disease and depression should be assessed regularly for suicidal ideation, because this phenomenon occasionally occurs in terminally ill patients. Early recognition of depression and anxiety is critical because most cases respond to medications, psychotherapy, or a combination.

Severe anxiety can cause individuals to believe they have no control over the events in their lives. Helping the patient develop a schedule of activities may decrease anxiety and feelings of powerlessness. Explore opportunities for spiritual support and comfort. Community support groups for patients and significant others may contribute to healthy coping. Arrange to spend time with the patient and the support system, in hopes that this will decrease anxiety and promote better coping.

The use of therapeutic communication and helping patients find meaning in life are critical nursing interventions. Assisting families and significant others in providing support to the terminally ill patient despite their own anger and grief is a unique nursing challenge. Such care, although emotionally draining, can provide great satisfaction.

Minimizing Social Isolation

The psychosocial aspects of HIV infection can be devastating. Feelings may include denial, fear, depression, and anger. These are similar to those that may be seen in an individual who has been diagnosed with cancer. The first stressful issue faced by a patient with newly diagnosed HIV infection is disclosure of HIV status. A very real concern for HIV-positive patients is that family, significant others, and friends will be angry and may even reject or abandon the patients. Families and friends of a patient with newly diagnosed HIV infection may be misinformed about the disease. The patient and the family may benefit from sources of support such as a mental health provider with experience providing service to patients who are infected with HIV. Support groups for patients and significant others are often also available. HIV-infected individuals who have been exposed through contaminated blood or who contract HIV from their partner may experience feelings of anger and hostility. Showing support and providing education about the disease may help alleviate some of these feelings.

Assisting With Grieving

Many patients with HIV infection benefit simply from having another person listen and explore in detail the feelings, unfounded fears, and treatment options. However, many others need the more structured support found in therapeutic relationships or formal support groups. Significant others and family members also may need assistance to provide support to their loved one. Formal counseling can help a patient address issues such as continued employment, health insurance concerns, preparations for disability, and feelings related to death. Referral to medical or clinical social workers and appropriate community agencies is part of the nurse's responsibility in addressing psychosocial needs. For some patients, it is appropriate to refer them to clergy.

CONFIDENTIALITY

Respect for the patient's right to confidentiality is particularly important for a patient with HIV disease. The confidentiality of the diagnosis must be protected carefully and shared only with caregivers who need to know for the purpose of assessment and treatment.

Health care workers should use standard precautions with each patient to prevent exposure to the patient's blood or bodily fluids. Not every infected patient may know that he or she is seropositive for HIV. When this information is shared by the patient, the information should be shared with other health care workers who are managing this patient's care.

The patient should be in control of who is told of the diagnosis, but laws dictate the reporting of an HIV diagnosis to appropriate health agencies. As with any patient seeking health care services, guidelines of the Health Insurance Portability and Accountability Act (HIPAA) must be followed. Partner notification laws also must be considered when HIV infection is diagnosed. The health care provider must follow laws in his or her state regarding partner notification.

ACUTE INTERVENTION

Early intervention after detection of an HIV infection can promote health and limit or delay disability. Because the course of HIV infection is extremely variable, assessment is of primary importance. Nursing interventions are tailored to any patient needs noted during assessment. The nursing assessment of HIV disease should focus on the early detection of constitutional symptoms, opportunistic diseases, and psychosocial problems (Box 56.9).

HIV disease progression may be delayed by maintaining the health of the immune system. Useful interventions for an HIV-infected patient include (1) nutritional changes that maintain lean body mass, maintain weight in the range of ideal body weight, and ensure consumption of appropriate levels of vitamins and micronutrients; (2) elimination of smoking and drug use; (3) elimination or moderation of alcohol intake; (4) regular exercise; (5) stress reduction; (6) avoidance of exposure to new infectious agents; (7) mental health counseling; (8) involvement in support groups; and (9) safer sexual practices.

The patient should be taught to recognize clinical manifestations that may indicate progression of the disease; this will ensure that medical care is initiated promptly. Early manifestations that must be reported include unexplained weight loss, night sweats, diarrhea, persistent fever, swollen lymph nodes, oral hairy leukoplakia, oral candidiasis (thrush; Fig. 56.5), and persistent vaginal yeast infections. In addition, the patient should report unusual headaches, changes in vision, nausea and vomiting, and numbness or tingling

Box 56.9 Conducting a Risk Assessment

Risk assessment specific to HIV and sexually transmitted infections (STIs), as well as bloodborne diseases, is crucial in health care delivery today. Perform regular risk assessments on all patients and when evaluating any new patient. Determine sexual and drug use risks, along with other risks, during routine history taking. Advise the patient, and provide education and resources regarding risky behavior.

KEY QUESTIONS TO ASK

Any "yes" responses necessitate further assessment and evaluation.

- "Have you ever had a blood transfusion? Have you ever received any other kind of blood product? Before 1985?"
- "Do you now or have you ever shared injection equipment?"
- "Are you now or have you ever been sexually active?"

KEY POINTS TO CONSIDER

- Begin by assuring confidentiality and telling the patient why asking these questions is important:
  - "I am going to ask some personal questions. I ask all of my patients these questions so I can provide better care. All of your responses will be kept confidential. Is it okay to proceed?"
- Ask direct questions about specific behaviors:
  - "When was the last time you …?"
  - "How often do you …?"
  - "Have you ever exchanged sex for money or drugs?"
- Exploratory questions may help (especially with adolescents and young adults):
  - "Do your friends use condoms?"
  - "What happens at parties?"
  - "How easy is it to get drugs?"
- Honest responses may be more forthcoming if the behaviors are described in a nonjudgmental manner:
  - "Some of my patients who use drugs inject them. Do you inject drugs or other substances?"
  - "Sometimes people have anal intercourse. Have you ever had anal intercourse?"

DRUG USE ASSESSMENT

- It is important to be nonjudgmental and nonmoralistic:
  - Injection drug use is illegal in the United States and many patients are afraid to be honest unless trust is established.
- Start with less-threatening questions:
  - "What over-the-counter or prescription medications are you taking?"
  - "How often do you use alcohol? Tobacco?"
  - "Have you ever used drugs from a nonmedical source?"
  - "Have you ever injected any kind of drug?"
- Do not assume anything.
- Drug use occurs in all socioeconomic strata. Do not forget that people inject substances such as insulin, steroids, and vitamins. Any sharing, even one time, can result in HIV exposure.
- Look for other clues in the history and physical examination, including antisocial behavior, recurrent criminal arrests, and needle tracks.
- If the patient has a positive history of drug injection use, get more information:
  - "Do [did] you share needles or other equipment?"
  - "Is [was] the equipment you use [used] clean? How did you know it was clean?"
  - "What drugs did you inject?"

SEXUAL RISK ASSESSMENT

- Direct and nonjudgmental questions work best:
  - "Do you have sex with men, women, or both?"
  - "Do you have oral sex? Vaginal sex? Anal sex?"
  - "What do you know about the sexual activities of your partners?"
  - "What do you do to protect yourself during sex?"
  - "Do you use condoms? How often?"
  - "Have you ever had sex with someone you didn't know or just met?"
- Ask for an explanation of sexual practices:
  - "When you say you had sex, what exactly do you mean?"
  - "I don't know what you mean; could you explain …?"
- Do not assume anything.
- Marriage does not always mean an individual is monogamous or heterosexual.
- People who identify as homosexual may also have heterosexual sex.
- Use specific terms:
  - Use "men who have sex with men" or "women who have sex with women" instead of "gay."
  - Some men who practice anal insertive intercourse do not consider themselves "gay," but their receptive partners are considered to be gay (can be culturally related).

CLINICAL RISK ASSESSMENT

- Assess the patient for constitutional signs, history of chronic infection and HIV, and associated problems:
  - Headaches
  - Diarrhea
  - Fatigue
  - Shingles
  - History of STI, hepatitis, or tuberculosis
  - Fever, chills, night sweats
  - Skin lesions
  - Weight loss
  - Oral thrush
  - Generalized lymphadenopathy

HIV, Human immunodeficiency virus.
Modified from Mountain Plains AIDS Education and Training Center: *HIV risk assessment: A quick reference guide,* Denver, 2009, Author.

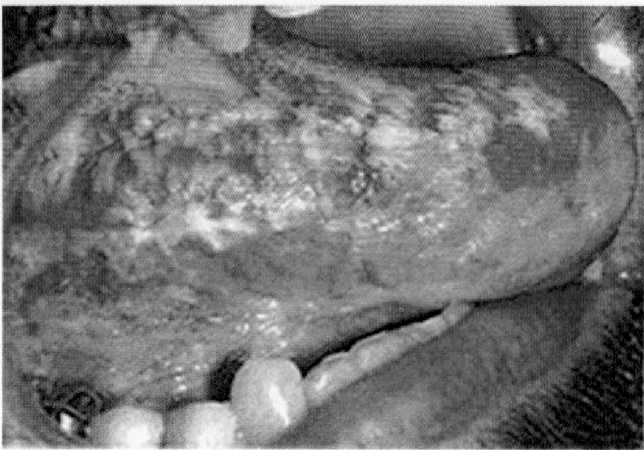

Fig. 56.5 Oral candidiasis, or thrush, manifests with a whitish, curdlike substance on the tongue or inside the mouth. (Courtesy Deborah Greenspan, DSC, BDS, University of California, San Francisco, and US Department of Veterans Affairs.)

in the extremities. Give the patient as much information as needed to make health care decisions. These decisions dictate the appropriate medical and nursing interventions.

Nursing interventions become more complicated as the patient's immune system deteriorates and new problems arise to compound existing difficulties. The nursing focus should be on quality-of-life issues and symptom management, rather than on issues regarding a cure.

When opportunistic diseases develop, provide symptom-based nursing interventions, education, and emotional support. For example, an acute case of *P. jiroveci* pneumonia necessitates intensive nursing interventions, including monitoring the respiratory status, administering medications and oxygen, positioning the patient to facilitate breathing, managing anxiety, promoting nutritional support, and helping the patient conserve energy to decrease oxygen demand. Because advanced HIV disease can lead to death, emotional support for the patient, caregiver, or significant other is particularly important (Nursing Care Plan 56.1).

Diarrhea is often a long-term problem for HIV-infected people. Damage to the intestinal villi, malabsorption, infections of the gastrointestinal tract, and the side effects of medications contribute to a large number of cases of diarrhea. Nursing interventions include recommending dietary interventions (Table 56.6), encouraging adequate fluid intake to prevent dehydration, instructing the patient about skin care, and managing excoriation around the perianal area. In some cases, antidiarrheal agents may help control diarrhea and prevent further complications. Recommend the use of incontinence products to prevent soiling of the clothes and bed linens. In addition, assess for factors that may trigger the diarrhea, such as anxiety, medications, or lactose intolerance.

HIV **wasting**—the loss of lean body mass as a result of illness—has been a common clinical manifestation of HIV disease since early in the epidemic. Wasting is caused by disturbances in metabolism, which interfere with the effective use of nutrients, resulting in the loss of lean (muscle) body mass, often without reduction of body fat. This loss of lean body mass is a primary cause of functional decline in wasting, which results in increased risk of opportunistic infections, reduced quality of life, and reduced length of survival. A person with HIV is considered to have wasting syndrome when he or she has lost 10% of body weight and has had either diarrhea or weakness and fever for 30 days. The person infected with HIV who has wasting syndrome has a more advanced form of HIV or AIDS (AIDSinfo, 1997).

The causes of wasting are probably multifactorial. Food intake may be inadequate because of mechanical difficulties (e.g., thrush or esophageal ulcers), loss of appetite (e.g., side effect of medications, nausea, or neurologic disease), or psychological factors such as depression and anxiety. Absorption in the intestine may be decreased as a result of infections and a damaged mucosal barrier, which may lead to diarrhea. Some patients stop eating to decrease the number of bowel movements per day. An increased metabolic rate with muscle catabolism contributes to wasting syndrome.

Wasting disturbs self-concept and self-image and can be one of the most difficult consequences of HIV infection to accept. Useful interventions for these disturbances include creating an atmosphere of acceptance and reassurance, encouraging a focus on past accomplishments and personal strengths, and facilitating the use of positive affirmations.

Decreased levels of testosterone have been reported in HIV-infected men. Testosterone has two distinct biologic properties: virilizing activity (androgenic effect) and protein building (anabolic effect). Because testosterone is an anabolic hormone, a deficiency may cause a loss of body cell mass, which contributes to HIV wasting. The role of gonadotropic hormones in women with wasting has not been studied sufficiently. Women with HIV wasting tend to lose a lot of body fat, but body cell mass is not significantly decreased. Conversely, men tend to lose a significant amount of lean body mass (e.g., exhibit skinny arms and legs), with preservation of fat, particularly in the truncal area.

With the advances in HIV treatment and opportunistic infection prophylaxis, serious malnutrition is less evident. However, nutrition does not return to normal after anti-HIV treatment begins. A syndrome of increased truncal obesity (visceral, abdominal), subcutaneous fat loss on the extremities and face (also called *lipoatrophy*), and metabolic abnormalities such as hyperlipidemia and insulin resistance have been reported in men and women.

The management of wasting and lipodystrophy is difficult and generally requires multiple nursing interventions. Diminished appetite and weight must be assessed and documented. Encourage nutritional supplementation (see Table 56.6) and increased protein intake, provide enteral supplements (through nasogastric or gastric tubes if necessary), and assist with total parenteral

Nursing Care Plan 56.1 The Patient Who Is HIV Positive

Ms. J. is a 20-year-old who comes to the emergency department, accompanied by her mother, with complaints of severe vomiting and recent weight loss of 10 pounds. Ms. J. went to the 24-hour clinic and learned that she is approximately 8 weeks pregnant and, because of risk factors for HIV exposure, gave informed consent for HIV antibody testing. The clinic determined that she is HIV positive according to ELISA and Western blot testing. Ms. J. is tearful and reluctant to answer questions about her recent HIV diagnosis and positive pregnancy test result. She states that she could not be HIV positive because she has had sexual intercourse only with her boyfriend of 5 years. In addition, Ms. J. is concerned about telling her mother about her HIV status and the pregnancy because she lives with her mother, who is also taking care of her sick elderly grandmother. Ms. J. does not have a job and depends on family members to help her meet financial obligations and needs. Ms. J. feels the added burden to her mother would "be too much" and is considering leaving home to live in a shelter.

PATIENT PROBLEM

Potential for Excessive Demand on Primary Caregiver, related to advancing disease in care receiver, inadequate caregiver coping pattern

Patient Goals and Expected Outcomes	Nursing Interventions	Evaluation
Caregiver will use available community and personal resources Caregiver will be able to complete necessary caregiving tasks Caregiver will receive effective support	Assess needs and capabilities of patient and caregiver. Assess factors that contribute to caregiver strain (unrealistic expectations, poor insight, inability to use resources, unsatisfactory relationship with care recipient, insufficient financial and psychosocial resources). Develop supportive and trusting relationship with caregiver. Enlist help of other family members or friends. Teach caregiver to perform care activities in a safe, efficient, and energy-conserving manner. Teach stress-reduction techniques. Encourage caregiver to attend to own personal and health needs.	The caregiver provides safe, supportive care to the HIV-infected patient. The caregiver acknowledges the need for personal support and accesses resources in family and community. The caregiver shares frustrations about difficulty of caring for a significant other. The caregiver receives assistance from family members and/or professional caregivers.

PATIENT PROBLEM

Insufficient Nutrition, related to chronic infections and/or malabsorption, nausea, vomiting, diarrhea, fatigue, or side effects of medications as evidenced by 10% or greater loss of ideal body mass

Patient Goals and Expected Outcomes	Nursing Interventions	Evaluation
Patient's weight will remain stable Patient's nutritional intake will exceed metabolic needs Patient will regain lost weight	Assist with diagnosis of underlying opportunistic infections. Assess patient's knowledge of optimal nutritional intake. Increase protein, calorie, and fat intake. Offer nutritional supplements (e.g., Carnation Instant Breakfast, Boost, Sustacal). Schedule procedures that are painful, stressful, or nauseating so that they do not interfere with mealtimes. Provide the patient with several small meals throughout the day, as opposed to three large meals. Provide referrals to dietitians, social workers, and case managers. Weigh patient daily.	Patient's weight remains stable or increases. Patient reports increased energy level. Patient is able to complete activities of daily living. Patient experiences increase in lean muscle mass.

CRITICAL THINKING QUESTIONS

1. Ms. J. is tearful and asks the nurse if there is any treatment to prevent her baby from becoming HIV positive. What should be included in the nurse's information to Ms. J.?
2. Ms. J. asks the nurse whether she can legally require her boyfriend to be tested for HIV infection. What is the most appropriate response?
3. Ms. J. asks the nurse when she will develop AIDS now that she is HIV positive. What is the correct answer?

AIDS, Acquired immunodeficiency syndrome; *ELISA*, enzyme-linked immunosorbent assay; *HIV*, human immunodeficiency virus.

Table 56.6 Nutritional Management: HIV Infection

CONDITION	DIETARY RECOMMENDATION	INTERVENTION
Diarrhea	Lactose-free, low-fat, low-fiber, and high-potassium foods	Instruct patient to avoid dairy products, red meat, margarine, butter, eggs, dried beans, peas, and raw fruits and vegetables. Provide cooked or canned fruits and vegetables, which provide needed vitamins. Encourage patient to eat potassium-rich foods such as bananas and apricot nectar. Instruct patient to discontinue foods, nutritional supplements, and medications that may make diarrhea worse (Ensure, antacids, stool softeners). Advise patient to avoid gas-producing foods. Serve warm, not hot, foods. Plan small, frequent meals. Encourage patient to drink plenty of fluids between meals.
Constipation	High-fiber foods	Instruct patient to eat fruits and vegetables (beans, peas), cereal, and whole wheat breads. Gradually increase patient's fiber intake. Encourage patient to drink plenty of fluids and to exercise.
Nausea and vomiting	Low-fat foods	Advise patient to avoid dairy products and red meat. Plan small, frequent meals. Prepare nonodorous foods. Encourage patient to eat dry, salty foods. Serve food cold or at room temperature. Instruct patient to drink liquids between meals. Advise patient to avoid gas-producing, greasy, spicy foods. Encourage patient to eat slowly in a relaxed atmosphere. Enable patient to rest after meals, with head elevated. Administer antiemetics 30 min before meals.
Candidiasis	Soft or pureed foods	Serve moist foods. Encourage patient to drink plenty of fluids. Instruct patient to avoid acidic and spicy foods. Advise patient to use straw and tilt head back and forth when drinking. To decrease discomfort, encourage patient to eat soft foods, such as puddings and yogurt.
Fever	High-calorie, high-protein foods	Administer nutritional supplements. Increase patient's fluid intake.
Altered taste	Diet as tolerated	Encourage patient to try adding herbs and spices, as well as salt and sugar. Advise patient to marinate meat, poultry, and fish. Serve food cold or at room temperature. Encourage patient to drink plenty of fluids. Introduce alternative protein sources.
Anemia	High-iron foods	Encourage patient to eat organ meats and raisins. Advise patient to drink orange juice when taking iron supplements, to facilitate absorption.
Fatigue	High-calorie foods	Advise patient or caregiver to cook in large quantities and freeze meal-size portions in packets. Suggest the use of microwaveable and convenience foods. Encourage the use of easy-to-fix snack foods. Advise patient to use social support system to assist with meal planning and preparation. Help patient access in-home homemaker services and Meals-on-Wheels programs.

HIV, Human immunodeficiency virus.

nutrition when it is needed. Medications to stimulate appetite, such as dronabinol (Marinol), can help; unfortunately, these medications tend to increase body fat and not lean muscle mass. Testosterone (anabolic steroid) can be administered by mouth, intramuscularly, or transdermally to increase lean body mass and weight. The effect of testosterone can be enhanced by a low-weight resistance-training program (e.g., weight-lifting), which maintains muscle tone and improves appetite.

Nutrition counseling is vital to ensure that individuals with HIV disease maintain a well-balanced diet, including supplements if necessary. The dietitian can assist in counseling, provide the patient with high-protein and high-calorie diets, and suggest meal plans that fit the patient's lifestyle. Smaller, more frequent meals can be less overwhelming than larger meals. Teaching about food safety is of paramount concern because enteric infections (e.g., cryptosporidiosis, microsporidiosis, and amebas) in HIV disease are often not treatable or are relapsing. In some cases, enteral or parenteral feeding becomes necessary.

Management of elevated triglyceride and lipid (cholesterol) levels is common in HIV disease. The HIV infection and some types of HIV medications are responsible for the hyperlipidemia. As in other patient populations, these elevations can lead to cardiovascular disease and gallbladder disease, pancreatitis, and diabetes (AIDSinfo, 2018). Lipid-lowering agents such as the statins may be effective in treating this complication. However, because the liver metabolizes many of the antilipid agents, it is important to choose a drug that is safer than those that must pass through the liver to be activated; safer anticholesterol drugs include pravastatin (Pravachol), fluvastatin (Lescol), and possibly atorvastatin (Lipitor). A program of diet, exercise, and medications can lower lipids safely and reduce the chances of a cardiovascular event.

Insulin resistance or diabetes sometimes responds to oral hypoglycemic agents (e.g., metformin or rosiglitazone [Avandia]). In some cases, the anti-HIV therapy must be changed. All medications belonging to the protease inhibitor class increase lipid levels. Efavirenz (a NNRTI), abacavir, stavudine, zidovudine (NRTIs), and stibild (combination medication) have been linked to hyperlipidemia. Diet management, smoking cessation, weight loss, reduced alcoholic intake, and exercise can help control the elevations in blood glucose that can occur with the use of anti-HIV medications.

Unfortunately, as with any overwhelming viral infection, HIV infection increases the patient's metabolic needs. This hypermetabolism and consequent higher energy expenditure frequently exceed the number of calories taken in by the patient. Malnutrition, weight loss, and generalized wasting are common problems in patients with HIV disease (see Nursing Care Plan 56.1). Many patients with HIV disease experience wasting. Malnutrition contributes to wasting, and wasting hastens the negative immune consequences of HIV infection. HIV wasting contributes to slower recovery from infection, impaired wound healing, increased risk of secondary infection, and decreased cardiac and respiratory function. Wasting can lead to an earlier death. The weight loss associated with HIV disease is often severe and debilitating, producing a vicious cycle of anorexia, malnutrition, loss of tissue mass, muscle wasting, profound fatigue, and increased susceptibility to infections and drug interactions. Although typically seen in later stages of HIV disease, malnutrition and wasting can occur in the early stages of HIV infection.

NEUROLOGIC COMPLICATIONS

HIV-Associated Related Cognitive Issues

AIDS dementia complex (ADC), also known as HIV-associated dementia, is the term used to describe a common central nervous system complication of HIV disease. This condition is a complex combination of signs and symptoms, including dementia; impaired motor function; and, at times, characteristic behavioral changes that resemble those accompanying a stroke or head trauma. The disease generally does not cause alterations in the level of consciousness. It usually is described as a triad of cognitive, motor, and behavioral dysfunction that slowly progresses over a period of weeks to months. The cognitive changes involve primarily a mental slowing and inattention. Affected patients typically lose their train of thought and complain of slowed thinking. They may miss appointments and find themselves making lists of tasks and chores that need completing. The signs and symptoms of motor dysfunction ordinarily develop after those of cognitive impairment. They include poor balance and coordination (e.g., falling and tripping, dropping things); slower manual activities (e.g., writing, eating); and, ultimately, leg weakness that can limit ambulation. This type of dementia can be diagnosed through a simple physical examination, neurologic testing, magnetic resonance imaging and computed tomography, and cerebrospinal fluid analysis. Another less severe form of HIV-related cognitive issues is referred to as minor cognitive motor disorder. It manifests with forgetfulness, slowed movements, poor coordination, personality changes, and difficulty concentrating (Thomas, 2018).

Nursing interventions for neurocognitive dysfunction include administration of ART, antidepressants, psychostimulants, anticonvulsants, anti-dementia medications, benzodiazepines, and psychotherapy. Supervision of the patient, which includes a home safety assessment, is imperative. Ensure that orientation cues such as clocks and calendars are present, hallways and living areas are brightly lit, walkways are clear of electrical cords or throw rugs, and potentially dangerous objects (e.g., knives, poisons) are stored safely away from the patient.

Caring for patients with dementia is a collaborative effort between the health care provider and family. It is advisable to seek advice from a social worker, the home health care department, and a psychologist in developing a plan to care for an impaired individual.

Peripheral neuropathy. Neuropathies are diseases that affect the peripheral nervous system. They can affect sensory, motor, or autonomic nerves. The causes of neuropathies can be related to HIV disease or, more frequently, the side effects of many anti-HIV medications. Symptoms include numbness, localized tingling, hypesthesia (diminished sensitivity to stimulation) or anesthesia, loss of sense of vibration and position (proprioception), and decreased or increased sensitivity to pain. In most cases, patients complain of numbness in the fingers, the hands, and the feet and pain on walking. Patients also may experience autonomic neuropathy. Symptoms such as mild positional hypotension, cardiovascular collapse, and chronic diarrhea are suggestive of autonomic neuropathy.

Management of Opportunistic Infections

With the advent of effective ART and better understanding of opportunistic infection prophylaxis, the frequency of such infections has decreased dramatically. Opportunistic infections still occur in severely immunocompromised patients, so become familiar with the recognition, treatment, and prophylaxis of these diseases. Opportunistic infections typically are seen in individuals who are nonadherent to their antiretroviral regimen, nonadherent to prophylactic regimens against opportunistic infections, or at the end stage of HIV disease and in individuals who do not consistently access the health care system. (See Table 56.3 and Box 56.4 for common opportunistic infections, treatment, and prevention.)

Health Care Promotion

Because patients with HIV disease are living longer and more productive lives, attention to the promotion of health and healthy behaviors is important (see the Health Promotion box). Patients should be encouraged to eat well-balanced meals, stop smoking or at least reduce the number of cigarettes smoked, get adequate sleep and rest periods if possible, use stress-reduction modalities (e.g., biofeedback, referral for counseling), obtain dental care regularly, and keep scheduled appointments with all health care providers. Attention to comorbid conditions, such as hypertension and diabetes, helps minimize additional health problems. Encourage patients to get all immunizations and keep them up to date; female patients should regularly receive gynecologic examinations. If hospitalizations are necessary, encourage the patient and significant others to participate in treatment decision making, and arrange for home care follow-up if indicated.

Although some pets can pose risks for transmission of opportunistic infections, they are, overall, therapeutic and healing for the patient. Only minor modifications must be made for HIV-infected pet owners (e.g., birdcage and cat litter box cleaning). If possible, pet visits to the hospital or care facility should be arranged if a long separation is anticipated; the idea of benefit should not be dismissed just because this practice is not acceptable at the nurse's health care facility. Speak with managers and supervisors to obtain permission or help develop policies and procedures that allow the visitation of pets.

 Health Promotion

The Patient Infected With HIV

- Remind patients that a positive diagnosis is not an immediate "death sentence." Patients are living increasingly longer, high-quality lives after diagnosis because of medications, more specialized care, and decreased morbidity and mortality related to opportunistic diseases.
- Stress the importance of health-promoting behaviors to reduce the risk of comorbidity.
- Encourage patients to maintain good nutritional status by eating regular, well-balanced meals that are high in protein and calories. Increased protein is necessary for cell and tissue repair, especially in patients who may be hypermetabolic.
- Encourage patients to limit their intake of alcoholic beverages and avoid the use of illicit or recreational drugs.
- Encourage patients to maintain an adequate sleep schedule.
- Encourage patients to use stress-reduction practices, such as biofeedback, massage, or progressive relaxation. They also should engage in relaxing or pleasurable activities.
- Advise patients to use safer sexual practices to avoid reinfection and exposure to other STIs.
- Encourage patients to establish an exercise regimen that includes aerobic activity and low-resistance weight-lifting if possible.
- Of most importance, support patients in setting short- and long-term goals and assist them in achieving those goals.

PREVENTION OF HIV INFECTION

HIV disease is *preventable.* However, prevention requires the cooperation and efforts of public health care providers, medical providers, nurses in all specialties, families, communities, churches, and schools (Box 56.10). Education on prevention is currently our best way to help reduce infection rates. Many patients admitted to acute care facilities have unrecognized HIV disease or are at risk for HIV infection. Assess each patient's risk, and counsel those at risk about HIV testing, the behaviors that put them at risk, and how to reduce or eliminate those risks. Today, every nurse is potentially an HIV nurse; that is, all nurses may find themselves responsible for teaching patients methods to reduce the risk of transmission. Nurses must be able to discuss, in a nonjudgmental way, behaviors related to sexual activity

Box 56.10 HIV Prevention Options

SEXUAL

No Risk

- Abstain from sexual contact that involves exchange of semen, vaginal secretions, or blood.
- Stay in a mutually monogamous relationship (the state of having one mate) in which neither partner is at risk of infection through injecting drug use and in which neither partner was previously exposed to HIV.

Reduced Risk

- Limit the number of partners, even though a potential risk exists if there was sexual contact with only one infected partner.
- Use protective measures through consistent and correct use of latex condoms with a spermicide in every act of sexual intercourse that would involve exchange of semen, vaginal secretions, or blood. The correct use of condoms is as follows:
    - Put on the condom as soon as erection occurs and before any sexual contact (anal, vaginal, oral).
    - Leave space at the tip of the condom.
    - Use only water-based lubricants.
    - Hold the condom firmly to keep it from slipping off; withdraw from partner immediately after ejaculation.

USE OF INJECTION DRUGS

No Risk

- Stop using injectable drugs; drug treatment opportunities should be provided.
- If drugs are going to be injected, use sterile needles and equipment.

Reduced Risk

- If needles and equipment are going to be shared, follow instructions on cleaning.
- Fill the syringe with sodium hypochlorite 5.25% (Clorox) bleach two times; empty two times. Fill the syringe with clean water two times; empty two times.

PERINATAL

No Risk

- Avoid pregnancy; this is the only certain way to prevent transmission of HIV to a fetus or infant.
- Women of childbearing age of unknown HIV status should be counseled about behaviors that would put them and their partners or spouses at risk for HIV infection. If risk factors are determined in either case, both individuals should be counseled about testing for HIV.

Reduced Risk

- Adhere to barrier birth control measures, including use of condoms, to avoid pregnancy.
- Use antiretroviral therapy given during pregnancy and to infant for first 6 weeks of life.

HIV, Human immunodeficiency virus.

and substance use (e.g., condom application, using clean needles). Establish rapport with patients before asking sensitive, explicit questions related to behaviors typically not discussed.

Harm-reduction education is a fundamental element of HIV prevention methods. Harm reduction does not completely eliminate the risk of HIV transmission, but it minimizes the social harms and costs associated with certain behaviors. For example, attempts to quit smoking two packs of cigarettes per day all at once almost always result in failure. A harm-reduction approach may involve suggesting that the patient reduce the number of cigarettes smoked from 40 to 30 a day. Although the ultimate goal is for the patient to stop smoking altogether, the patient has at least reduced the risk of long-term effects by limiting the number of cigarettes smoked. The same is true for HIV prevention. Encouraging patients to use protective barriers such as male and female condoms helps reduce the risk of HIV transmission.

HIV TESTING AND COUNSELING

An important part of preventing HIV transmission is HIV screening tests and follow-up education and counseling (see Box 56.3). However, patients must not be coerced into having an HIV screening test. Nurses and health care providers should counsel their patients before and after HIV testing. HIV tests necessitate informed consent per state law before blood is collected. The informed consent always is accompanied by an explanation about the testing and implications of results. The limitations of the test also must be explained.

Performing HIV testing early in the course of the disease is important for increasing survival rates of HIV-infected patients and preventing the transmission to other people through high-risk behaviors. Guidelines from the CDC (2018j) mandated that all patients in health care agencies be informed about HIV screening and then be screened for HIV. However, these patients are allowed to refuse the test. HIV antibody testing should be offered to all patients, regardless of patient-specific risk factors. Also, test results should be made available rapidly to the patient so that education can be given to the patient, if needed. The CDC's recommendations state that informed consent is not needed. However, patients may opt out of testing if they wish. In rare emergency situations in which health care providers need to know a patient's HIV status to make a decision regarding health care and the patient is unable to speak, the patient may be tested without his or her consent.

Increasing numbers of people with HIV can be identified with the continued push for routine HIV screening. The antibody screening test (immunoassay) is the most common type of HIV test. It is used to test for the antibodies present when someone is infected with HIV. Blood or oral fluid may be tested. There are several blood tests available that can identity antigens and antibodies associated with HIV infection (HIV.gov, 2017b). There is a rapid test available that can detect antibodies to HIV in 30 minutes or less. Oral fluids or blood may be used. Positive tests should be followed up with an antibody differentiation test to distinguish between HIV-1 and HIV-2 infections, an HIV-1 nucleic acid test to detect HIV, or a Western blot, which is used to identify antibodies. RNA tests can identify the virus directly. It can be used to detect the virus approximately 10 days after infection before the body's ability to develop antibodies. RNA tests are more expensive than antibody tests and typically are not used to screen. OraQuick and Home Access HIV-1 Test System are in-home, over-the-counter HIV tests approved by the FDA. OraQuick involves swabbing the mouth to collect oral fluid and can produce results in 20 minutes. This test is not as sensitive as other tests and can produce false-negative results if low levels of antibodies are present in the oral fluid (AIDS.gov, 2015).

HIV antibody testing may take place in a physician's office or at designated HIV counseling and testing sites. Many patients feel more comfortable being tested by someone who knows their medical and social history, but others prefer to be tested in a location where they are unknown. Be aware of the various options for HIV antibody testing in his or her state or community to advise patients appropriately.

HIV antibody testing can be done one of two ways: confidentially or anonymously. In *confidential testing,* patients provide identifying information, including a name; an address; and often demographic information such as age, sex, race, and occupation. Using this information, care providers can locate and provide information to an individual who does not return for the test results or counseling. All records are strictly confidential, and testing in physicians' offices, clinics, and hospitals is conducted in a confidential manner. Health care providers who share or use this information inappropriately can be sued for negligence and invasion of privacy, and they may be disciplined by licensing boards for unauthorized disclosure or breach of confidentiality. Patients should be informed that the results of their HIV antibody test will be linked to the patient's medical record.

In *anonymous testing,* individuals are not asked to provide identifying information. Records are kept through assigned numbers, and the patient must retain this number to receive test results. It is not possible to locate and provide information to an individual who does not return for test results and counseling. In either form of testing, the nurse can perform pretest and post-test counseling.

RISK ASSESSMENT AND RISK REDUCTION

Testing for HIV is an important part of the public health response to HIV disease. Risk assessment should be patient centered, a joint process between the nurse and patient. The patient should take "ownership" of the risk for HIV infection. The nursing assessment should include an evaluation of risky behaviors by the patient or a history of STIs. A patient will not get tested unless he or she perceives a need for testing and feels safe doing so. Help the patient assess the risks by asking some basic questions:

- Have you ever had a transfusion or used clotting factors? Was it before 1985?
- Have you ever shared needles, syringes, or other injecting equipment with anyone?
- Have you ever had a sexual experience in which your penis, vagina, rectum, or mouth came into contact with another person's penis, vagina, rectum, or mouth?

A positive response to any of these questions requires further exploration with the patient. Be prepared to refer the patient to centers that provide testing and counseling services. All testing should include pretest and posttest counseling (see Boxes 56.3 and 56.9).

HIV infection in women has been overlooked frequently for several reasons. In the United States, the disease initially occurred mostly in men, and treatment models were developed accordingly. Providers did not assess the risks for women, and women did not seek testing and counseling because of denial or ignorance; thus interventions have not been implemented effectively. Heterosexual intercourse surpassed injection drug use as a vector for HIV transmission in women in the second decade of this pandemic and globally continues to be the highest risk factor in women. The CDC case definition includes at least one female-specific disease: cervical carcinoma. Women now need to be assessed for different manifestations, such as vaginal candidiasis, a common presenting condition for HIV-positive women (CDC, 1993).

BARRIERS TO PREVENTION

HIV prevention has numerous barriers, not the least of which is a denial of risk, an attitude that "it won't happen to me." Because the virus infects the MSM population in the United States, members of many other subpopulations have ignored their risks. Fear, misunderstanding, and the potential for social isolation and social stigma are significant barriers. Some individuals are so fearful that they no longer give blood or eat at a restaurant if they think a homosexual food handler works there. Such reactions reinforce the need for consistent, accurate information about the virus, the risks of transmission, and HIV disease.

Cultural and community attitudes, values, and norms can affect the success of prevention efforts. A community may be opposed to HIV education in the local school district because of the fear that certain values will be compromised. Those values may include views on sexuality, abstinence, the use of condoms, the use of drugs, and the provision of instructions about cleaning needles and syringes. Community organizations, churches, educators, and leaders can determine the community's expectations or norms. Cooperative efforts are essential for successful prevention of HIV transmission. The issues related to the HIV epidemic—sex, drug use, death, and homosexuality—are not easy issues for most cultures or communities.

Fear of alienation and discrimination are significant additional barriers to prevention. Some individuals are reluctant even to pick up a pamphlet about HIV because they fear that someone will believe they are gay or using illicit drugs. Some people will not go to a physician or to a testing and counseling site for HIV testing for fear of being seen there by people they know. This fear may be further compounded in smaller communities. Fear of discrimination includes fear of losing family, friends, prestige, job, housing, and insurance. Fortunately, many states have statutes to protect individuals with HIV disease from discrimination. Protection also is afforded by the Americans With Disabilities Act.

REDUCING RISKS RELATED TO SEXUAL TRANSMISSION

When patients have acute HIV disease and high viral loads, they are 10 times more likely to transmit HIV during sexual intercourse than during the chronic stage of HIV. Infection risk also is increased when sex is forceful or when mucosal membranes are disrupted (situations often associated with STIs). Most HIV infections are transmitted during the primary stage of the infection. This is when most people are unaware of their infection because they have no symptoms. Men are less likely to be infected with HIV during heterosexual intercourse than are women because women have more mucosal surface that can be exposed to infected body fluids in comparison to men. Male circumcision also can minimize a man's risk of becoming infected with HIV via heterosexual intercourse, according to the WHO (2018).

Safer sexual activities reduce the risk of exposure to HIV through semen, rectal secretions, and cervicovaginal secretions. Abstaining from all sexual activity is the most effective way to accomplish this goal. Limiting sexual behavior to activities in which the mouth, penis, vagina, or rectum do not come into contact with the partner's mouth, penis, vagina, or rectum is also safe because there is no contact with blood, semen, or cervicovaginal secretions. These activities may include massage and masturbation. Insertive sex is considered safe only in a mutually monogamous relationship with a partner who is not infected with, or at risk of becoming infected with, HIV. The problem with mutual monogamy is that both partners need to follow all of the rules all of the time. Unfortunately, cases of HIV infection occur in individuals who are not aware that their partner has not remained monogamous. Serial monogamy (maintaining a monogamous relationship, often including unprotected intercourse, with one partner for a short time, followed by another relationship, and then another) also increases the risk of HIV exposure (Box 56.11).

ART can be provided to people who have been exposed to HIV through unwanted sexual intercourse (rape) or through injection drugs. The US Department of Health and Human Services (USDHHS) has developed some recommendations regarding these types of nonoccupational exposures. This is referred to as postexposure prophylaxis, or PEP. When a person has been exposed to body fluids from an HIV-infected person during high-risk activity less than 72 hours before seeking treatment, the exposed person should receive a 28-day supply of ART. This is recommended even if the HIV-infected source of the exposure has an undetectable viral load. However, if the activity is deemed to be low-risk exposure to body fluids, or if the exposed person seeks health care after the 72-hour window, ART is not recommended. Cases should be examined on an individual basis to determine the need for PEP, counseling, treatment, and education about preventing future exposures (CDC, 2018k).

The use of barriers (Fig. 56.6) reduces the risk of contact with HIV during sexual activity. Barriers should be used when a person engages in sexual activity with a partner whose HIV status is not definitely known or with a partner who is known to be infected with HIV. The most commonly used barrier is the male condom. Although not 100% effective, male condoms are very effective in the prevention of HIV transmission when used correctly and consistently. Other barriers include female condoms and latex dental dams. Female condoms consist of a vinyl sheath with two spring-form rings. The smaller ring is inserted into the vagina and holds the condom in place internally. The larger ring surrounds the opening to the condom. It keeps the condom in place externally while also protecting the external genitalia. The use of the female condom is complicated and cumbersome, and practice may be necessary to use this method effectively. Female condoms also can be used for anal sex, in men and women. Dental dams or microwave-safe plastic wrap can be used to cover the external genitalia or anus during oral sexual activity ("rimming"). Although the risk of HIV transmission is reduced significantly with the use of latex barriers, other STIs, such as human papillomavirus, warts, and HSV, can still be transmitted.

REDUCING RISKS RELATED TO DRUG ABUSE

The use of illicit or recreational drugs can cause immunosuppression, malnutrition, and emotional difficulties. Although using illicit drugs can increase a person's risk for acquiring HIV infection, drug use is not to blame. The major risks of HIV transmission are related to sharing injection equipment and having unsafe sexual experiences while under the influence of mood-altering chemicals. Essentially, people can reduce the risk of HIV infection by not using drugs. If drugs are injected, equipment should not be shared with other people. People should not engage in sexual activity while under the influence of any drug, including alcohol, that impairs decision making.

Abstaining from drugs is not always a viable option for a user who has no access to drug treatment services or who chooses not to quit. The risk of HIV for these individuals can be eliminated if they can find alternatives to injecting, such as smoking, snorting, or ingesting

Box 56.11 Risk of HIV Transmission

HIV is spread primarily by the following:

- Not using a condom when having sex with a person who has HIV. All unprotected sex with someone who has HIV contains some risk. However:
  - Unprotected anal sex is riskier than unprotected vaginal sex.
  - Among men who have sex with other men, unprotected receptive anal sex is riskier than unprotected insertive anal sex.
  - Having multiple sex partners or the presence of other sexually transmitted diseases (STDs). Unprotected oral sex can also carry risk for HIV transmission, but it is a much lower risk than that with anal or vaginal sex.
- Sharing needles, syringes, rinse water, or other equipment used to prepare illicit drugs for injection.
- Being born to an infected mother: HIV can be passed from mother to child during pregnancy, birth, or breast-feeding.

Less common modes of transmission include the following:

- Being "stuck" with an HIV-contaminated needle or other sharp object. This risk pertains mainly to health care workers.
- Receiving blood transfusions, blood products, or organ/tissue transplants that are contaminated with HIV. This risk is extremely remote, however, as a result of the rigorous testing of the US blood supply and donated organs/tissue.
- Unsafe or unsanitary injections or other medical or dental practices. However, the risk is also remote with current safety standards in the United States.
- Eating food that has been prechewed by an HIV-infected person. The contamination occurs when infected blood from a caregiver's mouth mixes with food while chewing. This appears to be a rare occurrence and has been documented among only infants whose caregiver gave them prechewed food.
- Being bitten by a person with HIV. Each of the very small number of cases has included severe trauma with extensive tissue damage and the presence of blood. There is no risk of transmission if the skin is not broken.
- Contact between broken skin, wounds, or mucous membranes and HIV-infected blood or blood-contaminated body fluids. Reports of these incidents also have been extremely rare.
- "French" or deep, open-mouth kissing with an HIV-infected person if the HIV-infected person's mouth or gums are bleeding. This chance, too, is extremely remote.
- Tattooing or body piercing. However, no cases of HIV transmission from these activities have been documented. Only sterile equipment should be used for tattooing or body piercing.
- Unsafe injections. There have been a few documented cases in Europe and North Africa in which infants have been infected by unsafe injections and then transmitted HIV to their mothers through breast-feeding. No cases of this mode of transmission have been documented in the United States.

HIV cannot reproduce outside the human body. It *is not* spread by any of the following:

- Air or water.
- Insects, including mosquitoes. Studies conducted by CDC researchers and others have shown no evidence of HIV transmission from insects.
- Saliva, tears, or sweat. No case of HIV being transmitted by spitting has been documented.
- Casual contact such as shaking hands or sharing dishes.
- Closed-mouth or "social" kissing.

All reported cases suggesting new or potentially unknown routes of transmission are thoroughly investigated by state and local health departments with assistance, guidance, and laboratory support from CDC.

HIV, Human immunodeficiency virus.
Modified from Centers for Disease Control and Prevention (CDC): HIV Transmission, 2018. Retrieved from *https://www.cdc.gov/hiv/basics/transmission.html.*

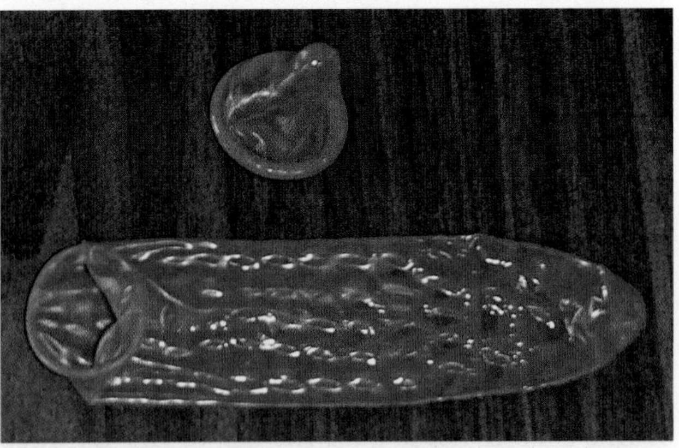

Fig. 56.6 Male condoms.

drugs. Risk also can be eliminated if the user does not share injection equipment, including needles, syringes, cookers, cotton, and rinse water. The safest tactic is for the user to have ready access to sterile equipment. Many states have laws that prohibit over-the-counter sale of needles and syringes, such as diabetic supplies. Some communities have needle exchange programs that supply sterile equipment to users to help reduce the risk of HIV transmission. The fear that needle exchange programs will result in increased illicit substance use has led to a lack of community support. However, studies have shown that in communities that have established exchange programs, drug use does not increase and rates of HIV infection are controlled (Wodak and Cooney, 2006).

REDUCING RISKS RELATED TO OCCUPATIONAL EXPOSURE

As previously discussed, the risk of acquiring HIV through occupational exposure is low. The CDC and the Occupational Safety and Health Administration have instituted policies to protect employees from exposure to blood and other potentially infectious fluids (CDC, 2013e). The use of standard precautions and body substance isolation has been shown to reduce the risk of bloodborne pathogens, the risk of transmission of other diseases between the patient and the health care worker, and the risk of transmission between patients. Hand hygiene in the form of handwashing still remains the most effective means of preventing the spread of infection.

Results of epidemiologic and laboratory studies suggest that several factors may affect the risk of HIV transmission after an occupational exposure. In a retrospective study of health care workers who had percutaneous exposure to HIV, the CDC (2001) found that the risk of HIV infection was increased with exposure to a larger quantity of blood from the source patient, as indicated by (1) a device visibly contaminated with the patient's blood, (2) a procedure that involved a needle being placed directly in a vein or artery, or (3) a deep injury. The risk also is increased for exposure to blood from a patient with terminal illness, which possibly reflects the higher viral load of the patient late in the course of HIV disease (CDC, 2001). Information about primary HIV infection (seroconversion) indicates that a systemic infection does not occur immediately. This leaves a brief window of opportunity during which initiation of antiretroviral PEP may prevent or inhibit systemic infection by limiting the proliferation of the virus in the initial target cells or lymph nodes.

For best prophylactic effect, PEP must be initiated within 36 hours but preferably as soon as possible after the exposure. PEP should include three or more ART medications (Kuhar et al, 2013). In addition to possible exposure to an antiretroviral-resistant strain of HIV, other factors that may contribute to failures include a high titer or large volume of inoculum exposure, delayed initiation or short duration of PEP, and factors related to the exposed health care personnel (e.g., immune status).

Completion of a 4-week course of therapy after an occupational exposure is fundamental. The medications used have many side effects, and health care workers may stop PEP prematurely because of these. It is important to consult with experts in occupational exposure if side effects (headache, nausea, vomiting, diarrhea) become unbearable. The use of PEP regimens has been associated with new-onset diabetes mellitus, hyperglycemia, hypertriglyceridemia, pancreatitis, elevated levels of lipids (cholesterol, low-density lipoproteins), liver dysfunction, and kidney stones. Despite these serious side effects, the exposed health care worker must continue therapy for 4 weeks or until it is determined that the source patient is not infected with HIV.

Hospitals or agencies should have policies that specifically address occupational HIV exposure, inasmuch as chemoprophylaxis must be undertaken immediately, even before testing of the source patient's and health care worker's blood for HIV or other bloodborne pathogens. Serial testing of the health care worker for HIV occurs immediately, 6 weeks, 3 months, and 6 months after the exposure.

Maintaining confidentiality for the exposed health care worker and the source patient is paramount. Many states and health care organizations have separate, distinct consent forms that are required before HIV antibody testing can be performed. Only in rare circumstances, such as the inability to give consent, can HIV antibody testing be completed without the patient's informed consent. Many ethical and legal issues surround HIV antibody testing; therefore nurses must be informed of the applicable laws in the state in which they practice. In many states, charges of assault and battery can be brought against health care workers who perform HIV testing against a patient's will. Appropriate counseling and referrals should be made for the health care worker and patient when HIV testing is indicated.

OTHER METHODS TO REDUCE RISK

HIV-infected people must be instructed not to give blood, donate organs, or donate semen for artificial insemination. They should not share razors, toothbrushes, or other household items that may contain blood or other body fluids. They also should avoid infecting sexual and needle-sharing partners, consider using birth control measures, and eliminate breast-feeding to avoid spreading the virus to infants.

OUTLOOK

During the HIV pandemic, much has been learned about transmission of the virus and ways to prevent infection. With no cure in sight, prevention of infection through education, prevention of mother-to-child transmission, and in some cases PEP or preexposure prophylaxis for people with a very high risk of becoming infected but are not currently infected can limit the effect of this disease on the human population.

The dynamics of the pandemic also have changed dramatically. In the United States, HIV disease has the characteristics of any other chronic illness, in that (1) it currently cannot be cured, (2) it continues throughout the patient's life, (3) it causes increasing physical disability and dysfunction if not treated, and (4) it ultimately results in significant morbidity and mortality. Chronic diseases are characterized by acute exacerbations of cyclic problems that compound each other. Despite a significant decrease in the number of opportunistic infections, new complications have emerged. Health care providers today must address body composition changes, cardiac disease, neuropathies, and the long-term effects of the very medications that have kept HIV at bay.

Since the discovery of HIV, knowledge about the viral cycle, resulting immune response, and disease progression of HIV has made significant advances. New medication treatments are very effective and can help the host manage the disease by limiting replication of the virus, which can allow the immune system to continue to function. Rates of survival among patients with late-stage HIV (and who have access to ART and are being cared for by health care providers with expertise in dealing with HIV) have increased dramatically. Patients who previously would have become disabled, quit jobs, and tended to end-of-life decisions are now reevaluating goals, returning to work, and rediscovering relative health. Now, couples with different HIV statuses have the option of having children with the use of sperm "washing" and in vitro fertilization.

For no other disease has there been such a rapid understanding and attempts at developing therapies as with HIV infection. The HIV research arena has provided insight into other diseases and scientific fields, including virology, immunology, and oncology. At this point, however, scientists' ability to develop new therapies depends on the patient's being nearly 100% adherent to regimens that are sometimes toxic. Adherence is poor even when therapy consists of only one pill per day. Even though treatment options for HIV have advanced, disease progression varies widely. Research is continuing into determining how psychological and social stressors alter immune system responses.

Minority MSM have become the fastest-growing segment of the population with HIV disease. Underdeveloped countries in Africa and Southeast Asia have been hardest hit; in fact, many villages have been destroyed because of HIV. The global threat of HIV is enormous, and nurses play a key role in the care and treatment of HIV-infected individuals. For the best possible outcomes, always seek guidance from HIV specialists when treating an individual with HIV disease because the care is very complex and multiple needs arise.

The field of HIV and AIDS nursing changes frequently, and nurses constantly must refresh their base of knowledge. Resources include local AIDS service organizations and state and regional AIDS education and training centers. As new therapies emerge, nurses are in a unique position to educate patients and the public about what is undoubtedly the most challenging infectious disease discovered in the 20th century.

Get Ready for the NCLEX® Examination!

Key Points

- HIV, a retrovirus, is the agent that causes HIV disease and AIDS.
- Education on prevention is the best method for preventing HIV disease and AIDS.
- In the United States, HIV most commonly is spread by sexual activities and sharing injection equipment.
- AIDS is the third and final stage of HIV infection.
- When HIV enters the body, its primary target is the immune system.
- HIV is transmitted by three major routes: (1) anal and vaginal intercourse, (2) injecting drugs with contaminated needles or works, and (3) from infected mother to child.
- Blood, semen, vaginal secretions, rectal secretions, and breast milk are the body fluids that most readily transmit HIV.
- Each patient's risks for HIV infection must be assessed, and those at risk must be counseled about testing, behaviors that put them at risk, and how to eliminate or reduce those risks.
- A positive result of an HIV antibody test does not mean the patient has AIDS.
- A multidisciplinary care approach in which the patient is a primary member of the team is the most appropriate method of caring for patients with HIV disease because of their complex needs.
- As HIV infection progresses, the immune system loses its ability to fight infectious agents and cancer cells.
- Patients at risk for HIV infection should be encouraged to learn their HIV status.
- A person infected with HIV virus can transmit the virus, regardless of whether signs and symptoms are present.
- Barriers to HIV prevention include denial, fear, misinformation, and cultural and community norms.
- $CD4^+$ counts are important markers of disease progression and the status of the immune system.
- The stigma of HIV disease, because of its association with drug use, homosexuality, and sexual transmission, is a major concern.
- The 1993 expanded case definition of AIDS includes all HIV-infected people who have $CD4^+$ T lymphocyte counts of less than 200/mm^3; includes all people who have one or more of more than 20 opportunistic infections regardless of CD4 count.
- Measuring viral load in the blood helps assess effectiveness of therapy and possibly adherence.
- Adherence to medications is essential.

Additional Learning Resources

SG Go to your Study Guide for additional learning activities to help you master this chapter content.

evolve Be sure to visit the Evolve site at *http://evolve.elsevier.com/Cooper/foundationsadult/* for additional online resources.

Review Questions for the NCLEX® Examination

1. What is responsible for causing the majority of HIV disease and AIDS?
   1. Human immunodeficiency virus type 1
   2. Human immunodeficiency virus type 2
   3. African immunodeficiency virus type 1
   4. *Pneumocystis jiroveci* deficiency virus
2. How does vertical transmission of HIV occur? *(Select all that apply.)*
   1. Mother to fetus during breast-feeding
   2. Mother to fetus during pregnancy
   3. Mother to fetus during delivery
   4. Mother to fetus during the postpartum period
   5. Mother to fetus during the first year of the infant's life
3. The nurse is assessing a patient who has requested HIV testing. What would be considered to be the most risky behavior?
   1. Dry kissing a casual date
   2. Sharing a soda with an infected person
   3. Swimming with an infected person
   4. Having more than three sex partners in a year
4. The student nurse is giving a presentation on the transmission of HIV to his class. The student is correct by sharing which information? *(Select all that apply.)*
   1. Health care workers are at a high risk for contracting HIV.
   2. Risk for transmission of HIV is higher with anal intercourse than with other types of sexual intercourse.
   3. People who use injection drugs and share needles have an elevated risk for being infected with HIV.
   4. The leading mode of transmission of HIV worldwide is sexual intercourse, despite sexual preference.
   5. During sexual intercourse, the partner who is being penetrated is least likely to contract HIV.
5. An 8-year-old boy receives a diagnosis of hemophilia. His mother is upset about his risk of acquiring HIV from blood products. What would be the nurse's best response?
   1. "All blood and blood products are screened for bloodborne diseases, so it is impossible for your son to be infected."
   2. "Many blood products are treated with heat or chemicals to inactivate the HIV virus."
   3. "We can talk about this if your son requires transfusions or blood products."
   4. "All blood donors are asked about HIV status and risk factors before giving blood."
6. A 34-year-old patient comes to the clinic requesting HIV testing. He is a gay man with two significant others in his lifetime. His partner recently received a diagnosis of HIV infection. The patient asks the nurse how long it will take before the infection could show up in him. What would be the nurse's best response?
   1. "Antibodies may be detected in the blood within 1 to 12 weeks of exposure."
   2. "It takes at least a year to know if you will be infected with HIV."
   3. "You'll have to ask your doctor the next time you go in for an appointment."
   4. "We don't know how long it will take for a person to seroconvert to being HIV positive."
7. The patient is concerned that he may be infected with HIV. Which sign or symptom is most commonly associated with an HIV infection?
   1. Night sweats
   2. Rash on the legs only
   3. Constipation
   4. Pruritus
8. A patient receives a diagnosis of HIV disease. She visits the physician today for her prescriptions. What medication does the nurse expect the physician to order for the patient?
   1. Tenofovir and emtricitabine (Truvada)
   2. Efavirenz (Sustiva)
   3. Lopinavir and ritonavir (Kaletra)
   4. Combination of these drugs
9. What diet should the patient with HIV follow?
   1. High calorie, high fiber, low protein
   2. Low calorie, low fiber, high protein
   3. High calorie, high protein, low residue
   4. Low calorie, high fiber, high protein
10. What are the most common opportunistic infection and malignant neoplasm in the patient with advanced HIV disease (AIDS)?
    1. Streptococcal pneumonitis, myeloma
    2. *Pneumocystis jiroveci* pneumonia, Kaposi's sarcoma
    3. *Streptococcus pneumoniae,* malignant melanoma
    4. *Mycoplasma* pneumonitis, Kaposi's sarcoma
11. For most people who are HIV positive, marker antibodies are usually present 10 to 12 weeks after exposure. What is the development of these antibodies called?
    1. Immunocompetence
    2. Seroconversion
    3. Immunodeficiency
    4. Viral load

12. What is the expanded definition of AIDS?
    1. The patient has HIV infection.
    2. The patient has a dysfunction of the immune system and is HIV positive.
    3. The patient is HIV positive and has an opportunistic disease.
    4. The patient is HIV positive with a $CD4^+$ lymphocyte count lower than 200/mm^3 or has an AIDS-related opportunistic infection.
13. What is the purpose of performing a viral load study once every 3 to 4 months in an HIV-positive person?
    1. To determine the $CD4^+$ lymphocyte count
    2. To determine the progression of the disease
    3. To determine the effectiveness of the medication regimen
    4. To determine the results of the Western blot test
14. The health care provider asks the nurse to talk with a patient about how HIV is transmitted. Which routes of transmission are most important for the nurse to discuss with the patient?
    1. Receiving blood, donating blood
    2. Food, water, air
    3. Sexual intercourse, sharing needles, mother-to-child transmission
    4. Dirty toilets, swimming pools, mosquitoes
15. The patient asks the nurse, "How does HIV cause AIDS?" What is the nurse's best response?
    1. "HIV attacks the immune system, a system that protects the body from foreign invaders, and thus makes it unable to protect the body from organisms that cause diseases."
    2. "HIV breaks down the circulatory system, which makes the body unable to assimilate oxygen and nutrients."
    3. "HIV attacks the respiratory system, which makes the lungs more susceptible to organisms causing pneumonia."
    4. "HIV attacks the digestive system, which causes a decrease in the absorption of essential nutrients and results in weight loss and fatigue."

Care of the Patient With Cancer

57

http://evolve.elsevier.com/Cooper/foundationsadult/

Objectives

1. Discuss the incidence rates of cancer in the United States.
2. Identify the three most common sites of cancer in men and women.
3. Discuss development, prevention, and detection of cancer.
4. List seven risk factors for cancer.
5. Discuss the American Cancer Society's recommendations for preventive behaviors and screening tests for men and women.
6. List seven warning signs of cancer.
7. Define the terminology used to describe cellular changes, characteristics of malignant cells, and types of malignancies.
8. Describe the pathophysiologic features of cancer, including the characteristics of malignant cells.
9. Describe the process of metastasis.
10. Define the systems of tumor classification: grading and staging.
11. List common diagnostic tests used to identify cancer.
12. Explain why biopsy is essential in confirming a diagnosis of cancer.
13. Describe nursing interventions for the individual undergoing surgery, radiation therapy, chemotherapy, bone marrow transplantation, or peripheral stem cell transplantation.
14. Describe the major categories of chemotherapeutic agents.
15. Explain the causes, pathophysiologic features, clinical manifestations, and medical management of tumor lysis syndrome, and describe the diagnostic tests, nursing interventions, and prognosis.
16. Discuss six general guidelines for pain relief in the patient with advanced cancer.

Key Terms

alopecia (ăl-ō-PĒ-shē-ă, p. 1999)
autologous (ăw-TŎL-ŏ-gŭs, p. 2003)
benign (bĕ-NĪN, p. 1988)
biopsy (BĪ-ŏp-sē, p. 1989)
cachexia (kă-KĔK-sē-ă, p. 2004)
carcinogenesis (kăr-sĭn-ō-JĔN-ĕ-sĭs, p. 1983)
carcinogens (kăr-SĬN-ō-jĕnz, p. 1983)
carcinoma (kăr-sĭn-Ō-mă, p. 1988)
differentiated (dĭf-ĕr-ĔN-shē-ā-tĕd, p. 1987)
dysgeusia (dis-gyū-zē-ă, p. 2006)
germline mutations (JĔRM-līn mū-TĀ-shănz, p. 1984)
immunosurveillance (ĭm-yū-nō-sĕr-VĀ-lĕns, p. 1988)
leukopenia (lū-kō-PĒ-nē-ă, p. 1997)
malignant (mă-LĬG-nănt, p. 1988)
metastasis (mĕ-TĂS-tă-sĭs, p. 1988)
neoplasm (NĒ-ō-plăz-ĕm, p. 1988)
oncology (ŏn-KŎL-ŏ-jē, p. 1981)
palliative (PĂL-ē-ă-tĭv, p. 1994)
Papanicolaou's (Pap) test or smear (pă-pĕ-NĬK-ō-lūz [PĂP] tĕst, smēr, p. 1989)
sarcoma (săr-KŌ-mă, p. 1988)
stomatitis (stō-mă-TĪ-tĭs, p. 2000)
thrombocytopenia (thrŏm-bō-sīt-ō-PĒ-nē-ă, p. 1999)
tumor lysis syndrome (TŪ-mŏr LĪ-sĭs SĬN-drōm, p. 2002)

ONCOLOGY

Oncology is the branch of medicine concerning study of tumors. An oncology nurse is a nurse with specialized training who cares for patients in whom cancer has been diagnosed.

Until the appearance of HIV, no other medical diagnosis produced as much fear as a diagnosis of cancer. The word *cancer* is thought by many people to be synonymous with death, pain, and disfigurement. However, advances in the treatment and control of cancer have outdistanced attitudes toward cancer. Education of health care professionals and the public is essential for promoting more positive and realistic attitudes about cancer and cancer treatment. The National Cancer Institute indicates that in the United States, 39% of women and men living in the United States will be diagnosed with at some point in their lifetime (NCI, n.d.a.). The leading sites of primary cancer in men are the prostate, lungs, and colon and rectum (Centers for Disease Control and Prevention [CDC], n.d.). The leading sites of primary cancer in women are the breasts, lungs,

Leading New Cancer Cases and Deaths – 2018 Estimates

Estimated New Cases*		Estimated Deaths*	
Breast	268,670	Lung and bronchus	154,050
Lung and bronchus	234,030	Colorectum	50,630
Prostate	164,690	Pancreas	44,330
Colorectum	140,250	Breast	41,400
Melanoma of the skin	91,270	Liver and intrahepatic bile duct	30,200
Urinary bladder	81,190	Prostate	29,430
Non-Hodgkin lymphoma	74,680	Leukemia	24,370
Kidney and renal pelvis	65,340	Non-Hodgkin lymphoma	19,910
Uterine corpus	63,230	Urinary bladder	17,240
Leukemia	60,300	Brain and other nervous system	16,830
Pancreas	55,440	Esophagus	15,850
Thyroid	53,990	Kidney and renal pelvis	14,970
Oral cavity and pharynx	51,540	Ovary	14,070
Liver and intrahepatic bile duct	42,220	Myeloma	12,770
Myeloma	30,770	Uterine corpus	11,350
Stomach	26,240	Stomach	10,800
Brain and other nervous system	23,880	Oral cavity and pharynx	10,030
Ovary	22,240	Melanoma of the skin	9,320
Esophagus	17,290	Soft tissue (including heart)	5,150
Cervix	13,240	Cervix	4,170
Larynx	13,150	Gallbladder and other biliary	3,790
Soft tissue (including heart)	13,040	Larynx	3,710
Gallbladder and other biliary	12,190	Thyroid	2,060
Small intestine	10,470	Bones and joints	1,590
Testes	9,310	Small intestine	1,450
Anus, anal canal and anorectum	8,580	Vagina and other female genital	1,330
Hodgkin lymphoma	8,500	Vulva	1,200
Vulva	6,190	Anus, anal canal and anorectum	1,160
Vagina and other female genital	5,170	Hodgkin lymphoma	1,050
Ureter and other urinary organs	3,820	Ureter and other urinary organs	960
Eye and orbit	3,540	Testes	400
Bones and joints	3,450	Penis and other male genital	380
Penis and other male genital	2,320	Eye and orbit	350

Fig. 57.1 Cancer: 2018 estimates. (Data from American Cancer Society, Inc.)

and colorectal (CDC, n.d.). Of every five deaths in the United States, one is from cancer, which makes cancer the second leading cause of death, after heart disease (Fig. 57.1).

Cancer is any one of a group of diseases characterized by the uncontrolled growth and spread of abnormal cells in the body. Early detection and prompt treatment can cure some cancers and slow the progression of others. If not detected and controlled, cancer can result in death. Overall, it affects people of all ages, but most cases are diagnosed in people older than 55 (see the Lifespan Considerations box). Cancer incidence is higher among African Americans than among members of any other race (CDC, n.d.; see the Cultural Considerations box). In 2018 over 1.7 million new cancer diagnoses were anticipated, and 609,640 Americans were expected to die from cancer (NCI, 2018). Cancer death rates have been decreasing since 1991 in men and since 1992 in women. In comparison with the peak rates in 1990 for men and in 1991 for women, the cancer death rate for all sites combined in 2004 was 18.4% lower in men and 10.5% lower in women. The 5-year survival rate is 67% (NCI, n.d.a.).

Lung cancer is the leading cause of cancer-related death in men and women. Other cancers, such as breast and prostate, occur more often than lung cancer, but they have better cure and survival rates because of early detection and treatment.

 Lifespan Considerations

Older Adults

Cancer

- More cases of cancer occur among older adults than among people of any other age group.
- The incidence of cancer increases with aging, possibly as a result of decreased effectiveness of the immune system and changes in DNA.
- The most common types of cancers observed in older adults are prostate, lung, breast, and colorectal cancer. Cancers of the skin, urinary bladder, vagina, and vulva are seen primarily in older adults. Chronic lymphocytic leukemia and multiple myeloma are seen more frequently in older adults than in younger people.
- Many early signs and symptoms of cancer may be misdiagnosed as normal changes of aging. Stress the importance of routine medical screening and self-examination.
- Because of fear or experience, older adults may adopt a fatalistic frame of mind after hearing the diagnosis of cancer. Use of the terms *tumor* or *growth* may be more acceptable.
- The type of treatment for cancer should be based on the older person's wishes and overall state of health. Older individuals, their family members, and significant others should be presented with all options so that they can make informed decisions regarding treatment.

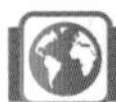 Cultural Considerations

Cancer in the United States

- The incidence of cancer is higher among African Americans than among white people.
- The death rate from the four most common cancers (lung, colorectal, breast, prostate) is higher among members of minority groups (except Asian Americans) than among white people.
- Of all ethnic groups, Asian Americans have the lowest rate of death from cancer.
- In comparison with white men, African American men have almost twice the rate of prostate cancer and are more than twice as likely to die from the disease.
- Hispanic women have the highest rate of invasive cervical cancer of any ethnic group other than Vietnamese, and the incidence rate is twice as high as that in non-Hispanic white women.
- Although African American women are less likely than white women to develop breast cancer, they are more likely to die from the disease if they develop it.
- Native Americans have a lower incidence of cancer than any other ethnic group in the United States but have the poorest survival rate when they do develop cancer.

DEVELOPMENT, PREVENTION, AND DETECTION OF CANCER

Carcinogenesis is the process by which normal cells are transformed into cancer cells. Cancer may be caused by external factors (infection, chemicals, radiation, and tobacco use) and internal factors (genetic mutations, immunologic conditions, and hormones).

Primary prevention of cancer consists of changes in lifestyle habits to eliminate or reduce exposure to **carcinogens,** substances known to increase the risk for developing cancer. Risk factors include the following:

- *Smoking:* According to the American Cancer Society, smoking is the most preventable cause of death from lung cancer. It is estimated that 80% of people who die from lung cancer are smokers. Other cancers associated with smoking are acute myeloid leukemia and cancers of the bladder, kidney, mouth, lip, stomach, colorectum, nasopharynx, larynx, paranasal sinuses, esophagus, pancreas, uterus, ovary, and cervix.
- *Dietary habits:* Nutrition is suspected to be a contributing factor to an estimated one-third of cancer deaths. Diets that are high in fat and low in fiber, as well as inadequate nutrient intake, are associated with cancer development. The National Cancer Institute (NCI) (2015) estimates that dietary modifications could prevent as many as one-third of all cancer deaths in the United States. Excessive body weight and inactivity are also linked (NCI, 2015); obesity is a risk factor for breast, endometrium, colon, rectum, esophagus, pancreas, kidney, and gallbladder cancer. Fruit and vegetable consumption may protect against cancers of the mouth and pharynx, esophagus, lung, stomach, and colon and rectum (see the Health Promotion box). In 2013 fewer than 25% of adults reported eating the recommended servings (Moore and Thompson, 2015). Currently, the majority of the US population consumes less than two and a half cups of fruits and vegetables each day.
- *Ultraviolet radiation:* Excessive exposure to the sun's ultraviolet rays is a factor in the development of basal and squamous cell skin cancers and melanoma. Indoor tanning beds also emit ultraviolet rays and confer the same risks as does sunlight. (In addition, the effects of radiation commonly used for medical diagnosis and treatment are known to be carcinogenic. Exposure should be limited and monitored.)

Health Promotion

Foods to Reduce Cancer Risk

- Vegetables from the cabbage family, such as the following:
  - Broccoli
  - Cauliflower
  - Brussels sprouts
  - All types of cabbage and kale
- Vegetables and fruits high in beta-carotene, such as the following:
  - Carrots
  - Peaches
  - Apricots
  - Squash
  - Broccoli
- Rich sources of vitamin C, such as the following:
  - Grapefruit
  - Watermelon
  - Apricots
  - Oranges
  - Cantaloupe
  - Strawberries
  - Red and green peppers
  - Broccoli
  - Tomatoes

The National Cancer Institute has recommended including at least five servings of fruits and vegetables in the daily diet. In addition are the following recommendations:

- Eat foods from protein sources such as lean meat, fish, and skinned poultry.
- Choose low-fat dairy products, including white cheese rather than yellow.
- Eat whole grains.
- Include beans in the diet.
- Avoid salt-cured, smoked, or nitrite-cured foods.
- Limit intake of saturated fat and added sugars.

- *Smokeless tobacco:* Use of smokeless tobacco increases the risk of cancer of the mouth, larynx, pharynx, and esophagus. Long-term snuff users have an increased risk for cheek and gum cancers (ACS, 2017a).
- *Environmental and chemical carcinogens:* Some of these include fumes from rubber and chlorine and dust from cotton, coal, nickel, chromate, asbestos, and vinyl chloride. The incidence of bladder cancer is higher among people who live in urban areas and among those who work with dyes, rubber, or leather.
- *Frequent heavy consumption of alcohol:* Alcohol use is linked to cancers of the mouth, larynx, pharynx, esophagus, colorectum, breast, and liver. The patient's risk increases significantly when the patient consumes more than two alcoholic drinks per day (American Cancer Society [ACS], 2017b).

HEREDITARY CANCERS

About 5% to 10% of cancers are hereditary (ACS, 2018a). Hereditary cancers arise from **germline mutations,** which are changes in egg or sperm cells that are then incorporated into the DNA of each body cell of the children produced (NCI, 2017a). Gene mutations occurring in specific genes are thought to be associated with more than 50 different hereditary cancer syndromes (NCI, 2017a). Hereditary cancers usually are diagnosed 15 to 20 years earlier than cancers that are not inherited. Often several relatives have the same or related cancers. In location, they are more likely to be bilateral, and the same person may have multiple cancers. These multiple cancers are often seen in unusual organ combinations, such as breast cancer and sarcoma, breast and thyroid cancers, and leukemia and brain tumors.

GENETIC SUSCEPTIBILITY

Scientific research has focused on genetic patterns in the most common cancer sites. The following patterns have emerged:

- *TP53* is the most commonly mutated gene found in all cancers. This gene is responsible for the synthesis of a protein that suppresses tumor growth. Germline mutations of this gene can produce Li-Fraumeni syndrome. This is an inherited and rare disorder that can lead to an elevated risk of developing specific cancers (NCI, 2017a).
- The incidence of postmenopausal breast cancer is three times higher and the incidence of premenopausal breast cancer is five times higher in women with a family history of this disease. An estimated 12% of the general female population develop breast cancer during their lifetime. In comparison, women who have either of the genes *BRCA1* and *BRCA2* have as much as an 80% risk of having breast cancer during their lifetime (ACS, 2017c). These genes also increase a person's risk for developing pancreatic, prostate (men), and male breast cancer (NCI, 2017a). Breast cancer is rare in Asian women and more common in white women.
- *PTEN* is a gene that assists with the production of another tumor growth suppressor. Mutations to *PTEN* can produce Cowden syndrome. This is an inherited disorder that can increase a patient's risk for developing endometrial, thyroid, and breast cancer (NCI, 2017a).
- The incidence of lung cancer is greater among smokers with a family history of this disease than in smokers without a family history of the disease.
- The incidence of leukemia is higher in an identical twin of a person with the disease.
- The frequency of neuroblastoma is increased among siblings.
- Colon cancer is more likely to occur in women who have a history of breast cancer.

CANCER RISK ASSESSMENT AND GENETIC COUNSELING

When an individual or family has characteristics suggestive of a hereditary cancer (such as cancers that occur in several generations of a family, multiple primary cancers in one person, or rare cancers associated with birth defects), a cancer risk assessment is performed.

The assessment begins with a comprehensive family history, including information on first-, second-, and third-degree relatives. Medical records, death certificates, and autopsy reports may be obtained to help confirm the cancer diagnoses previously identified in the family history.

Genetic counseling is an essential component of the genetic evaluation. The nurse who may be involved with the genetic counseling and genetic testing provides health care promotion education and support to individuals and families facing the uncertainty of hereditary cancer. Informed consent must be obtained before genetic testing.

CANCER PREVENTION AND EARLY DETECTION

The American Cancer Society (2012) advises specific preventive behaviors and screening tests for men and women (Table 57.1). Education regarding early detection of cancer includes recognition of warning signs (Box 57.1). The nurse plays an important role in prevention and detection of cancer. Early detection and prompt

Table 57.1 Screening Guidelines for the Early Detection of Cancer in People With No Symptoms and Average Risk

CANCER SITE	POPULATION	TEST OR PROCEDURE	FREQUENCY
Breast	Women, ages 20+	Breast self-examination (BSE)	It is acceptable for women to choose not to do BSE or to do BSE regularly (monthly) or irregularly. Beginning in their early 20s, women should be told about the benefits and limitations of BSE. Whether a woman ever performs BSE, the importance of prompt reporting of any new breast symptoms to a health care professional should be emphasized. Women who choose to do BSE should receive instruction and have their technique reviewed on the occasion of a periodic health examination.
		Clinical breast examination (CBE)	For women in their 20s and 30s, it is recommended that CBE be part of a periodic health examination, preferably at least every 3 years. Asymptomatic women ages 40+ should continue to receive a CBE as part of a periodic health examination, preferably annually.
Mammography		Begin annual mammography at age 40.[a]	
Cervix	Women, ages 21–65	Pap test and HPV DNA test	Cervical cancer screening should begin at age 21. For women ages 21–29, screening should be done every 3 years with conventional or liquid-based Pap tests. For women ages 30–65, screening should be done every 5 years with both the HPV test and the Pap test (preferred), or every 3 years with the Pap test alone (acceptable). Women ages 65+ who have had ≥3 consecutive negative Pap tests or ≥2 consecutive negative HPV and Pap tests within the past 10 years, with the most recent test occurring within 5 years, and women who have had a total hysterectomy should stop cervical cancer screening. Women should not be screened annually by any method at any age.
Colorectal	Men and women, ages 50+	Fecal occult blood test (FOBT) with at least 50% test sensitivity for cancer, or fecal immunochemical test (FIT) with at least 50% test sensitivity for cancer, **or**	Annual, starting at age 50. Testing at home with adherence to manufacturer's recommendation for collection techniques and number of samples is recommended. FOBT with the single stool sample collected on the clinician's fingertip during a DRE in the health care setting is not recommended. Guaiac-based toilet bowl FOBT tests also are not recommended. In comparison with guaiac-based tests for the detection of occult blood, immunochemical tests are more patient-friendly, and are likely to be equal or better in sensitivity and specificity. There is no justification for repeating FOBT in response to an initial positive finding.
		Stool DNA test, **or**	Every 3 years, starting at age 50
		Flexible sigmoidoscopy (FSIG), **or**	Every 5 years, starting at age 50. FSIG can be performed alone, or consideration can be given to combining FSIG performed every 5 years with a highly sensitive guaiac-based FOBT or FIT performed annually.
		Double-contrast barium enema (DCBE), **or**	Every 5 years, starting at age 50

Continued

Table 57.1 Screening Guidelines for the Early Detection of Cancer in People With No Symptoms and Average Risk—cont'd

CANCER SITE	POPULATION	TEST OR PROCEDURE	FREQUENCY
		Colonoscopy	Every 10 years, starting at age 50
		CT Colonography	Every 5 years, starting at age 50
Endometrial	Women, at menopause		At the time of menopause, women at average risk should be informed about the risks and symptoms of endometrial cancer and strongly encouraged to report any unexpected bleeding or spotting to their physicians.
Lung	Current or former smokers (quit within past 15 years) ages 55–74 in good health with at least a 30 pack-year history	Low-dose helical CT (LDCT)	Clinicians with access to high-volume, high-quality lung cancer screening and treatment centers should initiate a discussion about lung cancer screening with apparently healthy patients aged 55–74 who have at least a 30 pack-year smoking history, and who currently smoke or have quit within the past 15 years. A process of informed and shared decision making with a clinician related to the potential benefits, limitations, and harms associated with screening for lung cancer with LDCT should occur before any decision is made to initiate lung cancer screening. Smoking cessation counseling remains a high priority for clinical attention in discussions with current smokers, who should be informed of their continuing risk of lung cancer. Screening should not be viewed as an alternative to smoking cessation.
Prostate	Men, ages 50+	Digital rectal examination (DRE) and prostate-specific antigen test (PSA)	Men who have at least a 10-year life expectancy should have an opportunity to make an informed decision with their health care provider about whether to be screened for prostate cancer, after receiving information about the potential benefits, risks, and uncertainties associated with prostate cancer screening. Prostate cancer screening should not occur without an informed decision-making process.
Cancer-related checkup	Men and women, ages 20+	On the occasion of a periodic health examination, the cancer-related checkup should include examination for cancers of the thyroid, testicles, ovaries, lymph nodes, oral cavity, and skin, as well as health counseling about tobacco, sun exposure, diet and nutrition, risk factors, sexual practices, and environmental and occupational exposures.	

From http://www.cancer.org/acs/groups/content/@research/documents/webcontent/acspc-045101.pdf.
[a]Beginning at age 40, annual clinical breast examination should ideally be performed before mammography.
CT, Computed tomography.

Box 57.1 Eight Warning Signs of Cancer

If you have a warning sign, see your health care provider.

1. Changes in bowel or bladder habits
2. Sores that don't heal
3. White patches inside the mouth or on the tongue
4. Unusual bleeding or discharge
5. Thickening or lump in breast or elsewhere
6. Indigestion or difficulty swallowing
7. Recent change in warts, moles, or skin
8. Nagging cough or hoarseness

Modified from American Cancer Society (ACS): Signs and symptoms of cancer, 2014. From *https://www.cancer.org/cancer/cancer-basics/signs-and-symptoms-of-cancer.html.*

treatment are directly responsible for increased rates of survival among patients with cancer (see the Health Promotion box).

Beginning in high school, all women should be taught to perform breast self-examination (BSE) each month, 2 or 3 days after the menstrual period ends. After menopause, a woman should choose a specific day to help her remember, such as the first day of each month. A woman needs to become familiar with the appearance and feel of her breasts. This will help her identify any change from one month to the next. Any abnormality—such as discharge from the nipples; puckering, dimpling, peau d'orange (skin appearance of an orange peel) (Fig. 57.2), or scaling of the skin; and the palpation of a lump or thickness—is significant (see Chapter 52 for instructions on BSE). Teach BSE to all patients (men and women), emphasizing that any identifiable problem should be brought to the attention of a health care provider. Any delay is a waste of valuable time if cancer is present.

Teach boys, beginning at puberty, and men to check the scrotum for enlargement, thickening, and the presence of a lump in the testicles. This should be done monthly, after a warm bath or shower. Emphasize that any changes from the normal, smooth consistency of the testes should be brought to the attention of a health

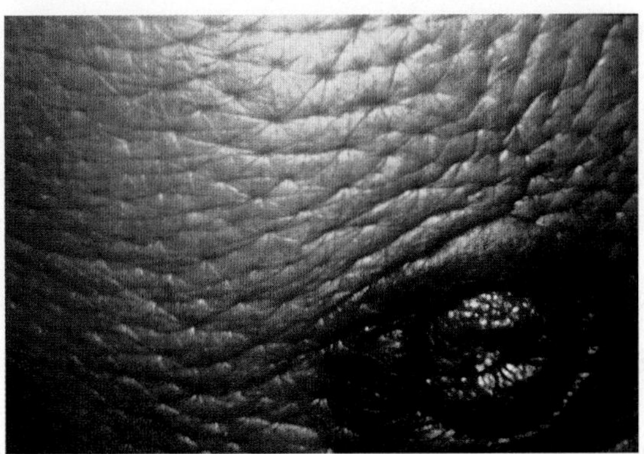

Fig. 57.2 Appearance of peau d'orange in the breast. (From Swartz MH: *Textbook of physical diagnosis*, ed 5, Philadelphia, 2006, Saunders.)

Health Promotion

Prevention and Detection of Cancer

- Reduce or avoid exposure to known or suspected carcinogens and cancer-promoting agents, including cigarette smoke and excessive sunlight.
- Eat a balanced diet that includes green, deep yellow, and orange vegetables; cruciferous vegetables (cabbage, broccoli, cauliflower, and Brussels sprouts); fresh fruits; allium vegetables (onion and garlic); nuts; legumes; soy products; whole grains; and adequate amounts of fiber. Reduce the amount of fat and preservatives, including smoked and salt-cured meats. Limit the consumption of processed foods and red meats.
- Exercise regularly. The American Cancer Society recommends that adults engage in at least 150 minutes of moderate physical activity or 75 minutes of vigorous activity each week (ACS, 2014).
- Obtain adequate, consistent periods of rest (at least 6 to 8 hours per night).
- Schedule regular health examinations that include a health history, a physical examination, and specific diagnostic tests for common cancers in accordance with the guidelines published by the American Cancer Society (see Table 57.1).
- Eliminate, reduce, or change the perceptions of stressors, and enhance the ability to cope effectively with stressors.
- Enjoy consistent periods of relaxation and leisure.
- Identify the eight warning signs of cancer (see Box 57.1).
- Learn and practice self-examination (e.g., skin examination, breast self-examination, testicular self-examination).
- Seek immediate medical care if you notice a change in what is normal for you and if cancer is suspected. Early detection of cancer has a positive effect on prognosis.

care provider (see Chapter 52). Some clinical manifestations of testicular cancer include a lump in or enlargement of either testicle, a heavy feeling in the scrotum, dull aching in either the groin or the lower abdomen, fluid collection in the scrotum, and tenderness or enlargement of the breasts (this results from hormones produced by cancer cells) (ACS, 2018b).

Advise men older than 50 to discuss the prostate-specific antigen test with their health care provider and undergo a rectal examination once a year. Populations at high risk for prostate cancer (African Americans and men who have positive family history for the disease) are urged to begin screening at ages 40 to 45 years. Blood in the urine, difficulty starting to urinate, a weak flow of urine, and other urination problems should be reported to the health care provider for evaluation.

PATHOPHYSIOLOGY OF CANCER

CELL MECHANISMS AND GROWTH

The basic unit of structure and function in all living things is the *cell.* The adult human body contains approximately 60,000 billion cells. Although there are many different types of cells, all of them have certain common characteristics. For example, all cells need nourishment to maintain life, and all cells use almost identical nutrients. All cells use oxygen, which combines with fat, protein, or carbohydrates to release the energy needed for cells to function. The mechanisms for changing nutrients into energy are generally the same in all cells, and all cells deliver their end product of chemical reactions into the nearby fluids.

Most cells are able to reproduce. When cells are destroyed, the remaining cells of the same type reproduce until the correct number has been replenished. This orderly replacement of cells is governed by a control mechanism that stops when the loss or damage has been corrected. Dynamic, active, and orderly, the healthy cell is a small powerhouse, laboratory, factory, and duplicating machine, copying itself over and over. The immune system aids in preventing the development of cancer by destroying the abnormal cells. On occasion, the immune system fails to recognize these abnormal cells, and cancer develops.

Cancer cells are not subject to the usual restrictions placed on cell proliferation by the host. When malignant cells change, they become unlike parent cells; they are not **differentiated** (recognizable as being the same in size or shape as normal cells). Cancer cells can divide and multiply, but not in a normal manner. Instead of limiting their growth to meet specific needs of the body, they continue to reproduce in a disorderly and unrestricted manner. The cellular features of cancer cells are a local increase in the number of cells, loss of normal cellular arrangement, variation in cell shape and size, increased nuclear size, increased miotic activity, and abnormal mitosis and chromosomes.

Proliferation is not always indicative of cancer, however. Abnormal cellular growth is classified as nonneoplastic growth and neoplastic growth. The four common nonneoplastic growth patterns are hypertrophy, hyperplasia, metaplasia, and dysplasia. Although not neoplastic conditions, these may precede the development of cancer. *Anaplasia* means "without form" and

Table 57.2 General Characteristics of Neoplasms

BENIGN TUMORS	MALIGNANT TUMORS
Slow, steady growth	Rate of growth varies; usually rapid
Remains localized	Metastasizes
Usually contained within a capsule	Rarely contained within a capsule
Smooth, well defined; movable when palpated	Irregular; more immobile when palpated
Resembles parent tissue	Little resemblance to parent tissue
Crowds normal tissue	Invades normal tissue
Rarely recurs after removal	May recur after removal
Rarely fatal	Fatal without treatment

is an irreversible change in which the structures of adult cells regress to more primitive levels.

Neoplasm is a group of cells whose growth is uncontrolled or abnormal. Neoplasms may be **benign** (not recurrent or progressive; nonmalignant) or **malignant** (abnormal cell growths with a loss of normal role and function). Malignant neoplasms have the ability to spread to other body sites and resist treatment, as in cancerous growths (Table 57.2). Growths also are referred to as *tumors,* which means "swelling" or "enlargement." They may be localized or invasive. Benign tumors may become problematic because their increased size damages surrounding tissues, as in a benign brain tumor. Malignant neoplasms may progress and destroy surrounding tissues. They also may metastasize from the primary site of origin to distant sites.

Metastasis is the process by which tumor cells spread from the primary site to a secondary site. Once cancer cells have moved to another area of the body, secondary tumors may grow in that area. Metastasis can occur by (1) diffusion to other body cavities or (2) circulation via blood and lymphatic channels.

In addition to the identified carcinogenic factors that may cause malignant cellular changes, certain viruses have been suspected. Viruses linked to the development of cancers include human papillomavirus, Epstein Barr virus (EBV), hepatitis B virus, hepatitis C virus, and human immunodeficiency virus (HIV). There is also evidence to suggest that particular genetic factors result in a predisposition to the development of cancer (ACS, 2016a).

The body's immune system is responsible for recognizing and destroying malignant cells. The immune system may be weakened by cancer-producing substances, tumor cells, and the aging process. Some T cells are responsible for **immunosurveillance** (the immune system's recognition and destruction of newly developed abnormal cells). When a cell becomes malignant, its membranes carry a tumor-specific antigen that is recognized by the body as nonself and is destroyed. If T cell function is suppressed by age, drugs (e.g., corticosteroids), poor nutrition, alcohol, serious infections, or certain disease processes (e.g., neoplastic invasion of bone and lymph tissue), the risk of cancer increases. To suppress T cell rejection of a transplanted organ, steroids and other drugs are given. The resultant loss of immunosurveillance increases the risk of certain cancers.

DESCRIPTION, GRADING, AND STAGING OF TUMORS

Cancers are described according to the original site of the primary tumor. A **carcinoma** is a malignant tumor composed of epithelial cells, which tend to metastasize. Carcinomas originate from embryonal ectoderm (skin and glands) and endoderm (mucous membrane linings of the respiratory tract, gastrointestinal [GI] tract, and genitourinary tract). A **sarcoma** is a malignant tumor of connective tissues; sarcomas originate from embryonal mesoderm, such as muscle, bone, or fat, usually manifesting as a painless swelling. Sarcomas may affect bone, bladder, kidneys, liver, lungs, parotid glands, and the spleen. *Lymphomas* and *leukemias* originate from the hematopoietic system.

A tumor may be named for its location, its cellular makeup, or the person by whom it was originally identified.

Grading of Tumors

Tumors are classified as grades 1 to 4 by the degree of malignancy. Grade 1 tumors are the most differentiated (most like the parent tissue) and the least malignant. Grade 4 tumors are the least differentiated (unlike parent tissue) tumor and the most malignant (Box 57.2).

Extent of Disease Classification

Classifying the extent and spread of disease is termed *staging.* This classification system is based on a description of the extent of the disease rather than on cell appearance. Although different types of cancer are staged similarly, there are many differences, based on a thorough knowledge of the natural history of each specific type of cancer.

Clinical staging. The clinical staging classification system is used to determine the extent of the disease process of cancer by stages:

Stage 0: Cancer in situ
Stage I: Tumor limited to the tissue of origin; localized tumor growth
Stage II: Limited local spread
Stage III: Extensive local and regional spread
Stage IV: Metastasis

TNM classification system. The *TNM classification system* represents the standardization of the clinical staging of cancer. This classification system is used to determine the extent of the disease process of cancer according to three parameters: tumor size *(T)*, degree of regional spread to the lymph nodes *(N)*, and metastasis *(M)* (see Box 57.2). This system is used to direct treatment, predict prognosis, and contribute to cancer research by ensuring reliable comparison of different patients.

Bethesda system. Exfoliative (pertaining to the shedding of something) cytologic study (e.g., **Papanicolaou's [Pap] test or smear**) is a means of studying cells that the body has shed during the normal sequence of growth and replacement of body tissues. If cancer is present, cancer cells also are shed. The method is used most commonly to detect cancers of the cervix, but it may be used for tissue specimens from any organ.

- *Normal:* Inconclusive or ASC-US (atypical squamous cells of undetermined cause): cells don't look normal
- *Abnormal:* Cell changes most likely related to presence of human papilloma virus, may progress to cancer over a period of time, dysplasia
- *Low-grade squamous intraepithelial lesion (LSIL) or intraepithelial neoplasia (CIN):* Abnormal cells are found, but typically this issue resolves on its own
- *High-grade squamous intraepithelial lesion (HSIL) or CIN2 or CIN3:* Moderately to severely abnormal cells, may indicate cancer is present (Association of Reproductive Health Professionals, 2012)

Box 57.2 TNM Cancer Staging Classification System

T SUBCLASSES: PRIMARY TUMOR	
T_x	Tumor cannot be adequately assessed
T_0	No evidence of primary tumor
T_{is}	Carcinoma in situ
T_1-T_4	Size and/or extent of the primary tumor
N SUBCLASSES: REGIONAL LYMPH NODES	
N_x	Regional lymph nodes cannot be assessed
N_0	No regional lymph node metastasis
N_1-N_4	Degree of regional lymph node involvement (number and location of lymph nodes)
M SUBCLASSES: DISTANT METASTASIS	
M_x	Distant metastasis cannot be evaluated
M_0	No distant metastasis
M_1-M_4	Distant metastasis present, specify site(s)
HISTOPATHOLOGY	
G_x	Grade cannot be assessed (undetermined grade)
G_1	Well-differentiated grade (low grade)
G_2	Moderately differentiated (intermediate grade)
G_3	Poorly differentiated (high grade)
G_4	Undifferentiated (high grade)

From the National Cancer Institute. *Fact sheet: Cancer staging,* 2013. Retrieved from *www.cancer.gov/cancertopics/factsheet/detection/staging;* and the National Cancer Institute. (2013). *Fact sheet: Tumor grade,* 2013. Retrieved from *www.cancer.gov/cancertopics/factsheet/detection/tumor-grade.*

DIAGNOSIS OF CANCER

BIOPSY

People who develop symptoms consistent with cancer should undergo diagnostic testing to confirm or rule out the diagnosis. The only definitive way to determine the presence of malignant cells is to perform a tissue **biopsy** (the removal of a small piece of living tissue from an organ or other part of the body for microscopic examination).

A biopsy is used to confirm or establish a diagnosis, establish prognosis, or follow the course of a disease. A variety of methods are used to perform a biopsy (Fig. 57.3). The *needle biopsy* is used to obtain fluid or to obtain tissue samples from the lesion. *Needle aspiration biopsy* is the aspiration of fluid or tissue by means of a needle (breast biopsy is performed with an aspiration needle). Transcutaneous needle aspiration biopsy has eliminated the need for most of the exploratory laparotomies for diagnosing metastatic cancer of the liver or for primary inoperable pancreatic cancer. Structures accessible to thin-needle biopsy under guidance of palpation include the breasts, skin, thyroid gland,

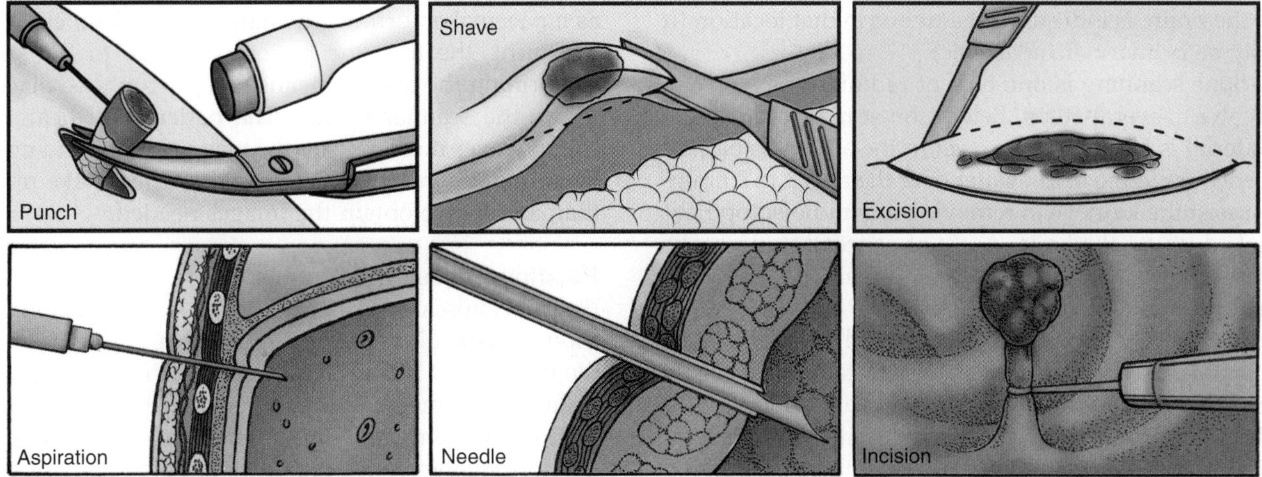

Fig. 57.3 Types of biopsy.

prostate, palpable lymph nodes, and salivary glands. *Excisional biopsy* is the removal of the complete lesion, with little or no margin of surrounding normal tissue removed, as in polypectomy. Another example of excisional biopsy is the dissection of peripheral lymph nodes, such as those of the axilla for staging of breast cancer or those of the peritoneal region for staging of various abdominal cancers. *Incisional biopsy* is the removal of a portion of tissue for examination, such as the bite biopsy performed during endoscopy. *Skin biopsy* is used to assess suspect lesions of integument (e.g., shave biopsy, punch biopsy).

ENDOSCOPY

Cells or tissue also can be obtained by means of an *endoscope* to visualize an internal structure directly through a body cavity or a small incision. Endoscopes are rigid or flexible tubes containing a magnifying lens and a light. Endoscopes vary in diameter and length according to the structure being examined. The bronchoscope is used to visualize the tracheobronchial tree; upper GI endoscopy allows direct visualization of the upper GI tract (esophagus, stomach, duodenum); the colonoscope is used to visualize the entire colon; and the sigmoidoscope is used to examine the sigmoid colon, the rectum, and the anus.

DIAGNOSTIC IMAGING

Additional diagnostic studies may be used to determine the depth of the specific lesion and identify other structures that may have been invaded. These include radiography and scanning procedures. Commonly ordered radiographic studies are chest radiography, mammography, bone scanning, GI series, barium enema study, and intravenous pyelography.

Radioisotope Studies

Radioisotope studies require the injection or ingestion of a radioactive substance. A scanning device then is used to identify the distribution of the substance in different areas of the body. Concentration of the radioisotope in a specific organ, such as the thyroid gland or the brain, is indicative of a tumor in that location (it may be primary or metastatic).

Bone scanning is one type of radioisotope study. It involves several steps. Before the scan, a radioactive material is injected into a vein in the arm. The patient is encouraged to drink water over the next 1 to 3 hours to assist the kidneys in removing any radioisotope not picked up by the bone. Areas of concentrated uptake may represent a tumor or an abnormality. These areas of concentration can be detected days or weeks before an ordinary radiograph could reveal a lesion. Bone scanning is indicated to detect metastatic tumors that have spread into the bone. All malignancies capable of metastasis may reach the bone, especially malignancies of breasts, kidneys, lungs, prostate, thyroid gland, and urinary bladder.

Computed Tomography

In *computed tomography* (CT), radiographs and a computed scanning system are used to record images of specific structures at different angles. The entire body can be scanned to detect any abnormal lesion. CT is especially helpful in detecting small lesions that were missed on radiography or other types of diagnostic tests.

Ultrasonography

Ultrasonography is a noninvasive procedure in which high-frequency sound waves are used to examine internal structures. As a transducer is moved over the area being studied, an ultrasound beam is directed through the tissues and is reflected back to the transducer. The sound waves are converted into electrical impulses, which produce an image on a display screen. Ultrasonography can show the size, consistency, and shape of the structure being studied. It is most helpful in distinguishing between cystic and solid tumors. Ultrasonography is not used to examine bones or air-filled organs. Although the procedure is painless, people undergoing ultrasonography feel the transducer moving over their skin and may need to hold their breath or remain still for brief periods.

Magnetic Resonance Imaging

Magnetic resonance imaging (MRI) is a painless diagnostic procedure that does not involve any exposure to radiation. The patient reclines on a narrow surface that moves into a cylindrical tunnel containing magnetic coils; radiofrequency energy waves produce signals that are processed by a computer and displayed as images on a video monitor. This test currently is used in the diagnosis of intracranial and spinal lesions and of cardiovascular and soft tissue abnormalities. The procedure also provides information about changes within the cells of soft tissues, arteries, veins, the brain, and the spinal column.

During the test, the patient must not have any metallic materials on the body, including jewelry. MRI cannot be performed on patients with metallic implants, such as a pacemaker, orthopedic nail, or aneurysm clip.

During the test, the patient can talk to the staff performing the test by means of a microphone placed inside the scanner tunnel. The patient will hear the sound waves thumping on the magnetic field and must lie still while the test is being done; it may take more than an hour to obtain the images needed.

Position Emission Tomography

Positron emission tomography (PET) is useful in many aspects of oncology. A radioactive chemical is given to the patient just before the procedure. PET can demonstrate glucose metabolism, oxygenation, blood flow, and tissue perfusion for any designated area. Alterations in the normal metabolic process in pathologic conditions are diagnosed during PET (Cancer.net, 2016).

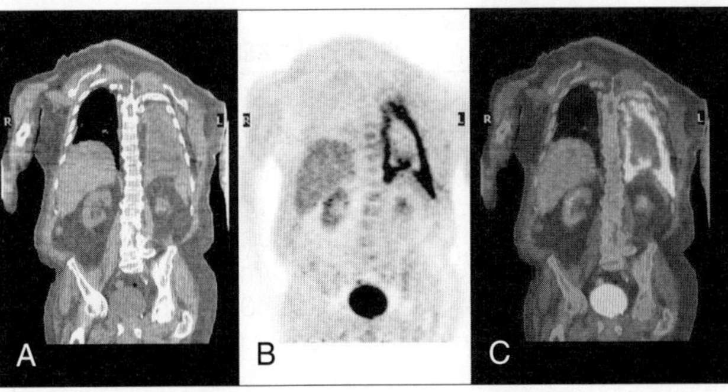

Fig. 57.4 Tomographic scans. A, Computed tomography (CT). B, Positron emission tomography (PET). C, Combined CT and PET. (From Christian PE, Waterstram-Rich KM: Nuclear medicine and PET/CT: Technology and techniques, ed 7, St. Louis, 2012, Mosby.)

PET is useful for visualizing fast-growing tumors and specifying their anatomic location. PET also helps note tumor response to therapeutic intervention, helps identify a recurrence of a tumor after surgical intervention, and assists in differentiating a tumor from other abnormal conditions such as an infection. PET is extremely useful in visualizing regional and metastatic extension of a specific tumor. Oncologic staging is more accurate with PET than with CT. The CT scan is used to take detailed images of organs and tissues within the patient's body, whereas the PET scan can be used to identify abnormal activities. PET also is used to determine the specific site for performing a biopsy of a suspected tumor (Cancer.net, 2016) (Fig. 57.4).

LABORATORY AND DIAGNOSTIC EXAMINATIONS

Measurement of Alkaline Phosphatase Blood Levels

The level of alkaline phosphatase is elevated in the presence of liver disease or metastasis to the bone or liver.

Serum Calcitonin Level

Calcitonin is a hormone secreted by the thyroid gland in response to a rise in serum calcium level. The level is increased in the blood of people who have cancer of the thyroid. It may be elevated with breast cancer and oat cell cancer of the lung. Calcitonin stimulation testing may be used in addition to the baseline level testing to confirm a diagnosis. Instruct the patient not to eat or drink anything the night before the test.

Carcinoembryonic Antigen Serum Level

Normally, production of carcinoembryonic antigen (CEA) stops before birth, but it may begin again if a neoplasm develops. Results of this test cannot be used as a general indicator of cancer, because CEA level can be elevated for other reasons, such as smoking cigarettes or the presence of inflammation. CEA is found in increased amounts in the blood of people with colorectal cancer. The test may assist in the evaluation of cancer treatment, in which a rising CEA level may indicate tumor recurrence or metastatic disease. This test is used less frequently today because it is less accurate than was thought previously.

Tumor Markers

Several different tumor markers may be identified with laboratory studies of blood or urine to help with cancer screening and diagnosis. Tumor markers are substances that are present in the body when the patient has cancer. Three examples are the prostate-specific antigen (PSA) for prostate cancer, CA-125 for ovarian cancer, and CA-19-9 for pancreatic or hepatobiliary cancer.

PSA is a biologic marker, specific for cellular activity in the prostate gland. PSA is the only tumor marker for prostate cancer. The American Cancer Society suggests that men discuss this test with their physician. Not all men should be screened routinely for this tumor marker. Men with a high risk of developing prostate cancer (family history, African American) should speak with their health care provider about this test beginning as early as the age of 40.

Although PSA levels usually are elevated when cancer is present, PSA level alone is not diagnostic of prostate cancer. Other common conditions, such as benign enlargement of the prostate, also can elevate PSA level. The finding of elevated PSA level necessitates further evaluation to determine the cause of increase. This may involve transrectal ultrasonography of the prostate gland.

The PSA assay requires a physician's interpretation. No specific level of PSA signals the presence or absence of prostate cancer. The PSA test is produced by different manufacturers, and the different products yield different results. In men with benign prostatic enlargement, levels defined as normal are different from those in men with normal prostate glands.

CA-125 is a cancer antigen detected in the blood and peritoneal ascites. The normal level is 35 units/mL. The CA-125 level may be elevated in patients with gynecologic cancers (including ovarian cancer) and cancer of the pancreas. A monoclonal antibody has been developed that reacts with this antigen, which gives physicians a method to measure the amount of CA-125 in blood samples. This test is used mainly to signal a recurrence of ovarian cancer. It is not a way to detect primary ovarian cancer, because other conditions (e.g., endometriosis, hepatitis, pelvic inflammatory diseases, or pregnancy) also may increase CA-125 levels in the blood.

CA-19-9 antigen, a tumor marker, is used in the diagnosis, monitoring, and surveillance of patients with pancreatic or hepatobiliary cancer. The CA-19-9 level is elevated in 70% of patients with pancreatic cancer and 65% of patients with hepatobiliary cancer. Measurement of CA-19-9 is not an effective screening tool for pancreatic or biliary tumors in the general population because of its lack of sensitivity and specificity (Pancreatic Cancer Action Network, n.d.). The following is a more comprehensive list of various tumor markers and how to interpret results of these tests (Vachani, 2018).

TUMOR MARKER	CANCERS ASSOCIATED WITH ELEVATED RESULTS	NONCANCEROUS REASONS FOR ELEVATED LEVELS	"NORMAL" RESULTS
Blood test (blood serum marker), except where noted	*([a]) indicates the most common association, if one exists*		*Different labs may have different high/low values*
AFP Alpha-fetoprotein	Germ cell cancers of ovaries and testes[a] (nonseminomatous, particularly embryonal and yolk sac, testicular cancers) Some primary liver cancers (hepatocellular)	Pregnancy (clears after birth), liver disease (hepatitis, cirrhosis, toxic liver injury), inflammatory bowel disease	Low levels present in men and nonpregnant women (0–15 IU/mL); generally results >400 are caused by cancer (half-life 4–6 days)
Bence-Jones Proteins (urine test) or **Monoclonal Immunoglobulins** (blood test)	Multiple myeloma[a] Waldenstrom's macroglobulinemia, chronic lymphocytic leukemia	Amyloidosis	Generally, a value of 0.03–0.05 mg/mL is significant for early disease
B2M Beta-2-Microglobulin	Multiple myeloma,[a] chronic lymphocytic leukemia (CLL), and some lymphomas (including Waldenstrom's macroglobulinemia)	Kidney disease, hepatitis	<2.5 mg/L
BTA Bladder tumor antigen (urine test)	Bladder cancer,[a] cancer of kidney or ureters	Invasive procedure or infection of bladder or urinary tract	None normally detected
CA 15-3 Cancer antigen 15-3 or carbohydrate antigen 15-3	Breast[a] (often not elevated in early stages of breast cancer), lung, ovarian, endometrial, bladder, gastrointestinal	Liver disease (cirrhosis, hepatitis), lupus, sarcoid, tuberculosis, noncancerous breast lesions	<31 U/mL (30% of patients have an elevated CA 15-3 for 30–90 days after treatment, so wait 2–3 months after starting new treatment to check)
CA 19-9 Cancer antigen 19-9 or carbohydrate antigen 19-9	Pancreas[a] and colorectal, liver, stomach and biliary tree cancers	Pancreatitis, ulcerative colitis, inflammatory bowel disease, inflammation or blockage of the bile duct, thyroid disease, rheumatic arthritis	<37 U/mL is normal >120 U/mL is generally caused by tumor
CA 125 Cancer antigen 125 or carbohydrate antigen 125	Ovarian cancer[a] breast, colorectal, uterine, cervical, pancreas, liver, lung	Pregnancy, menstruation, endometriosis, ovarian cysts, fibroids, pelvic inflammatory disease, pancreatitis, cirrhosis, hepatitis, peritonitis, pleural effusion, after surgery or paracentesis	0–35 U/mL
CA 27.29 Cancer antigen 27.29 or carbohydrate antigen 27.29	Breast[a] (best used to detect recurrence or metastasis) Colon, gastric, liver, lung, pancreatic, ovarian, prostate cancers	Ovarian cysts, liver and kidney disorders, noncancerous (benign) breast problems	<40 U/mL Generally, levels >100 U/mL signify cancer (30% of patients have elevated CA 27.29 for 30–90 days after treatment, so wait 2–3 months after starting new treatment to check)
Calcitonin	Medullary thyroid cancer[a]	Chronic renal insufficiency, chronic use of proton-pump inhibitors (medications given to reduce stomach acid)	<8.5 pg/mL for men <5.0 pg/mL for women

TUMOR MARKER	CANCERS ASSOCIATED WITH ELEVATED RESULTS	NONCANCEROUS REASONS FOR ELEVATED LEVELS	"NORMAL" RESULTS
CEA Carcinoembryonic antigen	Colorectal cancers,[a] breast, lung, gastric, pancreatic, bladder, kidney, thyroid, head and neck, cervical, ovarian, liver, lymphoma, melanoma	Cigarette smoking, pancreatitis, hepatitis, inflammatory bowel disease, peptic ulcer disease, hypothyroidism, cirrhosis, COPD, biliary obstruction	<2.5 ng/mL in nonsmokers <5 ng/mL in smokers Generally, >100 signifies metastatic cancer
Chromogranin A	Neuroendocrine tumors,[a] carcinoid tumors, neuroblastoma, and small cell lung cancer	Proton-pump inhibitors (medications given to reduce stomach acid)	Normal varies on how tested, but typically <39 ng/L is normal
Cytokeratin fragment 21-1 (blood test)	Lung, urologic, gastrointestinal, and gynecologic cancers	Lung disease	0.05–2.90 ng/mL
HCG Human chorionic gonadotrophin or beta-HCG (B-HCG)	Germ cell, testicular cancers,[a] gestational trophoblastic neoplasia	Pregnancy, marijuana use, hypogonadism (testicular failure), cirrhosis, inflammatory bowel disease, duodenal ulcers	In men: <2.5 U/mL In nonpregnant women: <5.0 U/mL
5-HIAA 5-Hydroxy-indol acetic acid (24-hour urine collection)	Carcinoid tumors	Celiac and tropical sprue, Whipple's disease, dietary: walnuts, pecans, bananas, avocados, eggplants, pineapples, plums, and tomatoes; medications: acetaminophen, aspirin, and guaifenesin	Normal 6–10 mg over 24 hours
LDH Lactic dehydrogenase	Lymphoma, melanoma, acute leukemia, seminoma (germ cell tumors)	Hepatitis, MI (heart attack), stroke, anemia (pernicious and thalassemia), muscular dystrophy, certain medications (narcotics, aspirin, anesthetics, alcohol), muscle injury	Normal values are 100–333 U/L
NSE Neuron-specific enolase	Small cell lung cancer,[a] neuroblastoma	Proton-pump inhibitor treatment, hemolytic anemia, hepatic failure, end stage renal failure, brain injury, seizure, stroke	Normal <9 ug/L
NMP 22 (urine test)	Bladder cancer[a]	BPH (benign prostatic hypertrophy), prostatitis	Normal <10 U/mL
PAP Prostatic acid phosphatase	Metastatic prostate cancer[a] Myeloma, lung cancer, osteogenic sarcoma	Prostatitis, Gaucher's disease, osteoporosis, cirrhosis, hyperparathyroidism, prostatic hypertrophy	Normal: 0.5 to 1.9 U/L
PSA Prostate-specific antigen	Prostate[a]	BPH (benign prostatic hypertrophy), nodular prostatic hyperplasia, prostatitis, prostate trauma/ inflammation, ejaculation	Normal <4 ng/mL (half-life 2–3 days)
Tg Thyroglobulin	Thyroid cancer	Antithyroglobulin antibodies	<33 ng/mL; if entire thyroid removed <2 ng/mL
Urine catecholamines:			
VMA Vanillylmandelic acid (24-hour collection of urine; it is a catecholamine metabolite)	Neuroblastoma,[a] pheochromocytoma, ganglioneuroma, rhabdomyosarcoma, PNET	Dietary intake (bananas, vanilla, tea, coffee, ice cream, chocolate), medications (tetracyclines, methyldopa, MAOIs)	8–35 mmols over 24 hours

TUMOR MARKER	CANCERS ASSOCIATED WITH ELEVATED RESULTS	NONCANCEROUS REASONS FOR ELEVATED LEVELS	"NORMAL" RESULTS
HVA Homovanillic acid (24-hour collection of urine; it is a catecholamine metabolite)	Neuroblastoma[a]	Same as VMA, in addition: psychosis, major depression, dopamine (a medication)	Up to 40 mmols over 24 hours

PNET, primitive neuroectodermal tumors.

Stool Examination for Occult Blood

The cause of blood in the stool must be identified to rule out the possibility of cancer. The *guaiac test* is used commonly to detect occult (hidden) blood in the stools. Other commonly used tests for occult blood in the stool are fecal occult blood test (FOBT), *fecal immunochemical test, hematest,* and *hemoccult test.* Early detection self-tests are available for home use. If blood is found, the person should seek immediate medical attention. Before these types of tests, it is essential that the person not ingest red meat, horseradish, uncooked broccoli, turnips, melons, aspirin, or vitamin C for 4 days before the test because this may result in a false-positive result. The test must be performed on three consecutive bowel movements. Urge patients to follow through with diagnostic tests recommended by their health care provider to screen for cancer.

CANCER THERAPIES

SURGERY

By the time it is decided that surgery is needed to remove a cancerous lesion, cancer cells already may have spread to other areas. The goal of surgery is to remove all malignant cells; this may include removal of the tumor, surrounding tissue, and regional lymph nodes. The combination of surgery with chemotherapy, radiation therapy, or both may destroy a higher number of cancer cells. The effects of cancer drugs and radiation treatments administered before, during, and after surgery are being investigated. A surgical cure may result from removal of an isolated lesion in the very early stages, as in cancer of the skin, testicle, breast, or cervix. Surgery may be performed for many reasons: preventive, diagnostic, curative, and **palliative** (designed to relieve uncomfortable symptoms but not producing a cure).

Polyps in the colon may be removed during a colonoscopy before malignant changes occur. A prophylactic mastectomy may be performed to help prevent the development of breast cancer in patients identified to be at increased risk because of their family history or other factors. If a cancerous lesion has metastasized already, surgery may provide palliation by relieving some of the associated problems, such as obstruction, ulceration, hemorrhage, and pain. The pituitary, adrenal glands, ovaries, or testes may be removed surgically to help control the growth and spread of malignancies caused by hormonal stimulation.

A radical surgical approach to operable tumors is no longer routinely used because of more sensitive and accurate diagnosing methods, a greater variety of surgical procedures, more sophisticated staging techniques, and more available advanced treatment options. The more conservative surgical management of breast cancer (i.e., lumpectomy instead of total mastectomy) is one example of this trend.

Reconstructive surgery may be needed after some types of resection, such as modified radical mastectomy. Breast reconstruction is an option for women whose disease and treatment enable the surgeon to implant a prosthesis or to transplant tissue from other areas of the body to recreate a more natural-looking breast. In many cases, the oncology surgeon and the plastic surgeon work together. When this is anticipated, preoperative counseling by the surgeons and the nurse helps the patient consider the long-range outcome instead of the immediate surgical procedure.

The use of laser beams, as an alternative to some types of oncologic surgical procedures, is increasing. The laser beam destroys tissue with little bleeding and low risk of infection. Laser surgery is used more commonly in the fields of ophthalmology, gynecology, urology, neurosurgery, and otolaryngology. The chief drawback with laser surgery is that the patient must lie very still while the laser is in use.

Nursing Interventions

If you are not present when the health care provider explains recommendations for care, ask the health care provider what he or she has told the patient and the family. This is essential to be able to reinforce the information given. Patients and families are usually anxious and may not remember everything that the health care provider has explained for them.

Patients should have confidence and trust in the health care professionals responsible for their care. Positive feelings and attitudes promote relaxation and help reduce anxiety and fear (see the Communication box). The patient should be encouraged to ask the health care provider any questions concerning potential risks of a given treatment. A patient needs to feel comfortable with the decision to follow through with the physician's recommendations.

The following are nursing guidelines to ensure that patients have the information needed to make an informed decision:

 Communication

Nurse-Patient Therapeutic Dialogue Before Modified Radical Mastectomy

Nurse: Good afternoon, Mrs. S. My name is J., and I will be your nurse this evening. How are you feeling? [Introduction and general lead]
Patient: I'm feeling all right now. It's tomorrow I'm dreading.
Nurse: You're dreading tomorrow? [Restatement]
Patient: Yes. My doctor told me he has to remove my entire breast. I hate thinking that I'll look so different.
Nurse: You're anxious about the fact that you won't look the same. [Reflection]
Patient: I'll be embarrassed to undress in front of my husband. He may think I'm no longer attractive.
Nurse: Have you had a chance to discuss your feelings with your husband? [Clarification]
Patient: No, he's out of town but will be back tonight. I guess I could talk to him then. Maybe he will accept it better than I think.
Nurse: We'll talk more after you've had a chance to talk to him about your feelings. Is there anything else on your mind that you'd like to talk about now? [Showing acceptance and general lead]

- Be present when the patient and health care provider are discussing treatment decisions.
- Assess the patient's progression in grieving for the loss of health and function related to the cancer diagnosis.
- If necessary, clarify explanations of treatments, including benefits and side effects, and help the patient formulate questions and voice concerns. Address patient or family concerns and questions concerning alternative treatments.
- Afterward, talk to the patient and the family about the information the health care provider presented; assess their understanding of the treatment, as well as identify their goals and needs.
- Report any misunderstandings, unrealistic expectations, or other problems to the health care provider.
- Communicate with the patient to verify that his or her questions were answered.
- Accept and support the patient's choice, regardless of personal opinion.

Preparing the patient for a surgical procedure must include an explanation of what to expect postoperatively. Preoperative teaching is discussed in Chapter 42.

Regardless of the surgical procedure, assess the patient's nutritional status before and after surgery. Nutritional status has been found to be a significant factor in the amount of surgery that can be tolerated, the rate of recovery, the patient's role performance, and the adequacy of wound healing.

When surgery may produce a change in the patient's body image, as in mastectomy, laryngectomy, or the formation of an ostomy, the patient may benefit from talking with another person who has undergone the same type of surgery. The American Cancer Society sponsors support groups and prepares volunteers to visit patients who need these types of surgical procedures. Some of the special groups available in some communities are Reach to Recovery; the Lost Chord Club; I Can Cope; Look Good, Feel Good; and local chapters of the United Ostomy Associations of America.

RADIATION THERAPY

Radiation therapy can be used to cure or control cancer that has spread to local lymph nodes or to treat tumors that cannot be removed surgically. Radiation may be used preoperatively to reduce the size of a tumor. Postoperative radiation therapy may be indicated to destroy malignant cells not removed by surgery. Radiation also may be used to slow the growth of malignant tumors.

Radiation may be delivered externally or internally. External therapy may be directed toward superficial lesions or toward deeper structures within the body. Malignant cells lack the capacity for repair, so more cancer cells than normal cells are damaged by radiation, and normal cells are able to recover more easily. However, normal cells can tolerate radiation only up to a certain amount before irreversible damage occurs. Treatment plans are designed to minimize the radiation dose to normal structures. Meticulous planning and recording of the doses are essential.

External Radiation Therapy

Radiation therapy is associated with skin damage and burning. Skin atrophy, changes in pigmentation, and chronic dermatitis may result. Frequent assessment and monitoring of the skin's condition are needed. When external radiation is planned, the specific area on the body is marked to indicate the port at which external radiation will be directed. These markings must not be washed off. Patients may be distressed about the presence of these markings. In a nonjudgmental manner, allow the patient the time to discuss these feelings. Management of the skin area marked for radiation should include the following:

- Keep the skin dry. If the area becomes wet during bathing, pat the skin dry with an absorbent towel.
- Do not apply lotions, ointments, creams, or powders in marked areas. Any lotions or creams designed specifically to manage drying skin must be prescribed by the physician.
- Protect the radiated area from direct sunlight.
- Avoid applications of heat or cold, because these would increase erythema, drying, and pruritus of the skin, which is common over an irradiated area.

Maintaining health during the treatment phase is important. Dietary interventions should focus on the ingestion of foods high in protein and calories. This helps promote healing and tissue regeneration. Fluid intake to maintain hydration is needed. The patient is encouraged to drink 2 to 3 L of fluid per day, unless this is contraindicated. In the event the patient experiences severe anorexia or is unable to tolerate food and fluid intake, the health care provider should be notified to evaluate dietary needs and prescribe accordingly. Reassure the patient undergoing radiation therapy that lethargy and fatigue are common during treatment and that frequent rest periods are helpful.

Many people with cancer are treated with radiation therapy at some point. Sometimes, radiation therapy is the only therapy needed to destroy the cancer.

Internal Radiation Therapy

Treatment with a radioactive implant (brachytherapy) is the insertion of *sealed radioactive materials* temporarily or permanently into hollow cavities, within body tissues, or on the body's surface. The radioactive source delivers a specific radiation dose continuously over hours or days. A highly concentrated radiation dose is delivered into or near a tumor. This technique generally is combined with a course of external radiation therapy to increase the dosage to a specific site. Certain organs, such as the uterus and vagina, are natural receptacles for the placement of an applicator that can be loaded with radioactive material. Radioactive needles, wires, seeds, beads, or catheters may be inserted directly into tumor tissue.

Unsealed internal radiation is administered intravenously or orally so that it is distributed throughout the patient's body. Special precautions are needed to prevent exposure to the nurse of the sources of radiation during periods of patient care or disposal of care-related items (Box 57.3). Assemble materials needed to provide care. Provide several nursing interventions at the same time when you enter the patient's room. Stand as far away as possible from the site where an internal radiation device is in the patient's body. In addition, limit the time needed for close contact near the irradiated site. If direct, prolonged care is needed, wear a lead apron.

Children younger than 18 years and pregnant women should not be allowed to visit implant recipients. Periods of visitation are limited to 10 minutes. Visitors are asked to stand as far away from the patient as possible.

When cancer of the cervix is treated with the use of an applicator containing a radioactive material, the applicator is placed in the vagina. The following special nursing measures are indicated:

1. Place "Radiation in Use" sign on the patient's door.
2. Prevent dislodgment. Keep the patient on strict bed rest. Instruct the patient not to turn from side to side or onto the abdomen. Do not raise the head of the bed more than 45 degrees.
3. Do not give a complete bed bath while the applicator is in place, and do not bathe the patient below the waist. Do not change bed linen unless it is necessary.
4. Encourage the patient to do active range-of-motion (ROM) exercises with both arms and mild foot and leg exercises to minimize the complications that can result from immobility. The patient also wears antiembolism stockings (thromboembolic disease hose) or pneumatic compression boots to prevent stasis of blood in the lower extremities.
5. Monitor vital signs every 4 hours, and be alert for elevations in temperature, pulse, and respirations. A temperature higher than 100°F (37.7°C) should be reported to the patient's health care provider.
6. Assess for and report any rash or skin eruption, excessive vaginal bleeding, or vaginal discharge.

Box 57.3 Instructions for Nursing Interventions for Patients Treated With Unsealed Internal Radiation for Thyroid Cancer

Spend as little time as possible for ordinary nursing care. The patient must be as self-sufficient as possible. The patient is radioactive and exposes the nurse to radiation while caring for the patient. The radioactive iodine-131 (^{131}I) leaves the patient through urine and perspiration. Therefore the patient contaminates everything he or she touches and can spread contamination to the nurse in this way.

PRECAUTIONS TO REDUCE EXPOSURE TO MEMBERS OF THE HEALTH CARE TEAM

1. Assign patient to a private room.
2. Limit the time spent in the patient's room. Work quickly, and enter only as necessary.
3. When in the room, maintain as much distance from the patient as possible. A few feet of distance makes a lot of difference in the amount of exposure to the nurse.
4. Wear personal protective equipment as indicated by the Radiation Safety Officer (RSO).
5. Wear dosimeter when in patient room.
6. The patient is confined to the room.
7. Removal of trash, linen, and equipment from the room must be approved by the RSO.
8. Pregnant and breast-feeding personnel will not enter the area.
9. All clothes and bed linens used by the patient should be placed in the laundry bag provided and should be left in the patient's room.
10. No housekeeping staff is allowed until the room is officially released.
11. Food is delivered only by nursing staff. It is delivered to the door and picked up by the patient. Mail, flowers, and other items are delivered in the same way.
12. Whenever possible, only disposable items may be used in the care of these patients. These items should be placed in the designated waste container. Contact the RSO/designee for proper disposal of the contents of the designated waste container.
13. If a nurse, attendant, or anyone else knows or suspects that his or her skin or clothing (including shoes) is contaminated, that person should notify the RSO/designee immediately.

Policies may vary depending upon dosage and patient condition. Review individual facility policy and procedures for specifics concerning patient and environmental management.

7. Maintain an accurate intake and output record. Encourage the patient to consume at least 3 L of fluid intake daily. An indwelling urinary catheter is placed to reduce the size of the bladder and decrease the effects of radiation on the bladder. Monitor patency of catheter. Ensure that it continues to drain well.
8. Monitor the patient's dietary intake. Encourage low-residue selections to minimize peristalsis and bowel movement, which may lead to dislodgment of the applicator.
9. Check the position of the applicator every 4 hours.
10. Keep long-handled forceps and a special lead container in the patient's room for use by the radiologist, should the implant become dislodged. If an applicator or any other materials become dislodged or fall out of the patient, never touch them because the material may be radioactive. Any bed linens, dressings, or pads that have been changed for the patient must be checked with a radiation safety officer before they are removed from the patient's room.
11. After the applicator is removed, the indwelling catheter usually is removed, and a douche and enema commonly are prescribed.
12. Precautions are no longer needed after removal of the applicator. Encourage the patient to ambulate and gradually resume activities.
13. Sexual intercourse is usually delayed for 7 to 10 days.
14. Instruct the patient to notify the health care provider of nausea, vomiting, diarrhea, frequent or painful urination, or a temperature higher than 100°F (37.7°C).

CHEMOTHERAPY

Chemotherapy drugs are used to reduce the size or slow the growth of cancer. Most chemotherapeutic agents work by interfering with the cells' *replication* process (ability to multiply or reproduce). These drugs damage the cell and cause cellular death. Malignant and normal cells are affected by chemotherapy. Cells that multiply rapidly, such as cells of the *hematopoietic system, hair follicles,* and *GI system,* are affected the most. The majority of the side effects from chemotherapeutic agents result from the destruction of normal cells in these systems. Common manifestations include alopecia, nausea, and vomiting. The damage to tissue is not limited to the cancerous cells, and nephrotoxicity is a common adverse effect of the therapies.

Neurologic System

Chemo brain. Chemo brain is a mental fog or cloudiness that affects some patients following chemotherapy (ACS, 2016b). Some patients experience these mental changes for a short period of time and others experience this for years after treatment. Patients with chemo brain commonly experience difficulty remembering things, poor concentration, slowed and disorganized thinking, and difficulty remembering common words. The condition can be worsened by the cancer itself, other types of medications used to treat the patient (such as antiemetics and pain medications), depression, poor nutrition, hormone changes, anxiety, surgery, infections, stress, insomnia, and anemia (ACS, 2016b),

Patients with chemo brain should be encouraged to use daily planners to help them remember appointments and schedules. Physical activity and mental puzzles can help. These patients should consume a nutritious diet, increase their intake of vegetables, try to get enough sleep, establish routines, and avoid attempting to multitask. Research studies currently are being performed to help prevent and protect the brain during chemotherapy (ACS, 2016b).

Hematopoietic System

Leukopenia. **Leukopenia** (reduction in the number of circulating white blood cells [WBCs] as a result of depression of the bone marrow) is a common problem for patients receiving chemotherapy. It can lead to life-threatening infections. The normal number of WBCs ranges from 5000/mm^3 to 10,000/mm^3. A patient with a total WBC count of less than 4000/mm^3 is considered to be leukopenic. Lack of neutrophils, the type of WBC most often found to be suppressed in the differential WBC count, is called *neutropenia.* The normal number of neutrophils ranges from 60% to 70%, or 3000/mm^3 to 7000/mm^3. When the neutrophil count is less than 1000/mm^3, neutropenia is considered present, and when the count is less than 500/mm^3, neutropenia is severe. A patient with neutropenia should be placed on neutropenic precautions, which sometimes is referred to as *protective precautions* or *reverse isolation.* Without enough neutrophils, the body's first line of defense collapses, paving the way for the development of pneumonia, septicemia, or other potentially overwhelming infections.

Protect the patient from pathogens, monitor the patient for signs of infection, and react quickly if an infection occurs. The patient's vital signs should be monitored every 4 hours. Notify the health care provider if the patient's temperature is elevated. A temperature of 100.4°F (38°C) or higher is considered a possible sign of infection (see the Safety Alert box).

Use the following systematic approach to assess the patient for infection.

Assessing the mouth. Stomatitis (inflammation of the oral mucosa) is one of the most common complications of chemotherapy and can lead to severe swallowing problems and systemic infections (Fig. 57.5). To assess for the presence of lesions, ulcers, or white plaque, a penlight and tongue blade may be used. Stomatitis may develop 5 to 14 days after chemotherapy and resolve after the end of treatments (Cancer.net, 2017a).

Teaching the patient the importance of performing regular but gentle mouth care is important. Discuss the

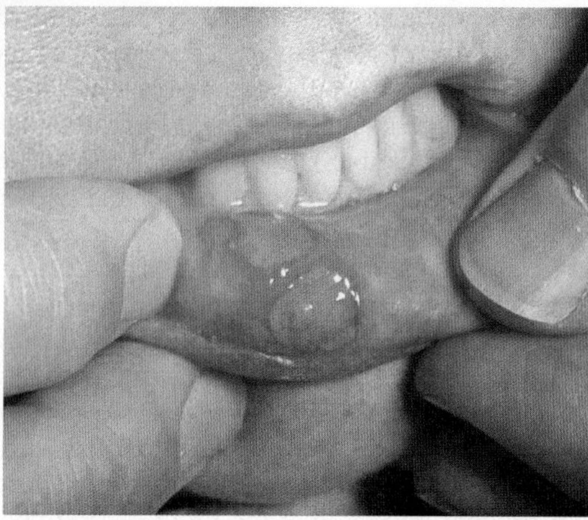

Fig. 57.5 Stomatitis. (Copyright Centers for Disease Control and Prevention/Robert E. Sumpter.)

> **Safety Alert**
>
> **Neutropenic Precautions**
>
> - Monitor neutrophil count to identify signs of infection.
> - Assess for presence of chills. Measure vital signs every 4 hours because fever may be the only indication of infection and septic shock.
> - Report temperature elevations of more than 100.4°F (38°C) to the health care provider immediately so that antibiotic therapy can be initiated promptly to help avoid the rapidly lethal effects of infection.
> - Ensure good hand hygiene techniques are used by all people in contact with patient; place patient in private room; limit or screen visitors and hospital staff members with colds or potentially communicable illnesses to prevent transmission of pathogens to patient.
> - Teach patient and family necessary personal hygiene techniques (e.g., hand hygiene, oral care, skin hygiene, pulmonary hygiene, and potential infection risks).
> - Avoid invasive procedures (e.g., venipuncture, urinary catheter) as much as possible.
> - Administer hematopoietic growth factors (e.g., granulocyte colony–stimulating factors such as filgrastim [Neupogen] or pegfilgrastim [Neulasta]) to increase patient's WBC count and reduce infection risk during periods of neutropenia. Provide neutropenic diet (avoid fresh fruits and vegetables because of presence of microscopic pathogens in uncooked produce). The patient's visitors should be discouraged from bringing fresh flowers or live plants to the patient's room. Mites, gnats, and other microscopic organisms could be a potential source of infection for the patient.

signs and symptoms of mouth infection, encourage the use of a soft toothbrush, and have the patient rinse the mouth with normal saline or sodium bicarbonate solution every 2 to 4 hours. A sponge-tipped applicator (toothette) may help prevent the patient's gums from bleeding during or after mouth care.

To reduce the risk of an oral *Candida* infection, the health care provider may prescribe prophylactic antifungal medications such as an oral nystatin (Mycostatin) suspension, clotrimazole (Lotrimin) lozenges, or fluconazole (Diflucan). A bland soft or liquid diet also may be ordered.

Assessing the skin. A rash or eruption may indicate that the patient has an infection or is predisposed to one. Bacteria may flourish in skinfolds, such as those in the groin and axillae; ensure that these areas are cleaned twice a day with soap and water. Water-soluble moisturizers may be used to keep the patient's skin from drying. To prevent cuts, advise the patient to shave with an electric razor.

Vascular access sites are common portals of entry for infectious organisms. The sites of central and peripheral intravenous catheters must be monitored carefully. Check routinely for the presence of edema, drainage, erythema, or pain around catheter entry sites. Organisms also can grow along catheter tracts and infect the blood, resulting in septicemia. Signs and symptoms of a central line–associated infection in the bloodstream include tenderness around the catheter site and pain.

Drugs should be administered orally whenever possible. Subcutaneous or intramuscular injections should be limited because they may cause abscesses in patients with neutropenia. These patients are also at risk for excessive bleeding because of the potential for an associated decrease in platelets and other formed elements in the blood.

Puncturing the skin is sometimes unavoidable, as when the patient needs a bone marrow biopsy. After a biopsy, carefully assess the site, clean the site with a facility-approved antiseptic, and apply a dressing over the site until the skin heals.

Assessing pulmonary function. Neutropenic patients with lung infections do not exhibit common clinical manifestations, such as sputum production or infiltrates demonstrable on chest radiographs. Assess the patient for other indications of a possible infection, such as changes in breath sounds, elevated respiratory rate and rhythm, and labored breathing. The patient also may complain of pain during inspiration or expiration.

To help prevent the patient from developing a lung infection, encourage the patient to perform deep-breathing and coughing exercises and to be as active as possible. Use of an incentive spirometer can help by maximizing ventilatory capacity.

Assessing urinary and bowel function. Changes in a neutropenic patient's urinary function are another indicator that the patient has developed an infection. Assess for decreased urinary output, changes in the odor or color of the urine, hematuria, or glycosuria. The patient also may complain of urinary frequency, urgency, or pain.

To reduce the risk of urinary tract infection, urinary catheterizations should be avoided in neutropenic patients. If catheterization is indicated absolutely, follow strict aseptic technique when inserting the catheter and must perform catheter care according to the facility's guidelines.

Assess the patient's bowel function. Chemotherapy can produce diarrhea or constipation. Characteristics of the stool include color, consistency, and the presence of blood. Dates of bowel movements should be recorded. The patient is instructed to report any changes in bowel habits.

If the patient needs to strain when defecating, the health care provider may prescribe a stool softener such as docusate (Colace). Straining can cause ulcerations or fissures in the rectum, which creates ports of entry for bacteria. Avoid the use of enemas, rectal medications, and rectal thermometers. They can abrade the mucosal lining creating an entrance for pathogens. Neutropenia also predisposes patients to rectal abscesses. If the patient complains of perirectal pain, notify the health care provider immediately.

Medical management. Colony-stimulating factors (CSFs) have been very helpful when treating patients with neutropenia. CSFs are commercially made. They are the only therapy that can prevent and manage neutropenia. CSFs are given subcutaneously or intravenously. Although CSFs are extremely expensive, they are administered prophylactically to patients at increased risk for neutropenia, such as those with a history of developing severe or prolonged neutropenia after chemotherapy.

Anemia. Anemia is a reduction in the number of circulating red blood cells (RBCs), hemoglobin, or hematocrit as a result of depression of the bone marrow. Normal values are as follows:

TYPE	MALE	FEMALE
Erythrocytes (RBCs)	4.7–6.1 million/ mm^3	4.2–5.4 million/ mm^3
Hemoglobin	14–18 g/dL	12–16 g/dL
Hematocrit	42%–52%	37%–47%

Hemoglobin levels of 10 to 14 g/dL indicate mild anemia, levels of 6 to 10 g/dL indicate moderate anemia, and levels lower than 6 g/dL indicate severe anemia. Patients with anemia often experience fatigue because of the decreased oxygenation to tissues. The plan of care should include a balance of activities to promote rest and prevent increased oxygen expenditure and hypoxemia. Such patients at home need to plan activities of daily living to allow for rest periods.

Recombinant human erythropoietin, or epoetin alfa (EPO; Epogen, Procrit), initially was approved by the US Food and Drug Administration (FDA) in 1987 for management of chronic anemia associated with end-stage renal disease. In 1993 the FDA approval was expanded to include management of chemotherapy-related anemia. EPO is administered subcutaneously or intravenously. Darbepoetin alfa (Aranesp) is a protein that stimulates erythropoiesis and also is identified as a synthetic form of erythropoietin.

Transfusion of packed RBCs is indicated if there is evidence of cardiac decompensation or if hemoglobin levels are low in combination with low platelet counts. The transfusion improves the patient's oxygen-carrying capacity, allows for a more efficient use of blood components, and lowers the risk of volume overload.

Thrombocytopenia. **Thrombocytopenia** is a reduction in the number of circulating platelets as a result of the depression of the bone marrow. Normal platelet values are 150,000 to 400,000/mm^3. When the platelet count is less than 20,000/mm^3, spontaneous bleeding can occur. Platelet transfusions may be necessary.

Patient teaching measures to prevent injury and hemorrhage caused by a decrease in platelets include (1) using a soft toothbrush or swab for mouth care; (2) keeping the mouth clean; (3) avoiding intrusions into rectum (such as rectally administered medications or enemas); (4) using an electric shaver; (5) applying direct pressure for 5 to 10 minutes if any bleeding occurs; (6) avoiding contact sports, elective surgery, and tooth extraction; (7) avoiding picking or blowing the nose forcefully; (8) avoiding trauma, falls, bumps, invasive procedures, and cuts; (9) avoiding the use of aspirin or aspirin preparations; and (10) using adequate lubrication and gentleness during sexual intercourse.

Integumentary System

Alopecia. **Alopecia** is loss of hair as a result of the destruction of hair follicles. It may occur by two mechanisms. If the hair roots are affected and have atrophied, alopecia occurs readily. The hair falls out either spontaneously or during hair combing, often in large clumps. If the hair shaft is affected, the hair breaks off very near the scalp. The root remains in the scalp, and a patchy, thinning pattern of hair loss occurs. Elsewhere on the body, other hair may be lost, such as eyebrows and eyelashes. Loss of leg, arm, pubic, axillary, and facial hair is less common.

The pattern and extent of hair loss is not predictable. When treatment involves a drug known to cause alopecia, education to the patient must include a frank discussion about the potential for hair loss that may begin within a few days or weeks of treatment and the fact that partial or complete baldness may occur rapidly. Drug-induced alopecia is temporary. The patient may note that the hair color or texture is different as the hair grows back. On occasion, hair growth may return while chemotherapy treatment continues. The loss of hair is a potential source of anxiety for the patient because it affects body image. Many patients tolerate this type of hair loss with minimal distress because the medication is necessary to control or cure the patient's cancer.

To meet the patient's needs, provide an education program that includes written materials and educational sessions with a hair stylist. The patient needs information about health care measures for scalp protection, such as using gentle shampoos; avoiding hair dryers, curling irons, permanents, and hair coloring; protecting the scalp; and wearing protective covering when outdoors (to reduce heat loss). A patient with long or thick hair may wish to trim or cut hair short before losing hair. There are organizations whose primary purpose is the provision of human replacement hair to patients in need. Express sincere concern and provide emotional support for the patient.

Gastrointestinal System

Stomatitis. **Stomatitis** is a condition that develops as a result of destruction of normal cells of the oral cavity, which results in the development of inflamed, sore, ulcerated areas within the patient's mouth. It may range from erythema of the oral mucosa to mild or severe ulceration. Methotrexate, 5-fluorouracil, doxorubicin, and bleomycin are the chemotherapeutic drugs that are associated most frequently with the development of stomatitis (NCI, 2016). Patients also may develop a superimposed fungal infection of the mouth and esophagus, and oral nystatin or fluconazole usually is prescribed. Excellent oral hygiene is important.

Viscous lidocaine (Xylocaine) is used when stomatitis becomes intolerable. A light topical application can decrease pain so that the patient may eat and drink. Patients who suffer from stomatitis usually benefit from a soft or liquid diet.

Nausea, vomiting, and diarrhea

Risk of nausea and vomiting from chemotherapy and targeted therapy. Some drugs used for cancer treatment are more likely to cause nausea and vomiting than other drugs (Cancer.net, 2017b). The table below lists the likelihood that a certain cancer drug will cause nausea and vomiting.

NEARLY ALWAYS CAUSES NAUSEA AND VOMITING (HIGH RISK)	USUALLY CAUSES NAUSEA AND VOMITING (MODERATE RISK)	SOMETIMES CAUSES NAUSEA AND VOMITING (LOW RISK)	RARELY CAUSES NAUSEA AND VOMITING (MINIMAL RISK)
Carmustine *(BiCNU)* Cisplatin Cyclophosphamide at higher doses	Alemtuzumab *(Campath)* Azacitadine *(Vidaza)* Bendamustine *(Treanda)*	Bortezomib *(Velcade)* Cabazitaxel *(Jevtana)*	Bevacizumab *(Avastin)* Bleomycin *(Blenoxane)* Busulfan *(Busulfex, Myleran)*
Dacarbazine Dactinomycin *(Cosmegen)* Daunorubicin *(Cerubidine)* when combined with cyclophosphamide	Carboplatin Clofarabine *(Clolar)* Cyclophosphamide at lower doses	Cytarabine at lower doses Docetaxel *(Taxotere)* Doxorubicin HCL liposome injection *(Doxil)*	Cetuximab *(Erbitux)* 2-Chlorodeoxyadenosine Fludarabine
Doxorubicin *(Adriamycin)* when combined with cyclophosphamide	Cytarabine *(Cytosar-U)* at higher doses	*(Etopophus, Toposar, VePesid)*	Pralatrexate *(Folotyn)*
Epirubicin *(Ellence)* when combined with cyclophosphamide	Daunorubicin	Fluorouracil *(5-FU, Adrucil)*	Rituximab *(Rituxan)*
Idarubicin *(Idamycin)* when combined with cyclophosphamide	Doxorubicin	Gemcitabine *(Gemzar)* Etoposide	Vinblastine
Mechlorethamine *(Mustargen, Valchlor)*	Epirubicin	Ixabepilone *(Ixempra)*	Vincristine
Streptozotocin *(Zanosar)*	Idarubicin	Methotrexate *(multiple brand names)* Fludarabine	Vinorelbine *(Navelbine)*
	Ifosfamide *(Ifex)* Irinotecan *(Camptosar)* Oxaliplatin *(Eloxatin)*	Mitomycin Mitoxantrone Paclitaxel *(Taxol, Abraxane)* Panitumumab *(Vectibix)* Pemetrexed *(Alimta)* Temsirolimus *(Torisel)* Topotecan *(Hycamtin)* Trastuzumab *(Herceptin)*	

Nausea, vomiting, and diarrhea are disorders of the GI tract that can be caused by the excessive breakdown of normal GI cells. There are several different types of nausea that can occur in the patient with cancer who is receiving chemotherapy. Nausea that occurs for this patient is referred to as chemotherapy-induced nausea and vomiting (CINV). Some patients experience breakthrough emesis, which can occur on any day of chemotherapy even with appropriate medications used to prevent its occurrence. Others experience refractory emesis, which occurs with continued failure to prevent the nausea and vomiting using prophylactic techniques. Some patients develop anticipatory nausea and vomiting. This is triggered by negative experiences associated with chemotherapy and poor control of nausea and vomiting in the past. The prevention of nausea and vomiting during the early stages and cycles of chemotherapy is the best treatment. Nausea and vomiting are among the most uncomfortable and distressing side effects of chemotherapy. The onset and duration vary greatly among patients and with the drug given. For the ambulatory patient, nausea may interfere with the ability to continue working. Persistent vomiting may result in fluid and electrolyte imbalance, general weakness, and weight loss. Decline of nutritional status renders the patient more susceptible to infection and perhaps less able to tolerate therapy. Such physiologic symptoms can accompany or precipitate psychological responses such as depression and withdrawal. Use nursing interventions and ordered medications to help minimize chemotherapy-induced nausea and vomiting.

Antiemetics vary in success. There are several medication classes used to prevent and treat CINV. Serotonin receptor antagonists include ondansetron (Zofran) and granisetron. Neurokinin-1 receptor antagonists include aprepitant and fosaprepitant (Emend). Dopamine receptor antagonists (butyrophenones, phenothiazines, and metoclopramide) also are used. Common corticosteroids used to treat CINV are methylprednisolone and dexamethasone. Other medication classes that are used include benzodiazepines and cannabinoids. Cannabinoids are chemical compounds of cannabis, and they activate receptors in the body to reduce nausea and vomiting. Two of the commercially prepared cannabinoids are nabilone and dronabinol (NCI, 2017b). The patient may receive antiemetics orally, intramuscularly, rectally, or intravenously.

Changes in bowel habits commonly occur but usually do not necessitate intervention. If diarrhea becomes marked or persistent, an antidiarrheal medication such as diphenoxylate with atropine (Lomotil) may be prescribed.

Nursing interventions. Combinations of chemotherapy agents, as well as chemotherapy combined with other treatments, have increased the remissions and survival rates among patients with cancer. Some problems experienced by patients undergoing chemotherapy are similar to those that may result from radiation therapy (depending on the target site and amount of radiation). Help the patient realize that some of the problems are merely the result of the therapy and not a sign that the cancer is getting worse.

Patient problems and interventions for patients undergoing chemotherapy include but are not limited to the following:

Patient Problem	Nursing Interventions
Compromised Tissue Integrity: Oral Mucous Membrane, related to • *Stomatitis (inflammation of the mouth)* • *Xerostomia (reduced salivation, "dry mouth")*	Assist with frequent, careful oral hygiene and hydration; use very soft toothbrush Provide meticulous mouth care Administer prescribed antifungal medication such as fluconazole Give soothing oral lozenges, ice chips, and frequent sips of ice water; do not give hot beverages; apply lip balm for lip dryness
Insufficient Nutrition, related to • *Anorexia (from changes in taste and smell)* • *Nausea and vomiting* • *Dysphagia (difficulty swallowing)* • *Aspiration* • *Diarrhea* • *Malabsorption* • *Cachexia*	Provide adequate, easily digestible, soft, bland diet; avoid spicy foods Keep room free of odors and clutter Administer prescribed antiemetic medications Provide small, frequent, highly nutritional meals to meet the extra demands placed on the body by rapidly dividing malignant cells Provide pleasant surroundings in which to eat, and allow plenty of time for meal
Potential for Infection, related to • *Weakened immune system* • *Leukopenia*	Protect against infections Limit visitors Discourage visits by people who are ill or have been recently exposed to a communicable disease Advise patient to avoid crowds Discourage eating fresh fruit or placing fresh-cut flowers or live plants in room Observe and promptly report any signs of inflammation at injection sites or insertion sites of any peripheral or central intravenous lines; report any temperature higher than 100°F (37.7°C) Use sterile technique whenever possible Initiate reverse isolation as indicated Monitor temperature and leukocyte count Avoid areas with indwelling catheters, and avoid performing rectal procedures or examinations Administer antibiotics as prescribed

Tumor Lysis Syndrome

Tumor lysis syndrome (TLS) is an oncologic emergency with rapid lysis of malignant cells.

Etiology and pathophysiology. TLS may occur spontaneously in patients with inordinately heavy tumor cell burdens. However, it is usually a result of chemotherapy or, less commonly, radiation therapy. It may occur anywhere from 24 hours to 7 days after antineoplastic therapy is initiated. Patients most at risk are those who have heavy tumor cell burdens (e.g., high-grade lymphomas) or markedly elevated WBC level (acute leukemias). TLS also occurs in chronic lymphocytic leukemia and metastatic breast cancer.

The syndrome develops when chemotherapy or irradiation causes the destruction (or lysis) of a large number of rapidly dividing malignant cells. As malignant cells are lysed, intracellular contents are released quickly into the bloodstream. This results in high levels of potassium (hyperkalemia), phosphate (hyperphosphatemia), and uric acid (hyperuricemia). These conditions, plus secondary hypocalcemia, increase the risk for renal failure and alterations in cardiac function.

Clinical manifestations. Early clinical manifestations include nausea, vomiting, anorexia, diarrhea, muscle weakness, and cramping. Later signs and symptoms may include tetany, paresthesias, seizures, anuria, and cardiac arrest.

Diagnostic tests. TLS is diagnosed by assessment of the signs and symptoms and by confirmation of abnormal laboratory values. Early symptoms of TLS may not be readily apparent, and clinical manifestations may appear rapidly. The syndrome is detected most frequently from abnormalities in blood chemistry. Other important values include serum creatinine, blood urea nitrogen, and urine pH.

Medical management. The best way to prevent TLS is to recognize which patients are at risk and to initiate prophylactic measures before antineoplastic therapy begins. This includes pretreatment *hydration* to maintain a urinary output of 150 mL/h. Hydration should begin 24 to 48 hours before treatment and continue for at least 72 hours after treatment. *Diuretics* may be used to promote the excretion of phosphate and uric acid, to prevent volume overload, and to promote the excretion of potassium in the urine. *Allopurinol* prevents uric acid formation; administration is initiated a few days before treatment and should be continued for 3 to 5 days after treatment is completed. *Sodium bicarbonate* is used to maintain alkalinity of the urine (pH over 7), which prevents uric acid crystallization. Cation-exchange resins, such as sodium polystyrene, bind with potassium, and so their administration enables excretion of potassium through the bowel. *Calcium gluconate* is administered intravenously to correct hypocalcemia. Cardiac monitoring is required. Phosphate-binding gels, such as aluminum hydroxide, form an insoluble complex that is excreted by the bowel. When these measures are not successful, renal failure may occur, and renal dialysis is necessary.

Nursing interventions. Nursing interventions include identifying patients at risk for TLS and initiating hydration 24 to 48 hours before chemotherapy. Allopurinol is administered before and during chemotherapy to maintain alkalinity of the urine. Determine which medications contain phosphate or spare potassium and discuss discontinuation with the health care provider. Monitor potassium, phosphorus, calcium, and uric acid levels. Assess the patient for signs and symptoms of TLS, including the following:

- *Hyperkalemia:* electrocardiographic changes, muscle weakness, twitching, paresthesia, paralysis, muscle cramps, nausea, vomiting, lethargy, and syncope
- *Hyperphosphatemia:* azotemia, oliguria, hypertension, and renal failure
- *Hypocalcemia:* electrocardiographic changes (heart block, dysrhythmias, and cardiac arrest), tetany, confusion, and hallucinations
- *Hyperuricemia:* renal failure, nausea, vomiting, flank pain, gout, and pruritus

If hyperuricemia is detected, diuretics, sodium bicarbonate, cation-exchange resins, and phosphate-binding gels are administered as appropriate. Monitor intake and output and notify the health care provider if urinary output is less than 100 mL/h. Urine pH is monitored and maintained at higher than 7 with sodium bicarbonate. Prepare the patient and family for dialysis if other measures are not effective.

Prognosis. When treating TLS, health care providers must focus on preventing renal failure. TLS typically resolves within 7 days, once appropriate treatment is initiated.

Chemotherapy has proved to be an effective treatment for many patients with cancer. Chemotherapy can be used to cure the cancer, control the cancer, or help reduce cancer-related pain. Learn about each drug being administered, anticipate the side effects, and monitor the plan of care, making modifications as needed with condition changes.

Safety guidelines in accordance with facility policy must be followed when chemotherapeutic agents are prepared and administered. Because of their potential for absorption or inhalation, they are potentially dangerous for the people who administer the agents.

TARGETED CANCER THERAPY

Sometimes, in addition to standard chemotherapy, oncologists may prescribe targeted cancer therapy. They are medications that can interfere with specific molecules that allow for the cancer's growth and its ability to spread to other tissues. This medication is cytostatic, meaning that it blocks cancer cell proliferation. Targeted cancer therapy also is known as molecularly targeted therapies and precision medicines. Standard chemotherapy is used to kill cancer cells, but it also kills other types of rapidly dividing normal cells. Standard chemotherapy is cytotoxic. Research studies currently are being performed regarding precision medicine so that oncologists can one day use information a patient's proteins and genetic makeup to treat cancer (NCI, 2018).

There are some significant side effects that are experienced by patients using targeted cancer therapy. Patients may develop problems with diarrhea and liver, skin changes (rash, dry skin, depigmentation of hair, and changes to their nails). Some have difficulty with wound healing, blood clotting, and hypertension (NCI, 2018).

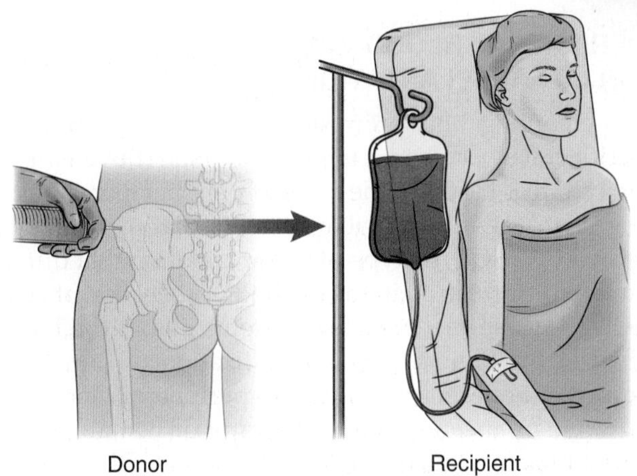

Fig. 57.6 The process of bone marrow transplantation. (Copyright We Care Health Services. [n.d.]. *Bone marrow transplant in India.* Retrieved from *www.wecareindia.com/cancer-treatment/bone-marrow-transplant.html.*)

BIOTHERAPY

The observation of interactions between the immune system and malignant cells led to the development of therapies that could manipulate this natural process. Traditionally, this field has been known as *immunotherapy.* It has led to the modern era of biotherapy. Since the 1980s, biotherapy, or biologic therapy, has emerged as an important fourth modality for treating cancer. *Biotherapy* may be defined as treatment with agents derived from biologic sources or affecting biologic responses.

Biologic response modifiers (BRMs) work against the cancer in three different ways. One type of BRM increases, restores, or modifies the host defenses against the tumor (CSFs, filgrastim, erythropoietin, GM-CSFs). Other BRMs are directly toxic to tumors (interleukins, bacille Calmette-Guérin vaccine [BCG]) or modify biologic features of the tumor (interferons alpha, beta, and gamma).

Most of these therapies are given via intramuscular or subcutaneous injection and must be administered to the patient over an extended time. While providing emotional support, help ensure that the patient remains compliant with treatment. Common side effects in patients receiving BRMs include fatigue, flulike symptoms, leukopenia, nausea, and vomiting.

Health care professionals must understand these therapies to help give the patient with cancer the best care available. These therapies and research are leading to the development of gene therapy today; this will improve outcomes for patients with cancer in the future.

BONE MARROW TRANSPLANTATION

Bone marrow transplantation (BMT) is the process of replacing diseased or damaged bone marrow with normally functioning bone marrow. BMT is used in the treatment of a variety of diseases and offers a chance for long-term survival.

Stem cell transplants are being used in some solid tumor cancers, such as high-risk breast cancer. Bone marrow harvests are becoming less frequent because many centers have turned to peripheral blood stem cells for hematopoietic support after high-dose chemotherapy.

Most bone marrow used for transplantation is obtained by multiple needle aspirations from the posterior iliac crest while the patient is under general or spinal anesthesia. The anterior iliac crest and sternum also may be used. The amount of marrow extracted ranges from 600 to 2500 mL for the average adult. After processing, the marrow is given to the patient intravenously through a transfusion bag, or it can be frozen (cryopreservation). Marrow may be kept for 3 years or more. When the bone marrow is infused, it is via a central line without a filter over 1 to 4 hours (Fig. 57.6).

Bone marrow may be removed from an individual for personal use (**autologous,** indicating something that originates within the patient, especially a factor present in tissues or fluids) at a later time. Alternatively, a patient may be given *allogenic* bone marrow (meaning the transplant came from someone else). Three types of allogenic bone marrow transplants are (1) *syngeneic* (donation from the patient's identical twin), (2) *related* (donation from a relative, usually a sibling), and (3) *unrelated* (donation from a nonrelative). The patient is at increased risk for developing infection during the process of transplantation because the immune defenses are weakened. Transplant recipients are cared for in special bone marrow units so that they can be monitored closely and carefully protected.

Interventions to prevent infections include protective isolation or laminar airflow rooms; prophylactic systemic antibiotics and antiviral agents (primarily acyclovir); and routine cultures of blood, urine, throat, and stool. Despite these and other interventions, the patient can become septic in hours, with multisystem failure.

Survival after BMT depends on the patient's age, remission, and clinical status at the time of transplantation.

PERIPHERAL BLOOD STEM CELL TRANSPLANTATION

An emerging and promising alternative to BMT is peripheral blood stem cell transplantation (PBSCT). This procedure is based on the fact that peripheral or circulating stem cells are capable of repopulating the bone marrow. PBSCT is a type of transplantation that differs from BMT primarily in the method of collection of stem cells. Because there are fewer stem cells in the blood than in the bone marrow, mobilization of stem cells from the bone marrow into the peripheral blood can be done by means of chemotherapy or hematopoietic growth factors, such as GM-CSF and G-CSF.

Vascular access from the donor is initiated. Tubing from the donor enters a cell separator machine that is used to remove the peripheral stem cells; then the blood is returned to the donor. This procedure, called *leukapheresis,* usually takes 2 to 4 hours. In autologous transplantation, the stem cells are purged to kill any cancer cells and then frozen and stored until used for transplantation. Although many of the same steps (harvesting, intensive chemotherapy, reinfusion) of BMT are used in PBSCT, the hematologic recovery period in PBSCT is shorter, and complications are less severe.

NURSING INTERVENTIONS

When discussing the expectations of specific treatments for the patient, communicate genuine concern. Encourage the patient to verbalize concerns and provide reinforced education as needed. Patients may become discouraged by toxic side effects and other problems they experience while undergoing conventional cancer treatment. Allow extra time to listen to patients with cancer express their feelings and encourage them to follow the guidelines of conventional medical practice that offer the most hope.

ADVANCED CANCER

PAIN MANAGEMENT

Patients with cancer may have pain at any point during the course of the disease and its treatment. In fact, of the 8.2 million people throughout the world who die from cancer each year, most experience pain as a primary symptom (CDC, 2018). Unfortunately, some patients seek care only after pain develops. Pain is usually a late symptom and indicates tumor obstruction, nerve damage, or invasion of bone.

It is estimated that in 85% of patients with cancer, pain can be managed effectively with appropriate therapy. The American Cancer Society, the American Pain Society, the World Health Organization, the Oncology Nursing Society, and other organizations consider pain control to be a significant issue for patients with cancer.

One of the many challenges in caring for the patient with pain is the assessment. The patient's communication of pain must be accepted. Remain nonjudgmental regarding the patient's complaints of pain and provide appropriate management interventions.

Cultural and religious practices in the patient's family play an important role in the perception of pain or expression of suffering. Some cultures tend to minimize pain, and patients with those cultural backgrounds may be less likely to express pain. Other cultures expect the expression of pain, and patients with such cultural backgrounds may exhibit a greater overt expression of pain.

Opioids used in the management of cancer pain include morphine, hydromorphone (Dilaudid), fentanyl, and methadone. Sustained-release morphine in an oral form—such as MS Contin, Kadian, or morphine sulphate—is particularly effective in the management of the terminally ill person with pain. Administering opioids via transdermal method, inhalation, intravenous drips, intrathecally, and epidurally enhances the analgesic effect. The nurse can provide more consistent pain relief for the patient by administering bolus injections to the patient. Often the most effective regimen involves round-the-clock dosage scheduling for effective pain control. Fixed dosage schedules of an adequate amount of pain medication provide more constant blood levels and predictable pain relief. Some patients have breakthrough pain that necessitates additional doses, but the fixed dosage schedule should be maintained. Monitor the patient for the development of any opioid-related side effects such as constipation, vomiting, and respiratory and central nervous system depression.

In addition to opioids, valuable nonopioid analgesics used in the treatment of certain levels of cancer pain are acetaminophen; aspirin; and nonsteroidal antiinflammatory drugs (NSAIDs), such as ibuprofen, indomethacin, and naproxen.

The patient should be educated about nonpharmacologic pain management methods such as distraction and relaxation. Acupuncture, biofeedback, hypnosis, guided imagery, and massages also may be used to help manage the patient's pain. Many patients find that nonpharmacologic measures enhance the effectiveness of other prescribed pain interventions. The patient with cancer should receive enough sleep and rest. This can be challenging when the patient is admitted to an acute care setting. The patient with advanced cancer may experience **cachexia,** a profound state of ill health and malnutrition, marked by weakness and emaciation (Fig. 57.7). Additional comfort measures include frequent position changes, meticulous skin care, nutritious foods and fluids, and the use of comfort measures to promote relaxation and reduce the perception of pain. The nurse's unique role in pain management for the patient with cancer involves acting as an advocate and a liaison between the patient and other members of the health care team. Spending time with the patient, assessing the patient's response to the pain, evaluating the

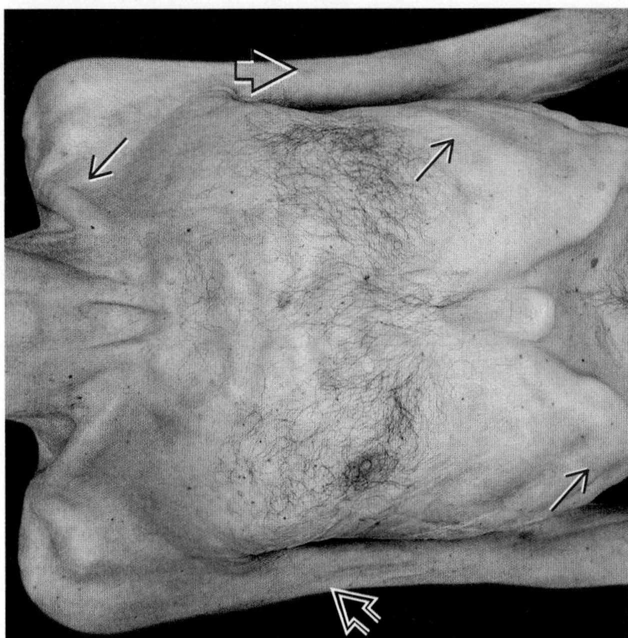

Fig. 57.7 Marked cachexia with severe loss of adipose tissue and muscle mass as noted here by prominent bony protrusions and marked muscular atrophy. (From Fyfe B, Miller D: *Diagnostic pathology: Hospital autopsy.* St. Louis, 2016, Elsevier.)

effectiveness of the pain management plan of care, revising the plan of care as indicated, and educating the patient and the family are important for providing the patient with the best pain relief possible. Be able to monitor the patient's pain effectively and address patient and family concerns regarding the pain management strategies. Some patients and their families have opioid phobia, the irrational fear that even the appropriate use of opioids will result in addiction. This fear of addiction may contribute to undertreatment of pain. A goal for the patient and family includes the verbalization of understanding of the need for opioids in the care of ill patients. Appropriate use of pain management strategies enables patients and families to accept the therapeutic value of drugs such as opioids to ensure that patients do not suffer from potentially controllable pain.

Planning interventions to manage pain in the patient with cancer is challenging. Some general guidelines must be followed. The best management involves a variety of pain relief measures. These include medications and nursing interventions to promote comfort. Pain should be managed before it becomes unbearable. Assessing the patient's past history or pain management is vital. Be certain to determine what relief measures have been effective in the past. The best plan for pain management includes patient participation and engagement. Activities that the patient believes will be helpful should be incorporated. Debilitating pain can leave the patient feeling defeated. Encourage the patient to share concerns and make suggestions. Be aware of fears that the patient may have. Fear and anxiety may increase the perception of pain. Patients with cancer may feel that increased pain is a sign that their condition is worsening and death is imminent. The most effective pain relief is often a combination of pharmacologic and nonpharmacologic methods.

NUTRITIONAL THERAPY

Nutritional problems that most frequently occur in patients with cancer are malnutrition, anorexia, altered taste sensation, nausea, vomiting, diarrhea, stomatitis, and mucositis. These problems can be caused by a combination of factors, including drug toxicity, effects of radiation therapy, tumor involvement, side effects of medication, recent surgery, emotional distress, and difficulty with ingestion or digestion of food. If the patient is malnourished, the patient's normal cells cannot recover well from the effects of therapy, and the immune system may be compromised because of the depletion of protein stores.

Malnutrition

Patients with cancer are at increased risk for protein and calorie malnutrition, characterized by fat and muscle depletion. Encourage the patient to eat foods high in protein to facilitate repair and regeneration of cells, as well as high-calorie foods that provide energy and minimize weight loss.

The patient must be weighed daily. A 5% weight loss or other indications that the patient is at risk for developing malnutrition are signals for the nurse to confer with the health care provider concerning the patient's nutritional needs. Once a 10-pound (4.5-kg) weight loss occurs, it is difficult for the patient to maintain adequate nutritional status. A nutritional supplement may be necessary. The nursing assessment should include review of albumin and prealbumin levels. The patient may choose to use nutritional supplements in place of milk when cooking or baking. Nutritional supplements can be added easily to scrambled eggs, pudding, custard, mashed potatoes, cereal, and cream sauces. Packages of instant breakfast can be used as indicated or sprinkled on cereals, desserts, and casseroles. If the patient's malnutrition cannot be treated with dietary intake, it may be necessary to use enteral or parenteral nutrition as an adjunct nutritional measure.

Anorexia

Anorexia experienced by a patient with cancer can be a challenging problem. An intervention may be effective one day and ineffective the next. Continue to assess the patient and use interventions as necessary to help manage this problem. Nursing care should be geared to prevent or minimize anorexia. Evaluate the effectiveness of interventions and modify the plan of care as indicated to promote continuation of the interventions that are most successful. Megestrol (Megace) may be prescribed to manage anorexia and stimulate the appetite.

Altered Taste Sensation

Cancer treatments may cause the patient to experience an alteration in the sweet, sour, bitter, and salty taste sensations. This change in taste is known as **dysgeusia.** The patient needs information about this phenomenon. Discuss dietary selections that will incorporate foods preferred by the patient and help maintain caloric intake. The patient may feel compelled to eat certain foods because they are "healthy." Advise the patient to experiment with spices and other seasoning agents to mask the taste alterations. Lemon juice, onion, mint, basil, and fruit juice marinades may improve the taste of certain meats and fish. Bacon bits, onion, and pieces of ham may enhance the taste of vegetables.

COMMUNICATION AND PSYCHOLOGICAL SUPPORT

The patient and the family may become irritable and angry with caregivers when the patient is suffering and experiencing progressive problems. Remember that these feelings are not directed toward the caregivers personally but have developed as a result of the circumstances associated with the patient's disease. A display of anger toward the staff may be caused by deep-seated frustration or anxiety. Continue to use therapeutic communication techniques during these types of situations. The patient may not be able to accept or comprehend the explanations that are given when the patient's stress level has escalated. Administering kind, gentle nursing care may communicate more effectively than words. Touch also may be used to indicate awareness of the patient's emotional distress.

Nurses are able to help make the effects of cancer less psychologically traumatic through sensitivity and creativity. The health care system can foster dependency by stripping away the powers of decision making and the patient's personal identity. Care can be individualized by including the patient and family in the planning process. This also promotes compliance inasmuch as the patient feels more involved in the decision making. Offer as many areas of control in the decision-making process as possible. This fosters feelings of independence and increases self-esteem in the patient.

Psychological support of the patient is an important aspect of cancer care. Because of the effectiveness of cancer treatment, many cases of cancer are cured or controlled for long periods. Thus emphasis must be placed on maintaining an optimal quality of life after the diagnosis of cancer. If the patient, family, and caregivers have a positive attitude toward cancer and cancer treatment, then it may have a significant positive effect on the quality of life that the patient experiences. A positive attitude also may influence the patient's prognosis positively.

Most people view the diagnosis of cancer as a crisis. Cancer affects the quality of life of all affected patients in some way. Four quality-of-life factors affecting patients with cancer and their families are social, psychological, physical, and spiritual. The most common concerns voiced by the patient are (1) fear of recurrence, (2) chronic or acute pain, (3) sexual problems, (4) fatigue, (5) guilt for delaying screening or treatment, (6) behavior that may have increased the risk for cancer, (7) changes in physical appearance, (8) depression, (9) sleep problems, (10) change in role performance, and (11) being a financial burden on his or her loved ones.

Coping with these fears produces a range of emotions within the patient: denial, anger, bargaining, depression, and eventually acceptance. Some patients experience feelings of helplessness and hopelessness. These feelings may occur at any time during the process of cancer. However, some patterns appear to occur more frequently or at a greater intensity at certain stages of the disease process. The following factors may determine how the patient will cope with the diagnosis of cancer:

- *Ability to cope with stressful events in the past* (e.g., loss of job, major disappointment): Assess the patient's past coping abilities. Review stressors in the patient's history, and review the coping skills demonstrated.
- *Availability of significant others:* Patients who have effective support systems tend to cope more effectively than do patients without such support systems.
- *Ability to express feelings and concerns:* Patients who are able to express their feelings and to ask for help usually cope more effectively than do patients who internalize these types of feelings.
- *Age at the time of diagnosis:* Age determines the coping strategies to a great degree. For example, an adolescent and an elderly person may employ different coping strategies to psychologically manage the stress of the disease.
- *Extent of disease:* Cure or control of the disease process is usually easier to cope with than the reality of terminal illness.
- *Disruption of body image:* Disruption of the body image (e.g., radical neck dissection, alopecia, mastectomy) may intensify the psychological effect of cancer.
- *Presence of symptoms:* Symptoms such as fatigue, nausea, diarrhea, and pain may intensify the psychological effect of cancer.
- *Experience with cancer:* If the patient's previous experiences with cancer have been negative, the patient will probably view his or her current status as negative.
- *Attitude associated with cancer:* A patient who feels a sense of control and has a positive attitude regarding his or her health care and treatment is better able to cope with the diagnosis and treatment than one who feels hopeless, helpless, or out of control.

To facilitate the development of a hopeful attitude about cancer and to support the patient and the family during the various stages of the process of cancer, continue to be available, especially during difficult times. Exhibit a caring attitude and listen actively to fears and concerns. The nurse-patient relationship should be based on trust and confidence; be open, honest, and caring in the approach. Touch may be used to exhibit caring;

touching the patient's hand may be more effective than words.

Essential information regarding cancer and cancer care should be provided. Provide relief from distressing symptoms. Assist the patient in setting realistic, reachable short- and long-term goals and in maintaining usual lifestyle patterns. Above all, maintain hope, which is the key to effective cancer care. The patient's perception of hope varies and is dependent on the patient's status. The patient may hope that the symptoms are not serious, hope that the treatment is curative, hope for independence, hope for relief of pain, hope for a longer life, or hope for a peaceful death. Recent research does not show a link between attitude and emotional states and the prevention of cancer growth.

TERMINAL PROGNOSIS

Coping with the multiple problems associated with advanced cancer can lead to a sense of helplessness and hopelessness in spite of all efforts. The patient and the family may look forward to death as a relief from unrelenting suffering.

Many patients with advanced cancer know that they are dying. They may be able to recognize attempts to avoid the truth and may distrust and feel hostile toward people who make such attempts. Honesty and openness are the best approaches. Patients frequently express relief at a caregiver's willingness to discuss death. Remaining open and honest with patients as they near the end of life can be difficult for the nurse. It requires the nurse be honest with his or her own personal feelings.

Spiritual activities may provide mental and emotional strength in spite of physical deterioration. The patient may ask the nurse to read the Bible or to pray with him or her, or the patient may request that a minister, priest, imam, or rabbi visit. Spiritual strength may help the patient and family cope with the continuing problems encountered in the cancer experience.

If the patient wishes to die at home, the hospital social worker or discharge planner assists the patient and family in planning for home care. Arrangements for any special supplies and equipment are made before discharge. The nurse plays a major role in teaching the patient and at least one family member or significant other how to continue any special care needed at home, such as dressing changes, irrigations, the management of a feeding tube, or the care of a central venous line for administration of parenteral nutrition or medications.

Throughout the patient's hospital stay, take advantage of time available to promote self-care to the greatest extent possible. Assess the patient's readiness to learn and ability to participate actively in self-care. If necessary, consult advanced clinical nursing specialists to provide individualized guidelines for teaching patients. Plans for patient education should be included in the nursing care plan. Evidence of the patient's ability to manage self-care should be documented, and any assistance needed from others should be planned. Continuity of care is the goal in discharge planning. Hospice services can be arranged in most communities for patients who have advanced cancer. There are freestanding hospices, hospices within a hospital or skilled nursing facility, or at-home arrangements. The primary focus of a hospice is enhancing the patient's quality of life, not prolonging it. Efforts are directed toward relief from pain and other problems. Skilled professional care and voluntary support services are provided to assist the patient and the family in living life to the fullest each day.

Get Ready for the NCLEX® Examination!

Key Points

- Cancer is the second leading cause of death in the United States (after heart disease).
- There is strong evidence that what people eat or drink and their lifestyle choices may predispose them to the development of cancer.
- The American Cancer Society recommends specific preventive behaviors and screening tests for cancer prevention and early detection for men and women.
- People must perform specific types of self-examination to detect any changes and report them to their health care provider immediately.
- It is important to have periodic physical examinations and to seek medical attention promptly if a person develops any warning signs of cancer.
- A common reason for a delay in diagnosing cancer is that early malignant changes are not accompanied by pain.
- Seeking medical attention when warning signs occur also is delayed frequently because people fear the possible diagnosis of cancer and hope the signs and symptoms will just go away.
- The diagnosis of cancer has a profound effect on family members, as well as on the patient. They may experience denial, anger, fear, and depression.
- Most of the side effects from chemotherapeutic agents result from the destruction of normal cells of the hematopoietic system, hair follicles, and the GI system.
- TLS is an oncologic emergency that occurs in patients with cancer who have heavy tumor cell burdens after they receive chemotherapy or irradiation, which causes rapid lysis of malignant cells.
- The American Cancer Society sponsors organized support groups for individuals with the same types of cancer; some of these are Reach to Recovery; the Lost Chord Club; I Can Cope; Look Good, Feel Good; and the Ostomy Club. Prepared volunteers are available

in most communities to visit a patient with newly diagnosed cancer.

- Spiritual strength assists the patient and the family in coping with the problems experienced as a result of cancer.
- The American Cancer Society, the American Pain Society, the World Health Organization, and the Oncology Nursing Society consider pain control a major issue in the management of a person with cancer.
- The concept of rehabilitation should be applied in the planning of care for the patient with cancer to promote the highest level of functioning possible.

Additional Learning Resources

SG Go to your Study Guide for additional learning activities to help you master this chapter content.

evolve Be sure to visit the Evolve site at *http://evolve.elsevier.com/Cooper/foundationsadult/* for additional online resources.

Review Questions for the NCLEX® Examination

1. A 58-year-old patient with colon cancer is receiving combined radiation therapy and chemotherapy. He has developed diarrhea. The patient asks the nurse why he is now having diarrhea. What nursing response is most accurate?
   1. "Your diagnosis of colon cancer has caused diarrhea."
   2. "Because you are unable to eat or drink much during treatment, you are having loose stools."
   3. "Radiation is very irritating to the lining of your GI tract, which has caused diarrhea."
   4. "You most likely have an imbalance in your fluid and electrolyte levels."

2. A patient has terminal lung cancer and reports constant pain. To maintain optimal pain control, when should analgesics be administered? *(Select all that apply.)*
   1. At scheduled intervals
   2. Mainly when the patient is active
   3. As requested with prn pain medication orders
   4. Every 2 hours as long as respirations are within normal limits
   5. Before the patient's pain is at its worst

3. Which is true regarding cancer prevention and health care promotion behaviors for patients with a diagnosis of cancer?
   1. They will not decrease the risk of developing a second malignancy.
   2. They will not be affected by personal choices related to diet and smoking.
   3. They are increasingly important with the growing population of cancer survivors.
   4. They would include only routine physical examinations.

4. A patient has received a diagnosis of stage I breast cancer. She is receiving adjuvant chemotherapy and radiation therapy after a lumpectomy. What teaching point should be included in this patient's plan of care? *(Select all that apply.)*
   1. Chemotherapy-related hair loss is usually temporary.
   2. All chemotherapeutic agents result in alopecia.
   3. Hair that grows back may have a different texture and color.
   4. Hair loss is most often related to radiation treatments.
   5. Avoid the use of lotions on the skin at and near the site of radiation treatment

5. A 61-year-old patient is receiving chemotherapy. The patient becomes anemic and has petechiae and ecchymoses scattered over her upper trunk, especially her arms. What side effect is the patient experiencing?
   1. Bone marrow suppression
   2. Cardiac suppression
   3. Liver toxicity
   4. Pulmonary toxicity

6. Before the insertion of a cervical implant, the nurse tells the patient what to expect while it is in place. Which statement is accurate? *(Select all that apply.)*
   1. "Nurses will always be available, but they will spend only a short time at your bedside."
   2. "Personal cleanliness is essential, so you will be given a complete bed bath each day."
   3. "Nausea and vomiting is a common side effect of this type of radiation."
   4. "Your bed linens will be completely changed each day to minimize radioactive contamination."
   5. "Visitors will be limited during the time you are being treated with the internal radiation therapy."

7. A 24-year-old patient has been receiving chemotherapy for acute lymphoblastic leukemia and has developed leukopenia. Which patient statement indicates that he understands discharge teaching concerning leukopenia? *(Select all that apply.)*
   1. "I am cured and have no limitations."
   2. "My family can catch leukopenia, so I need to be careful to not get too close to any of them."
   3. "I should avoid close contact with people who might give me an infection."
   4. "I need to be careful not to cut myself when shaving because I may not be able to stop the bleeding."
   5. "I should avoid being in large crowds until my white blood cell count raises to an acceptable level."

8. A 42-year-old patient has palpated a small lump in her left breast during her monthly BSE. She has scheduled an appointment with her health care provider. Which test will be used to make a definite diagnosis of a benign or malignant tumor of her breast?
   1. Biopsy
   2. Mammography
   3. Tomography
   4. Ultrasonography

9. The nurse educator is discussing the importance of the reduction of carcinogens in primary prevention of cancer. Which risk factor is considered significant in many types of cancer?
 1. Diet low in fat
 2. Occasional moderate use of alcohol
 3. High pollen count in the environment
 4. Smoking

10. The patient has been diagnosed with terminal cancer. Which of the following is the most therapeutic approach by the nurse?
 1. Antiinflammatory agents are effective analgesics for severe pain.
 2. Opioids should be withheld because they are addictive.
 3. Pain is what the patient says it is.
 4. One can increase one's tolerance for pain.

11. A patient is receiving chemotherapy and has a low WBC count. What patient statement indicates the need for further teaching?
 1. "I check my mouth after each meal."
 2. "Fresh fruits and vegetables will help me get better."
 3. "My husband and I have been using a vaginal lubrication before intercourse."
 4. "My lips are dry and cracking. I need some lubricant."

12. According to the American Cancer Society, what would have the greatest influence in reducing the risk of lung cancer?
 1. Five fruits and vegetables a day
 2. Yearly chest radiograph for people age 50 years and older
 3. Cessation of smoking
 4. Reduction of exposure to environmental carcinogens

13. The patient is receiving chemotherapy and has the patient problem of *Insufficient Nutrition.* What are likely reasons for this lack of nutrition? *(Select all that apply.)*
 1. The patient indicates that she doesn't feel hungry.
 2. The patient complains that she has developed small sores in her mouth.
 3. The patient has developed diarrhea.
 4. The patient complains that she has been nauseated.
 5. The patient has been having experiencing episodes of choking during meals.

14. A patient has a vaginal radiation implant in place. What nursing intervention should be added to the patient's plan of care?
 1. Instruct her to turn from side to side for comfort.
 2. Restrict fluid intake to prevent bladder distention.
 3. Promote intake of a high-fiber diet to prevent constipation.
 4. Monitor vital signs every 4 hours and report temperature higher than 100°F.

15. A patient has a history of oat cell carcinoma of the lung and is being treated with chemotherapy. His WBC count is 2.5/mm^3. What is the nurse's primary concern?
 1. Prevention of hemorrhage
 2. Prevention of infection
 3. Prevention of dehydration
 4. Prevention of electrolyte imbalance

16. A 63-year-old patient has a diagnosis of cancer of the prostate gland with metastasis and is experiencing cachexia. How is cachexia best described?
 1. Poor health, malnutrition, weakness, and emaciation
 2. Increased appetite and nervousness
 3. Irritability and anger
 4. Depression, fear, and anxiety

58 Professional Roles and Leadership

http://evolve.elsevier.com/Cooper/foundationsadult/

Objectives

1. Discuss the processes used to look for and secure employment.
2. Describe the traditional work shifts of a licensed nurse.
3. Discuss confidentiality.
4. List the advantages of membership in professional organizations.
5. Discuss certification programs and programs that further educational goals.
6. Discuss the computerized adaptive testing (CAT) in the National Council Licensure Examination (NCLEX®) for the licensed practical nurse or licensed vocational nurse (LPN/LVN) candidate (NCLEX-PN® examination).
7. Discuss nurse practice acts.
8. Identify three important functions of a state board of nursing.
9. Discuss mentoring.
10. Discuss career opportunities for the LPN/LVN.
11. Discuss the guidelines and duties for being an effective leader in nursing.
12. Discuss styles of leadership for nurses.
13. Discuss delegating nursing tasks.
14. Discuss nursing informatics.
15. List the three types of health care provider's orders, and discuss the legal aspects of each.
16. List three ways to ensure accuracy in transcribing health care providers' orders.
17. List the pertinent data necessary to compile an effective change-of-shift report.
18. Discuss the importance of malpractice insurance.
19. Identify strategies for burnout prevention.
20. Discuss the chemically impaired nurse.

Key Terms

advancement (ăd-VĂNS-mŭnt, p. 2015)
articulate (ăr-TĬK-yū-lāt, p. 2011)
as necessary (prn) (ĂS NĔS-ŭ-sĕr-ē, p. 2015)
burnout (BŬRN-out, p. 2032)
certification (sŭr-tĭf-ĭ-KĀ-shŭn, p. 2017)
contract (KŎN-trăkt, p. 2013)
endorsement (ĕn-DŌRS-mŭnt, p. 2020)
interview (ĬN-tŭr-vyū, p. 2011)
negligence (NĔG-lĭ-jĕns, p. 2021)
nurse practice act (NŬRS PRĂK-tĭs, ĂKT, p. 2021)
per diem (PŬR DĒ-ŭm, p. 2015)
preceptor (prē-SĔP-tŭr, p. 2017)
reciprocity (rĕs-ĭ-PRŎS-ĭ-tē, p. 2020)
resignation (rĕz-ĭg-NĀ-shŭn, p. 2016)
résumé (REZ-ū-mā, p. 2011)
transcribes (trăn-SKRĪBZ, p. 2029)

FUNCTIONING AS A GRADUATE

There are ample options for employment in today's health care system for a licensed practical/vocational nurse (LPN/LVN). It is important for the newly licensed LPN/LVN to consider career plans and options that best fit his or her strengths, skills, and areas of interest. The role of a graduate nurse is exciting and challenging, and a career-planning tool or career planning resource (e.g., *http://nalpn.org*) helps the recent graduate navigate the road toward gainful employment. This chapter provides some guidelines for being a conscientious nurse while assuming this new role, as well as methods to assist in securing a job, including a cover letter, a résumé, and the interview process. In addition, most colleges and universities offer career placement services to graduates. Box 58.1 provides an eight-step tool for helping the new nurse in career planning.

FINDING AND SECURING A JOB

Cover Letters

Cover letters are a means of introducing a job applicant to a potential employer. Key components of the cover letter include identification of interest in employment, a brief statement of qualifications, and availability for the position being sought. It is important to personalize

Box 58.1 Eight-Step Career Planning Tool

1. *Take stock:* the most important step of the career-planning process
   a. Read, listen, watch, learn; find out as much as possible about the trends in health care.
   b. Assess your professional strengths and weaknesses honestly and objectively.
   c. Ask yourself whether you hold certain beliefs that have any potential to undermine your attitude; such beliefs—myths, even—sometimes interfere with job performance and satisfaction.
2. *Explore the options.*
   a. Consider what kind of nursing positions are likely to enhance your strengths.
   b. Discuss your options with a mentor.
3. *Gather more information.*
   a. Attend health care job fairs.
   b. Research different nursing positions.
   c. Visit with colleagues who are doing the kinds of work you are interested in doing.
   d. Call nurse recruiters.
   e. Read professional journals and newspapers.
4. *Narrow your focus.*
   a. Take into account the education and skills required for each position.
   b. Evaluate the responsibilities involved in each position.
   c. Consider salary range, days and hours, travel time, and availability of that job in your area.
5. *Make a decision:* List the pros and cons of each position, and narrow the field to two or three possibilities.
6. *Get specific:* Learn as much as you can about other candidates for a nursing position.
   a. Obtain additional training if needed.
   b. Investigate the possibility of tuition reimbursement.
   c. Find out if on-the-job training is available.
7. *Map your strategy.*
   a. Record each step of your strategy.
   b. Develop a résumé.
   c. Develop interviewing skills.
   d. Practice interviewing by role-playing with a mentor or friend.
8. *Manage your career:* Periodically review where you are in your career and your life; choose a special date each year (e.g., your birthday) to make your reassessment.

Remember that successful careers do not happen accidentally. You make choices and changes along the way.

the cover letter and to emphasize strengths and desired qualities applicable to the position. When writing the cover letter, consider the fit of the prospective position for your personal skills and strengths. This aids in the development of a document that identifies you more clearly to the interview team. The cover letter should not exceed a single page. It also should contain contact information and a signature line. Cover letters (Fig. 58.1) may be mailed to the employer or uploaded as an attachment if the applicant is completing an online application.

Résumé

The **résumé** is a one- or two-page summary of educational and professional experiences, activities and honors, and concrete skills and interests. A concise, comprehensive, well-prepared résumé will impress future employers; therefore it should be well organized, neat, and accurate. The applicant should be certain to use a variety of descriptive terms (e.g., "highly motivated," "exceptional ability," or "outstanding skills") when preparing the résumé. The résumé is the tool used by the employer to preview job candidates and select candidates to interview.

The three primary types of résumés are the chronologic, functional, and combination. In the chronologic résumé, the applicant's job history is listed in reverse chronologic order, with the most recent job listed first. The chronologic résumé often is considered the easiest to prepare because it requires a recall of work- and education-related activities. Critics of the chronologic résumé report it does little to highlight a candidate's skillset. It also can emphasize gaps or a lack of experience. The functional résumé promotes the applicant's skills and experiences. It does not reference dates of the experiences listed. The combination type of résumé blends the two types. It allows a systematic, easily followed recall of work history and also allows a focus on skills and experiences. The applicant should choose the résumé style that best demonstrates his or her strengths and abilities. The employer is seeking the employee with the most potential for the job, and the résumé is likely to be one of the first means by which the employer obtains an impression of the applicant (Fig. 58.2).

Personal Interview

The **interview** is a face-to-face meeting, an online meeting via a webcam or Skype, or a telephone call during which the employer assesses the potential candidate's qualifications and personality. The interview is a vital part of the application process. It is important for the applicant to be prepared for the interview process (Box 58.2). First impressions have a lasting effect, so it is imperative to make the most of the initial contact with a potential employer (Box 58.3). Applicants should **articulate** (speak clearly, distinctly, and to the point) and present themselves with clarity and effectiveness to make a good first impression.

Processes used for interviews vary by organization. The interview may be conducted by a single person or a panel. Members of the interviewing team may include the department's management team as well as representation from the work unit. The interview process may consist of a single meeting or a multistep series of contacts. In some settings an initial screening may

July 1, 2017

Ms. Kelly Horrall
Nurse Recruiter
Kell-Russell Health and Rehabilitation Center
1650 East Health Valley Lane
Terre Haute, IN 47805

Dear Ms. Horrall,

In the next few weeks I will be completing my course work and graduating from the Practical Nursing program at Indiana College of Health and Nursing. I plan to sit for my licensure examination shortly after. During my nursing education, I was assigned clinical rotations at your facility. The experience provided me with a close view of the quality of care and the collegiality displayed by the health care team. As I begin my career these are qualities I will value in my nursing practice and I would like to have in my employer.

I have noted your website indicates there are open positions for licensed practical nurses on the memory care unit and I would like to meet with members of your team to discuss opportunities for employment. I will contact you next week to discuss this matter.

Sincerely,

Kim Dennis
3917 Marquette Ave
Terre Haute, IN 47805
Kimdennis555@qualitynurse.com
(811) 555-0011

Fig. 58.1 Sample cover letter.

Box 58.2 Preparing for a Successful Interview

1. *Build contacts.* Employers fill a majority of positions through personal contacts.
2. *Know the institution.* Learn everything possible about the institution to which you are applying.
3. *Take your personal inventory.* Record your strengths.
4. *Write or review your résumé.* Prepare or update your work history and professional accomplishments.
5. *Rehearse questions and answers.* Some standard interview questions are as follows:
   a. "Would you tell me about yourself?"
   b. "What are your major strengths and weaknesses?"
   c. "How do you think you will fit into this position?"
   d. "Give an example of when you have shown leadership skills or initiative."
6. *Make a good impression.* You have only a very short time to make a good impression.
7. *Understand the goal.* Interviewers need to determine four things about a job applicant: qualifications, attitude, adaptability, and affordability.
8. *Market yourself.* Think of a job interview as a sales pitch; you are assertively promoting yourself and your skills.
9. *Answer effectively.* How you answer a question is often more important than what you say.
10. *Practice role-playing.* Have different friends practice interviewing with you; video-record these role-plays, and review the recording.

be performed by a member of the human resources staff or a nurse recruiter. The initial screening is often by telephone. The next stage of the interview process consists of meetings between the applicant and the nursing division.

For a good working relationship, it is best if the applicant's skills and nursing care values are in harmony with the objectives of the job description (Boxes 58.4 and 58.5).

Job Shadowing

The entry into practice can be a frightening transition. School-based clinical experiences provide an introduction to the nursing care environment but do not often give a full picture of the culture of some nursing units. New graduates may have apprehension about the clinical environment and work expectations. There may be concerns about which units would best meet their needs and goals. Job shadowing provides a means for the individual to follow a nurse during a normal shift. This gives a snapshot of the unit culture, types of patients cared for, and expectations of the licensed caregiver. In addition, the opportunity provides an invaluable contact for the individual's professional network. Shadowing may begin before graduation. Multiple shadow opportunities provide experiences for comparison. Shadow experiences normally are coordinated by the human resources department.

Katelyn Bieser
2012 Putt Drive, Cottage Grove, MN 55301 (651) 555-2728 • ktbieser@star.com

PROFESSIONAL SUMMARY

Key Strengths

• Cardiac-oriented LPN	• Rudimentary Spanish	• Patient oriented
• Sterile Tech knowledge	• Strong clinical judgment	• Available night shift
• Willing to move	• Quality assurance	• Hardworking

PROFESSIONAL EXPERIENCE

St. Michael Hospital, Minneapolis, Minnesota — Spring 2014

PN School Rotation, Cardiac Unit

• Interdisciplinary health care team	• Basic data collection
• Time management	• Facilitated sterile techniques
• Medication administration	• Vital sign measurement
• Quality assurance	• Patient/family education
• Charted data	• Positive attitude
• Solicited supplemental feedback	• Assisted staff as needed

Forest View Nursing Home, Hastings, Minnesota — 2 Years

Certified Nursing Aide, Memory Unit

• Health care intervention	• Direct patient care
• Resident feeding/hygiene	• Promoted ADLs
• Charted vital signs	• Performed room sanitization
• Coordinated with 10 staff	• Monitored patient activity
• Positive communication	• Patient turning/lifting, etc.
	• Duties as assigned

The Small Town Café, Bloomington, Minnesota — 1½ Years

Waitress, Full Time

• Active customer service	• Promotion of specials
• 20% Sales increase	• Cashier and inventory
• Time management/memory development	• Assisted with food preparation
• Worked holidays, etc.	• Cleaned restaurant
	• Duties as assigned

LICENSE/CERTIFICATION

State of Minnesota Board of Nursing, St. Paul, Minnesota — 2014 to present
Practical Nursing License (LPN)

American Red Cross, St. Paul, Minnesota — 2011 to present
Cardiopulmonary Resuscitation
Certification

School District 916, White Bear Lake, Minnesota — Spring 2014
Hmong Cultural Awareness Class

EDUCATION

Rainy Lakes Technical College, International Falls, Minnesota — Diploma
Practical Nursing — 2014

Fig. 58.2 Sample résumé. (From Hill SS, Howlett HA: *Success in practical/vocational nursing: From student to leader*, ed 7, St. Louis, 2013, Saunders.)

CONTRACTS AND STARTING OUT

A **contract** is a promise or a set of promises between two or more people that creates a legal relationship with legal obligation between them. The usual contract that LPN/LVNs encounter is the employment contract. Today the contract between the employee and employer is often verbal and implied. Under the employment contract, it is the nurse's obligation to perform nursing functions with the skill and knowledge that is in accordance with the standards of the profession under that state's nurse practice act. The employer is responsible for providing a safe working environment, sufficient and competent fellow workers, and safe equipment. Failure on the part of the nurse or the employer to perform these duties is a breach of contract. It is possible for breach of contract to result in a lawsuit, in which the court may order the breaching party to perform the obligations of the contract or to pay money to the party who suffered damage because of the breach. Because the contract is one for personal services, a nurse usually is not forced to work for the employer. Rather, the nurse may be liable for money damages to an employer for breach of contract.

The employment contract properly specifies the length of the contract period; hours that the nurse is to work; salary; vacation; sick leave pay; medical, maternal, disability, and liability insurance coverage; educational benefits; and any other benefits or working conditions to which the nurse and employer agree. The employment

Box 58.3 Steps to a Successful Interview

1. Be well groomed. Dress conservatively and appropriately.
2. Arrive at the interview 10 minutes earlier than the appointment; if a receptionist or secretary greets you, identify yourself, and give the name of the person you are to see.
3. Be cheerful and polite.
4. Be knowledgeable about the position for which you are applying.
5. Be patient while waiting for an interview.
6. Smile and give your name distinctly when greeting the interviewer.
7. Use a firm handshake.
8. Address interviewer by last name, using "Mr.," "Mrs.," or "Ms."
9. Have at least three extra copies of your résumé and reference list and a neatly typed list of references.
10. Do not slouch or fidget; sit upright, and be attentive. Do not chew gum.
11. Maintain eye contact with the interviewer.
12. Allow the interviewer to take the initiative; be an attentive listener.
13. Put purses or portfolios on the floor beside you, not in your lap. Avoid looking at your watch.
14. Answer questions concisely. Try to make the interview interesting and informative. Use the time effectively.
15. Be prepared to be interviewed by a group or committee or to have the interview recorded. Look at each member of the interview team. Shake hands with each one, using his or her name.
16. Articulate your speech.
17. Be factual.
18. Avoid being critical.
19. Convey genuine interest and enthusiasm.
20. Avoid discussing personal problems unless they are applicable to the job.
21. Be prepared to relate qualifications and experiences.
22. Inquire about job description, work schedule, and benefits.
23. If you are asked, state desired salary; if salary offered is unacceptable, do not mislead the interviewer.
24. Inquire about starting salary, pay increases, and maximum salary allowed.
25. If you are asked, indicate your preference of positions (if more than one position is open, or if the interviewer invites you to "dream a little").
26. Look for clues when the interview is over. Usually an employer asks, "Do you have any more questions?" Hold any questions not covered until this time. If you do not have questions, this is probably a good time to say, "No, thank you, but I enjoyed our interview and hope that you will consider me for the position with your company."
27. Express appreciation for the interview.
28. Suggest when and where you may be contacted, if necessary.
29. Send additional information promptly on request.
30. Be aware that most beginning nursing positions require rotating shifts, even night shifts and working every other weekend. Many facilities require that you have medical-surgical experience before they will assign you to a specialty area such as obstetrics or pediatrics.
31. Follow up the interview with a thank-you letter or an e-mail to the interviewer within 48 hours.

Box 58.4 Common Interview Questions

1. Tell me about yourself.
2. What are your top strengths and weaknesses?
3. Tell me about your last position.
4. Do you prefer working with others or independently?
5. What are your travel or relocation limitations?
6. How would you prefer people to criticize you, and how do you criticize others?
7. How many hours per week do you think someone should spend on the job?
8. What do you know about our facility?
9. Why do you want to work for us?
10. What important trends do you see in our industry?
11. What are your three most important accomplishments thus far in your career?
12. Give an example of your creativity.
13. How do you define success?
14. Is your current (or past) income commensurate (in proportion to or adequate) with your abilities?

Box 58.5 What an Interviewer Can and Cannot Ask

CAN ASK	CANNOT ASK
• Criminal history • Hobbies • Community or social activities • Future professional goals • Education • Work experience • Strengths and weaknesses • Reason(s) for leaving previous job • Reason(s) why applicant thinks he or she is qualified • Reason(s) for applying for this job	• Financial or credit status • Sexual preferences • Marital status • Age • Color • Religious beliefs • Race • Creed • Nationality

contract can be terminated legally, without a breach, by completion of all obligations under the terms of the contract or by consent of all parties to the termination.

New employees usually find that facilities provide orientation programs, which vary in length, depending on the facility policy. Many facilities also require newly graduated nurses to take examinations or tests to assess competencies in medication and math skills.

Recent graduates also are often required to serve a probationary period before acquiring the status of a benefit-earning member of the staff. Internships or residency programs sometimes are offered by employers to nurses who have graduated recently. An internship helps with the transition to professional nursing. Some facilities provide a mentor or preceptor (person who supports a new or transferred employee through clinical orientation) to assist the new graduate during this internship period. Probationary policies such as internships or orientation should be discussed during the interview process.

Encountering Problems

Despite the best intentions, problems may arise during employment. It is important to follow the chain of command. Be aware of the organizational chart of your facility, as well as the grievance process for circumstances that cannot be resolved easily or if treatment is perceived to be unfair. Open communication is the best way to resolve most disagreements.

Work Schedule

Flexible scheduling is offered in most health care facilities. Common options include part-time and full-time schedules, straight evenings or straight nights, weekends only, shared jobs, **per diem** shifts or as needed or **as necessary (prn)** shifts, 12-hour shifts, 10-hour shifts, and 8-hour shifts. Eight-hour shifts are common in clinics, health care providers' offices, and care environments such as rehabilitation and long-term care facilities, in which continuity of care is key to the health and stability of the patient population.

Many employers offer sign-on incentives or bonuses, as well as tuition reimbursement for nurses who choose to further their education. Nurses working flex time sometimes are allowed to set their own hours, which enables them to fit their work schedule around personal or family responsibilities. Nurses working the 12-hour shift may work three 12-hour shifts per week; some employers consider this a full-time schedule. Twelve-hour shifts are traditionally from 7 a.m. to 7 p.m. or 7 p.m. to 7 a.m. Care units such as the emergency department or surgery may have a variety of other shifts designed to provide increased coverage during peak activity times. Patient care is not limited to weekdays. Most care units require some type of weekend rotation by employees. Some nurses find satisfaction working a "weekend only" shift option. Mandatory overtime is sometimes a concern. If no nurses are available for the oncoming shift, those who worked the preceding shift are obliged to remain on duty. Some hospitals have been forced to turn away patients because they did not have adequate staffing. In an effort to provide an adequate number of care providers, facilities may opt to require a "call schedule." Call schedules require nurses to remain available to the unit on day or shifts in which they are scheduled off. The amount of call shifts or hours required of a nurse varies by agency policy. Nurses continue to express their concerns and negotiate to improve patient care and working conditions.

Frequently, newly hired nurses in acute and long-term care facilities find themselves working the night shift, to which it may be difficult for some nurses to adapt. For nurses required to work the night shift, some suggestions on how to best adapt to working this shift are listed in Box 58.6.

Box 58.6 How to Cope With the Night Shift

STAYING ALERT AT WORK

- Sleep and eat well before your shift.
- Determine when and how many caffeinated beverages work for you.
- Eat light, balanced meals.

GETTING TO SLEEP

- Make your sleeping area cool, comfortable, quiet, and dark, with blackout shades or blinds, a sleep mask, earplugs, or a white noise machine. Unplug the phone, and turn down the doorbell volume.
- Stop drinking caffeinated beverages at a time before you plan to go to sleep that is most beneficial for you, and avoid eating large, greasy meals after work.
- Do not use alcohol or a sedative to get to sleep.
- Allow time to unwind after work. Eat a light breakfast, watch a morning show, read, go for a walk, or take a warm bath. Try to follow the same routine every day.
- If you exercise, determine how much time you need to wind down before you go to sleep.
- Wear sunglasses on the drive home to reduce the melatonin-inhibiting effect of sunlight.

BALANCING YOUR LIFE

- Eat right, exercise regularly, and get some fresh air and sunlight.
- Take short naps as needed, especially before driving home from work if necessary.
- Engage family and friends to help with sleep and work schedules.

Data from American College of Emergency Physicians. Circadian rhythms and shift work, 2003. Retrieved from *www.acep.org/practres.aspx?id=30560.*

ADVANCEMENT

Advancement (a rise in rank or importance; a promotion; progress; improvement) is a possible result of additional preparation or additional experience. A nurse may achieve advancement by learning the position more thoroughly and by assuming new and greater responsibilities. Advancements, together with the difficulties and obstacles that they bring, stimulate interest and enthusiasm. They usually are based on a person's qualifications, behavior, performance, and preparation. Facilities may employ a career ladder. Career ladders allow nurses who seek increasing responsibility and committee involvement to receive recognition for their contributions. Agency policies govern the application process and advancement. Nurses who seek to advance along the ladder may find financial compensation or other benefits provided for their participation.

TERMINATING EMPLOYMENT

Resigning from a position properly is another skill with which the LPN/LVN should be familiar. Employers sometimes raise questions about a résumé that reflects frequent job changes; therefore it is in your best interest to remain at the first place of employment at least 1 year. If this is impossible, follow the proper procedure for **resignation** (the act of resigning to give up a position of employment). A verbal statement and a written resignation, providing at least a 2-week notice, is considered professional courtesy and maintains a good relationship with the employer. The letter should be kept brief, with concise terms stating the reason for leaving the position, and provide the last planned date of employment. Some organizations may request an exit interview with the individual who is leaving. This traditionally is conducted by a representative from human resources. The exit interview may include returning any items that have been assigned to you, such as an identification badge or cell phone, discussing areas of improvement suggested for the organization, and reviewing benefits available after termination such as insurance. Failing to provide adequate notice may harm your reputation or leave the employer with an inadequate amount of time to find a replacement for the position. Positive references may be difficult to obtain from employers who feel they were abandoned or where the nurse did not act in a professional manner.

TRANSITION FROM STUDENT TO GRADUATE

KNOW YOUR ROLE

Sometimes it is difficult to understand clearly the exact responsibilities of each health team member. The LPN/LVN is responsible to a registered nurse (RN) or to the health care provider. The role of the LPN/LVN, like the roles of other health care professionals, is changing constantly. As the services of health care facilities attempt to meet the increasing demand of the population, the role of the LPN/LVN does not remain static. Many technical and scientific changes in the health care system have resulted in a multiplicity and complexity of responsibilities placed in nurses' job descriptions. In view of these developments, the LPN/LVN must continue to keep the patient as the focus of care. Patients quickly recognize a nurse's genuine concern for their individual needs.

Box 58.7 Confidentiality Reminders

1. Discuss patient information only in conferences or reports. Be mindful of conversations in the cafeteria and at the nurses' station.
2. Keep confidential all information gathered from medical records, reports, or conferences.
3. Be nonjudgmental in observations of patients, hospital staff, family members, and other personnel.
4. Do not store patient statistics on any retrievable or permanent computer system unless authorized.
5. Do not keep or copy any patient information except when necessary for required report. All notes should be shredded after use.
6. Never copy any original medical records for any reason unless a health care provider orders it done.
7. Do not leave a patient chart or electronic health record where unauthorized people are able to access it.
8. It is generally not the nurse's responsibility to release patient information to the police, media, relatives, or visitors.
9. Familiarize yourself with how patient information is to be handled within the facility.
10. You are obligated ethically to treat information about your patient as confidential.
11. Be aware of the actions of unlicensed personnel with whom you work. If necessary, teach others the importance of safeguarding a patient's privacy.

CONFIDENTIALITY

All patient information must remain confidential. Patient information should be exchanged only with other members of the health care team responsible for the care of the patient. Release of information to anyone other than the health care team without the consent of the patient is a violation of the right to privacy. Refer to Chapter 2 for additional information regarding confidentiality (Box 58.7).

ROLE OF THE LICENSED PRACTICAL/ VOCATIONAL NURSE IN THE COMMUNITY

The LPN/LVN participates in activities that promote the community's positive attitude toward health care. The LPN/LVN uses community resources to promote a better understanding of the health services available to the general public and promotes and participates in community health projects and other health-oriented activities such as maternal and child health clinics, disabled children clinics, mental health clinics, blood pressure clinics, and community health fairs.

PROFESSIONAL ORGANIZATIONS

To have a voice in one's profession, join a professional organization. No organization has the power to be any more active or effective than its members. Some professional health care organizations provide opportunities for continuing education to their members and associated allied health staff.

Two national organizations exist to support and meet the needs of the LPN/LVN: the National Association for Practical Nurse Education and Service (NAPNES) and the National Federation of Licensed Practical Nurses (NFLPN).

The purpose of NAPNES, founded in 1941, is to promote an understanding of practical nursing schools and continuing education for LPN/LVNs. The organization also developed a position on the education of the practical nurse, defines ethical conduct, and publishes standards of practical and vocational nursing practice. The *Journal of Practical Nursing* is its official publication, and *NAPNES Forum* is the newsletter that informs members of activities. Membership is open to students, graduates, faculty, and other people who are interested in practical or vocational nursing. NFLPN, founded in 1949, serves the interests specifically of LPN/LVNs. It restricts membership to only LPN/LVN students and graduates. It informs members of the most current issues of interest and makes available to its members insurance coverage for malpractice, personal liability, health, and accident. The NFLPN also lobbies on the state and national levels for issues that are of interest and concern to its members. *Licensed Practical Nurse* is its official publication. For further information about NAPNES, visit its website *(www.napnes.org)* or write to NAPNES, 2701 N. Bechtle Ave. #307, Springfield, OH 45504-1583. For further information about NFLPN, visit its website *(www.nflpn.org)* or write to NFLPN, 3801 Lake Boon Trail, Suite 190, Raleigh, NC 27607. Members of these two organizations share the common goals of the LPN/LVN.

CONTINUING EDUCATION

The health care system is changing constantly as a result of rapidly developing technology and research, and keeping current with nursing trends and issues is crucial. There are abundant avenues by which to gain additional nursing skills and knowledge. Facilities frequently offer employees continuing education through seminars, conferences, or workshops (Box 58.8). Continuing education credit is also available through some nursing journals.

To renew nursing licenses, some states require a given number of hours per year in continuing education units (CEUs). These requirements are intended to improve the quality of patient care by educating nurses about the most recent trends in nursing interventions. Not all continuing education opportunities are accepted by all state boards of nursing for renewal of licensure. The LPN/LVN is responsible for acquiring the required number of CEUs and for ensuring that the credits are attained from approved providers.

Box 58.8 Continuing Education

ORIENTATION TO THE FACILITY

Provides an opportunity to learn about variations in routine and a review of selected previously learned information and skills. Orientations vary in length, depending on the type of facility; orientation periods may last from days to weeks. The new employee may be assigned a **preceptor** to work with during the orientation period.

IN-SERVICE EDUCATION

Information chosen to meet specific needs within a facility. Attendance at some in-service programs, such as a yearly update on bloodborne pathogens, is required. Usually a specified amount of time is required for in-service programs, such as 1 hour a month or three times a year, according to the agency policy. Depending on the credentials of the instructor, continuing education credits or units may be earned.

WORKSHOPS

Forum in which information is presented, discussed, and practiced. Workshops provide excellent opportunities to learn new skills. The length varies according to the content. Some agencies pay the workshop fee or expenses if the topic is specific to and enhances the employee's nursing skills. Workshops are also a major source of continuing education credits or units required by many states as a part of relicensure.

CONTINUING EDUCATION CLASSES

There are often classes on complex nursing skills such as intravenous therapy, physical assessment, LPN/LVN charge nurse responsibilities, mental health concepts, nursing process for LPN/LVNs, and so on. Some vocational schools and community colleges provide courses that a nurse is interested in if the nurse requests them and if there are enough potential students to make up the required minimum enrollment. Many of these classes provide continuing education credits, as opposed to course credit. A certificate is awarded when course work is completed satisfactorily.

SHARING INFORMATION

One of the most valuable benefits of continuing education classes is the opportunity to meet with other working LPN/LVNs. Networking allows for the exchange of ideas and practices among nurses. Keep a personal record of all in-service programs, seminars, and workshops offered, including dates, credits, and topics, for future reference. Ensure that the employer includes these records in personnel files at your place of employment.

LPN/LVN, Licensed practical nurse or licensed vocational nurse.

CERTIFICATION OPPORTUNITIES

Certification is a process by which the nurse is granted recognition for competency in a specific area of nursing. Various certification opportunities are available to LPN/LVNs through seminars or self-guided study courses and successful completion of examinations. Knowledge is the basis for improved nursing skills and safety in patient care. Presently certification is available for the LPN/LVN in pharmacology, long-term care, and intravenous therapy. In many states or agencies, certification is also the basis for salary increases and advancement. Information on certification courses for the LPN/LVN can be found on the NAPNES website (*www.napnes.org*).

Certification in Managed Care

The American Board of Managed Care Nursing offers curriculum and testing that certifies the nurse in delivery of care that is patient centered. The nurse certified in managed care develops and puts into practice wellness and disease prevention/management programs, as well as quality management programs. The certification examination is a national examination, and recertification is required every 3 years.

Certification in Pharmacology

NAPNES pharmacology certification addresses principles of pharmacology and medication administration, including dosage calculation. The LPN/LVN has the option of taking the challenge examination without benefit of a course. Courses are available, however, and some sponsoring agencies mandate the course as an initial step. Recertification is required every 3 years.

Certification in Long-Term Care

NAPNES offers certification in long-term care that addresses issues across the lifespan for individuals faced with chronic illness and for elderly patients. Once the examination is successfully completed, the certification allows the nurse the extended title of certified in long-term care (CLTC).

Certification in Intravenous Therapy

For nurses who desire to enhance their practice skills in intravenous (IV) therapy and phlebotomy, NAPNES offers IV therapy certification. This certification is offered through an examination, as well as course work if desired. Nurses must consider the limits of their state's nurse practice act when seeking IV therapy certification.

LPN/LVN Refresher Course

For LPN/LVNs who seek to enhance their knowledge and skills, NAPNES offers an online self-study and self-paced refresher course. LPN/LVNs who have been inactive in their profession, are seeking reactivation of their license, or are seeking to update their knowledge and skills may benefit from this course. Information for the LPN/LVN refresher course can be found on the NAPNES website (*www.napnes.org*).

Further Education: LPN/LVN-to-RN Programs

Many community colleges, private schools, and universities have programs that offer a specialized curriculum that leads to obtaining an RN license for LPN/LVNs who wish to further their education or career. There are *degree* programs such as the associate of science in nursing (ASN) and baccalaureate of science in nursing (BSN). Further degree outcomes for the LPN/LVN offer opportunities of completion for master's of science in nursing (MSN). Some programs offer an accelerated pace for completion of the degree and may offer an online curriculum or a combination of classroom and online courses. These programs build on the education obtained in the LPN/LVN program. The state board of nursing is an excellent source of information about programs in each area. Colleges vary in their admission requirements and offer differing credits for previous education.

LICENSURE EXAMINATION

REGISTRATION FOR THE EXAMINATION

Completion of the nursing program's course of study results in the conferment of a degree. The type of degree varies by institution. Graduation from the program of nursing does not provide licensure. Licensure is granted by the state. Completion of the nursing program does not automatically provide eligibility to sit for the licensure examination. Most state boards require a criminal background check and fingerprinting before permission is granted for a candidate to take the NCLEX-PN. If there is a question about the candidate's work history or criminal background, an individual state board hearing may take place. A person who is knowledgeable about the candidate sometimes writes a recommendation regarding the candidate's moral character. The state board has the authority to accept or reject a candidate's request to take the licensure examination.

Each state enforces its own nurse practice act that addresses various issues, including licensure. The board of nursing in the jurisdiction where the candidate will take the NCLEX-PN approves the candidate's application. The state board of nursing has the authority to refuse any candidate the right to take the examination.

TEST PREPARATION

Some nursing programs administer an exit examination before graduation that will provide the graduate with an estimated likelihood of passing the National Council Licensure Examination for Practical Nurses (NCLEX-PN) Examination. The score on an exit examination is a good indicator of how much preparation the graduate will need for success on the NCLEX-PN.

Review courses are available to assist the graduate nurse in preparing for the NCLEX-PN. Before registering for a review course, the graduate should evaluate which course will be most beneficial. In considering a review course, the graduate must remember that the objective is not primary learning but review. Faculty members from the graduate's program may be able to provide recommendations for a reputable review course. Review material also may be found at the learning extension website of the National Council of State Boards of Nursing (NCSBN; *www.learningext.com*).

The graduate should take the following steps:

- Plan ahead, and make an intelligent decision regarding a review course.

- Carefully evaluate your need for a review course.
- Look for a course that uses faculty from outside your school.
- Know the course modality. Some are taught in a classroom setting and others online.
- Consider the cost; review courses may range from $250 to $500.
- Know the following: how long the course will last, where the course is held, the size of the class, and when the course is offered.
- Find out what guarantees the review vendor places on the review with regard to NCLEX success on the initial attempt.
- Determine if the review will provide a probability score tied to the likelihood of exam success.

Review books, online sources, and smartphone applications are available to aid the new graduate in preparing for the NCLEX-PN. It is important to select a review resource that meets individual study needs. Review resources undergo revision approximately every 3 years. Students should be sure to use current review resources because they follow the current NCLEX test plan. Nursing faculty frequently can offer suggestions for quality review resources.

Testing centers are available in each state, as well outside of the United States. After submitting an application to the state board of nursing, the candidate, if approved, registers with Pearson VUE to receive an authorization to test. The candidate also receives information that describes the test, the protocol for making an appointment for the examination, and a list of available centers and their contact information. Test times can be reserved by Internet or telephone, and testing times vary by site.

TAKING THE TEST

The NCSBN adopted computerized adaptive testing (CAT) for the NCLEX in 1994. The maximum time length for administration of the NCLEX-PN is 5 hours. Some candidates are able to complete the examination in less time.

CAT test centers are quiet and comfortable, with specially designed workstations to enhance security while providing a personal testing environment. Upon entry candidates are required to provide identification and have their fingerprints and photograph taken. The candidate sits at an individual computer terminal and answers questions that appear on the screen. Test staff maintain security by directly observing the testing session, in addition to continuous monitoring. The proctor is able to observe all candidates simultaneously and continuously during testing without entering the room, which eliminates the noise and distraction of people moving about the room.

In April 2005 test administrators revised the test format by introducing *alternate format items.* An alternate-item format is an examination item that takes advantage of new technology through the use of a format to assess candidate ability that differs from the standard one of four multiple-choice options with one correct response. Possible alternate-item formats include questions with multiple correct responses, fill-in-the-blank questions (including calculation and ordered-response item types), and "hot-spot" items, for which a candidate is to identify an area, picture, or graphic. All NCLEX-PN item formats, including current standard multiple-choice items, sometimes include charts, tables, or graphic images; the intent of alternate-item formats is to assess each candidate's ability to critically think in a way that is more flexible than with standard multiple-choice items.

Each test unfolds in an interactive way as the candidate proceeds through the material, but each one covers the same subject content (each test is based on the test plan). The goal of CAT is to determine competence on the basis of the difficulty of questions, not on how many questions are answered correctly. The interactive computerized format makes it possible to match the test questions posed to each candidate's demonstrated competence level. This makes for greater efficiency in the testing process: The program poses only questions that offer the best measurement of the candidate's competence, rather than a one-size-fits-all set that includes questions not relevant to a given candidate's situation.

Testing experts have ascertained the difficulty level of each of the thousands of questions in the computer's item bank by trying them out on thousands of candidates and then statistically analyzing the results. In the actual testing situation, the program uses a candidate's answers to calculate a competence estimate based on the known level of difficulty. It then scans through the test item bank, classified by test plan area and level of difficulty, and determines the question that will measure the candidate in the next test plan area most precisely and appropriately. It presents this selection on the computer screen as the successive test question to the candidate. This process continues, creating as it goes an examination tailored to the individual candidate's knowledge and skills and at the same time fulfilling all NCLEX-PN plan requirements.

Questions are ranked by the level of difficulty from easiest to hardest. If asked the easiest questions, most candidates answer most of them correctly. If asked only the hardest, they probably answer most incorrectly. As the examination questions progress from easy to hard, there comes a point at which an individual candidate is answering 50% of the questions correctly. Questions further along the difficulty continuum are likely to receive wrong answers (i.e., although some answers will be right, more will be wrong), and easier questions are likely to elicit correct answers. The goal of CAT is to find that point, which is different for everyone. That point is the competence level.

The minimum number of questions for the NCLEX-PN is 85 (60 "real" questions and 25 pilot, or "try-out," questions). The scores on the try-out questions are not counted toward the competence level of the candidate. If a candidate is able to answer the difficult questions correctly, there is no point wasting the candidate's time with a lot of easy questions. Likewise, if a candidate is not able to answer the easy ones correctly, there is no point in continuing with the difficult ones because the candidate is unlikely to be able to answer them. In fact, the system often has enough data to make a decision after less than the minimum of 60 questions, but a minimum of 60 scored questions is necessary to ensure coverage of the test plan. It is important that the candidates get the opportunity to answer several questions in each of the test plan content areas.

After the candidate has answered 85 questions, the system compares the competence level with the passing standard and determines (1) whether the candidate is clearly above the passing standard (the candidate passes), (2) whether the candidate is clearly below the passing standard (the candidate fails), or (3) whether the competence level is not clear. If it is not clear whether the candidate has passed, the system continues to ask questions. The system stops asking questions when the competence level is clearly above or clearly below the passing standard, when the maximum number of questions has been answered (265 for the NCLEX-RN and 205 for the NCLEX-PN), or when the candidate runs out of time.

There is no random selection of which candidates get a long examination. The length of the NCLEX-PN is based on the performance of the individual candidate.

Candidates who are accustomed to knowing most of the answers on tests sometimes find a CAT test difficult because they know the answers to only about half the questions. However, it is in fact possible that these candidates are doing well: Because they are answering the most difficult questions in the item bank, even 50% correct scores reflect a high competence level.

The most current and complete information about the NCSBN and the NCLEX-PN is available from its website *(www.ncsbn.org)*.

AFTER THE TEST

The test scores are pass or fail. Test administrators print score reports and send them to the board of nursing in each jurisdiction within 24 hours. Each board of nursing schedules its own notification timetable. Most test results are received by candidates in 1 week or less.

Candidates who have failed their licensure examination in most states are allowed to retake the test after waiting 45 days. Additional guidelines from the state board of nursing include (1) the number of times a candidate is allowed to retake the test before being required to seek reeducation and (2) the amount of time allowed between graduation from nursing school and taking the licensure examination.

On successful completion of the examination, the candidate has the right to practice as an LPN/LVN. The licensed LPN/LVN is responsible for license renewal and keeping the state board informed of any changes of address, name, and employment (i.e., active or inactive) status. The LPN/LVN is not allowed to practice without a license. Licensure permits nurses to offer special skills to the public, but it also provides legal guidelines for protection of the public.

ENDORSEMENT AND RECIPROCITY

The NCLEX-PN makes it possible to practice nursing in states other than the one in which the nurse first qualifies (see Chapter 2). If the nurse moves after successfully passing the examination and fulfilling the educational requirements, it is necessary to apply for a license or temporary practice permit before practicing nursing. Licensure that transfers this way from one state to another is called **endorsement** (a statement of recognition of the license of a health practitioner in one state by another state; the applicant needs to meet the current state's licensing requirements). Some states called this licensure **reciprocity;** this is a mutual agreement to exchange privileges, dependence, or relationships, such as an agreement between two governing bodies to accept the credentials of caregivers licensed in each other's state. True reciprocity means that an individual licensed in one state automatically can receive licensure in the other, even if the licensing requirements of the states differ. In either case, the nurse must have a license that is unencumbered. Some states also offer temporary licensure to individuals seeking endorsement in that state. This allows the applicant endorsement to work while the application for licensure is being reviewed.

Nurse Licensing Compact and Mutual Recognition

To date, 25 states have adopted mutual recognition licensure or an interstate compact. Those states (known as *compact states*) are listed in the NCSBN's website *(https://www.ncsbn.org/nurse-licensure-compact.htm)*.

Because mutual recognition licensure is based on the primary state of residence, every nurse is required to declare his or her primary state of residence. The primary state of residence is defined as a declared, fixed, permanent, and principal home for legal purposes (domicile). Indicators of a domicile include, but are not limited to, where real property is located and where the nurse pays state taxes, votes, and is licensed to operate a motor vehicle.

For example, if the LPN/LVN's primary state of residence is Missouri and the LPN/LVN's nursing practice is confined totally to the state of Missouri—that is, the LPN/LVN does not physically leave the state to care for patients and the LPN/LVN does not use technology (telephone, computer interface, interactive closed circuit television) to assess or provide advice to patients living outside of Missouri—this does not affect how the LPN/LVN is licensed.

If an LPN/LVN travels with a patient from one state to the other or to Canada, the LPN/LVN's license is valid for the length of the stay in the other state or Canada.

If the LPN/LVN's primary state of residence is Missouri and the state (or states) in which the LPN/LVN practices is on the list of compact states, the LPN/LVN's license entitles him or her to practice in that state after Missouri's effective date and the other compact state's effective date have passed. The LPN/LVN must be sure to maintain the Missouri license on active status. After Missouri and the other compact state's effective dates have passed, the LPN/LVN no longer needs to maintain a license in the other compact state.

If the LPN/LVN's primary state of residence is Missouri but the state in which he or she practices is not on the list of compact states, the LPN/LVN needs to maintain a license in the other state. If the LPN/LVN's primary state of residence is Missouri but the LPN/LVN practices in one or more states that are on the compact state list and one or more states that are not on the compact state list, the LPN/LVN is permitted to practice in the compact states because of the Missouri license, but the LPN/LVN must maintain a separate license in any states that are not on the list. Also the LPN/LVN should consider maintaining the Missouri license in anticipation of other states' adopting mutual recognition licensure.

Nurses who are on active duty in the armed forces or employed by the US Public Health Service, the US Department of Veterans Affairs, or any other federal institution must meet the licensure requirements of those federal institutions. The nurse licensure compact does not replace the federal requirements and thus does not necessarily affect licensure status. However, the LPN/LVN still is required to declare his or her primary state of residence. If the LPN/LVN is a federal employee and holds a second (civilian) job in nursing, the compact does not apply to the civilian position, and the LPN/LVN must obtain licensing by the usual route of applying to the state board of nursing. Some states that do not accept mutual recognition still require endorsement or reciprocity.

State boards of nursing differ, so contact the board of nursing in the state where licensure is being sought for the specific requirements of that state.

NURSE PRACTICE ACTS

The nurse practice act is a statute enacted by the legislature of any of the states or by appropriate officers of the districts or possessions.

A **nurse practice act** is the licensing law. It defines the title and the regulations governing the practice of nursing. The act delineates the legal scope of the practice of nursing within the geographic boundaries. Its provisions assist the nurse in staying within the legal scope of nursing practice in each state. Some states have separate governing boards for professional and practical or vocational nursing. The nurse practice act defines the regulations for practical nursing and includes requirements for an approved school of nursing. It also states the requirements for licensure and conditions under which a license may be revoked or suspended (see Chapter 2).

STATE BOARD OF NURSING

Each state has a board of nursing. The composition of the boards is determined by individual state statute. The majority of state boards are composed of LPN/LVNs and RNs. A few states have separate boards for the different practices. Boards are appointed by the state's governor or designee. The duties of the state boards have a focus on the promotion of public safety and the oversight of nursing licenses and educational programs. The duties may vary but generally include the following:

- Interpretation and enforcement of the state nurse practice act
- Administration and development of nurse licensure policies
- Discipline as determined of nurse licenses
- Development of nurse practice standards
- Accreditation and monitoring activities for nursing education programs

The purpose of the board is to protect the public by administering the nurse practice act. The board is responsible for approving schools of nursing and for renewing and issuing licenses. The board also has the authority to suspend or revoke a license. Some of the conditions under which a nurse's license is suspended or revoked include inability to perform competently as a result of drug addiction, alcohol abuse, and lack of mental or physical well-being. A nursing license may also be revoked for **negligence** in patient care (the commission of an act that a prudent person would not have committed or the omission of a duty that a prudent person would have fulfilled, resulting in injury or harm to another person; proof is necessary that other prudent members of the same profession would ordinarily have acted differently under the same circumstances), for endangering a patient's life, or for failing to comply with the standard and requirements of the nurse practice act of the state in which the nurse is practicing (see Chapter 2). Sanctions also may be taken in response to criminal actions that are outside of the realm of nursing practice.

MENTORING AND NETWORKING

A mentor is a nurse with more experience and knowledge who is willing to help a novice nurse learn the skills of the profession through counseling, role modeling, and teaching. Nurses need to demonstrate caring behaviors for themselves, each other, and patients. Much attention has been given to the benefits of mentoring in nursing. Retention rates for new graduates, and for

Box 58.9 Cost of Nursing Turnover

- Advertising and recruitment
- Vacancy costs (e.g., paying for agency nurses, overtime, closed beds, hospital diversions, etc.)
- Hiring
- Orientation and training
- Decreased productivity
- Termination
- Potential patient errors, compromised quality of care
- Poor work environment and culture, dissatisfaction, distrust
- Loss of organizational knowledge
- Additional turnover

From Jones C, Gates M: The costs and benefits of nurse turnover: A business case for nurse retention, *OJIN Online J Issues Nurs* 12(3):4, 2007.

nurses in general, have been found to increase for agencies that have a mentoring program in place (Cottingham et al, 2011; Ketola, 2009). The loss of a nurse from a position results in significant cost to the employer. Cost estimates vary but can add up to thousands of dollars. The loss is not limited to the care that would have been administered by the nurse but extends to include the cost of sharing the message of the open position, interviewing, loss of productivity, and impact of morale of the remaining members of the health care team (Box 58.9).

If a facility does not have a mentoring or preceptor program, the new graduate (mentee) should locate a nurse (mentor) who demonstrates similar clinical interests and displays actions and behavior that are desirable. The mentee should evaluate how receptive to questions the potential mentor seems and whether he or she seems likely to take time to explain and clarify information.

If the new graduate is unable to identify a mentor or the facility does not have a mentoring program, there are some ways to self-mentor. Suggestions include the following:

- Interact with nurses. Ask questions, listen, and clarify what you know with other nurses to enhance your understanding.
- Discover and use references. Read books and journal articles.
- Observe other nurses who are knowledgeable and insightful.
- Enroll in educational programs, especially those that include skill practices.
- Determine solutions for yourself, reflect on them, and work through them on your own.

Another strategy is networking, which is an effective method for interacting with and gaining support from other people employed in the same setting. Information and suggestions are shared when a nurse is networking with others in the same field. In addition to networking within a facility, there are various Internet resources through which nurses network with each other.

Box 58.10 LPN/LVN Demographics in the United States in 2017

1. Median pay: $45,030 per year ($21.65 per hour)
2. Number of jobs: 724,500
3. Job outlook from 2016 to 2026: 12% increase (faster than average occupations)
4. Projected employment change in number of jobs from 2016 to 2026: +88,100
5. Places of employment:
   Skilled nursing care facilities: 38%
   General medical and surgical care in hospitals: 16%
   Home health care services: 12%
   Community care facilities for the elderly: 7%
6. Work schedules: The majority of LPN/LVNs worked full time in their place of employment; the remainder worked part time.

LPN/LVN, Licensed practical nurse/licensed vocational nurse.
Modified from US Department of Labor, Bureau of Labor Statistics: Licensed practical and licensed vocational nurses: Occupational outlook handbook, 2018. Retrieved from *https://www.bls.gov/ooh/healthcare/licensed-practical-and-licensed-vocational-nurses.htm*.

CAREER OPPORTUNITIES

Never before has nursing been so exciting. Today the new graduate has an unprecedented variety of job opportunities available. Making the correct career decision requires considerable thought for the graduate. The job opportunities for the LPN/LVN extend beyond those in the long-term care facility and the hospital. When entering the field of nursing, the new graduate should be aware of the average wage, number of jobs available, and the job outlook for the LPN/LVN. This demographic information better prepares the new graduate for employment opportunities (Box 58.10).

Some nurses believe that it is better for the LPN/LVN to seek employment first in a hospital or long-term care facility with a subacute unit. This provides the opportunity to sharpen clinical skills and solidify the LPN/LVN's knowledge base, providing a strong foundation. This decision depends on the individual's goals and personal situation. For example, if the LPN/LVN knows that he or she can work only days and needs weekends off, a health care provider's office or clinic may be a preferable first job.

HOSPITALS

Because of health care economics, hospitals are responsible for providing quality care as economically as possible. Under the supervision of an RN, the LPN/LVN is legally able to provide most bedside care to patients in the hospital setting. Because the LPN/LVN salary is lower than that of the RN, it makes economic sense to employ a number of LPN/LVNs. It also makes sense because the LPN/LVN is prepared to give excellent bedside care.

The LPN/LVN has opportunities in various departments throughout the hospital, including coronary care, intensive care, emergency department, surgery scrub, outpatient surgery, and pediatrics. Policies vary by facility and locality. In the hospital setting, the LPN/LVN has responsibility for supervising nursing assistants, whereas overall management of a unit is the responsibility of an RN.

Salaries in a hospital setting may include shift differential and extra pay for holidays and perhaps weekends. Benefits tend to be good in hospitals, and some provide for 12-hour shifts and special schedule plans such as a 3-day weekend work schedule. Other opportunities in the hospital setting include work in infection control and employee health, as well as serving on various committees.

When seeking employment, the LPN/LVN should consider a number of different types of hospitals. Some have a wide range of services, and some are more specialized. Common specialized hospitals include pediatric facilities, orthopedic facilities, and rehabilitation facilities. Some hospitals operate in conjunction with a university and are the site of a great deal of teaching and research.

LONG-TERM CARE FACILITIES

LPN/LVN work is the backbone of long-term care facilities (previously called *nursing homes*). LPN/LVNs in this setting frequently advance to charge nurse and supervisory capacity with RN supervision. The LPN/LVN in the long-term care setting often is involved in staff development and recruitment and serves on various committees. Management and leadership skills have ample opportunity for development in the long-term care setting (Fig. 58.3).

Salaries for LPN/LVNs vary by clinical environment and regional location. The LPN/LVN earns the most amount of money in governmental agencies. Slightly lower earnings were reported in ambulatory settings such as physician practices. In 2017 the median salary was $45,030. In long-term care facilities salaries are currently similar to those in the hospital setting (Bureau of Labor Statistics, 2018). Shift differential pay and scheduling alternatives may be available. Benefit packages also tend to be good in the long-term care setting.

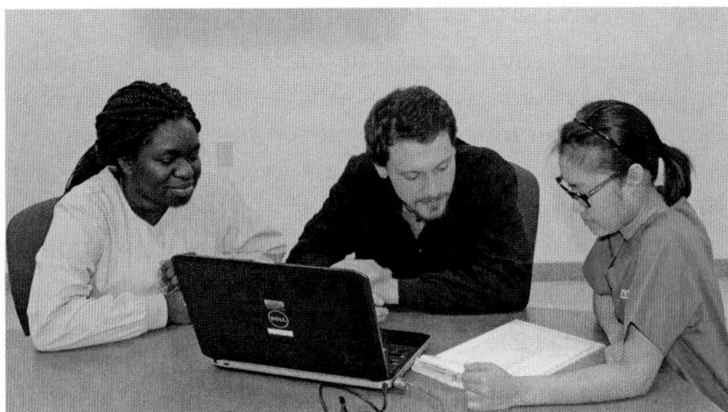

Fig. 58.3 Various positions on the health care team are available in the long-term care setting.

Many positive changes have occurred in the facilities. The long-term care facility is just that: a facility for patients who require long-term care. Hospitals no longer are an option for patients after the period of acute illness. Alternatives include rehabilitation hospitals if patients meet the qualifications, home health care, or a long-term care facility. Residents are of any age, and the level of care depends on the unit. Subacute units provide care that in years past was possible only in the hospital setting. Physical, speech, occupational, and other therapies are available. Many patients receive therapy and are able to return home.

HOME HEALTH

The degree to which home health care opportunities are available to LPN/LVNs varies in different parts of the United States. The LPN/LVN is capable of providing much of the care required, but RN supervision must be available. The advantages of home health care include patient preference, nurse autonomy, and the lower cost of care in comparison with hospital stays. Home health care also allows for continuity of care inasmuch as the nurse often is assigned a caseload that he or she follows during the entire time the patient is receiving home health care.

HEALTH CARE PROVIDER'S OFFICE OR CLINIC

Health care providers' offices and clinics are a common place of employment for LPN/LVNs. It is important for the LPN/LVN to be aware that certain skills may be required in these settings that were not included in his or her educational program, such as phlebotomy and electrocardiography. In some cases, the health care provider teaches these skills, or certification classes may be available. The LPN/LVN should check his or her state's nurse practice act to ensure that any additional skills are within the scope of practice. Computer skills are essential in virtually every health care setting, and insurance coding skills may be necessary in smaller offices.

Salary in offices tends to be lower than that in hospitals and long-term care facilities. Often the benefits package is not as complete as in the other settings. The schedule of primarily days with minimal weekend work is a definite advantage. There is an opportunity to focus on prevention in these settings, as well as opportunities for patient teaching.

INSURANCE COMPANIES

Insurance companies may employ LPN/LVNs in their preadmission and claims departments. These positions are office positions with few requirements involving manual dexterity. Companies usually require prior experience in medical-surgical nursing. The nurse's role may include performing basic physical examinations for potential policyholders or consultation for current policyholders. Practice environments largely determine the earning potential of the LPN/LVN in this field. Regional variables also determine earning capabilities.

TEMPORARY AGENCIES

There are opportunities to work for staffing agencies. These agencies provide nurses to meet the staffing needs in a variety of health care facilities. The salary is usually very good, but sometimes the benefits package is limited. The LPN/LVN must be very flexible to adjust to various work settings when working for a temporary agency.

Advantages of employment with a temporary agency are the right to refuse an assignment and the variety of assignments available. When employed by a temporary agency, the LPN/LVN has the right to say no on a given day when called upon to work, which provides flexibility in one's personal schedule. The nursing experiences are more varied than when working every day at the same facility on the same unit.

A disadvantage is the uncertainty that work is available. If the number of patients is low in a facility, temporary employees are not called to work, so it is important for the new LPN/LVN to budget appropriately in the event of no work. Another disadvantage is that it may be difficult to create friendships or obtain the feeling of being the part of a team.

TRAVEL OPPORTUNITIES

Experienced nurses may explore opportunities to travel and work for specified periods in areas in need of nurses through a type of temporary agency with an expanded area of service. These agencies match employers' needs with nurses' experience and interest in living in that area for a time. Lodging usually is provided in addition to salary. This affords nurses who have the flexibility to travel the chance to visit an area and work there for a period of time.

PHARMACEUTICAL SALES

Pharmaceutical sales companies sometimes employ nurses as sales representatives. These companies usually require experience in specific areas and an expertise in science and pharmacology. Salary usually is based on sales. There is no direct patient care. Sales representatives contact health care providers, pharmacists, and nurses in various clinical settings to present the advantages of products and to teach about side effects and precautions.

OTHER MEDICAL SALES

Opportunities are also available for nurses with companies selling medical supplies. Responsibilities and compensation are similar to those in pharmaceutical sales. Sometimes nurses in this line of work hold in-service programs at facilities to demonstrate product use. Products vary widely, from such items as incontinence products to surgical equipment.

MILITARY

Opportunities are available for the LPN/LVN in military service. Active duty and the reserves are options. Local recruiters can provide information regarding a military career. Benefits of serving in the military as a nurse include the opportunity to serve one's country and educational opportunities. Various programs assist with tuition if the LPN/LVN chooses to further his or her education.

ADULT DAY SERVICES

Some communities may provide adult day services that require nursing supervision. These facilities are designed for individuals who require medical supervision while their family members work or take a break from the responsibility of care. The pace is relaxed, and the schedule is excellent. Many nurses find it to be a rewarding experience to work in a facility providing this kind of service to the adults and their family members who need it.

SCHOOLS

Opportunities are available in some communities to work as a school nurse. Health screening, emergency care, and health teaching are the major responsibilities. The nurse may work in one school or travel to different schools. Working only during the school year and during school hours is an advantage for nurses who themselves have children.

PUBLIC/COMMUNITY HEALTH

There are sometimes opportunities for LPN/LVNs with the public health department. Responsibilities usually include working in clinics and home visits. The nurse sometimes also participates in health inspections. Teaching is a major area of responsibility. The focus is on prevention. Day schedules are usually available. Salaries tend to be lower than in hospitals and long-term care facilities. In addition, community health opportunities include employment in areas such as weight-loss clinics, Head Start programs, and camp programs.

OUTPATIENT SURGERY

Work in a large number of outpatient facilities, especially for outpatient surgery, is available. The LPN/LVN is sometimes employed to prepare patients for surgery, as a scrub nurse, or to work in the recovery room under the supervision of an RN. This is typically a Monday-through-Friday position. Some facilities are freestanding, and others are part of a hospital complex.

PRIVATE DUTY

The private duty nurse gives total care to one patient. The setting for the private duty nurse changes from patient to patient, but the job description is basically the same. This type of nursing is totally independent nursing care service when the nurse self-contracts. Private duty nursing takes place in the hospital, the home, or other facility and during travel abroad or in the United States. When performing private duty nursing, the LPN/LVN cares not only for the patient but also for the family. The nurse is paid directly by the patient or responsible person. When the setting for private duty nursing is in a health care facility, the nurse is expected to follow the policies and procedures of that facility.

In private duty nursing, the nurse is legally responsible for his or her own actions. If the nurse ever has any doubt about an order or procedure, he or she must obtain clarification from the health care provider before carrying out the order or procedure. It is important to keep charts carefully. In the home, the nurse can set up a type of record in which to list necessary items, such as medications given, vital sign measurements, and the conditions of the patient. This home record is sometimes requested by and released to the health care provider. The nurse returns any narcotics not used to the health care provider before leaving the assignment.

The major disadvantages of private duty nursing are the irregularity of assignments and the economic aspects. In private duty nursing, there is no certainty of work or payment. Also, the private duty nurse must keep accurate records for tax and Social Security purposes.

An advantage of private duty nursing is the option of working as many days as desired and the opportunity to accept an assignment for as long a period as desired. There are also more freedom and fewer restrictions in the workday.

GOVERNMENT (CIVIL SERVICE)

Some LPN/LVNs work in a Veterans Administration (VA) hospital or other government hospitals. Advantages are competitive salary, benefits, retirement plans, and tuition reimbursement programs. In addition, many VA nurses feel rewarded by caring for veterans who have served their country in the military (US Department of Veterans Affairs, 2012).

OCCUPATIONAL HEALTH

The focus in occupational health nursing is on promoting wellness and preventing accidents. The emphasis is on safety and administering first aid care. Job responsibilities include physical assessment, health surveys, insurance form preparation, and health education, as well as nursing intervention for patients injured in industrial accidents. The LPN/LVN works under the supervision of an RN or a health care provider. Depending on the size of the industrial or facility site, this type of nursing sometimes offers shifts and benefits different from those of other career opportunities.

REHABILITATION

This field requires responsibility for guiding the patient toward health and independence. The role of the rehabilitation nurse includes assisting patients to meet maximum functioning capabilities, caring for patients with disabilities or chronic disease, and working closely with not only the patient but also the patient's family. An important aspect of rehabilitation nursing is collaboration with the rehabilitation team (Association of Rehabilitation Nurses, 2012).

MENTAL HEALTH–PSYCHIATRIC NURSING

Mental health–psychiatric facilities employ LPN/LVNs in a variety of settings. Venues for this type of nursing vary from inpatient units in a general hospital to outpatient clinics, mental health agencies, and psychiatric hospitals. Residential rehabilitation facilities are another site in which the LPN/LVN works with patients experiencing mental health or psychiatric issues.

HOSPICE

Hospice nursing offers the opportunity to care for terminally ill patients in either an institution or a home setting. The qualifications for hospice nurses are to have a clear understanding of their own feelings concerning death and to understand the philosophy of the hospice setting. The nurse closely supports the patient and family without interfering with family interpersonal relationships. Advantages of hospice nursing are steady employment, an environment that is less formal, and opportunities to provide good bedside care that is concerned with pain relief and comfort measures. Disadvantages are the fact that the nurse cares only for dying patients and the possibility of having to travel to more than one home each shift (see Chapter 40).

CORRECTIONAL FACILITY NURSING

Employment in correctional facilities is a growing field for nursing. Nurses work in county and city jails, as well as state and federal prisons. Duties vary from basic first aid care to extensive nursing care. Some larger state and federal prisons are finding it more beneficial and economical to house all medical services within the facility rather than transporting inmates to surrounding hospitals and clinics. This trend will increase the number of correctional nurses needed to adequately staff such units. Certifications in correctional nursing are available for nurses and nurse managers.

LEADERSHIP AND MANAGEMENT

Leadership is the art of getting other people to want to do something that the leader believes must be done. One root of the word *lead* means "to go." Leaders typically have a vision of where to go: a direction in which they influence other people to follow. Leaders are the ones who show the way and envision the "big picture."

Management is closely related. The word *management* comes from a word meaning "hand." Managers handle the day-to-day operations to achieve a desired outcome. Successful organizations require leadership and management (see the Coordinated Care box for responsibilities of the nurse manager).

When determining rules of supervision, team members typically supervise other team members who have a lesser scope of practice. Understandably, an LPN/LVN would not supervise the RN but could be responsible for other LPN/LVNs. Other members of the health team who would be managed by the LPN/LVN would include medical assistants, certified medical assistants, orderlies or transport workers, clerks, and technicians. The majority (38%) of LPN/LVNs are employed in long-term or assistive care facilities (US Department of Labor, Bureau of Labor Statistics, 2018). In these settings nurses may work in a position of leadership or management. In addition, some states may view LPN/LVNs as supervisors or they may have waivers that allow them to have increased supervisory responsibilities (Greenwood, n.d.).

 Coordinated Care

Supervision

Responsibilities of the Nurse Manager

- Assist staff in establishing annual goals for the unit and determining the systems needed to accomplish goals.
- Monitor professional nursing standards of practice on the unit.
- Develop an ongoing staff development plan, including one for new employees.
- Recruit new employees (interview and hire).
- Conduct routine staff evaluations.
- Establish yourself as a role model for positive customer service (customers include patients, families, and other members of the health care team).
- Submit staffing schedules for the unit.
- Conduct regular patient rounds, and help resolve patient or family complaints.
- Establish and implement a quality improvement plan for the unit.
- Review and recommend new equipment needs for the unit.
- Conduct regular staff meetings.
- Conduct rounds with health care providers.
- Establish and support necessary staff and interdisciplinary committees.

Leadership is an important factor in determining the effectiveness of any undertaking. Management style is the approach or manner that a leader uses to influence the behavior of other people in various situations. Leadership styles relate to the amount of control or freedom the manager allows the group. Such styles range from total control by the manager to extreme permissiveness. The most common styles are autocratic, democratic, and laissez-faire.

AUTOCRATIC STYLE

The autocratic leader retains all authority and responsibility and is concerned primarily with tasks and goal accomplishment. This type of leader assigns clearly defined tasks and establishes one-way communication with the group. The input of other team members is not sought or considered. The autocratic leader is firm, insistent, and dominating. Such a leader stresses prompt, orderly performance and uses power to intimidate or pressure employees who fail to adhere to expectations. This leader displays little trust or confidence in employees and therefore makes all the decisions. Because employees generally fear this type of manager, there tends to be some stifling of individual initiative and creativity.

The autocratic style of leadership is appropriate in certain situations. In situations in which immediate action is required and there is no time for group decisions, the autocratic leader is able to take quick action. Autocratic leaders excel in times of crisis (e.g., cardiac arrest) and in situations of disorder (e.g., natural disaster); they often have the reputation for being able to get difficult assignments completed. In situations in which safety is of concern this style of leadership is beneficial (AANAC, 2014).

DEMOCRATIC STYLE

The democratic style is a people-centered approach that allows employees more control and individual participation in the decision-making process. The emphasis is on team building and on collaboration through the joint effort of all team members. Democratic leaders function to facilitate goal accomplishment while stressing the self-worth of each individual. These leaders treat each staff member as an adult and expect the same in return. Criticism focuses on behaviors, not on personality, and its purpose is to promote growth and development of the staff.

The democratic style works best with mature employees who work well together in a group. This style sometimes does not work as well with ancillary staff, who in many cases need more direction. The group decision-making process sometimes seems slow and frustrating to those who expect prompt action on an issue. Disagreements are more likely and sometimes require more time to resolve. This style tends to demand more of the leader, but many employees value it for the sake of the professional growth and development of the staff that it facilitates. The results of the democratic leadership style in health care settings are evident in shared governance (an organized, systematic approach to decision making that enables nurses at all levels to participate), self-directed work teams, and staff committees concerned with quality improvement.

LAISSEZ-FAIRE STYLE

This leadership style often is referred to as the "free-run style" or "permissive leadership." This type of leader relinquishes control completely and chooses to avoid responsibility by delegating all decision making to the group. Laissez-faire leaders want everyone to feel free to "do their own thing," and as a result there is no sense of direction unless provided by the group or an informal leader. This style sometimes works well with highly motivated professional groups (e.g., a research staff), but it seldom works well in health care settings because of the complexity of the work environment.

SITUATIONAL LEADERSHIP

Situational leadership is a comprehensive approach to the issue of management that takes into account the style of the leader, the group being managed, and the situation at hand. Supporters of situational leadership contend that no single leadership style is best but rather that the best style for the manager to use is contingent on the situation at hand.

The basis of situational leadership theory is the flexibility of the manager in adapting to the needs of the individual or the work group. In a typical work setting, the manager may be directive in dealing with staff who are in orientation and simultaneously act as a coach for those on another shift who are more experienced but still need some guidance. For seasoned staff nurses, the manager is more of a support person. The situational leadership style enables professional growth for manager and staff (Hill and Howlett, 2013).

TEAM LEADING

Sometimes an LPN/LVN is assigned the role of team leader. This role entails assisting and guiding the nursing team in providing care for a select group of patients. The team leader assigns patients to each team member and takes responsibility for the delivery of care to patients, as well as for supervision of all members of the team, including nursing assistants. Duties of a team leader include the following:

- Receiving reports on assigned patients
- Making assignments for team members
- Making rounds and assessing all assigned patients
- Giving team members reports about assigned patients
- Assisting in administering medications and treatments
- Providing time in the early part of the shift to have a conference with team members on priority patients (those with the most urgent needs) to keep everyone informed of progress in patient care, provide continuity of care, and allow the team member to answer questions and resolve problems

An advantage of team nursing is the collaborative style that encourages each member of the team to help others.

DELEGATION

Delegation of tasks is an important aspect of patient care. Delegation of care refers to the act of making another individual responsible for a specific task. One of the benefits of delegation is that licensed personnel are allowed more time to focus on higher level tasks.

Delegation mandates clear communication of all aspects of the delegated care to the person completing the task. Consider the job description, the legal responsibility, the educational level, the ability, and the licensure of the person to whom you are delegating complete care. The staff member performing the care must be able to perform tasks independently and must have the ability and knowledge to complete the task (see the Coordinated Care box on the five rights of delegation). Do not assign care to an unqualified staff member. For example, the LPN/LVN may delegate ambulation of a patient to a certified nursing assistant, but the LPN/LVN is responsible for determining the degree of assistance necessary for the patient.

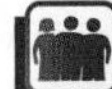 Coordinated Care

Delegation

The Five Rights of Delegation

RIGHT TASK

The right task refers to delegating care for a specific patient and ensuring that the task delegated is within the health care professional's scope of practice. If a task is delegated to unlicensed assistive personnel, the task should be a skill that is repetitive, requires little supervision, is relatively noninvasive, has predictable results, and poses minimal risk to the patient.

RIGHT CIRCUMSTANCES

Consider the appropriate patient setting, available resources, and other relevant factors. In an acute care setting, patients' conditions often change quickly. Good clinical decision making is necessary to determine what to delegate.

RIGHT PERSON

The right person is delegating the right tasks to the right employee for performance on the right patient.

RIGHT DIRECTION AND COMMUNICATION

Give a clear, concise description of the task, including its objective, limits, and expectations. It is essential for communication to be ongoing between the registered nurse (RN) and assistive personnel during a shift of care.

RIGHT SUPERVISION AND EVALUATION

Provide appropriate monitoring, evaluation, intervention as needed, and feedback. Assistive personnel must feel comfortable asking questions and seeking assistance.

Be aware that accountability remains with the delegating nurse in many situations. A major advantage of delegation is that tasks are completed in a more timely manner when all staff are working together to reach the common goal for the patient (Fig. 58.4).

Data from American Nurses Association: Joint statement on delegation: American Nurses Association (ANA) and National Council of State Boards of Nursing (NCSBN), 2005. Available at *https://www.ncsbn.org/Delegation_joint_statement_NCSBN-ANA.pdf*.

TIME MANAGEMENT

Time management is an aspect that is sometimes difficult for the new LPN/LVN. For a new nurse, the patient load is often heavier than that during nursing school and there are added responsibilities as a licensed professional. It is important for the new LPN/LVN to evaluate his or her time management skills to determine whether time is being used effectively. Suggestions for time management

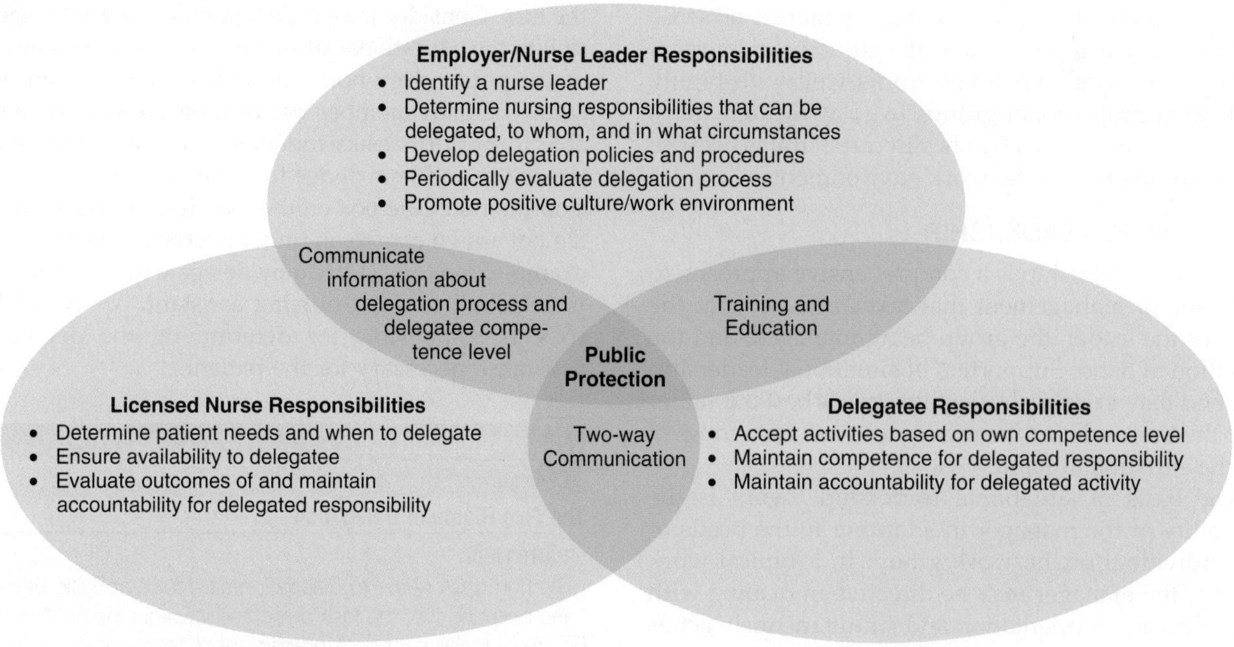

Employer/Nurse Leader Responsibilities
- Identify a nurse leader
- Determine nursing responsibilities that can be delegated, to whom, and in what circumstances
- Develop delegation policies and procedures
- Periodically evaluate delegation process
- Promote positive culture/work environment

Communicate information about delegation process and delegatee competence level

Training and Education

Public Protection

Licensed Nurse Responsibilities
- Determine patient needs and when to delegate
- Ensure availability to delegatee
- Evaluate outcomes of and maintain accountability for delegated responsibility

Two-way Communication

Delegatee Responsibilities
- Accept activities based on own competence level
- Maintain competence for delegated responsibility
- Maintain accountability for delegated activity

Fig. 58.4 Delegation model. (From National Council of State Boards of Nursing: National guidelines for nursing education. *J Nurs Reg,* 7:5-14, 2016.)

are listed in the Coordinated Care box on prioritization and time management.

NURSING INFORMATICS

Nursing informatics has become a well-recognized term since it first was introduced. The American Nurses Association (2008) recognized nursing informatics as a specialty that "integrates nursing science, computer science, and information science to manage and communicate data, information, knowledge, and wisdom in nursing practice." Numerous computer systems are available in the health care setting, so nurses are trained on the particular system used at their place of employment. Nurses incorporate nursing informatics into the daily routine in various ways, including entering health care information into the patient's *electronic medical record (EMR),* documenting medication administration, and researching medical information from online sources. Both certifications and graduate degrees in nursing informatics are available.

TRANSCRIBING HEALTH CARE PROVIDERS' ORDERS

Health care providers convey orders for patient care through writing, telephoning, or verbalizing the orders to the nurse. The health care providers' order may be handwritten in the patient's records by the health care provider. In an attempt to prevent errors in transcription, many facilities are now requiring the health care provider to submit orders directly into the computer system of

Coordinated Care

Prioritization

Principles of Time Management

GOAL SETTING
Review the patient's goals of care for the day and your goals for activities such as completing documentation, attending a patient care conference, giving the staff report on time, or preparing medications for administration.

TIME ANALYSIS
Reflect on how you use your time. While you work in a clinical area, keep track of how you use your time in different activities. Such tracking often provides valuable information and reveals how well organized you really are.

PRIORITY SETTING
Schedule the priorities that you have established for patients within set time frames. Determine the best time for activities such as conducting teaching sessions, planning ambulation, and providing times for rest.

INTERRUPTION CONTROL
Everyone needs time to socialize or to discuss issues with colleagues. However, do not let this interrupt important patient care activities. Use time during reports, meal breaks, or team meetings to the best advantage. Also, plan time to assist colleagues so that it complements your patient care schedule.

EVALUATION
At the end of each day, take time to think about how effectively you used your time. If you are having difficulties, discuss them with a more experienced colleague.

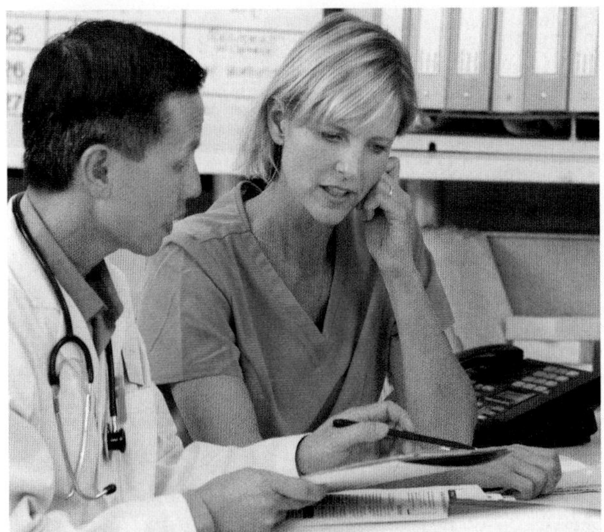

Fig. 58.5 Clarifying the health care provider's order. (Copyright 1999–2012 Thinkstock. All rights reserved.)

the facility. Some acute care facilities employ ward clerks, ward secretaries, or unit secretaries to transcribe the health care providers' orders. Conversely, in most long-term care facilities, there are no unit secretaries. In facilities that do employ unit secretaries, the secretaries usually do not work at night. In many facilities an expectation of the nurse is to transcribe the order from the patients' record if it was not submitted electronically. Some orders are difficult to read. If in doubt, clarify the order with the health care provider. Review the orders while the health care provider is on the unit so that clarification can be obtained in person immediately rather than later over the phone (Fig. 58.5). Also, if the written order seems unusual or does not seem congruous with the patient's condition, clarify the order with the health care provider. It is imperative to understand each order before carrying it out.

The health care provider is in charge of directing the patient care, and nurses carry out these orders for care, unless the nurse believes that the orders are in error or will be harmful to the patient. In this case, contact the health care provider to confirm or clarify the orders. If you still believe the orders to be inappropriate, immediately contact the nursing supervisor and put in writing why the orders are not being carried out. A nurse who carries out an erroneous or inappropriate order is at risk of being held liable for harm experienced by the patient. Nurses are responsible for their actions regardless of who told them to perform those actions.

The policies for verbal or telephone orders vary in different facilities. Check the facility's policy for accepting verbal or telephone orders. Orders given by telephone or verbal communication are more subject to error. If you are responsible for accepting this type of order, be certain of its accuracy. Clarify the order by repeating it to the person giving it and document that this was done. This gives both people a chance to hear the order. A telephone or verbal order always must be written down immediately. If the order is given too rapidly, ask the giver to repeat it more slowly. When the correct spelling of a medication is questionable, refer to a list of commonly ordered medications or to the *Physicians' Desk Reference.* Be cautious about medications whose spellings look alike or similar and those that sound alike. Several medications sound alike but have very different actions (e.g., Xanax [alprazolam] and Zantac [ranitidine]; Xanax is an antianxiety agent, and Zantac is a histamine antagonist for the treatment of ulcers).

When the nurse **transcribes** (writes or types a copy of) health care providers' orders, a number of precautions must be used to prevent errors (see the Medication Safety Alert box on precautions for transcribing orders).

! Medication Safety Alert

Precautions for Transcribing Orders

The following information applies to all health care providers' orders:

1. Check that written/computer entry orders correspond correctly to the intended chart.
2. If there is more than one order, read through all orders before beginning to transcribe them.
3. Process stat orders first. (A stat order is for a single dose of medication to be administered immediately and only once.)
4. If there is some confusion during a telephone order, have another nurse listen for clarification.
5. When you take telephone or verbal orders, write the order on the order sheet, read the order back to the person giving it, and document that you read the order back.

The following items are basic guidelines and sometimes vary from one facility to another. The LPN/LVN should refer to agency policy.

6. Order the medication needed from the pharmacy per facility policy; include date, patient's name and identification number, date of birth, room number, time of administration, medication, route of administration, dosage, and frequency.
7. Record the orders in the required areas, such as the medication administration record (MAR), unless the orders are computer generated. Be certain to include the date.
8. Make very certain that all orders have been carried out and recorded in the proper record. (The new graduate should have a second nurse verify for accuracy until experience is obtained.)
9. Check off each order on the health care providers' order sheet if it is handwritten; otherwise follow the policy of the facility for computerized systems. Most facilities require the nurse's signature or initials to verify that orders have been transcribed.
10. Make sure to notify the nurses responsible for administering medications of any new order.
11. Follow the facility policy for identifying new orders for the staff.

When there is an order to discontinue or change a medication, take the steps in the Medication Safety Alert box on the procedure for discontinuing or changing a medication (this procedure varies in different facilities).

Medication Safety Alert

Procedure for Discontinuing or Changing a Medication

1. If the medication administration record (MAR) is not on the computer, the discontinued medication should be marked off on the MAR by crossing through with a highlighter and documenting the discontinue date on the MAR. If the order is being changed, a new order should be written. If the MAR is a computerized system, follow the policy of the program or facility.
2. Notify the nurse responsible for carrying out new orders about discontinued and newly ordered medications.
3. On the health care provider's order sheet, verify that the order has been carried out.

Orders requiring transcription are those concerning diet, preoperative and postoperative instructions, all medical treatments, activity, procedures, medications, diagnostic imaging and other diagnostic studies, and laboratory tests. When a patient undergoes surgery, all preoperative orders are canceled automatically. The health care provider must rewrite the orders postoperatively if continuation of the orders is desired. Many health care providers have routine postoperative orders, which have been prepared beforehand. There is a protocol for each order according to the facility's policy. When transcribing any order, follow through all steps completely as described previously with medication orders.

Some drugs may be distributed as floor stock. Floor stock are medications distributed to the nursing unit in bulk (either individually wrapped or in bottles). In general, medications appropriate for floor stock are those that health care providers tend to prescribe routinely on an as-needed (prn) basis. Medication dispensing systems, such as computer-assisted or electronic devices, are variations of unit-dose and floor stock systems. For example, the Pyxis MedStation (Care Fusion Products) (Fig. 58.6) has the capacity to carry a variety of medications, housed in individual compartments, that the nurse can access after requesting the medication from a computerized screen. The MedStation often houses medications that are used frequently, such as floor stock and narcotics, as well as individual patient medication bins. All medications that nurses retrieve from the MedStation must be recorded in the system's computer. (See Chapter 17 for more detailed discussion of medication administration.)

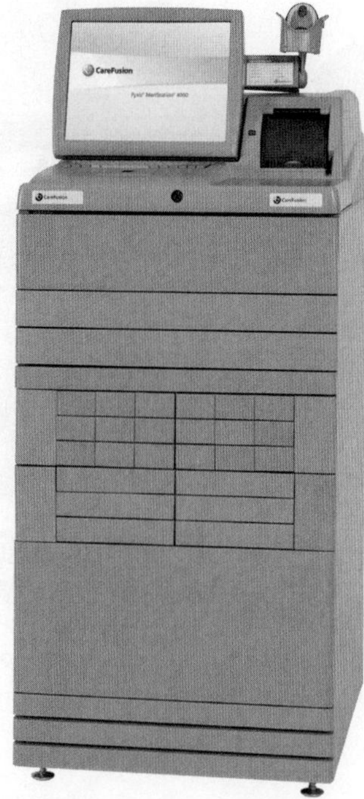

Fig. 58.6 The MedStation, a computerized system for narcotics distribution. A variety of medications are housed in individual compartments that the nurse can access. (Courtesy CareFusion Corporation.)

CHANGE-OF-SHIFT REPORT

The LPN/LVN is often responsible for giving a change-of-shift report. The purpose of the change-of-shift report is to provide the staff on the next shift with pertinent information about the patient. The quality of nursing care that the patient receives is contingent on how well the staff on each shift communicate with the staff on other shifts.

The change-of-shift report may be given in person or documented on a recording device, or the report may be given by making rounds from patient to patient (Fig. 58.7). Oral reports are given in a conference room with nurses from both shifts participating. When a recording device is used, the report is recorded before the end of the shift. This allows the nurses who are preparing to leave to finish last-minute tasks while the oncoming staff listens to the report. Allow time for clarification or updates before nurses leave the unit. Giving reports in person or on rounds allows immediate feedback. In all cases, maintain patient confidentiality.

Before beginning the report, consider what information regarding the patient is important to communicate and avoid reporting unnecessary information.

Typically, information that is considered important includes vital sign measurements (if abnormal), type of IV fluids (including rate of infusion, amount left to infuse, and IV site), intake, and output of feces, urine, and gastric secretions. The following should be reported using accepted medical and nursing terminology (Boxes 58.11 and 58.12):

- Output from all drainage tubes and appearance of drainage
- Any prn medications, including the time of administration and the effect, as well as the presence and amount of patient-controlled analgesia used

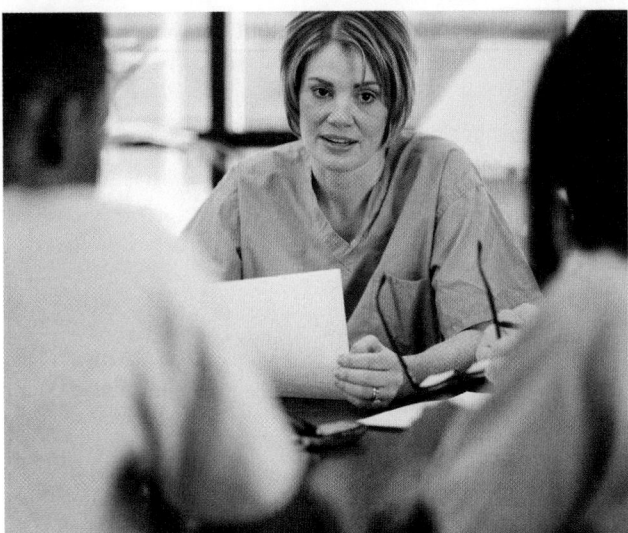

Fig. 58.7 Giving a change-of-shift report. (Copyright 1999–2012 Thinkstock. All rights reserved.)

Box 58.11 Information for Change-of-Shift Report

1. State patient's room and bed number, name, age, health care provider, all diagnoses, and date of surgery if patient is in a postoperative period.
2. Summarize patient's day (or evening or night).
3. Report all pertinent nursing care.
4. Describe change in patient's condition. Usually, most facilities report only abnormal vital sign measurements except for first postoperative day, when the last set of vital signs is measured.
5. Report special medications, intravenous (IV) solutions, infusion rate, amount of fluid remaining, and IV site. State time, method, and dosage of analgesics given and the effect.
6. Report all intake and output.
7. Report status of lungs and bowel sounds.
8. Report patient's mental status and level of consciousness.
9. Report circulatory checks, pedal pulses, and skin abnormalities in turgor or color.
10. State diagnostic procedures, such as computed tomography scans, x-ray studies, magnetic resonance imaging, endoscopy, proctoscopy, thoracentesis, and surgery. Report diet changes, special permits, preoperative procedures, daily weights, activity status, blood glucose measurements, blood in stools, clean-catch urine for analysis or culture and sensitivity (C&S), sputum specimen for C&S, respiratory therapy, and physical therapy orders. Report all nursing interventions, such as dressings, ostomy care, and oxygen.
11. Discuss patient and family education.
12. Note other services, such as social services, pastoral care, and discharge planning.
13. State any pertinent information helpful in patient care.
14. Report "no code" or do-not-resuscitate (DNR) status.
15. Present the report in an unbiased, nonjudgmental manner.

Box 58.12 Sample of a Change-of-Shift Report

Room 348A Mabel L., age 87, patient of Dr. B., in with heart failure and stasis ulcer of the right leg. She is alert and cheerful, has had a comfortable day. Edema in her ankles bilaterally has decreased from +2 to +1 after she received an additional 40 mg of Lasix orally at 1000 [10 AM]; weight is 165 lb [75 kg], down 10 lb [4.5 kg] since admission 2 days ago. Vital signs unremarkable except BP 168/100 mm Hg. Has an IV infusion of D_5W with 20 mEq of KCl infusing at 60 mL/h with 600 mL remaining. IV site in right forearm is without edema or erythema. Patient has been up about 1 hour today. Appetite has been good; ate 75% of breakfast and lunch. Received Vicodin [hydrocodone] tablets two at 1400 [2 p.m.] for pain in right leg. Intake 480 mL IV, 350 mL oral; voided 650 mL of clear, amber urine. Lung sounds clear except for fine crackles in base of right lung. She is expectorating a small amount of clear mucus. No dyspnea noted. Bowel sounds present; abdomen soft. Had moderate amount soft brown stool. Pedal pulses 2+ in strength bilaterally. Has a 2- to 3-cm stasis ulcer of right leg, treated with whirlpool and Hydrogel dressing. The dressing is to be changed every 24 hours; antiembolic hose are on. There is an order for Hematest of stools ×3, midstream urine for C&S, and a chest x-ray. She is to be NPO after midnight for surgery at 900 [9 a.m.] for débridement of the ulcer of her right leg. A preoperative consent form is needed. Social services will be seeing the patient and her daughter Ann Z. for discharge planning a few days after surgery.

BP, Blood pressure; *C&S*, culture and sensitivity (testing); *D_5W*, dextrose 5% in water solution; *IV*, intravenous; *KCl*, potassium chloride; *NPO*, nothing-by-mouth status.

- Assessment data that are pertinent to the patient
- Dressing changes, amount and color of exudate, and the condition of any incisions or wounds
- Any abnormal signs and symptoms, such as dyspnea, tachycardia, or abnormal mental status or level of consciousness
- Neurologic deficits

MALPRACTICE INSURANCE

Malpractice insurance for nurses is becoming increasingly important in a society that has become litigious. Paying for the defense of a lawsuit and any possible judgment is beyond the financial means of most people. To protect their employees and themselves against any legal and financial consequences that have potential to arise from provision of services, institutional employers carry malpractice liability insurance. Because individuals are responsible for their own actions, it is still possible for an employee to be sued personally. This is true even in states in which charitable immunity—the protection of nonprofit hospitals from legal liability—applies.

Some nurses choose to obtain a personal professional liability (malpractice) insurance policy separate from the employer's policy. The decision about whether to carry malpractice insurance is a personal choice. When making this decision, consider your state's malpractice compensation law, as well as the amount and type of malpractice insurance that your facility carries. Enlist the help of a knowledgeable expert to determine what, if any, additional amounts (dollar value) and type (occurrence or claims-based) of personal coverage is necessary or desired. (See Chapter 2 for further discussion of liability and professional liability insurance.)

BURNOUT

The term *burnout* has been used frequently over the years in health care. Maslach and Jackson (1986) identified **burnout** as a state of emotional exhaustion, depersonalization (responding in an impersonal manner toward patients/clients), and reduced sense of personal accomplishment in one's work, seen among human service, education, business, and government professions. The symptoms of burnout may include physical, psychological, and behavioral changes. Burnout in nursing today often is attributed to higher acuity levels in facilities, less available support staff, and the nursing shortage. Burnout may lead to more job turnover and patients' dissatisfaction with care being received from nurses. In one study an estimated 60% of staff interviewed reported feelings consistent with burnout (Monegain, 2013). The significance of burnout on the health care workplace can be underscored by the reports that the greatest challenge for health care administrative teams is the need to uplift the morale of the care team. This was prioritized above the recruitment and compensation of workers.

Signs and Symptoms of Burnout

Be aware of your feelings and emotional state to be alert to signs of burnout.

Box 58.13 identifies physical, psychological, and spiritual symptoms of burnout. Burnout is characterized by constant exhaustion, depression, irritability, insomnia, negative feelings toward one's job, difficulty focusing, becoming emotionally detached, and believing that one's actions do not make a difference to other people.

For the nurse experiencing burnout, it becomes increasingly difficult to delegate responsibility because of the fear that others may not perform a task as well. There seems to be less and less time available, and the nurse finds little time for replenishing the self. Time for other people (e.g., family or friends) is limited, and every demand on the nurse's time seems like an intrusion. The nurse is always tired and preoccupied with work and rarely experiences emotional pleasure.

Self-needs become buried by rationalizations, such as "As soon as I get the unit staffed…" or "As soon as I get my degree…" Despite working harder and enjoying it less, the nurse feels alone and isolated, misunderstood, and unappreciated. Repressed self-needs find maladaptive expression in overeating, overspending, addictions, snapping at family, or avoiding friends. Insomnia during the week, preoccupation with tasks, and utter exhaustion on the weekend or days off suggest a serious imbalance in lifestyle.

Box 58.13 Symptoms of Burnout

PHYSICAL
- Fatigue
- Changes in sleeping, eating
- Lack of energy
- Loss of interest in sex

PSYCHOLOGICAL
- Irritability
- Hypersensitivity
- Frustration
- Negative outlook
- Forgetting

SPIRITUAL
- Loss of commitment
- Loss of meaning
- Loss of integrity

Strategies for Burnout Prevention

Awareness. The first step in burnout prevention is awareness. Deliberately reflecting on the stress in one's life immediately puts it in perspective. If in doubt, ask colleagues as well as family and friends if they perceive any signs or symptoms of burnout. Solutions become possible once the problem is identified.

Balance. Another important step in dealing with or preventing burnout is restoring balance to one's life. A *healthy balance* among work, family, leisure, and lifelong learning enhances personal judgments, satisfaction, and productivity. Actively scheduling time for each of these activities is the best way to ensure that time will be made for them.

Choice. People experiencing burnout usually do not think they have any choice other than to keep doing what they have been doing, but life is a series of choices and negotiations. Nurses are especially fortunate in that there are a number of career paths in nursing. Transfers within facilities are usually available for the nurse who experiences burnout while working on a particular unit or department in a facility. Another option is employment in a totally different field of nursing by leaving the current place of employment for another. Choosing not to delegate tasks is another cause of burnout, so it is important for the nurse to learn to delegate appropriately.

Compartmentalizing. Being able to compartmentalize responsibilities helps the nurse complete as much of a job at hand as possible. Focusing on a job or project to the best of one's ability and then, at the end of the day or the time designated to the project, dropping it completely helps prevent burnout. Saying to oneself that something is "sufficient for the day" is a stress management strategy that puts boundaries on life tasks.

Altruistic egoism. Potential burnout victims generally put everyone and everything ahead of themselves. They ignore their own needs or minimize their importance. *Altruistic egoism* simply means paying as much attention to your own personal needs as you do to the needs of others. Although this seems obvious, many nurses consider paying attention to their own needs as being selfish. Nothing is further from the truth. In the long run, a balance between self-needs and the needs of others enhances the quality of care that the nurse is able to give to patients.

Focus. People who are focused are often able to achieve their goals more easily than other people. Focusing full energy on one thing at a time and finishing one project before starting another has several benefits: It is more likely that a person will enjoy each activity more, and being able to give full attention will make for a better product. A powerful contributor to the development of burnout is having several unfinished projects all demanding similar amounts of one's attention.

Goals. This step is closely aligned with focus, with an emphasis on outcome. An excellent burnout prevention strategy is identifying goals that are realistic, achievable, and in line with one's personal values. Being able to identify goals and the path to achieve goals enhances the chance for success.

Hope. People who feel burned out experience helplessness and hopelessness about changing their situation. The despair that accompanies emptiness and futility can be reversed by simply seeking out connections with other people who are empathetic. Their advice and caring support, even in one encounter, is a considerable antidote to inner emptiness. However, be sure to seek support from people who will help in developing solutions and not merely sympathize with how horrible the situation is. A solution-focused, rather than problem-oriented, approach is essential in the development of hope.

Integrity. Restoring personal integrity is important in the process of combating burnout. It is easy for the nurse experiencing burnout to lose sight of personal values. The nurse forgets what is important to him or her and instead tries to conform to others' expectations. Recognizing and reversing this process can go a long way in reversing burnout.

CHEMICALLY IMPAIRED NURSES

Chemical impairment is a concern for the nursing profession. At any given time an estimated 10% to 15% of nurses are impaired or in a recovery program. The number of nurses who illegally use drugs and abuse alcohol will continue to increase as addiction to drugs and alcohol increases in the general population (Thomas, 2011). Some of the excuses that nurses give for resorting to using drugs, alcohol, or both include job-related stress, inability to cope with changes in the workplace, overwhelming personal responsibilities, a feeling of frustration and helplessness in their personal and professional lives, and easy access to drugs. Addiction may begin as a workplace injury, requiring medications to manage, which eventually spiral out of control. The work environment of nurses allows a unique level of access to addictive medications.

Addiction is a chronic disease much like diabetes or hypertension. It requires the same care and ongoing attention and management. Nurses should receive the same care and support as other people with an addiction. With proper treatment, nurses can remain employed in their field and be able to provide quality care to their patients.

Each state's board of nursing has implemented nurse assistance programs to meet the needs of chemically impaired nurses. The makeup and monitoring of each state's program varies by statute. Many programs are abstinence based. This means that upon entry to the program full compliance requires that all addicting substances be discontinued. This can be a challenge because a nurse may have a chronic condition that is managed by a prescription medication that is not allowed for a nurse in monitoring. In this case efforts are made using a team approach between the nurse's physician and the nurse assistance program. Monitoring of the nurse in recovery includes counseling; random, unannounced urine drug screenings; worksite monitor reports; and participation in group activities such as Alcoholics Anonymous. There is often a change to the status of the nurse's license to practice nursing. If the addiction is deemed to be out of control and the nurse a danger to him- or herself, the license may be suspended. Probation commonly is imposed to allow the nurse the opportunity to work while providing oversight safeguards.

It is the nurse's responsibility to himself or herself and to the patients being cared for to avoid the abuse of prescription or nonprescription medications. If a nurse or a coworker does become addicted to drugs or alcohol, the only option is to seek immediate assistance. Referring oneself or someone else to the state board of nursing for voluntary treatment and a rehabilitation program may not only save a career but also save a life. See Chapter 36 for further discussion of chemical dependency.

Get Ready for the NCLEX® Examination!

Key Points

- Today's health care system is complex with a highly competitive job market.
- A well-prepared résumé broadens interview opportunities.
- An interview is important; every effort should be made to guarantee a successful one.
- Learning does not cease after graduation; it is a continuous process. The LPN/LVN must stay current with new concepts and technologies.
- Various job opportunities are available to new graduates. Each option requires considerable thought.
- A mentor is a nurse with more experience and knowledge who is able and willing to assist a novice nurse to learn the skills of the profession.
- Nursing care continues 24 hours a day in facilities to ensure continuity of care for all patients.
- LPN/LVNs are legally liable for their actions; therefore they need to understand the legal framework within which they are practicing.
- Endorsement or reciprocity enables the nurse to practice in another state without retaking the NCLEX-PN.
- The National Council of State Boards of Nursing has adopted computerized adaptive testing for the NCLEX-PN.
- The nurse practice act is the licensing law.
- It is a good idea for the LPN/LVN to take advantage of the knowledge available from certification seminars or self-guided study courses.
- The main function of a state board of nursing is to ensure safety for consumers of nursing services.
- Licensure permits people to offer special skills to the public, but it also provides legal guidelines for protection of the public.
- Leadership skills are an important aspect of nursing today.
- Although no single leadership style is always best, the overall approach of a leader has to foster the professional growth of other people and facilitate their professional development so that they become less dependent on the leader.
- The more that nurse managers adapt their leadership styles to work situations and the needs and abilities of staff, the more effective they are as managers.
- Effective problem-solving skills are key for providing quality nursing care.
- Nursing informatics continues to influence the delivery of nursing care.
- Correct procedure and facility policy should be followed in transcribing health care providers' orders.
- The health care provider is in charge of directing the patient's care, and nurses carry out the health care provider's orders, unless they believe that the orders are in error or will be harmful to the patient.
- The purpose of the change-of-shift report is to communicate pertinent patient information accurately from staff of one shift to staff of another.
- Burnout occurs more often in people who have excessive expectations of themselves and who believe that they need to do everything correctly. Nurses are especially prone to this characteristic.
- Malpractice insurance is available to nurses.

Additional Learning Resources

SG Go to your Study Guide for additional learning activities to help you master this chapter content.

evolve Be sure to visit the Evolve site at *http://evolve.elsevier.com/Cooper/foundationsadult/* for additional online resources.

Review Questions for the NCLEX® Examination

1. Which are functions of the state board of nursing? *(Select all that apply.)*
   1. Assisting health care facilities in the training of nursing staff
   2. Imposing discipline on a nursing license
   3. Monitoring the schools of nursing within the state
   4. Approving the students admitted to nursing programs in the state
   5. Enforcement of the state's nurse practice act
2. Which organizations are totally committed to practical and vocational nursing and its continuing education? *(Select all that apply.)*
   1. APNES
   2. ANA
   3. NFLPN
   4. NCSBN
3. The LPN/LVN has been hired at a long-term care facility. The nurse questions if the role will include supervision of other staff members. What response is most correct? *(Select all that apply.)*
   1. "You will be expected to organize and delegate as needed the care of patients on the unit of care."
   2. "You will be expected to supervise any nurse on your assigned wing who has less seniority."
   3. "The limit of charge or supervisory roles expected of the LPN/LVN is low."
   4. "In the long-term care setting you may find you are in a leadership role."
   5. "It is expected that you would supervise those staff members having less scope of practice than the LPN/LVN."
4. What is the main purpose of state requirements that nurses be licensed to practice nursing?
   1. To protect the LPN/LVN employer and the nurse
   2. To provide legal guidelines to protect the public
   3. To protect the patient and employer
   4. To protect the LPN/LVN from malpractice lawsuits

5. The style of leadership that takes into account the style of the leader, the maturity of the groups, and the circumstances at hand is which type of leadership style?
  1. Autocratic
  2. Situational
  3. Democratic
  4. Laissez-faire

6. When transcribing orders, the LPN/LVN knows that which health care provider order takes priority?
  1. prn orders
  2. One-time-only orders
  3. Routine orders
  4. Stat orders

7. Which act of the state legislature delineates the legal scope of the practice of nursing within the geographic boundaries of the jurisdiction?
  1. NLN Act
  2. Nurse practice act
  3. NCLEX Act
  4. JCOAH Act

8. In the change-of-shift report, which information should the outgoing nurse pass on to the receiving nurse? *(Select all that apply.)*
  1. The number of visitors that the patient has had during the shift
  2. The amount of time the patient has been able to nap during the shift
  3. The list of patient problem statements found in the care plan
  4. The patient's blood glucose levels for the shift
  5. The patient's total intake and output for the shift

9. Which statement best reflects the autocratic style of leadership?
  1. "Everyone knows their work assignment, so let's not meet together unless we have an unexpected crisis."
  2. "Let's discuss this case study thoroughly and decide on a plan of action as a group."
  3. "I'll consider each of your requests and then give you the guidelines for establishing new acuity ratings for our patients."
  4. "I'll try to pair you in comparable work teams, and we'll evaluate the success of this approach in 2 weeks."

10. Which actions demonstrate effective time management skills for the nurse? *(Select all that apply.)*
  1. Meeting all of the patient's major needs in the early morning hours
  2. Anticipating possible interruptions in the plan of care for the day
  3. Doing each of the patient's assessments and treatments individually at separate times
  4. Leaving each day unplanned to allow for adaptations in treatments
  5. Planning care based on prioritizing the needs of the patient

11. To settle a conflict between two staff members, the nurse manager should focus on which strategy?
  1. Developing a compromise solution to solve the conflict
  2. Investigating what the conflict parties want to achieve as an outcome
  3. Identifying the real issues and assisting in solving them
  4. Limiting the number of possible solutions to the conflict

12. Why is it beneficial to become certified in other areas after becoming an LPN/LVN?
  1. The certifications are designed to increase nursing knowledge and skill.
  2. The nurse will gradually be able to assume the work of an RN without becoming an RN.
  3. Use of the extended title(s) will improve the nurse's status among other employees and peers.
  4. Unless the state board of nursing acknowledges the certification, it serves no purpose.

13. Which is a primary function of the LPN/LVN?
  1. Teaching professional and practical nursing students
  2. Providing direct patient care
  3. Being in charge in various health care settings
  4. Directing nurses and other personnel who are employed in the hospital setting

14. The student nurse demonstrates understanding of the NCLEX-PN with which statement?
  1. "The NCLEX-PN measures the LPN/LVN student's ability to compete in the job market."
  2. "The NCLEX-PN measures the LPN/LVN student's entry-level competencies."
  3. "The NCLEX-PN measures the LPN/LVN student's proficiency-level competencies."
  4. "The NCLEX-PN measures success of the nursing program."

15. What will a new graduate include on a résumé? *(Select all that apply.)*
  1. Person to notify in an emergency
  2. Review of professional experience
  3. Grade transcripts from nursing schools
  4. Education history
  5. Only current work experience

16. What is a quality of an effective mentor?
  1. Inconsistent
  2. Unaccountable
  3. Inaccessible
  4. Informative

17. What will the nurse wish to consider when obtaining malpractice insurance?

1. Malpractice insurance is becoming less important for the nurse in today's health care environment.
2. If the employer has a claims-based policy in force, a personal policy is not necessary.
3. Most employers carry insurance for the employee, which will more than cover any expenses that will be incurred.
4. A separate personal malpractice insurance policy in addition to the employer's policy is a personal choice.

18. The nurse coworker of an LPN/LVN confides in the LPN/LVN that he is abusing alcohol. What is the best initial action for the LPN/LVN to take?

1. Talk to the coworker about the state's nurses assistance program for chemically impaired nurses.
2. Immediately report this information to the nurse manager.
3. Encourage the coworker to take a leave of absence from his current position.
4. Report the coworker to the state board of nursing.

appendix

A

Abbreviations

http://evolve.elsevier.com/Cooper/adult/

Common Abbreviations

ABBREVIATION	MEANING	ABBREVIATION	MEANING
°C	degrees Centigrade	CPR	cardiopulmonary resuscitation
°F	degrees Fahrenheit	CT	computed tomography
@	at	dL	deciliter
≥	greater than	DNR	do not resuscitate
≤	less than	DTR	deep tendon reflex
↑	increase	Dx, dx	diagnosis
↓	decrease	ECG, EKG	electrocardiogram
1°	primary	EEG	electroencephalogram
2°	secondary	elix	elixir
Δ	change	ER/ED	emergency room/department
ABGs	arterial blood gases	ESR	erythrocyte sedimentation rate
ac	before meals	ETOH	ethyl alcohol
ad lib	freely as desired	FUO	fever of unknown origin
ADL	activities of daily living	Fx, fx	fracture
AED	automated external defibrillator	g	gram
AIDS	acquired immunodeficiency disease syndrome	GI	gastrointestinal
		gr	grain
ama, AMA	against medical advice	gt; gtt	drop; drops
BE	barium enema	GTT	glucose tolerance test
bid	two times a day	h, hr	hour
BM	bowel movement	H&P	history and physical examination
BMI	body mass index	HCT, Hct	hematocrit
B/P, BP	blood pressure	Hgb	hemoglobin
BRP	bathroom privileges	HIV	human immunodeficiency virus
BSA	body surface area	hs	at bedtime
BUN	blood urea nitrogen	I&O	intake and output
C&S	culture and sensitivity	IM	intramuscular
$\bar{c}$	with	IV	intravenous
cap	capsule	IVP	intravenous push; intravenous pyelogram
CBC	complete blood count		
cc	cubic centimeter	K	potassium
CDC	Centers for Disease Control and Prevention	kg	kilogram
		KUB	kidney, ureters, and bladder (radiograph)
cm	centimeter		
c/o	complains of	KVO	keep vein open
CO	carbon monoxide	L	liter
CO_2	carbon dioxide	LLL	left lower lobe

Continued

Common Abbreviations—cont'd

ABBREVIATION	MEANING	ABBREVIATION	MEANING
LLQ	left lower quadrant	PO, po	orally, per os
LUL	left upper lobe	prn	as often as necessary, when required
LMP	last menstrual period	q	every
LOC	level of consciousness	qid	four times a day
LUQ	left upper quadrant	RLL	right lower lobe
M	meter	RLQ	right lower quadrant
mcg	microgram	ROM	range of motion
mg	milligram	RUL	right upper lobe
mL	milliliter	RUQ	right upper quadrant
mm	millimeter	Rx	treatment
mm Hg	millimeters of mercury	$\bar{s}$	without
MRI	magnetic resonance imaging	Sub-Q, subcut	subcutaneous
NG	nasogastric	$\dot{\bar{s}}\dot{s}$	half
NKA	no known allergies	SSE	soapsuds enema
NPO	nothing per os, nothing by mouth	stat	immediately
O_2	oxygen	tid	three times a day
OD	optical density; overdose	TKO	to keep open
oz	ounce	TPN	total parenteral nutrition
pc	after meals	TPR	temperature, pulse, and respirations
PERRLA	pupils equal, round, and reactive to light and accommodation	TX	treatment
pH	hydrogen ion concentration (acidity and alkalinity)	WBC	white blood cell

The Joint Commission "Do Not Use" Abbreviation List*

DO NOT USE	POTENTIAL PROBLEM	USE INSTEAD
U, u (unit)	Mistaken for "0" (zero), the number "4" (four), or "cc"	Write "unit"
IU (International Unit)	Mistaken for IV (intravenous) or the number 10 (ten)	Write "International Unit"
Q.D., QD, q.d., qd (daily)	Mistaken for each other	Write "daily"
Q.O.D., QOD, q.o.d., qod (every other day)	Period after the Q mistaken for "I" and the "O" mistaken for "I"	Write "every other day"
Trailing zero (X.0 mg)[†]	Decimal point is missed	Write X mg
Lack of leading zero (.X mg)	Decimal point is missed	Write 0.X mg
MS	Can mean morphine sulfate or magnesium sulfate	Write "morphine sulfate"
MSO_4 and $MgSO_4$	Confused for one another	Write "magnesium sulfate"

*Applies to all orders and all medication-related documentation that is handwritten (including free-text computer entry) or on preprinted forms.

[†]EXCEPTION: A "trailing zero" may be used only where required to demonstrate the level of precision of the value being reported, such as for laboratory results, imaging studies that report size of lesions, or catheter/tube sizes. It may not be used in medication orders or other medication-related documentation.

appendix B

Laboratory Reference Values*

Reference Intervals for Hematology

TEST	CONVENTIONAL UNITS	SI UNITS
Acid hemolysis (Ham test)	No hemolysis	No hemolysis
Alkaline phosphatase, leukocyte	Total score, 14–100	Total score, 14–100
Cell counts		
Erythrocytes		
Males	4.6–6.2 million/mm^3	4.6–6.2 × 10^{12}/L
Females	4.2–5.4 million/mm^3	4.2–5.4 × 10^{12}/L
Children (varies with age)	4.5–5.1 million/mm^3	4.5–5.1 × 10^{12}/L
Leukocytes, total	4500–11,000/mm^3	4.5–11.0 × 10^9/L
Leukocytes, differential counts*		
Myelocytes	0%	0/L
Band neutrophils	3%–5%	150–400 × 10^6/L
Segmented neutrophils	54%–62%	3000–5800 × 10^6/L
Lymphocytes	25%–33%	1500–3000 × 10^6/L
Monocytes	3%–7%	300–500 × 10^6/L
Eosinophils	1%–3%	50–250 × 10^6/L
Basophils	0%–1%	15–50 × 10^6/L
Platelets	150,000–400,000/mm^3	150–400 × 10^9/L
Reticulocytes	25,000–75,000/mm^3	25–75 × 10^9/L
Coagulation tests	(0.5%–1.5% of erythrocytes)	
Bleeding time (template)	2.75–8.0 min	2.75–8.0 min
Coagulation time (glass tube)	5–15 min	5–15 min
D-Dimer	<0.5 mcg/mL	<0.5 mg/L
Factor VIII and other coagulation factors	50%–150% of normal	0.5–1.5 of normal
Fibrin split products (Thrombo-Welco test)	<10 mcg/mL	<10 mg/L
Fibrinogen	200–400 mg/dL	2.0–4.0 g/L
Partial thromboplastin time, activated (aPTT)	20–25 sec	20–35 sec
Prothrombin time (PT, Pro-time)	12.0–14.0 sec	12.0–14.0 sec
International normalized ratio (INR)	0.8–1.1	
Coombs' test		
Direct	Negative	Negative
Indirect	Negative	Negative
Corpuscular values of erythrocytes		
Mean corpuscular hemoglobin (MCH)	26–34 pg/cell	26–34 pg/cell
Mean corpuscular volume (MCV)	80–96 mm^3	80–96 fL
Mean corpuscular hemoglobin concentration (MCHC)	32–36 g/dL	320–360 g/L

Continued

*From Rakel RE, Bope ET: *Conn's current therapy,* Philadelphia, 2009, Saunders.

Reference Intervals for Hematology—cont'd

TEST	CONVENTIONAL UNITS	SI UNITS
Haptoglobin	20–165 mg/dL	0.20–1.65 g/L
Hematocrit		
Males	40–54 mL/dL	0.40–0.54
Females	37–47 mL/dL	0.37–0.47
Newborns	49–54 mL/dL	0.49–0.54
Children (varies with age)	35–49 mL/dL	0.35–0.49
Hemoglobin		
Males	13.0–18.0 g/dL	8.1–11.2 mmol/L
Females	12.0–16.0 g/dL	7.4–9.9 mmol/L
Newborns	16.5–19.5 g/dL	10.2–12.1 mmol/L
Children (varies with age)	11.2–16.5 g/dL	7.0–10.2 mmol/L
Hemoglobin, fetal	<1.0% of total	<0.01 of total
Hemoglobin A_{1C}	3%–5% of total	0.03–0.05 of total
Hemoglobin A_2	1.5%–3.0% of total	0.015–0.03 of total
Hemoglobin, plasma	0.0–5.0 mg/dL	0.0–3.2 μmol/L
Methemoglobin	30–130 mg/dL	19–80 μmol/L
Erythrocyte sedimentation rate (ESR)		
Wintrobe		
Males	0–5 mm/hr	0–5 mm/hr
Females	0–15 mm/hr	0–15 mm/hr
Westergren		
Males	0–15 mm/hr	0–15 mm/hr
Females	0–20 mm/hr	0–20 mm/hr

*Conventional units are percentages; SI units are absolute cell counts.
SI, International System of Units.

Reference Intervals* for Clinical Chemistry (Blood, Serum, and Plasma)

ANALYTE	CONVENTIONAL UNITS	SI UNITS
Acetoacetate plus acetone		
Qualitative	Negative	Negative
Quantitative	0.3–2.0 mg/dL	30–200 μmol/L
Acid phosphatase, serum (thymolphthalein monophosphate substrate)	0.1–0.6 units/L	0.1–0.6 units/L
ACTH (see Corticotropin)		
Alanine aminotransferase (ALT, serum (SGPT)	1–45 units/L	1–45 units/L
Albumin, serum	3.3–5.2 g/dL	33–52 g/L
Aldolase, serum	0.0–7.0 units/L	0.0–7.0 units/L
Aldosterone, plasma		
Standing	5–30 ng/dL	140–830 pmol/L
Recumbent	3–10 ng/dL	80–275 pmol/L
Alkaline, phosphatase (ALP), serum		
Adult	35–150 units/L	35–150 units/L
Adolescent	100–500 units/L	100–500 units/L
Child	100–350 units/L	100–350 units/L
Ammonia nitrogen, plasma	10–50 mmol/L	10–50 μmol/L
Amylase, serum	25–125 units/L	25–125 units/L

Reference Intervals* for Clinical Chemistry (Blood, Serum, and Plasma)—cont'd

ANALYTE	CONVENTIONAL UNITS	SI UNITS
Anion gap, serum calculated	8–16 mEq/L	8–16 mmol/L
Ascorbic acid, blood	0.4–1.5 mg/dL	23–85 µmol/L
Aspartate aminotransferase (AST), serum (SGOT)	1–36 units/L	1–36 units/L
Base excess, arterial blood, calculated	0 ±2 mEq/L	0 ±2 mmol/L
Bicarbonate		
Venous plasma	23–29 mEq/L	23–29 mmol/L
Arterial blood	21–27 mEq/L	21–27 mmol/L
Bile acids, serum	0.3–3.0 mg/dL	0.8–7.6 µmol/L
Bilirubin, serum		
Conjugated	0.1–0.4 mg/dL	1.7–6.8 µmol/L
Total	0.3–1.1 mg/dL	5.1–19.0 µmol/L
Calcium, serum	8.4–10.6 mg/dL	2.10–2.65 mmol/L
Calcium, ionized, serum	4.25–5.25 mg/dL	1.05–1.30 mmol/L
Carbon dioxide, total, serum or plasma	24–31 mEq/L	24–31 mmol/L
Carbon dioxide tension (PCO_2), blood	35–45 mm Hg	35–45 mm Hg
β-Carotene, serum	60–260 mcg/dL	1.1–8.6 µmol/L
Ceruloplasmin, serum	23–44 mg/dL	230–440 mg/L
Chloride, serum or plasma	96–106 mEq/L	96–106 mmol/L
Cholesterol, serum or EDTA plasma		
Desirable range	<200 mg/dL	5.20 mmol/L
Low-density lipoprotein (LDL) cholesterol	60–180 mg/dL	1.55–4.65 mmol/L
High-density lipoprotein (HDL) cholesterol	30–80 mg/dL	0.80–2.05 mmol/L
Copper	70–140 mcg/dL	11–22 µmol/L
Corticotropin (ACTH), plasma, 8 AM	10–80 pg/mL	2–18 pmol/L
Cortisol, plasma		
8:00 AM	6–23 mcg/dL	170–630 nmol/L
4:00 PM	3–15 mcg/dL	80–410 nmol/L
10:00 PM	<50% of 8:00 AM value	<50% of 8:00 AM value
Creatine, serum		
Males	0.2–0.5 mg/dL	15–40 µmol/L
Females	0.3–0.9 mg/dL	25–70 µmol/L
Creatine kinase (CK), serum		
Males	55–170 units/L	55–170 units/L
Females	30–135 units/L	30–135 units/L
Creatinine kinase MB isoenzyme, serum	<5% of total CK activity	<5% of total CK activity
	<5% of ng/mL by immunoassay	<5% of ng/mL by immunoassay
Creatinine, serum	0.6–1.2 mg/dL	50–110 µmol/L
Erythrocytes	145–540 ng/mL	330–120 nmol/L
Estradiol-17β, adult		
Males	10–65 pg/mL	35–240 pmol/L
Females		
Follicular	30–100 pg/mL	110–370 pmol/L
Ovulatory	200–400 pg/mL	730–1470 pmol/L
Luteal	50–140 pg/mL	180–510 pmol/L

Continued

Reference Intervals* for Clinical Chemistry (Blood, Serum, and Plasma)—cont'd

ANALYTE	CONVENTIONAL UNITS	SI UNITS
Ferritin, serum	20–200 ng/mL	20–200 mcg/L
Fibrinogen, plasma	200–400 mg/dL	2.0–4.0 g/L
Folate, serum	3–18 ng/mL	6.8–4.1 nmol/L
Follicle-stimulating hormone (FSH), plasma		
Males	4–25 mU/mL	4–25 units/L
Females, premenopausal	4–30 mU/mL	4–30 units/L
Females, postmenopausal	40–250 mU/mL	40–250 units/L
Gastrin, fasting, serum	0–100 pg/mL	0–100 mg/L
Glucose, fasting, plasma or serum	70–115 mg/dL	3.9–6.4 nmol/L
γ-Glutamyltransferase (GGT), serum	5–40 units/L	5–40 units/L
Growth hormone (hGH), plasma, adult, fasting	0–6 ng/mL	0–6 mcg/L
Haptoglobin, serum	20–165 mg/dL	0.20–1.65 g/L
Immunoglobulins, serum (see table of Reference Intervals for Tests of Immunologic Function)		
Iron, serum	75–175 mcg/dL	13–31 mmol/L
Iron-binding capacity, serum		
Total	250–410 mcg/dL	45–73 mmol/L
Saturation	20%–55%	0.20–0.55
Lactate		
Venous whole blood	5.0–20.0 mg/dL	0.6–2.2 mmol/L
Arterial whole blood	5.0–15.0 mg/dL	0.6–1.7 mmol/L
Lactate dehydrogenase (LD), serum	110–220 units/L	110–220 units/L
Lipase, serum	10–140 units/L	10–140 units/L
Lutropin (LH), serum		
Males	1–9 units/L	1–9 units/L
Females		
Follicular phase	2–10 units/L	2–10 units/L
Midcycle peak	15–65 units/L	15–65 units/L
Luteal phase	1–12 units/L	1–12 units/L
Postmenopausal	12–65 units/L	12–65 units/L
Magnesium, serum	1.3–2.1 mg/dL	0.65–1.05 mmol/L
Osmolality	275–295 mOsm/kg water	275–295 mOsm/kg water
Oxygen, blood, arterial, room air		
Partial pressure (PaO_2)	80–100 mm Hg	80–100 mm Hg
Saturation (SaO_2)	95%–98%	95%–98%
pH, arterial blood	7.35–7.45	7.35–7.45
Phosphate, inorganic, serum		
Adult	3.0–4.5 mg/dL	1.0–1.5 mmol/L
Child	4.0–7.0 mg/dL	1.3–2.3 mmol/L
Potassium		
Serum	3.5–5.0 mEq/L	3.5–5.0 mmol/L
Plasma	3.5–4.5 mEq/L	3.5–4.5 mmol/L
Progesterone, serum, adult		
Males	0.0–0.4 ng/mL	0.0–1.3 mmol/L
Females		
Follicular phase	0.1–1.5 ng/mL	0.3–4.8 mmol/L
Luteal phase	2.5–28.0 ng/mL	8.0–89.0 mmol/L

Reference Intervals* for Clinical Chemistry (Blood, Serum, and Plasma)—cont'd

ANALYTE	CONVENTIONAL UNITS	SI UNITS
Prolactin, serum		
Males	1.0–15.0 ng/mL	1.0–15.0 mcg/L
Females	1.0–20.0 ng/mL	1.0–20.0 mcg/L
Protein, serum, electrophoresis		
Total	6.0–8.0 g/dL	60–80 g/L
Albumin	3.5–5.5 g/dL	35–55 g/L
Globulins		
α_1	0.2–0.4 g/dL	2.0–4.0 g/L
α_2	0.5–0.9 g/dL	5.0–9.0 g/L
β	0.6–1.1 g/dL	6.0–11.0 g/L
γ	0.7–1.7 g/dL	7.0–17.0 g/L
Pyruvate, blood	0.3–0.9 mg/dL	0.03–0.10 mmol/L
Rheumatoid factor	0.0–30.0 IU/mL	0.0–30.0 kIU/L
Sodium, serum or plasma	135–145 mEq/L	135–145 mmol/L
Testosterone, plasma		
Males, adult	300–1200 ng/dL	10.4–41.6 nmol/L
Females, adult	20–75 ng/dL	0.7–2.6 nmol/L
Pregnant females	40–200 ng/dL	1.4–6.9 nmol/L
Thyroglobulin	3–42 ng/mL	3–42 mcg/L
Thyrotropin (hTSH), serum	0.4–4.8 mIU/mL	0.4–4.8 mIU/L
Thyrotropin-releasing hormone (TRH)	5–60 pg/mL	5–60 ng/L
Thyroxine (FT_4), free, serum	0.9–2.1 ng/dL	12–27 pmol/L
Thyroxine (T_4), serum	4.5–12.0 mcg/mL	58–154 nmol/L
Thyroxine-binding globulin (TBG)	15.0–34.0 mcg/mL	15.0–34.0 mg/L
Transferrin	250–430 mg/dL	2.5–4.3 g/L
Triglycerides, serum, after 12-hr fast	40–150 mg/dL	0.4–1.5 g/L
Triiodothyronine (T_3), serum	70–190 ng/dL	1.1–2.9 nmol/L
Triiodothyronine uptake, resin (T_3RU)	25%–38%	0.25–0.38
Troponin I	0.05–0.50 ng/mL	0.05–0.5 ng/mL
Urate		
Males	2.5–8.0 mg/dL	150–480 μmol/L
Females	2.2–7.0 mg/dL	130–420 μmol/L
Urea, serum or plasma	24–49 mg/dL	4.0–8.2 nmol/L
Urea, nitrogen, serum or plasma	11–23 mg/dL	8.0–16.4 nmol/L
Viscosity, serum	1.1–1.8 × water	1.1–1.8 × water
Vitamin A, serum	20–80 mcg/dL	0.70–2.80 mcmol/L
Vitamin B_{12}, serum	180–900 pg/mL	133–664 pmol/L

*Reference values may vary depending on the method and sample source used.
EDTA, Ethylenediaminetetraacetic acid; *SI,* International System of Units.

Reference Intervals for Therapeutic Drug Monitoring (Serum or Plasma)*

ANALYTE	THERAPEUTIC RANGE	TOXIC CONCENTRATIONS	PROPRIETARY NAME(S)
Analgesics			
acetaminophen	10–40 mcg/mL	>150 mcg/mL	Tylenol, Datril
salicylate	100–250 mcg/mL	>300 mcg/mL	Aspirin, Bufferin
Antibiotics			
amikacin	20–30 mcg/mL	*Peak* >35 mcg/mL *Trough* >10 mcg/mL	Amkin
gentamicin	5–10 mcg/mL	*Peak* >10 mcg/mL *Trough* >2 mcg/mL	Garamycin
tobramycin	5–10 mcg/mL	*Peak* >10 mcg/mL *Trough* >2 mcg/mL	Nebcin
vancomycin	5–35 mcg/mL	*Peak* >40 mcg/mL *Trough* >10 mcg/mL	Vancocin
Anticonvulsants			
carbamazepine	5–12 mcg/mL	>15 mcg/mL	Tegretol
ethosuximide	40–100 mcg/mL	>250 mcg/mL	Zarontin
phenobarbital	15–40 mcg/mL	40–100 ng/mL (varies widely)	Luminal
phenytoin	10–20 mcg/mL	>20 mcg/mL	Dilantin
primidone	5–12 mcg/mL	>15 mcg/mL	Mysoline
valproic acid	50–100 mcg/mL	>100 mcg/mL	Depakene
Antineoplastics and Immunosuppressives			
cyclosporine A	150–350 ng/mL	>400 ng/mL	Sandimmune
methotrexate, high-dose, 48 hr	Variable	>1 µmol/L, 48 hr after dose	
sirolimus (within 1 hr of 2-mg dose)	4.5–14 ng/mL	Variable	Rapamune
sirolimus (within 1 hr of 5-mg dose)	10–28 ng/mL	Variable	Rapamune
tacrolimus (FK-506), whole blood	3–20 mcg/L	>15 mcg/L	Prograf
Bronchodilators and Respiratory Stimulants			
caffeine	3–15 ng/mL	>30 mcg/mL	Elixophyllin
theophylline (aminophylline)	10–20 mcg/mL	>30 mcg/mL	Quibron
Cardiovascular Drugs			
amiodarone (obtain specimen more than 8 hr after last dose)	1.0–2.0 mcg/mL	>2.0 mcg/mL	Cordarone
digoxin (obtain specimen more than 6 hr after last dose)	0.8–2.0 mcg/mL	>2.4 ng/mL	Lanoxin
disopyramide	2–5 mcg/mL	>7 mcg/mL	Norpace
flecainide	0.2–1.0 mcg/mL	>0.1 mcg/mL	Tambocor
lidocaine	1.5–5.0 mcg/mL	>6 mcg/mL	Xylocaine
mexiletine	0.7–2.0 mcg/mL	>2 mcg/mL	Mexitil
procainamide	4–10 mcg/mL	>12 mcg/mL	Pronestyl
procainamide plus NAPA (*N*-acetyl procainamide)	8–30 mcg/mL	>30 mcg/mL	
propranolol	50–100 ng/mL	Variable	Inderal
quinidine	2–5 mcg/mL	>6 mcg/mL	Cardioquin, Quinaglute
tocainide	4–10 ng/mL	>10 ng/mL	Tonocard

Reference Intervals for Therapeutic Drug Monitoring (Serum or Plasma)*—cont'd

ANALYTE	THERAPEUTIC RANGE	TOXIC CONCENTRATIONS	PROPRIETARY NAME(S)
Psychopharmacological Drugs			
amitriptyline	120–150 ng/mL	>500 ng/mL	Elavil, Triavil
bupropion	25–100 ng/mL	Not applicable	Wellbutrin
desipramine	150–300 ng/mL	>500 ng/mL	Norpramin
imipramine	125–250 ng/mL	>400 ng/mL	Tofranil
lithium (obtain specimen 12 hr after last dose)	0.6–1.5 mEq/L	>1.5 mEq/L	Lithobid
nortriptyline	50–150 ng/mL	>500 ng/mL	Aventyl, Pamelor

*Values may vary depending on the method and sample collection device used. Always consult the reference values provided by the laboratory performing the analysis.

Reference Intervals* for Clinical Chemistry (Urine)

ANALYTE	CONVENTIONAL UNITS	SI UNITS
Acetone and acetoacetate, qualitative	Negative	Negative
Albumin		
Qualitative	Negative	Negative
Quantitative	10–100 mg/24 hr	0.15–1.5 µmol/day
Aldosterone	3–20 mcg/24 hr	8.3–55 nmol/day
D-Aminolevulinic acid (d-ALA)	1.3–7.0 mg/24 hr	10–53 µmol/day
Amylase	<17 units/hr	<17 units/hr
Amylase-to-creatinine clearance ratio	0.01–0.04	0.01–0.04
Bilirubin, qualitative	Negative	Negative
Calcium (regular diet)	<250 mg/24 hr	<6.3 nmol/day
Catecholamines		
Epinephrine	<10 mcg/24 hr	<55 nmol/day
Norepinephrine	<100 mcg/24 hr	<590 nmol/day
Total free catecholamines	4–126 mcg/24 hr	24–745 nmol/day
Total metanephrines	0.1–1.6 mg/24 hr	0.5–8.1 µmol/day
Chloride (varies with intake)	110–250 mEq/24 hr	110–250 mmol/day
Copper	0–50 mcg/24 hr	0.0–0.80 µmol/day
Cortisol, free	10–100 mcg/24 hr	27.6–276 nmol/day
Creatine		
Males	0–40 mg/24 hr	0.0–0.30 mmol/day
Females	0–80 mg/24 hr	0.0–0.60 mmol/day
Creatinine	15–25 mg/kg/24 hr	0.13–0.22 mmol/kg/day
Creatinine clearance (endogenous)		
Males	110–150 mL/min/1.73 m^2	110–150 mL/min/1.73 m^2
Females	105–132 mL/min/1.73 m^2	105–132 mL/min/1.73 m^2
Cystine or cysteine	Negative	Negative
Dehydroepiandrosterone		
Males	0.2–2.0 mg/24hr	0.7–6.9 µmol/day
Females	0.2–1.8 mg/24hr	0.7–6.2 µmol/day
Estrogens, total		
Males	4–25 mcg/24 hr	14–90 nmol/day
Females	5–100 mcg/24 hr	18–360 nmol/day
Glucose (as reducing substance)	<250 mg/24 hr	<250 mg/day

Continued

Reference Intervals* for Clinical Chemistry (Urine)—cont'd

ANALYTE	CONVENTIONAL UNITS	SI UNITS
Hemoglobin and myoglobin, qualitative	Negative	Negative
Hemogentisic acid, qualitative	Negative	Negative
17-Hydroxycorticosteroids		
Males	3–9 mg/24 hr	8.3–25 µmol/day
Females	2–8 mg/24 hr	5.5–22 µmol/day
5-Hydroxyindoleacetic acid		
Qualitative	Negative	Negative
Quantitative	2–6 mg/24 hr	10–31 µmol/day
17-Ketogenic steroids		
Males	5–23 mg/24 hr	17–80 µmol/day
Females	3–15 mg/24 hr	10–52 µmol/day
17-Ketosteroids		
Males	8–22 mg/24 hr	28–76 µmol/day
Females	6–15 mg/24 hr	21–52 µmol/day
Magnesium	6–10 mEq/24 hr	3–5 mmol/day
Metanephrines	0.05–1.2 ng/mg creatinine	0.03–0.70 mmol/mmol creatinine
Osmolality	38–1400 mOsm/kg water	38–1400 mOsm/kg water
pH	4.6–8.0	4.6–8.0
Phenylpyruvic acid, qualitative	Negative	Negative
Phosphate	0.4–1.3 g/24 hr	13–42 mmol/day
Porphobilinogen		
Qualitative	Negative	Negative
Quantitative	<2 mg/24 hr	<9 µmol/day
Porphyrins		
Coproporphyrin	50–250 mcg/24 hr	77–380 nmol/day
Uroporphyrin	10–30 mcg/24 hr	12–36 nmol/day
Potassium	25–125 mEq/24 hr	25–125 mmol/day
Pregnanediol		
Males	0.0–1.9 mg/24 hr	0.0–6.0 µmol/day
Females		
Proliferative phase	0.0–2.6 mg/24 hr	0.0–8.0 µmol/day
Luteal phase	2.6–10.6 mg/24 hr	8–33 µmol/day
Postmenopausal	0.2–1.0 mg/24 hr	0.6–3.1 µmol/day
Pregnanetriol	0.0–2.5 mg/24 hr	0.0–7.4 µmol/day
Protein, total		
Qualitative	Negative	Negative
Quantitative	10–150 mg/24 hr	10–150 mg/day
Protein-to-creatinine ratio	<0.2	<0.2
Sodium (regular diet)	60–260 mEq/24 hr	60–260 mmol/day
Specific gravity		
Random specimen	1.003–1.030	1.003–1.030
24-hr collection	1.015–1.025	1.015–1.025
Urate (regular diet)	250–750 mg/24 hr	1.5–4.4 mmol/day
Urobilinogen	0.5–4.0 mg/24 hr	0.6–6.8 µmol/day
Vanillylmandelic acid (VMA)	1.0–8.0 mg/24 hr	5–40 µmol/day

*Values may vary depending on the method used.
SI, International System of Units.

Reference Intervals for Toxic Substances

ANALYTE	CONVENTIONAL UNITS	SI UNITS
Arsenic, urine	<130 mcg/24 hr	<1.7 µmol/day
Bromides, serum, inorganic	<100 mg/dL	<10 mmol/L
Toxic symptoms	140–1000 mg/dL	14–100 mmol/L
Carboxyhemoglobin, blood	Saturation, percent	
Urban environment	<5%	<0.05
Smokers	<12%	<0.12
Symptoms		
Headache	>15%	>0.15
Nausea and vomiting	>25%	>0.25
Potentially lethal	>50%	>0.50
Ethanol, blood	<0.05 mg/dL, 0.005%	<1.0 mmol/L
Intoxication	>100 mg/dL, 0.1%	>22 mmol/L
Marked intoxication	300–400 mg/dL, 0.3%–0.4%	65–87 mmol/L
Alcoholic stupor	400–500 mg/dL, 0.4%–0.5%	87–109 mmol/L
Coma	>500 mg/dL, 0.5%	>109 mmol/L
Lead, blood		
Adults	<20 mcg/dL	<1.0 µmol/L
Children	<10 mcg/dL	<0.5 µmol/L
Lead, urine	<80 mcg/24 hr	<0.4 µmol/day
Mercury, urine	<10 mcg/24 hr	<150 nmol/day

SI, International System of Units.

Reference Intervals for Tests Performed on Cerebrospinal Fluid

TEST	CONVENTIONAL UNITS	SI UNITS
Cells	<5 mm^3; all mononuclear	<5 × 10^6/L; all mononuclear
Protein electrophoresis	Albumin predominant	Albumin predominant
Glucose	50–75 mg/dL (20 mg/dL less than in serum)	2.8–4.2 mmol/L (1.1 mmol/L less than in serum)
IgG		
Children, <14 yr	<8% of total protein	<0.08 of total protein
Adults	<14% of total protein	<0.14 of total protein
IgG index	0.3–0.6	0.3–0.6
Oligoclonal banding on electrophoresis	Absent	Absent
Pressure, opening	70–180 mm H_2O	70–180 mm H_2O
Protein, total	<15–45 mg/dL	150–450 mg/L

SI, International System of Units.

Reference Intervals for Tests of Gastrointestinal Function

TEST	CONVENTIONAL UNITS
Bentiromide	6-hr urinary arylamine excretion .57% excludes pancreatic insufficiency
β-Carotene, serum	60–250 ng/dL
Fecal fat estimation	
Qualitative	No fat globules seen by high-power microscope
Quantitative	<6 g/24 hr (>95% coefficient of fat absorption)
Gastric acid output	
Basal	
Males	0.0–10.5 mmol/hr
Females	0.0–5.6 mmol/hr
Maximum (after histamine or pentagastrin)	
Males	9.0–48.0 mmol/hr
Females	6.0–31.0 mmol/hr
Ratio: basal/maximum	
Males	0.0–0.31
Females	0.0–0.29
Secretion test, pancreatic fluid	
Volume	>1.8 mL/kg/hr
Bicarbonate	>80 mEq/L
D-Xylose absorption test, urine	>20% of ingested dose excreted in 5 hr

Reference Intervals for Tests of Immunologic Function

TEST	CONVENTIONAL UNITS	SI UNITS
Autoantibodies, Serum, Adult		
Anti-CCP antibody	0–19 units	
Anti-dsDNA antibody	0–40 IU	0–40 IU
Antinuclear antibody	<1:40	
Rheumatoid factor (total IgG, IgA, IgM)	0–30 mg/dL	
Complement, Serum		
C3	85–175 mg/dL	0.85–1.75 g/L
C4	15–45 mg/dL	150–450 mg/L
Total hemolytic (CH_{50})	150–250 units/mL	150–250 units/mL
Immunoglobulins, Serum, Adult		
IgA	70–310 mg/dL	0.70–3.1 g/L
IgD	0.0–6.0 mg/dL	0.0–60 g/L
IgE	0.0–430 mg/dL	0.0–430 mg/L
IgG	640–1350 ng/dL	6.4–13.5 mcg/L
IgM	90–350 mg/dL	0.90–3.5 g/L

Anti-CCP, Anticyclic citrullinated peptide; *dsDNA*, double-stranded DNA; *Ig*, immunoglobulin; *SI*, International System of Units.

Reference Intervals for Lymphocytes Subsets, Whole Blood, Heparinized

ANTIGEN(S) EXPRESSED	CELL TYPE	PERCENTAGE	ABSOLUTE CELL COUNT
CD2	E rosette T cells	73–87	860–1880
CD3	Total T cells	56–77	140–370
CD3 and CD4	Helper-inducer cells	32–54	550–1190
CD3 and CD8	Suppressor-cytotoxic cells	24–37	430–1060
CD3 and DR	Activated T cells	5–14	70–310
CD16 and CD56	Natural killer (NK) cells	8–22	130–500
CD19	Total B cells	7–17	140–370

Helper-to-suppressor ratio: 0.8–1.8.

Reference Values for Semen Analysis

TEST	CONVENTIONAL UNITS	SI UNITS
Volume	2–5 mL	2–5 mL
Liquefaction	Complete in 15 min	Complete in 15 min
pH	7.2–8.0	7.2–8.0
Leukocytes	Occasional or absent	Occasional or absent
Spermatozoa		
Count	60–150 × 10^6 mL	60–150 × 10^6 mL
Motility	>80% motile	>0.80 motile
Morphology	80%–90% normal forms	>0.80–0.90 normal
Fructose	>150 mg/dL	>8.33 mmol/L

SI, International System of Units.

appendix C

Answers to Review Questions for the NCLEX® Examination

Chapter 1

1. 1
2. 4
3. 4
4. 4
5. 1
6. 3
7. 2
8. 3
9. 4
10. 3
11. 1
12. 2
13. 1
14. 2
15. 4
16. 1, 2, 5
17. 2, 4, 5

Chapter 2

1. 3
2. 3
3. 2
4. 4
5. 3
6. 1
7. 2
8. 1
9. 3
10. 2
11. 2
12. 1
13. 1
14. 4
15. 2
16. 3, 4
17. 1, 3, 4
18. 2, 4

Chapter 3

1. 1
2. 4
3. 3
4. 2, 5
5. 1
6. 3
7. 1
8. 4
9. 3, 5
10. 4
11. 4
12. 1
13. 2
14. 1, 4
15. 4
16. 1, 3, 5
17. 2
18. 1
19. 4

Chapter 4

1. 1
2. 4
3. 2
4. 2
5. 3, 5
6. 2
7. 4
8. 4, 5
9. 1, 5
10. 2
11. 2
12. 1
13. 2
14. 2
15. 1, 5
16. 2
17. 1
18. 4
19. 3, 5
20. 3

Chapter 5

1. 2, 5
2. 3
3. 3, 5
4. 1
5. 3
6. 4, 5
7. 4
8. 3
9. 2
10. 4
11. 3
12. 4
13. 4
14. 1
15. 3, 5
16. 3
17. 4
18. 2, 4

Chapter 6

1. 3
2. 3
3. 2
4. 2
5. 3
6. 3
7. 2
8. 3
9. 2
10. 2
11. 3
12. 4
13. 1
14. 4
15. 2, 3
16. 2
17. Cultural competence

Chapter 7

1. 1
2. 3
3. 1
4. 3
5. 4
6. 4
7. 2
8. 4
9. 1, 5
10. 1
11. 1
12. 1
13. 1, 2, 4, 3
14. 3
15. 2
16. 2
17. 4
18. 3
19. 1
20. 2

Chapter 8

1. 3
2. 1
3. 2
4. 1
5. 3
6. 2
7. 1
8. 4
9. 4
10. 3
11. 2
12. 2
13. 1, 2
14. 4
15. 1
16. 3
17. 2, 3, 5
18. 1, 3, 4, 5
19. 1
20. 4

Chapter 9

1. 2, 3
2. 3
3. 2
4. 4
5. 4
6. 2, 5
7. 1
8. 1
9. 4
10. 3
11. 3
12. 4
13. 3, 4, 5
14. 4
15. 3
16. 3
17. 3
18. 4
19. 2
20. 1, 4

Chapter 10

1. 3, 5
2. 1
3. 2
4. 1, 2, 5
5. 1
6. 1, 4
7. 4
8. 3, 5
9. 4
10. 1
11. 4
12. 2
13. 1
14. 4
15. 4

Chapter 11

1. 1, 5
2. 1
3. 4
4. 4
5. 1
6. 4
7. 2

8. 4, 5
9. 2
10. 4
11. 1, 5
12. 4
13. 3, 5
14. 2
15. 1, 4, 3, 2

Chapter 12

1. 2
2. 2
3. 3
4. 2
5. 2
6. 4
7. 2
8. 4
9. 4
10. 4, 5
11. 38
12. 3
13. 1
14. 2, 3, 1, 4
15. 2
16. 4, 5
17. 4
18. 1
19. 3
20. 2
21. 2
22. 1
23. 2, 5
24. 1
25. 2, 5
26. 1
27. 1 liter

Chapter 13

1. 1, 2, 3, 5
2. 1
3. 3
4. 3
5. 2
6. 1
7. 1, 2, 3, 5
8. 1
9. 2
10. 2
11. 3
12. 3, 5
13. 3
14. 1
15. 4, 5
16. 1, 2, 3, 4
17. 1, 2
18. 2

Chapter 14

1. 1, 2
2. 4
3. 1
4. 1
5. 1
6. 2, 3, 5
7. 3, 4
8. 1
9. 1
10. 2, 3, 5
11. 3
12. 1, 4, 3, 2
13. 2
14. 2
15. 1, 2, 4, 5

Chapter 15

1. 2
2. 3, 4
3. 3
4. 3
5. 3
6. 2, 3, 5
7. 4
8. 2
9. 4
10. 2, 3
11. 3
12. 1, 2, 5
13. 2
14. 4, 5
15. 3
16. 1, 2, 3, 4
17. 2
18. 4

Chapter 16

1. 2
2. 2
3. 3
4. 3
5. 3
6. 4
7. 5, 4, 3, 1, 2
8. 2
9. 1
10. 1, 3, 5
11. 3
12. 2, 3, 5
13. 3
14. 1, 3, 5
15. 1

Chapter 17

1. 2 mL
2. 0.25 mL
3. 13.6 kg
4. 125 mL/hr
5. 6.7 hours
6. 4
7. 0.02 mg
8. 2 mg
9. 3
10. 4
11. 2
12. 1, 2
13. 4
14. 3
15. 2
16. 4
17. 4
18. 3
19. 1
20. 3
21. 2, 5

Chapter 18

1. 1
2. 4
3. 1
4. 4
5. 3
6. 2
7. 1, 2, 3
8. 4
9. 1, 2, 4, 5
10. 1
11. 3
12. 1, 2, 3
13. 4
14. 2
15. 1
16. 7.35–7.45
17. 4
18. 3
19. 2, 3, 4
20. 2, 3
21. 1, 4, 5
22. 1
23. 1
24. 2
25. 3
26. 1
27. 2, 5
28. 1
29. 1
30. 1

Chapter 19

1. 3
2. 3
3. 2
4. 4
5. 3
6. 3
7. 2
8. 1
9. 1
10. 2
11. 1
12. 2
13. 3
14. 2, 3
15. 3
16. 1
17. 1, 2, 3, 4

Chapter 20

1. 1
2. 3
3. 1
4. 3
5. 1
6. 3
7. 2
8. 3, 4, 5
9. 3
10. 2, 4, 5
11. 3
12. holistic
13. 1
14. 3
15. 1, 3, 5
16. 3, 4, 5

Chapter 21

1. 3
2. 1
3. 3
4. 1
5. 3, 4, 5
6. 4
7. 1
8. 4
9. 2
10. 2
11. 3
12. 3
13. 1
14. 3
15. 3
16. 2, 3, 4
17. 2, 4, 5

Chapter 22

1. 4
2. 4
3. 1
4. 3
5. 4
6. 4
7. 3
8. 4
9. 3
10. 3
11. 1, 5
12. 4
13. 2, 3, 4, 5
14. 3
15. 2
16. 3
17. 4
18. 1
19. 2

Chapter 23

1. 3
2. 2
3. 4
4. 1
5. 3, 4, 1, 2, 5
6. 4
7. 3

8. 1, 4, 5
9. 2
10. 1
11. 1, 3, 4, 5, 6, 2
12. 3, 4, 1, 5, 2
13. 2
14. 1, 5
15. 3
16. 2
17. 1

Chapter 24
1. 2
2. 1
3. 1, 2, 3, 4
4. 3
5. 2
6. 3
7. 4
8. 3
9. 2
10. 2
11. 1, 3
12. 4
13. 3
14. 1, 2, 4
15. 2
16. 1, 2, 4
17. 2, 5
18. 1
19. 3
20. 2
21. 3
22. 1
23. 3

Chapter 25
1. 2
2. 2
3. 4
4. 1
5. 1
6. 4, 5
7. 2
8. 1, 5
9. 3
10. 3
11. 3
12. 3
13. 2
14. 3
15. 4
16. 1, 2, 3, 4
17. 1, 4, 5
18. 2, 3, 5
19. 1
20. 4
21. 1
22. 4
23. 1, 3, 6

Chapter 26
1. 4
2. 3
3. 1
4. 3
5. 1
6. 2, 5
7. 1
8. 1, 5
9. 1, 2, 4, 5
10. 4
11. 3
12. 2
13. 1
14. 2, 5
15. 2, 4
16. 3
17. 1
18. 4
19. 2
20. 2
21. Gravida
22. Primigravida
23. Multigravida
24. Viability

Chapter 27
1. 3
2. 3
3. 1
4. 2
5. 3
6. 2
7. 3
8. 4
9. 2
10. 4
11. 2
12. 1
13. 1
14. 4
15. 1
16. 1, 2, 3, 4
17. 1, 2, 3, 4

Chapter 28
1. 1, 4, 5
2. 3
3. 1
4. 1, 2
5. 3
6. 1, 3, 5
7. 3
8. 1
9. 1, 2, 3
10. 2
11. 4
12. 1, 2, 5
13. 1
14. 2
15. 1
16. 3, 4
17. 2

Chapter 29
1. 2, 3, 5
2. 2, 3, 4, 5
3. 4
4. 2
5. 3
6. 1, 3, 4
7. 2
8. 4
9. 2
10. 3
11. 4
12. 2, 3
13. 2
14. 4
15. 2, 3, 5

Chapter 30
1. 1, 2, 3
2. 3
3. 2
4. 1, 2, 5
5. 2
6. 1, 2, 3
7. 3
8. 4
9. 2, 4
10. 2, 3, 4, 5
11. 1, 2, 4
12. 1, 4, 5
13. 1, 2, 3, 5

Chapter 31
1. 2
2. 1, 2, 4
3. 3
4. 4
5. 2
6. 3
7. 3, 5
8. 3
9. 3
10. 4
11. 5th
12. 3
13. 1, 5
14. 2, 5
15. 1
16. 2, 3, 7
17. scoliosis
18. 4

Chapter 32
1. 3
2. 1, 5
3. 2
4. 1
5. 1
6. 1
7. 2
8. 1
9. 1
10. 2, 4, 5
11. 2, 3, 4, 5
12. 1, 3, 5
13. 2
14. 2
15. 1, 2, 4
16. 1
17. 2
18. 1
19. 3
20. 2
21. suicidal thoughts
22. 2
23. 4
24. 1, 2, 3, 4
25. 1
26. 2
27. 3
28. 1, 2, 3, 5

Chapter 33
1. 1, 4
2. 2, 3, 5
3. 2
4. 1, 2, 3
5. 1
6. 2
7. 4
8. 1, 3, 4
9. 2, 3, 5
10. 2
11. 1
12. 2
13. 2, 3, 4
14. 4
15. 3
16. 2

Chapter 34
1. 2
2. 3
3. 2
4. 4, 5
5. 1
6. 3
7. 2
8. 1, 3
9. 4
10. 2
11. 3
12. 1
13. 4
14. 4
15. 2, 5
16. 4
17. 3
18. 3, 4
19. 1, 3, 5
20. 2, 3

Chapter 35
1. 2
2. 3, 5
3. 2
4. 1
5. 2, 5
6. 1
7. 2
8. 3

9. 1
10. 4
11. 2
12. 4
13. 3
14. 2
15. 3
16. 1
17. 3, 1, 2, 4
18. 4
19. 4
20. 3
21. 3
22. 4
23. 1, 2, 3, 4

Chapter 36

1. 2
2. 4
3. 1
4. 2
5. 2
6. 1, 3, 4, 5
7. 2
8. 2
9. 1
10. 3, 5
11. 4
12. 2
13. 2
14. 3
15. 2
16. 1, 5
17. 1
18. 3, 5
19. 2, 4
20. 2

Chapter 37

1. 2
2. 3
3. 2
4. 3
5. 3
6. 3, 4, 5
7. 2, 3, 5
8. 3, 4
9. 1
10. 3
11. 1
12. 2, 4, 5
13. 3, 4, 5
14. tele-monitoring or telehealth
15. 2

Chapter 38

1. 4
2. 2
3. 2
4. 4
5. 1
6. 1, 5
7. 2
8. 4
9. 3
10. 3
11. 1, 2, 3, 4, 5

Chapter 39

1. 2
2. 1
3. 3
4. 1
5. 1
6. 1, 2
7. 3, 4
8. 4
9. 2
10. 4
11. 2, 3, 4
12. 1
13. 2
14. 1, 5
15. 2

Chapter 40

1. 1
2. 2
3. 1, 3, 4, 2
4. 3
5. 3
6. 1, 3, 4, 5
7. 2
8. 2
9. 2
10. Medical director
11. 2
12. 3
13. 3
14. 1
15. 1, 3, 5
16. 3
17. 1, 2, 3

Chapter 41

1. 2
2. 1, 2, 4, 5
3. 1
4. 4
5. 2
6. 4
7. 1
8. 3
9. 2
10. 2
11. 1, 3
12. 2, 5
13. 2
14. 1, 2, 3, 5
15. e
16. d
17. a
18. c
19. b
20. f
21. k
22. a
23. i
24. b
25. g
26. c
27. j
28. d
29. e
30. h

Chapter 42

1. 2
2. 3, 5
3. 1
4. 2
5. 4
6. 3
7. 2
8. 1
9. 2
10. 3
11. 2, 5
12. 3
13. 3, 5
14. 1, 2, 3, 5
15. 4
16. 2
17. 2
18. 3
19. 2

Chapter 43

1. 1
2. 2
3. 3
4. 2
5. 1
6. 1
7. 1, 5
8. 4
9. 2
10. 1, 5
11. 2
12. 1
13. 1
14. 2
15. 1
16. 1, 2
17. 2
18. 2
19. 1
20. 2
21. 1, 2, 3, 5
22. 1
23. 3
24. 2
25. 4, 5

Chapter 44

1. 4
2. 4
3. 1, 2, 5
4. 3
5. 4
6. 2, 5
7. 4
8. 3
9. 2
10. 2
11. 1
12. 2
13. 2
14. 3
15. 4
16. 1
17. 4, 5
18. 3, 4, 5
19. 4

Chapter 45

1. 4
2. 2
3. 3, 4, 5
4. 2, 5
5. 2
6. 1
7. 3
8. 4
9. 1
10. 3
11. 1
12. 2, 3, 4
13. 3
14. 4
15. 1
16. 4
17. 4
18. 2, 4, 5
19. 1, 2, 4

Chapter 46

1. 2, 3, 4, 5
2. 4
3. 2
4. 3
5. 2
6. 3
7. 3
8. 2, 3
9. 2
10. 3
11. 1
12. 2
13. 4
14. 4
15. 1
16. 1, 3, 4, 5
17. 3

Chapter 47

1. 3
2. 4
3. 2
4. 2
5. 4
6. 3
7. 1

8. 4
9. 3
10. 2
11. 3
12. 2
13. 2
14. 2
15. 4, 5
16. 3
17. 1
18. 2
19. 1
20. 1, 2, 3
21. 1, 2, 3, 5
22. 1, 2, 3, 5

Chapter 48

1. 1
2. 3
3. 4, 5
4. 1
5. 3
6. 3, 4, 5
7. 4
8. 1, 3
9. 4
10. 2, 5
11. 2
12. 2
13. 1
14. 1
15. 1
16. 2
17. 1
18. 2, 3, 4
19. 3
20. 2
21. 2, 4, 5
22. 2
23. 4
24. 3
25. 1, 3, 4, 5

Chapter 49

1. 2
2. 4
3. 4
4. 1
5. 2
6. 3
7. 2, 3
8. 3
9. 1
10. 3
11. 4
12. 1
13. 1, 2, 3
14. 1
15. 3
16. 3
17. 1, 3, 4, 5
18. 2, 4, 5
19. 2, 3, 5
20. 1, 2, 5
21. 2, 5
22. 1, 3, 4, 5
23. 2, 3
24. 1, 2, 3, 4
25. 1, 2, 4, 5
26. 1, 2, 3, 5

Chapter 50

1. 4, 5
2. 3
3. 2
4. 4
5. 1
6. 3
7. 4
8. 1
9. 1, 2, 3
10. 1, 4
11. 2
12. 3
13. 1
14. 3
15. 1
16. 4
17. 2
18. 4
19. 1
20. 1
21. 2
22. 1, 2
23. 2, 3, 5
24. 1, 2, 5
25. 2, 5
26. 1, 3, 4
27. 1
28. 2
29. 3

Chapter 51

1. 3
2. 1
3. 4
4. 2
5. 4
6. 1
7. 3
8. 4
9. 4
10. 1
11. 1
12. 2
13. 2
14. 4
15. 3
16. 1, 2
17. 1
18. 1, 2, 3, 4
19. 2
20. 1, 2, 3
21. 1
22. 1
23. 3

Chapter 52

1. 1
2. 2
3. 3
4. 4, 5
5. 3
6. 3, 4, 5
7. 2
8. 1, 5
9. 4
10. 2
11. 1
12. 3
13. 4
14. 4
15. 3
16. 4, 5
17. 2, 3
18. 2
19. 4
20. 1
21. 1, 3
22. 3
23. 1, 2, 4
24. 2
25. 2
26. 4

Chapter 53

1. 3
2. 1
3. 1
4. 4
5. 3
6. 4
7. 3, 4, 5
8. 1
9. 2
10. 1, 2, 3
11. 2, 3, 5
12. 2
13. 1
14. 1
15. 3
16. 2
17. 3, 4, 5
18. 2, 3, 4
19. 1
20. 4
21. 3
22. 1
23. 2
24. 4
25. 4

Chapter 54

1. 3
2. 1, 2, 4, 5
3. 1, 2, 3, 4
4. 4
5. 1
6. 4
7. 1, 3
8. 1, 4, 5
9. 3
10. 3
11. 2
12. 1
13. 1
14. 2
15. 1
16. 4
17. 1
18. 3
19. 1, 2, 3
20. 2, 4, 5
21. 3
22. 4
23. 3
24. 4
25. 3

Chapter 55

1. 4
2. 2
3. 1, 3, 6
4. 2, 4
5. 2
6. 2
7. 3
8. 3
9. 4
10. 2
11. 1
12. 1
13. 2, 3, 4, 5
14. 3
15. rubber latex proteins
16. 2, 3, 4
17. 1, 3, 4
18. 4
19. 3, 4

Chapter 56

1. 1
2. 1, 2, 3
3. 4
4. 2, 3, 4
5. 2
6. 1
7. 1
8. 4
9. 3
10. 2
11. 2
12. 4
13. 3
14. 3
15. 1

Chapter 57

1. 3
2. 1
3. 3
4. 1, 5
5. 1

6. 1, 5
7. 3, 5
8. 1
9. 4
10. 3
11. 2
12. 3
13. 3, 5
14. 4
15. 2
16. 1

Chapter 58

1. 2, 3, 5
2. 1, 3
3. 1, 2, 4, 5
4. 2
5. 2
6. 4
7. 2
8. 4, 5
9. 3
10. 2, 5
11. 3
12. 1
13. 2
14. 2
15. 2, 4
16. 4
17. 4
18. 1

References

CHAPTER 1

Agency for Healthcare Research and Quality: Women's health, 2011. Retrieved from: www.ahrq.gov/research/findings/factsheets/women/index.html.

American Association of Colleges of Nursing: Nursing shortage, 2012. Retrieved from: www.aacn.nche.edu/media-relations/factsheets/nursing-shortage.

American Hospital Association: *The patient care partnership: understanding expectations, rights and responsibilities*, Atlanta, 2003, Author.

Bureau of Labor Statistics (BLS): Occupational employment statistics, 2016. Retrieved from: https://www.bls.gov/oes/current/oes292061.htm.

Bureau of Labor Statistics (BLS): Licensed Practical and Licensed Vocational Nurses, 2018. Retrieved from: https://www.bls.gov/ooh/healthcare/licensed-practical-and-licensed-vocational-nurses.htm#tab-6.

Centers for Medicare and Medicaid Services: Resident rights, n.d. Retrieved from: www.medicare.gov/what-medicare-covers/part-a/rights-in-nursing-home.html.

Commonwealth Fund, The: U.S. health care from a global perspective, 2015. Retrieved from: http://www.commonwealthfund.org/publications/issue-briefs/2015/oct/us-health-care-from-a-global-perspective.

Early J: The Nurse Pinning Tradition, 2015. Retrieved from: http://www.nursinghistory.org/pinning-tradition/.

Ellis H: Florence Nightingale: creator of modern nursing and public health pioneer, *J Perioper Pract* 18(9):404–406, 2008.

The Henry J. Kaiser Family Foundation (KFF): Total number of professionally active nurses, 2017. Retrieved from: http://kff.org/other/state-indicator/total-registered-nurses/?currentTimeframe=0&selectedDistributions=licensed-practical-nurse-lpn.

Medscape Today News: Celebrating nurses: What happened to the cap? Part 2: Losing our tradition. slideshow, n.d. Retrieved from: www.medscape.com/features/slideshow/nurse-caps-pt2.

National Association for Practical Nurse Education and Service (NAPNES): Standards of practice and educational competencies of graduates of practical/vocational nursing programs, 2007. Retrieved from: http://napnes.org/drupal-7.4/sites/default/files/pdf/standards/standards_read_only.pdf.

NLN Board of Governors: NLN Vision Series, 2014. A Vision for Recognition of the Role of Licensed Practical/Vocational Nurses in Advancing the Nation's Health. A Living Document from the National League for Nursing. Retrieved from: http://www.nln.org/docs/default-source/about/nln-vision-series-(position-statements)/nlnvision_7.pdf.

Payne C: More men entering nursing profession, USA Today, 2013. Retrieved from: http://www.usatoday.com/story/news/nation/2013/02/25/men-nursing-occupatins/1947243.

Smith T: A policy perspective on the entry into practice issue, *Online J Issues Nurs* 15(1):2009. Retrieved from: www.nursingworld.org/MainMenuCategories/ANAMarketplace/ANAPeriodicals/OJIN/TableofContents/Vol152010/No1Jan2010/Articles-Previous-Topic/Policy-and-Entry-into-Practice.html.

US Army Heritage Center Foundation: Soldier stories, n.d. Retrieved from: www.armyheritage.org/education-and-programs/educational-resources/soldier-stories/130-army-nurses-of-worldwar-one-service-beyond-expectations.html.

US Census Bureau: Income, poverty, and health insurance coverage: 2011 Highlights, 2011. United States Department of Commerce, 2011. Retrieved from: www.census.gov/hhes/www/hlthins/data/incpovhlth/2011/highlights.html.

CHAPTER 2

American Nurses Association (ANA) and National Council of State Boards of Nursing (NCSBN): ANA and NCSBN unite to provide guidelines on social media and networking for nurses, 2011. Retrieved from: http://www.nursingworld.org/FunctionalMenuCategories/MediaResources/PressReleases/2011-PR/ANA-NCSBN-Guidelines-Social-Media-Networking-for-Nurses.pdf.

Cornell University Law School: Cruzan v. Director, Missouri Department of Health, (88-1503), 497 U.S. 261 (1990), 1990. Retrieved from: https://www.law.cornell.edu/supct/html/88-1503.ZO.html.

InfoNurses: ICN: Nurses and social media, 2015. Retrieved from: http://www.infonurses.com/2015/05/icn-nurses-and-social-media.html/.

Levin SM: H.R.4449–Patient Self-Determination Act of 1990, 1990. Retrieved from: https://www.congress.gov/bill/101st-congress/house-bill/4449.

Missouri Department of Health & Senior Services: Negligence and malpractice, n.d. Retrieved from: http://health.mo.gov/living/lpha/phnursing/negligence.php.

Motacki K, Burke K: *Nursing delegation and management of patient care*, ed 2, St. Louis, 2017, Elsevier.

National Council of State Boards of Nursing (NCSBN): Filing a complaint, n.d. Retrieved from: https://www.ncsbn.org/filing-a-complaint.htm.

Reising DL, Allen PN: Protecting yourself from malpractice claims, *Continuing Education* 2(2):2007. Retrieved from: www.americannursetoday.com/article.aspx?id = 4186.

Stokowski LA: Social media and nurses: promising or perilous? 2011. Retrieved from: https://www.medscape.com/viewarticle/753317_3.

CHAPTER 3

American Hospital Association: Communicating with patients, n.d. Retrieved from: www.aha.org/advocacy-issues/communicatingpts/index.shtml.

Centers for Medicare and Medicaid Services: Home Health Agency Center, n.d. Retrieved from: https://www.cms.gov/Center/Provider-Type/Home-Health-Agency-HHA-Center.html

The Joint Commission: National Patient Safety Goals, 2018. Retrieved from: https://www.jointcommission.org/standards_information/npsgs.aspx

Kaiser Permanente: Shifting perspectives, 2007. Retrieved from: http://xnet.kp.org/newscenter/clinicalexcellence/2007/030107perspectives.html.

The Office of the National Coordinator for Health Information Technology: EMR vs. EHR. What's the difference? Retrieved from: https://www.healthit.gov/buzz-blog/electronic-health-and-medical-records/emr-vs-ehr-difference/

US National Library of Medicine (NLM): Personal health records, 2017. Retrieved from: https://medlineplus.gov/personalhealthrecords.html.

CHAPTER 4

Balzer Riley J: *Communication in nursing*, ed 8, St. Louis, 2017, Elsevier.

Krauss Whitbourne S: Polish off your personal space. PsychologyToday, 2012. Retrieved from: www.psychologytoday.com/blog/fulfillment-any-age/201211/polish-your-personal-space.

Maier-Lorentz MM: Transcultural nursing: its importance in nursing practice, *J Cultural Divers* 15(1):37–43, 2008.

Old N, Kai T: Survival of the funniest: using therapeutic humour in nursing, *Nurs N Zealand* 18(8):17–19, 2012.

Scudder RH: Eye contact: what does it communicate in various cultures? 2014. Retreived from: http://www.brighthubeducation.com/social-studies-help/9626-learning-about-eye-contact-in-other-cultures/.

CHAPTER 5

American Nurses Association (ANA): *Nursing: scope and standards of practice*, Silver Spring, Md, 2010, Author.

American Nurses Association (ANA): What is nursing? n.d.a. Retrieved from: http://nursingworld.org/EspeciallyForYou/What-is-Nursing.

American Nurses Association (ANA): The nursing process, n.d.b. Retrieved from: http://nursingworld.org/EspeciallyForYou/What-is-Nursing/Tools-You-Need/Thenursingprocess.html.

Bulechek GM, Butcher HK, Dochterman JM: *Nursing interventions classification (NIC)*, ed 7, St. Louis, 2019, Mosby.

Carpenito LJ: *Nursing diagnosis: application to clinical practice*, ed 14, Philadelphia, 2016, Lippincott Williams & Wilkins.

Moorhead S, Johnson M, Maas M, et al: *Nursing outcomes classification (NOC)*, ed 6, St. Louis, 2018, Mosby.

National League for Nursing: *Think tank on critical thinking*, New York, 2000, Author.

North American Nursing Diagnosis Association–International (NANDA-I): Nursing diagnoses: glossary of terms, 2018. Retrieved from: http://www.nanda.org/nanda-international-glossary-of-terms.html.

CHAPTER 6

Giger JN: *Transcultural nursing: Assessment and intervention*, ed 7, St. Louis, 2017, Elsevier.

US Census Bureau: Census data 2010, 2010. Retrieved from: www.census.gov/2010census/data.

US Census Bureau: Most children younger that age 1 are minorities, 2012. Retrieved from: https://www.census.gov/newsroom/releases/archives/population/cb12-90.html.

CHAPTER 7

Association of periOperative Registered Nurses (AORN): *Perioperative standards and recommended practices*, Denver, 2013, Author.

Boyce JM, Pittet D, HICPAC/SHEA/APIC/IDSA Hand Hygiene Task Force, CDC Healthcare Control Practices Advisory Committee: Guideline for hand hygiene in health-care settings, *Infect Control Hosp Epidemiol* 23(12 Suppl):S3–S40, 2002.

Centers for Disease Control and Prevention (CDC): *Updated U.S. Public Health Service guidelines for the management of occupational exposure to HIV and recommendations for postexposure prophylaxis*, Washington, D.C., 2005, Author.

Centers for Disease Control and Prevention (CDC): Management of multi-drug-resistant organisms in health care settings, 2006. Retrieved from: www.cdc.gov/ncidod/dhqp/pdf/ar/mdroGuide line2006.pdf.

Centers for Disease Control and Prevention (CDC): Isolation precautions, 2007. Retrieved from: https://www.cdc.gov/infectioncontrol/guidelines/isolation/index.html.

Centers for Disease Control and Prevention (CDC): Handwashing: clean hands save lives: show me the science–how to wash your hands, 2015a. Retrieved from: https://www.cdc.gov/handwashing/show-me-the-science-handwashing.html.

Centers for Disease Control and Prevention: Healthcare associated infections: preventing healthcare-associated infections, 2015b. Retrieved from: www.cdc.gov/ncidod/dhqp/pdf/isolation2007.pdf.

Centers for Disease Control and Prevention (CDC): Bioterrorism, 2016. Retrieved from: https://www.cdc.gov/anthrax/bioterrorism/index.html.

Centers for Disease Control and Prevention (CDC): Food safety: keep food safe, 2017. Retrieved from: http://www.cdc.gov/foodsafety/groups/consumers.html.

Centers for Disease Control and Prevention (CDC): HAI data and statistics, 2018a. Retrieved from: https://www.cdc.gov/hai/surveillance/index.html.

Centers for Disease Control and Prevention (CDC): Healthcare-associated infections: types of healthcare-associated infections, 2018b. Retrieved from: http://www.cdc.gov/hai/surveillance/index.html.

(The) Joint Commission: National Patient Safety Goals, 2017. Retrieved from: https://www.jointcommission.org/assets/1/6/NPSG_Chapter_NCC_Jan2017.pdf.

Mayo Clinic: Drugs and supplements: anthrax vaccine (intramuscular route, subcutaneous route), 2017. Retrieved from: https://www.mayoclinic.org/drugs-supplements/anthrax-vaccine-intramuscular-route-subcutaneous-route/description/drg-20074564.

Mayo Clinic: Handwashing: do's and don'ts, 2018. Retrieved from: https://www.mayoclinic.org/healthy-lifestyle/adult-health/in-depth/hand-washing/art-20046253.

Potter PA, Perry AG, Stockert P: *Essentials for nursing practice*, ed 9, St. Louis, 2019, Elsevier.

Siegel JD, Rhinehart E, Jackson M, et al; Healthcare Infection Control Practices Advisory Committee: Guideline for isolation precautions: Preventing transmission of infectious agents in healthcare settings, 2007. Retrieved from: www.cdc.gov/ncidod/dhqp/pdf/isolation2007.pdf.

US Food and Drug Administration: Safety alerts for human medical products, 2016. Retrieved from: http://wayback.archive-it.org/7993/20170110235327/http://www.fda.gov/Safety/MedWatch/SafetyInformation/default.htm.

US Food and Drug Administration: Emergency preparedness (drugs), 2017. Retrieved from: https://www.fda.gov/drugs/emergencypreparedness/default.htm.

CHAPTER 8

Ackley BJ, Ladwig GB: *Nursing diagnosis handbook*, ed 11, St. Louis, 2017, Mosby.

Centers for Disease Control and Prevention (CDC), National Institute for Occupational Safety and Health (NIOSH): Safe patient handling and mobility (SPHM), 2017. Retrieved from: https://www.cdc.gov/niosh/topics/safepatient/default.html.

National Library of Medicine (NLM): Compartment syndrome, 2014. Retrieved from: https://medlineplus.gov/ency/article/001224.htm.

Potter PA, Perry AG, Stockert PA, et al: *Fundamentals of nursing: Concepts, process, and practice*, St. Louis, 2017, Mosby.

CHAPTER 9

Agency for Healthcare Research and Quality(AHRQ): Preventing pressure ulcers in hospitals: A toolkit for improving quality of care, 2014. Retrieved from: www.ahrq.gov/professionals/systems/hospital/pressureulcertoolkit/index.html.

Medscape: A closer look at pressure ulcers: "Reasonably preventable," 2008. Retrieved from: www.medscape.org/viewarticle/574206_2.

National Pressure Ulcer Advisory Panel (NPUAP): National Pressure Ulcer advisory panel NPUAP announces a change in terminology from pressure ulcer to pressure injury and updates the stages of pressure injury, 2016. Retrieved from: http://www.npuap.org/

national-pressure-ulcer-advisory-panel-npuap-announces-a-change-in-terminology-from-pressure-ulcer-to-pressure-injury-and-updates-the-stages-of-pressure-injury/.

CHAPTER 10

Campbell R: Fires in health care facilities, 2017. Retrieved from: http://www.nfpa.org/news-and-research/fire-statistics-and-reports/fire-statistics/fires-by-property-type/health-care-facilities/fires-in-health-care-facilities.

Centers for Disease Control and Prevention (CDC): Sharps injuries: Bloodborne pathogens, 2011. Retrieved from: www.cdc.gov/niosh/stopsticks/bloodborne.html.

Centers for Disease Control and Prevention (CDC): NCHS drug poisoning mortality: United States, 1999–2015, 2016. Retrieved from: https://blogs.cdc.gov/nchs-data-visualization/drug-poisoning-mortality/.

Centers for Disease Control and Prevention (CDC): Vaccine information for adults: recommended vaccines for health-care workers, 2017. Retrieved from: https://www.cdc.gov/vaccines/adults/rec-vac/hcw.html.

Environmental Protection Agency (EPA): Radionuclides in drinking water, 2015. Retrieved from: https://cfpub.epa.gov/safewater/radionuclides/radionuclides.cfm?action=Rad_Disposal%20Options.

The Joint Commission (TJC): Sentinal event, n.d. Retrieved from: www.jointcommission.org/sentinel_event.aspx.

The Joint Commission (TJC): Emergency management resources—security/violence/active shooter, 2016. Retrieved from: https://www.jointcommission.org/emergency_management_resources_violence_security_active_shooter/.

Occupational Safety and Health Administration (OSHA): Decontamination, n.d. Retrieved from: https://www.osha.gov/SLTC/hazardouswaste/training/decon.html.

Poison Control: Poison statistics: national data 2016, 2016. Retrieved from: http://www.poison.org/poison-statistics-national.

Stobart-Gallagher MA: Needle-stick guideline, 2017. Retrieved from: http://emedicine.medscape.com/article/784812-overview#a6.

US Department of Homeland Security: Active shooter: how to respond, 2008. Retrieved from: https://www.dhs.gov/xlibrary/assets/active_shooter_booklet.pdf.

US Department of Labor: Workplace violence, n.d. Retrieved from: https://www.osha.gov/SLTC/healthcarefacilities/violence.html.

CHAPTER 11

The Joint Commission (TJC): Standards FAQ details: Nursing assessments—Licensed practical nurse, n.d. Retrieved from: https://www.jointcommission.org/standards_information/jcfaqdetails.aspx?StandardsFaqId=771&ProgramId=46.

Kind AJH, Smith MA: Documentation of mandated discharge summary components in transitions from acute to subacute care, n.d. Retrieved from: https://www.ahrq.gov/downloads/pub/advances2/vol2/Advances-Kind_31.pdf.

Maslow A: *Motivation and personality*, ed 2, New York, 1970, Harper & Row.

CHAPTER 12

American Heart Association: Heart-health screenings, 2017. Retrieved from: http://www.heart.org/HEARTORG/Conditions/Heart-Health-Screenings_UCM_428687_Article.jsp#.WI1OvvIsOSo.

Goldman LR, Shannon MW, Committee on Environmental Health: Technical report: mercury in the environment: implications for pediatricians, *Pediatrics* 108:1, 2001.

CHAPTER 13

Center for Disease Control and Prevention (CDC): Clinical guidance for carbon monoxide poisoning after a disaster, 2017a. Retrieved from: https://www.cdc.gov/disasters/co_guidance.htmlhttps://www.cdc.gov/disasters/co_guidance.html.

Centers for Disease Control and Prevention (CDC): Standard precautions for all patient care, 2017b. Retrieved from: https://www.cdc.gov/infectioncontrol/basics/standard-precautions.html.

CHAPTER 16

American Burn Association: Burn Incidence Fact Sheet, 2016. Retrieved from: http://ameriburn.org/who-we-are/media/burn-incidence-fact-sheet/.

American Heart Association (AHA): Hands Only CPR Factsheet, 2017a. Retrieved from: https://cpr.heart.org/idc/groups/ahaecc-public/@wcm/@ecc/documents/downloadable/ucm_493890.pdf.

American Heart Association (AHA): CPR and ECG Guidelines, 2017. Updated November 2017. Retrieved from: https://eccguidelines.heart.org/index.php/circulation/cpr-ecc-guidelines-2/.

Centers for Disease Control and Prevention: Rabies, 2016. Retrieved from: http://www.cdc.gov/rabies/medical_care/.

Harrison L: Should POLICE replace RICE as the ankle therapy of choice? 2014. Retrieved from: http://www.medscape.com/viewarticle/823217_2.

Immunization Action Coalition: Rabies: Questions and answers: Information about the disease and vaccines, n.d. Retrieved from: www.immunize.org/catg.d/p4216.pdf.

Keany JE: Femur fracture clinical presentation, 2015. Retrieved from: https://emedicine.medscape.com/article/824856-clinical.

Li J: Hypothermia treatment and management, 2017. Retrieved from: http://emedicine.medscape.com/article/770542-treatment#d11.

Life Alliance Organ Recovery Agency: American Academy of Neurology Guidelines for Brain Death Determination, n.d. Retrieved from: http://surgery.med.miami.edu/laora/clinical-operations/brain-death-diagnosis.

Mareedo RK, Grandhe NP, Gangineni S, et al: Classic EKG changes of hypothermia, *Clin Med Res* 6(3–4):107–108, 2008.

Mayo Clinic: Hypothermia, 2018. Retrieved from: https://www.mayoclinic.org/diseases-conditions/hypothermia/symptoms-causes/syc-20352682.

National Library of Medicine (NLM): Snake Bites, 2017. Retrieved from: https://medlineplus.gov/ency/article/000031.htm.

University of Maryland Medical Center: Frostbite, 2010. Retrieved from: www.umm.edu/altmed/articles/frostbite-000065.htm.

Vyas KS, Wong LK: Oral rehydration solutions for burn management in the field and underdeveloped regions: A review, *Int J Burns Trauma* 3(3):130–136, 2013.

Wheeless CR, editor: *Wheeless' textbook of orthopaedics*, 2016, Duke Orthopaedics and Data Trace Internet Publishing. Retrieved from: www.wheelessonline.com.

Zonnoor B: Frostbite treatment and management, 2018. Retrieved from: https://emedicine.medscape.com/article/926249-treatment.

CHAPTER 17

American Nurses Association (ANA): Safe needles save lives, n.d. Retrieved from: https://www.nursingworld.org/practice-policy/work-environment/health-safety/safe-needles/safe-needles-law/.

Belle DJ, Singh H: Genetic factors in drug metabolism, *Am Fam Physician* 77(11):1553–1560, 2008.

Bollinger MB: How do patients determine that their metered dose inhaler is empty? *Pediatrics* 116(Suppl 2):2005. Retrieved from: http://pediatrics.aappublications.org/content/116/Supplement_2/563.1.

The Joint Commission: Official "do not use" list, 2018. Retrieved from: https://www.jointcommission.org/assets/1/18/dnu_list.pdf.

Kee JL, Hayes ER: *Pharmacology: a nursing process approach*, ed 7, St. Louis, 2012, Elsevier.

US Food and Drug Administration (FDA): What are generic drugs? 2009. Retrieved from: www.fda.gov/Drugs/ResourcesForYou/Consumers/BuyingUsingMedicineSafely/Understanding GenericDrugs/ucm144456.htm.

CHAPTER 18

American Red Cross: A compendium of transfusion practice guidelines, ed 3, 2017. Retrieved from: http://success.redcross.org/success/file.php/1/TransfusionPractices-Compendium_3rdEdition.pdf.

Clinical Transfusion Medicine Committee of the AABB: Red blood cell transfusion: a clinical practice guideline, *Ann Intern Med* 157(1):2012. Retrieved from: http://annals.org/article.aspx?articleid+1206681.

Infusion Nurses Society: Infusion nursing standards of practice, *J Intraven Nurs* 34(1S):S65, 2011.

CHAPTER 19

American Diabetes Association: Diabetes basics: Facts about type 2, n.d.a. Retrieved from: www.diabetes.org/diabetes-basics/type-2/facts-about-type-2.html.

American Diabetes Association: Diabetes basics: Type 1 diabetes, n.d.b. Retrieved from: www.diabetes.org/diabetes-basics/type-1.

American Heart Association: Trans fat, 2017. Retrieved from: https://healthyforgood.heart.org/Eat-smart/Articles/Trans-Fat.

Centers for Disease Control and Prevention (CDC): Hip fractures among older adults, 2013. Retrieved from: www.cdc.gov/homeandrecreationalsafety/falls/adulthipfx.html.

March of Dimes: Caffeine in pregnancy, 2015. Retrieved from: https://www.marchofdimes.org/pregnancy/caffeine-in-pregnancy.aspx.

The National Academies of Sciences, Engineering, Medicine: Dietary reference intakes (DRIs): recommended dietary allowances and adequate intakes, Elements, n.d. Retrieved from: http://nationalacademies.org/hmd/activities/nutrition/summarydris/dri-tables.aspx?_ga=2.139664307.1693095242.1531251493-1603260316.1531251493.

US Department of Health and Human Services (USDHHS), National Institutes of Health (NIH), National Heart, Lung and Blood Institute (NHLBI): Calculate your body mass index, n.d.a. Retrieved from: https://www.nhlbi.nih.gov/health/educational/lose_wt/BMI/bmicalc.htm?source=quickfitnesssolutions.

US Department of Health and Human Services (USDHHS), National Institutes of Health (NIH), National Heart, Lung and Blood Institute (NHLBI): DASH eating plan, n.d.b. Retrieved from: https://www.nhlbi.nih.gov/health/health-topics/topics/dash.

US Department of Health and Human Services (USDHHS), National Institutes of Health (NIH), National Heart, Lung, and Blood Institute (NHLBI): Your guide to lowering cholesterol with TLC, 2005. Retrieved from: https://www.nhlbi.nih.gov/files/docs/public/heart/chol_tlc.pdf.

US Department of Health and Human Services (USDHHS), National Institutes of Health (NIH), National Institute of Diabetes and Digestive and Kidney Diseases (NIDDK): Bariatric surgery, n.d.a. Retrieved from: https://www.niddk.nih.gov/health-information/weight-management/bariatric-surgery#SurgAdult.

US Department of Health and Human Services (USDHHS), National Institutes of Health (NIH), National Institute of Diabetes and Digestive and Kidney Diseases (NIDDK): Lactose intolerance, n.d.b. Retrieved from: http://digestive.niddk.nih.gov/ddiseases/pubs/lactoseintolerance.

US Department of Health and Human Services (USDHHS), National Institutes of Health (NIH), Office of Dietary Supplements: Calcium Fact Sheet for Health Professionals, 2017. Retrieved from: https://ods.od.nih.gov/factsheets/Calcium-HealthProfessional/.

US Department of Health and Human Services (USDHHS), National Institutes of Health (NIH), Office of Dietary Supplements: Chromium Fact Sheet for Health Professionals, 2018a. Retrieved from: http://ods.od.nih.gov/factsheets/Chromium-HealthProfessional.

US Department of Health and Human Services (USDHHS), National Institutes of Health (NIH), Office of Dietary Supplements: Folate Fact Sheet for Health Professionals, 2018b. Retrieved from: http://ods.od.nih.gov/factsheets/Folate-HealthProfessional.

US Department of Health and Human Services (USDHHS), National Institutes of Health (NIH), Office of Dietary Supplements: Iron: Fact Sheet for Health Professionals, 2018. Retrieved from: https://ods.od.nih.gov/factsheets/Iron-HealthProfessional/.

US Department of Health and Human Services (USDHHS), National Institutes of Health (NIH), Office of Dietary Supplements: Potassium Fact Sheet for Health Professionals, 2018d. Retrieved from: https://ods.od.nih.gov/factsheets/Potassium-HealthProfessional/.

US Department of Health and Human Services (USDHHS), National Institute of Health (NIH), Office of Dietary Supplements: Vitamin E Fact Sheet for Health Professionals. 2018e. Retrieved from: https://ods.od.nih.gov/factsheets/VitaminE-HealthProfessional.

US Department of Health and Human Services (USDHHS), National Institutes of Health (NIH), Office of Dietary Supplements: Vitamin B12 Fact Sheet for Health Professionals, 2018f. Retrieved from: https://ods.od.nih.gov/factsheets/VitaminB12-HealthProfessional/.

US Department of Health and Human Services (USDHHS), National Institutes of Health (NIH), Office of Dietary Supplements: Vitamin C Fact Sheet for Health Professionals, 2018g. Retrieved from: https://ods.od.nih.gov/factsheets/VitaminC-HealthProfessional/.

US Department of Health and Human Services (USDHHS), National Institutes of Health (NIH), Office of Dietary Supplements: Vitamin D Fact Sheet for Health Professionals, 2018h. Retrieved from: https://ods.od.nih.gov/factsheets/VitaminD-HealthProfessional/.

US Department of Health and Human Services (USDHHS), National Institutes of Health (NIH), Office of Dietary Supplements: Vitamin K Fact Sheet for Health Professionals, 2018i. Retrieved from: https://ods.od.nih.gov/factsheets/VitaminK-HealthProfessional/.

US Department of Health and Human Services (USDHHS) and US Department of Agriculture (USDA): 2015–2020 Dietary Guidelines for Americans, 8th Edition. December 2015. Available at: http://health.gov/dietaryguidelines/2015/guidelines/.

CHAPTER 20

American Cannabis Nurses Association (ACNA). n.d. Retrieved from: https://cannabisnurses.org.

American Optometric Association: Head-down yoga poses increase eye pressure in glaucoma patients, 2016. Retrieved from: http://www.aoa.org/news/clinical-eye-care/head-down-yoga-poses-increase-eye-pressure-in-glaucoma-patients?sso=y.

Clark TC, Black LI, Stussman BJ, et al: Trends in the use of complementary health approaches among adults: United States, 2002-2012, *Natl Health Stat Report* 79:2015.

Johnson C: DEA rejects attempt to loosen federal restrictions on marijuana, 2016. Retrieved from: http://www.npr.org/2016/08/10/489509471/dea-rejects-attempt-to-loosen-federal-restrictions-on-marijuana.

Leafscience.com: Can you overdose on marijuana, 2014. Retrieved from: http://www.leafscience.com/2014/08/26/can-you-overdose-on-marijuana/.

Mayo Clinic: Biofeedback: Using your mind to improve your health, 2012. Retrieved from: www.mayoclinic.com/health/biofeedback/MY01072.

Mayo Foundation for Medical Education and Research: Pet therapy: Man's best friend as healer, 2016. Retrieved from: www.mayoclinic.com.

The Medical Cannabis Institute (TMCI): About TMCI Global (TMCI), 2018. Retrieved from: https://themedicalcannabisinstitute.org/about/.

National Center for Complementary and Integrative Health (NCCIH): Paying for complementary and integrative health approaches, 2016. Retrieved from: https://nccih.nih.gov/health/financial.

National Center for Complementary and Integrative Health (NCCIH): Magnets for pain, 2017. Retrieved from: https://nccih.nih.gov/health/magnet/magnetsforpain.htm.

Patients Out of Time, n.d. Retrieved from: http://patientsoutoftime.org/.

Russo EB: Synthetic and natural cannabinoids: the cardiovascular risk, *British J Cardiol* 22(1):7–9, 2015. Retrieved from: https://www.researchgate.net/publication/273203570_Synthetic_and_natural_cannabinoids_The_cardiovascular_risk.

Russo EB, Hohmann AG: Role of cannabinoids in pain management. In Deer TR, et al, editors: *Comprehensive treatment of chronic pain by medical, interventional, and integrative approaches*, Chicago, 2013, American Academy of Pain Medicine.

Russo EB, Mead AP, Sulak D: Current status and future of cannabis research, 2015. Retrieved from: http://cannabisclinicians.org/wp-content/uploads/2015/04/Russo-et-al-Current-status-and-future-of-cannabis-research-Clin-Researcher-2015.pdf.

University of Michigan Health System: Guided imagery, 2017. Retrieved from: http://www.uofmhealth.org/health-library/aa84044spec.

Yang Y, Zhiqiang F, Schlageal R: *Taijiquan: the art of nurturing—the science of power*, ed 2, Champaign, Ill, 2008, Zhenwu.

CHAPTER 21

McCaffery M: Your patient is in pain. Here's how you respond, *Nursing* 32(10):35–2002, 2002.

McCaffery M, Pasero C: *Pain: clinical management*, ed 3, St. Louis, 2003, Mosby.

Meinhart NT, McCaffery M: *Pain: a nursing approach to assessment and analysis*, New York, 1983, Appleton-Century-Crofts.

The Joint Commission: Joint Commission Statement on Pain Management, April 18, 2016. Retrieved from: https://www.jointcommission.org/joint_commission_statement_on_pain_management/.

CHAPTER 23

Infusion Nurses Society: Infusion nursing standards of practice, *J Infus Nurs* 39(suppl 1), 2016.

Occupational Safety and Health Administration (OSHA): Quick Reference Guide to the Bloodborne Pathogens Standard, n.d. Retrieved from: https://www.osha.gov/SLTC/bloodbornepathogens/bloodborne_quickref.html.

CHAPTER 24

American Academy of Child & Adolescent Psychiatry (AACAP): TV violence and children, 2014. Retrieved from: http://www.aacap.org/AACAP/Families_and_Youth/Facts_for_Families/FFF-Guide/Children-And-TV-Violence-013.aspx.

American Academy of Child & Adolescent Psychiatry (AACAP): Adopted children, 2015. Retrieved from: http://www.aacap.org/aacap/families_and_youth/facts_for_families/fff-guide/The-Adopted-Child-015.aspx.

American Academy of Pediatric Dentistry: Frequently asked questions, n.d. Retrieved from: http://www.aapd.org/resources/frequently_asked_questions/.

American Cancer Society (ACS): Recommendations for prostate cancer early detection, 2016. Retrieved from: https://www.cancer.org/cancer/prostate-cancer/early-detection/acs-recommendations.html.

American Cancer Society (ACS): Recommendations for the early detection of breast cancer, 2017. Retrieved from: https://www.cancer.org/cancer/breast-cancer/screening-tests-and-early-detection/american-cancer-society-recommendations-for-the-early-detection-of-breast-cancer.html.

Centers for Disease Control and Prevention (CDC): Healthy weight, 2015. Retrieved from: https://www.cdc.gov/healthyweight/assessing/bmi/childrens_bmi/about_childrens_bmi.html.

Centers for Disease Control and Prevention (CDC): Understanding bullying, 2016. Retrieved from: http://www.cdc.gov/violenceprevention/pdf/bullying_factsheet.pdf.

Chin B, Chan E, Goldman R: Early exposure to food and food allergy in children, *Can Fam Physician* 60(4):338–339, 2014. Retrieved from: https://www.ncbi.nlm.nih.gov/pmc/articles/PMC4046529/.

Generations United: Raising the children of the opioid epidemic: Solutions and support for grandfamilies, 2016. Retrieved from: http://www.grandfamilies.org/Portals/0/2016%20State%20of%20Grandfamilies%20Report%20FINAL.pdf.

Livingston G: Fewer than half of U.S. kids today live in a "tradional family", 2014. Retrieved from: http://www.pewresearch.org/fact-tank/2014/12/22/less-than-half-of-u-s-kids-today-live-in-a-traditional-family/.

Mather M, Jacobsen L, Pollard K: Aging in the United States, *Popul Bull* 70(2):2015. Population Reference Bureau. Retrieved from: https://www.prb.org/wp-content/uploads/2016/01/aging-us-population-bulletin-1.pdf.

National Children's Alliance: Fact sheet, 2014. Retrieved from: http://www.nationalchildrensalliance.org/media-room/media-kit/fact-sheet.

National Institutes of Health (NIH): Calcium, 2016. Retrieved from: https://ods.od.nih.gov/factsheets/Calcium-HealthProfessional/.

Stibich M: What is the genetic theory of aging? How genes affect aging and how you may "alter your genes", 2018. Retrieved from: https://www.verywellhealth.com/the-genetic-theory-of-aging-2224222.

Stotzer RL, Herman JL, Hasenbush A: Transgender parenting: A review of existing research, 2014. Retrieved from: http://williamsinstitute.law.ucla.edu/wp-content/uploads/transgender-parenting-oct-2014.pdf.

US Department of Health and Human Services, Administration for Children and Families, Administration on Children, Youth and Families: Recent demographic trends in foster care, 2013. Retrieved from: http://www.acf.hhs.gov/sites/default/files/cb/data_brief_foster_care_trends1.pdf.

US Department of Health and Human Services, Office of Disease Prevention and Health Promotion: Healthy People 2020, 2014. Retrieved from: https://www.healthypeople.gov/2020/About-Healthy-People.

World Health Organization (WHO): Life expectancy at birth (years), 2000-2015, 2016. Retrieved from: http://gamapserver.who.int/gho/interactive_charts/mbd/life_expectancy/atlas.html.

CHAPTER 25

Aging With Dignity: Five Wishes, 2015. Retrieved from: https://www.agingwithdignity.org/five-wishes.

Centers for Disease Control and Prevention (CDC): Suicide and self-inflicted injury, 2017a. Retrieved from: https://www.cdc.gov/nchs/fastats/suicide.htm.

Death With Dignity: Death with dignity acts, n.d. Retrieved from: https://www.deathwithdignity.org/learn/death-with-dignity-acts/.

Eskanazi Health: No One Dies Alone, 2016. Retrieved from: http://www.eskenazihealth.edu/our-services/palliative-care-program/noda.

Kapel S: *Dying boy's letter pleads for empathy*, Kansas City, March 8, 1974, Kansas City Times.

National Consensus Project for Quality Palliative Care: *Clinical practice guidelines for quality palliative care*, Pittsburg, 2013, National Consensus Project for Quality Palliative Care.

National Organ Transplantation Act, Public Law 98-507, 10-14, 1984. Retrieved from: https://history.nih.gov/research/downloads/PL98-507.pdf.

NICU Helping Hands, The Angel Gown Program, n.d. Retrieved from: http://www.nicuhelpinghands.org/programs/angel-gown-program/.

Now I Lay Me Down to Sleep: Mission and history, n.d. Retrieved from: https://www.nowilaymedowntosleep.org/about/mission-and-history/.

The Oregon Death With Dignity Act, 1997. Retrieved from: http://public.health.oregon.gov/ProviderPartnerResources/EvaluationResearch/DeathwithDignityAct/Documents/statute.pdf.

ProCon.org: Opinion Polls/Surveys, 2011. Retrieved from: http://euthanasia.procon.org/view.resource.php?resourceID=000134.

Worden JW: *Grief counseling and grief therapy: a handbook for the mental health practitioner*, ed 4, New York, 2009, Springer.

World Health Organization: WHO definition of palliative care, n.d. Retrieved from: http://www.who.int/cancer/palliative/definition/en/.

CHAPTER 26

Behrman RE, Butler AS, editors: *Preterm births: Causes, consequences, and prevention. Institute of Medicine (US) Committee on Understanding Premature Birth and Assuring Healthy Outcomes*, Washington, D.C., 2007, National Academies Press. Retrieved from: www.ncbi.nlm.nih.gov/books/NBK11382.

Gabbe SG, Niebyl JR, Simpson JL, et al: *Obstetrics: normal and problem pregnancies*, ed 6, Philadelphia, 2012, Saunders.

May KA: Three phases of father involvement in pregnancy, *Nurs Res* **31**(6):337–342, 1982.

National Institutes of Health (NIH): Nuchal translucency test, 2018a. Retrieved from: https://medlineplus.gov/ency/article/007561.htm.

National Institutes of Health (NIH): Pica, 2018b. Retrieved from: https://medlineplus.gov/ency/article/001538.htm.

US National Library of Medicine (NLM): Nuchal translucency test, A.D.A.M. Medical Encyclopedia, 2012. Retrieved from: www.ncbi.nlm.nih.gov/pubmedhealth/PMH0002884.

CHAPTER 27

Centers for Disease Control and Prevention (CDC): National vital statistics reports: Birth: Final data for 2013, 2015. Retrieved from: https://www.cdc.gov/nchs/data/nvsr/nvsr64/nvsr64_01.pdf.

Cheyney M, Bovbjerg M, Everson C, et al: Outcomes of care for 16,924 planned home births in the United States: the Midwives Alliance of North America Statistics Project, 2004 to 2009, *J Midwifery Womens Health* 59:17–47, 2014.

Friedman AM, Ananth CV, Prendergast E, et al: Variation in and factors associated with use of episiotomy, *JAMA* 313:197–199, 2015.

CHAPTER 28

American Academy of Pediatrics (AAP), Task Force on Circumcision: Circumcision policy Statement, 2012. Retrieved from: http://pediatrics.aappublications.org/content/130/3/585.

Centers for Disease Control and Prevention (CDC): Longer hospital stays for childbirth, 2015. Retrieved from: https://www.cdc.gov/nchs/data/hestat/hospbirth/hospbirth.htm.

Centers for Disease Control and Prevention (CDC): Sudden unexpected infant death and sudden infant death syndrome, 2018. Retrieved from: https://www.cdc.gov/sids/parents-caregivers.htm.

Gagandeep, Sagar Nidhi, Mamta, Kaur Jasbir: Efficacy of cabbage leaves in relief of breast engorgement among postnatal mothers, 2013, *Int J Nurs Educ* 5(2):76–79, 2013.

Governors Highway Safety Association: Child passenger safety laws, 2014. Retrieved from: www.ghsa.org/html/stateinfo/laws/childsafety_laws.html.

Healthychildren.org: Swaddling: Is it safe? 2017. Retrieved from: https://www.healthychildren.org/English/ages-stages/baby/diapers-clothing/Pages/Swaddling-Is-it-Safe.aspx.

CHAPTER 29

American College of Obstetricians and Gynecologists (ACOG): Frequently asked questions: pregnancy, 2017. Retrieved from: https://www.acog.org/Patients/FAQs/Having-a-Baby-After-Age-35#childbearing.

Centers for Disease Control and Prevention (CDC): Behind international rankings of infant mortality: How the United States compares with Europe, 2009. Retrieved from: www.cdc.gov/nchs/data/databriefs/db23.htm.

Centers for Disease Control and Prevention (CDC): Birthweight and gestation, 2017a. Retrieved from: https://www.cdc.gov/nchs/fastats/birthweight.htm.

Centers for Disease Control and Prevention (CDC): Preterm birth, 2017b. Retrieved from: https://www.cdc.gov/reproductivehealth/maternalinfanthealth/pretermbirth.htm.

Centers for Disease Control and Prevention (CDC): National Center for Health Care Statistics: Multiple births, 2017c. Retrieved from: https://www.cdc.gov/nchs/fastats/multiple.htm.

Centers for Disease Control and Prevention (CDC): Infant mortality, 2018. Retrieved from: www.cdc.gov/reproductivehealth/MaternalInfantHealth/InfantMortality.htm.

Davidson MC, London ML, Ladewig PW: *Olds' maternal-newborn nursing & women's health across the lifespan*, ed 9, Upper Saddle River, NJ, 2012, Pearson Prentice Hall.

Khan FH: Hyperemesis gravidarum in emergency medicine treatment and management, 2016. Retrieved from: http://emedicine.medscape.com/article/796564-treatment#d10.

Lowdermilk DL, Perry SE: *Maternity and women's health care*, ed 9, St. Louis, 2007, Mosby.

Moore LE: Hydatidiform mole, 2016. Retrieved from: http://emedicine.medscape.com/article/254657-overview#a6.

Smith JR: Postpartum hemorrhage, 2017. Retrieved from: http://emedicine.medscape.com/article/275038-overview.

Statista: Infant mortality in the United States from 2006 to 2016, 2018. Retrieved from: https://www.statista.com/statistics/263738/infant-mortality-in-the-usa/.

CHAPTER 30

American Academy of Child and Adolescent Psychiatry (AACAP): Children and watching TV, 2011. Retrieved from: www.aacap.org/AACAP/Families_and_Youth/Facts_for_Families/Facts_for_Families_Pages/Children_And_Wat_54.aspx.

American Cancer Society (ACS): Health risks of smokeless tobacco, 2015. Retrieved from: https://www.cancer.org/cancer/cancer-causes/tobacco-and-cancer/smokeless-tobacco.html.

American Psychological Association (APA): Violence in the media: Psychologists help protect children from harmful effects, 2004. Retrieved from: www.apa.org/research/action/protect.aspx.

Centers for Disease Control and Prevention (CDC): Youth and tobacco use, 2013. Retrieved from: www.cdc.gov/tobacco/data_statistics/fact_sheets/youth_data/tobacco_use/index.htm.

Centers for Disease Control and Prevention (CDC): State Laws prohibiting sales to minors and indoor use of electronic nicotine delivery systems — United States, November 2014, 2014. Retrieved from: https://www.cdc.gov/mmwr/preview/mmwrhtml/mm6349a1.htm.

Centers for Disease Control and Prevention (CDC): Hookahs, 2016. Retrieved from: https://www.cdc.gov/tobacco/data_statistics/fact_sheets/tobacco_industry/hookahs/index.htm.

Centers for Disease Control and Prevention (CDC): Childhood overweight and obesity, 2017. Retrieved from: https://www.cdc.gov/obesity/childhood/index.html.

Chapman L: AAP changes milk recommendations for children under 2, 2008. Retrieved from: http://www.findingdulcinea.com/news/health/July-August-08/AAP-Changes-Milk-Recommendations-for-Children-Under-2.html.

Federal Communications Commission (FCC): Children's educational television, 2017. Retrieved from: https://www.fcc.gov/consumers/guides/childrens-educational-television.

Gray P: The many benefits, for kids, of playing video games, Psychology Today, 2012. Retrieved from: www.psychologytoday.com/blog/freedom-learn/201201/the-many-benefits-kids-playing-videogames.

Guttmacher Institute: Adolescent sexual and reproductive health in the United States, 2017. Retrieved from: https://www.guttmacher.org/fact-sheet/american-teens-sexual-and-reproductive-health.

Herrick KA, Fakhouri T, Carlson S, et al: TV watching and computer use in U.S. youth aged 12 to 15, 2012, 2014. Retrieved from: https://www.cdc.gov/nchs/data/databriefs/db157.htm.

Hockenberry MJ, Wilson D: *Wong's nursing care of infants and children*, ed 8, St. Louis, 2007, Mosby.

Kullgren JT, McLaughlin CG, Mitra N, et al: Nonfinancial barriers and access to care for US adults, Health Services Research, 2011. Retrieved from: https://www.rwjf.org/en/library/research/2012/02/special-issue-of-health-services-research-links-health-care-rese/nonfinancial-barriers-and-access-to-care-for-us-adults.html.

Lenhart A: Teens, social media & technology overview, 2015. Retrieved from: http://www.pewinternet.org/2015/04/09/teens-social-media-technology-2015/.

Mayo Clinic: Childhood obesity, 2012. Retrieved from: www.mayoclinic.com/health/childhood-obesity/DS00698/DSECTION=causes.

National Institute of Allergy and Infectious Diseases (NIAID): Human papilloma virus (HPV) and genital warts, 2009. Retrieved from: http://www3.niaid.nih.gov/topics/genitalWarts.

News Medical Life Sciences: AAP report addresses new phenomenon, "Facebook depression", 2012. Retrieved from: https://www.news-medical.net/news/20120131/AAP-report-addresses-new-phenomenon-Facebook-Depression.aspx.

Office of Disease Prevention and Health Promotion (ODPHP): Health.gov: Children and adolescents, 2018. Retrieved from: https://health.gov/paguidelines/guidelines/children.aspx.

Office of Disease Prevention and Health Promotion (ODPHP): Healthypeople.gov: Immunization and infectious diseases, 2014. Retrieved from: https://www.healthypeople.gov/2020/topics-objectives/topic/immunization-and-infectious-diseases/objectives#4722.

Office of Disease Prevention and Health Promotion (ODPHP): Healthypeople.gov: 2020 LHI topics, 2018. Retrieved from: https://www.healthypeople.gov/2020/leading-health-indicators/2020-LHI-Topics.

Parents Television Council: Facts and TV statistics, 2018. Retrieved from: http://w2.parentstv.org/main/Research/Facts.aspx.

Schurgin O, Keeffe G, Clarke-Pearson K: Clinical report – the impact of social media on children, adolescents, and families, Retrieved from: http://pediatrics.aappublications.org/content/pediatrics/early/2011/03/28/peds.2011-0054.full.pdf.

Stopbullying.gov: Facts about bullying, n.d. Retrieved from: https://www.stopbullying.gov/media/facts/index.html#stats.

Unite for Sight: Module 2: Unique barriers to health care for children and adolescents, n.d. Retrieved from: http://www.uniteforsight.org/women-children-course/barriers-children.

University of Michigan: Television and children, 2010. Retrieved from: www.med.umich.edu/yourchild/topics/tv.htm.

US Department of Agriculture (USDA): Choosemyplate.gov, 2016. Retrieved from: https://www.choosemyplate.gov/physical-activity-amount.

US Department of Agriculture (USDA): Dietary guidelines for Americans, 2010. Retrieved from: www.cnpp.usda.gov/Publications/DietaryGuidelines/2010/PolicyDoc/Chapter4.pdf.

US Food and Drug Administration (US FDA): Cervarix: Product information: Package insert, 2009. Retrieved from: www.fda.gov/downloads/BiologicsBloodVaccines/Vaccines/ApprovedProducts/UCM186981.pdf.

Victoria State Government: What is bullying? 2017. Retrieved from: http://www.education.vic.gov.au/about/programs/bullystoppers/Pages/what.aspx.

Whitten L: Brief intervention helps adolescents curb substance use, 2013. Retrieved from: www.drugabuse.gov/news-events/nida-notes/2013/01/brief-intervention-helps-adolescents-curbsubstance-use.

CHAPTER 31

American Academy of Pediatrics (AAP): Breastfeeding and the use of human milk, *Pediatrics* 129(3):e827–e841, 2012. Retrieved from: http://pediatrics.aappublications.org/content/129/3/e827.full.pdf+html.

American Academy of Pediatrics (AAP): Reduce the risk of SIDS and suffocation, 2017. Retrieved from: https://www.healthychildren.org/English/ages-stages/baby/sleep/Pages/Preventing-SIDS.aspx.

American Nurses Association (ANA): *Nursing's social policy statement*, MD, 2003, Silver Springs. Nursesbooks.org.

American Nurses Association (ANA): *Nursing's social policy statement: the essence of the profession*, MD, 2010, Silver Springs. Nursesbooks.org.

Centers for Disease Control and Prevention (CDC): Achievements in public health 1990-1999: healthier mothers and babies, *MMWR Morb Mortal Wkly Rep* 48(38):849–858, 1999. Retrieved from: https://www.cdc.gov/mmwr/preview/mmwrhtml/mm4838a2.htm.

Centers for Disease Control and Prevention (CDC): Community water fluoridation: questions & answers, 2016. Retrieved from: https://www.cdc.gov/fluoridation/index.html.

Cleveland Clinic: Should your child be screened for high cholesterol? 2016. Retrieved from: https://health.clevelandclinic.org/2016/02/should-your-child-be-screened-for-high-cholesterol.

Forum on Child and Family Statistics: America's children in brief: key national indicators of well-being, 2012. Retrieved from: http://childstats.gov/americaschildren/glance.asp.

Hockenberry MJ, Wilson D: *Wong's nursing care of infants and children*, ed 10, St. Louis, 2015, Mosby.

National Institute of Child Health and Human Development (NICHD): What are the recommendations for breastfeeding? n.d. Retrieved from: https://www.nichd.nih.gov/health/topics/breastfeeding/conditioninfo/recommendations.

Robertson J, Robertson J: *Separation and the very young*, London, 1990, Free Association Books.

Spitz RA: Hospitalism—an inquiry into the genesis of psychiatric conditions in early childhood, *Psychoanal Study Child* 1:53–74, 1945.

Spitz RA: Hospitalism; a follow-up report on investigation described in volume I, 1945, *Psychoanal Study Child* 2:113–117, 1946.

US Department of Health and Human Services (US DHHS): Child maltreatment, 2015. Retrieved from: www.acf.hhs.gov/sites/default/files/cb/cm11.pdf.

US Department of Health and Human Services (US DHHS): Trends in teen pregnancy and childbearing, 2016. Retrieved from: https://www.hhs.gov/ash/oah/adolescent-development/

reproductive-health-and-teen-pregnancy/teen-pregnancy-and-childbearing/trends/index.html.

CHAPTER 32

American Cancer Society: Prognostic factors in childhood leukemia (ALL or AML), 2016a. Retrieved from: https://www.cancer.org/cancer/leukemia-in-children/detection-diagnosis-staging/prognostic-factors.html.

American Cancer Society: What are the key statistics about Wilms tumor? 2016b. Retrieved from: https://www.cancer.org/cancer/wilms-tumor/about/key-statistics.html.

American Cancer Society: Key statistics about neuroblastoma, 2018. Retrieved from: https://www.cancer.org/cancer/neuroblastoma/about/key-statistics.html.

American Diabetes Association: Statistics about diabetes, 2018. Retrieved from: http://www.diabetes.org/diabetes-basics/statistics/.

American Kidney Fund: Childhood nephrotic syndrome, n.d. Retrieved from: www.kidneyfund.org/kidney-health/kidneyproblems/childhood-nephrotic-syndrome.html.

Anxiety and Depression Association of America (ADAA): Depression, n.d. Retrieved from: https://adaa.org/understanding-anxiety/depression.

Asthma and Allergy Foundation of America (AAFA): Allergy facts and figures, n.d. Retrieved from: http://www.aafa.org/page/allergy-facts.aspx.

Autism Speaks: What is autism? 2018. Retrieved from: https://www.autismspeaks.org/what-autism.

Boston Children's Hospital: Congenital HIV symptoms and causes, n.d. Retrieved from: http://www.childrenshospital.org/conditions-and-treatments/conditions/c/congenital-hiv/symptoms-and-causes.

Centers for Disease Control and Prevention (CDC): Attention deficit/hyperactivity disorder, 2013. Retrieved from: www.cdc.gov/ncbddd/adhd/data.html.

Centers for Disease Control and Prevention (CDC): Lead: Prevention tips, 2014. Retrieved from: https://www.cdc.gov/nceh/lead/tips.htm.

Centers for Disease Control and Prevention (CDC): Autism spectrum disorder: Screening and diagnosis, 2015. Retrieved from: https://www.cdc.gov/ncbddd/autism/screening.html.

Centers for Disease Control and Prevention (CDC): Epilepsy fast facts, 2016. Retrieved from: www.cdc.gov/epilepsy/basics/fast_facts.htm.

Centers for Disease Control and Prevention (CDC): Sickle cell disease (SCD): Data and statistics on sickle cell disease, 2017a. Retrieved from: https://www.cdc.gov/ncbddd/sicklecell/data.html.

Centers for Disease Control and Prevention (CDC): Asthma, 2017b. Retrieved from: https://www.cdc.gov/nchs/fastats/asthma.htm.

Centers for Disease Control and Prevention (CDC): Facts about cleft lip and cleft palate, 2017c. Retrieved from: https://www.cdc.gov/ncbddd/birthdefects/cleftlip.html.

Centers for Disease Control and Prevention (CDC): Cerebral palsy: Data & statistics for cerebral palsy, 2017d. Retrieved from: https://www.cdc.gov/ncbddd/cp/data.html.

Centers for Disease Control and Prevention (CDC): HIV among pregnant women, infants, and children, 2018a. Retrieved from: https://www.cdc.gov/hiv/group/gender/pregnantwomen/.

Centers for Disease Control and Prevention (CDC): Facts about Down syndrome, 2018b. Retrieved from: https://www.cdc.gov/ncbddd/birthdefects/downsyndrome.html.

Cystic Fibrosis Foundation: About cystis fibrosis, n.d. Retrieved from: https://www.cff.org/What-is-CF/About-Cystic-Fibrosis/.

HIV.gov: Lab tests and why they are important, 2017. Retrieved from: https://www.hiv.gov/hiv-basics/staying-in-hiv-care/provider-visits-and-lab-test/lab-tests-and-results.

Hockenberry MJ, Wilson D: *Wong's nursing care of infants and children*, ed 10, St. Louis, 2015, Mosby.

Johns Hopkins: Diagnosis: Testing: Sweat Test, 2018. Retrieved from: http://www.hopkinscf.org/what-is-cf/diagnosis/testing/sweat-test.

Leas DP: Atlantoaxial instability, 2017. Retrieved from: http://emedicine.medscape.com/article/1265682-overview#a5.

Maraqa NF: Bronchiolitis, 2018. Retrieved from: http://emedicine.medscape.com/article/961963-overview#a6.

Mayo Clinic: Intussusception, 2015. Retrieved from: http://www.mayoclinic.org/diseases-conditions/intussusception/diagnosis-treatment/diagnosis/dxc-20166997.

March of Dimes: Neural tube defects, 2016. Retrieved from: https://www.marchofdimes.org/baby/neural-tube-defects.aspx.

Marshall BC: Survival trending upward, but what does this really mean? Cystic Fibrosis Foundation, 2017. Retrieved from: https://www.cff.org/CF-Community-Blog/Posts/2017/Survival-Trending-Upward-but-What-Does-This-Really-Mean/.

Mayo Clinic: Iron deficiency in children: prevention tips for parents, 2016. Retrieved from: http://www.mayoclinic.org/healthy-lifestyle/childrens-health/in-depth/iron-deficiency/art-20045634?pg=2. Nov. 29, 2016.

Mayo Clinic: Congenital heart defects in children, 2018a. Retrieved from: https://www.mayoclinic.org/diseases-conditions/congenital-heart-defects-children/symptoms-causes/syc-20350074.

Mayo Clinic: *Hemophilia* 2018b. Retrieved from: http://www.mayoclinic.org/diseases-conditions/hemophilia/basics/tests-diagnosis/con-20029824.

Mayo Clinic: Intususception, 2018c. Retrieved from: http://www.mayoclinic.org/diseases-conditions/intussusception/diagnosis-treatment/diagnosis/dxc-20166997.

Mayo Clinic: Autism spectrum disorder, 2018d. Retrieved from: https://www.mayoclinic.org/diseases-conditions/autism-spectrum-disorder/symptoms-causes/syc-20352928.

Medscape: Cerebral palsy medication, 2016. Retrieved from: http://emedicine.medscape.com/article/1179555-medication#2-#4.

Munoz FM, Ralston SL, Meissner HC: RSV recommendations unchanged after review of new data, *AAP News* 2017. Retrieved from: http://www.aappublications.org/news/2017/10/19/RSV101917.

My Child Without Limits (MCWL): Down syndrome prognosis, 2018. Retrieved from: http://www.mychildwithoutlimits.org/understand/down-syndrome/down-syndrome-prognosis.

National Center for Education Statistics (NCES): Children and youth with disabilities, 2018. Retrieved from: https://nces.ed.gov/programs/coe/indicator_cgg.asp.

National Heart, Lung, and Blood Institute: Expert panel report 3: Guidelines for the diagnosis and management of asthma, 2007. Retrieved from: www.nhlbi.nih.gov/guidelines/asthma/asthgdln.pdf.

National Hemophilia Foundation: Hemophilia A (factor VIII deficiency), n.d. Retrieved from: www.hemophilia.org/NHFWeb/MainPgs/MainNHF.aspx?menuid=180&contentid=45&rptname=bleeding.

National Institutes of Health (NIH): Diabetes, type 1, n.d. Retrieved from: http://report.nih.gov/NIHfactsheets/ViewFactSheet.aspx?csid=120.

National Institutes of Health (NIH): Safe to sleep: Fast facts about SIDS, 2017. Retrieved from: https://www.nichd.nih.gov/sts/about/SIDS/Pages/fastfacts.aspx.

National Institutes of Health (NIH): Office of Dietary Supplements: Iron: Fact sheet for health professionals, 2018a. Retrieved from: https://ods.od.nih.gov/factsheets/Iron-HealthProfessional/#h2%20March%202,%202018.

National Institutes of Health (NIH): Encephalitis, 2018b. Retrieved from: https://medlineplus.gov/ency/article/001415.htm.

National Institutes of Health (NIH), National Cancer Institute: Childhood Hodgkin lymphoma treatment (PDQ)—Patient version, 2018. Retrieved from: https://www.cancer.gov/types/lymphoma/patient/child-hodgkin-treatment-pdq.

National Institute of Mental Health: Major depressive disorder in children, n.d. Retrieved from: www.nimh.nih.gov/statistics/1MDD_CHILD.shtml.

National Kidney Foundation: Childhood nephrotic syndrome, n.d. Retrieved from: https://www.kidney.org/atoz/content/childns.

National Library of Medicine: Death among children and adolescents, n.d. Retrieved from: https://medlineplus.gov/ency/article/001915.htm.

National Marrow Donor Program: Severe aplastic anemia transplant outcomes, n.d. Retrieved from: http://bethematch.org/Patient/Disease_and_Treatment/About_Your_Disease/Aplastic_Anemia/Transplant_Results.aspx.

Nowicki R, et al: Atopic dermatitis: current treatment guidelines, *Postepy Dermatol Alergol* 32(4):239–249, 2015. Retrieved from: https://www.ncbi.nlm.nih.gov/pmc/articles/PMC4565838/#_ffn_sectitle.

Patel M: Clubfoot, 2017. Retrieved from: http://emedicine.medscape.com/article/1237077-overview#a7.

Raghupathy P: Diabetic ketoacidosis in children and adolescents, *Indian J Endocrinol Metab* 19(Suppl 1):S55–S57, 2015. Retrieved from: https://www.ncbi.nlm.nih.gov/pmc/articles/PMC4413392/.

Regalado A: Gene therapy is curing hemophilia, 2016. Retrieved from: https://www.technologyreview.com/s/601651/gene-therapy-is-curing-hemophilia/.

Schwarz SM: Pediatric gastroesophageal treatment and management, 2017. Retrieved from: http://emedicine.medscape.com/article/930029-treatment.

UNAIDS: Global HIV & AIDS statistics — 2018 fact sheet. Retrieved from: http://www.unaids.org/en/resources/fact-sheet.

Wagner JP: Hirschsprung disease, 2017. Retrieved from: http://emedicine.medscape.com/article/178493-overview#a2.

CHAPTER 33

American Heart Association: The skinny on fats, 2017. Retrieved from: http://www.heart.org/HEARTORG/Conditions/Cholesterol/PreventionTreatmentofHighCholesterol/Know-Your-Fats_UCM_305628_Article.jsp .

American Heart Association/American Stroke Association (AHA/ASA): Heart disease and stroke statistics 2018 at-a-glance, 2018. Retrieved from: https://www.heart.org/-/media/data-import/downloadables/heart-disease-and-stroke-statistics-2018—at-a-glance-ucm_498848.pdf.

AssistedLivingFacilities.org: Assisted living costs: review the average costs of assisted living by state, n.d. Retrieved from: https://www.assistedlivingfacilities.org/resources/assisted-living-costs/.

Centers for Disease Control and Prevention (CDC): Cost of falls among older adults, 2016. Retrieved from: https://www.cdc.gov/HomeandRecreationalSafety/Falls/fallcost.html.

Centers for Disease Control and Prevention (CDC): Immunization schedule for adults (19 years of age and older), 2018. Retrieved from: https://www.cdc.gov/vaccines/schedules/easy-to-read/adult.html.

Ignatavicius DD, Workman ML: *Medical-surgical nursing: Patient centered collaborative care*, ed 8, St. Louis, 2016, Saunders.

Mayo Clinic: Calcium and calcium supplements: Achieving the right balance, 2015. Retrieved from: http://www.mayoclinic.org/healthy-lifestyle/nutrition-and-healthy-eating/in-depth/calcium-supplements/art-20047097.

Mayo Clinic: Unexplained weight loss, 2018. Retrieved from: http://www.mayoclinic.org/symptoms/unexplained-weight-loss/basics/definition/sym-20050700.

Mitchell SL, Mor V, et al: Tube feeding in U.S. nursing home residents with advanced dementia, 2000-2014, *JAMA* 316(7):769–770, 2016. Retrieved from: https://www.ncbi.nlm.nih.gov/pmc/articles/PMC4991625/.

National Eye Institute: Facts about glaucoma, 2015. Retrieved from: https://nei.nih.gov/health/glaucoma/glaucoma_facts.

National Institute on Deafness and Other Communication Disorders: Hearing loss and older adults, 2017. Retrieved from: https://www.nidcd.nih.gov/health/hearing-loss-older-adults.

National Pressure Ulcer Awareness Panel (NPUAP): Pressure ulcer awareness day is November 16, 2012. Retrieved from: www.npuap.org/pressure-ulcer-awareness-day-is-november-16-2012.

National Stroke Association: Minorities and stroke, n.d. Retrieved from: http://www.stroke.org/understand-stroke/impact-stroke/minorities-and-stroke.

Stibich M: What causes glaucoma? 2017. Retrieved from: https://www.verywell.com/glaucoma-aging-and-glaucoma-2223623.

Tan S: Myths of aging, 2011. Retrieved from: https://www.psychologytoday.com/blog/wise/201101/myths-aging.

Traywick LS: Exercise recommendations for older adults, n.d. Retrieved from: http://www.todaysgeriatricmedicine.com/news/ex_092210_03.shtml.

US Census Bureau: Profile America: Facts for features: Older Americans month: May, 2012. Retrieved from: www.census.gov/newsroom/releases/archives/facts_for_features_special_editions/cb12-ff07.html.

US Census Bureau: An aging nation: The older population in the United States, 2014a. Retrieved from: https://www.census.gov/prod/2014pubs/p25-1140.pdf.

US Census Bureau: Fueled by Baby Boomers, nation's older population to nearly double in next 20 years, census bureau reports, 2014b. Retrieved from: http://www.census.gov/newsroom/press-releases/2014/cb14-84.html.

US Department of Health and Human Services (USDHHS): Key features of the Affordable Care Act, by year, n.d.a. Retrieved from: www.healthcare.gov/law/timeline/full.html#top.

US Department of Health and Human Services (USDHHS), Administration for Community Living: National family caregiver support program, 2017. Retrieved from: https://www.acl.gov/node/314.

US Department of Health and Human Services (USDHHS): Development of the National Health Promotion and Disease Prevention Objectives for 2030, 2018a. Retrieved from: https://www.healthypeople.gov/2020/About-Healthy-People/Development-Healthy-People-2030.

US Department of Health and Human Services (USDHHS), Administration for Community Living: Services for Native Americans (OAA Title VI), 2018b. Retrieved from: https://www.acl.gov/programs/services-native-americans-oaa-title-vi.

US National Library of Medicine: Aging changes in the senses, 2018. Retrieved from: https://medlineplus.gov/ency/article/004013.htm .

World Health Rankings: United States: Life expectancy, 2015. Retrieved from: http://www.worldlifeexpectancy.com/united-states-life-expectancy.

CHAPTER 34

Beers CW: *A mind that found itself*, New York, 1908, Longmans, Green & Co.

Centers for Disease Control and Prevention (CDC): CDC report: Mental illness surveillance among U.S. adults, 2011. Retrieved from: www.cdc.gov/mentalhealthsurveillance.

National Alliance on Mental Illness (NAMI): Mental health investment by states slowed in 2014, 2014. Retrieved from: https://www.nami.org/Blogs/NAMI-Blog/December-2014/Mental-Health-Investment-By-States-Slowed-in-2014.

National Institute of Mental Health: Mental illness, 2017. Retrieved from: https://www.nimh.nih.gov/health/statistics/prevalence/any-mental-illness-ami-among-us-adults.shtml.

Thornton SP: Sigmund Freud (1856–1939). Internet Encyclopedia of Philosophy, n.d. Retrieved from: www.iep.utm.edu/freud/#H3.

CHAPTER 35

Alzheimer's Association: Alzheimer's and dementia facts and figures, 2018. Retrieved from: https://www.alz.org/alzheimers-dementia/facts-figures.

American Psychiatric Association: *Diagnostic and statistical manual of mental disorders*, ed 5, Arlington, VA, 2013, American Psychiatric Publishing.

Centers for Disease Control and Prevention (CDC): Leading causes of death, 2017. Retrieved from: https://www.cdc.gov/nchs/fastats/leading-causes-of-death.htm.

Centers for Disease Control and Prevention (CDC): Mental health conditions: depression and anxiety, 2018. Retrieved from: https://cdc.gov/tobacco/campaign/tips/diseases/depression-anxiety.html.

Maslow AH: *Motivation and personality*, New York, 1970, Harper & Row.

National Institute of Mental Health: Depression, 2018. Retrieved from: https://www.nimh.nih.gov/health/topics/depression/index.shtml.

CHAPTER 36

American Nurses Association: Impaired nurse resource center, n.d. Retrieved from: http://nursingworld.org/MainMenuCategories/WorkplaceSafety/Healthy-Work-Environment/Work-Environment/ImpairedNurse.

American Society of Addiction Medicine: n.d. Retrieved from: www.asam.org.

Burns MJ: Delirium tremens (DTs), *Medscape* 2013. Retrieved from: http://emedicine.medscape.com/article/166032-overview#aw2aab6b2b4aa.

Centers for Disease Control and Prevention (CDC): Illegal drug use, 2017a. Retrieved from: www.cdc.gov/nchs/fastats/druguse.htm.

Centers for Disease Control and Prevention (CDC): Prescription opioid data, 2017b. Retrieved from: https://www.cdc.gov/drugoverdose/data/prescribing.html?CDC_AA_refVal=https%3A%2F%2Fwww.cdc.gov%2Fdrugoverdose%2Fdata%2Foverdose.html.

Helpguide.org: Teenage drinking, n.d. Retrieved from: www.helpguide.org/harvard/alcohol_teens.htm.

National Council on Alcoholism and Drug Dependence (NCADD): FAQs/facts, n.d. Retrieved from: www.ncadd.org/index.php/learn-about-alcohol/faqsfacts.

National Institute on Alcohol Abuse and Alcoholism: Alcohol facts and statistics, 2018. Retrieved from: https://www.niaaa.nih.gov/alcohol-health/overview-alcohol-consumption/alcohol-facts-and-statistics.

National Institute on Drug Abuse: Heroin, 2018. Retrieved from: https://www.drugabuse.gov/publications/research-reports/heroin/scope-heroin-use-in-united-states

National Institute on Drug Abuse: MDMA (ecstasy/Molly), 2013b. Retrieved from: www.drugabuse.gov/drugs-abuse/mdmaecstasymolly.

Office of Disease Prevention and Health Promotion: Subst Abus, 2018. Retrieved from: https://www.healthypeople.gov/2020/leading-health-indicators/2020-lhi-topics/Substance-Abuse/data.

CHAPTER 37

Bureau of Labor Statistics: Occupational outlook handbook: occupational therapists, 2015. Retrieved from: https://www.bls.gov/ooh/healthcare/occupational-therapists.htm.

Center for Medicare Advocacy: Medicare home health benefit's face-to-face encounter requirement, 2016. Retrieved from: http://www.medicareadvocacy.org/medicare-home-health-benefits-face-to-face-encounter-requirement/

Centers for Medicare & Medicaid Services (CMS): CMS manual system Department of Health & Human Services (DHHS), Pub 100-01, Medicare general information, eligibility, and entitlement, 2011. Retrieved from: www.cms.gov/Regulations-and-Guidance/Guidance/Transmittals/downloads/R68GI.pdf.

Centers for Medicare & Medicaid Services (CMS): Home health prospective payment system (PPS), 2018a. Retrieved from: https://www.cms.gov/Medicare/Medicare-Fee-for-Service-Payment/HomeHealthPPS/index.html.

Centers for Medicare & Medicaid Services (CMS): Home health quality reporting program, 2018b. Retrieved from: https://www.cms.gov/Medicare/Quality-Initiatives-Patient-Assessment-Instruments/HomeHealthQualityInits/index.html.

Federal Interagency Forum on Aging-Related Statistics: *Older Americans 2012: key indicators of well-being*, Washington, D.C., 2012, United States Government Printing Office. Retrieved from: www.agingstats.gov/agingstatsdotnet/Main_Site/Data/2012_Documents/docs/Population.pdf.

HealthIT.gov: Telemedicine and telehealth, 2017. Retrieved from: https://www.healthit.gov/telehealth.

HealthIT.gov: Health IT and health information exchange basics, 2018. Retrieved from: https://www.healthit.gov/providers-professionals/electronic-medical-records-emr.

Jones AL, Harris-Kojetin L, Valverde R: Characteristics and use of home health care by men and women aged 65 and over.

Medicare.gov: Home health services, n.d. Retrieved from: https://www.medicare.gov/coverage/home-health-services.html.

Morse, S: Medicare proposed changes would cut home health reimbursement, 2017. Retrieved from: https://www.healthcarefinancenews.com/news/home-health-agencies-concerned-about-cuts-proposed-medicare-payments.

National Association for Homecare and Hospice: What types of services do home care providers deliver? 2014. Retrieved from: www.nahc.org/faq/#99.

National health statistics reports; no. 52, Hyattsville, MD, 2012, National Center for Health Statistics.

Nelson R, Staggers N: *Health informatics: an interprofessional approach*, St. Louis, 2014, Mosby.

US Government Publishing Office: Title 42 CFR 484.36—Condition of participation: Home health aide services, 2011. Retrieved from: https://www.gpo.gov/fdsys/granule/CFR-2011-title42-vol5/CFR-2011-title42-vol5-sec484-36/content-detail.html.

CHAPTER 38

AARP: About continuing care retirement communities, n.d. Retrieved from: www.aarp.org/relationships/caregiving-resourcecenter/info-09-2010/ho_continuing_care_retirement_communities.html.

Administration for Community Living (ACL): A statistical profile of older Hispanic Americans, 2015. Retrieved from: https://www.acl.gov/sites/default/files/news%202017-03/A_Statistical_Profile_of_Older_Hispanics.pdf.

Caffrey C, Harris-Kojetin, L, Sengupta M: Variation in Operating Characteristics of Residential Care Communities, by Size of Community: United States, 2014, 2015. Retrieved from: https://www.cdc.gov/nchs/data/databriefs/db222.htm.

Centers for Disease Control and Prevention (CDC): National Center for Health Statistics: Nursing home care, 2017. Retrieved from: https://www.cdc.gov/nchs/fastats/nursing-home-care.htm.

Healthypeople.gov: Health-related quality of life and well-being, 2010. Retrieved from: www.healthypeople.gov/2020/about/QoLWBabout.aspx.

Johnson JH Jr, Appold SJ: U.S. older adults: demographics, living arrangements, and barriers to aging in place, 2017. Retrieved from: http://www.kenaninstitute.unc.edu/wp-content/uploads/2017/06/AgingInPlace_06092017.pdf.

The Joint Commission (TJC): Nursing care center: 2018 national patient safety goals, 2017. Retrieved from: https://www.jointcommission.org/ncc_2017_npsgs/.

Medicare.gov: Long-term care, n.d.a. Retrieved from: https://www.medicare.gov/coverage/long-term-care.html

Medicare.gov: PACE, n.d.b. Retrieved from: https://www.medicare.gov/your-medicare-costs/help-paying-costs/pace/pace.html.

National Center for Assisted Living (NCAL): Communities: number and size of communities, n.d.a. Retrieved from: https://www.ahcancal.org/ncal/facts/Pages/Communities.aspx.

National Center for Assisted Living (NCAL): Residents, n.d.b. Retrieved from: https://www.ahcancal.org/ncal/facts/Pages/Residents.aspx

Statista: Population aged 65 years and over in the United States in 2016, sorted by state, 2018. Retrieved from: https://www.statista.com/statistics/301935/us-population-aged-65-years-and-over-by-state/.

US Census Bureau: Quick facts, 2017. Retrieved from: https://www.census.gov/quickfacts/fact/table/US/PST045217.

CHAPTER 39

ADA National Network: What is the definition of disability under the ADA? n.d. Retrieved from: https://adata.org/faq/what-definition-disability-under-ada.

American Association of Physiatrists: About the AAP, 2013. Retrieved from: www.physiatry.org.

American Lung Association: How pulmonary rehab helps you breathe, 2018. Retrieved from: http://www.lung.org/about-us/blog/2016/03/pulmonary-rehab-helps-breathe.html.

American Physical Therapy Association (APTA): Early rehab in ICU generates net financial savings in hospitals, PT in Motion, 2014. Retrieved from: www.apta.org/PTinmotion/newsnow/2014/1/15/earlyrehabstudy.

American Psychiatric Association (APA): *Diagnostic and statistical manual of mental disorders*, ed 3, Washington, D.C., 1980, American Psychiatric Press.

Anxiety and Depression Association of America (ADAA): How to prevent trauma from becoming PTSD, 2017. Retrieved from: https://adaa.org/learn-from-us/from-the-experts/blog-posts/consumer/how-prevent-trauma-becoming-ptsd.

Association of Rehabilitation Nurses: Definitions and scope of practice, 2016. Retrieved at: www.rehabnurse.org/certification/content/Definition-and-Scope.html.

Bamm EL, Rosenbaum P: Family-centered theory: origins, development, barriers, and supports to implementation in rehabilitation medicine, *Arch Phys Med Rehab* 89(8):1618–1624, 2008.

Barclay W: *Letters to the hebrews (the new daily study bible)*, London, 1976, Westminster John Knox Press.

Centers for Disease Control and Prevention (CDC): *The power of prevention, chronic disease … the public health challenge of the 21st century*, 2009, National Center for Chronic Disease Prevention and Health Promotion. Retrieved from: www.cdc.gov/chronicdisease/pdf/2009-Power-of-Prevention.pdf.

Centers for Disease Control and Prevention (CDC): Health and economic costs of chronic disease, 2018. Retrieved from: https://www.cdc.gov/chronicdisease/about/costs/index.htm.

Clark CC: Posttraumatic stress disorder: how to support healing, *Am J Nurs* 97(8):27–33, 1997.

Cultural Competency Advisory Group: *Establishing a culturally competent master's and doctorally prepared nursing workforce*, Washington, D.C., 2009, American Association of Colleges of Nursing.

Glass AJ: Introduction. In Bourne PG, editor: *The psychology and physiology of stress*, New York, 1969, Academic Press. Handicap [definition], n.d. Retrieved from: www.yourdictionary.com/handicap#medical.

Lipshutz AKM, Engel H, Thornton K, et al: Early mobilization in the intensive care unit, 2012. Retrieved from: www.icu.sagepub.com.

Mayo Clinic: Post-traumatic stress disorder, 2018. Retrieved from: https://www.mayoclinic.org/diseases-conditions/post-traumatic-stress-disorder/symptoms-causes/syc-20355967.

Medscape: Blast injuries, 2016. Retrieved from: http://emedicine.medscape.com/article/822587-overview.

National Center for PTSD: Treatment of PTSD, 2013. Retrieved from: www.ptsd.va.gov.

National Heart, Lung, and Blood Institute: What is cardiac rehabilitation? 2013. Retrieved from: www.nhlbi.nih.gov.

National Rehabilitation Information Center (NARIC): Can a chronic disease diagnosis motivate healthy lifestyle changes? 2016. Retrieved from: http://www.naric.com/?q=en/rif/can-chronic-disease-diagnosis-motivate-healthy-lifestyle-changes.

Pennardt A: Blast injuries, 2016. Retrieved from: http://emedicine.medscape.com/article/822587-overview.

Rehabilitation Institute of Chicago: The role of nurses in rehabilitation care, 2013. Retrieved from: www.ric.org/about/people/nurses.

Rosenfeld JV, Ford NL: Bomb blast, mild traumatic brain injury and psychiatric morbidity: A review, 2013. Retrieved from: www.noninvasiveicp.com.

Stevenson C: Evolving mechanisms and patterns of blast injury and the challenges for military first responders, *J Mil Vet Health*, 17(4):17–21, 2009.

Smeltzer SC, Bare BG, Hinkle JL, et al: *Textbook of medicalsurgical nursing*, ed 12, Philadelphia, 2010, Wolters Kluwer Health/Lippincott, Williams, & Wilkins.

US Department of Health and Human Services (USDHHS): 2020 Topics and objectives, 2013. Retrieved from: http://healthypeople.gov/2020/topicsobjectives2020/default.aspx.

CHAPTER 40

Goldstein LG, Glaser DI: Pain management in nursing homes and hospice care, 2011. Retrieved from: https://www.practicalpainmanagement.com/resources/hospice/pain-management-nursing-homes-hospice-care.

Gordon A: End of life issues. *Caring* 20(21):6, 2001.

Medicare.gov: Your Medicare coverage: Hospice and respite care, n.d. Retrieved from: https://www.medicare.gov/coverage/hospice-and-respite-care.html.

Morrow A: The 4 common myths about hospice, 2018a. Retrieved from: https://www.verywellhealth.com/hospice-myths-1132617.

Morrow A: How to become a hospice volunteer, 2018b. Retrieved from: https://www.verywellhealth.com/lend-a-caring-hand-1132290.

National Comprehensive Care Network: NCCN Guidelines for patients: Nausea and vomiting, 2016. Retrieved from: https://www.nccn.org/patients/guidelines/nausea/files/assets/common/downloads/files/nausea.pdf.

National Hospice and Palliative Care Organization (NHPCO): Facts and figures: Hospice care in America, 2018. Retrieved from: https://www.nhpco.org/sites/default/files/public/Statistics_Research/2017_Facts_Figures.pdf.

National Palliative Care Research Center: Guidelines for using the Edmonton Symptom Control Assessment, 2013. Retrieved from: http://www.npcrc.org/files/news/edmonton_symptom_assessment_scale.pdf.

National POLST Paradigm: Program designations, n.d. Retrieved from: http://polst.org/programs-in-your-state/.

Vidal M, Hui D, Williams J, Bruera E: A perspective study of hypodermoclysis performed by caregivers in the home setting. *J Pain Symptom Manage* 2016;October 4.

World Health Organization (WHO): 10 facts on palliative care, 2017. Retrieved from: http://www.who.int/features/factfiles/palliative-care/en/.

CHAPTER 41

famousscientists.org: Robert Hooke, 2014. Retrieved from: https://www.famousscientists.org/robert-hooke.

Lincoln D: Smaller than small: looking for something new with the LHC, 2014. Retrieved from: http://www.pbs.org/wgbh/nova/blogs/physics/2014/10/smaller-than-small/.

Moskowitz C: What is the smallest thing in the universe? LiveScience, 2012. Retrieved from: www.livescience.com/23232-smallest-ingredients-universe-physics.html.

Patton KT, Thibodeau GA: *Anatomy and physiology*, ed 10, St. Louis,, 2019, Mosby.

CHAPTER 42

Asthma and Allergy Foundation of America (AAFA): Types of latex reactions, n.d. Retrieved from: www.aafa.org/display.cfm?id = 9&sub = 21&cont = 428.

Blanchard JC, Denholm B: Association of operating room nurses, *AORNJ* 95(5):658–667, 2012.

Centers for Disease Control and Prevention (CDC): Promoting cultural sensitivity: A practical guide for tuberculosis programs that provide services to persons from Vietnam, 2010. Retrieved from: www.cdc.gov/tb/publications/guidestoolkits/Ethnographic-Guides/Vietnam/default.htm.

Centers for Disease Control and Prevention (CDC): Top CDC recommendations to prevent healthcare-associated infections, 2012. Retrieved from: www.cdc.gov/HAI/prevent/top-cdc-recs-preventhai.html.

Harris LJ, Moudgill N, Hager E, et al: Incidence of anastomotic leak in patients undergoing elective colon resection without mechanical bowel preparation: our updated experience and two-year review, *American Surgeon* 75(9):828–833, 2009.

The Joint Commission (TJC): Facts about the Universal Protocol, 2013. Retrieved from: www.jointcommission.org/assets/1/18/Universal_Protocol_1_3_13.pdf.

Kowalski TJ, Kothari SN, Mathiason M, et al: Impact of hair removal on surgical site infection rates: a prospective randomized noninferiority trial, 2016. Retrieved from: http://www.journalacs.org/article/S1072-7515(16)30035-7/fulltext?rss=yes.

Mayo Clinic Staff: Latex allergy, n.d. Retrieved from: https://www.mayoclinic.org/diseases-conditions/latex-allergy/symptoms-causes/syc-20374287.

National Council on Patient Information and Education (NCPIE): Medication management for older adults, 2018. Retrieved from: http://www.bemedwise.org/medication-safety/medication-therapy-management-for-seniors.

Nursing Interventions and Rationales: Latex allergy response, 2013. Retrieved from: http://nursinginterventionsrationales.blogspot.com/2013/07/latex-allergy-response.html.

Scabini S, Rimini E, Rairone E, et al: Colon and rectal surgery for cancer without mechanical bowel preparation: Onecenter randomized prospective trial, *World J Surg Oncol* 10:196, 2012.

CHAPTER 43

American Burn Association: Publications, 2016. Retrieved from: www.ameriburn.org/resources_publications.php.

American Cancer Society: Survival rates for melanoma skin cancer, by stage, 2016. Retrieved from: https://www.cancer.org/cancer/melanoma-skin-cancer/detection-diagnosis-staging/survival-rates-for-melanoma-skin-cancer-by-stage.html.

American Family Physician: STEPS New drug reviews: retapamulin (altabax) 1% topical ointment for the treatment of impetigo, 2007. Retrieved from: http://www.aafp.org/afp/2007/1115/p1537.html.

Carteret M: Traditional Asian health beliefs and healing practices. Dimensions of Culture, 2011. Retrieved from: www.dimensionsofculture.com/2010/10/traditional-asian-health-beliefshealing-practices.

Centers for Disease Control and Prevention (CDC): Parasites—lice, 2013. Retrieved from: https://www.cdc.gov/parasites/lice/index.html.

Centers for Disease Control and Prevention (CDC): Genital HSV infections, 2015. Retrieved from: https://www.cdc.gov/std/tg2015/herpes.htm.

Centers for Disease Control and Prevention (CDC): Vaccines and preventable diseases: what everyone should know about Zostavax, 2016. Retrieved from: https://www.cdc.gov/vaccines/vpd/shingles/public/zostavax/.

Centers for Disease Control and Prevention (CDC): Shingles (herpes zoster): preventing varicella-zoster virus (VZV) transmission from zoster in healthcare settings, 2017. Retrieved from: https://www.cdc.gov/shingles/hcp/hc-settings.html.

Centers for Disease Control and Prevention (CDC): Shingles (herpes zoster): overview, 2018a. Retrieved from: https://www.cdc.gov/shingles/about/overview.html.

Chrysopoulo, MT: Tissue flap classification. 2017. Retrieved from: https://emedicine.medscape.com/article/1284474-overview.

Lewis LS, Steele RW: Medscape: Impetigo medication, 2017. Retrieved from: https://emedicine.medscape.com/article/965254-medication.

Lupus Foundation of America: Lab tests for lupus, 2013. Retrieved from: http://www.lupus.org/answers/entry/lupus-tests.

Lupus Foundation of America: What is lupus? 2017. Retrieved from: http://www.lupus.org/answers/entry/what-is-lupus.

Mayo Clinic: Lupus, 2014. Retrieved from: http://www.mayoclinic.org/diseases-conditions/lupus/basics/tests-diagnosis/CON-20019676.

Mayo Clinic: Pityriasis rosea, 2015. Retrieved from: https://www.mayoclinic.org/diseases-conditions/pityriasis-rosea/symptoms-causes/syc-20376405.

Mayo Clinic: Acne, 2017a. Retrieved from: http://www.mayoclinic.org/diseases-conditions/acne/basics/causes/con-20020580.

Mayo Clinic: Self-injury/cutting, 2017b. Retrieved from: http://www.mayoclinic.org/diseases-conditions/self-injury/symptoms-causes/dxc-20165427.

Melanoma Research Foundation: Facts and stats, 2017. Retrieved from: https://www.melanoma.org/.

National Library of Medicine (NLM): Genital herpes. A.D.A.M Medical Encyclopedia, 2012b. Retrieved from: www.ncbi.nlm.nih.gov/pubmedhealth/PMH0001860.

National Library of Medicine (NLM): MedlinePlus.gov: Retapamulin, 2016. Retrieved from: https://medlineplus.gov/druginfo/meds/a607049.html.

National Library of Medicine (NLM): MedlinePlus.gov: Cellulitis, 2018. Retrieved from: https://medlineplus.gov/ency/article/000855.htm.

National Psoriasis Foundation: Fact sheet library, 2016. Retrieved from: https://www.psoriasis.org/publications/patient-education/fact-sheets.

National Pressure Ulcer Advisory Panel: National Pressure Ulcer Advisory Panel (NPUAP) announces a change in terminology from pressure ulcer to pressure injury and updates the stages of pressure injury, 2016. Retrieved from: http://www.npuap.org/national-pressure-ulcer-advisory-panel-npuap-announces-a-change-in-terminology-from-pressure-ulcer-to-pressure-injury-and-updates-the-stages-of-pressure-injury/

NutritionMD: Burns: nutritional considerations, n.d. Retrieved from: http://www.nutritionmd.org/health_care_providers/integumentary/burns_nutrition.html.

US Food & Drug Administration (FDA): Integra® dermal regeneration template, n.d. Retrieved from: www.accessdata.fda.gov/cdrh_docs/pdf/P900033S008d.pdf.

WebMD: Dermatitis medicamentosa on back, 2017. Retrieved from: http://www.webmd.com/skin-problems-and-treatments/picture-of-dermatitis-medicamentosa-back.

CHAPTER 44

American Academy of Orthopedic Surgeons: Osteoporosis and spinal fractures, 2016. Retrieved from: http://orthoinfo.aaos.org/topic.cfm?topic=A00538.

Arthritis Foundation: Rheumatoid arthritis symptoms, 2017. Retrieved from: http://www.arthritis.org/about-arthritis/types/rheumatoid-arthritis/symptoms.php.

Bethel MB: Osteoporosis treatment and management: Dietary measures, 2017a. Retrieved from: http://emedicine.medscape.com/article/330598-treatment#d10.

Bethel MB: Osteoporosis treatment and management: Pharmacologic therapy, 2017b. Retrieved from: http://emedicine.medscape.com/article/330598-treatment#d8.

Bethel MB: Osteoporosis treatment and management: Vertebroplasty and kyphoplasty, 2017c. Retrieved from: http://emedicine.medscape.com/article/330598-treatment#d9.

Cauley JA: Defining ethnic and racial differences in osteoporosis and fragility fractures, *Clin Orthop Relat Res* 469(7):1891–1899, 2011. Retrieved from: https://www.ncbi.nlm.nih.gov/pmc/articles/PMC3111798/.

Centers for Disease Control and Prevention (CDC): Fibromyalgia, 2015. Retrieved from: https://www.cdc.gov/arthritis/basics/fibromyalgia.htm.

Centers for Disease Control and Prevention (CDC): Osteoporosis, 2016. Retrieved from: https://www.cdc.gov/nchs/fastats/osteoporosis.htm.

Cleveland Clinic: Osteomyelitis, 2014. Retrieved from: http://my.clevelandclinic.org/health/articles/osteomyelitis.

International Osteoporosis Foundation: Diagnosing osteoporosis, 2015. Retrieved from: https://www.iofbonehealth.org/diagnosing-osteoporosis.

Kirkland L: Fat embolism clinical presentation. Medscape, 2013. Retrieved from: http://emedicine.medscape.com/article/460524-clinical#a0217.

Kishner S: Osteomyelitis treatment and management, 2016. Retrieved from: http://emedicine.medscape.com/article/1348767-treatment#d9.

Mayo Clinic of America: Carpal tunnel syndrome, 2016a. Retrieved from: http://www.mayoclinic.org/diseases-conditions/carpal-tunnel-syndrome/basics/treatment/con-20030332.

Mayo Clinic of America: Osteoporosis, 2016b. Retrieved from: http://www.mayoclinic.org/diseases-conditions/osteoporosis/symptoms-causes/dxc-20207860.

Mayo Clinic of America: Ankylosing spondylitis, 2017. Retrieved from: http://www.mayoclinic.org/diseases-conditions/ankylosing-spondylitis/symptoms-causes/dxc-20261125.

National Institute of Arthritis and Musculoskeletal and Skin Diseases: Osteoporosis and Hispanic women, 2015. Retrieved from: https://www.niams.nih.gov/Health_Info/Bone/Osteoporosis/Background/hispanic_women.asp.

National Institute of Arthritis and Musculoskeletal and Skin Diseases: Osteoarthritis, 2016. Retrieved from: https://www.niams.nih.gov/Health_Info/Osteoarthritis/default.asp#3.

National Institute of Arthritis and Musculoskeletal and Skin Diseases: Arthritis, 2016. Retrieved from: https://www.niams.nih.gov/Health_Info/Osteoarthritis/default.asp#3.

National Institutes of Health: Bed rest and immobilization: Risk factors for bone loss, 2016. Retrieved from: https://www.niams.nih.gov/Health_Info/Bone/Osteoporosis/Conditions_Behaviors/bed_rest.asp#a.

National Institutes of Health: Osteoarthritis, 2016. Retrieved from: https://www.niams.nih.gov/Health_Info/Osteoarthritis/default.asp#3.

National Library of Medicine (NLM): Glucosamine sulfate. Medline Plus, 2016. Retrieved from: https://medlineplus.gov/druginfo/natural/807.html.

Rheumatoid Arthritis Support Network: Rheumatoid arthritis facts and statistics, 2016. Retrieved from: https://www.rheumatoidarthritis.org/ra/facts-and-statistics/.

Spondylitis Association of America: Overview of psoriatic arthritis, 2017. Retrieved from: https://www.spondylitis.org/Psoriatic-Arthritis/.

University of Maryland Medical Center: Fibromyalgia, 2016. Retrieved from: http://umm.edu/health/medical/ency/articles/fibromyalgia.

US Food and Drug Administration (US FDA): Drug: FDA Drug Safety Communication: FDA to evaluate increased risk of heart-related death and death from all causes with the gout medicine febuxostat (Uloric), 2017a. Retrieved from: https://www.fda.gov/Drugs/DrugSafety/ucm584702.htm.

US Food and Drug Administration (US FDA): Medical devices: hip implants, 2017b. Retrieved from: http://www.fda.gov/MedicalDevices/ProductsandMedicalProcedures/ImplantsandProsthetics/MetalonMetalHipImplants/ucm241594.htm.

CHAPTER 45

Aberra FN: Clostridium difficile colitis treatment & management, 2016. Retrieved from: http://emedicine.medscape.com/article/186458-treatment.

American Cancer Society (ACS): Survival rates for oral cavity and oropharyngeal cancer by stage, 2014a. Retrieved from: https://www.cancer.org/cancer/oral-cavity-and-oropharyngeal-cancer/detection-diagnosis-staging/survival-rates.html.

American Cancer Society (ACS): What are the key statistics about Kaposi sarcoma? 2014b. Retrieved from: https://www.cancer.org/cancer/kaposi-sarcoma/about/what-is-key-statistics.html.

American Cancer Society (ACS): Colorectal cancer screening tests, 2016a. Retrieved from: https://www.cancer.org/cancer/colon-rectal-cancer/early-detection/screening-tests-used.html.

American Cancer Society (ACS): What are oral cavity and oropharyngeal cancers? 2016b. Retrieved from: https://www.cancer.org/cancer/oral-cavity-and-oropharyngeal-cancer/about/what-is-oral-cavity-cancer.html.

American Cancer Society (ACS): What are the survival rates for colorectal cancer, by age? 2016c. Retrieved from: https://www.cancer.org/cancer/colon-rectal-cancer/detection-diagnosis-staging/survival-rates.html.

American Cancer Society (ADS): Tests for stomach cancer, 2016d. Retrieved from: https://www.cancer.org/cancer/stomach-cancer/detection-diagnosis-staging/how-diagnosed.html.

American Cancer Society (ACS): Key statistics for colorectal cancer, 2017a. Retrieved from: https://www.cancer.org/cancer/colon-rectal-cancer/about/key-statistics.html.

American Cancer Society (ACS): Key statistics for oral cavity and oropharyngeal cancers, 2017b. Retrieved from: https://www.cancer.org/cancer/oral-cavity-and-oropharyngeal-cancer/about/key-statistics.html.

American Cancer Society (ACS): Key statistics for stomach cancer, 2017c. Retrieved from: https://www.cancer.org/cancer/stomach-cancer/about/key-statistics.html.

American Cancer Society (ACS): Survival rates for esophageal cancer rates by stage, 2017d. Retrieved from: https://www.cancer.org/cancer/esophagus-cancer/detection-diagnosis-staging/survival-rates.html.

American Cancer Society (ACS): Treatments and side effects, 2017e. Retrieved from: https://www.cancer.org/treatment/treatments-and-side-effects.html.

Anand BS: Peptic ulcer disease, 2017. Retrieved from: http://emedicine.medscape.com/article/181753-overview.

Aroniadis OC, Brandt LJ: Fecal microbiota transplantation, 2013. Retrieved from: http://www.medscape.com/viewarticle/776501.

Celiac Disease Foundation: What is celiac disease? 2017. Retrieved from: https://celiac.org/celiac-disease/understanding-celiac-disease-2/what-is-celiac-disease/.

Centers for Disease Control and Prevention (CDC): E. coli (Escherichia coli), 2013a. Retrieved from: www.cdc.gov/ecoli.

Centers for Disease Control and Prevention (CDC): Clostridium diffi cile infection, 2013b. Retrieved from: www.cdc.gov/HAI/organisms/cdiff/Cdiff_infect.html.

Centers for Disease Control and Prevention (CDC): Inflammatory bowel disease (IBD), 2014. Retrieved from: https://www.cdc.gov/ibd/index.htm.

Crohn's and Colitis Foundation of America (CCFA): Crohn's diagnosis & testing, n.d.. Retrieved from: http://emedicine.medscape.com/article/176319-overview.

Daley BJ: Peritonitis and abdominal sepsis, 2017. Retrieved from: http://emedicine.medscape.com/article/180234-overview#a7.

Drugs.com: Gastrografin, 2018. Retrieved from: https://www.drugs.com/pro/gastrografin.html.

Guandalini S: Diarrhea, 2016. Retrieved from: http://emedicine.medscape.com/article/928598-overview.

Hidalgo JA, Bronze MS: Candidiasis treatment & management, 2017. Retrieved from: http://emedicine.medscape.com/article/213853-treatment.

International Foundation for Functional Gastroinestinal Disorders (IFFGD): Statistics, 2016. Retrieved from: http://www.aboutibs.org/facts-about-ibs/statistics.html.

Johns Hopkins University: Barium swallow. Johns Hopkins Health Library, n.d.a.. Retrieved from: www.hopkinsmedicine.org/healthlibrary/test_procedures/gastroenterology/barium_swallow_92,P07688.

Johns Hopkins University: Peptic ulcer disease, n.d.b.. Retrieved from: www.hopkinsmedicine.org/healthlibrary/conditions/adult/digestive_disorders/peptic_ulcer_disease_22,PepticUlcerDisease.

Johns Hopkins University: Pyloroplasty. Johns Hopkins Health Library, n.d.c. Retrieved from: www.hopkinsmedicine.org/gastroenterology_hepatology/_pdfs/esophagus_stomach/peptic_ulcer_disease.pdf.

Kahrilas PJ: Clinical manifestations and diagnosis of gastroesophageal reflux in adults. UpToDate, 2012. Retrieved from: www.uptodate.com/contents/clinical-manifestations-and-diagnosis-of-gastroesophageal-refl ux-in-adults?source = search_result&search = Clinical + manifestations + and + diagnosis + of + gastroesophageal+ reflux + in + adults&selectedTitle = 1~150.

Mayo Clinic: E. coli, 2014a. Retrieved from: http://www.mayoclinic.org/diseases-conditions/e-coli/basics/causes/con-20032105.

Mayo Clinic: Gastroesophageal reflux disease: overview, 2014b. Retrieved from: http://www.mayoclinic.org/diseases-conditions/gerd/basics/symptoms/con-20025201.

Mayo Clinic: Capsule endoscopy: Overview, 2015a. Retrieved from: http://www.mayoclinic.org/tests-procedures/capsule-endoscopy/basics/definition/PRC-20012773.

Mayo Clinic: Inflammatory bowel disease, 2015b. Retrieved from: http://www.mayoclinic.org/diseases-conditions/inflammatory-bowel-disease/basics/treatment/con-20034908.

Mayo Clinic: Esophageal cancer, 2018a. Retrieved from: http://www.mayoclinic.org/diseases-conditions/esophageal-cancer/basics/treatment/con-20034316.

Mayo Clinic: Stomach cancer: symptoms and causes, 2018b. Retrieved from: http://www.mayoclinic.org/diseases-conditions/stomach-cancer/home/ovc-20202327.

MedlinePlus: Hiatal hernia; [updated 2018 Apr 30; reviewed 2017 May 30]. Retrieved from: https://medlineplus.gov/hiatalhernia.html.

Medscape: Misoprostol (Rx), 2010. Retrieved from: https://reference.medscape.com/drug/cytotec-misoprostol-341995#90.

Mounsey A, Raleigh M, Wilson A: Management of constipation in older adults, *Am Fam Physician* 92(6):500–504, 2015.

National Cancer Institute: Oral cancer. National Institutes of Health, n.d.a. Retrieved from: www.cancer.gov/cancertopics/types/oral.

National Institutes of Health: Virtual colonoscopy, 2016. Retrieved from: https://www.niddk.nih.gov/health-information/health-topics/diagnostic-tests/virtual-colonoscopy/Pages/diagnostic-test.aspx.

National Library of Medicine (NLM): Abdominal x-ray. Medline Plus, 2013. Retrieved from: www.nlm.nih.gov/medlineplus/ency/article/003815.htm.

National Library of Medicine (NLM): Bernstein test, 2014. Retrieved from: https://medlineplus.gov/ency/article/003897.htm.

National Library of Medicine (NLM): Helicobacter pylori infections, 2016. Retrieved from: https://medlineplus.gov/helicobacterpyloriinfections.html.

National Library of Medicine (NLM): Achalasia. MedlinePlus, 2018a. Retrieved from: https://medlineplus.gov/ency/article/000267.htm.

National Library of Medicine (NLM): Gastroesophageal reflux disease, MedlinePlus, 2018b. Retrieved from: https://medlineplus.gov/ency/article/000265.htm.

Nelson R: FDA approves Cologuard for colorectal cancer screening, 2014. Retrieved from: https://www.medscape.com/viewarticle/829757.

Noar MD: The rapidly evolving GERD universe: expanding the understanding of the pathogenesis, spectrum of disease, and therapeutic options of the 21st century and beyond, 2015. Retrieved from: http://s3.gi.org/wp-content/uploads/2015/03/15ACG_LGS_Regional_Course_0008-3.pdf.

Punnoose AR, Kasturia S, Golub RM: Intussusception, *JAMA* 307(6):628, 2012.

Rahman MA, Parash MH: A postmortem study of the number of germinal centers in the vermiform appendix of Bangladeshi people in different age groups, *Am J Med Sci Med* 1(5):94–97, 2013.

Skin Cancer Foundation: Lip cancer: not uncommon, often overlooked, 2016. Retrieved from: http://www.skincancer.org/skin-cancer-information/lip-cancer-not-uncommon.

University of Rochester Medical Center (URMC): Stomach cancer: your chances for recovery (prognosis), 2017. Retrieved from: https://www.urmc.rochester.edu/encyclopedia/content.aspx?ContentTypeID=34&ContentID=BStoD7.

CHAPTER 46

American Cancer Society (ACS): What is liver cancer? 2016a. Retrieved from: https://www.cancer.org/cancer/liver-cancer/about/what-is-liver-cancer.html.

American Cancer Society (ACS): Tests for liver cancer, 2016b. Retrieved from: https://www.cancer.org/cancer/liver-cancer/detection-diagnosis-staging/how-diagnosed.html.

American Cancer Society (ACS): Liver cancer survival rates, 2016c. Retrieved from: https://www.cancer.org/cancer/liver-cancer/detection-diagnosis-staging/survival-rates.html.

American Cancer Society (ACS): Pancreatic cancer survival rates, by stage, 2016d. Retrieved from: https://www.cancer.org/cancer/pancreatic-cancer/detection-diagnosis-staging/survival-rates.html.

American Cancer Society (ACS): About pancreatic cancer, 2017. Retrieved from: https://www.cancer.org/cancer/pancreatic-cancer/about.html.

American Liver Foundation: Liver transplant, 2016. Retrieved from: http://www.liverfoundation.org/abouttheliver/info/transplant/.

Centers for Disease Control and Prevention (CDC): Chronic liver disease and cirrhosis, 2016a. Retrieved from: https://www.cdc.gov/nchs/fastats/liver-disease.htm.

Centers for Disease Control and Prevention (CDC): Vaccine information statements: Hepatitis A VIS, 2016b. Retrieved from: https://www.cdc.gov/vaccines/hcp/vis/vis-statements/hep-b.html.

Centers for Disease Control and Prevention (CDC): Liver Cancer, 2018. Retrieved from: https://www.cdc.gov/cancer/liver/index.htm.

Mathew A: Pancreatic necrosis and pancreatic abscess, 2017. Retrieved from: http://emedicine.medscape.com/article/181264-overview.

Mayo Clinic: Hepatitis A, 2014. Retrieved from: http://www.mayoclinic.org/diseases-conditions/hepatitis-a/basics/prevention/con-20022163.

Mayo Clinic: Esophageal varices, 2016a. Retrieved from: http://www.mayoclinic.org/diseases-conditions/esophageal-varices/diagnosis-treatment/treatment/txc-20206471.

Mayo Clinic: Pancreatitis, 2016b. Retrieved from: http://www.mayoclinic.org/diseases-conditions/pancreatitis/symptoms-causes/dxc-20252598.

National Institutes of Health (NIH): Cirrhosis: What is cirrhosis?, 2014. Retrieved from: https://www.niddk.nih.gov/health-information/liver-disease/cirrhosis.

Peralta R: Liver abscess, 2016. Retrieved from: http://emedicine.medscape.com/article/188802-overview#a5.

CHAPTER 47

American Cancer Society (ACS): About multiple myeloma, 2016a. Retrieved from: https://www.cancer.org/content/dam/CRC/PDF/Public/8738.00.pdf.

American Cancer Society (ACS): High-dose chemotherapy and stem cell transplant for non-Hodgkin lymphoma, 2016b. Retrieved from: https://www.cancer.org/cancer/non-hodgkin-lymphoma/treating/bone-marrow-stem-cell.html.

American Cancer Society (ACS): Signs and symptoms of Non-Hodgkin lymphoma, 2016c. Retrieved from: https://www.cancer.org/cancer/non-hodgkin-lymphoma/detection-diagnosis-staging/signs-symptoms.html.

American Cancer Society (ACS): Hodgkin lymhoma [sic] early detection, diagnosis, and staging, 2017a. Retrieved from: https://www.cancer.org/content/dam/CRC/PDF/Public/8651.00.pdf.

American Cancer Society (ACS): Treating multiple myeloma, 2017b. Retrieved from: https://www.cancer.org/content/dam/CRC/PDF/Public/8741.00.pdf.

American Cancer Society (ACS): Key statistics for acute lymphocytic leukemia, 2018. Retrieved from: https://www.cancer.org/cancer/acute-lymphocytic-leukemia/about/key-statistics.html.

American Pregnancy Association: HELLP syndrome, 2015. Retrieved from: http://americanpregnancy.org/pregnancycomplications/hellpsyndrome.html.

Cattan D: Pernicious anemia: what are actual diagnostic criteria? *World J Gastroenterol* 17(4):543–544, 2011.

Centers for Disease Control and Prevention (CDC): Pneumococcal vaccination: Who needs it? 2013. Retrieved from: www.cdc.gov/vaccines/vpd-vac/pneumo/vacc-in-short.htm.

Centers for Disease Control and Prevention (CDC): Sickle cell disease, 2016. Retrieved from: https://www.cdc.gov/healthcommunication/toolstemplates/entertainmented/tips/SickleCell.html.

Chand NK, Subramanya HB, Rao GV: Management of patients who refuse blood transfusion, *Indian J Anaesth* 58(5):658–664, 2014.

Hemophilia Federation of America: Joint damage, 2017. Retrieved from: http://www.hemophiliafed.org/bleeding-disorders/complications/.

Kessler CM, Sandler SG: Immune thrombocytopenic purpura treatment & management, 2013. Retrieved from: http://emedicine.medscape.com/article/202158-treatment.

Leukemia and Lymphoma Society: Non-Hodgkin lymphoma, n.d. Retrieved from: https://www.lls.org/lymphoma/non-hodgkin-lymphoma.

Leukemia and Lymphoma Society: Leukemia, 2013. Retrieved from: www.lls.org/diseaseinformation/getinformationsupport/factsstatistics/leukemia.

Lewis SL, Bucher L, Heitkemper MM, et al: *Medical-surgical nursing: assessment and management of clinical problems*, ed 10, St. Louis, 2017, Elsevier.

Lindstrom E, Johnstone R: Acute normovolemic hemodilution in a Jehovah's Witness patient: a case report, *AANA J* 78(4):326–330, 2010.

Maakaron JE: Sickle cell treatment & management, 2017. Retrieved from: http://emedicine.medscape.com/article/205926-treatment?src=refgatesrc1.

Marcel ML, Schmaier AH: Disseminated intravascular coagulation treatment & management, 2012. Retrieved from: http://emedicine.medscape.com/article/199627-treatment.

Mayo Clinic: Thrombocytopenia, 2015. Retrieved from: http://www.mayoclinic.org/diseases-conditions/thrombocytopenia/basics/treatment/con-20027170.

Mayo Clinic: Lymphedema, 2016. Retrieved from: http://www.mayoclinic.org/diseases-conditions/lymphedema/basics/treatment/con-20025603.

Mayo Clinic: Hodgkin's lymhoma (Hodgkin's disease), 2017. Retrieved from: http://www.mayoclinic.org/diseases-conditions/hodgkins-lymphoma/symptoms-causes/dxc-20341203.

Mayo Clinic. Leukemia, 2018. Retrieved from: https://www.mayoclinic.org/diseases-conditions/leukemia/symptoms-causes/syc-20374373.

Medline Plus: Aplastic anemia, 2018. Retrieved from: https://medlineplus.gov/aplasticanemia.html.

Merck Manual for Health Care Professionals: Polycythemia vera, 2012. Retrieved from: www.merckmanuals.com/professional/hematology_and_oncology/myeloproliferative_disorders/polycythemia_vera.html.

National Cancer Institute: SEER stat fact sheets: Non-Hodgkin lymphoma, n.d. Retrieved from: http://seer.cancer.gov/statfacts/html/nhl.html.

National Cancer Institute: Pediatric supportive care (PDQ ®), 2013a. Retrieved from: www.cancer.gov/cancertopics/pdq/supportivecare/pediatric/healthprofessional.

National Cancer Institute: Multiple myeloma, 2013b. Retrieved from: www.cancer.gov/cancertopics/wyntk/myeloma/page1/All-Pages#3.

National Cancer Institute: Lymphedema (PDQ ®), 2013c. Retrieved from: www.cancer.gov/cancertopics/pdq/supportivecare/lymphedema/patient.

National Heart, Lung, and Blood Institute (NHLBI): How is hemophilia treated? 2013. Retrieved from: www.nhlbi.nih.gov/health/healthtopics/topics/hemophilia/treatment.html.

National Heart, Lung, and Blood Institute (NHLBI): Sickle cell disease, 2017. Retrieved from: https://www.nhlbi.nih.gov/health/health-topics/topics/sca/signs.

National Hemophilia Foundation: HIV/AIDS, 2017. Retrieved from: https://www.hemophilia.org/Bleeding-Disorders/Blood-Safety/HIV/AIDS.

National Institutes of Health: Polycythermia vera, 2017. Retrieved from: https://rarediseases.info.nih.gov/diseases/7422/polycythemia-vera.

National Institutes of Health Clinical Center: Procedures/diagnostic tests: Gastric analysis, 2016. Retrieved from: www.cc.nih.gov/ccc/patient_education/procdiag/gastricanaly.pdf.

National Library of Medicine (NLM): Sickle cell disease, PubMed Health, 2013. Retrieved from: www.ncbi.nlm.nih.gov/pubmedhealth/PMH0001554.

Phillips N: Lymphangitis, 2012. Retrieved from: www.healthline.com/health/lymphangitis.

Pollak ES, Nagalla S: von Willebrand disease, Medscape, 2017. Retrieved from: http://emedicine.medscape.com/article/206996-overview.

Szczepiorkowski ZM, Dunbar NM: Transfusion guidelines: when to transfuse. In *ASH education book*, vol 2013, No. 1, Dec 6, 2013, pp 638–644. Retrieved from: http://asheducationbook.hematologylibrary.org/content/2013/1/638.full.

University of Maryland Medical Center: Iron, 2013. Retrieved from: www.umm.edu/altmed/articles/iron-000309.htm#ixzz2Vvga1O9Z.

US Food and Drug Administration (USFDA): Hemophilia treatments have come a long way, 2014. Retrieved from: https://www.fda.gov/ForConsumers/ConsumerUpdates/ucm392954.htm.

Vaqas B, Ryan TJ: Lymphoedema: pathophysiology and management in resource-poor settings: relevance for lymphatic fi lariasis control programmes, *Filaria J* 2:4, 2003.

Vorvik LJ, Zieve D: Lymph nodes. MedlinePlus, 2016. Retrieved from: https://medlineplus.gov/ency/anatomyvideos/000083.htm.

Wade T: Estimating blood loss in a trauma patient based on vital signs according to ATLS, 2013. Retrieved from: http://www.tomwademd.net/estimating-blood-loss-in-a-trauma-patient-based-on-vital-signs-according-to-atls/.

Williams LS, Hopper PD: *Understanding medical surgical nursing*, ed 5, Philadelphia, 2015, F.A. Davis.

CHAPTER 48

American Heart Association: Hispanics/Latinos & cardiovascular diseases, 2013d. Retrieved from: https://www.heart.org/idc/groups/heart-public/@wcm/@sop/@smd/documents/downloadable/ucm_319572.pdf.

American Heart Association: Angina in women can be different than men, 2015. Retrieved from: http://www.heart.org/en/health-topics/heart-attack/angina-chest-pain/angina-in-women-can-be-different-than-men.

American Heart Association: Cardioversion, 2016a. Retrieved from: https://www.heart.org/HEARTORG/Conditions/Arrhythmia/PreventionTreatmentofArrhythmia/Cardioversion_UCM_447318_Article.jsp.

American Heart Association: Devices for arrhythmia, 2016b. Retrieved from: https://www.heart.org/HEARTORG/Conditions/Arrhythmia/PreventionTreatmentofArrhythmia/Devices-for-Arrhythmia_UCM_301994_Article.jsp.

American Heart Association: Restritive myocardiomyopathy, 2016c, Retrieved from: www.heart.org.

American Heart Association: Prevention and treatment of PAD, 2016d. Retrieved from: http://www.heart.org/en/health-topics/peripheral-artery-disease/prevention-and-treatment-of-pad.

American Heart Association: How to get your cholesterol tested, 2017a. Retrieved from: http://www.heart.org/HEARTORG/Conditions/Cholesterol/HowToGetYourCholesterolTested/How-To-Get-Your-Cholesterol-Tested_UCM_305595_Article.jsp#.Waihc9EpBPY.

American Heart Association: Ablation for arrhythmias, 2017c. Retrieved from: https://www.heart.org/HEARTORG/Conditions/Arrhythmia/PreventionTreatmentofArrhythmia/Ablation-for-Arrhythmias_UCM_301991_Article.jsp.

American Heart Association: Classes of heart failure, 2017d. Retrieved from: http://www.heart.org/HEARTORG/Conditions/HeartFailure/AboutHeartFailure/Classes-of-Heart-Failure_UCM_306328_Article.jsp#.WajCAdEpD7M.

American Heart Association: Types of blood pressure medications, 2017e. Retrieved from: https://www.heart.org/en/health-topics/high-blood-pressure/changes-you-can-make-to-manage-high-blood-pressure/types-of-blood-pressure-medications.

American Heart Association: Heart disease and aspirin therapy, 2018a. Retrieved from: http://www.heart.org/en/news/2018/07/19/heart-disease-and-aspirin-therapy.

American Heart Association: The facts about high blood pressure, 2018b. Retrieved from: http://www.heart.org/HEARTORG/Conditions/HighBloodPressure/GettheFactsAboutHighBloodPressure/The-Facts-About-High-Blood-Pressure_UCM_002050_Article.jsp#.WajZy9EpD7M.

American Heart Association: Heart transplant, n.d. Retrieved from: http://www.heart.org/en/health-topics/congenital-heart-defects/care-and-treatment-for-congenital-heart-defects/heart-transplant.

Botta DM: Heart transplantation, 2016. Retrieved from: http://emedicine.medscape.com/article/429816-overview#a3.

Centers for Disease Control and Prevention (CDC): African Americans heart disease and stroke fact sheet, 2014. Retrieved from: https://www.cdc.gov/dhdsp/data_statistics/fact_sheets/fs_aa.htm.

Centers for Disease Control and Prevention (CDC): Diabetes, heart disease and you, 2016a. Retrieved from: https://www.cdc.gov/features/diabetes-heart-disease/index.html.

Centers for Disease Control and Prevention (CDC): Heart failure fact sheet, 2016b. Retrieved from: https://www.cdc.gov/dhdsp/data_statistics/fact_sheets/fs_heart_failure.htm.

Centers for Disease Control and Prevention (CDC): Defining adult overweight and obesity, 2016c. Retrieved from: www.cdc.gov/about/default.

Centers for Disease Control and Prevention (CDC): Venous thromboembolism, 2017. Retrieved from: https://www.cdc.gov/ncbddd/dvt/data.html.

Centers for Disease Control and Prevention (CDC): Preventing high cholesterol, 2018. Retrieved from: https://www.cdc.gov/cholesterol/prevention.htm.

Kattoor A, Mehta JL: Marijuana and coronary heart disease, 2016. Retrieved from: http://www.acc.org/latest-in-cardiology/articles/2016/09/22/08/58/marijuana-and-coronary-heart-disease.

Lin K: Aspirin for primary prevention: 2016 USPSTF recommendations, 2016. Retrieved from: http://www.medscape.com/viewarticle/861772.

Mayo Clinic: Claudication, 2015. Retrieved from: http://www.mayoclinic.org/diseases-conditions/claudication/basics/treatment/con-20033581.

Mayo Clinic: Endocarditis, 2017a. Retrieved from: http://www.mayoclinic.org/diseases-conditions/endocarditis/symptoms-causes/dxc-20338073.

Mayo Clinic: Myocarditis, 2017b. Retrieved from: http://www.mayoclinic.org/diseases-conditions/myocarditis/symptoms-causes/dxc-20335631.

Mayo Clinic: Myocarditis: diagnosis and treatment, 2017c. Retrieved from: http://www.mayoclinic.org/diseases-conditions/myocarditis/diagnosis-treatment/diagnosis/dxc-20335638.

Mayo Clinic: Buergers' disease, 2017d. Retrieved from: http://www.mayoclinic.org/diseases-conditions/buergers-disease/symptoms-causes/dxc-20179162.

Mayo Clinic: Raynaud's disease, 2017e. Retrieved from: https://www.mayoclinic.org/diseases-conditions/raynauds-disease/symptoms-causes/syc-20363571.

Mayo Clinic: Deep vein thrombosis, 2017f. Retrieved from: http://www.mayoclinic.org/diseases-conditions/deep-vein-thrombosis/diagnosis-treatment/treatment/txc-20336858.

Mayo Clinic: Isolated systolic hypertension: a health concern? 2018. Retrived from https://www.mayoclinic.org/diseases-conditions/high-blood-pressure/expert-answers/hypertension/faq-20058527.

Muller ML: Cocksackieviruses, 2017. Retrieved from: http://emedicine.medscape.com/article/215241-overview.

Nassiri N: Thromboangiitis obliterans (Buerger disease), 2017. Retrieved from: http://emedicine.medscape.com/article/460027-overview#a6.

National Heart, Lung and Blood Institute: Aneurysm, 2011. Retrieved from: www.nhlbl.nih.gov.

Rabito MJ, Kaye AD: Complementary and alternative medicine and cardiovascular disease: an evidence-based review, 2013. Retrieved from: https://www.hindawi.com/journals/ecam/2013/672097/.

Shrivastava AK, Singh HV, Raizada A, et al: C-reactive protein, inflammation, and coronary heart disease, *Egypt Heart J* 67(2):89–97, 2015.

St. Luke's Health System: Chemical cardioversion, n.d. Retrieved from: https://www.saintlukeshealthsystem.org/health-library/chemical-cardioversion.

Spinler SA: 2014 NSTE-ACS Clinical Practice Guidelines – What's New? 2014. Retrieved from: https://professional.heart.org/professional/ScienceNews/UCM_466977_2014-NSTE-ACS-Clinical-Practice-Guidelines—Whats-New.jsp.

Texas Heart Institute: Smoking and your heart, n.d. Retrieved from: https://www.texasheart.org/heart-health/heart-information-center/topics/smoking-and-your-heart/.

US Department of Health and Human Services (USDHHS), National Institutes of Health, National Heart, Lung, and Blood Institute: Heart attack, n.d. Retrieved from: https://www.nhlbi.nih.gov/health-topics/heart-attack.

CHAPTER 49

American Association for Respiratory Care: Sleep apea facts, 2017. Retrieved from: http://www.yourlunghealth.org/lung_disease/sleep_apnea/facts/.

American Cancer Society: Treatment types, n.d. Retrieved from: www.cancer.org/treatment/treatmentsandsideeffects/treatmenttypes/index.

American Cancer Society: Lung cancer, 2017. Retrieved from: www.cancer.org/cancer/lungcancer/index.

American Cancer Society: About laryngeal and hypopharyngeal cancer, 2018. Retrieved from: https://www.cancer.org/content/dam/CRC/PDF/Public/8664.00.pdf.

American Lung Association: About COPD, n.d.a. Retrieved from: www.lung.org/lung-disease/copd/about-copd.

American Lung Association: Bronchiectasis, n.d.b. Retrieved from: www.lung.org/lung-disease/bronchiectasis.

American Lung Association: Lung cancer fact sheet, n.d.c. Retrieved from: http://www.lung.org/lung-health-and-diseases/lung-disease-lookup/lung-cancer/resource-library/lung-cancer-fact-sheet.html.

American Lung Association: Multidrug resistant tuberculosis (MDR-TB) fact sheet, n.d.d. Retrieved from: ww.lung.org/lungdisease/tuberculosis.

American Lung Association: Understanding severe acute respiratory syndrome, n.d.e. Retrieved from: www.lung.org/lungdisease/severe-acute-respiratory-syndrome/understanding-sars.html.

Centers for Disease Control and Prevention (CDC): Severe acute respiratory syndrome (SARS), 2013. Retrieved from: www.cdc.gov/sars/index.html.

Centers for Disease Control and Prevention (CDC): Treatment of LTBI and TB for persons with HIV, 2016a. Retrieved from: https://www.cdc.gov/tb/topic/treatment/tbhiv.htm.

Centers for Disease Control and Prevention (CDC): Trends in Tuberculosis, 2016b. Retrieved from: https://www.cdc.gov/tb/publications/factsheets/statistics/tbtrends.htm.

Centers for Disease Control and Prevention (CDC): When and how to wash your hands, 2016c. Retrieved from: https://www.cdc.gov/handwashing/when-how-handwashing.html.

Centers for Disease Control and Prevention: Anthrax: Emergency use instructions for doxyclycline and ciproflaxin for post-exposure prophylaxis of anthrax. 2017a. Retrieved from: https://www.cdc.gov/anthrax/medical-care/cipro-eui-recipients.html.

Centers for Disease Control and Prevention (CDC): Legionella (legionnaires' disease and Pontiac fever): diagnosis, treatment, and complications, 2017b. Retrieved from: https://www.cdc.gov/legionella/about/diagnosis.html.

Centers for Disease Control and Prevention (CDC): Vaccines and preventable diseases: Pneumococcal vaccination, 2017c. Retrieved from: https://www.cdc.gov/vaccines/vpd/pneumo/index.html.

Centers for Disease Control and Prevention: Asthma: Most recent asthma data. 2018. Retrieved from: https://www.cdc.gov/asthma/most_recent_data.htm.

Dartmouth-Hitchcock Norris Cotton Cancer Center: Asthma and GERD, 2013. Retrieved from: http://cancer.dartmouth.edu/pf/health_encyclopedia/hw161526.

Koenig JI: Regulation of the hypothalamo-pituitary axis by neuropeptide Y, *Ann N Y Acad Sci* 611:317–328, 1990.

Mayo Clinic: Pneumonia, 2013. Retrieved from: www.mayoclinic.com/health/pneumonia/DS00135.

Mayo Clinic: Pulmonary edema, 2014. Retrieved from: http://www.mayoclinic.org/diseases-conditions/pulmonary-edema/basics/causes/con-20022485.

Mayo Clinic: Anthrax, 2017a. Retrieved from: http://www.mayoclinic.org/diseases-conditions/anthrax/diagnosis-treatment/treatment/txc-20320695.

Mayo Clinic: Asthma and acid reflux: are they linked? 2017b. Retrieved from: http://www.mayoclinic.org/diseases-conditions/asthma/expert-answers/asthma-and-acid-reflux/FAQ-20057993.

Mayo Clinic: ARDS, 2018a. Retrieved from: www.mayoclinic.com/health/ards/DS00944.

Mayo Clinic. Obstructive Sleep Apnea. March 6, 2018b. Retrieved from: https://www.mayoclinic.org/diseases-conditions/obstructive-sleep-apnea/symptoms-causes/syc-20352090.

MD Anderson Cancer Center: Lung cancer diagnosis. University of Texas, 2013. Retrieved from: www.mdanderson.org/patient-andcancer-information/cancer-information/cancer-types/lung-cancer/diagnosis/index.html.

Medline Plus: Pulmonary ventilation/perfusion scan, 2012. Retrieved from: www.nlm.nih.gov/medlineplus/ency/article/003828.htm.

Medline Plus: Severe acute respiratory syndrome (SARS), 2013. Retrieved from: www.nlm.nih.gov/medlineplus/ency/article/007192.htm.

National Cancer Institute: Lung cancer prevention, 2012. Retrieved from: www.cancer.gov/cancertopics/pdq/prevention/lung/Patient/page3#Keypoint18.

National Heart, Lung and Blood Institute: What is pulmonary embolism? 2011. Retrieved from: www.nhlbi.nih.gov/health/health-topics/topics/pe/.

National Heart, Lung and Blood Institute: How is sleep apnea diagnosed? 2012. Retrieved from: www.nhlbi.nih.gov/health/health-topics/topics/sleepapnea/diagnosis.html.

National Institutes of Health (NIH): COPD, 2017. Retrieved from: https://www.nhlbi.nih.gov/health/health-topics/topics/copd.

National Library of Medicine: RAST test, 2012. Retrieved from: www.nlm.nih.gov/medlineplus/ency/imagepages/19334.htm.

Pain, 2013b. Retrieved from: www.drugs.com/condition/pain.html.

Woodruff D: Take these 6 easy steps to ABG analysis, *Nursing Made Incredibly Easy* 4(1):4–7, 2006.

World Health Organization (WHO): Use of interferon-y release assays (Igras). In *tuberculosis control in low- and middle-income settings*, Geneva, Switzerland, 2011, Author.

World Health Organization (WHO): Tuberculosis: Key facts, 2018. Retrieved from: http://www.who.int/mediacentre/factsheets/fs104/en/.

CHAPTER 50

Cleveland Clinic: Urinary retention, 2014. Retrieved from: http://my.clevelandclinic.org/health/articles/urinary-retention.

Cheuck L: Brachytherapy (radioactive seed implantation therapy) in prostate cancer, 2017. Retrieved from: http://emedicine.medscape.com/article/453349-overview#a1.

Hinkle JL, Cheever K: *Brunner & Suddarth's textbook of medical-surgical nursing*, ed 14, Philadelphia, 2017, Lippincott, Williams & Wilkins.

Mayo Clinic: Urinary incontinence, n.d. Retrieved from: http://www.mayoclinic.org/diseases-conditions/urinary-incontinence/basics/definition/CON-20037883?p=1.

Mayo Clinic: Cystitis, 2012. Retrieved from: www.mayoclinic.com/health/cystitis/DS00285/DSECTION = symptoms.

Mayo Clinic: Urinary Incontinence, 2017. Retrieved from: https://www.mayoclinic.org/diseases-conditions/urinary-incontinence/symptoms-causes/syc-20352808

Medline: Coude-Tip, 2017. Retrieved from: http://www.medline.com/product/Coude-100-Silicone-Foley-Catheters/Z05-PF02115.

Medscape: Specific gravity, 2014. Retrieved from: http://emedicine.medscape.com/article/2090711-overview.

Merck Manual for Health Care Professionals: Acquired renal cysts, 2013. Retrieved from: www.merckmanuals.com/professional/genitourinary_disorders/cystic_kidney_disease/acquired_renal_cysts.html.

National Cancer Institute (NCI): Hormone therapy for prostate cancer, 2014. Retrieved from: https://www.cancer.gov/types/prostate/prostate-hormone-therapy-fact-sheet.

National Institute of Diabetes and Digestive and Kidney Diseases (NIDDK). Urinary retention. 2014. Retrieved from: https://www.niddk.nih.gov/health-information/urologic-diseases/urinary-retention#sec3

National Kidney Foundation: End stage renal disease in the United States, 2013. Retrieved from: www.kidney.org/news/newsroom/factsheets/End-Stage-Renal-Disease-in-the-US.cfm.

National Library of Medicine (NLM): Creatine blood test, 2017a. Retrieved from: https://medlineplus.gov/ency/article/003475.htm.

National Library of Medicine (NLM): Creatinine clearance test, 2017b. Retrieved from: https://medlineplus.gov/ency/article/003611.htm.

New York Times: Urinary tract infection—adults, 2017. Retrieved from: http://www.nytimes.com/health/guides/disease/urinary-tract-infection/overview.html.

Prostate Cancer Treatment Guide: Prostate cancer treatment overview, n.d. Retrieved from: http://prostate-cancer.com/prostatecancer-treatment-overview/overview-gleason.html.

PubMed: Interstitial cystitis. *A.D.A.M. Medical Encyclopedia*, 2012. Retrieved from: www.ncbi.nlm.nih.gov/pubmedhealth/PMH0001508.

SEER: Cancer stat facts: kidney and renal pelvis cancer, n.d. Retrieved from: https://seer.cancer.gov/statfacts/html/kidrp.html.

WebMD: Blood urea nitrogen, 2010. Retrieved from: www.webmd.com/a-to-z-guides/blood-urea-nitrogen.

CHAPTER 51

Alkhalili E, Tasci Y, Aksoy E, et al: The utility of neck ultrasound and sestamibi scans in patients with secondary and tertiary hyperthyroidism, *World J Surg* 39(3):701–705, 2015.

American Cancer Society (ACS): Thyroid cancer, 2013. Retrieved from: www.cancer.org/cancer/thyroidcancer/detailedguide/thyroid-cancer-risk-factors.

American Diabetes Association (ADA): Eye complications, 2013. Retrieved from: www.diabetes.org/living-with-diabetes/complications/eye-complications.

American Diabetes Association (ADA): Hypoglycemia, 2015. Retrieved from: http://diabetes.org/living-with-diabetes/treatment-and-care/blood-glucose-control/hypoglycemia-low-blood.html.

Bass A, Will T, Todd M, et al: The latest tools for patients with diabetes, *RN* 70(6):39–43, 2007.

Bryant E: Male and female sexual dysfunction, *Voice of the Diabetic* 19(1):2004.

Daniel MS, Postellon DC: Congenital hypothyroidism, 2013. Retrieved from: http://emedicine.medscape.com/article/919758-overview#a0199.

Funnel M, Barlage D: Managing diabetes wh "agent oral," *Nursing* 34(3):36, 2004.

Gonzalez-Iglesias AE, Freeman ME: Brain control over pituitary gland hormones. In *Neuroscience in the 21st century*, New York, 2013, Springer, pp 1633–1681.

Lewis SL, Heitkemper MM, Dirksen SR, et al: *Medical-surgical nursing: Assessment and management of clinical problems*, ed 8, St. Louis, 2011, Mosby.

Marks AR: Calcium and the heart: A question of life and death, *J Clin Invest* 111(5):597–600, 2003.

Mayo Clinic: Hyperparathyroidism, 2011a. Retrieved from: www.mayoclinic.com/health/hyperparathyroidism/DS00396/DSECTION = risk-factors.

Mayo Clinic: Pheochromocytoma, 2011b. Retrieved from: www.mayoclinic.com/health/pheochromocytoma/DS00569/DSECTION = symptoms.

Mayo Clinic: Hypothyroidism (underactive thyroid), 2012a. Retrieved from: www.mayoclinic.com/health/hypothyroidism/DS00353/DSECTION = causes.

Mayo Clinic: Addison's disease, 2012b. Retrieved from: www.mayoclinic.com/health/addisons-disease/DS00361/DSECTION =causes.

Mayo Clinic: Gestational diabetes, 2017. Retrieved from: https://www.mayoclinic.org/diseases-conditions/gestational-diabetes/symptoms-causes/syc-20355339.

Mayo Clinic: Acromegaly, 2018a. Retrieved from: https://www.mayoclinic.org/diseases-conditions/acromegaly/diagnosis-treatment/drc-20351226.

Mayo Clinic: Dwarfism, 2018b. Retrieved from: https://www.mayoclinic.org/diseases-conditions/dwarfism/diagnosis-treatment/drc-20371975.

National Institute for Diabetes and Digestive and Kidney Diseases (NIDDKD): Acromegaly, 2012. Retrieved from: https://www.niddk.nih.gov/health-information/endocrine-diseases/acromegaly.

National Institute of General Medical Sciences (NIGMS): Circadian rhythms, 2018. Retrieved from: https://www.nigms.nih.gov/education/pages/Factsheet_CircadianRhythms.aspx.

National Library of Medicine (NLM): Calcitriol. Medline Plus, 2010. Retrieved from: www.nlm.nih.gov/medlineplus/druginfo/meds/a682335.html.

National Library of Medicine (NLM): Calcium: urine. Medline Plus, 2011. Retrieved from: www.nlm.nih.gov/medlineplus/ency/article/003603.htm.

National Library of Medicine (NLM): Goiter: Simple. Medline Plus, 2013. Retrieved from: www.nlm.nih.gov/medlineplus/ency/article/001178.htm.

National Library of Medicine (NLM): Growth hormone suppression test. 2018. Retrieved from: https://medlineplus.gov/ency/article/003376.htm.

Norman J: Thyroid cancer. Endocrineweb, 2012. Retrieved from: www.endocrineweb.com/conditions/thyroid-cancer/thyroid-cancer.

National Library of Medicine (NLM): Acromegaly. A.D.A.M Medical Encyclopedia, 2011a. Retrieved from: www.ncbi.nlm.nih.gov/pubmedhealth/PMH0001364.

Office of Dietary Supplements: Dietary supplement fact sheet: Iodine. National Institutes of Health, n.d. Retrieved from: http://ods.od.nih.gov/factsheets/Iodine-HealthProfessional.

Walker RA: Identifying diseases that mimic strokes, *J Emerg Med Serv* 36(3):2011. Retrieved from: http://www.jems.com/articles/print/volume-36/issue-3/patient-care/identifying-diseases-mimic-str.html.

CHAPTER 52

American Cancer Society (ACS): The American Cancer Society guidelines for the prevention and early detection of cervical cancer, 2016a. Retrieved from: https://www.cancer.org/cancer/cervical-cancer/prevention-and-early-detection/cervical-cancer-screening-guidelines.html.

American Cancer Society (ACS): Signs and symptoms of endometrial cancer, 2016. Retrieved from: https://www.cancer.org/cancer/endometrial-cancer/detection-diagnosis-staging/signs-and-symptoms.html.

American Cancer Society (ACS): American Cancer Society recommendations for the early detection of breast cancer, 2017a. Retrieved from: https://www.cancer.org/cancer/breast-cancer/screening-tests-and-early-detection/american-cancer-society-recommendations-for-the-early-detection-of-breast-cancer.html.

American Cancer Society (ACS): Survival rates for cervical cancer, by stage, 2017b. Retrieved from: https://www.cancer.org/cancer/cervical-cancer/detection-diagnosis-staging/survival.html.

American Cancer Society (ACS) Cancer Statistics Center: Uterine corpus: at a glance, 2017c. Retrieved from: https://cancerstatisticscenter.cancer.org/?_ga=2.117657742.645591719.1534695958-1601909998.1503257182#!/cancer-site/Uterine%20corpus.

American Cancer Society (ACS): Breast cancer survival rates, 2017d. Retrieved from: https://www.cancer.org/cancer/breast-cancer/understanding-a-breast-cancer-diagnosis/breast-cancer-survival-rates.html.

American Cancer Spociety (ACS): Key statistics for endometrial cancer, 2018a. Retrieved from: https://www.cancer.org/cancer/endometrial-cancer/about/key-statistics.html.

American Cancer Society (ACS) Cancer Statistics Center: Ovary: at a glance, 2018b. Retrieved from: https://cancerstatisticscenter.cancer.org/?_ga=2.117657742.645591719.1534695958-1601909998.1503257182#!/cancer-site/Ovary.

American Cancer Society (ACS): Key statistics for breast cancer in men, 2018c. Retrieved from: https://www.cancer.org/cancer/breast-cancer-in-men/about/key-statistics.html.

American Cancer Society (ACS): Key statistics for testicular cancer, 2018d. Retrieved from: https://www.cancer.org/cancer/testicular-cancer/about/key-statistics.html.

American Cancer Society (ACS): Testicular survival rates, 2018e. Retrieved from: https://www.cancer.org/cancer/testicular-cancer/detection-diagnosis-staging/survival-rates.html.

Breastcancer.org: TRAM flap reconstruction: What to expect, 2015. Retrieved from: http://www.breastcancer.org/treatment/surgery/reconstruction/types/autologous/tram/what-to-expect.

Breastcancer.org: Breast MRI for screening, 2016a. Retrieved from: http://www.breastcancer.org/symptoms/testing/types/mri/screening.

Breastcancer.org: Halotestin, 2016b. Retrieved from: http://www.breastcancer.org/treatment/druglist/halotestin.

Breastcancer.org: Femara, 2017. Retrieved from: http://www.breastcancer.org/treatment/hormonal/aromatase_inhibitors/femara.

Breastcancer.org: U.S. breast cancer statistics, 2018. Retrieved from: https://www.breastcancer.org/symptoms/understand_bc/statistics.

Cancer.org: Key statistics for ovarian cancer, 2017. Retrieved from: https://www.cancer.org/cancer/ovarian-cancer/about/key-statistics.html.

Cancereffects.com: Pamidronate disodium AREDIA, 2013. Retrieved from: www.cancereffects.com/Pamidronate-Disodium-(AREDIA)-Indication-and-Side-Effects-Information.html.

Centers for Disease Control and Prevention (CDC): 2014 Sexually transmitted diseases surveillance, Chlamydia, 2015. Retrieved from: https://www.cdc.gov/std/stats14/chlamydia.htm.

Centers for Disease Control and Prevention (CDC): 2015 Sexually transmitted diseases surveillance: gonorrhea, 2016a. Retrieved from: https://www.cdc.gov/std/stats15/gonorrhea.htm.

Centers for Disease Control and Prevention (CDC): CDC fact sheet: Reported STDs in the United States, 2016, 2017a. Retrieved from: https://www.cdc.gov/nchhstp/newsroom/docs/factsheets/std-trends-508.pdf.

Centers for Disease Control and Prevention (CDC): Cervical cancer statistics, 2017b. Retrieved from: https://www.cdc.gov/cancer/cervical/statistics/index.htm.

Centers for Disease Control and Prevention (CDC): Chlamydia - CDC Fact Sheet, 2017d. Retrieved from: https://www.cdc.gov/std/chlamydia/stdfact-chlamydia.htm.

Centers for Disease Control and Prevention (CDC): HPV (Human papilloma virus) Vaccine information statements (VIS), 2016b. Retrieved from: https://www.cdc.gov/vaccines/hcp/vis/vis-statements/hpv.html.

Centers for Disease Control and Prefenction (CDC): Trichomoniasis: CDC fact sheet, 2017c. Retrieved from: www.cdc.gov/std/trichomonas/STDFact-Trichomoniasis.htm.

Centers for Disease Control and Prevention (CDC): What are the risk factors for breast cancer, 2018. Retrieved from: https://www.cdc.gov/cancer/breast/basic_info/risk_factors.htm.

Cleveland Clinic: Dysmenorrhea, 2014. Retrieved from: http://my.clevelandclinic.org/health/articles/dysmenorrhea.

Guenin: Stereotactic breast biopsy, 2017. Retrieved from: http://www.radiologyinfo.org/en/info.cfm?pg=breastbixr.

Internet Health Resources (IHR): IVF costs, 2018. Retrieved from: https://www.ihr.com/infertility/ivf/ivf-in-vitro-fertilization-cost.html.

Johns Hopkins: Breast biopsy, n.d. Retrieved from: http://www.hopkinsmedicine.org/healthlibrary/test_procedures/gynecology/breast_biopsy_92,P07763/.

Komen.org: Breast cancer tumor characteristics, 2018a. Retrieved from: http://ww5.komen.org/BreastCancer/TumorCharacteristics.html.

Komen.org: Deciding between mastectomy or lumpectomy, 2018b. Retrieved from: http://ww5.komen.org/BreastCancer/DecidingBetweenMastectomyandLumpectomy.html.

Kumar S, Kekre NS, Gopalakrishnan G: Vesicovaginal fi stula: an update, *Indian J Urol* 23(2):187–191, 2007.

Mayo Clinic: Cytoscopy, n.d. Retrieved from: http://www.mayoclinic.org/tests-procedures/cystoscopy/basics/what-you-can-expect/prc-20013535.

Mayo Clinic: Male infertility, 2015a. Retrieved from: http://www.mayoclinic.org/diseases-conditions/male-infertility/basics/causes/CON-20033113.

Mayo Clinic: Colposcopy, 2018a. Retrieved from: https://www.mayoclinic.org/tests-procedures/colposcopy/about/pac-20385036.

Mayo Clinic: Hot flashes: diagnosis and treatment, 2018b. Retrieved from: https://www.mayoclinic.org/diseases-conditions/hot-flashes/diagnosis-treatment/drc-20352795.

Mayo Clinic: Infertility, 2018d. Retrieved from: www.mayoclinic.com/health/infertility/DS00310.

Mayo Clinic: Erectile dysfunction, 2018c. Retrieved from: http://www.mayoclinic.org/diseases-conditions/erectile-dysfunction/basics/treatment/con-20034244.

Mayo Clinic: Vaginal atrophy: diagnosis and treatment, 2018e. Retrieved from: https://www.mayoclinic.org/diseases-conditions/vaginal-atrophy/diagnosis-treatment/drc-20352294.

Mayo Clinic: Uterine prolapse, 2018f. Retrieved from: http://www.mayoclinic.org/diseases-conditions/uterine-prolapse/home/ovc-20343708.

National Cancer Institute (NCI): Sentinel lymph node biopsy, 2011. Retrieved from: www.cancer.gov/cancertopics/factsheet/detection/sentinel-node-biopsy.

National Cancer Institute (NCI): Endometrial cancer screening (PDQ)—health professional version, 2018. Retrieved from: https://www.cancer.gov/types/uterine/hp/endometrial-screening-pdq.

National Institute on Aging: What is menopause? 2017. Retrieved from: https://www.nia.nih.gov/health/publication/menopause.

National Institutes of Health (NIH): Infertility and fertility, 2017. Retrieved from: https://www.nichd.nih.gov/health/topics/infertility/Pages/default.aspx.

National Kidney and Urologic Diseases Information Clearinghouse (NKUDIC): Erectile dysfunction, 2015. Retrieved from: http://kidney.niddk.nih.gov/KUDiseases/pubs/ED/index.aspx.

National Library of Medicine (NLM): Infertility, A.D.A.M Medical Encyclopedia, 2013. Retrieved from: www.ncbi.nlm.nih.gov/pubmedhealth/PMH0002173.

National Library of Medicine: Endometriosis Overview, 2017. Retrieved from: https://www.ncbi.nlm.nih.gov/pubmedhealth/PMH0072685/.

National Library of Medicine, MedlinePlus: Toxic shock syndrome, 2018a. Retrieved from: https://medlineplus.gov/ency/article/000653.htm.

National Library of Medicine (NLM): Endometrial cancer, Medline Plus, 2018b. Retrieved from: www.nlm.nih.gov/medlineplus/ency/article/000910.htm.

Ollendorff AT: Cervicitis treatment & management, Medscape, 2017. Retrieved from: https://emedicine.medscape.com/article/253402-treatment#d9.

Osayande AS, Mehulic S: Diagnosis and initial management of dysmenorrhea, *Am Fam Physician* 89(5):341–346, 2014. Retrieved from: https://www.aafp.org/afp/2014/0301/p341.html.

Puscheck EE: Infertility, 2016. Retrieved from: http://emedicine.medscape.com/article/274143-overview#a2.

Spratto GR: *2013 Delmar nurse's drug handbook*, ed 22, Boston, 2012, Cengage Learning.

University of Miami/Jackson Memorial Medical Center: Sexuality in spinal injury: The spinal cord injured female: Orgasm. Louis Calder Memorial Library, 2009. Retrieved from: http://calder.med.miami.edu/pointis/orgasm.html.

US Department of Health and Human Services (USDHHS) Office on Women's Health: Premenstrual dysphoric disorder (PMDD), 2018. Retrieved from: https://www.womenshealth.gov/menstrual-cycle/premenstrual-syndrome/premenstrual-dysphoric-disorder-pmdd.

US Food and Drug Administration (FDA): Timeline of breast implant activities, 2004. Retrieved from: www.fda.gov/MedicalDevices/ProductsandMedicalProcedures/ImplantsandProsthetics/BreastImplants/ucm064242.htm.

US Food and Drug Administration (FDA): Cervarix, 2018. Retrieved from: http://www.fda.gov/BiologicsBloodVaccines/Vaccines/ApprovedProducts/ucm186957.htm.

US Preventive Services Task Force (USPSTF): Screening for breast cancer, 2009. Retrieved from: www.ahrq.gov/clinic/USpstf/uspsbrca.htm.

Winchester Hospital: Health library: Symptoms of premenstrual syndrome, 2016. Retrieved from: http://www.winchesterhospital.org/health-library/article?id=20026.

CHAPTER 53

American Foundation for the Blind, FamilyConnect: Functional visual assessment (FVA), 2018. Retrieved from: http://www.familyconnect.org/info/education/assessments/functional-vision-assessment-fva/135

American Optometric Association (AOA): Dry eye, 2018. Retrieved from: www.aoa.org/dry-eye.xml.

Centers for Disease Control (CDC): Why is Vision Loss a Public Health Problem? 2009. Retrieved from: www.cdc.gov/visionhealth/basic_information/vision_loss.htm.

Chin, C: Assistive technology devices for the blind and visually impaired, n.d. Retrieved from: http://chinchin.hubpages.com/hub/Assistive-Technology-for-the-Blind.

Ciancaglini E, Fazil P, Sforza GR: The use of a differential flourescent staining method to detect bacteriuria. *Clin Lab* 2004;50(11-12): 685–688. Retrieved https://www.ncbi.nlm.nih.gov/pubmed/15575310.

Glaucoma Research Foundation: Glaucoma facts and stats, 2017. Retrieved from: https://www.glaucoma.org/glaucoma/glaucoma-facts-and-stats.php.

Krishnadev N, Meleth AD, Chew EY: Nutritional supplements for age-related macular degeneration. *Curr Opin Ophthalmol* 2010;21(3):184–189.

Lewis SL, Heitkemper MM, Dirksen SR, et al.: *Medical-surgical nursing: Assessment and management of clinical problems*, ed 7, St. Louis, 2007, Mosby.

Mayo Clinic: Cataract surgery: Risks, 2010. Retrieved from: www.mayoclinic.com/health/cataract-surgery/MY00164/DSECTION=risks.

Mayo Clinic: Dry eyes, 2015. Retrieved from: https://www.mayoclinic.org/diseases-conditions/dry-eyes/diagnosis-treatment/drc-20371869

Mayo Clinic: Diabetic retinopathy, 2018. Retrieved from: https://www.mayoclinic.org/diseases-conditions/diabetic-retinopathy/diagnosis-treatment/drc-20371617

Munson, B: Now, listen up! Understanding hearing loss and deafness. *Nursing Made Incredibly Easy* 4 (2): 38, 2006.

National Eye Institute (NEI): National Institutes of Health (NIH). Age-Related Eye Disease Study: Results, 2008. Retrieved from: www.nei.nih.gov/amd.

National Library of Medicine (NLM): Tonometry. *Medline Plus,* 2012. Retrieved from: www.nlm.nih.gov/medlineplus/ency/article/003447.htm.

National Library of Medicine (NLM): Visual Field. *Medline Plus,* 2013a. Retrieved from: www.nlm.nih.gov/medlineplus/ency/article/003879.htm.

National Library of Medicine (NLM): Slit-lamp exam. *Medline Plus,* 2013b. Retrieved from: www.nlm.nih.gov/medlineplus/ency/article/003880.htm.

National Library of Medicine (NLM): Genetics Home Reference: *Sjögren syndrome*, 2016a. Retrieved from: https://ghr.nlm.nih.gov/condition/sjogren-syndrome.

National Library of Medicine (NLM): PubMed Health: How does our sense of taste work? 2016. Retrieved from: https://www.ncbi.nlm.nih.gov/pubmedhealth/PMH0072592/

National Library of Medicine (NLM): Fluorescein angiography. *Medline Plus,* 2018. Retrieved from: https://medlineplus.gov/ency/article/003846.htm.

Rhee DJ: Drug-induced glaucoma. Medscape, 2012. Retrieved from: http://emedicine.medscape.com/article/1205298-overview.

US Food and Drug Administration (US FDA): INTACS® prescription inserts for keratoconus: H040002, 2012. Retrieved from: www.fda.gov/MedicalDevices/ProductsandMedicalProcedures/DeviceApprovalsandClearances/Recently-ApprovedDevices/ucm080953.htm.

CHAPTER 54

Ahmed A, Simmons Z: Drugs which may exacerbate or induce myasthenia gravis: a clinician's guide, *Internet J Neurol* 10(2):2009. Retrieved from: http://archive.ispub.com/journal/theinternet-journal-of-neurology/volume-10-number-2/drugs-whichmay-exacerbate-or-induce-myasthenia-gravis-a-clinician-s-guide.html#sthash.pPOYqXmc.m8beVacX.dpuf.

American Brain Tumor Association: Brain tumor FAQs, n.d. Retrieved from: https://www.abta.org/about-brain-tumors/brain-tumor-faqs/.

American Heart Association/American Stroke Association (AHA/ASA): About stroke: treatment, n.d. Retrieved from: http://www.strokeassociation.org/STROKEORG/AboutStroke/Treatment/Stroke-Treatment_UCM_492017_SubHomePage.jsp.

American Heart Association/American Stroke Association (AHA/ASA): Ischemic strokes, 2018. Retrieved from: http://www.strokeassociation.org/STROKEORG/AboutStroke/TypesofStroke/IschemicClots/Ischemic-Strokes-Clots_UCM_310939_Article.jsp#.WJdf-DYiyM8.

American Speech-Language-Hearing Association: Swallowing disorders (dysphagia) in adults, n.d. Retrieved from: www.asha.org/public/speech/swallowing/Swallowing-Disorders-in-Adults/#tx.

BrainandSpinalCord.org: Brain injury FAQs, 2017. Retrieved from: http://www.brainandspinalcord.org/brain-injury-faqs/.

Centers for Disease Control and Prevention (CDC): Division of vector-borne infectious diseases: West Nile virus, 2008. Retrieved from: www.cdc.gov/ncidod/dvbid/westnile/index.htm.

Centers for Disease Control and Prevention (CDC): Rates of TBI-related emergency department visits by sex-United States,,2001-2010, 2016a. Retrieved from: https://www.cdc.gov/traumaticbraininjury/data/rates_ed_bysex.html.

Centers for Disease Control and Prevention (CDC): Stroke, 2016b. Retrieved from: https://www.cdc.gov/stroke/facts.htm.

Centers for Disease Control and Prevention (CDC): Vaccines and preventable diseases: Meningococcal vaccination, 2017. Retrieved from: https://www.cdc.gov/vaccines/vpd/mening/index.html.

Centers for Disease Control and Prevention (CDC): West Nile virus, 2018. Retrieved from: https://www.cdc.gov/westnile/faq/genquestions.html.

Cruz-Flores S, Chaisam T: Stroke anticoagulation and prophylaxis, 2018. Retrieved from: https://emedicine.medscape.com/article/1160021-overview#a3.

Epilepsy Foundation: About epilepsy: The basics, 2014. Retrieved from: https://www.epilepsy.com/learn/about-epilepsy-basics.

Glasgow Coma Scale: The Glasgow structured approach to the assessment of the Glasgow coma scale, 2014. Retrieved from: www.glascowcomascale.org.

Jalali R, Rezaei M: A comparison of the glasgow coma scale score with full outline of unresponsiveness scale to predict patients' traumatic brain injury outcomes in intensive care units, *Crit Care Res Pract* 2014:2014. Article ID 289803. 4 pages.

Lewis SL, Heitkemper MM, Dirksen SR, et al: *Medical-surgical nursing: assessment and management of clinical problems*, ed 7, St. Louis, 2007, Mosby.

Mayo Clinic: Amyotrophic lateral sclerosis, 2017. Retrieved from: http://www.mayoclinic.org/diseases-conditions/amyotrophic-lateral-sclerosis/diagnosis-treatment/treatment/txc-20247219.

Mayo Clinic: Epilepsy: diagnosis and treatment, 2018a. Retrieved from: https://www.mayoclinic.org/diseases-conditions/epilepsy/diagnosis-treatment/drc-20350098.

Mayo Clinic: Stroke: diagnosis and treatment, 2018b. Retrieved from: https://www.mayoclinic.org/diseases-conditions/stroke/diagnosis-treatment/drc-20350119.

Mosby's dictionary of medicine, nursing & health professions, ed 10, St. Louis, 2017, Elsevier.

Myasthenia Gravis Foundation of America: Clinical overview of myasthenia gravis, 2015. Retrieved from: http://www.myasthenia.org/healthprofessionals/clinicaloverviewofmg.aspx.

National Institutes of Health (NIH): All about ALS: Understanding a devastating disorder, 2015. Retrieved from: https://newsinhealth.nih.gov/issue/aug2015/feature2.

National Institute on Aging: Health care costs for dementia found greater than for any other disease, 2015. Retrieved from: https://www.nia.nih.gov/news/health-care-costs-dementia-found-greater-any-other-disease.

National Institute on Aging: Putting exercise to the test in people at risk for Alzheimer's, 2017. Retrieved from: https://www.nia.nih.gov/news/putting-exercise-test-people-risk-alzheimers.

National Institute of Neurological Disorders and Stroke: Questions and answers about carotid endarterectomy, 2016. Retrieved from: https://www.ninds.nih.gov/Disorders/Patient-Caregiver-Education/Hope-Through-Research/Stroke-Hope-Through-Research/Questions-Answers-Carotid-Endarterectomy.

National Institute of Neurological Disorders and Stroke: Bell's palsy fact sheet, 2017. Retrieved from: https://www.ninds.nih.gov/Disorders/Patient-Caregiver-Education/Fact-Sheets/Bells-Palsy-Fact-Sheet.

National Institutes of Neurological Disorders and Stroke: Guillan Barre sndrome fact sheet, 2018. Retrieved from: https://www.ninds.nih.gov/Disorders/Patient-Caregiver-Education/Fact-Sheets/Guillain-Barré-Syndrome-Fact-Sheet#3139_9.

National Library of Medicine (NLM): Migraine, 2014. Retrieved from: https://medlineplus.gov/migraine.html.

National Library of Medicine (NLM): Cluster headache, 2018. Retrieved from: https://medlineplus.gov/ency/article/000786.htm.

National Library of Medicine (NLM): Basal ganglia dysfunction, 2018a. Retrieved from: https://medlineplus.gov/ency/article/001069.htm.

National Library of Medicine (NLM): CSF leak, 2018b. Retrieved from: https://medlineplus.gov/ency/article/001068.htm.

National Library of Medicine (NLM): Guillain-Barre syndrome, 2018c. Retrieved from: https://medlineplus.gov/ency/article/000684.htm.

National Spinal Cord Injury Statistical Center: Spinal cord injury: facts and figures at a glance, 2016. Retrieved from: https://www.nscisc.uab.edu/Public/Facts%202016.pdf.

National Stroke Association: Stroke 101 fact sheet, 2014. Retrieved from: www.stroke.org/site/DocServer/STROKE101_2009.pdf?docID=4541.

Pappu S, Lerma J, Khraishi T: Brain CT to Assess Intracranial Pressure in Patients with Traumatic Brain Injury, *J Neuroimag* 26(1):37–40, 2016. doi:10.1111/jon.12289.

Parkinson's Foundation: Understanding parkinson's: Causes and statistics: environmental factors, n.d.a. Retrieved from: http://parkinson.org/Understanding-Parkinsons/Causes-and-Statistics/Environmental-Factors.

Parkinson's Foundation: Orthostatic hypertension, n.d.b. Retrieved from: http://toolkit.parkinson.org/content/orthostatic-hypotension#Common_Causes.

Potgieser ARE, Roosma E, Beudel M, et al: The Effect of Visual Feedback on Writing Size in Parkinson's Disease, *Parkinsons Dis* 2015:2015. doi:10.1155/2015/857041. Article ID 857041. 4 pages.

PubMed Health: Childhood brain tumors, 2016. Retrieved from: https://www.ncbi.nlm.nih.gov/pubmedhealth/PMHT0024761/.

CHAPTER 55

American College of Asthma, Allergy and Immunology: Latex allergy, 2014. Retrieved from: https://acaai.org/allergies/types/skin-allergies/latex-allergy.

American Latex Allergy Association: About latex allergy: statistics, 2018. Retrieved from: http://latexallergyresources.org/statistics.

Buelow B, Routes JM: Immediate hpersensitivity reactions, 2015. Retrieved from: https://emedicine.medscape.com/article/136217-overview.

Centers for Disease Control and Prevention (CDC): Vaccines and immunizations: immunity types, 2017. Retrieved from: https://www.cdc.gov/vaccines/vac-gen/immunity-types.htm.

Centers for Disease Control and Prevention (CDC): Vaccines and preventable conditions, 2018. https://www.cdc.gov/vaccines/vpd/shingles/index.html.

Fagundes CP, Gillie BL, Derry HM, et al: Chapter 2: resilience and immune function in older adults, *Ann Rev Gerontol Geriatr* 3229–3247, 2012. doi:10.1891/0198-8794.32.29.

Felix T, Hughes K, Stone E, et al: Age-specifi c variation in immune response in *Drosophila melanogaster* has a genetic basis, *Genetics* 191(3):989–1002, 2012.

Fernandez J: Overview of immunodeficiency disorders, 2018. Retrieved from: https://www.merckmanuals.com/home/immune-disorders/immunodeficiency-disorders/overview-of-immunodeficiency-disorders.

Kalokerinos EK, von Hippel W, Henry JD, et al: The aging positivity effect and immune function: positivity in recall predicts higher CD4 counts and lower CD4 activation, *Psychology & Aging* 29(3):636–641, 2014. doi:10.1037/a0037452.

Lewis SL, Bucher L, Heitkemper MM, et al: *Medical-surgical nursing: Assessment and management of clinical problems*, ed 10, St. Louis, 2017, Mosby.

Micans PA: The thymus gland, immune health, and aging, 2017. Retrieved from: https://www.antiaging-systems.com/articles/229-thymus-gland-immune-health-aging.

National Institute of Allergy and Infectious Diseases: Immune system: T cells, 2008. Retrieved from: www.niaid.nih.gov/topics/immunesystem/immunecells/pages/tcells.aspx.

National Institute for Occupational Safety and Health (NIOSH): Latex allergy: a prevention guide, 2014. Retrieved from: https://www.cdc.gov/niosh/docs/98-113/.

National Library of Medicine (NLM): Aging change in immunity, 2018. Retrieved from: https://medlineplus.gov/ency/article/004008.htm.

Salam N, et al: T cell ageing: effects of age on development, survival & function, *Indian J Med Res* 138(5):595–608, 2013.

Wein H: Shaking out clues to autoimmune disease, *National Institute of Health: Research Matters* 2013. Retrieved from: www.nih.gov/researchmatters/march2013/03182013autoimmune.htm.

CHAPTER 56

ACGT: Clinical trials: about participation, n.d. Retrieved from: https://actgnetwork.org/clinical-trials/about-trial-process/about-participation.

AIDSinfo: HIV wasting syndrome, 1997. Retrieved from: https://aidsinfo.nih.gov/news/362/hiv-wasting-syndrome.

AIDSinfo: When to start retroviral therapy, 2018. Retrieved from: https://aidsinfo.nih.gov/education-materials/fact-sheets/21/52/when-to-start-antiretroviral-therapy.

AIDSinfo: Preventing mother-to-child transmission of HIV, 2018a. Retrieved from: https://aidsinfo.nih.gov/education-materials/fact-sheets/20/50/preventing-mother-to-child-transmission-of-hiv.

AIDSinfo: The HIV life cycle, 2018b. Retrieved from: https://aidsinfo.nih.gov/education-materials/fact-sheets/19/73/the-hiv-life-cycle.

AIDSinfo: Stages of HIV infection, 2018c. Retrieved from: https://aidsinfo.nih.gov/education-materials/fact-sheets/19/46/the-stages-of-hiv-infection.

AIDSinfo: Side effects of HIV medicines, 2018d. Retrieved from: https://aidsinfo.nih.gov/education-materials/fact-sheets/22/66/hiv-and-hyperlipidemia.

AVERT: Global HIV and AIDS Statistics, 2018a. Retrieved from: https://www.avert.org/global-hiv-and-aids-statistics.

AVERT: HIV and AIDS in the United States of America, 2018b. Retrieved from: http://www.avert.org/professionals/hiv-around-world/western-central-europe-north-america/usa.

Buonaguro L, Tornesello ML, Buonaguro FM: Human immunodeficiency virus type 1 subtype distribution in the worldwide epidemic: Pathogenetic and therapeutic implications, *J Virol* 81(19):10209–10219, 2007.

Centers for Disease Control and Prevention (CDC): Global HIV/AIDS, n.d. Retrieved from: www.cdc.gov/globalaids.

Centers for Disease Control and Prevention (CDC): MMWR: recommendations and reports, *MMWR Morb Mortal Wkly Rep* 30(RR–21):1–3, 1981.

Centers for Disease Control and Prevention (CDC): 1993 Revised classification system for HIV infection and expanded surveillance case definition for AIDS among adolescents and adults, *MMWR Morb Mortal Wkly Rep* 41(RR–17):1–3, 1993.

Centers for Disease Control and Prevention (CDC): Updated U.S. Public Health Service guidelines for the management of occupational exposures to HBV, HCV, and HIV and recommendations forpostexposure prophylaxis, *MMWR Morb Mortal Wkly Rep* 50(RR–11):1, 2001.

Centers for Disease Control and Prevention (CDC): Revised surveillance case definitions for HIV infection among adults, adolescents, and children aged < 18 months and for HIV infection and AIDS among children aged 18 months to < 13 years—United States, 2008, *MMWR Morb Mortal Wkly Rep* 57(RR10):1–8, 2008.

Centers for Disease Control and Prevention (CDC): HIV transmission through transfusion—Missouri to Colorado, 2008, *Morbidity and Mortality Weekly Report* 59:1335–1339, 2010. Retrieved from: https://www.cdc.gov/mmwr/preview/mmwrhtml/mm5941a3.htm.

Centers for Disease Control and Prevention (CDC): Occupational HIV transmission and prevention among health care workers, 2011. Retrieved from: www.cdc.gov/hiv/resources/factsheets/hcwprev.htm.

Centers for Disease Control and Prevention (CDC): HIV in the United States: At a glance, 2013a. Retrieved from: www.cdc.gov/hiv/statistics/basics/ataglance.html.

Centers for Disease Control and Prevention (CDC): HIV among gay, bisexual, and other men who have sex with men, 2013b. Retrieved from: www.cdc.gov/hiv/risk/gender/msm/facts/index.html.

Centers for Disease Control and Prevention (CDC): HIV among African Americans, 2013c. Retrieved from: www.cdc.gov/hiv/pdf/risk_HIV_AAA.pdf.

Centers for Disease Control and Prevention (CDC): HIV among pregnant women, infants, and children, 2013d. Retrieved from: www.cdc.gov/hiv/risk/gender/pregnantwomen/facts/index.html.

Centers for Disease Control and Prevention (CDC): Blood/body fluid exposure option, 2013e. Retrieved from: https://www.cdc.gov/nhsn/PDFs/HPS-manual/exposure/3-HPS-Exposure-options.pdf.

Centers for Disease Control (CDC): HIV/AIDS: Testing, 2014. Retrieved from: www.cdc.gov/hiv/basics/testing.html.

Centers for Disease Control and Prevention (CDC): HIV risk behaviors, 2015. Retrieved from: http://www.cdc.gov/hiv/risk/estimates/riskbehaviors.html.

Centers for Disease Control and Prevention (CDC): Today's HIV/AIDS epidemic, 2016. Retrieved from: https://www.cdc.gov/nchhstp/newsroom/docs/factsheets/todaysepidemic-508.pdf.

Centers for Disease Control and Prevention (CDC): High-Impact HIV Prevention: CDC's approach to reducing HIV infection in the United States, 2017. Retrieved from: http://www.cdc.gov/hiv/policies/hip/hip.html.

Centers for Disease Control and Prevention (CDC): About HIV/AIDS, 2018a. Retrieved from: http://www.cdc.gov/hiv/basics/whatishiv.html.

Centers for Disease Control and Prevention (CDC): HIV among people aged 50 and over, 2018b. Retrieved from: http://www.cdc.gov/hiv/group/age/olderamericans/.

Centers for Disease Control and Prevention: Living with HIV, 2018c. Retrieved from: https://www.cdc.gov/hiv/basics/livingwithhiv/.

Centers for Disease Control and Prevention (CDC): HIV among African Americans, 2018d. Retrieved from: http://www.cdc.gov/hiv/group/racialethnic/africanamericans/.

Centers for Disease Control and Prevention (CDC): HIV among women, 2018e. Retrieved from: https://www.cdc.gov/hiv/group/gender/women/index.html.

Centers for Disease Control and Prevention (CDC): HIV testing, 2018e. Retrieved from: http://www.cdc.gov/hiv/guidelines/testing.html.

Centers for Disease Control and Prevention (CDC): HIV among Hispanics/Latinos, 2018f. Retrieved from: http://www.cdc.gov/hiv/group/racialethnic/hispaniclatinos/.

Centers for Disease Control and Prevention (CDC): HIV in the United States: At a glance, 2018g. Retrieved from: http://www.cdc.gov/hiv/statistics/overview/ataglance.html.

Centers for Disease Control and Prevention (CDC): Vaginal sex and HIV risk, 2018h. Retrieved from: http://www.cdc.gov/hiv/risk/vaginalsex.html.

Centers for Disease Control and Prevention (CDC): Injection drug use and HIV risk, 2018i. Retrieved from: http://www.cdc.gov/hiv/risk/idu.html.

Centers for Disease Control and Prevention (CDC): PEP, 2018k. Retrieved from: http://www.cdc.gov/hiv/basics/pep.html.

Coffin J: *HIV pathogenesis. 11th International AIDS Conference*, Vancouver, 1996, British Columbia.

Garry RF, Witte MH, Gottlieb AA, et al: Documentation of an AIDS virus infection in the United States in 1968, *JAMA* 260(14):2085–2087, 1988.

Henry J. Kaiser Family Foundation: People living with HIV/AIDS (adults and children), 2013. Retrieved from: http://kff.org/globalindicator/people-living-with-hivaids.

Henry J. Kaiser Family Foundation: The HIV/AIDS epidemic in the United States: The basics, 2018. Retrieved from: http://kff.org/hivaids/fact-sheet/the-hivaids-epidemic-in-the-united-states/.

HIV.gov: Preventing sexual transmission of HIV, 2016. Retrieved from: https://www.hiv.gov/hiv-aids-basics/prevention/reduce-your-risk/understanding-risk-activities/.

HIV.gov: HIV treatment overview, 2017a. Retrieved from: https://www.aids.gov/hiv-aids-basics/just-diagnosed-with-hiv-aids/treatment-options/overview-of-hiv-treatments/.

HIV.gov: Who should get tested?, 2017b. Retrieved from: https://www.aids.gov/hiv-aids-basics/prevention/hiv-testing/hiv-test-types/.

Ho DD, Neumann AU, Perelson AS, et al: Rapid turnover of plasma virions and CD4 lymphocytes in HIV-1 infection, *Nature* 373(6510):123–126, 1995.

Holmberg SD: The estimated prevalence and incidence of HIV in 96 large US metropolitan areas, *Am J Public Health* 86(5):642–654, 2008, 1996.

Ironson G, Hayward H: Do positive psychosocial factors predict disease progression in HIV? A review of the evidence, *Psychosomat Med* 70(5):546–554, 2008.

Kalichman SC: Co-occurrence of treatment nonadherence and continued HIV transmission risk behaviors: Implications for positive prevention interventions, *Psychosomat Med* 70(5):593–597, 2008.

Kuhar DT, Henderson DK, Struble KA, et al: Updated US Public Health Service guidelines for the management of occupational exposures to human immunodeficiency virus and recommendations for postexposure prophylaxis, *Infect Control Hosp Epidemiol* 34(9):875–892, 2013. Retrieved from: https://www.cambridge.org/core/journals/infection-control-and-hospital-epidemiology/article/updated-us-public-health-service-guidelines-for-the-management-of-occupational-exposures-to-human-immunodeficiency-virus-and-recommendations-for-postexposure-prophylaxis/FACD234C788E0D541E37BC3DEFB4C248.

Leserman J: Role of depression, stress, and trauma in HIV disease progression, *Psychosomat Med* 70(5):539–545, 2008.

Nayamweya S, Hegedus A, Jaye A, et al: Comparing HIV-1 and HIV-2 infection: Lessons for viral immunopathogenesis, 2013. Retrieved from: http://onlinelibrary.wiley.com/doi/10.1002/rmv.1739/abstract;jsessionid=6A7F5352382E943A337A548E92EDDDD4.f01t04.

Panel on Antiretroviral Guidelines for Adult and Adolescents: Guidelines for the use of antiretroviral agents in adults and adolescents living with HIV, 2018. Department of Health and Human Services, 2018. Retrieved from: https://aidsinfo.nih.gov/contentfiles/lvguidelines/adultandadolescentgl.pdf.

SciDevNet: African HIV trials could create world's first vaccine, 2016. Retrieved from: http://www.scidev.net/sub-saharan-africa/hiv-aids/news/african-hiv-trials-could-create-world-s-first-vaccine.html.

Sherman D: Palliative care. In Kirton CA, Talotta D, Zwolski K, editors: *Handbook of HIV/AIDS nursing*, St. Louis, 2001, Mosby.

Temoshok LR, Wald RL, Synowski S, et al: Coping as a multisystem construct associated with pathways mediating HIV-relevant immune function and disease progression, *Psychosomat Med* 70(5):555–561, 2008.

Thomas, FP: Dementia due to HIV infection, 2018. Retrieved from: https://www.emedicinehealth.com/dementia_due_to_hiv_infection/article_em.htm#pictures_of_brains_with_aids_dementia_complex.

US Department of Health and Human Services, Office of Minority Health: HIV/AIDS and African Americans, 2016. Retrieved from: http://minorityhealth.hhs.gov/omh/browse.aspx?lvl=4&lvlid=21.

US Department of Health and Human Services (USDHHS): Guidelines for the Use of Antiretroviral Agents in Adults and Adolescents Living with HIV. Developed by the DHHS Panel on Antiretroviral Guidelines for Adults and Adolescents – A Working Group of the Office of AIDS Research Advisory Council (OARAC). 2017. Retrieved from: https://aidsinfo.nih.gov/contentfiles/lvguidelines/adultandadolescentgl.pdf.

US Department of Health and Human Services (USDHHS), AIDSInfo: HIV AIDS glossary: antiviral pregnancy registry, 2018a. Retrieved from: https://aidsinfo.nih.gov/understanding-hiv-aids/glossary/793/antiretroviral-pregnancy-registry.

US Department of Health and Human Services (USDHHS), AIDSInfo: HIV treatment: medication adherence, 2018b. Retrieved from: https://aidsinfo.nih.gov/understanding-hiv-aids/fact-sheets/21/54/hiv-medication-adherence.

US Department of Health and Human Services (USDHHS), AIDSInfo: HIV overview: HIV testing, 2018c. Retrieved from: https://aidsinfo.nih.gov/understanding-hiv-aids/fact-sheets/19/47/hiv-testing/.

United States Food and Drug Administration (US FDA): Blood and blood products, 2013. Retrieved from: www.fda.gov/BiologicsBloodVaccines/BloodBloodProducts/default.htm.

Wei X, Ghosh SK, Taylor ME, et al: Viral dynamics in humanimmunodeficiency virus type 1 infection, *Nature* 373(6510):117–122, 1995.

Wodak A, Cooney A: Do needle syringe programs reduce HIV infection among injecting drug users: a comprehensive review of the international evidence, *Subst Use Misuse* 41(6–7):777–813, 2006.

World Health Organization (WHO): Mother-to-child transmission of HIV, 2013a. Retrieved from: www.who.int/hiv/topics/mtct/en/index.html.

World Health Organization (WHO): WHO-UNAIDS HIV vaccine initiative, 2013b. Retrieved from: www.who.int/immunization/research/forums_and_initiatives/HIV_vaccine_initiative/en/index.html.

World Health Organization (WHO): WHO definition of palliative care, 2013c. Retrieved from: www.who.int/cancer/palliative/definition/en.

World Health Organization (WHO): *Consolidated Guidelines on HIV Testing Services: 5Cs: Consent, Confidentiality, Counselling, Correct Results and Connection 2015*, Geneva, 2015 Jul. 3, World Health Organization, PRE-TEST AND POST-TEST SERVICES. Available from: https://www.ncbi.nlm.nih.gov/books/.

World Health Organization (WHO): Zoonoses: Managing public health risks at the human-Animal-environmental interface, 2016a. Retrieved from: http://www.who.int/zoonoses/en/.

World Health Organization (WHO): Global Health Observatory (GHO) data: HIV/AIDS, 2016b. Retrieved from: http://www.who.int/gho/hiv/en/.

World Health Organization (WHO): HIV/AIDS Key Facts, 2018. Retrieved from: http://www.who.int/en/news-room/fact-sheets/detail/hiv-aids.

CHAPTER 57

American Cancer Society (ACS): Make Exercise Work For You, 2014. Retrieved from: https://www.cancer.org/healthy/eat-healthy-get-active/get-active/make-exercise-work-for-you.html.

American Cancer Society (ACS): Viruses that can lead to cancer, 2016a. Retrieved from: http://www.cancer.org/cancer/cancercauses/othercarcinogens/infectiousagents/infectiousagentsandcancer/infectious-agents-and-cancer-viruses.

American Cancer Society (ACS): Chemo brain, 2016b. Retrieved from: http://www.cancer.org/treatment/treatmentsandsideeffects/physicalsideeffects/chemotherapyeffects/chemo-brain.

American Cancer Society (ACS): Cancer prevention and early detection: Facts and figures 2017-2018, Atlanta, 2017a, American Cancer Society. Retrieved from: https://www.cancer.org/content/dam/cancer-org/research/cancer-facts-and-statistics/cancer-prevention-and-early-detection-facts-and-figures/cancer-prevention-and-early-detection-facts-and-figures-2017.pdf.

American Cancer Society (ACS): Alcohol use and cancer, 2017b. Retrieved from: http://www.cancer.org/cancer/cancercauses/dietandphysicalactivity/alcohol-use-and-cancer.

American Cancer Society (ACS): Breast cancer risk factors you cannot change, 2017c. Retrieved from: http://www.cancer.org/cancer/breastcancer/moreinformation/breastcancerearlydetection/breast-cancer-early-detection-risk-factors-you-cannot-change.

American Cancer Society (ACS): Genetic counseling and testing, 2018a. Retrieved from: http://www.cancer.org/cancer/cancercauses/geneticsandcancer/heredity-and-cancer.

American Cancer Society (ACS): Signs and symptoms of testicular cancer, 2018b. Retrieved from: https://www.cancer.org/cancer/testicular-cancer/detection-diagnosis-staging/signs-and-symptoms.html.

Association of Reproductive Health Professionals: Health matters fact sheets: Understanding cervical cancer screening test results, 2012. Retrieved from: https://www.arhp.org/Publications-and-Resources/Patient-Resources/fact-sheets/Understanding-Pap-Test-Results.

Cancer.net: Positron emission tomography and computed tomography (PET-CT) scans, 2016. Retrieved from: http://www.cancer.net/navigating-cancer-care/diagnosing-cancer/tests-and-procedures/positron-emission-tomography-and-computed-tomography-pet-ct-scans.

Cancer.net: Nausea and vomiting, 2017a. Retrieved from: http://www.cancer.net/research-and-advocacy/asco-care-and-treatment-recommendations-patients/preventing-vomiting-caused-cancer-treatment.

Cancer.net: Side effects of chemotherapy, 2017b. Retrieved from: http://www.cancer.net/navigating-cancer-care/how-cancer-treated/chemotherapy/side-effects-chemotherapy.

Centers for Disease Control and Prevention (CDC): United States cancer statistics: digital visualizations, n.d. Retrieved from: http://www.cdc.gov/cancer/dcpc/data/types.htm.

Centers for Disease Control and Prevention (CDC): Cancer prevention and control, 2018. Retrieved from: http://www.cdc.gov/cancer/international/statistics.htm.

Moore LV, Thompson FE: Adults meeting fruit and vegetable intake recommendations—United States, 2013, *MMWR Morb Mortal Wkly Rep*, 64(26):709–713, 2015. Retrieved from: http://www.cdc.gov/mmwr/preview/mmwrhtml/mm6426a1.htm.

National Cancer Institute (NCI): Cancer stat facts: Cancer of any site, n.d.a. Retrieved from: https://seer.cancer.gov/statfacts/html/all.html.

National Cancer Institute (NCI): Obesity, 2015. Retrieved from: https://www.cancer.gov/about-cancer/causes-prevention/risk/obesity.

National Cancer Institute (NCI): Oral complications of chemotherapy and head/neck radiation (PDQ)—health professionals version, 2016. Retrieved from: https://www.cancer.gov/about-cancer/treatment/side-effects/mouth-throat/oral-complications-hp-pdq.

National Cancer Institute (NCI): The genetics of cancer, 2017a. Retrieved from: https://www.cancer.gov/about-cancer/causes-prevention/genetics.

National Cancer Institute (NCI): Cannabis and cannabinoids (PDQ)—health professionals version, 2017b. Retrieved from: https://www.cancer.gov/about-cancer/treatment/cam/hp/cannabis-pdq.

National Cancer Institute (NCI): Cancer Statistics, 2018. Retrieved from: https://www.cancer.gov/about-cancer/understanding/statistics.

National Cancer Institute (NCI): Targeted cancer therapies, 2018. Retrieved from: https://www.cancer.gov/about-cancer/treatment/types/targeted-therapies/targeted-therapies-fact-sheet.

Pancreatic Cancer Action Network: Learn about pancreatic cancer, n.d. Retrieved from: www.pancan.org/section_facing_pancreatic_cancer/learn_about_pan_cancer/diagnosis/CA19_9.php.

Vachani C: Patient guide to tumor markers, 2018. Retrieved from: https://www.oncolink.org/cancer-treatment/procedures-diagnostic-tests/blood-tests-tumor-diagnostic-tests/patient-guide-to-tumor-markers.

CHAPTER 58

American Association of Nurse Assessment Coordination (AANAC): Nursing leadership: Management and leadership styles, 2014. Retrieved from: http://www.aanac.org/docs/white-papers/2013-nursing-leadership—management-leadership-styles.pdf?sfvrsn=2.

American Nurses Association (ANA): *Nursing informatics: Scope and standards of practice*. Silver Springs, Md, 2008, Author.

American Nurses Association (ANA) and National Council on State Boards of Nursing (NCSBN): Joint statement on delegation, n.d. Retrieved from: https://www.ncsbn.org/Delegation_joint_statement_NCSBN-ANA.pdf.

Association of Rehabilitation Nurses: About ARN: History, 2012. Retrieved from: www.rehabnurse.org/about/content/History.html.

Cottingham S, Dibartolo MC, Battistoni S, et al: Partners in nursing: A mentoring initiative to enhance nurse retention, *Nurs Educ Perspect* 32(4):250–255, 2011.

Greenwood B: Can an LPN be a nurse manager? n.d. Retrieved from: http://work.chron.com/can-lpn-nurse-manager-13874.html.

Hill S, Howlett H: *Success in practical/vocational nursing*, ed 7, St. Louis, 2013, Mosby.

Ketola J: An analysis of a mentoring program for baccalaureate nursing students: does the past still influence the present?, *Nurs Forum* 44(4):245–255, 2009.

Maslach C, Jackson SE: *Burnout inventory manual*, ed 2, Palo Alto, Calif, 1986, Consulting Psychologists Press.

Monegain B: Burnout rampant in healthcare, 2013. Retrieved from: http://www.healthcareitnews.com/news/burnout-rampant-healthcare.

Thomas CM: The impaired nurse, 2011. Retrieved from: http://www.medscape.com/viewarticle/748598.

US Department of Labor, Bureau of Labor Statistics: Occupational outlook handbook: Licensed practical and vocational nurses, 2018. Retrieved from: https://www.bls.gov/ooh/healthcare/licensed-practical-and-licensed-vocational-nurses.htm#tab-3.

US Department of Veterans Affairs: VA careers: Nursing, 2012. Retrieved from: www.vacareers.va.gov/careers/nurses/index.asp.

Glossary

A

abduction Movement of an extremity away from the midline of the body.
ablation Amputation or excision of any part of the body; removal of a growth or harmful substance.
abortion Loss of a pregnancy before 20 weeks' gestation.
abuse Misuse, as of an addictive substance such as alcohol, tobacco, nicotine, and so forth.
accountability Being answerable for one's own actions.
accreditation Process whereby a professional association or nongovernmental agency grants recognition to an institution or agency for demonstrated ability in a special area of practice.
achalasia Abnormal condition characterized by the inability of a muscle, particularly the cardiac sphincter of the stomach, to relax.
achlorhydria Abnormal condition characterized by the absence of hydrochloric acid in the gastric secretions.
acid-base balance Homeostasis of the hydrogen ion (H^+) concentration in the body fluids.
acquired heart disorder Abnormality occurring after birth that compromises heart function.
acquired immunodeficiency syndrome (AIDS) Acquired condition that impairs the body's ability to fight infection; the end stage of the continuum of HIV infection, in which the infected person has a CD_4^+ (lymphocyte) count of ≤200 cells/mm^3.
acrocyanosis Peripheral cyanosis; the blue discoloration of the hands and feet in most infants at birth that sometimes persists for 7 to 10 days.
active listening Giving full attention and a concerted effort to understand the message being sent.
active transport The movement of materials across the cell membrane by means of chemical activity (the energy of metabolism), which allows the cell to admit molecules larger than would otherwise be able to enter.
activities of daily living (ADLs) Those activities of daily life, such as toileting, bathing, dressing, and grooming, that promote maintenance of functional abilities and independence in the environment.
actual nursing diagnosis Statement of a health problem that a nurse is licensed and competent to treat.
acupressure Complementary and alternative therapy that uses gentle pressure at points on the body; used primarily to prevent and relieve symptoms of muscle tension.
acupuncture Complementary and alternative therapy that stimulates certain points on the body by the insertion of special needles to modify the perception of pain, normalize physiologic functions, and to treat or prevent disease.
acute Having a short and relatively severe course; a disease process characterized by a relatively short duration of signs and symptoms that are usually severe and begin abruptly.
acute coryza Acute rhinitis, also known as the common cold; an inflammatory condition of the mucous membranes of the nose and accessory sinuses.
acute pain Intense, unpleasant sensation of short duration, lasting less than 6 months.
adaptation Adjustment to changing life situations by using various strategies.
adaptive immunity Protection that provides a specific reaction to each invading antigen and has the unique ability to remember the antigen that caused the attack.
addiction Excessive use or abuse of a substance or practice, displayed by psychological disturbance, decline of social and economic function, and uncontrollable consumption, indicating dependence.
addictive personality One who exhibits a pattern of compulsive and habitual use of a substance or practice to cope with psychological pain from conflict and anxiety.
adduction Movement of an extremity toward the axis of the body.
adenosine triphosphate A substance produced in the mitochondria from nutrients and capable of releasing energy that in turn enables the cell to work.
adherence Following a prescribed regimen of therapy or treatment for disease.
adjuvant Additional, as in additional drug or treatment.
admission Entry of a patient into a health care facility.
adoptive family Family unit with adoptive children who are chosen and taken into the family by legal process and raised as the family's own.
adult daycare A community-based program designed to meet the needs of functionally or cognitively impaired adults through an individualized plan of care.
advance directives Signed and witnessed documents providing specific instructions for health care treatment in the event that the individual is unable to make those decisions personally at the time they are needed.
advancement Rise in rank or importance; a promotion, progress, improvement.
adventitious Abnormal sounds superimposed on breath sounds.
adverse drug reaction A harmful, unintended reaction to a drug administered at a normal dosage.
advocate A person who acts on behalf of another person.
affect External manifestation of inner feeling or emotions, often reflected by facial expression.
against medical advice (AMA) Charting notation when a patient leaves a health care facility without a physician's order for discharge.
ageism Process of systematic stereotyping of and discriminating against people because of their advanced age.
aggressive communication Interacting with another in an overpowering and forceful manner to meet one's own needs at the expense of others.
agnosia Total or partial loss of the ability to recognize familiar objects or people through sensory stimuli; results from organic brain damage.
agonist Drug that produces a predictable response at the intended site of action.
agoraphobia An anxiety disorder characterized by a fear of being in an open, crowded, or public place such as a field, tunnel, bridge, congested streets, or busy stores, where escape may be difficult or help unavailable if anxiety incapacitates the person. If untreated, the individual often refuses to leave the home.

air embolism An abnormal circulatory condition in which air travels through the bloodstream and becomes lodged in a blood vessel.
akinesia Abnormal state of motor and psychic hypoactivity.
Alcoholics Anonymous (AA) Nonprofit organization founded in 1935, consisting of abstinent alcoholics helping other alcoholics to become and stay sober through group support.
alcoholism Addiction to alcohol.
alignment Relationship of various body parts to one another.
allergen A substance that can produce a hypersensitive reaction in the body but that is not necessarily inherently harmful.
allopathic medicine Traditional or conventional Western medicine.
allow natural death *See* do-not-resuscitate.
alopecia Loss of hair resulting from destruction of hair follicles.
alpha-fetoprotein (AFP) Antigen present in the human fetus; can be used to evaluate fetal development.
altered cognition A decrease or lack of cognitive ability to receive, process, and send information.
alternative therapies Nontraditional therapies that may include the same interventions as complementary therapies but that often become the primary treatment modalities that replace allopathic (traditional) medicine. Examples are exercise, massage, acupuncture, and herbalism.
Alzheimer's disease A presenile dementia characterized by confusion, memory failure, disorientation, restlessness, agnosia, speech disturbances, inability to carry out purposeful movements, and hallucinosis. Also called *senile dementia—Alzheimer's type (SDAT).*
amblyopia Lazy eye; reduction or dimness of vision, especially when there is no apparent pathologic condition of the eye.
amenorrhea Absence of menstrual flow.
amino acids Building blocks out of which proteins are constructed; the end products of protein digestion.
amniocentesis Obstetric procedure in which a small amount of amniotic fluid is removed for laboratory analysis; usually performed between the 16th and 20th weeks of gestation to aid in the diagnosis of fetal abnormalities.
amniotomy Artificial rupture of the fetal membranes (AROM).
amotivational cannabis syndrome Follows the use of cannabis and is characterized by decreased goal-directed activities, abrupt mood swings, abnormal irritability, etc.
anabolism The building aspect on which the energy released from catabolism allows the cells to build more complex, usable forms of nutrients; the building and repairing phase of metabolism; opposite of catabolism.
anaphylactic shock Severe, life-threatening hypersensitivity reaction to a previously encountered antigen.
anasarca Severe, generalized edema.
anastomosis Surgical joining of two ducts or blood vessels to allow flow from one to the other.
anatomy The study, classification, and description of structures and organs of the body.
anemia Blood disorder characterized by red blood cell, hemoglobin, and hematocrit levels below normal range.
anesthesia Absence of sensation (*an-*, meaning "without," and *-esthesia,* meaning "awareness or feeling").
aneurysm A localized dilation of the wall of a blood vessel, usually caused by atherosclerosis, hypertension, and less commonly by a congenital weakness in a vessel wall.
angina pectoris Paroxysmal thoracic pain and choking feeling caused by decreased oxygen (anoxia) of the myocardium.
anion Negatively charged ion that, when in solution, is attracted to the positive electrode.
ankylosis Fixation of a joint, often in an abnormal position, usually resulting from destruction of articular cartilage and subchondral bone.
anorexia nervosa A psychoneurotic disorder characterized by a prolonged refusal to eat; self-imposed starvation.
antagonist Drug that will block the action of another drug.
antepartal First stage of the maternity cycle. Also called the *prenatal* or *antenatal* period.
anterior fontanelle A diamond-shaped space covered by tough membranes between the bones of an infant's cranium. The posterior fontanelle is triangular.
anticipatory grief Expectation of or preparation for the loss of one or more valued or significant others; accomplishment of part of the grief work before the actual loss occurs.
anticipatory guidance Psychological preparation of a patient for an event expected to be stressful, such as preparing a child for surgery by explaining what will happen and what it will feel like. It is also used to prepare parents for normal growth and development of their children.
antigen A substance recognized by the body as foreign that can trigger an immune response.
antioxidant Chemical or other agent that delays or prevents the breakdown of a substance by oxygen.
antiseptic A substance that tends to inhibit the growth and reproduction of microorganisms; may be used on humans.
anuria Urinary output of less than 100 to 250 mL in 24 hours.
anxiety Condition in which an individual experiences a vague feeling of apprehension resulting from a real or perceived threat to the self.
aphasia Abnormal neurologic condition in which language function is defective or absent because of an injury to certain areas of the cerebral cortex.
apical pulse Heartbeat as measured with the bell or disk of the stethoscope placed over the apex of the heart; represents the actual beating of the heart. Most authentic of all pulses.
aplasia In hematology, a failure of the normal process of cell generation and development.
apnea The absence of breathing.
approved program Program that meets minimum standards established by the state agency responsible for overseeing education programs.
apraxia Impairment of the ability to perform purposeful acts; inability to use objects properly.
aromatherapy An alternative therapy that uses essential oils produced from plants to provide health benefits.
arteriosclerosis Common arterial disorder characterized by thickening, loss of elasticity, and calcification of arterial walls, resulting in a decreased blood supply.
arthrocentesis Puncture of a joint with a needle to withdraw fluid; performed to obtain synovial fluid for diagnostic purposes.
arthrodesis Surgical fusion of a joint.
arthroplasty Surgical repair or refashioning of one of both sides, parts, or specific tissues within a joint.
articulate Speaking clearly, distinctly, and to the point; presenting yourself with clarity and effectiveness.
as necessary (prn) The completion of activities as the condition demands; as needed.
ascites An accumulation of fluid and albumin in the peritoneal cavity.
asepsis Free of pathogenic microorganisms.
assertive communication Interaction that takes into account the feelings and needs of the receiver.
assessment Evaluation or appraisal of a condition; includes observing, gathering, verifying, and communicating pertinent data, usually information about the patient.
assisted living Residential care whereby the adult patient rents a small one-bedroom or studio apartment and can receive personal care services such as assistance with bathing, dressing, eating, etc.

asterixis Hand-flapping tremor usually induced by extending the arm and dorsiflexing the wrist; frequently seen in patients who are in a hepatic coma.
asthenia General feeling of tiredness and listlessness.
astigmatism Defect in the curvature of the eyeball surface.
ataxia Abnormal condition characterized by impaired ability to coordinate movement.
atelectasis Collapse of lung tissues, preventing the respiratory exchange of carbon dioxide and oxygen.
atherosclerosis A common arterial disorder characterized by yellowish plaques of cholesterol, lipids, and cellular debris in the inner layer of the walls of large and medium-sized arteries.
atony Lack of normal tone or strength.
attention deficit/hyperactivity disorder (ADHD) A group of behaviors—hyperactivity, inattentiveness, and impulsivity—that appear early in a child's life, persist throughout childhood and adolescence, and may extend into adulthood.
attenuation The process of weakening the degree of virulence of a disease organism.
attitude In obstetrics, the relationship of fetal body parts to one another.
audiometry Testing of hearing acuity.
auditors People appointed to examine patient charts and health records to assess the quality of care.
aura Sensation, as of light or warmth, that may precede the onset of a migraine or an epileptic seizure. An epileptic aura may be psychic, or it may be sensory with olfactory, visual, auditory, or taste hallucinations.
auscultate/auscultation To listen for sounds within the body to evaluate the condition of the heart, lungs, pleura, intestines, or other organs or to detect fetal heart sounds.
autism A complex developmental disorder of brain function accompanied by a broad range of severity of intellectual and behavioral deficits that impairs the child's ability for appropriate social interaction, communication skills, and behavior.
autocratic family pattern Family unit with unequal relationships; parents attempt to control with strict, rigid rules and expectations.
autograft Surgical transplantation of any tissue from one part of the body to another location in the same individual.
autoimmune/autoimmunity Immune response (autoantibodies or cellular immune response) to one's own tissues.
autologous Something that has its origin within an individual, especially a factor present in tissues or fluids.
autolysis Self-dissolution or self-digestion in tissues or cells by enzymes in the cells.
automated perimetry test Test places the patient in front of a computer-like device and asked to stare at a screen and to press a button when flashes of light enter the field of vision.
autopsy Examination performed after a person's death to confirm or determine the cause of death.
axilla Underarm area or armpit.
azotemia Retention of excessive amounts of nitrogenous compounds in the blood.

B

baby boomers The segment of the population who were born between 1945 and 1964.
bacteriuria Presence of bacteria in the urine.
ballottement Technique of palpating an organ or floating structure by bouncing it gently and feeling it rebound. Ballottement of a fetus within the uterus is a probable objective sign of pregnancy.
bandage A strip or roll of cloth or other material that may be wound around part of the body in a variety of ways for multiple purposes.
basal metabolic rate (BMR) Amount of energy used by the body at rest to maintain vital functions such as respiration, circulation, temperature, peristalsis, and muscle tone.
base of support Area on which an object rests; a stance with feet slightly apart.
basic life support (BLS) The role of cardiopulmonary resuscitation (CPR) and emergency cardiac care (ECC) to preserve circulatory or respiratory function or both in the emergency treatment of a victim of cardiac or respiratory arrest.
bedpan Device for receiving feces or urine from a patient who is confined to bed; may be used for specimen collection.
behavior Manner in which a person acts or performs. Any or all of the activities of a person, including physical actions, that are observed directly, and mental activity that is inferred and interpreted. Kinds of behavior include abnormal, automatic, invariable, and variable.
benign Not recurrent or progressive; opposite of malignant.
bereavement Common depressed reaction to the death of a loved one.
bereavement overload The individual's experience of an initial loss compounded with an additional loss before resolution of the initial loss.
bicarbonate A main anion of the extracellular fluid.
biliary atresia The absence of or underdevelopment of biliary structures that is congenital in nature.
binder Bandage made of large pieces of material to fit a specific body part (e.g., abdominal or breast binder).
biofeedback A technique that is nonpharmacological and noninvasive used to control body responses.
biographic data The facts and events of a person's life.
biologic death Results from permanent cellular damage caused by a lack of oxygen.
biomedical health belief system A belief that health and illness are controlled by a series of physical and biochemical processes that can be analyzed and manipulated by humans. Primary health belief in the United States.
biopsy The removal of a small piece of living tissue from an organ or another part of the body for microscopic examination to confirm or establish a diagnosis, estimate a prognosis, or follow the course of a disease.
bioterrorism Use of biologic agents to create fear and threat in a terrorist act.
bipolar hip replacement (hemiarthroplasty) Prosthetic implant used to replace the femoral head and neck in hip fractures when the vascular supply to the femoral head is or may become compromised.
birth defect (congenital anomaly) Any abnormality present at birth, particularly a structural one that may be inherited genetically, acquired during gestation, or inflicted during parturition (process of giving birth).
bladder training Development of the use of the muscles of the perineum to improve voluntary control over voiding.
blanching test A test of the rate of capillary refill; blanching means to cause to become pale by applying digital pressure.
blastocyst Embryonic form that is a spherical mass of cells having a central fluid-filled cavity (blastocele) surrounded by two layers of cells; the outer layer forms the placenta, and the inner layer later forms the embryo.
blended (reconstituted) family Family unit formed by parents who bring unrelated children from prior marriages into a new joint living situation. Also called a *stepfamily.*
blood buffers Compounds that work to enable the body to maintain homeostasis in the body's pH. These compounds include carbon dioxide, carbonic acid, and bicarbonate acid.
blood pressure Pressure exerted by the circulating volume of blood on the arterial walls, veins, and chambers of the heart.
body mass index (BMI) An estimate used to determine if a person may be at health risk because of excessive weight.

body mechanics Physiologic study of the muscular actions and the functions of muscles in maintaining the posture of the body.
body surface area (BSA) Total area exposed to the outside environment.
bonding *See* parent-child attachment. Emotional attachment between parent and child.
borborygmi Loud, gurgling sounds that accompany increased motility of the bowel.
botulism An often fatal food poisoning that results from ingestion of the toxin produced by the bacillus *Clostridium botulinum.*
bradycardia Slow cardiac rhythm characterized by a pulse rate of fewer than 60 beats per minute.
bradykinesia An abnormal condition characterized by slowness of voluntary movements and speech.
bradypnea A slow respiratory rate of fewer than 12 breaths per minute.
brain death Irreversible form of unconsciousness characterized by a complete loss of brain function while the heart continues to beat. The legal definition of this condition varies from state to state.
Braxton Hicks contractions Irregular tightening of the pregnant uterus that begins in the first trimester and increases in frequency, duration, and intensity as pregnancy progresses. Near term, strong Braxton Hicks contractions are often difficult to distinguish from real labor.
bronchoscopy Visual examination of the larynx, trachea, and bronchi using a standard rigid, tubular metal bronchoscope or a narrower, flexible fiberoptic bronchoscope.
brown fat Source of heat unique to the neonate; it is capable of greater thermogenic (heat-producing) activity than ordinary fat. Deposits are formed around the adrenal glands, kidneys, and neck; between scapulas; and behind the sternum, and they remain for several weeks after birth.
bruit Abnormal swishing sound heard over organs, glands, and arteries.
bruxism Teeth grinding.
B-type natriuretic peptide (BNP) A neurohormone secreted by the heart in response to ventricular expansion.
buccal In or directed toward the cheek.
buffer Chemical compound that neutralizes excess acids or bases by contributing or accepting hydrogen ions to form a weaker acid or base; can be considered chemical sponges.
bulimia nervosa An eating disorder involving an insatiable craving for food, often resulting in continual eating followed by periods of depression, self-deprivation, and/or purging. Also called *bulimia.*
burnout Physical, emotional, and spiritual exhaustion among caregivers.
burping Belching or eructation.

C

CABs Mnemonic for assessing status of an emergency patient: Circulation, *A*irway, *B*reathing; used in one- or two-rescuer CPR.
cachexia General ill health and malnutrition marked by weakness and emaciation; usually associated with a serious disease such as cancer.
calcium Silvery yellow metal; the most abundant mineral in the body; a positively charged ion, called a cation.
callus Bony deposits formed between and around the broken ends of a fractured bone during healing.
candidiasis Mild fungal infection that appears in men and women; usually caused by *Candida albicans* and *C. tropicalis.*
cannabidiol A cannabis compound purported to have anti-inflammatory effects.
cannabinoid Compounds found in marijuana. There are more than 60 of these compounds. It is responsible for the feelings of being "high" that are associated with the use of marijuana.
cannabis Marijuana.
canthus Angle at the medial and lateral margins of the eyelid (inner and outer corners of the eye).
carcinoembryonic antigen (CEA) Oncofetal glycoprotein antigen found in colonic adenocarcinoma and other cancers; also found in nonmalignant conditions.
carcinogen Substance known to increase the risk for the development of cancer.
carcinogenesis Various factors that are possible origins of cancer.
carcinoma The term used for a malignant tumor composed of epithelial cells; it displays a tendency to metastasize.
carcinoma in situ Preinvasive, asymptomatic carcinoma that can be diagnosed only by microscopic examination of cervical cells.
cardiac arrest Sudden cessation of functional circulation.
cardinal movements of labor Seven movements in sequence that the fetus undergoes in the process of labor, delivery and birth. These movements include engagement, descent, flexion, internal rotation, extension, externa rotation and expulsion.
cardiopulmonary resuscitation (CPR) Basic emergency procedure for life support, consisting of artificial respiration and manual external cardiac massage.
cardioversion Restoration of the heart's normal sinus rhythm by delivery of a synchronized electric shock through two metal paddles placed on the patient's chest.
career A profession for which one trains and is undertaken as a permanent calling.
carrier Person or animal who harbors and spreads an organism, causing disease in others but does not itself become ill.
case management The assignment of a health care provider to oversee the case of an individual patient.
catabolism Breakdown or destructive phase of metabolism. Catabolism occurs when complex body substances are broken down to simpler ones; opposite of anabolism.
cataract Opacity or clouding of the lens.
catheterization Introduction of a rubber or plastic tube through the urethra and into the bladder.
cation Positively charged ion that, when in solution, is attracted to the negatively charged electrode.
$CD4^+$ lymphocyte A type of white blood cell; a protein on the surface of cells that normally helps the body's immune system combat disease.
cell The fundamental unit of all living tissue.
cellular immunity Acquired immunity characterized by the dominant role of small T lymphocytes. Also called *cell-mediated immunity.*
Centers for Disease Control and Prevention (CDC) Federal agency that provides facilities and services for investigation, identification, prevention, and control of disease; headquartered in Atlanta, Georgia.
cephalocaudal Growth and development that proceeds from the head toward the feet. The infant's head is large compared with the rest of the body.
cephalopelvic disproportion The head of the fetus is larger than the pelvic outlet. Also called *pelvic disproportion.*
cerclage Technique that uses suture material to constrict the internal os of the cervix. Aids in preserving the pregnancy.
certification Process in which an individual or institution, agency, or educational program is evaluated and recognized as meeting certain predetermined standards.
cerumen Yellowish or brownish waxy secretion produced by vestigial apocrine sweat glands in the external ear canal; earwax.
chancre Painless erosion of a papule that ulcerates superficially with a scooped-out appearance.
chart (health care record) Legal record that is used to meet many demands of the health accreditation, medical insurance, and legal systems.

charting Process of recording information on a patient's chart.
charting by exception Recording only new data or changes in patient status or care; charting the exceptions to the previously recorded data.
charting, documenting, or recording Process of noting data in a patient record, usually at prescribed intervals.
chelation therapy In toxicology, use of a compound to group a toxic substance and make it inactive and thus nontoxic. Chelating agents are used in the treatment of metal poisoning.
chevron A method of applying tape to secure an intravenous line; a narrow piece (0.5-inch wide) of sterile tape is placed under the hub of the catheter with adhesive side up and then crisscrossed over the hub to form an inverted V. This method is no longer frequently used.
Cheyne-Stokes respiration An abnormal pattern of respiration characterized by alternating periods of apnea and deep, rapid breathing.
child maltreatment Physical and emotional neglect, and physical, emotional, and sexual abuse of children.
children with special needs Infants and children with congenital abnormalities, malignancies, gastrointestinal diseases, and central nervous system anomalies.
chiropractic therapy Nontraditional therapy that includes manipulation of the musculoskeletal system.
Chlamydia trachomatis A gram-negative intracellular bacterium that causes several common sexually transmitted diseases.
chloride Negatively charged extracellular anion; a salt of hydrochloric acid.
cholesterol Fat-soluble sterol found in animal fats and oils, organ meats, and egg yolk.
chorionic villi Tiny vascular protrusions of the chorionic surface that project into the maternal blood sinuses of the uterus and help form the placenta. This occurs when conception has occurred.
chorionic villus sampling Aspiration of a small amount of tissue from the placenta to test for genetic disorders of the fetus.
chromosomes Threadlike structures in the nucleus of a cell that function in the transmission of genetic information.
chronic Developing slowly and persisting for a long period, often for the remainder of an individual's life.
chronic illness An irreversible presence, accumulation, or latency of disease states or impairments that involve the total human environment for supportive care, function, and prevention of further disability.
chronic pain Pain lasting longer than 6 months; can be as intense as acute pain; can be continuous or intermittent.
chronologic age Age of an individual expressed as time elapsed since birth.
Chux Waterproof, disposable underpad.
Chvostek's sign Abnormal spasm of the facial muscles elicited by light taps on the facial nerve in patients who are hypocalcemic; seen in tetany.
circumcision Surgical procedure in which a part of the foreskin is removed, leaving the glans penis uncovered.
circumorbital Around an orbit; often referring to the eye.
clarifying Restating the patient's message in a manner that asks the patient to verify that the message received is accurate.
claudication Weakness of the legs accompanied by cramp-like pain in the calves caused by poor circulation of the blood to the leg muscles.
climacteric Phase of the aging process marking the transition from the reproductive phase to a nonreproductive stage of life.
clinical death Occurs when heartbeat and respiration have ceased.
clinical pathway Multidisciplinary plan that schedules clinical interventions over an anticipated time frame for a high-risk, high-volume, high-cost type of case.
closed posture A formal, distant body position, generally with the arms and possibly the legs tightly crossed.
closed question Focused question that seeks a particular answer (e.g., yes or no).
club drugs Drugs taken for euphoric effect at parties, concerts, dance clubs, and raves.
code System of notification that allows information to be transmitted rapidly.
cognitive impairment Significantly subaverage general intellectual functioning; existing concurrently with deficits in adaptive behavior and manifested during developmental period (formerly referred to as mental retardation).
cohabitation *See* social contract family.
collaborative problem Actual or potential health problem (complication) that focuses on the pathophysiologic response of the body for which nurses are responsible and accountable for identification and treatment in collaboration with the physician.
collagen Fibrous, insoluble protein found in connective tissue, including skin, bone, and ligaments.
Colles' fracture A fracture of the distal portion of the radius within 1 inch of the joint of the wrist.
colostomy A procedure in which the large intestine is brought through the abdominal wall for evacuation of stool.
colostrum Breast fluid that may be excreted from the second trimester of pregnancy onward but is most evident in the first 2 or 3 days after birth and before the onset of true lactation. This thin, yellowish fluid is rich in proteins and calories in addition to antibodies and lymphocytes.
colporrhaphy Surgical correction of cystocele and rectocele by shortening the muscles that support the bladder and repairing the rectocele.
colposcopy Examination of the cervix and vagina using a colposcope.
Commission on Accreditation of Rehabilitation Facilities (CARF) A not-for-profit, private, international standards–setting and accreditation body. Its mission is to promote and advocate delivery of quality rehabilitation. It is governed by a board of trustees who are responsible for accreditation decisions. Surveyors are peers involved in administrative or professional positions within an organization that is eligible for CARF accreditation.
communication Use of words and behaviors to construct, send, and interpret messages.
compartment syndrome Pathologic condition caused by progressive development of arterial compression and reduced blood supply to an extremity. Increased pressure from external devices (casts, bulky dressings) causes decreased blood flow, resulting in ischemic tissue necrosis; most often occurs in the extremities.
compatibility Quality or state of existing together in harmony.
complementary therapies/complementary and alternative therapies Therapies that are used in addition or as a complement to nontraditional therapies. Examples are exercise, massage, reflexology, acupuncture, and herbalism.
complicated grieving *See* dysfunctional grieving.
comprehensive rehabilitation plan An overall individualized plan of care that is initiated within 24 hours of admission and ready for review and revision by the team within 3 days of admission for each individual; a planned, orderly sequence of services for a disabled individual designed to help the patient realize maximum potential.
compress A soft pad, usually made of cloth, used to apply heat, cold, or medication to the surface of a body area, or over a wound to help control bleeding.
compulsion Irresistible, repetitive, irrational impulse to perform an act that is usually contrary to one's ordinary judgments or standards yet results in overt anxiety if not completed.

computer on wheels, or COWs Point-of-care systems housed on wheeled carts.
conception (fertilization) Beginning of pregnancy.
concrete operational phase Phase of Piaget's theory in which thoughts become increasingly logical and coherent so that the child is able to classify, sort, and organize facts while still being incapable of generalizing or dealing with abstractions; occurs between 7 and 10 years of age.
conflict Mental struggle, either conscious or subconscious, resulting from the simultaneous presence of opposing or incompatible thoughts, ideas, goals, or emotional forces, such as impulses, desires, or drives.
congenital heart disease (CHD) An abnormality or anomaly of the heart, present at birth.
conjunctivitis Inflammation of the conjunctiva.
connotative meaning Reflects the individual's perception or interpretation of a given word.
conscious sedation Central nervous system depressant drugs and/or analgesia given to relieve anxiety and/or provide amnesia during surgical, diagnostic, or interventional procedures.
contamination Condition of being soiled, stained, touched, or otherwise exposed to harmful agents by the entry of infectious or toxic material into a previously clean or sterile environment; making an object potentially unsafe for use as intended.
continuing care retirement community Offers complete range of housing and health care accommodations from independent to 24-hour skilled nursing care.
continuity of care Continuing of established patient care from one setting to another.
contract Promise or a set of promises between two or more people that creates a legal relationship between them and a legal obligation that one or more of them must fulfill.
contracture Abnormal, usually permanent condition of a joint characterized by flexion and fixation and caused by atrophy and shortening of muscle fibers.
contusion An injury that does not break the skin, is caused by a blow, and is characterized by edema, discoloration, and pain.
coping responses Voluntary patterns of behavior used to relieve stress or anxiety.
cor pulmonale Abnormal cardiac condition characterized by hypertrophy of the right ventricle of the heart as a result of hypertension of the pulmonary circulation.
coronary artery disease (CAD) Variety of conditions that obstruct blood flow in the coronary arteries.
coronary occlusion The partial or complete obstruction of a coronary artery.
coryza Acute inflammation of the mucous membranes of the nose and accessory sinuses, usually accompanied by edema of the mucosa and nasal discharge.
costovertebral angle Pertaining to a rib and a vertebra; one of two angles that outline a space over the kidneys.
cotyledon One of the 15 to 28 visible segments of the placenta on the maternal surface, each made up of fetal vessels, chorionic villi, and intervillous space.
crackle(s) Short, discrete, interrupted crackling or bubbling adventitious breath sounds heard on auscultation of the chest, most commonly upon inspiration. They are produced by passage of air through the bronchi that contain secretions of exudate or are constricted by spasms or thickening; usually heard during inspiration; formerly called rales.
crepitus Sound that resembles the crackling noise heard when rubbing hair between the fingers or throwing salt on an open fire. It is associated with gas gangrene, the rubbing of bone fragments, or the crackles of a consolidated area of the lung in pneumonia.
crime Breaking of any law; an offense to society that is punishable.
crisis Time of change or turning point in life when patterns of living must be modified to prevent disorganization of the person or family.
crown-rump length The measurement from the top of the fetal head to the buttocks.
cryosurgery Procedure to "freeze" the border of a retinal hole with a frozen-tipped probe.
cryotherapy A procedure in which a topical anesthetic is used so that a cryoprobe can be placed directly on the surface of the eye.
cryptorchidism Failure of testes to descend into the scrotum.
cue Word, phrase, or symptom that indicates the nature of something perceived. Cues are grouped to assist the nurse in interpretation of data, as in formulating the patient's plan of care.
culdoscopy Diagnostic procedure that provides visualization of the uterus and adnexa (uterine appendages that include the ovaries and fallopian tubes).
cultural competence Awareness by the nurse of his or her own cultural belief practices and an understanding of the limitations that these beliefs put on the nurse when dealing with those from other cultures. This understanding should give the nurse the ability to react to others with openness to and understanding and acceptance of cultural differences between them.
cultural healing beliefs Beliefs that reflect a specific culture's concept of health and illness.
culture (1) A set of learned values, beliefs, customs, and practices that are shared by a group and passed from one generation to another. (2) A laboratory test involving cultivation of microorganisms or cells in a special growth medium.
cumulative A drug that builds up in the body; can lead to a toxic or even lethal (deadly) effect.
curative treatment Aggressive care with the goal and intent of curing the disease and prolonging life at all costs.
curettage Scraping of material from the wall of a cavity or other surface; performed to remove tumors or other abnormal tissue for microscopic study.
Curling's ulcer Duodenal ulcer that develops 8 to 14 days after severe burns on the surface of the body; the first sign is usually vomiting of bright red blood.
"currant jelly" stools Feces mixed with blood and mucus from the intestinal mucosa.
customs Habitual practices; the usual way of acting under given circumstances.
cyanosis Slightly bluish, gray, slatelike, or dark purple discoloration of the skin resulting from the presence of abnormally reduced amounts of oxygenated hemoglobin in the blood.
cyclothymic disorder A pattern that involves repeated mood swings of hypomania and depression that are less intense than with bipolar disorder. There are no periods of "normal function" with this condition. It is thought to be a muted version of bipolar disorder.
cytology/cytologic evaluation Study of cells and their formation, origin, structure, biochemical activities, and pathology.
cytoplasm "Living matter"; a substance that exists only in cells, composed largely of a gel-like substance that contains water, minerals, enzymes, and other specialized materials.

D

database Large store or bank of information, as in forming the patient's nursing diagnosis.
death Cessation of life.
débridement Removal of damaged cellular tissue from a wound or burn to prevent infection and promote healing.

deciduous teeth Set of 20 teeth that normally appear during infancy.
deep brain stimulation (DBS) Involves placing an electrode in either the thalamus, globus pallidus, or subthalamic nucleus and connecting it to a generator placed in the upper chest (like a pacemaker).
defecation Elimination of bowel waste.
defense mechanisms Unconscious, intrapsychic reactions that offer protection to the self from stressful situations.
defibrillation The termination of ventricular fibrillation by delivering a direct electrical countershock to the precordium.
defining characteristics Clinical signs and symptoms that a problem exists.
dehiscence Partial or complete separation of a surgical incision or rupture of a wound closure.
deinstitutionalization Release of institutional psychiatric patients to be treated in the community setting.
delirium An acute, organic mental disorder characterized by confusion, disorientation, clouding of consciousness, incoherence, fear, anxiety, excitement, and often illusions and hallucinations. Symptoms are of short duration and reversible with treatment of the underlying cause, such as fever or electrolyte imbalance.
delirium tremens (DTs) An acute psychotic reaction that is a complication of alcohol withdrawal.
delusion A persistent, aberrant belief or perception held inviolable by a person despite evidence to the contrary.
dementia A slowly progressive, organic mental disorder characterized by chronic personality disintegration, deterioration of intellectual capacity and function, and memory loss that leads to confusion, disorientation, and stupor. An example is Alzheimer's disease.
democratic family pattern Family style in which the adult members are considered equal and children are treated with respect and recognized as individuals.
dendrite Branching process that extends from the cell body of a neuron and receives impulses.
denominator Bottom number of a fraction.
denotative meaning The commonly accepted definition of a particular word.
dentures Artificial teeth not permanently fixed or implanted.
deposition Out-of-court, under-oath statement of a witness.
depressant A drug that depresses the central nervous system, such as alcohol, sedative-hypnotic medications, and opioid analgesics.
depression An emotional disorder brought on by an imbalance of the neurotransmitter serotonin in the brain, which brings about exaggerated feelings of sadness, melancholy, emptiness, worthlessness, and frustration. Fatigue, inability to concentrate, short-term memory loss, and sleep pattern disturbance, as well as slowed body functions, can be seen with this disorder.
descent In obstetrics, the downward progress of the presenting part belonging to the fetus. The amount of progress measured by comparing the lowest point of the presenting part with the ischial spines of the mother.
detoxification Removal of poisonous effects of a substance from a patient.
development Gradual process or change and differentiation from a simple to a more advanced level of complexity.
diabetes mellitus *See* type 1 diabetes mellitus; type 2 diabetes mellitus.
diabetic retinopathy Disorder of retinal blood vessels characterized by capillary microaneurysms, hemorrhage, exudates, and formation of new vessels and connective tissue.
diagnose To identify a disease or condition by a scientific evaluation of physical signs, symptoms, history, laboratory tests, and procedures.
diagnosis-related group (DRG) System that classifies patients by age, diagnoses, and surgical categories; used to predict the use of hospital resources, including the length of stay.
dialysis Medical procedure for the removal of certain elements from the blood or lymph by virtue of the difference in their rates of diffusion through an external semipermeable membrane or, in the case of peritoneal dialysis, through the peritoneum.
diaphoresis The secretion of sweat, especially the profuse secretion of sweat.
diastole The period of time between contractions of the atria or the ventricles, during which blood enters the relaxed chambers from the systemic circulation and the lungs.
diastolic pressure The second number recorded in the blood pressure reading; represents the minimum level of blood pressure measured between the contractions of the heart.
dietary fiber Generic term for nondigestible chemical substances in plants.
differentiated Describes a tumor that is most like the parent tissue.
differentiation Process of cellular development in which unspecialized cells or tissues are systematically modified to achieve specific and characteristic physical forms, physiologic functions, and chemical properties.
diffusion A process in which solid particles in a fluid move from an area of higher concentration to an area of lower concentration.
dilemma Situation requiring a choice between two equally desirable or undesirable alternatives.
dimensional analysis A method of dosage calculation that employs the use of three factors, which include the drug label factor, conversion factor, and drug order factor.
diplopia Double vision.
direct Coombs' test Laboratory blood test to detect foreign antibodies that have adhered to red blood cells, which can cause cellular damage. These antibodies result in hemolytic anemia. Normal findings: negative, no agglutination.
disability Any restriction or lack (resulting from an impairment) of an ability to perform an activity in the manner or within the range considered normal for a human being.
disaster manual Written agency instructions specifying departmental responsibilities, chain of command, callback procedures for the receipt and management of casualties, and policies related to the overall management of supplies and equipment.
disaster situation Uncontrollable, unexpected, psychologically shocking event.
discharge Release of a patient from a health care facility.
discharge planning Schedule of events often planned by a multidisciplinary team leading to the return of a patient from hospital confinement to life at home or another health care setting.
disease Any disturbance of a structure or function of the body; a pathologic condition of the body.
disengagement stage Period of family life when the grown children depart from the home. In some family units this stage is brief because the adult children return to live in the family home.
disinfectant A chemical that can be applied to objects to destroy microorganisms.
disinfection Process by which pathogens, but not necessarily their spores, are destroyed.
disorientation Mental confusion characterized by inadequate or incorrect perceptions of place, time, and identity.
disoriented Having lost awareness or perception of space, time, or personal identity and relationships.
disseminated intravascular coagulation (DIC) Acquired hemorrhage syndrome of clotting, cascade overstimulation, and anticlotting processes.

disuse syndrome A condition that results from an extended period of physical activity. The resulting condition impacts both the physical and mental capabilities of the individual.
diuresis Secretion and passage of large amounts of urine.
dizygotic Of or pertaining to twins from two fertilized ova.
doctrine of informed consent The requirements on a physician to provide information to the patient about a procedure that will include both the risks and benefits of the intervention planned.
documenting Process of adding information to the chart, usually at prescribed intervals.
dominant group Group of people exercising authority or influence; ruling or prevailing group.
do-not-resuscitate (DNR) A note written in a patient's record and signed by a qualified attending physician instructing the staff of the institution not to attempt to resuscitate the patient in the event of cardiac or respiratory failure. Also called *no code.*
Dorothea Dix A retired teacher who was appalled by the care of the mentally ill. In 1841, she began her crusade for placing individuals with mental illnesses in specially built hospitals. Her efforts brought millions of dollars toward developing mental hospitals in the United States.
dorsal Toward the back.
dorsal (supine) Lying horizontally on the back.
dorsal recumbent Supine position with patient lying on the back, with head, shoulders, and extremities moderately flexed and legs extended.
dorsiflexion Bending or flexing backward, as in upward bending of the fingers, wrist, foot, or toes.
double bagging Infection control practice of placing a bag of contaminated items into another bag that is clean and held outside the isolation room by a second staff member.
Down syndrome A congenital condition usually resulting from having three copies of chromosome 21 and characterized by varying degrees of cognitive disability and multiple physical defects.
drainage Free flow or withdrawal of fluids from a wound or cavity by some sort of system (such as a urinary catheter or T-tube).
DRG *See* diagnosis-related group.
drip factor A method that is used to deliver measured amounts of intravenous solutions at specific flow rates based on the size of drops of the solution.
drug interaction Modification of the effect of a drug when administered with another drug.
dullness Low-pitched thudlike sound upon percussion of the body.
dumping syndrome A condition that results when food passes too rapidly from the stomach to the small intestine. It is often associated with high sugar containing foods. It may be the result of gastrointestinal surgery or it may be an independent condition.
durable powers of attorney A signed and notarized document that appoints another person to make decisions in the event of the patient's incompetence. Usually completed by the patient while still able to function.
dysarthria Difficult, poorly articulated speech resulting from interference in the control over the muscles of speech.
dysfunctional grieving Unresolved grief or complicated mourning.
dysgeusia A distortion to the sense of taste.
dysmenorrhea Painful menstruation.
dyspepsia Vague feelings of epigastric discomfort.
dysphagia Difficulty swallowing.
dyspnea Shortness of breath or difficulty in breathing; may be caused by disturbances in the lungs, certain heart conditions, and hemoglobin deficiency.
dysrhythmia Any disturbance or abnormality in a normal rhythmic pattern, specifically irregularity in the normal rhythm of the heart. Also called *arrhythmia.*
dysuria Painful or difficult urination.

E

ecchymosis Discoloration of an area of the skin or mucous membrane caused by the extravasation of blood into the subcutaneous tissues. Also called a *bruise.*
eclampsia Most severe form of pregnancy-induced hypertension, characterized by toxic and grand mal convulsions, coma, hypertension, albuminuria, and edema. Also called *gestational hypertension (GH).*
ectoderm Outer layer of embryonic tissue that gives rise to skin, nails, and hair.
ectopic pregnancy Implantation of the fertilized ovum outside the uterine cavity, such as in the abdomen, fallopian tubes, or ovary.
edema Abnormal accumulation of fluids in interstitial spaces of tissue; a combining form meaning swelling.
effacement Thinning and shortening of the cervix as it is stretched and dilated by the fetus. This occurs during late pregnancy, labor, or both.
electrocardiogram (ECG) Graphic representation of electrical impulses generated by the heart during a cardiac cycle.
electrolyte Substance that is sometimes called a mineral or salt; it develops tiny electrical charges when dissolved in water and breaks up into particles known as ions.
electronic health record An electronic patient record designed for health information exchange between facilities.
electronic medical record An electronic patient record designed for health information exchange only within a facility.
elopement Leaving the care agency/provider by a patient without medical approval and support. The action may be intentional or unintentional.
embolism An abnormal circulatory condition in which an embolus (e.g., a foreign substance, blood clot, fat, air, or amniotic fluid) travels through the bloodstream and becomes lodged in a blood vessel.
embolus A foreign object, quantity of air or gas, bit of tissue or tumor, or a piece of thrombus that circulates in the bloodstream until it becomes lodged in a vessel.
emergency medical services (EMS) National network of services coordinated to provide aid and medical assistance from primary response to definitive care, involving personnel trained in the rescue, stabilization, transportation, and advanced treatment of traumatic or medical emergencies.
empathy Ability to recognize and, to some extent, share the emotions and states of mind of another and to understand the meaning and significance of that person's behavior.
empyema Accumulation of pus in a body cavity, especially the pleural space, as a result of infection.
en face position Position in which the adult's face and the infant's face are approximately 8 inches apart, as when the mother holds the infant up in front of her face or when she nurses the infant.
endarterectomy Surgical removal of the intimal lining of an artery.
endemic A characteristic or condition that is associated with a group.
endocrinologist Physician who specializes in hormone imbalances and alterations in related body systems.
endoderm Innermost cell layer; from the endoderm arises the lining of cavities and passages of the body and covering for most internal organs.
endogenous Growing within the body; originating from within the body, or produced from internal causes, such as a

disease caused by the structural or functional failure of an organ or system.
endometriosis Condition in which endometrial tissue appears outside the uterus.
endorphin Any one of the neuropeptides composed of many amino acids, elaborated by the pituitary gland and acting on the central and peripheral nervous systems to reduce pain.
endorsement Statement of recognition of the license of a health practitioner in one state by another.
endotracheal tube The placement of a tube through the mouth or nose into the trachea. The purpose is to maintain a patent airway.
enema The instillation of a solution into the rectum of the sigmoid colon for the purpose of evacuating the bowel or introducing a medication.
engagement Fixation of the presenting part of the fetus in the maternal pelvis. The lowest part of the presenting part is at or below the level of the ischial spines.
engagement or commitment stage Period when the couple prepares for marriage and becomes free of parental domination.
engorgement Swelling of the breast tissue brought about by an increase in blood and lymph supply to the breast; occurs about 48 hours postpartum and usually reaches a peak between the third and fifth days after delivery.
enteral Within, or by way of, the intestine.
enteral nutrition Administration of nutrients into the gastrointestinal tract; usually referred to as *tube feeding*.
enteric-coated Encasement of a tablet in a candylike shell to prevent medications from being absorbed in the stomach; absorption takes place in the intestine.
enucleation Surgical removal of the eyeball.
enzyme-linked immunosorbent assay (ELISA) Antibody test that uses a rapid enzyme immunochemical assay method to detect HIV antibodies.
epidemic A large, unchecked spread of an infectious condition through a population.
epididymitis Infection of the cordlike excretory duct of the testicles.
episiotomy Surgical incision of the perineum at the end of the second stage of labor to facilitate delivery and avoid laceration of the perineum.
epistaxis Hemorrhage from the nose; nosebleed.
epistaxis digitorum Self-inflicted local digital trauma (i.e., from nose-picking).
ergonomics Processes geared toward the movements in a manner that takes into consideration ways to avoid injury and undue fatigue.
erythema Redness or inflammation of the skin or mucous membranes resulting from dilation and congestion of superficial capillaries. Examples are mild sunburn, nervous blushes, injury resulting from trauma or infection.
erythematous Pertaining to erythema (redness).
erythroblastosis fetalis Hemolytic anemia in newborns resulting from maternal-fetal blood group incompatibility, especially involving the Rh factor and ABO blood groups.
erythrocytosis Abnormal increase in the number of circulating red blood cells.
erythropoiesis The process of red blood cell production.
eschar Black, leathery crust; a slough that the body forms over burned tissue.
esophageal varices A complex of longitudinal, twisted veins at the lower end of the esophagus.
essential nutrient Carbohydrates, proteins, fats, minerals, vitamins, and water necessary for growth, normal function, and body maintenance. These substances must be supplied by food; they are not synthesized by the body in the quantities required for normal health.
establishment stage Period in a couple's life between their wedding and the birth of their first child.
ethical dilemma Situation that does not have a clear correct or incorrect answer.
ethics The way one should behave; how a person ought to act.
ethnic stereotype A fixed concept of how all members of an ethnic group act or think.
ethnicity A shared common social and cultural heritage based on traditions, national origin, and physical and biologic characteristics. It often includes social practices such as language, religion, dress, music, and food.
ethnocentrism A perception that the practices and beliefs of one's own culture are superior to those of other cultures.
etiology The study of all factors that may be involved in the development of a disease; the cause of disease.
euthanasia Deliberately bringing about the death of an individual suffering from an incurable disease or condition; can be done actively or passively.
evaluation The determination made about the extent to which the established outcomes have been achieved in the nursing care plan.
evisceration Protrusion of an internal organ through a disrupted wound or surgical incision.
exacerbation An increase in the seriousness of a disease or disorder; marked by greater intensity in the signs or symptoms of the patient being treated.
excoriation Injury to the surface layer of skin caused by scratching or abrasion.
exogenous Outside the body; originating outside the body or produced from external causes, such as a disease caused by a bacterial or viral agent foreign to the body.
exophthalmos An abnormal condition characterized by a marked protrusion of the eyeballs.
expectant stage The period of family life that begins when conception occurs and continues through the pregnancy.
expectorate To eject mucus, sputum, or fluids from the trachea and lungs by coughing or spitting.
expressive aphasia A physiologic condition in which an individual is unable to communicate a desired message.
expulsion Having the tendency to drive out or expel.
extended family A family group consisting of the parents, their children, the grandparents, and other family members.
extension Movement allowed by certain joints of the skeleton that increases the angle between two adjoining bones.
external rotation Occurs as the head and body move through the birth canal, using the same maneuvers as the head. The shoulders are delivered similarly to the fetal head, with the anterior shoulder pressing under the symphysis pubis, which again acts as a leverage point and assists in delivery of the posterior shoulder.
extracellular Fluid outside the cells of the body.
extravasation The escape of fluids into surrounding tissue.
extremes Outer terms of the proportion. Very severe or drastic.
extrinsic Caused by external factors.
extubate To remove an endotracheal tube from an airway.
exudate Fluid, cells, or other substances that have been slowly exuded or discharged from body cells or blood vessels through small pores or breaks in cell membrane.

F

failure to thrive The abnormal retardation of growth and development of the infant resulting from conditions that interfere with normal metabolism, appetite, and activity.
family-centered care Philosophy of care that recognizes the family as the constant in the child's life and holds that systems and personnel must support, respect, encourage, and enhance the strengths and competence of the family.

febrile Body temperature above normal.
fecal impaction The presence of stool that is obstructive and not passed without intervention to relieve it.
feces Waste from the intestine; bowel movement (BM).
fetal lie Relationship existing between the long axis of the fetus and the long axis of the mother.
fetal position The relationship of the occiput, sacrum, chin, or scapula on the presenting part of the fetus to its location in the front, back, or sides of the maternal pelvis.
fetal presentation The part of the fetus that enters the pelvis first and lies over the inlet; head, face, feet, or shoulders.
fetopelvic disproportion The head of the fetus is larger than the pelvic outlet. Also called *cephalopelvic disproportion.*
fibromyalgia A musculoskeletal chronic pain syndrome of unknown etiology that causes pain in muscles, bones, or joints.
filtration The transfer of water and dissolved substances from an area of higher pressure to an area of lower pressure.
fistula Abnormal opening between two organs.
fixative Any substance used to preserve gross or histologic specimens of tissue for examination.
flaccid Weak, soft, and flabby; lacking normal muscle tone.
flagellation Whiplike movement.
flail chest Two or more ribs fractured in two or more places resulting in instability in part of the chest wall with associated hemothorax, pneumothorax, and pulmonary contusion.
flatness Soft, high-pitched, flat sound produced by performing percussion over tissue such as muscle tissue.
flatulence Excessive formation of gases in the stomach or intestine.
flatus Air or gas in the intestine that is passed through the rectum.
flexion Movement of certain joints that decreases the angle between two adjoining bones.
flow meter A device to measure the outflow of a gas, such as oxygen.
focus charting Expansion of the data and need columns in nurses' notes to include topics concerning the whole patient, such as behavior or treatment and response. The charting format is data, action, response (DAR).
focused assessment Concentration of attention on the part of the body where signs and symptoms are localized or most active in order to determine their significance.
focusing A communication technique used when more specific information is needed to accurately understand the patient's message.
folk health belief system Belief that health and illness are controlled by supernatural forces. May use native healers, plants, religious rituals, and prayers.
fomite Nonliving material, such as bed linens, stethoscope, needles, and many other objects that may host and transfer pathogenic microorganisms.
fontanelle Broad area or soft spot consisting of a strong bond of connective tissue between an infant's cranial bones.
formal operational thought phase Piaget's phase that begins during adolescence, permitting abstract reasoning and systematic scientific problem solving.
foster family Family unit that cares for, supervises, and nurtures children whose parents are unable to care for them.
Fowler's Known as the standard patient position. The patient is lying with legs straight or bent at the knees and the head of the bed is elevated between 30 and 90 degrees.
fraction of inspired oxygen (FiO_2) The percentage of oxygen being breathed in.
frustration Emotional response to anything that interferes with a goal-directed activity.
functional assessment The assessment of the functional status of the patient, which is the ability of an individual to perform normal, expected, or required activities of daily living.
functional disease May be manifested as an organic disease, but careful examination fails to reveal evidence of structural or physiologic abnormalities.
functional limitation Any loss or ability to perform tasks and obligations of usual roles and normal daily life.
fundus Top part of uterus.

G

gate control theory Suggests that pain impulses can be regulated or even blocked by gating mechanisms located along the central nervous system.
gateway drug A drug, for example, alcohol, that is the first drug of abuse, later followed by other drugs.
gauge A standard or scale of measurement.
genupectoral Patient kneels so weight of body is supported by knees and chest.
germline mutations A variation in the composition of a germline cell.
gerontologic rehabilitation nursing Specialty practice that focuses on the unique requirements of elderly rehabilitation patients.
gestational diabetes mellitus (GDM) Disorder characterized by an impaired ability to metabolize carbohydrates, usually caused by a deficiency of insulin; occurs in pregnancy and disappears after delivery but in some cases returns years later.
gestational hypertension (GH) *See* pregnancy-induced hypertension.
gestures Movements used to emphasize the idea being communicated.
Glasgow Coma Scale A quick, practical, standardized system for assessing the degree of conscious impairment in the critically ill; also used for predicting the duration and ultimate outcome of coma, primarily in patients with head injuries.
glaucoma An abnormal condition of elevated pressure within an eye because of obstruction of the outflow of aqueous humor.
global cognitive dysfunction Generalized impairment of intellect, awareness, and judgment.
glomerular filtration rate A measure of kidney function that captures the rate of blood passing through the glomeruli each minute.
glomerulonephritis Inflammation of the glomeruli of the kidney.
gluten A protein primarily found in wheat, rye, and barley grains and products.
glycogen Polysaccharide that is the major carbohydrate stored in animal cells.
glycosuria Abnormal presence of sugar, especially glucose in the urine.
glycosylated hemoglobin This test produces an accurate long-term index of the patient's average blood glucose level by measuring the patient's glycohemoglobin (GHB). Glycohemoglobin is a minor hemoglobin that makes up 4% to 8% of the total hemoglobin. It is a combination of hemoglobin and blood glucose. This test can have a blood sample drawn at any time because it is not affected by short-term variations. This test reflects the average blood sugar level for the 100- to 120-day period before the test.
goal The purpose to which an effort is directed.
Goldmann tonometry A device used to assess ocular pressure.
Good Samaritan law Legal stipulation for protection of those who give first aid in an emergency situation.
Goodell's sign Softening of the uterine cervix; a probable sign of pregnancy.
Gowers' sign Classic sign of Duchenne's muscular dystrophy; the child positions on all fours and uses the hands to walk up the thighs.
graduated Container that has interval markings of measurement.

grandfamilies Families with children under the age of 18 years who live with or in the custody of grandparents.
granulation Soft, pink, fleshy projection consisting of capillaries surrounded by fibrous collagen that slowly fills the incision during the process of healing.
gravida A pregnant woman.
grief A pattern of physical and emotional responses to bereavement, separation, or loss; a natural response to loss.
grief therapy Mental treatment aimed at helping an individual deal with the pain of loss; a program in assisting the bereaved to cope with their loss.
grief work Adaptation process of mourning a loss.
group therapy Provides a caring, emotionally supportive atmosphere for a patient in a recovery program.
growth Increase in the size of an organism or any of its parts.
Guillain-Barré syndrome (GBS) An immune disorder characterized by attacks on the peripheral nervous system. Symptoms may vary in intensity.
gynecomastia Development of abnormally large mammary glands in a male that sometimes may secrete milk. When observed in the newborn, it is in response to maternal hormones; may be noted in either sex of the newborn.

H

hallucination A sensory experience without a stimulus trigger that occurs in the waking state. It can occur in any of the senses.
hallucinogen A drug that alters perception and thinking.
harlequin sign Rare color change of no pathologic significance occurring between the longitudinal halves of the newborn's body; when the infant is placed on one side, the dependent half is noticeably pinker than the superior half.
Hazard Communication Act Requires hospitals to inform employees about the presence of or potential for harmful exposures and how to reduce the risk of exposures.
health A condition of physical, mental, and social well-being and the absence of disease or other abnormal conditions.
health care facility Agency or institution that provides health care.
health care system The complete network of agencies, facilities, and all providers of health care in a specific geographic area.
Healthcare Integrity and Protection Data Bank (HIPDB) National data bank created in 1999 to which federal and state agencies report all final adverse actions taken against a health care provider.
heart failure (HF) Syndrome characterized by circulatory congestion due to the heart's inability to act as an effective pump; it should be viewed as a neurohormonal problem in which pathology progresses as a result of chronic release in the body of substances such as catecholamines (epinephrine and norepinephrine).
Hëgar's sign Softening of the isthmus of the uterine cervix early in gestation; a probable sign of pregnancy.
Heimlich maneuver An emergency procedure for dislodging a bolus of food or other obstruction from the trachea to prevent asphyxiation.
hemarthrosis Bleeding into a joint space, a hallmark of severe disease usually occurring in the knees, ankles, and elbow.
hematemesis Vomiting blood.
hematuria Blood in the urine.
hemianopia Defective vision or blindness in half of the visual field.
hemiplegia Paralysis of one side of the body.
Hemoccult test Detects occult (hidden) blood in the feces.
hemophilia Hereditary coagulation disorder; caused by a lack of antihemophilic factor VIII, which is needed to convert prothrombin to thrombin through thromboplastin component.
hemoptysis Expectorating blood from the respiratory tract.
hemothorax Collection of blood into the pleural space.
hepatic encephalopathy A type of brain damage caused by a liver disease and consequent ammonia intoxication.
hepatitis Inflammation of the liver resulting from several causes, including several types of viral agents or exposure to toxic substances.
herbal therapy An alternative therapy that uses herbs to provide health benefits.
heterograft (xenograft) Tissue from another species, used as a temporary graft.
heterozygous Having two different genes.
high-risk pregnancy Condition in which the life or health of the mother or infant is jeopardized by a disorder coincidental with or unique to pregnancy.
HIPAA The federal law governing patient privacy is the Health Insurance Portability and Accountability Act (HIPAA) of 1996, which went into effect on April 14, 2003. It mandates national standards for protecting all verbal or documented health information from improper alteration, access, or loss. The goal is to ensure the security and privacy of this data.
hirsutism Excessive body hair in a masculine distribution.
HIV disease Symptomatic human immunodeficiency virus (HIV) infection that is not severe enough for a diagnosis of acquired immunodeficiency syndrome (AIDS); symptoms of HIV disease are persistent unexplained fever, night sweats, diarrhea, weight loss, and fatigue.
HIV infection The state in which HIV enters the body under favorable conditions and multiplies, producing injurious effects.
holistic Pertaining to the total patient care that considers the physical, emotional, social, economic, and spiritual needs of the person.
holistic health belief system Belief that forces of nature must be kept in natural balance or harmony.
holistic health care A system of comprehensive or total patient care that considers the physical, emotional, social, economic, and spiritual needs of the person; the response to the illness and the effect of the illness on the person's ability to meet self-care needs.
holistic nursing The practice of nursing that focuses on the entire person.
Homans' sign Early sign of thrombophlebitis of the deep veins of the calf in which there are complaints of pain when the leg is in extension and the foot is dorsiflexed.
home health agency An organization that provides health care in the home.
home health care Services that enable individuals of all ages to remain in the comfort and security of their homes while receiving health care.
homeostasis A relative constancy in the internal environment of the body, naturally maintained by adaptive responses that promote healthy survival.
homograft (allograft) The transfer of tissue between two genetically dissimilar individuals of the same species, such as a skin transplant between two humans who are not identical twins.
homosexual family Family group made up of same-sex adults who share bonds of emotional commitment and roles of childrearing.
homozygous Having two identical genes, inherited from each parent, for a given hereditary characteristic.
hospice From the Latin word *hospitum,* meaning hospitality; a resting place for travelers on a difficult journey; philosophy of care that provides support to terminally ill people and their families.
host A person or group who, because of risk factors, may be susceptible to disease or illness; an organism in which another, usually parasitic, organism is nourished and harbored.
huffing Typically in a group setting, breathing in solvents from a cloth, paper, or plastic bag.

human immunodeficiency virus (HIV) An obligate virus; a retrovirus that causes AIDS.
humoral immunity One of the two forms of immunity that respond to antigens such as bacteria and foreign tissue. It is mediated by B cells.
humoral theory A theory dating back to Hippocrates. He viewed mental illness as an imbalance of humors (the fundamental elements of the world: air, fire, water, and earth). Each basic element was represented in the body by certain fluids: blood, yellow bile, black bile, and phlegm.
hydramnios Abnormal condition of pregnancy characterized by an excess of amniotic fluid.
hydrogenation Process in which hydrogen is added to vegetable oil to make it more solid and stable to rancidity.
hydronephrosis The dilation of the renal pelvis and calyces.
hydrostatic pressure The outward force exerted on a vessel wall.
hygiene The science of health and its maintenance; system of principles for preserving health and preventing disease.
hyperbilirubinemia An excess of bilirubin in the blood of the newborn.
hypercapnia Greater than normal amounts of carbon dioxide in the blood.
hyperextension Position of maximum extension; extreme or abnormal stretching.
hyperglycemia A greater than normal amount of glucose in the blood.
hyperopia Farsightedness; inability to see objects at close range.
hyperreflexia Neurologic condition characterized by increased reflex reactions.
hypersensitivity An abnormal condition characterized by an excessive reaction to a particular stimulus.
hypertension Occurs when the elevated blood pressure is above normal.
hyperthermia Condition of abnormally high body temperature.
hypertonic A solution of higher osmotic pressure.
hypocalcemia A deficiency of calcium in serum.
hypoglycemia A lower than normal amount of glucose in the blood; usually caused by administration of too much insulin, excessive secretion of insulin by the islet cells of the pancreas, or dietary deficiency.
hypokalemia A condition in which an inadequate amount of potassium, the major intracellular cation, is found in the circulatory bloodstream.
hypomanic episode The early phase of a manic episode when symptoms are not severe.
hypotension Occurs when the blood pressure is below normal.
hypothermia Condition of abnormally low body temperature.
hypotonic A solution of lower osmotic pressure.
hypoventilation An abnormal condition of the respiratory system that occurs when the volume of air is not adequate for the metabolic needs of the body.
hypoxemia An abnormal deficiency of oxygen in the arterial blood.
hypoxia An inadequate, reduced tension of cellular oxygen.

I

idiopathic Cause unknown.
idiopathic hyperplasia Increase, without any known cause, in the number of cells.
idiosyncratic An individual's unique hypersensitivity to a particular drug.
ileal conduit Ureters are implanted into a loop of the ileum that is isolated and brought to the surface of the abdominal wall.
ileostomy The placement of the end of the small intestine through an opening in the abdominal wall and creating a stoma.
illness An abnormal process in which aspects of the social, emotional, or intellectual condition and function of a person are diminished or impaired.
illusion A false interpretation of an external sensory stimulus, usually visual or auditory, such as a mirage in the desert or voices on the wind.
imagery Visualization techniques to create mental images to evoke physical changes in the body, improve perceived well-being, and enhance self-awareness.
immobility Inability to move around freely, caused by any condition in which movement is impaired or therapeutically restricted.
immunity The quality of being unsusceptible to or unaffected by a particular disease condition.
immunization A process by which resistance to an infectious disease is induced or increased.
immunocompetence/immunocompetent The ability of an immune system to mobilize and deploy its antibodies and other responses to stimulation by an antigen.
immunodeficiency An abnormal condition of the immune system in which cellular or humoral immunity is inadequate and resistance to infection is decreased.
immunogen Any agent or substance capable of provoking an immune response or producing immunity.
immunology Study of the immune system; the reaction of tissues of the immune system of the body to antigenic stimulation.
immunosuppression/immunosuppressive Administration of agents that significantly interfere with the ability of the immune system to respond to antigenic stimulation by inhibiting cellular and humoral immunity.
immunosurveillance The immune system's recognition and destruction of newly developed abnormal cells.
immunotherapy A special treatment of allergic responses; involves the administration of increasingly larger doses of the offending allergens to gradually develop immunity.
impaction Condition of being tightly wedged into a part, such as eruption of a tooth blocked by other teeth; the presence of a large or hard fecal mass in the rectum or colon which the patient is unable to pass.
impairment Any loss or abnormality of psychological, physical, or anatomic structure or function.
implantation Embedding of the fertilized ovum in the uterine mucosa.
implementation The phase of the nursing process that includes ongoing activities of data collection, prioritization, and performance of nursing intervention and documentation.
incentive spirometry A procedure in which a device (spirometer) is used at the bedside at regular intervals to encourage a patient to breathe deeply.
incision Surgical cut produced by a sharp instrument to create an opening into an organ or space in the body.
incompetent cervix Passive and painless dilation of the cervix during the second trimester of pregnancy; it is variable and exists as a continuum that is determined in part by cervical length.
incontinence The inability to control urination or defecation.
indirect Coombs' test Laboratory blood test that detects circulating antibodies against red blood cells (RBC). The test can detect Rh antibodies in maternal blood and is used to anticipate hemolytic disease of the newborn.
induration Hardening of a tissue, particularly the skin, because of edema, inflammation, or infiltration by neoplasm. May be seen with an IV infiltrate.
infant mortality The death of a child who is under 1 year of age.
infant mortality rate The number of deaths of children who are under 1 year of age. It is measured per 1000 children born.

infarct Localized area of necrosis in tissue, a vessel, or an organ resulting from tissue anoxia; caused by an interruption in the blood supply to an area.
infection Caused by an invasion of microorganisms such as bacteria, viruses, fungi, or parasites that produce tissue damage.
infection control The policies and procedures of a hospital or other health care facility to minimize the risk of nosocomial or community-acquired infection spreading to patients or other members of the staff.
infection prevention and control Activities geared toward stopping and limiting the transmission of infection.
infectious process Condition caused by the invasion of the body by pathogenic microorganisms.
infiltration The process whereby a fluid passes into the tissues.
inflammation Protective response of body tissues to irritation, injury, or invasion by disease-producing organisms. The cardinal signs include erythema, edema, heat, and loss of function.
inflammatory response A tissue reaction to injury.
informatics The process of retrieving, storing, and transmitting data.
informed consent Permission obtained from the patient to perform a specific test or procedure.
informed consent doctrine A legal doctrine that requires the patient to fully understand any proposed treatment and consent to it; this document gives the competent adult the choice to accept or reject any treatment modalities.
inhalant A volatile chemical that can alter thinking and feeling when inhaled.
innate immunity The body's first line of defense; provides physical and chemical barriers to invading pathogens and protects the body against the external environment.
inquest A legal inquiry into the cause or manner of a death.
inspection Visual examination of the external surface of the body and of its movements and posture, including observation of moods and all responses and nonverbal behaviors.
instrumental activities of daily living (IADLs) Daily tasks that are more complex than ADLs, such as shopping or using the telephone.
intelligence quotient (IQ) Index of relative intelligence determined through the subject's answers to arbitrarily chosen questions.
interdisciplinary When health care professionals work together as a team to meet the needs of a patient.
interdisciplinary hospice team Multiple-professional health team, such as physicians, nurses, social workers, and pastors, working together in caring for the terminally ill patient.
interdisciplinary rehabilitation team Team that collaborates to identify an individual's goals and is characterized by a combination of expanded problem solving beyond discipline boundaries and discipline-specific work toward goal attainment.
interdisciplinary team A diverse team of professionals from several disciplines who collaborate to optimize care and decrease fragmentation services.
intermittent claudication A weakness of the legs accompanied by cramplike pains in the calves; caused by poor arterial circulation of the blood to the leg muscles.
intermittent venous access device An intravenous infusion device with a male adapter covered by a rubber diaphragm for intermittent intravenous therapy. Also called *heparin* or *saline lock.*
internal rotation In obstetrics, when the largest diameter of the fetal head aligns with the largest diameter of the pelvis. This allows the fetal head to progress through the maternal pelvis.
interstitial Fluid between the cells or in the tissues of the body.
interview Meeting people for an evaluation or for questioning a job applicant.
intracellular Fluid inside the cells of the body.
intraoperative Pertaining to a period of time during a surgical procedure.
intrapartal Period that begins with the onset of labor and ends with the delivery of the placenta. Also called *perinatal.*
intravascular Fluid or plasma within the vessels of the body.
intravenous (IV) Pertaining to the inside of a vein, as of a thrombus, or an injection, infusion, or catheter.
intrinsic Caused by internal factors.
introitus An entrance to a cavity (e.g., the vaginal introitus).
intussusception Infolding of one segment of the intestine into the lumen of another segment; occurs in children.
involution Reduction in size of the uterus after delivery and return to its normal size.
ion Electronically charged particle resulting from the breakdown of an electrolyte; negatively or positively charged.
irrigation A gentle washing of an area with a stream of solution delivered through an irrigating syringe.
ischemia Decreased blood supply to a body organ or part; often marked by pain and organ dysfunction.
isolation precautions Practices of infection control to reduce or eliminate the transmission of pathogens; precautions include wearing protective apparel such as gowns, gloves, and masks and following the procedure for double bagging.
isotonic Having equal tension of a salt solution. Having the same osmotic pressure as blood.

J

jargon Commonplace language or terminology unique to people in a particular work setting.
jaundice Yellowish discoloration of the skin, mucous membranes, and sclera of the eyes caused by greater than normal amounts of bilirubin in the blood.
joint Any one of the connections between bones.

K

Kaposi's sarcoma (KS) Rare cancer of the skin or mucous membranes; characterized by blue, red, or purple raised lesions and seen mainly in middle-aged Mediterranean men and those with HIV disease.
Kardex/Rand A card system used to consolidate patient orders and care needs in a centralized, concise way.
Kegal exercises A series of contraction movements to the musculature of the perineum. The movements are intended to strengthen the pelvic floor.
keloids Overgrowths of collagenous scar tissue at the site of a skin wound.
keratitis An inflammation of the cornea.
keratoplasty Excision of the corneal tissue, followed by surgical implantation of a cornea from another human donor.
keratotomy A surgical procedure to correct myopia. The procedure involves making tiny incisions into the outer ring of the cornea.
kernicterus Abnormal toxic accumulation of bilirubin in central nervous system tissue caused by hyperbilirubinemia (an excess of bilirubin in the blood of the newborn).
ketoacidosis Acidosis accompanied by an accumulation of ketone in the blood resulting from faulty carbohydrate metabolism.
ketone bodies Normal metabolic products, beta-hydroxybutyric and aminoacetic acid, from which acetone may spontaneously arise.
kick count Daily counting of fetal movements felt in 1 hour while the mother is resting.
kilocalorie Unit that denotes the heat expenditure of an organism and the fuel or energy value of food; often abbreviated kcalorie or kcal.

Korotkoff sounds Sounds heard while measuring blood pressure when using a sphygmomanometer and stethoscope.
kyphosis An abnormal condition of the vertebral column; characterized by increased convexity in the curvature of the thoracic spine.

L

labia majora Two large folds of tissue extending from the mons pubis to the perineal floor; lip.
labia minora Smaller fold of tissue covered by the labia majora; lip.
labile Liable to change; unstable. As in unstable blood pressure.
labyrinthitis Inflammation of the labyrinthine canals of the inner ear.
lactation Function of secreting milk from the breasts for the nourishment of an infant or breastfeeding child.
lanugo Downy, fine hair characteristic of the fetus between 20 weeks of gestation and birth; most noticeable over the shoulders, forehead, and cheeks, but found on nearly all parts of the body except for the palms of the hands and the soles of the feet.
laparoscopy The examination of the abdominal cavity with a laparoscope through a small incision beneath the umbilicus.
latch-on The process by which the baby attaches to the nipple for the purpose of breastfeeding.
law The reference of a rule, principle, or regulation established and made known by a government to protect or restrict the people affected.
Legg-Calvé-Perthes disease A disorder caused by decreased blood supply to the femoral head that results in epiphyseal necrosis or degeneration of the femoral head followed by regeneration or calcification.
leukemia Malignant disorder of the hematopoietic system in which an excess of leukocytes accumulates in the bone marrow and lymph nodes.
leukopenia An abnormal decrease in the number of white blood cells to fewer than 5000 cells/mm^3 due to depression of the bone marrow.
leukoplakia A white patch in the mouth or on the tongue.
liability A legal concept that holds a person legally responsible for harm caused to another person or property.
licensure The granting of permission by a competent authority (usually government agency) to an organization or individual to engage in a practice or activity that would otherwise be illegal.
lichenification Hypertrophy of the epidermis, resulting in rough, thickened, leathery skin.
life expectancy Average number of years an individual will probably live.
lightening Sensation of decreased abdominal distention produced by uterine descent into the pelvic cavity as the fetal presenting part settles into the pelvis. It usually occurs 2 weeks before the onset of labor in nulliparas.
Linda Richards Practiced in the 1880s and has been credited as the first psychiatric nurse.
lipids Group name for organic substances of a fatty nature, including fats, oils, sterols (such as cholesterol), phospholipids, waxes, and related compounds.
lipodystrophy Abnormality in the metabolism or deposition of fats. Insulin lipodystrophy is the loss of local fat deposits in diabetic patients as a complication of repeated insulin injections.
lipohypertrophy An abnormal mass under the subcutaneous tissue of the abdomen. It is associated with repeated insulin injections.
lipoprotein A protein-and-lipid molecule that facilitates transport of lipids in the bloodstream.
lithotomy Incision of a duct or organ, especially the bladder, for removal of a stone.
lithotomy position Position assumed by the patient lying supine with the hips and knees flexed and the thighs abducted and rotated externally.
living will A legal document drawn up by a person who is not yet near death detailing how much medical care he or she wants to receive if terminally ill.
LOC Level of consciousness.
lochia Vaginal discharge during the puerperium consisting of blood, tissue, and mucus; following childbirth.
long-term care The range of services—physical, psychosocial, spiritual, social, and economic—needed to help people attain, maintain, and regain their optimum level of functioning.
lordosis An increase in the curve at the lumbar space region that throws the shoulder back, making the appearance "lordly or kingly."
loss When any aspect of self is no longer available to a person, that person suffers loss.
lumen Space within an artery, vein, intestine, or tube such as a needle or catheter.
lymphangitis Inflammation of one or more lymphatic vessels or channels; usually results from an acute streptococcal or staphylococcal infection in an extremity.
lymphedema Primary or secondary disorder characterized by the accumulation of lymph in soft tissue and edema.
lymphocytes White blood cells that occur in two forms—B cells and T cells.
lymphokine One of the chemical factors produced and released by T lymphocytes that attract macrophages to the site of infection or inflammation and prepare them for attack.

M

macules Small, flat, discolored blemishes; flush with the skin surface.
magnesium The second most abundant cation in the intracellular fluid of the body.
malignant Growing worse, resisting treatment; said of cancerous growths. Also tending or threatening to produce death; harmful.
malpractice (in law) Professional misconduct; behavior that fails to meet the standard of care.
mammogram X-ray examination of the breast; use of radiography of the breast to diagnose breast cancer.
mammography Radiography of the soft tissue of the breast to allow identification of various benign and neoplastic processes.
managed care A health care system that involves administrative control over primary health care services in a medical group practice. Redundant facilities and services are eliminated, and costs are reduced. Health education and preventive medicine are emphasized.
mania A state characterized by an expansive emotional state, extreme excitement, excessive elation, hyperactivity, flight of ideas, increased psychomotor activity, and sometimes violent, destructive, and self-destructive behavior.
Martha Mitchell Nurse educator and clinical specialist in psychiatric mental health nursing, appointed to the President's Commission on Mental Health, established in 1978.
mastoiditis Infection of one of the mastoid bones.
matriarchal family pattern A style in which the female assumes primary dominance in areas of child care and homemaking. Also called *matrilocal.*
maturational loss A loss from normal life transitions.
means Inner terms of the proportion; halfway between extremes.
meconium First stools of the infant; viscid, dark greenish brown, almost black; sterile; odorless.

Medicaid A federally funded, state-operated program of medical assistance to people with low income; authorized by Title XIX of the Social Security Act.
medical asepsis A group of techniques that inhibit the growth and spread of pathogenic microorganisms. Sometimes referred to as clean technique.
medical diagnosis The identification of a disease or condition by scientific evaluation of physical signs, symptoms, history, laboratory tests, and procedures.
medical nutrition therapy The use of specific nutrition services to treat an illness, injury, or condition.
Medicare A federally funded national health insurance for certain people older than 65 years of age.
medicine The art and science of the diagnosis, treatment, and prevention of disease and the maintenance of good health.
melena Abnormal, black, tarry stool containing digested blood.
membrane Thin sheet of tissue that serves many functions in the body; it covers surfaces, lines and lubricates hollow organs, and protects and anchors organs and bones.
meniscus Curved upper surface of a column of liquid as in a mercury column.
menorrhagia Excessive menstrual flow.
mental health One's ability to cope with and adjust to the recurrent stresses of everyday living.
mental health continuum Range of behaviors from adaptive (constructive) to maladaptive (destructive).
mental illness May be evidenced by behavior that is conspicuous, threatening, and disruptive of relationships or that deviates significantly from behavior that is considered socially acceptable. It is a manifestation of dysfunction (behavioral, psychological, and biologic).
meridians Channels of energy.
mesoderm Embryonic middle layer of germ cells giving rise to all types of muscles, connective tissue, bone marrow, blood lymphoid tissue, and all epithelial tissue.
metabolite Substance produced by metabolic action.
metastasis The process by which tumor cells are spread to distant parts of the body.
metrorrhagia Excessive spotting between cycles.
microorganism Any tiny (usually microscopic) entity capable of carrying on living processes; kinds of microorganisms include bacteria, fungi, protozoa, and viruses; seen only by a microscope.
micturition Urination.
midstream urine specimen Urine collected after voiding is initiated and terminated before voiding is complete.
milliequivalent (mEq) Number of grams of soluble substance dissolved in 1 mL of normal solution.
mind-body link Connection between the physiologic and the mental as applied to healing.
minimal encouragement A subtle communication technique that communicates to the patient that the nurse is interested and wants to hear more.
minimum data set (MDS) A part of the patient assessment instrument (PAI) that incorporates many of the same assessment factors as a functional assessment tool and requires input from nursing and social services within a specific time frame.
minority group A racial, religious, ethnic, or political group smaller than and differing from the larger, controlling group in a community or nation.
miotic Causing constriction of the pupil of the eye.
mitosis Type of cell division of somatic (i.e., nonreproductive) cells in which each daughter cell contains the same number of chromosomes as the parent cell.
mobility A person's ability to move around freely in his or her environment.
monozygotic Originating or coming from a single fertilized ovum, such as identical twins.
morbidity An illness or an abnormal condition or quality; the rate at which an illness occurs in a particular area of a population.
mores Accepted traditional customs, moral attitudes, or manners of a particular social group.
mortality The condition of being subject to death; number of deaths in a specific population, usually expressed as deaths per 1000, 10,000, or 100,000.
mortician Person trained in the care of the dead.
morula Development stage of the fertilized ovum in which there is a solid mass of cells resembling a mulberry.
motivation Inner drive to complete a task or reach a goal.
mourning Reaction activated by a person to assist in overcoming a great personal loss.
MUGA scanning A nuclear medicine scan that is used to photograph the heart.
multiaxial system A system that classifies mental disorders; used by most hospitals and health care professionals in the United States. Various disorders and descriptive references are outlined.
multidisciplinary rehabilitation team Team characterized by discipline-specific goals, clear boundaries between disciplines, and outcomes that are the sum of each discipline's efforts.
multidisciplinary setting A group of health care workers who are members of different disciplines, each one providing specific services to the patient.
multiple myeloma A malignant neoplastic immunodeficiency disease of the bone marrow; the tumor is composed of plasma cells.
mummification Mortification producing a dry, hard mass.
musculoskeletal disorders (MSDs) Conditions that impact the muscles, bones, and connective tissue.
mydriatic Causing pupillary dilation.
myeloproliferative Excessive bone marrow production.
myocardial infarction An occlusion of a major coronary artery or one of its branches; it is caused by atherosclerosis or an embolus resulting in necrosis of a portion of cardiac muscle.
myopia Condition of nearsightedness; inability to see objects at a distance.
myringotomy A surgical incision of the tympanic membrane to relieve pressure and release purulent exudate from the middle ear.

N

NANDA-I North American Nursing Diagnosis Association–International.
narrative charting Traditional system of charting in which the nurse documents in story form all pertinent patient observations, care, and responses in the nurse's notes section of the patient's records.
nasal cannula A device for delivery of oxygen by way of two small tubes that are inserted into the nares.
nasogastric tube A pliable tube that is inserted through the patient's nasopharynx and into the stomach.
negligence Failure to act as a responsible, prudent person would act in the given situation; applies to professionals and laypeople.
neoplasm Uncontrolled or abnormal growth of cells.
neoplastic Any abnormal growth of new tissue, benign or malignant.
nephrotoxin Substances with specific destructive properties for the kidneys, such as certain antibiotics, heavy metals, solvents, and chemicals.
neural tube Tube formed from the fusion of the neural folds from which the brain and spinal cord arise.
neuropathy Any abnormal condition characterized by inflammation and degeneration of the peripheral nerves.
neurosis A term describing difficulty with stress that causes mild interpersonal disorganization. There is no loss of reality

perception; the individual has insight that he or she has a problem.
neurotoxic Toxic or damaging to the brain.
nevi Pigmented, congenital skin blemishes that are usually benign but may become cancerous.
Nissen fundoplication A surgical procedure to wrap the fundus of the stomach around the distal esophagus to prevent reflux of the stomach contents to the esophagus.
nitrogen balance Difference between intake and output of nitrogen in the body. If intake is greater, a positive nitrogen balance exists and anabolism occurs. If output is greater, a negative nitrogen balance exists and catabolism occurs. When nitrogen intake equals output, the body is in zero nitrogen balance.
nocturia Excessive urination at night.
nomenclature The process of assigning names.
nonmaleficence Ethical principle meaning "to do no harm."
non–rapid eye movement (NREM) One of two highly individualized sleeping states divided into four stages through which a sleeper progresses during a typical sleeping cycle; represents three-fourths of a period of typical sleep.
non-rebreather mask A device used to deliver oxygen to the patient. The patient can breath on his or her own. The mask is used to deliver precise concentrations of oxygen.
nontherapeutic communication Communication techniques, both verbal and nonverbal, that hinder the nurse-patient relationship.
nonverbal communication The transmission of messages without the use of words.
nosocomial infection An infection acquired in a hospital or any other health care facility; an infection acquired at least 72 hours after admission.
noxious A stimulation of the sensory nerve endings that is harmful, injurious, or detrimental to physical health.
nuchal rigidity Pain and stiffness of the neck when flexed.
nuchal translucency screening Ultrasound screening to measure fetal nuchal folds to assess for potential Down syndrome.
nuclear family A family unit consisting of the parents and their offspring.
nucleus Largest organelle within the cell; it is responsible for cell reproduction and control of the other organelles.
numerator Top number of a fraction.
nurse practice act A statute enacted by the legislature of any of the states or by the appropriate officers of the district's possessions. The act delineates the legal scope of the practice of nursing within the geographic boundaries of jurisdiction.
nursing bottle caries Tooth decay caused by bottle feeding during sleep.
nursing care plan Plan of care based on a nursing assessment and a nursing diagnosis; lists nursing actions necessary to meet a patient's needs.
nursing diagnosis A clinical judgment about individual, family, or community responses to actual or high-risk (potential) health problems or life processes.
nursing health history Data collected about the patient's level of wellness, changes in life patterns, sociocultural role, and mental and emotional reactions to illness.
nursing intervention Activity performed by nurses that should promote the achievement of the desired patient outcome.
nursing notes The form on the patient's chart on which nurses record their observations, care given, and the patient's responses.
nursing physical assessment Identification by a nurse of the needs, preferences, and abilities of a patient. Assessment provides the scientific basis for a complete nursing care plan.
nursing process Systematic method by which nurses plan and provide care for patients.
nursing-sensitive outcomes The results or outcomes of nursing interventions. These outcomes or indicators are influenced by nursing and can be used to judge effectiveness of care and determine best practices.
nutrient A dietary element that is used to nourish the body.
nutrient density Nutrients relative to calories.
nutrient-dense foods Foods providing a high quantity of one or more nutrients in a small number of calories are nutrient dense.
nystagmus Involuntary, rhythmic movement of the eyes. Oscillations may be horizontal, vertical, rotary, or mixed.

O

obesity Abnormal increase in the proportion of fat cells, mainly in the viscera and subcutaneous tissues of the body; grossly overweight.
objective data Of or pertaining to a clinical finding that is observed, palpated, or auscultated. Laboratory findings, as well as radiologic and other studies, are included; observable and measurable signs.
obsessions Persistent thoughts and ideas that are recurrent, intrusive, and suggest an irrational act. The mind is continually and involuntarily preoccupied. These thoughts are anxiety producing and distressing in that they are uncontrollable.
occlusion An obstruction or closing off in a canal, vessel, or passage of the body.
occult Hidden.
occult blood Blood that is hidden or obscured from view.
Occupational Safety and Health Administration (OSHA) Federal agency responsible for monitoring safety and health standards in the workplace.
oligohydramnios Abnormally small amount or absence of amniotic fluid; often indicative of fetal urinary tract defect.
oliguria A diminished capacity to form and pass urine (less than 500 mL in 24 hours); result is that the end products of metabolism cannot be excreted efficiently.
Omnibus Budget Reconciliation Act (OBRA) Federal legislation that mandates specific standards governing the care of older adults in U.S. nursing facilities and prohibits routine use of safety reminder devices (SRDs; restraints) in nursing homes.
oncology The sum of knowledge regarding tumors; the branch of medicine that deals with the study of tumors.
one-way communication A structured form of communication in which the sender is in control.
open posture A relaxed stance with uncrossed arms and legs while facing another individual.
open reduction with internal fixation (ORIF) A surgical procedure allowing fracture alignment under direct visualization while using various internal fixation devices applied to the bone.
open-ended question A question that does not require a specific response and allows the individual to elaborate freely on a subject.
opportunistic Disease characteristic caused by a normally nonpathogenic organism in a host whose resistance has been decreased by a disorder such as AIDS.
oral hygiene Care of the oral cavity (mouth).
organ A group of several different kinds of tissue arranged so that they can work together to perform a special function.
organic disease Results in a structural change in an organ that interferes with its functioning.
orthopnea An abnormal condition in which a person must sit or stand to breathe deeply or comfortably.
orthopneic Pertaining to the posture assumed by the patient sitting up in bed at a 90-degree angle; patient may also lean forward supported by a pillow or over a bed table.

orthostatic hypotension A drop of 25 mm Hg in systolic pressure and a drop of 10 mm Hg in diastolic pressure when moving from a lying to sitting position.
osmosis Passage of water across a selectively permeable membrane; the water moves from a less concentrated solution to a more concentrated solution.
ostomy A surgical opening in the body. Some ostomies are created to allow the body to eliminate wastes.
outcome Description of the specific measurable behavior (outcome criteria) that the patient will be able to exhibit after the nursing interventions.
oxytocin Hormone produced in the hypothalamus and stored in the posterior pituitary gland; when needed, promotes the release of breast milk and stimulates uterine contractions during labor.

P

pain assessment An evaluation of the factors that alleviate or exacerbate a patient's pain.
palliative Designed to relieve pain and distress and to control the signs and symptoms of disease; not designed to produce a cure.
palliative care Preventing, relieving, reducing, or soothing symptoms of disease or disorders without effecting a cure. Extends the principles of hospice care to a broader population that could benefit from comfort care earlier in their illness or disease process.
palpation A technique used in physical examination in which the examiner feels the texture, size, consistency, and location of certain parts of the body with the hands.
pancytopenia Deficient condition of all three major blood elements (red cells, white cells, and platelets); results from the bone marrow being reduced or absent.
panhysterosalpingo-oophorectomy Removal of the uterus, fallopian tubes, and ovaries. Also called *total abdominal hysterectomy with bilateral salpingo-oophorectomy.*
panic disorder An anxiety disorder that exhibits a sudden onset of acute, extreme anxiety. Feelings of terror and intense apprehension are accompanied with physical manifestations such as dyspnea, palpitations, sweating, trembling, and dizziness. An attack may last for several minutes and may be triggered again in certain situations.
Papanicolaou test (Pap smear) A simple smear method of examining stained exfoliative cells; used most commonly to detect cancers of the cervix.
papules Palpable, circumscribed, red solid elevations in the skin; smaller than 0.5 cm.
para- A combining form meaning "similar, beside." Also a combining form meaning a woman who has given birth after 20 weeks' gestation (e.g., nonpara, unipara, bipara).
paracentesis A procedure in which fluid is withdrawn from the abdominal cavity.
paralytic (adynamic) ileus Most common type of intestinal obstruction; a decrease in or absence of intestinal peristalsis and bowel sounds that may occur after abdominal surgery.
paraphilia Sexual perversion or deviation. One of three main clusters of sexual and gender identity disorders.
paraphrasing A communication technique that involves restating the patient's message in the nurse's own words to verify that the nurse's interpretation of the message is correct.
parenchyma Tissue of an organ as distinguished from supporting or connective tissue.
parent-child attachment (bonding) Initial phase in a relationship characterized by strong attraction and a desire to interact.
parenteral Pertaining to treatment other than through the digestive system.
parenteral nutrition Administering nutrients by a route other than the alimentary canal, such as intravenously.
parenthood stage Begins at the birth or adoption of the first child.
paresis A lesser degree of movement deficit from partial or incomplete paralysis.
paresthesia Any subjective sensation, such as a prickling "pins and needles" feeling or numbness.
partial rebreather mask A device used for oxygen delivery of 50-70%. The devise includes a collection bag for exhaled air.
PASS A mnemonic used to outline the steps needed to use a fire extinguisher. (*P*ull the pin, *A*im low, *S*queeze handle, *S*weep the unit).
passive listening Receiving a message without any response or indication of understanding.
passive transport The movement of small molecules across the membrane of a cell by diffusion; no cellular energy is required.
passivity The acceptance of the actions of others with no active response or resistance.
patency A condition of being opened and unblocked.
pathogenic Capable of causing disease.
pathognomonic Sign or symptom specific to a disease condition.
patient A recipient of a health care service, usually thought of as a recipient who is ill or hospitalized.
patient assessment instrument (PAI) A method of patient assessment and care plan development prescribed by OBRA in 1987.
patient-controlled analgesia (PCA) A drug delivery system that dispenses a preset intravenous dose of an opioid analgesic into a patient's vein when the patient pushes a switch on an electric cord.
patriarchal family pattern A family style in which the male assumes the dominant role.
pediatric rehabilitation nursing Specialty practice that focuses on the care of children with disabilities or other chronic conditions and their families.
pediculosis Lice infestation.
peer assistance program Administers contract agreements requiring a nurse to undergo treatment and monitoring to keep his or her license in good standing.
peer review An appraisal by professional co-workers (of equal status) of the way an individual nurse conducts practice, education, or research.
per diem An agreed upon daily rate of payment for a service.
percent Hundredths; symbolized as %.
percussion Using fingertips to tap the body's surface to produce vibration and sound.
percutaneous Through the skin or mucous membrane.
perimenopause The changes in the female body that lead the transition into menopause. Symptoms may include hot flashes, impaired sleep patterns, and weight gain.
perinatal Period during pregnancy that begins with the onset of labor and ends with delivery of the placenta; sometimes called intrapartal.
perineal care Care given to the genitalia.
perioperative Entire surgical inpatient period occurring immediately before, during, and immediately after surgery.
peripheral Pertaining to the outside, surface, or surrounding area of an organ, other structure or field of vision.
pernicious Capable of causing great injury or destruction; deadly, fatal.
pernicious anemia A progressive megaloblastic, macrocytic anemia that results from a lack of intrinsic factor essential for the absorption of vitamin B_{12}.
personal health record An electronic record in which patients are allowed to input and update their own health information.
personal hygiene Self-care measures that people use to maintain their health.

personality Refers to the relatively consistent set of attitudes and behaviors particular to an individual; it consists of a pattern of mental, emotional, and behavioral tracts of a person.
pessary A device that can be inserted into the vagina to support the bladder and reduce pressure on the bladder from the uterus in cases of prolapse.
pesthouse A home or hospital used to house and care for patients with infections.
phagocytes White blood cells that are able to surround, engulf, and digest microorganisms and cellular debris.
phagocytic Refers to the ingestion and digestion of bacteria.
phagocytosis The process that permits a cell to surround or engulf any foreign material and digest it.
pharmaceuticals Drugs, or drug-based products or preparations.
pharmacology Study of drugs and their actions on the living body.
phimosis A condition in which the prepuce is too small to allow retraction of the foreskin over the glans penis.
phobia An anxiety disorder characterized by obsessive, irrational, and intense fear of a specific object or activity.
phosphorus Chiefly, an intracellular anion in fluid of the body.
photocoagulation Use of a laser beam to destroy new blood vessels, seal leaking vessels, and help prevent retinal edema.
phototherapy Treatment for hyperbilirubinemia and jaundice in the newborn that involves the exposure of light; accelerates the excretion of bilirubin in the skin, decomposing it by photooxidation.
physiologic jaundice Jaundice usually occurring 48 hours or later after birth, gradually disappearing by the 7th to 10th day; caused by the normal reduction in the number of red blood cells. The infant is otherwise well.
physiology Explanation of the processes and functions of the various structures of the body and how they interrelate.
pica Craving to eat nonfood substances.
pinocytosis The process by which extracellular fluid is ingested by the cells.
placebo effect Positive response to treatment that has no known medical effect.
placental barrier Obstruction, boundary, or separation provided by the placental tissue between the fetal and maternal circulation; substances of small size, excluding blood cells, may cross this barrier.
planning In the five-step nursing process, a category of nursing behavior in which a strategy is designed for the achievement of the goals of care for an individual patient, as established in assessing and analyzing. Planning includes developing and modifying a care plan for the patient, cooperating with other personnel, and recording relevant information.
plasmapheresis Removal of plasma that contains components causing or thought to cause disease. Also called *plasma exchange* because when the plasma is removed, it is replaced by substitution fluids such as saline or albumin.
pleural effusion An abnormal accumulation of fluid in the thoracic cavity between the visceral and parietal pleurae.
pleural friction rub Low-pitched, grating, or creaking lung sounds that occur when inflamed pleural surfaces rub together during respiration.
pleural space The potential space between the visceral and parietal layers of the pleurae.
***Pneumocystis jiroveci* (formerly *carinii*) pneumonia (PCP)** An unusual pulmonary disease caused by a parasite that is primarily associated with people who have suppressed immune systems, especially in people with AIDS.
pneumothorax A collection of air or gas in the pleural space, causing the lung to collapse.
point-of-care (POC) Computer electronic health record systems that are located at the patient's bedside.
poison A substance that is toxic.
poisoning The condition or physical state produced by the ingestion, injection, inhalation, or exposure of a poisonous (toxic) substance.
polycythemia Abnormal increase in the number of red blood cells in the blood.
polydactyly More digits (finger or toes) than normal.
polydipsia Excessive thirst.
polyphagia Eating to the point of gluttony.
polyuria Excretion of an abnormally large quantity of urine.
POMR *See* problem-oriented medical record.
portfolio A file of items accumulated that highlight an individual's educational and professional accolades.
postictal period A rest period of variable length after a tonic-clonic seizure.
postmortem care Care of the body after death.
postoperative Pertaining to a period of time after surgery.
postpartal The final stage of the maternity cycle; from Latin *post*, "after."
posture The position of the body. It may refer to the position when standing, sitting or lying.
potassium The dominant intracellular cation.
potentiation When one drug increases the action or effect of another drug.
preceptor Person assigned to support a new or transferred employee through clinical orientation.
preeclampsia An abnormal condition of pregnancy characterized by the onset of acute hypertension after the 24th week of gestation.
pregnancy-induced hypertension (PIH) A disease encountered during pregnancy or early in the puerperium, characterized by increasing hypertension, albuminuria, and generalized edema. Also called *gestational hypertension (GH)*.
prenatal Before birth; occurring or existing before birth; referring to both the care of the woman during pregnancy and the growth and development of the fetus.
preoperational thought stage Piaget's phase of child development during the period of 2 to 7 years of age, when the child focuses on the use of language as a tool. The child has the emerging ability to reason.
preoperative Pertaining to a period of time before surgery.
presbycusis A normal loss of hearing acuity, speech intelligibility, auditory threshold, and pitch associated with aging.
presbyopia Defect in vision in advancing age involving loss of accommodation or recession of near vision; due to loss of elasticity of crystalline lens.
priapism Persistent penile erection.
primary (deciduous) teeth Baby teeth that normally appear during infancy.
primary caregiver One who assumes ongoing responsibility for health maintenance and therapy for the ill.
primary intention A wound that has been made surgically and has little tissue loss; skin edges are close together and minimal scarring results.
problem Any health care condition that requires diagnostic, therapeutic, or educational action.
problem list Prioritized master list of the patient's active, inactive, temporary, and at-risk medical or other problems; serves as an index to the rest of the record.
problem-oriented medical record (POMR) Method of recording data about the health status of a patient in a problem-solving system. Parts included are the database, problem list, initial plan, and progress notes.
procidentia Protrusion of the entire uterus through the introitus.
prodromal Early sign of a developing condition or disease.

prolactin A hormone secreted from the anterior pituitary gland that is responsible for stimulating milk production in the mammary alveolar cells.
proliferation Reproduction or multiplication of similar forms.
pronation Palm of the hand turned down.
prone Lying face down on the abdomen.
proportion Shows that the relationship between two ratios has equal value.
proprioception Sensation pertaining to stimuli originating from within the body regarding spatial position and muscular activity stimuli or to the sensory receptors that those stimuli activate. This sensation gives one the ability to know the position of the body without looking at it and the ability to "know objectively the sense of touch."
prostatodynia Pain in the prostate gland.
prosthesis Artificial replacement for a missing body part.
proximodistal Growth and development that moves from the center toward the outside. The infant gains control of the shoulders before developing control of the hands and fingers.
pruritus The symptoms of itching; an uncomfortable sensation leading to the urge to scratch; scratching often leads to secondary infection. Some causes of pruritus are allergy, infection, elevated serum urea, jaundice, and skin irritation.
pseudomenstruation Discharge of blood-tinged mucus from the vagina of the newborn, which occurs in response to maternal hormones.
psychoactive drugs Drugs that make the user feel good but have the potential to be abused or addicting.
psychogenic Relating to causes that are emotional, psychological, or nonorganic in origin.
psychosis Any major disorder characterized by gross impairment in reality testing; the affected person exhibits moderate to severe personality disintegration.
psychosocial A combination of psychological and social factors.
puerperium Period of time after the third stage of labor and lasting until involution of the uterus takes place, usually about 3 to 6 weeks.
pulmonary edema Accumulation of extravascular fluid in lung tissues and alveoli; caused most commonly by left-sided heart failure.
pulse A rhythmic beating or vibrating movement; regular recurrent expansion and contraction of an artery produced by waves of pressure caused by the ejection of blood from the left ventricle of the heart as it contracts.
pulse deficit A condition that exists when the radial pulse rate is less than the ventricular rate as auscultated at the apex of the heart.
pulse pressure Difference between the systolic and diastolic blood pressures, usually 30 to 40 mm Hg.
pulverized Crushed to a powder.
puncture A perforation that my be the result of an accidental or intentional action.
purulent Producing or containing pus.
pustulant vesicles Small, circumscribed pus-containing elevations of the skin.
pyuria Pus in the urine.

Q

Qi Life force.
quality assurance/assessment/improvement In health care, any evaluation of services provided and the results achieved as compared with accepted standards.
quality of life A measure of the optimum energy that endows a person with the power to cope successfully with the full range of challenges encountered in the real world.
quarks The building blocks of protons and neutrons that comprise the atom.

R

RACE A formula to enable nurses to be prepared when safety is threatened by fire; *R*escue the patient, sound the *A*larm, *C*onfine the fire, *E*xtinguish or *E*vacuate.
race A group of people who share biologic and physical characteristics.
racism Any ethnocentric activity—cultural, individual, or institutional, deliberate or not—that is based on a belief in the superiority of one racial group over other racial groups; the oppression of, thus maintaining control over, these groups.
radial keratotomy Microscopic incisions on the surface of the cornea outside the optical area. These eight spokelike incisions flatten the cornea to a more normal curvature, thus reducing or eliminating myopia.
range of motion (ROM) Normal movement that any given joint is capable of making. Any body action involving the muscles, joints, and natural directional movements.
rapid eye movement (REM) One of the two highly individualized sleeping states that follows NREM state. May last from a few minutes to a half an hour and alternate with NREM periods; dreaming occurs during this time.
ratio Relationship of one number or quantity to another number or quantity.
raves All-night parties or "trances"; often the scene of club drug use.
receiver The individual or individuals to whom a message is conveyed.
receptive aphasia A physiological condition in which an individual cannot recognize or interpret the message being received.
receptivity Willingness to take in and accept new experiences.
receptors Molecules that recognize or respond to specific invaders.
reciprocity Mutual agreement to exchange privilege, dependence, or relationships as an agreement between two governing bodies to accept the credit of caregivers licensed in each state. True reciprocity means that individuals licensed in one state can automatically receive licensure in the next, even if the licensure requirements of the states differ.
recording Process of adding written information to the chart, usually at prescribed intervals.
Reed-Sternberg cells Atypical histiocytes; large, abnormal, multinucleated cells in the lymphatic system, found in Hodgkin's lymphoma.
referred pain Pain that is felt at a site other than in the injured or diseased organ or part of the body.
reflecting A communication technique that assists the patient to "reflect" on inner feelings and thoughts rather than seeking answers or advice from someone else.
reflexology A form of complementary and alternative medicine based on the premise that zones and reflexes in different parts of the body correspond to all parts, glands, and organs of the entire body. In reflexology it is thought that the entire body can be reached by applying pressure to specific areas on the feet.
refraction Light rays are bent as they pass through the colorless structures of the eye, enabling light from the environment to focus on the retina.
Reiki A form of alternative health treatment that originated in Japan. It is focused on the promotion of health and wellness through relaxation techniques.
relaxation The state of generalized decreased cognitive, physiologic, or behavioral arousal.
relaxin Ovarian hormone that softens and relaxes joints and ligaments to facilitate labor and delivery.
remission A decrease in the severity of a disease or any of its symptoms.
renal colic Abdominal pain that is associated with disorders of the kidney.

reservoir Any natural habitat of a microorganism that promotes growth and reproduction.
resident assessment instrument (RAI) A comprehensive tool that includes the minimum data set, resident assessment protocols, and guidelines for functional assessment of the resident.
residential care A care setting for older adults, providing a wide range of services, such as assisted living and continuing care.
residual urine Urine remaining in the urinary tract after voiding.
residue Bulk in the colon that includes undigested food, fiber, bacteria, body secretions, and cells.
resignation Act of resigning; giving up a position of employment.
respirations The taking in of oxygen, its use in the tissues, and the giving off of carbon dioxide; the act of breathing (i.e., inhaling and exhaling).
respite care Period of relief from responsibilities for the care of a patient.
restating A communication technique that involves the nurse repeating to the patient what the nurse believes to be the main point that the patient is trying to convey.
restitution In obstetrics, the turning of the fetal head to the left or right after it has completely emerged from the introitus of the vagina as it assumes a normal alignment with the infant's shoulders.
restorative nursing care Basic concepts of physical therapy for maintenance of functional mobility and physical activity.
résumé A summary of educational and professional experiences, including activities and honors, to be used in seeking employment for biologic citations on professional meeting programs or related purposes; curriculum vitae.
retention The inability to void even in the presence of an urge to void.
retinal detachment Separation of the retina from the choroid in the posterior of the eye.
retrovirus Lentivirus that contains reverse transcriptase, which is essential for reverse transcription (the production of a deoxyribonucleic acid [DNA] molecule from a ribonucleic acid [RNA] model).
risk nursing diagnosis A clinical judgment that an individual, family, or community is more vulnerable to develop the problem than others in same or similar situation.
role A socially expected behavior pattern associated with an individual's function in various social groups.
rule of nines Division of the body into multiples of nine; used to determine the total body surface area (BSA) involved in burn trauma.

S

safety reminder device (SRD) Any one of numerous devices used to immobilize a patient; formerly referred to as a restraint.
sandwich generation A group of people who find themselves captured between caring for their own children and their aging parents.
sanguineous Pertaining to blood.
sarcoma Malignant tumor of connective tissues such as muscle or bone; usually presents as a painless swelling.
satiety Feeling of fullness and satisfaction from food.
savants Children with autism who excel in particular areas such as art, music, memory, mathematics, or perceptual skills such as puzzle building.
SBAR (Situation, Background, Assessment, Recommendation) A common communication tool used in health care between the care team. It focuses on identifying pertinent issues related to the situation, background, assessment, and recommendation.
schema Innate knowledge structure that allows a child to organize his or her mind.
schizophrenia Any one of a large group of psychotic disorders characterized by gross distortion of reality, disturbances of language and communication, and disorganized and fragmented thought, perception, and emotional reaction.
school avoidance Repeated absence from school of a child who is physically healthy.
school violence Anything that physically or psychologically injures schoolchildren or damages school property.
sclerotherapy Chemicals used to cause inflammation, followed by fibrosis and destruction of the vessels causing the bleeding.
scoliosis Curvature of the spine usually consisting of two curves: the original abnormal curve and a compensatory curve in the opposite direction.
secondary intention Healing that occurs when skin edges of the wound are not close together or when pus is formed.
self A complex concept comprising four distinct parts: personal identity, body image, role performance, and self-esteem.
self-concept How an individual views the self; pertains to personal identity, body image, role, and self-esteem.
semi-Fowler's position The position a patient assumes while lying in bed; the head of the bed is raised to about 30 degrees, and the foot of the bed is raised slightly.
sender The person conveying a message.
senescence stage The last stage of the life cycle that requires the older adult to cope with a long range of changes.
senile The state of physical and mental deterioration associated with aging.
senility Pertaining to or characteristic of old age or the process of aging.
sensitivity A laboratory method of determining the effectiveness of antibiotics. A report of resistance means that the antibiotic is not effective in inhibiting the growth of a pathogen, whereas use of an effective antibiotic results in a sensitive report.
sensorimotor stage The developmental phase of childhood encompassing the period from birth to 2 years of age, according to Piaget's psychology. In this stage, an infant's knowledge of the world comes about primarily through sensory impressions and motor activities.
sensory deprivation An involuntary loss of physical awareness caused by detachment from external sensory stimuli.
sentinel event Any unexpected occurrence involving death or serious physical or psychological injury, or the risk thereof.
sentinel lymph node mapping Diagnostic tool used before therapeutic surgery, which identifies the first lymph node most likely to drain cancerous cells; used in axillary lymph node biopsy, specifically in breast cancer staging.
separation anxiety Fear and apprehension caused by separation from familiar surroundings and significant people.
sequestrum A fragment of necrotic bone that is partially or entirely detached from the surrounding or adjacent healthy bone.
seroconversion The development of detectable levels of antibodies; a change in serologic tests (e.g., ELISA and Western blot) from negative to positive as antibodies develop in reaction to an infection.
seronegative Negative result on serologic examination. The state of lacking HIV antibodies; confirmed by blood tests.
seroprevalence The overall frequency of findings of a disorder in a population as determined by blood testing.
serosanguineous Thin, red exudate composed of serum and blood.
serotonin syndrome A potentially life-threatening condition that can occur as a result of an interaction between a selective

serotonin reuptake inhibitor (SSRI) and another serotonergic agent.
serous Thin, watery exudate composing the serum portion of blood.
severe preeclampsia An elevation in blood pressure of 160/100 or higher accompanied by severe proteinuria in a pregnant woman that results after 20 weeks' gestation. The elevated blood pressure readings must be on at least two occasions 6 hour apart.
shearing forces Applied forces or pressure exerted against the surface and layers of the skin as tissue slides in opposite but parallel planes.
shock Abnormal condition of inadequate blood flow to peripheral tissues, with life-threatening cellular dysfunction, hypotension, and oliguria.
sibilant wheeze Musical, high-pitched, squeaking, or whistlelike sound caused by the rapid movement of air through narrowed bronchioles.
sickled cell Erythrocyte whose characteristic round shape has altered to an elongated crescent shape.
sign An objective finding as perceived by the examiner; a sign can be seen, heard, measured, or felt by the examiner.
simple face mask A device used to administer oxygen at a rate of 5 to 8 L/min.
Sims' position Lying on the left side with the right knee and thigh drawn upward toward the chest; the chest and abdomen are allowed to fall forward.
single-parent family Family group that occurs when one parent leaves the nuclear family because of divorce, separation, desertion, or death. May also be the result of an unwed parent living alone or the decision of a single person to adopt a child.
singultus Hiccup.
situational loss Loss occurring suddenly in response to a specific external event.
Sjögren syndrome Dry eye syndrome; an immunologic disorder characterized by low fluid production by lacrimal (tear), salivary, and other glands, resulting in abnormal dryness of mouth, eyes, and other mucous membranes.
skilled nursing care The provision of care by a team of trained and/or licensed heath care providers.
skilled nursing facility Houses a subacute unit with a stronger rehabilitative focus and shorter length of stay than a long-term facility.
Snellen's test Eye chart test for visual acuity; letters, numbers, or symbols are arranged on the chart in decreasing size from top to bottom.
SOAPE Charting format used in POMR. Components include subjective data *(S)* reported by the patient; objective data *(O)* acquired by inspection, percussion, auscultation, and palpation and by tests, usually measurable findings; assessment *(A)* of the problem; plan *(P)* of care; and evaluation *(E)* of the patient's response to the treatment plan.
SOAPIER Same as SOAPE charting except that intervention *(I)* and revision *(R)* are added. Interventions are specific actions carried out, and revisions are the changes to be made to the original plan.
social contract family/cohabitation Unmarried couple living together and sharing roles and responsibilities similar to those of the nuclear family structure.
society A nation, community, or broad group of people who establish particular aims, beliefs, or standards of living and conduct.
sodium The most abundant electrolyte in the body; the major extracellular electrolyte; it is a cation.
somatization A disorder characterized by recurrent, multiple, physical complaints and symptoms for which there is no organic cause.
sonorous wheeze Low-pitched, loud, coarse, snoring sound.
souffle cup Ungraduated, disposable paper cup.
spastic Involuntary, sudden movements or muscular contractions with increased reflexes.
specimen A small sample of something, intended to show the nature of the whole, such as a urine specimen.
sphygmomanometer Device for measuring arterial blood pressure.
spider telangiectases Dilated superficial arterioles.
spinal cord injury (SCI) An injury in which the spinal cord is compressed by fractures or displaced vertebrae, bleeding, or edema.
spore The reproductive cell of some microorganisms such as fungi or protozoa. These cells are highly resistant to heat and chemicals. Under proper environmental conditions they may revert to an actively multiplying form of bacterium (e.g., gas gangrene or tetanus).
stages of dependence The three characteristic stages of dependence, which are chronic, incurable, and progressive.
standard precautions A set of guidelines set forth by the CDC to reduce the risk of transmission of bloodborne pathogens and pathogens for moist body substances. These precautions promote handwashing and use of gloves, masks, eye protection, and gowns when appropriate for patient contact. These precautions are designed to reduce the risk of transmission of microorganisms from both recognized and unrecognized sources of infection.
standardized languages A structured vocabulary that provides nurses with a common means of communication.
standards of care Those acts that are permitted to be performed or prohibited from being performed by a prudent person working within the limits of the training, licensing, experience, and conditions existing at the time of the duty to give care.
stapedectomy The removal of the stapes of the middle ear and insertion of a graft and prosthesis.
steatorrhea Excessive fat in the feces.
stereotype A generalization about a form of behavior, an individual, or a group.
sterilization A process by which all microorganisms, including their spores, are destroyed.
stertorous Pertaining to a respiratory effort that is strenuous and struggling, which provokes a snoring sound.
stethoscope Instrument placed against patient's body to hear heart, lung, or bowel sounds.
stimulants Drugs that affect the central nervous system.
stoma Combining form meaning a mouth or opening.
stomatitis Inflammation of the mouth due to destruction of normal cells of the oral cavity that may result from infection by bacteria, viruses, or fungi from exposure to certain chemicals or drugs, vitamin deficiency, or systemic inflammatory disease.
strabismus Condition in which the eyes are unable to focus in the same direction. Also called *cross-eyed.*
street drugs Substances (drugs) sold to users illegally by drug dealers and that are manufactured without strict controls, illegally obtained prescription drugs, or drugs not approved for use in the United States.
stress The nonspecific response of the body to any demand made on it.
stressor A situation, activity, or event that produces stress.
stridor Harsh sound made during respirations; high pitched and resembling the blowing of wind; due to obstruction of air passages.
stroke An abnormal condition of the blood vessels of the brain characterized by hemorrhage into the brain; formation of an embolus or thrombus resulting in ischemia of the brain tissues normally perfused by the damaged vessels. The sequelae depend on the location and extent of ischemia.

subacute unit Institutional setting that provides a less expensive alternative to acute care; a bridge between acute care and long-term care.
subculture A group that shares many characteristics with the primary culture but has characteristic patterns of behavior and ideals that distinguish it from the rest of a cultural group.
subjective data Symptoms; verbal statements provided by the patient. That which arises from within or is perceived by the individual and related to the examiner.
sublingual Under the tongue.
subluxation Partial dislocation.
sundowning syndrome Sometimes referred to as nocturnal delirium. Manifested by increased disorientation and agitation only during the evening and nighttime. Seen more often in older adults.
supination Kind of rotation that allows the palm of the hand to turn up.
supine Being in the horizontal position, lying face upward.
suppuration To produce purulent material.
surfactant Lipoprotein necessary for normal respiratory function that prevents alveolar collapse (atelectasis); may be necessary for preterm infants.
surgery Branch of medicine concerned with diseases and trauma requiring operative procedures.
surgical asepsis A group of techniques that destroy all microorganisms and their spores (sterile technique).
surrogacy The agreement a woman makes to be artificially inseminated, voluntarily or for a fee, to bear a child and then relinquish parental rights to the baby's natural father or another couple.
surveillance Exercise of continuous scrutiny of and watchfulness over the distribution and spread of infections and factors related thereto, of sufficient accuracy and completeness to be effective control.
symptom Subjective indication of a disease or a change in condition as perceived by the patient.
syncope A transient loss of consciousness due to inadequate blood flow to the brain (fainting).
syndactyly Malformation of digits, commonly seen as a fusion of two or more toes to form one structure.
syndrome nursing diagnosis Used when a cluster of actual or risk nursing diagnoses are predicted to be present in certain circumstances.
synergistic Action of two or more substances or organs to achieve an effect of which each is capable.
system An organization of varying numbers and kinds of organs arranged so that they can work together to perform complex functions for the body.
systolic The number or reading that represents ventricles contracting, forcing blood into the aorta and pulmonary arteries. In blood pressure readings, it is the higher of the two readings.

T

T'ai chi/Taiji Martial arts practice that emphasizes relaxing the body and focusing the mind; Tai chi movement is performed slowly, accentuating the intention, mechanics, accuracy, and precision of motion.
tachycardia An abnormal condition in which the myocardium contracts regularly but at a rate greater than 100 beats per minute.
tachypnea An abnormally rapid rate of breathing.
temperature Relative measure of sensible heat or cold.
tenesmus Persistent, ineffectual spasms of the rectum or bladder, accompanied by the desire to empty the bowel or bladder.
teratogen Any substance, agent, or process that interferes with normal prenatal development, causing the formation of one or more developmental abnormalities in the fetus.
teratogenic agent *See* teratogen.
terminal illness An advanced stage of disease with no known cure and poor prognosis.
terrorism Use or threats of violence by individuals or organized groups using biological, chemical, or nuclear weapons against society or government for political gain.
tertiary intention Healing that occurs by primary intention with delayed suturing of a wound in which two layers of granulation tissue are sutured together.
tetanus toxoid Active agent prepared from detoxified tetanus toxin that produces an antigenic response in the body, conferring permanent immunity to tetanus infection.
tetrahydrocannabinol A compound of marijuana.
thanatologist One who studies dying and death.
thanatology The study of dying and death.
therapeutic Beneficial.
therapeutic communication A form of communication that facilitates the formation of a positive nurse-patient relationship.
therapeutic diet A diet used as a medical treatment.
therapeutic massage The manipulation of the soft tissues of the body to assist with healing.
third-party payers Entities (persons or elements) other than the giver or receiver of service responsible for payment (e.g., Medicare or an insurance company).
thoracentesis The surgical perforation of the chest wall and pleural space with a needle for the aspiration of fluid for diagnostic or therapeutic purposes.
thrill Fine vibration sensation along the artery, which is palpated by the examiner.
thrombocytopenia An abnormal hematologic condition in which the number of platelets is reduced to fewer than $100{,}000/mm^3$.
thrombus Of or pertaining to a clot.
tinnitus A subjective noise sensation in one or both ears; ringing or tinkling sound in the ear.
tissue An organization of many similar cells that act together to perform a common function.
titrate Slowly increasing the amount of drug to find the therapeutic dose.
tolerance A state that develops as the amount and frequency of use of an addicting substance increases to achieve the same effect.
tophi Calculi containing sodium urate deposits that develop in periarticular fibrous tissue; typically found in patients with gout.
topical application Applied to the skin.
TORCH (*T*oxoplasmosis, *O*ther, *R*ubella virus, *C*ytomegalovirus, and *H*erpes simplex viruses) Group of agents that can infect the fetus or the newborn infant, causing a constellation of morbid effects called TORCH syndrome.
total parenteral nutrition (TPN) The administration of a hypertonic solution into a large central vein, usually the superior vena cava, via a catheter threaded through either the subclavian or internal jugular vein.
tourniquet Constricting device applied to control bleeding.
toxicity The level of exposure to a substance that the body will experience detriment.
toxicologic analysis Scientific study of poisons, their detection, and their effects.
tracheostomy A surgical opening into the trachea through which an indwelling tube may be inserted; created by a tracheotomy.
traditional (block) chart Conventional patient chart broken down into sections or blocks; included are admission data, physicians' orders, history and physical examination, nursing care plan, nurses' notes and graphics, progress notes, and test data.
transcribe To write or type a copy.

transcultural nursing An integration of the nurse's understanding of culture into all aspects of nursing care.
transcutaneous electrical nerve stimulation (TENS) A type of pain control that is managed with a pocket-sized, battery-operated device that provides a continuous, mild electrical current to the skin via electrodes.
transdisciplinary rehabilitation team Team characterized by the blurring of boundaries between discipline and by cross-training and flexibility to minimize duplication of effort toward individual goal attainment.
transfer Moving a patient from one unit to another (intra-agency transfer) or moving a patient from one health care facility to another (interagency transfer).
transgender family A family unit that is composed of one or both of the parents who have undergone gender reassignment or who are nonconforming to their gender as identified at birth.
traumatic brain injury Head injury classified as either penetrating or closed; may also be classified as mild, moderate, severe, or catastrophic.
Trendelenburg's position A position in which the patient is lying supine with the head lower than the body with body and legs elevated and on an incline.
triage Process of classifying a group of patients as to the severity of injury and need of care.
trichomoniasis A sexually transmitted disease caused by the protozoan *Trichomonas vaginalis.*
trimester One of the three periods of approximately 3 months into which pregnancy is divided.
Trousseau's sign A test for latent tetany in which carpal spasms are induced by inflating a sphygmomanometer cuff on the upper arm to a pressure exceeding systolic blood pressure for 3 minutes; used in hypocalcemia and hypomagnesemia.
T-tube A tube inserted through the skin to provide drainage from a wound or cavity.
tube feeding Administration of nutritionally balanced liquefied food or formula through a tube inserted into the stomach, duodenum, or jejunum by way of nasoenteric or a feeding ostomy.
tumor lysis syndrome Oncologic emergency that occurs with rapid lysis of malignant cells; most frequently associated with chemotherapy treatment. It is most commonly a result of treatment-related malignant cell death in patients with large tumor cell burdens.
turgor The normal resiliency of the skin caused by the outward pressure of the cells and interstitial fluid; may be assessed as increased or decreased skin turgor.
two-way communication A form of communication that requires that both the sender and the receiver participate equally in the interaction.
tympanic Membranous eardrum.
tympanoplasty One of several operative procedures on the eardrum or ossicles of the middle ear designed to restore or improve hearing in patients with conductive hearing loss.
tympany A high-pitched drumlike sound produced by performing percussion over a hollow organ such as the stomach.
type 1 diabetes mellitus Condition in which impaired glucose tolerance results because of destruction of beta cells in the pancreatic islets; results in deficient insulin production, but the patient retains normal sensitivity to insulin action. Also called *insulin-dependent diabetes mellitus.*
type 2 diabetes mellitus Condition in which impaired glucose tolerance results from an abnormal resistance to insulin action. Also called *non–insulin-dependent diabetes mellitus.*

U

ultrasonography The process of imaging deep structures of the body by measuring and recording the reflection of pulsed or continuous high-frequency sound waves. Also called *sonography.*
umbilicus Point on the abdomen at which the umbilical cord joined the fetus. In most adults it is marked by a depression.
unassertive communication A style of communication in which the sender sacrifices legitimate personal rights to meet the needs of the receiver, often resulting in feelings of resentment.
unilateral neglect Condition in which an individual is perceptually unaware of and inattentive to one side of the body.
unresolved grief A disturbance in the normal progression toward resolution.
urinal A device for receiving urine; may be used with male or female; may be used for specimen collection.
urinary catheter A hollow, flexible tube that can be inserted into the bladder through the meatus and urethra to withdraw urine or instill medication or an irrigant.
urinary retention The inability to completely empty the bladder.
urolithiasis Formation of urinary calculi.
urostomy An opening through the skin created to provide an outlet for urinary elimination.
urticaria Itching skin eruption characterized by welts of varying sizes with well-defined inflamed margins and pale centers. Also called *hives.*
uterine inertia Absence or weakness of uterine contractions during labor.

V

Vacutainer Container used in blood collection.
vacuum-assisted closure An intervention used to provide wound healing and closure by withdrawing fluids from the cavity and pulling the wound closed by use of negative pressure.
value clarification A process of self-inspection to identify one's own beliefs, morals, and values.
values Individual's intrinsic (or personal) beliefs about the importance of a particular idea, object, or custom that will influence behavior.
variance The unexpected event that occurs during the use of a clinical pathway; can be positive or negative.
vasoconstriction When the lumen of the blood vessel narrows, thus hindering blood flow and resulting in less edema.
vasodilation When the lumen of the blood vessel widens, thus increasing the blood flow.
vastus lateralis muscle Located on the anterior (front) of thigh, this site is preferred for injections in children.
vector A living carrier for transmission of microorganisms.
vegan Vegetarian whose diet excludes all foods of animal origin.
vehicle The means by which organisms are carried about.
venipuncture Most common method of drawing a blood sample, involving inserting a hollow-bore needle into the lumen of a large vein.
ventral Facing forward; the front of the body.
venturi mask An oxygen delivery device used to administer a precise concentration of oxygen to a patient.
verbal communication A form of communication that involves the use of spoken or written words or symbols.
verdict Decision rendered based on the facts of a case, evidence and testimony presented, credibility of witnesses, and laws pertaining to the case.
vernix caseosa Protective, gray-white fatty substance of cheesy consistency covering the fetal skin at birth.
verruca Benign, viral, warty skin lesion with a rough, papillomatous (nipplelike) growth.

vertical transmission Transmission of HIV from a mother to a fetus; can occur during pregnancy, during delivery, or through postpartum breastfeeding.
vertigo The sensation that the outer world is revolving about oneself or that one is moving in space.
vesicle Circumscribed elevation of skin filled with serous fluid.
villi Short vascular processes or protrusions clustered over the entire mucous surface of the small intestine.
viral load Amount of measurable HIV virions.
virulent Having the power to produce disease; of or pertaining to a very pathogenic or rapidly progressive condition.
visual analog scale An objective means of assessing pain severity; it consists of a straight line, representing a continuum of intensity, and has visual descriptors at each end.
vital signs Measurement of temperature, pulse, respiration, and blood pressure.
vitrectomy The removal of excess vitreous fluid caused by hemorrhage and replacement with normal saline.
Volkmann's contracture A permanent contracture with clawhand, flexion of wrist and finger, and atrophy of the forearm; can occur as a result of compartment syndrome.
volvulus Twisting of the bowel on itself, causing intestinal obstruction.

W

wasting The loss of lean body mass as a result of illness.
weaning Gradually eliminating breastfeeding or bottle feedings, replaced by cup and table feeding.
wellness A dynamic state of health in which an individual progresses toward a higher level of functioning, achieving an optimum balance between internal and external environments.
wellness nursing diagnosis A clinical judgment about an individual, group, or community in transition from a specific level of wellness to a higher level of wellness.
Western blot A laboratory blood test to detect the presence of antibodies to a specific antigen; used in diagnosing HIV.
Wharton's jelly Gelatinous tissue that remains when the embryonic body stalk blends with the yolk sac within the umbilical cord.
wheals Irregularly shaped, elevated areas, white in the center with a pale red periphery, with superficial localized edema; vary in size (hives, mosquito bite).
wheeze Adventitious breath sounds that have a whistling or sighing sound resulting from narrowing of the lumen of a respiratory passageway. May be heard both on inspiration and expiration. Wheezes characteristically clear on coughing.
wound An injury to body tissue. The injury may be intentional or accidental.

Y

yoga Holistic system of mind-body connection that includes control of the body through correct posture and breathing, control of the emotions and mind, and meditation and contemplation.

Z

zygote Cell formed by the union of two reproductive cells; the fertilized ovum resulting from the union of a sperm and ovum from the time it is fertilized until, as a blastocyst, it is implanted in the uterus.

Index

Note: Page numbers followed by *f*, *t*, or *b* indicate figures, tables, or boxes, respectively.

B

C

E

G

J

M

Q

R

S

T

U

W

X

Y